Child Health Nursing
Partnering with Children & Families
Jane W. Ball
Ruth C. Bindler

Dear Future Nurse:

SUCCESS IS AS EASY AS 1, 2, 3!

We wrote this textbook to empower you as leaders and advocates in pediatric nursing—working with children and families in a variety of settings. In fact, the subtitle, **Partnering with Children & Families**, reflects a core value of the textbook—emphasizing family-centered care, recognition of the family as the central influence in each child's life, and respect for families of all cultures. Families are viewed as case managers, partners with healthcare providers, and as integral participants in care in all pediatric nursing settings. Likewise, partnership and collaboration with other healthcare providers is another key concept of the textbook. We believe that students need to master partnership in order to provide competent and effective nursing care.

With this in mind, we are thrilled to have the opportunity to partner with **you** and to offer you a new and fresh textbook, certain to help you succeed in pediatric nursing! If you read this textbook, attend class, and work hard, you will build the knowledge and skills you need to be successful in the classroom, in clinical, and on the NCLEX-RN®. Here's how you can use this textbook to your benefit:

1. ***READ THE BOOK***

As a nursing student, you have many demands on your time. However, it is important to prepare for class by doing the assigned readings. We use many tools throughout this textbook to facilitate your reading and understanding of key concepts. You will be amazed at how much more you get out of class by preparing ahead of time.

2. ***USE THE BOXES IN THE BOOK***

Some students tell us they only read the boxes, some tell us they skip the boxes and read only the text. This textbook is designed so that helpful information is presented in a format that will enhance your ability to comprehend and remember what you have read. This unfolding guide tells you how to make the most of this textbook. Take some time to review the guide and familiarize yourself with the features.

3. ***USE THE RESOURCES ACCOMPANYING THIS BOOK***

A wealth of materials accompanies this textbook to help you master the course material and apply the concepts using your critical thinking skills. Additionally, there are numerous opportunities to practice NCLEX-RN® questions and case studies, as well as many animations and videos that help bring the textbook concepts to life. Use the free Student CD-ROM or the free Companion Website at **www.prenhall.com/ball** to access these resources.

Finally, as you enter your pediatric nursing course, you may or may not be considering a career in this field. We encourage you to look at the unit openers that explore the field of pediatric nursing and its diverse opportunities. Nursing is a valuable and noble profession, and we applaud your desire to become a successful nurse. We wish you the best of luck as you embark on your life-long journey of rewards and successes in your nursing career.

Sincerely,

Jane W. Ball   Ruth C. Bindler

Jane W. Ball   **Ruth C. Bindler**

Open this guide to learn how this textbook and its resources will help you become successful in the classroom, in the clinical setting, on the NCLEX-RN® examination, and ultimately in your nursing practice!

② Success in Clinical!

The classroom is only part of the learning experience in nursing school. This textbook provides you with numerous learning tools that will help you prepare for clinical encounters with children and families in a variety of settings.

a Important Clinical Considerations

DEVELOPING CULTURAL COMPETENCE
Asthma Management

Asthma attack prevalence (having at least one asthma attack in the past 12 months) varies greatly among children under 18 years by race/ethnicity. In 1998, non-Hispanic Black children had the highest prevalence at 68.1% per 1,000 children, non-Hispanic White children had a prevalence of 52.1%, and Hispanic children had a prevalence of 47.4% (Centers for Disease Control and Prevention, 2000). A recent study investigating these disparities compared children in the above race/ethnicity groups and found a difference in the use of preventive medications for asthma. Among variables studied, specialist use, preventive visits, pets, and smoking in the home were found to be equal among the study population, indicating that these differences did not account for the asthma prevalence. Findings also revealed that Black and Hispanic children with similar insurance and sociodemographic characteristics to White children were 31% and 42%, respectively, less likely to be using inhaled anti-inflammatory medications to prevent the beginning or worsening of an asthma episode. This study suggests that factors such as differences in health beliefs, fear of steroids, or communication issues, rather than financial barriers, may play a role in the use of preventive medications (Lieu, Lozano, Finkelstein, et al., 2002).

Developing Cultural Competence boxes challenge you to explore differences among racial, ethnic, and social groups.

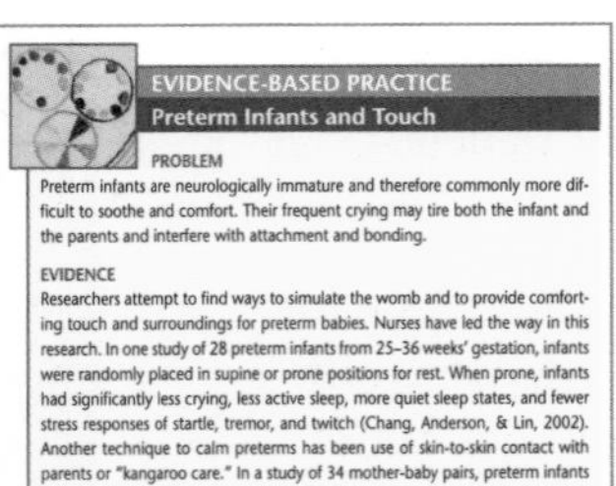

EVIDENCE-BASED PRACTICE
Preterm Infants and Touch

PROBLEM
Preterm infants are neurologically immature and therefore commonly more difficult to soothe and comfort. Their frequent crying may tire both the infant and the parents and interfere with attachment and bonding.

EVIDENCE
Researchers attempt to find ways to simulate the womb and to provide comforting touch and surroundings for preterm babies. Nurses have led the way in this research. In one study of 28 preterm infants from 25–36 weeks' gestation, infants were randomly placed in supine or prone positions for rest. When prone, infants had significantly less crying, less active sleep, more quiet sleep states, and fewer stress responses of startle, tremor, and twitch (Chang, Anderson, & Lin, 2002). Another technique to calm preterms has been use of skin-to-skin contact with parents or "kangaroo care." In a study of 34 mother-baby pairs, preterm infants with skin-to-skin contact were able to control temperature better and experienced more quiet sleep and less crying (Chwo, Anderson, Good, et al., 2002).

IMPLICATIONS
Nurses who care for preterm infants need to integrate knowledge of touch, positioning, and other modalities that provide neurologic comfort for babies.

CRITICAL THINKING APPLICATION
How will you integrate this information in the neonatal intensive care unit and with babies who have left the hospital and are at home with parents? How will your practice and the teaching you provide to parents be altered?

Do the critical thinking activity in the **Evidence-Based Practice** box to see how you would apply the evidence to a scenario.

COMPLEMENTARY THERAPY
Alternative Asthma Treatments

Parents of children from different cultures may have concerns about daily medication regimens. Some prefer to use folk medicines such as rubbing oils or camphor (Vicks VapoRub) preparations on the child's chest. Learn about the family's cultural beliefs and practices (Sydnor-Greenberg & Dokken, 2000). Up to 80% of Hispanic, African American, and immigrant adolescents attending an inner-city high school reported the use of complementary therapies for the treatment of asthma that included rubs, teas (chamomile, ginger, wild root, and eucalyptus), prayer, and massage. There was no association between complementary therapy use and ethnicity or immigrant status. Nearly all adolescents indicated that they would repeat the use of the complementary therapy. It is important to ask about complementary therapy use by children and adolescents with asthma, and how it is used in conjunction with traditional therapy (Reznik, Ozuah, Franco, et al., 2002).

Complementary Therapy boxes describe therapies that may be used by children and families and alert you about information to gather from the family when planning care.

b Applying the Nursing Process

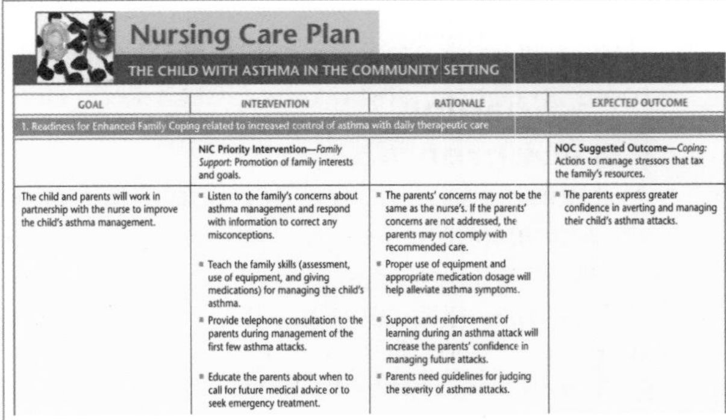

Nursing Care Plan
THE CHILD WITH ASTHMA IN THE COMMUNITY SETTING

GOAL	INTERVENTION	RATIONALE	EXPECTED OUTCOME
1. Readiness for Enhanced Family Coping related to increased control of asthma with daily therapeutic care			
	NIC Priority Intervention—*Family Support:* Promotion of family interests and goals.		**NOC Suggested Outcome—***Coping:* Actions to manage stressors that tax the family's resources.
The child and parents will work in partnership with the nurse to improve the child's asthma management.	▪ Listen to the family's concerns about asthma management and respond with information to correct any misconceptions. ▪ Teach the family skills (assessment, use of equipment, and giving medications) for managing the child's asthma. ▪ Provide telephone consultation to the parents during management of the first few asthma attacks. ▪ Educate the parents about when to call for future medical advice or to seek emergency treatment.	▪ The parents' concerns may not be the same as the nurse's. If the parents' concerns are not addressed, the parents may not comply with recommended care. ▪ Proper use of equipment and appropriate medication dosage will help alleviate asthma symptoms. ▪ Support and reinforcement of learning during an asthma attack will increase the parents' confidence in managing future attacks. ▪ Parents need guidelines for judging the severity of asthma attacks.	▪ The parents express greater confidence in averting and managing their child's asthma attacks.

Use these **Nursing Care Plans** to customize your own in preparation for the children and families you will encounter during your clinical experience.

c Important Memory Tools

CLINICAL MANIFESTATIONS of Pneumonia by Causative Organism

ETIOLOGY	CLINICAL MANIFESTATIONS	CHEST RADIOGRAPH FINDINGS
Mycoplasma pneumoniae	Insidious onset, malaise, muscle aches, headache, fever, sore throat, rhinorrhea, dry hacking cough that becomes productive, fine crackles, anorexia.	Patchy infiltrates and mild pleural effusions
Viral pneumonia	Sudden or insidious onset, rhinitis, slight cough that may become productive, fever and chills, crackles, and wheezes.	Hyperinflation and diffuse, patchy infiltrates
Streptococcus pneumoniae	Sudden onset, high fever, cough, shaking, chills, chest pain, nasal flaring, retractions, fine crackles, dullness on percussion, fremitus.	Lobar consolidation
Staphylococcus aureus	Upper respiratory infection and abrupt change in condition, high fever, cough, shaking, chills, lethargy, chest pain, nasal flaring, retractions, fine crackles, dullness on percussion, fremitus.	Limited patchy infiltrate, usually only right lung involved.
Chlamydia pneumoniae	Insidious onset, minimal or absent fever, tachypnea, malaise, persistent cough, pharyngitis.	Pleural effusions and lobar infiltrates

Clinical Manifestations boxes link etiology, clinical manifestations, and clinical therapy for specific conditions.

CLINICAL TIP
Coach the child to give the best effort each time. Encourage the child to seal the lips tightly around the mouthpiece. The child is then instructed to breathe out as hard as possible, and then to breathe in deeply.

Clinical Tips are "pearls of wisdom" from experienced nursing experts.

MEDICATIONS Used for Symptomatic Treatment of Laryngotracheobronchitis

MEDICATION	ACTION/INDICATION	NURSING CONSIDERATIONS
Beta-agonists and beta-adrenergics (e.g., albuterol, racemic epinephrine): aerosolized through face mask	Rapid-acting bronchodilator, decreases bronchial and tracheal secretions and mucosal edema, used to decrease symptoms of moderate to severe respiratory distress; and constriction of subglottic mucosa and submucosal capillaries. Used until dexamethasone begins working.	Provides only temporary relief; improvement in 30 minutes which lasts about 2 hours, it gives time for the steroid to work; the child may experience tachycardia (160–200 beats/min) and hypertension; dizziness, headache, and nausea may necessitate stopping medication; reduces the need for artifical airway.
Corticosteroids (e.g., dexamethasone): IM, PO Nebulized budesonide	Anti-inflammatory, used to decrease edema; has a long half-life of 36–54 hours.	The child may experience cardiovascular symptoms (hypertension): requires close observation for individual response; children less frequently need emergency airways; stridor resolves faster.

The boxes list medications used to treat certain conditions, present the actions and indications, and list important nursing implications.

PRACTICE ALERT
The depth and location of retractions is associated with the severity of respiratory distress. Isolated intercostal retractions indicate mild distress. Subcostal, suprasternal, and supraclavicular retractions indicate moderate distress. These retractions accompanied by use of accessory muscles in the neck indicate severe distress.

Practice Alerts warn you of safety precautions and other nursing alerts to consider for providing safe care.

③ Success on NCLEX-RN®!

This textbook and its accompanying resources provide you with numerous opportunities to practice NCLEX-RN® questions, including the new test item format questions.

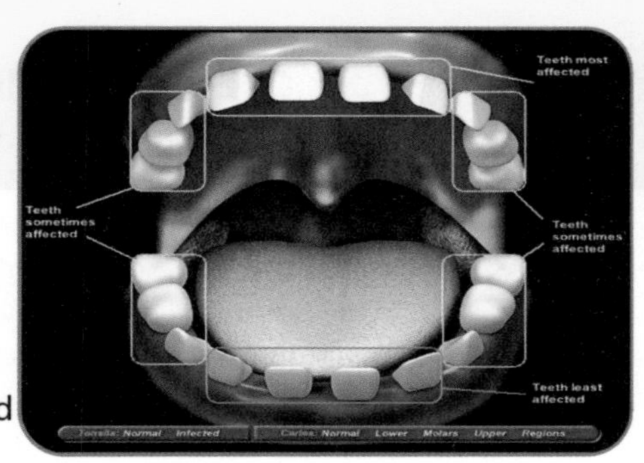

Student CD-ROM

Packaged free with the textbook, it provides an interactive study program that allows you to practice answering NCLEX-style questions with rationales for right and wrong answers. A unique activity called **Nursing in Action** shows brief video clips of real nurses and clients, and asks you to respond to critical thinking questions about these scenarios. It also contains an audio glossary, animations, and videos.

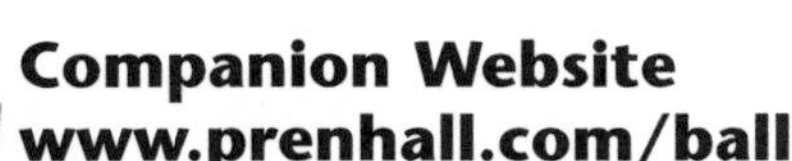

Companion Website www.prenhall.com/ball

This free online study guide is designed to help you apply the concepts presented in the book. Each chapter specific module features chapter objectives, audio glossary, chapter summary for lecture notes, NCLEX-RN® review questions, case studies, care plan activities, MediaLink applications, links, and useful tools, such as growth charts, food guide pyramid, assessment tools, and more.

MediaLink

At the beginning of each chapter, a MediaLink box lists specific animations or videos, NCLEX-RN® Review questions, and other interactive exercises that appear on the accompanying free Student CD-ROM and the Companion Website. The **EXPLORE MediaLink** box at the end of the chapter reminds you to use the media resources. MediaLink will further enhance your learning experience, build upon knowledge gained from this textbook, prepare you for the NCLEX-RN®, and foster critical thinking.

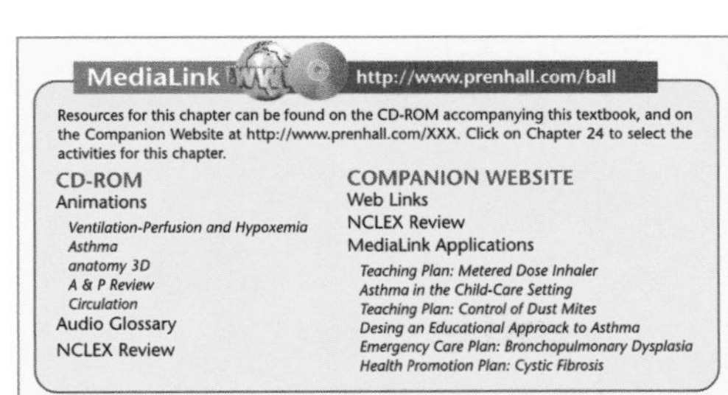

MediaLink http://www.prenhall.com/ball

Resources for this chapter can be found on the CD-ROM accompanying this textbook, and on the Companion Website at http://www.prenhall.com/XXX. Click on Chapter 24 to select the activities for this chapter.

CD-ROM
Animations
Ventilation-Perfusion and Hypoxemia
Asthma
anatomy 3D
A & P Review
Circulation
Audio Glossary
NCLEX Review

COMPANION WEBSITE
Web Links
NCLEX Review
MediaLink Applications
Teaching Plan: Metered Dose Inhaler
Asthma in the Child-Care Setting
Teaching Plan: Control of Dust Mites
Desing an Educational Approack to Asthma
Emergency Care Plan: Bronchopulmonary Dysplasia
Health Promotion Plan: Cystic Fibrosis

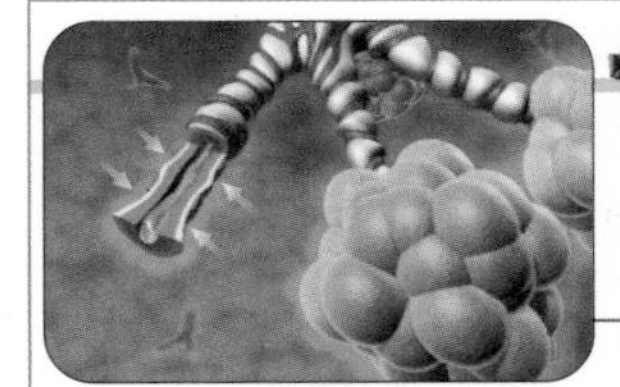

EXPLORE MediaLink

- NCLEX review, case studies, and other interactive resources for this chapter can be found on the Companion Website at **www.prenhall.com/ball**. Click on Chapter 26 to select the activities for this chapter.
- For animations, more NCLEX review questions, and an audio glossary, access the accompanying CD-ROM in this book.

http://www.prenhall.com/ball

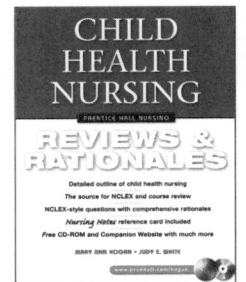

Reviews & Rationales: Child Health Nursing

Mary Ann Hogan, Judy White

ISBN: 0-13-030452-2

This resource provides a core content and NCLEX-RN® review of pediatric nursing in outline format. The CD-ROM, pre-test, and post-test guide you through a self-paced review.

Additional Resources for Success

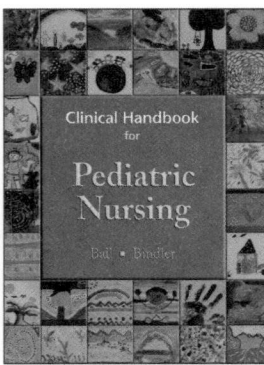

Clinical Handbook for Pediatric Nursing
ISBN: 0-13-113316-0
This quick-reference handbook provides general information on growth & development, vital signs, and assessment information specific to the care of children in the community or hospital, such as dosage calculations, pain charts, immunization schedules, and an overview of primary for conditions organized by body systems.

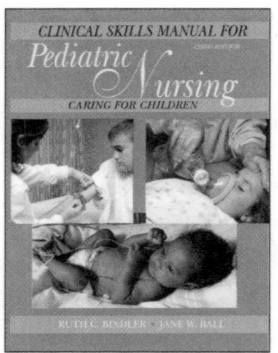

Clinical Skills Manual for Pediatric Nursing
Ruth Bindler, Jane Ball
ISBN: 0-13-048352-4
This manual guides you through more than 70 pediatric skills using full-color photographs and rationales. Throughout ***Child Health Nursing***, special cross-reference icons refer you to the complete skill presentation in this manual.

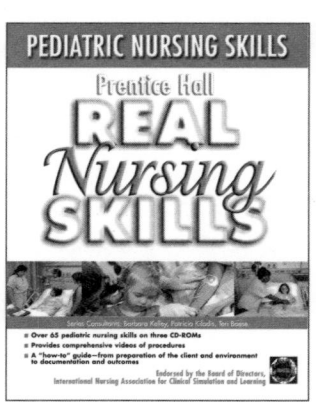

Prentice Hall Real Nursing Skills: Pediatric Nursing
ISBN: 0-13-191524-X
This set of interactive CD-ROMs offers you ***the*** complete foundation for competency in performing pediatric nursing skills. It provides comprehensive procedures and rationales demonstrated in hundreds of realistic video clips, animations, illustrations, and photographs.

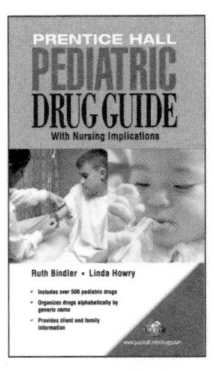

Prentice Hall Pediatric Drug Guide
Ruth Bindler, Linda Howry
ISBN: 0-13-119615-4
This guide provides easy access to over 500 drugs administered to children, organized alphabetically by generic name.

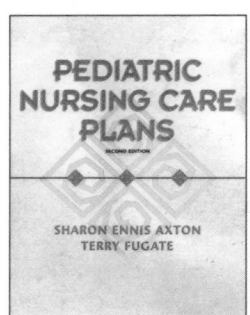

Pediatric Nursing Care Plans, 2nd Edition
Sharon Axton, Terry Fugate
ISBN: 0-13-098969-X
This unique reference begins with a foundation of medical diagnosis and pathophysiology before detailing the preparation of individualized nursing care plans tailored to meet the special needs of children.

Resources for Instructor Success

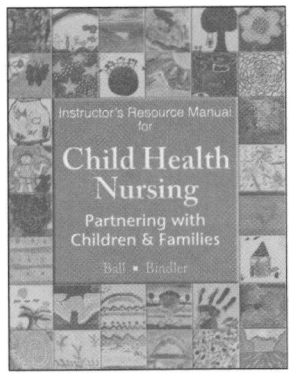

Instructor's Resource Manual

ISBN: 0-13-113318-7

This manual contains a wealth of material to help faculty plan and manage the pediatric nursing course. It includes chapter overviews, detailed lecture suggestions and outlines, learning objectives, a complete test bank, teaching tips, and more for each chapter. The IRM also guides faculty on how to assign and use the text-specific Companion Website, www.prenhall.com/ball, and the Student CD-ROM that accompany the textbook.

Instructor's Resource CD-ROM

This cross-platform CD-ROM provides several tools to aid faculty in teaching. It includes illustrations and lectures in PowerPoint for use in the classroom. It also contains an electronic test bank and animations and videos from the Student CD-ROM.

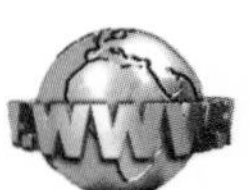

Companion Website Syllabus Manager

www.prenhall.com/ball

Faculty adopting this textbook have ***free*** access to the online **Syllabus Manager** feature of the Companion Website, www.prenhall.com/ball. It offers a whole host of features that facilitate the students' use of the Companion Website, and allows faculty to post syllabi and course information online for their students.

Instructors: *For packaging options with any Prentice Hall textbook, please contact your representative or check online at www.prenhall.com/nursing.*

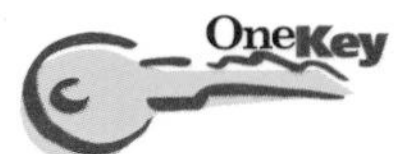

Online Course Management Systems

OneKey is an integrated online resource that brings a wide array of supplemental resources together in one convenient place for both students and faculty. OneKey features everything you and your students need for out-of-class work, conveniently organized to match your syllabus. OneKey's online course management solution features interactive modules, text and image PowerPoints, animations, videos, case studies, and more. OneKey also provides course management tools so faculty can customize course content, build online tests, create assignments, enter grades, post announcements, communicate with students, and much more. Testing materials, gradebooks, and other instructor resources are available in a separate section that can be accessed by instructors only. OneKey content is available in three different platforms. A nationally hosted version is available in the reliable, easy-to-use **CourseCompass** platform. The same content is also available for download to locally hosted versions of **BlackBoard** and **WebCT**. Please contact your Prentice Hall Sales Representative for a demonstration or go online to **http://myphlip.pearsoncmg.com/OneKey/index.html**

OneKey is all you need.
Convenience. Simplicity. Success.

Powered by

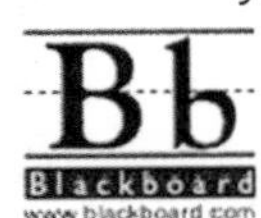

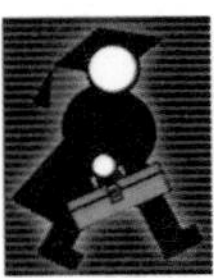

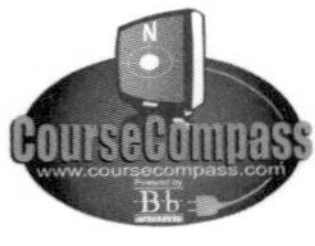

Research Navigator™

www.researchnavigator.com

Prentice Hall's **Research Navigator**™ is the easiest way for students to start a research assignment or research paper. Complete with extensive help on the research process and two exclusive databases of credible and reliable source material, **Research Navigator**™ helps students quickly and efficiently make the most of their research time.

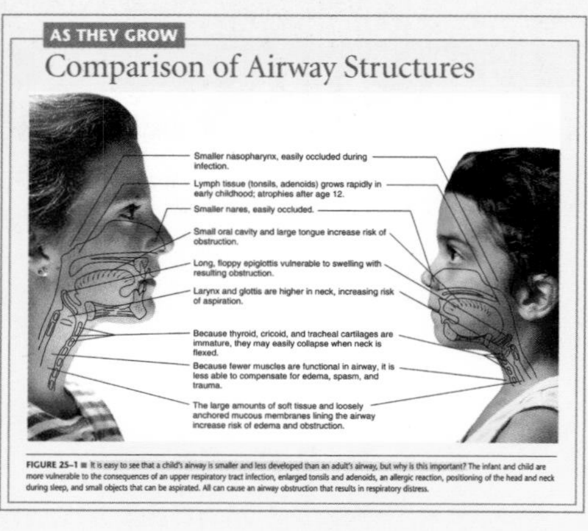
AS THEY GROW

Comparison of Airway Structures

Smaller nasopharynx, easily occluded during infection.

Smaller nares, easily occluded.

Larynx and glottis are higher in neck, increasing risk of aspiration.

FIGURE 25–1 ■ It is easy to see that a child's airway is smaller and less developed than an adult's airway, but why is this important? The infant and child are more vulnerable to the consequences of an upper respiratory tract infection, enlarged tonsils and adenoids, an allergic reaction, positioning of the head and neck during sleep, and small objects that can be aspirated. All can cause an airway obstruction that results in respiratory distress.

b Visuals That Teach

As They Grow boxes show you how children differ from adults, both anatomically and physiologically.

Pathophysiology Illustrated boxes allow you to see into the body so you can visualize the causes and effects of various conditions in children.

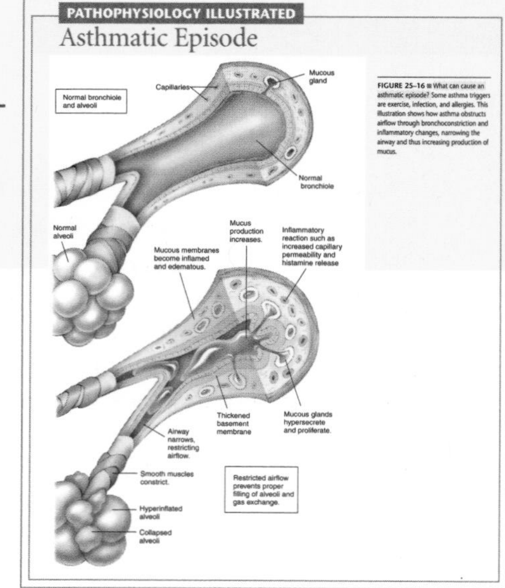
PATHOPHYSIOLOGY ILLUSTRATED

Asthmatic Episode

Normal bronchiole and alveoli

Mucous gland
Normal bronchiole
Normal alveoli

Thickened basement membrane
Mucous glands hypersecrete and proliferate.
Airway narrows, restricting airflow.
Smooth muscles constrict.
Restricted airflow prevents proper filling of alveoli and gas exchange.
Hyperinflated alveoli
Collapsed alveoli

FIGURE 25–16 ■ What can cause an asthmatic episode? Some asthma triggers are exercise, infection, and allergies. This illustration shows how asthma obstructs airflow through bronchoconstriction and inflammatory changes, narrowing the airway and thus increasing production of mucus.

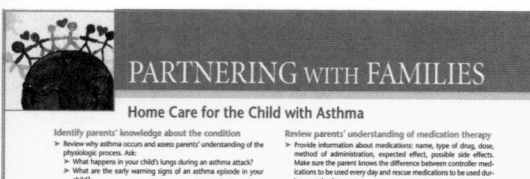
MediaLink Anatomical Landmarks Animation

Sudden Infant Death Syndrome

Sudden infant death syndrome (SIDS) has been the sudden death of an infant under 1 year of age th unexplained after a complete autopsy, a death scene tion, and review of the history. It remains a leadin death in infants between 1 month and 1 year of age, with 90% of cases occ fore 6 months of age (American Academy of Pediat mittee on Child Abuse and Neglect, 2001). SIDS occu infants less than 2 weeks. It is currently unpredictab preventable. The first symptom is cardiopulmonary a

SIDS is referred to as a "syndrome" because of the varied autopsy and clinical findings that characteriz fants who die of the disorder. The autopsy typically identify a disease process that caused the death. Clinic include evidence of a struggle or change in positio presence of frothy, blood-tinged secretions from the n nares. SIDS occurs more often in the fall and winter a periods of sleep. Most deaths are unobserved. Typica find the infant dead in the crib in the morning and r

MediaLink tabs appear wherever topics in the text are further explained visually on the student CD-ROM or Companion Website in specific videos, animations, or activities—watch an animation of an otoscope examination inside a child's ear.

c Partnering with Children and Families

PARTNERING WITH FAMILIES

Home Care for the Child with Asthma

Identify parents' knowledge about the condition

- Review why asthma occurs and assess parents' understanding of the physiologic process. Ask:
  - What happens in your child's lungs during an asthma attack?
  - What are the early warning signs of an asthma episode in your child?
  - What are your child's symptoms and how does he or she respond to them? Does your child use the peak expiratory flow meter to evaluate symptoms?
  - To help toddlers learn how to use a peak flow meter, have them practice by blowing into party favors (i.e., noisemakers).
  - Determine if the parents or child understands that asthma is a chronic condition that needs daily medication and environmental management to be controlled.
- Help parents explore and understand how asthma affects their child.
  - Does the child wake up at night?
  - Does the child cough a lot? When?
  - Does the child avoid sports practice? What physical activities does the child like to do? If none, why?
  - Does asthma interfere with social activities or activities with friends?
- Identify asthma triggers and assess parents' understanding of how to prevent, avoid, or minimize their effect in a timely manner. Ask:
  - Do you know your child's personal asthma triggers? (Suggest that the parents and child keep a notebook to track episodes so they can learn more about these triggers.) Where do most episodes begin—home, school, outdoors, with exercise?
  - What steps can you take to minimize or eliminate your child's exposure to indoor pollutants (cigarette smoke, molds, dust mites, allergens, furry animals, etc.)?

Set up a schedule for parents to learn asthma management

- Make sure the parents understand the need for daily management and how that enables the family and child to have control over asthma.
- Ensure that the family knows when and where to seek emergency medical help? Describe actions the family can take before seeking medical assistance.

Review parents' understanding of medication therapy

- Provide information about medications: name, type of drug, dose, method of administration, expected effect, possible side effects. Make sure the parent knows the difference between controller medications to be used every day and rescue medications to be used during an episode.
  - Color labels to match the peak flow meter zones can be used to help children and parents tell the difference between their medications. A green label can be used on controller medications, to be used every day. Yellow and red labels can be used on the rescue medications with the number of puffs to use when the childs's peak flow meter reading is in either color zone.
- Evaluate the child's technique for the use of an inhaler. To help children use a metered-dose inhaler, let them practice breathing in slowly through a straw. To help children use a dry powder inhaler, obtain a practice inhaler from the pharmaceutical representative so the child learns to listen for the whistle corresponding to correct use for that inhaler. (Some inhalers have a whistle when the inspiration is too fast or when the inspiration is the correct rate.)
  - To help parents provide a nebulizer treatment to the infant or young child, suggest different types of diversion that might be used to help the child cooperate during the 8- to 10-minute treatment.
- Make sure the parent and child have a written action plan that includes daily management and steps to take when an episode begins.

Address associated issues

- Do parents know how to store and properly transport medications?
- What are the financial considerations of medication cost and lifestyle changes?
- Has the child's school or teacher been notified? What arrangements have been made for the child's use of medications at school?
- Has a medical identification bracelet or medallion been obtained for the child to facilitate assistance when away from home?

Identify need for follow-up care

- Do parents know when to see a physician? When drug levels need to be checked?
- Does child need to see an allergist?
- Do the child and parents have special emotional needs?
- Would a self-help group or camp experience be helpful for the child?

You can apply the concepts of family-centered care by providing approaches in a format you can use when you work with families.

d Focus on Health Promotion

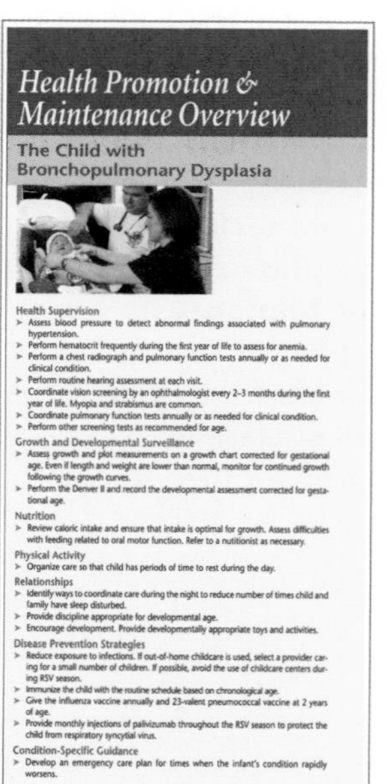
Health Promotion & Maintenance Overview

The Child with Bronchopulmonary Dysplasia

Health Supervision

- Assess blood pressure to detect abnormal findings associated with pulmonary hypertension.
- Perform hematocrit frequently during the first year of life to assess for anemia.
- Perform a chest radiograph and pulmonary function tests annually or as needed for clinical condition.
- Perform routine hearing assessment at each visit.
- Coordinate vision screening by an ophthalmologist every 2–3 months during the first year of life. Myopia and strabismus are common.
- Coordinate pulmonary function tests annually or as needed for clinical condition.
- Perform other screening tests as recommended for age.

Growth and Developmental Surveillance

- Assess growth and plot measurements on a growth chart corrected for gestational age. Even if length and weight are lower than normal, monitor for continued growth following the growth curves.
- Perform the Denver II and record the developmental assessment corrected for gestational age.

Nutrition

- Review caloric intake and ensure that intake is optimal for growth. Assess difficulties with feeding related to oral motor function. Refer to a nutritionist as necessary.

Physical Activity

- Organize care so that child has periods of time to rest during the day.

Relationships

- Identify ways to coordinate care during the night to reduce number of times child and family have sleep disturbed.
- Provide discipline appropriate for developmental age.
- Encourage development. Provide developmentally appropriate toys and activities.

Disease Prevention Strategies

- Reduce exposure to infections. If out-of-home childcare is used, select a provider caring for a small number of children. If possible, avoid the use of childcare centers during RSV season.
- Immunize the child with the routine schedule based on chronological age.
- Give the influenza vaccine annually and 23-valent pneumococcal vaccine at 2 years of age.
- Provide monthly injections of palivizumab throughout the RSV season to protect the child from respiratory syncytial virus.

Condition-Specific Guidance

- Develop an emergency care plan for times when the infant's condition rapidly worsens.

Health Promotion and Maintenance summarizes the needs of children with specific chronic conditions, such as asthma or diabetes. These overviews teach you to look at the chronically ill child like any other child, with health maintenance needs for prevention, education, and basic care.

e Hone Your Critical Thinking Skills

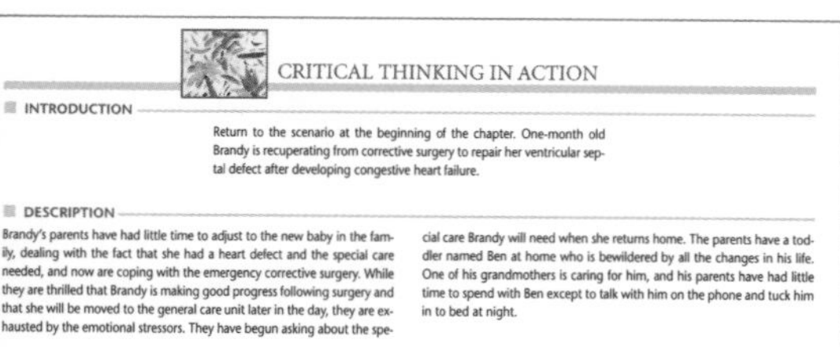
CRITICAL THINKING IN ACTION

INTRODUCTION

Return to the scenario at the beginning of the chapter. One-month old Brandy is recuperating from corrective surgery to repair her ventricular septal defect after developing congestive heart failure.

DESCRIPTION

Brandy's parents have had little time to adjust to the new baby in the family, dealing with the fact that she had a heart defect and the special care needed, and now are coping with the emergency corrective surgery. While they are thrilled that Brandy is making good progress following surgery and that she will be moved to the general care unit later in the day, they are exhausted by the emotional stressors. They have begun asking about the special care Brandy will need when she returns home. The parents have a toddler named Ben at home who is bewildered by all the changes in his life. One of his grandmothers is caring for him, and his parents have had little time to spend with Ben except to talk with him on the phone and tuck him in to bed at night.

DISCUSSION

1. Outline the nursing care that Brandy will need on the general care unit and describe how Brandy's parents can play an active role in her care.
2. Describe the care that Brandy will need in the first couple of weeks at home and develop a discharge plan. Identify the signs that might indicate an urgent need to return for medical evaluation.
3. Talk with the parents about their toddler's potential responses to all the changes in the family over the past month. Collaborate with the parents to outline strategies to meet Ben's developmental needs for attention, comfort, and security once Brandy returns home.
4. What information can you share with Brandy's parents to help them understand her prognosis so they begin to see her as a healthy child rather than a vulnerable child with a chronic condition?

At the end of the chapter, you revisit the child and family from the scenario at the beginning, and now you can apply the concepts you learned from the chapter and respond to the discussion questions.

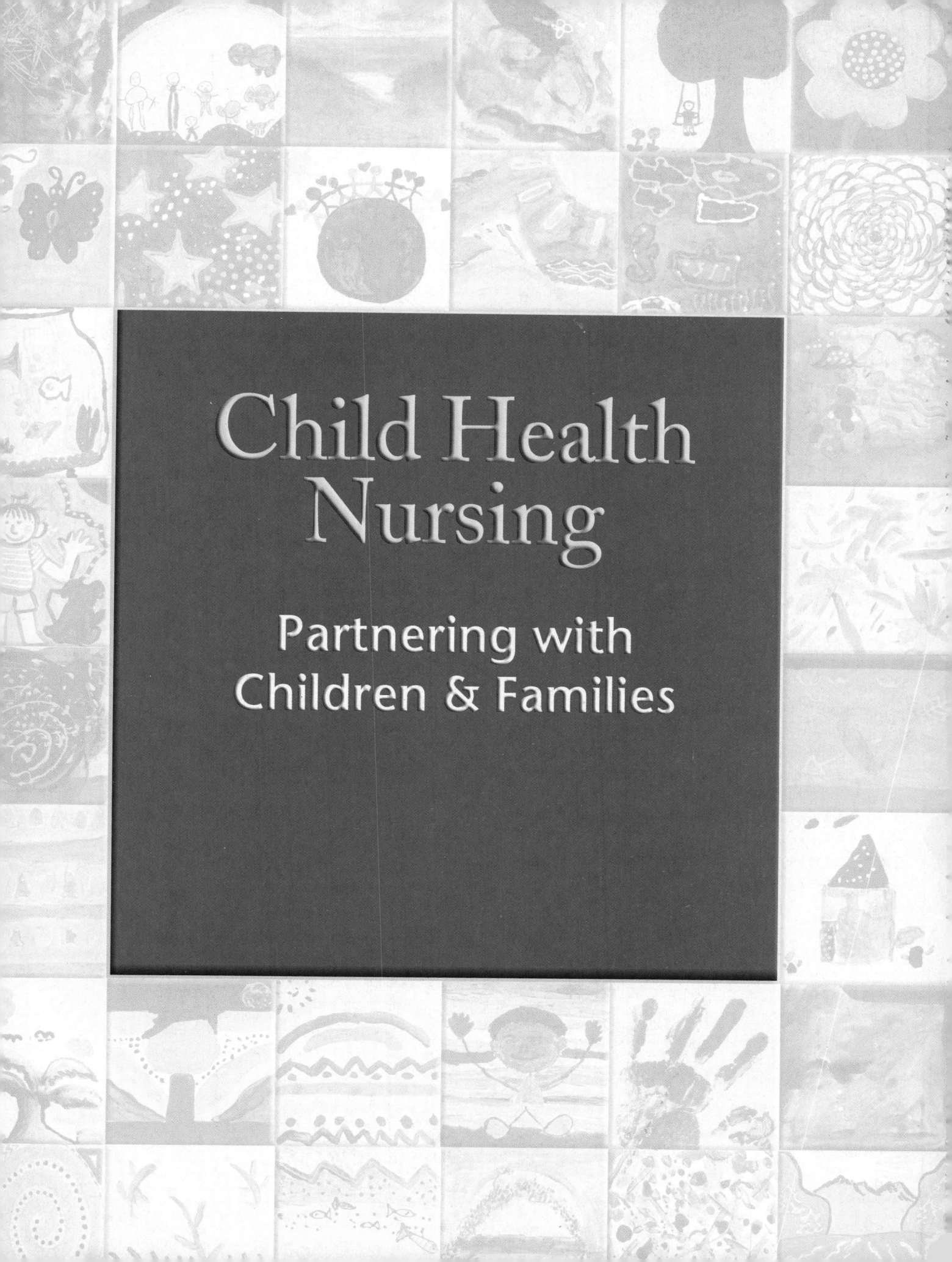

Child Health Nursing

Partnering with Children & Families

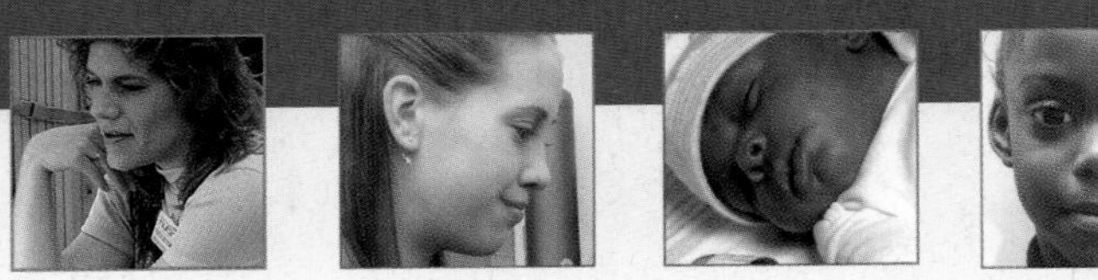

Brief Contents

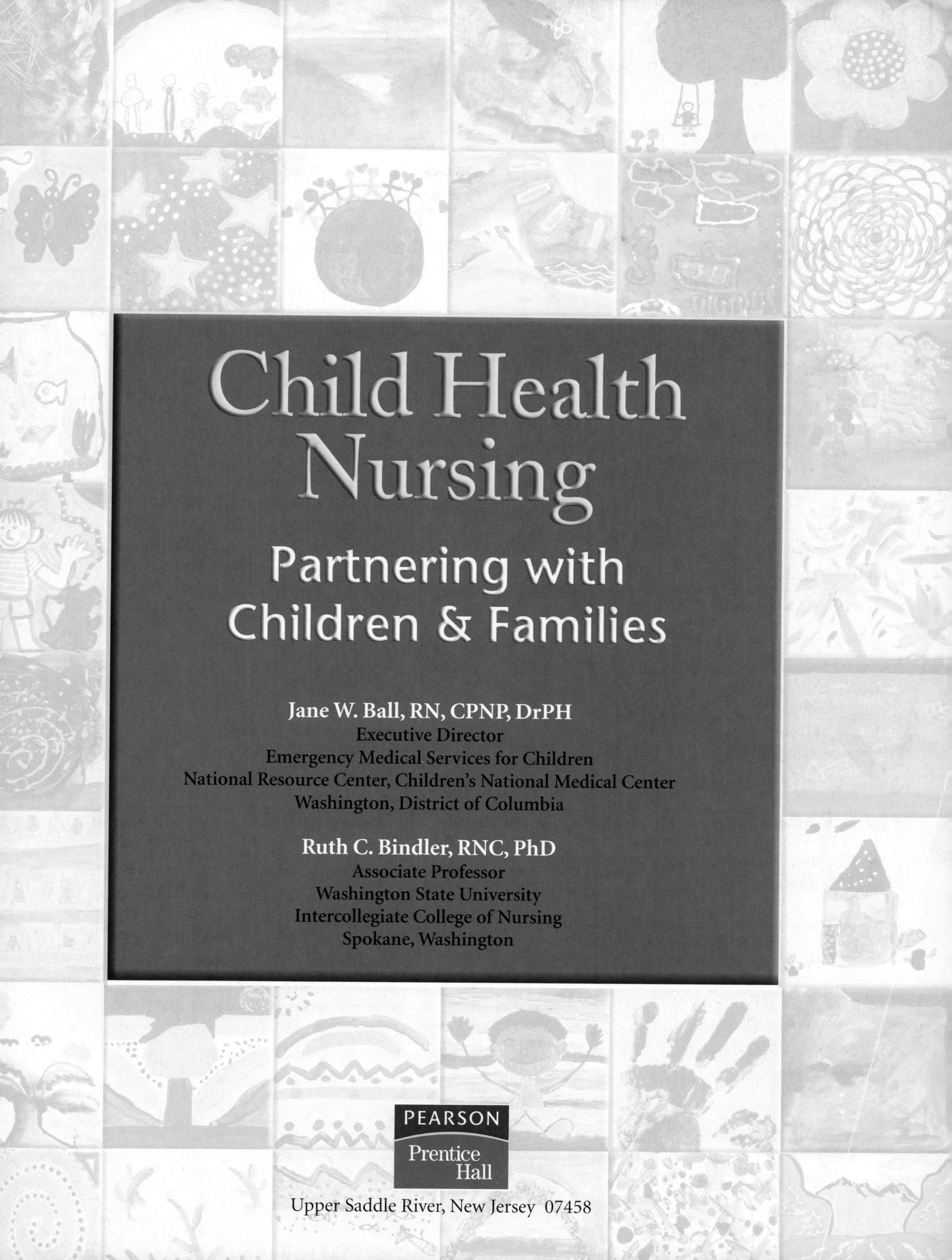

Child Health Nursing

Partnering with Children & Families

Jane W. Ball, RN, CPNP, DrPH
Executive Director
Emergency Medical Services for Children
National Resource Center, Children's National Medical Center
Washington, District of Columbia

Ruth C. Bindler, RNC, PhD
Associate Professor
Washington State University
Intercollegiate College of Nursing
Spokane, Washington

PEARSON
Prentice Hall

Upper Saddle River, New Jersey 07458

Library of Congress Cataloging-in-Publication Data
Ball, Jane.
Child health nursing : partnering with children and families / Jane W. Ball, Ruth C. Bindler.
p. cm.
Includes bibliographical references and index.
ISBN 0-13-113320-9
1. Pediatric nursing. I. Bindler, Ruth McGillis. II. Title.
RJ245.B344 2006
618.92'00231—dc22 2005007368

Notice: Care has been taken to confirm the accuracy of information presented in this book. The authors, editors, and the publisher, however, cannot accept any responsibility for errors or omissions or for consequences from application of the information in this book and make no warranty, express or implied, with respect to its contents.

The authors and publisher have exerted every effort to ensure that drug selections and dosages set forth in this text are in accord with current recommendations and practice at time of publication. However, in view of ongoing research, changes in government regulations, and the constant flow of information relating to drug therapy and drug reactions, the reader is urged to check the package inserts of all drugs for any change in indications or dosage and for added warnings and precautions. This is particularly important when the recommended agent is a new and/or infrequently employed drug.

Publisher: Julie Levin Alexander
Assistant to Publisher: Regina Bruno
Editor-in-Chief: Maura Connor
Senior Managing Editor: Marilyn Meserve
Development Editor: Kim Wyatt
Associate Editor: Danielle Doller
Assistant Editor: Sladjana Repic
Director of Production & Manufacturing: Bruce Johnson
Managing Production Editor: Patrick Walsh
Production Liaison: Nicholas Radhuber
Production Editor: Lori Dalberg, Carlisle Publishers Services
Manufacturing Manager: Illene Sanford
Design Director: Cheryl Asherman
Design Coordinator: Maria Guglielmo, Mary Siener
Interior Designer: Janice Bielawa
Cover Designer: Cheryl Asherman, Mary Siener
Electronic Art Creation: Precision Graphics, Imagineering Media Services
Photographers: George Dodson, Roy Ramsey
Senior Media Project Manager: John Jordan
Manager of Media Production: Amy Peltier
New Media Project Manager: Stephen Hartner
New Media Production: Hector Grillone, Anne Lukens, Jody Small, Kate Stillings, Video Productions Services; Stethographics, Inc.; Red Frog, Inc.
Director of Marketing: Karen Allman
Marketing Manager: Nicole Benson
Marketing Coordinator: Michael Sirinides
Marketing Assistant: Patricia Linard
Senior Channel Marketing Manager: Rachele Strober
Composition: Carlisle Communications, Ltd.
Cover Printer: Phoenix Color Corp.
Printing and Binding: Quebecor World

Cover and interior tile art reproduced from Shands Hospital at the University of Florida, Gainesville, Florida

---

Pearson Education Ltd.
Pearson Education Singapore, Pte. Ltd.
Pearson Education Canada, Ltd.
Pearson Education—Japan
Pearson Education Australia PTY, Limited
Pearson Education North Asia Ltd.
Pearson Educacíon de Mexico, S.A. de C.V.
Pearson Education Malaysia, Pte. Ltd.
Pearson Education, Upper Saddle River, New Jersey

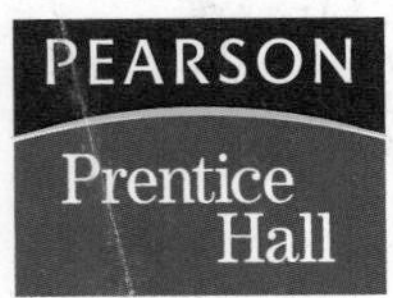

10 9 8 7 6 5 4 3
ISBN: 0-13-113320-9

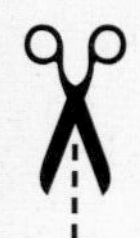

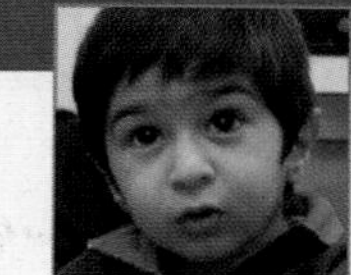
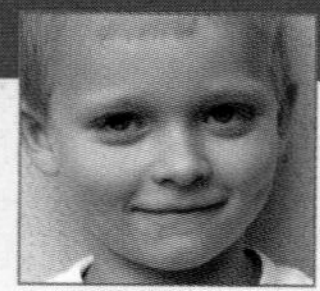
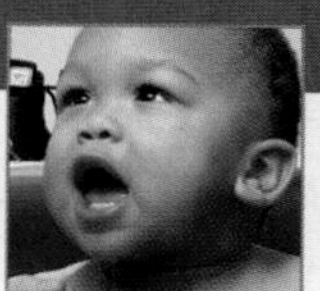
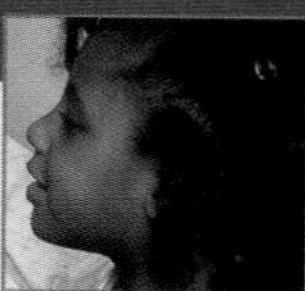

Make a Difference with Pearson Prentice Hall!

Simply by purchasing this textbook, you can have a positive impact on the health of children in your community. Here is an opportunity for you to have an even greater impact. Pearson Prentice Hall is pleased to contribute a portion of the revenue from this textbook to one of the child health organizations listed below. We are proud that together we can make a difference.

DIRECTIONS: Please complete the information below and then check the box next to the organization to which you would like Pearson Prentice Hall to make a contribution. Carefully cut this page from your book (would need to be the original page, not a photocopy) and mail the original page to: *Editor-in-Chief, Prentice Hall Nursing, Pearson Prentice Hall, One Lake Street, Suite 5E, Upper Saddle River, NJ 07458.*

Name ______________________________

School ______________________________

Email ______________________________

This information will be used to confirm that your school is using this textbook, and to contact you via email to thank you for participating in this donation program. Your contact information will not be released to third parties.

✓**Please send a $1 contribution to the organization I have indicated below (check only one):**

❑ March of Dimes

❑ Starlight Starbright Children's Foundation

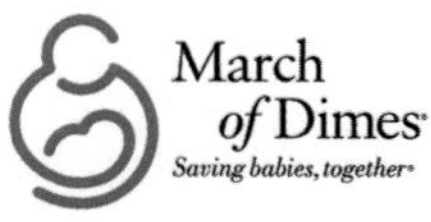

The March of Dimes focuses on the health of babies. Whether that means funding scientific research to find the causes of premature birth and birth defects, educating families about having healthy babies, or answering questions from parents-to-be and new parents, we're here to help. To find out more, visit marchofdimes.com today.

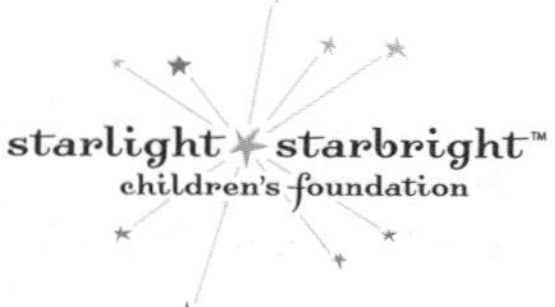

Starlight Starbright Children's Foundation seeks to transform the experience of childhood illness through programs that heal children's spirits, foster a sense of community and help alleviate pain and fear. Children laugh. Parents relax. The family feels together. Because even though we're focused on the child, we're helping the whole family. Learn more at www. starlight.org.

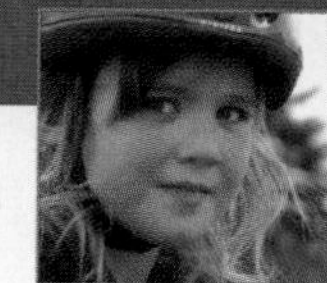
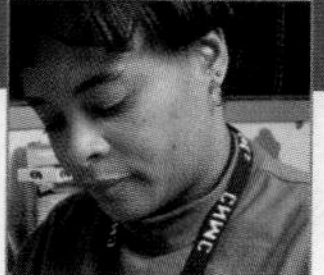
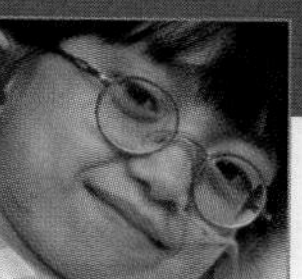
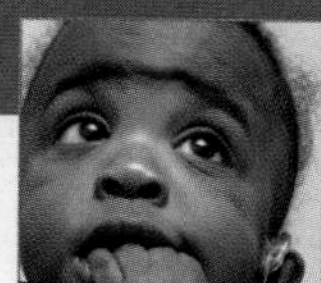

About the Authors

Jane W. Ball

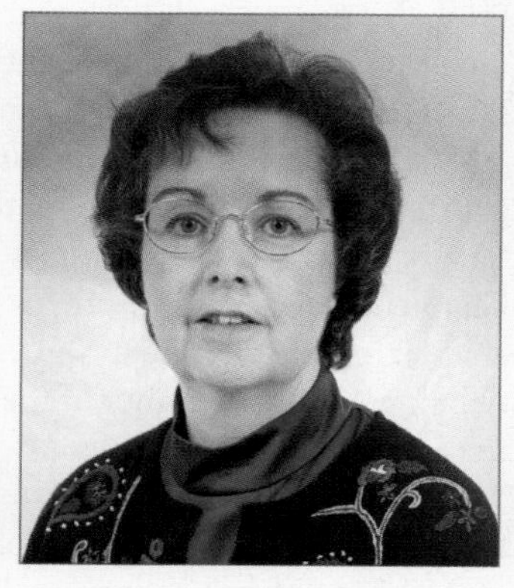

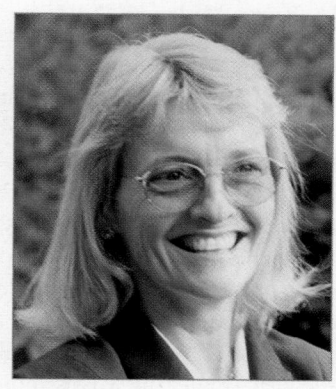

Jane W. Ball graduated from the Johns Hopkins Hospital School of Nursing, and subsequently received a BS from the Johns Hopkins University. She worked in the surgical, pediatric emergency, and outpatient units of the Johns Hopkins Children's Medical and Surgical Center, first as a staff nurse and then as a pediatric nurse practitioner. Thus began her career as a pediatric nurse and advocate for children's health needs. Jane obtained both a Master of Public Health and Doctor of Public Health degree from the Johns Hopkins University Bloomberg School of Public Health with a focus on Maternal and Child Health. After graduation she became the Chief of Child Health Services for the Commonwealth of Pennsylvania Department of Health. In this capacity she oversaw the state-funded well child clinics and explored ways to improve education for the state's community health nurses. After relocating to Texas, she joined the faculty at the University of Texas at Arlington School of Nursing to teach community pediatrics to RNs returning to school for a BSN. During this time she became involved in writing her first textbook, *Mosby's Guide to Physical Examination,* currently in its sixth edition. After relocating to the Washington, DC area, she joined Children's National Medical Center to manage a federal project to teach instructors of Emergency Medical Technicians from all states about the special care children need during an emergency. Exposure to the shortcomings of the emergency medical services system in the late 1980s with regard to pediatric care was a career-changing event. With federal funding, she developed educational curricula for emergency medical technicians and emergency nurses to help them provide improved care for children. A textbook entitled *Pediatric Emergencies, A Manual for Prehospital Providers* was developed from these educational ventures. For the past 14 years she has managed the federally funded Emergency Medical Services for Children National Resource Center. As executive director, Dr. Ball directs the provision of consultation and resource development for state health agencies, health professionals, families, and advocates about successful methods to improve the healthcare system so that children get optimal emergency and trauma care in all healthcare settings.

Ruth C. Bindler

Ruth Bindler received her BSN from Cornell University New York Hospital School of Nursing in New York. She worked in oncology nursing at Sloan Kettering Cancer Center in New York, and then moved to Wisconsin and became a public health nurse in Dane County, Wisconsin. Thus began her commitment to work with children as she visited children and their families at home, and served as a school nurse for several elementary, middle, and high schools. Due to this interest in child healthcare needs, she earned a Master of Science degree in Child Development from the University of Wisconsin. A move to Washington State was accompanied by a new position as a faculty member at the Intercollegiate Center for Nursing Education in Spokane, WA. Dr. Bindler has been fortunate to be involved for over 30 years in the growth of this nursing education consortium, which is a combination of public and private universities and colleges and is now the Washington State University/Intercollegiate College of Nursing. She has taught the theory and clinical courses in child health and a course on cultural diversity and health, as well as serving as lead faculty for the theory and clinical components of child health nursing. She teaches graduate research and works with both graduate and undergraduate nursing majors. Her first professional book, *Pediatric Medications,* was published in 1971, and she has continued to publish articles and books in the areas of pediatric medications and pediatric health. Special research interests are in the area of cardiovascular and type II diabetes risk factors in children, a topic that was the focus of her Ph.D. dissertation in Human Nutrition at Washington State University. Ethnic diversity has been another theme in her work. She facilitates international and other diversity experiences for students, performs research with culturally diverse children, and volunteers for Habitat for Humanity. Dr. Bindler believes that her role as a faculty member has enabled her to learn continually, to foster the development of students in nursing, and to participate fully in the profession of nursing. In addition to teaching, research, publication, and leadership, she enhances her life by service in several professional and community commitments, and by activities with her family.

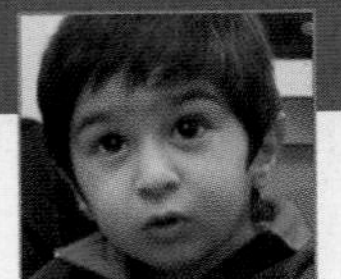
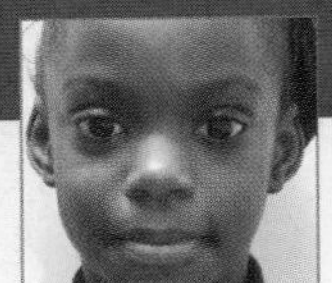
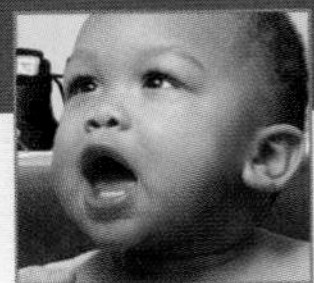
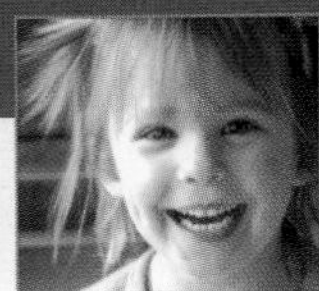

Consulting Editor

Joseann Helmes DeWitt

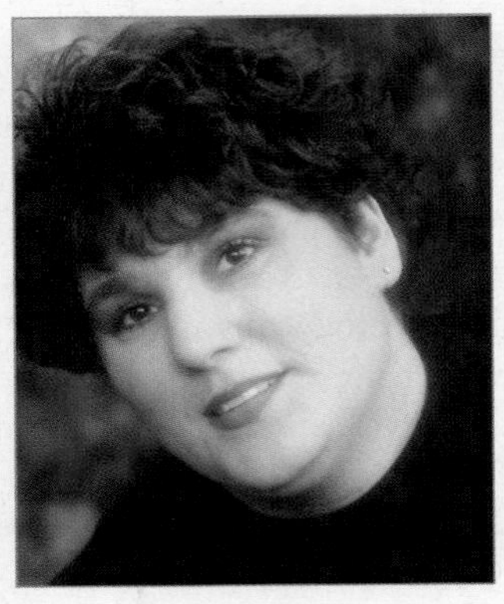

Joseann DeWitt received her Associate of Science in Nursing in 1988 and subsequently received her Bachelor of Science in Nursing from Northwestern State University in Natchitoches, Louisiana in 1996. She worked as a staff nurse in the intensive care unit and emergency department at Natchez Regional Medical Center in Mississippi. During that time, she became an instructor for Advanced Cardiac Life Support, Basic Life Support, and telemetry, and she developed and taught the critical care course for the medical center. She also served as a critical care preceptor for new nurses and nursing, paramedic, and respiratory students during their critical care clinical rotations.

Ms. DeWitt obtained her Master of Science in Nursing, with a focus on nursing education, from the University of Mississippi in 1998. Teaching nursing since 1994, she is an Assistant Professor of Nursing at Our Lady of the Lake School of Nursing in Baton Rouge, Louisiana and is the course coordinator and lead instructor of pediatrics. She is also currently a doctoral student in the Educational Leadership program at Louisiana State University.

Ms. DeWitt is involved in numerous professional nursing organizations. She has served on the executive board and as secretary of the Mississippi Nurses Association (MNA) District 1 Chapter. She served briefly as acting president of the district chapter of Sigma Theta Tau International Honor Society of Nursing. She is a member of the Society of Pediatric Nurses and the Louisiana State Nurses Association. Additionally, Ms. DeWitt served as faculty advisor to nursing students in the Mississippi Student Nurses Association chapter for nine years.

Ms. DeWitt has contributed numerous chapters in nursing textbooks and review books on topics including musculoskeletal, oncologic, endocrine, and genitourinary disorders, as well as eye and ear medication administration, special considerations in child health nursing. Her research interests are diabetes in children and end-of-life issues. She is certified as a Pediatric Nurse through the American Nurses Credentialing Center (AACN), and is a Certified Legal Nurse Consultant (CLNC). Ms. DeWitt and her husband, Kenneth, have two children, Justin and Gage.

Contributors

Textbook Contributors

Nancy R. Bowers, RN, MSN, CNS
Associate Professor of Nursing
University of Cincinnati Raymond Walters College
Cincinnati, Ohio

Kay Cowen, RN, MSN
Clinical Associate Professor
University of North Carolina at
Greensboro, North Carolina

Mary Kisting, RN, MS
Instructor
Michigan State University
East Lansing, Michigan

Andrea Kline, RN, MS, PCCNP, PNP, CCRN
Pediatric Critical Care Nurse Practitioner
Children's Memorial Hospital
Chicago, Illinois

Anita Kyle, MS, RNC, CNS
Associate Clinical Professor
Texas Woman's University
Houston, Texas

Sara Mitchell, RN, PhD, CPNP
Assistant Professor
Mercer University
Atlanta, Georgia

Pat Nosel, MN, RN
Assistant Professor and Chairperson
Edinboro University of Pennsylvania
Edinboro, Pennsylvania

Lynn B. Rasmussen, PhD, RNC, NNPn
Assistant Professor
University of Missouri
Kansas City, Missouri

Deborah Roberts, RN, EdD
Assistant Professor
Humboldt State University
Arcata, California

Jeanette Zaichkin, RNC, MN
Neonatal Nurse Consultant
Olympia, Washington

Student CD-ROM

Kay Cowen, RN, MSN
Clinical Associate Professor
University of North Carolina at
Greensboro, North Carolina

Sheri Curtis, MSN, ARNP
Clinical Assistant Professor
University of Florida
Gainesville, Florida

Mary Dowell, PhD
Professor
University of Mary Hardin Baylor
Belton, Texas

Jayne Howell, RN, BSN
Faculty
Florence Darlington Technical College
Florence, South Carolina

Patricia Kiladis, MS, RN
Associate Clinical Specialist
Northeastern University
Boston, Massachusetts

Virginia Rogers, MSN
Associate Professor
Oakton Community College
Des Plains, Illinois

Kathleen Walker, MSN, RN
Assistant Professor
Roberts Wesleyan College
Rochester, New York

Marilyn Weitzel, PhD, RN
Assistant Professor
Cleveland State University
Cleveland, Ohio

Instructor's Resource Manual and Instructor's Resource CD-ROM

Wendy Bowles, MSN, CPNP
Clinical Instructor
Kettering College of Medical Arts
Kettering, Ohio

Stephanie C. Butkus, MSN, RN, CPNP, IBCLC
Assistant Professor
Kettering College of Medical Arts
Kettering, Ohio

Kay Cowen, RN, MSN
Clinical Associate Professor
University of North Carolina
Greensboro, North Carolina

Sheri Curtis, MSN, ARNP
Clinical Assistant Professor
University of Florida
Gainesville, Florida

Mary Dowell, PhD
Professor
University of Mary Hardin Baylor
Belton, Texas

Sharon Falkenstern, PhD, CRNP, MSN, RN
Nursing Instructor
The Pennsylvania State University
University Park, Pennsylvania

Marcia Gardner, MA, RN, CPNP, CPN
Assistant Professor
Drexel University
Philadelphia, Pennsylvania

Donna Hallas, PhD
Associate Professor and Chairperson of
Undergraduate Studies
Pace University
Pleasantville, New York

Mary Jo Konkloski, RNC, MSN, ANP
Nursing Instructor
Arnot Ogden Medical Center
Elmira, New York

Brenda Ludwig, BSN, MS, RNCS, FNP, EdD
Nursing Faculty
Bob Jones University
Greenville, South Carolina

Karen Schneider, RN, MS
Nursing Faculty
Clackamas Community College
Oregon City, Oregon

Kathleen Taylor, BS, MAT
Mathematics Instructor
Clackamas Community College
Oregon City, Oregon

Angela Wood, RNC, MSN, PhD
Faculty and Chairperson of Undergraduate
Nursing Program
Carson-Newman College
Jefferson City, Tennessee

Companion Website

Wendy Bowles, MSN, CPNP
Clinical Instructor
Kettering College of Medical Arts
Kettering, Ohio

Kay Cowen, RN, MSN
Clinical Associate Professor
University of North Carolina at
Greensboro, North Carolina

Sharon Falkenstern, PhD, CRNP, MSN, RN
Nursing Instructor
The Pennsylvania State University
University Park, Pennsylvania

Joan Fleitas, EdD, RN
Associate Professor
Lehman College
Bronx, New York

Rebecca Gesler, MSN, RN
Assistant Professor
Spalding University
Louisville, Kentucky

Pamela Pranke, RN, MSN
Adjunct Associate Professor
Jamestown College
Jamestown, North Dakota

Karen Schneider, RN, MS
Nursing Faculty
Clackamas Community College
Oregon City, Oregon

Kathleen Taylor, BS, MAT
Mathematics Instructor
Clackamas Community College
Oregon City, Oregon

Julie Will, RN, MSN
Instructor
Ivy Tech State College
Terre Haute, Indiana

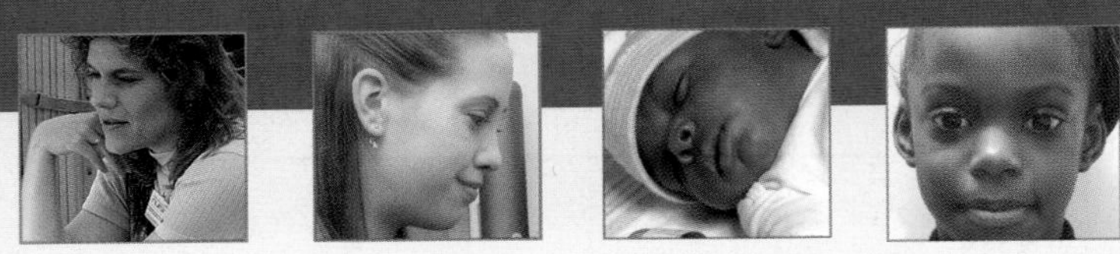

Thank You

We would like to express our deep gratitude to more than 125 of our colleagues from schools and hospitals across the country who provided us with hundreds of hours of their time over the past three years. These individuals assisted us in developing this book in one or more of the following activities—reviewed manuscript chapters, participated in focus groups, reviewed illustrations, class tested sample chapters, and patiently answered our questions—up until the time of publication. **Child Health Nursing: Partnering with Children & Families** has benefited immeasurably from your efforts, insights, objections, encouragements, and your selfless willingness to share your expertise as teachers and nurses.

Academic Reviewers

Becky Althaus, University of Texas-Arlington
Margaret Arieta, University Massachusetts-Dartmouth
Sandra Averitt, Kennesaw State University
Lawrette Axley, University of Memphis
Celeste Baldwin, University of Toledo
Janet Banks, University of Texas San Antonio Health Sciences
Jane Barnsteiner, University of Pennsylvania
Joanna Basuray, University of North Carolina-Greensboro
Teresa Berry, Piedmont College
Janice Bidwell, San Diego State University
Nancy Bingaman, Monterey Peninsula College
Wanda Bradshaw, Duke University
Vera Brancato, Kutztown University
Kitty Carmichael, Seattle University
Ellen Chiocca, Loyola University-Chicago
Kay Cowen, University of North Carolina-Greensboro
Vera Cull, University of Alabama-Birmingham
Sheri Curtis, University of Florida-Gainesville
Cheryl DeGraw, Florence-Darlington Technical College
Susan Dickey, Temple University
Pam Dinapoli, University of New Hampshire
Cheryl Dipretoro, California State University-San Bernardino
Carol Doane, University of Southern Maine
Laurie Doerner, Oral Roberts University
Edna Domingo, California State University-San Bernardino
Michele D'Arcy Evans, Lewis Clark State College
Karen Faison, Norfolk State University
Hobie Etta Feagai, Hawaii Pacific University
Missy Fleck, University of Nebraska Medical Center
Joseph Foley, University of Akron
Janelle Gardner, California State University-Chico
Pamela M. Gardner, Truman State University
Mary Jo Gay, Missouri Western State College
Theresa Turick-Gibson, Hartwick University
Lynn Gilbert, University of Colorado Health Science Center
Myra Goldman, Bellarmine University
Brigit Van Graafeiland, University of Maryland
Renee Granados, California State University-Hayward
Linda Grinstead, Grand Valley State University
Mary Jane Hamilton, Texas A&M University
Pamela Hamre, College of St. Catherine
Debra Hearington, Virginia Commonwealth University
Peg Heinzer, Case Western Reserve University
Marcia Hern, University of Cincinnati
Karrie Ingalsbe, Illinois State University
Ritamarie John, Columbia University
Amy Johnson, University of Delaware
Wendee Johnson, Arizona State University
Lorie Judson, California State University-Los Angeles
Anne Keith, University of Southern Maine
Vickie Keller, Ball State University
Sheila Kenning, Skagit Valley College
Ellen Christian Keogh, University of Massachusetts-Dartmouth
Sherry Knoppers, Grand Rapids Community College
Marie Kodadek, George Mason University
Anita Kyle, Texas Woman's University
Fred Lege, Washington State University
Kim Litwack, Grand Valley State University
Marcia London, Beth El College of Nursing/University of Colorado
Faith Lowe, Delaware Technical College
Lea Melvin, University of Texas-Arlington
Sara Mitchell, Mercer University
Sandra Mott, Boston College
Linda Aveni Murray, Anne Arundel Community College
Diana Neal, St. Olaf College
Louise M. Niemer, Northern Kentucky University
Patricia Nosel, Edinboro University of Pennsylvania
Jane Overbay, Purdue University
Donna Patterson, University of Pennsylvania
Deborah Persell, Arkansas State University
Mary Anne Peters, LaSalle University
Gloria Plascak, Indiana State University
Debbie Poling, Regis University
Sharon Pontious, Miami University/University of Phoenix
Deborah Popovich, University of Florida-Gainesville
Lynn Rasmussen, University of Missouri-Kansas City
Elisabeth Rettew, Malone College
Mary Reus, University of Maryland
Nicole Robert, McNeese State University
Deborah Roberts, Humboldt University
Katherine Roberts, Lamar University
Sue Robsel, North Central State College
Karen Saenz, University of Central Florida
Barbara Schaffner, Otterbein College
Susan Schultz, Angelo State University
Kimberly Serroka, Youngstown State University

JoAnne Solchany, University of Washington
Mary Stec, Abington Memorial Hospital-Dixon School of Nursing
Kathy Thornton, Georgia Southern University
Mary Ann Van Dam, San Francisco State University
Diane Van Os, Westminster College
Nancy Wagner, Youngstown State University
Maureen Waller, College of DuPage
Jacquelyn Williams, New Mexico State University
Amy Swango-Wilson, University of Alaska-Anchorage
Barbara Woodring, University of Alabama-Birmingham
Sue Yadro, University of Wisconsin-Madison
Kelly Zinn, Clarkson College

Clinical Reviewers

Fran Blayney, Children's Hospital, Los Angeles, CA
Dianne Cella, Children's Hospital, Boston, MA
Isabel Couto, Clinical Coordinator-Endocrinology, Children's National Medical Center, Washington, DC
Beth Devenis, Children's Hospital, Los Angeles, CA
Jennifer DuVal, Clinical Instructor, Children's National Medical Center, Washington, DC
Jill Fragoso, Children's Memorial Hospital, Chicago, IL
Pamela Gampetro, Family Nurse Practitioner, Children's Memorial Hospital, Chicago, IL
Cindy George, Nurse Practitioner, Children's National Medical Center, Washington, DC
Lisa Halbur, Pediatric Nurse Practioner, Children's Hospital, Omaha, NE
Erin Hanson, Pediatric Nurse Practitioner, Rainbow Babies & Children's Hospital, Cleveland, OH
Peter Keenan, Pediatric Nurse Practitioner, Children's Hospital, Boston, MA
Mary O'Neil Kinler, Advanced Practice Specialist, Respiratory Care Unit, Children's National Medical Center, Washington, DC
Andrea Kline, Pediatric Critical Care Nurse Practitioner, Children's Memorial Hospital Chicago, IL
Linda Larson, Case Manager-Neonatal Intensive Care, Children's National Medical Center, Washington, DC
Louise Minnich, Patient Resource Manager, Duke University Medical Center, Durham, NC
Dianne Molsberry, PALS & Pediatric Outreach Education Coordinator, Sacred Heart Children's Hospital, Spokane, WA
Nancy J. Morwessel, Pediatric Nurse Practitioner, Diabetes Center, Cincinnati Children's Hospital, Cincinnati, OH
Marijo Miller Ratcliffe, Pediatric Nurse Practitioner, Children's Hospital and Regional Medical Center, Seattle, WA
Kathy Ruccione, Nursing Administrator/Co-Director, Health Promotion & Outcomes Program, Center for Cancer and Blood Diseases, Children's Hospital, Los Angeles, CA
Joanna Spahis, Genetic Clinical Nurse Specialist, Children's Medical Center of Dallas, TX
Elizabeth Suddaby, Pediatric Cardiovascular Clinical Nurse Specialist, Inova Fairfax Hospital for Children, Falls Church, VA
Barbara Suplit, Children's Memorial Hospital, Chicago, IL
Nancy Weichler, Research Coordinator-Nephrology, Children's Hospital, Pittsburgh, PA
Judy White, Director of Nursing and Nurse Educator, Vital Care, Inc., Meridian, MO
Molly Winterich, Rainbow Babies and Children's Hospital, Cleveland, OH

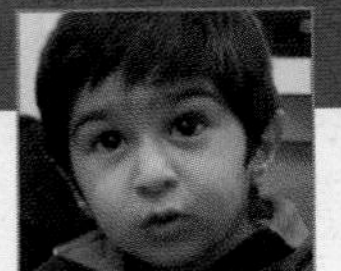
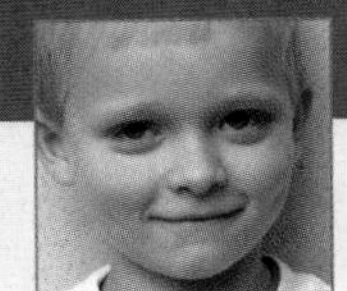
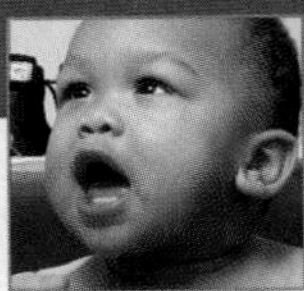
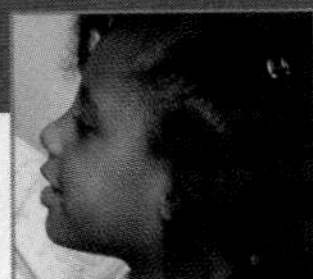

Preface

The world children grow up in today is vastly different from the world we experienced in our early years. Our evolving social environment has resulted in diverse family structures and roles. Multiple racial and ethnic groups now commonly share communities, work environments, and recreation. Television, computers, and video games are part of children's routines, and nutritional patterns have changed due to the complexity of daily lives. The physical structure of communities, including schools, modes of transportation, and degree of safety in neighborhoods, has altered physical activity habits. Life in complex societies offers new challenges to mental health, and home environments provide different risk and protective factors in managing the health and illness of child family members.

These changes in our society create a need for new paradigms in nursing and nursing education, as well as for a new, contemporary pediatric nursing textbook. Nursing care is the primary focus of *Child Health Nursing: Partnering with Children & Families.* Excellence in pediatric nursing care, whether it is in the acute care setting or in the community, is the major aim of the authors. You, as a student, will be challenged to synthesize previous and new knowledge, apply nursing research findings, and integrate current knowledge to use critical thinking skills in planning pediatric nursing care. You, as a nurse, will be challenged to lead, examining ways in which you can positively influence the healthcare of children and their families in all settings.

Child Health Nursing responds to the need for new approaches to child and adolescent healthcare and nursing education in several ways. Themes in this book include:

- Partnering with Children and Their Families
- The Roles of the Nurse
- Health Promotion and Health Maintenance
- The Child Healthcare Continuum
- Critical Thinking

The subtitle, *Partnering with Children & Families*, reflects the core value of our textbook—emphasizing family-centered care, recognition of the family as the central influence in each child's life, and respect for families from all cultures. Families are viewed as case managers, partners with healthcare providers, and as integral participants in care in all pediatric nursing settings. Partnership and collaboration with interdisciplinary healthcare providers is another key concept of our textbook. This approach supports the model and philosophy of family-centered care as the standard of practice in pediatric nursing (Lewandowski & Tesler, 2003).

This textbook also introduces a new paradigm with which to view healthcare of children. The *Bindler-Ball Child Healthcare Model* illustrates an important core value—that all children need health promotion and health maintenance interventions, no matter where they seek healthcare or what health conditions they may be experiencing. Families may visit offices or other community settings, specifically to obtain health supervision care; or nurses may integrate health promotion and health maintenance into the care for children with acute and chronic illness in a variety of inpatient and outpatient settings. The Bindler-Ball Healthcare Model places health promotion and health maintenance at the foundation of a pyramid to demonstrate the need to apply these concepts with all children. See Chapter 1 for an introduction to this model.

ORGANIZATION

The six units in this textbook have a unifying theme. The first unit, *Nurses, Children, and Families*, lays the foundation for a thorough understanding of pediatric nursing in today's world. It discusses the nurse's roles in caring for children in the hospital, community and home, as well as the concept of family-centered care. The unit also includes chapters exploring cultural, genetic, and hereditary influences on the child.

The second unit focuses on *Child Concepts and Application*, melding theory with application so that concepts can be applied to pediatric nursing care in any healthcare setting. We describe concepts of growth and development and communication with child and family in separate chapters, and examine their applications to pediatric nursing. A chapter on social and environmental influences addresses contemporary topics pertinent to children and their families in today's world. The pediatric assessment chapter provides basic and detailed information that will be applied in all pediatric healthcare settings. Lastly, we include a separate chapter for nutrition of the infant, child, and adolescent, including normal nutritional needs and some common disruptions.

The third unit focuses on *Health Promotion and Health Maintenance Through Childhood.* The first chapter introduces basic concepts and each of the remaining five chapters applies health promotion and health maintenance concepts with specific approaches for children at each developmental stage from newborn through adolescence. Nurses assess children thoroughly, establish goals in partnership with the family, intervene to promote and maintain health and foster development, and evaluate the outcomes of care. This unique approach minimizes repetition throughout the book, and provides the student a lens through which to approach care that underscores the need for all children to receive routine health promotion and health maintenance to achieve optimal health.

The fourth unit, *Child Healthcare Settings and Considerations*, explores the various settings in which care occurs. In addition to the hospital, nurses and nursing students are more likely than ever before to provide care in community settings, such as clinics, offices, out-patient centers, schools and homes, where health promotion and health maintenance activities predominate. Shorter hospitalizations have become the norm, thereby increasing the need for more comprehensive care in community settings. Therefore, the nurse's roles in caring for children in the community and the hospital are the focus of two separate chapters. A chapter on pain assessment and management, which is sometimes overlooked in children, provides general pediatric nursing care concepts that are woven through the remainder of the book.

The fifth unit discusses *Health Conditions: Episodic to End-of-Life.* Technology and mobility have radically changed the healthcare needs of children, as well as healthcare delivery. Children with chronic illness are living longer, and children, in general, are exposed to a greater variety of diseases. Prevention and treatment of infectious and communicable diseases is a significant role in pediatric nursing care, as addressed in the initial chapter. The remaining chapters in the unit focus on nursing care of the child with a chronic condition, nursing care of the child with a life-threatening illness or injury, and end-of-life care and bereavement. With continuous improvement in healthcare technology, children who once succumbed to illnesses and conditions are now living into adulthood. Accompanying the resultant growth in complex healthcare challenges is the need to improve care and outcomes for children with chronic conditions from infancy to adolescence and ease the transition to adulthood.

The sixth unit consists of 14 chapters that address *Nursing Care of Specific Health Conditions.* Information about health conditions, including both illnesses and injuries, is grouped by body systems, eliminating the need for duplication at various places in the text. This streamlined approach builds on previous concepts rather than repeating them, integrating a developmental approach with pertinent conditions affecting all age groups from newborn to adolescent.

The chapters fully describe diseases and injuries beginning with significant pediatric anatomical and physiological differences. This is followed by a discussion of the etiology, pathophysiology, clinical manifestations, and **collaborative care**, including diagnostics and clinical therapy sections. **Nursing management** of major conditions contains detailed sections on assessment and diagnosis, planning and intervention, and evaluation of care.

Sample nursing care plans will assist you in applying developmental, psychosocial, and physiological concepts to the care of children with specific conditions. North American Nursing Diagnosis Association (NANDA International) diagnoses are used, as well as the current Nursing Intervention Classifications (NIC) and Nursing Outcomes Classifications (NOC).

VISUALS THAT TEACH

When developing the first edition of a pediatric nursing textbook, the authors and the publisher painstakingly identify how the new book will differ from other existing textbooks—What key concepts should be emphasized for students, and what type of presentation will call attention to those key concepts? The result of such discussions is an art program that uses a thoroughly integrated approach, beginning with the cover and carried through the interior of the textbook. The cover of *Child Health Nursing* features hand-painted tiles from the Shands Children's Hospital at the University of Florida. The tiles on the Healing Wall at Shands express the "hope, life, and love" of children and family members. We have partnered with Shands to incorporate the children's expressions about life, healthcare, and their experiences throughout this book. Art is both a method of expression and a healing modality, and the feelings, design, and colors of the tiles integrated throughout this book will help you identify with children and their families, and understand their experiences. We acknowledge and thank Shands Children's Hospital, as well as the children and family members, for allowing us to reprint these tiles throughout this textbook.

The belief that art can teach is evident throughout the book. In addition to the tiles, you will see hundreds of contemporary photographs of children and families in healthcare and related settings throughout the textbook.

- **Photo Stories** help bring information and concepts "alive" so that you develop a deeper understanding about the effect of a specific condition on the child and family. These stories include photographs of a child or situation to demonstrate the progression of a condition or the various settings and the challenges a child and family may face.

- While the text explains in-depth pathophysiology of pediatric conditions, the **Pathophysiology Illustrated** figures allow you to see into the body in order to visualize the causes and effects of conditions on children. These elaborate drawings illustrate conditions on a cellular or organ level, and may also portray the step-by-step process of a disease. Drawings or photos with artistic overlays relate disease to its anatomical location and action.

- **As They Grow** illustrations help you visualize the important anatomical and physiological differences between a child and an adult. These features illustrate the important ways that a child's development influences health care needs and how the child progresses through developmental stages.

The photographs and drawings throughout the textbook do more than illustrate concepts and examples. You will find **Critical Thinking Highlights** among the figure captions. These unique highlights, also appearing in the text itself, encourage you to apply information and analyze the nursing implications needed to provide care for children and their families, thus adding true learning value to the visuals.

In addition, unit openers set the tone of the textbook, expressing the dynamic roles of the nurse through a collage of images that correlate to the chapters in that unit. One goal is for the book to serve as a portal through which students can visualize and explore the rich and varied career opportunities in the specialty area of pediatric nursing.

FEATURES THAT HELP YOU USE THIS BOOK SUCCESSFULLY

Nursing students face challenges in their education—demands on their time, the need to apply research findings, evaluating components of evidence-based practice, and developing their critical thinking skills. Thus instructors and students alike value the in-text learning aids that we include in our textbooks to meet the challenges of pediatric nursing in today's world. We developed a textbook that is easy to learn from and easy to use as a professional reference. The following guide will help you use the features and resources from *Child Health Nursing* to succeed in the classroom, in the clinical setting, on the NCLEX-RN® examination, and in nursing practice.

- **Practice Alerts** warn you of safety precautions and other nursing alerts to consider in providing safe care.
- **Clinical Tips** are "pearls" from clinical nursing experts embedded throughout the textbook.
- At the beginning of each chapter, a **MediaLink** box lists specific animations or videos, NCLEX-RN® Review questions, and other interactive exercises that appear on the accompanying free **Student CD-ROM** and the **Companion Website. The EXPLORE MediaLink** box at the end of the chapter reminds you to use the media resources. The MediaLink feature will further enhance your learning experience, build upon knowledge gained from this textbook, prepare you for the NCLEX-RN®, and foster critical thinking.
- **Case Scenarios** and photos at the beginning of the chapter engage you with a child's real-life experience with a specific health challenge. Additional information about the child and family appears throughout the chapter to illustrate application of nursing care. Use the questions embedded in each scenario to apply pathophysiological, psychosocial, family, culture, developmental, or nursing process considerations. At the end of the chapter, a detailed **Critical Thinking in Action** exercise picks up the opening scenario and asks you to apply what you have read to conclude the chapter.
- **Developing Cultural Competence** boxes challenge you to explore differences among racial, ethnic, and social groups, and to plan nursing care that addresses the issues of health disparity.
- The **Complementary Therapy** boxes present approaches other than traditional medical prescriptions that may be used by children and families to maintain health or treat diseases. These boxes discuss research when it is present to support or refute the efficacy of these modalities. At other times, they alert you about information to gather from the family and to consider when planning care.
- **Medications Used to Treat** boxes list the actions, indications, and important nursing implications for medications.
- **Evidence-Based Practice** boxes further enhance the approach to research. We describe a particular nursing problem and investigate the evidence from several studies that explore solutions to the problem. We emphasize nursing research, provide an interpretation explaining the implications of the studies, and then invite you to apply critical thinking skills to further identify nursing care approaches.
- **Partnering with Families** boxes help you to apply the concepts of family-centered nursing care by providing approaches and teaching in a format directly applicable when you work with families.
- **Health Promotion and Maintenance Overviews** summarize the needs of children with specific chronic conditions, such as asthma or diabetes. These overviews teach you to look at the chronically ill child like any other child, with health maintenance needs for prevention, education, and basic care.
- **Clinical Manifestations** boxes link etiology, clinical manifestations, and clinical therapy for specific conditions.
- **Nursing Care Plans** are present in every chapter dealing with health conditions. They illustrate the conceptual approach that nurses need in approaching care for children, including assessment, NANDA nursing diagnoses, goals, plans, interventions (with NIC) and evaluation (with NOC).

RESOURCES THAT INSPIRE SUCCESS—FOR THE STUDENT AND THE INSTRUCTOR

To enhance the teaching and learning process, the following supplements have been developed in close correlation with the new textbook. The full complement of supplemental teaching materials is available to all qualified instructors from your Prentice Hall Health sales representative.

Student CD-ROM—Packaged ***free*** with the textbook, it provides an interactive study program that allows students to practice answering NCLEX-style questions with rationales for right and wrong answers. A unique activity, *Nursing in Action,* shows brief video clips of real nurses and clients, and asks you to respond to critical thinking questions about these scenarios. It also contains an audio glossary, animations, videos, and a link to the Companion Website (an Internet connection is required).

Companion Website @ www.prenhall.com/ball—This ***free*** online study guide is designed to help you apply the concepts presented in the book. Each chapter–specific module features chapter objectives, audio glossary, chapter summary for lecture notes, NCLEX-RN® review questions, case studies, care plan activities, MediaLink applications, links, and useful tools, such as growth charts, food guide pyramid, assessment tools, and more. Additional modules include review of A&P, medications, clinical manifestations, and pediatric dosage calculations.

Clinical Handbook for Pediatric Nursing—Provides general information on growth and development, vital signs, and assessment; information specific to the care of children in the community or hospital, such as dosage calculations, pain charts, immunization schedules; and an overview of primary for conditions organized by body systems.

Clinical Skills Manual for Pediatric Nursing *(by Ruth Bindler and Jane Ball)*—Guides you through more than 70 pediatric skills using full-color photographs and rationales. Throughout *Child Health Nursing*, special cross-reference icons refer you to the complete skill presentation in this manual.

Prentice Hall Real Nursing Skills: Pediatric Nursing —This set of CD-ROMs offers you the complete foundation for competency in performing pediatric nursing skills. It provides comprehensive procedures and rationales demonstrated in hundreds of realistic video clips, animations, illustrations, and photographs.

Prentice Hall Pediatric Drug Guide *(by Ruth Bindler and Linda Howry)*—Provides easy access to over 500 drugs administered to children, organized alphabetically by generic name.

Pediatric Nursing Care Plans *(by Sharon Axton and Terry Fugate)*—This unique reference begins with a foundation of medical diagnosis and pathophysiology before detailing the preparation of individualized nursing care plans tailored to meet the special needs of children.

Reviews & Rationales: Child Health Nursing *(by Mary Ann Hogan and Judy White)*—Provides a core content and NCLEX-RN® review of pediatric nursing in outline format. The CD-ROM, pre-test and post-test guide you through a self-paced review.

Instructor's Resource Manual—Contains a wealth of material to help faculty plan and manage the pediatric nursing course. It includes chapter overviews, detailed lecture suggestions and outlines, learning objectives, a complete test bank, teaching tips, and more for each chapter. The IRM also guides faculty to assign and use the text-specific Companion Website, **www.prenhall.com/ball**, and the Student CD-ROM that accompany the textbook.

Instructor's Resource CD-ROM—Provides several tools to aid faculty in teaching. It features complete PowerPoint presentations—including animations, videos, illustrations, and text slides—for use in the classroom. It also contains an electronic test bank of NCLEX-RN®-style items and pediatric dosage calculation questions, as well as animations and videos from the Student CD-ROM. This resource is available to faculty free upon adoption of the textbook.

Companion Website Syllabus Manager @ www.prenhall.com/ball—Faculty adopting this textbook have ***free*** access to the online Syllabus Manager feature of the Companion Website, **www.prenhall.com/ball**. It offers a whole host of features that facilitate the students' use of the Companion Website, and allows faculty to post syllabi and course information online for their students. For more information or a demonstration of Syllabus Manager, please contact a Prentice Hall sales representative.

Prentice Hall's Research Navigator™—Provides the easiest way for students to start a research assignment or research paper. Complete with extensive help on the research process and two exclusive databases of credible and reliable source material, *Research Navigator*™ helps students quickly and efficiently make the most of their research time.

Online Course Management Systems—*Prentice Hall OneKey* is an integrated online resource that brings a wide array of supplemental resources together in one convenient place for both students and faculty. OneKey features everything you and your students need for out-of-class work, conveniently organized to match your syllabus. OneKey is an online course management solution that features interactive modules, text and image PowerPoint presentations, animations, videos, and case studies. OneKey also provides course management tools so faculty can customize course content, build online tests, create assignments, enter grades, post announcements, communicate with students, and much more. Testing materials, gradebooks, and other instructor resources are available in a separate section that can be accessed by instructors only. OneKey content is available in three different platforms. A nationally hosted version is available in the reliable, easy-to-use CourseCompass platform. The same content is also available for download to locally hosted versions of BlackBoard and WebCT. Please contact your Prentice Hall sales representative for a demonstration or go online to **http://myphlip.pearsoncmg.com/OneKey/index.html**.

Lewandowski, L.A. & Tesler, M.D. (2003). Family-centered care: Putting it into action: the SPN/ANA guide to family-centered care. Washington, DC: Society of Pediatric Nurses & American Nurses Association.

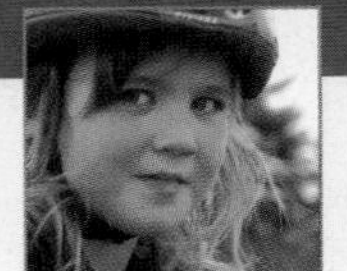
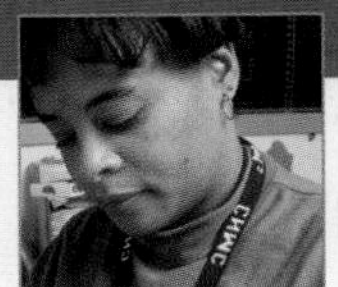
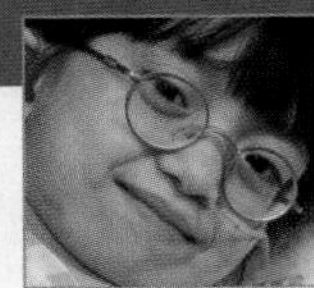
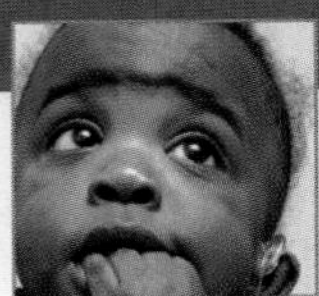

Acknowledgments

It is both an honor and a significant responsibility to develop and write a new pediatric textbook. We have had the privilege of collaborating with Prentice Hall Health to share our vision for a creative and inviting textbook to educate students about the nursing care of children and their families.

The development of a new textbook requires a team that is fully committed to the vision from the initial ideas and concepts discussed through the final production process. We were fortunate to have a close collaborative relationship with our publishing company, Prentice Hall Health, and our nursing editor, Maura Connor. Because of our relationship, we became full partners in the development of the textbook's conceptual framework, features, and design. Maura accepted our ideas and took the next steps of ensuring that we had the resources to make this a truly special book—reviewers and consultants to assure that our content focus was appropriate, new art to make the textbook come alive, and a developmental editor to act as our liaison and advocate throughout the process. Vice President & Publisher Julie Alexander enthusiastically supported this venture on behalf of Prentice Hall Health. We are also grateful to Robin Baliszewski, President of Prentice Hall's Careers, Health, Education, and Technology Division, and to Tim Bozik, President of Prentice Hall Higher Education, for their dedication and investment of the special development needs for this textbook.

Kim Wyatt, Developmental Editor, has been a steadfast partner throughout the venture of developing this textbook. She understood the vision and conceptual framework and applied her multiple talents to make this team project successful. She solved problems before we knew they existed, interpreted our desires and concerns to the publisher, and helped ensure that we achieved our goals. Without her unwavering support, this textbook would not have been as special for all of us.

Managing Editor Marilyn Meserve was an important liaison for editorial consultation. Former Assistant Editor Sladjana Repic was essential in cultivating our relationship with hundreds of reviewers—her pleasant and competent manner was outstanding. We thank Danielle Doller, Associate Editor, for analyzing reviews and developing the many resources accompanying this book, including the student CD-ROM, the companion website, the clinical handbook, and the many instructor resources. We thank Nick Radhuber, Production Editor, Patrick Walsh, Production Managing Editor, and Nicole Benson, Executive Marketing Manager, for their expertise and valuable contributions. Our thanks also go to Cheryl Asherman, Maria Guglielmo, and Mary Siener for creating the fresh textbook design. Media Project Manager John Jordan helped bring our media ideas to fruition. At Carlisle Communications, we thank Lori Dalberg for coordinating production, and Carey Lange for her copyediting skills.

A number of other individuals made major contributions to this textbook. George Dodson and Roy Ramsey are dedicated and meticulous photographers who have worked with us over many years. They have an amazing talent in capturing beautiful and creative images of children and families. Several agencies allowed us to photograph children. New images for this textbook were captured in Jackson, Mississippi at the University of Mississippi Medical Center, Blair Batson Children's Hospital; in Washington, D.C. at Children's National Medical Center; and in Spokane, Washington at the Shriner's Hospital for Children, Sacred Heart Children's Hospital, Peoples' Clinic, and many community sites. Above all, we sincerely thank the children and families who allowed us to illustrate development, pediatric healthcare conditions, and nursing care by photographing children in hospital, home, and community settings.

The tiles featured on the cover and throughout the textbook were created by children and families. We are grateful to Shands Hospital in Gainesville, Florida for allowing us to incorporate them into our book to illustrate our theme of partnering with children and their families. The tiles make up the Healing Wall located in the atrium at Shands at the University of Florida and the Cancer Center. Each tile reflects the individual artist's expression of hope, life, and love.

Two chapters in the book were written by experts in specialized fields. We particularly thank Nancy Bowers and Jeanette Zaichkin for their contributions on genetics and newborn health promotion, respectively. We would like to thank Joseann DeWitt for her assistance during photo shoots in Mississippi and for her contributions to the book while serving as consulting editor. We would also like to acknowledge the academic- and clinical-based pediatric nurses who served as reviewers and consultants. Their valuable feedback enabled us to more appropriately focus our chapters for today's student nurses and the practice of pediatric nursing.

This is a book that emphasizes partnering with families in order to provide comprehensive care for children. We also consider our families a critically important part of our lives. Without them we could not reach our own personal and professional goals and we depend on them every day for support, love, and caring. We thank them for their enduring partnerships with us in making this book a reality.

Jane W. Ball
Ruth C. Bindler

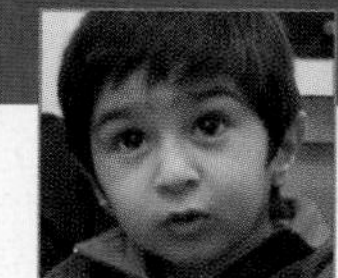
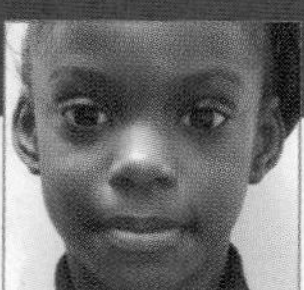
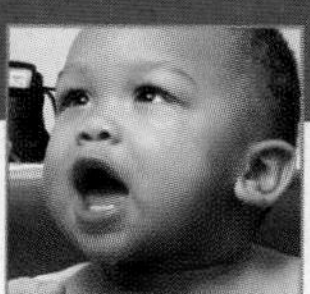
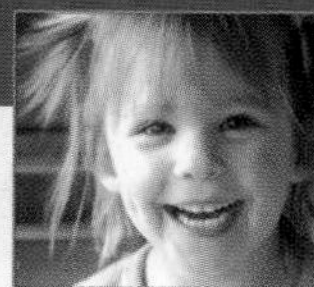

Detailed Contents

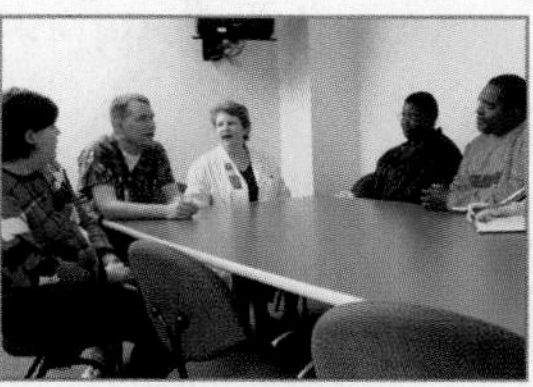

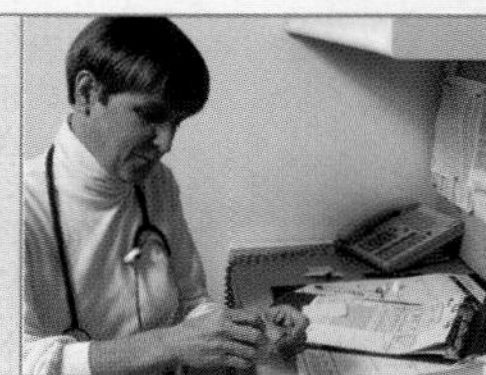

UNIT VI
Nursing Care of Specific Health Conditions 723

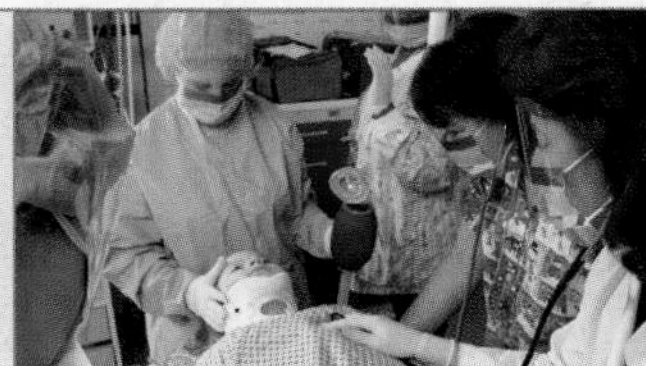

Chapter 23
Alterations in Fluid, Electrolyte, and Acid–Base Balance 724

Chapter 29
Alterations in Cellular Growth 1036

Chapter 30
Alterations in Gastrointestinal Function 1090

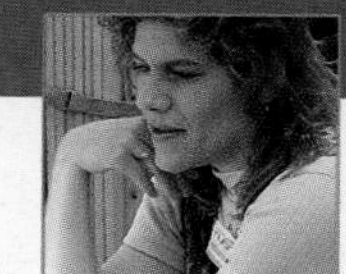
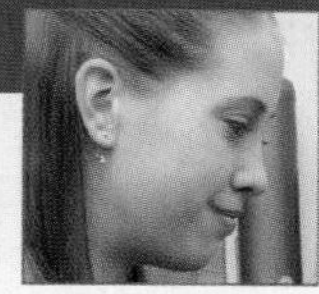
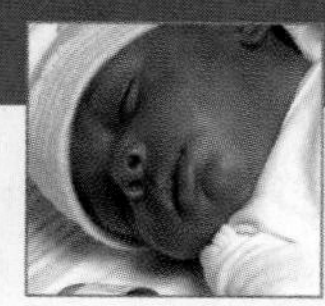
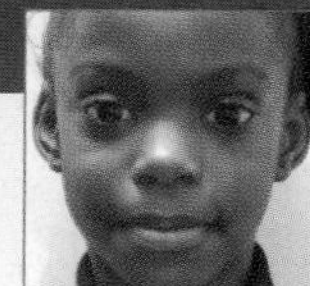

Special Features

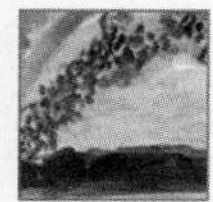

As They Grow

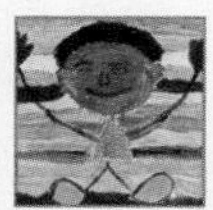

Photo Story

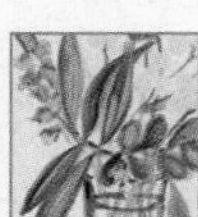

Health Promotion and Maintenance Overview

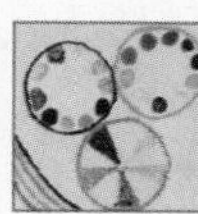

Evidence-Based Practice

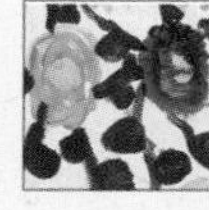

Nursing Care Plan

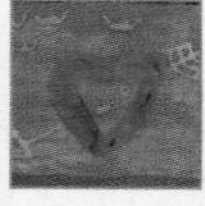

Clinical Manifestations

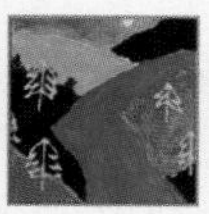

Complementary Therapy

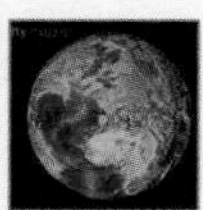

Developing Cultural Competence

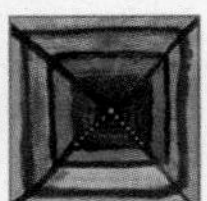

Medications Used to Treat . . .

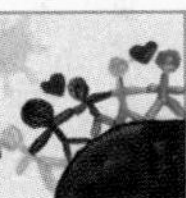

Partnering with Families

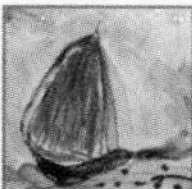

Pathophysiology Illustrated

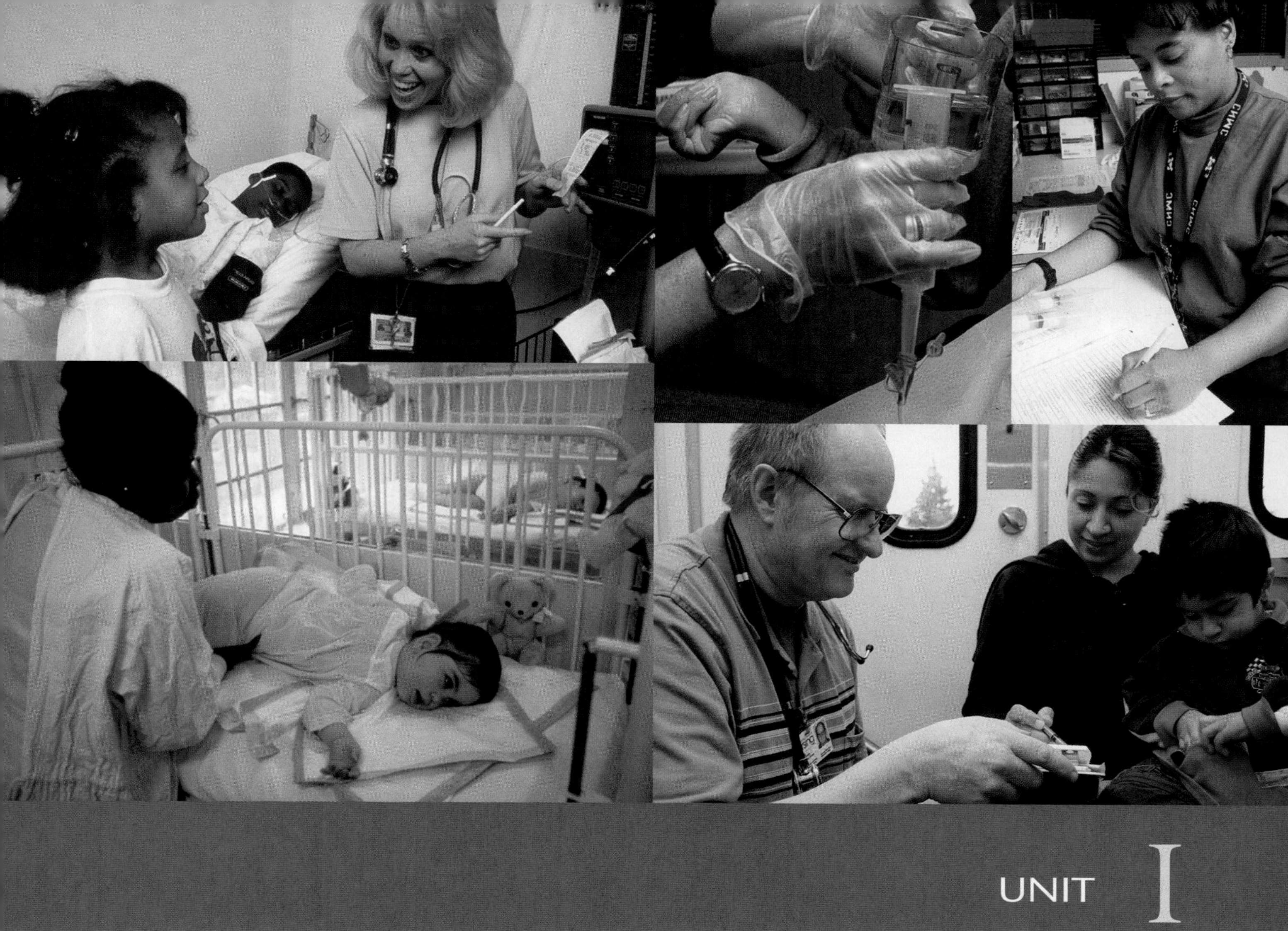

UNIT I

Nurses, Children, and Families

Pediatric nurses care for children and their families in many different settings, including the hospital, healthcare centers, physicians' offices, specialty care centers, the home, schools, and the community. Pediatric nurses develop partnerships with children and their families to address the child's acute or chronic health condition, to prevent disease, or to promote the child's growth and development. The partnerships formed enable the pediatric nurse to learn about the family's culture and belief system, potential genetic or hereditary influences, family strengths and resources, and preferences for care; this information will provide the foundation for the nursing care plan, developed in collaboration with the child and family. Pediatric nurses will implement the nursing care plan by providing direct care and education. In some cases, the pediatric nurse functions as the advocate for the child and family in the healthcare system and serves as case manager for children with complex health conditions.

Chapter 1

Nurse's Role in Care of the Child: Hospital, Community Settings, and Home

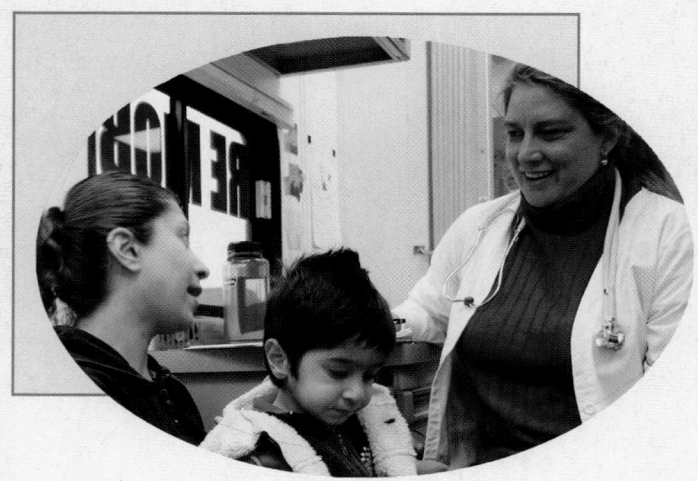

Drew Santo is a 3-year-old boy who has a seizure disorder that until a week ago was fairly well controlled by medication. He and his family receive healthcare at the center serviced by their health plan. A pediatric nurse and pediatrician collaborate in providing Drew's healthcare and monitoring his developmental progress.

Drew had a seizure in the last week. His phenytoin blood level, taken the day of the seizure, was slightly lower than the therapeutic range. This likely indicates that his parents have given Drew his medication fairly regularly, but perhaps he needs a higher dosage or a different medication. Because of the recent seizure, an electroencephalogram is ordered to identify any change in the electrical pattern in the brain. Other laboratory tests are also ordered, following the guidelines of the health center's clinical pathway for children with seizure disorders.

Over the past 2 years, Drew's family and the pediatric nurse have worked in partnership to ensure that Drew is treated as a healthy child with a chronic condition. The nurse has helped his parents to obtain information about his condition, to understand the action of his medication, and to take appropriate measures when he has a seizure. Drew's parents are upset that he has again had a seizure, especially when they have done everything they could to keep the seizures under control. They have been able to think of him as a normal boy because he had not had a seizure for a long time. Now they wonder if they will be able to keep treating him that way.

"Drew's seizure was scary, so I called Mom. He was shaking all over and wouldn't wake up. He even wet his pants, and he has not done that for a long time."

—Kevin, age 8

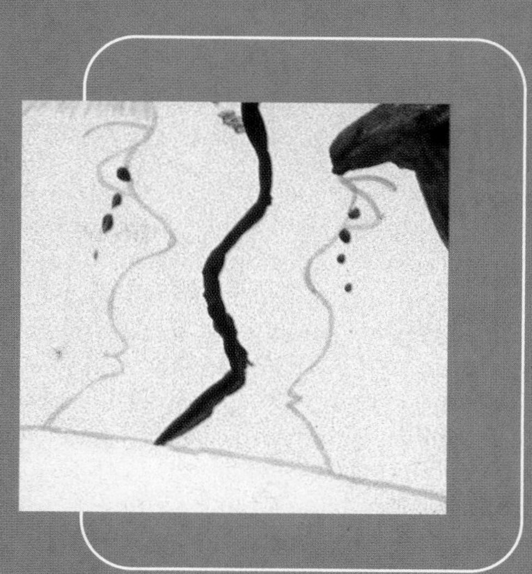

Learning Outcomes

After completing this chapter, you will be able to:

- Describe and differentiate between the general and advanced practice nurse roles in child health nursing.
- Understand the historical and current societal influences on pediatric healthcare and nursing practice.
- Analyze the current causes of child morbidity and mortality and identify opportunities for nurses to intervene.
- Contrast the policies for obtaining informed consent of minors with policies for adults.
- Identify unique pediatric legal and ethical issues in pediatric nursing practice.

Key Terms

advance directives/26
advocacy/7
assent/24
autonomy/27
beneficence/27
case management/7
clinical practice guidelines/12
competent/24
confidentiality/25
continuity of care/7
critical pathways/12
emancipated minors/24
evidence-based practice/13
family-centered care/14
informed consent/24
justice/27
mature minors/24
medical home/healthcare home/14
moral dilemma/26
morbidity/18
nonmaleficence/27
partnership/13
privacy/25
quality improvement/22
risk management/22

MediaLink http://www.prenhall.com/ball

Resources for this chapter can be found on the CD-ROM accompanying this textbook, and on the Companion Website at http://www.prenhall.com/ball. Click on Chapter 1 to select the activities for this chapter.

CD-ROM

Videos

The Role of the Pediatric Nurse

NCLEX Review

Audio Glossary

COMPANION WEBSITE

NCLEX Review

MediaLink Applications

Determine Eligibility for Health Programs
Develop an Educational Brochure
Ethical Dilemmas and the Decision-Making Process
Understanding Policies and Practices

PEDIATRIC HEALTHCARE OVERVIEW

Nurses provide care to healthy children, as well as to those with illnesses, injuries, and chronic conditions, in a wide variety of settings. Fortunately, most children in the United States and Canada are healthy, experiencing only occasional short-term health problems, and nurses have the opportunity to partner with them to prevent disease and promote a healthy lifestyle. However, children with special healthcare needs require frequent contact with the healthcare system to achieve and maintain their optimal level of health.

In all cases, nurses working with children have the pleasure of watching children grow, achieve milestones in development, and adapt to and manage their health conditions. As nurses, they find reward in knowing they made a contribution to the health and welfare of these children.

Nurses who choose to specialize in pediatrics need all of the foundational knowledge provided during nursing education such as the nursing process, anatomy and physiology, physical assessment, healthcare condition recognition and management, and a range of nursing skills. Building upon the principles, knowledge, and skills already learned, pediatric nurses integrate additional competencies related to the care of children and their families into their practice. The special knowledge and skills that nurses caring for children must acquire and apply are listed in Box 1–1.

Pediatric healthcare occurs along a continuum that reflects not only the various settings of care, but also the complexity and range of care required by individual children. For example, all children need health promotion and health maintenance services, but some children will need care for chronic conditions, acute illnesses and injuries, and even end-of-life care. See Figure 1–1 ■ for the model of pediatric healthcare upon which this text is based.

The range of healthcare services provided by nurses specializing in pediatrics leads to many exciting professional opportunities in a wide variety of clinical settings and nursing roles. The array of settings where pediatric nurses work includes the following:

- Hospital units, such as pediatric wards, intensive care units, newborn nursery, emergency department, radiology, and specialty clinics
- Physicians' offices, clinics, and healthcare centers
- Home of the child
- Rehabilitation centers and residential treatment centers
- Schools, childcare centers, and camps
- In the community

Many different healthcare providers collaborate in the provision of pediatric healthcare, such as nurses, physicians, social workers, pharmacists, optometrists, psychologists, dentists, nutritionists, emergency medical technicians, speech therapists, and physical and occupational therapists. Nurses play a significant role in the provision of healthcare for children, with varied responsibilities in different settings.

Think about the role of the nurse in working with children who have seizures. In how many different settings could you find nurses providing care to children with this condition? Does the type of nursing care provided to children by nurses differ among these settings? Regardless of the setting in which nurses work, assessment, nursing care interventions, education, and advocacy are universal roles. This chapter reviews concepts important to pediatric nursing: the role of the nurse in pediatrics, historical highlights of pediatric healthcare, the contemporary climate of pediatric healthcare, and legal and ethical issues.

BOX 1–1 Expected Competencies of the Pediatric Nurse

The Society of Pediatric Nurses has put forth these standards for pediatric prelicensure and early professional development for the generalist pediatric nurse.

- An understanding of the unique anatomical, physiological, and developmental differences among neonates, infants, children, and adolescents, as well as the needs unique to the growth and development of children who have chronic conditions and their families;
- The ability to care for children and promote their health in the context of their families;
- The ability to communicate effectively with children, families, and other healthcare providers, demonstrating sensitivity to cultural issues, especially those related to how the family and healthcare providers tend to children's healthcare needs;
- The provision of safety assurance and injury prevention to children and their families;
- The ability to provide for the exceptional needs of children with episodic injuries or illnesses;
- An understanding of the economic, social, and political influences outside the family that have an impact on children's health and development and family functioning; and
- An understanding of the ethical, moral, and legal dilemmas involving children, families, and healthcare professionals.

Note: Adapted from Society of Pediatric Nurses & American Nurses Association. (2003). Scope and standards of pediatric nursing practice. *(pp. 7–8) Washington, DC: nursesbooks.org*

ROLE OF THE NURSE IN THE CARE OF CHILDREN

Pediatric nursing focuses on protecting children from illness and injury, assisting them to attain optimal levels of health, regardless of health problems, and rehabilitation. This focus fits with the American Nurses Association (1998) definition of the scope of nursing practice: "the diagnosis and treatment of human responses to actual or potential health problems." The predominant nursing roles in caring for children and their families include direct care, education, advocacy, and case management.

Direct Care Provider

The primary role of pediatric nurses is to provide direct nursing care to children and their families. The nursing process provides the framework for delivery of direct pediatric nursing care. The nurse assesses the child and identifies the nursing diagnoses that describe the responses of the child and family to the health promotion and health maintenance plan and to any illness or injury experienced. The nurse then implements and evaluates nursing care. This care is designed to meet the child's physical and emotional needs. It is offered in a manner sensitive to and compatible with the child's and family's cultural beliefs (see Chapter 3∞). It is tailored to the child's developmental stage, giving the child ad-

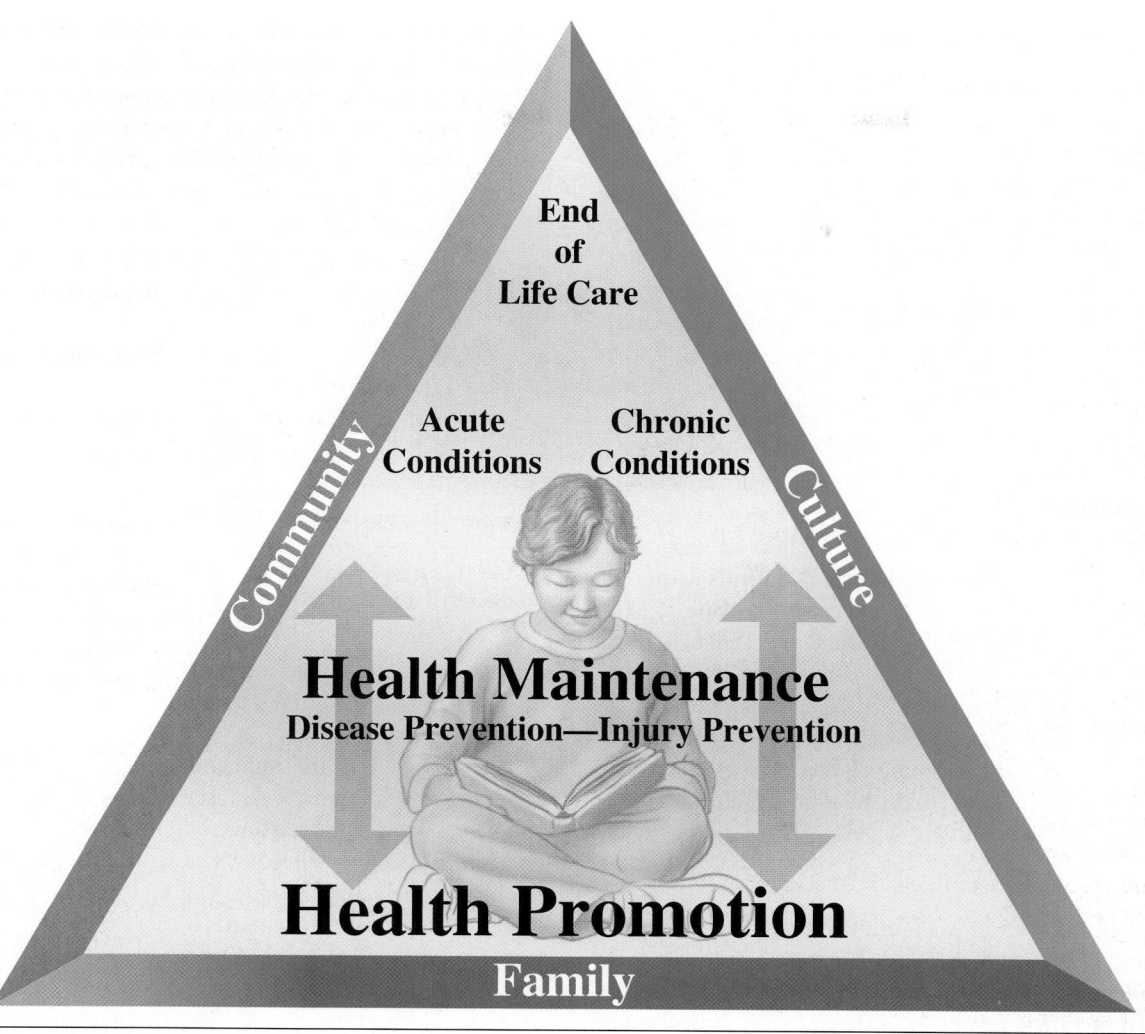

FIGURE 1–1 ■ The Bindler-Ball Continuum of Pediatric Healthcare for Children and Their Families

The outer bars represent the family, cultural, and community influence on the care that the child receives, either through the services sought by the family or the services provided in the community. Cultural influences include the family's decision to seek healthcare and follow recommendations, as well as the healthcare provider's cultural competence in caring for a child and family.

The inner categories represent the different types of healthcare needed by children. All children need health promotion and health maintenance services, represented by the base of the triangle. Notice the arrows representing the upward and downward movement between the levels of care as the child's condition changes.

Children may be healthy with episodic acute illnesses and injuries. Some children develop a chronic condition for which specialized healthcare is needed. A child's chronic condition may be well controlled, but acute episodes (such as with asthma) or other illnesses and injuries may occur, and the child also needs health promotion and health maintenance services to continue. Some children develop a life-threatening illness and ultimately need end-of-life care. A healthy child can also experience a catastrophic injury that causes death and the family needs supportive end-of-life care.

ditional responsibility for self-care with increasing age, and ultimately assisting the adolescent with transition to adult healthcare. This care is also provided in partnership with the family, embracing the principles of family-centered care (see Chapter 2∞).

Nurses play an important role in minimizing the psychological and physical distress experienced by children and their families. Providing support to children and their families is one component of direct nursing care. This often involves listening to the concerns of children and parents, being present during stressful or emotional experiences, and implementing strategies to help children and family members cope. Nurses can help families by suggesting ways to support their children in the hospital, in out-of-hospital settings, and in the home. Nurses also suggest ways to support the families with informational resources, family support groups, referrals for healthcare services, and in some cases respite care.

As a member of the child's healthcare team, the nurse is responsible for collaborating with other health professionals and ensuring that the nursing care is coordinated with that of other professionals. In many cases, experienced pediatric nurses or those with graduate level education assume a leadership role in coordinating the collaboration of a team of interdisciplinary health professionals. In some cases the nurse recognizes that the child and family need care that is outside of the nurse's scope of practice or specific skill level, so a referral must be initiated. In other cases, an interdisciplinary team will meet to jointly develop a care plan for a child with a chronic condition. See the case management section on page 7.

Nurses at differing levels of experience or nursing education expand the range of direct care provided. Once the pediatric nurse has developed experience and has a comfort level in the care of children typically seen in one setting, the pediatric nurse is often ready to move to a different setting or specialty area or to accept a leadership position. In some cases the experienced nurse may be given supervisory responsibility for nursing care provided by other members of the nursing care team. The experienced nurse may also become a preceptor for new nurses, serving as a role model and promoting their clinical skills development.

Advanced practice nurses (e.g., clinical nurse specialists and pediatric nurse practitioners) have a graduate level nursing education, and they are prepared to practice in a specialty area or at a higher level of responsibility. Clinical nurse specialists serve as educators and role models, members of the clinical research team, consultants to the healthcare team, and change agents within the healthcare system. They often have a specialty nursing practice such as respiratory, cardiovascular, or oncology. Pediatric nurse practitioners, in collaboration with physicians and other healthcare team members, perform assessment, diagnosis, and management of health conditions in office settings, schools, and hospitals. Nurse practitioners are now assuming a larger role within hospital settings in the management of children with acute illnesses or the exacerbation of chronic health problems.

Educator

Education of children and their families or caregivers improves treatment results. In pediatric nursing, patient education is especially challenging, because nurses must be prepared to work with children at various levels of understanding. It is also important to do more than give simple facts; the goal of the education is to help the child and family make informed choices about health and healthy behavior. Depending on the needs of the child and family at any particular time, education can focus on health promotion, health maintenance, self-care, and management of a health condition.

Most hospitals encourage a parent to stay with the child and to provide much of the direct and supportive care. Nurses teach parents to watch for important signs and responses to therapies, to increase the child's comfort, and even to provide advanced care. Taking an active role prepares and empowers the parent to assume total responsibility for care after the child leaves the hospital.

Education can be direct teaching to the child and family members about the medications needed to treat a specific health condition and other therapies that will be needed once the child is discharged. Patient education can also be indirect, such as nurses helping children adapt to the hospital setting and preparing them for procedures (Figure 1–2 ■).

Planning and preparation is required to be an effective educator. An understanding of the child's developmental capabilities is important. The nurse needs to become fully informed about the condition and information to be taught, and then to think about strategies and resources that will help the child and family learn about the health condition. See Developing Cultural Competence: Lowering the Reading Level of Patient Education Materials for guidelines about assessing and writing patient education materials.

MediaLink Critical Thinking: Develop an Educational Brochure

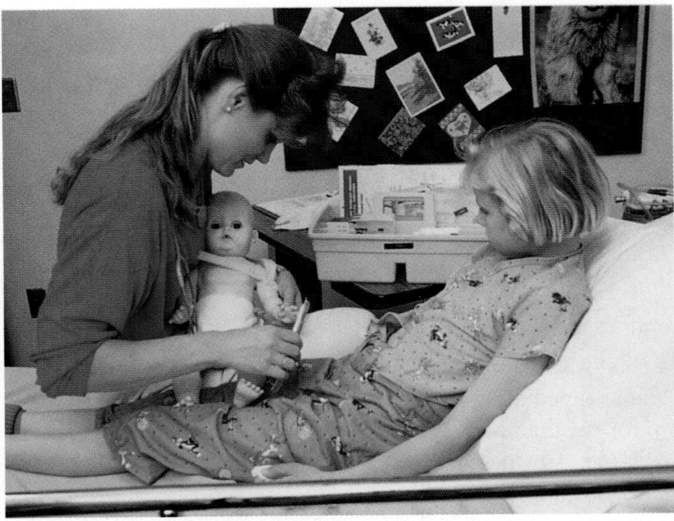

FIGURE 1–2 ■ Explaining procedures can reduce patient and family fears and anxieties about what to expect, as well as how to provide proper home care.

An assessment of the child and family's knowledge about the condition or health practices, past experiences, and their attitudes and beliefs provide the starting point for education. Rapport with the child and family will make it easier to provide education, and family members and the child will be more comfortable asking questions. Then the nurse needs to determine strategies to reinforce the information taught. Outcomes of education can be evaluated during future visits, particularly for children receiving ongoing health promotion and health maintenance care and for those with a chronic condition that requires home management.

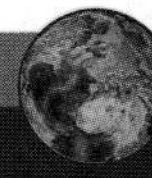

DEVELOPING CULTURAL COMPETENCE
Lowering the Reading Level of Patient Education Materials

Almost 25% of the adult population in the United States and Canada is functionally illiterate. Printed information to educate children and families about a health condition might be readily available, but they often are written at an 11th or 12th grade level. Most Internet patient education information is written at a 10th grade level. You need to evaluate each resource to determine the reading level before giving it to your patient and family. The average adult in the United States cannot read above an 8th grade level, and Medicaid enrollees generally read at a 5th grade level (Winslow, 2001). In addition, the materials need to be evaluated for cultural appropriateness. Because printed material may be available in the primary language of the patient and family, do not assume that the family has reading skills in that language. Some tips to developing patient education material with a lower reading level are as follows:

- Use short, familiar words with one or two syllables.
- Substitute simple language that defines a medical term rather than using the term.
- Use short sentences.
- Use active voice rather than passive voice.
- Use numerals rather than spelling out the number.

Support for the emotional needs of the child and family can also be provided during educational sessions. Children and families are encouraged to express their feelings and thoughts about the impact of the health condition that may result in the exploration of potential strategies that could improve the psychological aspects of living with the condition. Advanced practice nurses and experienced pediatric nurses often have responsibility for providing education and counseling that is directed toward helping the child or family solve a problem or deal with an acute crisis.

Experienced pediatric nurses and advanced practice nurses who enjoy teaching may choose to become nurse educators. Experienced pediatric nurses can serve as mentors to new nurses, supporting their professional development and enhancing nursing skills. Advanced practice nurses may join a faculty in a school of nursing to teach pediatrics or support the nursing education programs provided in clinical health settings.

Advocate

Advocacy—acting to safeguard and advance the interests of another—is directed at enabling the child and family to adjust to the changes in the child's health in their own way. To be an effective advocate, the nurse must be aware of the child's and the family's needs, the family's resources, and the healthcare services available in the hospital and the community. The nurse can then assist the family and the child to make informed choices about these services and to act in the child's best interests. For example, the nurse works to make sure the family member and child, to his or her level of understanding, have adequate information about treatment options to make an informed decision. The nurse must also protect the child and family by taking appropriate actions related to any potential or actual incidents of incompetent, unethical, or illegal practices by any member of the healthcare team.

As advocates, nurses also ensure that the policies and resources of healthcare agencies meet the psychosocial needs of children and their families. This sometimes requires nurses to become active participants on committees that develop policies or guidelines for either care or modernizing the healthcare facility design. In each case, the knowledge that the pediatric nurse contributes about the developmental and psychosocial needs of children is important in ensuring that the needs of children are appropriately addressed in their healthcare facility.

Pediatric nurses are also active at the community level, advocating for legislative and regulatory changes that improve the health of children. For example, community health statistics may reveal that several children have died from drowning in home swimming pools. The nurse may partner with other interested groups to enact regulations that require the installation of fencing around all four sides of home swimming pools. Such a barrier reduces the risk of toddlers and young children accessing the pool directly from the house. Nurses also advocate for improved health through community education about important health measures. Some pediatric nurses choose to obtain advanced education to specialize in ethics, public policy, or to become an attorney. In these roles, the nurse then takes a leadership position to promote and implement ethical practices and policy changes that benefit children and their families.

Case Manager

What happens when a child has significant health problems? When a child has a significant health problem or disabling condition, healthcare professionals (physicians, nurses, social workers, physical and occupational therapists, and other specialists) create an interdisciplinary plan to meet the child's medical, nursing, developmental, educational, and psychosocial needs. Because nurses spend large amounts of time providing nursing care for the child and family, they often know more than other healthcare professionals about the family's wishes and resources. As a member of the interdisciplinary care plan team, one important role for the nurse as the family's advocate is to ensure that the care plan considers the family's wishes and contains appropriate services. An experienced pediatric nurse or advanced practice nurse often becomes the child's case manager, coordinating the implementation of the interdisciplinary care plan. Sometimes the parent or a social worker becomes the case manager.

Case management is a process of coordinating the delivery of healthcare services in a manner that focuses on both quality and cost outcomes. This is often a collaborative practice with other healthcare providers that helps optimize the patient's self-care abilities, promotes **continuity of care** (an interdisciplinary process facilitating a patient's transition between and among settings based on changing needs and available resources), and effective utilization of resources. The family is integrated into the planning and decision-making process, adhering to the family-centered care philosophy described in Chapter 2∞. It involves regular interaction between the case manager and the child and family to develop an individualized care plan in collaboration with the healthcare team. The case manager is also responsible for communication with all health team members for care coordination and advocating for the child and family. The nurse case manager has control over the use of healthcare resources that are considered appropriate for the patient's condition and links the child and family to these services. The goal is to help the child and family have the best healthcare outcome and decrease fragmentation of care, while controlling the cost of healthcare services. Case management may be used for care of the patient when hospitalized as well as for long-term care of chronic conditions.

Discharge planning is a form of case management. Good discharge planning promotes a smooth, rapid, and safe transition into the community and improves the results of treatment begun in the hospital. To be a discharge planner, the nurse needs to know about community medical resources, home care agencies qualified to care for children, healthcare services offered in the school setting, educational interventions, and services reimbursed by the child's health plan or other financial resources.

Research

Research on pediatric healthcare is conducted to determine the most effective methods for treating a condition or providing care. Research evaluates innovations in care to determine if practice is improved, and it provides a scientific basis for nursing practice. Pediatric nurses are responsible for keeping current with new pediatric research findings and identifying when changes in practice are needed. Such findings may improve healthcare outcomes for children or reduce the cost of care. This research is also used in developing specific healthcare facility evidence-based practice guidelines. Pediatric nurses also identify issues in patient care processes that need to be explored, involving clinical practice, education, ethical issues, and specific needs of particular populations of children. In collaboration with advanced practice nurse researchers or other health professionals, pediatric nurses can help identify research questions, assist with the design of research studies, and collect data. With advanced education the pediatric nurse can become a nurse researcher. See page 24 for issues related to consent and assent.

HISTORY OF CHILD HEALTHCARE

An historical overview of child health services demonstrates the roots of pediatric nursing and how certain nursing roles evolved. It also provides a foundation for examining current child health issues and pediatric nursing practice. See the Photo Story on pages 10–11 for the early roles of child health nurses.

Historic Legislation

The first U.S. program supporting health services to mothers and infants was the Sheppard-Towner Child Welfare Act, enacted in 1920. It provided $1.2 million to improve health services for all classes of children and their families, such as education about proper methods of infant care and feeding (Velsor-Friedrich, 2003). Despite a significant reduction in the infant mortality rate, Congress did not reauthorize the program because it was thought to be socialist. The American Medical Association opposed the program because it was viewed as unsound in policy, extravagant, and unproductive. The loss of support for these services and the Great Depression led to major reductions in funding of maternal and child health program efforts. See Box 1–2 for a timeline of other significant federal legislation that has benefited children.

BOX 1–2 Significant Federal Legislation Affecting Child Health

1920 – Sheppard-Towner Act supported services to mothers and infants.

1935 – Social Security Act included two important programs for children: Aid to Families with Dependent Children (AFDC), now called Temporary Assistance to Needy Families (TANF), and Title V of this act initiated programs to improve the health of mothers and children.

1946 – National School Lunch Act created the modern school lunch program.

1965 – Medicaid, under Title XIX of the Social Security Act, enabled indigent pregnant women and children to have access to healthcare.

1966 – Child Nutrition Act initiated the school breakfast program.

1972 – Women, Infant, and Children (WIC) program began providing supplemental food for low-income pregnant women, infants, and children.

1973 – Rehabilitation Act required that accommodations be made for children with disabilities to have access to schools and other public programs.

1975 – Education for All Handicapped Children Act mandated that children with disabilities receive a free and appropriate education in the least restrictive environment. This act was reauthorized as the Individuals with Disabilities Education Act (IDEA) in 1997 and stated that children with disabilities must have educational opportunities and benefits equivalent to their nondisabled peers.

1984 – Emergency Medical Services for Children program was created to improve the quality of and access to emergency care for children with acute illnesses and injuries.

1997 – State Children's Health Insurance Program (SCHIP) legislation expanded health coverage to children through 19 years of age in families with an income too high to qualify for Medicaid.

In 1935, as part of the Social Security Act, child welfare was addressed through the establishment of the Aid to Families with Dependent Children program to support needy children without fathers. Title V of the Social Security Act focused on promoting and improving the health of mothers and children nationwide. Because the Title V program was created as part of a broad-sweeping social legislation rather than health legislation, the development and impact of this program has been extensive. The Title V Maternal and Child Health program legislation has been amended over the years to respond to changing maternal and child health as well as public health issues. Major landmarks are described in the following paragraphs (Maternal and Child Health Bureau, 2002).

The initial Title V legislation provided grants to states for maternal and child welfare, and public health was one of the programs supported. As a result state agencies, such as departments of health or public welfare, were established to address the needs of pregnant women and children. The funds were used to pay for physicians, dentists, public health nurses, social workers, and nutritionists who provided services in health centers, schools, and homes. Efforts were made to improve the health of historically underserved groups of mothers and children. By 1938, a Crippled Children's program (now known as the Children with Special Health Care Needs program or CSHCN) existed in all but one state.

In the 1950s, new programs responded to knowledge about the causes of infant mortality and risks. Special funding was also targeted to "mentally retarded children," now known as children with cognitive disabilities.

In the 1960s and 1970s, comprehensive child healthcare services were provided through Children and Youth Projects to millions of low-income children, becoming models for well-child care. Improved Pregnancy Outcome projects were supported in 34 states with high infant mortality rates. In 1972, the supplemental food program for Women, Infants, and Children (WIC) began to provide food and nutrition education to low-income pregnant and lactating women and infants and children up to 5 years of age.

In the 1980s, several categorical Title V maternal and child health programs were consolidated and states were given priorities and guidelines for addressing healthcare needs of mothers and children. See Box 1–3. States were also encouraged to adopt injury prevention as a public health issue. See pages 16–17 to

MediaLink Critical Thinking: Child Health History Review

BOX 1–3 Federal Goals for the Use of Maternal and Child Health Block Grant Funds Provided to States

- Provide and ensure mothers and children (especially those with low income or limited availability of services) access to quality maternal and child health services.
- Reduce infant mortality and the incidence of preventable diseases and handicapping conditions among children.
- Reduce the need for inpatient and long-term care services.
- Increase the number of children appropriately immunized against disease.
- Increase the number of children receiving health assessments and follow-up diagnostic and treatment services.
- Promote the health of children by providing preventive and primary care services for low-income children.
- Provide rehabilitation services for blind and disabled children under 16 years of age receiving benefits through the Title XVI program when health services are not covered by Medicaid.
- Provide and promote (or facilitate development of) family-centered, community-based, coordinated care for children with special healthcare needs.

Maternal and Child Health Bureau. (2002). Understanding the Title V of the Social Security Act. *Rockville, MD: Department of Health and Human Services, Health Resources and Services Administration, Maternal and Child Health Bureau.*

understand why injury prevention became a new major focus for maternal and child health programs (see also Figures 1–9 to 1–14 later in the chapter).

In the 1990s, the Healthy Start program targeted concerns about the rate of infant mortality in many states. The program promoted community development of culturally appropriate strategies to reduce infant mortality and low birth weight. Abstinence education was added as a categorical program to Title V in 1996.

In the current decade, the Maternal and Child Health Bureau was given responsibility for administering the newborn hearing screening program. Services provided by states through the Title V program are expected to be consistent with the health status goals and national health objectives established by the secretary of the Department of Health and Human Services, including *Healthy People 2010* and *Healthier U.S.*

The Title V program has supported many landmark projects over the past 65 years to improve the health of pregnant women and children. National guidelines have been developed for child health supervision from infancy through adolescence. Nutrition care during pregnancy and lactation has been enhanced. Successful strategies for childhood injury prevention have been identified. Safety standards for out-of-home childcare facilities have been developed.

Other Advances Contributing to Improved Child Healthcare

Other significant advances in society have had a major impact on the health of children.

- The development of antibiotics and vaccines in the 1940s and 1950s has saved the lives of thousands of children who would have died of infectious diseases.
- Technological advances have enabled new treatments for children with conditions that would have proven fatal, such as the heart-lung machine in the 1950s that made possible new surgical treatments for children with congenital heart defects.
- The National Aeronautic Space Administration (NASA) engineered miniaturized equipment that could be carried into space to monitor the astronauts. That equipment was then modified for use in healthcare, as seen in Figure 1–3 ■. Much of the portable equipment used for pediatric healthcare is based on this research and engineering.
- Access to health information by computers (publications, patient data, and scientific studies) has enabled health professionals to collect, contrast, and analyze information about the care of children with specific conditions in different settings. Significant advances in the treatment and outcomes of children with many conditions are constantly being made.

Nurses have been instrumental in the development of pediatric healthcare and the specialty of pediatric nursing. They continue to help the specialty develop and to make sure that the needs of children are addressed in all settings. Examples of the exciting contributions being made by pediatric nurses today include the following:

- Conducting research to improve the care of children, in areas such as pain assessment and management and brain injury rehabilitation
- Identifying strategies to provide health services to homeless children

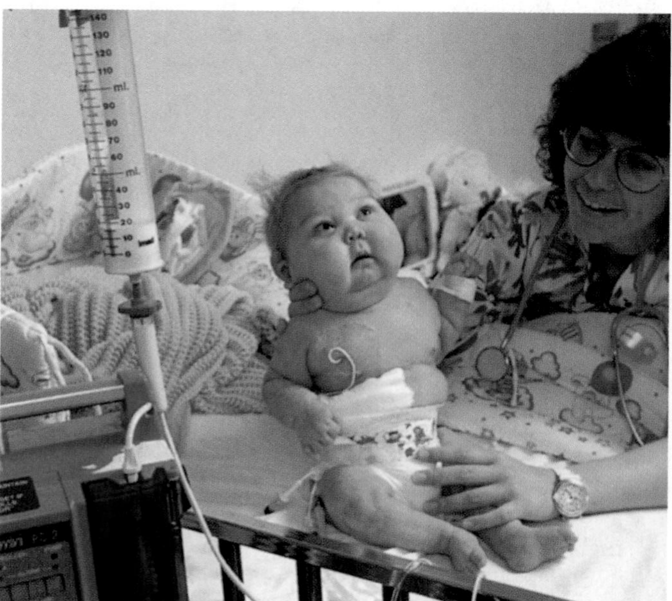

FIGURE 1–3 ■ This child is dependent on the latest technology for necessary nutrients.

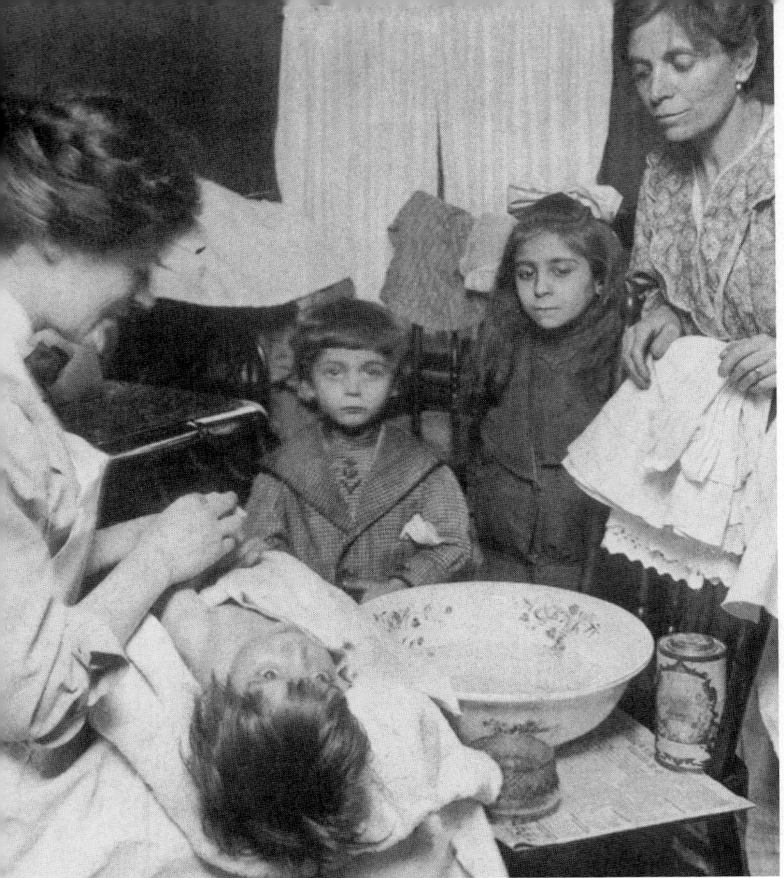

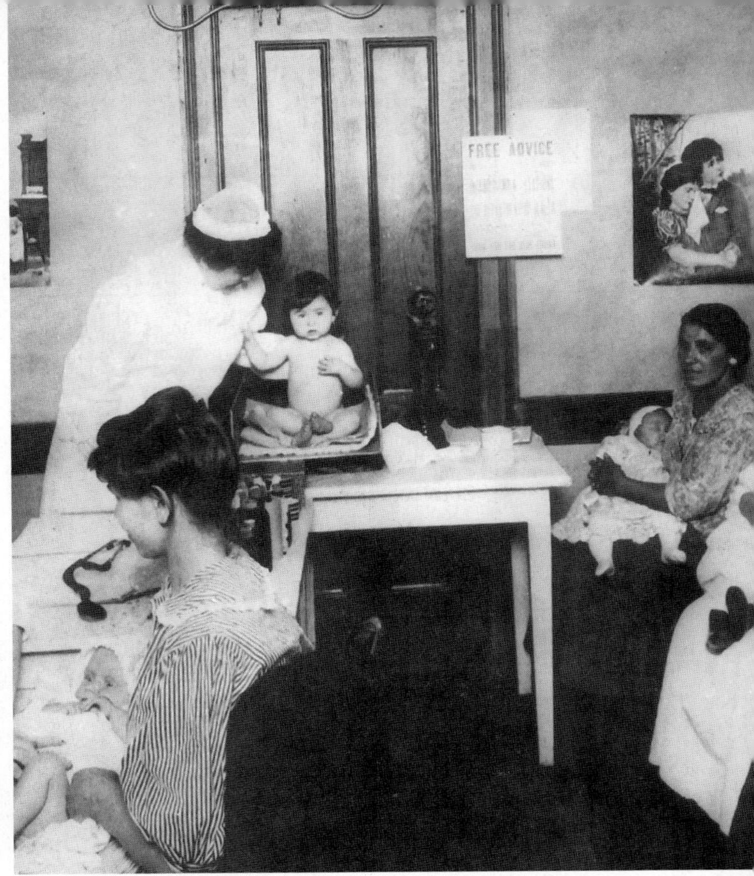

A community health nurse visits a family at home. ***(top left)*** *Photo courtesy of the Visiting Nurses Association of Boston.*

A well-baby clinic for recently immigrated mothers and their babies, circa 1912. ***(top right)*** *Photo courtesy of the National Archives, photo no. 90-G-5-1.*

PHOTO Story...

The beginnings of child health nursing

Significant efforts to address child health were initiated in 1880 to improve the infant mortality rate. No refrigeration and milk from sick cows often resulted in infantile diarrhea and tuberculosis. Regulations to improve the sanitation of milk, provision of clean, cheap milk to infants in poor families in milk stations, and the development of artificial infant formulas all occurred during this period. Dispensaries, freestanding medical clinics, became training grounds for physicians interested in the care of children and provided the model for future well-baby examinations.

In the 1890s, a nurse, Lillian Wald, recognized the need for health promotion and disease prevention among New York City's poor immigrant population, and she organized nursing services to children and their families at the Henry Street Settlement. While the nurses in these settings could not overcome poverty, they did actively seek improvements in social conditions affecting their health. The nurses made home visits, taught parents about nutrition and hygiene, and made arrangements for sick children to see a physician at a dispensary or hospital. In the early 1900s, some hospitals had pediatric dedicated wards.

Improving the health conditions for children attending public schools became a focus in the 1890s and early 20th century. Many children were absent or sent home from school because of illness. Physicians inspected schools and examined students in New York, Boston, Chicago, and Philadelphia to identify infectious disease and to quarantine students as necessary. In 1902, Lillian Wald assigned a nurse to a school for a pilot project that was successful in improving the health of children and reducing absenteeism. School nursing was thus initiated in New York City, and the model soon spread to other cities in the United States and Canada. Children and their parents were educated about personal hygiene and disease prevention in these school health programs.

Many advocates were as concerned about child labor as they were about child health. During the early 20th century, thousands of children worked in sweat shops or factories, working with machinery before they were physically and developmentally prepared to do such labor. Efforts by physicians, nurses, and other social activists during the first decade of the 20th century increased the awareness of child health and welfare issues at the federal level. The first White House Conference on Children was held in 1909, and it addressed the care of dependent children and working conditions of children. One outcome of that conference was the establishment of the Children's Bureau as part of the Department of Commerce and Labor in 1912 to investigate and report on the welfare of children and infant mortality.

Between 1850 and 1880, for every 1000 children born annually in the United States, an estimated 200 died before their first birthday (Markel, 2000). Causes of death included communicable diseases, poor nutrition, and epidemics of "summer diarrhea." By 1915, the infant mortality rate was estimated to be 100 per 1000 live births. With the development of a special focus of national legislation on the prenatal care and infant health services, infant mortality rates have declined dramatically. ■

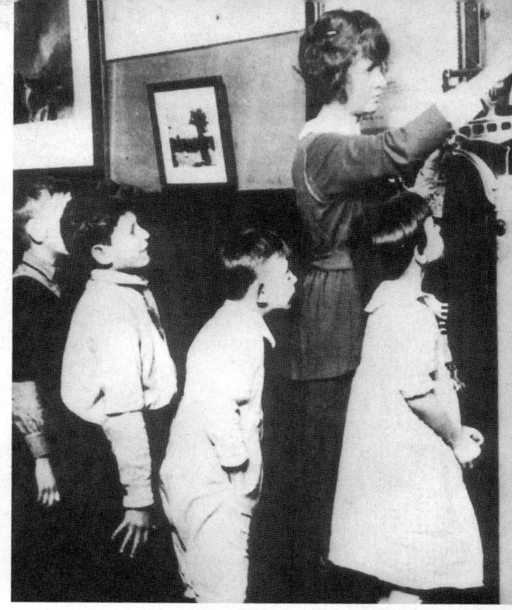

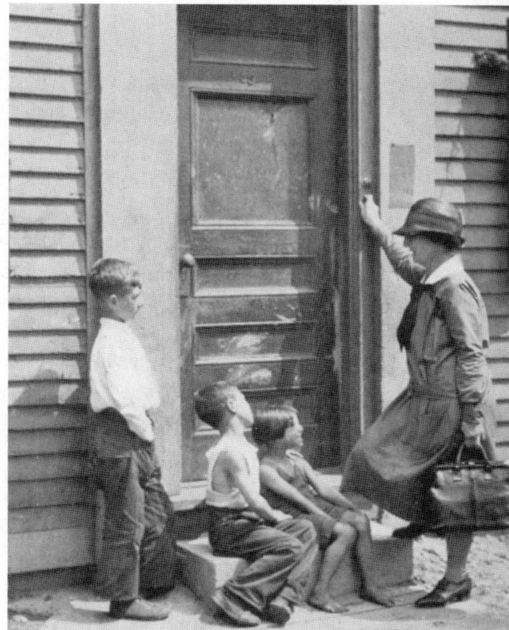

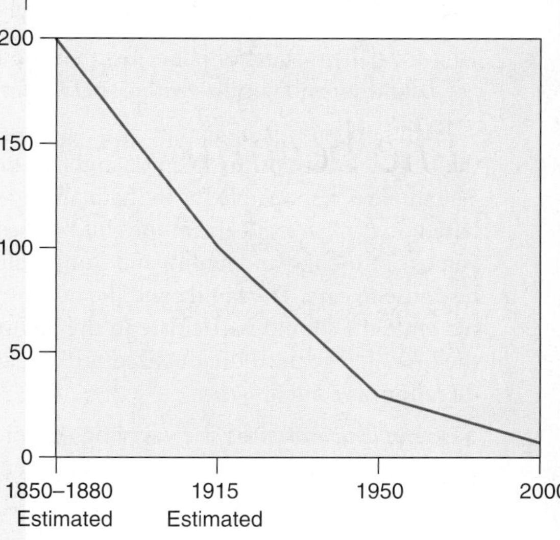

*A school nurse lines up children for height and weight measurement. (**top**) Photo courtesy of the National Archives, photo no. 90-G-5-20.*

*A community health nurse visits children who are not attending school due to a communicable disease. (**middle**) Photo courtesy of the Visiting Nurses Association of Boston.*

*Historical decline in the annual infant mortality rate per 1000 births in the United States. (**bottom**)*

- Promoting healthy behaviors and lifestyles for children to reduce their risk of chronic diseases as adults
- Developing strategies to reduce medication errors
- Improving emergency medical systems to assure access to appropriate and high-quality care

NURSING PROCESS IN PEDIATRIC CARE

Pediatric nurses use the nursing process to identify and solve problems and to plan patient care. The systematic framework for practice that the nursing process provides is the same for pediatric patients as for other patients. Consider how the five steps of the nursing process relate to children.

- *Assessment* involves collecting patient and family data and performing physical examinations during community-based health services, at admission, periodically during the child's hospitalization, and when home care services are provided. The nurse analyzes and synthesizes data to make a judgment about the patient's problems.
- *Nursing diagnoses* describe the health promotion and health patterns that nurses observe in the child and family and for which specific nursing actions can be planned, implemented, and evaluated. The North American Nursing Diagnosis Association (NANDA) has responsibility for endorsing the standard language for these nursing diagnoses to describe the health promotion and health patterns that nurses can independently manage. Each nursing diagnosis has defining characteristics and related factors or risk factors.
- *Nursing care plans* are based on goals that will improve the child's or family's health and health conditions. Specific expected outcomes should be realistic. Nursing care plans have nursing interventions classifications (NICs) and nursing outcome classifications (NOCs). NIC provides a standard language for general nursing actions that are specific for a nursing diagnosis. NOC provides a standard language for patient states or behaviors that should be monitored in children and families with a specific nursing diagnosis.

Standard care plans for specific diagnoses are often used in the pediatric unit of the hospital and by home health agencies. The nurse is responsible for individualizing standard care plans based on data collected from the child's assessment, the cultural values of the child and family, and from evaluation of the child's response to care. The family and the nurse (and the child, when old enough) should participate in the planning and agree with the care plan goals. Individualized nursing action plans provide directions for nursing care.

- *Implementation* is the carrying out of interventions outlined in the nursing care plan. Interventions may be modified if the child's responses are incomplete.
- *Evaluation* is the use of specific objective and subjective measures (often called outcome measures or criteria) to assess the progress of the child and family in reaching the goals defined in the nursing care plan. Following the evaluation of their progress toward the goals, the nursing care plan may be modified. For example, as the child's condition improves and goals are attained, new goals and nursing action plans must be defined. Data from ongoing assessments are collected to guide the revision of the care plan.

Specific examples of the nursing process used in nursing care plans are provided for health promotion activities and the management of a child with a specific condition in several chapters throughout this textbook.

Critical Thinking

Thinking critically plays an important role in the nursing process and clinical judgment that is used to meet the needs of children and families. This is an individualized, creative thinking or reasoning process that the nurse uses to solve problems. The process of critical thinking involves identifying the specific problem or issue that needs to be addressed or the goal to be achieved. The issue may be associated with care to a specific child and family, a quality improvement issue for the healthcare system, or a community health program. Information is then collected from multiple sources, including the child, family, health facility, and community, in addition to research, experts, and published literature. The nurse then creatively analyzes all of the information to make judgments about clinical actions. Additional considerations such as professional standards, ethics, and cultural values of the child and family are integrated into the thought and problem-solving process. Once a solution or action is identified, the nurse then must evaluate the impact or outcome of that action to improve the strategy or care provided (Alfaro-LeFevre, 2004).

Nursing Integrated into Other Care Processes

Clinical Practice Guidelines

Clinical practice guidelines are comprehensive interdisciplinary care plans for a specific condition, which describe the sequence and timing of interventions that should result in expected patient outcomes. Practice guidelines are most valuable when there are gaps in scientific evidence, a moderate degree of uncertainty, or a wide variation in practice patterns or differing opinions among experts about the care to be provided for a specific condition (Callender, 1999). The overall goal is to improve quality of care.

Clinical practice guidelines are increasingly evidence based—using research findings, the judgments of healthcare experts, and group consensus to identify the most effective practices for a specific health condition. Often a national organization will develop clinical practice guidelines to address a specific health condition with recommendations of its adoption. An example would be the asthma guidelines developed by the National Asthma Education Program based in the National Institutes of Health. Practice guidelines promote uniformity in care so that patient outcomes and health professional performance can be measured.

Critical Pathways

Critical pathways (clinical pathways) outline key events and timing for the management of a child with a specific disease or health problem during the hospital admission. With today's focus on healthcare costs, many hospitals have discovered that variations in care provided by its employees often result in different outcomes, such as length of hospital stay. To reduce the variation in care, and improve quality and efficiency of care, personnel in many healthcare settings have mapped out specific healthcare interventions to be provided by all health professionals during the hospital stay. Scientific evidence and the judgments of experts about the interventions needed for children with specific health conditions are integrated into the plan. Various categories of interventions for all health professionals caring for the child are addressed in critical pathways, including the following:

- Nutrition
- Assessment and monitoring
- Safety and activity
- Diagnostic tests
- Medications, IV fluids, and other treatments
- Consultations
- Equipment and supplies
- Patient teaching
- Discharge planning

Critical pathways usually integrate roles for physicians, nurses, respiratory therapists, physical therapists, speech therapists, social workers, case managers, and others. The ideal sequence and timing of the interventions are specified for the different health professionals. Critical pathways are developed by and uniformly adopted within a healthcare setting to reduce variation in the management of children with specific health conditions, to limit costs of care, and to evaluate the effectiveness of care (Melnyk, Fineout-Overholt, Stone, et al., 2000; Merritt, Palmer, Bergman, et al., 1997). Many nurses are engaged in the process of developing critical pathways.

Evidence-Based Practice

Evidence-based practice is the integration of the best research evidence with an individual's clinical expertise and the patient's values or preferences. This is one method used to keep nursing practice current and to promote positive outcomes for children and their families. Individual healthcare providers, such as nurse practitioners and physicians, may choose to modify their practice based on independent searches of evidence for clinical decision making. Health professionals in hospitals, clinics, and other settings may collaborate on collecting research evidence and recommending modifications to clinical practice guidelines or critical pathways. It is important to differentiate evidence-based practice from research-based practice. *Research-based practice* involves use of knowledge following a systematic search for the best evidence, but it does not integrate the health professional's expertise or individual patient preferences (Barnsteiner & Prevost, 2002).

To integrate the best research evidence, the health professional must analyze and evaluate all clinical studies related to a specific health condition or clinical problem. This method ensures that the latest information known about providing care (both nursing care and medical care) to children with a particular health problem can be built into the nursing care plan. However, clinical judgment is needed to determine if the research findings fit the population of care served by the health professional or in the healthcare setting. As partners in the healthcare process, the preferences of the child and family must be considered in any care provided.

The new evidence may alter the way care is provided because it has been revealed that the children have a better outcome or the cost of care is reduced with a new procedure or treatment. Once the nursing care plan, clinical practice guideline, and critical pathway are modified based on the new evidence, data need to be collected to determine if the expected outcomes are seen in the population served by the healthcare setting. The framework for organizing an evidence-based practice report includes the following: background information, statement of a focused clinical question, description of the evidence from research and clinical practice, evaluation of the evidence, and nursing practice implications.

CONTEMPORARY CLIMATE FOR PEDIATRIC NURSING CARE

More than 86 million children under the age of 21 live in the United States. They account for 31.2% of the population (U.S. Bureau of the Census, 2000). (See Figure 1–4 ■ for a distribution of the population by age group.) At one time, children were valued primarily as laborers. Over the past century, however, their unique needs and qualities have been recognized. In today's society, children are considered to have special value.

Partnering with Families: Family-Centered Care

Recognizing the family as the constant influence and support in the child's life is the foundation for development of a trusting relationship and partnership with families. A **partnership** is a relationship in which participants join together to ensure healthcare delivery is provided in a way that recognizes the critical roles and contributions of each partner in promoting health, preventing illness, and managing healthcare conditions.

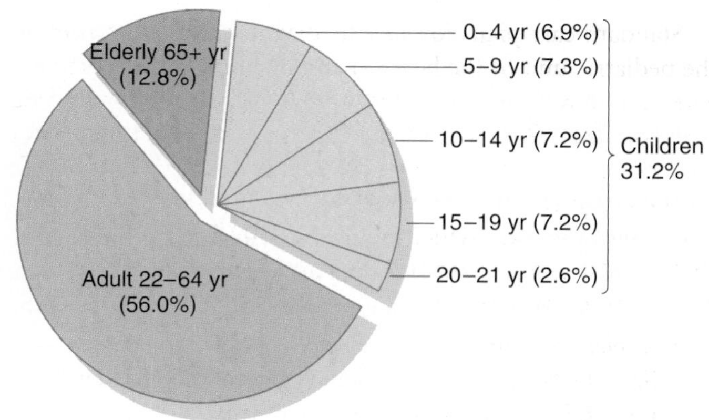

FIGURE 1–4 ■ In 2000, children from birth to 21 years of age accounted for 31.2% of the total population in the United States.

Note: From U.S. Bureau of the Census. (2000). Resident population estimates of the United States by age and sex, April 1, 1990 to July 1, 1999 with short-term projection to November 1, 2000. *Washington, DC: U.S. Government Printing Office.*

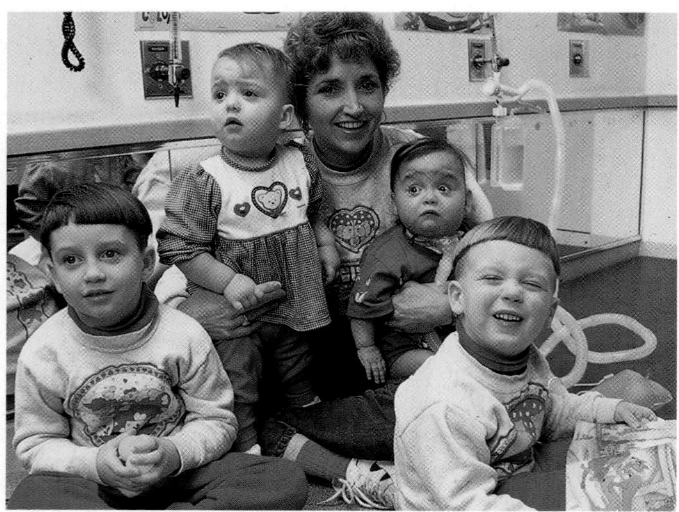

FIGURE 1–5 ■ Many facilities now encourage family visitation for children with health problems that require long-term hospitalization. Extended family visits enable parents to learn about the child's care, and provide siblings with opportunities to interact with the hospitalized child.

The family is the principal caregiver and center of strength and support for the child (Figure 1–5 ■). Partnerships with families are important in all healthcare settings because of the vital role that families play in meeting the emotional, social, and developmental needs of their children and in ensuring their health and well-being. **Family-centered care** is a dynamic, deliberate approach to building collaborative relationships between health professionals and families that is respectful of their diversity and beliefs about the nature of the child's condition and ways to manage it. See Chapter 2∞ for methods of implementing family-centered care and building partnerships with families.

All children need a **medical home** or **healthcare home**—a continuous, comprehensive, family-centered, and compassionate source of healthcare provided throughout the child's developmental years (National Association of Pediatric Nurse Practitioners, 2002). When a family has an established relationship with a care provider, a partnership between the parent and healthcare provider enables the child to receive health services based on the family's risks and protective factors. See Chapters 10 and 16∞ for more information about the role of nurses in the medical or healthcare home model of care.

Culturally Competent Care

The U.S. population has a varied mix of cultural groups, with ever increasing diversity. More than 33% of all children less than 20 years of age are from families of minority populations (U.S. Bureau of the Census, 2001). Consider the current issues:

- In 2001, 19% of children in the United States lived with at least one parent who was foreign born.
- In 1999, 5% (2.6 million) of all school-age children in the United States spoke another language other than English, and had difficulty speaking English.
- In 2000, 8% of the U.S. population 5 years of age and older spoke another language other than English and spoke English less than "very well."

The 2000 U.S. census offered individuals the opportunity to select an ethnic classification (e.g., Hispanic) in addition to race. Many statistical reports now show findings with both race and ethnic classifications. In the 2000 census, 64% of U.S. children were non-Hispanic White, 16% Hispanic, 15% non-Hispanic Black, 4% Asian or Pacific Islander, and 1% Native American or Alaska Native. The racial and ethnic diversity is expected to increase significantly over the next few decades. By the year 2020, it is expected that one in five children in the United States will be of Hispanic origin; 6% will be Asian or Pacific Islander. Increases in these two population groups reflect higher fertility and immigration rates than in the other groups (Federal Interagency Forum on Child and Family Statistics, 2002). It is also important to recognize the diversity among the non-Hispanic White population as they represent many cultural groups, such as immigrants from the former Soviet bloc countries.

Culture develops from socially learned beliefs, lifestyles, values, and integrated patterns of behavior that are characteristic of the family, cultural group, and community. Cultural values are beliefs, behaviors, and ideas that a group of people share and expect to be observed in their dealings with other people (Flores, 2000). The cultural background and values of children and their parents are often quite different from those of the nurse. This lack of knowledge about the family's cultural values may lead to practices that either inadvertently offend the family or result in less than optimal outcomes of care. Awareness of differences in cultural values is the first step in developing cultural competence. See Developing Cultural Competence: Integrating Tradition for initial steps in integrating culture into nursing care plans.

Specific cultural groups often practice complementary and alternative therapies. Information about these practices needs to be obtained during the history. While some therapies are beneficial or cause no harm, other therapies may interact with prescribed medications and have the potential to harm. See Chapter 3∞ for more information about complementary and alternative therapies.

When the family's cultural values are incorporated into the care plan, the family is more likely to accept and comply with the needed care, especially in the home care setting. Avoid imposing your personal cultural values on the children and families in your care. By learning about the values of the different ethnic groups in the community—religious beliefs that have an impact on healthcare practices, beliefs about common illnesses, and their specific healing practices—you can develop an individualized nursing care

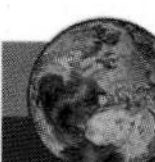

DEVELOPING CULTURAL COMPETENCE
Integrating Tradition

Conflicts can occur within a family when traditional rituals and practices of the family's elders do not conform to current healthcare practices. Nurses need to be sensitive to the potential implications for the child's healthcare, especially when the child is being cared for in the home. When cultural values are not part of the nursing care plan, parents may be forced to decide whether the family's beliefs should take priority over the healthcare professional's guidance. Make an effort to understand traditional health practices and to integrate them into the care plan.

plan for each child and family. See Chapter 3 for guidelines in developing a culturally competent practice in pediatric nursing.

Pediatric Health Statistics

Infant Mortality

Children have different healthcare problems than adults, and the problems may depend on age and development. The leading causes of infant mortality (death occurring during the first year of life) vary according to the age and race of the infant (Figure 1–6 ■). For example, the highest rates of infant mortality per 100,000 live births in the United States during 2000 occurred in the non-Hispanic Blacks (13.6), followed in decreasing order by American Indian and Alaskan Natives (8.3), non-Hispanic Whites (5.7), Hispanics (5.6), and Asian or Pacific Islanders (4.9) (Mathews, Menaker, & MacDorman, 2002).

The leading causes of death in neonates (birth to 28 days of age) are congenital anomalies, low birth weight, respiratory distress syndrome, and maternal complications of pregnancy. Nearly two thirds of all deaths to infants during the first year of life occur in the first 28 days of life. See Figure 1–6 for a comparison of the neonatal mortality rates in 2000 and 1989. Since low birth weight is such an important cause of neonatal mortality, it is important to see which populations contribute to the higher number of low-birth-weight infants. See Table 1–1. Such information helps target public health programs to reduce the infant mortality rate to population groups of highest risk.

TABLE 1–1 Percentage of Low-Birth-Weight Infants by Race in the United States, 2000

RACE	<2500 GRAMS	<1500 GRAMS
Hispanic	6.4	1.1
White	6.5	1.1
American Indian	6.8	1.2
Asian American	7.3	1.0
Black	13.0	3.1

Note: From Martin, J. A., Hamilton, B. E., Ventura, S. J., Menacker, F., & Park, M. M. (2002). Births: Final data for 2000. National Vital Statistics Report, 50(5). Hyattsville, MD: National Center for Health Statistics.

Sudden infant death syndrome accounts for nearly 28% of deaths to infants in the postneonatal period (between 1 and 12 months of age). Figure 1–7 ■ shows the relative frequency of major causes of death in the neonatal and postneonatal period in 2000 and 1989. What could account for homicide as the fifth leading cause of death in infants? See Chapter 7 for an answer.

Despite the historical success in reducing the infant mortality rate, the United States does not compare well to the infant

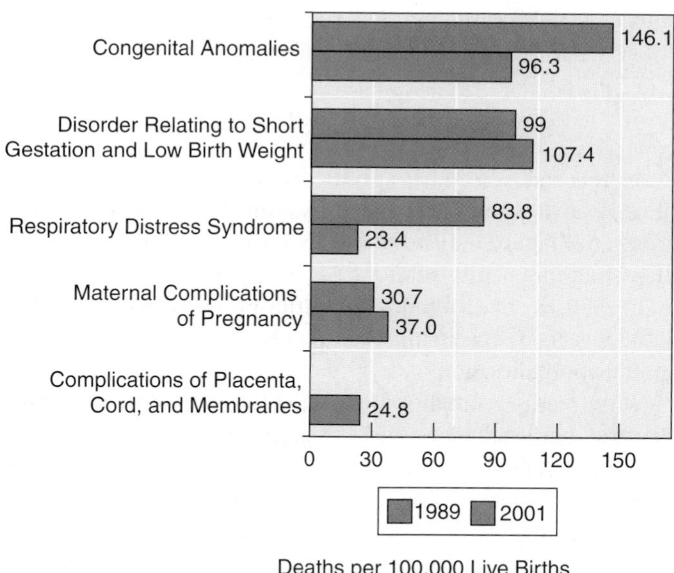

FIGURE 1–6 ■ Leading causes of death in the United States in the neonatal period (in infants up to 28 days of age) in 1989 and 2001. Why do you think the neonatal mortality rate associated with short gestation and low birth weight was higher in 2000 than in 1989? What could account for the dramatic reduction in mortality due to respiratory distress syndrome? Consider the impact of advances in healthcare technology on the changes in mortality rates during the decade illustrated. The neonatal intensive care nurseries have collaborated in multicenter research trials to identify the medical interventions associated with the best outcomes for low-birth-weight infants and those with respiratory distress syndrome. New technology and new knowledge have improved survival of infants with respiratory distress syndrome, but there are increasing numbers of very-low-birth-weight infants alive at birth who die in the first days of life.

Note: From National Center for Health Statistics. (1989). Vital statistics of the United States, vol. 2: Mortality. Part A. *Hyattsville, MD: Public Health Service; Anderson, R. N. & Smith, B. L. (2003). Deaths: Leading causes for 2001.* National Vital Statistics Reports, *52(9), 71.*

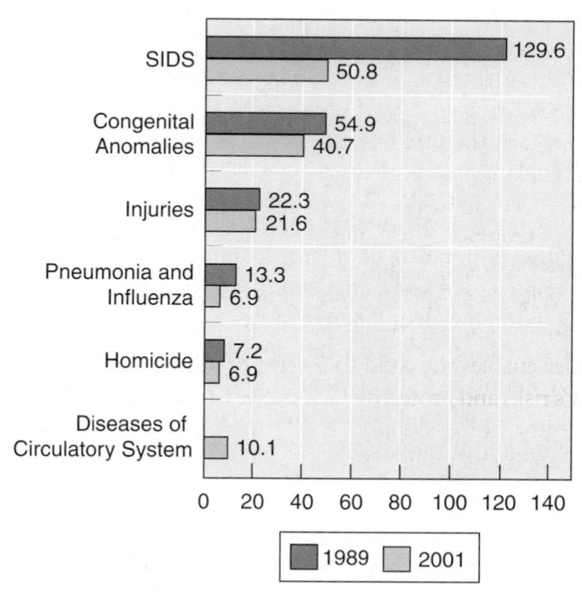

FIGURE 1–7 ■ Leading causes of death in the United States in the postneonatal period, 1989 and 2001 (in infants between 28 days and 1 year old). In 1989, the mortality rate for sudden infant death syndrome was 129.6 per 100,000 live births in contrast to 2001 when the mortality rate was 50.8 per 100,000 live births. The change in recommended sleep position for newborns and infants from the stomach to the back has been credited with much of this decreased rate of SIDS. See Chapter 24 for more information.

Note: From National Center for Health Statistics. (1989). Vital statistics of the United States, vol. 2: Mortality. Part A. *Hyattsville, MD: Public Health Service; Anderson, R. N. & Smith, B. L. (2003). Deaths: Leading causes for 2001.* National Vital Statistics Reports, *52(9), 74.*

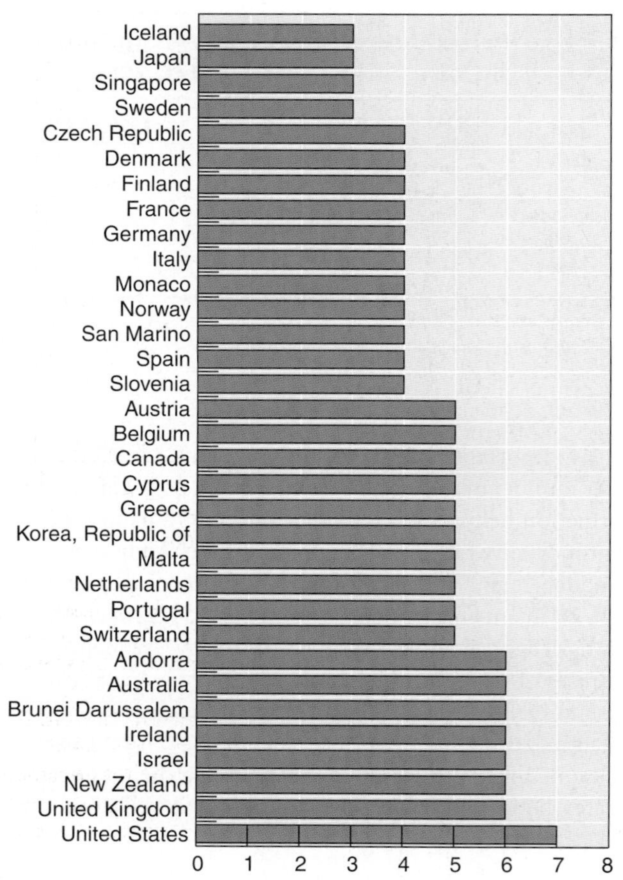

FIGURE 1–8 ■ Ranking of infant mortality rates in 2001 among world nations. Note the ranking of the United States, far behind Canada, European nations, and many Asian nations. What could account for the poorer ranking?

Note: From UNICEF. (2003). Official summary: The state of the world's children 2003 *(pp. 14–18). New York: United Nations Publications.*

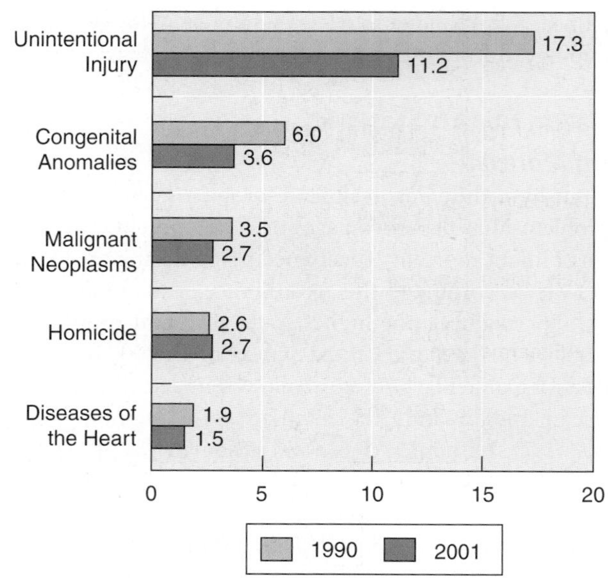

FIGURE 1–9 ■ Age-specific death rate per 100,000 children in the United States in 1990 and 2001 for children 1 to 4 years of age. Throughout the decade the leading cause of death in children between the ages of 1 and 4 years was unintentional injury. Why do you think that is? Do you think these data still apply today? Which type of injury has the highest rate of death? Drowning? Fires and burns? Motor vehicle crashes? See Figure 1–11 for the answer.

Note: From National Center for Health Statistics. (1993). National Vital Statistics System, unpublished data; America's Children 2004, http://childstats.gov/ac2004/tables/health7a.asp, accessed 2/9/2005.

mortality rates found in other industrialized or developed countries with a population of at least 1 million. In 2001, the United States ranked 33rd and Canada ranked 16th behind such nations as Singapore, Sweden, Japan, France, and Germany (UNICEF, 2003). See Figure 1–8 ■ for the comparison of infant mortality rates by nation in 2001. Research and perinatal care programs for high-risk pregnant women and infants are directed at reducing the infant mortality rate.

Child Mortality

The most common cause of death in 2001 for U.S. children between 1 and 4 years of age was unintentional injury. Congenital anomalies, cancer, diseases of the heart, homicide, pneumonia and influenza, and septicemia are the other major causes of death in children between 1 and 4 years of age. The major causes of death to children in this age group have not changed over the last decade; however, some progress has been made in lowering the rates of mortality for these causes. See Figure 1–9 ■. Significant reductions in the causes of death by type of injury have occurred over the past decade. Injury prevention became a major focus of maternal and child health programs in the United States in the 1980s, and along with the efforts of many national groups, the number of preventable injuries was reduced. What specific injury prevention interventions do you think contributed to reduced deaths in this age group? See Figure 1–10 ■ for the answers. See Box 1–4 for Canadian child injury information.

In 2000, the five leading causes of death for children between 5 and 9 years of age included unintentional injury, cancer, congenital anomalies, homicide, and diseases of the heart. In 2000, the seven leading causes of death for children between 10 and 14 years of age included unintentional injury, cancer, suicide, homicide, congenital anomalies, diseases of the heart, and chronic lower respiratory disease (National Center for Health Statistics Vital Statistics System, 2003). Figure 1–11 ■ shows the 2000 mortality rates for causes of death in the 5 to 14 year age group, contrasted with data from 1990. The major causes of death from unintentional injury in childhood include motor vehicle crashes (passengers and pedestrians), drowning, fires and burns, firearms, and suffocation (Health Resources and Services Administration, 2002). Figure 1–12 ■ shows how the injury rates have changed over the past decade due to various injury prevention programs.

Unintentional injury continues to be the leading cause of death in adolescents 15 through 19 years. Homicide, suicide, cancer, and diseases of the heart were the other leading causes of death in this age group in 2000 (Figure 1–13 ■). Of all deaths from unintentional and intentional injury, motor vehicle crashes are the leading cause, followed by firearms, suffocation, drowning, and poisoning (Figure 1–14 ■).

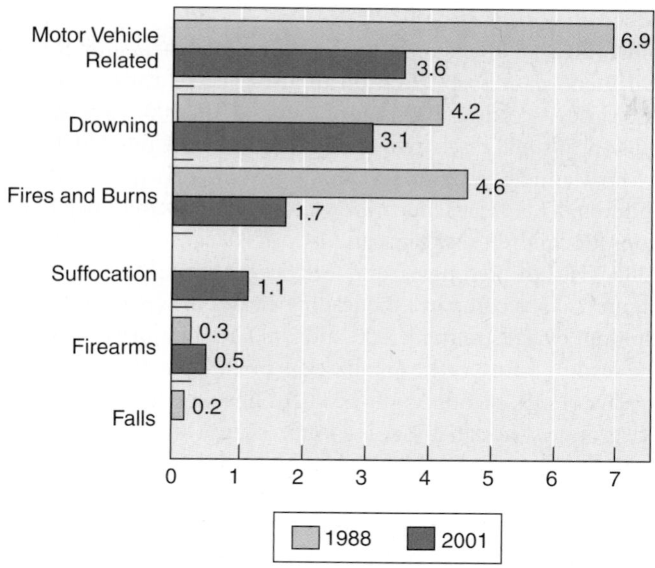

FIGURE 1–10 ■ Death rates from unintentional and intentional injuries per 100,000 children ages 1 to 4 years in the United States in 1988 and 2001. Interventions such as car safety seats, enforcement of fences around swimming pools, and working smoke detectors in homes all contributed to reductions in unintentional injury deaths. Which types of injuries are unintentional (unplanned or accidental) and intentional (violence or homicide related)?

Note: From Children's Safety Network. (1991). A data book of child and adolescent injury. *Washington, DC: National Center for Education in Maternal and Child Health; America's Children 2004, http://childstats.gov/ac2004/tables/health7a.asp, accessed 2/9/2005.*

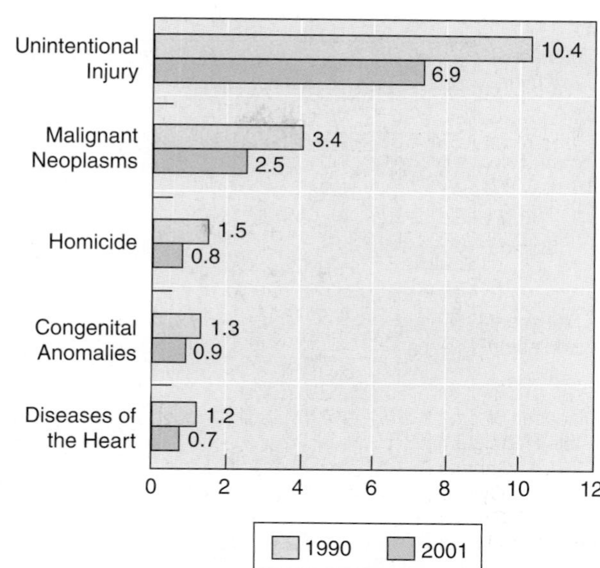

FIGURE 1–11 ■ Age-specific death rate per 100,000 children in the United States in 1990 and 2001 for children 5 to 14 years of age. Throughout the decade unintentional injury continued to be the leading cause of death in children between the ages of 5 and 14 years. Which type of injury has the highest rate of death? Drowning? Fires and burns? Motor vehicle crashes? See Figure 1–13 for the answer.

Note: From National Center for Health Statistics. (1993). National Vital Statistics System, unpublished data; America's Children 2004, http://childstats.gov/ac2004/tables/health7b.asp, accessed 2/9/2005.

Healthy People 2010

The U.S. government set objectives to improve the health of children and young adults in the 21st century in the report entitled *Healthy People 2010*. See Chapter 16∞ for a listing of national health goals and objectives that relate to children. These objectives focus on reducing the incidence of death and disability from the major causes of death shown in Figures 1–6 through 1–14. Federal funding is available to healthcare organizations for the development of programs aimed at reducing the number of deaths from these factors in specific high-risk groups.

BOX 1–4 Canadian Child Injury Mortality Statistics

Injuries are the leading cause of death for children in Canada between the ages of 1 and 19 years, accounting for 30.5% of all deaths in this age group.

- Injury rates were highest among the 15 to 19 year age group.
- Unintentional injuries accounted for 69.6% of all deaths at a rate of 11.1 per 100,000 population.
- Motor vehicle traffic deaths were the leading cause of unintentional injury deaths.
- Other major causes of injury deaths included suffocation in infants, suicide, and homicide.
- The highest homicide rates were seen in infants less than 1 year of age.

Note: From Health Canada. (2000). Statistical report on the health of Canadians, 2000. *Ottawa: Minister of Public Works and Government Services Canada.*

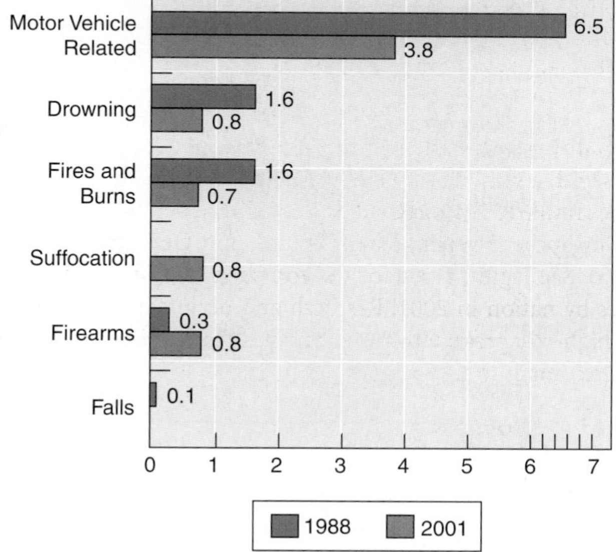

FIGURE 1–12 ■ Death rates from unintentional and intentional injuries per 100,000 children ages 5 to 14 years in the United States in 1988 and 2001. Intensive focus on infant and child passenger safety in motor vehicles has contributed to the reduction in motor vehicle–related deaths. What could be causing the increased rate of deaths due to firearms noted in 2001? See Chapter 7∞.

Note: From Children's Safety Network. (1991). A data book of child and adolescent injury. *Washington, DC: National Center for Education in Maternal and Child Health; America's Children 2004, http://childstats.gov/ac2004/tables/health7b.asp, accessed 2/9/2005.*

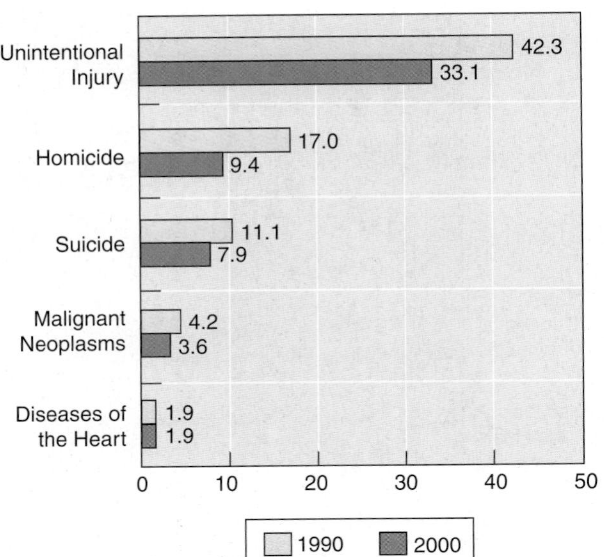

FIGURE 1–13 ■ Death rates per 100,000 adolescents 15 to 19 years in the United States in 1990 and 2000. What proportion of the deaths are preventable?

Note: From National Center for Health Statistics. (1993). National Vital Statistics System, unpublished data; Health Resources and Services Administration, Maternal and Child Health Bureau. (2002). Child Health USA 2002. *Rockville, MD: U.S. Department of Health and Human Services.*

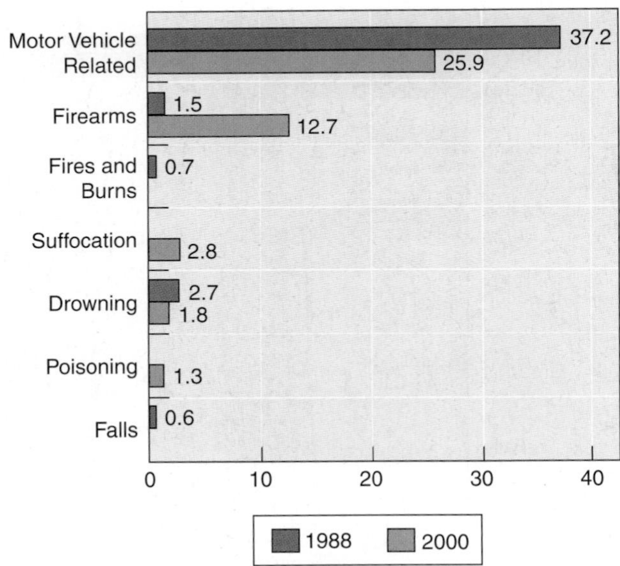

FIGURE 1–14 ■ Death rates from all injuries per 100,000 adolescents 15 to 19 years in the United States in 1988 and 2000. While the rate of motor vehicle–related deaths has decreased, a greater proportion of injury deaths is now due to firearms. How can you use these data with patients and families during patient teaching and when providing care?

Note: From Children's Safety Network. (1991). A data book of child and adolescent injury. *Washington, DC: National Center for Education in Maternal and Child Health; Health Resources and Services Administration, Maternal and Child Health Bureau. (2002).* Child Health USA 2002. *Rockville, MD: U.S. Department of Health and Human Services.*

Morbidity and Hospitalization

Morbidity, an illness or injury that limits activity, requires medical attention or hospitalization, or results in a chronic condition, also varies according to the age of the child. In 2000, there were 3.4 million hospital discharges for children in the United States between 1 and 21 years of age, an average of 4 discharges per 100 children. This represents a 38% decrease in overall hospitalizations for children between 1 and 14 years of age between 1985 and 2000 (Health Resources and Services Administration, 2002). Figure 1–15 ■ compares the leading causes of hospitalization of children by age group in 1993 and 2000. Respiratory diseases are the leading cause of hospitalization in children between 1 and 9 years of age, accounting for 33% of hospital discharges in this age group. Although injury is a leading cause of death in children 1 to 14 years of age, it accounted for only 9% of hospital discharges in 2000. Mental disorders were the leading cause of hospitalization in children between 10 and 14 years of age. Pregnancy and childbirth was the leading cause of hospitalization for adolescents between 15 and 21 years of age, followed by hospitalization for mental disorders (Health Resources and Services Administration, 2002). See Chapter 7∞ for potential reasons for the increase in hospital discharges for mental disorders in children and adolescents 10 to 21 years. See Box 1–5 for the leading causes of hospitalization among children in Canada.

In 2000, chronic illnesses and impairments limited the activities of 7% of children between 5 and 17 years of age; however, this rate varied by sex. Males (9%) had more activity limitations than females (4%) in the 5 to 17 year age group. Children who have activity limitations are more likely to have one or more chronic conditions with duration of 3 months or more, miss more days from school, and incur higher medical costs (Federal Interagency Forum on Child and Family Statistics, 2002).

Healthcare Financing

Not all children in the United States have access to healthcare. In 2000, 8.4 million children, 11.6% of those below 18 years of age, had no health insurance and 23.3% were covered by public insurance programs such as Medicaid and the State Children's Health Insurance Program (SCHIP). Private insurance covered 70.6% of children less than 18 years of age (Health Resources and Services Administration, 2002) (Figure 1–16 ■). Family members pay approximately 21% of their children's healthcare expendi-

BOX 1–5 Ten Leading Causes of Hospitalization in Canada in Children Under 15 Years

1. Diseases of the respiratory system
2. Injury and poisoning
3. Diseases of the digestive system
4. Symptoms, signs, and ill-defined conditions
5. Conditions originating in the perinatal period
6. Infectious and parasitic diseases
7. Congenital anomalies
8. Diseases of the nervous system and sense organs
9. Diseases of the genitourinary system
10. Endocrine, nutritional, metabolic, and immunity diseases

Note: From Statistics Canada, http://www.statcan.ca/english/Pgdb/health18a.htm, *accessed 6/6/2003.*

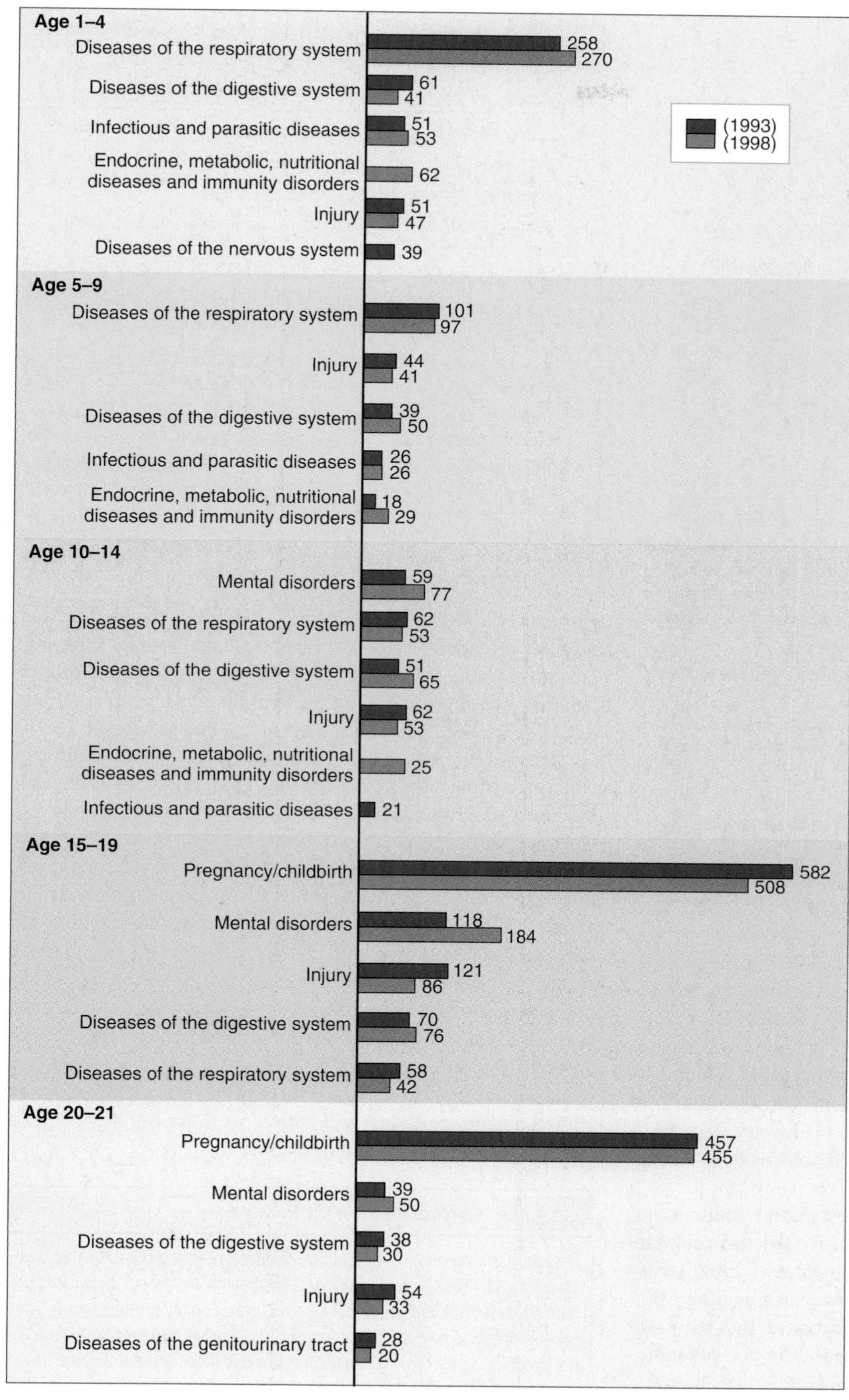

FIGURE 1–15 ■ The leading causes of hospitalization in the United States in 2000 are much the same as those in 1993 in those 21 years of age and younger, but the number of hospital discharges (in 1000s) have changed for some causes. What do you think might account for the rise in hospital discharges for mental disorders? What do you think the current hospital discharge numbers are today?

Note: From Child Health USA '95 *(DHHS Publication No. HRSA-M-DSEA-96–5). Washington, DC: Government Printing Office; Health Resources and Services Administration, Maternal and Child Health Bureau. (2002).* Child Health USA 2002. *Rockville, MD: U.S. Department of Health and Human Services.*

tures out of pocket. A considerably higher proportion of healthcare expenditures are paid out of pocket by families of uninsured children (McCormick, Weinick, Elixhauser, et al., 2001).

In contrast, of all children who lived in poverty in 2000, 22.3% had no health insurance and 59.6% were covered by public insurance (Health Resources and Services Administration, 2002). Most of these children had difficulty obtaining basic preventive healthcare, including immunizations. In many cases the difficulty in obtaining preventive health services results in uninsured children having poorer health outcomes than insured children (Kempe, Renfew, Barrow, et al., 2001). Efforts to provide universal access to healthcare for children continue. Congress passed legislation to

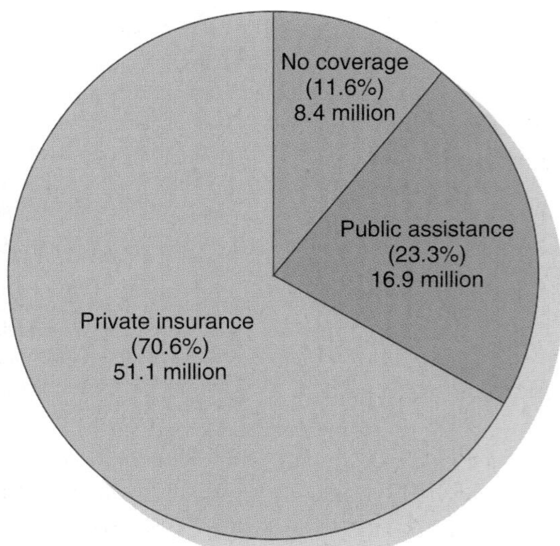

FIGURE 1–16 ■ In the United States, how is healthcare of children paid for? These data from 2000 show that our taxes support 35% of the costs. What can you do to help? Something as simple as counseling parents about injury prevention and providing immunizations while a child is under care for other problems can prevent potential health problems. Part of good nursing care is supporting the well-being of the child in addition to caring for the presenting problem.

*Percents do not add to 100 because some children have more than one source of coverage.

Note: From Frontin, P., Employee Benefit Research Institute. (2001). Sources of health insurance and characteristics of the uninsured: Analysis of the March 2001 current population survey *(EBRI Issue Brief No. 240). Washington, DC: EBRI.*

MediaLink Application: Determine Eligibility for Health Programs

create SCHIP in 1997 to enable more children to obtain access to essential healthcare services. States are allocated federal funds to encourage enrollment of children up to 200% of the federal poverty level (Smith, Wise, Chavkin, et al., 2000). In 2002, the family income eligibility level for a family of four was $34,100 per year (Centers for Medicare and Medicaid Services, 2003). Children enrolled must be provided with health benefits coverage that is substantially equal to the benefits coverage in the federal or state employee health benefits plan or the plan of the largest health maintenance organization in the state. As of the end of September 2002, 5.3 million children were enrolled (Centers for Medicare and Medicaid Services, 2003). Small gains were made in getting more children covered by Medicaid and SCHIP because of the strong economy and low unemployment rate.

Despite the availability of SCHIP, many eligible children are not enrolled. Reasons families have not enrolled their eligible children may include a belief that their income is too high to qualify, they have obtained other insurance such as Medicaid, they have difficulty with application procedure and required documentation, and they lack skills in negotiating the system to get coverage. Nurses can play an important role in encouraging families to investigate their eligibility for the program. Obtain current guidelines in your state about eligibility requirements and coverage benefits. For example, some states require a monthly premium or co-pay for healthcare visits.

Medicaid provides coverage to children and individuals with disabilities who meet income level qualifications set by the state. Children covered under the Temporary Assistance to Needy Families (TANF) are usually eligible. Children enrolled in Medicaid are provided services through the Early Periodic Screening, Diagnostic, and Treatment (EPSDT) service. This is a comprehensive and preventive child health program for individuals under 21 years. See Box 1–6 for a list of covered services.

Managed care is an effort to coordinate and provide quality care while preventing unnecessary care and controlling costs. Some state Medicaid programs have converted to a managed-care process. Children with relatively minor special healthcare needs often have two or three times the healthcare costs of healthy children. Approximately 5% of children with complex health conditions consume about 35% of total dollars spent on healthcare for all children and adolescents (Committee on Children with Disabilities, American Academy of Pediatrics, 1998). Managed care focuses on the control of the spiraling costs of healthcare, but now efforts are also targeted to children with complex health conditions. Many children's hospitals are using utilization review procedures and developing care management models to reduce the cost of care, such as through clinical practice guidelines and critical pathways. See Box 1–7 for a comparison of the Canadian health system.

BOX 1–6 Preventive Health Services Covered Under Medicaid's Early Periodic Screening, Diagnostic, and Treatment Service

- Comprehensive health and developmental history
- Comprehensive unclothed physical examination
- Appropriate immunizations
- Laboratory tests (statewide screening requirements and lead toxicity screening)
- Health education
- Vision services—screening, treatment for defects in vision, including eyeglasses
- Dental services—dental screening, relief of pain and infection, restoration of teeth, and maintenance of dental health
- Hearing services—diagnosis and treatment of hearing defects, including hearing aids
- Other necessary healthcare — to correct or ameliorate defects, physical and mental illnesses, and conditions discovered by the screening process

Note: From Centers for Medicare and Medicaid Services. (2003). Medicaid and EPSDT. www.cms.gov/medicaid/epsdt/default/asp, *accessed 7/7/2003.*

BOX 1–7 Canadian Health System

Canada has a predominantly publicly financed healthcare system that was established by the Canada Health Act. The healthcare system is primarily financed by federal and provincial income taxes. Eligible residents have reasonable access to medically necessary insured services on a prepaid basis and no direct charges from the healthcare provider. The Canadian federal government sets the national standards for the healthcare system and assists with financing healthcare services that are coordinated in the provinces. The initial contact for care is generally the primary care physician who coordinates referrals to specialists, arranges hospital admissions and diagnostic testing, and orders medications. Other supplemental health benefits include prescription drugs, vision care, medical equipment, and appliances for individuals with disabilities. Canadians may pay for private insurance to cover noninsured benefits such as cosmetic surgery (Health Canada, 2002).

Healthcare Technology

Research and technology have enabled many children with congenital anomalies and low birth weights to survive, with and without chronic conditions. However, lifesaving technology has also created such burdens as high healthcare costs and stresses on the functioning of the child's family. Technologic advances have resulted in the design of portable medical and infusion therapy equipment for home care. Many children are dependent upon or assisted by technology for physiologic functions. Examples of technology used in children in the home include ventilators, feeding tubes and intravenous or central lines along with their associated pumps, cardiorespiratory monitors, peritoneal dialysis, and pacemakers. The number of children assisted by technology continues to increase as scientific and technological advances continue.

After studies in the 1980s found that home healthcare was substantially less expensive than hospital care, Congress amended laws to permit payment of home care services with federal funds, such as through Medicaid (U.S. General Accounting Office, 1989). While some children with chronic conditions or complications of acute illnesses and injuries are managed in long-term care facilities, most of these children are now managed in home care programs and in school settings. In 1998, more than 400,000 children under 18 years were discharged by hospitals to a home care program. Nearly 300,000 of these children were under 6 years of age (National Center for Health Statistics, 2000). Some families have regained control over their lives by creating intensive care units in their homes (Figure 1–17 ■). Children who 10 years ago would have died from respiratory, neurological, or other medical conditions are thriving with home care and are participating in family, community, and school life.

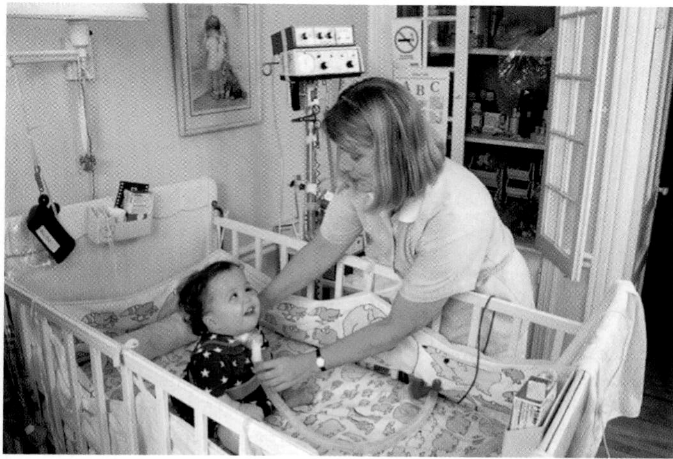

FIGURE 1–17 ■ It is often desirable from a family and cost perspective to provide healthcare in the home, and technologic advances have made this possible. But is it really less costly to provide care in the home for a child with technology assistance? How does one factor in parents' out-of-pocket expenses for medical supplies that are not reimbursed? Lost time from work or the need for a parent to discontinue employment to care for the child? The emotional strain on families who care for their child 24 hours a day, 7 days a week? What support is needed by these families to continue providing this level of care at home? See Chapters 16 and 20∞.

LEGAL AND ETHICAL CONCEPTS AND RESPONSIBILITIES

Regulation of Nursing Practice

Because nurses are accountable for their professional actions, each state regulates nursing practice with a nurse practice act. "Nursing is the protection, promotion, and optimization of health and abilities, prevention of illness and injury, alleviation of suffering through the diagnosis and treatment of human response, and advocacy in the care of individuals, families, communities, and populations" (American Nurses Association, 2003). A state's nurse practice act defines the legal roles and responsibilities of nurses. Become familiar with this act in your state.

As professionals, nurses set standards for education and practice that conform to state regulations. Professional nursing organizations and state agencies that accredit nursing programs modify the standards for nursing education as the science of nursing progresses. Nurses in professional organizations develop standards of nursing practice. These standards describe the public and patient responsibilities for which nurses are accountable.

Standards of clinical nursing practice developed by the American Nurses Association in 2004 define standards for both nursing care and performance. Standards of care describe the competent level of nursing care using the nursing process and form the foundation of clinical decision making. Standards of performance describe the nurse's behavior in the professional role and include such criteria as quality of care, performance appraisal, collegiality, resource utilization, ethics, research, education, and collaboration. The Society of Pediatric Nurses in collaboration with the American Nurses Association has also developed specific standards for pediatric clinical nursing practice. See Box 1–8.

Accountability and Risk Management

Accountability

The family entrusts the child's care to the healthcare team. Family members expect this team to provide good medical and nursing care and to avoid mistakes that cause harm. Nurses are personally accountable for expanding their knowledge base, staying current regarding changes in medical and nursing care for specific conditions, recognizing important changes in the child's condition that require intervention, and taking action as necessary to protect the child.

Patient Safety

Children are at a higher risk for medical error than other patients and also may be more vulnerable to harm from errors made. Most errors in medical care within hospitals are "systems" errors related to equipment, complex procedures, fragmented care, and lack of standardized procedures. The Joint Commission on Accreditation of Healthcare Organizations (JCAHO) has identified *patient safety* as an important responsibility, and the seven goals established as requirements for accreditation in

MediaLink Professional Nursing Organizations

BOX 1–8 Professional Practice Standards for Pediatric Nursing Practice

STANDARDS OF CARE FOR THE PEDIATRIC NURSE INCLUDE

- Collecting health data.
- Analyzing the assessment data in determining diagnoses.
- Identifying expected outcomes individualized to the child and family.
- Developing a plan of care that prescribes interventions to attain expected outcomes.
- Implementing the interventions identified in the plan of care.

STANDARDS OF PERFORMANCE FOR THE PEDIATRIC NURSE INCLUDE

- Systematically evaluating the quality and effectiveness of pediatric nursing practice.
- Evaluating own nursing practice in relation to professional practice standards and relevant statutes and regulations.
- Acquiring and maintaining current knowledge and competence in pediatric nursing practice.
- Interacting with and contributing to the professional development of peers, colleagues, and other healthcare providers.
- Making assessments and recommendations and taking action on behalf of children and their families in an ethical manner.
- Collaborating with the child, family, and other healthcare providers in providing patient care.
- Contributing to nursing and pediatric healthcare through the use of research methods and findings.
- Considering factors related to safety, effectiveness, and cost in planning and delivering care.

Note: From American Nurses Association & the Society of Pediatric Nurses. (2003). Scope and standards of pediatric nursing practice. *Washington, DC: nursesbooks.org. American Nurses Association, 600 Maryland Ave SW, Suite 100W, Washington, DC 20024-2571.*

2004 are listed in Box 1–9. Reasons for the increase in medical error among children include the following:

- Medication dosage calculations are more complex. Dosages are based on weight whereas adults are given standard doses. This means the optimal dose is based on mg/kg and divided by number of doses to be given a day. An additional problem is that children often need suspensions or liquid preparations adding to the dosage calculation complexity. Not only must the correct dose be calculated, but also the amount of liquid preparation with that dose.

BOX 1–9 2004 JCAHO National Patient Safety Goals

1. Improve the accuracy of patient identification.
2. Improve the effectiveness of communication among caregivers.
3. Improve the safety of using high-alert medications.
4. Eliminate wrong-site, wrong-patient, and wrong-procedure surgery.
5. Improve the safety of using infusion pumps.
6. Improve the effectiveness of clinical alarm systems.
7. Reduce the risk of healthcare-acquired infection.

Note: From JCAHO, www.jcaho.org/accreditated+organizations/patient+safety/npsg/04_npsg.htm, *accessed 9/5/2003.*

- The misplacement of a decimal in the medication dosage calculation can result in an overdose that can cause harm to the child or even death.
- Many drug preparations require dilution to achieve the small dosage required by infants.
- Medications not yet approved by the Food and Drug Administration for use in children are sometimes prescribed.
- Young children cannot communicate well if they are having a reaction to the medication.
- Children who are critically ill and injured do not have the reserves to deal with an overdose of medication like a healthy older child or adult.

Another cause of potential medical error involves families with limited English proficiency that are at risk for errors in interpretation of what the health professional or family member says. Even when using a hospital interpreter, errors such as omitting instructions on dose, frequency, and duration of medications have potential clinical consequences (Flores, Laws, Mayo, et al., 2003). Healthcare facilities are challenged to implement strategies that will reduce medical errors in all child patients.

Risk Management

Healthcare institutions make every effort to promote optimal patient care and reduce liability by various activities. **Risk management** is a process established by a healthcare institution to identify, evaluate, and reduce the risk of injury to patients, staff, and visitors, and thus reduce the institution's liability. This involves the study of causes of medical errors within a healthcare institution and implementing system changes to prevent future errors. Several strategies have been developed to reduce medication errors in children. Policy and procedure manuals should be current and provide guidance on patient care and the use of technology specifically related to potentially serious situations. See Evidence-Based Practice: Medication Errors and Children.

Quality improvement is the continuous study and improvement of the processes and outcomes of providing healthcare services to meet the needs of patients, by examining the systems and processes of how care and services are delivered. Nurses caring for children participate in the development of institutional policies and standards of pediatric nursing practice. Hospitals and home health agencies encourage the development of diagnosis-specific nursing care plans or interdisciplinary clinical practice guidelines or critical pathways that serve as minimal institutional standards of care.

During the development of institutional standards of care, indicators of effective care by pediatric nurses and other providers are identified. These indicators may measure either the process of care, the institution's systems, or the expected outcome of care for a specific patient condition. Patient records are regularly reviewed to identify deviations from the institutional standards or clinical practice guidelines/critical pathways. When deviations from expected processes and outcomes are identified, opportunities to improve the system or processes of care provision are explored with all care providers. Recommendations for the revision of institutional standards to further improve care by pediatric nurses and other health providers in the institution often result.

MediaLink Critical Thinking: Understanding Policies and Practices

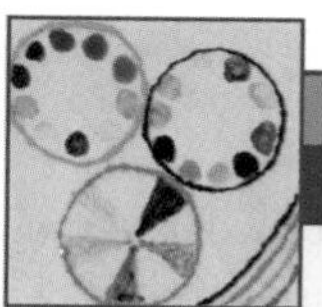

EVIDENCE-BASED PRACTICE
Medication Errors and Children

PROBLEM

Medication errors are a serious problem in pediatrics because dosages are calculated by the weight of the child, and an error in the placement of a decimal results in a potential overdose or underdose. Confusion about the medication ordered can occur due to similarity in medication names or difficulty in reading a physican's handwriting.

FOCUSED CLINICAL QUESTION

For children cared for in the pediatric intensive care unit, is there a better method of reducing medication errors than a weight-based dosing reference for commonly used medications?

EVIDENCE

An epidemiologic study was conducted at two urban teaching hospitals to determine the rates of medication errors and adverse drug events among hospitalized children. Medication errors were defined as errors in drug ordering, transcribing, dispensing, administering, and monitoring. Adverse drug events were medication errors with the potential to injure the patient. Errors were found in 5.7% of all medication orders, and medication error rates were similar across different types of pediatric units. The majority of errors were related to doses, followed by administration errors. Errors occurred most commonly at the stage of drug ordering. Errors with the greatest potential for harm occurred in infants cared for in the neonatal intensive care unit (Kaushal, Bates, Landrigan, et al., 2001). Medication errors occur more frequently in seriously ill children who are hospitalized longer and undergo more medical procedures. Both of these factors increase the child's likelihood of being affected by a medication error (Slonim, LaFleur, Ahmed, et al., 2003). A study examining the role of nurses and pharmacists in identifying prescribing errors prior to drug administration was conducted at a British hospital over two 2-week periods. Data obtained included information about who initiated the intervention (nurse or pharmacist), type of problem identified, and action taken. Two life-threatening drug errors were detected, one by the nurses and one by the pharmacists. Nurses identified almost 50% of the interventions in each study period. In 50% of cases of nurse intervention, the prescription was amended, versus 80% of the cases of pharmacist intervention. This study illustrates the importance of nurses and pharmacists in identifying errors in prescribed medications (Guy, Persaud, Davies, et al., 2003).

Methods to improve the accuracy of medication administration have not been extensively evaluated for the pediatric population. Computerized physician order entry with decision support reduced medication errors by 81% in a larger tertiary adult hospital (Bates, Teich, Lee, et al., 1999). Unit dosing has been used in many settings successfully. Bar coding for medication administration is now supported by the Food and Drug Administration, along with systems that electronically monitor each step of medication administration (U.S. Food and Drug Administration, 2003).

EVALUATION OF EVIDENCE

Studies on various systems to reduce neonatal and pediatric medication errors are needed so that healthcare facilities can take proactive steps in reducing errors. Nurses play an important role in reducing errors by verifying medications ordered and administering the correct dosage on time and in the correct manner (e.g., rate of IV infusion).

PRACTICE IMPLICATIONS

Until more evidence exists about ways to reduce medical error, several strategies have been proposed.

- Do not rely on memory; verify medication dosages and their calculations.
- Every prescription should include the child's weight and age, as well as the calculated dose and mg/kg dose. The dosage form (vial, tablet, or ampule) should not be used on the prescription, as medication preparations and concentrations may vary by pharmaceutical company.
- Prescription information should be written in legible printed letters to prevent confusion with other drugs having similar names.
- Abbreviations for medications and frequency of administration should not be used.
- The administration rate for all IV medications should be specified.
- A zero should not be used after a whole number (e.g., 5.0 could be misread as 50 which can potentially result in a 10-fold dosage increase).
- Drug interactions and patient allergies cause adverse drug events when the inappropriate medication is ordered. A computerized physician order system with clinical decision support can improve the system, reducing errors from poor handwriting and checking for drug interactions and allergies.
- Bar coding for medications and timers and alarms to remind nurses to administer medications are other strategies in development.
- Unit dose dispensing systems should be used.

CRITICAL THINKING APPLICATION

Identify the medication error reduction policies and strategies that exist in each health setting used for clinical practice. What other medication safety practices do nurses use routinely in these settings? Identify any potential areas of improvement in medication safety practice in these settings.

Documentation of nursing care is an essential part of risk management and quality assurance. The patient's record is a legal document that is admissible evidence in court. If a patient record is subpoenaed, documented care is considered the only care provided, regardless of the quality of undocumented care. Information in the patient's record must be legibly written in objective terms or appropriately recorded in the computerized medical record. The patient assessment, the nursing care plan, and the child's responses to medical therapies and nursing care, including the regularly scheduled evaluation of the patient's progress toward nursing goals, must be documented accurately and sequentially. When recording a patient's response to therapy, the nurse must include physiologic responses and exact quotes. The date, time, and nurse's signature and title are required. Nurses must also report any untoward incidents that could inhibit the patient's recovery

Legal and Ethical Issues in Pediatric Care

Shanti, a 15-year-old girl with acute myelocytic leukemia, has come out of her second remission with an acute onset of fever, joint pain, and petechiae. A bone marrow transplant is one of the few remaining therapeutic options. Although Shanti has agreed to a transplant if a suitable donor is found, she does not want to be resuscitated and placed on life support equipment should she have a cardiac arrest. She has talked extensively with the hospital chaplain and social worker and feels comfortable with her decision. Her parents want an all-out effort to sustain her life until a donor is located.

Shanti's case illustrates the legal and ethical dilemmas in caring for children. At what age can children make an informed decision about whether to accept or refuse treatment? At what age do children have the right to participate in the healthcare decision process? What happens when the parents and child have conflicting opinions about treatment? How are ethical decisions resolved?

Informed Consent

Informed consent is a formal preauthorization for an invasive procedure or participation in research. Informed consent was originally a principle to ensure the disclosure of information, but now informed consent also focuses on the comprehension by the patient or parents of the disclosed information. The physician is legally responsible for obtaining informed consent. In the case of research, the investigative researcher may formally designate a person to obtain informed consent. Information that must be provided to obtain informed consent includes an explanation of the condition, a detailed description of the treatment (such as surgical procedures, blood products, sedation, anesthesia, and certain diagnostic procedures), possible benefits and significant risks associated with the proposed treatments, possible alternative treatments, answers to questions, and notification of a parent's or guardian's right to refuse treatment on behalf of the child.

The nurse's role in obtaining informed consent includes the following:

- Alerting physicians to the need for informed consent
- Verifying that informed consent has been obtained prior to any procedure or research participation
- Responding to questions asked by parents and children
- Serving as a witness when parents or guardians sign consent forms or give verbal consent by telephone

Consent must be given knowingly, intelligently, and voluntarily (Beidler & Dickey, 2001). Because children are not considered competent to make healthcare decisions, parents, as the legal custodians of minor children, are customarily requested to give informed consent on behalf of a child. Both children and parents must understand that they have the right to refuse treatment at any time. In an emergency, consent for treatment to preserve life or limb is not required. When parents are divorced, some states limit the parental rights to give informed consent to the parent with custody. When parents have joint custody, in most cases either may give consent. Many children live in homes with a parent and other adult (stepparent, cohabitating unmarried adults, or grandparent) who does not have legal authority to sign consent. Proxy consent can be granted in writing by the parent to another adult so that children can obtain healthcare when needed (Berger & Committee on Medical Liability, 2003). Obtain information about your state law regarding custody and who can provide informed consent for healthcare procedures and treatments. Obtain legal advice for complex family issues related to guardianship, divorced parents disagreeing over care, or a caregiver who is not the legal guardian.

When is a child considered **competent?** This requires an ability to be involved in healthcare decisions requiring a certain degree of intellect, an ability to communicate, and an ability to remember. The individual must be able to understand a therapy or procedures, to consider the major risks and benefits, and to make a decision after deliberating. Competence is closely related to cognitive capacity that involves abstract reasoning, and inductive and deductive logical processes related to complex issues. The formal operations stage of development, occurring during early adolescence (11 to 13 years), is when mental functioning using abstract concepts in problem solving occurs (Beidler & Dickey, 2001).

Children under 18 or 21 years of age, depending on state law, are considered minors, and consent from the parent or guardian is required to perform a medical or surgical procedure or treatment. In some states minors can often legally give informed consent in the following circumstances.

- When they are minor parents of the child patient
- When they are **emancipated minors** (self-supporting adolescents under 18 years of age, not subject to parental control)
- When they are between 16 and 18 years of age seeking birth control, mental health counseling, testing and treatment of HIV and other sexually transmitted diseases, or substance abuse treatment (Dickey & Deatrick, 2000)
- Oregon permits minors of 15 years of age or older to give consent to hospital care, medical or surgical diagnosis, or treatment without the consent of the parent or guardian, and Alabama has a similar law for minors 14 years or older (Maradiegue, 2003)

Mature minors (14- and 15-year-old adolescents who are able to understand treatment risks) are permitted in some states to give consent for treatment or to refuse treatment. In some cases the minor must convince a judge that he or she is mature enough to make an independent judgment about consent for treatment.

Children should become more actively involved in decision making about treatment procedures as their reasoning skills develop. Each child needs to be evaluated individually to determine how extensive a role he or she should have in the decision-making process. Assuming a larger role in the decision-making process with increasing age helps the child develop into a self-determining person. Research is needed to develop valid and reliable tools to assist health professionals in identifying those children with more advanced problem-solving skills that should have a larger role in the decision making about their own care.

Assent, the voluntary agreement to participate in a research project or to accept treatment or dissent, is the ability to have a basic understanding of what will be done, what is required for participation, and then agree or disagree with the proposed treatment or research. Children too young to give informed consent can be given age-appropriate information about their condition and asked about their care preferences. Their parents, however, make ultimate decisions regarding their care (Figure 1–18 ■). Elements of assent are provided in Box 1–10.

With regard to participation in research, federal guidelines state that children 7 years of age and older must receive information about a research project with developmentally appropriate methods and with terms that are appropriate to the

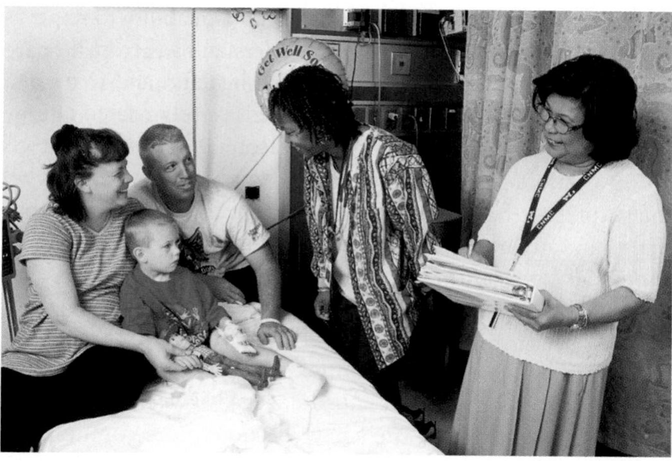

FIGURE 1–18 ■ Children need to be actively involved in decisions regarding their care when appropriate. Here, the family and staff come together to discuss the child's care in a positive and honest manner.

child's comprehension. Children should be given adequate time to ask questions and be told that they have the right to refuse to participate in the study. Assent from approached children must be obtained before they are enrolled (U.S. Department of Health and Human Services, 1983; Lindeke, Hauck, & Tanner, 2000). The number of children asked to participate in research is expected to increase because of Food and Drug Administration regulations requiring manufacturers to assess the safety and effectiveness of new drugs and biological products in pediatric patients associated with the Best Pharmaceuticals for Children Act of 2003 (Lewin & Dale, 2003; Food and Drug Administration, 1998).

Child's Rights Versus Parents' Rights

Parents or guardians have absolute authority to make choices about their child's healthcare except in the following cases.

- When the child and parents do not agree on major treatment options
- When the parents' choice of treatment does not permit lifesaving treatment for the child
- When there is a potential conflict of interest between the child and parents, such as with suspected child abuse or neglect
- When the parents are incapacitated and cannot make a decision (e.g., critically injured in the same motor vehicle crash) (Dickey & Deatrick, 2000)

In cases when the child and parents do not agree on major treatment options, negotiation and compromise may be tried as a first step to avoid destruction of family relationships. Medical consultation may be sought to identify other treatment options that might be acceptable to both the child and parents. An ethics committee usually becomes involved to help resolve the issue. In some cases, the court may be requested to appoint a proxy decision maker for the child or to determine that the child is capable of making a major treatment decision.

BOX 1–10 Steps to Gaining Assent by Children for Research or Treatment

- Help the child gain a developmentally appropriate awareness of the nature of his or her condition.
- Tell the child what to expect with the tests or treatment.
- Determine if the child understands the situation and what could be influencing responses to the proposed participation, such as the appropriate amount of pressure given to accept testing or treatment.
- Obtain the child's willingness to accept the proposed test or treatment. If the medical care will be provided despite the child's objections, that information should be given honestly.

Note: Reprinted from Bernat, J. L. (2002). Informed consent in pediatric neurology. Seminars in Pediatric Neurology, *9(1), 13. With permission from Elsevier.*

Confidentiality

Confidentiality is an agreement between a patient and a provider that information discussed during the healthcare encounter will not be shared without the permission of the patient. Concerns about privacy and the fear of disclosure of sensitive information to parents are a major reason adolescents do not seek healthcare (Ford, Bearman, & Moody, 1999). When the child is an emancipated or mature minor, many states permit healthcare providers to provide birth control and treatment for sexually transmitted diseases including HIV and AIDS, pregnancy, and substance abuse without informing the child's parents (Dickey & Deatrick, 2000). However, the issue of minors giving consent is complicated by the healthcare system that holds the parents responsible for the financial costs of the healthcare services sought in confidence. See Partnering with Families: Adolescents and Confidentiality.

Breaching confidentiality is a potential problem for adolescents, who are just learning whom they can trust in the healthcare system. Make sure you openly discuss the limits of confidentiality for topics such as mandatory reporting requirements with the patient and family. Inadvertent disclosure of personal information may lead to psychological, social, or physical harm in some patients.

PRACTICE ALERT

If the child has a reportable disease, confidentiality may create a public health hazard. In such cases, the healthcare professional is obligated to report the presence of the disease to the appropriate state or county agency. Suspected cases of child abuse must be reported to the appropriate agency specified by state law.

HIPAA and Confidentiality. In the current healthcare system, the complexities of treatment, the numbers of healthcare providers involved, and the ability to transmit information electronically make it more difficult to maintain confidentiality. However, the Health Insurance Portability and Accountability Act (HIPAA), Public Law (PL) 104-191 enacted by Congress in 1996, now requires the confidential management of patient medical record data. The goal of the law is to protect the **privacy**

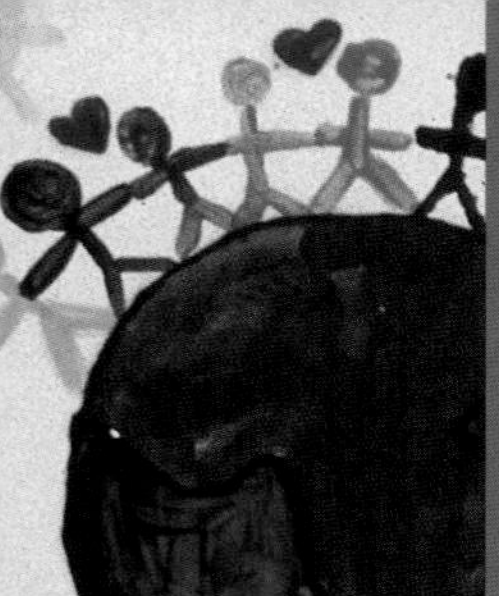

PARTNERING WITH FAMILIES

Adolescents and Confidentiality

Adolescents need a safe environment to discuss healthcare issues so that they seek health care when needed. Ways to promote confidentiality include the following actions:

- Assure that adolescents and parents talk separately to the healthcare provider about their concerns.
- Display and offer educational materials on confidentiality to adolescents and parents.
- Make sure all the doors are closed when collecting an adolescent's medical history or discussing sensitive issues.
- Ask if the adolescent is comfortable receiving messages and mail from the health professional using the contact information provided.
- Create a comfortable atmosphere and environment for adolescents to discuss private concerns regarding their health.
- Make sure clinic literature distributed is small enough to fit into a purse or wallet.
- Make sure you and your health professional colleagues are fully informed about the laws in your state about the rights of adolescents to receive care without their parent's consent.
- Explain the parameters of confidentiality between you and the adolescent and his or her parents at the beginning of the healthcare visit.
- Discuss situations in which you need to breech confidentiality.

Note: From Simmons, M., Shalwitz, J., & Pollack, S. (2002). Understanding confidentiality and minor consent in California: An adolescent provider toolkit. *San Francisco: Adolescent Health Working Group, San Francisco Health Plan.*

(the ability of an individual to maintain information in a protected manner) of citizens by establishing privacy standards for confidential medical information. HIPAA was designed to protect patient information transmitted electronically for the purpose of insurance payments. The rules developed for implementation of this law affect all persons who use medical and financial information in the healthcare system (Maradiegue, 2002). The privacy regulations cover protected health information, individually identifiable health information maintained or transmitted in any form—oral, written, or electronic. The protected health information applies to past, present, and future physical and mental health, provision of healthcare, and provision of payment for healthcare. Each healthcare provider or organization has been required to develop policies to prevent the disclosure of protected health information. There are serious fines and penalties for healthcare facilities and providers who do not conform to the HIPAA regulations. Patients have the right to access their health information (Maliszewski, 2003). Breaching confidentiality puts the nurse at risk for liability and legal action.

MediaLink Critical Thinking: Ethical Dilemma

Patient Self-Determination Act

The federal Patient Self-Determination Act directs healthcare institutions to inform hospitalized patients about their rights, which include expressing a preference for treatment options and making **advance directives** (writing a living will or authorizing a durable power of attorney for healthcare decisions on the patient's behalf). Nurses often discuss these issues with patients and their families. Minor children and their parents should also be informed of their rights. Adolescents with serious acute or chronic conditions with a higher risk of death should be encouraged to talk with their parents about their healthcare wishes and to jointly prepare advance directives (Dickey & Deatrick, 2000).

Do Not Resuscitate orders have become more common for children with terminal illnesses in which no further treatments are possible or desired. In many cases, these children are cared for at home or in a hospice program, but some still attend school. Implementation of Do Not Resuscitate orders for such children then becomes a community issue, to ensure that no resuscitation measures are initiated by any emergency care provider when the child has a life-threatening event. State health policies must be developed so children with these signed orders are easily identified and appropriate documentation of the orders is on file. See Chapter 22∞ for issues related to end-of-life care.

Ethical Concepts and Issues

Ethics is the philosophic study of morality, and the analysis of moral problems and moral judgments. Ethics has become a prominent discipline associated with the delivery of medical care and research due to significant developments (Mappes & DeGrazia, 2001).

- Major advances in medical research and resulting development of medical technology, for example, the ability to save the lives of severely impaired newborns, genetic testing, and gene therapy, have resulted in challenges in making the best decision for the child and family.
- Healthcare is provided in an increasingly complex environment with multiple disciplines involved in patient care, consumer rights, managed care and the economic constraints associated with healthcare costs, and legal liability.

Ethical issues may arise from a **moral dilemma,** a conflict of social values and ethical principles that supports different courses of action that could be correct (e.g., performing or refraining from performing a therapy), depending upon an individual's values and beliefs. Problems may develop because physicians, nurses, and parents have differing opinions about treatments for an infant or child with a serious or fatal condition. Approaches to ethical decision making take into account social-political philosophy, philosophy of law, moral philosophy, and moral theology as well as the concrete realities that medicine and biology contribute. An ethical theory or framework for decision making is often used in healthcare institutions to guide individuals to determine an appropriate action. Theories focus on different outcomes, such as the consequences of the decision, the greatest happiness or avoidance of suffering, or utilitarianism (a merger of the consequences and greatest happiness for the greatest number).

The four general ethical principles used in the development of decision-making framework include:

- **Beneficence**—an obligation to act or to make a decision to benefit the patient, promoting the child's well-being in addition to working with parents and other family members
- Respect for patient's **autonomy**—right for self-determination or decision making, to protect the informed choices (consent and refusal) of patients capable of decision making
- **Nonmaleficence**—to prevent harm
- **Justice**—fairness in the use of scarce resources

All individuals must be treated without prejudice, regardless of race, gender, religious preference, cultural or educational background, financial status, or sexual orientation (Cassidy & Fleischman, 1996). Professional integrity with regard to telling the truth and keeping promises is also important. Challenges arise because healthcare professionals may have different values from patients, based on their culture and life experiences, or there are differences in values between members of the healthcare team caring for the child. They want to do things for a child that can be a benefit, rather than do things to a child that cannot be of benefit and may seem harmful. Parents also want to protect the child, and they have their vision of what is good for the child.

Children commonly have their rights and autonomy compromised because they often are not capable of making a fully informed healthcare decision. Pediatric nurses have a responsibility to become knowledgeable about the moral and legal rights of their patients and families and to protect and support those rights. Some nurses have specialized in ethics by taking graduate education to become an ethics consultant or nurse ethicist.

The four ethical principles previously stated should direct nursing practice along with virtues such as honesty, compassion, courage, wisdom, confidentiality, and respect for privacy (White, 2001). Learn about the mechanism in your healthcare facility for requesting an ethical consultation. The consultation may be used to help nurses and other health professionals clarify if an ethical dilemma exists and how to respond once adequate information is collected. The consultation may also be requested by family faced with difficult decisions or conflict about the treatment options proposed.

PRACTICE ALERT

A therapeutic alliance is needed to foster positive outcomes for the child and family. Rather than let conflict erupt when the family's values and health professional's values do not match, it is better to look for shared values and opportunities for negotiation. Questions to ask to identify what is important to the family include (Glover, 2000):

- What is important to you in the care of your child?
- What do you fear and wish to avoid?
- What are your sources of support?
- What is your understanding of your child's condition?

BOX 1–11 Steps in Ethical Problem Solving

- Recognize that a potential or actual ethical dilemma exists.
- Collect as much information as possible:
  - About the medical facts and the physician's goals
  - About the child's and family's wishes or preferences
  - About your values and beliefs
- Identify if surrogate decision makers exist (e.g., a court-appointed guardian).
- State the dilemma as clearly as possible.
- Seek consultation on all possible courses of action or inaction.
- Identify the strengths and weaknesses of each therapeutic action.
- Identify the realistic expectations and benefits of each potential therapeutic action or inaction.
- Set goals and establish a decision-making process, and implement a plan of action.
- Evaluate the results.

Healthcare institutions have an ethics committee to resolve conflicts about treatment decisions that function in one of the following ways:

- Performing individual case consultations to resolve a conflict between health professionals and the child and family
- Resolving a dispute between health professionals about the care to provide to a child
- Serving as a forum to discuss policies about ethics within the healthcare facility
- Educating health professionals and the community about ethical concepts

The committees often make treatment decisions using the process of data collection and evaluation outlined in Box 1–11. Courts should make ethical decisions only when healthcare professionals and parents are unable to agree about providing or withholding treatment.

Terminating Life-Sustaining Treatment

Infant John, at 5 days of age, has a birth weight of 1200 g, acute respiratory distress, and a severe intraventricular hemorrhage. His physicians are seeking his parents' consent for surgical placement of a ventriculoperitoneal shunt. Regardless of intensive medical care and planned surgical intervention, the infant is expected to have a severe handicap. The infant's condition is critical, and it is not certain how well the infant will respond to surgery. The parents, after much consideration and discussions with their family and pastor, have requested that comfort measures only be provided. They want life-sustaining treatment to be withheld, because they believe the additional procedures will cause excessive suffering for the infant, especially when the outcome is uncertain.

Conflict often arises between health professionals and parents when parents choose to refuse therapy on behalf of their child. The ethical principle of autonomy in making an informed decision is especially challenging when parents choose to refuse treatment rather than accept treatment. In most cases parents are responsible for choosing what is best for their children. When they choose to refuse treatment in these cases, their rights to make such a decision may be challenged by the healthcare system. See Developing Cultural Competence: Jehovah's Witnesses and Use of Blood Products.

What happens when the parents' request differs from the opinion of physicians? Are the rights of the child violated? How do federal regulations for care of infants with severe defects affect current healthcare practice? How is the best interest of the child with an unknown future (mild or severe handicap) determined?

Federal "Baby Doe" regulations were developed to protect the rights of infants with severe defects. These rules mandated that treatment be provided for impaired newborns unless they are permanently comatose, any treatment would only prolong their death, or treatment would not be effective or humane (Morrow, 2000). These regulations created a standard of care that the prospect of a handicap should not play a role in treatment decisions (Fost, 1999). Parents of such infants are usually the ultimate decision makers about the child's care. They may want to terminate treatment because of the tremendous social, emotional, and financial burden (Schrode, 2000). Physicians may believe treatment will help the child and improve the quality of life (sometimes defined as a meaningful existence or an ability to develop human relationships). Federal regulations recommend a formalized ethical decision-making process before physicians accept or reject parents' wishes. The most common question brought before ethics committees is whether to terminate life-sustaining treatment.

Justifications for withholding, withdrawing, or limiting therapy include the following:

- The treatment in question will not work.
- The burdens of the treatment outweigh the benefits, or the quality of life is poor after treatment.
- The burdens of the disease outweigh the benefits of continued survival, or the quality of life is poor before the treatment (Cassidy & Fleischman, 1996).

Each of these conditions is considered by the members of the ethics committee according to their individual beliefs, their perceptions of the value of specific interventions for an individual child, and the ethical theory used to guide decision making. Treatment to save the infant's life is elected if it has the potential for improving the quality of life as well. In cases such as Infant John, the decision to withhold surgery may be made when the child's condition potentially would not be improved and additional pain and suffering would occur. Physicians are not obligated to offer interventions that cause extreme pain and suffering when there is no or limited potential benefit. Treatments that only prolong life without improving quality of life are often considered to represent a misuse of expensive healthcare resources.

Genetic Testing of Children

With advances in genetics research, it is now possible to conduct genetic testing and screening of children for the presence of carrier status or to the susceptibility for late onset of a condition, such as Huntington disease and some cancers. This testing is now possible for some conditions for which there is no definitive treatment or prevention of the condition.

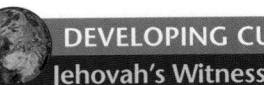

DEVELOPING CULTURAL COMPETENCE
Jehovah's Witnesses and Use of Blood Products

Jehovah's Witnesses oppose blood transfusions for themselves and their children because they believe transfusions are equivalent to the oral intake of blood, which is morally and spiritually wrong according to their interpretation of the Bible (Leviticus 17:13–14). A Jehovah's Witness who receives a transfusion believes he or she has committed a sin and may have forfeited everlasting life. Transfusions of any blood products, including plasma and the patient's own blood, are forbidden. While adults are permitted to make decisions to refuse blood products even when death may occur, most healthcare institutions have developed policies to address the care of children who need blood products. Every effort to avoid the use of blood products with alternative therapies is usually attempted before seeking a judicial order to administer a blood product when it will be lifesaving.

Important ethical issues are associated with genetic testing.

- What is the benefit of screening when no therapy can be offered?
- What is the potential risk (psychological harm, social stigma, discrimination in employment or insurance benefits) if an individual knows of the risk of developing a significant health condition or being a carrier of a health condition?
- Should newborn screening programs be mandatory or voluntary with informed consent required?

Genetic screening of newborns, such as for cystic fibrosis, is recommended only when the identification of the genetic condition will have a clear benefit to the child, a system is in place to confirm the diagnosis, and treatment and follow-up must be available to affected newborns. Informed consent for genetic testing should be required (Committee on Bioethics, American Academy of Pediatrics, 2001). See Chapter 24∞ for recent research on the benefits of newborn genetic screening for cystic fibrosis. See Chapter 4∞ for more information about ethical issues regarding genetic testing.

Organ Transplantation Issues

The death of a child can benefit another child through organ transplantation. The National Organ Transplant Act (PL 98–507) generated laws, regulations, and guidelines for organ collection and transplantation (Frader & Thompson, 1994). For example, the transplant team cannot provide care to the potential donor. The institution has specific requirements to approach family members when brain death is suspected or confirmed to request organ donation. Regulations are important because too few organs are available for patients needing transplantation, especially young children.

The limited supply of organs has created numerous ethical issues. Which patients on the waiting list should receive the organs available? Should a patient with multiple congenital anomalies or abnormal chromosomes be eligible for a transplant? Should families be permitted to pay donor families for organs? Should the family's ability to pay for an organ transplant give a child higher priority for an organ? Should a patient receive a second organ transplant, replacing an organ deteriorating because of rejection? Each institution performing organ transplants develops guidelines for ethical decision making regarding these questions.

Research Issues

While legal issues regarding informed consent and assent for research have been discussed, there are additional ethical questions related to conducting research with children as subjects. Because of the ethical principles of beneficence and nonmaleficence, it is imperative that there be a risk-benefit ratio that is favorable to the individual child or to children in general. Harm must be considered from the perspective of the child and be sensitive to the child's reduced capacity to understand what is happening, and the effects of disruption, inconvenience, and novel situations on the child and family (Shevell, 2002).

PARTNERING WITH CHILDREN AND THEIR FAMILIES

As illustrated throughout this chapter, partnering with parents and children is the foundation for our interactions with families for all pediatric nursing care. Developing relationships is challenging, exciting, and ultimately gratifying for nurses who choose to specialize in pediatrics. Partnering is essential every step of the way:

- Obtaining informed consent and assent
- Respecting that the parent is the expert with regard to the child's care
- Acknowledging and supporting cultural values in the provision of care
- Preparing parents to assume ongoing complex healthcare responsibilities for their child

Use the information in Partnering with Families boxes provided in other chapters to enhance your relationships with families and to provide appropriate care in a supportive environment that promotes the family unit and the child's development.

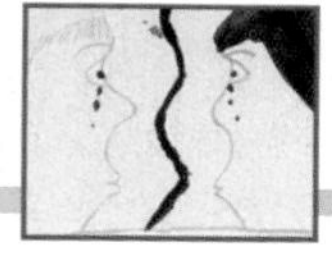

CHAPTER HIGHLIGHTS

- Roles of nurses in caring for children include providing direct care (health promotion, health maintenance, and nursing care for health conditions), patient education, patient advocacy, and case management, and minimizing the psychological and physical distress experienced by children and their families.
- Nurses care for children in many different settings. Within the hospital, these settings include the emergency department, observation or short-stay unit, postanesthesia unit, intensive care unit, general pediatric inpatient unit, and various outpatient clinics. Other settings include schools, childcare centers, physician offices, community health centers, rehabilitation centers, and the home.
- Family-centered care is a method designed to meet the emotional, social, and developmental needs of children and families needing healthcare.
- Nurses must identify culturally relevant facts about their patients to provide appropriate and competent care to an increasingly diverse population.
- Unintentional injury is the leading cause of death for children between 1 and 19 years of age.
- Efforts to provide all children with access to healthcare include the State Children's Health Insurance Program (SCHIP) currently being implemented nationwide.
- Documentation of nursing care is essential for risk management and quality improvement. Documentation must include the patient assessment, the nursing care plan, the child's responses to medical therapies and nursing care, and the regular evaluation of the child's progress toward nursing goals.
- Informed consent is the formal preauthorization for an invasive procedure or participation in research. Parents typically give informed consent for children under 18 years of age unless the child is an emancipated minor, a self-supporting adolescent not subject to parental control.
- Children need to become more actively involved in decisions about their care as their decision-making abilities develop. Even though they cannot provide informed consent, federal guidelines mandate that children as young as 7 years of age receive information about treatment procedures and research project participation and give their assent.
- Because adolescents fear disclosure of confidential information, they may avoid seeking healthcare. When the adolescents have a reportable disease, it is important to inform them that confidentiality cannot be maintained, as a report must be made to a public health agency.
- Adolescents at a higher risk of death due to a serious acute or chronic condition should be encouraged to talk with their parents and jointly prepare advance directives.
- Federal regulations require a formalized ethical decision-making process to assist healthcare providers and families in making important decisions about withholding, withdrawing, or limiting a child's therapy.

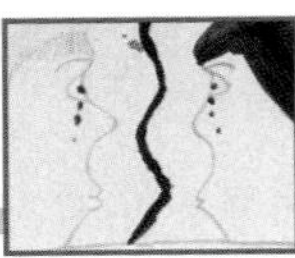

CRITICAL THINKING IN ACTION

INTRODUCTION

Return to the scenario about Drew at the beginning of the chapter. Despite his seizure disorder Drew has been developing normally, meeting expected developmental milestones as evaluated by the Denver II.

DESCRIPTION

The pediatric nurse has worked closely with the family to ensure that all of Drew's healthcare needs are addressed during health promotion and health maintenance visits. Prior to the seizure, the nurse had been helping the parents to ensure that all healthcare requirements were met for Drew to attend a new childcare center. The pediatric nurse will now modify her nursing care plan to integrate the needed diagnostic procedures and treatment for Drew's seizure disorder, and to help the parents manage their increased concerns about his seizure disorder.

DISCUSSION

1. Identify all the roles of Drew's nurse in working with this child and his family. What other roles could nurses have within this healthcare center and in other settings to support the nursing care provided to Drew and his family? Consider the roles of a nurse manager in the healthcare setting, a nurse consultant to the childcare center, and a nurse in the emergency department.
2. Informed consent is often needed before diagnostic procedures are performed and prior to releasing healthcare information. What is the process for obtaining informed consent in your healthcare setting? What is the nurse's role in the process? What needs to happen before health information is released to the childcare center? How does this healthcare facility ensure compliance with HIPAA?
3. The healthcare setting where Drew receives care has an evidence-based critical pathway for the management of children with seizures. Identify a critical pathway that has been developed for a pediatric healthcare condition in your healthcare setting. How is the critical pathway used and how does this process differ from implementation of a nursing care plan?
4. Describe the nursing interventions for the modified nursing care plan for diagnostic procedures, treatment, and family concerns.

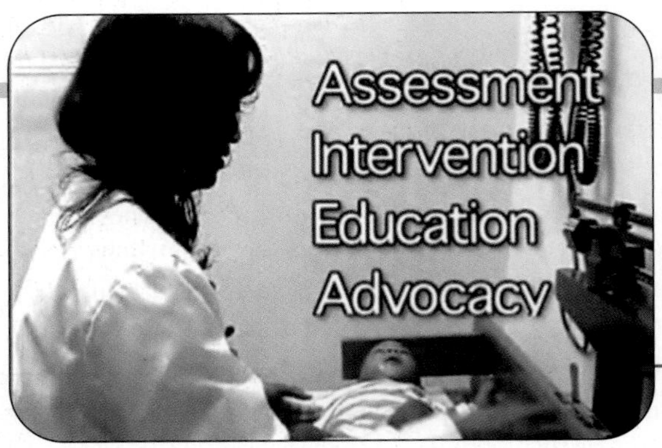

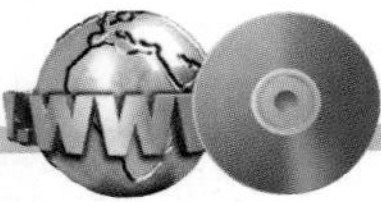

EXPLORE MediaLink

- NCLEX review, case studies, and other interactive resources for this chapter can be found on the Companion Website at **http://www.prenhall.com/ball**. Click on Chapter 1 to select the activities for this chapter.
- For animations, more NCLEX review questions, and an audio glossary, access the accompanying CD-ROM in this book.

http://www.prenhall.com/ball

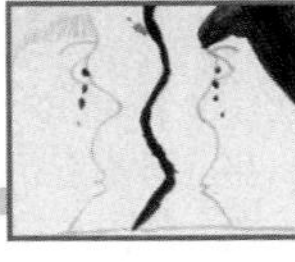

REFERENCES

Alfaro-LeFevre, R. (2004). *Critical thinking and clinical judgment* (3rd ed., pp. 4–8). Philadelphia: W. B. Saunders.

American Nurses Association. (2003). *Nursing's social policy statement.* Washington, DC: nursesbooks.org.

American Nurses Association. (2004). *Scope & Standards of Practice.* Washington, DC: nursesbooks.org.

American Nurses Association & Society of Pediatric Nurses. (2003). *Scope and standards of pediatric nursing practice.* Washington, DC: nursesbooks.org.

Arias, E., & Smith, B. L. (2003). Deaths: Preliminary data for 2001. *National Vital Statistics Reports, 51*(5), 1–29.

Barnsteiner, J., & Prevost, S. (2002). How to implement evidence-based practice: Some tried and true pointers. *Reflections on Nursing Leadership, 28*(2), 18–21.

Bates, D. W., Teich, J., Lee, J., et al. (1999). The impact of computerized physician order entry on medication error prevention. *Journal of American Informatics Association, 6,* 313–321.

Beidler, S. M., & Dickey, S. B. (2001). Children's competence to participate in healthcare decisions. *JONA's Healthcare Law, Ethics, and Regulation, 3*(3), 80–87.

Berger, J. E., & Committee on Medical Liability. (2003). Consent by proxy for nonurgent pediatric care. *Pediatrics, 112*(5), 1186–1195.

Bernat, J. L. (2002). Informed consent in pediatric neurology. *Seminars in Pediatric Neurology, 9*(1), 10–18.

Callender, D. (1999). Pediatric practice guidelines: Implications for nurse practitioners. *Journal of Pediatric Health Care, 13*(3), 105–111.

Cassidy, R. C., & Fleischman, A. R. (1996). *Pediatric ethics—From principles to practice.* Amsterdam, The Netherlands: Harwood Academic Publishers.

Centers for Medicare and Medicaid Services. (2003). State children's health insurance program. www.cms.gov/schip/schip02.pdf, accessed 7/07/2003.

Committee on Bioethics, American Academy of Pediatrics. (2001). Ethical issues with genetic testing in pediatrics. *Pediatrics, 107*(6), 1451–1455.

Committee on Children with Disabilities, American Academy of Pediatrics. (1998). Managed care and children with special health care needs: A subject review (RE9814). *Pediatrics, 102*(3), 657–660.

Dickey, S. B., & Deatrick, J. (2000). Autonomy and decision making for health promotion in adolescence. *Pediatric Nursing, 26*(5), 461–467.

Federal Interagency Forum on Child and Family Statistics. (2002). *America's children: Key national indicators of well-being 2002.* Washington, DC: U.S. Government Printing Office.

Flores, G. (2000). Culture and the patient-physician relationship: Achieving cultural competency in healthcare. *Journal of Pediatrics, 136,* 14.

Flores, G., Laws, M. B., Mayo, S. J., Zuckerman, B., Abreu, M., Medina, L., & Hardt, E. J. (2003). Errors in medical interpretation and their potential clinical consequences in pediatric encounters. *Pediatrics, 111*(1), 6–14.

Food and Drug Administration. (1998, December 2). Regulations requiring manufacturers to assess the safety and effectiveness of new drugs and biological products in pediatric patients. *Federal Register, 63*(231), 66631–66672. www.fda.gov/ohrms/dockets/98fr/120298c.txt

Ford, C. A., Bearman, P. S., & Moody, J. (1999). Foregone health care among adolescents. *Journal of American Medical Association, 282*(23), 2227–2234.

Fost, N. (1999). Decisions regarding treatment of seriously ill newborns. *Journal of the American Medical Association, 281*(21), 2041–2043.

Frader, J., & Thompson, A. (1994). Ethical issues in the pediatric intensive care unit. *Pediatric Clinics of North America, 41*(6), 1405–1421.

Glover, J. J. (2000). Pulling the plug on futility language. *Pediatric Ethiscope, 11*(2), 1–4.

Guy, J., Persaud, J., Davies, E., & Harvey, D. (2003). Drug errors: What role do nurses and pharmacists have in minimizing risk? *Journal of Child Health Care, 7*(4), 277–290.

Health Canada. (2000). *Canadian perinatal health report.* Ottawa, CA: Minister of Public Works and Government Services.

Health Canada. (2002). Canada's health care system at a glance. http://www.hc.sc.gc.ca/english/media/releases/ 2002/health_act/glance.html, accessed 9/4/2003.

Health Resources and Services Administration, Maternal and Child Health Bureau. (2002). *Child Health USA 2002.* Rockville, MD: U.S. Department of Health and Human Services.

Hefland, W. H., Lazarus, J., & Theerman, P. (2000). The Children's Bureau and public health at mid-century. *American Journal of Public Health, 90,* 1703.

Hoyert, D. L., Smith, B. L., Arias, E., & Murphy, S. L. (2001). *Deaths: Final data for 1999. National Vital Statistics Reports, 49*(8). Hyattsville, MD: National Center for Health Statistics.

Kaushal, R., Bates, D. W., Landrigan, C., McKenna, K. J., Clapp, M. D., Federico, F., & Goldmann, D. A. (2001). Medication error and adverse drug events in pediatric patients. *Journal of the American Medical Association, 285*(16), 2114–2120.

Kempe, A., Renfew, B. L., Barrow, J., Cherry, D., Jones, J. S., & Steiner, J. F. (2001). Barriers to enrollment in a state child health insurance program. *Ambulatory Pediatrics, 1*(3), 169–177.

Lewin, L., & Dale, J. (2003). Research considerations with children and adolescents. *Journal of Pediatric Health Care, 17*(5), 268–270.

Lindeke, L. L., Hauck, M. R., & Tanner, M. (2000). Practical issues in obtaining child assent for research. *Journal of Pediatric Nursing, 15*(2), 99–104.

MacPhee, M. (2002). Evidence-based practice in action. *Journal of Pediatric Nursing, 17*(4), 313–320.

Maliszewski, S. C. (2003). HIPAA privacy regulations. *Advance for Nurse Practitioners, 11*(1), 16.

Mappes, T. A., & DeGrazia, D. (2001). *Biomedical ethics* (5th ed.). Boston: McGraw Hill.

Maradiegue, A. (2002). The Health Insurance Portability and Accountability Act and adolescents. *Pediatric Nursing, 28*(4), 417–420.

Maradiegue, A. (2003). Minor's rights versus parental rights: Review of legal issues in adolescent health care. *Journal of Midwifery Womens Health, 48*(3), 170–177.

Markel, H. (2000). For the welfare of children: The origins of the relationship between U.S. public health workers and pediatricians. *American Journal of Public Health, 90*(6), 893–899.

Martin, J. A., Hamilton, B. E., Ventura, S. J., Menaker, F., & Park, M. M. (2002). *Births: Final data for 2000. National Vital Statistics Reports, 50*(5). Hyattsville, MD: National Center for Health Statistics.

Maternal and Child Health Bureau. (2002). *Understanding the Title V of the Social Security Act.* Rockville, MD: Department of Health and Human Services, Health Resources and Services Administration, Maternal and Child Health Bureau.

Mathews, T. J., Menaker, F., & MacDorman, M. (2002). Infant mortality statistics from the 2000 period linked birth/infant death data set. *National Vital Statistics Reports, 50*(12), Tables 3 and B.

McCormick, M. C., Weinick, R. M., Elixhauser, A., Stagnitti, M. N., Thompson, J., & Simpson, L. (2001). Annual report on access to and utilization of health care for children and youth in the United States—2000. *Ambulatory Pediatrics, 1*(1), 3–15.

Melnyk, B. M., Fineout-Overholt, E., Stone, P., & Ackerman, M. (2000). Evidence-based practice: The past, the present, and recommendations for the millennium. *Pediatric Nursing, 26*(1), 77–80.

Merritt, T. A., Palmer, D., Bergman, D. A., & Shiono, P. H. (1997). Clinical practice guidelines in pediatric and newborn medicine. Implications for their use in practice. *Pediatrics, 99*(1), 100–114.

Morrow, J. (2000). Making mortal decisions at the beginning of life: A case of impaired and imperiled infants. *Journal of the American Medical Association, 284*(9), 1146–1147.

National Association of Pediatric Nurse Practitioners. (2002). NAPNAP position statement on the health care home. www.napnap.org/practice/positions/healthcarehome.html, accessed 3/23/2004.

National Center for Health Statistics. (2000). *1998 National Home and Hospice Care Survey*, CD-ROM Series 13(27). Hyattsville, MD: Author.

National Center for Health Statistics Vital Statistics System. (2003). http://webapp.cdc.gov/cgi-bin/broker.exe, accessed 7/2/2003.

Schrode, K. (2000). Baby Doe and the Baby Doe regulations. *Children's National Medical Center Pediatric Ethicscope, 11*(1), 1–4.

Shevell, M. I. (2002). Ethics of clinical research in children. *Seminars in Pediatric Neurology, 9*(1), 46–52.

Simmons, M., Shalwitz, J., & Pollack, S. (2002). *Understanding confidentiality and minor consent in California: An adolescent provider toolkit.* San Francisco: Adolescent Health Working Group, San Francisco Health Plan.

Slonim, A., LaFleur, B. J., Ahmed, B. S., & Joseph, J. G. (2003). Hospital-reported medical errors in children. *Pediatrics, 111*(3), 617–621.

Smith, L. A., Wise, P. H., Chavkin, W., Romero, D., & Zuckerman, B. (2000). Implications in welfare reform for child health: Emerging challenges for clinical practice and policy. *Pediatrics, 106*(5), 1117–1125.

Teicher, S., Crawford, K., Williams, B., Nelson, B., & Andrews, C. (2001). Emerging role of the pediatric nurse practitioner in acute care. *Pediatric Nursing, 27*(4), 387–390.

UNICEF. (2003). *Official summary: The state of the world's children 2003* (pp. 14–18). New York: United Nations Publications.

U.S. Bureau of the Census. (2000). *Resident population estimates of the United States by age and sex, April 1, 1990 to July 1, 1999 with short term projection to November 1, 2000.* Washington, DC: U.S. Government Printing Office.

U.S. Bureau of the Census. (2001). Statistical abstract of the United States: 2001. www.census.gov/prod/2002pubs/01statab/pop.pdf

U.S. Department of Health and Human Services. (1983). *Protection of human subjects: Code of federal regulations* (45 CFR 46, Subpart D). Washington, DC: U.S. Government Printing Office.

U.S. Department of Health and Human Services. (2000). *Healthy People 2010* (2nd ed.). Washington, DC: U.S. Government Printing Office. www.healthy people.gov

U.S. Food and Drug Administration. (2003). *FDA proposes drug bar code regulation.* http://www.fda.gov/oc/initiatives/barcode-sadr/fs-barcode.html, accessed 6/4/2003.

U.S. General Accounting Office. (1989). *Home care experiences of families with chronically ill children.* Washington, DC: Author.

Velsor-Friedrich, B. (2003). Federally sponsored insurance progams for children: The state children's health insurance program. *Journal of Pediatric Nursing, 18*(2), 134–136.

White, G. (2001). The code of ethics for nurses. *American Journal of Nursing, 101*(10), 73–75.

Winslow, E. H. (2001). Patient education materials: Can patients read them or are they ending up in the trash? *American Journal of Nursing, 101*(10), 33–38.

Chapter

2

Family-Centered Care: Theory and Application

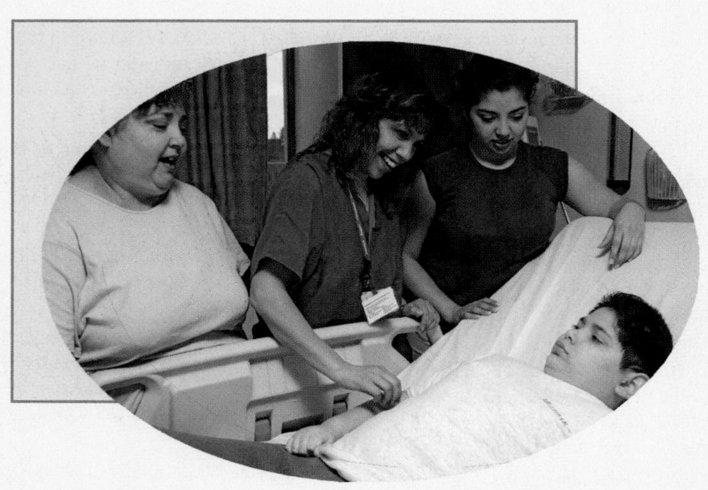

Casey DeProspero, a 14 year old, is recuperating from injuries sustained in a motor vehicle crash in which he was the passenger. He was not wearing a seat belt and experienced a brain injury after striking the windshield. His cognitive and motor functions are impaired. Following a 7-day acute care hospital stay, he was moved to the inpatient rehabilitation hospital where he has been for the past 5 days. He is much more responsive to stimuli and to family members 12 days after his injury. Physical therapy is provided twice a day to promote range of motion and muscle tone and to prevent contractures. Plans are being made to discharge him home with outpatient rehabilitation care within the next 5 days. A case manager will be assigned to coordinate his healthcare services.

Casey lives with his mother, sister, two half-brothers (10 and 6 years old) and stepfather. Both his mother and stepfather are employed full time and are trying to determine how to manage care for Casey once he returns home. Casey's father has not been actively involved in his life since the divorce 12 years ago. Casey's grandparents reside in the same town and may provide some support to the family.

What family supports will Casey need as he continues his rehabilitation from the brain injury? What family assessment information is needed to effectively plan nursing care for this adolescent and his family? Does this family have strengths and coping strategies that will help them adapt to Casey's disability?

"Mom and Dad are so worried about Casey. They were scared that he was going to die, and now they wonder if he will ever be normal again. We have been talking about how to take care of him when he comes home and how we will all have to help out more around the house."

—Casey's sister Teresa, 16 years old

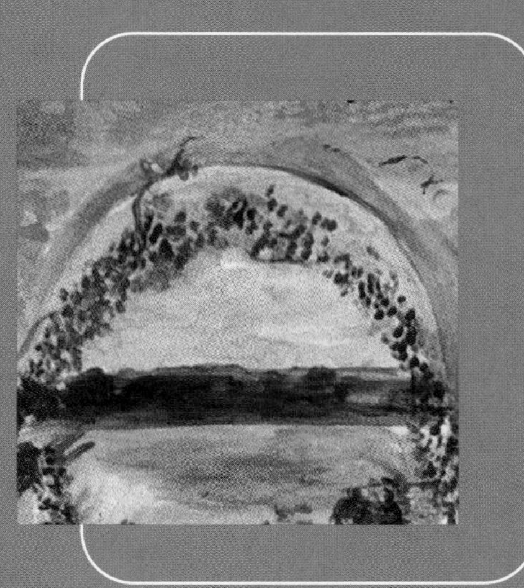

Learning Outcomes

After completing this chapter, you will be able to:

- Describe family-centered care and develop a nursing care plan for the child and family that integrates key concepts.
- Describe characteristics of different types of families.
- Identify four different parenting styles and analyze their impact on child personality development.
- Describe the effect of major family changes on children, including divorce, gaining a stepparent, being placed in foster care, and adoption.
- Review various family theories and identify their application to the nursing process.
- Delineate the advantages of using a family assessment tool.
- Identify a variety of family support services that might be available in a community.

Key Terms

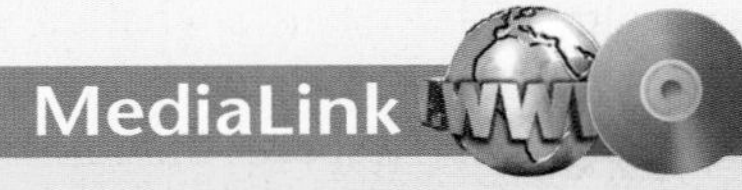

MediaLink http://www.prenhall.com/ball

Resources for this chapter can be found on the CD-ROM accompanying this textbook, and on the Companion Website at www.prenhall.com/ball. Click on Chapter 2 to select the activities for this chapter.

CD-ROM
Video
Defining Family
NCLEX Review
Audio Glossary

COMPANION WEBSITE
NCLEX Review
Care Plan: Needs of the Adopted Child
MediaLink Applications
Facility Assessment
Identifying Family Support
The Nursing Process and Family-Centered Care

FAMILY ROLES

The U.S. Census Bureau defines a **family** as individuals who are joined together by marriage, blood, adoption, or residence in the same household (Friedman, Bowden, & Jones, 2003). More broadly, however, a family may be a self-identified group of two or more persons joined together by sharing resources and emotional closeness (Figure 2–1 ■). Family members can also include "honorary relatives" of the family, whether or not they are related by blood, marriage, or adoption, or even living in the same household. The family as defined by its members is likely to be dynamic, because membership often changes over time. For example, second marriages often integrate children into a newly formed family; and spouses of married children are integrated into an existing family while the newly married couple begins a new family. In today's world it is even more likely that families will live in different cities, states, or even countries than their extended families. So, there is no *typical* family.

Generally, family members depend on each other for emotional, physical, and economic support. Families are guided by a common set of values or beliefs about the worth and importance of certain ideas and traditions. These values often bind family members together, and these values are greatly influenced by external factors including cultural background, social norms, education, environmental influences, socioeconomic status, and beliefs held by peers, coworkers, political and community leaders, and other individuals outside the family unit. Because of the influence of these external factors, a family's values may change considerably over the years, or members within a family may hold values that conflict with those of other family members.

A family is generally understood to be a safe haven for its members as they learn group values, norms, and acceptable behaviors. However, child abuse and neglect is a significant problem and can occur within any family configuration (see Chapter 7∞). Individual family members take on certain social and gender roles and hold a designated status within the family based on the values and beliefs that bind extended families together. These values and beliefs may evolve from the family's cultural background, social norms, education, and other influences to which parents were exposed during childhood, adolescence, and early adult years. Parental roles are usually learned through a socialization process during childhood and adolescence. Roles of the family are listed in Box 2–1.

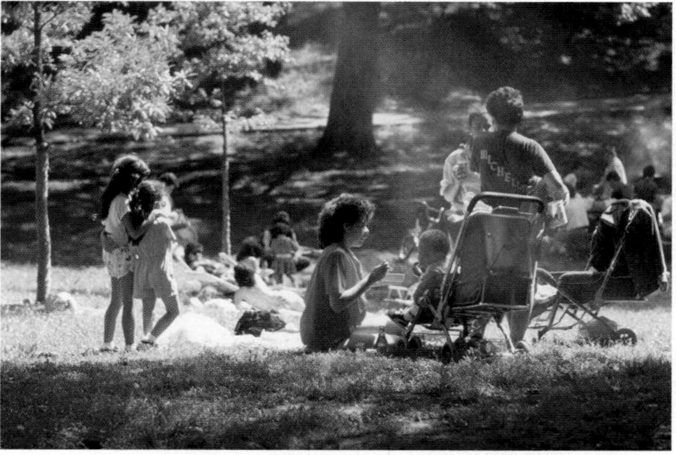

FIGURE 2–1 ■ Families are diverse in their composition. In this case, the extended family has gathered for a picnic in the park.

BOX 2–1 Roles of the Family

- Caring, nurturing, and educating children
- Maintaining the continuity of society by transmitting its knowledge, customs, values, and beliefs to children
- Receiving and giving love
- Preparing children to become productive members of society
- Meeting the needs of its members
- Serving as a buffer between its members and environmental and societal demands while addressing the interests and needs of the individual family members

Parents have important roles that involve childrearing and the long-term care of children until they reach adulthood. Depending on their other roles in society, parents work to successfully nurture and rear children, helping them to meet role expectations. Parents must also meet the needs of the family unit and provide economical support for the family. Children also learn specific roles through a socialization process. Parents set expectations of behavior with discipline and modeling of appropriate behavior.

Ideally the family is a child's source of strength and support, the major constant in the child's life. Families are intimately involved in their children's physical and psychological well-being, and they play a vital role in the health promotion and health maintenance of their children. By respecting the family's role, strengths, and experiences with the healthcare system, nurses have an opportunity to develop an effective partnership with the child and family as they make healthcare decisions that promote the child's health. This partnership between nurses and families is known as family-centered care.

FAMILY-CENTERED CARE

Family-centered care is a philosophy of healthcare in which a mutually beneficial partnership develops between families and the nurse, and also other health professionals, so that the priorities and needs of the family are addressed when the family seeks healthcare for the child. Each party respects the knowledge, skills, and experience that the other brings to the healthcare encounter. This is in contrast to family-focused care in which health professionals provide care from the position of being the expert. In family-focused care, the expert health professional directs care, tells the family what to do, and intervenes for the child and family as a unit.

History of Family-Centered Care

Family-centered care became integral to the nursing care of children when it was recognized that families had a significant role in promoting the psychosocial and developmental needs of children in the hospital. During the 1950s, parents were separated from children during hospitalization, and allowed to visit 1 to 2 hours per week. Evidence of the negative psychosocial consequences of this practice resulted in permitting families to first visit daily for a few hours, and then to "room in" during the child's hospitalization. As parents were allowed to stay with hospitalized children, nurses and other health professionals noticed that children were quieter, happier, and recovering sooner. Research began to confirm findings such as children experiencing decreased anxiety during procedures, needing less pain medication following surgery, and demonstrating improved coping and adjustment during hospitalization (American Academy of Pediatrics, 2003).

Hospital administrators became supportive when parent satisfaction improved as they gained greater involvement in the child's care. This support led to more nursing unit resources for families participating in their child's care. Eventually "rooming in" became a standard for hospital credentialing. Families and consumers continued to pressure the healthcare industry to permit more involvement of families (including fathers and siblings) in the child's care during hospitalization. Gradually it was recognized that parental presence during certain medical procedures, and sometimes resuscitation, was also beneficial to children (Box 2–2). Parents are now invited to participate in patient conferences, serve on hospital advisory committees, and to help educate health professionals about how to improve family-centered care (Figure 2–2 ■).

Nurses have long embraced the family-centered care philosophy. This philosophy is becoming more widely accepted by other health professionals caring for children and their families as noted by a recent policy statement on family-centered care by the American Academy of Pediatrics (2003). The Society of Pediatric Nurses and the American Nurses Association have developed nursing practice guidelines for family-centered care (Table 2–1).

Promoting Family-Centered Care

Partnering with families in the provision of healthcare is essential to promote the best outcome when caring for children. Families have important knowledge to share about their child, their child's health condition, and how their child responds to various actions and events. They also need access to information that will make it possible for them to fully participate in planning and decision making (Box 2–3). Parents need to assess their strengths in managing their ongoing caregiving responsibilities within the family and to consider how to fit additional caregiving responsibilities within this routine. Strategies that the nurse and parents develop in partnership for the care of the child must mesh with the family's cultural and ethnic illness-related behaviors, experiences, and beliefs (Sullivan-Bolyai, Sadler, Knafl, et al., 2004). See Developing Cultural Competence: Family-Centered Care. The child's opinions should also be integrated in the strategies for care. In almost all cases, the child leaves the healthcare setting and the family assumes responsibility for provision of needed care in the home. The family caregivers must not feel alienated from a healthcare system they need for continuing assistance. See Partnering with Families: Guidelines for Effective Partnership on page 38.

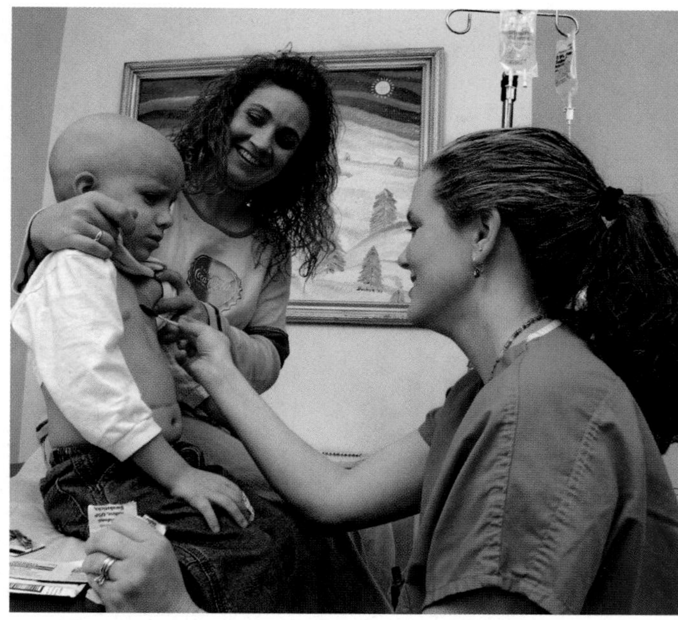

FIGURE 2–2 ■ Health facility policies that permit parents to be present during a procedure performed on their child are an example of a family-centered care policy. The parent plays an important role in providing security and comfort to this child who is having his port accessed for an IV infusion treatment.

BOX 2–2 Research: Parental Presence During Procedures

Increasingly, parents are permitted to be present during medical procedures performed on their children. Resistance to parental presence has been based on the fear that parents would delay the procedure, interfere with the procedure or distract the health professional, increase the anxiety of the health professionals performing the procedure, and increase their own anxiety. Studies have investigated parental presence in various situations involving medical procedures, such as venipuncture, anesthesia induction, IV starts, and even resuscitation (Munro & D'Errico, 2000; Powers & Rubenstein, 1999; Wolfram & Turner, 1996; Meyers, Eichhorn, & Guzzetta, 1998). Health professionals' attitudes regarding parental presence are often tied to their practice goal of efficiency or family-centered care (Jefferson & Paterson, 2001). In most cases, parents are less anxious and the ability of health professionals to perform procedures is not affected (Lewandowski & Tesler, 2003).

CLINICAL TIP

When providing care to children, recall that the family is central to all healthcare interventions with parents and child as the partners in care. It is important to consider how a healthcare setting's written policies, procedures, and literature for families refer to families and what attitudes these materials convey. Words like *policies, allowed,* and *not permitted* imply that hospital personnel have authority over families in matters concerning their children. Words like *guidelines, working together,* and *welcome* communicate an openness and appreciation for families in the care of their children.

In addition to partnering with families in the provision of the nursing care of the child, consider the value of child and parent

MediaLink Critical Thinking: The Nursing Process and Family-Centered Care

TABLE 2–1 Elements of Family-Centered Care and Recommendations for Nursing Practice

ELEMENTS	NURSING PRACTICE RECOMMENDATIONS
The Family at the Center	
Incorporate into policy and practice the recognition that the family is the constant in a child's life, while the service systems and support personnel within those systems fluctuates, and that the illness or injury of a child affects all members of the family system.	➤ Establish a therapeutic relationship with the family. ➤ Perform a comprehensive family assessment in collaboration with the family, identifying both strengths and needs. ➤ Use the family assessment when working with the family to plan, implement, and evaluate care, considering the impact of the child's illness or injury on the entire family, with special attention to the siblings. ➤ Provide siblings with information about their sibling's illness/injury at an appropriate developmental level and answer questions honestly. ➤ Promote sibling visitation in hospital settings and participation in home care activities. ➤ Identify extended family members who should receive information and be included in the educational process.
Family-Professional Collaboration	
Facilitate family-professional collaboration at all levels of hospital, home, and community care for: ➤ Care of an individual child ➤ Program development, implementation, evaluation, and evolution ➤ Policy formation	➤ Use a mutual-participation model for provider-family relationships, guided by goals and expectations of both the family and the provider. ➤ Ensure that parents are integral and critical collaborators in the decision-making process about their child's care. Involve children and adolescents in decision-making process as appropriate for their cognitive and emotional development. ➤ Assure parents 24-hour access to their children and facilitate their participation in the child's care. ➤ Provide parents with the option to stay with their child during procedures and tests, and provide ways for the parent to support the child during the procedure. ➤ Provide comfort and hygiene facilities for families who spend long hours at the facility or travel great distances. ➤ Promote the development of expertise in the special care of the child, fostering family independence and empowerment. ➤ Incorporate parents and children into the quality assessment/improvement process. ➤ Integrate family members into institutional and community advisory groups and in policy development.
Family-Professional Communication	
Exchange complete and unbiased information between families and professionals in a supportive manner at all times.	➤ Provide information about the child's problem, prognosis, and needs in a manner that respects the child and family as individuals and promotes two-way dialogue. ➤ Encourage the family to share information about the child and the illness/injury so that care planning and decisions are made in the most informed and collaborative manner.
Cultural Diversity of Families	
Incorporate into policy and practice the recognition and honoring of cultural diversity, strengths, and individuality within and across all families, including ethnic, racial, spiritual, social, economic, educational, and geographic diversity.	➤ Practice family-centered care in a culturally competent manner with respect and sensitivity for the wide range of families with diverse values and beliefs. ➤ Seek to understand the family's beliefs and practices related to race, culture, and ethnicity when developing relationships and collaborating in the child's healthcare. ➤ Seek to understand and respect the family's religious/spiritual beliefs and practices and integrate these into the child's care, as the family desires. ➤ Work with the family to address issues in care related to socioeconomic status, geographic considerations, access to healthcare, and insurance status. ➤ Integrate training programs on diversity, cultural understanding, and culturally competent care into staff development programs.
Coping Differences and Support	
Recognize and respect different methods of coping and implement comprehensive policies and programs that provide families with the developmental, educational, emotional, spiritual, environmental, and financial supports needed to meet their diverse needs.	➤ Assess the strengths and weaknesses of the family's coping strategies and their resiliency factors and characteristics. Identify maladaptive coping mechanisms and assist the family to augment their coping efforts. ➤ Assess and support the family's needs and desires for support and assist the family in accessing and accepting assistance from support networks as needed or desired.

TABLE 2–1 Elements of Family-Centered Care and Recommendations for Nursing Practice (continued)

ELEMENTS	NURSING PRACTICE RECOMMENDATIONS
Family-Centered Peer Support	
Encourage and facilitate family-to-family support and networking.	➤ Educate parents about parent-to-parent and family support resources and assist them to access such resources in the institution and community. ➤ Provide access to psychoeducational groups that might be useful to parents, siblings, or ill/injured children.
Specialized Service and Support Systems	
Ensure that hospital, home, and community service and support systems for children needing specialized health and developmental care and their families are flexible, accessible, and comprehensive in responding to diverse family-identified needs.	➤ Provide collaborative, flexible, accessible, comprehensive, and coordinated services to children and their families. ➤ Provide comprehensive case management/care coordination for children and families with ongoing care needs. ➤ Along with families, take an active role in advocating for the needs of ill and injured children.
Holistic Perspective of Family-Centered Care	
Appreciate families as families and children as children, recognizing that they possess a wider range of strengths, concerns, emotions, and aspirations beyond their need for specialized health and developmental services and support.	➤ Encourage attention to the normal developmental needs and developmental tasks of the entire family unit and individual family members. ➤ Encourage and facilitate the development of individual and family identities beyond a focus on illness or injury. ➤ Facilitate "normalization" as valued and desired by the family.

Adapted from Lewandowski, L.A., & Tesler, M.D. (Eds.). (2003). Family-centered care: Putting it into action. The SPN/ANA guide to family-centered care. *Washington, DC: American Nurses Association.*

participation in the development of policies and guidelines for family-centered care in all types of healthcare settings. The experience that children and families gain in the healthcare setting during care often leads them to have valuable insights worth sharing. Parents may help by serving as "pulse points" to the parents' perspectives and realities of hospital life for staff and hospital administrators. Listening to parents' perspectives is critical to providing quality patient care and achieving successful patient satisfaction. Parents who have been supported to develop leadership skills can be empowered to serve on advisory boards or councils and represent the family and community perspective. Examples of roles they may play include assisting in the design and evaluation of programs and systems; assessing a healthcare setting for its family-centered policies and care practices, as well as its cultural appropriateness; participating in the renovation or construction of healthcare facilities; recommending changes that will ultimately improve the quality of care; and educating health professionals about working effectively with families as partners in the child's care.

Feedback regarding the provision of family-centered care that can be valuable for all parents and children are responses such as (Hanson & Randall, 1999):

- How well care providers met their needs
- If information provided was complete and understood
- What attitudes they sensed from healthcare providers
- How accessible the needed services were
- How comfortable they felt in the setting

Parents can also serve a valuable role in family-to-family support networks by serving as mentors to new families entering the healthcare system for a new chronic condition. Parents may also help raise awareness about specific healthcare issues, serve as advocates for public policy issues, and assist with fundraising activities.

Guidelines for working with families as advisors and tools for assessing the family-centered policies in various healthcare settings are available from the Institute of Family-Centered Care.

MediaLink Critical Thinking: Facility Assessment

BOX 2–3 Family Resource Center

Some healthcare facilities are developing patient and family resource centers to provide information and support. In most cases, the resource center is a consumer-oriented health library with staffing. Benefits of such a resource center within the framework of family-centered care include the following (Institute for Family Centered Care, 2004):

- ➤ Families can be supported to access useful information from print and video resources, various databases, and the Internet. This helps families to become informed participants in decision making about their child's care.
- ➤ Resources can be provided in the preferred language and at an appropriate reading level.
- ➤ Peer support services may be coordinated through the resource center.
- ➤ The resource center may make it possible for parents to become involved as advisors for healthcare facility policies and programs.

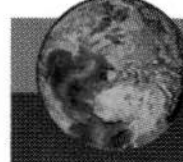

DEVELOPING CULTURAL COMPETENCE
Family-Centered Care

When working to establish a partnership with families of various ethnic groups, consider the potential that an extended family may need to be included. The parents may be supported by an extended family, and healthcare planning for the ill or injured child may need to be developed in partnership with the parents and representatives of the extended family. This enables the nurse to learn more about the strengths of the family network and to better assist the family in planning the child's care at home (Ochieng, 2003).

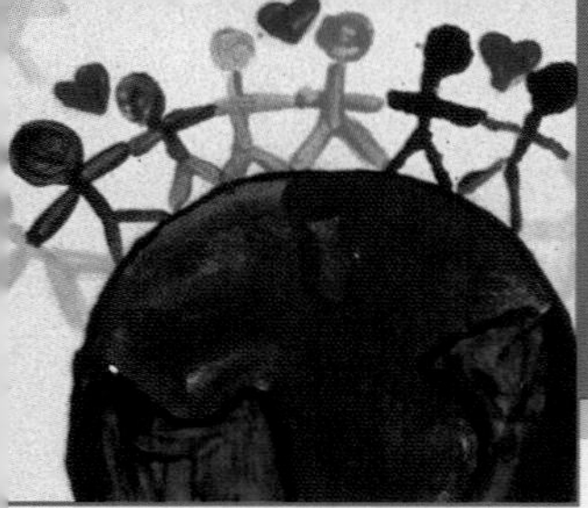

PARTNERING WITH FAMILIES

Guidelines for Effective Partnership

Parents have a role in making the partnership with nurses and other health professionals effective. Parents, especially those with children who have special healthcare needs, become experts in their child's disease. They learn to become an effective advocate for their child. They also must learn to communicate effectively with the health professionals caring for their child, and in the process develop a trusting relationship.

Tips for parents include (Allshouse & Goldberg, 2003):

- Be realistic about what you can expect from your child's nurses and doctors. They cannot solve all your problems or answer all your questions.
- You have responsibilities for communicating effectively with the healthcare professionals, keeping records, and following up.
  - Keep a journal that includes your observations about your child's behavior, eating habits, illness, temperature, or anything else that might be helpful to the healthcare providers caring for your child.
  - Keep a copy of your child's medical records, including test and procedure results.
  - Write out questions and do not hesitate to ask for clarification if you do not understand an answer provided.
- Recognize that health professionals are human. They can become frustrated at times by the child's condition or lack of answers to questions. Try to let your healthcare providers know you appreciate their time and efforts on behalf of your child.
- Prepare your child for what to expect at each health visit by describing who the child will see and tests that will be performed. Take comfort items (blanket, stuffed animal, favorite toy) along to the visit.

Tips for nurses include:

- Provide information and honestly discuss issues of concern to both the family and healthcare providers.
- Creatively problem solve and identify options for needed care that conform to the family's values and functioning.
- Demonstrate respect for the family's choices and methods for providing needed care.
- Continue to collaborate with the child and family and be willing to continue problem solving as new issues arise.

FAMILY COMPOSITION

Various types of families—both those considered traditional and nontraditional—exist in contemporary American society. This section identifies common types of family structure.

Traditional Nuclear Family

The nuclear family that popular culture considers *traditional* consists of a husband provider and a wife who stays home to rear the children. Less commonly the wife is the provider and the husband stays home with the children. In addition, the children live with both biological parents, and no other relatives or persons live in the household. Although this nuclear family was the norm in the United States, it is no longer the most common type of family. Important nursing considerations include respect for the parent who stays home to rear the children and an appreciation for the value of childrearing.

Two-Income Nuclear Family

Today, the majority of all two-parent families have both parents working, either by choice or necessity. Dual-career/dual-earner families are now considered the norm in modern society. In cases of excessive job demands and lack of control over the job, the parental stress can have a negative impact on the family. Two-income families must address important issues such as childcare arrangements, household chores, and how to assure quality family time. These families often find it difficult to find time to meet family and individual child needs as well as career demands. Important nursing considerations include helping parents to develop strategies to ensure that the child's health promotion needs are met, such as a nutritious diet with appropriate calories and adequate physical exercise.

Blended or Reconstituted Family

The blended or reconstituted nuclear family includes two parents and their children. Parents with biologic children from a previous marriage or relationship may marry or cohabitate. This family structure has become increasing common due to high rates of divorce and remarriage. Potential advantages to the children may include better financial support and a new supportive role model. Stressors can include lack of a clear role for the stepparent, lack of acceptance of the stepparent, financial stresses when two families must be supported by stepparents, and communication challenges. Parents in the blended family may have difficulties overcoming differences in parenting styles, discipline strategies, and values. These stressors can cause challenges in forming a cohesive family unit. Important nursing considerations include directing families to resources that may help reduce the potential conflicts associated with different parenting styles, discipline, and manipulative behaviors by children that can develop with the blended family. See the discussion on page 47 regarding stepparenting.

Another type of blended family is two parents with adoptive or foster children, sometimes including biologic children. Many parents choose adoption because of infertility. In other cases, a couple or single adult chooses to adopt a child or take in foster children for personal, religious, or family reasons. The adoptive or foster parent may be a relative of the child. This is often the case when grandparents raise children due to the inability of parents to care for children. Grandparents endure emotional, physical, and financial stresses when taking on this role. See the discussion beginning on page 48 regarding foster care and adoption.

Extended Family

Extended families exist when one parent or a couple shares expenses as well as household and child rearing responsibilities with grandparents, the sibling of a parent, or other relatives. According to the U.S. Bureau of Census, 4.1 million children live in an extended family with at least one parent and usually a grandparent (U.S. Census Bureau, 2002). This type of family is common in recent immigrant families as well as working class families. For example, in a multigenerational (three generations in same household) family living arrangement, the grandparents may be invited to live in the family home, or the family moves into the grandparents' home on a temporary basis. Families may reside together to share housing expenses and childcare. However, in many cases, the child may be residing with the grandparent and one parent because of issues associated with unemployment, parental separation, parental death, or parental substance abuse (Figure 2–3 ■).

Another example of an extended family is the extended relative network family in which two nuclear families of primary relatives or unmarried relatives live in close proximity to each other. The family shares a social support network in which chores, goods, and services are exchanged. This type of family model is common in the Latino community.

Single-Parent Family

The family of a single parent is formed when the mother or father is widowed, divorced, abandoned, or separated. According to the 2000 census, of the 11.3 million single-parent families with children under 18 years in the United States, approximately 30% are single-father families (Annie E. Casey Foundation, 2004). Single mother households make up 7% of all households (Council on Contemporary Families, 2003). In 2000, 26.7% of children less than 18 years lived with a single parent, and almost 1 in 10 children lived with a never-married parent (U.S. Bureau of the Census, 2002; U.S. Department of Health and Human Services, 2001). See Figure 2–4 ■ for the distribution of children

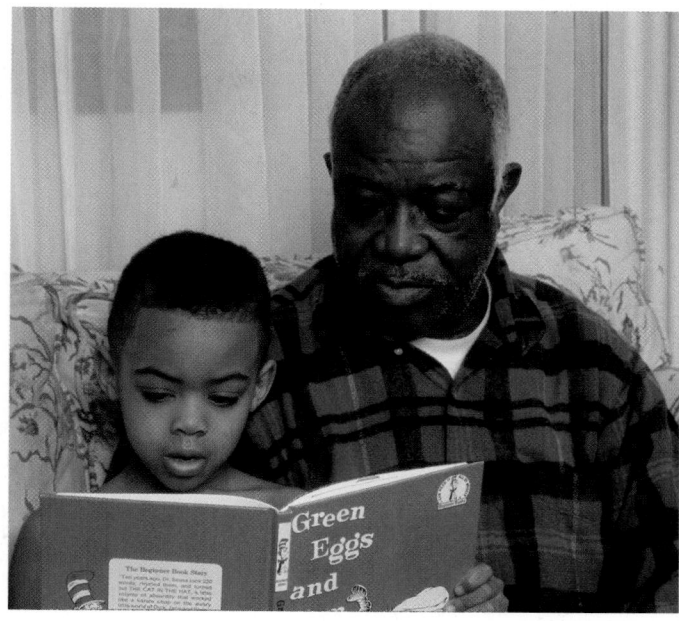

FIGURE 2–3 ■ This child lives with his mother and grandparents following the divorce of his parents. The special attention provided by his grandfather is helping him to adapt to the change in his family, and it enables the mother to work feeling confident that her son is safely cared for before and after school.

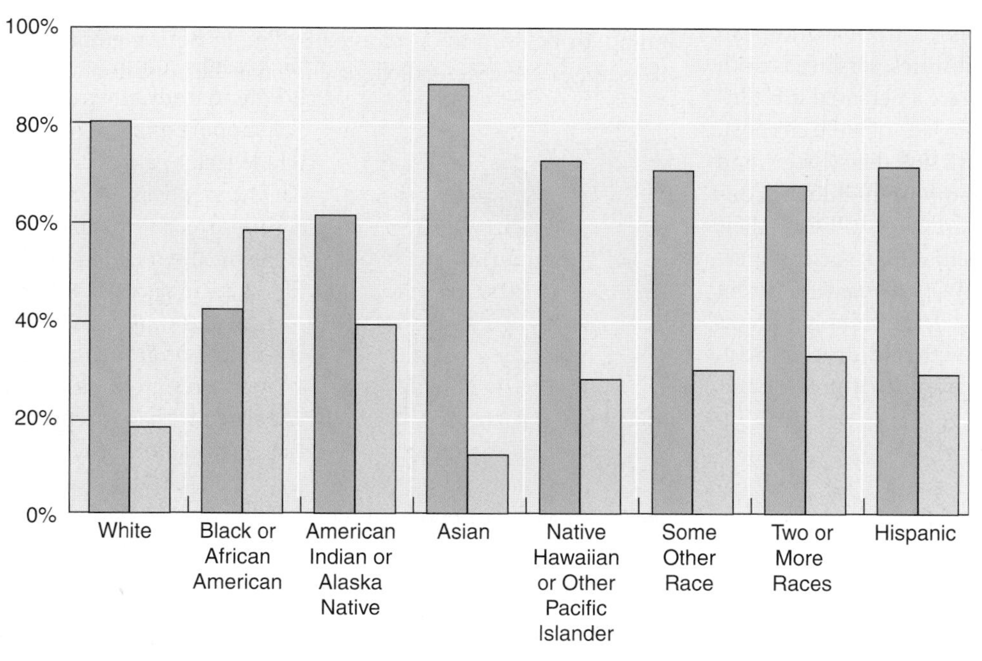

FIGURE 2–4 ■ Percentage of children living in married-couple and single-parent families by race and ethnic origin in the 2000 census.

From: Population Reference Bureau, U.S. Census Bureau (2003). Analysis of data from the U.S. Census, 2000 Census summary file 1 (Tables P28A–P28H).

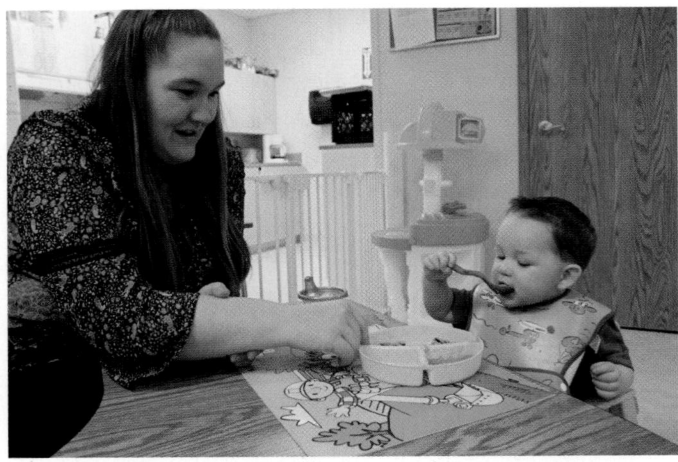

FIGURE 2–5 ■ Adolescents who become single parents often have challenges with balancing school, personal time, and care of the infant.

living in married-couple and single-parent family homes. Reasons for the increasing rate of single-parent families include the following (Friedman et al., 2003):

- High rates of divorce
- The large amount of financial aid to one-parent families with dependent children
- The loss of stigma associated with unwed motherhood
- The growth in number of births to never-married mothers

Single-parent families often face difficulties because the sole parent may lack social and emotional support, need assistance with child rearing issues, and face financial strain. Children may experience multiple living arrangements during childhood. Changes in family structure or living arrangements can undermine the child's psychological development due to stresses associated with lack of stability (Graefe & Lichter, 1999). Depending on social support and family resources, the single parent may be stressed from working to support the family, household responsibilities, serving as both mother and father, and attempting to have a personal life. Single mothers are often impoverished due to lack of child support, inequitable pay for work performed, work skill deficiencies, and cutbacks in social welfare programs. An important nursing consideration when working with single parents is to assess their strengths and needs in providing care to the child, such as after-school and backup childcare arrangements that enable to parent to fulfill work commitments. Determine if the child has access to all resources available to support growth and development, such as school breakfast and lunch programs that provide nutritional support (Figure 2–5 ■).

Binuclear Family

In a postdivorce family the biologic children can be members of two nuclear households, with parenting shared by the father and the mother. The children alternate between the two homes, spending varying amounts of time with both parents in a situation called co-parenting, usually involving joint custody. Joint custody is a legal situation in which both parents have equal responsibility and legal rights, regardless of where the children live. The binuclear family is a model for effective communication. It enables both biological parents to be involved in a child's upbringing and provides additional support and role models from extended family members. Special nursing considerations in this family type involve ensuring that health promotion guidance and education for care of the child with an acute or chronic condition are communicated effectively to both biological parents.

Heterosexual Cohabitating Family

In this family type, a heterosexual couple who may or may not have children lives together outside of marriage. This may include never-married individuals as well as divorced or widowed persons. According to the 2000 U.S. census, approximately 2.9 million children under 18 years of age live with a parent and unmarried partner (Peterson, 2003). Cohabitation is sometimes considered a step in the relationship that will result in marriage. Biologic children may result from the relationship, or in some cases children of one parent are present and help form a blended type of cohabitating family. Special concerns exist regarding the increased likelihood of the couple separating—approximately 50% in 5 years versus 20% for married couples (Peterson, 2003). An important nursing consideration for children who live in informal stepfamilies is that the nonbiologic parent has no legal authority to seek emergency medical care for the child. However, in the case of a true emergency that could result in loss of life or diminished functioning, health professionals are obligated to provide care and obtain consent as soon as possible afterwards. The nonbiologic parent also may not have knowledge of the child's medical history.

Gay and Lesbian Family

A gay or lesbian family involves two adults of the same sex who live together as domestic partners with or without children, or a gay or lesbian single parent rearing a child (Figure 2–6 ■). Children in these families may be from a previous heterosexual union, or be born to or adopted by one or both member(s) of the same-sex couple. A biologic child may be born to one of the

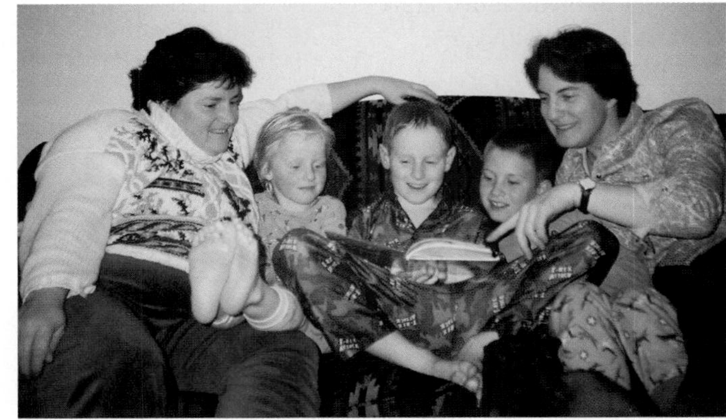

FIGURE 2–6 ■ No evidence exists to indicate that children raised in a homosexual family are at any greater developmental or dysfunction risk than a child raised in a heterosexual family (Ariel & McPherson, 2000). These parents are as dedicated as heterosexual families to promoting the growth and development of their children.

partners through artificial insemination or through a surrogate mother.

According to the 2000 U.S. census, 96% of all U.S. counties have at least one gay or lesbian couple with children under 18 years in the household (Urban Institute, 2003a). Lesbian and gay couples function much like heterosexual couples, and children who are adopted or born into the family are highly valued. Small studies that have evaluated children reared by same-sex couples found no significant differences in child rearing or in the children's adjustment from children reared in other types of families. These children have been found to have the same advantages and expectations for health, adjustment, and development as children born into heterosexual families (American Academy of Pediatrics, 2002a). Children raised by same-sex parents may face unique issues and challenges when interacting with peers, usually around the revelation of their parents' sexual orientation. In cases in which the biologic parents divorced or separated because of one parent's sexual orientation, children may be particularly vulnerable to concerns about relationships with their parents during the adjustment phase (Wald, 1999).

Children in these families sometimes have only one biologic or adoptive legal parent. The other partner is the co-parent and has no legal parental status in the majority of states. Only seven states (California, Connecticut, Massachusetts, New Jersey, New York, Pennsylvania, Vermont) and the District of Columbia have considered legislative actions to ensure the security of children whose parents are gay or lesbian by guaranteeing access to second-parent joint adoption rights (Urban Institute, 2003a). Co-parent adoption would help maintain the child's rights to a continuing relationship if the legal parent dies or becomes incapacitated, or if the parents separate. Either parent could then provide consent for healthcare and make other important decisions on behalf of the child. Financial support of the child is more assured if one parent dies or parents separate. Nursing considerations in this type of family involve respect for the relationship between partners and recognition of the nurturing capacity in these families. It is important to identify the biologic or adoptive parent, or a caregiver's legal documentation proving the right to medical decision making, when obtaining consent for the child's healthcare.

FAMILY FUNCTIONING

Transition to Parenthood

Choosing to become a parent is a major life change for adults. Couples experience significant family and cultural pressure to have a child. Mothers may be eager to have a child, but be concerned about fulfilling all of the expectations of others (father, the baby, other children, her parents, close friends, and employer). Fathers anticipate increased responsibility and are concerned about their ability to provide adequate support for the family.

However, the changes and adjustment caused by the birth of a child are rarely fully anticipated. Couples without children often have freedom to enjoy social events, recreational activities, and personal time, as there is no child to care for. If both partners are working, they can more freely spend money, as there are fewer expenses such as a college fund, childcare expenses, or life insurance bills. Having the first child leads to the transition that establishes the family. Many rapid changes occur during this transition to parenthood, including the following (Craig & Baucum, 1999):

- Each parent's sense of self and ideas about how family life works
- Division of labor and roles within the relationship, and decisions about new responsibilities regarding child rearing
- Relationships with parents of the couple who become grandparents
- Changes in work relationships (The mother or father who may choose to temporarily modify career goals to spend more time with the child. In other cases the mother's attitude about her job may change, but because of a better health insurance benefit package, she must continue working.)

At the time of birth the parents experience stresses and challenges along with feelings of pride and excitement. Mothers and fathers both make adjustments to their lifestyles to give priority to parenting. The baby is dependent for total care 24 hours a day and this often results in sleep deprivation, irritability, less personal time, and less time for the couple's relationship. In addition the family often experiences a change in financial status.

CLINICAL TIP

Eligible parents of newborns and adopted children are entitled to 12 weeks of unpaid leave during any 12-month period initially authorized under the federal Medical and Family Leave Act of 1993. Vacation or sick leave may often be used to pay for time away from work. This act also applies if a child, spouse, or parent of the employee develops a serious health condition. The employee is entitled to return to the previous position or an equivalent position with all the same pay, benefits, and other conditions (Family and Medical Leave, 1993).

Several factors influence how well the parents adjust to their new role. Social support provided to the mother, especially by the father, is important for the mother's adjustment. Marital happiness during pregnancy is an important adjustment factor for both parents. Parents with a higher self-esteem are more likely to have a better adjustment (Craig & Baucum, 1999). Infants with significant health conditions or those with difficult temperaments can cause extra stress for the parents and affect their adjustment to the parenting role.

With the birth of the first child, mothers and fathers both have challenges related to renegotiating their employment to accommodate family and childcare time. Fathers are sometimes additionally challenged to develop closeness with the infant and to learn how to care for the infant, especially when they may not have had role models or any childcare experience. Some fathers find that it takes longer than expected to develop closeness with the infant and to develop infant caregiving skills (Barclay & Lupton, 1999). Most parents find that caring for infants and children takes more time than anticipated.

Nurses can help parents through this important transition by listening to the challenges described by the parents during the infant's first health visits. Encourage fathers and mothers to attend and participate in health promotion visits with the healthcare provider so that positive parenting can be supported. Answer questions and offer ideas to address described problems that the parents may be too tired to solve on their own. Help them recognize that frustrations and feelings they have regarding the challenges of infant care are normal. Encourage both parents to become active in caring for the infant and to gain comfort in that care. Help each parent find activities that they enjoy with regard to infant care to encourage interaction and bonding with the infant.

Parental Influences on the Child

The qualities of family relationships and family behaviors are important aspects of family strengths and family functioning. Positive family relationships are characterized by parent–child warmth and supportiveness. Warm parent–child relationships can buffer children from stress and promote positive cognitive and social outcomes. Parents who are warm and place high demands on their children for appropriate behavior have children who tend to be content, self-reliant, self-controlled, and open to learning in school. Evidence of positive family processes or family functioning includes the following:

- Parents are mentally healthy.
- Family and household routines are well organized and they promote academic achievement, self-esteem, and behavioral and emotional development in children.
- Parents use time effectively to share activities with children.
- Communication between the parents and children reflects an interest in the child's opinion and praise.
- Children are monitored, supervised, and given help.

Mothers and fathers each contribute to the psychological, emotional, and social health and development of their children. Both parents provide affection, nurturing, and comfort. They teach children life skills and healthy lifestyles. Fathers play an important role in the sexual identity and gender role development of their children. They promote social competence, academic achievement, and problem-solving abilities of their children (American Academy of Pediatrics, 2004).

Family Size

The size of the family influences the amount of attention given to children. In small families, parents often have more time to give attention to the children, to encourage achievement, and to support involvement in community activities. Individual development is promoted and children are encouraged to meet family expectations. Democratic participation in family decision making may be supported.

Children in larger families are encouraged to be cooperative so that the family group functions well. The child usually receives less personal attention from the parents and must often turn to others in the family to get the support needed. Family organization and administration may be more pronounced, and there may be more limited space and finances. Children may adopt a specialized family role to gain family recognition, such as the "responsible one," "the clown," or "the black sheep."

Sibling Relationships

Siblings are the first peers of a child and often have a lifelong relationship lasting up to 70 or more years. Siblings, especially those of the same gender, who are closer in age, tend to have a closer relationship because they often share many common experiences through childhood and adolescence. In general, the parents have greater influence than siblings on children who are more widely spaced in age. However, the older sibling may be a very strong role model for younger siblings. Depending on relationships that develop among and between siblings, the child's relationships may be equally as strong with some siblings and with the parents.

Siblings serve many roles in their interactions with each other. Within the family children learn to share, compete, and compromise. Sibling rivalry exists between children at times in all families. Some siblings take on other roles such as protector, problem solver, friend, and supporter for dealing with issues in the family and in the environment. Some siblings learn to work well together to maintain privacy or to form a coalition for negotiating with the parents. An older sibling helps reinforce rules and roles in the family by prompting and inhibiting certain patterns of behavior in the younger siblings. However, one sibling may initiate a process whereby a previously implicit rule is broken, testing the waters and determining what rule flexibility is allowed in the family (Figure 2–7 ■).

Children develop different personalities because of a need to establish distinct identities for themselves. Earlier research findings that birth order was associated with specific personality traits of individual children in a family have not been replicated (Craig & Baucum, 1999). Other explanations have developed for the unique personalities of siblings within a family and roles they tend to play within the family. An individual child sees and experiences the personality traits of siblings and wants to be seen as special within the

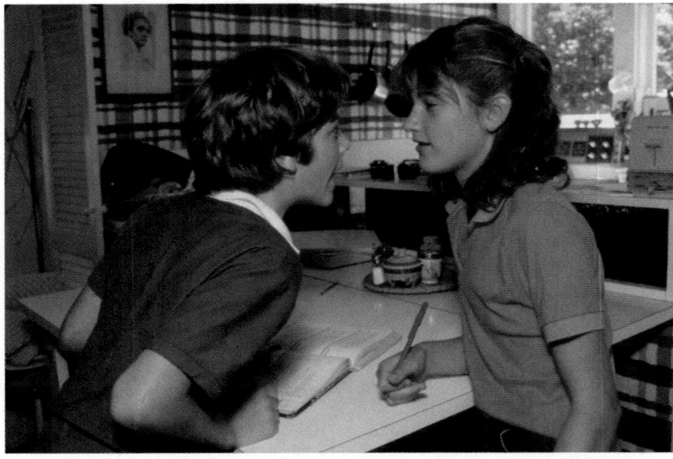

FIGURE 2–7 ■ Siblings often work together to persuade the parents to provide a treat or privilege.

family. The child works to find a particular role or develop a personality that is unique. Siblings also share some experiences, but there are also other experiences that are not shared. Thus siblings are exposed to different environmental experiences that also help shape their personalities (Craig & Baucum, 1999).

First-born children do have some advantages, such as more favorable treatment in the family. First-born children do have slightly higher IQs and greater achievement in school and in their careers (Craig & Baucum, 1999). Their intellectual development may be enhanced through experiences of teaching their younger siblings.

Parenting

The family is an important component in the lives of all children, and it plays an essential role in fostering the development of infants, children, and youth. A significant concept in families is that of parenting. **Parenting** is a leadership role in the family in which children are guided to learn acceptable behaviors, beliefs, morals, and rituals of the family and to become socially responsible, contributing members of society. The manner in which children are parented, in combination with their individual personality traits and characteristics, influences their developmental outcomes.

Parents have responsibility for providing stability to children with nurturance, safety, and structure in a family that undergoes frequent changes over time. The child needs to have physical and emotional space to grow and develop. This space enables the child to personally find the relationship balance between closeness and distance, as well as safety and risk. Parents also enculturate their children with the values, beliefs, rituals, and behaviors learned and transmitted across family generations. To be successful in parenting, parents must have a certain flexibility that enables the family to adapt and adjust to family changes with time and other significant stressors and challenges (Figure 2–8 ■).

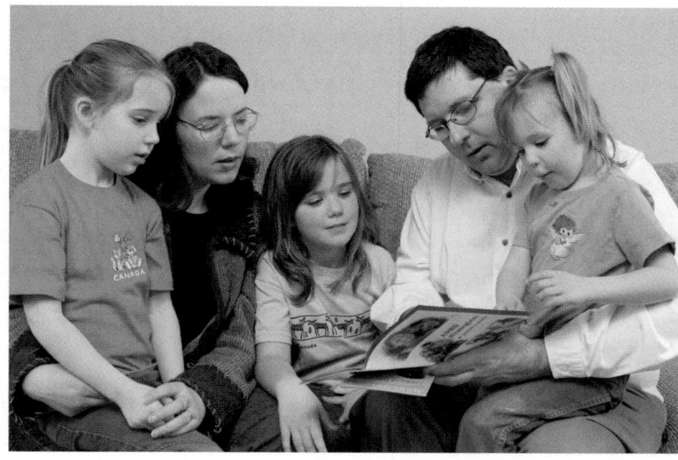

FIGURE 2–8 ■ Family time is important, especially during those times when all members of the family need to work together toward a common goal. In this family, everyone is learning more about the condition of one child and what each can do to help.

To be successful as parents, children should have reasonable **limit setting** (established rules or guidelines for behavior) on their autonomy, while learning values and self-control. Yet at the same time, parents need to foster the child's curiosity, initiative, and sense of competence. Parents use different styles to parent their children. Parental warmth and control are two major factors that are important in the development of children. Parental warmth refers to the amount of affection and approval displayed. Parental control refers to how restrictive the parents are. See Table 2–2 for the characteristics associated with parental warmth and control.

Diana Baumrind (1971), an important contemporary child developmentalist, proposed classifications of parenting styles that are still well accepted today. She identified three main types of parenting styles (*authoritarian, authoritative*, and *permissive*) and described the influences each style has on children. One additional parenting style, called *indifferent*, exists in some families. While families will generally tend to use one style, they may vary their style for certain situations. See Table 2–3 for characteristics or parenting styles by levels of warmth and control.

Authoritarian Parents

Authoritarian parents tend to be punitive and adhere to rigid rules. Parents who use this style might say, "Because I'm your parent, that's why," "A rule is a rule," or "Just do what I say." While this style sets firm limits, those limits or rules are not negotiable or open to any discussion. Parents expect family beliefs and principles to be accepted without question. Children have no opportunity to participate in the family decision-making process. Children with authoritarian parents do not develop the skills to examine why a certain behavior is desirable or how

TABLE 2–2 Characteristics of Significant Parenting Attributes

PARENTING ATTRIBUTE	PARENTAL WARMTH	PARENTAL CONTROL
High level	Warm, nurturing Express affection and smile at children frequently Limit criticism, punishment Express approval of child	Restrictive control of behavior Survey and enforce compliance with rules Encourage children to fulfill their responsibilities May limit freedom of expression
Low level	Cool, hostile Quick to criticize or punish Ignore children Rarely express affection or approval Rejection may be seen	Permissive, minimally controlling Make fewer demands Fewer restrictions on behavior or expression of emotion Permit freedom in exploring environment

TABLE 2–3 Parenting Styles by Level of Warmth and Control

PARENTING STYLE	WARMTH/CONTROL	BEHAVIOR OF PARENTS
Authoritarian	High control Low warmth	Issue commands and expect them to be obeyed Little communication with children, avoid lengthy verbal discussion with children Inflexible rules Permit little independence
Authoritative	Moderately high control High warmth	Accept and encourage growing autonomy of children Open communication with children Flexible rules
Permissive	Low control High warmth	Few or no restraints Unconditional love Communication from child to parent Much freedom and little guidance No limit setting
Indifferent	Low control Low warmth	No limit setting Lack affection for children Parents focused on stress in own life Parents may show hostility or neglect

From Craig, G. J., & Baucum, D. (1999). Human development *(8th ed., p. 264). Upper Saddle River, NJ: Prentice Hall.*

their actions might influence others. Children do not develop skills of communication, negotiation, or the ability to direct and initiate their own activities. Children become frustrated in their efforts to achieve autonomy. They may become withdrawn, fearful, and unassertive. Girls often become passive and dependent during adolescence, while boys often become rebellious and aggressive.

Authoritative Parents

Authoritative parents use firm control to set limits, but they establish an atmosphere with open discussion. Limits for behavior are clear and reasonable, but the child is encouraged to talk about why certain behaviors occurred and how the situations might be handled differently another time. Parents provide explanations about inappropriate behaviors at the child's level of understanding. Children are allowed to express their opinions and objections, and some flexibility is permitted when appropriate. However, parents make it clear that they are the ultimate authority for decisions. Children with authoritative parents develop a sense of social responsibility since they converse about their responsibilities and approaches. Children managed with this style of parenting tend to be more self-reliant, self-controlled, and socially competent. They have been found to have higher self-esteem and better school performance.

Permissive Parents

Permissive parents show a great deal of warmth, but set few controls or restraints on the child's behavior. Parents are so intent on showing unconditional love that they fail in performing some important parenting functions. Children are allowed to regulate their own behavior. Discipline is inconsistent and parents may threaten punishment but not follow through. Both extremes result in excessive permissiveness, and the child does not learn socially acceptable limits of behavior. As the parent does not impose any controls on the child, the child ends up controlling the parents. The child of a permissive parent is often unable to cooperate and negotiate with others. Depending on the child's personality, the child may become rebellious and aggressive, or socially inept, self-indulgent, or impulsive. Some have difficulty being accepted by peers or later being accepted and effective in a work setting. In some cases, the child may be creative, active, and outgoing.

Indifferent Parents

Indifferent parents display little interest in their children or in their roles as parents. They do not demonstrate affection or approval of the children, and they do not set limits or controls on the children. This may occur because of disinterest, or because their lives are so stressed that there is no time or energy left for the children. Children who experience this style of parenting often have the worst outcomes, such as destructive impulses and delinquent behavior. If the parents are also hostile, the child often develops delinquent behavior (Craig & Baucum, 1999).

Parent Adaptability

Parents who are able to adapt their behavior to meet the needs of children at different developmental stages are also more effective. Eleanor Maccoby (1980) expanded upon Baumrind's perspectives on parenting style by examining how parents and children interact during the parenting process. Parenting styles may change as the child grows older. For example, parents may use negotiation to help the child develop problem-solving skills and to learn how to compromise, which is necessary to get along with others. This enables the child to have more self-control and self-responsibility over time. Parents and some children can potentially develop shared goals and participate in decision making without a significant struggle for control or negotiation. In other cases parents may need to engage in constant negotiation, as shared goals cannot be agreed upon with a child or all children in the family. Either of these parenting styles can help promote a smoother transition for the child from family dependence to independence and close peer relationships

(Craig & Baucum, 1999). See Partnering with Families: Guidelines for Promoting Acceptable Behavior in Children.

Assessing Parenting Styles

Nurses assess parenting styles by asking families how they handle situations that require limit setting. As described, an authoritative style is preferred because of its positive outcomes for child behavior and learning. The nurse in all settings is often in a position to discuss parenting styles and to offer suggestions for managing certain types of child behaviors that are frustrating to the family. Keep in mind that children are all different and parents often must vary their parenting styles for different children in the family. For example, the child's temperament is often tied to their behavioral style. See Chapter 5∞ for more information on child temperament. One child may need clear limits set with discussion and reinforcement needed, whereas a sibling may immediately respond to the parents' limit setting without a need for discussion of the situation. See Developing Cultural Competence: Cultural Influences on Parenting.

Discipline

Discipline is a method for teaching the rules that govern behavior or conduct, or the action taken to enforce the rules when the child misbehaves. Parenting styles play an important role in the type of discipline used with children. When clear limits are set and consistently maintained, as with authoritative parenting, discipline may be needed less often. Limit setting and firm control of those limits are important for the child to learn to what extent they can safely and independently operate within the environment. Firm limits also help children to feel secure because they are reassured by consistency and the sense of protection perceived by the limits. Discipline helps children learn that there are consequences for misbehavior, and that other individuals may be affected by that behavior. This helps children develop a sense of responsibility for their behavior.

Various strategies are used for discipline, and these strategies change as the child grows older and understands more.

- *Reasoning*—explaining why a behavior or action is inappropriate
- *Behavior modification*—giving positive rewards or reinforcement for good behavior encourages children to behave in specified ways; consistently ignoring inappropriate behavior to minimize the behavior

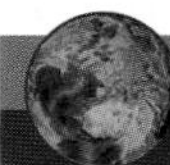

DEVELOPING CULTURAL COMPETENCE
Cultural Influences on Parenting

Some cultural influences on parenting are associated with chosen lifestyle. For example, living in a predominantly ethnic neighborhood makes it possible to participate in special ethnic events that help teach the child about the culture. Parents use the community for social contacts that help to reinforce patterns of parenting and to establish behavioral expectations of their children. Frequent contact or living with the extended family helps the child learn family and ethnic traditions, behaviors, and values. Children may be sent to religious or parochial schools that foster values important to the family.

PARTNERING WITH FAMILIES

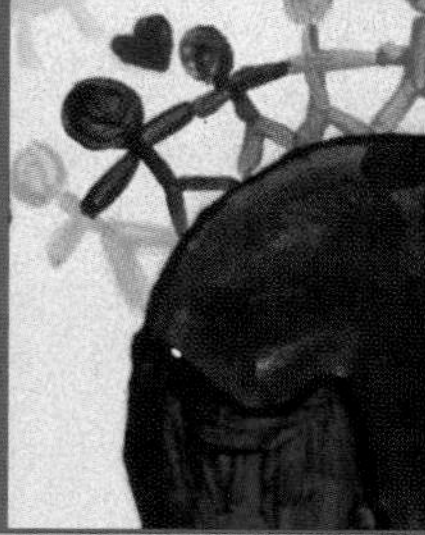

Guidelines for Promoting Acceptable Behavior in Children

- Set realistic expectations and directions for behavior based on the child's age and understanding; enforce the expected directions and behaviors consistently.
- Focus on promoting appropriate and desirable behaviors in the child.
  - Model or suggest appropriate behavior.
  - Review expected behavior for special situations, such as a family party, going to the movies, or other social event.
  - Help the child distinguish between inside and outside voice and behaviors.
  - Praise or reward the child using appropriate behaviors.
- Tell the child about his or her inappropriate behavior as soon as it begins and offer guidelines for behavior change or provide a distraction.
- When reprimanding the child, focus on the behavior rather than stating that the child is bad. Explain how the behavior is inappropriate, how it makes you as the parent and any other person involved feel. Avoid ridicule or accusation that can take the form of shame or criticism. These actions can have an impact on the child's self-esteem if repeated often enough.
- Be alert for situations when the child could potentially misbehave, such as when tired or overexcited. Use a distraction to control or calm the child.
- Help children gain self-control with friendly reminders (count to three, as soon as the clothes are on the doll, as soon as you finish the game) regarding the timing for transition to the next event of the day, such as bedtime, putting the toys away, or washing hands before dinner.
- Discuss reasons and social rules for expected behaviors when the child is old enough to understand.

- *Time-out*—a method of placing the child in a location away from toys and attention as a consequence of misbehavior (Figure 2–9 ■)
- *Experiencing consequences*—allowing the child to learn important lessons associated with misbehavior, such as by using a time-out, withdrawing privileges, providing no dessert if the child misses dinner or does not eat nutritious foods
- *Corporeal punishment*—spanking or inflicting pain with a paddle, whip, or other object (This form of discipline is not recommended as it teaches children that violence is acceptable. If parents are out of control or in a rage, the child may be seriously injured.)

See Chapters 12 through 15∞ for age-specific discipline strategies.

Discussion of inappropriate behaviors and the reason for limit setting or discipline will help the child to understand why certain behaviors are wrong. Personal stories and fables can also

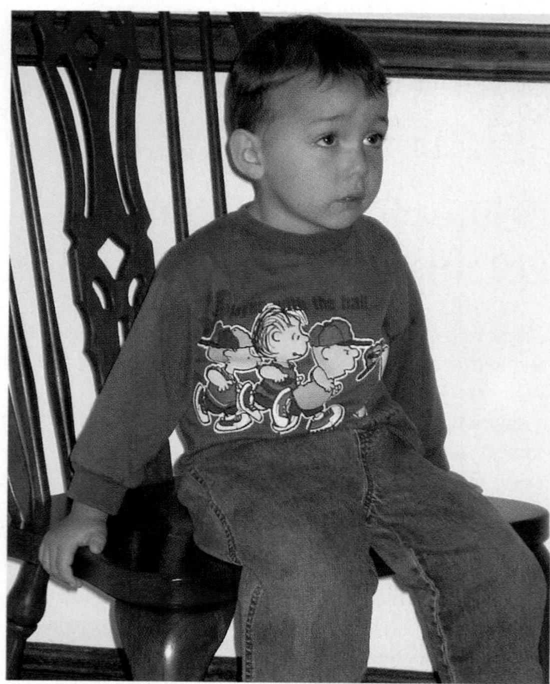

FIGURE 2–9 ■ One effective discipline method is to remove the child to an isolated area where no interaction with children and adults can occur and no toys are present. This is used to demonstrate that there is a consequence to misbehavior. For older children, consider the loss of phone, computer, or other privileges.

be used to help children understand social and moral values or to better understand acceptable behavior.

SPECIAL FAMILY CONSIDERATIONS

Divorce and Its Effects on Children

The average age of children at the time of divorce in the United States is 7 years (Sammons, 2003). Approximately 1 million children per year are involved in divorce (Equality in Marriage Institute, 2000). Children are affected in many ways when the family breaks apart due to divorce, even though there have often been many periods of stress and tension in the home before the actual separation and divorce occur. Many children believe they are at fault for the separation and divorce, that they said or did something to make the parent leave. When one parent leaves, the children may feel abandoned and divorced by that parent. They may fear being abandoned by the remaining parent. See Box 2–4 for behaviors of children experiencing separation and divorce.

Children may become engaged in the disputes of parents, and experience conflicts of loyalty when parents fight for their affection. Sometimes parents are so stressed their customary parenting styles are not maintained consistently, and they may not be capable of providing the warmth, affection, and support that the children need during this time. When the divorce involves a lot of conflict and hostility, the children may have increased problems with adjustment. Battles over custody, child support, property division, and visitation rights all cause more distress for the children. When children must make a lot of changes in their lives in addition to the parents' separation (new home, different school), their adjustment is made more difficult as their sense of order is upset. Predictable routines have changed and children may test limits to see if they still apply. The more changes they must make in the period immediately after the divorce, the more challenging is their adjustment. See Box 2–5.

Nurses can assist families experiencing divorce by inquiring about the circumstances and changes that the child is experiencing.

- Remind parents that even infants and toddlers can sense tensions in the home.
- Talk with parents about the child's fears of abandonment and concerns.
- Help parents recognize their children's needs for love and security during this difficult period.
- Remind parents about the need to keep children out of the middle of confrontations, and to maintain limits of acceptable behavior.

BOX 2–4 Behaviors of Children Experiencing Divorce by Age Group

The disruption associated with divorce is linked to academic and behavior problems among children, including depression, antisocial behavior, impulsive/hyperactive behavior, and school behavior problems (Amato, 2000).

- Infants and toddlers sense the tensions in the home and respond with increased irritability or tantrums, disturbance in eating and sleeping patterns, and regression in toilet training.
- Preschoolers and school-age children exhibit their anxiety and distress about the separation and divorce by "acting out," pestering siblings, becoming overly demanding of either parent, being clingy or regressive, or defiant, argumentative. They may also develop nervous habits, and begin bed-wetting.
- Older school-age children and adolescents may become angry, take risks with drugs or sex, develop school problems, disengage or withdraw from family and friends, or display other signs of depression or distress. Some children develop extremely destructive behavior such as suicide, drug abuse, and violence.

BOX 2–5 Research: Interventions for Adolescents Experiencing Divorce

An intervention program for divorced mothers and adolescents was evaluated using outcome variables as mental health problems, school drop-out, and adolescent pregnancy. Two intervention programs and a control group composed of 218 families with adolescents 15 to 19 years of age were interviewed 6 years after the intervention. One intervention group targeted mothers with 11 group and 2 individual sessions. A second intervention group targeted both mothers and adolescents with the mother program used in the first intervention group, plus 11 group sessions for the adolescents. The control group received books on postdivorce adjustment. Adolescents in the intervention groups were found to have reduced symptoms of mental disorders; lower rates of mental disorder diagnosis; reduced use of marijuana, alcohol or other drugs; and a lower number of sexual partners (Wolchik, Sandler, Millsap, et al., 2002).

- Encourage parents to avoid saying negative statements about the other parent and encourage parents to make every effort to maintain the relationship with the children.

The quality of the relationship between the divorced parents has an important impact on the future relationships their children have with them as adults. When divorced parents are able to minimize the conflict and continue sharing parenting (even in a minimal way), better maintenance of family and kinship ties (e.g., grandparents, stepparents, and half siblings) results (Ahrons, 2003).

Fathers who do not live with their children but live nearby are more likely to have involvement with their children if they have a good relationship with the child's mother, financial resources, and work experience. The relationship between father and child may be improved when the father can interact with the child in a conflict-free environment. Factors that negatively affect ongoing involvement with the child include conflicts with the mother, lack of financial resources, geographic distance, and a new spouse or partner (Halle & Le Menestrel, 2002). See Partnering with Families: Promoting Relationships with Parents Following Separation and Divorce.

PARTNERING WITH FAMILIES

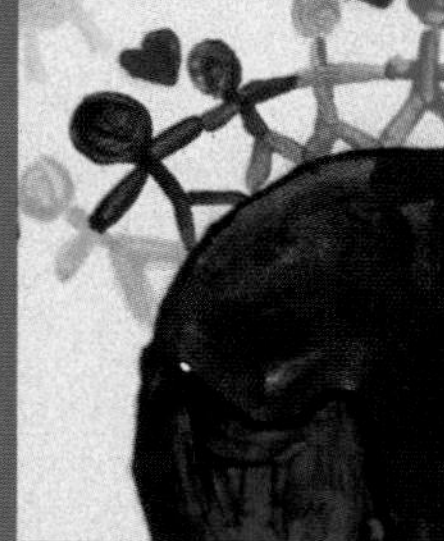

Promoting Relationships with Parents Following Separation and Divorce

Guidelines that may help to reduce conflict and to foster maintenance of a close relationship between the child and each parent include the following:

- Develop a way to stay in touch with the child even when apart, such as phone calls, faxes, or email.
- Encourage a liberal visitation schedule so that each parent has time to be a normal parent. Overnight stays rather than a few hours at a time allow for more normal interactions.
- When parents have difficulty minimizing conflict in front of the child, transition the child to the other parent after school or childcare, or from a friend's home. This keeps the child from feeling responsible for the conflict.

Stepparenting

When divorced or widowed parents remarry, the child may respond with ambivalence, divided loyalty, anger, or uncertainty. Many changes in lifestyles, routines, and interaction patterns for the child and entire family should be anticipated and addressed early in the formation of the new family relationship. When a stepparent joins a ready-made family, opportunities for improved emotional and financial support of the child can result, but the development of a new cohesive family requires many adjustments on the part of all family members. Stepparents must adjust to the habits and personality of the child and then work to gain trust and acceptance. If the child has not accepted the divorce or loss of a biological parent, developing a trusting, affectionate, and respectful relationship with the stepparent is more challenging. Discussing and gaining an understanding of the child's perceptions of loss or feared loss (close relationship with noncustodial parent, neighborhood friends if a move was required, loss of contact with grandparents, family traditions) may help the family develop plans that ease the transition to the new family structure.

Blending of two families often results in the need to identify or negotiate new customs, traditions, rituals, and routines for the family. Determining acceptable stepparent roles and the role of the joint or noncustodial parent needs to be discussed and negotiated. Discipline is a challenge in most stepparent families. Standards of behavior, as well as who, when, and how discipline is used need to be agreed upon within the family, and those guidelines need to be consistently maintained. Sharing in childrearing decisions and responsibilities is an important task for stepparents. Discipline by a stepparent is challenging until a bond develops between the stepparent and stepchild. Feelings and development of this bond cannot be forced. Time and honest communication are needed to make a successful transition to stepparenting and to gain the child's trust.

Stepparents are additional parents, not replacement parents. Adjustment of the child to the stepparent and the stepparent to the child are needed. The stepparent should try to establish a position in the child's life that is different from that of the missing biological parent, rather than competing with the biological parent. Men who live with their biological children and stepchildren, and those men who become stepparents when the children are young tend to be more involved in parenting their stepchildren (Halle & Le Menestrel, 2002). Stepmothers often have more challenges than stepfathers adjusting to their new role. This may be because they spend more time with the children.

Contact with the biological parent often continues through custody arrangements, financial support, and visitation. Children may actually move between two households adding to the complexity and stressors in their lives. Children may have divided loyalties between the two sets of parents. Power conflicts may emerge if the biological parents do not make efforts to cooperate in parenting decisions. A parenting coalition between all parents in the two families can reduce the conflicts and tensions that can emerge when parents agree to work together for the child's benefit.

CLINICAL TIP

Identify the parent who can legally provide consent for medical treatment when there has been a divorce and potentially a remarriage. In some states, the noncustodial parent cannot give consent. The stepparent cannot give consent unless the custodial parent grants written permission. Stepparents or other family members may also not know the child's medical history. Identify the legal framework for informed consent with regard to these children so that care is provided in an appropriate and responsible manner.

Foster Care

Foster care is the provision of protection and shelter for a child in an approved living situation away from the family of origin that is legally coordinated by the state's child welfare system. Children enter the foster care system for many varied and complex reasons. Neglect, often as a consequence of poverty, is a major reason children are placed in foster care (Gottesman, 2001). The goal of foster care is to ensure the safety and well-being of vulnerable children. Approximately 556,000 children were in foster care at the end of 2000, a substantial increase over the 302,000 children in foster care in 1980. Of the approximate 1.4 million children who do not live with either a parent or a grandparent, 40% are in foster care (U.S. Department of Health and Human Services, 2002).

The average length of stay in foster care is approximately 33 months; however, some children stay for shorter or longer times. An estimated 275,000 children were placed in foster care as a result of child abuse investigations or assessments, and the most common reason for placement in foster care is neglect. Racial distribution of children in foster care is 38% African American, 37% Caucasian, 17% Latino, 2% Native American, 1% Pacific Islander, and 5% of unknown race (Chipungu & Bent-Goodley, 2004).

Each state has guidelines regarding qualifications and standards for foster care parents and the process for becoming a foster parent. These guidelines include such things as interviewing and investigating the interested adults for readiness to be a foster parent, health of all family members, legal background checks, and safety of the residence in an effort to ensure that the child is placed in a safe and nurturing environment. Foster parents are also required to have initial training and annual continuing education.

Foster care parents may be relatives (kinship care) or unrelated families with whom the child has a strong emotional bond, but increasingly, more children are placed with relatives. More children needing foster care are currently placed in extended families, as there are fewer suitable nonkinship family foster homes. While there are psychologic benefits in keeping the child within the extended family, especially for helping the child learn and understand cultural and family values, the kinship foster parents have more challenges than other foster parents. They may be older, in poorer health, have less income, and be less educated. In many states, kinship foster parents receive less funding than licensed foster care parents, even though their costs are identical (Gottesman, 2001). In addition, they tend to receive less supervision and family service support than in nonkinship foster care (Green, 2004). See Box 2–6.

BOX 2–6 Grandparents Raising Grandchildren

Approximately 2.5 million grandparent-headed households are raising 3.9 million children, sometimes in association with the parents. Of these children, 1.3 million are being raised completely by the grandparents, in an effort to keep the children out of the foster care system. Challenges faced by these grandparents include no health insurance for the children, personal stress related to caring for an infant or young child, strained relationships with parents due to custody issues, challenges in enrolling the children in school, difficulty in providing needed transportation, and lack of affordable and appropriate housing (FRIENDS National Resource Center for Community-based Family Resource and Support Programs, 2001).

Foster Parenting

Foster parenting is very demanding. Children placed in foster care often have more problems than other children from the same socioeconomic background, such as chronic medical conditions, birth defects, emotional or mental health disorders, and school-related problems (Sobel & Healy, 2001). Foster parents must provide for the daily needs of children, support them emotionally, and provide appropriate responses to their behaviors. They provide transportation to medical appointments, mental health counseling, and court hearings. They coordinate visits with birth parents and caseworkers, and they also advocate for the child in school settings. When the child has complex problems or needs, the challenge of caring for the foster child is even greater. Foster parents receive some funding to care for children, but it is often inadequate for the child's needs, and the family often subsidizes the child's care from their own funds. Many parents become frustrated with the challenges and stop serving as foster parents after 1 year (Chipungu & Bent-Goodley, 2004). These challenges include complicated and time-consuming paperwork for health and other financial resources, negative perceptions about foster parents who use food stamps, and being required to open the home to social services and court services personnel (Sobel & Healy, 2001). When the child must be moved to a different foster family, this may further exacerbate the ongoing stress that the individual child has in the foster care system.

Much of the child's adjustment rests with the stability of the family and available resources. Even though foster care is intended to be a temporary short placement—until the child can be returned home or an adoptive home is found—placed children may actually reside with the foster family for a lengthy time. For children who have come from an environment that has been unstable, abusive, or neglectful, the foster care home can be supportive to the child's health status, development, and academic achievement. Children who have experience with the foster care system are more likely to have compromised development (behavioral problems, emotional problems, poor school adjustment) and higher levels of risky sexual behavior (Wertheimer, 2002). Many of the problems are thought tied to the reason foster care was sought, such as physical or sexual abuse, neglect, or abandonment. For the optimal psychologic outcome of children placed in foster care, efforts should be made for permanent placement of the child as rapidly as possible so the child perceives a sense of belonging and develops psychologic ties.

Foster parents caring for children need to provide continuity, consistency, and predictability. Foster parents should be encouraged to do the following (American Academy of Pediatrics, 2000):

- Give the child lots of love and attention.
- Be consistent with love, stimulation, and discipline.
- Use developmentally appropriate methods to stimulate the child such as holding, conversation, reading, music, and toys.
- Help the child develop language skills.

Children in Foster Care

Children in foster care have a high prevalence of chronic and complex health conditions and may be in poor health if prior healthcare needs have not been addressed. Efforts to ensure that children receive appropriate healthcare while in foster care are challenged by various barriers, such as an incomplete health history obtained from the parents, insufficient funding for needed health services, prolonged waits for community-based medical and mental health services, poor coordination of services with lack of communication between health professionals, and poor communication between health and community welfare professionals (American Academy of Pediatrics, 2002b). Every child entering foster care should receive an initial health screening, followed by a more comprehensive health assessment within a month. Findings and recommendations from the health assessment and additional health evaluations should be incorporated into the child's social service case plan. Nurses can play an important role in partnering with foster parents to arrange for and obtain the services needed by the child. Foster parents need to be supported in their efforts to be the caring adult for these children, helping them to develop self-esteem and resilience.

While some children are reunited with birthparents, it is not possible for other children. Foster care is not intended to be a long-term solution for a safe and secure home for the child. The Adoption and Safe Families Act of 1997 (PL 105-89) was passed to encourage states to find permanent homes for children who could not be reunited with birth parents. See Box 2–7 for more information about the provisions of this legislation. Foster parents have accounted for more than 50% of the adoptions of children in foster care, likely because they have a relationship already established with the child (Urban Institute, 2003b). For those children with kinship foster care, adoption is often not perceived as the best option. **Adoption** is a legal relationship between the child and parents not related by birth in which the adoptive parents assume all legal and financial responsibility for the child. All ties with the birth family are legally severed. **Legal guardianship** is an alternative permanent arrangement for the child, often with relatives. Parental rights are not terminated. In this case the child retains legal connections with the birth family and relationship with the extended family. The guardian assumes limited financial liability for the child's care. Legal guardianship can be reversed at a future point in time if the birth parents petition the court.

Many children stay in foster care until they reach 18 and are no longer eligible for services. The Foster Care Independence Act of 1999 (PL 106-169) requires states to provide youth 18 to 21 years of age with services to help them make the transition to self-sufficiency—training and education with services to help them gain employment, mentors for personal and emotional support, as well as financial, housing, counseling, and other support and services. States are required to track outcomes for the youth served (Barbell & Freundlich, 2001).

BOX 2–7 Adoption and Safe Families Act

The national Adoption and Safe Families Act of 1997 (PL 105-89) led to significant changes in child welfare. Provisions of this law include:

- Shortened timelines for making decisions about permanent placement of children
- Eliminated long-term foster care as a permanent option for nonkinship foster care, but permitted it to continue for kinship foster care to promote stability for children involved
- Established legal guardianship as a permanency option
- Required action to terminate parental rights in certain situations
- Clarified when states do not have to make reasonable efforts to reunite children with birthparents
- Recognized kinship caregivers as a placement option
- Established incentives for states to encourage adoption
- Increased emphasis on state accountability

Since passage of this law, adoptions of children previously in foster care have increased dramatically.

Adapted from Bass, S., Shields, M. K., & Behrman, R. E. (2004). Children, families, and foster care: Analysis and recommendations. The Future of Children, *14(1), 8–9.*

Adoption

Adoption is a legal relationship between the child and parents not related by birth in which the adoptive parents assume all legal and financial responsibility for the child. Motivations for adoption of a child vary with the families seeking adoption. In some cases, couples have infertility problems and are unable to have a biological child. In other cases, the family already has one or two biological children, and the reasons could include the following:

- A humanitarian perspective—providing a home to a child who needs one
- Fertility issues requiring invasive medical procedures that are too extensive, expensive, or psychologically too overwhelming for a subsequent pregnancy
- Adoption of a foster child with whom the family has established strong bonds
- Adoption by a family relative or stepparent
- A desire for a larger family but without additional biological children

The supply of healthy infants available for adoption is much smaller than the number of families who want to adopt. The majority of children in the United States available for adoption are older children, often of minority populations or of mixed races, and those with special healthcare needs. As of September 2001, 126,000 children under 16 years of age were awaiting adoption from the foster care system (U.S. Department of Health and Human Services, 2003). Because most families choosing to adopt children prefer to have an infant, many children have been adopted from foreign nations. Since 1995, the nations that have provided the largest number of orphans for adoption in the United States include mainland China, Russia, Guatemala, and South Korea (U.S. Department of State, 2004).

Legal Aspects of Adoption

Adoption is controlled by individual state law. Adoption may be arranged through an authorized agency, such as a licensed social service agency. Any family who wants to adopt a child is required

MediaLink Care Plan: Needs of the Adopted Child

BOX 2–8 Home Study Information for Adoption

- Personal and family background, including upbringing, siblings, key events, and what was learned from them (This may be in the form of an autobiography.)
- Significant people in the lives of the applicants
- Marriage and family relationships
- Motivation to adopt, type of child desired, ability to bond with an adopted child
- Expectations for the child
- Feelings about infertility (if this is an issue)
- Parenting and integration of the child into the family, considering how extended family members will respond to an adopted child
- Family environment, ordinary routines, hobbies, leisure activities, neighborhood, community resources, religion
- Physical and health history of the applicants
- Education, employment, and finances, including insurance coverage and childcare plans
- References and criminal background clearances
- Summary of home study data and the social worker's recommendation

by state laws to undergo a home study. This is a process in which parents are interviewed about a large number of topics and issues, as well as being provided education and guidelines to prepare for the adoption. See Box 2–8 for information generally included in a home study. Some adoptions are arranged through independent agencies in collaboration with physicians, lawyers, nurses, and members of the clergy. The family home study may not be conducted in the case of independent adoptions, which may not be in the best interest of the child. The National Adoption Information Clearinghouse provides information about state adoption laws.

Birth mothers and birth fathers are each required to relinquish legal rights to a child before an adoption can occur. States vary regarding the legal period that must exist between the child's birth and when the birth mother relinquishes legal rights. Every effort must be made to ensure that the birth mother is not coerced into relinquishing legal rights to the child immediately after birth. In an open adoption, the birth mother and adoptive parents often have contact with each other prior to the birth and have jointly planned potential future contacts between the child and biological mother. In some adoptions, birth mothers write a letter to the child that is given to the child at an appropriate age.

MediaLink Adoption Resources

Preparation for Adoption

Parents often benefit from preadoption counseling to prepare for receiving the child. Such counseling may help provide the support and reassurance needed about parenting, the adoptive process, and a connection to support groups or other families with adopted children. Parents may wonder about their ability to love and parent the child, and have concerns about the responses of relatives, other children, and friends, especially if the child is from a different ethnic or racial group. Children already present in the family need to be reassured that they will not be displaced by the new child. Families need information about the child's understanding of what adoption means and guidance to help inform the child about being adopted (Box 2–9). See Partnering with Families: Informing the Child About Adoption.

Children who are older when adopted must also make the commitment to the family relationship. They often have a memory of parents and other caregivers, so developing a close relationship with the adoptive parents takes more time. It may also be more challenging for parents to develop as close an emotional bond to the adopted older child than to an adopted infant. Even when a serious commitment has been made to adopt an older child, adjustment of the family and child may be difficult for everyone. Counseling may be helpful to some families during the transition process. See Box 2–10 for family resources related to adoption.

International Adoptions

Internationally adopted children often need special healthcare services. These children may be at risk for medical, developmental, and emotional problems that are uncommon in children born in the United States. Nurses work with families that have adopted children from other countries to provide a comprehensive evaluation of the child to detect potential developmental problems and health conditions as soon as the child is brought into the country (see Chapter 5∞). Examples of health problems that could potentially exist include infectious diseases (tuberculosis, hepatitis B, HIV infection, congenital syphilis) and parasites; various medical conditions such as fetal alcohol syndrome, anemia, lead poisoning; and incomplete immunizations (Miller, 1999).

BOX 2–9 Understanding of and Responses to Adoption by Children at Various Ages

- Children under 3 years of age do not recognize a difference between being adopted into a family versus being a biologic child in the family.
- Starting at about 3 years of age children like to hear more about their adoption story and they begin to ask what adoption means. Children adopted at this age may experience the separation from their other family and relatives. They are aware of physical differences between themselves and the adoptive family when they are of a different race or ethnic group. They may also be fearful of abandonment by the adoptive family.
- By 5 years of age adopted children begin to recognize they are different from most of their peers who were not adopted. Some children develop a feeling of responsibility for their biologic parent's decision not to keep them.
- School-age children may fantasize about their biologic family and what their life might have been like if they were not adopted. Their self-esteem may be affected as they think there was a flaw in them that led biologic parents to give them up for adoption.
- Adolescents may continue to fantasize about the "ideal" biologic family and try out identities similar to what they know or imagine about their biologic parents. They may also become angry that their own life experience is different from societal norms. They may choose to seek information about their biologic family through a reunion registry.

Data from Borchers and Committee on Early Childhood, Adoption, and Dependent Care, American Academy of Pediatrics. (2003). Families and adoption: The pediatrician's role in supporting communication. Pediatrics, 112*(6), 1437–1441.*

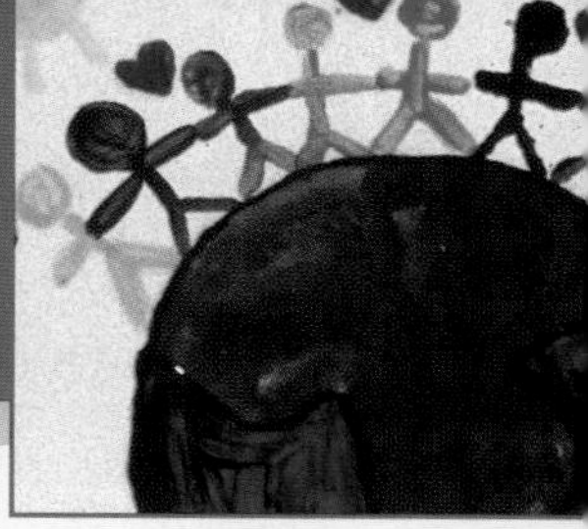

PARTNERING WITH FAMILIES

Informing the Child About Adoption

Most parents have anxiety about when and how to tell the child that he or she is adopted. There is no perfect age to tell the child about the adoption, so consider the child's age and developmental stage when sharing information.

- Some authorities believe the child should be told at such a young age that the child will always know that he or she is adopted. This may be especially important when the child is of a different ethnic or racial group, or has very different physical characteristics than the parents.
- The terms *adoption, adopted, birth family*, or *biologic family* should be part of the family's natural conversation (Borchers, 2003).
- Decide when you and the child are most ready to introduce the topic of adoption—such as when a discussion of babies and where they come from occurs. However, avoid waiting for "just the right moment" because children may wonder what other information has not yet been shared.
- Make sure the child is told before a third party is likely to say something. The chances of this happening increase as the child enters school.
- Tell the child in a matter-of-fact manner about the adoption. Let the child know how much he or she was wanted and that some personal qualities of the child made the selection special to them. Avoid phrases such as "given up" for adoption. A more positive phrase to use is that the biologic family made an adoption plan in the best interest of the child's future.
- Share the adoption story that includes the child's birth. Then the story can continue with the adoptive family's desire to adopt a child and that the adopted child was specifically chosen.
- Make sure the child understands that his or her place in the family is permanent. The adoptive family's commitment to the child should be repeated frequently.
- Maintain honesty and an open opportunity for discussion about adoption with the child. Be willing to discuss the child's biologic family and the adoption process so the child feels comfortable asking questions. This helps make the adoption a positive process. More discussion about adoption will be needed as the child grows older, especially when the child begins to ask at about 5 to 6 years of age why the he or she was not wanted by the biologic parents. Anticipate that the child will grieve the loss of the birth parents.
- As the child grows older and asks for more information about the birth parents, provide what information is known and try to help the child deal with difficult-to-hear information. If requested information is not available, be honest and admit it. Help the child decide what information to share with strangers, friends, and extended family members.
- Recognize that the adolescent may fantasize about the birth parents and want to find them. Listening to concerns and providing support during this challenging time of development is important.

Emotional and psychological problems may be the result of long-term institutionalization in an orphanage, such as inconsistency in interpersonal development and delayed developmental milestones. The child and family may need counseling and support to help the child adjust to being part of a family. The initial response of the child who has been in an orphanage to the new parents may be crying or turning away. Children need a transition period of several months to adjust to a different daily routine and to bond with the parents. Exposing the child to large numbers of family members or to busy environments may be stressful for the child. The nurse may become involved in providing counseling to the family trying to integrate the adoptive child into the family's life and routine. As the child grows, efforts to help the child understand the cultural birth heritage are also important (Figure 2–10 ■). See Developing Cultural Competence: Adopting a Child from a Different Culture.

Family Support Services

Family support services exist in all communities with a purpose of supporting families in the rearing of healthy children. Contemporary lifestyles (divorced parents, single parents, mothers in the labor force, more time away from children, and parents separated from extended families and natural support systems) stress families trying to provide for their children's needs. In other cases, families are stressed due to economics, living in or near poverty, or even being homeless. Many communities have worked to develop social support programs to support the health and development of children

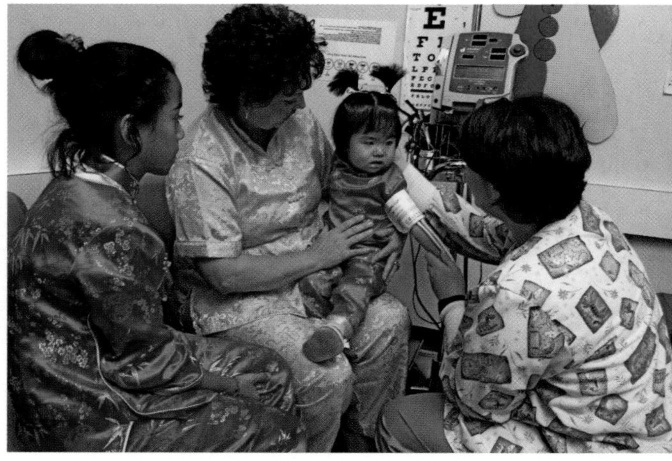

FIGURE 2–10 ■ Adopted children who are of mixed race or a different ethnic group than the parents may cause a few additional challenges for the adoptive parents. Family members may be less supportive of the adoption initially. Because the children may have different physical characteristics, the family may capture more attention than it wishes. The family needs to learn to appreciate the different cultures represented in the newly formed family.

BOX 2–10 Adoption Resources for Families

Adamec, C. (1993). *Explaining adoption to your child.* Rockville, MD: National Adoption Information Clearinghouse.

Bunin, C., & Bunin, S. (1992). *Is that my sister?* Wayne, PA: Our Child Press.

Howe, J. (1993). *Pinky and Rex and the new baby.* New York: Atheneum.

Keck, G. C., & Kupecky, R. M. (1995). *Adopting the hurt child: Hope for families with special needs kids. A guide for parents and professionals.* Colorado Springs, CO: Pinon Press.

Keefer, B., & Schooler, J. E. (2000). *Telling the truth to your adopted or foster child: Making sense of the past.* Westport, CT: Bergin & Garvey.

Matthew, T. (1999). *Our own: Adopting and parenting the older child.* Longmont, CO: Snowcap Press.

Melina, L. R. (1998). *Raising adopted children: Practical reassuring advice for every adoptive parent.* New York: Harper Perennial.

Pelligrini, N. (1991). *Families are different.* New York: Holiday House.

Register, C. (1991). *Are those kids yours? American families with children adopted from other countries.* New York: The Free Press.

Root, M.P.P., & Kelley, M. (Eds). (2003). *Multiracial child resource book: Living complex identities.* Seattle: Mavin Foundation. www.mavinfoundation.org

Stein, S. (1992). *Lacy's feet.* Indianapolis: Perspectives Press.

Steinberg, G., & Hall, B. (2000). *Inside transracial adoption.* Indianapolis: Perspectives Press.

Watkins, M., & Fisher, S. (1993). *Talking with young children about adoption.* New Haven, CT: Yale University Press.

Wright, S. (1994). *Real sisters.* Chalottetown, P.E.I., Canada: Ragweed Press.

Mister Rogers' Neighborhood Adoption Programs (two 30-minute videos), available from Family Communications with Adoptive Families of America, 2309 Como Ave., St. Paul, MN 55108, 612–535–4829. $12.95 each

and to promote family positive relationships. Examples of these family support services include the following:

- Head Start and Early Head Start
- Before- and after-school programs for children of working parents
- School-based health and counseling services
- Play groups for preschool children
- Peer support groups
- Social service programs offered by the faith community
- Home visiting programs for high-risk children and parents
- Job skills training, adult education, and literacy programs
- Crisis care and respite care programs

Many of these family support services work to promote positive family relationships, parental competencies, and behaviors that contribute to the health and development of the children and family. Most programs are designed with the premise that no family is entirely self-sufficient and most can benefit from some external support.

MediaLink Critical Thinking: Identifying Family Support

Think about the formal and informal family support services in your community. Nurses play an important role in helping to link families to the types of community support services they need after performing a family assessment and collaborating with families to identify and seek assistance most beneficial to their needs.

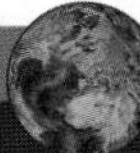

DEVELOPING CULTURAL COMPETENCE
Adopting a Child from a Different Heritage

Families adopting a child of another race or culture often want to learn about the cultures and traditions of the child's birth culture so they can show respect for that culture and promote an understanding of that culture in the child. This information also helps promote the child's development of identify and self-esteem. Strategies to learn and foster an understanding of the child's culture of origin include the following:

- Interact with people of the child's heritage or race—join a cultural association or church and make friends.
- Identify successful professionals from the child's culture who can be role models. Discuss ways to help the child develop an identity within the culture and to interact effectively with members of the culture.
- Live in a multicultural neighborhood. Enroll the child in a school with diversity of students and faculty.
- Learn about the culture through books, magazines, and movies targeted to the cultural group. Identify Internet sites with information and discussions to understand important issues.
- Celebrate special holidays of the cultural group.
- Take family field trips to learn about historical events important to the culture and encourage cultural pride. Help all members of the family develop a bicultural view.

FAMILY THEORIES

Families must be understood in their own context. It is important to understand each family's strengths and uniqueness and how the family and its members respond to the complex and often conflicting demands for time and attention. Many families live in a stressed state due to inadequate finances, healthcare concerns, relationship challenges, and other pressures. Nurses need to be able to assess family strengths and support mechanisms, to identify coping strategies, and to determine when families have overextended their resources and need additional support. Nurses can provide additional support as needed, and at other times referral to other health professionals is appropriate to address the family's needs.

Family social system theories are helpful in understanding family functioning, environment–family interchange, family changes over time, and family response to health and illness. A brief review of family theories provides a context about family functioning that can assist with planning nursing care and developing future partnerships with families and their children.

Each family has structure and functions to help it maintain stability while responding continuously to various stresses and strains within the family and in the family's interactions and functioning within the community. Families develop and modify their responses and functioning over time to adapt or be tolerant of family, community, and environmental changes. Family processes include the behaviors and strategies that help to regulate space, time, energy, and other aspects of family functioning to promote family stability, growth, and control.

Family Development Theory

Family development refers to the dynamic changes that a family experiences over time, including changes within the family and in response to societal pressures. Family development includes relationships, communication patterns, roles, and changes in interactions. Over the years many models and frameworks of family development have been proposed. These developmental frameworks observe a family's progression over time by identifying specific typical stages in family life. There are predictable stages in the life cycle of every family, but they follow no rigid pattern. Duvall's (1977) eight stages in the family life cycle of a traditional nuclear family have been used as the foundation for contemporary models of the family life cycle that describe the developmental processes and role expectations for different family types. Table 2–4 lists Duvall's eight stages to illustrate important developmental transitions that occur at some point in most families. However, life cycle stages have been developed for the more contemporary blended families, dual career families, and others (Friedman, Bowden, & Jones, 2003).

Although each family is unique, the members experience fairly predictable, similar, and consistent changes (Friedman, Bowden, & Jones, 2003). Developmental tasks, goals, or challenging issues for the family in each stage have been defined for different family types. Using these frameworks, families can be assessed by their development stage, how well they are fulfilling the tasks of that stage, and the availability of resources to accomplish developmental tasks. The stages provide a method for anticipating transitions and potential stressors with family role changes that occur at different points along the developmental continuum for different family types.

It is helpful to understand the family's developmental stage because it enables the nurse to analyze the family growth and health promotion needs. Understanding developmental transitions and potential stressors can then help the nurse identify the types of teaching and anticipatory guidance that might be needed.

TABLE 2–4 Eight-Stage Family Life Cycle

STAGES	CHARACTERISTICS
Stage I	Beginning family, newly married couples *
Stage II	Childbearing family (oldest child is an infant through 30 months of age)
Stage III	Families with preschool children (oldest child is between 2.5 and 6 years of age)
Stage IV	Families with school children (oldest child is between 6 and 13 years of age)
Stage V	Families with teenagers (oldest child is between 13 and 20 years of age)
Stage VI	Families launching young adults (all children leave home)
Stage VII	Middle-aged parents (empty nest through retirement)
Stage VIII	Family in retirement and old age (retirement to death of both spouses)

*Keep in mind that this was the norm at the time the model was developed, but today families form through many different types of relationships.

Adapted from: Duvall, E. M. (1977). Marriage and family development *(5th ed.), Philadelphia: Lippincott; Duvall, E. M. & Miller, B. C. (1985).* Marriage and family development *(6th ed.), New York: Harper Row; Craig, G. J. & Baucum, D. (1999).* Human development *(8th ed.). Upper Saddle River, NJ: Prentice Hall; Murray, R. B. & Zentner, J. P. (2001).* Health promotion strategies through the life span *(7th ed.) Upper Saddle River, NJ: Prentice Hall; and Craig, G. J. & Baucum, D. (2002).* Human development. *(9th ed.), Upper Saddle River, NJ: Prentice Hall.*

Family Systems Theory

Family systems theory evolved from "general systems theory" in which there is interaction between the components (family members) of the system (family) and between the system and the environment. A family is a living social system, consisting of a small group of individuals who are closely interrelated and interdependent while collaborating to attain family functions and goals; therefore, the family is more than the sum of its members. In family systems theory, due to the amount of interrelationship and interdependence in the family, it is recognized that any change or stressor experienced by one or more family members has an impact on the entire family and causes disruption. Families are adaptable, and can change interactions and behaviors associated with the disruption in response to positive feedback. The family is a system that may or may not exchange materials, energy, and information with its physical, social, and cultural environments. An *open family* seeks information and resources, and actively interacts with the community to solve problems. A *closed family* views change and offered support as a threat, and resistance to outside influences is a strategy used to maintain control. These attributes have an effect on the capacity of the family to adapt—to modify behavior and change as the situation demands.

This theory encourages nurses to see the child and parents as participating members of a whole family. It encourages looking at the processes within the family and the relationships between subsystems (spouse, parent–child, and siblings) and suprasystems (the community within which it is embedded). Stress and crises motivate the family to mobilize its resources and to begin problem solving.

Using this information, the nurse can assess the effects of illness or injury on the entire family system and the reciprocal effects of the family on the illness or injury. Assessing the interactions and interdependence within the family, the nurse recognizes the need to work with the family and the following subsystems in the provision of healthcare:

- Multiple dyad relationships (or lack thereof) between the parents, between the mother and child, and between the father and child
- Triad relationship between the two parents and child

Assessing how open or closed the family is to information and resources is important in planning nursing care. Open families will be more receptive to referrals and interventions from health professionals. The nurse will need to work with the closed family to establish trust and acceptance before the family is receptive to ideas and interventions proposed.

Family Stress Theory

Families experience many stressors as an inevitable part of life. Some stressors are positive, such as the birth of a child that leads to transitions within the family. Other stressors are unexpected and not considered positive, such as learning that a child has a serious health condition. All stressors demand a response from family members that can lead to change within the family's interactions among its members and with the environment. Stressors are also cumulative and can come from many sources (work demands, school issues, extended family demands, achieving quality family time, and community roles). Most families have developed coping strategies to deal with daily routine stressors. Unexpected events are often more stressful as the family has not had time to review resources and prepare a response.

Identifying how families respond to the stress of illness or injury of a child or other family member is important due to the potential hardships it causes the entire family. In determining how a family responds to stress, it is important to identify strengths and resources within the family that make coping with the stressors possible. Potential resources include religious faith, finances, social support, physical health, family flexibility, and family coping mechanisms. Another factor in the family's response to the stressors is how much of a hardship the stressor is perceived to be for the family. If resources are diminished and the family defines the stressor as significant enough to cause a crisis, then the family will be susceptible to more serious disruption by the event. The impact of a child's unexpected serious health condition, in addition to another hardship and usual stressors, can potentially cause a crisis in the family if coping mechanisms are overwhelmed. Functional families use a variety of coping strategies for stress management and they successfully reduce stress. Coping strategies of dysfunctional families are defensive and do not effectively manage the stress. See Table 2–5 for coping strategies used by functional and dysfunctional families.

Identifying the family's **resilience**—the family's capacity to develop strengths and abilities, to "bounce back" from the stresses and challenges faced, and to eliminate or minimize negative outcomes—is an important focus for family assessment prior to planning nursing interventions. The resilience of children will be discussed in Chapter 5∞.

The Resiliency Model of Family Stress, Adjustment, and Adaptation

The resiliency model of family stress, adjustment, and adaptation emphasizes the strength and resilience of families to adjust and adapt to stressful life situations such as those described in the family stress theory. It can be used to help identify why families respond in different ways to similar stressors. Families develop strengths and capabilities to foster the family members' and family unit's growth and development to help protect the family from major disruptions during family transitions and changes. These family-specific strengths and capabilities help to protect the family from unexpected or normative stresses, and they can help the family to adapt after a crisis or major change (McCubbin & McCubbin, 1991). The resiliency model has two phases: an adjustment phase and an adaptation phase, which are activated in response to stressors of differing severity.

Adjustment Phase

The adjustment phase is activated when there are minor changes needed in family functioning, such as a child's brief illness and complete recovery. The patterns of family interaction are relatively stable and predictable. The adjustment phase may also be the initial response when the family has a more significant stressor or crisis. Families respond by using the established family functioning processes, including use of existing resources, family problem solving, and coping strategies.

Adaptation Phase

The adaptation phase is activated when family functioning and resources are inadequate to manage the stressor or crisis situation. Actions are taken to regain a sense of balance by either acquiring new resources or coping behaviors, reducing the demands the family faces, or changing the meaning or perceptions associated with an incident. The family must make some structural or systematic changes in functioning to adapt to the

TABLE 2–5 Coping Strategies Used by Functional Families and Dysfunctional Families

FUNCTIONAL FAMILY COPING STRATEGIES	DYSFUNCTIONAL FAMILY COPING STRATEGIES
➤ Family relationships—increased structure and organization within the home and family, strengthening family cohesion, and increased role flexibility of family members	➤ Denial of family problems
➤ Gathering information and knowledge, family joint problem solving	➤ Exploitation of family members such as by scapegoating (negatively labeling and stigmatizing a family member, often a child) to avoid examining the real problem in the family
➤ **Normalization**—the process of family management that involves acknowledging a life-changing situation such as the child has a chronic health problem, but family makes an effort to lead a normal life. Family life is normal because the impact of the condition on the family functioning is minimized as demonstrated by behaviors, rituals, and routines that show others that the family is normal.	➤ Use of threat or withdrawal of affection and support to keep family members together at the expense of the emotional health of its members
➤ Passive acceptance about an event or situation about which little or nothing can be done and determining that it will take care of itself over time	➤ Myths or images the family has of itself that obscure reality and enable the family to deny some of its problems
➤ Direct, open, honest and clear communication	➤ Extreme dominance and submission patterns
➤ Use of humor and laughter	➤ Family addictions (drug or alcohol)
➤ Maintaining active linkages with the community and using social support networks	➤ Domestic violence (partner, child, sibling to sibling, and elder abuse)
➤ Spiritual supports	

Data from Friedman, M. M., Bowden, V. R., & Jones, E. G. (2003). Family nursing: Research, theory, and practice *(5th ed., pp. 476–494). Upper Saddle River, NJ: Prentice Hall.*

situation and restore stability to the family member and family unit functioning. In some cases the family must accept what cannot be changed and share control with others.

As described in the family stress theory, most families deal with more than one situational stressor at a time. Consider Casey and his family in the opening scenario. Casey has a significant brain injury following a motor vehicle crash in which his best friend was driving. The family is also dealing with its fears regarding Casey's potential for significant disability, fears expressed by Casey's siblings and their need to attend school and recreational activities, the stepfather's employer demands for increased seasonal work hours, and the mother's need to take a leave of absence from her job to care for Casey once he is discharged from rehabilitation. The number of stresses experienced by this family will require adaptation in family functioning.

Responses during both the adjustment and adaptation phases are related to the family functioning pattern, such as the family's flexibility and emotional closeness between family members. Resources available to the family can come from individual members and the family unit, as well as the community, such as the following (Friedman, et al., 2003):

- Individual family member knowledge, personality traits, intelligence, physical health, and self-esteem
- Family unit organization, decision-making skills, and conflict resolution skills
- Community resources such as relatives or healthcare services outside the family that can provide social support in addition to institutional support

During the adaptation phase, families assess the impact of the stressor on the family by defining how significant it is and how much of an impact it will have on the family's functioning. The family then conducts an appraisal of how well the family is responding to the demands of the stressor, as well as how it fits into the family's view of shared values, goals, and expectations. Once the family completes its appraisal and recognizes the significance of the situation, it begins implementing problem-solving and coping strategies. The outcome of family adaptation is an acceptance of the changes needed in family functioning to work together as a unit, based on family strengths. Adaptation is made between the individual family members and the family unit, as well as between the family unit and the community. When families cannot adapt successfully at the family unit and community level, another crisis can emerge.

Family Strengths

Family strengths are the relationships and processes that support and protect families and family members during times of adversity and change. These strengths help maintain family cohesion while supporting the development and well-being of individual family members (Moore, Chalk, Scarpa, et al., 2002). There are four types of strengths that enable families to develop, adapt to change, and cope with challenges (Feeley & Gottlieb, 2000):

- Individual or family traits, such as optimism or resilience
- Individual or family assets, such as finances
- Individual or family capabilities, skills, competencies, such as problem solving
- Another quality less permanent than a trait or asset, such as motivation

Recognition of family strengths is one method that can be used to develop a rapport and relationship with the family. Focus on family competence and acknowledge and validate family members' emotions. See Box 2–11 for types of family strengths. Once the family recognizes the strengths it brings to the management of their child's healthcare problem, the more likely the family will become an effective partner in the process. The nurse can often help families recognize that the strengths used in prior life experiences may transfer to the current healthcare experience.

When a family can control and deal with events satisfactorily, they gain a sense of competence, making them more resilient, in contrast to families who are overwhelmed by traumatic experiences. Characteristics of a resilient family include the following (Patterson, 1991):

- Balancing the child's illness with other family needs
- Forming collaborative relationships with healthcare professionals
- Maintaining a professional relationship rather than a friendship relationship with providers
- Developing competence in communication skills
- Maintaining family flexibility and adapting to changing circumstances
- Maintaining a commitment to the family as a unit
- Attributing positive meaning to the situation
- Maintaining supportive relationships outside the family
- Engaging in active coping efforts with effective and efficient problem-solving abilities

Most families do not naturally develop resilience. Often nursing support is needed to help family members learn new skills, make adaptations, and gain confidence in their abilities to manage the challenges they face. Nurses need to help families identify their strengths and areas for improvement that will lead to increased resiliency.

BOX 2–11 Family Strengths Helpful in Managing Stressors

- **Communication skills**—the ability of family members to listen and to discuss their concerns
- **Shared family values and beliefs**—the family's common perceptions of reality and willingness to have hope and to appreciate that change is possible
- **Intrafamily support**—the provision of support and reinforcement by extended family members, as well as establishing an atmosphere of belonging
- **Self-care abilities**—the family's ability to take responsibility for health problems and the demonstrated willingness of individual members to take good care of themselves
- **Problem-solving skill**—the family's use of negotiation in problem solving, using everyday experiences as resources, and focusing on the present rather than past events or disappointments

No one theory is sufficient for viewing the needs and behaviors of all families. The theories described herein continue to evolve as researchers identify new or broadened explanations for behaviors, so it is difficult to attach one specific theorist to each family theory. When assessing families, you may also find it useful to consider more than one of these theories for particular families to help you understand the full set of behaviors associated with individual families and to plan effective nursing interventions. Nurse theorists such as Friedman, Wright, and Leahy use elements from multiple theories as the conceptual framework for their family assessment tools.

FAMILY ASSESSMENT

Children and families live their lives within a variety of settings and interact with those settings in ways that directly or indirectly influence behaviors and learning. Urie Bronfenbrenner formulated the ecologic theory of child development that addresses the influences of various close and remote social systems on the developing child (Bronfenbrenner & Morris, 1998). See Chapter 5 for more information on Bronfenbrenner's theory. Due to these environmental influences on the family, it is important to consider the relationship of the family with the social networks within the community.

The family should still be the central focus in care of children as the family is an interdependent network of individuals who mutually influence each other.

- The family is vital in assuring that children and other family members seek and receive healthcare.
- Any dysfunction in the family can affect other family members.
- The child's illness or injury impacts the entire family.
- A strong interrelationship exists between the family and the health status of its members—such as health promotion lifestyle choices, nutritional status, activity level, and communicable diseases.

The strength, resilience, coping skills, and resources of a child's family play a major role in fostering the child's growth and development, as well as in managing the child's health problems. When providing care to children in all settings, taking time to assess the family's strengths and needs will help you to plan and provide nursing care that corresponds to the family's values, resources, and abilities.

Collecting Data

To obtain an accurate and concise family assessment, the nurse needs to establish a trusting relationship with the child and family. It is important to ask about the greatest concern of both parent and child. This concern will vary depending on which parent responds, and the child's concern will probably be different as well. In providing nursing care, acknowledge that these multiple perceptions and concerns are present and demonstrate respect for the diversity of the family. The goal is to obtain family information that will be helpful in planning nursing interventions that will help the family care for the child and improve the child's outcomes while valuing each person within the family.

Information about the family is collected continuously during the healthcare process, through interviews, observations of the family interactions, reports from other healthcare providers or agencies working with the family, and with a family assessment tool. See Box 2–12 for family assessment information to collect. (See Chapter 8, page 231, for suggested psychosocial history data collection and Box 8–3, Daily Living Patterns, as family assessment information is also obtained during the child's health history.) Observation of the home and family members is recommended in some cases to obtain valuable information about family functioning.

Family Assessment Tools

Family assessment tools can be used to gather additional information about the family's functioning and can place particular focus on family stresses, coping strategies, and family strengths. Information about the way the family functions in nurturing its members, problem solving, and communicating may help identify strategies that are potentially more effective for management of the child's healthcare. They enable the nurse to work more effectively with the family, such as collaborating with the family in planning for health maintenance and health promotion strategies.

Genogram

Information about family structure can be illustrated on a **genogram** or pedigree which incorporates information about the family member's significant life events, health, and illness status over at least three generations. See Figure 4–13 on page 120. A genogram is used most often to focus on the health history of a family, although additional identifying features such as social class, occupation, place of residence, religion, and ethnicity may be added for the family assessment process.

Family Ecomap

An **ecomap** illustrates the family's relationships and interactions with social networks in the community, enabling the nurse and other healthcare providers to visualize the family's social network. Family participation in the preparation of the ecomap may reveal information about how the family perceives or receives social support, as well as the strength of family relation-

BOX 2–12 Family Assessment Information to Collect

- Name, age, sex, and family relationship of all people residing in the household
- Family type, structure, roles, and values
- Cultural associations, including cultural norms and customs related to child rearing and infant feeding
- Faith-based affiliations
- Support systems network, including extended family, friends, and faith-based and community associations
- Communication patterns, including language barriers
- Environmental data—place of residence, condition of housing, number of persons living in the residence, sleeping arrangements, play areas, neighborhood characteristics

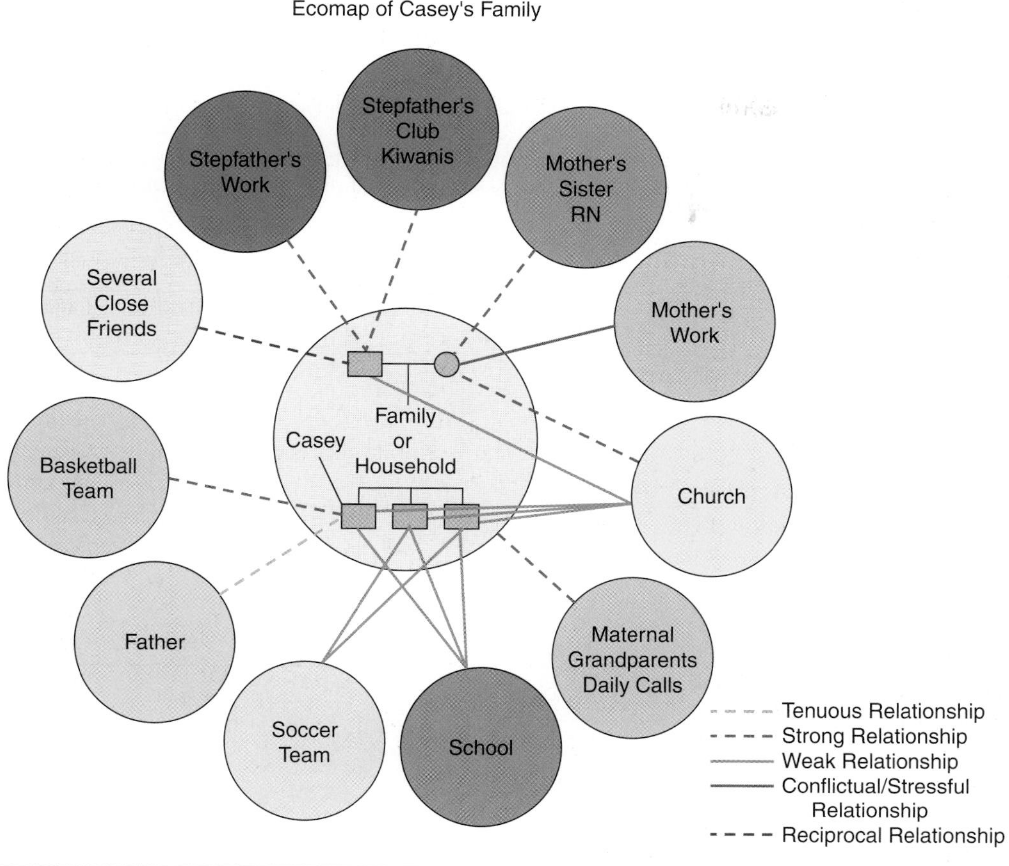

FIGURE 2–11 ■ An ecomap illustrates the family's relationships and interactions with groups and individuals in the immediate external environment.

ships with significant other persons and organizations. The ecomap provides an opportunity to identify the community resources being used by the family and to highlight any potential community resources that may help promote the family's health. Figure 2–11 ■ shows a sample ecomap for Casey's family.

Family APGAR

The Family APGAR is a quick five-item questionnaire that may be used as an initial screening tool for family assessment (Table 2–6). The five family concepts measured are family adaptability, partnership, growth, affection, and resolve. The five-item questionnaire can be administered quickly to family members over 10 years of age. Ask all family members to complete a separate copy of the questionnaire to gain a picture of the family's perspective on family functioning. Be more concerned if the majority of responses fall in the "hardly ever" category or responses vary widely among family members. This may indicate a family that needs much more support to cope with the demands of daily life and management of the child's condition.

Friedman Family Assessment Model

Friedman Family Assessment Model (FFAM), developed by Marilyn Friedman, is based on general systems theory, developmental theory, and structural-functional theory to provide a macroscopic view of families. This tool views the family as an open system and attention is directed to the family structure, functions, and the interplay of relationships with the social systems (Tarko & Reed, 2004). The FFAM has six broad categories (Friedman et al., 2003).

1. Identifying information
2. Developmental stage and developmental history of the family
3. Environmental data
4. Family structure
5. Family functions
6. Family stress, coping, and adaptation

A family genogram and ecomap are considered helpful in analyzing the data collected. See Box 2–13 for the short form of the FFAM.

Calgary Family Assessment Model

The Calgary Family Assessment Model, developed by Lorraine Wright and Maureen Leahy, is rooted in general systems theory in its approach for working with families (Wright & Leahy, 2000). The tool has three categories of information collected to help assess the family's strengths and problems.

- *Structural* family data include such information as family composition, extended family, and social aspects such as ethnicity and spirituality
- *Developmental* family data include information about the stages of the family's life cycle

TABLE 2–6 The Family APGAR Questionnaire

Directions

The following questions have been designed to help us better understand you and your family. You should feel free to ask questions about any item in the questionnaire.
The space for comments should be used when you wish to give additional information or if you wish to discuss the way the question is applied to your family. Please try to answer all questions. *Family* is defined as the individual(s) with whom you usually live. If you live alone, your family consists of persons with whom you now have the strongest emotional ties.[a]

For each question, check only one box.

	ALMOST ALWAYS 2	SOME OF THE TIME 1	HARDLY EVER 0
I am satisfied that I can turn to my family for help when something is troubling me. Comments: ______			
I am satisfied with the way my family talks over things with me and shares problems with me. Comments: ______			
I am satisfied that my family accepts and supports my wishes to take on new activities or directions. Comments: ______			
I am satisfied with the way my family expresses affection and responds to my emotions, such as anger, sorrow, and love. Comments: ______			
I am satisfied with the way my family and I share time together. Comments: ______			

[a] *According to which member of the family is being interviewed, the interviewer may substitute for the word* family *either* spouse, significant other, parents, *or* children. *Responses are scored either (2, 1, 0) and summed. The total score ranges from 0 to 10. The larger the score, the greater amount of satisfaction with family functioning.*

Note: Reprinted with permission from Smilkstein, G. (1978). The family APGAR: A proposal for a family function test and its use by physicians. Journal of Family Practice, *6(6), 1231–1239.*

- *Functional* family data include routines of daily living as well as roles and interactions involved in usual family activities.

The model enables assessment of extensive information about the family, but the originators of the model encourage focusing on specific data collection that matches the challenges that exist in the family, such as transitions of a child through adolescence or problems in managing a treatment plan within the family's routines. A family genogram or ecomap is also considered helpful in completing the assessment and ultimately in promoting a positive working relationship with the family.

Family Adaptability and Cohesion Evaluation Scales III

The Family Adaptability and Cohesion Evaluation Scales III (FACES III) provides an assessment of how individuals perceive their family and the description of their ideal family. The tool has 20 items that measure **family cohesion** (the level of attachment and emotional bonding between family members) and **family adaptability** (the ability of the family to change in power, structure, roles, and relationships to adjust to various situational stressors). Cohesion is graded as disengaged, separated, connected, and enmeshed. Adaptability is graded as rigid, structured, flexible, and chaotic. It can be used with diverse social and cultural groups to guide clinical practice.

The tool is self-administered twice, once to identify the ideal description and then to identify the individual's perceived description of his or her family. Children over 12 years can complete the scale for comparison with other family members. Examples of statements about the actual family include: "Family members ask

BOX 2–13 The Friedman Family Assessment Model (Short Form)

The following form is shortened for ease in assessing a family. If you are not sure what data should be covered in each of the assessment areas below, please refer to the original reference where more detailed questions/areas are presented.

Before using the following guidelines in completing family assessments, note that not all areas included below will be germane for each of the families visited. The guidelines are comprehensive and allow depth when probing is necessary. Do not feel that every subarea needs to be covered when the broad area of inquiry poses no problems to the family or concern to the health worker. Second, by virtue of the interdependence of the family system, one will find unavoidable redundancy. The assessor should try not to repeat data, but to refer the reader back to sections where this information has already been described.

IDENTIFYING DATA

1. Family Name
2. Address and Phone
3. Family Composition: The Family Genogram
4. Type of Family Form
5. Cultural (Ethnic) Background
6. Religious Identification
7. Social Class Status
8. Social Class Mobility

DEVELOPMENTAL STAGE AND HISTORY OF FAMILY

9. Family's Present Developmental Stage
10. Extent of Family Developmental Tasks Fulfillment
11. Nuclear Family History
12. History of Family of Origin of Both Parents

ENVIRONMENTAL DATA

13. Characteristics of Home
14. Characteristics of Neighborhood and Larger Community
15. Family's Geographical Mobility
16. Family's Associations and Transactions with Community

FAMILY STRUCTURE

17. Communication Patterns
    Extent of Functional and Dysfunctional Communication (types of recurring patterns)
    Extent of Emotional (Affective) Messages and How Expressed
    Characteristics of Communication Within Family Sub-systems
    Extent of Congruent and Incongruent Messages
    Types of Dysfunctional Communication Processes Seen in Family
    Areas of Closed Communication
    Familial and Contextual Variables Affecting Communication
18. Power Structure
    Power Outcomes
    Decision-making Process
    Power Bases
    Variables Affecting Family Power
    Overall Family System and Subsystem Power (Family Power Continuum Placement)
19. Role Structure
    Formal Role Structure
    Informal Role Structure
    Analysis of Role Models (optional)
    Variables Affecting Role Structure
20. Family Values
    Compare the family to American core values or family's reference group values and/or identify important family values and their importance (priority) in family.
    Congruence Between the Family's Values and the Family's Reference Group or Wider Community
    Disparity in Value Systems
    Presence of Value Conflicts in Family
    Effect of the Above Values and Value Conflicts on Health Status of Family

FAMILY FUNCTIONS

21. Affective Function
    Mutual Nurturance, Closeness, and Identification
    Separateness and Connectedness
    Family's Need–Response Patterns
22. Socialization Function
    Family Child-rearing Practices
    Adaptability of Child-rearing Practices for Family Form and Family's Situation
    Who Is (Are) Socializing Agent(s) for Child(ren)?
    Value of Children in Family
    Cultural Beliefs That Influence Family's Child-rearing Patterns
    Social Class Influence on Child-Rearing Patterns
    Estimation About Whether Family Is at Risk for Child-Rearing Problems and if So, Indication of High-Risk Factors
    Adequacy of Home Environment for Children's Needs to Play
23. Health Care Function
    Family's Health Beliefs, Values, and Behavior
    Family's Definitions of Health–Illness and Its Level of Knowledge
    Family's Perceived Health Status and Illness Susceptibility
    Family's Dietary Practices
    Adequacy of family diet (recommended 3-day food history record)
    Function of mealtimes and attitudes toward food and mealtimes.
    Shopping (and its planning) practices.
    Person(s) responsible for planning, shopping, and preparation of meals.
    Sleep and Rest Habits
    Physical Activity and Recreation Practices
    Family's Therapeutic and Recreational Drug, Alcohol, and Tobacco Practices
    Family's Role in Self-care Practices
    Medically Based Preventive Measures (physicals, eye and hearing tests, immunizations, dental care)
    Complementary and Alternative Therapies
    Family Health History (both general and specific diseases—environmentally and genetically related)
    Health Care Services Received
    Feelings and Perceptions Regarding Health Services
    Emergency Health Services
    Source of Payments for Health and Other Services
    Logistics of Receiving Care

FAMILY STRESS, COPING, AND ADAPTATION

24. Family Stressors, Strengths, and Perceptions
    Stressors Family Is Experiencing
    Strengths That Counterbalance Stressors
    Family's Definition of the Situation
25. Family Coping Strategies
    How the Family Is Reacting to the Stressors
    Extent of Family's Use of Internal Coping Strategies (past/present)
    Extent of Family's Use of External Coping Strategies (past/present)
    Dysfunctional Coping Strategies Utilized (past/present; extent of use)
26. Family Adaptation
    Overall Family Adaptation
    Estimation of Whether Family Is in Crisis
27. Tracking Stressors, Coping, and Adaptation Over Time

MediaLink Family Assessment Tools

each other for help" and "It is hard to identify the leaders in our family." Examples of statements about the ideal family include: "Family members would ask each other for help" and "We would know who the leader is in the family" (Olson, 1985). Differences in the scores identify how satisfied the individual is with his or her family. It can be used to assess changes in family functioning over time based on these two interrelated concepts.

Home Observation for Measurement of the Environment

The Home Observation for Measurement of the Environment (HOME) is an assessment tool developed to measure the quality and quantity of stimulation and support available to the child in the home environment (Caldwell & Bradley, 1984). Four age-specific scales are available (birth to 3 years, 3 to 6 years, 6 to 10 years, and 10 to 15 years). Examples of subscales within each age-specific scale include parental responsivity, acceptance of child, the physical environment, learning materials, variety in experience, and parental involvement. Data are collected during an informal, low-stress interview and observation over 45 to 90 minutes in the home setting. The child's primary caregiver and child must be present and awake during the interview. Observation of the parent–child interaction is an essential part of the assessment. The intent is to allow family members to act normally. Assessment of the home environment will help to identify factors that promote the child's growth and development. Examples of nursing interventions that could result from the HOME assessment include items that can be used in the home for toys and strategies for interacting with the child to promote learning.

NURSING MANAGEMENT

The goal of family-centered nursing management is to assess and help families recognize their strengths and resiliency. This information can then be used to collaboratively plan the nursing care with children and families.

Nursing Assessment and Diagnoses

The presence of a newly acquired disability, as occurred in Casey's family, adds a dimension of developmental risk for Casey and his family. The child and family members may respond with either psychologic or behavior problems, or they may respond in a more positive manner.

Collect the psychosocial history and daily living patterns data from the family and child. Select the appropriate family assessment tool to collect information that can help evaluate the family's strengths and resources. Analyze the information collected and focus on key information that will help develop a plan of care for Casey and his family.

- Determine how this condition influences family functioning.
- Identify how all of the family members have responded to the child's acute condition and disability.
- Obtain information about how the family is considering management of Casey's care at home.
- Determine if other family issues or stressors must be integrated into the plan of care.
- Identify the family's expectations of different health professionals and facilities to help manage Casey's care.
- Prepare an ecomap and genogram.

Examples of nursing diagnoses that may result from the family and home assessment include:

- Compromised Family Coping related to multiple simultaneous stressors
- Interrupted Family Processes related to child with a significant disability requiring alteration in family functioning
- Risk for Caregiver Role Strain related to child with a newly acquired disability and the associated financial burden
- Impaired Social Interaction (parents and child) related to lack of family or respite support

Planning and Implementation

Families need support to increase their resources and coping behaviors so they can successfully manage the multiple stressors, strains, and problems of daily living along with the child's chronic condition.

Establishing a therapeutic relationship with the family is an important intervention. This relationship should be characterized by empathy and trust, as well as the development of mutually identified goals for the child's care. To help families develop resiliency, focus on family competence and strengths. Acknowledge and validate their emotions. Provide information in a clear, timely, and sensitive manner. Ask questions that help direct the family's thinking rather than providing them with all of the answers. Work with families to create solutions until they are able to solve problems independently (Patterson, 1995). Linkage with other families who have faced similar situations may be helpful.

Assist the family to begin planning for ongoing care using family-centered principles.

- Discuss the family's goals for managing Casey's care in the home setting.
- Consider how the family's strengths and previous family problem-solving experiences can be integrated into the intervention.
- Consider the family's ethnic and religious background in developing intervention recommendations.
- Offer the family one or more potential interventions rather than trying to force one intervention. Be open to modifying the intervention or devising an alternate intervention to better match the family's lifestyle preferences.
- Identify what type of support or assistance the family would like to have.

Identify potential resources in the community that match the child's and the family's needs for support. Collaborate with the family to discuss those resources and to select those that are acceptable to the family. Make sure the family has a care coordinator, especially when a family member seems to be unable to assume the case management role initially. Assist families in obtaining resources through such actions as role rehearsal, providing instructions and support when making an initial call, or connecting with another family support person who can help with resource linkage. Refer families with moderate or severe dysfunction to community resources for social support and counseling as appropriate.

Evaluation

Expected outcomes of nursing care include:

- The family assumes the role of case manager or works effectively with an assigned case manager to implement the interventions recommended by nurse and healthcare team.
- The care needed by the child with an acquired disability is provided by the family according to recommended guidelines.

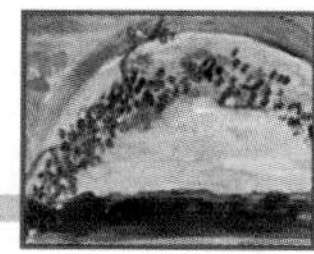

CHAPTER HIGHLIGHTS

- A family is composed of individuals who are joined together by marriage, blood, adoption, or residence in the same household, sharing resources and emotional closeness. Family membership often changes over time.
- Family-centered care is the development of a mutually beneficial partnership between families and the nurse, and also other health professionals. Each party respects the knowledge, skills, and experience that the other brings to the healthcare encounter. Partnering with families in the provision of health care is essential to promote the best outcome when caring for children.
- Various family composition models are common in today's society, such as the following: nuclear families, extended families, blended or reconstituted families, single-parent families, binuclear families, heterosexual cohabitating families, and gay and lesbian families.
- The changes and adjustment caused by the birth of a child cause unexpected stresses for the parents, such as changed relationships with their parents, attitudes and changes regarding employment, and lifestyle changes.
- Positive family relationships are characterized by parent-child warmth and supportiveness, and these traits help buffer children from stress while promoting positive social and cognitive outcomes.
- Parenting is a leadership role in the family in which children are guided to learn acceptable behaviors, beliefs, morals, and rituals of the family, and to become socially responsible contributing members of society.
- Discipline is a method for teaching the rules that govern behavior or conduct, or the action taken to enforce the rules when a child misbehaves.
- The quality of the relationship between the divorced parents has an important impact on the future relationships their children. Better maintenance of family and kinship ties results when divorced parents are able to minimize the conflict and continue sharing parenting.
- Stepparenting that involves the blending of two families leads to the need to identify and renegotiate new customs, traditions, rituals, and routines for the family. Adjustment of the child to the stepparent and the stepparent to the child are necessary.
- The goal of foster care is to ensure the safety and well-being of vulnerable children by placing them in an approved living situation away from the family of origin that is legally coordinated by the state's child welfare system.
- Adoption is a legal relationship between a child and parents not related by birth in which the parents assume legal and financial responsibility for the child. Many children are adopted from foreign nations.
- Family social systems theories help in understanding the family functioning, environment-family interchange, family changes over time, and family response to health and illness.
- Resilience is the family's capacity to develop strengths and abilities to bounce back from the stresses and challenges faced, and to eliminate or minimize negative outcomes.
- Family strengths are the relationships and processes that support and protect families and family members during times of adversity and change. These strengths enable families to develop, adapt to change, and cope with challenges.
- Family assessment tools are used to gather information about the family's functioning with regard to characteristics such as nurturing its members, problem solving, and communication. Information gathered helps the nurse work more effective with the family in meeting the child's health care needs.

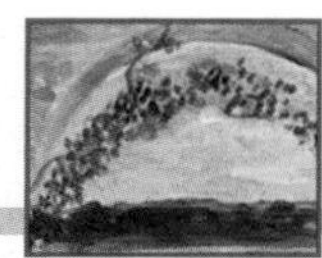

CRITICAL THINKING IN ACTION

INTRODUCTION

Reflect back to the scenario about Casey and his family at the beginning of the chapter, and review the ecomap on page 57. Casey's family is coping with his initial survival of a serious brain injury, and facing a long rehabilitation process. Family members are just now recognizing that life as they have known it is changing.

DESCRIPTION

Casey is totally dependent on others for care including bathing, toileting, feeding, and mobilizing. While he is expected to regain self-care abilities, the impact of the injury on his cognitive ability and future functioning is unknown.

Casey's extended family has provided support to the family during the past 12 days, but the level of support in the future weeks will decrease because of other family obligations. Casey's aunt, a nurse, has been especially helpful to his family during the initial crisis. Casey's mother has already initiated a leave of absence from work so she can care for him when he returns home; however, this will mean the family has reduced income during that time period. Casey's sister, Teresa, will try to earn more money babysitting to help the family out. Casey's younger brothers have been able to visit him, but they are very anxious because Casey cannot talk with them. They have been trying to avoid bothering their mother and father during this time, but they wonder when life will be more normal and they can again participate in their usual after-school activities.

DISCUSSION

1. What information about family strengths, needs, and resilience can be identified from the scenario, the information on page 55, the ecomap on page 57, and the information above?
2. What additional information would be helpful to know about family strengths and needs prior to developing a nursing care plan?
3. Based on your assessment of the family and challenges facing them, list at least one nursing diagnosis (in addition to those listed on page 60) that addresses an issue important for planning nursing care for Casey and his family.
4. Describe the use of family-centered care principles in planning Casey's nursing care in collaboration with the family.
5. What potential parenting issues could this family anticipate for Casey and his brothers?

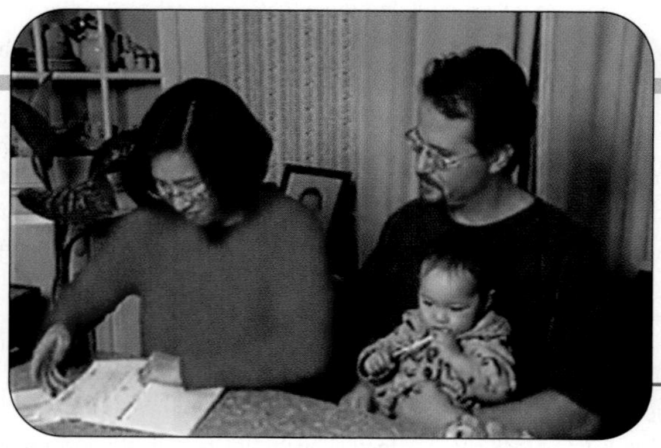

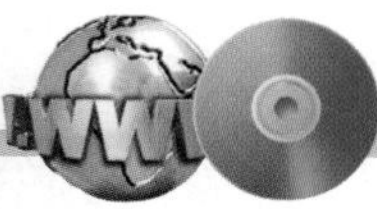

EXPLORE MediaLink

- NCLEX review, case studies, and other interactive resources for this chapter can be found on the Companion Website at **www.prenhall.com/ball**. Click on Chapter 2 to select the activities for this chapter.
- For animations, more NCLEX review questions, and an audio glossary, access the accompanying CD-ROM in this book.

http://www.prenhall.com/ball

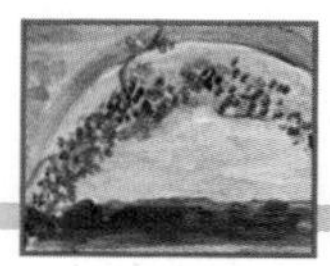

REFERENCES

Ahrons, C. R. (2003). *The facts about divorce.* Council on Contemporary Families. www.contemporaryfamilies.org/public/fact2.php, accessed 3/24/2004.

Allshouse, C., & Goldberg, P. F. (2003). *Working with doctors: A parent's guide to navigating the health system.* Minneapolis: Pacer Center, Inc.

Amato, P. R. (2000). The consequences of divorce for adults and children. *Journal of Marriage and the Family, 62*(4), 1269–1287.

American Academy of Pediatrics. (2004). Fathers and pediatricians: Enhancing men's roles in the care and development of their children. *Pediatrics, 113*(5), 1406–1411.

American Academy of Pediatrics, Committee on Psychosocial Aspects of Child and Family Health. (2002a). Coparent or second parent adoption by same-sex parents. *Pediatrics, 109*(3), 339–340.

American Academy of Pediatrics, Committee on Early Childhood, Adoption, and Dependent Care. (2002b). Health care of young children in foster care. *Pediatrics, 109*(3), 536–541.

American Academy of Pediatrics, Committee on Early Childhood, Adoption, and Dependent Care. (2001). The pediatrician's role in family support programs. *Pediatrics, 107*(1), 195–197.

American Academy of Pediatrics, Committee on Early Childhood, Adoption, and Dependent Care. (2000). Developmental issues for young children in foster care. *Pediatrics, 106*(5), 1145–1150.

American Academy of Pediatrics, Committee on Hospital Care and the Institute of Family Centered Care. (2003). Family-centered care and the pediatrician's role. *Pediatrics, 112*(3), 691–696.

Annie E. Casey Foundation. (2004). 2000 Census data—Living arrangements profile for United States. KIDS COUNT census data online. www.aecf.org, accessed 3/1/2004.

Ariel, J. & McPherson, D. (2000). Therapy with lesbian and gay families and their children. *Journal of Marital and Family Therapy, 26*(4), 421–432.

Barbell, K., & Freundlich, M. (2001). Foster care today. Washington, DC: Casey Family Programs. www.casey.org, accessed 2/11/2004.

Barclay, L., & Lupton, D. (1999). The experiences of new fatherhood. A socio-cultural analysis. *Journal of Advanced Nursing, 29*, 1013–1020.

Bass, S., Shields, M. K., & Behrman, R. E. (2004). Children, families, and foster care: Analysis and recommendations. *The Future of Children, 14*(1), 5–29.

Baumrind, D. (1971). Current patterns of parental authority. *Developmental Psychology, 4*, 1–103.

Borchers and Committee on Early Childhood, Adoption, and Dependent Care, American Academy of Pediatrics. (2003). Families and adoption: The pediatrician's role in supporting communication. *Pediatrics, 112*(6), 1437–1441.

Bronfenbrenner, U., & Morris, P. A. (1998). The ecology of developmental processes. In W. Damon & R. M. Lerner (Eds.), *Handbook of child psychology, Vol. 1: Theoretical models of human development* (5th ed., pp. 993–1028). New York: John Wiley.

Caldwell, B. M., & Bradley, R. H. (1984). *The home observation for measurement of the environment*. Little Rock: University of Arkansas.

Chipungu, S. S., & Bent-Goodley, T. B. (2004). Meeting the challenges of contemporary foster care. *The Future of Children, 14*(1), 75–93.

Council on Contemporary Families. (2003). America's changing families: The 2000 census. www.contemporaryfamilies.org/public/families.php, accessed 3/24/2004.

Craig, G. J., & Baucum, D. (1999). *Human development* (8th ed.). Upper Saddle River, NJ: Prentice Hall.

Duvall, E. M. (1977). *Marriage and family development* (5th ed.). New York: Harper & Row.

Duvall, E. M., & Miller, B. L. (1985). *Marriage and family development* (6th ed.). New York: Harper & Row.

Equality in Marriage Institute, 2000, www.equalityinmarriage.org, accessed 7/22/2004.

Family and Medical Leave Act of 1993, Public Law 103-3. 5 U.S.C. Chapter 63 6381–6387; 5 CFR part 630, subpart L. www.cpms.osd.mil/vip/per_data/586.htm, accessed 7/12/2004.

Feeley, N., & Gottlieb, L. N. (2000). Nursing approaches for working with family strengths and resources. *Journal of Family Nursing, 6*(1), 9–24.

Friedman, M. M., Bowden, V. R., & Jones, E. G. (2003). *Family nursing: Research, theory, and practice* (5th ed.). Upper Saddle River, NJ: Prentice Hall.

FRIENDS National Resource Center for Community-based Family Resource and Support Programs. (2001). Family support and intergenerational programming (Fact Sheet No. 5). Chapel Hill, NC: Author. www.friendsnrc.org, accessed 2/11/2004.

Gottesman, M. M. (2001). Children in foster care: A nursing perspective on research, policy, and child health issues. *Journal of the Society of Pediatric Nurses, 6*(2), 55–64.

Graefe, D. R., & Lichter, D. T. (1999). Life course transitions of American children. Parental cohabitation, marriage, and single motherhood. *Demography, 36*(2), 205–217.

Green, R. (2004). The evolution of kinship care policy and practice. *The Future of Children, 14*(1), 131–149.

Halle, T., & Le Menestrel, S. (2002). How do social, economic, and cultural factors influence fathers' involvement with their children? Child Trends Research Brief. www.childtrends.org, accessed 12/5/2003.

Hanson, J. L., & Randall, V. F. (1999). Evaluating and improving the practice of family-centered care. *Pediatric Nursing, 25*(4), 445–449.

Institute for Family Centered Care. (2004). Patient and family resource centers. www.familycenteredcare.org/special_topics/familyresource/main.html, accessed 3/12/2004.

Jefferson, R., & Paterson, B. (2001). Efficient or family-centered? Practitioners goals in decisions regarding parental presence during invasive procedures. *Dynamics, 12*(3), 14–20.

Lewandowski, L. A. & Tesler, M. D. (Eds.). (2003). Family-centered care: Putting it into action. *The SPN/ANA guide to family-centered care*. Washington, DC: American Nurses Association.

Liao, E., & Beery, J. (2001). *Working with the family to enhance emergency medical services for children* (2nd ed.). Washington, DC: Emergency Medical Services for Children National Resource Center.

Maccoby, E. E. (1980). *Social development: Psychological growth and the parent-child relationship*. New York: Harcourt Brace Jovanovich.

McCubbin, M. A. & McCubbin, H. I. (1991). Family stress theory and assessment: The resiliency model of family stress, adjustment and adaptation. In H. I. McCubbin & A. Thompson (Eds.), Family assessment inventories for research and practice (pp. 3–32). Madison, WI: University of Wisconsin-Madison.

Meyers, T. A., Eichhorn, D. J., & Guzzetta, C. E. (1998). Do family members want to be present during CPR? A retrospective study. *Journal of Emergency Nursing, 24*(5), 400–405.

Miller, L. C. (1999). Caring for internationally adopted children. *New England Journal of Medicine, 341*(20), 1539–1540.

Moore, K. A., Chalk, R., Scarpa, J., & Vandivere, S. (2002). Family strengths: Often overlooked, but real. Child Trends Research Brief. www.childtrends.org, accessed 12/5/2003.

Munro, H., & D'Errico, C. (2000). Parental involvement in perioperative anesthetic management. *Journal of PeriAnesthesia Nursing, 15*(6), 397–400.

Murray, R. B., & Zentner, J. P. (2001). *Health promotion strategies through the lifespan* (7th ed.). Upper Saddle River, NJ: Prentice Hall.

Nelson, S., Clark, R. L., & Acs, G. (2001). Beyond the two-parent family: How teenagers fare in cohabitating couple and blended families (Series B, No. B-31). Washington, DC: The Urban Institute www.urban.org, accessed 1/28/2004.

Ochieng, B. M. N. (2003). Minority ethnic families and family-centered care. *Journal of Child Health Care, 7*(2), 123–132.

Olson, D. H. (1985). FACES III (Family Adaptation and Cohesion Scales). St. Paul: University of Minnesota. www.clas/uiuc.edu/special/evaltools/c100945.htm, accessed 3/1/2004.

Patterson, J. (1991). A family systems perspective for working with youth with disability. *Pediatrician, 18*, 129–141.

Patterson, J. M. (1995). Promoting resilience in families experiencing stress. *Pediatric Clinics of North America, 42*(1), 47–63.

Peterson, K. S. (2003, September 18). Unmarried with children: For better or worse? *USA Today*, 1A, 8A.

Powers, K. S., & Rubenstein, J. S. (1999). Family presence during invasive procedures in pediatric intensive care unit: A prospective study. *Archives of Pediatric and Adolescent Medicine, 153*, 955–958.

Sammons, W. (2003). Divorce: How you can help the family. *Contemporary Pediatrics, 20*(9), 33–35.

Sobel, A., & Healy, C. (2001). Fostering health in the foster care maze. *Pediatric Nursing, 27*(5), 493–497.

Sullivan-Bolyai, S., Sadler, L., Knafl, K. A., & Gillis, C. L. (2004). Great expectations: A position description for parents as caregivers: Part II. *Pediatric Nursing, 30*(1), 52–56.

Tarko, M. A., & Reed, K. (2004). Family assessment and intervention. In P. J. Bomar, *Promoting health in families* (3rd ed., pp. 274–298). Philadelphia: Saunders.

Urban Institute. (2003a). Gay and lesbian families in the census: Couples with children. Washington, DC: Author. www.urban.org, accessed 01/28/2004.

Urban Institute. (2003b). Who will adopt the foster care children left behind. Washington, DC: Author. www.urban.org, accessed 2/1/2004.

U.S. Bureau of the Census. (2002). Living arrangements of children under 18 years of age: 1960 to present. www.census.gov/population/hh-fam/tabCH-1.xls, accessed 01/28/2002.

U.S. Department of Health and Human Services. (2001). Indicators of welfare reform. Annual report to Congress 2001. Table Birth 4. Washington, DC: Author.

U.S. Department of Health and Human Services. (2002). The AFCARS Report, No. 7: Interim FY 2000 estimates. www.acf.hhs.gov/programs/cb, accessed 12/28/2003.

U.S. Department of Health and Human Services. (2003). National Adoption and Foster Care Statistics. www.acf.hhs.gov/progrmas/cb/dis/afcars/publications/afcars.htm, accessed 2/11/2004.

U.S. Department of State. (2004). Immigrant visas issued to orphans coming to the U.S. http://travel.state.gov/orphan_numbers.html, accessed 2/11/2004.

Wald, M. S. (1999). *Same-sex couples: Marriage, families, and children.* Stanford, CA: Stanford Law School.

Wertheimer, R. (2002). Youth who "age out" of foster care: Troubled lives, troubling prospects. Child Trends Research Brief. www.childtrends.org, accessed 12/5/2003.

Wolchik, S. A., Sandler, I. N., Millsap, R. E., Plummer, B. A., Greene, S. M., Anderson, E. R., Dawson-McClure, S. R., Hipke, K., & Haine, R. A. (2002). Six-year follow-up of preventive interventions for children of divorce: A randomized controlled trial. *Journal of the American Medical Association, 288*(15), 1874–1881.

Wolfram, R. W., & Turner, E. D. (1996). Effects of parental presence during children's venipuncture. *Academic Emergency Medicine, 3*, 58–64.

Wright, L., & Leahy, M. (2000). *Nurses and families: A guide to family assessment and intervention* (3rd ed.). Philadelphia: FA Davis.

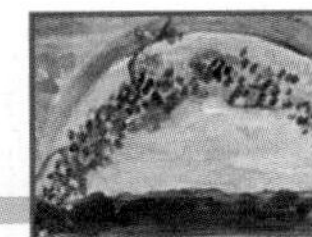

ADDITIONAL REFERENCES

Alperson, M. (2001). *Dim sum bagels and grits: A sourcebook for multicultural families.* New York: Farrar, Straus and Giroux.

Hallas, D. (2002). A model for successful foster child–foster parent relationships. *Journal of Pediatric Health Care, 16*(3), 112–118.

Chapter 3

Cultural Influences

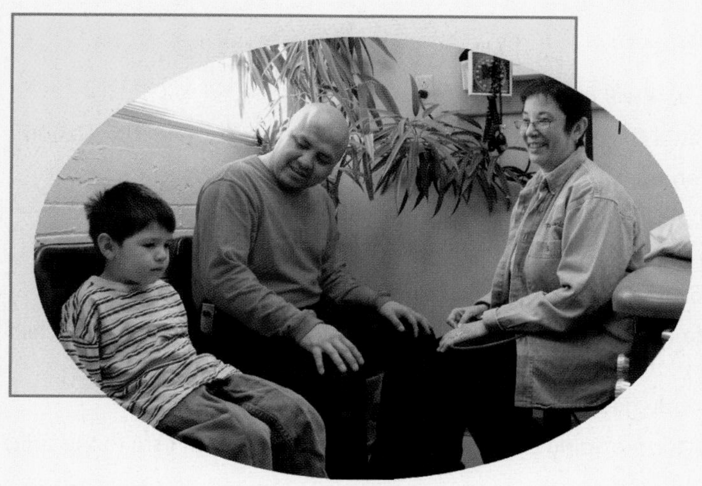

Raven Roanhorse is a 4-year-old male brought to the health clinic by his father, Alex. He is a Native American boy growing up on a reservation and is one of four children in the family who recently began to go to the clinic in a nearby town for healthcare. The nurse there has formed a positive relationship with Raven's family. Alex appreciates Carol's concern and rapport with the family and asks to see her when he brings in his children.

The purpose for the visit to the clinic is to evaluate Raven due to complaints of an earache. Alex also requests that Raven receive a thorough health examination and asks the nurse to identify and provide intervention for any health concerns. Alex acknowledges that the family has never taken Raven to a conventional healthcare facility, and that his care has always been given by the family or tribal healer. Some immunizations have been administered at a tribal clinic on the reservation. He adds that Raven has never experienced any major illnesses, but has been treated routinely by the tribal healer for "usual childhood illnesses" such as colds, fever, and stomachaches.

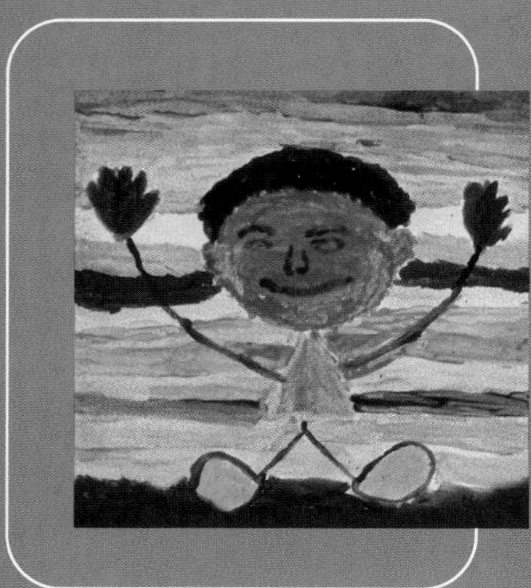

"I don't want to talk to her . . . I want Mimi, she makes me feel better."

—Raven, age 4

Key Terms

acculturation/70
alternative medicine/83
assimilation/70
complementary medicine/83
cultural competence/71
culture/67
curandero/a/80
ethnicity/69
ethnocentrism/70
faith-based belief/82
folk healers/80
holistic health belief/80
immigrant/70
magico-religious belief view/80
prejudice/70
race/69
refugee/71
religion/82
scientific or biomedical health belief/80
spirituality/82
stereotyping/70

Learning Outcomes

After completing this chapter, you will be able to:

- Discuss specific concepts related to culture such as diversity, race, ethnicity, and assimilation.
- Describe cultural influences on the family's beliefs about health, illness, and treatments.
- Identify cultural disparities in healthcare and barriers to healthcare for the child and family.
- Describe the various uses of complementary and alternative medicine in child healthcare.
- Describe and examine the role of the nurse in promoting cultural competence.
- Apply strategies for nurses to achieve cultural competence when providing care to the child and family.
- Identify nursing assessment strategies for various components of culture.
- Discuss nursing interventions for providing culturally sensitive and competent care to the child and family.

MediaLink 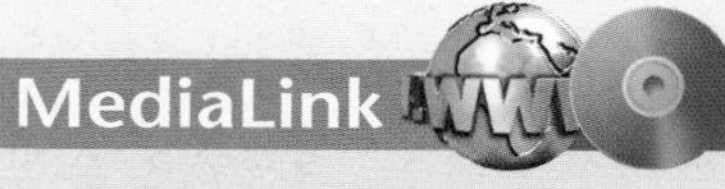 **http://www.prenhall.com/ball**

Resources for this chapter can be found on the CD-ROM accompanying this textbook and on the Companion Website at www.prenhall.com/ball. Click on Chapter 3 to select the activities for this chapter.

CD-ROM

Videos

Deaf Culture
Developing Cultural Competence

NCLEX Review

Audio Glossary

COMPANION WEBSITE

NCLEX Review

MediaLink Applications

Examine Your Cultural Influences

The United States and Canada are undergoing demographic shifts resulting in increasingly varied ethnic and cultural groups. Improved transportation capabilities, sponsorship of individuals and families from countries with limited opportunities for work or with dangerous political situations, and assistance from family members already in North America are some of the reasons for immigration. Nurses will come into contact with families of diverse backgrounds who seek healthcare for their children. Children, in turn, meld and reflect the cultures of both parents, in their own specific adaptation and manifestation. In response, nurses must continually strive to provide culturally competent care to children and their families. While it is impossible to know all of the mores (customs) and values of each culture, the nurse who possesses an understanding of the cultural factors that influence the child and family can accurately assess those factors and incorporate them into an individualized plan to deliver culturally competent, family-centered care to individual children.

Culture is not strictly defined by race, ethnicity, and geography. Culture is far broader: Many groups form customs, ways of viewing the world, and patterns of behavior and therefore can be described as cultures. Examples of these groups might include those with hearing impairments, gays and lesbians, and professional groups such as nurses.

This chapter provides an overview of culture and related concepts and the associated influences on health and healthcare for the child and family. Cultural competence is described as an essential element of nursing care, and specific examples are provided in the nursing management section to assist in applying the nursing process when working with culturally diverse children, families, and populations.

CULTURE—DEFINITIONS AND BASIC CONCEPTS

Culture has many definitions and is currently described as "the thoughts, communication, actions, customs, beliefs, values, and institutions of racial, ethnic, religious, or social groups" (Office of Minority Health, 2001, p. 131). Culture is important to study since it determines how people perceive health and healthcare. Specifically, culture informs people about how to view the body, mind, and spirit; what to do to maintain health; and what is acceptable as healthcare treatment. The child's concept of health is formed while growing up in a culture with its unique approaches and belief systems.

An overview of definitions of culture according to several common theories is provided in Table 3–1. These theories offer threads that, when woven together, create a foundation which nurses can utilize to understand and integrate culture into nursing care of children and families. They all involve partnering and collaborating with families in order to include cultural approaches into planned interventions. Several distinct theories and approaches are discussed throughout this chapter.

TABLE 3–1 Definitions of Culture

THEORIST	DEFINITION
Giger & Davidhizar (2004)	A patterned behavioral response that develops over time as a consequence of imprinting the mind through social and religious structures and intellectual and artistic manifestations
Leininger (2002)	The learned, shared, and transmitted values, beliefs, norms, and lifeways of a particular group
Purnell & Paulanka (2003)	The totality of socially transmitted behavioral patterns, arts, beliefs, values, customs, lifeways, and all other products of human work and thought characteristics of a population that guide their worldview and decision making
Spector (2004)	The nonphysical traits, such as values, beliefs, practices, habits, attitudes, and customs, that are shared by a group of people and passed from one generation to the next

Culture and Nurse Theorists

Although numerous theories about culture have been developed and described to provide a framework for understanding and assessment, four theories developed by and directly applicable to nursing are described here. One important theory is *culture care diversity and universality*, developed by nurse anthropologist Dr. Madeleine Leininger. In the 1950s, Leininger predicted that nurses in the future would need to understand more about culture to provide nursing care, and that care was foundational to nursing but would change in the next decades. She developed her visionary concepts by travel and work with various cultural groups; many of her views were formed by caring for children in these cultures. Leininger views care as an essential part of nursing and believes that all care must be culturally based in order to contribute to the well-being, healing, growth, and survival of healthcare recipients (Leininger, 2001, 2002). Leininger's "sunrise model" suggests the importance of certain factors in understanding one's sense of holistic health. Its components are useful assessment guides for nurses.

- Cultural values and lifeways
- Political and legal factors
- Economic factors
- Education factors
- Kinship and social factors
- Religious and philosophical factors
- Technological factors

Dr. Larry Purnell is another nurse theorist who has developed a useful approach to assessing and planning culturally based nursing care. Purnell's *model for cultural competence* describes important components of the individual, family, and community with the larger global society (Purnell, 2002; Purnell & Paulanka, 2003). He identified 12 major concepts that are common to all cultures and that can be assessed to provide important information about an individual child and family. They are:

- Overview, inhabited localities, topography
- Communication
- Family roles and organization
- Workforce issues
- Biocultural ecology
- High-risk health behaviors
- Nutrition

MediaLink Deaf Culture Video

- Pregnancy and child-bearing practices
- Death rituals
- Spirituality
- Healthcare practices
- Healthcare practitioners

You may choose to use these categories to focus your questions during assessments of children from various cultures. For a family recently immigrated to this country, you might ask about the life history: "What places have you lived in? What did those countries or geographic areas look like? Were you in a temporary shelter? How did you travel here? What do you miss about your native land?" Consider the area of family roles. When caring for a child recently diagnosed with type 1 diabetes, what questions about family roles are important to plan teaching that fits within the family's cultural patterns?

Dr. Joyce Newman Giger and Dr. Ruth Davidhizar are nurse theorists who have examined transcultural nursing. Giger and Davidhizar (2002, 2004) developed the *transcultural assessment model* in direct response to student need for a framework that would provide structure for assessments of health clients. In this framework, the client is the center of care and culturally unique; knowledge of the cultural heritage, beliefs, attitudes, and behaviors of the client is required to provide culturally competent care. This model is based on six phenomena that must be assessed by nurses. They are:

- Communication
- Space
- Social organization
- Time
- Environmental control
- Biological variations

For example, the concept of space involves information about the distance or proximity that is comfortable for persons during interactions with others, information about visual and auditory perception, skin membranes, and body movements or positions. The nurse is alert for the child's eye contact patterns, ability to hear and see, positioning in the bed or chair, and response to touch. Such observations, combined with data from the health record and responses of the child and family members, will help the nurse to structure the space to best support healing in the child. What do you know about differences in eye contact among cultural groups? Look back to Raven in the opening scenario. Many Native American groups are uncomfortable with prolonged eye contact, and will look away even while speaking or listening to someone. How will you adapt your care when dealing with a child who does not return eye contact? What are your own cultural patterns regarding eye contact, proximity to other people, and touch? In the next section we will explore more fully concepts such as time and communication, in addition to their links to healthcare provision.

An additional view of health is provided by the nurse Dr. Rachel Spector. According to Spector (2004), HEALTH (written in this manner to indicate the model) reflects the balance of the person—physical, mental, and spiritual—in the outside world. The *HEALTH traditions model* is predicated on the concept of holistic health and describes practices that can be used to maintain, protect, and restore health (Table 3–2). According to Spector, health is a complex, interrelated, and balanced state of the body, mind, and spirit. These facets of health are as follows:

- The *body*—all physical aspects, such as gender, age, nutrition, genetic inheritance, body chemistry, and physical condition
- The *mind*—cognitive processes, such as memories, thoughts, and knowledge of such emotional processes as feelings, self-esteem, and defenses
- The *spirit*—both positive and negative learned spiritual practices and teachings, dreams, stories, symbols; protecting forces; and metaphysical or innate forces

Contexts must also be considered, including the person's family, culture, work, community, history, and environment. The person must be in a state of balance within all personal and contextual parts. Illness occurs as a result of imbalance of one or all parts of the person (mind, body, spirit). When applying this theory, the nurse assesses the child's physical, cognitive, and spiritual states and examines all of the contexts in which the child has experiences.

TABLE 3–2 Spector's Facets of Health (Physical, Mental, and Spiritual) and Personal Methods of Maintaining, Protecting, and Restoring Health

	PHYSICAL	MENTAL	SPIRITUAL
MAINTAIN HEALTH	Proper clothing Proper diet Exercise/rest	Concentration Social and family support systems Hobbies	Religious worship Prayer Meditation
PROTECT HEALTH	Special foods and food combinations Symbolic clothing	Avoid certain people who can cause illness Family activities	Religious customs Superstitions Wearing amulets and other symbolic objects to protect from the "evil eye" or defray other sources of harm
RESTORE HEALTH	Homeopathic remedies, lineaments Herbal teas Special foods Massage Acupuncture/moxibustion	Relaxation Exorcism Curanderos and other traditional healers Nerve teas	Religious rituals, special prayers Meditation Traditional healings Exorcism

From Spector, R. (2004). Cultural diversity in health and illness *(p. 76). Upper Saddle River, NJ: Prentice Hall.*

This theory directly relates to activities that are described in the unit on health promotion (which Spector calls health protection) and health maintenance later in this text. See Chapter 10∞ for further description of health promotion and health maintenance.

Application of Cultural Theories

The previous section describes four frameworks that can be used as you assess cultural influences and work with children and families. Although there are many descriptions of culture, key elements are common to many of the theories. Some of these components are explored in this section.

- *Culture is based on shared values and beliefs.* Each culture identifies and articulates its shared values and beliefs. A view of the world develops that determines actions. Expected behaviors and roles emerge that are consistent with those values and beliefs. This belief system suggests what preventive health measures and treatment for diseases are sought and accepted. It may also state the importance of children, the family, other individuals, and the collective group, all of which can influence the choices people in the culture make regarding health.
- *Culture is learned and dynamic.* A child is born into a culture and starts learning the beliefs and practices of the group from birth. Children who are members of two cultural groups, such as African and immigrant, learn about both groups as they grow and develop. Immigrants may face challenges when integrating the rules of the dominant culture. Children who have family members from two or more cultural groups integrate parts of the worldview from each group. Therefore, although culture is connected with groups, each individual's manifestation of his or her own cultural background will be unique. Culture is therefore dynamic and constantly changing. It evolves and adapts as new members are born into or join the group, and as the surrounding social and physical environments change. For example, as first generation immigrants enter a new country they generally closely follow the cultural patterns of their native lands. As their children grow, the youth maintain some of the family cultural patterns but begin to incorporate some of the new culture (Figure 3–1 ■).
- *Culture is integrated into life and uses symbols.* Culture is integrated through social institutions such as schools, friendships, families, and occupations (Figure 3–2 ■). This provides a variety of opportunities for learning about one's culture. The sense of integration may be disrupted or harder to maintain as individuals move frequently and as cultures intertwine with each other. Symbols are an important way that many cultures communicate with each other and with the outside world. Language, dress, music, tools, and nonverbal gestures are symbols a culture uses to display and transmit the culture.

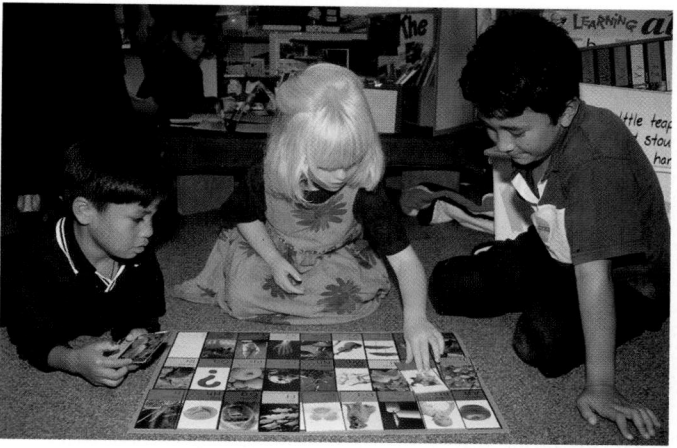

FIGURE 3–1 ■ A group of preschoolers from various cultural backgrounds plays together. When do children typically learn there are differences in cultures? How do they learn those differences? How can nurses partner with families to assist children to understand and respect cultural differences?

Definitions Related to Culture

It is important to understand several definitions related to culture. It is assumed that you have had prior courses and discussions about culture, so terms are briefly defined here and related to pediatric nursing. **Race** refers to a group of people who share biological similarities such as skin color, bone structure, and genetic traits. Examples of races include White (sometimes called Caucasian or European American), Black, Hispanic, Natives (such as Native Americans, Alaskan Native, Hawaiian Native, and First Nation people of Canada), and Asian. **Ethnicity** describes one's cultural background and a sense of identity to a group within the social system that has distinct characteristics of language, ancestry, race, national origin, or religion (Office of Minority Health, 2001). Examples of ethnic groups include African Americans, Hmong, Jewish, and Irish Americans. Ethnicity is the group's identity, or perception, of itself. It may be demonstrated when a group's members feel different from other groups; come from a common ancestry, country, or region; enjoy certain foods; speak a distinct language; practice a certain religious faith; have dances, music, or other pastimes; dress in a distinct way; or share other practices and background with group members. Even the mainstream or majority

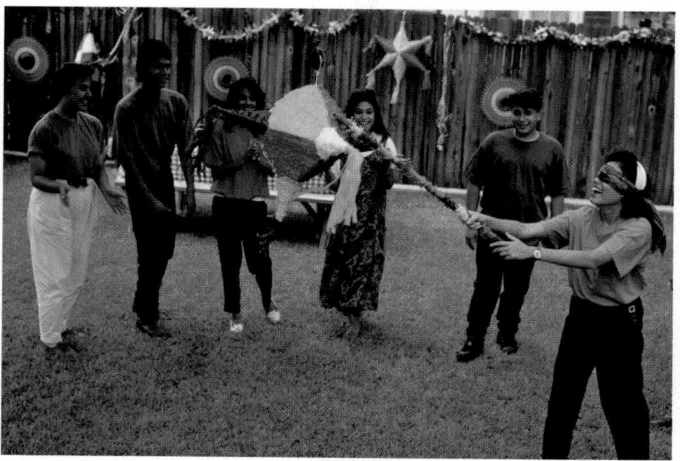

FIGURE 3–2 ■ These children are engaged in a cultural birthday tradition of breaking the piñata. Maintaining cultural traditions is one way families can continue their cultural heritage. Can you think of other common cultural traditions related to special occasions?

groups usually identify with some ethnic group. How would you describe your own ethnic identity? Is it based on your race, the country of origin of your parents, or the place where you live? How does your ethnic group determine your views of health and the type of healthcare you seek?

Think of some of the children you are working with in clinical settings. What are predominant ethnic groups in your area? What languages are spoken? Do children and their parents speak the same languages? What countries are represented? Are certain holidays commonly celebrated? Is there a common faith-based practice? Are certain ethnic groups more receptive in general to healthcare teaching and other interventions? Do some practice herbal medicine or other approaches? Some of these practices will be discussed later in the chapter.

Stereotyping is assuming that all members of a group have the same characteristics. When caring for a Hispanic child, a nurse who stereotypes would assume that the child speaks Spanish or that the parents are migrant farm workers. Each situation must be individually assessed to see which characteristics common to a group are possessed by a particular child rather than ascribing all traits to the child. **Prejudice** is a negative stereotype about certain groups that are applied to all individuals within the group. All people at times demonstrate **ethnocentrism,** or believing that one's own ethnic perspective and way of thinking is best. This belief necessarily affects all relationships with others. Think about how you treat a cold, what food you think is best to eat if you have an upset stomach, or how you think a child should be toilet trained. How can you work with children and families in a way that honors their beliefs and health practices rather than simply presenting the practices that are common in your ethnic group? **Acculturation** refers to modifying one's culture to fit within the new or dominant culture. **Assimilation** is related to acculturation and is described as adopting and incorporating traits of the new culture within one's practices (Spector, 2004). Awareness of these cultural concepts will enhance your ability to learn about diverse cultural groups, understand their concepts of health, work with individuals in the culture to evaluate their particular health practices, and become effective in planning nursing care for children of many racial and ethnic backgrounds.

DEMOGRAPHICS AND CULTURAL DIVERSITY IN THE UNITED STATES AND CANADA

According to the U.S. census of 2000, the White, non-Hispanic majority comprises 75.1% of the population, whereas it was 80.3% in 1990, and 83% in 1980 (U.S. Census Bureau, 2003). Changing demographics are apparent by examining these statistics. Considering current data, minority groups now represent approximately 25% of the population and are steadily growing. It is predicted that by the year 2020, there will be more people of color than Whites in the United States. Canada has shown a similar demographic shift. While over 13% of the Canadian census is now from minority populations, the number is growing and the youngest age groups demonstrate the highest percentages of minority members (Statistics Canada, 2004). The populations of children by race in the United States and Canada are identified in Figure 3–3 ■.

During the 1990s, the United States experienced an influx of millions of immigrants and refugees. **Immigrants** are individuals who are foreign born (anyone who is not born a U.S. citizen)

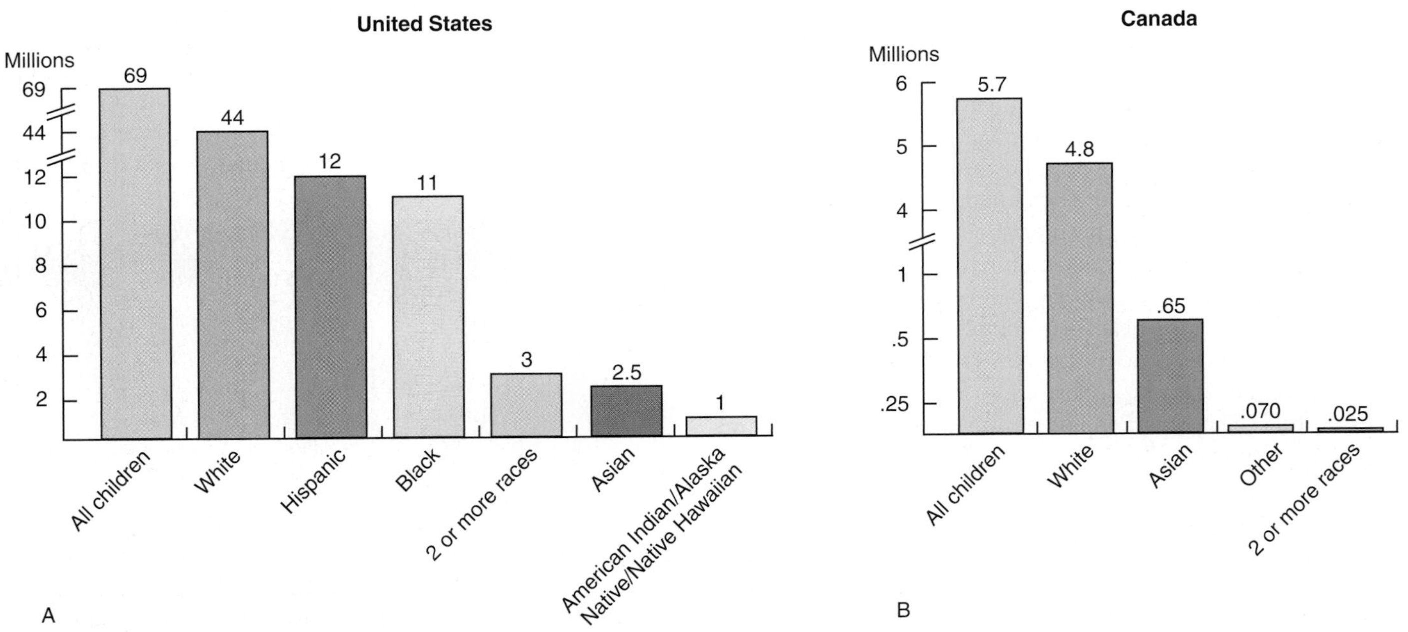

FIGURE 3–3 ■ Population of children in the U.S. and Canadian census. *A,* Population of children under 18 years by race in the 2000 U.S. census. U.S. Census Bureau. (2001). *Data from: Population by age, sex, race, and Hispanic or Latino origin for the United States: 2000. www.census.gov/population/cen2000/ phc-td/tab01.xls. B,* Population of children under age 15 years by race in the 2001 Canadian census. *Data from: Canadian Statistics. (2001). Visible minority population by age group. http://www.statcan.ca/engish/Pgdb/demo50a.htm.*

Note: Numbers are rounded to nearest million.

and are admitted as permanent residents to the United States to live and work. **Refugees** are those who leave their country based on fear of persecution due to race, religion, nationality, social group membership, or political opinion (U.S. Citizenship and Immigration Services, 2004). The foreign-born population of the United States has grown from 8% in 1990 to 11% in 2000. In 2000, of the 281.4 million people in the United States, 31.1 million (11.1%) were foreign born (U.S. Census Bureau, 2003). The immigrant population of Canada comprises about 18% of the total. Among Canadian immigrants, 42% are from Europe and 37% are from Asia (Statistics Canada, 2004). While most immigrants were formerly from Europe, since 1999, Asia and the Pacific were the most common homelands of immigrants to Canada, followed by Europe, and then Africa and the Middle East (Health Canada, 2000).

Community and world demographics are important for nurses to consider. All nurses must have an understanding of the major cultural groups found in their regions and be able to perform culturally sensitive assessments and plan interventions that are appropriate for the children and families in clinical settings. Immigrants may have different healthcare needs related to understanding of the majority healthcare system, variations in immunizations given to children in native countries, and mental health issues related to integration within a new country. See Developing Cultural Competence: Culture Shock.

Although about 25% of the U.S. population consists of minority and ethnic groups, only 12% of registered nurses in the country are from minority groups (American Nurses Association, 2004). Other health professionals are even less diverse, with 6% of physicians and 5% of dentists from minority groups (Sullivan Report, 2004). This general lack of diversity among healthcare providers has contributed to a lack of adequate healthcare for some minority groups, and resulting health disparities. Nurses from the majority cultural group may not fully understand the views of health and the healthcare practices of other groups. It is therefore important for all nurses to increase their knowledge about groups in their communities in order to provide culturally competent care. Go to your state, provincial, and local websites to find information about the cultural groups in your community; focus your learning and research on these groups as you continue to read this chapter.

DEVELOPING CULTURAL COMPETENCE
Culture Shock

The experience that a person has in attempting to understand or adapt to a culture that is fundamentally different from his or her own culture is known as culture shock. The person may experience feelings of discomfort, powerlessness, anxiety, and disorientation. Immigrants to the United States and Canada may experience culture shock when differences or conflicts arise between their own values, beliefs, and customs and the ways of their new surroundings. The nurse should assess children and their families who have recently immigrated for indications of culture shock. Referring the family to counseling and/or support from representatives of the child and family's culture, such as a translator or community group, may be helpful.

The nursing shortage is a critical concern of all people providing healthcare; however, the lack of adequate numbers of nurses from minority groups is another critical factor to consider (Nugent, Childs, Jones, et al., 2002). While about 72% of the U.S. population is White, about 87% of registered nurses are from that race. About 11% of the population is Hispanic but only about 2% of registered nurses are Hispanic. Likewise, 12% of the population is Black but only 5% of registered nurses are Black (Division of Nursing, 2004). Nurses who are members of minority groups offer distinct skills by being able to understand and interpret both healthcare institutions and the healthcare needs of certain minority groups. Do you work with student peers from various ethnic and racial groups? How can you learn from them and how can you share your cultural knowledge with others? All nurses have the responsibility to work within the profession to increase diversity of the profession and augment diverse knowledge of healthcare providers.

CULTURAL COMPETENCE IN NURSING

Cultural competence refers to the ability of the nurse to understand and effectively respond to the cultural needs of the child and family (Spector, 2004; Health Care Network, 2000) (Figure 3–4 ■). It involves identification and integration into care of the family's beliefs about health and cultural values, and of disease incidence, health disparities, and efficacious treatments for the cultural group (Office of Minority Health, 2001). To be culturally competent, nursing care must be both culturally sensitive and appropriate (Spector, 2004). It must include knowledge of cultural groups, attitudes that honor various cultures and seek to increase competence, and skills to ensure appropriate assessments and interventions. The Office of Minority Affairs of the U.S. Department of Health and Human Services and the Agency for Healthcare Research and Quality have been primary agencies in investigating issues regarding

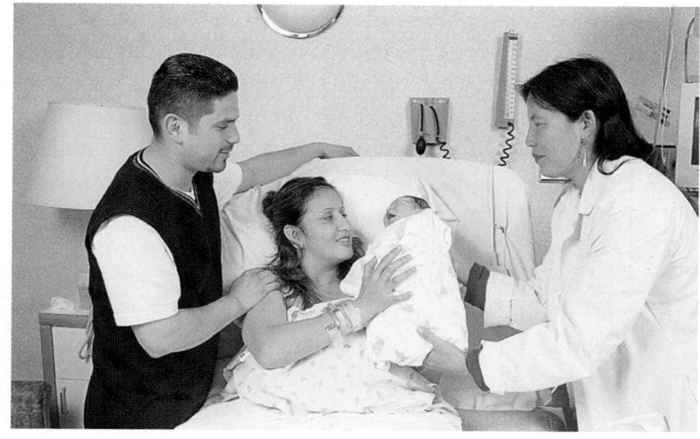

FIGURE 3–4 ■ Nurses increasingly have opportunities to provide culturally competent care as demographics continue to evolve; however, there continues to be disparity among ethnicity of nurses and the populations they serve. Nurses, such as this nurse providing care to the family of a newborn, must develop an understanding of the cultural beliefs and practices of the population. How can nurses improve their understanding of the individuals representing various cultures?

cultural competence and setting standards for healthcare providers. See Table 3–3 for the Office of Minority Health Standards and examples of application to pediatric nursing.

The Canadian government has also focused on cultural competence and provided guidelines for the healthcare provider specific to pediatric healthcare (Health Canada, 2000). The need for increased education to enhance knowledge of care providers is cited, with immigrant groups, language minorities, and gay/lesbian/bisexual/two-spirited communities given as examples of groups that are often misunderstood in healthcare. Health Canada notes that cultural competence requires self-awareness of value system by the nurse, understanding of culture and its relationship to healthcare, sensitivity to health clients, and ability to apply techniques to work with cultural issues.

A theory of cultural competence has been offered by Campinha-Bacote (1999, 2002). This model views the healthcare professional as always becoming more culturally competent. It is not a state that is ever achieved, but one toward which we can all move by increasing our knowledge and sensitivity. The major components of the Campihna-Bacote (2002) model of care are as follows:

- *Cultural awareness*—This cognitive process helps healthcare providers to become cognitively aware and sensitive to their own values, beliefs, assumptions, biases, prejudices, and problem-solving strategies regarding health. Gaining this awareness is an important first step in cultural competence because nurses who are not aware of their own approaches may impose them on others. Try to identify at least three beliefs or biases that might influence your care of children and discuss these with a classmate. For example, do you have beliefs about how a child should be treated to reduce obesity? What biases do you have about how a child with chronic pain should be managed? Do you believe that certain herbs can be used to treat common childhood illnesses? Which ones?
- *Cultural knowledge*—The nurse should seek and obtain knowledge about the worldviews of different cultures. This involves information about the beliefs and values of the culture, the specific physiologic and biologic variations among ethnic groups, and treatments that are effective for the groups. Identify one cultural group that you do not understand fully and investigate the beliefs, biological variations, and treatments chosen by and effective in that group. Include an investigation of beliefs and practices about child bearing and child rearing, and list ways that you will apply that information in pediatric nursing.
- *Cultural skill*—This component emphasizes the importance of collecting relevant cultural data regarding the child's health history and problems. Nurses must accurately perform a culturally specific physical assessment. For example, see Chapter 8 for descriptions of skin and hair variations among cultural groups. How would you identify and describe skin pallor or cyanosis in both fair- and dark-complexioned children? Do you have the language skills needed to work within your community?
- *Cultural encounters*—The nurse gains knowledge best by interacting directly with people from culturally diverse backgrounds. Seek out clinical experiences that will enable you to have encounters with children from many cultural backgrounds. While learning about the specific cultures, realize that each person is an individual who takes on only some of the common characteristics of the group. Use your encounters with children to learn about their backgrounds. Ask questions: "What do you do in your family when you have a cold?" "What do you already know about cystic fibrosis? What do you think will help you stay healthy since you have this disease?"
- *Cultural desire*—This component refers to the nurse's desire to engage in the process of becoming culturally competent. When you approach children and families with a caring attitude and demonstrate your desire to learn about them, they are usually receptive and willing to establish a meaningful relationship to focus on health issues. Spending time with the child, rocking a baby, asking opinions, and inquiring how you can help are all ways to demonstrate caring to the child and family.

MediaLink Critical Thinking: Examine Your Cultural Influences

You may be wondering how you can increase your cultural competence. What are your responsibilities? What are the steps you can take to achieve competence? The first essential step to developing cultural competence is for you, the nurse, to examine your own perceptions, stereotypes, and prejudices regarding various cultures. You can begin to identify individual beliefs that are ethnocentric, biased, or prejudiced through an examination of your own personal heritage and values. Complete a cultural assessment on yourself. Describe heritage, beliefs and values, language, and exposure to diverse cultures. Examine your childhood and the practices and beliefs of your family. Through this understanding of your own background, you establish a foundation for the appreciation of the values and beliefs of others. Additionally, this examination assists you in identifying similarities and differences of cultures other than your own.

HEALTHCARE AND CULTURE

Culture influences concepts of health and healthcare in many ways. The worldview of people in the family determines how health is viewed. Is an illness seen as fate or punishment for actions? Is preventive care viewed as important and an essential part of life? The family and cultural views influence the child, who gradually takes on parts of the culture during development. This section explores some of the important ways in which culture and healthcare interact.

Disparities in Health and Barriers to Healthcare

Research indicates that racial and ethnic minorities in the United States receive lower quality healthcare than the White population, despite comparable insurance status, income, age, and severity of condition (Smedley, Stith, & Nelson, 2002). The morbidity and mortality for these populations is also disproportionate as compared to Caucasians. For example, although there was

TABLE 3–3 National Standards for Culturally and Linguistically Appropriate Services in Healthcare

STANDARD	NURSING IMPLICATIONS FOR CHILD HEALTH
1. Healthcare organizations should ensure that patients/consumers receive from all staff members effective, understandable, and respectful care that is provided in a manner compatible with their cultural health beliefs and practices, and preferred language.	Ask about cultural health beliefs of the family and child. Inquire about desired language. Integrate these assessment areas into all care for the child.
2. Healthcare organizations should implement strategies to recruit, retain, and promote at all levels of the organization a diverse staff and leadership representative of the demographic characteristics of the service area.	Turn to diverse staff members for guidance in working with members of their groups. Collaborate with family and community members to plan care for children, decide on location, types and timing of services.
3. Healthcare organizations should ensure that staff at all levels and across all disciplines receive ongoing education and training in culturally and linguistically appropriate service delivery.	Request training in cultural approaches for groups in your area. Invite community members to participate in training for cultural competence. Partner with your agency and families to enhance care for children.
4. Healthcare organizations must offer and provide language assistance services, including bilingual staff and interpreter services, at no cost to each patient/consumer with limited English proficiency at all points of contact, in a timely manner during all hours of operation.	Investigate agency resources. Collaborate to assemble lists of translators and other resources. Arrange to have brochures and other health materials translated and available for children and families.
5. Healthcare organizations must provide to patients/consumers in their preferred language both verbal offers and written notices informing them of their right to receive language assistance services.	Post signs in the common languages used at health clinics, vans, hospitals, and other settings where children receive care to describe language services provided.
6. Healthcare organizations must ensure the competence of language assistance provided to patients/consumers with limited English proficiency by interpreters and bilingual staff. Family and friends should not be used to provide interpretation services (except on request by the patient/consumer).	Consider taking language classes to increase proficiency with children and families. Do not use children as translators for other family members.
7. Healthcare organizations must make available easily understood patient-related materials and post signage in the languages of the commonly encountered groups and/or groups represented in the service area.	Materials essential in care must be translated and available for families, including consent forms, health histories, and treatment instructions. See www.hhs.gov/ocr/lep for suggestions of documents that should be translated.
8. Healthcare organizations should develop, implement, and promote a written strategic plan that outlines clear goals, policies, operational plans, and management accountability/oversight mechanisms to provide culturally and linguistically appropriate services.	Ask in your clinical settings about services that are available for culturally diverse populations and what goals the agencies have for dealing with children and families from diverse groups.
9. Healthcare organizations should conduct initial and ongoing organizational self-assessments of activities and are encouraged to integrate cultural and linguistic competence-related measures into their internal audits, performance improvement programs, patient satisfaction assessments, and outcomes-based evaluations.	Ask questions of each child and family to evaluate their satisfaction with the services that they have received. Were their expectations for service met?
10. Healthcare organizations should ensure that data on the individual patient's/consumer's race, ethnicity, and spoken and written language are collected in health records, integrated in the organization's management information systems, and periodically updated.	Collect data on written health histories and verbal questions about the child's race, ethnicity, and languages. Record the information and note its application within care for the individual child.
11. Healthcare organizations should maintain a current demographic, cultural, and epidemiological profile of the community as well as a needs assessment to accurately plan for and implement services that respond to the cultural and linguistic characteristics of the service area.	Consult your national, state, provincial, and regional websites and documents to learn what childhood health conditions and healthcare needs are present in your communities. Integrate your knowledge of these needs as you approach children and parents; partner with them to plan care to meet healthcare needs.
12. Healthcare organizations should develop participatory, collaborative partnerships with communities and utilize a variety of formal and informal mechanisms to facilitate community and patient/consumer involvement in designing and implementing cultural activities.	Invite parents to participate in health teaching and screening programs at schools. Suggest that members of the community could assist with design of waiting areas in clinics and hospitals. Engage children and parents in projects that involve translation of signs.
13. Healthcare organizations should ensure that conflict and grievance resolution processes are culturally and linguistically sensitive and capable of identifying, preventing, and resolving cross-cultural conflicts or complaints by patients/consumers.	Ask children and parents to review care received. Refer them to appropriate sources for follow-up as needed. Be sensitive to situations when people are concerned that you were not aware of cultural concerns of a family; openness to one's biases and methods of interaction is the first step in increased sensitivity.
14. Healthcare organizations are encouraged to regularly make available to the public information about their progress and successful innovations in implementing these standards and to provide public notice in their communities about the availability of this information.	Post information about new cultural services available to families. Consider the use of community flyers, radio, or other approaches to inform families about culturally sensitive services in your facility.

Source: U. S. Department of Health and Human Services, Office of Minority Health (2001). National Standards for Culturally and Linguistically Appropriate Services in Health Care. Washington, DC: Author.

an overall 45.2% decline in infant mortality rates from 1980 to 2000, disparities still exist as the decline was greater for Whites (10.9% to 5.7%) than for Blacks (22.2% to 14%) (Umar, 2003). Native Americans and Alaskan Native groups have an infant death rate about twice that for Whites (National Institutes of Health, 2002). See Developing Cultural Competence: Health Disparities and Hispanics.

One of the two major goals of *Healthy People 2010* was to eliminate health disparities among segments of the population (U.S. Department of Health and Human Services, 2000). Health disparity populations are those groups with significant differences in disease incidence, prevalence, morbidity, mortality, or survival rates as compared to the general populations. Disparities in relation to gender, race, ethnic group, education, income, disability, geographic location, and sexual orientation are common. For example, while about 10% of White children are living in households below the poverty level, in African American and Hispanic groups about 40% of children live in households below the poverty level (U.S. Department of Health and Human Services, 2000). Poverty level is a major reason that families do not access healthcare. Insurance is lacking, preventive health services are not available, risk of disease and injury is greater, and limited resources may not be directed toward healthcare among poor families. African Americans, Hispanics, Native Americans, Alaskan and Hawaiian Natives, Asians, and Pacific Islanders have high rates of morbidity and mortality associated with diseases such as birth defects, asthma, infant mortality, mental illness, cancer, diabetes, and cardiovascular disease (National Institutes of Health, 2002). To address health and healthcare disparities, the *Strategic Plan to Reduce and Ultimately Eliminate Health Disparities* was developed by the National Institutes of Health (2002). This document and plan coordinates all of the institutes in regard to disparity research. It supports research that will lower rates of disparity and disseminate knowledge to health professionals. Six diseases are targeted due to the disproportionate burden of these diseases that is borne by minority groups.

- Infant mortality
- Heart disease and stroke
- Cancer
- Mental health
- Diabetes
- HIV and AIDS

These conditions have direct relevance to pediatric nurses. Infant mortality is directly related, while some other conditions such as heart disease and diabetes have their roots in youth due to a high rate of overweight among several minority youth groups. Mental health is a growing and serious condition among young people (see Chapter 34∞ for further discussion of mental illness in children).

Why do disparities exist? There are many reasons, and some known causes are addressed next.

Access and Barriers

One reason disparities exist among cultural groups relates to access and barriers to care. Access ensures that children of all races, ethnic groups, and income levels can obtain preventive care and treatment for illness or injury. Barriers delay or prevent healthcare for the child. In a literature review about barriers to care for young children, common themes creating barriers were lack of health insurance among low-income families, communication difficulties such as those experienced when families did not speak English, lack of knowledge about cultural approaches to healthcare on the part of care providers, transportation problems, and parental stress (Kataoka-Yahiro & Munet-Vilaro, 2002). See Evidence-Based Practice: Investigating Culture and Healthcare Barriers.

Families need access to healthcare services in their own communities and have means of transportation to the services. Obtaining even basic or emergency services for children in rural areas may be difficult due to the lack of providers. Service hours need to meet the needs of the population served. Language translators should be readily available. A welcoming atmosphere, pleasant surrounding, and reasonable wait time will all enhance use of healthcare. Pediatric nurses are instrumental in surveying families and planning approaches that welcome them to healthcare settings.

Lack of health coverage is a major barrier for children in many groups; those in immigrant families are at particular risk. Recall the earlier discussion about growing numbers of immigrants in both the United States and Canada. Approximately one in every five American children is now a member of an immigrant family. While less than 20% of all U.S. children are now uninsured, about 27% of children who are citizens but whose parents are not citizens are uninsured, and nearly 50% of children who are not citizens have no health insurance (Lessard & Ku, 2003). In addition to lack of health insurance, some of the common barriers in immigrant families include language differences, high degree of mobility, lack of information about healthcare services in this country, and lack of a pediatric or healthcare home. Recall the discussion in Chapter 1∞ that encouraged all families with children to seek a "home" that they can turn to for care and with questions. Identification of that pediatric healthcare home makes it more likely that preventive care is received, that early diagnosis of healthcare problems can occur, and that prompt treatment or referral takes place.

DEVELOPING CULTURAL COMPETENCE
Health Disparities and Hispanics

Hispanics make up one of the largest minority groups of U.S. citizens, with 35.3 million members. This large group experiences many ethnic disparities such as lack of health insurance, low immunization rates, limited prenatal care, high rates of homicide, and extremely high rates of obesity. Certain diseases such as stroke, liver disease, diabetes, human immunodeficiency virus (HIV), and cancer of stomach and cervix are more common (MMWR, 2004). Many of these problems affect children. When working with Hispanic groups, perform accurate weight and height measurements and plot on growth grids. Include additional nutritional assessment and guidance if overweight is evident. Ask about access to health insurance and healthcare. Investigate the immunization record for all children and update as needed. At the same time, recognize that healthcare needs may vary according to location and group. Look at each person and your area individually.

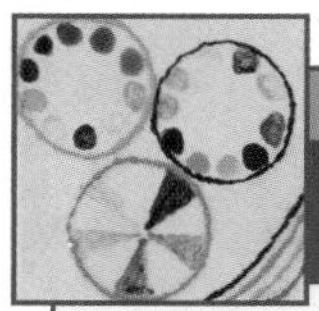

EVIDENCE-BASED PRACTICE
Investigating Culture and Healthcare Barriers

PROBLEM

Health disparities exist among various cultural groups. Although examination of factors in adults has identified some barriers to care, there has been little research about barriers that exist among families with children. An understanding of the factors that improve healthcare access and those that act as barriers is needed to provide accessible care for children from minority ethnic groups.

EVIDENCE

An interview with 62 Haitian family members about care for their school-aged children revealed that the major reason for not obtaining care was cost. About 42% of the children did not have healthcare coverage because families did not believe they were eligible for care, could not get transportation to the office to complete applications for care, had lack of knowledge about programs available, were opposed to the detailed questions asked on forms, or had general distrust of government (Schantz, Charron, & Folden, 2003).

In another study of immigrants, Korean children were examined for completion of the hepatitis B vaccination series. Perception that hepatitis B was a serious disease was an incentive for completion of the series, although difficulty paying the cost was a major barrier to completion (Kim, 2004).

A study was conducted of 42 family members with Latino children and 42 family members of Euro-Americans with special healthcare needs. Both groups cited frustrations in care related to access to rehabilitation, and lack of integration of care within school systems. Latino families often cited need for more information and access to a support group, whereas Euro-American families cited a need for referral to day care and respite care resources (Gannotti, Kaplan, Handwerker, et al., 2004).

NURSING IMPLICATIONS

A theme in two of the previous studies was cost of care. Nurses need to refer families to sources for healthcare services and then follow up to be sure the families were able to access care. Referrals to neighborhood clinics and instructions for transportation to the health setting are important for many families. A need for information is another theme among most groups. Explaining why an immunization is needed as well as providing information about the child's condition are important nursing roles. Referring the family to others from the same group and assisting them in navigating complex systems such as school and social services may also be necessary.

CRITICAL THINKING APPLICATION

What is the process that immigrant families in your state or province must follow to secure healthcare for their children? How would you help to guide someone through this process?

What cultural groups are common in your community? Do you speak their language? If not, what measures should you take to ensure that they understand the teaching offered in clinical settings? What type of support groups will be helpful for families when they have a child with special healthcare needs?

Lack of trust of healthcare providers can also be a barrier to care. Historically, groups such as Blacks and Native Americans were the recipients of inferior care and even unethical research studies. Members of these groups may continue to distrust healthcare providers. If inadequate care was received at some time or if care providers appear rude or noncaring, some families may prefer to treat children at home and seek care only in emergency situations. Trust can be enhanced when children and families of all races, ethnic groups, religious groups, and other populations are treated fairly and with respect. Collaborate with families to learn their healthcare goals and provide relationships with a stable group of health professionals when possible.

Biological Differences

Genetic and physical differences occur among cultural groups (Figure 3–5 ■) and can lead to disparity in needs and care. Differences include blood type, body build, skin color, drug metabolism, and susceptibility to certain diseases. Some variations between the genders occur and are presented in discussions of various conditions throughout this text. For example, male children are more likely to manifest pyloric stenosis and attention deficit disorder, whereas female children more often have slipped femoral epiphysis and systemic lupus erythematosus. Age provides another biological variation as infants are more likely to manifest the cancer neuroblastoma, whereas adolescents have a higher incidence of lymphoma. Race is also connected with certain disease processes. Blacks are more likely to experience diabetes and sickle cell anemia (see chapters throughout this text for a discussion of these conditions). Thalassemia, another type of anemia, is most common in Mediterranean people. Blacks and Native Americans tend to have higher rates of tuberculosis than the general population. Whites from certain geographic origins are more likely to manifest cystic fibrosis, celiac disease, and Crohn's disease. Hispanics have high rates of diabetes and lactose intolerance. Asians and Native Americans often do not metabolize alcohol readily and are more prone to either injury after alcohol ingestion or to alcohol abuse. Otitis

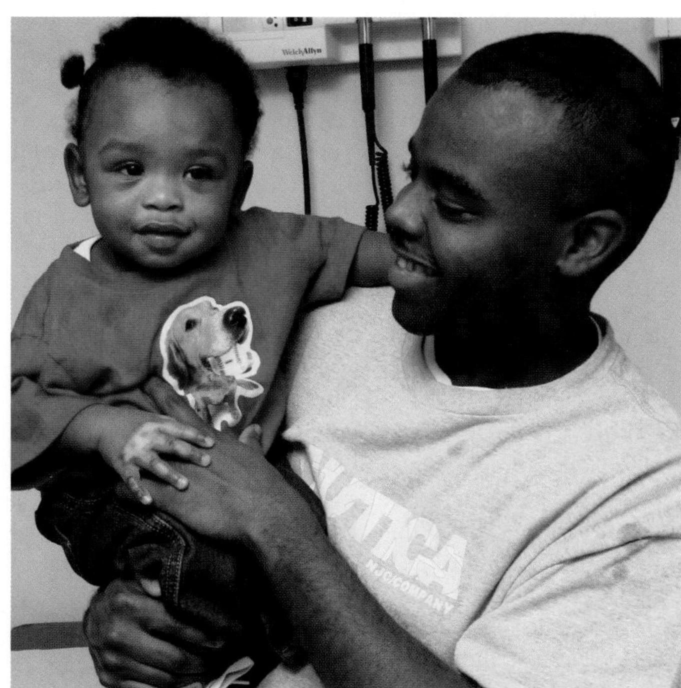

FIGURE 3–5 ■ Children manifest physical characteristics related to their ethnic groups. How will you integrate this knowledge into developmental assessments of children?

media, infection of the middle ear, is common in Native American and Alaskan Native children.

CLINICAL TIP

Although certain conditions are more common in various racial or ethnic groups, it is best to approach each group individually. There are marked differences in rates of diabetes among Native American tribes, so knowing the most common conditions for a race in general may not be directly applicable to the specific location and group in your area.

Metabolism of drugs is linked to genetic traits in certain groups. Polymorphisms, or variations in genes, encode either receptors to certain medications or enzymes that metabolize medications. One common example is isoniazid, a drug commonly used to treat tuberculosis. Whereas less than half of Whites and only 7% to 34% of Japanese and Chinese metabolize the drug slowly, over half of Blacks and up to 90% of Native Americans metabolize it slowly, resulting in drug overdose and resultant neuropathy (Giger & Davidhizar, 2004; Burroughs, Maxey, & Levy, 2002). Some cardiovascular drugs, seizure medications, and psychotropics are further examples of medications in which ethnic variations in metabolism have been noted. In addition, research has shown that some minority groups do not receive the same medications and therapy for similar conditions as the majority population. While some of the disparity relates to inaccessibility of healthcare, healthcare professionals treat African Americans with fewer drugs for HIV and cardiovascular disease and prescribe fewer antipsychotics for mental illness in Hispanics and African Americans (Burrough et al., 2002). Nurses can be alert to treatment regimens, refer minority groups to healthcare facilities where individualized treatment will occur, and question drug regimens when they seem different from recommended treatments.

Nurses must understand other genetic characteristics in order to perform culturally competent nursing assessments and interventions. Differences in skin color and tones may make cyanosis, pallor, and jaundice difficult to recognize and describe. Mongolian spots are darkened skin on the lower back and buttocks of some babies with dark skin tones. Variations in texture of hair require different approaches to hygiene among various racial groups. See Chapters 4 and 8∞ for more detail about biological variations and implications for assessment.

Environmental Differences

Some of the conditions mentioned in the previous section are clearly genetic in origin, such as sickle-cell anemia; however, it is obvious that some conditions are linked to environmental conditions. Native Americans have a high rate of injury related to suicide. These injuries may be directly related to the high unemployment rates common on some reservations, which leads to poor self-esteem and promotes depression. It is often hard to separate biological and environmental factors as they are closely interrelated. Native Americans or Hispanics who eat traditional diets have low rates of obesity and diabetes, but those who eat the "typical American diet," which is high in fat and low in fruits and vegetables, have high rates of these conditions. Likewise, the medication metabolism differences discussed in the previous section are sometimes further altered by exposure to environmental pollution, alcohol, and a particular diet. Biological and environmental factors interact in many cases to create certain healthcare risks.

Another environmental problem that can create healthcare needs is socioeconomic status. (See Chapter 7∞.) Families with inadequate finances are more likely to live in crowded conditions and experience more infectious disease. Conditions in their neighborhoods can be unsafe and result in injury to children. Homicide, falls, fires, and other hazards may be common. Peeling paint may result in conditions such as lead poisoning. Lack of knowledge about transmission, poor access to treatment, and use of intravenous drugs can increase incidence of human immunodeficiency virus (HIV) in populations with high rates of poverty. Socioeconomic effects were discussed above in the section on disparity. Lower access to healthcare, lower rates of immunization, poor nutritional status, and lack of transportation may all interact with ethnic factors to promote high incidence of certain disease states.

Cultural Practices that Influence Healthcare

Family Roles and Organization

A family's roles and organization are largely dependent upon cultural influence. The family structure defines acceptable roles and behavior of family members. For example, culture may determine who has authority (head of household) and is the primary decision maker for other members of the family. Additionally, the role of decision maker may change according to specific decisions. For example, in some cultures, decisions regarding the healthcare of children are primarily the responsibility of the female, whereas other decisions are male dominated. Family dominance patterns may be patriarchal, as seen in some Appalachian cultures; matriarchal, as seen in some African American cultures; or more egalitarian, as seen in some European American cultures. Nurses should be alert for roles and functions in families since teaching may need to be directed to those responsible for decision making in order to effectively promote child health.

Culture also defines gender roles, the role of the elderly, and the role of the extended family. For example, Native Americans may consult tribal elders (considered part of the extended family) before agreeing to medical care for their child. In some cultures, major decisions for the family, including a child's healthcare, include input from grandparents and other extended family members (Figure 3–6 ■). Grandparents may even assume responsibility for care of the children in the family (see Chapter 2∞). In these cases, nurses must direct teaching for health promotion and demonstration for treatment procedures to the grandparent.

Family goals are also determined by cultural values and practices, as are family member roles and child rearing practices and beliefs. In some families, children are expected to take on responsibilities early and may be expected to take on tasks such as management of their own chronic disease and nutritional intake. In other families, children are given long periods to grow up and are not expected to manage healthcare needs. Direct teaching to a child with diabetes in the latter family type may not

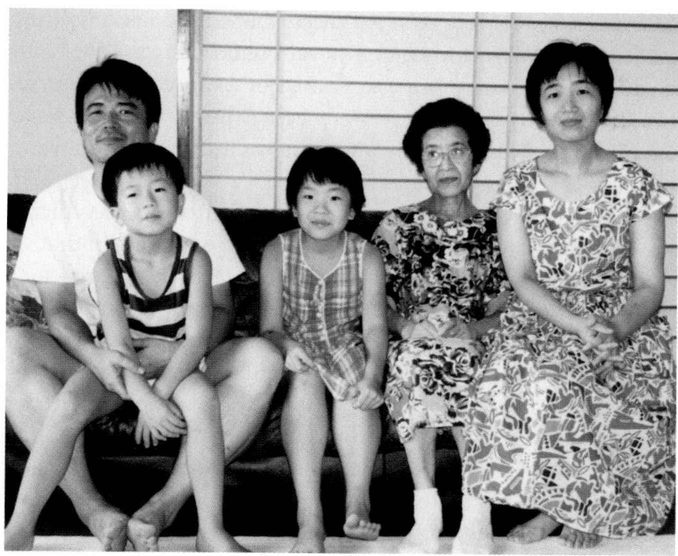

FIGURE 3–6 ■ Many cultures value the input of grandparents and other elders in the family or group. For example, in this multigenerational family, the grandmother's guidance is highly valued and significantly influences the family's child rearing practices.

be appropriate. Nurses often provide information and ask about developmental milestones for children; however, there may be variations in family goals and it is not unusual that families accomplish these tasks with children at younger or older ages. For example, it is commonly expected that children are weaned by 1 year of age and toilet trained at about 2 years of age, but this is not always the case. Ask about the norms in the family and whether the child is developing according to the parents' expectations. As long as the child is progressing in motor, language, and social tasks, some variation is expected due to cultural norms. Views about alternative lifestyles such as sexual orientation and single parenting are also established by the family's values and beliefs. Understanding such values assists the nurse in providing sensitive care. Examples of child rearing practices common to particular cultures are listed in Table 3–4. (See Chapter 2∞ for further discussion of family structures.)

TABLE 3–4 Child Rearing Practices of Selected Cultures

CULTURE	CHILD REARING PRACTICES
African American	Children may be raised by grandparent (typically grandmother) Children are expected to demonstrate respectfulness, conformity to rules, obedience, and good behavior May use belly band or coin on umbilicus to prevent protrusion of umbilicus
Amish	Children are expected to continue with the Amish tradition Grandparents often provide care to children Family may not seek prenatal care Children are expected to follow the rules as prescribed by the church district
Appalachian	Large families are common Strict parenting practices Grandparents frequently provide care to children
Arab American	Father is typically the disciplinarian The child's character is considered a reflection of the family's influence Aggression toward parents and authority is strongly disapproved Discipline may include physical punishment and shaming Preference may be noted toward male children
Chinese American	Family may lavish resources on child Children typically depend on family for all needs and may not be expected to earn their own money as adolescents Male children are often more valued than female children Children may be taught to avoid displaying their emotions/feelings Children are expected to assist parents in the home (chores) High educational achievement is expected
Mexican American	Children are closely protected and are not encouraged to leave the home Godparents are included in care of the child; considered "co-parents" Children are expected to demonstrate respect for parents and elder family members Discipline may include physical punishment
Navajo Indian	Children's name may not be revealed until their first laugh Infants may be kept in a cradleboard to protect them Grandmothers frequently are responsible for toilet training, disciplining, and weaning Older children may be taught to be stoic and uncomplaining

Data from Purnell, L. D., & Paulanka, B. J. (Eds.). (2003). Transcultural health care: A culturally competent approach *(2nd ed.). Philadelphia: F. A. Davis.*

Communication

Communication is the method by which members of cultural groups share information and preserve their beliefs, values, norms, and practices. Information is transmitted through both verbal and nonverbal methods. Verbal communication consists of spoken or written words. It may include tone and level of voice, language, verbal style and dialect, and written material. Nonverbal communication refers to body language such as posture, gestures, facial expressions, eye contact, and touch, as well as the use of silence. Included in communication are the concepts of time orientation, spatial distancing (space orientation) practices, and the use of names.

One obvious need related to verbal communication is to have a healthcare provider who speaks the same language. Recall the national standards related to language assistance services (see Table 3–3). Children are most likely to speak both the language of the parents and the healthcare providers and may appear to be likely translators. However, it is recommended that children never be used to translate in healthcare situations due to the confidentiality needs of both parent and child. Signs, posted literature, and brochures should also be available in the languages of the children and families served. Even when children speak the language of the healthcare providers, written material must be provided at a level that the family can read and understand.

CLINICAL TIP

Speaking and reading may not occur in the same language. For example, an immigrant may read and speak fluently in a primary language and speak but not read the language of the new country. The immigrant's child may read and speak the language of the present country and speak but not read the native language of the family. Always ask about both reading and speaking preferences.

Language can also affect health literacy skills. There are a large number of instructions given in writing. Examples include prescriptions and directions on medication bottles, signs hanging in health facilities, consent forms for procedures and surgery, insurance forms, directions for techniques or procedures, future appointment dates, and health promotion materials. Verify what the child and family can read and whether alternate methods should be used. Nurses can verbally give the information and provide paper and pencil so that the family can take notes in their own language. Translation services should be available in all healthcare settings, including the pharmacy, the appointment desk, and for phone calls, in order to ensure access to services for all clients served.

Variations in communication among cultures are reflected in word meaning, voice inflection and quality, and verbal styles. Culture not only influences the manner in which feelings are expressed, but also which verbal and nonverbal expressions of communication are considered appropriate. An individual's willingness to discuss certain topics or to express or conceal certain thoughts and feelings are also influenced by the cultural norms. Some groups, such as Asians and Native Americans, may be expected to remain quiet when experiencing pain; other cultures, such as Italians, Jews, and Hispanics, may loudly and dramatically express pain. Watch for the cues that family members give to children in pain, such as "Oh, you're all right—be a big boy," or "You go ahead and cry. How can you take that pain?" Remember that culture is constantly evolving, so children commonly exhibit communication patterns seen in their parents as well as reflecting the patterns of the majority culture and of childhood peers.

Use of names varies among cultural groups. Assuming that each person in healthcare wishes to be called by a first name can be disrespectful. Always ask upon admission to any facility what the child wishes to be called. Address family members respectfully, usually using terms such as Mr, Mrs, and Ms. If the person has a title such as doctor, judge, or senator, it should be used. Ask what the person prefers to be called and record this in the health record for future reference. In the Korean, Cambodian and Filipino cultures, the first name used is actually the family name. Asking for the "family name" rather than the "last name" may clarify this practice.

Nonverbal communication patterns may hinder or help communication. For example, gestures and body language may be misunderstood or misinterpreted. Eye contact has different meanings among cultures. European Americans, for example, value eye contact with communication and interpret this as a sign of sincerity and interest. In other cultures, sustained eye contact may be considered rude or disrespectful. Silence is considered a sign of respect in some cultures. Among those groups, offering an immediate response to a question may be viewed as being disrespectful because an instant reply could indicate that no thought was given to the matter. Watch for patterns in various cultures and alter your own approach to be more congruent. For example, many nurses commonly nod and say "yes" or "oh, I see" when a patient is speaking. This may seem disruptive to some cultures. If you note that the listener is silent and does not use such patterns of agreement, alter your own response to match more closely the acceptable method of communication for the child or family. Learn that silence and quiet listening can be perceived as positive approaches.

Touch is another form of nonverbal communication. The appropriateness of touch varies with each culture. For example, an Asian may consider touching an unfamiliar person of the opposite gender to be inappropriate, while touch between men and women may be viewed as appropriate by another culture. Adults commonly feel that it is acceptable to touch children of all ages; this may not be accurate. Look for responses from the child and family to touch. Does the parent touch the child, stroke the crying baby, or put an arm around a school-age child? What is the response as the nurse touches the child to take a blood pressure or pulse? If you think it might be reassuring to stroke an arm during a painful procedure and are unsure of the child's response, ask if it would help them to do that. Refer to Chapter 6∞ for further information on communication.

Depending on an individual's specific culture, the use of space has different definitions and meanings. Space, as defined in this context, refers to the relationship between the individual and other persons and objects in the environment. Cultures may have specific spatial preferences, such as personal distance and social distance. Some cultures tend to prefer close contact with less space since they use touch as a form of communication (Box 3–1). Be alert for how close a child comes to you and other individuals. Try to maintain this space in your interactions. Realize that nursing procedures often cause the space barrier to be broken. We must touch children to weigh them, take blood pressures, and give immunizations. This does not mean that close touch is appropriate at all times. Tell all children when you will touch them for procedures so they understand what is happening.

BOX 3–1 Zones of Personal Space

Four "zones" of personal space to consider during communication are as follows:

- The *intimate zone* is within 18 inches of the body. This zone is for close personal contact and is generally reserved for those who have a close relationship. Nurses often bridge this zone for weighing, taking blood pressure, and performing other procedures.
- The *personal zone* is 18 inches to 3 feet from the body. This zone is used when talking to the family and child during interviews and history assessment. Be alert that some people have closer or more remote distances for personal interactions. Try to maintain the comfort zone of the child and family.
- The *social zone* is 3 to 6 feet from the body. This zone is used for impersonal communication and is usually the first zone nurses use before entering the personal zone, such as when calling someone in from a waiting room.
- The *public zone* is greater than 6 feet from the body. This zone is used when giving speeches or lectures to a group of people.

Time Orientation

Cultures have specific values and meanings regarding time orientation. Cultural groups may place emphasis on the events of the past, those events that occur in the present, or those that will occur in the future. Children reflect the time orientation of their families and of the cultures in which they live. Time is also influenced by development so that young children sometimes do not understand the use of clocks, the importance ascribed to being "on time," or other time orientations.

Cultures that are oriented predominantly to the past may want to begin healthcare encounters with lengthy descriptions of past healthcare treatments, family history of diseases, or individual past experiences with health. There may be little interest in learning methods of adapting to or maintaining a new plan of care.

For cultures that are oriented predominantly to the present, little consideration may be given to either the past or the future. For example, adolescents commonly focus on the present, and may not engage in preventive health practices for long-term health. Short-term goals often provide more incentive to adolescents.

Cultures that are oriented predominantly to the future, such as European Americans, may not focus on what is important at the present time. For example, the family focusing on the future may dream of a child's education or sports performance and have trouble setting present goals for treatment of a disease such as juvenile rheumatoid arthritis. One commonly hears that it was a big adjustment to learn to "take one day at a time." Not living up to the family's expectation for future success may be difficult for a child who has developed an illness that has a chronic course.

Time also refers to punctuality regarding schedules and appointments. In the United States and Canada, the predominant culture respects being on time and considers time valuable and not to be wasted. Other cultures may not emphasize the concern for time. This may be manifested by a family's inability to follow timed medication schedules or treatments, or to show up as scheduled for an appointment. In these cases, it is not intended as a sign of disrespect.

Nutrition

Nutritional practices begin even before birth as many cultural groups have beliefs that determine foods that are healthy to eat or should be avoided during pregnancy. Nutritional habits and patterns vary among cultures and are related to both religious practices and health beliefs. Certain cultures and religions have restrictions on or prescriptions about specific foods and preparation methods. Ritualistic behaviors involving eating and drinking, for example on special occasions and holidays, are observed by most cultures (Figure 3–7 ■). Many religions recommend fasts during specific holiday seasons, such as Lent for Roman Catholics, Yom Kippur for Jews, and Ramadan for Muslims; however, in most cases, small children, pregnant women, and sick individuals are not required to fast.

Additionally, some cultures value large size or may associate a healthy child with being "large." Other cultures value slimness and look down upon overweight individuals. Both of these views influence family eating patterns and expectation for the child; the child's self-esteem can therefore be influenced. The U.S. and Canadian cultures honor being slim in the media but reinforce eating and large size by the availability of fast food and positive image of large sports stars such as some football players, which can result in confusion about health and body image.

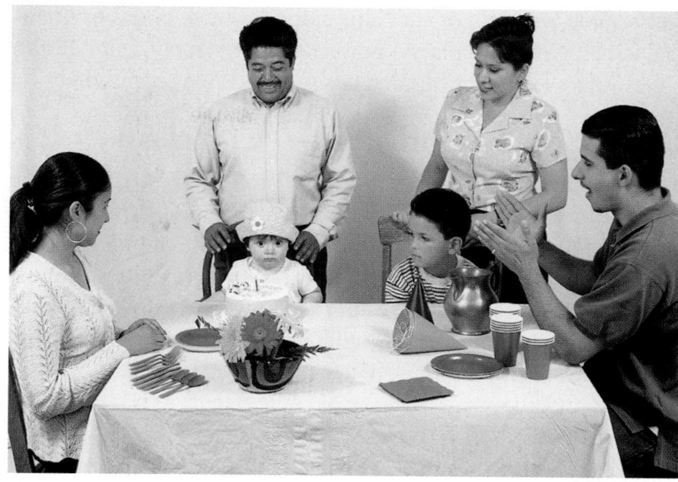

FIGURE 3–7 ■ Food traditions are common in many cultures and are often associated with rituals and celebrations. This family is celebrating the youngest child's birthday with traditional foods.

Nutrition may also be essential to the culture's practices for health promotion and care during illness. Specific food preferences are identified in Table 3–5. Health problems associated with specific cultures which may require dietary changes are also identified. Recognize that nutrition can be closely related to environmental situations so that families with few resources may

TABLE 3–5 Food Preferences of Selected Cultures

CULTURE	FOOD PREFERENCES	HEALTH CONDITIONS THAT MAY REQUIRE MODIFIED DIETARY HABITS
African American	Pork Rice Fried foods Greens	Hypertension Coronary heart disease Obesity
Hispanic/ Latin American	Beans Chili Cheese Fried foods Carbonated beverages	Coronary heart disease Obesity Diabetes
Native American	Fish Game Blue cornmeal Fruits such as berries	Malnutrition Diabetes
Asian American	Raw fish Soy sauce Rice	Coronary heart disease Ulcers Liver disease

Adapted from Andrews M. M., Boyle, J. S., & Carr, T. J. (2003). Transcultural concepts in nursing care *(4th ed.). Philadelphia: Lippincott Williams & Wilkins; Giger, J. N., & Davidhizar, R. (2004).* Transcultural nursing: Assessment and intervention *(4th ed.) St. Louis: Mosby-Yearbook.*

not be able to obtain or eat cultural foods due to access or financial issues. Nutrition plays a powerful role in maintaining health so resources for nutritious and desired foods may be needed.

Health Beliefs, Approaches, and Practices

Health beliefs and practices have a profound impact on the health of a child. Those beliefs influence the family's healing approaches and practices. They determine what the family perceives as the cause of the child's illness, the purpose of illness, and how illness should be treated. Moreover, because beliefs and practices vary, not all families will seek traditional Western medical care for their children.

Health Beliefs

Three views of health beliefs described by Andrews, Boyle, and Carr (2003) are magico-religious, scientific, and holistic. In reality, many people ascribe to a view that combines more than one of these belief systems, but it is helpful to examine them separately. In the **magico-religious belief view,** health and illness are determined by supernatural forces such as God, gods, magic, spirits, or fate. Illness of a child may be perceived as a punishment for actions. Children of preschool age usually have this view of illness; some adults also believe that higher or supernatural powers determine health and illness. It is wise to ask both children and their families what they think caused an illness or how they believe they can stay well. People who believe in this paradigm may gain comfort from prayer, healing rituals, and faith healing. Young children who believe that they have caused their own illness because of their developmental level (usually preschool and early school age) can be expressly told that it was not something they did that caused the illness in order to decrease their feelings of guilt.

The **scientific** or **biomedical health belief** assumes that physiology explains all illness and life itself (Andrews et al., 2003). Biochemical reactions and the genomic code are used to explain all health states, and a child's illness is always caused by viruses, bacteria, or damage to the body. This approach is often called Western medicine. Families who hold this view expect a traditional Western medical intervention, such as medication, treatment, or surgery, to treat the child's health problems. Parents may be dissatisfied with care if they are told that the child is to rest, drink fluids, and use comfort measures; they feel a medication is most likely to help. Within this belief system it is difficult to understand certain health conditions. Families may struggle to "explain" an illness by wondering if the child was exposed to something harmful during fetal life, or has an environmental exposure; a reason for the condition is needed in order to understand it. Most physicians, nurses, and other healthcare professionals adhere primarily to the biomedical or scientific theories to explain and treat illnesses. However, certain therapies such as therapeutic touch, biofeedback, and other nontraditional methods that are more common in a holistic health paradigm are gaining popularity within these professions. For the family with scientific or biomedical health beliefs, health professionals sometimes need to emphasize that certain conditions have no known cause, and to suggest treatments other than traditional Western medicine if other approaches may be helpful.

Balance and harmony of the body and nature are important concepts in the **holistic health belief.** It is believed that the child's illness results when the natural balance or harmony is disturbed. Infection and other illness gain entry into the body when it is not in balance. This health belief is most common in Eastern worldviews and in Native American and First Nation people. Increasingly, the ideas of holism are being integrated into Western healthcare and combined with other approaches. An example of integration of approaches is use of a medication or radiation for illness in combination with adequate rest and a diet that is designed to increase immune function. An associated holistic health belief is the hot and cold theory of disease, which subscribes to the thought that illnesses and diseases are a result of disruption in the hot and cold balance of the body. Therefore, consuming foods of the opposite variety can cure or prevent specific hot and cold illnesses. Hot and cold therapies related to healing are practiced in some African American, Indian, Hispanic, Arab, and Southern Anglo-American cultures. See page 83 for further information.

Health Approaches and Practices

The family's health beliefs influence their approaches and practices regarding health and illness. The young child has a view of health and illness connected with developmental understanding and gradually takes on the family's cultural view while growing older.

Additionally, some families, when faced with a life-threatening illness of their child, may seek alternate health practices that are not considered part of their cultural heritage. This is especially true if the family becomes frustrated with traditional biomedical treatments that are unable to cure their child. See Table 3–6 for examples of health practices common to specific cultures.

Healthcare Practitioners. The family seeking care for the child may choose one or a combination of magico-religious, holistic, or biomedical healthcare providers. Recall Raven in the opening scenario. His family has used a combination of a native healer and Western care. Nurses and other healthcare professionals seek to learn about the family's belief system and to integrate all types of care that the family wishes as long as there is no danger offered to the child (Box 3–2).

The use of **folk healers** varies according to the culture. Though the healer's role and position in the community differ among cultures, healers do share commonalities. Healers speak the language of the cultural group, use common methods of communication for the culture, and live in the same community. They most often conduct healing in their homes or the homes of the patients. Cost is usually reasonable for the family or some type of bartering may be common (Roy, Torrez, & Dale, 2004). Several types of healers are specific to certain groups.

Mexican American and some Hispanic cultures may seek healing by a **curandero** (male healer) or **curandera** (female healer), who deals with all levels of illness, from minor colds to cancer (Spector, 2004). The curandero's holistic treatment may include use of herbs, laying on of hands, massaging the afflicted area, cleansing the body with herbs, preparing an amulet to be worn, burning a candle with a specific prayer

TABLE 3–6 Health Practices of Selected Cultures

CULTURE	HEALTH PRACTICES
African American	Religious healing (laying on hands) Talismans Herbal remedies/Oils Use of healers: "Old Woman" healers Voodoo healers Shaman Spiritualist Root doctor
Asian American	Acupuncture/Acupressure Coin rubbing Cupping Herbs Hot and cold foods Massage Meditation Moxibustion Qi Restoring energy between yin and yang T'ai chi Tiger balm Use of healers: Physician Herbalist Acupuncturist
European American	Amulets Healing rituals Dietary modifications Exercise Traditional medicine Use of healers: Traditional healthcare providers: physician, nurse, and nurse practitioners
Hispanic or Latin American	Hot and cold foods Herbs Massage Prayers Religious medals Use of healers: Curandero/curandera Yerbero (herbalist) Brujo (uses witchcraft to heal) Espiritualista Sobadora Santiguadora
Native American	Ceremony Counseling Herbs and plants Laying on hands Medicine bundle Music Pipe ceremony Prayer/chanting Smudging-purification Sweatlodge Use of healers: Medicine man or woman Shaman

Data from Huebscher, R., & Shuler, P. A. (2004). Natural, alternative, and complementary health care practices. *St. Louis: Mosby; Fontaine, K. L. (2000).* Healing practices: Alternative therapies for nursing. *Upper Saddle River, NJ: Prentice Hall.*

BOX 3–2 Health Approaches and Safety

Families often combine treatments from more than one healthcare approach, both in seeking practitioners and in applying treatments such as medicines. Most often that is helpful to them and to the child. Nurses must be alert, however, to any practices that would be unsafe for the child. For example, the child with type 1 diabetes must be treated with insulin, and to rely only on a folk healer or herbs places the child in a life-threatening situation. Certain herbs may be harmful to young children and should not be used. In cases when the family's cultural practice is placing the child in a hazardous situation, civil courts may intervene to provide care for the child, for example, mandating a life-preserving blood transfusion for a child even when the family is opposed to transfusions. Support families in their beliefs and healthcare practices but remain alert for any care that could be harmful for the child and report it promptly.

printed on the candle jar, or calling the spirit of a saint to bless the patient. Essential to the curandero/a and patient relationship is the faith the child and family have in his or her abilities. Families may combine curanderismo (Hispanic medical system) with a Western approach for some conditions. For example, a child with seizures may be given medications for the disorder obtained from Western care and may be fed a tea that the healer believes will treat the condition.

African Americans often combine Western and traditional beliefs about illness. Some believe in spirits as causes of illness and may use powders, oils, and ceremony to maintain health.

Native Americans may seek healing from a shaman, healer, or medicine man or woman. Because Native Americans generally believe in the balance of nature and a state of harmony, they seek advice to identify what they have done to disrupt their body harmony. The healer will then prescribe the required treatment for restoration of balance and harmony. Teas, other herbal products, sweats, smudges, meditation, and other approaches are common (Box 3–3). Returning to one's family, home, and roots may produce a sense of balance. Children who are ill and hospitalized may be surrounded and cared for by family members and tribal elders.

Faith-Based Belief and Spirituality. Faith-based belief and practice is an integral part of culture for some families. Views of religion and spirituality can shape their approaches and responses to a child's illness and guide practices to maintain health. Religious beliefs may influence the family's explanation of the cause of a child's illness, their perception of the severity of the illness, and choices of treatments for the illness, and can

BOX 3–3 Smudging

Smudging is a process used by many Native Americans and First Nation people for cleansing and blessing the person. The smudge is usually performed by an elder who lights a fire in a natural product such as sweet grass or sage. The flame is blown out and the material smokes, creating the smudge. If families wish to conduct a smudge, provide a quiet and private place. Be sure that the smoke detector will not activate during the procedure. Alert other staff members so that they understand the purpose and need for the ceremony.

offer solace to the family and child. For these reasons, it is important to determine the influence of religion and spirituality on the child's health.

For many families of children who are ill, faith and spirituality can be a source of great comfort and support for the child and family. Conversely, conflicts may arise between the family's religion or spirituality and biomedical care for the child. For example, the family's pursuit of specific religious therapies can serve as a barrier to biomedical care, because some parents may believe that their spiritual practices can substitute for medical treatment of the child. Additionally, some parents may not adhere to biomedical therapies as they may believe that the use of biomedicine is an indication of a lack of faith (Barnes, Plotnikoff, Fox, et al., 2000).

Religion, commonly referred to as **faith-based belief,** is an organized system of shared beliefs regarding the significance of the nature, cause, and purpose of life and of the universe. **Spirituality** refers to the individual's experience and own interpretation of his or her relationship with a supreme being. Religion is usually centered on the belief in or the worshiping of a supernatural or supreme being (such as God). Religion may provide the child structures for moral development, and may also influence the child's concepts about illness, suffering, healing, and coping (Barnes et al., 2000). Prayer, one of the most common expressions of religious faith, is a frequently used therapy in which many children and families engage.

Although spirituality and faith-based beliefs are generally positive means of support for children and families in maintaining and restoring health, at times they can have potentially negative effects for children. Certain groups may blame individuals for their own illnesses and children may develop guilt as a result. If prejudice against other groups occurs, unhealthy responses may interfere with the child's psychosocial development. Abuse may result from parental religious beliefs regarding corporal punishment and discipline. If lifesaving treatments are denied by a religious group, courts may intervene to ensure care for the child. Children involved in cult groups may suffer emotional and psychological harm. Adolescents who are gay or lesbian may be the target of negative feedback and response from their religious communities (Barnes et al., 2000). This may lead them to avoid healthcare that could be potentially beneficial. (See Chapter 5∞ for a further discussion of gay and lesbian teen healthcare needs.)

The three most common faith traditions in the United States are Christianity, Judaism, and Islam (Fosarelli, 2003) (Figure 3–8 ■). Although adherence to a religious tradition is predominant in the United States, it should not be assumed that all individuals believe in or practice organized religion. Always ask family members if they follow a faith and would like a representative from that faith to visit when in the hospital. Adolescents may follow different faith traditions than their parents and should be asked the question individually.

Collaboration between the healthcare team and family is essential to providing care congruent with the child and family's expectations. While spirituality is important for many families, it is often overlooked as a healing strategy. Illness and injury may cause the family to turn to spiritual guidance as a method of understanding and coping. Trust in a higher being or purpose provides meaning for many children that assists them as they deal with health problems (Elkins & Cavendish, 2004). At all times, the nurse must respect the family's view and avoid being judgmental toward their beliefs. Partner with the child and family to incorporate their traditional practices and beliefs with prescribed therapies to ensure the delivery of safe and effective care for the child.

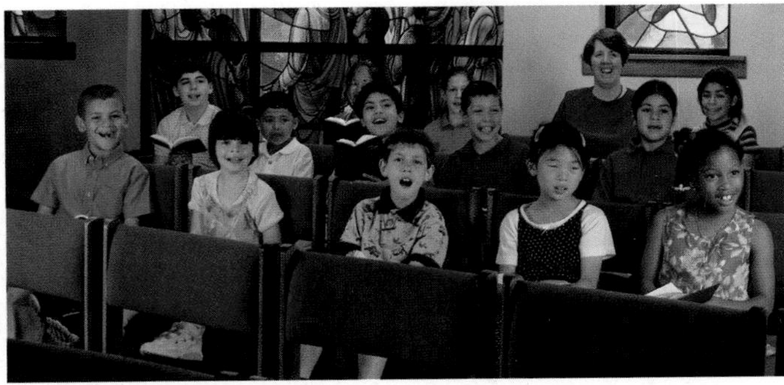

FIGURE 3–8 ■ No longer are communities limited to one culture. The children in this multicultural choir are representative of the changes in demographics in the United States and Canada. Even though they may differ in cultural background, a common thread is found in their religious preference. Can you identify other ways in which multicultural groups interact?

Healing Approaches. Most health professionals in the United States practice traditional Western medicine; however, healers are preferred by some families. There are multiple approaches and some families and practitioners will choose alternative treatments. Several other medical approaches are described here and further explored in the section on complementary and alternative modalities later in the chapter. One way to treat illness is by *homeopathy*, or treating a person with small doses of medicines that would cause illness when given to someone who is healthy. Traditional Western (or *allopathic*) medicine generally gives medicine or treatments that suppress symptoms. Analgesics for pain or antibiotics for infection are examples of such treatments. In homeopathy, the symptoms are viewed as the body's method of healing and small doses of medications are given to enhance the symptoms. For example, medications are chosen to promote fever and inflammation since they are thought to be healing forces (Fontaine, 2005; Spector, 2004).

Another approach to treatment is that of *osteopathic medicine*, which integrates many of the approaches of Western medicine with a belief that many of the body's disorders can be treated by mechanical correction of body imbalances. Several osteopathic medical schools are based in the United States and doctors of osteopathy (DO) may practice in the same health facilities as other physicians.

Naturopathy is a form of medicine that ascribes to the healing forces of nature. Naturopathic physicians treat the entire person using preventive care and treatments that involve natural products from animals, plants, and minerals. Treatments seek to bolster the immune system and a wide array of methods such as aromatherapy and nutritional supplements may be used. Certain medications, treatments, and immunizations may be refused in this approach (Atwood, 2003).

TABLE 3–7 Hot and Cold Conditions and Foods

HOT CONDITIONS	COLD FOODS USED TO TREAT HOT CONDITIONS	COLD CONDITIONS	HOT FOODS USED TO TREAT COLD CONDITIONS
Diarrhea	Barley water	Cancer	Beef
Fever	Chicken	Earaches	Cheese
Gastrointestinal disturbances	Dairy products	Headaches	Eggs
Infection	Dried fruits	Musculoskeletal conditions	Grains
Kidney problems	Fish	Pneumonia	Liquor
Sore throats	Fresh fruits		Onions
	Fresh vegetables		Spicy foods
	Goat meat		Vitamins

Data from Purnell, L. D. (2003). Mexican Americans. In L. D. Purnell & B. J. Paulanka (Eds.), Transcultural health care: A culturally competent approach *(2nd ed.). Philadelphia: F. A. Davis.*

Chiropractic medicine focuses on the relationship between bodily structure (primarily that of the spine) and function, and how that relationship affects the preservation and restoration of health. Chiropractors use manipulative therapy as an integral treatment tool.

Nutrition is another healing approach used by nearly all cultural groups. You may have heard the statement "Feed a cold and starve a fever." Some ascribe to certain foods for illness and health promotion while other foods may be withheld in certain situations. Recall the description of the need for balanced nutrition to treat disease in many cultures. Hot and cold conditions and foods and their links to culture are explained on page 80 and in Table 3–7. Dietary intake and food patterns are integrally connected to culture and so it is logical that food is used to maintain health, restore balance, and treat illness. As children become older, they often practice a combination of food patterns that derive from their cultural group and the larger society in which they live. Diet recalls, food frequencies, and questions about what foods are recommended for certain conditions are good approaches to learn about nutritional intake. (See Chapter 9 for examples of assessment techniques.) As long as a child is receiving fluids needed and no part of intake is contraindicated for the illness, cultural patterns should be honored.

Complementary and Alternative Modalities. Complementary and alternative medicine (CAM) refers to a group of diverse medical and healthcare systems, practices, and products that are not presently considered to be part of conventional Western medicine (National Center for Complementary and Alternative Medicine [NCCAM], 2002). For the purposes of this text we refer to CAM as complementary and alternative modalities, recognizing that not all are medical approaches and most are not applied by traditional medical doctors. A wide array of practitioners use CAM techniques; several types of CAM have already been discussed in this chapter, such as homeopathy and nutrition. The use of CAM therapies in the United States and Canada is widespread and is observed in some manner within all cultures (Figure 3–9 ■).

Though the terms *complementary* and *alternative* are often used interchangeably, they have different meanings and applications. **Complementary medicine** is used in combination with conventional biomedicine. An example of a complementary therapy is the use of massage therapy in conjunction with biomedical therapy, such as narcotic analgesics, for a child with cancer pain.

Alternative medicine is used in place of conventional biomedicine. An example of an alternative therapy is the use of herbal medicines instead of biomedicines for the treatment of a child's health condition. In other words, the child would not receive traditional Western medical care for the condition, such as surgery, radiation, prescribed medications, or other medical interventions.

The NCCAM (2002) classifies complementary and alternative medicine therapies into five categories or domains: alternative medical systems, mind–body interventions, biologically based therapies, manipulative and body-based methods, and energy therapies. Table 3–8 provides an overview of these domains. Most families use some type of CAM even when using traditional Western medicine. Always ask what therapies they believe are helpful, and facilitate the approaches when not contraindicated. Descriptions of common types of complimentary and alternative medicines (NCCAM, 2002) are provided in Table 3–9.

Safety Issues Concerning CAM Therapies. The ANA *Code of Ethics* (2001) mandates that the nurse must promote and protect the health, safety, and rights of patients. Nurses must become knowledgeable in CAM in order to be able to maximize its benefits and also protect the child from any possible harm (Cuellar, Cahill, Ford, et al., 2003). The use of CAM in the care of children must be addressed because of the limited research with this age group and

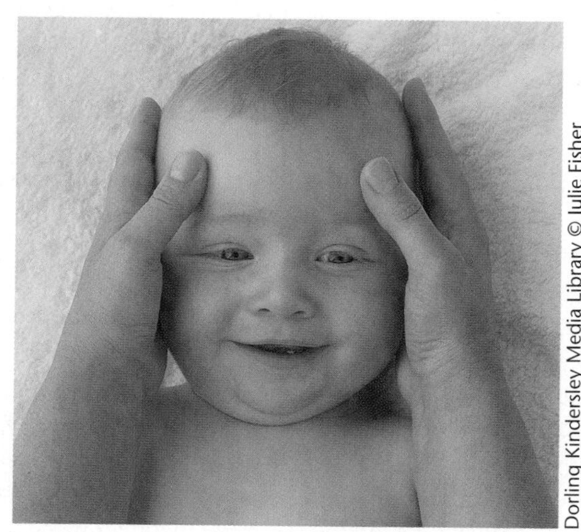

Dorling Kindersley Media Library © Julie Fisher

FIGURE 3–9 ■ Infant massage.

TABLE 3–8 Domains of Complementary and Alternative Medicine

ALTERNATIVE MEDICAL SYSTEMS	MIND–BODY INTERVENTIONS	BIOLOGICALLY BASED THERAPIES	MANIPULATIVE AND BODY-BASED METHODS	ENERGY THERAPIES
Alternative medical care based on theory and practice. They often evolved apart from and earlier than the Western medical approach (allopathic) used in the United States and Canada. Examples of alternative medical systems include naturopathic, homeopathic, osteopathic, and chiropractic medicine. See pages 82–83 for further explanations of these types of medicine.	Mind–body medicine uses a variety of techniques designed to enhance the mind's capacity to affect bodily function and symptoms. Some techniques that were considered CAM in the past have now become conventional therapies (e.g., biofeedback and cognitive-behavioral therapy). Other mind–body techniques are still considered CAM, including meditation, spiritual healing and prayer, mental healing, hypnotherapy, yoga, and therapies that use creative outlets such as art therapy, music therapy, or dance therapy.	Biologically based therapies in CAM use substances found in nature, such as herbs, foods, and vitamins. Some examples include herbal products, dietary supplements, and the use of other so-called natural but as yet scientifically unproven therapies (e.g., using shark cartilage to treat cancer).	Manipulative and body-based methods in CAM are based on manipulation and/or movement of one or more parts of the body. Some examples include massage and chiropractic or osteopathic manipulation. Other examples include acupressure, acupuncture, tai chi, and qi gong.	Energy therapies involve the use of energy fields. They are of two types, biofield therapies and bioelectromagnetic-based therapies. Biofield therapies are intended to affect energy fields that purportedly surround and penetrate the human body. The existence of such fields has not yet been scientifically proven. Some forms of energy therapy manipulate biofields by applying pressure and/or manipulating the body by placing the hands in, or through, these fields. Examples include reiki and therapeutic touch. Bioelectromagnetic-based therapies involve the unconventional use of electromagnetic fields, such as alternating current or direct current fields, magnetic fields, or pulsed fields. Examples include diathermy, where high-frequency electrical currents are used; light therapy using ultraviolet, low-intensity, or colored light; magnetic therapy, and neuroelectric therapy.

Data from National Center for Complementary and Alternative Medicine (2002). What is complementary and alternative medicine (CAM)? *(NCCAM Publication No. D156). http://www. nccam.nih.gov, accessed 11/22/204.*

developmental variations that may influence efficacy and safety. While many CAM therapies may have been proven effective in adults, they may have little effect on children, or even be harmful. The National Institutes of Health and the Agency for Healthcare Research and Quality have set research agendas to investigate the effectiveness of CAM therapies for treatment.

Complementary and alternative medicine practices must be assessed for safety, including positive and negative benefits, cost, efficacy, and clinical usefulness. The standards of products, misleading claims, safety related to megadoses of some products, and standardization of natural products are just a few of the issues raised with the use of herbs and natural products.

Determine the family's use of complementary and/or alternative medicine by asking the following questions:

- What types of home remedies are used? Treatments? Herbs? Teas? Other?
- What healthcare practices are used? Massage? Relaxation? Healer? Other?
- How long has the family used these therapies with the child?
- What are the benefits to the child when these CAMs are used?

Also determine the side effects, risks, and other implications to the child receiving this type of therapy. Partner with the family to ensure safe practices with the use of complementary and/or alternative modalities. See Partnering with Families: Discussions about CAM Therapies.

NURSING MANAGEMENT

The focus of nursing care is assessment of cultural influences on the child's health. The nurse providing culturally competent care to the child and family considers all facets of their culture. Identification of cultural influences as well as cultural barriers will enable the nurse to provide culturally competent nursing care in the management and support of the culturally diverse child and family.

■ Nursing Assessment

Assessment of the child and family includes determining the family's cultural healthcare beliefs and practices.

TABLE 3–9 Selected Types of Complementary and Alternative Medicines

THERAPY	DESCRIPTION	POTENTIAL USE IN CHILDREN	NURSING IMPLICATIONS
Aromatherapy	Involves the use of essential oils (extracts or essences) from flowers, herbs, and trees to promote health and well-being.	The family may use candles or oils to promote a child's pain relief or to encourage the child's relaxation.	Some families erroneously use certain aromatherapies for disorders such as asthma, which can actually worsen the child's symptoms. Caution families to avoid aromatherapy for pulmonary disorders such as asthma and cystic fibrosis.
Dietary supplements	A dietary supplement is a product (other than tobacco) taken by mouth that contains a "dietary ingredient" intended to supplement the diet. Dietary ingredients may include vitamins, minerals, herbs or other botanicals, amino acids, and substances such as enzymes, organ tissues, and metabolites. Dietary supplements come in many forms, including extracts, concentrates, tablets, capsules, gelcaps, liquids, and powders. They have special requirements for labeling.	Many parents administer daily multiple vitamins to their child. Other therapies used for children include the use of echinacea for colds.	Assess family's use of dietary supplements for child. Determine potential interactions between supplements and prescribed medications. Teach parents about safe dosages of vitamins for children.
Massage	Therapists manipulate muscle and connective tissue to enhance function of those tissues and promote relaxation, well-being, and relief from pain.	Families may seek massage therapy for children with musculoskeletal disorders or other chronic diseases.	Assess child for benefits of massage. Determine any potential contraindications to massage therapy (e.g., fractures).
Therapeutic touch	Derived from an ancient technique called laying on of hands. It is based on the premise that the healing force of the therapist affects the patient's recovery; healing is promoted when the body's energies are in balance; and, by passing the hands over the patient, the healer can identify energy imbalances.	The family may enlist a spiritualist or other practitioner to perform therapeutic touch on the child to promote pain relief or a quicker recovery.	Assess the benefits of therapeutic touch on the child (e.g., pain relief). Partner with family to establish other methods of pain relief if therapeutic touch is not effective.
Religious therapies	The most prevalent complementary and alternative therapy in the United States is religious practice such as prayer (Barnes et al., 2000). Religious therapies include faith healing, laying on hands, anointing, prayer, exorcism, pilgrimage, and visits to the sick.	Families may include a variety of religious therapies depending on the child's condition.	Provide the child and family a private environment for ritual practices. Assess for benefits of the therapies. Partner with family to determine alternative methods of therapy if needed.

Data from National Center for Complementary and Alternative Medicine (2002). What is complementary and alternative medicine (CAM)*? (NCCAM Publication No. D156). http://www. nccam.nih. gov, accessed 11/22/2004.*

Questions may include:

- What is your child's condition?
- What do you think caused the child's illness?
- How do you think the child could best be treated?
- Has your child had this condition before and how was it treated?
- What are the most important results you hope to achieve for your child?

When the family is new to the healthcare facility, ask about former healthcare providers and if cultural healers are used. Ask family members how they would like to partner with other healing practices and the goals they have for their interaction with you as the nurse.

Determine barriers to the child's healthcare:

- Do the child and family speak a language different from the healthcare providers?
- Is there adequate transportation to healthcare facilities?
- Is the living situation supportive of treatment and prevention of illness and injury?
- Do the child and family have adequate funds or coverage for healthcare?

Faith-based practice and spirituality may influence a child's health. Identify any religious or spiritual practices the child and family use, as well as the significance of religion and spirituality on health promotion and during the child's illness.

- Do the child and family have any religious or spiritual beliefs?
- How important are those beliefs in the child's life and health and other family members' life and health?
- Do the child and family belong to a religious/spiritual community (e.g., church, synagogue, mosque)?
- How do the child and family's religious/spiritual beliefs impact their practices for health and illness?
- What religious/spiritual healing rituals and practices are performed? By whom?
- Are any healthcare interventions forbidden by religious or spiritual beliefs?
- In what general religious practices (e.g., prayer, church attendance, meditation) does the family participate?

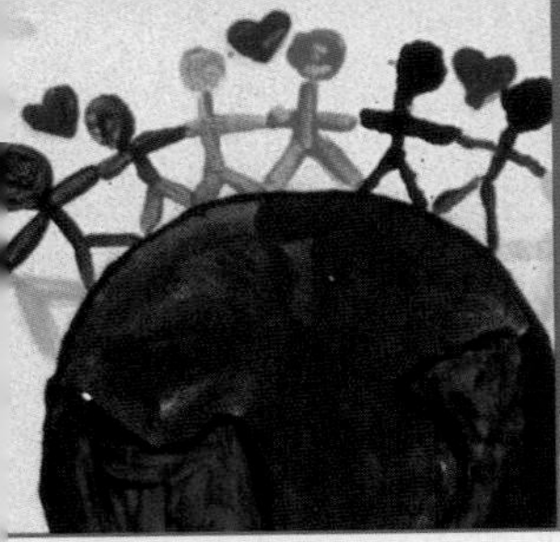

PARTNERING WITH FAMILIES

Discussions about CAM Therapies

Many families use CAM treatments for children. Nurses should always inquire about what therapies families have used in the past and what they intend to use for the present situation. Questions must be non-judgmental and open so that parents feel free to discuss and ask about therapies. Some questions include:

- What treatments do you use in your family for this condition? Do you think you will use them now?
- What are your goals for your child's condition? What combination of treatments do you believe will help you to reach the goal?

Nurses and families partner to examine findings related to CAM therapies and decide if a particular approach will be helpful or harmful. Some information that can help includes:

- Has the therapy been used in children and is it safe? If it involves a medication or supplement, are safe doses established for children? Does the child have a condition such as cancer, allergy, or diabetes that contraindicates use of a particular therapy?
- If an alternative health practitioner is being used, are there guidelines, certifications, or other standardization for the role? Does the individual maintain those verifications of ability to practice?
- Who will monitor the child's response to therapy and progress toward goals?

Families may use websites and other sources to obtain information about CAM therapies. Websites can provide valuable information, but some may have information that is unreliable or misleading. The nurse can provide families with the following key points about evaluating CAM and other medical sources on the web.

- Who sponsors and pays for the site?
- What is the purpose of the site? Is it educational or does it seek to raise money or sell products?
- What sources are used for the information?
- How current is the information?
- Does the site link to other sites? Are the sources reputable?
- What information about you does the site collect, and why?
- How does the site manage interactions with visitors?

Adapted from Dokken, D., & Sydnor-Greenberg, N. (2000). Exploring complementary and alternative medicine in pediatrics: Parents and professionals working together for new understanding. Pediatric Nursing, *26(4), 383–396;* NCCAM. *(2002, February 19). (Publication No. D142).*

Identifying the roles of family members and who is responsible for healthcare decisions is an integral part of the nurse during the initial assessment interview. Determine the following:

- What is the family's structure (e.g., nuclear, extended)?
- Is the family patriarchal, matriarchal, or egalitarian?
- Who is the primary decision maker for the child's healthcare?
- Are the family roles clearly delineated?
- Who does the child depend on for comfort and support?

To communicate effectively, the nurse assesses the communication patterns and needs of the child and family:

- What language(s) does the child speak?
- What language(s) do the parents speak?
- What language does the child read?
- What language do the parents read?
- Is an interpreter necessary or helpful?
- What language would the child and family prefer healthcare providers use to communicate with them?
- Who is doing the majority of the talking and answering of questions?
- What gestures, facial expressions, and body language are used?
- Are there specific ways of demonstrating respect or disrespect for the culture?
- How does the child learn best (e.g., demonstration, reading, hearing)?
- How do the parents learn best (e.g., demonstration, reading, hearing)?

To avoid misinterpretation of a child or family member's behavior, the nurse observes cues from the family to determine the appropriate spatial zone. Determine the following:

- What are the cultural preferences or restrictions related to spatial distancing, eye contact, touching, and other verbal and nonverbal forms of communication?
- Does the family plan for the future?
- Is being on time considered important to the family?
- How do the parent and other family members prefer to be addressed?
- How does the child prefer to be addressed (e.g., nicknames)?

Explore the meaning of food to the child and family. Identify the following:

- Acceptable foods and preparation practices
- Foods that are prohibited or taboo
- Specific food rituals (e.g., holidays, fasting)
- Dietary practices used in promoting the child's health and in treating the child's illnesses
- Foods the child typically likes to eat
- Foods the child dislikes
- The family's usual mealtimes
- The child's height, weight, and other developmental indicators of nutritional health

Refer to Chapter 9∞ for further discussion of nutrition assessment.

Assess the child's biological features for variations of physical characteristics of an ethnic or cultural group (e.g., bone structure, skin color). Assess the child's parental history for the existence of diseases such as hypertension, diabetes, and blood disorders. Determine if the child has been screened for ethnic or culturally specific diseases, for example, sickle-cell disease.

For the dying child or child who has died, determine culturally specific rituals. Determine the family's cultural beliefs regarding death and practices for care of the body. For a comprehensive discussion of care of end-of-life issues, including cultural considerations, refer to Chapter 22∞.

■ Nursing Diagnoses

The use of NANDA nursing diagnoses to describe situations specifically related to culture may be in itself culturally biased since the focuses of these diagnoses are based on Western cultural beliefs. Diagnoses such as "impaired verbal communication" or "deficient knowledge" should not be used solely because a person does not speak English. Is someone who speaks a different language "impaired" in communication?

Specific nursing diagnoses are dependent upon the reason the family seeks contact with healthcare professionals, ranging from the child's health promotion and health maintenance (e.g., immunizations) to the care of a child who is chronic or terminally ill. Examples include:

- Ineffective Therapeutic Regimen Management related to mistrust of healthcare personnel
- Fear related to separation from support system in stressful situation such as hospitalization
- Spiritual Distress related to discrepancy between spiritual beliefs and prescribed treatment
- Interrupted Family Processes related to shift in family roles due to illness

■ Planning and Implementation

The planning and implementation of nursing care for the culturally diverse child and family depends specifically on the findings of the previous assessments. Partner with the child and family to establish a safe, effective, and desirable plan of care. Establish access to an interpreter if needed and evaluate if the match with a particular interpreter is appropriate for the child and family. See Table 3–3 in this chapter and Chapter 6∞ for further guidelines for interpreters.

Recognizing the influence of culture on one's beliefs, values, and healthcare practices is essential for the nurse to deliver culturally competent care. The nurse who develops his or her own techniques in assessing the influence of culture on the child and family and incorporates that information into an individualized plan of care demonstrates appropriate strategies to delivering culturally sensitive care.

Partner with the child and family to assist them in determining how they can incorporate prescribed therapies with their healthcare practices. Ensure that the child and family understand the child's illness, treatment, or health promotion activities. Apply culturally sensitive techniques when dispelling any cultural myths.

Collaborate with a multidisciplinary team including social workers and language specialists to assist the family in receiving assistance for barriers to care such as transportation, financial issues, remote access, and others.

Partner with the family to determine the role traditional healthcare providers and other practitioners, such as folk healers, curandero or curandera, and spiritualists, will have in the care of the child. Encourage collaboration and communication between practitioners to ensure continuity of care.

Collaborate with the child and family to meet specific spiritual needs. This involves showing respect and allowing time and privacy for religious rituals. Offer to have a religious advisor visit and arrange for display and wearing of the child's religious symbols such as a cross in the room, a medicine bag around the neck or wrist, and wearing prayer shawls.

Establish a collaborative relationship with the child and family, recognizing the predominant decision maker of the child's healthcare. If culturally appropriate, encourage all family members to participate in the child's care.

Ensure that the child's nutritional preferences are available. Provide nutritional guidance for the child and family if necessary. Provide education to the family regarding high-risk dietary practices. Partner with the family to establish a well-balanced meal plan for the child. Incorporate cultural preferences in the diet plan. Refer the family to a nutritionist if necessary.

Encourage screening for child and other family members for disorders associated with specific ethnic groups (e.g., sickle-cell disease in African Americans, Tay-Sachs disease in Jews) if they have not been screened. Provide education regarding specific diseases of high incidence in specific populations. Determine the family's awareness of those specific diseases. Encourage early preventive care in children at risk for culturally specific diseases.

■ Evaluation

A desired outcome for the nurse is an awareness and understanding of the cultural influences on the health promotion and illness care of the child. Expected outcomes of care for the child and family include the following:

- Cultural influences on the health promotion and illness care of the child are identified and applied in the care plan.
- Collaboration between the nurse and the culturally diverse family and child occurs to ensure a true partnership in the delivery of nursing care.
- Culturally competent nursing care is provided for the child and family.
- The child and family goals for health promotion/health maintenance and illness/injury care are met.

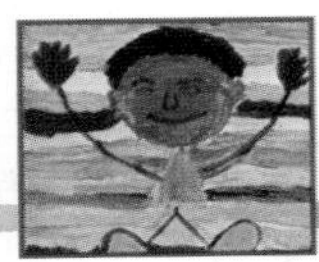

CHAPTER HIGHLIGHTS

- Culture is a significant determinant of an individual's beliefs, behavior, and response to health and illness. Parental beliefs and behaviors can either promote the child's healthcare or impede preventative care, delay or complicate medical care, or result in the use of ineffective or harmful remedies.
- The morbidity and mortality for culturally diverse populations is disproportionate as compared to the White population.
- Cultural barriers to healthcare include lack of cultural awareness and sensitivity in healthcare providers, health-seeking behaviors, perceptions of health and illness, how health information is communicated, lack of transportation, and inadequate access.
- Cultural competence refers to the ability of the nurse to understand and respond effectively to the cultural needs of the child and family.
- The development of cultural competence is an enduring process. Strategies include a self-assessment of one's own beliefs, changes in nursing school curriculum to reflect the diverse nature of the population, increasing diversity of nursing workforce, and increasing understanding through nursing research.
- Health beliefs of the family inform and determine its use of healthcare practitioners and therapies. A combination of Western and alternative practitioners and therapies is commonly used.
- Complementary and alternative modalities (CAM) are defined as diverse medical and healthcare systems, practices, and products that are not presently considered to be part of conventional medicine.

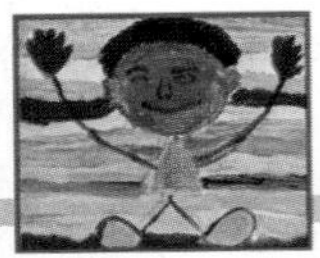

CRITICAL THINKING IN ACTION

INTRODUCTION

Recall Raven, the 4-year-old boy brought to the clinic for complaints of an earache. His father requests a health and physical examination to determine if any healthcare interventions are necessary. Raven does not seem to understand the purpose of the visit and indicates that he has no desire to talk to the nurse.

DESCRIPTION

As the nurse in this situation, you will implement developmentally and culturally appropriate interventions to communicate with Raven. You discuss Raven's living arrangements, education, and nutritional habits with his father, allowing Raven time to adjust to the surroundings of the examination room. Additional information collected relates to care provided for Raven's fever and pain, such as teas and herbs, prior to this visit to the clinic. Raven is observant of your communication with his father.

DISCUSSION

1. What are the most appropriate interventions for communicating with Raven?
2. What approach will you take to assess Raven?
3. How will you examine your cultural values in an effort to provide culturally competent care?
4. How will you demonstrate the role of the nurse to Raven, since his major experience with healthcare has been through his healer?
5. What short-term and long-term collaborative plans should you establish with this family?

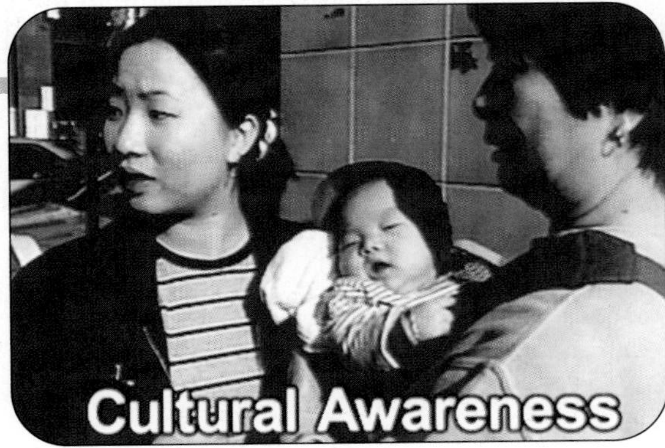

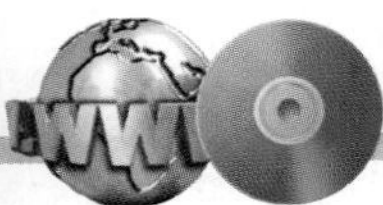

EXPLORE MediaLink

- NCLEX review, case studies, and other interactive resources for this chapter can be found on the Companion Website at **www.prenhall.com/ball**. Click on Chapter 3 to select the activities for this chapter.
- For animations, more NCLEX review questions, and an audio glossary, access the accompanying CD-ROM in this textbook.

http://www.prenhall.com/ball

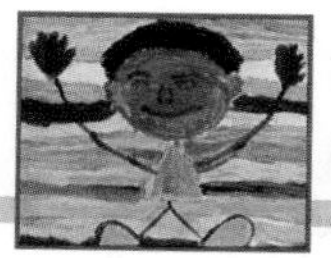

REFERENCES

American Nurses Association. (2001). *Code of ethics.* Washington, DC: Author.

American Nurses Association. (2004). Nursing facts: Today's registered nurses: Numbers and demographics. http://nursingworld/org/readroom/fsdemogrpt.htm, accessed 11/9/2004.

Andrews, M. M., Boyle, J. S., & Carr, T. J. (2003). *Transcultural concepts in nursing care* (4th ed.). Philadelphia: Lippincott Williams & Wilkins.

Atwood, K. C. (2003). Naturopathy: A critical appraisal. *Medscape General Medicine, 5*(4). http://www.medscape.com/viewarticle/465994, accessed 5/10/2004.

Barnes, L. L., Plotnikoff, G. A., Fox, K., & Pendleton, S. (2000). Spirituality, religion, and pediatrics: Intersecting worlds of healing. *Pediatrics, 106,* 899–908.

Burroughs, V. J., Maxey, R. W., & Levy, R. A. (2002). Racial and ethnic differences in response to medicine: Towards individualized pharmaceutical treatment. *Journal of the American Medical Association, 94*(10, suppl), 1–26.

Campinha-Bacote, J. (1999). A model and instrument for addressing cultural competence in health care. *Journal of Nursing Education, 38,* 204–207.

Campinha-Bacote, J. (2002). The process of cultural competence in the delivery of healthcare services: A model of care. *Journal of Transcultural Nursing, 13,* 181–184.

Centers for Disease Control and Prevention. (2004). Health disparities experienced by Hispanics—United States. *Morbidity and Mortality Weekly Report, 53,* 935–937.

Cuellar, N. G., Cahill, B., Ford, J., & Aycock, T. (2003). The development of an educational workshop on complementary and alternative medicine: What every nurse should know. *Journal of Continuing Education in Nursing, 34,* 128–135.

Division of Nursing. (2004). National sample survey of registered nurses. http://bhpr.hrsa.gov/nursing/images/raceth.jpg., accessed 11/9/2004.

Dokken, D., & Sydnor-Greenberg, N. (2000). Exploring complementary and alternative medicine in pediatrics: Parents and professionals working together for new understanding. *Pediatric Nursing, 26,* 383–396.

Elkins, M., & Cavendish, R. (2004). Developing a plan for pediatric spiritual care. *Holistic Nursing Practice, 18,* 179–184.

Fontaine, K. L. (2005). *Complementary & alternative therapies for nursing practice.* Upper Saddle River, NJ: Pearson Prentice Hall.

Fosarelli, P. (2003). Children and the development of faith: Implications for pediatric practice. *Contemporary Pediatrics, 20,* 85–98.

Gannotti, M. E., Kaplan, L. C., Handwerker, W. P., & Groce, N. E. (2004). Cultural influences on health care use: Differences in perceived unmet needs and expectations of providers by Latino and Euro-American parents of children with special health care needs. *Journal of Developmental and Behavioral Pediatrics, 25,* 156–165.

Giger, J. N., & Davidhizar, R. (2002). The Giger and Davidhizar transcultural assessment model. *Journal of Transcultural Nursing, 13,* 185–188.

Giger, J. N., & Davidhizar, R. (2004). *Transcultural nursing: Assessment & intervention* (4th ed.). St. Louis: Mosby-Yearbook.

Health Canada. (2000). *Introduction of cultural competence in pediatric health care.* Ottawa, Ontario: Publications Health Canada. http://www.hc-sc.gc.ca/hppb/healthcare/pubs/circumstances/partIV/doc1.html., accessed 11/16/2004.

Huebscher, R., & Shuler, P. A. (2004). *Natural, alternative and complementary health care practices.* St. Louis: Mosby.

Kataoka-Yahiro, M. R., & Munet-Vilaro, F. (2002). Barriers to preventive health care for young children. *Journal of the American Academy of Nurse Practitioners, 14,* 66–72.

Kim, Y. O. R. (2004). Access to hepatitis B vaccination among Korean American children in immigrant families. *Journal of Health Care for the Poor and Underserved, 15,* 170–174.

Leininger, M. (Ed.). (2001). *Culture care diversity and universality: A theory of nursing.* Boston: Jones and Bartlett Publishers.

Leininger, M. (2002). Culture care theory: A major contribution to advance transcultural nursing knowledge and practices. *Journal of Transcultural Nursing, 13,* 189–192.

Lessard, G., & Kum, K. (2003). Gaps in coverage for children in immigrant families. *The Future of Children, 13,* 101–115.

National Center for Complementary and Alternative Medicine (NCCAM). (2002). *What is complementary and alternative medicine (CAM)?* (NCCAM Publication No. D156). http://www.nccam.nih.gov, accessed 11/22/2004.

National Institutes of Health. (2002). *Strategic research plan and budget to reduce and ultimately eliminate health disparities.* Washington, DC: U.S. Department of Health and Human Services.

Nugent, K. E., Childs, G., Jones, R., Cook, P., & Ravenell, K. (2002). Call to action: The need to increase diversity in the nursing workforce. *Nursing Forum, 37*(2), 28–32.

Office of Minority Health. (2001). *National standards for culturally and linguistically appropriate services in health care.* Washington, DC: U.S. Department of Health and Human Services.

Purnell, L. (2002). The Purnell model for cultural competence. *Journal of Transcultural Nursing, 13,* 193–196.

Purnell, L. D., & Paulanka, B. J. (Eds.). (2003). *Transcultural health care: A culturally competent approach* (2nd ed.). Philadelphia: FA Davis.

Roy, L. C., Torrez, C., & Dale, J. C. (2004). Ethnicity, traditional health beliefs, and health-seeking behavior: Guardians' attitudes regarding their children's medical treatment. *Journal of Pediatric Health Care, 18,* 22–30.

Schantz, S., Charron, S. A., & Folden, S. L. (2003). Health seeking behaviors of Haitian families for their school aged children. *Journal of Cultural Diversity, 10,* 62–68.

Smedley, B., Stith, A., & Nelson, A. (2002). *Unequal treatment: Confronting racial and ethnic disparities in health care.* Washington, DC: National Academy Press.

Spector, R. E. (2004). *Cultural diversity in health and illness* (6th ed.). Upper Saddle River, NJ: Pearson Prentice Hall.

Statistics Canada. (2004). Visible minority population, by age group (2001 census). http://www.statcan.ca/english/Pgdb/demo50a.htm, accessed 11/15/2004.

Sullivan Report. (2004). *Missing persons: Minorities in the health professions.* Atlanta: The Sullivan Commission.

Umar, K. B. (2003, August). *Disparities persist in infant mortality: Creative approaches work to close the gap.* Washington, DC: Department of Health and Human Services, Office of Minority Health.

U.S. Census Bureau. (2003). *The foreign-born population: 2000.* Washington, DC: U.S. Department of Commerce. www.census.gov/population/www/socdemo/foreign.html, accessed 11/9/2004.

U.S. Department of Health and Human Services. (2000). *Healthy People 2010.* Washington, DC: U.S. Government Printing Office.

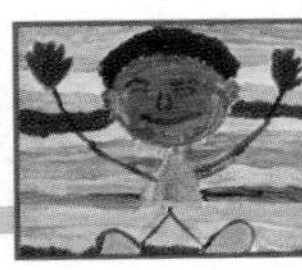

ADDITIONAL REFERENCES

Ahmann, E. (2002). Developing cultural competence in health care settings. *Pediatric Nursing, 28*, 133–137.

Chen, J. L., & Rankin, S. H. (2002). Using the resiliency model to deliver culturally sensitive care to Chinese families. *Journal of Pediatric Nursing, 17*, 157–166.

Dell'Orfano, S. (2002). The meaning of spiritual care in a pediatric setting. *Journal of Pediatric Nursing, 17*, 380–385.

Edmonds, V. M., & Brady, P. (2003). Health care for Vietnamese immigrants. *Journal of Multicultural Nursing & Health, 9*, 52–59.

Fiscella, K., Franks, P., Doescher, M. P., & Saver, B. G. (2002). Disparities in health care by race, ethnicity, and language among the insured. *Medical Care, 40*, 52–59.

Flores, G. (2004). Culture, ethnicity, and linguistic issues in pediatric care: Urgent priorities and unanswered questions. *Ambulatory Pediatrics, 4*, 276–282.

Flores, G., Rabke-Verani, J., Pine, W., & Sabharwal, A. (2002). *Pediatric Emergency Care, 18*, 271–284.

Jintrawet, U., & Harrigan, R. C. (2002). Beliefs of mothers in Asian countries and among Hmong in the United States about the causes, treatments, and outcomes of acute illnesses: An integrated review of the literature. *Issues in Comprehensive Pediatric Nursing, 26*, 77–88.

Loman, D. G. (2003). The use of complementary and alternative health care practices among children. *Journal of Pediatric Health Care, 17*, 58–63.

Luffy, R., & Grove, S. K. (2003). Examining the validity, reliability, and preference of three pediatric pain measurement tools in African-American children. *Pediatric Nursing, 29*, 54–60.

Nichols, L. A. (2004). The infant caring process among Cherokee mothers. *Journal of Holistic Nursing, 22*, 226–253.

Ochieng, B. M. N. (2003). Minority ethnic families and family-centered care. *Journal of Child Health Care, 7*, 123–132.

Sobo, E. J. (2004). Good communication in pediatric cancer care: A culturally-informed research agenda. *Journal of Pediatric Oncology Nursing, 21*, 150–154.

Tellep, T. L., Chim, M., Murphy, S., & Cureton, V. Y. (2001). Great suffering, great compassion: A transcultural opportunity for school nurses caring for Cambodian refugee children. *Journal of Transcultural Nursing, 12*, 261–274.

White, N., Richter, J., Koeckeritz, J., Lee, Y. A., & Munch, K. L. (2002). A cross-cultural comparison of family resiliency in hemodialysis patients. *Journal of Transcultural Nursing, 13*, 218–227.

Chapter

4

Genetic and Hereditary Influences

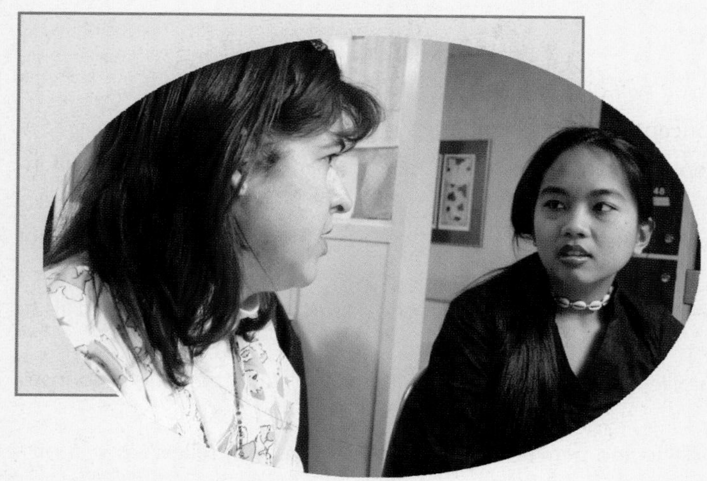

Sarah Hart is an intelligent, mature 17-year-old who arrives alone at the clinic for a sports physical. Sarah was raised by her mother, Diane, and does not know her father. Sarah appears anxious and tells the nurse about her concerns. Sarah has memories of her mother's father dying from Huntington disease when she was 8 years old and she has recently begun researching information. She knows Huntington disease is inherited in an autosomal dominant inheritance pattern with symptoms often manifesting by age 40, but that it often presents earlier as it is inherited from generation to generation. Sarah also knows there is no treatment or cure for Huntington disease. Diane will not discuss her father's death or the inheritance issues with Sarah even though they have a very close relationship. Sarah states that her mother is a free spirit and always "lives in the moment." Sarah, on the other hand, has told the nurse that she is concerned about whether or not she should save money, attend college, pursue a career, get married, have children, or just live in the moment herself, travel, and take on no responsibilities. Sarah would like to be tested to see if she has the altered gene and will have Huntington disease but her mother strongly objects. Diane is not interested in knowing if she has the altered gene and if Sarah were found to have the dominant gene that causes Huntington disease, it would be inferred that her mother also has the gene.

Does the nurse have enough knowledge about genetics to evaluate Sarah's knowledge and also to provide reinforcement of information and guidance to Sarah? Is Sarah able to give informed consent for genetic testing or is she too young to make a decision? Where can the nurse refer Sarah to find the answers to her questions in order to make an informed decision? If Sarah tests positive for the altered gene, will she blame her mother? How will a positive finding impact their roles and relationship?

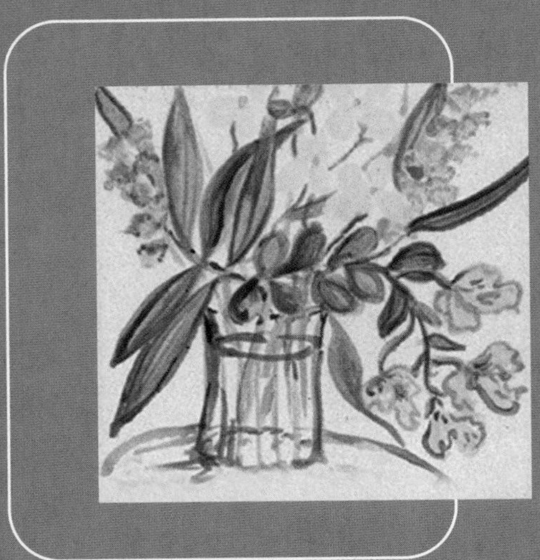

"If I know whether I have the gene alteration that causes Huntington disease, then I will be able to be honest with myself and plan my life with more straightforward choices."

—Sarah, age 17

Key Terms

alleles/100
autosome/96
carrier/107
cell/95
consanguinity/121
crossing over/96
dominant/103
dysmorphology/115
gene/100
gene expression/100
genotype/100
heterozygous/100
homologous chromosomes/96
homozygous/100
human genome/95
inversion/99
karyotype/96
major anomaly/115
meiosis/96
minor anomaly/115
mitosis/96
monosomic (monosomy)/97
mosaicism/97
multifactorial/101
nondisjunction/97
pedigree/118
penetrance/110
phenotype/100

Learning Outcomes

After completing this chapter, you will be able to:

- Discuss the role of genetic concepts in health promotion and health maintenance.
- Integrate basic genetic concepts into child and family education and the reinforcement of information provided to clients by genetic professionals.
- Integrate genetic physical assessment and the use of a pedigree family history into delivery of nursing care.
- Identify children or families with actual or potential genetic conditions and initiate referrals to a genetics professional.
- Prepare children and their families for a genetic evaluation and facilitate the genetic counseling process.
- Describe the significance of delivering genetic education and counseling follow-up in a professional manner.
- Identify the implications of genetic advances on the role of nurses with particular attention to spiritual, cultural, ethical, legal, and social issues.
- Identify the significance of recent advances in human genetics and the impact on healthcare delivery.

MediaLink 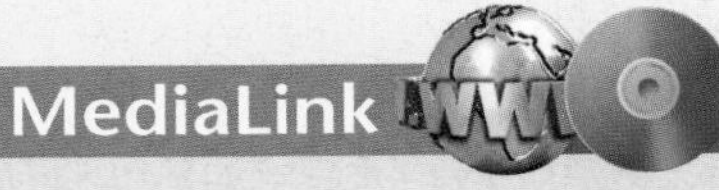 http://www.prenhall.com/ball

Resources for this chapter can be found on the CD-ROM accompanying this textbook, and on the Companion Website at www.prenhall.com/ball. Click on Chapter 4 to select the activities for this chapter.

CD-ROM

Animations/Videos

- *Cystic Fibrosis*
- *Gene Mutation*
- *Human Genome Project*
- *Sickle Cell Anemia*

NCLEX Review

Audio Glossary

COMPANION WEBSITE

NCLEX Review

Case Study: Genetic Testing

MediaLink Applications

- *Create a Family Pedigree*
- *Human Genome Project*

PARTNERING WITH FAMILIES: MEETING THE STANDARD OF GENETIC NURSING CARE DELIVERY

The genetic knowledge obtained from the Human Genome Project has changed not only the way disease treatment is approached but also, more importantly, how nurses look at health promotion and health maintenance. DNA is at the center of the state of our health (Figure 4–1 ■). We now know that good health is associated with genes functioning properly and if genes are functioning improperly, disease or an increased risk for disease can result. This includes the traditional genetic disorders as well as the common complex diseases such as heart disease, stroke, diabetes, and several kinds of cancer. The knowledge gained from the Human Genome research continues to have a profound impact on the prevention, diagnosis, and treatment of genetic disorders and complex diseases (Box 4–1).

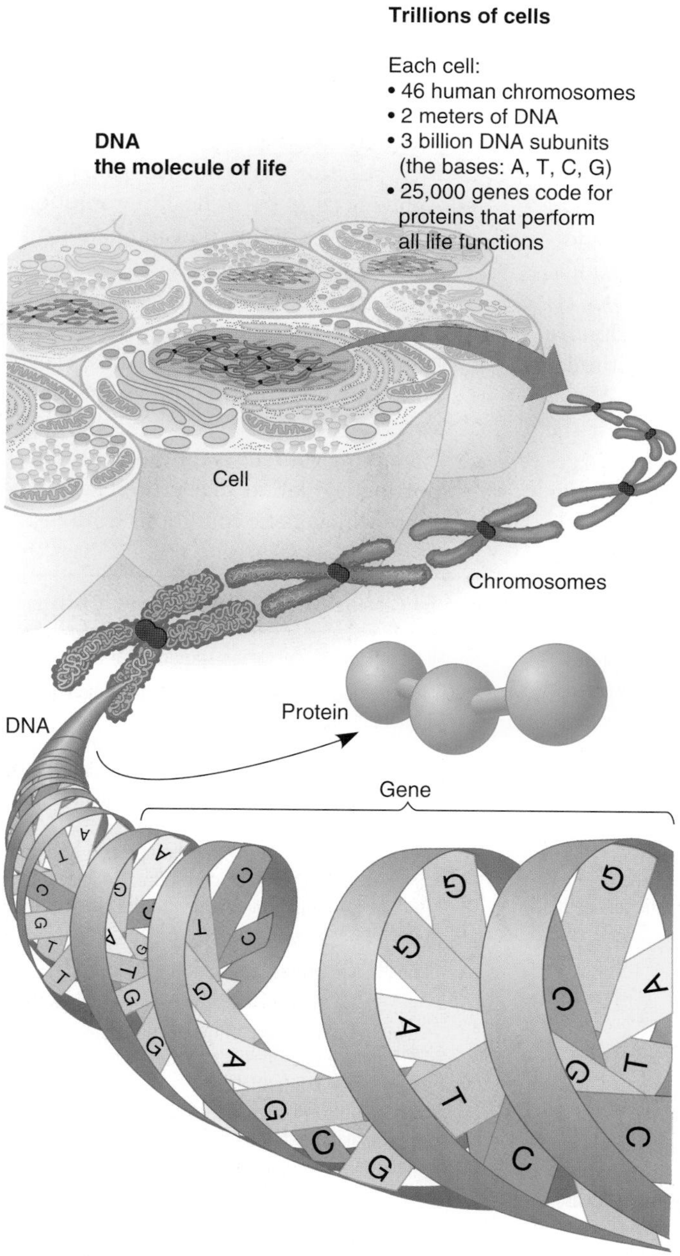

FIGURE 4–1 ■ Each cell nucleus throughout the body contains the genes, DNA, and chromosomes that make up the majority of an individual's genome. The remaining portion of the human genome is in the mitochondria.

Key Terms *(continued)*

polymorphism/102
recessive/103
sex chromosome/96
translocation/99
trisomic (trisomy)/97
wild type gene/95
X linked/108

BOX 4–1 Human Genome Project

In 1986, the United States Department of Energy (USDOE) announced the Human Genome Initiative, and in 1990 the USDOE joined with the National Institutes of Health (NIH) to develop the Human Genome Project (HGP). The ultimate goal was to sequence the human genome and to identify all human genes. The completion of a high-quality reference sequence was announced in April 2003. Information obtained through the sequencing of the human genome has had a tremendous impact on finding the genes associated with human disease. Future research will now be directed toward understanding the complex functions of cellular regulation, human variation, and the interplay of genes and environment and how all the cell organelles, genes, and proteins work together in life's functions (USDOE Genome Programs, 2003).

BOX 4–2 ANA/ISONG Standards of Genetics Clinical Nursing Practice Statement

ANA/ISONG *Statement on the Scope and Standards of Genetics Clinical Nursing Practice:*

> *All licensed registered nurses, regardless of their practice setting, have a role in the delivery of genetics services and the management of genetic information. Nurses require genetic knowledge to identify, refer, support, and care for persons affected by, or at risk for manifesting or transmitting, genetic conditions. As the public becomes more aware of the genetic contribution to health and disease, nurses in all areas of practice will be increasingly asked to address basic genetics-related questions, service needs, or both.*

Used with permission from American Nurses Association and International Society of Nurses in Genetics. Copyright 1998, p. 2. Washington, DC: American Nurses Publishing.

Genetic knowledge will continue to revolutionize how persons perceive themselves as well as their health status and their health potential. Therefore, nurses must integrate new genetic knowledge into their nursing practice. This expectation has been defined in the American Nurses Association/International Society of Nurses in Genetics (ANA/ISONG) *Statement on the Scope and Standards of Genetics Clinical Nursing Practice* (Box 4–2). In addition, a national interdisciplinary group known as the National Coalition for Health Professional Education in Genetics (NCHPEG) has developed competencies to encourage healthcare providers to integrate genetic knowledge, skills, and attitudes while delivering care to children and their families (Box 4–3).

Nurses must have basic genetic knowledge to care for the needs of patients and their families with known or suspected genetic disease. Basic-level nursing practice that meets the standard of genetic nursing includes:

- Identifying simple risk factors by completing a genetic-focused family history and also drawing a three-generation pedigree
- Incorporating a genetic focus into physical assessments
- Applying concepts of health promotion and health maintenance to assist the child and family make informed decisions and lifestyle choices
- Partnering with families to perform interventions that include advocacy, supporting the child and family's decisions, teaching, making referrals, clarifying information, and providing information about available resources and services
- Partnering with the community to educate the public; supporting legislation that protects genetic information and those with genetic conditions from discrimination

BOX 4–3 National Coalition for Health Professional Education in Genetics (NCHPEG) Core Competencies

In a national effort to promote the genetic education of healthcare professionals, these core competencies were formulated and endorsed by an interdisciplinary group made of leaders in more than 100 professional groups including professional organizations, consumers, voluntary groups, government agencies, private industries, managed-care organizations, and genetics professional societies.

Each healthcare professional should at a minimum be able to:

- Appreciate limitations of his or her genetic expertise
- Understand the social and psychological implications of genetic services
- Know how and when to make a referral to a genetic professional

Selected Competencies

All healthcare professionals should understand:

- Basic human genetic terminology
- Basic patterns of biological inheritance and variation, both within families and within populations
- The importance of family history (minimum three generations) in assessing predisposition to disease
- The role of genetic factors in maintaining health and preventing disease
- The history of misuse of human genetic information
- One's own role in the referral to genetic services, or provision, follow-up and quality review of genetic services

All healthcare professionals should be able to:

- Gather family history information, including appropriate multigenerational family history
- Identify clients who would benefit from genetic services
- Explain basic concepts of probability and disease susceptibility, and the influence of genetic factors in maintenance of health and development of disease
- Facilitate the genetic counseling process and prepare clients and families for what to expect, communicate relevant information to the genetics team, and follow up with the client after genetic services have been provided

All healthcare professionals should:

- Recognize philosophical, theological, cultural, and ethical perspectives influencing use of genetic information and services
- Appreciate the sensitivity of genetic information and the need for privacy and confidentiality
- Speak out on issues that undermine client's rights to informed decision making and voluntary action
- Recognize when personal values and biases with regard to ethical, social, cultural, religious, and ethnic issues may affect or interfere with care provided to clients
- Support client-focused policies

Adapted from National Coalition for Health Professional Education in Genetics (NCHPEG). (2001). Core competencies in genetics essential for all health-care professionals. www.nchpeg.org, *accessed 12/4/2004.*

MediaLink Human Genome Project Animation

- Completing an evaluation of the delivery of care for the child and family
- Applying knowledge of the ethical, legal, and social implications of genetic information

Through the application of fundamental genetic concepts, nurses can significantly improve the nursing care provided to children and their families.

Impact of Genetic Advances on Health Promotion and Health Maintenance

Health promotion and health maintenance of children and their families is viewed as the foundation of all nursing care. (See Chapter 10∞.) However, most individuals do not know their complete genetic makeup. Some know they carry an altered gene that causes a specific disease, but the majority do not know with certainty what their future health status will be. With no sure knowledge of genetic makeup or whether a certain alteration in health state will occur (heart disease, for example), healthy lifestyles are not always a priority. Imagine, then, if people knew their statistical risks for developing or inheriting disease by having complete access to the types of genes in their cells. Health promotion and health maintenance teaching and nursing interventions would be based on specific genes. Parents could provide proper diets and important lifesaving nutritional information for their children. Adolescents may give up their sedentary lifestyle, increase exercise, and decrease fast food intake. Lifestyle choices would become more personal and monitoring health may take on a new meaning.

With knowledge of genetic conditions, the pediatric nurse can ensure health teaching and early detection of complications from genetic conditions with emphasis on primary and secondary care interventions. For example:

- Nurses should stress to all teenage girls the importance of folic acid whether they consider themselves sexually active or not. The impact of taking folic acid on the reduction of the incidence of neural tube defects is well documented.
- A child who screens positive for scoliosis should be assessed for axillary freckling and café-au-lait spots, due to the relationship between scoliosis and the variably expressed neurofibromatosis.
- During a sports physical, screening for Marfan syndrome should occur due to its lethal cardiovascular complication of aortic dilation. This can be accomplished by assessing for common characteristics such as myopia, scoliosis, tall stature, long fingers and thumbs, a hollow chest, and an arm span that may be greater than the height.
- The importance of maintaining a PKU diet for life and children with sickle cell disease being maintained on penicillin is also essential to avoiding complications.
- When caring for the child with Down syndrome, the pediatric nurse can help the parents shift from the more expected and traditional focus of disease management to health promotion and health protection by teaching parents that there are established guidelines for exams and screenings.
- With late onset diseases such as Huntington, the pediatric nurse should be aware of the child's struggle to maintain a healthy lifestyle and meet society's moral expectations while struggling with the knowledge of having a lethal gene alteration. See Box 4–4.

Children receiving early intervention and health promotion–focused care are living longer and with a much better quality of life than those who do not (Van Riper & Cohen, 2001). The pediatric nurse must be able to identify both community-based and genetic-based resources that are available to assist the child or adolescent and the family in strategies to support both health promotion and health maintenance activities.

MediaLink Genetics Resources

GENETIC BASICS

A basic knowledge of the cell, DNA, cell division, chromosomes, and genes is essential to deliver the genetic standard of care to children, adolescents, and their families.

The **cell** is the basic unit of life and it is the working unit of all living systems. Life starts as a single cell but the developed human body is made up of trillions of cells. These cells share common features such as a nucleus that contains 46 chromosomes, and organelles such as mitochrondria. There are many different types of "specialized" cells which function differently depending on their location. For example, pancreatic cells function much differently than nerve cells.

All human cells, except mature red blood cells, contain a complete set of deoxyribonucleic acid (DNA) molecules. DNA molecules consist of long sequences of nucleotides or bases represented by the letters A, G, T, and C. The order of these sequences (bases) gives the exact instructions for the functioning of that particular cell. Writing the correct order of the bases using these abbreviations represents the sequence of the bases in DNA. The entire DNA in a human cell is referred to as the **human genome,** or the complete set of inheritance for an individual. The human genome includes the DNA in the cell nucleus as well as the DNA found in the mitochondria, which will be discussed later in this section. Each person's genome is one of a kind. The exception to this is the occurrence of monozygotic twins who are derived from only one

BOX 4–4 Using the People-First Approach

The nurse must incorporate a person-first philosophy and use genetic terminology that is sensitive to the maintenance of an individual's positive self-image. This can be accomplished by using "unaltered" or "**wild type**" **gene** instead of "normal" gene and "altered" gene, "altered, disease-producing gene," or "gene alteration," instead of the terms "mutated" or "abnormal" gene when communicating genetic concerns to children, families, other healthcare providers, or the public.

wild type = normal = expected = unaltered

versus

mutated = abnormal = defective = unexpected = altered

Likewise, newborn Sammy, who exhibits Down syndrome, should not be identified as the "Down baby" but Sammy who has Down syndrome.

fertilized ovum and share identical DNA (Guttmacher & Collins, 2002).

The cell nucleus contains about 6 feet of DNA that is tightly wound and packaged into 23 pairs of chromosomes, making a complete set of 46 chromosomes. There are two copies of each chromosome. One copy, or half of the complete set of these 46 chromosomes, is inherited from the mother and the other copy, or half of the 46 chromosomes, is inherited from the father. For example, an individual will have two chromosome 1s, one inherited from the mother and one inherited from the father. These two inherited copies or pairs are called **homologous chromosomes.** The sperm and ova are exceptions to these numbers. They contain only one chromosome of a homologous pair, or 23 chromosomes per cell. Chromosomes are numbered according to size, with chromosome 1 being the largest and chromosome 22 being the smallest. The 23rd pair determines an individual's gender. A female has two copies of the X chromosome (one copy inherited from each parent) and a male has one X chromosome (inherited from his mother) and a Y chromosome (inherited from his father). These X and Y chromosomes are known as **sex chromosomes.** The remaining 22 pairs of nonsex chromosomes that are alike in both males and females are called **autosomes.** The structure and number of chromosomes can be shown by karyotype. A **karyotype** refers to a picture of an individual's chromosomes (Figure 4–2 ■).

Cell Division

Mitosis and meiosis are the two types of cell division in human cells. **Mitosis** is how the body makes new cells and it takes place in somatic or tissue cells of the body. Cell division through mitosis fills in new skin to heal a scrape or cut. It also replaces cells such as those lost daily on the skin surfaces and in the lining of gastrointestinal and respiratory tracts. In addition, mitosis is responsible for the rapid growth of the human. The mitotic activity of the zygote and its daughter cells is the foundation for the human's growth and development. The zygote undergoes mitosis to form a multicellular embryo, then fetus, then infant. Cell division through mitosis results in two cells called daughter cells that are genetically identical to the original cell or mother cell, and each other.

Meiosis is also known as the reduction division of the cell. Meiosis occurs only in the sex cells of the testes and ovaries and results in the formation of the sperm and oocyte (gametes). Meiosis is similar to mitosis in that it is a form of cell division; however, through a series of complex mechanisms, the amount of genetic material is reduced to half (23 chromosomes). This is important because when the two sex cells combine during fertilization, the total number of chromosomes (46) is present in the offspring's cells. The purposes of meiosis are to produce gametes, to reduce the number of chromosomes by half, and to make new combinations of genetic material from crossing over and independent assortment processes which allow diversity in the human population. **Crossing over** results from a genetic exchange or reshuffling of materials between two homologous chromosomes or genetic materials inherited from the father and mother. There is an exchange of sections of DNA resulting in new intact chromosomes. An exception to chromosomal crossing over is the Y chromosome. The Y chromosome does not have the ability to cross over since it is only a single chromosome with no homologous mate. It is presently believed that the Y chromosome performs the phenomenon of gene conversion and exchanges genes within itself (National Human Genome Research Institute [NHGRI], 2003). Independent assortment results from the multiple chromosomal combinations that are possible at fertilization.

Chromosomal Alterations

Alterations in chromosomes often occur during cell division (meiosis or mitosis) and are classified as either structural alterations or alterations in the number of chromosomes. They involve either part of or the whole chromosome. The clinical

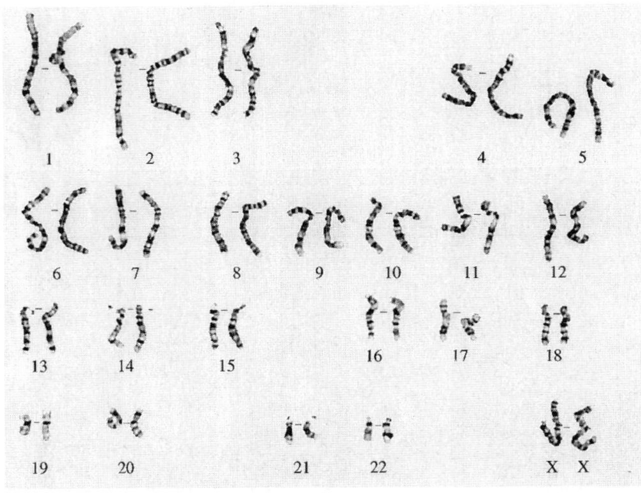

A Female

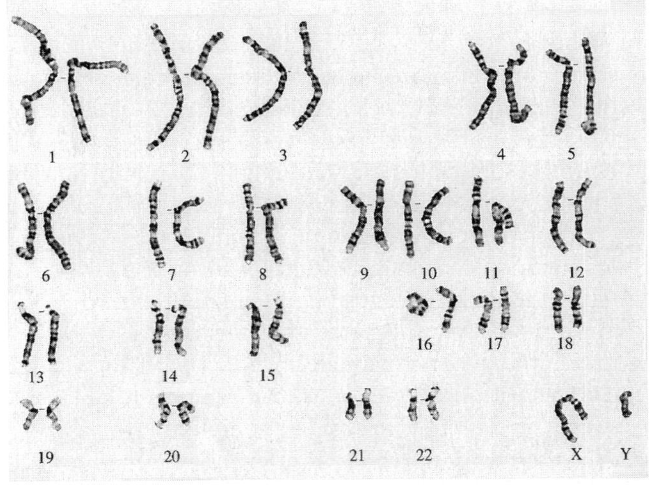

B Male

FIGURE 4–2 ■ A karyotype is a picture of an individual's chromosomes. It shows chromosomal structure and number of the 22 pairs of autosomes and the sex chromosomes.

Courtesy of the Greenwood Genetic Center, Greenwood, SC.

BOX 4–5 Variations in Chromosomal Number

Aneuploidy—the condition when extra or missing chromosomes exist; if there is an addition or deletion of chromosome number and the individual lives, physical abnormalities and/or mental retardation is common.

- **Monosomy**—the loss of a single chromosome from a pair; i.e., Turner syndrome (45,XO)
- **Trisomy**—the gain of a single chromosome, making a total of three copies of a certain chromosome; i.e., trisomy 21 or Down syndrome

Euploidy—the presence of the normal number of 46 chromosomes

Polyploidy—the condition when more than two pairs of all the chromosomes are present

consequences of structural and number changes in the chromosomes in an individual vary depending on the amount of DNA affected by the alterations.

Alterations in Chromosome Number

An increase or decrease in chromosomal numbers can occur during meiosis or mitosis (Box 4–5). Alterations occur often during meiosis because it is a highly specific and complex process and each new daughter cell must contain exactly one chromosome from each homologous pair of chromosomes. It is during these complex phases of meiosis that **nondisjunction** may occur (Figure 4–3 ■).

With nondisjunction, the paired homologous chromosomes do not separate and do not migrate properly into separate egg or sperm cells. This creates an egg or sperm cell with either two copies or no copies of a particular chromosome. When these egg or sperm cells are fertilized by a normal gamete that contains 23 copies of all of the chromosomes, a zygote that is **monosomic** (one member of the chromosome pair is missing) or **trisomic** (having three chromosomes instead of the usual two) results. These circumstances produce such conditions as Turner syndrome (monosomy) or trisomy 21 (Down syndrome). Although Turner syndrome is an exception, monosomic conceptions are not usually compatible with life and are lost through spontaneous abortions. Extra chromosomal material (as in trisomy) is not compatible with life the majority of the time. In most cases, products of conception with extra chromosomal materials are spontaneously lost. Trisomies 13, 18, and 21 demonstrate the clinical variations that present when different chromosomes are involved, particularly chromosomes that are not rich in genes. See Table 4–1.

Mosaicism. Monosomy and/or trisomy can also occur during mitosis which results in two separate cell lines with different chromosomal makeup, also known as **mosaicism.** The earlier the error occurs, the more cells that will be abnormal and the converse is also true. The degree to which a person is affected by this chromosomal error depends directly on the number or percentage of cells with the altered chromosomal number. For example, an

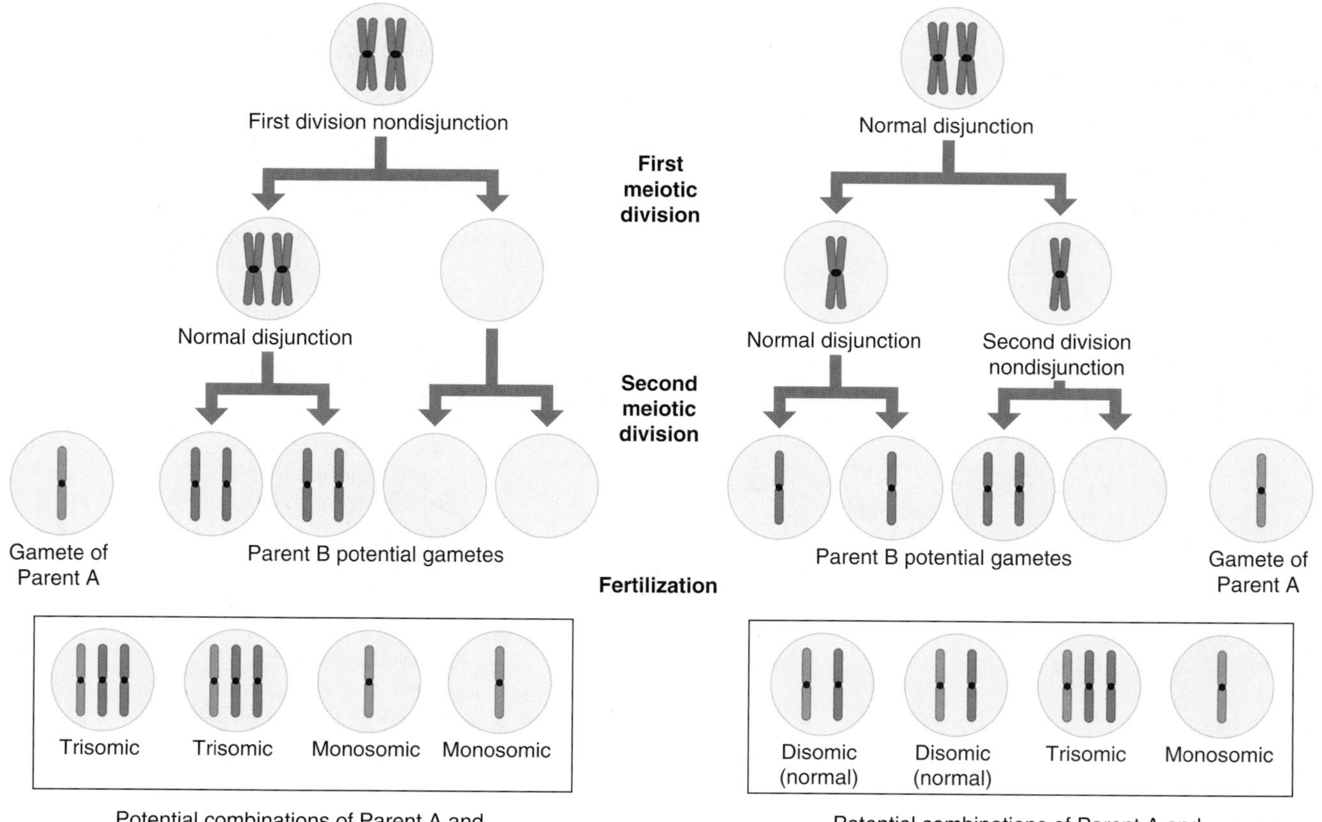

FIGURE 4–3 ■ Examples of nondisjunction—a random error which occurs when a chromosome pair fails to separate during cell division resulting in more (e.g., trisomy) or less (e.g., monosomy) than the expected number of chromosomes present in the new cell; nondisjunction is the most common cause of trisomy 21 (Down syndrome).

TABLE 4–1 Examples of Chromosomal Alterations

SYNDROME NAME	CHROMOSOMAL VARIATION	GENDER AFFECTED	CLINICAL MANIFESTATIONS
Cri du Chat			
Incidence: 1 in 20,000–50,000	Autosomal deletion syndrome 5p (large deletion on the short arm of chromosome 5)	Male and female	Low birth weight (<2.5 kg) Microcephaly Hypertelorism High-pitched, catlike cry Low-set and poorly formed ears Single transverse palmar crease Severe mental retardation Slow growth (Jones, 1997)
Down Syndrome			
Incidence: 1 in 800 Variable with maternal age Etiology: Nondisjunction 94% Mosaicism 2.4% Translocation 3.3%	Trisomy 21	Male and female	Flat occiput Hypotonia Congenital heart defects Single transverse palmar crease Short limbs High-arched palate that may cause protruding tongue Small nose
(See Chapter 34∞)	Epicanthal folds		Brushfield spots (white speckles on edge of iris) Absent Moro reflex Variable degrees of mental retardation (Nussbaum et al., 2001; Lashley, 1998)
Edwards Syndrome			
Incidence: 1 in 7,500 births	Trisomy 18	Male and female	Low-set malformed ears Hands held in a clenched fist Rocker bottom feet Small nails (hypoplastic) Prominent forehead Weak cry Small jaw (micrognathia) Poor suck Failure to thrive (Klug & Cummings, 2003; Nussbaum et al., 2001; Lashley, 1998)
Patau Syndrome			
Incidence: 1 in 20,000–25,000 births	Trisomy 13	Male and female	Cleft lip and palate Hands held in a clenched fist Multiple fingers or toes (polydactyly) Small head (microcephaly) Small or absent eyes Rocker bottom feet Severe growth and mental retardation Multiple system anomalies (Klug & Cummings, 2003; Nussbaum et al., 2001; Lashley, 1998)
Klinefelter Syndrome			
Incidence: 1 in 500 males (See Chapter 32∞)	47, XXY Trisomy	Male	Small testes Long legs Slim, tall stature Infertility Gynecomastia in 1/3 of adolescents Fifth finger clinodactyly Appear physically normal until puberty, then show signs of hypogonadism (Jones, 1997)

TABLE 4–1 Examples of Chromosomal Alterations (continued)

SYNDROME NAME	CHROMOSOMAL VARIATION	GENDER AFFECTED	CLINICAL MANIFESTATIONS
Triple X Syndrome			
Incidence: 1 in 1,000 females	47, XXX (Trisomy)	Female	Usually physically normal May be above average in stature May have behavioral problems during development transition from adolescent to early adulthood Usually have learning difficulties Mild depression (Jones, 1997)
Turner Syndrome			
Incidence: 1 in 2,000 females (See Chapter 32∞)	45, XO Monosomy	Female	Short, webbed neck Loose skin around neck in infancy Congenital lymphedema with residual edema over the dorsum of the fingers and toes that can be seen at any age Ovarian dysgenesis Infertility Short stature Broad chest with widely spaced nipples Low posterior hairline Low birth weight (2,900 g average) Delayed bone maturation Cardiovascular and renal abnormalities (Jones, 1997)

individual with mosaic Turner syndrome may have varying degrees of infertility or short stature and an individual with mosaic Down syndrome may have a higher intelligence level than children whose every cell has three copies of chromosome 21.

Structural Chromosomal Alterations

Inversion. A chromosomal **inversion** is a chromosomal rearrangement where a segment of a chromosome is reversed causing a change in the DNA sequence for that portion of the chromosome. The inversion occurs when a chromosome breaks in two places and the piece between the breaks turns upside down and reattaches within the same chromosome. The clinical consequences of an inversion depend on how much chromosomal material is involved, where the inversion occurs, and what type of inversion is present.

Deletion and Duplication. A chromosomal alteration that includes missing (deletion) or additional (duplication) parts of a whole chromosome or a segment of a chromosome is an *unbalanced* rearrangement. An unbalanced rearrangement can result in missing genes, confusing directions from the genes, or too much gene product which often results in a condition that is not compatible with life or an altered physical and/or mental development. An example is cri du chat syndrome (mental retardation, cry sounding like a cat mewing, and low-set ears) from a large deletion on chromosome 5.

Translocation. **Translocation** (chromosomal reshuffling) occurs when a segment of a chromosome transfers or moves and attaches itself to another chromosome. A translocation that includes the entire correct amount of chromosomal material but in a new arrangement is a *balanced translocation.* The individual who has a balanced rearrangement has all of the chromosomal material present and therefore does not usually have any physical or mental disabilities. However, the individual with a balanced translocation has an increased risk of pregnancy losses or having children with mental and/or physical disabilities from an unbalanced rearrangement. This increased risk for having children with chromosomal alterations is present with *all* future pregnancies. A common chromosomal rearrangement known as an *unbalanced translocation* is responsible for about 3.3% (Jones, 1997) of the children diagnosed with Down syndrome (Figure 4–4 ■). The rearrangement is between chromosome 14 and 21. One copy of chromosome 21 attaches itself to the end of chromosome 14 and is then considered "translocated." When fertilization occurs, there is the potential to have one single copy of chromosome 21 from parent A, one single copy from parent B and also the copy of chromosome 21 that is attached to chromosome 14 of the balanced carrier parent, making a total of three copies of chromosome 21. Thus, the child would inherit three copies of chromosome 21, resulting in Down syndrome. Because translocations can be inherited, chromosomal studies of each parent are suggested to determine the cause of a trisomy.

Genes

The nurse must also have knowledge of genes—what they are, the role genes play in homeostasis, and the consequences of gene alterations. Knowing how these gene alterations are inherited is also important for nursing interventions and teaching the child, adolescent, and family at risk for or with a known gene (DNA-based)

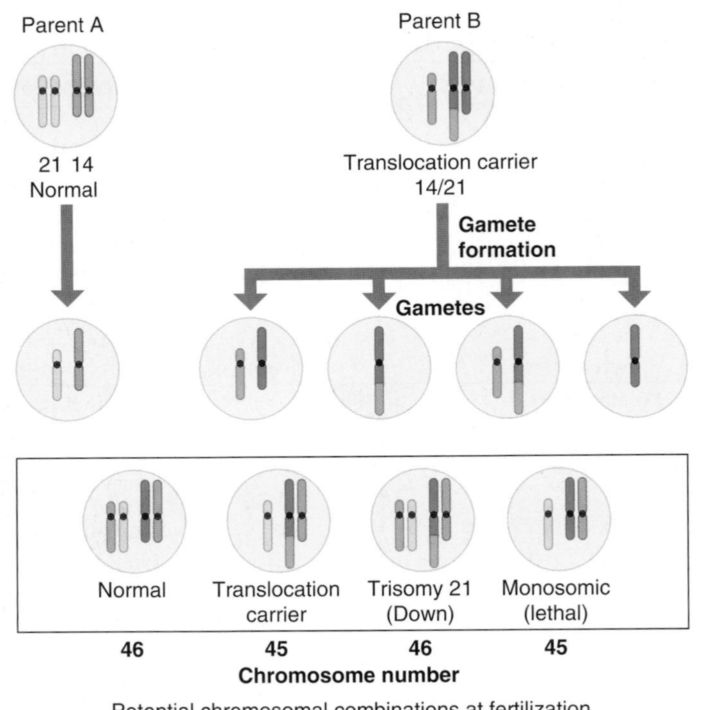

FIGURE 4–4 ■ *A*, Example of translocation which occurs when a segment of a chromosome transfers or moves and attaches itself to another chromosome. When meiosis occurs in the balanced carrier parent, an ovum or sperm has the potential to have one single copy of chromosome 21 plus the copy of chromosome 21 that is attached to chromosome 14, making a total of two copies of chromosome 21. When combined with the other parent's chromosome 21, the offspring then has three copies of chromosome 21. *B*, Chromosomal translocation is responsible for 3% to 4% of all Down syndrome occurrences.

condition. Knowledge of the function and inheritance of genes is implicit in health promotion as well as health maintenance of the child and family.

A **gene** is a small portion (segment) of the nucleotide (base) sequence of a chromosome DNA molecule that can be identified with a particular function or characteristic. These segments of DNA within each gene have specific directions for the functioning of the gene. This specific sequence of nucleotides (the genes and the variations therein) is referred to as the individual's **genotype.** Each chromosome contains numerous genes arranged in a linear order. It is currently believed that there are about 25,000 genes in the human genome. The number of genes present on each chromosome varies. Chromosome 1 is the largest chromosome and has the largest number of genes with 2,968. The Y chromosome has the smallest number of genes with 231 (United States Department of Energy [USDOE] Genome Programs, 2003). All genes come in pairs because chromosomes come in pairs. The only exception to all genes being paired are the genes on the sex chromosomes (X and Y) present in males. All genes have a specific location on a specific chromosome. This is known as *genetic locus.* For example, one of the many genes located on chromosome 19 is a gene for eye color. This gene is located at a specific site on chromosome 19. There may be slight variations or different forms of a gene, as in this case of green versus blue eye color, and these different forms or versions of genes are called **alleles.** An individual who has two identical forms (alleles) of a gene is said to be **homozygous** (*homo* = same). An individual who has two different forms (alleles) of the gene is said to be **heterozygous** (*hetero* = different). See Figure 4–5 ■. Genes can be described as *altered* or *mutated* when a change has taken place, or **expressed** when the gene has an impact on the outward appearance of an individual and/or the functioning of cells. The observable, outward expression of an individual's entire physical, biochemical, and physiologic makeup, as determined by the person's genotype and environmental factors is referred to as **phenotype.** Phenotype may be expressed or observed as curly or straight hair or the presentation of signs and symptoms of a disease.

Function and Distribution of Genes

Although the functions of over 50% of the genes in the human genome are unknown, it is known that about 2% of the genes give directions to parts of the cell for how to make proteins, what type of proteins to make, and how much of a protein to make (Lea, Jenkins, & Francomano, 1998). These protein-directing genes are important to life and functioning as a human being because proteins are highly specialized and perform a variety of

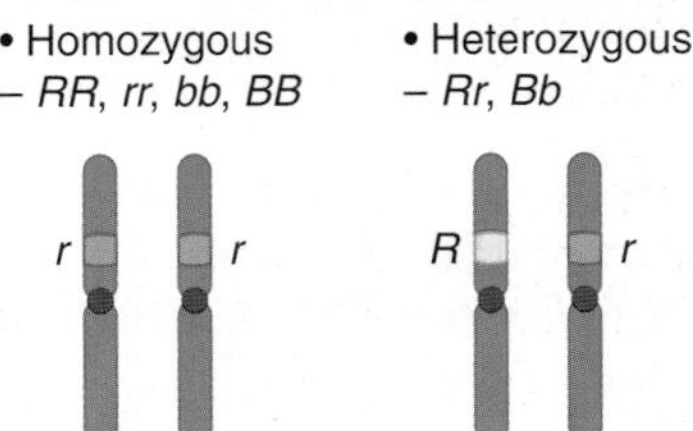

FIGURE 4–5 ■ Sample homozygous (two identical alleles of a gene) and heterozygous (two different alleles of a gene) genotypes. Genotype may be represented with two letters; capital letters are used to represent dominant forms of genes and small letters are used to represent recessive forms of genes in a genotype.

functions within the cell (Box 4–6). These functions include transmitting messages between cells, fighting infection, directing genes to turn on or off, forming structures, and sensing light, taste, and smell (Jegalian, 2000). Some gene activities change moment to moment, in response to tens of thousands of intra- and extracellular environmental signals (USDOE Genome Programs, 2003). An example is the feedback mechanism that stimulates a cell to produce insulin after eating a candy bar. After eating, a gene on chromosome 11 directs pancreatic cells to produce, modify, and secrete insulin. Although the gene for producing insulin is present in all nucleated cells of the body, it is only functional in insulin-secreting pancreatic cells. Genes are distributed unevenly across the chromosomes with random areas of gene concentrations. Chromosomes 13, 18, and 21 are the three autosomes with the fewest number of genes. It is not a coincidence then that chromosomes 13, 18, and 21 are also the three chromosomes for which the occurrence of trisomy (three copies of a chromosome) is compatible with life (Guttmacher & Collins, 2002).

Mitochondrial Genes

Chromosomes in the cell nucleus are not the only site where genes reside. Several dozen that are involved in energy metabolism are located in the cell mitochondria (the "powerhouse" of the cell). Mitochondria are concerned with energy production and metabolism. Some cells contain more mitochondria than others, but each mitochondrion contains its own copies of DNA identified as mitochondrial DNA (mtDNA). Because ova have many mitochondria and sperm do not (most mitochondria are located in the tail of the sperm that detaches after fertilization), mtDNA is usually inherited from the mother. Therefore mitochondrial genes and any diseases due to DNA alterations on those genes are transmitted through the mother in a *matrilineal* pattern. This pattern of inheritance is different from the pattern of inheritance of genes found in the nucleus of the cell (Guttmacher & Collins, 2002). Thus, an affected female will pass the mtDNA mutation to all of her children whereas an affected male will not pass the mtDNA mutation to any of his children (Nussbaum, McInnes, Willard, et al., 2001). Signs and symptoms of conditions as a result of mitochondrial gene alterations are primarily involved in high-energy organs such as skeletal muscles, brain, and heart muscle (Lashley, 1998). An example is Leber's hereditary optic neuropathy where there is a rapid loss of central vision in both eyes because of progressive optic nerve death that results in blindness in young adults (Lea et al., 1998; Nussbaum et al., 2001). Hypertrophic cardiomyopathy, heart block, seizures, and deafness are also associated with mtDNA gene alterations (Nussbaum et al., 2001).

BOX 4–6 Genes and Health or Disease

Person 1's DNA sequence for a certain gene is: A A **A T** T T and consequently a normal protein is produced.
Person 2's DNA sequence for that same gene is: A A **T A** T T and a low or nonfunctioning protein is produced and may have no negative effects.
Person 3's DNA sequence for that same gene is: A A **C A** T T and this mutation causes disease.

Gene Alterations and Disease

A protein will malfunction and in many cases cause disease if any kind of alteration (mutation or change) is present in the order of the DNA sequence within a gene. These gene alterations can be inherited from one or both parents or they can be acquired. Mutations inherited from a parent (hereditary mutations) are also known as germline mutations because the mutation exists in the reproductive sperm or ova of the parent. Consequently, the DNA in every cell of that offspring will have the gene alteration and also can be inherited from generation to generation.

The second kind of gene alteration is an acquired or a somatic mutation. These alterations occur in the DNA of cells of the individual throughout a lifetime. They can result from errors during cell division (mitosis) or from environmental influences such as radiation or toxins (National Institutes of Health [NIH] & National Cancer Institute, 1995). See Figure 4–6 A and B ■.

MediaLink Cystic Fibrosis Animation

Today it is known that gene alterations are responsible for approximately 6,000 hereditary diseases such as cystic fibrosis, Duchenne muscular dystrophy, and phenylketonuria. However, different gene alterations within a particular gene can result in a wide variety of signs and symptoms. For example, the CFTR gene for cystic fibrosis is a very large gene located on chromosome 7. More than 800 different mutations of this gene have been reported to cause cystic fibrosis (Wine, Kuo, Hurlock, et al., 2001). The area of the CFTR gene that controls mucous production can have more than 300 different gene alterations resulting in a variety of symptoms ranging from mild to severe, or no symptoms at all (NIH & National Cancer Institute, 1995).

Other situations when gene alterations cause illness and disease are through gene interactions with the environment. These genes and conditions are referred to as **multifactorial** (Jegalian, 2000). Alterations in regulatory genes may also occur. Regulatory genes play a part in maintaining homestasis or normal functioning. A regulatory gene mutation might lead to the loss of expression of a gene, to unexpected expression in a tissue in which it is usually silent, or a change in the time when a gene is usually expressed. An example of a regulatory gene mutation associated with disease is the insulin gene region that increases the risk of type 1 diabetes (Guttmacher & Collins, 2002).

Gene Alterations that Decrease Risk of Disease

Although it is common to associate gene mutations with disease, it is important to remember that gene mutations can also be helpful and decrease the risk of disease. Gene alterations and genetic variations may also have a protective role in the expression of diseases. A common example is the protective value of the gene alteration that causes sickle cell disease. Those individuals with this gene alteration have protection against malaria. Another, less common, example of a protective gene alteration is the one on the receptor gene named CCR5. This mutation consists of a deletion within the DNA sequence. Persons who are homozygous for the CCR5 mutation (have two copies of the altered gene) are almost completely resistant to infection with HIV type I, and those who

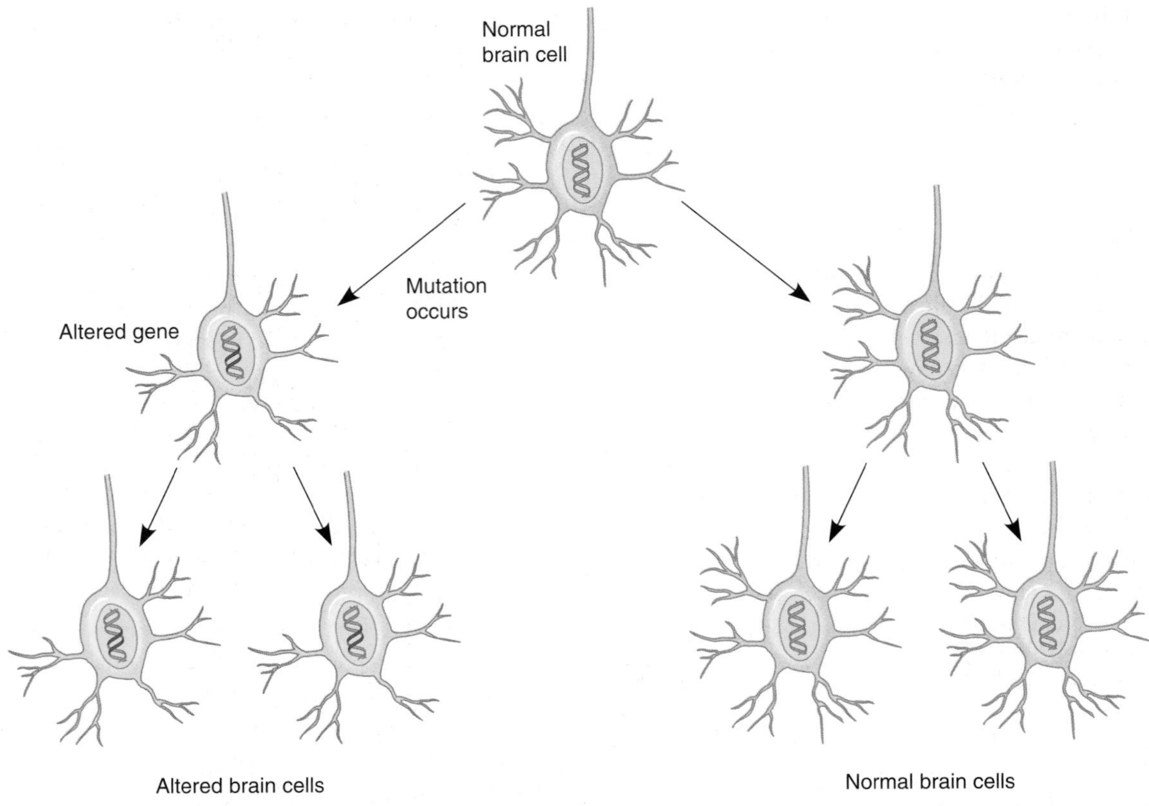

FIGURE 4–6A ■ Acquired DNA mutations may occur in the body's tissue (somatic) cells throughout an individual's lifetime. Consequently, all new cells resulting from cell division of the cell with the DNA mutation will have the same DNA alteration (mutation) in that tissue but these mutations are not inheritable. Some cancers result from acquired DNA alterations.

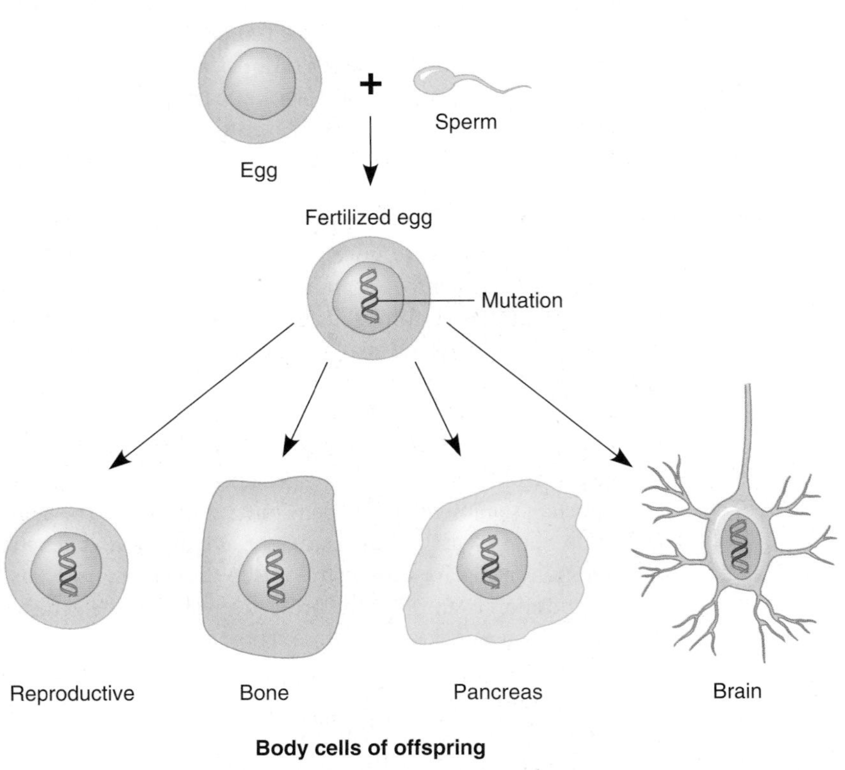

FIGURE 4–6B ■ A germline mutation can occur in the egg, sperm or the single-cell zygote (fertilized egg). A germline DNA alteration results in the DNA alteration being present in all cells throughout the body because of the cell division of the zygote.

are heterozygous for the deletion (have one copy of the altered gene) progress much slower from the stage of HIV infection to AIDS (Guttmacher & Collins, 2002). As genomic research continues, more of these types of beneficial gene alterations will be identified.

Single Nucleotide Polymorphisms

Single nucleotide polymorphisms (SNPs, pronounced "snips") are one-letter (base pair) variations in the DNA sequence. In all people, 99.9% of the DNA is identical but these SNPs are responsible for differences among individuals. **Polymorphisms** are DNA sequences that have many forms but give the genetic "directions" for the same thing. Most of these differences have no effect on the individual. Some cause subtle differences in numerous characteristics in appearance such as widow's peak, tongue rolling, and attached ear lobes. Other SNPs, however, affect an individual's risk for certain diseases and have a major impact on how the individual responds to environmental factors such as toxins, microbes, and medications. Scientists are mapping these areas of SNPs in order to move to the next step of identifying the multiple genes that are associated with diseases that are not caused by single gene alterations, but the complex diseases caused by multiple genes such as cancer, cardiovascular disease, and diabetes (USDOE Genome Programs, 2003; Jegalian, 2000).

PRINCIPLES OF INHERITANCE

Knowledge of inheritance allows the nurse to not only offer and reinforce genetic information to children, adolescents, and their families but also to assist them in managing their care and in making reproductive decisions. The basic underlying principles of inheritance that nurses can apply to inheritance risk assessment and teaching include (1) all genes are paired, (2) only one gene of each pair is transmitted (passed on) to an offspring, and (3) one copy of each gene in the offspring comes from the mother and the other copy comes from the father. Understanding the Mendelian patterns of inheritance is made easier by relating these principles.

Mendelian Pattern of Inheritance

Conditions that are caused by a mutation or alteration of a single gene are known as monogenic or single-gene disorders. There are more than 6,000 known single-gene disorders occurring in about 1 per 200 births (Human Genome Project [HGP] Information, 2003c). The most common gene alterations that result in genetic disorders are categorized into Mendelian inheritance patterns, as they are predictably passed on from generation to generation following Mendel's laws of inheritance. These single-gene mutations follow an autosomal dominant, autosomal recessive, X-linked recessive, or X-linked dominant inheritance pattern. The first three of these patterns are the most common. Modes of transmission or inheritance for thousands of conditions resulting from monogenic alterations have been identified (Online Mendelian Inheritance in Man [OMIM], 2003). See Table 4–2.

Recessive versus Dominant Disorders

The distinction between recessive and dominant phenotypes or disease presence (expression) is in the amount of gene product from the unaltered (wild type or normal) gene. When the individual is heterozygous (has one unaltered gene and one altered gene), the altered gene as well as the disease is classified as **recessive** *if* half of the product produced from the unaltered gene is enough to maintain homeostasis and perform the expected function. Therefore, two altered genes must be present to cause a diseased state. If the altered gene causes disease even though the unaltered gene is producing the gene product, then the altered gene and the disease are classified as **dominant** (Nussbaum et al., 2001).

Autosomal Dominant

More than half of the known Mendelian conditions are autosomal dominant (AD). Examples include neurofibromatosis, achondroplasia (dwarfism), Marfan syndrome, Huntington disease, and hypercholesterolemia. In autosomal dominant conditions, disease occurs in spite of the fact that there exists one unaltered or normal gene. Also, homozygous dominant conditions are generally much more severe than heterozygous dominant conditions and are often lethal. For example, the child who is born homozygous for achondroplasia (short stature; short-limbed dwarfism) is much more severely affected than a child who is heterozygous and usually will not survive early infancy. A homozygous fetus with a dominant disease-producing gene will often spontaneously abort. One exception to this is the individual with the gene alteration that causes Huntington disease (HD). There is no obvious difference between homozygous and heterozygous individuals with this gene alteration (Nussbaum et al., 2001). Because homozygous dominant conditions are usually lethal and would result from *both parents being affected*, the nurse should consider an individual exhibiting an autosomal dominant condition as heterozygous.

MediaLink Gene Mutation Animation

Inheritance Risk in Autosomal Dominant Conditions

Autosomal dominant conditions are the result of an altered gene on any of the 22 autosomes or nonsex chromosomes (Figure 4–7 ■). Because the gene alteration occurs on a nonsex chromosome, both males and females have an equal chance of inheriting the altered gene from their affected parent. There is a 50% chance that an affected parent will pass the altered disease-producing gene on to a child. Each pregnancy is an independent event and this probability percentage remains constant with each pregnancy, no matter how many of a couple's previous children have inherited the altered gene. Family histories will often reflect this 50% inheritance

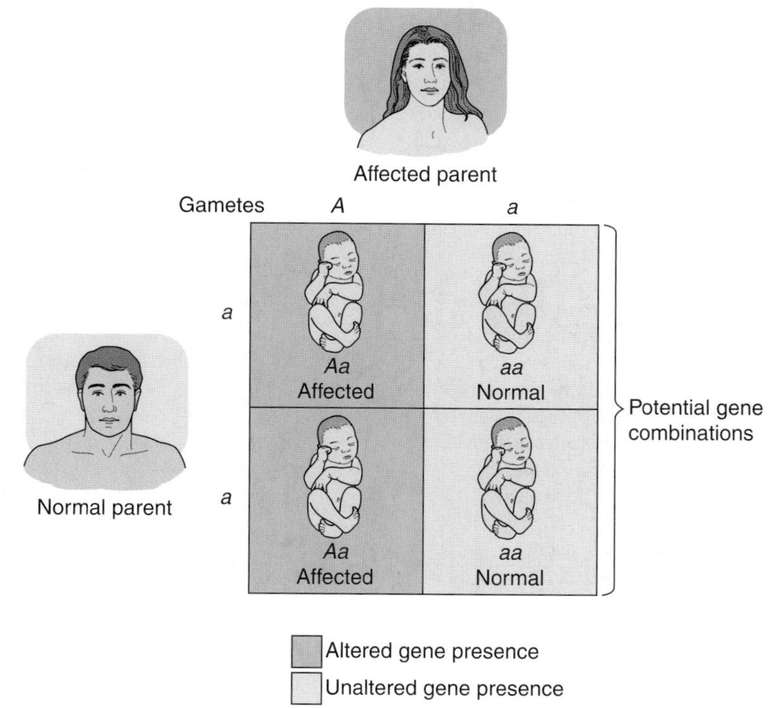

FIGURE 4–7 ■ This punnett square shows potential gene combinations (genotypes) and resulting phenotypes of children from parent genotypes with an **autosomal dominant altered gene**. Phenotypes are expressed (affected) when a male *or* female has one copy of the gene alteration. These are possible genotypes/phenotypes for each pregnancy.

TABLE 4–2 Selected Genetic Conditions That Follow a Mendelian Inheritance Pattern

GENETIC CONDITION	CLINICAL MANIFESTATIONS	INHERITANCE	DIAGNOSIS	CLINICAL THERAPY	PERTINENT CONSIDERATIONS
Achondroplasia (Francomano, 2003) (See Chapter 35)	Change in bone growth resulting in short stature Disproportionately short arms and legs Limited elbow extension Large head Frequent middle ear infections	Autosomal dominant 80% new mutation rate	Clinical findings DNA-based testing Prenatal testing is available	Monitor height, weight, and head circumference on growth curve standardized for achondroplasia Assess for history of sleep apnea Orthopedic care Speech evaluation/therapy Monitor social development	Life expectancy normal Increased risk (7.5%) of infant death from spinal cord and upper airway compression Obesity is a major concern
Beta-thalassemia (Cooley's anemia) (Cao & Galanello, 2003) (See Chapter 28)	Suspected in children (6–24 months) who present with severe microcytic anemia and hepatosplenomegaly Untreated children exhibit failure to thrive and growth retardation with pallor Diarrhea Irritability Unexplained fever Progressive enlargement of spleen	Autosomal recessive	Clinical presence of microcytic, hypochromic RBCs DNA-based analysis Prenatal testing is available	Regular transfusions maintained to keep hemoglobin at optimal level to maintain normal growth and development up to age 10–11 years After age 10–11 years iron overload can result from multiple transfusions so chelation therapy is necessary Chelation therapy should occur after 10–12 transfusions; administered 5–7 days a week by 12-h continuous SQ pump	Prevalent in population of Mediterranean, Middle East, Central Asia, the Far East, and the subcontinent of India. However, it is also seen in Northern Europe, North and South America, the Caribbean, and Australia Untreated children are seen for the most part in undeveloped countries
Cystic fibrosis (CF) (Moskowitz, Gibson, Sternen, Cheng, & Cutting, 2004) (See Chapter 25)	Pulmonary disease Chronic cough, sputum production, wheeze and air trapping Clubbing Malabsorption and pancreatic insufficiency, rectal prolapse Failure to thrive Chronic hepatobiliary disease Meconium ileus occurs in 10%–20% of newborns diagnosed with CF Obstructive azoospermia in 95% of males with CF Diabetes mellitus may be present in adolescents	Autosomal recessive	Multiple diagnostic criteria exist including degrees of the following: 1) Sweat test with adherence to strict guidelines 2) Transepithelial nasal potential difference (NPD) 3) DNA-based testing 4) Exhibiting phenotypic features of CF Newborn screening in some states Prenatal diagnosis is available	Referral to regional CF center Respiratory specialist—pulmonary function studies Oral, inhaled, and IV antibiotics, bronchodilators, anti-inflammatory and mucolytic agents and chest physiotherapy Heart/lung transplant may be needed Nutritional support—special formulas, supplemental feedings, additional fat-soluble vitamins, pancreatic enzyme replacement Infertility is treated with reproductive technologies Gene therapy is currently in research phase	Is the most common life-threatening AR disorder in the Caucasian population Incidence of 1 in 3,200 live Caucasian births Approximately 30,000 affected individuals alive in United States Carrier incidence in Caucasians is 1 in 22–28 Pulmonary disease is the primary cause of chronic illness and death A positive newborn screen must be further evaluated with molecular genetic testing
Duchenne muscular dystrophy (Korf, Darras, Urion, 2003)	Progressive muscle disease Presents by age 5 Developmental milestone not met—delays in sitting and standing (see next page)	X-linked recessive	DNA-based testing: identification of DMD gene alteration If DMD gene alteration not identified with testing, diagnosis made by (see next page)	Weight control Physical therapy Cardiology monitoring Surgical interventions for musculoskeletal complications	Carrier females may have clinical involvement including cardiomyopathy creatinine phosphokinase (CK) level 2–10 × normal

TABLE 4–2 Selected Genetic Conditions That Follow a Mendelian Inheritance Pattern (continued)

GENETIC CONDITION	CLINICAL MANIFESTATIONS	INHERITANCE	DIAGNOSIS	CLINICAL THERAPY	PERTINENT CONSIDERATIONS
Duchenne muscular dystrophy, (continued)	independently; walking Unsteady gait Wheelchair bound by age 12 Cardiomyopathy after age 18 Increased serum creatinine phosphokinase (CK) concentrations (> 10 times normal)		clinical findings, family history, muscle biopsy Prenatal testing is available		
Fragile X syndrome (fragile X mental retardation) (Saul & Tarleton, 2003) (See Chapter 34)	Moderate mental retardation in males Mild retardation in females There is normal growth and no associated malformations Delayed developmental milestones (sitting, walking) Delayed speech Abnormal temperament: autism, hyperactivity, tantrums IQ 30–50 Long face, prominent forehead and jaw, and large ears Macro-orchidism Shyness, gaze aversion Joint hyperextensibility Mitral valve prolapse Soft, smooth skin	X linked Anticipation is demonstrated	Mutation analysis and DNA-based testing for FMR1 gene on the X chromosome More than 99% of affected individuals have an alteration in one specific site of the X chromosome Mosaicism is present in 15%–20% of individuals Prenatal diagnosis is available	Behavioral management Pharmacologic management of behavioral issues that significantly interfere with social interactions Education interventions Small class size, avoidance of sudden change and individual attention	Chromosome analysis is no longer done for diagnosis due to low sensitivity and high costs Individuals who should be tested include those of either sex with mental retardation, developmental delay or autism of unknown origin A family history of fragile X Relatives with undiagnosed mental retardation Fetuses of mothers who are diagnosed carriers Incidence: 16–25 in 100,000 males Prevalence of unaffected female carriers is 1 in 259
Gaucher disease (type 1) (Pastores, 2003)	*Type 1* Clinical or radiographic signs of bone disease Hepatosplenomegaly Anemia Thrombocytopenia Absence of CNS complications which occur in type 2 and 3 *Type 2* Above manifestations plus neurologic disease Onset prior to age 2–4 years *Type 3* Above manifestations plus neurologic disease Onset prior to age 2 but progress slow Perinatal form is lethal Cardiovascular form is characterized by calcification of aortic and mitral valve, corneal opacities and mild splenomegaly	Autosomal recessive	Diagnosis is from deficient enzyme activity in peripheral blood leukocytes or other nucleated cells Carrier testing is unreliable Gene identification is available in a few laboratories for only a few common mutations Identification of altered gene within families can be accurately done Prenatal testing is available	Symptomatic care Physical exam every 6–12 months Assessment of liver and spleen size and volume Partial or total splenectomy Analgesics for bone pain Joint replacement surgery Enzyme replacement therapy administered intravenously every 2 weeks Bone marrow transplantation	Multiple types which vary from asymptomatic to a perinatal lethal form Type 1 is prevalent in the Ashkenazi Jewish population occuring in 1 in 855 live births As many as 1 in 18 are carriers Type 1 bone disease may lead to acute and chronic bone pain, pathologic fractures, and degenerative arthritis and often the most debilitating aspect of type 1 Spleen enlargement may reach 1,500–3,000 cc size compared to 50–200 cc size in normal adult

(continued)

TABLE 4–2 Selected Genetic Conditions That Follow a Mendelian Inheritance Pattern (continued)

GENETIC CONDITION	CLINICAL MANIFESTATIONS	INHERITANCE	DIAGNOSIS	CLINICAL THERAPY	PERTINENT CONSIDERATIONS
Hemophilia A (Johnson & Thompson, 2003) (See Chapter 28)	Deficiency of factor VIII results in prolonged bleeding as well as renewed bleeding after initial bleeding has stopped Hemarthrosis Deep muscle hematomas Excessive nose bleeds Excessive bruising	X-linked recessive High new mutation rate	Family history Clinical findings Low VIII clotting factor DNA-based testing identifies 98% of patients Prenatal testing is available	Factor VIII concentrate through home infusions used prophylactically Patient education	1 in 4,000 live male births Incidence the same in all ethnic groups About 10% of carriers have reduced factor VIII and prolonged bleeding time
Marfan syndrome (Dietz, 2003) (See Chapter 35)	Connective tissue disorder Myopia Lens displacement Bone overgrowth and joint laxity Extremities long compared to the trunk Scoliosis Lethal: dilation of aorta	Autosomal dominant 25% due to new mutation	Family history and multiorgan assessment findings Linkage studies available for several cases in a family Prenatal testing if linkage exists	Annual echocardiography Annual ophthalmic exams Orthopedist Cardiologist Ophthalmologist Geneticist Cardiothoracic surgeon	Prevalence 1 in 5,000 to 10,000 Not related to any particular ethnic group
Neurofibromatosis 1 (NF1, von Recklinghausen disease) (Friedman, 2002) (See Chapter 33)	Multiple café au lait spots Axillary and inguinal freckling Dermal neurofibromas Iris Lisch nodules Learning disability Optic and CNS gliomas	Autosomal dominant 50% due to new mutation	Clinical findings DNA-based testing Prenatal diagnosis available but used infrequently	Annual physical exam Annual ophthalmologic evaluation Blood pressure monitoring Developmental assessment	
Phenylalanine hydroxylase deficiency (PKU) (Ryan & Scriver, 2003) (See Chapter 32)	If untreated, severe cognitive impairment from impaired brain development Microcephaly Seizures Epilepsy Severe mental retardation Behavioral problems Musty body odor Eczema Decreased hair and skin pigmentation	Autosomal recessive	Biochemical testing DNA-based testing Newborn screening Prenatal testing is available	Restriction of intake of dietary phenylalanine and phe-free medical formula Must be started as soon as possible after birth Current philosophy is diet for life	Noncompliance with diet common in older child and adolescents and can result in reduced attention span and other decreased cognitive functioning even if diet was maintained prior to change *Incidence* Irish—1 in 4,500 Caucasian, East Asian—1 in 10,000, Turks—1 in 2,600 If contemplating pregnancy, the woman should start the phenylalanine-free diet prior to conception and maintain it throughout pregnancy
Sickle cell disease (Vichinsky & Schlis, 2003) (See Chapter 28)	Healthy at birth and become symptomatic later in infancy or childhood Variable degrees of hemolysis Pain Intermittent vascular occlusion Tissue ischemia Acute and chronic organ malfunction Infection Delayed growth and sexual maturation	Autosomal recessive	Clinical findings DNA-based testing Prenatal diagnosis is available	Hydration Immunizations including the influenzae, HIB, pneumococcal, and meningococcal vaccine Prophylactic penicillin Folic acid	Prevalance of sickle cell trait (HbAS) among African Americans is 8%–10% 2,000 infants are born annually with sickle cell anemia (HbSS) About 1 in 250–600 African American births in the United States have sickle cell disease

MediaLink Sickle Cell Anemia Animation

TABLE 4–2 **Selected Genetic Conditions That Follow a Mendelian Inheritance Pattern (continued)**

GENETIC CONDITION	CLINICAL MANIFESTATIONS	INHERITANCE	DIAGNOSIS	CLINICAL THERAPY	PERTINENT CONSIDERATIONS
Tay-Sachs disease (Kaback, 2004)	Neurogenerative disorder Loss of motor skills beginning 3–6 months Progressive neurodegeneration including seizures, blindness, death by age 4	Autosomal recessive	Serum enzyme studies DNA-based genetic testing Prenatal testing is available	Due to screening programs and reproductive choices the incidence has decreased > 90%	1 in 3,600 Ashkenazi Jewish births (descents from central and eastern Europe) Sephardic Jewish and non-Jewish incidence is 100 times less

Data from Gene Reviews. www.genetests.org, accessed 03/28/2004.

rate as well as both males and females being affected. An affected child always has an affected parent, who in turn also has an affected parent. Exceptions to the pattern expected with autosomal dominant inheritance can occur if the condition is due to a spontaneous new mutation. See Box 4–7.

Autosomal Recessive

A gene or genetic condition is considered autosomal recessive (AR) when two copies of altered genes are needed to express the condition. Examples include cystic fibrosis, phenylketonuria (PKU), sickle cell anemia, and Tay-Sachs disease. A child born with a recessive condition has inherited one altered gene from the mother and one from the father. In most cases, neither of the parents is affected and, therefore, each of the parents must have a single gene alteration on one chromosome of a pair and the normal, wild type, or unaltered form of the gene on the other chromosome. These parents would be known as **carriers** of the condition but do not usually exhibit signs and symptoms of the condition. Generally, conditions that are autosomal recessive are more severe and have an earlier onset than conditions with other patterns of inheritance. Most inborn errors in metabolism (IEM) or metabolic conditions are autosomal recessive. Many are enzyme defects and the functioning of the unaltered gene is sufficient to provide normal functioning in the person who is heterozygous or the carrier of one copy of the altered gene (Lashley, 1998).

Inheritance Risk in Autosomal Recessive Conditions. Autosomal recessive conditions are the result of an altered gene on any of the 22 autosomes or nonsex chromosomes. It is only when two copies of the altered gene are present that the condition is expressed and presents itself (Figure 4–8 ■). A gene alteration on one chromosome is not enough of a disturbance and the unaltered gene on the other chromosome of the pair is able to produce enough gene product. Therefore, the gene alteration is not expressed or disease is not produced. Because the gene alteration occurs on a nonsex chromosome, both males and females have an equal chance of inheriting the altered gene from their parent. Gene carriers are individuals who have one altered and one unaltered gene and, in most cases, are asymptomatic. A common exception to this is the individual who carries one altered gene that causes sickle cell anemia. Although the individual who is a carrier of the sickle cell trait usually has no symptoms, symptoms can occur in situations of extremely low oxygenation such as high altitudes. See Developing Cultural Competence: Ethnic or Population Groups and Autosomal Recessive Inheritance. When both parents are carriers of an autosomal recessive gene alteration, each pregnancy presents the same inheritance risks. A child born to carrier parents has a 25% chance of inheriting two copies of the altered

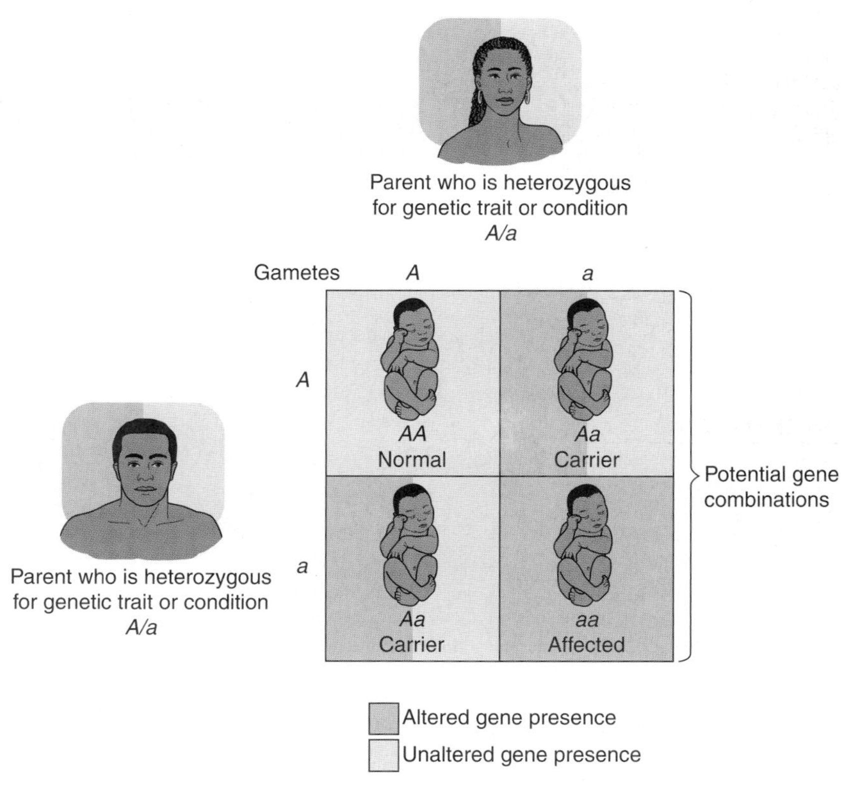

FIGURE 4–8 ■ This punnett square shows potential gene combinations (genotypes) and resulting phenotypes of children from parent genotypes with an **autosomal recessive altered gene.** Phenotypes are expressed (affected) when a male *or* female has two copies of the gene alteration. These are possible genotypes/phenotypes for each pregnancy.

BOX 4–7 Autosomal Dominant Mendelian Inheritance Characteristics

When gathering a family history, the nurse should assess for any of the following characteristics of autosomal dominant inheritance.

1. Both males and females are affected.
2. Males and females are usually affected in equal numbers.
3. An affected child will have an affected parent and/or all generations will have an affected individual (appearing as a vertical pattern of affected individuals on the family pedigree).
4. Unaffected children of an affected parent will have unaffected offspring.
5. A significant proportion of isolated cases are due to a new mutation.

disease-producing gene, a 50% chance of being a carrier with only one copy of the altered gene, and a 25% chance of inheriting both unaltered genes and thus not being affected nor being a carrier. Remembering that each pregnancy is an independent event, these probability percentages remain constant with each pregnancy, no matter how many times a child inherits the altered gene from the parent. This is often a difficult concept for parents to grasp and the nurse should carefully evaluate the parent's level of understanding of this detail about inheritance. See Box 4–8.

All occurrence percentages will change if only one parent is a carrier, unaffected, or affected with the condition. The nurse must be able to teach a parent about these simple inheritance percentages.

X-linked Recessive

X-linked conditions are the result of an altered gene on the X chromosome. Examples include hemophilia A and Duchenne muscular dystrophy. Unlike the autosomes, the sex chromosome, X, is unevenly distributed to males and females. The female has two X chromosomes and the male has only one. Thus, the family history and pattern of inheritance has a characteristic distribution pattern among the males and females in the family. Because the male has only one copy of any gene on the X chromosome, it becomes the only copy available to give direction for those particular functions of these genes regardless of whether it is considered dominant or recessive in the

BOX 4–8 Autosomal Recessive Mendelian Inheritance Characteristics

When gathering a family history, the nurse should assess for any of the following characteristics of autosomal recessive inheritance.

1. Both males and females are affected.
2. Males and females are usually affected in equal numbers.
3. An affected child will have an unaffected parent but may have affected siblings (appearing as a horizontal pattern of affected individuals on the family pedigree).
4. The condition may appear to skip a generation.
5. The parents of the affected child may be consanguinous (close blood relatives).
6. The family may be descendents of an ethnic group that is known to have a more frequent occurrence of a certain genetic condition.

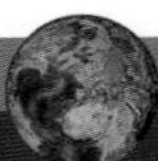

DEVELOPING CULTURAL COMPETENCE
Ethnic or Population Groups and Autosomal Recessive Inheritance

Because of the geographic origins where the gene alteration first occurred, certain recessive genetic conditions are more prevalent in particular ethnic populations. Common examples are as follows:

Ashkenazi Jewish—Tay-Sachs disease (infantile), Gaucher disease

Tay-Sachs is a progressive neurologic degenerative disorder that is usually fatal by age 2 to 3 years. Online Mendelian Inheritance of Man (OMIM) reports that it is approximately 100 times more common in infants of Ashkenazi Jewish ancestry (central-eastern Europe) than in non-Jewish infants. Symptoms include developmental regression or retardation followed by paralysis, blindness, dementia, and death.

Gaucher disease is a lysosomal storage disease that affects approximately 1 in 450 persons with Ashkenazi Jewish ancestry. This condition leads to gross hepatomegaly and splenomegaly. The bone marrow cells are replaced by Gaucher cells resulting in decreased production of erythrocytes and platelets producing anemia and thrombocytopenia. Some patients have CNS involvement.

Asian (Yemen), Polish, Irish—Phenylketonuria (PKU)

PKU is an enzyme defect resulting in increased levels of phenylalanine. If untreated with special diet, developmental delays, seizures, and irreversible mental retardation will result. The great majority of the cases are detected during newborn screening. The carrier rate for those of Irish descent is reportedly 1 in 33. Neural tube defect occurrences are more prominent in those individuals with an Irish descent.

Mediterranean (Italians, Greeks), Middle East, Far East, Africans—β-Thalassemia

Beta-thalassemia is caused by a gene alteration that causes premature destruction of red blood cells and results in anemia. Usually, the infant is symptomatic between 6 and 24 months of age with failure to thrive, feeding problems, diarrhea, irritability, repeat occurrences of fever and progressive enlargment of the abdomen due to splenomegaly. Children have a shortened life expectancy without treatment.

Northern European—Cystic fibrosis (CF)

CF is the most common life-limiting autosomal recessive condition in the Caucasian population. It affects cells of the respiratory tract, exocrine pancreas, intestine, male genital tract, hepatobiliary system, and the exocrine sweat resulting in complex multisystem disease. Incidence is 1 in 3,200 live Caucasian births.

Sub-Saharan African, South and Central American, Saudi Arabian, Indian—Sickle cell

Sickle cell is a severe hemolytic disease where the red cells become grossly abnormally sickle shaped during periods of low oxygen tension. These sickle-shaped cells clump and cause occlusion of capillaries in small bones of the extremities, lungs, spleen, kidneys, and other organs. Strokes and infarcts can occur with prolonged ischemia.

female. Thus, if any of these genes are altered, an unaltered counterpart is not present to "override" the altered functioning gene. The consequences of the altered gene on an X chromosome will be expressed in all males. The females, on the other hand, will have two copies and the unaltered gene generally compensates for the altered gene, making the female a carrier.

Inheritance Risk in X-linked Recessive Conditions. The male receives his X chromosome from his mother and his Y chromosome from his father. The female offspring receives an X chromosome from each of her parents. This means that all affected males will pass on the altered X chromosome to all of his daughters who will be carriers of the altered gene. A male can never transmit an altered gene on the X chromosome to his sons because the male will transmit only the Y chromosome to his sons. Because of these transmission patterns, the most common occuring transmission of an X-linked condition is through a female who is a carrier of an altered gene.

In X-linked recessive inheritance, a woman who is a carrier has a 50% chance of passing an altered gene to her male child, who would then be affected with the condition (Figure 4–9 ■). A woman would also have a 50% chance of passing the altered gene to her daughter who would then be a carrier, like her mother. This woman would also have a 50% chance of passing the unaltered gene to her son who would not be affected or her daughter who would not be affected nor a carrier. See Box 4–9.

BOX 4–9 X-linked Recessive Mendelian Inheritance Characteristics

When gathering a family history, the nurse should assess for any of the following characteristics of X-linked recessive inheritance.

1. More males will be affected than females; rarely seen in females.
2. An affected male will have all carrier daughters.
3. There is no male-to-male inheritance.
4. Affected males are related by carrier females.
5. Females may report varying milder symptoms of the condition.
6. A new sporadic case could be due to a new mutation.

X Inactivation

Early in embryonic life, soon after fertilization, the process of X inactivation occurs. This process is believed to be completed by the end of the first week of development. Each female receives an X chromosome from her mother (maternal X) and an X chromosome from her father (paternal X). The inactivation of either the maternal or paternal X chromosome is random. However, once that X has been inactivated in any given cell, all of the cell's descendents (through mitosis) contain the same inactive X chromosome. Because of the random process of inactivating an X chromosome, the amount of cells in a carrier female that are active and carry altered genes versus unaltered genes is variable. Therefore, expression of symptoms can vary from extremely mild to a full manifestation of the condition. For example, carriers of

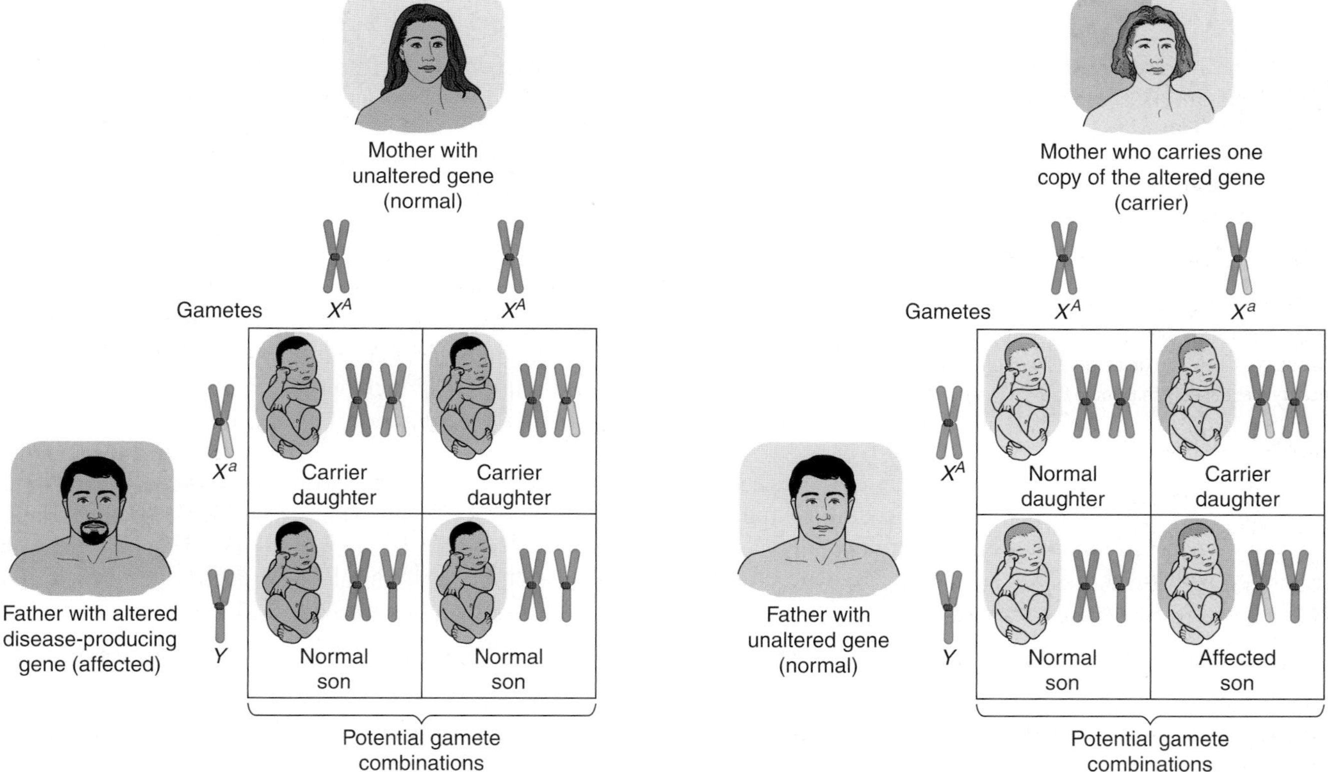

FIGURE 4–9 ■ These punnett squares show potential gene combinations (genotypes) and resulting phenotypes of children from different parent genotypes with an **X-linked recessive altered gene.** Phenotypes are expressed (affected) in a male with only one copy of the gene alteration and in a female with two copies of the altered gene. These are possible genotypes/phenotypes for each pregnancy.

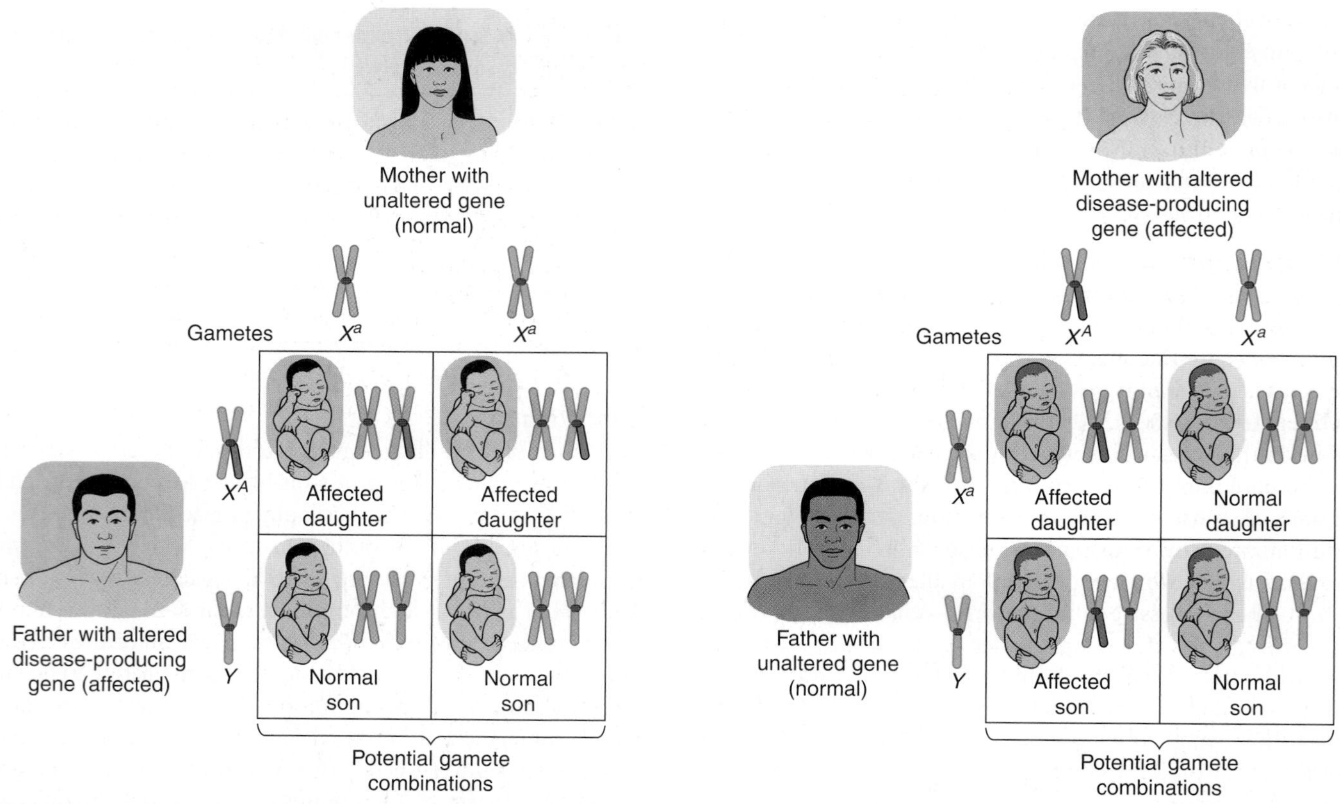

FIGURE 4–10 ■ These punnet squares show potential gene combinations (genotypes) and resulting phenotypes of children from different parent genotypes with an **X-linked dominant altered gene.** Phenotypes are expressed (affected) in a heterozygous female and in a male with only one copy of the gene alteration. These are possible genotypes/phenotypes for each pregnancy.

the X-linked recessive condition, hemophilia A, may exhibit prolonged bleeding times; and carriers of Duchenne muscular dystrophy may exhibit muscle weakness (Nussbaum et al., 2001).

X-linked Dominant

X-linked dominant conditions also exist but these conditions are rare. An example is hypophosphatemic rickets. If a male is affected, the condition is severe and often lethal. A family history of multiple male miscarriages may be a sign of an X-linked dominant condition. See Figure 4–10 ■.

Variability in Classic Mendelian Patterns of Inheritance

Along with understanding the classic Mendelian inheritance patterns are several concepts that are important for families to understand when the nurse is assisting children, adolescents, and parents with or at risk for inheriting a genetic disorder. These include the following exceptions or variations to the traditional Mendelian patterns of inheritance.

Penetrance

Penetrance is the probability that a gene will be expressed phenotypically. It is an "all or none" concept in that either the gene will be expressed (even if mildly expressed) or it will not be expressed at all. Penetrance can be measured in the following way. In a certain group of individuals with the same genotype, what percentage of them will exhibit at least some signs and/or symptoms of the condition? If the number is less than 100%, then that condition is said to show *reduced penetrance.* For example, the gene alterations that cause achondroplasia exhibit 100% penetrance and all individuals with one copy of the gene alteration will exhibit signs and symptoms of the disease (Nussbaum et al., 2001).

New Mutation

When there is no previous history of a condition including even subtle signs and symptoms of the disease in any other immediate or distant family member, the disease may be caused by a spontaneous new mutation, and is said to be *de novo.* New mutations of a gene are most frequently seen in autosomal dominant conditions because one copy of an altered gene is all that is necessary to elicit a state of altered health. Autosomal dominant diseases known to have high mutation rates include neurofibromatosis (NF-1), achondroplasia (dwarfism), and Marfan syndrome. New mutations are also possible in autosomal recessive diseases although rarely expressed because two altered genes are necessary for signs and symptoms to appear. Finally, new mutations are often seen in X-linked recessive disorders, such as hemophilia A, since the male with just one altered gene will demonstrate the disease.

Anticipation

Anticipation is said to occur when successive generations of a family exhibit more severe signs and symptoms of certain diseases and the disease often has an earlier onset. An example is myotonic dystrophy, an autosomal dominant condition characterized by myotonia, muscular dystrophy, cataracts, hypogonadism, and EKG changes. The congenital form is severe, causing mental retardation and possible death. Most children with this congenital form of myotonic dystrophy have a mildly affected mother who may not even be aware she has the disease (Nussbaum et al., 2001).

Variable Expressivity

Expressivity is used to describe the severity of the expression of the phenotype. When people with the same genetic makeup (genotype) exhibit signs and/or symptoms with varying degrees of severity, the phenotype is described as *variable expression* (Nussbaum et al., 2001).

Variable expression is common in the autosomal dominant condition, neurofibromatosis (NF-1). Although neurofibromatosis has 100% penetrance, variable expressivity can occur within family members with each family member exhibiting a variety of signs and/or symptoms.

Sex Limited Traits

Sex limited traits are those autosomal traits that are either expressed in males or females but not both. However, it is important to note that although one gender does not express the trait due to the individual's environment (created by estrogen or testosterone), the gene is present in the parent's genome and it can be inherited. Examples of these traits include milk production, beard growth, and breast size. A young girl has the gene for beard growth but does not develop beard growth as part of secondary sexual development and a young boy has the gene for development of breasts but does not develop breasts (Lashley, 1998).

Sex Influenced Traits

Sex influenced traits are those that act differently in males and females. Pattern baldness is an autosomal dominant trait in males and requires only one copy to be expressed. In females, however, the gene for pattern baldness acts recessive and is expressed when a woman has two copies of the gene (Lashley, 1998).

OTHER MEANS OF MONOGENIC INHERITANCE

Other single gene disorders that have been discovered in the past few decades include new types of inheritance patterns. They include mitochondrial inheritance, imprinting, and uniparental disomy (Guttmacher & Collins, 2002). Mitochondrial inheritance was discussed previously in this chapter.

Imprinting

The expression of some genetic conditions is dependent on whether the altered gene is inherited from the mother or the father. Some genes are inactivated when they are transmitted through one sex or another. Common examples include Prader Willi syndrome that presents in most cases because there is a deletion on chromosome 15 that is inherited from the father. With Angelman syndrome, there is a gene alteration in the same area of chromosome 15, but it is inherited from the mother (Nussbaum et al., 2001).

Uniparental Disomy

With uniparental disomy, the child inherits both copies of one pair of a person's 23 pairs of chromosomes from the same parent instead of the one copy of the pair being inherited from the mother and one copy of the pair being inherited from the father. In other words, the child has two paternal chromosomes or two maternal chromosomes. If there are no altered genes on these chromosomes, the child may not be affected by this event. However, if the chromosome contains an altered gene for an autosomal recessive disease, the child will express the disease. For instance, if a child inherits two copies of chromosome 7 from his mother who is a carrier for the altered gene that causes cystic fibrosis, the child will then have the two copies of the altered gene and the child will exhibit signs and symptoms of cystic fibrosis (Lashley, 1998).

MULTIFACTORIAL (POLYGENIC) DISORDERS

Many birth defects such as cleft lip and palate as well as many adult onset conditions such as cancer and heart disease have a multifactorial cause. Multifactorial conditions occur as a result of several gene (polygenic) variations and environmental influences that work together. Because the term *polygenic* does not infer the influence of the environment, the term *multifactorial* is the preferred terminology. Exactly how many environmental influences are enough to cause the presentation of the defect or disease is not known. The classic analogy is pouring water into a glass full of ice where the water represents the environmental factors and the ice represents the genes or the individual's genome. If enough water (environmental factors) is added to the glass containing the ice (the individual's genes), eventually the glass will overflow which represents the presentation of a multifactorial condition in that individual. If the water (environmental factors) is held within the glass, this represents the fact that the environmental factors are not enough to cause presentation of the disorder even though the same genes (amount of ice) is present in both situations.

Multifactorial conditions accumulate in families but these conditions do not follow the characteristic Mendelian pattern of inheritance seen with single-gene conditions. Inheritable recurrence risks vary in multifactorial conditions. Recurrence risks refer to whether a condition will occur again in subsequent pregnancies. Since a Mendelian pattern is not present, statistical percentages can be used to represent the chance that parents have for a condition occurring in another child. It is known that the risk of recurrence is higher when more than one family member is affected. The recurrence risk after the first affected child is 4% while the recurrence risk after a second affected child increases to 10%. It is also known that the recurrence risk increases with an increase in severity of the defect. The recurrence risk for a unilateral cleft lip is 2.6% and a bilateral cleft lip is 5.6%. See Table 4–3.

COLLABORATIVE CARE

Many health professionals work together in screening, diagnosis, identification, and treatment of genetic disorders. The goals

TABLE 4–3 Common Birth Defects and Conditions with a Multifactorial Cause

Condition	Description
Neural tube defects	A condition that occurs during fetal development with the incomplete closure of the neural tube. The neural tube is usually closed completely by day 28 of development. This malformation of the neural tube can result in clubfoot, hydrocephalus, and spina bifida depending on which part of the neural tube is not closed.
Pyloric stenosis	Hypertrophy and hyperplasia of the smooth muscle of the pylorus. The antrum of the stomach easily becomes obstructed and the infant has severe feeding problems and projectile vomiting.
Cleft lip and palate	Failure of fusion of the frontal process with the maxillary process at about day 35 of gestation.
Breast cancer, obesity, Alzheimer disease, diabetes, alcoholism, heart disease	In addition to causing multiple diseases, several inheritable traits are considered polygenic. These include fingerprint patterns, eye color, height, and skin color.

of collaborative care are early diagnosis through testing and assessment, and development of an effective treatment plan, combined with psychosocial support to enhance coping, and referral to a genetic specialist when needed.

Genetic Testing

Genetic testing is available for both chromosomal and DNA (gene)-based alterations. With knowledge of available genetic tests and the many implications related to genetic testing, the pediatric nurse can assist clients and their families as they weigh choices regarding genetic testing. As consumers of multimedia, clients and families often have unreliable sources for information related to genetic testing. They can form many misconceptions about the types of genetic tests available and what information these different types of genetic tests are able and not able to provide.

Recommendations for Genetic Testing

Presently, there may or may not be available formal recommendations or guidelines for certain genetic tests. Information regarding when to test and who should be tested is available for some genetic conditions. For example, in 1997, the National Institutes of Health published recommendations for cystic fibrosis (CF) genetic testing. These recommendations state genetic tests should be offered as an option to pregnant couples, those adults planning a pregnancy, those individuals with a family history of CF, and partners of individuals with CF.

Categories of Genetic Tests

There are several categories of genetic testing. Genetics tests have been used for some time for diagnosis. These include prenatal diagnostic tests or confirmation of diagnosis in a symptomatic child or adult. Another genetic test in this category is used for preimplantation genetic diagnosis. This involves the detection of disease-causing gene alterations in human embryos just after in vitro fertilization and before implantation in the uterus, thus providing an opportunity for preselection of unaffected embryos for implantation. Couples at risk for having a genetic disease such as Tay-Sachs commonly use preimplantation genetic diagnosis and preselection of unaffected embryos. Newborn screening is carried out on large sections of the newborn population and provides a means to identify children who have an increased risk for developing a genetic disease such as phenylketonuria (PKU), sickle cell disease, or maple syrup urine disease. See Chapter 11∞. There are criteria for conditions included in newborn screening programs. In order to meet the criteria, it must be established that the condition leads to permanent disability or death if left untreated and there must be available treatments for these conditions. If a screening test is positive, a diagnosis must be confirmed through more extensive testing. Another purpose of genetic testing is for carrier screening. This involves the identification of an individual who is asymptomatic but is suspected of being a carrier for an autosomal or X-linked recessive genetic disease. Carrier screening is often used with potential parents who want to make informed reproductive decisions. Predictive testing is the last category of genetic testing, and involves an asymptomatic individual for the presence of a late-onset genetic disease. Common examples are testing for adult onset cancers and Alzheimer and Huntington diseases. Prediction is tempered, however, by the fact that some conditions such as adult onset cancers are multifactorial. Consequently, there are no direct answers as to whether signs and symptoms will appear, or if they do appear when that will occur or how severe the signs and symptoms might be (Grady, 1999).

Diagnosing Chromosomal Alterations. Microscopic examination of chromosomes can reveal chromosomal alterations such as additions, deletions, gross breaks, and rearrangements or rejoinings (translocations) (USDOE Genome Programs, 2003). Prenatally, amniocentesis and chorionic villi sampling (CVS) are examples of diagnostic testing for some of these chromosomal alterations. Fluorescence in situ hybridization (FISH) analysis is a screening test for chromosomal alterations. After the child is born, chromosomal diagnostic examination can be accomplished with a simple blood sample and skin or buccal cell sampling.

Chromosome Alteration Diagnosis. Both amniocentesis and CVS provide cells from the fetus that can be examined by karyotype method. Fetal cells are available within the amniotic fluid as the fetus sloughs off cells. These cells contain the genome of the fetus and provide an opportunity to examine chromosomes for structure or number alterations. With the CVS, fetal cells are obtained directly from the chorionic villus of the fetus. These cells also contain the genome of the developing fetus. Whether the cells are from amniocentesis, CVS, or blood, a karyotype can be completed in a cytogenetics laboratory. Chromosomes can be identified by their size and unique light and dark banding patterns. The pairs of autosomal chromosomes are arranged from 1 to 22 according to each chromosome's size, unique banding patterns, and centromere position. The sex chromosomes complete the picture, with the X chromosome(s) first, then the Y chromosome (if present). The karyotype shows all of the chromosome pairs lined up and positioned on a piece of paper allowing for visual chromosomal analysis. The final report contains numerical data including the total number of chromosomes present. If there is an additional or deleted chromosome, it is identified with a plus (+) or minus (−) symbol. For example, the male individual with 47, XY, +18 has 47 chromosomes (instead of the expected 46) that includes an additional chromosome 18.

Chromosome Screening Test. Fluorescence in situ hybridization (FISH) analysis of amniotic fluid and other cells uses DNA probes that attach to specific chromosomes. FISH does not require growth of cells in an incubator so results can be obtained faster than with karyotyping. Cells can be analyzed within hours after the DNA probes are added. FISH screening can identify the number of chromosomes present. Specifically, this screening test can identify the total number of chromosomes present for chromosome numbers 13, 18, 21, X and Y. This procedure is possible because probes will attach themselves to a specific sequence of the chromosomes and a fluorescent signal within the cell becomes visible through the microscope. It can then be determined whether there are several copies of one of these specific chromosomes. For example, there may be three copies of chromosome 13 present suggesting the need for an accurate diagnostic chromosomal test. Numerical abnormalities of these five chromosomes represent about two thirds of the chromosomal abnormalities found during midtrimester amniocentesis (GeneCare, 2002). It is important for the nurse to evaluate the parents' understanding of what chromosomal studies can and cannot do. A chromosomal study will give information about chromosomal number, placement, and structure but it will not give specific information about each gene on the chromosomes.

Diagnosing Gene Alterations. With the advances in technology and the identification of genes in the human genome, the availability of genetic, DNA-based tests has grown tremendously. There are currently more than 900 genetic tests available with more being added each day (USDOE Genome Programs, 2003). DNA-based tests involve new, sophisticated technology than permits the examination of the DNA itself. Genetic testing that is DNA based can be obtained from blood, bone marrow, amniotic fluid, fibroblast cells of the skin, or buccal cells from the mouth. Other genetic tests include biochemical-based methods that examine enzymes and other protein products and also the microscopic examination of chromosomes that were discussed earlier in this chapter (HGP Information, 2003a).

Quality and Accuracy of Genetic Tests

There is a great deal of concern expressed by genetic nurses that genetic tests are becoming available too quickly with no regulation of the companies that are offering them. The quality, accuracy, and reliability of the genetic test results are not measured against any common standard. Individuals often make hard and irrevocable life-altering decisions after receiving test results, so accuracy and reliability are essential. Also, in most cases, minimal or no education is provided for the individual undergoing testing nor is there any quality counseling or follow-up after the results are given to the individual.

The Role of the Nurse in Genetic Testing

When managing information about genetic testing, the nurse must include education of the individual or family. Parents often will request genetic testing for their minor children. It is important that the family knows that genetic testing is not 100% accurate or a guarantee of a healthy outcome and that the primary focus of genetic testing in children is to promote the state of well-being of the child. Communication with the child and family about genetic testing should include an assessment of the positive and negative outcomes of the test. Are there existing treatments for the condition being tested? Psychologic issues should also be emphasized. Who will be affected by the test results? Will the test results be shared with extended family members?

A second area of focus for the nurse is the assessment of the decision-making ability of the child. Is the child cognitively or emotionally developed enough to make such a decision? Do the parents understand the impact the test results will have on the child throughout the child's lifespan? It is also imperative for the nurse to be an advocate for the child. By the age of 7 years, children usually are developmentally able to begin to participate in decisions. As the child grows and develops into an individual separate from the parents, the child's own genetic knowledge may exceed the parents' knowledge level. Older children and adolescents may be better prepared to participate in decision making and may disagree with their parents (American Society of Human Genetics [ASHG] & American College of Medical Genetics [ACMG], 1995). The pediatric nurse can help facilitate understanding on both sides of the issue or refer the family to experienced professionals.

Finally, the pediatric nurse has a responsibility to assure autonomy when decisions are made related to genetic testing. Each family member's decisions should be respected whether it is to participate in genetic testing or the refusal to participate. Not all family members will want to know their genetic health (Williams & Lessick, 1996). Above all, as with all aspects of delivering genetic nursing care, privacy and confidentiality is paramount.

Genetic Testing Issues of Minors. In order to support, advocate for, and educate children, adolescents, and their families, the pediatric nurse must have knowledge of the issues related to genetic testing of minor children. Parents may not be able to foresee the consequences associated with a positive finding for a disease-producing gene in a child. The nurse can educate and reinforce information and ensure adolescents or parents are making informed decisions.

Genetic testing issues of underage minors usually present in one of these four situations. First, the genetic testing offers an immediate medical benefit for the child. This would include carrier testing for familial hypercholesterolemia, a single-gene inherited condition which results in early death from extremely high cholesterol levels if left untreated. In this situation immediate lifestyle changes and pharmacologic treatment can improve the quality and length of the child's life. A second situation is when the genetic test offers no medical benefit to the child, but the adolescent is facing reproductive decisions. A sibling or offspring of a person affected with a genetic condition could present such a situation. The third situation would include a genetic test for a condition that offers no immediate benefit but the parent or child requests it for future planning. For example, an older child related to an individual affected with Huntington disease may need confirmation of whether they carry the altered gene in order to plan for a life career or to make relationship decisions such as marriage. Finally, a family member may request genetic testing for a child but the test results are entirely for the benefit of that family member and there is no related benefit to the child. This often occurs during DNA linkage studies where multiple blood samples taken from affected and unaffected individuals within a family must be analyzed and compared in order to produce a recognized DNA pattern for diagnosing the genetic condition in that particular family (Wertz, Fanos, & Reilly, 1994). The pediatric nurse must be aware of these potential situations and know that decisions to perform genetic tests on children and adolescents are not made easily. In order to justify a genetic test on minors, the outcome must be perceived as positive, otherwise genetic testing should be postponed until the child is capable of making an informed decision that often presents itself when an adolescent is making reproductive decisions.

Ensuring Informed Consent for Genetic Testing. The pediatric nurse is responsible for alerting children and their families of their right for making an informed decision prior to *any* genetic testing with consideration of the special circumstances arising from the family, culture, and community life. All genetic testing should be voluntary and it is the nurse's responsibility to ensure that the consent process includes discussion of the risks and benefits of the test including any physical harm as well as potential psychologic and societal injury by stigmatization, discrimination, and emotional stress (International Society of Nurses in Genetics [ISONG], 2000; Beskow, Burke, Merz, et al., 2001).

Ensuring Confidentiality and Privacy for Genetic Testing. Although confidentiality and privacy are an integral part of delivery of care for all nurses, this issue is of greater concern as it relates to genetic information. Results of genetic tests can be far reaching and can affect employment and insurance options. Will the results affect the child's or parents' ability to obtain and/or maintain insurance coverage? Can an employer refuse to hire or promote an individual because of genetic testing results? Can genetic information be released to the courts, military, schools, or adoption agencies? Would a child with a known gene alteration for Huntington disease be offered a college scholarship for the best law school? There is debate over whether genetic privacy is different from medical privacy. The pediatric nurse should inform the child and the family of their right and responsibility to know who will have access to the genetic test results. Those providing the genetic tests must provide the child and the family with assurance that the results will be handled confidentially, and that there will be no access to the genetic information by a third party without written permission of the individual being tested.

Psychosocial Issues. Although family and individual anxiety may be decreased with a negative test result, potential problems do exist and the pediatric nurse must be prepared to address them. Concerns about carrier status may interfere with development of intimacy and interpersonal relationships. A positive test result may lead to feelings of unworthiness and self-image disturbance. Survivor guilt may affect children with negative results if their siblings are positive. Younger children may blame themselves, thinking they did or said something to cause the gene alteration. The adolescent carrying a gene alteration for a late-onset disease may have an increased tendency for risky behaviors. The adolescent who has inherited an altered disease-producing gene may foster deep resentment toward the parent who carries the altered gene. Parental guilt may exist for passing the altered gene to the child. Finally, parent–child bonds may be altered as parents may become either overprotective or overly permissive and the parent and other family members may unconsciously form lowered expectations for the child or adolescent (Wertz et al., 1994).

Economic Issues

The nurse should keep in mind that the cost of genetic tests can range from hundreds to thousands of dollars, depending on the size of the gene being tested. Most insurance companies do not cover genetic tests but if there is insurance coverage, the individual must weigh the cost of allowing the insurance company to have access to the genetic information (HGP Information, 2003a).

NURSING MANAGEMENT

By simply integrating into practice the genetic aspects of assessment, observation, and history gathering, the pediatric nurse can improve the standard of care delivered and have a positive impact on the child and family. The pediatric nurse does not need to be a genetic expert, but with heightened awareness, appropriate inquiries and referrals to genetic specialists can be completed.

■ Family Risk Assessment

Family Intake and History

While gathering a family history, the nurse must assess the information that is provided by the family, looking for significant information that might indicate the need for a follow-up or a referral to genetic specialists. A family history that includes cataracts, cleft lip and/or cleft palate, congenital heart disease, contractures, diaphragmatic hernia, genital malformations, glaucoma, an asymmetric skull, missing limbs or fingers/toes, neural tube defects, or any other congenital anomalies would indicate the family may benefit from a genetic referral (US-DOE Biological and Environmental Research Source, 2003).

Genetic Physical Assessment

The pediatric nurse in any healthcare setting should incorporate the genetic aspects into the comprehensive assessment (see Chapter 8∞). An early finding by the nurse provides the child and the family an opportunity for a genetic referral and more comprehensive healthcare.

Major and Minor Anomalies

Dysmorphology refers to the study of human congenital defects or abnormalities of body structure that begin before birth. Dysmorphic anomalies can occur anywhere in the body. As a routine part of client assessment, the nurse should complete a screening for minor anomalies or malformations. A **minor anomaly** or malformation is an unusual or morphologic feature that in itself is of no serious medical or cosmetic concern to the individual or family. Minor abnormalities are either present or not, with no variation of severity. Some minor anomalies are merely family traits or are present in certain ethnic groups. Family traits include a low anterior hairline, preauricular (in front of the ears) pits and tags, broad face, or mild proportionate short stature. Examples of ethnic origin would include upward slanting or prominent epicanthal folds among individuals of Asian descent. A single transverse palmar crease across the hand without the presence of any other signs of Down syndrome is another example of a minor anomaly. However, minor anomalies may be important diagnostic cues especially if several are found in the same individual.

Between 13% and 40% of otherwise normal newborns will have one minor anomaly, and less than 1% will have two minor anomalies. If a newborn or older child has three or more minor anomalies, this would signal the nurse to the possibility of a major anomaly or an underlying genetic condition, and a genetic referral would be in order. About 3% of all children have a **major anomaly** or a serious structural defect at birth that may interfere with normal functioning of body systems, lead to a lifelong disability, or even an early death (Aase, 1992). Pyloric stenosis, cleft lip and/or palate, myelomeningocele, duodenal atresia, and cataracts are considered major anomalies. Some major anomalies are present at birth but are not apparent. These would include deafness, various skeletal dysplasias, and some types of congenital heart defects. With the inclusion of these less apparent groups of conditions, the incidence of major anomalies is believed to increase to 5% to 6% (Aase, 1992). See Table 4–4.

The nurse can pick up cues to genetic problems by inspecting the child, the parents, and other family members (Tables 4–5 and 4–6). Nurses should ask to look at family photographs and examine them for common dysmorphic features and family traits

TABLE 4–4 Estimated Incidence of Common Genetic Conditions per Number of Births

CONDITION/STRUCTURAL OR METABOLIC BIRTH DEFECT	ESTIMATED INCIDENCE PER NUMBER OF BIRTHS
Club foot	1 in 735
Cleft lip/palate	1 in 930
Anencephaly	1 in 8,000
Spina bifida	1 in 2,000
Chromosomal syndromes	1 in 600
Down syndrome (trisomy 21)	1 in 900
Metabolic disorders	1 in 3,500
Phenylketonuria (PKU)	1 in 12,000

Data from March of Dimes, (2003).

TABLE 4–5 Selected Dysmorphic Physical Assessment Findings*

Skull	Asymmetrical head/face Brachycephaly Flattened occiput Fontanels too large or small Micrognathia (small jaw) Overlapping sutures Prognathism (projection of jaw beyond that of the forehead)
Extremities	Abnormally positioned feet Arachnodactyly (long fingers or toes) Brachydactyly (small fingers) Camptodactyly (permanent flexion of fingers or toes) Clinodactyly (curved fingers or toes [most often 5th finger]) Extremely long, thin extremities Hypoplastic (very small) or absent nails Loose joints Single transverse palmar crease Polydactyly (extra fingers and/or toes) Rocker bottom feet Syndactyly (webbing between fingers and toes) Unusually tall or short stature
Ears	Ear tags or pits Ears that are posteriorly rotated Hearing loss Low-set ears Malformed ears
Hair	Excessive body hair Hairline and hair distribution Large section of white hair in otherwise pigmented hair Sparse or brittle hair
Eyes	Blue sclera Different colored eyes Down slanting eyes Epicanthal folds Extreme hyperopia (farsightedness) Extreme myopia (nearsightedness) Hypertelorism (widely spaced eyes) Hypotelorism (closely spaced eyes) Short palpebral fissures (distance between inner and outer canthus of eyes) Upslanting eyes
Skin	Axillary freckling Café au lait spots Excessive skin Extremely loose skin Hyperelastic skin Leaf-shaped white markings Syndactyly (webbing between fingers and toes)
Mouth	Large or small tongue Misshapen, missing, or extra teeth Early loss of teeth Late eruption of teeth Smooth or abnormal philtrum Thin upper lip
Other	Catlike mewing cry Hoarse, weak cry Hypogonadism Obesity Short, webbed neck Multiple fractures

**This list is not all-inclusive, but is meant to increase the nurse's awareness of assessment findings that may be significant and require a referral to genetic specialists.*

TABLE 4–6 Selected Assessment Findings or Anomalies and Associated Conditions

ASSESSMENT FINDING OR ANOMALY	ASSOCIATED CONDITION	ASSESSMENT FINDING OR ANOMALY	ASSOCIATED CONDITION
Abdominal wall defect	Trisomies 13, 18 CHARGE Association Down syndrome	Inguinal or umbilical hernia	Fetal hydantoin syndrome Hunter syndrome Hurler syndrome Ehlers-Danlos syndrome Marfan syndrome Williams syndrome
Ambiguous genitalia or hypospadias	Beckwith-Wiedeman syndrome Fetal hydantoin syndrome Trisomies 13, 18 XXY Kleinfelter syndrome	Low-set ears	Treacher Collins syndrome Trisomy 18 Down syndrome (occasionally) Fetal hydantoin syndrome Trisomy 13
Blue sclera	Osteogenesis imperfecta, types I and II Ehlers-Danlos syndrome Marfan syndrome	Macrocephaly	Achondroplasia Hunter syndrome Hurler syndrome Beckwith-Wiedeman syndrome Fragile X syndrome Neurofibromatosis
Brachydactyly	Achondroplasia Apert syndrome Down syndrome Fetal warfarin Prader Willi syndrome	Malformed auricles	Beckwith-Wiedeman syndrome (folded or creased lobes) Down syndrome (small) Ehlers-Danlos syndrome Fetal hydantoin syndrome Fragile X Trisomies 13, 18 XO Turner syndrome XYY (long) Fetal alcohol syndrome Marfan syndrome (large) Prader Willi syndrome
Clinodactyly of fifth finger	Down syndrome XXY Kleinfelter syndrome Prader Willi syndrome Triploidy syndrome Williams syndrome	Microcephaly	Angelman syndrome Fetal alcohol syndrome Maternal PKU fetal effects Trisomies 13, 18 Williams syndrome Beckwith-Wiedeman syndrome Fetal varicella effects Fetal warfarin syndrome Fetal hydantoin syndrome Prader Willi syndrome
Craniosynostosis	Apert syndrome Crouzon syndrome Fetal hydantoin syndrome Williams syndrome	Nail hypoplasia	Fetal alcohol syndrome Fetal hydantoin syndrome Fetal warfarin syndrome Trisomies 13, 18 XO Turner syndrome
Cryptorchidism	Trisomies 13, 18	Nipple	Fetal hydantoin syndrome (wide spaced) Trisomy 18 (small, occasionally wide spaced) XO Turner syndrome (wide spaced, small)
Deafness	Hurler syndrome Treacher Collins syndrome Trisomy 13 Cleft lip sequence Crouzon syndrome Osteogenesis imperfecta type 1	Obesity	Prader Willi syndrome XO Turner syndrome Down syndrome XXY Kleinfelter syndrome

TABLE 4–6 Selected Assessment Findings or Anomalies and Associated Conditions (continued)

ASSESSMENT FINDING OR ANOMALY	ASSOCIATED CONDITION
Edema of hands and feet	XO Turner syndrome
Epicanthal folds	Down syndrome Williams syndrome Trisomy 18
Flat, prominent occiput	Down syndrome Apert syndrome Trisomy 18
Fractures	Osteogenesis imperfecta Hypophosphatasia
Hirsutism	Fetal hydantoin syndrome Hunter syndrome Hurler syndrome Fetal alcohol syndrome XO Turner syndrome
Hypertelorism	Apert syndrome Cleft lip syndrome Fetal hydantoin syndrome
Hypogonadism	Prader Willi syndrome XXY Kleinfelter syndrome Down syndrome
Hypotelorism	Maternal PKU effects Trisomy 13 Fetal hydantoin syndrome Williams syndrome
Hypotonia	Achondroplasia Angelman syndrome Down syndrome Ehlers-Danlos syndrome Hypophosphatasia Marfan syndrome Prader Willi syndrome (infancy) Osteogenesis imperfecta type II
Other hair anomalies	Fetal hydantoin syndrome (coarse, profuse, low hairline) Prader Willi (blonde) Waardenburg syndrome (completely white forelock) XO Turner syndrome (low hairline)
Polydactyly	Trisomy 13 VATER Association
Scoliosis	Angelman syndrome Marfan syndrome Ehlers-Danlos syndrome Fetal warfarin syndrome Fragile X Neurofibromatosis Prader Willi syndrome XO Turner syndrome XXY Kleinfelter syndrome
Seizures	Tuberous sclerosis Neurofibromatosis Maternal PKU fetal effects
Short limbs	Achondroplasia Osteogenesis imperfecta type II Fetal warfarin syndrome
Single transverse palmar crease	Down syndrome Fetal alcohol syndrome Fetal hydantoin syndrome Trisomies 13, 18
Single umbilical artery	Trisomies 13, 18 VATER Association
Thin skin	Ehlers-Danlos syndrome
Unusual acne	XXY Kleinfelter syndrome
Web neck	XO Turner syndrome Trisomies 13, 18 Down syndrome Fetal alcohol syndrome Fetal hydantoin syndrome

Adapted from Jones, K. L. (1997). Smith's recognizable patterns of human malformation *(5th ed.). Philadelphia: Saunders.*

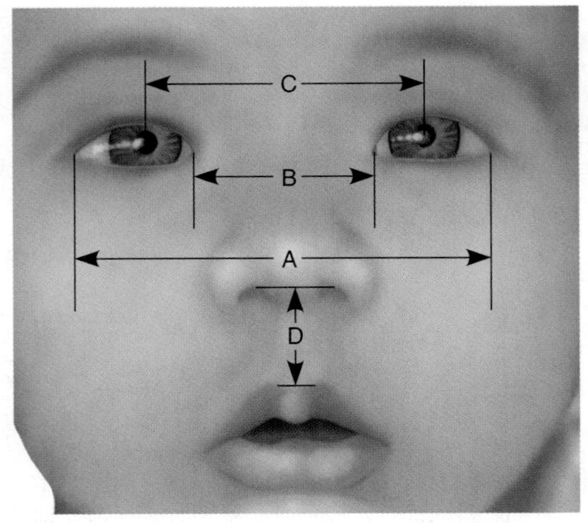

FIGURE 4–11 ■ Classic facial measurements for assessment with a genetic focus on faces/eyes, e.g., hypertylorism, hypotylorism, as described in Table 4–6.

(Figure 4–11 ■). By making a genetic referral, the pediatric nurse can make a difference in the child's state of health.

Pedigrees

Pediatric nurses should know how to take a family history, record the history in a pedigree, and think "genetic." A **pedigree** is a pictorial representation or diagram of the medical history of a family (Figure 4–12 ■). Multiple symbols are utilized to present this picture and the finished pedigree presents a family's medical data and biologic relationship information at a glance. A pedigree provides the nurse, genetic counselor, or geneticist with a clear, visual representation of relationships of affected individuals to the immediate and extended family. It can identify other individuals in the family who might benefit from a genetic consultation. A pedigree can also identify a single gene alteration pattern of inheritance or a cluster of multifactorial conditions and consequently a genetic referral and/or reproductive risk teaching for the individual and family can occur. A family's learning can be enhanced by the visual teaching contribution a pedigree can bring and also clarify any inheritance misunderstandings or misconceptions. If completed correctly and comprehensively a pedigree permits all healthcare professionals working with the child or family to quickly see what history and background information has been collected (Box 4–10).

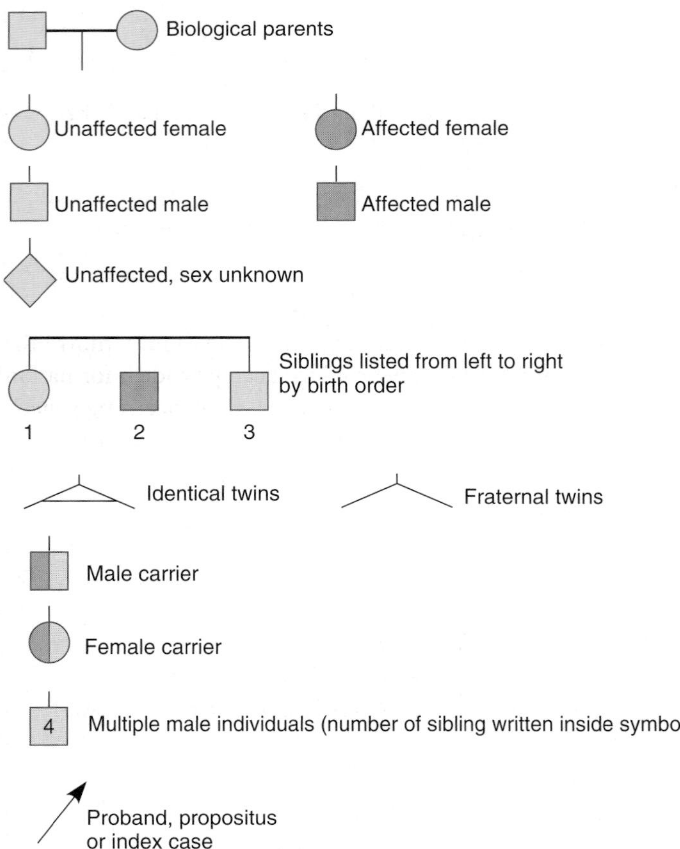

FIGURE 4–12 ■ Selected standardized symbols for use in drawing a pedigree.

It is important to gather a three-generation family pedigree even if the nurse believes this is a first occasion of the condition within a family (Figure 4–13 ■). A condition without any identifiable inheritance pattern on the pedigree may be due to a new mutation or variable expressivity. Throughout the process of gathering family history assessment data, the nurse must remember family confidentiality at all times: All information related to a pedigree is confidential information. The historian may reveal sensitive details that include infertility problems, elective termination of pregnancies, or nonpaternity. This information may not even be known by a current partner or immediate and extended family members. Other sensitive issues include pregnancies conceived by technology, a history of suicides, drug or alcohol abuse, and same-sex relationships. See Box 4–11.

Challenges inherent in recalling the family history include the parents' inability to remember any conditions that may have been surgically repaired and then forgotten, or reporting conditions that may have been attributed incorrectly to other causes. Also, the family history may contain information previously unknown to extended family members. Reproductive decisions may have been made that were against the family's religious or cultural beliefs. Both immediate and extended family members may be unaware of these "family skeletons" and the parent may be reluctant to reveal this information (Bowers, 2002; Bennett, 1999).

■ Planning and Implementation

The pediatric nurse is responsible for comprehensively delivering the standard of care to children and families, but at the same time being aware of the limitations of their own knowledge and expertise. In addition to the continuous integration of genetic aspects into the nurse's assessment of family history and physical assessment, the nurse is also responsible for carrying out interventions that include initiating referrals to genetic specialists and delivering care to the individual or family in any of the following ways.

Genetic Referrals and Counseling

After gathering assessment data that incorporate genetic concepts, the pediatric nurse is able to partner with children and

BOX 4–10 Steps in Drawing a Pedigree

I. How To
   1. Work in pencil
      a. Family historians often remember additional relatives and details only after questioning is almost completed

II. Organization
   1. Begin recording data in the middle of the sheet of paper
      a. Allows enough room for both the maternal and paternal sides of the family
   2. Use only standard pedigree symbols (see Figure 4–12)
      a. For example, males are represented by squares and females by a circle.
   3. The male individual in a couple is placed on the left of the relationship line and the paternal side of the family also goes on the left side of the paper.

III. Determining Family Relationships
   1. The nurse should determine the relationships within the family by asking questions such as:
      - Do you have a partner or are you married?
      - How many biological brothers and sisters do you have?
      - How many children do you have?
      - Do all the children have the same biological father?
      - Do all the children share the same mother and father?
   2. Referral to "the baby's father or mother" can be helpful until a relationship or marriage is established between the parents
   3. Referral to a "union" if marriage does not exist can also help communication

IV. Who Should or Should Not Be Included
   1. To ensure accuracy, the pedigree should include the parents, offspring, siblings, aunts, uncles, grandparents, and first cousins of the individual seeking counseling
   2. Detailed information about the spouses of the proband's family can be omitted unless there is a history of some kind of disorder or condition
   3. Eliminating persons or any information that does not contribute any valuable information can help keep the pedigree small and more manageable

V. Recording the Family History
   1. Determine the approximate size of the family
   2. Record the family's ethnic background at the top of the page
   3. The initial drawing should begin with the proband, or the person who is affected with the genetic condition
      a. Usually the reason someone is seeking a genetic referral
   4. The proband is marked with an arrow on the pedigree
   5. Draw and mark the symbols for the brothers and sisters of the proband, the relationship line is drawn, the line of descent, marriage or union line, and symbols for parents of proband
      a. Repeat this step for any children of the proband or children of the proband's brothers and sisters
   6. Continue with symbols for all immediate relatives drawn previously and then draw and mark symbols for paternal grandparents and indicated relatives followed by the same for the maternal grandparents and relatives
   7. A legend key should contain all of the correct symbols for each indicated disease
   8. The pedigree should include at least three generations
      a. Generations are symbolized by Roman numerals along the left side of the paper with the first generation marker, (I) at the top
      b. Each person in the generation should follow an imaginary horizontal line from left to right
   9. The name of each individual (maiden names in case of married women) and their date of birth should be included along with half-siblings, pregnancy losses, still births, previous marriages, and adopted children
   10. Causes of death, age at death, and current health problems are also very important to note

VI. Other
   1. Consanguinity may be suspected if the historian repeatedly gives the same last name on both sides of the family
      a. Consanguinity can be confirmed by asking if any relatives in the family have ever had a child together

VII. Completing the Pedigree
   1. When completed, the pedigree should be dated and signed with the name, credentials, and position of the person drawing it

Data from Bennett, R. L. (1999). The practical guide to the genetic family history. *New York: Wiley-Liss.*

their families by initiating a referral to genetic specialists if there are indicators for a genetic referral (Box 4–12). The nurse should provide the family with information about the advantages of a referral to genetic specialists, and the disadvantages of not following through with the referral. The nurse should inform the child and family that a genetic referral can provide information and answer many questions they may have concerning genetic health. Questions regarding the conditions, inheritance, avail-

BOX 4–11 Specific Facts and Health Information to Include in a Pedigree

- Age/birth date or year of birth
- Age of death (year, if known)
- Cause of death
- Age at diagnosis
- Full siblings versus half or step-siblings
- Pregnancy with gestational age (LMP) or estimated date of delivery (EDD)
- Infertility versus no children by choice
- Pregnancy complications with gestational ages noted (e.g., 6 wks, 32 wks)
- Miscarriage (SAB)
- Stillbirth (SB)
- Pregnancy termination (TOP)
- Relevant health information (e.g., height and weight)
- Affected/unaffected status—define shading of symbols in a legend key
- Ethnic background
- Consanguinity
- Date pedigree taken or updated
- Name of person who took pedigree and credentials
- Key or legend

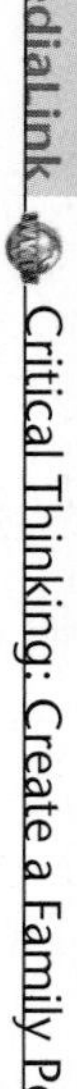

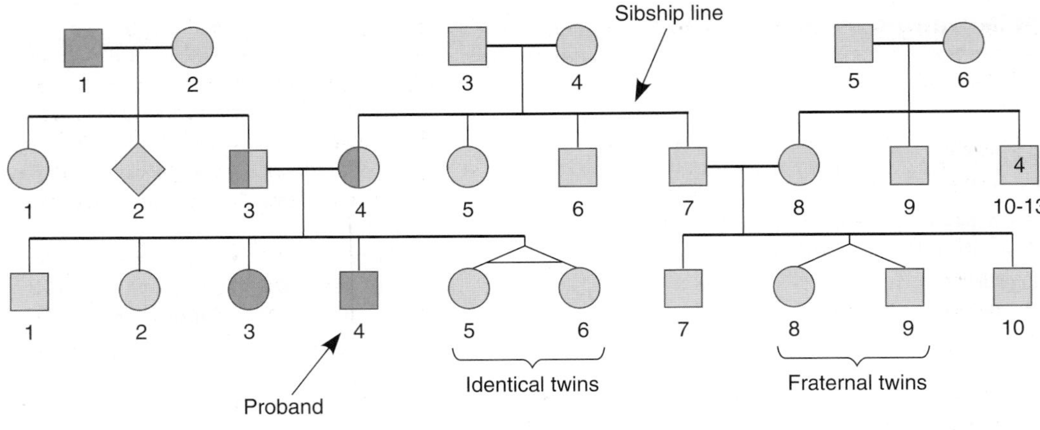

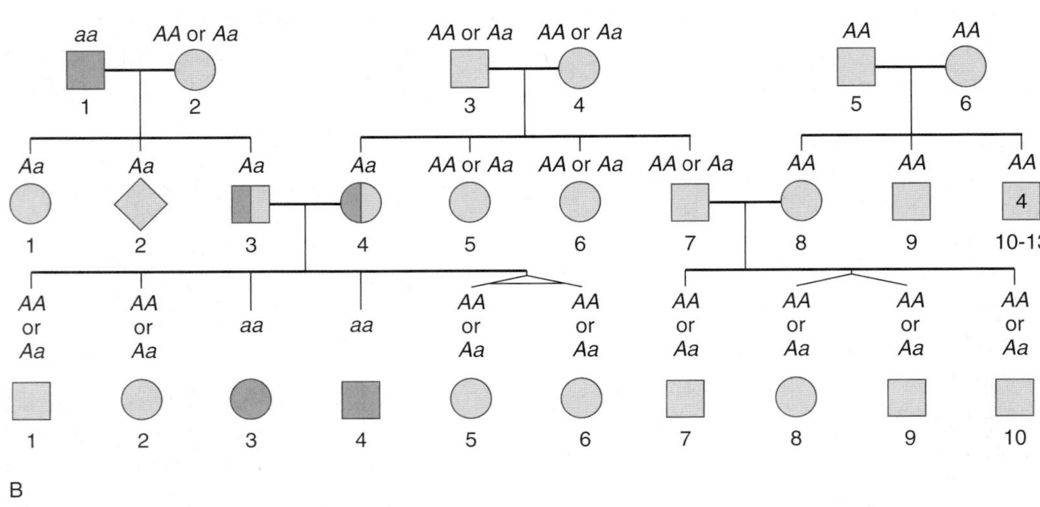

(a) A representative pedigree for a single character or genetic condition through three generations.
(b) The most probable genotypes of each individual in the pedigree for an autosomal recessive condition, represented by AA, Aa, or aa.

FIGURE 4–13 ■ Sample three-generation pedigree.

Redrawn from Klug, W. S., & Cummings, M. R. (2003). Concepts of genetics *(7th ed. p. 63). Upper Saddle River, NJ: Prentice Hall.*

ability of treatment, as well as economic, insurance, and future implications can be addressed. See Table 4–7.

Those who are concerned about genetic disease may benefit from a genetic consultation whether or not genetic testing is available for that condition. Many people seek information and coping strategies as much as they do test results. Referral of a child with a suspected genetic problem to geneticist, genetic clinical nurse specialist, or genetic clinic is an expected nursing responsibility in the same way as referrals to a dietitian or a social worker. When in doubt, the pediatric nurse should contact the advanced practice genetic clinical nurse, genetic counselor, or geneticist to discuss concerns.

FAMILY PREPARATION FOR GENETIC REFERRALS AND GENETIC COUNSELING

Not knowing what to expect from a genetic referral is common, and the fear of the unknown may cause anxiety for both the child and family. In order to facilitate the referral to genetic specialists, the pediatric nurse should educate the client and family so that they know what to expect during as well as after a genetic evaluation. See Partnering with Families: Ethical Implications of Genetic Information.

Usually before the first genetic evaluation visit, the parent will be contacted to provide a detailed medical and family history and to make an appointment for genetic consultation. The parent should be prepared to give as exact a family history as possible so that a detailed three-generation pedigree can be constructed. The parents should be informed that a genetic consultation usually lasts several hours. During the appointment, a genetic clinical nurse, genetic counselor, and/or physician will perform an initial interview with the parents and their child. A geneticist will examine the child and possibly the parent(s) in order to establish an accurate diagnosis. Tests may be ordered. These may include chromosome analysis, DNA-based testing, radiographs, biopsy, biochemical tests, developmental testing, and linkage studies (Lashley, 1998). After the exam and the completion of any applic-

BOX 4–12 Child or Family Indicators for a Referral to a Genetic Specialist

PRENATAL HISTORY INDICATORS FOR A GENETIC REFERRAL

- Infertility
- Repeated spontaneous abortions (usually 2–3 or more)
- Stillbirths or infant deaths due to unknown or genetic causes
- Females exposed to radiation, infectious disease, toxic agents, or certain drugs immediately before or during pregnancy
- Males exposed to radiation, toxic agents, or certain drugs who are contemplating *immediate* paternity

OTHER INDICATORS FOR A PRENATAL GENETIC REFERRAL

- Unexpected drug or anesthesia reactions
- If the child or family reports a known or "believed" genetic condition in the family
- Any anomaly affecting more than one member of a family
- Single or multiple congenital anomalies
- Familial occurrence of neoplasms
- The early onset of common complex disorders such as coronary heart disease or cancer
- Consideration of marriage to a blood relative (**consanguinity**)
- Women who are 35 years and older and are considering pregnancy or are already pregnant
- Men who are 45 years and older and are considering paternity
- Member of ethnic groups in which certain genetic disorders are frequent and screening, testing, or prenatal diagnosis is available
- History of chronic conditions such as bleeding disorders, sickle cell disease, cystic fibrosis, thalassemia, kidney or urinary tract infections, or childhood cancers
- Any other situation where suspicious signs and/or symptoms might suggest genetic disease and the nurse feels further evaluation may be needed

POSTNATAL DEVELOPMENTAL INDICATORS FOR A GENETIC REFERRAL

- Delayed or abnormal development
- Developmental regression
- Mental retardation
- Speech problems
- Learning disability

POSTNATAL PHYSICAL INDICATORS FOR A GENETIC REFERRAL

- Failure to thrive in an infant or child
- Delays in physical growth, usual body proportions, or low muscle tone
- Abnormal or delayed development of secondary sex characteristics or sex organs
- Short or extremely tall stature
- Blindness, cataracts in infants or children
- Deafness
- Hypotonia in an infant or child
- Seizures in newborns or infants
- Skin lesions such as café au lait spots

TABLE 4–7 Nursing Considerations for the Individual or Family with a Genetic Condition

Newborn/Infant	Disruption in parent–newborn bonding/attachment/relationship Implications for extended family members Implications for siblings Loss Parental depression Parental guilt Potential for impaired parenting Spiritual distress
Pediatric	Alteration in parent–child relationship Complex medical needs Family or individual coping Implications for siblings Potential for interruption of growth and development Potential for social stigmatization Risk for caregiver role strain Spiritual distress
Adolescent	Alteration in parent–child relationship Body image disturbance Health maintenance Hopelessness Impaired coping Knowledge deficit Lifestyle and reproductive choices Potential for interruption of growth and development Potential for social stigmatization Self-concept Social interaction

Adapted from Lea, D. H., Jenkins, J., & Francomano, C. (1998). Genetics in clinical practice: New directions for health care. *Boston: Jones and Bartlett.*

able testing, the geneticist and/or genetic counselor will discuss the findings with the parents and/or child and make recommendations. The discussion will include the natural history of the condition, the inheritance patterns, the current preventative or treatment options, and the risks to the client and/or family. The visit will also include opportunities for questions and answers as well as the assessment and evaluation of the family's understanding. It is typical for the information retention of a family facing a new genetic diagnosis to be very low. This makes it imperative for the nurse to take advantage of opportunities to reinforce genetic concepts at a later time when the individual or family is ready.

As the visit concludes, the child and parents can expect appropriate referrals to be made, discussion of available services, and a follow-up visit may be scheduled. A summary of the information is usually sent to the family and the child's healthcare provider will receive a report if requested by the individual or parents.

Genetic healthcare providers present the individual and the family with information to promote informed decisions. They are also sensitive to the importance of protecting the individual's autonomy. A challenge during any visit to a genetic specialist is in providing nondirective counseling. Families should be permitted to make decisions that are not influenced by any biases or values from the nurse, counselor, or geneticist. Many families are accustomed to practitioners and nurses providing direction and guidance in their decision making and families may be uncomfortable with the nondirectional approach of the nurse. They may believe that the nurse or healthcare provider is withholding very bad news. The nurse

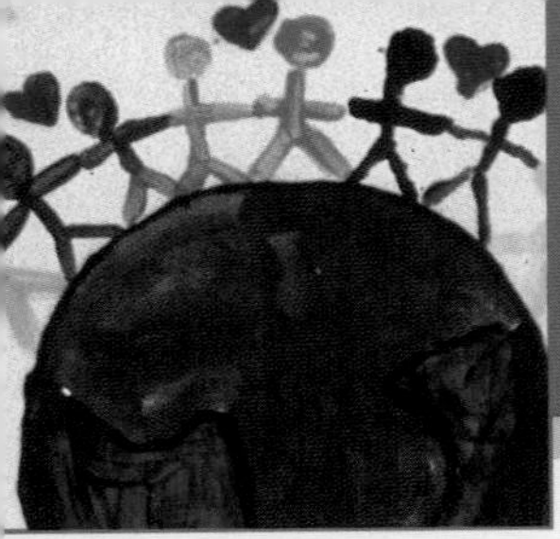

PARTNERING WITH FAMILIES

Ethical Implications of Genetic Information

The nurse must consider the enormity of the ethical issues facing all families who have knowledge of their genetic makeup. The ethical issues a nurse may have to discuss with the child and family are numerous. A few of the issues are listed below.

Access to Information

- Who should have access to personal genetic information, and how will it be used?
- Do insurers, employers, courts, law enforcement, schools, universities, adoption agencies, and the military have a right to access this information?

Self-Perception

- How does personal genetic information affect an individual's perception of self?
- How does personal genetic information affect society's perceptions of that individual?
- How does personal genetic information affect an individual's cultural identity?
- How is self-identity and self-worth affected by a confirmed genetic risk or condition?

Family Roles and Relationships

- Should an individual be tested for an autosomal dominant condition if the siblings and/or parents are opposed to knowing if they, themselves, have the altered gene?
- Should potential mates have genetic information?
- Should two people with increased genetic risk be prohibited from having children?
- Should a child be tested?
- Should the father be told if genetic testing and/or genetic counseling reveals nonpaternity?
- Should adoption records contain a complete genetic history of the biologic parents?
- Is there an obligation to tell other family members if an altered gene that demands a change in lifestyle (nutrition, exercise, smoking, etc.) is diagnosed?
- Is there an obligation to tell other family members if an altered gene that causes early debilitation and/or death is diagnosed?

Informed Consent

- Are all individuals receiving true informed consent and do they understand all of the consequences of agreeing to even a simple blood test in the doctor's office that may reveal a diagnosis or increased risk for a genetic condition?

Health and Life Insurance

- Should insurance companies have access to genetic test results?
- Should medical insurance costs be higher for persons with a known gene disease-producing alteration?
- Should medical insurance costs be higher for persons with a known increased risk for disease because of any gene alteration?
- Should medical insurance costs be higher for persons with known increased risk for disease because of any gene alteration if they make unhealthy lifestyle choices and do nothing to lower their risk?
- Should the individual be covered by medical insurance at all?
- Should individuals pay higher costs if they have children?
- Should individuals be required to have a large life insurance policy to financially protect their families?

Financial

- Should the child be eligible for government grants or any scholarship money?
- Should society be expected to financially support children through governments programs or private insurance?
- What is the motivation to save money for the future?

Employment

- Should an employer have access to an individual's genetic profile?
- Should a young adult be hired even though she/he will burden the company with multiple sick days, higher insurance financial support, etc.?
- Should the individual receive promotional opportunities and increased job responsibilities if the employer knows there will be a great deal of lost work days?
- Will the individual's productivity be affected by the genetic condition?

should discuss the positives and negatives of each decision and present as many options as possible through the use of therapeutic listening and communication skills (Cunniff, 2001).

Family Teaching

The pediatric nurse must be aware of available genetic resources and participate in the education of genetic disorders as well as health promotion and prevention. Informing children and their families of what to expect from a genetic referral as well as clarifying and/or reinforcing information obtained during a genetic referral or genetic test results is also important.

Cultural and religious beliefs and values of the individual and family must be assessed by the nurse prior to teaching. Are the gene alterations viewed as uncontrollable and believed to be occurring secondary to cultural beliefs such as a stranger looking at the infant? Or, are the gene alterations considered a "punishment"? A family's readiness to learn can be influenced by cultural or religious beliefs and values. Obtaining educational materials in the native language of the child or family will also help facilitate the teaching-learning experience.

The nurse must be aware of common inheritance misconceptions such as a parent's belief that with a 25% recurrence risk, after one child is affected, the next three children will be unaffected or with a 50% recurrence risk, every other child will be affected. The recurrence risk *for each pregnancy* should be continually stressed by the nurse. Families often believe that a family member has inherited the genetic condition because they look or "take after" a relative with a genetic condition. When new gene alterations or mutations are discussed, families will often exhibit surprise because no one else in the family has the condition so they perceive that the trait or condition cannot possibly be inherited (Bennett, 1999). Helping families to understand these genetic concepts is fundamental to delivering the standard of genetic nursing care.

Psychosocial Care

In order to meet the psychosocial needs of the child and family, the nurse should identify their expectations and needs as well as the cultural, spiritual, value, and belief systems. From where does the individual or family receive strength? Denial of the genetic diagnosis is common and nurses must be aware of the family's state of acceptance. Individuals and families often will not believe that a chronic genetic condition exists. Nurses must also provide care to help alleviate any anxiety and/or guilt in the child or family. Anxiety of the unknown is common when awaiting diagnosis or test results, but individuals also experience anxiety from not understanding the future implications of a confirmed genetic disease. Guilt may be associated with knowledge of the existence of a genetic condition being in a family. The nurse must support families as they contemplate telling extended family members, friends, and neighbors about a confirmed diagnosis. Immediate family members often do not want to tell extended family members until they are ready. It is important that the nurse reassures the parents that the genetic condition is not the result of something they did or did not do during pregnancy. The nurse should encourage open discussions and the expression of fears and concerns. Guilt and shame are common as a family deals with the loss of the expectation and dream of a healthy child, grandchild, niece, or nephew. Reinforce to parents that genetic alterations are caused by changes within a gene and not by superstitions related to sin or other cultural beliefs. It is important to remember that everyone has superstitions or beliefs and the pediatric nurse must remain nonjudgmental. As mothers, fathers, and extended family members provide continuous care for the individual with a genetic condition, depression can result. Depression also can occur in the individual with the chronic condition. The nurse must maintain awareness of the possibility of depression and be proactive in obtaining support for the individual or family. See Chapter 34∞.

The nurse also is responsible for assessing the family's coping mechanisms (see Chapter 2∞) as well as available family, spiritual, cultural, and community support systems. Genetic conditions can cause a permanent strain on family dynamics and relationships. The pediatric nurse may need to help the child and family reaffirm self-worth and value (Lashley, 1998). If seen in an academic setting, parents and children may feel they are part of a "production line" even though they are present for a very private problem (Cunniff, 2001). Nurses must be sensitive to these perceptions, provide open communication, and encourage discussion of feelings. Growth and development can be altered by actual or potential genetic disorders. Especially unique is the potential or actual inheritance of a late-onset condition such as Huntington disease, as discussed in the chapter opening scenario. Like Sarah, the adolescent with this altered gene may not meet any of the developmental tasks in moving toward adulthood. Should the adolescent attend college or worry about the future? The pediatric nurse must identify the impact of genetic knowledge on activities of daily living but also movement through developmental milestones. Both individual and family strengths need to be identified. See Chapter 5∞.

The nurse can refer the individual or family to a support group. However, it is important to have permission from the child or family if the nurse is providing a support group with the client's name and contact information.

Another key role for the nurse is to help families with the often difficult task of communicating genetic information such as inheritance patterns to extended family members. Cultural values of autonomy and privacy are impacted when a person must consider whether to communicate genetic information to extended family members who may also carry the altered gene. The history of a genetic alteration that may or may not cause disease can be extensive within a family, affecting multiple family members. Family members often have difficulty understanding that some genetic conditions have variable expressivity. Members of the extended family often are shocked and feel a profound sense of guilt that they are the one who has carried the gene alteration that caused their loved one to have a genetic condition.

Managing Care Through Advocacy

Careful self-assessment of feelings is essential for the nurse. The pediatric nurse must continually advocate for the child and family and support their decisions even if the decisions contradict the nurse's own ideals and morals. Coping with genetic revelations and making genetic-related treatment decisions are difficult activities for everyone. The nurse must remember that families will need resources and support, and also help in gathering information about reproductive options.

MediaLink Genetic Support Resources

■ Evaluation

Expected outcomes of delivering nursing care with a genetic focus include:

- The child and family will make informed and voluntary decisions related to genetic health issues.
- The child and family will accurately identify:
  - Basic genetic concepts and simple inheritance risk probabilities
  - What to expect from a genetic referral

- The influence of genetic factors in health promotion and health maintenance
- Social, legal, and ethical issues related to genetic testing

VISIONS FOR THE FUTURE

Nurses are often the primary caregivers that children and their families turn to for information, guidance, and clarification of ideas. This nursing role is essential not only in providing direct nursing care but also as a member of the community. As more information about the genetic revolution is available to consumers—in areas such as pharmacogenomics, gene transfer, ethics, genetic engineering, and stem cell research—the role of nurses remains not only vital but grows enormously. Nurses should remain educated, informed, knowledgeable, and ready to discuss trends and changes with children, adolescents, and their families.

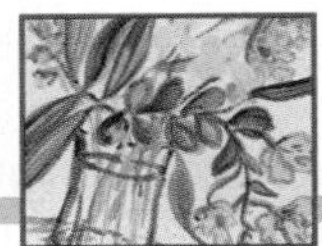

CHAPTER HIGHLIGHTS

- Nurses are responsible for basic genetic knowledge and delivering the expected standard of genetic nursing care.
- Genetic concepts can be applied to health promotion and health maintenance.
- When cell division does not occur as expected, chromosomal alterations on the autosomes or sex chromosomes can result.
- Mosaicism will present varied clinical manifestations of chromosomal alterations.
- Chromosomal alterations can be seen in a human karyotype.
- Protein-directing genes are important to life and functioning as a human being because proteins are highly specialized and perform a variety of functions within the cell.
- Different forms of a gene that occupy the same place on a pair of chromosomes are alleles.
- An individual may be identified as heterozygous or homozygous for a single gene.
- Some gene alterations cause disease and some protect individuals from disease.
- Mitochondrial gene alterations are inherited from the mother and are primarily involved in high-energy organs such as skeletal muscles, brain, and heart muscle.
- Knowledge of the principles of inheritance allows the nurse to not only offer and reinforce genetic information to children, adolescents, and their families but also to assist them in managing their care and in making reproductive decisions.
- Multifactorial inheritance does not follow Mendelian inheritance patterns.
- Basic genetic nursing care involves family risk assessment through a detailed family history, drawing a three-generation pedigree, and integrating genetic concepts into physical assessment.
- Basic genetic nursing involves initiating a referral to genetic specialists.
- Genetic healthcare providers present the individual and the family with information to promote informed decisions.
- There are several types of genetic tests available, all with special considerations related to the genetic testing of minors.
- The nurse must be aware of the social, ethical, cultural, and spiritual issues related to the delivery of genetic nursing care.

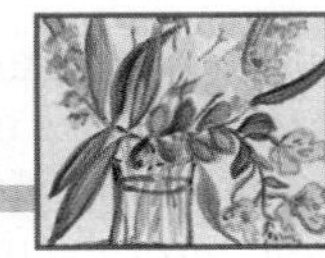

CRITICAL THINKING IN ACTION

INTRODUCTION

Recall 17-year-old Sarah from the chapter opening scenario. While at the sports clinic for a routine physical, she questions the nurse about the likelihood that she will acquire Huntington disease.

DESCRIPTION

Sarah's mother, Diane, is of western European Caucasian descent. Sarah's knowledge about her father is limited. She knows that he is a third generation Filipino American but has no medical information on him or his extended family.

Sarah's grandmother on her mother's side has three sisters and two brothers. The two brothers died of myocardial infarctions at the ages of 37 and 55 years, respectively. Sarah's maternal grandfather had no brothers but two sisters. Her maternal grandfather died at age 62 years of Huntington disease. The sisters are alive and well and have no medical problems.

Diane has two brothers and two sisters. She is the youngest of the siblings. Her oldest brother, Ken, was diagnosed 10 years ago with Huntington disease at age 41 years. Ken has two daughters ages 21 and 25 years.

Sarah is very close to these cousins and she knows that they have no medical problems beyond seasonal allergies and migraine headaches. Diane's other brother, Brian (age 38 years) has recently had bouts of depression and noticed slight difficulties in coordination and involuntary movements. Brian and his wife Sally adopted a son, Dave, with Down Syndrome, and he is 19 years old. All of Brian's other children (ages 10, 6 and 3 years) are alive and well. Diane's sister, Marion, has had two pregnancy losses at 22 weeks and 10 weeks gestation. Marion also has two children, ages 3 and 12 years, who are alive and well. She has informed the family that she has had genetic testing for the Huntington gene alteration with a negative result. Sarah's maternal aunt Kathy has daughter from a previous relationship and two sons from her current marriage. Her daughter was born with a cleft lip and palate. Sarah's brother is age 12 years and does not have any medical problems.

DISCUSSION

1. What further data would you gather from Sarah before referring her to a genetic specialist?
2. Search websites and other literature to learn more about Huntington Disease. What are the signs and symptoms? The prognosis? Is it linked to any ethnic group?
3. Create a family pedigree for Sarah based on the family information she has provided. What does the pedigree reveal, and what nursing actions would you plan for Sarah?
4. Based on a summary of Sarah's risk and protective factors (see Chapter 5∞), list three nursing diagnoses that encompass both physical and psychosocial health.
5. Should Sarah be tested at this time? Give a rationale for your answer.
6. How would Sarah's identity be affected by a positive or negative genetic testing result?
7. What key points should the nurse consider when developing a teaching plan for Sarah?

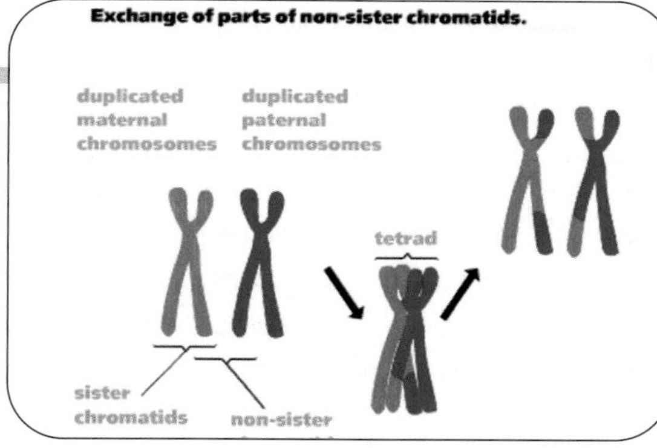

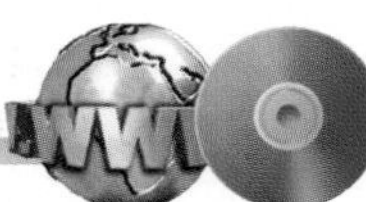

EXPLORE MediaLink

- NCLEX review, case studies, and other interactive resources for this chapter can be found on the Companion Website at **www.prenhall.com/ball**. Click on Chapter 4 to select the activities for this chapter.
- For animations, more NCLEX review questions, and an audio glossary, access the accompanying CD-ROM in this book.

http://www.prenhall.com/ball

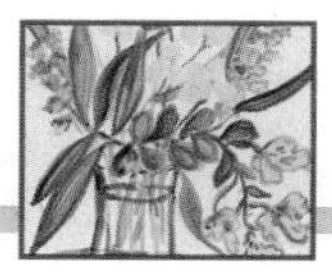

REFERENCES

Aase, J. (1992). Dysmorphic diagnosis for the pediatric practitioner. *Pediatric Clinics of North America, 39*, 135–156.

Aldhous, P. (2001). Can they rebuild us? [Electronic version]. *Nature, 410*, 622–625.

American Nurses Association & International Society of Nurses in Genetics, Inc. (1998). *Statement on the scope and standards of genetics clinical nursing practice*. Washington, DC: American Nurses Publishing.

American Society of Human Genetics (ASHG). (1998). ASHG Statement: Professional disclosure of familial genetic information. *American Journal of Human Genetics, 62*, 474–483.

American Society of Human Genetics (ASHG). (2000, April). ASHG Statement: Statement on gene therapy. *American Journal of Human Genetics, 67*, 272–273.

American Society of Human Genetics (ASHG) & American College of Medical Genetics (ACMG). (1995). Points to consider: Ethical, legal, and psychosocial implications of genetic testing in children and adolescents. *American Journal of Human Genetics, 57*, 1233–1241.

Bennett, R. L. (1999). *The practical guide to the genetic family history*. New York: Wiley-Liss.

Bennett, R. L., Steinhaus, K. A., Uhrich, S. B., O'Sullivan, C. K., Resta, R. G., Lochner-Doyle, D., Markel, D. S., Vincent, V., & Hamanishi, J. (1995). Recommendations for standardizing human pedigree nomenclature. *American Journal of Human Genetics, 56*, 745–752.

Beskow, L., Burke, W., Merz, J., Barr, P., Terry, S., Penchaszadeh, V., Gostin, L., Gwinn, M., & Khoury, M. (2001). Informed consent for population based research involving genetics. *Journal of the American Medical Association, 286*, 2315–2321.

Bowers, N. R. (2002). Meeting the standard of genetic nursing care. *JSPN: The Journal for Specialists in Pediatric Nursing, 7*, 123–126.

Centers for Disease Control and Prevention (CDC). (1992). Recommendations for the use of folic acid to reduce the number of cases of spina bifida and other neural tube defects. *Morbidity and Mortality Weekly Report, 41*(RR-14), 1–7.

Collins, F. S. (2000). Shattuck lecture—Medical and societal consequences of the human genome project. *The New England Journal of Medicine, 341*(1), 28–37.

Collins, F. S., Green, E. D., Guttamacher, A. E., & Guyer, M. S. (2003). A vision for the future of genomic research [Electronic version]. *Nature, 422*, 835–847.

Cunniff, C. (2001, October). *Culture and genetic health care.* Paper presented at the meeting of the International Society of Nurses in Genetics 14th Annual Educational Conference, San Diego, CA.

Fibison, W. J. (2000). Gene therapy. In S. O. Olsen, L. Baxendale-Cox, & V. Mock (Eds.), *The nursing clinics of North America: Clinical genetics* (Vol. 35[3], pp. 757–772). Philadelphia: W. B. Saunders.

Gaston, M. H., Verter, J. I., Woods, G., Pegelow, C., Kelleher, J., Presbury, G., et al. (1986). Prophylaxis with oral penicillin in children with sickle cell anemia. *The New England Journal of Medicine, 314,* 1593–1599.

GeneCare Medical Genetics Center. (2002). *FISH.* [Brochure]. Chapel Hill, NC: Author.

Georgetown University, National Reference Center for Bioethics Literature. (2003). Human gene therapy scope note 24. www.georgetown.edu/research/nrcbl/scopenotes/sn24.html, accessed 8/11/2003.

Grady, C. (1999). Ethics and genetic tesing. *Advances in Internal Medicine, 44,* 389–411.

Greendale, K., & Pyeritz, R. E. (2001). Empowering primary care health professionals in medical genetics: How soon? How fast? How far? *American Journal of Medical Genetics, 106,* 223–232.

Guttmacher, A. E., & Collins, F. (2002). Genomic medicine: A primer. *The New England Journal of Medicine, 347,* 1512–1527.

Guttmacher, A. E., Jenkins, J., & Uhlman, W. R. (2001). Genomic medicine: Who will practice it? A call to open arms. *American Journal of Medical Genetics, 106,* 216–222.

Human Genome Project Information. (2002). The Human Genome Project partners with minority community leaders for genomics education. www.ornl.gov/sci/techresources/Human_Genome/publicat/jmmbbag.pdf, accessed 8/11/2003.

Human Genome Project Information. (2003a). Gene testing. www.ornl.gov/TechResources/Human_Genome/ medicine/genetests.html, accessed 8/11/2003.

Human Genome Project Information. (2003b). Gene therapy. www.ornl.gov/TechResources/Human_Genome/ medicine/genettherapy.html, accessed 8/11/2003.

Human Genome Project Information. (2003c). Genetic disease information—Pronto! www.ornl.gov/TechResources/Human_Genome/medicine/assist.html, accessed 8/11/2003.

Human Genome Project Information. (2003d). Pharmacogenomics. www.ornl.gov/TechResources/Human_Genome/medicine/pharma.html, accessed 8/11/2003.

International Society of Nurses in Genetics (ISONG). (2000). Position statement: Informed decision-making consent: The role of the nurse. http://nursing.creighton.edu/isong/, accessed 6/28/2003.

Jegalian, K. (2000). *Genetics the future of medicine* (NIH Publication No. 00-4873). Washington, DC: National Human Genome Research Institute, National Institutes of Health.

Jenkins, J. F. (2000). *The present state of genetics in nursing. Report of the Expert Panel on Genetics and Nursing: Implications for education and practice* (pp. 31–37). Washington, DC: U.S. Department of Health and Human Resources.

Jones, K. L. (1997). *Smith's recognizable patterns of human malformations* (5th ed.). Philadelphia: Saunders.

Kline, R. M. (2001). Whose blood is it, anyway? *Scientific American,* 43–49.

Klug, W. S., & Cummings, M. R. (2003). *Concepts of genetics* (7th ed.). Upper Saddle River, NJ: Prentice Hall.

Lagay, F. (2003). Pharmacogenomics: Revolution in a bottle? www.ama-assn.org/ama/pub/printcat/7459 .html, accessed 8/11/2003.

Lashley, F. R. (1998). *Clinical genetics in nursing practice* (2nd ed.). New York: Springer.

Lea, D. H. (2000, September 30). A new world view of genetics service models. *Online Journal of Issues in Nursing, 5*(3), manuscript 6. www.nursingworld.org/ojin/topic13/tpc13_6.htm, accessed 10/11/2000.

Lea, D. H., Jenkins, J., & Francomano, C. (1998). *Genetics in clinical practice: New directions for health care.* Boston: Jones and Bartlett.

Lewin, M. B. (2000, August). The genetic basis of congenital heart disease. *Pediatric Annals, 8,* 469–480.

Lopez-Rangel, E. (1996). Latino culture. In N. L. Fisher (Ed.), *Cultural and ethnic diversity: A guide for genetic professionals* (pp. 19–35). Baltimore: Johns Hopkins University Press.

March of Dimes. (2003). *Data book for policy makers: Maternal, infant, and child health in the United States* (No. 50-1749-03). Washington DC: Office of Government Affairs March of Dimes.

National Center for Birth Defects and Developmental Disabilities, Center for Disease Control. (1999). *Folic acid for healthy babies: A primer* (NCEH Pub. No. 99-0093). cdc.gov/ncbddd/fact/babies.htm, accessed 11/7/2003.

National Coalition for Health Professional Education in Genetics (NCHPEG). (2001). Core competencies in genetics essential for all health-care professionals. www.nchpeg.org, accessed 12/4/2000.

National Human Genome Research Institute (NHGRI). (2003). Researchers discover use of novel mechanism preserves Y chromosome genes. www.genome.gov/11007628, accessed 8/5/2003.

National Institutes of Health (NIH). (1997). Genetic testing for cystic fibrosis. *NIH Consensus Statement, 15*(4), 1–37.

National Institutes of Health (NIH). (2000). Stem cells: A primer. www.nih.gov/news/stemcell/primer.htm, accessed 5/3/2001.

National Institutes of Health (NIH) & National Cancer Institute. (1995). *Understanding gene testing* (NIH Publication No. 96-3905). Washington, DC: U.S. Department of Health and Human Services, National Institutes of Health.

Nussbaum, R. L., McInnes, R. R., Willard, H. F., & Boerkoel, C. F. (2001). *Thompson & Thompson genetics in medicine* (6th ed.). Philadelphia: Saunders.

Online Mendelian Inheritance in Man, OMIM (TM). (2003). McKusick-Nathans Institute for Genetics Medicine, Johns Hopkins University (Baltimore, MD) and National Center for Biotechnology Information Library of Medicine (Bethesda, MD). www.ncbi.nlm.nih.gov/omim/

Orkin, S. H., & Morrison, S. J. (2002). Stem-cell competition [Electronic version]. *Nature, 418,* 25–27.

Roses, A. D. (2000). Pharmacogenetics and the practice of medicine [Electronic version]. *Nature, 405,* 857–865.

Scanlon, C., & Fibison, W. (1995). *Managing genetic information: Implications for nursing practice.* Washington, DC: American Nurses Publishing.

Secretary's Advisory Committee on Genetic Testing (SACGT), National Institutes of Health. (2000). A public consultation on oversight of genetic tests. www4.od.nih.gov/oba/sacgt/GTDocuments.html, accessed 8/15/2003.

Secretary's Advisory Committee on Genetic Testing (SACGT), National Institutes of Health. (2000). Enhancing the oversight of genetic tests: Recommendations of the SACGT. www4.od.nih.gov/oba/sacgt/GTDocuments.html, accessed 8/15/2003.

Spahis, J. (2002). Human genetics: Constructing a family pedigree. *American Journal of Nursing, 102*(7), 44–49.

United States Department of Energy Biological and Environmental Research Source. (2003). Gene gateway—Exploring genes and genetic disorders. www.ornl.gov/TechResources/Human_Genome/posters/chromosome/, accessed 6/28/2003.

United States Department of Energy Genome Programs. (2003). Genomics and its impact on science and society: The human genome project and beyond. www.ornl.gov/hgmis/publicat/primer/, accessed 6/28/2003.

Van Riper, M., & Cohen, W. I. (2001). Caring for children with Down syndrome and their families. *Journal of Pediatric Health Care, 15,* 123–131.

Veach, P. M., Bartels, D. M., & LeRoy, B. S. (2001). Ethical and professional challenges posed by patients with genetic concerns: A report of focus group discussions with genetic counselors, physicians, and nurses. *Journal of Genetic Counseling, 10,* 97–119.

Wertz, D., Fanos J., & Reilly, P. (1994). Genetic testing for children and adolescents: Who decides? *Journal of American Medical Association, 272,* 875–881.

Williams, J. K., & Lessick, M. (1996). Genome research: Implications for children. *Pediatric Nursing, 22*(1), 40–46.

Wine, J., Kuo, E., Hurlock, G., & Moss, R. (2001). Comprehensive mutation screening in cystic fibrosis center. *Pediatrics, 107,* 280–286.

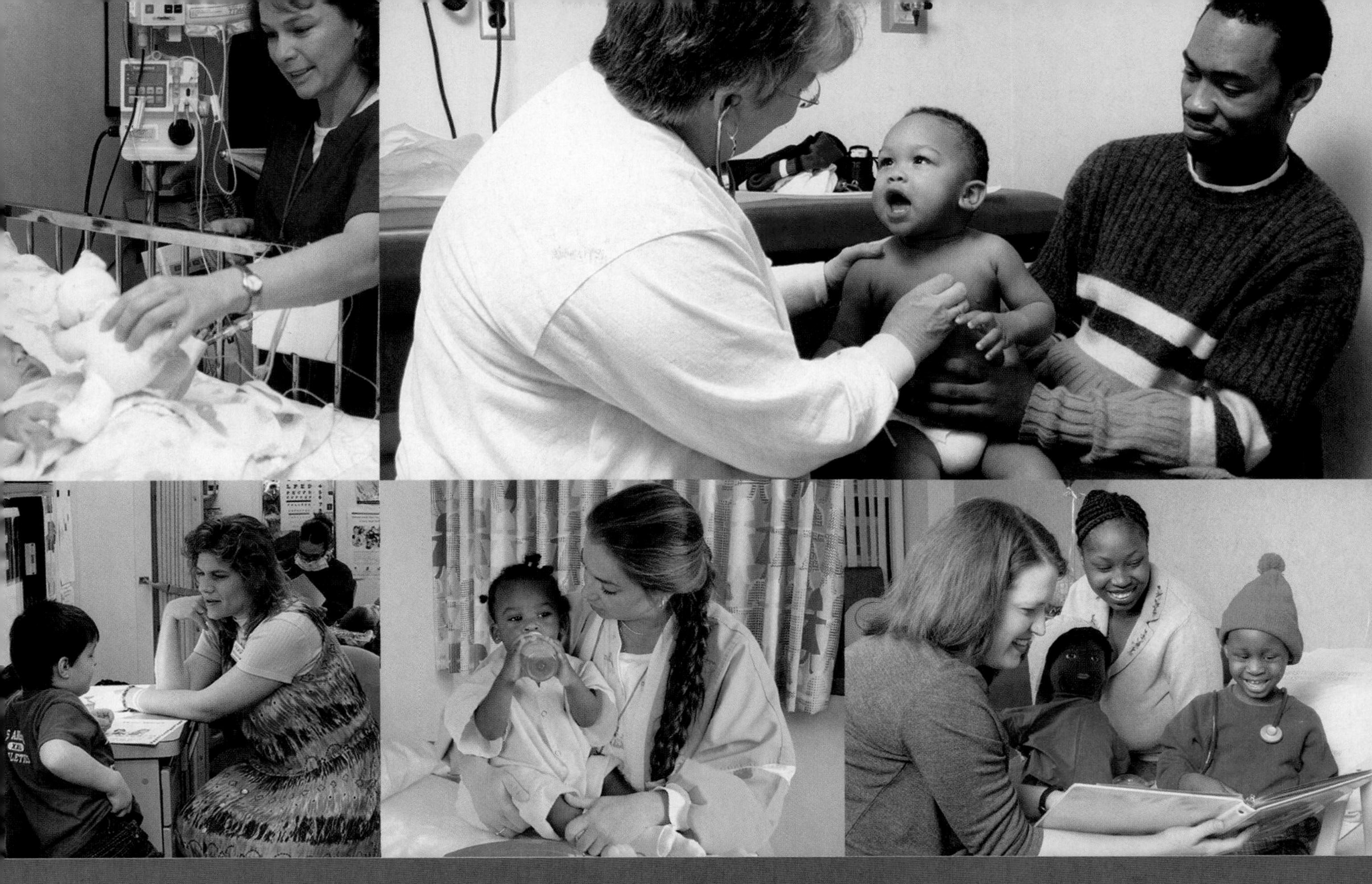

UNIT II

Child Concepts and Application

Pediatric nurses rely on a thorough knowledge base to formulate appropriate nursing interventions. Understanding the child's physical, cognitive, and psychosocial developmental stages is essential to providing care. The nurse applies communication principles when working with both children and their family members. While many of the child's characteristics are determined by developmental stages, the child's social and environmental settings are also significant influences that must be assessed and included in planning interventions. The nurse applies knowledge of growth and development, communication, and societal influences during physical and nutritional assessment of young children; describing findings and identifying abnormalities is crucial to providing effective nursing care.

Chapter 5

Concepts of Growth and Development

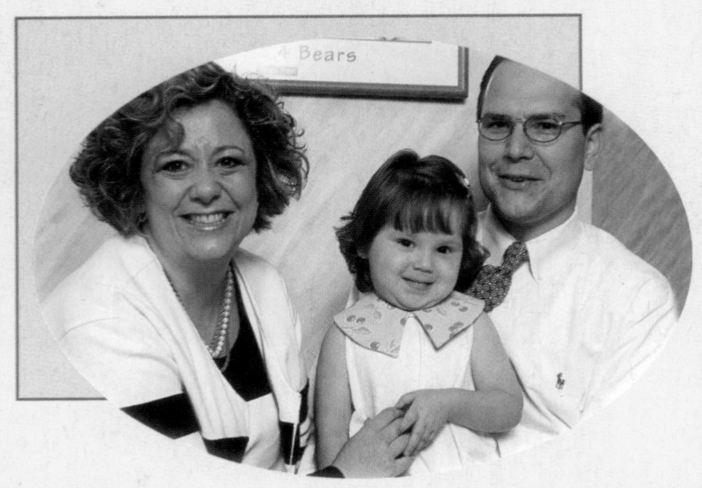

Michael and Alyssa Vann had tried for several years to have a biologic child. After an unsuccessful in vitro fertilization, they decided to adopt. They explored opportunities with adoption agencies, and learned that international adoption was possible for them. They adopted 2-year-old Irena from Romania several months ago. Despite a thorough investigation of Michael and Alyssa by the adoption agency, they received only scant information about Irena's history. She was left at an orphanage by her mother when she was about 7 months old; the mother stated that the pregnancy and delivery were normal. She was giving up the child because she had two older children to care for and her husband had left home nearly a year before and had not been heard from since. Irena appears small for her age, but is thriving in her new environment. She is learning to say a few English words and is responding appropriately to care and interactions. How can the nurse work with Michael and Alyssa to ensure special attention to Irena's growth and healthcare needs? What will Irena's cultural needs be as she grows older?

"We want to help Irena grow into a normal and special child. She has had challenges in her short life that we can only imagine. We worry about whether she'll want to go back to Romania when she's older to find her family."

—Alyssa, Irena's mother

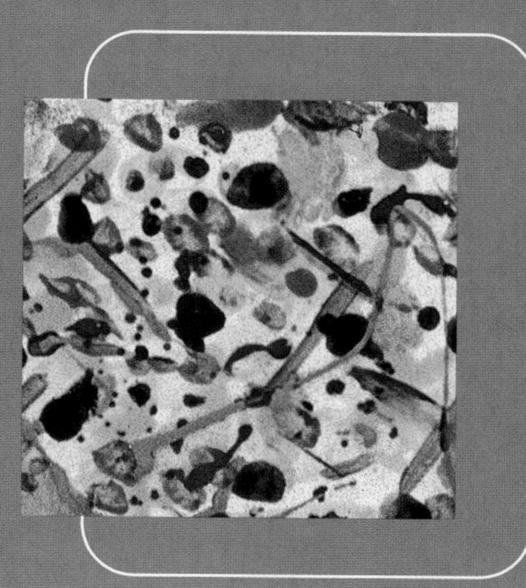

Learning Outcomes

After completing this chapter, you will be able to:

- Describe the major psychological theories of development (Freud, Erikson).
- Describe the major cognitive and moral theories of development (Piaget, Kohlberg).
- State major components of social learning theory, ecologic theory, and resiliency theory.
- Explore application of temperament characteristics to understanding the behavior of children.
- Apply physical, cognitive, and psychosocial theories when planning care for children from newborn through adolescent age groups.

Key Terms

MediaLink **http://www.prenhall.com/ball**

Resources for this chapter can be found on the CD-ROM accompanying this textbook, and on the Companion Website at http://www.prenhall.com/ball. Click on Chapter 5 to select the activities for this chapter.

CD-ROM

Video

Growth and Development

NCLEX Review

Audio Glossary

COMPANION WEBSITE

Case Study: Diabetic Risk Factors: School-Age Child

NCLEX Review

MediaLink Applications

Critical Thinking: Linking Theory and Research
Developing Values in Adolescence
Preparing a Preschooler for a Procedure

Key Terms *(continued)*

proximodistal development/131
puberty/163
receptive speech/153
resilience/144
risk factors/144
self-efficacy/140
solitary play/149
superego/132
transductive reasoning/138

Children develop as they interact with their surroundings. They learn skills at different ages, but the order in which they learn them is universal. Development is affected by factors such as nutrition and cultural practices, as well as the social situation in the country or neighborhood. While Irena will develop in a unique manner influenced by her genetic makeup, life experiences, and the interaction between these factors, certain principles of development can assist her parents and the nurse in fostering positive adaptations for her.

In this chapter, you will learn general principles of growth and development and will explore several theories related to childhood development, as well as their nursing applications. Each age group, from infancy through adolescence, is described in detail. Developmental milestones, physical and cognitive characteristics, psychosocial concerns, and communication strategies are presented. This basic information will help you provide developmentally appropriate care for children in each age group. You can apply these concepts to all children, including special situations such as the one described in the opening scenario. (See Developing Cultural Competence: International Adoptions.)

PRINCIPLES OF GROWTH AND DEVELOPMENT

It is essential to understand the concepts of growth and development when learning to care for children. Nurses who work with children must not only understand the pathophysiology of disease practices and the health promotion and health maintenance needs, but also must integrate knowledge of development into each encounter with a child. The pathophysiologic process, metabolism of medications, and healing process are influenced by the child's age and organ maturity. Health promotion needs regarding topics such as safety measures and immunizations are determined by age and developmental stage of the child, and these factors must also be considered for therapeutic communication to occur. The language used, explanations for procedures, and integration of approaches such as stories and pictures depend on the child's development. A skilled pediatric nurse therefore integrates knowledge of physical growth and psychosocial development into each child healthcare encounter.

Growth refers to an increase in physical size. Growth represents quantitative changes such as height, weight, blood pressure, and number of words in the child's vocabulary. **Development** refers to an increase in capability or function. Developmental skills unfold in a complex manner as a relationship between the child's innate, unfolding capabilities with the stimuli and support provided in the environment. Examples include the ability to sit without support or to throw a ball overhand. Growth and development or quantitative and qualitative changes in body organ functioning, ability to com-

DEVELOPING CULTURAL COMPETENCE
International Adoptions

Over 20,000 international adoptions occurred in 2001 in the United States, up from less than half that number one decade ago. China, Russia, Guatemala, South Korea, Ukraine, Kazakhstan, and Vietnam are presently the most frequent countries of origin for orphans being adopted in the United States (Chamberlain, 2003). Average age of adoptees is 2 years (Jenista, 2000). Although these children may have an array of medical conditions such as infectious diseases, inadequate immunizations, and nutritional disorders, the effects of their early life experiences on development can also be profound. Institutionalization and multiple foster care placements can result in emotional neglect, growth and developmental delays, and behavior problems (Chen, Barnett, & Wilson, 2003; Faber, 2000; Johnson, 2000; Miller, 2000; Aronson, 2000; Chamberlain, 2001).

Many international adoptees are small in size, due to poor nutrition of the mother during pregnancy and of the infant after birth, and to growth delay related to emotional issues. The child should be examined closely at the time of adoption for length, weight, and head circumference. Within 6 months of arrival, most children show improvement in growth patterns. If growth does not improve by this time, the child is further assessed for problems such as intestinal parasites, chronic diseases, or other medical problems (Chen, Barnett, & Wilson, 2003; Miller, 2000). The psychosocially based problem of eating disorder of infancy and childhood should also be considered (see Chapter 9 for a thorough discussion of this condition).

Although it is expected that international adoptees may have some developmental delays and often improve dramatically after adoption, testing of development, including verbal skills, upon arrival with their adoptive family is important. It provides a baseline upon which to measure future developmental test results and provides information needed to help parents encourage and stimulate the child appropriately (Miller, 2000).

Nurses perform careful developmental monitoring and assist adoptive parents in fostering normal growth and development.

municate, and performance of motor skills unfold over time and are key components in the process of planning pediatric healthcare.

Each child displays a unique maturational pattern during the process of development. Although the exact age at which skills emerge differs, the sequence or order of skill performance is uniform among children. Skill development proceeds according to two processes: from the head down and from the center of the body out to the extremities. Development that proceeds from the head downward through the body and toward the feet is called **cephalocaudal development** (Figure 5–1 ■). For example, at birth, an infant's head is much larger proportionately than the trunk or extremities. Similarly, infants learn to hold up their heads before sitting, and to sit before standing. Skills such as walking that involve the legs and feet develop last in infancy. Development that proceeds from the center of the body outward to the extremities is called **proximodistal development** (see Figure 5–1). For example, infants are first able to control the trunk, then the arms; only later are fine motor movements of the fingers possible. Pediatric nurses use these concepts of predictable and sequential developmental direction to analyze the infant's or child's present state and to partner with families to plan ways to encourage and support emerging developmental abilities.

During the childhood years, extraordinary changes occur in all aspects of development. Physical size, motor skills, cognitive ability, language, sensory ability, and psychosocial patterns all undergo major transformations. Nurses study normal patterns of development so they can perform thorough pediatric assessments and identify children who demonstrate slow or abnormal growth development. These assessments can guide the nurse in planning interventions for the child and family, such as referring the child for a diagnostic evaluation or rehabilitation, or teaching the parents how to provide adequate stimulation for the child. When development is proceeding normally, the nurse uses the knowledge of usual patterns to plan teaching approaches based on the child's cognitive and language ability, to offer appropriate toys and activities during illness, and to respond therapeutically during interactions with the child. These interventions form the basis of visits for health promotion and health maintenance (see Chapters 10 through 15∞ for detailed contents of these visits).

To highlight the important facets of development that are explored in this chapter, examine some of Irena's characteristics in the Photo Story on pages 132–133. These involve her physical growth and development, cognitive development, and psychosocial development, the latter including play patterns, temperament characteristics, and communication.

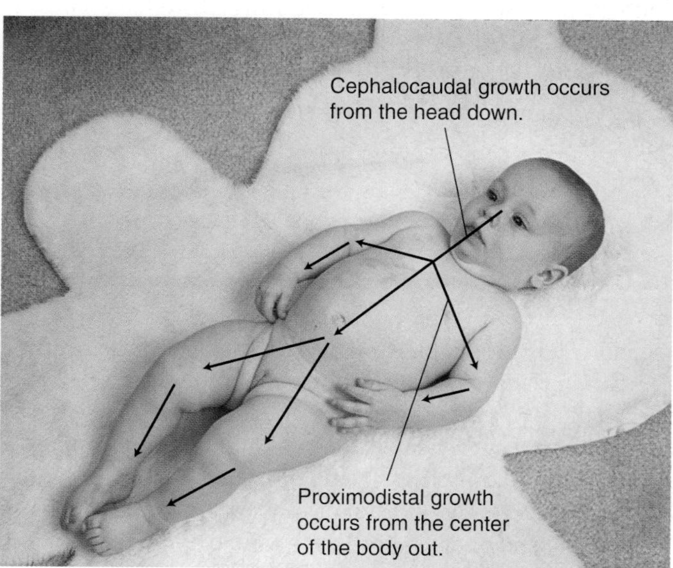
Cephalocaudal growth occurs from the head down.
Proximodistal growth occurs from the center of the body out.

FIGURE 5–1 ■ In normal cephalocaudal growth, the child gains control of the head and neck before the trunk and limbs. In normal proximodistal growth, the child controls arm movements before hand movements. For example, the child reaches for objects before being able to grasp them. Children gain control of their hands before their fingers; that is, they can hold things with the entire hand before they can pick something up with just their fingers.

MediaLink Growth and Development Video

MAJOR THEORIES OF DEVELOPMENT

Child development is a complex process. Many theorists have attempted to organize their observations of behavior into a description of principles or a set of stages. Each theory focuses on a particular facet of development. No one theory provides all necessary information and stages are not absolute. That is, there are differences in rates of progression among children and overlapping of stages within a specific child. Most developmental theorists separate children into age groups by common characteristics. Some of the age groups and developmental characteristics commonly used to group children include:

- *Prenatal period*—Includes the time from conception to birth; influenced by the genetics of the baby and the health of parents, particularly the mother.
- *Newborn*—From birth to 1 month of life. Although part of infancy, the first month is marked by the need for adaptation to extrauterine life and requires special support and care.
- *Infancy*—From 1 to 12 months. Includes infants or babies up to 1 year of age who require a high level of care in daily activities.
- *Toddlerhood*—From 1 to 3 years. Characterized by increased motor ability and independent behavior.
- *Preschool*—From 3 to 6 years. The preschooler refines gross and fine motor ability and language skills and often participates in a preschool learning program.
- *School age*—From 6 to 12 years. Begins with entry into a school system and is characterized by growing intellectual skills, physical ability, and independence.
- *Adolescence*—From 12 to 18 years. Begins with entry into the teen years. Mature cognitive thought, formation of identity, and influence of peers are important characteristics.

Freud's Theory of Psychosexual Development

Theoretical Framework

The psychoanalytic techniques used by Sigmund Freud (Box 5–1) led him to believe that early childhood experiences form the unconscious motivation for actions in later life. He developed a

PHOTOStory...

Developmental observations of a young child

Observing the activities of a child provides information about developmental status. Follow Irena as she goes about her daily activities.

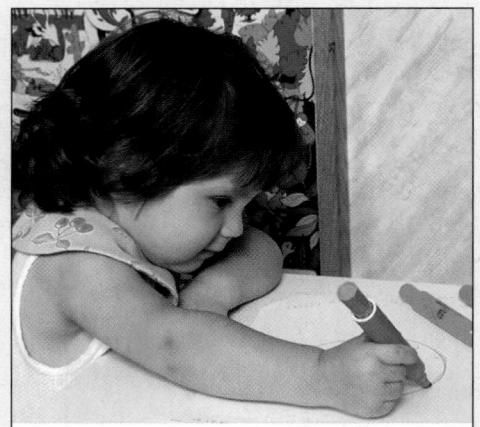

Irena shows fine motor skills as she begins to scribble and color in a circle provided by a parent.

PHYSICAL GROWTH AND DEVELOPMENT

Although many international adoptees are small for their age, Irena appears well nourished. (See Chapter 9 ∞ for a discussion of nutritional needs during toddlerhood.) Her gross motor skills, including walking up steps, running, and kicking a ball, are well developed. Fine motor skills are evident in her ability to brush teeth and dress with help, scribble on paper, and build a tower of cubes. As her physical abilities continue to develop, her family needs to integrate injury prevention to keep her safe from falls, car crashes, and other injuries.

COGNITIVE DEVELOPMENT

Cognitive development relates to intellectual or thinking processes. It is hard to identify Irena's cognitive stage at this time, as she knows only a few English words and is shy during interactions with strangers. As she adapts to her new home, frequent assessments of her cognitive development will be necessary.

PSYCHOSOCIAL DEVELOPMENT

Play

Irena is observed playing with toys and making sounds with her dolls. This is expected behavior, as toddlers often engage in solitary play. Toddlers also begin to enjoy the presence of other children, even though they do not yet play cooperatively with them. Irena's parents can encourage the emergence of parallel play commonly seen in toddlers by arranging to have Irena play with

---

theory that sexual energy is centered in specific parts of the body at certain ages. Unresolved conflict and unmet needs at a certain stage lead to a fixation of development at that stage (Lerner, 2002).

Freud viewed the personality as a structure with three parts: the **id,** the basic sexual energy that is present at birth and drives the individual to seek pleasure; the **ego,** the realistic part of the person, which develops during infancy and searches for acceptable methods of meeting impulses; and the **superego,** the moral and ethical system, which develops in childhood and contains a set of values and conscience (Craig & Baucum, 2001). He viewed all of these forces as largely out of conscious awareness.

BOX 5–1 Sigmund Freud (1856–1939)

Freud was a physician in Vienna, Austria. His work with adults who were experiencing a variety of nervous disorders led him to develop the approach called psychoanalysis, which explored the driving forces of the unconscious mind. Freud viewed these forces as largely due to unconscious childhood experiences.

Development and behaviors then unfold as the ego balances the tension between the two opposing forces of id and superego. The ego diverts impulses of the id and protects itself from excess anxiety created by the superego by use of **defense mechanisms.** These unconscious techniques distort reality to guide actions and prevent painful challenges to the personality. Examples of defense mechanisms used by children include regression to earlier stages of development, and repression or forgetting of

other children. The parents can be available at first so that Irena feels secure; once she shows comfort with other children, parents can gradually increase their absence during these playtimes.

Personality and Temperament

Irena has been demonstrating what experts term an "easy" temperament; that is, she has readily acquired a regular schedule for eating and sleeping, her mood is generally pleasant, and she is easily comforted when upset. These temperamental characteristics will form a critical link to communication with family, teachers, and friends.

Communication

Irena has only learned a few words. This is abnormal for a toddler, since most know several hundred words. However, it is expected that Irena will learn language quickly as she adapts. Michael and Alyssa should speak with Irena often, pointing out names of people and objects. Positive reinforcement for Irena's attempts at speech can involve smiles, phrases such as "that's right," and further elaboration such as "Yes, that is a bus; it's a big, yellow bus." *What else can you suggest to her parents as activities that will enhance speech development?* ■

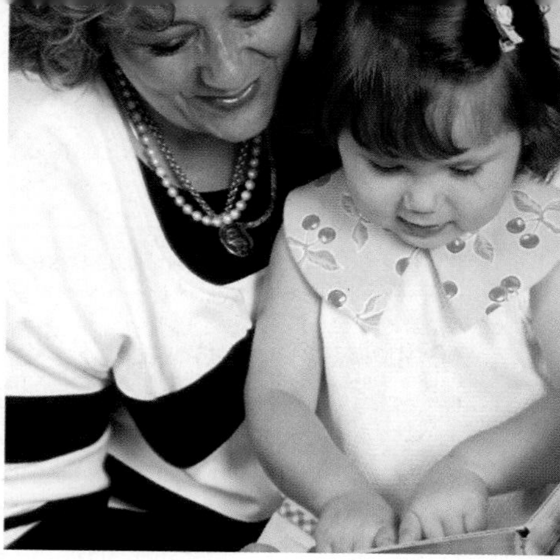

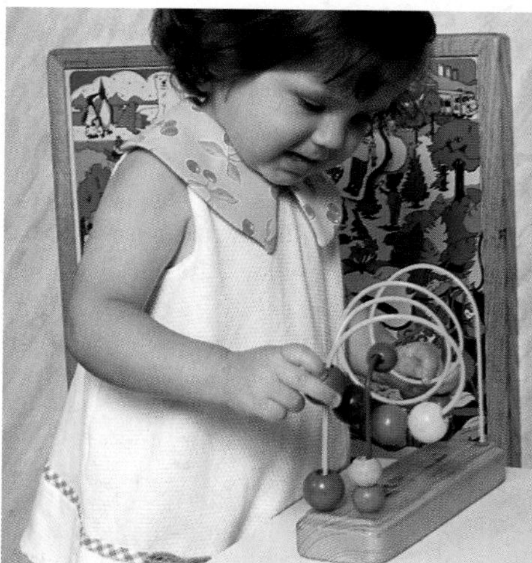

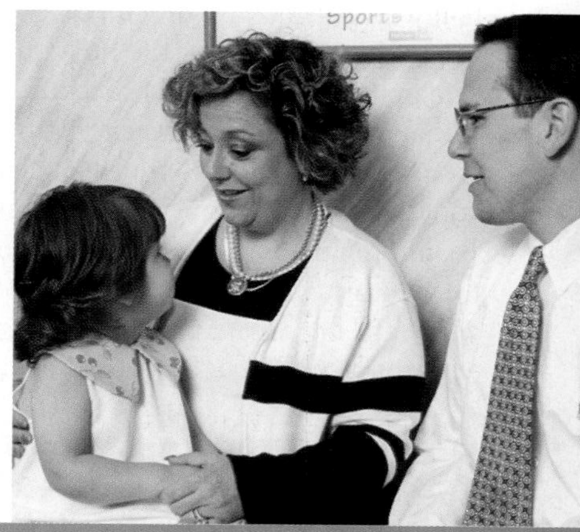

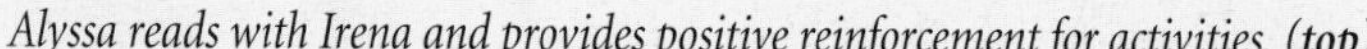

Alyssa reads with Irena and provides positive reinforcement for activities. ***(top)***

Cognitive development is enhanced as toddlers manipulate objects. What is Irena learning about color, texture, and spatial relationships? ***(middle)***

Irena's parents provide comfort and a trusting environment. This enhances her trust and helps her to feel secure, confident in her own abilities, and more autonomous. ***(bottom)***

painful experiences such as child abuse. See Table 5–1 for examples of defense mechanisms used in childhood.

Stages

Oral (Birth to 1 Year). The infant derives pleasure largely from the mouth, with sucking, eating, chewing, and mouthing objects as primary desires. These oral behaviors also release tension for the infant and play an important part in formation of the ego.

Anal (1 to 3 Years). The young child's pleasure is centered in the anal area, with control over body secretions as a prime force in behavior.

Phallic (3 to 6 Years). Sexual energy becomes centered in the genitalia and children explore touching their sexual organs. Freud also viewed this period as the time that the child works out relationships with parents of the same and opposite sexes. He believed that children love the parent of the opposite sex and want to take the place of the parent of their same sex. The child needs to accept the presence of both parents and begin to identify with the parent of the same sex.

Latency (6 to 12 Years). Sexual energy is at rest in the passage between earlier stages and adolescence. During this stage Freud believed that the child focused on other activities related to social and cognitive growth.

Genital (12 Years to Adulthood). Mature sexuality is achieved as physical growth is completed, sexual pleasure reemerges, and relationships develop with others outside the family.

TABLE 5–1 Common Defense Mechanisms Used by Children

DEFENSE MECHANISM	DEFINITION	EXAMPLE
Regression	Return to an earlier behavior	A previously toilet trained child becomes incontinent when separated from parents during a hospitalization.
Repression	Involuntary forgetting of uncomfortable situations	An abused child cannot consciously recall episodes of abuse.
Rationalization	An attempt to make unacceptable feelings acceptable	A child explains hitting another because "he took my toy."
Fantasy	A creation of the mind to help deal with unacceptable fear	A hospitalized child who is weak pretends to be Superman.

Nursing Application

Freud emphasized the importance of meeting the needs of each stage in order to move successfully into future developmental stages. His work has been criticized for several reasons—he developed a theory of childhood by his work with adults, primarily women, who sought help in dealing with emotional issues; he viewed males as dominant because of their possession of a penis; and he ignored the effects of culture and other external experiences. However, there are some aspects of his theory that appear to be supported by more current research and theory testing and can be applied in nursing.

The crisis of illness can interfere with normal developmental processes and add challenges for the nurse who is striving to meet an ill child's needs. For example, the importance of sucking in infancy guides the nurse to provide a pacifier for the infant who cannot have oral fluids. The preschool child's concern about sexuality guides the nurse to provide privacy and clear explanations during any procedures involving the genital area. It may be necessary to teach parents that masturbation by the young child is normal and to help parents deal with it. The adolescent's focus on relationships suggests that the nurse should include questions about significant friends during history taking. Table 5–2 and Figure 5–2 ■ summarize ways in which the nurse can apply these theoretical concepts to the care of children.

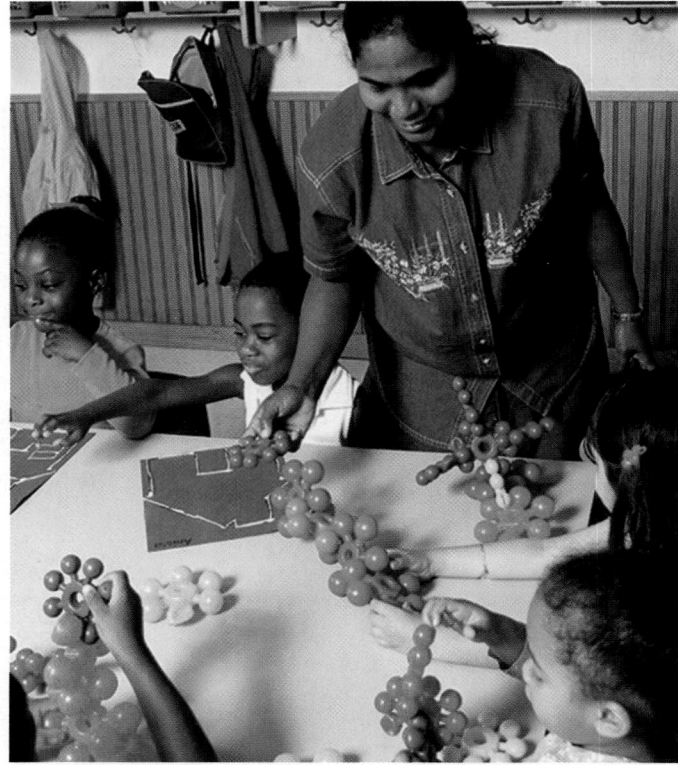

FIGURE 5–2 ■ Children exposed to pleasant stimulation and who receive positive feedback from an adult for engaging in activities will develop and refine their skills faster, demonstrating the importance of a nurturing environment. Group activities provide an opportunity for motor skill and psychosocial development. Which skills are being developed by children in this photograph?

Erikson's Theory of Psychosocial Development

Theoretical Framework

Erikson's theory establishes psychosocial stages during eight periods of human life. For each stage, Erikson identifies a crisis, that is, a particular challenge that exists for healthy personality development to occur (Erikson, 1963, 1968) (Box 5–2). The word *crisis* in this context refers to normal maturational social needs rather than to a single critical event. Each developmental crisis has two possible outcomes: When needs are met, the consequence is healthy and the individual moves on to future stages with particular strengths. When needs are not met, an unhealthy outcome occurs that will influence future social relationships.

BOX 5–2 Erik Erikson (1902–1994)

Erikson studied Freud's theory of psychoanalysis under Freud's daughter, Anna, but later established his own developmental theory emphasizing the psychosocial rather than psychosexual nature of individuals. Erikson's theory is one of the few that addresses development over the entire life span.

Stages

Trust Versus Mistrust (Birth to 1 Year). The task of the first year of life is to establish trust in the people providing care. Trust is fostered by provision of food, clean clothing, touch, and comfort. If basic needs are not met, the infant will eventually learn to mistrust others. Developing a sense of trust leads the child and eventually the adult to have confidence that the world is a good place and to approach life with a general sense of optimism. However, it is also important to have a balance between trust and mistrust with trust being the predominant characteristic. If a child is too trusting, child abuse or other poor

TABLE 5–2 Nursing Applications of Theories of Freud, Erikson, Piaget

AGE GROUP	DEVELOPMENTAL STAGES	NURSING APPLICATIONS
Infant (birth to 1 year)	Oral stage (Freud): The baby obtains pleasure and comfort through the mouth.	When a baby is NPO, offer a pacifier if not contraindicated. After painful procedures, offer a baby a bottle or pacifier or have the mother breast-feed.
	Trust versus mistrust stage (Erikson): The baby establishes a sense of trust when basic needs are met.	Hold the hospitalized baby often. **(1)** Offer comfort after painful procedures. Meet the baby's needs for food and hygiene. Encourage parents to room in. Manage pain effectively with use of pain medications and other measures.
	Sensorimotor stage (Piaget): The baby learns from movement and sensory input.	Use crib mobiles, manipulative toys, wall murals, and bright colors to provide interesting stimuli and comfort. Use toys to distract the baby during procedures and assessments.
Toddler (1–3 years)	Anal stage (Freud): The child derives gratification from control over bodily excretions.	Ask about toilet training and the child's rituals and words for elimination during admission history. Continue child's normal patterns of elimination in the hospital. Do not begin toilet training during illness or hospitalization. Accept regression in toileting during illness or hospitalization. Have potty chairs available in hospital and childcare centers.
	Autonomy versus shame and doubt stage (Erikson): The child is increasingly independent in many spheres of life.	Allow self-feeding opportunities. Encourage child to remove and put on own clothes, brush teeth, or assist with hygiene. **(2)** If restraint for a procedure is necessary, proceed quickly, providing explanations and comfort.
	Sensorimotor stage (end); preoperational stage (beginning) (Piaget): The child shows increasing curiosity and explorative behavior. Language skills improve.	Ensure safe surroundings to allow opportunities to manipulate objects. Name objects and give simple explanations.
Preschooler (3–6 years)	Phallic stage (Freud): The child initially identifies with the parent of the opposite sex but by the end of this stage has identified with the same-sex parent.	Be alert for children who appear more comfortable with male or female nurses, and attempt to accommodate them. Encourage parental involvement in care.
	Initiative versus guilt stage (Erikson): The child likes to initiate play activities.	Plan for playtime and offer a variety of materials from which to choose. Offer medical equipment for play to lessen anxiety about strange objects. **(3)** Assess children's concerns as expressed through their drawings. Accept the child's choices and expressions of feelings.
	Preoperational stage (Piaget): The child is increasingly verbal but has some limitations in thought processes. Causality is often confused, so the child may feel responsible for causing an illness.	Offer explanations about all procedures and treatments. Clearly explain that the child is not responsible for causing the illness.

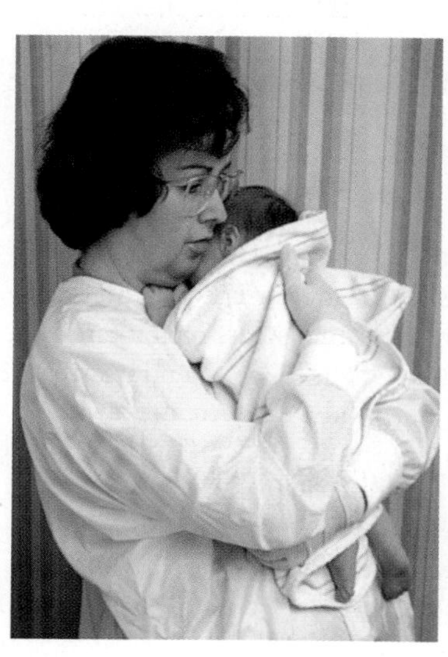

(1)

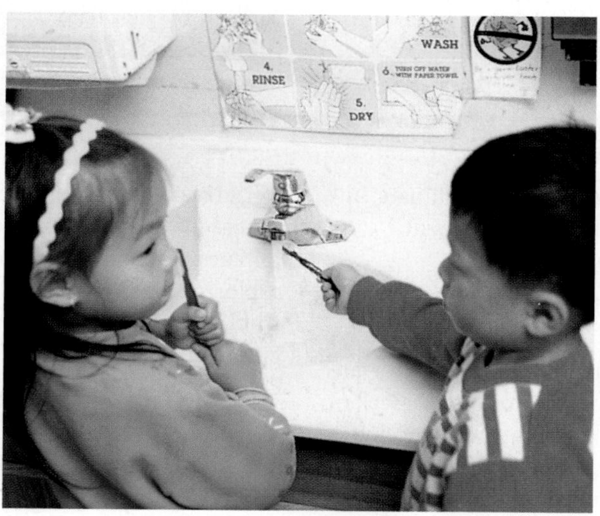

(2)

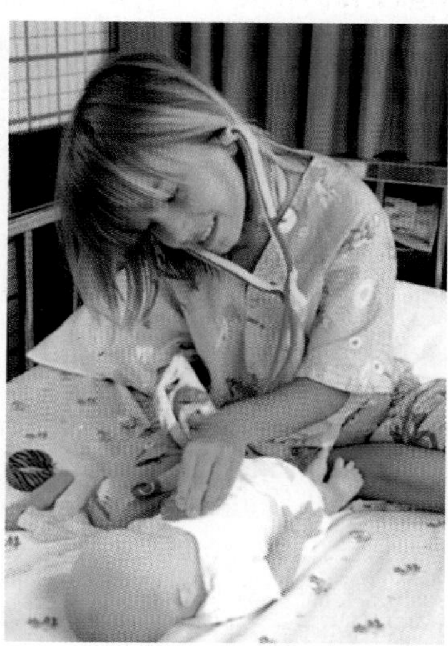

(3)

(continued)

TABLE 5–2 Nursing Applications of Theories of Freud, Erikson, Piaget (continued)

AGE GROUP	DEVELOPMENTAL STAGES	NURSING APPLICATIONS
School age (6–12 years)	Latency stage (Freud): The child places importance on privacy and understanding the body. Industry versus inferiority stage (Erikson): The child gains a sense of self-worth from involvement in activities. Concrete operational stage (Piaget): The child is capable of mature thought when allowed to manipulate and see objects.	Provide gowns, covers, and underwear. Knock on door before entering. Explain treatments and procedures. Encourage the child to continue school work while hospitalized. Encourage child to bring favorite pastimes to the hospital. **(4)** Help child adjust to limitations on favorite activities. Give clear instructions about details of treatment. Show the child equipment that will be used in treatment.
Adolescent (12–18 years)	Genital stage (Freud): The adolescent's focus is on genital function and relationships. Identity versus role confusion stage (Erikson): The adolescent's search for self-identity leads to independence from parents and reliance on peers. Formal operational stage (Piaget): The adolescent is capable of mature, abstract thought.	Ensure access to gynecologic care for adolescent girls. Provide information on sexuality. Ensure privacy during healthcare. Have brochures and videos available for teaching about sexuality. Provide a separate recreation room for teens who are hospitalized. **(5)** Take health history and perform examinations without parents present. Introduce adolescent to other teens with same health problem. Give clear and complete information about healthcare and treatments. Offer both written and verbal instructions. Continue to provide education about the disease to the adolescent with a chronic illness, as mature thought now leads to greater understanding.

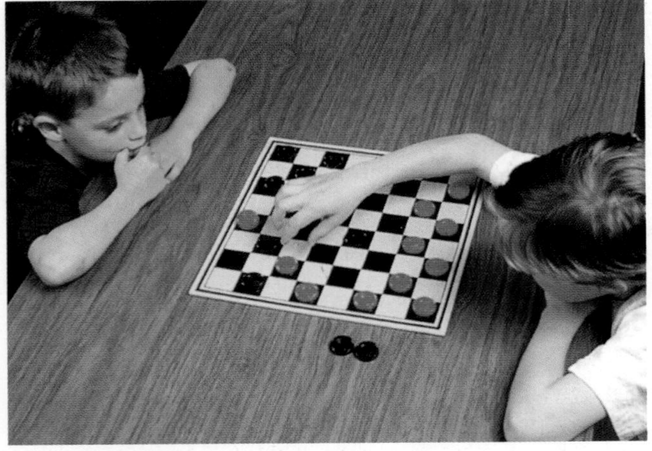

(4)

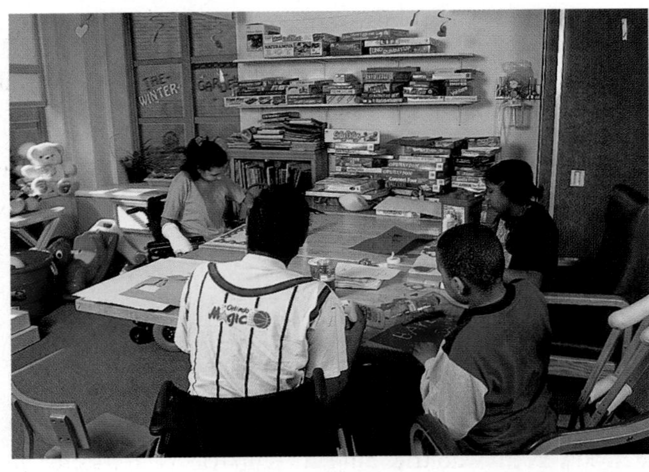

(5)

outcomes may occur. The sense of trust must predominate, but mistrust is also needed at times for healthy development.

Autonomy Versus Shame and Doubt (1 to 3 Years). The toddler's sense of autonomy or independence is shown by controlling body excretions, saying no when asked to do something, and directing motor activity. Children who are consistently criticized for expressions of autonomy or for lack of control—for example, during toilet training—will develop a sense of shame about themselves and doubt in their abilities. Developing a healthy sense of autonomy results in a person who can function with independence and self-direction. It is also important for the toddler to recognize feelings and needs of others; excessive autonomy could lead to disregard and inability to work with others.

Initiative Versus Guilt (3 to 6 Years). The young child is exposed to more people outside of the family and therefore initiates new activities and considers new ideas. This interest in exploring the world creates a child who is involved and busy. The child learns to assume new responsibilities and becomes aware of guiding principles for actions. Constant criticism for the child's activities, on the other hand, leads to feelings of guilt and a lack of purpose. Preschoolers' sense of initiative leads to the ability to start projects but they may not always see the value in completing them, a potentially frustrating situation for parents.

Industry Versus Inferiority (6 to 12 Years). The middle years of childhood are characterized by development of new interests and by a focus on intellectual or cognitive pursuits. The child takes pride in accomplishments in sports, school, home, and community. Developing a sense of industry provides the child with purpose and confidence in his or her ability to be successful. If the child cannot accomplish what is expected, however, the result will be a sense of inferiority. The child's sense of industry must be balanced by a realistic perspective gained over time, that there is always more to learn and that one cannot be the "best" at every activity.

Identity Versus Role Confusion (12 to 18 Years). In adolescence, as the body matures and thought processes become more complex, a new sense of identity or self is established. The adolescent tries out roles and examines what fits best for the self and family/society expectations. The self, family, peer group, and community are all examined and redefined. Identifying with values and roles provides guidance as the adolescent enters adulthood. The adolescent who is unable to establish a meaningful definition of self will experience confusion in one or more roles of life. On the other hand, a certain amount of role confusion is desirable as it is the impetus for self-examination and provides the basis for establishment of identity.

Although not discussed here, Erikson describes adulthood through three additional stages of development. They include intimacy versus isolation, generativity versus stagnation, and integrity versus despair.

Nursing Application

Erikson's theory is directly applicable to the nursing care of children. Health promotion and health maintenance visits in the community provide opportunities for helping caregivers to meet children's needs. The nurse asks for examples of the child's social interactions and self-concept. The child's behaviors can be explained within the perspective of developmental stages. Parents benefit from learning what the child's developmental tasks are at each stage, and from discussing ideas about how to encourage healthy psychosocial development. Such discussions also may highlight parental concerns and provide a forum for reassurance about normal developmental characteristics, such as a preschooler who does not follow through on each activity, or an adolescent who tries different hairstyles each month.

The child's usual support from family, peers, and others is interrupted by hospitalization. The challenge of hospitalization also adds a situational crisis to the normal developmental crisis a child is experiencing. Although the nurse may meet many of the hospitalized child's needs, continued parental involvement is necessary both during and after hospitalization to ensure progression through expected developmental stages (see Table 5–2). Asking parent's about the child's developmental progression provides clues to activities and provides information about what the child needs in the hospital. (See Chapter 17∞.)

Piaget's Theory of Cognitive Development

Theoretical Framework

Based on his observations and work with children, Jean Piaget formulated a theory of cognitive, or intellectual, development (Box 5–3). He believed that the child's view of the world is influenced largely by age, experience, and maturational ability. Given nurturing experiences, the child's ability to think matures naturally (Ginsberg & Opper, 1988; Piaget, 1972). The child incorporates new experiences via **assimilation** and changes to deal with these experiences by the process of **accommodation.** The child is an active participant in this cognitive building. For example, an infant first sucks or grasps by reflex. As feedback occurs (some things produce more satisfaction than others when sucking them and when grasping, one can shake to create sound, or let go to watch an object fall), the infant learns to change behaviors by sucking a breast, bottle, or fingers, and learns to shake a rattle or bring it to the face to examine. In these examples, can you describe which parts of the behaviors represent assimilation and which represent accommodation?

> **BOX 5–3 Jean Piaget (1896–1980)**
>
> Piaget was a 20th-century Swiss scientist who watched his own three children carefully and wrote detailed journals of their behaviors and verbalizations. He studied the intellectual abilities of children, focusing on child psychology and its application to education.

Some earlier theories viewed children as totally formed and shaped by adults around them. John Locke, a 17th-century theorist, formulated the theory of *tabula rasa*, or blank slate, to explain children. He believed that they entered the world with nothing but genetic potential and the way they developed was a result of experiences provided. While this theory is similar to Piaget's in recognizing the importance of experiences in building cognitive processes, Piaget believed that children were active participants in the unfolding of their inborn cognitive structures, taking in information and modifying behavior as a result.

Another important characteristic of Piaget's theory is that each of the stages he described is qualitatively different. By that, he means that a child does not simply learn by having *more* experiences. Instead, the child's mind unfolds so that the processes used to understand reality at different ages are unlike those of earlier stages. Piaget identified characteristics of thought that are found at various stages. Examine Table 5–3 as you read about the stages below.

Stages

Sensorimotor (Birth to 2 Years). Infants learn about the world by input obtained through the senses and by their motor activity. Six substages are characteristic of this stage.

Use of Reflexes (Birth to 1 Month). The infant begins life with a set of reflexes such as sucking, rooting, and grasping. By using these reflexes, the infant receives stimulation via touch, sound, smell, and vision. The reflexes thus pave the way for the first learning to occur.

Primary Circular Reactions (1 to 4 Months). Once the infant responds reflexively, the pleasure gained from that response causes repetition of the behavior. For example, if a toy grasped reflexively makes noise and is interesting to watch, the infant will grasp it again.

TABLE 5–3 Characteristics of Thought Identified by Piaget

CHARACTERISTIC	DEFINITION	DEVELOPMENT STAGE	NURSING IMPLICATIONS
Object permanence	Ability to understand that when something is out of sight it still exists	Sensorimotor period, especially in coordination of secondary schemes substage from 8–12 months	Before development of object permanence babies will not look for toys or other objects out of sight; as the concept is developing they are concerned when a parent leaves since they are not certain the parent will return.
Egocentrism	Ability to see things only from one's own point of view	Preoperational thought	Peers or others who have gone through an experience will not impress the preschooler; teaching should focus on what an experience will be like to the child.
Transductive reasoning	Connecting two events in a cause-effect relationship simply because they occur together in time	Preoperational thought	Ask the child what he or she thinks caused an occurrence; ask how the two events are connected; correct misconceptions to lessen child's guilt.
Centration	Focusing only on one particular aspect of a situation	Preoperational thought	Listen to the child's comments and deal with concerns in order to be able to present new concepts to the child.
Animism	Giving lifelike qualities to nonliving things	Preoperational thought	Ask preschool children to describe how a machine works, or how the trees move. Provide opportunities to learn about machines that may move and make noises (intravenous pumps, magnetic resonance imaging) to decrease fears.
Magical thinking	The belief that events occur because of one's thoughts or actions	Preoperational thought	Ask the young child how they became ill, what caused a parent or sibling's illness. Correct misconceptions when the child blames self for causing problems by wishing someone ill or having bad behavior.
Conservation	Knowledge that matter is not changed when its form is altered	Concrete operational thought	Before conservation of thought is reached, the child may think that gender can be changed when hair is cut; the leg under a cast is broken in separate pieces. Ask perceptions and clarify misconceptions.

Secondary Circular Reactions (4 to 8 Months). Awareness of the environment grows as the infant begins to connect cause and effect. The sounds of bottle preparation will lead to excited behavior. If an object is partially hidden, the infant will attempt to uncover and retrieve it.

Coordination of Secondary Schemes (8 to 12 Months). Intentional behavior is observed as the infant uses learned behavior to obtain objects, create sounds, or engage in other pleasurable activity. **Object permanence** (the knowledge that something continues to exist even when out of sight) begins when the infant remembers where a hidden object is likely to be found; it is no longer "out of sight, out of mind."

The concept of object permanence is not fully developed, however. The infant knows the parent well, objects to new people, and seems very worried when the parent leaves. Other caretakers may be rejected as the infant does not understand that the parent will return. This phase of "stranger anxiety" is quite common and heralds the infant's growing recognition of and desire to be cared for by the parent.

Tertiary Circular Reactions (12 to 18 Months). Curiosity, experimentation, and exploration predominate as the toddler tries out actions to learn results. Objects are turned in every direction, placed in the mouth, used for banging, and inserted in containers as their qualities and uses are explored.

Mental Combinations (18 to 24 Months). Language provides a new tool for the toddler to use in understanding the world. Language enables the child to think about events and objects before or after they occur. Object permanence is now fully developed as the child actively searches for objects in various locations and out of view. The child who has had successful separations from the parents followed by return, such as hours spent in another's home or childcare center, begins to understand that the missing parent will return.

Preoperational (2 to 7 Years). The young child thinks by using words as symbols, but logic is not well developed. During the preconceptual substage (2 to 4 years), vocabulary and comprehension increase greatly, but the child shows **egocentrism** (that is, an inability to see things from the perspective of another). In the intuitive substage (4 to 7 years), the child relies on **transductive reasoning** (that is, drawing conclusions from one general fact to another). For example, when a child disobeys a parent and then falls and breaks an arm that day, the child may ascribe the broken arm to bad behavior. Cause-and-effect relationships are often unrealistic or a result of

magical thinking (the belief that events occur because of thoughts or wishes). Additional characteristics noted in the thought of preschoolers include **centration,** or the ability to consider only one aspect of a situation at a time, and **animism,** or giving life to inanimate objects because they move, make noise, or have certain other qualities.

Concrete Operational (7 to 11 Years). Transductive reasoning has given way to a more accurate understanding of cause and effect. The child can reason quite well if concrete objects are used in teaching or experimentation. The concept of conservation (that matter does not change when its form is altered) is learned at this age.

Formal Operational (11 Years to Adulthood). Fully mature intellectual thought has now been attained. The adolescent can think abstractly about objects or concepts and consider different alternatives or outcomes. A certain amount of idealism, however, is characteristic at this age.

Nursing Application

Piaget's theory is essential to pediatric nursing. The nurse must understand a child's thought processes in order to design stimulating activities and meaningful, appropriate teaching plans. Presence of the parent as much as possible for the infant experiencing stranger anxiety is important, while providing links to peers may be important to the teen.

Health teaching is tailored to understanding of cognitive stages. For example, the teaching that a 6-year-old needs about newly diagnosed diabetes would focus on very different topics than the teaching provided for a 16-year-old with the same diagnosis. The nurse applies knowledge of the young child's magical thinking and egocentrism by asking about possible causes of the disease and planning teaching that focuses on the child's experiences. The adolescent will receive teaching with others of the same age or by teens who are managing the disease. Causation and possible outcomes can be addressed.

Understanding a child's concept of time suggests to the nurse how far in advance to prepare that child for procedures. Similarly, the nurse's decision to offer manipulative toys, read stories, draw pictures, or give the child reading material to explain healthcare measures depends on the child's cognitive stage of development (see Table 5–2).

What activities will you plan for Irena based on her expected cognitive level? How can you encourage her cognitive development?

Kohlberg's Theory of Moral Development

Theoretical Framework

Lawrence Kohlberg's focus is on a particular type of cognitive development concerned with moral decisions (Box 5–4). He presented stories involving moral dilemmas to children and adults and asked them to solve the dilemmas. For example, in one story a woman was very ill and the drug that would help her was too expensive for her family. The scientist who made that drug would not sell it for less money, so the woman's husband broke in to the store to steal the drug. Kohlberg asked a series of questions about whether it was right or wrong to steal the drug, and to charge a high price for it. Kohlberg then analyzed the motives people expressed when making decisions about the best course to take. Based on the explanations given, Kohlberg established three levels of moral reasoning. Although he provided age guidelines, he stated that they are approximate and that many people never reach the highest (postconventional) stage of development (Santrock, 2003).

BOX 5–4 Lawrence Kohlberg (b. 1927)

Kohlberg used Piaget's cognitive stage theory as the basis for his theory of moral development. He worked with children in his native Germany and in many other countries, including Kenya, Taiwan, and Mexico.

Kohlberg's work has been criticized for insensitivity to cultural differences in moral reasoning, lack of consideration of the family in moral development, an emphasis on moral reasoning rather than actual actions, and for sexual bias. However, it remains a useful framework for some to help understand moral decision making.

Stages

Preconventional (4 to 7 Years). Decisions are based on the desire to please others and to avoid punishment.

Conventional (7 to 11 Years). Conscience or an internal set of standards becomes important, but these standards are based on the beliefs and teachings of others such as parents. Rules are important and must be followed to please other people and "be good."

Postconventional (12 Years and Older). The individual has internalized ethical standards on which to base decisions, and uses awareness of the common good and ethical principles rather than relying on the standards of others. Social responsibility is recognized. The value in each of two differing moral approaches can be considered and a decision made.

Nursing Application

Decision making is required in many areas of healthcare. Children can be assisted to make decisions about healthcare and to consider alternatives when available. The nurse should keep in mind that young children may agree to participate in research simply because they want to comply with adults and appear cooperative. Guidelines for child participation in research are available (see Chapter 1∞).

Provide parents with information so that they can assist their children in moral judgments. Encourage talking with a child or adolescent about how a given decision was made. Parents can then add information and help the child learn to integrate more factors into decision making. Talking about the process is important in helping children progress to higher moral development stages. Focusing on the feelings of others, using positive discipline techniques, and clearly identifying positive and negative behaviors are important. See Chapters 13 through 15∞ for positive discipline techniques at each age.

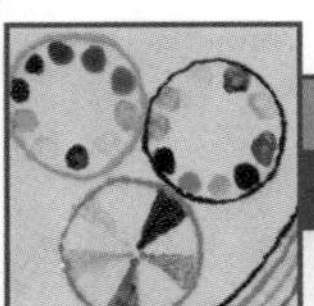

EVIDENCE-BASED PRACTICE
Self-Efficacy

PROBLEM

Nurses often provide information for parents and children that will encourage them to adopt healthy lifestyles. Providing information may not be enough; many of us know about healthy behaviors but do not consistently apply them. The concept of self-efficacy helps to explain why some people take on healthy behaviors while others do not. People who are convinced they can make a positive change are more likely to do so. A number of research projects test and apply self-efficacy in teaching about health. Two examples follow.

EVIDENCE

- Few effective interventions have been found that prevent or lower obesity rates in early adolescents. Nurses tested a health promotion program designed to increase self-efficacy and provide information in a group of 60 middle school youth, matched with 57 youth who did not receive the teaching. Children who had low self-efficacy scores tended to have greater consumption of high-fat foods. The intervention was associated with significantly lowered fat in the diet. Approaches that address diet choices, consciousness, efficacy, and other behavioral factors are more likely to contribute to dietary change than simple presentation of facts about dietary intake (Frenn, Malin, & Bansal, 2003).
- Violence among youth is a complex problem that presents challenges to nurses in many settings. The authors examined factors that influence extent and likelihood of youth violence among 318 middle school students. Self-efficacy was identified as a key concept for testing, and was defined as the confidence of students to avoid engaging in physically violent behaviors. Lower self-efficacy was associated with and a strong predictor of more frequent violent behaviors. Interventions can be targeted at increasing students' self-efficacy so that violent behaviors will decrease (Riner & Saywell, 2002).

IMPLICATIONS

In addition to providing information about health behaviors, nurses need to integrate methods to increase self-efficacy in teaching projects with youth. Choices, problem solving approaches, and increasing confidence should be parts of each teaching plan.

CRITICAL THINKING APPLICATION

Nurses can apply the concept of self-efficacy in teaching children and families. Plan a teaching project for school-age children to foster healthy eating. Include expected outcomes for the children and interventions. *Could your outcome be improved if you focus not just on getting the content across, but in increasing the belief and confidence that the children will be able to integrate the new behaviors into their lives? What activities could your teaching plan include that would be likely to improve the self-efficacy of these school-age children?*

Social Learning Theory

Theoretical Framework

Albert Bandura, a contemporary psychologist, believes that children learn attitudes, beliefs, customs, and values through their social contacts with adults and other children (Box 5–5). Children imitate (or model) the behavior they see; if the behavior is positively reinforced, they tend to repeat it. However, Bandura also believes that people can consciously choose how to act, such as deciding to handle problems by talking rather than hitting or yelling, even when some role models engage in the latter approach. The external environment (the behavior of others) and the child's internal processes and characteristics are thus both key elements in the behaviors a child manifests (Bandura, 1986, 1997a).

Bandura believes that an important determinant of behavior is **self-efficacy,** or the expectation that someone can produce a desired outcome. For example, if adolescents believe they can avoid use of drugs or alcohol, they are more likely to do so. A child who has confidence in his or her ability to exercise regularly or lose weight has a greater chance of success with these behavior changes. Parents who have confidence in their ability to care adequately for their infants are more likely to do so (Bandura, 1997b).

BOX 5–5 Albert Bandura (b. 1925)

Bandura is a Canadian who has conducted psychologic research at Stanford University for many years. He believes that children learn from their social environments, particularly by modeling the observed behaviors of others. His theories are the foundation of social learning theory which has been used extensively in nursing and psychological research.

Nursing Application

The importance of modeling behavior can readily be applied in healthcare. Children are more likely to cooperate if they see adults or other children performing a task willingly. A frightened child may watch another child perform vision screening or have blood drawn and then decide to allow the procedure to take place. Contact with positive role models is useful when teaching children and adolescents self-care for chronic diseases such as diabetes. Positive reinforcement should be given for desired performance.

Nurses can utilize the concept of self-efficacy to increase the chance of success with lifestyle behavior changes. For example, encouraging youth who are trying to quit smoking, providing them with role models, and pointing out parental successes with their children all demonstrate methods of fostering self-efficacy. See Evidence-Based Practice: Self-Efficacy in the box above.

Behaviorism

Theoretical Framework

John Watson (Box 5–6) studied the research of Pavlov and Skinner, who demonstrated that actions are determined by responses from the environment. Pavlov and, later, Skinner worked with animals, presenting a stimulus such as food and pairing it with another stimulus such as a ringing bell. Eventually the animal being fed began to salivate when the bell rang. As Skinner and

BOX 5–6 John Watson (1878–1958)

Watson was an American scientist who applied the work of animal behaviorists, such as Ivan Pavlov and B. F. Skinner, to children.

then Watson began to apply these concepts to children, they showed that behaviors can be elicited by positive reinforcement, such as a food treat, or extinguished by negative reinforcement, such as by scolding or withdrawal of attention. Watson believed that he could make of a child anyone he desired—from a professional to a thief or beggar—simply by reinforcing behavior in certain ways (Santrock, 2003).

Nursing Application

Behaviorism has been criticized for its simplicity and its denial of the inherent capability of persons to respond willfully to events in the environment. This theory does, however, have some use in healthcare. When particular behaviors are desired, positive reinforcement can be established to encourage these behaviors. Behavioral techniques are also used to alter behavior of children who misbehave or to teach skills to children who are physically challenged. Parents often use reinforcement in toilet training and other skills learned in childhood. Indeed, combining behaviorism with social learning theory can be beneficial. For example, children might have desired activities, such as tooth brushing, modeled by an adult or older child (social learning theory), and be rewarded (behaviorism) for carrying out the activity on a regular basis.

Ecologic Theory

Theoretical Framework

You may have noticed the controversy among theorists concerning the relative importance of heredity versus environment—or nature versus nurture—in human development (Box 5–7). **Nature** refers to the genetic or hereditary capability of an individual. **Nurture** refers to the effects of the environment on a person's performance. Piaget believed in the importance of internal cognitive structures that unfold at appointed times, given any environment that provides basic opportunities. He emphasized the strength of nature. The behaviorist John Watson, on the other hand, believed that behaviors are primarily shaped by environmental responses; he thus stressed the predominance of nurture. Contemporary developmental theorists increasingly recognize the interaction of nature and nurture in determining the child's development.

The ecologic theory of development was formulated by Urie Bronfenbrenner to explain the unique relationship of the child to all of life's settings, from close to remote (Bronfenbrenner, 1986; Bronfenbrenner, McClelland, Ceci, et al., 1996) (Box 5–8). **Ecologic theory** emphasizes the presence of mutual interactions between the child and these various settings. Neither nature nor nurture is considered of more importance. Bronfenbrenner believes each child brings a unique set of genes—and specific attributes such as age, gender, health, and other characteristics—to his or her interactions with the environment. The child then interacts in many settings at different levels or systems (Figure 5–3 ■).

> **BOX 5–7 Critical Thinking: Nature Versus Nurture**
>
> Does nature or nurture have primary importance in the theories of Erikson, Kohlberg, Freud, and social learning? Think about whether each of the theories emphasizes the role of heredity (nature) or the role of the environment (nurture) in influencing the development of children.

> **BOX 5–8 Urie Bronfenbrenner (b. 1917)**
>
> Bronfenbrenner, a professor at Cornell University, established the ecologic theory of development. He views the child as interacting with the environment at different levels, or systems.

Levels or Systems

Microsystem. The microsystem level is defined as the daily, consistent, close relationships such as home, childcare, school, friends, and neighbors. For the child with a chronic illness requiring regular care, the healthcare providers may even be part of the microsystem. In the ecologic model, the child influences each of these settings in addition to being influenced by them, with reciprocal interactions. Consider how Irena's microsystems have changed. Initially her mother and siblings were the important persons in her daily life, then the orphanage staff and other children, and finally Michael and Alyssa and their families and friends. How might these changes have influenced Irena? What stability is needed now to foster her ability to form relationships?

Mesosystem. The mesosystem level includes relationships of microsystems with one another. For example, two microsystems for most children are the home and the school. The relationships between these microsystems are shown by parents' involvement in their children's school. This involvement, in turn, influences the effects of the home and school settings on the children.

Exosystem. The exosystem level is composed of those settings that influence the child even though the child is not in close daily contact with the system. Examples include the parents' jobs and the governing board of the local school district. Although the child may not go to the parents' workplaces, he or she can be influenced by policies related to healthcare, sick leave, inflexible work hours, overtime, travel, or even by the mood of the boss (through its impact on the parent). The child's needs may influence a parent to give up a certain job or to work harder to obtain money for the child's education. Likewise, when a local school board votes to ban certain books or to finance a field trip, the child is influenced by these decisions; the child, in turn, can help establish an atmosphere that will guide future school board decisions.

Macrosystem. The macrosystem level includes the beliefs, values, and behaviors expressed in the child's environment. Culture is a powerful influence in the macrosystem, as is the political system. For instance, a democratic system creates different beliefs, values, and even eating practices than an anarchic system.

Chronosystem. The outer level, the chronosystem, brings the perspective of time to the previous settings. The time period during which the child grows up influences views of health and illness. For example, the experiences of children with influenza in the 19th versus 20th centuries were quite different.

Nursing Application

Nurses use ecologic theory when they assess the child's settings to identify influences on development. Table 5–4 provides an

MediaLink Critical Thinking: Linking Research and Theory

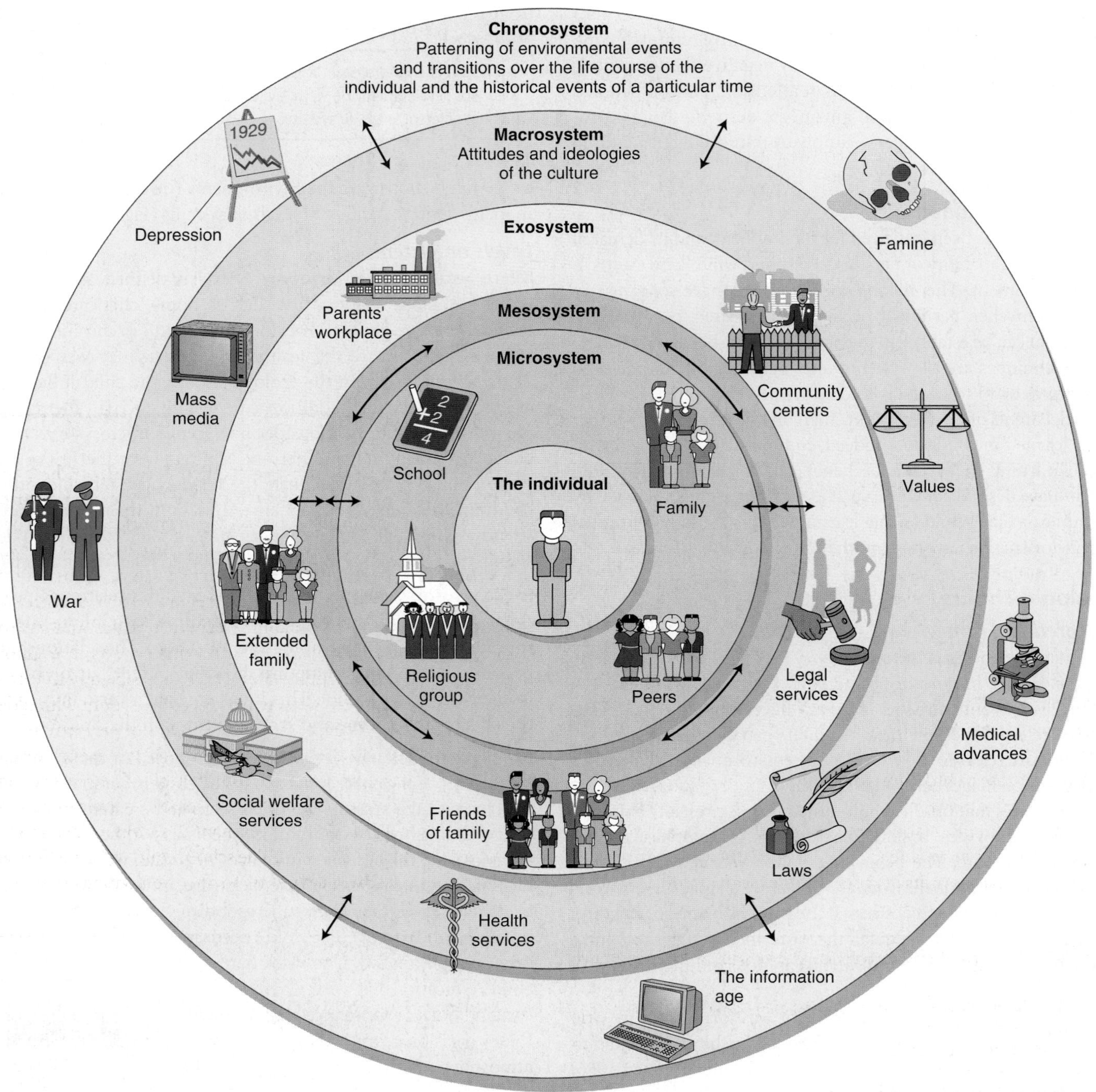

FIGURE 5–3 ■ Bronfenbrenner's ecologic theory of development views the individual as interacting within five levels or systems.

Note: Redrawn from Santrock, J. W. (1999). Life span development. Madison, WI: Brown & Benchmark. Based on Bronfenbrenner's (1979, 1986) works in Contexts of child rearing: Problems and prospects. American Psychologist, 34, 844–850; Ecology of the family as a context for human development: Research perspectives. Developmental Psychology, 22, 723–742.

assessment tool based on this theory. Interventions are planned to enhance the strengths of the child's settings and to improve on areas that are not supportive.

Temperament Theory

Theoretical Framework

In contrast to behaviorists such as Watson or maturational theorists such as Piaget, Stella Chess and Alexander Thomas recognized the innate qualities of personality that each individual brings to the events of daily life (Box 5–9). They, like Bronfenbrenner, believe the child is an individual who both influences and is influenced by the environment. However, Chess and Thomas focus on one specific aspect of development—the wide spectrum of behaviors possible in children, identifying nine parameters of response to daily events (Box 5–10). Infants generally display clusters of responses, which Chess and Thomas have classified into three major personality types (Box 5–11). Although most children do not demonstrate all behav-

TABLE 5–4 Assessment of Ecologic Systems in Childhood—Bronfenbrenner

MICROSYSTEMS	MESOSYSTEMS	EXOSYSTEMS	MACROSYSTEMS	CHRONOSYSTEMS
Parents Significant others in close contact Childcare arrangements School Neighborhood contacts Clubs Friends, peers Religious community (e.g., churches, synagogues, mosques)	Parents' involvement in child-care or school Parents' involvement in community Parents' relationships with significant others (e.g., grandparents, care providers) Influences of religious community (e.g., church, synagogue, mosque) or parents and school	Community centers Local political influences Parents' work Parents' friends and activities Social services Healthcare Libraries	Cultural group membership Beliefs and values of group Political structure	Child's age Parents' ages

BOX 5–9 Stella Chess and Alexander Thomas

Chess and Thomas are psychiatrists who began the New York Longitudinal Study in 1956 with 141 children, which they expanded in 1961 with 95 additional children. Most of these individuals are still being assessed periodically as adults. Their research has identified characteristics of personality and provides a basis for the ongoing study of temperament (Chess & Thomas, 1995).

iors described for a particular type, they usually show a grouping indicative of one personality type (Chess & Thomas, 1995, 1996).

Current research demonstrates that personality characteristics displayed during infancy are often consistent with those seen later in life. The ability to predict future characteristics is not possible, however, due to the complex and dynamic interaction of personality traits and environmental reactions.

Many other researchers have expanded the work of Chess and Thomas, developing assessment tools for temperament types. The concept of "goodness of fit" is an outgrowth of this theory. Goodness of fit refers to whether parents' expectations of their child's behavior are consistent with the child's temperament type. There is a "good fit" when the properties of the environment are in accord with the child's capabilities, characteristics, and style of behavior (Chess & Thomas, 1999; Turecki, 2003). As an example of lack of good fit, an active infant who reacts strongly to verbal stimuli may be unable to sleep when placed in a room with older siblings. A child who is slow to warm up may not perform well in the first few months at a new school, much to parents' disappointment. When parents understand a child's temperament characteristics, they are better able to shape the environment to meet the child's needs. The active infant described above should be put to sleep in a quiet room. The school child will benefit from meeting the teacher while parents are present, inviting classmates

BOX 5–10 Nine Parameters of Personality—Chess and Thomas

1. **Activity level.** The degree of motion during eating, playing, sleeping, bathing. Scored as high, medium, or low.
2. **Rhythmicity.** The regularity of schedule maintained for sleep, hunger, elimination. Scored as regular, variable, or irregular.
3. **Approach or withdrawal.** The response to a new stimulus such as a food, activity, or person. Scored as approachable, variable, or withdrawn.
4. **Adaptability.** The degree of adaptation to new situations. Scored as adaptive, variable, or nonadaptive.
5. **Threshold of responsiveness.** The intensity of stimulation needed to elicit a response to sensory input, objects in the environment, or people. Scored as high, medium, or low.
6. **Intensity of reaction.** The degree of response to situations. Scored as positive, variable, or negative.
7. **Quality of mood.** The predominant mood during daily activity and in response to stimuli. Scored as positive, variable, or negative.
8. **Distractibility.** The ability of environmental stimuli to interfere with the child's activity. Scored as distractible, variable, or nondistractible.
9. **Attention span and persistence.** The amount of time devoted to activities (compared with other children of the same age) and the degree of ability to stick with an activity in spite of obstacles. Scored as persistent, variable, or nonpersistent.

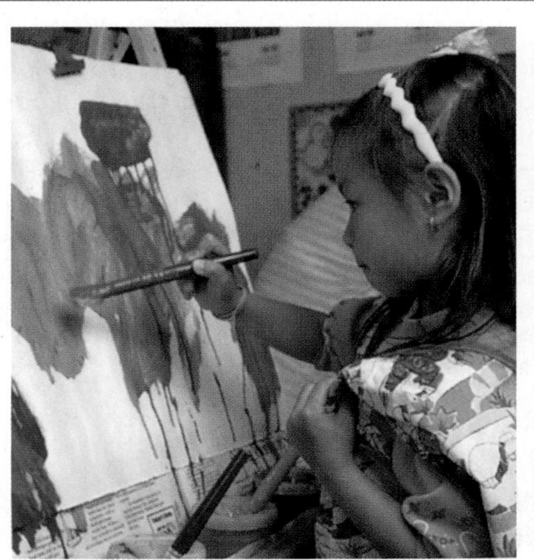

Data from Chess, S., & Thomas, A. (1996). Temperament: Theory and practice. *Philadelphia: Brunner/Mazel Publishers.*

BOX 5–11 Patterns of Temperament—Chess and Thomas

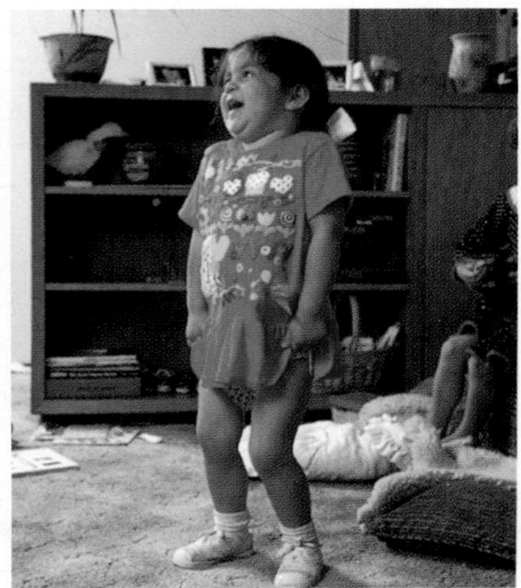

The "easy" child is generally moderate in activity; shows regularity in patterns of eating, sleeping, and elimination; and is usually positive in mood and when subjected to new stimuli. The easy child adapts to new situations and is able to accept rules and work well with others. About 40% of children in the New York Longitudinal Study displayed this personality type.

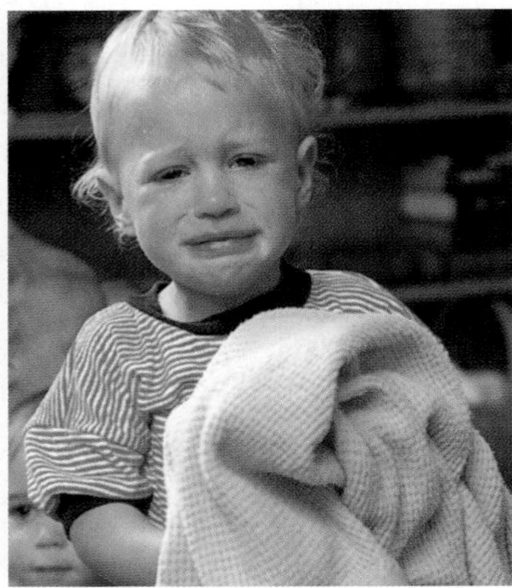

The "difficult" child displays irregular schedules for eating, sleeping, and elimination; adapts slowly to new situations and persons; and displays a predominantly negative mood. Intense reactions to the environment are common. About 10% of children in the New York Longitudinal Study displayed this personality type.

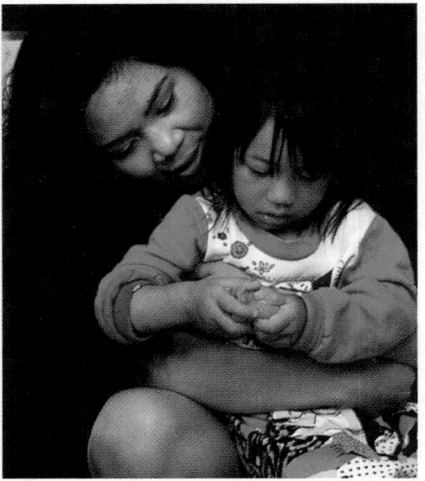

The "slow-to-warm-up" child has reactions of mild intensity and slow adaptability to new situations. The child displays initial withdrawal followed by gradual, quiet, and slow interaction with the environment. About 15% of children in the New York Longitudinal Study displayed this personality type.

The remaining 35% of children studied showed some characteristics of each personality type.

from the new school to play with the child at home, and asking the teacher to assign a special buddy to help out the new child.

Nursing Application

The concept of personality type or temperament is a useful one for nurses (Melvin, 1995). Nurses can assess the temperament of young children and alter the environment to meet their needs. This may involve moving a hospitalized child to a single room to ensure adequate rest if the child is easily stimulated, or allowing a shy child time to become accustomed to new surroundings and equipment before beginning procedures or treatments.

Parents are often relieved to learn about temperament characteristics. They learn to appreciate their children's qualities and to adapt the environment to meet the children's needs. A burden of guilt can also be lifted from parents who feel that they are responsible for their child's actions. The nurse can teach parents ways of enhancing goodness of fit between the child's personality and the environment (Table 5–5). See further suggestions for helping parents understand temperament during health promotion and health maintenance visits in Chapters 12 through 15∞.

Resiliency Theory

Theoretical Framework

Why do some children coming from similar backgrounds have such different behavioral outcomes? A theory that examines both the individual's characteristics and the interaction of these characteristics with the environment is the resiliency model. **Resilience** is the ability to function with healthy responses, even with significant stress and adversity (Stewart, Reid, & Mangham, 1997). In this model, the individual or family members experience a crisis that provides a source of stress, and the family interprets or deals with the crisis based on resources available. Families and individuals have **protective factors** that provide strength and assistance in dealing with crises, and **risk factors** that promote or contribute to their challenges. Risk and protective factors can be identified in children, in their families, and in their communities (see Chapter 7∞ for further description of the interplay of social and environmental factors with individual characteristics). A crisis for a young child might be a transfer to a new childcare provider. Protective factors could involve past positive experiences with new people, an "easy" tempera-

TABLE 5–5 Ways to Improve Goodness of Fit Between Parent and Child

CHILD'S BEHAVIOR	PARENT'S ACTIVITY
Extremely active	Plan periods of active play several times in day. Have restful periods before bedtime to foster sleep.
Shy	Allow time to adapt at own pace to new people and situations.
Easily stimulated	Have quiet room for sleeping as an infant. Have quiet room for homework for school-age child.
Short attention span	Provide projects that can be completed in a short period. Gradually encourage longer periods at activities.

TABLE 5–6 Components of Resiliency Model

COMPONENT	MEANING	EXAMPLE
A = Crisis Event or Health Challenge	Nature of health care challenge	Parent leaving home
V = Vulnerability; risk factors	Stresses and risks related to dealing with the health challenge	Prior abandonment; financial instability; child's developmental understanding of abandonment
T = Typology	Family methods of functioning	Reliance on extended family; parent alcoholism
B = Protective factors	Strengths for dealing with challenge	Child's desire to succeed in school; positive role modeling of maternal grandparents
C = Appraisal	Family's interpretation of crisis event	Abandonment by loved one; inability to trust others
PS = Problem-solving or coping techniques	Skills that help family work toward solution	Use of community resources; acceptance of school and community counselors; child's involvement in classroom activities
X = Response	Positive or negative response to tension created by the health challenge	Remaining parent using counseling available; child identifying with a teacher in school; establishment of sense of mutual interdependence among remaining family members

Data from Malone, J. A. (1998). The resiliency model of family stress, adjustment, and adaptation. In B. Vaughan-Cole, M. A. Johnson, J. A. Malone, & B. L. Walker, Family Nursing Practice. *Philadelphia: W.B. Saunders, pg 42. Adapted.*

ment, and awareness of the new childcare provider about adaptation needs of young children to new experiences. Risk factors for a similar child might be repeated moves to new care providers, limited close relationships with adults, and a "slow-to-warm-up" temperament.

Once confronted by a crisis, the child and family first experience the **adjustment phase,** characterized by disorganization and unsuccessful attempts at meeting the crisis. In the **adaptation phase,** the child and family meet the challenge and use resources to deal with the crisis (Malone, 1998). Adaptation may lead to increasing resilience as well when the child and family learn about new resources and inner strengths and develop the ability to deal more effectively with future crises. The model and examples are described in Table 5–6.

Nursing Application

Nurses gather information about the individual characteristics, prior life experiences, and environmental factors that act as protective and risk factors for children. Table 5–7 lists questions that can be helpful as the nurse gathers information from a child or family members. Nurses then use concepts of resiliency theory in planning interventions for children and families. Nursing strategies can target risk factors, such as encouraging family behaviors to ensure gun safety by teaching about use of gun trigger locks and locked gun cabinets in families with firearms. In addition, protective factors can be emphasized, such as encouraging holding and verbalization to parents of infants to provide an environment that meets needs for trust establishment and speech development.

INFLUENCES ON DEVELOPMENT

Family and Parenting

As we have seen, both nature and nurture are important in determining individual patterns of development. These two forces interact in distinctive ways in each individual, explaining differences in time frames for acquisition of developmental skills among children, personality variations between identical twins, and other unique characteristics of individuals. An environmental factor that is extremely important in the development of children is the profile of family characteristics. The family is an important component in the lives of all children, and plays an essential role in fostering the development of youth. A significant concept in families is that of parenting. How children are parented interacts with their individual characteristics to influence risk and protective factors, personality characteristics, and developmental outcomes. Chapter 2∞ discusses types of families, frameworks used to understand families, the roles of families in fostering the development of children, and types of parenting styles.

TABLE 5–7 Assessment Questions to Determine Resilience Capability

QUESTIONS TO DETERMINE RISK FACTORS

- Describe the event that occurred and what it has been like for your family.
- What other stressors do you have in your family right now?
- Are there financial worries?
- Are there things you think and worry about late at night?
- Describe your job, your friends.
- Describe your typical day.
- Describe your neighborhood.
- Do you have friends, people to call in emergencies?

QUESTIONS TO DETERMINE PROTECTIVE FACTORS

- What gives you strength?
- How do you deal with this stress?
- What do you think you do well in your family?
- Who do you call when you need help?
- Do you have a computer? Internet access?
- Are you religious? Spiritual?
- Do you exercise regularly?
- How do you spend free time?

MediaLink Resources for Families with Newborns or Infants

Culture

The traditional customs of the many cultural groups represented in North America influence the growth and development of the children in these groups. Genetic traits may predispose children for being at the upper or lower ranges of growth. Nutritional practices of various ethnic groups may influence the rate of growth for infants. Physical development is also influenced by genetic characteristics of ethnic groups (see Chapter 3∞). In addition, development may be influenced by child rearing practices. For example, the Native American practice of carrying infants on boards often delays walking when it is measured against the norm for walking on some developmental tests. These infants will begin walking later than other babies, but achieve other gross motor skills on schedule. Children who are carried by straddling the mother's hips or back for extended periods have a low incidence of developmental dysplasia of the hip, since the practice keeps their hips in an abducted position. There is no lasting delay in any milestone. The nurse needs to be aware of potential limitations of developmental tests when applied to various cultural groups.

While the sequence of cognitive and psychosocial development is the same for all children, the rates of acquiring new skills can vary. When the surrounding cultural group provides much stimulation, the child may achieve cognitive milestones at early ages. On the other hand, in cultures where self-exploration is valued, the child learns at a slower pace, but is more able to apply learning to new situations. In some cultures interactions are valued and the child is always with adults and other children; in other cultures independence is more valued and a child may be slower to develop cooperative psychosocial behaviors. What are the values of your cultural group and how have they influenced your development?

NEWBORN (UP TO 1 MONTH)

Physical Growth and Development and Prenatal Influences

Some Asian cultures calculate age from the time of conception. This practice acknowledges the profound influence of the prenatal period. The mother's nutrition and general state of health play a part in pregnancy outcome. Poor nutrition can lead to low-birth-weight infants and infants with compromised neurologic performance, slow development, or impaired immune status with resultant high disease rates. Low maternal stores of iron can result in anemia in the infant (Kleinman, 2004; UNICEF, 1998). Maternal smoking is associated with low-birth-weight infants. Ingestion of alcoholic beverages, including beer and wine, during pregnancy may lead to fetal alcohol syndrome (see Chapter 34∞ for further description of fetal alcohol syndrome). Illicit drug use by the mother may result in neonatal addiction, convulsions, hyperirritability, poor social responsiveness, and other neurologic disturbances (Children's Defense Fund, 2004).

Even prescription drugs may adversely affect the fetus. An example is the drug thalidomide, which was commonly used in Europe to treat nausea during the 1950s. This drug resulted in the birth of infants with limb abnormalities to women who used the drug during pregnancy. Other drugs can cause bleeding, stained teeth, impaired hearing, or other defects in the infant (Briggs, Freeman, & Yaffe, 2001). Some maternal illnesses are harmful to the developing fetus. An example is rubella (German measles), which is rarely a serious disease for adults but can cause deafness, vision defects, heart defects, and mental retardation in the fetus if it is acquired by a pregnant woman. A fetus can also acquire diseases, such as acquired immunodeficiency syndrome (AIDS) and human immunodeficiency virus (HIV) infection or hepatitis B from the mother. Paternal influence may be important as well. Either parent may have been exposed during war to Agent Orange, to toxins in the workplace, to stresses such as anxiety and violence, or to steroid or street drugs. Radiation, chemicals, and other environmental hazards may adversely affect a fetus when the parent is exposed to these influences. The best outcomes for infants occur when both parents have had minimal exposure to environmental toxins, have enjoyed general good health, and refrain from use of drugs, excessive alcohol, and tobacco. During pregnancy mothers should eat well, exercise regularly, seek early prenatal care, and refrain from harmful exposure to substances.

Babies are born with important physical characteristics, including a set of newborn reflexes (see Chapter 8∞ for their description) that help them receive input from the environment. The baby's sucking reflex provides food, physical contact with the mother, and a way to comfort the self. The grasp reflex creates a way to feel the world and its textures. The newborn takes in food through stimulation of the reflexes. This food enables the baby to grow and perform a gradually expanding array of motor skills. Developmental progression is monitored closely during the baby's first month of life, as the transition of all body systems to extrauterine life occurs.

Cognitive Development

Piaget's theory of cognitive development recognized the importance of the newborn reflexes in determining the newborn's cognitive development. Reflexes are not just a way to obtain food or maintain safety, but are the tools that help the newborn transition from the uterus to the external world. The baby uses reflexes and learns through them. Grasping opens the world to many objects that the baby will gradually learn to manipulate. When comfort needs are met, the baby learns from the experiences of eating and being clothed and held. The foundations of thought have been laid.

Psychosocial Development

Many people may believe that the newborn is incapable of anything but eating and sleeping. However, some observant researchers and care providers have noted that the newborn is particularly attuned to people in the environment, especially the parents. Relationships begin and will continue to develop throughout infancy. **Attachment** is a strong emotional bond between people and it can begin in the newborn period. When women hold their babies directly after birth, they tend to progress from touching them by fingertip, to full palm, and then enfolding them in hands and arms. Newborns are often alert after birth and follow the mother's face carefully with their eyes. This first interaction fosters attachment between the mother and baby. For many families, the process also involves attachment with the father, and sometimes siblings. The newborn learns quickly in the first month about safety and security, comfort when distressed, and food. These basic needs are associated with the primary caretakers and the infant forms a close attachment when needs are met; the foundations of trust are established. The baby who is fed by parents when hungry, held and comforted when in pain or distress, and played with several times daily learns that the parents and other caretakers can be trusted to meet basic needs. The infant learns how to trust, how to believe that people will provide care, and is free to move on to explore the environment more actively. Berry Brazelton, a pediatrician who has worked extensively with newborns and their parents, has shown that even in the first days of life infants can focus on the face of an adult, imitate behaviors such as smiling, frowning, or sticking out the tongue, and become totally engaged in the interaction with another person. The term *en face* is used to indicate the baby and adult gazing into each other's faces with their faces oriented in the same positions (Figure 5–4 ■). There are periods in the day when the baby's level of alertness supports the ability to focus on faces of caretakers, and learn positive aspects of the interpersonal relationship. Nurses support parents to recognize these times and use them to interact with the baby when possible (Figure 5–5 ■). See Table 5–8 for a description of infant states of alertness and suggested parental responses.

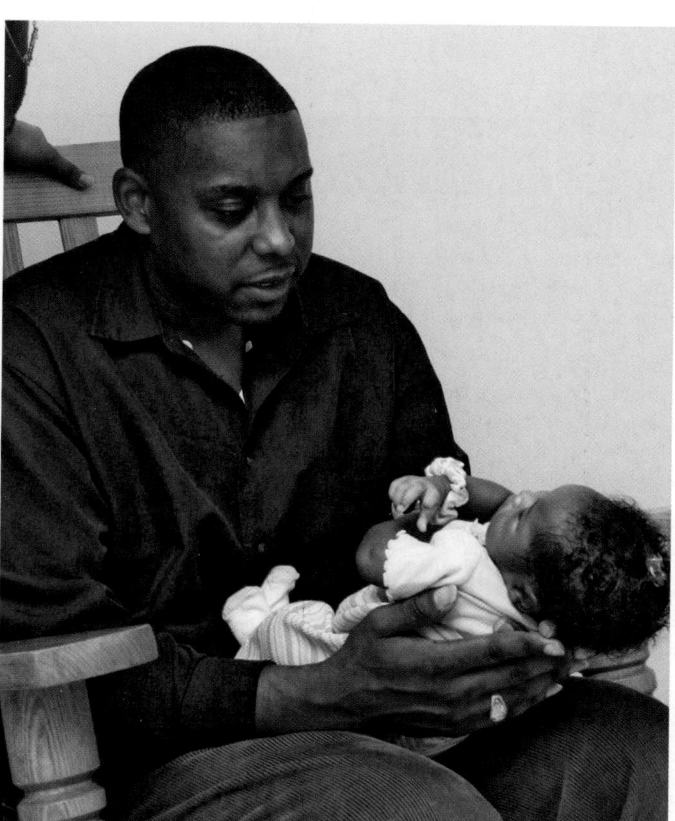

FIGURE 5–4 ■ Note that the parent and infant faces are in the same plane. This "en face" position enables both to examine each other's faces and establish eye contact, fostering attachment between parent and child.

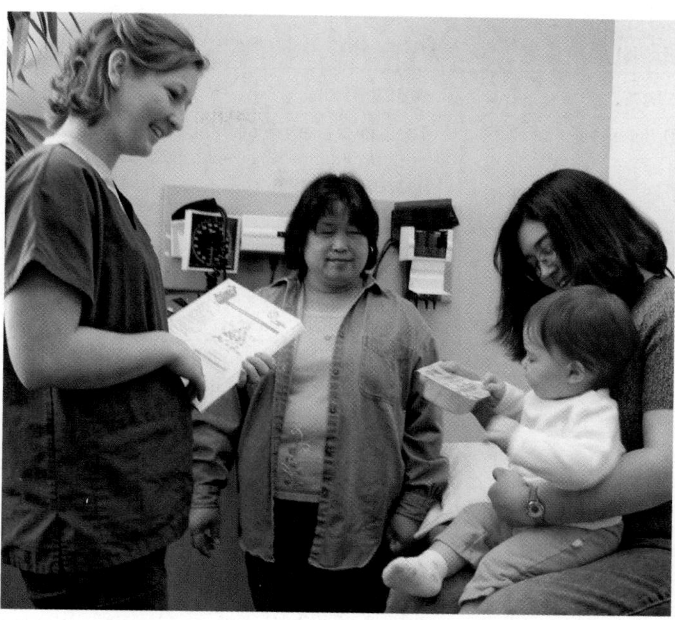

FIGURE 5–5 ■ Nurses in many settings with young children are applying the attachment facilitation techniques suggested by Dr. Berry Brazelton. Health professionals can teach parents to recognize the nonverbal cues of their infants and toddlers. The nurse can also model and positively reinforce the mother's interactions with her infant.

Nurses play an important role in helping new parents to learn about their babies' communication ability and responding appropriately. When there are risks, such as parents who are very young or have limited experience with babies, parents with mental health problems, or the birth of a premature newborn, parents may need ongoing help for a period of time to foster attachment with the child. Challenges for parents of a high-risk infant include:

- Guilt and grieving about the child's condition
- Worry upon hospital discharge about whether skills are present to be competent in care of the baby
- Concern about future development
- Constant adaptation to changes as the child grows and develops

Nursing interventions that can promote positive attachment with the high-risk infant include (Hummel, 2003):

- Encouraging frequent visits to the baby in the newborn care unit
- Promoting holding of the baby
- Providing for skin-to-skin contact of the baby and parent (Box 5–12)
- Pointing out baby's attributes and responses to voice or touch
- Involving parents in care of and decisions about the baby
- Advocating for healthcare agency policies that are supportive of attachment between infant and parents
- Giving information and repeating as needed; letting parents have a telephone number they can call at any time to get information about the baby or talk with a supportive person

See Evidence-Based Practice: Preterm Infants and Touch.

TABLE 5–8 Infant States of Alertness

STATE	DESCRIPTION	RECOMMENDED PARENTAL RESPONSES
Drowsiness or dozing	The baby's eyes are open or closed but there is not concentration on surroundings; the eyelids flutter, extremities move slowly and occasional startles occur. The baby either transitions to deeper sleep or wakefulness.	Parents can provide a quiet place for sleep or encourage wakefulness if that is desired.
Quiet alert	The baby is wide awake, follows objects, sounds, and faces; there is minimal motor movement. The infant is learning from the environment and will look away every few seconds and then look back at the face or object of interest.	Parents can talk with, sing to, assume the en face position, or provide objects for the baby to look at.
Active alert	The baby is very active with movements of extremities and head; responds to all stimuli with movement.	Parents may swaddle or quiet the infant if desired or allow the baby to move about, understanding that either crying or settling into quiet alert will likely occur next.
Crying	The baby cries and has movements of extremities.	Parents can look for reasons for the crying and intervene to provide comfort. The baby may be tired and need swaddling, hungry, having gastric distress, wet, or cold. Sometimes the source of crying is not known and an episode of crying, while annoying to parents, may continue to occur.

Note: Adapted from London, Ladewig, Ball, et al., (2003). Maternal-Newborn & child nursing. *Upper Saddle River, NJ: Prentice Hall Health.*

BOX 5–12 Kangaroo Care

"Kangaroo care" is used to describe skin-to-skin contact between infant and parent. This type of care developed in treatment of premature infants and involves clothing the baby in only a diaper and placing the infant against the skin of the parent's chest. The parent then wraps in warm clothes and holds the child close for several minutes daily. Premature infants having kangaroo care grow well, maintain temperature, and calm more easily. Parents usually feel close to the infant and appreciate the skin contact. Nurses have been instrumental in performing research on this technique and using it in hospitals and family homes.

INFANT (1 MONTH TO 1 YEAR)

Can you imagine tripling your present weight in a single year? Or becoming proficient in understanding fundamental words in a new language and even speaking a few? These and many more accomplishments take place in the first year of life. Starting the year as a mainly reflexive creature, the infant can walk and communicate by the year's end. Never again in life is development so swift (Figure 5–6 ■).

Physical Growth and Development

The first year of life is one of rapid change for the infant. The birth weight usually doubles by about 5 months and triples by the end of the first year (Figure 5–7 ■). Height increases by approximately 1 foot during this year. Teeth begin to erupt at about 6 months, and by the end of the first year the infant has six to eight deciduous teeth (see Chapter 8 for a full description of tooth eruption). Physical growth is closely associated with type and quality of feeding. See Chapter 9 for a discussion of nutrition in infancy.

Body organs and systems, although not fully mature at 1 year of age, function differently than they did at birth. Kidney and liver maturation helps the 1-year-old excrete drugs or other toxic substances more readily than in the first weeks of life. The changing body proportions mirror changes in developing internal organs. Maturation of the nervous system is demonstrated by increased control over body movements, enabling the infant to sit, stand,

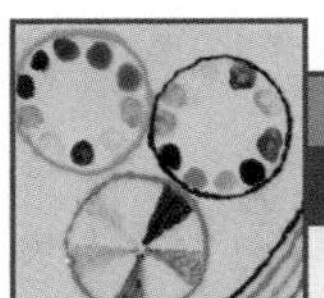

EVIDENCE-BASED PRACTICE
Preterm Infants and Touch

PROBLEM

Preterm infants are neurologically immature and therefore commonly more difficult to soothe and comfort. Their frequent crying may tire both the infant and the parents and interfere with attachment and bonding.

EVIDENCE

Researchers attempt to find ways to simulate the womb and to provide comforting touch and surroundings for preterm babies. Nurses have led the way in this research. In one study of 28 preterm infants from 25–36 weeks' gestation, infants were randomly placed in supine or prone positions for rest. When prone, infants had significantly less crying, less active sleep, more quiet sleep states, and fewer stress responses of startle, tremor, and twitch (Chang, Anderson, & Lin, 2002). Another technique to calm preterms has been use of skin-to-skin contact with parents or "kangaroo care." In a study of 34 mother-baby pairs, preterm infants with skin-to-skin contact were able to control temperature better and experienced more quiet sleep and less crying (Chwo, Anderson, Good, et al., 2002).

IMPLICATIONS

Nurses who care for preterm infants need to integrate knowledge of touch, positioning, and other modalities that provide neurologic comfort for babies.

CRITICAL THINKING APPLICATION

How will you integrate this information in the neonatal intensive care unit and with babies who have left the hospital and are at home with parents? How will your practice and the teaching you provide to parents be altered?

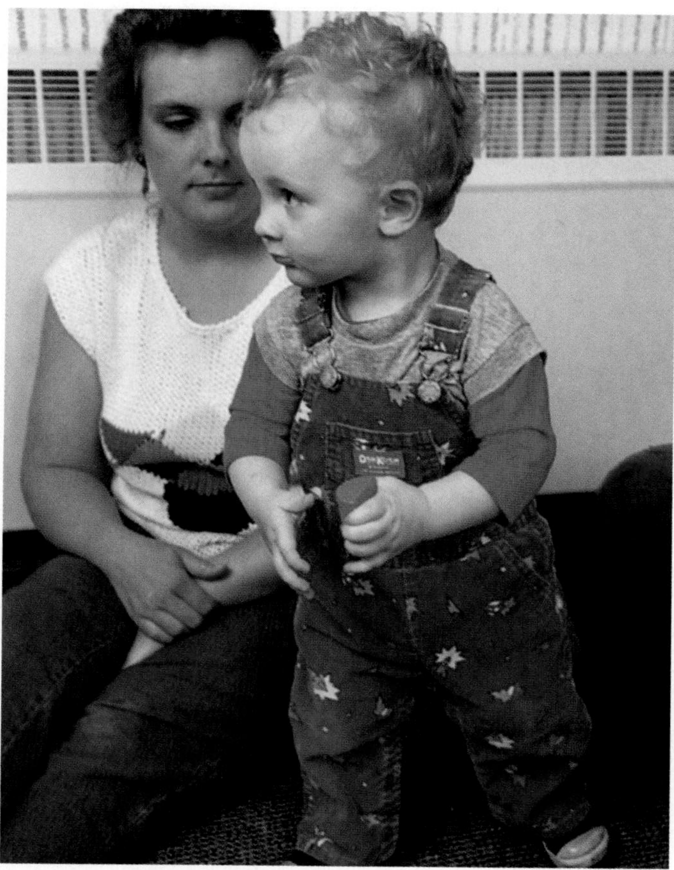

FIGURE 5–6 ■ A 12-month-old child will have tripled his birth weight, learned to walk, and will be beginning to talk.

and walk. Sensory function also increases as the infant begins to discriminate visual images, sounds, and tastes (Table 5–9).

Cognitive Development

The brain continues to increase in complexity during the first year. Most of the growth involves maturation of cells, with only a small increase in cell number. This growth of the brain is accompanied by development of its functions. One has only to compare the behavior of an infant shortly after birth with that of a 1-year-old to understand the incredible maturation of brain function. The newborn's eyes widen in response to sound; the 1-year-old turns to the sound and recognizes its significance. The 2-month-old cries and coos; the 1-year-old says a few words and understands many more. The 6-week-old grasps a rattle for the first time; the 1-year-old reaches for toys and self-feeds.

The infant's behaviors provide clues about thought processes. Piaget's work outlines the infant's actions in a set of rapidly progressing changes in the first year of life. The infant receives stimulation through sight, sound, and feeling, which the maturing brain interprets. This input from the environment interacts with internal cognitive abilities to enhance cognitive functioning.

Psychosocial Development

Play

An 8-month-old infant is sitting on the floor, grasping blocks and banging them on the floor. Infants spend much of their time engaging in **solitary play,** or playing by themselves. However, when a parent walks by, the infant laughs and waves hands and feet wildly, showing that periodic interactions with others are pleasureable (Figure 5–8 ■). Physical capabilities enable the infant to move toward and reach for objects of interest. Cognitive ability is reflected in manipulation of the blocks to create different sounds. Social interaction enhances play. The presence of a parent or other person increases interest in surroundings and teaches the infant different ways to play.

The play of infants begins in a reflexive manner. When infants move extremities or grasp objects, they experience the foundations of play. They gain pleasure from the feel and sound of these activities, and gradually perform them purposefully. For example, when a parent places a rattle in the hand of a 6-week-old infant, the infant grasps it reflexively. As the hands move randomly, the rattle makes an enjoyable sound. The infant learns to move the rattle to create the sound and then finally to grasp the toy at will to play with it.

The next phase of infant play focuses on manipulative behavior. The infant examines toys closely, looking at them, touching them, and placing them in the mouth. The infant learns a great

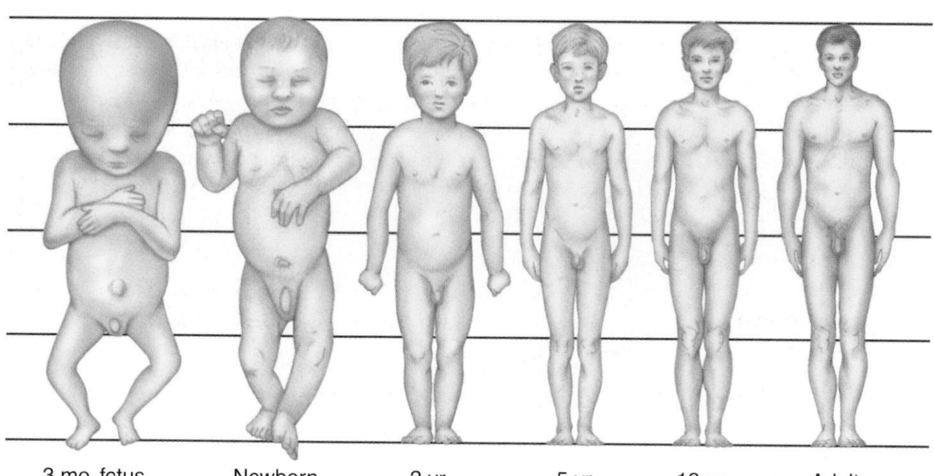

FIGURE 5–7 ■ Body proportions at various ages.

TABLE 5–9 Physical Growth and Development Milestones During Infancy

AGE	PHYSICAL GROWTH	FINE MOTOR ABILITY	GROSS MOTOR ABILITY	SENSORY ABILITY
Birth to 1 month	Gains 5–7 oz (140–200 g)/week Grows 1.5 cm (1/2 in.) in first month Head circumference increases 1.5 cm (1/2 in.)/month	Holds hand in fist **(1)** Draws arms and legs to body when crying	Inborn reflexes such as startle and rooting are predominant activity May lift head briefly if prone **(2)** Alerts to high-pitched voices Comforts with touch **(3)**	Prefers to look at faces and black-and-white geometric designs Follows objects in line of vision **(4)**

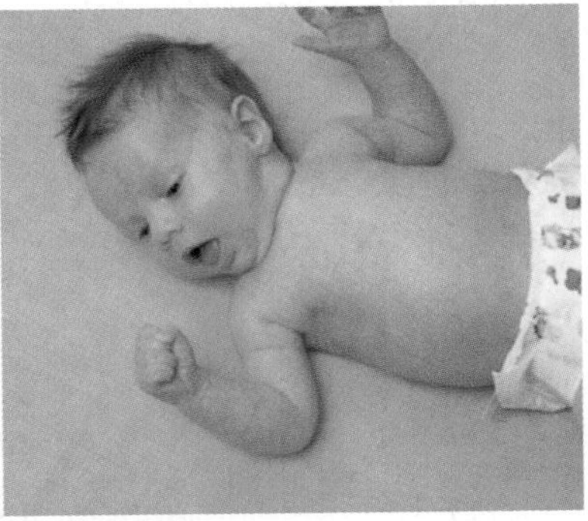

(1) Holds hand in fist

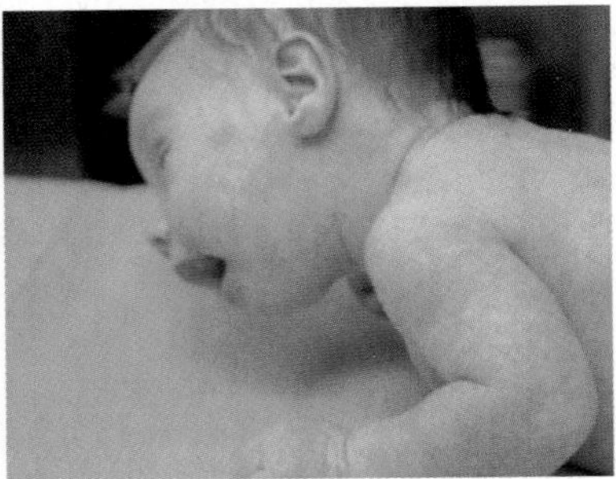

(2) May lift head

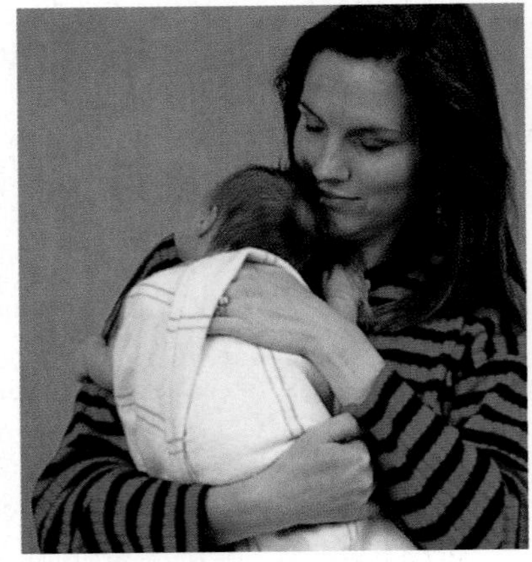

(3) Comforts with touch

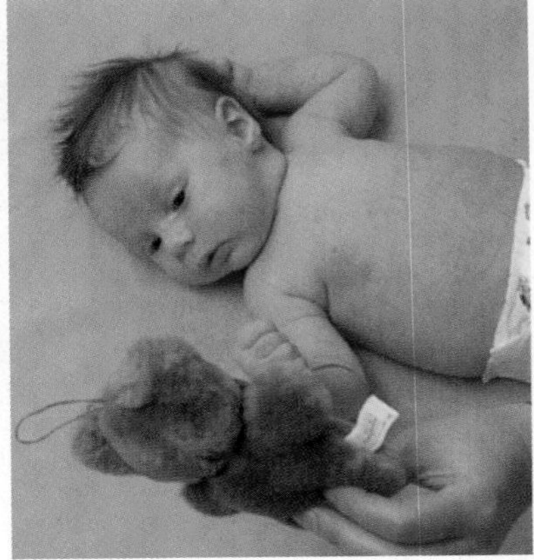

(4) Follows objects

AGE	PHYSICAL GROWTH	FINE MOTOR ABILITY	GROSS MOTOR ABILITY	SENSORY ABILITY
2–4 months	Gains 5–7 oz (140–200 g)/week Grows 1.5 cm (1/2 in.)/month Head circumference increases 1.5 cm (1/2 in.)/month Posterior fontanel closes Eats 120 mL/kg/24 hr (2 oz/lb/24 hr)	Holds rattle when placed in hand **(5)** Looks at and plays with own fingers Readily brings objects from hand to mouth	Moro reflex fading in strength Can turn from side to back and then return **(6)** Decrease in head lag when pulled to sitting; sits with head held in midline with some bobbing When prone, holds head and supports weight on forearms **(7)**	Follows objects 180 degrees Turns head to look for voices and sounds

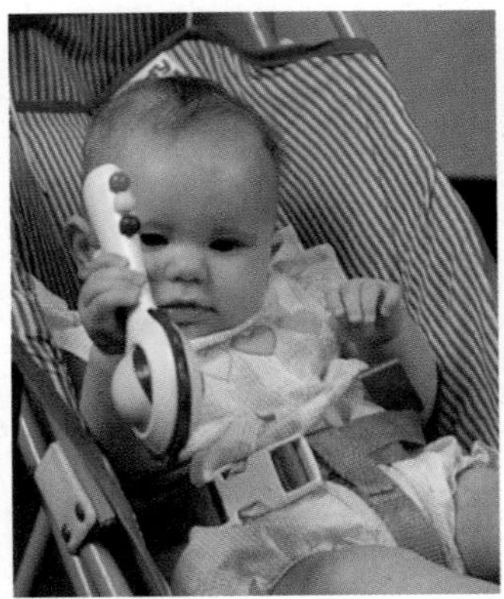

(5) Holds rattle

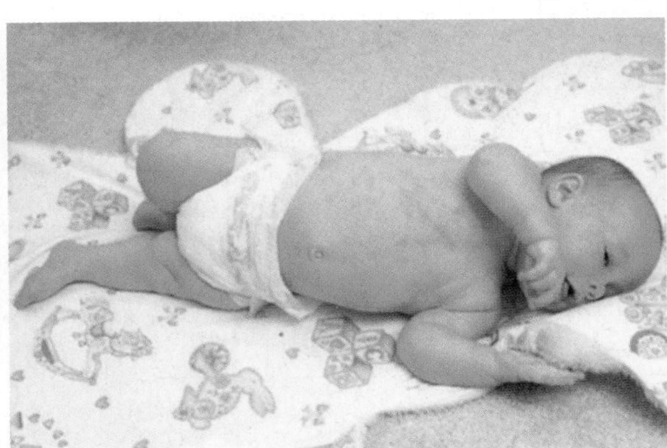

(6) Can turn from side to back

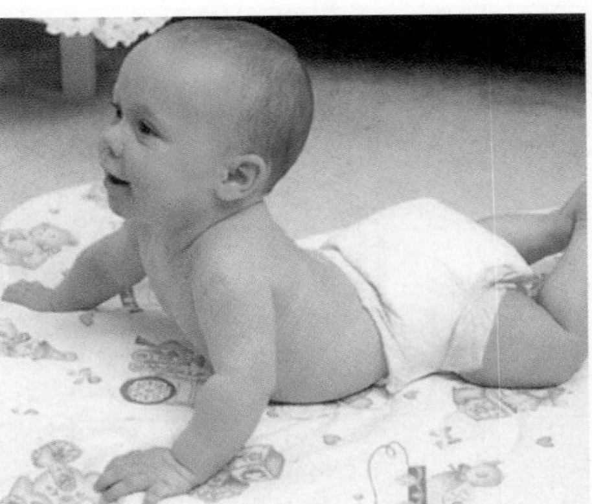

(7) Holds head up and supports weight with arms

TABLE 5–9 Physical Growth and Development Milestones During Infancy (continued)

AGE	PHYSICAL GROWTH	FINE MOTOR ABILITY	GROSS MOTOR ABILITY	SENSORY ABILITY
4–6 months	Gains 5–7 oz (140–200 g)/week Doubles birth weight 5–6 months Grows 1.5 cm (1/2 in.)/month Head circumference increases 1.5 cm (1/2 in.)/month Teeth may begin erupting by 6 months Eats 100 mL/kg/24 hr (1 1/2 oz/lb/24 hr)	Grasps rattles and other objects at will; drops them to pick up another offered object **(8)** Mouths objects Holds feet and pulls to mouth Holds bottle Grasps with whole hand (palmar grasp) Manipulates objects **(9)**	Head held steady when sitting No head lag when pulled to sitting Turns from abdomen to back by 4 months and then back to abdomen by 6 months When held standing supports much of own weight **(10)**	Examines complex visual images Watches the course of a falling object Responds readily to sounds

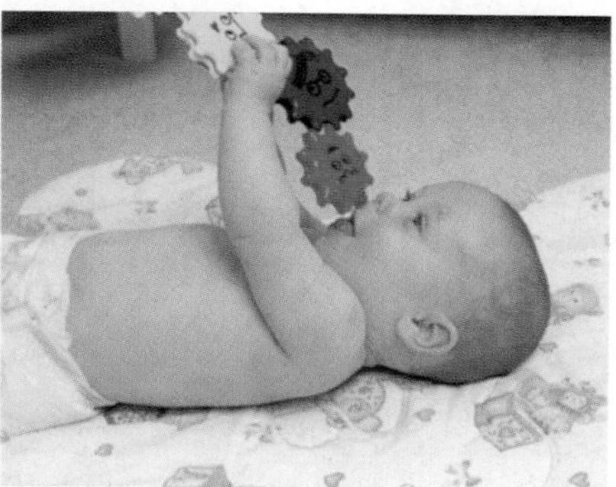

(8) Grasps objects at will

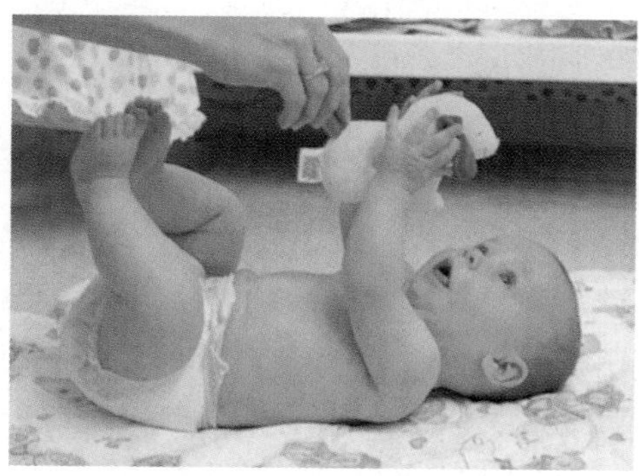

(9) Manipulates objects

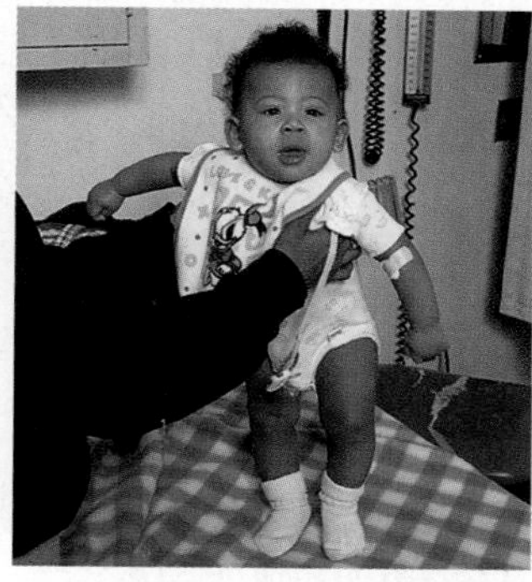

(10) Supports most of weight when held standing

AGE	PHYSICAL GROWTH	FINE MOTOR ABILITY	GROSS MOTOR ABILITY	SENSORY ABILITY
6–8 months	Gains 3–5 oz (85–140 g)/week Grows 1 cm (3/8 in.)/month Growth rate slower than first 6 months	Bangs objects held in hands Transfers objects from one hand to the other Beginning pincer grasp at times	Most inborn reflexes extinguished Sits alone steadily without support by 8 months **(11)** Likes to bounce on legs when held in standing position	Recognizes own name and responds by looking and smiling Enjoys small and complex objects at play

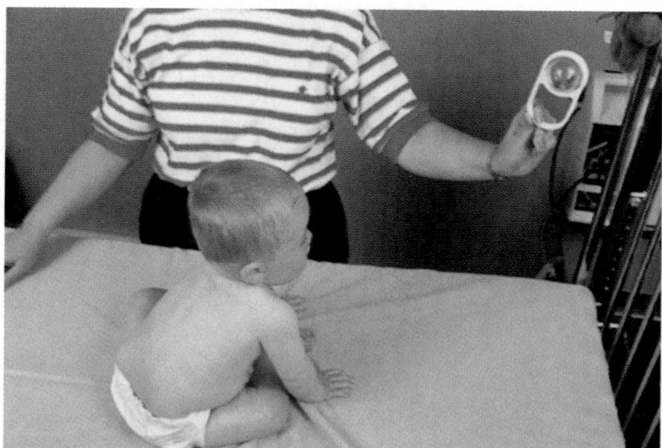

(11) Sits alone without support

(continued)

TABLE 5–9 Physical Growth and Development Milestones During Infancy (continued)

AGE	PHYSICAL GROWTH	FINE MOTOR ABILITY	GROSS MOTOR ABILITY	SENSORY ABILITY
8–10 months	Gains 3–5 oz (85–140 g)/week Grows 1 cm (3/8 in.)/month	Picks up small objects **(12)** Uses pincer grasp well **(14)**	Crawls or pulls whole body along floor by arms **(13)** Creeps by using hands and knees to keep trunk off floor Pulls self to standing and sitting by 10 months Recovers balance when sitting	Understands words such as "no" and "cracker" May say one word in addition to "mama" and "dada" Recognizes sound without difficulty
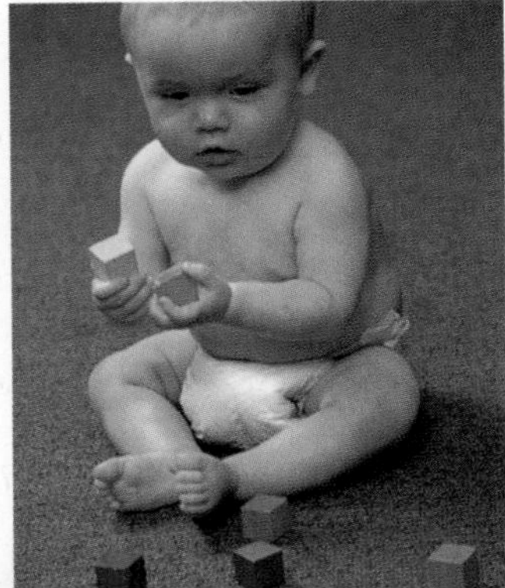 **(12)** Picks up small objects		 **(13)** Crawls or pulls body by arms		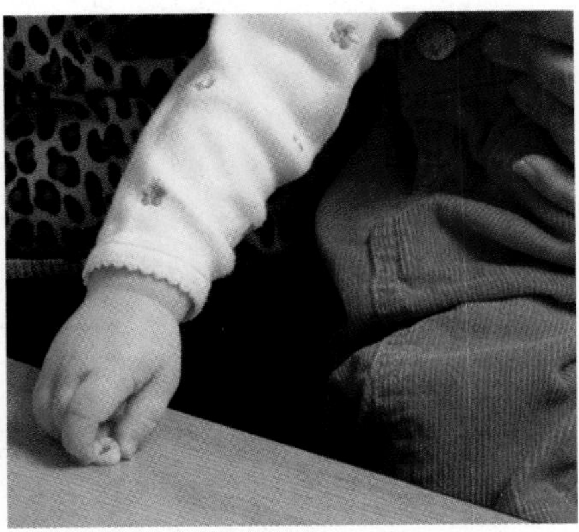 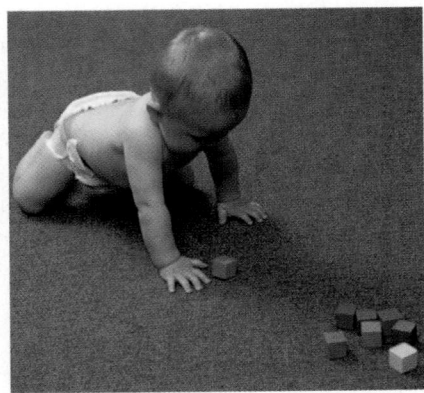 **(14)** Uses pincer grasp well
10–12 months	Gains 3–5 oz (85–140 g)/week Grows 1 cm (3/8 in.)/month Head circumference equals chest circumference Triples birth weight by 1 year	May hold crayon or pencil and make mark on paper Places objects into containers through holes **(15)**	Stands alone **(16)** Walks holding onto furniture Sits down from standing **(17)**	Plays peek-a-boo and patty cake
 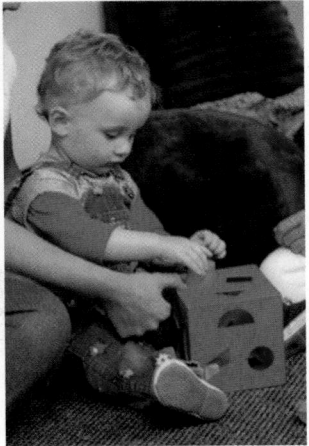 **(15)** Places objects in container through holes		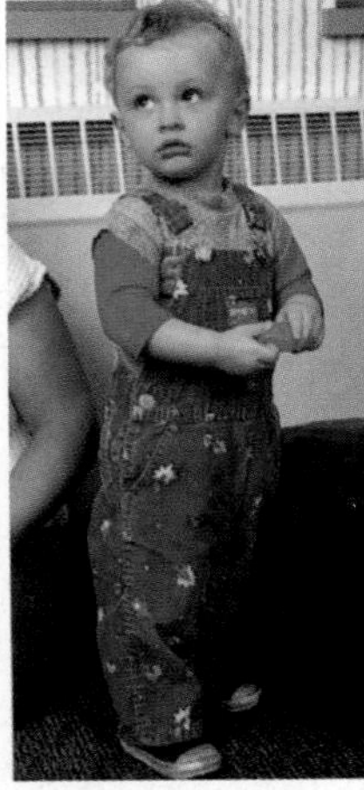 **(16)** Stands alone		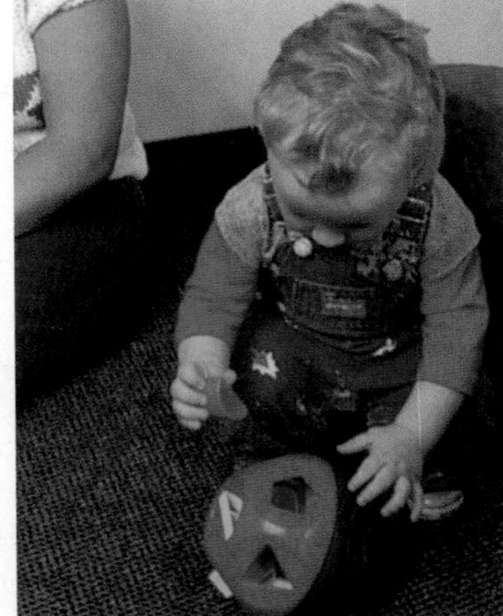 **(17)** Sits down from standing

deal about texture, qualities of objects, and all aspects of the surroundings. At the same time, interaction with others becomes an important part of play. The social nature of play is obvious as the infant plays with other children and adults.

Toward the end of the first year, the infant's ability to move in space enlarges the sphere of play. Once infants crawl or walk, they can get to new places, find new toys, discover forgotten objects, or seek out other people for interaction. Play is a reflection of every aspect of development, fostering psychosocial skills and enhancing learning and maturation (see Table 5–9).

Personality and Temperament

Why does one infant frequently awaken at night crying while another sleeps for 8 to 10 hours undisturbed? Why does one infant smile much of the time and react positively to interactions while another is withdrawn around unfamiliar people and fre-

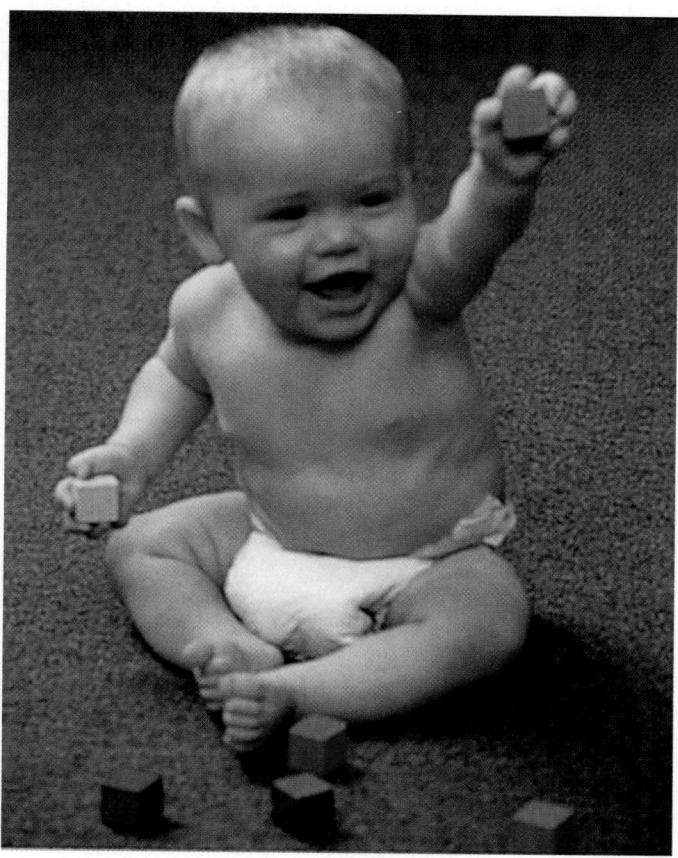

FIGURE 5–8 ■ Garrett shows us that an 8-month-old child can play with blocks, demonstrating physical, cognitive, and social capabilities.

quently frowns and cries? Such differences in responses to the environment are believed to be inborn characteristics of temperament. Infants are born with a tendency to react in certain ways to noise and to interact differently with people. They may display varying degrees of regularity in activities such as eating and sleeping, and manifest a capacity for concentrating on tasks for different amounts of time.

Nursing assessment identifies personality characteristics of the infant that the nurse can share with the parents. With this information, the parents can appreciate more fully the uniqueness of their infant and design experiences to meet the infant's needs. Parents can learn to modify the environment to promote adaptation. For example, an infant who does not adapt easily to new situations may cry, withdraw, or develop another way of coping when adjusting to new people or places. Parents might be advised to use one or two babysitters rather than engaging new sitters frequently. If the infant is easily distracted when eating, parents can feed the infant in a quiet setting to encourage a focus on eating. Although the infant's temperament is unchanged, the ability to fit with the environment is enhanced. See Chapter 12∞ for further ideas about how nurses apply information on infant temperament to health promotion and health maintenance visits.

Communication

Even at a few weeks of age, infants communicate and engage in two-way interaction, and express comfort by soft sounds, cuddling, and eye contact. Newborns respond best to a high-pitched voice, something that most parents inherently seem to know. Even fathers raise their voice to a higher pitch when talking with a young infant. The infant displays discomfort by thrashing the extremities, arching the back, and crying vigorously. From these rudimentary skills, communication ability continues to develop until the infant speaks several words at the end of the first year of life (Table 5–10).

Nurses assess communication to identify possible abnormalities or developmental delays. Language ability may be assessed with the Denver II Developmental Test and other specialized language screening tools (see Chapter 10∞). Normal infants and toddlers understand (**receptive speech**) more words than they can speak (**expressive speech**). Abnormalities may be caused by a hearing deficit, developmental delay, or lack of verbal stimulation from caretakers. Further assessment may be required to pinpoint the cause of the abnormality.

Nursing interventions focus on providing a stimulating and loving environment. Parents are encouraged to speak and sing to infants frequently and teach words. Descriptive verbalizations encourage the infant's speech. For example, when a 1-year-old says "bottle," the parent can say, "Oh you want your warm bottle of milk now? This is your blue bottle." Hospital nurses should include the infant's known words when providing care, and talk to infants using comforting and descriptive terminology. Security is communicated when care providers hold the infant for feedings, cuddle and play gently often during the day, and swaddle and hold the young infant securely during crying episodes. Parents may enjoy receiving information about how to swaddle the infant or perform infant massage. (See Complementary Therapy: Infant Massage below.)

TODDLER (1 TO 3 YEARS)

Toddlerhood is sometimes called the first adolescence. An infant only months before, the child from 1 to 3 years is now displaying independence and negativism. Pride in newfound accomplishments emerges.

Physical Growth and Development

The rate of growth slows during the second year of life. Parents may become concerned because the child has a limited intake and may need reassurance that this is normal. See Chapter 9∞

COMPLEMENTARY THERAPY

Infant Massage

Infant massage is a technique for communicating with and soothing infants that has been used in many cultures throughout history, but is not traditional within most families in the United States and Canada. It has many benefits both for infants and parents and can be taught to families who are interested. Some of the benefits for babies include improved sleep, soothability, and decreased stress hormones. Premature infants have been shown to have enhanced growth and motor ability (Field, 2002; Mainous, 2003). Massage periods of 10–15 minutes daily can be encouraged and facilitated. Such episodes will enhance bonding and attachment between parents and infant.

TABLE 5–10 Psychosocial Development During Infancy

AGE	PLAY AND TOYS	COMMUNICATION
Birth–3 months  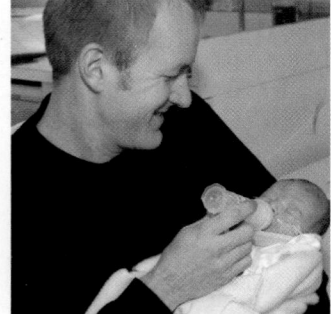	Prefers visual stimuli of mobiles, black-and-white patterns, mirrors Auditory stimuli are music boxes, tape players, soft voices Responds to rocking and cuddling Moves legs and arms while adult sings and talks Likes varying stimuli—different rooms, sounds, visual images	Coos Babbles Cries
3–6 months	Prefers noise-making objects that are easily grasped like rattles Enjoys stuffed animals and soft toys with contrasting colors	Vocalizes during play and with familiar people Laughs Cries less Squeals and makes pleasure sounds Babbles multisyllabically (mamamamama)
6–9 months	Likes teething toys Increasingly desires social interaction with adults and other children Soft toys that can be manipulated and mouthed are favorites	Increases vowel and consonant sounds Links syllables together Uses speechlike rhythm when vocalizing with others
9–12 months	Enjoys large blocks, toys that pop apart and go back together, nesting cups and other objects Laughs at surprise toys like jack-in-the-box Plays interactive games like peek-a-boo Uses push-and-pull toys	Understands "no" and other simple commands Says "dada" and "mama" to identify parents Learns one or two other words Receptive speech surpasses expressive speech

for further discussion of nutrition in toddlerhood. By age 2 years, the birth weight has usually quadrupled and the child is about one half of the adult height. Body proportions begin to change, with legs longer and head smaller in proportion to body size than during infancy (see Figure 5–7). The toddler has a potbellied appearance and stands with feet apart to provide a wide base of support. By approximately 33 months, eruption of deciduous teeth is complete, with 20 teeth present.

Gross motor activity develops rapidly (Table 5–11), as the toddler progresses from walking to running, kicking, and riding a tricycle (Figure 5–9 ■). As physical maturation occurs, the toddler develops the ability to control elimination patterns. See Chapter 13∞ for a discussion of the nurse's role in assisting parents in the process of toilet training toddlers, and Developing Cultural Competence: Toilet Training below.

DEVELOPING CULTURAL COMPETENCE
Toilet Training

In traditional Native American families, children are allowed to unfold and develop naturally at their own pace. Children thus wean and toilet train themselves with little interference or pressure from parents. Nurses should honor the beliefs and practices of families rather than suggesting that one approach, for example, that a single age for toilet training is right for all families and situations.

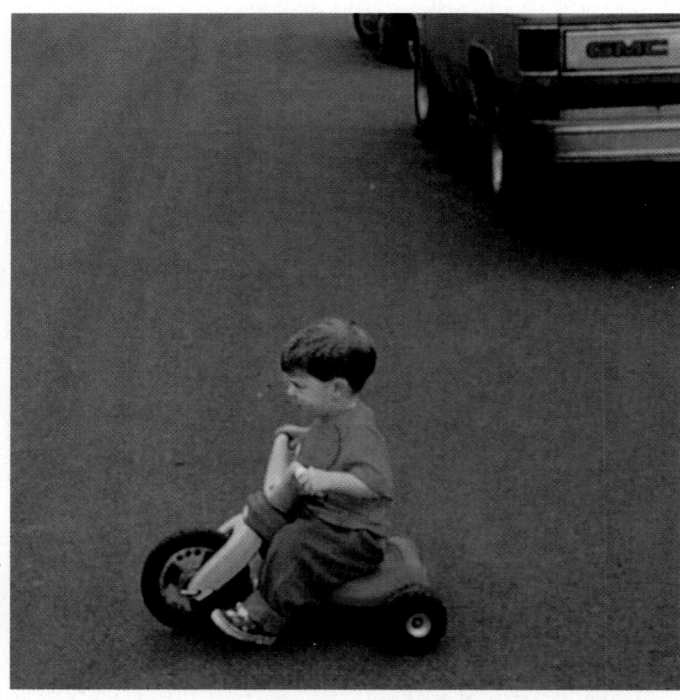

FIGURE 5–9 ■ This toddler has learned to ride a Big Wheel, which he is doing right into the street. Toddlers must be closely watched to prevent injury.

TABLE 5–11 Physical Growth and Development Milestones During Toddlerhood

AGE	PHYSICAL GROWTH	FINE MOTOR ABILITY	GROSS MOTOR ABILITY	SENSORY ABILITY
1–2 years	Gains 8 oz (227 g) or more per month Grows 3.5–5 in. (9–12 cm) during this year Anterior fontanel closes	By end of 2nd year, builds a tower of four blocks **(1)** Scribbles on paper **(2)** Can undress self **(3)** Throws a ball	Runs Walks up and down stairs **(5)** Likes push and pull toys	Visual acuity 20/50
2–3 years	Gains 1.4–2.3 kg (3–5 lb)/year Grows 5–6.5 cm (2–2.5 in.)/year	Draws a circle and other rudimentary forms Learns to pour Learning to dress self **(4)**	Jumps Kicks ball Throws ball overhand	

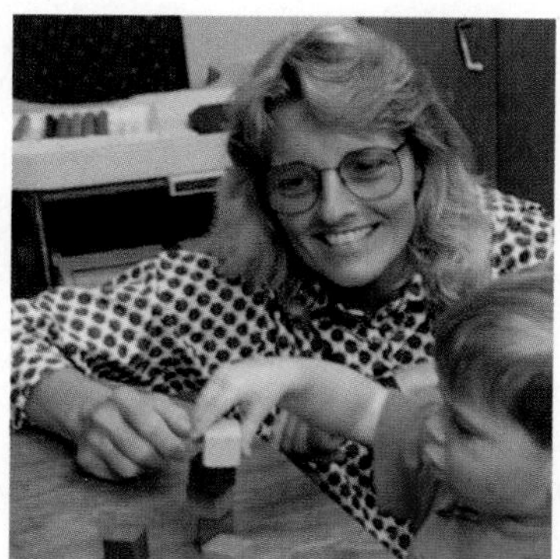

(1) Tower of four blocks

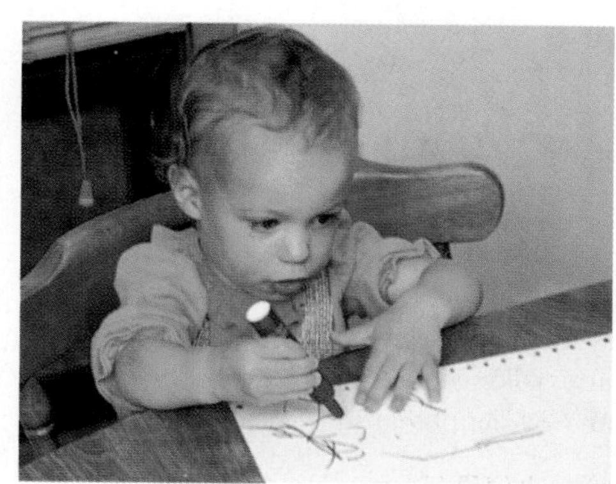

(2) Scribbles on paper

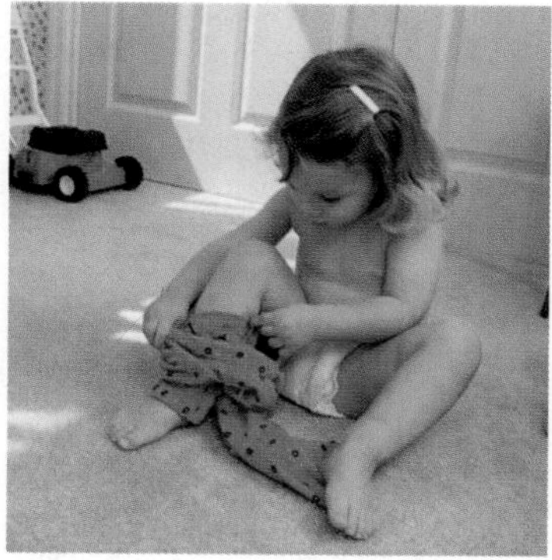

(3) Can undress self

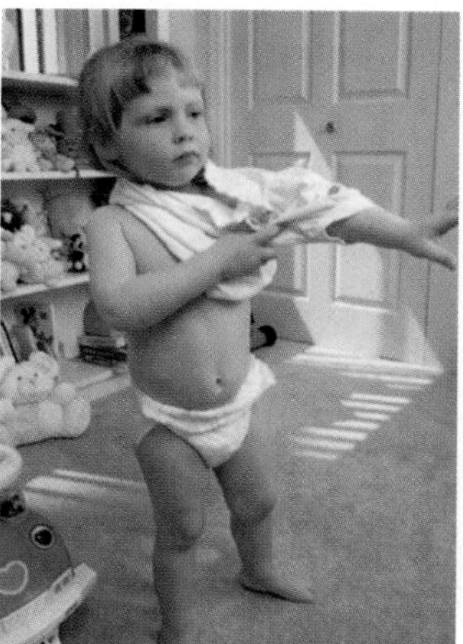

(4) Learning to dress self

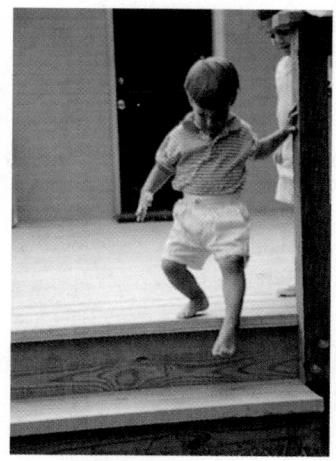

(5) Walks up and down stairs

Cognitive Development

During the toddler years, the child moves from the sensorimotor to the preoperational stage of development. The early use of language awakens in the 1-year-old the ability to think about objects or people when they are absent. Object permanence is well developed.

At about 2 years of age, the increasing use of words as symbols enables the toddler to use preoperational thought. Rudimentary problem solving, creative thought, and an understanding of cause-and-effect relationships are now possible.

Psychosocial Development

Play

Many changes in play patterns occur between infancy and toddlerhood. The toddler's motor skills enable him or her to bang pegs into a pounding board with a hammer. The social nature of toddler play is also readily seen. Toddlers find the company of other children pleasurable, even though socially interactive play may not occur. Two toddlers tend to play with similar objects side by side, occasionally trading toys and words. This is called **parallel play.** This playtime with other children assists toddlers to develop

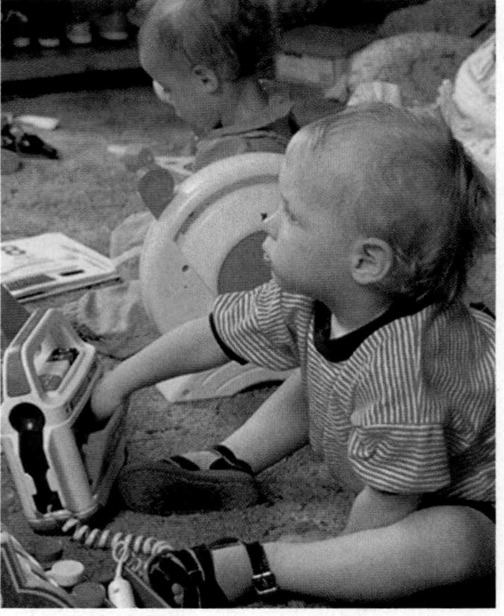

A

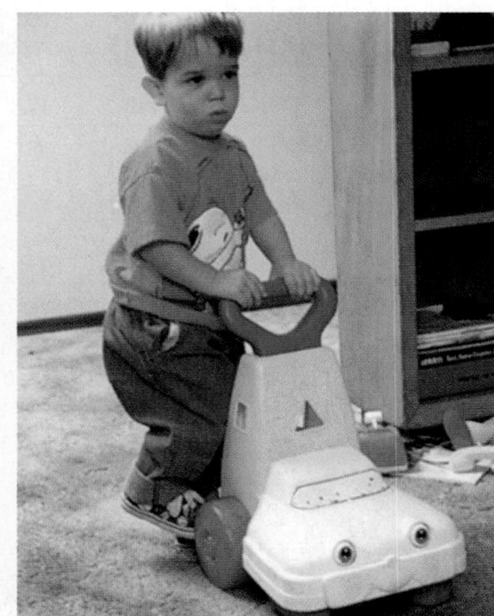

B

FIGURE 5–10 ■ *A,* Two children are displaying typical parallel play since they enjoy playing near other children, but are not engaging in social interactions with each other. Which cognitive and motor skills are these children developing? *B,* Imitative play such as pushing and pulling a vacuum allows this toddler to develop gross and fine motor skills.

social skills. Toddlers engage in play activities they have seen at home, such as pounding with a hammer and talking on the phone. This imitative behavior teaches them new actions and skills (Figure 5–10 ■).

Physical skills are manifested in play as toddlers push and pull objects, climb in and out and up and down, run, ride a Big Wheel, turn the pages of books, and scribble with a pen. Both gross motor and fine motor abilities are enhanced during this age period.

Cognitive understanding enables the toddler to manipulate objects and learn about their qualities. Stacking blocks and placing rings on a building tower teach spatial relationships and other lessons that provide a foundation for future learning. Various kinds of play objects should be provided for the toddler to meet play needs. These play needs can easily be met whether the child is hospitalized or at home (Table 5–12).

Personality and Temperament

The toddler retains most of the temperamental characteristics identified during infancy, but may demonstrate some changes. The normal developmental progression of toddlerhood also plays a part in responses. For example, the infant who previously responded positively to stimuli, such as a new babysitter, may appear more negative in toddlerhood. The increasing independence characteristic of this age is shown by the toddler's use of the word *no*. The parent and child constantly adapt their responses to each other and learn anew how to communicate with each other.

Communication

Because of the phenomenal growth of language skills during the toddler period, adults should communicate frequently with children in this age group. Toddlers imitate words and speech intonations, as well as the social interactions they observe.

At the beginning of toddlerhood, the child may use four to six words in addition to "mama" and "dada." Receptive speech (the ability to understand words) far outpaces expressive speech. By the end of toddlerhood, however, the 3-year-old has a vocabulary of almost 1,000 words and uses short sentences.

Communication occurs in many ways, some of which are nonverbal. Toddler communication includes pointing, pulling an adult over to a room or object, and speaking in **expressive**

TABLE 5–12 Psychosocial Development During Toddlerhood

AGE	PLAY AND TOYS	COMMUNICATION
1–3 years 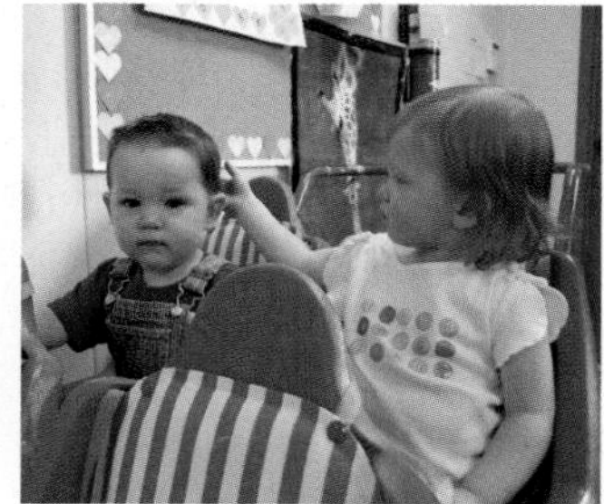	Refines fine motor skills by use of cloth books, large pencil and paper, wooden puzzles Facilitates imitative behavior by playing kitchen, grocery shopping, toy telephone Learns gross motor activities by riding Big Wheel tricycle, playing with soft ball and bat, molding water and sand, tossing ball or bean bag Cognitive skills develop by educational television shows, music, stories and books	Increasingly enjoys talking Exponential growth of vocabulary especially when spoken and read to Needs to release stress by pounding board, frequent gross motor activities, and occasional temper tantrums Likes contact with other children and learns interpersonal skills

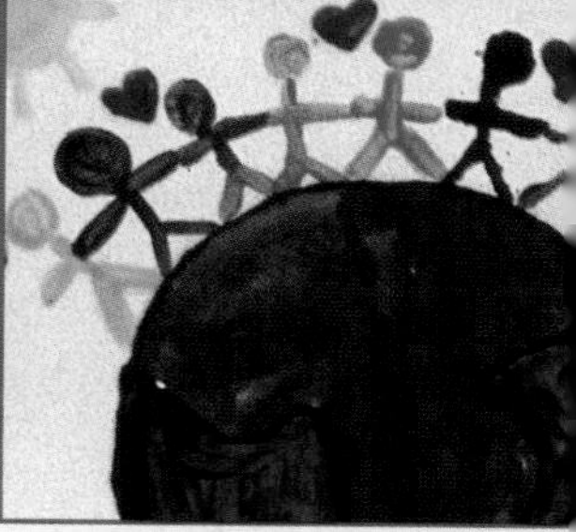

PARTNERING WITH FAMILIES

Communicating with a Toddler

Procedures such as drawing blood, getting immunizations, or even having ears checked can be frightening for a toddler. Parents and nurses can partner to provide effective communication that minimizes the trauma caused by such procedures.

- Avoid telling toddlers about the procedure too far in advance. They do not have an understanding of time and can become quite anxious. Telling them just before the procedure begins is most appropriate.
- Use simple terminology: "We need to get a little blood from your arm. It will help us to find out if you are getting better." If the parent is willing, say, "Your Mom will hold your arm still so we can do it quickly." Approach positively and confidently.
- Give short, clear instructions. Do not give choices if none exist. Offer a choice of two alternatives when possible. "Would you like apple or grape juice after you drink this medicine?"
- Tell the toddler what you are doing; name objects.
- Allow the toddler to cry. Acknowledge that it must be frightening and that you understand. Encourage parents to allow the child to cry out during a procedure or other frightening event.
- If in a hospital, perform the procedure in a treatment room so that the toddler's bed and room are a safe haven.
- Be sure the toddler is restrained, with the joints above and below the procedure immobilized so the procedure can be quickly accomplished with the least trauma.
- Use a Band-Aid to cover the site and to reassure the toddler that the body is still intact.
- Allow the toddler to choose a reward such as a sticker after the procedure.
- Praise the toddler for cooperation and acknowledge that you know this was difficult.
- Comfort the toddler by rocking, offering a favorite drink, playing music, and holding. If parents are present, they can offer the comfort needed.

jargon (using unintelligible words with normal speech intonations as if truly communicating in words). Another communication method occurs when the toddler cries, pounds feet, displays a temper tantrum, or uses other means to illustrate dismay. These powerful communication methods can upset parents, who often need suggestions for handling them. It is best to verbalize the feelings shown by the toddler, for example, by saying, "You must be very upset that you cannot have that candy. When you stop crying you can come out of your room," and then to ignore further negative behavior. The toddler's search for autonomy and independence creates a need for such behavior. Sometimes an upset toddler responds well to holding, rocking, and stroking.

Parents and nurses can promote a toddler's communication by speaking frequently, naming objects, explaining procedures in simple terms, expressing feelings that the toddler seems to be displaying, and encouraging speech. The toddler from a bilingual home is at an optimal age to learn two languages. If the parents do not speak English, the toddler will benefit from a childcare experience because both languages can then be learned. See Partnering with Families: Communicating with a Toddler.

The nurse who understands the communication skills of toddlers is able to assess expressive and receptive language and communicate effectively, thereby promoting positive healthcare experiences for these children.

PRESCHOOL CHILD (3 TO 6 YEARS)

The preschool years are a time of new initiative and independence. Most children are in a childcare center or school for part of the day and learn a great deal from this social contact. Language skills are well developed, and the child is able to understand and speak clearly. Endless projects characterize the world of busy preschoolers. They may work with play dough to form animals, then cut out and paste paper, then draw and color (Figure 5–11 ■).

Physical Growth and Development

Preschoolers grow slowly and steadily, with most growth taking place in long bones of the arms and legs. The short, chubby toddler gradually gives way to a slender, long-legged preschooler (Table 5–13).

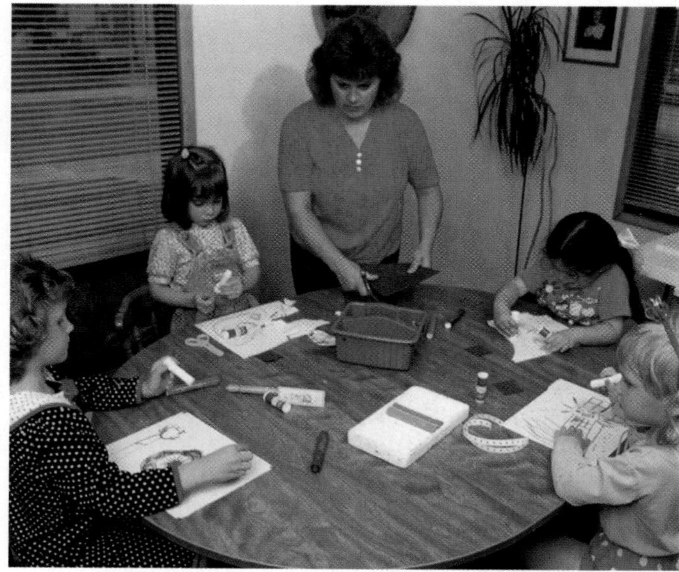

FIGURE 5–11 ■ Preschoolers have well-developed language, motor, and social skills, and they can work creatively together on an art project, as this group is doing at an in-home childcare center.

TABLE 5–13 Physical Growth and Development Milestones During the Preschool Years

PHYSICAL GROWTH	FINE MOTOR ABILITY	GROSS MOTOR ABILITY	SENSORY ABILITY
Gains 1.5–2/5 kg (3–5 lb)/year Grows 4–6 cm (1 1/2–2 1/2 in.)/year	Uses scissors **(1)** Draws circle, square, cross **(2)** Draws at least a six-part person Enjoys art projects such as pasting, stringing beads, using clay Learns to tie shoes at end of preschool years **(3)** Buttons **(4)** Brushes teeth **(5)**	Throws a ball overhand Climbs well **(6)** Rides tricycle **(7)**	Visual acuity continues to improve Can focus on and learn letters and numbers **(8)**

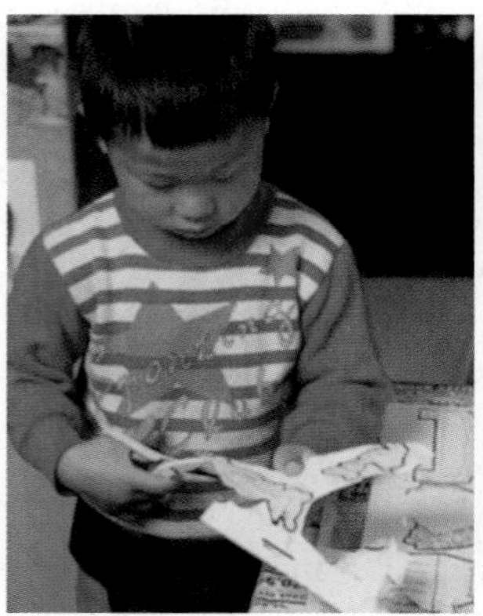
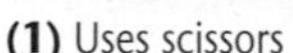

(1) Uses scissors

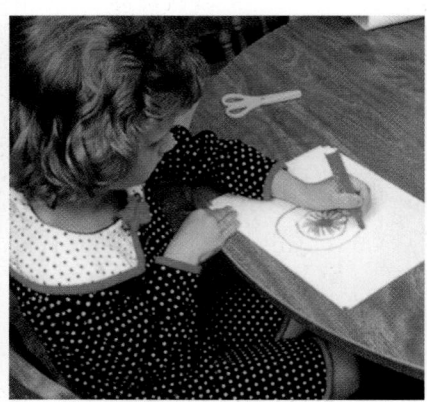

(2) Draws circle, square, cross

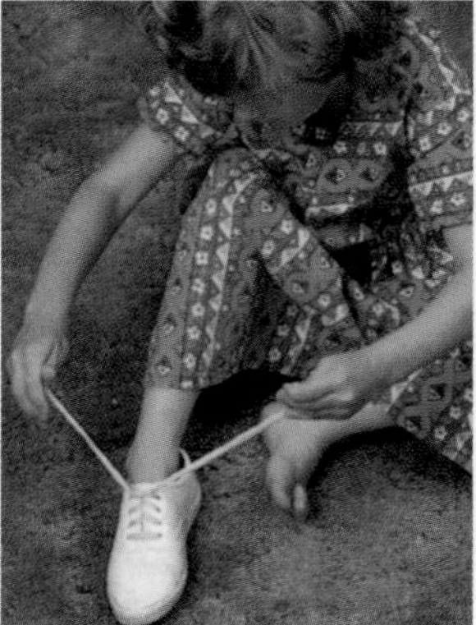

(3) Ties shoes

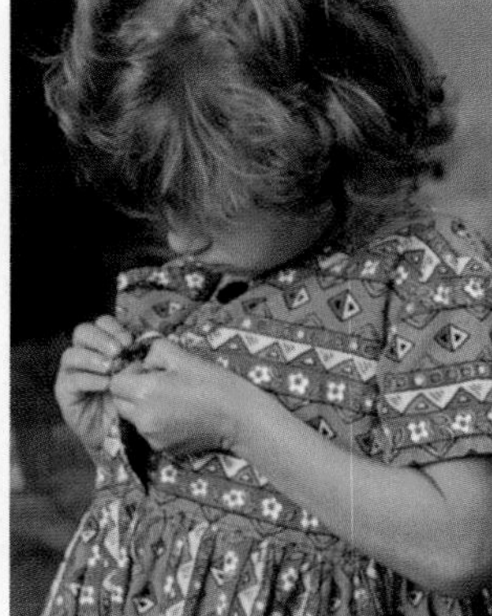

(4) Buttons clothes

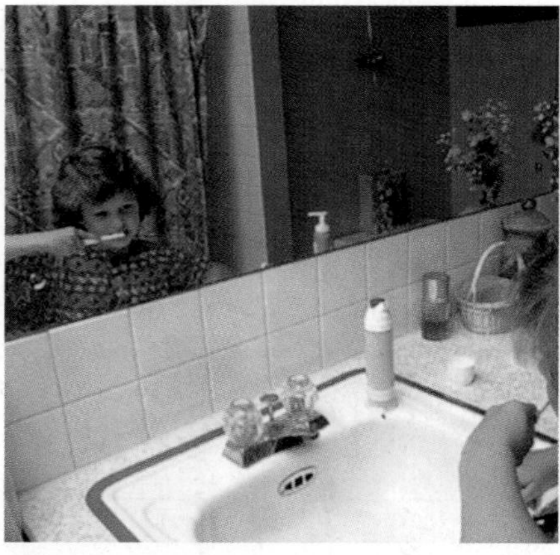

(5) Brushes teeth

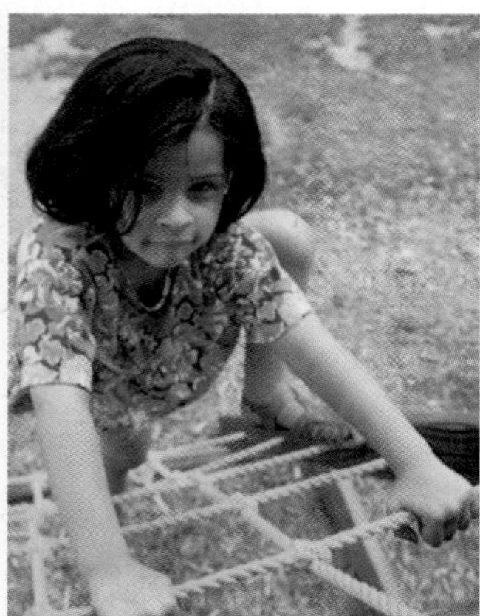

(6) Climbs well

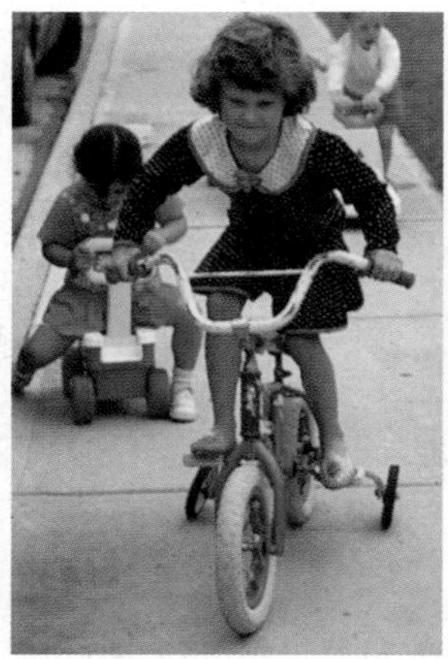

(7) Rides bicycle or bicycle with training wheels

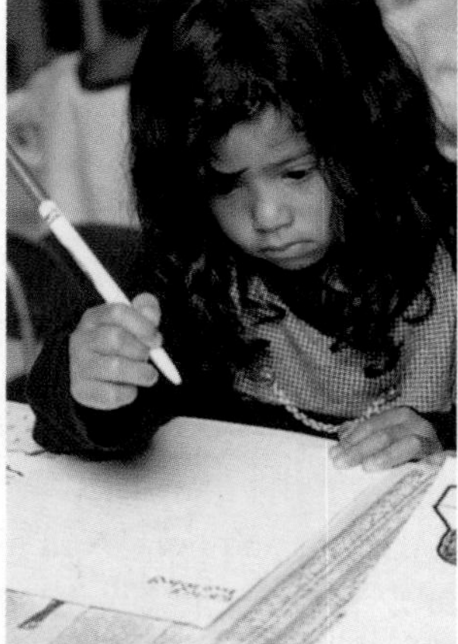

(8) Learns letters and numbers

Physical skills continue to develop (Figure 5–12 ■). The preschooler runs with ease, holds a bat, and throws balls of various types. Writing ability increases, and the preschooler enjoys drawing and learning to write a few letters. The preschooler becomes interested in the body and its function so the nurse can teach handwashing, general hygiene, dental care, and other health promotion topics to both parents and child. See Chapter 13∞ for further information about partnering with families to promote and maintain health of preschoolers.

Cognitive Development

The preschooler exhibits characteristics of preoperational thought. Symbols or words are used to represent objects and people, enabling the young child to think about them. This is a milestone in intellectual development; however, the preschooler still has some limitations in thought (Table 5–14). Recall that Piaget states that the young child does not have "less thought" than adults, but that the thought is qualitatively different. Understanding the child's thought will help you to explain procedures, conduct health teaching, and communicate

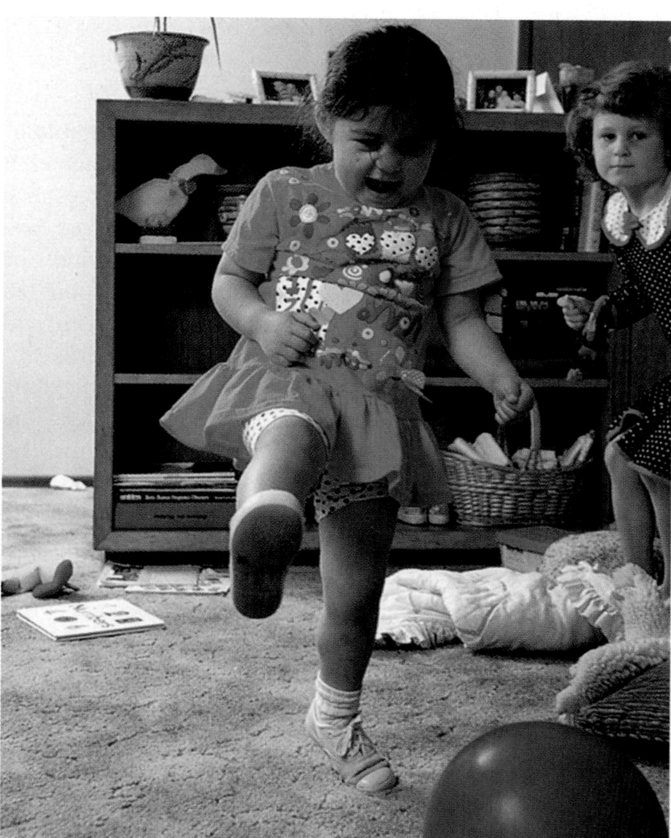

FIGURE 5–12 ■ Preschoolers continue to develop more advanced motor skills, such as kicking a ball without falling down.

more effectively with the preschooler. For example, as you plan to teach about how handwashing can prevent colds, what connections will you need to make for the preschooler? Consider the transductive reasoning of the child and formulate an effective teaching approach.

Psychosocial Development

Play

The preschooler has begun to play in a new way. Toddlers simply play side by side with friends, each engaging in his or her own activities; but preschoolers interact with others during play. One child cuts out colored paper while her friend glues it on paper in a design. This new type of interaction is called **associative play,** and it is characterized by children interacting in groups and participating in similar activities.

In addition to this social dimension of play, other aspects of play also differ. The preschooler enjoys large motor activities such as swinging, riding a tricycle, and throwing a ball. Increasing manual dexterity is demonstrated in greater complexity of drawings and manipulation of blocks and modeling. These changes necessitate planning of playtime to include appropriate activities. Preschool programs and child life departments in hospitals help meet this important need.

Materials provided for play can be simple but should guide activities in which the child engages. Because fine motor activities are popular, paper, pens, scissors, glue, and a variety of other such objects should be available. The child can use them to create important images such as pictures of people, hospital beds, or friends. A collection of dolls, furniture, and clothing can be manipulated to represent parents and children, nurses and physicians, teachers, or other significant people. Because fantasy life is so powerful at this age, the preschooler readily uses props to engage in **dramatic play,** that is, the living out of the drama of human life.

The nurse can use playtime to assess the preschooler's developmental level, knowledge about healthcare, and emotions related to healthcare experiences. Observations about objects chosen for play, content of dramatic play, and pictures drawn can provide important assessment data. The nurse can also use play periods to teach the child about healthcare procedures and offer an outlet for expression of emotions (see Table 5–14). See Chapter 17∞ for further information about use of play with hospitalized

TABLE 5–14 Psychosocial Development During Preschool Years

AGE	PLAY AND TOYS	COMMUNICATION
3–6 years 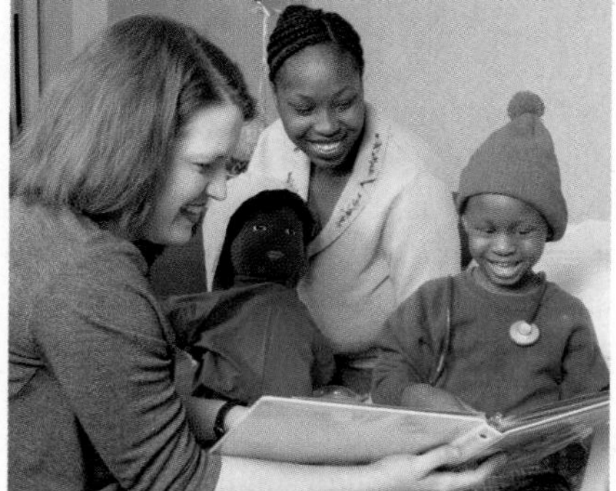	Associative play is facilitated by simple games, puzzles, nursery rhymes, songs Dramatic play is fostered by dolls and doll clothes, play houses and hospitals, dress-up clothes, puppets Stress is relieved by pens, paper, glue, scissors Cognitive growth is fostered by educational television shows, music, stories and books	All parts of speech are developed and used, occasionally incorrectly Communicates with a widening array of people Play with other children is a favorite activity Health professionals can ➤ Verbalize and explain procedures to children ➤ Use drawings and stories to explain care ➤ Use accurate names for bodily functions ➤ Allow the child to talk, ask questions, and make choices

children, and Chapter 34 for a description of play therapy with children who have psychiatric and mental health needs.

Personality and Temperament

Characteristics of personality observed in infancy tend to persist over time. The preschooler may need assistance as these characteristics are expressed in the new situations of preschool or nursery school. An excessively active child, for example, will need gentle, consistent handling to adjust to the structure of a classroom. Encourage parents to visit preschool programs to choose one that would best foster growth in their child. Some preschoolers enjoy the structured learning of a program that focuses on cognitive skills, whereas others are happier and more open to learning in a small group that provides much time for free play. Nurses can help parents to identify their child's personality or temperament characteristics and to find the best environment for growth.

Communication

Language skills blossom during the preschool years. The vocabulary grows to over 2,000 words, and children speak in complete sentences of several words and use all parts of speech. They practice these newfound language skills by endlessly talking and asking questions.

The sophisticated speech of preschoolers mirrors the development occurring in their minds and helps them to learn about the world around them. However, this speech can be quite deceptive. Although preschoolers use many words, their grasp of meaning is usually literal and may not match that of adults. These literal interpretations have important implications for healthcare providers. For example, the preschooler who is told she will be "put to sleep" for surgery may think of a pet recently euthanized; the child who is told that a dye will be injected for a diagnostic test may think he is going to die; mention of "a little stick" in the arm can cause images of tree branches rather than of a simple immunization, or the nurse's explanation that a shot is "like a mosquito bite" may signal the idea of buzzing and itching for a child.

The child may also have difficulty focusing on the content of a conversation. The preschooler is unable to consider the perspective of another and may be unable to move from individual thoughts to those the nurse is proposing, as the following conversation illustrates:

NURSE: I'd like to tell you about the operation that you will have tomorrow.

SHARISSE: OK. Did you know my brother just got a new squirt gun?

NURSE: That's nice. Now, first thing in the morning you will wake up early and your foot will be scrubbed with a special soap.

SHARISSE: The gun can spurt for about 40 feet—you have to pump it up.

NURSE: We'll talk about that later. Let me tell you about your operation now. After your foot is scrubbed, the nurse will measure your blood pressure and temperature and feel the pulse in your arm. Do you remember my doing those things today?

SHARISSE: Yes. And I got a sticker when I came into the hospital today, too. Do you know that my Mom is going to stay here tonight?

During this interchange, Sharisse engages in **collective monologue,** in which separate conversations occur even though each person waits for the other to speak. Though waiting for the nurse to speak, Sharisse is not generally responding to the nurse's content but is instead focusing on content from her own mind. She exhibits centration or a focus on just one aspect of a situation (the squirt gun). The nurse needs to respond to Sharisse's content and then reinsert more facts about the preparations for surgery.

Concrete visual aids such as pictures of a child undergoing the same procedure or a book to read together enhance teaching by meeting the child's developmental needs. Handling medical equipment such as intravenous bags and stethoscopes increases interest and helps the child to focus. Teaching may have to be done in several short sessions rather than one long session. Use short, directive approaches: "I know this hurts. It will be over soon. Hold your mom's hand and let's count while you get this shot. One, two, three, four, oh it's over!"

MediaLink Critical Thinking: Preparing a Preschooler for a Procedure

SCHOOL-AGE CHILD (6 TO 12 YEARS)

Errol, 10 years old, arrives home from school shortly after 3 P.M. each day. He immediately calls his friends and goes to visit one of them. They are building models of cars and collecting baseball cards. Hours are spent on these projects and on discussions of events at school that day (Figure 5–13 ■).

Nine-year-old Karen practices soccer two afternoons a week and plays in games each weekend. She also is learning to play the flute and spends her free time at home practicing. Although practice time is not her favorite part of music, Karen enjoys the performances and wants to play well in front of her friends and teacher. Her parents now allow her to ride her bike unaccompanied to the store or to a friend's house.

These two school-age children demonstrate common characteristics of their age group. They are in a stage of industry in which it is important to the child to perform useful work. Meaningful activities take on great importance and are usually carried out in the company of peers. A sense of achievement in these activities is important to develop self-esteem and to prevent a sense of inferiority or poor self-worth.

Physical Growth and Development

School age is the last period in which girls and boys are close in size and body proportions. As the long bones continue to grow, leg length increases (see Figure 5–7). Fat gives way to muscle, and the child appears leaner. Jaw proportions change as the first deciduous tooth is lost at 6 years and permanent teeth begin to erupt. Body organs and the immune system mature, resulting in fewer illnesses among school-age children. Medications are less likely to cause serious side effects, because they can be metabolized more easily. The urinary system can adjust to changes in fluid status. Physical skills are also refined as children begin to play sports, and fine motor skills are well developed through school activities (Table 5–15).

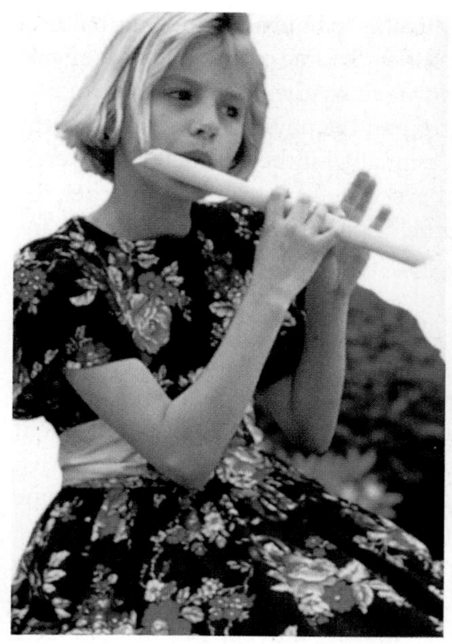

A

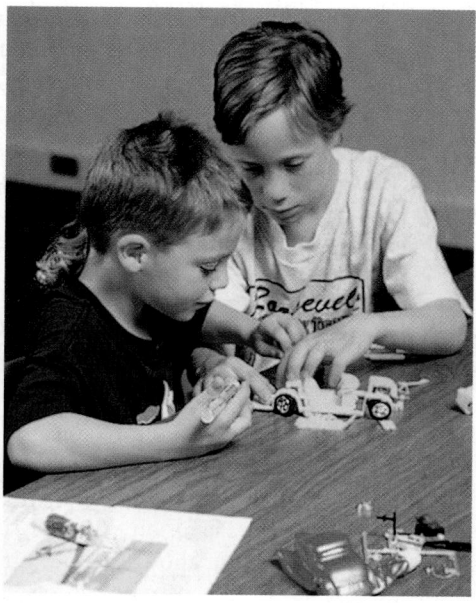

B

FIGURE 5–13 ■ *A,* School-age children may take part in activities that require practice. This is a consideration when children are hospitalized and unable to practice or perform. Why? *B,* School-age children enjoy spending time with others the same age on projects and discussing the activities of the day. This is an important consideration when they are in an acute-care setting. When you are in the clinical setting, look for examples of this type of interaction taking place.

Although it is commonly believed that the start of adolescence (age 12 years) heralds a growth spurt, the rapid increases in size commonly occur during school age. Girls may begin a growth spurt by 9 or 10 years and boys a year or so later (Figure 5–14 ■). Nutritional needs increase dramatically with this spurt.

The loss of the first deciduous teeth and the eruption of permanent teeth usually occur at about age 6, or at the beginning of the school-age period. Of the 32 permanent teeth, 22 to 26 erupt by age 12 and the remaining molars follow during the teenage years. The school-age child should be closely monitored to ensure that brushing and flossing are adequate, that fluoride is taken if the water supply is not fluoridated, that dental care is obtained to provide for examination of teeth and alignment, and that loose teeth are identified before surgery or other events that may lead to loss of a tooth.

TABLE 5–15 Physical Growth and Development Milestones During the School-Age Years

PHYSICAL GROWTH	FINE MOTOR ABILITY	GROSS MOTOR ABILITY	SENSORY ABILITY
Gains 1.4–2.2 kg (3–5 lb)/year Grows 4–6 cm (1 1/2–2 1/2 in.)/year	Enjoys craft projects Plays card and board games	Rides two-wheeler **(1)** Jumps rope **(2)** Roller skates or ice skates	Can read Able to concentrate for longer periods on activities by filtering out surrounding sounds **(3)**

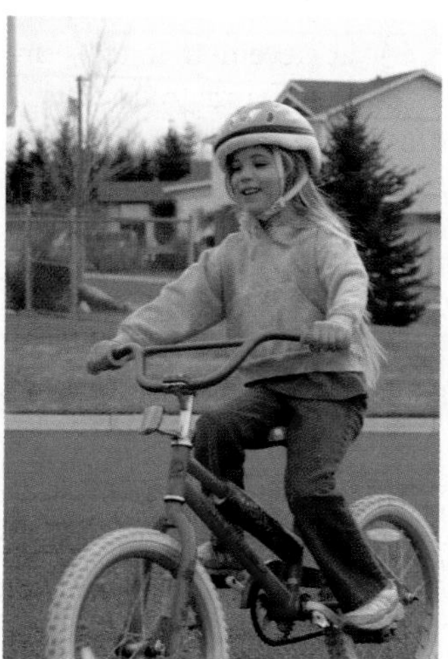

(1) Rides two-wheeler

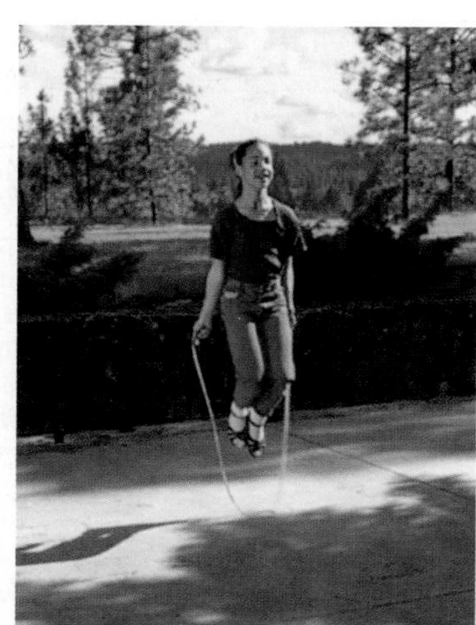

(2) Jumps rope

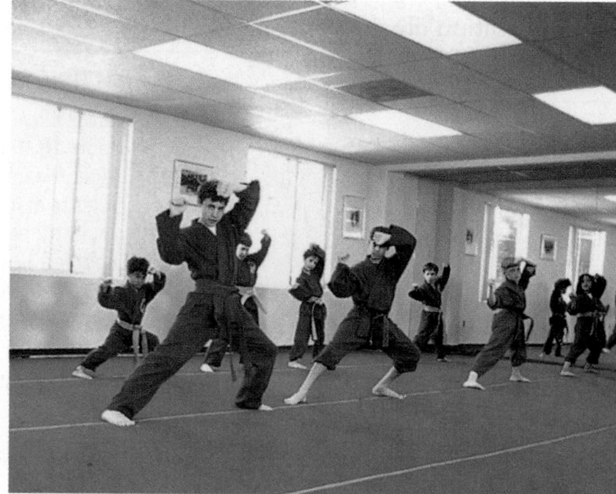

(3) Concentrates on activities for longer periods

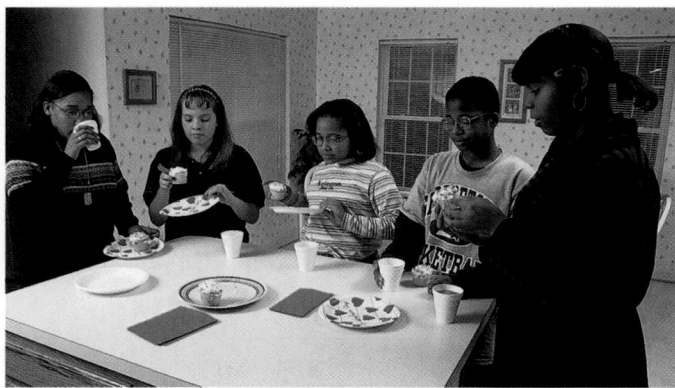

FIGURE 5–14 ■ Because girls have a growth spurt earlier than boys, girls often are taller than boys of the same age. Remember what it was like at your first dance?

Cognitive Development

The child enters the stage of concrete operational thought at about 7 years. This stage enables school-age children to consider alternative solutions and solve problems. However, school-age children continue to rely on concrete experiences and materials to form their thought content.

During the school-age years, the child learns the concept of **conservation** (that matter is not changed when its form is altered). At earlier ages, a child believes that when water is poured from a short, wide glass into a tall, thin glass, there is more water in the taller glass. The school-age child recognizes that although it may look like the taller glass holds more water, the quantity is the same. The concept of conservation is helpful when the nurse explains medical treatments. The school-age child understands that an incision will heal, that a cast will be removed, and that an arm will look the same as before once the intravenous infusion is removed.

Psychosocial Development

Play

When a preschool teacher tries to organize a game of baseball, both the teacher and the children become frustrated. Not only are the children physically unable to hold a bat and hit a ball, but they also seem to have no understanding of the rules of the game and do not want to wait for their turn at bat. By 6 years of age, however, children have acquired the physical ability to hold the bat properly and may occasionally hit the ball. School-age children also understand that everyone has a role—the pitcher, the catcher, the batter, the outfielders. They cooperate with one another to form a team, are eager to learn the rules of the game, and want to ensure that these rules are followed exactly (Table 5–16).

The characteristics of play exhibited by the school-age child are cooperation with others and the ability to play a part in order to contribute to a unified whole. This type of play is called **cooperative play.** The concrete nature of cognitive thought leads to a reliance on rules to provide structure and security. Children have an increasing desire to spend much of playtime with friends, which demonstrates the social component of play. Play is an extremely important method of learning and living for the school-age child. Active physical play has decreased in recent years as television viewing and playing of computer games have increased, leading to poor nutritional status and other health risks in children. See Chapter 9 for further discussion of nutrition and physical activity in children.

When a child is hospitalized, the separation from playmates can lead to feelings of sadness and purposelessness. School-age children often feel better when placed in multibed units with other children. Games can be devised even when children are using wheelchairs (Figure 5–15 ■). Normal, rewarding parts of play should be integrated into care. Friends should be encouraged to visit or call a hospitalized child. Discharge planning for the child who has had a cast or brace applied should address the activities in which the child can participate and those the child must avoid. Reinforce the importance of playing games with friends.

Personality and Temperament

The enduring aspects of temperament continue to be manifested during the school years. The child classified as "difficult" at an ear-

TABLE 5–16 Psychosocial Development During the School-Age Years

AGE	ACTIVITIES	COMMUNICATION
6–12 years 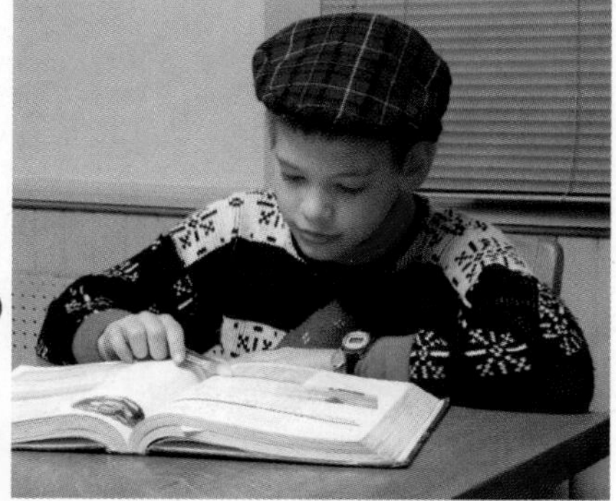	Gross motor development is fostered by ball sports, skating, dance lessons, water and snow skiing/boarding, biking A sense of industry is fostered by playing a musical instrument, gathering collections, starting hobbies, playing board and video games Cognitive growth is facilitated by reading, crafts, word puzzles, school work	Mature use of language Ability to converse and discuss topics for increasing lengths of time Spends many hours at school and with friends in sports or other activities Health professionals can: ➤ Assess child's knowledge before teaching ➤ Allow the child to select rewards following procedures ➤ Teach techniques such as counting or visualization to manage difficult situations ➤ Include both parent and child in healthcare decisions

MediaLink Case Study: Diabetic Risk Factors: School-Age Child

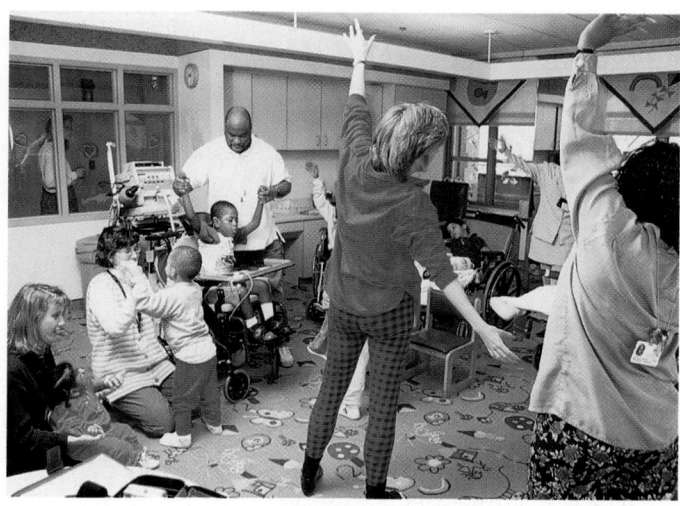

FIGURE 5–15 ■ The nurse can help the child and family accept and adjust to new circumstances. Encouraging the child in a wheelchair to participate in group activities can help build confidence in physical skills. Good self-esteem, goal attainment, personal satisfaction, and general health are the continued benefits.

lier age may now have trouble in the classroom. Advise parents to provide a quiet setting for homework and to reward the child for concentration. For example, after homework is completed, the child may play a game with the parent. Creative efforts and alternative methods of learning should be valued. Encourage parents to see their children as individuals who may not all learn in the same way. The "slow-to-warm-up" child may need encouragement to try new activities and to share experiences with others, whereas the "easy" child will readily adapt to new schools, people, and experiences.

Communication

During the school-age years, the child should learn how to correct any lingering pronunciation or grammatical errors. Vocabulary increases, and the child learns about parts of speech in school. School-age children enjoy writing and can be encouraged to keep a journal of their experiences while in the hospital as a method of dealing with anxiety. The literal translation of words characteristic of preschoolers is uncommon among school-age children; they understand the meaning of phrases such as being "put to sleep" or "getting a little stick in the arm."

Sexuality

Although children become aware of sexual differences between genders during preschool years, they deal much more consciously with sexuality during school age. As children mature physically, they need information about their bodily changes so that they can develop a healthy self-image and an understanding of the relationships between their bodies and sexuality. Children become interested in sexual issues and are often exposed to erroneous information on television shows, in magazines, or from friends and siblings. Schools and families need to use opportunities to teach school-age children factual information about sex and to foster healthy concepts of self and others. It is advisable to ask occasional questions about sexual issues to learn how much the child knows and to provide correct information when answers demonstrate confusion. Both friends and the media are common sources of erroneous ideas. Appropriate and inappropriate touch should be discussed, with lists of trusted people who can be approached (teachers, clergy, school counselors, family members, neighbors) to discuss any episodes with which the child feels uncomfortable. Recognize that even these trusted people can be implicated in inappropriate episodes, so encourage the child to go to more than one person, an important approach if the child is uncomfortable about a relationship with any individual.

ADOLESCENT (12 TO 18 YEARS)

Adolescence is a time of passage, signaling the end of childhood and the beginning of adulthood. Although adolescents differ in behaviors and accomplishments, they are in a period of identity formation. If a healthy identity and sense of self-worth are not developed in this period, role confusion and purposeless struggling will ensue. The adolescents in your care will represent various degrees of identity formation, and each will offer unique challenges.

Physical Growth and Development

The physical changes ending in **puberty,** or sexual maturity, begin near the end of the school-age period. The prepubescent period is marked by a growth spurt at an average age of 10 years for girls and 13 years for boys. The increase in height and weight is generally remarkable and is completed in 2 to 3 years (Table 5-17). The growth spurt in girls is accompanied by an increase in breast size and growth of pubic hair. Menstruation occurs last and signals achievement of puberty. In boys, the growth spurt is accompanied by growth in size of the penis and testes and by growth of pubic hair. Deepening of the voice and growth of facial hair occur later, at the time of puberty. See Chapter 8∞ for a description of the pubertal stages.

During adolescence children grow stronger and more muscular and establish characteristic male and female patterns of fat distribution. The apocrine and eccrine glands mature, leading to increased sweating and a distinct odor to perspiration. All body organs are now fully mature, enabling the adolescent to take adult doses of medications.

The adolescent must adapt to a rapidly changing body for several years. These physical changes and hormonal variations offer challenges to identity formation.

Cognitive Development

Adolescence marks the beginning of Piaget's last stage of cognitive development, the stage of formal operational thought. The adolescent no longer depends on concrete experiences as the basis of thought but develops the ability to reason abstractly. Concepts such as justice, truth, beauty, and power can be understood. The adolescent revels in this newfound ability and spends a great deal of time thinking, reading, and talking about abstract concepts.

The ability to think and act independently leads many adolescents to rebel against parental authority. Through these actions, adolescents seek to establish their own identity and values.

TABLE 5–17 Physical Growth and Development Milestones During Adolescence

PHYSICAL GROWTH	FINE MOTOR ABILITY	GROSS MOTOR ABILITY	SENSORY ABILITY
Variation in age of growth spurt During growth spurt, girls gain 7–25 kg (15–55 lb) and grow 2.5–20 cm (2–8 in.); boys gain approximately 7–29.5 kg (15–65 lb) and grow 11–30 cm (41/2–12 in.)	Skills are well developed **(1)**	New sports activities attempted and muscle development continues **(2)** Some lack of coordination common during growth spurt	Fully developed

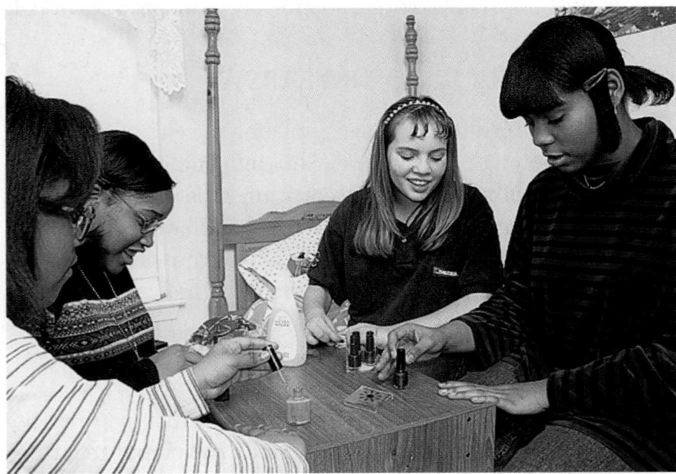

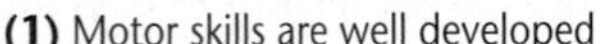

(1) Motor skills are well developed

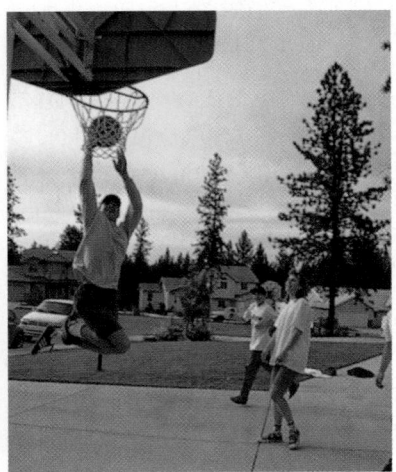

(2) New sports activities attempted

Psychosocial Development

Activities

Maturity leads to new activities. Adolescents may drive, ride buses, or bike independently. They are less dependent on parents for transportation and spend more time with friends. Activities include participation in sports and extracurricular school activities, as well as "hanging out" and attending movies or concerts with friends (Table 5–18). The peer group becomes the focus of activities, regardless of the teen's interests. Peers are important in establishing identity and providing meaning. Although same-sex interactions predominate, boy–girl relationships are more common than at earlier stages. Adolescents thus participate in and learn from social interactions fundamental to adult relationships.

Personality and Temperament

Characteristics of temperament manifested during childhood usually remain stable in the teenage years. For instance, the adolescent who was a calm, scheduled infant and child often demonstrates initiative to regulate study times and other routines. Similarly, the adolescent who was an easily stimulated infant may now have a messy room, a harried schedule with assignments always completed late, and an interest in many activities. It is also common for an adolescent who was an easy child to become more difficult due to the psychologic changes of adolescence and the need to assert independence.

Similar to the child's earlier ages, the nurse's role may be to inform parents of different personality types and to help them support the teen's uniqueness while providing necessary structure and feedback. Nurses can help parents to understand their teen's personality type and to work with the adolescent to meet expectations of teachers and others in authority.

Communication

All parts of speech are used and understood by the adolescent. Colloquialisms and slang are commonly used with the peer group. The adolescent often studies a foreign language in school, having the ability to understand and analyze grammar and sentence structure.

The adolescent increasingly leaves the home base and establishes close ties with peers. These relationships become the basis for identity formation. There is generally a period of stress or crisis before a strong identity can emerge. The adolescent may try out new roles by learning a new sport or other skills, experimenting with drugs or alcohol, wearing different styles of clothing, or trying other activities. It is important to provide positive role models and a variety of experiences to help the adolescent make wise choices.

The adolescent also has a need to leave the past, to be different, and to change from former patterns to establish a self-identity. Rules that are repeated constantly and dogmatically will probably be broken in the adolescent's quest for self-awareness. This poses difficulties when the adolescent has a health problem, such as diabetes or a heart defect that requires ongoing care. Introducing the adolescent to other teens who manage the same problem appropriately is usually more successful than telling the adolescent what to do.

Privacy should be ensured during the taking of health histories or interventions with teens. Even if a parent is present for part of a history or examination, the adolescent should be given the opportunity to relay information or ask questions alone with the healthcare provider. The adolescent should be given a choice of whether to have a parent present during an examination or while care is provided. Most information shared by an adolescent is confidential. Some states mandate disclosure of certain information to parents such as an adolescent's desire for an abortion. In these cases, the adolescent should be informed of what will be disclosed to the parent. (See Chapter 1∞ for further discussion.)

Setting up teen rooms (recreation rooms for use only by adolescents) or separate adolescent units in hospitals can provide necessary peer support during hospitalization. Most adolescents are not pleased when placed on a unit or in a room with young children. Choices should be allowed when possible, and include preference for evening or morning bathing, the type of clothes to wear while hospitalized, timing of treatments, and visitation guidelines. Use of contracts with adolescents may increase compliance. Firmness, gentleness, choices, and respect must be balanced during care of adolescent patients.

Sexuality

With maturation of the body and increased secretion of hormones, the adolescent achieves sexual maturity. This complex process involves growing interactions with members of the opposite sex, an interplay of the forces of society and family, and identity formation. The early adolescent progresses from dances and other social events with members of the opposite sex to the late adolescent who is mature sexually and may have regular sexual encounters. About half of all high school students in the United States have had intercourse, but only 63% of these youth used a condom at their last sexual encounter (Acquavella & MMWR, 2004).

Teenagers need information about their bodies and emerging sexuality. They should understand the interests and forces they experience. Including sex education in school classes and healthcare encounters is important. Information on methods to prevent sexually transmitted diseases is given, with most school districts now providing some teaching on AIDS. Far more common risks to teens, however, are diseases such as gonorrhea, herpes, and hepatitis. Health histories should include questions on sexual activity, sexually transmitted diseases, and birth control use and understanding. Most hospitals routinely perform pregnancy screening on adolescent girls before elective procedures.

Adolescents will benefit from clear information about sexuality, an opportunity to develop relationships with adolescents in various settings, an open atmosphere at home and school where problems and issues can be discussed, and previous experience in problem solving and self decision making. Sexual issues should be among topics that adolescents can discuss openly in a variety of settings. Alternatives and support for their decisions should be available.

Some adolescents identify with a sexual minority group such as lesbian, gay, bisexual, or transgendered. They are at particular risk of being stigmatized and harassed by other youth or adults. They are more likely to suffer a variety of problems such as isolation, rejection by significant others, violence, suicide, and taking sexual risks (Stevens & Morgan, 1999, 2001). Nurses are instrumental in helping these youths by providing information for them and their parents, integrating sexual minority content into sexual education curricula, and providing referrals for health and social care when needed. Nurses must examine their own beliefs and communication styles to provide culturally competent care. They can promote trust and acceptance among youth and in the general school community (Bakker & Cavender, 2003). See Chapter 7∞ for further information about the health issues related to homosexuality and other sexual minority practices.

MediaLink Critical Thinking: Developing Values in Adolescence

TABLE 5–18 Psychosocial Development During Adolescence

AGE	ACTIVITIES	COMMUNICATION
12–18 years 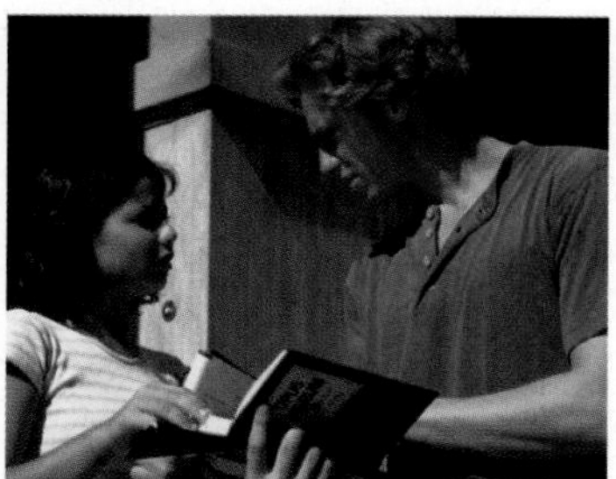	Sports—ball games, gymnastics, water and snow skiing/boarding, swimming, school sports School activities—drama, yearbook, class office, club participation Quiet activities—Reading, school work, television, computer, video games, music	Increasing communication and time with peer group—movies, dances, driving, eating out, attending sports events Applying abstract thought and analysis in conversations at home and school

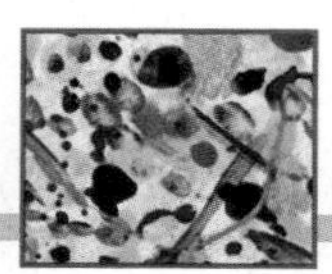

CHAPTER HIGHLIGHTS

- Development unfolds in a predictable pattern, but at different rates dependent on the particular characteristics and experiences of each child.
- Major theories of development encompass the psychosexual (Freud), psychosocial (Erikson), cognitive (Piaget), moral (Kohlberg), social learning (Bandura), and behavioral (Skinner and Watson) components of individuals.
- The ecologic theory of Bronfenbrenner and the temperament theory of Chess and Thomas emphasize the interactions of the individual within the environment.
- Resiliency theory examines risk and protective factors that hinder or help children and families when dealing with developmental and life crises.
- Influences on the developmental process include one's genetic potential and a series of environmental influences unique to each family and individual.
- The newborn period begins at birth and ends at about 1 month, and is characterized by adaptation to extrauterine life, establishing periods of varying alertness, and specific physical findings.
- Infancy spans the time from 1 month to 1 year, and is marked by rapid physical growth, mastery of basic fine and gross motor skills, and beginning cognitive and language skills.
- Toddlers range in age from 1 to 3 years, and become increasingly mobile and communicative. They master control over excretion and are known for exerting their own opinions and wishes to parents. Injury prevention and toilet training are specific parental teaching needs.
- Preschool years range from 3 to 6 and are marked by increasing social skills. Most preschool children attend childcare programs and learn to play with other children. Continued mastery of physical coordination and language occur.
- School age spans the years from 6 to 12, when children mature in many areas. They show slow, steady growth until reaching puberty between 9 and 12 years, when a growth spurt marks increased height and weight, as well as sexual maturation. School-age children play cooperatively with other children and participate in various school and community activities.
- Adolescence occurs from about 12 years of age through the teen years. Adolescents establish their own identities distinct from parents and other adults. They are mature physically and cognitively. The peer group exerts the major influence at this age.
- The nurse is involved in assessing development at each stage, and in providing anticipatory guidance to families to foster optimal development.

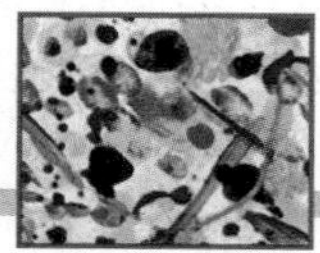

CRITICAL THINKING IN ACTION

INTRODUCTION

Consider Irena, who was introduced in the chapter opening scenario. She is 2 years of age and was recently adopted from Romania. Irena is adapting well, but her parents have many questions.

Although Irena has an easy temperment, she is quiet in her interactions with other toddlers. She has learned a few words in English, and is generally in a pleasant mood.

DESCRIPTION

Since they have no other children and have limited experience with children, Michael and Alyssa are essentially new parents. As parents of a toddler, they have unique information needs.

Irena is 32 inches (81 cm) (standing height) and weighs 23 lb (10.45 kg). Items she performs in the Denver II Developmental Test include:

- Personal social—washes and dries hands, brushes teeth with help, and removes garments
- Fine motor—builds a tower of six cubes
- Language—has six words (in English; unknown in native language), combines words, and points to two pictures
- Gross motor—kicks ball forward, jumps up, and throws ball overhand

DISCUSSION

1. Irena and her parents have many challenges and yet possess many strengths. Using the theory of resilience, list the child and family risks and protective factors.
2. Calculate Irena's height and weight percentiles. Consult the growth grids in Appendix A and the Skills Manual for correct analysis. What nutritional advice do you have for Irena's parents?
3. What developmental strengths are suggested by Irena's Denver II results? (Consult the Denver II form in Chapter 10.) Which area needs the most attention? What specific suggestions do you have for Irena's parents as they seek to encourage her development?
4. Michael and Alyssa are parenting a toddler. What special needs are they likely to have? What resources are available for adoptive parents? How could they preserve Irena's heritage as a Romanian as she grows older?

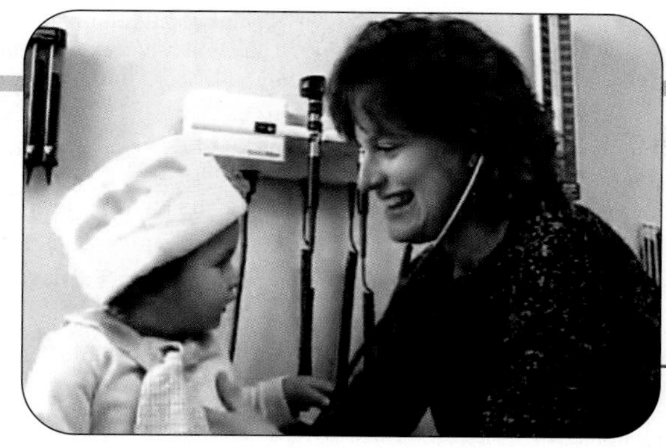

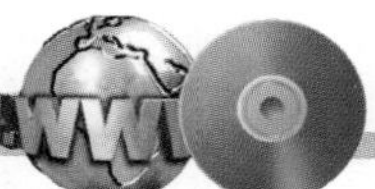

EXPLORE MediaLink

- NCLEX review, case studies, and other interactive resources for this chapter can be found on the Companion Website at **http://www.prenhall.com/ball**. Click on Chapter 5 to select the activities for this chapter.
- For animations, more NCLEX review questions, and an audio glossary, access the accompanying CD-ROM in this book.

http://www.prenhall.com/ball

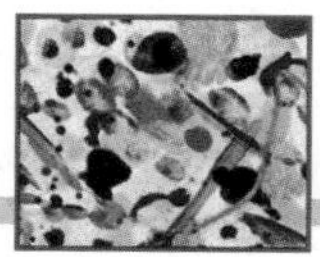

REFERENCES

Aronson, J. (2000). Medical evaluation and infectious considerations on arrival. *Pediatric Annals, 29*, 218–223.

Bakker, L. J., & Cavender, A. (2003). Promoting culturally competent care for gay youth. *Journal of School Nursing, 19*, 65–72.

Bandura, A. (1986). *Social foundations of thought and actions: A social cognitive theory*. Englewood Cliffs, NJ: Prentice Hall.

Bandura, A. (1997a). *Self-efficacy: The exercise of control*. New York: W. H. Freeman.

Bandura, A. (1997b). *Self-efficacy in changing societies*. New York: Cambridge University Press.

Baumrind, D. (1971). Current patterns of parental authority. *Developmental Psychology, 4*, 1–103.

Bosch, J., Sullivan, S., Van Dyke, D. C., Hongjun, S., Klockau, L., Nissen, K., Blewer, K., Weber, E., & Everly, S. S. (2003). Promoting a healthy tomorrow here for children adopted from abroad. *Contemporary Pediatrics, 20*, 69–86.

Briggs, G., Freeman, R., & Yaffe, S. (2001). *Drugs in pregnancy and lactation* (6th ed.). Baltimore: Lippincott, Williams & Wilkins.

Bronfenbrenner, U. (1986). Ecology of the family as a context for human development: Research perspectives. *Developmental Psychology, 22*, 723–742.

Bronfenbrenner, U., McClelland, P. D., Ceci, S. J., Moen, P., & Wethington, E. (1996). *The state of Americans*. New York: Free Press.

Chamberlain, L. J. (2001). Children adopted abroad could face life-long psychological problems. *Infectious Diseases in Children, 14*(1), 20.

Chamberlain, L. J. (2003). Initial medical examination important for international adoptees. *Infectious Diseases in Children, 16*(3), 52, 59.

Chang, Y. J., Anderson, G. C., & Lin, C. H. (2002). Effects of prone and supine positions on sleep state and stress responses in mechanically ventilated preterm infants during the first postnatal week. *Journal of Advanced Nursing, 40*, 161–169.

Chen, L. H., Barnett, E. D., & Wilson, M. E. (2003). Preventing infectious diseases during and after international adoption. *Annals of Internal Medicine, 139*, 371–378.

Chess, S., & Thomas, A. (1995). *Temperament in clinical practice*. New York: Guilford Press.

Chess, S., & Thomas, A. (1996). *Temperament: Theory and practice*. Philadelphia: Brunner/Mazel Publishers.

Chess, S., & Thomas, A. (1999). *Goodness of fit: Clinical applications from infancy through adult life*. Philadelphia: Brunner/Mazel Publishers.

Children's Defense Fund. (2004). *The state of America's children*. Washington, DC: Children's Defense Fund.

Chwo, M. J., Anderson, G. C., Good, M., Dowling, D. A., Shiau, S. H., & Chu, D. M. (2002). A randomized controlled trial of early kangaroo care for preterm infants: Effects on temperature, weight, behavior, and acuity. *Journal of Nursing Research, 10*, 129–142.

Craig, G. J., & Baucum, D. (2001). *Human development*. Upper Saddle River, NJ: Pearson Education.

Erikson, E. (1963). *Childhood and society*. New York: W.W. Norton.

Erikson, E. (1968). *Identity: Youth and crisis*. New York: W.W. Norton.

Faber, S. (2000). Behavioral sequelae of orphanage life. *Pediatric Annals, 29*, 242–248.

Field, T. (2002). Preterm infant massage therapy studies: An American approach. *Seminars in Neonatology, 7*, 487–494.

Finan, S. L. (1997). Promoting healthy sexuality: Guidelines for the school-age child and adolescent. *The Nurse Practitioner, 22*, 62–72.

Frenn, M., Malin, S., & Bansal, N. K. (2003). Stage-based interventions for low-fat diet with middle school students. *Journal of Pediatric Nursing, 18*, 36–45.

Ginsberg, H., & Opper, S. (1988). *Piaget's theory of intellectual development* (3rd ed.). Paramus, NJ: Prentice Hall.

Hummel, P. (2003). Parenting the high-risk infant. *NBIN, 3*, 88–92.

Jenista, J. A. (2000). Preadoption review of medical records. *Pediatric Annals, 29*, 212–217.

Johnson, D. E. (2000). Long-term medical issues in international adoptees. *Pediatric Annals, 29*, 234–241.

Kleinman, R. E. (Ed.). (2004). *Pediatric nutrition handbook* (5th ed.). Elk Grove Village, IL: American Academy of Pediatrics.

Lerner, R. M. (2002). *Adolescence*. Upper Saddle River, NJ: Pearson Education.

London, M. L., Ladewig, P. W., Ball, J. W., & Bindler, R. C. (2003). *Maternal-newborn & child nursing*. Upper Saddle River, NJ: Prentice Hall Health.

Mainous, R. O. (2003). Infant massage as a component of developmental care: Past, present, and future. *Holistic Nursing Practice, 17*, 1–7.

Malone, J. A. (1998). The resiliency model of family stress, adjustment, and adaptation. In B. Vaughan-Cole, M. A. Johnson, J. A. Malone, & B. L. Walker, *Family nursing practice* (pp. 49–60). Philadelphia: W. B. Saunders.

Melvin, N. (1995). Children's temperament: Intervention for parents. *Journal of Pediatric Nursing, 10*, 152–159.

Miller, L. C. (2000). Initial assessment of growth, development, and the effects of institutionalization in internationally adopted children. *Pediatric Annals, 29*, 224–233.

MMWR. (2004). Youth Risk Behavior Surveillance United States, 2003. 53(5502), 1–96.

Piaget, J. (1972). *The child's conception of the world*. Totowa, NJ: Littlefield, Adams Co.

Riner, M. E., & Saywell, R. M. (2002). Development of the social ecology model of adolescent interpersonal violence prevention (SEMAIVP). *Journal of School Health, 72*, 65–70.

Saiman, L. (2003). Evaluating internationally adopted children: An important skill to know. *Infectious Diseases in Children, 16*(3), 54.

Santrock, J. (2003). *Life-span development* (9th ed.). Boston: McGraw-Hill.

Stevens, P., & Morgan, S. (1999). Health of lesbian, gay, bisexual, and transgender youth. *Journal of Child and Family Nursing, 2*, 237–249.

Stevens, P., & Morgan, S. (2001). Health of lesbian, gay, bisexual, and transgender youth. *Journal of Pediatric Health Care, 15*, 24–34.

Stewart, M., Reid, G., & Mangham, C. (1997). Fostering children's resilience. *Journal of Pediatric Nursing, 12*, 21–31.

Turecki, S. (2003). The behavioral complaint: Symptom of a psychiatric disorder or a matter of temperament? *Contemporary Pediatrics, 20*, 111–119.

UNICEF. (1998). The state of the world's children 1998: A UNICEF report. Malnutrition: causes, consequences, and solutions. *Nutrition Reviews, 56*, 115–123.

Zacharyczuk, C. (2003). Think about country of origin when diagnosing GI illness in adoptees. *Infectious Diseases in Children, 16*(3), 57–58.

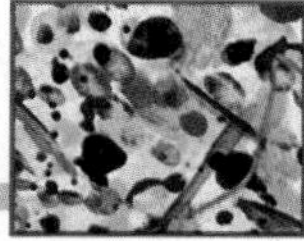

ADDITIONAL REFERENCES

Altemeier, W. A. (2000). Growth charts, low birth weight, and international adoption. *Pediatric Annals, 29*, 204–205.

Baker, E., Croot, K., McLeod, S., & Paul, R. (2001). Psycholinguistic models of speech development and their application to clinical practice. *Journal of Speech, Language and Hearing Research, 44*, 685–702.

Board on Children, Youth and Families, National Research Council and Institute of Medicine. (2001). *From neurons to neighborhoods*. Washington, DC: National Academy Press.

Carno, M. A., Hoffman, L. A., Carcillo, J. A., & Sanders, M. H. (2003). Developmental stages of sleep from birth to adolescence, common childhood sleep disorders: Overview and nursing implications. *Journal of Pediatric Nursing, 18*, 274–283.

Federal Interagency Forum on Child and Family Statistics. (2000). *America's children: Key national indicators of well-being*. Washington, DC: U.S. Government Printing Office.

Fields, J., Smith, K., Bass, L. E., & Lugaila, T. (2001). *A child's day: Home, school, and play (selected indicators of child well-being)*. Washington, DC: U.S. Department of Commerce.

Green, M., & Palfrey, J. S. (2000). *Bright futures: Guidelines for health supervision of infants, children and adolescents*, (2nd ed.). Arlington, VA: National Center for Education in Maternal and Child Health.

Healthy People 2010. (2000). *Healthy people 2010* conference edition. Washington, DC: United States Department of Health and Human Services.

Jana, L. A. (2003). Children's books about the body, its part, and how it works. *Contemporary Pediatrics 20*, 121–124.

Kessenich, M. (2003). Developmental outcomes of premature, low birth weight, and medically fragile infants. *NBIN 3*, 80–87.

Yont, K., Hewitt, L. E., & Miccio, A. W. (2002). "What did you say": Understanding conversational breakdowns in children with speech and language impairments. *Clinical Linguistics and Phonetics 16*, 265–285.

Chapter 6

Child and Family Communication

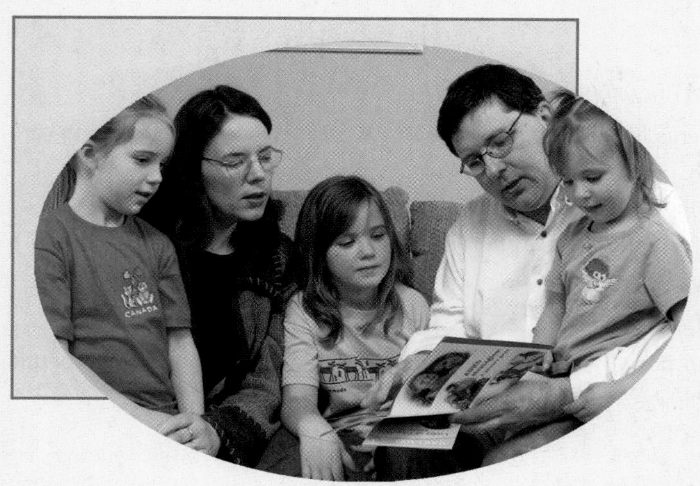

Madison Clarke has been discharged from the hospital after a workup and diagnosis of juvenile rheumatoid arthritis, a chronic condition. The nurse has worked with Madison and her family in the hospital, and now the focus shifts to meeting with the siblings, Brittney, age 9, and Madeline, age 4. The nurse is in their home to explain the disease process, the treatment regimen, how their lives might be impacted, and how they can be involved in Madison's care.

The nurse tells Brittney and Madeline that on some days Madison's knees may hurt more than others and she may not be able to play. She tells the girls that a physical therapist will be coming to the house to help Madison with some exercises for her legs, and will show them how to gently move Madison's knees to help her stay active. The nurse uses anticipatory guidance in communications with family members to assist them in developing coping mechanisms for the changes in routine. Effective communication can also assist Madison and her family to identify creative hobbies or activities to further her sense of self-worth.

What communication skills are required to explain the disease and treatment to children at various developmental stages? What factors influence communication? What are potential barriers to communication?

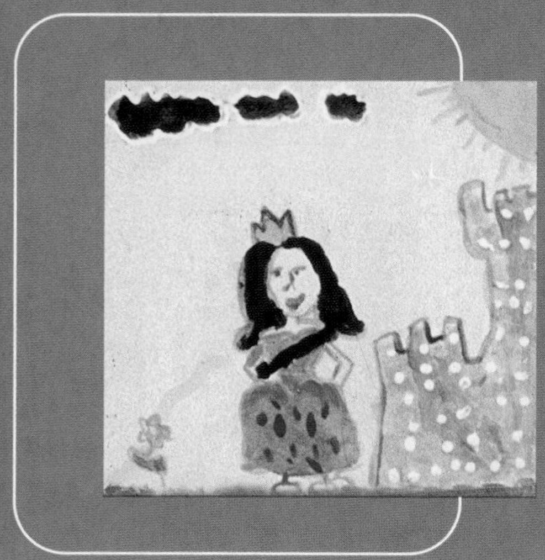

"I'm so glad that the nurse came to our house and talked to Brittney and Madeline about my arthritis. I think it helped my mom and dad, too."

—Madison, age 7

Key Terms

abstract communication/171
bibliotherapy/186
body language/173
caring/176
communication/171
decode/178
empathy/176
expressive language/171
medical jargon/175
nonverbal communication/171
paralanguage/172
receptive language/171
verbal communication/171

Learning Outcomes

After completing this chapter, you will be able to:

- Describe the major components of the communication process as they apply to nursing care of children and their families.
- Identify forms of communication and their related concepts.
- Identify factors influencing the communication process.
- Apply concepts of communication to the developmental levels of childhood.
- Identify barriers and challenges to communication with the child and family.
- Apply the nursing process to promote effective communication and establish a therapeutic nurse–child–family relationship.

MediaLink 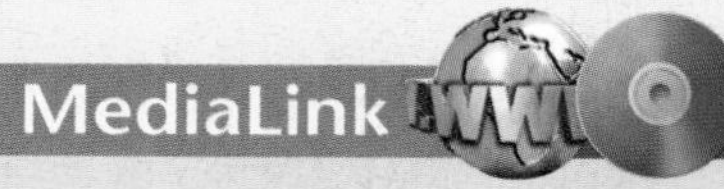 http://www.prenhall.com/ball

Resources for this chapter can be found on the CD-ROM accompanying this textbook, and on the Companion Website at www.prenhall.com/ball. Click on Chapter 6 to select the activities for this chapter.

CD-ROM

Videos

Alternative Communication Methods
Caring and Empathy
Nonverbal Communication

NCLEX Review

Audio Glossary

COMPANION WEBSITE

NCLEX Review

Case Study: A School-Age Child Who is Non-English-Speaking

Care Plan: An Infant with a Hearing Impairment

Care Plan: Preschooler Hospitalized for Diabetes

MediaLink Applications

Communicating with a Child: Create an IPR
Develop a Communication Strategy:
- *A 7-year-old Girl Hospitalized for Diabetes*
- *A 16-year-old Boy Hospitalized for Fractures*

Communication is an essential component of human interaction, as it provides the means by which individuals, from birth through adulthood, learn about the physical and social world through exchange of information.

The nurse–child–family relationship is dependent on effective communication. The nurse's communication with the child and family serves as a key connection between the family and the healthcare system, and establishing a therapeutic relationship with the child and family is essential to promote the health of the child. However, effective communication is a learned process. Pediatric nurses must understand and apply techniques of effective communication, including listening, interpreting the various forms of communication, and being aware of factors that can positively or negatively influence the process. Ongoing evaluation will help the nurse identify strategies to modify communication techniques for children at different ages and developmental stages.

This chapter provides an overview of the communication process, and factors that influence communication with the child and family. The chapter then addresses developmental considerations for communication, and considerations for special pediatric populations. The remainder of the chapter focuses on nursing management of communication with the child and family.

COMMUNICATION AND THE NURSE–CHILD–FAMILY RELATIONSHIP

Communication is the exchange of information, thoughts, and feelings. It is an ongoing cyclical process in which people constantly connect, either consciously or unconsciously, through verbal and nonverbal techniques. Major components of the communication process are the *sender, message, channel, receiver,* and *response* (Figure 6–1 ■).

Effective communication is essential in the nurse–child–family relationship, in that it secures trust in the healthcare professional, which can lead to a positive health outcome. Communication begins when the child and family enter the healthcare setting. As the child and family interact with the nurse, anxiety may be reduced as they become aware of the nurse's interest and caring. This feeling of security can generate open communication where families feel free to discuss their concerns.

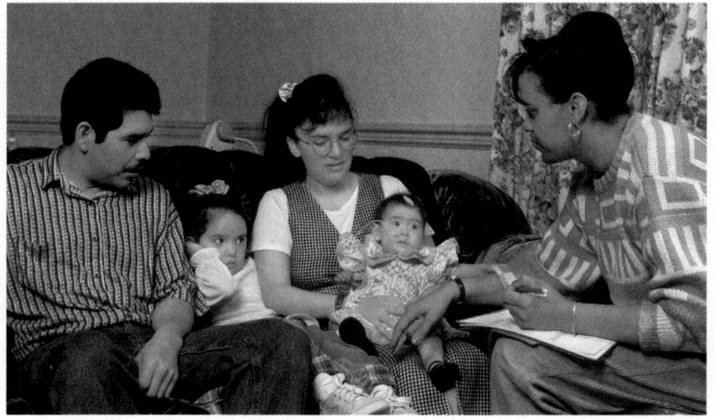

FIGURE 6–1 ■ The nurse is sending a message to the older child, the receiver. Notice the nonverbal communication expressed by the young girl. What message is she communicating? How should the nurse respond?

Parents need accurate information and assurance from someone they can trust, as they may be relinquishing the care of their child to strangers. The nurse is the one healthcare professional who will experience the majority of the interaction with the child and family and, therefore, the nurse is challenged to also meet the parent's psychological and educational needs. Including the parents in their child's care is crucial to validate their importance and their role in returning their child to a healthy state (Thompson, Hupcey, & Clark, 2003).

The overall goal of the nurse is to establish rapport with the child and family to assist them in identifying mutual goals and to facilitate positive health outcomes. Refer to the opening scenario. What indications are present to suggest that the nurse is establishing a therapeutic relationship with positive rapport?

FORMS OF COMMUNICATION

Communication occurs through different forms: verbal, nonverbal, and abstract. **Verbal communication** is the use of verbal and written words; vocalizations, such as laughter or crying; or the implication of what is not spoken to convey messages. **Nonverbal communication** is the use of body language that includes gestures, facial expressions, posture, touch, and reactions. **Abstract communication** is displayed through play, visual images, and even the selection of clothing to wear. While the younger child may choose to communicate through play, the adolescent may select specific clothes to "send the message."

Verbal Communication

The use of language—as well as nonverbal communication resources—is crucial to the nurse's assessment. However, the way the nurse frames the interaction verbally is of great importance to how the message is understood. For example, if the nurse states, "I will be back in a few minutes and we will draw your blood," then the young child may simply think that the nurse will return with paper and crayons and together the two of them will "draw blood" on the paper. An understanding and application of the developmental and cognitive stages of children is essential to ensure clear communication.

Developmental level and cognitive stage determine the child's vocabulary and means of expression as well. Use of language and verbal communication are determined also by the patterns in the child's family and individual differences among children. Recall that expressive and receptive language can be different (see Chapter 5∞). A child may understand more (**receptive language**) than he or she verbalizes (**expressive language**).

Consideration must be given to the cultural influences and tone of voice, inflection, and volume. When a language barrier is encountered, the nurse should allow adequate time or seek a translator to enable the child and parents to express their thoughts.

Nonverbal Communication

Nonverbal communication patterns provide meaningful clues to the intended messages, especially when working with a pediatric

MediaLink Nonverbal Communication Video

population. Children communicate by *what* they do and *how* they do it. Children naturally express themselves nonverbally. They may cling to a parent when frightened, cry when hungry or tired, or moan when attempting to communicate desires. A child's silence may indicate fear, shyness, or anger. Aggressive nonverbal behaviors include biting, kicking, banging fists, and hitting; they may signify anger, frustration, or fear. Nonverbal communication includes facial expressions, body language, eye contact, gestures, posture, spatial distancing, touch, and physical appearance (Table 6–1). Look back to the picture in the opening scenario. What nonverbal cues are the parents and children displaying?

Interpretation of nonverbal communication may be ambiguous depending on the culture and the context of the situation (Table 6–2). For example, a child may not understand the meaning of certain gestures in the nurse's culture and thus misinterpret them; likewise, it is essential for the nurse to be familiar with the cultures in his or her community and understand the communication patterns. (See Developing Cultural Competence: Periods of Silence During Communication.)

Of considerable importance to the receiver of nonverbal messages is perceived incongruence between verbal and nonverbal communication; the receiver may interpret the nonverbal message rather than the verbal. For example, if a nurse smiles while preparing to change a painful dressing, the child may interpret that to mean the nurse enjoys causing pain.

TABLE 6–1 Nonverbal Communication Patterns in Major Cultural Groups*

CULTURAL GROUP	NONVERBAL COMMUNICATION PATTERNS
African American	Touch common with family members and close friends Close personal space
Chinese	Avoid direct eye contact when listening Distant personal space Prefer not to be touched by strangers
Eastern Indian	Direct eye contact is considered disrespectful Handshake between men only
Hispanic/Latino	Touch used often, especially between members of the same sex Close personal space
Japanese	Direct eye contact is considered disrespectful Handshaking acceptable Not accustomed to intimate physical contact by casual acquaintances Distant personal space
Native American	Close personal space Limited eye contact during conversation Silence during communication allows thinking and demonstrates respect
European (Spanish, French)	Use firm eye contact and look for impact of what has been said

* *Behavioral patterns of nonverbal behavior vary within groups, so avoid stereotyping any one group with these communication characteristics.*
Data from Spector, R. E. (2004). Cultural diversity in health and illness *(6th ed.). Upper Saddle River, NJ: Prentice Hall; Flores, G., Rabke-Verani, J., Pine, W., & Sabharwal, A. (2002). The importance of cultural and linguistic issues in the care of children.* Pediatric Emergency Care, 18*(4), 271–284.*

Paralanguage, another essential aspect of nonverbal communication, is the tone and pitch of the voice, speed, pace, volume, and inflection of the conversation, as well as other vocalizations. Paralanguage has as much, if not more, significance to the receiver

TABLE 6–2 Forms of Nonverbal Communication

BEHAVIOR	NURSING IMPLICATIONS
Standing	
At the beginning or end of interaction	Can indicate initiation/termination of interaction
Over other person while talking	Can indicate intimidation or domination
	The nurse can invite (with open hands) patient or family member to sit while conversing
Sitting	
Face to face	Indicates interest
Side by side	Neutrality
Turned away	Termination of the interaction
At the edge of the chair	Anxiety or eagerness
	The nurse can encourage further communication by a caring and calming voice and facial expression
Body Posture	
Relaxed	Friendliness, warmth
Rigid or tense	Fear or anger
Leaning back	Withdrawal, distance
Leaning forward	Interest, friendliness
Arms and/or legs tightly crossed	Self-protection, withdrawal
Shrinking in	Depression, low self-esteem
Turned away	Distance, withdrawal
	Constant awareness of body language by the nurse can result in enhanced communication
Gestures	
Leg or foot shaking, finger tapping	Anxiety, frustration, anger
Fidgety, restless movements	Anxiety, embarrassment
Finger shaking, hands on hips	Authority, intimidation
Hiding hands	Shyness, insecurity
Fist clenching	Anger, frustration
Wringing hands	Hopelessness, helplessness
	The nurse can display an empathetic and caring attitude to help patient and families relax during stressful events. Listening is an effective tool for exhibiting support
Eyes	
Frequent eye contact	Interest, honesty
Minimal eye contact	Low self-esteem, shyness, boredom
Rapidly shifting eye contact	Confusion
Frequent blinking	Anxiety
	The type of eye contact can display positive as well as negative feelings from the patient/family
Touch	
Touching arm or hand	Gentle touch (often) with permission can display interest and concern

Adapted from Fontaine, K. L. (2003). Relating, communicating, and educating. In Mental health nursing *(5th ed., p. 56). Upper Saddle River, NJ: Prentice Hall.*

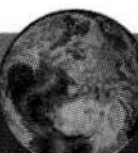

DEVELOPING CULTURAL COMPETENCE
Periods of Silence During Communication

Certain cultures, such as some Asian and Native American groups, consider the use of silence during conversations respectful. The nurse should avoid interruption of silence and allow the person time to reflect and formulate responses when communicating. In other cultures, silence may be utilized when the issue discussed is painful or sensitive. Be compassionate and recognize that parents and children will talk when they are ready (Seidel, et al., 2003). Refrain from saying something just to fill the silence with words.

as verbal messages do, especially with young children. From infancy, children understand paralanguage long before they know the meaning of the words. They sense anger and stress by the volume, the pitch, and the rate of the spoken word. Paying attention to the *rate* of speech is imperative when speaking to children, especially toddlers and preschoolers. The nurse who speaks hurriedly while instructing or informing the child likely will not capture the full attention or the cooperation that he or she would if speech were slower and more distinct.

Despite the significance of nonverbal communication, some pediatric studies concentrate on verbal, rather than nonverbal, communication. However, due to their level of verbal skills, children exhibit less verbal competence in interactions when compared to adults. To date, there are limited studies of child healthcare that include nonverbal interactions between children, parents, and pediatric nurses (Hyden & Baggins, 2004). This reveals a shortcoming in the overall implications of the child's presence in medical conversations.

Facial Expressions

The facial expressions of the nurse and child convey nonverbal messages more than any other body language (Figure 6–2 ■). Facial expressions include smiling, frowning, raising or lowering of eyebrows, and wrinkling of forehead. A child may be observed pouting or the lips may quiver, suggesting impending crying.

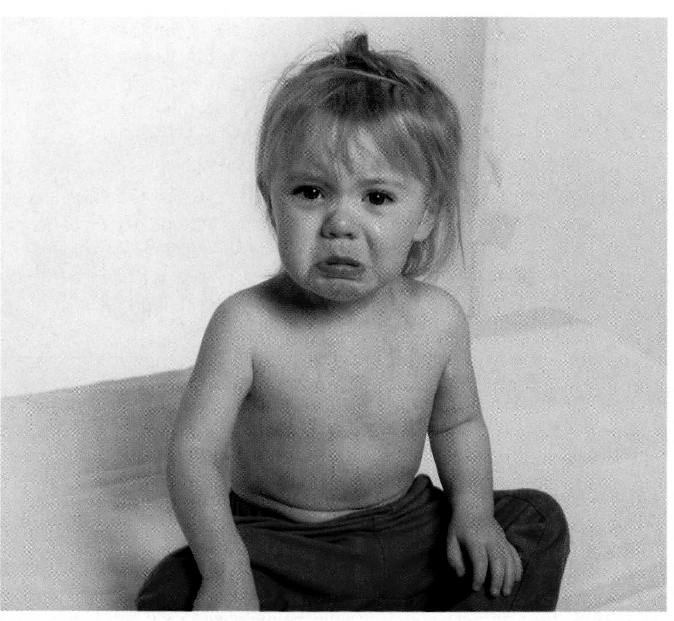

FIGURE 6–2 ■ Facial expressions are a powerful means of communication. What does this child's facial expression convey? What actions can the nurse take to reduce her distress?

Children with limited verbal expression are masters at using facial expression, eye contact, and gestures to send powerful messages about themselves, their feelings, and their needs; this method of communication can help guide the nurse when providing care. For example, while changing a dressing, the nurse observes the child's facial expressions for signs of pain and proceeds accordingly. Nonverbal communication offers a much wider context than verbal expression, which is often imprecise about the expression of emotion possible with body language. When nurses are sensitive to nonverbal communication, they can respond appropriately, and thus decrease the child's fears and anxieties (Chambers, 2003).

Body Language

Body language refers to movement of body parts and includes gestures and posture. Gestures often add emphasis to what is being said, for example, through shrugging of shoulders, shaking the head, tapping the feet, repetitive movement of feet or hands, and waving hands. The importance of understanding the cultural meaning of gestures may avoid misinterpretation when communicating.

The nurse's caring presence is conveyed in gestures as well as the patient's response to the communication (Godkin & Godkin, 2004). The nurse's posture can convey a positive or negative feeling to the child or parents. Sitting in a chair at the child's eye level and leaning forward is generally indicative of interest and a desire for open communication, whereas standing or leaning back in a chair with arms crossed can indicate disinterest or an unwillingness to communicate. An erect posture generally indicates self-assuredness, while a slouched posture can indicate a low self-esteem or not feeling well.

Eye Contact

The importance of maintaining eye contact varies according to cultural influences. For European Americans, maintaining eye contact during communication is essential to establishing trust and conveying interest, while in other cultures, such as Native American and some Asian cultures, sustained eye contact may be considered rude or disrespectful. Children in these cultures are taught from an early age to avert their gaze and to look downward when being addressed.

The eyes can also demonstrate emotions such as happiness or anger. Children often have a difficult time hiding their feelings, and their eyes tell the story. Tearing of the eyes can indicate sadness or sometimes happiness. Raising eyebrows may indicate confusion or astonishment. Rapid blinking may indicate anxiety, fear, or nervousness. Nurses need to recognize these nonverbal gestures and clarify what the child is experiencing at that time.

Touch

Nurses caring for infants and children routinely utilize touch with their young patients, both consciously and unconsciously. Therapeutic touch has been applied as a discipline in Western medicine since the 1970s, and has been used in other medical approaches over the centuries. A nurse, Dolores Krieger, was one of the first people to introduce therapeutic touch into mainstream contemporary practice (Kemper & Kelly, 2004). Therapeutic touch involves assessing and then mobilizing a child's energy fields to facilitate healing (Ireland & Olson, 2000). The most common pediatric conditions treated by therapeutic touch include asthma, anxiety, fatigue and insomnia, feelings of isolation, and pain (Kemper & Kelly, 2004). Healing touch is closely related to and derived from therapeutic touch. It is a specific type of touch that requires certification, and has been applied to alleviate specific health problems such as headache or menstrual pain.

Touch is used in many ways, however, and may not involve consciously applied techniques. Nurses use touch while performing procedures and treatments, but also use social, communicative touch especially with infants and young children. Touch conveys trust, compassion, caring, and can be calming to a parent and child. Touch may cause discomfort as a child grows older, and the nurse must be sensitive to the child and adolescent response. In addition, although often considered a demonstration of caring by nursing professionals, touch may be culturally inappropriate for some children and their families. Depending on these influences, touch can be perceived in some instances as a method of personalizing communication, while in others it is viewed as a violation of personal space. Various factors modify how, when, and even if touch should be utilized. These factors include the patient's age and physiological and psychological status, the setting, a variety of sociocultural factors, and the child's previous experience with touch, for example, if the child has experienced abuse or neglect.

Pediatric nurses should inform the parents and the child prior to touch, for example, when listening to the heart rate. Asking permission to touch is then perceived as a request. Constant observations of the response of the child to touch will help the nurse modify approach or technique. If a child is in pain, the nurse can ask if it is all right to rub the child's back or stroke a hand. Be sensitive to responses and whether the child settles with touch or pulls away. See Complementary Therapy: Research on Children and Touch.

Physical Appearance

The physical appearance of the child and family members can convey significant nonverbal messages to the nurse. Clothing style, grooming, and jewelry items such as religious artifacts can provide insight to the child's care and cultural beliefs. Children's clothing can often represent their values—what's important to them as represented by current fashion statements. The nurse should avoid making judgments based on how the child or family is dressed.

The nurse's physical appearance also communicates nonverbal messages to the child and family. The nurse in the pediatric setting typically wears colorful uniforms with lab jackets depicting children's favorite cartoon characters (Figure 6–3 ■). White uniforms are often avoided since children sometimes associate a white uniform with medical procedures, which may instill fear and block therapeutic communication.

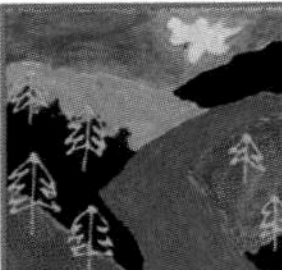

COMPLEMENTARY THERAPY

Research on Children and Touch

A review article described 14 studies of massage in children and 5 therapeutic touch studies. Massage is a form of tactile and kinesthetic stimulation, whereas therapeutic touch involves a skilled practitioner who assesses and mobilizes the child's energy fields to achieve relaxation or pain relief or to facilitate healing (Ireland & Olson, 2000). The authors concluded that massage therapy is related to growth and development achievements, decreased anxiety, improved sleep, and pain reduction.

Parasympathetic nervous response may be the explanation for these effects. The authors believe that similar physiologic mechanisms may be present in therapeutic touch but find that fewer studies in this area have been performed. Additional studies are recommended to determine the outcomes of both techniques in children, but the authors found that massage therapy, especially in premature babies and other infants, improves several parameters of health in young children.

FACTORS INFLUENCING COMMUNICATION WITH CHILDREN AND THEIR FAMILIES

Essentially every aspect of a child's life influences communication, from an infant's crying due to a wet diaper to a teen's explosion of anger when parents refuse permission to drive the family car. The child's style of communication is also influenced by his or her environment, spatial distancing, time, and culture (Table 6–3).

The nurse needs to consider factors unique to the family and situation that can act as blocks to effective communication. Barriers to communication can be physical and/or psychological. Physical factors include:

- Language used (such as medical jargon)
- Gender

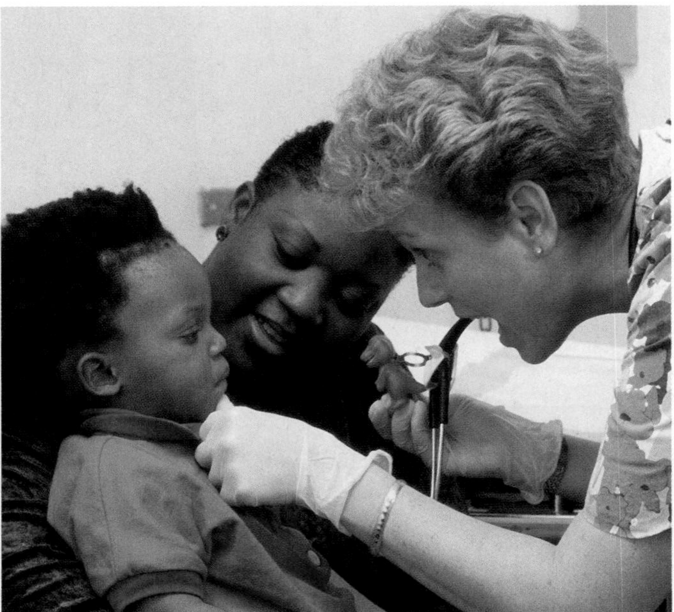

FIGURE 6–3 ■ Notice the nurse's brightly colored uniform and her attempts to allay the child's fears. She is showing a toy and is ready to quickly examine the mouth if the boy smiles.

TABLE 6–3 Factors Influencing Communication

FACTOR	NURSING IMPLICATIONS
Environmental Factors	
Surroundings and sensory stimuli noted during the communication process	➤ Physical environment should include a quiet, private room at a comfortable temperature and with adequate lighting. ➤ Adequate seating for the child and immediate family members should be readily available, with chairs facing each other to promote communication. ➤ For the small child, remove any unnecessary medical equipment that may be frightening to the child. ➤ Provide privacy and comfort for difficult conversations; the child and family's privacy are maintained at all times.
Spatial Distancing Patterns	
The distance between the participants in communication, often referred to as "personal space." Each person defines his or her own personal space zone and cultural influence is a key determinant in establishing this zone of comfort. The zone may also vary according to the specific situation and with whom the space is shared. (See Chapter 3 for further discussion of spatial distancing patterns.)	➤ Determine the appropriate spatial distancing pattern preference prior to session. ➤ Assess for nonverbal cues in level of comfort with personal closeness and contact.
Time	
Ample time is needed to communicate with the child and family. The appearance of being rushed may be perceived negatively.	➤ The nurse may have a difficult balance to respond to questions and provide information within the time available. ➤ Focus on the family and child for the time available and avoid giving signals concerning the need to move on to other tasks during that dedicated time.
Culture	
Culture influences the child and family's communication patterns. Linguistic barriers associated with culturally diverse populations provide a unique opportunity for the nurse to employ a variety of communication techniques.	➤ Assess the impact that culture has on communication to determine the best methods for communication. ➤ The use of interpreters, translators, foreign language dictionaries, and symbols or pictures from the family's native language can help to decrease a language barrier. ➤ An interpreter or translator may not be available at all times; however, be aware of when to have one available for significant conversations and consent for treatment. ➤ Prior to session, discuss with the interpreter the plan of care for the child and a list of possible questions from the nurse.

- Environment
- Linguistic barriers

Psychosocial barriers include:

- Child's health status
- Parents' emotions related to their child's health status
- Culture
- Spatial distancing patterns

Medical Jargon

The healthcare system has its own unique language. **Medical jargon** refers to the technical language associated with healthcare. Using this technical language when discussing information with the child and family can lead to major barriers in communication. This language may confuse the child and family members who have no prior experience with medical terminology.

The child and family may also experience powerlessness when faced with unfamiliar environments coupled with an unfamiliar language. Older adolescents and adults may feel embarrassed or offended because they are unable to understand the meaning of medical terminology and may even feel the offense was intentional. Jargon translated into more accessible terms fosters understanding.

Gender

Gender is an important consideration in establishing effective communication. A child may respond more positively to females than males if the child associates caring and nurturing with women. Furthermore, if the child associates negative experiences with a particular gender, such as a male physician who performed a bone marrow biopsy in which the child experienced pain, the child may also withdraw from other healthcare professionals who appear similar (e.g., a male wearing a white jacket).

In addition, some cultures place less value on the female's authority and others do not consider females to be experts or have authority, including the female nurse discussing health-related issues. The child taught that the female has no authority may not cooperate with the female nurse or follow instructions.

MediaLink Caring and Empathy Video

Child's Health Status

The family dealing with a child's illness and hospitalization may be experiencing stress, anxiety, confusion, or shock. Parental emotions regarding their child's illness may range from overt exhibition of anger to complete withdrawal. When the family is preoccupied with their child's condition they may be unable to communicate effectively and may even be unable to understand simple messages.

Families who have confidence in and trust the nurse caring for their child exhibit decreased anxiety. Nurses can decrease parental stress by providing parents with information and education in a nonjudgmental manner. Communication with the distraught family requires skill, patience, compassion, and the use of therapeutic techniques described later in the chapter.

Nursing Attitudes

The nurse's attitude transcends all actions and is key in establishing open lines of communication with child and family, who are astute at identifying the nurse who is caring, empathetic, and family centered versus the nurse who is indifferent or concerned with interests related only to nursing tasks. Comfort and reassurance can be provided to the child and family when the nurse's communication techniques are individualized according to developmental stage, abilities, and cultural influences.

Caring refers to the nurse's emotional investment in the child and family. The caring nurse evokes feelings of security and comfort in the child and family by perceiving the child's needs and concerns, displaying behaviors that indicate the child is valued, comforting, and offering presence of self. A caring environment provides the child and family the atmosphere needed for open communication.

Empathy is the ability to perceive another person's experience from his or her point of view, in other words, "putting oneself in another's shoes." Empathy differs from sympathy in that the nurse associates with the feelings of the child rather than understanding them. Sympathy is not always therapeutic in caring for a child as it can lead to emotional overinvolvement and possibly professional burnout. Some nurses are naturally empathetic; however, empathy can be learned by focusing on the child's developmental parameters and verbal and nonverbal language.

DEVELOPMENTAL AND COGNITIVE CONSIDERATIONS FOR COMMUNICATION WITH CHILDREN

By virtue of their developmental ages, children process information differently than adults. Children are egocentric and they often have difficulty in understanding another person's point of view. They expect those around them to understand what they are thinking or feeling without the prerequisite exchange of information; in other words, assuming that another's experiences are the same as theirs, others should understand how they feel.

Children may not necessarily comprehend what they hear, despite indicating that they do understand. Children also express themselves through nonverbal messages more frequently than adults, since by adulthood more control is exercised over nonverbal forms of communication. The nurse must consider the developmental and cognitive levels of the child for whom communication is intended. This section provides an overview of developmental factors affecting the child's communication. Discussion of language acquisition according to the child's developmental stage is discussed in Chapter 5∞.

Newborn

The primary mode of communication for the newborn is through nonverbal methods and crying. Newborns have no comprehension of words; however, they are attentive to human voice and presence. The newborn responds to touch through patting, stroking, rocking, and comforting. Touch has been shown to be a significant positive factor in the development of newborns and infants. Recent studies of premature infants in the NICU show that the use of touch, combined with massage, resulted in increased infant weight gain, improved developmental scores, and early hospital discharge (Beachy, 2003; Mainous, 2002). "Kangaroo care," or wrapping a baby to the mother's chest, has proven to be a positive influence on the infant's physiological outcomes. Nurses have conducted research studies on the importance of touch with infants. Early skin-to-skin contact between infant and mother is accomplished by putting the baby on the mother's chest soon after birth. An analysis of 17 studies that examined effects of this contact found positive effects on length and success of breastfeeding, infant regulation of temperature, amount of infant crying, infant blood glucose, and maternal attachment (Anderson, Moore, Hepworth, et al., 2003). Nurses can encourage infant touch by parents, can teach techniques of infant massage, and can use touch to comfort babies in healthcare encounters.

Infant

Like the newborn, young infants have no comprehension of words; however, they are also attentive to human voice and presence. The infant continues to respond to touch through patting, stroking, rocking, and comforting. Other stimuli such as singing and developmentally appropriate toys such as rattles elicit responses in the infant.

Infants initially communicate through nonverbal methods and crying. Facial expressions, quivering, and thrashing arms and legs may indicate distress or pain. Cooing, leg kicking, and arm waving may mean contentment and interest in engaging in interaction.

Over time, infants learn to communicate through touch, hearing, and sight. Verbal communication is demonstrated by cooing and crying. Infants will communicate hunger, pain, and other discomforts through crying. Infants develop a bonding relationship with parents, siblings, other family members, and caregivers through touch, as touch can convey safety and love. Nurses can facilitate the communication between an infant and parent, as well as model positive communication techniques.

The following may help to promote communication with the newborn or infant and family.

- Do not block the infant's view of parents.
- Do not remove the infant from parent's arms unless necessary.
- Speak in a high-pitched, soft tone.
- Establish eye contact with the baby but be sensitive that when the baby turns away a period of relaxation is needed.
- Avoid leaning over the infant's face and talking in a forceful tone.
- Use swaddling, rubbing, patting, cuddling, or rocking to quiet a crying baby.
- Communicate through play, such as peek-a-boo.
- Be aware that stranger anxiety may occur in infants age 6 to 12 months.

Toddler and Preschooler

The acquisition of language in the toddler is rapid. Toddlers begin using three to four words appropriately by 12 to 15 months. By 15 to 18 months, toddlers can typically use ten words including names, and are capable of naming objects. The use of short sentences of three to four words is observed by 18 to 24 months. Approximately 90% of the toddler's speech is comprehensible by 24 to 36 months (Seidel, Ball, Dains, et al., 2003).

Toddlers and preschoolers need the opportunity to express their thoughts. Adults are often tempted to interrupt toddlers and complete their sentences for them. This can lead to the child experiencing frustration or shame (Deering & Cody, 2002). When caring for toddlers, allow them time to verbalize. Ask parents questions initially and then direct questions at the toddler once they are comfortable with the setting.

The toddler and preschooler are egocentric, and interpret the world from their own points of view. The toddler is developing a sense of self and asserts independence. Allowing the toddler choices when possible promotes communication.

The preschooler is concrete and literal. Avoid using expressions and vocabulary that are likely to be misunderstood by the child. For example, the nurse may say, "We will put *dye* in your arm," and the child may interpret this statement as "the arm will *die.*" Instead, the nurse might state, "We will give you some medicine in your arm and it will feel warm." See Table 6–4.

Preschoolers also have short attention spans and limited memory of recent events, so asking them what they did yesterday would likely not reveal an accurate recounting. At about 3 years of age, preschoolers can state their name and address if they are taught this information. They can describe the names of toys and family members, but they may not be able to give details of an event unless it had special significance, such as a situation that caused them to feel happy or sad, or was painful.

Preschoolers ask numerous questions and they should be given ample opportunity to ask more questions if they desire. For the child to comprehend the information, the responses to these questions should be brief and honest.

Preschoolers engage in magical thinking and believe that inanimate objects, such as the blood pressure cuff, may come alive and harm them. The sounds of electronic equipment may seem to give the machine life as a "monster." The child can act out feelings and thoughts through dramatic play, puppets, and drawings (Deering & Cody, 2002).

TABLE 6–4 Language Alternatives when Communicating with Children

POTENTIALLY CONFUSING OR AMBIGUOUS WORDS OR STATEMENTS	ALTERNATE COMMUNICATION CHOICE
"We will give you some dye in your arm."	"We will put some warm medicine into your arm."
"I will give you a shot."	"I will give you some medicine through a small needle."
"This will hurt or burn."	"It might feel sore or very warm."
"The doctor will make a small cut/incision."	"The doctor will make a small opening."
"Gas, anesthesia"	"Medicine that you breathe or get through your arm to make you sleep"
"The medicine tastes bad."	"Some children say the medicine tastes different to them."

To promote communication with the toddler or preschooler:

- Acknowledge the child, but interact with parents before communicating with the child. This allows the child the opportunity to become accustomed to the nurse's presence.
- Communicate with the child at his or her eye level.
- Communicate using simple language and short sentences.
- Be honest in responses to the child.
- Avoid discussing frightening matters in front of the child.
- Encourage the child to engage in imaginative play with dolls, drawings, or puppets to allow the child to act out feelings and thoughts.
- Encourage toddlers to engage in parallel play.
- Encourage preschoolers to engage in dramatic and associative play (see Chapter 5∞ for further description of play in childhood).
- Allow the child the opportunity to ask questions.
- Allow additional time for the child to express thoughts without interruption.
- Offer the toddler choices when possible, such as "Do you want ice cream or a popsicle?" This helps the child assert his or her independence.

School-Age Child

The school-age child is able to use logic and understand certain events. School-age children also begin to understand the viewpoints of others, making them capable of empathy. School-age children begin to understand body parts and organs, which allows them the opportunity to better understand hospitalization and illness. Clear and developmentally appropriate explanations of procedures can facilitate the child's participation in the decision-making process concerning

MediaLink Care Plan: Preschooler Hospitalized for Diabetes

healthcare (Box 6–1). This participation decreases the child's anxiety and fears (Runeson, Hallstrom, Elander, et al., 2002).

School-age children possess a large vocabulary and can provide important information about what they are feeling. Due to their developmental level, however, school-age children may misinterpret information. The use of simple questions, such as "Why do you think you are in the hospital?" can reveal misconceptions and offer an opportunity for clarification (Deering & Cody, 2002). When explanations are offered, knowledge transferred to the child allows the child to feel some control over the situation.

The following may help to promote communication with the school-age child.

- Explain all procedures, techniques, and events.
- Speak directly to the child.
- Be honest in responses to the child.
- Encourage the child to express thoughts and feelings through drawing, writing, or painting.
- Provide the school-age child with third-person conversation prompts, such as "Sometimes kids have told me that they are afraid of having surgery." This may encourage the child to admit fears or learn about the situation by asking about the other children.

Adolescent

Adolescents pose a particular communication challenge in their quest to be viewed as adults, even though they have not yet achieved adult cognitive abilities. Adolescents have adequate cognitive capacity to understand and employ abstractions in communication, but their ability to **decode** or interpret medical terminology is limited to their past healthcare experiences.

Adolescents may feel that adults do not understand them and that they may not be treated with respect. Although communication between teen patients and their parents is strongly encouraged by the healthcare team, HIPAA privacy rule allows the adolescent in some cases to request special privacy protection and speak with the nurse in private, without the presence of parents (English & Ford, 2004). (See Chapter 1∞ for more on confidentially and consent.) To build an effective communication relationship with an adolescent, the nurse must allow time to build rapport and establish trust.

The following may help to promote communication with the adolescent.

- Use a straightforward approach and explain the purpose of the interaction.
- Encourage the adolescent's participation by initiating a topic unrelated to health, such as "Tell me about your favorite music."
- Reassure the adolescent that he or she does not have to talk about anything until ready.
- Do not interrupt and avoid comments or expressions that convey disapproval or surprise.
- Be aware of laws and limits regarding confidentiality. Inform the adolescent that anything affecting his or her immediate safety (such as suicidal ideation) must be communicated to the parent. Issues such as birth control vary from state to state, so clarify guidelines in the jurisdiction where the teen is seen for healthcare.
- Provide the adolescent the opportunity to interact with the nurse in private, without the parents present.
- Listen more than you talk (Deering & Cody, 2002).
- Offer the adolescent choices when possible (e.g., procedure times, lunch times).
- Do not assume that the adolescent is on the same cognitive level as adults even though he or she may appear to be.

See Table 6–5 for guidelines on preparing a child for procedures according to developmental level.

BOX 6–1 Clear Communication: A Child's Point of View

In a study of children ages 4–17 years, researchers determined, based on the children's previous experiences, what they prefer in terms of communication with healthcare providers (Sydnor-Greenberg & Dokken, 2001). Mothers were also interviewed and offered their opinions; the responses were categorized into five components, developing what the researchers identified as the CLEAR communication framework:

1. **Context**—see the child as more than a medical diagnosis
2. **Listening**—allow the child to speak without being interrupted and to not make disapproving comments
3. **Empowerment**—make the child feel important; speak directly to the child and not to the parents, using developmentally appropriate terms
4. **Advice**—give child the resources to assist him or her in managing the illness
5. **Reassurance**—recognize the child's ability to manage symptoms, to promote self-esteem

Adapted from Sydnor-Greenberg, N., & Dokken, D. L. (2001). Communicate in healthcare: Thoughts on the child's perspective. Journal of Child and Family Nursing, *4(3), 225–230.*

MediaLink Care Plan: Infant with a Hearing Impairment

The Child with Special Needs

Effective communication is reciprocal. Children who are unable to communicate verbally due to physical, developmental, or acquired disabilities such as cerebral palsy, brain injuries, or intubation may experience anxiety and frustration. Feelings of helplessness may be exacerbated in young children, who are at a developmental disadvantage as they are frightened by the unfamiliar sights and sounds of the hospital and at the same time, powerless to communicate to the people in charge of caring for them. Families may also become anxious due to their child's frustration with his or her communication impairment.

Positive communication strategies with the nonverbal child include signs or gestures, picture boards, or writing tablets. For children who may be neurologically impaired, the nurse must be sensitive to the child's nonverbal cues such as facial expressions, eye gaze, and body language. Direct eye contact, repeating the child's name, and speaking in a calm voice can help decrease the child's anxiety. To elicit responses from the child, a system such as head nods or eye blinks for "yes" or "no" can be established.

TABLE 6–5 Communication Strategies to Prepare Children for Procedures Based on Developmental Level

DEVELOPMENTAL LEVEL	PREPARATION AND RATIONALE
Newborn and infant	Talk to the newborn. *Newborns have no concrete understanding of verbal communication, but do respond to a soothing voice.*
Toddler	Integrate the toddler's own words into the explanation. *Using their limited vocabulary provides better comprehension.* Explain the procedures immediately before they are carried out. *Toddlers have limited attention span and will forget if explanations are given too early.*
Preschooler	Explain the procedures to the child 1 to 2 hours before they are carried out. *Although preschoolers have short attention spans, they remember longer than a toddler and are able to remember for several hours.* Utilize dolls, play, and storytelling to explain procedures. *These forms of play use verbal and physical interaction. Feelings can be expressed through a "third person," such as a doll.*
School-age child	Explain the procedures several days in advance if possible. *School-age children have concrete operational thought and can remember events and explanations; knowing in advance can help them to mobilize resources for dealing with the procedure.* Utilize reading materials, books, videos, and drawings to explain procedures. *These allow for use of the child's concrete thinking.*
Adolescents	Explain the procedures up to 1 week in advance. *The teen is able to comprehend concrete and abstract concepts. They may like to think about the procedure and plan for how to deal with it.* Utilize peer mentoring to assist in explaining procedures. *The teen often responds to those in their own age group. They may have a fear of adults, but identify with other teens with the same illness.* Utilize reading materials and videos to assist in explaining procedures. *Adolescents can read, comprehend, and are interested in the scientific information associated with their illness. Feeling informed increases their self-esteem.*

When the child is intubated, the tube blocks the vocal cords and speech is prohibited. Children experiencing oral surgery, dental surgery, oral trauma, or facial trauma may also not be able to verbally communicate. The nurse can decrease the child's anxiety by thoroughly explaining to the child that he or she will be able to speak when the tube is removed. Alternate means of communication such as a writing board, alphabet board, keyboard, symbol cards, or other methods of communication are essential for the child's physical and psychological well-being.

Communicating with a Child with an Alteration in Visual Perception

Nonsighted or children with limited visual perception are challenged when removed from their familiar environment, especially during hospitalization. Nurses can enhance communication with the child by the following:

- Identify self when entering the room; encourage others to do so.
- Orient the ambulating child to the objects in the room.
- Speak with a calm, slow voice—do not shout.
- Explain procedure before touching the child.
- Allow the child to handle the equipment when appropriate.
- Explain any unfamiliar sounds the child may hear.
- Encourage parents to stay with young children.
- Continually observe child's facial expression.
- Announce when exiting the room.

Communicating with the Child with an Alteration in Hearing Perception

Children with hearing deficits may be challenged in healthcare settings because they do not hear healthcare personnel or equipment; this can result in increased anxiety and stress. Nurses can enhance communication with a child who is hard of hearing or deaf by the following:

- Always enter the child's room slowly—sudden images may startle the child.
- Face child when speaking—to get his or her attention.
- Assess the degree of the hearing impairment—to consider the necessity of using a registered interpreter.
- Clarify the roles of the nurse and the interpreter—the nurse's awareness of how to use an interpreter will increase his or her credibility from the child's viewpoint.
- Inform the child that the interpreter is bound to confidentiality.

See Developing Cultural Competence: Suggested Guidelines for Communicating Using an Interpreter or Translator.

Communicating with the Child Who Does Not Speak English

Given the variety of cultures in the United States and a continued increase in refugees and immigrants, the nurse will likely come in contact with a child and family who do not speak English. (See Chapter 3∞ for a discussion of culture.) In a recent study looking at 13 "encounters" or translation sessions with patients, researchers found 396 errors in omission of information or false fluency when ad hoc interpreters (nurses, social workers, and a 11-year-old sibling) were used rather than a hospital or medical interpreter (Flores, Laws, Mayo, et al., 2003). The errors committed by the ad hoc interpreters were significantly more likely to have potential clinical consequences than those committed by hospital interpreters; the authors suggest third-party reimbursement for trained interpreter services for patients with limited English proficiency.

Children who are hospitalized and do not understand English are examined by people they do not know, and see and hear

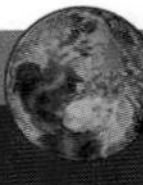

DEVELOPING CULTURAL COMPETENCE
Suggested Guidelines for Communicating Using an Interpreter or Translator

Nurses sometimes provide care to children and families with whom they cannot directly communicate. The family members may speak a language with which the nurse is not proficient, or the child may be deaf and might use sign language to communicate. Whatever the reason, certain guidelines can foster positive communication with the child and family. It is generally viewed as positive if the nurse can speak at least a few words in the child's language or is able to sign to introduce self. Other general guidelines are as follows:

- Obtain a skilled interpreter or translator who is adept at both languages or systems of communication.
- Arrange seating so that the nurse and child or family face each other and both can readily see the translator. Speak to the child and family, rather than to the interpreter.
- Ensure a situation that fosters communication such as soft and appropriate lighting, quiet environment, and comfort for all present.
- Ensure that all information is transmitted. If preliminary introductions occur with the translator, ask him or her to tell the child and family what was said. If the family has much to say to the interpreter but the interpreter relays only a few words to the nurse, ask for further explanation of content.
- Have the family evaluate the translation services at a later time so they can state positive and negative parts of the experience. Another interpreter may be needed to successfully accomplish this evaluation. Adjust use of translators as needed to meet the family's needs, considering their preference for gender, age, and other characteristics.
- Avoid using children as translators for family members because the family may not feel comfortable sharing all healthcare issues with the child, and it can be a burden for the child to translate for the family. Confidentiality is also an issue.
- Be sensitive to issues that are confidential such as child abuse, alcoholism, pregnancy, and others. Watch for nonverbal communication that shows discomfort with the discussions occurring.

Further guidelines can be found in National Standards for Culturally and Linguistically Appropriate Services in Health Care. (2001). Washington, DC: U.S. Department of Health and Human Services.

things which may make no sense to them, as they cannot benefit from the nurse's explanation. Therefore, when the nurse is interacting with a child who speaks another language, the goal is to minimize the possible negative outcomes related to the circumstances surrounding the child's treatment regimen. Studies have demonstrated that when the nurse speaks a few words or phrases in the child's language, the child interprets it as a desire to connect, which lessens the communication barrier, and invites trust (Green-Hernandez, Quinn, Denham-Vitale, et al., 2004).

Some basic tips for communicating with a child and/or family who do not speak English include:

- Determine the need for a medical or hospital translator and use the same translator for each interaction if possible (Figure 6–4 ■).
- Speak to the child in a normal tone of voice.
- Use a communication board with pictures and names of basic needs or requests printed in both languages (e.g., bathroom, water, food, pain, hot, cold).

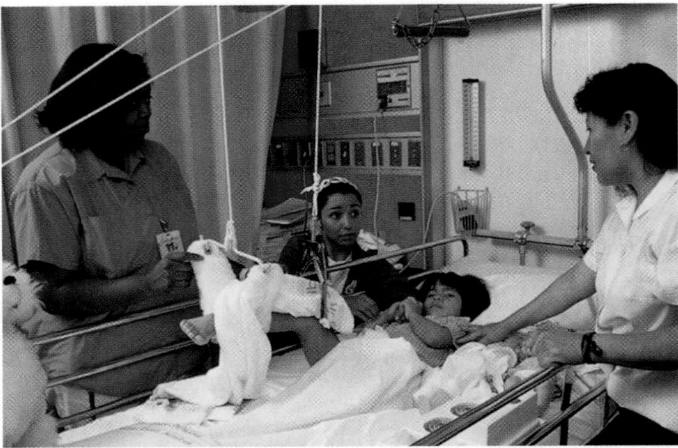

FIGURE 6–4 ■ Most hospitals have designated interpreters that you should use. If not available, find a professional interpreter whom you have identified beforehand and who knows medical terms and the cultural norms of the family. The interpreter (center) should be positioned to improve communication. Maintain eye contact with the parent or patient, not the interpreter. To ensure confidentiality of information for parents, avoid using a family member for history taking.

- Learn commonly used words in the child's language when possible.
- Allow all family members the opportunity to express their feelings.
- Encourage parents and other family members to participate in the child's care.
- Develop a plan of care that includes acknowledgment and respect of the child's culture.
- Offer the family appropriate reassurance.
- Acknowledge effective parenting.

NURSING MANAGEMENT

The goal of nursing management is to collaborate with the child and family in establishing effective communication in order to plan and provide nursing care.

■ Nursing Assessment and Diagnosis

A thorough assessment of the child's mental, physical, developmental, and cognitive abilities is necessary to identify the most effective method of communication with the child. Assess the child's developmental level, communication abilities, factors influencing communication, and potential barriers to communication. In addition, assess the language, communication skills, and level of understanding of the parent. (See Chapter 8∞ for assessment and interviewing techniques.)

Nursing diagnoses related to communication that may apply to the child and family include:

- Impaired Verbal Communication related to language development (toddler)

MediaLink Case Study: A School-Age Child Who Is Non-English Speaking

- Readiness for Enhanced Individual Coping related to communication about planned diagnostic procedures
- Disturbed Sensory Perception: Visual or Auditory related to alteration in reception, transmission, or integration
- Impaired Social Interaction related to verbal communication disability
- Readiness for Enhanced Communication related to availability of a medical interpreter or translator

■ Planning and Implementation

The focus of nursing interventions is facilitation of effective therapeutic communication with the child and family, and the resulting establishment of an effective nurse–child–family relationship (Table 6–6). The nurse accomplishes these tasks through the use of specific techniques, attitudes, and skills tailored to the needs of the child and family (Figure 6–5 ■). See Partnering with Families: Establishing Rapport with Children on page 185. Providing an appropriate environment will foster effective nurse–child–family communication Remember to provide privacy to ensure confidentiality.

Establish Trust

Trust plays a critical role for an effective nurse–child–family relationship. To establish an atmosphere of trust, the nurse should do the following:

- Follow through with promises to child and family—ensures secure feelings for family.
- Respect confidentiality—promotes protection of family.
- Be truthful with the child and family—they will respect the nurse, even if the truth is not what they want to hear.

If a child asks whether a procedure is painful, answer truthfully, but follow with positive words. For example, if a child asks if his "shot" is going to hurt, you might reply, "Yes, most people say that a shot hurts, but it will only hurt for a moment, and then it will be over. Your mother can hold your hand while I give you the medicine, if that will make you feel better."

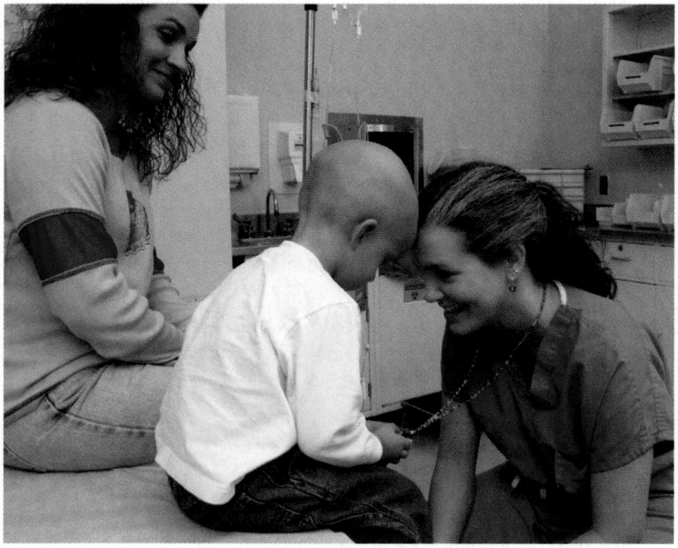

FIGURE 6–5 ■ Taking time to listen to the family members and child is important to the establishment of trust and developing a rapport with the child and family.

Maintain Confidentiality

Essential to the development of trust between the nurse, child, and family is an understanding of the confidentiality of shared information, especially when related to a sensitive nature. To foster trust, assure the child and family that information is shared only with those directly involved in the child's care. For the older child and adolescent, the nurse offers them the opportunity to discuss matters privately, without the presence of their parents. Explain any exceptions to confidentiality to the child or adolescent. Exceptions to confidentiality include situations such as the child potentially posing a danger to self or others, for example, with suicidal ideation or homicidal thoughts.

Practitioners are increasingly concerned about losing the trust of their patient if they disclose information gained in confidence; however, if the child has consented, either verbally or in writing, that the information may be shared, there is no breach of confidentiality. In other cases, the child needs to be informed that confidential information must be shared due to state reporting requirements or safety concerns for the child. The nurse should take the time to explain the rationale for sharing confidential information in an effort to gain the child's assent and maintain trust.

Convey Respect

Nursing behaviors that demonstrate respect for the child and family include:

- Knocking before entering the room to denote respectful attitude
- Addressing the child by first name and parents by "Mr" or "Ms"
- Looking at the child when asking questions to encourage response from child
- Considering the family's values, culture, and feelings, such as spatial distancing and eye contact, to enhance communication
- Explaining needed procedures before beginning assessments or interventions
- Encouraging their participation in discussions with the multidisciplinary team

Implement Appropriate Communication Strategies

Implement appropriate verbal and nonverbal communication strategies. Be aware of nontherapeutic communication techniques that can lead to communication barriers; they are often based in bias and/or judgment, and it is essential for the nurse to recognize his or her own feelings and separate those from the

TABLE 6–6 Using Therapeutic Communication Techniques with Children

COMMUNICATION TECHNIQUE	EXAMPLE	NURSING IMPLICATION
Accepting	"It is okay to cry, I know that this hurts."	The nurse should empathize with the child's thoughts and feelings. Conveying acceptance includes respecting the child's emotions by allowing the child to cry when in pain or letting the child know that crying is okay. Assist the child to channel aggression into a constructive outlet such as talking about feelings or play that is an outlet such as tossing a bean bag or using a punching bag.
Active listening	Pay attention to what the child says, acknowledge the child's feelings, and avoid interruption.	Involve children in the discussion and encourage them to relay their points of view. Face the child and parents when talking to let the child and family know that the nurse is listening and understands what is being communicated.
Broad openings	"What do you want to talk about right now?"	Use open-ended questions to allow the child to choose the discussion topic.
Clarifying	*Child*: "Whenever the doctor tells me I have to stay in the hospital longer, I get so mad." *Nurse:* "It sounds like you are very angry. What does that feel like?"	Communicate understanding by asking the child to clarify or elaborate on the thoughts expressed.
Collaborating	"Perhaps we can work together and figure out the best way to go about handling this."	Assist the child and family through the problem-solving process. The nurse first suggests collaboration with the child and/or family, and then assists them to work through each step of the problem-solving process.
Exploring	"Can you tell me more about how you feel after you receive your chemotherapy?"	Exploring helps the child to organize thoughts and focus on particular issues as well as encourages the child to freely discuss issue in more detail.
Focusing	"I do want to hear about your dog in a little while, but right now could you tell me about your stomachache?"	Utilize focusing to guide the direction of the conversation. This is useful for small children who often wish to discuss a variety of topics rather than focus on one topic. Do not interrupt the child while he or she is talking; allow the child to finish and then refocus the direction of the conversation. It is important to provide the child the opportunity to discuss various topics, so allow the child to talk freely at times.
Giving recognition	"That is a very colorful picture you are drawing."	Identify observed behaviors or cues of the child. This indicates an interest in the child.
Observations	"You tell me you aren't hurting, but your fists are clenched and your mouth is quivering." "You seem sad today."	Pay close attention to the behavioral aspect of communication. The nurse acknowledges behaviors of the child, which indicate their thoughts and feelings. The nurse may make observations about incongruence in the child's messages, and the meaning of these mixed signals can be explored with the child.
Offering self	"I will stay with you while your mother goes to the cafeteria to eat lunch."	The nurse is available to listen and be with the child.
Placing the event in time or sequence	"Which happened first. . . ?" "When did you first start feeling. . . ?"	Assist the child to determine what happened and in what order. The goal is to help the child and nurse understand the progression of events.
Reflection	*Adolescent*: "I keep thinking about what my friends are doing while I am in the hospital, and if they miss me." *Nurse:* "It is hard not being with your friends."	Repeat a phrase or sentence the child just said. By reflection, the nurse indicates an interest in the discussion, active listening, and a desire for further elaboration.
Restatement or paraphrasing	*Child:* "I think I should tell my mother that I have been smoking." *Nurse:* "You want to tell your mother about your smoking?"	The nurse repeats what the child has said using different words. By restating, the nurse is acknowledging to the child that he or she is listening to them and it also provides a means to validate the interpretation of the child's statement.

TABLE 6–6 Using Therapeutic Communication Techniques with Children (continued)

COMMUNICATION TECHNIQUE	EXAMPLE	NURSING IMPLICATION
Summarizing	"The two main issues that you want to address with your doctor this evening are. . . "	Highlight the key facts obtained in the conversation by condensing the information the child related. Summarizing provides the child and nurse an opportunity to consider further direction of the discussion or as a means to give the discussion closure. The nurse can summarize at various points during the conversation; it is not necessary to wait until the discussion is nearing completion.
Validating perceptions	"It sounds like you are sad about being sick. Is that correct?"	The nurse shares the conclusions drawn from the discussion with the child. Validating perceptions provides an opportunity for the child to confirm or deny the nurse's interpretation of the meaning of their communication.

Data from Fontaine, K. L. (2003). Relating, communicating, and educating. In Mental health nursing *(5th ed.). Upper Saddle River, NJ: Prentice Hall.*

child and family. Table 6–7 provides examples of ineffective communication techniques and nursing implications.

Encourage Communication Through Alternate Techniques

Children have the ability to communicate thoughts and feelings in ways other than verbal expression. Play, writing, drawing, journaling, storytelling, bibliotherapy, and humor are effective methods to encourage the child's communication.

PLAY

Play promotes growth and development and is crucial for the mental health of children. It has been described as the "work" of children in that it confirms what children know about their world and allows them to explore the rest. Play has been further described as the "language" of childhood; it is the talk, and the toys are its words.

Children have limited experience with stressful events; therefore, when illness or hospitalization occurs, their fears and anxieties rise. Where hospitalization forces a passive role on children, play allows them to take an active role, thus allowing them to gain an increased sense of independence. Role or fantasy play utilizing puppets, dolls, stuffed animals, skits, and visits from cartoon characters offer the child an opportunity to learn about health issues affecting them as well as providing an opportunity to communicate their feelings. Allowing children to play with unfamiliar equipment (that has been thoroughly inspected to ensure the child's safety) is another effective means of play. Handling the equipment and pretending to use the equipment, such as giving the doll a "shot," helps the child to understand what will happen and further allows expression of fears and concerns. Furthermore, especially for children engaged in magical thinking, through play the equipment loses some of its influence as a frightening object once the child observes that the equipment is not "alive" (Figure 6–6 ■).

EXPRESSIVE PLAY—PAINTING, DRAWING

Younger children have developed fine motor ability to draw with crayons, markers, chalk, and colored pencils. While drawings are used as an assessment tool to determine a child's developmental level, they are also a therapeutic activity in which the child is free to put into pictures that which he or she may not be able to put into words. Having children express themselves through drawing, poetry, songs, or pictures often reveals critical information that can change the direction of planned nursing care (Michael, Candela, & Mitchell, 2002). Although the stress of hospitalization and illness can easily be interpreted, other drawings, such as those related to abuse and trauma, should be interpreted by a certified play therapist who is specially trained in interpretation of children's drawings. Provide the child with opportunities and necessary equipment to draw or paint (Figure 6–7 ■). Ask if the child would prefer to draw or paint, though both approaches may be

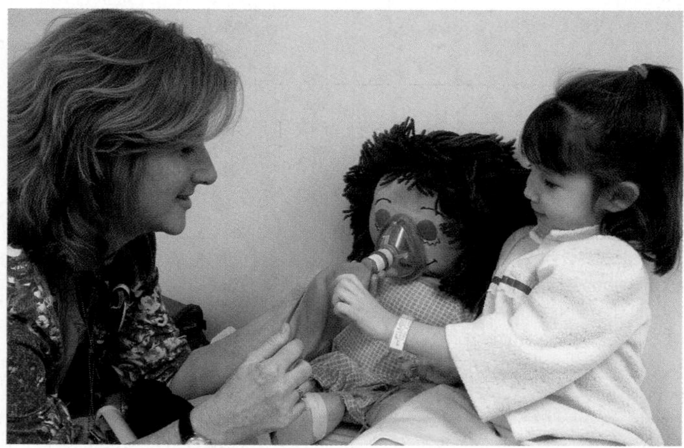

FIGURE 6–6 ■ Putting a mask on her doll gives this child some mastery over her coming surgical experience. It is important for children to see and touch medical equipment in order to allay fears of the unknown.

TABLE 6–7 Ineffective Communication Techniques

INEFFECTIVE COMMUNICATION TECHNIQUE	EXAMPLE	NURSING IMPLICATIONS
Advising (nurse tells the child what to do)	"If I were you, I would tell your parents that you have been drinking with your friends."	Advising prevents child (and family) from problem solving and makes nurse rather than family responsible for outcome.
Belittling expressed feelings (nurse may be ignoring the importance of the child's problems and not listening carefully)	"Don't you know that big boys don't cry?"	Common expressions may cause the child to "feel like a baby."
Challenging (arguing with the child indicates that his or her perceptions are not genuine or legitimate)	"Was that a good reason to become angry?"	Arguing or challenging the child or family may imply judgment. It is not productive to the progress of the communication.
Changing the topic (introduction of an unrelated topic to the child's discussion)	*Child:* "I wish that I would just die so I don't have to go through this pain anymore." *Nurse:* "Has your mom been in to see you yet today?"	Child may believe that his or her thoughts are not important. It interrupts the child's thought pattern and sponaneity. Allow the child to discuss feelings. Encourage further discussion.
Disagreeing (opposing the child's thoughts and emotions denies self-respect)	*Child's mother:* "That doctor doesn't know what he is doing—our child is sicker now than when he first came to the hospital." *Nurse:* "Your child's doctor is an expert in his field and he is a highly respected pediatrician. Your child is getting the best care around."	Encourage the child and family to express their thoughts. Limits the opportunity to establish rapport or to increase child's self-understanding.
False reassurance (telling the child how to feel ignores his or her real feelings of distress)	"You are going to be just fine." "You don't have anything to worry about."	Minimizes the child's situation and increases anxiety. Be caring and honest in responses to questions.
Imposing values (nurse applies own biases and prejudices to impose values, judgments, and morals)	*Nurse to parent:* "You should let your child have that transfusion!" *Nurse to child:* "You were bad to refuse to take your medicine." Terms imposing values are *should, good, bad, wrong, right.*	Biases and prejudices can impede open communication and cause child/family to mistrust nurse.
Multiple questions (asking more than one question at a time)	"When did you first start feeling bad? How did you feel when you first got sick? How do you feel now?	Expecting a young child to answer multiple questions results in the child's frustration and limits his or her participation.
Parroting (repeating the child's words)	*Child:* "I am so tired." *Nurse:* "You are so tired."	No further expectations of the child are required. Child often misunderstands meaning and ceases to respond. Rephrase the child's statement or ask questions for clarification.
Probing (failure of nurse to respect the child or family's decisions and privacy)	"Tell me what secrets you keep from your parents." "I won't be able to help you unless you tell me everything."	Implies secrecy or blame of one family member to another. The nurse should demonstrate respect for the child and family's decisions—unless the decision may cause harm to the child or delay his or her recovery.
Requesting an explanation (similar to challenging and begins with "why?")	"Why can't you just take your medicine like you are supposed to?"	Child interprets "why" as misbehavior. Also implies devaluation of his or her feelings and thoughts. Ask questions such as "Can you tell me the reason that you don't want to take your medication?"
Stereotypical comments or idiomatic expressions (an indication to the child and family that you may have little concern about their experiences; often references from folklore and proverbs, which means they may be culture specific)	"It is all water under the bridge." "That's the way the ball bounces."	Avoid expressions that children from different backgrounds may not understand.

Adapted from Fontaine, K. L. (2003). Relating, communicating, and educating. In Mental health nursing *(5th ed.). Upper Saddle River, NJ: Prentice Hall.*

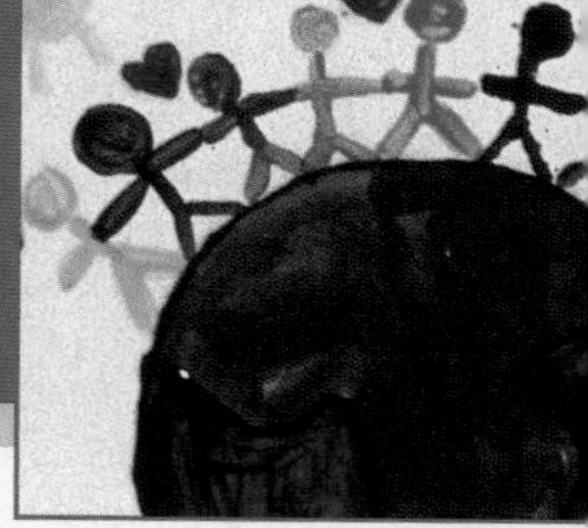

PARTNERING WITH FAMILIES

Establishing Rapport with Children

A child will be more responsive to the nurse when efforts are made to help the child feel like he or she is an important person in the interaction. Following these guidelines will help establish rapport with the child and encourage the child to share personal information and feelings.

- Sit or otherwise lower yourself so that you are at the child's eye level. *Sitting at eye level suggests that the nurse cares.*
- Note what the child is playing with or reading; ask about his favorite cartoon character. *Interest displayed by nurse encourages child's feeling of security.*
- Agree with the child when appropriate and share your feelings: "I don't like the taste of that medicine either, but sometimes I have to take it when I am sick—but then I have juice." *This statement offers encouragement to the child and family.*
- Compliment a physical feature or activity performed by the child: "You are really strong" or "You picked really nice colors for that picture." *This observational statement may reduce anxiety and imparts status for the child.*
- Use a calm tone of voice, with developmentally appropriate language. *Children want to talk and share information on their level of comprehension.*
- Pace the discussion or procedure in a nonhurried manner. *Trying to rush the child will only add to his or her anxiety.*
- Preschoolers have a limited concept of time. Explain concepts in terms they understand: "Your mother will be back after lunch." *This type of response provides them with a concrete time frame.*
- Include the adolescent in discussion about his or her care. *They have the cognitive ability to employ abstract communication and comprehend scientific terminology.*
- Listen more that you talk, and avoid distractions. *This attentive behavior of the nurse conveys an attitude of interest in the child.*
- Be truthful with the child. *They will respect your honesty.*

Data from Boggs, K. (1999). Communicating with children. In A. E. Boggs, Interpersonal relationships: Professional communication skills for nurses *(3rd ed., pp. 405–429). Philadelphia: Saunders; Adubato, S. (2004). Making the communication connection.* Nursing Management, *35(9), 33–36; Fleitas, J. (2003). The power of words: Examining the linguistic landscape of pediatric nursing.* MCN The American Journal of Maternal/Child Nursing, *28(6), 384–388.*

utilized. See Chapter 17∞ for further description of communication techniques with hospitalized children.

JOURNALING

Older children and adolescents may find journaling a good method to express their thoughts and feelings as well as to vent frustrations, fears, and the effects of their illness and treatments (Figure 6–8 ■). Provide the child or adolescent with a journal or notebook in which to write thoughts. Assure the child or adolescent that the journal is his or her property and assist in determining a safe place for the journal when not in use.

STORYTELLING

Storytelling is an effective means to communicate with the child. The child can engage in storytelling verbally, or by writing and drawing, providing the child an opportunity for self-expression. The nurse can begin a story by saying, "Once upon a time, there was a little girl named (child's name or another fictitious name) and she had to go to the hospital. . . " Then ask the child to tell what happens next or to finish the story. Another method is to have the child complete a sentence, for example, begin a sentence such as "What hurts me the most is. . . ." and have the child complete the sentence.

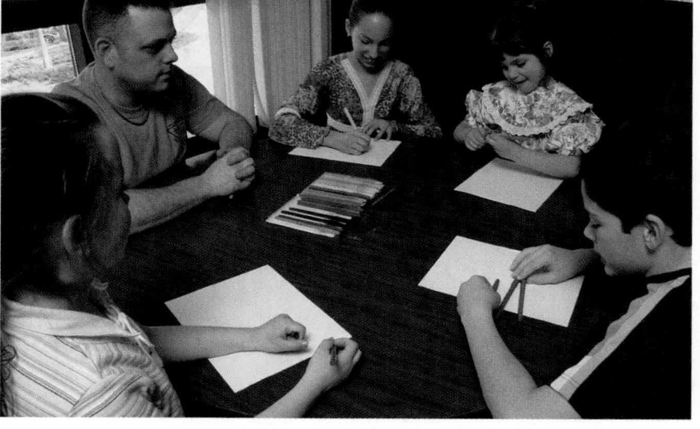

FIGURE 6–7 ■ The nurse is leading a group session for school-age children and has them complete both drawings and journals to describe their experiences.

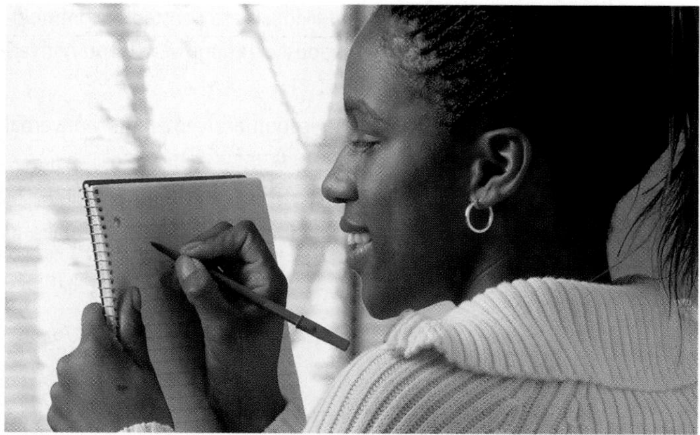

FIGURE 6–8 ■ Most teens are happy to keep a journal of important events and feelings. Ensure them confidentiality.

BIBLIOTHERAPY

Bibliotherapy describes the use of books related to topics and events the child is experiencing or will experience. Through books, the child can learn about life events such as illness, hospitalization, and the birth of a sibling. Children can be encouraged to draw and write their own stories. An abundance of developmentally appropriate books are available to explain a variety of illness, treatments, and other concepts such as those related to death and tragedy.

In collaboration with the family, the nurse determines the appropriate materials specific to the child's needs. The nurse assists the family in obtaining these resources either through the institution's sources or by other means such as websites, bookstores, and support groups.

Humor

The use of humor to communicate in the pediatric setting can serve to bridge communication gaps. It can help to reduce a child's fear of illness, injury, and hospitalization. Children age 3 to 4 years take great delight in distorting familiar concepts. Many children enjoy the verbal expressions of humor in stories like *The Cat in the Hat* (Seuss, 1957), *The Stinky Cheese Man* (Scieszka & Smith, 1992), and *Where the Sidewalk Ends* (Silverstein, 1974). Children age 7 to 8 years try to understand the incongruous nature of humor by responding seriously to riddles and telling jokes without a punch line. Using funny books to help the child relax and laugh can lessen anxiety and enhance relaxation in healthcare settings.

Knowing when to use humor is important. Three considerations to consider are timing, receptiveness, and context. First the nurse should establish a therapeutic relationship with the patient and/or family. Receptiveness to humor can be assessed after the nurse observes interactions between patient and family or assess their values and practices to humor. Thirdly, humor interventions need to respect patient values. Always avoid ethnic, racist, sexist, and ridiculing humor (Dowling, 2002).

Nurses can look for that particular time that laughter is appropriate for the child. Engaging in a familiar activity or task in an unfamiliar way such as wearing a lab or scrub jacket backwards can offer a coping strategy to a stressed child. Use humorous comments such as, "I'm going to use a light to look in your mouth because your mouth doesn't have windows" (Nevo & Shapira, 1989) or "Adolescence is that period in a child's life when his parents become more difficult" (Robinson, 1991).

Evaluation

Evaluation is dependent on assessment findings and specific interventions. General anticipated outcomes include the following:

- The nurse uses effective therapeutic techniques for communication.
- The nurse acknowledges and validates feelings and thoughts of child and family.
- A therapeutic nurse–child–family relationship is established.

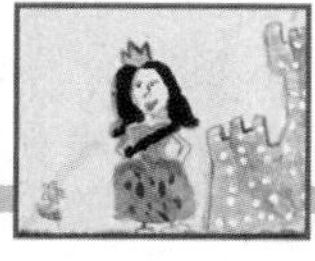

CHAPTER HIGHLIGHTS

- The nurse–child–family relationship is dependent on effective communication. The nurse's communication with the child and family serves as the connection between the family and the healthcare system.
- Communication is the exchange of information, thoughts, and feelings. It is an ongoing, cyclical process. Individuals are constantly communicating, either consciously or unconsciously, through verbal and nonverbal techniques.
- The two primary modes of communication are verbal and nonverbal communication.
- A child's communication ability and variety of techniques utilized to communicate directly corresponds with his or her developmental and cognitive levels.
- The challenge of communication with the child is compounded when the child has a sensory or other neurological impairment.
- Nursing care focuses on identifying communication patterns and needs of the child and family. A thorough assessment of the child's mental, physical, developmental, and cognitive abilities is necessary to determine the most effective method of communication with the child and family.
- Nursing techniques and skills in communication include establishing an appropriate environment, establishing rapport and trust, conveying respect, maintaining professional boundaries, maintaining confidentiality, and implementing appropriate verbal and nonverbal communication techniques.

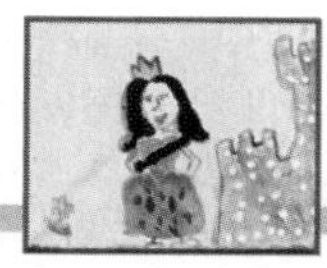

CRITICAL THINKING IN ACTION

INTRODUCTION

Recall the family in the opening vignette. Madison, age 7, was recently hospitalized and diagnosed with juvenile rheumatoid arthritis. A nurse is visiting the home to explain Madison's condition to her siblings, Brittney and Madeline, and to further develop a plan of care with Madison and her parents.

DESCRIPTION

The nurse will collaborate with the clinic's multidisciplinary team and the family to establish a plan of care for Madison. The nurse's first priority is to establish a therapeutic relationship with the family, and the home visit provides an opportunity to discuss Madison's condition with her siblings.

DISCUSSION

1. What developmental considerations will the nurse address when communicating with Madison?
2. What information do the parents need regarding Madison's understanding of the disease process based on her developmental level?
3. How will the nurse present information to Madison's 4-year-old sibling? What therapeutic communication techniques will the nurse implement? How do these techniques differ for this preschooler from that of school-age Madison?
4. How will the nurse present information to Madison's 9-year-old sibling? What therapeutic communication techniques will the nurse implement? How will the nurse evaluate the effectiveness of her teaching to Madison, her parents, and her siblings?
5. What are the benefits of involving the siblings in Madison's care? In what ways can they assist and participate?

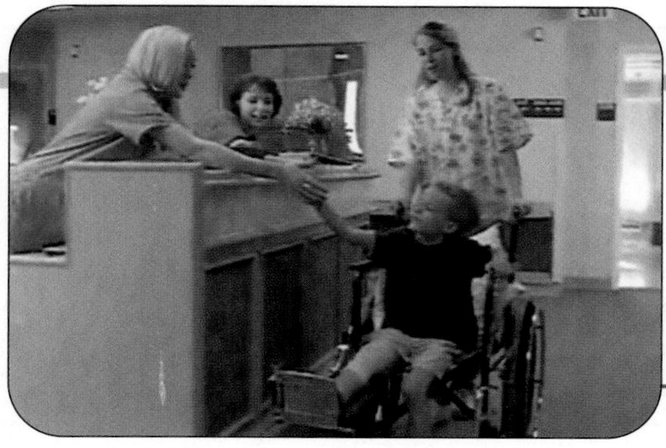

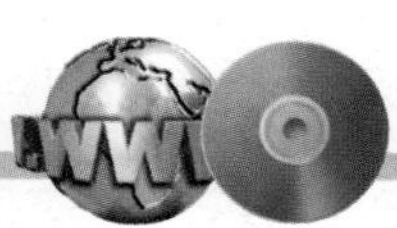

EXPLORE MediaLink

- NCLEX review, case studies, and other interactive resources for this chapter can be found on the Companion Website at **www.prenhall.com/ball**. Click on Chapter 6 to select the activities for this chapter.
- For animations, more NCLEX review questions, and an audio glossary, access the accompanying CD-ROM in this book.

http://www.prenhall.com/ball

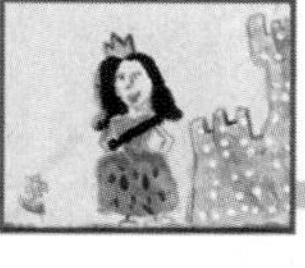

REFERENCES

Anderson, G. C., Moore, E., Hepworth, J., & Bergman, N. (2003). Early skin-to-skin contact for mothers and their healthy newborns and infants (Cochrane Review). In *The Cochrane Library*, Issue 2 (CD003519). Oxford: Update Software.

Beachy, J. M. (2003). Premature infant massage in the NICU. *Journal of Neonatal Nursing, 22*(3), 39–45.

Candlin, S. (2002). "Taking risks: An educator of expertise?" *Research in Language and Social Interactions, 35*, 173–193.

Chambers, S. (2003). Use of non-verbal communications to improve nursing care. *British Journal of Nursing, 12*(14), 874–881.

Deering, C. G., & Cody, D. J. (2002). Communicating with children and adolescents: 'Children are all foreigners,' Ralph Waldo Emerson said; but it need not always be the case. Here are some specific, age-appropriate tips for understanding the language of children. *American Journal of Nursing, 102*(3), 34–41.

Dowling, J. S. (2002). Humor: A coping strategy for pediatric patients. *Pediatric Nursing, 28*(2), 123–129.

English, A., & Ford, C. A. (2004). HIPAA privacy rule and adolescents: Legal questions and clinical challenges. *Perspectives on Sexual and Reproductive Health, 36*, 80–87.

Fleitas, J. (2003). The power of words: Examining the linguistic landscape of pediatric nursing. *MCN American Journal of Maternal Child Nursing, 28*, 389–390.

Flores, G., Laws, M. B., Mayo, S. J., Zuckerman, B., Abreu, M., Medina, L., & Hardt, E. J. (2003). Errors in medical interpreters and their potential clinical consequences in pediatric encounters. *Pediatrics, 111*, 6–14.

Fontaine, K. L. (2003). Relating, communicating, and educating. In *Mental health nursing* (5th ed.). Upper Saddle River, NJ: Prentice Hall.

Godkin, J., & Godkin, L. (2004). Caring behavior among nurses: Fostering a conversation of gestures. *Health Care Management Review, 29*, 258–268.

Green-Hernandez, C., Quinn, A. A., Denham-Vitale, S., Falkenstern, S. K., & Judge-Ellis, T. (2004). Making nursing care culturally competent. *Holistic Nursing Practice, 18*, 215–219.

Hemsley, B., Sigafoos, J., Balandin, S., Forbes, R., Taylor, C., Green, V. A., & Parmenter, T. (2001). Nursing the patient with severe communication impairment. *Journal of Advanced Nursing, 35*, 827–835.

Hyden, L., & Baggins, C. (2004). Joint working relationship: Children, parents, and child healthcare nurses at work. *Communication & Medicine, 1*, 71–83.

Ireland, M., & Olson, M. (2000). Massage therapy and therapeutic touch in children: State of the science. *Alternative Therapies, 6*(5), 54–63.

Kemper, K. J., & Kelly, E. A. (2004). Treating children with therapeutic and healing touch, *Pediatric Annals, 33*(4), 248–252.

Kneisel, C. R., Wilson, H. S., & Trigoboff, E. (2004). *Contemporary psychiatric-mental health nursing*. Upper Saddle River, NJ: Prentice Hall.

Kozier, B., Erb, G., Berman, A., & Synder, S. (2004). *Fundamentals of nursing: Concepts, process, and practice* (7th ed.). Upper Saddle River, NJ: Prentice Hall.

Mainous, R. O. (2002). Infant massage as a component of developmental care: Past, present, and future. *Holistic Nursing Practice, 16*(5), 1–7.

Michael, S. R., Candela, L., & Mitchell, S. (2002). Aesthetic knowing: Understanding the experience of chronic illness. *Nursing Educator, 27*, 25–27.

Nevo, O., & Shapira, J. (1989). The use of humor by pediatric dentist. In R. E. McGhee (Ed.), *Humor and children's development: A guide to practical applications* (pp. 171–178). New York: Haworth Press.

Robinson, V. R. (1991). *Humor and the health professionals* (2nd ed.). Thorofare, NJ: Slack Publishers.

Robshaw, M., & Smith, J. (2004). Concerns about confidentiality: The child protection jigsaw. *Paediatric Nursing: Harrow-on-the-Hill, 16*(5), 36–39.

Runeson, I., Hallstrom, I., Elander, G., & Hermeren, G. (2002). Children's participation in the decision-making process during hospitalization: An observational study. *Nursing Ethics, 9*(6), 583–598.

Seidel, H. M., Ball, J. W., Dains, J. D., & Benedict, G. W. (2003). *Mosby's guide to physical examination* (5th ed.). St. Louis: Mosby.

Spector, R. E. (2004). *Cultural diversity in health and illness* (6th ed.). Upper Saddle River, NJ: Prentice Hall.

Swallow, V., & Macfadyen, A. (2004). Nurses' communication skills: Are they effective research tools? *Paediatric Nursing, Harrow-on-the-Hill, 16*(5), 20–24.

Sydnor-Greenberg, N., & Dokken, D. L. (2001). Communicate in healthcare: Thoughts on the child's perspective. *Journal of Child and Family Nursing, 4*(3), 225–230.

Thompson, V. L., Hupcey, J. E., & Clark, M. B. (2003). The development of trust in parents of hospitalized children. *Journal of the Specialists in Pediatric Nurses, 8*(4), 137–147.

Wardell, D. W., & Weymouth, K. F. (2004). Review of studies of healing touch. *Journal of Nursing Scholarship, 36*, 147–154.

Social and Environmental Influences on the Child and Adolescent

Chapter

7

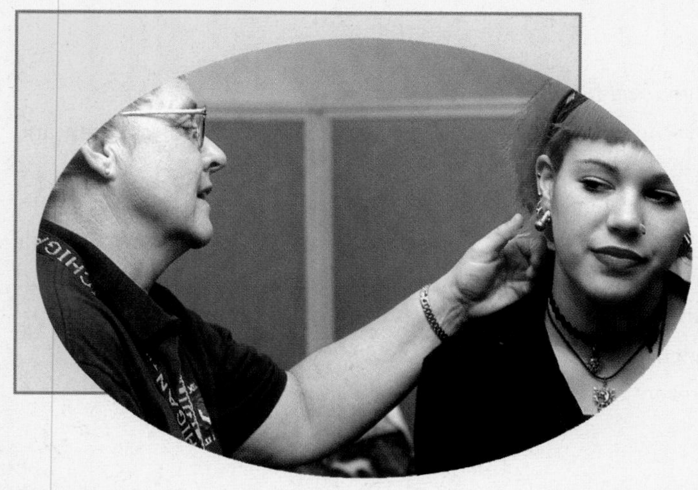

Amy Beckman is 15 years old and attends an alternative high school. She recently had an ear piercing and it is sore. She comes to the health room to ask the advice of the school nurse. Upon examination, the area around the piercing is inflamed and mildly edematous. After asking some questions, the nurse learns that Amy's ear was pierced by a friend, using a needle that had been "sterilized" by passing it through a match flame. She has had a slight fever, but otherwise feels fine.

In her home state, adolescents under 18 years of age must have the signature of a parent for body piercings and tattoos, so Amy chose to have the procedure done by a friend. She believes this is safe since her friend has done many piercings on others. She admits that her parents are not very pleased with her body art, but that they allow her to do it as long as she agrees to stay in high school. She had previously run away and spent several weeks living on the streets.

What healthcare and social needs does Amy have? How can you support both her and her parents? What signs of resilience does Amy show? This chapter examines the complex social contexts in which children live, learn, and grow, and explores the role of nurses in supporting them to reach their potentials. The challenges of providing comprehensive healthcare for all children and adolescents, no matter what their lifestyles, are discussed.

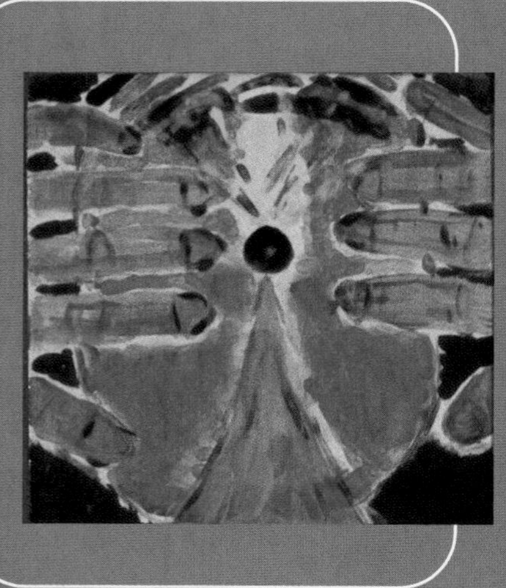

"This school is a lot better than the other one I was in. At least they try to understand you here. It is probably important to get through high school and my parents seem happier that I'm in school. It seems like you can trust the teachers and the nurse more here."

—Amy, 15 years old

Key Terms

branding/208
bullying/210
child sexual abuse/215
cutting/208
emotional abuse/215
emotional neglect/215
hazing/220
homosexuality/208
incest/215
LGBT/208
LGBQ/208
physical abuse/215
physical neglect/215
violence/208

Learning Outcomes

After completing this chapter, you will be able to:

- Identify major social and environmental factors that influence the health of children and adolescents.
- List external influences that can affect child and adolescent health.
- Apply the ecologic model and resilience theory to assessment of the social and environmental factors in children's lives.
- Examine the effects of substance use, physical activity, and other lifestyle patterns on health.
- Plan nursing interventions for children who experience violence.
- Explore the nursing role in prevention and treatment of child abuse and neglect.

MediaLink 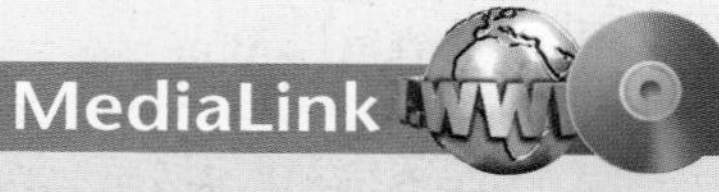 **http://www.prenhall.com/ball**

Resources for this chapter can be found on the CD-ROM accompanying this textbook, and on the Companion Website at www.prenhall.com/ball. Click on Chapter 7 to select the activities for this chapter.

CD-ROM

Videos

The Effects of Media on Children
Extreme Sports
Identifying Child Abuse
Identifying Youth Who Abuse Drugs & Alcohol Use
Smoking & Smoking Cessation

NCLEX Review

Audio Glossary

COMPANION WEBSITE

NCLEX Review

MediaLink Applications

Critical Thinking in Action: Music and Violence
Develop a Teaching Plan: Individualized Sport

Many of the major causes of mortality and morbidity in children are closely linked with social influences in the child's environment. The social contexts for young children growing up today are different from those of even a decade ago. Examining the social contexts in which children live and grow can provide insights into the behavior of children and adults, and present opportunities for nursing interventions. All nurses must examine social influences and apply the knowledge gained to plan healthcare that will benefit youth as they grow into adulthood.

What are the challenges of today's society, some of which children face at a very young age? How can nurses help children to face these challenges and to emerge as healthy and contributing members of society? What roles do nurses play in identifying the protective factors and in minimizing the risk factors of youth? This chapter will help you to examine and apply these concepts in a variety of nursing settings.

Consider the major causes of death for children from 1 year of age through adolescence that are presented in Chapter 1∞ (Figures 1–6 through 1–14). Note that most morbidity is related to preventable causes linked to present-day lifestyles, including car crashes, fires, drownings, and homicides.

Now examine the major reasons for hospitalization (Figure 1–16). By the time children are 5 years of age, injuries rank as the second cause, and by 10 years, mental disorders are the major cause of hospitalization. By the teen years, pregnancy and mental disorders are the most common admitting diagnoses to hospitals. These conditions are related, at least in part, to the social and environmental settings in which we live. These settings and their influences must be examined in order to understand how to best intervene with children. Theories that help us to examine the social and environmental contexts of children and families are discussed earlier in the text and reviewed below.

> **BOX 7–1 Research: The ADD Health Study**
>
> The ADD Health Study (National Longitudinal Study of Adolescent Health) was conducted during the latter 1990s with over 100,000 adolescents and helped to determine the family, school, and individual characteristics associated with risk factors. Parent–family connectedness, school connectedness, a belief in a higher being, and academic success were predictive of youth having the lowest health risks. Recall the concept of *attachment* discussed in Chapter 5∞. Attachment to family, school, and parents constitute strong protective factors for adolescence in preventing them from violent behavior such as shoplifting, stealing, fights, and physical injury incidents (Franke, 2003). Nurses can assist adolescents and their families in establishing a sense of attachment to each other. Encourage families to include adolescents in activities, attend their sports and other school events, have meals together regularly, and attend faith-based activities or other community events as a family.

THEORETICAL FRAMEWORKS

In this chapter, two main theories will be used to provide a framework in which to examine societal influences on children. These are the ecologic model and the resilience theory, as discussed in Chapter 5∞. Review them now to assist in evaluating the environmental settings that influence children (see Figure 5–3 and Tables 5–4, 5–6, and 5–7).

The ecologic theory views the child and the environment as interacting forces, with children influencing systems around them, while they are influenced by these systems (Lackey & Walker, 1998). Close systems providing daily contact are microsystems, but other systems such as parental work and political or cultural environments are also important. Understanding these systems, or the forces in which children function, can provide information that guides care providers. For example, if the parents' employment agencies do not provide healthcare insurance, their children may not obtain necessary healthcare such as immunizations, treatment for diseases, and growth monitoring.

Resilience theory examines risk and protective factors in the child's environment as they influence the child's adaptation to stressful events, and can be modified to lead to more productive and healthy outcomes (Box 7–1). For example, if a young child is hospitalized for treatment of an acute infectious illness, some protective factors might include ability of one parent to stay with the child at all times, the ability of a grandmother to care for siblings at home during this time, and the child's ability to adapt to new situations and communicate readily with staff members. On the other hand, risk factors might include lack of comprehensive health insurance to pay for the hospitalization, lack of an identified health care "home" (consistent care provider) for the child, and missing some immunizations.

Theoretical frameworks are useful when examining social and environmental influences on children because they guide us to examine certain factors that can be altered or understood. They will suggest assessment data to collect and pertinent nursing interventions. They also help foster partnerships with other care providers who use these and similar theories to plan social, psychological, and other care for children and their families.

EXTERNAL INFLUENCES ON CHILD HEALTH

While the genetic characteristics of a child can influence susceptibility to acute or chronic health conditions, the environment in which the child grows also has a powerful impact on health. The ecologic model recognizes the inborn characteristics of the child, as well as how these characteristics relate to the child's family, community, and culture. The resilience model suggests methods of evaluating all of the child and social characteristics in order to identify protective factors and risks. Some of the external factors that can directly or indirectly influence child health are discussed below.

Poverty

An important risk factor that influences the health of children is poverty. Conversely, basic financial stability is a protective factor that contributes to the general health and well-being of children. However, children are the poorest group in this country and more children are poor now than at any time in our past (Board on Children, Youth, and Families, 2001). One in six children is poor, or lives in a family earning less than $14,128 annually for a family of three persons or less than $18,104 for a family of four (Children's Defense Fund, 2004a).

Children who are poor are overrepresented in nearly every health indicator. Children who are poor are more likely to have unmet health needs, to have difficulty in school, to become teen parents, and to experience multiple health problems, including stunted growth and lead poisoning. Inadequate, unsafe housing, food insecurity, and poor dietary quality are more common. What is the face of poverty? Some statistics that may prove surprising include:

- The children most likely to be living in poor households are those below 6 years of age.
- About 39% of children living in a single-headed household are poor, while only 8% in married couple households are poor.
- Ethnic variations are startling: 9% of White, 27% of Hispanic, and 30% of Black children live in poverty.
- Poverty rates are higher in suburban and rural areas than in central cities.
- Nearly 80% of poor children have at least one parent working full time.

(Federal Interagency Forum on Child and Health Family Statistics, 2003)

Nurses should understand the demographics in the areas where they work. What is the poverty rate in the community? What ethnic groups are overrepresented among the poor? Locate resources such as food services, healthcare for the underserved, and enhanced school programs in order to refer poor families. Recognize that health promotion services may not be high priority when a family lacks adequate housing or food. When children are seen in any setting, such as in school or in an emergency room or hospital for acute care, refer to health promotion guidelines for the child's age (see Chapters 11 through 15∞). Measure growth, assess vision and hearing, evaluate dietary intake, and check immunization status. Find out the stresses the family experiences and what resources they need to meet basic necessities. Your nursing care plan should include these health promotion needs as well as identifying nursing diagnoses connected to the acute illness or other health problem.

Homelessness

Poverty leads to homelessness for some children. Children comprise over one fourth of the homeless, and families represent 39% of the homeless population. Families are the fastest growing group of homeless people; on any night, about 100,000 children are homeless in the United States (DeForge, Zehnder, Minick, et al., 2001). The reasons for homelessness are also common risks for a number of the other challenges to health discussed in this chapter. Homeless people often have poor finances, may have been abused or victims of other violence, and may experience mental instability.

Children who experience homelessness often have multiple physical and mental health problems, and lack health insurance to provide care for these problems. Some of the common problems faced by homeless children and families include trauma, alcoholism, respiratory and skin infections, tuberculosis and HIV,

TABLE 7–1 Common Health Problems and Nursing Management of Poor and Homeless Children

COMMON HEALTH PROBLEMS	NURSING MANAGEMENT
Lack of immunizations	Check immunization records. Provide immunizations at schools and in homeless shelters.
Common infectious diseases	Facilitate free clinics in shelters, schools, and community settings. Teach hygiene measures. Provide resources for disease management. Arrange for medications when needed. Provide information about resources for bathing, hygiene.
Sleep deficits	Inform parents about respite facilities. Arrange for children to have quiet sleep time in school if possible.
Vision and hearing deficits	Perform screening for deficits. Provide resources for eyeglasses, hearing aids, care for ear infections (e.g., service organizations such as Lion's Club).
Nutritional deficits	Perform height and weight checks and nutritional assessment. Evaluate family for food security (see Chapter 9∞). Be sure child is registered for school breakfast and lunch programs if available. Ensure that children are linked to summer food programs at end of academic year. Refer to Women, Infants, and Children (WIC) Nutrition Program. Inform about resources for meals and field gleaning in the community.
Dental care problems	Teach oral hygiene. Provide toothbrushes and toothpaste. Provide bottled water for use if child lives in a car or on the street. Perform oral assessment. Refer to dental programs for people with low incomes.
Injuries	Teach basic safety precautions. Visit the living situation if possible to assess for safety hazards. Teach "street safe" skills. Provide helmets, car seats, or other gear needed.
Adolescent pregnancy and sexually transmitted infections	Provide sexuality teaching. Inform about access to family planning services. Assess for child abuse and prostitution.
Mental illness	Assess for depression. Evaluate for suicide potential. Provide links to services. Plan programs to foster self-esteem. Arrange for Big Brother or Big Sister. Refer to extracurricular activities in the school and community. Arrange for a school bus stop away from a shelter so other students do not stigmatize the homeless child.

and nutritional disorders (Stratigos & Katsambas, 2003). Teens who have been homeless are more likely to engage in risky behavior, such as unprotected sex with multiple partners and substance abuse. They are more likely to need emergency care, to be depressed, and to become pregnant than other teens (Steele, Ramgoolam, & Evans, 2003).

Health problems related to homelessness and other family characteristics continue even after finding a place to live. After families leave homeless shelters, children frequently become separated from their mothers due to parent stress, lack of access to resources, and inability of parents to provide adequate settings for the children (Cowal, Shinn, Weitzman, et al., 2002). Complex ongoing care is needed. This may begin in a shelter for the homeless, but should continue while the family obtains a place to live, accesses other community services, enrolls the children in school, and attains financial and mental stability.

Adolescents who are homeless often have some similarities to younger children, but may be dealing with other issues of importance. While teens may be homeless because parents have lost jobs and homes, they may be homeless because they have had difficulties at home and have chosen to leave. Recall Amy, who was described in the scenario at the beginning of the chapter. She left home and lived on the streets for several weeks. Some teens begin taking drugs or become sexually active during periods when they are homeless. They may be subjected to violence in the areas they choose to live. As with younger children, they may lack adequate food, facilities to maintain hygiene, and healthcare. Problems that homeless teens deal with may include sexually transmitted diseases, pregnancy, substance abuse, poor performance or nonattendance at school, and physical or mental illness.

Nursing management for families with children who are poor or homeless focuses on identification of poverty and homelessness, careful assessment of health risks, and linking the family to resources that can assist with stability and health. There is often no way to identify poor or homeless children from appearance and they may hide their status when in school or at healthcare facilities. Addresses given may not be accurate, or the address of a shelter might be used. Children living at shelters or in cars and on the street may not take the school bus, but prefer to walk to avoid stigma. (See Evidence-Based Practice: Homelessness from the Viewpoint of Children.) Be alert for children who have multiple health problems and repeated infectious diseases. They are often hungry, tired, suffer from skin and other infections, and have varying degrees of personal hygiene depending on access to laundry and bathing facilities. See Table 7–1 for examples of nursing care needs for homeless children and families.

Stress

The adverse effect of stress on adults is well documented. More recently the impact of stress on children has been recognized. Children manifest stress in a variety of ways, including regressive behavior, interrupted sleep, hyperactive behavior, gastrointestinal symptoms, crying, and withdrawal from normal events. Common stressful events for children include moving to a new home or school, marital difficulties in the family, abuse, a parent deployment in the military, and being expected to achieve at an extremely high level in school or sports (Figure 7–1 ■). The busy pace of today's lifestyles and the impact of the media in encouraging early development of children may put undue stress upon some children and preteens (Elkind, 2001). Adolescents may be stressed by fulfilling many roles, such as student, part-time worker, and active family member. They may be in school all day, be in sport or music practice for 2 to 3 hours after school, and

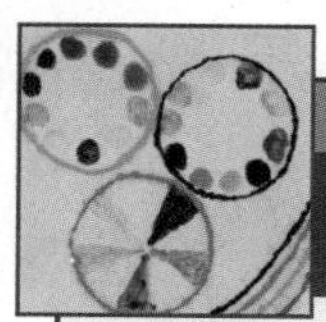

EVIDENCE-BASED PRACTICE
Homelessness from the Viewpoint of Children

PROBLEM

Children are the age group showing the fastest growth in homelessness, accounting for about 39% of the homeless population. Due to their ages, children are vulnerable to developmental delays, mental health problems, and effects of violence. Most nurses have not been homeless and do not understand the experience of homelessness for children.

EVIDENCE

A study by four nurses sought to describe the homeless experience from the perspective of children. They interviewed 14 children with an average age of 10 years who were located in shelters in a metropolitan area. The children had been in the shelters from 2 weeks to 6 months, and most had prior periods living in shelters, hotels, or with relatives. The researchers identified five themes common to the children:

- "I'm not homeless." The children viewed homelessness as having no resources, and having to live outside. They felt that they had resources and felt they might be ridiculed if people thought they were homeless.
- "I like living in a shelter sometimes." While the children had mixed feelings about living in shelters, most were glad to have food, a place to sleep, and a feeling of safety. They described friends in the shelter and were glad to have those relationships.
- "Living in a shelter is hard." The children complained about rules and rigid schedules in the shelters. They missed freedom of movement, play space, and privacy.
- "Stop the violence." All children described living in violent neighborhoods and the wish that violence would stop. Fighting back was perceived as important to protecting oneself.
- "I need approval." Children frequently described how important it was to be noticed and praised by teachers and other adults.

IMPLICATIONS

Although this study was small, there were important findings for nurses. The stigma of being homeless should be considered when interacting with children. The researchers suggest reading stories and describing families that lose a home to all children in schools so that the topic is addressed. Nurses can partner with teachers to plan collaborative approaches. The privacy of children should be considered and school buses should not stop directly in front of shelters to pick up children. Integrating positive reinforcement for children into shelter routines, school classrooms, and other settings is important for the child's sense of self-esteem (DeForge et al., 2001).

CRITICAL THINKING APPLICATION

Find at least two shelters in your community. Are nurses involved in planning healthcare? How long do families usually remain? Do the schools know that children are homeless? Do they strive to preserve the privacy of homeless children while supporting their needs for growth, health, and education? What is the nursing role in the shelter, in the school, in the community?

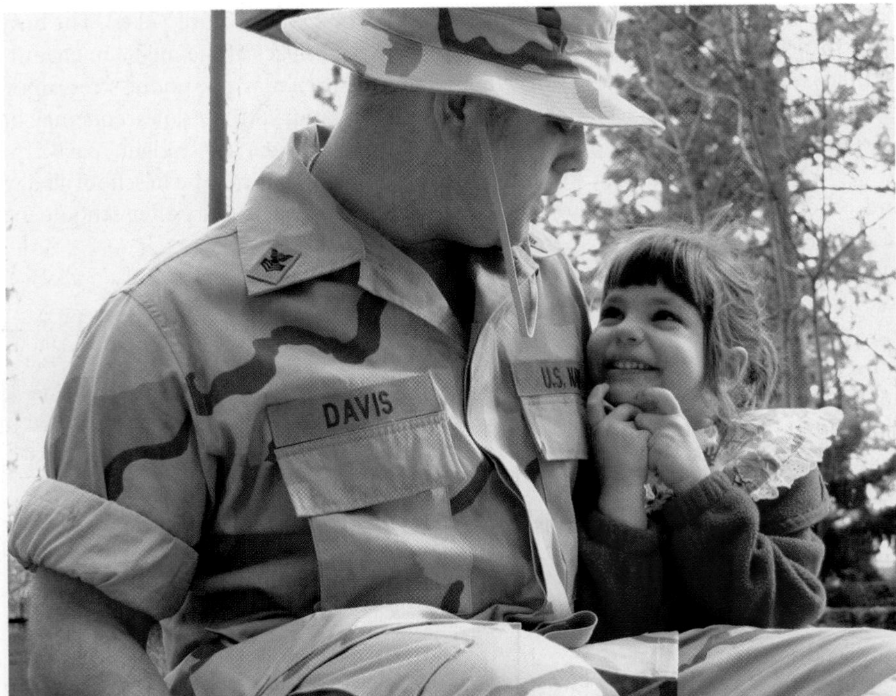

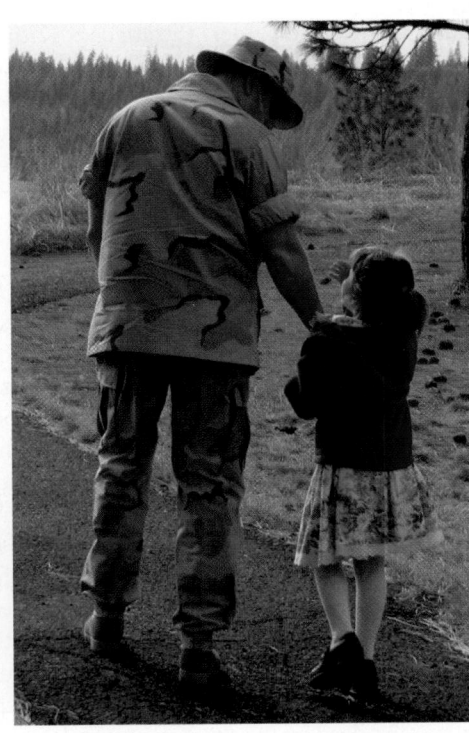

FIGURE 7–1 ■ The special relationship between a father about to be deployed in the military and his young daughter is clear. This father has two other children and is spending time with each of them, as well as with the family together, before leaving. The cycle of leaving and returning home can be stressful for families. Nurses can assist military families in making plans for healthcare, finances, and communication while gone and providing resources for emotional support for the entire family.

then have a job for several additional hours. Lack of adequate sleep can add further to stress, in addition to putting the teen at risk for car crashes and poor school performance. For poor families, commonly reported stressors are related to food provision, shelter, transportation, medical care, and personal-time needs.

The child experiencing stress has more frequent respiratory and gastrointestinal illnesses and is more likely to be the victim of an injury. The negative long-term effects of stress on body organs and systems suggest that children under stress are more likely to develop illnesses such as strokes, hypertension, and heart attacks later in life. Nurses help children to manage stress by encouraging good coping strategies. Healthy lifestyles including good nutrition, exercise, and plenty of sleep can be emphasized with all children. Integrate these topics into each health promotion/health maintenance visit, using some of the following ideas: Consult Chapters 11 through 15∞ for detailed interventions with each specific age group. The National Heart, Lung, and Blood Institute has launched a 5-year program to encourage children and adolescents to get at least 9 hours of sleep nightly. Refer to the Companion Website for information on the program and interactive exercises for children and teens.

Partner with military families to assist them as one or both parents are deployed for duty in a remote location. Connect parents with resources for childcare, psychological support, and arrangements that need to be made to prepare for the absence. Due to frequent moves, the family may not be strongly connected to resources in the community. Help families explain to children why and where the parents are going, and how they will keep in touch during the absence. Children need to know who they will stay with, whether they will attend the same school, and how food and other needs will be met (Stafford & Grady, 2003).

Parents can be encouraged to provide youth with activities that foster self-esteem and to avoid unrealistic expectations about performance in sports and other activities. Resources to assist with food acquisition, shelter, transportation, and medical care should be provided for families needing the assistance. Adolescents may benefit from various approaches for stress management such as massage, rest, physical activity, and yoga. See Complementary Therapy: Youth and CAM.

Family Structure

The families into which children are born influence them profoundly. Children are supported in different ways and acquire different worldviews depending on such factors as whether one or both parents work, how many siblings are present, and whether an extended family is nearby. Note should be made of variations in family structure such as adolescent parent, single parent, gay or lesbian parents, extended family, grandparents caring for grandchildren, and stepparents. Societal changes have impacted family life and the needs of children immensely. Working parents often raise children with little time for quality relationships and without the financial resources needed for optimum development (Board on Children, Youth, and Families, 2001). All factors influence the physical and mental health of children and can determine their needs for nursing intervention. See Chapter 2∞ for a

COMPLEMENTARY THERAPY
Youth and CAM

Many healthcare providers assume that youth use few complementary and alternative medicine (CAM) approaches. A study at a Texas university suggests that this may not be accurate. Researchers received a total of 913 questionnaires from college students who answered questions related to use of CAM; 66% of the students reported use of such therapy in the past year. The most common types were high-dose vitamin/nutritional supplements, herbal medicine, relaxation/meditation, and massage. Less common were chiropractic medicine, yoga, and acupuncture. Most students had positive attitudes about CAM and those engaging in the practices were more commonly female, holistic in approach to health, and expressed a sense of control over their own health. The researchers suggest that healthcare providers working with youth assess their use of CAM and provide written and other materials to provide information. Those who are self-directed and take control of their own health may benefit most from resources provided on CAM approaches (Chng, Neill, & Fogle, 2003).

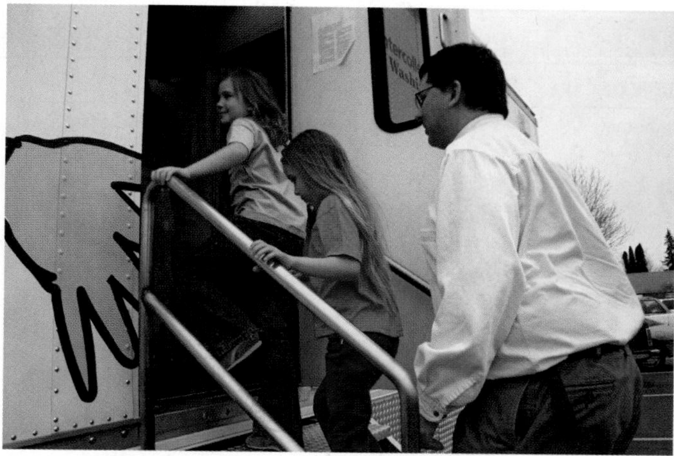

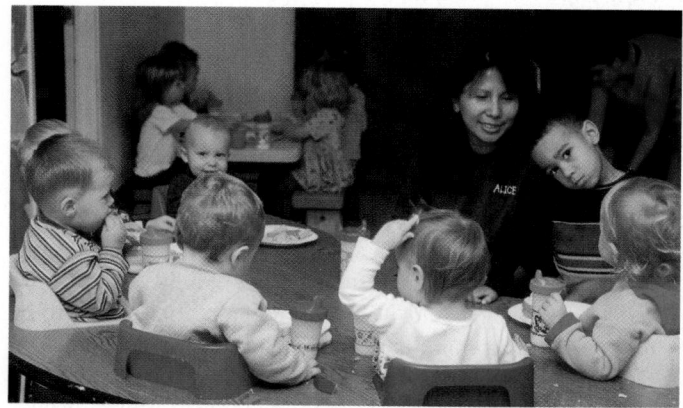

FIGURE 7–2 ■ This father is bringing his two daughters to a mobile van parked near a school to receive healthcare. Children may receive some of their healthcare from school-based services including school nurses, clinics, or mobile vans.

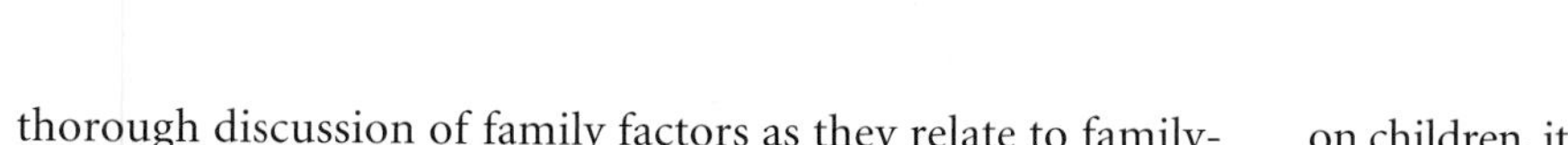

thorough discussion of family factors as they relate to family-centered care.

School and Childcare

Once a child is 5 or 6 years of age, several hours daily are spent in a school setting. Physical skills are developed through participation in education and sports. Psychosocial stages are met as the child interacts with children and adults and achieves social interaction patterns and pride in accomplishments. The presentation of concepts that challenge thought processes enhances cognitive development.

Although the primary role of schools is educational, they also perform several health-related functions. School health screening programs play an important role in identifying children with such health problems as hearing loss, visual impairment, and scoliosis. Nurses provide assessment, teaching, and clinical management related to some health problems. Consider the case of Amy in the opening scenario. She went to the school nurse when her body piercing was potentially infected; the nurse examined the site and made suggestions for cleaning and taught Amy the symptoms that could indicate serious infections. Some schools have clinics that examine and provide even more complete healthcare for children (Figure 7–2 ■). Many schools teach good nutrition, healthful living, safe sexual practices, and other health-related subjects. A school nurse may be present, at least part time, to plan these classes or to work with teachers. Nurses assist school districts in providing plans for emergency healthcare when needed. With the increase in mainstreaming, school staff now has the responsibility for administering medications, maintaining urinary catheters, and providing respiratory care and other treatments to ensure the child's proper growth and development. See Chapter 16∞ for a further discussion of school nurse activities. Some children spend part or nearly all of their days in childcare settings (Figure 7–3 ■). Nearly half of all children are in regular childcare by their first birthday (Fields, Smith, Bass, et al., 2001). While there has been debate about whether childcare has a positive or negative impact on children, it appears now that the closeness of the parent–child relationship, the quality of care, and the length of the childcare day are important in determining childcare effects on children (National Institute of Child Health and Human Development, 1997).

Nursing management involves helping parents to explore types of childcare options available and to evaluate programs in their communities (Table 7–2). Care options for young school-age children, either before or after school, can also be shared with parents. Early intervention programs with at-risk children, such as the Zero to Three Project and Head Start, have been influential in contributing to the health and welfare of children and should be recommended when available. Nurses frequently manage the health programs in early intervention, providing for screening and health evaluations and establishing early intervention education plans.

MediaLink Child Care Resources

Nurses assist families in evaluating childcare centers and share information about accreditation. (See Partnering with Families: Evaluation of Childcare.) The National Association for

FIGURE 7–3 ■ Most children will spend time in childcare settings. It is important to explore options and find the best fit for the child's needs.

TABLE 7–2 Types of Childcare

TYPE OF CARE	DESCRIPTION	ADVANTAGE/DISADVANTAGE
In home	Caretaker comes to home of the child	Child can remain at home Little exposure to infectious diseases No need for alternative care when child is ill Limited contact with other children to encourage development Most costly
Family childcare	Parent brings child to home of a caretaker	Limited number of children Some exposure to other children and encouragement of development Family-type atmosphere Little governmental regulation or examination
Center a. Private, nonprofit (e.g., church, YMCA) b. Public (e.g., Head Start) c. Private proprietary care	Parent brings child to a center where many children receive care	A learning curriculum plan is in place Contact with other children can enhance development Exposure to multiple children increases infectious disease risk

the Education of Young Children (2004) has established criteria related to the following:

- Interactions among teachers and children
- Curriculum
- Relationships among teachers and families
- Staff qualifications and professional development
- Administration
- Staffing
- Physical environment
- Health and safety
- Nutrition and food safety
- Evaluation

Community

The community in which a child lives may support the child's development or, conversely, expose the child to hazards. Social programs such as Head Start preschools, sports activities, after-school programs, and child abuse treatment centers offer valuable services that improve the experience of growing children. On the other hand, an economically depressed community with scant services and a high homicide rate is unsupportive and hazardous for growing children.

The physical environment is supportive when the child is provided with sidewalks on which to walk to school, open spaces in which to learn and play, and clean air to breathe. Children who must walk to school on unsafe roads, have access to contaminated drinking supplies, or live near polluting manufacturing companies or in crowded housing or old structures are at risk for injuries and health problems such as lead poisoning (see Chapter 30∞). The following developmental variations place children at high risk for environmental contaminant exposure.

- Children are of course smaller than adults and thus are closer to the ground. They are therefore more likely to be exposed to contaminants in soil and on floors, including lead-based paint dust, chemicals, and other pollutants.
- During infancy and toddlerhood, hand-to-mouth behaviors are common, so young children are more likely to ingest toxic substances.
- Higher metabolic rates and fluid turnover expose children to air, food, and water contaminants.
- The nervous system and growth/development of children are vulnerable to toxic insults during early developmental periods.

(Sattler, Afzal, Condon, et al., 2003)

See Table 7–3 for common contaminants in children's environments and nursing implications.

Nurses should be aware of the types of neighborhoods in the community. Learn about local resources and hazards. Assessment of every child involves information about the community and the healthcare that the family needs help to obtain. Refer children when appropriate for lead poisoning and safe programs after school, and teach them about injury prevention specific to their communities. See Chapter 16∞ for a thorough discussion of the nursing role regarding child health in the community.

Culture

The child's cultural group may influence the use of traditional and contemporary healthcare practices. If the parents or children are recent immigrants, they may still be learning the English language and finding out about healthcare resources. Even in families that have been in this country for some time, a combination of approaches to healthcare is common. Children of immigrants may feel stress as they combine their family's traditional culture with the new culture in which the family now lives. They may also have a great deal of responsibility to interpret for the family, since they may speak two languages and understand the practices of the new culture.

Recent immigrants may experience culture shock, a state of crisis related to the difference in values and lifestyle. This can lead to stress-related symptoms, and create a need for healthcare intervention. Children whose parents emigrated from another country may feel different than peers and develop conflict with their parents, particularly during adolescence.

All cultural groups have rules regarding patterns of social interaction. The number of languages spoken and the amount of speech in the home determine schedules of language acquisi-

PARTNERING WITH FAMILIES

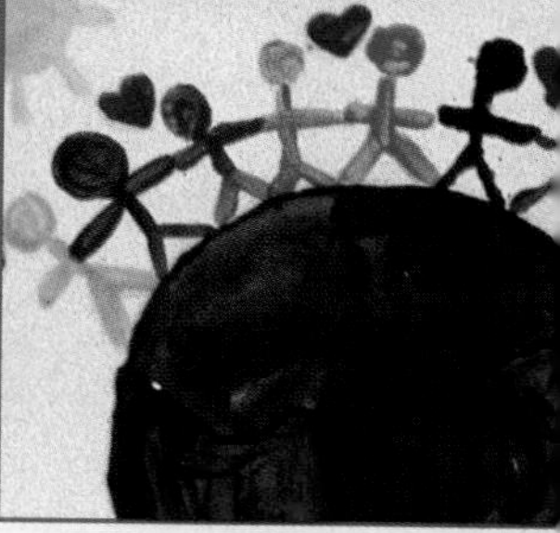

Evaluation of Childcare

The nurse can help parents to evaluate childcare options and make decisions about placement for their children. Parents should always be welcome to visit an agency or home childcare—this is essential so they can see the routines in action. Following are suggested questions for them to ask.

Administration

- Is the facility licensed?
- Who are the administrators? What is their training and experience?
- How many staff members are employed? What is their training?
- Is there a parent board? What part does the board play in administering the center?

Physical environment, health, and safety

- What is the neighborhood like? Is transportation to the center convenient?
- What is the condition of lighting, heat, cooling, ventilation system, play spaces (inside and out), and the building's general condition?
- Is playground equipment safe?
- Is there a soft material such as bark, sand, or rubber tiles under climbing equipment?
- Is there always supervision for the children?
- Are there emergency medical forms and signed forms for field trips?
- Who may pick up children? How are they signed in and out?
- What is the immunization policy and how are records examined and maintained?
- Are criminal background checks of staff done for potential child abuse and other problems?
- What is the policy for children with infectious diseases and other illness?
- How are foods prepared? Is staff licensed in food handling?
- What is the state of general cleanliness?
- Who changes diapers? Are recommendations for standard precautions to prevent pathogen transfer followed?
- What arrangements and routines are made for naps and quiet times?

Developmental approaches

- Is the curriculum appropriate for different age groups?
- Are there materials and plans for gross motor, fine motor, language, and social development?
- How much time do children spend in structured time? Free time?
- How is discipline handled?
- Do the children appear occupied and happy?
- What reading materials are available?
- What type and quantity of field trips are planned?
- What is the educational level and longevity of the childcare workers?
- Is there diversity among the children's backgrounds and experiences?

tion. The particular social roles assumed by men and women in the culture affect school activities and ultimately career choices. Attitudes toward touching and other methods of encouraging developmental skills vary among cultures.

Nurses must become aware of common characteristics of the cultural groups they are serving in order to establish culturally competent nursing care. Arrange for translators when needed. Be aware that traditional and Western healthcare may both be

TABLE 7–3 Examples of Environmental Contaminants

CONTAMINANT	EFFECTS	NURSING IMPLICATIONS
Radon	Lung cancer	Radon is a radioactive gas which can seep into homes undetected. Homes should be tested for radon presence. Ask if testing has been done and recommend home test kit or local contractor.
Carbon monoxide	Tissue anoxia from CO combination with hemoglobin, leading to its inability to transport oxygen	CO is formed during combustion. Newborns and infants are especially vulnerable. Check chimneys for proper burning and ventilation. Do not leave children in or around running cars or place them near exhaust of motor boat or other vehicle. Do not use charcoal grills inside.
Pesticides	Cancer, neurologic damage	Avoid infestations by storing food and pet supplies correctly. Teach families to follow directions on pesticides and avoid use around children. Wash clothes and skin after use before coming in contact with children. Store pesticides locked out of reach of children.
Food and water contaminants	Gastrointestinal distress, neurologic damage	Common contaminants are mercury (in household batteries and thermometers and in fish), lead (in older homes with peeling lead-based paint), and water (bacterial growth, especially in untreated well water). Assess the home environment for ingestible contaminants. Instruct in safe removal. Be alert for signs of gastrointestinal distress, neurologic changes, or slow development in young children. Newborns and infants are at greatest risk.

Data from Sattler, B., Afzal, B. M., Condon, M. E., Belka, E. K., & McKee, B. A. (2003). Children's health and the environment: Environmentally healthy homes and communities. *American Nurses Association. www.medscape.com/viewprogram/2660_pnt.*

accepted and applied; remain nonjudgmental about traditional healing practices. Provide ethnic foods in healthcare facilities. Evaluate youth in immigrant families for conflict between family and societal expectations. See Chapter 3∞ for a thorough discussion of cultural influences on health and the nurse's role in providing culturally competent care.

LIFESTYLE ACTIVITIES AND THEIR INFLUENCES ON CHILD HEALTH

Many of the patterns of daily life play a part in determining the length and quality of one's life. The child's use of tobacco products and controlled substances influences both physical and mental health. Patterns of exercise and use of protective gear help to avoid early disabilities. Media use can influence aggressive behaviors, interfere with need for physical activity, or be a positive force in teaching young children new concepts. Tattoos that can introduce pathogens are an example of a lifestyle pattern that influences mental and physical health, and body image.

Substance Abuse

Children use many substances that have the potential for harming health. These include tobacco, either smoked or chewed, alcohol, and a variety of drugs and other substances. Substance abuse is a maladaptive pattern of substance use that is characterized by adverse consequences and repeated use (American Psychiatric Association 2000). Children are more vulnerable than adults both to addiction and to negative effects of substances due to their developing organs and body systems.

MediaLink Identifying Youth Who Abuse Drugs and Alcohol Use Video

Tobacco Use

Tobacco use is the most preventable cause of adult death in the United States. It leads to 430,000 deaths annually, and will be responsible for the premature death of 5 million of today's youth as they reach adult years (*Healthy People 2010*, 2000). Major health problems linked to tobacco use include cardiovascular disease, cancer, chronic lung disease, low birth weight, and other newborn problems. Even passive smoking or environmental tobacco smoke (ETS) is linked to increased heart disease, blood pressure, and respiratory problems (Leone, 2003). Cigarettes are most common; however, chewing tobacco, snuff, cigars, and bidis may also be used, and also pose significant health hazards.

PRACTICE ALERT

Forms of tobacco other than cigarettes may be popular among certain groups or in specific parts of the country. Chewing tobacco may be used by adolescents in school without staff being aware of the behavior. Bidis are small, brown, hand-rolled cigarettes that are popular among some youths. These usually have more nicotine than traditional cigarettes and are therefore very addicting. Try to learn the types of tobacco most common in the local community and plan to integrate history questions during health exams to learn about cigarette and other tobacco use.

Many nurses view tobacco use as an adult issue. While sale of tobacco products to children and advertisements aimed at this age group are forbidden by federal law, many youths obtain and use tobacco. After steadily increasing rates of youth smoking for many years, rates began to decrease in 1997. However, a significant number of youth still continue to use tobacco, making this an important health topic. About 30% of high schoolers and 13% of middle schoolers in the United States smoked in the month prior to being surveyed (MMWR, 2003a); about 14% of students are frequent smokers (MMWR, 2002) (Box 7–2). When including children who have ever smoked, the numbers are even larger. About 64% have tried smoking before high school (MMWR, 2002). Significant numbers of youth also report using chewing tobacco and cigars in the month prior to being surveyed (*Healthy People 2010*, 2000). Approximately 3,000 youths per day try their first cigarette; the major ages for trying tobacco are 9 to 14 years, between sixth and ninth grade. Early initiation of smoking becomes an extremely risky behavior when it is recognized that 80% of current adult smokers began smoking before 18 years of age (MMWR, 2001). Nicotine is highly addictive, and most people become addicted to the substance in adolescent years.

BOX 7–2 Research: Youth Risk Behavior Surveillance System

The Youth Risk Behavior Surveillance System is conducted every other year on large representative numbers of youth by the Centers for Disease Control and Prevention. For example, in 2003, 43 states were included in reported results, including 22 large cities and a number of suburban and rural areas. About 15,240 students were included in that data set, representing a student response rate of 83% of those questioned in participating schools (MMWR, 2004). The categories of priority health-risk behaviors investigated in each survey are:

- Behaviors contributing to unintentional and intentional injury
- Tobacco use
- Alcohol and other drug use
- Sexual behaviors that contribute to unintended pregnancy and sexually transmitted diseases, including HIV infection
- Physical activity
- Overweight and weight control

Etiology and Pathophysiology. Certain characteristics contribute to the likelihood of tobacco use. They include increasing age, male gender, ethnic group, ease of obtaining tobacco products, and smoking among family members. (See Developing Cultural Competence: Smoking.) Low socioeconomic group membership, access to tobacco products, low price of products, advertising, and lack of parental involvement in the

DEVELOPING CULTURAL COMPETENCE
Smoking

Among youth in the United States, White youth are significantly more likely to smoke than either Hispanic or Black peers. About 32% of White students reported smoking in the previous month, while 27% of Hispanic and 15% of Black students reported this behavior (MMWR, 2002a). American Indian and Alaska Natives also have high smoking rates, while Asian Americans have low rates (*Healthy People 2010*, 2000).

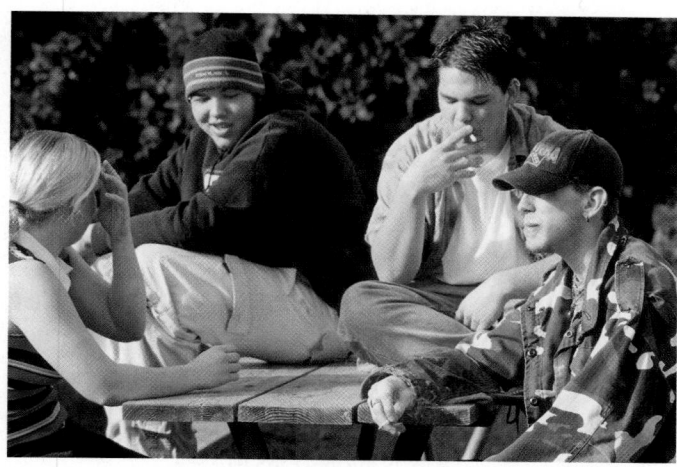

FIGURE 7–4 ■ Approximately 70% of children have tried smoking by their high school years. Early intervention can begin with discussions about smoking starting at 9 or 10 years of age.

youths' lives are also associated with tobacco use (*Healthy People 2010*, 2000). Cigarette use may be associated with use of alcohol and marijuana, suicidal thoughts, and younger age at first sexual intercourse (Busen, Modeland, & Kouzekanani, 2001). Girls commonly cite reasons for smoking as a desire to be slim and to appear mature, while boys more often view smoking as a method to be tough and rebellious. Both genders admit that smoking helps them to feel part of a group (Hanson, 1999) (Figure 7–4 ■).

COLLABORATIVE CARE

Many groups work together to both prevent and help tobacco users with cessation. Community activists, parents, nurses, school personnel, other health professionals, and even teens themselves join partner in youth programs. Successful programs combine several approaches:

- Youth-oriented mass media campaigns about hazards of tobacco use
- Increased tobacco taxes
- Smoke-free policies for schools, restaurants, and other community sites
- Increased regulation of tobacco
- Reduction in youth access to tobacco
- School-based programs in cessation

(*MMWR, 2002*)

Clinical Therapy

Several programs have been developed to encourage youth to avoid tobacco use. In addition, smoking cessation programs are available to assist youth who are already regular smokers, and are successful in achieving the goals of cessation or decrease in tobacco use (Coleman-Wallace, Lee, Montgomery, et al., 1999). About 55% of middle school smokers and 61% of high school smokers state they want to quit smoking cigarettes (MMWR, 2001), so cessation programs are needed to assist these age groups. Once a teen is identified as a smoker, using a biological marker such as urine cotinine (a by-product of tobacco) levels can help to identify the frequency of smoking. This information can be used to make suggestions to the teen about the potential outcomes of the behavior and the cessation program which is most likely to be helpful (Box 7–3).

BOX 7–3 Research: Youth and Smoking Cessation

It is not clear whether smoking cessation efforts for youth should be the same as those aimed at adults. In an attempt to examine the factors associated with adolescent smoking cessation, researchers surveyed 276 youth smokers in New Hampshire over a 3-year period, and found that nearly one third quit smoking. Smoking cessation rate was greatest in those who smoked occasionally versus daily, so researchers suggest that keeping occasional smokers from becoming regular smokers is essential (Sargent, Mott, & Stevens, 1998). Ask all youths about whether they smoke and how much. Target those who have tried but are not regular smokers by providing information about hazards of smoking, and role-play saying "no" to friends who suggest tobacco use. Smoking cessation programs may involve use of peer leadership and support, counseling, and computer instruction. When teens have become regular smokers, nicotine replacement therapy may be needed as they are likely addicted to nicotine (Donovan, 2000).

NURSING MANAGEMENT

Nursing management focuses on prevention of tobacco use, early identification of smokers, and referral to treatment and smoking cessation options.

■ Nursing Assessment and Diagnosis

Nurses are in a unique position to inquire about the incidence of smoking and other tobacco use among youth. Questions should be inserted into all well-child visits, beginning at about 9 to 10 years of age. Inquire about whether family members (especially parents and siblings) smoke or chew, and ask if some of the child's friends have tried smoking. Determine the child's knowledge and beliefs about the benefits and risks of tobacco use. Assess for associated risk behaviors such as alcohol and drug use, sexual behavior, and suicidal thoughts. As the child gets older, more direct and detailed questions are necessary. A nonjudgmental approach will be best to obtain a truthful response. School nurses can make observations about numbers of teens smoking and general attitudes about tobacco use. When children come to hospitals and other health facilities for care, use of tobacco should be part of general admission questions. Remember to include smokeless tobacco use in questioning (chewing tobacco, snuff, dip), and to ask about all forms of smoking. About 8% of youth have used smokeless tobacco in the preceding month, and 15% have smoked cigars (MMWR, 2002).

MediaLink: Smoking & Smoking Cessation Video

The following nursing diagnoses may apply to youth who smoke or show potential for this behavior.

- Activity Intolerance related to lowered oxygen supply
- Impaired Gas Exchange related to ventilation-perfusion imbalance
- Chronic Low Self-esteem related to negative self-appraisal

- Knowledge Deficient regarding dangers of tobacco use related to developmental focus on the present
- Imbalanced Nutrition, Less than Body Requirements related to effects of chemical dependence

Planning and Implementation

The roles of nurses in preventing and intervening in youth smoking are to inform youth, identify smokers, and implement programs (Table 7–4). Nurses should provide developmentally appropriate information about the hazards of tobacco use in all settings where youth are present. Posters, flyers, and speakers are particularly useful. Addicted teens who share their stories of difficult withdrawal from tobacco, and adults who have had cancer of the lungs or larynx may be effective speakers. Find out where teens obtain tobacco products in the community and where they engage in use of the products to target these places. Offer information on available prevention and cessation programs to youth and families in clinics, outpatient surgery centers, community activities, and in hospitals. Use opportunities such as adolescent pregnancy and presence of illness to reinforce the hazardous effects of tobacco on the individual and on those nearby. Speak to young athletes about the effects of tobacco on athletic performance. Show youth the ways in which this product can interfere with their meeting of life goals. Role-play how to tell other youth "no" when tobacco is offered. Establish programs that increase the sense of self-esteem without tobacco use. Be sure to include parents in the programs so that they see and acknowledge their role in setting an example about tobacco use, and in providing guidelines for the child. Influence of environmental tobacco (secondhand smoke) should be provided.

MediaLink Smoking Cessation and Support Resources

Adopt a nonjudgmental attitude when asking questions about smoking so that youth who are using tobacco can be identified. Ask questions without parents present and assure youth that the information will not be shared. Ask each smoker if they have tried to quit and if they want to "kick the habit." Encourage all youth to cut back and to quit use of tobacco products. Offer direct links to cessation programs to help them in these efforts.

Work with the schools and school districts to help establish preventive and cessation programs. There should be clear guidelines about school policies regarding smoking on school grounds. Keeping occasional youth smokers from becoming regular users should be a goal in order to avoid nicotine addiction. Find out what positive incentives can be offered to youth who are successful in quitting smoking. Contract with them to achieve their goals.

Evaluation

Expected outcomes of nursing interventions regarding tobacco use are lowered rates of regular use, delayed initiation of use, and success of cessation programs. Use the following *Healthy People 2010* (2000) objectives as guidelines.

- Reduce the proportion of children who are regularly exposed to tobacco smoke at home to 10%.
- Increase smoke-free and tobacco-free environments in schools, including all school facilities, property, vehicles, and school events, to 100%.
- Eliminate tobacco advertising and promotions that influence adolescents and young adults.
- Increase adolescents' disapproval of smoking to 95%.
- Reduce tobacco use by adolescents to 21%.
- Increase the average age of first use of tobacco products from 12 years to 14 years.

Alcohol and Drug Abuse

Substance abuse of alcohol and drugs occurs in children and adolescents of all socioeconomic levels and is a growing health problem. It is important to keep in mind that the use of any drug can pose a serious psychologic and physical risk to children and adolescents. Recent ability to examine the imaging of the brain by magnetic resonance imaging (MRI) and positron emission tomography (PET) shows that methamphetamine users have significant changes in brain blood flow and response times, even months after cessation of drug use (Swan, 2003).

Abuse of many substances—particularly marijuana, alcohol, cocaine, crack, and heroin—remains high among youth. Methamphetamine use continues to grow since it can be manufactured relatively easily and inexpensively in homes (Figure 7–5 ■). The Youth Risk Behavior Surveillance of high school seniors reported the following alarming statistics: 75% have had alcohol to drink, 45% had an alcoholic drink in the month prior to being surveyed, 28% engaged in binge drinking of alcohol, and the average age for beginning alcohol and cigarette use was 12 years (MMWR, 2004). Prevalence increases with advancing age and grade in school, while 47% of children have had their first drink by 9 years of age (Fetro, Coyle, & Pham, 2001). Over 40% of students have used marijuana; nearly 9% have used cocaine; 12% reported inhalant use of glue, paints, or other substances; 8% report methamphetamine use; 11% report ecstasy use; and 3% used heroin (MMWR, 2004). Syn-

TABLE 7–4 Nursing Role in Youth Smoking Prevention

INFORM	IDENTIFY	IMPLEMENT
➤ Hang posters, provide brochures, and facilitate presentations about smoking risks in all settings where youth are present. ➤ Target smokers with special information about the effects of nicotine on their bodies.	➤ Ask questions about smoking and other tobacco use at every health encounter beginning at about 9–10 years of age. ➤ For users, ask amount and type of tobacco. ➤ Learn where youth obtain tobacco and be proactive in stopping sales.	➤ Encourage youth tobacco users to quit. ➤ Facilitate referral to cessation programs. ➤ Arrange positive rewards for youth who are successful in cessation.

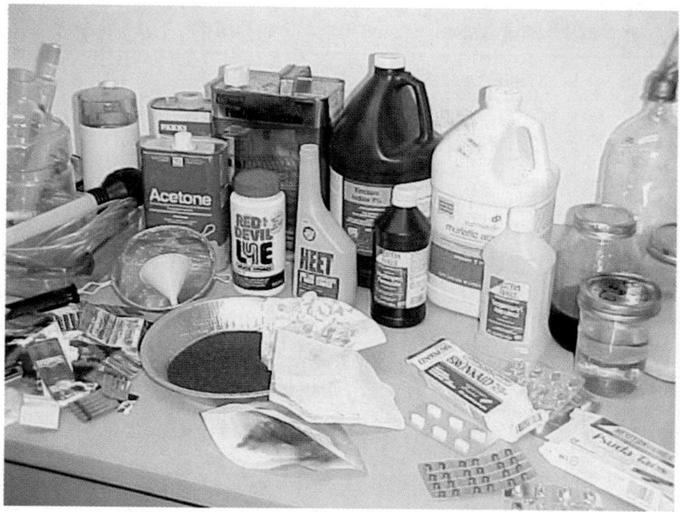

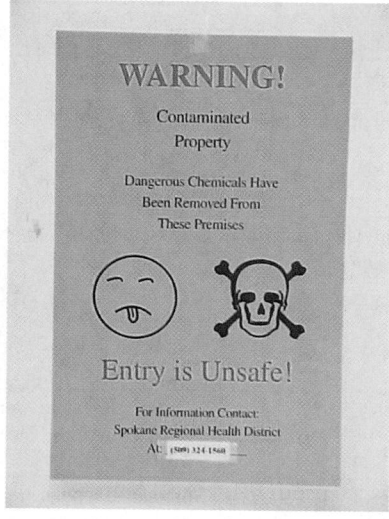

FIGURE 7–5 ■ *A,* Methamphetamine is a popular drug because it can be manufactured with items that are available to the lay public such as those shown in the picture on the left. Manufacture of the substance in homes has become a concern of health departments and communities at large. Children can be harmed by the chemicals produced, and may experience neglect and abuse. They may suffer even after the home is found and adults are apprehended as they must be placed in foster homes. *B,* Homes must be decontaminated in a lengthy and costly manner before future use after methamphetamine production. *(Photos courtesy of Spokane Regional Health District.)*

thetic drugs such as phencyclidine (PCP) (commonly referred to as "designer" drugs) mimic other narcotics, stimulants, and hallucinogens and are also dangerous. About 6% of students report use of illegal steroids (MMWR, 2004). Interestingly, all areas show slight decreases in use since the data from 2 years previously except steroid use, which has increased. See Developing Cultural Competence: Alcohol Use.

Over-the-counter medications are legal substances that are frequently abused. Easily obtainable at grocery stores and drugstores, these drugs include antihistamines, atropine, bromides, caffeine, ephedrine, pseudoephedrine, phenylpropanolamine, and amphetamine-like substitutes. Volatile inhalants such as glues are dangerous substances of abuse, and their use appears to be rising among school-age children and adolescents. Anabolic steroids are the drugs of abuse most commonly used by athletes. Some common contemporary drugs and street names are listed in Table 7–5. See Box 7–4 for common inhalant agents.

Etiology and Pathophysiology. In most cases, substance abuse represents a maladaptive coping response to the stressors of childhood and adolescence. A child may begin using drugs or alcohol to deal with stress because family members or peers do so. Children in families with a history of substance abuse are at higher risk of abusing drugs and alcohol. Other risk factors include rebelliousness, aggressiveness, low self-esteem, dysfunctional parental relationships, lack of adequate support systems, academic underachievement, poor judgment, and poor impulse control. Adolescents and young adults use "club drugs" to achieve greater satisfaction during nights dancing, drinking, and attending clubs. Use of these drugs with alcohol can lead to deadly consequences. See Table 7–5 for common club drugs.

Initial experimentation with alcohol or drugs may be unpleasant. With continued use, however, the adolescent learns to "achieve the high," an illusion of power and well-being. The

DEVELOPING CULTURAL COMPETENCE
Alcohol Use

In a study of middle school students, Asian students were least likely to drink alcohol (9%), with African Americans next (23%), followed by Hispanics (26%) and Whites (29%) (Fetro et al., 2001). Among high school students, Whites had highest alcohol use (47%), with Hispanics next (46%), and Blacks least (37%) (MMWR, 2004). In a survey of Bureau of Indian Affairs–funded high schools, the CDC has found that 49% of students reported current alcohol use and 38% reported episodic heavy drinking (MMWR, 2003b). Nurses can use this information to target groups most at risk of alcohol ingestion, even at these young ages. Incidence varies among the genders also, so learning about risks can assist in assessment and intervention. For example, Hispanic females had higher incidence of drinking in the previous month than Hispanic males (48% versus 43%) (MMWR, 2004). Include members of the ethnic groups to provide information to other members of those groups. Youth will be more likely to listen to someone from their own cultural group discuss importance of avoiding alcohol and resources for treatment of alcoholism.

BOX 7–4 Common Inhalant Agents

Aerosols	Solvents
Cooking spray	Nail polish remover
Whipped cream	Paint thinner or cleaner
Spray paint	Lighter fluid
Cosmetic sprays	Degreaser
Adhesives	**Other**
Model glues	Gasoline
Rubber cements	Helium

Adapted from Cook, K. R. (1999). Assessment of potential inhalant use by students. Journal of School Nursing, 15*(20), 20–23.*

TABLE 7–5 Common Contemporary Club Drugs, Street Names, and Drug Information

DRUG	ACTION	STREET NAMES	ROUTE	TIME OF ACTION
Methylenediosymethamphetamine (MDMA)	Stimulant; appetite suppressant; Increased pulse, BP, temperature, overhydration, hyponatremia, memory loss	Ecstasy, XTC, X, Adam, Clarity, Lover's speed	PO (tablets, capsules)	3–6 hours
Gamma-hydroxybutyrate (GHB)	CNS depressant, euphoria, growth hormone release	Grievous Bodily Harm, G., Liquid Ecstasy, Georgia Home Boy	PO (liquid, powder, tablets, capsules)	4 hours
Ketamine	Anesthetic; Decreased memory, attention, learning; Increased BP; Respiratory collapse	Special K, K, Vitamin K, Cat Valiums	IV, respiratory (injected, snorted or smoked; liquid or powder)	1–2 hours
Rohypnol (benzodiazepine)	Amnesia, sedative; Decreased BP, urinary retention; Given prior to sexual assault	Roffies, Rophies, Roche, Forget-me Pill	PO, respiratory, (snorted) (tablets)	8–12 hours
Methamphetamine	Stimulant; highly addictive; memory loss, violence, psychosis; Cardiac and neurologic damage	Speed, Ice, Chalk, Meth, Crystal, Crank, Fire, Glass	PO, respiratory, IV (smoked, snorted, injected)	Several hours; long-term permanent effects
Lysergic acid diethylamide (LSD)	Hallucinogen; Increased pulse, BP, temperature; psychosis, flashbacks	Acid, Boomers, Yellow Sunshines	PO (liquid, tablets, capsules)	1–2 hours; possible flashbacks later

Note: Data from National Institute on Drug Abuse. 2004. NIDA Community Drug Alert Bulletin—Club Drugs. Bethesda, MD: U.S. Department of Health and Human Services.

adolescent wants the high more frequently and actively seeks alcohol or drugs. Tolerance to the substance occurs with continued use, and ever-increasing amounts are required to achieve a pleasurable high. Physical and psychologic dependence ensues as the body's tissues require the substance to function properly. Withdrawal symptoms occur when the child or adolescent is deprived of the substance.

Clinical Manifestations. Substance abuse in children and adolescents is commonly overlooked and underdiagnosed by healthcare providers (Pagliaro & Pagliaro, 1996), due in part to the wide range of clinical presentations. These vary according to type of drug abused, amount, frequency, time of last use, and severity of drug dependence. See clinical manifestations of commonly abused drugs on page 203.

Common physical manifestations include alterations in vital signs, weight loss, chronic fatigue, chronic cough, respiratory congestion, red eyes, and general apathy and malaise. The mental status examination (refer to Chapter 8∞) may reveal alterations in level of consciousness, impaired attention and concentration, impaired thought processes, delusions, and hallucinations. Low self-esteem, feelings of guilt or worthlessness, and suicidal or homicidal thoughts are also common.

Poor school performance and changes in mood, sleep habits, appetite, dress, and social relationships are nonspecific characteristics of the substance-abusing child.

COLLABORATIVE CARE

Multiple psychiatric diagnostic criteria exist for each drug class. Children and adolescents who have other psychosocial disorders commonly use or abuse drugs or alcohol. Treatment should therefore focus not only on the substance use or abuse, but also on the issues underlying the problem. Intervention includes both the family and child or adolescent abuses substances.

Clinical Therapy

The primary goal of treatment is to teach the child and other family members to develop and sustain positive coping patterns, and to support them during this process. Most treatment programs offer inpatient and outpatient services, as well as aftercare programs. These programs usually consist of peer support focusing on the development of a lifestyle free of drugs or alcohol, healthy family relationships, and positive coping skills. Family involvement is strongly encouraged. Hospitalization is required if the physical dependence is significant and withdrawal places the child at risk for complications such as seizures, depression, or suicidal behavior.

NURSING MANAGEMENT

Nursing management focuses on prevention of substance abuse, early identification of users, and referral to treatment options.

Nursing Assessment and Diagnosis

Nurses may encounter the substance-abusing child or adolescent in the emergency department or outpatient clinic, in the school and other community settings, or during hospitalization

CLINICAL MANIFESTATIONS of Commonly Abused Drugs

DRUG	POTENTIAL FOR DEPENDENCE	CLINICAL MANIFESTATIONS
Depressants Alcohol, barbiturates (amobarbital, pentobarbital, secobarbital)	*Physical and psychologic:* High; varies somewhat among drugs	*Physical:* Decreased muscle tone and coordination, tremors *Psychologic:* Impaired speech, memory, and judgment; confusion; decreased attention span; emotional lability
Stimulants Amphetamines (e.g., Benzedrine), caffeine, cocaine	*Physical:* Low to moderate *Psychologic:* High; withdrawal from amphetamines and cocaine can lead to severe depression	*Physical:* Dilated pupils, increased pulse and blood pressure, flushing, nausea, loss of appetite, tremors *Phsychologic:* Euphoria; increased alertness, agitation, or irritability; hallucinations; insomnia
Opiates Codeine, heroin, meperidine (Demerol), methadone, morphine, opium, oxycodone (Percodan, Oxycontin)	*Physical and psychologic:* High; varies somewhat among drugs; withdrawal effects are uncomfortable but rarely life threatening	*Physical:* Analgesia, depressed respirations and muscle tone (may lead to coma or death), nausea, constricted pupils *Psychologic:* Changes in mood (usually euphoria), drowsiness, impaired attention or memory, sense of tranquility
Hallucinogens Lysergic acid diethylamide (LSD), mescaline, phencyclidine (PCP)	*Physical:* None *Psychologic:* Unknown	*Physical:* Lack of coordination, dilated pupils, hypertension, elevated temperature; severe PCP intoxication can result in seizures, respiratory depression, coma, and death *Psychologic:* Visual illusions and hallucinations, altered perceptions of time and space, emotional lability, psychosis
Volatile Inhalants Glues, typing correction fluid, acrylic paints, spot removers, lighter fluid, gasoline, butane	*Physical and psychologic:* Varies with drug used	*Physical:* Impaired coordination, liver damage (in some cases) *Psychologic:* Impaired judgment, delirium
Marijuana	*Physical:* Low *Psychologic:* Usually low; occasionally moderate to high	*Physical:* Tachycardia, reddened conjunctiva, dry mouth, increased appetite *Psychologic:* Initial anxiety followed by euphoria; giddiness; impaired attention, judgment, and memory

for an injury or other acute problem. Nursing assessment includes taking a thorough history from the parents and child, observing the child's behavior, and performing a physical examination. The history should include the age at which drug use began, pattern of use, length of time the drug has been used, amount of drug used, and psychologic state while on drugs. A history of parental drug use and noninvolvement in parenting the child puts the child at higher risk for substance abuse, reflecting the combined effects of genetic and environmental influences. Assessment tools provide useful information for the healthcare provider. These include the PACES tool (see clinical tip) and the HEEADSSS tool (see Chapter 1∞). See Partnering with Families: Identifying the Youth Who Is Abusing Substances.

CLINICAL TIP

PACES provides a framework for areas that should be assessed for each child to identify risk and protective factors related to substance use.

- P = Parents, peers
- A = Accidents, alcohol/drug use
- C = Cigarettes
- E = Emotional problems
- S = School, sexuality

(Data from Knight, 1997)

Physiologic Assessment

Look for physical signs and symptoms of substance abuse, including bloodshot eyes, dilated pupils, slurred speech, and weight loss. The adolescent may appear sleepy or restless, or may show signs of clumsiness or inconsistent behavior. Consider all types of substance abuse, including model glue, gasoline, and other sources. Assess for signs of withdrawal and current intoxication effects.

PRACTICE ALERT

Adolescents who have some or all of the following symptoms may be experiencing alcohol withdrawal: anxiety, headache, tremors, nausea and vomiting, malaise or weakness, insomnia, depressed mood or irritability, and hallucinations.

Psychologic Assessment

Changes in social habits may indicate substance abuse. Parents may report a drop in the school-age child's or adolescent's grades or decreased interest in school activities. New friends are not introduced to parents, and the adolescent has less contact with parents, teachers, and other adults who were previously important.

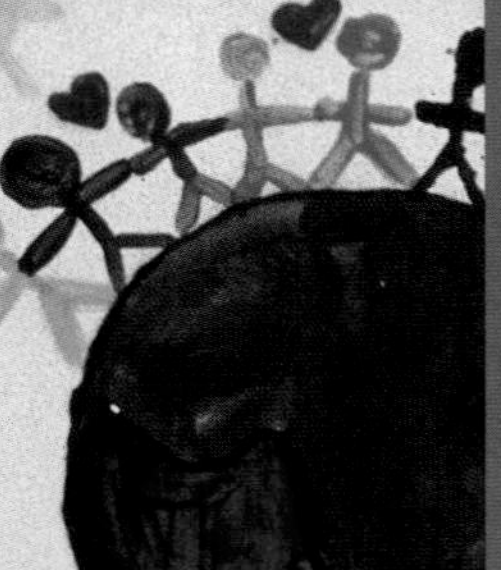

PARTNERING WITH FAMILIES

Identifying the Youth Who Is Abusing Substances

Families are often confused about the behavior of adolescents and unsure whether it represents normal development or abuse of substances. Some characteristics of normal development that help to differentiate these occurrences are listed here. When concerned about possible substance use, the parent can confront the child or talk with school nurses or counselors.

- Many youth are periodically distant with parents at times, but remain involved with peers in school sports and other activities. Withdrawal from all activities and friends may indicate substance abuse.
- Adolescents often complain about school, but when teachers report the student meets expectations and is consistently performing in the classroom this is normal behavior.
- Teens may be weepy on occasion when having a difficult time with friends or not performing as desired. Continued, consistent weepiness is more likely to indicate depression or substance abuse.
- Teens like to stay up late and are frequently tired in the morning, while abusing teens may "nod off" frequently during the day.
- Many adolescents like to achieve a disheveled look in clothing, but the teen who frequently neglects basic hygiene or does not seem to have the energy to wash and dress may be depressed or abusing substances.
- All teens get some infections, but abusing teens may have reddened eyes, oral sores, and constant respiratory discomfort from "snorting" substances.

MediaLink Substance Abuse Resources and Support

The child's current drug use, potential for violence, and motivation to make changes are noted. Assess the degree of family support available.

Following are possible nursing diagnoses for children and adolescents who abuse drugs or alcohol.

- Impaired Social Interaction related to altered thought processes
- Chronic Low Self-esteem related to dysfunctional family and social relationships
- Risk for Injury related to altered perceptions and sensorium
- Risk for Violence, Self-directed or Other-directed related to physiologic dependence on drugs, alcohol, and other substances

Planning and Implementation

Care of children and adolescents who abuse drugs, alcohol, and other substances is challenging and often frustrating. Long-term mental health counseling may be necessary to resolve underlying issues and foster lifestyle and behavioral changes.

Prevention is the most desirable intervention. The nurse can play a major role in teaching children and their families about substance abuse. Education should begin in primary school and continue with intensification during middle and high school years. Nurses also can play a major role in community education. Various prevention programs have been developed by federal and private organizations. Referral to support organizations may be beneficial for the child, parents, and other family members. Self-help groups, which are available in most communities, include Alcoholics Anonymous, Narcotics Anonymous, Al-Anon, Nar-Anon, and Ala-Teen. Parents may receive support from a group such as Parents Anonymous.

The youth's protective factors can be identified and used in planning appropriate interventions. For example, a child with goals related to a future career can be helped to see the way in which substance use will interfere with goal attainment. Identifying a strong role model through a program like Big Brothers or Big Sisters can assist children who lack that strength in their families.

Evaluation

Expected outcomes of nursing interventions regarding substance abuse include the following:

- Abstention from alcohol and street drugs
- Successful participation in substance abuse programs
- Developmentally normal social interactions
- School performance at level of potential
- Absence of injury

Physical Inactivity

In the past few decades, children have become increasingly physically inactive. This decrease is a reflection of lifestyles in which car travel is valued, computers and televisions are part of daily life, neighborhoods are sometimes unsafe places for play activities, and schools do not routinely require daily physical education classes (Figure 7–6 ■).

Children and adolescents spend an average of almost 3 hours a day watching television. This is 20 to 30 hours weekly, and may extend to 50 hours weekly for some children. When video game and computer time is added to this, the media total average is 6.5 hours daily (Committee on Public Education, American Academy of Pediatrics, 2001). Children who watch 4 or more hours of television daily get significantly less physical activity and have poorer sports performance than those who watch 1 hour or less (Crespo, Smit, Troiano, et al., 2001). There is often a high intake of fatty snacks during television viewing. Even at very young ages, children are immersed in various types of media (Box 7–5).

Physical inactivity leads to many health concerns. A primary outcome is overweight or obesity (see Chapter 9∞). Other outcomes can be an increased rate of type 2 diabetes (see Chapter 32∞), increased exposure to television and computer game violence and sexual activity at early ages, and early progression of cardiovascular disease (see Chapter 26∞).

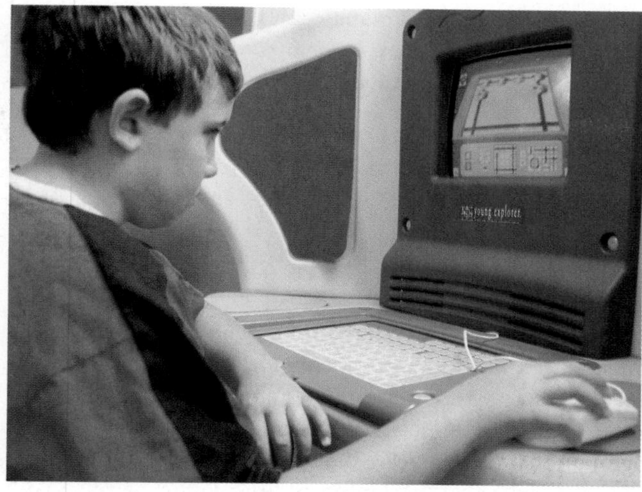

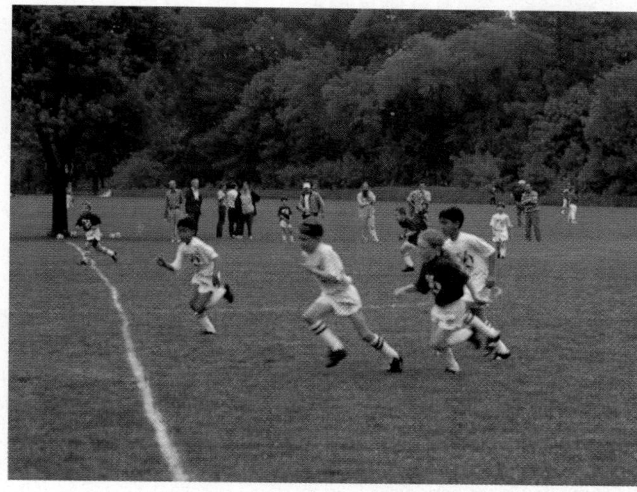

FIGURE 7–6 ■ Physical inactivity is a growing problem among children, and can contribute to poor health. It is important to balance sedentary activities, such as playing computer games, with physical and social activities. Sports are an excellent way for children to develop their psychosocial, cognitive, and motor skills.

Soccer photo courtesy of Rebecca Scheirer, Kensington, Maryland.

On the other hand, patterns of physical activity established in childhood can increase exercise behaviors in adulthood and contribute to lower rates of low back pain, overweight, osteoporosis, heart disease, diabetes, colon cancer, high blood pressure, and a more positive self-image.

Although many children demonstrate low levels of physical activity, a profound decrease in vigorous activity is common in grades 9 through 12, more pronounced in females than males. Boys who do remain active generally engage in team sports and weight training, while girls more commonly enjoy aerobics and dance classes (*Healthy People 2010*, 2000).

Health professionals can integrate assessment of physical activity into all healthcare, and make recommendations to children and families that will help to increase opportunities for physical activity. Nurses assess height, weight, and body mass index to look for signs of overweight (see Chapter 9∞). Ask what a typical day is like and include specific questions about television, computers, and video games. Suggest strategies to lessen the

BOX 7–5 Young Children and Media Effects

The increasing role of media in the daily schedules of children has been known for some time. However, little data examined the issue in very young children. The first study that examined the role of electronic media in the lives of infants, toddlers, and preschoolers found startling results. A nationally representative survey of 1,065 parents of children from 6 months to 6 years found the following:

- One in four children under 2 years of age has a television in the bedroom; 36% of children under 6 years have a television in their bedrooms, while 27% have a VCR or DVD, 10% have a video game player, and 7% have a computer.
- Those children who have a television in their bedrooms spend significantly less time reading or playing outside than other children.
- Sixty-five percent of young children live in a household where the television is on at least half of the time; 36% are in homes where the television is nearly always on.
- Young children spend the same amount of time with electronic media as they spend outdoors (about 2 hours each).
- In contrast, these children spend only 39 minutes daily reading or being read to.
- Half of children under 6 years, and 70% of those 4–6 years, have used computers.
- Much new media is targeted at this very young audience.
- Parents have generally positive views of media, with 72% saying computers mostly help child learning, and about half saying that television and videos are very important to the intellectual development of children.

(Rideout, Vandewater & Wartella, 2003)

These findings are critical for nurses to consider. Physical inactivity or sedentary behavior is linked to obesity, type 2 diabetes, and other chronic disease risks. Children's ready access to media in the home and other settings directly interferes with recommended levels of physical activity. In all settings with parents of young children, ask about exposure to media. Encourage parents to turn off the television in the house except for select and limited viewing times, avoid media use in the child's bedroom, limit exposure to media, and have the child engaged in physical activity for a greater part of the day than in quiet pursuits. Encourage reading and being read to for young children; parents can schedule reading time to at least equal media viewing. Carefully perform developmental testing on children when exposure to media is high (see Chapter 10∞).

CRITICAL THINKING APPLICATION

What other teaching can you identify to address this issue with parents of young children? How can parents integrate media concerns into evaluation of childcare settings? What might the effects be on child growth and development with excessive use of media?

MediaLink The Effects of Media on Children Video

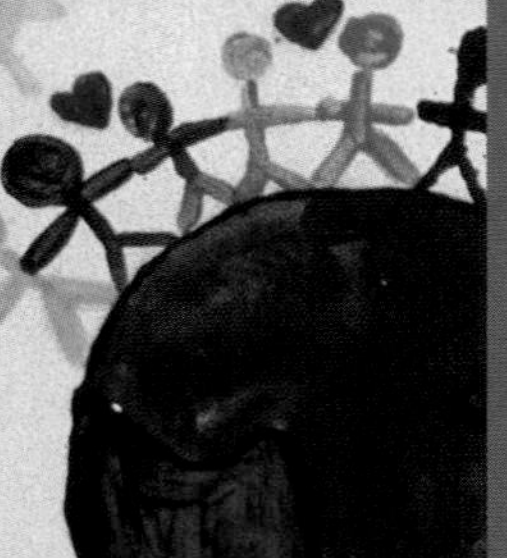

PARTNERING WITH FAMILIES

Physical Activity Guidelines for Youth

- Engage in moderate physical activity (bike riding, walking, baseball, roller blading) at least 30 minutes five times weekly.
- Engage in vigorous physical activity that causes sweating and hard breathing (soccer, running, ice hockey) at least 20 minutes three times weekly.
- Encourage schools to offer physical education to all students, and have students sign up when this is an elective.
- Encourage walking and bike riding to friends' homes and stores when safe.
- Plan physical activities together as a family.
- Get a pet and plan to walk the pet daily.
- Limit television and other similar sedentary activities to no more than 2 hours daily.
- On days home, allow the child to watch television for up to 1 hour, and then insist that 1 hour of reading, 1 hour of physical activity, and 1 hour of socializing with others take place before returning to more television.

hours spent with media such as increased physical activity and family meals.

Children should be asked about how they like to spend free time. Community and school activities should be encouraged and rewarded. Examples include fun runs, walks that benefit causes, aerobics classes, team sports, roadside cleanups, and fairs and carnivals. Examine the community in which the family lives. Is it possible to walk to the store, to ride a bicycle to school? Be sure suggestions are realistic for the particular situation. Help parents and children learn what they can do for physical fitness. Work with school physical education personnel to plan activities both in and out of physical education class that promote lifelong exercise routines. See Partnering with Families: Physical Activity Guidelines for Youth.

Injury and Protective Equipment

In the discussion of causes of childhood and adolescent morbidities and mortalities in Chapter 1∞, unintentional injuries are listed as a common problem. In fact, 71% of deaths from age 10 years onward result from four causes—motor vehicle crashes, other unintentional injury, homicide, and suicide (MMWR, 2004). (See Developing Cultural Competence: Unintentional Injury Rates.) Homicide is discussed in the violence section later in this chapter; suicide is discussed in Chapter 34∞. Chapters 11 through 15∞ discuss the frequent injuries seen in children at different developmental ages, and safety precautions to avoid injuries from car crashes, falls, poisonings, and other developmentally related injuries. Many common injuries are preventable with simple use of protective gear and following of safety guidelines (Figure 7–7 ■). These recommendations are explored in the following section.

CLINICAL TIP

Many sports and activities require safety gear. These include roller blading, skate boarding, roller hockey, ice hockey, football, soccer, baseball, scooters, and skiing or snow boarding fast or using jumps.

Eighteen percent of youth rarely or never wear seat belts in automobiles; 38% of those who ride motorcycles do not wear helmets (MMWR, 2004). The use of safe automobile and motorcycle behaviors must be emphasized again in adolescence, with the recognition that risks increase if driving is combined with use of alcohol and controlled substances, and risk-taking behaviors occur with all wheeled transportation. Adolescents sometimes engage in practices that put them at particular risk and nurses should be alert for activities in their communities. Examples include car surfing (standing on the trunk, hood, or roof of a moving vehicle) (Geiger, Drongowski, & Lenni, 2001) or street racing (racing cars down a street at extremely high speed).

Many children ride bicycles, but only about 14% are protected by helmet use, contributing to 23,000 bicycle-related head injuries annually. Bike helmets could prevent up to 88% of serious brain injuries from bicycle crashes (Committee on Injury and Poison Prevention, American Academy of Pediatrics, 2001). A recent increase in scooter use led to over 28,000 emergency room visits in 2000 (MMWR, 2000). Many of these injuries could be avoided by use of helmet, knee and elbow pads, riding only on smooth surfaces in areas without cars, and avoiding rid-

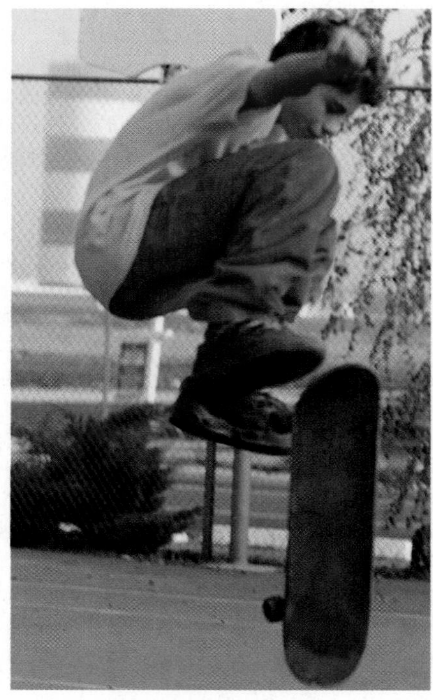

FIGURE 7–7 ■ What protective gear should children use for skate boarding? How would you convince them to use the protection?

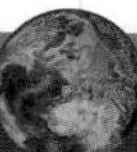

DEVELOPING CULTURAL COMPETENCE
Unintentional Injury Rates

Striking ethnic disparities exist in the rates of unintentional injury among children. These differences are due mainly to living in impoverished communities rather than any innate biological variations. While the unintentional injury rate in children under 14 years declined 39% from 1987 to 2000, the smallest reductions were among American Indian/Alaskan Natives (20% decline) and African American children (36% decline), while higher reductions were seen in Asian/Pacific Islanders (52% decline) and White children (39% decline) (National Safe Kids Campaign, 2003.) What are the major causes of unintentional injury in your community and state? What ethnic and age groups are at greatest risk? How can you integrate teaching in your practice that is specific to the findings in your community?

ing after dark. Strategies to make use of helmets and other protective gear more attractive to children and adolescents are needed (Figure 7–8 ■). Nurses can play a major role in programs to educate and reward children for helmet use, and can assist families to find helmets at a price they can afford (Behrman, Kliegman & Jenson, 2004).

Nurses can be active in identifying behaviors in youths in specific communities and working with schools and other community groups to establish educational programs. Efforts should also include adequate conditioning for sports, proper treatment of injuries, and prevention of overuse injuries (Committee on Sports Medicine and Fitness, American Academy of Pediatrics, 2001). See Box 7–6.

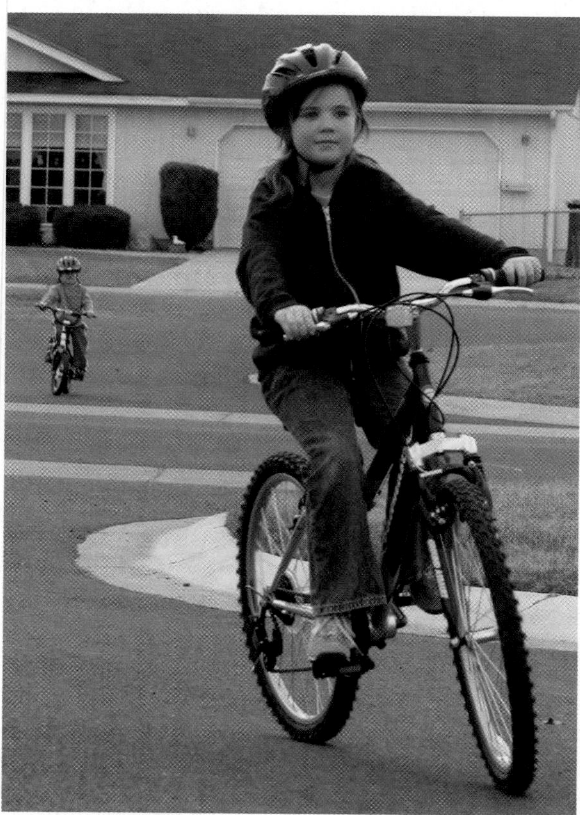

FIGURE 7–8 ■ Having parents insist on helmet use and having friends who also wear bicycle helmets can encourage use by young children.

BOX 7–6 Extreme Sports

A growing number of children engage in "extreme" sports, those that carry a high degree of risk and have not traditionally been common. Some examples are mountain biking, three wheeling, ski racing, snow boarding through trees and on courses with pikes and other challenges, ice climbing, rock climbing, and wake boarding. While the nurse is probably unable to dissuade youth from engaging in these activities, safety measures should be emphasized. Find out what protective gear the youth wears and what is recommended. Keep at hand examples of stories of youth who have been saved by use of such gear. Encourage the youth to engage in sports activities only when others are present and to have a plan for emergencies, including a working cell phone, leaving information with an adult about plans and expected return, and planning for harsh weather with items such as emergency blankets, gear, and food. Encourage the youth to talk with parents and other adults about the risks and benefits of the activities.

MediaLink Extreme Sports Video

Body Art

Body art in the form of painting, tattooing, and piercing has been donned by humans throughout history. There is a resurgence of interest in this decorative art, especially among teens and young adults. Many adolescents have multiple body piercings and tattoos and may even resort to performing these decorations on themselves or friends.

From 10% to 25% of adolescents have tattoos, and even more have at least one body piercing (Armstrong & Kelly, 2001). In some states, teens must be 18 years of age or have parental permission to obtain body art, but students often report that it is easy to have an adult present who signs and claims to be a parent. Only in some states are tattoo and body piercing businesses required to be licensed and comply with certain regulations. Remember that Amy, who is described in the opening scenario, had her piercing done by a friend. Amy demonstrates some common characteristics of teens who choose to use body art. It may be seen as a way to establish individualism and independence, and helps some teens to feel part of a peer group. Multiple tattoos and piercings are common, as is the case with Amy (Figure 7–9 ■).

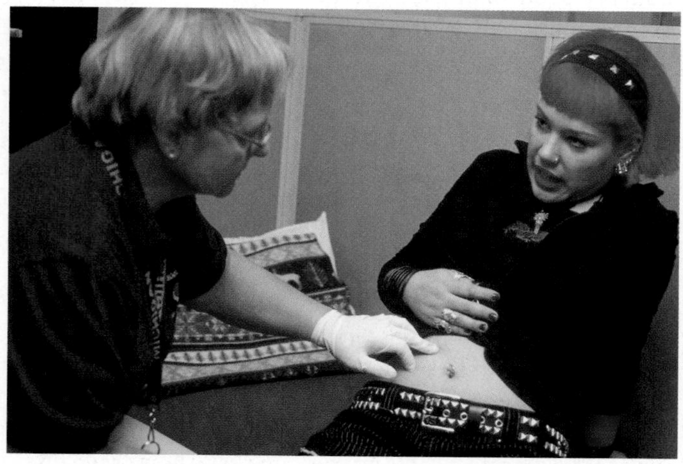

FIGURE 7–9 ■ Talk openly with adolescents about their health and teach them to avoid health risks connected with tattoos and piercing.

Body art is a common source of infections with skin pathogens, as well as hepatitis B and C. Body piercing is a major method of transmission of hepatitis C, a disease that may not even become manifested until years later. It can be a source of HIV if proper techniques are not followed. Piercings in parts of the body such as the mouth or navel are most prone to bacterial infection and continued redness and irritation. Serious systemic infections such as endocarditis have occurred after some piercings. The pierced site may not appear infected but transfer of organisms causes serious infection and heart damage. Common infective agents include *Neisseria* and *Staphylococcus.* When noting signs of systemic infection such as fever, weakness, malaise, and arthralgia (see Chapter 26∞ for full discussion of endocarditis), gather history about body piercings and refer for care to the primary healthcare provider (Goldrick, 2003). Pierced tongues can lead to chipped teeth or even be the cause of choking if dislodged from the site.

Another issue that the teen should consider prior to tattoo is the relationship of the tattoos to future lifestyle changes. Advise teens to avoid tattooing the name of a person or musical group since relationships change and tastes in music evolve. Be sure they know the meaning of phrases, foreign words, or symbols. Consider the visibility of the tattoo and its effect on future employment. Tattoos on the face, neck, or other readily visible places may be a detriment during employment interviews. Tattoos should always be considered permanent. Methods for removal may be costly, painful, and unsuccessful (Selekman, 2003).

Another form of body art that is regarded as disfigurement is **branding** or scarification. In this process, the skin is burned to result in a scar. Usually a desired sign, symbol, or word is inscribed. Results are usually not precise and do not adhere to expected designs. This procedure is done on the self or friend, using common household metal implements heated in fires or stoves. Others cut themselves in the form of a desired design, a process called **cutting.** These practices can result in infection, often do not yield the desired result, and may indicate underlying problems. They should be discouraged and the youth involved should be referred for further assessment by primary care providers or counselors.

Since teens may choose to obtain body art even if parents object and if there are state laws to prohibit or make it difficult, nursing care must focus on providing information to the teen, assessing sites, identifying infections, and referring if needed. See Partnering with Families: Care for Tattoos and Body Piercings. Care is almost always provided in community settings such as clinics or schools. Ask teens if they are considering body art, because they often do not seek advice before obtaining the art, and may therefore not get adequate teaching (Montgomery & Parks, 2001).

MediaLink LGBT/Q Resources and Support

Sexual Orientation

Adolescence is a time of identifying emerging sexuality. Most teens establish relationships with members of the opposite sex and learn how to interact in ways that are guided by their peer group, family, and culture. For some youth, the transition into adult sexuality is more challenging, as they feel emotional and sexual attraction to people of the same sex (**homosexuality**). The term *gay* is often used for homosexual males and *lesbian* for homosexual females. Other youth are *bisexual,* or attracted to both men and women, and some are *transgendered,* an imprecise term for individuals who cross gender lines. The initials **LGBT** are sometimes used to refer to these minority sexuality choices, while the acronym **LGBQ** is sometimes used for lesbian, gay, bisexual, or questioning. From 1% to 10% of youth self-identify as homosexual (Benton, 2003).

Sexual attractions and practices different from the mainstream are not deviant, but may be viewed as part of a continuum of sexual expression. No gene, early life experience, or other event causes homosexuality.

LGBT/Q youth are at risk for a variety of problems related to emotional and physical health. These include rejection by family members and peers, verbal harassment, sexual abuse and physical assault, a high rate of suicide, substance abuse, high rate of homelessness, and sexual risks of HIV and other sexually transmitted diseases (Stevens & Morgan, 2001). Their health risks need to be identified and appropriate care provided.

Nurses can provide healthcare for LGBT youth in a variety of settings. School nurses and clinics can display a sign that demonstrates they are accepting of persons with minority sexual preferences. These signs include rainbows and triangles, and can be obtained from local gay and lesbian community groups, and other groups such as PFLAG (Parents, Families, and Friends of Lesbians and Gays). Terminology in assessment should be gender free. Ask the youth, "Do you have one or more sexual partners?" rather than "Do you have a boyfriend?" When youth identify as LGBT, usual care of all kinds should be provided, including preventive care such as immunizations, sports assessments, and injury prevention teaching. Be alert that the youth may have additional health challenges. Ask about peer and parental support; refer to support groups if needed. When a youth is "coming out," or disclosing sexual preference to family or friends, there is often much stress and there may even be rejection by loved ones. The nurse is often able to provide support both to the youth and parents during this time. Offer to meet with family or friends if that will assist the teen. Many resources are available to help schools provide safe settings for LGBT/Q youth; nurses can be effective in obtaining such resources for school personnel. Provide resources when the teen is homeless, depressed, or suicidal (see Chapter 34∞). Perform testing for sexually transmitted diseases if sexual contact is occurring and teach preventive measures. Foster a positive sense of self-esteem through encouraging positive activities such as sports, music, and friendships with peers (Benton, 2003).

EFFECTS OF VIOLENCE

Violence is a threatened or actual use of physical force that leads to potential or actual physical or emotional trauma. In the past several years, adults and children alike have been shocked by violent episodes in schools. Although these incidents had much media coverage, they are just one type of violence to which children may be exposed on a regular basis. Children can be the recipients of violence during child abuse and homicides, and they

PARTNERING WITH FAMILIES

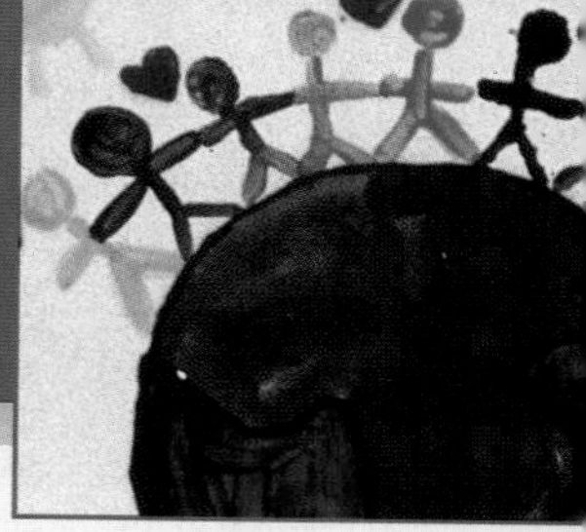

Care for Tattoos and Body Piercings

Before the procedure

- Visit several studios to make comparisons of technique, quality, and cleanliness.
- Ask to watch a tattoo or piercing done on someone else.
- What are the sterilization and hygiene practices of the artist?
- Is the artist licensed? Trained?
- Look at pictures of completed art and talk with former clients.
- Insist that new, sterile equipment be opened in front of the person to be decorated.
- Consider if this permanent body decoration is desired for a lifetime.
- Consider what the tattoo or piercing will look like in several years.
- Consider the possible side effects of infection, dislike for the art, allergy to dyes or metals.
- Be sure that hepatitis B vaccination is completed before the procedure.
- Be aware that no immunization is available to protect against the health risks of hepatitis C and HIV.

Care after the procedure

- Touch the area only after careful handwashing.
- Keep the area elevated and use ice for the first 2 days to minimize swelling.
- Avoid contact with other person's bodily fluids until well healed.
- Turn the piercing jewelry gently several times daily using washed hands.
- Use antibacterial mouthwash, cleaner, or ointment as recommended.
- Avoid pressure and rubbing on the site (such as belts on navel piercings).
- Watch carefully for signs of infection and report them to a health-care provider:
  - Increased redness
  - Swelling
  - Pain
  - Hot feeling
  - Discharge
- Ask the artist how long healing of a piercing will take. It varies from 2 months in the mouth to 6–8 months in the navel.
- Metal is dangerous during some medical procedures such as magnetic resonance imaging (MRI) or during surgery. Be sure to tell doctors and nurses about the piercings when hospitalized or receiving medical care, especially if they are not readily visible.
- If you decide to remove a piece of jewelry soon after placement, then the skin may heal with only a slight scar.

themselves can perform acts of violence on others. They may be touched by violence when parents, siblings, or other family members are killed in gang conflicts, in terrorist attacks, or in wars. The effects of violence are far reaching and ongoing; they permeate the child's entire lifetime. This section explores certain types of violence affecting children.

Schools and Communities

At a time when firearm deaths are decreasing overall, unintentional deaths and suicides have increased among children. About 75% of these deaths are committed with firearms found in the home. Forty percent of households with children have guns and in 25% of those homes the firearms are stored loaded or are not secured under lock (Society for Pediatric Nurses, SPN Public Policy Committee, 2000).

Homicide among children has gained attention in past years due to several shootings at schools. Although homicide is an extreme example, other types of violence exist. Children report being threatened verbally and with guns or knives at home, in schools, and neighborhoods. They may be beaten up, bullied, or harassed. They may view domestic violence in their own homes. They may be subjected to dangerous situations in their neighborhoods or during times of homelessness. About half of youths report experiencing serious threats to their well-being (Pratt & Greydanus, 2000). Date rape or other sexual violence is reported by up to 15% of teens (Spencer & Bryant, 2000).

PRACTICE ALERT

Nursing Alert

When a group of children is attacked or killed in a school shooting, this tragic occurrence gains media attention. Little do many realize that this tragedy is part of daily life, in separate settings all over the country. About 8 children are killed by a firearm every day in the United States, or about 56 children per week. An additional 200–300 children suffer from nonfatal firearm injuries (Children's Defense Fund, 2004b). Nurses must intervene in this national tragedy. Become familiar with firearm injury statistics in your community. Teach families about the dangers of firearms. Urge safe storage. Teach children and youth about the danger of firearms. Help schools establish programs to ensure safety for students.

Family risk factors have been identified as more commonly seen in situations when violence has been committed against children (Box 7–7). In addition, children who commit violence more commonly have ready access to firearms, are exposed to violence in the home or community, engage in violent media viewing, and have poor self-esteem or depression.

Another type of violence is terrorism. The events of September 11, 2001, in the United States, and other examples in various countries take a large toll on the mental health of children and adolescents. Likewise, children who live through wars or have a parent or sibling die in war can be permanently affected by these events. The response of children to terrorism is not well studied. Disasters such as the World Trade Center attack can lead to sleep

BOX 7–7 Risk Factors Common in Families with Child Victims of Violence

- History of mental illness, domestic violence, incarceration, or substance abuse in the home
- Family stresses
- Inadequate childcare or supervision
- Inadequate family social support
- Use of corporal punishment for the child
- Child abuse
- Access to firearms
- Gang membership in family or neighborhood
- High exposure to media violence
- Child hyperactivity and other developmental behavioral disorders

Note: Data from Elders, J. (2003). The role of the pediatrician in violence in the school. www.schoolhealth.org/reduviol.html, *accessed 1/30/2004.*

and eating problems, fears of entering tall buildings, regression in school performance and other behaviors, and posttraumatic stress disorder (see Chapter 34∞). Children and adolescents experience profound sadness, cling to adults who provide security, and have a variety of somatic complaints (Murray 2002). Several resources have been developed to help families and health professionals help children deal with war and violence. See the Companion Website for resources on the National Center for Children Exposed to Violence, Society of Pediatric Nurses, and American Academy of Child & Adolescent Psychiatry.

Bullying

One type of violence that frequently occurs in schools is **bullying,** or aggressive behavior that is intended to cause harm, exists in a relationship with imbalance of power, and occurs repeatedly (Limber, 2003). Bullying behaviors include verbal abuse (taunting, teasing), name calling, threats, spreading rumors, social exclusion, and physical abuse (hitting, shoving, kicking, tripping). About 16% of children in a large national survey had suffered bullying, most commonly in grades 6 through 8, and more frequently among males. Almost 30% of children age 11 to 15 years have been either a victim or perpetrator of bullying. Up to 160,000 U.S. children may miss school every day in efforts to avoid bullying (Limber, 2003; Nansel, Overpeck, Pilla, et al., 2001). Although bullying is most commonly reported in schools, it can occur in neighborhoods as children go to and from school, on school buses, on sports teams, and in other settings.

Bullies are more likely to smoke, drink alcohol, and perform poorly in school; and one in four bullies has a criminal record by 30 years (Health Resources and Services Administration [HRSA], 2003). Bullies are more likely to bring weapons to school, putting other children at risk (Fox, Elliot, Kerlikowske, et al., 2003), and bullying is associated with future delinquent behavior (van der Wal, de Wit, & Hirasing, 2003). Bullies are aggressive, impulsive, and need to dominate others.

On the other hand, children who are bullied are more commonly socially isolated and anxious (Nansel, et al., 2001). This social isolation has many negative outcomes. This includes feelings of depression, low self-esteem, loneliness, and suicidal ideation among those bullied. Health problems such as migraines, stomach pains, suicidal thoughts, and other problems can result. Academic performance commonly deteriorates and rates of school absenteeism increase (Limber, 2003; Children's Safety Network, National Injury and Violence Prevention Resource Center, 2003). Realizing the serious effects of such behaviors, a number of states have now passed legislation that reiterates the rights of all children to attend school in a safe and peaceful manner. Some state education departments mandate school district programs for students about bullying and clear school policies about dealing with the behavior.

Nurses can be active in setting up school policies about bullying and integrating assessment and interventions related to bullying into health promotion visits. School programs should do the following:

- Inform all students that bullying is not tolerated.
- Train teachers and other personnel about signs of bullying.
- Ensure adult supervision in hallways and playgrounds—sites where bullying is most common.
- Teach children to promptly report bullying that is experienced or observed.
- Set up peer support for those who are bullied.
- Arrange therapeutic treatment through school counselors and other resources for those who bully; involve parents in the treatment plan.
- Measure incidences of bullying and outcomes of policies; use data to evaluate policies in schools.

Nurses who are in clinics, offices, and other health promotion settings can do the following:

- Be alert for children with behavior changes (irritability, anxiety, poor self-concept).
- Consider bullying as a potential cause when fear or refusal to attend school is reported by child or parents.
- Ask questions during visits: "Have you ever been afraid to go to school?" "What are the best and worst things about going to your school?" "What are the other kids in your neighborhood like?"
- Ask parents what they have done about any situations identified. Partner with the parent to act as liaison to the school or other agency.
- Refer identified bullies and victims of bullying to mental health specialists.

A campaign is being developed by the Health Resources and Services Administration (HRSA) Maternal and Child Health Bureau, which will target youth 9 to 13 years old, to prevent bullying. Access the Companion Website for information about dealing with this issue in schools in your state.

Incarceration

A growing number of children are entering the judicial system and many are admitted at young ages. Juveniles were responsible for 12% of arrests for violent crimes in 2001 (Snyder, 2003). Girls represent an increasing number of children in juvenile justice. Children in detention, courts, and other facilities have frequently

MediaLink Critical Thinking in Action: Music and Violence

been victims as well as perpetrators of violence. They often have multiple risks such as substance abuse, early sexual activity, multiple sexual partners, lack of a healthcare home, and mental health issues (Guthrie, Hoey, Ravoira, et al., 2002). Nurses may work within the juvenile justice systems to provide episodic care for children or to partner with others to establish health-related programs within facilities. Youth need the following:

- Basic physical care such as immunizations, and vision and hearing screening
- Nutrition assessment and teaching
- Skin assessment and hygiene practice teaching
- Information about sexuality, sexual practices, abstinence and sexually transmitted diseases
- Assessment for substance abuse
- Teaching about hazards of substance use and assistance with quitting
- Mental health services
- Developmental assessment
- Individualized education plans to meet cognitive needs

NURSING MANAGEMENT

The focus of nursing management is to prevent violence, identify warning signs of violence, intervene with children to decrease effects of violence, and partner with families and other professionals to provide programs and enact legislation that will decrease violence. Realizing the impact of violence on and by children, several federal healthcare initiatives have begun to assist in lowering violence. Some programs have been helpful and incidents of homicides and most other forms of violence have begun to decrease. Programs that are most successful include individual children, parents, schools, and communities. School health professionals are instructed to identify signs of violence (Table 7–6).

Nursing Assessment and Diagnosis

Nurses are in key positions to prevent violence by identifying children who are at risk of being recipients and victims of violence. The ecologic framework can be used to assess children. Some questions that can be asked are listed in Table 7–6. It is important to detect both the risks that lead to vulnerability and the protective factors that can promote resilience and safety. Questions should be adapted to each age group and inserted in every healthcare encounter.

Nursing care for violence is discussed in the nursing care plan on the following pages. The following additional nursing diagnoses may be appropriate.

- Risk for Violence: Self-directed related to history of violence
- Chronic Low Self-esteem related to history of abuse
- Interrupted Family Processes related to situational crises
- Delayed Growth and Development related to environmental deficiencies

Planning and Implementation

Nurses intervene with individual children, with families, in schools, jails, and detention centers, and in other community settings to increase safety and decrease violence. Children and families are assisted in meeting basic needs and accessing resources to assist with finances, respite care, domestic violence, and other issues. Education is a key element of intervention.

Providing Information

The nurse can teach family members about the dangers of firearms and the necessity for use of gun locks, locked cabinets, storing guns unloaded, and storing guns and ammunition in separate places. Suggest alternative activities to minimize child exposure to violence in the media. Inform parents about rating systems for television and other media, and about lockout mechanisms for televisions and computers. Harmful effects of verbal and physical abuse to the child or other family members are discussed and alternatives explored. See Partnering with Families: Rating Systems for Media.

The school-age child and adolescent are presented with information about bullying and strategies for dealing with the problem. School and community resources are provided concerning where the child can go if there are threats of any kind. Date rape and violence are topics for discussion for all teens, as is the importance of reporting the situations when they occur.

TABLE 7–6 Assessment Questions to Identify Violence Risk and Protective Factors

MICROSYSTEM	MESOSYSTEM	EXOSYSTEM
Have you been hurt by your parents or anyone else at home? When was the last time you were teased or bullied at school? What did you do? Have you ever brought a gun, knife, or other weapon to school? Do you have access to guns and knives at home? At friends' houses? What stresses are there in your family now? Tell me about school—what do you like and dislike?	Do your parents attend school meetings? Talk with your teachers? Do you participate in any church, synagogue, or mosque services? Do you participate in any community activities? (Examples include clubs, volunteering at sporting events, helping at soup kitchens.)	What stresses do your parents have at work, in their families, with their health or finances? Do you feel like your school helps to keep you safe? Are there plans for handling violent episodes at your school if they were to occur? Do you feel safe in your neighborhood? Where would you go or who would you call if you felt unsafe or were hurt and no one was at home?

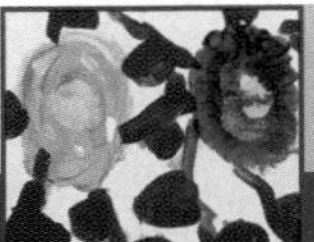

Nursing Care Plan

THE CHILD AND VIOLENT BEHAVIOR

GOAL	INTERVENTION	RATIONALE	EXPECTED OUTCOME
1. Risk for Violence: Other-directed related to history of family violence			
	NIC Priority Intervention— *Environmental Management:* Violence Prevention: Monitoring and manipulation of the environment to decrease the potential for violent behavior directed toward self, others, or the environment		**NOC Suggested Outcome—***Impulse Control:* Ability to restrain compulsive or impulsive behavior in child and others
The child demonstrates impulse control	■ Identify violent behaviors in the child ■ Provide a safe place for exploration of feelings by referral to school or other counseling, support groups, and other resources ■ Provide strategies for managing anger, alternative ways for coping with problems	■ Violence in the child usually develops over time ■ The child needs an opportunity to explore feelings and vulnerability ■ Coping strategies can be learned from others and can help in dealing with a stressful home or community situation	The child expresses ability to manage problems in acceptable ways
The child is secure in a safe environment	■ Perform thorough assessment of hazards to physical and emotional state in the child's home, neighborhood, and school ■ Institute actions that will result in removal of child from unsafe situations ■ Use community resources to provide respite care, teaching for families, and safety Instruction for the child	■ Hazards to physical and emotional health promote violence to and from the child ■ Removal from family, community, or school may be needed to ensure child safety ■ Stress reduction measures may help to decrease violent behaviors	The child expresses a sense of physical and emotional safety in daily life
2. Impaired Home Maintenance related to insufficient family organization			
	NIC Priority Intervention—*Home Maintenance Assistance:* Helping the family to maintain the home as a safe place to live		**NOC Suggested Outcome—***Role Performance:* Congruence of an individual's role behavior with role expectations
Family members are able to meet role expectations	■ Provide information on child's developmental needs ■ Provide ongoing assessment in the home via home healthcare visits ■ Assist the family in identifying hazards in the environment that can impair the child's growth and development ■ Evaluate ability of adults to provide a safe, secure, nurturing environment	■ Parents need to understand the developmental progression of their children ■ Early identification of hazards can lead to proper interventions to protect against harm to the child ■ Families may need respite care, information about child needs, financial assistance, or other resources in order to meet the needs of the child	Family members meet role expectations, contributing to making the home a safe and secure place for the child
3. Hopelessness related to long-term family stress			
	NIC Priority Intervention—*Hope Instillation:* Facilitation of the development of a positive outlook in the given situation		**NOC Suggested Outcome—***Hope:* Presence of internal state of optimism that is personally satisfying and life supporting

Nursing Care Plan THE CHILD AND VIOLENT BEHAVIOR (continued)

GOAL	INTERVENTION	RATIONALE	EXPECTED OUTCOME
3. Hopelessness related to long-term family stress (continued)			
The child will have adequate food, sleep, and express satisfaction with life	■ Monitor child's nutritional state and growth and daily patterns ■ Monitor child's developmental status ■ Determine adequacy of relationships and support systems	■ The child's nutrition, sleep, and other patterns provide clues to the family's ability to perceive hope and provide care for the child ■ The child needs close personal relationships in order to grow and learn	The child demonstrates normal growth patterns and meets expected developmental outcomes
The family will identify resources to achieve life goals	■ Monitor the family's decision making ability ■ Provide information on community resources ■ Refer for psychiatric and other services if needed ■ Assist in goal setting	■ Feeling overwhelmed by daily life events leads to an inability to set goals and make decisions to meet the goals ■ Resources can assist the family members in setting and achieving realistic goals	The family establishes realistic goals for growth and development of its members, and takes steps to meet the goals
4. Risk for Injury related to physical or psychological conditions in the environment			
	NIC Priority Intervention—*Safety Behavior:* Family actions to minimize risk of physical or emotional trauma		**NOC Suggested Outcome**—*Parenting: Social Safety:* Parental actions to avoid social relationships that might cause harm or injury; *Risk Control:* Actions to eliminate or reduce actual, personal, and modifiable health risks
Risk for physical and emotional injury to the child is decreased	■ Identify physical and psychological factors that affect child's safety ■ Assist family to deal with issues such as mental status challenges, fatigue, financial concern, substance abuse, lack of adequate childcare resources, and other factors ■ Instruct family on methods of keeping the child safe	■ Multiple factors in the family can contribute to risk of violence and lack of safety for the child ■ Families need information about the impact of unsafe settings on the child and methods that can decrease risk of injury	The child is not injured in physical or emotional ways in the home or other immediate settings
5. Post-Trauma Syndrome related to physical or psychosocial abuse			
	NIC Priority Intervention—*Counseling:* Use of an interactive helping process focusing on the needs, problems and feelings of the child who is a victim of abuse or other violence.		**NOC Suggested Outcome**—*Abuse/Violence Recovery:* Healing of psychologic and physical wounds of abuse or violence
The child demonstrates abuse or violence recovery	■ Assess the child's affect and behaviors ■ Evaluate social interactions and sense of trust in others ■ Assist the child in identifying feelings and coping strategies by providing counseling, art therapy, and other strategies	■ Disturbed child behaviors can demonstrate a sense of mistrust and insecurity ■ Establishment of close interactions with others demonstrates reestablishment of a sense of trust ■ A child who has experienced abuse or other violence needs a therapeutic relationship with a counselor to deal with the trauma and begin to rebuild trust, respect, and to learn coping mechanisms	The child identifies feelings related to violent episode(s) and expresses healing of the self

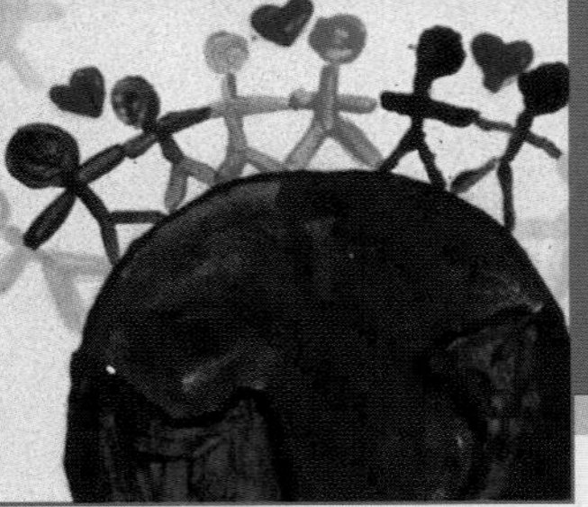

PARTNERING WITH FAMILIES

Rating Systems for Media

Television Rating	Television MA Categories	Video & Computer	Movies
TV-Y: for all	FV: fantasy violence	E: for everyone	G: general audience
TV-Y7: for older children	L: language	T: for teen	PG: parental guidance suggested
G: general audience	V: Violence	M: mature user	PG13: Parents strongly cautioned
TV-PG: parental guidance suggested	S: sexual situation	AO: adults only	R: restricted to above 18 years without adult
TV-14: parents strongly cautioned	D: sexual dialogue		NC17: no one under 18 years admitted
TV-MA: mature audience			

Care in the Community

Both in schools and community settings, nurses can plan peer mentoring to provide assistance to children at high risk of experiencing violence. School and community programs for children can be linked and coordinated by nurses to provide for parent involvement and child support. Discuss safety issues, both risks and protective actions, in schools and community groups. Report children who are at risk. Work to establish extended programs for children so that they are safe after school. Help children learn behaviors that will help them to be safe in their communities and at home. Teach positive problem solving and conflict management techniques to children and parents.

Youth with special needs are a concern of nurses. Jails and detention centers often have a nurse who visits youth on a regular basis or when health problems occur. Health teaching may be provided in some facilities. Halfway houses and homeless shelters are examples of settings where violence prevention and intervention can occur with youth. Mental health centers and other programs have nurses who work with either child victims of violence (for example, children who have witnessed domestic violence, have witnessed or had a family member murdered, have been abused at home or school) or perpetrators of violence. See Chapter 34∞ for a discussion of posttraumatic stress disorder and its effects on the child and adolescent.

Partner with families to assist them in dealing with children about war and terrorism. Recognize that youth who have experienced such events are more at risk for mental health disruptions with future events. Answer questions from children honestly, but reassure them that many people are trying to make the situation safe. Other suggestions for parents include:

- Limit television viewing and other media exposure due to constant replaying of the events of terrorism or war. Preschoolers may think the events continue to happen, rather than being a one-time occurrence. Watch with the child and talk with him or her about what is happening.
- Continue with structured family events such as meals, recreation, and faith-based activities. Spend time with the child.
- Take cues from the child about how much to discuss. Use words the child or adolescent can understand.
- Partner with the school so teachers know what parents have discussed and parents are aware of how events are discussed at school.
- If youth decide to become active by writing letters or joining campaigns, allow them to participate in this way.
- Be alert for regression in behavior, sleep and eating problems, or other indications of stress. Consider talking with the healthcare provider or a counselor in such situations.
- Expect that even after the child has adjusted, there may be delayed reactions. Anniversaries of events, holidays, and birthdays often bring renewed pain and sadness.
- Realize that adults must care for themselves, obtain stress relief, and talk with others in order to have strength and resources available for children.

Evaluation

Expected outcomes of nursing care for violence prevention include the following:

- A decrease in incidents of homicides, firearm injuries, abuse, date rape, bullying, and other violence among children
- Establishment and evaluation of programs to decrease violence and verbalization by all children of what to do if violence occurs, and how to solve problems without becoming violent
- Personal positive judgment of self-worth by youth
- Youth ability to make positive choices between alternative behaviors
- Family function to provide mutual support for each family member
- Healthy adjustment following violent events

Child Abuse

One of the most common types of violence against children is child abuse. This type of violence can have implications for both the physical and mental health of children, and can influence their health status long after the abuse has occurred. Awareness of the problem of child abuse is increasing. More cases are being reported; however, these are probably only a small percentage of the total. Approximately 10% to 20% of children between the ages of 3 and 17 years—about 2.8 million children—are physically abused each year (Murray, Baker, & Lewin, 2000).

Physical abuse is only one part of a larger problem. The definition of child abuse has expanded over the past 10 years to include physical neglect, emotional abuse and neglect, verbal abuse, and sexual abuse, as well as physical abuse. Many children who are sexually abused are under the age of 5 years, some as young as 3 months. The average age for sexual molestation is 4 years. The perpetrator is the parent or another person legally responsible who does the following:

- Inflicts or allows another to inflict physical or emotional pain or injury
- Creates or allows another to create a significant risk of serious physical or emotional pain or injury
- Commits or allows another to commit an act of sexual abuse, as defined by law, against the child

Abuse generally involves an act of commission, that is, actively doing something to a child physically, emotionally, or sexually, such as hitting, belittling, or molesting. Neglect more often involves an act of omission, such as not providing adequate nutrition, emotional contact, or necessary physical care. Because the evidence is often not visible, emotional abuse and neglect are more difficult to identify and prove than physical abuse or neglect. Risk factors for abuse and neglect are listed in Table 7–7.

Physical Abuse

Physical abuse is the deliberate maltreatment of another individual that inflicts pain or injury and may result in permanent or temporary disfigurement or even death. Common methods of physical abuse in children are listed in Table 7–8.

Physical Neglect

Physical neglect is the deliberate withholding of or failure to provide the necessary and available resources to the child. Behaviors constituting physical neglect include failure to provide for the following basic needs: adequate nutrition and hydration, hygiene (e.g., clean diapers and clothes, bathing and toileting facilities), shelter (e.g., warmth in winter), and appropriate healthcare (e.g., immunizations, dental care, medications, eyeglasses).

TABLE 7–7 Risk Factors for Child Abuse and Neglect

FACTORS INCREASING RISK FOR PHYSICAL ABUSE	FACTORS INCREASING RISK FOR SEXUAL ABUSE
Poverty Violence in the family Prematurity Unrelated male primary caretaker Parents who were abused as children Age less than 3 years Handicap or condition that requires a great deal of care (e.g., mental retardation, attention deficit hyperactivity disorder) Parental substance abuse or social isolation	Absence of natural father or having a stepfather Being female Mother's employment outside the home Poor relationship with parent Parental relationship characterized by conflict Parental substance abuse or social isolation

MediaLink Identifying Child Abuse Video

Emotional Abuse

Emotional abuse usually involves shaming, ridiculing, embarrassing, or insulting the child. It can also include the destruction of a child's personal property, such as tearing up the child's favorite family photographs or letters or harming, killing, or giving away the child's pet. These actions are frequently used as a means of frightening or controlling the child.

Verbal abuse is a common method of emotional abuse. Words can be a violent and volatile weapon against a child, eroding the child's fragile sense of self and destroying self-esteem. Common examples of verbal abuse include yelling obscenities at the child, calling the child names, threatening to "put the child away" or to give away or kill the child's pet, telling the child "I wish you were never born" or "You're worthless," and using words to humiliate, shame, or degrade the child.

Emotional Neglect

Emotional neglect is characterized by the caretaker's emotional unavailability to the child. The usual style of interaction is cold and lacking in sensitive personal attention. The child suffers from a lack of nurturance and failure of the parent or caretaker to meet basic dependency needs.

Sexual Abuse

Child sexual abuse is the exploitation of a child for the sexual gratification of an adult. Between 100,000 and 500,000 children in the United States are sexually abused each year. Of child sexual abusers, 75% to 80% are immediate family members, other relatives, friends, or neighbors. The word *child* in sexual abuse and molestation refers to anyone who has not reached the age of consent, even if a teenager. **Incest** is sexual activity between close family members, so that marriage would be legally or culturally prohibited. Male perpetrators are 92% to 98% of all abusers (Murray et al., 2000; Frederickson, 1999). Abusers often threaten to harm or kill the child or another family member if the child discloses the abuse (Box 7–8). Some abusers are pedophiles, people who have sexual impulses toward preadolescent children.

BOX 7–8 Common Forms of Sexual Abuse

- Oral–genital contact
- Fondling and caressing the genitals
- Anal intercourse
- Sexual intercourse
- Rape
- Sodomy
- Prostitution
- Forcing viewing of or participation in pornography

TABLE 7–8 Methods of Physical Abuse in Children

Hitting, slapping, kicking, or punching
Whipping with belts, shoes, or electrical cords **(1)**
Inflicting burns with a lit cigarette or lighter **(2)**
Immersing child or body part in scalding water (commonly legs, perineal area, hands, or feet: see Figure 36–23
Shaking the child violently ("shaken child" syndrome)
Tying the child to a fence, bed, tree, or other object
Throwing the child against a wall, down stairs, or against a window
Choking or gagging the child
Fracturing the legs, arms, ribs, or skull
Deliberately administering excessive doses of prescribed or nonprescribed drugs
Deliberately withholding prescribed medication

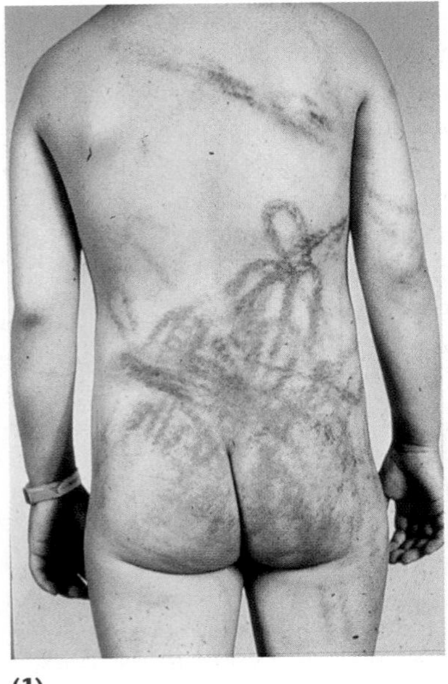
(1)

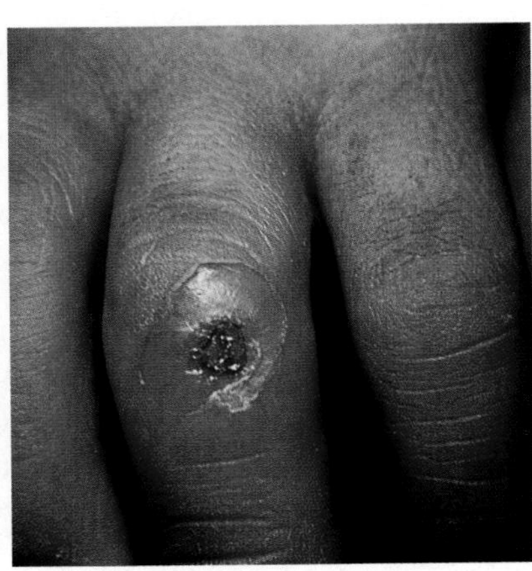
(2)

Used with permission of the American Academy of Pediatrics, Visual Diagnosis of Child Abuse Slide Kit. Photographs Copyright © AAP/Kempe.

The pedophile is at least 16 years of age, is at least 5 years older than the victim, and the victim is 13 years of age or younger. Another form of sexual abuse is exhibitionism, or obtaining sexual arousal by exposing one's genitals to a stranger.

Etiology and Pathophysiology. Regardless of the type of abuse, the most common abuser is the child's parent or guardian or the male friend of the child's mother. Risk factors associated with abusive behavior in adults include the following:

- Psychopathology, such as drug addiction or alcoholism, low self-esteem, poor impulse control, and other personality disorders
- Poor parenting experiences, such as abuse in the abuser's own childhood, rejection by the abuser's own parent(s), lack of knowledge of alternative methods of discipline, strong belief in or family tradition of harsh discipline, and lack of parental affection
- Marital stressors and problems with partners, such as hostile-dependent, abusive, or nonsupportive relationships, and one-sided decision making
- Environmental stressors, such as legal, financial, medical, or housing problems
- Social isolation, such as few friends and limited use of sitters, family, or other resources
- Inappropriate expectations for the developmental level of the child

Clinical Manifestations. Clinical manifestations of physical abuse are listed on page 217. Behaviors inconsistent with developmental stage may be apparent. For example, the toddler or preschooler may be indiscriminately friendly with unfamiliar adults, including healthcare providers, rather than demonstrating shyness or anxiety. For the infant or young child with "shaken baby syndrome" or "shaken child syndrome," the symptoms are those of central nervous system injury from repeated coup and contrecoup injury (see Chapter 33∞) and include vomiting, irritability, fatigue, poor feeding, bradycardia, apnea, enlarged fontanel, and seizures. Bruises are usually not present (Castiglia, 2001).

Manifestations of physical neglect include undernourishment (evidenced by constantly feeling hungry, hoarding or stealing food, and being underweight), unclean clothes and body, poor dental health (extensive cavities or generally poor condition of teeth), and inappropriate clothing for the season.

Manifestations of emotional abuse, verbal abuse, emotional neglect, and witnessing domestic violence include fear, poor physical growth, and failure to meet appropriate developmental milestones. The child may have difficulty relating to adults, impaired communication skills, and developmental delays. Behavioral manifestations include anxiety, fear, shame, aggression, delinquency, and depression (Frederickson, 1999).

Children who have been sexually abused may exhibit a variety of physical and behavioral signs and symptoms (see page 217). However, sexual abuse does not always result in apparent injury. Among the many long-term consequences of child sexual abuse are ongoing feelings of shame, guilt, anger, and hostility; decreased self-esteem, which leads to increased self-destructive behavior and risk of suicide; recurrence of victimization experiences; substance abuse; posttraumatic stress disorder (see Chapter 34∞); and eating disorders (see Chapter 9∞). Children who have been abused are more likely to abuse others in the future. Factors associated with greater psychologic harm to the child include (1) a long period of abuse, (2) use of violent force or threat of violence, (3) abuse involving penetration (intercourse or oral–genital sex), and (4) abuse involving family members, especially the father or stepfather (Walker, Scott, & Koppersmith, 1998).

CLINICAL MANIFESTATIONS of Child Abuse

- Multiple bruises in various stages of healing
- Scald burns with clear lines of demarcation and in a glove or stocking distribution (see Figure 36–23)
- Rope, belt, or cord marks, usually seen on the mouth, buttocks, back, legs, and arms (see Figure 1 in Table 7–8)
- Burn scars in various stages of healing
- Multiple fractures in various stages of healing
- Shortness of breath and distress upon being moved, indicating chest contusions and possible rib fractures
- Sedation from overmedication
- Exacerbation of chronic illness (such as diabetes or asthma) because of withholding of medication

COLLABORATIVE CARE

The diagnosis and management of child abuse is complicated and can involve partnerships among many individuals and groups. Often the child is identified in a healthcare setting with an injury and physicians, nurses, and others partner to analyze the situation. Sometimes parents suspect abuse by another care provider and seek assistance. At times, suspected abuse is reported to investigating agencies and social service workers or law enforcement officials investigate. School personnel identify and report suspected abuse. Once verified, treatment may also be complex, involving school counselors, nurses, mental health specialists, physicians, and family members. The child's risk situations and protective situations are identified in order to build a safety net and to manage the mental health issues involved.

CLINICAL MANIFESTATIONS of Sexual Abuse in Children and Adolescents

- Vaginal discharge
- Blood-stained underpants or diaper
- Genital redness, pain, itching, or bruising
- Difficulty walking or sitting
- Urinary tract infection
- Sexually transmitted disease
- Somatic complaints, such as headaches or stomachaches
- Excessively seductive behavior
- Sleeping problems, such as nightmares or night terrors
- Bedwetting
- Unwillingness to go to babysitter, family member, neighbor, or other person
- Fear of strangers
- New or excessive sexual curiosity or play
- Constant masturbation
- Curling into fetal position
- Phobias about particular places, people, or things
- Abrupt changes in school performance and attendance
- Changes in eating habits
- Abrupt changes in behavior (especially withdrawal)
- Child or adolescent female acts like a wife or mother

Diagnostic Tests

Diagnosis of abuse is made on the basis of a careful history and thorough physical examination. Radiograph, CT, and MRI studies may be ordered to identify signs of recurrent abuse such as healed fractures and other damaged tissues. Laboratory studies may involve urine culture for signs of infection or screening for sexually transmitted infections. Genitourinary examination may be performed if sexual abuse is suspected. Some children are admitted directly to the hospital with the diagnosis of suspected abuse or neglect. Less obvious as a victim of abuse is the child admitted with a skull fracture who parents report fell off a chair.

Neglect, which is more difficult to define and identify, frequently requires hospitalization with a comprehensive medical, social, and psychiatric evaluation. Five basic categories must be considered when attempting to diagnose neglect: (1) medical care neglect (lack of necessary medical care), (2) gross safety neglect (lack of appropriate supervision), (3) physical neglect (lack of food and shelter), (4) emotional neglect, and (5) educational neglect.

Interviews by mental health specialists may be performed in cases where the child is old enough to communicate verbally or through play techniques. All 50 states have extensive and complex statutes regarding reporting of child abuse and neglect. A specialist must be consulted, especially if the child's testimony will be used in court.

PRACTICE ALERT

Child Abuse Laws

Every state has a child abuse law specifying the particular behaviors that define each type of abuse. Any professional who works with children and reasonably suspects that a child has been abused is required to report this suspicion to the local agency for child protective services. Reports made in good faith are not liable to countersuits; however, professionals who suspect abuse and do not report it may be held responsible by the courts.

Children do not routinely make false allegations of abuse. If indeed there is reason to believe the allegations are false, a child and adolescent therapist (psychiatrist, psychologist, psychiatric clinical nurse specialist, or social worker) with special expertise should be consulted to determine the truth. Keep in mind that children who withdraw their accusations have often been threatened or coerced into doing so.

Clinical Therapy

Initial therapy focuses on providing safety. Physical injuries are treated and the child is removed from the abusive situation. Children who have been physically, emotionally, or sexually abused are at risk for major mental health problems, such as depression and posttraumatic stress disorder. They require skilled care by mental health professionals who are specially trained in this area. Initially the treatment goals include prevention of self-destructive or other dangerous acts. Children must be encouraged to express their fears and feelings in a safe and supportive environment. Equally important is the child's need to build coping skills and self-esteem. The child must be reassured and convinced that he or she is in no way responsible or to blame for what happened.

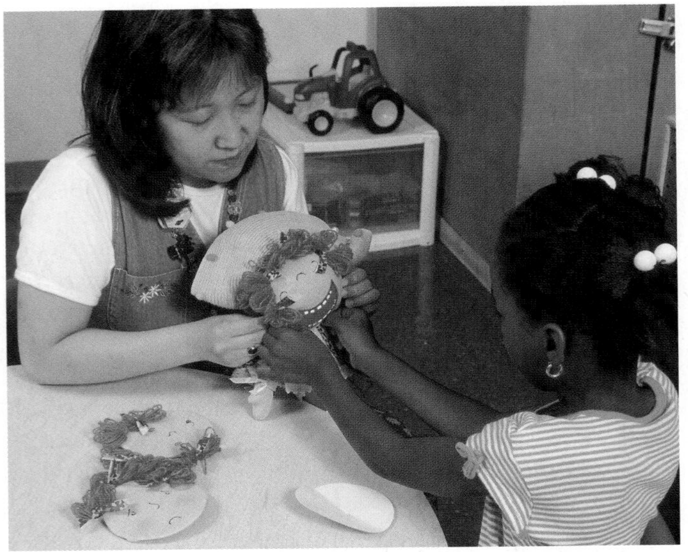

FIGURE 7–10 ■ Therapeutic strategies with young children involve various methods of communication, such as dramatic play and art.

Individual treatment with art therapy is often used initially because it is the least threatening method in the early stages of treatment, it can easily be tailored to meet the child's individual needs, and it prepares the child for other forms of treatment such as family and group therapy (Figure 7–10 ■). Family or group therapy may be of benefit in exploring the child's concerns and feelings. Anger is common, especially in children who were abused by a trusted adult such as the father or stepfather.

Some children are themselves sexual offenders. An adolescent sexual offender is a minor who commits any sexual act with a person of any age that is against the victim's will, without consent, and/or in an aggressive, exploitive, or threatening manner (Horner, 2003). Some common characteristics of these youth are prior violence, psychological/psychiatric problems, history as a victim of abuse, member of dysfunctional family, and personal characteristics such as loneliness and low self-esteem.

NURSING MANAGEMENT

■ Nursing Assessment and Diagnosis

Nursing assessment in instances of suspected child abuse or neglect requires a comprehensive history and physical examination, with documentation of findings. Consultation with social service agencies in the community is important if the family is receiving services.

Obtaining the history can be stressful for both the nurse and the parent. Use of therapeutic communication techniques and a quiet, unhurried environment are helpful. Maintaining a nonjudgmental attitude at all times is essential.

CLINICAL TIP

The nurse should communicate in an open manner. A clear statement of purpose is needed, for example, "Hello, Mr. S. My name is Joan T. I'm Jonathan's nurse. I will be talking with you and asking you some questions about his overall health."

It is important to differentiate true child abuse from cultural variations that might inaccurately be assumed to indicate abuse (Figure 7–11 ■). Obtaining information about abusive and neglectful behaviors requires the nurse to establish a trusting relationship with parents, who are often afraid to trust any professional.

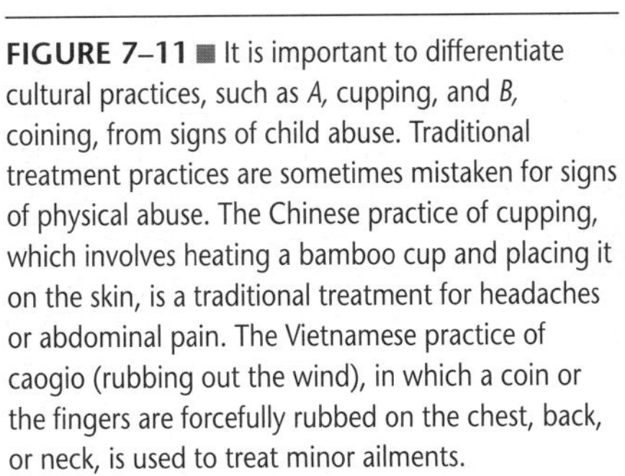

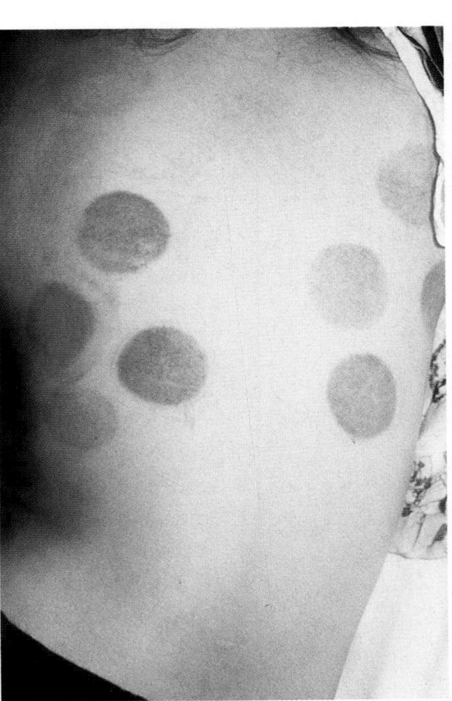

A

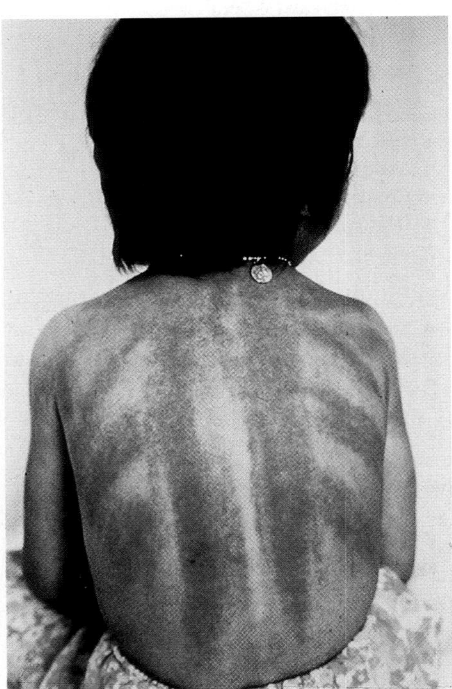

B

FIGURE 7–11 ■ It is important to differentiate cultural practices, such as *A,* cupping, and *B,* coining, from signs of child abuse. Traditional treatment practices are sometimes mistaken for signs of physical abuse. The Chinese practice of cupping, which involves heating a bamboo cup and placing it on the skin, is a traditional treatment for headaches or abdominal pain. The Vietnamese practice of caogio (rubbing out the wind), in which a coin or the fingers are forcefully rubbed on the chest, back, or neck, is used to treat minor ailments.

Used with permission of the American Academy of Pediatrics, Visual Diagnosis of Child Physical Abuse Slide Kit. Photographs copyright © AAP/Kempe.

The health history sequence should include (1) parental concerns, (2) general family history, and (3) specific child history. This sequence begins with nonthreatening topics and allows the nurse to demonstrate concern before asking abuse-related questions. Obtain details about how injuries occurred. The parents' and child's own words should be documented verbatim using quotation marks. Compare reports obtained from each family member for lack of consistency and details that change over time.

It is desirable to interview the parent and child both separately and together. Parent–child interaction during an intensive history-taking session provides an opportunity to observe the child's behavior and the parent's method of handling and responding to the child. Interviews may occur in school. The nurse should provide a confidential setting and use a nonjudgmental manner.

CLINICAL TIP

A suggested approach might be, "Many teens have had sexual experiences that they did not want, where someone forced them to do something sexually. So I ask everyone this: Have you ever had a sexual experience when you didn't want to?" (Saewyc, Pettingell, & Magee, 2003, p. 270.) Ask about relationships with younger children to identify adolescent sexual offenders (Horner, 2003).

Data gathered during history-taking are particularly important in light of physical findings. Are there discrepancies between the history and physical assessment data? Do the parents give a history of an uncontrollable, inattentive toddler when the nurse observes a child who is attentive throughout a 15-minute examination? Assess the child's general appearance, including dress and behavior during the assessment. How do the child's affect, behavior, and development compare with those of other children the same age? Be alert for the signs of shaken child syndrome; this most often appears as a subtle neurologic condition. Measure head circumference and perform a neurologic examination (see Chapter 8∞).

Be alert for signs of domestic violence; for example, a mother who brings in a child for care displays signs of abuse. Say to the mother, "I see you have a black eye. Can you tell me what happened?" or "You say you are afraid that your boyfriend may hurt Shandra. Has he been hurting you? Do you want to talk about that?"

Documentation of findings is important in all situations, but is essential in cases of suspected child abuse and neglect. Record physical findings as observed. Draw diagrams to document skin injuries. Document the location, nature, and extent of injuries with photographs.

PRACTICE ALERT

Documenting Handling of Child Abuse Evidence

Each person who handles a laboratory specimen or other item (e.g., clothing soiled with semen) in cases of suspected child abuse must be identified in the patient's record, and the specimen must never be left unattended. This documented chain of possession is necessary to ensure the admissibility of the evidence in court.

Following are nursing diagnoses that may be appropriate for the physically abused or neglected child.

- Defensive Coping related to psychological impairment
- Acute Pain related to inflicted injuries
- Impaired Skin Integrity related to inflicted injuries
- Altered Growth and Development related to lack of supportive parenting and environment
- Imbalanced Nutrition: Less than Body Requirements related to inadequate caloric intake
- Ineffective Health Maintenance related to lack of parental provision of child's essential needs
- Fear related to actual physical harm or repeated risk of injury
- Risk for Injury related to physical abuse
- Risk for Violence (parent), Other-directed related to inability to manage anger

Additional diagnoses that may apply to the emotionally abused or neglected child include the following:

- Defensive Coping related to psychological impairment
- Chronic Low Self-esteem related to lack of appropriate emotional support from parents
- Disabled Family Coping related to dysfunctional family dynamics and pattern of physical abuse

Diagnoses that may apply to the sexually abused child include the following:

- Anxiety related to potential separation from parent
- Rape-trauma Syndrome related to sexual exploitation
- Ineffective Role Performance related to domestic violence
- Personal Identity Disturbance related to disturbance of usual activities of childhood

■ Planning and Implementation

Nursing care focuses on helping to remove the child from an abusive environment, preventing further injury, providing supportive care, and reinforcing the importance of follow-up care and counseling.

Prevent Further Injury

Work with social services and community agencies to assess the child's home environment, individuals living in the home, and the actions surrounding the abuse. Assist in removing the child from the home to temporary custody of the court or foster care of another relative, if indicated. Counsel family members about abuse and refer for appropriate therapy. Be sure that all people of childbearing age know the law in your state regarding safe places to leave unwanted babies. Teach all dating youth how to deal with violence during dating. Have domestic violence resources in your community readily available at all settings where care is provided for children.

Provide Supportive Care

Protect and treat the child's injuries (e.g., fractures, burns). Include parents in the child's treatment plan and keep them informed about the child's progress. Even if suspected of inflicting injuries to the child, the parent is still the child's primary caretaker. Talk with the parent as you would with any parent. Be supportive of any guilt expressed. Encourage the parent to assist with the child's care. Observe parent–child interactions and document supportive behaviors and the child's response to the parent versus other care providers.

CLINICAL TIP

When children have been abused, they are often frightened in new situations. Sexually abused children may resist removing clothes for a physical examination or medical test. They may want to wear undergarments to the surgical suite. Members of the gender who abused them may be distrusted. When aware of a history of abuse, ask the parents or guardians how to best facilitate the child's healthcare. Be sensitive to fears and allow the child to wear clothing, have a support person present or whatever may provide a sense of security.

Interacting nonjudgmentally with a parent suspected of abusing his or her child can be difficult. Talk with a colleague about anger you feel toward the parents or about the child's injuries or specific actions surrounding the abuse. Use team meetings to develop strategies that enable you to work with the parents and child.

Home Care Teaching

If there is any question about the child returning to a potentially dangerous situation, support the child's removal from the situation. The child may receive supervised care in the home by court order. Childcare, home nursing, and social worker visits may need to be arranged. Parents should be referred to parent effectiveness classes, family therapy, and support groups as necessary. If a neighbor or friend is the abuser, then the family may need support and legal advice when a term of incarceration is finished and the perpetrator returns to the community. Some states and communities have sexual offender laws which require that the presence of an offender on parole within neighborhoods be publicized.

Encourage the family to inform other care providers when the child's abuse history may affect a response to care. They should be alert to signs of PTSD in order to seek assistance if the child has continuing problems (see Chapter 34∞).

■ Evaluation

Expected outcomes of nursing care for the child who has been abused or neglected include maintenance of normal growth and development, establishment of a positive sense of self-esteem, provision of parenting information and stress relief for parents, provision of a nurturing environment for the child, and absence of episodes of abuse.

ADDITIONAL ABUSIVE AND VIOLENT SITUATIONS

Abandoned Babies

There are no accurate statistics on numbers of babies that are abandoned in dumpsters, on doorsteps, and other locations. This tragedy has been addressed by "safe haven" laws in some states that allow women to drop unwanted babies at certain locations such as hospitals and fire stations without legal recrimination. Despite these laws, babies continue to be abandoned, perhaps because mothers do not know about the laws or because they do not believe they will not be found guilty. Young teen mothers may not want others to know they had a baby. In addition, placement of these babies in adoptive homes is difficult due to paternity suits. Nurses should know their state's safe haven law details. Inform adolescents and young women about the law and post information in community sites frequented by women. Partner with young pregnant women to link them to resources such as adoption agencies when they might not want to keep a baby.

Hazing

Hazing is an activity that is forced upon an individual, causes humiliation, and is required for membership in an organization or group. It can sometimes be potentially harmful. In the past 30 years, about 60 college students have died of events linked to hazing, and even middle and high school athletes commonly engage in hazing activities (Gershel, Katz-Sidlow, Small, et al., 2003). Activities might include removing clothes, drinking large amounts of alcohol, using snuff or other substances, being locked in small places, being beaten, and many other behaviors. In spite of its common practice, many coaches are not aware of it, and many students do not know what to do about hazing practices. Ask during health visits if the student has ever had to do something to belong to the group or team. Ask about "scary" things others have had them do. Assist schools and colleges in setting up antihazing policies. Encourage students to report hazing. Be aware of the possibility of hazing when seeing children with traumatic injuries.

Domestic Violence

Domestic violence or intimate partner abuse is that which occurs between adult partners in a family. It may involve the parents of a child, or one parent and the significant other. Even teens who are in a sexual relationship with another person can be direct victims in domestic violence. This type of abuse then injures the child or adolescent either by witnessing a loved one being abused, or by being the victim. About 3.3 million children annually in the United States are exposed to violence against their mothers or other female care providers; and children who live in homes where intimate partner abuse occurs are 10 times more likely to be abused themselves, so the behavior is often a precursor to child abuse (Regan, 2003). (See Chapter 11 and Chapter 12∞ for further descriptions of domestic violence.)

Dating Violence

Dating violence is another type of intimate partner abuse; this type occurs in relationships among youth. Most dating violence is directed at females and studies have focused largely on girls. In one questionnaire, over 9% of adolescent girls reported being victims of dating violence. African American girls more commonly report dating violence than Hispanic or White girls (Howard & Wang, 2003). In another study, about 20% of high school females reported dating violence (Silverman, Raj, Mucci, et al., 2001). Girls who report dating violence were also more likely to report other risk behaviors, such as feeling sad, having attempted suicide, or having used substances such as tobacco and drugs. Early sexual activity, having a higher number of sex partners, and being less likely to use birth control are also associated with higher incidence of dating violence. A cluster risk profile may therefore put adolescents more at risk for dating violence.

Date rape is a term used when dating violence takes the form of rape. This can be particularly harmful to females who often do not want to share the event or press charges against the attacker.

Nurses should screen for violence at each health promotion visit, including gynecologic visits and prenatal care. Ask what is going well and not going well in intimate relationships, and whether the person ever feels unsafe or is forced to do things she does not wish to do. Recognize that while not as common, males may even be victims of violence in close relationships. As alcohol and other drugs are often connected with violence in relationships, ask about their use. Organize peer discussion groups about intimacy in order to help youth develop a sense of self-confidence and self-efficacy which will empower them to refuse activities in relationships in which they do not wish to engage (Rickert, Vaughan, & Wiemann, 2002).

Munchausen Syndrome by Proxy

Munchausen syndrome by proxy is a potentially deadly form of child abuse that involves the fabrication of signs and symptoms of a health condition in a child. In 94% to 99% of cases, it is the mother who creates these fictitious signs in her child (the proxy). The victim is usually under 6 years, and commonly under 1 year of age (Paulk, 2001; Hettler, 2002). Frequently the child's symptoms of illness are used to gain entry into the medical system to meet the abuser's own needs.

The issues of abuse are multidimensional. The child is a victim of the feigned illness, repeated hospitalizations, and invasive procedures. Equally disruptive is the deprivation of the child's daily routine caused by the periodic medical crises.

Munchausen syndrome by proxy should be suspected when unexplained, recurrent, or extremely rare conditions occur; illness is unresponsive to treatment; and the history and clinical findings are inconsistent. The most commonly reported signs and symptoms are central nervous system dysfunction, apnea, diarrhea, vomiting, fever, seizures, signs of bleeding (in urine or stool), and rashes. The parent may overdose the child on medications, such as nonprescription drugs and even syrup of ipecac, causing a variety of side effects. Poisoning and suffocation are commonly found. The symptoms occur in the presence of the same caretaker and disappear when the child is separated from that caretaker.

The child often appears uncooperative, extremely anxious, fearful, and negative. The caretaker, who in contrast appears very cooperative, competent, and loving, often expresses a desire for the child to recover. The caretaker may even suggest diagnostic procedures to try to determine "what's wrong." Characteristically the caretaker thrives in the healthcare environment.

The cause of Munchausen syndrome by proxy is often complex and rooted in the caretaker's own abusive or neglectful childhood. The disorder occurs in all socioeconomic classes. Often the perpetrator has some type of healthcare background, such as nursing or another allied health profession. The abuser is often young, married, and of the middle socioeconomic class (Paulk, 2001).

A suspicion of Munchausen syndrome by proxy requires a coordinated evaluation by an interdisciplinary team. Members of the team must organize and communicate a strategic plan regarding collection of evidence, confrontation of the abuser, and management of the hospitalized child. The child's safety is the ultimate concern. The case must also be reported to the appropriate child protective services.

Nursing Management

Special care should be taken to maintain a trusting relationship with the caretaker so that he or she does not become suspicious and leave the hospital. Often the best person on the team to function in the role of "trusted other" is a member of the psychiatric consultation team.

Careful documentation of parent–child interactions, presence or absence of symptoms, and other pertinent observations is essential. The child must be closely monitored. If blood is present in the child's urine, stool, or vomitus, careful documentation is needed about whether the nurse was present or whether the sample was provided by the parent. Covert video surveillance may be ordered by the hospital when the syndrome is highly suspected in a particular situation. Expert consultants may be needed to ensure legal requirements for investigation are met. When enough evidence is collected to prove Munchausen syndrome by proxy, the caretaker is confronted by the physician or another member of the psychiatric team.

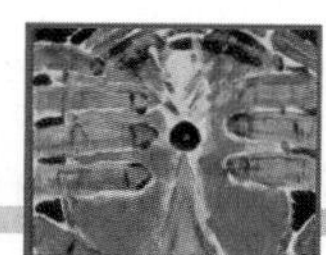

CHAPTER HIGHLIGHTS

- Many of the major morbidities and mortalities of childhood and adolescence are related to social and environmental factors.
- The theory of ecologic development provides a framework to use in assessing the interactions of children with factors in their environments.
- The theory of resilience examines risk and protective factors of children in order to formulate interventions to assist the child dealing with health problems related to social conditions.
- Poverty is a pervasive and important risk factor that influences many health outcomes.

- Some families that are poor experience homelessness and are at risk for a number of health problems.
- Stressful experiences, family structure, and the community all influence the health of children.
- Tobacco use is high among youths, and the most common time for initiation of tobacco use is middle school years.
- Tobacco prevention and cessation programs are needed throughout the school years.
- Substance abuse by alcohol and drugs occurs in childhood and adolescence and compounds many health risks.
- A major contributor to overweight and other health problems is the lack of physical activity among children.
- Protective equipment can reduce the number and severity of injuries during risky physical activities.
- Teens need information about body art safety procedures if they choose this method of self-expression.
- Violence can be directed at children, and children can be the perpetrators of violence.
- All families should be regularly assessed for violence and prevention strategies applied when needed.
- Child abuse can take the form of physical abuse or neglect, emotional abuse or neglect, or sexual abuse.
- The nurse plans interventions for an array of abusive situations such as abandoned babies, hazing, domestic violence, and Munchausen syndrome by proxy.

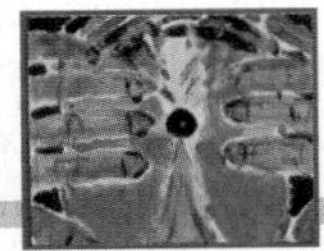

CRITICAL THINKING IN ACTION

INTRODUCTION

Recall 15-year-old Amy Beckman from the chapter opening scenario. She has visited the school nurse due to an ear that is painful after a piercing by a friend. The nurse examines all of Amy's piercings on her ears, face, and navel. Amy is talkative and willing to answer the nurse's questions about her body art and her life. She elaborates about her life when she ran away from school last year and seems to be analyzing her own motives and goals.

DESCRIPTION

The nurse finds that both of Amy's ears have multiple piercings and jewelry. They all appear clean and without inflammation or drainage. The ear that Amy had the nurse check has one new small earring about midway in the ear. Amy admitted that it was hard for her friend to get this piercing in the places desired so her ear was manipulated a great deal during the insertion about 2 days ago. Amy's vital signs are: temperature 99.8°F, pulse 76, respirations 18, blood pressure 118/62.

While gathering data, the nurse inquires about Amy's immunization status. She states that she has no idea what immunizations she has had. The last she remembers were when she was quite small. She had a diagnosis of mild asthma in the past but is not using any inhalers now and has had no exacerbations for about 2 years. She does not really know what asthma is, only that she occasionally had difficulty breathing.

Amy provides information about her weeks spent living on the streets. She left home and school because she felt like no one understood her and she did not like the rules that she had to follow. She spent a few nights with a friend, but left when the friend's mother was going to call Amy's mother to inform her of Amy's whereabouts. She slept under bridges at night and went to a mission for meals and showers. She began smoking and panhandled for money. After a few weeks, while speaking with a nursing student at the shelter, Amy decided that a life on the street was not for her. She "saw the light," as she describes it. She called her own mother and asked to come home. She describes her mother as concerned and caring, and her father as distant and removed. Amy has one older brother who is living and working in another state; she talks with him only on his infrequent visits home. She is sad that she is not closer to her father and older brother. She has a younger brother who is 6 years old, and feels like she needs to be around home for him. At the same time, she discusses her dislike of rules and states that it is hard to have her mother tell her what time to be home at night.

DISCUSSION

1. Amy seems to have some conflicting feelings. She yearns to be at home with her family members, but resists the rules that the family sets. She is distraught that there is not more closeness with her father and brother but has broken some family ties herself when she ran away. What is Amy's developmental stage, according to Erikson? What tasks does she need to accomplish for healthy development to occur? How is her present setting supportive of accomplishing her developmental tasks? How can the school nurse support Amy's developmental progression?
2. Amy clearly has demonstrated many risk and protective factors for physical and psychosocial health. Recall the theory of resilience described in this chapter and Chapter 5∞. Make a list of Amy's risk factors. What puts her at risk of disease or of developing an unhealthy lifestyle? Then make a list of Amy's protective factors. What strengths does she have? You will use this list to formulate nursing diagnoses and interventions for Amy.
3. Based on your summary of Amy's risk and protective factors, list three nursing diagnoses. Be sure that they encompass both physical and psychosocial health.
4. What immunizations should Amy have at her age? Consult the immunization schedule in Chapter 19∞ for ideas. Think also about the dis-

eases that are common with body art and learn which of these can be prevented by immunization.

5. Amy admitted that she began smoking while living on the street. Phrase some open-ended questions to determine both her present smoking habits and whether she has experimented with drugs.

6. Develop a series of nursing interventions that would enhance Amy's health and prevent disease and mental health problems.

7. Consider the roles played by the school nurse in an alternative school. Discuss the skills needed by that nurse in order to work effectively with teens, families, school, and the greater community. What partnerships should the nurse develop with each of these groups?

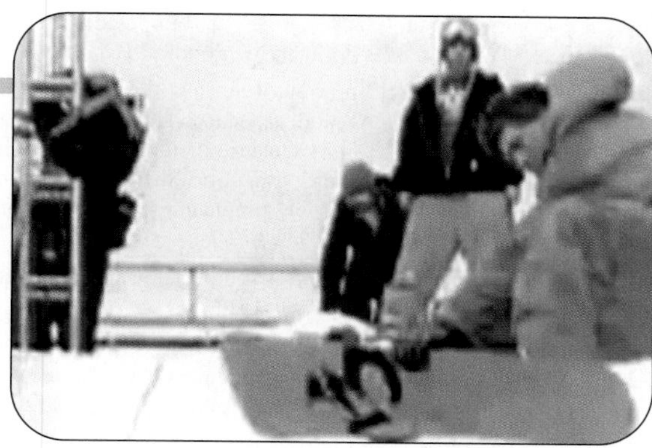

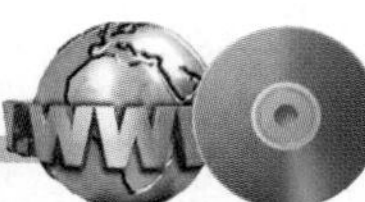

EXPLORE MediaLink

- NCLEX review, case studies, and other interactive resources for this chapter can be found on the Companion Website at **www.prenhall.com/ball**. Click on Chapter 7 to select the activities for this chapter.
- For animations, more NCLEX review questions, and an audio glossary, access the accompanying CD-ROM in this book.

http://www.prenhall.com/ball

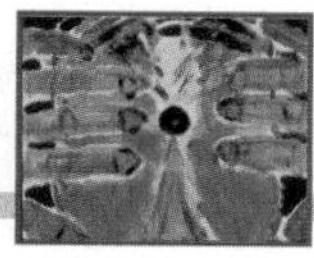

REFERENCES

American Psychiatric Association (2000). Diagnostic and Statistical Manual: DSM-IV-TR. Washington, DC: American Psychiatric Association.

Armstrong, M. L., & Kelly, L. (2001). Tattooing, body piercing, and branding are on the rise: Perspectives for school nurses. *Journal of School Nursing, 17*, 12–23.

Behrman, R. E. (Ed.). (2000). *The future of children: Unintentional injuries in childhood.* Los Altos, CA: The David and Lucille Packard Foundation.

Behrman, R. E., Kliegman, R. M., & Jenson, H. B. (2004). *Nelson textbook of pediatrics* (17th ed.). Philadelphia: Saunders.

Benton, J. (2003). Making schools safer and healthier for lesbian gay bisexual and questioning students. *Journal of School Nursing, 19*, 257–259.

Board on Children, Youth, and Families, National Research Council and Institute of Medicine. (2001). *From neurons to neighborhoods.* Washington, DC: National Academy Press.

Busen, N.H., Modeland, V. & Kouzekanani, K. (2001). Adolescent cigarette smoking and health risk behavior. *Journal of Pediatric Nursing 16*, 187–193.

Castiglia, P. T. (2001). Shaken baby syndrome. *Journal of Pediatric Health Care, 15*, 78–80.

Children's Defense Fund. (2004a). *Basic facts on poverty*. Washington, DC: Author. wysiwyg://main.10/http://www.childrensdefense.org/fs_cpfaq_facts.php, accessed 1/26/2004.

Children's Defense Fund (2004b). Data. Each day in America. http://www.childrensdefense.org/data/eachday.asp, accessed 8/16/2004.

Children's Safety Network, National Injury and Violence Prevention Resource Center. (2003). *Preventing bulleying: The role of the public health professional.* http://www/childrenssafetynetwork.org, accessed 1/23/2004. Coleman-Wallace, D., Lee, J. W., Montgomery, S., Blix, G., & Wang, D. T. (1999). Evaluation of developmentally appropriate programs for adolescent tobacco cessation. *Journal of School Health, 69*, 314–319.

Chng, C. L., Neill, K. & Fogle, P. (2003). Predictors of college students' use of complementary and alternative medicine. *American Journal of Health Education, 39*, 269–271.

Committee on Injury and Poison Prevention, American Academy of Pediatrics. (2001). Bicycle helmets. *Pediatrics, 108*, 1030–1032.

Committee on Public Education, American Academy of Pediatrics. (2001). Children, adolescents and television. *Pediatrics, 107*, 423–426.

Committee on Sports Medicine and Fitness, American Academy of Pediatrics. (2001). Risk of injury from baseball and softball in children. *Pediatrics, 107*, 782–784.

Cook, K. R. (1999). Assessment of potential inhalant use by students. *Journal of School Nursing, 15*(20), 20–23.

Cowal, K., Shinn, M., Weitzman, B. C., Stojanovic, D., & Labay, L. (2002). Mother-child separations among homeless and housed families receiving public assistance in New York City. *American Journal of Community Psychology, 30*, 711–730.

Crespo, C., Smit, E., Troiano, R., Bartlett, S. J., Macera, C. A., & Anderson, R. E. (2001). Television watching, energy intake and obesity in United States children. *Archives of Pediatric and Adolescent Medicine, 155*, 360–363.

DeForge, V., Zehnder, S., Minick, P., & Carmon, M. (2001). Children's perspectives of homelessness. *Pediatric Nursing, 27*, 377–383.

Donovan, K. A. (2000). Smoking cessation programs for adolescents. *Journal of School Nursing, 16*(4), 36–43.

Elkind, D. (2001). *The hurried child: Growing up too fast too soon.* Reading, MA: Perseus Books.

Federal Interagency Forum on Child and Family Statistics. (2003). *America's children: Key national indicators of well-being 2003.* Washington, DC: U.S. Government Printing Office.

Fetro, J. V., Coyle, K. K., & Pham, P. (2001). Health-risk behaviors among middle school students in a large majority-minority school district. *Journal of School Health, 71*, 30–37.

Fields, J., Smith, K., Bass, L. E., & Lugaila, T. (2001). *A child's day: Home, school, and play (selected indicators of child well-being).* Washington, DC: U.S. Department of Commerce.

Fox, J. A., Elliot, D. S., Kerlikowske, R. G., Newman, S. A., & Christeson, W. (2003). *Bullying prevention is crime prevention.* Washington, DC: Fight Crime: Invest in Kids.

Franke, T. M. (2003). The effect of attachment on adolescent violence. *The Prevention Researcher, 10*, 14–16.

Frederickson, D. (1999). Maltreatment of children. *Journal of Child and Family Nursing, 2*, 393–401.

Geiger, J. D., Drongowski, R. A., & Lenni, J. L. (2001). Car surfing: An underreported mechanism of serious injury in children and adolescents. *Journal of Pediatric Surgery, 36*, 232–234.

Gershel, J. C., Katz-Sidlow, R. J., Small, E., & Zandieh, S. (2003). Hazing of suburban middle school and high school athletes. *Journal of Adolescent Health, 32*, 333–335.

Goldrick, B. A. (2003). Endocarditis associated with body piercing. *American Journal of Nursing, 103*, 26–27.

Guthrie, B. J., Hoey, E., Ravoira, L. W., & Kintner, E. (2002). Girls in the juvenile justice system: Leave no girl's health un-addressed. *Journal of Pediatric Nursing, 17*, 414–423.

Hanson, M. (1999). Which straw will break the camel's back? *American Journal of Nursing, 99*, 63–69.

Health Resources and Services Administration (HRSA). (2003). *The national bullying prevention campaign*. Washington, DC: Author.

Healthy People 2010 (2000). Washington, DC: U.S. Department of Health and Human Services. www.health.gov/healthypeople/document/html, accessed 4/13/2001.

Hennes, H. (1998). A review of violence statistics among children and adolescents in the United States. *Pediatric Clinics of North America, 45*, 269–280.

Hettler, J. (2002). Munchhausen syndrome by proxy. *Pediatric Emergency Care, 18*, 371–374.

Horner, G. (2003). Adolescent sexual offenders: A challenge for primary care NPs. *American Journal for Nurse Practitioners, 7*(9), 37–45.

Howard, D. E., & Wang, M. Q. (2003). Risk profiles of adolescent girls who were victims of dating violence. *Adolescence, 38*, 1–14.

Knight, J. R. (1997). Adolescent substance use: Screening, assessment, and intervention. *Contemporary Pediatrics, 14*, 45, 51–56, 61–72.

Lackey, N., & Walker, B. L. (1998). An ecological framework for family nursing practice and research. In B. Vaughan-Cole, M. A. Johnson, J. A. Malone, & B. L. Walker, *Family nursing practice* (pp. 38–48). Philadelphia: WB Saunders.

Leone, A. (2003). Relationship between cigarette smoking and other coronary risk factors in atherosclerosis: Risk of cardiovascular disease and preventive measures. *Current Pharmacological Design, 9*, 2417–2423.

Limber, S. (2003). Youth development program: Olweus bullying prevention. Clemson University website: www.clemson.edu.scg/youth/IFNLbully.htm, accessed 1/20/2004.

MMWR. (2000). Unpowered scooter-related injuries—United States, 1998–2000. *Morbidity and Mortality Weekly Report, 49*, 1108–1110.

MMWR. (2001). Youth tobacco surveillance—United States, 2000. *Morbidity and Mortality Weekly Report, 50*(SS4), 1–84.

MMWR. (2002). Trends in cigarette smoking among high school students. *Morbidity and Mortality Weekly Report, 51*, 409–412.

MMWR. (2003a). Tobacco use among middle and high school students—United States, 2002. *Morbidity and Mortality Weekly Report, 52*, 1096–1098.

MMWR. (2003b). Tobacco, alcohol, and other drug use among high school students in Bureau of Indian Affairs—Funded schools, United States, 2001. *Morbidity and Mortality Weekly Report, 52*, 1070–1072.

MMWR. (2004). Youth Risk Behavior Surveillance—United States, 2003. *Morbidity and Mortality Weekly Report, 53*(SS2), 1–95.

Montgomery, D. F., & Parks, D. (2001). Tattoos: Counseling the adolescent. *Journal of Pediatric Health Care, 15*, 14–19.

Murray, J. S. (2002). Helping children cope with separation during war. *Journal of Specialists in Pediatric Nursing 7*, 127–130.

Murray, S. K., Baker, A. W., & Lewin, L. (2000). Screening families with young children for child maltreatment potential. *Pediatric Nursing, 26*, 47–54.

Nansel, T. R., Overpeck, M., Pilla, R. S., Ruan, W. J., Simons-Morton, B., & Scheidt, P. (2001). Bullying behaviors among US youth: Prevalence and association with psychosocial adjustment. *JAMA, 285*, 2094–2100, 2131–2132.

National Association for Education of Young Children (2004). NAEYC Earlychildhood Programs Standards. http://www.naeyc.org/accreditation. Retreived 8/10/04.

National Institute of Child Health and Human Development. (1997). The effects of infant child care on infant-mother attachment security. *Child Development, 68*, 860–879.

National Institute on Drug Abuse. (1999). *Some facts about club drugs*. Bethesda, MD: U.S. Department of Health and Human Services.

National Safe Kids Campaign (2003). *Report to the nation: Trends in international childhood injury mortality 1987–2000*. Washington DC: Author.

Pagliaro, A. M., & Pagliaro, L. A. (1996). *Substance use among children and adolescents*. New York: John Wiley & Sons.

Paulk, D. (2001). Munchausen syndrome by proxy. *Clinician Reviews, 11*(8), 51–56.

Pratt, H. D., & Greydanus, D. E. (2000). Adolescent violence: Concepts for a new millennium. *Adolescent Medicine, 11*, 103–125.

Regan, K. (2003, October). When daddy hits mommy. *Advance for Nurses*, 27–28.

Rickert, V. I., Vaughan, R. D., & Wiemann, C. M. (2002). Adolescent dating violence and date rape. *Current Opinions in Obstetrics and Gynecology, 14*, 495–500.

Rideout, V. J., Vandewater, E. A., & Wartella, E. A. (2003). Electronic media in the lives of infants, toddlers, and preschoolers. Mento Park, CA: Kaiser Family Foundation, Pub #3378.

Saewyc, E. M., Pettingell, S., & Magee, L. L. (2003). The prevalence of sexual abuse among adolescents in school. *Journal of School Nursing, 19*, 266–272.

Santrock, J. (1999). *Life-span development*. Boston: McGraw-Hill.

Sargent, J. D., Mott, L. A., & Stevens, M. (1998). Predictors of smoking cessation in adolescents. *Archives of Pediatric and Adolescent Medicine, 152*, 388–393.

Sattler, B., Afzal, B. M., Condon, M. E., Belka, E. K., & McKee, B. A. (2003). Children's health and the environment: Environmentally healthy homes and communities. American Nurses Association. www.medscape.com/viewprogram/2660_pnt

Scott, J. U., Hague-Armstrong, K., & Downes, K. L. (2003). Teasing and bullying: What can pediatricians do? *Contemporary Pediatrics, 20*, 105–120.

Selekman, J. (2003). A new era of body decorations: What are kids doing to their bodies? *Pediatric Nursing, 29*, 77–79.

Silverman, J. G., Raj, A., Mucci, L. A., & Hathaway, J. E. (2001). Dating violence in adolescent girls and associated substance use, unhealthy weight control, sexual risk behavior, pregnancy and suicidiality. *JAMA, 286*, 572–579.

Snyder, H. (2003, December). Juvenile arrests. *Juvenile Justice Bulletin*, 1–12.

Society for Pediatric Nurses, SPN Public Policy Committee. (2000). Gun accidents, suicides increase among children. *SPN News, 9*, 6.

Spencer, G. A., & Bryant, S. A. (2000). Dating violence: A comparison of rural, suburban, and urban teens. *Journal of Adolescent Health, 27*, 302–305.

Stafford, E. M., & Grady, B. A. (2003). Military family support. *Pediatric Annals, 32*, 111–115.

Steele, R. W., Ramgoolam, A., & Evans, J. (2003). Health services for homeless adolescents. *Seminars in Pediatric Infectious Diseases, 14*, 38–42.

Stevens, P. E., & Morgan, S. (2001). Health of lesbian, gay, bisexual, and transgender youth. *Journal of Pediatric Health Care, 15*, 24–34.

Stratigos, A. J., & Katsambas, A. D. (2003). Medical and cutaneous disorders associated with homelessness. *Skinmed, 2*, 168–172.

Swan, N. (2003). New imaging technology confirms earlier PET scan evidence: Methamphetamine abuse linked to human brain damage. *National Institute on Drug Abuse Notes (NIDA Notes), 18*(2), 1, 6–7.

Swerdlow, J. L. (2000). *Nature's medicine: Plants that heal*. Washington, DC: National Geographic Society.

Task Force on Violence, American Academy of Pediatrics. (1999). The role of the pediatrician in youth violence prevention in clinical practice and at the community level. *Pediatrics, 103*, 173–181.

Van der Wal, M. F., de Wit, C. A. M., & Hirasing, R. A. (2003). Psychosocial health among young victims and offenders of direct and indirect bullying. *Pediatrics, 111*, 1312–1317.

Walker, G. C., Scott, P. S., & Koppersmith, G. (1998). The impact of child sexual abuse on addiction severity and analysis of trauma processing. *Journal of Psychosocial Nursing, 36*(3), 10–18.

Youssef, N. N., & DiLorenzo, C. (2001). The role of motility in functional abdominal disorders in children. *Pediatric Annals, 30*, 24–30.

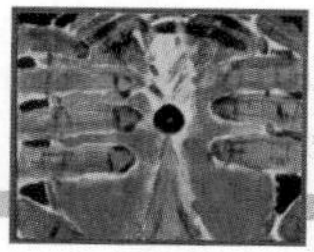

ADDITIONAL REFERENCES

Crook, W. P. (1998). The new sisters of the road: Homeless women and their children. *Journal of Family Social Work, 3*(4), 49–64.

Elgar, F. J., Knight, J., Worrall, G. J., & Sherman, G. (2003). Behavioural and substance use problems in rural and urban delinquent youths. *Canadian Journal of Psychiatry, 48*, 633–636.

Ensign, J., & Santelli, J. (1998). Health status and service use. *Archives of Pediatric and Adolescent Medicine, 152*, 20–24.

Frank, M. A. (2002). Traumatic injuries caused by hazing practices. *American Journal of Emergency Medicine, 20*, 228–233.

Hanze, D. (2002). How to help children and adolescents deal with the threat of terrorism. *Journal of Specialists in Pediatric Nursing, 7*, 42–44.

Kreiss, J. L., & Patterson, D. L. (1997). Psychosocial issues in primary care of lesbian, gay, bisexual, and transgender youth. *Journal of Pediatric Health Care, 11*, 266–274.

Murray, J. S. (2002). Helping children cope with separation during war. *Journal of Specialists in Pediatric Nursing, 7*, 127–130.

Muscari, M. E. (2003). From bullying to the big house: Child offenders. *Topics in Advanced Practice Nursing eJournal, 3*, www.medscape.com/iewarticle/457969.

Rew, L., Chambers, K. B., & Kulkarni, S. (2002). Planning a sexual promotion intervention with homeless adolescents. *Nursing Research, 51*, 168–174.

Scheiman, L., & Zeoli, A. M. (2003). Adolescents' experiences of dating and intimate partner violence: "Once is not enough." *Journal of Midwifery and Womens Health, 48*, 226–228.

Schonfeld, D. J. (2003). Supporting children after terrorist events. *Pediatric Annals, 32*, 182–187.

Thomas, S. P. (2003). Identifying and intervening with girls at risk for violence. *Journal of School Nursing, 19*, 130–139.

Vostanis, P., Grattan, E., & Cumella, S. (1998). Mental health problems of homeless children and families: A longitudinal study. *British Medical Journal, 346*, 899–902.

Chapter

8

Pediatric and Newborn Assessment

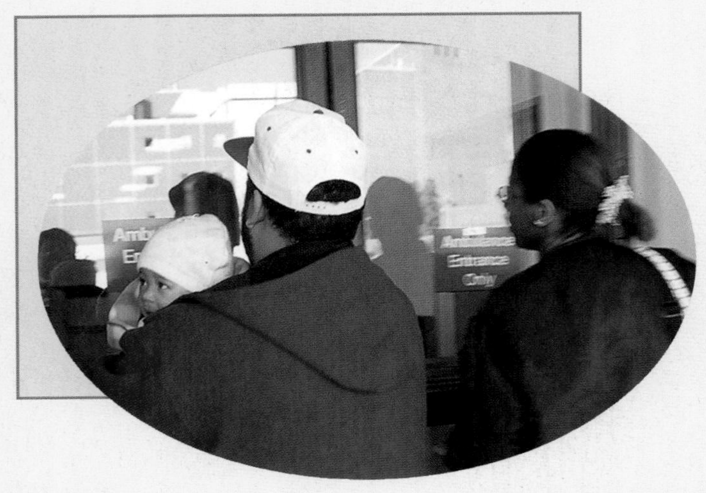

Latoya Pruitt, 6 months old, is brought by her mother and father to the emergency department. She is an emergency admission from the local pediatrician's office with a diagnosis of bronchiolitis. As Latoya's nurse, you are responsible for assessing her condition after she arrives on the pediatric nursing unit.

What information do you look for, and in what order do you gather this information? What techniques can you use to obtain information about Latoya's condition? How do you organize your findings to make sense of them?

The patient history and physical examination provide a structure and a sequence for collecting and analyzing relevant assessment data. The initial physical examination findings provide the baseline for monitoring Latoya's response to treatment. Analysis of the assessment data also enables you to form nursing diagnoses and to develop a nursing care plan to direct the nursing care that Latoya will receive.

"Mama and Daddy got really scared when Latoya's breathing got fast and noisy. She is so little, I hope she gets better fast."

—Monique, Latoya's 6-year-old sister

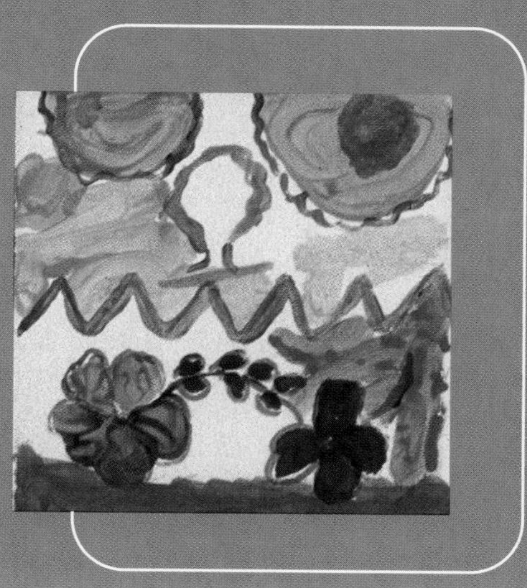

Learning Outcomes

After completing this chapter, you will be able to:

- Describe the elements of a health history for an infant and children of different ages.
- Describe strategies to gain cooperation of a young child for assessment.
- Modify physical assessment techniques according to the age and developmental stage of the child.
- Analyze findings from the assessment of multiple systems and recognize signs of a serious health condition.
- Describe differences in assessment techniques between newborns and older infants.

Key Terms

audiometry/254
auscultation/233
bronchophony/265
caput succedaneum/304
cephalhematoma/305
coloboma/249
crepitus/264
egophony/266
heave/268
hypertelorism/248
inspection/233
lanugo/304
molding/305
palpation/233
percussion/233
retractions/263
sexual maturity rating/281
stadiometer/240
strabismus/249
stridor/266
tactile fremitus/264
tympanometry/255
wheezing/266
whispered pectoriloquy/265

MediaLink http://www.prenhall.com/ball

Resources for this chapter can be found on the CD-ROM accompanying this textbook, and on the Companion Website at http://www.prenhall.com/ball. Click on Chapter 8 to select the activities for this chapter.

CD-ROM

Animations
- *Child's Ear*
- *Middle Ear*
- *Mouth and Throat Examination*
- *Movement of Joints*
- *Otoscopic Examination*
- *3D Eye*

Nursing in Action: Pediatric Assessment and Considerations

NCLEX Review

Audio Glossary

COMPANION WEBSITE

A & P Review

NCLEX Review

Case Study: Newborn Assessment

MediaLink Application
- *BMI Calculator*

Do examination techniques need to vary for children of different ages? How does the nurse gain cooperation for the examination from infants and toddlers? This chapter answers these questions and provides an overview of pediatric assessment, including communication and history taking followed by examination techniques geared to the unique needs of newborns and pediatric patients. Strategies for obtaining the child's history are presented first. The remainder of the chapter then outlines a systematic process for physical examination of the newborn, infant, child, and adolescent. The data obtained from an accurate and complete assessment is the foundation for the nursing process, development of a plan of care, and the implementation and evaluation of nursing interventions.

The techniques for the pediatric physical assessment are presented before the newborn assessment, as many of those skills and techniques are applicable to the newborn. As the focus and purpose of the newborn assessment is to assess transition to extrauterine life and to identify significant health alterations, application of the assessment skills and techniques for a comprehensive newborn assessment is presented in a separate section at the end of the chapter.

OBTAINING THE CHILD'S HISTORY

Communication Strategies

What makes communication effective? What does it mean when a parent or caretaker will not look you in the eye when speaking with you? What types of cues indicate that a parent may be withholding historical information?

The health history interview is a personal conversation with a parent, caretaker, or adolescent during which private concerns and feelings are shared. It takes place in many different healthcare settings—hospital, school, clinic, office setting, or home. Try to ensure that this exchange of information with the parent or the child is clearly understood by both parties, and that it is effective communication (Box 8–1). Effective communication is difficult to accomplish for many reasons: Parents and children may not correctly interpret what the nurse says; the nurse may not understand completely what the parent or child says; or parents are too stressed with life events or the child's condition to fully respond to questions. Additionally, people's interpretation of information is based on their life experiences, culture, and education.

BOX 8–1 Health Insurance Portability and Accountability Act (HIPAA)

Assure the parents and child that the information provided during the assessment is protected under the Health Insurance Portability and Accountability Act (HIPAA), a federal law that established guidelines for the electronic transmission of patient information. Written consent is required for the child's information to be shared with healthcare providers outside the facility. Healthcare facilities carefully guard the privacy of patient information. Be extremely careful and avoid revealing any patient information in casual discussions and to unauthorized individuals.

Strategies to Build a Rapport with the Family and Child

As you begin the history, make sure the parents understand the purpose of the interview and that the information will be used appropriately. To develop rapport, demonstrate your interest in and concern for the child and family during the interview by actively listening to the information shared. Communicate as a nonjudgmental and noncontrolling professional. This rapport forms the foundation for the collaborative relationship between the nurse and parent that will provide the best nursing care for the child. Refer to Chapter 6∞ for age-specific communication strategies. The following strategies help to establish rapport with the child's family during the nursing history.

- *Introduce yourself* (your name, title or position, and your role in caring for the child). To demonstrate respect, ask all family members present what name they prefer you to use when talking with them.
- *Explain the purpose of the interview* and why the nursing history is different from the information collected from other health professionals. For example, "The nurses will use this information to plan nursing care best suited for your child."
- *Provide privacy* and remove as many distractions as possible during the interview. If the patient's room does not offer privacy, attempt to find a vacant patient room or lounge.
- *Direct the focus of the interview* with open-ended questions. Use close-ended questions or directing statements to clarify information. Open-ended questions are useful to initiate the interview, develop a rapport, and understand the parent's perceptions of the child's problem; for example, "Tell me what problems led to Roberto's admission to the hospital." Close-ended questions are used to obtain detailed information; for example, "How high was Tommy's fever this morning?"
- *Ask one question at a time* so that the parent or child understands what piece of information you want and so that you know which question the parent is answering. "Does any member of your family have diabetes, heart disease, or sickle cell anemia?" is a multiple question. Ask about each disease separately to ensure the most accurate response. See Developing Cultural Competence: Q&A.
- *Use nonverbal behavior* such as nodding, smiling, and eye contact at appropriate times to communicate that you are hearing the information shared. Paraphrasing or providing a brief summary of the information shared often helps assure you and the parent and child that you have heard the information correctly.
- *Observe the parent-child interaction and behavior* during the interview and try to sense their feelings. Be alert for the emotional tone of the family and child during the interview. If two or more adults are present, consider who does the talking (mother or father, parent or grandparent, parent or child) and note areas of agreement or disagreement. Direct questions to the child when appropriate and look to

the child for verification after answers from the accompanying adult.

- *Be honest* with the child when answering questions or when giving information about what will happen. Children need to learn that they can trust you.
- *Choose the language style that is best understood* by the parent and child. Commonly used phrases can have different meanings to persons in various regions of the country or to different ethnic groups. Parents may have previously heard clinical terms and use them to describe the child's condition. Parents may not have a full understanding about the condition the terms describe, but think these terms match the signs noted in their child. To improve communication, clarify the parents' understanding of clinical terms or request frequent feedback from the parents or child to ensure you understand their meaning. For example, "You used the term hyperactivity. I think I know what you mean, but would you explain the behavior a bit more for me?"
- *Use an interpreter* to improve communication when you are not fluent in the family's primary language. Look at and direct questions to the family members rather than to the interpreter. This helps the family see themselves as the focus of care. (See Chapter 6 ∞.)

Subtle nonverbal and verbal cues often indicate that the parent has not provided complete information about the child's problem. Observe for behaviors such as avoiding eye contact, change in voice pitch, or hesitation when responding to a question. Being supportive and asking clarifying questions encourage further description or the expression of information that is difficult for the parent or child to share; for example, "It sounds like that was a very difficult experience. How did Latasha react?" (See Developing Cultural Competence: Eye Contact.)

Encourage parents to share information, even if it is private or sensitive, especially when it influences nursing care planning. Often parents avoid sharing some information because they want to make a good impression, or they do not understand the value of the missing information. If a hesitation to share information is detected, briefly explain why the question was asked, for example, to make their child's hospital experience more pleasant or to begin planning for the child's discharge and home care.

In some cases, the parent becomes too agitated, upset, or angry to continue responding to questions. When the information is not needed immediately, move on to another portion of the history to determine whether the parent is able to respond to other questions. Depending on the emotional status of the parent, it may be more appropriate to collect the remaining historical data at a later time.

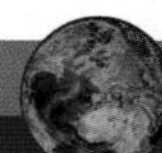

DEVELOPING CULTURAL COMPETENCE
Q & A

Some cultural groups, particularly Asians, try to anticipate the answers you want to hear, or they say yes even if they do not understand the question. This practice is done in an effort to please you or as an expression of politeness. Remember to phrase your questions in a neutral manner. It is also important to assess the family's understanding of English or the language used for history taking.

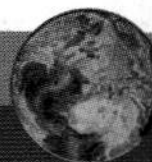

DEVELOPING CULTURAL COMPETENCE
Eye Contact

Understanding perceptions of various cultural groups regarding the use of eye contact will reduce the risk of misinterpreting behaviors when communicating with children and their families. Europeans such as the French and Spanish use firm eye contact and look for a response or impact regarding what has been said. Some Americans may make brief eye contact and then let the eyes wander (Seidel et al., 2003). However, eye contact with the interviewer may be avoided by many cultural groups (Asian, Native American, and Middle Eastern patients) because it is considered impolite, aggressive, or a sign of disrespect (Spector, 2000).

DATA TO BE COLLECTED

The child's health, medical, and personal-social history is collected and organized to plan the child's nursing care. A modification of the Burns Classification System is the data collection framework used (Burns, 1992; Byrnes, 1996). Physiologic, psychosocial, and developmental data are organized to help develop the nursing diagnoses and the nursing care plan. Be alert for nonverbal cues throughout the data gathering process (Figure 8–1 ■).

Patient Information

Obtain the child's name and nickname, age, sex, and ethnic origin. The child's birth date, race, religion, address, phone number, and cell phone number can be obtained from the admission form. Ask the parent for an emergency contact address and phone number, as well as a work phone number. Record the name of the person providing the patient history and that person's relationship to the patient. If the historian is not a parent,

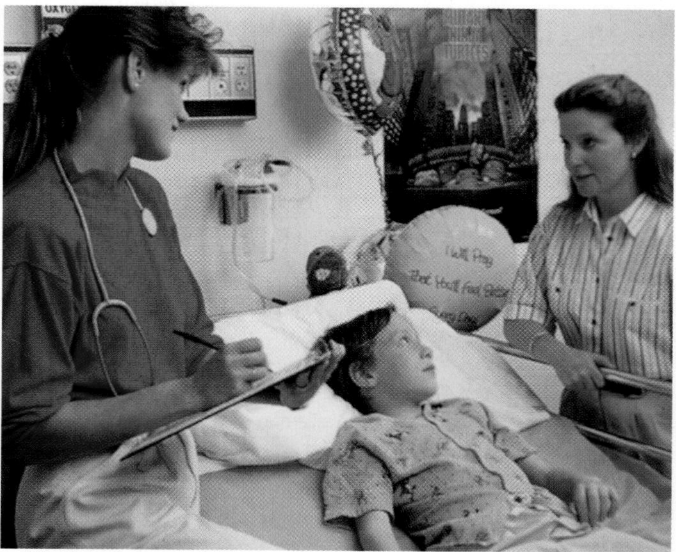

FIGURE 8–1 ■ Observe the behavior of children and family members while you are collecting historical and physiologic data.

determine if this individual has authority to consent for medical care for the child.

Physiologic Data

Information about the child's health problems and diseases is collected chronologically in a format similar to the traditional medical history.

Chief Complaint

The chief complaint is the child's primary problem or reason for hospital admission or visit to a healthcare setting, stated in the parent's or child's exact words.

History of Present Illness or Injury

The history of the present illness or injury is a detailed description of each current health problem. This includes the onset and sequence of events, characteristics of and changes in symptoms over time, influencing factors, and the current status of the problem. Each problem is described separately. Table 8–1 lists the specific data to be collected about each illness and injury.

Past History

The past history is a more detailed description of the child's prior health status. It includes the birth history and all major past illnesses and injuries. A detailed and complete birth history is obtained for a newborn or when the young child's present problem may be related to the birth history. Use the guidelines provided in Box 8–2 to obtain a birth history. Document the child's age at the time of each illness, injury, related surgery, or hospitalization. Obtain information about each specific diagnosis, treatment, outcome, complication or residual problem, and the child's reaction to the event.

Collect information about the child's past history and the child's age at each occurrence. Identify all major illnesses including common communicable diseases. Identify major injuries, their cause or mechanism, and their severity. For past surgeries obtain information about the specific type and if the surgery was performed as day surgery or required at least a night of hospitalization. For all hospitalizations, record the reason and length of hospitalization. If any transfusions (blood or blood products) have been given in the past, identify the circumstances, type and date of transfusion, and reactions to the transfusion. Obtain information about each specific diagnosis, treatment, outcome, complication or residual problem, and the child's reaction to the event.

BOX 8–2 Obtaining a Birth History

PRENATAL CONDITION

- Mother's age, health during pregnancy, prenatal care, weight gained, special diet, expected date of delivery
- Details of illnesses, radiograph findings, hospitalizations, medications, complications, and timing during pregnancy
- Prior obstetric history

INTRAPARTUM—DESCRIPTION OF DELIVERY

- Gestation at birth
- Site of delivery (hospital, home, birthing center)
- Labor induced or spontaneous
- Length of labor
- Time/duration of rupture of membranes
- Quantity and appearance of amniotic fluid
- Vaginal or cesarean section, forceps or suction used, vertex or breech position
- Single or multiple birth
- Medications or anesthesia used during labor/birth

CONDITION OF BABY AT BIRTH

- Weight, Apgar score, cried immediately
- Need for incubator, oxygen, suctioning, ventilator
- Any abnormalities detected, meconium staining

POSTNATAL CONDITION

- Difficulties in the nursery—feeding, respiratory difficulties, jaundice, cyanosis, rashes
- Length of hospital stay, special nursery, home with mother
- Breast or formula fed, weight lost/gained in hospital
- Medical care needed in first week—readmission to hospital

TABLE 8–1 History of Present Illness or Injury

CHARACTERISTIC	DEFINING VARIABLES
Onset	Sudden or gradual, previous episodes, date and time began
Type of symptom	Pain, itching, cough, vomiting, runny nose, diarrhea, rash, for example
Location	Generalized or localized—anatomically precise
Duration	Continuous or episodic, length of episodes
Severity	Effect on daily activities (e.g., interrupted sleep, decreased appetite, incapacitation)
Influencing factors	What relieves or aggravates symptoms, what precipitated the problem, recent exposure to infection or allergen
Past evaluation for the problem	Laboratory studies, physician's office or hospital where performed, results of past examinations
Previous and current therapies	Prescribed and over-the-counter drugs used, alternative and complementary therapies, other treatment measures tried (e.g., heat, ice, rest), response to treatments

Current Health Status

The current health status is a detailed description of the child's typical health status. Obtain information about allergies, current medications, immunization status, activities and exercise, sleep patterns, nutrition, safety measures used, and health maintenance care as follows:

Health Maintenance. Identify the name and when the last visit was made to the child's primary care provider, dentist, and other healthcare providers (such as specialty physicians, emergency department, or urgent care clinic).

Medications. Provide names of prescribed and over-the-counter medications (such as acetaminophen, cold medications, vitamins, ointments, creams) taken daily or frequently, their purpose, and their effectiveness. If the child is being assessed for an episodic illness or injury, inquire about the medications used for home management of conditions such as fever, colds, coughs, cuts, and rashes. Inquire about the use of plants, herbs, teas, or other complementary therapies used and their purpose and effectiveness.

Allergies. List the child's allergies to food, medication, animals, insect bites, or environmental exposure, and the type of reaction (e.g., respiratory difficulty, rash, hives, itching).

Immunizations. Record the types of immunizations, dates received, and any unexpected reactions. Identify any immunizations still needed. Chapter 19∞.

Safety Measures Used. Determine if age-appropriate safety measures are used, such as a car restraint system, window guards, medication storage, sports protective gear, smoke detectors, bicycle helmet, and firearm storage.

Activities and Exercise. Identify the child's play and/or sports activities; identify any physical mobility problem, limitations, and adaptive equipment used.

Nutrition. For infants, determine if the baby is formula fed or breastfed, and if breastfed, for how long. Determine the type and amount of formula intake each day, as well as any other liquids. Identify when solid foods were introduced, which ones, and the amounts eaten each day. Contrast to the appropriate food intake for age and weight as described in Chapter 9∞.

Inquire about enrollment in the Women, Infants, and Children (WIC) Program. For children, determine the amount of foods and milk consumed each day. Identify eating and snacking habits, the variety of foods consumed, "junk foods" eaten, and appetite. Inquire about the family eating patterns such as meals eaten together, food consumption in the childcare center or school, and during other social events.

Sleep. Identify the length and timing of naps and nighttime sleep, presence of nightmares or night terrors or other sleep disturbances, where the child sleeps, and bedtime rituals.

Family History

Obtaining a familial and hereditary disease history is important to identify any major familial and hereditary diseases that could potentially affect the child. Specific diseases the nurse inquires about are listed in Table 8–2. Information is collected for three generations of family members, including the parents, grandparents, aunts, uncles, cousins, child, and siblings. Collect information about the health status of each parent. If there is the potential for a hereditary disorder, a family pedigree will likely be constructed. See Chapter 4∞ for information about constructing a pedigree and important questions used in data collection.

Review of Systems

The review of systems provides a comprehensive overview of the child's health. This is an opportunity to identify additional signs and symptoms associated with the child's health or hospital admission problem. The review of systems may identify other problems that have no direct relationship to the child's significant health problem, but these problems could be factors complicating nursing care or home care. For example, asking about any urinary problems may reveal that a child still wets the bed at 7 years of age, although the admission is for a femur fracture. The nurse would then need to consider how bedwetting might cause problems with the spica cast. For each problem, obtain the treatment, outcomes, residual problems, and age at time of onset. Data collection guidelines are given in Table 8–3.

TABLE 8–2 Familial or Hereditary Diseases

CATEGORY OF DISEASES	EXAMPLES
Infectious diseases	Tuberculosis, HIV, hepatitis, varicella
Heart disease	Heart defects, myocardial infarctions, hypertension, hyperlipidemia, sudden childhood deaths
Allergic disorders	Eczema, hay fever, asthma
Eye disorders	Glaucoma, cataracts, vision loss
Ear disorders	Hearing loss
Hematologic disorders	Sickle-cell anemia, thalassemia, G6PD deficiency, leukemia
Lung disorders	Cystic fibrosis
Cancer	Type, i.e., retinoblastoma, early age of onset
Endocrine disorders	Diabetes mellitus, hypothyroidism, hyperthyroidism
Neurologic and mental disorders	Mental retardation, epilepsy, Huntington chorea, psychiatric disorders
Musculoskeletal disorders	Arthritis, muscular dystrophy
Gastrointestinal disorders	Ulcers, colitis, kidney disease
Problem pregnancies	Repeated miscarriages, stillbirths
Learning problems	Attention deficit disorder, Down syndrome

Psychosocial Data

Obtain information about family composition to establish a socioeconomic and sociologic context within which to plan care for the newborn or child in the hospital and at home. (See Chapter 7∞ to review societal and environmental issues that should be considered in data collection, such as food insecurity.) Include the following:

- Family composition, including family members living in the home, their relationship to the child, marital status of parents or other family structure, and persons participating in the care of the child; household members employed, family income, and financial resources or agencies used such as private health insurance, Medicaid, State Children's Health Insurance Program (SCHIP), food stamps, or Temporary Assistance for Needy Families (TANF)
- Description of the housing and home environment (atmosphere, emotional stresses, family activities), child's sleeping area, safe play area, pets, use of city or well water, and availability of electricity, heat, and refrigeration

TABLE 8–3 Data Collection Guidelines for Review of Systems

BODY SYSTEM	EXAMPLES OF PROBLEMS TO IDENTIFY
General	➤ General growth pattern, overall health status, ability to keep up with other children or tires easily with feeding or activity, fever, sleep patterns ➤ Allergies, type of reaction (hives, rash, respiratory difficulty, swelling, nausea), seasonal or with each exposure ➤ Alertness of child
Skin and lymph	➤ Rashes, dry skin, itching, changes in skin color or texture, tendency for bruising, swollen or tender lymph glands
Hair and nails	➤ Hair loss, changes in color or texture, use of dye or chemicals on hair ➤ Abnormalities of nail growth or color, clubbing
Head	➤ Headaches
Eyes	➤ Vision problems, squinting, crossed eyes, "lazy eye," wears glasses ➤ Eye infections, redness, tearing, burning, rubbing, swelling eyelids
Ears	➤ Ear infections, frequent discharge from ears, tubes in ears or myringotomy ➤ Hearing loss (no response to loud noises or questions, inattentiveness, was hearing test ever performed?) ➤ Hearing aids or cochlear implants
Nose and sinuses	➤ Nosebleeds, nasal congestion, colds with runny nose, sinus pain or infections ➤ Nasal obstruction, difficulty breathing, snoring at night
Mouth and throat	➤ Mouth breathing, difficulty swallowing, sore throats, strep infections ➤ Mouth odor ➤ Tooth eruption, cavities, braces ➤ Voice change, hoarseness, speech problems
Cardiac and hematologic	➤ Heart murmur, anemia, hypertension, cyanosis, edema, rheumatic fever, chest pain
Chest and respiratory	➤ Trouble breathing, choking episodes, cough, wheezing, cyanosis, exposure to tuberculosis, other infections
Gastrointestinal	➤ Bowel movements, frequency, color, regularity, consistency, discomfort, constipation or diarrhea ➤ Abdominal pain, bleeding from rectum, flatulence ➤ Nausea or vomiting, appetite
Urinary	➤ Frequency, urgency, dysuria, dribbling, enuresis, strength of urinary stream ➤ Toilet trained—age when day and night dryness attained
Reproductive Female Male Both	For pubescent children: ➤ Menses onset, amount, duration, frequency, discomfort, problems; vaginal discharge, breast development ➤ Puberty onset, emissions, erections, pain or discharge from penis, swelling or pain in testicles ➤ Sexual activity, use of contraception, sexually transmitted diseases
Musculoskeletal	➤ Weakness, clumsiness, poor coordination, balance, tremors, abnormal gait ➤ Painful muscles or joints, swelling or redness of joints, fractures
Neurologic	➤ Seizures, fainting spells, dizziness, numbness, brain injuries ➤ Cranial nerves functioning ➤ Learning problems, concentration, attention span, hyperactivity, memory problems

- School or childcare arrangements; description of the neighborhood, including playgrounds, transportation, lighting, sidewalks, and proximity to stores
- Changes in family or lifestyle since last seen; number of times the family has moved; how the child and family members have coped with the changes

Information about daily routines, psychosocial data, and other living patterns forms the basis for many nursing diagnoses and development of an individualized nursing care plan. Collection of information should focus on issues that have an impact on the quality of daily living, even if some data seem to overlap with disease data (Box 8–3). See Chapter 2∞ for tools that may be used for a family assessment.

Newborns

The psychosocial history for parents of newborns should focus on readiness to care for the newborn at home. Issues such as support for the parent in the initial postpartum period, safe transport, and a home environment that provides heat, refrigeration, and safe water supplies should be addressed. Determine if referral for WIC or TANF is needed to ensure adequate nutrition and financial support for the mother and newborn. See Chapter 11∞ for more information on newborn health promotion.

Adolescents

The psychosocial history for adolescents should focus on critical areas in their lives (home environment, education/employment, eating, activities, drugs, sexual activity/sexuality/sexual abuse, suicide/depression, and safety) that may contribute to a less-than-optimal environment for normal growth and development (Goldenring & Rosen, 2004). Possible screening questions can be found in Table 8–4. Refer to Chapters 7 and 15∞ for a more detailed assessment of these issues.

Developmental Data

The nurse records information about the child's motor, cognitive, language, and social development and indicates if the information was obtained by direct observation or reported by the caregiver. Some information is gained by observation of the child during the history and physical examination, as described in "Developmental Approach to the Examination" (later in the chapter). In other cases, ask the parent about the young child's developmental progress in categories such as language, fine and gross motor milestones, and current skills. Actual assessment of the child with the Denver II may also be used to collect this information (see Chapter 10∞). For school-age children, ask about academic performance to assess cognitive development. Ask the parent about the child's manner of interaction with other children, family members, and strangers. Alternatively, have the parent complete the Behavior Checklist to assess development of children between 7 and 11 years (Table 8–5). This 5-minute tool can be used to evaluate mood, play, school, friends, and family relations. For adolescents, ask about school performance and activities indicating development of independence and autonomy.

The developmental data will help the nurse plan nursing care that is appropriate for the child. Guidelines for a nursing assessment of development can be found in Chapter 5∞.

BOX 8–3 Daily Living Patterns

ROLE RELATIONSHIPS
- Family relationships/alterations in family process
- Peer relationships
- Social interactions: childcare, preschool, school, neighborhood
- Communication

SELF-PERCEPTION/SELF-CONCEPT
- Personal identity and role identity
- Self-esteem
- Body image/nonvisible disorder

COPING/STRESS TOLERANCE
- Temperament
- Coping behaviors
- Discipline methods used
- Any substance abuse

SPIRITUAL LIFE
- Formal religion practiced as a family
- Belong to any spiritual group or community
- Any foods or drinks not allowed according to spiritual beliefs
- Special food preparation required
- Prohibition of certain medical interventions
- Personal values/beliefs

HOME CARE PROVIDED FOR CHILD'S CONDITION
- Resources needed/available
- Knowledge and skills of parents, other family members
- Respite care available

SENSORY/PERCEPTUAL PROBLEMS
- Adaptations to daily living for any sensory loss (vision, hearing, cognitive, or motor)

Adapted from Burns, C. (1992). A new assessment model and tool for pediatric nurse practitioners. Journal of Pediatric Health Care, *6, 73–81. Used with permission from the National Association of Pediatric Nurse Practitioners.*

ANATOMIC AND PHYSIOLOGIC CHARACTERISTICS OF INFANTS AND CHILDREN

It is readily apparent that infants and children are smaller than adults. Significant differences in physiology also normally exist between children and adults. Knowledge of pediatric anatomic and physiologic differences will aid in recognizing normal variations found during the physical examination. It also assists with understanding the different physiologic responses children have to illness and injury. Figure 8–2 ■ on page 236 provides an overview of important anatomic and physiologic differences between children and adults.

PHYSICAL EXAMINATION TECHNIQUES

Inspection is the purposeful observation of the child's physical features and behaviors that continues through the entire physical examination. Physical feature characteristics include size, shape, color, movement, position, and location. Adequate lighting is essential. Detection of odors is also a part of inspection.

Palpation is the use of touch to identify characteristics of the skin, internal organs, and masses. Characteristics include texture, moistness, tenderness, temperature, position, shape, consistency, and mobility of masses and organs. Palpation with different areas of the hands is performed to enhance certain findings. The palmar surface of the fingers and finger pads is used for determining position, size, consistency, and masses. The ulnar surface of the hand is best for detecting vibrations.

Auscultation is listening to sounds produced by the airway, lungs, stomach, heart, and blood vessels to identify their characteristics. Auscultation is usually performed with a stethoscope to enhance the sounds heard in the chest and abdomen. Some sounds such as speech are heard directly by the ear.

Percussion is striking the surface of the body, either directly or indirectly, to set up vibrations that reveal the density of underlying tissues and borders of internal organs. As the density of the tissue increases, the percussion tone becomes quieter. The tone over air is the loudest and the tone over solid areas is soft. Percussion is most often used for the chest and abdomen.

Standard precautions are used during the physical examination. Good handwashing should be performed before contact with the child. Gloves should be worn for any contact with mucous membranes and body fluids.

MediaLink Nursing in Action: Pediatric Assessment and Considerations

TABLE 8–4 Adolescent Psychosocial Assessment Using the HEEADSSS Screening Tool

	SCREENING QUESTIONS
Home environment	➤ Who lives with you? Where do you live? Do you have your own room? ➤ What are relationships like at home? ➤ To whom are you closest at home? ➤ To whom can you talk at home? ➤ Is there anyone new at home? Has someone left recently? ➤ Have you ever had to live away from home? (Why?)
Employment and education	➤ Are you currently in school? ➤ What are your favorite subjects at school? Your least favorite subjects? ➤ How are your grades? Any recent changes? Any dramatic changes in the past? ➤ Have you changed schools in the past few years? ➤ What are your future education/employment plans/goals? ➤ Are you working? Where? How much? ➤ Tell me about your friends at school.
Eating	➤ What do you like and not like about your body? ➤ Have there been any recent changes in your weight? ➤ Have you dieted in the last year? How? How often? ➤ Have you done anything else to try to manage your weight? ➤ How much exercise do you get in an average day? Week? ➤ What do you think would be a healthy diet? How does that compare with your current eating patterns?
Activities	➤ What do you and your *friends* do for fun? (With whom, where, and when?) ➤ What do you and your *family* do for fun? (With whom, where, and when?) ➤ Do you participate in any sports or other activities? ➤ Do you regularly attend a church group, club, or other organized activity?
Drugs (substance use)	➤ Do any of your friends use tobacco? Alcohol? Other drugs? ➤ Does anyone in your family use tobacco? Alcohol? Other drugs? ➤ Do you use tobacco? Alcohol? Other drugs? ➤ Is there any history of alcohol or drug problems in your family? Does anyone at home use tobacco?
Sexuality	➤ Have you ever been in a romantic relationship? ➤ Tell me about the people that you've dated OR Tell me about your sex life. ➤ Have any of your relationships ever been sexual relationships? ➤ Are your sexual activities enjoyable? ➤ What does the term "safer sex" mean to you? ➤ Are you interested in boys? Girls? Both?
Suicide/depression	➤ Do you feel sad or down more than usual? ➤ Do you find yourself crying more than usual? ➤ Are you "bored" all the time? ➤ Have you thought a lot about hurting yourself or someone else?
Safety (savagery)	➤ Have you ever been seriously injured? (How?) How about anyone else you know? ➤ Do you always wear a seat belt in the car? ➤ Have you ever ridden with a driver who was drunk or high? When? How often? ➤ Do you use safety equipment for sports or other physical activities (e.g., helmets for biking or skateboarding)? ➤ Is there any violence in your home? Does the violence ever get physical? ➤ Is there a lot of violence at your school? In your neighborhood? Among your friends? ➤ Have you ever been physically or sexually abused? Have you ever been raped, on a date or at any other time? (if not asked previously)

Reprinted with permission from: Goldenring, J. M., & Rosen, D. S. (2004). Getting into adolescent heads: An essential update. Contemporary Pediatrics, 21*(1), 64–90.*

DEVELOPMENTAL APPROACH TO THE EXAMINATION

The sequence and approach to the examination varies by age. Provide a comfortable atmosphere for the examination with privacy so that modesty is respected. Explain the procedures as you begin to perform them. In young children, a foot-to-head sequence is often used so that the least distressing parts of the examination are completed first. This gives the child more time to become accepting of the procedures. In older cooperative children, the head-to-toe approach is generally used. The sequence is usually varied by experienced examiners to take advantage of opportunities for more optimal assessment, such as listening to heart, breath, and abdominal sounds when the infant or toddler is asleep or quiet. See the Photo Story on pages 238–239.

Newborns and Infants Under 6 Months of Age

Infants are among the easiest children to examine, as they do not resist the examination procedure. Keep the parent present to provide security to the infant. The young infant can be placed on the examining table as long as safety is assured. Provide physical comfort when needed during the examination by feeding, using a pacifier, cuddling, or changing the diaper to keep the infant calm and quiet. Other simple maneuvers for distraction such as rocking or clicking noises may help when the infant begins to get distressed. Observe the infant for general level of activity, overall mood, and responsiveness to handling.

The sequence of the examination should be flexible to capture opportunities for auscultating the lungs, heart, and abdomen when the infant is quiet or asleep. Make sure the hands and stethoscope are warmed and motions are gentle. If the infant continues to be quiet or can be quieted with a pacifier, palpate the abdomen while the muscles are relaxed. Then proceed to palpate the femoral pulses. The remainder of the examination can proceed in a head-to-toe sequence. Portions of the examination that will disturb the infant, such as the examination of the hips, should be performed at the end.

Infants over 6 Months of Age

Because of developing separation and stranger anxiety, the older infant often resists portions of the physical examination. For this reason, it is often best to keep the older infant with the parent. The infant and toddler can be examined on the parent's lap and then held against the parent's chest for some steps, such as the ear examination. If the infant must be placed on the examining table for any procedure, keep the parent close. The infant will not object to having clothing removed, but make sure the room is warm for the infant's comfort. Observe the infant's general level of activity, mood, and responsiveness to handling by the parent.

Smile and talk soothingly to the infant during the procedure, and use the various techniques of the exam to play with the child, such as during range of motion and reflex assessment. Use toys to distract the older infant. Use a pacifier, bottle, or a gloved finger to quiet the child when necessary. Because the infant may be fearful of being touched by a stranger, begin with the feet and hands before moving to the trunk. Be flexible in the sequence of the examination to take advantage of opportunities presented when the infant is sleeping or quiet to auscultate the heart and lungs.

Toddlers

Toddlers may be active, curious, shy, cautious, or slow to warm up. Because of stranger anxiety, toddlers do not like to be separated from their parents, so assessment on the parent's lap is usually preferred. Let the child hold a security object if it helps. Attempt to reduce the child's anxiety about the examination instruments by demonstrating their use on the parent or letting the parent hold the instrument first. Perform the cranial nerve assessment or developmental assessment as a method to gain cooperation for other procedures.

Avoid asking the child if you can perform a part of the examination as the typical response will be "no." Tell the child what you will do at each step of the examination, using a confident voice that expects cooperation. When a choice is possible, let the child have some control by selecting which part of the examination to do next, such as touching the chest or the abdomen or letting the child choose to stand or sit for a certain part of the examination. Begin the examination by touching the feet and then moving gradually toward the body and head. Instruments to examine the ears, eyes, and mouth are usually viewed as the most fearful and should be used at the end of the examination.

While much of the examination can be performed with the child sitting, it is possible to create a flat surface for the abdominal and genital examination by sitting close to the parent with knees together. For invasive procedures (ear, eye, and mouth exam) the parent can hold the child closely to the chest with legs between the parent's legs. (See Figure 8–24 later in the chapter.) Remember that much of the neurologic and musculoskeletal assessment can be conducted by observing the child play and walk around in the examining room.

TABLE 8–5 Behavior Checklist

BEHAVIOR	NEVER	SOMETIMES	OFTEN
1. Prefers to play alone			
2. Gets hurt in major accidents			
3. Does he/she ever play with fire?			
4. Has difficulties with teachers			
5. Gets poor grades in school			
6. Is absent from school			
7. Becomes angry easily			
8. Daydreams			
9. Feels unhappy			
10. Acts younger than other children his/her age			
11. Does not listen to parents			
12. Does not tell the truth			
13. Unsure of himself/herself			
14. Has trouble sleeping			
15. Seems afraid of someone or something			
16. Is nervous and jumpy			
17. Has a nervous habit			
18. Does not show feelings			
19. Fights with other children			
20. Is understanding of other people's feelings			
21. Refuses to share			
22. Shows jealousy			
23. Takes things that are not his/hers			
24. Blames others for his/her troubles			
25. Prefers to play with children not his/her age			
26. Gets along well with grownups			
27. Teases others			

Scoring: 0 = Never, 1 = Sometimes, 2 = Often. Scoring is reversed for items 20 and 26. Scores between 15 and 22 indicate a need to follow more closely; scores above 22 indicate a need for psychiatric referral and evaluation.

From Jellinek, M., Evans, N., & Knight, R. (1979). Use of a behavior checklist on a pediatric inpatient unit. J. Pediatrics, 94, *156–159. Used with permission from Elsevier.*

AS THEY GROW

Anatomic & Physiologic Characteristics of Children

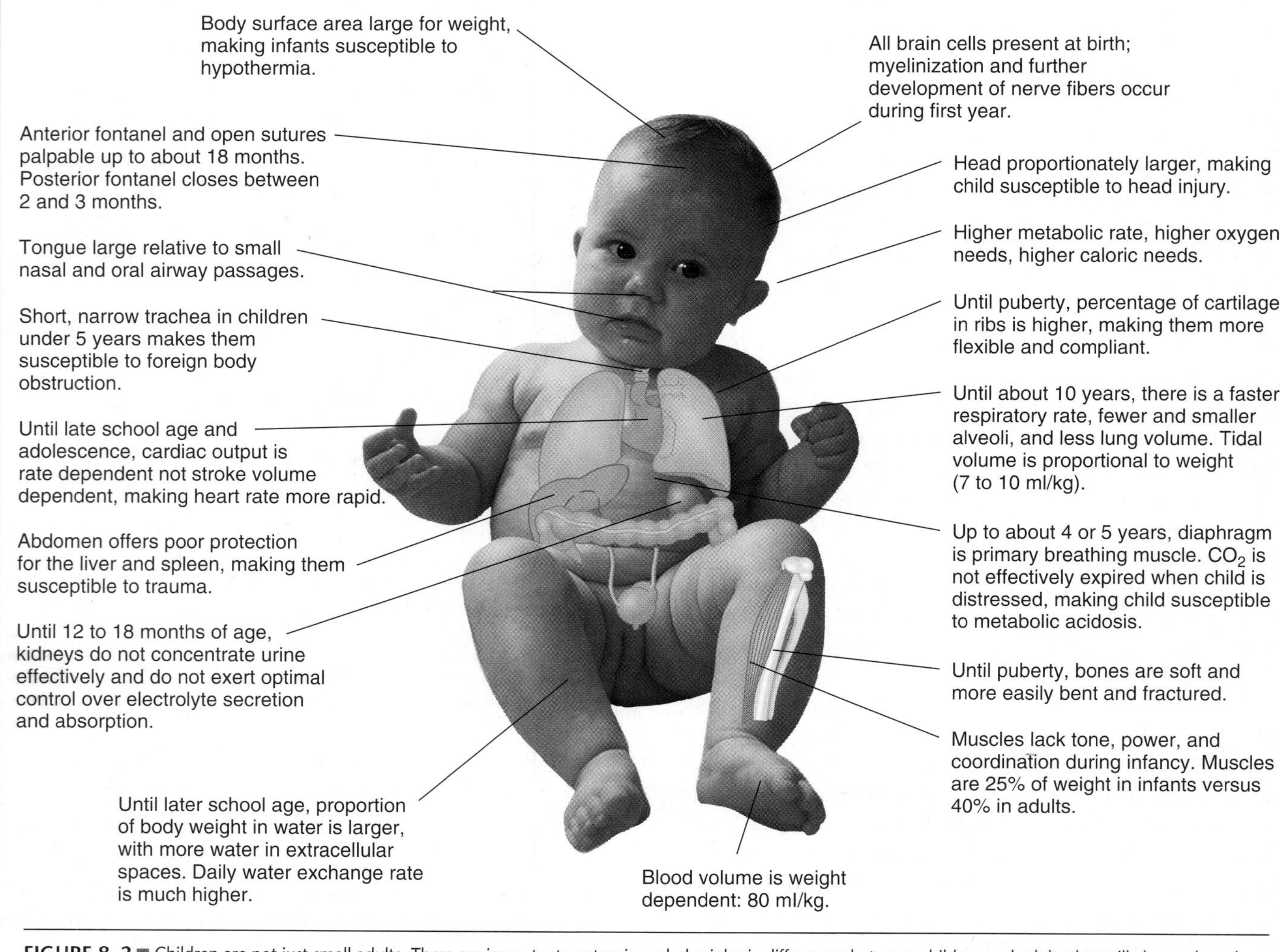

Body surface area large for weight, making infants susceptible to hypothermia.
Anterior fontanel and open sutures palpable up to about 18 months. Posterior fontanel closes between 2 and 3 months.
Tongue large relative to small nasal and oral airway passages.
Short, narrow trachea in children under 5 years makes them susceptible to foreign body obstruction.
Until late school age and adolescence, cardiac output is rate dependent not stroke volume dependent, making heart rate more rapid.
Abdomen offers poor protection for the liver and spleen, making them susceptible to trauma.
Until 12 to 18 months of age, kidneys do not concentrate urine effectively and do not exert optimal control over electrolyte secretion and absorption.
Until later school age, proportion of body weight in water is larger, with more water in extracellular spaces. Daily water exchange rate is much higher.
Blood volume is weight dependent: 80 ml/kg.
All brain cells present at birth; myelinization and further development of nerve fibers occur during first year.
Head proportionately larger, making child susceptible to head injury.
Higher metabolic rate, higher oxygen needs, higher caloric needs.
Until puberty, percentage of cartilage in ribs is higher, making them more flexible and compliant.
Until about 10 years, there is a faster respiratory rate, fewer and smaller alveoli, and less lung volume. Tidal volume is proportional to weight (7 to 10 ml/kg).
Up to about 4 or 5 years, diaphragm is primary breathing muscle. CO_2 is not effectively expired when child is distressed, making child susceptible to metabolic acidosis.
Until puberty, bones are soft and more easily bent and fractured.
Muscles lack tone, power, and coordination during infancy. Muscles are 25% of weight in infants versus 40% in adults.

FIGURE 8–2 ■ Children are not just small adults. There are important anatomic and physiologic differences between children and adults that will change based on a child's growth and development. Can you identify which of these differences are of greatest concern for the hospitalized child and why?

Preschoolers

Assess the willingness of the child to be separated from the parent. Younger children will often prefer to be examined on the parent's lap, while older children will be comfortable on the examining table. They are usually willing to undress, but leave the underpants on until conducting the genital examination. Most children in this age group are cooperative during the physical examination; however, consider which sequence of examination is best for the child. Some children will prefer to have the head, eyes, ears, and mouth over with first while others respond better if these procedures are postponed to the end of the examination.

Preschoolers like to be involved in the examination. Allow the child to touch and play with the equipment. Use games to reduce anxiety about the examination, such as listening to and looking in the ears of the child's stuffed animal first. Give the child simple explanations about the assessment procedures, and offer choice where there is one during the examination, such as which ear to look into first. Use distraction to gain the child's cooperation during the examination, such as asking the child to count, name colors, or talk about a favorite activity. Give positive feedback when the child cooperates.

School-Age Children

School-age children are willing to cooperate during the physical examination, so have the child sit on the examining table. Anticipate the development of modesty in school-age children and offer a patient gown to cover the underwear. Let the older school-age child determine if the examination will be conducted in privacy or with the parent or siblings present.

A head-to-toe sequence is usually well accepted by school-aged children. Demonstrate how the instruments are used and let the child handle them if so desired. As you perform the examination, tell the child what you are doing and why. Offer as many choices as possible to help the child feel empowered. The examination is a good opportunity to teach the child about how the body works, such as letting the child listen to heart and breath sounds.

Adolescents

Protect the adolescent's modesty by providing a private place to undress and put on the patient gown, and then during the examination by covering the parts of the body not being assessed. Use the head-to-toe sequence and the same procedures used for adults. Perform the examination in private without parent or siblings unless the adolescent specifically requests the parent's presence. Provide a chaperone when the parent or accompanying adult is not present during the examination.

Adolescents often have concerns regarding their developing bodies. When appropriate provide reassurance about the normal progression of secondary sexual characteristic development and what further changes to expect.

GENERAL APPRAISAL

The examination begins when you first meet the child in any setting (Figure 8–3 ■). Observe the child's general appearance and behavior. The child should appear well nourished and well developed. Infants and young children are often fearful and seek reassurance from their parents. The child may resist interacting with you until rapport is established.

Observe the behavior and tone of voice used by the parent when he or she is talking to the child. Is the child encouraged to speak? Is the child appropriately reassured or supported by the parent? The child should feel secure with the parent and perceive permission to interact with the nurse.

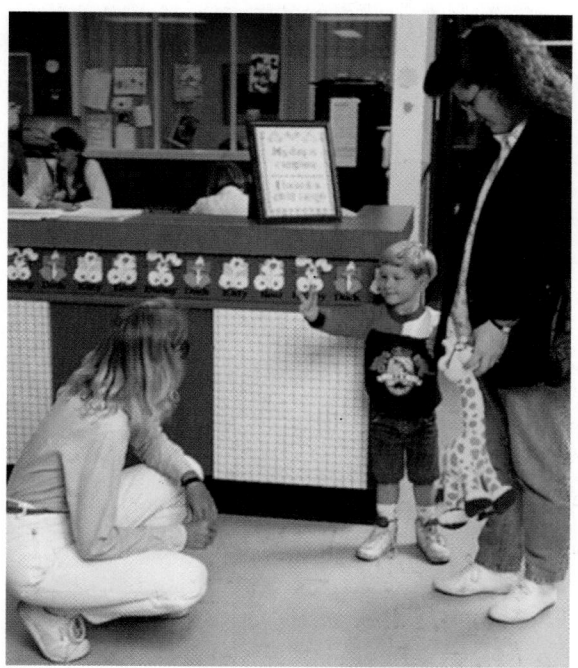

FIGURE 8–3 ■ Examination of the child begins from the first contact. You should be observing the behavior of the child and parent by using visual cues to make a proper assessment. Does the child appear well nourished? Does the child appear secure with the parent?

ANTHROPOMETRIC MEASUREMENTS

Measure the child's weight, length or height, and head circumference, if appropriate. The accurate assessment of growth and the plotting of growth measurements over time are important throughout childhood to assure health or to identify the impact of disease on the child. Accurate measurements are also important as medication dosage is calculated from weight (and sometimes height when the nomogram is used, see Appendix D∞). Growth charts for all ages of boys and girls are provided in Appendix A∞.

Infants and Toddlers

Length

The length measurement with the child in supine position is the standard for accurate assessment of growth in children under 2 years of age, even when they are able to stand independently. A calculation for difference in recumbent length and standing height measurements for children does exist. If height were plotted on a length-based growth chart, a true assessment of the child's growth over time could not be determined.

Use a measuring board and place the infant's head against the top of the board. Ask the parent or an assistant to hold the infant's head in the midline while you gently push down on the knees until the legs are straight. Position the heels of the feet on the footboard and record the length to the nearest 0.5 cm or 1/4 inch (Figure 8–4 ■). Repeat the measurement for accuracy. If a difference between the two readings is found take a third reading or average the readings for documentation. Plot the measurement for the child's age on the standardized growth curve. (Some facilities use a different type of measuring device.)

Weight

Infants are weighed on a platform scale (Figure 8–5 ■), either in a supine or sitting position, depending on their age. Take care to

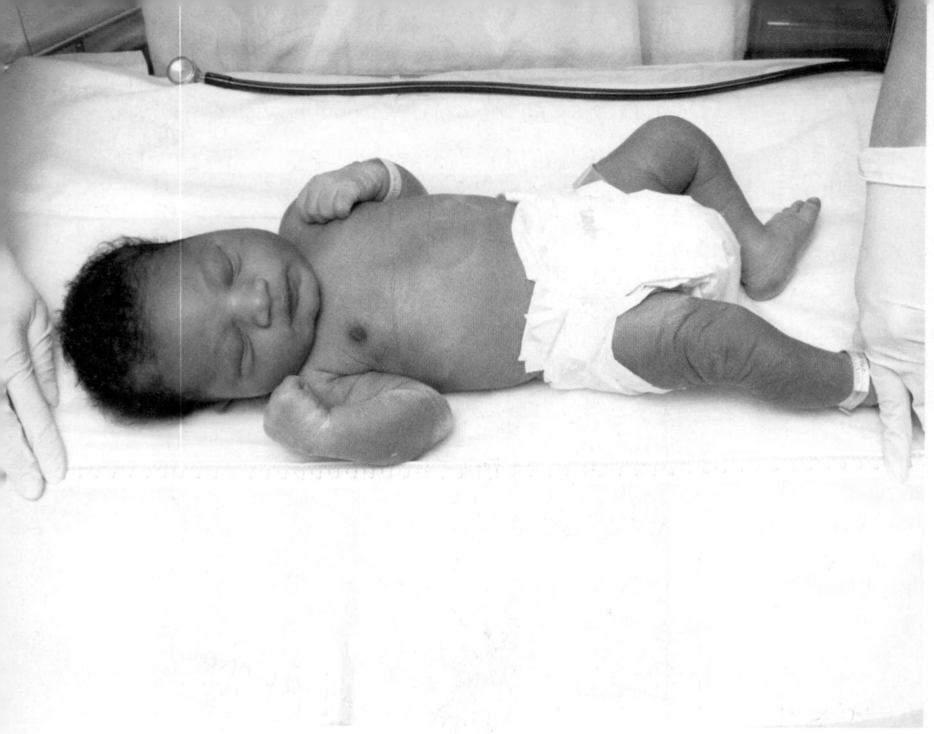

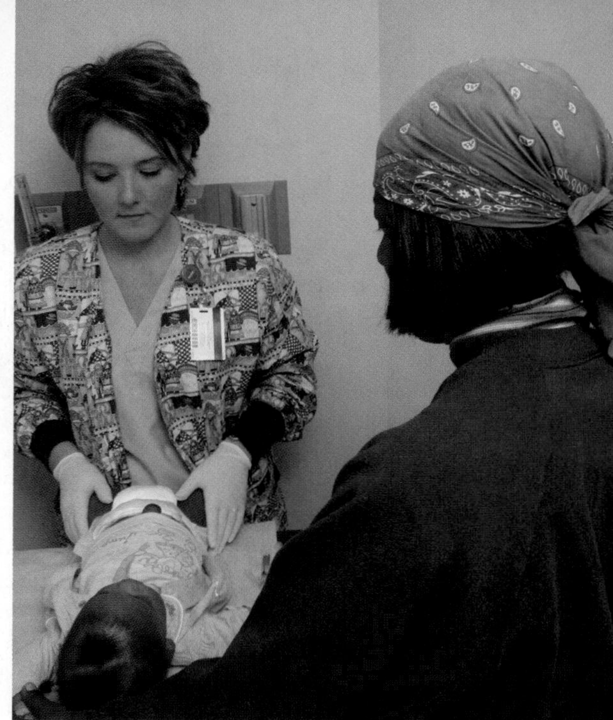

Keep the newborn warm during the examination. ***(left)***

Keep the parent close by when examining the infant. ***(right)***

PHOTOStory...

Assessment of the child at different ages

Developmental stages must be considered prior to assessment, as the needs of each child vary according to age and temperament.

The newborn is usually examined in the nursery on a warming table so that clothing may be removed. Maintaining the newborn's temperature is important during this early transition period.

The young infant is usually assessed on an examining table surface with the parent nearby. The infant does not resist examination procedures, and the parent can often assist by holding the arms or head when necessary.

Examine the toddler on the parent's lap. The child can be moved and positioned here to conduct a large majority of the examination. For example, when the child faces you, it is possible to interact with the child in an effort to reduce anxiety. The extremities can be examined, as well as the face and general body build of the child. Assessment of the eyes, nose, mouth, neck, heart, and lungs can take place in this position. The child can be positioned with the back or side to the examiner to allow auscultation of the posterior chest and head, and to inspect the ears. The toddler can also be positioned on the back across the parent's and examiner's legs so that the abdomen can be assessed.

The preschooler enjoys demonstrating skills and much of the musculoskeletal and neurologic examination can be conducted by requesting that the child perform specific actions. Asking the child to throw a ball, jump in place or hop, stand with arms out and eyes closed help make the child more eager to participate in the rest of the examination.

The school-age child is usually very cooperative when being assessed on the examining table. Explaining each step of the assessment helps the child know what is expected, such as taking a deep breath and holding it so the heart can be auscultated. The child still enjoys demonstrating certain abilities such as coordination of rapid alternating movements.

The adolescent is also very cooperative and appreciates knowing about each step in the assessment sequence. The adolescent is also interested in feedback about the assessment findings, particularly if pubertal changes are occurring as expected. The physical examination is an opportunity to teach about normal body changes and self-examination for breast or testicular masses. ■

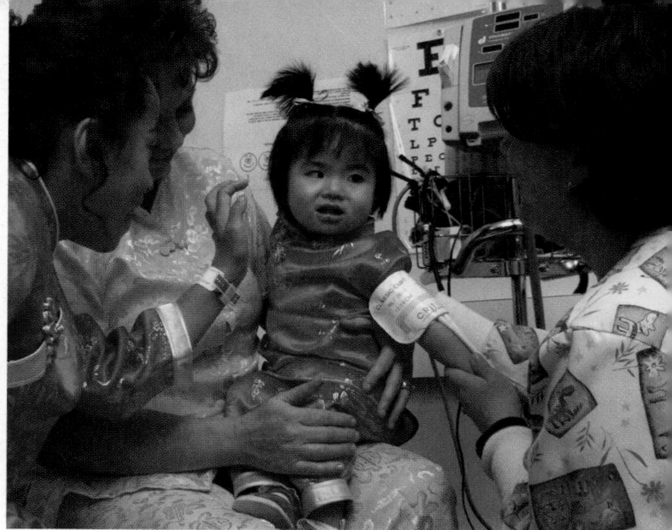

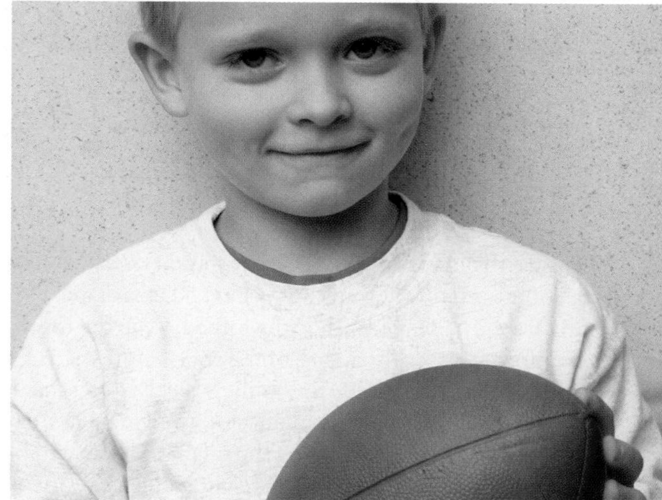

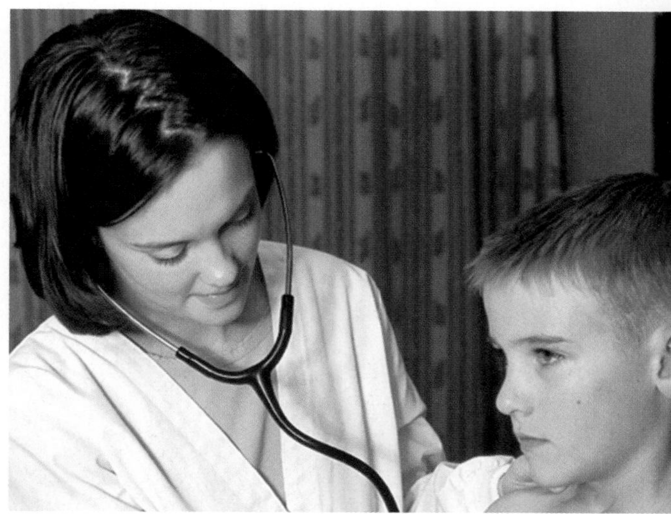

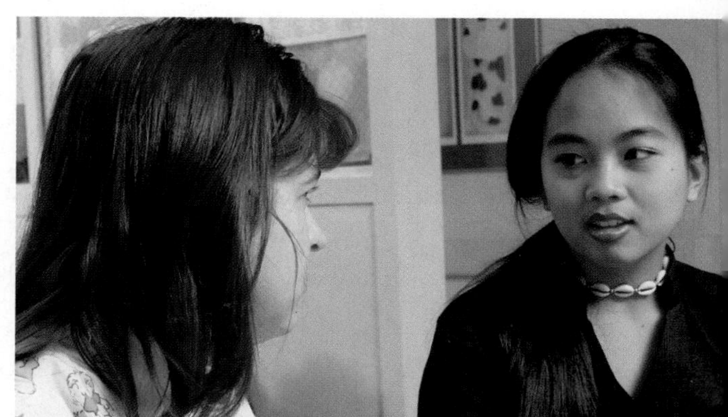

Examine the toddler on the parent's lap. ***(top)***

Preschoolers like to demonstrate skills, so use games to gain cooperation. ***(middle)***

School age children are receptive to directions about how they can help during the examination. ***(middle)***

Talk with the adolescent privately to learn about needs and concerns regarding health care. ***(bottom)***

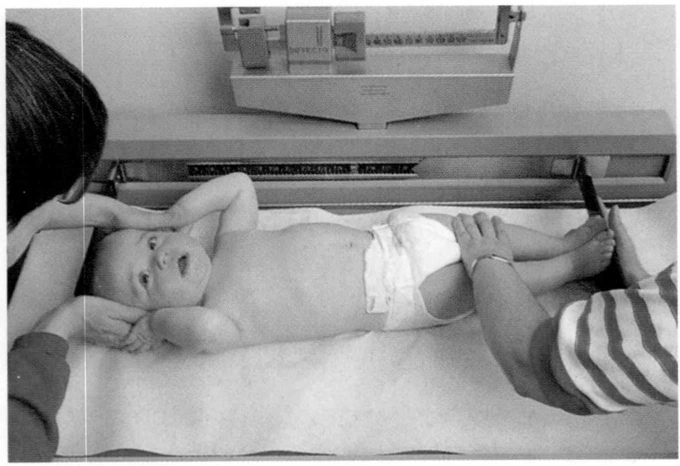

FIGURE 8–4 ■ Measuring infant length. Have an assistant hold the infant's head in the midline while you gently push down on the knees until the legs are straight. Position the heels of the feet on the footboard and record the length to the nearest 0.5 cm or 1/4 inch.

ensure the infant's safety. Ask the parent or assistant to remove all of the infant's clothing and diaper. Keep a diaper close at hand in case the baby voids while unclothed. Keep the room warm for comfort. Check the balance of the scale before placing the infant on it, and put a paper cover on the scale. Distract the infant, and take the reading when the infant stops moving. Place a hand close to the chest without touching the infant to be able to prevent the infant from falling. Record the weight in the nearest 10 g or 1/2 oz. Plot the measurement for the child's age on the standardized growth curve.

Head Circumference

Head circumference is measured at regular intervals until the child's second or third birthday because the brain is growing rapidly during this period and achieves 80% of adult size by age 2 years. Use a disposable paper tape, but take care to prevent the paper from cutting the infant. Wrap the tape around the head at the supraorbital prominence, above the ears, and around the occipital prominence, the point of largest circumference of the head (Figure 8–6 ■). The same position is used in newborns, although this may not be the largest circumference due to molding or swelling. Record the circumference in the nearest 0.5 cm or 1/8 inch. Repeat the measurement to confirm the reading. Plot the measurement for the child's age on the standardized growth curve.

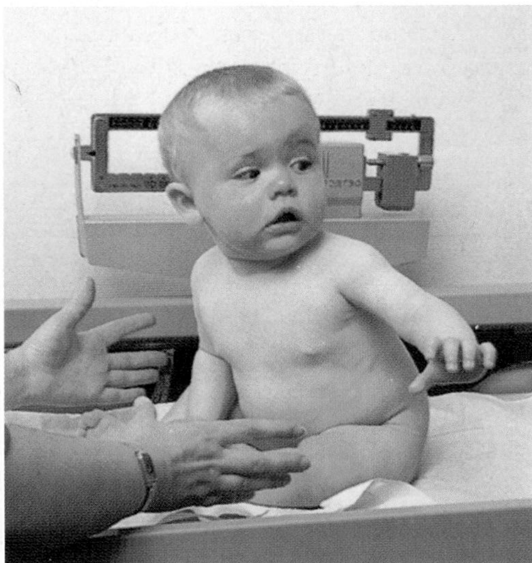

FIGURE 8–5 ■ Measuring infant weight. Place a hand close to the chest without touching the infant to be able to prevent the infant from falling. Record the weight in the nearest 10 g or 1/2 oz.

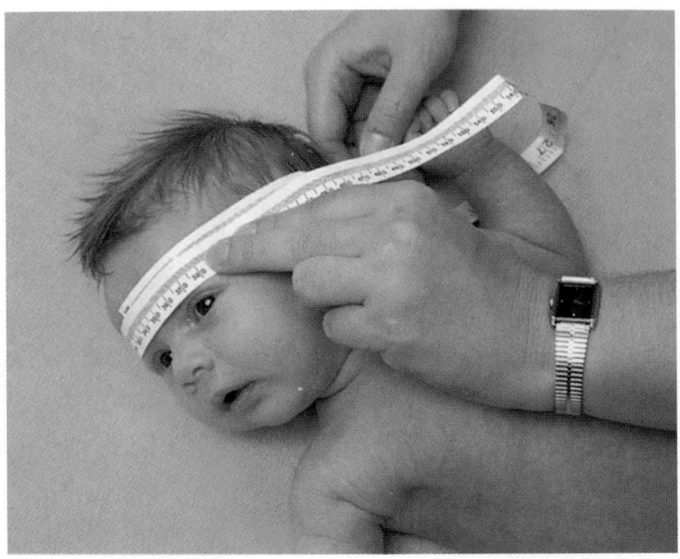

FIGURE 8–6 ■ Measuring head circumference. Wrap the tape around the head at the supraorbital prominence, above the ears, and around the occipital prominence, the point of largest circumference of the head.

Preschoolers and School-Age Children

Height

After the age of 2 to 3 years, a **stadiometer,** height measuring device attached to the wall, is used to improve the accuracy of the height measurement (Figure 8–7 ■). With shoes removed, have the child stand straight with the back to the wall. The head should be held erect and in the midline position. The shoulders, buttocks, and heels should touch the wall. The canthi of the eyes should be on the same horizontal plane as the stadiometer headpiece. Move the head piece down to touch the crown. Measure the height reading to the nearest 0.5 cm or 1/4 inch. Plot the measurement for the child's age on the standardized growth curve.

Weight

Measure the child's weight on a standing scale. Check the balance of the scale before use. Weigh young children in their underclothes. Weigh older children in their street clothes with heavy clothing and shoes removed. Record the weight to the nearest 0.1 kg or 1/4 lb. Provide privacy for the older child and adolescent. Plot the measurement for the child's age on the standardized growth curve.

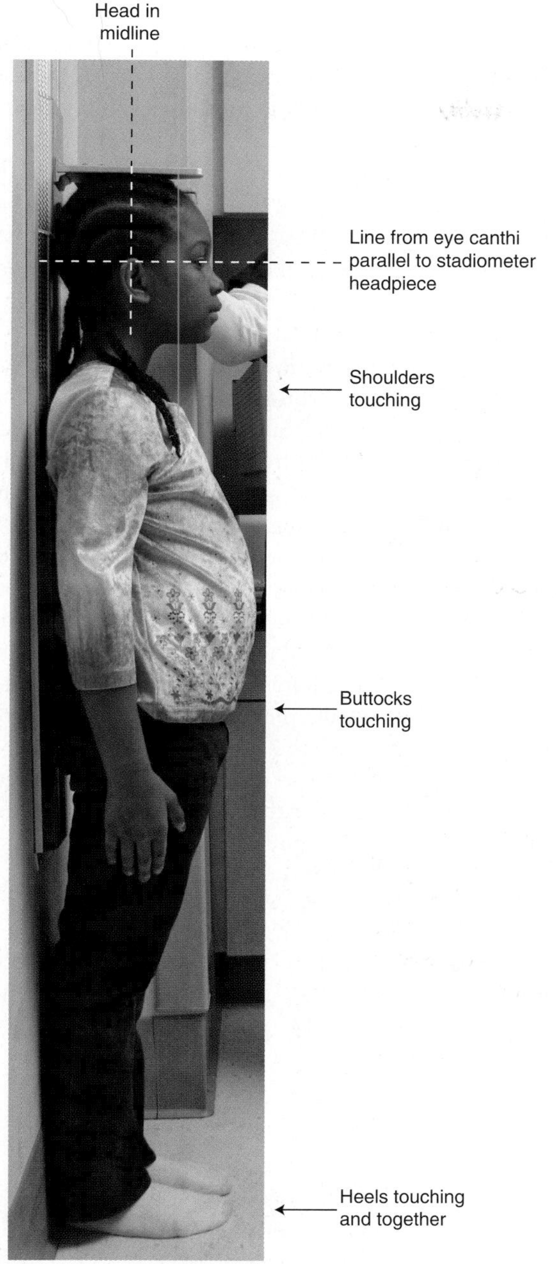

FIGURE 8–7 ■ Standing height measurements are taken routinely at each well-child visit to assess the child's rate of growth. Position the head in an erect and midline position while the shoulders, buttocks, and heels touch the wall. Move the head piece down to touch the crown. Measure the height reading to the nearest 0.5 cm or 1/4 inch.

Older Children and Adolescents

Height and Weight

Measure the height using a platform scale with an attached stature-measuring device. Have the child stand erect with the back to the scale. Move the stature-measuring device to the top of the head. Have the child step off the scale and read the height in centimeters or inches. Then measure the weight as described for school-age children.

Body Mass Index

The body mass index (BMI) is a formula used to assess total body fat and nutritional status. For children it helps determine if the child's height and weight are proportional. As children grow, their body fat changes, and differences also exist between boys and girls. Once the weight and height of children have been measured, the body mass index can be calculated and plotted on the growth curve. Interpretation of the BMI for children is as follows:

- BMI for age < 5th percentile—underweight
- BMI for age > 85th percentile—risk for overweight
- BMI for age > 95th percentile—overweight

The formula for calculation of the BMI is kilograms of weight divided by meters^2 of height. Be sure the weight measurement is in kilograms. Pounds can be converted to kilograms by dividing by 2.2. Next convert the height measurement to meters. Multiply the child's height in inches by 0.0254 (1 inch equals 0.0254 meter). If the child's height is in centimeters divide that number by 100. The height in meters is then squared. The BMI can now be calculated (Box 8–4). Alternatively you can go to the CDC website and enter the child's height and weight for an automatic calculation of the BMI. See Chapter 9 for a detailed discussion of BMI.

MediaLink BMI Calculator

Skinfold Thickness

Measurement of the skinfold thickness is a technique sometimes used to evaluate the nutritional status of adolescents and for children whose weight for stature is greater than 90th percentile. It is difficult to differentiate fat folds from lean muscle tissue in children. Follow guidelines for the use of skinfold thickness calipers and take the skinfold thickness measurement at middle of the upper arm over the triceps muscle (or alternatively the subscapular and abdominal areas). Repeat the measurement and use an average of the two readings. Compare the reading to the skinfold thickness curves for children, ages 2 to 18 years in Figure 8–8 ■. Approximately 50% of the body fat is present in the subcutaneous tissue layers, so there is a correlation between the triceps skinfold thickness and the body's fat content (Seidel, Ball, Dains, et al., 2003).

ASSESSING SKIN AND HAIR CHARACTERISTICS AND INTEGRITY

What is indicated when the child's skin is not uniform in color or when it feels spongy to the touch? What are each of the primary

BOX 8–4 Calculating Body Mass Index

Example: A 2 year-old boy weighs 26.5 lb. When divided by 2.2, the weight equals 12 kg. The child's height is 34.5 in. When multiplied by 0.0254, the height equals 0.8763 m. Next 0.8763 is squared equaling 0.7679. To calculate the BMI, 12 kg is divided by 0.7679 to equal 15.63. This measurement can be plotted on the standardized growth charts for age and sex to interpret the BMI. The BMI for this boy falls between the 10th and 25th percentiles.

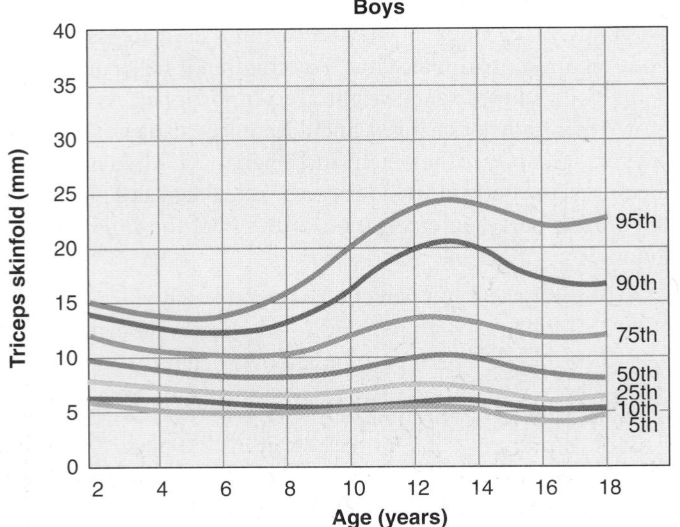

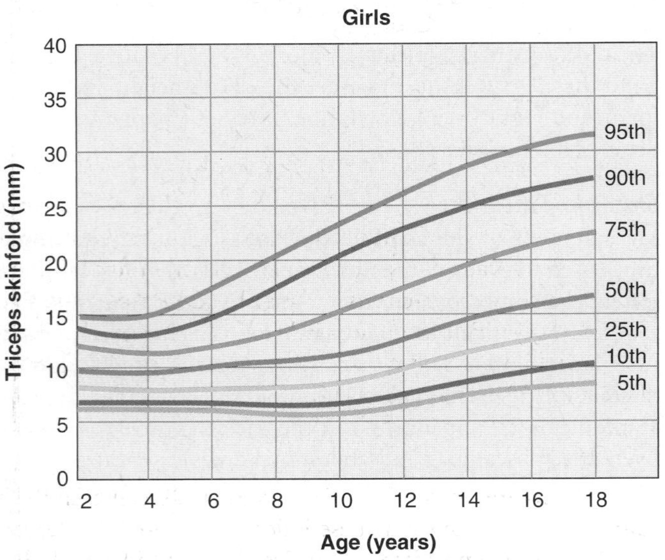

FIGURE 8–8 ■ Skinfold thickness percentiles for children age 2 to 18 years, boys and girls.

Redrawn From: Seidel, H. M., Ball, J. W., Dains, J. E., & Benedict, G. W. (2003). Mosby's Guide to Physical Examination, (5th ed., p. 120, Fig. 5–17). St. Louis: Mosby.

skin lesions called, and what characteristics are used to describe each of them? How can cyanosis and jaundice be detected in children of darker skin? Why is skin turgor assessed? How is the presence of head lice identified in a child?

Examination of the skin requires good lighting to detect variations in skin color and to identify lesions. Natural daylight is preferred when available. Rather than inspecting the entire skin surface of the child at one time, examine the skin simultaneously with other body systems as each region of the body is exposed.

Inspection of the Skin

The child's skin is inspected for color and the presence of imperfections, elevations, variations, or lesions.

Skin Color

The color of the child's skin usually has an even distribution. The skin is inspected for color variations—such as increased or decreased pigmentation, pallor, mottling, bruises, erythema, cyanosis, or jaundice—that may be associated with local or generalized conditions. The palms of the hands and soles of the feet are often lighter than the rest of the skin surface in darker skinned children. In addition, their lips may appear slightly bluish. Some variations in skin color are common and normal, such as freckles found in the white population and Mongolian spots found on infants with dark skin (Figure 8–9 ■).

Bruises are common on the knees, shins, and lower arms as children stumble and fall. Bruises on other parts of the body, especially in various stages of healing, should raise a suspicion of child abuse. Bruises often go through various skin color changes as the body resorbs the blood over several days. The transition of color often progresses through reddish blue, brownish blue, brownish green, greenish yellow, and yellow-brown before returning to normal skin color. Note any tattoos or body piercings.

When a skin color abnormality is suspected, the buccal mucosa and tongue should be inspected to confirm the color change. This is especially important in children of darker skin because the mucous membranes are usually pink, regardless of skin color. The gums are pressed lightly for 1 to 2 seconds. Any residual color, such as jaundice or cyanosis, is more easily detected in blanched skin. Jaundice may also be noticed in the sclerae of the eyes. Generalized cyanosis is associated with respiratory and cardiac disorders. Jaundice is associated with liver disorders. Infants who eat at lot of yellow vegetables may have a yellow or orange tint to the skin.

Palpation of the Skin

Palpation of the skin provides a sense of its characteristics: temperature, texture, moistness, and resilience or turgor. To

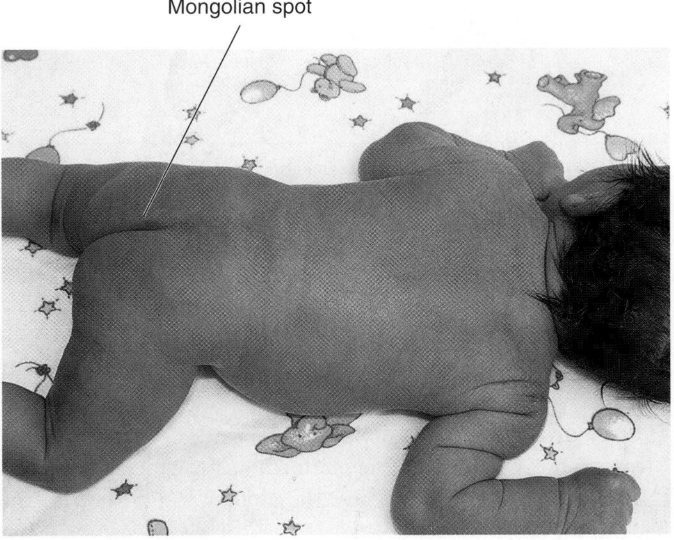

FIGURE 8–9 ■ Mongolian spots are large patches of bluish skin often seen on the buttocks. They are a normal occurrence in dark-skinned infants, but are sometimes incorrectly thought to be bruises.

evaluate these characteristics, the nurse lightly touches or strokes the skin surface. The nurse follows standard precautions by wearing gloves when palpating mucous membranes, open wounds, and lesions.

Temperature

The child's skin normally feels cool to the touch. A general evaluation of skin temperature can be obtained by placing the wrist or dorsum of the hand against the child's skin. Excessively warm skin may indicate the presence of fever or inflammation, whereas abnormally cool skin may be a sign of shock or cold exposure.

Texture

Children have soft, smooth skin over the entire body. Any areas of roughness, thickening, or induration (area of extra firmness with a distinct border) should be identified. Abnormalities in texture are associated with endocrine disorders, chronic irritation, and inflammation.

Moistness

The child's skin is normally dry to the touch. The skin may feel slightly damp when the child has been exercising or crying. Excessive sweating without exertion is associated with a fever or with an uncorrected congenital heart defect.

Resilience (Turgor)

The child's skin is taut, elastic, and mobile because of the balanced distribution of intracellular and extracellular fluids. To evaluate skin turgor, the examiner pinches a small amount of skin on the abdomen between the thumb and forefinger, releases the skin, and watches the speed of recoil (Figure 8–10 ■). If the skin rapidly returns to its previous contour, good skin turgor is indicated. When poor skin turgor is present, the skin tents or stands up rather than rapidly resuming its previous contour. Poor skin turgor is commonly associated with dehydration.

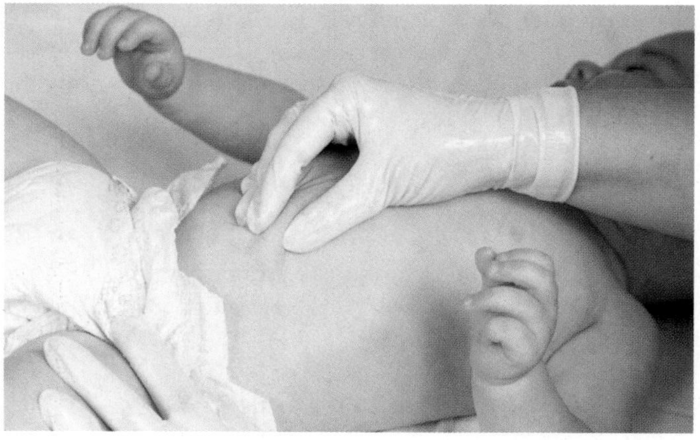

FIGURE 8–10 ■ Testing skin turgor. Tenting of the skin is associated with poor skin turgor. Pinch a small amount of skin on the abdomen between the thumb and forefinger. Release the skin, and watch the speed of recoil. Skin with normal turgor will quickly return to a flat position.

PRACTICE ALERT

The degree of dehydration, or weight loss caused by dehydration, can be estimated from the time it takes tented skin to return to its natural contour (Seidel et al., 2003).

Weight Loss	Time to Return from Tenting to Normal Contour
<5%	<2 seconds
5–8%	2–3 seconds
8–10%	3–4 seconds
>10%	>4 seconds

If edema, an accumulation of excess fluid in the interstitial spaces, is present, the skin feels doughy or boggy. To test for the degree of edema present, the examiner presses for 5 seconds against a bone beneath the area of puffy skin, releases the pressure, and observes how rapidly the indentation disappears. If the indentation disappears rapidly, the edema is "nonpitting." Slow disappearance of the indentation indicates "pitting" edema, which is commonly associated with kidney or heart disorders.

Capillary Refill and Small-Vein Filling Times

Two techniques are used to determine the adequacy of tissue perfusion (oxygen circulating to the tissues). When tissue perfusion is inadequate, immediately assess the child for shock or a physical constriction such as a cast or bandage that is too tight. The capillary refill time is normally less than 2 seconds (Figures 8–11A and B ■). The small-vein filling time is normally less than 4 seconds (Figures 8–11C and D ■).

Skin Lesions

Skin lesions are usually an indication of an abnormal skin condition. Characteristics of these lesions—location, size, type of lesion, pattern, and discharge, if present—provide clues about the cause of the condition. Inspect and palpate the isolated or generalized skin color abnormalities, elevations, lesions, or injuries to describe all characteristics present. See Chapter 36∞ for the characteristics of some common lesions.

Primary lesions (such as macules, papules, and vesicles) are often the skin's initial response to injury or infection. Mongolian spots and freckles are normal findings also classified as primary lesions. Primary lesions may appear in certain configurations or shapes that can help distinguish between lesions.

- Linear—occur in a line, e.g., poison ivy
- Annular—ring shaped with a central clearing, e.g., ringworm (When annular lesions run together they are polycyclic.)
- Archiform—semicircular, e.g., erythema multiforme
- Herpetiform—grouped lesions, e.g., herpes, chickenpox
- Reticulated—networked or interlaced, parvovirus B19
- Gyrate—twisted, spiral, coiled

Secondary lesions (such as scars, ulcers, fissures) are the result of irritation, infection, and delayed healing of primary lesions

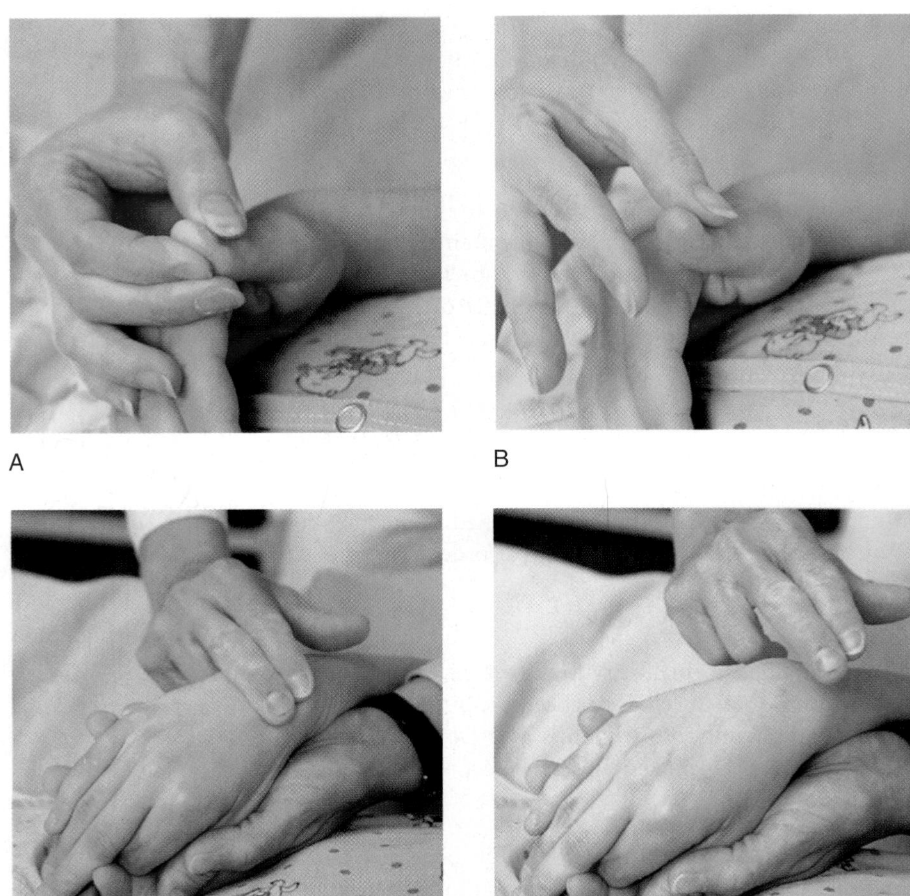

FIGURE 8–11 ■ Capillary refill technique: *A*, Pinch the end of a finger until the skin is blanched. *B*, Quickly release the finger and watch the blood return to the veins. Count the seconds it takes for the color to return or veins to fill. Slow color return or vein filling time could be related to shock or constriction due to a tight bandage or cast.

Small-vein filling time technique: *C*, Using the index finger, milk a vein on the dorsum of the hand or foot from proximal to distal. *D*, Release your pressure and color should return promptly.

(see Table 36–1∞). Figure 8–12 ■ describes common primary lesions.

Inspection of the Hair

Inspect the scalp hair for color, distribution, and cleanliness. The hair shafts should be evenly colored, shiny, and either curly or straight. Variation in hair color not caused by bleaching can be associated with a nutritional deficiency. Normally, hair is distributed evenly over the scalp. Investigate areas of hair loss. Hair loss in a child may result from tight braids or skin lesions such as ringworm (see Figure 36–11A)∞. Notice any unusual hair growth patterns. An unusually low hairline on the neck or forehead may be associated with a congenital disorder such as hypothyroidism.

Children are frequently exposed to head lice. Inspect the individual hair shafts for small nits (lice eggs) that adhere to the hair (Figures 8–13A and B ■). None should be present.

Observe the distribution of body hair as other skin surfaces are exposed during examination. Fine hair covers most areas of the body. The presence of body hair in unexpected places should be noted. For example, a tuft of hair at the base of the spine often indicates a spinal defect.

Pubic hair begins to develop in children between 8 and 12 years of age, and axillary hair develops about 6 months later. Facial hair is noted in boys shortly after axillary hair develops. Note the age at which pubic and axillary hair develops in the child. Development at an unusually young age is associated with precocious puberty.

Palpation of the Hair

Palpate the hair shafts for texture. Hair should feel soft or silky with fine or thick shafts. Endocrine conditions such as hypothyroidism may result in coarse, brittle hair. Part the hair in various spots over the head to inspect and palpate the scalp for crusting or other lesions. If lesions are present, describe them using the characteristics in Figure 8–12.

ASSESSING THE HEAD FOR SKULL CHARACTERISTICS AND FACIAL FEATURES

What can cause a child's head or face to be asymmetric? How does a normal fontanel feel? What does an unusually large or small head suggest in an infant?

Inspection of the Head and Face

Head

During early childhood, the skull's sutures permit expansion for brain growth. Infants and young children normally have a rounded skull with a prominent occipital area. See Figure 8–14 ■. The shape of the head changes during childhood, and the occip-

PATHOPHYSIOLOGY ILLUSTRATED

Common Primary Skin Lesions and Associated Conditions

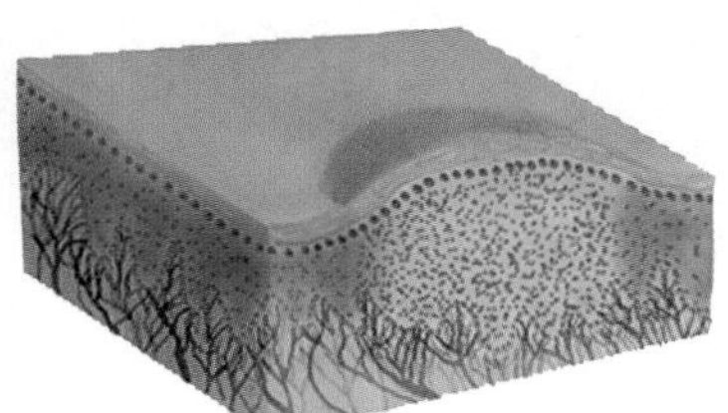

Lesion Name: Papule
Description: Elevated, firm, diameter <1 cm (1/2 in.)
Example: Warts, pigmented nevi

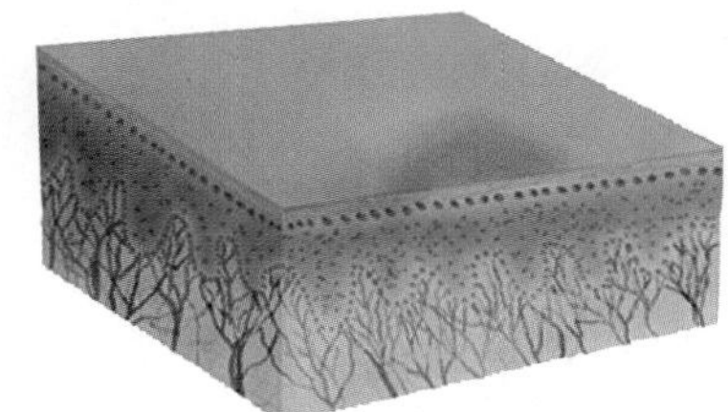

Lesion Name: Macule
Description: Flat, nonpalpable, diameter <1 cm (1/2 in.)
Example: Freckle, rubella, rubeola, petechiae

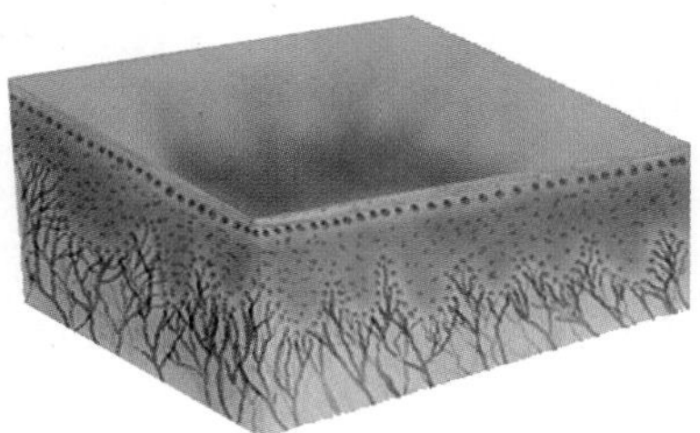

Lesion Name: Patch
Description: Macule diameter >1 cm (1/2 in.)
Example: Vitiligo, Mongolian spot

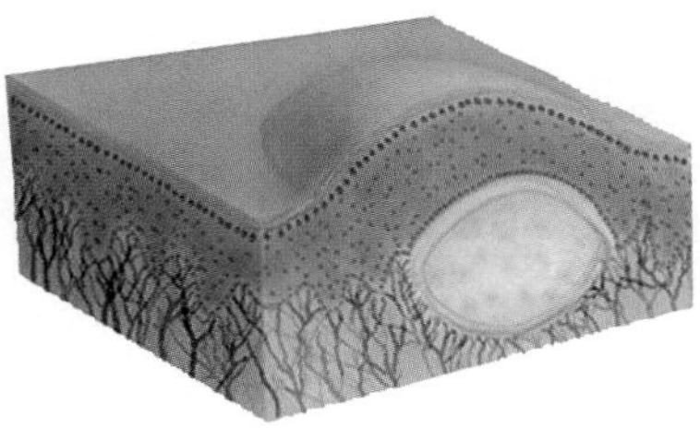

Lesion Name: Nodule
Description: Elevated, firm, deeper in dermis than papule, diameter 1–2 cm (1/2 in.-1 in.)
Example: Erythema nodosum

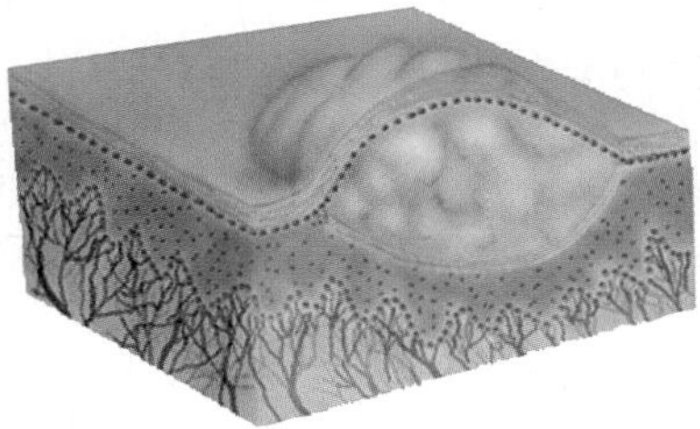

Lesion Name: Tumor
Description: Elevated, solid, diameter >2 cm (1 in.)
Example: Neoplasm, hemangioma

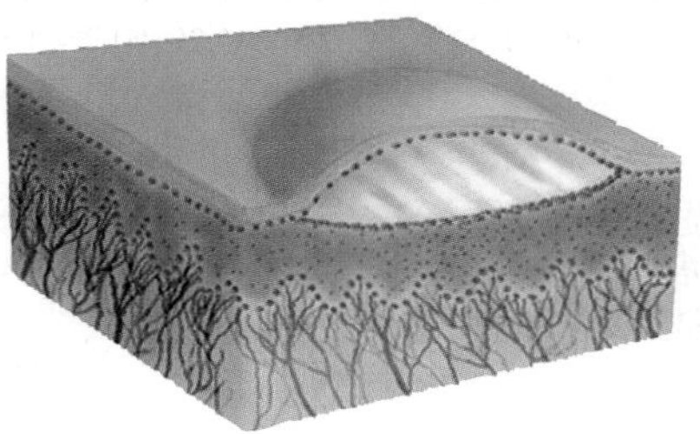

Lesion Name: Vesicle
Description: Elevated, filled with fluid, diameter <1 cm (1/2 in.)
Example: Early chickenpox, herpes simplex

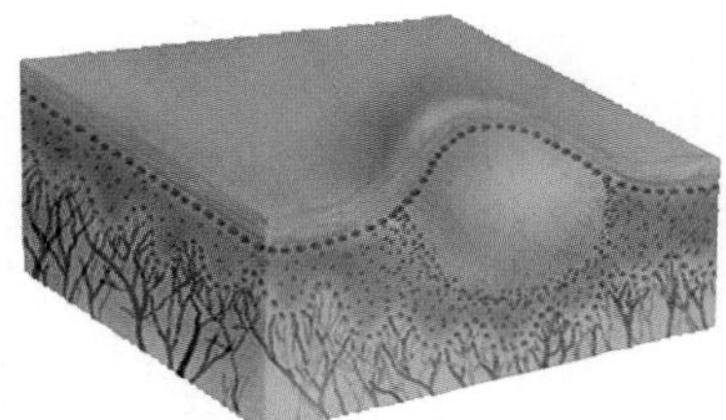

Lesion Name: Pustule
Description: Vesicle filled with purulent fluid
Example: Impetigo, acne

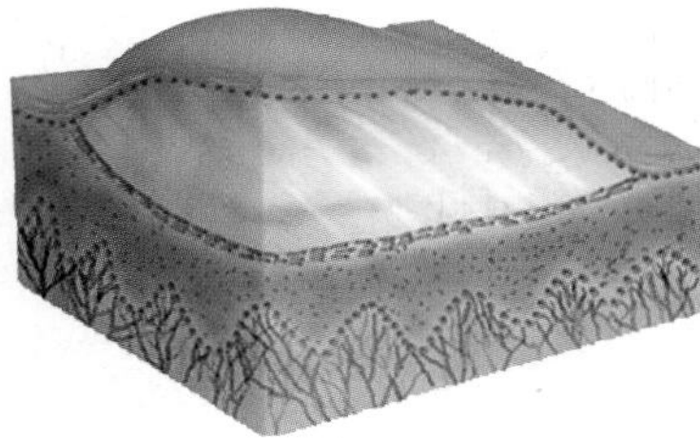

Lesion Name: Bulla
Description: Vesicle diameter >1 cm (1/2 in.)
Example: Burn blister

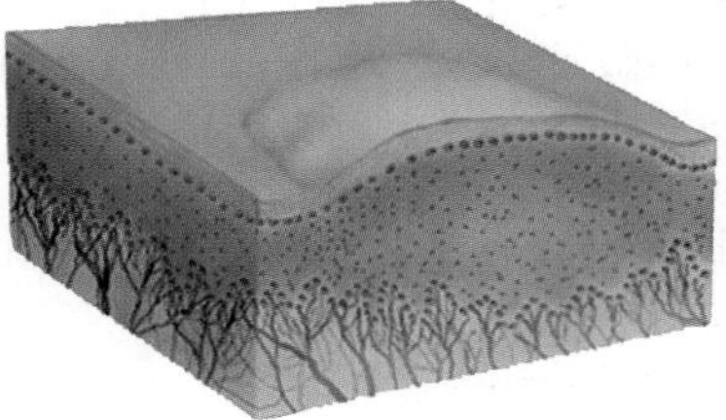

Lesion Name: Wheal
Description: Irregular elevated solid area of edematous skin
Example: Urticaria, insect bite

FIGURE 8–12 ■ Skin lesions usually indicate abnormal skin conditions. Identifying characteristics of these lesions can provide clues about the cause of the condition.

ital area becomes less prominent. An abnormal skull shape can result from premature closure of the sutures. Children who were low-birth-weight infants often have a flat, elongated skull because the soft skull bones were flattened by the weight of the head early in infancy. Head flattening is also associated with the side and back-lying positions in infants.

The head circumference of infants and young children is routinely measured until 2 to 3 years of age to ensure that adequate

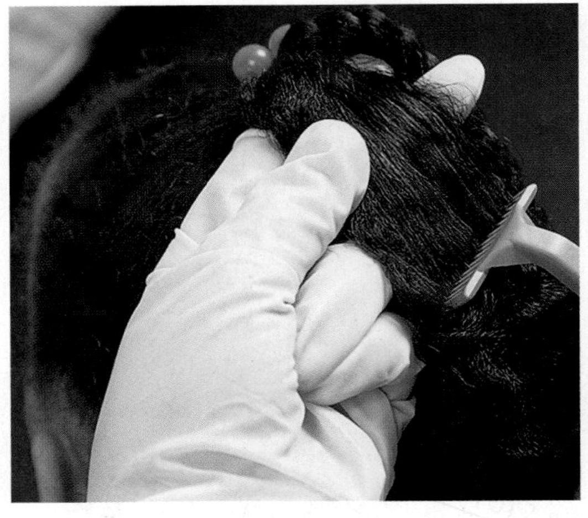

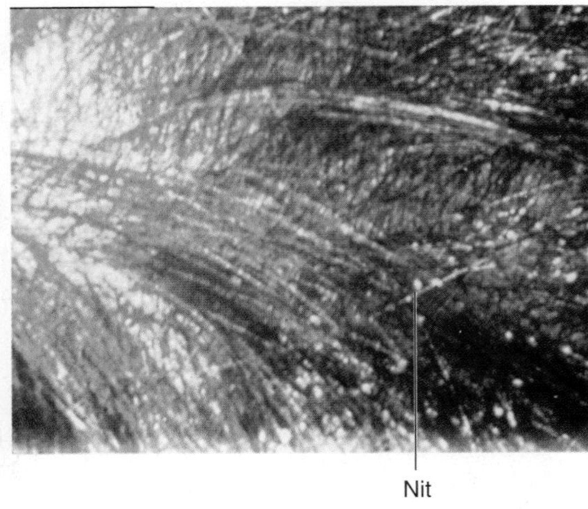

FIGURE 8–13 ■ *A*, Inspecting for head lice with a fine-tooth comb. *B*, Nits in the hair.
Courtesy of Centers for Disease Control

growth for brain development has occurred. A larger than normal head is associated with hydrocephalus, and a smaller than normal head suggests microcephaly.

Face

Inspect the child's face for symmetry during several facial expressions such as resting, smiling, talking, and crying (Figure 8–15 ■). Draw an imaginary line down the middle of the face over the nose and compare the features on each side. Significant asymmetry may result from paralysis of trigeminal or facial nerves (cranial nerves V or VII), in utero positioning, and swelling from infection, allergy, or trauma.

Next inspect the face for unusual facial features such as coarseness, wide eye spacing, or disproportionate size. Tremors, tics, and twitching of facial muscles are often associated with seizures.

Palpation of the Skull

Palpate the skull in infants and young children to assess the sutures and fontanels and to detect soft bones (Figure 8–16 ■). (See Developing Cultural Competence: Touching the Head.)

Sutures

Use your fingerpads to palpate each suture line. The edge of each bone in the suture line is felt, but normally there is no separation of the two bones. If additional bone edges are felt, it may indicate a skull fracture.

Fontanels

At the intersection of the sutures, palpate the anterior and posterior fontanels. The fontanel should feel flat and firm inside the bony edges. The anterior fontanel is normally

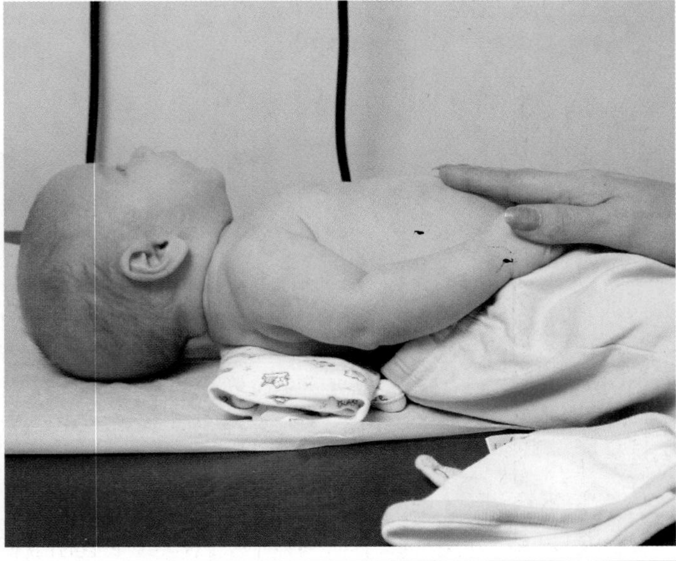

FIGURE 8–14 ■ Note the profile of the infant's head. The occipital area is prominent.

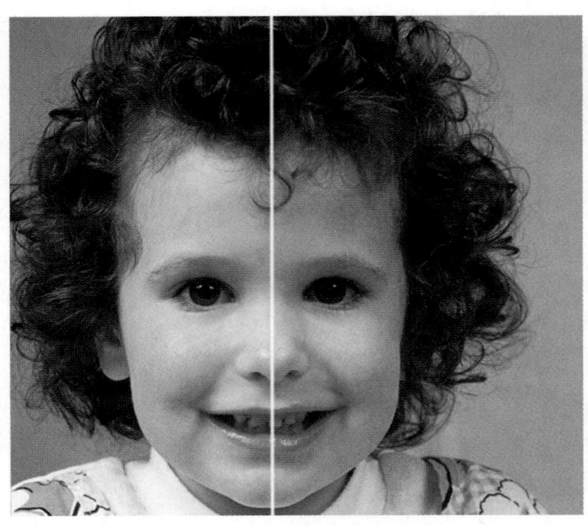

FIGURE 8–15 ■ Draw an imaginary line down the middle of the face over the nose and compare the features on each side. Significant asymmetry may be caused by paralysis of cranial nerve V or VII, in utero positioning, or swelling from infection, allergy, or trauma.

AS THEY GROW

Sutures and Fontanels of the Skull

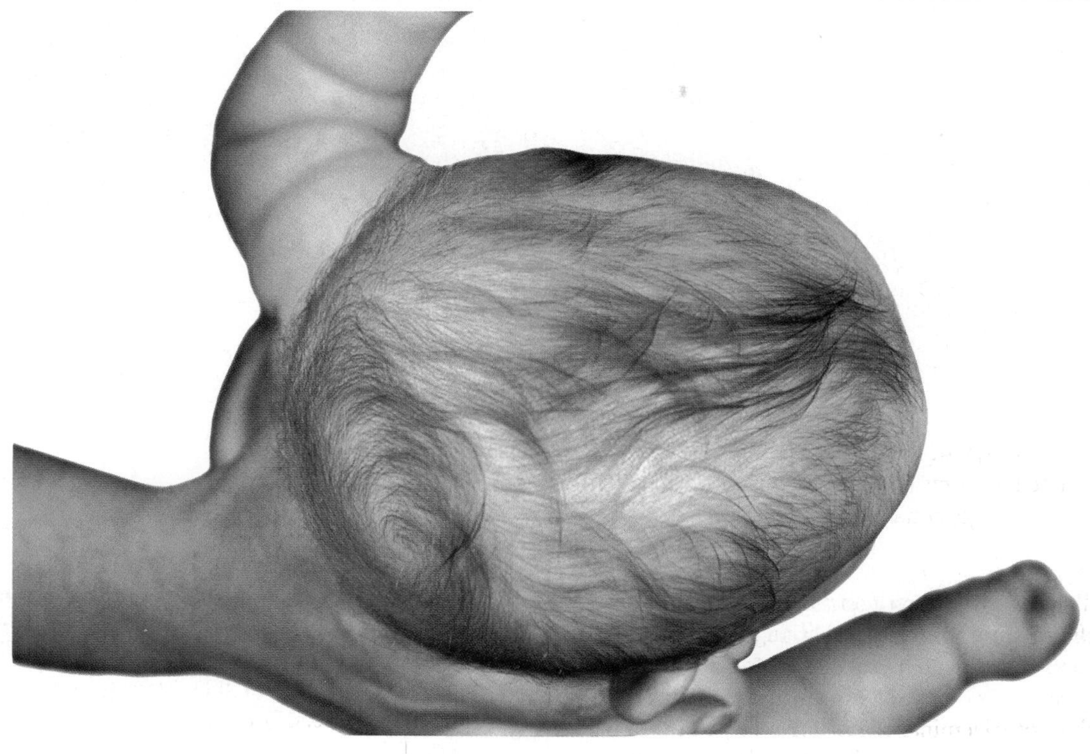

FIGURE 8–16 ■ The sutures are separations between the bones of the skull that have not yet joined. The fontanels are formed at the intersection of these sutures where bone has not yet formed. Fontanels are covered by tough membranous tissue that protects the brain. The posterior fontanel closes between 2 and 3 months. The anterior fontanel and sutures are palpable up to the age of 18 months. The suture lines of the skull are seldom palpated after 2 years of age. After that time, the sutures rarely separate.

diamond shaped and smaller than 5 cm (2 in.) in diameter at 6 months of age and then becomes progressively smaller. It closes between 12 and 18 months of age. The posterior fontanel closes between 2 and 3 months of age. The suture lines of the skull are seldom palpated after 2 years of age. After that time the sutures rarely split.

A tense fontanel, bulging above the margin of the skull, is an indication of increased intracranial pressure. If you suspect that the fontanel is tense, palpate when the child is quietly sitting to determine if the brain tissues bulge above the skull opening and feel tense. A soft fontanel, sunken below the margin of the skull with prominent margins of the skull, is associated with dehydration.

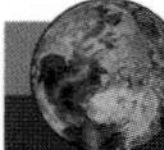

DEVELOPING CULTURAL COMPETENCE

Touching the Head

The head is a sacred part of the body to some Southeast Asians. Ask for permission before touching the infant's head to palpate the sutures and fontanels (Spector, 2000). When a Hispanic child is examined, however, not touching the head is considered bad luck by many families.

ASSESSING EYE STRUCTURES, FUNCTION, AND VISION

What is one of the most common eye problems that occurs during childhood? What do bulging or sunken eyeballs look like? What is the red reflex and what does it indicate? How is eye muscle balance tested? Is it normal for a child's visual acuity to be different at certain ages?

Inspection of the External Eye Structures

The function of the external and internal eye structures and related cranial nerves makes vision possible. The external eye structures, including the eyeballs, eyelids, and eye muscles, are inspected. The function of cranial nerves II, III, IV, and VI, which innervate the eye structures, is also tested (Figure 8–17 ■). Equipment needed for this examination includes an ophthalmoscope, vision chart, penlight, small toy, and an index card or paper cup.

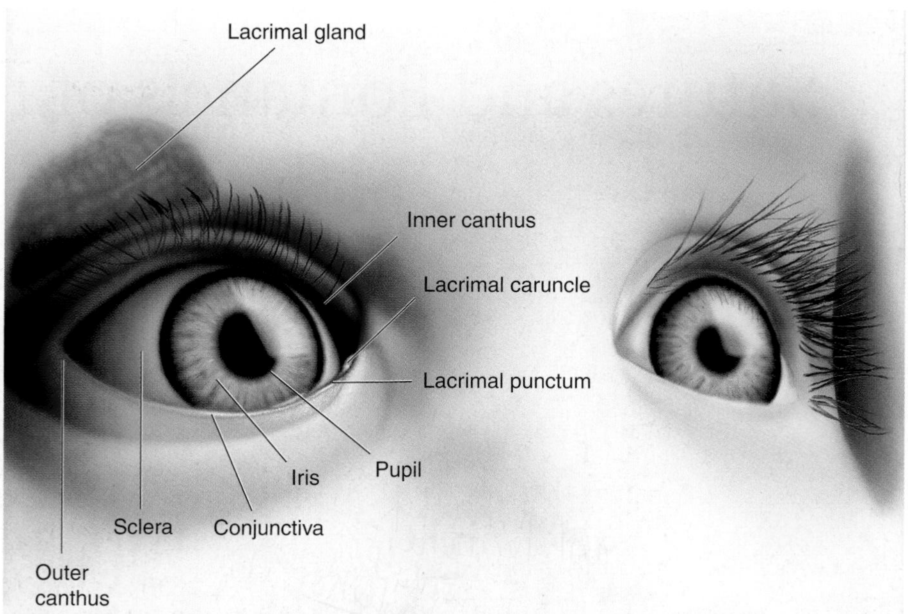

FIGURE 8–17 ■ External structures of the eye. Notice that the light reflex is at the same location on each eye.

Eye Size and Spacing

Inspect the eyes and surrounding tissues simultaneously when examining facial features. The eyes should be the same size but not unusually large or small. Observe for eye bulging, which can be identified by retracted eyelids or a sunken appearance. Bulging may be associated with a tumor, and a sunken appearance may reflect dehydration. Note the characteristics of the eyebrows.

Next inspect the eyes to see if they are appropriately distanced from each other. **Hypertelorism,** or widely spaced eyes, is associated with mental retardation, but it can be a normal variation in children.

Eyelids and Eyelashes

Inspect the eyelids for color, size, position, mobility, and condition of the eyelashes. Eyelids should be the same color as surrounding facial skin and free of swelling or inflammation along the edges. Sebaceous glands that look like yellow striations are often present near the hair follicles. Eyelashes curl away from the eye to prevent irritation of the conjunctivae.

Inspect the conjunctivae lining the eyelids by pulling down the lower lid and then everting the upper lid. The conjunctivae should be pink and glossy. The lacrimal punctum, the opening for the lacrimal gland on each lid, is located near the medial canthus. No redness or excess tearing should be present.

When the eyes are open, inspect the level at which the upper and lower lids cross the eye. Each lid normally covers part of the iris but not any portion of the pupil. The lids should also close completely over the iris and cornea. Ptosis, drooping of the lid over the pupil, is often associated with injury to the oculomotor nerve, cranial nerve III. Sunset sign, in which the sclera is seen between the upper lid and the iris, may indicate retracted eyelids or hydrocephalus.

Inspect the eyes for the palpebral slant (Figure 8–18 ■). The eyelids of most people open horizontally. An upward or Mongolian slant is a normal finding in Asian children; however, children with Down syndrome also often have a Mongolian slant (Figure 8–19 ■). A downward or anti-Mongolian slant is seen in some children as a normal variation. Children of Asian descent often have an extra fold of skin, known as the epicanthal fold, covering all or part of the medial canthus of the eye.

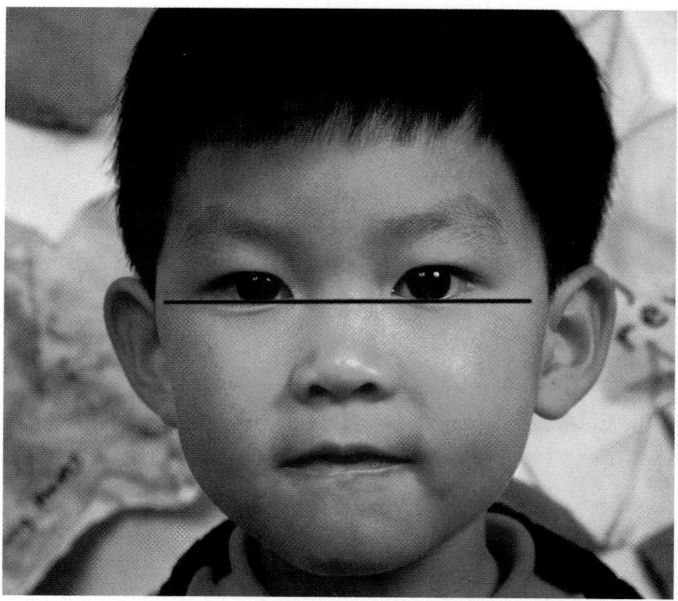

FIGURE 8–18 ■ Draw an imaginary line across the medial canthi and extend it to each side of the face to identify the slant of the palpebral fissures. When the line crosses the lateral canthi, the palpebral fissures are horizontal and no slant is present. When the lateral canthi fall above the imaginary line, the eyes have an upward or Mongolian slant. A downward or anti-Mongolian slant is present when the lateral canthi fall below the imaginary line. Epicanthal folds are present when an extra fold of skin partially or completely covers the caruncles in the medial canthi. What type of slant does this child have? Are epicanthal folds present?

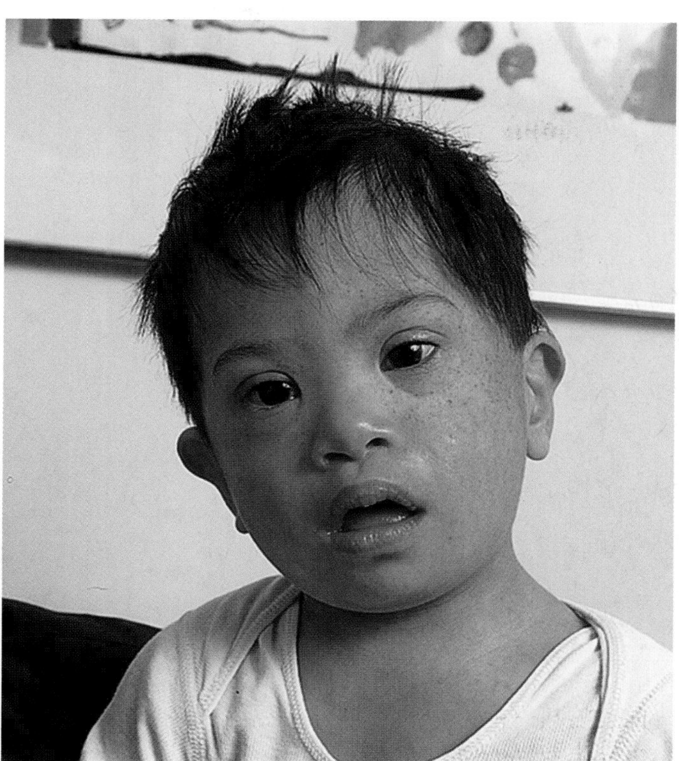

FIGURE 8–19 ■ The eyes of this boy with Down syndrome show a Mongolian slant.

Eye Color

Inspect the color of each sclera, iris, and bulbar conjunctiva. The sclera is normally white or ivory in children with darker skin. Sclerae of another color suggest the presence of an underlying disease. For example, yellow sclerae indicate jaundice. An excessive blue tinge to the sclerae may be associated with some types of osteogenesis imperfecta. Typically the iris is blue or light colored at birth and becomes pigmented within 6 months. Inspect the iris for the presence of Brushfield spots, white specks in a linear pattern around the iris circumference, which are often associated with Down syndrome. The bulbar conjunctivae, which cover the sclera to the edge of the cornea, are normally clear. Redness can indicate eyestrain, infection, allergies, or irritation.

Pupils

Inspect the pupils for size and shape. Normally the pupils are round, clear, and equal in size. Some children have a **coloboma,** a keyhole-shaped pupil caused by a notch in the iris. The presence of this sign can indicate that the child has other congenital anomalies.

To test the pupillary response to light, shine a bright light into one eye. A brisk constriction of both the pupil exposed to direct light and the other pupil is a normal finding.

To test pupillary response to accommodation, ask the child to look first at a near object (for example, a toy) and then at a distant object (for example, a picture on the wall). The expected response is pupil constriction with near objects and pupil dilation with distant objects. This procedure tests the optic nerve, cranial nerve II. See Box 8–5.

BOX 8–5 Positioning Infants for the Eye Assessment

Some infants resist having their eyes examined by keeping them closed. Often they will open their eyes if held in an upright position over the parent's shoulder. The examiner can then walk around behind the parent and use the ophthalmoscope as a penlight to assess pupil size, shape, and responsiveness to light as well as the corneal light reflex. Then the ophthalmoscope can be used to assess the red reflex.

Inspection of the Eye Muscles

A common pediatric eye disorder is *strabismus*, or crossed eyes. This condition is important to detect because, if uncorrected, it can cause vision impairment. Several tests are used to detect the presence of a muscle imbalance that can result in strabismus. These tests include the evaluation of extraocular movements, the corneal light reflex, and the cover–uncover test.

Extraocular Movements

For children of 3 years or older, seat the child at your eye level to evaluate the extraocular movements to detect a muscle imbalance or **strabismus.** Hold a toy or penlight 30 cm (12 in.) from the child's eyes and move it through the six cardinal fields of gaze illustrated in Figure 8–20 ■. You may need to hold the young child's head still until fine motor eye movement develops. Both eyes should move together, tracking the object in all directions. This procedure tests the oculomotor, trochlear, and abducens nerves (cranial nerves III, IV, and VI).

Corneal Light Reflex

To test the corneal light reflex, shine a light on the infant's or child's nose, midway between the eyes. Identify the location

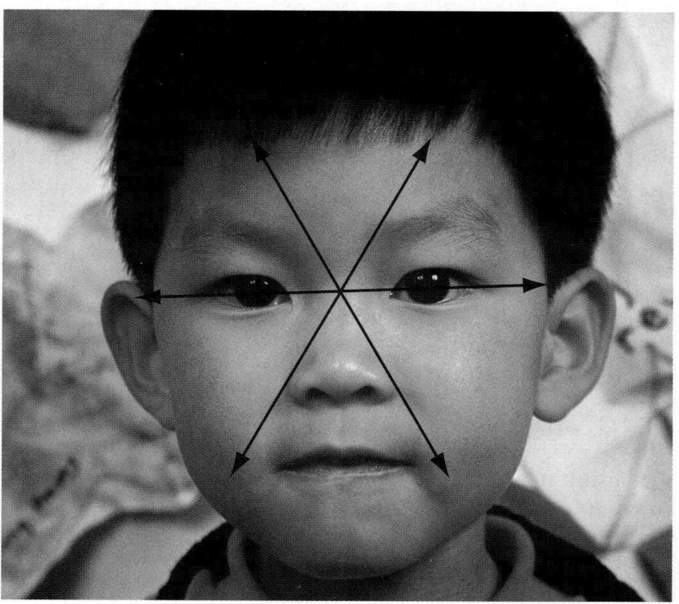

FIGURE 8–20 ■ Inspection of the extraocular movements. Have the child sit at your eye level. Hold a toy or penlight about 30 cm (12 in.) from the child's eyes and move it in all six directions indicated. Both eyes should move together, tracking the object.

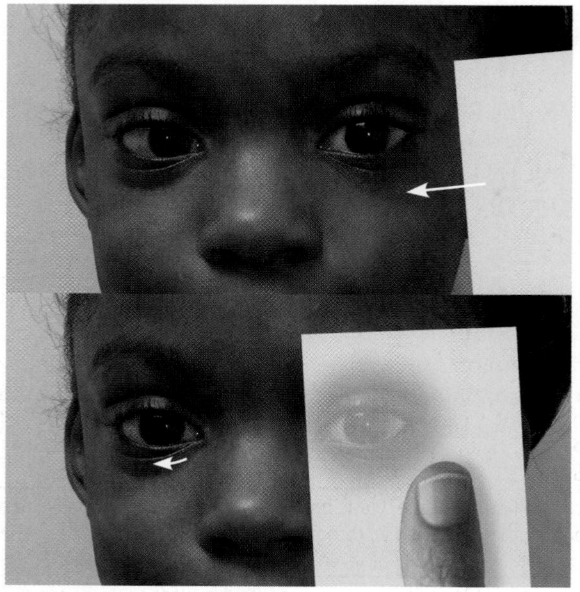
A Right, uncovered eye is weaker

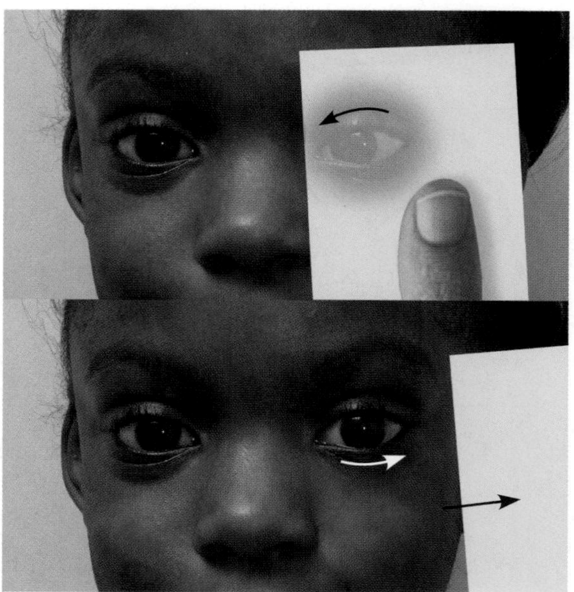
B Left, covered eye is weaker

FIGURE 8–21 ■ Cover–uncover test. With the child at your eye level, ask the child to look at a picture on the wall. *A*, As you cover one eye with an index card or paper cup, observe for any movement of the uncovered eye. If it jumps to fixate on the picture, the uncovered eye has a muscle weakness. *B*, As you remove the cover from the eye, observe the covered eye for any movement to fixate on the picture. If the eye has a muscle weakness, it will drift to a relaxed position once covered.

where the light is reflected on each eye. The light reflection is normally symmetric, at the same spot on each cornea (see Figure 8–17). An asymmetric corneal light reflex after 6 months of age indicates strabismus.

Cover–Uncover Test

The cover–uncover test can be used only for older, cooperative children. While standing slightly to one side, but in a position from which you are still able to see the child's eyes, ask the child to look at a picture on the wall or have the parent distract the child with a toy to look at. Cover one of the child's eyes with an index card or paper cup and simultaneously inspect the uncovered eye for movement as it focuses on the picture. Then remove the card from the covered eye and inspect it for movement as it focuses on the picture (Figure 8–21 ■). Repeat the procedure covering and uncovering the child's other eye. Because the eyes work together, no obvious movement of either eye is expected. Eye movement indicates a muscle imbalance.

Vision Assessment

Because vision is such an important sense for learning, assessment is essential to detect any serious problems. Vision is evaluated using an age-appropriate vision test, but no simple method exists. It is possible to assess the presence of vision in infants and children by observing their behavior in response to certain maneuvers and during play. Visual assessment techniques focus on light perception, visual acuity, and color perception.

Infants and Toddlers

When the infant's eyes are open, test the blink reflex by moving your hand quickly toward the infant's eyes. A quick blink is the normal response. Absence of the blink reflex can indicate that the infant is blind. If the supine infant will not open the eyes voluntarily, stand behind the parent who is holding the infant upright against the chest. The infant usually opens the eyes in this position.

To test an infant's ability to visually track an object, hold a light or toy about 15 cm (6 in.) from the infant's eyes. When the infant has fixated on or is staring at the object, move it slowly to each side. The infant should follow the object with the eyes and by moving the head.

Once an infant has developed skills to reach for and then pick up objects, observe play behavior to evaluate vision. The ability to easily find and pick up small toys is a good indicator of vision in children under 3 years of age. See Table 24–1∞.

Visual Fields

Peripheral vision is evaluated by a confrontation test in children over 3 years of age. Have the child look at your nose or chin and hold the head still. Move both hands beyond your field of vision and slowly move the hands toward the body with a wiggling finger. Tell the child to tell you when the moving fingers are seen. The child should see the fingers at the same time as the examiner. In the young child you may need to watch for the child's eye or head movement to see the moving fingers rather than depend upon the child to tell you when the moving fingers are seen.

Standardized Vision Charts

Standardized vision charts cannot be used to test vision until the child can understand directions and cooperate, usually at about 3 years of age. For preschool children several types of vision screening tools can be used until the alphabet is mastered. See Table 8–6. The Snellen letter chart is used for

TABLE 8–6 Standardized Vision Testing for Children and Adolescents

TEST	DESCRIPTION
Snellen Letter Chart	This alphabet chart is the most commonly used standardized assessment tool for visual acuity. It consists of lines of letters in decreasing size. Charts are designed for reading from a distance of 10 or 20 ft.
Snellen E Chart	This chart is used for children who have not yet mastered the alphabet. It consists of lines of decreasing-size capital Es shown facing in different directions. The child is asked to point in the direction of the "legs" of the E that the examiner indicates. Another option is to give the child a paper with an E on it and have the child turn it in the direction the E is pointing on the chart. Charts are designed for reading from a distance of 10 or 20 ft.
Blackbird Eye Test	This chart is a variation of the Snellen E chart in which a blackbird flies in a shape similar to an E. The child identifies which direction the bird is flying.
The Picture Chart	The picture chart has commonly identified silhouettes (e.g., house, apple, umbrella) placed on lines in decreasing size. The child is asked to identify the pictures either by naming them or by pointing to each one on a piece of paper.
HOTV Chart	This chart uses the letters *H, O, T,* and *V* on lines in decreasing size. The child is given a chart with the four letters to point to during the screening. There is no need to know the alphabet. The HOTV chart can also be used after a practice session with children who do not speak English.
Allen Cards	The picture cards contain seven familiar objects (birthday cake, teddy bear, tree, house, car, telephone, and horse with rider). Show the pictures to the child to be sure that the child can recognize them during the test. Then show the pictures again 15 ft away. The child should be able to name three of seven cards within three to five trials.
Stereograms (Titmus Stereograms or Random Dot E Game)	*Stereoacuity,* the ability of the eyes to work together for depth perception, is tested in older children. The child wears stereoscopic glasses and is asked to distinguish between cards that are blank, have a raised E, and a recessed E when held 16 in. from the eyes. The child should consistently be able to identify the cards with Es.
Jaeger or Rosenbaum Chart	This standardized card with graduated letters is used to test near vision in children who have mastered the alphabet. The card is held 12 to 14 in. from the face.
Ishihara Chart	This series of polychromatic cards is used to test color vision in boys as young as 4 years. A pattern of dots is printed against a background of many colored dots. Ask the child to identify the pattern. The boy who is color blind cannot identify the letter within the colored field. Boys are targeted for testing because of X-linked color blindness.

testing far vision in school-age children and adolescents. For all screening tools testing far vision, make sure the child is the appropriate distance from the chart, usually 10 or 20 feet. Cover one eye so each eye is evaluated separately before testing them together. Observe for squinting, moving the head forward, excessive blinking, or tearing. If the child wears glasses or contact lenses, test the child without corrective lenses before testing with lenses. When the child correctly reads the letters on the line designated "20 feet" while standing 20 feet away, vision is "20/20." If however, the child can only read the line labeled "40 feet" while standing 20 feet away, vision is "20/40." See Box 8–6.

PRACTICE ALERT

Criteria for referral is as follows:

- Newborn—not tracking an object or parent's face from midline to either side
- Age 3 to 5 years—20/40 or less in either eye
- Age 6 years and older—20/30 or less in either eye
- A difference in vision between the eyes is one line or more on the Snellen eye chart, for example, 20/20 in one eye and 20/40 in the other eye, even when one eye is within expected range
- Any problems with ocular alignment
- Any other indication of vision impairment, regardless of acuity

Data from: American Academy of Pediatrics Committee on Practice and Ambulatory Medicine and Section on Ophthalmology. (2003). Eye examination in infants, children, and young adults by pediatricians. Pediatrics, 111*(4), 902–907.*

BOX 8–6 Visual Acuity Development

Researchers have discovered that newborns can see well enough at birth to prefer faces to other patterns, and to follow a moving object. The child's visual acuity develops during early childhood (Seidel et al., 2003).

Age	Visual Acuity
3 years	20/40
4 years	20/40
5 years	20/30
6 years	20/20

Inspection of the Internal Eye Structures

The funduscopic examination allows you to inspect the structures of the internal eye—the retina, optic disc, arteries and veins, and macula (Figure 8–22 ■). This examination takes extensive practice because the ophthalmoscope is a complex instrument to master and because the examination is difficult to perform on uncooperative children. Most often it is performed by experienced examiners.

Darkening the room will cause the child's pupils to dilate. Explain the procedure to the child to gain full cooperation. Have a picture on the wall or have the parent or assistant hold a toy for the child to stare at so that the child's eye will not have to be held open forcibly.

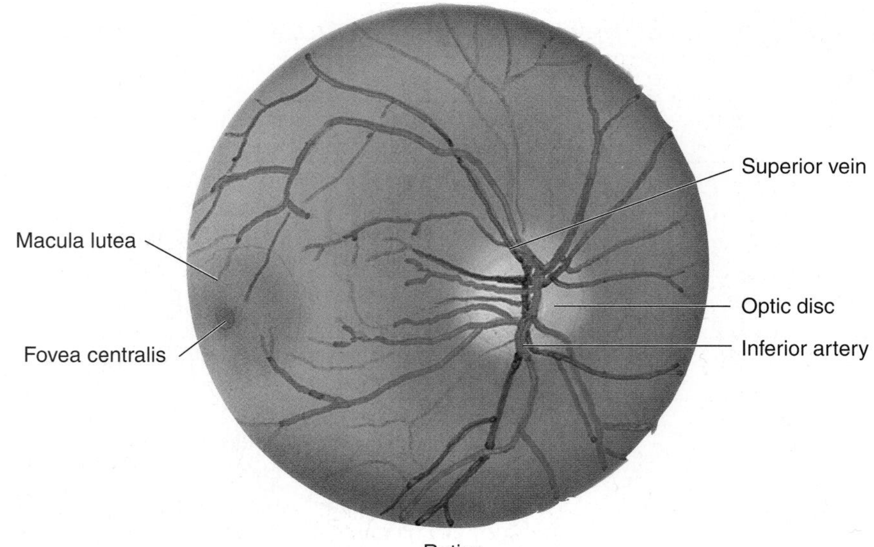

FIGURE 8–22 ■ Normal fundus. Only a portion of the fundus is seen through the ophthalmoscope with each view. Follow the blood vessels on the retina to see other areas of the fundus.

Using the Ophthalmoscope

The ophthalmoscope has a lens-and-mirror system and a bright light for inspecting the structures of the internal eye.

Turn the ophthalmoscope on and set the lens power at zero. Keep your forefinger on the disk to change the lens power as needed. Hold the ophthalmoscope so you can see through the lens. Rest the top against your eyebrow and the handle against your cheek to keep the instrument stabilized. The right eye is used to examine the child's right eye and the left eye to examine the child's left eye. This position is best for visualizing the eye, and it reduces direct exposure to infection. Place a hand on the child's head for stabilization.

Red Reflex

Shine the ophthalmoscope light at the child's eye from a distance of 30 cm (12 in.). The first image seen is the red reflex, the red glow of the vascular retina. When you see the red reflex, know that you are using the ophthalmoscope correctly and that the child's lens is clear.

> **CLINICAL TIP**
>
> Black spots or opacities within the red reflex are abnormal and may indicate congenital cataracts. If a white reflex is seen rather than a red reflex, a retinoblastoma may be present. See Chapter 24∞.

The red reflex can also be tested by shining a small flashlight into the eye.

Visualizing the Internal Eye Structures

Slowly move closer to the child, keeping the red reflex in view to make sure your head and the ophthalmoscope move as one unit. If you lose the red reflex when moving closer to the child, move back, find the red reflex, and start again. Deeper levels of the vitreous humor are inspected before the pink retina comes into view. The retina is a deeper pink in children with darker skin. A blood vessel is the first retinal structure usually seen. Continue moving closer to the child's eye and adjust the plus or minus lenses to focus on this blood vessel. Retinal arteries appear smaller and brighter red than veins. The blood vessels branch to spread and cover the retina.

Inspect and follow the branching of the blood vessels toward the nose until they merge into the optic disc. Dark areas along the blood vessels may indicate retinal hemorrhages. Carefully inspect sites where arteries and veins cross.

The optic disc margin is normally sharply defined, round, and yellow to creamy pink. Blurring of the disc margins or bulging of the optic disc is a sign of increased intracranial pressure. The diameter of the optic disc is used to identify the location of other landmarks on the retina.

The macula is located approximately two disc diameters lateral to the optic disc. To see the macula, ask the child to look at the light. It appears as a yellow dot surrounded by deep pink. The macula is inspected last because the bright light causes the child to blink and look away.

Assessing the Ear Structures and Hearing

How do you identify proper ear placement on the head? What is the significance of low-set ears? Why is otitis media the most common ear problem during early childhood? What play activities can be used to test hearing in young children? How do you evaluate the hearing of an older child?

Inspection of the External Ear Structures

The position and characteristics of the pinna, the external ear, are inspected as a continuation of the head and eye examination. Equipment needed for this assessment includes an otoscope, noisemakers (bell, rattle, tissue paper), and a tuning fork of 500 to 1000 Hz.

The pinna is considered "low set" when the top lies completely below an imaginary line drawn through the medial and

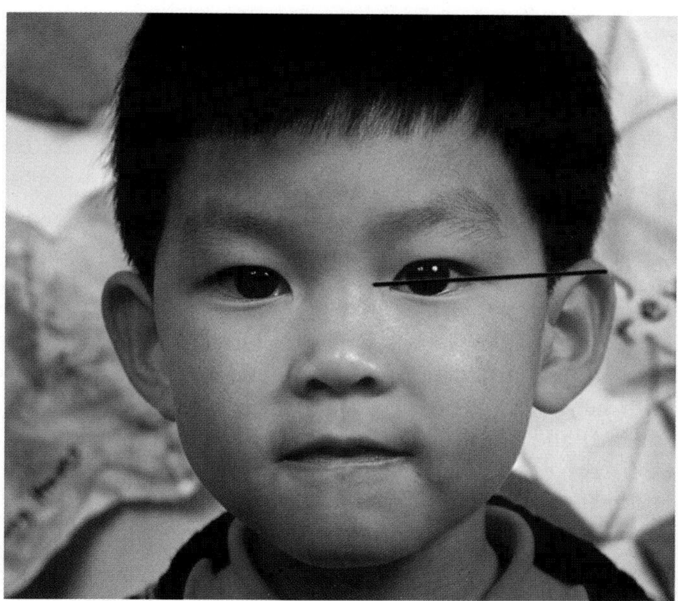

FIGURE 8–23 ■ To detect the correct placement of the external ears, draw an imaginary line through the medial and lateral canthi of the eye toward the ear. This line normally passes through the upper portion of the pinna. The pinna is considered "low set" when the top lies completely below the imaginary line. Low-set ears are often associated with renal disorders. Is this a normal ear placement? (Yes, it is.)

lateral canthi of the eye toward the ear. Low-set ears are often associated with congenital renal disorders (Figure 8–23 ■).

Inspect the pinna for any malformation. The pinna should be completely formed, with an open auditory canal. Next, inspect the tissue around the pinna for abnormalities. A pit or hole in front of the auditory canal may indicate the presence of a sinus. If the pinna protrudes outward, there may be swelling behind the ear, a sign of mastoiditis.

Inspect the external auditory canal for any discharge. A foul-smelling, purulent discharge may indicate the presence of a foreign body or an infection in the external canal. Clear fluid or a blood-tinged discharge may indicate a cerebrospinal fluid leak caused by a basilar skull fracture.

Inspection of the Tympanic Membrane

Examination of the tympanic membrane is important in infants and young children because they are prone to otitis media, a middle ear infection. The eustachian tubes are shorter, wider, and more horizontally positioned in infants and young children than in older children and adults. This positioning enables bacteria to move up the eustachian tube from the pharynx, causing an infection. (See Figure 24–2∞.)

The otoscope, an instrument with a magnifying lens, bright light, and speculum, is used to examine the internal auditory canal and tympanic membrane. Infants and young children often resist having their ears inspected with the otoscope because of past painful experiences. The otoscopic examination is often delayed until portions of the assessment requiring cooperation are completed. Use simple explanations to prepare the child. Let the child play with the otoscope or demonstrate how it is used on the parent or a doll. Figures 8–24A and B ■ illustrate different methods that can be used to restrain an uncooperative infant and child.

Using the Otoscope. To begin the otoscopic examination, hold the handle of the otoscope in the palm of your hand with your thumb pointed toward the base of the handle. If a pneumatic squeeze bulb is used, hold it between the index finger and the handle. Choose the largest ear speculum that fits into the auditory canal to form a seal for testing the movement of the tympanic membrane. A large speculum is also less likely to injure the auditory canal if the child moves suddenly.

Hold the otoscope in the hand closest to the child's face and when the child is cooperative rest the back of your hand against the child's head to stabilize it. Use your other hand to pull the pinna toward the back of the head either up or down, whichever position provides the best view. Pulling the pinna straightens the auditory canal and improves inspection of the tympanic membrane (Figure 8–25 ■).

Slowly insert the speculum into the auditory canal, inspecting the walls for signs of irritation, discharge, or a foreign body. The walls of the auditory canal are normally pink, and some cerumen is present. Children often put beads, peas, or other small objects into their ears. If cerumen or a foreign

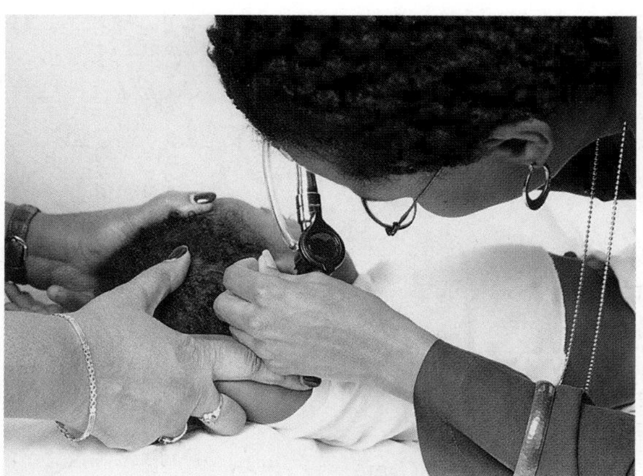

A

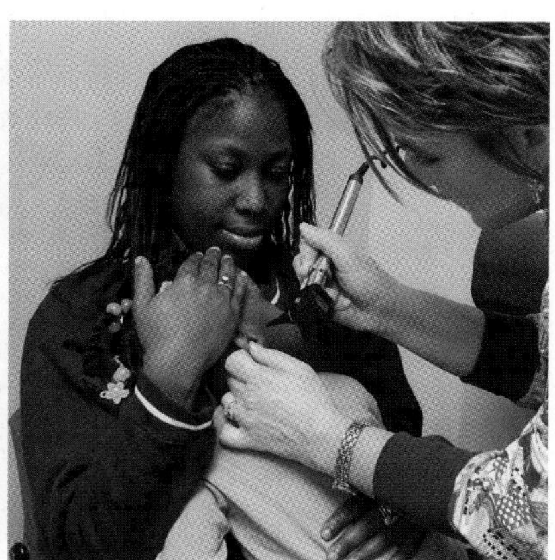

B

FIGURE 8–24 ■ *A,* To restrain an uncooperative infant, place the infant supine on the examining table. Have an assistant hold the child's arms next to the head to restrain the child's head movements. Restrain the child's body movements by lying across the child's body. Keep your hands free to hold the otoscope and position the external ear. *B,* Place the uncooperative toddler on the parent's lap with legs held between the parent's legs. One of the parent's arms hold the child's head to the chest and the other arm holds the child's arms and upper torso against the chest.

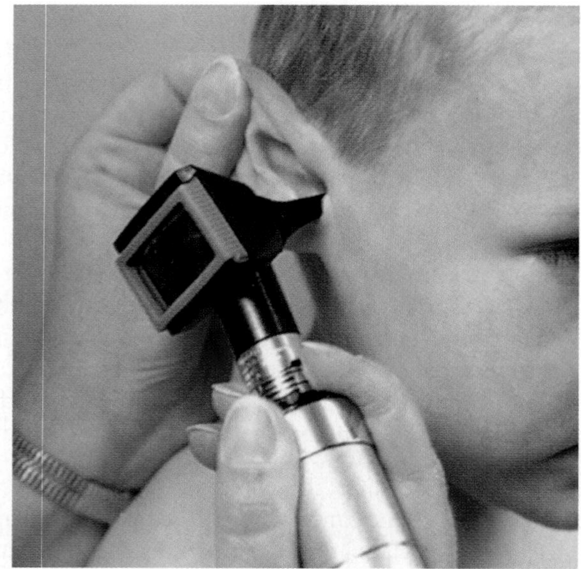

FIGURE 8–25 ■ To straighten the auditory canal: pull the pinna back and up for children over 3 years of age; pull the pinna down and back for children under 3 years of age.

body obstructs the auditory canal, irrigation with warm water can be used to clean the canal.

The tympanic membrane, which separates the outer ear from the middle ear, is usually pearly gray and translucent. It reflects light, and the bones (ossicles) in the middle ear are normally visible. When the pneumatic attachment is squeezed, the tympanic membrane normally moves in and out in response to the positive and negative pressure applied (Figure 8–26 ■). Table 8–7

CLINICAL TIP

Never irrigate the ear canal if any discharge is present, as the tympanic membrane may be ruptured. Irrigation would allow the water to enter the middle ear and potentially worsen the infection.

lists the abnormal findings of a tympanic membrane examination and their associated conditions. See Figure 24–9∞.

Hearing Assessment

Hearing evaluation is important in children of all ages because hearing is essential for normal speech development and learning. With new technology, even newborns can have their hearing screened, and many states require such screening prior to hospital discharge. (See Chapter 24∞ for newborn hearing screening information.) Often hearing must be evaluated by inspection of the child's responses to various auditory stimuli. Hearing loss may occur at any time during early childhood as the result of birth trauma, frequent otitis media, meningitis, or antibiotics that damage cranial nerve VIII. Documented hearing loss may be associated with other congenital anomalies and genetic syndromes.

Use hearing and speech articulation milestones as an initial hearing screen. Select an age-appropriate method to screen hearing. When a hearing deficiency is suspected as a result of screening, the child is referred for audiometry, tympanometry, or evoked response to obtain the most accurate evaluation of hearing. **Audiometry** is a screening procedure using air conduction that measures hearing for pure-tone frequencies and loudness. The high and low pitch sounds are presented through earphones testing different sound frequencies and the loudness needed to hear each sound. Hearing loss is determined when the child needs higher decibels to hear a tone.

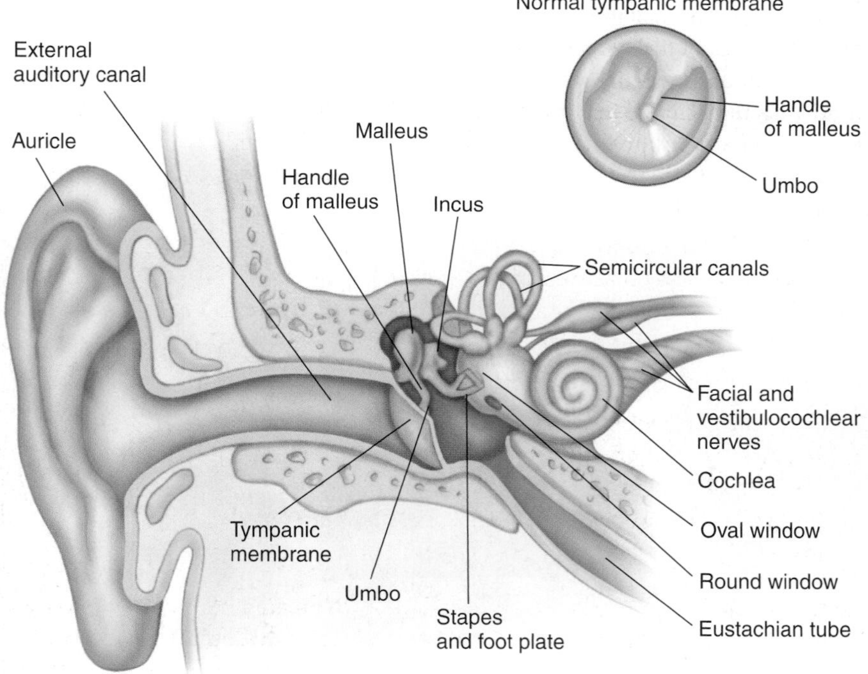

FIGURE 8–26 ■ Cross section of the ear. The tympanic membrane normally has a triangular light reflex with the base on the nasal side pointing toward the center. The bony landmarks, the umbo and handle of malleus, are seen through the tympanic membrane.

TABLE 8–7 Unexpected Findings on Examination of the Tympanic Membrane and Their Associated Conditions

CHARACTERISTICS OF TYMPANIC MEMBRANE	UNEXPECTED FINDINGS	ASSOCIATED CONDITIONS
Color	Redness Slight redness Amber Deep red or blue	Infection in middle ear Prolonged crying Serous fluid in middle ear Blood in middle ear
Light reflex	Absent Distorted, loss of triangular shape	Bulging tympanic membrane, infection in middle ear Retracted tympanic membrane, serous fluid in middle ear
Bony landmarks	Extra prominent	Retracted tympanic membrane, serous fluid in middle ear
Movement	No motility Excess motility	Infection or fluid in middle ear Healed perforation

Tympanometry is a test to estimate the pressure in the middle ear and an indirect measure of tympanic membrane movement. See Chapter 24∞ for more information. Refer to the Skills Manual ⊘ for procedures.

Infants and Toddlers. Select noisemakers with different frequencies, such as a rattle, bell, and tissue paper, that will attract the young child's attention. Ask the parent or an assistant to entertain the infant with a quiet toy, such as a teddy bear. Stand behind the infant, about 60 cm (2 ft) away from the infant's ear but outside the infant's field of peripheral vision, and make a soft sound with the noisemaker. Make sure that no air movement provides a clue to the child to turn the head. Have the parent or your assistant observe the child for any of the following responses when the noisemaker is used: widening the eyes, briefly stopping all activity to listen, or turning the head toward the sound. Repeat the test in the other ear and with the other noisemakers. Indicators of hearing loss in an infant include:

- No startle reaction to loud noises
- Does not turn toward sounds by 4 months of age
- Babbles as a young infant, but does not keep babbling or develop speech sounds after 6 months of age

Indicators of hearing loss in a young child include:

- No speech by 2 years of age
- Inability to follow age-appropriate directions, such as "bring me the block"
- Speech sounds are not distinct as expected at appropriate ages

Preschool and Older Children. Whispered words are used to evaluate the hearing of children over 3 years of age. Position your head about 30 cm (12 in.) away from the child's ear, but out of the range of vision so the child cannot read your lips. Use words easily recognized by the child, such as Mickey Mouse, hot dog, and Popsicle, and ask the child to repeat the words. Repeat the test with different words in the opposite ear. The child should correctly repeat the whispered words.

When the child will not repeat the whispered words, try an alternate procedure. As you whisper directions, ask the child to point to different body parts such as an eye, ear, and hand. Remember to stay out of the child's range of vision so the child cannot read your lips. The child should point to the correct body part each time.

Bone and Air Conduction of Sound. A tuning fork is used to evaluate the hearing of school-age children who can follow directions. Stroke the tines of the tuning fork to begin the vibration. Avoid touching the vibrating tines, which will dampen the sound. Bone conduction is tested when the handle of the tuning fork is placed on the child's skull. Air conduction is tested when the vibrating tines are held close to the child's ear (Figure 8–27 ■).

To perform the Weber test, place the vibrating tuning fork on top of the child's skull in the midline. Ask the child to tell you where the sound is heard the best, either in both ears equally or in one ear. The sound should be heard equally in both ears.

To perform the Rinne test, place the vibrating tuning fork handle on the mastoid process behind an ear. Ask the child to tell you when the sound is no longer heard. Immediately move the tuning fork, holding the vibrating tines about 2.5 to 5 cm (1 to 2 in.) from the same ear. Again, ask the child to indicate when the sound is no longer heard. The child normally hears the air-conducted sound twice as long as the bone-conducted sound. Repeat the Rinne test on the other ear. Table 8–8 provides an interpretation of the Weber and Rinne tests.

Assessing the Nose and Sinuses for Airway Patency and Discharge

What is the most common cause of a nasal obstruction in children? What does nasal flaring indicate? What signs indicate that a foreign body might be lodged in the nose? What does it mean if the child frequently wipes the nose upward with a hand?

Inspection of the External Nose

The external nose characteristics and placement on the face are examined simultaneously with the facial features. Inspect the external nose for size, shape, symmetry, and midline placement on the face. The nose should be proportional in size to other facial features and positioned in the middle of the face. A flattened nasal bridge is the expected finding in Asian and Black children.

The nasolabial folds are normally symmetric. Asymmetry of these folds may be associated with injury to the facial nerve (cranial nerve VII). A saddle-shaped nose is associated with congenital defects such as cleft palate.

Inspect the external nose for the presence of unusual characteristics. For example, a crease across the nose between the

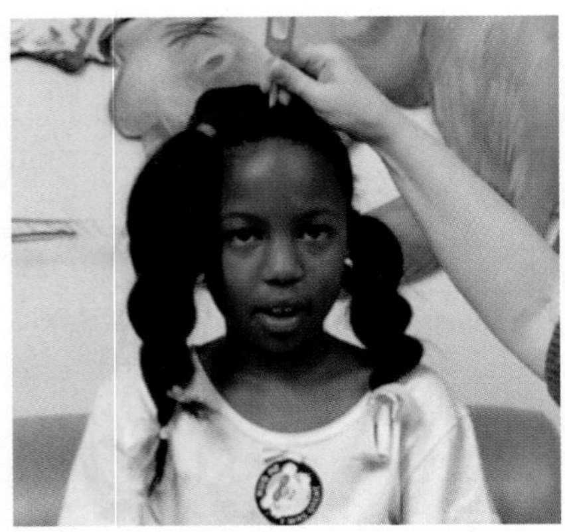
A

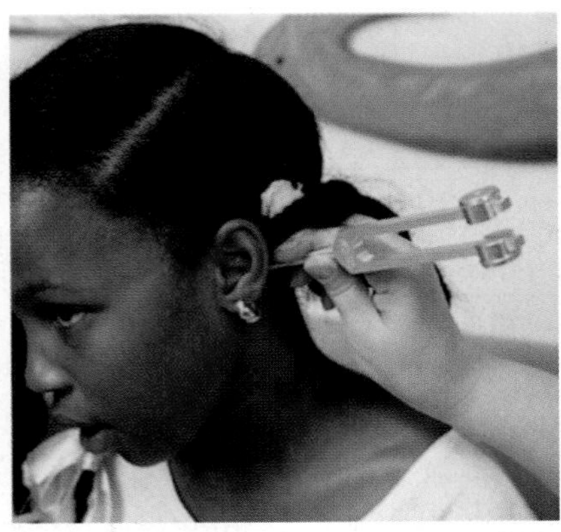
B

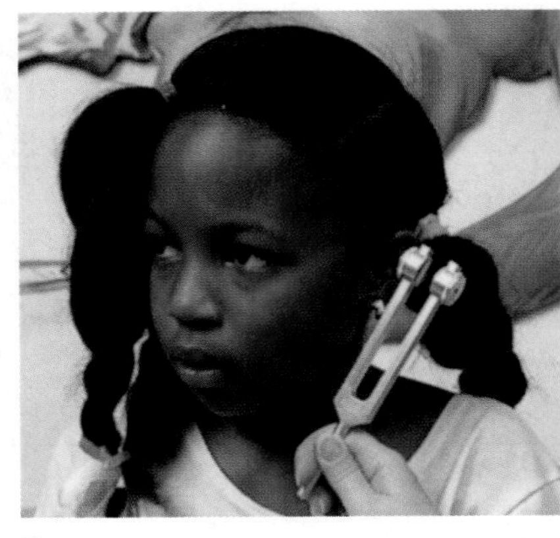
C

FIGURE 8–27 ■ *A*, Weber test. Place vibrating tuning fork on midline of the child's head. *B*, Rinne test, step 1. Place vibrating tuning fork on mastoid process. *C*, Rinne test, step 2. Reposition still vibrating tines between 2.5 and 5 cm (1 and 2 in.) from ear.

cartilage and bone is often caused by the allergic child's wiping an itchy nose upward with a hand.

Palpation of the External Nose

When a deformity is noted, gently palpate the nose to detect any pain or break in contour. No tenderness or masses are expected. Pain and a contour deviation are usually the result of trauma.

Nasal Patency

The child's airway must be patent to ensure adequate oxygenation. To test for nasal patency, occlude one nostril and observe the child's effort to breathe through the open nostril with the mouth closed. Repeat the procedure with the other nostril. Breathing should be noiseless and effortless. Nasal flaring, an effort the child makes to widen the airway, is a sign of respiratory distress and should not be present.

If the child struggles to breathe, a nasal obstruction may be present. Young infants under 6 months of age will not automatically open their mouths to breath when the nose is occluded, such as by mucus. Nasal obstruction may be caused by a foreign body, congenital defect, dry mucus, discharge, polyp, or trauma.

TABLE 8–8 Interpretation of the Weber and Rinne Tests of Hearing

TEST AND RESULT	ASSOCIATED CONDITION
Weber Test	
– Sound heard equally in both ears	No hearing loss
– Sound heard better in one ear (lateralized)	Conductive hearing loss if sound lateralized to deaf ear
Rinne Test	
– Sound heard by air conduction twice as long as bone conduction	No hearing loss
– Sound heard longer by bone conduction than air conduction	Conductive hearing loss in affected ear
– Sound heard longer by air conduction than bone conduction, but less than twice as long	Sensorineural hearing loss in affected ear

Young children commonly place objects up their nose, and unilateral nasal flaring is a sign of such an obstruction.

Assessment of Smell

The olfactory nerve (cranial nerve I) is rarely tested in preschool children, but it can be tested in school-age children and adolescents. When testing smell, choose scents the child will easily recognize such as orange, chocolate, and mint. When the child's eyes are closed, occlude one nostril and hold the scent under the nose. Ask the child to take a deep sniff and identify the scent. Use alternate odors between the nares. The child can normally identify common scents.

Inspection of the Internal Nose

Inspect the internal nose for color of the mucous membranes and the presence of any discharge, swelling, lesions, or other abnormalities. Use a bright light, such as an otoscope light or penlight. For infants and young children, push the tip of the nose upward and shine the light at the end of the nose (Figure 8–28 ■). The nasal speculum for the otoscope can be used in older children. Avoid touching the septum of the nose with the speculum. Injury to the septum can cause a nosebleed.

Mucous Membranes. The mucous membranes should be dark pink and glistening. A film of clear discharge may also be present. Turbinates, if visible, should be the same color as the mucous membranes and have a firm consistency. When the turbinates are pale or bluish gray, the child may have allergies. A polyp, a rounded mass projecting from the turbinate, is also associated with allergies.

Nasal Septum. Inspect the nasal septum for alignment, perforations, bleeding, or crusting. The septum should be straight. Crusting will be noted over the site of a nosebleed.

Discharge. Observe for the presence of nasal discharge, noting if the drainage is from one or both nares. Nasal discharge is not a normal finding unless the child is crying. Discharge may be watery, mucoid, purulent, or bloody. The character of the discharge depends on the condition present. A foul-smelling

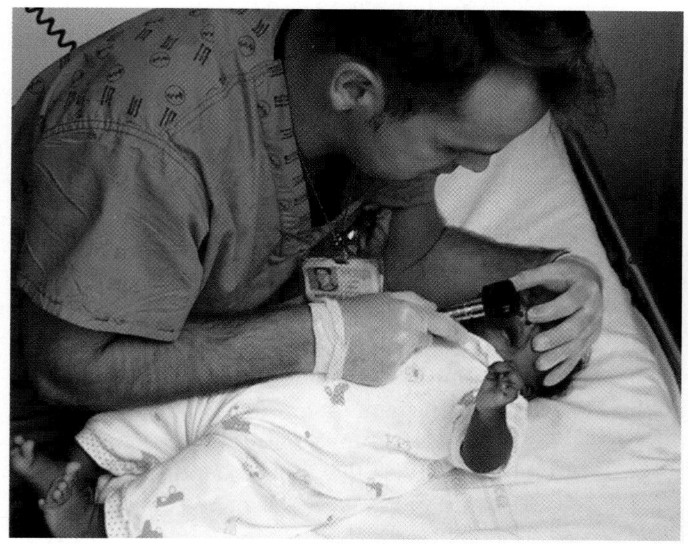

A

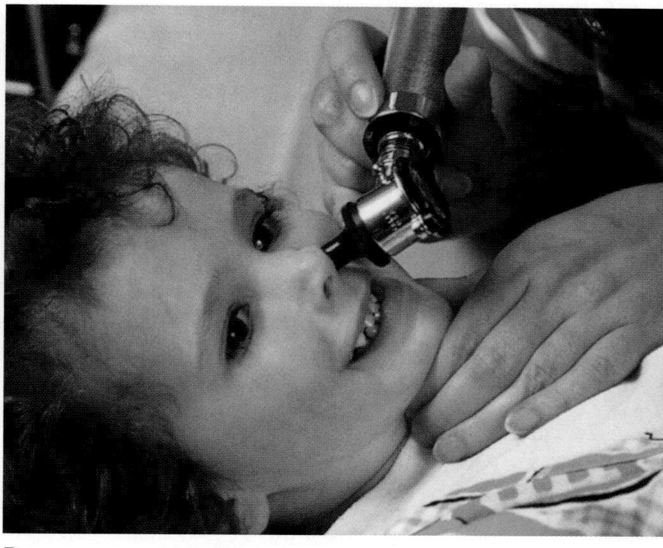

B

FIGURE 8–28 ■ Techniques for examining nose. *A,* Technique for infant or small child. *B,* Technique for older child.

discharge in only one nostril is often associated with a foreign body. Table 8–9 lists conditions associated with nasal discharge.

Inspection of the Sinuses

The maxillary and ethmoid sinuses develop during early childhood (Figure 8–29 ■). Sinus infections can occasionally occur in young children. Suspect a sinus problem when the child has a headache or pain and swelling around one or both eyes.

Inspect the face for any puffiness around one or both eyes. Puffiness and swelling are not normally present. To palpate over the maxillary sinuses, press up under both zygomatic arches with the thumbs. To palpate the ethmoid sinuses, press up against the bone above both eyes with the thumbs. No swelling or tenderness is expected. Tenderness may be an indication of sinusitis.

ASSESSING THE MOUTH AND THROAT FOR COLOR, FUNCTION, AND SIGNS OF ABNORMAL CONDITIONS

What is the best site to evaluate cyanosis in children? What is the expected sequence of tooth eruption? How is it determined that the tongue has adequate movement for all speech sounds? How can the throat be inspected without causing the child to gag?

TABLE 8–9 Nasal Discharge Characteristics and Associated Conditions

DISCHARGE DESCRIPTION	ASSOCIATED CONDITIONS
Watery	
Clear, bilateral	Allergy
Serous, unilateral	Spinal fluid from fracture of cribiform plate
Mucoid or purulent	
Bilateral	Upper respiratory infection
Unilateral	Foreign body
Bloody	Nose bleed, trauma

Inspection of the Mouth

Young children often need coaxing and simple explanations before they will cooperate with the mouth and throat examination. Most children readily show their teeth. If the child resists by clenching the teeth, the teeth can be gently separated with a tongue blade. Equipment needed for the examination of the mouth includes a tongue blade and penlight. Wear gloves when examining the mouth because of contact with mucous membranes. See Figure 8–30 ■ for structures of the mouth.

PRACTICE ALERT

Avoid examining the mouth if there are signs of respiratory distress, high fever, drooling, and intense apprehension. These may be signs of epiglottitis. Inspecting the mouth may trigger a total airway obstruction. See Chapter 25∞ for more information.

Lips

Inspect the lips for color, shape, symmetry, moisture, and lesions. The lips are normally symmetric without drying, cracking, or other lesions. Lip color is normally pink in white children and more bluish in children with darker skin. Pale, cyanotic, or cherry red lips are indicators of poor tissue perfusion caused by various conditions, such as anemia, respiratory distress, and carbon monoxide poisoning. Note any clefts or edema.

Teeth

Inspect and count the child's teeth. The timing of tooth eruption is often genetically determined, but it involves a regular sequence. Figure 8–31 ■ presents the typical sequence of tooth eruption for both deciduous and permanent teeth.

AS THEY GROW

Sinus Development

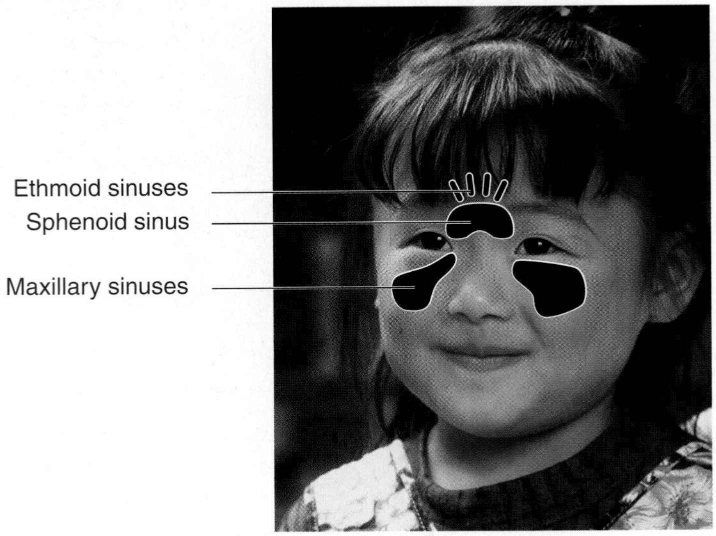

Ethmoid sinuses
Sphenoid sinus
Maxillary sinuses

FIGURE 8–29 ■ Sinuses grow and develop during childhood. Maxillary sinuses can be identified in 1-year-old children. Ethmoid sinuses have developed in children by 6 years of age. Sinus problems under 7 years occur infrequently.

Inspect the condition of the teeth, look for loose teeth, and note any spaces where teeth are missing. Compare empty tooth spaces with the child's developmental stage of tooth eruption. Once the permanent teeth have erupted, none should be missing. Teeth are normally white, without a flattened, mottled, or pitted appearance. Discoloration on the crown of a tooth may indicate caries. Discoloration of the tooth surface may be associated with some medications and fluorsis. See Chapter 24∞. Interruption of dentine can be associated with chronic vomiting with bulimia nervosa. See Chapter 9∞.

Mouth Odors

During inspection of the teeth, be alert to any abnormal odors that may indicate problems such as diabetic ketoacidosis, infection, or poor hygiene. In older children be alert for odors of alcohol that could indicate substance use.

Gums

Inspect the gums for color and adherence to the teeth. The gums are normally pink, with a stippled or dotted appearance. Use a tongue blade to help visualize the gums around the upper and lower molars. No raised or receding gum areas should be apparent around the teeth. When inflammation, swelling, or bleeding is observed, palpate the gums to detect tenderness. Inflammation and tenderness are associated with infection and poor nutrition.

Buccal Mucosa

Inspect the mucous membrane lining the cheeks for color and moisture. The mucous membrane is usually pink, but patches of hyperpigmentation are commonly seen in children with darker skin. The Stensen duct, the parotid gland opening, is opposite the upper second molar bilaterally. Normally pink, the duct opening becomes red when the child is infected with mumps. Small pink sucking pads can be present in infants. No areas of redness, swelling, or ulcerative lesions should be present.

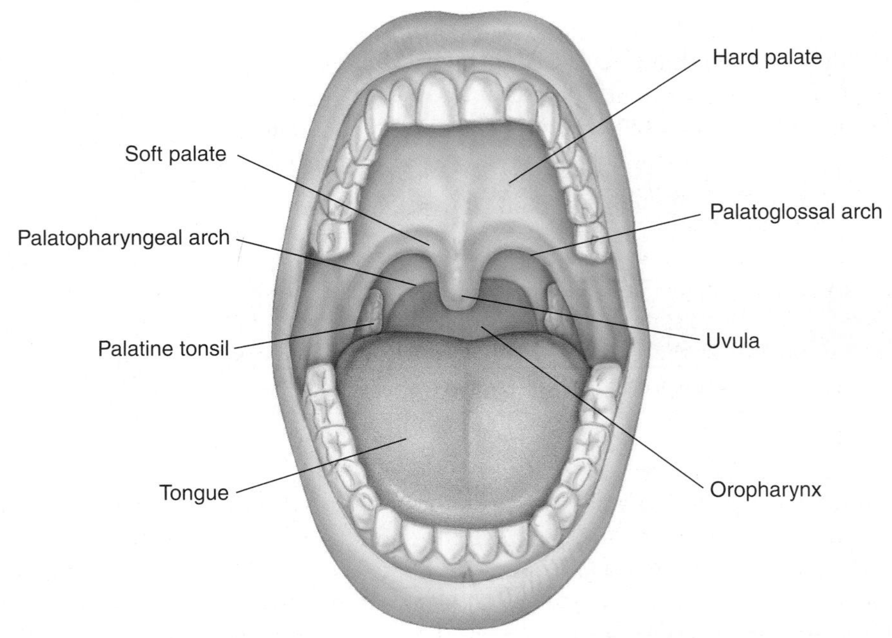

FIGURE 8–30 ■ The structures of the mouth.

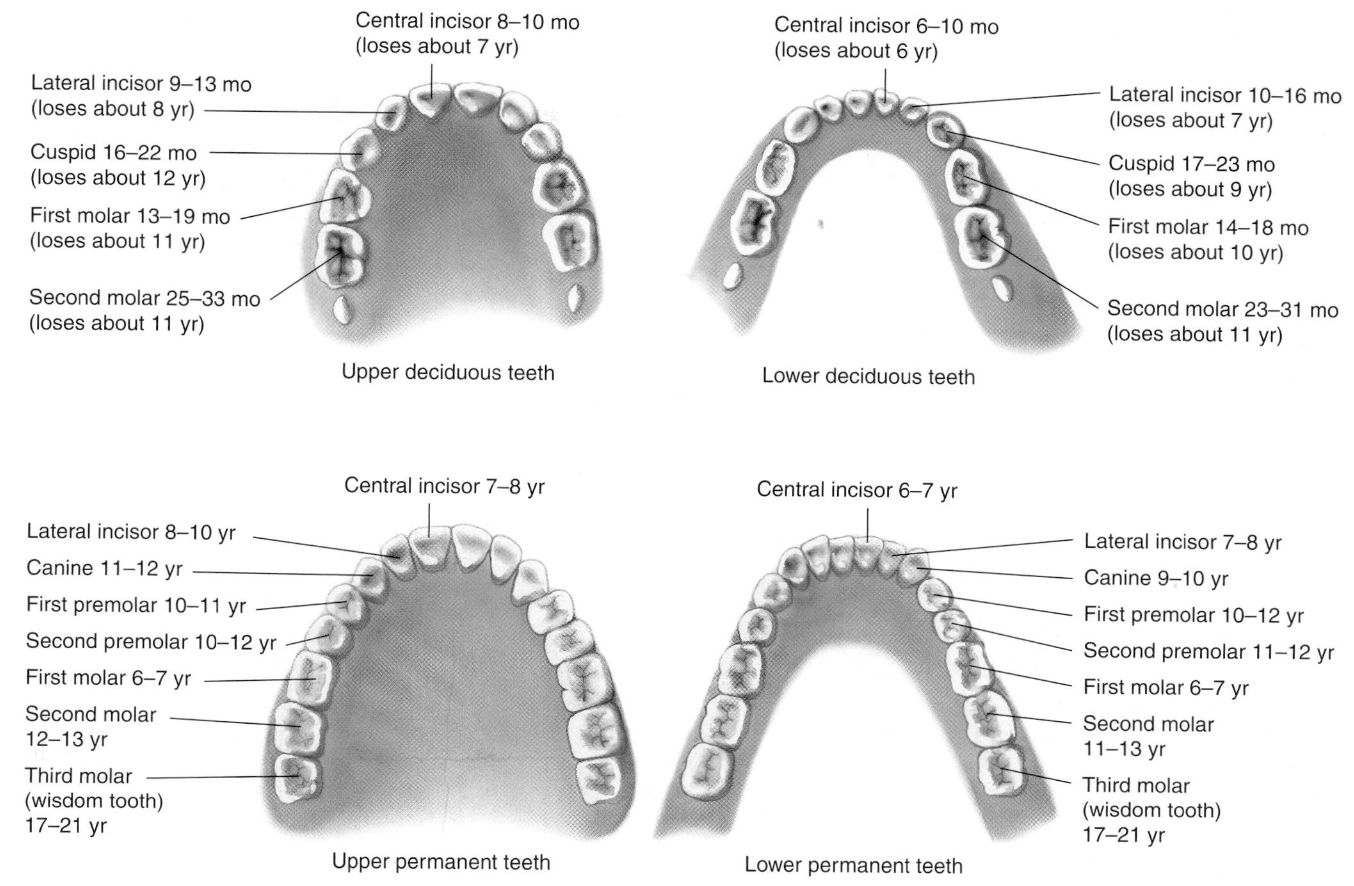

FIGURE 8–31 ■ Typical sequence of tooth eruption for both deciduous and permanent teeth. Notice that bottom teeth come in first for each kind of tooth, incisors, cuspids, and molars. They are lost in the same pattern.

Tongue

Inspect the tongue and floor of the mouth for color, moistness, size, tremors, and lesions. The child's tongue is normally pink and moist, without a coating. The tongue's size permits it to fit easily into the mouth. A protuberant tongue is associated with various genetic conditions, such as Down syndrome. A pattern of gray, irregular borders that form a design (geographic tongue) is often normal, but it may be associated with fever, allergies, or drug reactions. Tremors are abnormal. A white adherent coating on an infant's tongue and extending to the buccal mucosa may be caused by thrush, a Candida infection.

Observe the mobility of the tongue to assess the frenulum. The child should be able to touch the gums above the upper teeth with the tongue. This tongue movement is adequate to enunciate all speech sounds clearly. Ask the child to stick out the tongue and lift it so the underside of the tongue and the floor of the mouth can be inspected for distended veins.

Palate

Inspect the hard and soft palate to detect any clefts, masses, or an unusually high arch. The palate is normally pink, with a dome-shaped arch and no cleft. The uvula hangs freely from the soft palate. Newborns often have Epstein pearls, white papules in the midline of the palate that disappear in a few weeks. A high-arched palate can be associated with sucking difficulties in young infants.

Palpation of the Mouth Structures

Using a gloved finger, palpate any masses seen in the mouth to determine their characteristics, such as size, shape, firmness, and tenderness. No masses should be found.

Tongue

To assess the tongue's strength, simultaneously testing the hypoglossal nerve (cranial nerve XII), place the index finger against the child's cheek and ask the child to push against your finger with the tongue. Some pressure against the finger is normally felt.

Palate

To palpate the palate, insert the gloved little finger, with the fingerpad upward, into the mouth. While the infant sucks against your finger, palpate the entire palate. This procedure also tests the strength of the sucking reflex, innervated by the hypoglossal nerve (cranial nerve XII). No clefts should be palpated.

Inspection of the Throat

Inspect the throat for color, swelling, lesions, and the condition of the tonsils. Ask the child to open the mouth wide and stick out the tongue. A flashlight is used to illuminate the throat. A tongue blade can be used, if needed, to visualize the posterior pharynx. Moistening the tongue blade may decrease the child's

AS THEY GROW

Lymph Tissues

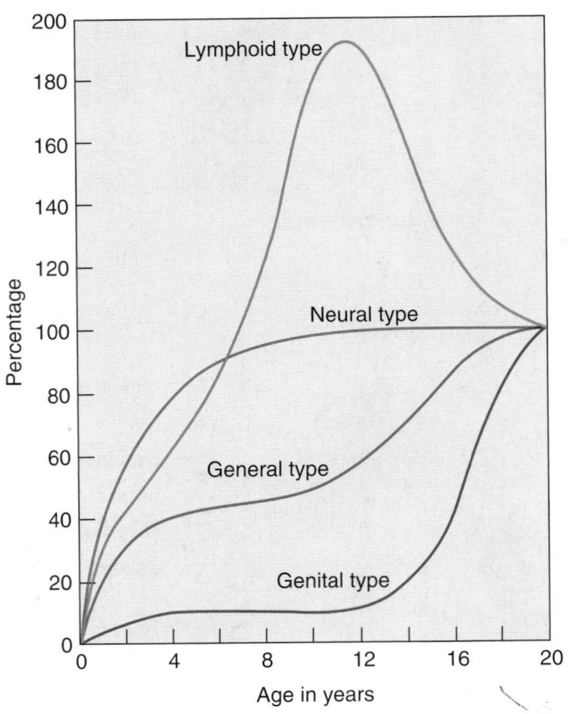

FIGURE 8–32 ■ The lymph tissues are well developed at birth and grow rapidly to reach adult dimensions by 6 years of age. They continue growing until 10 to 12 years when they reach their peak in size, and then decrease in size until adult size is achieved during late adolescence. Only the neurologic tissues grow faster than lymph tissue during early childhood, and in contrast, the genital and other body organs reach their peak in development during adolescence.

tendency to gag. The throat is normally pink without lesions, drainage, or swelling. Swelling or bulging in the posterior pharynx may be associated with a peritonsillar abscess.

Tonsils

During childhood the tonsils are large in proportion to the size of the pharynx because lymphoid tissue grows fastest in early childhood. See Figure 8–32 ■. The tonsils should be pink without exudate, but crypts (fissures) may be present as a result of prior infections. Significantly enlarged tonsils can cause respiratory distress. The size of tonsils can be graded as indicated in Figure 8–33 ■.

Gag Reflex

Use a tongue blade when you are unable to see the posterior pharynx or need to test the gag reflex. The gag reflex is tested at the end of the examination because children dislike the gagging sensation. Prepare the child for what will happen. Ask the child to say "Ah" and watch for the symmetric rising movement of the uvula. This reflex tests the glossopharyngeal and vagal nerves (cranial nerves IX and X). If the uvula does not rise or rises to one side, cranial nerves IX and X may be paralyzed. The epiglottis lies behind the tongue and is normally pink like the rest of the buccal mucosa.

ASSESSING THE NECK FOR CHARACTERISTICS, RANGE OF MOTION, AND LYMPH NODES

What does it mean when a child's head is tilting to one side? By what age should an infant be able to control his or her head? What does a lymph node feel like? What does an enlarged lymph node feel like?

Inspection of the Neck

Inspect the neck for size, symmetry, swelling, and any abnormalities. A short neck with skinfolds is normal for infants. The neck is normally symmetric. No swelling should be present. Swelling may be caused by local infections such as mumps or a congenital defect. The neck lengthens between 3 and 4 years of age.

Inspect the child's neck for any webbing, an extra skinfold on each side of the neck. Webbing is commonly associated with Turner syndrome. See Chapter 32∞.

Infants develop head control by 2 months of age. By this age, an infant can lift the head up and look around when lying on the stomach. A lack of head control can result from neurologic injury, such as an anoxic episode.

Palpation of the Neck

Face the child and use the fingerpads to simultaneously palpate both sides of the neck for lymph nodes, as well as the trachea and thyroid.

Lymph Nodes

To palpate the lymph nodes, slide the fingerpads gently over the lymph node chains in the head and neck. The sequence for lymph node palpation is as follows: around the ears, under the jaw, in the occipital area, and in the cervical chain of the neck (Figure 8–34 ■). Firm, clearly defined, nontender, movable lymph nodes up to 1 cm (1/2 in.) in diameter are common in young children. When a lymph node is palpated, a gentle circular motion helps define the characteristics of the node. Enlarged, firm, warm, tender lymph nodes indicate the presence of local infection. Enlarged, nontender, nonmovable lymph nodes can be associated with lymphomas.

Trachea

Palpate the trachea to determine its position and to detect the presence of any masses. The trachea is normally in the midline of the neck. It is difficult to palpate in children less than 3 years of age because of their short necks. To palpate the trachea, place the thumb and forefinger on each side of the trachea near the chin and slowly slide

PATHOPHYSIOLOGY ILLUSTRATED

Tonsil Size with Infection

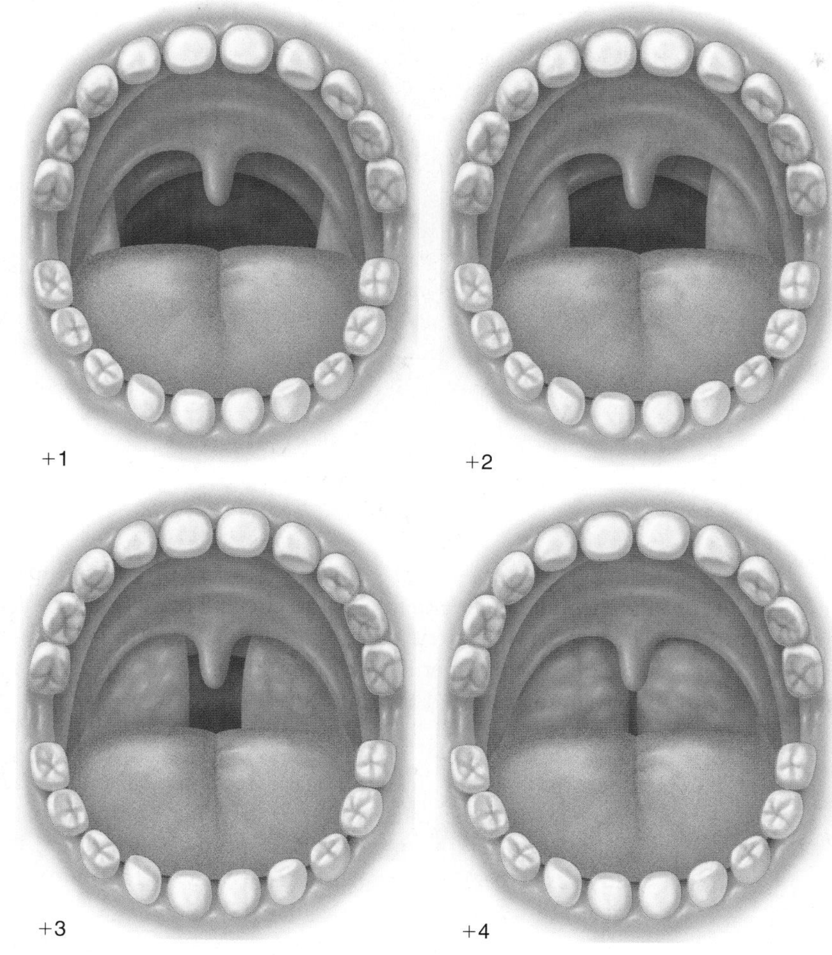

FIGURE 8–33 ■ Tonsil size can be graded from 1+ to 4+ in relation to how much of the airway is obstructed. Tonsil size of 1+ or 2+ is normal. Tonsil size of 3+ is common with infections such as strep throat. Tonsils that "kiss" or nearly touch each other (4+) significantly reduce the size of the airway.

them down the trachea. Any shift to the right or left of midline may indicate a tumor or a collapsed lung.

Thyroid

As the fingers slide over the trachea in the lower neck, attempt to feel the isthmus of the thyroid, a band of glandular tissue crossing over the trachea. The lobes of the thyroid wrap behind the trachea and are normally covered by the sternocleidomastoid muscle. Because of the anatomic position of the thyroid, the lobes of the thyroid are not usually palpable in the child unless they are enlarged.

Range of Motion Assessment

To test the neck's range of motion, ask the child to touch the chin to each shoulder and to the chest and then to look at the ceiling. Move a light or toy in all four directions when assessing infants. Children should freely move the neck and head in all four directions without pain.

When the child is unable to move the head voluntarily in all directions, passively move the child's neck through the expected range of motion. Limited horizontal range of motion may be a sign of torticollis, persistent head tilting. Torticollis results from a birth injury to the sternocleidomastoid muscle or from unilateral vision or hearing impairment. Pain with flexion of the neck toward the chest (Brudzinski sign) may indicate meningitis. See Chapter 33∞.

ASSESSING THE CHEST FOR SHAPE, MOVEMENT, RESPIRATORY EFFORT, AND LUNG FUNCTION

What terms are used to describe the location of specific sounds heard when auscultating the chest? What does it mean when a child's chest is rounded in shape? What are retractions and what do they indicate? How can normal and adventitious breath sounds be distinguished when auscultating the lungs?

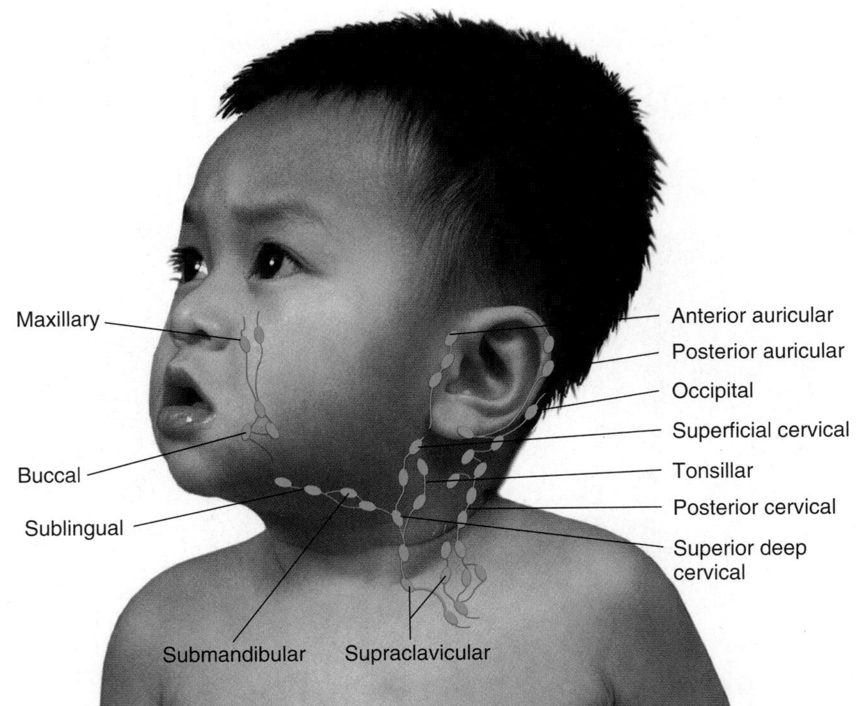

FIGURE 8–34 ■ The neck is palpated for enlarged lymph nodes around the ears, under the jaw, in the occipital area, and in the cervical chains of the neck.

Examination of the anterior and posterior chest includes the following procedures: inspecting the size and shape of the chest, palpating chest movement that occurs during respiration, observing the effort of breathing, and auscultating breath sounds. A stethoscope is needed for the chest examination.

Topographic Landmarks of the Chest

The chest skeleton provides most of the landmarks used to describe the location of findings during examination of the chest, lungs, and heart. The intercostal spaces are the horizontal markers. The sternum and spine are the vertical landmarks. When both a horizontal and a vertical landmark are used, the location of findings can be precisely described (Figures 8–35 ■ and 8–36 ■). Be sure to indicate whether the finding is on the right or left side of the patient's chest (Table 8–10).

Inspection of the Chest

Position the child on the parent's lap or on the examining table with all clothing above the waist removed to inspect the chest. The thoracic muscles and subcutaneous tissue are less developed in children than in adults, so the chest wall is thinner. As a result, the rib cage is more prominent.

In infants, the chest is rounded with the anteroposterior diameter approximately equal to the lateral diameter. By 2 years of age, the chest becomes more oval with growth, and the lateral diameter is greater than the anteroposterior diameter.

Chest Circumference

Chest circumference may be measured until 1 year of age, but it is not routinely performed. Chest circumference is a useful measurement in comparison with the head circumference if the growth of either the head or chest is of concern. See Figure 8–37 ■. Compare the chest circumference to the head circumference measurement. The head and chest circumferences are expected to be approximately equal until after 1 year of age, when the chest circumference begins to surpass head circumference.

Shape of the Chest

Inspect the chest for any irregularities in shape. A rounded chest is present when the anteroposterior diameter is approximately equal to the lateral diameter. If a rounded chest is found in a child over 2 years of age, a chronic obstructive lung condition such as asthma or cystic fibrosis may be present.

An abnormal chest shape results from two different structural deformities (Figure 8–38 ■ on page 265). If the sternum protrudes, increasing the anteroposterior diameter, pigeon chest (pectus carinatum) may be present. If the lower portion of the sternum is depressed, decreasing the anteroposterior diameter, funnel chest (pectus excavatum) may be present. Scoliosis, curvature of the spine, causes a lateral deviation of the chest (see Chapter 35∞).

Chest Movement and Respiratory Effort

Inspect for simultaneous chest expansion and abdominal rise. Chest movement is normally symmetric bilaterally, rising with

TABLE 8–10 Vertical Landmarks of the Chest

VERTICAL LINES FOR ASSESSING THE CHEST	LOCATION OF VERTICAL LINES
Midsternal	Through the middle of the sternum
Midclavicular	From the middle of the clavicle
Anterior axillary	From the anterior axillary fold
Midaxillary	From the middle of the axilla
Posterior axillary	From the posterior axillary fold
Spinal	Through the spinous processes of the vertebrae

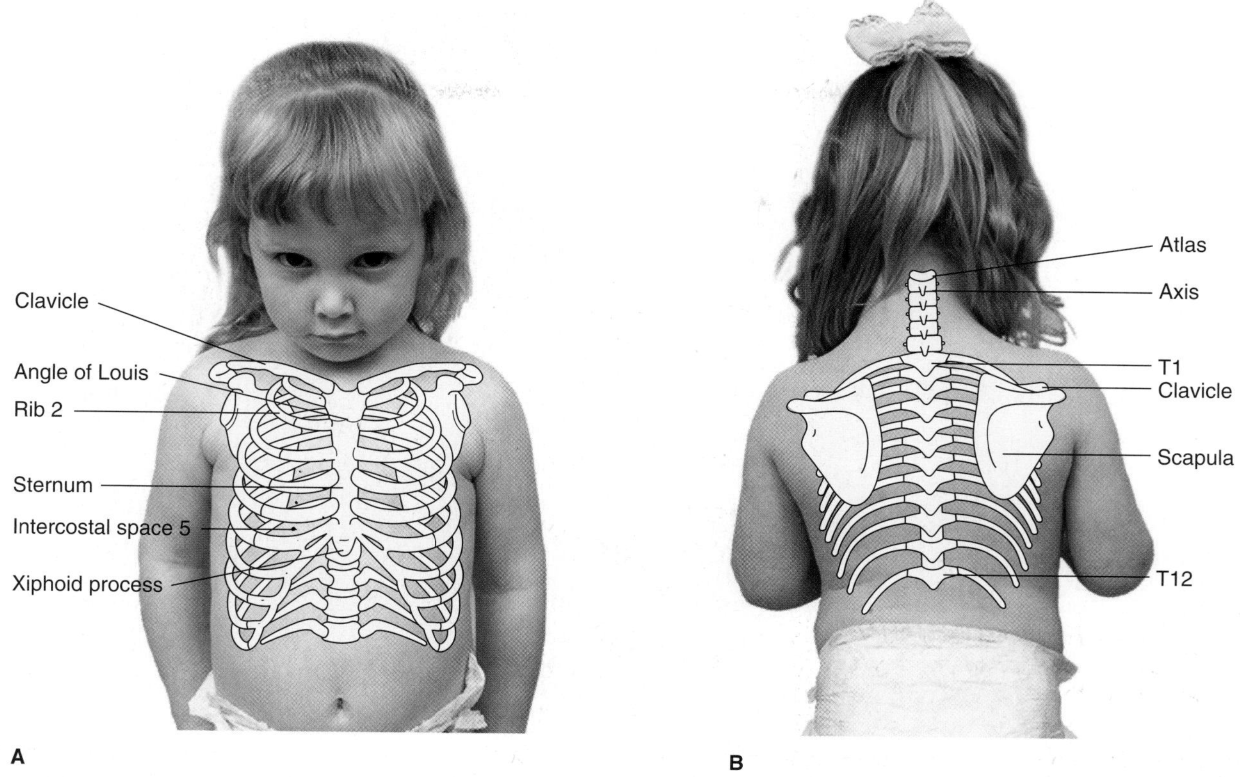

FIGURE 8–35 ■ Intercostal spaces and ribs are numbered to describe the location of findings. *A*, To determine the rib number on the anterior chest, palpate down from the top of the sternum until a horizontal ridge, the angle of Louis, is felt. Directly to the right and left of that ridge is the second rib. The second intercostal space is immediately below the second rib. Ribs 3–12 and the corresponding intercostal spaces can be counted as the fingers move toward the abdomen. *B*, To determine the rib number on the posterior chest, find the protruding spinal process of the seventh cervical vertebra at the shoulder level. The next spinal process belongs to the first thoracic vertebra, which attaches to the first rib.

inspiration and falling with expiration. The chest movement of infants and young children is less pronounced than the abdominal movement. The diaphragm is the primary breathing muscle in infants and children under 6 years old. The thoracic muscles are less developed and serve as accessory muscles in cases of respiratory distress. As the thoracic muscles develop, they become primarily responsible for ventilation. On inspiration the chest and abdomen should rise simultaneously. Asymmetric chest rise is associated with a collapsed lung. **Retractions,** indentations between the ribs during each inspiration, are seen when the accessory muscles are used for breathing in cases of respiratory distress.

Respiratory Rate. Because young children use the diaphragm as the primary breathing muscle, observe or feel the rise and fall of the abdomen to count the respiratory rate in children under age 6 years. Table 8–11 gives the normal respiratory rates for each age group. Make every effort to count the respiratory rate when the child is quiet. The respiratory rate rises in response to excitement, fear, respiratory distress, fever, and other conditions that increase oxygen needs.

Infants and children have a faster respiratory rate than adults because of a higher metabolic rate and need for oxygen. Young children are also unable to increase the depth of respirations because not all the alveoli are developed (Hazinski, 1999).

A sustained respiratory rate greater than 60 breaths per minute is an important sign of respiratory distress. At that rate, children develop hypoxemia if treatment is not started. The child's airway is very narrow, resulting in higher airway resistance than occurs in adults.

CLINICAL TIP

When the respiratory rate exceeds 60 breaths per minute, inadequate amounts of oxygen reach the alveoli for gas exchange because airway resistance prevents passage of oxygen into the lower airways (Eichelberger, Ball, Pratsch, et al., 1998).

TABLE 8–11 Normal Respiratory Rate Ranges for Each Age Group

AGE	RESPIRATORY RATE PER MINUTE
Newborn	30–60
1 year	20–40
3 years	20–30
6 years	16–22
10 years	16–20
17 years	12–20

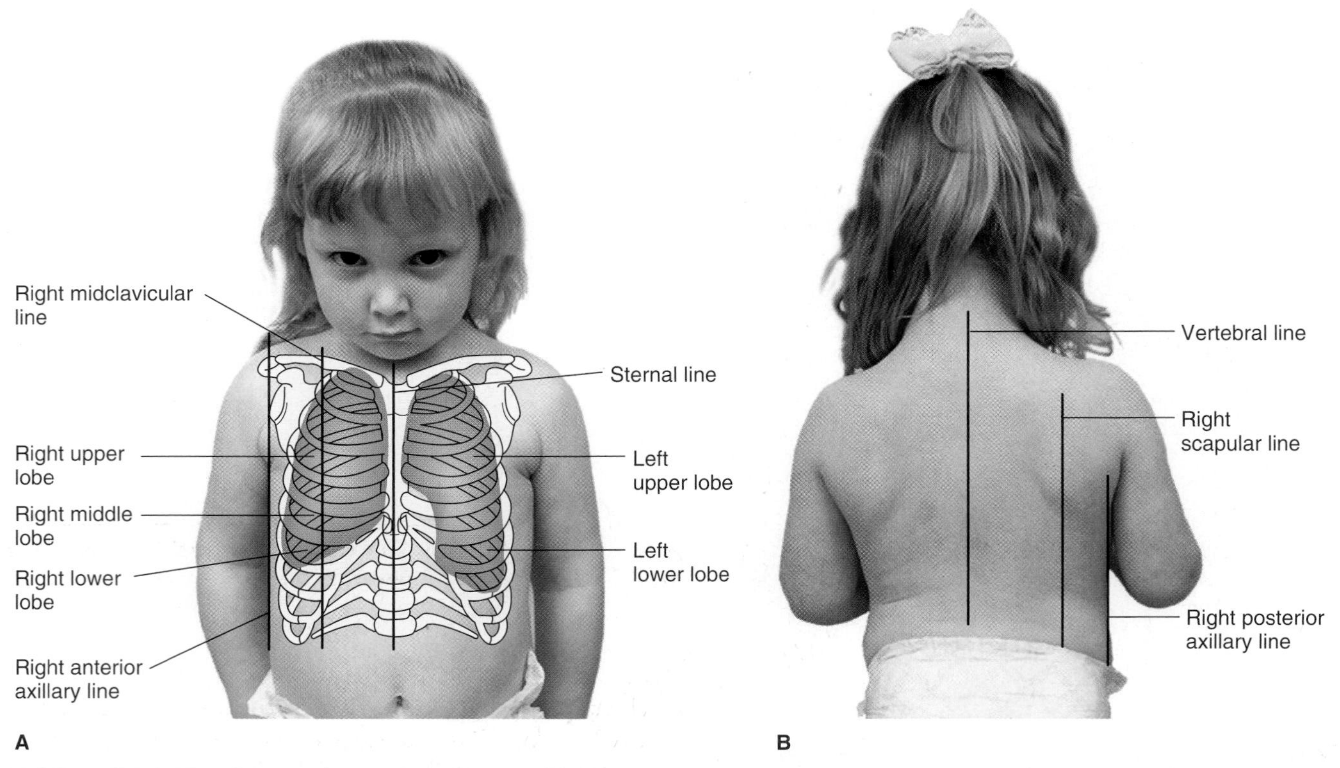

FIGURE 8–36 ■ The sternum and spine are the vertical landmarks used to describe the anatomic location of findings. The distance between the finding and the center of the sternum (midsternal line) or the spinal line can be measured with a ruler. Imaginary vertical lines, parallel to the midsternal and spinal lines, are used to further describe the location of the findings.

Palpation of the Chest

Palpation is used to evaluate chest movement, respiratory effort, deformities of the chest wall, and tactile fremitus.

Chest Wall

To palpate the chest motion with respiration, place the palms of your hands with fingers spread on each side of the child's chest. Confirm the bilateral symmetry of chest motion. Use your fingerpads to palpate any depressions, bulges, or unusual chest wall shape that might indicate abnormal findings such as tenderness, cysts, other growths, crepitus, or fractures. None should be found. **Crepitus,** a crinkly sensation palpated on the chest surface, is caused by air escaping into the subcutaneous tissues. It often indicates a serious injury to the upper or lower airway. Crepitus may also be felt near a fracture.

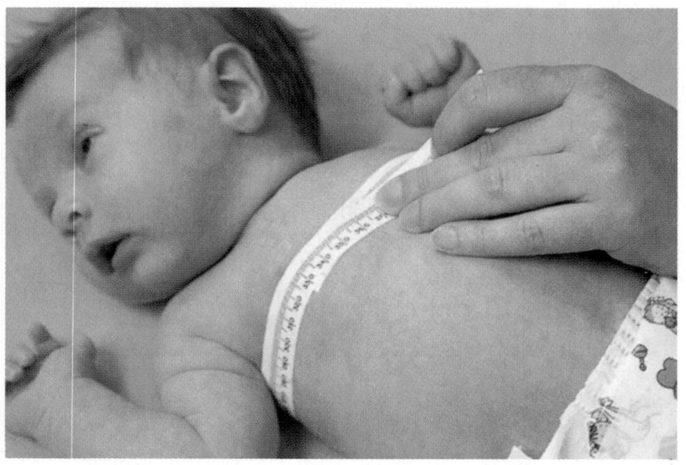

FIGURE 8–37 ■ Measure the chest with a tape measure placed just under the axilla and at the nipple line. Record the circumference to the nearest 0.5 cm or 1/8 inch.

Tactile Fremitus

Crying and talking produce vibrations, known as **tactile fremitus,** that can be palpated on the chest. Place the palms of your hands on each side of the chest to evaluate the quality and distribution of these vibrations. Ask the child to repeat a series of words or numbers, such as Mickey Mouse or ice cream. As the child repeats the words, move your hands systematically over the anterior and posterior chest, comparing the quality of findings side to side. The vibration or tingling sensation is normally palpated over the entire chest. Decreased sensations indicate that air is trapped in the lungs, as occurs with asthma. Increased sensations indicate lung consolidation, as occurs with pneumonia.

Auscultation of the Chest

Auscultate the chest with a stethoscope to assess the quality and characteristics of breath sounds, to identify abnormal breath sounds, and to evaluate vocal resonance. Use an infant or pediatric stethoscope when available to help you localize any unexpected breath sounds. Use the stethoscope diaphragm because it transmits the high-pitched breath sounds more clearly.

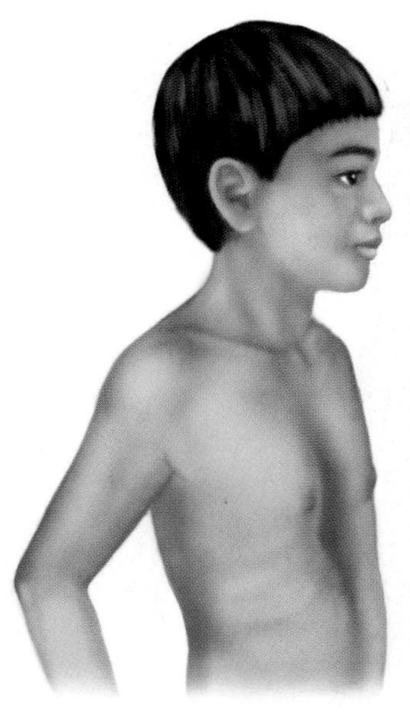

A

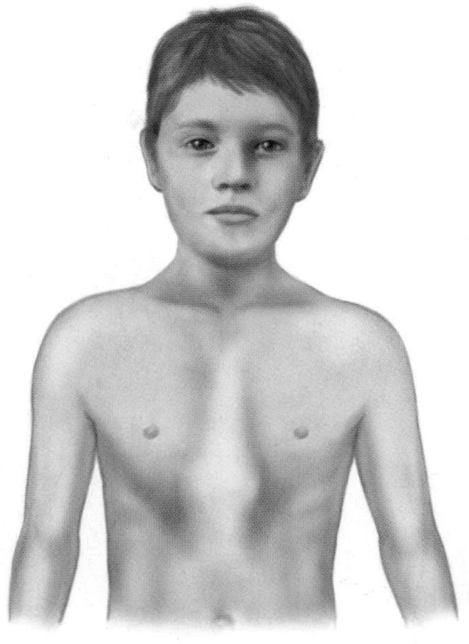

B

FIGURE 8–38 ■ Two types of abnormal chest shape. *A,* Pectus excavatum (Funnel chest) *B,* Pectus carinatum (Pigeon chest).

PRACTICE ALERT

Auscultation of breath sounds is difficult when an infant is crying. First try to quiet the infant with a pacifier, bottle, or toy. If the infant continues to cry, all is not lost. At the end of each cry the infant takes a deep breath, which you can use to assess breath sounds, vocal resonance, and tactile fremitus. Encourage toddlers and preschoolers to take slow, deep breaths by providing a pinwheel or mobile to blow.

Breath Sounds

Evaluate the quality and characteristics of breath sounds over the entire chest, comparing sounds between the sides. Select a routine sequence for auscultating the entire chest so you will consistently assess all lobes of the lungs and lateral lung fields. Figure 8–39 ■ shows one suggested chest auscultation sequence. Listen to an entire inspiratory and expiratory phase at each spot on the chest before you move to the next site. When trying to encourage the child to breathe normally while auscultating the chest, use suggestive language to increase cooperation: "You certainly are good at breathing slowly. Have you been practicing?" The child will often deepen and slow the breathing pattern as you draw attention to it and give praise.

CLINICAL TIP

Another method to gain cooperation for auscultation and to hear expiratory sounds is to have the child blow a piece of tissue off of your hand. This may enhance auscultation of subtle wheezes that occur at the end of expiration.

Three types of normal breath sounds are usually heard when the chest is auscultated. *Vesicular* breath sounds are low-pitched, swishing, soft, short expiratory sounds. They are usually heard in older children but not in infants and young children. *Bronchovesicular* breath sounds are medium-pitched, hollow, blowing sounds heard equally on inspiration and expiration in all age groups. The location of these sounds on the chest is related to the child's developmental status. *Bronchial/tracheal* breath sounds are hollow and higher pitched than vesicular breath sounds.

Breath sounds normally have equal intensity, pitch, and rhythm bilaterally. Absent or diminished breath sounds generally indicate a partial or total obstruction, such as from a foreign body or mucus that does not permit airflow.

PRACTICE ALERT

Infants and young children have a thin chest wall because of immature muscle development. The breath sounds of one lung are heard over the entire chest. It takes practice to accurately identify absent or diminished breath sounds in infants and young children. Because the distance is greatest between the apices and midaxillary areas in young children, these sites are best for identifying absent or diminished breath sounds in a lung. Carefully auscultate, comparing the quality of breath sounds heard bilaterally.

Vocal Resonance

Auscultate the chest to evaluate how well voice sounds are transmitted. Have the child repeat a series of words, either the same as or different from those used for evaluating tactile fremitus. Use the stethoscope to auscultate the chest, comparing the quality of sounds from side to side and over the entire chest. Voice sounds, with words and syllables muffled and indistinct, are normally heard throughout the chest.

If voice sounds are absent or more muffled than usual, an airway obstruction such as asthma may be present. When a lung consolidation condition such as pneumonia is present, the vocal resonance quality changes in characteristic ways. These abnormal characteristics are called whispered pectoriloquy, bronchophony, and egophony. **Whispered pectoriloquy** is present when syllables are heard distinctly in a whisper. **Bronchophony**

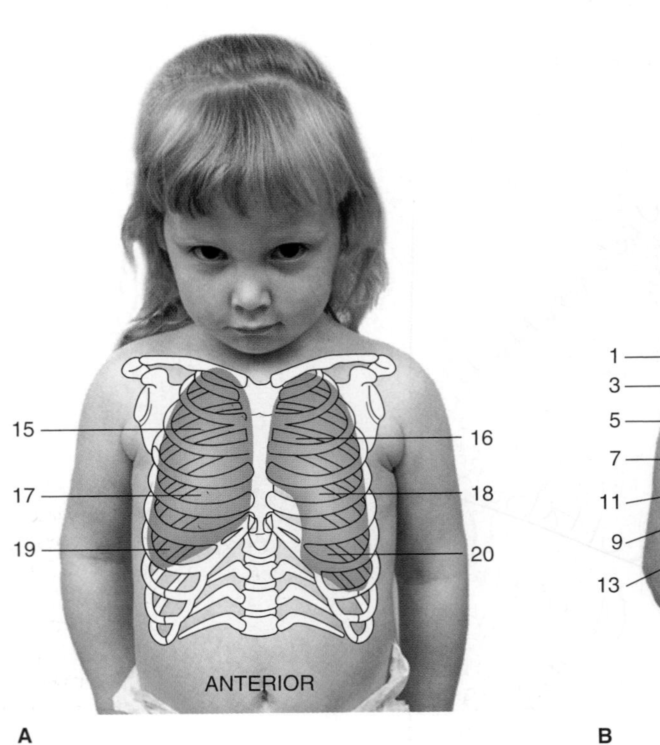

FIGURE 8–39 ■ One example of a sequence for auscultation of the chest.

is the increased intensity and clarity of sounds while the words remain indistinct. **Egophony** is the transmission of the "eee" sound as a nasal "ay" sound.

Abnormal Breath Sounds

Abnormal breath sounds, also called adventitious sounds, generally indicate the presence of a disease process. Examples of abnormal breath sounds are crackles, rhonchi, and friction rubs. To further assess abnormal breath sounds, determine their location, the respiratory phase in which they are present, duration, intensity, and whether they change or disappear when the child coughs or shifts position. To routinely identify these adventitious sounds takes practice. Absent or diminished breath sounds may indicate a pneumothorax or airway obstruction. Table 8–12 describes adventitious sounds.

Abnormal Voice Sounds

Observing the quality of the voice and other audible sounds is also important during an examination of the lungs. Examples of these sounds are hoarseness, wheezing, stridor, and cough. **Stridor** is a noise resulting from air moving through a narrowed trachea and larynx. It is a high-pitched crowing sound often associated with croup. **Wheezing** is a noise resulting from the passage of air through mucus or fluids in a narrowed lower airway; it is associated with asthma. A cough is a reflexive clearing of the airway associated with a respiratory infection. Hoarseness is associated with inflammation of the larynx.

Percussion of the Chest

Percussion is a method sometimes used to assess the resonance of the lungs and the density of underlying organs, such as the heart

TABLE 8–12 Description of Adventitious Sounds Heard When Auscultating the Chest

TYPE	DESCRIPTION	CAUSE
Fine crackles	High-pitched, discrete, noncontinuous sound heard at end of inspiration *(Rub pieces of hair together beside your ear to duplicate the sound.)*	Air passing through watery secretions in the smaller airways (alveoli and bronchioles)
Sibilant rhonchi	Musical, squeaking, or hissing noise heard during inspiration or expiration, but generally louder on expiration	Bronchospasm or an anatomic, narrowing of the trachea, bronchi, or bronchioles
Sonorous rhonchi	Coarse, low-pitched sound like a snore, heard during inspiration or expiration; may clear with coughing	Air passing through thick secretions that partially obstruct the larger bronchi and trachea

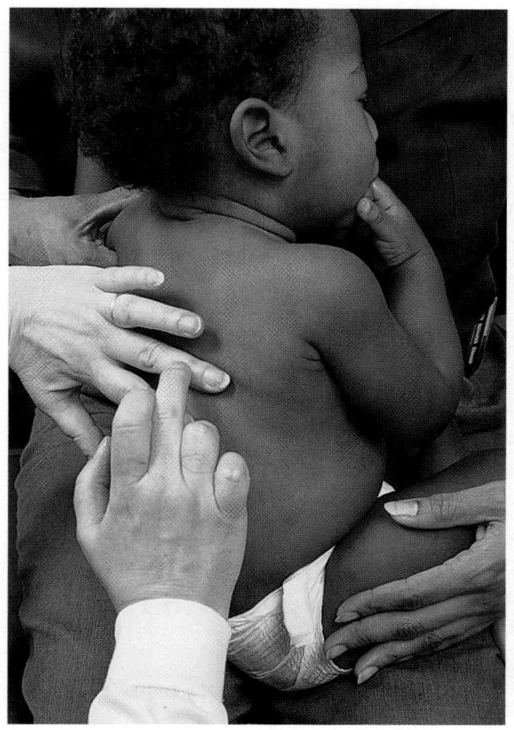
A

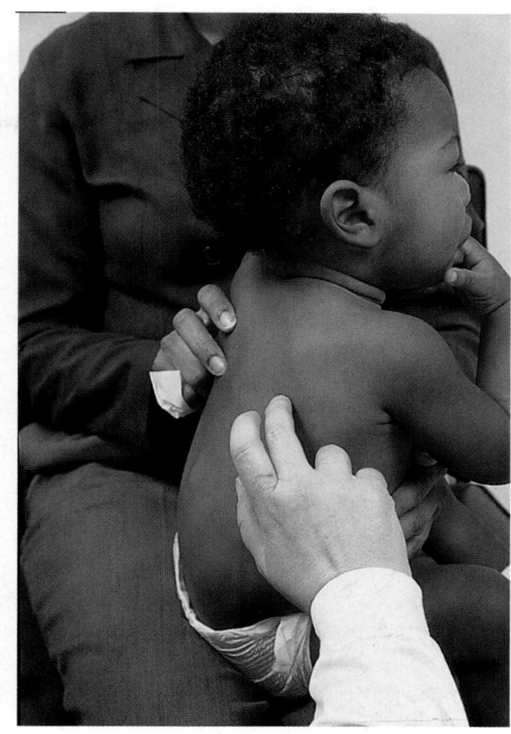
B

FIGURE 8–40 ■ *A*, Indirect percussion. Place the middle finger on the child's chest at an intercostal space with the other fingers off of the chest. Tap the finger with a springlike motion with the fingertip of the other hand. *B*, Direct percussion. Tap the infant's chest with the fingertip directly at an intercostal space.

and liver. There is currently less reliance on percussion to evaluate the lungs because of the frequent use of radiograph examination.

When percussing the anterior and posterior chest, choose a sequence that covers the entire chest and permits comparison bilaterally. The same sequence as that used for auscultation is effective. To perform *indirect percussion*, lay the middle finger of your nondominant hand on the child's chest at an intercostal space. Keep the other fingers off the chest. With a springlike motion, use the fingertip of your other hand to tap the finger in contact with the chest (Figure 8–40A ■). *Direct percussion* is a technique effective for infants. Tap the chest at an intercostal space with a fingertip to elicit the quality of resonance (Figure 8–40B ■).

Characteristic patterns of percussion resonance are expected (Figure 8–41 ■). Characteristic descriptions of sounds heard with percussion of the chest include tympany, flatness, dullness, resonance, and hyperresonance.

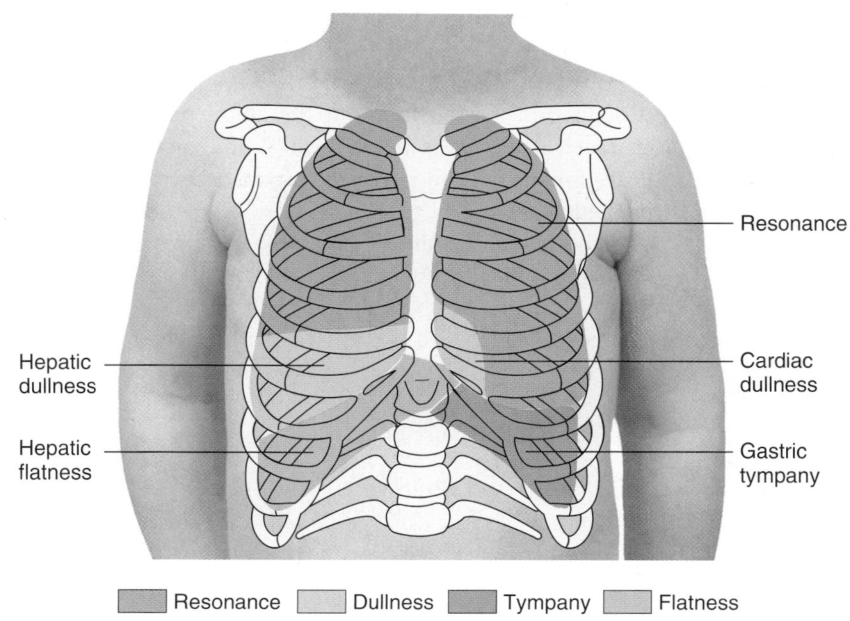

FIGURE 8–41 ■ Normal resonance patterns expected over the chest. *Tympany* is a loud, high-pitched sound, like a drum. It is usually heard over an air-filled stomach. *Flatness* is a soft, dull sound, like the sound made when percussing your thigh. It is heard over dense muscle and bone. *Dullness* is a moderately loud, thudlike sound. It is heard when percussing over the liver and heart, and at the base of the lungs (at the level of the diaphragm). *Resonance* is a loud, low-pitched, hollow sound, like the sound made when percussing a table. It is heard over the lungs. *Hyperresonance* is a loud, very low-pitched, booming sound. It is usually heard over superinflated lungs. However, because of the thin chest wall in young children, hyperresonance may be a normal finding.

Breasts

What does breast tissue feel like? Do boys have breast development during puberty? See page 281 for the assessment of pubertal development.

Inspection

The nipples of prepubertal boys and girls are symmetrically located near the midclavicular line at the fourth to sixth ribs. There is no palpable breast tissue. The areola is normally round and more darkly pigmented than the surrounding skin. Inspect the anterior chest for other dark spots that may be supernumerary nipples, which are small, undeveloped nipples and areola that may be mistaken for moles. Occasionally there may be a fully developed nipple and areola. Supernumary nipples can occur anywhere along the mammary line, from the neck to the pubic area. Their presence may be associated with congenital renal or cardiac anomalies.

Palpation

The developing breasts of adolescent females are palpated for abnormal masses or hard nodules. While the adolescent is lying down with one arm behind the neck, palpate the breast and axilla on that side. Palpate in a concentric pattern covering all quadrants of the breast including the axilla, all around the areola, and then around the nipple. Gently squeeze the nipple to assess for discharge. Repeat the procedure on the opposite breast. Breast tissue normally feels dense, firm, and elastic. Any masses need further investigation, but are usually not malignancies. The physical examination is a good opportunity to teach adolescent females how to perform self-breast examination.

The majority of boys have unilateral or bilateral breast enlargement during adolescence (gynecomastia), generally most noticeable around 14 years of age. The breast tissue generally regresses by the time of full sexual maturity. Palpate the tissue to differentiate actual breast tissue from fatty tissue in the pectoral area, and to detect any masses.

ASSESSING THE HEART FOR HEART SOUNDS AND FUNCTION

What is the point of maximum intensity and where is it located? Where are the pulse points to assess pulse quality? What heart sounds are associated with systole and diastole? What is the normal heart rate of infants and children? What is the difference between heart sounds and murmurs? Equipment needed for the heart examination includes a stethoscope and sphygmomanometer.

Inspection of the Precordium

Begin the heart examination by inspecting the precordium, or anterior chest. Place the child in a reclining or semi-Fowler's position, either on the parent's lap or on the examining table. Inspect the shape and symmetry of the anterior chest from the front and side views. The rib cage is normally symmetric. Bulging of the left side of the chest wall may indicate an enlarged heart.

Observe for any chest movement associated with the heart's contraction. The apical impulse, sometimes called the point of maximum intensity, is located where the left ventricle taps the chest wall during contraction. The apical impulse can normally be seen in thin children. A **heave,** an obvious lifting of the chest wall during contraction, may indicate an enlarged heart.

Palpation of the Precordium

Place the entire palmar surface of the fingers together on the chest wall to palpate the precordium. Systematically palpate the entire precordium to detect any pulsations, heaves, or vibrations. Palpating with minimal pressure increases the chance of detecting abnormal findings.

Apical Impulse

The apical impulse is the point at which the heart is closest to the anterior chest wall. Use the topographic landmarks of the chest to describe its location. (See Figures 8–35 and 8–36). See Figure 8–42 ■ to visualize the expected location of the apical impulse in infants and children. The apical impulse is sometimes seen on the anterior chest wall, but it is normally felt as a slight tap against one fingertip. Any other sensation palpated is usually abnormal.

Abnormal Sensations

A lift is the sensation of the heart lifting up against the chest wall. It may be associated with an enlarged heart or a heart contracting with extra force. A thrill is a rushing vibration that feels like a cat's purr. It is caused by turbulent blood flow from a defective heart valve and a heart murmur. If present, the thrill is palpated in the right or left second intercostal space. To describe a thrill's location, use the topographic landmarks of the chest (see Figures 8–35 and 8–36) and estimate the diameter of the thrill palpated.

Percussion of the Heart Borders

Percussion of the heart borders is rarely performed during physical examination. The borders of the heart are better identified by radiograph examination. Percussion of the heart may be performed by an experienced examiner.

Auscultation of the Heart

Auscultation is used to count the apical pulse, to assess the characteristics of the heart sounds, and to detect abnormal heart sounds. Use the bell of the stethoscope to detect lower pitched sounds.

To assess heart sounds completely, auscultate the heart with the child in both sitting and reclining positions. Differences in heart sounds caused by a change in the child's position or by a change in the position of the heart near the chest wall can then be detected. If differences in heart sounds are detected with a position change, then place the child in the left lateral recumbent position and auscultate again.

Heart Rate and Rhythm

The apical heart rate can be counted at the site of the apical impulse, either by palpation or by auscultation. Count the apical rate for 1 minute in infants and in children who have an irregular rhythm. The brachial or radial pulse rate should be the same

AS THEY GROW

Location of the Apical Impulse

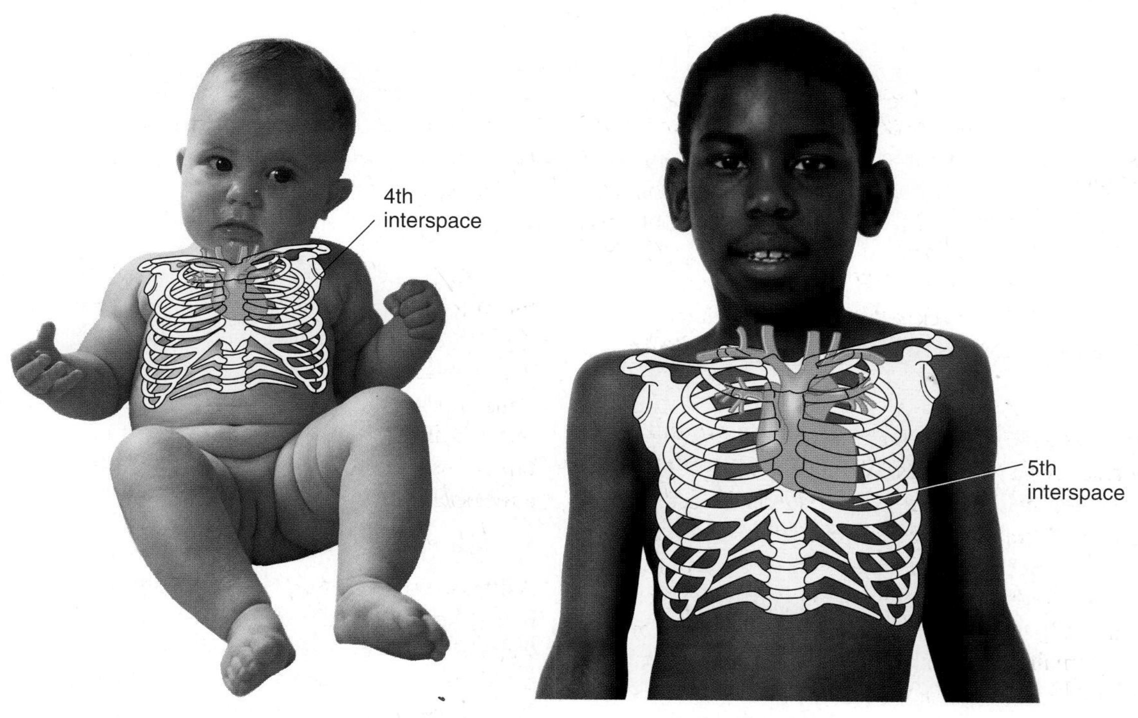

FIGURE 8–42 ■ The location of the apical impulse changes as the child's rib cage grows. In children under 7 years, it is located in the fourth intercostal space just medial to the left midclavicular line. In children over 7 years, it is located in the fifth intercostal space at the left midclavicular line.

as the auscultated apical heart rate. Table 8–13 gives normal heart rates in children of different ages.

Listen carefully to the heart rate rhythm. Children often have a normal cycle of irregular rhythm associated with respiration called *sinus arrhythmia*. With sinus arrhythmia, the child's heart rate is faster on inspiration and slower on expiration. When any rhythm irregularity is detected, ask the child to take a breath and hold it while you listen to the heart rate. The rhythm should become regular during inspiration and expiration. Other rhythm irregularities are abnormal (Box 8–7).

TABLE 8–13 Normal Heart Rates for Children of Different Ages

AGE	HEART RATE RANGE (BEATS/MINUTE)	AVERAGE HEART RATE (BEATS/MINUTE)
Preterm	100–180	110–160 when stabilized
Newborns	100–180	120–160 when stabilized
Infants to 2 years	80–130	110
2–6 years	70–120	100
6–10 years	70–110	90
10–16 years	60–100	85

Differentiation of Heart Sounds

Heart sounds are due to the closure of the valves and vibration or turbulence of blood produced by that valve closure. Two primary sounds, S_1 and S_2, are heard when the chest is auscultated.

S_1, the first heart sound, is produced by closure of the tricuspid and mitral valves when the ventricular contraction begins. The two valves close almost simultaneously; so only one sound is normally heard.

S_2, the second heart sound, is produced by the closure of the aortic and pulmonic valves. Once blood has reached the

BOX 8–7 Response of the Child's Heart Rate to Stresses

The child's heart rate varies with age, decreasing as the child grows older. The heart rate also increases in response to exercise, excitement, anxiety, and fever. Such stresses increase the child's metabolic rate, creating a simultaneous need for more oxygen. Children respond to the need for more oxygen by increasing their heart rate, a response called sinus tachycardia. They cannot increase their cardiac stroke volume to deliver more oxygen to the tissues as adults do.

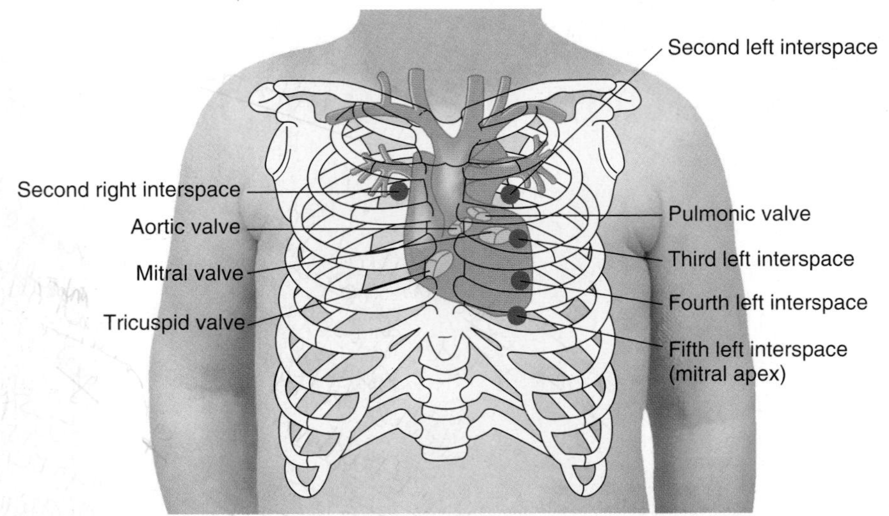

FIGURE 8–43 ■ Sound travels in the direction of blood flow. Rather than listen for heart sounds over each heart valve, auscultate heart sounds at specific areas on the chest wall away from the valve itself. These areas are named for the valve producing the sound. *Aortic*: Second intercostal space near the sternum. *Pulmonic*: Second left intercostal space near the sternum. *Tricuspid*: Fifth right or left intercostal space near the sternum. *Mitral (apical)*: In infants—third or fourth intercostal space, just left of the left midclavicular line; in children—fifth intercostal space at the left midclavicular line.

pulmonic and aortic arteries, the valves close to prevent leakage back into the ventricles during diastole. The timing of the valve closure varies with respirations. Sometimes S_2 is heard as a single sound and at other times as a split sound, that is, two sounds heard a fraction of a second apart.

Sound is easily transmitted in liquid, and it travels best in the direction of blood flow. Auscultate heart sounds at specific areas on the chest wall in the direction of blood flow, just beyond the valve (Figure 8–43 ■). The sounds produced by the heart valves or blood turbulence are heard throughout the chest in thin infants and children. Both S_1 and S_2 can be heard in all listening areas.

Auscultate heart sounds for quality (distinct versus muffled) and intensity (loud versus weak). First, distinguish between S_1 and S_2 in each listening area. Palpate the carotid pulse when auscultating the heart to distinguish between the two heart sounds. The heart sound heard simultaneously with the pulsation is S_1. Heart sounds are usually distinct and crisp in children because of their thin chest wall. Muffling or indistinct sounds may indicate a heart defect or congestive heart failure. Document the area where heart sounds are heard most clearly. Table 8–14 and Figure 8–43 review the location where each sound is normally heard most clearly for assessment of quality and intensity. In a child with a potential murmur, take care to auscultate the heart sounds when the child is in the sitting, reclining, and standing positions.

TABLE 8–14 Identification of the Sites for Auscultating the Quality and Intensity of Heart Sounds

HEART SOUND	LOCATIONS BEST HEARD	WHERE HEARD SOFTLY
S_1	Apex of the heart Tricuspid area Mitral area	Base of the heart Aortic area Pulmonic area
S_2	Base of the heart Aortic area Pulmonic area	Apex of the heart Tricuspid area Mitral area
Physiologic splitting	Pulmonic area	
S_3	Mitral area	

Record the differences in heart sounds auscultated with exercise, postural changes, respirations, or the Valsalva maneuver, as important diagnostic clues may be revealed about a heart condition.

Splitting of the Heart Sounds

After the first and second heart sounds are successfully distinguished, try to detect physiologic splitting. The split second heart sound is more apparent during inspiration when the child takes a deep breath. More blood returns to the right ventricle, causing the pulmonic valve to close a fraction of a second later than the aortic valve. To detect physiologic splitting, auscultate over the pulmonic area while the child breathes normally and then while the child takes a deep breath. Splitting is normally more easily detected after a deep breath. The splitting returns to a single sound with regular breathing. If splitting does not vary with respiration, then it is called fixed splitting, which is an abnormal finding associated with an atrial septal defect.

Third Heart Sound

A third heart sound, S_3, is occasionally heard in children as a normal finding. S_3 occurs when blood rushes through the mitral valve and splashes into the left ventricle. It is heard in diastole, just after S_2. It is distinguished from a split S_2 because it is louder in the mitral area than in the pulmonic area.

Murmurs

Occasionally abnormal heart sounds are auscultated. These sounds are produced by blood passing through a defective valve, great vessel, or other heart structure.

It takes practice to hear murmurs in children. Often murmurs must be very loud to be detected. For softer murmurs, normal heart sounds must be distinguished before an extra sound is recognized. Once a murmur is detected, define the characteristics of the extra sound. Murmurs are classified by the following characteristics.

- *Intensity.* How loud is it? Can a thrill also be palpated? See Table 8–15 for grades of murmur intensity.
- *Location.* Where is the murmur the loudest? Identify the listening area and precise topographic landmarks. Is the child sitting or lying down?

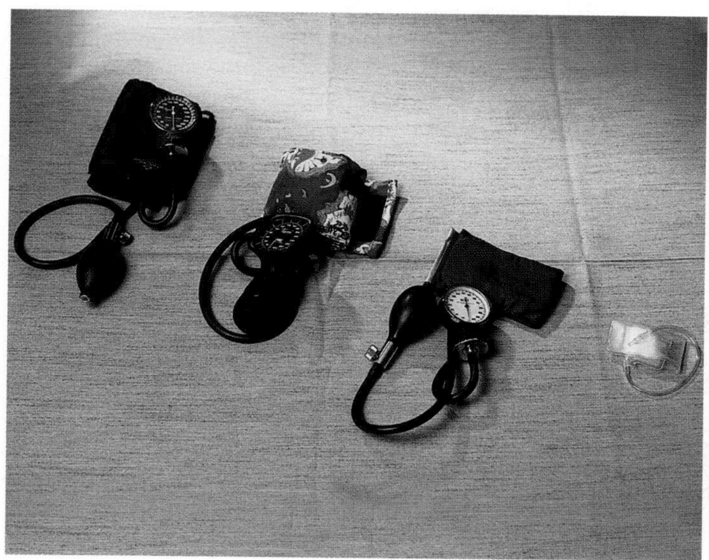

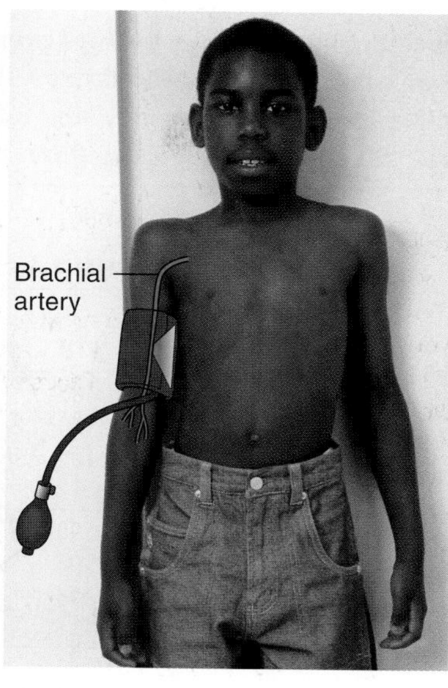

FIGURE 8–44 ■ Choose a cuff with a bladder width that is approximately 40% of the arm circumference of the upper arm. When the cuff is wrapped around the upper arm, the bladder length usually covers 80% to 100% of the arm's circumference.

- *Radiation or transmission.* Is the sound transmitted over a larger area of the chest, to the axilla, or to the back?
- *Timing.* Is the murmur heard best after S_1 or S_2? Is it heard during the entire phase between S_1 and S_2?
- *Quality.* What does the murmur sound like? For example, is it machinelike, musical, or blowing?

Auscultate for a venous hum over the supraclavicular fossa above the middle of the clavicle or over the upper anterior chest with the bell of the stethoscope. A venous hum is heard as a continuous low-pitched hum throughout the cardiac cycle, but it may be loudest during diastole or when the child stands. The hum does not change with respiration, but it may be quieted by having the child turn the neck or by occluding the jugular veins in the neck. A venous hum may be associated with anemia, but it has no pathologic significance.

Completing the Heart Examination

A complete assessment of cardiac function also includes measuring the blood pressure, palpating the pulses, and evaluating signs from other systems.

Blood Pressure

Assessment of blood pressure is important to detect conditions of hypertension or hypovolemic shock. The technique for obtaining the blood pressure in children involves selection of the appropriate cuff size for the size of the extremity used. (Figure 8–44 ■).

The recommended method of blood pressure determination is by auscultation. Use the right arm when possible as this is the arm used consistently for development of blood pressure standard tables. The child should be seated and quiet for 3 to 5 minutes before blood pressure measurement. (Figure 8–45 ■). Take the blood

TABLE 8–15 Guidelines for Grading the Intensity of a Murmur

INTENSITY	DESCRIPTION
Grade I	Barely heard in a quiet room
Grade II	Quiet, but clearly heard
Grade III	Moderately loud, no thrill palpated
Grade IV	Loud, a thrill is usually palpated
Grade V	Very loud, a thrill is easily palpated
Grade VI	Heard without the stethoscope in direct contact with the chest wall

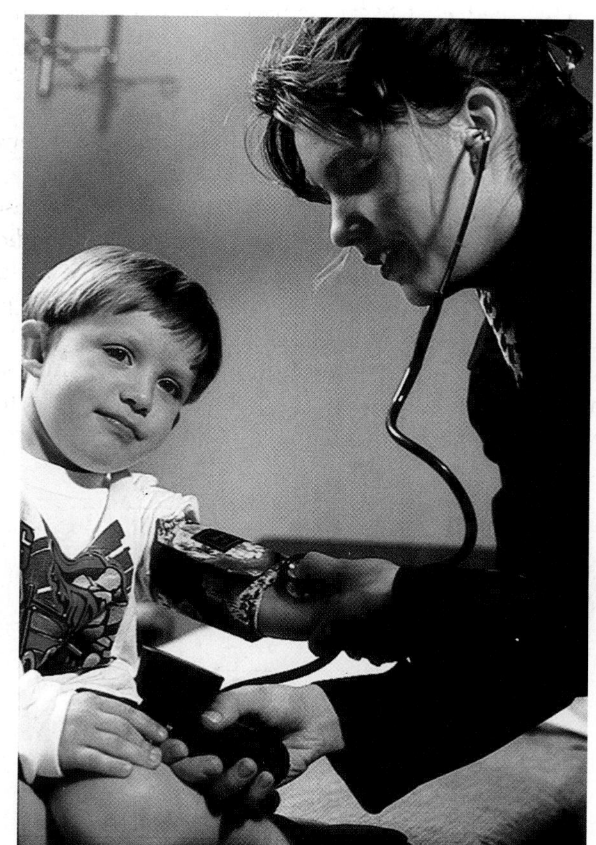

FIGURE 8–45 ■ With the cuff snugly wrapped around the arm, hold the arm with the cubital fossa at the level of the heart.

TABLE 8–16A Blood Pressure Levels for Boys by Age and Height Percentile. Use the child's height percentile for the age and sex from the standard growth charts found in Appendix A. A blood pressure value at 50th percentile for the child's age, sex, and height percentile is considered the midpoint of the normal range. A reading above the 95th percentile indicates hypertension.

		SYSTOLIC BP (mmHg)							DIASTOLIC BP (mmHg)						
		PERCENTILE OF HEIGHT							PERCENTILE OF HEIGHT						
AGE (YEAR)	BP PERCENTILE	5TH	10TH	25TH	50TH	75TH	90TH	95TH	5TH	10TH	25TH	50TH	75TH	90TH	95TH
1	50th	80	81	83	85	87	88	89	34	35	36	37	38	39	39
	90th	94	95	97	99	100	102	103	49	50	51	52	53	53	54
	95th	98	99	101	103	104	106	106	54	54	55	56	57	58	58
	99th	105	106	108	110	112	113	114	61	62	63	64	65	66	66
2	50th	84	85	87	88	90	92	92	39	40	41	42	43	44	44
	90th	97	99	100	102	104	105	106	54	55	56	57	58	58	59
	95th	101	102	104	106	108	109	110	59	59	60	61	62	63	63
	99th	109	110	111	113	115	117	117	66	67	68	69	70	71	71
3	50th	86	87	89	91	93	94	95	44	44	45	46	47	48	48
	90th	100	101	103	105	107	108	109	59	59	60	61	62	63	63
	95th	104	105	107	109	110	112	113	63	63	64	65	66	67	67
	99th	111	112	114	116	118	119	120	71	71	72	73	74	75	75
4	50th	88	89	91	93	95	96	97	47	48	49	50	51	51	52
	90th	102	103	105	107	109	110	111	62	63	64	65	66	66	67
	95th	106	107	109	111	112	114	115	66	67	68	69	70	71	71
	99th	113	114	116	118	120	121	122	74	75	76	77	78	78	79
5	50th	90	91	93	95	96	98	98	50	51	52	53	54	55	55
	90th	104	105	106	108	110	111	112	65	66	67	68	69	69	70
	95th	108	109	110	112	114	115	116	69	70	71	72	73	74	74
	99th	115	116	118	120	121	123	123	77	78	79	80	81	81	82
6	50th	91	92	94	96	98	99	100	53	53	54	55	56	57	57
	90th	105	106	108	110	111	113	113	68	68	69	70	71	72	72
	95th	109	110	112	114	115	117	117	72	72	73	74	75	76	76
	99th	116	117	119	121	123	124	125	80	80	81	82	83	84	84
7	50th	92	94	95	97	99	100	101	55	55	56	57	58	59	59
	90th	106	107	109	111	113	114	115	70	70	71	72	73	74	74
	95th	110	111	113	115	117	118	119	74	74	75	76	77	78	78
	99th	117	118	120	122	124	125	126	82	82	83	84	85	86	86
8	50th	94	95	97	99	100	102	102	56	57	58	59	60	60	61
	90th	107	109	110	112	114	115	116	71	72	72	73	74	75	76
	95th	111	112	114	116	118	119	120	75	76	77	78	79	79	80
	99th	119	120	122	123	125	127	127	83	84	85	86	87	87	88
9	50th	95	96	98	100	102	103	104	57	58	59	60	61	61	62
	90th	109	110	112	114	115	117	118	72	73	74	75	76	76	77
	95th	113	114	116	118	119	121	121	76	77	78	79	80	81	81
	99th	120	121	123	125	127	128	129	84	85	86	87	88	88	89

pressure twice and average the two readings. The systolic reading is the onset of Korotkoff sounds. The diastolic reading is the fifth Korotkoff sound or the disappearance of Korotkoff sounds in children and adolescents (National High Blood Pressure Education Program Working Group on Hypertension Control in Children and Adolescents, 1996). In some children, the Korotkoff sounds can be heard to 0 mm Hg which would be the diastolic reading. In this case there is usually a qualitative change in the sounds at some point that should be noted (i.e., 100/52/0). The systolic and diastolic blood pressure reading should be compared to the table of age, sex, and height-specific standard blood pressure values on Table 8–16A & B. Blood pressure values indicating hypertension should be confirmed with repeated readings on several visits.

Automated devices to measure blood pressure commonly use oscillometric methods to measure the systolic blood pressure and the mean arterial blood pressure. The diastolic blood pressure is calculated from these two values. While easy to use, it is important to remember that no blood pressure reference standards exist for these automated devices and they need frequent calibration for reliable readings.

For any child in which there is a concern about a heart condition, obtain a blood pressure reading in both an arm and a leg,

TABLE 8–16A Blood Pressure Levels for Boys by Age and Height Percentile. Use the child's height percentile for the age and sex from the standard growth charts found in Appendix A. A blood pressure value at 50th percentile for the child's age, sex, and height percentile is considered the midpoint of the normal range. A reading above the 95th percentile indicates hypertension. (continued)

		SYSTOLIC BP (mmHg)							DIASTOLIC BP (mmHg)						
		PERCENTILE OF HEIGHT							PERCENTILE OF HEIGHT						
AGE (YEAR)	BP PERCENTILE	5TH	10TH	25TH	50TH	75TH	90TH	95TH	5TH	10TH	25TH	50TH	75TH	90TH	95TH
10	50th	97	98	100	102	103	105	106	58	59	60	61	61	62	63
	90th	111	112	114	115	117	119	119	73	73	74	75	76	77	78
	95th	115	116	117	119	121	122	123	77	78	79	80	81	81	82
	99th	122	123	125	127	128	130	130	85	86	86	88	88	89	90
11	50th	99	100	102	104	105	107	107	59	59	60	61	62	63	63
	90th	113	114	115	117	119	120	121	74	74	75	76	77	78	78
	95th	117	118	119	121	123	124	125	78	78	79	80	81	82	82
	99th	124	125	127	129	130	132	132	86	86	87	88	89	90	90
12	50th	101	102	104	106	108	109	110	59	60	61	62	63	63	64
	90th	115	116	118	120	121	123	123	74	75	75	76	77	78	79
	95th	119	120	122	123	125	127	127	78	79	80	81	82	82	83
	99th	126	127	129	131	133	134	135	86	87	88	89	90	90	91
13	50th	104	105	106	108	110	111	112	60	60	61	62	63	64	64
	90th	117	118	120	122	124	125	126	75	75	76	77	78	79	79
	95th	121	122	124	126	128	129	130	79	79	80	81	82	83	83
	99th	128	130	131	133	135	136	137	87	87	88	89	90	91	91
14	50th	106	107	109	111	113	114	115	60	61	62	63	64	65	65
	90th	120	121	123	125	126	128	128	75	76	77	78	79	79	80
	95th	124	125	127	128	130	132	132	80	80	81	82	83	84	84
	99th	131	132	134	136	138	139	140	87	88	89	90	91	92	92
15	50th	109	110	112	113	115	117	117	61	62	63	64	65	66	66
	90th	122	124	125	127	129	130	131	76	77	78	79	80	80	81
	95th	126	127	129	131	133	134	135	81	81	82	83	84	85	85
	99th	134	135	136	138	140	142	142	88	89	90	91	92	93	93
16	50th	111	112	114	116	118	119	120	63	63	64	65	66	67	67
	90th	125	126	128	130	131	133	134	78	78	79	80	81	82	82
	95th	129	130	132	134	135	137	137	82	83	83	84	85	86	87
	99th	136	137	139	141	143	144	145	90	90	91	92	93	94	94
17	50th	114	115	116	118	120	121	122	65	66	66	67	68	69	70
	90th	127	128	130	132	134	135	136	80	80	81	82	83	84	84
	95th	131	132	134	136	138	139	140	84	85	86	87	87	88	89
	99th	139	140	141	143	145	146	147	92	93	93	94	95	96	97

BP, blood pressure

**The 90th percentile is 1.28 SD, 95th percentile is 1.645 SD, and the 99th percentile is 2.326 SD over the mean.*

National Heart, Lung, and Blood Institute. (2004). Blood pressure tables for children and adolescents from the fourth report on the diagnosis, evaluation, and treatment of high blood pressure in children and adolescents. www.nhlbi.nih.gov/guidelines/hypertension/child_tbl.htm, *accessed 6/11/2004.*

and then compare the readings. The blood pressure in the leg should be the same or up to 10 mm Hg higher than the arm reading. If the reading in the leg is lower than the arm, coarctation of the aorta may be present.

Palpation of the Pulses

Palpate the characteristics of the pulses in the extremities to assess the circulation. The technique and sites for palpating the pulse are the same as those used for adults (Figure 8–46 ■ on page 276). Infants have a low systolic blood pressure, and detecting the distal pulses is often difficult. Use the brachial artery in the arms and the popliteal or femoral artery in the legs to evaluate the pulses. The radial and tibial pulses are normally palpated easily in older children. Evaluate the pulsation for rate, regularity of rhythm, and strength in each extremity and compare your findings bilaterally.

Palpate the femoral arteries and compare their strength with the strength of the brachial or radial pulse. The femoral pulsations are usually stronger than or as strong as the brachial pulsations. A weaker femoral pulse is associated with coarctation of the aorta.

TABLE 8–16B Blood Pressure Levels for Girls by Age and Height Percentile. Use the child's height percentile for the age and sex from the standard growth charts found in Appendix A. A blood pressure value at 50th percentile for the child's age, sex, and height percentile is considered the midpoint of the normal range. A reading above the 95th percentile indicates hypertension.

		SYSTOLIC BP (mmHg)							DIASTOLIC BP (mmHg)						
		PERCENTILE OF HEIGHT							PERCENTILE OF HEIGHT						
AGE (YEAR)	BP PERCENTILE	5TH	10TH	25TH	50TH	75TH	90TH	95TH	5TH	10TH	25TH	50TH	75TH	90TH	95TH
1	50th	83	84	85	86	88	89	90	38	39	39	40	41	41	42
	90th	97	97	98	100	101	102	103	52	53	53	54	55	55	56
	95th	100	101	102	104	105	106	107	56	57	57	58	59	59	60
	99th	108	108	109	111	112	113	114	64	64	65	65	66	67	67
2	50th	85	85	87	88	89	91	91	43	44	44	45	46	46	47
	90th	98	99	100	101	103	104	105	57	58	58	59	60	61	61
	95th	102	103	104	105	107	108	109	61	62	62	63	64	65	65
	99th	109	110	111	112	114	115	117	69	69	70	70	71	72	72
3	50th	86	87	88	89	91	92	93	47	48	48	49	50	50	51
	90th	100	100	102	103	104	106	106	61	62	62	63	64	64	65
	95th	104	104	105	107	108	109	110	65	66	66	67	68	68	69
	99th	111	111	113	114	115	116	117	73	73	74	74	75	76	76
4	50th	88	88	90	91	92	94	94	50	50	51	52	52	53	54
	90th	101	102	103	104	106	107	108	64	64	65	66	67	67	68
	95th	105	106	107	108	110	111	112	68	68	69	70	71	71	72
	99th	112	113	114	115	117	118	119	76	76	76	77	78	79	79
5	50th	89	90	91	93	94	95	96	52	53	53	54	55	55	56
	90th	103	103	105	106	107	109	109	66	67	67	68	69	69	70
	95th	107	107	108	110	111	112	113	70	71	71	72	73	73	74
	99th	114	114	116	117	118	120	120	78	78	79	79	80	81	81
6	50th	91	92	93	94	96	97	98	54	54	55	56	56	57	58
	90th	104	105	106	108	109	110	111	68	68	69	70	70	71	72
	95th	108	109	110	111	113	114	115	72	72	73	74	74	75	76
	99th	115	116	117	119	120	121	122	80	80	80	81	82	83	83
7	50th	93	93	95	96	97	99	99	55	56	56	57	58	58	59
	90th	106	107	108	109	111	112	113	69	70	70	71	72	72	73
	95th	110	111	112	113	115	116	116	73	74	74	75	76	76	77
	99th	117	118	119	120	122	123	124	81	81	82	82	83	84	84
8	50th	95	95	96	98	99	100	101	57	57	57	58	59	60	60
	90th	108	109	110	111	113	114	114	71	71	71	72	73	74	74
	95th	112	112	114	115	116	118	118	75	75	75	76	77	78	78
	99th	119	120	121	122	123	125	125	82	82	83	83	84	85	86
9	50th	96	97	98	100	101	102	103	58	58	58	59	60	61	61
	90th	110	110	112	113	114	116	116	72	72	72	73	74	75	75
	95th	114	114	115	117	118	119	120	76	76	76	77	78	79	79
	99th	121	121	123	124	125	127	127	83	83	84	84	85	86	87

Other Signs

To assess the heart and tissue perfusion, other signs should be considered. These signs include skin color, capillary refill, and respiratory distress. The mucous membranes are usually pink. Cyanosis is most commonly associated with a congenital heart defect in children. Capillary refill is normally less than 2 seconds, indicating good circulation and perfusion of the tissues. Signs of respiratory distress, such as tachypnea, flaring, and retractions, may be associated with the child's attempts to compensate for hypoxemia caused by a congenital heart defect.

ASSESSING THE ABDOMEN FOR SHAPE, BOWEL SOUNDS, AND UNDERLYING ORGANS

What does a sunken abdomen indicate? What do bowel sounds normally sound like? How frequently should bowel sounds be heard in children? What do the various percussion tones indicate? What does a rigid abdomen indicate?

Topographic Landmarks of the Abdomen

The location of underlying organs and structures of the abdomen must be considered upon examination. The abdomen

TABLE 8–16B Blood Pressure Levels for Girls by Age and Height Percentile. Use the child's height percentile for the age and sex from the standard growth charts found in Appendix A. A blood pressure value at 50th percentile for the child's age, sex, and height percentile is considered the midpoint of the normal range. A reading above the 95th percentile indicates hypertension. (continued)

		SYSTOLIC BP (mmHg)							DIASTOLIC BP (mmHg)						
		PERCENTILE OF HEIGHT							PERCENTILE OF HEIGHT						
AGE (YEAR)	BP PERCENTILE	5TH	10TH	25TH	50TH	75TH	90TH	95TH	5TH	10TH	25TH	50TH	75TH	90TH	95TH
10	50th	98	99	100	102	103	104	105	59	59	59	60	61	62	62
	90th	112	112	114	115	116	118	118	73	73	73	74	75	76	76
	95th	116	116	117	119	120	121	122	77	77	77	78	79	80	80
	99th	123	123	125	126	127	129	129	84	84	85	86	86	87	88
11	50th	100	101	102	103	105	106	107	60	60	60	61	62	63	63
	90th	114	114	116	117	118	119	120	74	74	74	75	76	77	77
	95th	118	118	119	121	122	123	124	78	78	78	79	80	81	81
	99th	125	125	126	128	129	130	131	85	85	86	87	87	88	89
12	50th	102	103	104	105	107	108	109	61	61	61	62	63	64	64
	90th	116	116	117	119	120	121	122	75	75	75	76	77	78	78
	95th	119	120	121	123	124	125	126	79	79	79	80	81	82	82
	99th	127	127	128	130	131	132	133	86	86	87	88	88	89	90
13	50th	104	105	106	107	109	110	110	62	62	62	63	64	65	65
	90th	117	118	119	121	122	123	124	76	76	76	77	78	79	79
	95th	121	122	123	124	126	127	128	80	80	80	81	82	83	83
	99th	128	129	130	132	133	134	135	87	87	88	89	89	90	91
14	50th	106	106	107	109	110	111	112	63	63	63	64	65	66	66
	90th	119	120	121	122	124	125	125	77	77	77	78	79	80	80
	95th	123	123	125	126	127	129	129	81	81	81	82	83	84	84
	99th	130	131	132	133	135	136	136	88	88	89	90	90	91	92
15	50th	107	108	109	110	111	113	113	64	64	64	65	66	67	67
	90th	120	121	122	123	125	126	127	78	78	78	79	80	81	81
	95th	124	125	126	127	129	130	131	82	82	82	83	84	85	85
	99th	131	132	133	134	136	137	138	89	89	90	91	91	92	93
16	50th	108	108	110	111	112	114	114	64	64	65	66	66	67	68
	90th	121	122	123	124	126	127	128	78	78	79	80	81	81	82
	95th	125	126	127	128	130	131	132	82	82	83	84	85	85	86
	99th	132	133	134	135	137	138	139	90	90	90	91	92	93	93
17	50th	108	109	110	111	113	114	115	64	65	65	66	67	67	68
	90th	122	122	123	125	126	127	128	78	79	79	80	81	81	82
	95th	125	126	127	129	130	131	132	82	83	83	84	85	85	86
	99th	133	133	134	136	137	138	139	90	90	91	91	92	93	93

BP, blood pressure

**The 90th percentile is 1.28 SD, 95th percentile is 1.645 SD, and the 99th percentile is 2.326 SD over the mean.*

National Heart, Lung, and Blood Institute. (2004). Blood pressure tables for children and adolescents from the fourth report on the diagnosis, evaluation, and treatment of high blood pressure in children and adolescents. www.nhlbi.nih.gov/guidelines/hypertension/child_tbl.htm, *accessed 6/11/2004.*

is commonly divided by imaginary lines into quadrants for the purpose of identifying underlying structures (Figure 8–47 ■ on page 277). A stethoscope is needed to examine the abdomen.

Inspection of the Abdomen

Begin the examination of the abdomen by inspecting the shape and contour, condition of the umbilicus and rectus muscle, and abdominal movement. Inspect the child's abdomen from the front and side with good lighting. Inspection and auscultation of the abdomen are performed before palpation and percussion because touching the abdomen may change the characteristics of the bowel sounds.

Shape

Inspect the shape of the abdomen to identify an abnormal contour. The child's abdomen is normally symmetric and rounded or flat when the child is supine. A scaphoid or sunken abdomen is abnormal and may indicate dehydration or a diaphragmatic hernia in a newborn.

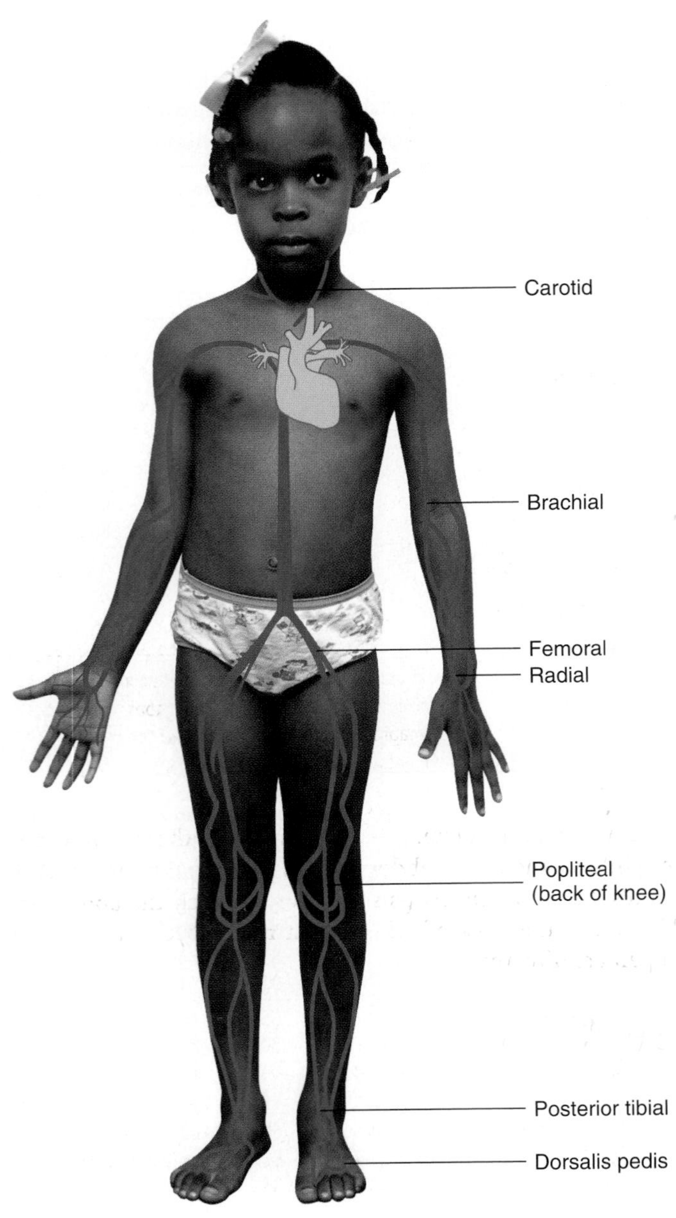

FIGURE 8–46 ■ The sites used to assess pulses in children.

Umbilicus

Inspect the umbilicus in older infants and toddlers. Children in these age groups often have an umbilical hernia, a protrusion of abdominal contents through an open umbilical muscle ring.

Rectus Muscle

Inspect the abdominal wall for any depression or bulging at midline above or below the umbilicus, indicating diastasis or separation of the rectus abdominis muscles. The depression may be up to 5 cm (2 in.) wide. Measure the width of the separation to monitor change over time. As abdominal muscle strength develops, the separation usually becomes less prominent. However, the splitting may persist if congenital muscle weakness is present.

Abdominal Movement

Infants and children up to 6 years of age breathe with the diaphragm. The abdomen rises with inspiration and falls with expiration, simultaneously with the chest rise and fall. When the abdomen does not rise as expected, peritonitis may be present.

Other abdominal movements such as peristaltic waves are abnormal. Peristaltic waves are visible rhythmic contractions of the intestinal wall smooth muscle, which move food through the digestive tract. Their presence generally indicates an intestinal obstruction, such as pyloric stenosis.

Auscultation of the Abdomen

To evaluate bowel sounds, auscultate the abdomen with the diaphragm of the stethoscope. Bowel sounds normally occur every 10 to 30 seconds. They have a high-pitched, tinkling, metallic quality. Loud gurglings (*borborygmi*) are heard when the child is hungry, and increased sounds are common after eating or drinking. Listen in each quadrant long enough to hear at least one bowel sound. Before determining that bowel sounds are absent, auscultate at least 5 minutes. Absence of bowel sounds may indicate peritonitis or a paralytic ileus. Hyperactive bowel sounds, as many as 15 to 30 sounds per minute, may indicate gastroenteritis or a bowel obstruction.

Next auscultate over the abdominal aorta and the renal arteries for a vascular hum or murmur. No murmur should be heard. A murmur may indicate a narrowed or defective artery.

Percussion of the Abdomen

Use indirect percussion to evaluate borders and sizes of abdominal organs and masses. Percussion is performed with the child supine. Choose a sequence that permits you to systematically percuss the entire abdomen (see Figure 8–48 ■).

Different tones are expected when the abdomen is percussed, depending on the underlying structures. *Dullness* is found over organs such as the liver, spleen, and a full bladder. *Tympany* is found over the stomach or the intestines when an obstruction is present. It may also be found over areas beyond the stomach in infants because of air swallowing. *Resonance* may be heard over other areas.

Organ size can be identified by listening for a percussion tone change at the border of an organ. For example, when you percuss down the chest, the upper edge of the liver is usually detected by a tone change from resonant to dull near the fifth intercostal space at the right midclavicular line. The lower liver edge is usually detected 2 to 3 cm (about 1 in.) below the right costal margin in infants and toddlers, but closer to the costal margin in older children. The expected liver span from the upper edge to the lower edge at the midclavicular line by age is found in Table 8–17.

Palpation of the Abdomen

Both light and deep palpation are used to examine the abdomen's organs and to detect any masses. *Light palpation* is used to evaluate the tenseness of the abdomen (how soft or hard it is), the liver, the presence of any tenderness or masses, and any defects in the abdominal wall. *Deep palpation* is used to detect

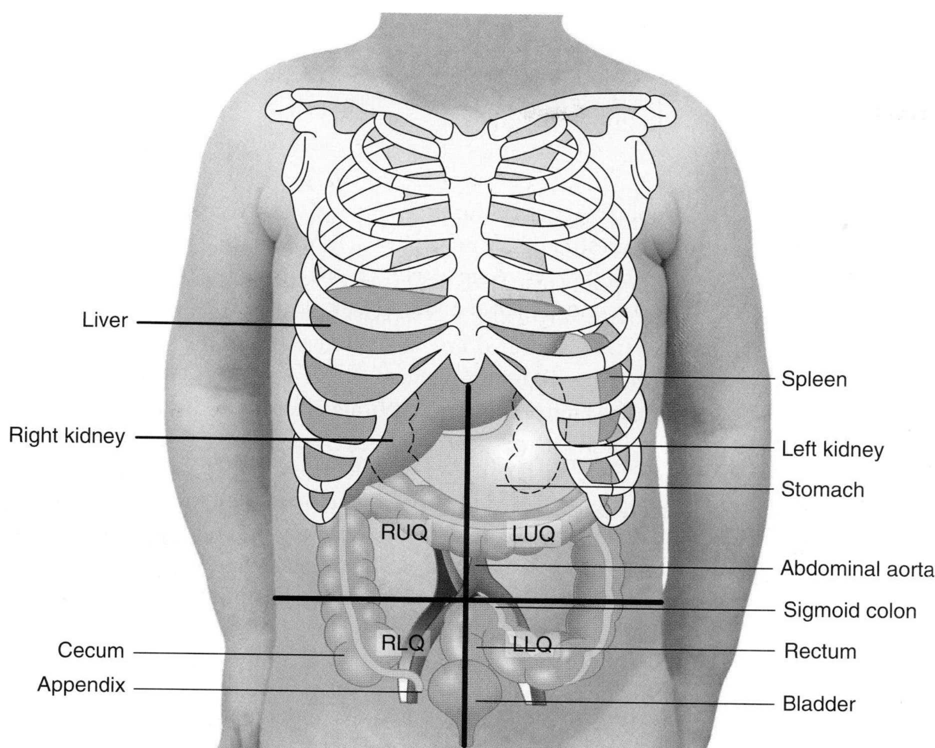

FIGURE 8–47 ■ Topographic landmarks of the abdomen. The abdomen is commonly divided by imaginary lines into quadrants for the purpose of identifying underlying structures.

masses, define their shape and consistency, and identify tenderness in the abdomen.

To make the most accurate interpretation, perform the abdominal examination when the child is calm and cooperative. Organs and other masses are more easily palpated when the abdominal wall is relaxed. Infants and toddlers often feel more secure lying supine across both the parent's and the examiner's laps. A bottle, pacifier, or toy may distract the child and improve cooperation for the examination. When the child is ticklish, some special approaches are needed to gain cooperation. Use a firm touch and do not pretend to tickle the child at any point during the examination. Alternatively, put the child's hand on the abdomen and place your hand over the child's. Let your fingertips slide over to touch the abdomen. The child has a sense of being in control, and you may be able to palpate directly.

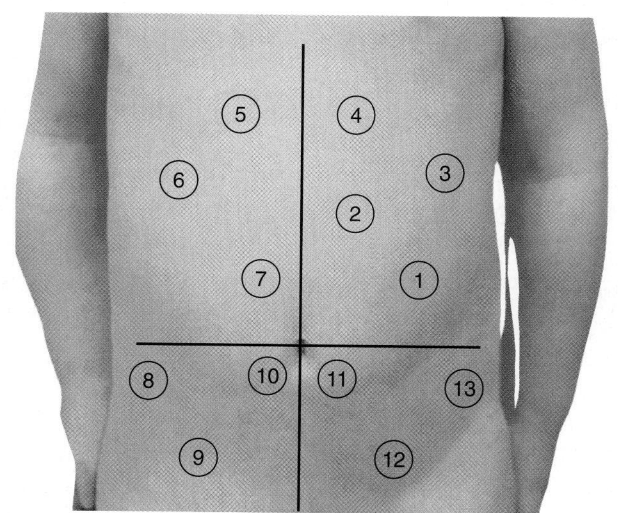

FIGURE 8–48 ■ Sequence for indirect percussion of the abdomen.

CLINICAL TIP

Use suggestive words to help the child relax so you can palpate the abdomen. "How soft will your tummy get when my hand feels it? Does it get softer than this? Yes. See, it softens as you breathe out. Will it also be softer here?" In this way, the child learns to relax the abdomen and is challenged to do it better.

To begin palpation, position the child supine with knees flexed. Stand beside the child and place your warmed fingertips across the child's abdomen. Palpate with the edge of your fingers, not just your fingerpads, and palpate in a sequence to examine the entire abdomen. Watch the child's face as you palpate for a grimace or constriction of the pupils, which indicates the presence of pain.

CLINICAL TIP

Older children often need distraction, especially when there is a question of abdominal tenderness and guarding or when the child is ticklish. Have the child perform a task that requires some concentration, such as pressing the hands together or pulling locked hands apart.

Light Palpation

For light palpation, use a superficial, gentle touch that slightly depresses the abdomen. Usually the abdomen feels soft and no tenderness is detected. Palpate any bulging along the abdominal

TABLE 8–17 Expected Liver Span by Age and Sex as Determined Through Percussion

AGE	MEAN ESTIMATED LIVER SPAN (CM) MALES	FEMALES
6 months	2.4	2.8
1 year	2.8	3.1
2 years	3.5	3.6
3 years	4.0	4.0
4 years	4.4	4.3
5 years	4.8	4.5
6 years	5.1	4.8
8 years	5.6	5.1
10 years	6.1	5.4
12 years	6.5	5.6
16 years	7.1	6.0
20 years	7.7	6.3

Modified from Lawson, E. E., Grand, R. J., Neff, R. K., & Cohen, L. F. (1978). Clinical estimation of liver span in infants and children. American Journal of Diseases in Children, *132, 474–476.*

wall, especially along the rectus muscle and umbilical ring, which could indicate the presence of a hernia. Measure the diameter of the muscle ring, rather than the protrusion, to monitor change over time. The muscle ring normally becomes smaller and closes by 4 years of age. An umbilical hernia that persists beyond this age may need surgical repair.

Liver. Locate and lightly palpate the lower liver edge. Place the fingers in the right midclavicular line at the level of the umbilicus and gently move them toward the costal margin during expiration. As the liver edge descends with inspiration, your finger usually feels a flat, narrow ridge. Measure the distance of the liver edge from the right costal margin at the right midclavicular line. The liver edge is normally palpated 2 to 3 cm (approximately 1 in.) below the right costal margin in infants and toddlers. It may not be palpable in older children. The liver is enlarged when the edge is more than 3 cm (1.25 in.) below the right costal margin. An enlarged liver may be associated with congestive heart failure or hepatic disease.

Deep Palpation

To perform deep palpation, press the fingers of one hand (for small children) or two hands (for older children) more deeply into the abdomen. Because the abdominal muscles are most relaxed when the child takes a deep breath, ask the child to take regular deep breaths when each area of the abdomen is palpated.

Spleen. Palpate for the spleen at the left costal margin in the midclavicular line. The spleen tip may be felt when the child takes a deep breath. The spleen is enlarged when it can be easily palpated below the left costal margin.

Kidneys. Palpate for the kidneys deep in the abdomen along each side of the spinal column. The kidneys are difficult to palpate in all children, except newborns, because of the deep layer of abdominal muscles and intestines. If a kidney is actually palpated, an abnormal mass may be present.

PRACTICE ALERT

If an enlarged kidney or mass is detected during abdominal palpation, do not continue to palpate the kidney. Pressure on the mass may release cancerous cells if the child has Wilms tumor.

Other Masses. Occasionally other masses, both normal and abnormal, can be palpated in the abdomen. A tubular mass commonly palpated in the lower left or right quadrant is often an intestine filled with feces. A distended bladder is often palpated as a firm, central, dome-shaped mass above the symphysis pubis in young children. Any fixed mass that moves laterally, pulsates, or is located along the vertebral column may be a neoplasm.

Assessment of the Inguinal Area

The inguinal area is inspected and palpated during the abdominal examination to detect enlarged lymph nodes or masses. The femoral pulse, a part of the heart examination, may be assessed simultaneously with the abdominal examination.

Inspection

Inspect the inguinal area for any change in contour, comparing sides. A small bulging noted over the femoral canal in girls may be associated with a femoral hernia. A bulging in the inguinal area in boys may be associated with an inguinal hernia.

Palpation

Palpate the inguinal area for lymph nodes and other masses. Small lymph nodes, less than 1 cm (0.5 in.) in diameter, are often present in the inguinal area because of minor injuries on the legs. Any tenderness, heat, or inflammation in these palpated lymph nodes could be associated with a local infection.

ASSESSING THE GENITAL AND PERINEAL AREAS FOR EXTERNAL STRUCTURAL ABNORMALITIES

What can a vaginal discharge indicate in a preadolescent girl? Is swelling in an infant's scrotum normal? Where is the proper location of the urethral meatus on the penis?

Preparation of Children for the Examination

Examination of the genitalia and perineal area can cause stress in children because they sense their privacy has been invaded. To make young children feel more secure, position them on the parent's lap with their legs spread apart. Children can also be positioned on the examining table with their knees flexed and the legs spread apart like a frog (Box 8–8).

BOX 8–8 Preparing Young Children for a Genital Assessment

Nurses may perform an external genital examination or assist another healthcare provider. Preschool-age children are often taught that strangers are not permitted to touch their "private parts." When a child this age actively resists examination of the genital area, ask the parent to tell the child that the nurse or doctor has permission to look at and touch these parts of the body. Some children develop modesty during the preschool period. Briefly explain what you need to examine and why. Then calmly and efficiently examine the child.

In younger children the genital and perineal examination is performed immediately after assessment of the abdomen. The genitals and perineum may be examined last in older children and adolescents. Gloves, lubricant, and a penlight are needed for the examination.

Inspection of the Female Genitalia

The external genitalia of girls are inspected for color, size, and symmetry of the mons pubis, labia, urethra, and vaginal opening (Figure 8–49 ■). Simultaneously look for any abnormal findings such as swelling, inflammation, masses, lacerations, or discharge.

> **PRACTICE ALERT**
>
> Signs of sexual abuse in young children include bruising or swelling of the vulva, foul-smelling vaginal discharge, enlarged opening of the vagina, and a rash or lesions in the perineal area.

Mons Pubis

Inspect the mons pubis for the presence of pubic hair and its characteristics. See page 283 for guidelines to assess the stage of pubic hair development.

Labia

The labia minora are usually thin and pale in preadolescent girls but become dark pink and moist after puberty. In young infants, the labia minora may be fused and cover the structures in the vestibule. These adhesions may need to be separated.

Hymen

Use the thumb and forefinger of one hand to separate the labia minora for viewing structures in the vestibule. The hymen is just inside the vaginal opening. In preadolescents it is usually a thin membrane with a crescent-shaped opening. The vaginal opening is usually about 1 cm (0.5 in.) in adolescents when the hymen is intact. Sexually active adolescents may have a vaginal opening with irregular edges.

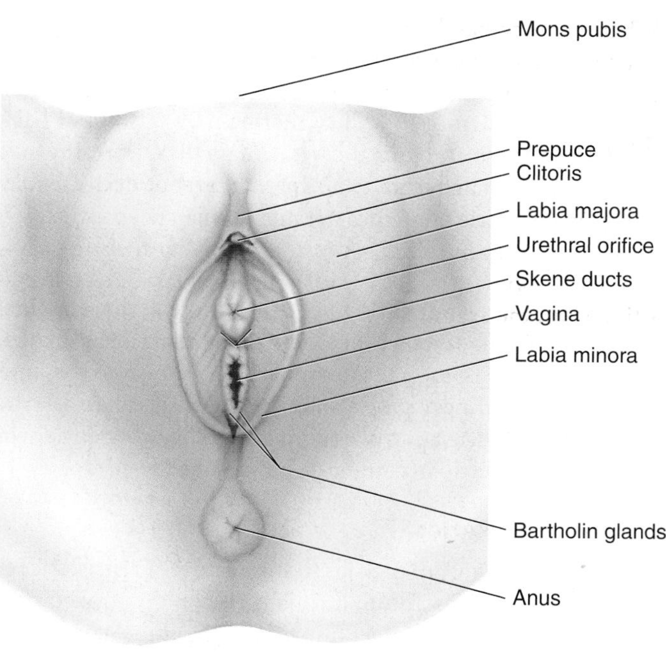

FIGURE 8–49 ■ Anatomic structures of the female genital and perineal area.

Urethral and Vaginal Openings

Inspect the vestibule for lesions. No lesions or signs of inflammation are expected around the urethral or vaginal opening. Redness and excoriation are often associated with an irritant such as bubble bath or pinworms.

Vaginal Discharge

Preadolescent girls do not normally have a vaginal discharge. Adolescents often have a clear discharge without a foul odor. Menses generally begin approximately 2 years after breast bud development. A foul-smelling discharge in preschool-age children may be associated with a foreign body. Various organisms may cause a vaginal infection in older children.

An internal vaginal examination is indicated when abnormal findings such as a vaginal discharge or trauma to the external structures is noted. Only an experienced examiner should perform the vaginal examination of the child. Refer to other assessment texts for guidelines in performing this examination.

Palpation of the Female Genitalia

Palpate the vaginal opening with a finger of your free hand. The Bartholin and Skene glands are not usually palpable. If these glands are palpated in preadolescent children this indicates enlargement because of an infection such as gonorrhea.

Inspection of the Male Genitalia

The male genitalia are inspected for the structural and pubertal development of the penis, scrotum, and testicles. Boys are placed in tailor position, seated with their legs crossed in front of them. This position puts pressure on the abdominal wall to push the testicles into the scrotum. Note the presence and characteristics of pubic hair. See page 283 for guidelines to assess the staging of pubic hair and external genital development.

Penis

The penis is inspected for size, foreskin, hygiene, and position of the urethral meatus. The length of the nonerect penis in the newborn is normally 2 to 3 cm (1 in.). The penis enlarges in length and breadth during puberty. The penis is normally straight. A downward bowing of the penis may be caused by a chordee, a fibrous band of tissue associated with hypospadias.

When the penis is circumcised, the glans penis is exposed. The glans penis is normally clean and smooth without inflammation or ulceration. The urethral meatus is a slit-shaped opening near the tip of the glans. No discharge should be present. A round, pinpoint urethral meatus may indicate meatal stenosis. Location of the urethral meatus at another site on the penis is abnormal, indicating hypospadias or epispadias. Inspect the urinary stream. The stream is normally strong without dribbling. (See Developing Cultural Competence: Circumcision.)

In the uncircumcised infant and child, avoid forcible retraction of the foreskin to prevent tearing of adhesions that could lead to fibrosis. Preputial adhesions are normal in infants and young boys and usually resolve on their own. Use gentle traction

> **DEVELOPING CULTURAL COMPETENCE**
> **Circumcision**
>
> Estimates of neonatal circumcision are 60% to 65%; however; the rate varies by racial and ethnic group. White infants have the highest rate of circumcision, followed by Blacks, and then Hispanics. Male infants in the Jewish culture are traditionally circumcised. See Chapters 11 and 31 ∞ for further information on circumcision.

to evaluate the degree of foreskin retraction and the meatal location and size. It is usually possible to visualize the meatus; however, a foreskin opening large enough for a good urinary stream is normal, even when the meatus cannot be seen. The foreskin normally retracts easily past the corona by 5 years of age in the majority of boys.

Phimosis is the presence of an abnormal ring of tissue distal to the glans that prevents retraction of the foreskin to allow visualization of the meatus. Erythema and edema of the glans (*balanitis*) may result from an infection or trauma. In the uncircumcised penis, purulent discharge and an edematous foreskin may be seen.

Scrotum

Inspect the scrotum for size, symmetry, presence of the testicles, and any abnormalities. The scrotum is normally loose and pendulous with rugae, or wrinkles. The scrotum of infants often appears large in comparison to the penis. A small, undeveloped scrotum that has no rugae indicates that the testicles are undescended. Enlargement or swelling of the scrotum is abnormal. It may indicate an inguinal hernia, hydrocele, torsion of the spermatic cord, or testicular inflammation. A deep cleft in the scrotum may indicate ambiguous genitalia. To distinguish between a hydrocele and an incarcerated hernia, place a bright penlight under the scrotum and look for a red glow or transillumination through the scrotum. A hydrocele transilluminates; a hernia does not.

Palpation of the Male Genitalia

Penis

Palpate the shaft of the penis for nodules and masses. None should be present.

Testicles

Palpate the scrotum for the presence of the testicles. Make sure your hands are warm to avoid stimulating the cremasteric reflex that causes the testicles to retract. Place your index finger and thumb over both inguinal canals on each side of the penis. This keeps the testicles from retracting into the abdomen (Figure 8–50 ■).

Gently palpate each testicle with only enough pressure to identify the shape and size. The testicles are normally smooth and equal in size. They are approximately 1 to 1.5 cm (0.5 in.) in diameter until puberty, when they increase in size. A hard, enlarged, painless testicle may indicate a tumor.

If a testicle is not palpated in the scrotum, the examiner palpates the inguinal canal for a soft mass. When the testicle is found in the inguinal canal, try to move it to the scrotum to palpate the size and shape. The testicle is descendable when it can be moved into the scrotum. An undescended testicle is one that does not descend into the scrotum or cannot be palpated in the inguinal canal.

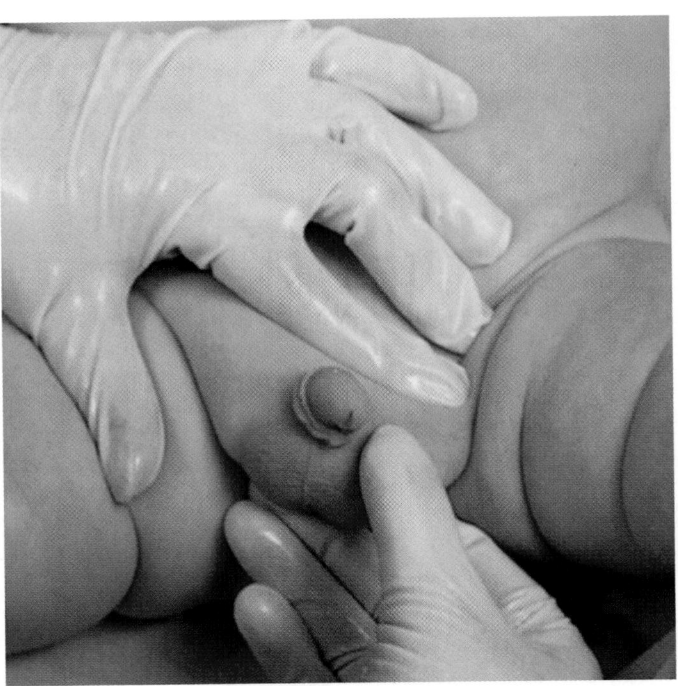

FIGURE 8–50 ■ Palpating the scrotum for descended testicles and spermatic cords.

Spermatic Cord

Palpate the length of the spermatic cord between the thumb and forefinger from the testicle to the inguinal canal. It normally feels solid and smooth. No tenderness is expected.

Enlarged Scrotum

When bulging or swelling of the scrotum is present, palpate the scrotum to identify the characteristics of the mass. Try to determine whether the mass is unilateral or bilateral. An experienced examiner may attempt to reduce the mass by pushing it back through the external inguinal ring. A mass that decreases may indicate an inguinal hernia. A mass that does not decrease may indicate a hydrocele or an incarcerated hernia.

Inguinal Canal

Attempt to insert your little finger into the external inguinal canal to determine whether the external inguinal ring is dilated. The inguinal ring is normally too small for the finger to pass into the canal. If the finger passes into the inguinal canal, ask the child to cough. A sensation of abdominal contents coming down to touch the fingertip may indicate an inguinal hernia.

Cremasteric Reflex

Stroke the inner thigh of each leg to stimulate the cremasteric reflex. The testicle and scrotum normally rise on the stroked side. This response indicates intact function of the spinal cord at the T12, L1, and L2 levels.

Inspection of the Anus and Rectum

Inspect the anus for sphincter control and any abnormal findings such as inflammation, fissures, or lesions. This exam is often done with the child in supine or prone position. If a more focused inspection is needed, the child can be placed in knee-chest position. The external sphincter is usually closed. Inflammation and scratch marks around the anus may be associated with pinworms. A protrusion from the rectum may be associated with a rectal wall prolapse or a hemorrhoid.

Palpation of the Anus and Rectum

Lightly touching the anal opening should stimulate an anal contraction or "wink." Absence of a contraction may indicate the presence of a lower spinal cord lesion.

Rectal Examination

A rectal examination is not routinely performed on children. It is indicated for symptoms of intraabdominal, rectal, bowel, or stool abnormalities. The rectal examination should be performed only by an experienced examiner. To reduce anxiety associated with this examination, distract the child with an age-appropriate toy or discussion when assisting with this procedure. Let the child know that the lubricant might feel cold. As the examiner's finger is positioned, help the child to relax the sphincter by "pushing out the poop."

ASSESSMENT OF PUBERTAL DEVELOPMENT AND SEXUAL MATURATION

What is the first stage of breast development in girls? How is the stage of pubertal development determined in girls and boys?

The age of onset of secondary sexual characteristics can vary with race and ethnicity, environmental conditions, geographic location, and nutrition. For example, sexual maturity begins earlier in taller and heavier girls. Black girls have an earlier onset of breast and pubic hair development than Whites (Herman-Giddens, Slora, Wasserman, et al., 1997).

Females

Breast development in females precedes other pubertal changes. See Figure 8–51 ■ for Tanner stages of breast development. *Thelarche* or breast budding is the first stage of pubertal development in the majority of girls, indicating breast Tanner stage II. Breast tissue is seen and palpated below a slightly enlarging areola. While breast budding normally occurs between 9 and 14 years of age, the mean age for breast development in Black girls is 8.87 years and for White girls is 9.96 years. Breast development before 6 years of age in Black girls and 7 years of age in White girls is abnormal and needs further evaluation (Herman-Giddens, et al., 1997; Kaplowitz, Oberfield, & the Drug and Therapeutics and Executive Committees of the Lawson Wilkins Pediatric Endocrine Society, 1999).

Inspect the adolescent's breasts while she is sitting to determine the stage of development. A girl's breasts often develop at different rates and appear asymmetric, and most teens have one breast slightly larger than the other. Catch-up growth of the smaller breast typically occurs during late adolescence (Alderman, 1999).

Next observe the development of pubic hair. Preadolescent girls have no pubic hair. Initial pubic hair is lightly pigmented, sparse, and straight, along the labia majora. Pubic hair develops in consistent stages for all girls, but the timing of pubic hair stages is individually determined (Tanner, 1962). The hair then becomes coarse and curly and extends over a larger area of the labia majora as development proceeds. Breast development usually precedes pubic hair development. The presence of pubic hair before 8 years of age is unusual. Compare the girl's pubic hair development with the stages illustrated in Figure 8–52 ■.

Males

Initial signs of pubertal development in males are enlargement of the testicles and thinning of the scrotum. This is followed by pubic hair development about 6 months later. Straight, downy pubic hair first develops at the base of the penis. The hair becomes darker, dense, and curly, extending over the pubic area in a diamond pattern by the completion of puberty. The presence of pubic hair before 9 years of age is uncommon, and delayed onset of testicular enlargement after 14 years of age needs evaluation. Penile enlargement generally follows testicular enlargement about 1 year later, genitalia Tanner stage III. Tanner stages of genital growth and pubic hair development follow a standard pattern, as illustrated in Figure 8–53 ■.

Sexual Maturity Rating

The **sexual maturity rating** (SMR) is an average of the breast and pubic hair Tanner stages in females and of the genital and pubic hair Tanner stages in boys. The rating is a number between 2 and 5, as stage I is prepubertal. The sexual maturity rating is then related to other physiologic events that happen during puberty. Compare the stage of the child's secondary sexual characteristics with information in Figure 8–54 ■ on page 283 to identify the SMR.

In females, menarche generally occurs in SMR 4 or breast stage III to IV. The peak height velocity usually occurs before menarche at a mean of 11.5 years. This staging provides an opportunity to educate the girl about her body and when to anticipate menarche.

In males ejaculation usually occurs at SMR 3, with semen noted between SMR 3 and 4. The peak height velocity usually occurs in SMR 4 or genital development stage IV to V, at about 13.5 years of age.

ASSESSING THE MUSCULOSKELETAL SYSTEM FOR BONE AND JOINT STRUCTURE, MOVEMENT, AND MUSCLE STRENGTH

What do extra skinfolds on an arm or leg indicate? What causes poor muscle tone? What condition does a rib hump indicate? At what age is it normal for children to be knock-kneed and bowlegged?

AS THEY GROW

Tanner Stages of Breast Development

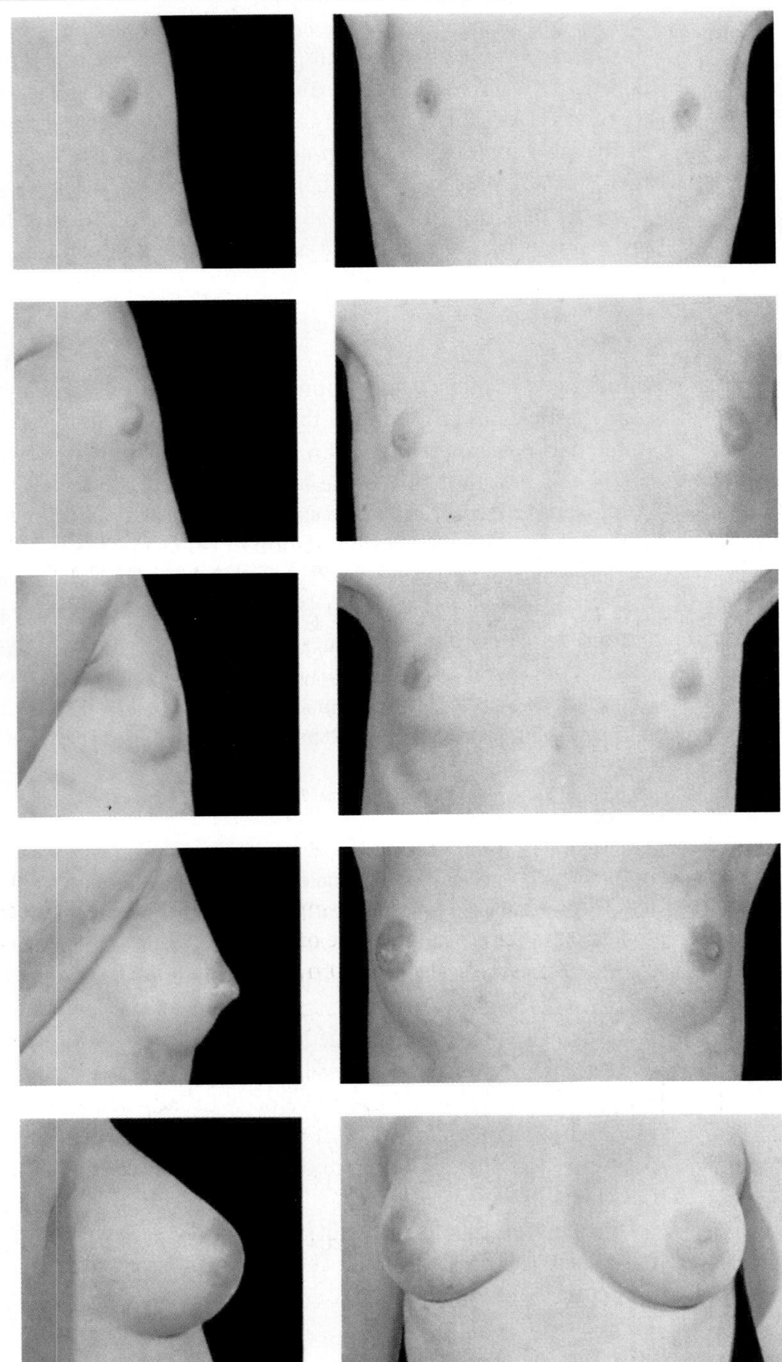

FIGURE 8–51 ■ *I*, Preadolescent. Only the nipple is raised above the level of the breast, as in the child. *II*, Budding stage. Areola increased in diameter and surrounding area slightly elevated. *III*, Breast and areola enlarged. No contour separation. *IV*, Areola forms a secondary elevation above that of the breast in half of girls. *V*, Areola is usually part of the general breast contour and is strongly pigmented. Nipple usually projects.

From Van Wieringen et al. (1971). Growth diagrams 1965 Netherlands. Groningen: Walters-Noardhof.

Inspection of the Bones, Muscles, and Joints

Bones and Muscles

Inspect and compare the arms and then the legs for differences in alignment, contour, skinfolds, length, and deformities. The extremities normally have equal length, circumference, and numbers of skinfolds bilaterally. Extra skinfolds and a larger circumference may indicate a shorter extremity.

Joints

Inspect and compare the joints bilaterally for size, discoloration, and ease of voluntary movement. Joints are normally the same

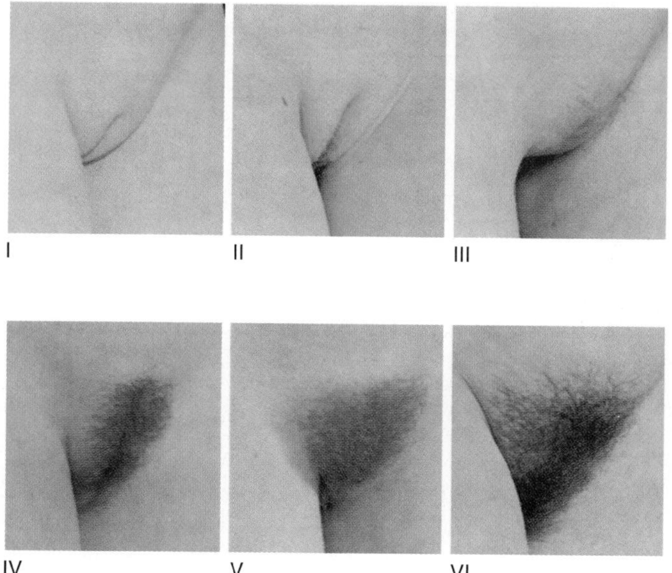

FIGURE 8–52 ■ The Tanner stages of female pubic hair development with sexual maturation. *I*, Preadolescent, no growth of pubic hair. *II*, Initial, scarcely pigmented straight hair, especially along medial border of the labia. *III*, Sparse, dark, visibly pigmented curly pubic hair on labia. *IV*, Hair coarse and curly, abundant but less than adults. *V*, Lateral spreading in triangle shape to medial surface of thighs. *VI*, Further extension laterally and upward.

From Van Wieringen et al. (1971). Growth diagrams 1965 Netherlands. Groningen: Walters-Noordhof.

color as surrounding skin, with no sign of swelling. Children should voluntarily flex and extend joints during normal activities without pain. Redness, swelling, and pain with movement may indicate injury or infection.

Palpation of the Bones, Muscles, and Joints

Bones and Muscles

Palpate the bones and muscles in each extremity for muscle tone, masses, or tenderness. Muscles normally feel firm, and

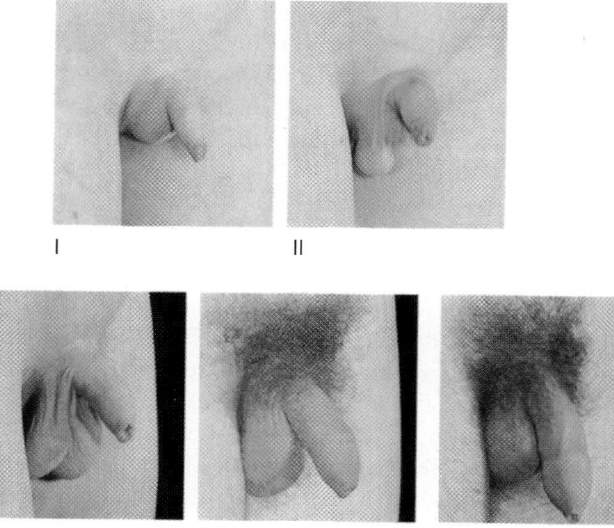

FIGURE 8–53 ■ The Tanner stages of male pubic hair and external genital development with sexual maturation. *I*, Preadolescent, hair present is no different than that on abdomen. Testes, scrotum, and penis are the same size and shape as young child. *II*, Pubic hair slightly pigmented, longer, straight hair, often still downy usually at base of penis, sometimes on scrotum; enlargement of scrotum and testes. *III*, Pubic hair dark, definitely pigmented, curly pubic hair around base of penis; enlargement of penis, especially in length, further enlargement of testes, descent of scrotum. *IV*, Pubic hair definitely adult in type but not in extent, spread no further than inguinal fold. Continued enlargement of penis and sculpturing of glans, increased pigmentation of scrotum. *V*, Hair spread to medial surface of thighs in adult distribution. Adult stage, scrotum ample, penis reaching nearly to bottom of scrotum.

From Van Wieringen et al. (1971). Growth diagrams 1965 Netherlands. Groningen: Walters-Noordhof.

bony masses are not normally present. Doughy muscles may indicate poor muscle tone. Rigid muscles, or hypertonia, may be associated with an active seizure or cerebral palsy. A mass over a long bone may indicate a recent fracture or a bone tumor.

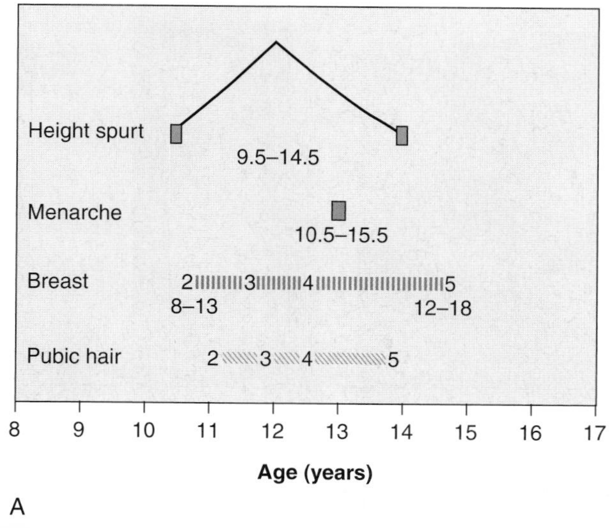

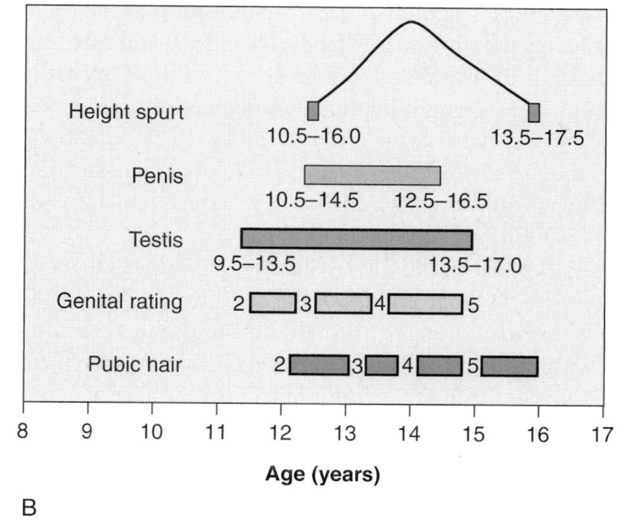

FIGURE 8–54 ■ Sexual maturity rating. Approximate timing of developmental changes. The numbers (2, 3, 4, 5) indicate stages of development. Range of ages during which some changes occur is indicated by the inclusive numbers below them. *A*, Females. *B*, Males.

A. Redrawn from *Marshall, W. A. & Tanner, J. M. (1969). Variations in pattern of pubertal changes in girls.* Archives of Disease in Childhood, 44, *291. B. Marshall, W. A. & Tanner, J. M. (1970). Variations in pattern of pubertal changes in boys.* Archives of Disease in Childhood, 45, *13.*

Joints

Palpate each joint and surrounding muscles to detect any swelling, masses, heat, or tenderness. None is expected when the joint is palpated. Tenderness, heat, swelling, and redness can result from injury or a chronic joint inflammation such as juvenile rheumatoid arthritis.

Range of Motion and Muscle Strength Assessment

Active Range of Motion

Observe the child during typical play activities, such as reaching for objects, climbing, and walking, to assess range of motion of all major joints. Children spontaneously move their joints through the full normal range of motion with play activities when no pain is present. Limited range of motion may indicate injury, inflammation of a joint, or a muscle abnormality.

Passive Range of Motion

When a joint is suspected of having limited active range of motion, perform passive range of motion. Flex and extend, abduct and adduct, or rotate the affected joint cautiously to avoid causing extra pain. Full range of motion without pain is normal. Limitations in movement may indicate injury, inflammation, or malformation. Increased passive range of motion may indicate muscle weakness.

Muscle Strength

Observe the child's ability to climb onto an examining table, throw a ball, clap hands, or move around on a bed. The child's ability to perform age-appropriate play activities indicates good muscle tone and strength. See Table 8–18 for age-appropriate motor development. Attainment of these skills is another indicator of good muscle strength.

To assess the strength of specific muscles in the extremities, engage the child in games. Muscle strength is compared bilaterally to identify muscle weakness. For example, ask the child to squeeze your fingers tightly with each hand; push against and pull your hands with his or her hands, lower legs, and feet; and resist extension of a flexed elbow or knee. Children normally have good muscle strength bilaterally. Unilateral muscle weakness may be associated with a nerve injury. Bilateral muscle weakness may result from hypoxemia or a congenital disorder such as Down syndrome. Asymmetrical weakness may be associated with conditions such as cerebral palsy.

When generalized muscle weakness is suspected in a preschool- or school-age child, ask the child to stand from the supine position. Children are normally able to rise to a standing position without using their arms as levers. Children who push their body upright using the arms and hands may have generalized muscle weakness, known as a positive Gower sign. This may indicate muscular dystrophy (see Chapter 35∞).

Posture and Spinal Alignment

Posture

Inspect the child's posture when standing from a front, side, and back view. The shoulders and hips are normally level. The head is held erect without a tilt, and the shoulder contour is symmetric. After beginning to walk, young children often have a pot-bellied stance because of a lumbar lordosis. This posture generally disappears by 5 years of age. The spine has normal thoracic convex and lumbar concave curves after 6 years of age. See Figure 8–55 ■ for the expected developmental sequence of posture and spinal curves by age.

TABLE 8–18 Selected Gross Motor Milestones for Age

GROSS MOTOR MILESTONES	AGE ATTAINED
Rolls over from prone to supine position	4 months
Sits without support	8 months
Pulls self to standing position	10 months
Walks around room holding onto objects	11 months
Walks alone well	15 months
Kicks ball	24 months
Jumps in place	30 months
Throws ball overhand	36 months

From Frankenburg, W. K., Dodds, J., Archer, P., Shapiro, H., & Bresnick, B. (1992). The Denver II: A major revision and restandardization of the Denver Developmental Screening Test. Pediatrics, 89, *91–97.*

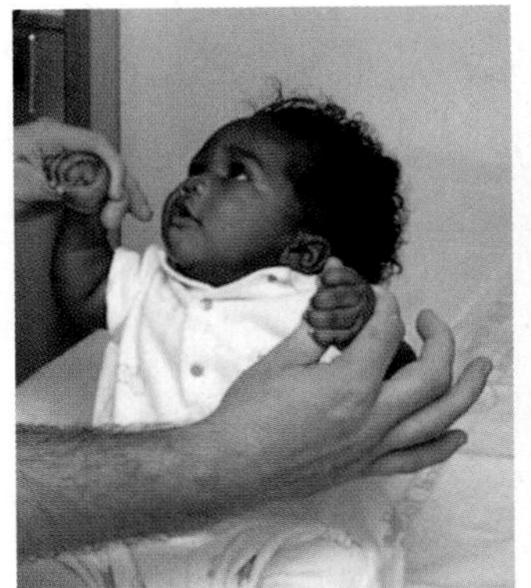
A

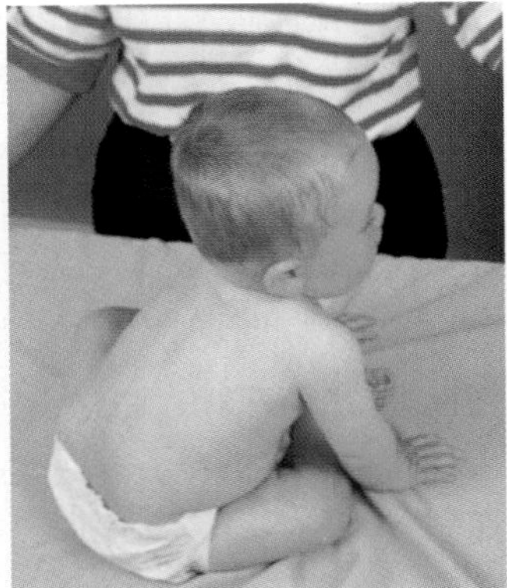
B

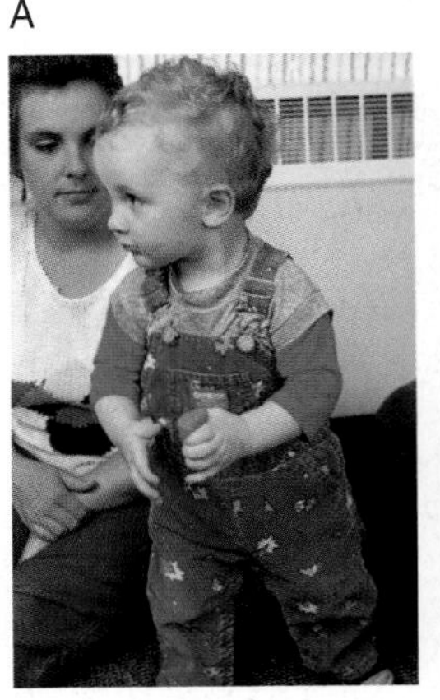
C

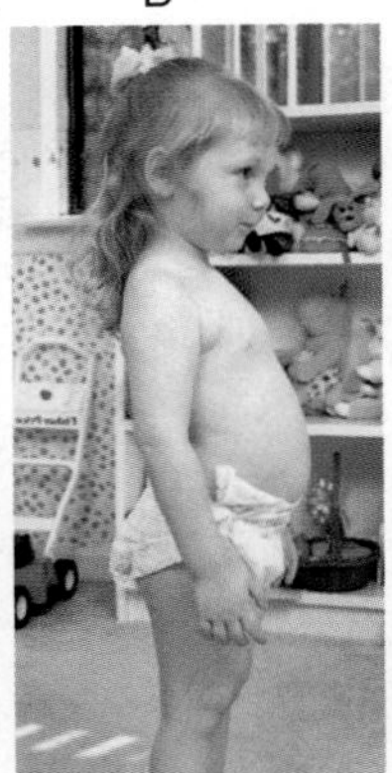
D

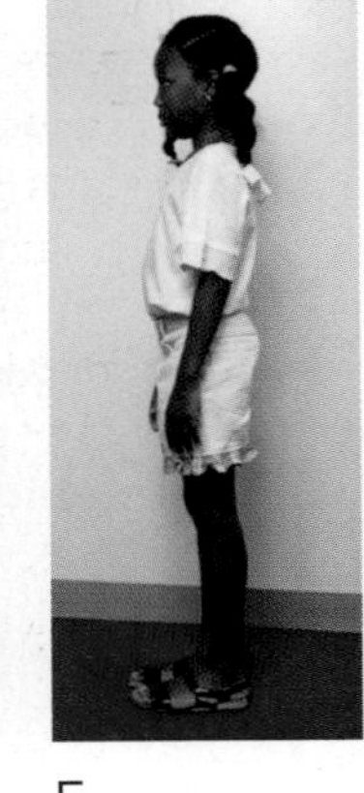
E

FIGURE 8–55 ■ Normal development of posture and spinal curves. *A,* Infant 2–3 months–Holds head erect when held upright; thoracic kyphosis when sitting. *B,* 6–8 months–Sits without support; spine is straight. *C,* 10–15 months–Walks independently; straight spine. *D,* Toddler–Protuding abdomen; lumbar lordosis. *E,* School-age child–Height of shoulders and hips is level; balanced thoracic convex and lumbar concave curves.

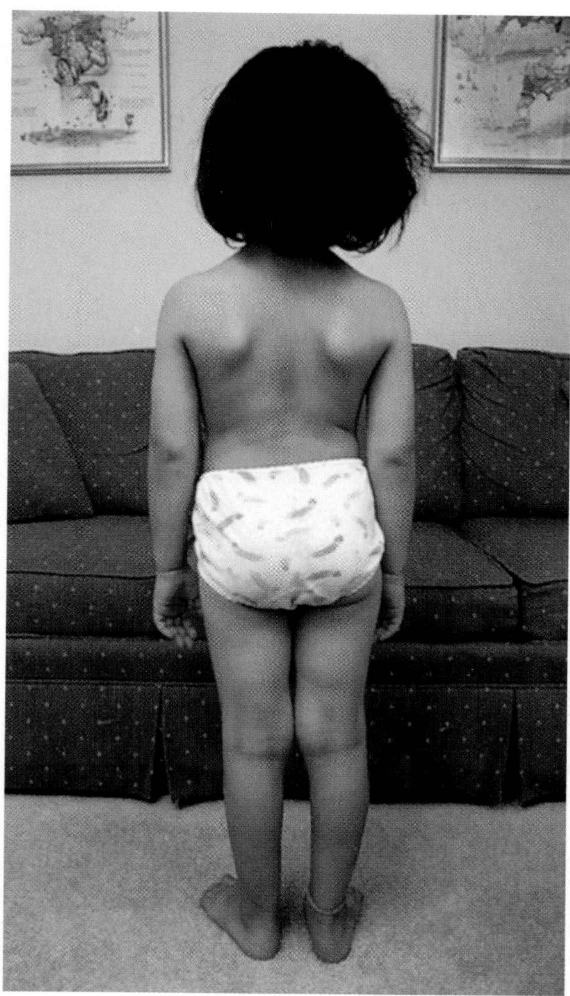

FIGURE 8–56 ■ Does this child have legs of different lengths or scoliosis? Look at the level of the iliac crests and shoulders to see if they are level. See the more prominent crease at the waist on the right side? This child could have scoliosis.

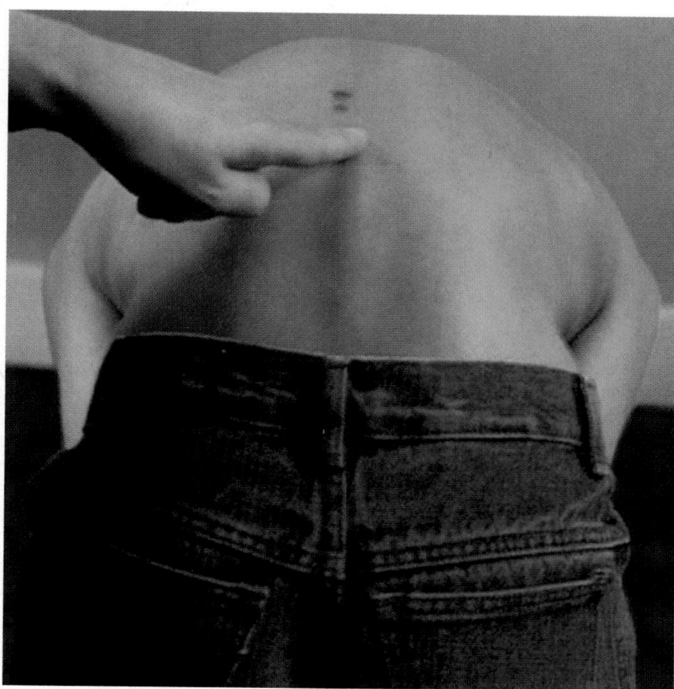

FIGURE 8–57 ■ Inspection of the spine for scoliosis. Ask the child to slowly bend forward at the waist, with arms extended toward the floor. Run your forefinger down the spinal processes, palpating each vertebra for a change in alignment. A lateral curve to the spine or a one-sided rib hump is an indication of scoliosis.

Spinal Alignment

Assess the school-age child and adolescent for scoliosis, a lateral spine curvature. Stand behind the child, observing the height of the shoulders and hips (Figure 8–56 ■). The shoulders and hips should be level. Ask the child to bend forward slowly at the waist, with arms extended toward the floor. No lateral curve should be present in either position. The ribs normally stay flat bilaterally. The lumbar concave curve should flatten with forward flexion (Figure 8–57 ■). A lateral curve to the spine or a one-sided rib hump is an indication of scoliosis (see Chapter 35∞).

Inspection of the Upper Extremities

Arms

The alignment of the arms is normally straight, with a minimal angle at the elbows, where the bones articulate.

Hands

Count the fingers. Extra finger digits (*polydactyly*) or webbed fingers (*syndactyly*) are abnormal. Inspect the creases on the palmar surface of each hand. Multiple creases across the palm are normal. A single crease that crosses the entire palm of the hand, a simian crease, may be associated with Down syndrome (Figure 8–58 ■).

Nails

Inspect the nails for size, shape, and color. Nails are normally convex, smooth, and pink. *Clubbing*, widening of the nailbed with an increased angle between the proximal nail fold and nail, is abnormal (see Figure 26–14∞). Clubbing is associated with chronic respiratory and cardiac conditions.

Inspection of the Lower Extremities

Hips

Assess the hips of young infants for dislocation or subluxation. The skinfolds on the upper legs are inspected first. The same number of skinfolds should be present on each leg. Uneven skinfolds may indicate a hip dislocation or difference in leg length (Allis sign). Check for a difference in knee height symmetry (Figure 8–59 ■). The Ortolani–Barlow maneuver is used to assess an infant's hips for dislocation or subluxation (Figure 8–60 ■).

The child is asked to stand on one leg and then the other. The iliac crests should stay level. If the iliac crest opposite the weight-bearing leg appears lower, the hip that is bearing weight may be dislocated.

Legs

Inspect the alignment of the legs. After a child is 4 years of age, the alignment of the long bones is straight, with minimal

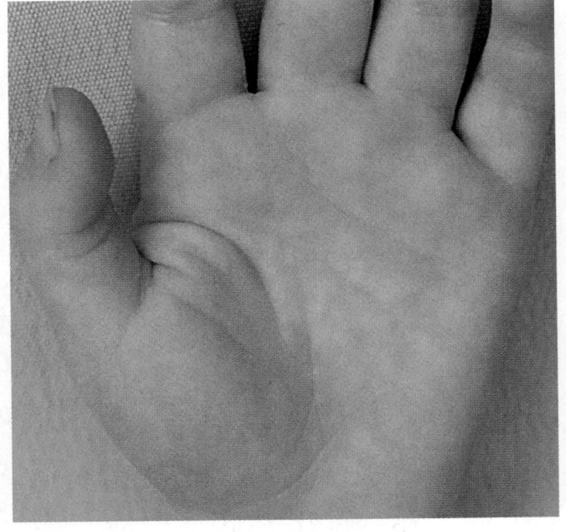

A

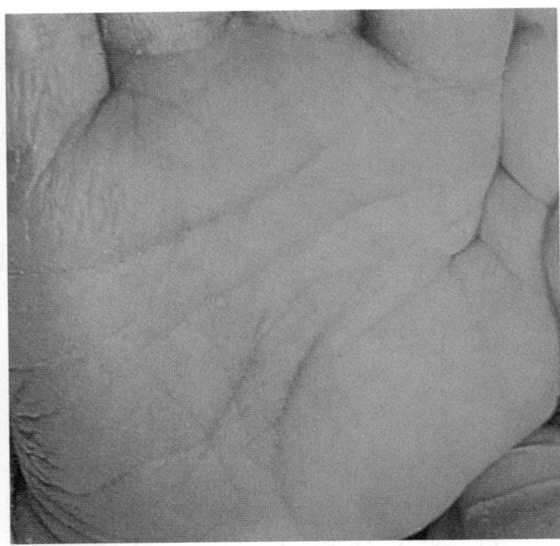

B

FIGURE 8–58 ■ *A*, Normal palmar creases. *B*, Simian crease associated with Down syndrome.

Photo B from Zitelli, B. J., & Davis, H. W. (Eds.). (2002). Atlas of pediatric physical diagnosis *(4th ed.). St. Louis: Mosby-Year Book.*

angle at the knees and feet where the bones articulate. Alignment of the lower extremities in infants and toddlers is assessed to ensure that normal changes are occurring. Infants are often born with a twisting of the tibia caused by positioning in utero (tibial torsion). The infant's toes turn in as a result of the tibial torsion. Toddlers go through a skeletal alignment sequence of bowlegs (genu varum) and knock-knees (genu valgum) before the legs assume a straight alignment. See Figure 8–61 ■.

To evaluate the toddler with bowlegs, have the child stand on a firm surface. Measure the distance between the knees when the child's ankles are together. No more than 3.5 cm (1.5 in.) between the knees is normal. To evaluate the child with knock-knees, have the child stand on a firm surface. Measure the distance between the ankles at the level of the medial malleoli when the child stands with the knees together. The normal distance is not more than 5 cm (2 in.) between the ankles.

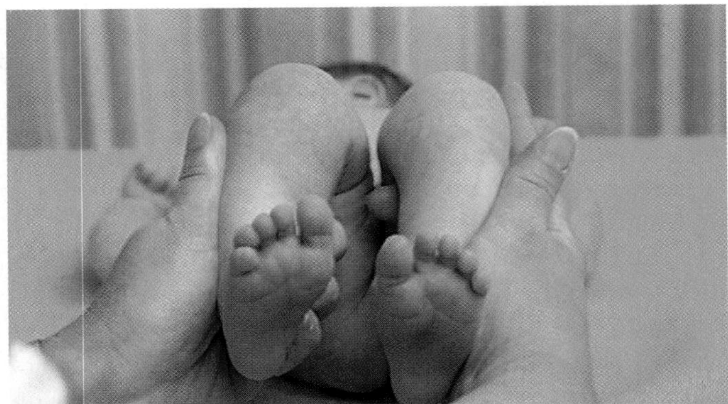

FIGURE 8–59 ■ Flex the infant's hips and knees so the heels are as close to the buttocks as possible. Place the feet flat on the examining table. The knees are usually the same height. A difference in knee height (Allis sign) is an indicator of hip dislocation (see also Chapter 35).

Courtesy of Dee Corbett, RN, Children's National Medical Center, Washington, DC.

Feet

Inspect the feet for alignment, the presence of all toes, and any deformities. The weight-bearing line of the feet is usually in alignment with the legs. Inspect the feet for the presence of an arch when the child is standing. Children up to 3 years of age normally have a fat pad over the arch, giving the appearance of flat feet. Older children normally have a longitudinal arch. The arch is usually seen when the child stands on tiptoe or is sitting. Inspect the nails on the feet in the same manner as the hands.

ASSESSING THE NERVOUS SYSTEM FOR COGNITIVE FUNCTION, BALANCE, COORDINATION, CRANIAL NERVE FUNCTION, SENSATION, AND REFLEXES

What aspects of developmental information are useful for assessment of cognitive function? How are the infant's and child's levels of consciousness evaluated? How are cranial nerves assessed in infants? A scissoring gait is associated with what condition? At what age does a Babinski response become abnormal? What response is expected when a deep tendon reflex is stimulated?

The neurologic examination provides an opportunity to develop rapport with the child. Many of the procedures can be presented as games that young children enjoy. Cognitive function can be assessed by how well the child follows directions for the game. As the assessment proceeds, the child develops trust and is more likely to cooperate with examination of other systems.

Cognitive Function

Observe the child's behavior, facial expressions, gestures, communication skills, activity level, and level of consciousness to assess cognitive functioning. Match the neurologic examination to the child's stage of development. For example, cognitive function is evaluated much differently in infants than in older children because infants cannot use words to communicate.

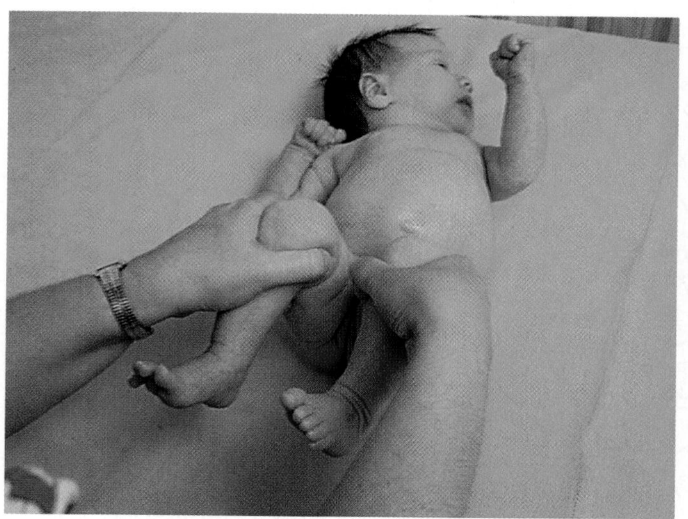

A

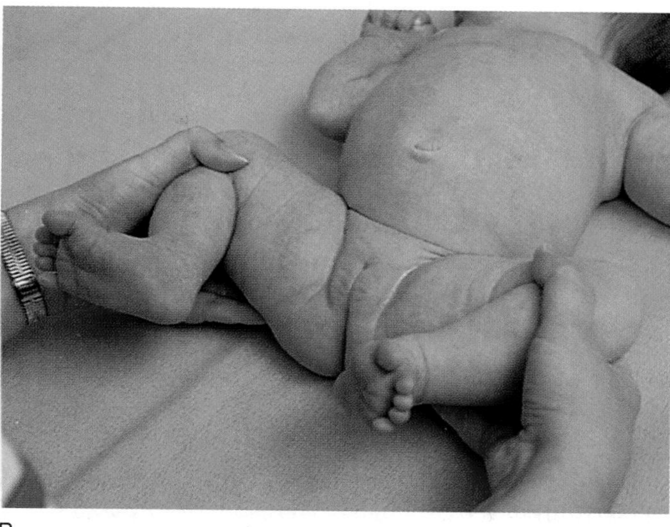

B

FIGURE 8–60 ■ Ortolani-Barlow maneuver. *A*, Place the infant on his or her back and flex the hips and knees at a 90-degree angle. Place a hand over each knee with the thumb over the inner thigh, and the first two fingers over the upper margin of the femur. Move the infant's knees together until they touch, and then put downward pressure on one femur at a time to see if the hips easily slip out of their joints or dislocate. *B*, Slowly abduct the hips, moving each knee toward the examining table. Keep pressure on the hip joints with the fingers in a lever-type motion. Equal hip abduction, with the knees nearly touching the examining table, is normal. Any resistance to abduction or a clunk felt on palpation can be an indication of a congenital hip dislocation.

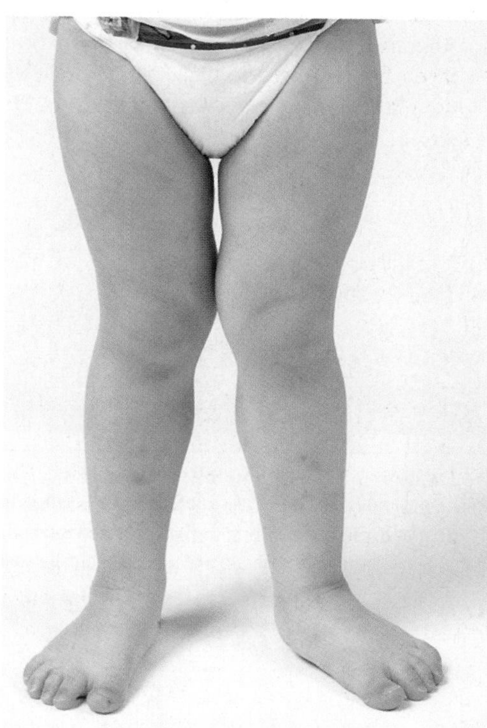

FIGURE 8–61 ■ To evaluate the child with knock-knees, have the child stand on a firm surface. Measure the distance between the ankles when the child stands with the knees together. The normal distance is not more than 5 cm (2 in.) between the ankles.

Behavior

The alertness of infants and children is indicated by their behavior during the assessment. Infants and toddlers are curious, but seek the security of the parent, either by clinging or by making frequent eye contact. Older children are often anxious and watch all of the examiner's actions. Lack of interest in assessment or treatment procedures may indicate a serious illness. Excessive activity or an unusually short attention span may be associated with an attention deficit hyperactivity disorder.

Communication Skills

Speech, language development, and social skills provide clues to cognitive functioning. Listen to speech articulation and words used, comparing the child's performance with standards of social development and speech articulation for the child's age (Table 8–19). Toddlers can normally follow simple directions such as "Show me your mouth." By 3 years of age, the child's speech should be easily understood. Delay in language and social skill development may be associated with mental retardation or hearing loss.

Memory

Immediate, recent, and remote memory can be tested in children starting at approximately 4 years of age. To evaluate recent memory, ask the child to remember a special name or object.

TABLE 8–19 Expected Language Development for Age

LANGUAGE MILESTONES	AGE ATTAINED
Understands mama and dada	10 months
Says mama, dada, 2 other words: imitates animal sounds	12 months
4–6 word vocabulary, points to desired objects	13–15 months
7–20 word vocabulary, points to 5 body parts	18 months
2-word combinations	20 months
3-word sentences, plurals	36 months

Reprinted with permission from Capute, A. J., Shapiro, B. K., & Palmer, R. B. (1987). Marking the milestones of language development. Contemporary Pediatrics, *4, 24–4. Contemporary Pediatrics is a copyrighted publication of Advanstar Communications. All rights reserved.*

BOX 8–9 Growth & Development

Immediate memory can be tested by asking the child to repeat a series of words or numbers, such as the names of Disney or Sesame Street characters. Children can remember more words or numbers with age.

Age	Recall Ability
4 years	3 words or numbers
5 years	4 words or numbers
6 years	5 words or numbers

Then 5 to 10 minutes later during the examination have the child recall the name or object. To evaluate remote memory, ask the child to repeat his or her address or birth date or a nursery rhyme. By 5 or 6 years of age, children are normally able to recall this information without difficulty (Box 8–9).

Level of Consciousness

When approaching the infant or child, observe his or her level of consciousness and activity, including facial expressions, gestures, and interaction. Children are normally alert, and sleeping children arouse easily. The child who cannot be awakened is unconscious. A lowered level of consciousness may be associated with a number of neurologic conditions such as a brain injury, seizure, infection, or brain tumor.

Cerebellar Function

Observe the young child at play to assess coordination and balance. Development of fine motor skills in infants and preschool children provides clues to cerebellar function. Equipment needed includes a reflex hammer, cotton balls, penlight, and tongue blades.

Balance

Observe the child's balance during play activities such as walking, standing on one foot, and hopping (Table 8–20). The Romberg procedure can also be used to test balance in children over 3 years of age (Figure 8–62 ■). Once balance and other motor skills are attained, children do not normally stumble or fall when tested. Poor balance may indicate cerebellar dysfunction or an inner ear disturbance.

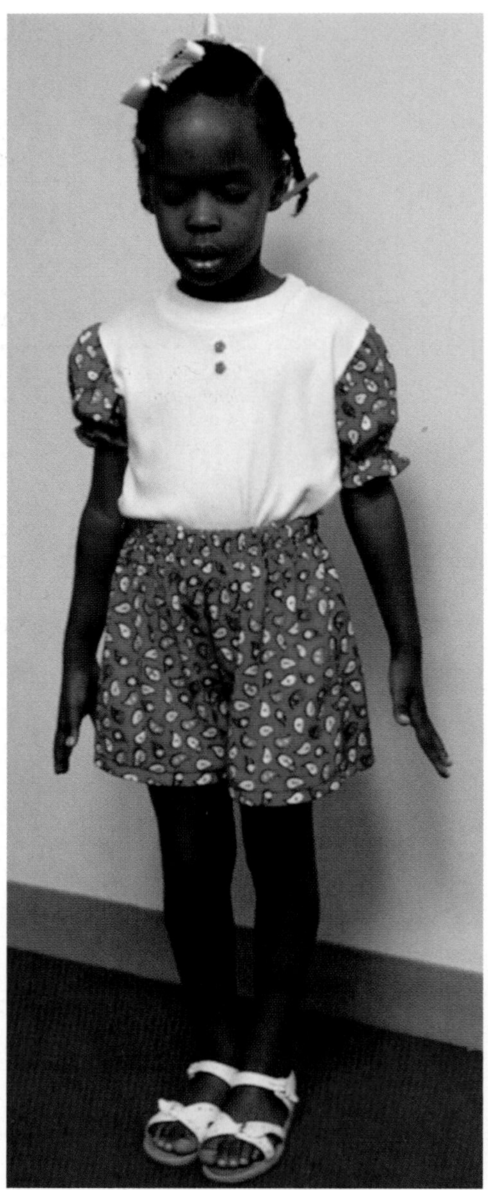

FIGURE 8–62 ■ Romberg procedure. Ask the child to stand with feet together and eyes closed. Protect the child from falling by standing close. Preschool children may extend their arms to maintain balance, but older children can normally stand with arms at their sides. Leaning or falling to one side is abnormal and indicates poor balance.

Coordination

Tests of coordination assess the smoothness and accuracy of movement. Development of fine motor skills can be used to assess coordination in young children (Table 8–21). After 6 years of age, the tests for adults (finger-to-nose, finger-to-finger, heel-to-shin, and alternating motion tests) can be used (Figure 8–63 ■). The child usually responds enthusiastically when these tests are presented as games. Jerky movements or inaccurate pointing (past pointing) indicates poor coordination, which can be associated with delayed development or a cerebellar lesion.

TABLE 8–20 Expected Balance Development for Age

BALANCE MILESTONES	AGE ATTAINED
Stands without support briefly	12 months
Walks alone well	15 months
Walks backwards	2 years
Balances on one foot for 5 seconds	4 years
Hops on one foot, heel-toe walking	5 years
Heel-toe walking backwards	6 years

Gait

A normal gait requires intact bones and joints, muscle strength, coordination, and balance. Inspect the child when walking from both a front and a rear view. The iliac crests are

TABLE 8–21 Expected Fine Motor Development for Age

FINE MOTOR MILESTONES	AGE ATTAINED
Transfers objects between hands	7 months
Picks up small objects	10 months
Feeds self with cup and spoon	12 months
Scribbles with crayon or pencil	18 months
Builds 2-block tower	24 months
Builds 4-block tower	30 months
Unfastens front buttons	36 months

From Frankenburg, W. K., Dodds, J., Archer, P., Shapiro, H., & Bresnick, B. (1992). The Denver II: A major revision and restandardization of the Denver Developmental Screening Test. Pediatrics, *89, 91–97.*

normally level during walking, and no limp is expected. Gait stance is related to the motor development of the child. Toddlers beginning to walk have a wide-based gait and limited balance. With practice, the toddler's balance improves and the gait develops a narrower base.

A limp may indicate injury or joint disease. Staggering or falling may indicate cerebellar ataxia. Scissoring, in which the thighs tend to cross forward over each other with each step, may be associated with cerebral palsy or other spastic conditions.

Cranial Nerve Function

To assess the cranial nerves in infants and young children, modifications can be made to the procedures used to assess school-age children and adults (Table 8–22). Abnormalities of cranial nerves may be associated with compression of an individual nerve, brain injury, or infection.

Sensory Function

To assess sensory function, compare the responses of both sides of the body to various types of stimulation. Equal responses bilaterally are normal. Loss of sensation may indicate a brain or spinal cord lesion. An infant's sensory function is not routinely assessed. Withdrawal responses to painful procedures indicate normal sensory function.

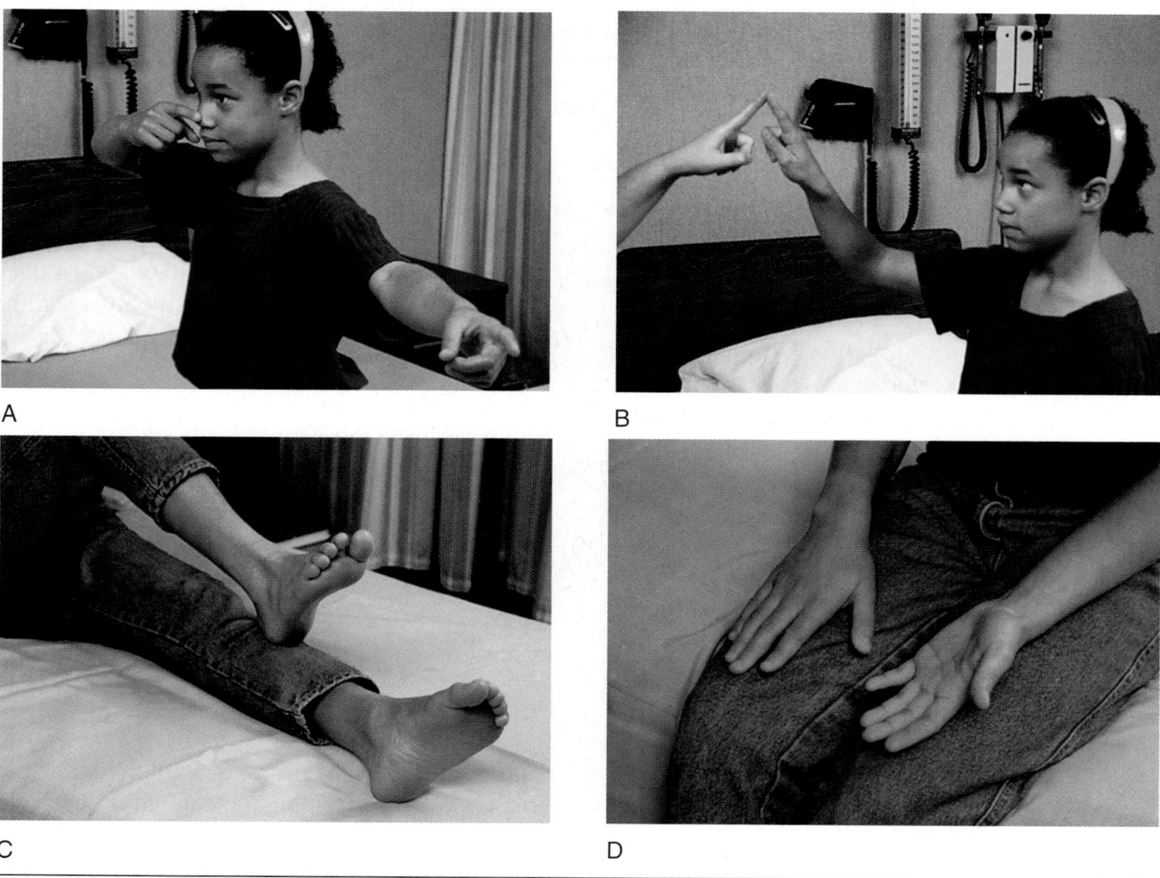

FIGURE 8–63 ■ Tests of coordination. A, *Finger-to-nose test.* Ask the child to close the eyes and touch his or her nose, alternating the index fingers of the hands. B, *Finger-to-finger test.* Ask the child to alternately touch his or her nose and your index finger with his or her index finger. Move your hand to several positions within the child's reach to test pointing accuracy. Repeat the test with the child's other hand. C, *Heel-to-shin test.* Ask the child to rub his or her leg from the knee to the ankle with the heel of the other foot. Repeat the test with the other foot. This test is normally performed without hesitation or inappropriate placement of the foot. D, *Rapid alternating motion test.* Ask the child to rapidly rotate his or her wrist so the palm and dorsum of the hand alternately pat the thigh. Repeat the test with the other hand. Hesitating movements are abnormal. Mirroring movements of the hand not being tested indicates a delay in coordination skill refinement.

TABLE 8–22 Cranial Nerve Assessment in Infants and Children

CRANIAL NERVE[a]	ASSESSMENT PROCEDURE AND NORMAL FINDINGS[b]
I Olfactory	Infant: Not tested. Child: Not routinely tested. Give familiar odors to child to smell, one naris at a time. *Identifies odors such as orange, peanut butter, and chocolate.*
II Optic	Infant: Shine a bright light in eyes. *A quick blink reflex and dorsal head flexion indicate light perception.* Child: Test vision and visual fields if cooperative. *Visual acuity appropriate for age.*
III Oculomotor IV Trochlear VI Abducens	Infant: Shine a penlight at the eyes and move it side to side. *Focuses on and tracks the light to each side.* Child: Move an object through the six cardinal points of gaze. *Tracks objects through all fields of gaze.* All ages: Inspect eyelids for drooping. Inspect pupillary response to light. *Eyelids do not droop and pupils are equal sized and briskly respond to light.*
V Trigeminal	Infant: Stimulate the rooting and sucking reflex. *Turns head toward stimulation at side of mouth and sucking has good strength and pattern.* Child: Observe the child chewing a cracker. Touch forehead and cheeks with cotton ball when eyes are closed. *Bilateral jaw strength is good. Child pushes cotton ball away.*
VII Facial	All ages: Observe facial expressions when crying, smiling, frowning, etc. *Facial features stay symmetric bilaterally.*
VIII Acoustic	Infant: Produce a loud sound near the head. *Blinks in response to sound, moves head toward sound, or freezes position.* Child: Use a noisemaker near each ear or whisper words to be repeated. *Turns head toward sound and repeats words correctly.*
IX Glossopharyngeal X Vagus	Infant: Observe swallowing during feeding. *Good swallowing pattern.* All ages: Elicit gag reflex. *Gags with stimulation.*
XI Spinal accessory	Infant: Not tested. Child: Ask child to raise the shoulders and turn the head side to side against resistance. *Good strength in neck and shoulders.*
XII Hypoglossal	Infant: Observe feeding. *Sucking and swallowing are coordinated.* Child: Tell the child to stick out the tongue. Listen to speech. *Torque is midline with no tremors. Words are clearly articulated.*

[a] *Bracketed nerves are tested together.*
[b] Italics indicate normal findings.

Superficial Tactile Sensation

Stroke the skin on the lower leg or arm with a cotton ball or a finger while the child's eyes are closed. Cooperative children over 2 years of age can normally point to the location touched.

Superficial Pain Sensation

Break a tongue blade to get a sharp point. After asking the child to close the eyes, touch the child in various places on each arm and leg, alternating the sharp and dull ends of the tongue blade. Children over 4 years of age can normally distinguish between a sharp and dull sensation each time. To improve the child's accuracy with the test, let the child practice telling you the difference between the sharp and dull stimulation.

An inability to identify superficial touch and pain sensation may indicate sensory loss. Identify the extent of sensory loss, such as all areas below the knee. Other sensory function tests (temperature, vibratory, deep pressure pain, and position sense) are performed when sensory loss is found. Refer to other texts for description of these procedures.

Infant Primitive Reflexes

Evaluate the movement and posture of newborns and young infants by the Moro, palmar grasp, plantar grasp, placing, stepping, and tonic neck primitive reflexes (Table 8–23). These reflexes appear and disappear at expected intervals in the first few months of life as the central nervous system develops. Movements are normally equal bilaterally. An asymmetric response may indicate a serious neurologic problem on the less responsive side.

Superficial and Deep Tendon Reflexes

Evaluate the superficial and deep tendon reflexes to assess the function of specific segments of the spine. The best response to deep tendon reflex testing is achieved when the child is relaxed or distracted. Children often anticipate the knee jerk and either tighten up or exaggerate the response. Making the child focus on another set of muscles may provide a more accurate response. When testing the reflexes on the lower legs, have the child press his or her hands together or try to pull them apart when gripped together.

Superficial Reflexes

Assess superficial reflexes by stroking a specific area of the body. The plantar reflex, testing spine levels L4 through S2, is routinely evaluated in children (see Figure 8–64 ■ on page 295). Assess the cremasteric reflex in boys (see page 280).

Deep Tendon Reflexes

To assess the deep tendon reflexes, tap a tendon near specific joints with a reflex hammer (or with the index finger for infants), comparing responses bilaterally. The biceps, triceps, brachioradialis, patellar, and Achilles tendons are usually evaluated in children. Inspect for movement in the associated joint and palpate the strength of the expected muscle contraction (Table 8–24). Table 8–25 outlines the numeric scoring of deep tendon reflexes. Responses are normally symmetric bilaterally. The absence of a response is associated with decreased muscle tone and strength. Hyperactive responses are associated with muscle spasticity.

TABLE 8–23 Techniques for Assessing Selected Primitive Reflexes, with Normal Findings and Their Expected Age of Occurrence

PRIMITIVE REFLEX	TECHNIQUE AND NORMAL FINDINGS[a]	NORMAL APPEARANCE AND DISAPPEARANCE
Moro 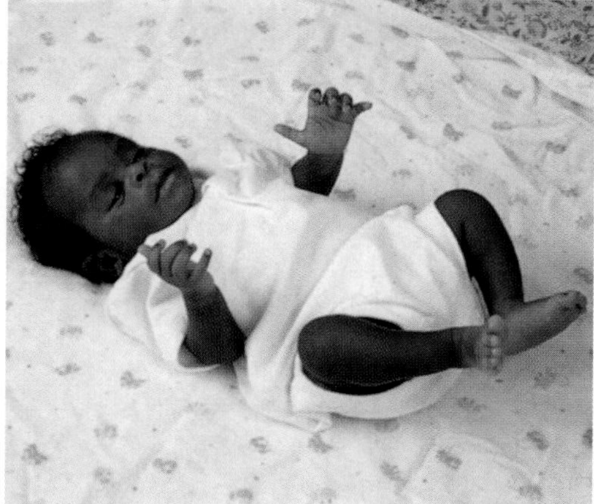	Startle the infant with a sudden noise or change in position. *The arms extend and the fingers form a C as they spread. The arms slowly move together as in a hug. The legs may make a similar motion.*	Present at birth. Decreases in strength by 4 months of age. Disappears by 6 months of age.
Palmar grasp 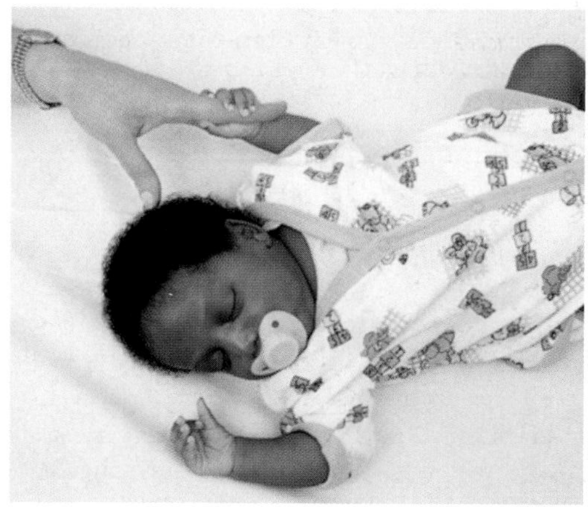	Place finger across the infant's palm and avoid touching the thumb. *A strong grip around the finger is normal.*	Present at birth. Disappears by 3 months of age.
Plantar grasp 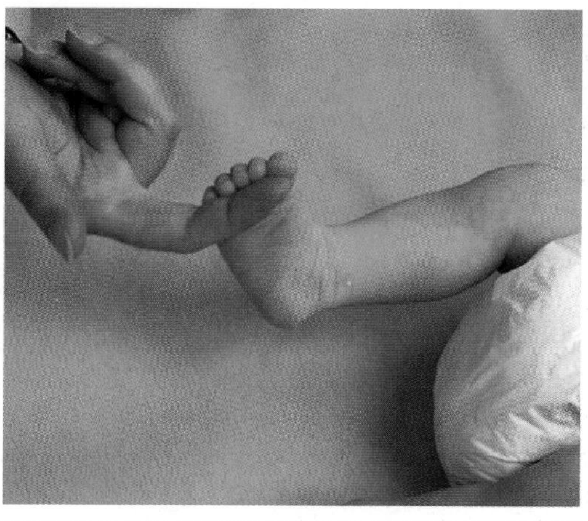	Place finger across the foot at the base of the toes. *The toes normally curl as if gripping the finger.*	Present at birth. Disappears at about 8 months of age.

[a] *Italics indicate normal findings.*

(continued)

TABLE 8–23 Techniques for Assessing Selected Primitive Reflexes, with Normal Findings and Their Expected Age of Occurrence (continued)

PRIMITIVE REFLEX	TECHNIQUE AND NORMAL FINDINGS[a]	NORMAL APPEARANCE AND DISAPPEARANCE
Placing 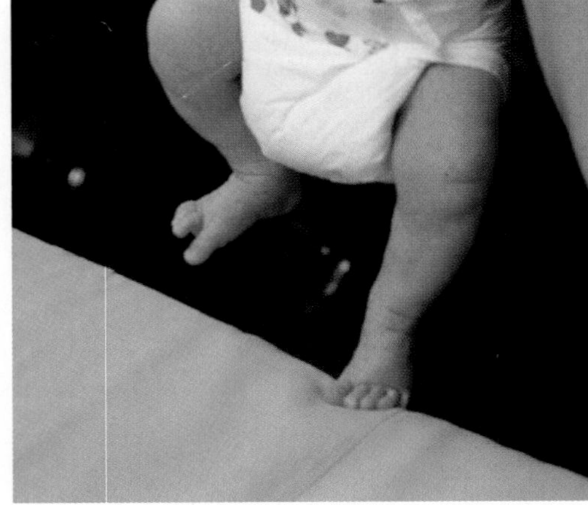	Hold the infant erect and touch the top of one foot with the edge of a table or chair. *The infant normally lifts the foot, as if to step up onto the surface.*	Present within days of birth. Disappears at various times.
Stepping 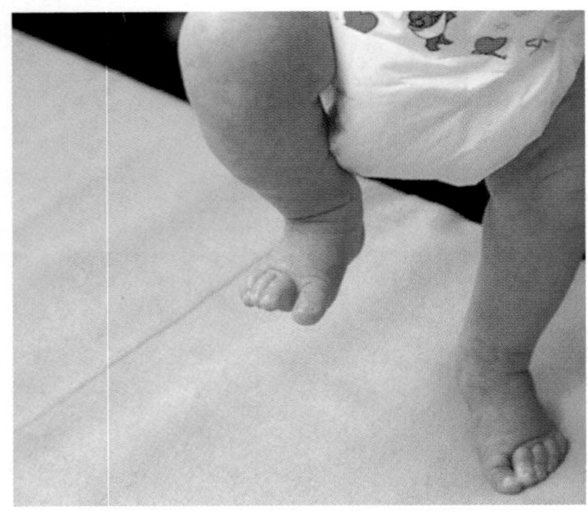	Hold the infant erect and touch the bottom of one foot on the surface of a table or chair. *The feet lift in an alternating pattern as if to walk.*	Present at birth. Disappears between 4 and 8 weeks of age.
Tonic neck 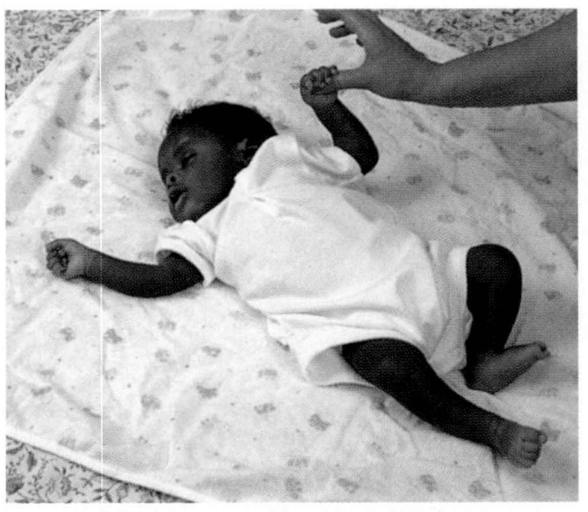	Place the infant in a supine position and, when relaxed, turn the head to one side. Repeat by turning the head to the opposite side. *The arm and leg on the face side normally extend and the opposite arm and leg flex, as if to assume a fencing position.*	Appears about 2 months of age. Decreases by 4 months of age. Disappears no later than 6 months of age. This reflex must disappear before the infant can turn over.

[a] *Italics indicate normal findings.*

TABLE 8–24 Assessment of Deep Tendon Reflexes and the Spinal Segment Tested With Each

DEEP TENDON REFLEX	TECHNIQUE AND NORMAL FINDINGS[a]	SPINE SEGMENT TESTED
Biceps 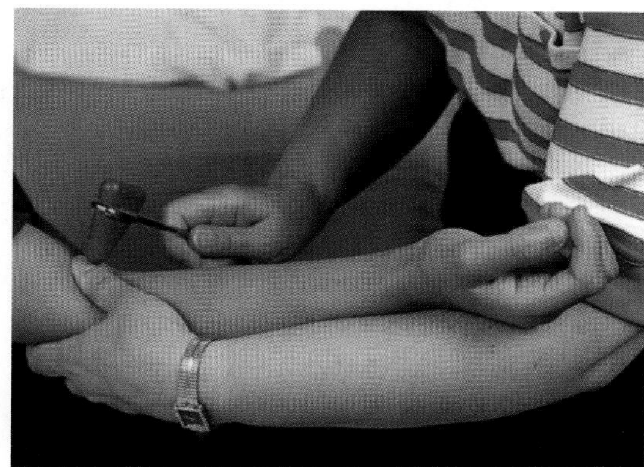	Flex the child's arm at the elbow, and place your thumb over the biceps tendon in the antecubital fossa. Tap your thumb. *Elbow flexes as the biceps muscle contracts.*	C5 and C6
Triceps 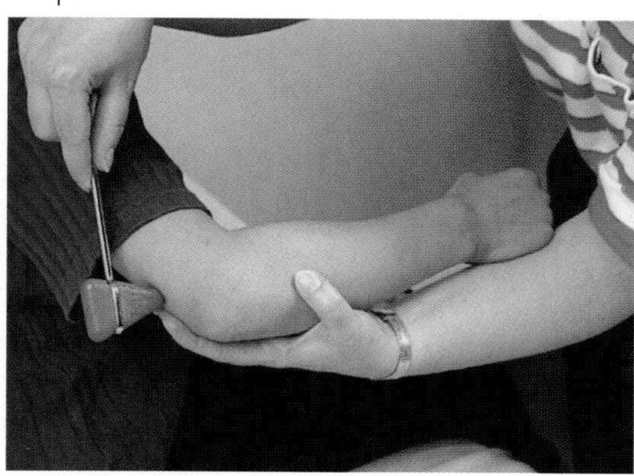	With the child's arm flexed, tap the triceps tendon above the elbow. *Elbow extends as the triceps muscle contracts.*	C6, C7, and C8
Brachioradialis 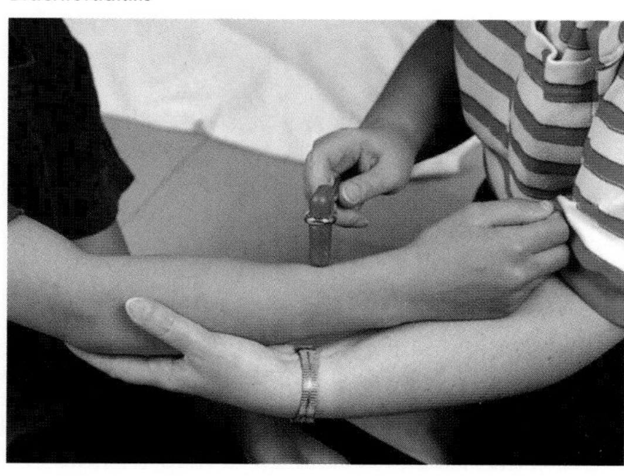	Lay the child's arm with the thumb upright over your arm. Tap the brachioradial tendon 2.5 cm (1 in.) above the wrist. *Forearm pronotes (palm facing downward) and elbow flexes.*	C5 and C6

(continued)

TABLE 8–24 Assessment of Deep Tendon Reflexes and the Spinal Segment Tested with Each (continued)

DEEP TENDON REFLEX	TECHNIQUE AND NORMAL FINDINGS[a]	SPINE SEGMENT TESTED
Patellar 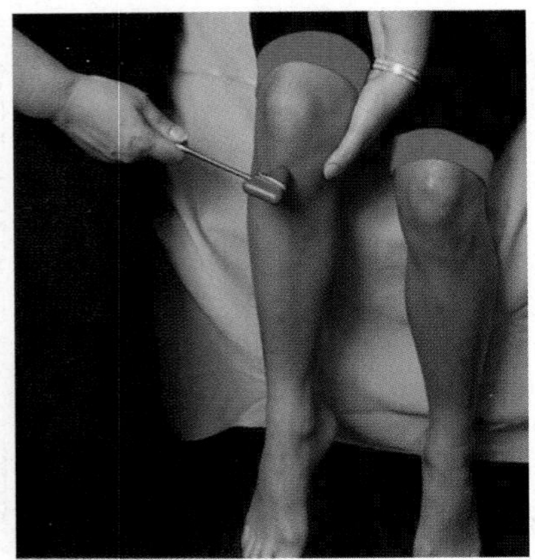	Flex the child's knees, and when the legs are relaxed, tap the patellar tendon just below the knee. *Knee extends (knee jerk) as the quadriceps muscle contracts.*	L2, L3, and L4
Achilles 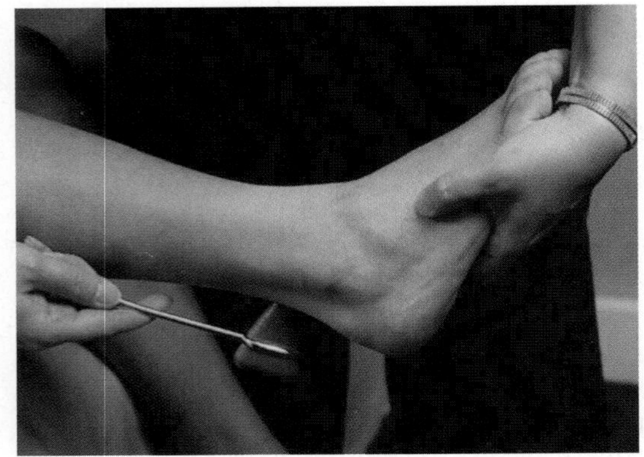	While the child's legs are flexed, support the foot and tap the Achilles tendon. *Plantar flexion (ankle jerk) as the gastrocnemius muscle contracts.*	S1 and S2

[a] *Italics indicate normal findings.*

ANALYZING DATA FROM THE PHYSICAL EXAMINATION

Once the physical examination has been completed, review all abnormal findings and group them together and contrast them with expected findings. Clinical judgment is used to identify common patterns of signs and physiologic responses that could be associated with medical conditions. Individual abnormal physiologic responses are also the basis of many nursing diagnoses.

Let us return to the vignette at the beginning of the chapter. Your thorough physical assessment of Latoya has revealed signs of respiratory difficulty and inadequate tissue perfusion from several body systems. These signs include mottled skin color, an increased resting respiratory rate, retractions, increased respiratory effort, nasal flaring, tachycardia, and lethargy. Based on these findings, you would be able to select nursing diagnoses appropriate for an infant with bronchiolitis, for example, Ineffective Breathing Pattern, use of accessory muscles to breathe related to respiratory muscle fatigue; and Caregiver Role Strain related to unpredictability of the care situation. These diagnoses, in turn, would direct your nursing care of this child.

NEWBORN ASSESSMENT

The newborn is examined at specific intervals while in the birthing facility due to the rapid transitions occurring from intrauterine to extrauterine life. It is important to know that the newborn is adapting to extrauterine life before discharge home. The primary changes that the newborn experiences are noted in the cardiovascular and respiratory systems, and these changes are triggered by the birthing process, exposure to the environment, and cutting the umbilical cord.

Newborn Transition

Prior to birth, the fetus was oxygenated by blood transferred from the placenta. At birth, the infant must initiate respirations. A series of mechanical, chemical, thermal, and sensory stimuli lead to the initiation of breathing.

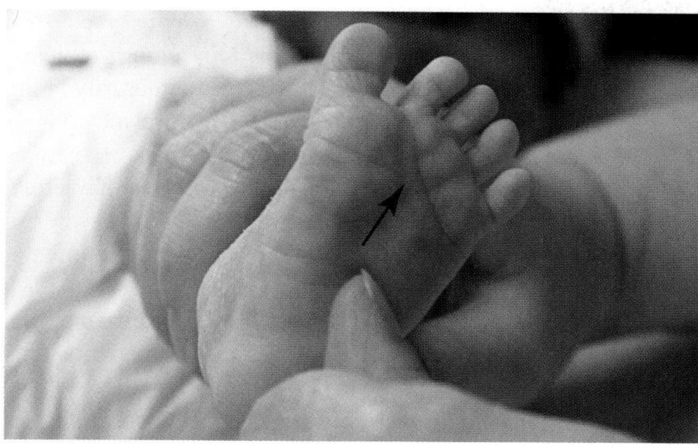

FIGURE 8–64 ■ To assess the plantar reflex, stroke the bottom of the infant's or child's foot in the direction of the arrow. Watch the toes for plantar flexion or the Babinski response, fanning and dorsiflexion of the big toe. The Babinski response is normal in children under 2 years of age. Plantar flexion of the toes is the normal response in older children. A Babinski response in children over 2 years of age can indicate neurologic disease.

- *Mechanical*—pressure on the thorax as the newborn passes through the birth canal forces some of the fluid out of the lungs. The negative pressure enables the lung to recoil and inspire a small amount of air to replace the fluid. The newborn exhales with crying against a partially closed glottis, leading to positive intrathoracic pressure. The air remaining in the lungs is distributed through the alveoli. With each succeeding breath the lungs continue to expand.
- *Chemical*—when the umbilical cord is clamped, the Po_2 level falls and the Pco_2 level rises. The aortic and carotid chemoreceptors are stimulated which triggers the respiratory center to initiate breathing. Lack of prostaglandin crossing the placenta facilitates closure of the ductus arteriosis.
- *Thermal*—The change in temperature between the uterus and external environment stimulates nerve endings that lead to rhythmic respirations.
- *Sensory*—various tactile, auditory, and visual stimuli also support the initiation of breathing.

The cardiovascular system begins transitioning after breathing has been initiated.

- The Po_2 rises in the alveoli after air enters the lungs and the pulmonary arteries relax leading to a decrease in pulmonary vascular resistance.

TABLE 8–25 Numeric Scoring of Deep Tendon Reflex Responses

GRADE	RESPONSE INTERPRETATION
0	No response
1+	Slow, minimal response
2+	Expected response, active
3+	More active or pronounced than expected
4+	Hyperactive, clonus may be present

- Blood flow to the lungs increases as pulmonary vascular resistance falls, making the transition from fetal circulation to newborn circulation.
- Blood flow to the extremities through the patent ductus arteriosis and foramen ovale is reduced as systemic vascular resistance increases. Functional closure of the ductus arteriosis occurs about 15 hours after birth. The foramen ovale is closed about 1 to 2 hours after birth. See Chapter 26∞ for more details of hemodynamic changes at birth.

MediaLink Case Study: Newborn Assessment

Assessment at Birth

Immediately after birth, the infant who is full term, pink, flexed, breathing spontaneously, and has no meconium staining may be moved to the mother's abdomen and be warmed with skin-to-skin contact and a warm blanket. The newborn needing initial assistance and support with breathing is moved to a radiant warming table for assessment to determine the need for resuscitation or other interventions. Decisions about the need for resuscitation are made and implemented quickly, often before the Apgar score is obtained. The Apgar score is used to determine the newborn's adaptation to extrauterine life at 1 and 5 minutes after birth. The heart rate, respiratory effort, muscle tone, grimace or irritability, and color are evaluated. The score for each physiologic response is 0, 1, or 2 according to criteria listed in Table 8–26. Total scores may range from 0 to 10. A score of 8 to 10 indicates the newborn is adapting to extrauterine conditions and needs routine supportive care. A score of 5 to 7 indicates an alteration in the newborn respiratory, cardiac, or nervous system, and the need for supportive measures. A score of 4 or less requires immediate and aggressive resuscitation. Extremely preterm infants have lower Apgar scores than full-term infants due to neuromuscular immaturity. Health professionals implement aggressive resuscitation without waiting for a 5-minute score. Newborns with a 5-minute Apgar score less than 7 are at greater risk for morbidity and ongoing organ system dysfunction.

PRACTICE ALERT

Because newborns have a large skin surface area for their body mass, they are at much greater risk of losing body heat. Special precautions to help the newborn conserve body heat are needed. Newborns lose body heat in four ways:

- **Evaporation**—water or liquid on the newborn's skin is converted to vapor and cools the newborn
- **Convection**—movement of cool air currents across the newborn's skin removes heat
- **Radiation**—body heat transfers to a cooler surface not in contact with the skin
- **Conduction**—body heat transfers to a cooler surface in contact with the skin

Immediately drying the infant after birth and moving the newborn to a warm location, such as the mother's abdomen or a radiant warmer, helps reduce heat loss at the time of birth. *What measures are used to conserve the newborn's body temperature in the newborn nursery?*

After the newborn is stable, a brief examination is conducted to identify the general condition of the cardiovascular, respiratory, neurologic, and gastrointestinal systems, as well as any congenital anomalies. With the newborn on a warming table,

TABLE 8–26 The Apgar Scoring System

	SCORING		
PHYSIOLOGIC SIGN	**0**	**1**	**2**
Heart rate	Absent	Slow, below 100	Above 100
Respiratory effort	Absent	Slow, irregular	Good crying
Muscle tone	Flaccid	Some flexion of extremities	Active motion
Reflex irritability	None	Grimace	Vigorous cry
Color	Pale blue	Body pink, blue extremities	Completely pink

From Apgar, V. (1966, August). The newborn (Apgar) scoring system, reflections and advice. Pediatric Clinics of North America, *13, 645. Used with permission from Elsevier.*

auscultate the heart and lungs and take the initial vital signs (temperature, heart rate, respiratory rate). Palpate the abdomen and examine the umbilical cord for the presence of three vessels. Inspect the head, face, oral cavity, extremities, genitalia, and perineum for the presence of any visible defects. Assess reactivity; the newborn's behavioral responses immediately after birth should be active and alert. The infant may appear hungry and have a strong sucking reflex. Bursts of random diffuse movements alternating with no movement may also be noted.

Assessment of the Newborn

The comprehensive newborn assessment, including a gestational age assessment, is conducted within the first few hours of birth to make sure the newborn's transition to extrauterine life is proceeding as expected or to identify specific problems that put the newborn at risk. The newborn assessment is repeated prior to discharge from the birthing facility. Most of the techniques of physical assessment used for the newborn were presented earlier in the chapter; however, their application to the newborn, special procedures, and newborn findings are described here.

Gestational Age Assessment

It is important to determine the gestational age of newborns to determine the risk for conditions associated with prematurity or postmaturity. When the mother's menstrual history is reliable, determination of gestational age can be calculated counting the number of completed weeks between the first day of the mother's last menstrual period and the date of birth. However, this method is not always correct. In many cases, prenatal ultrasound is used to assess gestation. The nurse can compare the mother's dates, ultrasound gestational assessment, and the Ballard assessment for the best estimate of the newborn's gestational age. Gestational ages of 37 to 41 completed weeks are considered to be term. Infants born before 37 weeks of gestation are preterm. Infants born after 41 completed weeks of gestation are postterm.

Gestational age assessment is performed on all newborns to assess the stage of newborn maturity. Knowledge of the birth weight and gestational age helps to determine if newborns are large, appropriate, or small for gestational age. Newborns found to be small or large for gestational age are at risk for greater morbidity. For example, preterm infants may be large for gestational age but still experience the problems of prematurity, such as respiratory distress syndrome, temperature instability, and feeding problems. A higher birth weight does not indicate increased maturity of the newborn. Conversely, a term or postterm newborn may have a low birth weight indicating a need for more careful assessment as they are at increased risk for respiratory distress, hypoglycemia, infection, and temperature instability. The preterm newborn's gestational age is also used to evaluate the infant's developmental progress during future health promotion visits.

The Ballard Gestational Age Assessment Tool evaluates six physical and six neuromuscular characteristics of maturity. This tool updates the earlier Dubowitz assessment of gestational age by expanding it to include extreme preterm newborn characteristics. The physical characteristics are assessed with the following guidelines.

- *Skin*—assess for thickness, transparency, and texture. The preterm infant's skin is thin, smooth, and has visible blood vessels. The extremely preterm infant has sticky, transparent skin. The term infant has thick skin that may have a flaky texture, and blood vessels are difficult to see.
- *Lanugo*—assess for the quantity of lanugo, the fine, soft hair covering the fetus during intrauterine development. This hair begins to appear at approximately 24 weeks' gestation and is mostly shed by 37 weeks' gestation. It first begins to thin over the lower back, and then disappears last from the shoulders.
- *Plantar surfaces*—assess the number of deep folds and creases over the sole of the foot. See Figure 8–65 ■. One to two creases appear at approximately 32 weeks' gestation, and by 36 weeks creases cover the anterior two thirds of the foot. At term, creases cover the entire foot. For extremely preterm infants, a measurement of the foot length from the tip of the great toe to the back of the heel is taken.
- *Breast*—assess the chest for the visibility of the nipple and areola. See Figure 8–66 ■. Then assess the size of the breast bud when grasped between the thumb and forefinger. The extremely preterm infant has no visible nipple and areola. The nipple and areola become more defined and raised by 34 weeks' gestation. A small breast bud appears by 36 weeks' gestation, and grows to 5 to 10 mm in term infants.
- *Eye/ear*—assess the formation of the ear cartilage and curving of the pinna. See Figure 8–67 ■. At earlier gestational ages the lack of cartilage allows the ear to fold easily and retain the fold. As gestational age increases, the resistance of the ear to folding increases and recoil is seen. In extremely preterm infants the pinnae are flat. Incurving proceeds from the top down toward the lobes with advancing gestational age. In extremely preterm infants the eyelids are examined with gentle flexion to determine the amount of fusion.
- *Genitals (male)*—assess whether testicles are in the scrotum and presence of scrotal rugae. See Figure 8–68 ■. The testicles are in the inguinal canal around 28 weeks' gestation and scrotal rugae are becoming visible. By 36 weeks, the testicles are in the upper scrotum and rugae cover the anterior third of the scrotum. At term, rugae cover the scrotum, and at postterm the testicles are pendulous.

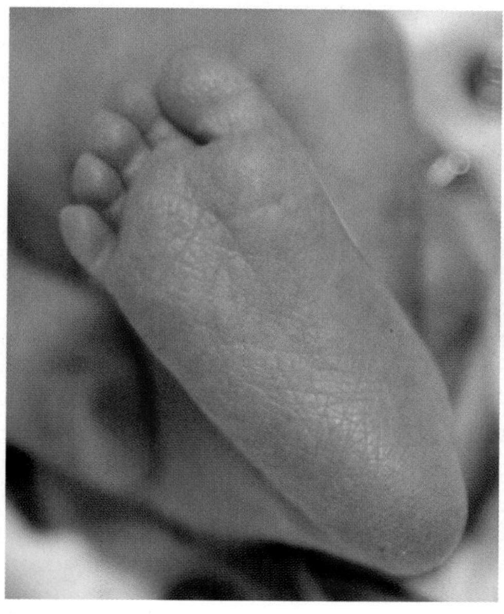
A

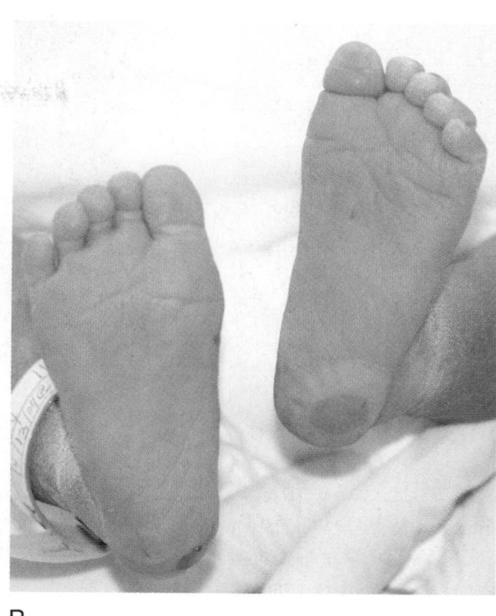
B

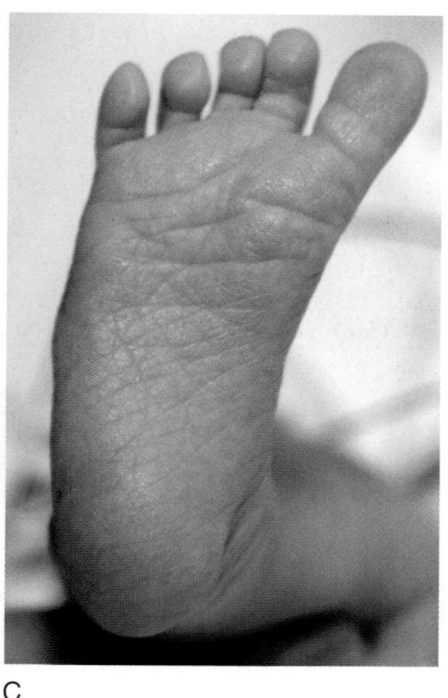
C

FIGURE 8–65 ■ Sole creases. *A,* At a gestational age of approximately 35 weeks, the newborn has few sole creases only on the anterior portion of the foot. *B,* At a gestational age of approximately 37 weeks, the newborn has a deeper network of sole creases on the anterior two thirds of the sole. *C,* At term, the newborn has deep creases down to and including the heel as the skin loses fluid and dries after birth.

- *Genitals (female)*—assess labial development. See Figure 8–69 ■. The clitoris is initially prominent and the labia minora are flat. By 36 weeks, the labia majora are larger and the clitoris is nearly covered.

The neuromuscular characteristics are assessed using the following guidelines.

- *Posture*—assess the position the infant assumes at rest in supine position. See Figure 8–70 ■ on page 299. The extremely preterm infant will lie with arms and legs extended or in any posture placed. With advancing gestational age, the infant has more flexion in the arms and legs. At term the infant lies with arms flexed to the chest, hands fisted, and legs flexed toward the abdomen.
- *Square window*—assess the angle of the wrist when the palm is flexed toward the forearm. See Figure 8–71 ■ on page 300. The preterm infant has poor flexion and is unable to flex the arm at the elbow more than 90 degrees. The extremely preterm infant has no flexor tone and cannot achieve a 90-degree angle. The term infant can achieve complete flexion against the forearm.
- *Arm recoil*—assess the amount of elbow flexion as illustrated in Figure 8–72 ■ on page 300. Term infants resist extension and briskly return their arms to flexed position.

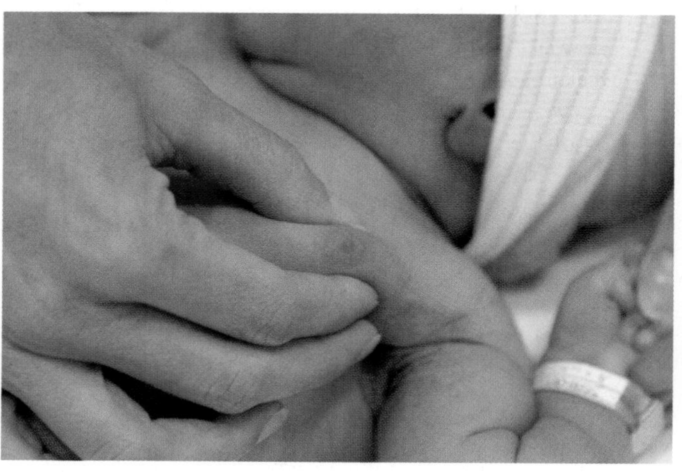
A

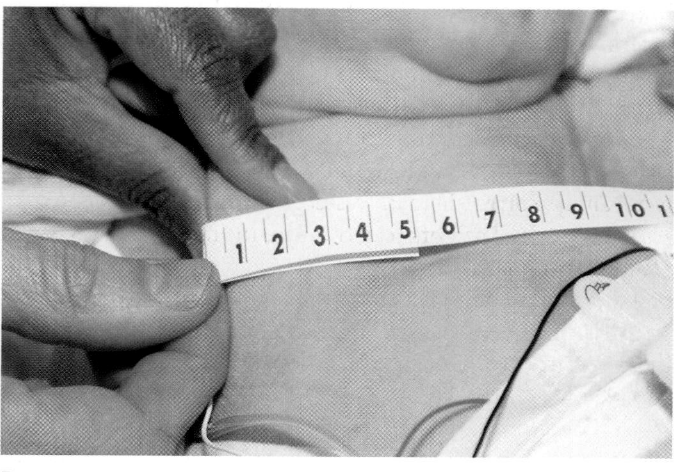

B

FIGURE 8–66 ■ Breast tissue. To assess breast tissue, gently compress the tissue between the middle and index fingers and measure the tissue in millimeters. *A,* At a gestational age of 38 weeks, the newborn has a visible raised area that is 4 mm in diameter on palpation. *B,* At a gestational age of 40–44 weeks, the newborn has 10 mm breast tissue.

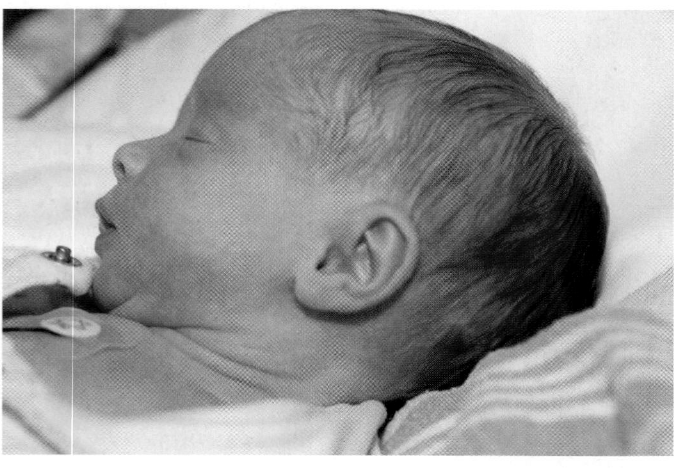

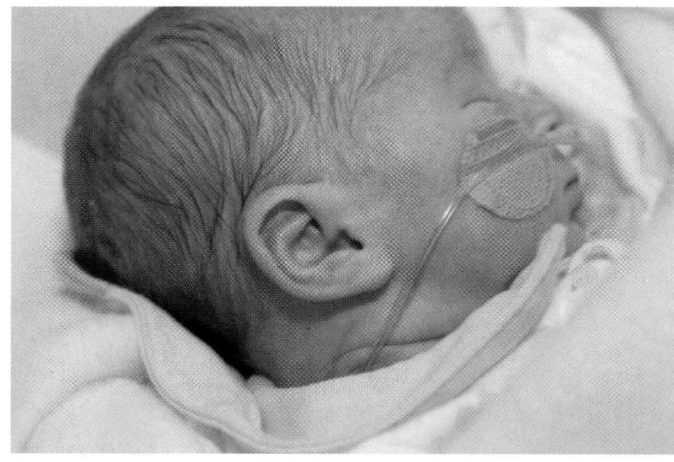

A B

FIGURE 8–67 ■ Ear form and cartilage. Press the pinna over to see how quickly it returns to original position. If it stays in the pressed position or returns slowly to the original position, the gestational age is usually less than 38 weeks. *A,* At a gestational age of approximately 36 weeks, the ear of the infant shows incurving of the upper two thirds of the pinna. *B,* At term, the ear of the infant shows well-defined incurving of the entire pinna.

Very preterm infants do not resist extension and respond with weak and delayed flexion in a small arc.

- *Popliteal angle*—assess the angle of the knee with the infant in supine position holding the pelvis flat as demonstrated in Figure 8–73 ■ on page 301. Estimate the angle of the knee. The infant with more advanced gestational age will have greater flexion.
- *Scarf sign*—assess the infant's resistance to pulling the arm across the chest toward the opposite shoulder when in supine position. See Figure 8–74 ■ on page 301. The term infant's elbow will not cross the midline of the chest. The preterm infant's elbow will move closer to the opposite shoulder with decreasing gestational age.
- *Heel-to-ear extension*—assess the amount of resistance to extension of the leg toward the ear without holding the knee or thigh in place as demonstrated in Figure 8–75 ■ on page 301. The infant's heel will come closer to the head with decreasing gestational age.

Specific criteria are used to score each characteristic as seen in Figure 8–76 ■ on page 302. Scores for each characteristic range from −1 to 4 or 5. Each of the 12 characteristics is scored according to criteria. In some facilities, 0.5 point is given when findings fall between criteria for the whole-number score. It is also important to note that newborns will not necessarily have consistent scores for each characteristic as maturity of different characteristics may vary in that newborn. Once the scoring for all criteria is completed, the scores are added together. The minimum score with this tool is −10, corresponding to a gestational age of 20 weeks. The maximum score is 50, corresponding to a gestational age of 44 weeks. The total score is then compared to the maturity rating table to identify the esti-

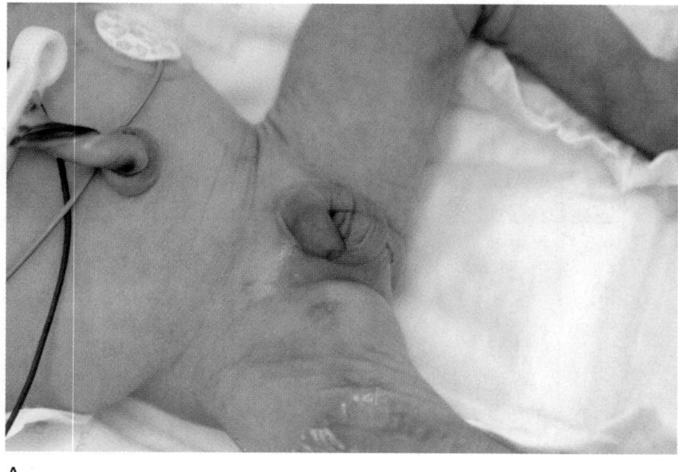

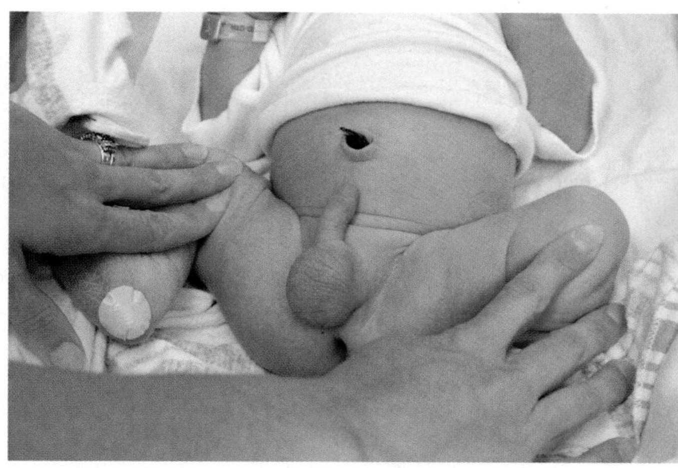

A B

FIGURE 8–68 ■ Male genitals. *A,* Note the absence of the testicles in the scrotum, and a scrotum with few rugae in the preterm newborn. *B,* In the term newborn, the testicles are usually descended into the scrotum, and the scrotum is covered by rugae.

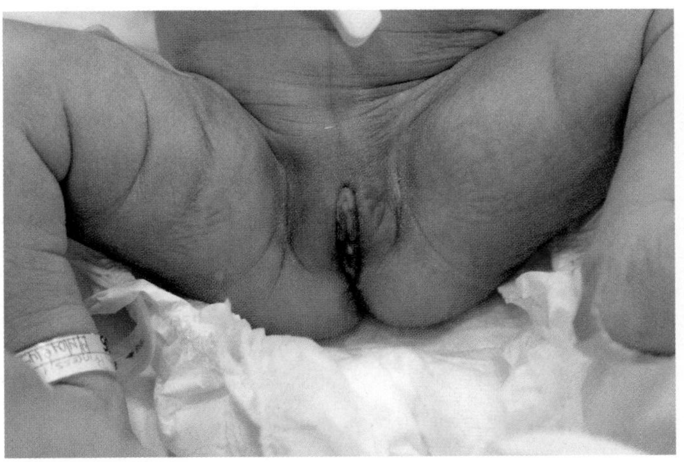

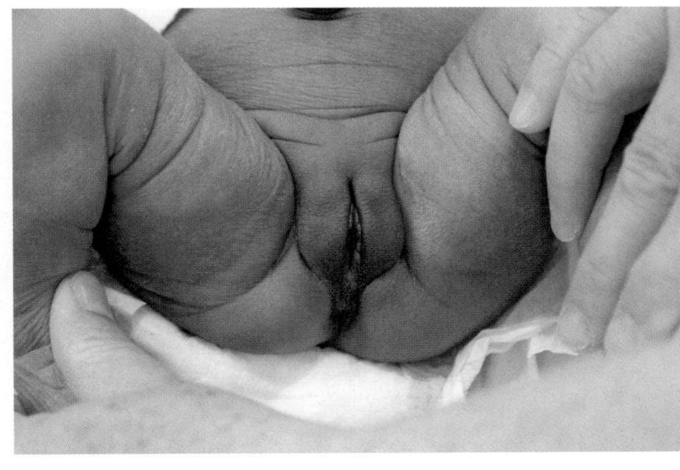

FIGURE 8–69 ■ Female genitals. *A,* At a gestational age of 30–36 weeks, the newborn has a prominent clitoris, widely separated labia majora, and labia minora protruding beyond the labia majora (when viewed laterally). *B,* At term, the labia majora are well developed and cover both the clitoris and labia minora.

mated gestational age. The findings of the assessment process are accurate within 2 weeks of the assigned gestational age. Scores for infants, especially those less than 26 weeks' gestation, are most accurate when performed within 12 hours of birth (Dodd, 1996). However, the Ballard Gestational Age Assessment Tool loses some accuracy in infants under 28 weeks' or over 43 weeks' gestation.

Size for Gestational Age

Once the gestational age is assessed, the newborn's birth weight is used to determine the size classification (small, appropriate, or large) for gestational age. A standardized intrauterine growth curve is used to plot the newborn's anthropometric measurements (birth weight) for the gestational age. See Figure 8–77 ■ on page 303 and Appendix A∞. Small-for-gestational-age infants fall below the 10th percentile. Appropriate-for-gestational-age infants fall between the 10th and 90th percentiles. Large-for-gestational-age infants fall above the 90th percentile.

Length is also measured, but it is difficult to obtain a reliable measurement because of the natural flexion of the newborn and molding of the head. One method of length measurement is to place the infant on his or her back with the legs extended as far as

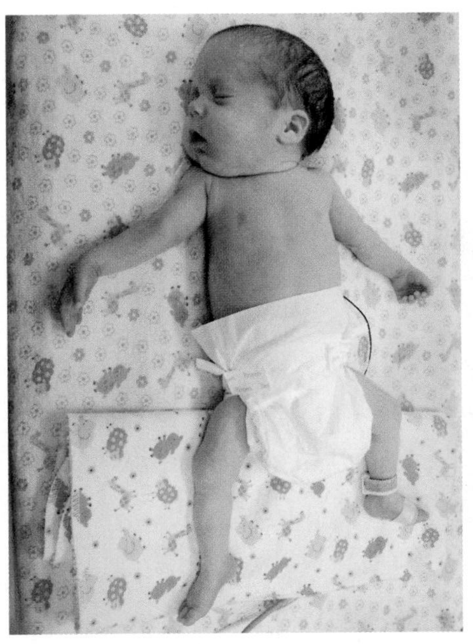

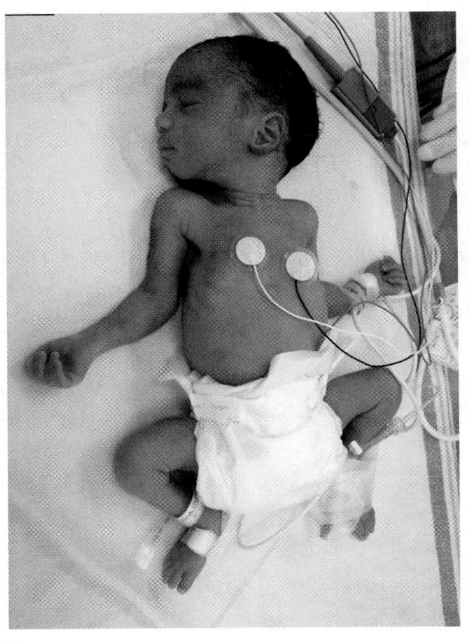

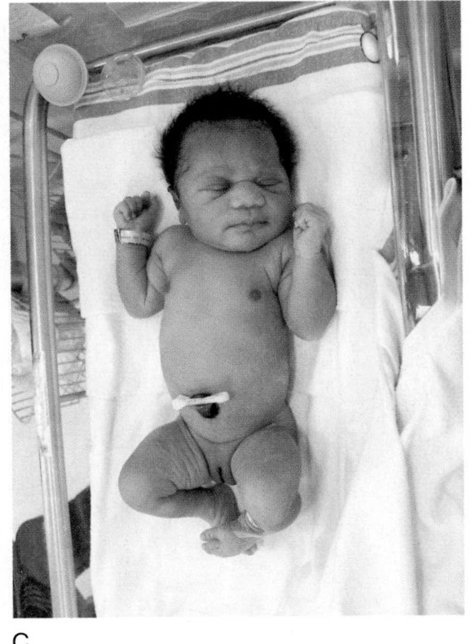

FIGURE 8–70 ■ Resting posture. *A,* At a gestational age of approximately 31 weeks, there is extension of the upper extremities and beginning flexion of the thighs. *B,* At a gestational age of approximately 35 weeks the newborn shows stronger flexion of the arms, hips, and thighs. *C,* At term, the newborn exhibits hypertonic flexion of all extremities.

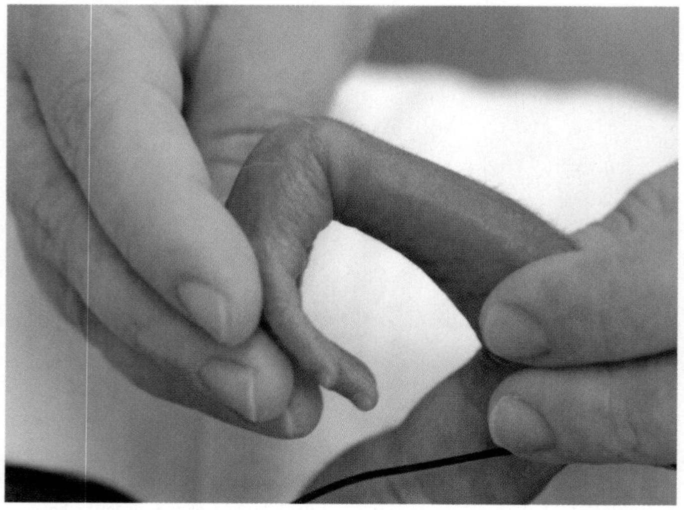

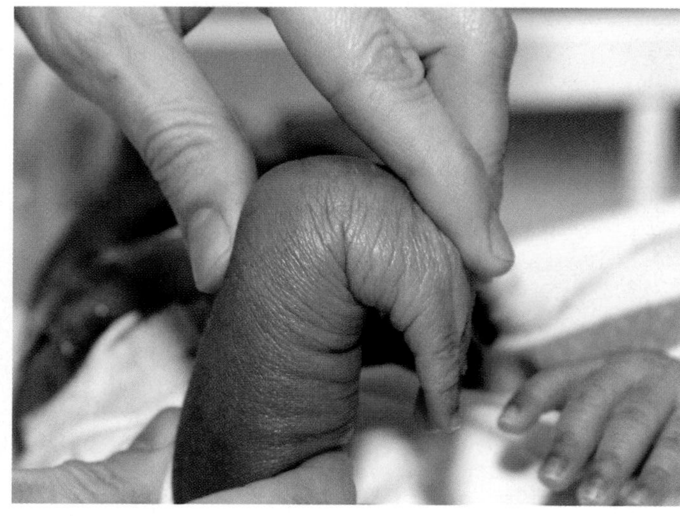

FIGURE 8–71 ■ Square window sign. *A,* At approximately 28–32 weeks' gestation, the angle is 90 degrees. *B,* At a gestational age of approximately 39–40 weeks, the angle is commonly 30 degrees.

possible. Place the top of the measuring tape at the top of the head and stretch the tape to the heel of the foot as shown in Figure 8–78 ■ on page 303. Each facility should use a consistent technique to increase the reliability between examiners. Verify the accuracy of the length with a second measurement (Johnson et al., 1999). Plot the length on the gestational age growth curve.

A weight-length ratio can also be calculated and plotted by gestational age growth curves to determine if weight and length are proportional. The formula is

$$100 \times \text{weight in grams/length}^3 \text{ in centimeters.}$$

Head circumference is measured as previously described and in some cases is contrasted to the chest circumference. The head circumference is generally 2 cm larger than the chest circumference. Plot the head circumference on the gestational age growth curve.

General Appearance

Following gestational age assessment, observe the newborn's general appearance, body proportions, posture, and movements. The newborn's head is about one fourth of the total body size. The body appears long with short extremities due to their flexed position. Full-term newborns generally lie in a symmetrical position with the limbs semiflexed similar to their position in utero. The legs are partially abducted at the hip. The chest appears rounded and the abdomen appears

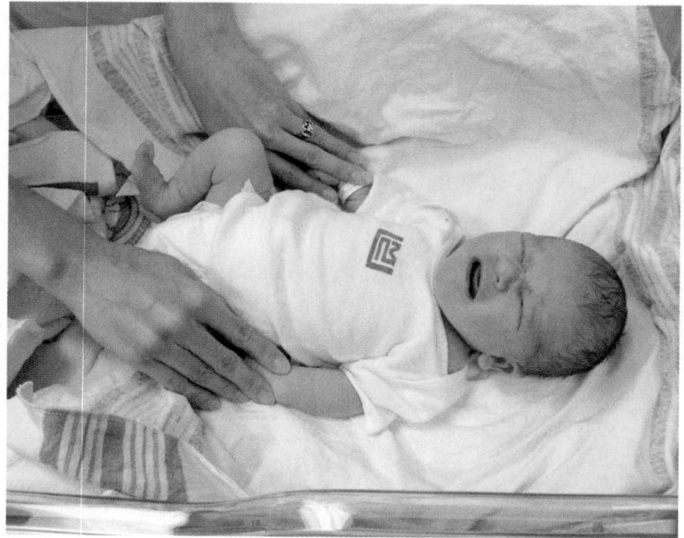

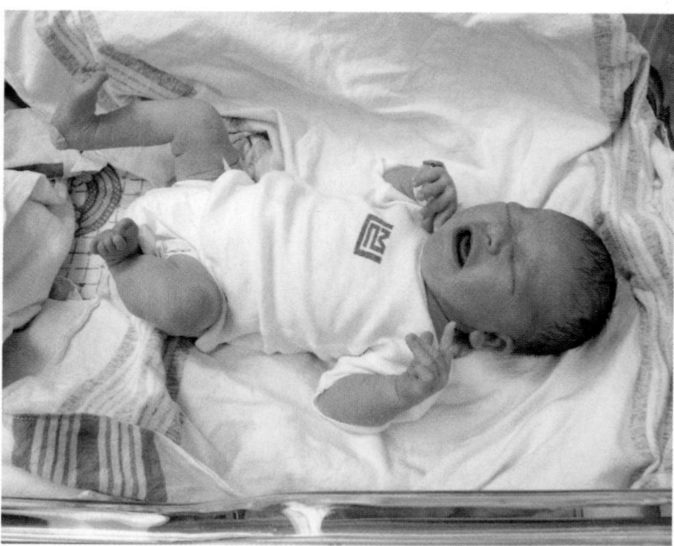

FIGURE 8–72 ■ Elicit the arm recoil by flexing the arms at the elbows to the chest for 5 seconds. *A,* Then extend the arms at the elbows. *B,* Release the arms to see the amount of recoil. In healthy newborns, the angle of flexion is usually less than 90 degrees followed by rapid recoil to the flexed position.

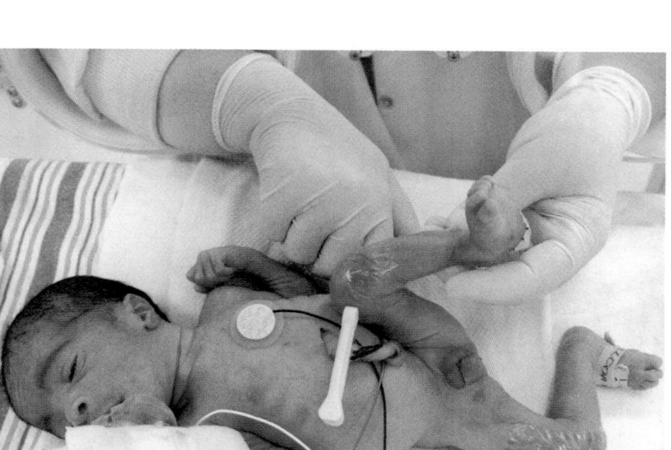

FIGURE 8–73 ■ To assess the popliteal angle, flex and hold the thigh to the abdomen while extending the leg at the knee.

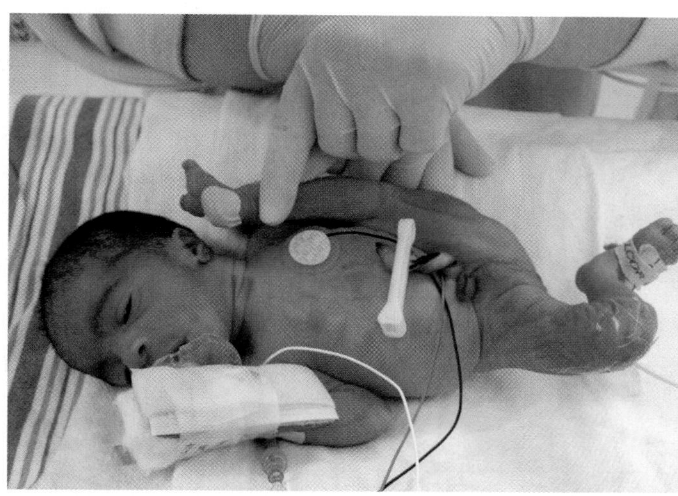

FIGURE 8–75 ■ Heel-to-ear scoring. Move the infant's foot as near to the head or ear as possible and determine the distance between the heel and head.

prominent. The head is slightly flexed and positioned in midline or turned to one side. The hands are held in a tight fist but they may occasionally extend the fingers. Infants of breech birth have legs and head extended. In frank breech, the legs are abducted and externally rotated, and the feet may be dorsiflexed.

The newborn typically has a second phase of reactivity lasting 4 to 6 hours that occurs following a short sleep phase. The newborn is awake and alert making this a good time to assess motor and neurologic responses such as sucking, rooting, and other primitive reflexes. Spontaneous motor activity with flexion and extension alternating between the arms and legs is common. Tremors of the arms, legs, and body may be seen with vigorous crying or at rest for the first 48 hours. Be alert for asymmetrical movements as they may indicate birth injuries, congenital anomalies, or a neurologic deficit.

Listen to the quality of the newborn's cry; it should be strong, lusty, and of medium pitch. A high-pitched cry with a shrill quality may indicate hypoglycemia or a neurologic condition. Grunting with respirations indicates respiratory distress.

Vital Signs. Regular temperature measurements are important as newborns are at risk for heat loss and are unable to stabilize their temperature in the first few hours after birth. Temperature is taken by an axillary thermometer. Axillary temperatures range from 36.4° to 37.2°C (97.5° to 99.0°F). A skin thermal sensor may be used for some newborns when temperature instability is a concern.

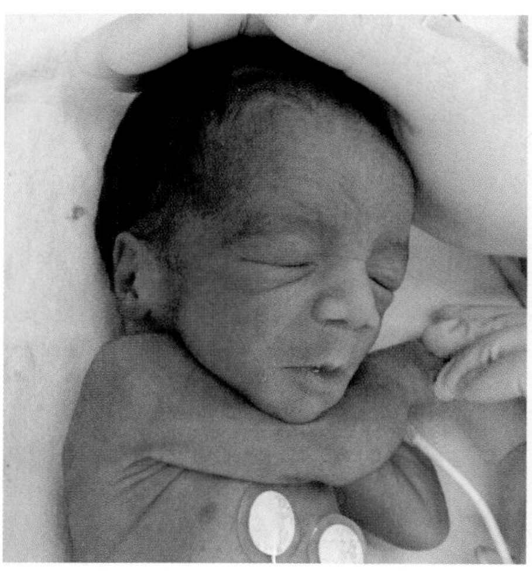

A

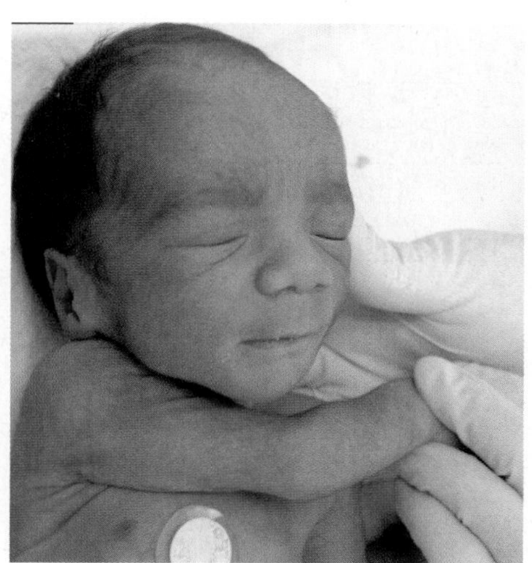

B

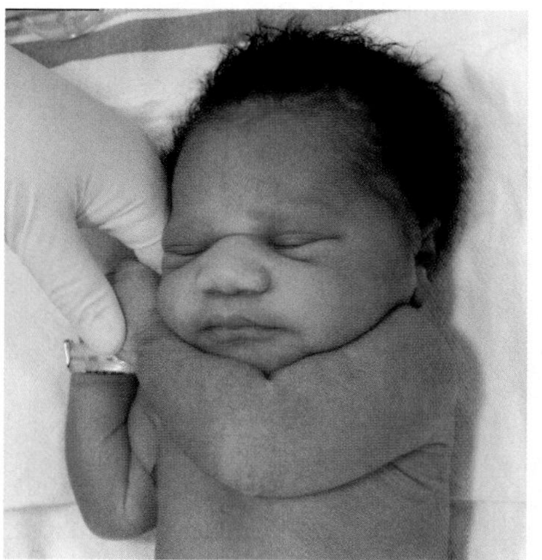

C

FIGURE 8–74 ■ Scarf sign. *A,* Until approximately 30 weeks' gestation, the elbow moves past midline with no resistance. *B,* At approximately 36–40 weeks' gestation, the elbow is at midline. *C,* The elbow will not reach midline after 40 weeks' gestation.

NEWBORN MATURITY RATING & CLASSIFICATION

ESTIMATION OF GESTATIONAL AGE BY MATURITY RATING
Symbols: X - 1st Exam O - 2nd Exam

NEUROMUSCULAR MATURITY

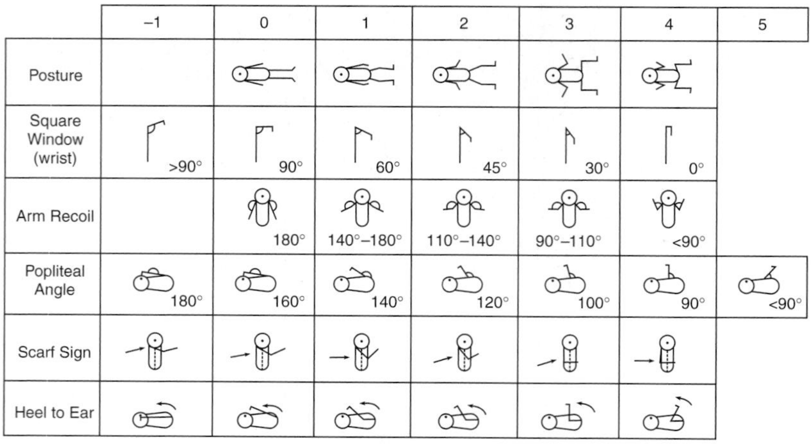

	−1	0	1	2	3	4	5
Posture							
Square Window (wrist)	>90°	90°	60°	45°	30°	0°	
Arm Recoil		180°	140°–180°	110°–140°	90°–110°	<90°	
Popliteal Angle	180°	160°	140°	120°	100°	90°	<90°
Scarf Sign							
Heel to Ear							

Gestation by Dates ____________ wks

Birth Date ________ Hour ________ am pm

APGAR ________ 1 min ________ 5 min

MATURITY RATING

score	weeks
−10	20
−5	22
0	24
5	26
10	28
15	30
20	32
25	34
30	36
35	38
40	40
45	42
50	44

PHYSICAL MATURITY

Skin	sticky friable transparent	gelatinous red, translucent	smooth pink, visible veins	superficial peeling &/or rash, few veins	cracking pale areas rare veins	parchment deep cracking no vessels	leathery cracked wrinkled
Lanugo	none	sparse	abundant	thinning	bald areas	mostly bald	
Plantar Surface	heel-toe 40-50mm:−1 <40mm:−2	>50mm no crease	faint red marks	anterior transverse crease only	creases ant. 2/8	creases over entire sole	
Breast	imperceptible	barely perceptible	flat areola no bud	stippled areola 1–2mm bud	raised areola 3–4mm bud	full areola 5–10mm bud	
Eye/Ear	lids fused loosely:−1 tightly:−2	lids open pinna flat stays folded	sl. curved pinna; soft slow recoil	well curved pinna, soft but ready recoil	formed & firm instant recoil	thick cartilage ear stiff	
Genitals male	scrotum flat, smooth	scrotum empty faint rugae	testes in upper canal rare rugae	testes descending few rugae	testes down good rugae	testes pendulous deep rugae	
Genitals female	clitoris prominent labia flat	prominent clitoris small labia minora	prominent clitoris enlarging minora	majora & minora equally prominent	majora large minora small	majora cover clitoris & minora	

SCORING SECTION

	1st Exam = X	2ndExam = 0
Estimating Gest Age by Maturity Rating	______Weeks	______Weeks
Time of Exam	Date ______ Hour ______ am pm	Date ______ Hour ______ am pm
Age at Exam	______ Hours	______ Hours
Signature of Examiner	______ M.D.	______ M.D.

FIGURE 8–76 ■ Ballard scoring system to assess gestational maturity.

Reprinted from Ballard, J. L., Khoury, J. C., Wang, L., Eilers-Walsmann, B. L., & Lipp, R. (1991). New Ballard score, expanded to include extremely premature infants. Journal of Pediatrics, *119(3), 417–423. Used with permission from Elsevier.*

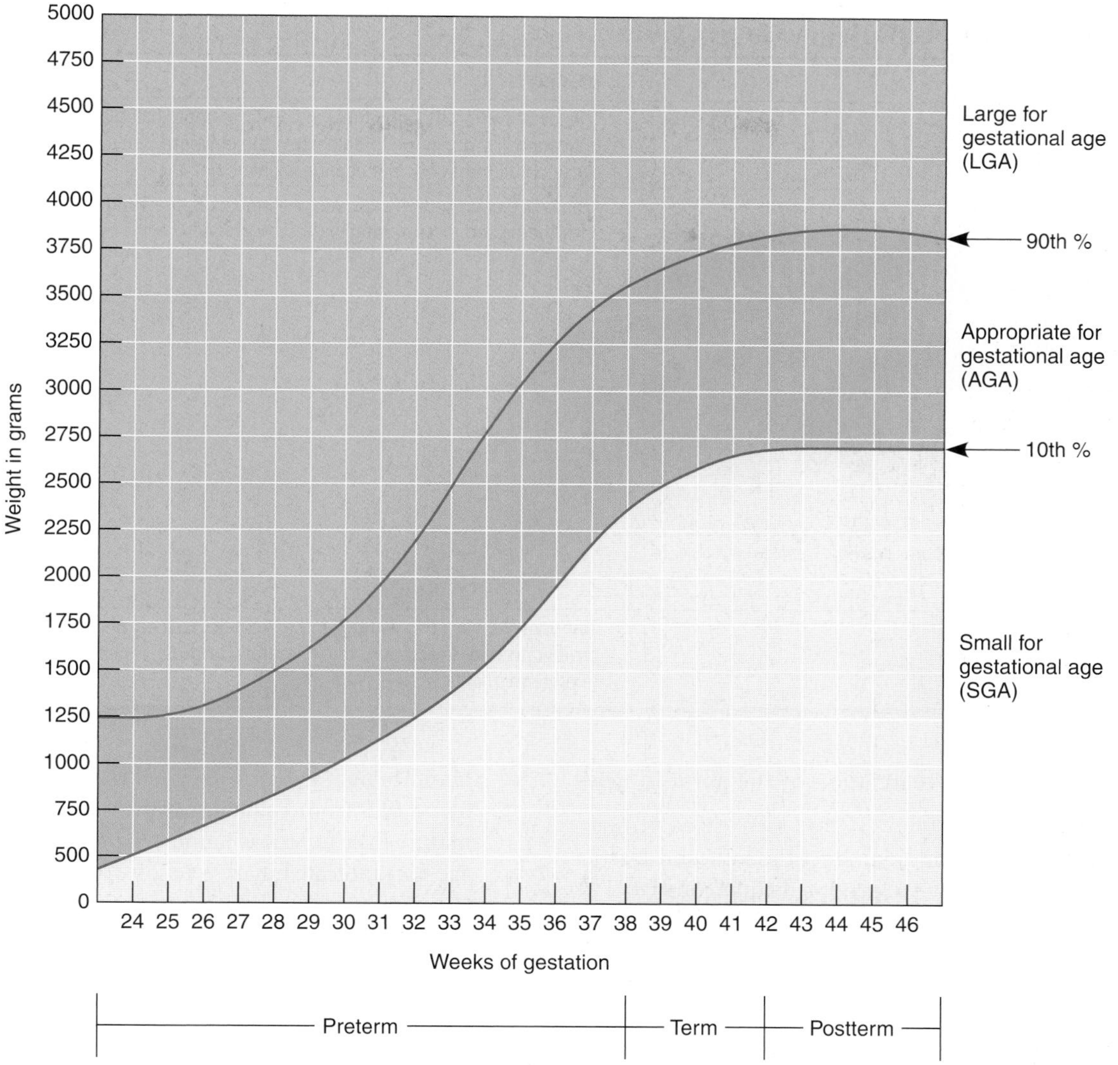

FIGURE 8–77 ■ Preterm infant growth chart to determine size (weight) for gestational age.

Reprinted from Battaglia, F. C., & Lubchenco, L. O. (1967). A practical classification of newborn infants by weight and gestational age. Journal of Pediatics, *71(2), 161. Used with permission from Elsevier.*

The respiratory rate should be counted for a full minute when the newborn is sleeping or resting quietly. Use the stethoscope to auscultate the rate or place your hand over the abdomen because the breathing is primarily diaphragmatic. The respiratory rate may range between 30 and 60 breaths per minute. Periods of apnea lasting less than 20 seconds duration are common, but no skin color changes or heart rate changes should accompany these episodes.

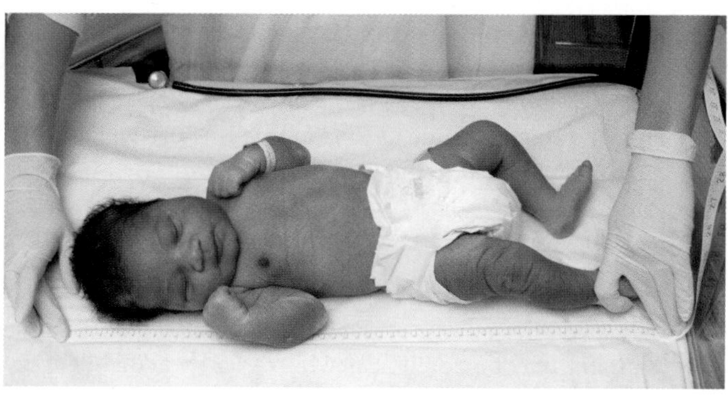

FIGURE 8–78 ■ Measuring the length of the newborn.

Count the heart rate with the stethoscope over the apical impulse for a full minute. The heart rate may range between 100 and 180 beats per minute immediately after birth, and it then stabilizes to between 120 and 160 beats per minute. The heart rate may increase to 180 beats per minute with cyring. Wider variations are seen in preterm infants.

The blood pressure is taken in both the arm and leg with a Doppler technique. Hold the extremity used during the procedure to reduce movement and improve the accuracy of the reading. An average blood pressure reading is 60/40 to 80/45 mm Hg at birth. Normal blood pressure ranges for preterm infants vary by gestational age and weight of the infant. Alternatively, the mean arterial pressure (MAP) is reported from the Doppler machine. Report the extremity in which the reading was taken. A difference in the pressure readings between the

TABLE 8–27 Transient Color Variations in Newborns

COLOR CHANGE	DESCRIPTION
Harlequin	The lower half of the body turns red and the upper half blanches with a distinct demarcation line down the middle when the newborn is in a side-lying position. The cause of the transient color change is unknown.
Acrocyanosis *Photo from Ladewig, P. W., London, M. L., Moberly, S. M., & Olds, S. B. (2002).* Contemporary maternal newborn nursing care. *(5th ed.) Upper Saddle River, NJ: Prentice Hall Health.*	A bluish color around the lips, hands, fingernails, feet, and toenails may occur, lasting a few hours and disappearing without warning.
Cutis marmorato (mottling)	Transient mottling of the trunk and extremities that occurs in response to cooler room temperatures or in response to environmental stress. It persists or is more pronounced in preterm infants.

arm and leg could indicate coarctation of the aorta in newborns. See Chapter 26∞.

Skin. The newborn's skin is thin, smooth, soft, and elastic; however, there are also defined areas of subcutaneous fat. The baby's skin dimples over the joints. The feet and hands may have peeling. **Lanugo** (fine downy hair) may be seen depending on the newborn's gestational age. Leathery skin with deep creases is seen in postterm newborns.

Assess the newborn for signs of skin disruptions related to the birth process such as forceps marks, site where the internal fetal monitor was attached, or lacerations sustained during the birth process.

The newborn's skin has a ruddy flush for the first 24 hours due to vasomotor instability. It gradually fades to its normal color. Black newborns initially have lighter toned skin than their parents because the pigment function is not yet in full production. The full melanotic color is seen in the nail cuticles and scrotal folds. Bruising over the buttocks of a breech presentation or over the eyes and forehead of a facial presentation may be seen. Identify and record the color, location, and size of all birthmarks, including the Mongolian spot. See Table 8–27 for common transient skin color changes in newborns that rarely indicate a pathologic condition.

The following color changes in the newborn are unexpected and cause for concern.

- Assess for jaundice by pressing the tip of the nose, forehead, or sternum to blanch the skin. A yellowish color to the skin immediately after blanching indicates the presence of jaundice. Jaundice appearing within 24 hours of birth is unexpected and may indicate hemolytic disease due to blood incompatibility. Immediate evaluation is needed. Jaundice may also be associated with the hemolysis of red blood cells from hematomas, bruises from forceps, or immature liver function. Jaundice appearing after 2 weeks of age may indicate biliary tract obstruction.
- Green-brown discoloration of the skin, nails, and cord results from meconium staining in utero, and may indicate fetal distress.
- Cyanosis or pallor can indicate respiratory or cardiac problem, cold stress, central nervous system damage, loss of blood volume, or infection.

Skin alterations that may be seen in newborns include the following:

- Milia, tiny white papules on the face, are due to occlusion of the hair follicles by sebum (Figure 8–79A ■).
- Erythema toxicum is a common rash (tiny red macules and papules on the cheeks, trunk, back, and buttocks) that appears in the first 3 to 4 days of life (Figure 8–79B ■).
- Storkbite or salmon patch (nevus flammeus), a vascular marking or common birthmark, is a flat irregularly shaped red or pink patch found on the back of the neck, forehead, eyelid, or upper lip. The mark fades by about 1 year of age.
- Hemangiomas include nevus flammeus (port-wine stain), nevus vasculosus (strawberry hemangioma), and cavernous hemangioma.
- Petechiae on the head and neck may be associated with a breech presentation or a cord around the neck.

Head. Inspect the contour of the head from all angles. A **caput succedaneum** may be noted in newborns with vaginal delivery (Figure 8–80 ■). This edematous swelling and ecchymosis occurs over the presenting part of the head due to birth trauma.

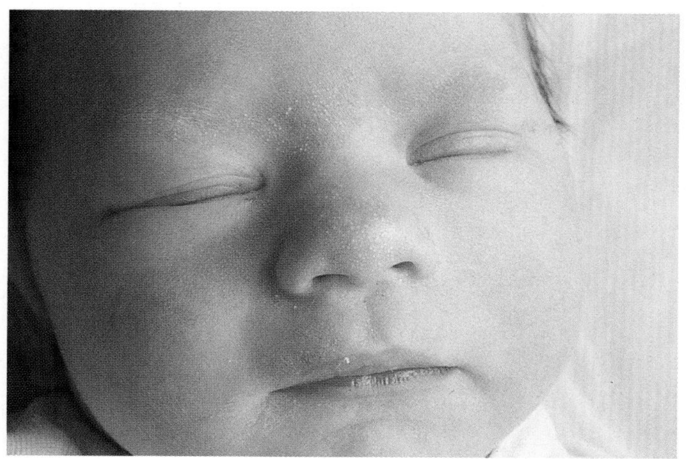

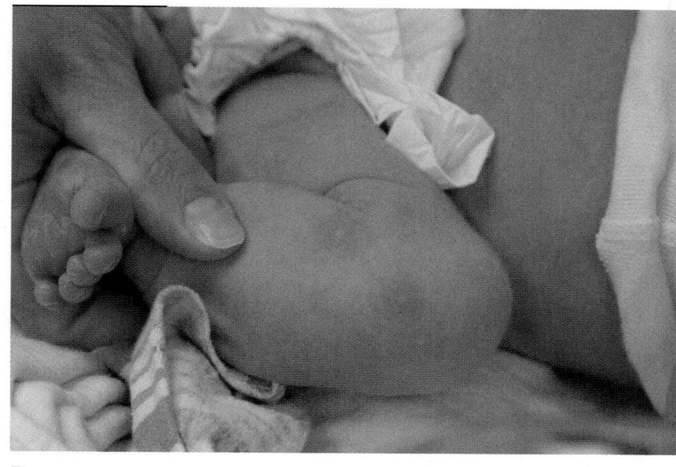

A B

FIGURE 8–79 ■ *A*, Milia. *B*, Erythema toxicum.

A, From Ladewig, P. W., London, M. L., Moberly, S. M., & Olds, S. B. (2002). Contemporary maternal newborn nursing care. *(5th ed.), Upper Saddle River, NJ: Prentice Hall.*

It feels soft and may extend across suture lines. It resolves over the first few days of life without treatment. A **cephalhematoma** is a subperiosteal hemorrhage that also results from birth trauma. It may take months to resolve. It is a soft, fluctuant elevation without discoloration that is well defined over one cranial bone (Figure 8–81 ■). **Molding**, an overriding of the cranial bones to accommodate the head's passage through the vaginal canal, may be noted in newborns with vaginal delivery and in those who experienced a long labor prior to cesarean birth. Molding resolves after a few days.

Palpate the head for suture lines. Suture lines may feel more like ridges and be more prominent if molding has occurred. Palpate the fontanels. The anterior fontanel is generally diamond shaped and 3 to 4 cm long by 2 to 3 cm wide. The posterior fontanel is 1 to 2 cm and triangular. A mild pulsation may be palpated over the anterior fontanel. Note the quality and distribution of hair.

Note the features of the face for spacing and symmetry of facial expression at rest and when crying. Asymmetry of facial features may indicate injury to the fifth cranial nerve (Figure 8–82 ■).

Eyes. Eye examination may be delayed for about 24 hours after birth when the eyelids are less edematous due to birth trauma or chemical conjunctivitis from antibiotics instilled in the eyes. A purulent discharge may be due to the chemical irritant or a bacterial or viral infection acquired during birth.

Use the ophthalmoscope to check for a red reflex or lens opacities bilaterally. The newborn's response to bright light should be a blink reflex. Dim the lights so that the infant opens the eyes or rock the newborn from upright to horizontal position to test the pupillary response to light.

The sclera should appear white and clear, but there may be a slight bluish tint due to their thinness. Subconjunctival hemorrhage may be present. No tears are generally seen when the newborn cries.

Vision is present and can be noted by the newborn's fixation on high-contrast geometric shape or a face that is held 8 to 12 inches from the face. Term newborn vision is 20/200. The eyes should track a moving object to the midline; however, a slight nystagmus may be seen.

A doll's eye phenomenon is an expected response within the first 10 days after birth. Hold the infant upright and as the head is moved from left to right, the eyes move in the opposite direction. This response disappears as head-eye coordination develops.

Ears. Inspect the pinna for position and any lesions. Note any preauricular skin tags. Hearing is present after mucus from the middle ear is absorbed and the eustachian tube is aerated. Note whether the infant awakens to loud noises or responds to sudden sounds with the Moro reflex as a gross hearing assessment.

Nose. Inspect the external nose that may appear flattened during the birth process. To assess for nasal patency, gently close the newborn's mouth and occlude one naris at a time and observe the baby's chest rise with inspiration. Newborns who become distressed with an occluded naris may have choanal atresia, a malformation of the bucconasal membrane resulting in an obstructed nasal passage. The presence of choanal atresia is confirmed by the inability to insert a small feeding tube from the naris into the hypopharynx. Choanal atresia may be unilateral or bilateral.

Observe for any flaring of the nares with respiration, a sign of respiratory distress. The newborn can smell after the nose is cleared of mucus and amniotic fluid, as noted by their search for milk.

Mouth. Inspect the mouth for any defects. The hard palate should be dome shaped and the uvula should be midline. Sucking pads should be present. The tongue should move freely and be proportionately sized for the mouth. Observe the newborn for coordinated sucking and swallowing. Palpate the hard and soft palate to detect any clefts using a gloved finger. Elicit the gag reflex but take care to avoid stimulating the vagal nerve to prevent the occurrence of reflexive bradycardia.

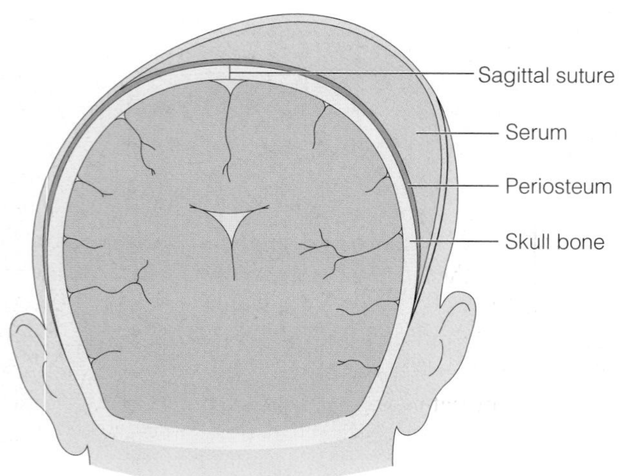

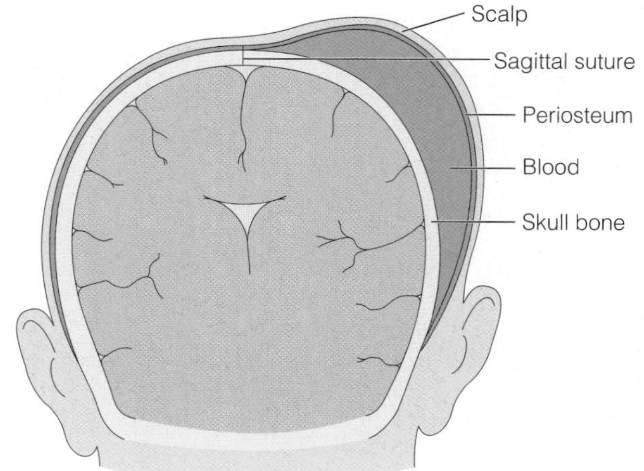

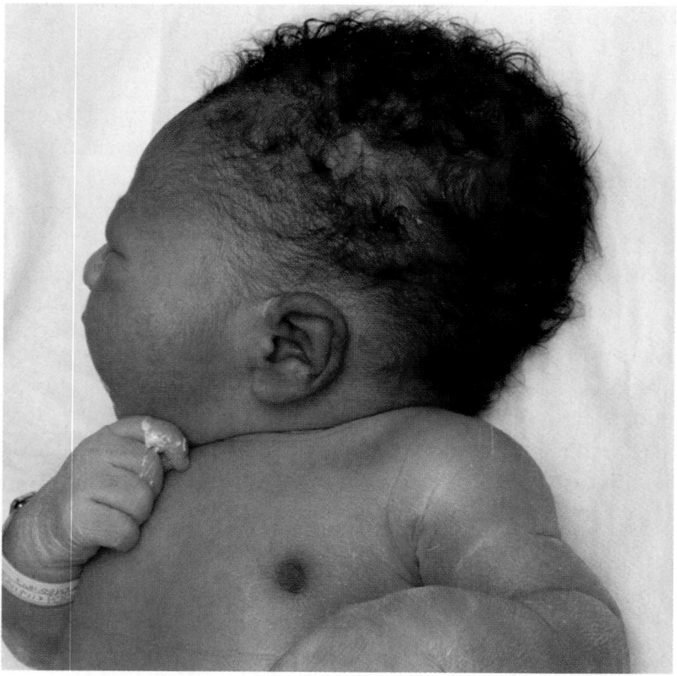

FIGURE 8–80 ■ Caput succedaneum. Following vaginal birth, some newborns develop swelling and a collection of serous fluid in the scalp due to birth trauma. The swelling often crosses the suture lines.

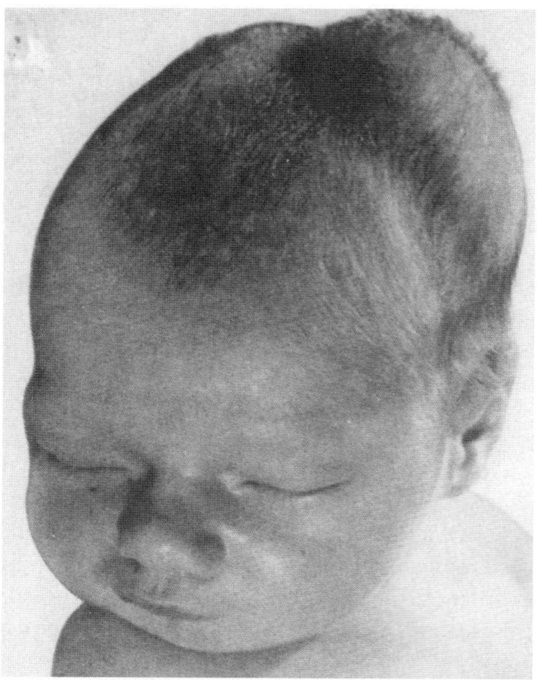

FIGURE 8–81 ■ Cephalhematoma. Following vaginal birth, some newborns develop a collection of blood between the surface of the cranial bone and the periosteal membrane due to birth trauma. The swelling is usually confined to one cranial bone and does not cross the suture lines. *From Potter, E. L., & Craig, J. M. (1975).* Pathology of the fetus and infant *(3rd ed.). Chicago: Year Book Medical Publishers. Used with permisison from Elsevier.*

Findings noted in the mouth include Epstein pearls, small white cysts containing keratin that feel hard to the touch. Occasionally a tooth may be noted. Inclusion cysts, gray-white lesions on the gums, may look like teeth.

Neck. Note the position of the head. The head should be positioned midline and there should be free movement through the range of motion. The neck is generally short and creased with skinfolds. The neck is not strong enough at birth to fully support the head. Generally, the newborn can raise the head slightly when in the prone position, but there is a noted head lag when the newborn is raised from supine to sitting position.

Move the newborn's head through a full range of motion. Limitation in movement may be associated with torticollis or a wry neck, resulting from injury to the sternocleidomastoid muscle during birth or to a congenital defect. Palpate the neck to verify that the trachea is in the midline position. Assess the thryoid for any enlargement and palpate the neck for masses. Note any webbing or extra folds of skin on the posterior neck that could be associated with Turner syndrome.

Palpate the entire length of the clavicles to detect any sign of a fracture, such as a ridge or mass over a clavicle or crepitus. If a fracture is present, the newborn will have limited range of motion of the arm on that side.

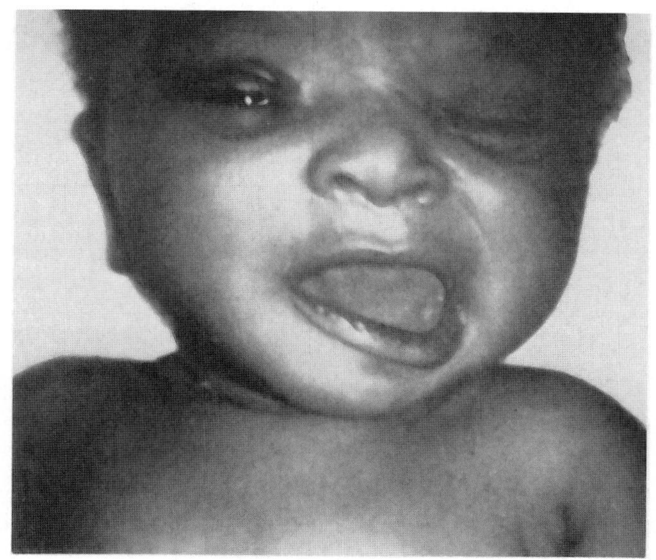

FIGURE 8–82 ■ Facial paralysis associated with injury to the right facial nerve.

Source: Courtesy of Dr. Ralph Platow. From Potter, E. L., & Craig, J. M. (1975). Pathology of the fetus and infant *(3rd ed.). Chicago: Year Book Medical Publishers. Used with permission from Elsevier.*

Chest and Lungs. The newborn has a rounded thorax with equal anteroposterior-to-transverse chest diameter. The xiphoid cartilage may appear to protrude because of the thinness of the tissue covering the chest. Observe for any unexpected shapes in the chest such as protrusion or depression of the sternum. The newborn's chest circumference ranges between 30 to 36 cm and is 2 cm smaller than the head circumference.

Breasts may be enlarged and visible in both males and females because of exposure to estrogen crossing the placenta. For a few days after birth, the breasts may also secrete a clear or white fluid, known as "witch's milk." See Figure 8–83 ■.

Observe the newborn's chest for respiratory effort. No retractions or paradoxical breathing should be present. During periods of rapid eye movement sleep, periods of apnea lasting less than 20 seconds are common. In cases of respiratory distress, retractions are an indication of accessory muscle use to inflate stiff, noncompliant lungs. If retractions are noted, determine if they are minimal (substernal) or marked (suprasternal and intercostal). See-saw respirations, another sign of respiratory distress, are seen when the chest flattens as the abdomen bulges.

Auscultate the anterior and posterior chest for breath sounds with an infant stethoscope. Breath sounds may be louder than in older children, and they are transmitted over the entire chest wall due to thin chest tissue. Localizing breath sounds will be very difficult, but adventitious sounds should clear when the newborn cries. Grunting is a mechanism used by newborns in respiratory distress to prevent atelectasis. The newborn exhales against a closed glottis to increase transpulmonary pressure, producing the sound. Indicate when grunting is heard with or without a stethoscope. Audible grunting without a stethoscope is indicative of greater respiratory distress.

Heart. Locate the apical impulse to identify the placement of the heart in the chest. It should be located in the upper left side with the point of maximum intensity in the third or fourth intercostal space along the left sternal border. Listen to the heart tones to ensure their appropriate location in the chest. Sounds heard nearer to the mediastinum or in the right side of the chest may indicate dextrocardia, diaphragmatic hernia, or a pneumothorax.

The transition from fetal to pulmonic circulation occurs in the immediate newborn period. See Chapter 26∞ for illustrations and explanation. Fetal shunts normally close within 10 to 15 hours, but may take up to 48 hours. Assess the heart sounds during the first 24 hours, and then frequently over the next 48 to 72 hours. Soft systolic murmurs (grade 1 to 2) are relatively common in the first 2 to 3 days with the closure of the fetal shunts. The low-pitched, continuous flow musical murmur of the patent ductus arteriosus is commonly heard at the second intercostal space along the midclavicular line in infants during the first couple of days of life. The murmur may also be heard posteriorly. Other significant murmurs may also be heard. See pages 270–271 for characteristics of murmurs and the assessment of the cardiovascular system in infants.

Palpate the peripheral pulses at the brachial, femoral, and pedal sites. Compare the strength and quality of the brachial pulses with the femoral pulses. Weak femoral pulses may indicate coarctation of the aorta. Note other unusual characteristics with regard to pulsations and quality.

Abdomen. Observe the abdomen while the newborn is quiet. Abdominal movement is synchronous with chest movement. It should appear rounded and slightly protruding. The abdominal muscles may appear relaxed. Note diastasis recti or the presence of an umbilical hernia. Few if any blood vessels should be seen. If distention is present or develops, be suspicious of a gastrointestinal congenital anomaly. If the abdomen is scaphoid or hollow, be concerned about the

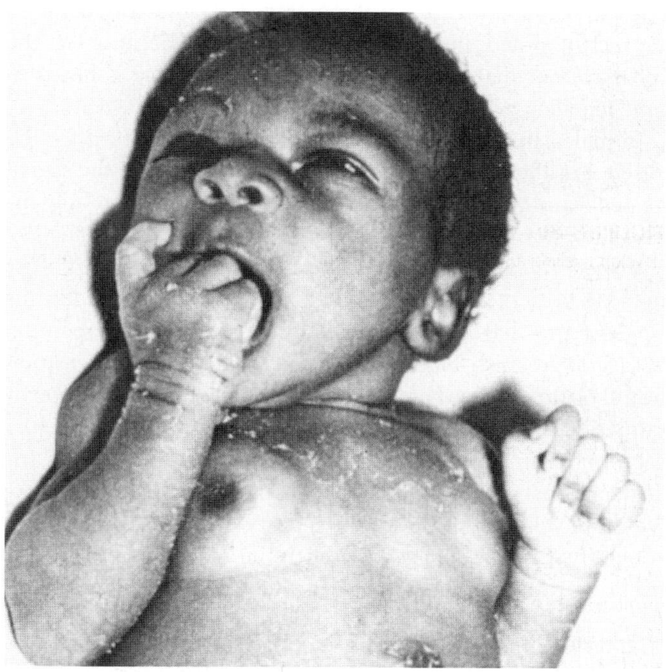

FIGURE 8–83 ■ Breast hypertrophy associated with maternal hormones.

Source: Korones, S. B. (1986). High-risk newborn infants *(4th ed.). St. Louis: Mosby. Used with permission from Elsevier.*

CLINICAL MANIFESTATIONS Associated with the Umbilical Cord

CLINICAL MANIFESTATION	ETIOLOGY	CLINICAL THERAPY
Bleeding from the cord	Cord clamp is loose or the cord has been pulled	Control bleeding with pressure and tighten or replace the cord clamp.
One artery (two-vessel cord)	Associated with congenital anomalies	Carefully examine the newborn for congenital anomalies such as trisomy 18.
Discharge and odor	Infection	Administer antibiotic therapy and monitor for signs of worsening infection.
Draining urine or moistness at the base of the cord	Patent urachus, abnormal connection between the bladder and the umbilicus	Surgery to remove the fistula. Monitor for urinary tract infection.
Serous or serosanguinous drainage after the cord falls off	Granuloma	Clean with alcohol several times a day, cauterization of granuloma with silver nitrate.

presence of a diaphragmatic hernia and that the abdominal contents are located in the chest cavity.

Auscultate the abdomen for bowel sounds that are present shortly after birth. Absent bowel sounds may indicate a bowel obstruction.

The umbilical cord should be clamped. Inspect the umbilical cord for the presence of two arteries and one vein. At birth these blood vessels are surrounded by mucoid connective tissue called Wharton's jelly. The stump dries quickly and is shriveled and blackened by the third day. See the clinical manifestations table above for various findings associated with the umbilical cord.

Palpate the abdomen for softness, tenderness, and the presence of masses. Feel the liver edge, the spleen tip, both kidneys, and the bladder.

GENITALIA AND ANUS. In females, inspect the external genitalia and compare to expected size for the newborn's gestational age. A thick white mucoid or blood-tinged vaginal discharge is commonly noted in newborns and occurs because of the withdrawal of maternal hormones. A hymenal tag is noted in some female newborns.

In males, inspect the penis and palpate the scrotum for the presence of the testes as described on page 280. Note the size of the penis and the location of the urethral meatus. Carefully inspect the external genitalia for signs of ambiguous genitalia.

Inspect the anus to ensure that it is patent and that no fissures are present. Observe stool passage to make sure the anus is patent and that the stool passed through the anal opening. Passage of greenish-black meconium, the newborn's first stool, should occur within the first 24 hours. When passage of meconium is delayed, a lubricated catheter can be inserted 1 cm (0.5 in.) into the anus. Resistance in passage of the catheter may indicate an obstruction. The stool transitions by the fourth day to a more yellow to yellow-brown pasty or firm consistency.

Lightly stroke the anal area to elicit the anal wink reflex. Constriction of the sphincter indicates it has good muscle strength.

EXTREMITIES. Inspect the arms and legs for any deformities in shape or position. Compare the length and skinfolds of arms and legs to detect differences that could indicate a potential problem. Inspect the hands and feet for extra digits (polydactyly), webbing (syndactyly), and creases. The hands are typically held in fisted position, but will open periodically.

Many newborns have a flexible forefoot inversion (metatarsus adductus) that results from uterine positioning. Any fixed deformity is abnormal. Move the feet toward midline position to identify any positional deformities such as clubfoot or metatarsus adductus. See Chapter 35∞.

Note any problems with movement of extremities. Paralysis of the arm may be associated with a difficult birth and injury to the brachial plexus. In Erb-Duchenne paralysis (Erb's palsy), injury to the fifth and sixth cervical roots of the brachial plexus, the upper arm is affected. The newborn is unable to raise the arm and the elbow is held in extension with the forearm pronated as illustrated in Figure 8–84 ■.

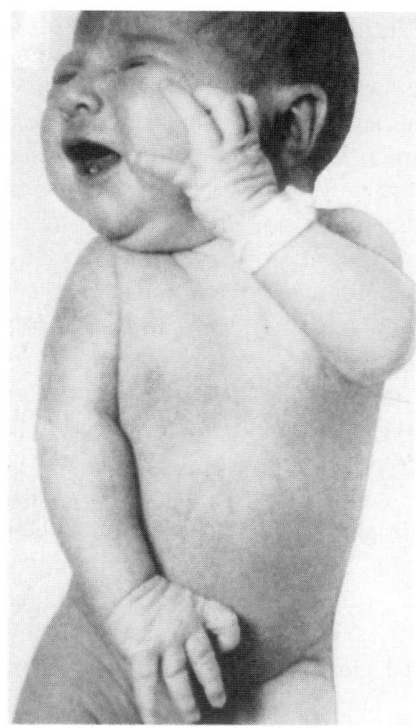

FIGURE 8–84 ■ Erb's palsy, associated with injury to the fifth and sixth cervical roots of the brachial plexus due to birth trauma.

From Potter, E. L., & Craig, J. M. (1975). Pathology of the fetus and infant (3rd ed.). Chicago: Year Book Medical Publishers. Used with permisison from Elsevier.

Note any asymmetry in skin creases on the legs. Check the hips for dislocation with the Ortolani-Barlow maneuver as described on page 287.

Inspect the spine for a dimple, cyst, mass, or tuft of hair in the midline that might indicate an underlying condition such as spina bifida, meningocele, or a dermoid sinus. Palpate each vertebrae of the spine to assess uniformity in shape. Assess the range of motion of the spine.

Note generalized muscle strength by holding a newborn upright between your hands. The newborn who starts to slip between your hands has weakened shoulder muscles. Assess muscle tone by observing the resting posture. The position is generally a symmetric flexed posture with extremities folded inward, hips slightly abducted, and fists flexed. Move all the extremities to determine the range of motion and resistance to extending the knee and elbow joints. The newborn should be slightly hypertonic and resist full extension of the legs and arms at the knees and elbows. See Table 8–28 for abnormal postures. Limpness or flaccidity is abnormal in a full-term newborn and may indicate a central nervous system disorder.

Assess head control by pulling the supine newborn a few inches off of the mattress by holding the arms. The newborn should hold the head in the same plane as the body. When the baby is held in a prone position with one hand under the chest, the newborn holds the head at an angle of 45 degrees or less from horizontal when the back is straight or slightly flexed.

TABLE 8–28 Abnormal Postures of the Newborn

POSTURE	DESCRIPTION
Frog position	Hips abducted and externally rotated, nearly flat against the table. Seen after a breech delivery.
Opisthotonos	Head is arched back, stiff neck, arms and legs extended, seen with meningeal or brainstem irritation and kernicterus
Extended limbs	Intracranial hemorrhage
Continuous asymmetry of upper extremity	Brachial plexus palsy

Neurologic System. The newborn should appear alert with eyes open after swelling subsides. A strong suck and coordinated swallow should be noted.

Occasional spontaneous, brief jerky or twitching tremors are common. Prolonged or repeated tremors may be caused by hypoglycemia, hypocalcemia, nicotine, or opiate withdrawal. Signs of seizures may be subtle, such as chewing or swallowing movements, lip smacking, deviations of the eyes, rigidity or flaccidity, or bicycling movement of the legs.

CLINICAL TIP

To help distinguish between a seizure and a tremor, gently hold the extremity in your hand. If the held extremity stops moving, the baby is jittery. If the extremity continues to shake, the newborn is more likely to be having a seizure.

Newborns have protective reflexes that may be observed during the assessment: blink, yawn, sucking, cough, sneeze, and withdrawal from pain. Yawns and sneezes often indicate the newborn has been overstimulated. Assessment of central nervous system evaluation can be performed with the following steps.

- Insert a gloved finger in the mouth to elicit the sucking reflex.
- When the newborn is sucking vigorously, note a change in sucking when exposed to a light, rattle, and a voice. A brief cessation of sucking is followed by continuous sucking with repetitious stimulation (Ladewig, London, Moberly et al., 2002).

Primitive reflexes are also used to assess the neurologic development of the newborn. See Table 8–23 for techniques to assess primitive reflexes and the expected findings.

At the conclusion of the assessment, carefully review the findings to determine if any cluster of findings indicates a particular health condition or determine if the newborn is adapting as expected to extrauterine life.

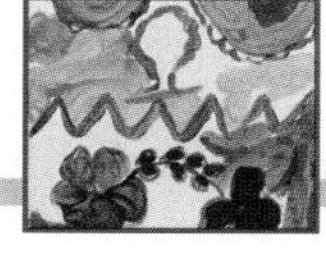

CHAPTER HIGHLIGHTS

- Establish a rapport with the family and use careful listening techniques to collect historical information about the child's health status.
- Collection of historical data includes the chief complaint, history of the present illness or injury, past history, current health status, review of systems, and family history. In addition, psychosocial and developmental data are collected.
- The physical examination sequence includes assessment of the following:
  - Skin and hair
  - Head, eyes, ears, nose, and mouth structures and function
  - Neck
  - Chest and lungs
  - Breasts
  - Heart and pulses
  - Abdomen
  - Inguinal area
  - Genitalia and perineal areas
  - Musculoskeletal system
  - Nervous system

- Assessment sequences vary by the age of the child and the child's cooperation with the procedures.
- Clinical judgment is used to identify common patterns of physiologic responses associated with medical conditions.
- The physiologic responses and family and child responses to health conditions become the basis for many nursing diagnoses.
- The initial newborn assessment at the time of birth includes the Apgar score to identify the need for immediate resuscitation.
- The comprehensive newborn assessment, including a gestational age assessment, is conducted within the first few hours of birth to make sure the newborn's transition to extrauterine life is proceeding as expected and to identify any specific problems that put the newborn at risk.
- Knowledge of the birth weight and gestational age helps to determine if newborns are large, appropriate, or small for gestational age and potentially at risk for morbidity.

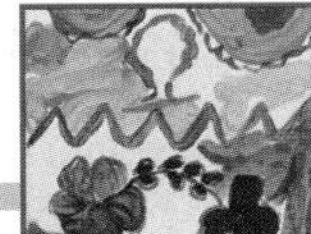

CRITICAL THINKING IN ACTION

INTRODUCTION

Return to the opening scenario involving 6-month-old Latoya, who has bronchiolitis. Her parents took her to the emergency department after a visit to their private pediatrician.

DESCRIPTION

Latoya had been sick with an upper respiratory infection for a couple of days, but overnight she got progressively worse with a fever, refusal to eat or drink formula or water, and difficulty breathing. After calling the advice nurse, Latoya's parents were told to come to the physician's office right away. It was determined that Latoya needed close observation in the hospital due to the viral infection. Her parents report that they have never had an experience with this type of illness before, as her 6-year-old sister Monique has always been healthy.

DISCUSSION

When Latoya is admitted to the hospital, a full nursing assessment is performed. Your thorough physical assessment of Latoya has revealed signs of respiratory difficulty and inadequate tissue perfusion from several body systems.

1. Latoya has a respiratory condition called bronchiolitis. Identify all the components of the physical assessment that revealed the signs of respiratory difficulty and inadequate tissue perfusion. Which body systems provided this information?
2. List the information that should be collected during a review of systems regarding the respiratory system.
3. What information should be collected about her past medical history that might have a direct connection to her current respiratory condition?
4. Complete the nursing assessment and develop two nursing diagnoses related to her physical condition.

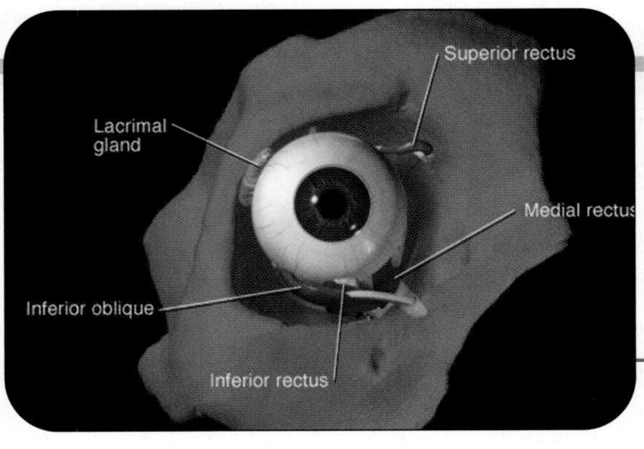

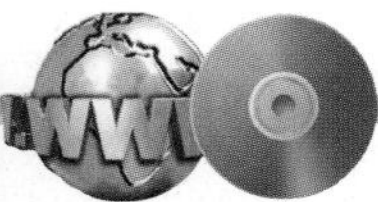

EXPLORE MediaLink

- NCLEX review, case studies, and other interactive resources for this chapter can be found on the Companion Website at **http://www.prenhall.com/ball**. Click on Chapter 8 to select the activities for this chapter.
- For animations, more NCLEX review questions, and an audio glossary, access the accompanying CD-ROM in this textbook.

http://www.prenhall.com/ball

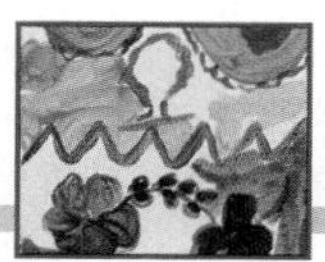

REFERENCES

Alderman, E. M. (1999). Breast problems in the adolescent. *Contemporary Pediatrics, 16*(9), 99–119.

Algranati, P. S. (1998). Effect of developmental status on the approach to physical examination. *Pediatric Clinics of North America, 45*(1), 1–23.

American Academy of Pediatrics Committee on Practice and Ambulatory Medicine and Section on Ophthalmology. (2003). Eye examination in infants, children, and young adults by pediatricians. *Pediatrics, 111*(4), 902–907.

Ballard, J. L., Khoury, J. C., Wang, L., Eilers-Walsmann, B. L., & Lipp, R. (1991). New Ballard score, expanded to include extremely premature infants. *Journal of Pediatrics, 119*(3), 417–423.

Battaglia, F. C., & Lubchenco, L. O. (1967). A practical classification of newborn infants by weight and gestational age. *Journal of Pediatics, 71*(2), 161.

Burns, C. (1992). A new assessment model and tool for pediatric nurse practitioners. *Journal of Pediatric Health Care, 6*, 73–81.

Byrnes, K. (1996). Conducting the pediatric health history: A guide. *Pediatric Nursing, 22*, 135–137.

Camille, C. J., Kuo, R. L., & Wiener, J. S. (2002). Caring for the uncircumcised penis: What parents (and you) need to know. *Contemporary Pediatrics, 19*(11), 61–72.

Dodd, V. (1996). Gestational age assessment. *Neonatal Network, 15*(1), 27–36.

Eichelberger, M. R., Ball, J. W., Pratsch, G. S., & Clark, J. R. (1998). *Pediatric emergencies: A manual for prehospital care providers* (2nd ed.). Upper Saddle River, NJ: Brady, Prentice Hall.

Ganel, A., Dudkiewicz, I., & Grogan, D. P. (2003). Pediatric orthopedic physical examination of the infant: A 5-minute assessment. *Journal of Pediatric Health Care, 17*(1), 39–41.

Goldenring, J. M., & Rosen, D. S. (2004). Getting into adolescent heads: An essential update. *Contemporary Pediatrics, 21*(1), 64–90.

Green, M., Sullivan, P., & Eichberg, C. (2002). Avoid a "Swiss cheese" history when psychosocial complaints are on the menu. *Contemporary Pediatrics, 19*(10), 115–125.

Hazinski, M. F. (1999). *Manual of pediatric critical care* (pp. 289–293). St. Louis: Mosby.

Herman-Giddens, M. E., Slora, E. J., Wasserman, R. C., Bourdony, C. J., Bhapkar, M. V., et al. (1997). Secondary sexual characteristics and menses in young girls seen in office practice: A study from the pediatric research in office setting network. *Pediatrics, 99*(4), 505–512.

Instone, S. L. (2002). Developmental strategies for interviewing children. *Journal of Pediatric Health Care, 16*(6), 304–305.

Johnson, T. S., Engstrom, J. L., Haney, S. L., & Mulcrone, S. L. (1999). Reliability of three length measurement techniques in term infants. *Pediatric Nursing, 25*(1), 13–17.

Kaplowitz, P. B., Oberfield, S. E., & the Drug and Therapeutics and Executive Committees of the Lawson Wilkins Pediatric Endocrine Society. (1999). Reexamination of the age limit for defining when puberty is precocious in girls in the United States: Implications for evaluation and treatment. *Pediatrics, 104*(4), 936–941.

Karpas, A., Hennes, H., & Walsh-Kelly, C. M. (2002). Utilization of the Ottawa ankle rules by nurses in a pediatric emergency department. *Academic Emergency Medicine, 9*(2), 130–133.

Ladewig, P. W., London, M. L., Moberly, S. M., & Olds, S. B. (2002). *Contemporary maternal-newborn nursing care* (5th ed.). Upper Saddle River, NJ: Prentice Hall.

McEvoy, M. (2000). An added dimension to the pediatric health maintenance visit: The spiritual history. *Journal of Pediatric Health Care, 14*(5), 216–220.

National Heart, Lung, and Blood Institute. (2004). Blood pressure tables for children and adolescents from the fourth report on the diagnosis, evaluation, and treatment of high blood pressure in children and adolescents.www.nhlbi.nih.gov/guidelines/hypertension/child_tbl.htm, accessed 6/11/2004.

National High Blood Pressure Program Working Group on Hypertension Control in Children and Adolescents (1996). Update of the 1987 task force report on high blood pressure in children and adolescents: A working group report from the National High Blood Pressure Education Program. *Pediatrics*, 98(4), 649–658.

Pomeranz, A. J., & Fairley, J. A. (1998). The systematic evaluation of the skin in children. *Pediatric Clinics of North America, 45*(1), 49–63.

Saphis, J. (2002). Human genetics: Constructing a family pedigree. *American Journal of Nursing, 102*(7), 44–49.

Seidel, H. M., Ball, J. W., Dains, J., & Benedict, G. W. (2003). *Mosby's guide to physical examination* (5th ed.). St. Louis: Mosby.

Spector, R. E. (2000). *Cultural diversity in health and illness* (5th ed.). Upper Saddle River, NJ: Prentice Hall Health.

Tanner, J. M. (1962). *Growth at adolescence* (2nd ed.). Oxford: Blackwell Scientific Publications, Inc.

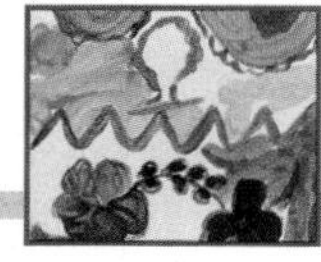

ADDITIONAL REFERENCES

American Academy of Pediatrics Section on Ophthalmology. (2002). Red reflex examination in infants. *Pediatrics, 109*(5), 980–981.

Leung, A. K. C., & Robson, W. L. M. (2004). Childhood cervical lymphadenopathy. *Journal of Pediatric Health Care, 18*(1), 3–7.

Marshall, W. A., & Tanner, J. M. (1969). Variations in pattern of pubertal changes in girls. *Archives of Disease in Childhood*, 44, 291.

Marshall, W. A., & Tanner, J. M. (1970). Variations in pattern of pubertal changes in boys. *Archives of Disease in Childhood*, 49, 13.

Muntner, P., He, J., Cutler, J. A., Wildman, R. P., & Whelton, P. K. (2004). Trends in blood pressure among children and adolescents. *Journal of American Medical Association, 291*(17), 2107–2113.

Unkin, J., Gazala, E., & Bar-David, Y. (2004). Cleaning earwax: Why you shouldn't play it be ear. *Contemporary Pediatrics*, 21(2), 73–86.

Chapter

9

Infant, Child, and Adolescent Nutrition

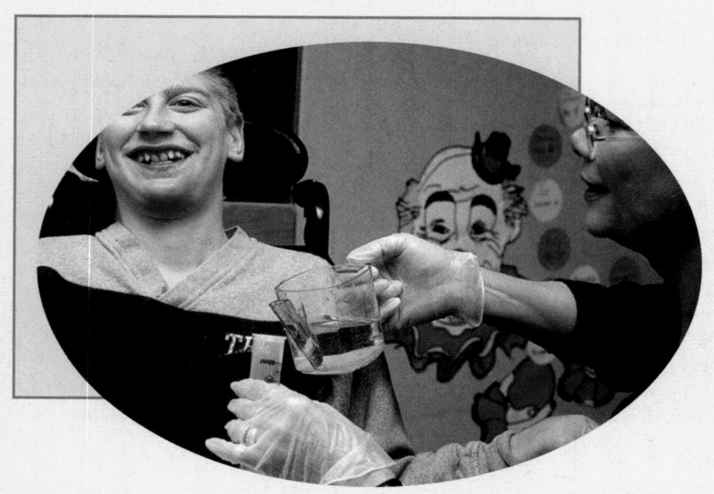

Joey Jenkins was diagnosed with cerebral palsy early in life. He is now 11 years old and has returned to school after surgery for scoliosis. When evaluated prior to surgery, Joey's nutritional status showed some caloric and nutritional deficits. Joey has limited ability to swallow, related to muscle weakness of cerebral palsy, and was therefore unable to ingest enough calories by mouth to ensure his optimal growth and development. A gastrostomy tube was inserted into his stomach to provide supplementary feedings and maximize his nutritional status prior to surgery. After several weeks of supplemental feedings, Joey was ready for surgery, and did well in his postoperative recovery.

Joey continues to have supplemental feedings throughout the day. The school nurse has met with his parents and home health nurse to learn about the amount and type of tube feedings he receives, as well as the texture of oral feedings he can manage. The nurse has planned the feeding schedule at school to facilitate adequate nutrition in that setting. In addition, careful ongoing nutritional assessment will be needed to evaluate if Joey is getting the calories and other nutrients he needs for growth and development. The school nurse is also educating the classroom teachers and other school personnel about Joey's unique nutritional requirements.

"I'm so glad to be back with my friends. I get tired sometimes, but it's worth it to be here. It's neat that the school nurse has shown my teacher how to do my tube feedings."

—Joey, 11 years old

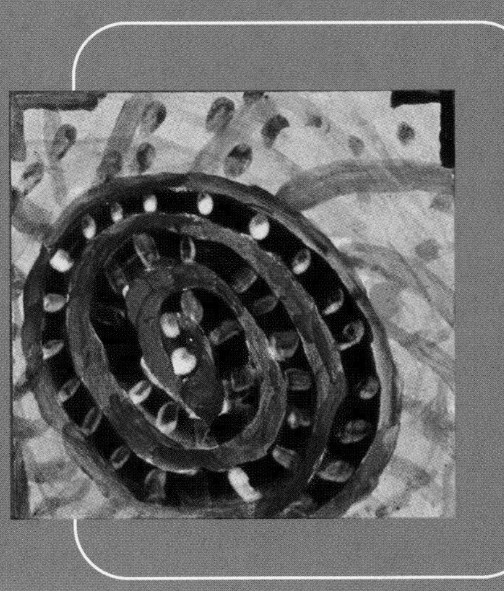

Learning Outcomes

After completing this chapter, you will be able to:

- Discuss major nutritional concepts pertaining to the growth and development of children.
- Describe and plan nursing interventions to meet nutritional needs for all age groups from preterm infants through adolescents.
- Integrate methods of nutritional assessment into care for children and adolescents.
- Discuss common nutritional concerns of children growing up in developed countries.
- Apply the nursing process to care for children or adolescents with feeding and eating disorders.
- Describe the nurse's role when children need unusual nutritional support due to illness or lifestyle.

MediaLink http://www.prenhall.com/ball

Resources for this chapter can be found on the CD-ROM accompanying this textbook, and on the Companion Website at http://www.prenhall.com/ball. Click on Chapter 9 to select the activities for this chapter.

CD-ROM

Videos

Anorexia Nervosa
Breastfeeding and First Foods
Children & Overweight
Nutritional Status

Nursing in Action: Administering a Gavage/Tube Feeding

NCLEX Review

Audio Glossary

COMPANION WEBSITE

A & P Review

Clinical Manifestations Review

NCLEX Review

Case Study: Manage a Child's Peanut Allergy at School

MediaLink Applications

Analyze Your Diet
Diet and Culture
Fast Food Analysis
Growth Chart Analysis
Preschoolers: Plan a Nutrition Teaching Session
Vegetarian Teens: Plan a 2-Day Menu

Key Terms

anabolism/315
anemia/343
anthropometric measurement/331
atopy/351
body mass index (BMI)/331
carbohydrate/314
catabolism/315
cholesterol/315
Dietary Reference Intakes (DRIs)/317
early childhood caries/325
essential amino acid/315
fats/315
fatty acids/315
fiber/315
food allergy/351
food insecurity/337
food intolerance (sensitivity)/351
food jags/328
food security/337
glycemic index/315
glycogen/315
kwashiorkor/315
lacto-ovovegetarian/354
lactovegetarian/354
lipoproteins/315
macronutrients/314
marasmus/315

Key Terms *(continued)*

- micronutrients/314
- nitrogen balance/315
- nonessential amino acid/315
- nutrition/314
- osteomalacia/343
- physiologic anorexia/326
- pica/344
- preterm/318
- protein/315
- radioallergosorbent test (RAST)/352
- small for gestational age/318
- triglycerides/315
- vegan/354
- vegetarian/354
- weaning/325

MediaLink A & P Review

Adequate nutrition is an essential component of growth and development. The child's nutritional status begins before birth and is related to the mother's nutritional state. After birth and throughout all of childhood, intake influences health. All children must be assessed for nutritional status, followed by teaching or other interventions to enhance health. Nurses are instrumental in providing families with information about normal nutritional needs of infants and young children. Common techniques to assess nutrition, such as measuring growth and monitoring hematocrit, provide needed information about whether intake of nutrients is adequate.

All children, parents, and other care providers can benefit from information about nutritional needs, but some children have additional issues that must be considered. The nurse recognizes the special intake requirements of children with conditions such as food allergies, cystic fibrosis, cerebral palsy, cancer, or diabetes. Nutrition monitoring is provided throughout childhood so that dietary counseling can be integrated with other teaching to promote development.

Some children have unique nutritional needs due to their social environments. Parents may not be knowledgeable about child nutritional requirements. Perhaps the family is vegetarian and needs extra help to ensure intake of essential nutrients. If finances are limited, the family may need resources such as access to food stamps, food banks, or budget planning. The nurse considers the high rate of childhood obesity and common nutritional deficits when applying concepts of health promotion with families. Whatever the setting in which the nurse is employed, knowledge of nutrition must be integrated within nursing care.

How can the nurse help parents to monitor food intake in various settings, such as home, child-care settings, schools, and hospitals? What interventions will assist families in establishing nutritional habits that foster health promotion? How can the nurse help the family prepare for meeting nutritional needs of a child who has special nutritional requirements during travel by car or plane? How can nurses intervene to help decrease rates of obesity among children? These are some of the topics that will be addressed in this chapter.

NUTRITION CONCEPTS

Major Dietary Components

Nutrition refers to taking in food and assimilating it metabolically for use by the body. It is an essential component of life and therefore an important topic to consider in discussions of child growth and development. The body requires a wide array of intake products. **Macronutrients** are the major building blocks of the body. **Micronutrients** are substances needed in small quantities for healthy body functioning. The need for nutrients is dependent on activity level, state of health and presence of disease or other stress, and age-related needs.

The essential macronutrients are carbohydrates, proteins, and fats. **Carbohydrates** are composed of carbon, hydrogen, and oxygen, arranged in various configurations to form saccharides (sugar molecules). The main function of carbohydrates in the body is production of energy, and indeed, 50% or more of our daily calories come from carbohydrates. See Table 9–1 for common sac-

TABLE 9–1 Carbohydrates in the Human Diet

SIMPLE CARBOHYDRATES	EXAMPLES
Monosaccharides	Corn syrup
Glucose	Honey
Fructose	Fruits
Disaccharides	
Sucrose	White sugar
Lactose	Molasses
Maltose	Milk
	Food sweetener
Complex Carbohydrates	
Polysaccharides	Grains (cereals, breads)
Starch	Pasta
Glycogen	Rice, corn, bulgur
	Legumes
	Potatoes

BOX 9–1 Health Promotion: Dietary Fiber

Dietary fiber has many health benefits, but North Americans commonly do not ingest enough fiber to obtain its beneficial effects. Dietary fiber is known to promote regular bowel movements, contribute to maintenance of healthy serum lipids and glucose, and to decrease rates of duodenal ulcer and colon cancer. Eating whole grains, fruits, vegetables, and legumes are easy ways to increase fiber intake.

charides. Digestion occurs in the mouth and small intestine, and monosaccharides are absorbed in the small intestine. These digestive products are turned into glucose in the liver and used for energy throughout the body. When there is an excess of glucose, the liver can convert glucose to **glycogen** and store it for use when the body requires energy and food is not being ingested. Remaining carbohydrates are converted to short-chain fatty acids and absorbed in the colon. **Fiber** represents indigestible carbohydrate components which ensure healthy movement of fecal contents through the bowel (Box 9–1). While some carbohydrates are quickly absorbed, causing a rapid rise in blood sugar after ingestion, others are more slowly absorbed, causing a more prolonged blood sugar increase without a high peak (Box 9–2). When insufficient carbohydrates are ingested, the deficiency disease **marasmus** can occur. See the section on dietary deficiencies for further discussion.

Proteins are made of amino acids, compounds that have nitrogen as an essential component, in addition to carbon, hydrogen, and oxygen. There are 20 amino acids that comprise the proteins in the body. Nine of these are **essential amino acids,** which cannot be manufactured by humans and must be ingested in the diet, while 12 are **nonessential amino acids,** which humans can manufacture when in good health. See Table 9–2 for a list of the amino acids in the body. Proteins are the building blocks of body tissues and are constantly being broken down (**catabolism**) and resynthesized (**anabolism**). When inadequate carbohydrates and fats are available, the body can break down protein, and use components to meet basic energy needs. Since nitrogen is an essential component of amino acids, protein balance is also referred to as **nitrogen balance.** *Positive nitrogen balance* is the term used when more nitrogen is taken into the body than excreted; it occurs during periods of growth during childhood, when additional body tissues are being manufactured, and when the body is replenished after illness or surgery. *Negative nitrogen balance* indicates that the body excretes more nitrogen than it retains; it occurs when dietary intake is limited. **Kwashiorkor** is a deficiency disease that occurs when insufficient protein is ingested. See the section on dietary deficiencies for further discussion.

BOX 9–2 Health Promotion: Glycemic Index

Glycemic index refers to the blood glucose response to 50 g of carbohydrate from any specific food, as compared to the glucose level after ingestion of white bread. A low glycemic index diet has been found to have beneficial effects such as reducing serum lipids, insulin levels, and improving serum glucose control. Beans are an example of a low glycemic index food, while potatoes have a high glycemic index, indicating that the glucose level rises very high after ingestion. Charts of glycemic index of common foods have been developed. Parents can be taught how to interpret resources so that glycemic index information about a particular food can be applied to dietary decisions.

TABLE 9–2 Amino Acids

ESSENTIAL AMINO ACIDS	NONESSENTIAL AMINO ACIDS
Isoleucine (Ile)	Alanine (Ala)
Leucine (Leu)	Arginine (Arg)
Lysine (Lys)	Aspartic acid (Asp)
Methionine (Met)	Asparagine (Asn)
Phenylalanine (Phe)	Glutamic acid (Glu)
Threonine (Thr)	Glutamine (Gln)
Tryptophan (Trp)	Glycine (Gly)
Valine (Val)	Proline (Pro)
Histidine (His)	Serine (Ser)
	Cysteine (Cys)
	Tyrosine (Tyr)

Fats (or lipids) are the third macronutrient group ingested in the diet. They are complex molecules of several types, consisting of carbon, hydrogen, and oxygen, arranged so that glycerol and fatty acids are the structural subcomponents. The major role of fats is production of body energy, but they are essential in many processes such as cell membrane function, cell signaling, and blood clotting. **Fatty acids** are major components of fats and are referred to as *saturated* (no additional hydrogen atoms could be absorbed by the structure) or *unsaturated* (some additional bonds with hydrogen are possible). Unsaturated fatty acids are further designated as *monounsaturated* (only one potential bond with hydrogen possible) or *polyunsaturated* (two or more potential bonds). *Trans fatty acids* are formed when food processing is applied to partially hydrogenate unsaturated fatty acids. Unsaturated fatty acids are commonly liquid at room temperature, and hydrogenation hardens them into spreads such as margarine. In recent years it has become evident that these artificially hydrogenated fatty acids (trans fatty acids) have similar actions to saturated fatty acids in the body; that is, they may raise levels of cholesterol and promote cardiovascular disease. The average intake of trans fat is 5 g daily, but since it is not separately noted on food labels, the intake for individuals is difficult to identify or modify. See Table 9–3 for major dietary sources of fatty acids. Many fats consist of three fatty acids connected to a glycerol base, and are called **triglycerides;** these are the major fats consumed by humans. Cholesterol and lipoproteins are two terms related to fats and are sometimes confused with fats. **Cholesterol** is actually a steroid or sterol compound found only in animal cells, and is essential to cell membranes. It may be ingested from foods and is also manufactured in the body. **Lipoproteins** are combinations of fat and protein that transport fats in the blood. Major lipoproteins included low-density lipoprotein (LDL), high-density lipoprotein (HDL), and very-low-density lipoprotein (VLDL). See Chapter 26∞ for further description of cholesterol levels in the body. See Table 9–4

TABLE 9–3 Fatty Acids

SATURATED FATTY ACIDS	SOURCES
Butyric Caproic Caprylic Capric Lauric Myristic Palmitic Stearic Arachidic Behenic	butterfat, coconut, peanut oil
Monounsaturated Fatty Acids	
Palmitoleic Oleic Elaidic (trans)	beef, fish, olive
Polyunsaturated Fatty Acids	
Linoleic Alpha-linolenic Arachidonic Eicosapentaenoic Docosahexaenoic	safflower, corn, soybean, cottonseed, canola, fish

for recommended amounts of dietary carbohydrate, protein, fat, and fiber in childhood and adolescence.

In addition to the macronutrients of carbohydrate, protein, and fat, the human body depends on a number of micronutrients, commonly vitamins and minerals. A few vitamins are fat soluble and must have dietary fat for absorption; these include vitamins A, D, E, and K. All other vitamins are water soluble, easily absorbed but readily excreted from the body. They include thiamin, riboflavin, niacin, biotin, vitamins B_6, B_{12}, and C. See the clinical manifestations table for a list of macronutrients, vitamins, minerals, their uses, and the clinical manifestations of deficiency in the body. See Appendix B∞ for recommended amounts of micronutrients in the daily diet of children and adolescents.

Nutrition Facts Labels

In 1990, the federal government first mandated information that must be supplied on labels for all foods in the Nutritional Labeling and Education Act. Since then the law has been updated to provide additional information that is helpful to the consumer. Some additional information is provided voluntarily by manufacturers of particular food products. The label must contain the name of the product, name and address of manufacturer, net contents, ingredients (most common first and then in descending order of amount), serving size, servings per container, amount per serving of calories, total fat, cholesterol, sodium, total carbohydrate, protein, vitamin A, vitamin C and iron, and % daily value for fat, cholesterol, carbohydrate, pro-

CLINICAL MANIFESTATIONS of Dietary Deficiencies/Excesses

NUTRIENT	DEFICIENCY MANIFESTATION	EXCESS MANIFESTATION
Vitamin A	Night blindness Skin dryness and scaling	Headache Drowsiness Hepatomegaly
Vitamin C	Abnormal hair (coiled shape) Skin abnormalities (dermatitis and lesions) Purpura Bleeding gums Joint tenderness Sudden heart failure	Usually none—excess is excreted in urine
Vitamin D	Rib abnormalities Bowed legs	Drowsiness
B vitamins	Weakness Decreased deep tendon reflexes Dermatitis	Usually none—excess is excreted in urine
Protein	Hepatomegaly Edema Scant, depigmented hair	Kidney failure
Carbohydrate	Emaciation Decreased energy Retarded growth and development	Overweight
Iron	Lethargy Slowed growth and developmental progression Pallor	Vomiting, diarrhea, abdominal pain Pallor Cyanosis Drowsiness Shock

TABLE 9–4 Recommended Dietary Allowances

	AGE	PROTEIN	CARBOHYDRATE	POLYUNSATURATED FATTY ACIDS n-6	POLYUNSATURATED FATTY ACIDS n-3	TOTAL FAT	FIBER
Infants	0–6 months 7–12 months	9.1 g/d or 1.52 g/kg/d* 1.5 g/kg/d	60 g/d* 95 g/d*	4.4 g/d 4.6 g/d	0.5 g/d 0.5 g/d	31 g/d 30 g/d	NE NE
Children	1–3 years 4–8 years	1.1 g/kg/d or 13 g/d 0.95 g/kg/d or 19 g/d	130 g/d 130 g/d	7 g/d (linoleic) 10 g/d (linoleic)	0.7 g/d (α-linolenic) 0.9 g/d (α-linolenic)	NE NE	19 g/d 25 g/d
Males	9–13 years 14–18 years	0.95 g/kg/d or 34 g/d 0.85 g/kg/d or 52 g/d	130 g/d 130 g/d	12 g/d (linoleic) 16 g/d (linoleic)	1.2 g/d (α-linolenic) 1.6 g/d (α-linolenic)	NE NE	31 g/d 38 g/d
Females	9–13 years 14–18 years	0.95 g/kg/d or 34 g/d 0.85 g/kg/d or 46 g/d	130 g/d 130 g/d	10 g/d (linoleic) 11 g/d (linoleic)	1.0 g/d (α-linolenic) 1.1 g/d (α-linolenic)	NE NE	26 g/d 26 g/d

**Values are Adequate Intakes (AIs) rather than Recommended Dietary Allowances (RDAs). All other values on charts are RDAs.*
NE = not established
All data from Institute of Medicine. (2002). Dietary Reference Intakes. *Washington DC: National Academy Press.* www.nap.edu/iom

Nutrition Facts

Serving Size 1 cup (228g)
Servings Per Container 2

Amount Per Serving	
Calories 250	Calories from Fat 110
	% Daily Value*
Total Fat 12g	**18%**
Saturated Fat 3g	**15%**
Cholesterol 30mg	**10%**
Sodium 470mg	**20%**
Total Carbohydrate 31g	**10%**
Dietary Fiber 0g	**0%**
Sugars 5g	
Protein 5g	
Vitamin A	4%
Vitamin C	2%
Calcium	20%
Iron	4%

*Percent Daily Values are based on a 2,000 calorie diet. Your Daily Values may be higher or lower depending on your calorie needs:

	Calories:	2,000	2,500
Total Fat	Less than	65g	80g
Sat Fat	Less than	20g	25g
Cholesterol	Less than	300mg	300mg
Sodium		2,400mg	2,400mg
Total Carbohydrate		300g	375g
Dietary Fiber		25g	30g

FIGURE 9–1 ■ The nutrition facts label of food is based on a typical serving and contains information about fat, cholesterol, sodium, carbohydrate, protein, and selected vitamins. However, the daily value information is based on a 2000–2500 calorie diet. What adjustments should be made if the diet has lower calories, such as with young children? *From Green, M., & Palfrey, J. S. (2000).* Bright futures: Guidelines for health supervision of infants, children and adolescents *(2nd ed.). Arlington, VA: National Center for Education in Maternal and Child Health, p. 6.*

BOX 9–3 DRI Age Groups

Pregnancy and Lactation	14–18 years
Birth to 6 months	19–30 years
6–12 months	31–50 years
1–3 years	51–70 years
4–8 years	Over 70 years
9–13 years	

tein, sodium, and potassium based on a 2,000 calorie diet. The labels are designed to provide information valuable to children from age 4 years through adulthood. However, it is obvious that some interpretation is needed for the young child not yet consuming a diet of about 2,000 calories. See an example of a nutrition facts food label in Figure 9–1 ■.

Recommendations for Dietary Intake

The **Dietary Reference Intakes (DRIs)** are a set of values for macronutrient and micronutrient intake established by the Food and Nutrition Board of the Institute of Medicine and the National Academy of Science which can be used to assess and plan intake for individuals of different ages. They commonly include four different values that can be considered by nurses, nutritionists, and other health personnel (Table 9–5). While the DRIs are the approach used in the United States, other countries have developed their own approaches to dietary standards. For example, Canada uses *Adequate Intake and Reference Nutrient Intake,* and the United Kingdom uses *Recommended Daily Nutrient Intakes.* The aim of these standards is to provide a method of evaluating individual and population diets, and of planning nutrition programs and education. DRIs are generally specific to males and females in several age categories (Box 9–3).

TABLE 9–5 Dietary Reference Intakes (DRIs)

TERM	DEFINITION	USE	EXAMPLE
Estimated Average Requirement (EAR)	Daily intake needed to meet the requirements of 50% of a certain age and gender group	Evaluate intake of a group; plan for intake of a group	Compare the daily intake of vitamin C of a class of children from 24-hour recalls to this number to learn how many do not meet average requirements; plan daily menu for a childcare center
Recommended Dietary Allowance (RDA)	Daily intake needed to meet the requirements of most people (97%–98%) of a certain age and gender group	Set goal for daily intake	Evaluate the dietary intake of an individual for a nutrient such as vitamin C; make recommendations to an individual for a daily menu
Adequate Intake (AI)	Used when limited information on the needs for a vitamin is known and EAR is not available, usually because studies on its metabolism in the body are hard to carry out; rather than metabolic studies, it is based on the average intake of that nutrient by a healthy group of people	Evaluate intake of a group; plan intake for a group	See EAR
Upper Intake (UI)	Upper tolerable intake level; maximum level unlikely to pose a health risk	Limit fortification levels of foods and provide information to limit dietary supplements	Consider intake of a fat-soluble vitamin such as vitamin A that is not readily excreted; include both food sources and supplements

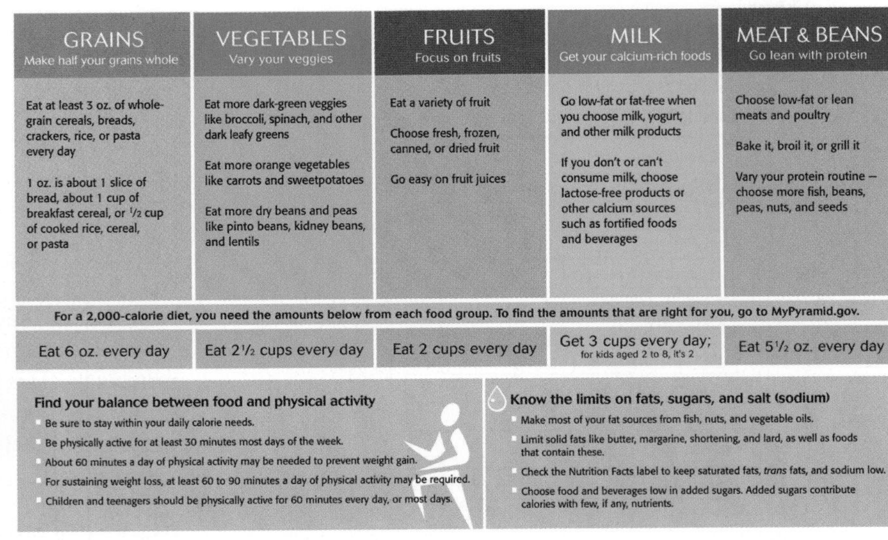

FIGURE 9–2 ■ The food guide pyramid and food rainbow are used to provide teaching about amounts of foods recommended for daily intake.

From U.S. Department of Agriculture and U.S. Department of Health and Human Services. (2005). http://www.mypyramid.gov/downloads/miniposter.pdf; *Canada's Food Guide to Healthy Eating. (2003).* www.hc-sc.gc.ca/hpfb-dgpsa/onpp-gppn/food_guide_rainbow_e.html, accessed 04/04/04. Reproduced with permission of the minister of Public Works and Government Services Canada, 2004.

Although the DRIs provide useful information when evaluating diets, their use can be time consuming. What "quick check" can be performed to provide feedback about the daily diets of children? Become familiar with the food guide pyramid if you are in the United States, and food rainbow if you are in Canada. Hang them in schools, clinics, and hospitals. These are fast methods of looking at children's intakes for a day and seeing if they meet most requirements. Instead of calculating amounts of nutrients ingested, the pyramid and rainbow focus on categories of foods, which readily reflect the actual intake. The numbers of servings from various categories stay constant throughout childhood while the serving sizes increase as the child gets older. See Figure 9–2 ■ for the food guide pyramid and rainbow, and consult websites for alternative pyramids for vegetarians and those from various ethnic groups, such as Hispanic and Native American. (See Developing Cultural Competence: The Mediterranean Diet and Box 9–4).

NUTRITIONAL NEEDS

Nutritional needs evolve during all of infancy and childhood. They support growth and development, and influence the progression of the child along the developmental path. Nutritional intake helps to maintain the health of the child and fosters a state of maximal potential or health promotion. Specific needs during each developmental stage are discussed in this section.

MediaLink Nutritional Resources and Tools

Preterm Infant

Preterm (< 37 weeks' gestation) and **small for gestational age** (< 2500 g) infants have special nutritional needs. They usually need a high calorie/kg intake to provide energy for necessary weight gain. At the same time, immaturity of body systems can make intake and absorption of needed nutrients a challenge. For example, the premature infant may lack the neuromuscular ability to adequately swallow and protect the airway, has a small stomach size, demonstrates gastrointestinal inability to absorb some nutrients, and lacks the renal maturity needed to handle osmolarity (concentration) of formula and to manage glucose, fluid, and electrolyte excretion dependent on intake. Acute medical problems related to a difficult birth and regulation of body homeostasis offer additional challenges.

To provide for energy needs, 50 to 60 kcal/kg per day (parenteral feeding) to 75 kcal/kg per day (oral feeding) are recommended just to support the infant's resting metabolism. To support growth and other activities, additional calories are added, so the total parenteral feeding should be 90 kcal/kg/day

> **DEVELOPING CULTURAL COMPETENCE**
> **The Mediterranean Diet**
>
> Some ethnic groups in Greece and southern Italy are renowned for the longevity of their members. As they have been studied, certain dietary characteristics have received much attention. The Mediterranean Diet is the term for the manner of eating that is found in these groups. The diet encompasses an area called the "Fertile Crescent" and includes sections of Greece, Italy, France, Spain, Portugal, and North Africa. Intake includes many fresh fruits and vegetables, whole grains, beans, nuts, olive oil, dairy products, moderate amounts of fish, poultry and meat, and moderate amounts of wine. In addition, daily physical activity is common. Research is being carried out to define the parts of this diet and lifestyle that make the greatest contribution to health. An abundance of fresh produce appears important and is a component of the diet that can be encouraged for all adults and children.

Canada's Food Guide to Healthy Eating

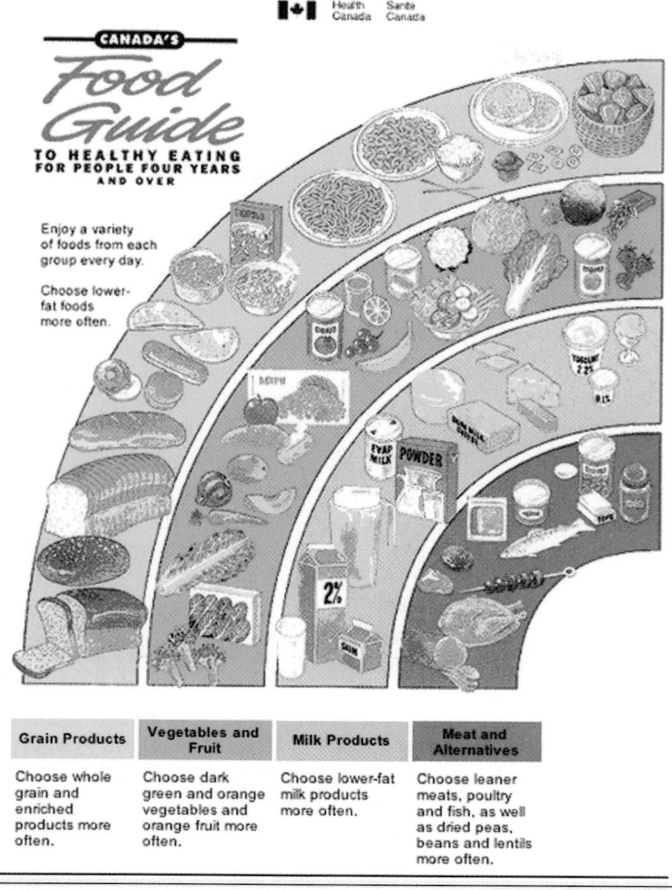

Health Canada Santé Canada
CANADA'S
Food Guide
TO HEALTHY EATING FOR PEOPLE FOUR YEARS AND OVER
Enjoy a variety of foods from each group every day.
Choose lower-fat foods more often.
Grain Products
Vegetables and Fruit
Milk Products
Meat and Alternatives
Choose whole grain and enriched products more often.
Choose dark green and orange vegetables and orange fruit more often.
Choose lower-fat milk products more often.
Choose leaner meats, poultry and fish, as well as dried peas, beans and lentils more often.

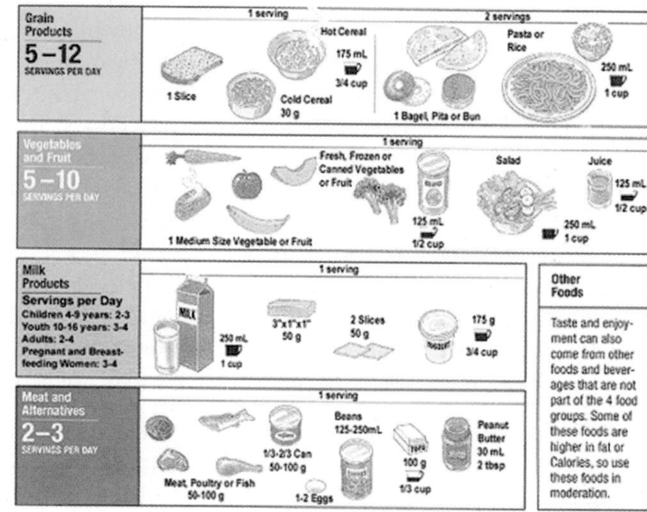

Different People Need Different Amounts of Food

The amount of food you need every day from the 4 food groups and other foods depends on your age, body size, activity level, whether you are male or female and if you are pregnant or breast-feeding. That's why the Food Guide gives a lower and higher number of servings for each food group. For example, young children can choose the lower number of servings, while male teenagers can go to the higher number. Most other people can choose servings somewhere in between.

FIGURE 9–2 ■ (continued)

or more, while the total recommended for the infant fed enterally is 120 kcal/kg/day or more (Trahms, 2000). The preterm baby who has illness such as bronchopulmonary dysplasia (see Chapter 25∞), sepsis (see Chapter 26∞), necrotizing enterocolitis (see Chapter 30∞), or other abnormalities often has increased metabolic demands. The need for catch-up growth should also be considered. Some preterm babies may have nutrient needs as high as 140 kcal/kg/day, making it very difficult to provide adequate breast or formula intake (Nevin-Folino, Loughead, & Loughead, 2001). Protein requirements range

BOX 9–4 **Food Guide Pyramid Debate**

Dr. Walter Willett, chair of the Department of Nutrition at Harvard Medical School, has long challenged the usefulness of the former USDA food guide pyramid, noting that since its introduction, the rate of obesity has climbed in this country. He believed it presented a static view of nutrition in which all fats are bad, all complex carbohydrates are good, dairy products are valuable in high amounts, and that all protein sources are the same (Willett, 2001). Dr. Willett proposed a pyramid that included daily exercise, and suggested a lesser importance for breads and cereals. His criticisms brought about debate and reexamination of the food guide pyramid. The new USDA food guide, seen in Figure 9–2, meets many of his recommendations. Consult the Companion Website for a link to the new pyramid.

In the last decade, there has been a doubling of obesity, even among youth. About a quarter of youth and one half of adults are now overweight. During this time, the food guide pyramid (U.S.) and food rainbow (Canada) have been the major methods chosen for displaying graphically to the public nutritional needs in daily life.

The food guide pyramid and food rainbow do not appear to have translated important nutritional information. Several methods may need to be used for informing families about foods to eat during each day. Portion sizes are not emphasized by the federal approaches and should be included in teaching. Limiting intake of fast foods and suggestions for healthy fast meals may be helpful approaches for today's families.

CRITICAL THINKING APPLICATION

What do you think are the positive aspects of the food guide pyramid or food rainbow? The negative aspects? How will you help families to interpret differences of opinion about nutritional intake in the press?

MediaLink Alternative Food Pyramids

from 3.5 to 4.0 g/kg daily, and fat intake should be 5 to 7 g/kg daily, or 40% to 55% of total energy ingested by enterally fed infants (American Academy of Pediatrics, 2004). Fluid needs range from 80 to 140 mL/kg/day and are adjusted in response to the infant's condition.

Breast milk is considered the best food and should be used whenever the baby can feed adequately to meet requirements. It provides factors that foster growth of the brain, eyes, and other organs; it enhances cognition and general development (Landers, 2003). In addition, babies who breastfeed have greater maintenance of temperature and oxygenation. While preterm formulas contain essential medium-chain triglycerides and polyunsaturated long-chain triglycerides, additional fatty acids found in breast milk include docosahexaenoic acid (DHA) and arachidonic acid (AA). DHA is generally 0.1% to 0.3% of total fatty acids in breast milk and AA is 0.4% to 0.6% of total fatty acids (American Academy of Pediatrics, 2004, pp. 268–269). These fatty acids are major components of neural tissue and retinal photoreceptor membranes, so some companies have started to add these fatty acids to their formulas. The lipids in human breast milk are well absorbed by the premature baby. Human milk contains the amino acids taurine, glycine, and cystine, which are needed by the premature (Aguayo, 2001). In addition, breast milk provides immunologic protection for the baby against some infections (such as sepsis and necrotizing enterocolitis) and feeding fosters positive bonding between mother and newborn.

If the mother is unable or unwilling to breastfeed, the baby can be given breast milk from a milk bank. Many hospitals now maintain such banks so that premature babies can have access to the benefits of breast milk. When the baby cannot nurse adequately or when the premature baby has major nutritional needs, human milk fortifiers can be added to breast milk. They can be tailored to meet the baby's particular needs, but can include nutrients such as protein, fat, carbohydrate, calcium, phosphorus, and vitamin D (Aguayo, 2001). Fortifiers commonly provide an increase of 11% in fat intake, 50% in protein, and 25% in carbohydrates. In addition, mineral content is increased, leading to positive outcomes such as improved calcium balance and bone growth (Landers, 2003). Fortifiers are in-

TABLE 9–6 Comparison of Preterm and Infant Formula, Early and Mature Breast Milk (Typical Ingredients per Liter of Liquid)

NUTRIENT	INFANT FORMULA	PRETERM FORMULA	EARLY MILK (< 28 DAYS)	MATURE MILK (≥ 28 DAYS)
Energy (kcal)	676–680	810–812	varies	650–700
Protein (g)	14.5–16	22–24	16	9–12.6
Fat (g)	34.5–37	41–44	varies	39
Polyunsaturated fat (%)	29–37	8.4–10.3	13	14–15
Monounsaturated fat (%)	16–26	4.6–4.8	NA	40
Saturated fat (%)	43–55	25–26	43–44	44–45
Carbohydrate (g)	72–74	86–90	42–55	80–82
Calcium (mg)	433–528	1340–1460	250	200–250
Iron (mg)	10.1–12.2	2–3	0.5–1.0	0.3–0.9
Vitamin A (mcg)	600–676	1658–3030	4	0.5–1.2
Vitamin D (mcg)	10–10.8	31–55	NA	0.33
Vitamin E (international unit)	8–20	32–51	8–12	3–8
Vitamin K (mcg)	54–55	65–100	2–5	2–3
Thiamine (mcg)	406–680	1620–2030	20	200
Riboflavin (mcg)	913–1020	2400–5030	NA	400–600
Pyridoxine (mcg)	406–507	1220–2030	NA	0.09–0.31
Vitamin B_{12} (mcg)	1.5–2	2–4.5	NA	0.5–1
Niacin (mg)	5.1–7.1	32–41	0.5	1.8–6
Folic Acid (mcg)	61–108	280–300	NA	80–140
Pantothenic acid (mg)	3–3.4	9.7–15.4	NA	2–2.5
Biotin (mcg)	15–30	32–300	NA	5–9
Vitamin C (mg)	54–81	162–300	NA	80–100
Choline (mg)	81–109	81–97	NA	NA
Inositol (mg)	32–122	45–138	NA	NA

Data summarized from American Academy of Pediatrics (1998, pp. 653–668); American Academy of Pediatrics (2004, pp. 880–883).

NA = values not available or highly variable

tended only for the preterm infant and should not be used in babies beyond 37 weeks' gestation.

Preterm formulas may be needed for some infants and are designed to meet the high-density nutrient needs and to supplement babies with necessary micronutrients. These preparations contain different amounts of some vitamins and minerals than other formulas. They may be used for variable amounts of time, depending on the condition of the baby. Some research has found that continuing preterm formulas during the first year of life enhances the growth of preterm infants (Carver, Wu, Hall, et al., 2001). Table 9–6 lists common amounts of ingredients in preterm and regular infant formula.

Feeding methods for premature babies may need to be altered until they have acquired necessary neuromuscular and gastrointestinal maturity (Figure 9–3 ■). Some infants need parenteral nutrition for a time, and receive a mixture of carbohydrate, amino acids, fats, electrolytes, vitamins, and minerals via a central line. As the baby gains maturity, enteral feedings begin. Sometimes these are initially through gavage or tube feeding of breast milk or formula, with gradual introduction of oral feedings by breast or bottle. Nurses assist the parents in learning how to successfully achieve enteral feedings for the baby, and perform thorough assessments of the infant's growth and feeding ability. (See Partnering with Families: Feeding the Preterm Infant.) Babies who have been exposed to drugs prenatally may suck a great deal to meet comforting needs. Careful monitoring of growth and self-consoling ability assists in providing the correct proportions of sucking for nutrition and nonnutritive sucking via pacifier.

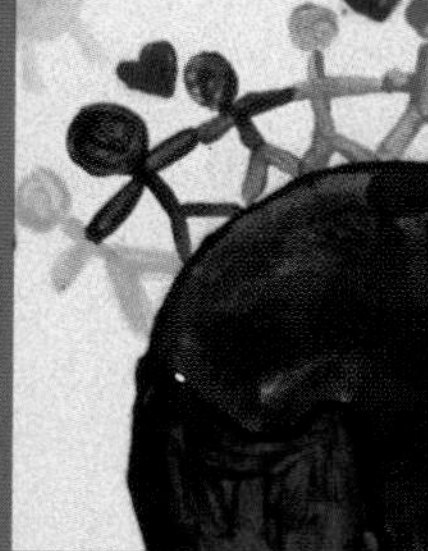

PARTNERING WITH FAMILIES

Feeding the Preterm Infant

Parents of preterm infants often need extra support to breastfeed successfully and to feed the infant adequately. Some suggestions include:

- Begin breast pumping by 6 hours postpartum to ensure adequate milk production.
- Pumping should be done five or more times daily.
- Babies can be held in skin-to-skin contact with the mother during feedings, even during gavage.
- Letdown (milk ejection) reflex can be induced before feeding by stimulation of the breast so the baby does not have to suck hard to obtain milk.
- Assist the baby to place the mouth over the entire areola for feedings, directing the nipple far back to the infant's upper palate.
- Consult local experts, books, and websites.

Adapted from Morton, J. A. (2003). The role of the pediatrician in extended breastfeeding of the preterm infant. Pediatric Annals, *32, 308–316.*

Infancy—Birth to 6 months

From the first feeding of a few ounces of breast milk to a meal of pureed baby foods with the family at 6 months of age, the infant demonstrates an amazing growth in ability to ingest and digest a wide variety of foods. Never again will the individual have such a high metabolic rate or high intake requirements in relation to size. Infants have an extremely fast rate of growth, since birth weight is usually doubled by about 5 months of age. Meeting nutritional needs is made difficult by the small size of the infant's stomach and the immaturity of the digestive system. The great physical activity also necessitates high caloric intake. Nutrient demands for protein and vitamins must be met for the cells of the nervous system and body organs to develop properly. Brain development and normal development depend on adequate nutritional intake. See Table 9–4 for macronutrient requirements of infants.

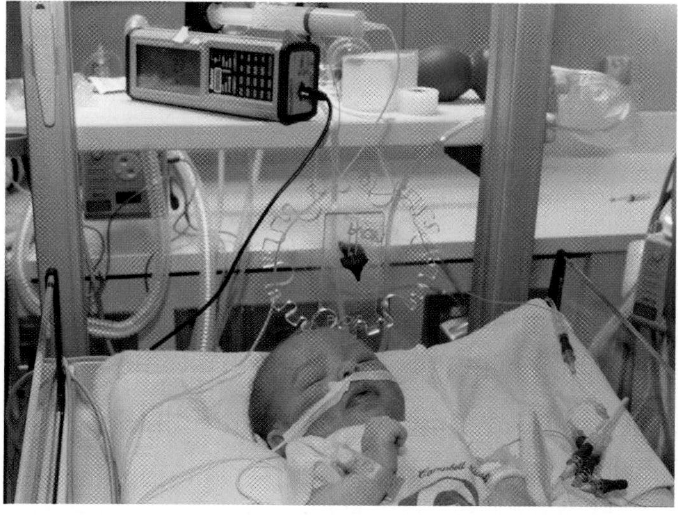

FIGURE 9–3 ■ This premature baby cannot yet coordinate suck and swallow. Gavage feeding is being used until the baby can effectively acquire nutrients.

Breast and Formula Feeding

The natural first food is breast milk and its intake should be encouraged for all infants (Figure 9–4 ■). It can be the only food for the first 6 months, and should continue through 12 months of age (Boxes 9–5 and 9–6). The many advantages to breastfeeding, include excellent nutritional balance, promotion of gastrointestinal function, fostering immune defense, psychological benefits, and economic advantage. Although breast milk is the best nutritional source for infants, there may be a need for limited supplements. Fluoride and sometimes vitamin D are recommended.

Breastfeeding rates have increased from a low of 20% in the 1970s, to about 68% at present (American Dietetic Association, 2001). However, many mothers do not breastfeed for more than

MediaLink Breastfeeding and First Foods Video

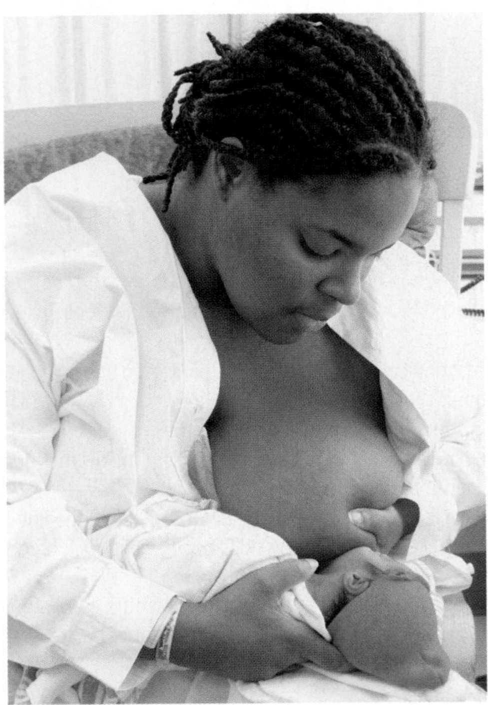

FIGURE 9–4 ■ Breastfeeding offers many physical and emotional benefits for the infant. This new mother is learning to breastfeed her baby. How can nurses encourage mothers to have positive breastfeeding experiences?

a few weeks, and interventions are needed to increase both rates and length of breastfeeding. Exclusive breastfeeding for the first six months, and having mother and baby sleep in close proximity are recommended (American Academy of Pediatrics, 2005). Nurses are uniquely positioned to encourage and foster breastfeeding. Providing breastfeeding information and instruction promotes health of infants by positively influencing the number of women who decide to breastfeed and increasing the number of months they choose to continue breastfeeding (Kramer, 2001). The most effective programs for encouraging breastfeeding are those that involve education and skill/problem-solving information given in at least one session by a health professional (U.S. Preventive Services Task Force, 2003). Some hospitals have

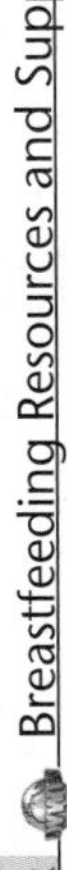

BOX 9–5 Statements on Breastfeeding

The American Academy of Pediatrics states that breastfeeding is the best source of nutrition for babies at least through the first birthday and longer when possible; exclusive breastfeeding for the first six months is recommended. Mothers should receive ongoing instructions and support from medical professionals to assist them in breastfeeding. The American Dietetic Association states that broad-based efforts are needed to break barriers to breastfeeding, citing that exclusive breastfeeding for 6 months and breastfeeding with complementary foods for at least 12 months is the ideal feeding pattern for infants. The U.S. Preventive Services Task Force recommends breastfeeding education and behavioral counseling in 30–90 minute individual or group sessions with specially trained nurses or lactation specialists. The Canadian Task Force on Preventive Health Care also recommends counseling for women to encourage breastfeeding.

BOX 9–6 Health Promotion: First Foods

Nurses should instruct parents that 4–6 months is the optimal time to begin supplementary or complementary foods. Many parents begin the first solid foods as early as a few weeks of life. They have often been told by others or read that early food enhances "sleeping through the night" and is more satisfying for the baby. Early feeding is not needed by the baby, nor does it enhance sleeping for longer periods, health, or any other benefits. Babies are more prone to developing allergies when fed early and they lack the tongue control and digestive enzymes to take in and metabolize many food products (American Academy of Pediatrics, 2004).

lactation specialists who assist breastfeeding mothers; in others, staff nurses provide this service. Home visits, phone calls from hospital nursing staff, early visits after the birth to obstetric and pediatric offices, and resources such as LaLeche League can provide mothers with needed breastfeeding information and problem-solving suggestions. Provide information so that the mother understands the importance of adequate nutritional intake and sufficient rest. Refer mothers to support programs if they have difficulty breastfeeding, feel unsure how it will fit into family and work life, are very young, or have an infant with problems related to feeding.

Teaching can emphasize the importance of breastfeeding to the child's well-being. Lower incidence of otitis media, other infections, type 2 diabetes, and, later, obesity are some reasons why mothers often are encouraged to breastfeed. The nurse can search out barriers in the population served and try to remove them. For example, Women, Infant, and Children (WIC) Program mothers have noted that incentives to feed formula such as free samples and coupons, or lack of family and physician support for breastfeeding, decrease the percentage of mothers who breastfeed (Walker, 2002). Teen mothers may lack information about breastfeeding (Leffler, 2000). Barriers for women of a specific culture such as Hispanic or Latino may relate to embarrassment about feeding in public, lack of printed materials showing members of the cultural group, or absence of family members with the breastfeeding mother in brochure photographs (Stopka, Segura-Perez, Chapman, et al., 2002). The nurse needs to identify barriers among women served and work to decrease them and foster increased incidence of breastfeeding. Barriers can be related to lifestyle, social and work needs, attitudes, and knowledge. See Chapter 11∞ for further guidelines on encouragement of breastfeeding and consult the American Academy of Pediatrics policy on breastfeeding and the use of human milk (American Academy of Pediatrics, 2005).

The mother of a hospitalized infant will need special support to continue breastfeeding. The mother should be encouraged to come to the hospital to feed her baby on the same schedule as at home. If the infant cannot breastfeed, the hospital can provide an electric pump so the mother can maintain lactation. Often hospitals provide meals for the mother of a hospitalized baby so that she can maintain good nutrition and quality breast milk while she stays in the hospital with the baby.

Some women decide not to breastfeed or are unable to do so. After several months of breastfeeding, some mothers begin to use

BOX 9–7 Common Baby Formulas

MILK-BASED FORMULAS
- Enfamil
- Good Start
- Similac

SOY-BASED FORMULAS
- Isomil
- Nursoy
- Prosobee
- Soyalac

SPECIALIZED FORMULAS
- Lofenalac (low phenylalanine)
- Nutramigen (casein hydrolysate)
- Pregestimil (casein hydrolysate)
- Alimentum (casein hydrolysate)
- Portagen (sodium caseinate)
- Lactofree (lactose free)
- Neocate (synthetic amino acids)

supplemental bottles of formula when they are away from the infant. Nurses provide these mothers with information about formula preparation and feeding. Three types of formula are available—ready to feed, concentrate, and powder (Table 9–7). All are nutritionally adequate for infants. The nurse can help parents decide which preparation of formula is best suited for their infant (Box 9–7). Iron-fortified infant formula should always be used during the first year of life.

PRACTICE ALERT

Formula can be mixed with tap water but must be refrigerated once mixed. Formula that the baby does not drink should be discarded after use and not kept for future feedings. This minimizes the chance for bacteria to grow and to cause illness in the baby. When the family lives in older housing, caution them to run tap water for about 2 minutes before using it, and to use only cold water for formula preparation. These practices will minimize the chance that lead is leached from the older pipes in the house (see Chapter 30 for further discussion of lead poisoning). If the family has a well, the water should be tested for microorganisms before being used for the baby.

Some infants, such as those with phenylketonuria, other metabolic disorders, or babies with cow milk allergy, require specialized formulas. For example, casein hydrolysate formula is specially treated (hydrolyzed) to decrease incidence of allergy to casein, the milk protein. Breast or formula feeding is discussed at each contact with health professionals to identify potential teaching needs. (See Partnering with Families: Health Promotion—Supplements for Breastfed Babies.)

PARTNERING WITH FAMILIES

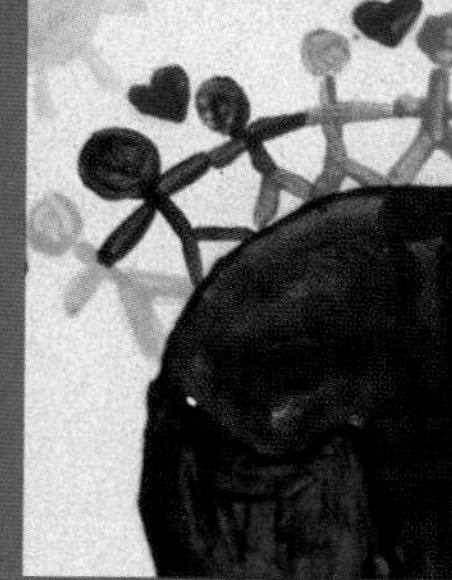

Health Promotion—Supplements for Breastfed Babies

- Each baby receives a vitamin K injection after birth to promote adequate blood clotting. After this time no further vitamin K is needed, as the baby manufactures this vitamin in the gut once he or she begins eating.
- The need for vitamin D is not fully established, but 400 international units per day is recommended for all infants, especially those who are breastfed, live in northern climates and urban settings especially in winter, are dark skinned, or kept well covered when outside.
- Iron is not needed unless the infant is not taking in other sources of food with iron by 6 months. The baby may need an iron source earlier if the mother was anemic during pregnancy or while breastfeeding.
- Fluoride 0.25 mg is given after 6 months of age if water is not fluoridated to a level of 0.3 parts per million (ppm), or the baby is not drinking any water.

CLINICAL TIP

Cow milk (including evaporated milk) can lead to bleeding and anemia (see Chapter 28), can interfere with absorption of some nutrients, and has a high solute load (concentration) which immature kidneys can have difficulty excreting. It should be avoided during infancy.

Emphasize to parents the need to hold babies for bottle feeding rather than propping up bottles. This promotes the relationship between parent and child since touch, voice, and eye contact are possible. Caution parents not to let the baby go to sleep with a bottle as this may increase potential for otitis media (see Chapter 24). Cereal should not be added to formula; the baby needs to learn to eat this more textured food from a spoon.

TABLE 9–7 Advantages and Disadvantages of Formula Preparations

FORMULA PREPARATION	HOW PACKAGED	ADVANTAGES	DISADVANTAGES
Ready to feed	Bottles or cans	No preparation needed	Most expensive type of formula
Concentrate	Cans of concentrated liquid	Easy to add equal amounts of formula concentrate and water directly into bottle and shake	Can be incorrectly measured, leading to inadequate or unsafe nutrition for infant; requires access to clean water supply such as city tap water or bottled water; well water may have too high a mineral concentration
Powder	Cans	Least expensive type of formula	Can be incorrectly measured, leading to inadequate or unsafe nutrition for infant; requires shaking to mix thoroughly; requires access to clean water supply such as city tap water or bottled water; well water may have too high a mineral concentration

Infancy—6 to 12 months

The second 6 months of life are marked by increasing ability to absorb foods and growing nutritional needs. Babies continue breast or formula feeding and gradually add soft and then more textured foods to the diet. Parents who are using formula should continue to select iron-fortified formula for the infant up to 12 months of age. When breastfed babies are not eating foods with iron adequate to meet RDA by 6 months, supplemental iron may need to be added in dosage of 1 mg/kg/day. Careful dietary assessment and discussion of intake by the nurse at health visits helps the practitioner decide if supplemental iron is needed.

Introduction of Supplemental Foods

When should other foods be added to the infant's diet? Although some parents add other foods when the infant is only days or weeks old, it is best to take cues from the infant's developmental milestones. The American Academy of Pediatrics (2004) recommends introducing semisolid foods at 4 to 6 months. At this age the extrusion reflex (or tongue thrust) decreases and the infant can sit well with support. The infant is also developing the ability to appreciate texture and to swallow nonliquid foods, and can indicate desire for food or turn away when full.

The first food added to the infant's diet is usually rice cereal. The advantages of introducing cereal first are that it provides iron at an age when the infant's prenatal iron stores begin to decrease, it seldom causes allergy, and it is easy to digest. One to 2 tablespoons are fed to the infant once or twice daily just before formula or breastfeeding. The infant may appear to spit out food at first because of normal back-and-forth tongue movement. Parents should not interpret this early feeding behavior as indicating dislike for the food. With a little practice, the infant becomes adept at spoon feeding.

Once the infant eats 1/4 cup of cereal twice daily, usually at 6 to 8 months of age, vegetables or fruits can be introduced (Table 9–8). By 8 to 10 months, most fruits and vegetables have been introduced and strained meats or other protein (e.g., tofu, cheese, mashed cooked beans) can be added to the infant's diet. Finger foods are introduced during the second half of the first year as the infant's palmar and then finger grasps develop and as teeth begin to erupt (Figure 9–5 ■). Infants enjoy toast, O-shaped cereal, finely sliced meats, cheese and tofu, and small pieces of cooked, softened vegetables. As food and juice intake increase, formula or breast feedings decrease in amount and frequency (Table 9–9). Certain foods are more commonly associated with development

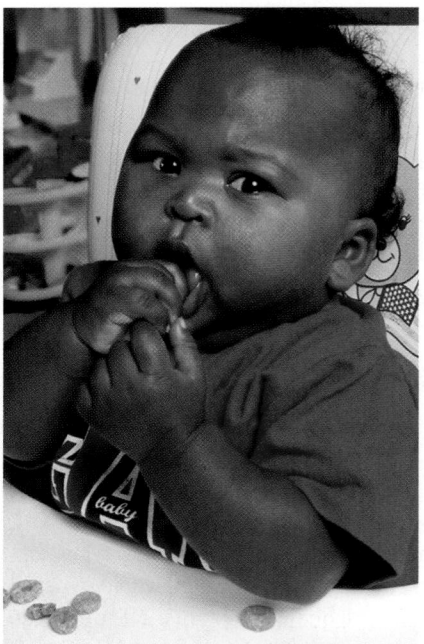

FIGURE 9–5 ■ The baby who has developed the ability to grasp with thumb and forefinger should receive some foods that can be held in the hand.

TABLE 9–8 Health Promotion—Introduction of Solid Foods in Infancy

RECOMMENDATION	RATIONALE
Introduce rice cereal at 4–6 months.	Rice cereal is easy to digest, has low allergenic potential, and contains iron.
Introduce fruits or vegetables at 6–8 months. Some healthcare providers recommend vegetable introduction before fruits.	Fruits and vegetables provide needed vitamins. Vegetables are not as sweet as fruits; introducing them first may enhance acceptability to the infant.
Introduce meats at 8–10 months.	Meats are harder to digest, have high protein load, and should not be fed until close to 1 year of age.
Use single-food prepared baby foods rather than combination meals.	Combination meals usually contain more sugar, salt, and fillers.
Introduce one new food at a time, waiting at least 3 days to introduce another. Delay feeding eggs, strawberries, wheat, corn, fish, and nut products until close to 1 year of age.	If a food allergy or intolerance develops, it will be easy to identify. The foods listed are those most commonly associated with food allergy.
Avoid carrots, beets, and spinach before 4 months of age. Have well water evaluated for nitrates.	Nitrates in these foods and in water near agricultural runoff can be converted to nitrite by young infants, causing methemoglobinemia.
Infants can be fed mashed portions of table foods such as carrots, rice, and potatoes.	This is a less expensive alternative to jars of commercially prepared baby food; it allows parents of various cultural groups to feed ethnic foods to infants.
Avoid adding sugar, salt, spices when mixing own baby foods.	Infants need not become accustomed to these flavors; they may get too much sodium from salt or develop gastric distress from some spices.
Avoid honey until at least 1 year of age.	Infants cannot detoxify *Clostridium botulinum* spores sometimes present in honey and can develop botulism.

TABLE 9–9 Infant Nutritional Pattern

Birth to 1 month	➤ Eats every 2–3 hours, breast milk or formula ➤ Eats 2–3 oz (60–90 mL) per feeding ➤ Has coordinated suck-swallow by 36 weeks' gestation
2–4 months	➤ Has coordinated suck-swallow ➤ Eats every 3–4 hours ➤ Eats 3–4 oz (90–120 mL) per feeding
4–6 months	➤ Begins baby food, usually rice cereal ➤ Eats 4 or more times daily ➤ Eats 4–5 oz (100–150 mL) per feeding
6–8 months	➤ Eats baby food such as rice cereal, fruits, and vegetables ➤ Eats 4 times daily ➤ Eats 6–8 oz (160–225 mL) per feeding
8–10 months	➤ Enjoys soft finger foods ➤ Eats 4 times daily ➤ Eats 6 oz (160 mL) per feeding ➤ Uses cup with lid
10–12 months	➤ Eats most soft table foods with family ➤ Attempts to feed self with spoon though spills often ➤ Eats 4 times daily ➤ Eats 6–8 oz (160–225 mL) per feeding

of food allergy and avoiding them in infancy may decrease allergy incidence. Recommendations for infants at risk due to family history are to delay feeding of cow milk until 1 year, eggs until 2 years, and peanuts, nuts, fish, and shellfish until 3 years (American Academy of Pediatrics, 2004).

PRACTICE ALERT

Advise parents to use caution when providing finger foods to the infant. Hard foods and some soft and malleable ones slip easily into the pharynx and may cause choking. Avoid hot dogs, hard vegetables, candy, whole grapes, and chunks of peanut butter. Infants and other young children should always be supervised while eating. Be sure parents are familiar with techniques for airway obstruction removal and have emergency numbers clearly listed on their phones.

Parents who want to make baby foods at home can be encouraged and instructed about how to do so. Some commercially prepared foods have unnecessary additives such as salt, sugar, and food starch, and they may be costly for some families. Parents can easily blend fruits and vegetables the family is eating before adding salt, sugar, or seasoning, as these additives should be avoided in the baby's foods.

CLINICAL TIP

Caution parents not to use honey in foods for infants, as it can lead to infant botulism.

Prepared foods should be used promptly and stored in the refrigerator between feedings. Foods can also be placed into ice cube trays and frozen; a cube or two can be defrosted at mealtime.

PRACTICE ALERT

If foods or fluids are microwaved for use with infants or children, there can be "hot spots" that lead to burning. Stirring, shaking, and checking temperature before feeding is needed to protect the child from burns to the mouth. Bottles of formula or breast milk should not be heated in a microwave because of the danger of hot spots, even when the outside of the bottle feels only warm. Placing the bottle in a pan of hot water or under hot tap water for a few minutes is a better alternative.

Weaning has come to be associated with a baby giving up breastfeeding or bottle feeding to drink from a cup, although it can be used to refer to any change in prior patterns. For example, in some cultures and eras, weaning meant to replace the breast with food as the primary nutritional source. Most babies begin to drink from cups sometime in the second half of the first year. By then they can sit upright, like to grasp objects and bring them to their mouths, and are interested in "drinking" in the same manner they see in others. Once most of their liquids are taken from a cup, they are "weaned." There is no perfect time for weaning, but it is good to offer a cup by 8 or 9 months of age. As the baby becomes more adept, the cup can replace or supplement one breast or bottle feeding. The process of weaning is gradual, with both parent and infant making the transition. Some babies prefer to have the comfort of being held for at least one feeding a day well into the second or third year, while others make the transition to cup quickly. Some mothers want to continue breastfeeding for as long as the young child is interested and should be supported in this decision. Others are interested in having the baby weaned by 1 year of age. Ask about the cultural patterns in a family, the parents' desires, and look for clues in the infant. Then provide information to assist the family in the best time and manner in which to wean the baby. See Partnering with Families: Weaning.

Dental Care

During infancy and toddlerhood, nurses should carefully examine the patterns of breast and bottle feeding. **Early childhood caries** is the presence of one or more decayed, lost, or filled tooth surfaces in a primary tooth from birth to 71 months of age (American Dental Association, 2000). This condition is frequently caused by drinking from a bottle or nursing for prolonged periods, especially when sleeping. Other terms that formerly defined the condition are nursing bottle mouth syndrome and baby bottle tooth decay (Figure 9–6 ■). The milk, juice, or other fluid pools around the upper anterior teeth, salivary flow decreases, and acid buffering is decreased, resulting in tooth decay. Teach parents to avoid putting the child to bed with a bottle and to avoid putting fruit juice into a bottle at any time. Encourage pacifier use or a bottle of water instead. Mothers who breastfeed should also be cautioned to limit nursing to specific times so that milk will not pool in the mouth during sleep. Other potential causes of early childhood caries are general poor nutrition and oral care, bacterial invasion of the gingiva, serious illness, lack of dental care, and genetic conditions influencing condition of the teeth.

Teach parents beginning dental care for the infant, which includes wiping the teeth off daily once they erupt with a piece of

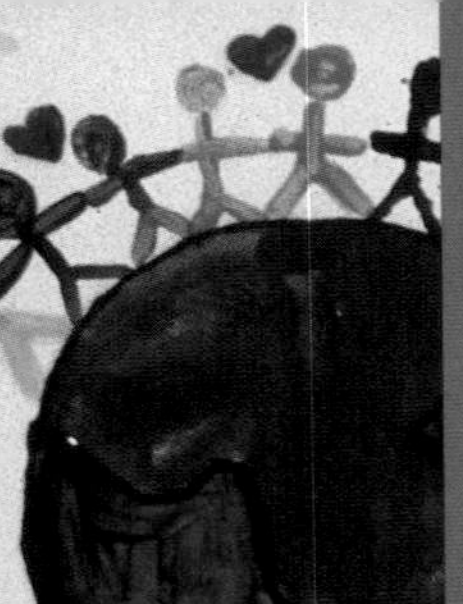

PARTNERING WITH FAMILIES

Weaning

Weaning is often easy to accomplish but some parents need assistance in deciding when and how to accomplish this developmental task. Some tips include:

- Once the infant likes to grasp and hold objects, offer water in a cup with lid.
- If the infant looks around and is preoccupied with other activities during feedings from the breast or bottle, a cup can be offered.
- Start by substituting the cup for one breast or bottle feeding daily and increase to other feedings as the baby seems ready.
- Never provide bottles or cups to carry around or to go to sleep; use them only during feeding times while being held to ensure good dental health.
- Expect the baby to prefer being held for breast or bottle feeding at night, when otherwise tired, or when upset or stressed for a longer period than at other times.

moist gauze or a small infant toothbrush. Some pediatric dentists like to see the child for a first dental visit at about 1 year of age while others wait until the child is older. Have the parents select and establish contact with a dental provider when the child is nearing the end of infancy. See Chapter 12 for further information about promoting dental health in infants.

PRACTICE ALERT

According to the National Center for Chronic Disease Prevention and Health Promotion, "Dental decay is one of the most common chronic infectious diseases among U.S. children. This preventable health problem begins early: 17% of children aged 2–4 years have already had decay. By the age of 8, approximately 52% of children have experienced decay, and by the age of 17, dental decay affects 78% of children. Among low-income children, almost 50% of tooth decay remains untreated, and may result in pain, dysfunction, underweight, and poor appearance—problems that can greatly reduce a child's capacity to succeed in the educational environment."

Dental care is one of the greatest healthcare needs of children, particularly in the national economic slowdowns, when parents often do not have dental insurance through jobs that cover their children or the financial resources to pay for the care. Ask about access to dental care at each child healthcare visit. Refer to low-cost dental programs in the community as appropriate. Keep a list of dental resources to share with families as needed. Some dentists offer care to a certain number of low-income families for reduced rates, and health departments or clinics may offer dental care to children not served by other programs.

Toddlerhood

Why do parents of toddlers frequently become concerned about the small amount of food their children eat? Why do toddlers seem to survive and even thrive with minimal food intake? The toddler often displays the phenomenon of **physiologic anorexia,** caused

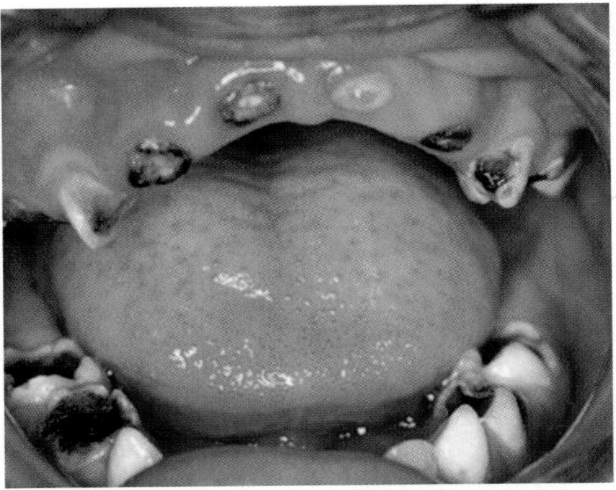

FIGURE 9–6 ■ Early childhood caries. This child has had major tooth decay related to sleeping as an infant and toddler while sucking bottles of juice and milk.

Courtesy of Dr. Lezley McIlveen, Department of Dentistry, Children's National Medical Center, Washington, DC.

when the extremely high metabolic demands of infancy slow to keep pace with the more moderate growth rate of toddlerhood. Although it can appear that the toddler eats nothing at times, intake over days or a week is generally sufficient and balanced enough to meet the body's demands for nutrients and energy.

Parents often need knowledge about types of foods that constitute a healthy diet. During the toddler period, parents play the major role in choosing food intake and socializing the child to eating patterns, and so nutritional patterns should be discussed at each healthcare visit. Some easy-to-prepare foods are high in salt and other additives, and can lead to exceeding the recommendation of *Healthy People 2010* for sodium intake. Provide alternatives to hot dogs, microwave meals, or fast foods with information about easy preparation of sliced meats, cheese, tofu, fruits, and vegetables. Healthy snacks for young children include yogurt, cheese, milk, slices of bread with peanut butter, thinly sliced fruits, and soft vegetables.

Advise parents to offer a variety of nutritious foods several times daily (three meals and two snacks) and let the toddler make choices from the foods offered. Offer foods only at meal-

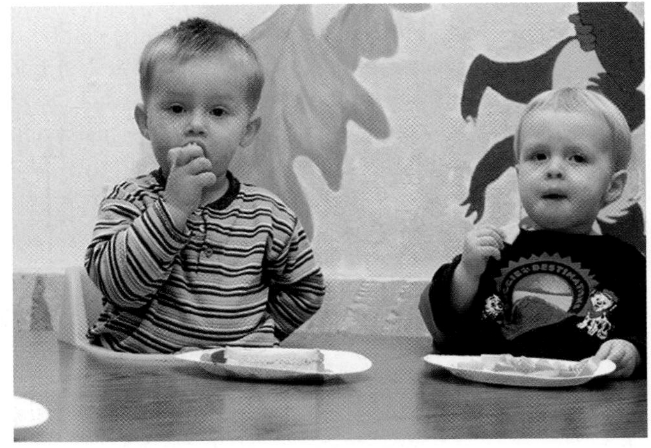

FIGURE 9–7 ■ Toddlers should sit at a table or in a high chair to eat, to minimize chance of choking and to foster positive eating patterns.

TABLE 9–10 Health Promotion—Typical Daily Intake at Various Ages

	BREAKFAST	SNACK	LUNCH	SNACK	DINNER	SNACK
Infant 6 months	2 T rice cereal with 2 oz (60 mL) formula	4 oz (120 mL) formula or breast milk	6 oz (180 mL) formula or breast milk	6 oz (180 mL) formula or breast milk	2 T rice cereal with 2 oz (60 mL) formula, then 6 oz (180 mL) formula or breast milk	4 oz (120 mL) formula or breast milk
12 months	1/4 to 1/2 cup (60–120 mL) apple juice 4 T rice cereal with 4 oz (120 mL) milk	3 crackers 1/2 cup (120 mL) milk	1 thin slice (1/2 oz [14 g]) of turkey 1/2 cup soft cooked carrots 1 cup (240 mL) milk	1/2 slice of cheese 1/2 cup (120 mL) milk or water	1/4 cup plain pasta 1/4 cup thin-sliced apple chunks 1/2 cup (120 mL) milk	1/2 cup yogurt
Toddler	1/4 cup (60 mL) orange juice 1/4 cup cereal with 1/2 cup (120 mL) milk 1/4 banana	5 crackers 1/2 cup (120 mL) milk	2 thin slices (1 oz [28 g]) of turkey with 1/2 slice of bread 1/2 cup soft cooked carrots 1 cup (240 mL) milk	1 slice cheese 1/2 cup (120 mL) juice	1/4 cup plain pasta 1/4–1/2 cup thin-sliced apple chunks 1/2 cup (120 mL) milk	1/2 cup yogurt
Preschooler	1/2 cup (120 mL) orange juice 1/3 cup cereal with 3/4 cup (180 mL) milk 1/2 banana	5 crackers 1/2 orange 1/2 cup (120 mL) milk	3 thin slices (1 1/2 oz [42 g]) of turkey with 1/2 slice bread 1/4 cup cooked carrots 3/4 cup (180 mL) milk	1 slice cheese 1/2 cup (120 mL) juice	1/4–1/2 cup plain pasta with meat sauce 1/2 cup thin-sliced apple chunks 1/2 cup (120 mL) milk	1/2 cup yogurt
School-age child	1/2 cup (120 mL) orange juice 3/4 cup cereal with 1 cup (240 mL) milk 1/2 bagel with jam		4 thin slices (2 oz [56 g]) of turkey with 1 slice bread and condiments Apple 1 cup (240 mL) milk 1 oatmeal cookie	1 1/2 cups popcorn 1 cup (240 mL) lemonade	1/2 cup pasta with meat sauce Dinner salad 1 slice garlic bread 1 cup (240 mL) milk	1 cup pudding or yogurt
Adolescent	1/2 cup (120 mL) orange juice 1 cup cereal 1 cup (240 mL) milk 1 bagel with 1 T peanut butter and jam		3 oz (84 g) meat with 2 slices of bread plus condiments Apple 1 cup (240 mL) milk 1 oatmeal cookie	3 cups popcorn 1 cup (240 mL) lemonade	1 1/2 cup pasta with meat sauce 1 slice garlic bread Salad with dressing 1 cup (240 mL) milk	1 cup pudding Fruit

times and have the child eat in a high chair or on a special seat at the table (Figure 9–7 ■). Small portions are most appealing to the toddler. A general guideline for food quantity at a meal is 1 tablespoon of each food per year of age (see Table 9–10 for common serving sizes at various ages). The toddler should drink 16 to 24 ounces (1/2 to 3/4 L) of milk daily. Caution parents against giving the toddler more than 1 quart (1 L) of milk daily, since this interferes with the desire to eat other foods. Too much milk leads to dietary deficiencies (Box 9–8). Recall that the child should not be placed to bed with a bottle or allowed to carry a bottle of milk or juice around during the day, due to the risk of early childhood caries (see previous discussion in chapter).

BOX 9–8 Growth & Development

Toddlers can drink 2% milk starting at 2 years of age. A maximum of 1 L of milk per day should be consumed. Larger amounts can contribute to obesity, and may interfere with the toddler's consumption of a variety of foods, leading to iron deficiency anemia. Cups are recommended for milk and other drinks; bottle use should have been discontinued before this age. The child is learning to use utensils (spoons are best) but may prefer fingers and still needs small serving sizes. Mild flavors are preferred, with minimal spices and bitter tastes.

Parents should be cautioned to limit fruit juice to 4 to 6 oz daily for children ages 1 to 6 years to decrease the opportunity for overweight, dental caries, and abdominal discomfort (American Academy of Pediatrics Committee on Nutrition, 2001). Using water to drink in combination with whole fruits, which provide fiber, is a healthier alternative. Avoid more than one meal weekly from a fast-food restaurant due to the generally high-fat and low-fiber content of such meals.

CLINICAL TIP

Unpasteurized juice should never be used since it may contain pathogens particularly harmful to young children.

Learning how to eat with others is an important task of toddlerhood. The toddler displays characteristic autonomy or independence during mealtime. Advise parents to provide opportunities for self-feeding of food with fingers and utensils, and to allow some simple choices, such as type of liquid or cup to use. Young children should eat at a table with others, not be allowed to run and play while eating, and eat at specified meal and snack times. Because social skills are developing, the hospitalized toddler may eat better if allowed to have meals with parents or other hospitalized children. See Chapter 17∞ for further suggestions about management of nutrition in hospitalized children.

Preschool

The diet of the preschooler is similar to that of the toddler, but mealtime is now a more social event, and the child increasingly makes food choices. Preschoolers like the company of others while they eat, and they enjoy helping with food preparation and table setting (Figure 9–8 ■). Involving them in these tasks can provide a forum for teaching about nutritious foods and principles of preparation such as the need for refrigeration, safety around stoves, and cleanliness. Limit visits to fast-food restaurants to about one weekly and use the opportunity to assist the child in making wise choices of nutritionally adequate foods in that setting.

Although the rate of growth is slow and steady during the preschool years, the child has periods of **food jags** (eating only a few foods for several days or weeks) and greater or lesser intake. Advise parents to assess food intake over a 1- or 2-week period rather than at each meal to obtain a more accurate impression of total intake. Food jags can be handled by providing the desired food along with other foods to foster choice. The child who chooses not to eat at snack or mealtime should not be given other foods in between. Hunger will develop and the child will become accustomed to eating when food is provided. Three meals and two or three snacks daily are the norm (see Table 9–10). Limit fruit juice to 8 to 12 oz daily, but begin teaching the "5-a-day" program that supports having five servings of fruits/vegetables each day. Children often spend part of the day in a childcare center or school. Parents need to examine the food provided in these settings, and decide how to provide food at home that will supplement the school intake. Times for home meals may need to be altered if the child eats very early or late in the day at school.

The preschool period is a good time to continue encouraging good dental habits. Children can begin to brush their own teeth with parental supervision and help to reach all tooth surfaces. See Chapter 13∞ for recommended doses of fluoride when the water supply is not fluoridated. If the child has not yet visited a dentist, the first dental visit should be scheduled so the child can become accustomed to the routine of dental care. Nurses in childcare centers can teach tooth brushing techniques and encourage the routine of having all children brush after meals and snacks at the center.

School Age

The school-age years are a period of gradual growth when energy requirements remain at a steady level, although sometime during these years, most children experience a preadolescent growth spurt. Girls may begin a growth spurt by 10 or 11 years, and boys a year or so later (Box 9–9). Nutritional needs increase dramatically with this spurt, with large numbers of calories and increased amounts of other nutrients required (see Table 9–4 and Appendix B∞ for RDAs).

School-age children are increasingly responsible for preparing snacks, lunches, and other meals. These years are a good time to teach children how to choose nutritious foods and how to plan a well-balanced meal. Because school-age children operate at the concrete level of cognitive thought, nutrition teaching is best presented by using pictures, samples of foods, videotapes, handouts, and hands-on experience.

School-age children often prefer the types of foods eaten at home and may be resistant to new food items. A hospitalized child may refuse to eat, slowing the recuperative process. Encourage family members to bring favorite foods from home that meet nutritional requirements. This can be especially helpful when the hospital serves food only from the dominant cultural group. A child accustomed to a diet of rice, tofu, and vegetables may not enjoy a hospital meal of hamburger and fries. By school age, food has become strongly associated with social interaction, so it is beneficial to have children eat together or to invite family members to take the child off the unit to eat or to bring in food from home and eat with the child. Many hospitals allow children to plan a pizza night or sponsor other events to encourage eating in a social atmosphere.

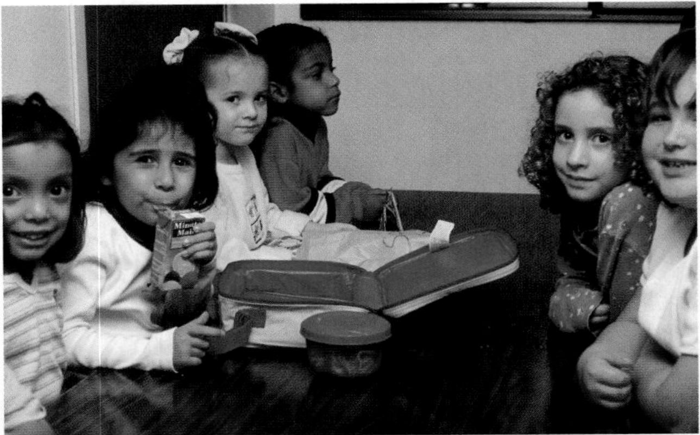

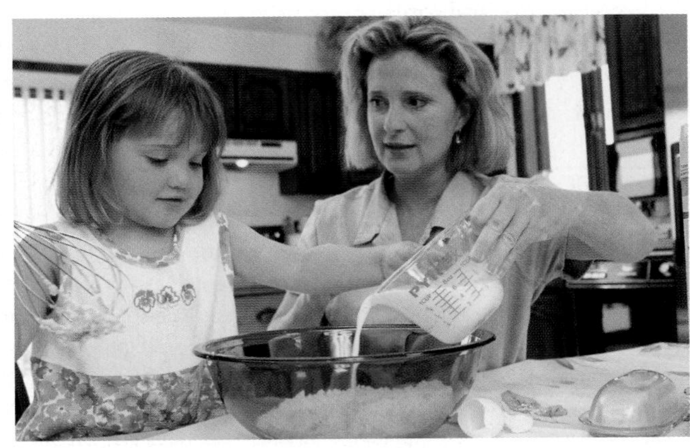

FIGURE 9–8 ■ Preschoolers learn food habits by eating with others. Engaging them in food preparation enhances knowledge of food and promotes intake at meals.

BOX 9–9 Research: Early Menarche

When girls experience menarche before 11 years of age, they are more frequently overweight. Early weight control and being alert for early menarche can help identify young girls in need of obesity prevention. Such prevention efforts are needed to decrease risks such as type 2 diabetes (Adair & Gordon-Larsen, 2001).

BOX 9–10 School Vending Machines

Over the last decade, many school systems in the United States have allowed vending machines for carbonated sweetened beverages and snacks to be installed in public schools. Part of the profits from such machines has enabled revenue-strapped school districts to enhance their incomes. However, schools are increasingly challenged about the presence of the machines, especially in light of the growing problem of overweight among youth. Some school districts have now limited the number of machines or the hours during which they can be used by students. Nurses are able to provide information for districts about the problem of obesity and healthy foods for youth. Parents may need assistance in organizing to work with school districts to ensure healthy food access for school-age children.

Find evidence to support your decisions about the following questions.

- Should public schools allow vending machines to be placed within schools?
- Is their an age limit for accessibility (should machines be in high schools, middle schools, elementary schools)?
- Should carbonated sweetened beverages and snacks be sold all day or only at certain times such as after lunch periods or after school?
- What alternatives exist for fund raising for districts with insufficient funds for school programs?

Most children consume at least one meal daily in school. Although they may bring lunches to school, many children participate in the school lunch program, and perhaps the school breakfast program. Become familiar with the school district's policies in your area for providing foods, snacks, and reduced-price food to students in need. Realize that schools are an excellent setting for educating children about the 5-a-day and other nutritional programs. Classroom teaching and environmental clues in hallways and cafeterias can be used. Establish creative ways to inform and involve parents in nutritional education programs, so that teaching may be reinforced at home (Reynolds, Franklin, Leviton, et al., 2000). This is also a good age to teach emergency care for choking, since persons of any age can choke and some have been saved by children who learned airway obstruction removal. Nurses working in clinics, offices, and other community settings can partner with school nurses to promote nutritionally adequate services within the school setting. The loss of the first deciduous teeth and the eruption of permanent teeth usually occur at about 6 years, or at the beginning of the school-age period. Of the 32 permanent teeth, 22 to 26 teeth erupt by age 12, and the remaining molars follow in the teenage years. (See Chapter 8 for the typical sequence of tooth eruption, Chapter 14 for health promotion regarding oral care, and Chapter 24 for emergency care for accidental tooth evulsion.) The school-age child should be closely monitored to ensure that brushing and flossing are adequate, that fluoride is taken if the water supply is not fluoridated, that dental care is obtained to provide for examination of teeth and alignment, and that loose teeth are identified before surgery or sports participation. Ask about tooth hygiene, fluoride intake (when pertinent), and loss of teeth at each health maintenance visit.

Adolescence

Most adolescents need well over 2,000 calories daily to support the growth spurt, and some adolescent boys require nearly 3,000 calories daily. When teenagers are active in a variety of sports, these requirements increase further. Because adolescents prepare much of their own food and often eat with friends, they need to learn about good nutrition. Developing a diet that includes a large number of calories, meets vitamin and mineral requirements, and is acceptable to the teen may be a challenge. An adolescent who does not like the hospital lunch and reaches for a soft drink and chips may be receptive to juice and pizza, a more nutritious meal. Small improvements should be viewed positively as they may lead to further changes. The pregnant adolescent has complex nutritional needs; refer to maternity nursing texts for information on working with this population.

Fast food represents a significant intake for many adolescents. Commonly fast food is high in fat, calories, and sodium, and low in essential nutrients such as calcium, folic acid, riboflavin, vitamins A and C, and fiber. Assisting teens to make nutritious selections at fast-food restaurants can be helpful in controlling weight and enhancing intake of nutrients. Some high schools are intervening to improve the health of youth by encouraging students to eat at school rather than at nearby fast-food restaurants, decreasing availability of vending machines in schools, and making the school cafeteria a more enticing place to eat (Box 9–10). While a la carte food items have been integrated into many school lunch programs and are popular with teens, they are often high in fat and calories. Adding fruit items and salads can be healthy alternatives (Calderon, 2002). School nurses play a vital role in helping to tailor a healthy school nutrition program (Figure 9–9 ■).

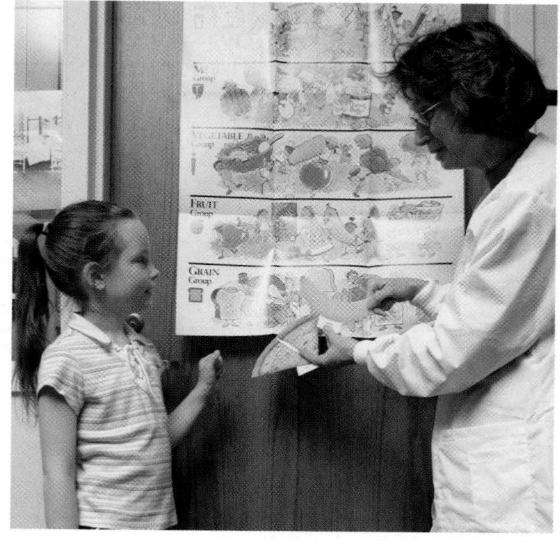

FIGURE 9–9 ■ The school nurse provides nutrition posters for the classroom and teaches school children about healthy food choices.

Remember that peer group influence is important, so group sessions in which adolescents eat lunch together can provide a forum for influencing food habits. What other methods can encourage positive nutritional habits among teens?

Nutritional Challenges

Nutrition is vital for growth and development of all children. Ensuring adequate nutrition, however, is not always as simple as teaching families about dietary needs at various ages. Challenges exist for all families as they strive to obtain and ingest healthy foods. Social, cultural, and political influences all play a part in determining the intake available and acceptable to children and families. Lack of adequate financial resources, widespread availability of fast foods, and mental health problems are discussed throughout this chapter. Nurses can partner with other health professionals to combine knowledge of dietary needs to promote normal growth and development, and the special stresses of particular families, to assess and intervene in this important health promotion topic. *Healthy People 2010* recognizes the importance of nutrition and has established several goals related to childhood nutrition. See Table 9–11 for examples of *Healthy People* goals and related health promotion activities of nurses.

NUTRITIONAL ASSESSMENT

What is the best indication that the child's nutrition is adequate? Which data collection methods provide the most accurate information about a child's dietary intake? The nurse plays an important role in assessing the diets of children and in seeking additional evaluation from dietitians and nutritionists in complex situations.

TABLE 9–11 *Healthy People 2010* Goals Related to Nutrition

GOAL	*BASELINE DATA	*TARGET	HEALTH PROMOTION NEEDS
19.3 Reduce the proportion of children and adolescents who are overweight or obese.	11%	5%	➤ Dietary intake teaching ➤ Encouragement of physical activity
19.4 Reduce growth retardation among low-income children under age 5 years.	8%	5%	➤ Consistent monitoring of growth parameters ➤ Provision of information and resources about child intake needs
19.5 Increase the proportion of persons aged 2 years and older who consume at least two daily servings of fruit.	28%	75%	➤ Teaching about benefits and accessibility of fruits ➤ Ensuring accessibility to fruits in schools, childcare, and other settings
19.6 Increase the proportion of persons aged 2 years and older who consume at least three daily servings of vegetables, with at least one-third being dark green or orange vegetables.	3%	50%	➤ Teaching about benefits and accessibility of vegetables ➤ Ensuring accessibility to vegetables in schools, childcare, and other settings
19.7 Increase the proportion of persons aged 2 years and older who consume at least six daily servings of grain products, with at least three being whole grains.	7%	50%	➤ Teaching about benefits and accessibility of grains ➤ Ensuring accessibility to whole grains in schools, childcare, and other settings
19.8 Increase the proportion of persons aged 2 years and older who consume less than 10% of calories from saturated fat.	36%	75%	➤ Teaching about sources of fats and alternatives
19.9 Increase the proportion of persons aged 2 years and older who consume no more than 30% of calories from total fat.	33%	75%	➤ Teaching about sources of fats and alternatives
19.10 Increase the proportion of persons aged 2 years and older who consume 2,400 mg or less of sodium daily.	21%	65%	➤ Teaching about sources of sodium and alternatives
19.11 Increase the proportion of persons aged 2 years and older who meet dietary recommendation for calcium.	46%	75%	➤ Teaching about benefits and sources of calcium
19.12 Reduce iron deficiency among young children and females of childbearing age.	1–2 yrs: 9% 3–4 yrs: 4% over 12 yrs: 11%	1–2 yrs: 5% 3–4 yrs: 1% over 12 yrs: 7%	➤ Teaching about benefits and sources of dietary iron
19.15 Increase the proportion of children and adolescents whose intake of meals and snacks at school contributes to good overall dietary quality.	Not established		➤ Ensuring dietary guidelines are met in school lunch programs ➤ Ensuring school snack machines have healthy alternatives
19.18 Increase food security among U.S. households and in so doing reduce hunger.	88%	94%	➤ Assessing food security in all healthcare settings ➤ Teaching about resources for acquisition of foods

Goals, baseline, and target from Healthy People 2010 *(2000).*
**Baseline is established from national data available in 2000, and goals are desired targets to reach by 2010.*

MediaLink Nutritional Status Video

Nursing assessments form the basis for establishing health promotion and health maintenance interventions related to nutrition.

Physical and Behavioral Measurement

Growth Measurement

A common method used to evaluate the adequacy of diet is measurement of growth. Preterm infants need a special combination of nutritional assessment techniques (Table 9–12). **Anthropometric measurement** is the term used to refer to assessment of various parts of the body. Anthropometry of young children commonly includes weight, length, and head circumference. Standing height is substituted for length once the child can stand. Head circumference, also known as occipital-frontal circumference (OFC), is measured until the child is about 5 years of age. Additional measurements that may be included in special circumstances include chest circumference, mid-upper arm circumference, and skinfold measurement at sites such as triceps, abdomen, and subscapular regions. See Chapter 8 and the Skills Manual for detailed descriptions of measurement techniques.

Once the measurements are collected, plot the readings on the appropriate standardized growth curves for weight, length or height, head circumference, and **body mass index (BMI)** (Figure 9–10 ■). BMI is a calculation based on the child's weight and height, or length, and is calculated as kilograms of weight/m^2 of height (Box 9–11). This is a useful calculation for determining if the child's height and weight are in proportion. Identify on the grids where the child

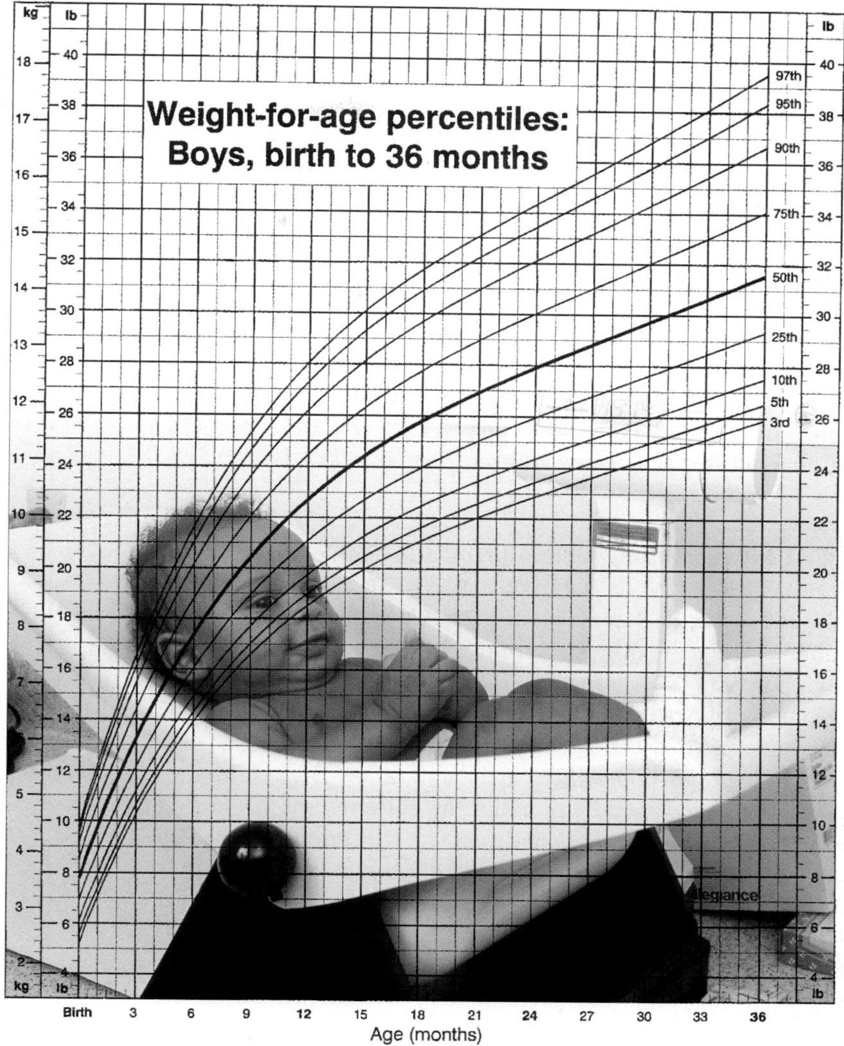

FIGURE 9–10 ■ The nurse accurately measures the child and then places height and weight on appropriate growth grids for the child's age and gender.

TABLE 9–12 Preterm Newborn Nutrition Assessment Techniques

GROWTH MEASUREMENT	FEEDING PATTERNS	SERUM MEASUREMENTS	OTHER
➤ Daily weight ➤ Weekly length, crown-heel length, and head circumference ➤ Use of special growth charts for preterm infants* ➤ Periodic mid-upper arm circumference or skinfold measurement	➤ Abdominal distention/girth ➤ Gastric residual ➤ Emesis ➤ Stool frequency ➤ Blood in stool	➤ Serum glucose ➤ Weekly or more often serum electrolytes ➤ Weekly serum alkaline phosphatase, phosphorus, calcium (to detect ostopenia or low bone mass) ➤ Weekly hematocrit, hemoglobin, reticulocyte count ➤ Periodic serum proteins and BUN ➤ Weekly serum bilirubin, alanine amino transferase (AST) if on total parenteral nutrition ➤ Serum vitamins or minerals if indicated	➤ Periodic dual-energy X-ray absorptiometry (DEXA) to evaluate lean-, fat-, and bone-mineral mass

Adapted from Rigo, J., De Curtis, M., & Pieltain, C., (2002); Nutritional assessment in preterm infants with special reference to body composition. Seminars in Neonatology, *6, 383–391; Anderson, D. M. (2002). Nutritional assessment and therapeutic interventions for the preterm infant.* Clinics in Perinatology, *29, 313–326.*

**Special growth charts available in Ehrenkranz, R. A., Younes, N., Lemons, J. A. et al. (1999). Longitudinal growth of hospitalized very low birth weight infants.* Pediatrics, *104, 280–289.*

BOX 9–11 Growth Measurement

To calculate body mass index (BMI), you must:

1. Be sure that weight is in kilograms. If it is in pounds, divide that number by 2.2 to get kilograms.
2. Change height measurement to meters. Because 1 m = 39.37 in. (or 0.0254 m = 1 in.), you must multiply the child's height in inches by 0.0254 to obtain height in meters.
3. Now square the number of meters.
4. You are ready to calculate BMI. Put kilograms of weight/height in meters squared and divide appropriately.

If a child weighs 26.5 lb, convert to kilograms = 12 kg. The child's height is 34.5 in. = 0.8763 m. Because $m^2 = 0.7679$, BMI = 15.63.

Alternatively, see the Centers for Disease Control and Prevention website for direct calculation of BMI using metric or English units (www.cdc.gov/growthcharts).

falls in percentile for each measurement. Children normally fall between the 10th and 90th percentiles. A measurement below the 5th percentile, especially for BMI, may indicate undernutrition, whereas one over the 85th to 95th percentile can indicate overnutrition (see discussion of overweight later in this chapter). It is important, however, to look at the differences between measurements. A child in the 90th percentile for length and weight is proportional and may be a naturally large child; the body mass index will be in about the 50th percentile. On the other hand, a child who is consistently in the 10th percentile for all measurements, but is growing steadily and is at a normal development level, may simply be a small child, and will also be at the 50th percentile for body mass index. The BMI numbers change as children grow. While adults with a BMI of 30 or above are obese, the specific numbers are not descriptive for the child, only the BMI percentile is used to evaluate growth (Table 9–13).

Much cultural and individual variation exists regarding size. See Appendix A∞ for standardized growth curves by gender and age for infants, children, and adolescents. Visit this chapter's Companion Website to find out more about the growth curves and to access the Centers for Disease Control and Prevention website course in accurate assessment techniques. Plot your measurements on the same growth curve with earlier percentiles for the child (Figure 9–11 ■). When measurements follow the same percentile over time, growth is generally normal for the child and nutrition is likely adequate (Box 9–12). However, a sudden or sustained change in per-

BOX 9–12 Growth Patterns

If you measure a child and find him or her to be either in very low or high percentiles, try the following:

1. Measure again to check for accuracy.
2. Examine if length or height, weight, and head circumference are in similar percentiles. Is the child proportional?
3. Observe if the parents are very large or very small.
4. Look at the child's chart to see if the patterns have continued over time or if they represent a sudden change.

TABLE 9–13 Body Mass Index Percentiles for Boys and Girls from 5–17 Years

AGE	BMI PERCENTILE	BMI FOR BOYS	BMI FOR GIRLS
5	5th	13.7	13.1
	50th	15.6	15.1
	85th	17.2	16.9
	95th	18.3	18.5
6	5th	13.8	13.4
	50th	15.6	15.2
	85th	17.4	17.2
	95th	19.0	19.3
7	5th	13.9	13.6
	50th	15.8	15.4
	85th	17.8	17.9
	95th	20.0	20.4
8	5th	14.1	13.6
	50th	16.2	15.8
	85th	18.6	18.9
	95th	21.5	21.7
9	5th	14.3	13.7
	50th	16.6	16.4
	85th	19.7	20.1
	95th	23.1	23.0
10	5th	14.6	14.0
	50th	17.2	17.1
	85th	20.9	21.4
	95th	24.6	24.5
11	5th	14.9	14.5
	50th	17.8	17.9
	85th	21.9	22.6
	95th	25.7	26.1
12	5th	15.3	15.1
	50th	18.4	18.8
	85th	22.6	23.6
	95th	26.5	27.5
13	5th	15.9	15.9
	50th	19.1	19.6
	85th	23.2	24.4
	95th	27.1	28.6
14	5th	16.5	16.6
	50th	19.8	20.2
	85th	23.7	24.9
	95th	27.8	29.3
15	5th	17.2	17.1
	50th	20.6	20.6
	85th	24.5	25.2
	95th	28.7	29.6
16	5th	17.9	17.4
	50th	21.3	20.9
	85th	25.4	25.5
	95th	29.8	29.9
17	5th	18.3	17.7
	50th	21.8	21.2
	85th	25.9	25.9
	95th	30.1	31.3

Adapted from Rosner, B., Prineas, R., Loggie, J., & Daniels, S. R. (1998). Percentiles for body mass index in U.S. children 5 to 17 years of age. Journal of Pediatrics, *132, 211–222.*

centile may indicate a chronic disorder, emotional difficulty, or a nutritional intake problem. Further assessment of physical status and dietary intake will be needed. See Developing Cultural Competence: Growth Grids.

Additional Physical Measurement

Observations from the physical assessment provide clues to nutritional status. Every body system can be affected by dietary intake, and a combination of certain symptoms may suggest specific nutritional problems (Box 9–13). Common clinical manifestations of deficient and excess nutritional intake are outlined in the clinical manifestations table on page 316.

Laboratory measurements can provide useful information when nutritional status is questionable. Some common studies include hematocrit and hemoglobin, serum glucose and fasting insulin, lipids and lipoproteins, and liver and renal function studies. Adding further measurements such as chest circumference and skinfolds (measurement of fat at certain body sites such as triceps, scapular, and abdominal areas) may also be useful (Bessler, 1999).

Dietary Intake

The mother's dietary intake during pregnancy may provide information about the child's nutritional state and it can be assessed for pertinent information. Obtain detailed information about the child's dietary intake when there is a potential for nutritional deficiency due to disease, knowledge deficit, or socioeconomic status (Hensrud, 1999). After the information is collected, compare the dietary intake with the recommended levels for a child of that age and gender (see Figure 9–2, Table 9–4, and Appendix B∞ for Recommended Dietary Allowances). The 24-hour recall of intake, food frequency questionnaire, and a dietary screening history provide a good overview of the infant's or child's intake and eating patterns. A food diary provides information about the child's precise food intake.

24-Hour Recall of Food Intake

The 24-hour diet recall is frequently used to assess the adequacy of the diet. People can generally remember their intake in the past day, so results are fairly accurate; it is easy to gather the data and analyze results; only a few minutes are needed. Ask the parent or child to list all foods eaten during the past 24 hours (Figure 9–12 ■). It is usually helpful to ask for a description of activities in the last day. Then start with the most recent event and move backwards, integrating food intake into the daily schedule. For example, you might begin by saying, "You mentioned you got up early to come to the clinic today. What did Sam eat at home before you left? Did he have a snack as you traveled

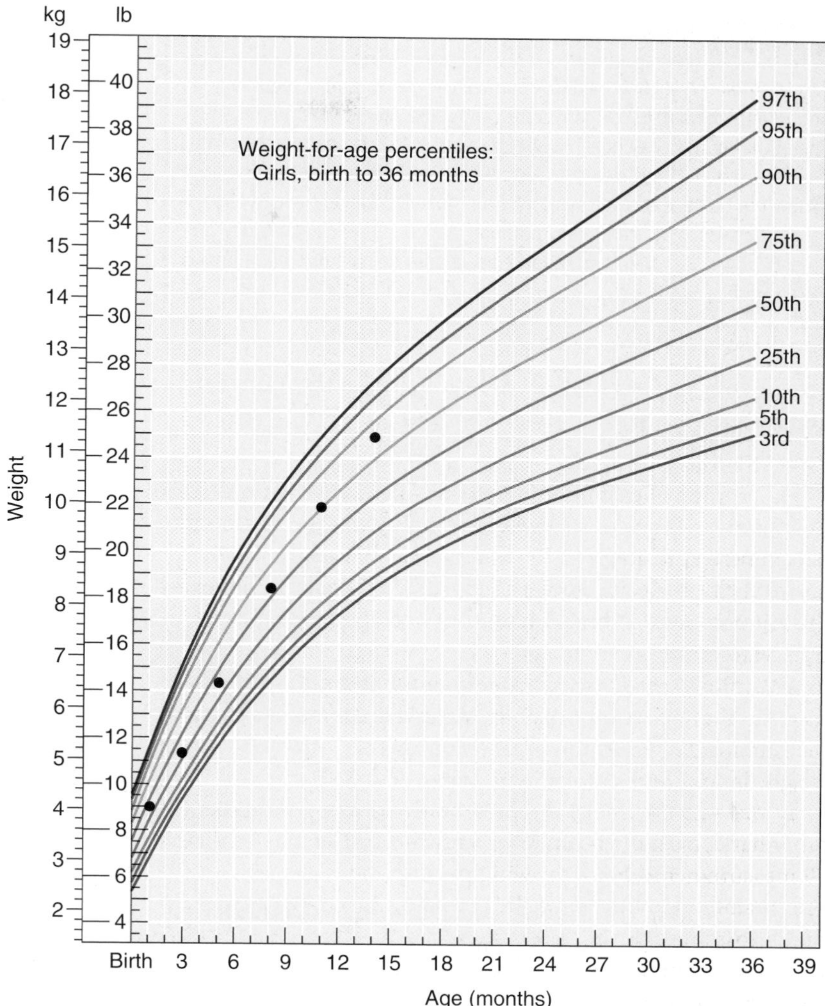

FIGURE 9–11 ■ Growth chart with first few entries in same channel and then a change indicated. The growth for the child indicated on this chart remained steady and in the same channel (75th percentile) for some months. Then the weight measurement decreased to another channel. What kind of dietary assessment will you complete with the parents? What could be the possible causes?

DEVELOPING CULTURAL COMPETENCE
Growth Grids

The revised growth grids now in use were standardized using a cross section of the U.S. population and are generally reflective of most children. However, children from some other countries or cultures may fall outside of these curves. For example, new immigrants or adoptees may be in lower percentiles, and catch up over several months or years. Children of immigrants from developing countries tend to be larger than their parents. Even when small, children should follow normal growth patterns. For example, a child may remain at the 10th or 25th percentile for height, but continue to slowly grow and not fall to a lower percentile.

MediaLink Growth Grids

BOX 9–13 Brain Development Research

Many studies have confirmed that normal brain development requires good nutrition. Amino acids, carbohydrates, and some vitamins are precursors for neurotransmitters. Essential fatty acids are essential elements in the central nervous system. Trace elements such as zinc are found in the brain and are known to be necessary for memory. Iron is needed for central nervous system myelinization. Clearly, early nutrition plays a part in cognitive development and the importance of a good diet cannot be minimized (Wauben & Wainwright, 1999).

here or after you arrived?" While asking about the foods eaten, inquire specifically about the following:

- All meals and snacks
- Amounts of each food item consumed (have various sizes of measuring cups, bowls, and plates so accurate amounts can be indicated)
- Types of specific foods used, such as whole milk versus nonfat or 2%, brand names of cereals, specific types of margarine or butter
- Additives used, such as condiments, table salt, spices
- Food preparation methods, including adding fats to cook, removal or retention of fats on meats
- Vitamins and supplements, types, and doses
- Whether the intake is representative of the typical diet (in situations such as illness or vacation, intake may be different than usual)

Once the 24-hour recall is obtained, intake analysis is next. First, a quick check can be done to compare servings of various food types with the food guide pyramid, as described earlier. Next, a detailed analysis is done to compute calories, carbohydrate, protein, and fat intake and compare them with recommended amounts. All major vitamins and minerals are also computed and comparisons made to the DRIs. This computation may be done by hand, using a book of nutrients in common foods, or may be done on the computer. Several computer programs are available, and the federal government has a website that provides intake levels and comparisons to the RDAs—try computing your own 24-hour recall or that of a child in your clinical setting with the Healthy Eating Index.

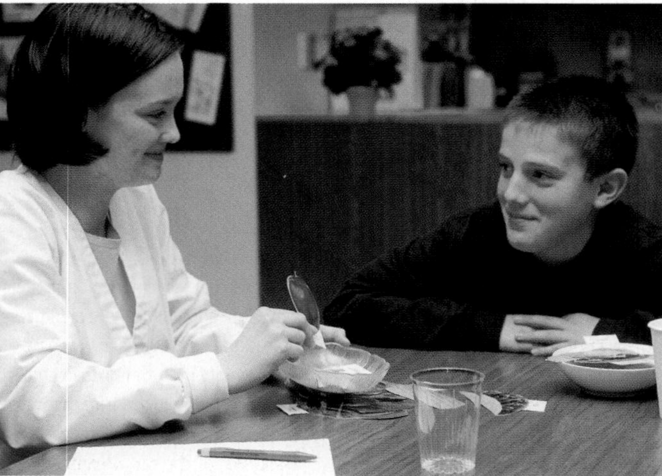

FIGURE 9–12 ■ The nurse is interviewing a child about foods eaten in the last day. Note the models of food and dishes for accurate assessment of serving sizes.

MediaLink Analyze Your Diet

Food Frequency Questionnaire

Food frequency questionnaires are available that can be easily administered to parents or children. Usually they ask about how often certain types of foods are eaten in a specified period such as a week or month. Food frequencies provide information about dietary trends for an individual or a group of children. For example, it can answer questions about whether milk or fruit intakes are close to recommended, or whether sugared cereals are commonly ingested. Questionnaires can be long and evaluate a total diet, or short to focus on specific items such as fruit and vegetable intake. A short questionnaire about milk intake or fruit and vegetable intake may be helpful before the start of a teaching project on nutrition to a class of school-age children. Knowing their usual intake of a food item can provide helpful information for the project. One example of types of questions asked on a food frequency questionnaire is shown in Box 9–14.

BOX 9–14 Sample Questions—Youth Adolescent Questionnaire (YAQ)

1. Where do you usually eat breakfast?
   - Home
   - School
   - Don't eat breakfast
   - Other
2. Which cold breakfast cereal do you usually eat?
3. What type of milk do you usually drink?
   - Whole milk
   - 2% milk
   - 1% milk
   - Skim/nonfat milk
   - Don't know
   - Don't drink milk
4. How much milk (glass or with cereal) do you drink?
   - Never/less than 1 glass per month
   - 1 glass per week or less
   - 2–6 glasses per week
   - 1 glass per day
   - 2–3 glasses per day
   - 4 glasses per day
5. How often do you eat pizza (2 slices)?
   - Never/less than once per month
   - 1–3 times per month
   - Once per week
   - 2–4 times per week
   - 5 or more times per week
6. Do you eat peanut butter sandwiches (plain or with jelly, marshmallow fluff, etc.)?
   - Never/less than 1 sandwich per month
   - 1–3 sandwiches per month
   - One sandwich per week
   - 2–4 sandwiches per week
   - 5 or more sandwiches per week

From Youth/Adolescent Questionnaire. (1995). Harvard Medical School. Channing Laboratory, 181 Longwood Avenue, Boston, MA 02115. Used with permission.

BOX 9–15 Dietary Screening History for Infants

OVERVIEW QUESTIONS

What was the infant's birth weight?

At what age did the birth weight double and triple?

Was the infant premature?

Does the infant have any feeding problems such as difficulty sucking and swallowing, spitting up, fatigue, or fussiness?

IF INFANT IS BREASTFED

How long does the baby nurse at each breast?

What is the usual schedule for nursing?

Does the baby also take any milk or formula? Amount and frequency? What type?

IF INFANT IS FED OTHER FOODS

What formula is used? Is it iron fortified?

How is it prepared?

Do you hold or prop the bottle for feedings?

How much formula is taken at each feeding?

How many bottles are taken each day?

Does the baby take a bottle to bed for naps or nighttime? What is in the bottle?

IF INFANT IS FORMULA FED

At what age did the baby start eating other foods?

Cereal	Finger foods
Fruit/juices	Meats
Vegetables	Other protein sources

Do you use commercial baby food or make your own?

Does the baby eat any table foods?

How often does the baby take solid foods?

How is the baby's appetite?

Do you have any concerns about the baby's feeding habits?

Does the baby take a vitamin supplement? Fluoride?

Have there been any allergic reactions to foods? Which ones?

Does the baby spit up frequently?

Have there been any rashes?

What types of stools does the baby have? Frequency? Consistency?

Dietary Screening History

Ask the parent about the infant's or child's eating habits using questions in Boxes 9–15, 9–16, and 9–17. Responses provide information about the family's eating habits and food beliefs beyond that collected on a 24-hour dietary recall or food frequency questionnaire. See Developing Cultural Competence: Dietary Patterns.

BOX 9–16 Dietary Screening History for Children

- What foods or beverages does the child dislike?
- What types of food or beverage does the child especially like?
- What is the child's typical eating schedule? Meals and snacks?
- Does the child eat with the family or at separate times?
- Where does the child eat each meal?
- Who prepares the food for the family?
- What method of cooking is used? Baking? Frying? Broiling?
- What ethnic foods are commonly eaten?
- Does the family eat in a restaurant frequently? What type?
- What type of food does the child usually order?
- Is the child on a special diet?
- Does the child need to be fed, feed himself or herself, need assistance eating, or need any adaptive devices for eating?
- What is the child's appetite like?
- Does the child take any vitamin supplements (iron, fluoride)?
- Does the child have any allergies? What types of symptoms?
- What types of regular exercise does the child get?
- Are there any concerns about the child's eating habits?

CLINICAL TIP

Parents seldom control all of the food a child eats. To help parents record an accurate food diary, remind them about all the places a child might be fed or obtain food. Older children often get snacks independently and obtain food from friends. Younger children may be fed in childcare centers.

Food Diary

Parents are asked to keep a food diary when the child has a nutrition problem or disorder, such as malnutrition, obesity, or diabetes, which requires dietary management. All meals and snacks, with food preparation method and quantities eaten over a 1- to 7-day period, are recorded. Eating patterns change significantly for holidays or family gatherings, so ask parents to select typical days for the food diary or to record specific events affecting food intake. Food diaries can provide a great deal of

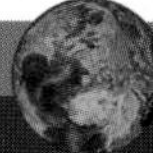

DEVELOPING CULTURAL COMPETENCE
Dietary Patterns

Each culture has eating practices that influence dietary intake. Some groups eat three meals daily and sit with each other for conversation and sharing. Some religious groups may fast at certain parts of the year. Certain foods are more commonly eaten by specific groups. It is important to understand the eating patterns and foods commonly eaten by each cultural group and their contribution to the total nutrition of the child. For example, immigrants from Mexico commonly make their own cheese; Native Americans may eat traditional foods such as roots, berries, and wild game or fish; Asian groups commonly consume rice as the major carbohydrate source. Nurses should know common food patterns in cultural groups where they work in order to ask appropriate dietary questions and perform effective teaching.

BOX 9–17 Dietary Screening for Adolescents

1. Which of these meals or snacks did you eat yesterday?
   ___ Breakfast
   ___ Morning snack
   ___ Lunch
   ___ Afternoon snack
   ___ Dinner/supper
   ___ Evening snack
2. Do you skip breakfast three or more times a week?
   ___ Yes ___ No
3. Do you skip lunch three or more times a week?
   ___ Yes ___ No
4. Do you skip dinner/supper three or more times a week?
   ___ Yes ___ No
5. Do you eat dinner/supper with your family four or more times a week?
   ___ Yes___ No
6. Do you fix or buy the food for any of your family's meals?
   ___ Yes ___ No
7. Do you eat or take out a meal from a fast-food restaurant two or more times a week?
   ___ Yes ___ No
8. Are you on a special diet for medical reasons?
   ___ Yes ___ No
9. Are you a vegetarian?
   ___ Yes ___ No
10. Do you have any problems with your appetite, like not feeling hungry, or feeling hungry all the time?
    ___ Yes ___ No
11. Which of the following did you drink last week?
    ___ Regular soft drinks
    ___ Diet soft drinks
    ___ Fruit-flavored drinks
    ___ Whole milk
    ___ Reduced fat (2%) milk
    ___ Low-fat (1%) milk
    ___ Fat-free (skim) milk
    ___ Flavored milk (for example, chocolate, strawberry)
    ___ Coffee/tea
    ___ Tap/bottled water
    ___ Juice
    ___ Sports drinks
    ___ Beer/wine, hard liquor
12. Which of these foods did you eat last week?

    Grains
    ___ Bread ___ Cereal/grits
    ___ Rolls ___ Popcorn
    ___ Bagels ___ Noodles/pasta/rice
    ___ Crackers ___ Tortillas
    ___ Other: ___________________

    Vegetables
    ___ Corn ___ Greens (collard, spinach)
    ___ Peas ___ Green salad
    ___ Potatoes ___ Broccoli
    ___ French fries ___ Green beans
    ___ Tomatoes ___ Carrots
    ___ Other: ___________________

    Fruits
    ___ Apples/juice ___ Peaches
    ___ Oranges ___ Pears
    ___ Grapefruit/juice ___ Berries
    ___ Grapes/juice ___ Melon
    ___ Bananas
    ___ Other: ___________________

    Milk and Other Dairy Products
    ___ Whole milk ___ Yogurt
    ___ Reduced-fat (2%) milk ___ Cheese
    ___ Low-fat (1%) milk ___ Ice cream
    ___ Fat-free (skim) milk ___ Flavored milk
    ___ Other:

    Meat and Meat Alternatives
    ___ Beef/hamburger ___ Sausage/bacon
    ___ Pork ___ Peanut butter/nuts
    ___ Chicken ___ Eggs
    ___ Turkey ___ Dried beans
    ___ Fish ___ Tofu
    ___ Cold cuts
    ___ Other: ___________________

    Fats and Sweets
    ___ Cake/cupcake ___ Chips
    ___ Pie ___ Doughnuts
    ___ Cookies ___ Candy
    ___ Other: ___________________
13. Do you have a working stove, oven, and refrigerator where you live?
    ___ Yes ___ No
14. Were there any days last month when your family didn't have enough food to eat or enough money to buy food?
    ___ Yes ___ No
15. Are you concerned about your weight?
    ___ Yes ___ No
16. Are you on a diet now to lose weight or to maintain your weight?
    ___ Yes ___ No
17. In the past year, have you tried to lose weight or control your weight by vomiting, taking diet pills or laxatives, or not eating?
    ___ Yes ___ No
18. Did you participate in physical activity (for example, walking or riding a bike) in the past week? If yes, on how many days and for how long?
    ___ Yes ___ No
19. Do you spend more than 2 hours per day watching television and videotapes or playing computer games? If yes, how man hours per day?
    ___ Yes ___ No
20. Do you take vitamin, mineral, herbal, or other dietary supplements (for example, protein powders)?
    ___ Yes ___ No
21. Do you smoke cigarettes or chew tobacco?
    ___ Yes ___ No
22. Do you ever use any of the following?
    ___ Alcohol/beer/wine
    ___ Steroids (without a doctor's prescription)
    ___ Street drugs (marijuana/speed/crack/heroin)

From Story, M., Holt, K., & Sofka, D. (Eds). (2002). Bright futures in practice: Nutrition *(2nd ed.). Arlington, VA: National Center for Education in Maternal and Child Health, Nutrition Tools Appendix.*

helpful information, but take time and motivation to complete accurately (Lee & Nieman, 2002). Be sure instructions are thorough and that the form has a place to record amounts, preparation, events occurring, and where food was eaten. The nurse or parent may need to obtain the school lunch menu and talk with the school lunch personnel to add accurate school intake.

The nurse analyzes data obtained during the assessment. The information is integrated in order to determine if the child demonstrates risk for nutritional problems. See Box 9–18 for a list of risk alerts. The nurse may consult with or refer the family to a dietitian or nutritionist for additional assessment and teaching.

COMMON NUTRITIONAL CONCERNS

Childhood Hunger

Although most Americans live in a "land of plenty," significant numbers of children periodically experience hunger. **Food security** is access at all times to enough nourishment for an active, healthy life (Federal Interagency Forum on Child and Family Statistics, 2000). In contrast, **food insecurity** indicates an inability to acquire or consume adequate quality or quantity of foods in socially acceptable ways, or the uncertainty that one will be able to do so (Boyle & Morris, 1999).

BOX 9–18 Risk Alerts for Nutrition

- Consumes
  - fewer than 2 servings of fruits daily
  - fewer than 3 servings of vegetables daily
  - fewer than 6 servings of grains daily
  - fewer than 2–3 servings of dairy products daily
  - fewer than 2 servings of meat/meat alternative daily
  - excessive amount of fat
  - food from fast food restaurants 3 or more times weekly
- Has poor appetite
- Skips breakfast, lunch, or dinner 3 or more times weekly
- Has food jags (eating just a few foods and refusing others for extended periods)
- Has inadequate financial resources to buy food, has insufficient access to food, or lack of access to cooking facilities
- Uses chronic dieting, vomiting, or pills to lose weight
- Is excessively concerned about body size or shape
- Has had significant weight change in past 6 months
- Has BMI < 5th or > 95th percentile
- Is physically inactive (physical activity < 5 days weekly)
- Participates in excessive physical activity
- Has chronic disease or condition
- Is taking prescription or nonprescription medication
- Uses alcohol, tobacco, or other drugs
- Takes dietary supplements
- Has hyperlipidemia, iron deficiency anemia, or other abnormal serum values
- Has dental caries
- Is pregnant

Adapted from Story, M., Holt, K., & Sofka, D. (Eds). (2002). Bright futures in practice: Nutrition *(2nd ed. p. 249–254). Arlington, VA: National Center for Education in Maternal and Child Health.*

The major cause of hunger in children is poverty, and since one in five children is poor, their families may be unable to provide sustainable nutrition at all times (Children's Defense Fund, 2004). Many single-income families have a head of household moving into the workforce, so incomes are often not sufficient to provide for family food needs (see Chapter 1∞ for a description of Temporary Assistance for Needy Families [TANF]). Families may be ineligible for food assistance programs even though they are unable to purchase enough food for all their members. Children with special nutritional needs are at particular risk because it may be more costly to buy and prepare formula or foods for a child with allergies, diabetes, or an immune disorder.

Children who have insufficient dietary intake are at risk for a wide array of health problems. They may become anemic, experience a high rate of infectious disease due to lowered immune response, have slowed developmental maturation, delayed or stunted physical growth, and learning disorders, and be at greater risk of overweight, cardiovascular disease, and diabetes in adulthood (American Academy of Pediatrics, 2004; Hanson, Dahlman-Hoglund, Lundin, et al., 1997; Walter, Olivares, Pizarro, et al., 1997). Subsequently, the national and individual cost of childhood hunger is great.

Nurses are well positioned to partner with other health professionals such as dietitians and physicians in evaluation of families for food insecurity in a variety of hospital, clinic, school, and home settings. In addition to the assessment of the individual child's nutritional status, further questions can determine families with potential problems. Administer the screening tool to identify risk in families (Box 9–19). Most parents go without food themselves in order to feed their children, so food insecurity may not necessarily have directly impacted all children. However, anxiety over providing food can be a very stressful event in families and diet quality deteriorates as insecurity increases. If families have experienced food insecurity or may be likely to at some time, be sure to provide them

BOX 9–19 Food Insecurity Screening

1. Does your household ever run out of money to buy food to make a meal?
2. Do you or members of your household ever eat less than you feel you should because there is not enough money for food?
3. Do you or members of your household ever cut the size of meals or skip meals because there is not enough money for food?
4. Do your children ever eat less than you feel they should because there is not enough money for food?
5. Do you ever cut the size of your children's meals or do they skip meals because there is not enough money for food?
6. Do your children ever say they are hungry because there is not enough food in the house?
7. Do you ever rely on a limited number of foods to feed your children because you are running out of money to buy foods for a meal?
8. Do any of your children ever go to bed hungry because there is not enough money to buy food?

Scoring: 5–8 yes = hungry; 1–4 yes = risk of hunger

From the Washington State Department of Health.

with access to community agencies and programs that can be of assistance. What resources are available in your community to help families with food insecurity? See Table 9–14.

Overweight and Obesity

After several decades of stable statistics regarding overweight in children, the numbers are now skyrocketing. The current incidence of overweight in the United States has been called an epidemic and is associated with a wide array of health problems, such as the appearance of type 2 diabetes in youth (Ludwig & Ebbeling, 2001). See Chapter 32∞ for a discussion of diabetes. Overweight can also influence self-image, dietary quality, and amount of physical activity. The Third National Health and Nutrition Examination Survey has found that 11% to 15% of child and adolescent groups are now overweight or fall at or above the 95th percentile for BMI (*Healthy People 2010*, 2000). When using the 85th percentile of BMI as indicator for risk of overweight, from 20% to 33% of youth in different age groups are affected (Ogden, Flegal, Carroll, et al., 2002). Even higher rates are seen among specific ethnic groups, with non-Hispanic Blacks and Mexican Americans showing very high rates. Since overweight in childhood and adolescence frequently tracks into adulthood, the implications for healthcare are obvious.

There are many reasons cited for the increase in overweight children. The number of calories consumed is not increasing, but children tend to exercise less, particularly on a daily basis. They infrequently walk or ride bikes, either because of the convenience of driving or due to unsafe neighborhoods. Television viewing is very high among youth and contributes to overweight both from the inactivity associated with it and the pattern of snacking during commercial time. As many as 60% of obese children view excessive television, defined as more than 4 hours daily; over one fourth of all children watch 4 or more hours of television daily, and 67% watch at least 2 hours daily (Crespo, Smit, Troiano, et al., 2001). When television is combined with other "screen activities" such as videos, computers, and handheld games the numbers are even higher. The percentage of calories from fat consumed in the United States is among the highest in the world. Although no more than 25–35% of calories should come from total dietary fat, and no more than 10% from saturated fat, about 35% of calories consumed in the United States are supplied by fat and 12% by saturated fat (National Cholesterol Education Program, 1991; Krauss, Eckel, Howard, et al., 2001). Most fats should be from polyunsaturated and monounsaturated fatty acids, but current diets contain low amounts of those fats and high amounts of trans-fatty acids (Dietary Guidelines for Americans, 2005). High levels of dietary fat, particularly trans-fat, are associated with higher cholesterol levels and decreased activity. The high rate of dietary fat is related to the large amount of fast food consumed, as fast-food restaurants are convenient and fit well into today's lifestyles. Another contributing factor to overweight is poor snacking habits, which have been on the increase in the last decade. Snacks of choice are often nutrient poor and calorie dense (Zizza, Siega-Riz, & Popkin, 2001).

COLLABORATIVE CARE

The goal of collaborative care is identification of children with overweight and partnering with youth and their families to develop healthy lifestyles. Several diagnostic tests may be indicated when the child is overweight. Height, weight, and body mass index (described earlier in this chapter) are key to accurate diagnosis. Once the child is identified as overweight, a thorough nutrition assessment should be performed. Gather information about physical activity patterns, family history of overweight, cardiovascular disease, hypertension, diabetes, and hypercholesterolemia. Serum cholesterol, triglycerides, glucose, hemoglobin A_{1c}, and insulin may be measured to evaluate cardiovascular and type 2 diabetes risk. Blood pressure must be carefully measured and evaluated with norms to determine presence of hypertension. See Chapter 26∞ for cardiovascular measurements and Chapter 32∞ for a discussion of type 2 diabetes in children.

In the United States, national goals for obesity prevention in children and youth have been established. For all youth, goals include a reduction in incidence of obesity, reduction in average BMI, increase in number of children meeting Dietary Guidelines for Americans and the number meeting physical activity guidelines. For individual children and youth, goals include a healthy weight trajectory, using BMI charts, a diet that is healthful in quantity and quality, appropriate amount and type of physical activity, and achieving physical, psychosocial, and cognitive growth and development milestones (Institute of Medicine, 2005) .

TABLE 9–14 Health Promotion—Community Resources for Food

Food Stamp Program	Eligibility based on household size and income; refer students and those with low incomes, especially when they have young children; education services often available
Child Nutrition Programs	School lunch, breakfast, and milk programs; free and lowered cost meals in schools; assist parents to apply
Special Child Programs	Summer programs, Head Start, childcare centers, and homeless children programs may provide nutritional support in some communities
Women, Infants, and Children (WIC)	Supplemental foods and nutrition education to pregnant, breastfeeding, and postpartum women and to their young children; assessment of child growth often included
Nutrition Education and Training Program	Nutrition education for teachers and school food service personnel
Community Services	May include food banks, field gleaning, and other programs

What services are available to provide food and nutrition education in your community? Make a list for use in clinical settings with families.

NURSING MANAGEMENT

The goal of nursing management is to prevent new cases of overweight, identify children who are overweight, and support youth and families to establish healthy lifestyles that promote weight loss and maintenance of recommended weights. Assessment includes height, weight, body mass index at each health promotion visit, along with plotting findings on growth charts. Any child who is at or above the 85th percentile for BMI, or who has a change in growth channels, needs further nutritional analysis. Measure and plot blood pressure. Risks for poor health often cluster in individuals and families, so the nurse can be alert for situations in which parents and siblings are overweight, have elevated blood pressure, exercise infrequently, or are in upper percentiles for weight, BMI, or skinfold. Ask about smoking in a nonjudgmental manner and inquire about exposure to environmental tobacco smoke. History also includes information about number of daily hours of television viewing and other screen activities. Ask about sports, how often and for how long the child engages in them, and how vigorously.

Based on the history, the nurse identifies children who are overweight and establishes a profile of the child's associated risks (Box 9–20). Nursing diagnoses are established based on this data. Several examples are listed in the accompanying nursing care plan. Interventions are directed at all children to promote healthy lifestyles and at children with identified risks to lower the risks for overweight and associated chronic diseases. Nurses can assist parents and children in building good nutritional and exercise habits throughout life, thus decreasing the incidence of overweight and its attendant health risks. Patterns of eating fast foods and meals on the run, and eating while watching television, should be addressed in early health maintenance visits. Caution parents that television viewing and other screen activities should be limited to a maximum of 2 hours total daily, and that television and video games should not be placed in children's bedrooms. Daily exercise routines starting at 30 minutes and increasing to 60 minutes can be included in most families. This includes walking to school or in the neighborhood, working out with an exercise video, bike riding, taking physical education in school, and performing other similar activities. Also, teach about the food guide pyramid and its integration into a healthy life. Healthy snacks include fruits, vegetables, grains, and nuts. "Super sizing" fast foods and eating out often should be avoided. Recognize that the nurse is often an important role model for healthy eating and physical activity, both for youth and their families. See Developing Cultural Competence: Overweight.

BOX 9–20 Research: Overweight and Family History

When a child has one obese parent, chances of the child being overweight are increased by 220%. In families where both parents are overweight, the incidence of obesity in children increases by 320%. Finally, the child who has obese parents and is overweight as an adolescent has about an 80% risk of becoming an obese adult (Whitaker, Wright, Pepe, et al., 1997). Be alert for families with overweight adults and begin prevention early with the children in these families.

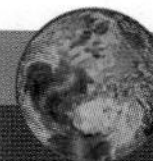

DEVELOPING CULTURAL COMPETENCE
Overweight

Overweight is more common among some ethnic and socioeconomic groups. Lack of knowledge about foods and physical activity, limited access to fresh produce and safe places to exercise, easy access to increasing numbers of fast foods, and ethnic differences in metabolism may constitute risk factors. Lower income and Hispanic, African American, and Native American ethnic identities are associated with higher incidence of overweight, especially among women. National goals to eliminate health disparities in income and ethnic groups have been set (*Healthy People 2010*, 2000).

Nurses can partner with families to encourage weight management. See resources such as "Helping Your Overweight Child" and "Take Charge of Your Health: A Teenager's Guide to Better Health." Some important suggestions include:

MediaLink Children and Overweight Video

- Plan the desired weight goal with your healthcare provider.
- Make changes slowly and one or two at a time.
- Always eat breakfast.
- Include vegetables with each meal.
- Have plenty of fresh fruits, vegetables, and whole grains in the home.
- Limit chips, cookies, carbonated beverages, and other sweetened and fatty snacks.
- Plan meals ahead and eat together as a family.
- Integrate daily physical activity into daily life.
- Consult with healthcare provider regularly.

The child who is overweight should be followed closely. Desired outcomes may include weight loss, integration of at least five fruits and vegetables and six servings of whole grains daily, lack of risk factors for cardiovascular disease or type 2 diabetes, and daily exercise of 60 minutes. Consult dietary guidelines for Americans (2005) for further recommendations. See the nursing care plan for the child who is overweight for additional information on nursing management.

Food Safety

Every year in the United States, about 76 million people contract foodborne illnesses. Some are quite mild, whereas others can be severe. Children are at greater risk of severe illness and death from food and water than adults, due to their immature gastrointestinal and immune systems. The most common pathogens are *Campylobacter, Salmonella, Shigella,* and *E. coli*; infants under 1 year are at extremely high risk of *Campylobacter, Rotavirus*, and *Salmonella* illness (Morbidity and Mortality Weekly Report [MMWR], 2001a). A potential cause of food-related illness is hepatitis A. Although still prevalent in some parts of the country, effective management and prevention through immunization has decreased its general incidence (see Chapter 19∞).

PRACTICE ALERT

Worldwide, over 3 million people die of illness related to unsafe drinking water each year and most of those deaths are among children. The World Health Organization is focusing on this important health problem. Children are more prone to illnesses such as diarrhea and dehydration when drinking contaminated water. Caution families with children to be sure water supplies are safe during travel and to use bottled or purified water.

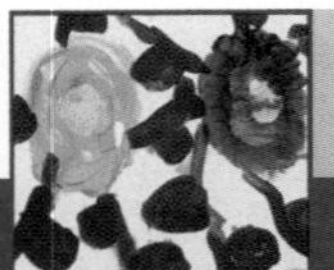

Nursing Care Plan

THE CHILD WHO IS OVERWEIGHT

GOAL	INTERVENTION	RATIONALE	EXPECTED OUTCOME
1. Imbalanced Nutrition: More than Body Requirements related to excessive intake in comparison to metabolic needs			
	NIC Priority Intervention—*Weight Reduction Assistance:* Facilitating loss of weight and body fat		**NOC Suggested Outcome**—*Weight Control:* Personal actions resulting in achievement and maintenance of optimum body weight for health
Child will demonstrate adequate intake of all nutrients without excessive energy intake	▪ Perform thorough nutritional assessment of child	▪ Assessment assists in identification of dietary risks and strengths as well as health conditions related to nutrition	Child meets all dietary requirements while achieving weight and body mass index goal
	▪ Share results of assessment with child and family by showing weight, height, and body mass index grids	▪ Many families do not consider their child overweight. Concrete information about the child's size in comparison with recommendations assists in establishing the importance of weight management	
	▪ Identify with the child and family 2–3 target areas to begin weight management. Examples might include: ▪ Eating fast food only once weekly ▪ Switching to low-fat dairy products ▪ Keeping 2 more fresh fruits and vegetables in the house and 2 less snack foods	▪ Changing dietary patterns drastically is difficult and may lead to giving up the attempt at weight management. Partnering with the family to set goals enhances chances of success.	
	▪ Integrate nutrition information into each visit. Examples of topics include: ▪ Dietary requirements for age group ▪ Effects of simple sugar and fat intake on weight ▪ Beneficial effects of fruits, vegetables, whole grains, and nonfat dairy ▪ Reading food labels ▪ Healthy choices in fast-food restaurants ▪ Calculation of fat content of foods	▪ Nutrition information is best learned in an ongoing program	
	▪ Use growth grids to help child and family establish a weight reduction or maintenance goal	▪ Goals motivate families to achieve desired health behaviors. The goal for a young child may be weight maintenance so that as the child grows in height, the correct proportion is reached, while weight reduction may be needed for older children or youth who are very obese.	
2. Readiness for Enhanced Family Coping related to need to foster health of family member			
	NIC Priority Intervention—*Health System Guidance:* Facilitating child's use of appropriate nutrition and health services to foster weight control		**NOC Priority Outcome**—*Health Promoting Behavior:* Actions to promote, sustain, and increase wellness
Family will assist child to manage stressors and to develop new strategies to support weight control goals	▪ Include key family members in some of the counseling sessions with the overweight child	▪ Key members of the family are those who purchase foods, provide support for the child, and participate in decisions about health	Child expresses satisfaction with family understanding and support of weight management goals

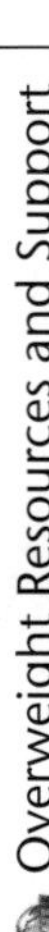

MediaLink Overweight Resources and Support

Nursing Care Plan THE CHILD WHO IS OVERWEIGHT (continued)

GOAL	INTERVENTION	RATIONALE	EXPECTED OUTCOME
2. Readiness for Enhanced Family Coping related to need to foster health of family member (continued)			
	■ Encourage the family to eat together at least once daily if possible or to increase number of meals eaten together weekly	■ The family is an important support system in weight loss programs. Eating as a family or in a social situation can provide a chance to promote healthy foods; intake is generally lower fat and calorie than when eating alone	
	■ Seek a resource for the child to be monitored about twice monthly; this may be a health care provider office, nutritionist, school nurse or other person	■ Provides opportunity to monitor the child's progress, offer support, additional information, and problem solving techniques	
3. Activity Intolerance related to sedentary lifestyle			
	NIC Priority Intervention—*Exercise Promotion:* Facilitating regular exercise to maintain and increase endurance and energy use		**NOC Priority Outcome**—*Endurance:* Extent that energy enables the child to sustain activity
Demonstrated activity tolerance by adequate oxygenation, respiratory effort, and ability to speak during brisk walking, biking, or other activity	■ Establish daily exercise routine beginning with 15–30 minutes daily of walking	■ Starting with brief amounts of exercise makes the child feel comfortable and enhances potential for success	Child demonstrates ability to engage in moderate activity for 60 minutes with minimal respiratory discomfort
	■ Gradually increase activity over 1–2 months until 60 minutes of daily exercise is maintained	■ Gradual increase as the cardiovascular and respiratory systems adapt is generally comfortable for children; 60 minutes of moderate activity daily is recommended for children	
	■ Use activities enjoyed by the child and suggest options as necessary; refer the family to community resources such as swimming pools, organized sports, and biking groups	■ Activities the child enjoys will be more likely to remain in usual activity patterns; exercising with others in groups increases motivation	
	■ Have families plan at least 1–2 activities they can do together weekly	■ This fosters family relationships and provides support and motivation for the child	
	■ Limit screen activities to a maximum of 2 hours daily	■ Increased use of screen activities is related to poor dietary habits and increased sedentary behaviors and excess weight	
	■ Have child keep a log of hours of television, video games, computer and other similar activities		
	■ Tell child never to snack while doing screen activities		
	■ Ask about use of tobacco in children in 5th grade or higher	■ Most adults who smoke began the habit in childhood; middle school years are the most common age for smoking initiation	
	■ Inquire about exposure to environmental tobacco smoke at all ages	■ Smoking by others in the household can be harmful to children	
	■ Perform teaching to discourage tobacco use or offer cessation programs as needed	■ Smoking decreases respiratory reserves and worsens several cardiovascular disease risks	

(continued)

Nursing Care Plan THE CHILD WHO IS OVERWEIGHT (continued)

GOAL	INTERVENTION	RATIONALE	EXPECTED OUTCOME
4. Chronic Low Self-Esteem related to weight			
	NIC Priority Intervention—*Self-Esteem Enhancement:* Assisting the child to increase personal judgment of self-worth		**NOC Priority Outcome**—*Quality of Life and Self-Esteem*: Expressed satisfaction with life circumstances and positive judgment of self-worth
Child expresses positive perception of self-worth and confidence in ability to deal with issues related to weight	■ Facilitate development of a positive outlook by exposing child to others who have been successful with weight loss	■ Increases motivation and feelings of self efficacy	Child speaks positively about accomplishments in weight control management
	■ Praise child for weight loss, weight maintenance, increased physical activity, and other achievements	■ Enhances judgment of self worth and pride in accomplishments	
	■ Help the child establish rewards for meeting goals, such as purchase of new clothing		
	■ Partner with parents so that they understand the value of praise and never label the child by derogatory words such as "fat"	■ Family members are usually the most intimate support system for the child	

Foodborne illness is relayed by food preparation and storage practices, lack of adequate training of retail employees regarding foods and hygiene, and increasing amounts and types of foods being imported from other countries. Some examples of contaminated foods in the last few years include undercooked hamburger meat, cross contamination of salad bar from meats, unpasteurized apple cider, green onions, prepackaged salad and delicatessen meat, and sprouts. While most infected persons experience acute bloody diarrhea, some can develop serious complications such as hemolytic uremic syndrome (see Chapter 31∞) or thrombocytic purpura (see Chapter 28∞). Health personnel should integrate teaching regularly so that families can decrease risks of foodborne illness transmitted at home. See Partnering with Families: Health Promotion Food Safety Guidelines.

Food may carry products other than microorganisms that can be harmful. An example is mercury, which may be concentrated in certain types of fish. This metal can cause harm to the developing nervous system of fetuses, infants, and young children when consumed in large quantities. The U.S. Food and Drug Administration (FDA) and Environmental Protection Agency (EPA) note that fish are an important part of a healthy diet, but that certain recommendations should be followed to lower risk of mercury's detrimental effects. Women who may become pregnant, are pregnant or nursing, and young children should take care to do the following:

- Eliminate shark, swordfish, king mackerel, and tilefish from the diet.
- Eat up to 12 oz (two average meals) a week of a variety of low-mercury fish and shellfish such as shrimp, canned light tuna, salmon, pollock, catfish. Albacore or white tuna has more mercury than light tuna, so limit white tuna to one meal weekly.
- Check for local advisories about the safety of fish caught in local waters in your area. In the absence of advice, up to 6 oz (one meal) weekly may be eaten from local waters. Do not eat other fish during that week.

(FDA, 2004)

Dietary Deficiencies

Although there can be deficits in nearly all nutrients, certain deficiencies are more common in childhood. Either limitations in the food supply or patterns of dietary intake are the cause of most deficiencies, while children with certain disease processes, such as metabolic diseases, may have difficulty absorbing or using nutrients ingested (see Chapter 32∞ for a discussion of inborn errors of metabolism and Chapter 4∞ for other genetic conditions that can influence intake or metabolism of food). The nutrient deficiencies present in a population are a result of genetic factors and characteristics of the food supply and intake patterns of particular groups. See Developing Cultural Competence: Vitamin A.

Iron

Newborns have a store of iron obtained from their mothers in utero, if the maternal nutritional state was satisfactory and the baby is normal gestational age. Breast milk contains little iron, but the iron it does contain has high bioavailability. By 4 to 6 months of age, however, the baby's iron stores begin to decrease and a dietary source of iron must be added. Enriched rice cereal is commonly used to meet these initial iron needs. In babies who do not have adequate iron stores or do not take in enough iron, **anemia** (a reduction in the number of red blood cells) can result (Figure 9–13 ■). Feeding cow milk during infancy can also cause anemia by irritating the gut and leading to small but consistent

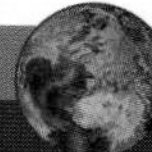

DEVELOPING CULTURAL COMPETENCE Vitamin A

Vitamin A deficiency is common in developing countries. The vitamin is found in liver, dairy products, and fish. Provitamin A sources are yellow and dark green vegetables. The vitamin is fat soluble and stored in the liver. When deficient, children develop night blindness, vision loss, and high rates of infection. Public health efforts have been directed at identifying children with low vitamin A status and in providing the vitamin in capsule form or in commonly ingested foods. Nurses should be aware of this health risk when caring for children who have been adopted or otherwise move from developing countries. Adequate nutrition is needed to promote recommended vitamin A intake.

loss of blood from the gastrointestinal tract. When formulas are used, they should be iron fortified to help avoid iron deficiency anemia (Box 9–21).

The other group most commonly deficient in iron is adolescent females, related to loss of blood in menses, metabolic need of the growth spurt, and poor dietary balance due to sporadic dieting. Further discussion of the symptoms and treatment of iron deficiency anemia can be found in Chapter 28∞.

Calcium

Calcium is an essential nutrient for bone development during childhood and adolescence. An increased intake of sweetened carbonated beverages and fruit juices is related to a decrease in calcium intake, especially among adolescents. In addition to displacing milk intake, a high intake of sweetened carbonated beverages may decrease calcium absorption because of the high phosphorus content of the beverages. During the adolescent growth spurt, almost 40% of the adult bone mass is accumulated (Trahms, 2000). Inadequate intake puts the person at risk for osteoporosis later in life, as there is no ability to make up for earlier deficits. Although genetic variables account for some of the influence on adult bone mass, increasing calcium intake has been shown to promote bone formation. While the recommended daily intake for adolescents is 1,500 mg, the average intake for adolescent males is 1,169 mg and for females is only 753 mg—only half of the recommended level (Food and Nutrition Board, 2001). See Box 9–22.

Adolescents at highest risk for impaired bone development include female athletes and others who diet to a great degree to maintain slimness. These teens manifest the "female athlete triad" of excessive thinness, excessive exercise, and amenorrhea (Rumball & Lebrun, 2004). A high rate of fractures and **osteomalacia** (softening of bones) can result, in addition to an extreme risk of osteoporosis in adulthood (Box 9–23). Asking about menstrual patterns, as well as exercise and diet, can be combined with physical measurements of height and weight to obtain pertinent information about the teen athlete. See the discussion of the eating disorders anorexia nervosa and bulimia nervosa later in this chapter.

Vitamin D

Vitamin D deficiencies are rare because the vitamin can be synthesized in the skin upon exposure to sunlight. However, an increased

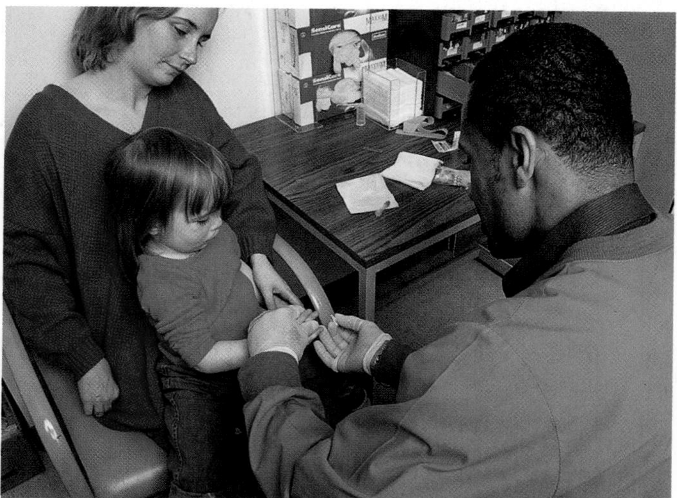

FIGURE 9–13 ■ Most Head Start centers participate in screening programs to identify children at risk for anemia. The child is comfortable sitting on the mother's lap while the nurse does a fingerstick to measure hematocrit.

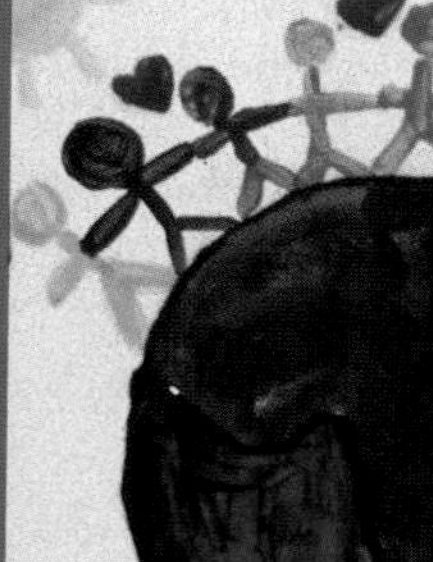

PARTNERING WITH FAMILIES

Health Promotion Food Safety Guidelines

Four key food preparation safety practices are to:

1. **Clean**: Wash hands and surfaces often.
2. **Separate**: Avoid cross contamination.
3. **Cook**: Cook to proper temperatures.
4. **Chill**: Refrigerate promptly.

Data from Healthy People 2010. *(2000).* Healthy people 2010. *Washington, DC: U.S. Department of Health and Human Services. www.health.gov/healthypeople/document.html, accessed 4/13/2004.*

BOX 9–21 Sources of Iron

- Meats
- Iron-fortified formula
- Iron-fortified baby cereal
- Iron absorption is enhanced by vitamin C intake if taken together.
- Iron is present in breast milk in a small amount, but is very well absorbed.

BOX 9–22 Sources of Calcium

- Milk and milk products
- Egg yolks
- Grains
- Legumes
- Nuts
- Soybeans

incidence in cases of vitamin D–deficient rickets has recently been observed. This vitamin is needed to enhance absorption of calcium so a lack of vitamin D can contribute to calcium deficiency as well. Human milk contains little vitamin D, and if infants are exclusively breastfed for long durations, kept wrapped when outside, live in northern climates and rarely get outside in winter months, have extensive sunscreens applied, or are dark in skin color, vitamin D deficiency can result. This has led to a recommendation by the American Academy of Pediatrics that all breastfed infants receive a daily supplement of 400 international units of vitamin D. Formula-fed babies receive adequate amounts in commercial formulas. When rickets is suspected, laboratory studies should include serum calcium, phosphorus, 25-OH vitamin D, alkaline phosphatase, parathyroid hormone, and hematocrit (Oken & Lightdale, 2001). See Box 9–24.

Folic Acid

Epidemiologic evidence has linked increasing folic acid (the most common form of folate in the human body) intake with decreased incidence of neural tube defects such as spina bifida in offspring of mothers. More recently cleft lip and palate incidence has also been found to decrease when folate intake increases. Folate levels are low among adolescents, putting them at particular risk of birth defects when they have babies. The Food and Drug Administration approved fortification of cereals and breads with folate to decrease the population risk of related congenital anomalies. All women from 15 to 45 years should consume 0.4 mg of folic acid daily and pregnant women should consume 0.6 mg. Teaching for all teens and women of childbearing age should include common sources and the importance of folate (Box 9–25).

Protein-Energy Malnutrition

While micronutrient deficiencies as described are the most common problems in developed countries, macronutrient deficiencies are the most common nutritional problems worldwide.

BOX 9–23 Growth & Development: Female Athlete Triad

The "female athlete triad" is commonly assumed to occur only in females performing sports that emphasize thinness, but others are also affected. Anorexics often exercise excessively in an effort to lose weight. Males may diet because of anorexia or due to participation in a sport with a weight category such as wrestling or horse racing. Good history questions will help you to elicit information about factors influencing extremely thin adolescents.

BOX 9–24 Growth & Development: Vitamin D

Vitamin D rickets had virtually disappeared from the United States, but several cases have recently been identified. Suggested reasons for the resurgence include failure to provide vitamin D supplementation when breastfeeding is the sole source of intake for over 6 months, use of nonfortified products such as soy milk, and use of sunscreens or covers when infants are outside. Be alert for infants and toddlers with neurologic conditions such as seizures, low height for age, slowness in learning to walk, and malformations (bowing) of spine, legs, and arms. Encourage sunscreen use, but be aware that children who are dark skinned or are kept covered due to religious beliefs may be at higher risk. Be certain that breastfed babies receive vitamin D supplements until other vitamin D sources are added to the diet (MMWR, 2001b).

Whereas kwashiorkor indicates protein deficiency and marasmus a lack of energy producing calories, both deficiencies often occur together and are referred to as *protein-energy malnutrition (PEM)*. Protein deficiency manifests with edema, leading to the large abdomens and rounded faces seen in severely malnourished children. Other symptoms include scant, depigmented hair, skin changes, and decreased serum proteins. It can occur following severe diarrhea or other infection in susceptible children. Caloric deficiency results in emaciation, decreased energy levels, and retarded development (see the clinical manifestations table on page 316). PEM may occur when a child is weaned in order for the mother to provide breast milk to a new baby. Adoptees and immigrants to developed countries sometimes manifest with at least mild PEM so careful nutritional assessment is needed in order to provide adequate nutrition.

FEEDING AND EATING DISORDERS

Deficiencies in food intake related to available nutrients and safety of the food supply were discussed in the previous section. In addition to these issues of availability, nutrient intake is affected by psychologic issues of individuals as well. Disorders of food intake span the entire developmental spectrum, and can affect pregnant women, young children, and adolescents. Some of the most common feeding and eating disorders are discussed here.

Pica

Pica is an eating disorder characterized by ingestion of nonfood items or food items consumed in abnormal quantities or forms. Examples of ingested items include starch, peeling paint, paper,

BOX 9–25 Sources of Folate

- Bread and other products made with or containing flour
- Yeast
- Spinach, avocado, green leafy vegetables
- Beans and peas
- Liver
- Fruits

soil components, flour, and coffee grounds. Clinical manifestations include zinc and iron deficiencies as well as symptoms of lead or other poisoning (see Chapter 30∞) if these substances are contained in peeling paint or other ingested material. The disorder most commonly manifests in pregnancy when women have abnormal cravings for nonfood products and can seriously impair the developing fetus. Some children also manifest ingestion of abnormal amounts of nonfood items and fail to take in adequate nutrients from food. Treatment for children involves removing them from the substances, ensuring an adequate and nutritious diet, and treating any dietary deficiencies noted.

Feeding Disorder of Infancy and Early Childhood (Failure to Thrive)

Feeding disorder of infancy and early childhood, or failure to thrive (FTT), describes a syndrome in which infants or young children fail to eat enough food to be adequately nourished. This disorder accounts for 1% to 5% of pediatric hospitalizations in children under 1 year of age, and many more children are managed in community settings. From 5% to 10% of low-birth-weight infants are affected (Behrman, Kliegman & Jenson, 2004).

Etiology and Pathophysiology

The cause of FTT can be organic, as in congenital acquired immunodeficiency syndrome (AIDS) (see Chapter 27∞), inborn errors of metabolism (see Chapter 32∞), neurologic disease, and esophageal reflux (see Chapter 30∞). However, most cases of FTT are nonorganic in origin. FTT resulting from nonorganic causes is called feeding disorder of infancy or early childhood.

Infants and children whose parents or caretakers experience depression, substance abuse, mental retardation, or psychosis are at risk for this disorder. Parents may be socially and emotionally isolated, or may lack knowledge of infant nutritional and nurturing needs. A reciprocal interaction pattern may exist whereby the parent does not offer enough food or is not responsive to the infant's hunger cues, and the infant is irritable, not soothed, and does not give clear cues about hunger (Corrales & Utter, 1999). Premature and small-for-gestational-age babies more commonly have eating disorders.

Clinical Manifestations

The characteristics of this feeding disorder are persistent failure to eat adequately with no weight gain or with weight loss in a child under 6 years of age, which is not associated with other medical conditions or mental disorders, and is not caused by lack of or unavailability of food (American Psychiatric Association Working Group on Eating Disorders, 2000). Infants with feeding disorders refuse food, may have erratic sleep patterns, are irritable and difficult to soothe, and are often developmentally delayed (Figure 9–14 ■).

COLLABORATIVE CARE

A thorough history and physical examination are needed to rule out any chronic physical illness. The infant or child may be hospitalized so that healthcare providers can establish a routine for feeding and sleeping. The goals of treatment are to provide adequate caloric and nutritional intake, promote normal growth and development, and assist parents in developing feeding routines and responding to the infant's cues of physical and psychologic hunger.

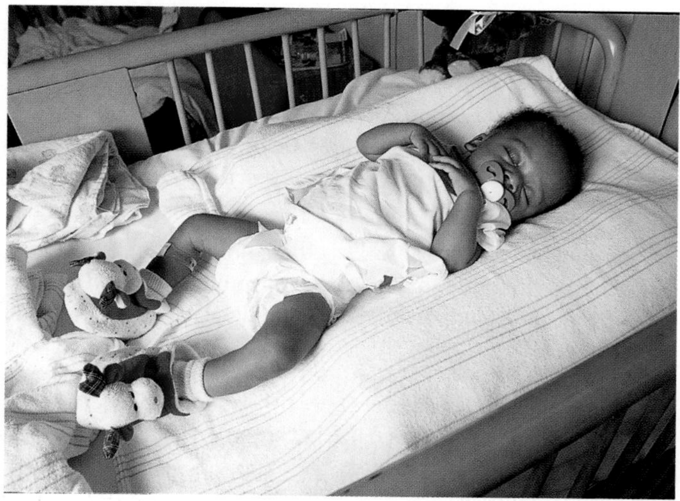

FIGURE 9–14 ■ Infants with failure to thrive may not look severely malnourished, but they fall well below the expected weight and height norms for their age. This infant, who appears to be about 4 months old, is actually 8 months old. He has been hospitalized for feeding disorder of infancy.

NURSING MANAGEMENT

■ Nursing Assessment and Diagnosis

Assessment of the child by the nurse is essential for establishing the best intervention plan. Accurate measurement of weight and height each time any child is seen for healthcare provides an important record of growth patterns over time. This helps in identification of the child with an eating disorder. The child's activity level, developmental milestones, and interaction patterns provide important information. When feeding the child, the nurse observes how the child indicates hunger or satiety, the ability of the child to be soothed, and general interaction patterns such as eye contact, touch, and cuddliness. See Developing Cultural Competence: Growth Measurement.

Parents are questioned about stresses in their lives; these may prevent appropriate interaction with the child. Asking about the pregnancy and delivery can elicit information about early disturbances in the child–parent relationship. Are there other children

DEVELOPING CULTURAL COMPETENCE
Growth Measurement

Each child should maintain a height and weight growth pattern similar to the population standard. Asian American children may normally be below the 5th percentile on growth charts and not have an eating disorder. Suspect an eating disorder when the infant or child falls one standard deviation below his or her own curve and either fails to gain weight or loses weight over several months.

in the family and have eating problems occurred with them? Are depression, mental illness, or substance abuse present? Observe the child and parent behaviors while they feed the child; cues given by each person and interactional modes such as rocking, singing, talking, and body postures are important.

Following are nursing diagnoses pertinent for the young child with an eating disorder.

- Imbalanced Nutrition: Less than Body Requirements related to inability to ingest proper amounts of food
- Delayed Growth and Development related to inadequate intake
- Risk for Impaired Parenting related to lack of knowledge about nutritional needs
- Fatigue related to malnutrition

Planning and Implementation

Nursing care centers on performing a thorough history and physical assessment, observing parent–child interactions during feeding times, and providing necessary teaching to enable parents to respond appropriately to their child's needs. The child is often hospitalized initially and evaluated for physical growth while staff members feed the child. Accurate weights, nutritional assessments, and developmental evaluation should be done to see if the child grows more normally. Additional diagnostic tests may be carried out at this time to rule out organic causes of the poor growth.

Once a diagnosis of nonorganic failure to thrive is confirmed, parents become involved in feeding the child. Observations of feeding and continued careful physical assessments are needed. The child's intake is accurately recorded at each meal or feeding. Parents are taught how to understand and respond to the child's cues of hunger and satiety. They are taught to hold, rock, and touch the infant during feedings, and to establish eye contact with infants and older children.

Upon discharge, referral to an agency that can continue monitoring of the home situation is needed. This provides an opportunity to observe feeding during a home visit and evaluate stresses and behavior patterns among family members. Frequent growth measurement and developmental assessment must be ensured. Parents may need referral to community resources to help them manage stressful situations in their lives and to enhance their parenting skills. Finding a nurturing relationship for the parent may provide the support needed to enhance their parenting of the child.

Evaluation

Expected outcomes of nursing care include the following:

- Adequate growth and normal development of the infant is achieved.
- An improved parent–child relationship is established.

Anorexia Nervosa

Anorexia nervosa is a potentially life-threatening eating disorder that occurs primarily in teenage girls and young women, affecting an estimated 5% of young women and 1% of young men in the United States (American Dietetic Association, 2001). The typical patient is White and from a middle- to upper middle-class family. Age at onset varies, and incidence peaks at 12 to 13 years and again at 17 to 18 years.

Etiology and Pathophysiology

Many causes are now thought to contribute to the onset of anorexia. Cultural overemphasis on thinness may contribute to the overconcern with dieting, body image, and fear of becoming fat that is experienced by many adolescents. Chemical changes have been found in the brain and blood of anorectic patients, leading to theories about a biologic cause. Often a significant life stress, loss, or change precedes the onset of anorexia. Stress hormones are commonly elevated in anorectics and immune system function may be disturbed (Brambilla, 2001; White, 2000).

Many authorities view family issues as contributory to anorexia. Intrafamilial conflicts and dysfunctional family patterns may occur when parents are overcontrolling and perfectionistic. The adolescent's eating behaviors may be an attempt to exercise independence and resolve internal psychologic conflicts.

The adolescent may engage in lengthy and vigorous exercise (up to 4 hours daily) to prevent weight gain. Laxatives or diuretics may be used to induce weight loss. As the disorder progresses, the adolescent perceives the ever-thinner body as becoming more beautiful. Youth may share weight-loss techniques with anorectic friends and search out Internet sites which praise anorexia. The body responds to the abnormal eating behaviors as if starvation were occurring. Leukopenia, electrolyte imbalance, and hypoglycemia develop as a result of protein-energy malnutrition. Once the body mass decreases below a critical level, menstruation ceases.

Clinical Manifestations

Anorectic adolescents are characterized by extreme weight loss accompanied by a preoccupation with weight and food, excessive compulsive exercising, peculiar patterns of eating and handling food, and distorted body image. They may prepare elaborate meals for others but eat only low-calorie foods. Characteristically, the fear of becoming fat does not decrease with continued weight loss. Accompanying signs and symptoms of depression, crying spells, feelings of isolation and loneliness, and suicidal thoughts and feelings are common. The disorder is often associated with mental illness such as obsessive-compulsive disorder, anxiety disorders (see Chapter 34∞), and history of abuse (Herpertz-Dahlmann, Muller, Herpertz, et al., 2001).

Physical findings include cold intolerance, dizziness, constipation, abdominal discomfort, bloating, irregular menses, and malnutrition (see the Photo Story on pages 348–349). Hypothalamic suppression can lead to disturbances of gynecologic function, osteoporosis, decreased bone density, and fractures (Seidenfeld & Rickert, 2001). Lanugo (fine, downy body hair) may be present. Fluid and electrolyte imbalances, especially potassium imbalances, are common. The child or adolescent is usually energetic despite significant weight loss. Extreme weight loss often leads to cardiac arrhythmias (bradycardia).

COLLABORATIVE CARE

Diagnosis is based on a comprehensive history, physical examination revealing characteristic clinical manifestations, and the DSM-IV criteria included in Box 9–26. Diagnostic tests commonly include hematocrit and hemoglobin, serum electrolytes, and serum vitamins and vitamin precursors.

The goal of treatment is to address the physiologic problems associated with malnutrition, as well as the behavioral and cognitive components of the disorder. A firm focus is placed on reaching a targeted weight with a gradual weight gain of 0.1 to 0.2 kg/day (0.25 to 0.5 lb/day). Enteral feedings or total parenteral nutrition (TPN) may be necessary to replace lost fluid, protein, and nutrients, although the adolescent often perceives these feedings as a punitive measure.

Individual treatment and family therapy are used to address dysfunctional family patterns and assist the family to accept and deal with the adolescent as an independent and less-than-perfect individual. Family involvement is crucial to effect a lasting change in the adolescent. Nurses, psychologists, family therapists, and dietitians commonly partner to plan and implement therapy.

Long-term outpatient treatment, in either an individual or a group setting, is frequently necessary. Counseling may be continued for 2 to 3 years to ensure that weight gain and self-image are maintained. Antidepressant drugs such as imipramine (Tofranil) or desipramine (Norpramin) may be prescribed for coexisting conditions such as depression, anxiety, or obsessive-compulsive disorders.

Indications for hospitalization include loss of 25% to 30% of body weight, fluid and electrolyte imbalances or arrhythmias, or the need to provide a more intense period of therapy if outpatient treatment fails to produce improvement. Behavior modification techniques are used extensively in combination with counseling and other methods in care of the hospitalized anorectic adolescent.

BOX 9–26 DSM-IV Criteria for Anorexia Nervosa

A. Refusal to maintain body weight at or above a minimally normal weight for age and height (e.g., weight loss leading to maintenance of body weight less than 85% of that expected; or failure to make expected weight gain during period of growth, leading to body weight less than 85% of that expected).

B. Intense fear of gaining weight or becoming fat, even though underweight.

C. Disturbance in the way in which one's weight or shape is experienced, undue influence of body weight or shape on self-evaluation, or denial of the seriousness of the current body weight.

D. In postmenarcheal females, amenorrhea, i.e., the absence of at least three consecutive menstrual cycles.
(A woman is considered to have amenorrhea if her periods occur only following hormone, e.g., estrogen administration.)

NURSING MANAGEMENT

Nursing Assessment and Diagnosis

Obtain a thorough individual and family history. Ask about usual eating patterns, daily caloric intake, exercise patterns, and menstrual history. Ask about medication use; include prescription, nonprescription, and herbal products. Is there a family history of eating disorders? Assess for signs of malnutrition. Obtain height and weight measurements and compare with norms for the general population. Because the anorectic patient often wears layers of clothes when being weighed, strive to obtain an accurate measurement.

Nursing diagnoses for the adolescent with anorexia nervosa include the following:

- Imbalanced Nutrition: Less than Body Requirements related to inadequate intake
- Risk for Deficient Fluid Volume related to inadequate fluid intake or fluid volume loss from overuse of laxatives and diuretics
- Risk for Imbalanced Body Temperature related to excessive weight loss and absence of subcutaneous fat
- Constipation related to inadequate food intake and overuse of laxatives
- Disturbed Body Image related to distorted perception of body size and shape
- Chronic Low Self-Esteem related to dysfunctional family dynamics
- Compromised Family Coping related to parental tendency to be overcontrolling and perfectionistic

Planning and Implementation

Nursing care centers on meeting nutritional and fluid needs, preventing complications, administering medications, and providing referral to appropriate resources. Specific treatment measures vary depending on physical complications, length and degree of illness, emotional symptoms accompanying the disorder, and family dynamics. Resistance to treatment is common, and nurses who care for anorectic adolescents must deal with their own feelings of frustration and anger.

Meet Nutritional and Fluid Needs

Monitor nutritional and fluid intake, encourage consumption of food, and observe eating behaviors at mealtime. Elimination patterns may be altered as a result of increased intake during hospitalization. Monitor for possible problems, including abdominal distention, constipation, or diarrhea. Daily monitoring of serum electrolytes is necessary.

If TPN is administered, watch for complications such as circulatory overload, hyperglycemia, or hypoglycemia. Use strict aseptic technique when changing tubing or dressings.

Administer Medications

Monitor vital signs if the adolescent is receiving antidepressants. Watch for signs of hypertension and tachycardia. Administering

MediaLink Anorexia Nervosa Video

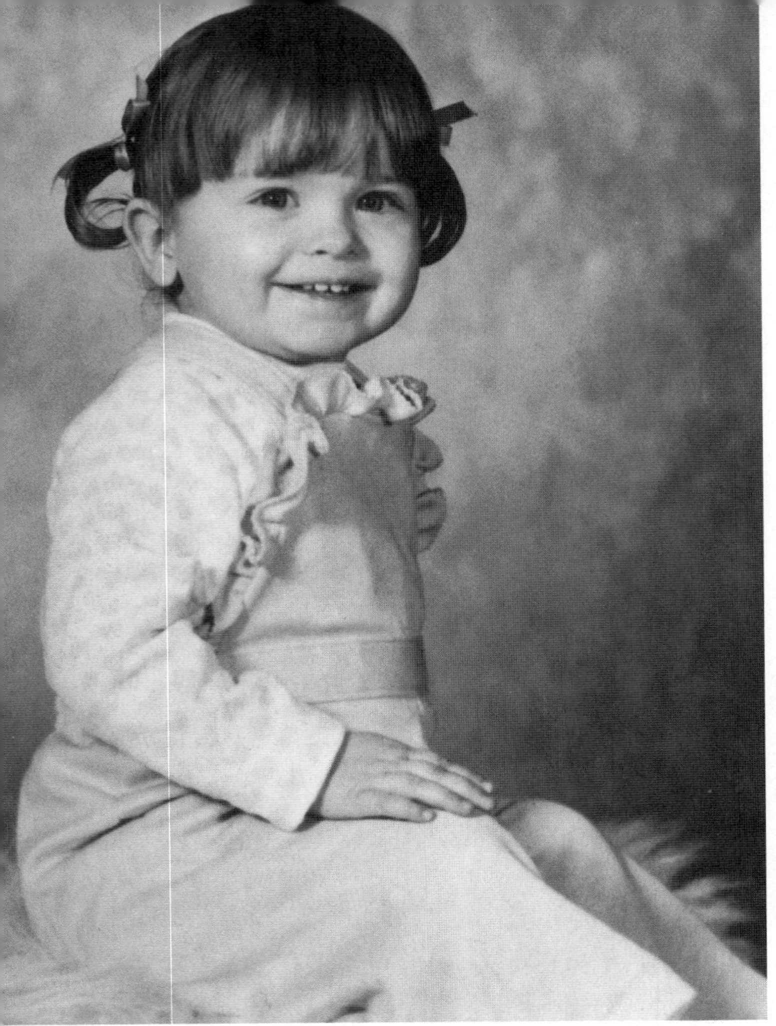

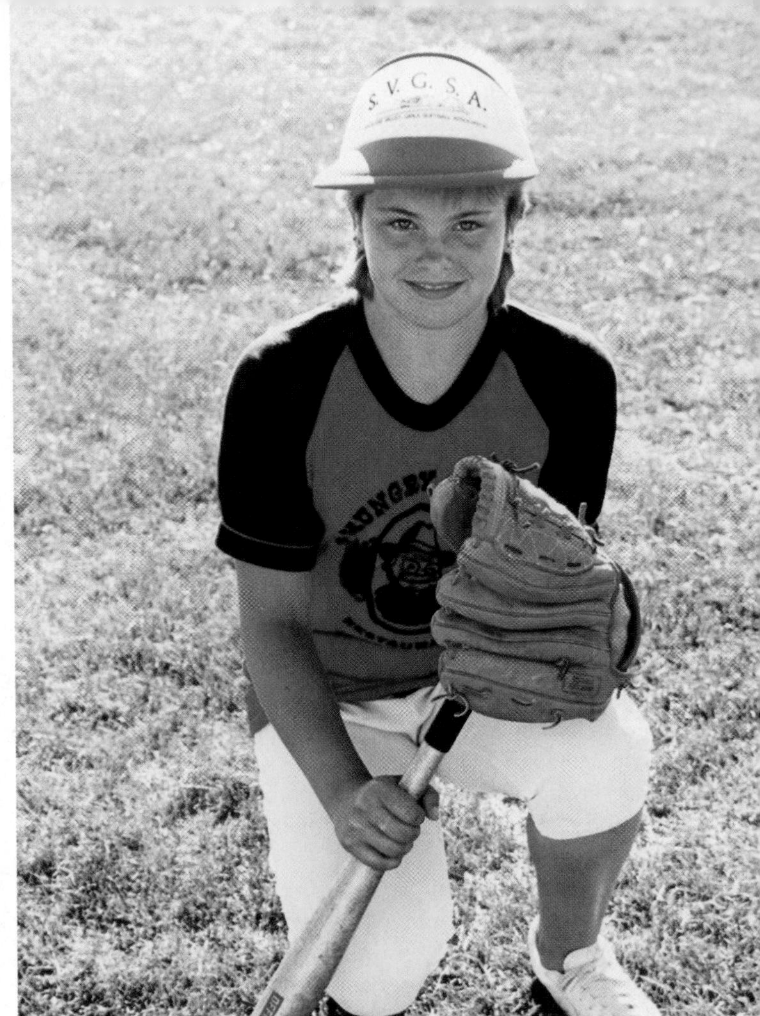

Stacia was a happy child who played an important part in the lives of her parents, brother, and grandparents. She was an outgoing and active young child. ***(left)***

During her school years, Stacia was active in many sports, as demonstrated here in a baseball picture. She had many friends, was popular with classmates, and had an engaging personality. ***(right)***

PHOTOStory...

Stacia: A young woman's struggle with anorexia nervosa

While anorexia nervosa is successfully treated among many youth and adults, at times the disease can lead to death. This is the story of a young woman who died of anorexia after what many would call a normal childhood. Stacia lived in a suburban area and had a loving family and many close friends. She was active in sports, engaged in school and extracurricular activities, and had a busy schedule.

Stacia first became ill with bulimia nervosa at age 12 years. She successfully concealed the disease from her parents until she was about 15 years of age. At that point her weight was normal and no outward signs of disturbance were evident. Teens can easily cover up disturbed eating patterns by stating that they are eating with friends during a study time, or that they had a large lunch and will not eat dinner with the family. Such patterns of increasing independence in food choices and schedules are common and expected, although they can easily mask an eating difficulty. Later, her parents discovered that she had undergone several traumatic episodes with neighbors and friends that were not known to them during the early teen years. They believe these traumatic events were held inside, and became a major reason for Stacia's eating disorder.

As time progressed, Stacia's bulimia evolved into anorexia nervosa. As her disease became more obvious to her family, she was confronted and agreed to counseling. She continued to tell her family that she could stop being anorexic at any time she wanted and that it was just helpful to be thin in her chosen roles of cheerleader and model. Stacia's concerned family continued to talk with her and she was finally placed in a residential treatment program. Her parents attended family sessions and attempted to establish a supportive but curative family environment.

Stacia began college and working. She had many friends and a close relationship with a boyfriend. However, as time progressed, she began to show more signs of depression and her anorexia clearly worsened. Her boyfriend broke up with her because it was too painful to see her harming herself. She moved back home and gradually had fewer and fewer friends. She became too weak to work and was obsessed with maintaining control over her food intake. Although she continued to see a therapist, there was no improvement, but rather, a constant deterioration of her condition. Stacia was hospitalized for electrolyte imbalance, dehydration, and other effects of anorexia. She took many medications to treat sleep abnormalities, depression, gastric distress, and other symptoms. Stacia died at age 25 years, weighing 62 lb.

Stacia's mother tells nurses that eating disorders should be confronted and faced early; as the disease progresses, cognition is altered by poor nutrition so treatments are less likely to be successful. She also alerts nurses to websites that encourage and support anorexia; these are very harmful to young people. We are so grateful to Stacia's family for sharing her story.

Consider the effects of this chronic disorder on Stacia and her family and friends. What are the many roles of the nurse in eating disorders, beginning with prevention and early identification, and progressing through treatment phases and the support of family members? How can you help health professionals, school personnel, parents, and youth to understand and deal with eating disorders? What resources are available for you to discuss a friend who may think may have an eating disorder? ■

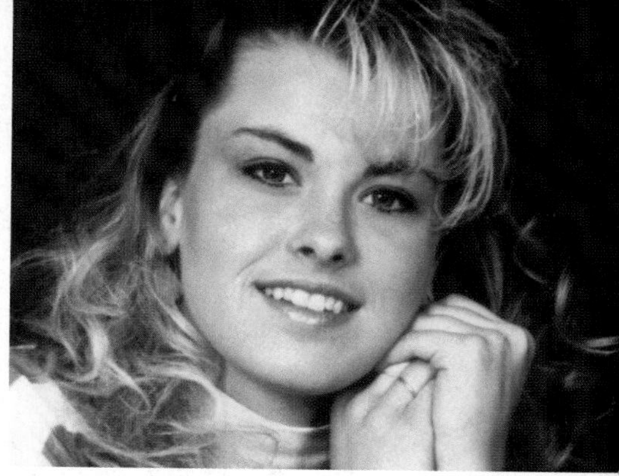

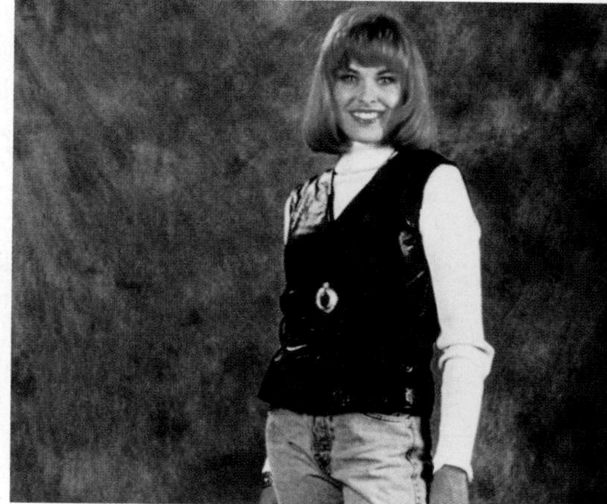

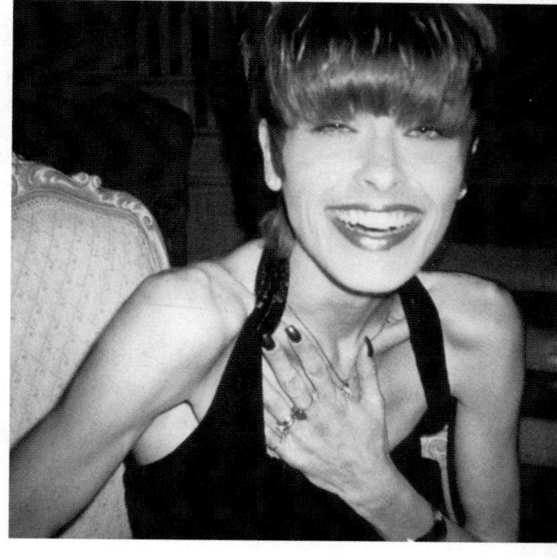

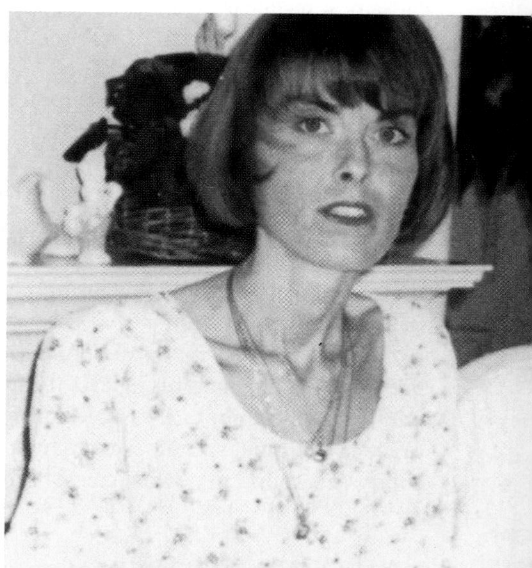

Stacia was 15 years of age in this picture. Her parents had seen no outward signs to cause alarm, but learned at this time that she had been bulimic since she was 12 years of age. Her mother found vomitus concealed in her room and confronted Stacia who admitted she had engaged in bulimia but that it was "under control." ***(top)***

In this photo in her late teen years, Stacia is shown modeling. Most youth who see a photo like this admire the thin appearance of the model and emulate this "look." The praise that thin models receive may positively reinforce anorexic behaviors. ***(middle)***

Stacia continued to lose weight slowly over many years. She still looked like an outgoing and fun-loving person, but her cachexia is obvious. ***(middle)***

In this photo taken a short time before her death, Stacia demonstrates many symptoms of starvation. She has downy hair on various parts of her body, her skin is pale, eyes are sunken, and her despair and depression are obvious. ***(bottom)***

medications after meals helps to prevent gastric irritation. Be alert for substance abuse. Anorectics often use products such as excess laxatives or ephedra (also known as ma huang) to induce weight loss. Changes in the central nervous system, vital signs, and other findings may indicate over-the-counter or herbal drug use.

Provide Referral to Appropriate Resources

Refer parents and other family members to the American Anorexia and Bulimia Association, National Anorectic Aid Society, and National Association of Anorexia Nervosa & Associated Disorders for further information about the disorder and a list of support groups in their area.

Evaluation

Expected outcomes for nursing care include weight gain, maintenance of adequate fluid volume, beginning of positive sense of self-esteem, intake of nutritionally balanced diet, and use of psychologic counseling to understand the disorder.

Bulimia Nervosa

Bulimia nervosa is an eating disorder characterized by binge eating (a compulsion to consume large quantities of food in a short period of time). Usually the episodes of bingeing are followed by various methods of weight control (purging), such as self-induced vomiting, large doses of laxatives or diuretics, or a combination of methods. Bulimia affects 5% or more of young women. Like anorexia, it affects mainly adolescent girls and young women who are White and in the higher socioeconomic classes (Orbanic, 2001). The disorder usually begins in middle to late adolescence, frequently emerging during college.

Etiology and Pathophysiology

Causes of bulimia nervosa are similar to those of anorexia nervosa: sensitivity to social pressure for thinness, body image difficulties, and long-standing dysfunctional family patterns. Families may be chaotic and distant from the girl, rather than overinvolved as with the anorectic. Many bulimic individuals experience depression. It is not clear whether the depression is a cause or a result of the bulimic individual's inability to control the bingeing and purging cycles. A bulimic adolescent often binges after any stressful event.

Bingeing usually occurs in secret for several hours until the individual is stopped by abdominal discomfort, by another person, or by vomiting. At first the episodes of binge eating are pleasurable. Immediately following the binge episode, however, feelings of guilt, shame, anger, depression, and fear of loss of control and weight gain arise. As these feelings intensify, the bulimic adolescent becomes increasingly anxious. This usually initiates the purge behaviors.

Purging eliminates the discomfort from bloating and also prevents weight gain. This relieves the feelings of depression and guilt, but only temporarily. Adolescents with bulimia commonly practice the binge–purge cycle many times a day, losing their ability to respond to normal cues of hunger and satiety.

Clinical Manifestations

Bulimic adolescents, like anorectics, are preoccupied with body shape, size, and weight. They may appear overweight or thin and usually report a wide range of average body weight over the years. Physical findings depend on the degree of purging, starvation, dehydration, and electrolyte disturbance. Erosion of tooth enamel, increased dental caries, and gum recession, which result from vomiting of gastric acids, are common findings. The back of a hand can have callouses from inducing vomiting. Abdominal distention is often seen. Esophageal tears and esophagitis may also occur.

COLLABORATIVE CARE

A comprehensive history is necessary because most bulimic adolescents appear normal in weight or only slightly underweight. Diagnostic tests include hematocrit, hemoglobin, and serum electrolytes; they may identify signs of altered electrolyte and hematologic status. The diagnosis is confirmed by the presence of specific DSM-IV criteria (Box 9–27).

Treatment includes management of physiologic problems, behavior modification, and psychotherapy. Such management involves a variety of healthcare providers such as physicians, nurses, and therapists. Behavior modification focuses on modifying the dysfunctional eating patterns and restoring a normal pattern. Until the episodes of bingeing and purging are under control, feelings of discouragement and hopelessness prevail. Thus, the focus early in treatment is on initiating an immediate behavioral change. Once initial interventions have been successful, group therapy sessions work well for persons with bulimia nervosa. Specific treatment measures may include the following:

- Educating the adolescent about good nutrition (including food choice and caloric content)

BOX 9–27 DSM-IV for Bulimia Nervosa

A. Recurrent episodes of binge eating. An episode of binge eating is characterized by both of the following:
  1. Eating, in a discrete period of time (e.g., within any 2-hour period), an amount of food that is definitely larger than most people would eat during a similar period of time and under similar circumstances
  2. A sense of lack of control over eating during the episode (e.g., a feeling that one cannot stop eating or control what or how much one is eating)

B. Recurrent inappropriate compensatory behavior in order to prevent weight gain, such as self-induced vomiting; misuse of laxatives, diuretics, enemas, or other medications; fasting; or excessive exercise.

C. The binge eating and inappropriate compensatory behaviors both occur, on average, at least twice a week for 3 months.

D. Self-evaluation is unduly influenced by body weight and shape.

E. The disturbance does not occur exclusively during episodes of anorexia nervosa.

- Encouraging the adolescent to keep a log or food journal and assisting the adolescent to make connections between emotional states and stress and the impulse to binge or purge
- Setting up a daily dietary routine of three meals and three snacks a day (using the same foods for each meal and snack every day to change misconceptions about the weight-gaining potential of certain foods and to decrease anxiety about what food must be eaten at the next meal)

Once these initial measures have been taken, the underlying psychosocial issues are explored. The goals of therapy are to provide the bulimic adolescent with adaptive coping skills and to improve self-esteem.

Most bulimic adolescents do not require hospitalization. Serious abnormalities in fluid and electrolyte levels caused by uncontrollable cycles of bingeing and vomiting, accompanied by depression or suicidal activity, are indications of the need for hospitalization. The prognosis is good with long-term therapy.

NURSING MANAGEMENT

■ Nursing Assessment and Diagnosis

Obtain a thorough individual and family history, including daily dietary intake and weight fluctuations. Inquire about problems such as abdominal pain or distention, which may indicate an abnormal eating or elimination pattern. Assess the oral mucosa for signs of damage to tooth enamel caused by purging; examine hands for evidence of vomiting-induced callouses.

Following are nursing diagnoses that may be appropriate for the adolescent with bulimia nervosa.

- Imbalanced Nutrition: Less than or More than Body Requirements related to inadequate intake
- Risk for Deficient Fluid Volume related to fluid volume loss
- Impaired Oral Mucous Membrane related to chemical effects of vomited gastric acids
- Deficient Knowledge (child) related to health risks of excessive use of laxatives and diuretics
- Anxiety related to discomfort with weight and eating patterns
- Chronic Low Self-Esteem related to dysfunctional family dynamics
- Ineffective Individual Coping related to life stressors

■ Planning and Implementation

Nursing care includes monitoring nutritional intake and elimination patterns, preventing complications, and providing appropriate referrals.

During hospitalization, the patient should keep a food diary. Be alert to the adolescent who hides, gives away, or discards food from the tray or who exits to use the bathroom after meals. The adolescent should be monitored for at least 30 minutes after meals by remaining in a central area in the company of the nurse or other responsible individuals. Withdrawal from laxatives and diuretics is managed with careful observation for alterations in fluid and electrolyte status. Cardiac monitoring may be necessary if potassium levels are seriously altered. Esophageal tearing or esophagitis is treated to promote mucosal healing. Medications such as antidepressants may be administered. Encourage continuation of group and other therapy sessions.

Bulimic adolescents and their families can be referred to organizations such as those listed in the section on anorexia for assistance and information about the disorder.

■ Evaluation

Expected outcomes for nursing care for the adolescent with bulimia include healthy mucous membranes and skin, adequate intake of fluids and food, balanced food intake, maintenance of normal weight, and absence of bingeing and purging.

FOOD REACTIONS

Food reaction encompasses any adverse reaction to foods or substances ingested in foods. The most common food reaction is **food intolerance,** or an abnormal physiologic response to a food that is not IgE mediated. Examples include indigestion or flatulence upon eating certain foods, or a sweating reaction to some spices (Burks, 2000). Milk and grain products are common causes of food intolerance. Chemical additives, antibiotics, preservatives, and food colorings also can cause food sensitivity reactions.

Food allergy is an IgE-mediated reaction that is potentially systemic, characteristically rapid in onset, and may be manifested as swelling of the lips, mouth, uvula, or glottis, generalized urticaria, and, in severe reactions, anaphylaxis. Food allergies are the most common cause of anaphylaxis and are most prevalent in children with a family history of allergic reactions to various substances and foods (**atopy**). The foods that most commonly cause a reaction are fish, shellfish, peanuts, tree nuts, eggs, soy, wheat, corn, strawberries, and milk. Children who have both food allergy and asthma are most at risk of death from anaphylaxis due to a food allergy. Children with allergies may experience urticaria of the lips, mouth, and throat upon eating certain foods; reddened cheeks; circulatory problems such as hypotension or irregular heartbeat; gastrointestinal discomfort; respiratory problems such as sneezing, congestion, coughing, laryngeal edema, recurrent ear infections; neurologic disorders such as fatigue, depression, headache, hyperactive behavior, or sleep disturbance; and skin disorders such as urticaria and hives (Pongracic, 2000; Bendelius, 2002). Allergic individuals need to be aware of "hidden" substances in prepared foods. For example, the child who is allergic to peanuts will experience a reaction to a food if peanut extracts were used in preparation of another food in the kitchen at the same time, or if dishes previously containing peanut extract were not adequately washed before preparation of the present food.

Delayed hypersensitivity reactions are attributed to digestive products of food and require a thorough diet history over several

MediaLink Case Study: Peanut Allergy at School

days to identify the offending food. These reactions are more difficult to diagnose, because the reaction can occur up to 24 hours after ingestion of the food. There may also be biphasic reactions that occur 1 to 30 hours after an initial anaphylaxis. Such reactions can be severe and life threatening. For these reasons every child with a food allergy who ingests the allergen should be promptly treated with epinephrine and transported to an emergency facility for further management and monitoring.

Note that certain foods can cause either allergy or intolerance so accurate diagnosis is needed. An example is cow milk that can cause an allergy with IgE-mediated systemic reaction, or an intolerance from gastrointestinal response to milk proteins (diarrhea, vomiting, abdominal pain) as a result of lack of the enzyme lactase in the gastrointestinal tract. Diagnostic tests to identify suspected food allergies include measurement of serum IgE levels, scratch tests, and the **radioallergosorbent test (RAST),** in which radioimmunoassay is used to measure IgE antibodies to specific allergens (see Chapter 27∞). A diet diary helps to track the date, types of foods eaten, and reaction(s), if any. Treatment consists of eliminating the offending foods from the child's diet. See Developing Cultural Competence: Lactose Intolerance.

NURSING MANAGEMENT

Prevention is the first step. Instruct parents of infants to introduce new foods at a rate of not more than one new food every 3 to 5 days. If an intolerance is noted, the causative food can be easily identified. Discuss any changes in diet or preparation of formula. Reassure parents that the child's symptoms will disappear when the offending foods are removed from the diet.

Be alert for skin, respiratory, and other characteristic manifestations of allergy. Refer such cases to an allergist for diagnosis and assist in testing and instruction. Nursing care of a child with food allergy recognizes that the responsibility for preventing ingestion of an allergenic food for a particular child is shared by the child (when old enough to participate), the family, and the school or other setting. Help the family to identify and eliminate the offending foods. Emphasize the importance of reading food labels for hidden foods that can trigger an allergic reaction (Bock, Munoz-Furlong, & Sampson, 2001). School personnel should know that children should not be given foods at school without parental permission. See Table 9–15 for examples of ingredients and food preparation methods that can indicate presence of a food allergen. Some schools have identified peanut-free tables or sections of lunch rooms, or peanut-free classrooms to try to prevent any exposure of susceptible children to peanut products.

Explain to parents all tests, use of a food diary, and care of the child should a reaction occur. The home and school should have an Epipen® or other emergency treatment for the allergic child. It should be available in an accessible place at all times (Figure 9–15 ■). The child with a food allergy should wear a medical alert tag. Be sure that school personnel know about the allergy and to avoid giving the child the food product. Refer the family to the Food Allergy Network and other resources. Recognize that food allergies can be life threatening and plan carefully with the family, childcare facilities, schools, and other community contacts to ensure avoidance of food and fast treatment if needed. See Table 9–16 for the responsibilities when a child has a food allergy. Be certain that the food allergy plan is in place in each setting where the child spends time.

DEVELOPING CULTURAL COMPETENCE
Lactose Intolerance

Some ethnic groups have a high incidence of lactose intolerance due to low amounts of the enzyme lactase in the gut. During childhood, most members of all ethnic groups have adequate amounts of lactase to metabolize milk products, but by adulthood 70%–100% of some groups have become lactose intolerant. African Americans, Native Americans, and Asians often have lactase deficiency which may begin to emerge during childhood. When intolerance to milk products develops, suggest alternative sources of calcium and other nutrients found in milk. Some people who have indigestion with milk are able to eat yogurt without problems.

NUTRITIONAL SUPPORT

Providing adequate nutrition for all children can be a challenge for families. Nutritional needs change as children grow and develop, family patterns must be integrated into the child's intake, and many social influences intervene to influence dietary patterns. Some children require even more careful management to ensure that they receive necessary nutrients, either due to increased needs, or the difficulty in ingesting adequate foods. Several of these particular challenges are discussed here.

TABLE 9–15 Food Ingredients

ALLERGEN	POTENTIAL "HIDDEN" FOOD SOURCE EXAMPLES
Milk	Simplesse (fat substitute), pareve kosher designation, goat milk (similar protein to cow milk), deli slicers may be used for both meat and cheese so contamination with milk products common
Eggs	Simplesse (fat substitute), baking powder, egg substitutes, cooked pastas, deli meats and cold cuts, baked goods
Fish	Imitation crab or lobster (surimi), Worcestershire sauce, sauces, salad dressings
Soy	Canned tuna, cereals, crackers, infant formula, sauces, soups, peanut butter, baked goods
Wheat	Baked goods, imitation crab meat, ice cream, hotdogs, labels listing bulgur, durum, farina, flour, graham flour, malt, modified wheat starch, semolina, wheat bran, wheat germ, wheat starch, vegetable gum, vegetable starch, bread crumbs, gelatinized starch, modified vegetable protein, natural flavoring, gluten, cereal extract
Peanuts	Artificial nuts, ice cream, candy, cookies, many processed foods, preparation bowls and utensils often contain trace amounts of peanuts used in prior batches and cross contamination readily occurs

Adapted from Bendelius, J. (2002, May). Food allergies and label reading: A healthy relationship. School Nurse News, *24–26.*

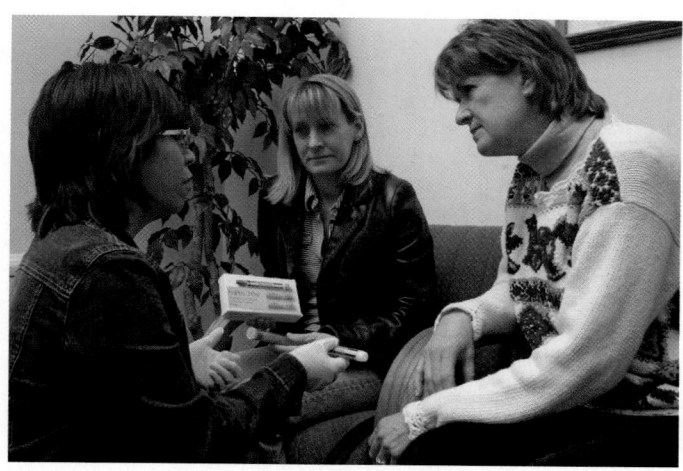

FIGURE 9–15 ■ The school nurse is providing instruction for a mother and teacher about the use of the Epipen © which may be needed for treatment of a child with food allergy. They have both received prior instruction and practice but need to review techniques before a field trip.

Sports Nutrition

Regular physical activity should be encouraged for all children, with at least 30 to 60 minutes of activity recommended daily. However, during vigorous or prolonged exercise, or during hot weather, there may be special nutritional needs of child and adolescent athletes. A well-balanced diet, reflective of the food pyramid, is needed. A wide variety of fresh fruits and vegetables, grains, and complex carbohydrates usually provides for adequate caloric intake. When the child is hungry, extra calories should come from the food groups listed there, rather than from increased intake of fat. When the child or teen is very active, sports bars or drinks can provide the additional needed calories in a nutritionally balanced manner. Consumption of carbohydrates soon after an athletic event assists in restoring glycogen stores. As always, the height, weight, and BMI percentiles are the best assurance that the individual is growing adequately over time. Adequate energy to perform the sport as well as be attentive and productive at school and for other activities should also be considered.

Water should be increased during activity both to minimize chance of dehydration and to maximize performance. About 1 hour before vigorous exercise, the child should drink one or two glasses (8 to 16 oz) of water, and should repeat the same amount of fluid just before the exercise begins. Young children may not feel thirsty, and should be encouraged to drink 4 to 6 oz of fluid every 15 minutes during exercise (Trahms, 2000). Water is usually the best replacement, but during extended exercise, sports drinks may be a good alternative for some of the fluid intake. Additional water is needed after activity. Weight loss of 1 lb indicates a loss of about 0.5 quart of fluid. Be sure the child takes in fluid to replace all losses.

Some common nutrients that may be deficient in all teens, but even more often in the athlete, are calcium and iron. The increased blood volume common in the well-conditioned person necessitates greater intake. Calcium foods such as milk products and dark green vegetables, and iron foods such as adequate meats and grains, can guard against deficiencies. Many adolescents

TABLE 9–16 Food Allergies—Shared Responsibility

FAMILY RESPONSIBILITY	CHILD RESPONSIBILITY	SCHOOL RESPONSIBILITY
➤ Notify and work with school to develop an allergy plan for the child ➤ Provide written documentation, instructions, and medications; update and replace as needed (e.g., Epipen) ➤ Provide a current photo of child for the allergy plan ➤ Educate the child to the level possible depending on age and cognition ➤ Institute review of plan after any reaction	➤ Do not trade food with other children ➤ Do not eat anything known to contain the allergen or when ingredients are unknown ➤ Notify an adult immediately if an allergen may have been ingested ➤ Know location of emergency medication (e.g., Epipen)	➤ Inform all personnel and follow federal, state, and district laws relevant to allergies and sharing medical information ➤ Review health records of all students ➤ Identify core team to work with parents and child to establish prevention plan ➤ Implement treatment upon possible ingestion of allergen; do not wait for a reaction ➤ Teach all staff interacting with child the recognition of food allergy, actions to take in emergency, and elimination measures of allergen from meals, educational tools, arts and craft, incentives, etc. ➤ Allow for safe and accessible storage of emergency medicines; arrange instruction for personnel in administration of medication ➤ Include field trips, transportation on school bus, sports outings in action plan ➤ Ensure emergency communication from all buses, school events, field trips ➤ Be alert for and deal appropriately with threats or harassment against an allergic child ➤ Institute review of plan after any reaction

Adapted from Food Allergy Network. School guidelines for managing students with food allergies. www.foodallergy.org/school/guidelines.html

believe that they need extra protein during athletic seasons; however, most Americans ingest adequate protein to meet even the increased needs of sports, although the vegetarian child or adolescent may need assistance to plan a diet with adequate protein.

Many teens ingest a wide variety of dietary supplements, believing that they enhance performance during sports. Most of the claims of these products are unproven, and their safety has not usually been investigated, especially in the young. Offer guidance and help the family and teen to investigate claims before choosing to use a product. Be sure they know doses, desired effects, and potential side effects of supplements. Be aware that some sports and coaches may encourage small body size and dieting. Consider that children and adolescents in activities such as ballet, figure skating, wrestling, track or running, and horse racing may have health risks associated with inconsistent or poor intake.

Some common amino acid nutritional supplements include creatine, carnitine, and glutamine. Although side effects to these substances are minimal, their possible enhancement of performance is temporary and outcomes of long-term use are unknown. Increasing overall nutritional intake to meet needs during high activity is a better alternative. Creatine has been studied more than most supplements; it is made by the body and is present in many protein sources. Supplemental creatine increases the creatine level in muscle and may help to increase performance in short bursts of activity, while not affecting endurance sports. The increase in muscle mass that can occur is actually due to water and will be lost quickly when the supplement is discontinued (Johnson, 2001). Some athletes obtain steroids, which can cause serious side effects, lead to endocrine disturbance, and interfere with growth; their use is also illegal in sports. Minerals such as chromium, iron, and calcium are used by some youths. The nurse can ask careful and sensitive questions, such as "Many athletes take supplements to aid in performance in sports. What supplements do you take or are you considering?" Information can then be provided to enhance the youth's understanding of nutrition and sports performance. Generally, intake of a balanced diet with adequate carbohydrate, protein, and fat will meet the needs of most athletes and lead to maximal sport performance

Health-Related Conditions

Many health conditions influence the nutritional state of the child. Conversely, the child's nutritional state can influence the state of health. Figure 9–16 ■ shows some common conditions that influence nutritional needs. These conditions are discussed in various chapters throughout the text. When you read about them, discuss with classmates how you will adjust normal nutritional assessment and teaching due to the presence of a healthcare concern. Which conditions influence absorption of nutrients? Which cause changes in nutritional intake requirements? Some children benefit from special dietary aids, such as eating utensils and cups that are easy to grasp. Therapists can evaluate and make recommendations about devices that can assist the child at meals. Some genetic conditions affect food intake and metabolism. For example, Prader-Willi syndrome is most commonly caused by a deletion in chromosome 15, and causes obesity, hypotonia, and abnormal ingestion of large amounts of food (see Chapter 4∞). Nurses work with families to plan for food access and intake patterns of the child. Some families use herbal products in order to treat conditions. Nurses inquire about supplements, herbs, and homeopathic remedies and search resources to provide information for families about the effects of these treatments in children. See Complementary Therapy: Nutrition and Homeopathy.

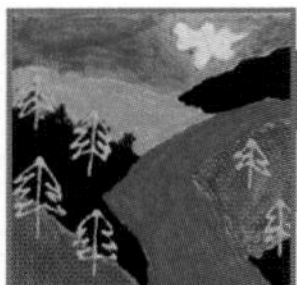

COMPLEMENTARY THERAPY
Nutrition and Homeopathy

Many families use food products to promote health and treat diseases. These include herbal products that may be acquired from health food stores or the Internet, and homeopathy which uses small amounts of natural substances as treatment for conditions such as otitis media and diarrhea in children. Herbs are not tested nor regulated by the government, so amounts of ingredients are often not known. Homeopathy, on the other hand, uses dilute amounts of remedies, and prepares them uniformly as described in the *Homeopathic Pharmacopoeia*. Some studies have shown effective treatment of minor childhood illnesses by homeopathy. Ask families how they are treating conditions at home and inquire about whether they will give the child a medicine if one is prescribed. Sometimes families use Western medicine to obtain a diagnosis and then treat it at home. Most homeopathy will not harm the child, but in some cases treatment is needed to prevent dehydration or treat serious disease. Nurses are more able to work effectively with parents using a variety of treatments if questions about home remedies are clear, nonjudgmental, and inserted into every healthcare visit (Kemper & Jacobs, 2003).

Vegetarianism

Some families choose to eat vegetarian diets and can be helped and encouraged in their endeavors. Several variations of intake occur. **Vegetarians** eat no poultry, meat, or fish. **Lacto-ovovegetarians** eat eggs and dairy products, while **lactovegetarians** eat dairy products. In contrast, **vegans** are strict vegetarians and eat no animal products. When someone says they are vegetarian, it is best to ask specific questions about what they will and will not eat (Box 9–28).

The vegetarian can be very healthy, but may need some additional help to ensure nutritional adequacy. Some common deficiencies exist; assessment and planning are needed to avoid them. Deficiencies sometimes experienced by vegans include vitamin D and calcium, vitamin B_{12}; minerals such as zinc and iron; fiber; calories; protein; and fat. Completing a 24-hour diet recall for the pregnant or lactating woman, and for vegetarian children, with analysis for RDAs, can be helpful. Be sure to routinely assess growth and other nutritional measures as well. Provide ideas of various foods to meet nutritional needs and perform other general nutritional teaching. When a vegetarian

BOX 9–28 Growth & Development: Vegetarian Diet

When a pregnant teen follows a vegetarian diet, additional help will be needed to encourage adequate nutrition (Rudys-Shapard, 2001). A 24-hour or 2-day diet record will help identify nutritional needs. Consider additional pregnancy needs for protein, iron, and calcium, and note that vitamin B_{12} is recommended as a supplement. Use the vegetarian food guide pyramid available through the American Dietetic Association.

child is hospitalized, plan with the nutrition department and the child's family to meet intake needs.

Enteral Therapy

Enteral therapy is a form of nutritional support provided when a child cannot take in enough food orally to sustain health. Since it is the closest form of nutritional support to the natural method of eating, it has the least untoward effects and greatest rate of success. Infants, especially preterm or those with medical problems, may need enteral therapy if they cannot ingest adequate nutrients. Some of the children who use enteral therapy are those with cerebral palsy or other neurologic conditions which lead to weakness of the throat and mouth, children with neoplasm or immune dysfunction, those with acute or chronic problems of the gastrointestinal tract, and those in acute states of recovery from accidents or illness. A tube can be inserted into the nasal opening and placed through the esophagus into the stomach; however, a tube that is surgically placed into the stomach through an abdominal opening (gastrostomy), or a jejunal tube, may be chosen for long-term use. As long as the child can absorb and use nutrients, enteral therapy can be successful in providing calories and essential nutrients. Commercially prepared formulas are available and specially formulated solutions can be adapted for children with specific dietary needs. The gastrostomy tube and entry site are cared for to prevent infection and skin breakdown. See Chapter 30∞ for suggestions on management of nursing care during tube feedings.

Total Parenteral Nutrition

Parenteral nutrition has made it possible to provide intravenous nutritional support for individuals who cannot eat or are unable to absorb nutrients from the intestinal tract in a normal manner and are at risk of severe malnutrition (Matarese & Gottschlich, 2002). Examples of children who benefit from this method of nutrition are those with congenital malformation of the gastrointestinal tract, head injury, severe burns, or for support after bone marrow transplant, sepsis, or other critical conditions. A catheter is inserted so that a sterile nutrition solution is infused directly into the bloodstream. A central venous catheter is inserted to promote safe infusion. Fluids usually contain glucose; electrolytes such as sodium, potassium, calcium, magnesium, phosphate, and chloride; vitamins; and proteins. Lipid emulsions are another type of TPN used in some children. Meticulous care is needed, whether in the hospital or at home, to ensure safe TPN infusion and treatment. Possible complications involve infection acquired at the site of infusion or air emboli causing respiratory problems. The nurse performs initial assessment and ongoing evaluation and monitoring of treatment, ensures solution storage recommendations are followed, and administers the solutions in hospital or other settings (Skipper, 1998).

PATHOPHYSIOLOGY ILLUSTRATED

Conditions That Influence Nutritional Needs

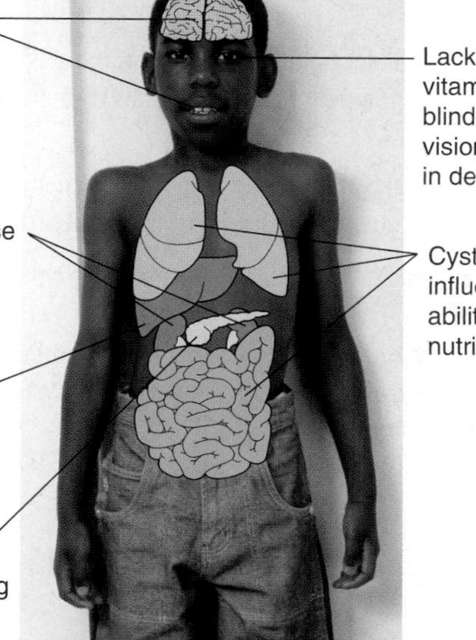
Cerebral palsy or other brain damage can influence the child's ability to chew and swallow food.
Lack of sufficient vitamin A intake causes blindness or impaired vision in many children in developing countries.
Child with renal disease may have trouble regulating fluids and proteins in the body.
Cystic fibrosis influences the child's ability to absorb nutrients.
Liver disease alters the child's ability to break down metabolic waste products.
Child with diabetes needs close monitoring and regulation of dietary intake.

FIGURE 9–16 ■ While a child's nutritional status influences health, it is also important to consider conditions that may affect the child's nutrition and include this knowledge in your assessment.

PRACTICE ALERT

Total parenteral nutrition (TPN) is expensive, complicated to administer, and can have adverse side effects. How are decisions made about when to institute this type of nutritional support? Should it be used in all situations? If someone is unconscious or dying, should this method of nutrition be started? These ethical issues are often difficult and have no easy answers. Nurses usually administer TPN in the home and hospital and may feel stressed if families, the patient, and other health professionals do not agree on its use (Breier, 2000). Guidelines are available to help healthcare professionals make decisions about treatments, and nurses should seek the guidance of ethics professionals in their agencies when needed.

See the protocols for TPN management in the Skills Manual ∞.

MediaLink: Nursing in Action: Administering a Gavage/Tube Feeding

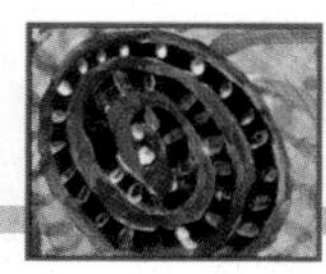

CHAPTER HIGHLIGHTS

- Adequate nutritional intake is necessary for the normal growth and development of children.
- Children with medical or psychosocial conditions require additional nutritional support.
- Dietary intake patterns vary throughout childhood as the child grows, is able to metabolize different types of food, and gains greater gross and fine motor control.
- Nutritional assessment is an essential part of nursing care and may involve approaches such as growth measurement and intake records.
- Common nutritional concerns in childhood include hunger, overweight, foodborne illness, and dietary deficiencies.
- The child with feeding disorder of infancy and childhood requires comprehensive assessment and ongoing management to foster parent–child interaction and adequate nutritional intake.
- The most common eating disorders of adolescents are anorexia nervosa and bulimia nervosa.
- A combination of behavioral management, counseling, and medication is often used in treatment programs for eating disorders.
- Food allergy represents a life-threatening condition for children, while food sensitivity can lead to uncomfortable but non-life-threatening symptoms.
- Children engaging in sports and those who eat vegetarian diets may need guidance to meet nutritional needs.
- Alternative feeding methods such as enteral and parenteral feedings are required by some children.

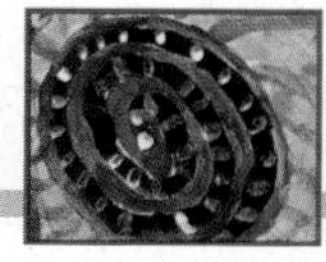

CRITICAL THINKING IN ACTION

INTRODUCTION

Recall Joey in the opening scenario. He has cerebral palsy which makes it difficult for him to swallow. This difficulty, in addition to recent surgery for scoliosis, has created nutritional challenges for him. A gastrostomy tube has been inserted so that he can receive supplemental feedings at home and school.

DESCRIPTION

Children with cerebral palsy are often unable to ingest enough nutrients to remain in a healthy nutritional state. The disorder makes it hard to chew and swallow food and the excess muscular movements of the disorder use extra calories. Surgery has taken an additional toll on Joey. He was unable to eat for several days after the operation for scoliosis and blood loss of surgery creates negative protein balance. While he has healed well, nutritional analysis by a nutritionist demonstrated a shortage of calories, calcium, iron, and several other nutrients. Joey can eat soft foods that require little chewing and are easy to swallow. Supplemental feedings by gastrostomy tube have been planned to meet the deficiencies. The feedings will be given every few hours both at home and during school. The family learned how to administer the feedings for Joey in the hospital and they have partnered with the school nurse so that the teacher can administer them in school. Joey has a hematocrit of 29% and hemoglobin of 10 g/dL.

DISCUSSION

Joey has some nutritional problems but his care is enhanced by the presence of a supportive family, school nurse, and nutritionist. His teacher has shown competence and understanding in administering feedings in school.

1. Since Joey cannot stand or walk, he is at risk of osteoporosis. What is this disorder and which children are at risk of developing the disorder?
2. What nutrients are especially important to prevent osteoporosis?
3. Formulate nursing interventions that will enhance intake of the nutrients that Joey needs. Consider Joey's age and the school setting as you list realistic interventions.
4. How can the school nurse collaborate with the nutritionist and family to plan for Joey's nutritional needs and evaluate outcomes of his care?
5. If Joey's family decides to go on a summer car trip and will need to take feeding solutions and equipment with them, what suggestions can you provide about how to accomplish this?
6. Analyze Joey's hemoglobin and hematocrit. What levels would you expect at his age? How can you foster normal hemoglobin and hematocrit levels? What other nutritional observations can you observe that provide clues about Joey's nutritional status?

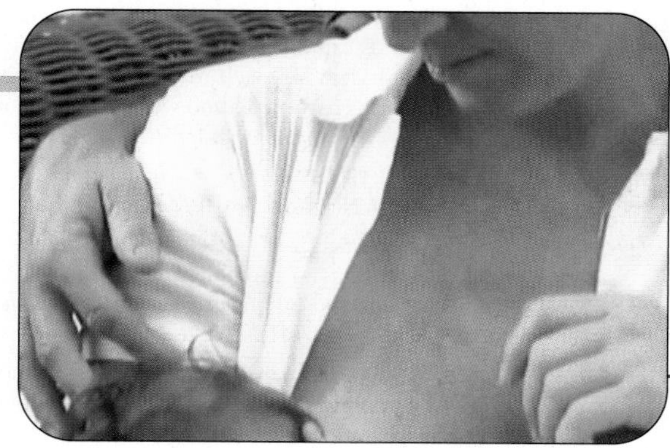

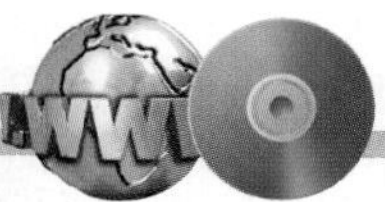

EXPLORE MediaLink

- NCLEX review, case studies, and other interactive resources for this chapter can be found on the Companion Website at **http://www.prenhall.com/ball**. Click on Chapter 9 to select the activities for this chapter.
- For animations, more NCLEX review questions, and an audio glossary, access the accompanying CD-ROM in this textbook.

http://www.prenhall.com/ball

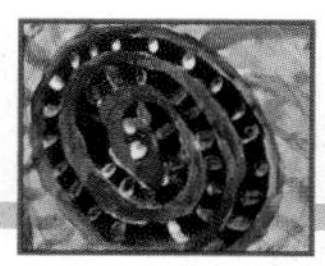

REFERENCES

Adair, L. S., & Gordon-Larsen, P. (2001). Maturational timing and overweight prevalence in U.S. adolescent girls. *American Journal of Public Health, 91*, 642–644.

Aguayo, J. (2001). Maternal lactation for preterm newborn infants. *Early Human Development, 65*(Suppl), S19–S29.

American Academy of Pediatrics, Committee on Nutrition. (2001). The use and misuse of fruit juice in pediatrics. *Pediatrics, 107*, 1210–1213.

American Academy of Pediatrics, Committee on Nutrition. (2004). *Pediatric nutrition handbook* (5th ed.). Elk Grove Village, IL: American Academy of Pediatrics.

American Academy of Pediatrics, Section on Breastfeeding (2005). Breastfeeding and the use of human milk. *Pediatrics* 115, 496–506..

American Dental Association. (2000). ADA statement on early childhood caries. www.ada.org/prof/resources/positions/statements/caries.asp, accessed 6/7/2004.

American Dietetic Association. (2001). Position of the American Dietetic Association. Breaking the barriers to breastfeeding. *Journal of the American Dietetic Association, 101*, 1213–1220.

American Dietetic Association. (2001). Position of the American Dietetic Association. Nutrition intervention in the treatment of anorexia nervosa, bulimia nervosa, and eating disorders not otherwise specified (EDNOS). *Journal of the American Dietetic Association, 101*, 810–819.

American Psychiatric Association Working Group on Eating Disorders. (2000). Practice guidelines for the treatment of patients with eating disorders. *American Journal of Psychiatry, 157*, 1–39.

Anderson, D. M. (2002). Nutritional assessment and therapeutic interventions for the preterm infant. *Clinics in Perinatology, 29*, 313–326.

Behrman, R. E., Kliegman, R. M., & Jenson, H. B. (2004). *Nelson textbook of pediatrics* (17th ed.). Philadelphia: Saunders.

Bendelius, J. (2002, May). Food allergies and label reading: A healthy relationship. *School Nurse News*, 24–26.

Bessler, S. (1999). Nutritional assessment. In P. Q. Samour, K. K. Helm, & C. E. Lang, *Handbook of pediatric nutrition* (2nd ed., pp. 17–42). Gaithersburg, MD: Aspen.

Bock, S. A., Munoz-Furlong, A., & Sampson, H. A. (2001). Fatalities due to anaphylactic reactions to foods. *Journal of Allergy and Clinical Immunology, 107*, 191–193.

Boyle, M. A., & Morris, D. H. (1999). *Community nutrition in action* (2nd ed.). Belmont, CA: West/Wadsworth.

Brambilla, F. (2001). Social stress in anorexia nervosa: A review of immuno-endocrine relationships. *Physiology and Behavior, 73*, 365–369.

Breier, S. J. (2000). Ethics and total parenteral nutrition. *Journal of Intravenous Nursing, 23*, 52–57.

Burks, W. (2000). Diagnosis of allergic reactions to food. *Pediatric Annals, 29*, 744–752.

Calderon, L. (2002). Promoting a healthful lifestyle and encouraging advocacy among university and high school students. *Journal of American Dietetic Association 102*(3 suppl), S71–S72.

Carver, J. D., Wu, P. Y., Hall, R. T., Ziegler, E. E., Sosa, R., Jacobs, J., Baggs, G., Auestad, N., & Lloyd, B. (2001). Growth of preterm infants fed nutrient-enriched or term formula after hospital discharge. *Pediatrics, 107*, 683–689.

Children's Defense Fund. (2004). *The state of America's children*. Washington, DC: Author.

Corrales, K. M., & Utter, S. L. (1999). Failure to thrive. In P. Q. Samour, K. K. Helm, & C. E. Lang, *Handbook of pediatric nutrition* (2nd ed., pp. 395–412). Gaithersburg, MD: Aspen.

Crespo, C. J., Smit, E., Troiano, R. P., Bartlett, S. J., Macera, C. A., & Anderson, R. E. (2001). Television watching, energy intake, and obesity in U.S. children: Results from the third National Health and Nutrition Examination Survey. *Archives of Pediatric and Adolescent Medicine, 155*, 360–365.

Dietary Guidelines for Americans (2005). United States Department of Health and Human Services and United States Department of Agriculture. Washington DC: U.S. Government Printing Office or http://www.healthierus.gov/dietaryguidelines/

Failla-Tommasino, J. (2002). E. coli 0157:H7: An emerging bacterial threat. *Clinician Reviews, 12*(7), 48–54.

Federal Interagency Forum on Child and Family Statistics. (2000). *America's children: Key national indicators of well-being, 2000*. Washington, DC: Author.

Food and Drug Administration. (2004). Backgrounder for the 2004 FDA/EPA consumer advisory: What you need to know about mercury in fish and shellfish. Washington, DC: Department of Health and Human Services. www.fda.gov/oc/opacom/ hottopics/mercury/backgrounder.html, accessed 6/8/2004.

Food and Nutrition Board. (2001). *Dietary reference intakes*. Washington DC: National Academy Press.

Green, M., & Palfrey, J. S. (2000). *Bright futures: Guidelines for health supervision of infants, children and adolescents* (2nd ed.). Arlington, VA: National Center for Education in Maternal and Child Health.

Hanson, L. A., Dahlman-Hoglund, A., Lundin, S., Karllson, M., Dahlgren, U., Ahlstedt, S., & Telemo, E. (1997). Early determinants of immunocompetence. *Nutrition Reviews, 55*, S12–S17.

Healthy People 2010. (2000). *Healthy people 2010*. Washington, DC: U.S. Department of Health and Human Services. www.health.gov/healthypeople/document.html, accessed 4/13/2001.

Hensrud, D. D. (1999). Nutrition screening and assessment. *Medical Clinics of North America, 83*, 1525–1546.

Herpertz-Dahlmann, B., Muller, B., Herpertz, S., Heussen, N., Hedebrand, J., & Remschmidt, H. (2001). Prospective 10-year follow-up in adolescent anorexia nervosa—course, outcome, psychiatric comorbidity, and psychosocial adaptation. *Journal of Child Psychology and Psychiatry, 42*, 603–612.

Institute of Medicine (2005). Preventing Childhood Obesity. Washington DC: National Academics Press.

Johnson, W. A. (2001). Nutritional supplements: What you need to know. *Contemporary Pediatrics, 18*(7), 63–74.

Kemper, K. J., & Jacobs, J. (2003). Homeopathy in pediatrics—No harm likely, but how much good? *Contemporary Pediatrics, 20*, 97–111.

Kramer, M. S. (2001). Promotion of breastfeeding intervention trial (PROBIT). *Journal of the American Medical Association, 285*, 413–420.

Krauss, R. M., Eckel, R. H., Howard, G., Appel, L. J., Daniels, S. R., Deckelbaum, R. J., Erdman, J. W., Kris-Etherton, P., Boldberg, I. J., Kotchen, T. A., Lichtenstein, A. H., Mitch, W. E., Mullis, R., Robinson, K., Wylie-Rosett, J., St. Jeor, S., Suttie, J., Tribble, D. L., & Bazzarre, T. L. (2001). AHA scientific statement: AHA dietary guideline. *Journal of Nutrition, 131*, 132–146.

Landers, S. (2003). Maximizing the benefits of human milk feeding for the preterm infant. *Pediatric Annals, 32*, 298–306.

Lee, R. D., & Nieman, D. C. (2002). *Nutrition assessment* (3rd ed.). Boston: McGraw-Hill.

Leffler, D. (2000). U.S. high school age girls may be receptive to breastfeeding promotion. *Journal of Human Lactation, 16*, 36–40.

Ludwig, D. S., & Ebbeling, C. B. (2001). Type 2 diabetes in children. *Journal of the American Medical Association, 286*, 1427–1430.

Matarese, L. E., & Gottschlich, M. M. (2002). *Contemporary nutrition support practice*. St. Louis: Elsevier.

MMWR. (2001a). Preliminary FoodNet data on the incidence of foodborne illnesses. *Morbidity and Mortality Weekly Report, 50*, 241–246.

MMWR. (2001b). Severe malnutrition among young children—Georgia, January 1997 to June 1999. *Morbidity and Mortality Weekly Report, 50*, 224–227.

National Cholesterol Education Program. (1991). *Report of the expert panel on blood cholesterol levels in children and adolescents*. Washington, DC: U.S. Department of Health and Human Services.

Nevin-Folino, N. L., Loughead, J. L., & Loughead, M. K. (2001). Enhanced-calorie formulas: Considerations and options. *Neonatal Network, 20*, 7–15.

Ogden, C. L., Flegal, K. M., Carroll, M. D., & Johnson, C. L. (2002). Prevalence and trends in overweight among US children and adolescents, 1999–2000. *JAMA, 288*, 1728–1732.

Oken, E., & Lightdale, J. R. (2001). Updates in pediatric nutrition. *Current Opinions in Pediatrics, 13*, 280–288.

Orbanic, S. (2001). Understanding bulimia. *American Journal of Nursing, 101*, 35–41.

Pongracic, J. A. (2000). Is it food allergy? *Contemporary Pediatrics, 17*, 101–112, 117–121.

Reynolds, K. D., Franklin, F. A., Leviton, L. C., Maloy, J., Harrington, K. F., Yaroch, A. L., Person, S., & Jester, P. (2000). Methods, results, and lessons learned from process evaluation of the high 5 school-based nutrition intervention. *Health Education & Behavior, 27*, 177–186.

Rigo, J., De Curtis, M., & Pieltain, C. (2002). Nutritional assessment in preterm infants with special reference to body composition. *Seminars in Neonatology, 6*, 383–391.

Rudys-Shapard, R. (2001). Adolescent, pregnant, and vegetarian: A turbulent time for a teen. *Journal of Pediatric Health Care, 15*, 35–40.

Rumball, J. S., & Lebrun, C. M. (2004) Preparticipation physical examination: Selected issues for the female athlete. *Clinical Journal of Sports Medicine 14*, 153–160.

Seidenfeld, M. E., & Rickert, V. I. (2001). Impact of anorexia, bulimia and obesity on the gynecologic health of adolescents. *American Family Physician, 64*, 445–450.

Skipper, A. (1998). *Dietitian's handbook of enteral and parenteral nutrition* (2nd ed.). Gaithersburg, MD: Aspen.

Stopka, T. J., Segura-Perez, S., Chapman, D., Damio, G., & Perez-Escamilla, R. (2002). An innovative community-based approach to encourage breastfeeding among Hispanic/Latino women. *Journal of the American Dietetic Association, 102*, 766–767.

Trahms, C. M. (2000). *Nutrition in infancy and childhood* (7th ed.). New York: WCB/McGraw-Hill.

U.S. Preventive Services Task Force. (2003). Behavioral interventions to promote breastfeeding: Recommendations and rationale. *American Journal for Nurse Practitioners, 7*(11), 23–32.

Walker, M. (2002). Expanding breastfeeding promotion and support in the special supplement nutrition program for women, infants and children (WIC). *Journal of Human Lactation, 18*, 115–124.

Walter, T., Olivares, M., Pizarro, F., & Munoz, C. (1997). Iron, anemia, and infection. *Nutrition Reviews, 55*, 111–124.

Wauben, I. P., & Wainwright, P. E. (1999). The influence of neonatal nutrition on behavioral development: A critical appraisal. *Nutrition Reviews, 57*, 35–44.

Whitaker, R., Wright, J. A., Pepe, M. S., Seidel, K. D., & Dietz, W. H. (1997). Predicting obesity in young adulthood from childhood and parental obesity. *New England Journal of Medicine, 337*, 869–873.

White, J. H. (2000). The prevention of eating disorder: A review of the research on risk factors with implications for practice. *Journal of Child and Adolescent Psychiatric Nursing, 123*, 76–88.

Willett, W. (2001). *Eat, drink, and be healthy*. New York: Simon & Schuster.

Zizza, C., Siega-Riz, A. M., & Popkin, B. M. (2001). Significant increase in young children's snacking between 1977–1978 and 1994–1996 represents a cause for concern! *Preventive Medicine, 32*, 303–310.

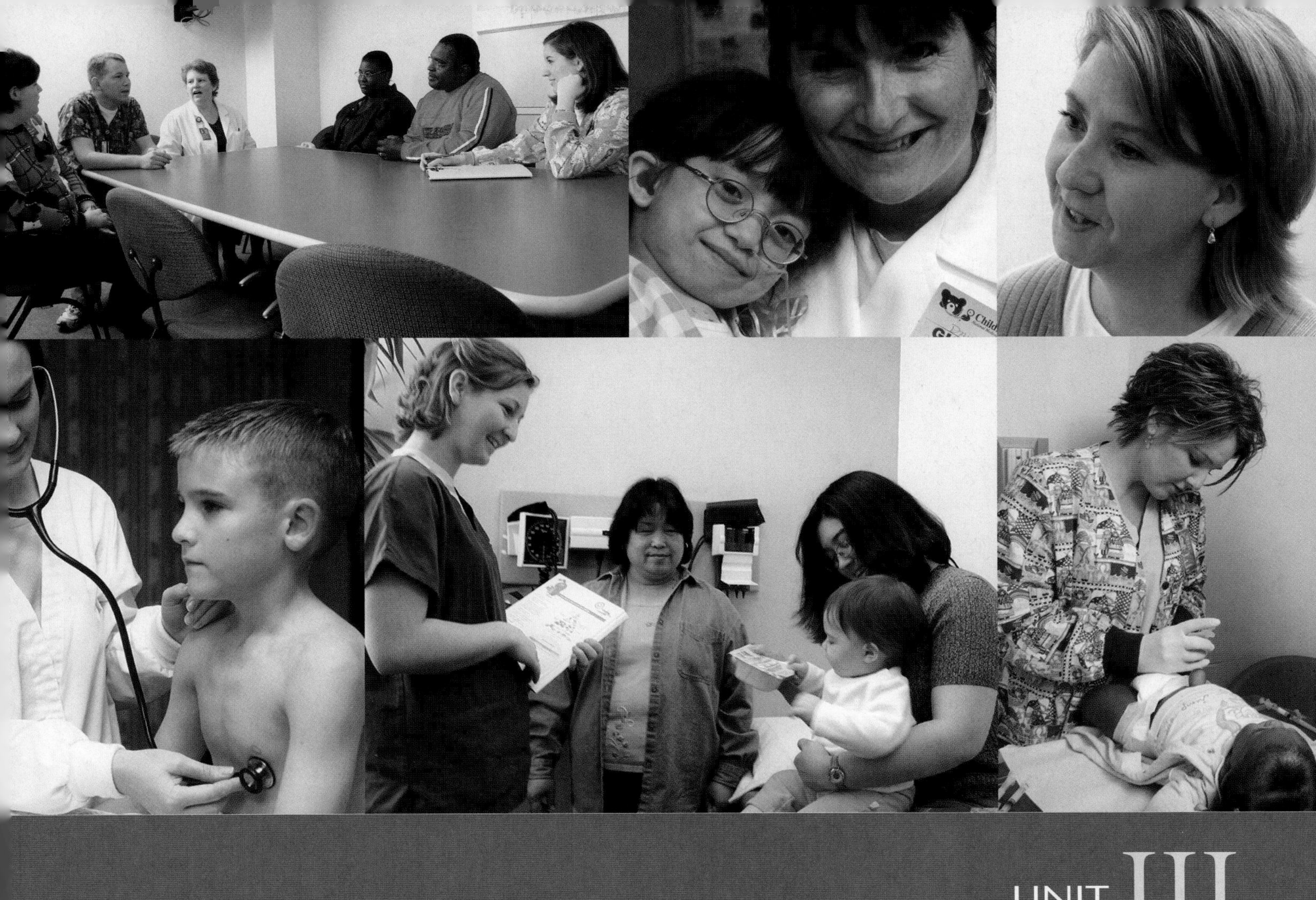

UNIT III

Health Promotion and Health Maintenance Through Childhood

Concepts of health promotion and health maintenance are critical components of all pediatric healthcare. During healthcare encounters, the nurse applies the ecologic model and resilience theory when assessing growth and development, nutrition, physical activity, oral health, mental and spiritual status, and relationships with families and other people. Pediatric nurses partner with other health professionals to provide health promotion and health maintenance for children from the newborn through adolescent age groups. The nurse plans interventions to enhance the child's health status. Disease and injury prevention strategies are applied during interactions that occur in well-child visits, schools, hospitalizations, and other encounters with children.

Chapter

10 Concepts of Health Promotion and Health Maintenance

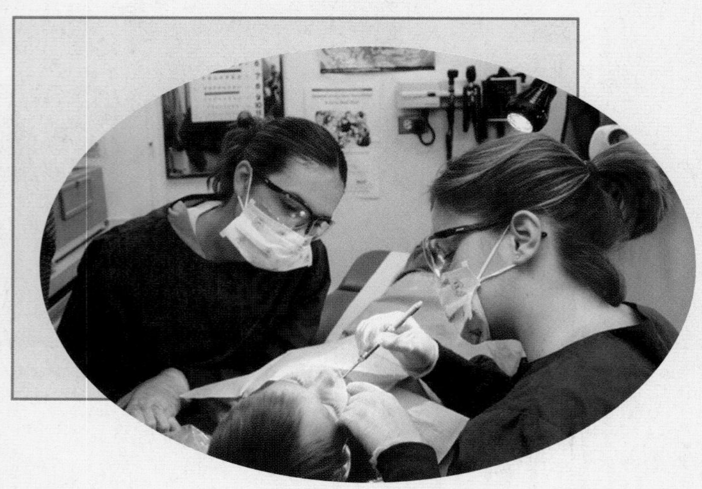

Mr. and Mrs. Yevteshenko have brought their two young sons to a mobile van for care. Tony and Ilya are 7 and 5 years of age. The nurse has arranged to have a translator present to assist in history taking, explaining procedures, and teaching. The family came from Lithuania about 9 months ago, sponsored by a local ministry. The mother is caring for the children at home, although she worked in an office in her native country. Mr. Yevteshenko had a job in the computer industry, but now he works as a custodian. The parents are devoted to the health and well-being of their children and are eager to learn more English so they can understand the clinic personnel. The school nurse recommended that the family consider using the van, locally managed by nurse practitioners. In addition to offering health promotion and health maintenance visits, a dentist and dental hygienists come weekly to the van to provide dental care. Nurses and dental personnel partner with the family to provide care and perform necessary teaching for the family.

The nurse focuses not only on health screening and immunization, but also on the stress of adaptation to life in a new country for each family member. Links are made to community resources that can help the family with basic necessities, educational needs, and provide a sense of belonging.

How will the needs of the family change as they spend more time in the country? What are the major health promotion and health maintenance needs for each child? How can nurses in various settings such as schools and mobile health-care facilities partner with each other to promote health of families in the community?

"It's kind of fun to come to the van. We've never been to the dentist before. We just moved from Lithuania and my parents don't speak English very well. I like the nurses here. They're always nice to me and my brother."

— Tony, age 7

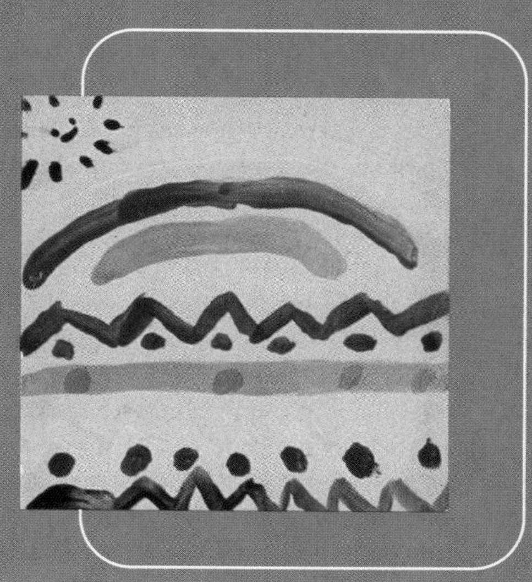

Learning Outcomes

After completing this chapter, you will be able to:

- Define health promotion and health maintenance.
- Describe how health promotion and health maintenance are addressed by partnering with families during health supervision visits.
- Describe the components of a health supervision visit.
- Explore the nurse's role in providing health promotion and health maintenance for children of different ages in a variety of settings.
- Apply principles of health promotion and health maintenance to children of different ages in a variety of settings.

Key Terms

MediaLink http://www.prenhall.com/ball

Resources for this chapter can be found on the CD-ROM accompanying this textbook, and on the Companion Website at http://www.prenhall.com/ball. Click on Chapter 10 to select the activities for this chapter.

CD-ROM

Videos

Health Promotion and Health Maintenance
Healthy People 2010

NCLEX Review

Audio Glossary

COMPANION WEBSITE

NCLEX Review

MediaLink Applications

Define Personal Health
Determine Tool Validity

One of the two major goals of *Healthy People 2010* is to help individuals of all ages to increase life expectancy and improve their quality of life. The concepts of health promotion and health maintenance provide for nursing interventions that contribute to meeting this goal. Many students in health professions begin their studies with a strong interest in the care of ill individuals. However, as time progresses, they learn that "well" people need care also. They need teaching to improve diet, reduce stress, and obtain immunizations. They may seek information about how to exercise properly or ensure a safe environment for their children. These examples of care and teaching are components of health promotion and health maintenance.

Nursing is a holistic profession that examines and works with all aspects of the lives of individuals, and has a strong focus on family and community as well. Nurses therefore are uniquely positioned to provide health promotion and health maintenance activities, and indeed these activities should be a part of each encounter with families.

What is the difference between health promotion and health maintenance? When should nurses engage in activities that focus on health? How are these activities integrated into health supervision visits? How do nurses partner with other healthcare professionals to offer comprehensive health services in settings accessible to parents and children? How can nurses help children and their families to maximize length and quality of life? These are some of the questions that will be explored in this chapter, with specific activities for certain age groups following in the next five chapters.

DEFINITIONS

In order to understand health promotion and health maintenance it is important to develop a definition of health. The World Health Organization defines **health** as a "state of complete physical, mental, and social well-being and not merely the absence of disease and infirmity" (World Health Organization, 1996). Even individuals with chronic disease can be viewed as healthy if they are successfully adapting to their conditions. Health is viewed as dynamic, changing, unfolding; it is the realization of a state of actualization or potential (Pender, Murdaugh, & Parsons, 2002). It is a basic human right and is necessary for development of societies (Box 10–1).

Health promotion refers to activities that increase well-being and enhance wellness or health (Pender et al., 2002). These activities lead to actualization of positive health potential for all individuals, even those with chronic or acute conditions. Examples include providing information and resources in order to:

- Enhance nutrition at each developmental stage
- Integrate physical activity into the child's daily events
- Provide adequate housing
- Promote oral health
- Foster positive personality development

Health promotion emerged in nursing literature following a Canadian document, the Lalonde Report (Young & Hayes, 2002; Lalonde, 1974). The concept has subsequently been developed by the World Health Organization through conferences and statements about health promotion (Table 10–1), in the United States through documents such as the *Healthy People 2010* and *Bright Futures* publications and through the Healthier US program, and in many other countries.

Health promotion is concerned with development of sets of strategies that seek to foster conditions that allow populations to be healthy and to make healthy choices (World Health Organization, 2001). Nurses engage in health promotion by partnering with children and families to promote family strengths in the areas of lifestyles, social development, coping, and family interactions. You will provide **anticipatory guidance** for families when you understand the child's upcoming developmental stages and teach families how to provide an environment to assist in meeting the milestones of the stages. This concept is explored more fully later in this chapter.

Health maintenance (or **health protection**) refers to activities that preserve an individual's present state of health and that prevent disease or injury occurrence. Examples of these activities include performing developmental screening or surveillance to identify early deviations from normal development, providing immunizations to prevent illnesses, and

BOX 10–1 Prerequisites for Health

The World Health Organization has established fundamental conditions that are needed for health: peace, shelter, education, food, income, stable ecosystem, sustainable resources, social justice, and equity. When nurses work with families who cannot meet one of these fundamental resources, activities should first be directed at security for the absent condition, and then other health activities will be more successful. For example, assisting a family to identify resources for adequate food if they are hungry will increase the family's ability to respond to teaching about safety or immunizations.

TABLE 10–1 World Health Organization Conferences on Health Promotion

DATE	LOCATION	MAJOR FOCUS
1986	Ottawa, Canada	Health promotion is viewed as a new movement to promote public health
1988	Adelaide, Australia	Public policy is examined as critical to health promotion
1991	Sundsvall, Sweden	Supportive environments are viewed as key components of health
1997	Jakarta, Indonesia	Partnerships between health professionals, public and private sectors, and other constituencies are essential to promote health
2000	Mexico City, Mexico	Measures must be taken to bridge the inequality gap in access to health promotion services

MediaLink Health Promotion and Health Maintenance Video

TABLE 10–2 Levels of Preventive Health Maintenance Activities

LEVEL	DESCRIPTION	EXAMPLE OF NURSING ACTIONS
Primary prevention	Activities that decrease opportunity for illness or injury	Giving immunizations Teaching about car safety seats
Secondary prevention	Early diagnosis and treatment of a condition to lessen its severity	Developmental screening Vision and hearing screening
Tertiary prevention	Restoration to optimum function	Rehabilitation activities for child after a car crash

Adapted from Murray, R. B., & Zentner, J. P., (2001). Health promotion strategies through the life span *(7th ed.). Upper Saddle River, NJ: Prentice Hall. p. 53.*

teaching about common childhood safety hazards (see the Photo Story on pages 364–365). Health maintenance activities are commonly preventive in nature and terminology common to community or public health nursing explains the levels and aims of preventive actions. Prevention levels are identified as **primary prevention**, **secondary prevention**, and **tertiary prevention** (Table 10–2).

While it is clear that health promotion and health maintenance activities are closely linked and often overlap, certain differences exist. Health maintenance focuses on known potential health risks and seeks to prevent them, or identify them early so that intervention can occur. Health promotion looks at the strengths and goals of individuals, families, and populations, and seeks to use them to assist in reaching higher levels of wellness. It involves partnerships with the family as health goals are set, and with other health professionals and resources to provide for meeting the goals. The nurse must apply both health promotion and health maintenance concepts when providing healthcare, recognizing that the concepts overlap. See Figure 10–1 ■ for examples of the application of each concept and how they relate to each other.

Health promotion and health maintenance are integrated into healthcare visits for children, with the care provider applying both knowledge of health maintenance concepts and adding information the family has identified that will assist in increasing health or wellness (health promotion). These activities commonly take place at well-child or health supervision visits. (See a detailed description of health supervision later in the chapter.)

Consider the opening scenario. Tony and his brother have come to a mobile van that is parked near their school. The nurse identifies a need for immunizations and connection to resources to assist the newly relocated family. At the same setting, dental care is provided and teaching is performed for these children who have never had a dental visit before. What nursing activities represent health promotion? Which represent health maintenance? With what other professionals must the nurse partner to provide culturally competent care for the family?

APPLICATION OF RESILIENCE AND ECOLOGIC THEORIES

Two theories that provide useful approaches to children and families have been described. See Chapter 5∞ for a description of resilience and the ecologic theory. Both of these theories can be linked to concepts of health promotion and health maintenance; they both suggest questions to ask families and data to gather.

You may recall that the concept of resilience focuses on the ability of children to use their protective factors or strengths to overcome risks and emerge as healthy and strong individuals. Nurses assess both the protective factors and the risk factors of individual children and their families, and use this information in planning appropriate health-related activities. For example, you may identify the following protective factors for a toddler.

- Both parents are present in home and share in childcare activities.
- Parents express interest in learning about how to limit television time and plan alternative activities for the child.
- Toddler has been weaned from a bottle, is eating family table foods, and has a body mass index in the 50th percentile.

Health Promotion and Health Maintenance Overlap

Health Promotion	Overlap	Health Maintenance
• Nutrition to meet all RDAs and enhance health and well-being, with emphasis on whole grains, fruits, vegetables. • Activities to promote self-concept formation including body image and decision-making skills.	• Nutrition that provides for growth and energy needs also helps prevent chronic diseases. • Integrating positive activities will both promote self-image and decrease potential for injury.	• Nutrition to prevent obesity or growth retardation. • Limiting television viewing to decrease exposure to violence which may lead to disturbed sleep and aggressive behaviors.

FIGURE 10–1 ■ While the focus and goals for health promotion and health maintenance differ, there is often overlap in nursing activities and expected outcomes, as demonstrated in these examples

PHOTO Story...

Health maintenance visits

Health maintenance begins at birth and is a part of every healthcare visit throughout childhood. The nurse is instrumental in integrating teaching and performing other interventions that help to prevent disease or injury.

Recall that developmental surveillance entails observation of the child's progress in fine motor, gross motor, language, social skills, and cognition. In the first photograph, the nurse is administering a Denver II Developmental Screening Test to Jarad. *Why do you think the nurse is sitting on the floor? How does the nurse ensure that she gets Jarad's best performance so that his developmental skills are accurately evaluated?*

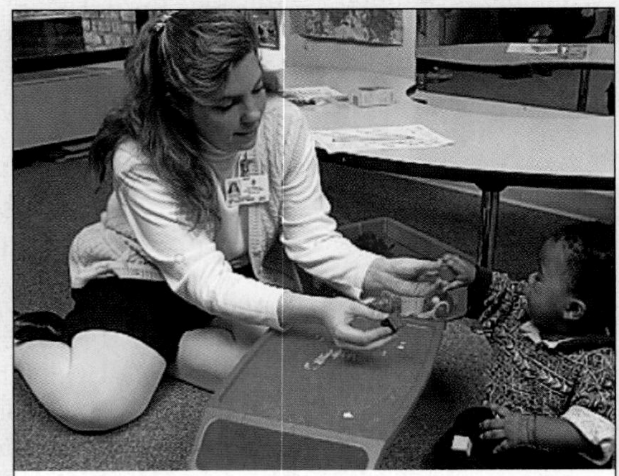

A nurse administers the Denver II to Jarad when he is an infant.

Jarad grows and develops normally. As he prepares to attend kindergarten, his mother brings him to the pediatric healthcare home and he receives immunizations needed for school entry. Recall that immunization administration is an example of a disease prevention activity. *What immunizations are most likely needed*

You also have identified the following risks.

- The grandmother who cares for the toddler three times weekly smokes in her home.
- The family has recently moved and expresses concern that their new jobs do not provide adequate healthcare insurance.
- The toddler has recently been biting and hitting the parents when frustrated.

The nurse uses the information gathered to plan health promotion and health maintenance activities.

- Information is provided about the effects of environmental tobacco smoke and ideas are discussed with the parents about ways to suggest that the grandmother not smoke when the toddler is present (*health maintenance*).
- The nurse finds low-cost but comprehensive healthcare resources and presents them to the family (*health maintenance*).
- Information is provided on setting limits for common toddler behaviors and a local support group for parents of toddlers is recommended; ideas for activities appropriate for the age group are discussed and parents choose their favorites (*health promotion*).
- Parents are praised for their management of the child's weight; teaching to enhance health nutritional knowledge is integrated into the visit (*health promotion*).

The nurse uses the list of protective factors and risk factors to plan topics for the visit. Information is provided that parents need to keep the child safe and prevent injury (health maintenance). Goals that the family has set are recognized and resources are provided that will help the family to meet these goals (health promotion). The family and the nurse establish a health partnership to maintain and promote the health of the young toddler in the family.

Using the ecologic model, the nurse also assesses the child, and then progresses on to assess several systems in the child's life. (See Table 5–4∞ on page 143.) The *microsystem* involves those settings in which the child has close contact. These involve the parents and the grandmother for the toddler described

at the time of school entry (see Chapters 14 and 19)? How will you apply your knowledge of development of children who are 5 years old to administer the immunizations safely and with as little trauma as possible? What other health maintenance activities might be implemented during this prekindergarten visit?

During Jarad's visit before kindergarten, you notice that his mother is pregnant. She is being seen for prenatal care but has many questions about how to manage her new baby when it arrives. You tell her about a class for new mothers at the clinic and she begins attending once the baby is born. During the class Jarad's mother learns with other mothers about safe transport of their infants. Safety teaching about strollers, car seats, grocery carts, and many other items can prevent injury to young children.

Many clinics have lists of health maintenance topics that can be addressed at each visit. This list and the results of assessment of individual children and families guides the nurse in addressing topics to prevent injury and disease. See Chapters 11–15∞ for specific ideas for health maintenance at specific ages. ■

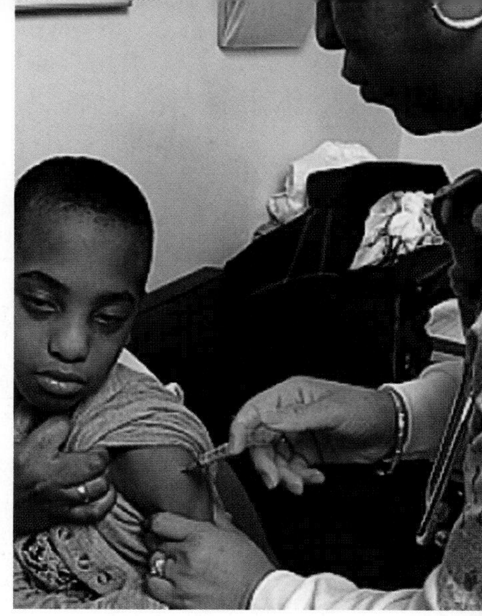

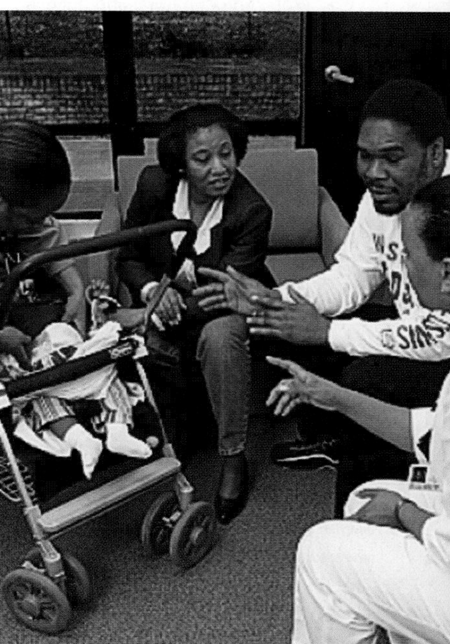

Later, Jarad receives an immunization as part of health maintenance. **(top)**

Jarad's mother receives injury prevention teaching for Jarad's younger sibling. **(bottom)**

above. The *mesosystem* involves relationships between the microsystems. At this point, the nurse can seek additional information about the relationship between the parents and the grandmother that will provide clues to methods of dealing with the issue of smoking near the child. The *exosystem* is outside of the child's daily contacts but influences the child indirectly. It is reflected in the family concern about lack of healthcare resources due to a recent move and job change. The child is part of a *macrosystem* or society that provides ready access to television and other media, necessitating health teaching about wise use of media and planning for alternative activities.

The ecologic theory provides guidance that is particularly useful in health promotion activities. Several components of health promotion have been established that relate to the systems of the ecologic model. See Table 10–3 for examples.

Using one or both of the theories described will assist you in the assessment of children and families, and point you toward other data to gather. Use the information obtained to plan appropriate health promotion and health maintenance activities. Remember that guidelines for topics at various ages are just guidelines; using your assessment data wisely will help you to individualize the specific information needed by a particular family.

HEALTH SUPERVISION

Health supervision is the provision of services that focus on disease and injury prevention (health maintenance), growth and developmental surveillance, and health promotion at key intervals during the child's life. What health promotion and health maintenance activities are parts of health supervision visits? How can these activities be integrated into all settings where care is provided for children? What are the recommended times for health visits to occur and what care is provided at certain times? How can you organize a health supervision visit to accomplish goals of family and health professionals? These and other questions will be answered in this section and the section that focuses on nursing management.

TABLE 10–3 Socioecologic Approach to Health Promotion Objectives

HEALTH PROMOTION OBJECTIVES	ECOLOGIC MODEL SYSTEM
Develop personal skills ➤ Enhance life skills ➤ Provide information	Individual in microsystems
Strengthen community action ➤ Enable resources to work together ➤ Enhance systems for public participation ➤ Improve self-help and social support	Mesosytems
Create supportive environments ➤ Assess health impacts of rapidly changing environments ➤ Protection of natural and built environments	Exosystems
Reorient health services ➤ Embrace an expanded role to address health promotion as well as disease treatment ➤ Health research and training for health promotion	Macrosystems
Build healthy public policy ➤ Inform policy makers of health consequences of decisions and policies ➤ Foster equity and eliminate disparities among diverse groups ➤ Identify obstacles to health public policy	Macrosystems

Adapted from Bronfenbrenner, U., McClelland, P. D., Ceci, S. J., Moen, P., & Wethington, E. (1996). The state of Americans. *New York: Free Press; World Health Organization. (1999).* Ottawa charter for health promotion. *www.who.int/hpr/archive/docs/ottawa.html, accessed 5/30/2003.*

All children need a medical home, where ongoing health supervision is provided during the developmental years. A medical home or **pediatric healthcare home** is the site of comprehensive healthcare by a pediatric healthcare professional in order to ensure optimal health (National Association of Pediatric Nurse Associates and Practitioners [NAPNAP], 2002). See Chapter 16∞ for a further description of medical home or pediatric healthcare home. When a family has an established partnership with a care provider, comprehensive, family-centered health services can be provided based on the family's risks and protective factors. These services may be provided at physician offices, community health clinics, in the home, schools, childcare centers, shelters, or mobile vans (Figure 10–2 ■). National guidelines for preventive health services have been developed for infants, children, and adolescents by the U.S. Department of Health and Human Services (DHHS), the American Academy of Pediatrics (AAP), and the American Medical Association (Box 10–2). The National Association of Pediatric Nurse Associates and Practitioners supports the list of comprehensive services identified by the AAP (Box 10–3).

BOX 10–2 National Guidelines for Health Promotion

- *Bright Futures,* Maternal and Child Health Bureau, Health Resources and Services Administration, DHHS (*Bright Futures* recently partnered with the American Academy of Pediatrics for future editions of their recommendations.
- *Put Prevention into Practice,* Office of Disease Prevention and Health Promotion, Public Health Service, DHHS.
- *Guidelines for Adolescent Preventive Services,* American Medical Association.

The health supervision visit is individualized to the family and child. Standardized screenings and examinations are included, and time is provided for the family's specific concerns and questions about the child's health. Nurses play an integral part in these comprehensive visits, and they partner with other healthcare providers to accomplish health supervision.

A tracking system in the pediatric healthcare home site helps to identify appropriate health supervision activities for each child at

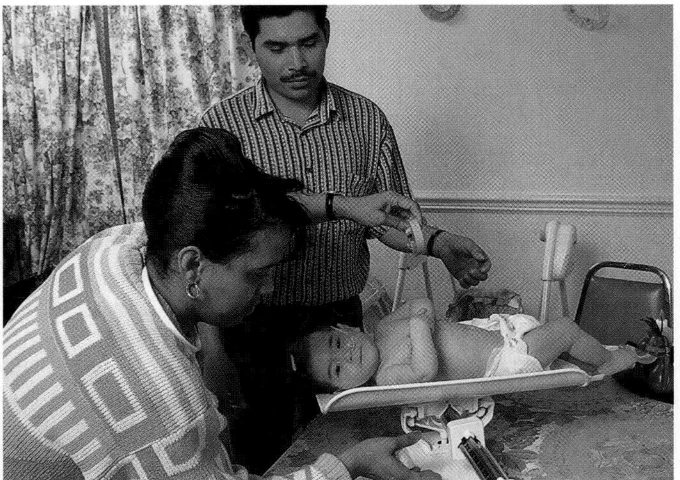
A

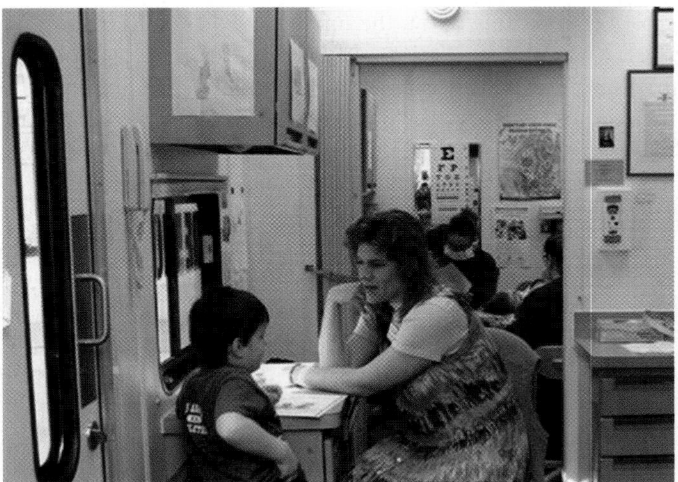
B

FIGURE 10–2 ■ *A,* The nurse is providing a health supervision visit in the child's home after discharge from the hospital for an acute illness. *B,* A nurse is providing information to a child visiting a mobile healthcare van.

MediaLink Health Promotion National Guidelines

BOX 10–3 Elements of a Pediatric Healthcare Home

The American Academy of Pediatrics and the National Association of Pediatric Nurse Associates and Practitioners concur that a pediatric healthcare home should offer:

- Family-centered care and trusting partnership
- Sharing of unbiased and clear information
- Provision of primary care to include acute and chronic care, breastfeeding promotion, immunizations, growth and development, screenings, healthcare supervision, counseling about health, nutrition, safety, parenting, and psychosocial issues
- Continuous available care
- Continuity of care
- Referral to specialists as needed
- Referral to early intervention and childcare
- Coordination of services
- Maintenance of a comprehensive central record
- Provision of developmentally appropriate and culturally competent care

Data from American Academy of Pediatrics. (2002). The medical home. Policy statement. Pediatrics, 110, *184–186; National Association of Pediatric Nurse Associates and Practioners [NAPNAP]. (2002). NAPNAP position statement on the pediatric health care home. www.napnap.org/practice/positions/healthcarehome.html, accessed 8/25/2003.*

every visit. Most often computers are used to list appropriate topics for visits at specific ages. If a child misses a visit, the family can be contacted by phone and encouraged to come in for the recommended care. A family may be called if the young child is lacking immunizations. Recognizing that not all families get into the healthcare home for each visit, every health visit, including an episodic illness visit or care for a chronic illness, an opportunity to complete health promotion and health maintenance activities. For example, if the child has missed a prior health supervision visit, immunizations may be given during a visit for an acute condition such as otitis media. When caring for children in hospitals, emergency rooms, or other settings, ask about their pediatric healthcare home, and when the last visit occurred. Identify children who need basic health supervision services and provide them, or refer to other settings to meet these needs at another time.

Nurses play an important role in managing health supervision visits (Figure 10–3 ■). Depending on the setting, the nurse may provide all services or support other care providers by obtaining an updated health history, screening for diseases and other conditions, conducting a developmental assessment, and providing immunizations, anticipatory guidance, and health education. And nurses in all settings are instrumental in identifying children who need health supervision and are not obtaining recommended care (Box 10–4).

While health supervision visits can address many health-related topics, there is generally a limited time in which to engage a child or family. The nurse needs to direct the encounters and have ideas for pertinent agendas. *Bright Futures* booklets provide guidance about how the nurse can manage health supervision visits. The following six concepts should be integrated into care.

First, the nurse *builds effective partnerships* with the family. A **partnership** is a relationship in which participants join together to ensure healthcare delivery in a way that recognizes the critical roles and contributions of each partner in promoting health and preventing illness. The partners in child health include the child, family, health professional, and the community. Strategies the nurse can use to build partnerships include:

- Modeling and encouraging open, supportive communication
- Recognizing and respecting family strengths
- Using open-ended questions to identify health issues
- Mutually identifying goals for the health encounter
- Mutually establishing a plan of action to meet goals
- Sustaining the partnership and evaluating the goals

Second, the nurse *fosters family-centered communication* by:

- Showing interest in the family and their concerns
- Conveying understanding and empathy
- Clarifying information as needed

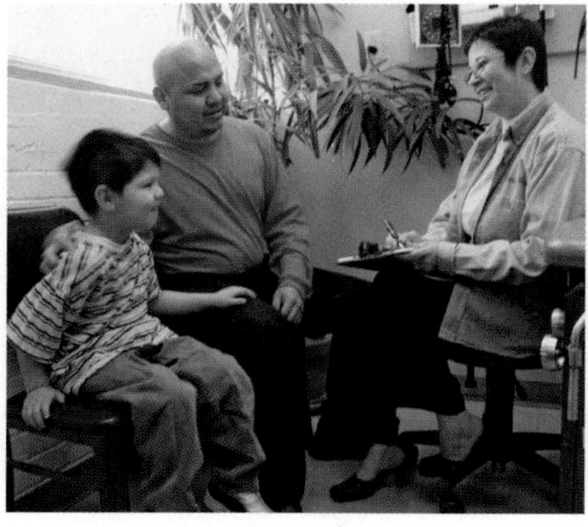
A

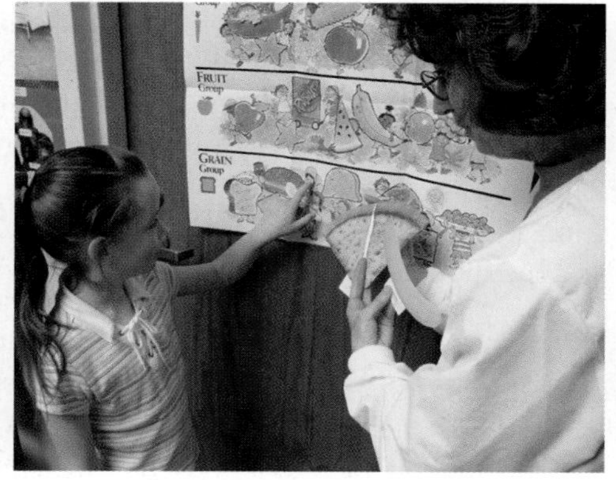

B

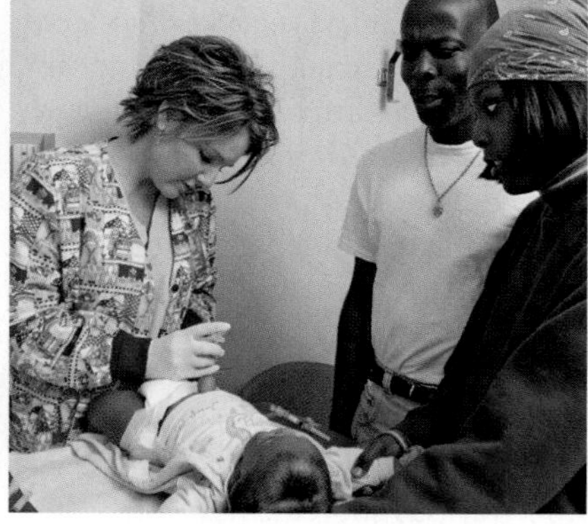
C

FIGURE 10–3 ■ The nurse plays many roles in providing health promotion and health maintenance for children. *A,* Data are collected from the time a nurse calls the child and family to the examination room and during the history taking phase. The nurse asks questions while observing the child's behaviors and the relationship between parent and child. The nurse also performs screening tests, including blood pressure, tuberculosis, vision and hearing, and developmental screening. *B,* Interventions that include teaching may take place. *C,* A nurse may administer immunizations as parents watch and assist by holding the child. Nurses also play important roles in teaching families information to enhance health.

BOX 10–4 Nursing Goals in Health Supervision

- Build effective partnerships with families
- Foster family-centered communication
- Address health promotion and health maintenance needs
- Manage time to provide for health promotion during routine healthcare visits
- Educate in family's teachable moments
- Advocate for children and their families

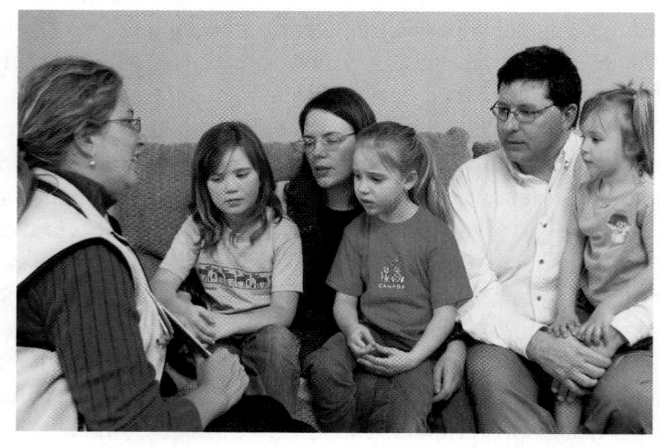

TABLE 10–4 Advocating for Children and Families

HEALTH NEED	NURSE ADVOCACY ACTIONS
Members of the community need to learn about places to obtain immunizations.	➤ Make a list of agencies that provide immunizations. ➤ Check on cost and special programs. ➤ Obtain financial assistance from a local foundation to print your findings. ➤ Make copies available in childcare centers and other community agencies.
A local homeless shelter has little in the way of self-image amenities for the clients.	➤ Obtain donations of hotel lotions, soaps, and shampoos from classmates and faculty that can be given to the shelter. ➤ Visit several local hotels and ask if they will each donate a box of small toiletries for the residents.
Your state has a law protecting the rights of any woman to bring her unwanted newborn baby to certain sites, and give the child up without legal recriminations. Many women do not know about the law and babies are abandoned in unsafe locations.	➤ Find a local newspaper reporter who is willing to write an article about the law. ➤ Run off copies of the article to distribute. ➤ Make posters with necessary information for several community sites.

What local child healthcare issues could benefit from advocacy in your community?

(See Chapter 6∞ for a thorough discussion of communication with children and families.)

Third, the nurse *focuses on health promotion and health maintenance topics during visits*, recognizing that families may not initiate these discussions. (Further discussion of topics follows.) Fourth, the nurse *can manage the time to enable health promotion topics to be addressed*. This may involve:

- Preparing for the visit by reviewing the child's health record and selecting topics appropriate for the child's age
- Clarifying key health promotion topics for the family
- Planning together for meeting of goals not accomplished in the visit due to lack of time or the need to focus only on certain high-priority concerns

Fifth, the nurse *educates the family during "teachable moments."* Large teaching plans are not always needed. Children and families often learn best when presented with small bits of information. The family may not need a large amount of information on preschool nutrition, but may benefit from knowing simply the recommendations for limiting fruit juice intake (see Chapter 9∞). These bits of information are geared to a specific question or topic the family has brought up, or an observation you have made during history or other conversation.

Sixth, the nurse *becomes an advocate for child health issues*. When an issue arises as you care for a child, seek additional data from various sources. Talk with others and strategize how the problem could be solved. Obtain the support you need and begin to advocate on the issue (Table 10–4).

As stated, the nurse identifies and isolates pertinent topics for health promotion and health maintenance during health supervision visits. You will apply your knowledge of areas that need to be addressed to a particular age and developmental stage, and then make general observations of the child and family to guide you to additional topics. Although categories to consider vary depending on the age of the child, the family's particular needs, and community resources, common topics generally require attention. Start with this list, integrating general observations as you progress with the visit, and add to it as needed. Topics for health promotion and health maintenance include:

- Growth and developmental surveillance
- Nutrition
- Physical activity
- Oral health
- Mental and spiritual health
- Relationships
- Disease prevention strategies
- Injury prevention (safety) strategies

General Observations

As a pediatric nurse, you will be making observations of children and their families whenever you encounter them. Be observant during the health supervision visit, and you will have many opportunities for assessing the family. These general observations begin as you call the family in and welcome them to the facility. They continue as you weigh and measure the child, and throughout the visit. Key observations include the following:

- Do the child and care provider have close physical contact, eye contact, and vocalization frequently during the visit?
- Do the parents appear relaxed or stressed?
- What are the child's behaviors? Are they what you would expect?

- If a sibling is present, can the parent attend to both children appropriately?
- What responses are you able to elicit in the baby related to eye contact, interest in voice, motor movements? What verbal and nonverbal behaviors do you see in the child or adolescent? Are they within expected norms?

Use your general observations to guide questions. Include additional examination if you have concerns about your observations. For example, if a 2-month-old sleeps for most of the visit, ask questions about the baby's amount of sleep and usual state of alertness. If a mother seems impatient with a crying infant, ask how she usually calms the baby at home. Her answer may reveal that she needs information about how to comfort an infant. If a father is nervously trying to quiet an active child, ask if the child's behavior is typical in new settings. Inquire about how the family sets limits, how much physical activity the child gets daily, and what concerns the father has about child behavior. As you progress in your child health nursing experiences, you will become more skilled at integrating your knowledge of development into observations during the visit. Practice these skills and check your observations with more experienced nurses.

Growth and Developmental Surveillance

Growth and development provide important clues about the child's condition and environment. Adequate growth suggests good nutrition and positive relationships with parents or other care providers. Poor growth could indicate lack of food, lack of a supportive environment, or an underlying child illness. In order to evaluate growth, child height, weight, and body mass index are calculated at each health supervision visit, and results are placed on percentile charts (see Chapter 8 and Chapter 9∞). Parents are given the information in written form and it is interpreted for them. Physical assessment is performed to ensure that the child is growing as expected and has no abnormal or unexplained physical findings (see Chapter 8∞). Health maintenance activities focus on disease prevention and might involve teaching parents of an infant or an adolescent athlete proper methods for avoiding fluid imbalance in these two vulnerable groups. Health promotion activities related to growth involve encouraging at least five servings of fruits and vegetables daily and switching to low-fat dairy products at about 2 years of age.

Developmental surveillance is a flexible, continuous process of skilled observations that also provides data about the child's capabilities, allows for early identification of any neurologic problems, and helps to verify that the home environment is stimulating. Information may be collected from several sources, for instance, a questionnaire that the parent completes, trigger questions asked during the interview, or observation of the child during the visit. Parents can also be interviewed to identify any developmental concerns they may have about the child or adolescent. To initiate general health supervision and developmental surveillance, ask questions about what skills the child is able to perform. Specific examples of questions to ask at particular ages are provided in each of the health promotion/health maintenance chapters that follow (Chapters 11 through 15∞).

When talking with parents, review physical, social, and communication milestones for infants, young children, older children, or adolescents. Detailed milestones for each age group are found in Chapter 5∞. Be aware that parents' recall of past developmental milestones is often faulty. The child is often reported to have achieved milestones at ages earlier than actually occurred. When accuracy of developmental milestones is critical, ask to see the child's baby diary or review the past health history at ages closer to the milestone achievement. The parents' report of current skills and achievements is usually accurate.

Review school performance for older children and adolescents, including report cards, school achievement records, and any performance on psychoeducational tests when indicated. Inquire about the child's participation in sports and other activities, as well as noted abilities.

Standardized developmental questionnaires are effective for developmental surveillance of most children, especially when time for health supervision visits is limited. These questionnaires are easy to administer, do not require the child's cooperation, and can be completed by parents in the waiting area. Children in need of more extensive developmental surveillance can be identified. See Table 10–5 for a list of commonly used developmental screening questionnaires that have been tested for validity and reliability. **Validity** of a test or tool refers to its ability to measure the characteristics it is established to measure. **Reliability** of a test or tool is measured by its ability to achieve similar results over time or when administered by various examiners. If a developmental delay or abnormality is suspected, a specific developmental screening test is needed to document developmental progress. See Table 10–6 for a list of commonly used developmental screening tests. Some healthcare providers actually use the Denver II as a developmental chart, like a growth curve, to monitor the child's developmental progress (Figures 10–4 ■ and 10–5 ■). However, remember that developmental screening tests are not diagnostic tests. They simply help to confirm that most children are progressing along an age-appropriate norm, and they help document suspicions or patterns of developmental problems. Each test addresses a unique combination of **domains,** which are categories or foci of developmental progression. Some common domains tested include fine motor, gross motor, language, self-help skills, social skills, and reading.

To perform developmental screening with any of the standardized screening tools, make sure all directions are followed:

- Choose the proper test for the child's age and desired information.
- Read directions thoroughly or utilize specific training tools available.
- Practice as needed until proficient with the test.
- Calculate the infant's or child's age correctly, especially if premature.
- Attempt to develop rapport with the infant or child to get the best performance.
- In some cases, parents can be asked if a child demonstrates specific skills at home, especially if the child is not cooperative.
- Note the behavior and cooperativeness of the child during the screening process.
- Analyze the findings using the test instructions to make the correct interpretation.

TABLE 10–5 Developmental Surveillance Questionnaires

QUESTIONNAIRE	GUIDELINES FOR ADMINISTRATION
Parent's Evaluation of Developmental Status[a] (birth to 8 years)	Consists of 10 questions for parents to answer in interview; based on research on parents' concerns. Requires less than 5 minutes to complete. English and Spanish forms are available.
Prescreening Development Questionnaire (PDQ and Revised-PDQ)[b] (birth to 6 years)	Parents complete one of age-specific forms. Helps identify children who need Denver II assessment. Requires less than 10 minutes to complete. PDQ is available in English, Spanish, and French versions; R-PDQ in English only.
Ages and Stages Questionnaire[c] (4–48 months)	Questionnaires for 11 specific ages, with 10–15 items each in areas of fine motor, gross motor, communication, adaptive, personal, and social skills. Parents try each activity with the child. Requires less than 10 minutes to complete. English and Spanish versions are available.
Child Development Inventories[d] (3–72 months)	Consists of 60 yes-no descriptions for three separate instruments to identify children with developmental difficulties. Requires about 10 minutes to complete.

[a]Frances P. Glascoe, Ellsworth & Vandermeer Press Ltd, P.O. Box 68164, Nashville, TN 37206.
[b]Denver Developmental Material, Inc., P.O. Box 371075, Denver, CO 80237-5075.
[c]Brookes Publishing Co., P.O. Box 10624, Baltimore, MD 21285-0625.
[d]Behavior Science Systems, Box 580274, Minneapolis, MN 55458.

Failure to perform an item in a single domain does not mean the child has failed the test (see Developing Cultural Competence: Developmental Testing). The child should be reevaluated at a future visit. Schedule the appointment at a time of day when the child is awake and rested. Provide parents with guidance on specific methods for stimulating the child. Failure of multiple items within one domain or across multiple domains is of greatest concern. When poor development patterns in one or more domains are revealed, referral for diagnostic developmental assessment is needed.

Both health promotion and health maintenance activities relate to developmental surveillance. Health promotion during a health supervision visit could involve teaching about the next milestones the child will be learning and how to provide an environment where that can occur. This type of anticipatory guidance helps to foster the child's developmental progression. Health maintenance seeks to prevent developmental delay and activities are focused on deficits found during the visit. For example, if parents of a preschooler have arranged no playmates, the child is likely to have problems with language and social interaction skills. To avoid these health problems, the nurse suggests ways to add social interactions to the child's experience.

Nutrition

Nutrition is a vital part of each health supervision visit, and is closely linked to both health promotion and health mainte-

TABLE 10–6 Developmental Screening Tests for Infants and Young Children

SCREENING TEST	GUIDELINES FOR ADMINISTRATION
Denver II[a] (birth to 6 years)	Consists of observation of the child in four domains; personal social, fine motor-adaptive, language, and gross motor. Requires 30 minutes to complete. A training video is available.
Bayley Infant Neurodevelopmental Screener (BINST)[b] (3–24 months)	Consists of observation of child with 10–13 items for each of six age-specific scales to assess neurological processes, neurodevelopmental skills, and developmental accomplishments. Requires 10–15 minutes to complete.
McCarthy Scales of Children's Abilities[b] (2.5–8.5 years)	Consists of observation of child in domains of motor, verbal, perceptual-performance, quantitive, general cognition, and memory. Requires 45 minutes to complete.
Denver Articulation Screeening Exam (DASE)[a] (2.5–6 years)	Consists of observation of child's articulation of 30 sound elements and intelligibility. Requires 5 minutes to complete.
Early Language Milestone Scale—2 (ELM)[c] (birth to 36 months)	Consists of observation of child to assess auditory expressive, auditory receptive, and visual components of speech. Requires 5–10 minutes to complete.

[a]Denver Development Materials, Inc., P.O. Box 371075, Denver, CO 80237–5075.
[b]Harcourt Assessment: The Psychological Corporation, 19500 Bulverde Rd., San Antonio, TX 78259.
[c]PRO-ED, Inc., 8700 Shoal Creek Blvd., Austin, TX 78758-6897.

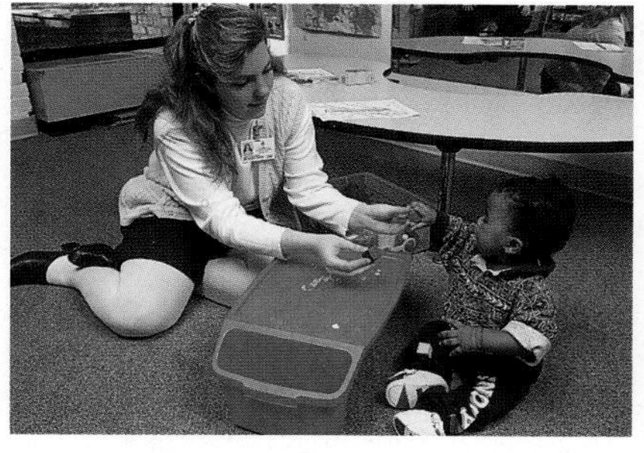

A

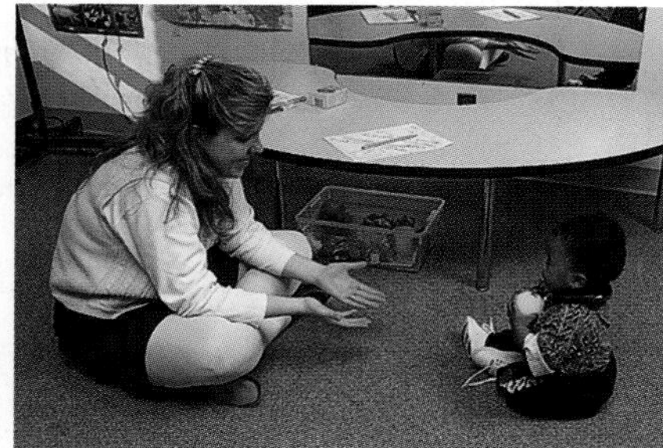

B

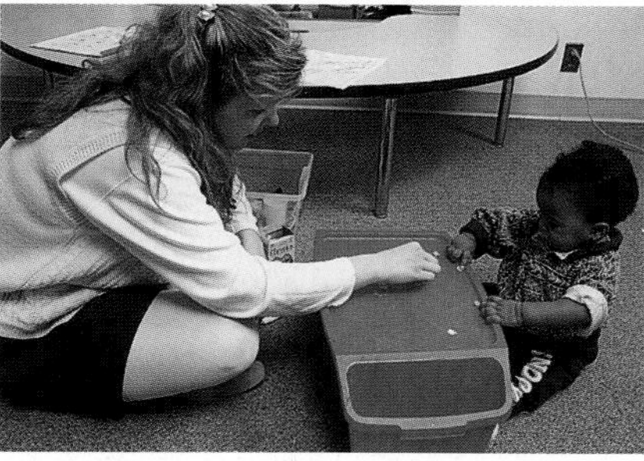

C

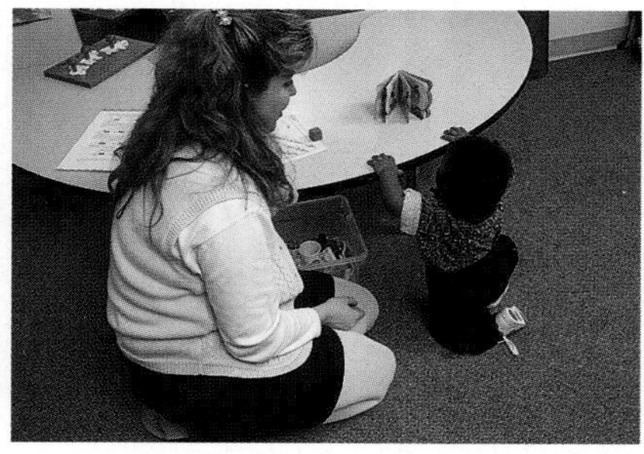

D

FIGURE 10–4 ■ Follow all directions for performing the Denver II assessment and for interpreting responses. Develop rapport with the child and approach the assessment as fun. This often helps the child participate more actively during the entire Denver II assessment. This 9-month-old boy is able to perform the following age-appropriate behaviors: Banging two cubes, *A;* playing ball with the examiner, *B;* using a thumb-finger grasp, *C;* and pulling to stand, *D.*

nance. Good nutrition makes important contributions to general health and fosters growth and development. Eating the proper foods for age and activity level ensures that children have the energy for proper growth, physical activity, cognition, and immune function. Enhancing one's diet with more fruits and vegetables can lead to a stronger immune system and sense of well-being, thus promoting health. It can also contribute to health maintenance by preventing problems such as obesity and some cancers.

For infants, monitoring type and amounts of feedings is essential. Food introduction, infant ability to eat, and integration of food intake and developmental skills are important to ascertain. Good nutrition requires balance and should be woven into all aspects of daily life (Story, Holt, & Sofka, 2002).

Once the baby has become older, food patterns of the family become important. Consider childcare settings as well. School-age children and adolescents are establishing food patterns that are most likely to remain with them for life. Ask if the child or adolescent eats breakfast and/or lunch at school. Inquire about vending machine presence in the school and how much the child uses them. How often does the family or the adolescent eat out at fast-food restaurants? Analyze growth patterns carefully and ask sensitive questions. Find out if the child or adolescent or parents have any concerns about weight or nutrition.

See Chapter 9∞ for detailed nutritional assessment recommendations, and Chapter 11 through Chapter 15∞ for specific nutritional questions to ask for each age group. Include observations and screening relevant to nutritional intake at each health supervision visit. Determine what questions parents have about feeding their children. Use the information gathered to provide both health promotion and health maintenance interventions. In the area of nutrition there is much overlap—information provided is likely to both promote a general state of health and prevent disease in the future.

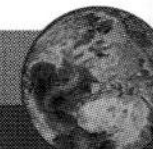

DEVELOPING CULTURAL COMPETENCE
Developmental Testing

Be alert that children who have recently come from other countries and even some born in this country who live in families from minority ethnic groups may have difficulty with some items on developmental tests. For example, children who are not skilled in the English language may not understand some instructions or be able to answer questions about definitions of words. If an item such as "wave good-bye" or "plays patty-cake" represents a practice not common in another culture, the child may not have had exposure to the skill. Be alert for cultural variations, allow the child time to learn a developmental skill, and retest on other occasions.

Physical Activity

Physical activity provides many physical and psychologic health benefits. However, there is growing disparity between recommendations and reality among most of our children (Patrick, Spear, Holt, et al., 2001) (Box 10–5). The physical activity of infants and young children gives clues to gross motor development status. Observe the infant for symmetrical movement, flexion and extension of extremities when excited, and ability to engage with objects and play. Developmental milestones such as sitting, walking, and throwing a ball are important. Ask what activities the child prefers and amount of time that is spent in activity during the day. As the child grows older, ask questions about sedentary activities such as number of hours spent watching television or playing computer games. Determine if the child plays sports at school or in the community. Ask about activities in a typical day to measure amount of activity. Are parents satisfied with the

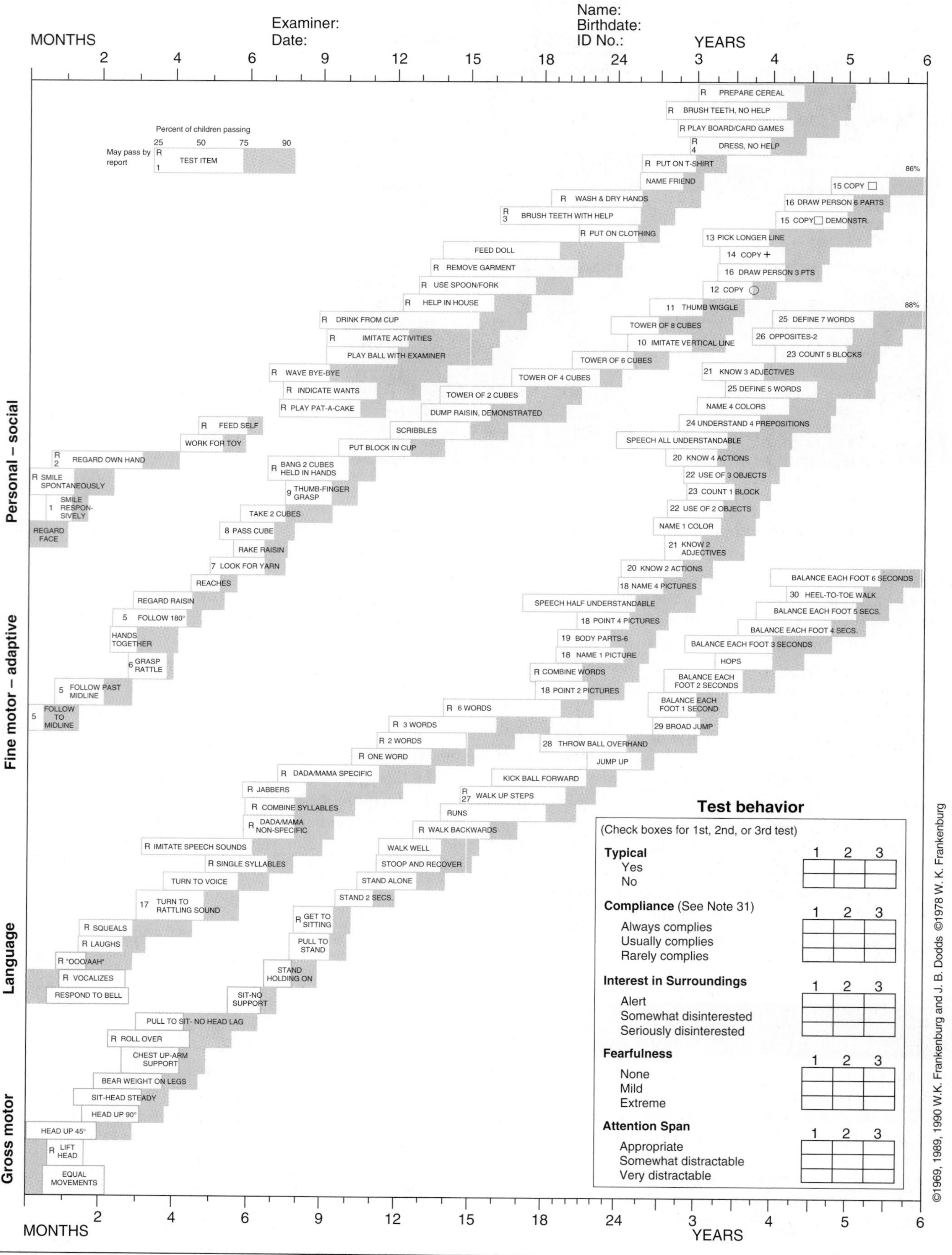

FIGURE 10–5A ■ Denver II.

From W. K. Frankenburg, Denver, CO.

DIRECTIONS FOR ADMINISTRATION

1. Try to get child to smile by smiling, talking or waving. Do not touch him/her.
2. Child must stare at hand several seconds.
3. Parent may help guide toothbrush and put toothpaste on brush.
4. Child does not have to be able to tie shoes or button/zip in the back.
5. Move yarn slowly in an arc from one side to the other, about 8" above child's face.
6. Pass if child grasps rattle when it is touched to the backs or tips of fingers.
7. Pass if child tries to see where yarn went. Yarn should be dropped quickly from sight from tester's hand without arm movement.
8. Child must transfer cube from hand to hand without help of body, mouth, or table.
9. Pass if child picks up raisin with any part of thumb and finger.
10. Line can vary only 30 degrees or less from tester's line.
11. Make a fist with thumb pointing upward and wiggle only the thumb. Pass if child imitates and does not move any fingers other than the thumb.

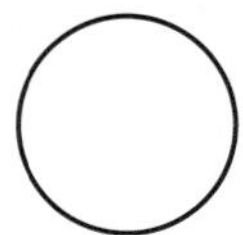

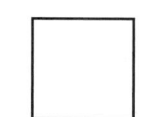

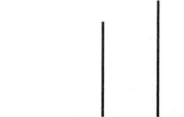

12. Pass any enclosed form. Fail continuous round motions.

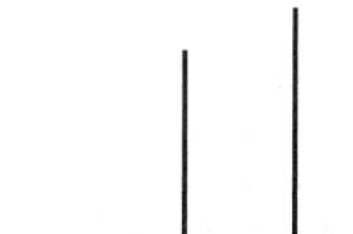

13. Which line is longer? (Not bigger.) Turn paper upside down and repeat. (pass 3 of 3 or 5 of 6).

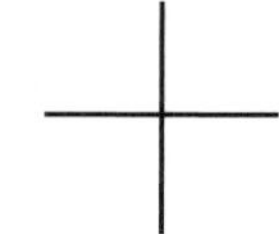

14. Pass any lines crossing near midpoint.

15. Have child copy first. If failed, demonstrate.

When giving items 12, 14, and 15, do not name the forms. Do not demonstrate 12 and 14.

16. When scoring, each pair (2 arms, 2 legs, etc.) counts as one part.
17. Place one cube in cup and shake gently near child's ear, but out of sight. Repeat for other ear.
18. Point to picture and have child name it. (No credit is given for sounds only.) If less than 4 pictures are named correctly, have child point to picture as each is named by tester.

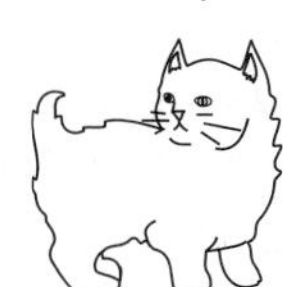 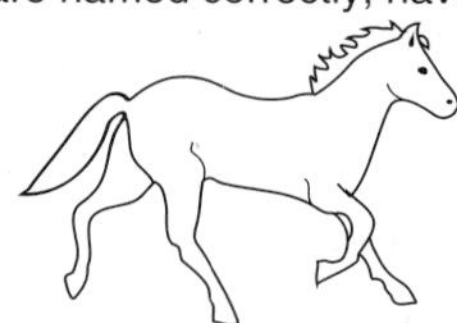 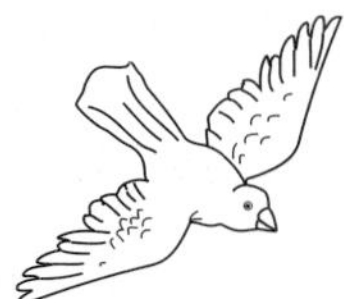 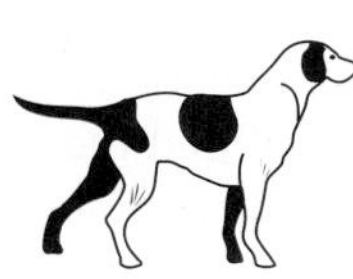 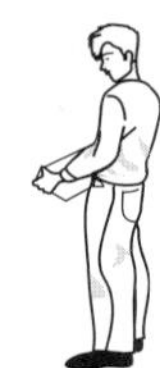

19. Using doll, tell child: Show me the nose, eyes, ears, mouth, hands, feet, tummy, hair. Pass 6 of 8.
20. Using pictures, ask child: Which one flies?... says meow?... talks?... barks?... gallops? Pass 2 of 5, 4 of 5.
21. Ask child: What do you do when you are cold?... tired?... hungry? Pass 2 of 3, 3 of 3.
22. Ask child: What do you do with a cup? What is a chair used for? What is a pencil used for? Action words must be included in answers.
23. Pass if child correctly places and says how many blocks are on paper. (1, 5).
24. Tell child: Put block **on** table; **under** table: **in front of** me, **behind** me. Pass 4 of 4. (Do not help child by pointing, moving head or eyes.)
25. Ask child: What is a ball?... lake?... desk?... house?... banana?... curtain?... fence?... ceiling? Pass if defined in terms of use, shape, what it is made of, or general category (such as banana is fruit, not just yellow). Pass 5 of 8, 7 of 8.
26. Ask child: If a horse is big, a mouse is_____? If fire is hot, ice is_____? If sun shines during the day, the moon shines during the ____? Pass 2 of 3.
27. Child may use wall or rail only, not person. May not crawl.
28. Child must throw ball overhand 3 feet to within arm's reach of tester.
29. Child must perform standing broad jump over width of test sheet (8 1/2 inches).
30. Tell child to walk forward, ⊂⊃⊂⊃⊂⊃⊂⊃ → heel within 1 inch of toe. Tester may demonstrate. Child must walk 4 consecutive steps.
31. In the second year, half of normal children are non-compliant.

OBSERVATIONS:

FIGURE 10–5B ■ (continued)
Directions for administration of Denver II.
From W. K. Frankenburg, Denver, CO.

BOX 10–5 Research: Physical Activity Levels

Recent research by the Centers for Disease Control and Prevention (CDC) using the Youth Media Campaign Longitudinal Survey (YMCLS) of parents and children found that 61.5% of children 9 to 13 years of age report that they do not participate in any organized physical activity during hours outside of school. While organized activities are important and consistent forms of exercise, not all children can participate or desire to do so. However, 22.6% of these children reported that they do not engage in ANY physical activity outside of school. Parents noted that barriers to physical activities included transportation problems, lack of opportunities in area, expense, lack of parental time, and lack of neighborhood safety (MMWR, 2003). Adding more physical activity to the leisure time of children is important. Ask questions of all children to learn about their activity levels, and find out what barriers to activity exist. This will provide you with the data needed to plan interventions to increase activity for individual children.

child's activity level, or do they have questions about sports, athletics, other physical activity, and sedentary behaviors? Do the child's weight or body mass index percentile and reported activity level correspond? Once the nurse gathers data about physical activity, interventions are implemented to enhance activity patterns. Examples of health promotion include suggestions for allowing safe infant crawling and other gross motor activities for periods each day, recommending places to provide sports for a child interested in soccer or hockey, or encouraging a teen to register for a local fun run. These activities will lead the child to a higher state of wellness. The purpose of health maintenance activities is to prevent disease and injury; include provision of information about safety gear for sports and safe practices such as warm-ups and adequate fluid to prevent injury. Adequate physical activity will contribute to prevention of obesity and its related diseases. See Chapter 5∞ for further discussion of data gathering and interventions related to physical activity.

Oral Health

While oral health may seem to require the knowledge of a specialist, there are many implications that relate to general healthcare. Oral health is important because teeth assist in language development, impacted or infected teeth lead to systemic illness, and teeth are related to positive self-image formation. Between 4 and 5 million children in the United States are affected by tooth decay and pain that interfere with activities of daily living such as eating, sleeping, attending school, and speaking (Ryan, 2003). When families have financial challenges, dental care is often not obtained; low-income children account for 80% of all childhood dental decay. A family of four will need to pay almost $1,000 annually in the United States just for basic dental examinations and preventive care. When decay has already occurred, care is more costly and difficult for the child. Nurses address oral health issues by performing oral assessments during health supervision visits, asking about dental care access, and referring families to other resources as needed (Box 10–6).

Clearly, health promotion is needed for dental health. Nurses teach about oral care and access to dental visits so that general health is enhanced. Health maintenance activities relate to prevention of caries and illness related to dental disease. Use of fluoride to strengthen teeth and referral for care when poor dental care is apparent are examples of these activities.

Mental and Spiritual Health

Families usually are accustomed to questions about physical status of the child, but may be unprepared to discuss mental health. Encourage parents to keep a record of mental health issues to bring to health supervision visits. This helps them understand that the healthcare professional is willing to partner with them to assist in dealing with mental health. Suggest topics such as child and parental mood, child temperament, stresses and ways that family members manage stress, or sleep patterns. Make notes in the record as a reminder of questions to ask at the next visit (Jellinek, Patel, & Froehle, 2002).

The child and family are both observed for appropriateness of affect and mood. Be alert for signs of depression, stress, or anxiety (see Chapters 5 and 34∞ for more detail). Signs of abuse, neglect, or domestic violence are noted.

Spiritual health is seen in the larger context of entities that provide meaning in life. For some, this may be membership in a faith-based group; for others, it may be feeling part of a society with a purpose of greater good, or setting goals for the future (Box 10–7, Box 10–8). Ask about the family's meaningful activities. Provide links to faith-based groups as needed.

The nurse establishes both health promotion and health maintenance goals related to child and family mental health. Health promotion goals relate to adequate resources to meet family challenges, protective factors such as involvement in extended family and the community. Teaching stress reduction techniques such as meditation, relaxation, and imagery, as well as providing resources for yoga or other techniques is helpful. See Chapter 3∞ for further discussion. Health maintenance goals relate to prevention of mental health problems. Examples include providing resources when domestic violence occurs, or referring cases of suspected child abuse or neglect. The sleep-deprived child needs help to establish healthy sleep patterns to prevent psychologic and physical problems.

Relationships

The relationships that a child establishes with others begin at birth. The first and most important set of relationships develops

BOX 10–6 Dental Care Resources

Children in homes with low incomes are especially prone to poor dental health, so efforts are being extended to help families receive care. Many of the State Children's Health Insurance Programs (SCHIPs) offer dental services (VanLandeghen, Bronstein, & Brach, 2003). All children in the Medicaid program are eligible for dental coverage in the Early and Periodic Screening, Diagnostic, and Treatment (EPSDT) services. Private and public clinics in many communities provide low cost or free care for families with limited financial resources (Ryan, 2003). Many families do not realize their children could receive these services. Find out what resources are available in your state and community, and refer as needed. See Chapter 1∞ for further description about programs mentioned here.

BOX 10–7 Spiritual Dimension

The **spiritual dimension** is a connection with a greater power than that in the self, and guides a person to strive for inspiration, respect, meaning, and purpose in life (Murray & Zentner, 2001). Some individuals develop and reinforce the spiritual dimension through membership in a religious group while others study or honor positive human and moral qualities.

with the family. The mother, father, siblings, and perhaps extended family are the contexts in which the baby learns to relate with others. As the child grows, the world widens to encompass other children, friends of the family, peers, school, and the larger community network. Analyzing the child's relationships at all ages provides important clues to social interactions.

From the moment the family is called in from a waiting area, be alert for clues to family interactions. Who brought the child to the visit? What was the family doing when you called them from the waiting room? Were they reading to the child or interacting in some way? Do the parents talk with the child? What is the child's response? Are developmentally appropriate interactions apparent? For example, the parent of a 5-year-old might hold the child's hand, but this would rarely be seen with an adolescent. Does the parent of an older child or adolescent let the child answer your questions?

Likewise, other social interactions are important to evaluate. Does the young infant interact in an age-appropriate manner with the healthcare provider or other children in the area? See Chapter 5∞ for social milestones at various ages.

Ask the parents questions about family and social interactions. What is easy and difficult in caring for the infant? What kind of temperament does the child have? **Temperament** is the characteristic behavioral style of the infant. Babies' temperaments represent inborn characteristics about responses to the environment, such as regularity of sleeping and eating, and response to new people and situations. See Chapter 5∞ for a detailed description of temperament. Does the older child have playmates? What are they like? What activities do the children do together? Ask older children to describe their best friends and how they spend time. Common tools to assess temperament during health supervision visits are Carey Infant and Child Questionnaires.

BOX 10–8 Mental and Spiritual Health Components

There are many components to mental health. Some areas that can be focused upon during health supervision visits include:

- Mood, especially evidence in any family member of depression, anxiety, anger
- Sleep patterns, especially of the child
- Presence of domestic violence
- Presence of substance abuse
- Family stresses such as illness, incarceration, financial concerns, marital discord, deaths, recent moves, job loss
- Spiritual health and meaning in life
- Participation in faith-based groups

Apply resilience theory by asking about both risk and protective factors. What are the mental health issues and how do family members handle them? One family may have financial concerns, but has the resources to face and solve problems while another family resorts to fighting and other behaviors that influence the child's environment.

MediaLink: Temperament Assessment Tools

Once assessment has taken place, establish goals and interventions related to family and social interactions. Health promotion issues include anticipatory guidance for parents of young children about needs for socialization of the child with others and discipline techniques to be used at various ages. Health promotion for the older child may involve teaching related to how to show friends you care, and how to solve disputes in a positive manner. Health maintenance activities are aimed at preventing family and social interaction problems. Provide information to children about bullying in schools and dealing with conflict at home. Specific examples for different age groups can be found in Chapters 11 through 15∞.

Disease Prevention Strategies

Disease prevention strategies focus mainly on health maintenance, or prevention of disease. Some health disruptions can be detected early and treatment for the condition can begin. **Screening** is a procedure used to detect the possible presence of a health condition before symptoms are apparent. It is usually conducted on large groups of individuals at risk for a condition and represents the secondary level of prevention (see Table 10–2). Most screening tests are not strictly diagnostic, but are followed by further diagnostic tests if the screening result is positive. Once a screening test identifies the existence of a health condition, early intervention can begin, with the goal of reducing the severity or complications of the condition. For example, all newborns are screened within 1 week of birth for at least two genetic diseases, congenital hypothyroidism and phenylketonuria. Appropriate interventions (medication or diet therapy) reduce the chances or severity of mental retardation if either of these conditions is present. (See Chapters 4 and 11∞ for more information about newborn screening.)

Screening tests are administered at times when children are most likely to develop a condition or to identify the greatest number of children at highest risk for the condition. Screening tests are also expected to correctly identify children who do have the condition. Some children are at greater risk of contracting certain conditions due to their environment. For example, young children living in housing built before 1960 are screened more frequently for lead poisoning than children who live in newer houses where only lead-free paints have been used (see Chapter 30∞ for a discussion of lead poisoning). Table 10–7 outlines the recommended screening tests by age for infants, children, and adolescents (Box 10–9).

Infants are commonly screened for diseases and growth parameters, young children for growth and disorders such as anemia, and school-age children for growth, blood pressure, hearing, and vision. In addition, adolescents may be screened for scoliosis, substance abuse, and sexually transmitted diseases.

Another way to prevent diseases is to immunize children against common communicable diseases. See Chapter 19∞ for

TABLE 10–7A Recommendations for Preventive Pediatric Health Care, Committee on Practice and Ambulatory Medicine, American Academy of Pediatrics, U.S.

Each child and family is unique; therefore, these **Recommendations for Preventive Pediatric Health Care** are designed for the care of children who are receiving competent parenting, have no manifestations of any important health problems, and are growing and developing in satisfactory fashion. **Additional visits may become necessary** if circumstances suggest variations from normal.

These guidelines represent a consensus by the Committee on Practice and Ambulatory Medicine in consultation with national committees and sections of the American Academy of Pediatrics. The Committee emphasizes the great importance of **continuity of care** in comprehensive health supervision and the need to avoid **fragmentation of care**.

	INFANCY[4]									EARLY CHILDHOOD[4]				
AGE[5]	PRENATAL[1]	NEWBORN[2]	2-4d[3]	By 1mo	2mo	4mo	6mo	9mo	12mo	15mo	18mo	24mo	3y	4y
HISTORY														
Initial/Interval	•	•	•	•	•	•	•	•	•	•	•	•	•	•
MEASUREMENTS														
Height and Weight		•	•	•	•	•	•	•	•	•	•	•	•	•
Head Circumference		•	•	•	•	•	•	•	•	•	•	•		
Blood Pressure													•	•
SENSORY SCREENING														
Vision		S	S	S	S	S	S	S	S	S	S	S	O[5]	O
Hearing		O[7]	S	S	S	S	S	S	S	S	S	S	S	O
DEVELOPMENTAL/ BEHAVIORAL ASSESSMENT[8]		•	•	•	•	•	•	•	•	•	•	•	•	•
PHYSICAL EXAMINATION[9]		•	•	•	•	•	•	•	•	•	•	•	•	•
PROCEDURES-GENERAL[10]														
Hereditary/Metabolic Screening[11]		←	•	→										
Immunization[12]		•	•	•	•	•	•	•	•	•	•	•	•	•
Hematocrit or Hemoglobin[13]								•	→	★	★	★	★	★
Urinalysis														
PROCEDURES-PATIENTS AT RISK														
Lead Screening[16]								★	→			★		
Tuberculin Test[17]									★	★	★	★	★	★
Cholesterol Screening[18]												★	★	★
STD Screening[19]														
Pelvic Exam[20]														
ANTICIPATORY GUIDANCE[21]	•	•	•	•	•	•	•	•	•	•	•	•	•	•
Injury Prevention[22]	•	•	•	•	•	•	•	•	•	•	•	•	•	•
Violence Prevention[23]	•	•	•	•	•	•	•	•	•	•	•	•	•	•
Sleep Positioning Counseling[24]	•	•	•	•	•	•	•							
Nutrition Counseling[25]	•	•	•	•	•	•	•	•	•	•	•	•	•	•
DENTAL REFERRAL[26]									←				•	

	MIDDLE CHILDHOOD[4]				ADOLESCENCE[4]										
AGE[5]	5y	6y	8y	10y	11y	12y	13y	14y	15y	16y	17y	18y	19y	20y	21y
HISTORY															
Initial/Interval	•	•	•	•	•	•	•	•	•	•	•	•	•	•	•
MEASUREMENTS															
Height and Weight	•	•	•	•	•	•	•	•	•	•	•	•	•	•	•
Head Circumference															
Blood Pressure	•	•	•	•	•	•	•	•	•	•	•	•	•	•	•
SENSORY SCREENING															
Vision	O	O	O	O	S	O	S	S	O	S	S	O	S	S	S
Hearing	O	O	O	O	S	O	S	S	O	S	S	O	S	S	S
DEVELOPMENTAL/ BEHAVIORAL ASSESSMENT[8]	•	•	•	•	•	•	•	•	•	•	•	•	•	•	•
PHYSICAL EXAMINATION[9]	•	•	•	•	•	•	•	•	•	•	•	•	•	•	•
PROCEDURES-GENERAL[10]															
Hereditary/Metabolic Screening[11]															
Immunization[12]	•	•	•	•	•	•	•	•	•	•	•	•	•	•	•
Hematocrit or Hemoglobin[13]	★				←		•[14]								→
Urinalysis	•				←					•[15]					→
PROCEDURES-PATIENTS AT RISK															
Lead Screening[16]															
Tuberculin Test[17]	★	★	★	★	★	★	★	★	★	★	★	★	★	★	★
Cholesterol Screening[18]	★	★	★	★	★	★	★	★	★	★	★	★	★	★	★
STD Screening[19]					★	★	★	★	★	★	★	★	★	★	★
Pelvic Exam[20]					★	★	★	★	★	★	★	★ ←	★[20]	★	→ ★
ANTICIPATORY GUIDANCE[21]	•	•	•	•	•	•	•	•	•	•	•	•	•	•	•
Injury Prevention[22]	•	•	•	•	•	•	•	•	•	•	•	•	•	•	•
Violence Prevention[23]	•	•	•	•	•	•	•	•	•	•	•	•	•	•	•
Sleep Positioning Counseling[24]															
Nutrition Counseling[25]	•	•	•	•	•	•	•	•	•	•	•	•	•	•	•
DENTAL REFERRAL[26]															

TABLE 10–7A Recommendations for Preventive Pediatric Health Care, Committee on Practice and Ambulatory Medicine, American Academy of Pediatrics, U.S. (continued)

1. A prenatal visit is recommended for parents who are at high risk, for first-time parents, and for those who request a conference. The prenatal visit should include anticipatory guidance, pertinent medical history, and a discussion of benefits of breastfeeding and planned method of feeding per AAP statement "The Prenatal Visit" (1996).
2. Every infant should have a newborn evaluation after birth. Breastfeeding should be encouraged and instruction and support offered. Every breastfeeding infant should have an evaluation 48-72 hours after discharge from the hospital to include weight, formal breastfeeding evaluation, encouragement, and instruction as recommended in the AAP statement "Breastfeeding and the Use of Human Milk" (1997).
3. For newborns discharged in less than 48 hours after delivery per AAP statement "Hospital Stay for Healthy Term Newborns" (1995).
4. Developmental, psychosocial, and chronic disease issues for children and adolescents may require frequent counseling and treatment visits separate from preventive care visits.
5. If a child comes under care for the first time at any point on the schedule, or if any items are not accomplished at the suggested age, the schedule should be brought up to date at the earliest possible time.
6. If the patient is uncooperative, rescreen within 6 months.
7. All newborns should be screened per the AAP Task Force on Newborn and Infant Hearing statement, "Newborn and Infant Hearing Loss: Detection and Intervention" (1999).
8. By history and appropriate physical examination: if suspicious, by specific objective developmental testing. Parenting skills should be fostered at every visit.
9. At each visit, a complete physical examination is essential, with infant totally unclothed, older child undressed and suitably draped.
10. These may be modified, depending upon entry point into schedule and individual need.
11. Metabolic screening (eg, thyroid, hemoglobinopathies, PKU, galactosemia) should be done according to state law.
12. Schedule(s) per the Committee on Infectious Diseases, published annually in the January edition of *Pediatrics*. Every visit should be an opportunity to update and complete a child's immunizations.
13. See AAP *Pediatric Nutrition Handbook* (1998) for a discussion of universal and selective screening options. Consider earlier screening for high-risk infants (eg, premature infants and low birth weight infants). See also "Recommendations to Prevent and Control Iron Deficiency in the United States". *MMWR*. 1998;47 (RR-3):1-29.
14. All menstruating adolescents should be screened annually.
15. Conduct dipstick urinalysis for leukocytes annually for sexually active male and female adolescents.
16. For children at risk of lead exposure consult the AAP statement "Screening for Elevated Blood Levels" (1998). Additionally, screening should be done in accordance with state law where applicable.
17. TB testing per recommendations of the Committee on Infectious Diseases, published in the current edition of *Red Book: Report of the Committee on Infectious Diseases*. Testing should be done upon recognition of high-risk factors.
18. Cholesterol screening for high-risk patients per AAP statement "Cholesterol in Childhood" (1998). If family history cannot be ascertained and other risk factors are present, screening should be at the discretion of the physician.
19. All sexually active patients should be screened for sexually transmitted diseases (STDs).
20. All sexually active females should have a pelvic examination. A pelvic examination and routine pap smear should be offered as part of preventive health maintenance between the ages of 18 and 21 years.
21. Age-appropriate discussion and counseling should be an integral part of each visit for care per the AAP *Guidelines for Health Supervision III* (1998).
22. From birth to age 12, refer to the AAP injury prevention program (TIPP*) as described in *A Guide to Safety Counseling in Office Practice* (1994).
23. Violence prevention and management for all patients per AAP Statement "The Role of the Pediatrician in Youth Violence Prevention in Clinical Practice and at the Community Level" (1999).
24. Parents and caregivers should be advised to place healthy infants on their backs when putting them to sleep. Side positioning is a reasonable alternative but carries a slightly higher risk of SIDS. Consult the AAP statement "Changing Concepts of Sudden Infant Death Syndrome: Implications for Infant Sleeping Environment and Sleep Position" (2000).
25. Age-appropriate nutrition counseling should be an integral part of each visit per the AAP *Handbook of Nutrition* (1998).
26. Earlier initial dental examinations may be appropriate for some children. Subsequent examinations as prescribed by dentist.

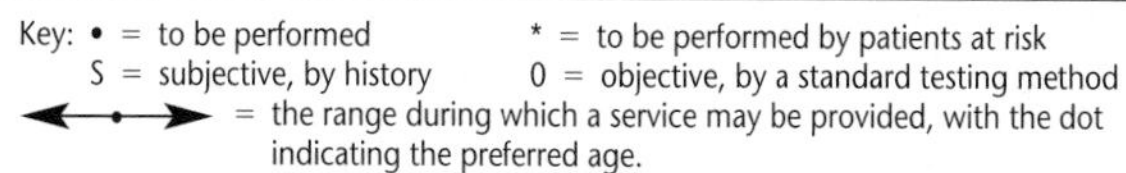

Key: • = to be performed
* = to be performed by patients at risk
S = subjective, by history
0 = objective, by a standard testing method
= the range during which a service may be provided, with the dot indicating the preferred age.

American Academy of Pediatrics

NB: Special chemical, immunologic, and endocrine testing is usually carried out upon specific indications. Testing other than newborn (eg. inborn errors of metabolism, sickle disease, etc) is discretionary with the physician.

Used with permission of the American Academy of Pediatrics (2004).

TABLE 10–7B Components of Well-Child Assessments at Various Ages, Pediatric Clinical Practice Guidelines for Nurses in Primary Care, Health Canada

HEALTH PARAMETER	MOST IMPORTANT AGES FOR ASSESSMENT
Height, weight	Every visit from birth to 16 years of age
Head circumference	Every visit in the first 2 years of life
Growth chart plotting	Every visit
Blood pressure	Once in the first 2 years, once at 4-6 years, during school-age years only if there is a risk or concern about high blood pressure, and every second year during adolescence
Eye assessment	Every visit in the first year of life
Strabismus assessment	Every visit in the first year of life
Visual acuity testing	Initial screening (e.g., Snellen chart) at 3–5 years of age; every 2 years between 6 and 10 years of age, then every 3 years until 18 years of age
Dental assessment	Every visit
Speech assessment	Every visit
Developmental assessment	Every visit
Sexual development	Every visit
School adjustment	Every visit after child reaches school age
Chemical abuse	Consider during assessments of children >8 years of age
Immunizations	According to schedule: at 2, 4, 6, 12 and 18 months and at 4–6 and 14–16 years
Hemoglobin	Screen at 6–12 months
Safety counseling	Every visit
Nutrition counseling	From birth to 5 years, and for teenagers
Parenting counseling	Every visit

Health Canada (2004). Pediatric Clinical Practice Guidelines for Nurses in Primary Care. Ch.1 Guidelines for Pediatric Health Assessment. Downloaded 7/15/04 from http://www.hc-sc.gc.ca/fnihb/ons/nursing/resource/pediatric_guidelines/Chapter_1.htm. Reproduced with the permission of the Minister of Public Works and Government Services Canada, 2004.

BOX 10–9 Screening Test Interpretation

Sensitivity is the ability of the test to accurately identify those with the condition. High sensitivity is seen in a test that is able to detect the condition when only a small amount of the indicator is present, or early in the disease process. Some children who test positive for a condition do not actually have it; they are classified as false positives.

Specificity is the ability of the test to exclude those who do not have the condition. Some children who test negative may actually have the disease; they are classified as false negatives. The best screening tests have both high sensitivity and high specificity. In addition to this accuracy, other considerations include cost, ease of administration, and acceptability.

Adapted from Clark, M. J. (2003). Community health nursing: Caring for populations *(4th ed.). Upper Saddle River, NJ: Prentice-Hall.*

the complete list of childhood immunizations and schedules for administration, and Chapters 11 through 15∞ for usual immunization needs at specific ages. The nurse who administers immunizations is performing a health maintenance activity. However, even health promotion activities can occur when a parent expresses interest in learning more about certain immunizations, how they act, and the risks and benefits of immunizations and corresponding diseases. Meeting the parent goal to understand more and make intelligent choices and healthcare decisions is an example of health promotion activity.

Injury Prevention (Safety) Strategies

Most childhood mortality and hospitalization is related to injury (see Chapter 1∞). Therefore, it is important for the nurse to integrate injury prevention strategies in all health supervision visits. These strategies represent health maintenance activities because they recognize injury risks and aim to prevent potential injuries.

The family is constantly challenged to maintain a safe environment as the child grows older, reaches more advanced developmental levels, is exposed to a widening world outside of the family, and has less supervision. Asking parents to bring their questions about safety to each visit can be a good starting point for discussion. Safety teaching should be integrated with developmental progression. For example, as the child begins to crawl, the family needs to be aware of hazards on the floor of the house. When the school-age child is riding a bicycle to school, traffic patterns and helmet use should be discussed. Ask the teen driver about drinking patterns in self and friends.

The nurse considers knowledge about the age of the child and information from the health supervision visit to plan health maintenance interventions related to injury. Teaching is performed, resources are made available, and parents and children who have experienced injury are invited to present their experiences. What other activities and approaches would you plan to prevent injuries at specific ages?

Additional Topics

Many other topics might be discussed during health supervision visits. They may relate to either health maintenance activities designed to preserve health, or health promotion activities intended to enhance or improve the state of wellness. They include topics such as extended family members and their role in the child's life, cultural variations or inclusion, or development of moral values and ethical behaviors. The nurse should be alert for clues to potential areas for discussion and should invite the family several times during a visit to ask any questions that they might have. See Developing Cultural Competence: Culture and Disease.

NURSING MANAGEMENT

Nursing Assessment and Diagnosis

During health supervision visits, a portrait of the child and family will emerge. Observe the parent-child interaction in the waiting room and throughout the examination. If siblings are present, watch for interactions among all family members. Observe affect and mood of child and parents. Nursing assessment of the child and family at each visit for health supervision then focuses on the following:

- Interviewing the family and child to update the health history, to ask about the child's developmental or educational progress, to identify dietary habits, physical activity, and safety practices
- Eliciting questions and concerns that the parent or child may have
- Conducting developmental surveillance assessments, including review of questionnaires completed by parent in waiting room
- Performing age-appropriate screening tests (Figure 10–6 ■)
- Performing a physical assessment

Following a thorough assessment, the nurse derives nursing diagnoses that are pertinent to the health status of the child, and which consider the family needs. Nursing diagnoses are developed jointly with the family as an essential component of the partnership between nurse and family. Examples of nursing diagnoses for an 18-month-old child who is brought by parents

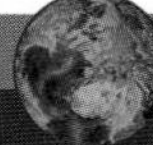

DEVELOPING CULTURAL COMPETENCE
Culture and Disease

Culture and health are intimately linked. Some ethnic groups may have a greater incidence of certain diseases and screening for these diseases should be more commonly performed (see Chapter 3∞). For example, type 2 diabetes is common in African Americans and Native Americans, and ischemic heart disease is at low risk in Chinese Americans. Fair-skinned people are more likely to get skin melanoma.

At other times the perception of health or illness may differ among cultures. Certain Asian cultures may view illness as an imbalance in the body and will need to have certain ceremonies or other procedures done to restore balance. Bad dreams are believed to be responsible for mental illness in some cultural groups. There is varying acceptance of screening tests such as blood work among various groups; and health takes on different meanings for various people—it may be the absence of disease, or the ability to be active in spite of illness, or a state of complete balance.

Be familiar both with common diseases in the groups you see in clinical settings and with the beliefs about health and illness within the groups. Honor the beliefs of others and learn from them, as you share your knowledge in a respectful manner.

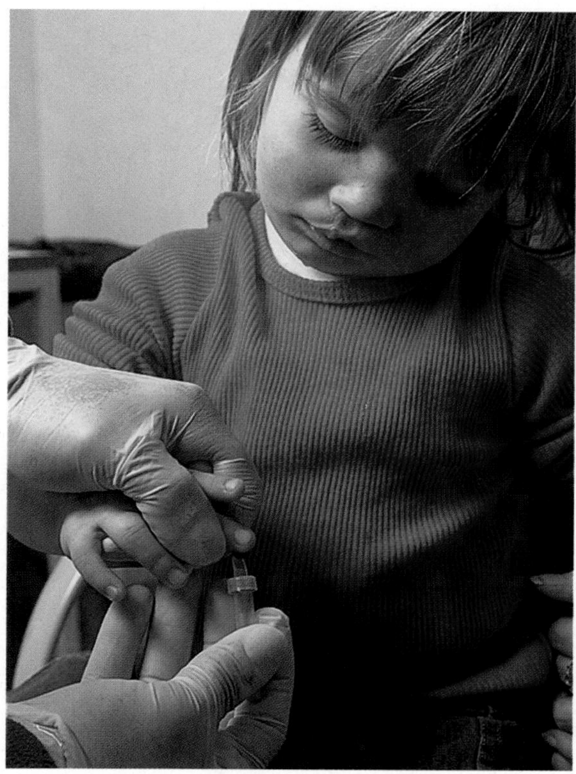

FIGURE 10–6 ■ This 18-month-old toddler is having a blood screening test to detect iron deficiency anemia. Children are often screened for adequate levels of iron in later infancy and during toddlerhood.

for regular health supervision and immunizations may include the following:

- Imbalanced Nutrition: More than Body Requirements related to lack of basic nutritional knowledge
- Risk for Poisoning related to lack of proper precautions with increased mobility to reach and climb
- Health-seeking Behaviors related to needed immunizations
- Risk for Caregiver Role Strain related to mother's plans to return to full-time work

■ Planning and Implementation

Nursing management for health supervision visits begins with collaborative planning with the family. They share their concerns and questions, and the nurse also lists procedures and discussion topics to be addressed. These may include providing immunizations, offering anticipatory guidance about discipline, educating parents and children about healthy behaviors, addressing health promotion regarding nutrition, suggesting ways to prevent disease and injury, and providing referrals for follow-up care. For more information about the recommended schedule for immunizations and the nurse's role in ensuring full immunization status for children, refer to Chapter 19∞.

Most parents want to know how to contribute to their child's growth and development. Discussions at the conclusion of the health supervision assessments should focus on building family strengths by promoting the development of competence, confidence, and self-esteem in the growing child. Offering examples of health promotion activities such as these provides a positive ending for the visit.

Although health supervision most likely takes place only in an office or clinic setting, most of the nursing management for health supervision can occur in any setting. The nurse recognizes that health promotion and health maintenance activities are key to any nurse-family relationship. For example, if the child is seen in an emergency room for treatment of a fracture, the nurse should ask about immunization status and safety issues. A child with a chronic disorder such as cerebral palsy may obtain most health promotion and health maintenance service in the outpatient clinic at an orthopedic hospital. A child hospitalized for an acute respiratory illness often has a parent present and the nurse should explore the health promotion questions that parent has, and perform some teaching about developmental findings. Indeed, health promotion is a constant and foundational aspect of all pediatric care. Viewing it as essential ensures that this part of healthcare, which most closely reflects a partnership with families, will be part of every healthcare encounter. Health maintenance information is included to lessen disease and injury risk. See Figure 10–7 ■. Some specific nursing actions for health supervision are described next.

Provide Anticipatory Guidance

Anticipatory guidance involves prediction of the upcoming developmental tasks or needs of a child and gears teaching to those needs. It provides the family with information on what to expect during the child's current and next stage of development. Topics for each visit should include age-appropriate information about healthy habits, prevention of illness and injury, prevention of poisoning, nutrition, oral health, and sexuality. Use health promotional guidance to help the child and family develop strategies that support and enhance social development, family relationships, parental health, community interactions, self-responsibility, and school or vocational achievement.

Because the time for each visit is limited, build upon the parents' current knowledge and care practices, and start with a topic about which they expressed interest. Time can be used to focus on anticipatory guidance to introduce new information, to reinforce what the family is doing well, and to clear up any poorly understood concepts.

Take advantage of other sources of information in the community to enhance the guidance provided. For example, state and local SAFE KIDS Coalitions help inform families about injury prevention strategies. School health programs such as the National Fire Prevention Association's "Risk Watch" may educate children about injury prevention, and other school programs may educate students about smoking and drug avoidance. Keep informed about the types of health education provided in different community settings so it is easier to reinforce the concepts already being taught.

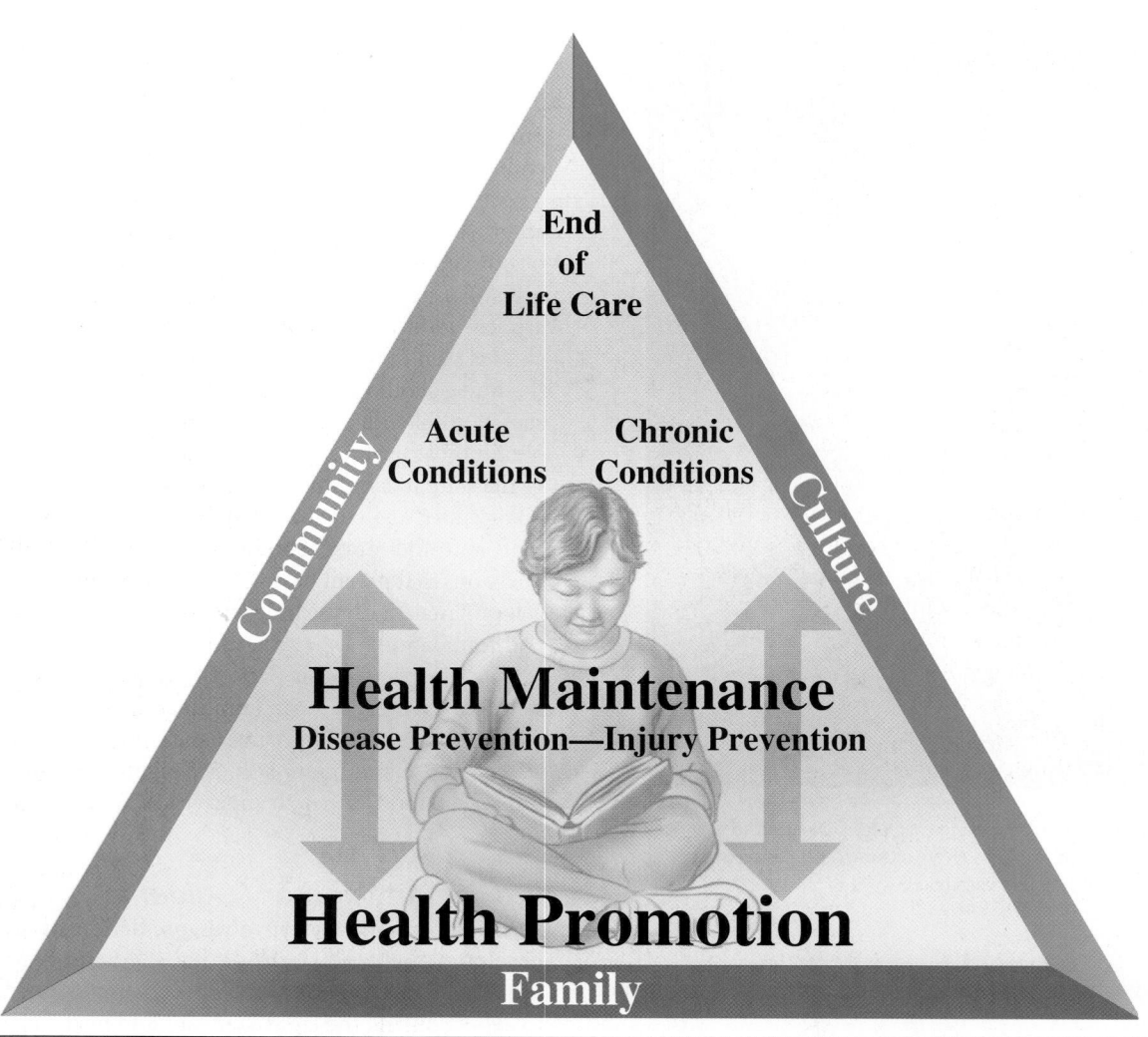

FIGURE 10–7 ■ The Bindler-Ball Continuum of Pediatric Healthcare for Children and Their Families. Health promotion is foundational to all care in pediatric nursing. Health promotion and health maintenance activities take place at health supervision visits and provide the strong foundation for health as the infant grows into childhood and adolescence. The influences from these activities are carried forward as the child experiences any chronic or acute conditions. Likewise, health promotion and maintenance activities can take place at any health encounter. Health promotion goals of balance and spiritual peace may even be met at end of life. Notice that the family is the strong foundation upon which the child's health encounters rest. The family is an integral part of the child's health and has a strong influence upon it. The community and culture must also be examined to understand their ramifications regarding the child's health status.

Encourage Health Promotion Activities

Families often need health education and counseling to promote healthy behaviors in their own children. Examples of focused health education and counseling may be information about environmental control to limit sedentary behaviors, dietary changes to increase fruit and vegetable intake, and switching to low-fat dairy products. Counseling in the case of the 18-month-old toddler for whom nursing diagnoses were previously stated could focus on childcare arrangements and the anticipation and management of potential behavior problems. Partner with the parents to learn what concerns they have and how they want to improve their parenting.

Patient education and counseling are most effective when the family understands the relationship between a behavior change and the resulting health outcome. The parents and child can then work in partnership with the nurse or healthcare provider and make a commitment to the change or changes needed. The Health Belief Model (Glanz, Lewis, & Rimer, 1997; Young & Hayes, 2002) helps to explain how people decide whether to participate in programs or activities to prevent disease or enhance health (Table 10–8). They consider whether the health problem is serious and whether they are likely to get the condition. For example, in a family with several members with diabetes, a father is more likely to believe his overweight child will develop diabetes. He is aware of the seriousness of the disease from direct observation. He may weigh the benefits of his child's weight loss and activity increase (disease prevention) against the barriers (child fighting with him over food, difficulty managing teen's intake). Then several modifying factors

TABLE 10–8 Health Belief Model

INDIVIDUAL PERCEPTION OF HEALTH THREAT	INFLUENCES ON MOTIVATION TO TAKE ACTION	MODIFYING FACTORS	LIKELIHOOD OF ACTION
Susceptible to disease or condition	Benefits (i.e., prevent pain and maintain activity)	Social, psychologic, community factors (i.e., age, social class, media, previous experiences with condition)	Perceived benefits minus perceived barriers
Disease or condition is serious	Barriers (i.e., time or change required for new behavior)	**Self-efficacy** (i.e., confidence in one's own ability to make change)	

How might the child's self-efficacy (confidence in ability to change) affect the likelihood that the child will adapt increased physical activity?
How can you decrease barriers to health behavior changes?

Note: Data from Glanz, K., Lewis, F. M., & Rimer, B. (Eds.). (1997). Health behavior and health education: Theory, research, and practice *(2nd ed.) San Francisco: Jossey-Bass and Young, L. E., & Hayes, V. (2002).* Transforming health promotion practice: Concepts, issues, and applications. *Philadelphia: F.A. Davis Company.*

may influence the situation. The family may have healthcare so that the child can get screened and enter a weight-loss program, or media announcements may have been made about diabetes, and the teen's motivation to change and confidence in her ability to alter her diet may affect decision making. When finding a family that would benefit from a change in health behavior, consider their perceptions, modifying factors, barriers, and benefits and plan interventions to enhance the possibility for change.

Steps in promoting patient education and counseling are as follows:

- Clarify learning needs of child and family.
- Set a limited agenda.
- Prioritize needs with family.
- Select teaching strategy (explaining, showing, providing resources, questioning, practicing, giving feedback).
- Evaluate effectiveness. (Green & Palfrey, 2002)

Perform Health Supervision Interventions

After all of the information from the interviews, physical assessment, and screening tests is collected and analyzed, specific health and developmental achievements should be summarized for the parents and child. Immunizations are provided as appropriate. Anticipatory guidance may be offered at various points during the health supervision visit.

When a child is found to be at risk for a health condition, integrate health maintenance interventions to lessen the possibility of disease or injury. If an actual health problem is detected, follow-up care must be arranged. The child may need to return for another visit to the primary care provider for further evaluation, or referral to another provider may be needed. The nurse needs to learn about all of the available community resources to make appropriate referrals. The range of such services may include the following:

- Hospital- and community-based healthcare specialists from a variety of disciplines (dentists, physicians, physical therapists, speech therapists, nutritionists, social workers)
- Community-based programs (childcare centers, developmental stimulation programs, home visitor programs, early intervention programs, mental health centers, diagnostic and evaluation centers, schools, family support centers, food and nutrition referral centers, public health clinics, churches, and other organizations that support families and children)

Evaluation

Expected outcomes of nursing care include the following:

- The child and family collaborate in a partnership with the healthcare provider in joint problem solving and decision making regarding the management of the child's healthcare needs after appropriate education and counseling.
- The child and family prepare for future health supervision visits by identifying questions or concerns they want to discuss.

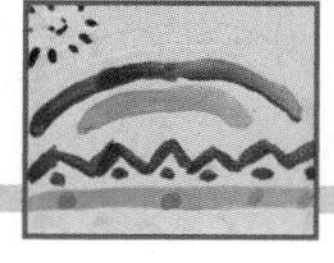

CHAPTER HIGHLIGHTS

- Health is a state of physical, mental, and social well-being and is the objective of health promotion and health maintenance activities.
- Theories of resilience and ecology provide guidance in health promotion and health maintenance activities.
- Health supervision visits are healthcare encounters designed to provide assessment, screening, developmental surveillance, immunizations, and health information.

- Partners in providing health supervision are the child, family, health professional, and community.
- Families are best educated in "teachable moments" with small bits of information.
- Developmental surveillance is an essential part of health supervision that provides for observations of children's fine and gross motor skills, language, and psychosocial behavior milestones.
- Nutrition, physical activity, and oral health are essential topics during health supervision visits.
- Mental and spiritual status, as well as the relationships in the family and larger community, are assessed at each health supervision visit.
- The nurse establishes diagnoses based on a thorough assessment of the child and family during healthcare visits.
- The nurse establishes goals for visits collaboratively with families, and plans interventions to meet goals.
- Health promotion and health maintenance interventions are essential components of all child healthcare, even during periods of acute or chronic illness.

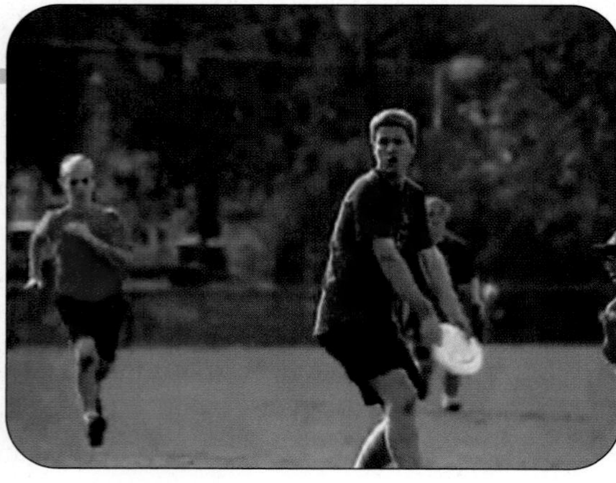

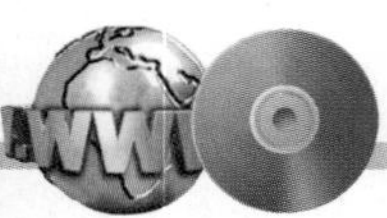

EXPLORE MediaLink

- NCLEX review, case studies, and other interactive resources for this chapter can be found on the Companion Website at **http://www.prenhall.com/ball**. Click on Chapter 10 to select the activities for this chapter.
- For animations, more NCLEX review questions, and an audio glossary, access the accompanying CD-ROM in this book.

http://www.prenhall.com/ball

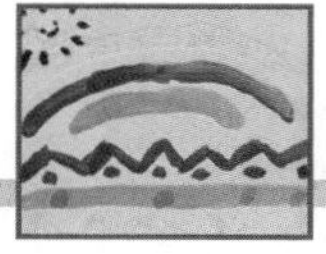

CRITICAL THINKING IN ACTION

INTRODUCTION

Recall the Yevteshenko family in the opening scenario. Tony is receiving dental care for the first time as a 7-year-old and his 5-year-old brother is waiting his turn. The family recently emigrated from Lithuania and is adjusting to life in this country.

DESCRIPTION

The nurse in the mobile van finds that Tony has well-developed English skills and often acts as translator when his parents do not understand questions. He states that he and his brother Ilya like school and that the school nurse is nice to them. She had referred the family to the mobile van for health and oral care. The boys had medical visits and immunizations in Lithuania, but never had been to a dentist. They are excited about this visit and interact positively with all staff members. The children and parents appear well nourished and state that they have a comfortable home, adequate clothing, and are able to find foods they like to eat.

DISCUSSION

1. With the father's limited employment, what health and dental care insurance needs might the family have? Are there programs for emigrants in your community or state to which a family such as the Yevteshenkos could be referred?
2. The family has several protective factors such as their willingness to make an appointment and come to the van for care. What other protective factors can you identify? What risk factors?
3. Relationships are an important part of development for school-age children. How will you assess the relationships that Tony and Ilya have at school with peers? How can you as the nurse in the mobile van partner with the school nurse to provide comprehensive health promotion and health maintenance for these boys?
4. Plan a teaching session to include Tony and Ilya that demonstrates tooth brushing and flossing and allows for return demonstration. How can you and the dental hygienist partner with the family to be sure oral care at home is adequate, and access to professional dental care occurs on a regular basis?

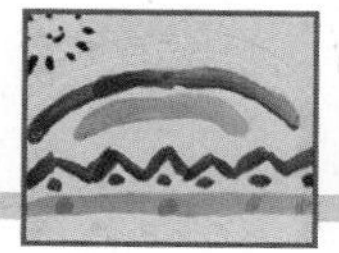

REFERENCES

American Academy of Pediatrics. (2002). The medical home. Policy statement. *Pediatrics, 110,* 184–186.

Bronfenbrenner, U., McClelland, P. D., Ceci, S. J., Moen, P., & Wethington, E. (1996). *The state of Americans.* New York: Free Press.

Clark, M. J. (2003). *Community health nursing: Caring for populations* (4th ed.). Upper Saddle River, NJ: Prentice Hall.

Deloian, B. J. (1997). Screening tests. In J. A. Fox (Ed.), *Primary health care of children* (pp. 148–157). St Louis: Mosby.

Glanz, K., Lewis, F. M., & Rimer, B. (Eds.). (1997). *Health behavior and health education: Theory, research, and practice* (2nd ed.). San Francisco: Jossey-Bass.

Green, M., & Palfrey, J. S. (2000). *Bright futures: Guidelines for health supervision of infants, children, and adolescents* (2nd ed.). Washington, DC: U.S. Department of Health and Human Services.

Jellinek, M., Patel, B. P., & Froehle, M. C. (Eds.). (2002). *Bright futures in practice: Mental health* (Vol. I and II). Arlington, VA: National Center for Education in Maternal and Child Health.

Lalonde, M. (1974). *A new perspective on the health of Canadians.* Ottawa: Health and Welfare Canada.

MMWR. (2003). Physical activity levels among children aged 9–13 years—United States, 2002. *Morbidity and Mortality Weekly Report, 52,* 785–788.

Murray, R. B., & Zentner, J. P. (2001). *Health promotion strategies through the life span* (7th ed.). Upper Saddle River, NJ: Prentice Hall.

National Association of Pediatric Nurse Associates and Practitioners [NAPNAP]. (2002). NAPNAP position statement on the pediatric health care home. www.napnap.org/practice/positions/healthcarehome.html, accessed 8/25/2003.

Office of Public Health and Science and Office of Disease Prevention and Promotion. (1998). *Put prevention into practice: Clinician's handbook of preventive services* (2nd ed.). Washington, DC: U.S. Department of Health and Human Services, Public Health Services.

Patrick, K., Spear, B., Holt, K., & Sofka, D. (Eds.). (2001). *Bright futures in practice: Physical activity.* Arlington, VA: National Center for Education in Maternal and Child Health.

Pender, N. J., Murdaugh, C. L., & Parsons, M. A. (2002). *Health promotion in nursing practice* (4th ed.). Upper Saddle River, NJ: Prentice Hall.

Ryan, J. (2003). Improving oral health: Promise and prospects. *National Health Policy Forum Background Paper.* Washington, DC: The George Washington University.

VanLandeghen, L., Bronstein, J., & Brach, C. (2003). *Children's dental care access in Medicaid. The role of medical care use and dentist participation* (CHIRI Issue Brief 2) (AHRQ Publication No. 03-0032). Rockville, MD: Agency for Healthcare Research and Quality. www.ahrq.gov/about/cods/chirident.htm, accessed 6/30/2003.

World Health Organization. (2001). *Background information about health promotion.* www.who.int/hpr/backgroundhp/, accessed 6/6/2003.

World Health Organization. (1996). *Basic document* (36th ed.). Geneva, Switzerland: WHO.

World Health Organization. (1999). *Ottawa charter for health promotion.* www.who.int/hpr/archive/docs/ottawa.html, accessed 5/30/2003.

Young, L. E., & Hayes, V. (2002). *Transforming health promotion practice: Concepts, issues, and applications.* Philadelphia: F.A. Davis Company.

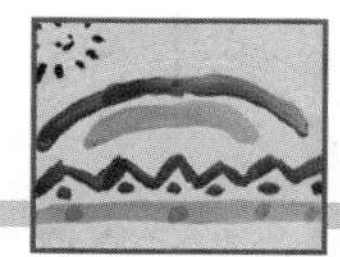

ADDITIONAL REFERENCES

Boyle, M. A., & Morris, D. H. (1999). *Community nutrition in action* (2nd ed.). Belmont, CA: West/Wadsworth.

Denehy, J. (1999). Health promotion: A golden opportunity for school nurses. *Journal of School Nursing, 15,* 4–5.

Edelman, C. L., & Mandle, C. L. (2002). *Health promotion throughout the life span* (5th ed.). St. Louis: Mosby.

Glanz, K., Rimer, B. K., & Lewis, F. M. (Eds.). (2002). *Health behavior and health education: Theory, research, and practice* (3rd ed.). Boston: John Wiley.

Hammermeister, J., & Peterson, M. (2001). Does spirituality make a difference? Psychosocial and health-related characteristics of spiritual well-being. *American Journal of Health Education, 32,* 293–297.

Lipman, T. H., & Hayman, L. L. (2000). Celebrating 25 years of pediatric nursing research: Progress and prospects. *MCN, 25,* 331–335.

Rice, A. H. (2000). Interdisciplinary collaboration in health care: Education, practice, and research. *National Academies of Practice Forum, 2,* 59–73.

Sessanna, L. (2003). Teaching holistic child health promotion using Watson's theory of human science and human care. *Journal of Pediatric Nursing, 18,* 64–68.

Story, M., Holt, K., & Sofka, D. (Eds.). (2002). *Bright futures in practice: Nutrition* (2nd ed.). Arlington, VA: National Center for Education in Maternal and Child Health.

Chapter

11

Health Promotion and Health Maintenance of the Newborn

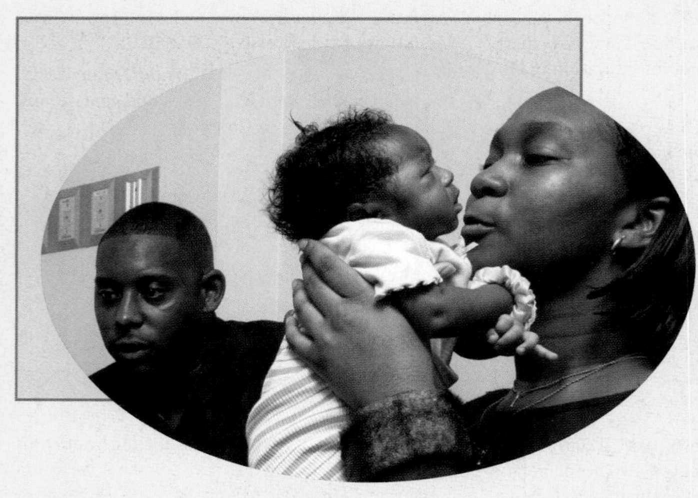

Shannon Regis comes to the pediatric health services clinic with her 10-day-old daughter, Rhonda. Shannon is a 22-year-old single mother who lives with her 5-year-old daughter and boyfriend of 2 years. Shannon had an uncomplicated pregnancy and birth. Rhonda was born at 37 weeks' gestation. She required phototherapy for newborn jaundice and had initial difficulties breastfeeding. Rhonda was discharged at 5 days of age in good health. The nurse weighs and measures Rhonda, and notices that she weighs just 1 oz more than her birth weight. Shannon voices concerns that Rhonda sleeps very little, cries a lot at night, and makes sleep difficult for her boyfriend, who has to get up early for work. The nurse asks Shannon how she knows when Rhonda is ready to feed. Shannon recognizes only Rhonda's crying as a feeding cue. The nurse gives Shannon information on newborn states and cues, and encourages Shannon to notice more subtle feeding cues. The nurse calls the lactation consultant and together they assess the effectiveness of Rhonda's breastfeeding. The lactation consultant works with Shannon on a feeding plan to ensure that Rhonda is getting enough milk to gain weight. Then the pediatric nurse partners with Shannon to strategize how to help Rhonda sleep for longer periods, recognizing that newborns often do not settle into a schedule until well into the second month. What ongoing assessment will Rhonda and her parents need? How can the nurse encourage shared parenting between Shannon and her boyfriend? What coordinated follow-up is required between the pediatric nurse and the lactation consultant?

"I'm a big sister! Mommy says she's excited, but she takes naps a lot. She says new babies are mixed up about sleeping. Rhonda sleeps in the daytime and the nighttime."

—Denise, 5 years old

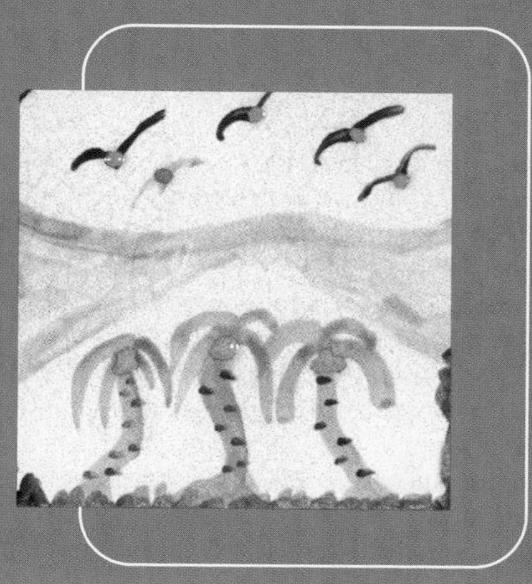

Learning Outcomes

After completing this chapter, you will be able to:

- Verbalize the important link between prenatal care and health promotion and health maintenance of the family and newborn.
- Define term, preterm, and postterm newborn.
- Identify the major health concerns of the newborn.
- Describe physical and developmental milestones expected by the end of the first month of life.
- Apply assessment skills to gather data regarding nutrition, physical activity, mental health status, and growth and development of newborns.
- Apply therapeutic communication skills with the newborn and family during health supervision visits.
- Intervene with newborns and their families to integrate activities to promote health and to prevent disease and injury.
- Synthesize data from history and examination of the newborn and family to plan approaches useful with the family during health supervision encounters.
- Describe the advantages of breastfeeding and the nurse's role in breastfeeding promotion.

MediaLink http://www.prenhall.com/ball

Resources for this chapter can be found on the CD-ROM accompanying this textbook, and on the Companion Website at www.prenhall.com/ball. Click on Chapter 11 to select the activities for this chapter.

CD-ROM

Videos

Making the Pacifier Decision
Responding to a Baby's Cry

NCLEX Review

Audio Glossary

COMPANION WEBSITE

NCLEX Review

Case Study: Newborn Weight Loss

MediaLink Applications

Develop an Agency Plan: Newborn Abduction Prevention
Plot Weight and Measurements to Assess Size

Key Terms

appropriate for gestational age (AGA)/393
attachment behaviors/393
continuum of care/391
corrected age/397
co-sleeping/406
dental caries/398
dental home/398
developmental delay/394
domestic violence/386
infant cues/398
infant mental health/398
infant state/399
large for gestational age (LGA)/393
metabolic screening/403
postpartum/386
postpartum blues/400
postpartum depression/400
postpartum mood disorder (PPMD)/400
postpartum psychosis/400
prenatal care/386
self-regulation/398
shaken baby syndrome (SBS)/406
SIDS (sudden infant death syndrome)/407
small for gestational age (SGA)/393
temperament/393

A healthy pregnancy usually results in the birth of a healthy newborn. The expectant mother focuses on her pregnancy and the major event of labor and birth. Often the expectant mother is so focused on her pregnancy and anticipated labor experience that the responsibilities and demands of parenthood come as a shock after she gives birth and realizes that she is now a mother.

For a healthy woman, prenatal care, labor, and birth may be her first experience of an ongoing relationship with healthcare professionals. The quality of that experience is key to ensuring a continuing partnership between her and her child's healthcare providers.

The month following delivery is a time of huge transition for the new mother and her family. Not only is the mother coping with hormonal shifts and a **postpartum** (after giving birth) body, but roles and relationships are also changing. The role of the nurse is to assess knowledge about self-care and newborn care, teach health promotion and maintenance activities, promote parental confidence in newborn caregiving, and promote a partnership among healthcare professionals and the family.

EARLY CONTACTS WITH THE FAMILY

Prenatal

The nurse who sees the expectant woman during **prenatal care,** healthcare supervision during pregnancy, has the unique opportunity to help parents prepare for their new roles. The nurse listens attentively and provides information and support. During prenatal visits, parents learn to value health supervision and an active partnership with healthcare professionals.

Prenatal Assessment of Risk and Protective Factors

The nurse who interacts with the family in the prenatal period assesses risk and protective factors. A pregnant woman is more likely to change risky behaviors, such as smoking, during pregnancy than at any other time in her life (Orleans, Barker, Kaufman, et al., 2000). The motivation to give birth to a healthy newborn is usually strong, and the nurse can use maternal readiness for change to promote behaviors that improve maternal and newborn health.

Risk factors should be assessed throughout pregnancy. The nurse begins with the questions that demonstrate interest in the woman's health and well-being. The more sensitive questions, such as use of drugs and alcohol and **domestic violence,** a pattern of assaultive or coercive behaviors, are asked after the nurse establishes rapport with the woman. Questions to assess risk factors include:

- "Is this a good time for you to be pregnant?"
- "How does your family feel about having a new baby?"
- "How has your pregnancy been for you so far? Have you had any physical or emotional problems?"
- "What is the most exciting part of becoming parents? The most worrisome part?"
- "How do you think a baby will change your lives?"
- "How were you raised? Will you raise your baby the same way, or what things would you change?"
- "Who will help you with caring for the baby in the first few weeks?"
- "Do you plan to breastfeed or formula feed? How did you make that decision? Do you need more information?"
- "Do you have concerns about labor and giving birth? What are they?"
- "If your newborn is a boy, are you considering circumcision?" (See Developing Cultural Competence: Circumcision and Partnering with Families: Circumcision.)
- "Are you considering umbilical cord blood collection?" (See Box 11–1.)
- "Are you ready at home for your baby? Do you have clothing, diapers, a crib, a car safety seat that is intended for a newborn? Do you know how to use your newborn's car safety seat?"
- "Do you have financial worries? Do you worry about being able to pay your rent, for food or baby supplies?"

BOX 11–1 Umbilical Cord Blood Collection

Umbilical cord blood is a rich source of stem cells, unspecialized blood cells that produce all other blood cells. In some cases, cord blood is an alternative to bone marrow transplant and has been used to treat a number of oncologic, hematologic, and immunologic disorders (AAP, 1999b). At this time, about 45 disorders can be treated with stem cells retrieved from the umbilical cord at birth (March of Dimes, 2004b).

Pregnant women may receive direct mail information from commercial blood banks about cord blood banking and wonder if they should collect and bank their newborn's cord blood in case the newborn or family member develops a condition in the future for which the stem cells in cord blood would be a lifesaving treatment. A woman also has the option of donating cord blood to a public bank, which makes their cord blood available to any appropriately matched individual in need of a stem cell transplant. Private cord blood banking comes at a price: An initial fee of $250 to $1,500 and an annual storage fee of $50 to $100 (March of Dimes, 2004b).

Parents may be influenced by the emotional appeal to collect umbilical cord blood for future healthcare usage in their families. Who should consider umbilical cord blood banking?

The American Academy of Pediatrics acknowledges that it is difficult to estimate the likelihood of a family needing cord blood cells for transplantation. The estimate of need ranges from 1 in 1,000 to 1 in 200,000. Therefore, private storage of cord blood as "biological insurance" is not recommended for most families at this time (AAP, 1999b).

Umbilical cord blood banking should be considered if the family has a child with a genetic disorder that is potentially treatable with stem cell transplantation. Research is ongoing and the list of diseases that are potentially treatable with cord blood transplantation is growing. Treatable disorders include severe combined immune deficiency, thalassemia, sickle cell anemia, leukemia, lymphoma, and metabolic storage disorders such as Hurler syndrome (Mills, 2000).

Arrangements for umbilical cord blood collection must be made well before labor and birth. Consent for the procedure should be obtained during a prenatal visit (AAP, 1999b). The parent is responsible for making arrangements with the umbilical cord blood bank of their choosing. A member of the delivery room staff attempts to collect approximately 3 to 5 oz of cord blood immediately after delivery using a collection kit provided by the cord blood storage agency. The cord blood is then shipped to the designated laboratory, processed, and stored for potential future use (March of Dimes, 2004b).

PARTNERING WITH FAMILIES

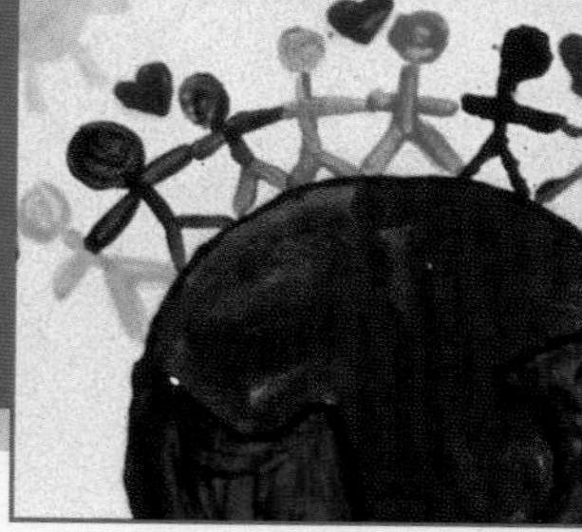

Circumcision

Circumcision is the surgical removal of the foreskin from the tip of the penis. Parents of all male newborns should be given accurate and unbiased information about circumcision, an opportunity to discuss the decision, and decide what is in the best interests of the child. In addition to cultural, religious, and ethnic traditions, parents should take into account medical factors when making this decision. The American Academy of Pediatrics does not recommend routine newborn circumcision (AAP, 1999a). There is little evidence to suggest that circumcision prevents penile problems such as phimosis, penile inflammation, or balanitis. The true frequency of these problems is unknown; however, penile problems may develop in both circumcised and uncircumcised males.

- Research demonstrates that uncircumcised males have an increased risk of urinary tract infection (UTI), with the greatest risk in infants younger than 1 year of age. However, studies vary in methodology, samples of infants used, determination of circumcision status, method of urine collection, UTI definition, and assessment of confounding variables such as prematurity and breastfeeding.
- The risk of developing penile cancer is higher in uncircumcised men than circumcised men; however, the overall risk is low. In the United States the annual penile cancer rate is 9 to 10 cases of penile cancer per year per 1 million men. Some research suggests a relationship among hygiene, phimosis, and penile cancer and that good hygiene (attainable without circumcision) prevents phimosis and penile cancer.
- Research regarding the relationship between circumcision and acquisition of sexually transmitted infections (STI) is conflicting. Studies suggest that circumcision reduces the risk of syphilis and HIV infection in the male; however, behavioral risk factors are more important in the acquisition of HIV than circumcision status.
- There is little evidence that circumcised males have better penile hygiene than uncircumcised males.
- Research is inconclusive regarding whether uncircumcised males have more varied sexual practice, less sexual dysfunction, and better tactile discrimination than circumcised males.
- Complications of newborn circumcisions are rare, and most are minor. The most frequent complication is bleeding, which occurs in approximately 0.1% of circumcision. Infection is the second most common complication and most of these infections are minor.

Adapted from American Academy of Pediatrics. (1999a) Circumcision Policy Statement. Pediatrics, *103(3), 686–693.*

- "Do you have a gun at home? Is the gun unloaded and locked up? Where is the ammunition stored? Would you consider getting rid of the gun because of the danger to children and other family members?"
- "Are you safe in your relationships? Does your partner ever kick, slap, shove, hit you, or yell at you?" (Ask this question to the woman when she is alone, never when her partner is in the room with her.)
- "How many cigarettes do you smoke in a day? Did you use alcohol before you knew you were pregnant? How many drinks do you drink in a day (or in a week) now? Tell me about any street drugs or prescription drugs that you take now. Does your partner use any street drugs?"

(Green & Palfrey, 2002)

Most obstetrical care providers encourage the expectant mother to choose her newborn's care provider prior to the baby's birth. Pediatric care providers usually welcome a short office visit, sometimes at no charge, to allow the expectant mother and care provider to assess their "fit" prior to committing to this important relationship (American Academy of Pediatrics [AAP], 2001) (see Partnering with Families: Prenatal Visit to the Pediatric Care Provider). Most pediatric care providers have written information for expectant parents, explaining their professional philosophy of care as well as information about services.

At Birth

The hospital length of stay for a healthy mother and newborn is short, approximately 48 hours for a vaginal birth and 72 to 96 hours for an uncomplicated cesarean birth; a hospital stay of less than 48 hours requires that certain criteria be met prior to newborn discharge (AAP, 2004b). During the hospital stay, the nurse provides ongoing physical assessment of the mother and newborn, while providing education and anticipatory guidance to prepare the mother to care for herself and her newborn following hospital discharge.

DEVELOPING CULTURAL COMPETENCE
Circumcision

Circumcision is uncommon in Asia, South and Central America, and most of Europe. About 48% of Canadian newborns are circumcised (AAP, 1999a). Based on available data, it is believed that a majority of newborn males in the United States are circumcised; however, the rate of circumcision varies by region, religion, and socioeconomic status. In the United States, Whites are more likely to be circumcised (81%) than Blacks (65%) or Hispanics (54%) (AAP, 1999a, p. 2).

PRACTICE ALERT

Standard precautions should be observed when handling the newborn immediately after birth. Most blood and fluids are wiped from the baby's skin at birth with a towel or blanket to prevent further heat loss and reduce the risk of bloodborne infection from mother to infant and from infant to care provider. However, to protect the care provider from residual blood and amniotic fluid on the newborn's skin, gloves must be worn when handling the newborn for any reason prior to the newborn's first bath. Wash hands immediately before gloving and after gloves are removed (AAP & ACOG, 2002).

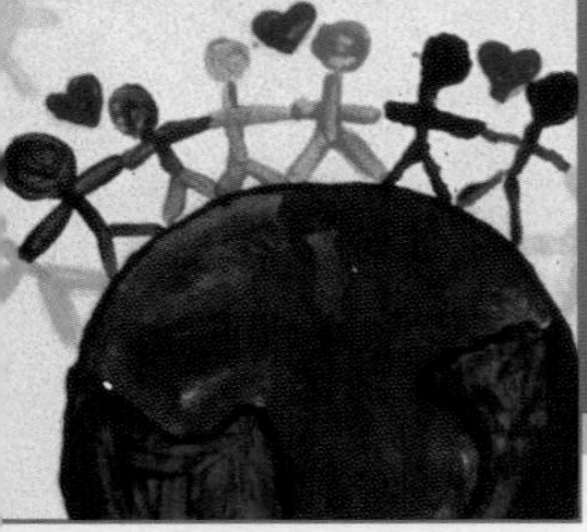

PARTNERING WITH FAMILIES

Prenatal Visit to the Pediatric Care Provider

Encourage parents to visit the pediatric healthcare home before the baby is born. This will ensure that the home will provide the type of care they want for their infant. Assist parents to prepare questions and make an appointment to visit the provider they are interested in interviewing.

Questions they can ask the provider include:

- How soon after birth will the baby be seen? Can parents be present during the initial physical examination? Will you speak with us again before hospital discharge?
- What is your philosophy about male circumcision? Do you perform circumcision? If not, who does this procedure? Is circumcision performed in the hospital before discharge or in the office after discharge?
- What if our baby needs intensive care? Under what circumstances would our baby need to be transported to a different hospital? Would you continue to provide the baby's care, during the hospital stay and after discharge?
- When is our newborn's first office visit? Do we call for that appointment or is it made for us while we are in the hospital?
- As our baby's provider, what can I expect from you? What do you think is your most important job? What do you enjoy most about your work?
- As the parent of a new baby, what do you expect from me? What is my most important job?
- What are the costs of care? Do you accept my method of payment/insurance/government assistance?
- What are office hours? Do you take emergency calls from your own patients at night? What number do we call if we have a question or if we think the baby is sick outside of office hours?
- Who covers your office when you are unavailable? Do you have partners in the office or colleagues in the community who cover for you when you are out? May I have a list of their names and phone numbers?
- Who else answers our questions about routine baby and childcare? What is that person's training? May we meet that person today?
- How much time is usually spent on an office visit? How much time will we have to ask questions?
- If our child needs hospitalization, what hospital do you prefer to use? Would you be our baby's doctor, or would you refer the hospital care to someone else? Why?
- What do you think are the most important things you offer to new families like us? Do you have resources to support breastfeeding mothers? Working mothers?
- If we disagree about a childcare issue or a course of treatment, how would we come to an understanding?

After the interview, parents can ask themselves the following questions.

- Was I comfortable talking with this person? Did this person listen to me?
- Did I get clear answers to my questions?
- Do I feel that I could trust this provider with my child's care?
- Was I comfortable in the office? Did I feel welcome?
- Were all staff members friendly and helpful? Did all staff members seem good at their jobs?
- Did I feel like this provider would be a good "fit" for my family?

Data from American Academy of Pediatrics. (2001). The prenatal visit. Pediatrics, 107*(6) and Shelov, S. P. (Ed.). 2004, 4th edition.* The American Academy of Pediatrics: Caring for your baby and young child: Birth to age 5. *New York: Bantam Books.*

The birth experience and first few postpartum days can be busy and distracting for new mothers, making it difficult for them to focus on self-care and newborn care instructions. Most hospitals offer discharge instructions in a variety of formats in the hope that parents will retain the most essential information. To facilitate learning for parents with different learning styles and literacy levels, nurses use bedside teaching, return demonstration, and written pamphlets for parent education. Many hospitals and birthing centers have a series of videotapes, DVDs, or closed-circuit TV channels with information for new families. Parents can watch when it is convenient and the nurse can discuss their questions and thoughts after they view. In addition, some hospitals send parents home with a video or DVD of postpartum and baby care instructions which enables parents to see and hear instructions at home.

Although challenging, the nurse incorporates many newborn health promotion and maintenance activities into this short stay. Starting at the moment of birth, the newborn is continuously assessed and procedures are performed to ensure newborn health. For the healthy newborn, basic activities usually include:

- First bath (to remove blood and amniotic fluid from the newborn's skin and prevent transmission of microorganisms to others)
- Umbilical cord care (Figure 11–1 ■ and Box 11–2)
- Vitamin K injection (to prevent vitamin K deficiency bleeding [VKDB])
- Eye prophylaxis (administration of ophthalmic antibiotic ointment to prevent gonococcal ophthalmia neonatorum)
- Physical assessment (see Chapter 8∞)
- Feeding assessment (see Chapter 9∞)
- Metabolic screening (see page 404∞)

BOX 11–2 Umbilical Cord Care

Cord care practices vary according to region and are often based on institutional tradition rather than evidence-based practice. The objective of cord care is to prevent infection and promote cord separation. Cord care practices include no care, application of triple dye, and application of povidone-iodone, isopropyl alcohol, or antimicrobial ointments. Aseptic cord care decreases bacterial colonization but delays cord separation (Blackburn, 2003, p. 538).

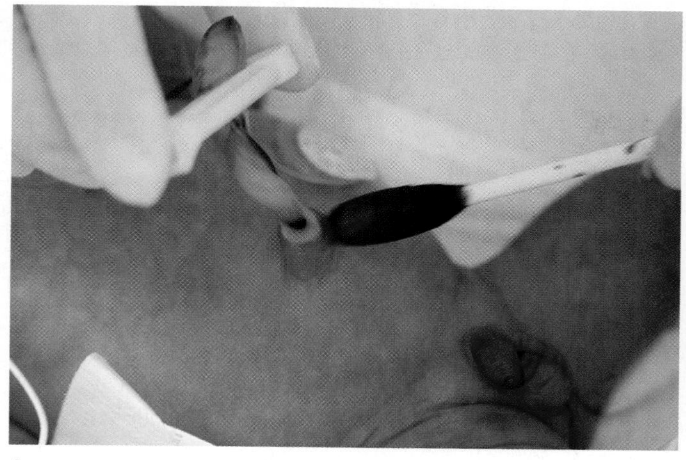

A

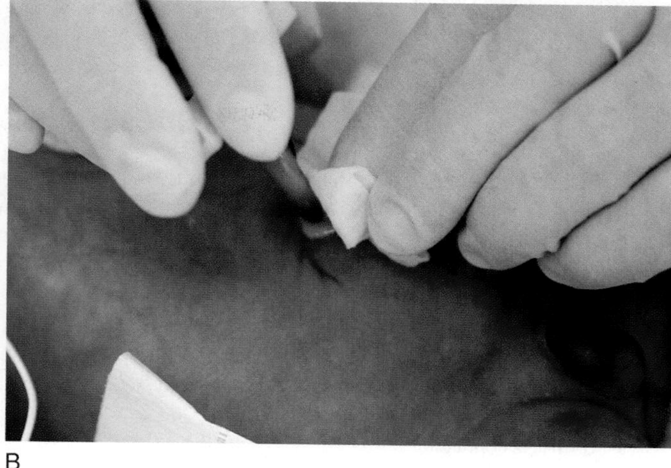

B

FIGURE 11–1 ■ Two different methods for cord care, *A*, betadine cleaning and *B*, alcohol cleaning.

- Hepatitis B vaccination (see Chapter 19∞)
- Hearing screening (see Chapter 24∞)
- Maternal syphilis screen reviewed
- Other screening test results reviewed as indicated by maternal-newborn risk factors and state regulations, including screening for human immunodeficiency virus infection (AAP, 2004b)
- Assessment of parental ability to adequately care for the newborn, recognize and report signs of illness

(AAP & American College of Obstetricians and Gynecologists [ACOG], 2002)

See the medication table on page 390 and Partnering with Families: Discharge Teaching for New Parents.

CLINICAL TIP

Administration of medications can be stressful for the newborn and parents.

- Administer eye prophylaxis before, or at a different time, than the vitamin K injection. The newborn may cry after the vitamin K injection, making it difficult to administer ophthalmic ointment.
- Administer eye prophylaxis when the newborn is calm. Do not attempt to pry the newborn's eyes open when the newborn is crying, or supine and facing bright overhead lights. Dim the room, swaddle or contain the newborn's limbs, and hold the newborn semi-upright. If the newborn is awake or drowsy, the eyes will usually open, allowing easier administration of the ophthalmic ointment.
- The newborn is less likely to cry during the vitamin K injection if the nurse lays the newborn on a firm surface and the parent gently holds the newborn's arms across the newborn's chest during the injection. This "containment" helps the newborn stay calm during the procedure.

Assessment of Risk and Protective Factors

During this short period of hospitalization, the nurse must establish rapport with the mother and family to accurately assess not only physical recovery and well-being but also psychosocial status and preparation for parenthood. Risk and protective factors are assessed and appropriate referrals are made if necessary. Discussion includes the following:

- "How are you feeling?"
- "Was labor and birth what you had expected? What was different?"
- "What do you think of your new baby? Are you surprised by anything about her?"
- "Does your baby seem easy to comfort? What seems to calm the baby when she is crying?"
- "Are you ready to take your baby home? What supplies do you have for baby care (diapers, blankets, and clothing)? Do you have a car safety seat? Will the person who brings you home have the seat in the car today?"
- "Do you have help at home? Who will answer your questions?"
- "Who will you call if you have concerns about yourself or your new baby?"
- "How is feeding your baby going so far? Do you have questions about feeding your baby? Who will you call for breastfeeding questions? OR What formula will you use? How will you prepare the bottles, nipples, and formula?"
- "Do you have concerns about going home today?"

The nurse works closely with both the mother's and newborn's healthcare provider in order to provide coordinated services. For many families, few referrals are necessary and may be routine; for example, all first-time breastfeeding mothers may receive a referral to a lactation consultant, or for a follow-up visit in a hospital-sponsored postpartum/newborn follow-up clinic. For families with complex needs, a multidisciplinary team of nurses, physicians, social workers, mental health professionals, and staff from involved community agencies may be involved in providing comprehensive and coordinated services.

When the nurse assesses a need for referral, the assessment information should be discussed with the primary care provider and documented in the mother's and/or newborn's chart. The nurse's scope of responsibilities for making referrals varies with hospital policy and state regulations. Some referrals require a written order from the mother's primary healthcare provider.

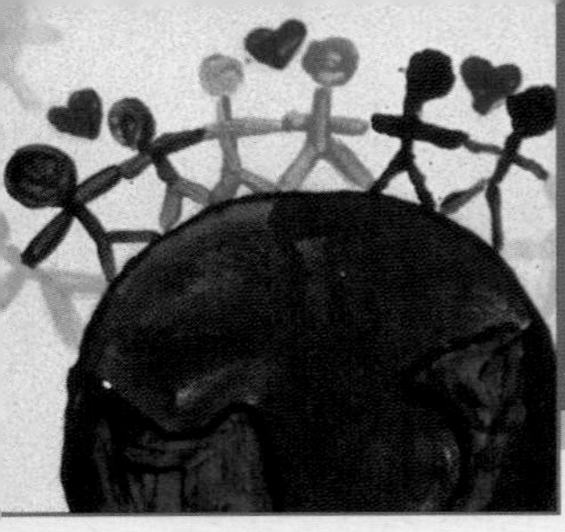

PARTNERING WITH FAMILIES

Discharge Teaching for New Parents

Parents should be taught prior to hospital discharge, and have access at home, to education materials to help ensure adequate care of the newborn and instructions regarding how to access healthcare providers for consultation.

Discharge teaching includes:

- Breastfeeding technique (position, latch, adequacy of urine and stool, lactation referral and resources) or formula feeding technique (formula type, preparation, safety, feeding)
- Umbilical cord care
- Bathing and skin care
- How to diaper and dress a newborn
- Temperature assessment using a thermometer
- Signs of newborn illness
  - Rectal temperature higher than 101°F
  - Abdominal swelling, especially if accompanied by no bowel movement for 1 or 2 days and/or vomiting
  - Blue skin coloring, especially of the face, lips, or tongue (blue hands and feet are normal in the newborn.)
  - Persistent coughing or choking during feedings
  - Unusually long period of crying that will not stop despite comfort measures
  - Jaundice (yellow coloring of the skin) that appears head to toe
  - Sleeping through feedings or baby is too tired or uninterested to eat
  - Infected umbilical cord (pus or red skin at base of cord, crying when skin near the cord is touched with your finger)
  - Respiratory distress
    - Fast breathing (more than 60 breaths/minute)
    - Retractions (muscles between ribs suck in with each breath)
    - Flaring of nose
    - Grunting while breathing
    - Persistent blue skin color
- Immediate newborn safety
  - Infant car seat use
  - Supine sleeping position

Adapted from American Academy of Pediatrics & The American College of Obstetricians and Gynecologists. (2002). Guidelines for perinatal care (5th ed.). *Elk Grove Village, IL: Author, and Shelov, S. P. (Ed.). (2004, 4th edition).* The American Academy of Pediatrics: Caring for your baby and young child: Birth to age 5. *New York: Bantam Books.*

To help ensure that the mother follows through with the referral, the nurse and/or primary care provider should involve the mother in decision making, discuss the purpose of the referral, and state how the mother and/or newborn will benefit from the service.

Newborn Visit Following Hospital Discharge

The American Academy of Pediatrics (2004b and c) recommends that if the newborn is discharged from the hospital in less than 48 hours, an experienced healthcare professional who is competent in newborn assessment should examine the newborn in the clinic or home setting within 48 hours of discharge. For newborns discharged between 48 and 72 hours of age, the first follow-up visit should occur by 5 days of age. The purpose of this visit is to ensure that the newborn is continuing to progress normally and that no previously undiscovered problems have surfaced.

The nurse who assesses the newborn in the clinic or home setting reviews the prenatal and birth history and continues her assessment of the newborn and of ongoing maternal recovery and postpartum adjustment. The nurse weighs the newborn and calculates weight loss; assesses general health, feeding, voiding

PROPHYLACTIC MEDICATIONS Used to Treat Newborns

MEDICATION	PROPHYLACTIC ACTION/IMPLICATION	METHOD/APPLICATION
Vitamin K (phytonadione)	To prevent vitamin K–dependent hemorrhagic disease of the newborn	1 mg IM within 6 hours of birth (AAP, 2005)
Sterile ophthalmic ointment containing tetracycline (1%) or erythromycin (0.5%) or one of a variety of topical agents, including ophthalmic solution of povidone-iodine (2.5%)	As prophylaxis against gonococcal ophthalmia neonatorum	1–2 cm ribbon along the conjunctival sac of each eye within 1 hour of birth, taking care that the agent reaches all areas of the conjunctival sac
Hepatitis B virus (HBV) immunoprophylaxis	• All women should be screened for hepatitis B as part of routine prenatal care • The first hepatitis B vaccination for the newborn is preferably received prior to hospital discharge; however, managed care plans may prefer to vaccinate the newborn beginning with the first outpatient visit.	• For babies of HBsAg-negative women, first dose of HBV vaccine is administered during the newborn period or by age 2 months; second dose 1–2 months later, and third dose by age 6–18 months. • Babies of HBsAg-positive women receive HBV vaccine shortly after birth AND receive one dose of HBIG preferably within 12 hours of birth. Can be given concurrently, in different thighs.

Adapted from American Academy of Pediatrics & The American College of Obstetricians and Gynecologists. (2002). Guidelines for perinatal care *(5th ed.). Elk Grove Village, IL: Author.*

and stooling patterns; and observes mother–infant interaction. This is also an important opportunity to assess the degree of newborn jaundice to prevent the occurrence of newborn kernicterus (Box 11–3).

At this initial contact, the nurse promotes maternal confidence in caregiving and offers education and anticipatory guidance. Following hospital discharge, most new mothers are extremely open to learning about infant care (bathing, diapering, soothing) and breastfeeding. The nurse ensures that the parent knows how to contact the obstetric and pediatric care provider for questions and confirms follow-up appointments. The nurse communicates any concerns about the newborn to the primary care provider on the same day as the visit and interventions are agreed upon (such as an immediate clinic appointment) or referrals are made (for example, to a lactation specialist).

Routine Health Supervision Visits

The schedule for routine infant health supervision visits varies somewhat; however, an assessment by a physician, nurse practitioner, or nurse is recommended at 3 to 5 days of age, with subsequent follow-up visits for newborns at risk for hyperbilirubinemia or feeding problems (AAP, 2004c). Health supervision visits should then occur at 1, 2, 4, 6, 9, and 12 months (Behrman, 2004). (See Chapters 10 and 12.) Pediatric office visits are frequent in the first year of life, and the partnership among the baby's family members and office staff remains essential to ensuring a **continuum of care,** an ongoing relationship between the healthcare provider and family.

The parent must believe that health supervision and surveillance are important to the child's health in order to keep appointments and follow through with suggested health promotion and maintenance activities. Clear communication with parents in a culturally competent setting helps establish trust and impart the value of frequent interactions with providers in the pediatric healthcare home. See Developing Cultural Competence: Effective Care in the Outpatient Setting.

The first outpatient visits influence the tone and effectiveness of future visits (Jellinek, Patel, & Froehle, 2002). The office staff should welcome the baby and family to the office in an unhurried and genuine manner. It is important to convey that the family's and baby's needs are a high priority for the entire staff. The nurse takes time to comment on the baby and validate good parenting ("I like the way you talk to your baby when he makes noises. He really responds to your voice"). The nurse models nurturing behavior as she handles the baby gently and respectfully, and responds to any distress appropriately. Parents should be involved in decreasing the newborn's stress, such as allowing the parent to hold and comfort the baby during immunizations. Clinical findings, such as the baby's current weight and growth percentile, should be explained to parents. Provide pamphlets and reading materials to reinforce information and discussion. Include parents in decision making when possible, such as discussing the need for referrals and making follow-up appointments.

MediaLink Case Study: Newborn Weight Loss

BOX 11–3 Prevention of Kernicterus

Kernicterus is a lifelong neurologic syndrome caused by severe and untreated hyperbilirubinemia (jaundice) during the neonatal period. Kernicterus may result in cerebral palsy, mental retardation, hearing loss, and gaze paresis. Because hyperbilirubinemia can be treated with phototherapy and exchange transfusions, kernicterus is a preventable condition (MMWR, 2001). (See Chapter 30 for more information about newborn hyperbilirubinema.)

All birth settings should provide information for parents about newborn jaundice and when to call their pediatric provider. The pediatric nurse must be alert to parents' reports of signs indicating hyperbilirubinemia in the newborn's first few weeks of life and facilitate immediate medical evaluation. Signs of hyperbilirubinemia in the newborn include (AAP, 2004d):

- Skin more yellow than at discharge
- Yellow abdomen, arms, or legs
- Yellow whites of the eyes
- Yellow skin and is hard to wake, fussy, or not feeding well from the breast or bottle

Newborns 35 weeks' gestation or more who are most at risk for development of severe hyperbilirubinemia include those with (AAP, 2004c):

- Bilirubin level at hospital discharge in the high-risk zone
- Jaundice in the first 24 hours following birth
- Blood group incompatibility
- Gestational age 35–36 weeks
- Sibling received phototherapy for treatment of hyperbilirubinemia
- Cephalhematoma or significant bruising
- Exclusive breastfeeding, particularly if nursing is not going well and weight loss exceeds 10% or more of birth weight
- East Asian race

A newborn's bilirubin level usually peaks at 3–5 days of age, which is when the newborn should be assessed by a healthcare provider. The timing of the first visit depends on the newborn's hospital length of stay and the newborn's risk factors for developing hyperbilirubinemia (AAP, 2004d).

GENERAL OBSERVATIONS

At the first health promotion visit, the nursing assessment begins with general observations of the newborn and family

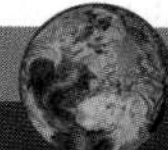

DEVELOPING CULTURAL COMPETENCE: Effective Care in the Outpatient Setting

In the United States, nurses care for families from increasingly diverse cultures. To help ensure that services are welcome and effective for these families, the pediatric nurse must be aware and respectful of families' values, beliefs, traditions, customs, languages, and religious convictions.

- Identify the ethnocultural composition of the practice population and learn about the cultural practices of the families. Ask about parenting practices.
- Attempt cultural diversity within the staff that reflects the racial and ethnic makeup of the practice population.
- Provide language-appropriate materials.
- Have ready access to interpreter services.
- Furnish and decorate waiting rooms and exam areas to reflect the ethnocultural composition of the practice population.
- Conduct staff training in cultural competence.
- Solicit family feedback on cultural competence issues.
- Access resources for working with families from diverse communities.

Adapted from Jellinek M., Patel, B. P., & Froehle, M. C. (Eds). (2002). Bright futures in practice: Mental health *(Vol. I). Arlington, VA: National Center for Education in Maternal and Child Health.*

(Figure 11–2 ■). This often occurs as the family is called in from the waiting area. See Table 11–1.

Welcome the family to the facility and comment on the newborn. Ask how the family is adjusting. In the first month of the newborn's life, parents are usually exhausted and experiencing stressful adjustments in their relationship with each other. The nurse gathers information in order to assess the needs of the family, to invite discussion, to validate positive parenting efforts, and to promote partnership between the family and the health-care team. Questions for new parents may include:

- "How are you feeling these days?"
- "How is Rhonda doing? What do you enjoy most about her?"
- "How can you tell when Rhonda wants to eat? To sleep? What calms her when she's crying?"
- "How is breastfeeding going? How often does Rhonda breastfeed? How long are feedings? What questions or concerns do you have?"
  or, if formula feeding:
- "How much formula does Rhonda drink at a feeding? How often? What questions or concerns do you have about feeding?"
- "Do you have an infant car safety seat? What questions do you have about using the car seat?"
- "How do you position Rhonda for sleep?"

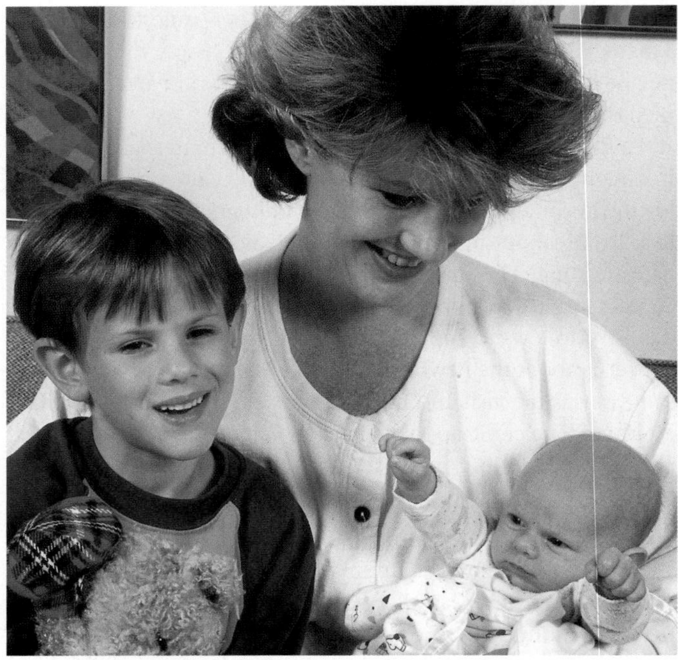

FIGURE 11–2 ■ Observation of the newborn and family begins at first contact during the health supervision and maintenance visit.

TABLE 11–1 General Observations and Implications for Newborn and Family During Health Promotion and Health Maintenance Visits

ASSESSMENT PARAMETER	NORMAL FINDING	OBSERVATION THAT REQUIRES FURTHER ASSESSMENT
Who brings the baby in for care?	Mother and/or father or partner, baby's grandparent(s) and siblings in attendance.	Baby's mother is absent.
Is the parent on time (or nearly on time) for the appointment? Does the parent have adequate transportation? Does the parent share the care provider's philosophy of the importance of timeliness or do cultural differences make timeliness less important to the family than to the care providers?	Parent is on time or nearly on time. Parent calls to say she will be late or reschedules appointment if necessary. Parent may be late if common in culture.	Parent misses appointment and does not reschedule.
Are family members, including the newborn, dressed appropriately for weather conditions?	Family members and the newborn are dressed appropriately for current weather conditions.	Baby, siblings, or parent are overdressed or underdressed.
Is interaction among parents and siblings relaxed and appropriate for the setting?	Parent is attentive to the child's needs. Parent speaks to the newborn in a soothing voice. Parent makes appropriate comments to the baby, such as "You're such a good boy!" or "Let's see how much you weigh today."	Parent ignores the child's needs or requests for attention. Parent is verbally or physically abusive. Parent makes abusive comments to the baby or sibling(s) such as "You always want something!" or "You're as stupid as your father!"
Is the parent's behavior appropriate?	Parent is engaged in the activity, alert, and interactive with newborn and office staff.	Parent is apathetic, lethargic, depressed, hallucinating, belligerent or aggressive, has alcohol on breath, slurred speech, frantic behavior, uncontrollable crying, suicidal ideology.
Does the baby appear healthy, well nourished, and cared for?	Baby appears to be in good health with no respiratory distress, little or no evidence of newborn jaundice, flexed with good muscle tone, responsive to the environment and parent's efforts to calm baby. Baby is clean and appropriately dressed. Parent holds baby protectively and supports baby's head.	Baby is limp, lethargic, or crying excessively. Baby is working hard to breathe or has central cyanosis. Baby is markedly jaundiced. Baby is not appropriately dressed or cleaned, parent places baby in unsafe situations, such as leaving the baby unattended on a chair or exam table, does not hold the newborn in a supportive manner, baby has injuries or bruises unrelated to birth.

Adapted from Jellinek M., Patel, B. P., & Froehle, M. C. (Eds). (2002). Bright futures in practice: Mental health *(Vol. I). Arlington, VA: National Center for Education in Maternal and Child Health.*

- "How is your 5 year old doing? What do you do with her individually?"
- "How do you and your partner manage some time for yourselves?"
- "Have you been feeling sad? All the time or for short periods? What seems to help?"
- "This first month can be really stressful. What do you do when problems really get to you? Who do you turn to for help?"
- "Describe your transportation situation. Is transportation a problem for you? Do you have enough money for food and housing?"
- "What is the most helpful thing we can do for you today?"

(Jellinek et al., 2002)

Through these questions the nurse assesses development of **attachment behaviors** (behaviors that demonstrate an emotional connection between newborn and caregiver), parental perception of infant **temperament**, (characteristic style of activity, mood, and reaction), feeding status, safety, family integration, parental mental health, and parental coping mechanisms. The nurse may determine that further assessment is required, for example, if the parent states that breastfeeding is so painful she wants to switch to formula, she is continuously depressed, has started smoking again, or cannot calm her crying baby. The nurse in the pediatric setting is aware that pediatric health is closely connected to health of the entire family. Many concerns require referral for parents outside the pediatric care setting; therefore, the office or clinic should have a system in place and ready access to referrals and resources for parents in need.

GROWTH AND DEVELOPMENTAL SURVEILLANCE

At Birth

Assessment of growth and development begins at birth. An experienced neonatal or labor nurse can accurately assess many parameters of newborn health within a few moments of the infant's birth. The nurse notes posture, flexion, reflexes, and a battery of physical attributes that help the nurse assess appropriate development for gestation. The nurse determines, by physical assessment findings and prenatal history, if the newborn is preterm (born prior to 37 weeks' gestation), term (born between 37 completed weeks and 42 weeks), or postterm (born after 42 weeks' gestation). See Figure 11–3 ■. In addition, the nurse determines if the newborn is the expected size and weight for the time spent in utero. This is done by plotting the baby's weight and measurements on a standard intrauterine growth chart to determine if the newborn is:

- **appropriate for gestational age (AGA)**—a newborn whose weight, length, and head circumference fall between the tenth and ninetieth percentiles when plotted on a standard intrauterine growth/gestational age chart.
- **small for gestational age (SGA)**—a newborn whose weight (and possibly length and head circumference) falls below the tenth percentile when plotted on a standard intrauterine growth/gestational age chart.
- **large for gestational age (LGA)**—a newborn whose weight (and possibly length and head circumference) falls above the 90th percentile when plotted on a standard intrauterine growth/gestational age chart.

The combination of head circumference, body length, and weight, in relation to the length of pregnancy, is an important factor in newborn health and development. The healthy newborn is the product of an uncomplicated pregnancy and birth, is term, and appropriate for gestational age. Newborns who are not term and/or not appropriately grown require careful nursing and medical management to prevent or manage complications such as respiratory distress, infection, hypoglycemia, feeding problems, and temperature instability. (See Chapters 8, 9, 19, 25, and 32∞ for specific conditions.)

Assessing Growth and Development in the Outpatient Setting

The first outpatient visit usually occurs 3 to 5 days following the birth of a healthy term newborn who was discharged more than 48 hours after vaginal birth (AAP, 2004c). At this visit, the baby's current weight, length, and head circumference are measured and plotted on a growth chart (see Appendix A∞), and a basic physical examination is performed (see Chapter 8∞).

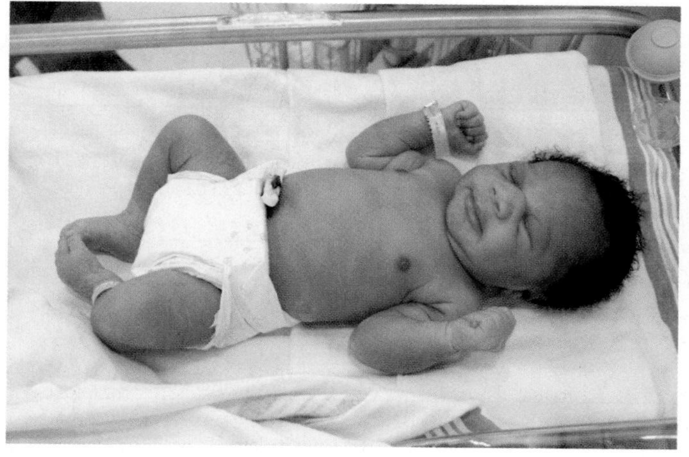

A

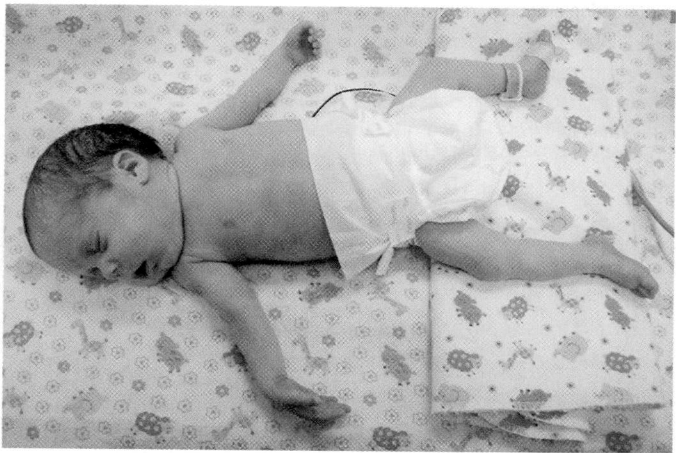

B

FIGURE 11–3 ■ The pediatric nurse can determine from the initial observation of position and muscle tone that one baby is *A*, term, and the other is *B*, preterm.

In the first week of life, most babies lose about one tenth of their birthweight. For example, a 3,500 g baby (7 lb, 12 oz) could lose up to 350 g (nearly 12 oz). Growth spurts are evident at around 7 to 10 days, and again between 3 and 6 weeks of age. By day 10, most babies are back to their original birth weight and gaining about 2/3 oz per day. Length increases by 1 to 1.5 inches in the first month, and head circumference increases about 1 inch (Shelov, 2004).

Developmental surveillance includes assessment of the baby's ability to calm when being held or spoken to, and respond to sounds by blinking, crying, quieting, or startling. The baby should be able to fixate on a human face and follow it with his or her eyes. The baby should be able to lift his or her head momentarily when placed prone, demonstrate a flexed position, and move all extremities. Most babies will sleep for 3 or 4 hours at a time and stay awake for an hour or longer (Green & Palfrey, 2002). See Box 11–4.

CLINICAL TIP

Preterm infants do not reach developmental milestones at the same chronologic age as their full-term counterparts. A baby born at 32 weeks' gestation (8 weeks early) may reach developmental milestones approximately 8 weeks later than if he or she had been born full term. For example, a 4-week-old, full-term baby should be able to move the head from side to side while lying prone. A baby born at 32 weeks' gestation should not be expected to meet this milestone until about 12 weeks of age (Gregory, 2002).

It is normal for parents to compare their newborn's developmental skills with others of the same age. Every baby develops according to his or her own timetable; however, when a baby falls far behind, fails to reach a developmental milestone, or loses a previously acquired skill, the baby requires further evaluation (Shelov, 2004). In the first month of life, signs of **developmental delay**—a delay in mastering functions, such as motor coordination and behavioral skills—in a full-term infant usually merit immediate investigation by a pediatrician, pediatric developmental specialist, pediatric neurologist, or a multidisciplinary team of professionals. Parents require additional emotional support, clear and honest communication, and resources to cope with the stress of this situation (see Chapter 20∞).

Table 11–2 summarizes some growth and developmental milestones that can commonly be observed in the first month of life.

BOX 11–4 Signs of Developmental Delay

During the second, third, or fourth week of life, the following signs of potential developmental delay require a complete medical and developmental evaluation to determine if a disability exists and to plan interventions and future management. The pediatric nurse observes the newborn for these signs and may have opportunity to assess for problems through discussing the newborn's abilities and behaviors with the caregiver.

- Sucks poorly and feeds slowly.
- Does not blink when shown a bright light.
- Does not focus and follow a nearby object moving side to side.
- Rarely moves arms and legs; seems stiff.
- Seems excessively loose in the limbs, or floppy.
- Lower jaw trembles constantly.
- Does not respond to loud sounds.

Adapted from Shelov, S. P. (Ed.). (2004, 4th edition). The American Academy of Pediatrics: Caring for your baby and young child: Birth to age 5. *New York: Bantam Books. Used with permission.*

NUTRITION

Breastfeeding

Breastfeeding is a valuable contributor to infant health. Breast milk is the perfect food for infants, and breastfeeding offers lifelong benefits for both mother and baby. The American Academy of Pediatrics recommends exclusive breastfeeding (no water, juice, or other foods) for the first 6 months of life. Solid foods may be introduced in the second half of the first year to complement the breast milk diet, with breastfeeding continuing at least until the infant's first birthday, and beyond if mutually desired (AAP, 2005).

Advantages of breastfeeding for the infant include decreased incidence and/or severity of the following:

- Ear infections (otitis media)
- Allergies
- Diarrhea
- Vomiting
- Respiratory tract infection
- Meningitis and other infections

Breastfeeding may also provide the infant protection against the following:

- Sudden infant death syndrome (SIDS)
- Insulin-dependent (type 1) and non-insulin dependent (type 2) diabetes mellitus
- Obesity and overweight
- Asthma
- Lymphoma and leukemia

Despite obvious health and developmental advantages of breastfeeding, efforts are needed to promote breastfeeding in the United States. Currently, it is thought that only 8% to 24% of women report that their prenatal provider talked with them about infant feeding (Meek, 2001). Other barriers to breastfeeding include insufficient

TABLE 11–2 Newborn Growth and Developmental Milestones Observed in Health Promotion and Health Maintenance Visits

Growth	➤ Weight: baby may lose up to one tenth of birthweight in the first week; birthweight should be reattained by day 10; weight gain is about 2/3 oz ounce per day thereafter. ➤ Length increases by 1 to 1.5 inches. ➤ Head circumference increases by about 1 inch.
Vision	➤ Focuses 8–12 inches away. ➤ Eyes wander and may cross. ➤ Prefers black and white or high-contrast patterns. ➤ Prefers the human face to all other patterns.
Hearing	➤ Hearing is fully mature. ➤ Recognizes some sounds. ➤ May turn toward familiar sounds and voices.

(Shelov, 2004).

PARTNERING WITH FAMILIES

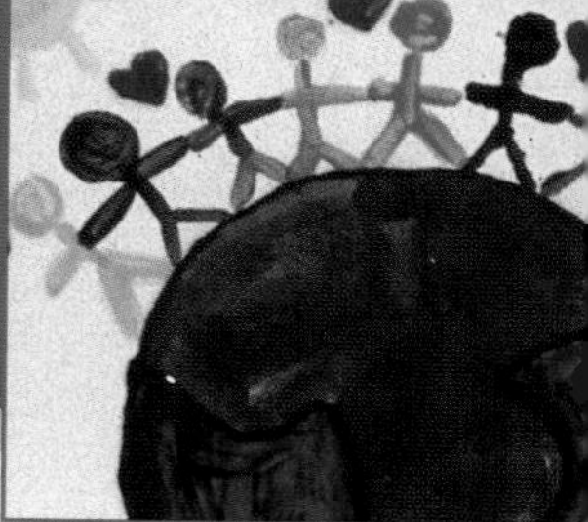

The Nurse's Role in Breastfeeding Promotion

Because breastfeeding offers many health benefits for both mother and newborn, the nurse promotes and supports the practice of breastfeeding in the prenatal period, at birth, and in the outpatient setting.

Prenatal period:

- Promote breastfeeding prenatally by discussing infant feeding and advantages of breastfeeding.
- Encourage attendance at prenatal breastfeeding classes.
- Provide educational resources to expectant parents.
- Identify women at risk for lactation risk factors (flat or inverted nipples, breast surgery, no change in breast size during pregnancy), recommend appropriate interventions, and encourage early follow-up after delivery.

At birth:

- Encourage initial breastfeeding in the first 30 minutes to 1 hour after delivery unless medically contraindicated.
- Discourage separation of mother and infant (baby should room in with mother at all times).
- Teach infant feeding cues to breastfeeding mothers and promote breastfeeding on demand.
- Observe at least one breastfeeding period and assess technique and adequacy of breastfeeding.
- Discourage use of artificial nipples and pacifiers until breastfeeding is well established.
- Evaluate state of hydration and jaundice.
- Avoid distribution of discharge packages that contain formula.
- Provide referral to lactation support group and/or lactation specialist as necessary.
- Schedule early follow-up after discharge.

In the outpatient setting:

- Provide anticipatory guidance about breastfeeding at every infant health screening visit.
- Educate all staff on aspects of breastfeeding support and management of common breastfeeding problems.
- Use visual images and slogans in the office that depict breastfeeding as normative behavior by women and families of diverse backgrounds.
- Post signs in waiting rooms and exam rooms encouraging mothers to breastfeed wherever they are comfortable and whenever they desire.
- Use culturally appropriate educational resources (pamphlets, books, videotapes).
- Remove commercial logos and other indirect formula endorsement (e.g., note pads, pens, calendars) and store formula out of view.
- Meet literacy and language needs of mothers.
- Identify at least one breastfeeding resource person on staff and encourage continuing education for breastfeeding management skills.
- Identify community resources and establish office referral guidelines.
- Ensure that office practices do not interrupt or discourage breastfeeding during visits.
- Coordinate with hospital maternity units to promote consistent information and resources.
- Promote good working relationships with lactation specialists in area hospitals and in the community.
- Commend breastfeeding mothers at every visit for continuing to breastfeed.

Adapted from American Academy of Pediatrics. (1999d). Ten steps to support parents' choice to breastfeed their baby. www.aap.org/advocacy/bf/tensteps.pdf. Used with permission.

prenatal breastfeeding education, disruptive hospital practices, media portrayal of bottle feeding as normative and advertising of infant formula, and lack of routine follow-up and home visits (AAP, 2005).

The decision about whether to breastfeed or formula feed the newborn is usually made prior to birth. Expectant mothers pondering this decision are influenced by previous experience with breastfeeding, support (or lack of support) from friends and family members, cultural norms, and current knowledge regarding differences between breastfeeding and formula feeding.

Healthcare providers in the prenatal setting play a vital role in educating expectant mothers about the health benefits of breastfeeding and providing anticipatory guidance prior to childbirth. The nurse in the birth setting promotes breastfeeding by facilitating nursing in the first 30 to 60 minutes following birth, and providing supportive guidance as the mother begins to develop this skill prior to discharge. Continued assessment, encouragement, and support of breastfeeding are vital to the continued success of breastfeeding mothers, as many mothers initiate breastfeeding and discontinue after a few days or weeks (Lawrence, 1999). See Partnering with Families: The Nurse's Role in Breastfeeding Promotion.

There are very few contraindications to breastfeeding. Mothers who should not breastfeed are usually aware, prior to giving birth, of the reasons formula feeding is a safer choice for them than breastfeeding. Communication should be clear and coordinated between prenatal care providers and pediatric care providers to ensure that the mother visiting the pediatric care provider is not asked how breastfeeding is going, counseled about the benefits of breastfeeding versus formula feeding, or repeatedly asked about her decision to formula feed instead of breastfeed.

PRACTICE ALERT

For some women, formula feeding is a safer choice than breastfeeding. Nursing is contraindicated in women who:

- Use drugs of abuse ("street drugs")
- Have uncontrolled alcohol use
- Have an infant with classic galactosemia
- Have HIV infection
- Take certain medications (cytotoxic drugs, some psychotrophic drugs)
- Have untreated active tuberculosis
- Are receiving or have exposure to radioactive isotopes or materials
- Are receiving antimetabolites or chemotherapeutic agents
- Have herpes simplex lesions on a breast

(AAP 2005 and AAP & ACOG 2002, p. 223)

The decision to breastfeed or formula feed may be influenced more by economic and social factors than health information (Wolf, 2003). Despite evidence that breastfeeding reduces health-care costs and employee absenteeism due to infant illness (AAP, 2005), there is almost no evidence that employers accommodate breastfeeding mothers. Only 10% of full-time working mothers breastfeed at 6 months compared to almost 33% of stay-at-home mothers. This is true for all ethnic, education, and age groups (Meek, 2001). Pediatric care providers can promote breastfeeding through partnering with employers in the community, educating them about the economic benefits of supporting breastfeeding mothers, and supporting their efforts to do so.

Although breastfeeding initiation rates vary among states, the overall rate of breastfeeding initiation for all women is 64%; the *Healthy People 2010* goal for breastfeeding initiation is 75% (U.S. Department of Health and Human Services, 2000). See Box 11–5. The highest rates of breastfeeding occur in higher income, college-educated women living in the Mountain and Pacific regions of the United States. Racial and ethnic disparities in breastfeeding rates are of grave concern throughout the United States. See Developing Cultural Competence: Ethnic Disparities in Breastfeeding Rates.

Nurses play a vital role in assisting and supporting breastfeeding mothers. The nurse who encounters breastfeeding mothers should understand the basics of breastfeeding management (Figure 11–4 ■). See Partnering with Families: Breastfeeding Basics. Ideally, the pediatric setting has a lactation specialist or resource person who can assess breastfeeding and problem-solve with the mother. Referrals to a community lactation specialist or support group may be necessary. See Chapter 9 for more information.

DEVELOPING CULTURAL COMPETENCE
Ethnic Disparities in Breastfeeding Rates

Breastfeeding is an important contributor to infant health, yet racial and ethnic disparities in breastfeeding rates are wide. Because breastfeeding contributes significantly to the health of mothers and babies, public health initiatives such as *Healthy People 2010* aim to increase awareness of these disparities and promote culturally appropriate strategies to increase breastfeeding rates among all women. See the following table.

Breastfeeding in Early Postpartum Period	1998 Baseline %	*Healthy People 2010* Target
All women	64	75% goal for all groups
Black or African American	45	
Hispanic or Latino	66	
White	68	
At 6 months		
All women	29	50% goal for all groups
Black or African American	19	
Hispanic or Latino	28	
White	31	
At 1 year		
All women	16	25% goal for all groups
Black or African American	9	
Hispanic or Latino	19	
White	17	

(U.S. Department of Health and Human Services, 2000)

BOX 11–5 *Healthy People 2010* National Goals for Breastfeeding

Breastfeeding offers important long-term health benefits for both mother and baby. *Healthy People 2010*, a national public health initiative, has set the following goals for breastfeeding initiation and duration.

- Increase the proportion of women who initiate breastfeeding to 75%.
- Increase the proportion of women who continue breastfeeding their babies until 6 months of age to 50%.
- Increase the proportion of women who breastfeed their babies until 1 year of age to 25%.

(U.S. Department of Health and Human Services, 2000).

Formula Feeding

Formula is not the same as breast milk. Breast milk is specifically for the needs of the human infant, and provides ideal nutrition for brain growth in the first 12 months of life. Breast milk, in contrast to formula, has elements available from the mother's bloodstream that are immediately available for infant nutrition. Breast milk contains elements that work together to enhance absorption; formula is a mix of isolated single nutrients that do not guarantee the same nutritional benefits of breast milk (Lawrence, 1999).

In some cases, formula feeding is a safer choice than breastfeeding. Mothers who use infant formula should feed iron-fortified formula (containing between 4 and 12 mg/L of iron)

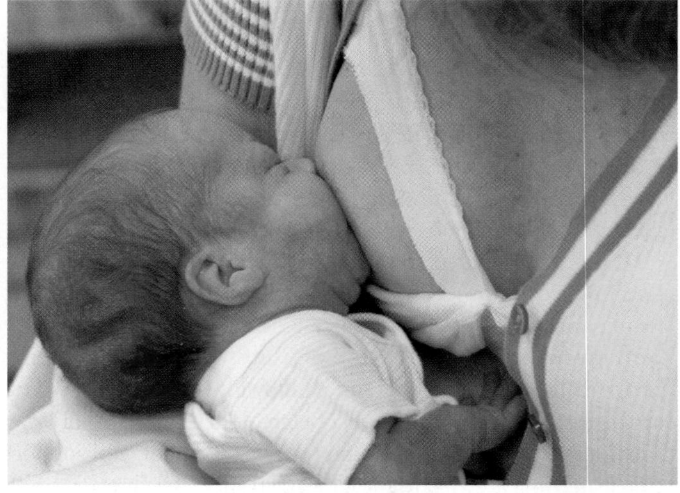

FIGURE 11–4 ■ Breastfeeding has lifelong benefits for the mother and child and should be promoted prenatally, in the hospital, and through the first year of health supervision visits.

PARTNERING WITH FAMILIES

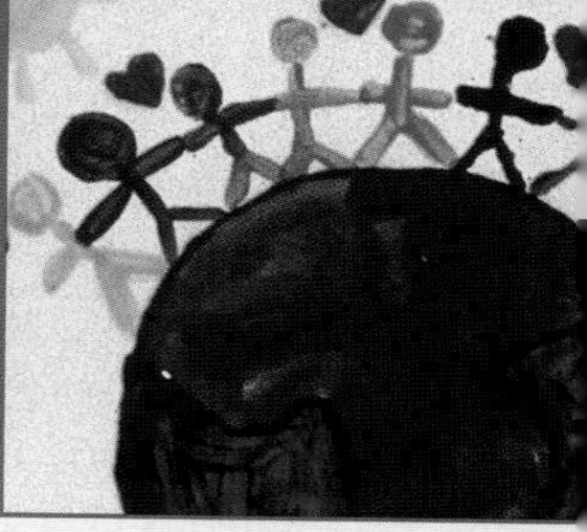

Breastfeeding Basics

The pediatric nurse in the outpatient setting receives numerous questions about breastfeeding, especially from new mothers in the first month of their breastfeeding experience. Responsibilities for counseling and referring nursing mothers to lactation resources vary according to office protocols; however, the new mother may simply need reassurance and basic information. The nurse may use these two lists as a start for assessing breastfeeding effectiveness and to answer two common questions asked by new breastfeeding mothers: "How do I know my baby is getting enough milk?" and "Is my baby positioned correctly at my breast in order to get enough milk and prevent sore nipples?"

Signs that your baby is well fed

- Your baby is alert and active.
- Your baby is happy and satisfied after breastfeeding.
- Your baby breastfeeds at least 8 times in every 24 hours.
- You hear or see your baby swallow when he breastfeeds.
- Your baby loses less than 7% of his birth weight during the first 5 days.
- Your baby is back to his birth weight by 10 days of age.
- Your baby gains 4–8 ounces each week after the first week.
- Your baby has 3 or more stools a day after day 1, increasing to 4 or more stools a day by day 5.
- Your baby's stool changes from black to yellow by day 5.
- Your baby has clear or pale yellow urine and 6 or more wet diapers a day by day 5.

Signs that your baby is positioned well

- Your baby's chin, chest, and knees face your breast.
- Your baby's mouth is opened wide like a yawn.
- Your baby's tongue is over her lower gum.
- Your baby's lips curl out like a fish.
- Your baby's chin firmly touches your breast.
- You hear or see your baby swallow when she breastfeeds.
- Your nipples are the same shape before and after you breastfeed.
- You feel pain only at the start of a feeding.

Used with permission from Spangler, A. (2000). Breastfeeding: A parent's guide *(7th ed.). Danbury Hospital, The Family Birth Center.*

from birth to 12 months (AAP, 1999c). This helps ensure adequate iron stores and very low rates of iron deficiency between 6 and 18 months of age. (See Chapter 9∞ for more information about formulas.)

PHYSICAL ACTIVITY

Muscle development begins early in fetal life. Buoyed by amniotic fluid and contained within the uterus, fetal movements are usually smooth and limited in range. After birth, however, gravity exerts a strong effect and newborn movements are often weak and jerky (Blackburn, 2003). Even so, strong muscle tone is evident in the term newborn. The flexed position of the newborn demonstrates development of the flexor muscles and relaxation of the extensor muscles. This flexed position protects the newborn, conserves energy by reducing movement, and reduces heat loss (Blackburn, 2003).

Parents may need to be reminded that a preterm infant will develop according to his or her **"corrected age."** If the baby was born 8 weeks premature, at 32 weeks' gestation, parents can expect their otherwise healthy preterm baby to reach developmental milestones about 8 weeks later than if the baby had been born at term (Gregory, 2002).

During the first month of life, the newborn gradually "unfolds" and the body straightens. Movements begin to change from reflexive to purposeful. By the end of the first month, the newborn should be able to do the following:

- Bring hands to eyes and mouth
- Move head side to side when lying on abdomen
- Attempt to lift head when prone

In addition, the newborn's hands are kept in tight fists and reflexes are strong (see Chapter 8∞) (Shelov, 2004).

Health promotion teaching for the family includes the following activities.

- Position baby on stomach for supervised play periods. This allows the newborn to lift the head and turn it from side to side, make crawling motions, and push up on arms. Allowing supervised "tummy time" is also important for prevention of flat spots on the back of the baby's head caused by constant supine positioning (Persing, James, Swanson, et al., 2003). Be sure to place the baby in a supine position when tiring and starting to fall asleep.
- Allow the baby free movement of arms and hands. If the baby is swaddled, allow the hands to be outside the blanket and positioned in midline. This allows flexion and extension of arms, brings hands into line of vision, and brings hands to mouth.
- Encourage appropriate toys such as a mobile with contrasting colors and patterns, a plastic mirror, music boxes and exposure to soft music on the radio, tape recorder, or CD player, and soft toys with colors, patterns, and gentle sounds.
- Encourage switching positions when bottle feeding. It may be most comfortable for the mother to hold the baby in cradle position with the bottle in her right hand (or left hand if left-handed); however, switching arms encourages newborn muscle development and control on each side of the baby's body. Breastfeeding babies automatically feed from both sides. Parents who bottle feed may need to be reminded to promote this skill in their newborn.

- Beginning at birth, prevent flat spots on the newborn's head from supine positioning by nightly alternating the head position from left to right during sleep and occasionally changing the orientation of the newborn in relation to the activity at the doorway of the room (Persing et al., 2003).

ORAL HEALTH

Ideally, pediatric oral health begins with prenatal oral health counseling for parents (American Academy of Pediatric Dentistry [AAPD], 1999). If not already established, promotion of healthy oral hygiene practices and routine preventive dental care for parents establishes a foundation for a lifetime of good oral health for their children.

Protective factors for good oral health include good general health, appropriate use of fluoride in family members more than 6 months of age (either topically, in community water systems, or systemically as deemed appropriate by healthcare professionals), high socioeconomic status, family intake of simple sugars occurring primarily at mealtime, and regular use of dental care in an established **dental home**, a specialized primary dental care provider who manages and facilitates all aspects of oral healthcare. Risk factors include infant's siblings with **dental caries** (cavities, or tooth decay) in the past 12 months, active caries present in the mother, suboptimal fluoride exposure, frequent between-meal exposure of family members to simple sugars, low socioeconomic status, no usual source of dental care, and children with special healthcare needs (AAPD, 2002).

Parents can help prevent decay in their new baby by practicing good oral health habits from birth. In the first month of life, parents should be warned against propping the bottle in the baby's mouth while the baby falls asleep. Babies who sleep with their teeth exposed to juice, formula, or breast milk can develop early childhood caries (ECC), formerly known as "baby bottle tooth decay" in primary teeth, even before they emerge. (See Chapter 9∞.)

Oral disease may be prevented if strategies are applied early enough in the child's life. The nurse plays an important role in assessing risk factors for dental disease, promoting oral hygiene beginning in infancy, and providing anticipatory guidance to help parents ensure good oral health for their children.

MENTAL AND SPIRITUAL HEALTH

The first 3 years of a child's life are critically important to the child's development of skills that allow for learning, thinking, responding, and solving problems. The environment that parents create for their baby and young child influence the way the child develops and how nearly the child achieves her or his full potential. A "child-centered" environment provides for basic needs such as adequate nutrition, loving family members and caregivers, a feeling of safety and predictability, opportunities for play, positive reinforcement, exchange of ideas through conversation, exposure to books and music, and a balance of freedom and limits (Shelov, 2004).

An **infant's mental health**—the developing capacity of the child to experience emotions, form attachments, and learn—is also affected by physical health, temperament, and resiliency. Through a combination of genetic attributes and the environment provided by the newborn's parents, the baby develops personality, strategies for **self-regulation** (the ability to maintain state and self-console), attachments to the family, and cognitive abilities (Jellinek et al., 2004).

In the first year of life, infants form emotional attachments and learn to trust caregivers to meet their needs (Figure 11–5 ■). Newborns begin to meet these goals by making their needs known through verbal and nonverbal **cues** (see Partnering with Families: Newborn Engagement and Disengagement Cues). The parent who can interpret these signals and respond to the newborn's needs in a timely and appropriately manner strengthens attachment and promotes optimal infant mental health. In addition, the parent benefits from understanding infant sleep-wake states and the activities most appropriate to the newborn's level of attention (Table 11–3). The mature newborn demonstrates neural organization by moving smoothly from one state to another, and a parent who knows the behavioral implications of each state is able to respond appropriately to the baby's cues and elicit responses that make the parent feel successful in meeting the baby's needs. A newborn with Down syndrome, a biochemical disturbance, brain malformation, or birth asphyxia may demonstrate difficulty with state control and move unpredictably from one state to another (Blackburn, 2003). These babies are more difficult to parent and the family is at risk for poor parent–infant attachment.

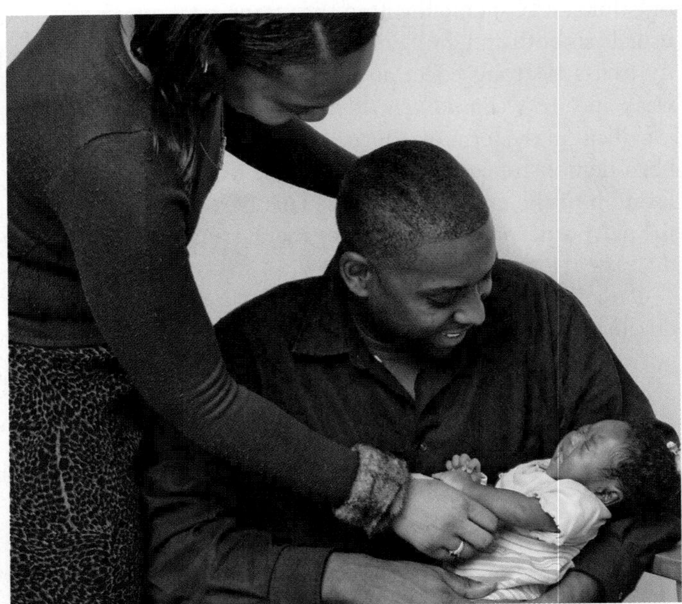

FIGURE 11–5 ■ A healthy parent forms strong attachments to the newborn and is motivated to ensure physical and mental health for the child.

TABLE 11–3 Infant Sleep and Awake States

STATE*	BODY ACTIVITY	EYE MOVEMENTS	FACIAL MOVEMENTS	BREATHING PATTERN	LEVEL OF RESPONSE	IMPLICATIONS FOR CAREGIVING
Sleep States						
Quiet Sleep (also called deep sleep)	Nearly still, except for occasional startle or twitch	None	None, except for occasional sucking movement at regular intervals	Smooth and regular	The infant's threshold to stimuli is very high; only very intense and disturbing stimuli will arouse the infant.	Quiet sleep is restorative and anabolic. The threshold to sensory stimuli is very high during quiet sleep. Caregivers trying to feed an unresponsive infant in quiet sleep will find the experience frustrating. Feeding will be more pleasant if nurses and parents respect the infant's needs by waiting until the infant moves to a higher, more responsive state. Even if caregivers use disturbing stimuli, chances are the infant will arouse only briefly, then return to quiet sleep.
Active sleep (also called light sleep or rapid eye movement (REM sleep)	Some body movements	Rapid eye movements (REM); fluttering of eyes beneath closed eyelids	May smile and make brief fussy or crying sounds	Irregular	The infant is more responsive to internal stimuli (hunger) and external stimuli (handling) than when in quiet sleep. When stimuli occur, the infant may remain in active sleep, return to quiet sleep, or arouse.	Active sleep is associated with processing and storing of information and has been linked to learning. It accounts for the highest proportion of newborn sleep and usually precedes wakening. Due to brief fussy or crying sounds during this state, caregivers who are not aware that these sounds normally occur may try to feed infants before they are ready to eat.
Awake States						
Drowsy	Variable activity level with mild startles interspersed; movements usually smooth	Eyes occasionally open and close, are heavy-lidded or slit-like	May have some facial movements. Often none, and face appears still.	Irregular	Infants react to sensory stimuli, although their responses are delayed. A change to quiet alert, active alert or crying after stimulation is frequently noted.	To awaken infants, caregivers can provide something for infants to see, hear, or suck. If infants are left alone without stimuli, they may return to a sleep state.
Quiet alert	Minimal	Eyes brighten and widen	Attentive appearance	Regular	During this state, infants are most attentive to the environment, focusing attention on any stimuli present.	Immediately after birth, many newborns experience intense alertness before a long sleeping period. As infants become older, they spend more time in this state. Providing something for infants to see, hear, or suck will often maintain this state or help them enter a quiet-alert state from a drowsy or active-alert state. Infants in this state provide pleasure and positive feedback to caregivers. This is a good time to feed the infant.
Active alert	Variable activity level with mild startles interspersed. Movements usually smooth.	Eyes are open, with dull, glazed appearance	May have some facial movements. Often none, and face appears still.	Irregular	Infants react to sensory stimuli, although responses are delayed. With stimulation, the infant may change to quiet alert or crying.	Infants may fuss and become increasingly sensitive to disturbing stimuli (hunger, fatigue, noise, excessive handling). Infants may become more active and cry. Fatigue or caregiver interventions often interrupt this state, allowing infants to return to a drowsy or sleep state.
Crying	Increased motor activity. Skin color darkens or changes to red or ruddy.	Eyes may be tightly closed or open	Grimaces	More irregular than in other states	Infants are extremely responsive to unpleasant external or internal stimuli	An infant cries in response to unpleasant stimuli. The infant's limits have been reached. Sometimes infants can console themselves; at other times they need help from caregivers.

**__State__ is a group of characteristics that regularly occur together; body activity, eye movements, facial movements, breathing pattern, and level of response to external stimuli (e.g., handling) and internal stimuli (e.g., hunger).*

Blackburn, S., & Blakewell-Sachs (2003). Understanding the Behavior of Term Infants. *White Plains, NY: March of Dimes Birth Defects Foundation, https://www.marchofdimes.com/nursing/index.bm2?cid=00000003&spid=ne_s1_1&tpi, Accessed 3-29-05, Adapted by pemission of the March of Dimes.*

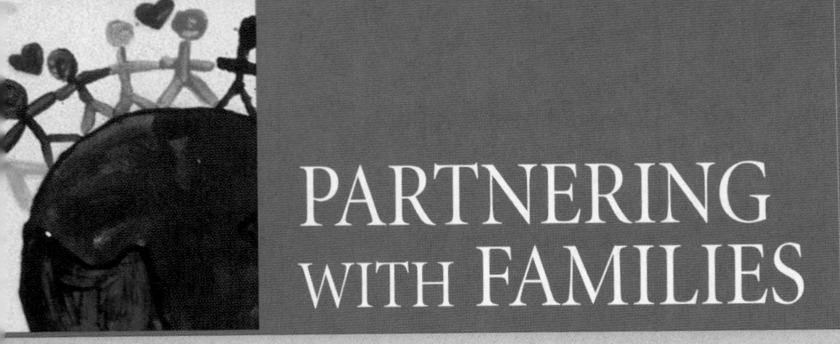

PARTNERING WITH FAMILIES

Newborn Engagement and Disengagement Cues

Newborns use verbal and nonverbal cues to communicate with caregivers. When a newborn is interested in eliciting care and attention, he demonstrates engagement cues:

- Turns toward caregiver
- Reaches toward caregiver
- Opens eyes and gazes at caregiver

When the newborn needs to stop interaction, he demonstrates disengagement cues:

- Turns head away
- Begins to hiccup or drool
- Falls asleep
- Begins to cry

Adapted from Jellinek M., Patel, B. P., & Froehle, M. C. (Eds.). (2002). Bright futures in practice: Mental health *(Vol. I, p. 29). Arlington, VA: National Center for Education in Maternal and Child Health.*

The nurse assesses signs of a growing secure attachment between parent and child in the first month of life by making the following observations.

- Parent looks at the newborn frequently.
- Parent has specific questions and observations about the individual characteristics of the newborn.
- Parent touches, massages, or gently rubs the newborn.
- Parent attempts to soothe the newborn when the newborn is upset.
- Newborn looks content.
- Newborn signals needs.
- Newborn feeds well.
- Newborn responds to parent's attempts to soothe.

The newborn's mental health and development is highly dependent on the mental and spiritual health of the primary caregiver, usually the mother. The mother who is emotionally whole and fully present in her newborn's life is best able to provide the nurturing environment necessary for optimal growth and development (Jellinek et al., 2002).

Promoting Maternal Mental Health

Bringing a newborn home can be an overwhelming emotional experience for the mother, her partner, and other family members. An immediate shift in roles and responsibilities must occur within the family. In addition to meeting the needs of the newborn, the new mother must also deal with meeting other family members' needs, rapidly shifting emotions, and her postpartum body.

Assessing Postpartum Mental Health Status

The nurse in the pediatric care setting may be the first healthcare provider encountered by the postpartum woman. Because the mother's and newborn's health are so closely intertwined, the nurse should be alert to signs and symptoms of marked maternal psychosocial stress and mood disorders.

Most women experience **postpartum "blues"** or temporary sadness in the first week after delivery due to hormonal shifts and sleep deprivation. This usually resolves without intervention after a few hours to several days. **Postpartum depression** is a more serious and debilitating **postpartum mood disorder (PPMD)** that usually occurs 2 to 3 months after delivery. Counseling and medication originating from the mother's primary care provider may be necessary interventions. **Postpartum psychosis** is a serious condition that can occur at any point postpartum and is considered a psychiatric emergency (Jellinek et al., 2002). See Table 11–4.

Activities that Promote Newborn Mental Health

Beginning at birth, parents can take advantage of the newborn's short periods of wakefulness to communicate and play together. Following are suggestions for parents to promote newborn mental health.

- Encourage your newborn to look at your face while feeding. Imitate the baby's soft sounds and accommodate his or her movements.
- Respond quickly to your baby's feeding cues and avoid rigid feeding schedules. Feeding times are unpredictable, especially in the first few months.
- Identify ways to soothe your crying newborn. Babies cry for reasons other than hunger. See Partnering with Families: Responding to Your Baby's Cry.
- Learn infant massage. For healthy infants, massage reportedly facilitates bonding, helps induce sleep in the baby, and makes parents feel good while massaging their baby. Chapter 5∞.
- Allow your baby to suck fingers and hands or a pacifier. See Box 11–6 and Partnering with Families: Making the Pacifier Decision.
- Make eye contact with your baby, hold and rock the baby frequently, and read and sing to your baby. If you cannot think of what to say to the baby, tell him about your day, or talk about what is happening, for example, "Are you hungry now?" "Is that milk nice and warm?" "Do you hear that dog barking outside?" "You are very alert. I like it when you look at me that way."
- Be consistent and predictable in the way you respond to the newborn's needs.

(Jellinek et al., 2002; Shelov, 2004).

During the health supervision visit, the nurse models behavior for parents that promotes positive infant mental health, such as handling the newborn gently, speaking in a soft voice, noticing attributes ("Look how you hold your head up today! You're really getting strong!"), and noticing likes and dislikes. The nurse strengthens parental confidence by asking the parent what the

TABLE 11–4 Postpartum Mood Disorders

DISORDER	SYMPTOMS	ONSET
Postpartum blues	Predominantly positive mood punctuated by: ➤ labile and intense episodes of tearfulness, irritability, sadness, reactivity to slights ➤ exaggerated sense of empathy (Miller & Rukstalis, 1999).	Begins during first few weeks after delivery (usually peaks at 3–5 days)
Postpartum depression	Five or more of the following symptoms present for at least 2 weeks: ➤ Consistently depressed mood ➤ Loss of pleasure/interest ➤ Poor concentration or indecisiveness ➤ Feelings of worthlessness or guilt ➤ Recurrent thoughts of death ➤ Psychomotor agitation or retardation ➤ Fatigue or loss of energy ➤ Insomnia or hypersomnia* ➤ Significant decrease or increase in appetite*	Can be insidious, but starts within the first 2–3 months after delivery
Postpartum psychosis	Early signs typically include: ➤ Restlessness ➤ Irritability ➤ Insomnia ➤ Rapidly evolving or shifting depressed or elated mood ➤ Disorganized behavior, with confusion and disorientation ➤ Hallucinations or delusions (frequently focused on the infant)	Usually starts within 2–4 weeks of delivery, but can start as early as 2–3 days after delivery; onset can be dramatic and abrupt

**Symptoms are often difficult to assess in the postpartum period.*

Adapted from Jellinek, M., Patel, B. P., & Froehle, M. C. (Eds.). (2002). Bright futures in practice: Mental health (Vol. I). *Arlington, VA: National Center for Education in Maternal and Child Health.*

baby likes, such as, "How does he like to be carried, in your arms or up on your shoulder?" and then following the parent's advice. The nurse also promotes nurturing behavior by parents during procedures, such as allowing the parent to hold and comfort the baby while the nurse administers immunizations or draws blood.

BOX 11–6 Research: Breastfeeding and Pacifier Use

Breastfeeding mothers and infants were studied to ascertain the effect of pacifier introduction by 6 weeks of age on breastfeeding duration (Howard, Howard, Lanphear, et al., 1999). A cohort of 265 breastfeeding mother–infant couples was studied prospectively. Of this group, 181 mothers (68%) introduced a pacifier before 6 weeks postpartum. This practice was associated with a significantly increased risk for shortened duration of full and overall breastfeeding. Women who used pacifiers breastfed their infants fewer times per day, and at 12 weeks postpartum were more likely to report that breastfeeding was inconvenient and reported problems consistent with infrequent feeding, such as insufficient milk supply. This study suggests that pacifier use may be associated with less frequent breastfeeding and a subsequent decline in breastfeeding duration.

Many factors influence breastfeeding duration, such as cultural practices, prenatal education, hospital practices, and postpartum support; therefore, it is unclear whether pacifier use should be discouraged. Until more conclusive research is available, expectant and postpartum mothers should be educated about methods to calm an infant other than pacifier use, the importance of frequent feeding to establish and maintain milk supply, and the benefits of full breastfeeding in the first 6 months of life with addition of appropriate foods to complement the breast milk diet in the second 6 months of life.

RELATIONSHIPS

Family adaptation to a new baby begins in pregnancy, and evidence of initial family adaptation to pregnancy may be predictive of future parental coping (Green & Palfrey, 2002). In the prenatal period, the nurse has the opportunity to gather information about the family and their concerns, educate the family about newborn care and characteristics, provide support and strategies for the immediate postpartum period, and begin to develop a trusting relationship between the family and healthcare professionals.

After the newborn has spent some time with the parent at home, the nurse assesses current protective factors and risks (Table 11–5). A healthy newborn with normal behavior and mature engaged parents has fewer risks than a newborn with special needs and family dysfunction. Based on assessment of the newborn and family, the pediatric nurse may need to coordinate services and resources for families at risk, or work with resources already in place, such as those begun prior to discharge from the neonatal intensive care nursery. (See Chapter 2∞ for more discussion about family assessment and interventions.)

New parents may need assistance in identifying activities that promote family health and positive parent–newborn interaction. Activities could include the following:

- Share newborn care activities. Recognize that you may do things differently than your partner, such as the way you change a diaper or give a bath, but if the baby is cared for, safe and secure, these differences in technique do not matter.

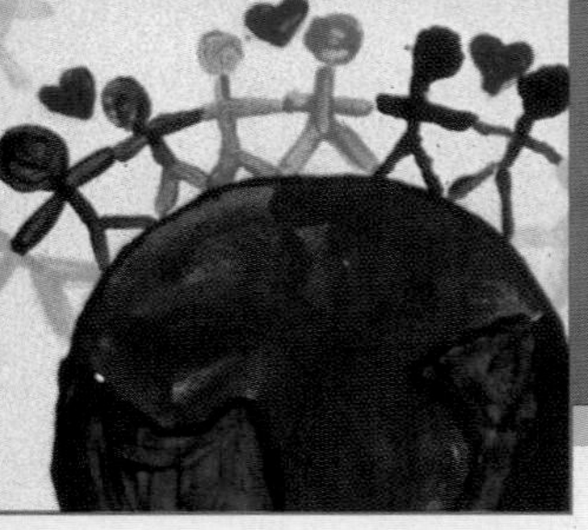

PARTNERING WITH FAMILIES

Responding to Your Baby's Cry

Babies cannot be spoiled by having their cries answered each time during the newborn period and in the first 6 months of life. Babies cry for multiple reasons; they may be tired, hungry, hot, cold, uncomfortable, overexcited, bored, lonely, or sick. The parent can try several approaches to calm the crying infant. As the baby progresses through infancy, techniques to enhance self-regulation should also be integrated (see Chapter 12∞).

When parents answer cries swiftly, consistently, and completely, infant crying has been reduced by 60% (Ludington-Hoe, Cong, & Hashemi, 2002). In response to their newborn's cries, parents should:

- **Answer the cry as soon as possible.** The sooner the cry is answered, the sooner the crying will stop.
- **Answer the cry consistently.** Research suggests that answering a cry each time teaches newborns that their needs will be met, and lessens infant crying later. Infants who had their cries answered consistently in the first 6 months of life were secure infants who were more likely to use vocalization rather than crying to communicate with caregivers after 6 months of life.
- **Answer the cry completely.** When the parent responds to the cry, the parent should be within the newborn's visual field (10–13 inches from the face), the parent should speak to the newborn in a reassuring tone, and use gentle but firm touch. If the newborn does not stop crying, the parent should hold the newborn chest to chest with knees flexed, providing containment and flexion.

Try one thing at a time to calm a crying newborn:

- Change the newborn's diaper.
- Feed the newborn, especially if it has been an hour or more since the last feeding.
- If the newborn's back or stomach feels too hot or cold, remove or add a layer of clothing or blankets.
- Gently pat or stroke the newborn's back or bottom in a rhythmic pattern.
- Wrap the newborn in a blanket to keep arms and legs close to body.
- "Wear" the newborn in a sling or front-pack carrier.
- Rock the newborn forward and backward, as if in a swing.
- Lay the baby's bare skin against your bare skin.
- Dim the lights and rock the baby in a quiet room.
- Give the baby a warm bath. A parent and baby may bathe together. Babies are comforted by skin-to-skin contact.

Crying can be a sign of illness. If a baby continues to cry despite all efforts to calm him, contact the baby's healthcare provider. If you feel frustrated with the baby and need help, contact your health care provider immediately.

Adapted from Jellinek, M., Patel, B. P., & Froehle, M. C. (Eds) (2002). Bright futures in practice: Mental health *(Vol. II, p. 68). Arlington, VA: National Center for Education in Maternal and Child Health; Ludington-Hoe, S. M., Cong, X., & Hashemi, F. (2002). Infant crying: Nature, physiologic consequences, and select interventions. Neonatal Network, 21(2), 29–36.*

- Compliment one another on newborn caregiving strengths, such as the mother's ability to breastfeed, the partner's ability to calm the crying baby.
- Attend health supervision visits together as much as possible.
- Be sensitive to when your partner is overstressed and overtired. Ask how you can help and then follow through with suggested activities. Sometimes listening is the most helpful thing you can do.

TABLE 11–5 Risk and Protective Factors in Newborn and Family Relationships

NEWBORN PROTECTIVE FACTORS	NEWBORN RISK FACTORS
Good health	Preterm birth, congenital disabilities, chronic illness
Normal eating, bowel, and sleep patterns	Feeding and sleep problems
Positive temperament	Fussing, crying, irritability, difficulty consoling
Responds to parents' attention	Diminished social interactions and responsiveness
Normal growth and development	Undernutrition, developmental delay
PARENTAL PROTECTIVE FACTORS	**PARENTAL RISK FACTORS**
Welcome baby at birth	Baby unplanned and unwanted at birth; potential for neglect and/or rejection
Meet newborn's basic needs for food, shelter, clothing, healthcare	Financial insecurity, homelessness, lack of knowledge about how to care for newborn
Provide a strong nurturing environment	Cannot promote strong nurturing environment due to serious problems such as abusive behavior, depression, mental illness, substance abuse
Parents have strong relationship with one another, share care of newborn	Severe marital problems, absent parent, or frequent change of partners
Strong self-esteem, developmental maturity, developing knowledge of infant development	Lack of parenting skills, lack of parenting self-esteem, inability to cope with multiple roles, inappropriate coping strategies
No history of maltreatment as a child	History of maltreatment as a child (risk increases with positive history)

Adapted from Green, M., & Palfrey, J.S. (Eds.). (2002). Bright futures: Guidelines for health supervision of infants, children, and adolescents *(2nd ed., rev.). Arlington, VA: National Center for Education in Maternal and Child Health.*

MediaLink Responding to Your Baby's Cry Video

- Rest and take time for yourself. Make decisions about what must be done (paying bills, laundry, grocery shopping) and what could wait (traveling to visit grandparents, painting the house, cleaning closets). Accept help from family and friends.
- Discuss how you will raise your baby in a loving, supportive, and respectful environment.
- Discuss how you were raised and what you would like to be different in your new family. Learn about parenting strategies and try out what feels comfortable for you.
- Keep in contact with family and friends. Maintain community ties that are important to you, such as social, religious, cultural, or recreational organizations or programs.
- Leave the baby with a trusted friend or family member and take time to be alone occasionally. Talk about something other than the baby.
- Prepare siblings for the new baby prior to the baby's arrival. Allow sibling to "help" care for the new baby in age-appropriate ways. Praise siblings for positive attention they give to the baby, and allow siblings to express their feelings about the new baby and changes in the family.
- Support one another in seeking and using community resources to strengthen parenting skills, such as classes and parenting groups.
- Cuddle, hold, and rock the baby as much as possible. Babies cannot be spoiled by too much attention.
- Take advantage of baby's awake time to play with baby. Singing, reading, and simply talking to the baby about what is happening provides the baby with developmental stimulation.

Family assessment should include screening for domestic violence, substance abuse, and child neglect or abuse (Box 11–7). See Chapter 7∞. Problems with parental bonding and attachment may also be apparent and require further assessment and interventions. The nurse should seek consultation and coordination of services when encountering serious problems with family dynamics. For instances in which the children are in immediate jeopardy, the nurse needs to be aware of reporting mandates and protocols for child protective services and how to access assistance with interventions.

The setting in which the family seeks care should be aware of resources and how to refer family members in a timely and culturally appropriate fashion. For example, an interpreter from the family's community may know the family, causing mutual discomfort between the family members and the interpreter when discussing culturally sensitive or intensely private matters, such as domestic violence or substance abuse.

DISEASE PREVENTION STRATEGIES

Over two thirds of all babies in the United States (about 71%) are born and discharged from the hospital without clinical problems or complicating diagnoses (Owens, Thompson, Elixhauser, et al., 2003). The most common neonatal conditions that require extension of the newborn hospital stay or return to the hospital are conditions associated with bilirubin metabolism, prematurity (including respiratory distress), respiratory problems, infections, and birth defects (Owens et al., 2003).

PARTNERING WITH FAMILIES

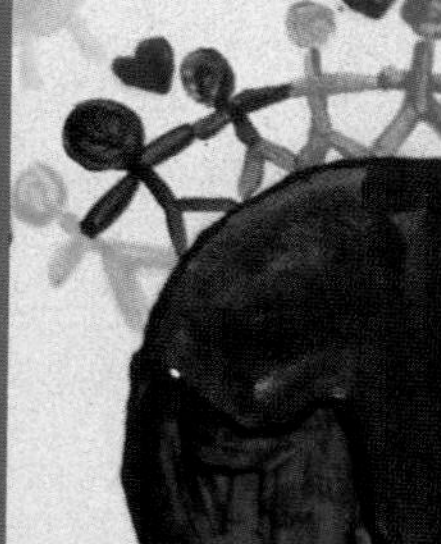

Making the Pacifier Decision

In the preterm infant, pacifiers are used for nonnutritive sucking, which means that the baby sucks for reasons other than to provide nutrition. In the preterm infant, pacifier use facilitates self-consolation and self-reguation and provides positive oral stimulation in preparation for nutritive sucking and feeding. However, pacifier use in the healthy full-term infant is controversial.

- Pacifiers do not cause medical or psychologic harm.
- Sucking on a pacifier can satisfy a baby's need to suck beyond breastfeeding or bottlefeeding.
- For some newborns, pacifier use may cause interference with proper sucking at the breast (Lawrence, 1999).
- Pacifier use may induce early weaning from the breast (Lawrence, 1999).
- Parents may incorrectly use a pacifier to soothe a newborn who is actually hungry and needs to feed (Shelov, 2004).
- A newborn who grows accustomed to falling asleep with a pacifier may awaken and cry frequently when it falls from the mouth, necessitating around-the-clock assistance from parents (Shelov, 2004).
- A newborn who uses a pacifier is at risk for gastrointestinal illness from bacteria on the pacifier. Until the baby is 6 months old and has a more mature immune system, the pacifier should be washed frequently in the dishwasher or boiled. After age 6 months, the pacifier can be washed with soap and rinsed with clear water (Shelov, 2004).

Pacifier use is a parental decision. Nurses should not introduce a pacifier to a healthy newborn in the hospital setting unless the mother requests it (Lawrence, 1999). Breastfeeding mothers should be informed about the possibility of pacifier use interfering with effective breastfeeding.

Parents who choose to offer their newborn a pacifier should be taught to use the pacifier after or between feedings, and never in place of a feeding. Parents should be cautioned about tying the pacifier to the baby with a string or cord that could cause suffocation. Parents should purchase a one-piece pacifier with ventilation holes, and never use a home-made pacifier from a bottle nipple that could come loose and choke the newborn (Shelov, 2004).

Disease prevention in the first month includes the following health maintenance activities.

- **Metabolic screening**—all states require screening for congenital metabolic diseases such as phenylketonuria (PKU) (see Figure 11–6 ■ and Box 11–8)
- Hearing screening (see Box 11–9 and Chapter 24∞)
- Eye examination
- Immunizations
- Prevention of secondhand smoke exposure
- SIDS risk reduction (Figure 11–7 ■)
- Formula safety (see Chapter 9∞)
- Handwashing (see Partnering with Families: Handwashing)

BOX 11–7 Screening for Domestic Violence

Domestic violence is a pattern of assaultive and coercive behaviors, including physical, sexual and psychological attacks, as well as economic coercion, that adults or adolescents use against their intimate partners to gain or maintain power and control. Domestic violence occurs in heterosexual, gay, lesbian, bisexual, and trans-intimate relationships and crosses all socioeconomic, religious, racial, ethnic, cultural, disability status, class, and age groups. However, domestic violence is primarily a crime against women. Women in abusive relationships may be more motivated to disclose domestic violence during pregnancy and postpartum than at other times. This may be due to an increase in abuse during pregnancy or postpartum, or they may seek help for the sake of their baby (HealthCanada, 1999). Women abused before or during pregnancy are at increased risk of abuse after the baby is born. The newborn is then at risk for child abuse and the long-term effects of violence and anger in the child's future relationships.

HOW TO ASK ABOUT ABUSE

Asking the question is in and of itself an intervention. The nurse's role is to identify abuse and assist women who are pregnant or have babies and young children to obtain the help they need to remain safe and keep the children safe. Questions about violence should be a part of each prenatal and newborn care visit. Nursing implications include:

- Ask about domestic violence ("Have you ever been scared or hurt by your partner?")
- Acknowledge the client's response and validate her experience ("I'm so sorry this is happening. It must be hard for you.")
- Assess the immediate physical safety of mother and children ("Is it safe for you to go home today?")
- Refer to local domestic violence program for safety plan and support
- Ensure medical follow-up and support
- Document findings in the chart
- Report to appropriate agencies when the safety of a child is at risk (see Chapter 12∞ for further discussion of domestic violence and Chapter 7∞ for a discussion of child abuse).

Conversations should be respectful, private, and confidential:

- Children should not be present
- Use an interpreter when necessary
- Never use children to interpret
- Never ask about domestic violence in front of the woman's partner

Washington State Department of Health. (2004). Domestic Violence and Pregnancy: Guidelines for Screening and Referral *http://www.doh.wa.gov/cfh/mch/documents/dv_for_web.pdf accessed 2/25/05.*

- Minimizing the newborn's exposure to disease by avoiding infant exposure to large crowds, especially in cold and flu season; covering coughs and sneezes and using good handwashing technique especially if parent/caregiver is ill; alerting baby's caregiver if newborn is exposed to varicella, pertussis, or other serious communicable disease

Detailed immunization recommendations can be found in Chapter 19∞. For further information on SIDS risk reduction, see Partnering with Families: SIDS Risk Reduction and Developing Cultural Competence: SIDS.

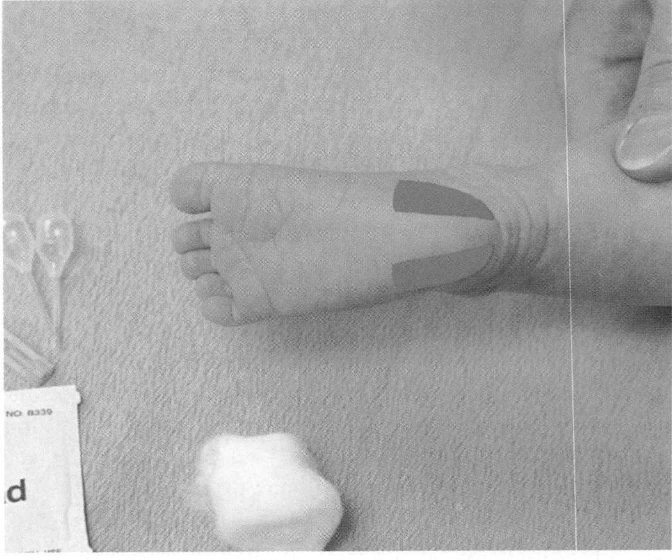

FIGURE 11–6 ■ Heel sites for capillary puncture.

INJURY PREVENTION STRATEGIES

New parents are sometimes unaware of sources of potential injury for the newborn. Some aspects of injury prevention are pertinent to the newborn's immediate care and other topics promote discussion and provide opportunities for anticipatory guidance. In the immediate newborn period, the nurse should assess the parents' knowledge of injury prevention strategies, and promote healthy and safe habits. Injury prevention strategies include proper and consistent use of an infant car seat, and strategies to prevent falls, burns, choking, drowning, and suffocation (see Box 11–10 and Table 11–6).

Newborn safety awareness begins in the birth setting. Parents should be cautioned against laying the baby on the mother's bed instead of in the bassinet, taught to use the bulb syringe in the event that the baby spits up a large amount of fluid, and taught to position the baby supine instead of side-lying or prone. Parents should also be oriented to procedures in place to prevent newborn abduction and to their critical role in assuring newborn safety and security.

BOX 11–8 Newborn Metabolic Screening

The purpose of newborn metabolic screening is to identify those newborns who require further diagnostic testing for an array of genetic diseases and metabolic disorders. The test involves a small amount of blood, usually taken by heelstick sample, which is then analyzed for indicators of specific disorders. The baby's healthcare provider is notified of the screening results, and should be alert to these results at the newborn's first outpatient visit. The department of health in each state regulates newborn metabolic screening, including the timing of the test, the need for repeat testing, and which tests are included in the screen.

The March of Dimes (2004a) recommends that all babies are screened for at least 29 specific disorders. Visit our Companion Website for more information.

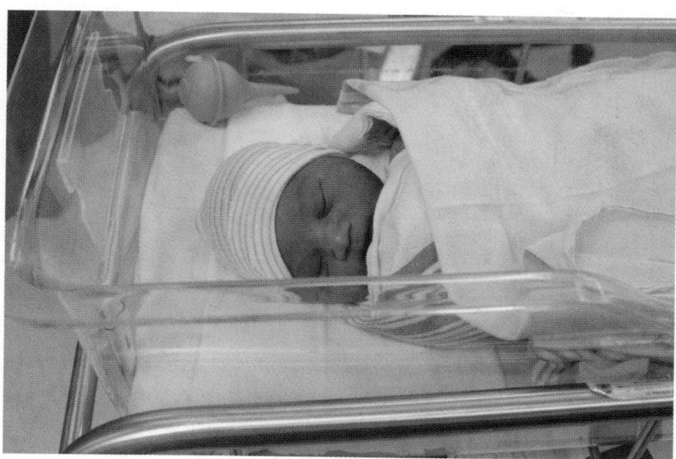

FIGURE 11–7 ■ Parents are more likely to place their newborn in the back-sleeping postion when they see it used in the hospital.

BOX 11–9 Newborn Hearing Screening

Hearing loss occurs in 1 of every 1,000 healthy newborns and 20–40 newborns requiring intensive care (AAP & ACOG, 2002). Universal hearing screening (all newborns tested regardless of risk factors) prior to hospital discharge is becoming the standard of care; however, universal hearing screening is not mandated by law in some states.

Newborn hearing screening is not diagnostic. A baby who "fails" the initial screen may be retested prior to hospital discharge. Parents should be advised that a "failed" screen is only an indication for referral to an audiologist for more conclusive testing. The evaluation should occur as soon as possible, but no later than 3 months of age. If treatment is delayed for longer than 6 months, permanent developmental delays can occur in an otherwise healthy infant (AAP & ACOG, 2002, p. 209). Encourage parents to return for follow-up screening, and provide suggestions about observing for infant hearing loss.

Following hospital discharge, the nurse promotes safety by encouraging parents to think about the hazards that the child could encounter and how to eliminate them. In the newborn period, the parent or caregiver is uniquely responsible for ensuring that the newborn is not placed in a dangerous situation. The newborn cannot turn on a hot water faucet or run with a sharp object, but it is possible for the parent to inadvertently place the newborn in danger. The newborn is capable of twisting and rolling off any surface higher than the floor, falling out of an infant carrier seat, or drowning while left unattended for a moment in a bathtub filled with only an inch or two of water.

BOX 11–10 Car Seat Assistance and Education

Nurses should use caution when teaching or assisting parents with infant car safety seats. Nurses who go beyond their level of expertise could face legal action if a subsequent car crash results in injury to the baby. Refer parents to a local trained child passenger safety technician for assistance, or use 1–866-SEAT-CHECK (www.seatcheck.org) to find a car seat inspection location.

(From Child Restraints, 2004)

PARTNERING WITH FAMILIES

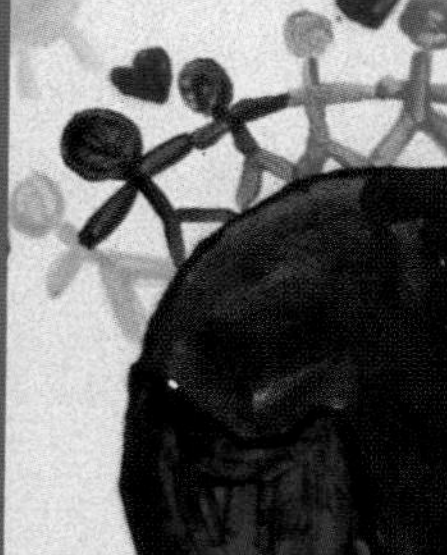

Handwashing

Handwashing is the key to preventing illness in the newborn and family members. Parents and family members should be taught about the importance of washing hands with soap and warm water.

- After diaper changes
- Before feeding the newborn
- After using the bathroom or assisting someone to use the bathroom
- Before preparing food or eating
- When returning home after being out in the community (e.g., at work, daycare, church, playing with friends, the mall)
- After handling pets
- After blowing nose or sneezing

Parents might find it helpful to be aware that most pediatric injuries occur when the parents are under stress; for example, when a parent is hungry and tired (the hour before dinner), during pregnancy, during illness or death in the family, when there is tension between parents, and during changes in the environment, such as a change in the child's caregiver or the family's living environment

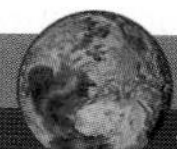

DEVELOPING CULTURAL COMPETENCE
SIDS

Since 1994, the Back to Sleep campaign has focused on increasing awareness among parents, healthcare providers, and childcare providers about the benefits of placing the baby to sleep in a back-lying position. (Figure 11–7). The Back to Sleep campaign is an ongoing nationwide public health effort to disseminate information on this health topic.

Even though there has been an almost 50% drop in the number of SIDS deaths among African American and White babies, a significant disparity still exists among racial and ethnic groups (HRSA, 2004). SIDS rates are highest for African Americans and American Indians and lowest for Asian and Hispanics. In 2001, the rate of SIDS among African Americans was more than twice that of Whites, and more than three times greater among American Indians than Whites (HRSA, 2004).

To promote the use of supine sleeping position for African American babies, the Back to Sleep campaign partners with the National Black Child Development Institute and other historically Black organizations to develop materials for a new initiative to reduce SIDS in African American communities.

Another culturally competent effort to reduce SIDS deaths among American Indians and Alaskan Natives comes from the Department of Health and Human Services Office of Minority Health and the Indian Health Service. Supported by the Robert Wood Johnson Foundation, these partners designed a tool for use by health and medical service providers, and community health trainers to expand SIDS risk reduction activities aimed at the Native American community. The SIDS Risk Reduction Resource Kit, titled "Face Up to Wake Up ™" includes culturally appropriate educational materials including posters, brochures, PSAs, radio spots, videos and CD-ROMs to enhance Back to Sleep campaigns.

TABLE 11–6 Injury Prevention Topics for Parents of Newborns

TOPIC	INJURY PREVENTION TEACHING TOPICS
Car safety seat	➤ Choose an infant-only seat or a convertible seat suitable for an infant. ➤ Infant rides rear-facing until at least 1 year of age and more than 20 lb. ➤ The safest place for all children to ride is in the back seat. Never place a rear-facing car safety seat in the front seat with an active passenger airbag. ➤ Use a car safety seat every time the infant is in the car. ➤ Read and follow the manufacturer's instructions for the car safety seat and the vehicle owner's manual for installation information. ➤ Dress the infant in clothes that allow the straps to go between the legs. Never place blankets under the baby. Buckle the baby into the seat, and place blankets over the baby. ➤ To make sure the car safety seat is installed correctly and the baby is positioned correctly, go to a car seat inspection station. A certified child passenger safety technician will assist you. Find a list of certified CPS technicians and safety seat inspection stations by state or zip code on the National Highway Traffic Safety Administration website or 1–866-SEAT-CHECK. (AAP, 2004a)
Shaken baby syndrome	Never shake a baby. Recognize that sometimes you will not be able to console your baby. Shaking a baby, even for only a few seconds, can cause serious brain damage and death. One of four shaken babies dies.
Crib	Use a safety approved crib. Slats should be no more than 2 3/8 inches apart. Mattress should be firm and fit snugly into the crib. Keep crib rails raised.
Co-sleeping	The AAP discourages co-sleeping due to the risk of SIDS (with overheating as a possible factor) and the danger of suffocation. Sleep with the baby nearby, but not in the parental bed. If the parent must sleep with the baby, ensure that the infant is supine; separated from any soft surfaces such as pillows; ensure that no blankets will cover the infant's head; beware of spaces between the mattress and the wall, headboard, or footboard; and do not sleep with the baby under the influence of drugs or alcohol. The infant should never sleep in the same bed with siblings due to the high risk of suffocation.
Baby toys	Use age-appropriate baby toys. Check toys for sharp edges or loose parts. Keep older siblings' toys out of baby's reach. Do not use toys with loops or string cords.
Drowning	Never leave baby alone in the bathtub. If you must turn your back on the baby or leave the room, take the baby out of the tub.
Suffocation	Keep plastic bags and wrappings away from baby (take the plastic bag off the crib mattress). Shake baby powder into your hand first then apply it so the baby does not inhale it. Do not allow a baby or sibling to play with a latex balloon. Keep small objects (such as safety pins, coins, small toys) out of baby's reach. Do not attach pacifiers, medals, or other objects to the crib or to the baby's body with a string or cord. Do not put the crib near blinds, curtains, or anything with a hanging cord. Do not let baby wear clothing with strings near the neck (such as a sweatshirt hood that ties with a cord) or a headband that could slip down and wrap around baby's neck. Use a tight-fitting crib sheet that does not come loose when the corner is pulled.
Burns	Set the hot water heater thermostat lower than 120°F. Do not smoke or drink hot liquids while holding the baby. Do not microwave bottles of formula or breast milk due to uneven heating. Do not expose baby to direct sunlight.
Falls	Keep a hand on the baby while dressing or diaper changing on a surface other than the floor. Never leave the baby unsupervised on any high surface such as a bed, changing table, or sofa. Always keep one hand on the baby.
Pet safety	Keep some distance between the newborn and the pet until the pet's initial reaction to the new baby is assessed. Never leave the baby unsupervised with the family dog or cat, or any animal capable of harming the newborn.
Sibling supervision	Never leave the baby alone with a young sibling. When young children hold the baby, seat the child on a large soft surface, such as the couch and supervise closely. Watch siblings for aggressive behavior toward the newborn, such as hitting or biting. Siblings may take on a caregiving role and imitate adults; watch for "feeding" of nonfood items or choking hazards.
Fire safety	Install working smoke detectors on every floor of the house and in every sleeping area. Have a fire escape plan from the house and practice it.
Poisoning	Post the universal phone number for the poison control center near your telephone: 1-888-222-1222.
Gun safety	Keep the household guns unloaded and locked up. Keep the ammunition locked up separately from the gun. Consider not keeping a gun in the household due to safety hazards for family members.
In case of emergency	➤ Know when and how to call the pediatric care provider. ➤ Know when it is appropriate to go to the emergency department. ➤ Take a first-aid class and learn CPR for children and adults.

Data from Green & Palfrey, 1998; Shelov, 2004; Child Restraints, 2004; AAP, 2004a; Carbaugh, 2004.

(Shelov, 2004). At these times, the parent should be particularly vigilant and supervise children closely.

NURSING MANAGEMENT

Nursing Assessment and Diagnosis

An essential skill for the nurse in the hospital, clinic, or community setting is the ability to assess the family and newborn and identify potential health promotion and health maintenance activities. Many health promotion and health maintenance activities are pertinent to prenatal health as well as the postpartum period. If maternal and pediatric care providers are located at different agencies, nurses must coordinate and integrate services so that the new mother and family benefit from a seamless continuum of care.

Based on nursing assessments, the nursing diagnoses form the basis for subsequent interventions. Possible nursing diagnoses for the family and newborn in the first month following birth might include:

- Anxiety (parent) related to change in role status
- Risk for Impaired, Attachment, Parent/Infant/Child related to relationship factors
- Risk for Impaired Attachment related to parental exhaustion or lack of knowledge of infant cues
- Risk for Impaired Parenting related to premature birth
- Effective Breastfeeding related to basic breastfeeding knowledge
- Ineffective Breastfeeding related to inadequate sucking by infant
- Readiness for Enhanced Parenting

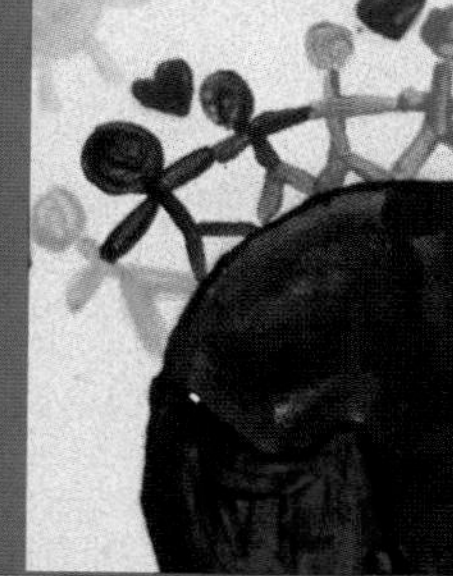

PARTNERING WITH FAMILIES

SIDS Risk Reduction

SIDS is defined as the sudden unexpected death of an infant less than 1 year of age, with onset of the fatal episode apparently occurring during sleep, that remains unexplained after a thorough investigation, including performance of a complete autopsy and review of the circumstances of death and the clinical history (Krous, Beckwith, Byard, et al., 2004). SIDS is the major cause of death in infants from 1 month to 1 year of age, with most deaths occurring between 2 and 4 months (Health Resources and Services Administration, 2004). See Chapter 24∞.

Currently, there is no way to prevent SIDS, but parents and caregivers can reduce the risk of a SIDS death. Prenatal behavior and maternal health can influence the occurrence of SIDS. Parents should know the following rules for basic sleep safety to reduce the risk of SIDS.

- Always place the baby in a supine (back-lying) position.
- Use a safe crib and a firm mattress.
- Remove all fluffy objects from the crib, such as quilts, stuffed animals, and pillows.
- Make sure the baby's face and head stay uncovered during sleep. Use a blanket sleeper instead of blankets in the crib.
- Avoid overheating the baby. A room temperature that is comfortable for the parent is fine for the newborn.
- Never smoke or allow anyone to smoke around the baby.
- Breastfeed your baby.

Planning and Implementation

Newborn health maintenance and promotion begins in the prenatal period. In most cases, the expectant mother is highly motivated to engage in activities that result in a healthy newborn, and the healthcare team has a unique window of opportunity to promote maternal and newborn health.

In the prenatal period, the nurse's goal is to promote an optimal outcome for both mother and newborn. Comprehensive quality prenatal care is outside the scope of this text; however, important health maintenance and health promotion activities include interventions to help ensure healthy diet and exercise; avoidance of alcohol, tobacco, and drugs; and establishment or maintenance of a dental home. The nurse may assess the need for assistance with food, clothing, and safe housing, which entails numerous referrals and advanced skills to ensure coordinated community services. The nurse provides anticipatory guidance regarding newborn care and safety, and the nurse may assist the woman with choosing a pediatric healthcare provider. The nurse in the prenatal setting plays an important role in educating the woman about the lifelong benefits of breastfeeding and in guiding her toward an informed infant feeding decision.

Hospital-Based Care

The hospital length of stay is short for the healthy mother and newborn. The nurse in the birth setting is responsible for assessing and implementing nursing care during a time of dramatic physiologic changes in both mother and newborn, as well as helping the new parents learn basic newborn care skills. Consistent and accurate breastfeeding information is essential to ensure continued efforts at home, and referral to a lactation specialist or support group is helpful. The nurse assesses and refers the mother to community resources as needed for domestic violence and drug, alcohol, or tobacco use. The nurse may coordinate interventions such as access to the Women, Infant, Child Nutrition Program (WIC) to help ensure adequate food and nutritional support, and refer the mother to parenting classes or support groups. Through listening to the family's concerns, providing nurturing responses, respecting cultural differences, and validating parental efforts to learn parenting skills, the nurse further develops the partnership between the family and the healthcare providers.

Prior to discharge the newborn has blood taken for metabolic screening, may have initial hearing screening, and may receive the first hepatitis B vaccination. Follow-up after these interventions requires communication among multiple community agencies and the pediatric care provider to ensure that the newborn receives appropriate continuing care.

Care in the Community

In the outpatient setting, the goal of the pediatric healthcare team is to "help the parents gain knowledge and confidence in caring for the physical, intellectual and emotional needs of their infant, and to encourage their personal growth as parents and the family's development as a unit" (Green & Palfrey, 2002). In the first month of the newborn's life, health promotion and maintenance activities may include teaching the parents how to interact with their baby to promote attachment, provide a safe sleeping environment, continue development and validation of baby care activities, especially breastfeeding, and begin to learn about the newborn's temperament in order to respond quickly and correctly to needs in order to promote infant mental health.

The relationship between the family and pediatric healthcare team must be nurtured. Time should be allowed for parents' questions. Cultural differences in perspectives must be considered. Results of screening and testing should be explained. When the nurse involves the parent in healthcare activities of the infant in these ways, it is more likely that parents will be cooperative and interested in promoting and maintaining their child's health.

Evaluation

Expected outcomes for the family and healthy newborn by the end of the first month are as follows:

- The newborn makes a successful transition from intrauterine to extrauterine life.
- Risk factors are identified in the prenatal and newborn period, and nursing assessment coordinates with medical intervention to prevent or manage complications.
- The newborn achieves expected physical and developmental milestones.
- Breastfeeding is established and the mother has identified sources of support to continue breastfeeding.
- The family begins successful integration of the newborn into the family.
- Parents demonstrate newborn care skills and beginnings of healthy attachment behaviors.
- Parents recognize the importance of health promotion and health maintenance activities and partner with healthcare professionals to promote and maintain the physical and mental health of the newborn and family.

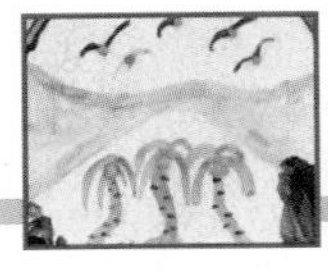

CHAPTER HIGHLIGHTS

- Health promotion and maintenance of the newborn begins with good prenatal care.
- The expectant mother is encouraged to choose her baby's care provider prior to the baby's birth.
- Family partnership is promoted when family has warm and supportive interactions with healthcare professionals who respect the parent's ability to learn about and participate in decisions related to the child's pediatric healthcare.
- The initial pediatric visits focus on infant growth and development, identification of problems not discovered at birth, parent teaching and support, and assessment of family–infant interaction.
- Breastfeeding advocacy is one of the most important health promotion activities that occurs during prenatal care and the first year of life.
- Infant mental health is promoted by parents who create a "child-centered" environment that allows the infant to develop a full set of skills for learning, thinking, responding, and solving problems.
- Infant mental health is largely dependent on the mental health of the primary caregiver, usually the infant's mother.
- Infant mental health and parent–infant attachment are promoted by such activities as responding quickly to the infant's expressed needs, holding, rocking, singing, talking to, and providing consistent and predictable responses to baby's needs.
- Disease prevention strategies include immunizations, back sleeping position, preventing secondhand smoke exposure, handwashing, screening, and minimizing newborn exposure to disease.
- Injury prevention strategies include proper and consistent use of an infant car seat, and strategies to prevent falls, burns, choking, drowning, and suffocation.

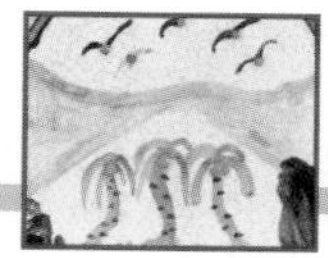

CRITICAL THINKING IN ACTION

INTRODUCTION

Recall 22-year-old Shannon who is described at the beginning of the chapter. She is a single mother with two daughters, 5-year-old Denise and 10-day-old Rhonda. Shannon lives with her boyfriend of the past 2 years. Rhonda was born at 37 weeks' gestation, weighed 2,800 g (6 lb, 3 oz) at birth, required phototherapy for newborn jaundice, and had initial difficulties breastfeeding. She was discharged from the nursery at 5 days of age.

DESCRIPTION

Rhonda is an active and fussy baby who reacts strongly to everything that happens around her. Shannon carries her into the exam room in her car seat. Rhonda is dressed appropriately for the weather and appears clean and well cared for. As the nurse undresses Rhonda, the baby arches and screams. Her diaper is dry. Shannon strokes her head and speaks quietly to her. Rhonda now weighs 2,830 g (6 lb, 4 oz). The nurse swaddles Rhonda in a blanket. She quiets, and the nurse places her in Shannon's arms. The nurse learns that Rhonda sleeps for only an hour or two at a time, then fusses. Shannon tries to feed her each time she stirs, but sometimes she has short drowsy feedings and does not seem hungry. Rhonda has about four wet diapers and two stools per day. Shannon's boyfriend is increasingly irritable as Rhonda is keeping him awake at night. Shannon states that Rhonda is a much more difficult baby than Denise was. She is exhausted, and feels like a bad mother and partner.

DISCUSSION

1. Shannon is an experienced mother, yet this newborn poses unexpected challenges. List the risk factors in the family, as well as the protective factors.
2. Based on the risk and protective factors, list three or four nursing diagnoses related to the family. What interventions will assist the family to better integrate Rhonda into their lives?
3. Lack of sleep is a major issue for Shannon's family. Describe infant states and determine what sleep state Rhonda is in when she stirs and fusses and makes crying sounds. How could Shannon extend the time between feedings so that Rhonda is more awake and interested in breastfeeding well 8 to 10 times per day? What other strategies could Shannon use to calm her sensitive newborn?
4. What questions would the pediatric nurse and lactation consultant ask Shannon to assess the adequacy of breastfeeding at this time? Calculate the percentage of Rhonda's weight loss since birth. Is this concerning? What other factors should be assessed at this visit?
5. Shannon feels sad and discouraged about her life at this point. What factors could be influencing her mood? What questions should be asked to assess Shannon's coping strategies? What interventions might be suggested? What positive aspects of Shannon's parenting could be noted and validated?

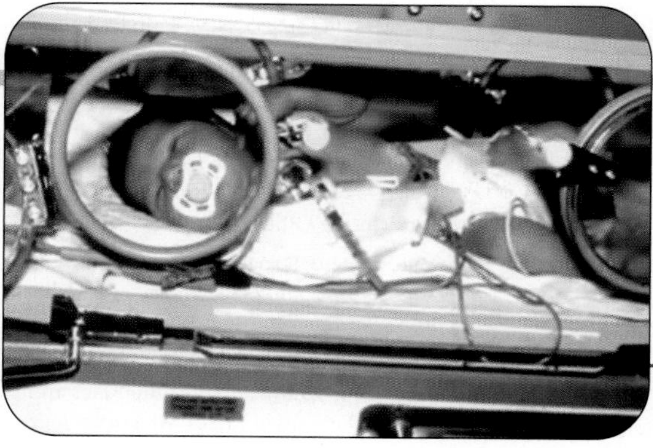

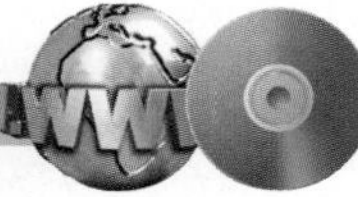

EXPLORE MediaLink

- NCLEX review, case studies, and other interactive resources for this chapter can be found on the Companion Website at **http://www.prenhall.com/ball**. Click on Chapter 11 to select the activities for this chapter.
- For animations, more NCLEX review questions, and an audio glossary, access the accompanying CD-ROM in this book.

http://www.prenhall.com/ball

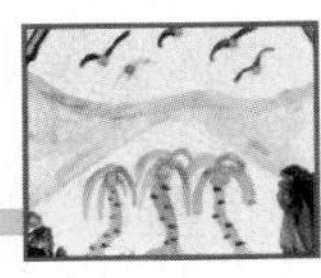

REFERENCES

American Academy of Pediatric Dentistry. (1999). Oral health policies. *Pediatric Dentistry, 21*, 18–37.

American Academy of Pediatrics. (2005). Policy statement: Breastfeeding and the use of human milk. *Pediatrics, 115*(2), 496–506.

American Academy of Pediatrics. (1999a). Circumcision policy statement. *Pediatrics, 103*(3), 686–693.

American Academy of Pediatrics. (1999b, July 6). News release: AAP: Cord blood banking for future transplantation not recommended. www.aap.org/advocacy/archives/julcord.htm, accessed 5/2/2004.

American Academy of Pediatrics. (1999c). Policy statement: Iron fortification of infant formulas. *Pediatrics, 104*(1), 119–123.

American Academy of Pediatrics. (1999d). Ten steps to support parents' choice to breastfeed their baby. www. aap.org/advocacy/bf/tensteps.pdf, Accessed 5/10/2004.

American Academy of Pediatrics. (2001). The prenatal visit. *Pediatrics, 107*(6).

American Academy of Pediatrics. (2002). Policy on use of a Caries-risk Assessment Tool (CAT) for infants, children, and adolescents. Oral Health Policies http://www.aapd.org/members/referencemanual/pdfs/02-03/p_CariesRiskAssess.pdf(9/5/04).

American Academy of Pediatrics. (2004a). *Car safety seats: A guide for families 2004*. Chicago: Author.

American Academy of Pediatrics. (2004b). Hospital stay for healthy term newborns. *Pediatrics, 113*(5), 1434–1436. http://aappolicy.aappublications.org/cgi/content/full/pediatrics;113/5/1434

American Academy of Pediatrics. (2004c). Management of hyperbilirubinemia in the newborn infant 35 or more weeks of gestation. *Pediatrics, 114*(1), 297–316. http://aappolicy.aappublications.org/cgi/content/full/pediatrics;114/1/297.

American Academy of Pediatrics. (2004d). Question and answers: Jaundice and your newborn. www.aap.org/family/jaundicefaq.htm, accessed 6/25/2004.

American Academy of Pediatrics & The American College of Obstetricians and Gynecologists. (2002). *Guidelines for perinatal care* (5th ed.). Elk Grove Village, IL: Author.

Blackburn, S. T., (2003). *Maternal, fetal, and neonatal physiology: A clinical perspective* (p. 538). St Louis: Saunders.

Blackburn, S. T., & Kang, R. (1991). *Early parent-infant relationships* (2nd ed.). White Plains, NY: March of Dimes Birth Defects Foundation.

Carbaugh, S. F. (2004). Understanding shaken baby syndrome. *Advances in Neonatal Care, 4*(2), 105–114.

Child restraints for newborn infants: A health care provider's guide. (2004). Seattle, WA: Safe Ride News Publications.

Dixon, S., & Stadtler, A. (2002). Age-specific observations of the parent–child interaction. In M. Jellinek, B. P. Patel, & M. C. Froehle (Eds.), *Bright futures in practice: Mental health* (Vol. II, p. 24). Arlington, VA: National Center for Education in Maternal and Child Health.

Green, M., & Palfrey, J. S. (Eds.). (2002). *Bright futures: Guidelines for health supervision of infants, children, and adolescents* (2nd ed., rev.). Arlington, VA: National Center for Education in Maternal and Child Health.

Gregory, S. (2002). Homeward bound. In J. Zaichkin (Ed.), *Newborn intensive care: What every parent needs to know* (2nd ed., p. 286). Santa Rosa, CA: NICU Ink Book Publishers.

Health and Human Services. (2000). *Blueprint for action on breastfeeding*. Washington, DC: U.S. Department of Health and Human Services, Office on Women's Health.

HealthCanada. (1999). A handbook for health and social service professionals responding to abuse during pregnancy. www.hc-sc.gc.ca/hppb/familyviolence/html/femexpose_e.html

Health Resources and Services Administration (HRSA), U.S. Department of Health and Human Services. (2004). *SIDS deaths by race and ethnicity 1995–2001*. Vienna, VA: National Sudden Infant Death Syndrome/Infant Death Resource Center.

Holditch-Davis, D., Blackburn, S.T., & VandenBerg, K. (2003). Newborn and infant neurobehavioral development. In C. Kenner & J. W. Lott (Eds.), *Comprehensive neonatal nursing: A physiologic perspective*. (3rd ed., p. 259). Philadelphia: Saunders.

Howard, C. R., Howard, F. M., Lanphear, B., deBlieck, E. A., Eberly, S., & Lawrence, R. (1999). The effects of early pacifier use on breastfeeding duration. *Pediatrics, 103*(3), e33. http://pediatrics.aappublications.org/cgi/content/full/103/3/e33

Jellinek, M., Patel, B. P., & Froehle, M. C. (Eds). (2002). *Bright futures in practice: Mental health* (Vol. I). Arlington, VA: National Center for Education in Maternal and Child Health.

Krous, H. F., Beckwith, B., Byard, R. et al. (2004). Sudden infant death syndrome and unclassified sudden infant deaths: A definitional and diagnostic approach. *Pediatrics, 114*(1), 234–238.

Lawrence, R. A. (1999). *Breastfeeding: A guide for the medical profession* (5th ed., p. 259). St Louis: Mosby.

Ludington-Hoe, S. M., Cong, X., & Hashemi, F. (2002). Infant crying: Nature, physiologic consequences, and select interventions. *Neonatal Network, 21*(2), 29–36.

March of Dimes. (2004a). Newborn screening tests: Professionals and researchers. www.marchofdimes.com/professionals/681_1200.asp accessed 2/25/05.

March of Dimes. (2004b) Umbilical cord blood. www.marchofdimes.com/professionals/681_1160.asp, accessed 5/12/2004.

Meek, J. Y. (2001). Breastfeeding in the workplace. *Pediatric Clinics of North America, 48*, 461–474.

Miller, L.J., & Rukstalis, M. 1999. Beyond the "blues": Hypotheses about postpartum reactivity. In L.J. Miller (Ed). *Postpartum mood disorders*, (pp. 65–82). Washington, DC: American Psychiatric Press.

Mills, L. (2000). Umbilical cord blood banking: Helping our patients make the best choices. *Genetics Northwest* (Oregon Health Science University), *14*(1), 5.

MMWR. (2001). Kernicterus in full-term infants—United States, 1994–1998. *MMWR, 50*(23), 491–494.

National Center for Missing & Exploited Children. (2003). *For healthcare professionals: Guidelines on prevention of and response to infant abductions* (7th ed.). Alexandria, VA: Author.

Orleans, C. T., Barker, D. C., Kaufman, N. J., & Marx, J. F. (2000). Helping pregnant smokers quit: Meeting the challenge in the next decade. *Tobacco Control, 9*(Suppl III), iii6–iii11.

Owens, P. L., Thompson, J., Elixhauser, A., & Ryan, K. (2003). *Care of children and adolescents in U.S. hospitals*. (HCUP Fact Book No. 4, AHRQ Publication No. 04–0004). Rockville, MD: Agency for Healthcare Research and Quality.

Persing, J., James, H., Swanson, J., & Kattwinkel, J. (2003). Prevention and management of positional skull deformities in infants. *Pediatrics, 112*(1), 199–202.

Shelov, S. P. (Ed.). (2004, 4th edition). *The American Academy of Pediatrics: Caring for your baby and young child: Birth to age 5*. New York: Bantam Books.

Spangler, A. (2000). *Breastfeeding: A parent's guide* (7th ed.). Danbury Hospital, The Family Birth Center.

U.S. Department of Health and Human Services. (2000). *Healthy People 2010: Understanding and improving health* (2nd ed.). Washington, DC: U.S. Government Printing Office.

Washington State Department of Health. (2004). *Domestic Violence and Pregnancy: Guidelines for Screening and Referral.* http://www.doh.wa.gov/cfh/mch/documents/dv_for_web.pdf accessed 2/25/05.

Wolf, J. H. (2003). Low breastfeeding rates and public health in the United States. *American Journal of Public Health, 93*(12).

Chapter 12

Health Promotion and Health Maintenance of the Infant

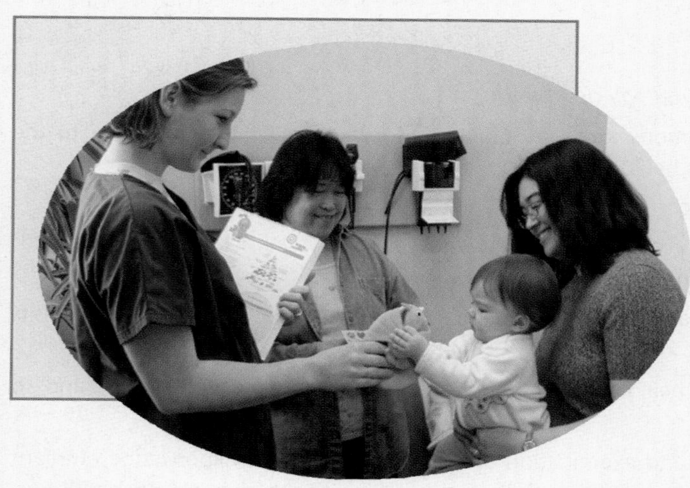

Colleen Agamata arrives at the Women, Infant, and Children's (WIC) clinic with her 7-month-old infant Amanda. Colleen works full time, so her mother accompanies her to take Amanda home by bus after the examination by the nurse and a meeting with the dietitian.

It has been hard for Colleen to manage with Amanda and her four-year-old Melody, but she is determined to support them. She was recently referred to the WIC program to receive screening and examination of her infant, and teaching related to nutrition. The eligibility card enables her to purchase food for herself and her children. She has had several episodes of food insecurity when she did not have enough money to buy food for herself or Melody. Now, with a new infant, the challenges are even more difficult to meet. Colleen's mother helps as much as possible, but has impaired vision, and also needs assistance with some tasks.

The nurse screens Amanda for hematocrit to measure her iron intake, and weighs and measures her so that growth can be monitored. The nurse and dietitian collaborate to teach Colleen health promotion information related to the benefits of nutritious intake, and health maintenance data about ways that food intake can help to prevent such diseases as iron deficiency anemia. They make an appointment to have Colleen bring in both Melody and Amanda for a visit in 2 months.

What ongoing assessment will Melody and Amanda need? How can the nurse in the WIC clinic work with Colleen and the rest of her family to ensure food security and food intake that will both ensure healthy growth and prevent disease?

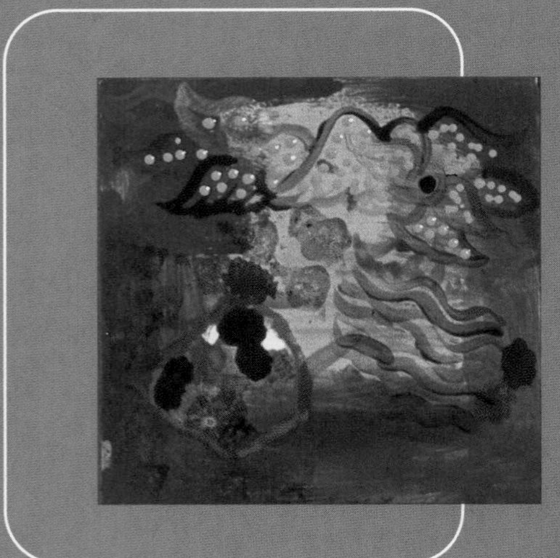

"Mommy was really glad to go see the nurse today. She took our baby and grandma said that they would give us a card that would help us buy food. Mommy said we could get some milk and juice."

—Melody, age 4

Key Terms

Learning Outcomes

After completing this chapter, you will be able to:

- Describe the general observations made of infants and their families as they come to the pediatric healthcare home for health supervision visits.
- Identify the major health concerns of infancy.
- Apply assessment skills to gather data regarding nutrition, physical activity, mental health status, and growth and development of infants.
- Apply therapeutic communication skills with infant and family during health supervision visits in infancy.
- Intervene with infants and their families to integrate activities to promote health and to prevent disease and injury.
- Synthesize data from history and examination of infant and family with knowledge of infant development to plan approaches useful with the family during health supervision encounters.

MediaLink 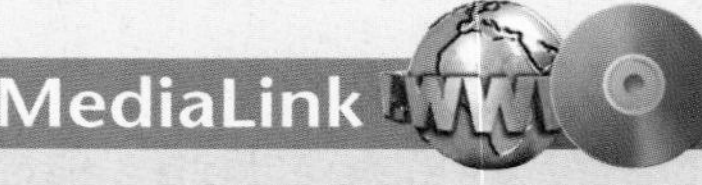 **http://www.prenhall.com/ball**

Resources for this chapter can be found on the CD-ROM accompanying this textbook, and on the Companion Website at www.prenhall.com/ball. Click on Chapter 12 to select the activities for this chapter.

CD-ROM

Videos

Helping the Infant Sleep
Infancy: A Major Life Transition

NCLEX Review

Audio Glossary

COMPANION WEBSITE

NCLEX Review

Case Study: Recognize Domestic Abuse

MediaLink Applications

Evaluate Immunizations Resources
Infant Percentile Measurements

Infancy is a major life transition for the infant and parents. The infant accomplishes phenomenal physical growth and many developmental milestones while the family adapts to the addition of a new member and establishes new goals for each of its existing members. Infant health supervision visits are important to support the health of the infant and the family unit. These visits begin after the newborn period, at about 1 month of age. This is the time when parents establish an ongoing partnership with a healthcare provider. A "medical home" or "pediatric healthcare home" is identified to serve the infant's health needs. (See Chapters 1 and 10∞ for further description of the medical or pediatric healthcare home.) The goals of health supervision visits are to identify and address the health promotion and health maintenance (or health protection) needs of the infant. Health promotion activities focus on promoting the highest level of wellness possible for the infant. Facilitating breastfeeding, helping parents to understand their infant's temperament, and employing strategies to ensure adequate sleep by the infant and parents are examples of health promotion activities. Health maintenance activities focus on disease and injury prevention. Some examples of these interventions include administering immunizations and teaching about infant car seats. Both health promotion and health maintenance interventions are integrated into each health supervision visit.

Recall the Bindler-Ball Continuum of Pediatric Healthcare from Chapters 1 and 10∞. All children require health promotion and health maintenance activities, even if they have frequent acute health conditions or chronic health diagnoses. The Health Resources and Services Administration of the U.S. Maternal and Child Health Bureau has partnered with the American Academy of Pediatrics to sponsor an initiative to ensure access to a medical home or pediatric healthcare home for all children, including those with children with special healthcare needs (CSHCN). While these children often receive specialty care related to their conditions, routine healthcare is sometimes lacking. The components of this care include:

- *Access to a consistent place to go for both sick and well-child care.* This will enhance preventive services and health outcomes.
- *Personal doctor or nurse.* This relationship influences family satisfaction and access to care.
- *Referrals for specialty care as needed.* Prompt identification of the need for specialty care and coordination with the primary care provider are needed.
- *Care coordination as a distinguishing characteristic of the pediatric healthcare home.* This involves knowledge of other types of care received and a focused time to discuss all care.
- *Family-centered care which is essential for all children.* For CSHCN, families are recognized as care coordinators and case managers; it involves partnership with the family to plan for the best care options for the child.

(Strickland, McPherson, Weissman, et al., 2004)

Establishment of the relationship with a healthcare provider and agency is important so that trust develops and the family feels comfortable turning to professionals for information and guidance as the infant grows. Nurses play a vital role in welcoming new families into office and clinic settings, establishing rapport, and applying principles of communication so that trust and positive partnerships develop between providers and families. Infancy is a time when the child grows in physical, psychological, and cognitive ways; health supervision visits play a key role in fostering healthy growth and development. When should the infant be seen for health supervision visits? What are key components of these visits? How can the nurse best assess and intervene to ensure the infant's health and safety? These are some of the questions that will be answered in this chapter.

MediaLink Infancy: A Major Life Transition Video

EARLY CONTACTS WITH THE FAMILY

Health promotion and health maintenance occur in a series of health supervision visits during the first year of life. Schedules vary among facilities, but a common pattern includes visits at about 1 month, 2 months, 4 months, 6 months, 9 months, and 1 year of age. In addition, most children have some episodic illnesses such as gastrointestinal illness or otitis media and visit the facility at other times for treatment of these illnesses. A few children have chronic or serious healthcare problems during the first year, and have extensive contact with the healthcare home and other services.

Since the family relies on the healthcare provider for support and interventions during infancy, the family has preferably established contact with the provider before the infant is born. If the family has not chosen a care provider during pregnancy and the newborn period, they can visit potential agencies when the baby is an infant and ask questions related to the services, personnel, and other components of care. (See Chapter 11∞ for questions the parents can ask at this visit and for clues about how to evaluate their fit with the care provider.) At whatever time it occurs, the purpose of the visit is to ensure that the family understands the services offered and the policies related to provision of care, and feels comfortable with the personality of the providers. Sometimes parents visit two or more providers and choose the best fit for the family.

Chapter 11∞ discusses the first health supervision visits in the immediate newborn period and up to 1 month of life. At about 1 month, the visits of infancy begin. During these first visits, assess the family for protective factors and risks. Protective factors might include parental knowledge level of infant needs, support from family and friends, and the mother's good health and nutritional state during pregnancy. Risk factors could include limited financial resources, lack of preparation for the infant, and illness or other stress among family members. Knowledge of these factors will shape the nursing interventions in health supervision in infancy. The nurse applies health promotion principles by building on strengths and fosters health maintenance by intervening to minimize risks. Many examples of these activities follow throughout this chapter.

GENERAL OBSERVATIONS

When the family comes to the clinic or office for care with an infant, general observations should begin at first contact (Figure 12–1 ■). This often occurs as the family is called in from the waiting area. The nurse can observe factors such as:

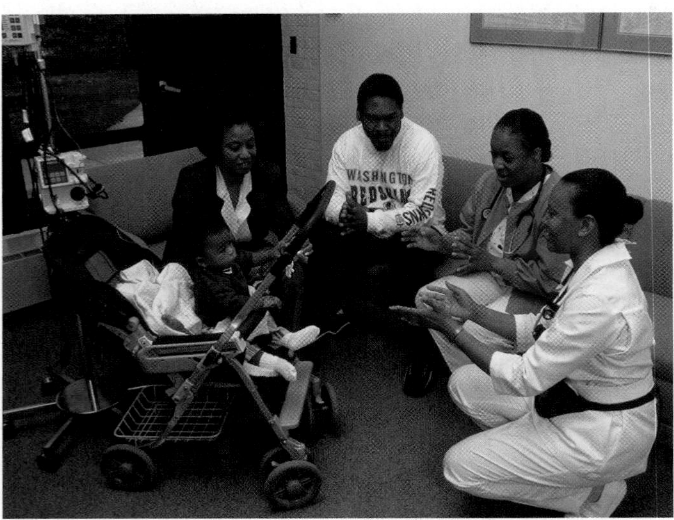

FIGURE 12–1 ■ The nurse begins assessment of the infant's family when they are seen in the waiting room and called in for care. What observations can you make of the infant's general appearance? Developmental accomplishments? Interaction of parents with the baby?

- Who is bringing the infant in for care?
- What are interactions like between the adults present or adults, other siblings, and the infant?
- Is the infant awake or sleeping?
- If awake, is the infant's body posture and alertness appropriate for age and developmental level?
- Does the infant look well nourished and cared for?

Welcome the family warmly to the facility and comment on the infant. Ask how the family is doing with the baby and how the adjustment is going. Be alert for signs of fatigue or depression in the parents, as these can occur when caring for an infant and can interfere with bonding and positive transition (Box 12–1). Postpartum blues and postpartum depression are two specific types of mood disorders sometimes observed in new mothers; postpartum psychosis is more serious and less common. These conditions are discussed in Chapter 11∞, and are referred to later in this chapter.

Upon entering the examination room, it is helpful to explain the plans for the visit, such as "I will weigh and measure Sarah now and show you how she is growing. Then I'll ask a few questions about her eating, sleeping, and other things. Then the nurse practitioner will be in to do Sarah's physical examination. Do you have any questions as we start? Will you undress Sarah now so we can weigh her accurately?"

BOX 12–1 Signs of Sleep Deprivation in Parents

- Confusion
- Forgetfulness
- Lack of alertness and coordination
- Fatigue
- Increased injuries
- Anxiety
- Decreased motivation
- Disturbed appetite

Data from Murray, R. B., & Zentner, J. P. (2001). Health promotion strategies through the life span *(7th ed.). Upper Saddle River, NJ: Prentice-Hall.*

GROWTH AND DEVELOPMENTAL SURVEILLANCE

Physical growth and meeting of developmental milestones provide important information about infants. The infant is measured for accurate length, weight, and head circumference (see the Skills Manual and Chapter 8∞). The measurements should be placed on growth grids and interpreted. (See Appendix A∞.) Parents enjoy seeing how the infant is progressing and are usually eager to learn about the child's weight gain and growth percentiles (Figure 12–2 ■). Be alert for an infant who demonstrates a change in percentile range. For example, if the infant was in the 75th percentile for length and weight at birth, but has fallen to below the 50th percentile for weight, additional assessment will be needed about the infant's feedings. Likewise, if the head circumference is much lower or higher than the length and weight percentiles, further neurologic and developmental assessment should be done. See Partnering with Families: Percentile Measurements.

In some settings, other growth measurements may be taken, such as chest circumference. If the infant was premature or has specific healthcare needs, particular attention must be paid to physical growth measurements.

Growth measurement is followed by a physical assessment. The nurse may complete parts of the assessment, with the remainder performed by the physician, nurse practitioner, or other primary care provider. The assessment evaluates each body system, with particular attention paid to heart, skin, musculoskeletal system, abdomen, and neurologic status. See Chapter 8∞ for a thorough discussion of physical assessment.

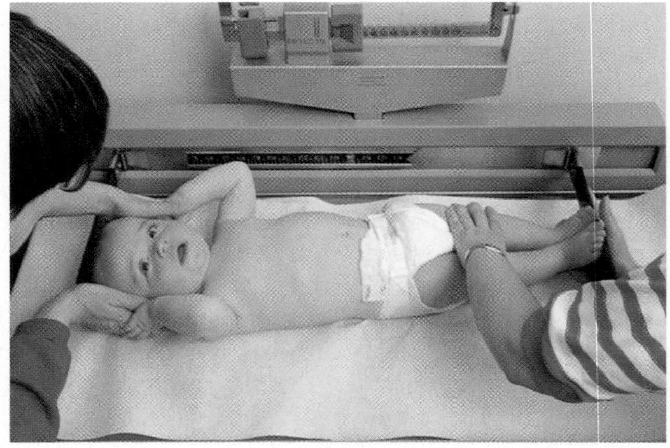

FIGURE 12–2 ■ Weighing and measuring length during health supervision visits provides important information about the child's nutrition and general development. This young infant was measured and then while the parents dressed the child the nurse placed the findings on the growth grid.

TABLE 12–1	Developmental Milestones Observed in Health Promotion and Health Maintenance Visits
AGE	**DEVELOPMENTAL MILESTONES**
1 month	Responds to sound by startle or increased alertness Follows objects and human face with eyes Has periods of alertness and restfulness Comforted by touch or feeding by parent Has symmetrical movements and generally has arms and legs flexed Lifts head momentarily when prone
2 months	Above characteristics Makes noises such as cooing in response to interaction with adult Smiles Lifts head, neck, upper chest when prone Has increasing head control when held in sitting position
4 months	Increasing cooing and babbling Smiles, laughs, makes other noises during interactions Supports self on hands when prone Rolls front to back Touches objects and grasps rattle placed near hand
6 months	Uses sounds in repeated speech such as "bababa, dadadada" Interested in surroundings and toys When pulled to sitting has no head lag Sits with support Grasps objects easily and places in mouth Transfers objects from one hand to other Bears weight on legs when held in standing position
9 months	Understands simple words and uses more sounds in babbling Responds to name Enjoys interactive games with parent Moves when placed on floor by crawling, creeping, or rolling repeatedly Sits without support Stands holding on to support Plays with toys Feeds self readily with fingers and tries to use cup
12 months	Has one or more words Imitates sounds readily Increasing interactions and interest in surroundings Follows directions such as saying "bye-bye" or waving goodbye Pulls to standing, walks a few steps holding on Well-developed pincer grasp Able to drink from cup

During the assessment, ask about care of the infant, observing areas where the family feels comfortable and those where the family needs assistance.

- Ask about the infant's bath routine and general skin and nail care. If the infant is a boy, do the parents have questions about care for the circumcised or uncircumcised penis?
- Find out about bowel patterns and if the family has questions about normal bowel movements for infants. (See Chapter 30∞ for a description of bowel movements in infants.) While breastfed babies rarely become constipated, they may not have daily bowel movements.

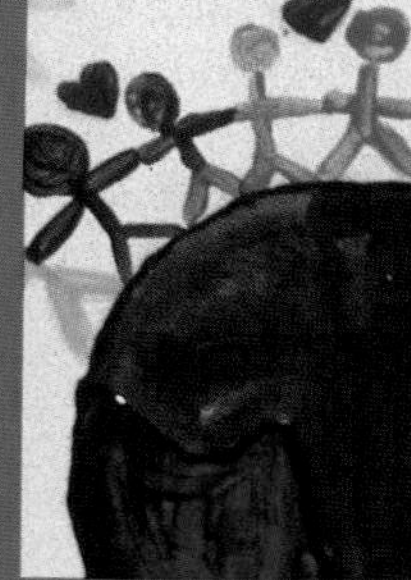

PARTNERING WITH FAMILIES

Percentile Measurements

Parents commonly do not understand what the term *percentile* means. When you tell them that their infant is in the 50th percentile for length, it is good to tell them, "If there were 10 babies of the same age, about half would be longer than your baby and about half would be shorter." Then explain that each baby has individual characteristics and that percentile measurements help to see if the baby is staying in approximately the same percentile range over time and growing at the expected rate. Show them the grid on which the percentile ranking is placed.

- Was the infant wrapped appropriately for the temperature? Some parents wrap babies in many layers of clothing even in very hot weather.
- Does the parent have a nonmercury thermometer and know how to take the baby's temperature?

Developmental surveillance is integrated into each visit (see Chapter 10∞). Begin by observing developmental milestones in the infant (see Chapter 5∞ for a summary of milestones expected at different ages). Table 12–1 summarizes some developmental milestones that can commonly be observed during infant healthcare visits.

PRACTICE ALERT

If an infant is observed to fail to meet an expected developmental milestone during a healthcare visit, inquire about this with the parents. Examine the results of any developmental questionnaire the parents may have completed. Plan to administer the Denver II or other developmental test to obtain further information. Observe the infant carefully. For example, if a 4-month-old baby fails to hold the head erect when sitting or prone, ask the parents if the baby has ever done so. Inquire about how the baby is positioned at home. Have the baby follow an object to see if the eyes can track. Observe the infant in the prone position and observe how far the head is held and whether the body is supported on the hands.

When there is no opportunity to observe a skill directly, ask parents about whether the infant performs the skill (Box 12–2). In addition to direct observation, parents are usually requested to fill in a form that asks questions about common developmental tasks. (Table 10–5∞ lists some commonly used questionnaires.) Review the results and determine if additional questions should be asked. When some milestones have not been met, make an appointment for the infant to have a developmental test by a certified examiner. (See Developing Cultural Competence: Developmental Milestones.) Tests commonly used with young children are listed in Table 10–6∞ on page 370.

The nurse establishes health promotion and health maintenance interventions related to growth and development assessment data. Anticipatory guidance related to development is a

BOX 12–2 Communication Techniques

When inquiring about a child's performance of a skill, begin with open-ended questions. Parents want their children to perform well, so they may answer that the child can do any skill about which the nurse inquires. Open-ended questions can help avoid this problem. For example, rather than asking "Does Jeremiah reach for a rattle with his hand?" it is better to say "Describe what Jeremiah does if you hold a rattle in front of him."

major component of health promotion. The nurse anticipates the next milestones the infant will be meeting, and recommends ways for the parents to support the infant in progression. Health promotion activities include the following:

- Teaching about food introduction that will foster growth
- Encouraging toys and activities that will assist in meeting the next developmental milestones
- Demonstrating gross and fine motor skills that the infant has achieved
- Demonstrating to parents how the child will focus on their faces and mimic their vocal sounds

Other interventions are focused on health maintenance or disease and injury prevention. For example, a 6-month-old is reaching for objects, readily places things in the mouth, and is able to move around on the floor; these characteristics make certain accidents more likely to occur. Ask if the parents have handed the infant any finger foods. Suggest foods that would be appropriate and discuss foods that commonly cause choking and should be avoided (see Chapter 9∞). Likewise, since the infant is becoming more mobile, parents should get onto the floor and look for hazards at the infant's eye level. Safety hazards and ways to avoid them are discussed, and parents are given brochures, websites, or videotapes to enhance injury prevention information. Can you outline additional health promotion and health maintenance interventions that relate to the infant's growth and development?

NUTRITION

The importance of nutrition during the first year of life cannot be overestimated. The infant will triple in birth weight by 1 year of age, and has a need for nutritional balance. From the first sips of breast milk or formula as a newborn, to eating the family meal at 1 year of age, the fast progression of nutritional intake patterns is obvious (Figure 12–3 ■). See Chapter 9∞ for a thorough description of nutritional needs during infancy.

During each visit, the nurse seeks to learn what the infant is eating, and whether the family has any questions or concerns related to intake (Story, Holt, & Sofka, 2002). Once again, open-ended questions are a good way to begin, with more specific questions inserted after the parent's perceptions are known. Examples are as follows:

- Describe Kara's breastfeeding.
- How do you know when Kara is hungry? Satisfied?
- Describe how often Kara eats and for how long.
- Do you think she eats enough? Too much?
- Is there anything you would change about the eating patterns?
- What does your baby do when you hold him on your lap and are eating?
- Which foods are more likely to cause a baby to choke?
- Describe your diet, weight, and energy level.
- What questions and concerns do you have related to your breastfeeding?
- Does your family always have access to adequate foods? Are you ever hungry or worried about having enough food for yourself or your family? Do you ever go without food so your children have enough to eat?
- What is the source of your drinking water? Describe how and when you give fluoride to your baby.

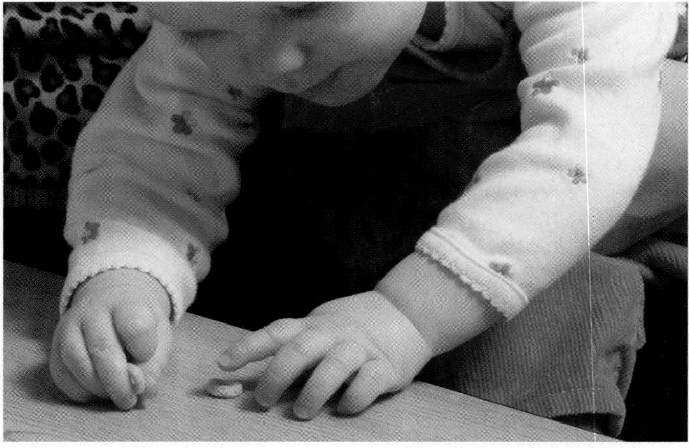

FIGURE 12–3 ■ During the first year of life nutritional intake patterns reflect the developmental progression of the infant. The baby first receives all nutrition from milk and closely bonds with the parent during feeding. As the baby becomes able to take in and metabolize other foods, parents begin to feed soft foods. When the infant can sit, reach for objects, and place them in the mouth, finger foods are introduced. The baby in this picture has developed the pincer grasp and is able to feed foods to self using this ability. Choices should include nutritionally sound food that helps to meet the baby's recommended allowances. By the first birthday, the child has developed the social and motor ability to eat most of the food commonly consumed in the family. Eating has been a mirror of social, metabolic, and developmental progression throughout the first year.

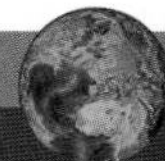

DEVELOPING CULTURAL COMPETENCE
Developmental Milestones

Be alert for differences in cultural practices and beliefs that may influence developmental milestones. For example, if a child is kept on a cradleboard for much of the time, the baby may be slow in learning to crawl. This baby may progress directly to standing by furniture without demonstrating as much creeping or crawling as other infants. In addition, when parents do not have English as a primary language and the examiner uses English, common terms might be misinterpreted. Parents might not understand what is meant if you ask, "Does your baby have a mobile over the crib at home?" or "Is she starting to be afraid of strangers?" How can you be alert for language differences and become sensitive to miscommunication? Refer to Chapter 3∞ for additional examples of cultural influences.

Once the infant is in the second half of the first year, food patterns of the family become more important. Consider childcare settings as well. Questions could include:

- Kara goes to an infant care center each day. Do you know what they feed her there?
- What unusual reactions has your baby shown to foods? Are there foods she dislikes?

Observations from other portions of the visit can provide clues about additional questions to ask. If an infant has not gained weight as expected and has fallen into a lower channel of weight percentile, more specific analysis of intake is needed. Ask for a recall of the infant's intake in the previous day. When the infant does not meet developmental milestones on schedule or is lethargic, intake may be inadequate for age. In these cases support may be needed to ensure adequate intake; a thorough description of feeding may be the first step in analyzing the problem and planning interventions. When the child's ability to take in nutrients or the parent's ability to feed the infant is questioned, an observation of a feeding might take place, either at the healthcare setting or during a home visit. Tools are available to evaluate the feeding interactions of infants and their parents. One example is the Feeding Scale, which is part of the Nursing Child Assessment Satellite Training (NCAST) program. Such tools require training and provide the nurse with a method to make reliable observations about the child's feeding patterns and the corresponding interaction with the parent.

On the other hand, for the infant who has gained more weight than expected it is important to ask how often the child is eating and what types of foods are consumed. The family may need information about the recommended number of feedings and types of foods appropriate for the child.

Babies with health conditions such as cerebral palsy often have difficulty eating and may need additional support. Other health conditions can create the need for increased intake of certain nutrients. For example, a premature infant might need milk enhancers for breast milk or preterm formulas during infancy. Whatever the health condition, the principles of health promotion and health maintenance visits are still followed, with addition of approaches specific for the child's health needs.

As the infant grows, the nurse asks questions about the types of foods the infant has been offered. Parents are invited to describe feedings and any concerns they have. Other family members may have provided information about how to feed infants, and the parents need an opportunity to ask about the family's recommendations. Ask about fluid intake of the infant and assess the parent's knowledge of signs of dehydration (see Chapter 23∞). Integrate your knowledge of infant nutritional needs (see Chapter 9∞) to develop a set of questions specific to each health supervision visit. How will nutritional concerns of the 9-month-old infant differ from those of the 4-month-old infant?

Additional nutritional assessment measures are used at certain points in the first year. A hematocrit or hemoglobin is generally performed between 9 and 12 months of age. Lead screening may be needed in certain population groups (see Chapter 30∞). Food security screening can be used when appropriate (see Chapter 9∞). Recall that food security relates to the family's access at all times to adequate food.

Each visit includes nutritional teaching about important items. The topics for discussion vary according to age group. See Table 12–2 for suggested teaching topics at specific ages. Can you identify which topics are mainly health promotion and which are mainly health maintenance? Most of the activities listed are

TABLE 12–2 Nutrition Teaching for Health Promotion and Health Maintenance Visits

AGE	NUTRITION TEACHING
1 month	Support breastfeeding efforts Teach correct formula types and preparation if used Teach burping and rate of feeding information Suggest water during hot weather or if family wants to use a bottle at baby's bedtime Encourage families to view feedings as social interactions; emphasize importance of holding the infant and not propping bottles
2 months	Continue above Review fluid needs of infants Reinforce food safety for partially used bottles of breast milk or formula Use warm water for heating bottles rather than microwave to avoid burning Warn against feeding honey in the first year of life Begin cleaning of infant gums daily Provide information about any supplements needed (e.g., iron for premature infant, vitamin D for babies not exposed to adequate sunlight)
4 months	Continue above Discuss introduction of first foods between 4–6 months, and surveillance for symptoms of allergy or intolerance Discuss changing food patterns such as increasing amounts and decreasing numbers of daily milk feedings
6 months	Continue above Reinforce proper introduction of new foods, to include rice cereal, fruits, vegetables Discuss any unusual food reactions observed Introduce cup for drinking Introduce soft finger foods Serve juice only in a cup and limit to no more than 6 ounces daily Caution about common choking foods and items Provide information about fluoride supplement if water supply is not fluoridated
9 months	Continue above If mother does not continue to breastfeed, teach family to use iron-fortified formula for the first year of life Encourage self-feeding of finger foods, integrating common foods for the family Introduce source of protein such as tofu, cheese, mashed beans, slivers of meat
12 months	Continue above Support mother who wishes to continue breastfeeding beyond 1 year of age Encourage cups for all feedings other than breast

MediaLink Developmental Tools

related to health promotion; however, a few relate to health maintenance as they are directed at disease prevention. Offering adequate fluids helps to prevent dehydration. Using only cups for juice limits amounts of juices, thereby helping to prevent obesity, and limits the exposure, thus preventing dental caries in newly erupting teeth. Do you see any other health maintenance interventions for nutrition teaching in Table 12–2?

Desired outcomes for nutrition in infancy include adequate growth, normal nutritional assessment findings, and knowledge by parents of the nutritional needs of the infant.

PHYSICAL ACTIVITY

Physical activity is needed for adequate development of fine and gross motor skills in infancy. Unlike other times of life, the focus is on providing only the opportunities for activity, without a need to focus on motivation. As long as infants are meeting developmental milestones and have a stimulating environment that provides opportunity for fine and gross motor activity, they will use their motor skills, thus enhancing their performance. Time should be provided each day for the infant to reach for objects, exercise legs and arms freely, and increasingly use head control. Playing with parents or others and being surrounded by toys and other stimulating items will encourage motor behavior in all body parts. Ask the parents for a description of the infant's typical day and listen for these types of play periods. Observe the physical skills of the infant (see Chapter 5∞ for motor developmental norms), ask questions about play periods provided, and compose a list of the family protective factors and risk factors in this area. Table 12–3 lists risk and protective factors related to physical activity during infancy.

When the child has a special health or developmental condition such as mental retardation or neuromuscular disease, physical activity is important to evaluate. General guidelines for the child with a disability include the following:

- Focus on assessment of usual routines and skills needed to accomplish daily tasks such as eating and moving the head to follow objects.

TABLE 12–3 Risk and Protective Factors Regarding Physical Activity in Infancy

RISK FACTORS	PROTECTIVE FACTORS
➤ Premature birth ➤ Delayed developmental milestones ➤ Limited stimulation by family or other care providers ➤ Lack of knowledge by family about infant's physical activity needs ➤ Limited community resources for families with infants	➤ Meets developmental milestones at expected ages ➤ Has contact with parents, siblings, and others for significant time each day ➤ A supportive environment with room to play safely, stimulating surroundings ➤ Physically active family ➤ Family knowledge about infant's physical activity needs ➤ Community programs that promote physical activity in infants and information for families

Data from Patrick, K., Spear, B., Holt, K., & Sofka, D. (Eds.). (2001). Bright futures in practice: Physical activity. *Arlington, VA: National Center for Education in Maternal and Child Health.*

- Consider assessing the child in the natural environment of home or childcare to ensure validity.
- Search out and use tools designed to measure physical performance of infants with developmental delay.
- Include the family in the assessment process.

(Miller & Robinson, 1996)

Based on the results of assessment and using the concept of anticipatory guidance, the nurse plans appropriate teaching for the family. Health promotion teaching for the family includes the following:

- Frequent and supervised play opportunities are needed.
- Holding the infant in various positions, helping the older infant to stand, and providing positive feedback for the infant's accomplishments are encouraged.
- Toys should be placed to encourage movement.
- Participation in parent-infant play groups provides stimulation for the child and social interaction with other infants, and increases the parent's knowledge of the child's abilities.
- Discussion of the next fine and gross motor skills are anticipated.

(Patrick, Spear, Holt, et al., 2001).

Health maintenance deals with prevention of physical development delays. When an infant is developing more slowly than expected, was premature, or has a diagnosed condition such as cerebral palsy, additional support may be needed. Explain physical activities that the child will be learning next. Make specific suggestions to foster stimulation, ensure adequate range of motion, and maximize developmental progression. The nurse may partner with a physical therapist or other specialist during the health supervision visit to enhance the physical activity of the infant. Referral for developmental screening or to infant programs that work with developmentally delayed infants should be considered. The Zero-to-Three Project: National Center for Infants, Toddlers and Families works to promote the healthy development of infants and toddlers by supporting and strengthening families, communities, and those who work on their behalf. Locate this resource or other services in your community to assist with health maintenance of infants with physical delays.

The nurse evaluates success of interventions by the child's progression in physical activity milestones at the next health supervision visit. Adequate parental understanding of the importance of physical activity and the means of supporting the child's activities is an important outcome of care.

ORAL HEALTH

The first teeth begin to erupt about midway during infancy. Two front teeth are common at about 6 months of age. However, even before this, parents lay the foundation for good oral health. The mother's intake during pregnancy and breastfeeding are essential to ensuring adequate availability of calcium and other nutrients that will be used as the infant's teeth develop. The nurse in child health supervision settings ensures that the infant has adequate intake of these nutrients via breastfeeding and other foods. A dietary recall of the mother's and infant's intake is one way of assessing for nutrients. When the water supply is not fluoridated, inquire about use of fluoride drops.

PRACTICE ALERT

Be sure that parents do not give the child excessive fluoride since it can permanently discolor the teeth. For example, parents may administer fluoride drops each morning if their water supply has no fluoride, but then have the child at a childcare center several days each week where the water supply is fluoridated. This could cause an overdosage of fluoride.

One challenge during infancy is to help the family establish healthy dental habits. Not only will this lead to clean and attractive teeth (*health promotion*), but it will also help to prevent dental caries (*health maintenance*). The parents should wipe the infant's gums with soft moist gauze once or twice daily. This helps to clean residues of food from the gums and gets the infant accustomed to having something wiping the gums, a practice that may assist when tooth brushing begins. Families are also cautioned to avoid having the infant nurse when sleeping, to avoid use of bottles in bed, and not to allow the infant to drink at will from a bottle during the day. These practices are linked to early childhood caries (see Chapter 9∞) and can lead to tooth decay. While some parents are convinced that this involves "baby teeth" that will be lost, teach that these teeth are needed for healthy food intake and for maintaining proper spaces for permanent teeth eruption.

Nurses assess for the presence of teeth and whether patterns are similar to those expected (see Chapter 8∞). It is wise to ask if the infant has had any difficulty with teeth eruption. Many babies have increased crying and parents have disrupted sleeping during these periods. Suggest comfort measures such as offering cool beverages and safe "teething toys" for the baby. While most infants do not need to have a dental visit, partner with parents to identify a dental care facility for use by the time the child is 3 years of age. Refer families to resources such as Medicaid, State Children's Health Insurance Program, and local resources for dental care.

There is a good deal of overlap in health promotion and health maintenance activities related to oral health. Many interventions are designed to prevent caries and infections, which relate to health maintenance. At the same time, they contribute to health promotion by improving dentition, language development, appearance, and self-image. Desired outcomes of care include the eruption of a set of healthy teeth.

MENTAL AND SPIRITUAL HEALTH

How do you assess the mental health of an infant? What characteristics indicate that an infant is developing the resources needed for future mental health? The infant's mental health is related to early experiences, inborn characteristics such as temperament and resilience, and relationships with caregivers. The first year of life provides many opportunities for the infant to develop positive mental health; interventions during this important period can enhance the child's future mental status.

One way to evaluate mental health is to look carefully at growth and developmental surveillance data, as described earlier. Children who feel secure and have nurturing environments usually grow as expected and perform milestones at usual times. Slow growth and delayed development are sometimes related to feeding disorder of infancy and early childhood (see Chapter 9∞). In these cases, a disturbed relationship with the primary caregiver influences the psychologic state of the infant and results in decreased food intake. Growth is slowed, energy is not available for activity, and development is therefore delayed.

Another way to assess mental health is to observe the child and parent interacting. Does the parent hold the infant securely and does the child cuddle and settle into the parent's arms (Figure 12–4 ■)? Is there eye contact between parent and child? Does the parent appear comfortable in holding and comforting the infant? These interactions indicate bonding or positive attachment (see Chapter 11∞ for further discussion of these topics). During the first year, the infant learns to identify parents; beginning at about 6 months of age, infants may cry or protest when another person holds them. This so-called **stranger anxiety** indicates expected attachment to parents. Similarly, in the second half of the first year of life, infants may exhibit **separation anxiety** by inconsolable crying and other signs of distress when parents are not present. Recognize that these behaviors are normal, demonstrate healthy attachment to primary caregivers, and indicate good mental health. Help

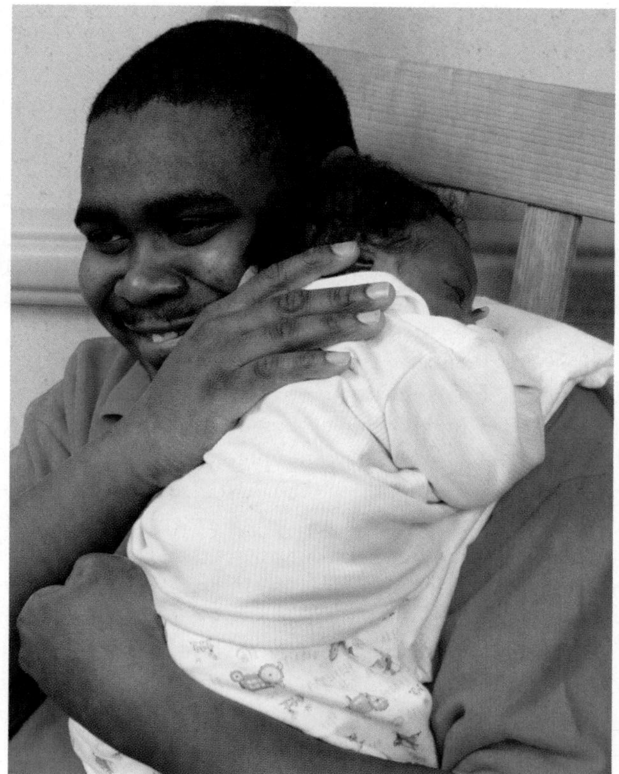

FIGURE 12–4 ■ Interactions between the parent and infant provide clues to mental health. Do the adult and child appear comfortable with each other? Is eye contact and vocalization present? Are their bodies soft and relaxed or tense?

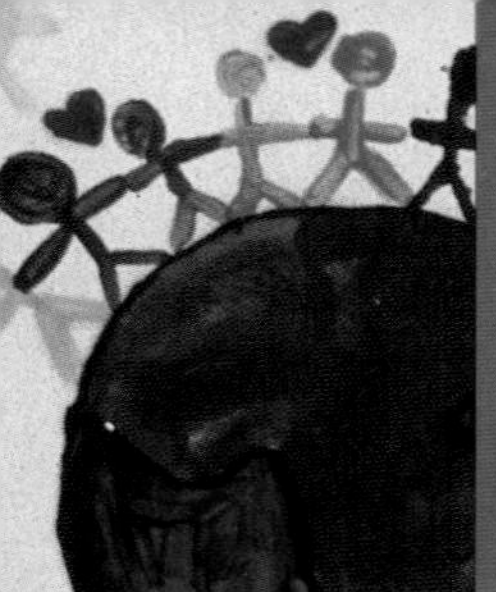

PARTNERING WITH FAMILIES

Comforting the Distressed Infant

Teen parents and those with little prior experience with babies need help to develop a repertoire of interventions to try when a baby is crying. Ask about how they comfort the baby. Suggest the following interventions if the parent does not state them:

- Offer a breast or bottle feeding, especially if the last feeding was more than 2 hours ago.
- If feeding was recent, hold the baby in a sitting position and rub or pat the back to help expel gastric gas.
- Change the diaper if wet or dirty.
- Place a hand on the abdomen and feel for movement. If movement or passing gas is present, hold the baby against the chest, walk slowly, and pat the back.
- Swaddle the baby securely in a blanket and hold horizontally while rocking.
- Hold the baby on your lap, secure the hands in yours, and talk softly.
- Never shake or throw the baby, no matter how long the crying. Call your healthcare provider for suggestions if you feel like nothing works and you are very frustrated.

See Chapter 11 ∞ for further details about responding to the cries of newborns and young infants.

parents to recognize them as expected occurrences. Provide them ideas of how to deal with this behavior. Parents can remain in sight and talk to the infant during health supervision examinations. They should be encouraged to hold and comfort the infant after painful procedures such as immunizations. Further techniques for dealing with separation during hospitalization can be found in Chapter 17∞. Once the infant has experienced that the parent leaves and returns, security in the care of others can emerge.

The infant provides a series of cues about feelings and needs. These include a different type of cry when hungry, wet, or in pain; clearly seeking the nipple when hungry; and readily establishing eye contact when desiring interaction. Parents who are aware of these cues respond to them and meet the infant's needs for contact and comfort, thus increasing trust and a positive state of mental balance. Watch to see how parents respond when an infant cries, or falls asleep, or appears hungry. Parents who have a selection of options promote their infant's health. That is, they are most likely to promote infant mental health if they attempt to rock an infant who continues to cry, then change to swaddling and holding securely, or perhaps try feeding or changing the infant. If you notice that the parent is not responding to the infant, point out your observations of the infant's cues. "Look at how your son is watching your face. That usually means that a baby is eager to be talked to and looked at directly." "Your son seems really unhappy right now. Let's try to wrap him securely in the blanket and see if that helps. This is something you can try at home when he is unable to calm himself." See Partnering with Families: Comforting the Distressed Infant.

Another important indication of infant mental health is the ability to comfort oneself. **Self-regulation** is the process of dealing with feelings, learning to soothe oneself, and focusing on activities for increasing periods of time. Infants learn early how to comfort and calm themselves. Ask parents if the child sucks a finger, softly rocks, or otherwise comforts self when distressed. Some babies prefer to be alone and quiet when tired or distressed; others calm better when held, rocked, or placed in an infant swing. Help the parents to identify and reinforce the infant's methods of self-soothing. Teach swaddling and rocking techniques.

PRACTICE ALERT

Many infants are assisted in soothing themselves when they are swaddled or tightly wrapped (see the Skills Manual). Start by placing the baby on a blanket on a flat surface. Securely take the bottom edge of the blanket and pull it tightly over the feet and up to the chest. Wrap the sides of the blankets around the baby so the arms are secured. Many babies will immediately quiet once swaddled, and will either sleep or become quietly alert. Be aware of the baby that finds this position uncomfortable. If they fight the blanket and try to free themselves, this may not be an approach that works for quieting those particular babies.

Self-regulation is needed by the infant when learning to go to sleep while tired and agitated. Most parents have periods when an infant is not sleeping well and some infants regularly stay awake for long periods at night; parents consequently become sleep deprived and have little energy left to deal with the challenges and responsibilities of the family. Nurses use health promotion principles to teach about sleep patterns in infants, and implement health maintenance when partnering with families to deal with problem sleep behaviors that lead to infant and parent fatigue (Boxes 12–3 and 12–4). See Partnering with Families: Helping the Infant Sleep and Evidence-Based Practice: Infant Sleep.

The infant is born into a family with spiritual strengths and limitations. The nurse assesses the family and provides additional resources when needed. Although the infant is not mature enough to understand the family's spiritual framework, the atmosphere in the family that relates to nurturing, valuing children, providing a safe and secure environment, and recognizing mental balance is conveyed readily to the infant. The infant's social and psychological health are closely related to these factors. For many parents, membership in a faith-based congregation provides spiritual sustenance and an important sense of belonging. This group may also provide food, clothing, and care for the new infant. Sometimes parents who have not attended institutionalized services will choose to do so in order to offer a significant spiritual home for their new child. Services such as christening and blessing an infant welcome the child formally into the family and provide meaning to parents and extended family members. Having a baby often helps parents to feel that they have an important meaning and purpose in life, regardless of a faith-based membership. An atmosphere where the infant is valued and offers meaning to the lives of the adults present is a positive atmosphere for emotional

BOX 12–3 Infant Sleep Patterns

BIRTH–3 MONTHS

10–16 hours of sleep daily in about five sleep periods of 30 minutes to 3 hours

3–6 MONTHS

14 hours of sleep daily with a longer sleep at night plus two or three naps daily

By 4–6 weeks, a consistent sleep pattern should emerge

6–12 MONTHS

12–14 hours of sleep daily with a longer sleep at night plus one or two naps daily

Data from Green, M., & Palfrey, J. S. (Eds.). (2002). Bright futures: Guidelines for health supervision of infants, children, and adolescents *(2nd ed.). Arlington, VA: National Center for Education in Maternal and Child Health.*

growth. Assess the family's meaningful activities, practices, and engagement in faith-based rituals. Ask about needs or desires for referrals in the community such as to an organized religious body or other meaningful activities.

While there are risks to mental health there are also protective factors. The partnership that is developing between the health professional and the parents is an important resource. It leads to increased knowledge, support, and parenting skills. The family knowledge and skills leads them to face challenges with courage and resilience. When mental health topics related to the infant and parents are included in each visit, parents are more likely to share with professionals the stresses and challenges that inevitably emerge. Acknowledge in a nonjudgmental manner the parent's feelings of fatigue and frustration with an infant who does not sleep well. Help parents identify with the strengths and resources they have to meet their challenges. Assure them that their child will learn from them a positive sense of self and the feeling that a positive outcome is possible.

Many of the nurse's interventions are aimed at positive mental health development in the infant. Health promotion activities focus on teaching parents the needs of infants for security and interaction. Suggest healthy sleep patterns and how they can be achieved. Teach self-regulation skills so that the parents can help the child become quiet and calm.

BOX 12–4 Types of Infant Sleep

- Drowsy—Flaccid posture, eyes slowly closing and then opening, random movements
- REM (rapid eye movement) or active sleep—body activity, eye movements with eyes open or closed, irregular respirations, sucking motions
- NREM (nonrapid eye movement) or quiet (or deep) sleep—little body activity, eyes are quiet, respirations regular, no sucking motions

(Data from Green & Palfrey, 2002)

See Table 11–3 for further details about the characteristics of newborn and infant sleep and wake states.

PARTNERING WITH FAMILIES

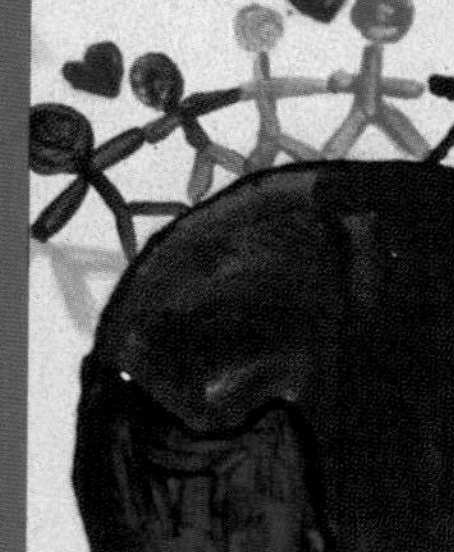

Helping the Infant Sleep

Helping an infant to self-regulate and be able to sleep for longer periods of time is often a stressful challenge for families. Parents need to have substantial sleep periods themselves in order to be refreshed and able to deal with daily life. When up several times during the night with a baby, parents may become irritable and fatigued. Question the family about the baby's sleep routine. The infant passes into light sleep several times at night and may awaken; self-regulation will assist in helping the infant get back to sleep. Suggestions helpful for the family are as follows:

- Place the baby to sleep in a quiet and darkened room.
- Have similar bedtime routines each night.
- Provide a consistent transitional object, such as a favorite blanket each night.
- Put the baby to bed while still awake rather than after falling asleep nursing so he or she becomes accustomed to getting to sleep without nursing.
- Do not try to awaken the baby in NREM (quiet) sleep.
- Establish a regular sleep routine and time; routine may involve some cuddling and rocking time but should not be vigorous, stimulating play.
- For the baby who has trouble going to sleep, remain in the room for a few minutes but do not establish eye contact; place a hand on the abdomen or chest or gently hold flailing arms and legs.

Data from Green & Palfrey, 2000; Jellinek et al., 2002, Mindell, 2003.

Health maintenance seeks to identify babies with disruptions in mental health status, often manifested by growth or interaction abnormalities. When the infant has disturbed sleep patterns, difficulty calming self when upset, or the parents do not interpret infant cues related to hunger or discomfort, the nurse plans interventions to help prevent further problems. Teaching, demonstrations, and acknowledging parent success are all health maintenance actions. An expected outcome for these activities is the reestablishment of expected growth and development, and age-appropriate interactions of the infant with others.

MediaLink Helping the Infant Sleep Video

RELATIONSHIPS

Family

The family is the primary unit where the infant learns to interact with other people. Therefore, family dynamics must be examined during health supervision visits. See Chapter 2∞ for more discussion about the role of the family in child health, and techniques of family assessment. Identify strengths of the family and positively reinforce them. Suggest

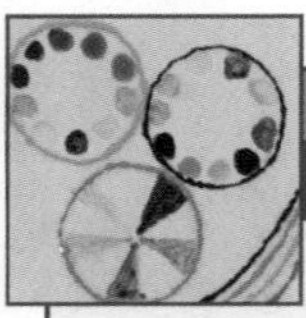

EVIDENCE-BASED PRACTICE
Infant Sleep

PROBLEM

Many babies have limited sleeping periods during the night, and their night awakenings disturb parents' sleep. Parents may have busy days and be unable to nap for adequate sleep to perform at a safe and productive level during the day. In an effort to increase sleep, some parents may feed the infant frequently during the day, believing that if the baby has fed well, longer night sleep periods may occur.

EVIDENCE

It had been noted that infants with more than 11 feeds in 24 hours at 1 week of age were nearly 3 times more likely to have night wakenings than infants who had less feedings. A group of 316 newborns with more than 11 feedings daily and their families participated in a study and were randomly assigned to receive one of three interventions:

- Three-step behavioral program
- Educational booklet
- Helpline for sleeping problems

After 12 weeks, 82% of babies in the behavioral program slept through the night, compared with 61% for the other two interventions. The behavioral program taught parents to minimize light and social interaction at night, avoid feeding or cuddling at night, and beginning at 3 weeks of age, delay feeding when the baby awoke at night (Nikolopoulou & St. James-Roberts, 2003).

NURSING IMPLICATIONS

This evidence-based practice provides implications for nursing practice. Ask parents of young newborns to keep track of the number of daily feedings and nighttime awakenings of the infant. For infants with 11 or more feedings, teach parents about how to minimize stimulation and interaction at night, as described above. Provide opportunities to review results at future health supervision visits.

CRITICAL THINKING APPLICATION

What reasons might working parents have for responding eagerly and interacting with an infant who awakens at night? Do you think there are other reasons why babies awake at night? What clues help you to decide if an infant sleep problem exists?

these ideas when performing health promotion. Strengths might include the following:

- Playing with the infant each day
- Vocalizing frequently to the infant
- Reading to the infant (provide books so parents are encouraged to do this)
- Providing for basic physical and emotional needs of infant and other family members
- Sharing infant care among parents and other family and friends
- Encouraging positive relationships among parents and other children
- Knowing infant needs
- Accessing adequate community services and resources

On the other hand, certain risk factors in every family adversely interfere with family interaction patterns. Questions that may help to identify risk are as follows:

- What do you do when you are frustrated? Do you ever get away together (parents) and can you maintain your own special relationship?
- (For a teen parent) Are you able to do things with your friends each week? Do friends maintain contact and visit?
- All parents experience fatigue related to childrearing. Is there a resource to provide help when you need it? Can you sleep through the night occasionally while someone else bottle-feeds the infant for a night feeding? Can you nap during the day while the infant sleeps?
- Babies each have a unique temperament (see Chapter 5∞). What are the challenges and the positive aspects of your baby's temperament?

Evaluate if the parents are able to laugh about the infant who is very social and wants to be part of everything happening in the house. Be alert to learn if parents have developed mechanisms to quiet the infant's environment so the baby can rest and parents can get a break from care, or if everyone in the family is chronically fatigued.

Factors in the mental health of the parents directly affect the atmosphere in the home, and the resulting health of the infant. Depression in parents or other family members is an important condition that has the potential to influence the infant's health. Interactions with parents who are depressed will be altered; caretaking, both physical and emotional, can be impaired. See Chapter 11∞ for further discussion of postpartum blues and postpartum depression.

Depression in the mother or other caretaker can have serious implications for the infant. The baby may not get the physical care that is needed, leading to poor nutrition, an inadequate state of cleanliness and health, or influencing other basic needs (see Chapter 7∞ for a description of child neglect). These babies may appear in unkempt conditions to healthcare providers and may cry and appear uncomfortable. In addition, the social interactions may be disrupted and the infant may show decreased vocalization, lack of interest in the environment or in people, and may be fussy and irritable or withdrawn and nonengaging (Jellinek, Patel, & Froehle, 2002). Without positive interactions with caretakers, babies may develop a feeding disorder and fail to gain adequate weight (see Chapter 9∞ for a description of feeding disorder of infancy and childhood).

The nurse's role in depression for families with young children relates to health maintenance goals, and involves recognizing the condition and referring for care. The safety and well-being of the infant is important, so resources for childcare may be needed while the parent obtains treatment. Other family members can assist by caring for the infant until the parent is able to do so. Be alert for parents who are sad, cry readily, fail to interact during the visit, and show little emotion in caring for the infant. Likewise, as described in the section on the infant mental health, identify infants who do not establish eye contact or interactions with adults, who are withdrawn or seem sad, or are unkempt. See Chapter 34∞ for further information about depression.

Another challenge to the mental health of families and the infants in these families is that of domestic violence. (See Chapter 11∞.) Domestic violence is a situation in which parents or adult care providers commit violent acts toward one another. These actions most commonly occur by men toward their female companions, but females also are sometimes violent toward men. Approximately 2 to 4 million women are assaulted annually by male partners, and over 3 million children witness such assaults in their families (Kerker, Horowitz, Leventhal, et al., 2000). Women who are abused may be reluctant to tell about such violence either out of fear for safety or due to mental health needs. Be alert for women who appear with bruises, black eyes, or other conditions common with violence. Routine screening for domestic violence should be part of clinic and hospital questionnaires and history forms. Ask questions at each health supervision visit about domestic violence, such as:

- What happens in your family if you and the baby's father disagree about something?
- Has your partner ever threatened you or made you feel afraid for your safety?
- I see you have a black eye. Sometimes people are hurt in their family. Can you tell me how it happened?

Domestic violence makes it difficult for the mother to provide loving and secure care, and as the infant gets older, witnessing such episodes can be harmful. Learn about shelters and other resources that provide services for domestic violence victims in your community. Provide resources to parents as needed. Recognize that these situations are reportable by law and must be referred to departments of social and health services for investigation.

Another risk that occurs in some families with infants is child abuse or maltreatment. This problem is a serious issue that causes disturbed mental status in the infant. See Chapter 7∞ for a detailed description of child abuse and its effect on infants and older children. Suspected child abuse must be reported to legal authorities in order to protect children.

Social Interactions

The infant's social interactions both within and outside the family display remarkable growth in the first year. See Chapter 5∞ for a full description of social milestones. The newborn tracks with eyes over part of the visual field, focuses on the human face, and even mimics facial movements of adults. By 6 weeks of age, the infant smiles responsively and soon after that coos in response to parental vocalizations. By 4 months, the infant babbles and laughs, gets excited about toys in the environment, and recognizes the parent's voice. By 6 months, the infant imitates sounds, is aware of and shows anxiety about strangers, and has definite personality characteristics. In the remainder of the first year, the infant continues to develop some words, with the first words usually representing people ("mama" or "dada"), builds strong relationships with siblings in the family, and has a well-established temperament. An environment is needed to support the infant in establishment of positive social skills during the first year.

One aspect of the child's personality that influences social interactions, both within and outside of the family, is temperament. See Chapter 5 ∞ for detailed descriptions of temperament. Help the parents to identify if the infant's temperament is primarily:

- Easy (moderate activity, easy to console, regular sleep and eating patterns)
- Slow to warm up (slow adaptation to new events and people or to changes in environment and schedule)
- Difficult (high activity, difficult to console, irregular sleep and eating patterns)

Point out the positive aspects of the child's temperament: "Your daughter has already established the ability to sleep through the night. That shows she is able to comfort herself." "Your son does have difficulty sleeping, but he is so interactive and learns a lot from everyone around him." Evaluate the "goodness of fit" between the child's temperament characteristics and the parents' expectations and lifestyle (see Chapter 5∞). Parents who are on flexible schedules and available much of the day may not find it difficult to care for an infant with irregular sleeping and eating habits, while other families have trouble adapting to the infant's patterns. When the fit is not good, parents will need more support and suggestions as they and the infant adapt to each other.

The role of the nurse related to infant social interactions in health supervision visits is to evaluate the social skills of the infant, learn what parents have noticed about the infant's temperament and how it fits with their lives, and make suggestions for positive social development. These are primarily health promotion activities since they aim to enhance the infant's developing social skills. Be aware of health maintenance needs also if any signs of abnormal social interactions are noted. Questions to help identify problems early might include:

- What happens when you are close to your baby's face and smile at him? And if you coo and make sounds?
- What sounds has he made so far?
- Does he go to sleep at the same time each night or does his schedule vary?
- How do your other children respond to your new baby? What does the baby do when he is near your other children?
- You say that you are interested in getting your daughter into a childcare center. What experience has she had with other children? What are you expecting in terms of her relationships with other children? How do you think she might respond when you first leave her? Has she shown any anxiety or crying so far when she meets new people?

Remember that social skills are closely linked with both physical capabilities and mental health status. For example, an infant who is not smiling responsively may have a visual impairment or may have parents who are not interacting appropriately with him. An infant who is not babbling may have a hearing impairment or might have a lack of vocal stimulation from care providers. Gather as much information as possible in order to complete a thorough assessment that provides clues to possible risk factors.

It is clear that family and other social interactions play an important role in development in the first year of life. Concepts related to these interactions must be inserted in every health supervision visit. Examples of health promotion activities are:

- Encourage parents to hold, read to, and talk to babies. Positively reinforce these behaviors when observed.
- Point out the infant's abilities to respond to faces and voices, to smile and laugh, to reflect the mood of adults in the home.

- Review sleep patterns and make recommendations for methods to plan bedtime routines.
- Be sure that parents have resources to turn to when needing assistance with infant care or other household responsibilities.

Health maintenance activities are designed to prevent disturbed mental health in the infant. Examples include:

- Report suspected child abuse immediately.
- Provide resources in cases of domestic violence.
- Refer infants for further diagnostic workup who do not appear to respond to sound, do not follow objects with their eyes, or do not have normal vocalization.

Desired outcomes for the infant include establishment of close relationships with parents and other family members, a stimulating home environment that is responsive to the infant's temperament, and developmental progression in social interactions.

DISEASE PREVENTION STRATEGIES

Infants are prone to many infectious diseases, especially once passive immunity from the mother wanes at about 6 months of age (see Chapters 19 and 26∞). Recommended immunizations are administered on schedule to provide protection from some diseases. Recommended immunizations for infancy are listed in Table 12–4. Further details on immunizations can be found in Chapter 19∞. Instruct parents about upcoming immunizations and when the infant should be seen again. Be sure the parent understands the risks and benefits of each immunization. Answer their questions truthfully and have resources on hand such as brochures and videotapes for interested parents.

Infants may also have other conditions that have not yet been identified, so screening is helpful for these conditions. During each health supervision visit, the nurse performs screenings recommended by the American Academy of Pediatrics and other child health organizations, and counsels the parents about why such screening is important. Vision and hearing screening are consistently performed. Screening for anemia and lead poisoning are added at particular times or with certain groups. Families with certain genetic diseases such as sickle cell disease or cystic fibrosis may choose to have screening for the infant so that supportive care could begin early if the child has the disease (Table 12–5).

Parents benefit from teaching about common diseases and conditions of young children and measures for their prevention (Box 12–5). Ask about environmental tobacco smoke (ETS) and encourage smoking parents to quit. This will lower the chance of sudden infant death syndrome, tooth decay, and asthma (see Chapter 25∞). Teach parents to put babies to sleep on their backs to assist in lowering the chance of sudden infant death syndrome.

When an infant is in a childcare setting or has siblings at home, common infectious diseases such as ear infection, gastroenteritis, and skin infection could be discussed. Provide par-

TABLE 12–4 Routine Immunizations Recommended During Infancy

IMMUNIZATION	AGE RECOMMENDED
Hepatitis B	After birth up to 2 months (#1) 1–4 months (#2) 6–18 months (#3)
Diphtheria, tetanus, pertussis	2, 4, and 6 months (3 doses)
Haemophilus influenzae type b	2, 4, and 6 months (3 doses; last dose is not needed if PRP-OMP [Pedvax HIB or ComVax] are used for primary series)
Inactivated poliovirus	2, 4, and 6–18 months (3 doses)
Pneumococcal	2, 4, and 6 months (3 doses)

TABLE 12–5 Screening During Health Promotion and Health Maintenance Visits

AGE	RECOMMENDED SCREENING TESTS
1 month	Vision (follow objects, red reflex) Hearing (response to sound; screening by machine if not completed in the hospital) Physical examination with special attention to skin problems, hip dysplasia, foot position and range of motion, mouth, abdomen, cardiac abnormality, tearing of eyes, neurologic (including child abuse), anthropometric measurements Developmental milestones Dietary screening and stool/urine pattern assessment Review immunization record
2 months	As above
4 months	As above Vision (add cover-uncover test for strabismus)
6 months	As above Vision (add ability to follow object bilaterally, corneal light reflex) Physical examination with special attention to muscle tone, extremities, appearance of first teeth, tympanic membrane, testicle descent for males
9 months	As above Lead exposure and levels if appropriate Anemia Physical examination with special attention to symmetry of movement
12 months	As above Tuberculosis test if indicated Physical examination with special attention to condition of teeth

Data from Green, M., & Palfrey, J. S. (Eds.). (2002). Bright futures: Guidelines for health supervision of infants, children, and adolescents *(2nd ed.). Arlington, VA: National Center for Education in Maternal and Child Health.*

BOX 12–5 Common Health Conditions of Infants

- Otitis media (see Chapter 24∞)
- Respiratory infection (see Chapter 25∞)
- Gastrointestinal infection (see Chapter 30∞)
- Skin conditions (see Chapter 36∞)

ents with needed information about prevention and treatment of conditions. Be sure they have a phone number to call when they have questions about conditions or whether the infant should be seen by the healthcare provider (Box 12–6).

If the infant has had a health condition, evaluate with the parents how they managed the situation. Did they have the resources needed? Could they call and get needed information? Did they have access to fluid and electrolyte solution, medication, or transportation to get care for the child? Did they have insurance or other coverage for bills? Did the childcare center provide necessary information about a child at the center who had an infectious disease? What situations need to be altered for more successful management of health threats in the future?

Disease prevention strategies focus on health maintenance. These activities are designed to identify diseases in early stages (such as vision impairment or cystic fibrosis) so that they can be managed effectively. This prevents complications and additional health issues. This is a type of secondary prevention (see Table 10–2∞). In addition, teaching regarding topics such as immunizations and management of communicable diseases prevents serious diseases from occurring.

Desired outcomes for disease prevention strategies include adequate management of health problems, integration of immunization and other preventive measures into care of the infant, and family understanding of preventive measures recommended for infants.

INJURY PREVENTION STRATEGIES

During the first year of life, injury becomes an increasingly common cause of mortality. Strategies must be included in each health supervision visit to lower the risk of injury. Nurses should never assume that parents understand how to insert an infant car seat correctly or what types of toys and foods can lead to choking. Know the most commons hazards at each age and teach parents methods of avoiding them (see Tables 12–6 and 12–7). Review at each visit the recommendation to place babies to sleep on their backs to lower the risk of sudden infant death syndrome (see Chapter 25∞).

BOX 12–6 When to Contact Healthcare Provider

Instruct parents to contact a provider if the child has:

- Rectal temperature ≥ 100.4°F (38.0°C)
- Seizure
- Skin rash, purplish spots, petechiae
- Change in activity or behavior that makes the parent uncomfortable
- Unusual irritability, lethargy
- Failure to eat
- Vomiting
- Diarrhea
- Dehydration
- Cough

Data from Green, M., & Palfrey, J. S. (Eds.). (2002). Bright futures: Guidelines for health supervision of infants, children, and adolescents *(2nd ed.). Arlington, VA: National Center for Education in Maternal and Child Health.*

PARTNERING WITH FAMILIES

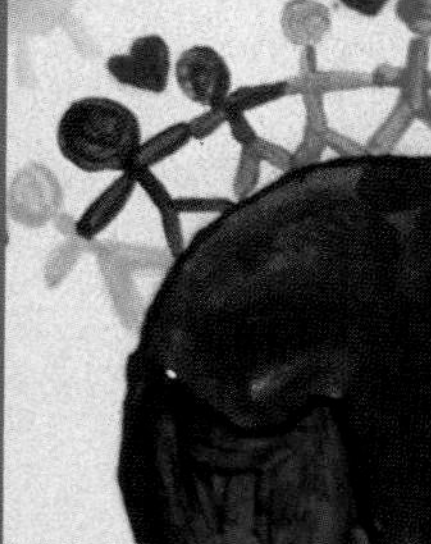

Car Seats for Infants

Review the family's routines for transporting an infant by car at every health supervision visit. Recommendations for infants from birth to 1 year or 2–22 lb include:

- Use infant-only or rear-facing convertible seat.
- The seat is always placed in the back seat in the rear-facing position.
- Harness straps should be at or below shoulder level.
- Be sure to follow guidelines for every trip, no matter how short.
- Have car seat and car checked at examiner station and evaluated for correct technique.
- If car seat is changed between two or more cars, it should be checked for proper installation in each car.

Data from National Highway Traffic Safety Administration (NHTSA).

MediaLink Car Seat Safety

Begin the conversation by asking parents what safety hazards they are aware of in the child's environment. Use this information as the starting point for discussion. Give positive feedback for their awareness of hazards and measures they have taken to prevent them. Consider using a home assessment survey that assists parents in identifying hazards that may be present in their homes. When infants visit friends, relatives, or neighbors, they may be exposed to other hazardous situations. Grandparents may not have a home that is "babyproofed" and the infant could have access to electrical cords, machinery, medicines, or other hazards. Help the parents to evaluate the childcare home or center. Are babies adequately supervised? Do older children have toys that could be harmful to the babies present? Do infants have access to cooking areas, hot water, or heaters? Can they crawl into bathrooms where there is access to toilets or other water sources?

Focus on car safety, as this is a frequent cause of injury for infants. Provide brochures and other types of information about recommendations. Become a certified car seat examiner if possible and ask to view the infant's car seat. If this is not possible, locate examination centers in your community (frequently fire or police stations) and refer every family for a car seat examination. Provide resources for car seats if the family is not able to afford one. Discuss other possible safety hazards such as extensions on the parent bicycle and use of infant strollers in areas where cars are present. See the Photo Story on pages 428–429 and Partnering with Families: Car Seats for Infants.

Injury prevention assessment and teaching strategies are examples of health maintenance activities. They are designed to minimize the exposure to hazardous environmental materials and practices.

TABLE 12–6 **Injury Prevention in Infancy**

HAZARD	DEVELOPMENT CHARACTERISTICS	PREVENTIVE MEASURES
Falls	Mobility increases in first year of life, progressing from squirming movements to crawling, rolling, and standing.	Do not leave infant unsecured in infant seat, even in newborn period. Do not place on high surfaces such as tables or beds unless holding child. **(1)** Once mobile by crawling, keep doors to stairways closed or use gates. Standing walkers have led to many injuries and are not recommended.
Burns	Infant is dependent on caretakers for environmental control. The second half of the first year is marked by crawling and increased mobility. Objects are explored by touching and placing in mouth.	Check temperature of bath water and food/liquids for drinking. Cover electrical outlets. Supervise infant so that play with electrical cords cannot occur.
Motor vehicle crashes	Infant is dependent on caretakers for placement in car. On impact with another motor vehicle, an infant held on a lap acts as a torpedo.	Use only approved restraint systems (according to federal Motor Vehicle Safety Standards). The seat must be used for every trip, even if very short. The seat must be properly buckled to the car's lap belt system. **(2)**
Drowning	Infant cannot swim and is unable to lift head.	Never leave infant alone in a bath of even 2.5 cm (1 in.) of water. Supervise when in water even when a life preserver is worn. Flotation devices such as arm inflatables are not certified life preservers.
Poisoning	Infant is dependent on caretakers to keep harmful substances out of reach.	Keep medicines out of reach. Teach proper dosage and administration of medicines to parents. Cleaning products and other harmful substances should not be stored where the infant can reach them. Remove plants from play areas. Have poison control center number by telephone.
Choking	The second half of infancy is marked by exploratory reaching and mouthing objects. Infant explores objects by placing them in the mouth. **(3)**	Avoid foods that commonly cause choking. Keep small toys away from infants, especially toys labeled "not intended for use by those under 3 years."
Suffocation	Young infant has minimal head control and may be unable to move if vomiting or having difficulty breathing.	Position infant on back for sleep. **(4)** Do not place pillows, stuffed toys, or other objects near head. Do not use plastic in crib. Avoid latex balloons.
Strangulation	Infant is able to get head into railings or crib slats but cannot remove it.	Be sure older cribs have slats spaced 6 cm (2 3/8 in.) or less apart. The mattress must fit tightly against the crib rails.

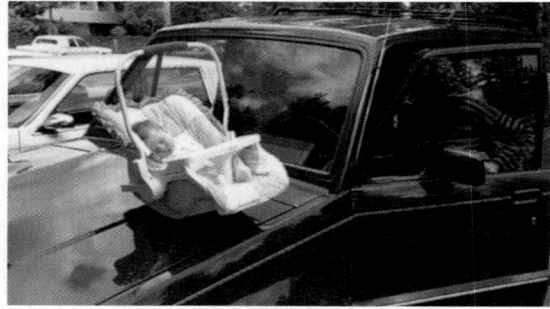

(1) Never leave infant unsecured or on high surface.

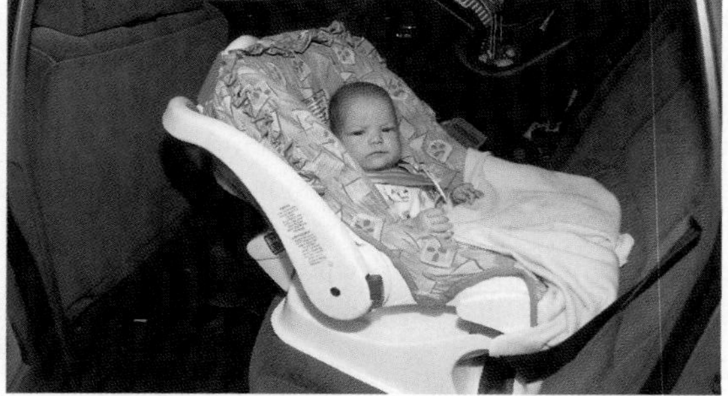

(2) Always use approved restraint system. Place infant in rear-facing seat in backseat of car

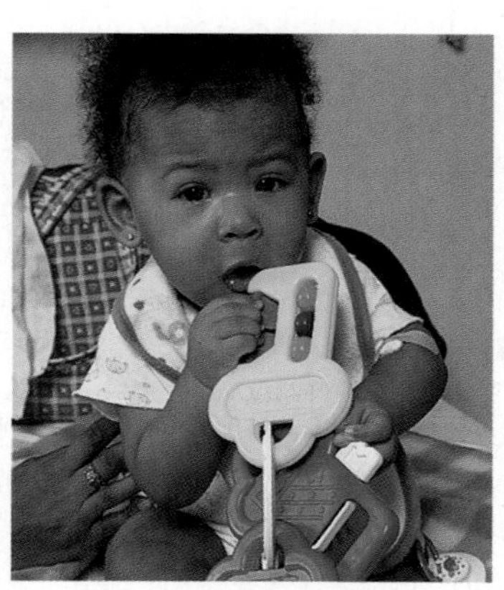

(3) Explores objects with mouth.

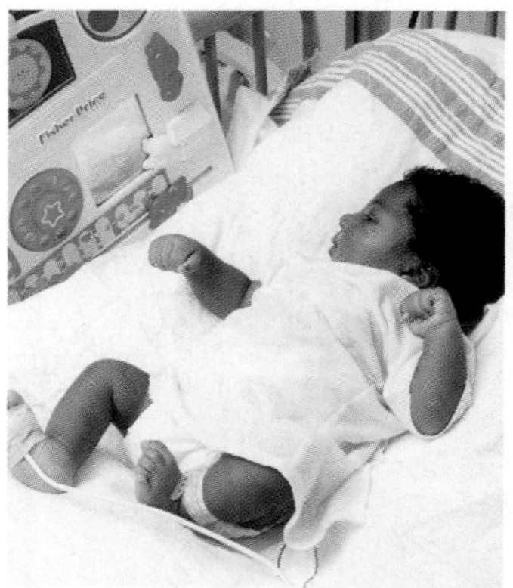

(4) Place infant on back for sleeping, keep toys clear.

TABLE 12–7 Injury Prevention Topics by Age

AGE	INJURY PREVENTION TEACHING TOPICS
1 month	Infant car safety seat Put baby to sleep on back Avoid loose bedding and toys in crib Avoid tobacco use in the environment Provide adult supervision of the baby at all times by trusted individuals Test bath water temperature and never leave baby alone in bath Never place baby on high object such as counter, table, or bed; always keep one hand on the baby during such activities as diaper changes to prevent falling Wash hands correctly and often Avoid contact with persons with communicable diseases Have smoke alarms and avoid fire hazards Learn infant CPR and airway obstruction removal Never shake the baby Have plans for emergency care
2 months	As above Use only recommended playpens or cribs and keep sides up Avoid moldy environments Keep baby toys clean Avoid direct sunlight for the baby Keep sharp and small objects out of baby's environment Keep hot water heater lower than 120°F Review emergency plan with all care providers
4 months	As above Get all poisonous substances out of baby's view and reach; install locks to keep them inaccessible Do not use latex balloons or plastic bags near the baby
6 months	As above If an infant-only car seat was used, switch to rear-facing convertible safety seat (intended for babies up to 40 lb) when baby is 20–30 lb or 26 inches Empty containers of water immediately after use; be sure pools or other bodies of water are locked and not accessible to baby Use sunscreen, hat, and long sleeves when baby is in the sun Keep heavy and sharp objects out of reach; check that all poisons are locked away including in homes visited; keep pet food and cosmetics out of reach Do not drink hot liquids or eat soup while holding the baby Have poison control number by phones and programmed into cell phones Be alert for dangers of hot curling irons and other appliances Have electrical cords out of reach and not hanging down Have home and environment checked for lead hazards Lower infant crib mattress if still in upper position Install gates and guards on stairs and windows Never use an infant walker
9 months	As above Crawl on the floor and look for hazards at baby's eye level Pad sharp corners on tables and other furniture Watch for tables, chairs, and other devices the baby may use for climbing to unsafe places
12 months	As above Change to forward-facing car safety seat if baby is at least 20 lb; install correctly and have installation checked; place in back seat and never in front seat with a passenger air bag Start showing the child how to wash hands frequently Provide own personal items such as clothing and blankets to childcare providers; wash often Change batteries in home smoke alarms and check system Turn handles to back of stove; use back rather than front burners; watch for hot liquids Check care provider setting for safety hazards Remember that responsible adults should always supervise your infant, not other children Peruse home once again for hazards now that the child is more active, climbing, and walking

Data from Green, M., & Palfrey, J. S. (Eds.). (2002). Bright futures: Guidelines for health supervision of infants, children, and adolescents *(2nd ed.). Arlington, VA: National Center for Education in Maternal and Child Health.*

PHOTOStory...

Placement of infant in a car safety seat

"I thought I had the seat in correctly but wanted to check. They showed me that it was not attached right, so it could actually have allowed Sammie to be thrown and injured in a crash. I'm so glad it got checked. We've changed where and how I put the seat in the car."

This mother attends a high school alternative program that offers child-

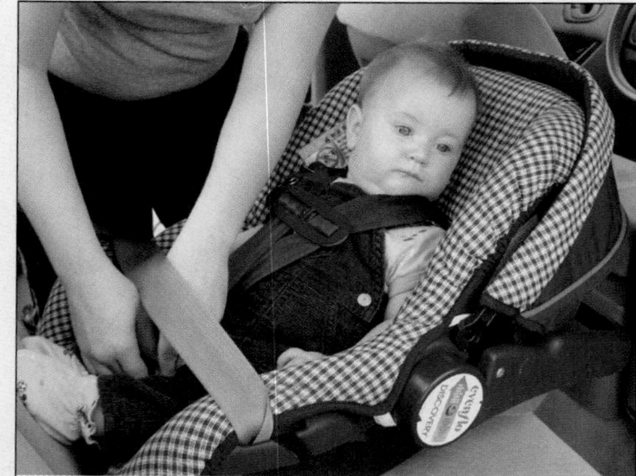

To ensure a proper fit, slide hand under harness and secure belt tightly.

care for her infant son. The local police station was invited to send the car seat examiner to the program to evaluate car safety seats for the children. This mother learned where to place the seat securely in the back seat and facing to the rear of the car, and how to lift her child in, adjust the harness to fit him properly, and fasten the belt. Many parents do not correctly install and use car seats. Intentions are good, but seats may be

NURSING MANAGEMENT

Nursing Assessment and Diagnosis

The nurse working in clinics, offices, and other settings that offer primary care for infants should be skillful in assessing health promotion and health maintenance. The infant's growth, developmental level, general physical health, and mental/social health are assessed. Family interactions and other settings where the infant spends time are evaluated for risks and protective factors that influence the child's development. Assess the health of siblings and patterns of integrating the infant into the rest of the family. Particular attention is directed at assessment of risk for diseases and injuries. The data-gathering phase always provides parents with the opportunity to ask questions and relay concerns. Further assessment may need to be directed at these areas.

Based on the assessment data, the nurse establishes nursing diagnoses that become the basis for nursing interventions. Both areas of strength and need are included; often the family strengths can be used to further promote health. Possible nursing diagnoses established during a health supervision visit of an infant are as follows:

- Breastfeeding, Effective related to the mother's confidence and knowledge
- Breastfeeding, Interrupted related to mother's resumption of employment outside the home
- Family Coping: Compromised related to recent role changes
- Risk for Altered Parent/Child Attachment related to anxiety associated with parenting role
- Sleep Pattern Disturbance (infant) related to frequently changing sleep routines and cycles
- Impaired Skin Integrity (infant) related to developmental factors
- Risk for Infection (infant) related to inadequate acquired immunity
- Risk for Injury (infant) related to design of environment
- Risk for Altered Growth and Development related to parental substance abuse

Planning and Implementation

The nurse plays a vital role in successful health promotion and health maintenance activities. Explain to the parents what procedures are being performed and their purpose. Encourage them to ask questions and share their perceptions of the infant's

old and not meet current standards, instructions for installation in cars may be hard to follow, and the care needed may not be taken. Young parents like the teen mother whose baby is shown here are at particular risk. They may not be able to afford a seat, may rely on "hand me downs" from friends, and may not realize the importance of securing the child in a manner that meets current standards. What are the benefits of having someone come to an alternative school to teach and evaluate car safety? What programs are available in your community for providing car seats for parents who have difficulty affording them? ■

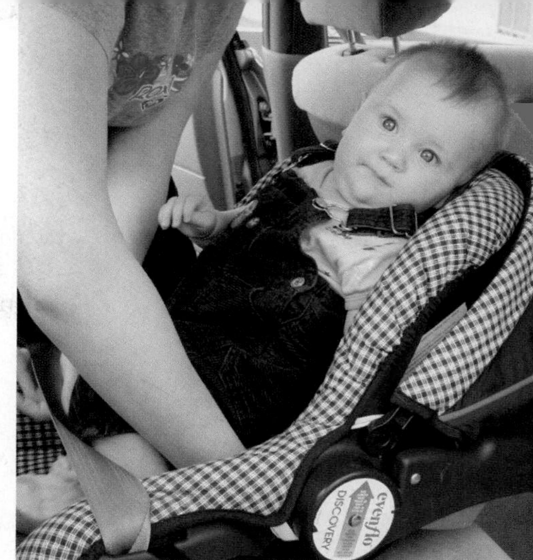

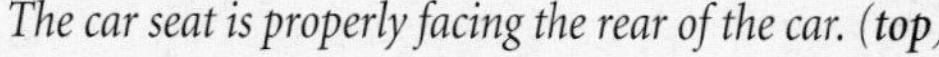

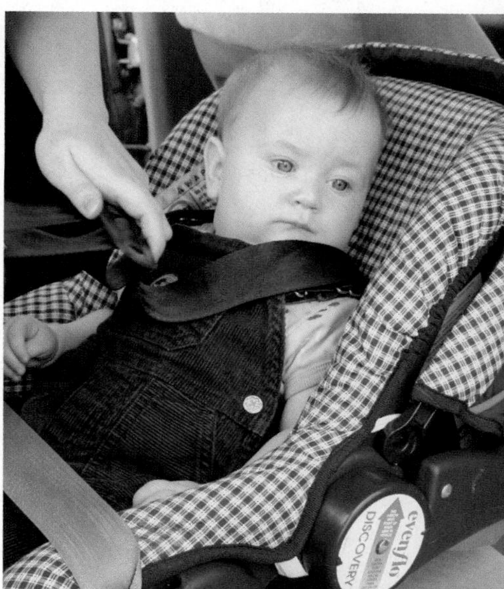

The car seat is properly facing the rear of the car. **(top)**

The child must be rear facing and securely harnessed. **(bottom)**

personality, development, and other traits. This will enhance their understanding that healthcare involves a partnership between them and the care providers. It will lead to trust that promotes their ability to share concerns honestly. Recognize that the first year of the infant's life is a key time for establishing a trusting relationship with health professionals.

Recognize the importance of data provided by simple assessments such as length and weight. Analyze all findings to learn if the child is developing as expected. Much of the visit is spent in teaching parents about topics such as safety measures, providing anticipatory guidance related to development, assisting with integration of the new infant into the family, and relaying resources for support of the family in the community, Internet, or other areas (Box 12–7). Parenting classes, childcare facilities, and family planning resources are examples of common parental needs. Perform recommended physical and developmental assessment, administer screening tests, and give immunizations (Figure 12–5 ■). Be sure parents understand the need for tests and treatments, and relay the results of tests to them.

Nurses who work in hospitals, emergency services, and other facilities also are an important link in health supervision. Ask where and how often the child is seen for care. Check

BOX 12–7 Research: Health Promotion Strategies

Two nurses reported on a study that attempted to identify health promotion strategies most preferred by mothers of infants. Their goal was to use evidence-based practice to find the intervention approaches that would most likely lead to positive infant health outcomes. A sample of 138 mothers of 4-month-old infants ranked eight intervention approaches for care *(Gaffney & Altieri, 2001)*. The most preferred to least preferred methods were as follows:

1. Nurse home visitation
2. Group session with mothers, led by a nurse
3. Community lay worker home visitation
4. Classes in the clinic
5. Health diary
6. Videotape viewing at home
7. Brochures
8. Videotape viewing in the clinic

The nurses concluded that the preferred intervention approaches use interpersonal communication. Commonly employed methods such as brochures and videotapes were least preferred because they did not involve discussion and a chance to ask questions.

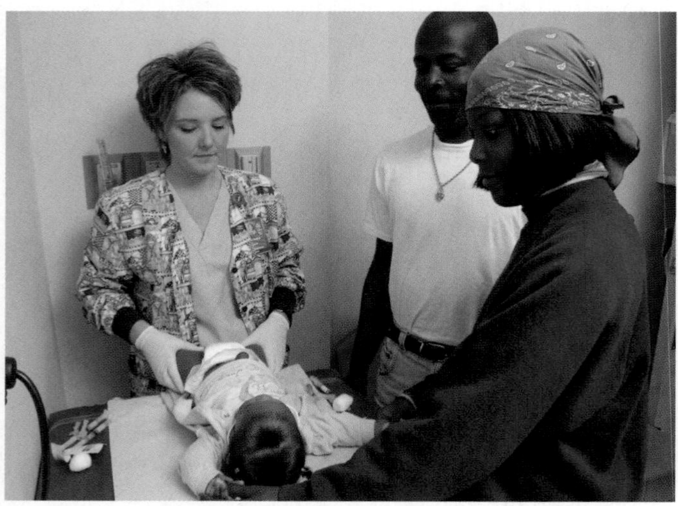
A

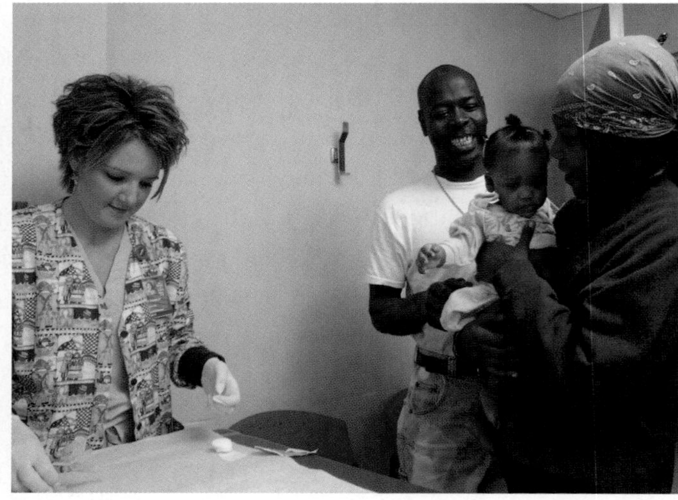
B

FIGURE 12–5 ■ The nurse positions the baby on the edge of the examination table to isolate the vastus lateralis muscle used for immunization administration. *A,* The mother holds the baby's arms out of reach. *B,* After the immunization the parents comfort the infant and are reassured that all is well.

immunization schedules to be sure they are up to date. When the child is not being seen regularly, find out if the family does not understand the importance of these visits or lacks resources to obtain the necessary care. Refer them to resources as needed so that they can identify a pediatric healthcare home. Agencies that provide health supervision are equipped to perform home visits on a regular basis or in case of special need. When nurses make regular home visits to families with risk factors, health outcomes are improved. Seeing the family in the natural setting enables the nurse to tailor interventions to the specific situation. Nutrition, safety, and other teaching is more effective when it matches the family needs. For example, showing how to set up a stimulating environment with safe materials, even if toys are limited, is an effective nursing strategy. Ensure that home visits are performed when appropriate and available, either through the pediatric healthcare home or other community agency.

Before the family leaves the facility, be sure they have the next appointment scheduled. Summarize content of the present visit, emphasizing the family's strengths and the infant's newly acquired developmental skills. Sensitively list any areas that require work in the coming weeks, such as "babyproofing" the home or encouraging the infant to reach for objects. Provide a journal or notebook in which the parents can record the infant's development and write down questions to ask in future visits. Suggest possible topics for the parents to think about and provide books, brochures, and other printed material.

Evaluation

Expected outcomes of nursing care for the infant and family in health promotion and health maintenance are as follows:

- The infant demonstrates normal patterns of growth and progression in developmental milestones.
- The infant is well adjusted, showing positive response to the environment and interactions with significant others.
- The infant remains free of disease and injury.
- Parents state common safety hazards at the child's present and upcoming ages.

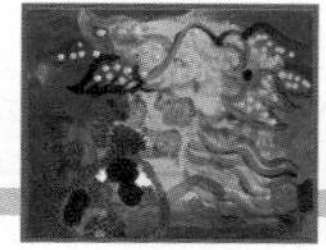

CHAPTER HIGHLIGHTS

- The first contact between the infant's primary healthcare provider and the parents should occur prior to birth.
- A trusting relationship between the family and the care provider fosters a partnership that is influential in promoting the development of the infant.
- Health supervision visits begin with careful observations of the infant and parent–child interactions.
- Surveillance of growth and development provides important clues to the infant's well-being.
- Nutrition assessment and teaching are important to provide for the very challenging nutritional needs of the first year of life.
- The mental health of parents influences the atmosphere in the home and the development of the infant.
- Patterns of interaction between parent and child as well as relationships with other adults and children provide the infant with strong emotional bonds that are essential to normal development.
- Disease and injury prevention strategies are integrated into each infant healthcare supervision visit.

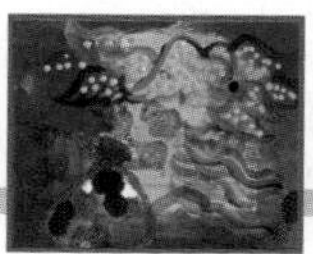

CRITICAL THINKING IN ACTION

INTRODUCTION

Recall the opening scenario. Colleen has come to the WIC clinic with her 7-month-old daughter Amanda. A nutritional assessment is performed, teaching begins, and an appointment is made for a follow-up visit in 2 months for both Amanda and her 4-year-old sister Melody. The children's grandmother is a support person for Colleen, who is a single mother; however, her impaired vision limits her somewhat in interactions with the children.

DESCRIPTION

Upon examination, Amanda appears adequately nourished. Her skin is well hydrated and in good condition. She is alert and shows expected developmental progression. Her hematocrit is 33%, weight is 17 lb 8 oz, length is 26.5 in. Colleen drives Amanda and Melody to a home childcare each morning on her way to work; they spend afternoons with their grandmother. Colleen is motivated to provide safe and stimulating care for the children and has a supportive group of neighbors and friends.

DISCUSSION

Colleen clearly has many strengths or protective factors to draw from as she cares for her family. The nurse can address several areas of Amanda's development to enhance the family's strengths.

1. Evaluate Amanda's physical findings. Is the hematocrit within expected norms? What percentiles are her height and weight? What foods are recommended at her age?
2. What questions will you ask and what suggestions will you make to ensure that Amanda is safely transported to childcare each day in Colleen's car? How will you ensure a safe environment for Amanda at the grandmother's home when she provides childcare for the children?
3. Suggest several toys and activities that are appropriate for Amanda at her age. What developmental milestones do you expect to observe in areas of language, fine motor, gross motor, and social interactions?

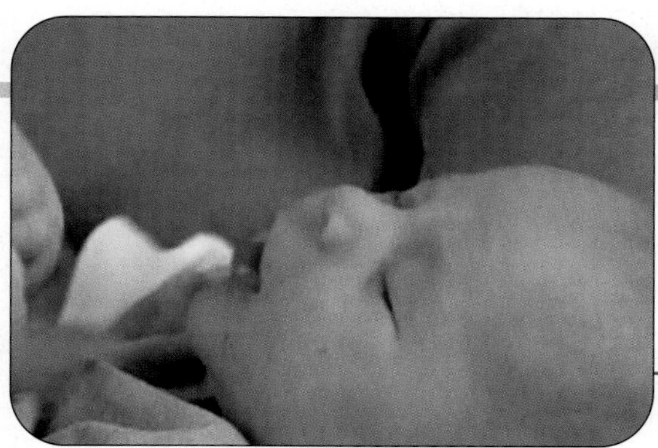

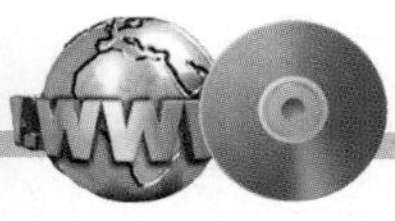

EXPLORE MediaLink

- NCLEX review, case studies, and other interactive resources for this chapter can be found on the Companion Website at **www.prenhall.com/ball**. Click on Chapter 12 to select the activities for this chapter.
- For animations, more NCLEX review questions, and an audio glossary, access the accompanying CD-ROM in this textbook.

http://www.prenhall.com/ball

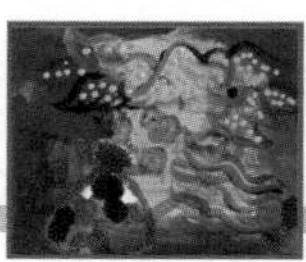

REFERENCES

Gaffney, K. F., & Altieri, L. B. (2001). Mothers' ranking of clinical intervention strategies used to promote infant health. *Pediatric Nursing, 27,* 510–515.

Green, M., & Palfrey, J. S. (Eds.). (2002). *Bright futures: Guidelines for health supervision of infants, children, and adolescents* (2nd ed.). Arlington, VA: National Center for Education in Maternal and Child Health.

Jellinek, M., Patel, B. P., & Froehle, M. C. (Eds.). (2002). *Bright futures in practice: Mental health* (Vols. I and II). Arlington, VA: National Center for Education in Maternal and Child Health.

Kerker, B., Horowitz, S. M., Leventhal, J. M., et al. (2000). Identification of violence in the home: Pediatric and parental reports. *Archives of Pediatric and Adolescent Medicine, 154,* 457–462.

Miller, L. J., & Robinson, C. C. (1996). Strategies for meaningful assessment of infants and toddlers with significant physical and sensory difficulties. In S. J. Meisels & E. Fenichel (Eds.), *New visions for the developmental assessment of infants and young children* (pp. 313–328). Washington, DC: Zero to Three: National Center for Infants, Toddlers, and Families.

Mindell, J. (2003). *Sleep, infants, and parents.* National Sleep Foundation. www.sleepfoundation.org/ask/infantsandparents, accessed 8/28/2003.

Murray, R. B., & Zentner, J. P. (2001). *Health promotion strategies through the life span* (7th ed.). Upper Saddle River, NJ: Prentice Hall.

Nikolopoulou, M., & St. James-Roberts, I. (2003). Preventing sleeping problems in infants who are at risk of developing them. *Archives of Diseases in Children, 88,* 108–111.

Patrick, K., Spear, B., Holt, K., & Sofka, D. (Eds.). (2001). *Bright futures in practice: Physical activity.* Arlington, VA: National Center for Education in Maternal and Child Health.

Story, M., Holt, K., & Sofka, D. (Eds.). (2002). *Bright futures in practice: Nutrition.* Arlington, VA: National Center for Education in Maternal and Child Health.

Strickland, B., McPherson, M., Weissman, G., van Dyck, P., Huang, Z. J., & Newacheck, P. (2004). Access to the medical home: Results of the National Survey of Children with Special Health Care Needs. *Pediatrics, 113,* 1485–1492.

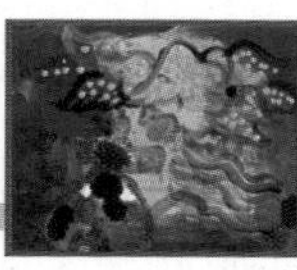

ADDITIONAL REFERENCES

Borghese-Lang, R., Morrison, L., Ogle, A., & Wright, A. (2003). Successful bottle feeding of the young infant. *Journal of Pediatric Health Care, 17,* 94–101.

Colyar, M. R. (2003). *Well-child assessment for primary care providers.* Philadelphia: FA Davis.

Edelman, C. L., & Mandle, C. L. (2002). *Health promotion throughout the life span* (5th ed.). St. Louis: Mosby.

Glascoe, F. P. (2003). How you can implement the AAP's new policy on developmental and behavioral screening. *Contemporary Pediatrics, 20,* 85–95.

Halfon, N., McLearn, K. T., & Schuster, M. A. (Eds.). (2002). *Child rearing in America.* Cambridge, UK: Cambridge Press.

Hammermeister, J., & Peterson, M. (2001). Does spirituality make a difference? Psychosocial and health-related characteristics of spiritual well-being. *American Journal of Healthy Education, 32,* 293–297.

Pender, N. J., Murdaugh, C. L., & Parsons, M. A. (2002). *Health promotion in nursing practice* (4th ed.). Upper Saddle River, NJ: Prentice Hall.

Squires, J., & Nickel, R. (2003). Never too soon: Identifying social-emotional problems in infants and toddlers. *Contemporary Pediatrics, 20,* 117–125.

Thompson, K. M. (2003). The role of bath seats in unintentional infant bathtub drowning deaths. *Medscape General Medicine, 5.* www.medscape.com/viewarticle/450989, accessed 4/2/2003.

Young, L. E., & Hayes, V. (2002). *Transforming health promotion practice: Concepts, issues, and applications.* Philadelphia: F. A. Davis.

Chapter 13

Health Promotion and Health Maintenance of the Toddler and Preschooler

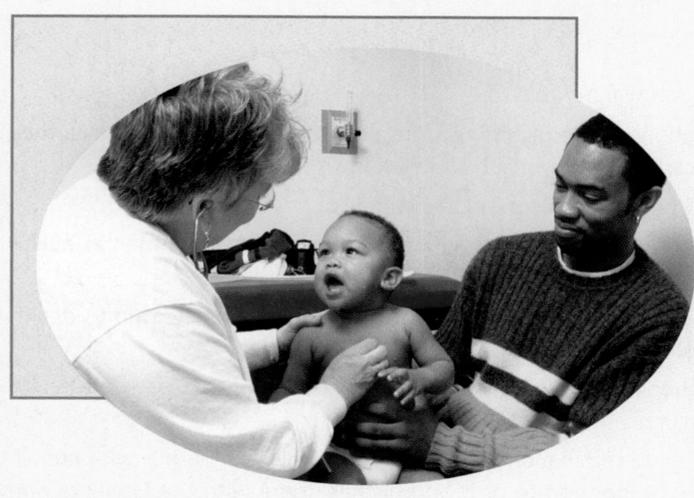

Clarence Kaufman has been brought in for his 15-month-old health supervision visit by his parents. Clarence is a healthy toddler, but his parents have questions about his development. They are concerned about his high activity level and need for constant supervision. As both parents work while Clarence is at childcare, they are busy in the evening trying to spend time with him and meet other family obligations. You notice on the record that Clarence missed his 12-month health supervision visit and was last seen when he was 9 months old.

What health promotion activities will be appropriate for this visit? How will you integrate his parents' questions about Clarence's activity level into the visit? Since Clarence has not been seen in healthcare for some time, what are some likely health maintenance needs?

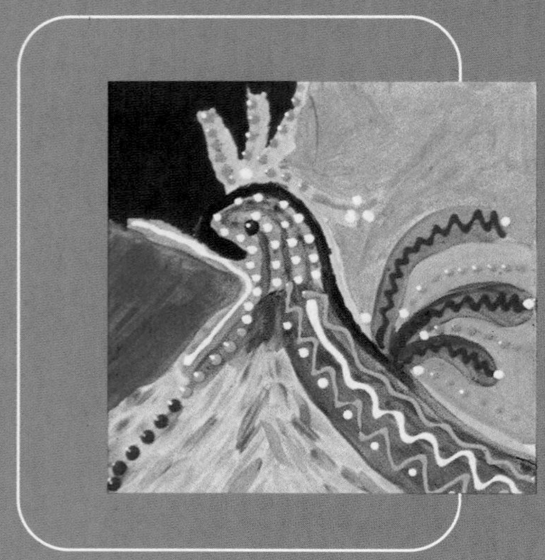

"Clarence is so busy! I babysit for all my cousins and he is the hardest one. He's always moving and does not stay interested in anything for very long."

—Clarence's cousin Miranda, age 14

Key Terms

deciduous teeth/442
dysfluency/447
early childhood caries (ECC)/442
food jags/440
growth channel/439
kinesthesia/441
nightmares/444
night terrors/444

Learning Outcomes

After completing this chapter, you will be able to:

- Describe the general observations made of toddlers/preschoolers and their families as they come to the pediatric healthcare home for health supervision visits.
- Identify the major health concerns of toddlers and preschoolers.
- Apply assessment skills to gather data regarding nutrition, physical activity, mental health status, and growth and development of toddlers and preschoolers.
- Apply therapeutic communication skills with toddler/preschooler and family during health supervision visits in toddlerhood/preschool.
- Intervene with toddlers/preschoolers and their families to integrate activities to promote health and to prevent disease and injury.
- Synthesize data from history and examination of toddler/preschooler and family with knowledge of toddler/preschooler development to plan approaches useful with the family during health supervision encounters.

MediaLink  **http://www.prenhall.com/ball**

Resources for this chapter can be found on the CD-ROM accompanying this textbook, and on the Companion Website at www.prenhall.com/ball. Click on Chapter 13 to select the activities for this chapter.

CD-ROM

Videos

- *Drowning Precautions*
- *Handling Temper Tantrums*

NCLEX Review

Audio Glossary

COMPANION WEBSITE

NCLEX Review

Case Study: Single-Parenting Challenges and Nutrition

The years following infancy are challenging for parents as the child grows and acquires new developmental skills. The child progresses from the first tentative steps and words at a year of age through the "terrible twos" of toddlerhood and into preschool age when most children attend some type of educational program, have well developed verbal communication, and acquire many gross and fine motor skills. Toddler and preschool ages are often grouped as "young childhood," as the family remains the primary system within which the child interacts, and there are many common concerns such as nutrition, sleep, and growing independence. Facing consistent changes in development, parents rely on the pediatric healthcare home (medical home) for advice and information. Nurses apply concepts of anticipatory guidance during visits for health promotion and health maintenance to assist parents in the transitions they face. See Partnering with Families: Health Promotion and Health Maintenance Visits.

What are some of the unique concerns of the family with a toddler or preschooler? How can the nurse facilitate health growth and development during these stages? What resources can parents use to provide support in their task of raising a young child and providing experiences to ready them for school entry? These are some of the topics that will be addressed in this chapter.

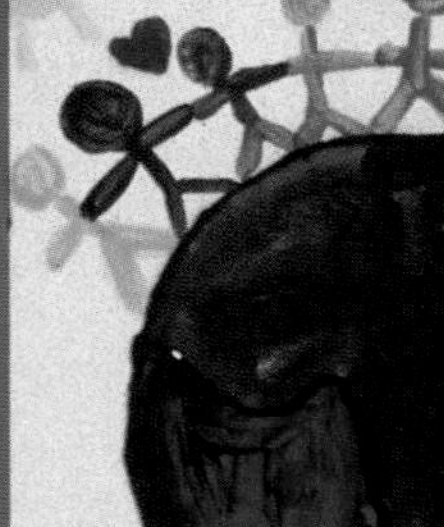

PARTNERING WITH FAMILIES

Health Promotion and Health Maintenance Visits

It is important for parents of toddlers and preschoolers to know the ages when children should be examined for health promotion and health maintenance. List these ages and at each visit, make the next appointment or provide written information about where and when to call for the next visit. Encourage families who speak languages other than English to bring an interpreter or arrange for one to be present in the visit. Be sure they understand the information provided about future visits. The recommended ages for care are:

- 12 months
- 15 months
- 18 months
- 2–3 years
- 3–4 years
- 4–5 years

See Table 13–6 for recommended screening tests at each of these visits.

GENERAL OBSERVATIONS

While calling the 18-month-old child in from the waiting room, remember the child just 1 year before. This young child is now a toddler who is able to walk in, even if with a bit of help. Watch for the child's desire for independence or signs of continuing reliance on the parent. Does the child strike out independently or cling to the parent once a stranger is seen? Make note of this temperament characteristic, comment about it to the family, and learn how they describe the child's temperament (see Chapter 5 for a description of child temperament). In addition to temperament, observations should be made about mobility. Does the child walk independently? What other means are used for locomotion? Again, verify your observations of mobility with the parents during the visit.

Health supervision visits are adapted for older toddlers and preschoolers to include observations of parental discipline and interaction style. Does the parent respond to the child's questions? Were age-appropriate toys or activities brought to the visit to help occupy the child while waiting? Is the child observant of the environment and alert? By preschool age, the child is walking independently and usually engages in conversations easily. The nurse welcomes the child warmly, and assesses social skills and motor activities. Direct greetings or questions to the child to evaluate stranger anxiety and ability to understand simple commands or questions. What verbal skills are observed? The parent usually allows the child some independence in answering questions and provides support for the child who is quiet and appears apprehensive. Watch for these interactions.

The relationship with the family should now be established as a partnership in care of the child. If, however, a family is new to the care provider, reach out to welcome them and express interest in them as individuals and parents. Families often feel uncomfortable in healthcare settings and it is important to establish positive rapport so they will be able to ask questions and bring up concerns about the child. Recall Ben and Karie, described in the opening scenario. They are concerned about the impact of their son's activity level and their busy lives on his development. Since the family has not been at the facility for some time, they will need to be welcomed and shown that the healthcare providers are eager to work with them in a partnership to provide care to benefit their child.

Most parents enjoy talking about their children, so asking questions and commenting positively about a child's traits will encourage them to share thoughts about the child. The following questions promote opportunities to educate.

- "Your son is really able to walk so well now, isn't he?"
- "Your daughter has grown so much and she is talking a lot. What is she interested in?"

Once they answer, respond appropriately and ask for additional specific information pertinent to the visit.

- "Yes, it is a challenge now that your son can walk and climb. We'll talk about some safety precautions that are advised at this age."
- "Preschoolers who are outgoing like your daughter are a real pleasure. At the same time, it is sometimes hard to keep them occupied. What do you do to keep her busy?"

What questions could you ask Clarence's parents, described in the opening scenario, about their son? Remember that he is 15 months old; include your knowledge of development into the questions.

The mental health of the parents influences the environment in which the child is growing and learning. It is therefore important to ask questions about the parent who comes with the child and the family in general. Inquire about how the family is adjusting to the growing child. If there are other children, ask about their health and the challenges they bring to the family. Were there recent job or insurance changes, or has the family moved? Are there parental concerns about the neighborhood or resources for the child? Does the parent want to talk about any personal problems such as depression, substance use, illness, or stress? These topics will be explored later in the chapter.

Recommendations for developmental health supervision of young children includes four main categories. Use this framework to plan health supervision visits.

1. *Assessment* is performed, using screening tests, evaluations, and observations.
2. *Education* provides information about parent–child interactions, sleep, discipline, and other developmental tasks.
3. *Intervention* includes counseling the parent, making home visits, and ensuring ongoing contacts with health professionals.
4. *Care coordination* between the office setting and community resources ensures that proper referrals occur.

(Halfon, Regalado, McLearn, et al., 2003)

BOX 13–1 Health Conditions Related to Growth in Young Children

Growth Pattern	Possible Conditions
Low percentile for weight, height, and BMI, especially decreasing percentile channels	➤ Cardiac defect ➤ Cystic fibrosis ➤ Gastrointestinal anomaly or parasites ➤ Malabsorption ➤ Cerebral palsy ➤ Endocrine disorder ➤ Eating disorder of infancy and childhood (failure to thrive)
High percentile for weight and BMI, especially increasing percentile channels	➤ Excess caloric intake ➤ Low physical activity ➤ Endocrine disorder

GROWTH AND DEVELOPMENTAL SURVEILLANCE

The first assessment skill integrated into the visit is generally measurement of growth. Weight and length measurement are described in Chapter 8∞, and expected patterns of growth are discussed in Chapter 5∞. Once the child can stand to be measured, sometime between 2 to 3 years of age, charts for standing height rather than recumbent length are used. Body mass index (BMI) is first calculated at 2 years of age and provides information about the relationship of height and weight (see Chapter 9∞). Head circumference is usually measured until between 1 and 2 years of age. Consult growth grids in Appendix A∞. Growth continues to be a primary way of evaluating the child's nutritional status. It may also provide clues about conditions that have not yet been identified or evaluated (Box 13–1). Depending on the results of growth measurement, additional data may be gathered. For a child under the 5th percentile for weight or BMI, detailed nutritional intake records should begin. Laboratory studies such as hematocrit and hemoglobin can be performed. Patterns of family growth can be examined. What size are the parents and siblings? Ask if the child has had any illness or hospitalization.

The physical assessment is performed, with some parts conducted by the nurse and others by the primary care provider such as a physician or nurse practitioner. See Chapter 8∞ for a thorough discussion of physical examination. The order of the examination and the approaches to the child are particularly important at this age. Leave intrusive procedures such as ear and eye exam and visualization of genitalia until the end of the exam. Integrate techniques such as allowing the child to play with the stethoscope, "blow out" the light from the otoscope, or make a game of pushing the legs against the examiner to measure symmetry of strength (Figure 13–1 ■). Preschoolers are generally interested in their bodies and teaching about parts of the examination is helpful. Ideas include comments such as:

- "Do you know what your heart sounds like? Do you want to listen to it?"
- "When you take a deep breath, where does the air go?"
- "This is your tummy. Your food goes here when you eat, then into your blood, and all around your body to make it strong."

During the physical examination, ask the parents pertinent questions. Consider the young child's expected developmental milestones (see Chapter 5∞) and ask questions related to them. Important questions include:

- "What are Jim's sleep patterns like now? Is he consistently sleeping through the night?"
- "How often does Cassandra have a bowel movement? Are you concerned that they are too frequent or not often enough? Does she ever appear constipated? What are the symptoms she displays?"
- "You mentioned that Jim is in a Head Start program. How often does he go? Has he had any illnesses that have kept him home?"
- "Do you have a thermometer at home? What type is it? Do you know how to take a temperature?"

Remember that some parents understand child growth and development, and your questions give them an opportunity to discuss observations or concerns, as well as help the child to see that the parent trusts and has positive rapport with the examiner. When parents answer questions readily and bring up concerns, move into a discussion of these topics during the examination. This encourages the child to relax and establish trust also. Teaching related to topics such as sleep and nutrition are discussed later in this chapter.

Developmental surveillance is integrated throughout the visit and developmental screening and testing are performed. See Table 13–1 for developmental milestones that can commonly be observed during health promotion and health maintenance visits of

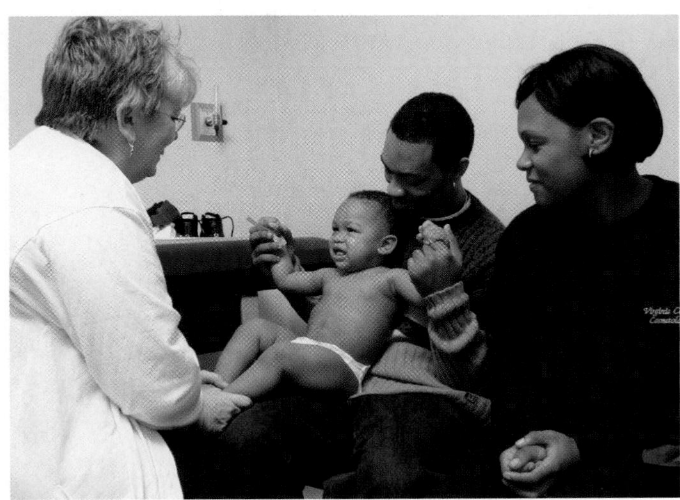
A

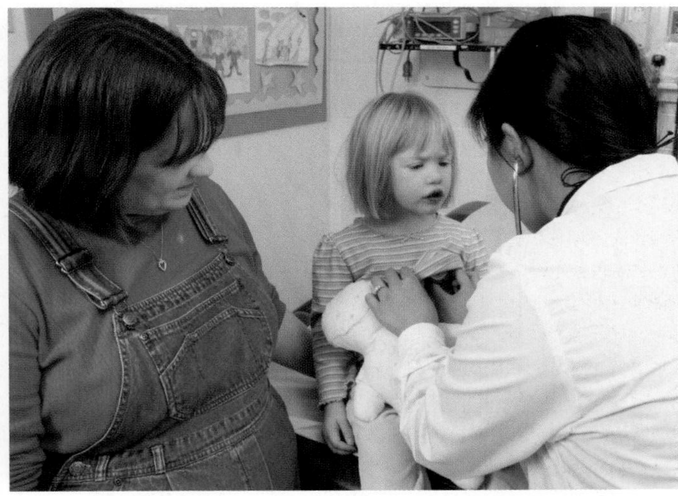
B

FIGURE 13–1 ■ The approach to examination of the toddler or preschooler is important in order to elicit cooperation. *A,* The toddler may accept parts of the examination best when seated on the parent's lap such as shown in this photo of Clarence. *B,* The preschooler likes the opportunity to touch and become comfortable with equipment used, or in this instance, holds a doll that receives the same examinations as the child.

TABLE 13–1 Developmental Milestones Observed During Health Promotion and Health Maintenance Visits of Toddlers and Preschoolers

AGE	DEVELOPMENTAL MILESTONES
12 months	➤ Walks alone or with help ➤ Enjoys social games and interactions ➤ Speaks 1–3 words and understands simple commands ➤ Drinks from cup and feeds self
15 months	➤ Walks by self, crawls or walks up stairs ➤ Stacks two blocks ➤ Points to one or more body parts ➤ Is increasingly interactive ➤ Explores environment
18 months	➤ Walks with ease ➤ Pushes or pulls toy ➤ Stacks three or more blocks ➤ Uses spoon to eat, spilling often ➤ Follows directions and uses 15–20 words
2–3 years	➤ Goes up and down steps ➤ Kicks ball ➤ Scribbles and draws lines on paper ➤ Imitates words and actions of adults
3–4 years	➤ Jumps ➤ Rides tricycle ➤ Draws precise lines on paper; attempts to imitate circle, line, and cross ➤ Always feeds self ➤ Dresses self though sometimes clothes are backwards ➤ Has friends and plays with others
4–5 years	➤ Recites rhymes and songs ➤ States name ➤ Draws a rudimentary person ➤ Builds tower of blocks and bridges with blocks ➤ Throws ball overhand

toddlers and preschoolers. Ask if the child has had developmental testing done at a childcare agency or another site. While health promotion and health maintenance visits commonly address issues such as immunizations, nutrition, and sleep positions, research has demonstrated that pediatricians are less likely to address topics such as child communication, reading, parental stress, or other issues related to developmental progression (Halfon et al., 2003). Nurses generally have in-depth knowledge of child development, through growth and development courses and pediatric nursing curricula, and are thus well positioned to ensure that parental concerns related to child development are addressed (Table13–2). Watch for the inclusion of development in child health visits, identify deficits in your agency, and take steps to meet the needs of parents and children (Box 13–2).

BOX 13–2 Pediatric Service Satisfaction

Several researchers have examined the satisfaction of parents with the pediatric services received by their children. These studies include the 1996 Commonwealth Fund Survey of Parents with Young Children (Young et al., 1998; Schuster et al., 2000), the 2000 National Survey of Early Childhood Health (Halfon, 2002), and the American Academy of Pediatrics survey (AAP, 2000). Topics that have been identified by parents in these surveys as needing more attention in child healthcare visits include:

- Sleep issues
- Discipline
- Toilet training
- Learning/reading
- Child communication
- Parent substance use, emotional state, supports

Nurses can be influential in ensuring that each of these topics is inserted appropriately into each health promotion/health maintenance visit. See Table 13–2 for examples of questions to ask and teaching to perform during the early childhood healthcare visits.

TABLE 13–2 Sample Questions and Teaching Topics Pertinent to Early Childhood Visits

TOPIC	QUESTIONS	TEACHING
Sleep	How long does Cassandra sleep at night? Does she take naps? Does Jim ever wake at night crying? Do you have trouble consoling him? Is your daughter able to concentrate on preschool and stay alert during the hours she is there? What concerns do you have about your son's sleep patterns?	Normal amounts of sleep at various ages Establishment of consistent sleep routines Types of sleep disruptions and their treatment
Discipline	Does Cassandra ever misbehave? When it happens, what does she typically do? How do you respond to her behavior? Have you tried using "time out" when she seems out of control? How does the childcare center deal with inappropriate behavior? Do you agree with the center's techniques?	Consistency and limit setting Appropriate consequences for behaviors Evaluating methods of discipline Adapting methods to individual children
Toilet training	Have you thought about beginning to toilet train your toddler? How do you think you will do it? What signs have you seen that he might be ready soon? You mentioned that Cassandra has occasional accidents. How often are they and are you concerned about them? What rewards do you use when your son is successful in using the toilet? Do you have a small toilet for him to use?	Readiness cues for toilet training (see Chapter 5) Introducing toilet training Positive reinforcement for children Transitions to childcare and other settings away from home
Learning/reading	Describe the things that Jim is learning now. Is he progressing as you would expect or like? How often do you read to Jim? How does he like reading with you? Have you been able to get books to keep for him at home? Do you ever visit the library together? Does your library have a story time for young children?	Providing stimulating environments for learning Importance of reading to children Importance of providing books for children to look at during play time Pointing out letters to preschool children
Communication	What is Cassandra's language like now? Are you concerned or particularly pleased about any of her ways of communicating? How does she get along with other children in Head Start? What has she been learning about getting along with other children?	Expected language skills Social interaction with adults and other children
Parental issues	How is your life going right now? Do you or does anyone else in your family drink more than two drinks per day, smoke, or take street drugs? How is your general mood? Are you often tired, sad, or depressed? Who helps out when you need something? Are there friends or family close to call upon? What resources that you do not have would be helpful to you (e.g., more food, counseling, other parents)?	Effects of parental substance abuse on children Need for healthy mental status to meet child's developmental needs Referrals to needed community resources to meet basic mental status needs

Developmental screening and testing were addressed in Chapters 10 through 12 and the principles continue for toddlers and preschoolers. (See Table 10–6 for a list of suggested tests.) During the early childhood years, common areas addressed on developmental screening tests include social skills, continuing gross and fine motor activity, and language skills.

MediaLink Childcare Resources

Many children, especially by preschool age, attend a childcare center. Ask about the experience and whether developmental skills are a focus of activity. Governmental programs include Early Head Start and Head Start (federal) or Early Childhood Education and Assistance Program (ECEAP) (state); nonprofit centers may be in schools, YMCA or YWCA, or related to religious entities; for-profit centers may be run by individuals or as cooperative ventures. See Chapter 5 for further information about types of childcare. Ask if the parent is pleased with childcare experience or requires further resources. Payment for care can be problematic for some families and should be explored. Resources to assist families with promotion of the social, intellectual, and emotional development of young children are available. Refer families to Zero to Three or other appropriate resources (Box 13–3).

Health promotion growth and development issues for toddlers and preschoolers are addressed at each visit. Examples include:

- Explaining growth patterns and what is expected in the months ahead

BOX 13–3 Zero to Three

Zero to Three is a national center for infants, toddlers, and families that seeks to promote the healthy development of the nation's babies and toddlers by supporting and strengthening families, communities, and those who work on their behalf. The results of research are used to establish policies and practices that integrate the latest research into practice. Zero to Three works closely with Early Head Start centers, trains program employees, provides information to parents and health professionals, and publishes results in professional and lay journals. Find out how Zero to Three activities influence your community.

- Providing toys that encourage development of the coming developmental milestones (see Chapter 5 for specific suggestions)
- Showing parents the child's developmental progression on a screening tool

Likewise, health maintenance activities are included in health supervision visits, with the primary purpose being prevention of disease and injury. Specific examples are included throughout the chapter, but general areas addressed are as follows:

- Connecting developmental skills with risks for injury such as drowning and car crashes
- Recognizing the possibility of infectious diseases as the child begins a childcare experience and addressing recognition and treatments for common diseases

Expected outcomes for the child include normal growth and development patterns for motor, language, and social skills; parental knowledge of stimulating activities for the child; awareness of the family about risks to growth and development; and healthy body systems for the child.

PRACTICE ALERT

When you examine growth grids you will find that the percentiles can be grouped along the lines presented. The channels commonly seen are:

Below 5th percentile (needs nutritional assessment)
5th–10th percentile
10th–25th percentile
25th–50th percentile
50th–75th percentile
75th–95th percentile
Above 95th percentile (needs nutritional assessment)

A child who generally falls between the 25th and 50th percentile may have weight closer to the 25th percentile at one visit and closer to the 50th percentile on the next, which simply reflects normal patterns of fluctuation. On the other hand, going from the 25th–50th weight percentile channel on one visit to the 75th–95th percentile channel on a visit a few months later may indicate nutritional problems. Weigh the child a second time to verify your findings, add dietary questions to the health supervision visit, collect additional nutritional data, and refer to the physician or nurse practitioner in the facility. See Chapter 9 for further information about nutritional assessment.

NUTRITION

The child's nutritional status continues to play an important part in promoting health and preventing health disruptions during toddler and preschooler years. Good nutrition fosters normal growth patterns, promotes developmental progression, and helps prevent disorders such as anemia, tooth decay, and immune dysfunction. In addition, intake of food takes on an increasingly social dimension during early childhood as children interact more with adults and other children at mealtimes.

As with infants, the measurements of weight and height form the basis of the nutritional assessment. When the child is able to stand for height measurements, the percentile grid for standing height is used rather than the recumbent length grid. Once the child is 2 years of age, the height and weight proportion are the basis for body mass index (BMI) calculation. Then weight, height, and BMI percentiles are all considered. See Chapter 9 for further explanation of evaluation of these percentiles and Appendix A for the percentile grids. Children usually stay within the same **growth channel,** or percentile range over time, even though their rates of growth vary somewhat from child to child. For example, if an infant is consistently between the 25th and 50th percentiles for length and weight, the percentiles generally remain about the same as the child gets older. When children change percentile channels, or when the BMI percentile increases or decreases, additional nutritional data will be collected. The child may be consuming too many calories for activity if the length stays in the same channel and the weight increases, or may not be consuming enough energy if the weight percentile decreases while the length stays in the same channel. While some variation in percentile is expected, staying in the same growth channel or percentile range demonstrates expected growth patterns. Other physical assessment data that provide information about nutrition include energy level of the child, condition of hair, nails, and skin, and meeting developmental milestones.

For toddlers, questions for the family focus on introduction of foods, child's eating patterns, and transition from breast or bottle to other liquids. The toddler often consumes small amounts of foods and parents consequently worry about the change in appetite. Showing them that the child is growing normally can help allay their anxiety about this common developmental variation.

Preschoolers increasingly interact with others during food preparation and meal consumption. Questions focus on the child's likes and dislikes for particular foods, behavior at the table, and establishment of healthy family eating patterns. Ask how often the family eats out, especially at fast-food restaurants. Excess intake of fat and salty foods, as well as large portion sizes, is associated with eating out frequently. See Chapter 9 for further discussion of the issues related to fast foods.

When parents are busy and older siblings are in activities, both toddlers and preschoolers may be eating foods such as French fries or milk shakes several times weekly. Suggest alternative approaches to the busy lifestyle, such as bringing fresh fruit slices along when an older sibling is at a sporting event, keeping a cooler in the car to maintain cool items, and limiting fast-food meals to no more than one or two each week. Encourage the family to establish times to eat together, even if only a few times weekly. If children help with preparations for this family meal, and then eat together, nutritional knowledge and intake can be positively enhanced. When the child is in a childcare center, encourage the parents to find out what food is provided for the child in that setting. If the parents would prefer to send food or have particular food requests, assist them in dealing with the childcare personnel.

Questions that provide information to be used as the basis for nutritional teaching include:

- "What type of milk is Jim drinking now? How much does he drink each day? How much juice does he drink each day?"

MediaLink Case Study: Single-Parenting Challenges and Nutrition

- "Does your son like to eat with the family at the table? What foods does he like? Dislike?"
- "What types of foods are served at Cassandra's childcare center? Do children eat together at tables there?"
- "What kinds of things does Cassandra like to do with you in the kitchen? How often do you prepare meals at home each week? Which meals do you most commonly prepare? How often does your family eat together? How often do you eat at fast-food restaurants? What are the major times when it is hard to feed your family the foods you would like to or that are good for them? Does your family eat breakfast each day? What do you eat for breakfast?"
- "Are you giving your children any vitamins? Fluoride?"
- "What questions do you have about your child's food needs and patterns?"
- "What access do you have to fresh fruits and vegetables at your local market or farmer's market? Are they affordable? Do you feel like you know how to prepare the foods that are healthy to offer your children?"

During the toddler and preschool years, children are gaining much more independence about food choices and patterns of eating. At the same time, their eating patterns depend mainly on the family and so assessment should involve the entire family unit. See Developing Cultural Competence: Family Nutrition.

Parents can benefit from receiving information about nutrition in young children (Table 13–3). Health promotion interventions are designed to focus on leading the child and family to a higher state of wellness, and may include actions such as supporting breastfeeding for young toddlers and being sure preschoolers have a role in selecting foods for healthy snacks. Important health promotion teaching to include with every family is the importance of including "5 a day," or five servings of fruits and vegetables into the daily diet. (See Chapter 14 for further description of the 5-a-day program.) Inclusion of adequate fruits and vegetables promotes health by boosting the immune system, providing for regular elimination patterns, and leading to healthy hair and nails. Nurses and parents partner together to ensure that the young child establishes healthy eating habits at home and in other daily settings.

DEVELOPING CULTURAL COMPETENCE
Family Nutrition

Families integrate their own cultural backgrounds and past experiences into food preparation and choices. Ask what foods are common in the child's cultural group and help the family learn when to introduce each food. For example, rice may be a first food for an Asian baby, rather than rice cereal. Simply be sure the child also takes in adequate iron sources in the first foods offered. Tofu or bean paste may be a common protein source in some diets. A Native American child may eat fish or wild game, along with berries and roots. Ask and learn about each family's cultural patterns. Learn what you can about cultural groups in your community. Encourage the family to offer the young child their usual foods, as long as they meet needs for requirements, are prepared with minimal salt and seasoning, and are soft enough to avoid choking. Perform diet recalls and analyses to identify specific teaching needs.

TABLE 13–3 Nutrition Teaching for Health Promotion and Health Maintenance Visits

AGE	NUTRITION TEACHING
1 year	Support mother who continues to breastfeed Wean child from bottle by substituting cup If beginning to use cow milk, use whole milk Limit juice to 4–6 oz daily; offer water several times daily Encourage safety measures—use high chair with strap, secure child and use caution in grocery carts, do not allow foods to be eaten in car Provide information on choking and airway obstruction removal training Provide food and water safety guidelines (see Chapter 9) Be sure all major food groups have been introduced Limit high-fat and high-sugar foods Review amounts of food commonly consumed and frequency of feedings Review use of fluoride if water supply is not fluoridated
2 years	Encourage total removal of bottle if still in use Ensure that all foods common to family have been offered Offer child-size eating utensils Child can change to low-fat or skim milk if family desires Limit milk to two servings daily Teach parents methods for dealing with temper tantrums over food—make food available at meal and snack times only, do not force intake, offer a variety of foods Teach that child may have days of very low intake due to slowing growth rate
3 years	Teach normal intake and decreasing number of snacks Engage child in food preparation and pouring liquids from small pitcher Recognize that **food jags** (periods when only one or two foods are eaten) are common Recognize importance of social nature of eating; expect child to sit for a short period at meals with family Meals and snacks should not be eaten while watching television
4 years	Encourage involving child in snack selection and preparation Start to teach food groups and importance of nutrition for the body Alter intake as appropriate depending on weight and BMI Dairy products consumed should all be low or reduced fat

Health maintenance activities are those that focus primarily on disease and injury prevention, with examples of feeding practices that do not include common choking foods, and limiting daily fruit juice intake to prevent dental caries and excessive caloric intake.

Desired outcomes related to nutrition include meeting normal growth and development milestones, maintenance of recommended weight, increasing understanding of healthy food patterns, and prevention of nutrition-related disorders.

PHYSICAL ACTIVITY

The toddler and preschooler consistently show gains in fine and gross motor abilities. They move around independently and have more physical activity away from the home base. They commonly visit parks, swim, attend childcare centers, and help with some household tasks. These activities are important, both because they assist the child to continue to develop motor skills and limit the amount of time spent in sedentary behavior. The toddler and preschool years are an important time for setting the habits for physical activity during all of childhood.

During toddler years, the main emphasis is on providing experiences that encourage further motor development. The child needs to walk, run, hop, push and pull objects, and throw balls. Motor activity is a major component in all play times and activities should engage the child's large and small muscle groups.

By the preschool years, coordination becomes increasingly important (Figure 13–2 ■). Physical activity is important for all children, including those with developmental disabilities. The preschooler learns to balance, walk on one foot, skip, and throw and catch with greater accuracy. **Kinesthesia,** or the sense of one's body position and movement, develops during these years. Eye-hand coordination improves at the same time that visual acuity matures (Patrick, Spear, Holt, et al., 2001). The social component plays an important role as children learn to engage in games and activities cooperatively with others.

The nurse applies the concept of resilience by identifying both risk and protective factors related to physical activity (Table 13–4). This assessment becomes the basis for nursing interventions, both to reinforce positive physical activity and to make recommendations for changes where needed. When the family has many responsibilities or lives in an unsafe neighborhood, suggest methods to integrate physical activity into daily life. Nurses working in inner-city settings help teachers to add physical activity to childcare center activities, and seek to keep schools open for toddler and preschool programs in early mornings and late afternoons and evenings. Soft beach balls and other items can be provided to assist the family in designing activities that foster the young child's physical capacities. Safety is always a concern and nurses teach about safety gear, safe playground construction, and emergency care in case of injury. Encourage families to limit television and other "screen" activities like computers and games to a total of no more than 2 hours daily. As these sedentary behaviors decrease, physical activity will naturally have to increase.

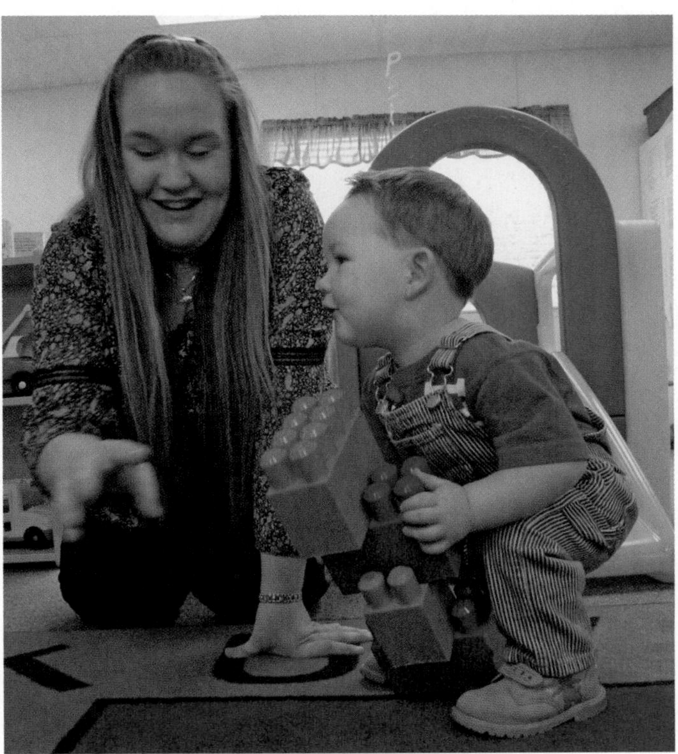

FIGURE 13–2 ■ This toddler enjoys motor activity that uses large muscle groups. The preschooler begins to spend increasing amounts of time in coordination of both small and large muscle mass. List several physical activities that you can suggest for the parents of children in each of these age groups.

Children who have special healthcare needs often have particular physical activity limitations or requirements. The toddler or preschooler with diabetes may require glucose monitoring and insulin adjustment during activity (see Chapter 32∞). The child with cystic fibrosis or asthma may need respiratory

TABLE 13–4 Risk and Protective Factors Regarding Physical Activity in Toddlerhood and Preschool

RISK FACTORS	PROTECTIVE FACTORS
➤ Limited stimulation by family or other care providers ➤ Long work hours by parents ➤ Parents who have little physical activity on a daily basis ➤ Limited social time with other children ➤ Limited access to balls, slides, balance beams, tricycles, and other materials that foster physical activity ➤ Adequate safety gear for activities is not available ➤ Reluctance to try new physical activity ➤ Television or other screen activities are engaged in for more than 2 hours daily ➤ Developmental delay ➤ Slow development of social skills ➤ Lack of knowledge by family about child physical activity needs ➤ Limited community resources for childcare and physical activity ➤ Unsafe neighborhood and lack of lawns, parks, and other facilities	➤ Expected developmental progression ➤ Daily contact with other young children ➤ Easily engaged socially with others ➤ Eagerness to try new physical activity ➤ Access to balls, slides, balance beams, tricycles, and other materials that foster physical activity ➤ Adequate safety gear that properly fits child is available ➤ Family members engage in daily physical activity ➤ Family members spend time daily in physical activity with child ➤ Family understands motor developmental milestones and importance of physical activity in childhood ➤ Television and other screen activities are limited to no more than 2 hours daily ➤ Neighborhood contains access to childcare which integrates physical activity ➤ Neighborhood is safe, and contains lawns, parks, and other facilities

Adapted from Patrick, K., Spear, B., Holt, K., & Sofka, D. (Eds.). (2001). Bright futures in practice: Physical activity. *Arlington, VA: National Center for Education in Maternal and Child Health.*

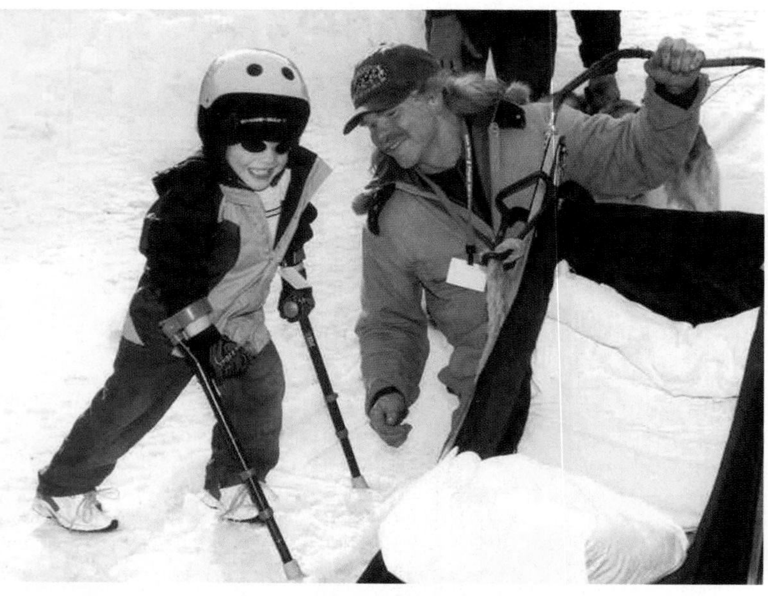

A

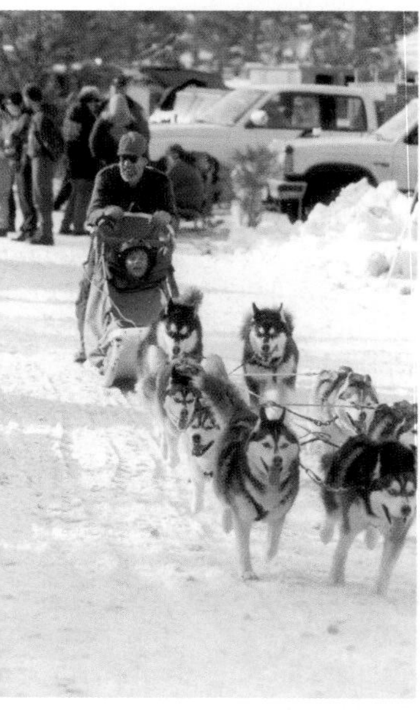

B

FIGURE 13–3 ■ *A,* Children with developmental disabilities or other health problems still need physical activity. *B,* Special events such as this dog sled ride for children with disabilities ensure that children experience movement and learn to enjoy physical activity. *Courtesy of Shriners Hospital, Spokane, WA.*

support or monitoring during exercise (see Chapter 25∞). The child with a musculoskeletal abnormality may require special shoes or other devices to promote activity (see Chapter 35∞ and Figure 13–3 ■). The nurse partners with the family to plan for the child's special health needs while engaging in physical activity.

Because both children and adults are commonly overweight and sedentary in today's society, emphasis on physical activity should be a part of each health supervision visit. Nurses and parents are partners in planning activities for the young child; patterns set in motion at this early age will continue into the rest of childhood and into adulthood. Suggestions for the family may include setting guidelines to limit television and other screen activities to a maximum of 2 hours daily to facilitate adequate physical activity time. Children should not have television and computers in their bedrooms. Health promotion teaching imparts to parents the benefits of activity, such as a healthy immune and cardiovascular system, positive self-concept of the child, and the child's learning of important motor skills. Health maintenance teaching focuses on disease prevention, such as avoidance of overweight, and injury prevention, with use of protective gear for sports.

Expected outcomes of health promotion and health supervision related to physical activity are daily inclusion of at least 60 minutes of activity into life patterns, normal developmental progression of musculoskeletal system, growth in coordination, and appropriate balance between dietary intake and physical activity so that normal weight is maintained.

ORAL HEALTH

The early childhood years play an important part in the child's future oral health, and yet dental care remains one of the most preventable and common unmet healthcare needs for children in developed countries (VanLandeghen, Bronstein, & Brach, 2003). **Early childhood caries (ECC)** is defined as one or more decayed, missing, or filled tooth surfaces in a child less than 5 years of age (American Academy of Pediatric Dentistry, 2000). This condition is caused by inadequate preventive care, which can include diet, brushing, and feeding habits. ECC is serious because young children with the condition are more likely to have continuing dental problems that can influence speech, cause pain, and delay development. Teaching prevention at an early age is key to preventing the problem. See Chapter 9∞ for further information about this condition.

By 1 year of age the child should have made a first visit to the dentist. By about 2 years of age, the toddler has a full set of 20 teeth. Evaluate these teeth for condition and number. They help to maintain space for the permanent teeth, foster positive eating habits, and are needed for language development. Inquire about how the family cleans the teeth and ask them to demonstrate if the child has any dental decay. At the end of preschool, the first of these **deciduous teeth** are lost, an important developmental event for most children. (See Chapter 8∞.)

The nurse assists the family to ensure oral health for the young child. Some questions during the health promotion visit elicit important information.

- "How many teeth does your toddler have? Did they all come in without problems? What comfort measures have helped when he is teething? Do you have any concerns about his teeth?"
- "What is the source of your drinking water? Do you know if it is fluoridated? If not, does your child take fluoride? How much? How often?"

- "Describe how Cassandra's teeth get brushed and how often? Do you use toothpaste? What type? How much? Is it hard for you to afford toothbrushes?"
- "Are there any loose teeth?"
- "How much juice or sweetened drinks does Jim have each day? How does he drink these (bottle, cup)? How many sweet foods such as candy, gum, cookies, cake, doughnuts are eaten daily?"
- "Has Jim been to the dentist? When was the last time? Do you have dental insurance? If not, do you have a resource for dental care or are financial concerns limiting dental visits?"

Based on the results of the assessment of the child's teeth, observation of language skills, and answers to questions directed at parents, plan interventions that will foster maintenance of oral health, thus preventing dental disease. (See Chapter 24∞ for emergency treatment of dental injury.) These may include referral to low-cost dental clinics, provision of toothbrush and toothpaste, demonstration to the parents and young child about proper brushing technique, and teaching about limiting sweet snacks and drinks. Remember to positively reinforce health promotion practices such as good oral hygiene for toddlers and preschoolers who brush, visit the dentist, and are careful to limit intake of sweets. See Partnering with Families: Oral Care.

Desired outcomes for oral health are eruption of a normal set of deciduous teeth, regular dental care, nutrition and hygiene practices that foster dental health, and knowledge of child and parent about oral health.

MENTAL AND SPIRITUAL HEALTH

In Chapter 12∞, the relationship of normal growth and development to the child's mental health is described. This relationship continues into the toddler and preschool years, since young children with a sense of security and self-worth generally grow and develop as expected. During toddler and preschool years, the child develops a conscious sense of self during interactions with others and in play activities. Be sure the office or clinic setting is set up to provide space and activities for young children in order to promote a positive sense of self (Jellinek, Patel, & Froehle, 2002).

PRACTICE ALERT

While toddlers and preschoolers are waiting for a health supervision visit, they should be in a pleasant setting with age-appropriate activities. As you visit various clinics and offices evaluate the setting:

- Are the colors bright and yet restful?
- Are there books for young children, child-sized chairs and tables, crayons, paper, and other activities provided?
- Can parents sit and observe the child in play activities?
- Is the setting safe, without hazards such as glass that can be pulled down and break, sharp corners, or access to street or other unsafe places?
- Are there stimulating surroundings that include a variety of items to look at and to do?
- Can surfaces and toys be easily cleaned frequently to discourage transfer of microorganisms?

PARTNERING WITH FAMILIES

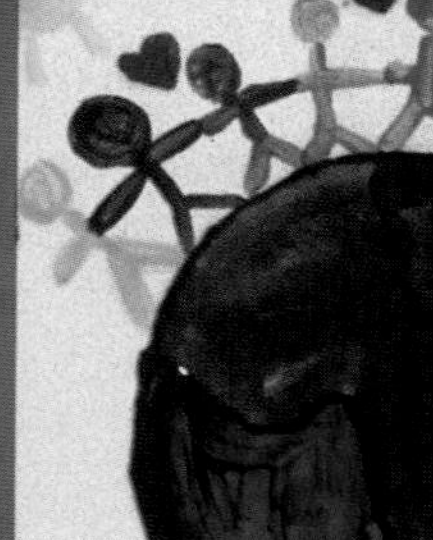

Oral Care

Ask parents to describe their child's oral hygiene practices and enhance with teaching as needed. Recommendations of the American Dental Association include the following:

- Help the child to brush twice daily with a pea-sized amount of fluoride toothpaste, using a small, soft children's brush. Brush for the time it takes to think about the words to a favorite song such as the ABC song. The toddler and preschooler need help to brush for the proper time and to use the right amount of toothpaste. Be sure the child spits out the toothpaste to avoid ingesting too much fluoride which can discolor the teeth.
- Once the child has two teeth together that are nearly touching, use dental floss once daily.
- Limit sweet snacks and drinks to once daily, followed by brushing.

The family is key in fostering a positive self-image and setting the stage for the child's mental health. As the family is called in for the visit, begin your assessment of the family's methods of influencing mental health.

- Do parents communicate readily with the child?
- Are interactions generally warm, caring, and loving, or are there constant criticisms of behavior?
- Does the parent seem willing to point out the child's accomplishments, or have trouble making any positive statements about the child?
- Does the child appear at ease with the parent? Is the child at ease in the healthcare setting? Toddlers often still have some stranger anxiety and may show discomfort, while preschoolers are more often eager and excited to meet you.

Next ask for a description of a typical day or what the child has recently begun to do. The child's sense of self and mental status are related to new accomplishments. Inquire about toilet training, toothbrushing, choosing clothes and getting dressed, using crayons, or other developmental tasks. See the Denver II Developmental Test and a list of tasks in Chapter 5∞. Direct questions or comments to the child. If the toddler or preschooler appears nervous or shy, return to questioning the parent and quietly offer a toy or book to the child. Once the nurse appears to be trusted by the parent, rapport can often be established with the child. Toddlers tend to have some continuing stranger anxiety and to take longer to warm up to new individuals, while preschoolers more often engage in new relationships readily.

Self-regulation by the infant was described earlier as the ability to soothe and comfort the self. By the toddler and preschool periods, the young child self-regulates other activities to control

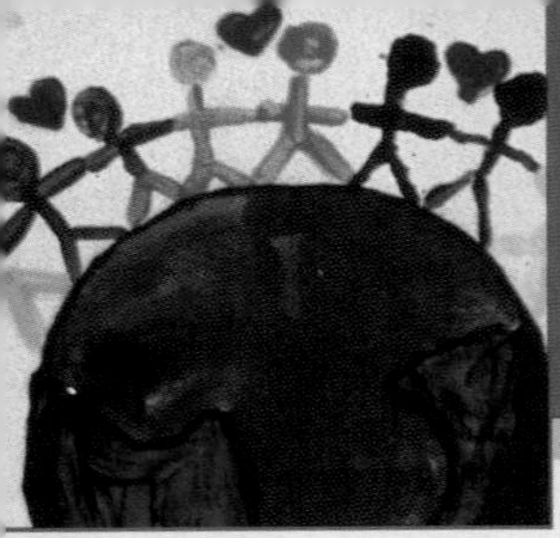

PARTNERING WITH FAMILIES

Positive Discipline

To provide structure that enhances the possibility of desirable behaviors:

- Limit rules to those that are essential. It will be easier to enforce a few important rules than many that are nonessential.
- Provide an environment where the child is mainly free to explore safely in order to avoid constant cautions. For example, have adequate play space for toddlers with limited fragile glassware in the usual daily environment. It is easier for the toddler to learn not to touch a few objects when adequate objects are provided for play.
- Spend time interacting with the child several times each day. Praise positive behaviors frequently. Preschoolers often like to have charts with stars to record picking up toys, helping a parent, and performing other positive behaviors. Once preschoolers obtain a certain number of stars they earn a reward such as stickers or an outing with the parent.

When the child shows undesirable behaviors:

- Use distraction as the first approach and praise the child for selecting the new activity suggested by the parent.
- Tell the child one time that the behavior is unsatisfactory and what will happen if the behavior persists.
- Separate the child from a setting in which behavior is undesirable. Place the child in "time out," a separate place that is safe. Toddlers can be placed in a play pen or crib, while preschoolers are told to sit on a chair. One minute of time out per year of age is a good length of time. Once time out is over, provide a positive activity and move the child directly toward the activity.

When undesirable behaviors include other people, such as biting or hitting:

- Tell the child clearly that it is not appropriate to hurt another person.
- Separate the child immediately from the situation and use time out.
- If there are repeated episodes, be sure the child is getting adequate sleep and food, has opportunities for active play that releases energy, has positive attention from many people in the environment, and be sensitive to stresses such as a recent trauma or a new sibling.
- Encourage children to "use words" instead of hitting or biting. Until able to do so on their own, parents can model this behavior. "You feel like saying 'I am really upset that you took my toy away.' Let's use words instead of hitting so your sister knows that."

anger, desires for objects or foods, and other behaviors. To assist the child in developing the ability to control and regulate self, parents often use discipline techniques. Ask about how the parent responds to the child who is having a temper tantrum or showing other undesirable behaviors. Reinforce positive ways of helping the child set limits for self and make suggestions when parents need assistance. Spanking or other physical forms of discipline are not more effective than less physical methods, and can have negative outcomes, such as increased child anger, aggression, and decreased self-esteem (Jellinek et al., 2002). Parents who were spanked often use this technique and do not know that other methods work well and have more positive outcomes. Share principles that can be used for positive limit setting. Model positive limit setting when the child is in the office. "Oh, here's a book you can look at. This instrument on the wall is just for the nurse to use." (See Partnering with Families: Positive Discipline.) The goal of discipline is to help the child develop a sense of right and wrong, and to learn acceptable ways of dealing with other people. Help parents of the toddler with temper tantrums to learn specific management techniques for these behaviors. (See Partnering with Families: Handling Temper Tantrums.)

Adequate sleep and rest are needed for children to master self-regulation. Most toddlers have established regular sleeping patterns with occasional night awakenings. They sleep about 10 to 12 hours at night with one or two daytime naps (Murray & Zentner, 2001). Parents have usually learned to establish clear routines such as reading a story, rubbing a back, and then leaving the child alone. Occasionally parents who work during the day may feel guilty about putting the child to bed. Encourage them to spend quality time with the child after arriving home, and then to establish clear sleeping expectations. Transitional objects such as blankets or toys are important for the toddler and can be used during childcare experiences to provide comfort and help maintain normal routines. Some families prefer to have children sleep in the bed with parents. If this is the parent's decision, be sure they are aware of safety hazards such as excessive bedding, falling between headboard and frame, parental smoking that could lead to fire, or parental alcohol and drug use which can lead to being not attuned to the child's needs.

The preschooler sleeps about 9 to 11 hours and may have one or no naps each day (Murray & Zentner, 2001). Some quiet playtime can be beneficial even for the preschooler who does not nap. At this age, some children develop awakenings at night and may need some assistance in falling back to sleep. **Nightmares** are frightening dreams that awaken the child who is often crying and upset. Parents can reassure the child, rub the back, provide some repeat of a bedtime routine such as reading a story, and then allow the child to settle into sleep again. It is not advisable to bring the child to the parental bed because the child may start to awaken at night in order to continue this practice. **Night terrors** are characterized by a child who cries out and appears frightened. However, in contrast to nightmares, the child having a night terror is not fully awake, and may appear disoriented (Edelman & Mandle, 2002). Parents should quietly talk to and comfort the child, allowing them to return to sleep. There is no recollection of these events the next morning.

The toddler gains more independence in many aspects of life such as mobility and speech. Control over toileting is another milestone that signals greater independence and can lead to a sense of self-control. Ask parents if the toddler has shown interest in toilet training and how they intend to work with the child to attain control over bowel and bladder. See Partnering with Families: Toilet Training, and refer to Chapter 5∞ for further discussion of readiness for toilet training.

Preschoolers are generally well trained for bowel and bladder with only occasional accidents. These should be treated with understanding rather than blame in order for healthy self-concept to develop. Preschoolers are increasingly aware of gender and sexuality issues. They may ask questions about kissing, love, or their genitals. These questions should be truthfully answered, leaving the child with a positive sense of sexuality. Exploration of genitals can occur, and children should be told simply that it is something that should take place in private; offer other activities to engage them when with other people.

For some toddlers or preschoolers, extraordinary stresses can cause challenges to mental health. Traumatic events such as witnessing or being involved in a car crash or losing a parent to death have profound effects on young children. If it is learned during a health supervision that a toddler or preschooler has experienced a severe trauma or has ongoing stress, refer the family to specialized services such as psychiatric and mental health experts for care. See Chapter 34∞ for further descriptions of these challenges to mental health.

In all families, toddlers and preschoolers are learning about moral codes, what is right and wrong, and the rules that guide behaviors. (See Chapter 5∞ for further description of moral development in young children.) The family's spiritual orientation takes on additional meaning for the toddler and preschooler. They can participate in the family's faith-based practices, which enlarge their microsystem influences to include that of the religious group, thus reinforcing the child's learning about right and wrong. The nurse assesses the family's faith-based or spiritual beliefs and provides support for the family's approach, whether it be in established religious organizations or in the family's other meaningful activities.

Identify strengths and risks in the mental and spiritual health of toddlers and preschoolers. Examples of strengths include:

- Child has adapted positively to both family and childcare routines.
- The toddler is generally able to quiet within a few moments after a temper tantrum.
- The preschooler is showing increasing ability to identify undesirable behavior and readily goes to time out when needed.
- Family patterns have established a sleep routine that is working well and providing adequate rest for the child.
- Parents have time each day to spend individually with their children, and provide much positive feedback for desirable behaviors.
- Family attends regular religious activity meaningful to them.

PARTNERING WITH FAMILIES

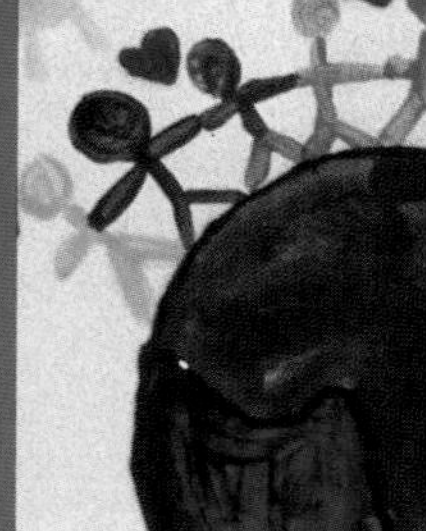

Handling Temper Tantrums

Temper tantrums are common in toddlers and are manifested as episodes of screaming, crying, pounding objects, kicking, and otherwise showing anger. Toddlers may be expressing frustration with something that has occurred. They have learned that they are independent individuals and have an effect by showing their dismay. Temper tantrums should gradually decrease in number as the child grows into the preschool years. Parents can learn that although tantrums are normal, techniques exist that can assist in handling them successfully. The approaches are similar to those used when the child bites or hits. Some specific suggestions for tantrums include:

- Learn the signals that a tantrum is about to occur. Most toddlers become increasingly agitated and upset. Holding and distracting them at that point may help avoid a tantrum.
- Separate the child from others if possible ("time-out") to eliminate reinforcement by attention given.
- If not possible, be sure the child is safe and not throwing self against objects that could cause injury.
- Remain calm, holding the child firmly still if needed.
- Do not "give in" to the child's demands by giving them a food treat or toy; avoid this positive reinforcement of the behavior.
- Talk calmly to the child, verbalizing his or her feelings and what the child needs to do to calm down.
- Reward the child briefly after control is gained. "It was really good that you could calm down and say you were sorry. Now let's go back to the living room."

Adapted from Colyar, M. R. (2003). Well-child assessment for primary care providers. *Philadelphia: FA Davis.*

Risk factors that may indicate the need for more teaching and problem solving with the family include:

- Parents express guilt about expecting that the toddler will be able to sleep through the night.
- Preschooler frequently awakens with night terrors.
- Child was recently in a car accident.
- Preschooler is having several episodes daily at the childcare center of biting or hitting other children.
- Parents commonly spank the child for undesirable behaviors but report that the behaviors are increasing.
- Parents express interest in having others help the child learn right from wrong, but do not have ideas about how to access such assistance.

Health promotion activities focus on development of a healthy self-concept in the toddler and young child by helping parents to set up successful play experiences, to praise the child for successes, to use effective limit-setting techniques,

MediaLink: Handling Temper Tantrums Video

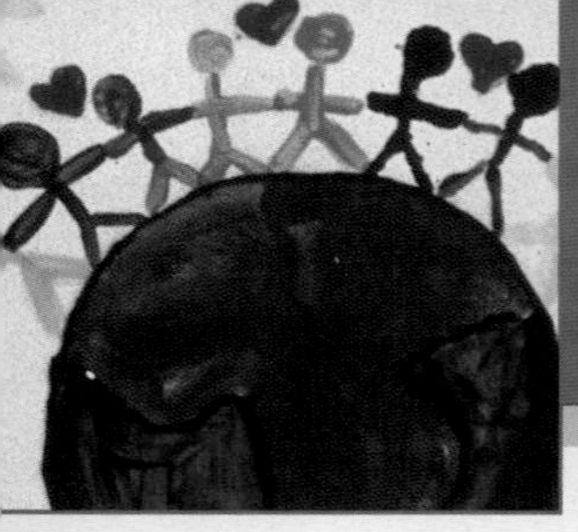

PARTNERING WITH FAMILIES

Toilet Training

When are children ready to learn toileting? Are parents responsible for the differences in ages at which toilet training is accomplished? Does toilet training provide clues to a child's intellectual ability?

We know that children are not ready for toilet training until several developmental capabilities exist: to stand and walk well, to pull pants up and down, and to recognize the need to eliminate and then to be able to wait until in the bathroom. Once this readiness is apparent, the child can be given a small potty chair and the procedure explained.

Children often prefer their own chair on the floor to using the large toilet. The child should be placed on the chair at regular intervals for a few moments and can be given reward or praise for successes. If the child seems not to understand or does not wish to cooperate, it is best to wait a few weeks and then try again. Just as all of development is subject to individual timetables, toilet training occurs with considerable variability from one child to another. Identify for parents the developmental characteristics of their child and encourage them to appreciate without anxiety the unfolding of skills. These timetables are not predictive of future development.

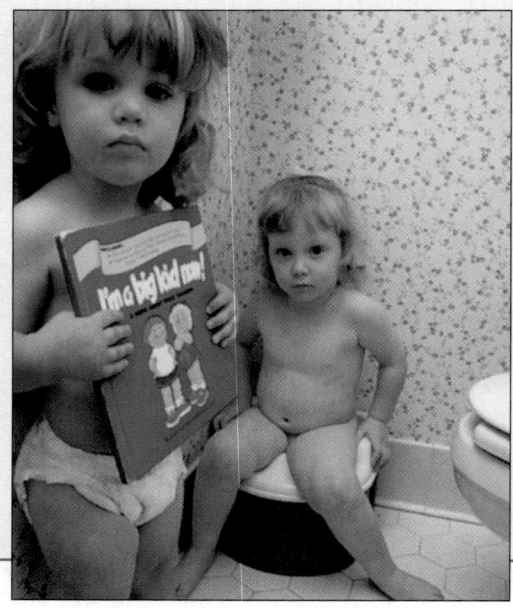

The child who is ill or hospitalized or has other stress often regresses in toilet training activities. It is best to quietly reinstitute attempts at training after the trauma. Potty chairs should be available on pediatric units and toileting habits identified during initial assessment so that regular routines can be followed and the child's usual words for elimination can be used.

and to realize and appreciate the child's unique characteristics. Health maintenance seeks to avoid poor self-image that can occur with constant criticism or expectations not in alignment with the toddler or preschooler developmental capabilities. Further examples of family interactions that can influence the child's self-concept are provided in the following section on relationships.

Desired outcomes for the child related to mental and spiritual health include emergence of a positive self-esteem, ability to self-regulate behaviors, and emergence of methods to handle daily stressors, and normal developmental progression in tasks such as toilet training and sleep.

RELATIONSHIPS

Family members are part of the microsystem for the toddler and preschooler, and as such, form a vital part of the child's environment. Families with members who handle stress well and have healthy lifestyle patterns offer security for the young child. As described in Chapter 12∞, when parents are stressed or depressed, the mental status of all family members can be affected. Ask how things are going for the family in general. Inquire about siblings and whether there are any issues of concern that might influence the toddler or preschooler. Illness or behavior problems in a sibling can decrease the parent's ability to deal with other children. The focus on a sibling in need can be confusing to a toddler or preschooler. Further information about concerns of children who have a sibling hospitalized are discussed in Chapter 17∞.

Mental health issues discussed above often relate directly to family members. As you inquire about discipline techniques and whether there has been violence in the family or neighborhood, realize that these family-related events can have profound influence on the child. Be alert for signs of child abuse and for substance abuse in family members. See Chapter 7∞ for further discussion of both child abuse and substance abuse. Have the parents become separated or divorced? Is there a new stepparent? (See Box 13–4.)

During questions and observations, the nurse identifies family risk and protective factors. Reinforce strengths and provide services and referrals to deal with risks. Strengths include:

- Family time together each day
- Parents proud of child's accomplishments and knowledgeable about developmental progression

BOX 13–4 Divorce and Children

Children may experience stress, sadness, and loss when parents become separated or divorced. However, one research project has demonstrated that some children have positive outcomes from divorce, such as increased maternal involvement with their lives, close proximity, communication, and support. Identify both the risk and protective factors when a family experiences separation or divorce (Arditti, 1999). Ask parents to identify things that are stressful for the child, such as changes in living situation or being present during fighting. Ask also what positive outcomes there are for the family, such as increased time with the custodial parent, decreased parental stress, and no fighting.

- Childcare center personnel and family members interact regularly to plan consistent approaches for the toddler and preschooler
- Teen mother of toddler enrolled in high school continuation program with childcare component

Examples of risks to mental health include:

- Parent diagnosed with depression
- Relative in home uses street drugs
- Child awakens with night terrors
- Teen mother estranged from own family and has few goals and resources

Temperament of the toddler and preschooler plays an important part in how they respond to people and events, and how others perceive them. Remember that the child is usually classified as primarily easy, difficult, or slow to warm up (see page 144). The concept of goodness of fit with the environment still warrants consideration. If there was a good fit between the infant and expectations of those in the surroundings, the fit may change as the child grows older. For example, most people appreciate "easy" infants because they are generally positive, adaptable, and regular in routines. However, in some families there may be a value on independent behaviors as children grow into toddlerhood and preschool age. Parents who were pleased with the infant's temperament may not value the same characteristics in the preschooler; they might prefer the child to be more outgoing and less accepting of changes in others. Assist parents in identifying their child's characteristic temperament and learning to appreciate it. They may need help to structure the difficult child's environment to establish routines to facilitate more regular schedules, or the slow to warm up child's environment to provide more time to adapt to new settings and care providers.

Toddlers continue to grow in social abilities, while preschoolers demonstrate large strides in socializing with others. Expect that most toddlers will enjoy playing with other children, although they play "side by side" and not cooperatively. They also engage in play with adults for short periods, such as throwing a ball. On the other hand, preschoolers begin to engage in activities that involve other children directly. They play "house," with one child playing the mother or father, and another the child. They engage in simple games where each plays a separate role. Their interactions with adults display similar maturity as they take on tasks such as setting the table for dinner, or picking up books from the floor. Social skills involve getting along with others. Ask the parents how this child does with siblings or other children. While a few arguments are common, a growing ability to share toys and communicate with others is expected. Ask parents about the child's favorite activities with other children. Preschoolers themselves are usually old enough to name their best friend and what they like to play together. See Chapter 5∞ for a thorough description of the developmental social activity of toddlers and preschoolers.

Young children exhibit increasing skill in language development, a primary medium for social exchange. From just a few words at 1 year, the child has progressed to stating three-word sentences by 3 years of age. Although all parts of speech are not in place, young children certainly have the ability to make needs and thoughts known. Assessment of language skills provides a mirror into this important means of socializing. One example of a language screening tool is the Early Language Milestone Scale (Figure 13–4 ■). The Denver II Developmental Screening Test described in Chapter 10∞ also has a language component. As the child nears school entry, communication skills should be assessed again. By that time, the child should be easy to understand, should use plurals readily, answers questions with ease, and interacts readily with others. These skills are necessary for success in kindergarten classrooms. School readiness tools include language components as parts of their testing. Recognize that children who speak a different language at home from that in the dominant culture may need extra time to learn language skills. When children display slow language development or problems such as stuttering they should be referred to a language specialist (Box 13–5).

Successful social skills involve separating from the parent at times. During toddlerhood, most children spend some time away from parents. Initially, they may be fearful and display crying, but gradually learn to adapt to the new person and place. Preschoolers need to begin developing relationships with other adults and children in order to adapt to the school setting at about 5 years of age. Ask how many people the child has contact with each week, and how the child manages separation from the parent. Encourage parents to see separation as a skill the child is learning rather than something that is guilt-producing for them. When they leave the child in a secure setting, they should hug, provide a favorite object, and leave. Short periods initially will teach the child that the parent can be trusted to return.

Expected outcomes of health promotion and health maintenance activities with young children include increasing social skills with parents, siblings, and other children and adults; successful management of temperament characteristics; adjustment to time away from the home; and improving language/communication skills.

DISEASE PREVENTION STRATEGIES

Toddlers remain prone to many infectious diseases due to immature immune systems. By the preschool age, immune defenses are more mature and communicable diseases are less common. Some immunizations are given during this age period to complete the basic series. For the child who has not had all immunizations,

BOX 13–5 Stuttering

All children have some episodes of **dysfluency**, or a disruption in the smooth transition between sounds, syllables, and words. Examples include repeating a word or phrase or inserting sounds such as "um" in sentences. The child who has more than three of these dysfluencies in 100 words of conversation is often displaying stuttering (Zebrowski, 2003). Stuttering is often accompanied by other behaviors such as frowning, blinking, or squeezing the eyes. About 75% of preschool stutterers will improve on their own. However, when stuttering is suspected, the child should be referred to a speech and language pathologist since assessment and effective interventions can best be carried out by this specialist.

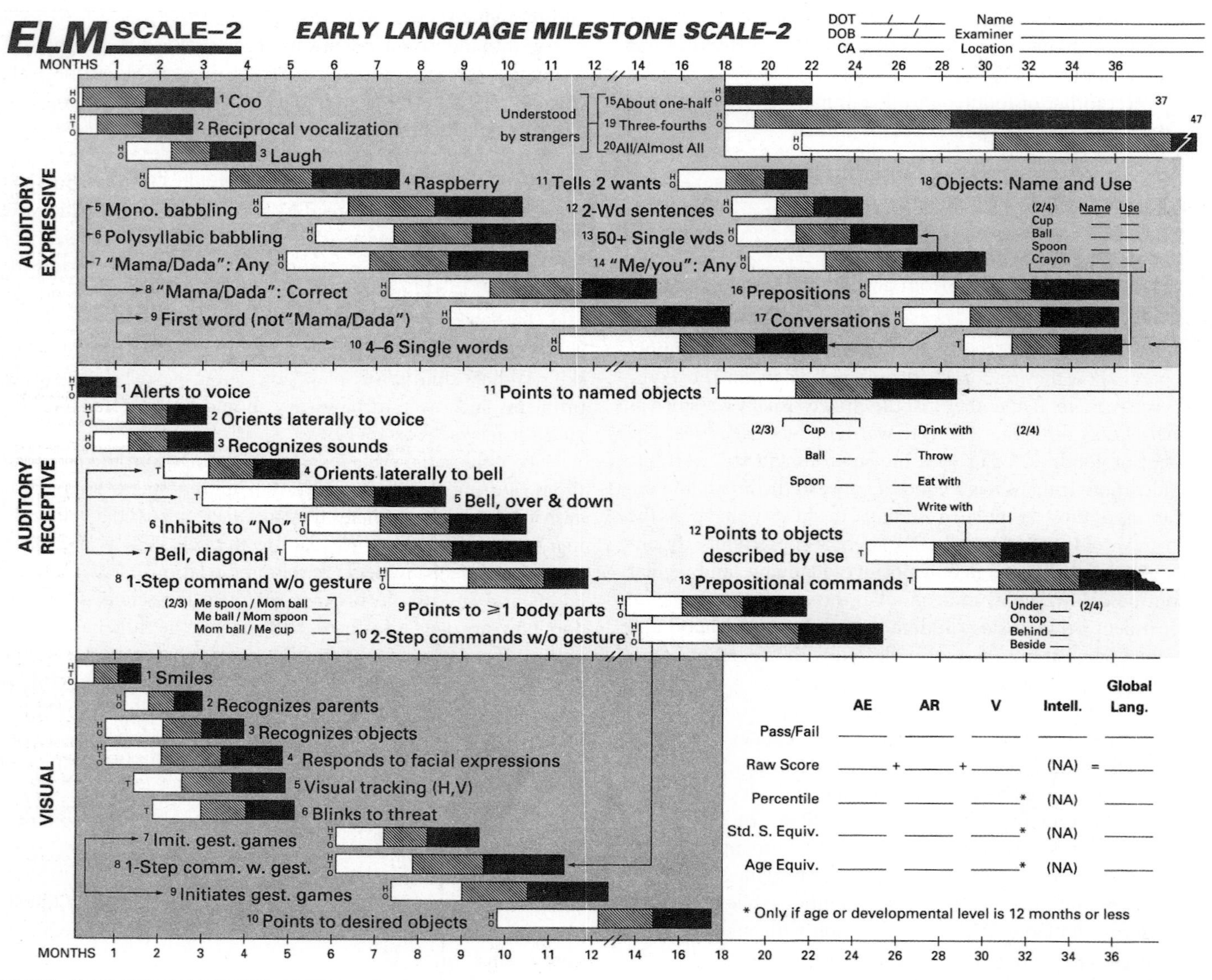

FIGURE 13–4 ■ The Early Language Milestone (ELM) Scale is one method of evaluating speech in young children. It differentiates receptive from expressive speech, recognizing that children may understand some language even though they do not speak to their level of understanding. Examine this tool to see what receptive and expressive language you would expect to see in 15-month-old Clarence in the opening scenario. Used with permission.

extra visits to catch up to recommended levels may be needed. At the end of the preschool period, the child has a complete review of the immunization record so any needed injections are given before school entry. See Table 13–5 for immunizations recommended during toddlerhood and preschool; detailed immunization recommendations can be found in Chapter 19∞.

Toddlers and preschoolers also need screening for several health conditions. See Table 13–6 for recommended screening at each visit. Earlier visits may have failed to identify a problem due to the child's young age, so areas such as vision, hearing, and developmental milestones are always included. Ascertain any concerns the parents have about the child's health and assess the child as needed for these conditions.

Recognize that the environment is a powerful influence on the health of children. Ask if parents or others in the home smoke. Discourage this practice and describe the health implications for the child. Is the neighborhood generally safe? Are there air, water, or other toxic exposures? Ask about lead exposure in the home. How much television and other screen time is common in the home? Older siblings who allow the preschooler to play violent video games or watch many hours of inappropriate television can be affecting the mental health of the young child. Do parents watch the evening news, even when it involves violence, in front of young children? Do they discuss television shows with the child?

Ask if the child has had any diseases, whether common ones such as middle ear infection, or less common ones such as a serious respiratory infection. Has the child been diagnosed with a chronic disorder such as cystic fibrosis or hemophilia? How has that impacted the child's general health and family functioning?

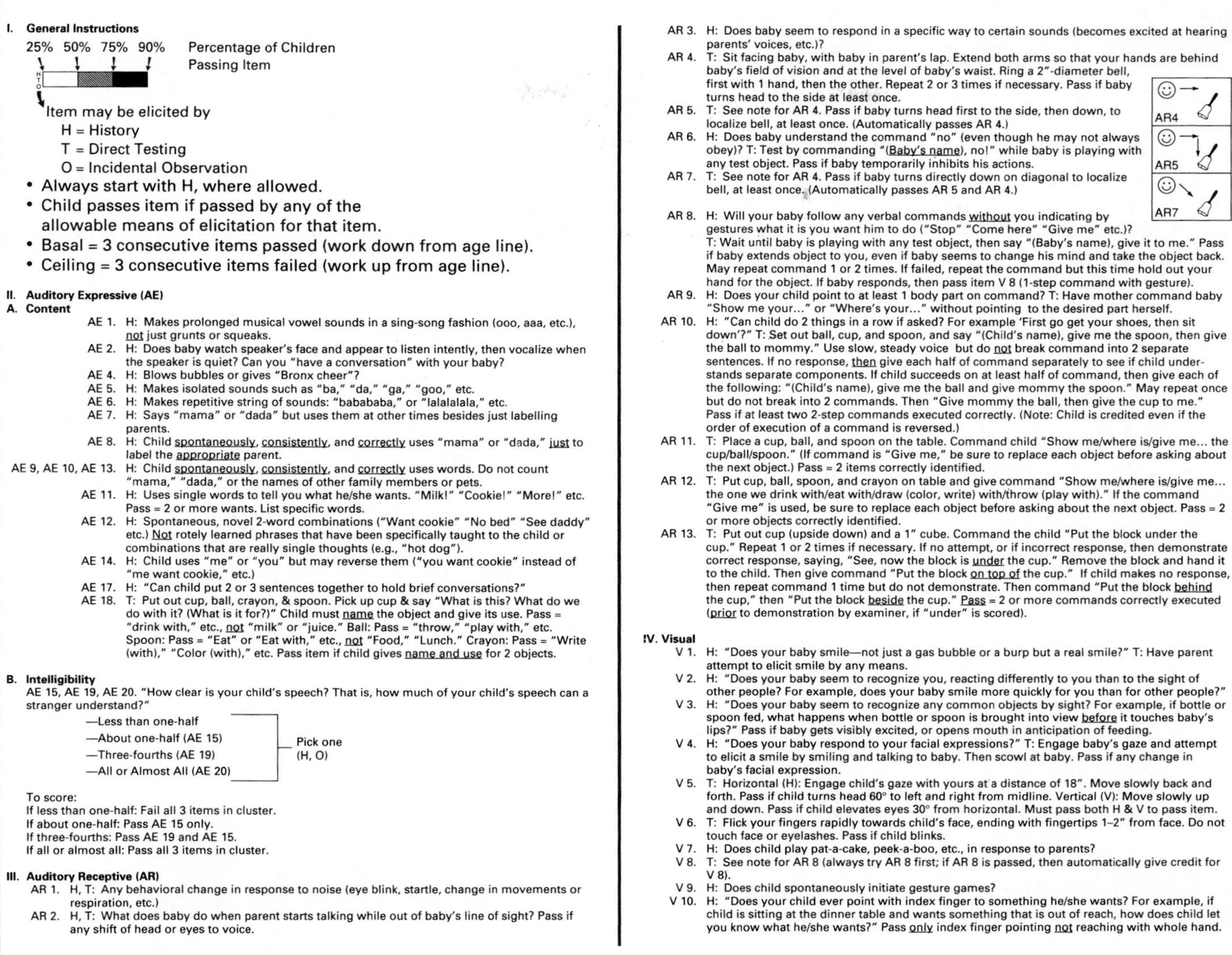

I. General Instructions

25% 50% 75% 90% Percentage of Children Passing Item

H
T
O

Item may be elicited by
H = History
T = Direct Testing
O = Incidental Observation

- Always start with H, where allowed.
- Child passes item if passed by any of the allowable means of elicitation for that item.
- Basal = 3 consecutive items passed (work down from age line).
- Ceiling = 3 consecutive items failed (work up from age line).

II. Auditory Expressive (AE)

A. Content

AE 1. H: Makes prolonged musical vowel sounds in a sing-song fashion (ooo, aaa, etc.), not just grunts or squeaks.
AE 2. H: Does baby watch speaker's face and appear to listen intently, then vocalize when the speaker is quiet? Can you "have a conversation" with your baby?
AE 4. H: Blows bubbles or gives "Bronx cheer"?
AE 5. H: Makes isolated sounds such as "ba," "da," "ga," "goo," etc.
AE 6. H: Makes repetitive string of sounds: "babababa," or "lalalalala," etc.
AE 7. H: Says "mama" or "dada" but uses them at other times besides just labelling parents.
AE 8. H: Child spontaneously, consistently, and correctly uses "mama" or "dada," just to label the appropriate parent.
AE 9, AE 10, AE 13. H: Child spontaneously, consistently, and correctly uses words. Do not count "mama," "dada," or the names of other family members or pets.
AE 11. H: Uses single words to tell you what he/she wants. "Milk!" "Cookie!" "More!" etc. Pass = 2 or more wants. List specific words.
AE 12. H: Spontaneous, novel 2-word combinations ("Want cookie" "No bed" "See daddy" etc.) Not rotely learned phrases that have been specifically taught to the child or combinations that are really single thoughts (e.g., "hot dog").
AE 14. H: Child uses "me" or "you" but may reverse them ("you want cookie" instead of "me want cookie," etc.)
AE 17. H: "Can child put 2 or 3 sentences together to hold brief conversations?"
AE 18. T: Put out cup, ball, crayon, & spoon. Pick up cup & say "What is this? What do we do with it? (What is it for?)" Child must name the object and give its use. Pass = "drink with," etc., not "milk" or "juice." Ball: Pass = "throw," "play with," etc. Spoon: Pass = "Eat" or "Eat with," etc., not "Food," "Lunch." Crayon: Pass = "Write (with)," "Color (with)," etc. Pass item if child gives name and use for 2 objects.

B. Intelligibility

AE 15, AE 19, AE 20. "How clear is your child's speech? That is, how much of your child's speech can a stranger understand?"

—Less than one-half
—About one-half (AE 15)
—Three-fourths (AE 19)
—All or Almost All (AE 20)

Pick one (H, O)

To score:
If less than one-half: Fail all 3 items in cluster.
If about one-half: Pass AE 15 only.
If three-fourths: Pass AE 19 and AE 15.
If all or almost all: Pass all 3 items in cluster.

III. Auditory Receptive (AR)

AR 1. H, T: Any behavioral change in response to noise (eye blink, startle, change in movements or respiration, etc.)
AR 2. H, T: What does baby do when parent starts talking while out of baby's line of sight? Pass if any shift of head or eyes to voice.
AR 3. H: Does baby seem to respond in a specific way to certain sounds (becomes excited at hearing parents' voices, etc.)?
AR 4. T: Sit facing baby, with baby in parent's lap. Extend both arms so that your hands are behind baby's field of vision and at the level of baby's waist. Ring a 2"-diameter bell, first with 1 hand, then the other. Repeat 2 or 3 times if necessary. Pass if baby turns head to the side at least once.
AR 5. T: See note for AR 4. Pass if baby turns head first to the side, then down, to localize bell, at least once. (Automatically passes AR 4.)
AR 6. H: Does baby understand the command "no" (even though he may not always obey)? T: Test by commanding "(Baby's name), no!" while baby is playing with any test object. Pass if baby temporarily inhibits his actions.
AR 7. T: See note for AR 4. Pass if baby turns directly down on diagonal to localize bell, at least once. (Automatically passes AR 5 and AR 4.)

AR4
AR5
AR7

AR 8. H: Will your baby follow any verbal commands without you indicating by gestures what it is you want him to do ("Stop" "Come here" "Give me" etc.)? T: Wait until baby is playing with any test object, then say "(Baby's name), give it to me." Pass if baby extends object to you, even if baby seems to change his mind and take the object back. May repeat command 1 or 2 times. If failed, repeat the command but this time hold out your hand for the object. If baby responds, then pass item V 8 (1-step command with gesture).
AR 9. H: Does your child point to at least 1 body part on command? T: Have mother command baby "Show me your..." or "Where's your..." without pointing to the desired part herself.
AR 10. H: "Can child do 2 things in a row if asked? For example 'First go get your shoes, then sit down'?" T: Set out ball, cup, and spoon, and say "(Child's name), give me the spoon, then give the ball to mommy." Use slow, steady voice but do not break command into 2 separate sentences. If no response, then give each half of command separately to see if child understands separate components. If child succeeds on at least half of command, then give each of the following: "(Child's name), give me the ball and give mommy the spoon." May repeat once but do not break into 2 commands. Then "Give mommy the ball, then give the cup to me." Pass if at least two 2-step commands executed correctly. (Note: Child is credited even if the order of execution of a command is reversed.)
AR 11. T: Place a cup, ball, and spoon on the table. Command child "Show me/where is/give me... the cup/ball/spoon." (If command is "Give me," be sure to replace each object before asking about the next object.) Pass = 2 items correctly identified.
AR 12. T: Put cup, ball, spoon, and crayon on table and give command "Show me/where is/give me... the one we drink with/eat with/draw (color, write) with/throw (play with)." If the command "Give me" is used, be sure to replace each object before asking about the next object. Pass = 2 or more objects correctly identified.
AR 13. T: Put out cup (upside down) and a 1" cube. Command the child "Put the block under the cup." Repeat 1 or 2 times if necessary. If no attempt, or if incorrect response, then demonstrate correct response, saying, "See, now the block is under the cup." Remove the block and hand it to the child. Then give command "Put the block on top of the cup." If child makes no response, then repeat command 1 time but do not demonstrate. Then command "Put the block behind the cup," then "Put the block beside the cup." Pass = 2 or more commands correctly executed (prior to demonstration by examiner, if "under" is scored).

IV. Visual

V 1. H: "Does your baby smile—not just a gas bubble or a burp but a real smile?" T: Have parent attempt to elicit smile by any means.
V 2. H: "Does your baby seem to recognize you, reacting differently to you than to the sight of other people? For example, does your baby smile more quickly for you than for other people?"
V 3. H: "Does your baby seem to recognize any common objects by sight? For example, if bottle or spoon fed, what happens when bottle or spoon is brought into view before it touches baby's lips?" Pass if baby gets visibly excited, or opens mouth in anticipation of feeding.
V 4. H: "Does your baby respond to your facial expressions?" T: Engage baby's gaze and attempt to elicit a smile by smiling and talking to baby. Then scowl at baby. Pass if any change in baby's facial expression.
V 5. T: Horizontal (H): Engage child's gaze with yours at a distance of 18". Move slowly back and forth. Pass if child turns head 60° to left and right from midline. Vertical (V): Move slowly up and down. Pass if child elevates eyes 30° from horizontal. Must pass both H & V to pass item.
V 6. T: Flick your fingers rapidly towards child's face, ending with fingertips 1–2" from face. Do not touch face or eyelashes. Pass if child blinks.
V 7. H: Does child play pat-a-cake, peek-a-boo, etc., in response to parents?
V 8. T: See note for AR 8 (always try AR 8 first; if AR 8 is passed, then automatically give credit for V 8).
V 9. H: Does child spontaneously initiate gesture games?
V 10. H: "Does your child ever point with index finger to something he/she wants? For example, if child is sitting at the dinner table and wants something that is out of reach, how does child let you know what he/she wants?" Pass only index finger pointing not reaching with whole hand.

FIGURE 13–4 ■ (Continued)

Nursing interventions for disease prevention involve health maintenance activities. They are designed to stop disease occurrence and prevent further problems. Reinforce teaching from earlier visits about recognition of infectious disease, particularly if the child is in a new setting for childcare or other activities. Provide sources for clean water and information about food safety if these seem to be areas of concern. Draw blood for lead screening if the child is exposed to lead sources. Give the immunizations recommended for the age of the child. If parents smoke, review the possible problematic effects on young children such as increased incidence of otitis media and asthma. Refer parents who wish to quit smoking to resources for cessation. Recommend that children not be exposed to more than 2 hours of television or other screen activities each day. Teach parents to avoid violent shows and video games, watch television with the child, and discuss programs together.

The results of the examination should be summarized for parents. They need to know the normal findings and whether there are concerns that will need further evaluation. Provide time for parents to ask questions about health conditions. Verify that they have financial resources and transportation to continue obtaining healthcare for the child. Now that visits are further apart, write down the next recommended appointment date, arrange for a telephone reminder, and provide the phone and contact information for questions or emergencies that may occur in the interim.

Desired outcomes for disease prevention include integration of prevention methods into the family's daily lives, prompt treatment of acute conditions, and individualization of all

MediaLink Car Seat Safety

TABLE 13–5 Routine Immunizations Recommended During Toddlerhood and Preschool Age

IMMUNIZATION	AGE RECOMMENDED
Hepatitis B	6–18 months: Administer #3 if series not completed during infancy
Diphtheria, tetanus, pertussis	15–18 months (#4) 4–6 years (#5)
Haemophilus influenzae type b	12–15 months (#4 or will be #3 for PRP-OMP type that requires only 3 doses for whole series)
Inactivated poliovirus	4–6 years (#4)
Measles, mumps, rubella	12–15 months (#1)
Varicella	12–18 months (only 1 dose needed at this age)
Pneumococcal	12–15 months (#4)

Note: Schedule may need to be adapted if child did not receive all recommended immunizations during infancy. See CDC and American Academy of Pediatrics for recommended catch-up schedules.

health supervision topics for the child with a chronic condition or special healthcare need.

INJURY PREVENTION STRATEGIES

Injuries remain a common healthcare problem for children during the toddler and preschooler years. The child's mobility, physical skills, and lack of understanding about the presence of hazards put the child at particular risk. In addition, children are generally left to play alone for short periods and toddlers and preschoolers can quickly get into dangerous situations. Every healthcare visit needs to include an assessment of risks and teaching to prevent injuries. Tables 13–7 and 13–8 list injury hazards during these age periods.

Ask parents to name the most common hazards for the age of their child, and add other hazards to their awareness. Reinforce car safety, as the types of seats change when the child reaches 20 lb and then 40 lb. Be certain that parents provide children from 20 to 40 lb the following:

- A convertible forward-facing seat that has been placed in the back seat
- Harness straps at or above the shoulders

Children over 40 lb should be placed in a belt-positioning booster seat:

- In the back seat
- That uses both lap and shoulder belts
- With the lap belt low and tight across the lap/upper thigh area and shoulder belt snug across the chest and shoulder

Recommend that parents have their car seat checked by a childcare inspector. Give them the addresses of the closest inspection stations, which you can locate through the National Highway Traffic Safety Administration (www.nhtsa.dot.gov) (Figure 13–5 ■).

Other common and serious safety hazards are falls and drowning. In addition to providing general guidelines about

TABLE 13–6 Screening During Health Promotion and Health Maintenance Visits

AGE	RECOMMENDED SCREENING TESTS
15 months	Vision Hearing Anemia (if not previously done) Tuberculosis (if at risk) Teeth present and condition Physical examination with special attention to skin, gait, bruising, and other signs of possible abuse Developmental milestones Dietary screening Review immunization record
18 months	As above
2–3 years	As above Language development Lead exposure risk Hyperlipidemia risk
3–4 years	As above Blood pressure Behavioral abnormalities
4–5 years	As above Dental malocclusion problems

Adapted from Green, M., & Palfrey, J. S. (Eds.). (2002). Bright futures: Guidelines for health supervision of infants, children and adolescents *(2nd ed.). Arlington, VA: National Center for Education in Maternal and Child Health.*

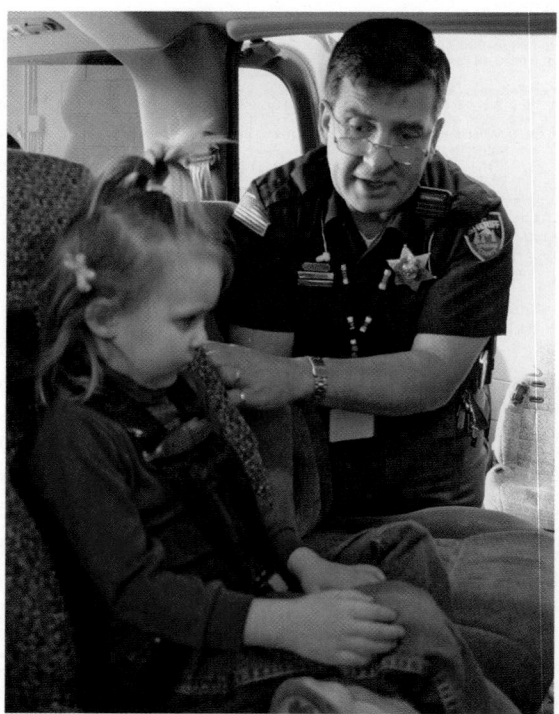

FIGURE 13–5 ■ The officer at this police station is certified to examine car seats for children and make recommendations for parents. He is examining a preschooler in a booster seat for proper fit and alignment. Many car seats are improperly installed or not the proper type for a specific age of child, so centers that check seats provide an important service.

TABLE 13–7 Injury Prevention in Toddlerhood

	HAZARD	DEVELOPMENTAL CHARACTERISTICS	PREVENTIVE MEASURES
	Falls	Gross motor skills improve: Toddler is able to move chairs to counters and can climb up ladders.	Supervise toddler closely. Provide safe climbing toys. Begin to teach acceptable places for climbing.
	Poisoning	Gross motor skills enable toddler to climb onto chairs and then cabinets. Medicines, cosmetics, and other poisonous substances are easily reached.	Keep medicines and other poisonous material locked away. Use child-resistant containers and cupboard closures. Have poison control center number (1–800–222–1222) by telephone.
 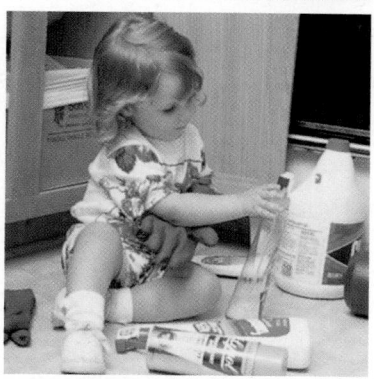	Burns	Toddler is tall enough to reach stove top. Toddler can walk to fireplace and may reach into fire.	Keep pot handles turned inward on stove. Do not burn fires without close supervision. Use a fire screen.
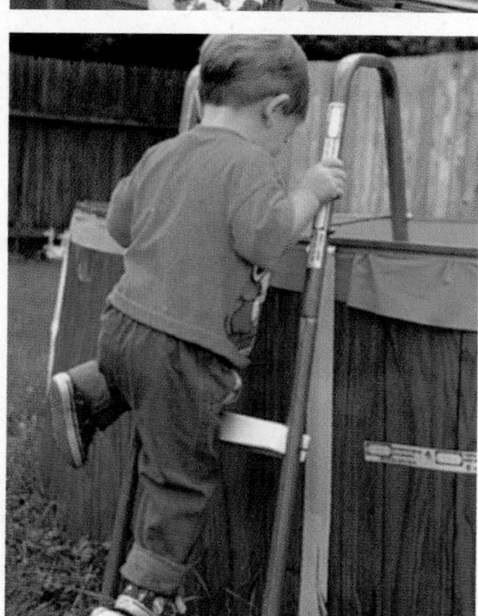 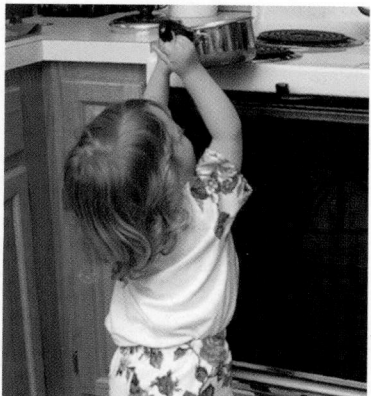	Drowning	Toddler can walk onto docks or pool decks. Toddler may stand on or climb seats on boat, Toddler may fall into buckets, toilets, and fish tanks and be unable be get top of body out.	Supervise any child near water. Swimming classes do not protect a toddler from drowning. Use child-resistant pool covers. Use approved child life jackets near water and on boats. Empty buckets when not in use.
	Motor vehicle crashes	Toddler may be able to undo seat belt, may resist using car seat, demonstrating characteristic negativism and autonomy.	Insist on safety seat use for all trips. Use approved safety only, such as forward-facing convertible seat. Toddler is not large enough to use car seat belts.

TABLE 13–8 Injury Prevention in the Preschool Years

	HAZARDS	DEVELOPMENTAL CHARACTERISTICS	PREVENTIVE MEASURES
	Motor vehicle crashes	Older preschooler independently gets into car and puts on seat bell. Child may forget to belt up or may do so incorrectly.	Verify that child is belted in properly before starting car. Child restraint systems must be used until child weighs 18 kg (40 lb) and is 100 cm (40 in.) tall.
 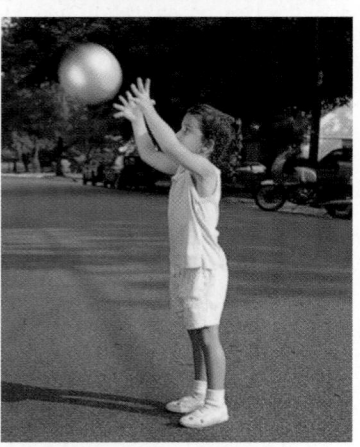	Motor vehicle and pedestrian accidents	Preschooler increasingly plays outside alone or with friends. Preschooler is unable to judge speed of moving car and assumes driver knows that he or she is present.	Teach child never to go into road. A safe, preferably enclosed, play yard is recommended.
	Drowning	Preschooler who has had swimming lessons may choose to go into a lake or pool.	Teach child never to go into water without an adult. Provide supervision whenever child is near water.
 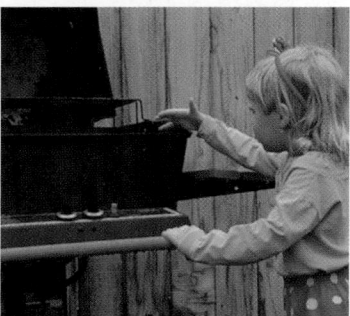	Burns	Preschooler can understand the hazards of fire.	Teach child to stop, drop, and roll if clothes are on fire. Practice escapes from home are useful. A visit to a fire station can reinforce learning. Teach child how to call 911.
	Needle sticks in hospital	Preschooler can ambulate and is interested in new objects.	Keep needles out of reach. Remove from unit immediately after use.
	Electrical injury in hospital	Preschooler is mobile and may trip over cords and equipment or may choose to examine them.	Avoid use of electrical cords if possible. Keep equipment out of major traffic areas. Keep beds away from electrical outlets. Monitor child closely.

safety, these most common injuries should be directly addressed. Children often fall down stairs, from counters where they have been placed or crawled, and from grocery carts. (See Evidence-Based Practice: Grocery Shopping Cart Falls.) Drowning episodes occur when toddlers and preschoolers are not watched every moment while at a lake or ocean, fall from boats without personal flotation devices on, fall into a backyard pool, or drown in a bathtub or other body of water. While all young children should begin to take swim lessons, this does not guarantee their safety around water. (See Evidence-Based Practice: Drowning.) Nursing interventions concentrate on relaying to parents the severity of the risk of falls and drowning for children. Teach parents to be aware of the dangers and to avoid them, both at home and in other settings. Refer them to classes on first aid and cardiopulmonary resuscitation.

The child spends increasing time away from the parent. Childcare situations should provide the same supervision the child receives at home. Help parents to ask questions and feel confident in safety at other settings. For example, while parents may be cautious about gun safety at home, few of them inquire if a home the child is visiting has guns and how they are stored.

Preschoolers are generally interested in health and their bodies. This is a time when teaching can become directed at both the parents and the child. Preschoolers are receptive to

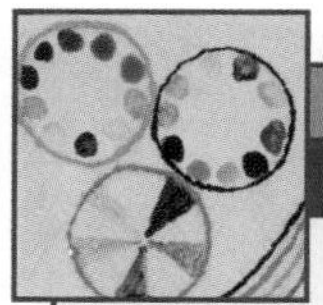

EVIDENCE-BASED PRACTICE
Grocery Shopping Cart Falls

PROBLEM

Over 10,000 children less than 5 years of age annually fall from shopping carts, even though adults are usually very close to the cart and child.

EVIDENCE

In a sample of almost 400 families in Edmonton, Alberta, about half were exposed to a warning sign in the grocery cart about the need to prevent children from standing in the cart, while the other half were not exposed to carts with warnings (Harrell, 2003). No differences were observed on incidence of the child standing in the cart or on the seat, or climbing the cart, or in the parent supervision related to the warning signs in carts. About 8% of children in the cart seat stood up, while 55% in the cart basket stood. Seven percent of children actually climbed out of the cart and 66% stood on the ends or sides. About 5% of adults lost sight of children at least once and 25% were 10 feet or more away from the children, a distance thought to be too far to prevent a fall.

NURSING IMPLICATIONS

The study indicated that toddlers and preschoolers are commonly at danger in and around grocery carts and that the level of parental supervision may not be sufficient, even when warnings about the hazard are visible in the cart.

CRITICAL THINKING APPLICATION

What techniques can you suggest to teach parents about the risk of falling from grocery carts? What other types of falls are common for children in this age group?

practicing street crossing and tricycle/bicycle riding skills. It may be helpful to have a place in the clinic or office where they can be taught basic skills such as handwashing or street crossing. Consider the time of year and geographic location and teach appropriately. Spring is often a good time to teach bicycle and water safety, while winter hazards may include wood stoves or other heating devices. See Table13–9 for additional listings of toddler and preschooler hazards and safety teaching needed. Injury prevention efforts represent health maintenance activities since they are aimed at preventing injuries from occurring.

Desired outcomes for the child are integration of safe practices into car restraints and other daily activities, progression through toddlerhood and preschool with no serious injuries, prompt care for minor injuries, and increasing understanding by child, parent, and other care providers of the common safety hazards at this age.

NURSING MANAGEMENT

■ Nursing Assessment and Diagnosis

Nurses partner with other healthcare professionals such as physicians, nurse practitioners, and speech therapists to assess health promotion and health maintenance status of young children. The toddler and preschool years are characterized by much developmental progression and strategies need to be constantly adapted to meet the particular needs of the child and family. Parents are partners in the care of the child and every health supervision visit should address their questions and concerns; their observations of the child are an invaluable part of the process. As the preschooler becomes more verbal, another partner is added to the healthcare team. Ask preschoolers what they want to learn, what they want to know about staying well, and other pertinent questions.

Toddlers and preschoolers are examined for growth, physical health status, and mental/social characteristics. Development is an area that many pediatricians feel ill-prepared to address, but which parents commonly want addressed (Halfon et al., 2003). Nurses are adept at describing normal developmental milestones, evaluating the progression of children, and using anticipatory guidance to address parental developmental concerns.

Based on a thorough assessment, you will establish nursing diagnoses that are appropriate for the young child and family. Potential nursing diagnoses established during a health supervision of a toddler or preschooler might include:

- Anxiety related to change of environment (new care provider)
- Parental Role Conflict related to lack of support from significant others
- Risk for Delayed Growth and Development related to lead exposure
- Health-seeking Behaviors related to parental desire for safety information
- Impaired Skin Integrity related to hyperthermia (sunburn)

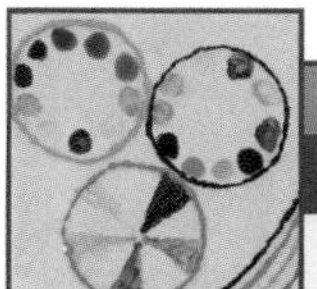

EVIDENCE-BASED PRACTICE
Drowning

PROBLEM

Drowning is the leading cause of unintentional injury death among toddlers, and the second leading cause in all children. Many other children suffer serious nonfatal submersion events, leaving them with permanent disabilities. See Chapters 1 and 25∞. Drownings occur more often on Saturday and Sunday than other days. More data are needed about drownings to provide parents with information about the hazard.

EVIDENCE

The most common characteristic of drownings is inadequate adult supervision *(Brenner & the Committee on Injury, Violence, and Poison Prevention, 2003)*. Leaving a young child alone in the bath or swimming in an area without lifeguards are common examples. Strategies to prevent drowning include four-sided locked fencing around pools, adult supervision, using pools or other sites with lifeguards for additional safety, using personal flotation devices when boating or near bodies of water, and having parents and other adults prepared to do resuscitation at the scene of a submersion before emergency medical personnel arrive.

NURSING IMPLICATIONS

Teach parents major safety hazards around water and how to avoid them. Emphasize that a toddler or preschooler must never be left alone in or around water, even for a few seconds.

CRITICAL THINKING APPLICATION

How will you convince parents that children should learn to swim but that swimming does not guarantee safety around water? How can you help a family to identify risks to drowning that may be present in their home or neighborhood?)

MediaLink Drowning Prevention Video

TABLE 13–9 Disease and Injury Prevention Topics by Age

AGE	INJURY PREVENTION TEACHING TOPICS
15 months	Wash adult and toddler hands frequently Clean toys with soap and water regularly Provide child's own bedding for childcare setting and wash weekly Use forward-facing car safety seat if child is 20 lb; install correctly and have installation checked; place in back seat and never in front seat with a passenger air bag Empty containers of water immediately after use; be sure pools or other bodies of water are locked and not accessible Use sunscreen, hat, and long sleeves in the sun Keep heavy and sharp objects out of reach; check that all poisons are locked away including in homes visited; keep pet food and cosmetics out of reach Have poison control number by phones and programmed into cell phones Be alert for dangers of hot curling irons and other appliances Have electrical cords out of reach and not hanging down Keep water temperature from being too hot to touch Have home environment checked for lead hazards Secure the child in shopping carts Do not let child have access to alcoholic drinks Remember that responsible adults should always supervise their own child, not other children Know CPR, airway obstruction removal, and other first aid
18 months	As above Bolt heavy objects that might be pulled down securely to the wall Be cautious of the toddler near machinery in the yard (e.g., lawn mowers, farm equipment) Use a helmet on the child when on the back of a bicycle Check batteries in home smoke alarms and check system Ask care providers about discipline methods; do not allow corporal punishment
2–3 years	As above When the child is 40 lb, switch to a belt-positioning booster seat, using vehicle lap and shoulder belt; place in rear seat Teach handwashing after toileting and other activities Clean potty chair thoroughly Keep guns unloaded and locked away in a different locked place than ammunition; have trigger locks installed Teach how to cross streets Provide a helmet for riding tricycles Check playgrounds for safety hazards and hard surfaces under equipment
3–4 years	As above Do not let child play unsupervised Know CPR, airway obstruction removal, and other first aid for the child who has become a preschooler
4–5 years	As above Continue teaching safety skills to the child Continue supervising when near streets, water sources Teach safety around strangers (never go with a stranger; find a trusted person such as a parent or police officer)

Adapted from Green, M., & Palfrey, J. S. (Eds.). (2002). Bright futures: Guidelines for health supervision of infants, children and adolescents *(2nd ed.). Arlington, VA: National Center for Education in Maternal and Child Health.*

Planning and Implementation

Based on the nursing diagnoses established the nurse works with others to plan strategies to meet the needs of the family. Explain that assessment questions are asked in order to provide a picture of the child that can be helpful in partnering with parents to plan healthcare. Reinforce the importance of the family coming to health supervision visits with their own list of issues. Work with other healthcare professionals to ensure all needs of a particular child and family are addressed.

Some teaching takes place as the examination occurs. Explain the height and weight measurements and what they mean. Relate them to questions about dietary intake and family food patterns. During the physical examination, insert information about common infections such as otitis media (middle ear infection) and share immunization information.

If the family has been reluctant to ask questions, reflect on the child's development. "Many children have trouble sleeping through the night; is that the case for Cassandra? What helps her to sleep? What is it like at her bed time?" Developmental areas such as sleep, discipline, toilet training, and expected developmental milestones should be addressed. If the parents were provided in an earlier visit with a journal to record observations and questions, ask if they have brought it with them.

A key part of the visit involves health promotion activities. It is essential to apply concepts of anticipatory guidance as you address the child's coming developmental progression. If the child will soon be toilet trained, provide information about possible approaches. If the child is learning to swim or has access to water, reinforce safety precautions near water. For the child going to a new childcare center, provide the parents with a list of questions they can ask the care provider, and tips to assist in the transition to a new setting (see Chapter 7∞).

Health maintenance activities are added to the visit as you give immunizations and screen for tuberculosis, lead screening, or problems with language, vision, or hearing. The focus of these activities is to prevent disease or to find it early before there are serious consequences. When you find information that may indicate a problem, be sure to refer the child to the primary care provider, such as physician or nurse practitioner. You may even recommend that the child be seen by another specialist such as a speech pathologist or dentist. Other health maintenance activities that must be part of each visit with a toddler or preschooler involve teaching about common hazards and how to avoid them. Emergency care in case of injury is also helpful information for parents, so first-aid classes can be recommended.

Conclude the visit with some words of praise about the parent and child accomplishments. Provide the date for the next visit. List any resources helpful to the family, including the clinic/office contact information and emergency services.

Evaluation

Parents should be asked occasionally to evaluate the care they are receiving at the health promotion and health maintenance site. Use these comments to monitor and adjust procedures as needed. The expected outcomes for nursing care of the toddler and preschooler include the following:

- The child demonstrates normal patterns of growth and progression in developmental milestones.
- The child remains free of disease and injury.
- Parents relay satisfaction with the pediatric healthcare home.
- The child manifests positive physical, social, and emotional adjustment.

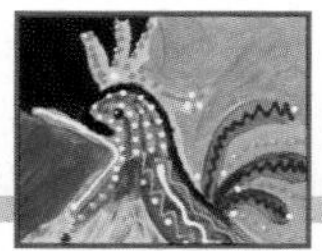

CHAPTER HIGHLIGHTS

- General observations of physical ability and social interactions are made as the toddler and preschooler are called back for the healthcare visit.
- Questions about growth and information related to physical health are integrated during the physical examination.
- The approaches and order of the physical examination should be adapted to minimize threats to the young child.
- Developmental surveillance is integrated within each health promotion/health maintenance visit.
- Toddlers and preschoolers gradually take on mature eating patterns; assessment of nutritional status involves growth, food eaten, and family food patterns.
- Physical ability progresses steadily in young children. Opportunities for daily active periods are necessary for healthy growth.
- By 2 years of age a full set of primary teeth is present; they will be kept until the first one is lost at about 6 years.
- Early years are essential to development of a healthy sense of self and positive social interactions with others.
- Screening for common diseases is performed during routine care. Immunizations are administered to prevent infectious diseases.
- Safety hazards for toddlers and preschoolers are addressed at each visit, with suggestions given to parents to provide safe environments.

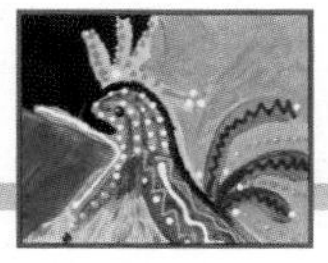

CRITICAL THINKING IN ACTION

INTRODUCTION

Recall the parents of 15-month-old Clarence. They are working parents who are overwhelmed by the activity level of their son. They express concern about how to spend time with and ensure safety for Clarence, while having some time to spend with each other.

DESCRIPTION

During the examination of Clarence, he is constantly moving and squirming. However, he is a pleasant and happy child who interacts appropriately with adults. His parents are loving and patient with him, but express that they are often tired and wonder how to manage such an active child. They recognize that some children are normally active and request information about how to handle his activity, and particularly how to keep their home a safe place for him. Clarence naps at the childcare center each day and does not go to sleep until 10 P.M. each evening. Since the parents are up early, they get him ready to leave at about 6 A.M. The parents have only lived in this city for 2 years. Extended family visit occasionally, but they socialize mainly with other employees at work. As you examine the record you find that Clarence has had three doses of DTaP, three doses of hepatitis B, three doses of *Haemophilus influenzae* type b, and two doses of pneumococcal vaccine.

DISCUSSION

1. Clarence's mother and father show many strengths as parents. List the protective factors that you identify in their parenting.
2. How would you classify Clarence's temperament? Consult Chapter 5 for a description of the different types of temperament in children.
3. What techniques can the nurse use in examining Clarence that will contribute to his cooperation?
4. As you review the safety hazards that the parents have identified for Clarence, what injury prevention is essential to address?
5. How much should Clarence be sleeping at night? What questions will you ask parents about the sleeping situation and what recommendations might you suggest to enhance sleep patterns?
6. What immunizations should Clarence receive today? What history questions will you ask and what teaching will you perform related to immunizations? (Consult this chapter and Chapter 19 for information about immunizations.)

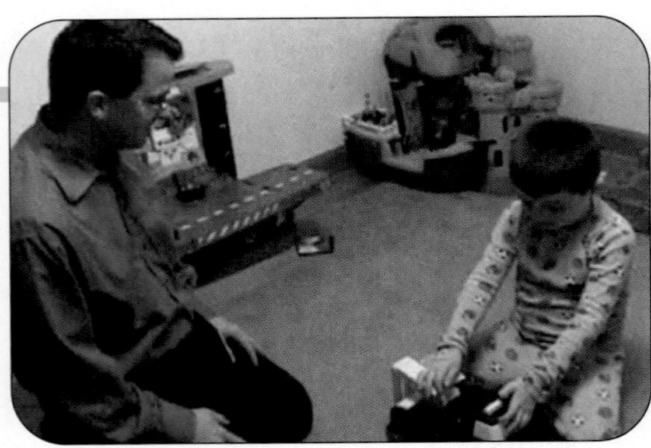

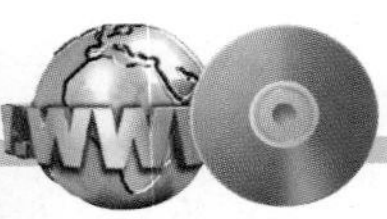

EXPLORE MediaLink

- NCLEX review, case studies, and other interactive resources for this chapter can be found on the Companion Website at **www. prenhall.com/ball**. Click on Chapter 13 to select the activities for this chapter.
- For animations, more NCLEX review questions, and an audio glossary, access the accompanying CD-ROM in this book.

http://www.prenhall.com/ball

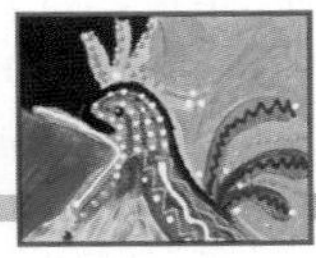

REFERENCES

American Academy of Pediatric Dentistry. (2000). *Policy on early childhood caries (ECC): Unique challenges and treatment options.* www.aapd.org, accessed 8/31/2003.

American Academy of Pediatrics. (2000). *Fellows survey.* Elk Grove Village, IL: Author.

Arditti, J. A. (1999). Rethinking relationships between divorced mothers and their children: Capitalizing on family strengths. *Family Relations, 48,* 109–119.

Brenner, R. A., & the Committee on Injury, Violence, and Poison Prevention. (2003). Prevention of drowning in infants, children, and adolescents. *Pediatrics, 112,* 440–445.

Colyar, M. R. (2003). *Well-child assessment for primary care providers.* Philadelphia: FA Davis.

Edelman, C. L., & Mandle, C. L. (2002). *Health promotion throughout the life span* (5th ed.). St. Louis: Mosby.

Green, M., & Palfrey, J. S. (Eds.). (2002). *Bright futures: Guidelines for health supervision of infants, children, and adolescents* (2nd ed.). Arlington, VA: National Center for Education in Maternal and Child Health.

Halfon, N. (2002). *Child rearing in America: Challenges facing parents with young children.* New York: Cambridge University Press.

Halfon, N., Regalado, M., McLearn, K. T., Kuo, A., & Wright, K. (2003). *Building a bridge from birth to school: Improving developmental and behavioral health services for young children.* New York: The Commonwealth Fund.

Harrell, W. A. (2003). Effect of two warning signs on adult supervision and risky activities by children in grocery shopping carts. *Psychological Reports, 92,* 889–898.

Jellinek, M., Patel, B. P., & Froehle, M. C. (Eds.). (2002). *Bright futures in practice: Mental health* (Vols. I and II). Arlington, VA: National Center for Education in Maternal and Child Health.

Murray, R. B., & Zentner, J. P. (2001). *Health promotion strategies through the life span* (7th ed.). Upper Saddle River, NJ: Prentice Hall.

Patrick, K., Spear, B., Holt, K., & Sofka, D. (Eds.). (2001). *Bright futures in practice: Physical activity.* Arlington, VA: National Center for Education in Maternal and Child Health.

Schuster, M. A., Duan, N., Regalado, M. & Klein, D. J. (2000). Anticipatory guidance: What information do parents receive: What information do they want? *Archives of Pediatric and Adolescent Medicine, 154,* 1191–1198.

Story, M., Holt, K., & Sofka, D. (Eds.). (2002). *Bright futures in practice: Nutrition.* Arlington, VA: National Center for Education in Maternal and Child Health.

VanLandeghen, K., Bronstein, J., & Brach, C. (2003, June). *Children's dental access in Medicaid. The role of medical care use and dentist participation.* (CHIRI Issue Brief 2, AHRQ Publication No. 03–0032). Rockville, MD: Agency for Healthcare Research and Quality. www.ahrq.gov/about/chirident.htm, accessed 6/30/2003.

Young, K. T., Davis, K., Schoen, C., & Parker, S. (1998). Listening to parents: A national survey of parents with young children. *Archives of Pediatric and Adolescent Medicine, 152,* 255–262.

Zebrowski, P. M. (2003). Developmental stuttering. *Pediatric Annals, 32,* 453–458.

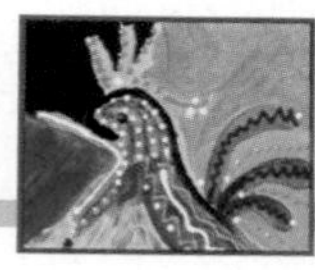

ADDITIONAL REFERENCES

Bloom, L. (1998). Language development and emotional expression. *Pediatrics, 102,* 1272–1277.

Grossman, L. B. (2003). *Infection control in the child care center and preschool* (6th ed.). Philadelphia: Lippincott Williams and Wilkins.

Kerker, B., Horowitz, S. M., Leventhal, J. M., et al. (2000). Identification of violence in the home: Pediatric and parental reports. *Archives of Pediatric and Adolescent Medicine, 154,* 457–462.

O'Donnell, G. W., & Mickalide, A. D. (1998). *SAFE KIDS at home, at play and on the way: A report to the nation on unintentional childhood injury.* Washington, DC: National SAFE KIDS Campaign.

Pender, N. J., Murdaugh, C. L., & Parsons, M. A. (2002). *Health promotion in nursing practice* (4th ed.). Upper Saddle River, NJ: Prentice Hall.

Young, L. E., & Hayes, V. (2002). *Transforming health promotion practice: Concepts, issues, and applications.* Philadelphia: FA Davis.

Chapter 14

Health Promotion and Health Maintenance of the School-Age Child

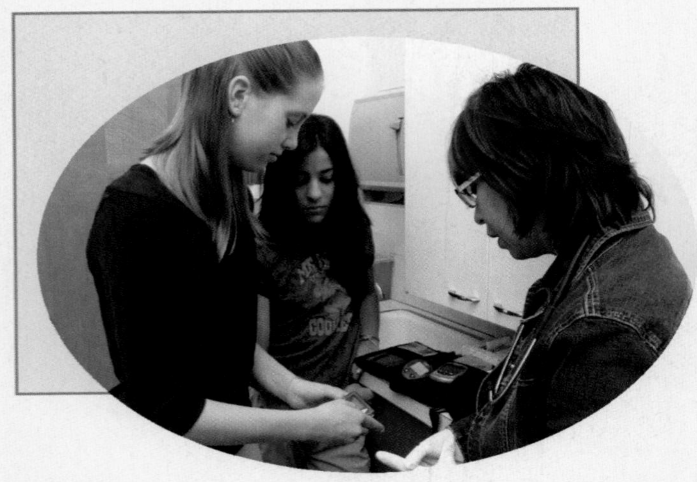

Jessalyn McIntyre is 12 years old and in sixth grade. She and her friend Kelly Gutierrez both have type 1 diabetes and need to test their blood glucose each day during school. They also both use insulin pumps. When they started using the pumps the school nurse met with their parents and talked with the endocrinologist in order to be able to help them manage in school. Their close management of diabetes has enabled Jessalyn and Kelly to participate in sports and other school activities. The school nurse performs many of the girls' health supervision activities, such as nutrition assessment, growth monitoring, physical assessment, and fostering relationships with other children. She partners with other healthcare providers to plan comprehensive care for Jessalyn and Kelly.

Youth such as Jessalyn and Kelly require the same health promotion and health maintenance activities as all school-age children. They need teaching about nutrition and physical activity, their immunization records should be reviewed, and safety needs addressed. In addition, due to their chronic disease they need additional growth monitoring, teaching regarding dietary management, and assistance in monitoring and managing their insulin needs. The chronic disease may also cause mental health challenges due to differences from peers. What health promotion interventions will you plan for Jessalyn and Kelly? How will you adapt usual needs of school age children when a chronic disease is being managed? What adaptations will parents have to make as a child with diabetes grows older and begins to manage the disease on their own?

"Our school nurse is really great. She answers our questions about diabetes without making us feel like we're different from other kids. We can keep equipment like syringes in her office and she helps us program our insulin pumps."

—Jessalyn, age 12

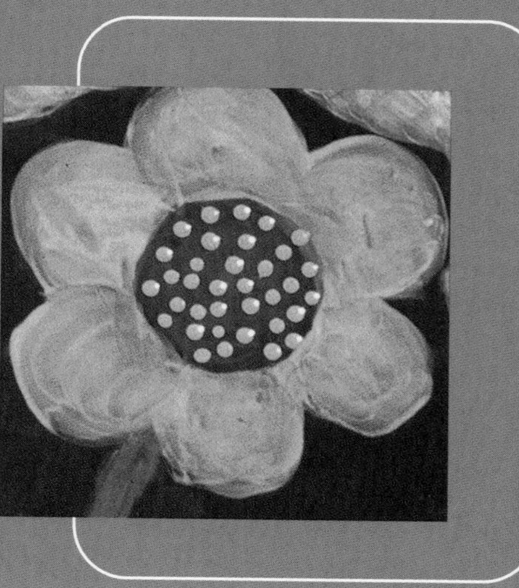

Learning Outcomes

After completing this chapter, you will be able to:

- Describe the general observations made of school-age children and their families as they come to the pediatric healthcare home for health supervision visits.
- Identify the major health concerns of school age.
- Apply assessment skills to gather data regarding nutrition, physical activity, mental health status, and growth and development of school-age children.
- Apply therapeutic communication skills with the school-age child and family during health supervision visits during school age.
- Intervene with school-age children and their families to integrate activities to promote health and to prevent disease and injury.
- Synthesize data from history and examination of school-age child and family with knowledge of school-age development to plan approaches useful with the family during health supervision encounters.

Key Terms

body image/466
individualized approach/473
latchkey children/463
population-based approach/473
self-concept/466
self-esteem/466
sexuality/466
spiritual health/469

MediaLink http://www.prenhall.com/ball

Resources for this chapter can be found on the CD-ROM accompanying this textbook, and on the Companion Website at www.prenhall.com/ball. Click on Chapter 14 to select the activities for this chapter.

CD-ROM
Videos
Health Maintenance for School-Age Children
The Importance of Physical Activity
NCLEX Review
Audio Glossary

COMPANION WEBSITE
NCLEX Review
MediaLink Applications
Develop a Teaching Plan: Healthy Blood Pressure
Develop a Teaching Plan: Smoking Education
Risk Evaluation: Bicycling

School age spans several years, beginning when most children enter kindergarten at about 5 years of age, and progressing until adolescence, approximately 12 to 13 years of age. Even though health promotion and health maintenance needs continue during this time, less frequent visits to the pediatric healthcare home are recommended. In addition, most children are relatively healthy and need few immunizations, which may lead to only sporadic visits for care. When school-age children are seen in healthcare, even for illness or emergency care, ask for the date of the last well-child or health supervision visit, and encourage the parents to make an appointment if the child is due for a visit. See Partnering with Families: Health Promotion and Health Maintenance Visits for recommended ages for healthcare visits.

Visits during the school-age years will focus on establishing good health habits related to issues such as nutrition, physical activity, and mental health; learning the importance of avoiding tobacco and drugs; ensuring success in school, family, and extracurricular activities; and fostering good decision-making and problem-solving skills. Health supervision concepts are applied to children with special healthcare needs, such as Jessalyn and Kelly, described in the opening scenario. What are common sites for health visit provision for school-age children? What resources are available for working with parents and children? How can nurses assist young children in establishing positive health practices? What special challenges do children face today that readily impact health? These are some of the questions that will be discussed in this chapter.

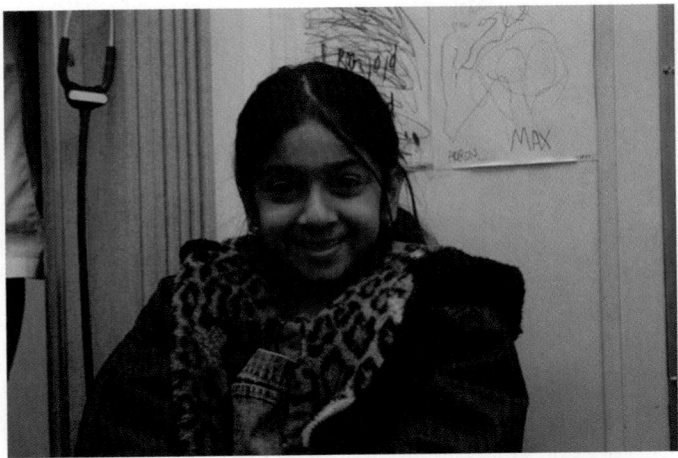

FIGURE 14–1 ■ Children generally interact readily with healthcare providers and appear at ease when welcomed and engaged in interactions. Notice the pleasant setting with child art posted on the wall.

GENERAL OBSERVATIONS

MediaLink Health Maintenance for School-Age Children Video

The first school-age visit usually occurs just before entry into kindergarten. During this visit, the child receives a thorough examination to be certain that physical development is normal, developmental milestones have been met for fine and gross motor skills, school readiness is displayed in social skills and language, and final sets of basic immunizations are completed (see Chapter 19∞ for immunization schedule). The child is often excited about the visit because it is associated with beginning school; anxiety is often felt as it may be the first time the child is aware of getting "shots." As with earlier visits, your observations begin as the child is called in for the visit. Speak to the child first, introducing yourself and welcoming the child and parents to the office or clinic. Many children of this age actively participate in conversations, making teaching and gathering data easy (Figure 14–1 ■). For children who are quiet or look to the parents, allow more time for them to get to know the personnel, directing most initial questions to parents. This may be the first visit where the child is old enough to be a partner in the healthcare visit. Establishing positive rapport with the child will enhance health teaching efforts.

Observe the interaction between the parents and the child. What types of speech tones are used? Is there mutual respect or are parents and child ignoring each other or having disagreements? The child should walk showing symmetry and ease of movement, follow instructions about where to go and taking off shoes for weighing, and demonstrate clear language skills with parent or healthcare personnel.

By the time children come for the 6–8 year visit and 8–10 year visits, they are expected to be increasingly active in sports, school activities, music, or other interests. Look for clues about their interests as they arrive. Did they bring books or a CD player? What are the book topics or favorite types of music? Ask what they are doing during the summer, or what the two favorite after-school activities entail. What two subjects do they like best in school? Which do they not like? Have they learned to swim? What activities would they like to do that they have not been able to engage in yet? Who are their best friends? How would they describe their best friends? Do they have brothers and sisters? What are the best things and worst things about having siblings? Have them describe a typical day to obtain clues about the child's life. The questions serve both to put the child at ease and to learn about the child's interests and activities. Compare the child's answers with your understanding of school-age development (see Chapter 5∞). If you have concerns about an answer, follow it up later in the visit. For example, if the child does not know how to swim, suggest to the parent that this is an important skill and offer resources for swim classes. Further examples of information requiring follow-up are discussed throughout this chapter.

Not all children go to clinics, offices, or other settings for health supervision visits. School nurses or nurse practitioners in school-based clinics sometimes offer health promotion/health maintenance activities in the school setting. Children with special healthcare needs, such as Jessalyn and Kelly, may need more frequent monitoring of health, which can be performed in the school setting. A major focus of school nurses is making the environment conducive to health for groups of children (see Chapter 16∞ for further discussion of the role of the school nurse). Schools may offer specific examinations to individual children, such as growth and developmental surveillance and health screening like vision, hearing, or scoliosis; may work with food service personnel and administration to improve meal and snack quality and minimize unhealthy choices in vending machines; and may work with teachers to integrate concepts such as physical activity and self-esteem into classroom activities (Wainwright, Thomas, & Jones, 2000). The nurse often links children with healthcare needs to other community services. While not a substitute for health supervision visits, such health approaches can be important to provide both health promotion and health maintenance services to children. Parents are welcomed to discuss health issues with the school nurse to explore further options for receiving additional health services.

Parents are generally proud of their children. During health supervision visits, watch the parents' responses as children answer questions. Be alert for the parent who interrupts the child or constantly "corrects" what is said. Suggestions for dealing with this communication pattern will be addressed later in this chapter. Comments by the parent should involve praise of the child or looking to the child for opinions on certain topics. This indicates that a partnership is developing in the family and that family members work together and value each other. Direct questions to the parents also. Ask if they came with specific concerns that should be addressed. If the child has an individualized education or health plan (see Chapter 20∞), ask if the parent brought a copy, if the plan is still appropriate, or if it needs updating. Allow the parent an opportunity to meet with the physician, nurse practitioner, or other professional in a private place and without the child present if desired. Be alert for family dynamics that can influence mental health status. Ask if there have been any important changes in the family and how they have influenced the child. During conversations, be alert for reports of separation, divorce, remarriages, ill siblings or grandparents, recent or upcoming moves, parent job changes, substance abuse, incarceration of family members in jail, custody disputes, or other issues. Such topics can be followed up with further questions, as described later in the mental health section, to learn how they influence the child.

GROWTH AND DEVELOPMENTAL SURVEILLANCE

As the child comes into the health supervision site, height and weight are measured. Be sure to have the child remove shoes and coat. Ask the child and parents if they know the child's current height and weight, and if they have any questions. Plot the percentiles for these measurements, calculate body mass index (BMI) and its percentile, and explain the meaning of these findings later in the visit. See Partnering with Families in Chapter 12∞ for an example of how to explain percentiles to parents. Watch for children who have changed channels on a growth grid. For example, if the child was in the 25th percentile for height in earlier visits, and is presently in the 50th percentile, a growth spurt might be occurring. Most children do not grow uniformly; they have periods of slow growth followed by fast spurts. School age is a time when overweight can begin to be a problem, so look for significant differences in weight and height percentiles, as reflected in a high BMI percentile, and gather additional data as needed (see Chapter 9∞ for nutritional assessment approaches). Health promotion

PARTNERING WITH FAMILIES

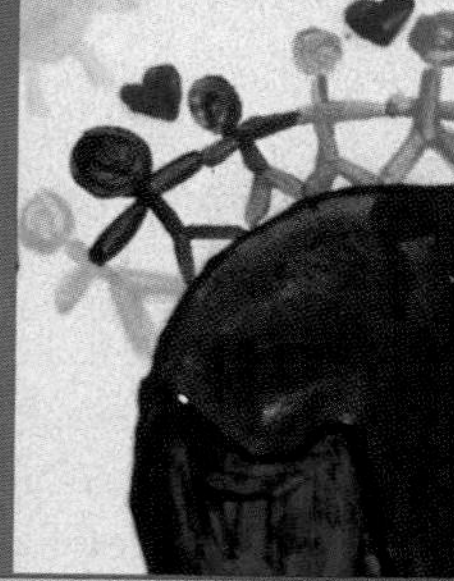

Health Promotion and Health Maintenance Visits

The frequency of health promotion visits decreases throughout childhood. Find out when the last visit was made and encourage an appointment if one is due. Teach parents the ages recommended for these visits by the American Academy of Pediatrics and U.S. Department of Health and Human Services (Green & Palfrey, 2000). They are:

- 5 years
- 6–8 years
- 8–10 years
- 10–12 years

and health maintenance needs regarding growth are addressed further in the nutrition section of this chapter.

School-age children have logical thought processes and are learning about their bodies. They should be active participants in the physical examination. Explain what you are doing and why. "I'm listening to your heart with this stethoscope and counting how many times it beats in a minute. Have you heard your heart? When have you noticed it beating hard?" Ask if they are nervous about any part of the examination. Verbalizing this anxiety allows you to explain what will be done and why it is important. Most children understand the purpose of the examination; a few will be very nervous, possibly related to a negative experience in healthcare at a younger age. They can be helped to verbalize their concerns and will often work through the feelings of insecurity or worry by talking about the prior experience. Young children generally want parents present during the examination, while children of 9 to 10 years may choose to have a parent wait outside. Allow children to choose what is comfortable, explaining to parents and meeting with parents to relay the findings from the examination.

A head-to-toe examination is carried out, with particular attention to systems and skills that influence success in school. Vision, hearing, muscular strength, and coordination are examples of areas that impact school performance. See Chapter 8∞ for detailed information about the physical examination. Remember to provide feedback about the findings; families appreciate knowing that the child's vision is normal and strength is well developed. They should be told what is normal as well as areas that may need more assessment or intervention. Inquire about the child's sleep patterns. During the examination, ask for a description of any illnesses the child has had. Children of school age are generally healthy, with only a few upper respiratory infections or other minor illnesses annually. Unusual complaints may indicate a need for further testing; examples will be discussed in the disease prevention section later in this chapter.

School-age children frequently have minor injuries. These might include falls from bicycles, skin rashes from exposure to plants on a hiking trip, bruises from a ball sport, and other minor mishaps. Be alert for more serious problems that may indicate a need for additional detailed data gathering and teaching. Examples are discussed in the injury prevention section later in the chapter.

Developmental surveillance continues to be an important part of the examination for school-age children. Some milestones can be observed during the visit while other information is obtained by report of parent and child. This information is combined with reports about school and other activities in order to establish that the child is developing as desired. You can ask parents:

- "Does your daughter seem like most 8-year-olds to you? Tell me about her school performance. Do you have any questions or concerns about her behavior or school performance?"
- "Describe your son's best friends and what they like to do."
- "What are the ways that he has been growing up this year?"

While milestones for development are quite different than at earlier ages, it is still important to evaluate progression. Direct observations, history questions, and questionnaires that parents complete are possible methods for development data collection. See Table 14–1 for developmental milestones of school-age children.

Once children attend school, parents may need to alter childcare arrangements. Ask about whether the child comes home after school on a school bus, public transportation, rides in a car, or walks. Is someone at home to supervise the young child? Do the parents feel that the child's after-school activities are safe? If the child goes to a childcare center, are parents satisfied with the program offered? Provide resources as needed to after-school programs that may be available in the school, and at other childcare providers. Search your community resource directories to learn about local sites. Help the parent to decide when the child is able to stay alone for a period of time after school. (See Partnering with Families: After-School Care.)

Desired outcomes for growth and developmental surveillance include normal progression with developmental tasks, absence of physical and psychosocial abnormalities or trauma, and integration of safe practices into daily life.

TABLE 14–1 Developmental Milestones Observed During Health Promotion and Health Maintenance Visits of School-Age Children

AGE	DEVELOPMENTAL MILESTONES
5 years	➤ Independent in bathroom and dressing activities ➤ Ties shoes, buttons ➤ Runs well, jumps, may skip, balances on one foot 10 seconds ➤ Pours fluids well, uses hands to catch ball ➤ Prints some letters, first name ➤ Draws triangle, square, 3–5 part person ➤ Knows full name, address, phone
6–8 years	➤ Skilled in physical activities such as running, skipping, jumping, hopping ➤ Learns to ride bicycle ➤ Can cut, paste, write all letters ➤ Reads
8–10 years	➤ Has increasingly longer periods of concentration for both physical activity and school or other quiet activity ➤ Can throw objects far and with accurate aim ➤ Increased coordination ➤ Develops hobbies such as model building, musical instrument, video production, building with wood, needle work
10–12 years	➤ Fine and gross motor skills similar to adult in ability ➤ Writes well, adept at computer use ➤ Some clumsiness may develop as prepubertal growth spurt begins

NUTRITION

Key concepts related to nutrition in school-age children are independence and formation of habits that influence the future. First, children are increasingly independent in food choices. They usually have strong likes and dislikes of certain foods. They may come home alone and prepare snacks. During school, they choose what to eat from the school lunch or the sack lunch sent by family. They may even have access to vending machines or sales of snacks during school hours. While independence in food choices is growing, the child is greatly influenced in those choices by friends and the media. Foods that may be rejected often include fresh vegetables and fruits, since they get little media attention, and friends may not prefer them.

At a time when the child chooses many of the foods in the daily diet, habits are being formed that will impact nutrition and health in general in the years to come. Good choices will help to promote health, maintain weight at a recommended level, provide nutrients for adequate growth and activity, and prevent onset of some chronic diseases. On the other hand, poor choices can lead to overweight and its accompanying problems, lack of adequate calcium and resultant osteoporosis, eating disorders, or lack of energy for brain growth and optimal performance in school. The patterns established during this period of time are influential in later nutritional status. Knowledge about foods, family participation in good nutritional practices, and access to healthy foods can all be enhanced by nursing intervention during this critical formative period.

The first nutritional status assessment includes height and weight measurement, body mass index calculation, and examination of percentiles for each measurement on growth grids (see Chapter 9 and Appendix A∞). See the discussion of measurement in the previous growth and developmental surveillance section. Slow, steady growth is the norm during the early school-age years; it will be followed by a growth spurt when the child nears puberty.

During the visit, observations provide information about nutritional status. What is the condition of the nails, skin, hair? What is the energy level and reported physical activity? Does the child look lean or overweight? As the child nears puberty, there may be an increase in fat stores as a preparation for the pubertal growth spurt (Story, Holt, & Sofka, 2002). Integrate

PARTNERING WITH FAMILIES

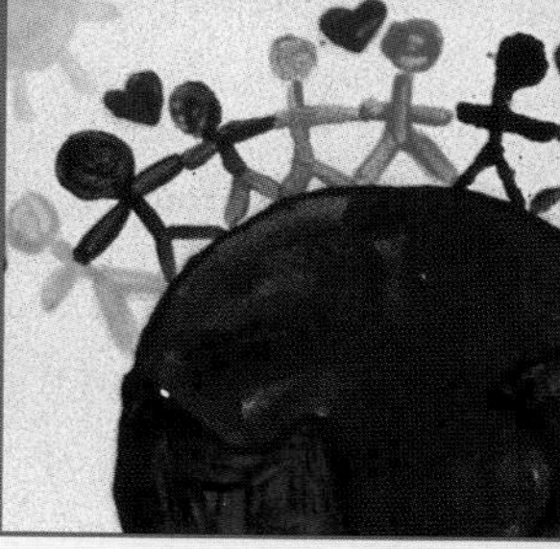

After-School Care

Children who come home to an empty house after school are called **latchkey children.** The age at which children are ready for this responsibility varies. Parents need help to decide when the child can come home and stay alone, and then plan for safety precautions for the child. Characteristics that indicate a child may be ready to stay alone for 1 to 3 hours include the following:

- The child has had opportunities to stay alone for shorter periods and has successfully planned appropriate activities and felt secure.
- The child has several activities and interests that can be pursued at home after school (e.g., music, model building, reading).
- The neighborhood and the route home are considered safe.
- The child understands major safety hazards such as not taking rides and not talking on the phone to strangers.
- The child understands fire, firearm, water, and other safety hazards and what to do in emergencies.
- Someone is always directly available by phone.
- A neighbor or other close resource is available.

Provide guidelines that a parent can use to help prepare the child to stay alone. These include the following:

- Teach the child where to keep a key so that it is not available to others, such as pinned inside a backpack. Alternatively, a touch pad key code may be used; be sure the child does not give the code to anyone, even friends. Have alternative plans of a place the child is to go in case the child loses a key or the power is off.
- Teach the child to never get in a car with a stranger, open the door of the home, or leave windows or doors unlocked.
- Review the amount of time that can be spent on television, computer, or games. Place a child control on the computer and television to limit access to adult viewing.
- Tell the child that other children are not to come home and stay while an adult is not present.
- Review fire safety, such as avoiding use of matches, open flames, or small appliances. Microwave ovens may be safest for preparing snacks.
- Be sure firearms are locked, with guns unloaded and ammunition in a separate place. The child should not have access to the key to firearm cabinets; remember that children know the house and often are successful in finding parent's hiding places.
- Review first aid for scratches or minor incidents.
- Review use of 9–1–1 and other resources. Keep these numbers by the phones.
- Be sure the child makes good decisions about what to do in case of fire, someone seeking entry to house, power outage, or severe weather. Provide scenarios and ask the child what should be done. Reinforce teaching as needed.
- Arrange for friends, family members, or neighbors who the child can call if lonely, scared, in need of help, or in danger. Be sure the child knows that it is alright to feel afraid sometimes. Some communities have phone services that help with homework or talk to children who are home alone. Find out if such a service is available in your community.
- Call the child every hour or so during the first few months of staying alone. Consider getting a cell phone so the child can use that phone and does not need to answer the family phone. If the home phone is answered, the child should tell callers that their parents are busy, rather than not at home.

Adapted from Murray, R. B., & Zentner, J. P. (2001). Health promotion strategies through the life span (7th ed., pp. 469–470). Upper Saddle River, NJ: Prentice Hall.

questions for the parent and child into the visit that provide clues about diet.

- "Do you eat school lunch, or pack a lunch from home?"
- "Do you eat breakfast? What do you usually eat in the morning?"
- "You mentioned that you are without a car now, Mrs. Jennings. How are you able to get your groceries?"
- "What did you have to eat so far today?"
- "Do you every worry that you do not have enough food to feed your family?"
- "Do you use WIC (Women, Infant, and Child Nutrition Program), food banks, farmers' markets, or other resources?"
- "Do you have a garden? Would you like to?"
- "What is your favorite grocery store? Why?"
- "You mentioned that all of your children are in activities after school. How do you usually fit in an evening meal for everyone? How often do you eat fast food? How often does the whole family eat together?"
- "How do you feel about your weight and the way you look?"

As you observe the child and family and ask dietary questions, list risks and protective factors related to nutrition. Perhaps protective factors relate to adequate access to nutritious foods, a family garden, and weight and height within normal limits. Reinforce the positive practices of the family and inform the child of how food choices relate to energy level, school performance, and general health. Risk factors become the basis for teaching and planning with the family for necessary change. It is difficult to tackle several nutritional changes at one time, so concentrate on those most needing attention, and on those the family agrees are important. Provide information about healthy snacks to keep at home, ways to improve calcium intake, limitation of soda pop to one can daily, and the importance of family meals (Box 14–1). Nutrition teaching can take place during visits, at schools, and in other settings with school-age youth (Figure 14–2 ■).

It is clear that teaching regarding nutrition can promote health of children. Desired outcomes for health maintenance include absence of overweight and future chronic disease, adequate intake of all nutrients, and increasing child and family knowledge about nutrition.

BOX 14–1 5-a-Day Program

The 5-a-day program is a comprehensive, coordinated national nutrition program designed to increase the consumption of at least five servings of fruits and vegetables daily. The National Cancer Institute and the Produce for Better Health Foundation joined together to launch the program; now many states and local areas have initiatives to raise awareness of the benefits of fruits and vegetables for health.

Most children do not consume this ideal, so concentrating on this topic may help families. Explain that fruits and vegetables contain vitamins necessary for good health, and have been associated with lower rates of several cancers, diabetes, and obesity. Ask what vegetables and fruits are available and which they like. Apples, oranges, and bananas comprise the most commonly selected fruits, while carrots, potatoes (most in the form of fries), and tomatoes are common vegetables. Recognize that likes may relate to cultural group. Compose a list, including both common fruits and vegetables, and less commonly eaten items such as beets, beans, corn, mangoes, pineapple, kiwi, cantaloupe, berries, and other seasonal or geographically related foods. Ask families to choose two or three fruits and two or three vegetables that everyone in the family likes and teach them to purchase those foods weekly. Recommend that fresh fruits and vegetables always be cut and readily available in the refrigerator; this encourages their consumption when a child comes home alone and is hungry. Add berries and other fruits to cereals. Make shakes with nonfat frozen yogurt and added fruit. Recognize that frozen and canned fruits and vegetables are a good way to get these food groups. See if local food programs like WIC provide vouchers to obtain foods in local farmers' markets; this is often a good resource for produce in low-income families. Are there field gleaning programs if you live in an agricultural area? Set the goal with a family of increasing by one to two servings daily the intake of fruits and vegetables. Ask them to keep a log and invite them to call and tell you how they are doing. Health promotion programs in schools can offer incentives and prizes to children who eat five servings a day. Work with school nurses to facilitate these programs.

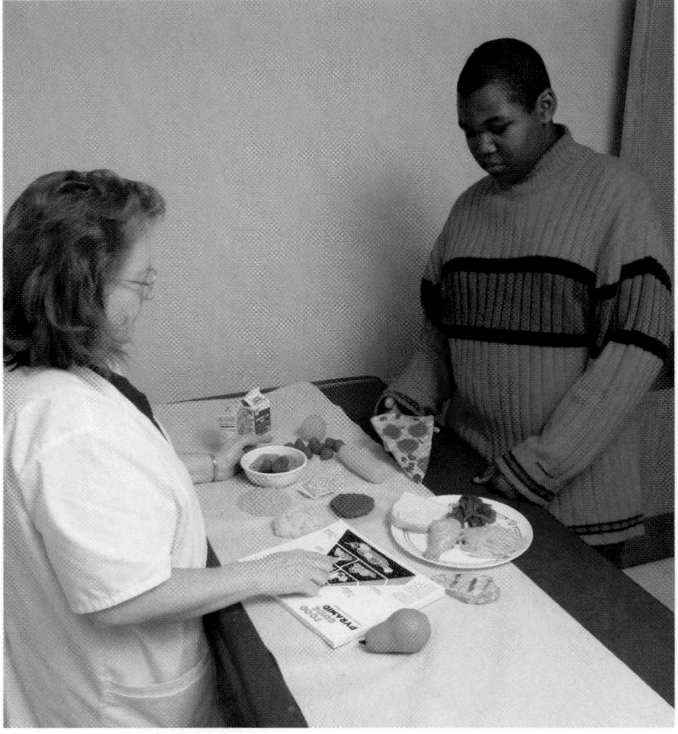

FIGURE 14–2 ■ This school-age child is receiving teaching from the nurse about food choices. What benefit do the food models provide in this situation? What other teaching techniques can you suggest?

PHYSICAL ACTIVITY

MediaLink The Importance of Physical Activity Video

Just as food choices during the school-age years are likely to influence the child's future nutrition, physical activity during these years is often crucial to development of lifelong exercise. During these years, the child who is physically active continues to refine skills such as eye-hand coordination, muscular strength, agility, and speed. Some children become skilled at ball sports such as basketball, football, soccer, or baseball. Others focus on gymnastics, wrestling, horseback riding, or hockey (Figure 14–3 ■). Some do not like team or organized sports but choose skate boarding, skiing, or biking. Whatever the interest, it is important that children identify some physical activity and continue to develop motor skills. The benefits include socialization, positive sense of accomplishment and self-esteem, weight control, and increasing physical ability (Figure 14–4 ■). Children who do not have an activity of importance often fall behind their peers in agility and skill, making future attempts at an activity very difficult and less likely to be successful.

Similar to earlier periods in life, the nurse lists risk and protective factors related to school-age physical activity (Table 14–2). Families are often significant in promoting physical activity for children. Find out what the parents do for physical activity and how often. Do they attend a sports club after work or does the child see them engaging in exercise? Most families can include some walking, yard work, or other activity that is done together to engage the child. Do they walk to a neighbor's house or a nearby store rather than driving? Do they take elevators or choose the stairs in buildings? What is the activity level of siblings? When older siblings are involved in sports, the younger child often is encouraged to develop skills in the same sport.

The child spends much of the day in school; therefore, this setting is important to consider. In an effort to conserve financial resources, some schools have decreased physical education (PE) programs. Children may not have regular PE classes, and there may be few standards of performance. In addition, many states and provinces have established tests and standards for performance in certain cognitive areas. In an attempt to increase teaching time to meet these standards, some schools have cut recess and other breaks. Schools are sometimes located in unsafe areas and outside recreation is not advisable. However, it is unrealistic to expect children to sit for long periods without physical activity, and such practice reinforces the poor habits of inadequate exercise among children. Nurses are influential members of school committees and can encourage the integration of activity in the school day. You may be able to serve on a school or community committee, educating other committee members of the benefits of exercise to enhance cognitive performance and general health. Teachers and school administrators can be supplied with models of successful school activity programs.

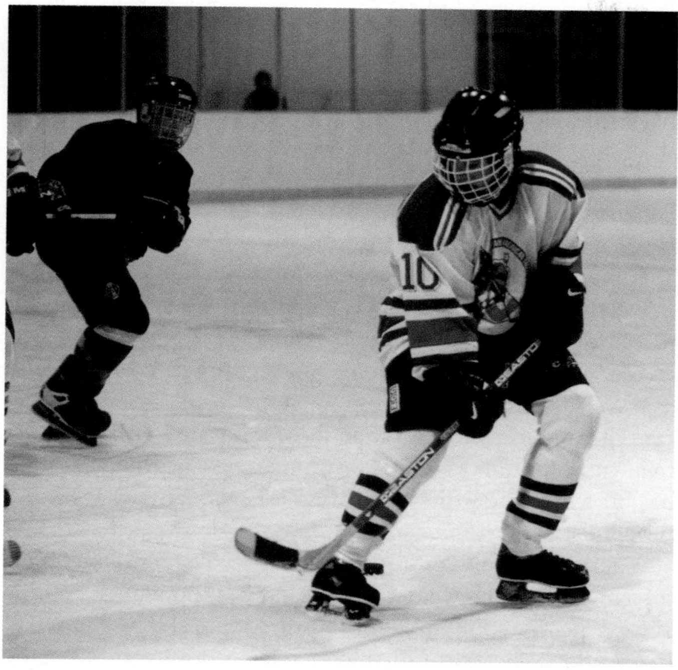

FIGURE 14–3 ■ Everyone needs to be physically active. Some children participate in school sports. Others, such as these boys playing hockey, choose a sport that is available in the community. Other children prefer to walk, ride a bike, or engage in other more solitary activities. Determine what is enjoyable for a particular child and provide assistance in integrating desirable exercise into daily routines.

Some schools offer sports programs in after-school settings. When these organized sports have tryouts and eliminations, the children who most need activity may be those eliminated. The child who has a pubertal growth spurt early (see Chapter 5∞) is often better at certain organized sports and has many more opportunities to engage in them. Eliminating smaller children or those less adept at sports means that they are then unable to learn the skills necessary to play the sport; some of them may actually become better at the sport as they grow older and bigger. It is best if there are levels so that all interested children can play and learn the physical skills needed to improve. Again, school finances make this difficult, so nurses can often be influential in finding community volunteers to work with teams of students. Student nurses, physical education students, senior citizens, and others are often able to help young children play baseball, tennis, or soccer. Other volunteers may teach stretching or warm-up activities. Community partners such as businesses may provide protective gear or uniforms for school sports, especially if the business name can be displayed. In addition, schools can offer alternative activities that some children might prefer to traditional organized sports. Can the school obtain a climbing wall? Is there a skate park near? Will a local ski resort sponsor a weekly or monthly bus of children from the school? Is swimming available at a nearby city or YMCA/YWCA pool? What can you do in your local community schools to ensure equal access to sports for all children? How can you help parents to become influential in the community to improve options for their children?

It is essential to consider physical activity for the child who has special healthcare needs. It may be difficult for schools to plan an activity for the child with cerebral palsy, visual impairment, or developmental delay. Search for other community resources and help the family to access them. There may be programs for children to ride horses, swim, ski, and engage in other physical activities. Imagine the thrill that waits a child who has rarely moved quickly when riding a sled or sliding on skis.

In summary, the nurse plays an important role in meeting desired outcomes of health promotion by suggesting activities that

TABLE 14–2 Risk and Protective Factors Regarding Physical Activity in School-Age Children

RISK FACTORS	PROTECTIVE FACTORS
➤ Limited role modeling of daily physical activity by parents and other family members ➤ Limited facilities in the neighborhood to encourage activity, such as parks, skate board facilities, rinks, ball courts/fields ➤ Inadequate financial resources to join clubs or pay for organized sports ➤ School cuts to physical education programs and recess ➤ School tryouts for sports that eliminate all but the best players in certain sports ➤ Reluctance to try new activity ➤ Worry about competence and physical appearance ➤ Television viewing or other screen activities for more than 2 hours daily ➤ Developmental delay and special needs	➤ Expected developmental skill level ➤ Feels self-confident in ability and physical appearance ➤ Willing to try new activities ➤ Sets goals for learning physical skills ➤ Parents exercise daily and exercise with the child some of this time in setting the child can see ➤ Parents set expectation that everyone in family will choose a physical activity and engage in it regularly ➤ Schools provide physical education each day with a variety of offerings; student gets to choose and set goals for some activities ➤ Schools schedule recess or physical activity breaks twice daily ➤ Sports teams are leveled so that all students desiring to play a particular sport, such as soccer, are able to do so ➤ Adequate safety gear that properly fits child is available ➤ Neighborhood provides access to parks, skate board facilities, rinks, ball courts, and other facilities ➤ Family has adequate financial resources to pay for health club or organized sports ➤ Television viewing and other screen activities limited to no more than 2 hours daily

Adapted from Patrick, K., Spear, B., Holt, K., & Sofka, D. (Eds.). (2001). Bright futures in practice: Physical activity. *Arlington, VA: National Center for Education in Maternal and Child Health.*

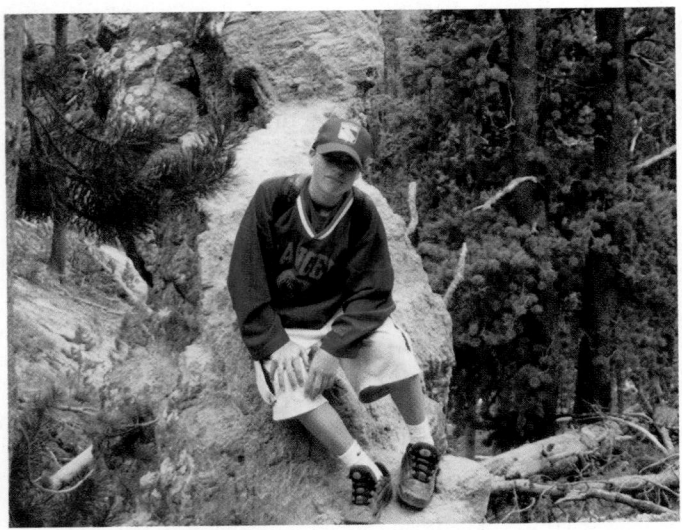

FIGURE 14–4 ■ School-age children often enjoy hikes with family, clubs, or other groups. What are the physical and mental health benefits to this physical activity?

families can do together, becoming active in physical education programs in schools, acting as a positive role model, and helping interested children to partner with community resources for activity. Health maintenance outcomes include use of safety gear and correct techniques to prevent injury from sport participation.

ORAL HEALTH

Many changes occur in the mouth during the school-age years, necessitating periodic examination. About 6 years of age, most children lose a tooth, usually in the front. Following that, all 20 of the deciduous or primary teeth will be lost, and the permanent teeth will simultaneously begin to erupt. See Chapter 8∞ for the schedule of tooth loss and tooth eruption (see Developing Cultural Competence: Tooth Loss). In addition, the jaw line elongates and teeth move into new positions. Periodic dental visits focus on both the placement of teeth and oral hygiene.

During the health promotion visit, examine the teeth. Look to see how many deciduous and permanent teeth are present. Describe the child's oral hygiene. Ask how often the child brushes, flosses, and visits the dentist. The child should have learned how to brush and floss during preschool years but is now performing the skills independently. If there are caries or poor oral hygiene is apparent, ask the child to demonstrate brushing and flossing. Reinforce the need for brushing twice daily and flossing once daily. Provide toothpaste and toothbrushes as gifts during health supervision visits. Local dentists will often provide these supplies so that you can encourage oral hygiene.

Dental visits are recommended every 6 months, so if the child is not visiting on that schedule, ask if finances or transportation are issues, or if the family needs a referral to a dentist, or if there is some other reason. If caries or malocclusion is present, stress the need for a dental appointment. Inquire about use of fluoride if the water supply is not fluoridated. Ask if the child has had sealants applied to the permanent teeth; these will help to prevent future caries.

Many children have a high intake of sugared foods and snacks. If this is apparent from the nutritional assessment, discuss the importance of limiting these foods and brushing after their consumption. Frequent brushing is needed when the child has braces. Ask how they are caring for them and what the orthodontist has recommended.

The nurse's health promotion activities include positive reinforcement of good hygiene habits, and health maintenance involves teaching about need for improved care and limiting food that furthers the formation of caries. Desired outcomes include good oral hygiene, attendance at recommended dental visits, and absence of dental caries.

DEVELOPING CULTURAL COMPETENCE
Tooth Loss

In the mainstream U.S. and Canadian cultures, lost teeth signal growing up and are celebrated events. It is common for the tooth lost at school or in the hospital to be sent home to the parents with a note about when it was lost. Many children place the lost tooth under the pillow at night and expect the "tooth fairy" to leave a small gift. Parents remove the tooth while the child sleeps and place a gift. Ask about how tooth loss is handled in the family.

MENTAL AND SPIRITUAL HEALTH

The school-age years are marked by the emergence of new cognitive skills, ability to interact cooperatively with others, and a feeling of accomplishment in achievements. The child's self-concept and mental health are linked to these important developmental tasks (see Chapter 5∞ for further discussion of developmental tasks).

Self-concept is the mental idea that one has of the self. School age is an important period of time in the development of one's self-concept. **Self-esteem** reflects a positive self-concept; it includes the feelings and beliefs of children about their competence and worth as individuals, ability to meet challenges, and to learn lessons from success and failure (Jellinek, Patel, & Froehle, 2002, p. 90). The aim is to establish a positive sense of self-esteem, even in the face of adversity and challenge. The child who believes in his or her ability to face good times and bad has a lowered chance of mental illness such as depression, eating disorder, and anxiety. Parents are encouraged to evaluate and help to build the child's sense of self-esteem (see Partnering with Families: Evaluating and Fostering Self-Esteem).

Self-concept and self-esteem include all parts of the person such as cognitive, spiritual, sexual, and physical. **Body image** refers to a specific part of the self-concept, the idea that one forms about one's body. **Sexuality** is another part of the self-concept and refers to the person's view of self as a sexual being.

Many of the areas discussed already in this chapter provide clues to the child's self-concept. Does the child engage in sports or other physical activities? The child may then reflect a positive self-concept and body image. On the other hand, if the child is forced to do these sports by parents and feels inadequate in performance, he or she may promote a negative self-concept and body image. Ask both about the child's activities and feelings about them. Does the child enjoy them? How does the child rate his or her performance? Inquire about school performance and best friends. Is there an increasing independence and responsibility for self? Success in achieving developmental milestones leads to a positive sense of self-esteem in the child.

A low sense of self-esteem is noted when the child states a disinterest in exercise, school clubs, and family activities. This can lead to loneliness, depression, and mental health problems such as eating disorders (Jellinek et al., 2002). When these feelings are noted during a health supervision visit, the nurse should recommend that the child see a counselor at school or another setting, and should recommend that parents be included in the sessions so that they can best help the child.

It is obvious that the family plays a critical part in the child's developing self-esteem and mental health. To understand the child, it is necessary to ask questions about and explore dynamics in the family. Several protective factors have been identified for families.

- Communication is open and clear, and parents use problem-solving skills.
- Members are encouraged and appreciated.
- Family is committed to each other, including spending time together.
- Religious or spiritual orientation is present.
- Social connectedness or support are available.
- Resilience or the ability to adapt to new situations is present.

(Wertlieb, 2003)

Ask about and observe the family's relationships when you are with them. Evaluate the effect of family interactions on the child. Model respectful interchanges by listening carefully to the child, as well as the parent. Gently recognize the child if parents answer for them or seem to put them down. You might say, "Jared seems to have something to say and I'd like to hear his opinion. What were you saying, Jared, about what you do not enjoy at school?" Provide brochures and examples of ways to show children their importance. Encourage both parents to come to child healthcare visits and support the involvement of both parents in child rearing (Task Force on the Family, 2003). Ask about family stressors such as job changes, financial concerns, illness, substance abuse, and domestic violence. About one half of marriages end in divorce, so be prepared to offer suggestions to deal with this situation (see Partnering with Families: Divorce and the School-Age Child). Ask about risk factors and protective factors. Remember that resilience is the ability to use strengths to help deal with adversity (see Chapter 5∞ for a detailed description of resilience theory). Look for risk and protective factors in the family and suggest ways to use protective factors to foster resilience. The child's strengths are used to assist the family functioning and will, in turn, give the child a sense of accomplishment. Examples include the following:

- A child who is able to act independently can be given responsibility for parts of the home or family function, such as planning the menu for dinner two evenings weekly.
- A creative child can be given the task of planning books and other activities for a younger sibling.

PARTNERING WITH FAMILIES

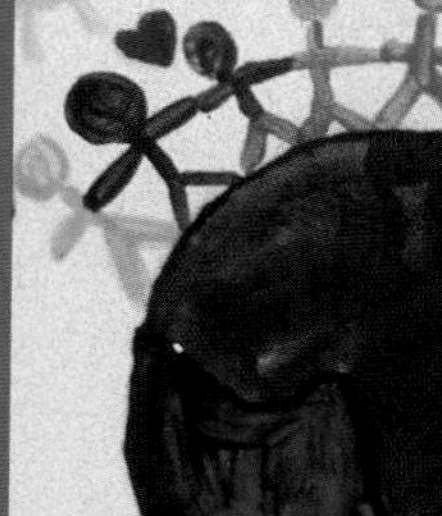

Evaluating and Fostering Self-Esteem

Parents play an important part in fostering the child's self-esteem. The nurse can ask parents to evaluate the child and provide suggestions about positive actions.

Evaluation Questions	Positive Actions
What does your child do well?	Build on the child's strengths and talents; point out the child's abilities
How does your child respond to failure?	Assist the child to assess performance; help the child see that mistakes are expected and have lessons to teach
Does your child have close friends?	Arrange structured play times such as going to a movie or cooking with a friend
How does your child respond to new challenges?	Give the child responsibilities at home; encourage your child to try new experiences; help the child feel a sense of control over outcomes
How does your own personality compare to your child's?	Recognize differences in style; appreciate the unique qualities of the child; tailor expectations to the child and not to self or other children
Are you setting reasonable and attainable expectations for your child?	Ask the child what is attainable; establish goals for behaviors together

Adapted from Spratt, E. (2002). Assessing and reinforcing your child's self-esteem. In M. Jellinek, B. P. Patel, & M. C. Froehle, (Eds.), Bright futures in practice: Mental health—Volume II. Tool kit *(p. 94). Arlington, VA: National Center for Education in Maternal and Child Health.*

- A child with a talent for design can be asked to set the table for dinner guests.

The school-age child is developing a sense of body image and sexuality. Look at the child's appearance and dress. Some children may have poor posture, display a sense of insecurity, and seem uncomfortable with themselves. Others may dress as if they were much older, seem sophisticated, and are clearly assuming the role identification with their gender group. Ask the parents in a private setting what observations they have about the child's body image and sexuality. Inquire about friends of the opposite sex and whether the parent has concerns. Questions related to sexuality will emerge during school years. They should be answered truthfully and fully. Even children who do not ask questions usually need information related to sexuality education. They may receive information in school beginning

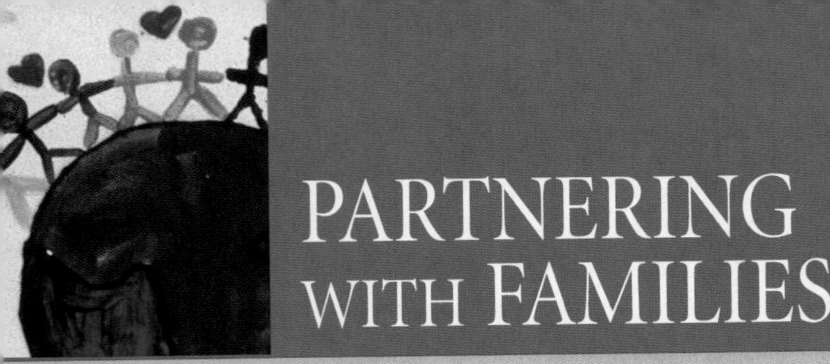

PARTNERING WITH FAMILIES

Divorce and the School-Age Child

Divorce is a common stressful event for school-age children. While parents are engaged in their own stresses, they may benefit from help to plan for ways to lessen the strain on children. They can:

- Be sure the child understands that the divorce is not the child's fault and is only related to the parents' relationship to each other.
- Assert that the child is loved by both parents and will not be abandoned. Spend time with the child regularly to reinforce his or her central role in the family.
- Do not share marital concerns with the child or place the child in a position of having to choose between relationships with one parent or the other. Conflicts between parents should not take place in front of the children.
- Recognize that the child will feel hurt, sad, and lonely.
- Maintain stability when possible for the child, such as attendance at the same school, using the same childcare settings, and arranging visits with friends and family members.
- Continue household routines, rules, and discipline.
- Arrange for support for the child from religious clergy, family, friends, or counselors.

Adapted from Jellinek, M., Patel, B. P., & Froehle, M. C. (2002). Bright futures in practice: Mental health—Volume II. Tool kit *(pp. 113–114). Arlington, VA: National Center for Education in Maternal and Child Health.*

in approximately fourth grade, but often have misconceptions about the bodies of men and women, sexual intercourse, how babies are born, and other topics. Suggest that parents read books with their children that deal with these issues at an appropriate developmental level. If books are available at home, children will be likely to look at them and ask questions. Many young girls have bodily changes as early as 9 or 10 years of age (see Chapter 5∞), and reading material can put both parent and child at ease and open the door to discussion. Parents should be advised to talk with teachers to learn what is presented in school and be able to supplement and clarify this information. Having discussions at a young age will help open the door to further discussion as the child gets older.

Suggest to parents that computer and other media provide information that can confuse children. Encourage them to watch movies with children, encourage frank discussions related to sexuality observed, and answer questions truthfully. Children generally learn about topics such as sexual intercourse, sexual orientation, and childbirth from school discussions and the media. A few moments alone with parents and child at healthcare visits may help to identify the concerns of each related to sexuality.

By approximately grades 4 to 6, most girls have started to have prepubertal body changes and may begin to menstruate. This is another opening to discussions about mature bodies of men and women and the transformation from childhood to greater maturity. Boys mature about 2 years later than girls, and without an event such as menstruation, parents may be less likely to start discussions with male children. Suggest that parents consciously begin conversations with boys periodically to explain changes they see in themselves and their peers. See Chapters 5 and 8∞ for further discussion of the body changes seen in the prepubertal period and during puberty.

School-age children continue to develop an ability to self-regulate activities and responses to situations. At this age, the abilities to solve problems and assume more responsibility for self are important. Encourage parents to discuss issues with the child and to seek solutions together when appropriate. For example, the parent may tell the child that there is enough money to sign up for one summer camp and let the child help to choose which one it should be. If the child is having difficulty in getting homework done, they can be included in a discussion about possible solutions. If the child suggests doing homework when first coming home, or limiting television time on weeknights, it is more likely that the solution will work. The child assumes more responsibility for assisting with meal preparation and home chores, coming home alone after school, and caring for younger siblings. Encourage the parents to praise the child for assuming more family responsibilities and recognize that the child will need some guidance when taking on new tasks.

Sleep is still important for children in order for them to have the energy to perform well in school and other activities. They generally take charge of bedtime routines with reminders about the time to go to sleep, and they sleep through the night. Sleep time varies from 8 to 12 hours, depending on child and activity level. Busy schedules may interrupt this pattern, leading to irritability, lack of concentration, or even hyperactive behavior (Colyar, 2003). Help children and families plan what the bedtime should be.

Sleepwalking and sleep talking sometimes occur at this age, but usually decrease as the child nears adolescence. Children who have stress at home, such as parental fighting, ill family members, or inadequate food or shelter, may not get enough sleep and fall asleep at school. Ask the child if he or she falls asleep in class, and seek additional information about family stressors. This can lead to interventions such as recommending family counseling or referring to resources to obtain better housing or more stable food sources.

School is a major microsystem influence in the lives of children, and plays a role in self-concept and mental health formation. Ask the child to describe a best friend; if unable to do so, isolation may be occurring. Inquire about what the three best and three worst things are about school. Children with low self-concepts often have trouble talking about and evaluating school. Find out where the child attends school, if the area is generally safe, and how the child gets to school. Are there clubs, after-school sports, or school performances for parents on occasion? What are the child's grades like? Do parents and child feel that the child is challenged intellectually but not unduly stressed? Encourage the parents to meet the child's teachers, to become active in school activities, and to be available to solve problems with school personnel when needed. Partner with the parents and child when interventions are needed. An office nurse may contact a school nurse when the child needs support in the school environment. This may occur if the child has become ill and missed school, has family stressors, does not get along well with a teacher, or has a condition such as attention deficit disorder. Identify the risk and protective factors in the school environment and plan interventions to support the child when risks are present. See the following section in this chapter and Chapters 7 and 34∞ for more information about attention deficit disorder, bullying, and other issues in the school environment.

Certain mental health disorders are commonly seen during the school years. One example includes anxiety problems that result in worries, fears, physical symptoms, stress, and sleep disorder, without significantly impairing daily functioning. On the other hand, anxiety disorders affect functioning and have more striking characteristics such as clinging, abdominal pain and headache, and refusal to attend school (American Psychiatric Association, 2000). Posttraumatic stress syndrome and depression may also be seen. See Chapter 34∞ for further description of these disorders. Anxiety disorder, posttraumatic stress, and depression should be referred to a mental health specialist for treatment. However, all children worry at times and this type of anxiety can be helped by learning coping skills and relaxation techniques.

Spiritual health is the ability to develop a spiritual nature, including awareness of a life purpose and fulfillment (Pender, Murdaugh, & Parsons, 2002). School age is a time when children learn more about the people and the world around them, and begin to find their place in that world. Connection with faith-based groups assists some children and families in defining the purpose of life, while others may do so through social activity or a strong moral sense of responsibility. Ask children what brings happiness, how they help other people, or if they are members of a church, synagogue, or mosque. If families seem to have little purpose, parents are withdrawn or depressed, or the child has difficulty answering questions about meaningful activities, suggest methods of engagement in the community. These might include providing contacts at local religious events, posting flyers about community events designed to bring unity to various cultural groups, or suggesting services needing volunteers in the community. Families who spend time together and find meaning in supporting each other nurture the spiritual health of their members. Suggest that every family plan a "family night" weekly when they play games, talk, eat, or engage in other activities together.

The nurse has an important role in fostering the mental and spiritual health of school-age children. Health promotion fosters strengths of families and children, leading to healthy self-concept and positive self-esteem. Some strengths to consider in health promotion include:

- Family spends time together in activities several times weekly.
- Child is able to verbalize school and home activities that are important and meaningful.
- Family is engaged in religious and/or community activities on a regular basis.
- There are adequate resources for housing, food, and other basic necessities.

Health maintenance seeks to prevent mental health disruptions. Be alert for risk factors in families since they represent the need for intervention. Some examples include:

- Family schedules are chaotic with little chance for interaction among family members.
- Family is isolated and feels little connection to the community.
- Basic necessities are often not met, whether for food, housing, or healthcare.
- Child has no school or community activities such as sports or clubs.

Expected outcomes for health promotion and health maintenance activities with school-age children include formation of a positive sense of self-esteem and healthy body image, use of coping skills to deal with stress, sleep patterns that meet needs for rest, and a growing purpose and meaning in life.

RELATIONSHIPS

While the school-age child is gradually moving away from the family as the center of life, the family remains an important anchor. The previous section discusses several issues where the parents foster development. Ask also about siblings, grandparents, and other extended family members. Sometimes these persons assist in the child's formation of a self-concept. Peers are increasingly important to the school-age child's self-identity. School age is a time of cooperative engagement with others (see Chapter 5∞). All children need to be able to learn how to make and maintain friendships and work with others on projects and in recreation.

As mentioned, you can inquire about the child's best friends at school. Ask parents if they are comfortable with the child's selection of friends. Find out if the parents facilitate friendships by allowing other children to come to the home and providing transportation as needed. When the child experiences a risk factor such as a move to a new town or school, role-play how to meet new children and how to make friends. If the child feels like an outcast or outsider among peers at school, explore how the family can create a safe and secure place for the child in extracurricular activities with children who have similar interests. When children are home schooled, the family may need to plan social events and contacts after usual school hours.

Since peers are important to the school-age child, pressure begins to appear like others, to fit in, and to do what others encourage. Although such pressures are often associated with teen years, they usually begin earlier, at least by 8 or 9 years of age. Ask children what things friends try to get them to do that they know they should not do, or if friends have tried to get them to smoke. Middle school years are the most common age for smoking to begin, so always ask if the child has tried smoking. The child may tell you about activities when parents are not in the room, such as playing with guns, trying alcohol or other substances, or partaking in other risky behavior. It is best to ask what the child does in these situations, what the child wants to do, and to whom the child can turn to talk about these events. Offer information about the risks connected with behaviors that are described, and suggest people such as parents, teachers, counselors, or clergy who are possible resources. If the child's health is at risk, be sure to report the activity to the physician or other healthcare provider so that it can be pursued and the child's safety can be assured. Activities such as playing with firearms or visiting a friend whose parents are making methamphetamine, for example, place children in extreme danger.

School age is often a time when children first experience violence in relationships with others. Some children are bullied, while others are the bullies. Anger and aggression can occur, and children get in fights with each other. Ask children to describe when they last had a disagreement with someone and how the problem was solved. Have they ever been hit, called names, or had fights? How did it make them feel? What did they do about it? Suggest people like school nurses, teachers, and counselors who can help, and be sure that children feel safe in schools, neighborhoods, and homes. Ask parents how they resolve arguments between children at home and what help they need to help children learn problem-solving skills. Find out what policies the schools have in your community to assist in decreasing harassment of and by children. As you progress in your career, become active on school committees that help children learn how to solve problems peacefully and how to respond to episodes of violence. See Chapter 7∞ for further discussion of violence in children and a detailed discussion of bullying.

The child's temperament still plays a part in response to situations and the ability to self-regulate (see page 144). The "difficult" child may have trouble getting to sleep or in being quiet in the classroom. Have parents plan more physical activity for this child, and teach the child that bedtime routines are helpful, and that sitting near the front of the class can help with concentration. The "slow to warm up" child may need ideas about what to say when meeting new people. Parents of this child can help the child prepare for a new school by visiting with the child, talking about it, and meeting with the teacher so that a warm welcome can occur. The "easy" child is usually adaptable in most situations and is regular in activities. However, this child may object when other children interrupt in conversation, fail to take turns, or otherwise "break the rules" of behavior. Children may need help to understand differences in temperament in order to be more tolerant of classmates and their behaviors. Often nurses in schools address the issue of individual differences by speaking with classes or small groups of children.

Once again, the nurse takes an active role in promoting the child's health by anticipating developmental issues and preparing parents and child to deal with them. Health maintenance outcomes include preventing problems in interactions with others.

DISEASE PREVENTION STRATEGIES

School-age children are generally healthy. The immune system is mature (see Chapter 27∞), personal hygiene practices are more mature than at earlier ages, and immunizations are usually complete. Engage school-age children in active pursuit of their own health. Teach strategies that can enhance the prevention of diseases. Nurses in offices and schools can teach children how to wash hands effectively, how respiratory infections are transmitted, and what can cause gastrointestinal illness. Ask children in your settings what topics are of most interest to them and be prepared to suggest common areas of concern (Box 14–2). Children are interested in their bodies and can understand the connection between eating well and avoiding illness, maintaining normal weight and preventing type 2 diabetes, avoiding smoking to prevent cancer and other respiratory diseases, and exercising to prevent hypertension. Recall Jessalyn in the opening scenario. How will you integrate exercise, nutrition knowledge, and management of her diabetes to prevent related diseases such as high blood pressure, retinal damage, renal damage, or cardiovascular disease? See Figure 14–5 ■.

School-age children are in the concrete stage of intellectual development (see Chapter 5∞). This means that teaching is most effective when opportunities are provided to touch, feel, and otherwise become actively engaged in learning. When teach-

BOX 14–2 Research: Health Promotion Topics

Middle school students participating in a research study were presented with a list of health topics and asked to rank their need for more information about the topics. The top 10 learning needs identified are as follows:

1. Hair care
2. Safety (fire, poison, auto, bicycle)
3. Prevention of mouth infections
4. Skin care
5. Physical fitness
6. Dental care
7. Hearing protection
8. Eye protection
9. Care of minor skin injuries
10. Why people use drugs

The researchers suggest that nurses examine these interests of youth to plan appropriate health promotion teaching. Personal care and safety are primary themes of importance identified by these middle school students (Adderly-Kelly & Green, 2000).

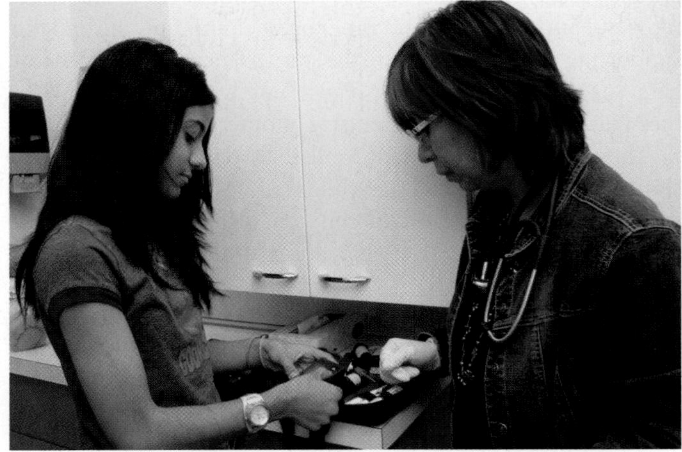

FIGURE 14–5 ■ Jessalyn is showing the school nurse how she programs her insulin pump. The nurse has partnered with nurses in the endocrinologist office to learn about the type of pump Jessalyn is using. Such collaboration enhances chances that diabetes will be well monitored and managed.

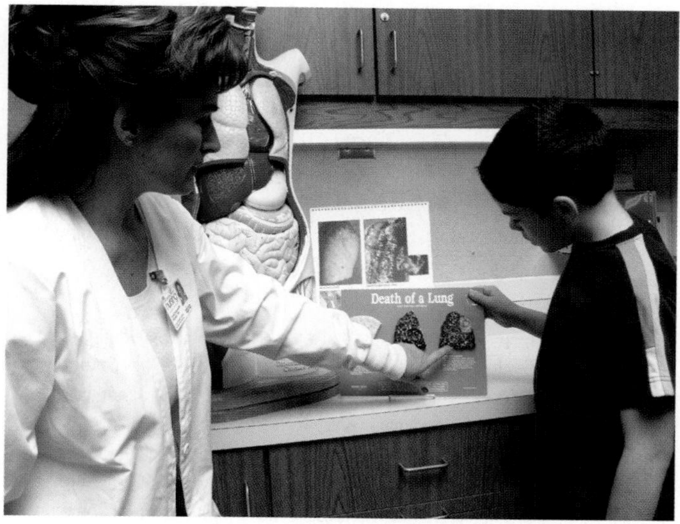

FIGURE 14–6 ■ This boy is learning about the effects of smoking on the body through the concrete experience of examining a model of the lungs. Why does this type of hands-on technique help school-age children to learn concepts?

ing about smoking, provide models of lungs and have students breathe through a straw to demonstrate the effects of airway narrowing. These concrete activities will teach them concepts better than simple lecture or reading (Figure 14–6 ■). Concepts of health promotion tend to be abstract since they deal with supporting one's highest potential for wellness. Thus it becomes even more important to provide concrete methods of learning.

Immunizations are generally up to date for school-age children. However, some children may have missed earlier doses due to illness or missed healthcare visits. Evaluate the immunization record to be sure it meets all recommendations. The most common immunization needs at this time are as follows:

- Hepatitis B (whole series or a missed third shot)
- Hepatitis A (if in state with recommendation for immunization)
- Tetanus-diphtheria, polio, or measles-mumps-rubella (if booster dose was not given prior to school entry)
- Varicella if not given earlier and the child has not had the disease
- Certain vaccines for children at high risk, such as pneumococcal, influenza, meningococcal (see Chapter 19∞)

Screening for health risks should occur during the visit (Table 14–3). Unusual complaints such as the following may indicate a need for further testing.

- Pain other than brief discomfort after an injury
- Headaches
- Bruising
- Lack of coordination
- Repeated infections
- Decreasing vision or hearing
- Problems or changes in school performance or behavior

Children who have an identified health problem or developmental disability may have additional needs for screening and for interventions to assist with health maintenance. For example, the child with cystic fibrosis will need information to lessen risk of respiratory infection, and the child with diabetes may need additional blood studies. The child who has difficulty reading will need alternative approaches to teaching correct handwashing; demonstration with explanation may be the best approach. A family history of diseases increases the child's risk and necessitates testing. For example, if a parent has had early cardiovascular disease (before age 55 years), a lipid profile should be performed on the child.

Parents should receive explanations about the screening tests performed and the results obtained. Inform them about vision and hearing results. Send home or call in results of blood tests when available. Be sure they understand the findings and have resources to assist in preventing or treating the specific disease in their children. Encourage parents to call with questions about health problems the child develops, and provide information about lowering risks of diseases. Be sure that families know when to keep children home from school (elevated temperature, active vomiting or diarrhea, coughing up brown or green mucus). Assist schools in setting guidelines for management of infectious diseases in that setting. Contact your local county and state health department for infectious disease guidelines for schools; consult Chapter 19∞ for further ideas.

Many disease prevention strategies are designed as health maintenance activities, since their objectives are to prevent health problems. Some health promotion is also integrated when teaching to children emphasizes how their bodies work

TABLE 14–3 Screening During Health Promotion and Health Maintenance Visits

AGE	RECOMMENDED SCREENING TESTS
5 years	Vision Hearing Lead exposure risk Anemia Hyperlipidemia risk Blood pressure Urinalysis Tuberculosis (if at risk)
6–8 years	Vision Hearing Lead exposure risk Hyperlipidemia risk Blood pressure Tuberculosis (if at risk)
8–10 years	Vision Hearing Hyperlipidemia risk Blood pressure Tuberculosis (if at risk)
10–12 years	Vision Hearing Hyperlipidemia risk Blood pressure Tuberculosis (if at risk)

Adapted from Green, M., & Palfrey, J. S. (Eds.). (2002). Bright futures: Guidelines for health supervision of infants, children and adolescents *(2nd ed.). Arlington, VA: National Center for Education in Maternal and Child Health.*

and how they can best promote their own health. Health promotion activities are important for children such as Jessalyn and Kelly, who have a disease that influences several body systems and the course of which can be altered by healthy lifestyles.

Desired outcomes for the school-age child include prevention of infectious diseases, prompt treatment for acute infections, and careful management of existing health conditions in order to maximize health potential.

INJURY PREVENTION STRATEGIES

Injuries are a common cause of morbidity and mortality among school-age children, and each health maintenance encounter should include injury prevention strategies. Children at this age are increasingly independent and may be harmed by activities they engage in without adults, such as playing with fire or firearms. They participate in many sports and other physical activities and may suffer related injuries. Some children unfortunately suffer harm due to physical abuse. See Chapter 7∞ for further discussion of violence prevention.

Many common injuries are preventable with simple use of protective gear and following safety guidelines. Eighteen percent of youth rarely or never wear seat belts in automobiles (MMWR, 2004). Many children ride bicycles, but only about 14% are protected by helmet use, contributing to 23,000 bicycle-related head injuries annually. Bike helmets could prevent up to 88% of serious brain injuries from bicycle crashes (Committee on Injury and Poison Prevention, American Academy of Pediatrics, 2001). Strategies to make helmet use more attractive and to ensure correct wearing of helmets are needed (see Evidence-Based Practice: Bicycle Helmet Effectiveness and Use). Other risky behaviors that require protective gear include:

- Roller blading
- Skate boarding
- Roller hockey
- Ice hockey
- Football
- Soccer
- Scooters
- Skiing or snowboarding
- Snowmobiling
- Motorcycle and all-terrain vehicle riding

Identify youth engaging in these activities and teach them safe practices. Partner with schools and community groups to establish education programs. Provide information about adequate conditioning for sports in order to decrease chance of overuse injury (Committee on Sports Medicine and Fitness, American Academy of Pediatrics, 2001).

Each visit should contain basic history questions related to injury prevention, and then pursue topics that appear to indicate problems. The following questions are appropriate.

- "How often does your daughter wear a seat belt in the car?" (If less than "always" this issue must be addressed.)
- "What sports or other physical activities do you like, Kelly?"

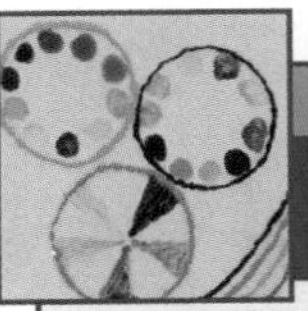

EVIDENCE-BASED PRACTICE
Bicycle Helmet Effectiveness and Use

PROBLEM
About 900 children die of bicycle-related injuries annually in the United States. Although helmets can reduce injury, many times they are not worn or are worn incorrectly.

EVIDENCE
Pender's Health Promotion Model was used in a nursing study that administered a bicycle helmet questionnaire to parents of school-age children. Those parents who received education had significantly higher knowledge scores. In another study, nearly 500 children visiting a pediatric office were asked to bring their helmets to their health supervision visits, or were supplied with one when they came. Although about 73% of the children claimed to wear a helmet when bicycling, only 4% were able to demonstrate correct fitting and wearing of the helmet. Commonly the helmets were worn too high on the head, were not properly strapped on, or were secured so that they moved around the head excessively. The researchers suggest that helmet assessment be integrated into health supervision visits.

NURSING IMPLICATIONS
Interventions can significantly increase parental knowledge about benefits of helmets and their correct use. Nurses should not assume that reports of safety precautions such as wearing helmets or seat belts means that children use these measures correctly. Teach about the benefits of helmets at each health supervision visit. Ask for demonstrations and provide suggestions to improve technique as needed. Common injury causes such as car and bicycle crashes necessitate including at least these evaluations as part of health maintenance activities (Lohse, 2003; Parkinson & Hike, 2003).

CRITICAL THINKING APPLICATION
Where will you find information about helmet safety? How do you determine if a child is wearing a helmet correctly? Plan educational materials and programs for children who bicycle.

- "Who would you go to if someone was touching you inappropriately or if you felt uncomfortable with anyone?"
- "Do you have firearms, Mr. Bonci? Describe how you store them in the house."
- "You say you come home after school now. How long do you spend at home before your parents or big brother get home? What do you do during that time?"
- "I see you're playing video games today. How long do you play at home each day? What are your favorite games? Do your parents have any rules about the types of games you can play?"

Once information is collected during the visit, plan two or three health maintenance topics that seem most important for injury prevention in this family. For the previous questions plan the following related interventions.

- Emphasize the importance of wearing a shoulder and lap belt for every car trip. Evaluate by demonstration whether the child wears the belts properly. Review Box 14–3 for recommendations for school-age children.
- Teach about protective gear necessary for any sport in which the child participates. Provide resources for financial assistance for such gear. Bike shops often provide

BOX 14–3 Car Safety for the School-Age Child

Recommendations include:

- For children over 40 lb (generally 4–8 years of age), use a belt-positioning, forward-facing booster seat located in the back seat. Always use both lap and shoulder belts. Make sure the lap belt fits low and tight across the lap/upper thigh area and the shoulder belt is snug across the chest and shoulder to avoid abdominal injuries.
- Children 4′9″ and taller can sit in a regular car seat restrained with lap and shoulder belt that are snug and correctly located across the lap and chest. Back seat is preferred for all children and necessary for children 12 years and younger.

Note: ALL children 12 years and younger should ride in the back seat.

discounts on helmets for low-income families, health fairs may provide gear, and local community groups will often make contributions.

- Teach all children safe resources such as teachers, school counselors, and police. If they do not feel safe with one person, even if in these groups, encourage them to contact someone else. Further information on child abuse is found in Chapter 7∞.
- Be sure parents store firearms locked, with ammunition locked in a separate place. Remind them that most school-age children can find keys that are stored in desks, drawers, and other locations at home. Have them get the keys out of accessible household locations, and to install trigger locks if they are not already in place as an additional safeguard.
- Suggest activities when alone and provide resources for the child. See Partnering with Families on page 463 for further suggestions for the child at home alone.
- Encourage parents to limit television and video game time to less than 2 hours daily. They should avoid violent television shows and games and can look at ratings on boxes to learn about violence and sexual content. Encourage children to begin self-monitoring to limit screen time and avoid violence.

When you have identified a history of injury in the child, partner with the family to plan ways to avoid repeated harm. Examples that indicate a need for specific discussion are:

- Firearm injury
- Fractures
- Known or suspected child abuse
- Dirt bike or motorcycle injury
- Burns from setting fires

See Table 14–4 for common injury hazards during the school years. See Table 14–5 for injury prevention teaching.

NURSING MANAGEMENT

Nursing Assessment and Diagnosis

Assessment of health promotion and health maintenance topics occurs in many settings with school-age children. They may be seen in offices or clinics, in settings designed to provide such care. They may come for episodic care for a fracture or infection, and health promotion and health maintenance can be easily integrated. They may be seen in the home or neighborhood center, and are frequently encountered by nurses in schools. Take advantage of opportunities for assessment and intervention when they occur. The individual child is examined, and the family, friends, school, and community are addressed. These visits provide an opportunity to identify early and intervene in health-related problems that emerge or become apparent during school age. Examples include:

- Anxiety
- Attention deficit hyperactivity disorder
- Child abuse
- Domestic violence
- Eating disorders
- Learning problems
- Mental retardation and developmental disabilities
- Mood disorders
- Aggression and violence
- Substance abuse
- Parental depression and other mental disorders

(Green & Palfrey, 2002, p. 121)

Assessment can be considered on two levels with school-age children. Individual children may be assessed for height and weight, for immunization status, and for use of protective gear during sports. Populations of children may also be assessed since school age is the first time that large numbers of children are together in certain settings. The findings from such assessments will become the basis of an **individualized approach** or a **population-based approach** to health promotion and health maintenance. For example, nurses commonly measure height and weight and calculate body mass index (BMI) for individual children seen in a clinic. The results are shared with the family, and appropriate teaching about weight control and nutritious intake can be addressed. In other settings, nurses may measure a classroom of children and use the collective data to plan appropriate interventions. If 40% of children in a school are classified as overweight by BMI percentile, much emphasis should be placed on teaching about dietary intake, physical activity, and the relationship of recommended weight levels to chronic disease risk. However, if only a small number of children are overweight, interventions may not be as extensive.

Research is needed to develop assessment techniques with groups of children (Lipman & Hayman, 2000). Such assessments and the related interventions consider the contexts or systems of a group of children and integrate them into care. Recall the theory of ecology of human development (see Chapter 5∞); see Table 14–6 for examples of how the ecologic theory application leads to assessments for specific populations of children. Another example of a data gathering tool for populations of children is the Youth Risk Behavior Surveillance. See Chapter 7∞ for further description of this tool, which is administered by the Centers for Disease Control and Prevention (CDC).

TABLE 14–4 Injury Hazards in the School-Age Years

	HAZARD	DEVELOPMENTAL CHARACTERISTICS	PREVENTIVE MEASURES
	Motor vehicle/ pedestrian/ biking crashes	Child plays outside; may follow ball into road; rides two-wheeler.	Teach child safe outside play, especially near streets. Reinforce use of bike helmet. Teach biking safety rules and provide safe places for riding.
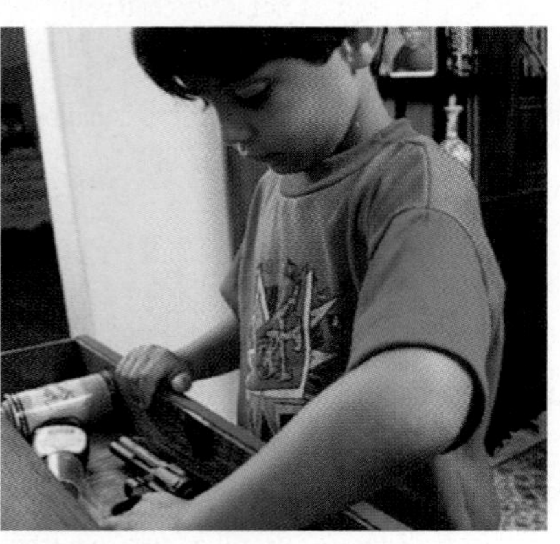	Firearms	Child may have been shown location of guns; is interested in showing them to friends.	Teach child never to touch guns without parent present. Guns should be kept unloaded and locked away. Guns and ammunition should be stored in different locations. Be sure guns have trigger locks.
	Burns	Child may perform experiments with flames or toxic substances.	Teach child what to do in case of fire or if toxic substances touch skin or eyes. Reinforce teaching about 911.
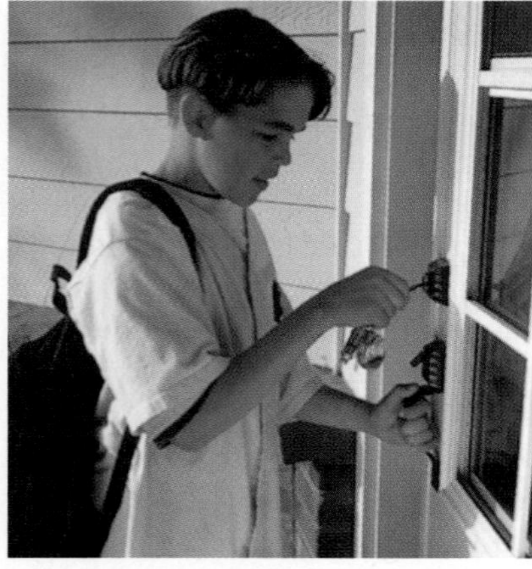	Assault	Child may be left alone after school and may walk, bike, or take public transportation alone.	Provide telephone numbers of people to contact in case of an emergency or if child feels lonely. Leave child alone for brief periods initially, and evaluate child's success in managing time. Teach child not to accept rides from or talk to or open doors to strangers. Teach child how to answer the phone.

Data can be analyzed geographically, by ethnic group, by age categories, or other criteria to describe the risks of groups of children. Nurses look to these national data, and to regional surveys to provide profiles of children in the populations they serve. These collective data can suggest areas that can be applied with groups of children in the local community, as well as with individual children. Many states, cities, and counties provide collective data about health of youth on their websites. Can you find such data for your geographic location on the Internet? How will you use these data to assist in planning assessment of groups of school-age children, or individual children?

Nurses perform growth assessment in school-age children, look for achievement of developmental tasks, assess physical and mental health, and note social characteristics. Based on the assessment of individual or populations of children, nursing diagnoses for child and families are established. Possible nursing diagnoses include the following:

- Delayed Growth and Development related to abuse
- Impaired Parenting related to lack of knowledge about child health maintenance
- Sleep Deprivation related to sleep terrors
- Risk for Violence Directed at Others related to history of witnessing family violence
- Risk for Loneliness related to long periods alone after school
- Health-Seeking Behaviors related to locating swimming classes

TABLE 14–5 Injury Prevention Topics by Age

AGE	INJURY PREVENTION TEACHING
5–8 years	Use a booster seat, properly positioned in the back seat of the car; use lap and shoulder belts Never place the child in a front car seat with a passenger air bag Be sure the child knows how to swim and works on this skill regularly Protect the child with sunscreen when outside Check smoke alarms and keep them in proper function Have an escape plan in case of fire in the home Keep poisons, electrical appliances, fire starters locked Keep firearms unloaded and locked; store ammunition in separate locked location; have trigger locks installed on guns; keep dangerous knives locked Provide protective gear for bicycling and other activities and insist that it be worn Teach safety precautions for bicycling and other activities Teach safety with strangers Provide list of people a child can approach if feeling threatened by touch or other experience Choose care providers carefully; occasionally pick up child earlier than expected; ask policies about discipline and do not leave child with someone who uses corporal punishment Be sure the child knows emergency numbers, names, and plans Review carefully any hazardous event that has occurred with the child and summarize what was done correctly and how response could be improved Limit screen time to 2 hours daily; do not allow violent games, videos, or television programs Review behavior with strangers regularly such as not getting in cars, not engaging in phone or Internet conversations
8–10 years	Car booster seat used until child sits upright against back seat with bent knees over edge of seat; insist on use of lap and shoulder belts Do not place child in front seat of car with a passenger air bag Do not allow child to operate power tools or machinery Continue to reinforce other teaching described above, including child more fully, and enlarging responsibility to the child with increasing age
10–12 years	Continue to reinforce teaching described above Parents and child should attend class on cardiopulmonary resuscitation and airway obstruction removal Avoid high noise levels such as when listening to music through earphones

Adapted from Green, M., & Palfrey, J. S. (Eds.). (2002). Bright futures: Guidelines for health supervision of infants, children, and adolescents *(2nd ed.). Arlington, VA: National Center for Education in Maternal and Child Health.*

■ Planning and Implementation

The nurse is instrumental in planning interventions to promote and maintain health in school-age children. When working with individuals, summarize the strengths and needs that you have identified during the visit, and ask child and family if they concur. Plan together to provide the needed information for topics you have identified as a group. Be sure to emphasize those areas where the family excels. For example, positively reinforce use of car seat belts, use of protective sports gear, and being current with immunizations. Summarize the next expected developmental tasks, such as increasing independence and growing self-responsibility for choosing snacks and television shows. Provide anticipatory guidance to assist with the child's growing independence. As peers are becoming more important, focus discussion on maintaining healthy social relationships through school peers, faith-based or community events, and sibling contacts. A combination of discussion and reading material or pertinent websites for later exploration are welcomed by most families. Provide telephone numbers of resources for questions and community contacts. Inform the parents of the next health promotion/maintenance visit recommendation. If you come in contact with school children for episodic care, ask when the last health maintenance visit occurred. If a child is seen for healthcare after a bicycling accident, the family may be receptive to teaching about safety precautions. When exposed to injuries to the skin a review of the last tetanus booster may reveal health maintenance needs. Use every opportunity to work with individual children and insert appropriate health promotion/maintenance topics.

TABLE 14–6 Application of Ecology of Development to Assessment of Child Populations

SYSTEM	ASSESSMENT EXAMPLES
Microsystem	➤ Types of common injuries in the community ➤ Neighborhood services for swimming, bicycle safety ➤ School curriculum offerings about abuse issues
Exosystem	➤ School board policies related to teaching health promotion and health maintenance activities ➤ Parks department offerings for youth ➤ Amount of involvement of adult volunteers and local businesses in area schools
Macrosystem	➤ State grants for smoking prevention and cessation among youth ➤ Insurance reimbursement for health promotion teaching ➤ Availability of results of Youth Risk Behavior Surveillance and other studies to local communities

When working with groups of children, health promotion should focus on known needs, interests, and risk areas. Nurses in school settings have used a variety of creative approaches to promote the health of youth, including development of a program to train students in health topics; these students then become

BOX 14–4 Recommended School Health Program Components

The Centers for Disease Control and Prevention (CDC) conducts the School Health Policies and Programs Study (SHPPS) periodically to measure programs at local and national levels. The components of the system include:

- Health education
- Physical education and activity
- Health services
- Mental health and social services
- Food service
- School policy and environment
- Faculty and staff health promotion
- Family and community involvement

See the Companion Website and Chapter 16 in this book for further information about health objectives in schools.
(Kolbe, Kann, & Brener, 2001)

peer coaches or health advocates in working with other students (Streng, 2000). Another activity is evaluating the components of school health programs and making recommendations for additions as needed (Box 14–4). A newsletter developed to inform school children about health topics has also been used by nurses (Tyrell & Eyles, 1999).

Bulletin boards, community newspapers, television, and community group membership may each be as effective as teaching in school classrooms. Stress reduction teaching should be provided on group and individual levels. Nurses can teach or assist in development of progressive relaxation, deep breathing, biofeedback, yoga, or meditation. See Chapter 3 for an overview of stress reduction techniques. Interventions will be most effective if they begin with an understanding of the population served. What is important to the families of children in your community or school? What are the values, beliefs, and motivation needed for children to make changes that will enhance health (Denehy, 1999)? See Chapter 16 for further analysis of the community that will help you to plan population-based interventions for health promotion and health maintenance.

Evaluation

Seek evaluation from parents during visits for care. Were their questions answered? Do they know where to turn for advice? Do they know when the child should be seen again for health promotion/maintenance?

The expected outcomes for nursing care of individual school-age children include:

- The child demonstrates normal patterns of growth and development.
- The child, family, and community provide a supportive and nurturing environment for the child.
- The child shows growing independence in directing own health promotion activities.

Expected outcomes of nursing care for groups of children include:

- Children identify lifestyle decisions that influence their health status.
- School and community offer resources that help to lessen risk factors related to health and disease/injury prevention.

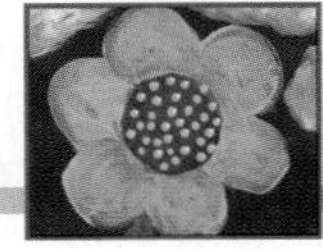

CHAPTER HIGHLIGHTS

- School-age health promotion and health maintenance visits begin with a prekindergarten examination.
- Health promotion should take place in any setting where the child is seen, even for episodic or emergency care.
- Growth measurement and developmental surveillance provide the basis for establishing risk and protective factors for an individual child.
- School children have increasing independence in making food choices; teaching is needed for child and family to promote healthy choices.
- Physical activity should be included in the home and school setting for every child.
- Establishment of self-esteem is an important mental health task of the school-age child.
- Peer relationships play an important role in the lives of school-age children, even though they still depend on families for support and nurturing.
- Injury prevention efforts focus on common causes of morbidity and mortality in young children, such as firearms, abuse, motor vehicle crashes, and sports-related injuries.
- The nurse integrates population-based health promotion activities into all settings where groups of children are seen; individualized approaches are used primarily in clinics and offices and focus on the particular needs of a given child.

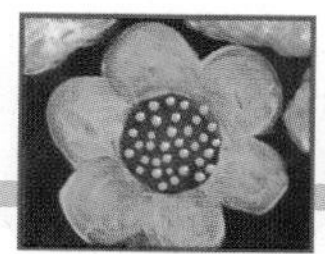

CRITICAL THINKING IN ACTION

INTRODUCTION

Recall the chapter opening scenario involving two sixth graders with type 1 diabetes. The school nurse meets with Jessalyn and Kelly regularly to monitor their management of diabetes and use of insulin pumps. She is in close contact with the endocrinologist who treats the girls, and with the parents of each of them.

DESCRIPTION

Jessalyn has had diabetes for 2 years and is still learning about the disease. She attended a summer camp for diabetics last year which gave her the confidence to try the insulin pump for constant infusion of insulin this academic year. Her parents were surprised about the diagnosis and are now worried about their younger son and whether he will develop the disease. There is no other diabetes history in their family. Recent blood lipid studies indicate a total cholesterol of 180 mg/dL, LDL of 120 mg/dL, and HDL of 32 mg/dL. Her most recent hemoglobin A_{1c} was 7%.

Kelly has an uncle and grandmother with type 1 diabetes and she has had the diagnosis for 7 years. For the last 4 years, she has been using an insulin pump. Her major issues with management of the disease are difficulty maintaining blood glucose at proper levels during a recent growth spurt, and integration of her basketball and volleyball activities into diabetic management.

DISCUSSION

1. Strengths for both Jessalyn and Kelly are their interest in disease management, access to a school nurse, and supportive families. What other protective factors can you identify?
2. What support and information would be helpful for the parents of Jessalyn and Kelly? How do their needs for information differ? How do these differences relate to the specific situations in the microsystems of their families?
3. Jessalyn and Kelly are in a transition stage between school age and adolescence. Consult Chapter 5 to examine their expected cognitive stages. How would you approach teaching for them based on their developmental level?
4. How might the physical growth patterns of 12-year-old girls affect management of diabetes?
5. Consider the psychosocial stages of Jessalyn and Kelly. Are there diabetic management issues that could be related to expected social interactions during older school age? What are the benefits of summer camp attendance for school-age children with a health problem?
6. Examine Jessalyn's lipid levels. Consult Chapter 26 and the laboratory values in Appendix C to evaluate these findings. Review your knowledge of pathophysiology to describe why lipid levels should be measured in diabetics.
7. What does hemoglobin A_{1c} measure? What is your evaluation of Jessalyn's level?
8. Outline health promotion related to nutrition and physical activity that you will plan for Jessalyn and Kelly.

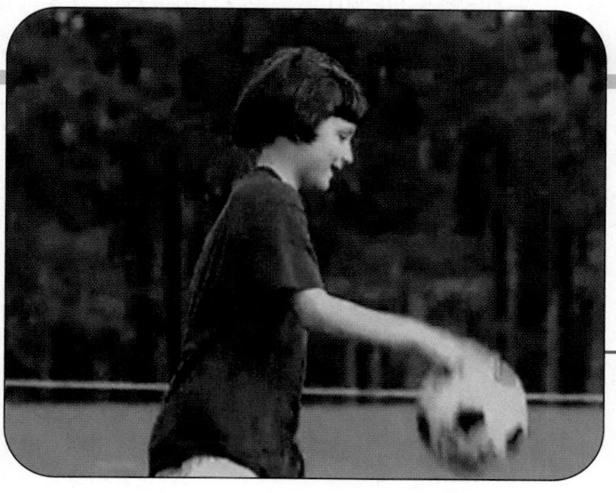

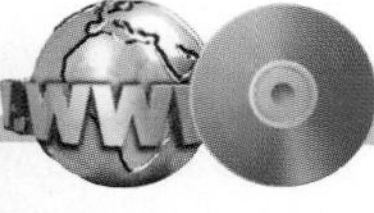

EXPLORE MediaLink

- NCLEX review, case studies, and other interactive resources for this chapter can be found on the Companion Website at **www. prenhall.com/ball**. Click on Chapter 14 to select the activities for this chapter.
- For animations, more NCLEX review questions, and an audio glossary, access the accompanying CD-ROM in this book.

http://www.prenhall.com/ball

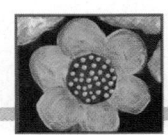

REFERENCES

Adderly-Kelly, B., & Green, P. M. (2000). Health promotion for urban middle school students: A survey of learning needs. *Journal of National Black Nurses Association, 22*, 34–38.

American Psychiatric Association (2000). *Diagnostic and statistical manual of mental disorders: DSM-IV-TR*. Washington, DC: American Psychiatric Association.

Colyar, M. R. (2003). *Well-child assessment for primary care providers*. Philadelphia: FA Davis.

Committee on Injury and Poison Prevention, American Academy of Pediatrics. (2001). Bicycle helmets. *Pediatrics, 108*, 1030–1032.

Committee on Sports Medicine and Fitness, American Academy of Pediatrics. (2001). Risk of injury from baseball and softball in children. *Pediatrics, 107*, 782–784.

Denehy, J. (1999). Health promotion: A golden opportunity for school nurses. *Journal of School Nursing, 15* (5), 4–5.

Dombrowski, M. A. (1999). Preventing disease with stress management in elementary schools. *Journal of School Health, 69*, 126–127.

Finney, J. W., Brophy, C. J., Friman, P. C., Golden, A. S., Richman, G. S., & Ross, A. R. (1990). Promoting parent-provider interaction during young children's health-supervision visits. *Journal of Applied Behavioral Analysis, 23*, 207–213.

Green, M., & Palfrey, J. S. (Eds.). (2002). *Bright futures: Guidelines for health supervision of infants, children, and adolescents* (2nd ed.). Arlington, VA: National Center for Education in Maternal and Child Health.

Jellinek, M., Patel, B. P., & Froehle, M. C. (Eds.). (2002). *Bright futures in practice: Mental health* (Vols. I and II). Arlington, VA: National Center for Education in Maternal and Child Health.

Kolbe, L. J., Kann, L., & Brener, N. D. (2001). Overview and summary of findings: School health policies and programs study 2000. *Journal of School Health, 71*, 253–259.

Lipman, T. H., & Hayman, L. L. (2000). Celebrating 25 years of pediatric nursing research: Progress and prospects. *MCN, 25*, 331–335.

Lohse, J. L. (2003). A bicycle safety education program for parents of young children. *Journal of School Nursing, 19*, 100–110.

MMWR. (2004). Youth Risk Behavior Surveillance—United States, 2003. *Morbidity and Mortality Weekly Report, 53*(SS-02), 1–96.

Murray, R. B., & Zentner, J. P. (2001). *Health promotion strategies through the life span* (7th ed.). Upper Saddle River, NJ: Prentice Hall.

Parkinson, G. W., & Hike, K. E. (2003). Bicycle helmet assessment during well visits reveals severe shortcomings in condition and fit. *Pediatrics, 112*, 320–323.

Patrick, K., Spear, B., Holt, K., & Sofka, D. (Eds.). (2001). *Bright futures in practice: Physical activity*. Arlington, VA: National Center for Education in Maternal and Child Health.

Pender, N. J., Murdaugh, C. L., & Parsons, M. A. (2002). *Health promotion in nursing practice* (4th ed.). Upper Saddle River, NJ: Prentice Hall.

Story, M., Holt, K., & Sofka, D. (Eds.). (2002). *Bright futures in practice: Nutrition*. Arlington, VA: National Center for Education in Maternal and Child Health.

Streng, N. (2000). A student health advocate program. *Journal of School Nursing, 16*, 50–53.

Task Force on the Family. (2003). Family pediatrics: Report of the Task Force on the Family. *Pediatrics, 111*(Supp), 1541–1571.

Tyrell, A., & Eyles, P. (1999). Health promotion in elementary schools: A newsletter as one strategy. *Journal of School Health, 69*, 341–343.

VanAntwerp, C. A. (1995). The Lifestyle Questionnaire for school-aged children: A tool for primary care. *Journal of Pediatric Health Care, 9*, 251–255.

Wainwright, P., Thomas, J., & Jones, M. (2000). Health promotion and the role of the school nurse: A systematic review. *Journal of Advanced Nursing, 32*, 1083–1091.

Wertlieb, D. (2003). Converging trends in family research and pediatrics: Recent findings for the American Academy of Pediatrics Task Force on the Family. *Pediatrics, 111*(Supp), 1572–1587.

Young, K. T. (1998). Listening to parents: A national survey of parents with young children. *Archives of Pediatric and Adolescent Medicine, 152*, 255–262.

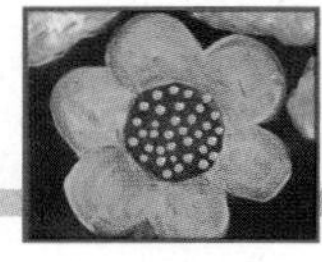

ADDITIONAL REFERENCES

Edelman, C. L., & Mandle, C. L. (2002). *Health promotion throughout the life span* (5th ed.). St. Louis: Mosby.

Halfon, N. (2002). *Child rearing in America: Challenges facing parents with young children*. New York: Cambridge University Press.

Halfon, N., Regalado, M., McLearn, K. T., Kuo, A., & Wright, K. (2003). *Building a bridge from birth to school: Improving developmental and behavioral health services for young children*. New York: The Commonwealth Fund.

Kerker, B., Horowitz, S. M., Leventhal, J. M., et al. (2000). Identification of violence in the home: Pediatric and parental reports. *Archives of Pediatric and Adolescent Medicine, 154*, 457–462.

O'Donnell, G. W., & Mickalide, A. D. (1998). *SAFE KIDS at home, at play and on the way: A report to the nation on unintentional childhood injury*. Washington, DC: National SAFE KIDS Campaign.

VanLandeghen, K., Bronstein, J., & Brach, C. (2003, June). *Children's dental access in Medicaid. The role of medical care use and dentist participation* (CHIRI Issue Brief 2, AHRQ Publication No. 03-0032). Rockville, MD: Agency for Healthcare Research and Quality. www.ahrq.gov/about/chirident.htm, accessed 6/30/2003.

Young, L. E., & Hayes, V. (2002). *Transforming health promotion practice: Concepts, issues, and applications*. Philadelphia: FA Davis.

Health Promotion and Health Maintenance of the Adolescent

Chapter

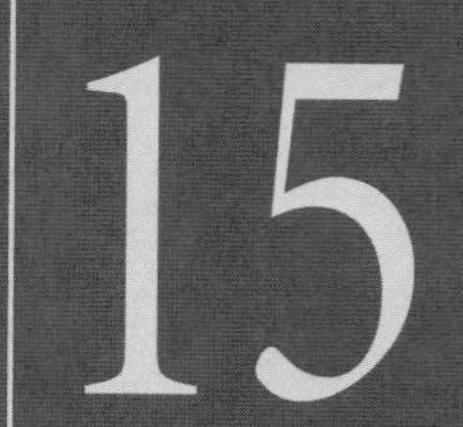

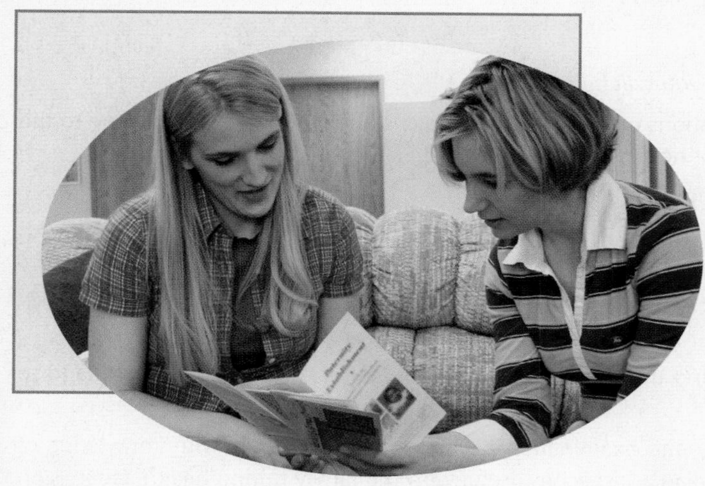

Kim Patterson is a sexually active 16-year-old female who has come to the clinic to obtain birth control pills. A history is taken and physical examination performed. Kim is found to be anemic, and states that she has trouble talking with her parents about her boyfriend and other important things. She wishes she could talk with them more freely. The nurse teaches Kim about the risks of sexually transmitted diseases, and helps Kim examine what makes it difficult to talk with her parents, and to identify where she can go to get support and discuss issues that she does not want to explore with her parents. A casual sofa is available for collecting history before the examination and for performing teaching; teens feel comfortable with this approach.

What should the nurse do for follow-up during the next visit with Kim? Which immunizations might Kim need for disease prevention? What special skills are needed to partner with an adolescent in health supervision visits? Consider these questions as you read this chapter.

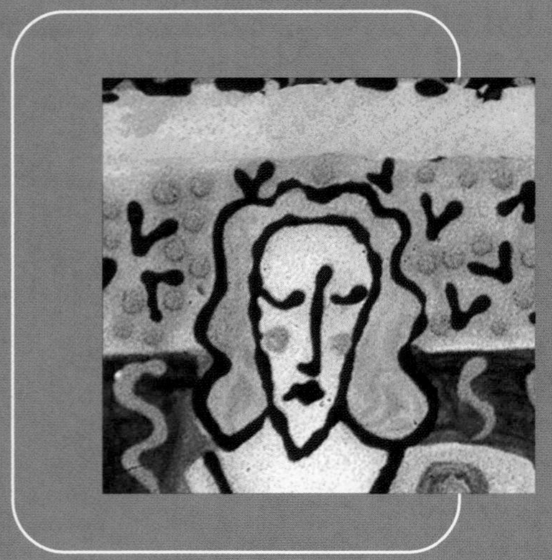

"I've never really liked going to see the doctor or nurse. But now that I need some birth control, I have to do it. They're actually pretty nice here and have helped me with a lot of things. It doesn't even seem like a doctor's office. It feels like I can ask questions and they won't just lecture me about what to do."

—Kim, age 16

Key Terms

modeling/482
outcome expectancy/482
self-efficacy/482

Learning Outcomes

After completing this chapter, you will be able to:

- Describe the general observations made of adolescents and their families as they come to the pediatric healthcare home for health supervision visits.
- Identify the major health concerns of adolescents.
- Apply assessment skills to gather data regarding nutrition, physical activity, mental health status, and growth and development of adolescents.
- Apply therapeutic communication skills with the adolescent and family during health supervision visits.
- Intervene with adolescents and their families to integrate activities to promote health and to prevent disease and injury.
- Synthesize data from history and examination of adolescent and family with knowledge of adolescent development to plan approaches useful with the family during health supervision encounters.

MediaLink 

http://www.prenhall.com/ball

Resources for this chapter can be found on the CD-ROM accompanying this textbook, and on the Companion Website at www.prenhall.com/ball. Click on Chapter 15 to select the activities for this chapter.

CD-ROM
Video
Teen Mental and Spiritual Health
NCLEX Review
Audio Glossary

COMPANION WEBSITE
NCLEX Review
Case Study: Immunization Update
MediaLink Applications
Develop a Teaching Plan: Smoking Education

Even though visits are recommended annually, adolescents are often seen only sporadically for healthcare (Box 15–1). They are usually healthy, may not need immunizations, and consequently do not often come for healthcare. If they have a minor illness, come in for birth control, have a chronic condition requiring periodic assessments, or need a sports examination, the visit should be viewed as a health supervision opportunity (Figure 15–1 ■). While all components of the usual visit may not be performed, at least those parts most important are inserted into care. If time is limited, the nurse has to decide which topics to address during a healthcare visit. It is advisable to start with the topic of most interest to the teen and then to insert injury prevention teaching, since injury is the greatest risk to teens. (See Chapter 1∞.) Health promotion topics such as dietary and exercise habits could be discussed if time permits. Mental health assessment and teaching are other areas of prime importance. If the teen suggests an immediate risk, such as considering suicide in response to depression, this must be dealt with immediately by collaborating with a mental health specialist.

What general principles can guide programs to promote health in adolescents? Researchers have analyzed theory application and approaches of programs, and others have suggested key elements of programs (Box 15–2). Programs that assist adolescents in taking on health promotion behaviors foster a sense of competence, confidence in the youth's own abilities, building of a sense of character and responsibility, connection to other youth and beneficial programs, and the qualities of caring and compassion (Lerner & Thompson, 2002). When establishing youth programs, whether with individual adolescents or with groups, the nurse includes evaluation of effectiveness and plan methods to enlarge and sustain successful approaches.

How does the nurse interact with the adolescent in order to be effective in health promotion and health maintenance activities? What are the major health supervision needs of adolescents? How does the nurse recognize the independence of the teen but yet include parents as partners in the youth's healthcare team? These are some of the questions that will be addressed in this chapter.

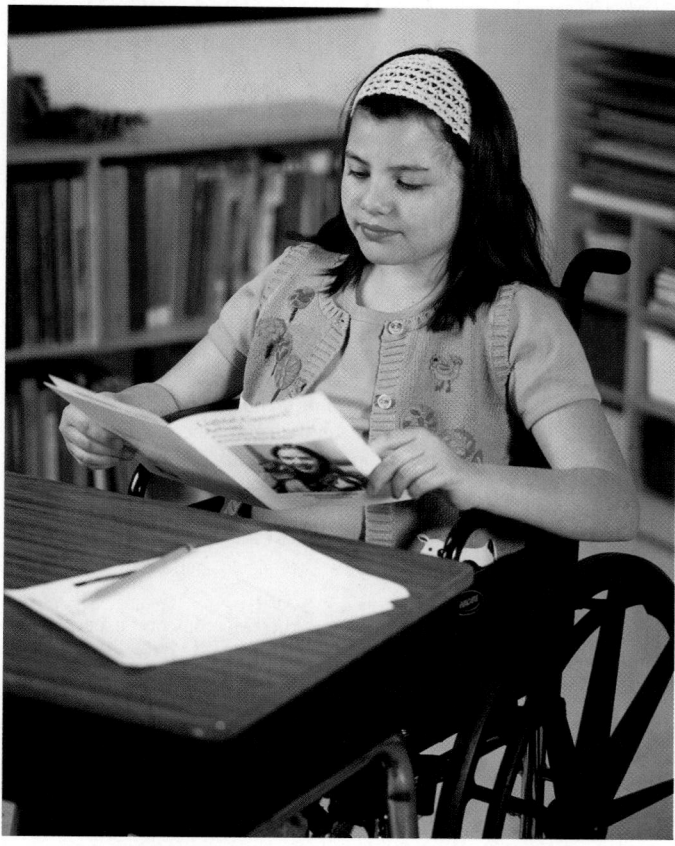

FIGURE 15–1 ■ This teen, who uses a wheelchair, does well in school and has many friends and activities. When she comes for periodic health care visits, health promotion and health maintenance activities should be integrated into the examinations.

BOX 15–1 Adolescents and Recommended Health Supervision Visits

The teenager often comes in for care only sporadically. However, it is recommended that health supervision visits occur annually during the teen years, since many health topics are important to address. The ages recommended for care by the American Academy of Pediatrics are:

- 12 years
- 13 years
- 14 years
- 15 years
- 16 years
- 17 years
- 18 years
- 19 years

When you see adolescents who come in for an illness or injury, or in a school or other setting, find out when the adolescent was last seen for a health supervision visit. Ask if they have a pediatric healthcare home and reinforce the need to make an appointment. If there is not an agency relationship established, suggest a resource in your community.

GENERAL OBSERVATIONS

The beginning of the visit with an adolescent can be an important source of information, just as it is with younger children. However, the adolescent is at a more advanced stage of development, and the observations you make will relate to this developmental stage.

Ideally, the facility has a waiting area that is designed for teens. Teens may not want to wait for healthcare with either young children or older adults. Teen waiting areas are popular because they provide a special place, thereby relaying that the teen is important, and can use video and other popular methods to impart health information while the teen waits. As you call the adolescent in for care, observe if parents or friends are present, or if the teen is alone. Young adolescents often come with parents to the facility, and parents may wait in the waiting room during the examination (Figure 15–2 ■). If the teen comes in for a specific problem such as a skin lesion or other health concern, the parent may accompany the adolescent into the examination room. If someone does come with the teen, be aware that you may need to provide private time by asking the other person to wait outside for a moment. Reassure the parents that they will have an opportunity to ask questions and discuss their concerns.

BOX 15–2 Research: Theories Used in Health Promotion Programs for Adolescents

A review that analyzed articles describing adolescent health promotion identified the most common theories used (Montgomery, 2002). Two major theories described are:

1. **Social cognitive theory.** This theory was developed by Walter Bandura, who is described in Chapter 5∞ (Bandura, 1985, 1997a, 1997b). The key components of his theory involve **self-efficacy** (the person's belief in his or her ability to perform a behavior) and **outcome expectancy** (what the person expects to get from performing a certain behavior). Learning a new behavior occurs through **modeling**, or imitation of the behavior of someone else. Bandura believes that individuals make decisions about health behaviors based on thought about the consequences and outcomes of those behaviors. The *person's characteristics*, such as self-efficacy and outcome expectancy, interact with the external *environment* and the *behavioral choices* available. All of these components interact to determine health behaviors, and all can be influenced to promote health. If you were seeking to promote physical activity behaviors in youth, some essential components would be:
   - Encourage youth to believe they could perform the activity (self-efficacy)
   - Point out the positive aspects of the behavior (outcome expectancy)
   - Show youth how to do the activity (modeling)
   - Provide a physical setting and opportunity for performing the behavior (environment)
   - Allow trial and error, choice in time and extent of activity (behavioral choices)
2. **Health belief model.** This theory attempts to explain why some individuals take actions to prevent disease or promote health while others do not. Factors that influence the likelihood of taking on preventive behaviors include the *perceived susceptibility to disease, seriousness of the disease, perceived benefits of preventive action*, and *barriers to preventive actions*. Modifying factors include knowledge, personality, and peer influence, while cues such as media or reminders by a healthcare professional also influence perception of the condition and therefore influence action (Becker, Haefner, Kasl, et al., 1977). When using this theory to encourage physical activity in youth, the program would include information about the following:
   - Necessity of exercise to prevent problems such as overweight, diabetes, and cardiovascular disease
   - Prevalence of serious diseases in those with low levels of activity
   - Benefits of physical activity to weight control, health, and sense of well-being
   - Common reasons people do not exercise along with methods to dispel these reasons

The adolescent is able to respond to questions and requests, and to state the reason for the visit. Be alert for teens who cannot perform these basic skills and examine them carefully as described in the next section of this chapter. Observe interactions with parents and others who accompany the child to the visit. Some teens are comfortable in healthcare settings and actively engage in conversation, while others are nervous and will need more explanations and reassurance as you progress with the first steps of measurement and blood pressure.

Your initial observations will guide some of the interactions with the teen. For example, if a teen is overweight, provide a quiet and private location while taking the weight, and do not announce the weight aloud. Being alert, quiet, and sensitive are all important qualities of the nurse working with adolescents.

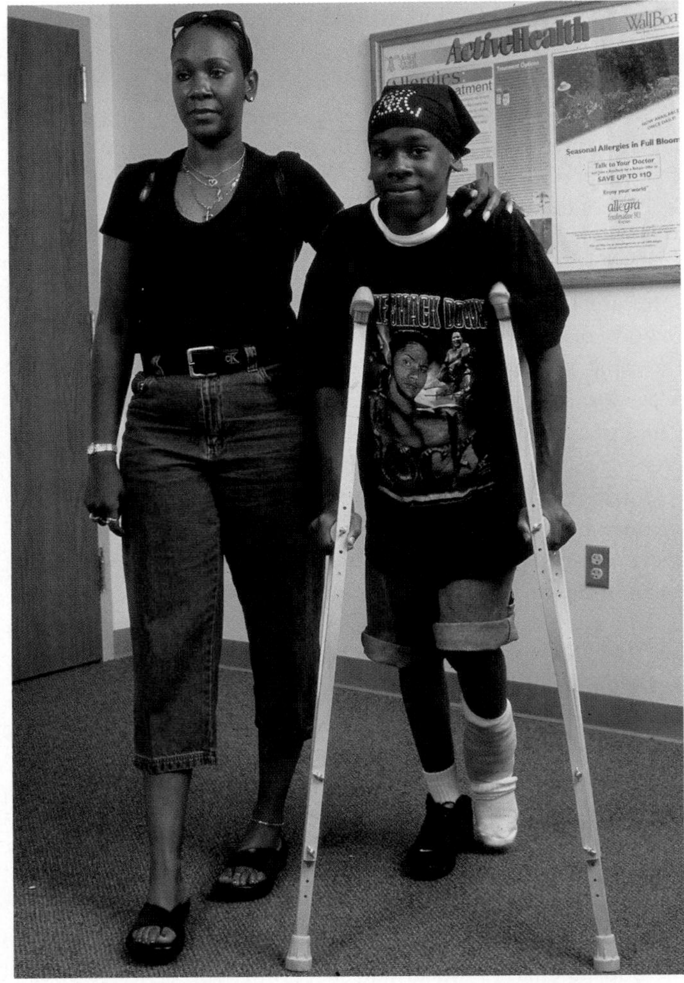

FIGURE 15–2 ■ Parents often accompany teens with a healthcare problem in for the examination. Provide an opportunity to see both the teen and parent privately and integrate general health promotion and health maintenance into the visit. What questions can you ask this teen? What teaching might be needed?

In our discussion on health promotion and health maintenance of the school-age child (see Chapter 14∞), we noted that the healthcare partnership grew from one with parents to one encompassing the child as a partner as well. By adolescence, children should be assuming more of a partnership role in their own healthcare. As the visit begins, greet adolescents warmly, ask about their concerns and questions, and ask for their opinions and reactions throughout the visit. This will demonstrate that their thoughts are important and that they play an important role in guiding the healthcare visits. When adolescents are visiting the same office or clinic that they came to during childhood, they usually know and feel comfortable with the care providers. If the setting is new to them, explain procedures and introduce personnel so they feel more at ease.

GROWTH AND DEVELOPMENTAL SURVEILLANCE

Adolescence spans several years, and growth and developmental issues vary throughout the period. For young adolescents, or those from about 12 to 13 years of age, growth measurement remains important. Many youth are still growing and use of percentile grids continues to be an important part of care. Growth should remain in the same percentile channel as during childhood (see description of growth channels in Chapter 14), with girls reaching nearly adult height at this age, and boys still continuing to grow. Be alert as always, for youth who have either increased or decreased channels, or are above the 85th percentile or below the 5th percentile for body mass index (BMI). They will need additional assessment of nutritional intake and physical activity (see Chapter 9).

By middle and late adolescence, adult growth is nearly achieved, earlier for girls than boys. While measurement continues to be performed, nurses assess the BMI more carefully to be sure the height and weight indicate appropriate intake and exercise. Overweight at this age is likely to continue into adulthood, particularly if parents are overweight, so early intervention will be needed to decrease this potential. Other youth may have eating disorders and should be referred to a specialist for care. Children from homes without sufficient financial resources may be hungry and lack food. Parents who were eligible for Women, Infant, and Child (WIC) Nutrition Program services when children were younger may not receive them once the child is an adolescent, so the increasing dietary intake needs of their teens cannot be met. If an adolescent is thin and has little energy, consider this possibility; administer the food security questionnaire found in Chapter 9.

There are few options for measuring the developmental competence of adolescents, but observations and questions during care provide information about the meeting of developmental milestones. Key tasks for adolescents involve separating from the parents and establishing positive relationships with peers. The young teen may come to an appointment with a parent and rely on that parent to answer some questions during the examination. However, the middle and late teen should be increasingly able to come alone, answer questions, and assume responsibility for healthcare decisions. Offer older teens the option of coming into the room alone, stating, "Your mom can wait here and we can come and get her later. Does that sound all right?" During your time with an adolescent, ask questions such as the following to learn about peer interactions and activities.

- "Describe your two best friends."
- "What are the two things you like best about school? What do you not like?"
- "Describe how you generally spend Friday and Saturday nights."
- "Describe what you do before and after school."
- "What do you like about the way your parents treat you? What do you not like?"
- "What are your plans for (the summer, the vacation coming up, after high school)?"

The adolescent receives a physical examination, often by the nurse practitioner or physician. See Chapter 8 for components of the examination. Some particular parts of the examination to include for teens are scoliosis screening, sexual maturity rating (Tanner stages), breast exam, testing for sexually transmitted diseases (among those sexually active), pelvic exam and Pap smear (for sexually active females), hematocrit for anemia annually in menstruating adolescents, hearing screening at 12, 15, and 18 years, blood pressure annually, lipid screening for those with family history of early heart disease or other risk factors, and tuberculosis for those in high-risk areas. Most adolescents do not want parents present during the examination, but occasionally will want a parent for something like a first pelvic examination or a blood draw. Ask them their wishes in a confidential setting so they can freely make the choice. They also may choose to have a healthcare provider of the same gender complete the genitourinary examination.

During all parts of the admission and measurement process, and during the physical examination, the nurse is aware of the teen's developmental progression. Teaching is applied throughout the entire visit. While details about essential components are discussed throughout this chapter, Table 15–1 provides a list of topics that should be addressed, along with questions to ask the adolescent and teaching to include. Health promotion approaches are used when the teaching emphasizes common teen issues and provides ideas for the adolescent and parent to deal with these concerns. Health maintenance issues are those designed to keep the youth healthy by avoiding disease and preventing injury.

Expected outcomes of care include screening and early identification for common health problems, normal patterns of growth, and meeting of developmental milestones.

NUTRITION

The young adolescent needs a well-balanced diet to support the growth of this period, and the late adolescent requires intake that supports physical activity and provides nutrients for metabolism and to promote the immune system. While nutritional intake is important, teens often do not eat well. They may be busy and do not want to plan meals, they like to eat foods that are popular with other teens so high fat and sugar intake can be common, they may be dieting to achieve weight loss, and some do not have enough financial resources to access proper foods.

Questions that can guide your data gathering include:

- "You mentioned while you were being weighed that you are trying to lose weight. What are you doing to lose the weight? Have you lost any weight yet? How much would you like to weigh? Describe how you exercise."
- "What is your favorite meal? What foods do you dislike or avoid? What do you eat for snacks? Do you drink milk? Do you ever eat cheese or ice cream or yogurt? How often?"
- "Do you take vitamins? Fluoride? Do you take any dietary supplements because of your weight lifting? Do you have to cut back on foods to get into your weight category in wrestling?"
- "Do you bring a lunch to school or eat school lunch? How often does your family eat together?"

TABLE 15–1 Sample Questions and Teaching Topics Pertinent to Adolescence

TOPIC	QUESTIONS	TEACHING
Sleep	"What time do you generally go to bed on school nights? On weekends? Do you feel rested when you get up? Do you have trouble getting to sleep?"	Importance of adequate sleep and rest to school performance, alertness, and safety Recommended hours of sleep Allowing time for bedtime routines and limiting caffeine intake, especially in the afternoon and evening
School performance	"Describe how school is going for you, Franco. Are you getting the grades you expected? What is most difficult for you? Are your teachers available for help when you need it?"	Study habits including adequate time and a quiet setting Resources for getting assistance such as meeting teachers before or after school
Peer interactions	"Describe your best friend. What do you like to do together? Do you usually hang out with one or two friends or in groups? Do you have dates? What do you do on them? Do you have a boyfriend/girlfriend?"	Importance of friends Influence of friends on decisions regarding studying, risky behaviors Sexuality education including decision making about close relationships with others Showing respect and concern for self and friends
Discipline	"What happens when you do something that your parents do not approve of, Carrie? Is it hard for you to set limits for yourself or to do things different than your friends?" (For parents): "How often do you have to discipline Carrie? What kinds of things does she do to get into trouble? How do you feel about your ability to handle discipline for Carrie?"	Establishing limits for self and still feeling accepted by friends (For parents): Deciding appropriate discipline methods such as withdrawing privileges such as driving Limiting rules to those necessary and then consistently enforcing them
Injury prevention	"What sports do you enjoy? What protective gear do you wear for this sport? Have you been hurt doing the sport?" "You have had your driver's license about a year now, Franco. Have you had any tickets? Any accidents? Do you ever drive after drinking? Do you ride with friends who have been drinking?" "So you have been helping with getting in the harvest this year. What part of that is your job?"	Protective gear and practices that decrease sports injury Bicycle and automobile safety Importance of avoiding drinking and driving or operating any machinery Farm safety measures
Planning for future	"You're a junior this year, Franco? Have you started to think about what you will do after graduation? What skills will you need to be able to get that type of job?" "It looks like you have managed well with your baby, Carrie. You will have your GED soon. Do you know what you will do then, and how you'll continue to care for your baby?"	Resources for future planning, such as school counselors, parents, and the Internet Suggesting a visit to potential job sites or colleges to get a realistic view Resources and realistic planning for the teen parent

Compare the information from measurement of the adolescent with the answers to questions about diet in order to identify possible areas for intervention. Determine any questions the teen has about foods, diet, maintaining desired weight, and topics like vegetarianism or supplements to enhance athletic performance. (See Chapter 9 for further detail about these special nutritional topics.) Health promotion plans focus on practices that lead to healthy growth and development, including topics such as:

- Consuming five fruits and vegetables daily
- Including whole grain products to replace refined products when possible
- Eating three meals each day including breakfast and lunch
- Eating together as a family several times weekly, which enhances quality food intake
- Planning menus and preparing foods for balanced intake

Health maintenance plans center on those practices that prevent disease including:

- Limiting refined sugar and high fat intake (such as soft drinks and fried foods) in order to maintain weight at recommended level
- Including two to three servings of dairy products daily to enhance bone formation and decrease chance of osteoporosis as an adult
- Using resources for treatment of eating disorders if they are identified (see Chapter 9)

While much of nutrition teaching should be aimed directly at the adolescent, parents are also included. They can be effective contributors to healthy intake by providing plenty of fruits and vegetables for snacks, having foods attractively prepared and ready for consumption when the teen is hungry, planning several meals together as a family each week, encouraging milk or other forms of calcium intake, and setting a good example for food intake. Help them to identify the youth with an eating disorder and provide resources for intervention in these cases (see Chapter 9 for a full discussion).

Consider as well the teen mother. The adolescent who is pregnant or nursing has even more need for nutritional teaching and may need financial resources to access sufficient food. How will you combine the growth and developmental needs of an adolescent with those of her infant when planning teaching? See the Photo Story on pages 486–487.

PHYSICAL ACTIVITY

Many adolescents suffer from the effects of inadequate physical activity. As children grow and enter the teenage years, physical activity decreases, particularly in girls. Only about 30–60% of adolescents report daily vigorous activity, and the percentage is lower among females and some ethnic groups (Epstein et al., 2001). The recommendation of *Healthy People 2010* (2000) is moderate, stating that adolescents get at least 20–30 minutes of vigorous activity 3–5 days weekly. At a time when teens are not very active as a group, physical education requirements in school are also decreasing, with only 19% of 12th grade students regularly attending a PE class (Lowry, Wechsler, Kann, et al., 2001).

Physical activity levels must therefore be assessed at each health supervision visit or in other contacts with adolescents. Apply resilience theory and assess youth, family, and community for risk and protective factors regarding physical activity (Table 15–2).

Some youth have established regular physical activity programs, and this behavior should be encouraged (Figure 15–3 ■). Be alert for those who exercise but have other health problems. Some athletes try to eat very little to remain a certain weight for wrestling, running, or other sports. Integrate nutritional teaching that includes the importance of adequate intake for sports performance. Other athletes use nutritional supplements to enhance performance (see Chapter 9∞ for a list of some popular products). While most are not harmful, few have proven benefits and their cost is not warranted.

Other youth have very little physical activity and feel incompetent in performing many sports. Work with them to find at least

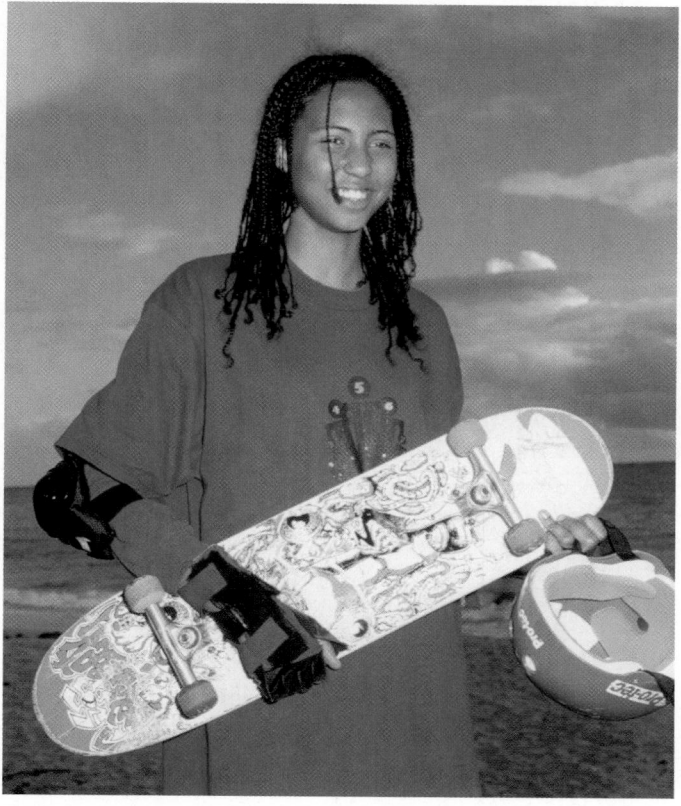

FIGURE 15–3 ■ This teen girl is an avid "boarder." How can you encourage and praise her for the activity? What clues do you have that she is using adequate safety measures?

TABLE 15–2 Risk and Protective Factors Regarding Physical Activity in Adolescence

RISK FACTORS	PROTECTIVE FACTORS
➤ Lives in isolated setting with little opportunity for contact with other teens ➤ Has a developmental disability that impairs physical movement ➤ Does not like physical activity ➤ Has a pattern and history of low activity levels ➤ Is overweight ➤ Does not feel competent in most sports ➤ Limited financial resources to pay registration fees or buy protective gear for sports ➤ Family members who have little physical activity ➤ Parents who are not active in school sports and committees ➤ Parents who do not like physical activity and have had low levels while their teen was growing up ➤ Parents who have little time or facilities for exercise, or always exercise at a club out of view of their family ➤ Lack of youth and parent knowledge about physical activity needs and benefits ➤ Lack of neighborhood programs for physical activity promotion ➤ Presence of neighborhood hazards and unsafe areas	➤ Has opportunities for participation in physical activity at home, at school, and in the community ➤ Likes physical activity ➤ Has exercised during all of childhood, often with parents ➤ Knowledgeable about benefits of activity; committed to maintaining exercise patterns ➤ Has many friends living close who participate in physical activity ➤ Youth and parents agree to a limit of 2 hours daily of screen time ➤ Availability of financial and other resources for sports gear and protective equipment ➤ Parents participate in regular physical activity and encourage the adolescent to do so also ➤ Neighborhood and community provide physical activity options ➤ Public policies maintain parks, green spaces, biking trails, playgrounds ➤ Programs are available for adolescents with developmental disabilities or other healthcare needs

What risk and protective factors for physical activity are present in your community? Go to the Companion Website to examine the positive effect community planning can have on its members' exercise levels.

Adapted from Green, M., & Palfrey, J. S. (2002). Bright futures: Guidelines for health supervision of infants, children, and adolescents *(2nd ed.). Arlington, VA: National Center for Education in Maternal and Child Health.*

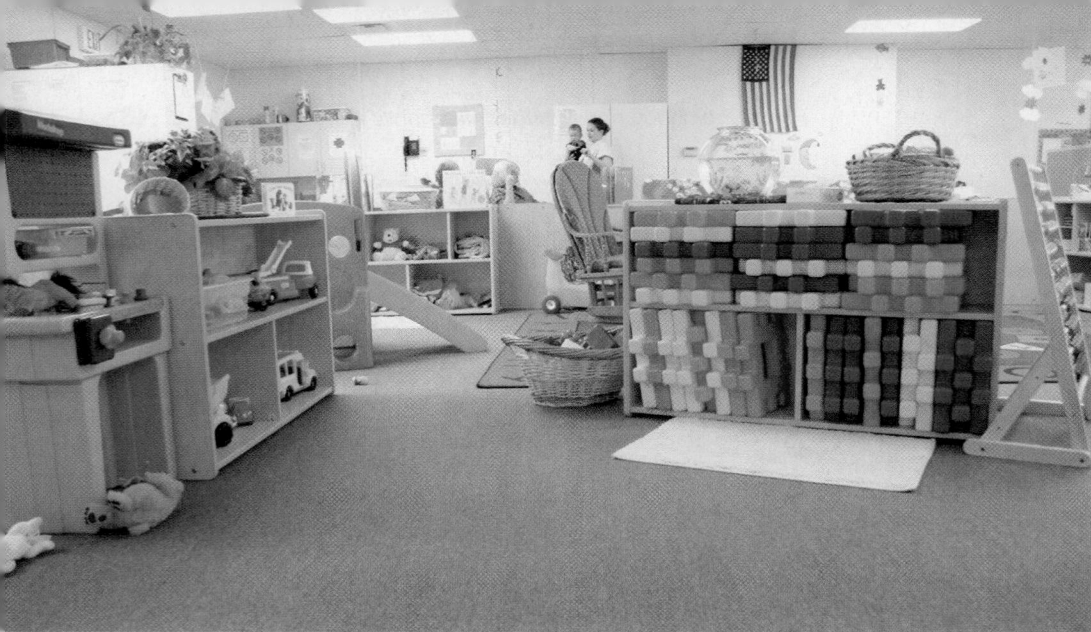

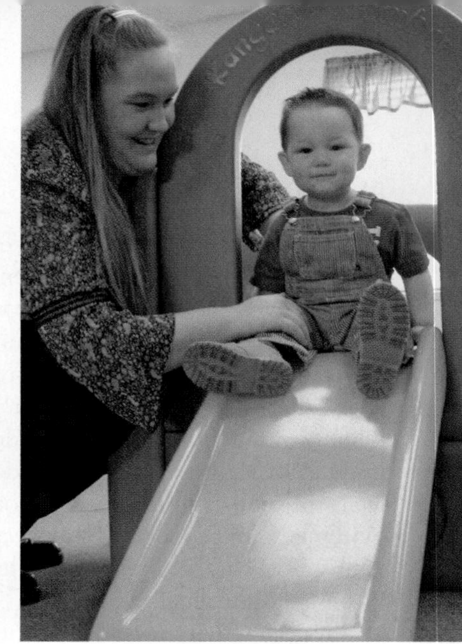

This alternative high school offers a place for teen mothers to continue their education, while sharing experiences and learning how to care for their children. (left)

Charisse and Jeremy take time to play together at the school's childcare center. ***(right)***

PHOTO Story...

Charisse and Jeremy at school

Charisse is the 17-year-old mother of Jeremy. She is enrolled in an alternative high school that supports teens in their education by providing childcare in a stimulating environment. The teens take child development courses as part of the curriculum and spend time each day in the childcare center. Charisse's baby Jeremy is an active, alert toddler who attends the childcare center at the high school, and both he and Charisse enjoy the time they spend together during the day. Charisse is often too busy with school and childcare to fix nutritious meals for her and her son, and she lacks knowledge of how to plan a diet. She wants to feed her baby well, but needs to learn that she influences her child's nutrition by her own example. At the center, she has learned to prepare nutritious food, and to join her son in eating so that he learns healthy eating patterns. Teachers work in the childcare center with the teens to enhance knowledge of child development. The teachers use discussion, show the teens how to find valuable information in books and magazines, help

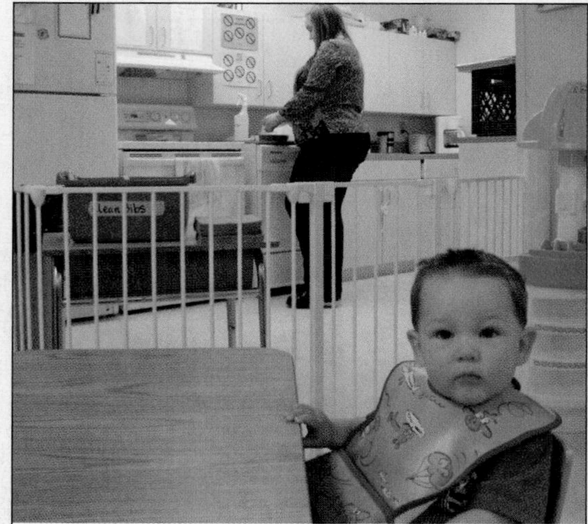

Charisse takes a nutrition course at the school, and is learning to prepare more nutritious meals for herself and Jeremy.

them analyze web sites for accuracy, and have many guests and speakers from the community so that the teens learn about local resources. When parents return to the classroom, the children prepare to take a ride outside with center personnel. Develop a plan for the ways in which the school nurse can partner with teachers and others to support young teens and their infants in a setting such as this.

Jeremy is just over one year of age and has begun to walk. Charisse was unfamiliar with safety hazards for one-year-olds and has benefited from demonstrations in the childcare center about hazardous toys, furniture, wall plugs and other parts of the environment. A teacher and the school nurse visit each teen's home every month. *What environmental assessment will you plan for Charisse's home in order to ensure a safe environment for Jeremy? What teaching is important to avoid some of the most common injuries of toddlers?* (See the section on injury prevention later in this chapter for ideas to integrate into your teaching plan.)

Plan a nutritious daily menu for Jeremy. Consult Chapter 9∞ for details about the recommended daily intake of nutrients and the types and amounts of food needed at Jeremy's age. *What common foods that teens like could be part of Jeremy's diet? Which foods that Charisse likes for herself might not be good choices for Jeremy?* In addition to nutrition, Jeremy's health depends on physical activity. Notice some of the large climbing toys at the child center. *Which gross and fine motor skills are expected at his age?* See Chapter 5∞ for ideas. ■

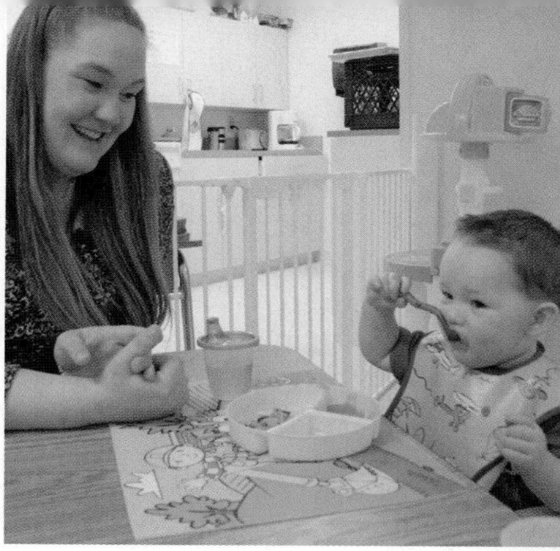

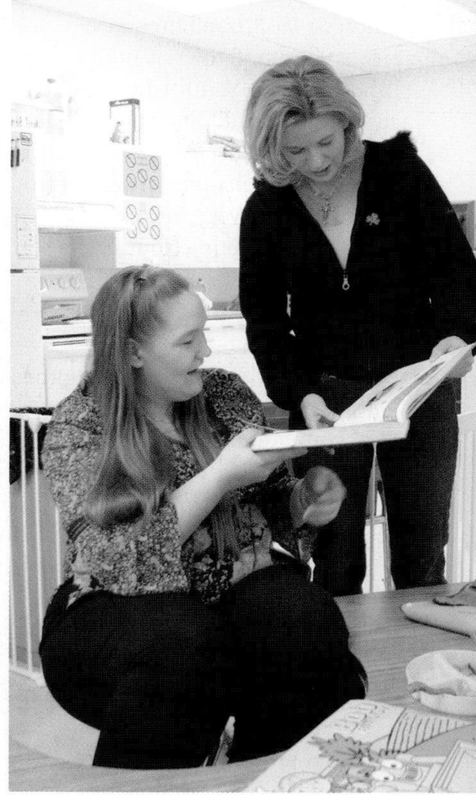

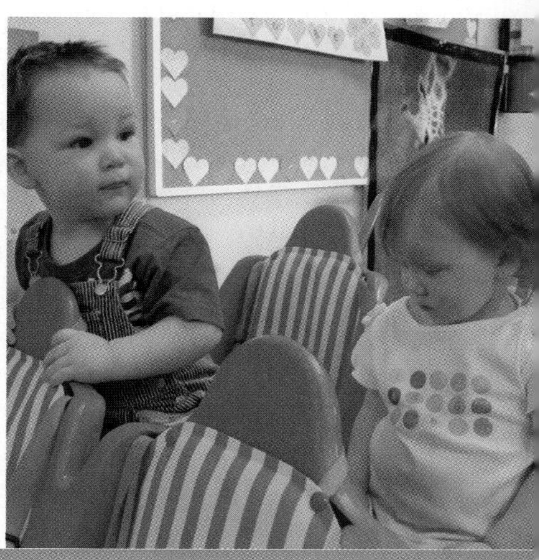

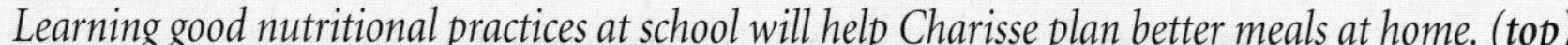

Learning good nutritional practices at school will help Charisse plan better meals at home. ***(top)***

The child development teacher discusses anticipatory guidance with Charisse, who has questions about Jeremy's growth. ***(middle)***

While Charisse is in class, Jeremy remains at the childcare center; knowing that her son is in a safe and nurturing environment allows Charisse to focus on her studies. ***(bottom)***

one thing they can do on a daily basis—walking their dog in the neighborhood, riding a bike to the store, using stairs instead of elevators when possible, parking on the far side of the school lot and walking farther, swimming at a club their parents belong to or at a local YMCA or YWCA, saving money to take lessons for horseback riding, or golf. Form interest groups at schools and community centers that provide an outlet for adolescents who cannot "make the team" for school sports. Encourage parents and adolescents to set goals together to integrate some physical activity daily.

The nurse's activities for health promotion concentrate on teaching the health and mental benefits of physical activity such as increased energy, weight control, and a feeling of control and success. Health maintenance focuses on viewing physical activity as a method to prevent disease such as cardiovascular disease and diabetes. Youth who have family members with these diseases or meet adults who have them are more likely to understand the importance of their own activity.

Desired outcomes include maintenance of weight within recommended level, daily exercise of 20 to 60 minutes, and establishment of lifetime routines for exercise.

ORAL HEALTH

Continued dental care during the adolescent years can ensure oral health. The recommendations remain the same as those for young children. The adolescent should floss daily, brush twice daily with a small amount of fluoridated toothpaste, and visit a dental provider every 6 months. By about 14 years of age, those who do not have fluoridated water and have been taking fluoride can stop this supplement. Even the molars have been formed by that age, so fluoride tablets are no longer needed. Continue to examine the condition of the teeth and the number of erupted permanent teeth present. Be alert for any unusual growths and ulcers in the mouth and refer for care as needed.

One potential concern that should be addressed includes the availability of dental insurance for the adolescent. The teen whose family does not have dental insurance needs referrals for care to affordable resources. Dental specialists clean off plaque that has formed, apply sealants to erupting molars, examine the teeth for caries, and perform restorative care. There are particular groups more at risk for inadequate dental care; see Developing Cultural Competence: Dental Care. When working with these populations, nurses can question access to care, and make recommendations that foster regular checkups. Some teens may wish to whiten the teeth or get orthodontia to improve appearance. The nurse helps the youth and parents to find resources for needed care. Expected outcomes are dental visits twice annually with recommended follow-up care for problems, and good oral health.

MENTAL AND SPIRITUAL HEALTH

Adolescents have many challenges to their mental health and need support to emerge from adolescence with mental and spiritual strengths. Mental health topics must be addressed at each health supervision opportunity to promote mental health among teens. Mental health is closely linked to developmental tasks such as growing independence, formation of close relationships with peers, becoming confident in accomplishments, becoming part of a social group, and setting goals for the future (Figure 15–4 ■).

As during other ages, the self-concept continues to develop and tailors reactions to the environment, and self-regulation in

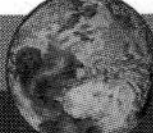

DEVELOPING CULTURAL COMPETENCE
Dental Care

An analysis of several national surveys such as the National Health and Nutrition Examination Survey (NHANES) reported that rural children were more likely (41%) to be uninsured for dental care than urban children (35%). They were also less likely to have visited a dentist in the last year (70%) than urban children (74%). More rural children (8%) had unmet dental needs than did urban children (6%) (Vargas, Ronzio, & Hayes, 2003). When children live in rural areas, be sure to ask about their access to dental care.

Another analysis of NHANES data examined African American respondents. Sixty-two percent reported that they only visit a dentist when needed rather than regularly. Those who were poor, unemployed, uninsured, or living in the South had poorer dental health. If you work with African American youth, be conscious of the need to integrate oral assessment into care, and to encourage utilization of services (Green, Person, Crowther, et al., 2003).

National Health Interview Survey (NHIS) data were analyzed for dental care utilization by Asians and native Hawaiian and other Pacific Islanders. Native Hawaiian and other Pacific Islander children were most likely (82%) to have had a dental visit in the last year, while Asian Indians were least likely to have a visit (60%). Once again, children with no insurance and who were poor were more likely to have less care. In addition, children living with a single parent or someone other than a parent, and those whose parents had under 12 years of education were more likely to have unmet dental needs (Qui & Ni, 2003).

When you work with these populations, be certain to include dental assessment in health supervision visits, and have resources for care readily available.

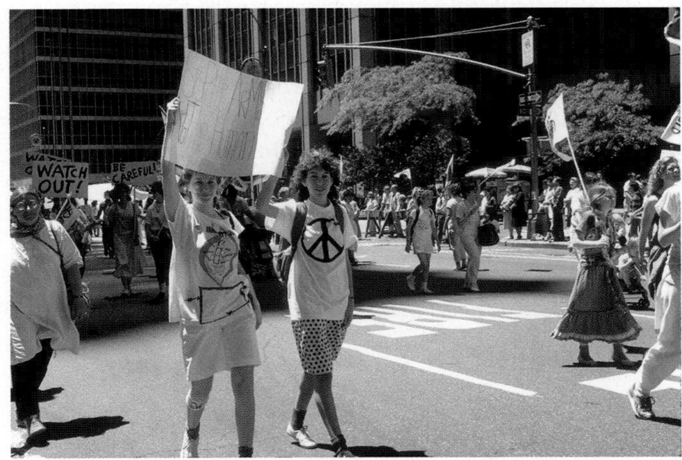

FIGURE 15–4 ■ Teens often become associated with causes. This helps them to feel part of a social group and also provides the opportunities to examine belief systems and make decisions about meaningful activities.

them analyze web sites for accuracy, and have many guests and speakers from the community so that the teens learn about local resources. When parents return to the classroom, the children prepare to take a ride outside with center personnel. Develop a plan for the ways in which the school nurse can partner with teachers and others to support young teens and their infants in a setting such as this.

Jeremy is just over one year of age and has begun to walk. Charisse was unfamiliar with safety hazards for one-year-olds and has benefited from demonstrations in the childcare center about hazardous toys, furniture, wall plugs and other parts of the environment. A teacher and the school nurse visit each teen's home every month. *What environmental assessment will you plan for Charisse's home in order to ensure a safe environment for Jeremy? What teaching is important to avoid some of the most common injuries of toddlers?* (See the section on injury prevention later in this chapter for ideas to integrate into your teaching plan.)

Plan a nutritious daily menu for Jeremy. Consult Chapter 9 for details about the recommended daily intake of nutrients and the types and amounts of food needed at Jeremy's age. *What common foods that teens like could be part of Jeremy's diet? Which foods that Charisse likes for herself might not be good choices for Jeremy?* In addition to nutrition, Jeremy's health depends on physical activity. Notice some of the large climbing toys at the child center. *Which gross and fine motor skills are expected at his age?* See Chapter 5 for ideas. ■

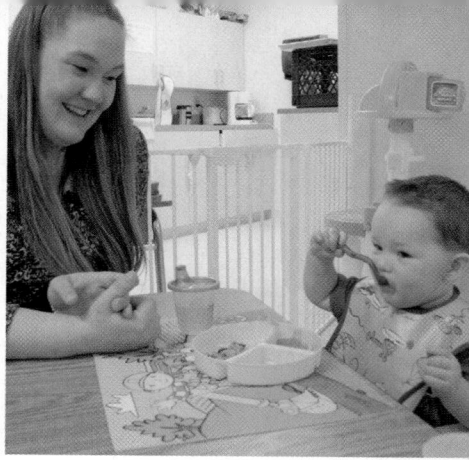

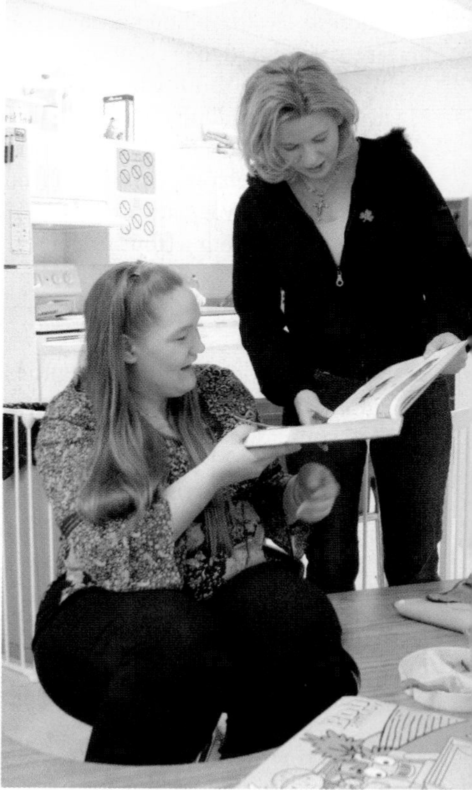

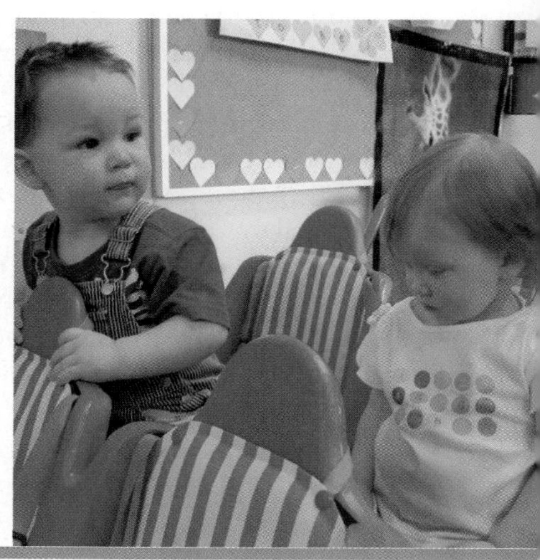

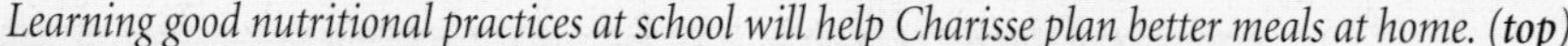

Learning good nutritional practices at school will help Charisse plan better meals at home. ***(top)***

The child development teacher discusses anticipatory guidance with Charisse, who has questions about Jeremy's growth. ***(middle)***

While Charisse is in class, Jeremy remains at the childcare center; knowing that her son is in a safe and nurturing environment allows Charisse to focus on her studies. ***(bottom)***

one thing they can do on a daily basis—walking their dog in the neighborhood, riding a bike to the store, using stairs instead of elevators when possible, parking on the far side of the school lot and walking farther, swimming at a club their parents belong to or at a local YMCA or YWCA, saving money to take lessons for horseback riding, or golf. Form interest groups at schools and community centers that provide an outlet for adolescents who cannot "make the team" for school sports. Encourage parents and adolescents to set goals together to integrate some physical activity daily.

The nurse's activities for health promotion concentrate on teaching the health and mental benefits of physical activity such as increased energy, weight control, and a feeling of control and success. Health maintenance focuses on viewing physical activity as a method to prevent disease such as cardiovascular disease and diabetes. Youth who have family members with these diseases or meet adults who have them are more likely to understand the importance of their own activity.

Desired outcomes include maintenance of weight within recommended level, daily exercise of 20 to 60 minutes, and establishment of lifetime routines for exercise.

ORAL HEALTH

Continued dental care during the adolescent years can ensure oral health. The recommendations remain the same as those for young children. The adolescent should floss daily, brush twice daily with a small amount of fluoridated toothpaste, and visit a dental provider every 6 months. By about 14 years of age, those who do not have fluoridated water and have been taking fluoride can stop this supplement. Even the molars have been formed by that age, so fluoride tablets are no longer needed. Continue to examine the condition of the teeth and the number of erupted permanent teeth present. Be alert for any unusual growths and ulcers in the mouth and refer for care as needed.

One potential concern that should be addressed includes the availability of dental insurance for the adolescent. The teen whose family does not have dental insurance needs referrals for care to affordable resources. Dental specialists clean off plaque that has formed, apply sealants to erupting molars, examine the teeth for caries, and perform restorative care. There are particular groups more at risk for inadequate dental care; see Developing Cultural Competence: Dental Care. When working with these populations, nurses can question access to care, and make recommendations that foster regular checkups. Some teens may wish to whiten the teeth or get orthodontia to improve appearance. The nurse helps the youth and parents to find resources for needed care. Expected outcomes are dental visits twice annually with recommended follow-up care for problems, and good oral health.

MENTAL AND SPIRITUAL HEALTH

Adolescents have many challenges to their mental health and need support to emerge from adolescence with mental and spiritual strengths. Mental health topics must be addressed at each health supervision opportunity to promote mental health among teens. Mental health is closely linked to developmental tasks such as growing independence, formation of close relationships with peers, becoming confident in accomplishments, becoming part of a social group, and setting goals for the future (Figure 15–4 ■).

As during other ages, the self-concept continues to develop and tailors reactions to the environment, and self-regulation in

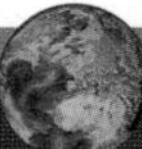

DEVELOPING CULTURAL COMPETENCE
Dental Care

An analysis of several national surveys such as the National Health and Nutrition Examination Survey (NHANES) reported that rural children were more likely (41%) to be uninsured for dental care than urban children (35%). They were also less likely to have visited a dentist in the last year (70%) than urban children (74%). More rural children (8%) had unmet dental needs than did urban children (6%) (Vargas, Ronzio, & Hayes, 2003). When children live in rural areas, be sure to ask about their access to dental care.

Another analysis of NHANES data examined African American respondents. Sixty-two percent reported that they only visit a dentist when needed rather than regularly. Those who were poor, unemployed, uninsured, or living in the South had poorer dental health. If you work with African American youth, be conscious of the need to integrate oral assessment into care, and to encourage utilization of services (Green, Person, Crowther, et al., 2003).

National Health Interview Survey (NHIS) data were analyzed for dental care utilization by Asians and native Hawaiian and other Pacific Islanders. Native Hawaiian and other Pacific Islander children were most likely (82%) to have had a dental visit in the last year, while Asian Indians were least likely to have a visit (60%). Once again, children with no insurance and who were poor were more likely to have less care. In addition, children living with a single parent or someone other than a parent, and those whose parents had under 12 years of education were more likely to have unmet dental needs (Qui & Ni, 2003).

When you work with these populations, be certain to include dental assessment in health supervision visits, and have resources for care readily available.

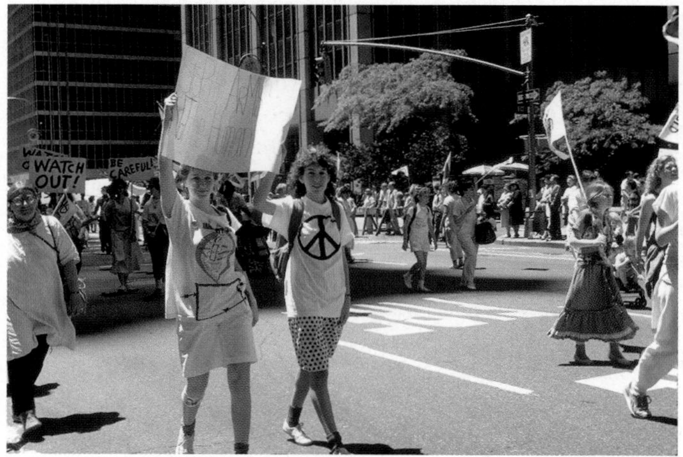

FIGURE 15–4 ■ Teens often become associated with causes. This helps them to feel part of a social group and also provides the opportunities to examine belief systems and make decisions about meaningful activities.

the form of making decisions to govern one's self is important. Self-esteem, or a positive feeling about the self, is key to meeting life's challenges. Questions that provide information about self-esteem are as follows:

- "What things have you accomplished that you feel proud about?"
- "What are some of your major disappointments? How have you dealt with them?"

Ask parents how the adolescent generally feels about himself/herself. Provide resources to deal with disappointments and give praise for the teen's accomplishments.

Another part of the self-concept that continues to develop is that of body image. Factors such as early or late maturation, overweight or underweight, or the role of the media can influence the teen's body image. A healthy image includes the realization that the body has positive and less positive attributes and that the individual can influence the body by healthy eating and physical activity. Be alert for the teen whose wish for a different body leads to eating disorders and excessive exercise or intake of nutritional supplements (see Chapter 9∞).

Sexuality involves both bodily changes that signal mature sexual development, and the mental concept of oneself as a sexual being. Bodily changes and mental concepts do not necessarily mature at the same time, and adolescents may not be ready for sexual maturity and the decisions about sexual behavior simply due to achieving sexual maturation. Most young adolescent girls have begun menstruating, and by early to middle adolescence, boys are having nocturnal emissions and ejaculations. Ask teens if they have received information about puberty, body changes, and sexuality. Inform young adolescents that most teens have questions and that you will talk with them about any areas of interest, including contraception and sexually transmitted diseases. Ask older adolescents directly if they have had sexual intercourse and if so, what they are doing to protect against pregnancy and sexually transmitted diseases. Provide support for the adolescent who has decided not to have sexual intercourse; reinforce that sexual feelings are normal, but that decisions about sexual intercourse are their right and privilege. Ask if the teen has confusion about sexuality. If teens identify as homosexual, let them know they are welcome and ask about decisions regarding sexual practices, reinforcing the need for protection against sexually transmitted diseases. Provide community resources to support gay, lesbian, or bisexual teens so that they can develop a social group in which they feel comfortable.

Some adolescents are seen for healthcare at the time they become sexually active. Use this opportunity to reinforce and correct prior knowledge about the body and protection against pregnancy and sexually transmitted diseases. Recall Kim in the opening scenario. How will you ensure that she gets the information she needs for safe sex? Since she has come for healthcare, what other information and interventions does she need? Has she received a tetanus booster in the last 10 years? Has she ever had hepatitis b vaccine? Kim is having trouble talking openly with her parents. What topics would she like to address? What resources might be available in her school or community to assist her?

PRACTICE ALERT

The nurse who works with adolescents dealing with sexuality issues may find that the values of some teens are very different from one's personal values. How do you react when a teen decides to have sexual intercourse or has become pregnant? Can you help teens to make wise decisions without telling them what they should do? It is important for adolescents to learn the importance of sexual intercourse and the meaning of close relationships. Teaching them early about this will enable them to respect others at the time they do have intimate relations. Nurses should also treat teens with respect, expecting them to consider options and make wise decisions. Nurses who cannot work with certain groups of teens due to differences in moral values have the obligation to refer the teens for care to resources where they can receive the information and services they are requesting.

Most adolescents require discipline or guidance from parents at certain times. Rather than a constant battle over daily events, it is best if there are just a few important rules, and parents have to enforce them only rarely. Guidelines that can help parents include the following:

- Gradually increase the teen's independence. If there is success with growing responsibility, the teen may be ready for more. If the teen misuses independence (perhaps by staying out too late, having a party at home without parents present, lying about location on an evening out), there should be clear limits and loss of privilege.
- Be willing to talk with and hear the teen's story. On the other hand, do not be talked out of consequences for the teen's bad decisions.
- Recognize that driving a car, staying out late, and other activities are not a given. They are privileges for responsibility displayed.
- Comment on a teen's behavior rather than making belittling comments about them as a person.
- Realize that the teen is establishing independence and that the relationship will change. Be consistent and loving as your adolescent tries out and learns about limits and the self.

MediaLink Teen Mental and Spiritual Health Video

Sleep is necessary for anyone to function safely and at a level of one's potential. Unfortunately many youth do not get the sleep needed for healthy functioning. Teens have an increased need for sleep due to their growth rates and activity levels. At the same time, their internal clocks change, making it more difficult to get to sleep at the usual time. It is thought that a decrease in secretion of melatonin occurs, so the teen does not feel tired in the late evening. However, they often have not received the number of hours of sleep needed by the time they wake up for school or work. The problem may be worsened if the student participates in sports or other activities. They may need to get to school early for music, sports, or other activities, or perhaps stay late into the evening for practices. Some adolescents work on weekends or evenings as well. Of course, social activities usually fill much of their time.

While about 9 hours of sleep are needed, most adolescents get about 6 hours (Mayo Clinic, 2003). The effects of sleep deprivation can be serious. Teens cannot perform to their potential in school or at work. Many parents state that adolescents are moody and difficult to communicate with when they are tired. There may be a connection between lack of sleep and substance abuse, and teens commonly use caffeinated beverages to stay awake. Some people tend to eat more when they are tired, and get less physical activity. Perhaps one of the most serious consequences deals with the danger of driving while sleepy; this is a common cause of accidents. Ask adolescents about what time they go to bed and when they awake. Inquire about whether the teen is frequently tired. Suggestions that may help include:

- Try to keep to similar hours for sleeping so the body becomes accustomed to a schedule.
- Avoid caffeine in the late afternoon and evening.
- Do homework early, and relax a bit before going to bed.
- Plan a day each weekend to simply relax and have few demands.

Temperament or personality type characteristics continue into adolescence but they generally do not change from earlier years. For example, the active infant and young child is usually an active teenager. The slow-to-warm-up baby may be the adolescent who needs more time to adjust to a new school or teachers. If the adolescent or parent has trouble with personality characteristics, it may be helpful to talk about these traits, help them to establish a positive sense about the attributes, and discuss ways to adapt the environment as needed. For example, parents should not expect a slow-to-warm-up teen to be interested in running for a class office. An adolescent with irregular sleep and eating habits will find it difficult to have a job at a set time and will need to set alarms and other reminders.

Spirituality offers comfort and support for the adolescent. Being a member of a teen group in a faith-based home can offer a peer group with similar values and bring meaning to life. Some adolescents reject the faith of their parents and seek a different group; others seek to leave religious practices totally while others become more committed to them. Ask teens if they have the resources they need to bring meaning to their lives; and provide referrals if needed. In addition to faith-based practices, participation in community food kitchens, raising money for causes, and other activities can provide meaning for many adolescents.

The nurse actively promotes the mental health of youth by understanding their developmental needs and providing information and resources. Gentle guidance and active partnership with youth help to provide the resources to ensure healthy self-concept, sexuality, and personality development. While most teenagers have many protective factors that can be identified and fostered, a few have risks that can harm mental health. It is important to identify the risks also, and to use health maintenance techniques to lessen the risk factors. Depression and substance use are two common risks to mental health. Depression is discussed in Chapter 34∞ and substance use in Chapter 7∞. See the checklists in Table 15–3 to help in identification of these problems during health supervision visits.

Although health promotion and health maintenance activities commonly occur in office or clinic settings, there are many other settings where nurses work with adolescents and mental health activities are often integrated into these settings. Consider offering health promotion/maintenance wherever you might see students. Some nontraditional settings include correctional facilities, school-based health centers, and programs for pregnant teens. Adolescents in these facilities can benefit from services to improve diet, physical activity, and lifestyle behaviors that influence mental health (Box 15–3).

The desired outcomes for mental and spiritual health promotion and maintenance include meaningful activities in the adolescent's life, emerging independence, good choices about lifestyle behaviors, and development of successful coping skills.

TABLE 15–3 Signs of Depression and Substance Abuse

DEPRESSION	SUBSTANCE USE
Changes in behavior, school performance, sleep, and appetite	Changes in behavior, school performance, sleep, and appetite
Physical complaints	Accidents and other unexplained events
Loss of interest in usual activities	Lack of responsibility
Difficulty in motivating self and setting goals	Labile mood and attitude
Change in friends	Hopelessness
Feelings of worthlessness	Depression
Consideration of death or suicide	Feelings of ambivalence
	A variety of physical changes depending on the substance

Adapted from Jellinek, M., Patel, B. P., & Froehle, M. C. (Eds.). (2002) Bright futures in practice: Mental Health *(Vols. I and II). Arlington, VA: National Center for Education in Maternal and Child Health.*

RELATIONSHIPS

Adolescents form stronger bonds with friends than at any time earlier in development; at the same time they need their parents for guidance and reassurance as they become more independent. However, as teenagers strive for independence they frequently strike out at parents, test limits, and engage in conflicts. Interactions in the family provide consistent and important ties at the same time that social interactions outside the family become a central part of life (Figure 15–5 ■). Health promotion helps teens to form strong friendships with peers and to continue to value and participate in the family, and helps parents to understand the developmental needs and their role in establishing a new type of relationship with the emerging young adult in the family. Partnerships with care providers are important to help families work together to achieve these outcomes.

When adolescents are seen for healthcare visits, assess relationships with others. Provide time alone with both the adolescent and the parents (if they are present) so that everyone has time to freely talk and ask questions. Some areas already discussed, such as school performance and activities, provide information about the adolescent's friends and how time is spent. Ask teens to describe their best friends and what they do together. Ask parents their opinions of the youth's friends.

Inquire about the youth's roles in the family. Does the teen have jobs and responsibilities? What freedom is allowed? What are relationships like with siblings and extended family members such as grandparents and cousins? What activities are done together as a family? Are there differences in the teen's and the parents' answers to these questions? What are the risk and pro-

BOX 15–3 Nurses Offering Health Promotion and Maintenance in Nontraditional Settings

Several examples of programs started by nurses to offer health promotion and health maintenance to adolescents are found in the literature. Examples include:

1. **A description of health programs for youth that are offered in youth correctional facilities.** Nurses performed risk assessment of incarcerated youth and provided health education programs and intervention services such as immunizations in regional correction facilities. Topics for discussion included alternatives to violence, feelings, and goal setting. Costs were minimal and the program promotes collaboration with corrections departments, health departments, and other professionals (Greene, Lucarelli, & Shocksnider, 1999).
2. **A proposal has been made to include expanded school mental health services in school-based health centers.** There has been a growth of school-based healthcare, but most of these centers have not yet integrated mental health services. The impetus for the proposal is that most children and adolescents with mental health needs do not receive adequate care for their conditions. Integrating services into school settings improves access, increases referrals, fosters collaboration among professionals, and provides screening of populations to find youth with mental health needs. Personnel are viewed by students as part of the school and often accept them more readily than they do professionals in offices or other settings. They can offer population-based interventions such as teaching in the classroom about topics like decision making and intimate relationships. Mental health professionals are then also available to offer an individualized approach for youth experiencing mental health concerns (Weist, Goldstein, Morris, et al., 2003).
3. **Nurses commonly work with pregnant adolescents in offices, clinics, and schools.** When providing services to these teens, nurses can focus on many health promotion and health maintenance topics. Youth are commonly interested in these topics since they realize that their behaviors may influence the fetus. A program that addresses smoking cessation for pregnant teenagers has been described. Nurses provide information about effects of smoking on the fetus, infants, and children, and assess teens' motivation to quit. Intervention strategies are carried out and their effectiveness in leading to smoking cessation is evaluated (Albrecht, Cassidy, Reynolds, et al., 1999).

What clinical settings are used in your nursing program to provide interactions with adolescents? How can you integrate health promotion and health maintenance interventions within these settings, whether they are in the hospital, in clinics, offices, schools, homes, or other settings?

tective factors in the teen-parent relationship? (Centers for Disease Control and Prevention, 2004).

Provide an opportunity alone with the teen to talk about issues such as domestic violence. Is the youth abused or is their violence between adults in the family? Are there stressors such as lack of sufficient finances, an ill parent, or a lost job? How have these occurrences affected the adolescent? Minor adjustments can be helped by discussion while some major problems will need referral to mental health specialists (see Chapter 34∞ for discussion of mental health problems and approaches).

Help families realize that the roles of all members change when a teenager is present. The following information may be useful for parents.

- It is common to feel rejected as the teen becomes more independent and critical of parents; talk about this with other parents; recognize that a new and positive relationship will likely emerge.

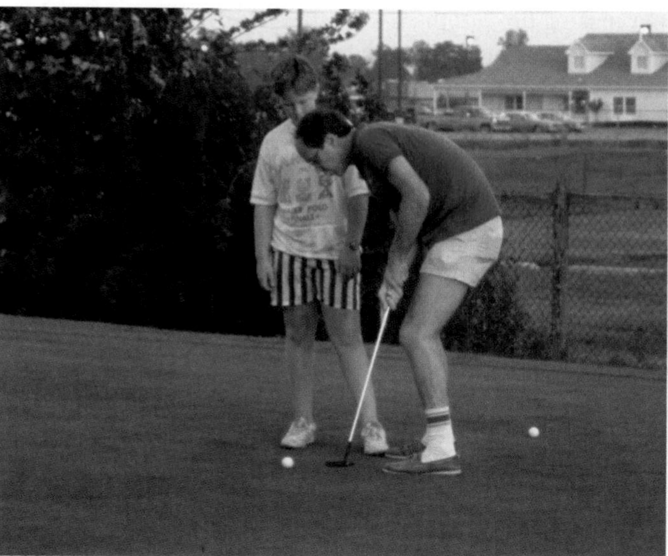

FIGURE 15–5 ■ This father and son have an opportunity to talk, share a common interest, and enjoy a bonding experience that can last for many years. The teen can transfer the relationship skills he has learned to many future interactions.

- Provide opportunities for your teen to talk but do not force the conversation.
- Use open-ended questions. Say, "Tell me something good that happened today." rather than "How was your day?"
- Recognize that it will take time for the teen to take on responsible mature behaviors and that guidance is needed throughout the teen years.
- Provide discipline by talking about the unacceptable behavior, rather than belittling the teen.
- Provide plenty of positive feedback for good grades, participation in activities, help at home, or other behaviors.
- Insist on few rules; important rules are to give respect to family members and other people and to avoid risky behaviors such as drinking and driving.

Some helpful tips for adolescents include:

- Most teens get frustrated with their parents at times; list some things you like and some you don't like about your family.
- Be sure to focus complaints on specific issues like wanting a later curfew rather than telling your parents they don't know anything.
- Most parents, like kids, want to know what they do right; tell your parents occasionally things that are going well or things that you appreciate.
- Talk to your parents; if you don't feel you can, find another adult you respect, like an older sibling, a teacher, counselor, clergy.

In their relationships with peers, adolescents often have many of the same issues that emerge with parents. They may have disagreements with friends or feel hurt by things that are said or done. Ask teens about how things are going with friends and what problems they have. Talk about negotiating, joining groups to form new friendships, and the importance of respecting and not making fun of others. Give them strategies for living up to their own standards even when friends are enticing them to do other things. Say "Most teenagers have trouble saying no when friends ask them to drink and drive, or smoke, or sneak into the house late. When has it been difficult to you to say no to friends?" Suggest that having friends one can trust and who have the same ideals can be very supportive in adolescent years.

Expected outcomes are the formation of strong relationships both within and outside of the family, along with independence in decision making.

DISEASE PREVENTION STRATEGIES

Teenagers typically do not have many diseases and most are minor illnesses such as respiratory and gastrointestinal illness. However, there are some diseases that occur and health professionals must be aware of signs of potential disease. Common adolescent health issues that are described throughout this book include:

- Acne and skin infections
- Body piercing and tattooing
- Sports overuse injuries
- Constipation and diarrhea
- Dental problems

Other observations may signal more serious health concerns and need to be referred for further evaluation. Examples include:

- Scoliosis
- Anemia
- Excessive tiredness
- Bruising
- Sexually transmitted diseases
- Eating disorder
- Abuse or severe bullying

There are several screening tests that should be performed during health supervision visits with adolescents. Physical examination is combined with mental health screening as described in the previous sections to provide a complete picture of the child's risks for diseases. See Table 15–4.

Screening tests with abnormal results require follow-up and intervention. For example, if the adolescent is anemic, iron tablets may be needed and teaching about high-iron foods should be performed (see Chapter 9∞). Vision impairment requires referral to an eye specialist. Presence of sexually transmitted diseases requires teaching and medication treatment. History of sexual activity will guide you to tests that should be included in the examination.

PRACTICE ALERT

Sexually active teens should be screened annually for:

- Chlamydia
- Gonorrhea
- Trichomoniasis
- Human papilloma virus
- Herpes simplex virus
- Bacterial vaginosis

Teens should be screened for syphilis and/or HIV/AIDS if requesting testing or meeting any of these criteria:

- History of STIs
- More than one sexual partner in past 6 months
- Intravenous drug use
- Sexual intercourse with a partner at risk
- Sex in exchange for drugs or money
- Homelessness
- Males—sex with other males
- Syphilis—residence in areas where disease is prevalent
- HIV/AIDS—blood or blood product transfusion before 1985

From Green, M., & Palfrey, J.S. (2002). Bright futures: Guidelines for health supervision of infants, children, and adolescents (2nd ed., p. 268). Arlington, VA: National Center for Education in Maternal and Child Health.

The adolescent should receive extensive information about ways to protect health and prevent disease. The hazardous outcomes of smoking are discussed, and smoking cessation programs

TABLE 15–4 Screening During Health Promotion and Health Maintenance Visits of Adolescents

AGE	RECOMMENDED MENTAL HEALTH/BEHAVIORAL SCREENING	RECOMMENDED PHYSICAL HEALTH SCREENING TESTS
11–14 years	Use of tobacco and alcohol History of abuse Unsatisfactory school performance History of depression or other mental health problems History of violence or risk taking History of multiple personal or family stresses Loneliness or lack of friends	Vision Hearing Anemia Lipids Blood pressure Urinalysis Tuberculosis (if at risk) Pap smear (for sexually active females) Breast exam Sexually transmitted disease risks
15–17 years	As above	As above
18–21 years	As above Difficulty with job	As above Offer pelvic exam for all females even if not sexually active

Adapted from Green, M., & Palfrey, J. S. (2002). Bright futures: Guidelines for health supervision of infants, children, and adolescents *(2nd ed.). Arlington, VA: National Center for Education in Maternal and Child Health.*

are encouraged for smokers. Unprotected sexual activity is presented as a serious health threat. Use of sunscreens to prevent burns and future skin cancer is encouraged. Females are taught breast self-exam and males are taught testicular exam. For youth who are overweight and sedentary, involve teaching about the possible outcomes such as type 2 diabetes and cardiovascular disease (see Health Belief Model discussion on page 482). While it is not advisable to threaten or frighten an adolescent with descriptions of diseases, an understanding of the potential serious outcomes like smoking or diabetes can be motivators for behavior change.

In addition to teaching disease prevention, the nurse also administers any needed immunizations. Many adolescents have not had immunizations since school entry; therefore, their record should be carefully reviewed. Common immunizations needed by adolescents are as follows:

- Last tetanus-diphtheria booster–It is recommended every 10 years if no wounds have required an update in the interim, so if the child received it at age 5 years, a booster is needed at 15 years.
- Second measles-mumps-rubella–A second dose may not have been routine when teens were younger so they may need it now.
- Is hepatitis A common in your state–If so, the teen needs to receive the vaccine.
- Hepatitis B vaccine–This is important for all youth and some may not have received it as infants.
- A clear history of varicella disease–If not, the vaccine is needed.
- Is the teen headed to college, or travel for sports or music in groups of other teens? Meningococcal vaccine is recommended.

See Chapter 19∞ for further discussion of immunizations.

The results of health screening are shared with the teen and with the parent as appropriate. Teaching and other interventions for disease prevention are examples of health maintenance activities. Expected outcomes are increasing knowledge of common diseases and methods of prevention among teen and parent, use of screening tests by the healthcare provider, and use of the healthcare home by the adolescent for treatment of diseases.

INJURY PREVENTION STRATEGIES

Injury is the greatest health hazard for adolescents; therefore, injury prevention must be integrated into every health contact with youth. The major hazard is automobile crashes (see Chapter 1∞). Many teens learn to drive and have a license by 16 years of age (Figure 15–6 ■). They often transport friends, get distracted by social interactions in the car, have little experience with actions to take if a car slides or has mechanical problems, may drink and drive, and are often tired when driving. Several states have instituted graduated driver licensing to help decrease some risks. Commonly, the youth cannot drive other youth for the first few months, cannot drive from approximately 1 A.M. to 6 A.M. and receives serious consequences for speeding or other infractions. Parents in states without these laws may wish to establish them for their own adolescents. Driving should always be presented as a privilege and a responsibility. Serious consequences such as losing the ability to drive for a time after any infraction can be suggested to parents (Box 15–4). Because of the great risk of injury and death from car crashes, ask at each health visit if the teen drives, rides with other teens, what rules parents have established about driving, and whether the teen ever drinks and drives or rides with someone who does. Reinforce the need to wear a lap and shoulder belt at all times and to never drink and drive.

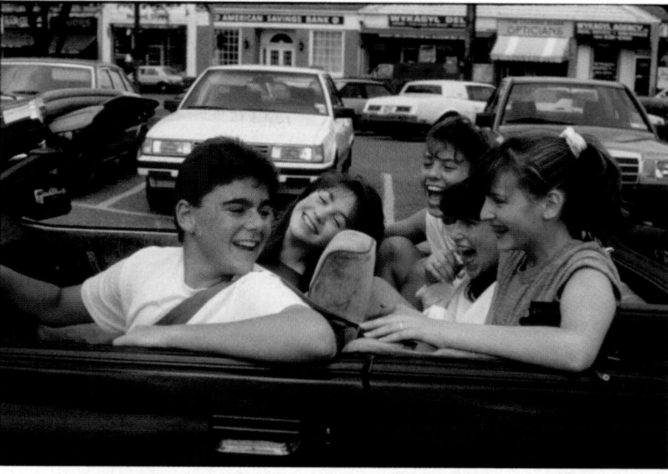

FIGURE 15–6 ■ Adolescents often drive motorized vehicles and may be at risk for injury if not properly prepared or protected. What teaching and experience do these youth need for safe enjoyment of the experience of driving and riding with friends? Do schools in your area offer driver education classes? What are the state requirements for driver licensure?

MediaLink Case Study: Immunization Update

Youth are at risk for injury with other motorized vehicles. Motorcycles, four-wheelers, boats, jet skis, farm machinery, and tools are other sources of injury. Ask about the youth's exposure, teach about avoiding alcohol and drug use, and encourage safety gear and precautions to be used. See Evidence-Based Practice: Farm Injury.

Every health visit should also include other questions that help to identify injury hazards:

BOX 15–4 Research: Parent Restrictions and Teen Driving

A group of 658 parents and their 16-year-old adolescents participated in a study that included a video and driving agreement between parent and teen. The video was viewed while the parent brought the teen to the motor vehicle department for the license test and was then sent home with them. Phone questioning showed that parental restrictions on youth driving resulted from the video and persisted until at least 4 months later. The short intervention in a motor vehicle department was thought to be successful (Simons-Morton, Hartos, & Beck, 2003). Since nearly all youth are brought to the driving test by a parent, it is easy to access them in this setting. What financial resources would be needed to make this intervention more widely available? How could nurses be active in political discussions to promote restrictions on teen driving to afford them the time to develop safe driving skills?

- "You mentioned that you like target practice. What type of gun do you have? Describe how you store it. Are there other guns in your home?"
- "What is your favorite summer activity? Oh, you jump from the cliffs. How often? Do you jump or dive? How do you know how deep the water is there? How would you describe your swimming skills? Do you ever go alone? Do your parents know you are jumping from the cliffs?"
- "People are sometimes hurt or abused by others. Has that happened to you, either at home or somewhere else?"
- "Do you know what date rape is? Has that ever happened to you?"

Once you have asked about common causes of injury, be sure to discuss and provide written material to perform injury prevention teaching. Such measures are important health maintenance activities. See Tables 15–5 and 15–6 for injury prevention topics and interventions. Desired outcomes for nursing care include absence of serious injury, the ability to state sources of risk for injury, and emergency plans for assistance when engaging in any risky activities.

NURSING MANAGEMENT

Nursing Assessment and Diagnosis

Nurses assess adolescents in a variety of settings, including offices, clinics, schools, home, correctional facilities, extended care facilities, in sports-related endeavors, and family planning clinics. A wide array of health concerns should be included in these assessments. They include measurement of growth; presence of any unusual findings on physical examination; lifestyle choices related to dietary intake, physical activity and oral hygiene; assessment of mental status, family interactions, and social connections with peers; any risky behaviors the adolescent engages in such as smoking, unprotected sexual relations, alcohol or drug use, or unsafe driving practices. The people and organizations around the adolescent such as family, school, and neighborhood are all assessed (Table 15–7). Remember to list both risks and protective factors. The protective factors can be used during implementation to enhance the youth's resilience.

TABLE 15–5 Injury Prevention in Adolescence

HAZARD	DEVELOPMENTAL CHARACTERISTICS	PREVENTIVE MEASURES
Motor vehicle crashes	Adolescents learn to drive, enjoy new independence, and often feel invulnerable.	Insist on driver's education classes. Enforce rules about safe driving. Seat belts should be used for every trip. Discourage drug and alcohol use. Get treatment for teenagers who are known substance abusers.
Sporting injuries	Adolescents may participate in physically challenging sports such as soccer, gymnastics, or football. They may be allowed to drive motorboats.	Encourage use of protective sporting gear. Teach safe boating practices. Perform teaching related to hazards of drug and alcohol use, especially when using motorized equipment.
Drowning	Adolescents overestimate endurance when swimming. They take risks diving.	Encourage swimming only with friends. Reinforce rules and teach them about risks.

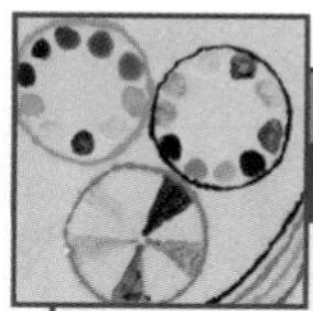

EVIDENCE-BASED PRACTICE
Farm Injury

PROBLEM

Injury is common in communities where children live and work on farms. Most injuries occur on weekends during the spring or summer. Before lunch and late afternoon are common times of the day for injury.

EVIDENCE

A study of trauma patients in the Midwest revealed an average age of 10.75 years for those with farm injuries. The most common injuries involved dislocations/fractures, lacerations/avulsions, concussions, contusions, and burns. Falls from high buildings, moving machinery, tractors, and cattle are common causes of these injuries (Walsh, 2000). The best outcomes were associated with being treated in a pediatric trauma center (Little, Vermillion, Dikis, et al., 2003). Because of the remote locations of some farms, children may not be promptly treated when injuries occur.

NURSING IMPLICATIONS

Nurses should intervene when working with families from rural areas to help them plan to promote safety for children on the farm (Figure 15–7 ■). Realize that many rural families seek healthcare in urban areas so even if you are working in a city, you may have rural families in the agency. Encourage parents to consult the North American Guidelines for Children's Agricultural Tasks to match the child's physical and mental abilities with the tasks on a farm. Then suggest that parents supervise children in farm tasks, know first aid to follow for injuries, realize that serious accidents can occur, have a cell phone to call for help, and know what facilities are available for phone advice and for emergency rescue. Help families plan ahead to keep rural children safe.

CRITICAL THINKING APPLICATION

What items would you include on a checklist for parents of children on a farm? How might pesticides or other chemicals used on a farm injure youth who work near them? Plan educational materials and programs for families that live on farms.

Based on a thorough assessment, you will establish nursing diagnoses that are appropriate for the adolescent and family. Possible nursing diagnoses include:

- Rape-Trauma Syndrome related to date rape
- Impaired Dentition related to ineffective oral hygiene
- Imbalanced Nutrition: More than Body Requirements related to lack of basic nutritional knowledge and obesity in both parents
- Disturbed Sleep Pattern related to frequently changing sleep/wake schedule
- Low Self-Esteem related to situational crisis of friends making fun of adolescent

■ Planning and Implementation

Whatever the setting, the nurse partners with the adolescent, the parents, and other persons such as teachers or school counselors to plan appropriate goals and related interventions. Nurses work with individual adolescents in offices, schools, and other settings, and often work with groups of adolescents to perform teaching. Apply communication skills effective with teens (see Chapter 6∞) such as listening to concerns, allowing for discussion, and bringing peers who have had experiences related to the topic being discussed.

Many of the interventions will involve teaching, so it is wise to develop a number of resources for working with teens. Consult the web resources on the Companion Website, and visit agencies in the community to gather appropriate materials. Teaching topics will be directed both at health promotion (providing information to enhance the adolescent's state of health) and health maintenance (sharing tips about how to avoid disease and injury). A good starting point is to have the adolescent identify a personal health goal and begin teaching there.

Recall Kim from the chapter opener. She wants help in talking with her parents, so providing tools at the beginning of the visit will make her receptive to other topics that need to be addressed.

TABLE 15–6 Injury Prevention Topics for Adolescents

TOPIC	TEACHING
Driving	Always wear seat and shoulder belt Do not drink and drive or ride with others who do Do not talk on a cell phone as you drive Do not drive when you are tired Drive with parents or other adults for several months in winter driving conditions if you live where there is snow, ice, or heavy rains Keep your car in good repair
Sun	Wear sunscreen Limit time outside especially early in summer
Machinery	Learn how to use power tools correctly Always have someone near when you use tools or machinery
Emergency care	Learn first aid, CPR, and airway obstruction removal
Water safety	Learn to swim well If you supervise younger children near water, never leave them alone, even for a minute
Fires	Do not play with fire Follow guidelines to avoid igniting gasoline Test smoke alarms in your house every 6 months and change batteries annually
Firearms	Know and follow rules to keep firearms locked, with ammunition locked in a separate place Never take out a gun to show a friend unless your parent is also present Take firearm safety classes if you hunt or target shoot
Hearing	Avoid loud music especially for long periods and through ear phones
Sports	Wear protective gear recommended for your sport
Abuse	Report any abuse to an adult you trust Date with other couples when possible and report date rape Do not drink or take drugs

Adapted from Green, M. & Palfrey, J. S. (2002). Bright Futures: Guidelines for health supervision of infants, children and adolescents *2nd ed. Arlington, VA: National Center for Education in Maternal and Child Health.*

TABLE 15–7 Application of Ecology of Development to Assessment of Adolescent Populations

MICROSYSTEM	EXOSYSTEM	MACROSYSTEM
➤ Incidence of adolescent injury for common problems like teen driving, boating, farm injury, firearms, drowning ➤ Neighborhood agencies that offer services to adolescents such as driver education, firearm training ➤ School curricula related to substance use and sexual behaviors ➤ Student and family behaviors related to nutrition and physical activity	➤ School board policies related to sexuality teaching, HIV education, and other risks for teens ➤ Community agencies providing jobs and other services for youth ➤ Availability of healthcare services that youth can access ➤ Integration of health promotion and health maintenance into community services ➤ Amount of involvement of adult volunteers and local businesses in area schools	➤ State grants for smoking prevention and cessation among youth ➤ Insurance reimbursement for health promotion teaching ➤ Availability of results of Youth Risk Behavior Surveillance and other studies to local communities

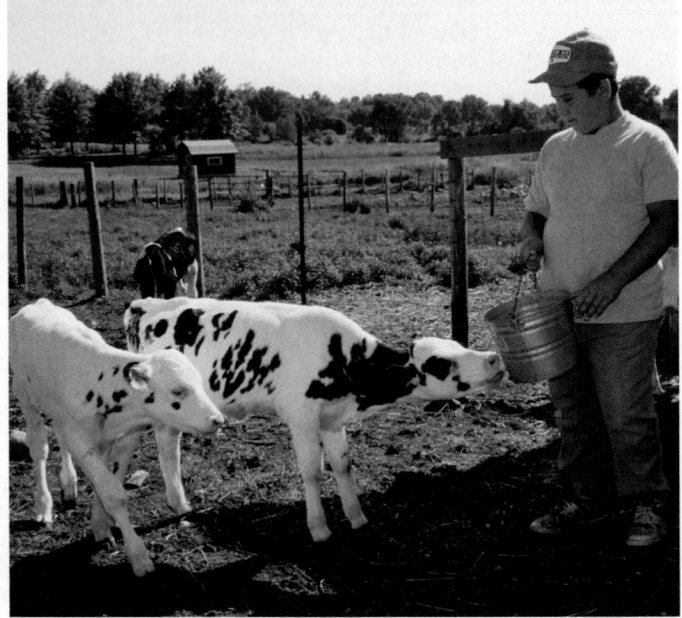

FIGURE 15–7 ■ What items would you include on a checklist for parents of children on a farm? How might pesticides or other chemicals used on a farm injure youth who work near them?

Her interest in birth control can lead to information about protection from sexually transmitted diseases. In addition to teaching, you will provide direct care when you administer immunizations, perform vision screening, and examine the spine and posture for scoliosis.

One challenge during health supervision for adolescents is including the right mix of teen and parent decision making and involvement. You will again apply communication skills by tactfully allowing time for both parent and adolescent to be seen alone. Realize that you are supporting and providing information for parents, like useful discipline techniques, recognition of common parental feelings about teens, and the need for growing independence by their youth. When you provide teaching to groups of teens in schools, there may be policies about what needs to be sent home to parents. Some schools require an outline of topics such as sexually transmitted diseases or substance use be sent home for parents to read. Parents may call you with questions about content and approach, or some may choose to attend and sit in on your presentation. This obviously requires that you partner with the school administration, teachers, parents, and others to be effective in your presentation. Collaboration with many individuals and agencies is an important skill.

Whether you see adolescents in offices or other private settings, or in schools, correction facilities, or other places with groups present, leave information about how you or another nurse or care provider can be contacted. Provide brochures, referral numbers, names, and email addresses related to the topics discussed. Encourage annual visits for health supervision visits and suggest a variety of places to obtain this care. For example, if a youth will soon graduate from high school, find out if he or she will be working or attending college and provide links to health insurance or care providers in the new location. Partner with other healthcare professionals to improve the environments of adolescents and help meet health goals (Centers for Disease Control and Prevention, 2004)

■ Evaluation

Inquire about the care received by teens and their families. They should feel comfortable with care providers and settings and believe that health care concerns are well-addressed.

Some expected outcomes for care of adolescents and their families include:

- Absence of debris and plaque on dental surfaces
- Approaching ideal weight
- Demonstration of amount and pattern of sleep for mental and physical rejuvenation
- Positive personal judgment of self-worth

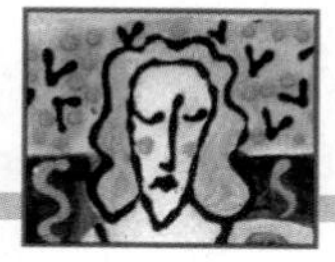

CHAPTER HIGHLIGHTS

- Health promotion and health maintenance of adolescents takes place in settings with individual youth as well as in facilities with groups of adolescents.
- Observations of youth and their parents provide valuable clues that assist the nurse in deciding which health issues need most attention during a given interaction.
- Growth measurement provides useful clues about nutrition status of teenagers. Further nutritional assessment provides information about the teen's food choices, knowledge, and nutritional intake.
- Physical activity is important for youth but large numbers do not get adequate amounts of exercise.
- The adolescent has many mental health challenges to meet in order to emerge with a positive self-concept and body image.
- Adolescents often have conflicts with parents as they begin to be more independent individuals and parents learn that family roles are changing during the teenage years.
- Peers form a primary source of companionship, self-worth, and influence for the adolescent.
- Since they are not seen often for healthcare, adolescents have needs for disease and injury prevention that must be met at any healthcare encounter.

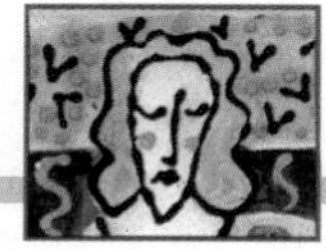

CRITICAL THINKING IN ACTION

INTRODUCTION

Recall 16-year-old Kim who was described in the opening scenario and has come to a health clinic for birth control. It is common to see adolescents for healthcare only when they come for a specific need. Nurses will maximize the opportunity by providing needed healthcare during this health encounter.

DESCRIPTION

When talking with Kim, you learn that she talks with her parents about most other health concerns and problems, but does not feel comfortable talking about her sexual activity. She feels that they will be disappointed in her. She also thinks they do not approve of her boyfriend because he is 2 years older and has dropped out of high school. Kim's partner has been using a condom and will continue to do so; she wants birth control pills to be sure she avoids pregnancy. Her tests for sexually transmitted infections are all negative.

DISCUSSION

1. What is Kim's psychosocial stage according to Piaget? Review these stages in Chapter 5 ∞ if necessary. How does her difficulty in telling her parents about her sexual activity relate to her development? To the roles of her and her parents in the family? What suggestions might be helpful to enhance Kim's communication with her parents?
2. What protective factors do you identify in Kim's sexual behaviors?
3. What nursing diagnoses can you develop based on the history given in the scenario and the description above?
4. Examine again the photograph in the opening scenario. How can the setting influence the receptivity of an adolescent to care? What do you see in this setting that would help to make the teen comfortable?
5. Plan the information that Kim needs about disease and injury prevention at her developmental stage. How can such information best be transmitted?
6. Kim is found to be anemic. What common dietary patterns of adolescents could contribute to this problem? What nutritional assessment will you perform? What interventions are appropriate?
7. List the immunizations that Kim might need. Which one directly protects against a sexually transmitted infection?

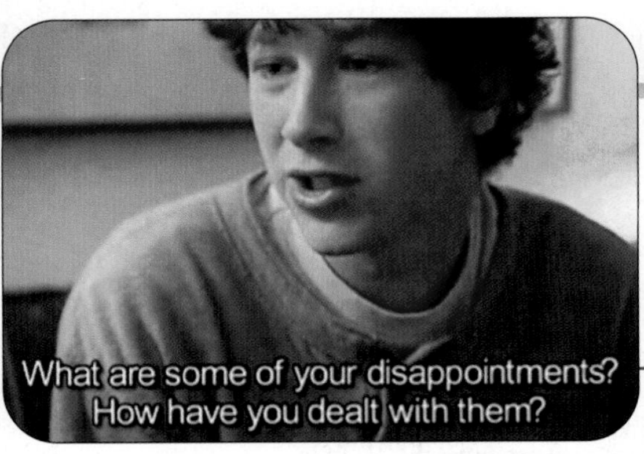

What are some of your disappointments?
How have you dealt with them?

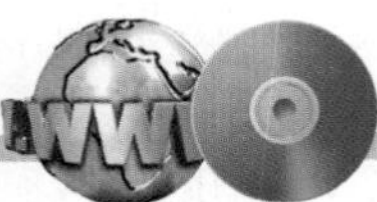

EXPLORE MediaLink

- NCLEX review, case studies, and other interactive resources for this chapter can be found on the Companion Website at **www. prenhall.com/ball**. Click on Chapter 15 to select the activities for this chapter.
- For animations, more NCLEX review questions, and an audio glossary, access the accompanying CD-ROM in this book.

http://www.prenhall.com/ball

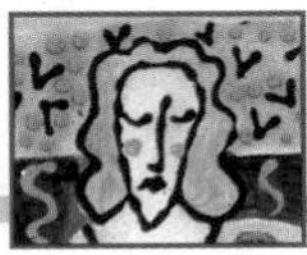

REFERENCES

Albrecht, S., Cassidy, B., Reynolds, J. D., Ketchem, S., & Abriola, D. (1999). Developing guidelines for smoking cessation interventions for pregnant adolescents. *Journal of Pediatric Nursing, 14*, 150–156.

Bandura, A. (1986). *Social foundations of thought and actions: A social cognitive theory*. Englewood Cliffs, NJ: Prentice Hall.

Bandura, A. (1977b). *Self-efficacy: The exercise of control*. New York: W. H. Freeman.

Bandura, A. (1977a). *Self-efficacy in changing societies*. New York: Cambridge University.

Becker, M. H., Haefner, D. P., Kasl, S. V., et al. (1977). Selected psychosocial models and correlates of individual health-related behaviors. *Medical Care, 15*, 27–46.

Centers for Disease Control & Prevention (2004). Improving the Health of Adolescents & Young Adults: A Guide for States and Communities. Atlanta, GA: CDC.

Epstein, L. H., Paluch, R. A., Kalakanus, L. E., Goldfield, G. S., Cerny, F. J., & Roemmich, J. N. How much physical activity do youth get? A Quantitative review of heart-rate measured activity. *Pediatrics, 108*, p. e44 (electronic article). http://pediatrics.aappublications.org/cgi/content/full/108/3/e44.

Green, B. L., Person, S., Crowther, M., Frison, S., Shipp, M., Lee, P., & Martin, M. (2003). Demographic and geographic variations of oral health among African Americans based on NHANES III. *Community Dental Health, 20*, 117–122.

Green, M., & Palfrey, J. S. (Eds.). (2000). *Bright futures: Guidelines for health supervision of infants, children, and adolescents* (2nd ed.). Arlington, VA: National Center for Education in Maternal and Child Health.

Greene, E., Lucarelli, P., & Shocksnider, J. (1999). Health promotion and education in youth correctional facilities. *Pediatric Nursing, 25*, 312–314.

(2000). *Healthy People 2010*. Washington, DC: U.S. Department of Health and Human Services. www.healthypeople.gov/document/html.volume2/22Physical.htm, accessed 9/1/2003.

Jellinek, M., Patel, B. P., & Froehle, M. C. (Eds.). (2002). *Bright futures in practice: Mental health* (Vols. I and II). Arlington, VA: National Center for Education in Maternal and Child Health.

Lerner, R. M., & Thompson, L. S. (2002). Promoting health adolescent behavior and development: Issues in the design and evaluation of effective youth programs. *Journal of Pediatric Nursing, 17*, 338–344.

Little, D. C., Vermillion, J. M., Dikis, E. J., Little, R. J., Custer, M. D., & Cooney, D. R. (2003). Life on the farm—children at risk. *Journal of Pediatric Surgery, 38*, 804–807.

Lowry, R., Wechsler, H., Kann, L., & Collins, J. S. (2001). Recent trends in participation in physical education among US high school students. *Journal of School Health, 71*, 145–152.

Mayo Clinic. (2003). Adolescents and sleep. www.cnn.com/HEALTH/library/CC/00019, accessed 9/7/2003.

Montgomery, K. S. (2002). Health promotion with adolescent: Examining theoretical perspectives to guide research. *Research and Theory for Nursing Practice: An International Journal, 16*, 119–134.

Murray, R. B., & Zentner, J. P. (2001). *Health promotion strategies through the life span* (7th ed.). Upper Saddle River, NJ: Prentice Hall.

Pate, R. R., Freedson, P. S., Sallis, J. F., Taylor, W. C., Sirard, J., Trost, S. G., & Dowda, M. (2002). Compliance with physical activity guidelines: Prevalence in a population of children and youth. *Annals of Epidemiology, 12*, 303–308.

Patrick, K., Spear, B., Holt, K., & Sofka, D. (Eds.). (2001). *Bright futures in practice: Physical activity*. Arlington, VA: National Center for Education in Maternal and Child Health.

Qui, Y., & Ni, H. (2003). Utilization of dental care services by Asians and native Hawaiian or other Pacific Islanders: United States, 1997–2000. *Advances in Data, 336*, 1–11.

Simons-Morton, B. G., Hartos, J. L., & Beck, K. H. (2003). Persistence of effects of a brief intervention on parental restrictions of teen driving privileges. *Injury Prevention, 9*, 142–146.

Vargas, C. M., Ronzio, C. R., & Hayes, K. L. (2003). Oral health status of children and adolescents by rural residence, United States. *Journal of Rural Health, 19*, 260–268.

Walsh, M. (2000). Farm accidents: Their causes and the development of a nurse led accident prevention strategy. *Emergency Nurse, 8*(7), 24–31.

Weist, M. D., Goldstein, A., Morris, L., & Bryant, T. (2003). Integrating expanded school mental health programs and school-based health centers. *Psychology in the Schools, 40*, 297–308.

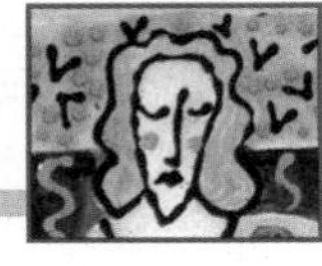

ADDITIONAL REFERENCES

Colyar, M. R. (2003). *Well-child assessment for primary care providers*. Philadelphia: FA Davis.

Dickey, S. B., & Deatrick, J. (2000). Autonomy and decision making for health promotion in adolescence. *Pediatric Nursing, 26*, 461–467.

Edelman, C. L., & Mandle, C. L. (2002). *Health promotion throughout the life span* (5th ed.). St. Louis: Mosby.

Eisenberg, M. E., Neumark-Sztainer, D., & Story, M. (2003). Associations of weight-based teasing and emotional well-being among adolescents. *Archives of Pediatrics and Adolescent Medicine, 157*, 733–738.

Kerker, B., Horowitz, S. M., Leventhal, J. M., et al. (2000). Identification of violence in the home: Pediatric and parental reports. *Archives of Pediatric and Adolescent Medicine, 154*, 457–462.

Nygard, P., Waiters, E. D., Grube, J. W., & Keege, D. (2003). Why do they do it? A qualitative study of adolescent drinking and driving. *Substance Abuse and Misuse, 38*, 835–863.

O'Donnell, G. W., & Mickalide, A. D. (1998). *SAFE KIDS at home, at play and on the way: A report to the nation on unintentional childhood injury*. Washington, DC: National SAFE KIDS Campaign.

Wilkinson, J. M. (2000). *Nursing diagnosis handbook* (7th ed.). Upper Saddle River, NJ: Prentice Hall Health.

Young, L. E., & Hayes, V. (2002). *Transforming health promotion practice: Concepts, issues, and applications*. Philadelphia: FA Davis.

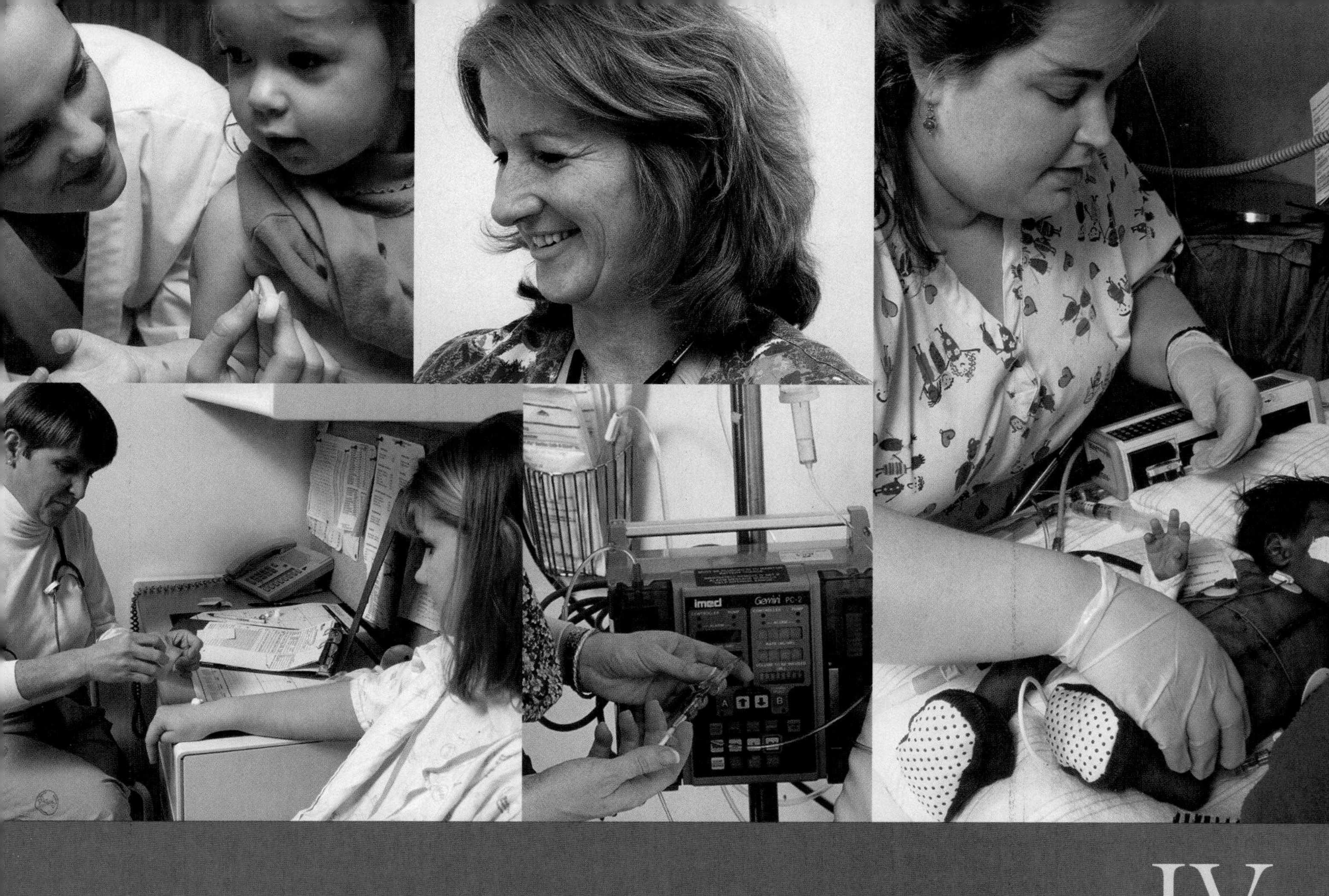

UNIT IV

Child Healthcare Settings and Considerations

Because children receive the majority of their healthcare in community settings, pediatric nurses have an important role in promoting the child's health and partnering with families to plan care for the child with episodic or chronic health conditions. In many cases, pediatric nurses develop long-term relationships with the children and families who return for continued care in a particular healthcare setting, such as a health center, physician's office, or school. When working with the hospitalized child and family, pediatric nurses additionally develop individualized nursing care plans that promote coping strategies to deal with the stressors of hospitalization and support the child's optimal growth and development. In all settings, the pediatric nurse serves as an advocate for pain assessment and management for any diagnostic or therapeutic interventions that cause pain or when pain is associated with the health condition.

Chapter 16

Nursing Care of the Child in the Community

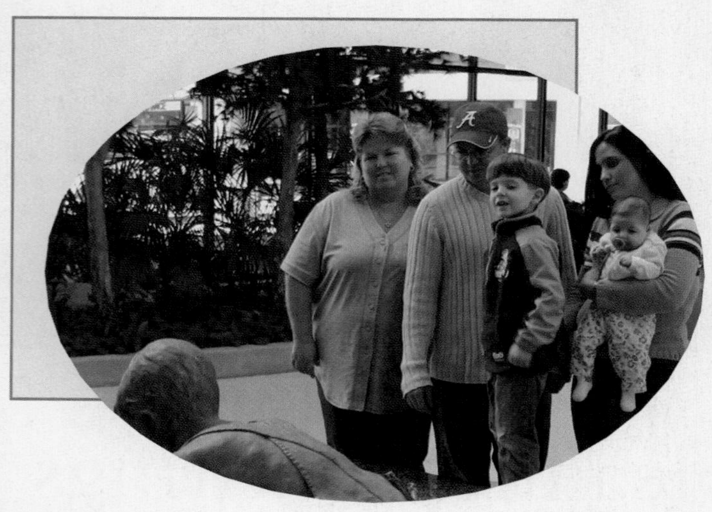

Jill Folsom is 4 months old and she has a congenital anomaly, a large ventricular septal defect. She has been successfully managed at home by her family while she grows enough to have surgery. Her mother returned to work 2 months ago, and her grandmother has provided childcare for Jill while her brother Ryan goes to kindergarten. In the last week, Jill has started to breathe more quickly, and it is taking nearly 30 minutes to drink her formula. Her mother has noticed sweat forming on her forehead during feeding. Her parents were taught to look for these signs, so they called the nurse at the cardiac clinic for advice. An immediate appointment was arranged for Jill to be evaluated for signs that her heart condition is worsening.

Jill's parents took her brother and grandmother to the cardiac clinic visit, anticipating the need for support and decision making. The outcome of the visit revealed that early signs of congestive heart failure are present, but not serious enough to require hospitalization. Jill's diuretic medication dose will be increased. More frequent visits to the cardiac clinic will now be needed. If possible, the surgeons would prefer to wait until Jill is at least 6 months old before performing corrective surgery. The parents are relieved that Jill's condition can still be managed at home. The family took a few moments to enjoy the indoor sculpture garden at the hospital before returning home.

"I am trying hard to help Mom and Dad take care of Jill. I know she is sick, so I help watch her when they leave the room, and I try to keep her happy with things for her to look at. She smiles at me a lot."

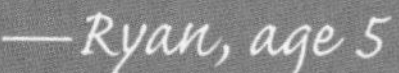
—Ryan, age 5

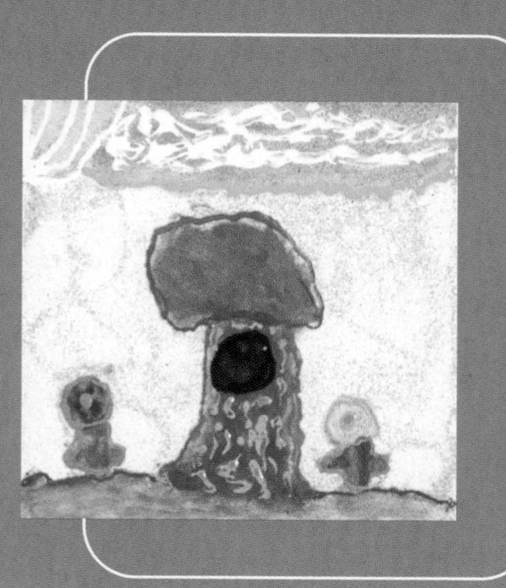

Learning Outcomes

After completing this chapter, you will be able to:

- List the variety of nursing roles in child healthcare settings outside the hospital.
- Outline the steps of a family-centered assessment for the child and family in a community setting and develop a nursing care plan that promotes the health of the child.
- Describe the potential roles of the pediatric nurse or school nurse in supporting a community assessment process.
- Describe the special needs of children that should be considered in disaster preparedness.

Key Terms

community assessment/515
disability/509
disaster preparedness/522
emergency preparedness/508
individualized health plan (IHP)/509
medical home/502
medically fragile/509
population/515
primary care/502
triage/506

MediaLink http://www.prenhall.com/ball

Resources for this chapter can be found on the CD-ROM accompanying this textbook, and on the Companion Website at http://www.prenhall.com/ball. Click on Chapter 16 to select the activities for this chapter.

CD-ROM

Videos
- *Disaster Preparedness*
- *EMS for Children*

NCLEX Review

Audio Glossary

COMPANION WEBSITE

NCLEX Review

MediaLink Applications
- *Community Assessment*
- *Complete an Emergency Information Form (EIF)*
- *Develop an Individualized Health Plan (IHP)*
- *Identifying Hazards*
- *Identifying Health Issues in Childcare Settings*
- *Plan a Health Supervision Visit*
- *Provide Health Education in the Schools*
- *School Policy Review*
- *Teaching Plan*
  - *Disasters and the Family with an Infant*
  - *Disasters and the Family with a School-Aged Child*
  - *Disasters and the Child Assisted by Technology*

THE CONTINUUM OF PEDIATRIC OUT-OF-HOSPITAL HEALTHCARE SETTINGS

The majority of pediatric healthcare occurs in community settings, as most children are healthy and need health promotion, health maintenance, and episodic acute care. Every child should have a healthcare home or **medical home,** a consistent, continuous, comprehensive, family-centered, and compassionate source of healthcare (Box 16–1). The healthcare providers in the healthcare home or medical home assume responsibility for coordinating the healthcare needed by the child. In some cases the primary care provider is a school nurse, community health nurse, or nurse practitioner working alone or in partnership with a physician. In other cases, the nurse collaborates with the physician or other healthcare providers in provision of care. While much of pediatric healthcare has always occurred in the community, care that was traditionally provided to children as hospital inpatients has shifted to ambulatory centers and community settings for many reasons.

- Children who are medically fragile or with serious chronic healthcare conditions now receive care in the community because of family willingness to care for the child at home and desire for the child to be integrated into the family and community. The healthcare system has supported the family preferences because care in the community is less costly. Community care for children with chronic conditions is possible because needed medical equipment is now small enough to be portable, so the child can be transported to different community settings.
- Invasive diagnostic procedures and surgery in outpatient surgical centers no longer require hospital admission for most children.
- Short-stay units associated with emergency departments have reduced the number of hospital admissions.

BOX 16–1 The Primary Healthcare Home or Medical Home

A primary healthcare home or medical home includes the following:

- A partnership with the family that involves a trusting relationship that respects their diversity and the importance of the family's role in the child's life
- Provision of family-centered health promotion and health maintenance care
- Assurance of ambulatory and inpatient care 24 hours a day
- Continuity of care from infancy to adolescence, and transition of adolescents with disabilities and chronic conditions to adult care (see Chapter 20∞)
- Appropriate use of subspecialty consultation and referrals
- Interaction with childcare center and school, as well as community agencies as needed, such as early intervention programs
- Development of a coordination of care approach with all health service providers
- A central record and database containing all pertinent information

Data from American Academy of Pediatrics (2002). The medical home. Pediatrics, 110*(1), 184–186; Green, M., & Palfey, J. S. (2000).* Bright futures: Guidelines for health supervision of infants, children, and adolescents *(2nd ed.). Arlington, VA: National Center for Education in Maternal and Child Health.*

- Long-term intravenous antibiotics can be provided with the support of home care nursing services.
- Pediatric hospice and palliative care is offered in the home setting more frequently as services specific to children and their families have emerged.

Health plans and healthcare providers continue to explore options to provide safe, high-quality care with fewer hospitalizations or shorter stays when hospitalization is needed.

Pediatric healthcare in the community occurs along a continuum that covers the entire child healthcare system. This continuum is reflected in the Bindler & Ball Continuum of Pediatric Health including health promotion and health maintenance services, care for chronic conditions, acute illnesses and injuries, and end-of-life care (see page 5 in Chapter 1∞). The settings for community care may offer a limited or extensive range of services.

- A healthcare center and a physician's office is the usual site of **primary care,** the range of health services that includes health promotion, health maintenance, episodic acute care, and health maintenance care for children with chronic conditions. See Chapters 11 through 15∞ for age-specific health promotion and health maintenance guidelines. Many children have a chronic health condition that needs ongoing nursing and medical management that is also often offered in these settings.
- A public health clinic may provide only health promotion and health maintenance services. A homeless shelter may also have the capacity to offer such services.
- A hospital outpatient center may provide specialized services to children with chronic conditions or a full range of services similar to a health center.
- Schools usually provide health promotion and health maintenance services at a minimum, plus first aid and emergency care as needed. School-based health centers may additionally provide counseling, health education, and care for acute conditions. Some school settings offer after-school respite services.
- Childcare centers provide first aid for emergencies and some health promotion services.
- Camp settings, particularly for children with specific health conditions, offer health promotion and education to promote self-care of the chronic condition.
- The home is a site for chronic condition management, rehabilitation, and end-of-life care. Children with acute illnesses and complex health conditions, including those with advanced disease states assisted by technology, can be cared for at home when their families are supported by home health services.

Other settings for community-based pediatric healthcare include:

- *Community events*—Many health education and injury prevention activities occur in the community, sponsored by hospitals, voluntary organizations, and the health department. Bike rodeos, for example, teach children about the need for bicycle helmets and bicycle riding safety. Health fairs offer opportunities to demonstrate correct car safety seat installation.

- *Urgent care centers, walk-in clinics, and emergency departments*—Care for acute illnesses and injuries is provided when other sources of acute healthcare are closed or unavailable.
- *Emergency Medical Services (EMS) System*—Children with a serious injury or illness may need to receive immediate care and transport to the hospital emergency department.
- *Disaster shelters*—Children and their families need food and safe shelter, health promotion, and occasionally acute care services within the community during a natural or man-made disaster. Children with dependence on technology will need access to healthcare in shelters.
- *Respite facilities*—Families with a child who has a special healthcare need (disability or chronic illness) often need periodic breaks from the constant stress of caring for the child, enabling them to keep the child at home. Respite care, matched to the family's and child's specific needs, can be provided in the home or in out-of-home respite facilities. For example, a crisis nursery allows the family of an infant with special healthcare needs to have a break from providing constant care, and offers counseling and linkage with other community services. Other respite services may be provided in a childcare or after-school program. The goal is to support families so the child can remain in the home. The Children's Disabilities Temporary Care Reauthorization Act (PL 101-127) authorizes federal funding to the states to develop and implement affordable respite care services and crisis nurseries. The Canadian Association of Community Care was funded by Health Canada to develop best practices for respite care for children with disabilities or chronic illness and their families; the provinces provide funds for respite care.

ROLES OF NURSES IN COMMUNITY SETTINGS

An individual child may receive care in all the above settings, or only a few. The nurse in any of the above settings has an important role in promoting the health and safety of the child, being a leader in setting policies in the center, as well as using the nursing process to help families meet the healthcare needs of their children.

Healthcare for individual children is improved when there is continuity of care and communication between settings in this continuum. The pediatric nurse working with families in a community setting is more successful when using knowledge of how the larger environment influences the child's health and development and the family's activities. (See Chapter 7∞.) That knowledge needs to be integrated into the nursing care plan.

Nurses have a variety of positions within these settings, such as community health nurse, home health nurse, school nurse, pediatric nurse in an office setting, nurse practitioner or advance practice nurse, emergency nurse, and nurse-paramedic. The nurse may assume the role of direct care provider, educator, advocate, or planner in any of these positions. To work effectively in the community, the nurse needs to gain experience and skills in the following areas.

- Partnering with families to conduct a child and family assessment and to plan individualized healthcare strategies, as well as implementing and evaluating nursing care strategies to match the family's economic, cultural, and social situation, and available resources.
- Assisting community agencies (e.g., schools, churches, and other community-based resources) to conduct a community assessment and then to plan, implement, and evaluate approaches addressing the healthcare needs of the community's children.

Role of the Pediatric Nurse in an Office or Health Center Setting

The nursing process is used when providing care for children in the primary care setting. The range of assessment responsibilities may vary by setting, as well as the preparation and experience of the nurse (Figure 16–1 ■). Specific functions of the pediatric nurse in primary care include the following:

- Providing telephone advice to families (Box 16–2)
- Collecting health history data
- Performing nursing assessments including vital signs, growth and development, nutritional status, immunization status, and family strengths and challenges
- Conducting physical examinations
- Performing screening tests to detect health problems such as vision or hearing loss, anemia, and lead poisoning
- Developing nursing diagnoses and implementing a plan of care
- Assisting with physician examinations and performing diagnostic tests
- Providing immunizations
- Providing information about procedures and offering reassurance

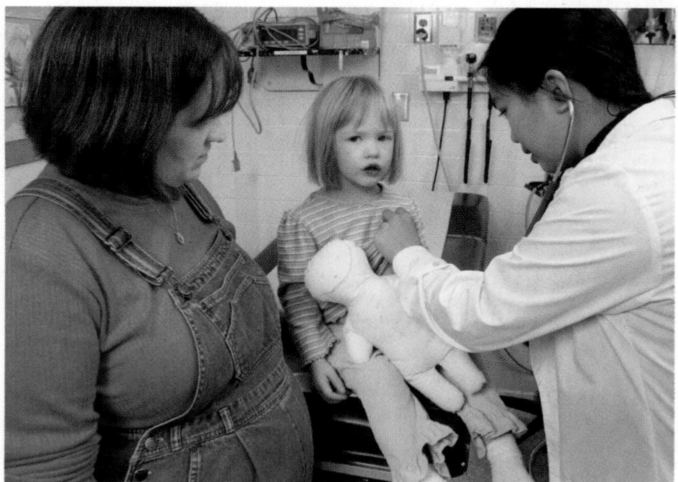

FIGURE 16–1 ■ Nurses carefully assess children in the office setting who present with an acute care illness. It is important to identify how serious the child's illness is and to monitor the child for progression of symptoms during the visit. This is also a time to gather information about the child's illness and to identify health information that will be needed for the family to care for the child at home.

- Providing patient education for health promotion or management of the health condition
- Linking families with community resources
- Assuring a safe environment and that infection control guidelines are followed

An important goal is to develop a positive partnership with the child and family so that optimal healthcare is provided. The relationship with the family grows over the months and years of providing care to the child and family. (See Partnering with Families: The First Interaction.)

Educating the Child and Family

Patient education regarding injury prevention, growth and development, nutrition, healthy lifestyles, and the home care of episodic illnesses and injuries are important nursing roles in primary care. In addition to working with individual children and families, the nurse may be responsible for selecting patient education materials that are provided in the waiting area and those specifically used for management of various conditions. Knowledge of community health problems and of the characteristics of the pediatric population served enables the nurse to select culturally and linguistically appropriate education materials.

Identifying Community Resources

Nurses in primary care settings are often involved in identifying community resources that are needed by the child and family that will help promote the child's health. Because of the range of issues that can present in the primary care setting, the knowledge of health-related resources in the community is important. Compiling a manual of community resources and regularly updating names and phone numbers of contacts will make it easier to provide information efficiently. For example, knowledge of how to access the community's early intervention programs for infants and toddlers ensures that families of children with developmental disabilities have educational services under PL 99-457, Education of the Handicapped Act Amendments of 1986. Other community resources that might be included are support groups, language and translation services, food banks, lead paint abatement services, social services, and mental health services.

The nurse may also be responsible for coordinating referrals for diagnostic or therapeutic services such as physical therapy, nutritionist consultation, or diagnostic testing. Because the child usually returns to the primary care provider after the consultant visit, the nurse has the opportunity to review the consultant's recommendation with the family and ensure that the family understands the results of diagnostic testing or recommended care. Reinforcing care recommendations may well improve the family's compliance with recommended care and the child's outcome.

Ensuring a Safe Environment for Children

Another responsibility of the nurse in the primary care setting is to ensure a safe environment for the child. The healthcare center and office settings have many potential hazards such as equipment, cleaning supplies, sharps, medications, and laboratory materials from which the child needs to be protected. Guidelines for infection control must be developed and implemented to reduce the transmission of infectious diseases between child patients and between the healthcare providers and children.

Role of the Pediatric Nurse in Episodic Care for Illnesses and Injuries

During childhood, most children have several episodes of illnesses and injuries that require a healthcare visit to the primary care provider. When the child with an episodic illness or injury arrives in the primary care setting, the nurse must assess the child to determine the urgency of care needed. The nurse performs many of the same functions as for a health promotion visit, such as collecting historical information and performing a nursing assessment, but the assessment may be abbreviated and specific to the presenting problem. It is important to recognize that the child's physical status needs to be monitored frequently during these visits to identify any worsening of condition and the potential need for emergency care intervention.

Readiness for Emergency Care

Approximately 25 to 50 emergencies occur in each primary care office setting per year, and the most common pediatric emergencies are seizures, status asthmaticus, respiratory distress, upper airway obstruction, hypovolemia or severe dehydration, sepsis, meningitis, and anaphylaxis (Wheeler, 1999). For example, the child could have an anaphylactic reaction to an immunization. The nurse is an important partner in the planning and rehearsal of emergency care that might be needed within the office setting until emergency medical services personnel arrive to transport the child to the emergency department. The nurse collaborates with the physician to ensure that guidelines are developed for recognizing children who need emergency care and for emergency response in the office setting. The nurse is often responsible for ensuring that

BOX 16–2 Telephone Triage Principles

Parents and caregivers placing telephone calls to the healthcare provider need assistance with determining the extent of the child's illness or injury, the urgency of a needed visit with the healthcare provider, and ideas for home care management. Before any advice can be given, the nurse must collect essential health information about the child and ensure that it gets recorded.

- Child's name, age, significant past medical history (chronic conditions, allergies, medications, treatments, recent immunizations)
- Reason for the call—chief complaint
- Present illness or injury—symptoms, duration, severity, pain, appetite, fever
- Review of systems related to the present illness

Once the information is collected and analyzed, the nurse may consult with the physician or follow specific written guidelines for telephone advice that match the child's condition. Parents will be directed to call 9-1-1 or the local emergency phone number if an emergency condition exists. An appointment may be made to see the healthcare provider, or guidelines for care at home are provided. Parents are routinely provided with information about signs of a worsening condition or when to call back because signs have not improved.

all emergency care equipment, supplies, and medications are organized and readily available in the central treatment room (Box 16–3). The nurse takes a leadership role in coordinating mock drills with all staff in the primary care setting so that all employees know and perform their designated role when a true emergency occurs in the setting.

Educating the Child and Family

Nurses teach families to help them provide the condition-specific care for the child at home (Figure 16–2 ■). Examples of information included are as follows:

- Signs that the condition is not improving as expected, indicating a need to return to the physician
- How and when to administer prescribed medications, and the potential side effects to monitor for and report to the healthcare provider
- Modifications in diet and activity
- Other supportive care for the child's condition
- Education to help the child and family recognize the need to initiate care for a new episodes (e.g., asthma, sickle-cell anemia, or hemophilia), to prevent the need for a healthcare visit, or to reduce the severity or progression of the condition

Role of the Pediatric Nurse in a Hospital Outpatient Setting

Pediatric nurses provide care for children with acute and chronic conditions within hospital outpatient or ambulatory settings. With experience, pediatric nurses working in a hospital ambulatory setting develop specialized knowledge and skills to meet the specific needs of the population of children they care for in that setting. Health promotion, health maintenance, and episodic illness care are provided in many hospital-supported clinics. The roles for nurses are similar to those described for office and healthcenter settings.

Specialty Care Ambulatory Clinics

Many children are referred to pediatric specialists based in specialty care ambulatory clinics for diagnostic workups and the long-term management of their chronic conditions. Nurses in these settings often collect health history data and perform nursing assessments that include vital signs, growth and development, nutritional status, immunization status, and family strengths and challenges. Advance practice nurses and nurse practitioners assume a larger role in patient assessment, implementing a care plan for the health condition, educating the child and family to manage the condition at home, and linking the child and family with community resources. For example, diabetic nurse educators teach parents and children with newly diagnosed diabetes how to manage their disease. See Figure 16–3 ■. Some advance practice nurses work as case managers of children with specific health conditions such as spina bifida, promoting coordination of care between all providers (including primary care), helping families get appropriately linked to community resources, and educating them about treatment options.

BOX 16–3 Emergency Equipment in an Office Setting

Essential equipment needed for managing an emergency in an office setting includes the following: oxygen and an oxygen delivery system, bag-valve mask resuscitator in pediatric and adult sizes, clear oxygen masks in various pediatric sizes (both breather and nonrebreather masks with a reservoir), oral airways in various sizes, suction devices, peak flow meter, and a nebulizer or metered-dose inhaler with a spacer/mask. Essential medications are epinephrine 1:1000 and albuterol (Committee on Pediatric Emergency Medicine, American Academy of Pediatrics, 1999). Locate the emergency equipment in every clinical setting where you have assignments so that you can quickly bring it to the site of an emergency if needed.

PARTNERING WITH FAMILIES

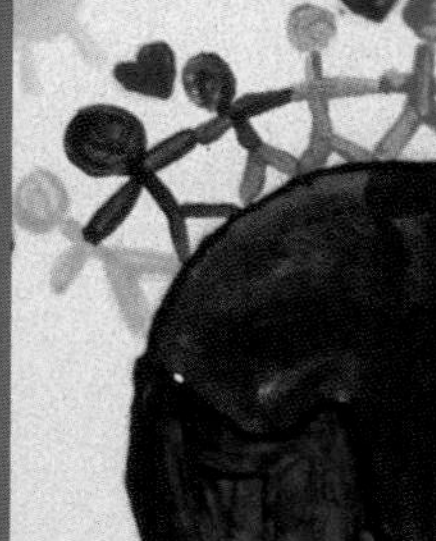

The First Interaction

Developing a relationship with the child and family in a community setting is equally as important as in the hospital. In many cases, the initial interaction sets the stage for the long-term relationship with the family that returns to the healthcare environment over many years. Remember to put aside the stressors you may be feeling before you approach the child and family. Take a few moments to play with the infant or child and to comment on a positive attribute of the child to the parents. The parent's, and perhaps the child's, stress level will also be reduced. This helps set the stage for a long-term partnership with the child and family.

Urgent Care or Emergency Department Settings

Children with acute illnesses may be seen by nurses in the emergency department or in an urgent care setting. Nurses working in

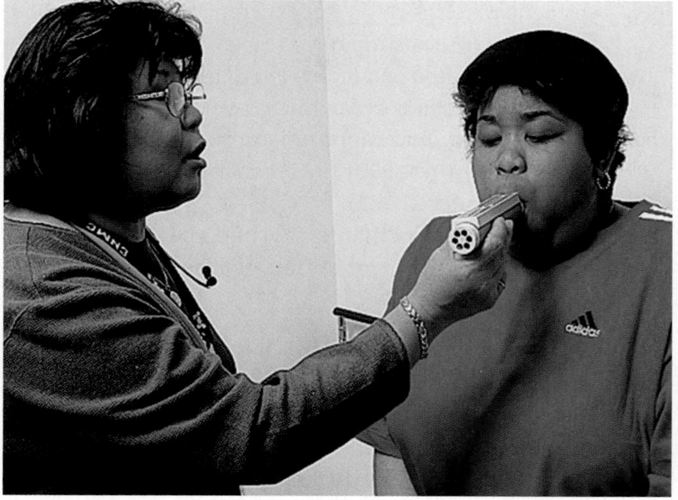

FIGURE 16–2 ■ Nurses provide patient education to help families learn to recognize the early stages of an asthma attack by using a peak flow meter. The child learns the proper method for taking a deep breath and blowing into the peak flow meter so the best reading is obtained.

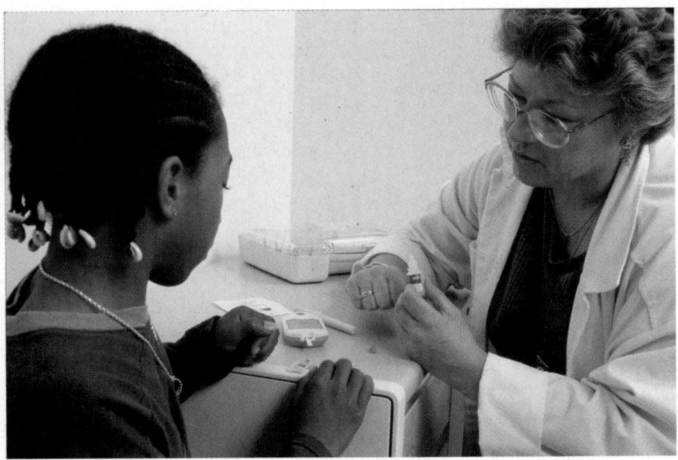

FIGURE 16–3 ■ Nurses often assume a larger role in working with children and families with a chronic health condition in the hospital ambulatory setting. Developing a care plan and educating the family to manage diabetes type 1 is an important role of this pediatric nurse, who is also a certified diabetes educator.

an emergency department or urgent care setting need advanced skills in assessment to identify subtle changes in physiologic status while these children receive treatment during the emergency department visit or in a 23-hour observation unit. Some of the nurses most experienced in care of children perform **triage** (rapid assessment to sort patients by the urgency of their condition) to identify those children most seriously ill and injured needing immediate care. Other important roles of nurses in emergency departments and urgent care settings include:

- Keeping the emergency department or urgent care setting in a state of readiness for care of children with life-threatening emergencies
- Frequently monitoring each child's health status and ensuring the child's safety during the visit
- Assisting with diagnostic procedures
- Collaborating with various health professionals providing treatments, such as respiratory therapists providing nebulizer treatments to asthmatics
- Educating the child and family about the diagnostic procedures and emergency department treatments implemented
- Providing emotional support because children and families are usually stressed by the urgency of the child's condition (see Chapter 21∞)
- Identifying and coordinating the child's need for follow-up healthcare and treatment for the emergent condition

Nursing in a School Setting

School nursing is a specialized practice of professional nursing that advances the well-being, academic success, and lifelong achievement of students. To that end, school nurses facilitate positive student responses to normal development; provide health promotion, health maintenance, and safety; intervene with actual and potential health problems; provide case management services; and actively collaborate with others to build student and family capacity for adaptation, self-management, self-advocacy, and learning (National Association of School Nurses, 1999). See Box 16–4 for the Standards of Professional School Nursing. Pediatric nurses interested in school nursing usually have a strong interest in community health and seek continuing education to learn more about nursing in a school environment. Many of them seek and maintain special certification status as a school nurse.

The school nurse practices independently as the only licensed healthcare provider in the setting. Depending on the school system, the nurse may be responsible for providing health promotion and health supervision to children in one or several schools, and for up to 3,000 children. The nurse has a physician consultant who provides standing orders for episodic and emergency care. A school nurse consultant may also be available to the school nurses in the education district to provide guidance and mentoring, especially for new school nurses. Many school nurses have obtained advanced education to practice as a school nurse practitioner, enabling them to better manage this independent practice. Some schools have school-based health centers in which the school nurse practitioner provides health promotion, health maintenance, and episodic acute care to children.

BOX 16–4 Standards of Professional School Nursing Practice

1. The school nurse collects client data.
2. The school nurse analyzes the assessment data in determining nursing diagnoses.
3. The school nurse identifies expected outcomes individualized to the client.
4. The school nurse develops a plan of care/action that specifies interventions to attain expected outcomes.
5. The school nurse implements the interventions identified in the plan of care/action.
6. The school nurse evaluates the client's progress toward attainment of outcomes.
7. The school nurse systematically evaluates the quality and effectiveness of school nursing practice.
8. The school nurse evaluates one's own nursing practice in relation to professional practice standards and relevant statutes, regulations, and policies.
9. The school nurse acquires and maintains current knowledge and competency in school nursing practice.
10. The school nurse interacts with and contributes to the professional development of peers and school personnel as colleagues.
11. The school nurse's decisions and actions on behalf of clients are determined in an ethical manner.
12. The school nurse collaborates with the student, family, school staff, community, and other providers in providing student care.
13. The school nurse promotes use of research findings in school nursing practice.
14. The school nurse considers factors related to safety, effectiveness, and cost when planning and delivering care.
15. The school nurse uses effective written, verbal, and nonverbal communication skills.
16. The school nurse manages school health services.
17. The school nurse assists students, families, school staff, and community to achieve optimal levels of wellness through appropriately designed and delivered health education.

From the National Association of School Nurses and American Nurses Association (2001). Scope and standard of professional school nursing practice. *Silver Spring, MD: American Nurses Publishing.*

The role of school nurses has changed over the past decade as the population of children attending school has changed. School nurses address a wide range of issues to help improve school performance, such as attention deficit hyperactivity disorder, learning differences, communicable diseases, obesity, chronic disease, and medically fragile children (Schainker, & Grant, 2003). The breadth of school health issues are illustrated in 13 national health objectives published in *Healthy People 2010* (Box 16–5).

Many children have no health insurance, and school health services often serve as the safety net for these children. Many children have a single working parent or both parents work. In these instances the parents may be limited in their ability to obtain primary healthcare for the child. The school nurse is often relied upon to provide nursing assessment and identification of potential or existing health problems that require medical intervention. School nurses are also in a position to refer families to community resources to support their children's development and health.

School nurses work to remove or minimize the health barriers to learning so students can perform academically. School health services include preventive services, health promotion and health maintenance, health education, emergency care, and the referral and management of acute and chronic health problems. The traditional tasks of screening, first aid, and monitoring immunization status are still important, but health services provided in schools settings have increased dramatically.

MediaLink Resources for School Nurses

BOX 16–5 ***Healthy People 2010* Objectives that Relate to School Health Issues**

- Increase high school completion rate.
- Increase the percentage of middle, junior high, and senior high schools that provide health education to prevent health problems in the following areas: unintentional injury; violence; suicide; tobacco use and addiction; alcohol and other drug use; unintended pregnancy; HIV/AIDS, and STD infection; unhealthy dietary patterns; inadequate physical activity; and environmental health.
- Increase the percentage of the nation's elementary, middle, junior high, and senior high schools that have a nurse-to-student ratio of at least 1 to 750.
- Increase the percentage of the nation's primary and secondary schools that have official school policies ensuring the safety of students and staff from environmental hazards, such as chemicals in special classrooms, poor indoor air quality, asbestos, and exposure to pesticides.
- Increase the percentage of public and private schools that require use of appropriate head, face, eye, and mouth protection for students participating in school-sponsored physical activities.
- Reduce weapon carrying on school property.
- Increase the percentage of children and adolescents age 6 to 19 years whose intake of meals and snacks at school contributes to good overall dietary quality.
- Increase the percentage of school-based health centers with an oral health component.
- Increase the percentage of the nation's public and private schools that require daily physical education for all students.
- Increase the percentage of adolescents who participate in daily school physical education.
- Increase the percentage of adolescents who spend 50% of school physical education time being physically active.
- Increase the percentage of the nation's public and private schools that provide access to their physical activity spaces and facilities for all persons outside of normal school hours.
- Reduce the number of school or workdays missed by persons due to asthma.

From U.S. Department of Health and Human Services. (2000). Healthy People 2010 *(2nd ed.). Washington, DC: U.S. Government Printing Office. www.healthypeople.gov*

Roles of the Nurse in the School Setting

Nursing roles in the school setting include the following (Robinson, 2002).

- Infection control management to reduce infectious disease transmission, to improve school attendance, and to ensure compliance with immunization requirements
- Health education to promote healthy behaviors and wellness for students, parents, faculty, and staff
- Healthcare provision to assess the health status and screening of children for health conditions that have an impact on health and learning (such as vision and hearing impairments, and scoliosis) (Figure 16–4 ■); this additionally involves referring and managing acute and chronic health conditions, and administering medications and assuring appropriate administration by health aides

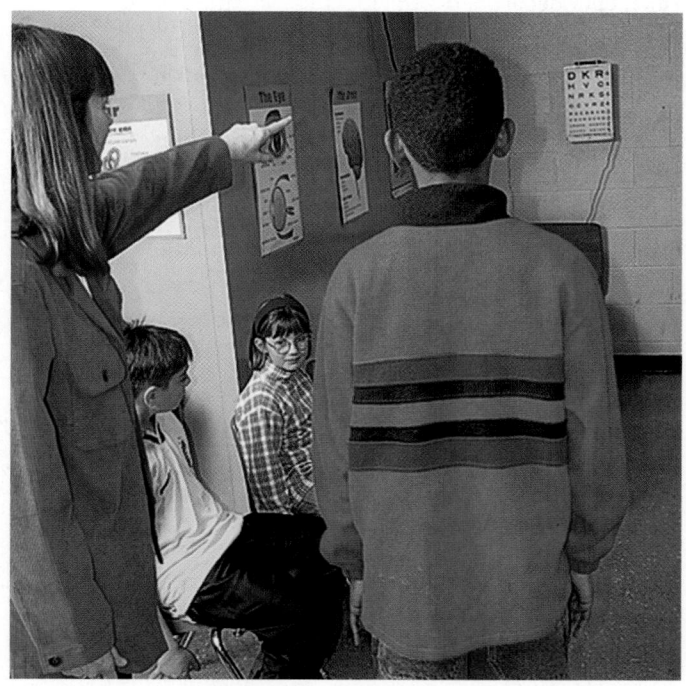

FIGURE 16–4 ■ The school is often the setting for screening tests of large groups of students at risk for a problem. Screening tests are often organized so all children in a particular grade are assessed, as in this test to detect vision problems. State laws mandate grades for screening and selected children who must be screened for conditions such as visual or hearing problems, and scoliosis screening in public schools.

- Special needs facilitation to make it possible for the child with complex health conditions to attend school; the nurse also participates as the health specialist on the team developing a child's individualized education plan (IEP) and individualized health plan (IHP) (see Chapter 20∞)
- Emergency care provider to ensure that children who are injured or who develop an acute illness while at school are assessed and provided the appropriate care until emergency medical services arrive (Figure 16–5 ■)
- Healthcare resource to guide development of a system for crisis intervention and other mental health problems
- Environmental safety officer to identify and control hazards in the school setting and promote a healthy school environment; documenting injury incidents that occur on school property can be analyzed to identify environmental and psychosocial behaviors that contribute to an unsafe setting
- Child advocate to promote a safer school environment, better nutrition, or increased physical activity for children to improve overall health
- Community resource to promote development of effective support systems between the student, family, school, and community

The 13 nurse activities that take the most time during the school year in one state are as follows: assessing health complaints, providing crisis intervention, documenting health room visits, administering medications, administering first aid, evaluating and counseling staff about their health needs, updating health records, ensuring immunization compliance, conferring with faculty, obtaining health and social histories, performing screening procedures, using the nursing process, and serving as a child advocate (Guilday, 2000).

Community Health Focus. The school nurse also plans, develops, manages, and evaluates healthcare services to all children in the educational setting. In many cases, the nurse works with families of the students to ensure that needed care is provided. Collaboration with the other health professionals in the community is becoming increasingly important to promote health in the school setting. Examples of such collaboration include the following:

- Partner with the physician consultant to discuss and update standing orders for the care of children. These standing orders usually address urgent and emergency care potentially needed by students as well as the variety of healthcare problems present in the population of students.
- Work with the parent-teacher association and other community organizations to organize health fairs and injury prevention programs for students.
- Communicate with the primary healthcare provider or with the pediatric specialist about children with specific health conditions that need to be effectively managed in the school setting. Because the school nurse has regular opportunities to monitor the health status of these children, the information shared helps primary healthcare providers with their ongoing management.

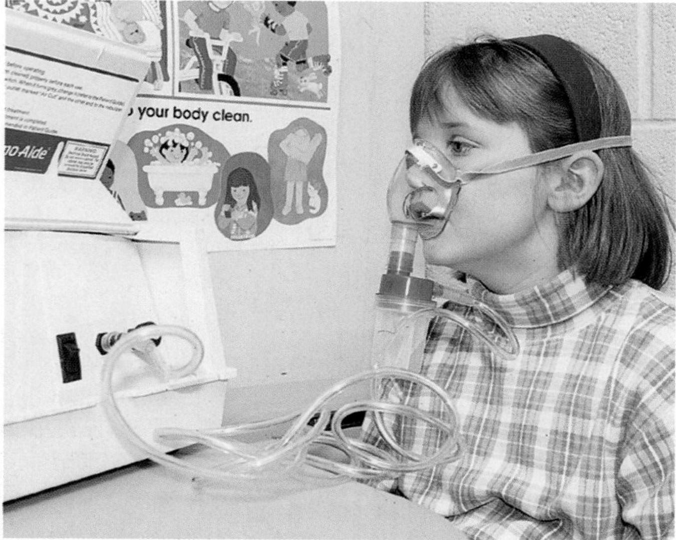

FIGURE 16–5 ■ The school nurse treats this child with a nebulizer to determine if the asthma attack can be controlled before calling the parent to come and pick up the child and seek care from the primary care provider.

Preparation for Emergencies. Injuries and acute illnesses occur frequently during school hours. An **emergency preparedness** plan, to ensure effective emergency intervention and transport for an acutely ill or injured child, is needed by every school. The school nurse often works with the school administrators, the physician consultant, and the local emergency medical services (EMS) agency to develop the plan of managing the emergency care of students. School personnel (administrators, secretaries, and health aides in the absence of the school nurse) need training to distinguish between a true emergency that requires activation of the local EMS system and an urgent problem that parents can be called to manage. Because the school nurse may not be employed at a school full time, other school personnel need to learn how to provide emergency care until the EMS providers arrive at the scene. See Box 16–6 for

BOX 16–6 Developing a School Emergency Preparedness Plan

1. Perform an emergency readiness needs assessment.
2. Invite a group of stakeholders (parents, teachers, community leaders, police, fire, EMS personnel) to participate in the initial meeting to form an emergency response plan.
3. Have a school walk-through.
4. Draft the emergency plan, then distribute and maintain the plan in the identified school or school system/district.
5. Develop training program goals and organize staff first-responder training.
6. Conduct a mock emergency with the local EMS agency before an emergency occurs.
7. Reevaluate the plan after each incident to identify ways to improve the plan.

Adapted from Hohenhaus, S. M. (2001). Pediatric emergency preparedness in schools: A report from the 2001 southeastern regional EMSC annual meeting. Journal of Emergency Nursing, *27(4)*, 355.

guidelines in developing an emergency care plan. (Table 9–16∞ on page 353 lists key points for an emergency healthcare plan for a child with a food allergy.)

Children with Special Healthcare Needs.

CHILDREN WITH COMPLEX HEALTHCARE CONDITIONS. Previously homebound children who are **medically fragile**—needing skilled nursing care with or without medical equipment to support vital functions—now attend school. Classifications of children who are medically fragile are as follows:

- Children with prolonged dependence on a medical device that is required to sustain life (mechanical ventilators, intravenous nutrition or drugs, tracheostomy, suctioning, oxygen, or tube feedings)
- Children with prolonged dependence on other medical devices that compensate for vital body functions who require daily or near daily nursing care such as apnea monitors, renal dialysis, urinary catheters, and colostomies (Office of Technology Assessment, 1987).

Federal law mandates that education be provided to all children with **disabilities,** impairment in one or more of five categories of function—cognition, communication, motor abilities, social abilities, or patterns of interactions, regardless of healthcare status. As a result, schools are now obligated to provide complex healthcare services to children (Box 16–7).

Some of these children have an assigned health aide or nurse because of the need for care and monitoring during the school day. The school nurses must be prepared to provide acute, episodic, chronic, and emergency care to medically fragile children. Examples of direct nursing care that is provided to these children are suctioning and tracheostomy care, IV medications, and gastrostomy feedings. See the skills manual for these procedures. The school nurse must also teach teachers and health aides to recognize when the child urgently needs care, and how to provide emergency care until help arrives. Because school nurses are unable to provide full-time care to medically fragile children in the classroom, they are responsible for training teachers and health aides to provide appropriate nursing care and monitoring the care provided.

CHILDREN WITH CHRONIC HEALTH CONDITIONS. Children with chronic conditions, such as asthma or diabetes, also need attention from the school nurse. These children may develop acute illnesses or become injured while at school and need nursing care. Some of these children need special accommodations in the school setting to fully participate in the learning environment. An **individualized health plan (IHP),** developed collaboratively by the parent, child, school nurse, school administrator, and teachers, is a formal mechanism to ensure that the child's health needs are managed in the school setting (Figure 16–6 ■).

BOX 16–7 Individuals with Disabilities Education Act

The 1975 Education for All Handicapped Children Act, PL 94-142, and the Education of the Handicapped Amendments of 1986, PL 99-457, guarantee a free and appropriate education for all children with disabilities between 3 and 21 years of age. This legislation was renamed the Individuals with Disabilities Education Act (IDEA) in 1991 and reauthorized by Congress in 1997. As a result of these laws, children with complex health conditions must receive a free and appropriate education regardless of their disability severity. The student must receive an individualized education based on their unique needs in the least restrictive educational environment.

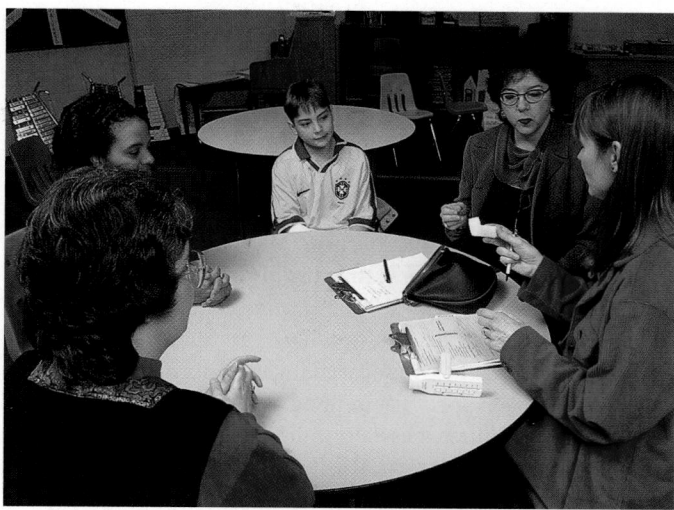

FIGURE 16–6 ■ Because some children need medications or other therapies during school hours, the parents and child, school nurse, teacher, and school administrators develop a plan to manage the child's condition during school hours. This document is the child's individual health plan.

The IHP is used when the student has a relatively complex health condition or when a need for modification of the school environment exists due to the child's health condition. For example when the child uses a wheelchair, arrangements must be made to use the elevator or the child must be assigned to classes only on the ground floor. The IHP helps ensure that all necessary information, needs, and procedures are considered to maximize the student's participation in the educational program. The parent provides medications, supplies, and equipment along with the physician's written instructions for care. The IHP may also include an emergency information form and emergency care plan.

CLINICAL TIP

Make sure the individualized health plan (IHP) includes directions for care of the child on the bus, on field trips, and during extracurricular activities.

The nursing process is the format used for development of the IHP. In many cases the health plan is integrated into the child's individualized education plan or individual family service plan. Treat the information in this plan as confidential, but make sure it is stored in an easily accessible area for personnel who must provide emergency care. Train the school personnel to care for the child who needs medications or has special equipment, including special precautions to use when providing care.

MediaLink Develop an IHP

Facilitating Child's Return to School. The school nurse also helps transition the child back into the classroom following an acute illness or injury, especially when environmental adaptation is required or following the diagnosis of a health condition or the significant change in status associated with a chronic condition. This transition is greatly assisted when the pediatric nurse in the hospital or community setting or the child's primary care provider contacts the school nurse to coordinate the child's return to school. Educational materials about the child's condition sent to the school assist with this transition. The school nurse then begins to work with the family to prepare teachers and school administrators for the child's special needs. The child's teacher and classmates can be prepared for the child's physical changes if appropriate. Often an IHP must be developed or modified.

Because the nurse has continuing contact with the child throughout the school year, it is possible to evaluate the effectiveness of the IHPs, the nursing care provided, and the administration's policies regarding school healthcare. Evaluation of the IHPs and emergency plans leads to future improvements in the school health program.

Nursing in Childcare Settings

Many young children are cared for in childcare settings while parents are at work, and different types of childcare arrangements are available. The most common settings include the following:

- In-home care by a family member, babysitter, or nanny; alternate arrangements may be made by babysitter cooperatives
- A licensed childcare family home setting in which up to five children are cared for by a single childcare provider
- A licensed childcare center that cares for six or more children

States establish minimum licensure requirements and guidelines for the safe operation of childcare settings that are based on the number of children cared for. The licensure requirements address the qualifications of staff, ratio of staff to number of children, training requirements for staff, safe food handling and safe health practices, and environmental safety. The goal is to promote the health and safety, as well as growth and development, of the children served. Guidelines for the safe operation of childcare centers are available through the National Resource Center for Health and Safety in Child Care.

Role of the Nurse in Childcare Settings

Although nurses are not often employed in childcare centers, they can have an important role in providing consultation for the health and safety of the center. Nurses can assume an important role in the establishment of the childcare center's policies for health practices, teaching staff about safe health practices, and monitoring health practices in the setting. The nurse consultant can also teach staff to identify children with illnesses and to provide first aid for injured children. In some cases, especially in childcare centers for ill children, nurses provide health screening and direct nursing care (Evers, 2002).

Reducing Disease Transmission. The nurse works with the childcare center administrators to develop guidelines and to assess childcare practices to identify opportunities for reducing infectious disease transmission among the staff and children. This is crucial, as children are close together in large numbers; they put things in their mouths; they may be contagious before symptoms occur; and they are susceptible to most infectious agents. Studies have found that children attending childcare centers are at increased risk for otitis media, bronchiolitis, and gastroenteritis (Donowitz, 1999). The nurse can also teach the childcare staff to assess children and provide care in a manner that reduces the transmission of infectious disease.

- Guidelines for review of each child's and staff member's immunization documentation should be developed. Nurses help childcare administrators understand the schedule of immunizations so that their assessment of appropriate immunization status is correct. Guidelines also need to be developed for the exclusion of unimmunized children when a vaccine-preventable disease occurs in the facility. See Chapter 19∞.
- Childcare workers are taught to conduct a daily health check of each child, looking for behavior changes, rashes, fever, complaints of not feeling well, and other signs and symptoms such as vomiting, diarrhea, or eye drainage. Guidelines for exclusion of children with different infectious conditions should be developed and followed.
- Guidelines for diapering infants and toddlers are important to reduce the transmission of diseases. Disposable diapers are used routinely unless the infant has a documented medical reason, such as an allergy, that allows an exception to the policy. Infants are checked for wet and soiled diapers at least hourly. A specific diaper-changing area is used and guidelines to reduce contact of urine and feces with various surfaces and staff clothing are followed. Handwashing and sanitizing the diaper-changing surface are also necessary (Box 16–8).

BOX 16–8 Childcare Procedure for Diaper Changing

1. Get organized. Before bringing the child to the diaper-changing area, wash your hands, gather what is needed, and bring it to the diaper-changing table.
2. Carry the child to the changing table, keeping soiled clothing away from you and any surfaces you cannot easily clean and sanitize after the diaper is changed.
3. Remove soiled clothing and the diaper. Place and securely tie soiled clothing in a plastic bag to send home with the child. Fold the soiled surfaces of the diaper inward and place in the covered diaper pan.
4. Clean the diaper area with disposable wipes. If gloves were used, remove the gloves and place them in the covered diaper pan. If gloves were not used, clean your hands with a disposable wipe.
5. Put on a clean diaper and dress the child. Wash the child's hands and return the child to the play area.
6. Clean and sanitize the diaper-changing surface and other potentially contaminated surfaces.
7. Wash your hands and record the diaper change on the child's daily log.

Adapted from National Resource Center for Health and Safety in Child Care Health Promotion and Protection in Child Care. http://nrc.uchsc.edu/CFOC/XMLVersion/Chapter_3.xml, *accessed 8/13/2003.*

- Guidelines for handwashing of all staff and children, managing nasal secretions, sanitizing toys and surfaces where children play, and managing cuts and scrapes to reduce exposure to bodily fluids are also important to reduce disease transmission. The nurse can work with childcare center staff to implement these guidelines and monitor how well they are followed.
- As it often takes a while to contact the parents of a sick child, teach childcare staff ways to provide care to the child and reduce exposure to the other children. Review immunization records of enrolled children to ensure that vaccine-preventable diseases are minimized.
- Guidelines are also needed for when to send home a child who is ill and when to permit the child to return after various types of illnesses.

Health Promotion. The nurse promotes healthy behaviors by designing and offering health education programs for the children. For example, teach proper oral hygiene, blowing the nose into a tissue, and handwashing after toileting and before eating. If childcare providers encourage these practices, they will become habits that the children use routinely.

Other health promotion actions that the nurse can encourage in the childcare center are monitoring the food eaten by the child to ensure that the child's essential nutritional needs are met in support of growth and development. Arrangements for rest periods and naps by young children are also important. Childcare providers need to place infants on their back to sleep to reduce the risk of sudden infant death syndrome. See Chapter 25∞.

Environmental Safety. The nurse should inspect the childcare environment to identify potential hazards that could cause injury to the children. Be sure that cleaning supplies and other toxins are stored in a locked cabinet to prevent children from gaining access to them. Toys used by children should be inspected to ensure that there are no sharp edges or points, small parts, or pinching parts. Check the playground equipment for safety (Figure 16–7 ■). See Evidence-Based Practice: Reducing Injuries in Childcare Centers.

Care for Children with Illnesses. Some childcare centers have the capacity to care for children with illnesses. The nurse can work as a consultant to develop plans to care for and manage children with communicable diseases. Additional guidelines for infection control are needed to prevent the spread of infection to other children in the center.

Emergency Care Planning. The nurse can help develop a guideline for assessment of children to identify an emergency health condition or when medical care is needed within an hour. The nurse should assist the childcare center in developing an

FIGURE 16–7 ■ Assess the childcare center's environment for safety hazards. Check the area around playground equipment, making sure that there are wood chips or cushioned tiles under the equipment. Inspect the playground equipment for loose nuts and bolts and instability at least monthly and make sure that no screws are protruding or exposed.

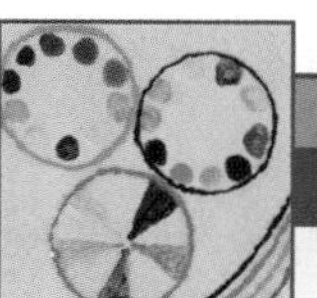

EVIDENCE-BASED PRACTICE
Reducing Injuries in Childcare Centers

BACKGROUND

Injuries are a major cause of morbidity and mortality in children. Limited information is known about the incidence of injury in childcare settings to design and implement injury prevention programs.

EVIDENCE

Data were collected for a full year about the types of injuries occurring to children in two urban childcare centers. A total of 131 children between 6 weeks and 7 years of age (mean age of 24 months) were enrolled full or part time in the centers. During the year, a total of 897 incident reports identified 1,023 injuries. The distribution of injuries was as follows: bites (39%), falls (23%), bumps and bruises (22%), and scratches, cuts, blisters, and fracture (16%). Only 2 children required medical attention, while the remainder received first aid on site. Infants and toddlers (0 to 36 months of age) had the highest frequency of injury, reflecting in large part the high frequency of biting reported. Approximately 60% of all injuries occurred in the morning hours (Waibel & Misra, 2003).

IMPLICATIONS

Understanding the type of injuries that happen in childcare centers, the age group most affected, and other information, such as time of day, provides important information for childcare center management in promotion of the health of enrolled children. Injury prevention strategies can potentially be developed based on collected data.

CRITICAL THINKING APPLICATION

Consider the distribution of injuries and identify potential strategies that could be used to reduce the number of biting and fall incidents. What actions could the childcare center workers take to reduce the number of incidents that occur during morning hours?

emergency care plan for instances when a child becomes acutely ill or injured. This plan should include the following elements:

- Giving first aid
- Calling 9-1-1 or the local emergency number for emergency medical response to transport the child to the emergency department
- Calling the parent or emergency contact person to notify someone about the child's condition
- accompanying the child to the emergency department to stay with the child until the parent arrives

Other Community Settings

In many other community settings, the nurse's role may be similar to that in a school setting. Promoting health, preventing disease, and preventing injury are equally important in childcare centers, camps, health department clinics, and disaster or homeless shelters. For example, nurses may work with homeless shelter administrators to address infection control issues and to assess the safety of the children's environment. See Chapter 7∞.

Role of the Nurse in Camp Settings

Nurses in camps assess and improve the safety of the children's environment, provide nursing care to children with acute illnesses and injuries, and plan activities to promote health. Some special camps for children with chronic conditions must have trained personnel to provide needed medical and nursing care while children are participating in recreational activities.

Home Healthcare Nursing

Home healthcare is a component of the continuum of comprehensive healthcare provided to children and families. Children with episodic or long-term health conditions can benefit from home health services, including health promotion, health maintenance, and health restorative care, to promote their optimal function and participation in the family. Children with complex healthcare needs can be cared for in their home because of technological advances, such as portable medical equipment. Home health services include the care to children with complex health conditions, short-term acute care conditions, and even for terminal conditions (Figure 16–8 ■). See Chapter 22∞ for more information about palliative and hospice care in the home setting.

Advances in medical technology have enabled many infants and children who would previously have died to survive very low birth weight, birth defects, and various health conditions. This has resulted in an increasing number of children with complex healthcare conditions cared for at home. The home environment is believed to be optimal for the long-term care of these children so they can participate as part of the family and have their growth and development promoted. The family gains some control over their lives by having the child in the home versus coordinating visits to the child and trying to maintain the family (Balinsky & Marié, 2001).

Home healthcare is costly, but less expensive than when the same care is provided in the hospital. Several studies have documented significantly lower monthly costs for the care of low-birth-weight infants, intravenous antibiotics for cellulitis, children dependent on respiratory technology, and children on chemotherapy (National Association of Home Care, 2001). Health insurers pay many of the costs associated with home care; however, the family ends up paying some costs out of pocket, such as some medications, supplies, and transportation, causing a financial burden. In some cases a parent must give up employment to provide care to the child.

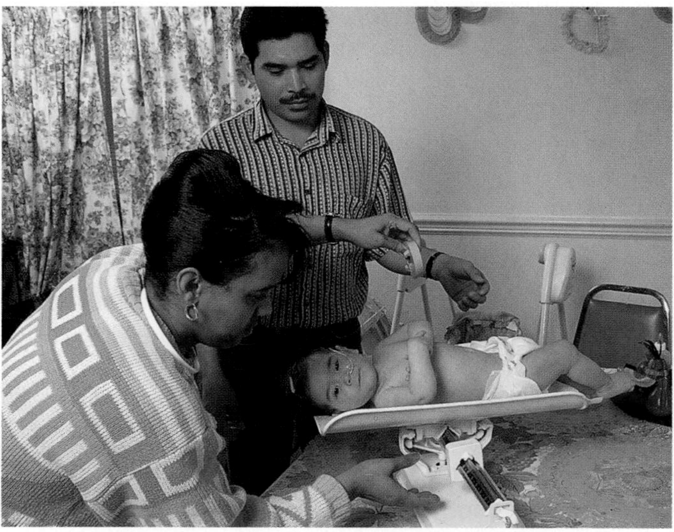

FIGURE 16–8 ■ Nurses provide both short-term and long-term services to families in the home setting. In some cases, families need support for a short time after the child is discharged from the hospital following an acute illness. In other cases, families need assistance with complex nursing care for the child dependent on technology for survival.

Many of the children needing home healthcare are medically fragile. Parents and other care providers without backgrounds in healthcare are given tremendous responsibilities to provide technology-assisted healthcare to their child. Technology-assisted care in the home may include any of the following: ventilators, tracheostomies, suctioning, cardiorespiratory monitors, nutritional support with enteral or intravenous feedings and feeding pumps, intravenous fluids, and medications with intravenous pumps. In some cases, families have created mini intensive care units in their home. Examples of some serious chronic conditions cared for by families in the home include children with congenital heart defects before corrective surgery, bronchopulmonary dysplasia, children on peritoneal dialysis, and cancer in its terminal stage.

Only a small number of these children have chronic conditions serious enough to need continuous (daily, or up to 24 hours a day) private duty care in the home. Nurses remain in the home for an 8- to 12-hour period providing direct nursing care to the child. Healthcare systems (healthcare providers and insurers) are challenged to simultaneously address the child's illness and developmental needs while providing the support needed by these families so that children do well in their environments. The family also needs help to support the growing child, particularly when of preschool and school age. Options for interaction with children the same age are also important. In these cases, the federal mandate for the education of children with disabilities provides an avenue to assure education in the preschool and school setting.

Most children receive intermittent skilled nursing visits to assess the child and to see how family members are managing the child's healthcare needs. Intermittent home healthcare services (one to several visits a week) may be provided to help families during the child's acute recovery, such as a child with osteomyelitis receiving home antibiotic infusion therapy.

Role of the Pediatric Nurse in Home Care

Home care nursing is focused on assisting a family to gain a greater ability to more independently manage the care of a child with a chronic condition. Following are two major goals of working with families in the home care setting.

- Promoting or restoring health while attempting to minimize the effects of the disability and illness, including terminal illness
- Promoting child or family self-care capacity in the home

Nurses develop strategies to support and partner with families who provide care to their children in the home. To work in the home care setting, nurses need a variety of skills:

- Knowledge and experience in acute care practice with various medical technologies (These skills enable nurses to provide direct care, teach the family and child self-care practices, and monitor the child's progress. This may involve collaboration with other healthcare team members.)
- Community assessment skills; an understanding of community resources, financing mechanisms, and multiagency collaboration; and good communication skills
- An understanding of the cultural diversity in the community and the specific cultural values of the families served
- An understanding of the community's healthcare resources to better assist families to find the most supportive services to match the child's and family's needs
- Skill in educating family members to assume care of the child

For most children, home healthcare is initiated after an acute hospitalization. Conditions associated with preterm births are the major reason for pediatric home care referrals (Madigan, Younglut, & Haruzivishe, 1999). The hospital nurse, discharge planner, or case manager usually has responsibility for coordinating the child's and family's transition from hospital to home care in collaboration with the home health agency and an assigned home health nurse. The home health nurse works in collaboration with hospital nurses by assessing the following caregiver readiness to care for the child at home (Figure 16–9 ■).

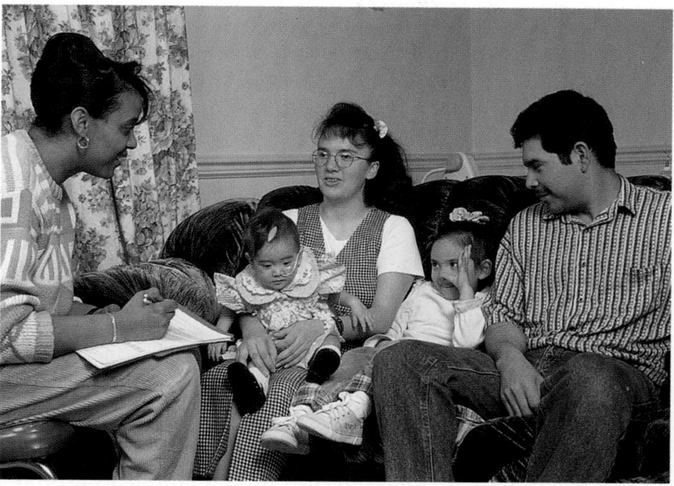

FIGURE 16–9 ■ A visit to the home when all family members are present provides the best information for assessing caregiver readiness to care for the child being discharged from the hospital with a complex health condition.

NURSING MANAGEMENT

■ Nursing Assessment and Diagnosis

Home health nurses assess the home, the child, and the family during intermittent skilled nursing visits. Assessment of the home is focused on safety of the environment for the child and the resources needed for the child's care. When working with the hospital discharge planner to initiate home health services, the following aspects of the home are assessed.

- Home readiness (safe sleeping arrangements, adequate supplies, ability to meet nutritional and fluid needs, telephone access, heat, electricity, refrigeration, and lack of any communicable diseases in the home)
- Potential hazards related to the child's age, condition, and requirements for technology-assisted care (if extension cords are needed to reach electrical outlets, the equipment may lose power if someone trips over the cord and disconnects it by mistake)
- Features in the home environment that could cause an acute illness, such as use of a woodstove or fireplace for heating that could cause respiratory distress or renovation of a house built before 1960 that could expose the child to lead dust. (Additionally, the nurse may identify family members who smoke.)

Assessment of the child is focused on the current health status, growth, developmental progress, and social interaction with family members and healthcare providers. Observation of the potential for abuse and neglect is an important ongoing assessment for these high-risk children.

The family is assessed for parenting skills, as well as their abilities in providing the child's needed medical procedures and monitoring the child's health status. Family strengths and coping abilities are evaluated using the family assessment guidelines in Chapter 2∞. The presence of siblings, their developmental and physical status, and their needs should also be assessed.

Examples of nursing diagnoses that could apply to the family as the child transitions from the hospital to home setting include the following:

- Impaired Home Maintenance related to ineffective family coping
- Impaired Adjustment (parents) related to multiple stressors in caring for a child with a complex health condition

- Ineffective Family Therapeutic Regimen Management related to complexity of medical interventions, information misinterpretation, and excessive demands made on the family
- Social Isolation related to demands on family members to care for child

Planning and Implementation

Nurses help families in the home setting in the following ways.

- Assuring competent care to the child
- Educating them about the child's condition and physical signs and symptoms that may indicate a change in health status
- Educating them and demonstrating methods to promote the child's development
- Linking them to community resources, including support groups, respite care, and therapeutic recreation
- Assisting families in time management skills and patient care management
- Advocating for increased insurance coverage or locating other sources of financial assistance

Partnering with the Family

The nurse and family work in partnership in the home to promote the health of the child and of the family as a unit. The nurse must recognize and accept that control belongs to the family in the home care setting. The parents are the employer with the ability to hire and fire. It is critical for the nurse to develop a respectful and trusting relationship with the family. Every interaction is negotiated with the family, or between the family and child, if there are differences in what they want. The nurse must be flexible and able to set aside power. Conflicts may occur when differences in opinion about the child's care become apparent. Open communication is essential so the nurse can learn what is important to the child and family, and then modify the nursing care plan when appropriate. House rules for such things as parking, private areas in the home, and routines may need to be negotiated, and then rules must all be followed (Box 16–9). Role expectations of the nurse must be clearly understood to reduce stress in the family. The success of home care is also based on effective cultural communication. For example, some Jewish families follow strict dietary guidelines that do not permit milk and meat to be mixed. The nurse needs to abide by the dietary guidelines and observe the family's food preparation practices. See Developing Cultural Competence: Integrating Family Preferences in the Care Plan.

When nurses provide home care, it is important for a parent to be present and work in partnership with the nurse. Informed consent is needed for invasive treatments and decisions for provision of emergency care to avoid serious risk for life and limb. When the caregiver is not present and the home care nurse provides such care, the home health agency and the nurse are at significant liability risk (Hogue, 1993).

The range of nursing care activities that may be included in a child's care plan in the home setting include sensory stimulation, routines of daily living, positioning and skin care with gentle handling, respiratory care, nutrition and elimination, medications, and other supportive therapies. Other providers, such as physical therapists, speech-language therapists, occupational therapists, and social workers, may provide other healthcare services in collaboration with the home health nurse. A plan for safe evacuation of the home is needed in case of fire. See Partnering with Families: Developing a Fire Escape Plan.

BOX 16–9 House Rules for Negotiation

When working with families in the home, be sure to discuss the following guidelines for expected behavior and role of the nurse, as well as the family's preferences for involvement in the care of the child (Messinger & Dolan, 1997).

- Access to the home: parking location, door to enter, where to store belongings, refrigerator use, private areas
- Care of child: routines for daily care, feeding, bathing, bedtime, clothing, discipline, division of labor
- Care of child's environment, child's laundry
- Safety: visitors who are permitted to enter the home, arrangement of furniture
- Breaks for meals, use of telephone, use of radio or television
- Discipline of other children

Emergency Preparedness

An emergency care plan should be developed for any child whose condition could worsen rapidly and become life threatening, beyond the care that the parents or home health nurse can provide. Examples of health conditions that fall into this category are serious congenital heart defects, tracheostomies, and apnea. Information should provide guidelines for when to call 9-1-1 or the local emergency number. The local emergency medical services squad should be called to visit so emergency medical technicians can become knowledgeable of the child's potential emergency care needs. The emergency care plan should include a written emergency medical history that provides the emergency healthcare provider with enough basic information to understand the child's health condition, to prevent delays in disease-specific treatment, and to minimize unnecessary interventions until the child's personal physician can be consulted. See Figure 16–10 ■ for a copy of the emergency information form recommended by emergency care providers.

DEVELOPING CULTURAL COMPETENCE
Integrating Family Preferences in the Care Plan

When providing care in the home, recognize potential conflicts between "mainstream" medical care and the family's cultural preferences after carefully listening to the parents' perspectives. Learn and use the family's perspectives of health and disease in discussions and in development of the plan of care. For example, the family may want an amulet to hang around the infant's neck to protect against witchcraft (Hopi Indians) or to have a child wear a jade charm to bring health (Chinese).

When the child is dependent upon technology, the family should notify the power company so that high priority can be given to getting resources to the child when needed. Backup generators may be needed if electrical power for life-sustaining equipment is essential. The child should also be registered for a disaster shelter that can accommodate the healthcare needs of the child and at least one caregiver.

Evaluation

Expected outcomes of nursing care include the following:

- Care of the child's medical needs is integrated into the family's routines when possible.
- The family has an emergency care plan for the child in the event of a disaster, a weather emergency, or if the child's condition suddenly worsens.
- The home health nurse and family work in partnership to promote the child's health, growth, and development.

Community Health Nursing

Community health nursing is the fusion of public health and nursing practice to promote the health of a **population,** the collection of individuals that make up a community. Public health practice promotes the health of populations rather than individuals with an emphasis on health promotion and disease prevention. This is often accomplished through assessment, policy development to promote the population's health, and assuring the availability of and access to those health services needed to sustain and improve health. One example of national public health goals and objectives for the U.S. population is *Healthy People 2010.* See Box 16–10 for overarching goals and objective categories. The document has 28 focus areas and 467 individual measurable objectives, each with a health indicator and target for improvement.

Community health nurses provide care to children in many settings. Depending upon the manner in which healthcare services are organized in a community, community health nurses may provide services in a variety of settings, such as the following:

- Public health clinics providing well-child care, immunizations, and care for other populations such as adolescents seeking family planning or treatment for sexually transmitted diseases
- Schools serving as school nurses or consultants on school health issues
- Childcare settings serving as consultants for the health and safety of enrolled children
- Home providing skilled nursing care through a visiting nurses service, or by assisting high-risk families with the transition of a newborn into the family
- Homeless shelters providing health promotion, health maintenance, and episodic illness care

Community health nurses take a leadership role in helping the population obtain health services through assessing community needs and resources, and then developing health programs to address the needs of children and their families.

PARTNERING WITH FAMILIES

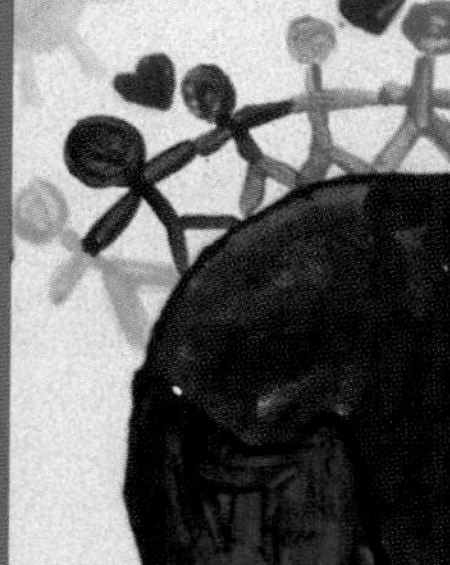

Developing a Fire Escape Plan

- Have working smoke detectors in the home and teach children what the alarm means.
- Draw a diagram of your house. Mark all windows and doors.
- Plan two routes out of every room.
- Think about an escape plan if the fire starts in the kitchen, bedroom, or basement.
- Figure out the best way to get infants and young children out of the house. Will you carry them? Is there more than one small child, and if so how will you get them out if you are the only adult?
- Teach preschool and school-age children to follow the escape plan by crawling, touching doors, and going to the window if the door is hot. Show children how to cover the nose and mouth to reduce smoke inhalation.
- Prepare an alternate fire escape plan in case you are alone with the child when the fire begins.
- Keep home exits clear of toys and debris.
- Select a safe meeting place outside the home. Teach children not to go back inside the burning home.

ASSESSMENT OF COMMUNITY NEEDS AND RESOURCES

Community Assessment

Community assessment is a process of compiling data about a community's health status and resources for the purpose of public health planning to address health needs. A community assessment may be used to identify the specific needs of a target population within that community. This could be for all children in a community or for a selected group of children

BOX 16–10 *Healthy People 2010* Goals and Objectives Categories

GOALS

- Increase quality and years of healthy life
- Eliminate disparities in health status among subpopulations

CATEGORIES OF OBJECTIVES

- Promoting healthy behaviors
- Promoting healthy and safe communities
- Improving systems for personal and public health
- Preventing and reducing diseases and disorders

From U.S. Department of Health and Human Services. (2000). Healthy People 2010 *(2nd ed.). Washington, DC: U.S. Government Printing Office. www.healthypeople.gov*

Last name:

Emergency Information Form for Children With Special Needs

American College of Emergency Physicians®

American Academy of Pediatrics 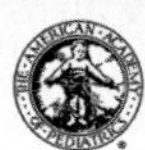

Date form completed By Whom	Revised	Initials
	Revised	Initials

Name:	Birth date: Nickname:
Home Address:	Home/Work Phone:
Parent/Guardian:	Emergency Contact Names & Relationship:
Signature/Consent*:	
Primary Language:	Phone Number(s):

Physicians:	
Primary care physician:	Emergency Phone:
	Fax:
Current Specialty physician: Specialty:	Emergency Phone:
	Fax:
Current Specialty physician: Specialty:	Emergency Phone:
	Fax:
Anticipated Primary ED:	Pharmacy:
Anticipated Tertiary Care Center:	

Diagnoses/Past Procedures/Physical Exam:	
1.	Baseline physical findings:
2.	
3.	Baseline vital signs:
4.	
Synopsis:	
	Baseline neurological status:

*Consent for release of this form to health care providers

FIGURE 16–10 ■ Emergency information form. Special medical emergencies can develop quickly in a child with severe and complex medical problems. An emergency information form should provide a summary of the child's medical history, baseline physical findings, and important and unique management requirements. (Used with permission of the American Academy of Pediatrics, Committee on Pediatric Emergency Medicine, 1999.)

Last name:

Diagnoses/Past Procedures/Physical Exam continued:

Medications:

1.
2.
3.
4.
5.
6.

Significant baseline ancillary findings (lab, x-ray, ECG):

Prostheses/Appliances/Advanced Technology Devices:

Management Data:

Allergies: Medications/Foods to be avoided	and why:
1.	
2.	
3.	

Procedures to be avoided	and why:
1.	
2.	
3.	

Immunizations

Dates					
DPT					
OPV					
MMR					
HIB					

Dates					
Hep B					
Varicella					
TB status					
Other					

Antibiotic prophylaxis: Indication: Medication and dose:

Common Presenting Problems/Findings With Specific Suggested Managements

Problem	Suggested Diagnostic Studies	Treatment Considerations

Comments on child, family, or other specific medical issues:

Physician/Provider Signature: **Print Name:**

FIGURE 16–10 ■ (continued)

(such as those who rely on technology to sustain life) who may have needs for special services. Knowledge of existing resources and programs permits health professionals to learn if the health needs of children are being met or if additional programs or resources are needed. A community assessment is a detailed and lengthy process that involves community partners, but follows the nursing process format. An overview of the community assessment process is provided below, but additional resources such as a community health nursing textbook are needed to complete a full assessment.

Community assessments are conducted for the following reasons.

- A request from interested community advocates or the local health department can identify health needs for a specific target population.
- Justification to fund for a new or expanded healthcare program occurs. Healthcare programs constantly compete for funding, so information about the program and its success in reaching children in one community may lead to support for the program's expansion to another community.
- Evaluation of responses to healthcare programs or interventions (such as immunizations, injury prevention program, or services targeted to new immigrants in the community) may provide the data to know if the children with greatest needs have been appropriately targeted and are benefiting equally from the intervention.

The focus of a community assessment is on the target population, such as the children in a specific community, rather than the needs of an individual patient. This ensures that all children, regardless of socioeconomic status and racial group, are considered when trying to assure access to care or specific interventions—such as injury prevention programs, getting all children immunized, and making sure all children have access to school health services or suicide prevention programs.

A community assessment is often initiated because one or more individuals (i.e., concerned parents, school nurse, or community leader) are concerned about a health or social issue, such as a child who is severely injured in a pedestrian crossing on the way to school. The concerned individuals then partner with others from the community to investigate if this is an isolated event, or if similar incidents have happened at other locations and to identify ways to protect other children. Community partners for this investigation and community assessment may include the following: a school nurse, parent-teacher association, Safe Kids Coalition, faith community, local trauma center, emergency department nurses, representatives of community organizations such as Kiwanis, health department statistician, community advocates, elected officials, and family members. A pediatric nurse and school nurse are important members of the group when pediatric health issues are being addressed. See Developing Cultural Competence: Integrating Cultural Groups into Community Assessments.

The first step in beginning a community assessment is to clearly define the purpose. Then the scope of the assessment is outlined to keep the community assessment focused. The purpose is usually associated with a specific problem that an advocate or community leader would like to have researched and addressed by the community. Example issues could be one of the following:

- Several child pedestrians and bicyclists have been injured or killed by motor vehicles over the past 6 months in the same neighborhood.
- Five teens riding in the back of a pickup truck are killed after a motor vehicle crash.
- Three teens from a local high school have committed suicide in the past 2 months.
- The number of children who are fully immunized on school entry has declined in the last year.

Once the group has determined the focus of the assessment to be conducted, the data resources are identified to study the problem. Various factors that influence the health of a community should be considered in the collection of data (Clark, 2003).

- *Biophysical characteristics*—demographic characteristics such as age composition of the community, birth statistics, age-specific and cause-specific mortality rates, racial composition, and morbidity (Incidence and prevalence of certain diseases as well as the immunization status of children in the community are also important characteristics.)
- *Psychological characteristics*—community prospects for continuing growth or economic challenges, cohesion of the community in dealing with past health problems or crises, existing tensions between various community groups, adequacy of personal safety services, communication networks, stresses in the community, and incident rates of homicide and suicide
- *Physical environment*—type of community (rural, urban, suburban), size, climate, topographical features, adequacy of housing, water supply, waste disposal, and potential hazards in community (chemical plant, nuclear reactor, pollution, trains carrying hazardous materials through community)
- *Sociocultural characteristics*—community government and informal community leadership, language as a barrier to healthcare and health education, transportation resources, income and education levels, employment levels, occupations and exposure to health hazards, number of homeless families and children, marital status, family composition, religion, recreational services, shopping, and local social service agencies

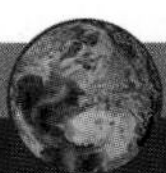

DEVELOPING CULTURAL COMPETENCE
Integrating Cultural Groups into Community Assessments

Community assessment leaders need to make sure members of the targeted community are involved in any assessment process. Community members representing the different cultural groups in the target population help balance out the experts who may have an organizational agenda. Cultural group representatives provide a more balanced perspective of the community's needs and help identify culturally appropriate and culturally acceptable strategies to address the problem.

- *Behavioral characteristics*—nutrition and specific dietary patterns (overweight, underweight, ethnic nutritional patterns) and use of harmful substances
- *Health system characteristics*—type of health services available to children in the community, their underuse or overuse, number of children covered by health insurance, Medicaid or State Children's Health Insurance Program (SCHIP), uninsured children, alternative healthcare services, and barriers to healthcare access

The types of data, where to obtain them, methods for obtaining the data, and the plans for data analysis are made. See Table 16–1 for suggestions for obtaining community data. Collect national, neighboring state, and state data for comparison with community data. Comparison will provide information about how similar or different the community statistics are for the health problem. Look at trends in data over several years to determine if the identified problem is a cluster of events that is part of a larger significant pattern. For example, the timing and clustering of events, such as the number of child pedestrians and bicyclists killed or injured, provide a clue to explore recent changes in the community environment that could be associated with the events. (Have traffic patterns changed because of construction? Does this happen every year as school sessions begin? Is it related to children enjoying spring weather after school?) Once the data are collected and analyzed, the community group can then develop a plan to address the problem and have baseline data for evaluation of the planned community intervention.

Key community assets should also be identified during the data collection stage. See Figure 16–11 ■ for a sample geographic map of a community and the location of its assets, such as its healthcare facilities and resources. The community assets map helps identify the presence of some community resources. Community organizations that are not associated with a specific healthcare facility may provide additional community health resources. Examples of such groups include the following:

- Kiwanis International has a community program focus called Young Children Priority One that supports education, trauma care, and injury prevention programs.
- Coalitions of the National SAFE KIDS Campaign have programs to reduce unintentional childhood injury.
- General Federation of Women's Clubs supports purchase of pediatric equipment for hospitals and emergency medical services.
- Lions Clubs support programs for visually impaired children.
- Shriner organizations support healthcare of children with musculoskeletal conditions, burns, and spinal cord injuries.

TABLE 16–1 Sources of Data for a Community Assessment

SOURCE OF COMMUNITY DATA	EXAMPLES
State vital records	Birth rate, age-specific death rate
Census	Age and racial composition of the population
Local agencies	Hospital trauma registry for number of injured children admitted to hospital, child abuse incidents from child protective services, number of infants receiving WIC services, number of children with type 1 diabetes
Local chapters of voluntary organizations	
Faith-based community	Number of refuge families sponsored, number of children in the families
Community surveys	Frequency of health services used, such as public health clinic for immunizations
Newspaper reports	Number of pediatric motor vehicle injuries
Telephone book	Numbers and types of healthcare providers
Law enforcement agencies	Motor vehicle accident reports, crime, homicides
Observation	Number of schools, recreational facilities
Interviews with key informants	Perception of personal/child health needs, perception of community health needs

Adapted from Clark, M. J. (2003). Community health nursing *(4th ed., p. 323). Upper Saddle River, NJ: Prentice Hall Health.*

Community Nursing Diagnoses

When the data have been collected, a careful analysis is conducted. The results are shared with the group performing the community assessment for interpretation and to begin setting priorities for action. School nurses and community health nurses may use these data to develop community or target group nursing diagnoses. The community nursing diagnoses should reflect existing, emerging, or potential threats to health, as well as community strengths and competencies. Examples include:

- Risk for Injury related to lack of safe bicycle paths in high traffic areas
- Ineffective Community Coping related to lack of disaster planning
- Ineffective Community Therapeutic Regimen Management related to inadequate resources for health promotion services to homeless children
- Impaired Health Maintenance related to knowledge deficit and non-English speaking or reading ability.

Planning and Intervention

Planning and implementation begins after collected data has been analyzed and the community health problem is more clearly described. The plan often involves brainstorming to identify several interventions that help the community improve the problem. The planning and selection of interventions continues to be a collaborative process with all the partners contributing ideas, developing

MediaLink Community Health Resources

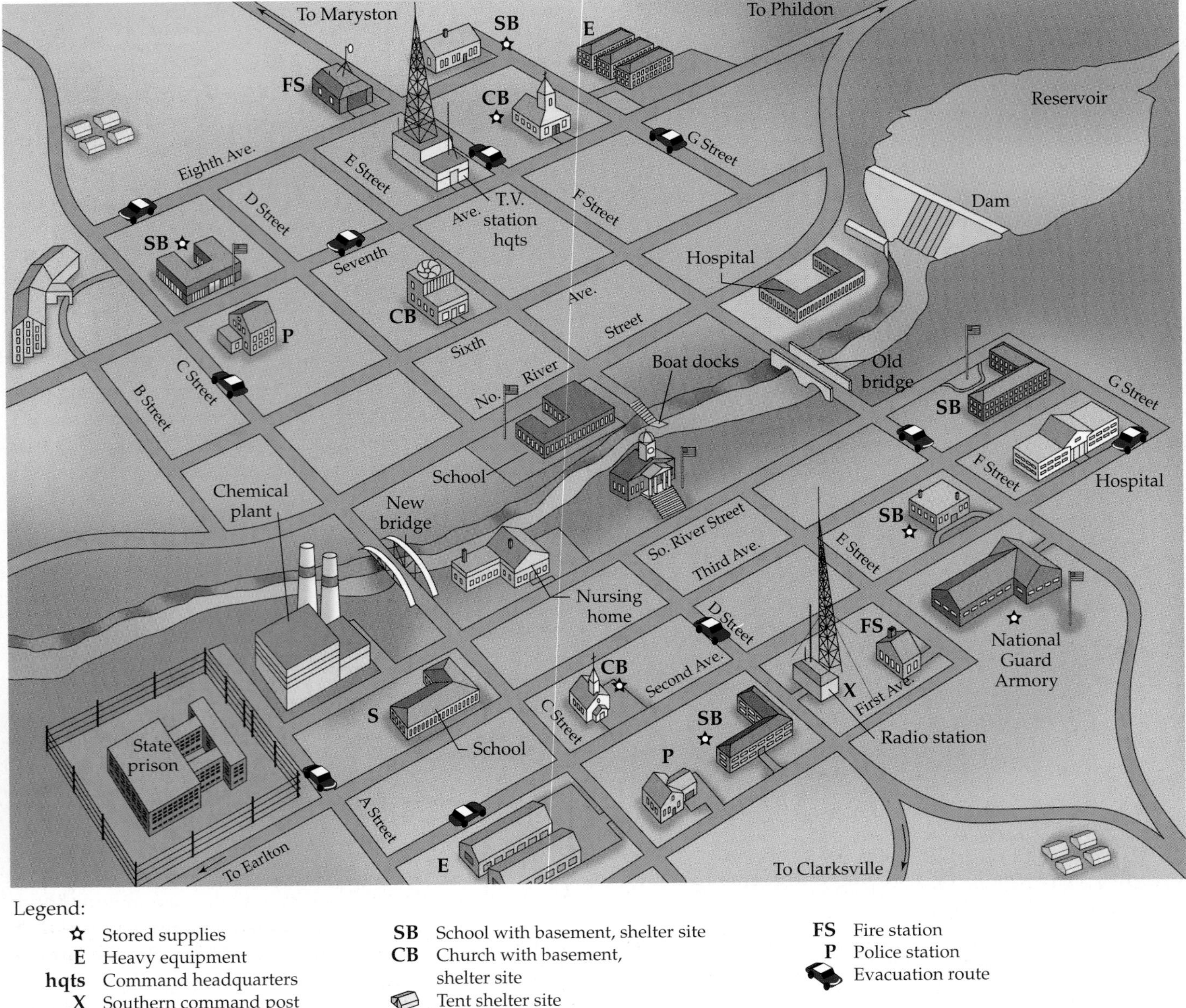

FIGURE 16–11 ■ Part of completing a community assessment is mapping the assets and resources in the community. Note the location of essential health resources and emergency preparedness resources.

strategies, considering funding sources, and ultimately promoting and advertising the plan in the community. The collaboration often has persons with different talents who can take leadership roles with different aspects of the interventions.

Information gained from the community assessment about the community, target population, and existing programs and resources is essential to design a health education program or other community intervention for the target population. Knowledge of the cultural beliefs, primary language, income levels, reading level, sources of community health education, and potential community partners are valuable in designing the intervention. Knowledge about potential community funding resources or barriers helps in determining potential strategies that may be approved and endorsed by community decision makers.

Community Plan and Intervention Example

In trying to improve the safety of children riding their bicycles to school, it was determined that constructing new bike paths in the high traffic areas was not possible unless state funding could be obtained. Funding for such a project could not be obtained without legislative action, so an alternate plan was needed. The nurse working with other community leaders identified a number of alternate routes with less traffic for children to use when bicycling to schools and other important destinations. Approval was obtained from the community government to mark and advertise these routes. Additional community actions that could result in implementation and use of the new bike routes include the following:

- Increase awareness of the alternate bike routes through the local media (radio, television, and newspapers), church bulletins, and flyers sent home from school. It is important to remember to promote awareness in all cultural groups, such as by using the local newspapers printed in other languages.

- Encourage the use of the alternate routes by working with local businesses to provide incentives to children (e.g., an ice cream cone) to use the alternate bike paths, especially to those wearing a bike helmet and riding safely. Local firefighters and police officers could be given coupons to distribute to children as rewards.
- Partner with local voluntary organizations to sponsor a bike rodeo to teach new riders safe biking skills and the rules of riding.

Community leaders can then work with the community government to develop the state transportation proposal for constructing bike paths in the high traffic areas.

Evaluation

Finally, an evaluation of the plan and intervention is needed. Data collected in the problem identification stage should serve as one comparison for the evaluation.

At the local level, evaluation of a plan should be part of the overall planning. Specific data and data sources should be identified and a community leader (sometimes the nurse) should be assigned the responsibility of evaluating the program. Evaluation should focus on the intervention and how well the target population accepted it, as well as the outcome, such as reduced injuries and deaths.

In the case of the bike routes, community leaders can monitor the use of the recommended bike routes versus the more dangerous routes. An increase in numbers of children using the recommended bike routes should be seen and sustained over an extended period of time. Nurses can monitor the newspapers, and local hospital emergency departments may be able to provide data on the number of children with bicycle-related injuries in the high traffic areas and the alternate bike routes. Actual comparison of bicycle-related injuries and deaths should be made between the preintervention phase and at annual intervals to determine if the intervention was associated with the desired outcome.

EMERGENCY MEDICAL SERVICES FOR CHILDREN

The emergency medical services (EMS) system is the organized community-based public health response to ensure that adults and children with acute illnesses and injuries receive emergency care and timely transport to the hospital emergency department. The EMS system at the local community level is composed of ambulance units and trained emergency medical personnel who respond to emergencies. In some communities, this EMS system is part of the fire department and in others it is a separate organization. Each local EMS system has a medical director who establishes the protocols used by emergency medical personnel when caring for ill and injured individuals. The public accesses the EMS system by placing a call to 9-1-1 or their local emergency phone number where a dispatcher directs the ambulance unit to respond, takes information, and provides information to the caller about how to manage the ill or injured person until the emergency personnel arrive. State EMS offices set the guidelines for training and certification of emergency medical personnel, equipment to be carried on ambulances, data collection of care provided, and communication systems used. In addition, the state EMS office works closely with hospital emergency departments and trauma centers to coordinate emergency care of patients transported by the EMS system. Federal legislation was enacted in 1984 to ensure that children's special needs were integrated into the overall EMS system.

Children have different physiologic responses to emergencies because of their smaller anatomy and developing organ systems (see Appendix E∞). Small children cannot communicate and describe their health problems, and they are dependent upon family members for security and recognition of the emergency. With the smaller anatomy, pediatric-size equipment and supplies are essential. EMS providers need education to assess the child and recognize the signs that the child's condition is a true emergency, and then to provide the appropriate medical intervention before and during transport to the hospital.

Hospitals are part of the EMS system and their emergency departments must be prepared to treat children as well as adults. Emergency departments need to have appropriately sized resuscitation equipment for children of all ages and well-trained emergency department physicians and nurses. In addition, clinical guidelines for a well-orchestrated response for serious trauma and medical emergencies are developed and rehearsed. Urgent care centers and smaller emergency departments need to have agreements with major medical centers to ensure that children with life-threatening injuries or illnesses can be transferred and transported to a more advanced level of care.

Nurses sometimes work as volunteer EMS providers in their community. Nurses also work as interfacility transport team members, providing care to critically ill children who need to be transferred by ground or air ambulance from a community hospital to a hospital with more advanced care. Figure 16–12 ■ shows the interconnection between the EMS system and hospitals for provision of emergency services.

DISASTER PREPAREDNESS

Many types of disasters occur each year in the United States. Natural disasters include floods, ice storms, hurricanes, earthquakes, tornados, and fires. Other types of disasters can occur when trains or trucks carrying toxic agents such as chemicals and nuclear waste crash or explode. Concerns of terrorism with infectious organisms, toxic chemicals, or radioactive agents have elevated the need for disaster and emergency preparedness. (See Chapter 19∞ for infectious agents used for bioterrorism.) State emergency management agencies, hospitals, and the EMS system are developing community plans for mass casualty events that will be effective for both natural and man-made disasters.

Children have special vulnerabilities during a disaster. Their developmental ability and cognitive levels may interfere with their ability to escape danger. They have unique psychological

MediaLink EMS for Children Video

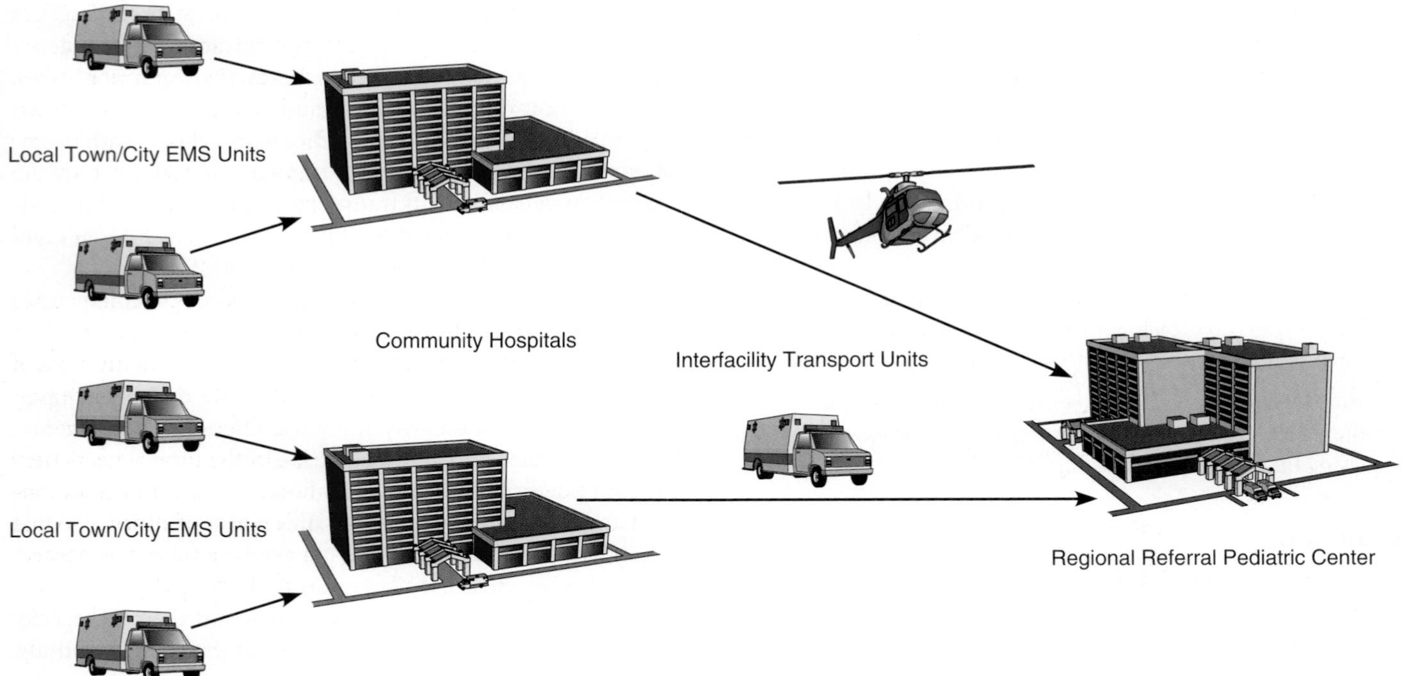

FIGURE 16–12 ■ The emergency medical services (EMS) system is a carefully linked set of resources in the community and region that enable children with serious illnesses and injuries to get the care needed in the most appropriate hospital. The continuum of emergency care includes the caregiver of the child at the scene, the communications center taking the call for help, the EMS personnel responding to the scene who provide immediate emergency care and transport the child to the emergency department, and the hospital emergency department. If the child is transported to a community emergency department, but needs more complex care, transfer to a larger hospital or trauma center is then coordinated. A team of specially trained pediatric emergency care providers often manages transfer in an ambulance, helicopter, or small plane. The goal is to get the child to the medical and specialty care resources needed to have the best chance of survival and optimal functional outcome.

vulnerabilities and need special plans for management. See Table 16–2 for the developmental responses to disasters.

The impact of disasters on the mental health of children is also significant. Consider the following:

- Children have developed fewer coping skills to help deal with the impact of witnessing injuries.
- Their understanding may be limited due to cognitive level and abilities.
- Their fear and anxiety is heightened with hoaxes, actual incidents, and the associated media coverage. They feel the fear and anxiety that their parents have, and therefore become fearful. They become more fearful after a disaster has occurred, fearing that it will happen again, that someone will be injured or killed, that they will be separated from their family or they will be left alone. Seeing the event repeatedly on television increases their fear because young children may believe the event is occurring again and again.
- The disruption of normal life patterns (reliability, cohesion, and predictability) may be prolonged and may cause stress.

MediaLink Disaster Preparedness Video

Because children spend many hours a day in school and childcare, they may be separated from the parents at the time of the disaster, resulting in more stress. See Chapter 7∞ for more information about promoting coping skills and resilience in children to promote healthier responses in the times of disasters.

Children are likely to have emergency needs different from adults due to their size and earlier stages of development. Because of their anatomy and physiology, they have different vulnerabilities in response of various terrorism agents. (See Table 19–7∞ on page 640.) Special developmental considerations that must be considered with young children include the following:

- They are unable to flee or take evasive action to escape danger.
- Caregivers or parents may become incapacitated and childcare with mental health support will be needed.
- They are unable to follow the instructions given to adults regarding evacuation or safe actions.
- They cannot distinguish between reality and fantasy. Young children may fear emergency responders in protective suits and hoods. Children may believe that repeated broadcasts of mass casualty events are additional events.

Other problems that must be considered in **disaster preparedness**, addressing the special needs of children during disasters, by ensuring that pediatric-size equipment and beds are available in shelters and that the national disaster medical response system has providers trained to care for children. Pedi-

TABLE 16–2 Responses to Disasters by Children of Different Age Groups

AGE GROUP	RESPONSES
Toddlers and preschoolers	Reaction reflects that of parents Regressive behaviors Decreased appetite Vomiting, constipation, diarrhea Sleep disorders (insomnia, nightmares) Tics, stuttering, muteness Clinging Reenactment by play Irritability Posttraumatic stress disorder
School age	Fear, anxiety Increased hostility with siblings Somatic complaints Sleep disorders School problems Social withdrawal Reenactment by play Apathy Decreased interest in peers, hobbies, school Posttraumatic stress disorder
Preadolescents	Increased hostility with siblings Somatic complaints Eating disorders Decreased interest in peers, hobbies, school Rebellion Refusal to do chores Interpersonal difficulties Posttraumatic stress disorder
Adolescents	Decreased interest in social activities, peers, hobbies, school Inability to experience pleasure Decline in responsible behaviors Rebellion, behavior problems Somatic complaints Sleep disorders Eating disorders Change in physical activity Confusion Lack of concentration Risk-taking behaviors

Adapted from Aghababian, R. V. (1999). Pediatric disaster life support—PDLS. Boston: University of Massachusetts Medical School.

atric medical treatment guidelines must be readily available to respond appropriately when an incident occurs. Pediatric dosages of drugs and antidotes needed in response to biologic or chemical events need to be readily available, and are gradually being integrated in the prepackaged kits from the Strategic National Stockpile maintained by the Department of Homeland Security. The Strategic National Stockpile contains enough pharmaceuticals and patient care materials for community disaster response. It is shipped to the community immediately after an emergency and the local healthcare system determines how to distribute the pharmaceuticals and supplies to the population in need.

Disaster response systems need the coordination of a wide variety of resources, such as communication systems, utilities, transportation, and medical and emergency response systems. Immediately following a disaster, the disaster response system will be activated. Initial efforts will be focused on security, care for casualties, setting up shelters, and then restoring services in the community. Families must prepare to manage on their own for at least 72 hours following a major disaster (unless the child needs special technology for life support). See Table 16–3.

MediaLink Disaster Preparedness Resources

Advance planning is needed to ensure that medically fragile children who need technology for survival or have the potential for life-threatening episodes have the resources needed in the event of a disaster. The designated shelter for such children with health professionals and electrical power for the needed equipment should be identified and known to the family. In the meantime, battery packs for power backup should be available at all times. Additionally, parents need to arrange for durable power of attorney so that consent for emergency medical care can be available as needed. The child and parents may become separated during the disaster, or the parents may become injured and unable to care for the child.

Pediatric nurses in schools and other community settings have a significant role in working with families in preparing for a disaster. They can help families use developmentally appropriate information to talk with their children about disaster planning and information about disasters when they occur. They can help the family develop a disaster plan. They can also help after the disaster by assessing the child for distress, posttraumatic stress disorder, and promoting security and stability (Ferguson, 2002).

TABLE 16–3 Resources for Surviving a Disaster for 72 Hours

CATEGORIES OF ITEMS NEEDED	EXAMPLES
Water	1 gallon of water per person per day, enough for 3 days needed
Food	3-day supply of nonperishable food that does not require cooking and little or no water
First aid kit	One for the home and one for the car
Nonprescription drugs	Pain reliever, antacid, antidiarrhea medication, laxative
Tools and supplies	Flashlight and batteries, battery-operated radio, cash or travelers checks, paper plates and utensils, etc.
Sanitary supplies	Soap, toilet paper, hygiene products, disinfectant, household chlorine bleach
Clothing and bedding	Rain gear, sturdy shoes, warm clothes, complete change of clothes per person
Special items	Prescription medications, baby formula, games and books for entertainment, family documents

Adapted from Federal Emergency Management Agency's Community and Family Preparedness Program. (1997). Your family disaster supplies kit *(FEMA L-189). Washington, DC: FEMA.* http://www.fema.gov

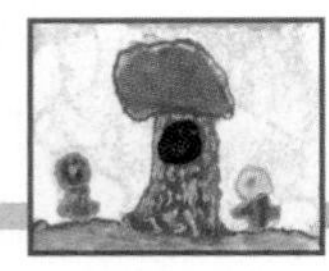

CHAPTER HIGHLIGHTS

- Pediatric care in the community occurs in the following settings: primary care settings, schools and childcare centers, urgent care centers, community events, outpatient departments, home, homeless shelters, and disaster shelters.
- Working with the child and family in the community setting requires an understanding of how the larger environment influences the child's health and development and integration of that knowledge into the nursing care plan.
- Every child should have a medical home, a continuous source of family-centered, comprehensive, and compassionate healthcare.
- During episodic care for illnesses and injuries, the nurse collects health information, assesses the child, assists the primary care provider with diagnostic or therapeutic procedures, and educates the child and family about care of the child at home.
- Pediatric nurses in hospital outpatient clinics assist with diagnostic workups and management of children with chronic health problems, including patient assessment, health education, and health promotion.
- School nursing focuses on removing or minimizing health barriers to learning so children can perform academically. Services include prevention, health promotion, health education, emergency care, and managing chronic health problems.
- An individualized school health plan describes the school-based care of the child with a chronic condition for optimal participation in school and class activities.
- Pediatric nursing in childcare settings focuses on reducing infectious diseases among children and caregivers, and assisting caregivers to identify and minimize hazards that could injure children.
- Nurses in camps assess and improve the safety of the children's environment and care for children with acute illnesses and injuries.
- Home care nursing is focused on helping the family gain the ability to manage the child with a chronic condition more independently.
- Community health nurses provide care to children in many settings. They take a leadership role in conducting community assessments and developing health programs to address identified needs.
- A community assessment is a process of compiling data about a community's health status and resources for the purpose of public health planning to address a population's health needs.
- The emergency medical services (EMS) system is the organized community-based public health response to ensure that children with acute illnesses and injuries receive emergency care and timely transport to the hospital emergency department.
- Pediatric nurses have a significant role in working with families in preparing for a disaster. They can help families develop a disaster plan and then use developmentally appropriate information to talk with their children about what to do when disasters occur.

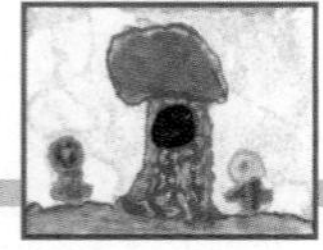

CRITICAL THINKING IN ACTION

INTRODUCTION

Return to the scenario at the beginning of the chapter. Jill, her parents, and 5-year-old brother Ryan live in a three-bedroom townhouse in the city. Jill's parents have health insurance and obtain regular healthcare for both children at the health center. Jill's parents both work and childcare is provided by Jill's grandmother.

DESCRIPTION

Until now, Jill's grandmother has felt comfortable and confident in providing childcare, but she is becoming concerned about her ability to continue providing care if Jill becomes increasingly sick.

DISCUSSION

1. Describe the primary roles for the nurse at the health center and the cardiac clinic in caring for Jill and her family. What information should be shared between the nurses to improve the nursing care each provides?
2. Describe the major nursing issues that need to be addressed for Jill's ongoing healthcare prior to surgery. Develop a home nursing care plan to help Jill's parents and grandmother provide optimal care.
3. Jill has a health condition that places her at higher risk for a medical emergency (respiratory distress due to congestive heart failure). What needs to be considered in the development of an emergency care plan? What information should be readily available for emergency care providers?

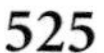

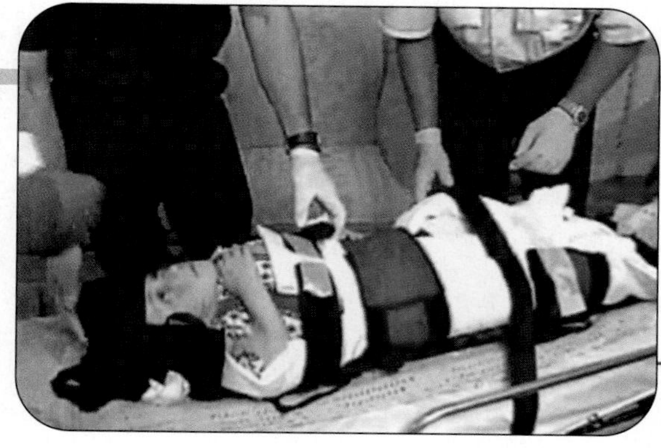

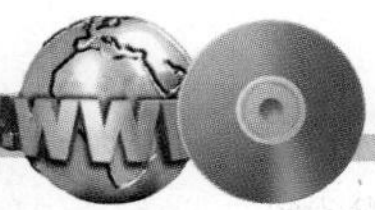

EXPLORE MediaLink

- NCLEX review, case studies, and other interactive resources for this chapter can be found on the Companion Website at **http://www.prenhall.com/ball**. Click on Chapter 16 to select the activities for this chapter.
- For animations, more NCLEX review questions, and an audio glossary, access the accompanying CD-ROM in this textbook.

http://www.prenhall.com/ball

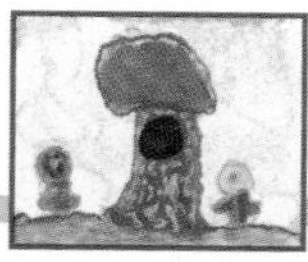

REFERENCES

American Academy of Pediatrics. (2002). The medical home. *Pediatrics, 110*(1), 184–186.

American Academy of Pediatrics, Committee on Pediatric Emergency Medicine. (1999). Emergency preparedness of children with special health care needs. *Pediatrics, 104*(4), e53.

Balinsky, W., & Marié, J. (2001, June). Pediatric home care: A cost benefit and cost effectiveness update. *Caring Magazine*, 16–19.

Cieslak, T. J., & Henretig, F. M. (2003). Ring-a-ring-a-roses: Bioterrorism and its peculiar relevance to pediatrics. *Current Opinion in Pediatrics, 19*, 107–111.

Clark, M. J. (2003). *Community health nursing* (4th ed.). Upper Saddle River, NJ: Prentice Hall.

Committee on Pediatric Emergency Medicine, Seidel, J. S., & Knapp, J. F. (Eds.). (2000). *Childhood emergencies in the office, hospital, and community: Organizing systems of care.* Elk Grove Village, IL: American Academy of Pediatrics.

Donowitz, L. G. (1999). At-a-glance guide to infection control in day care. *Contemporary Pediatrics, 16*(11), 127–138.

Evers, D. B. (2002). The pediatric nurse's role as health consultant to a child care center. *Pediatric Nursing, 22*(3), 231–235.

Farrior, K. C., Englelke, M. K., Collins, C. S., & Cox, C. G. (2000). A community pediatric prevention partnership: Linking schools, providers, and tertiary care services. *Journal of School Health, 70*(3), 79–83.

Ferguson, S. L. (2002). Preparing for disasters: Enhancing the role of pediatric nurses in wartime. *Journal of Pediatric Nursing, 17*(4), 307–308.

Green, M., & Palfey, J. S. (2000). *Bright futures: Guidelines for health supervision of infants, children, and adolescents* (2nd ed.). Arlington, VA: National Center for Education in Maternal and Child Health.

Guilday, P. (2000). School nursing practice today: Implications for the future. *Journal of School Nursing, 16*(5), 25–31.

Hogue, E. (1993). Care in the absence of primary caregivers. *Pediatric Nursing, 19*(1), 49–50.

Madigan, E. A., Younglut, J., & Haruzivishe, C. (1999). Pediatric home healthcare: Patients and providers. *Home Healthcare Nurse, 17*(11), 699–705.

Messinger, R., & Dolan, M. K. (1997). The parents' perspective on pediatric home care. In W. I. Votroubek, & J. L. Townsend, *Pediatric home care* (2nd ed., pp. 537–541). Gaithersburg, MD: Aspen.

National Association of Home Care. (2001). Basic statistics about home care. www.nahc.org/Consumer/hcstats.html, accessed 10/7/2003.

National Association of School Nurses. (1999). Definition of school nursing. *Journal of School Nursing, 15*(3), 5.

National Association of School Nurses and American Nurses Association (2001). *Scope and standards of professional school nursing practice.* Silver Spring: MD: American Nurses Publishing.

Office of Technology Assessment. (1987). *Technology-dependent children: Hospital vs. home care. A technical memorandum.* Washington, DC: Congress of the United States.

Robinson, J. (2002, October). The changing role of the school nurse: A partner in infection control and disease prevention. *Journal of School Nursing, 18* (Suppl.), 12–14.

Schainker, E., & Grant, L. (2003). Medical home meets educational home: How you can make the most of school health services. *Contemporary Pediatrics, 20*(3), 55–81.

U.S. Department of Health and Human Services. (2000). *Healthy People 2010* (2nd ed.). Washington, DC: U.S. Government Printing Office. www.healthy people.gov

Valluzzi, J. L. (1995). Safety issues in community-based settings for children who are medically fragile: Program planning for natural disasters. *Infants and Young Children, 7*(4), 62–76.

Vessey, J. A. (2000). Coordinated school health. *Pediatric Nursing, 26*(3), 303.

Waibel, R., & Misra, R. (2003). Injuries to preschool children and infection control practices in childcare programs. *Journal of School Health, 73*(4), 167–172.

Wheeler, D. S. (1999). Emergency medical services for children: A general pediatrician's perspective. *Current Problems in Pediatrics, 29*, 225–241.

Wolfe, L. C., & Selekman, J. (2002). School nurses: What it is and what it was. *Pediatric Nursing, 28*(4), 403–407.

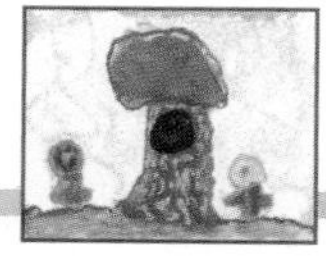

ADDITIONAL REFERENCE

Ahmann, E. (1996). *Home care for the high risk infant: A family centered approach* (2nd ed.). Gaithersburg, MD: Aspen Publishers.

Chapter

17 Nursing Care of the Hospitalized Child

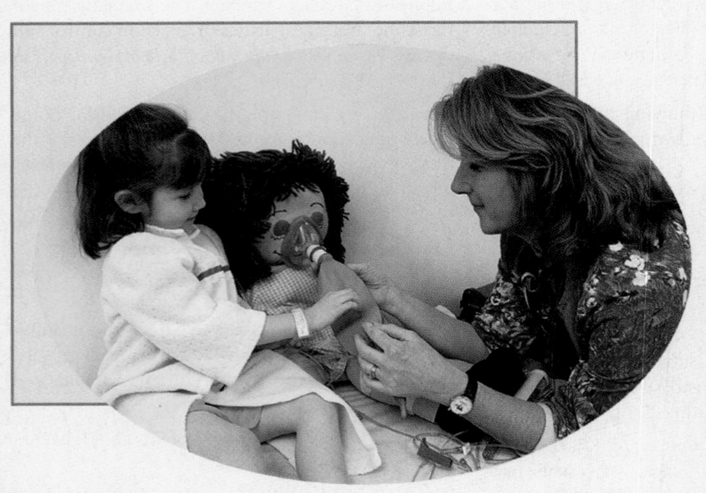

Four-year-old Sabrina Jambois has experienced several nosebleeds and fainting spells in the last few weeks. After an examination by the primary healthcare provider and an evaluation of diagnostic studies such as chest radiograph examination, echocardiography, and electrocardiography, coarctation of the aorta is diagnosed. Sabrina will be admitted to the hospital this week for a cardiac catheterization and scheduled for open heart surgery to correct the coarctation.

Sabrina and her family live approximately 50 miles from the medical center. Her parents have two other children, ages 9 and 7. The parents are both employed, but Sabrina's mother plans to take several days off at the time of surgery. Sabrina attends preschool, and she is used to spending time with other children.

Sabrina's experiences with healthcare professionals have been limited to immunizations, hearing, and vision screenings at the health clinic. Sabrina's parents, who are anxious about the heart surgery, are concerned about how their daughter will adapt to hospitalization.

How should you prepare Sabrina for the cardiac catheterization and for surgery? How far in advance should teaching take place? What teaching aids are helpful? How can Sabrina's parents be involved in and reinforce teaching? What kinds of support do her parents and siblings need during her hospitalization?

"I was screaming when my nose kept bleeding—it was going to all leak out."

—Sabrina, age 4

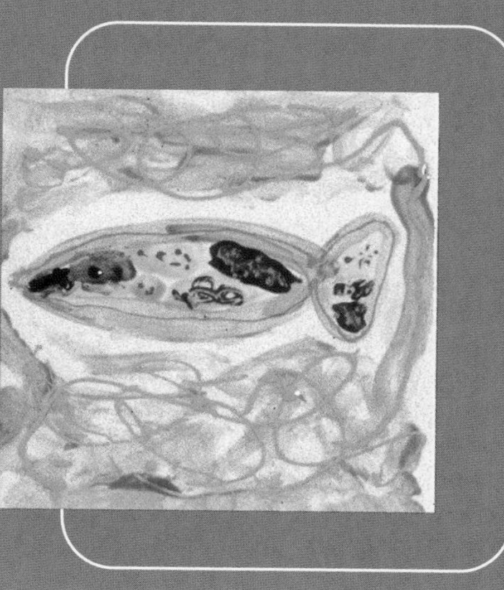

Learning Outcomes

After completing this chapter, you will be able to:

- Discuss the child's understanding of health and illness according to the child's psychosocial and developmental levels.
- Discuss the effects and response to illness and hospitalization on children and their families.
- Discuss the child's and family's adaptation to hospitalization.
- Identify nursing strategies to enhance the illness and hospitalization experience for children and their families.
- Identify nursing strategies to minimize the stressors related to hospitalization.

Key Terms

child life specialist/548
dramatic play/550
object permanence/530
pet therapy/551
rehabilitation/538
rooming in/548
separation anxiety/530
stranger anxiety/530
therapeutic play/549
therapeutic recreation/551
transitional objects/550
treatment room/541

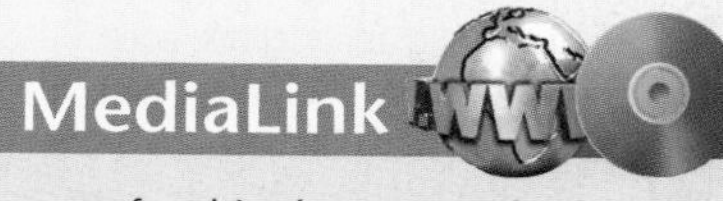

MediaLink **http://www.prenhall.com/ball**

Resources for this chapter can be found on the CD-ROM accompanying this textbook and on the Companion Website at www.prenhall.com/ball. Click on Chapter 17 to select the activities for this chapter.

CD-ROM

Video
Treatment Room
NCLEX Review
Audio Glossary

COMPANION WEBSITE

NCLEX Review
Case Study: Preparing an Adolescent for Surgery
Care Plan: Preparing a School-Age Child for Surgery
MediaLink Applications
Communication Strategy: Preparing a Toddler for Venipuncture

Hospitalization, whether it is elective, planned in advance, or the result of an emergency or trauma, is stressful for children of all ages and their families. Most pediatric conditions can be managed within the home and community setting; therefore, hospitalization is not necessarily a requirement to manage the child with an illness (Box 17–1). However, while fewer children require hospitalization, those who are hospitalized usually have a high level of illness acuity.

Hospitalized children experience a variety of emotions as they are in an unknown environment, surrounded by strangers, unfamiliar equipment, and frightening sights and sounds. These children are subjected to unfamiliar procedures, some of which are invasive or painful, and may even require surgery. For both children and families, routines are disrupted and normal coping strategies are tested.

Nurses today are challenged to provide individualized care for the hospitalized child with complex medical conditions, acute illnesses, or injury. A key role of nurses caring for hospitalized children and their families includes addressing the psychosocial concerns that accompany hospitalization. To minimize the stress of hospitalization, nurses provide support and education to children and their families before, during, and after hospitalization.

During hospitalization, nurses use a family-centered approach and work collaboratively with parents to implement various strategies to promote coping and adaptation and to prepare children for necessary procedures. Nurses are instrumental in ensuring that the developmental and educational needs of children are met, especially when hospitalization is prolonged. Nurses also collaborate with members of a multidisciplinary team and partner with families to assist them in preparation for discharge home or transfer to a long-term care or rehabilitation facility.

BOX 17–1 Education to Reduce Incidence of Pediatric Hospitalizations

A recent study revealed that many pediatric hospitalizations might be avoided if parents and children were better educated about the child's condition, medications, importance of avoiding known disease triggers, and the importance of follow-up care (Flores, Milagros, Chaisson, et al., 2003). Avoidable hospitalization conditions are those that can be avoided with timely, effective outpatient care. The most frequent conditions for which hospitalization could be avoided were asthma, dehydration and gastroenteritis, pneumonia, seizure disorder, and skin infections. Better education can lead to early treatment at home and decreased need for hospitalization. Nurses can partner with other healthcare providers to educate parents about the child's condition, proper administration of medications, need for outpatient follow-up, and avoiding known disease triggers.

By determining the child's and family's levels of understanding of the condition, the nurse can directly collaborate with the family to help reduce the number of avoidable hospitalizations.

EFFECTS OF HOSPITALIZATION ON CHILDREN AND THEIR FAMILIES

Children's Understanding of Health and Illness

Can you remember as a child thinking that yelling at your mother caused your strep throat? Perhaps as an adolescent you believed that you would never become ill or have an accident. Maybe you feared being in a car crash like that of a friend. Children have limited knowledge about the body and its relation to health and illness. Their understanding is based primarily on their cognitive ability at various developmental stages and on previous experiences with healthcare professionals. Table 17–1 provides a discussion of childrens' understanding of health and illness according to their developmental level.

TABLE 17–1 Childrens' Understanding of Health and Illness According to Developmental Level

INFANT	TODDLER AND PRESCHOOLER	SCHOOL-AGE CHILD	ADOLESCENT
By approximately 6 months of age, infants have developed an awareness of themselves as separate from their mother or father. They are unaware of the effects of illness. However, they are capable of sensing distress in their parents who may be experiencing anxiety related to the infant's hospitalization.	Toddlers and preschoolers are beginning to understand illness, but not its cause. Two unrelated events may appear to have a cause-and-effect relationship for young children, who may consider the sun, an animal, bad behavior, or even magic to be the cause of their illnesses. These children may blame other people, events, or themselves for becoming ill, especially if the other event occurs shortly before the illness. The child's concept of the body usually is limited to names and locations of some body parts. Although toddlers and preschoolers are not likely to understand how lungs, the heart, bones, or other body parts function, they are learning concepts of safety and other health-related issues.	The child's concept of body parts and function is maturing. School-age children between the ages of 5 and 8 years believe that the internal body consists of heart and bones. They view the digestive system as having two parts, the mouth and the stomach. Older school-age children have a more realistic understanding of the reasons for illness and are able to comprehend explanations.	After 11 years of age, adolescents become increasingly aware of the physiologic, psychologic, and behavioral causes of illness and injury. Young adolescents, aged 11 to 13 years, can describe the location and function of major organs such as the brain, nose, eyes, heart, and stomach. Adolescents are concerned with appearance and perceive an illness or injury in terms of its effect on their body image.

TABLE 17–2 Stressors of Hospitalization for Children at Various Developmental Stages

DEVELOPMENTAL STAGES	RESPONSES	NURSING IMPLICATIONS
Infant Separation anxiety Stranger anxiety Painful, invasive procedures Immobilization Sleep deprivation, sensory overload	Sleep–awake cycle disrupted Feeding routines disrupted Displays excessive irritability	Encourage parental presence Adhere to infant's home routine as much as possible Utilize topic anesthetics or preprocedural sedation as prescribed Promote a quiet environment and reduce excess stimuli
Toddler Separation anxiety Loss of self-control Immobilization Painful, invasive procedures Bodily injury or mutilation Fear of the dark	Is frightened if forced to lie supine Associates pain with punishment Wonders why parents don't come to the rescue	Encourage parental presence Allow choices when possible Utilize topic anesthetics or preprocedural sedation as prescribed Explain all procedures Provide a night-light or flashlight
Preschooler Separation anxiety and fear of abandonment Loss of self-control Bodily injury or mutilation Painful, invasive procedures Fear of the dark, ghosts, and monsters	Displays difficulty separating reality from fantasy Fears ghosts and monsters Fears body parts will leak out when skin is not intact Fears that tubes are permanent Demonstrates withdrawal, projection, aggression, regression	Encourage parental presence Allow choices when possible Utilize topic anesthetics or preprocedural sedation as prescribed Explain all procedures Provide a night-light or flashlight
School-age Child Loss of control Loss of privacy and control over bodily functions Bodily injury Painful, invasive procedures Fear of death	Displays increased sensitivity to the environment Demonstrates detailed recall of events to self and other patients	Encourage parental participation Allow the child choices when possible Explain all procedures and offer reassurance Utilize topic anesthetics or preprocedural sedation as prescribed Encourage peer interaction
Adolescent Loss of control Fear of altered body image, disfigurement, disability, and death Separation from peer group Loss of privacy and identity	Displays denial, regression, withdrawal, intellectualization, projection, displacement	Include the adolescent in the plan of care Encourage discussion of fears and anxieties Explain all procedures Ask the adolescent his or her desire for parental involvement Encourage peer interaction

Hospitalization and medical procedures are significant sources of stress for children (Lau, 2002). Hospitalization disrupts the child's and family's lifestyle. Infants, toddlers, and preschoolers lack the cognitive skills to understand hospitalization and are the most likely age groups to exhibit regressive behaviors. Hospitalized children may experience fears and anxieties about wild animals, darkness, and monsters, which are initiated by the strange hospital environment. In addition to dealing with these stressors, the hospitalized child may experience an intense emotional and physical threat to his or her well-being. Children commonly fear injections, human blood, and being touch by strangers.

The four most significant stressors for hospitalized children of all ages are:

- Separation from parents or the primary caretaker (or peers)
- Loss of self-control, autonomy, and privacy
- Painful and/or invasive procedures
- Fear of bodily injury and disfigurement

Table 17–2 highlights key stressors of hospitalization for children at each developmental stage. The effects of hospitalization according to developmental stage are discussed in the following section.

Nursing care of the hospitalized child focuses on minimizing the child's fears, anxieties, and disruption of routine associated with hospitalization, and supporting the family. Strategies include minimizing separation anxiety and loss of control, and promoting stress-reducing techniques. See Partnering with Families: Stress-Reducing Techniques.

Newborn

Newborns requiring hospitalization are admitted to the neonatal intensive care unit (NICU). At a time when the newborn is generally being held and comforted by parents in the safety of their own home, these newborns are instead in a busy, high-technology area being cared for by multiple healthcare professionals. Depending on the neonate's condition, ventilatory support and other technical equipment as well as the parent's fear of losing the neonate, may interfere with the parent–newborn attachment phase. Hospitalized neonates may have less physical contact and nurturing than

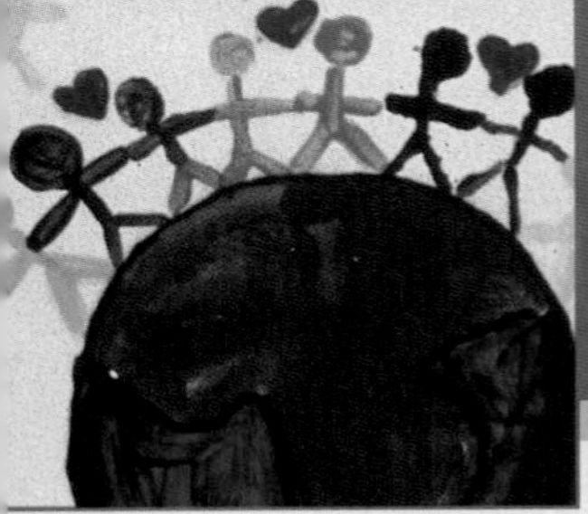

PARTNERING WITH FAMILIES

Stress-Reduction Techniques

Strategies the nurse and family can implement to reduce the hospitalized child's stress include encouraging recreation and physical activity (if appropriate for child and not restricted due to condition), obtaining sufficient rest, ensuring parental or other significant person's presence, and maintaining routines.

Recreation

Newborn and Infant

- Provide developmentally appropriate mobiles, rattles, and music boxes.
- If possible, hold the newborn or infant and talk soothingly to him or her.
- For the older infant, play "peek-a-boo" and similar games.

Toddler and Preschooler

- Provide developmentally appropriate toys.
- Encourage coloring, singing, use of music and games.
- Take toddler or preschooler to playroom if possible and encourage interaction with peers.

School-Age Child

- Encourage participation in peer group activities if possible.
- Provide favorite collection items or encourage new hobby (collecting stamps or coins, or building models and playing board games for the child that has activity restriction).
- Provide music, video games, or computer access.
- Encourage child to visit playroom or recreation room and interact with other hospitalized school-age children.

Rest

- Promote calm, quiet environment to allow for rest periods.
- Establish rituals to help child prepare for sleep at night. For example, reading a story at night, playing a quiet board game, or watching favorite TV show (if necessary, record show to play at appropriate time).

Relationships

- Arrange for visits from family members, including siblings.
- Encourage visits from friends.
- If friends are unable to visit, encourage writing, calling, email, or live-computer chat to maintain communication.
- Encourage school-age child and adolescents to attend peer support groups.

Routines

- Ask families to inform nursing staff of the child's normal routines.
- Provide transition objects from home, such as a blanket or favorite toy.
- Talk with the older school-age child and adolescent to determine his or her wishes regarding routines (e.g., if the child prefers to perform hygiene in the mornings or evenings).
- Inform the child or adolescent about anticipated changes to provide an opportunity to adapt.

the newborn at home. Failure to form parental-newborn attachment can have lifelong negative effects on the neonate.

Infant

Hospitalization can be a traumatic time for an infant, particularly during periods of parental absence. After 3 months of age, most infants have begun to develop a sense of **object permanence** (the knowledge that an object or person continues to exist when not seen, felt, or heard) and corresponding trust in parents, familiar caretakers, and environment. The most common stressor of hospitalization for the infant is separation from parents, which is manifested by **separation anxiety.** Three phases of separation anxiety were first identified in young children who were separated from their parents for long periods or permanently and lacked a close relationship with one caretaker after separation (Bowlby, 1960). Characteristic behaviors of children in the three phases of separation anxiety are listed in Table 17–3. Infants and toddlers who are hospitalized often display some of these behaviors, particularly if parents are unable to remain with the child. In addition to separation anxiety, infants between 6 and 18 months of age may display **stranger anxiety** (wariness of strangers) when confronted with strangers such as healthcare professionals.

Before the 1970s, healthcare professionals assumed that the despair and denial manifested by infants and young children after prolonged separation were signs of positive adaptation, since the child in these stages seemed calm and quiet. Infants sometimes protested when their parents visited, and parents were therefore advised not to visit often. However, the protest phase is now viewed as a healthy response to separation from loved ones and as an indication that the infant has meaningful, close relationships.

CLINICAL TIP

Parents often feel guilty for leaving their child, especially if the child protests adamantly or cries upon return. Support the parents and reassure them that this protest is a normal behavior and it represents healthy parent–infant attachment.

Other stressors to the infant include painful procedures, immobilization of extremities, and sleep deprivation caused by disruption of normal sleep patterns and routines.

Because parent–infant attachment is critical to the infant's developmental achievements (see Chapter 5∞), the nurse encourages the family to remain with and be active participants in care of the hospitalized infant. If parents are unable to remain at the hospital, encourage them to visit the newborn or infant as often as possible. Explain and emphasize the importance of parent–newborn attachment and bonding to the parents.

Parents are often frightened of the high-technology environment of neonatal intensive care or pediatric intensive care units. Explain the purpose of all equipment and procedures to the parent. Assist them in establishing physical contact with the infant or newborn. Demonstrate how to touch, hold, feed, and stimulate the newborn or infant. When possible, the parent is encouraged to hold the neonate or infant. Even neonates with numerous monitoring and supportive lines and tubes can be gently stroked and verbally stimulated.

The infant's satisfaction is achieved through meeting oral needs; therefore, the nurse provides sources for oral stimulation such as pacifiers and age-appropriate teething toys. The infant should be rocked and touched with light stroking to provide tactile stimulation for developmental growth. Excessive noise and stimuli in the hospital environment are minimized to allow the neonate or infant periods of rest.

Toddler

Toddlers are the group most at risk for a stressful experience as a result of illness and hospitalization. At this developmental stage, the child lacks the cognitive ability to understand the reason for hospitalization. Separation from parents is the major stressor and children protest vigorously when their parents depart. The toddler does not tolerate the disruption of normal routines. Having activities limited and being confined threatens the meeting of developmental tasks. Fear of pain, the dark, invasive procedures, change, and mutilation are additional common stressors for the toddler.

When a parent cannot be present, reminders can be left with the child. These might include a piece of cloth saturated with the mother's favorite perfume or father's cologne (unless the child has a respiratory condition or another contraindication for this intervention), an object belonging to the parent, or an audiotape or videotape with messages from the parents.

Disruption of routine also causes stress for the toddler. The nurse encourages parents to remain present as much as possible for important rituals such as toileting, carrying out bedtime routines, and singing favorite nursery rhymes. Autonomy is the developmental task of the toddler (see Chapter 5∞). When possible, maintain the toddler's normal home routines for bathing and other activities. Allow the toddler to have choices when possible, such as choosing the color of jello or which clothing to wear.

CLINICAL TIP

Toddlers may present challenges to the nurse regarding cooperation with treatments and procedures, including physical assessments. Interventions such as commenting, "Once I have listened to your heart, lungs, and stomach you can choose whether you want to ride in the wagon or be pushed in the big buggy to the play room." This gives the toddler some sense of control and encourages cooperation.

Preschooler

The greatest stressors for preschoolers are the fears of being alone, the dark, abandonment, loss of self-control related to the body and emotions, and bodily injury or mutilation. They may feel guilty about getting sick. Waking up in the pediatric intensive care unit (PICU) (discussed later in the chapter) and feeling the presence of an endotracheal, nasogastric, or chest tube, along with intravenous, arterial, and urinary catheters, is a terrifying experience for the preschooler.

As with the toddler, preschoolers desire maintenance of a normal routine. To promote a sense of initiative, the developmental task of the preschool child (see Chapter 5∞), the nurse partners with the family to maintain familiar routines as much as possible and to encourage the preschool child's independence through offering choices.

Preschoolers want to know when to expect their parents to return to the hospital. Responding with simple statements such as "after supper" or "before breakfast" gives the preschooler an understanding of the anticipated time since they do not understand "3:00" or "12:00." Encourage parents to make telephone calls to the preschooler if possible. Some parents are able make calls from work and hearing their parent's voice and confirming that they will return to the hospital offers the preschooler a sense of security.

Parents often believe it is better for the child to leave when the child is asleep. Actually, when children do not expect parents to be absent and they awaken to find them gone, they become anxious and may develop a lack of trust. Encourage parents to inform the child if they will not be there, and explain why (e.g., needing to go to work or go home) when the child wakes up. Providing honest information to the child gives the assurance that the parent or caregiver can be trusted.

School-Age Child

Major sources of stress for hospitalized school-age children are loss of control related to bodily functions, privacy issues, fear of bodily injury, pain, and concerns related to death. School-age

TABLE 17–3 Stages of Separation Anxiety

PROTEST	DESPAIR	DENIAL
Screaming, crying	Sadness, depression	Lack of protest when parents leave
Clinging to parents	Withdrawal or compliant behavior	Appearance of being happy and content with everyone
Withdrawal from other adults	Crying when parents appear	Close relationships not established
		Developmental delay possible

Adapted from Bowlby, J. (1960). Separation anxiety. International Journal of Psychoanalysis, 41, *89–113.*

children may also experience separation anxiety from family as well as school friends. The child relies on parents and others for support and understanding during stressful events and procedures. School-age children attempt to maintain their composure during painful or invasive procedures, but generally still require a great deal of support.

Concepts of time are well formed, and parents who cannot remain at the bedside are encouraged to tell the child when they will return. Parents are also encouraged to be available for telephone calls to provide support and comfort. As with the toddler and preschooler, stressful procedures can lead to regression or other behavioral changes. Inform the parents that this behavior is normal during stressful situations.

To promote a sense of industry (see Chapter 5∞) encourage the child to continue with school work and engage in creative outlets such as art or crafts. Allow the school-age child choices when possible.

Adolescent

Separation from peers, home, and school are major stressors experienced by hospitalized adolescents. Additional stressors for the hospitalized adolescent include fear of bodily injury or changes in body image, disability, pain, and even death. Loss of control, privacy, and independence are also major stressors. Preoccupation with appearance and body image are paramount in this age group. Education and discussions that focus on these issues will provide significant reassurance to the adolescent. The adolescent may experience more dependence on their parents, leading to frustration and anger. Adolescents often try to maintain rigid self-control when undergoing painful and invasive procedures.

The adolescent desires privacy and independence. The nurse who respects these desires and demonstrates interest is often successful in establishing a trusting relationship and assisting the adolescent to cope with the hospitalization and illness. The adolescent is encouraged to discuss thoughts and feelings about experiences, and careful listening by the nurse assists in establishing a positive rapport.

Educating the adolescent and the family about normal development helps alleviate stress and promote individuation. Treat the hospitalized adolescent as normally as possible, and assist him or her through the developmental tasks of adolescence by fostering learning of appropriate social and coping skills, allowing choices whenever possible, and enhancing self-esteem (Pinckney & Stuart, 2004).

Allowing choices in clothing, hair, and music acknowledges the importance of their self-identity. Privacy and modesty are major concerns of adolescents because their physical characteristics are rapidly changing. Nurses respect their feelings by knocking on the door before entering and asking permission before conducting assessments or other procedures.

Adolescents are in the process of establishing their identity and becoming independent of their parents' influence (see Chapter 5∞); therefore, control over aspects of their care is important. Partner with the family and multidisciplinary team to ensure the adolescent is an active participant in decisions and plan of care.

The peer group is a major influence in adolescent's lives. Encouraging participation in recreation and teen lounge facilities available during hospitalization provides the adolescent with peer group support opportunities.

Family Responses to Hospitalization

The illness and hospitalization of a child disrupt a family's usual routines. Sometimes roles are altered as one parent remains at the hospital with the child while the other parent or siblings takes on additional tasks at home. Family members may experience anxiety and fear, especially when the outcome is unknown or the reason for hospitalization is a potentially serious health condition. Parents who perceive their child is in pain find the experience difficult and require support. Coping is made more difficult by a serious emergency, lengthy illness, chronic condition, poor prognosis, lack of family support, and lack of financial or community services. The burden of missed work, additional expenses, and concern regarding care for children at home compound the stress the family experiences with a hospitalized child. (See Chapter 21∞ for a description of nursing support for the family of a child with life-threatening illness or injury.)

Research indicates that parents report greater satisfaction with their children's care when nurses tailor actions to the family's needs and preferences. Maintaining positive communication with medical personnel and viewing care as a partnership between parents and other key family members and clinicians are considered predictive of parental satisfaction with the child's hospital care (Marino & Marino, 2000). Nurses view families as the people who know and understand the child best; ask for their participation and partnership in care, and carefully explain all aspects of treatment. Information and modeling on how to talk with and touch the hospitalized child fosters participation that can be beneficial to the child and parent. Parents need this support to lessen their anxiety, because those with many fears may not be able to parent children effectively and perform protective, nurturing, and decision-making roles (Melnyk, 2000). (See Developing Cultural Competence: Family and Mexican Americans.)

Siblings' Experience

The siblings of a hospitalized child may receive little attention from the parents who are overwhelmed and anxious about their hospitalized child's health. Parents are preoccupied and may not consider taking the siblings to visit the child in the hospital. The siblings may fantasize about the illness or injury and the appearance of their brother or sister. Siblings who are not adequately informed about the hospitalized child's condition may

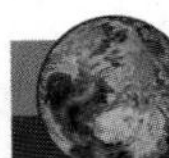

DEVELOPING CULTURAL COMPETENCE
Family and Mexican Americans

For many Mexican Americans, family is a strong support. Extended family and godparents may desire to be with a hospitalized child. Although the father of the child is often the spokesperson, mothers commonly are influential in decisions regarding child healthcare. The nurse should be inclusive of all people the family wishes to have present in the hospital and for explanations about healthcare.

fear that the child will be disabled or die, even when this is unlikely. Siblings may feel guilty about fighting with or being mean to their brother or sister in the past and believe that they played a role in causing his or her illness. Siblings often have nightmares about the illness or injury their brother or sister has sustained and about the ill child dying (see Chapter 22∞ for further discussion of siblings' responses to the dying child).

As family roles and routines continue to change, siblings may feel insecure and anxious. Behavioral problems may develop, or school performance may deteriorate. Siblings may feel jealous because the ill brother or sister seems to monopolize the parents' attention. Siblings of hospitalized children may demonstrate behaviors ranging from jealousy or envy to resentment, guilt, hostility, anger, insecurity, regression, and fear. Given support, however, the siblings of an ill child can manage well.

As the parents' focus shifts to the hospitalized child, they may need support in dealing with the healthy siblings. Siblings may feel left out when attention is focused on the ill child. Recognize that siblings may fear becoming ill themselves or believe that they played a role in the child's illness.

Inform siblings about their brother or sister's condition and hospitalization using language and concepts appropriate to their ages and developmental levels. As appropriate, encourage siblings to visit. Such a visit is especially encouraged if the child could potentially die; this allows the sibling the opportunity to say good-bye (see Chapter 22∞ for further discussion of the dying child). These visits contribute to the mental health of the hospitalized child and assist the sibling to overcome misconceptions or deal with emotions. Because children's fantasies are often worse than reality, unfounded fears may be relieved by a visit.

The nurse prepares the sibling before the visit by explaining sights and sounds likely experienced and by describing how the brother or sister will appear. If the hospitalized child acts, moves, talks, or appears different than usual, provide an explanation beforehand. Describe the hospital environment, including equipment, sounds, and smells. Using a doll, drawing pictures, or showing an actual picture of the child can help prepare the siblings. See Partnering with Families: Strategies for Working with the Sibling of a Hospitalized Child.

During the visit, demonstrate how to talk to and touch the ill child and encourage the siblings to do the same. After the visit, discuss with siblings what they saw and felt, and answer any questions they may have. When a sibling cannot visit, contact with the hospitalized child can be maintained by sending pictures, drawings, cards, and messages recorded on audiotapes or videotapes, and through email or instant messaging. Partner with the family to determine the most appropriate and effective method of communicating if the sibling is unable to visit.

If parents are staying at the hospital with the hospitalized child, partner with them to help establish a routine for the well siblings. For example, encourage them to call the siblings at home at a regular time each night. Allowing the siblings at home the opportunity to share their day, and to receive an update on the hospitalized child, provides a feeling of connectedness and may minimize feelings of worry and resentment. The phone call offers siblings a consistent link to the parent as well as the reassurance that they are important and loved.

PARTNERING WITH FAMILIES

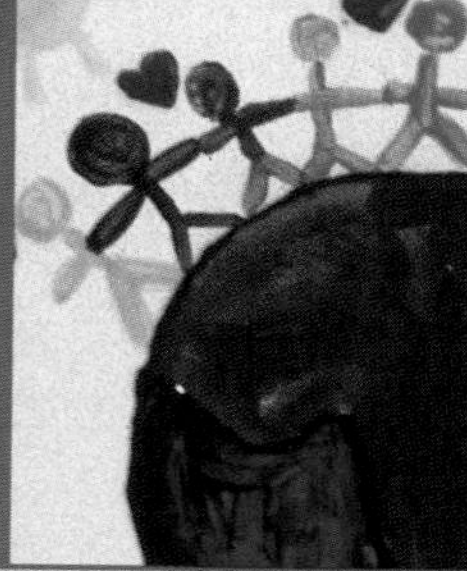

Strategies for Working with the Sibling of a Hospitalized Child

The nurse working with siblings of a hospitalized child can implement the following strategies to assist the siblings in understanding.

- **Be truthful.** Explain why the child is hospitalized, what the treatment involves, and how long the hospitalization is expected to last.
- **Assure siblings that they did not cause the illness and that the hospitalized child did nothing wrong.** If a sibling had some involvement in or responsibility for the health crisis, referral for mental health counseling is needed.
- **Allow siblings to ask questions and discuss fears and other feelings.**
- **Encourage siblings to visit if possible.** Cover tubes and wires with a sheet. Wash off blood or cover bloody bandages if possible. Prepare them for any equipment, dressing, and procedures they might see, and any sounds they might hear.
- **Warn siblings if the hospitalized child is not speaking.** Say something like, "John can't talk now. He seems to be sleeping deeply. He may be able to hear, though, so you can touch him and talk to him."
- **Encourage siblings to express their feelings related to the disruptive effect of the child's hospitalization on family life.**

Family Assessment

To support the hospitalized child and provide family-centered care, the nurse develops an understanding of the family dynamics and individualizes the nursing care according to the needs of the child and family. To develop a plan of care that involves all family members, the nurse assesses the impact of the child's illness or hospitalization on the family. Table 17–4 provides a list of questions to guide the nurse in determining the roles of family, knowledge of family, support systems, and effects on siblings.

Collaborate with the family to determine their resources. These resources include the coping strategies of family members, financial resources, access to healthcare, and availability of community services. One family may manage quite well with limited financial support because they have effective coping strategies; conversely, another family with greater financial resources may have difficulty caring for an ill child if their coping strategies are ineffective. Staying with a hospitalized child can be a financial drain for parents if they must take a leave of absence from work or miss scheduled workdays, and perhaps travel to another location and stay away from home. Additional expenses incurred may include hotel rooms, meals, parking fees, and childcare for other children. Assess the family's ability to manage these additional expenses. A multidisciplinary approach to

TABLE 17–4 Family Assessment

Family Roles

- What changes will the child's illness create in the family?
- Will household tasks need to be reallocated?
- Will a burden be placed on certain family members?
- Will one parent room in or spend a great deal of time in the hospital?

Knowledge

- What knowledge does the family have about the child's condition and treatment? Does the family need further information?
- At what time should discharge planning and teaching begin?

Support Systems

- Does the family have medical insurance? What percentage of costs will it cover? Will other financial support be needed?
- Are close friends or family available to provide care for other children, assist with family tasks, or help in other ways?
- Are there community services such as support groups, camps for children with disabilities, education sessions, or equipment and financial resources to which the nurses can refer the family?

Siblings

- Have siblings been informed of the ill child's condition and the expected outcome?
- Have they been reassured that they did not cause the illness?
- Do they understand the change in roles and family routines?
- Are they able to visit the ill child?
- Have their teachers been informed of the family stress?
- If the hospitalized child's life is threatened, are the siblings involved in a therapy plan to assist them in dealing with that stress?

evaluate the burden of hospitalization may lead to increased access to community resources and support for families.

The nurse also assesses the family dynamics and evaluates the quality of communication, methods of coping with stress, risk factors, and sources of strength. Partner with the family to identify coping mechanisms. Recognize that many children may be hospitalized far from home and their usual support systems. This creates stress for them and for their family members. Find out where family is staying, how far they are from home, and what support systems have been disrupted. Some parents in this situation have reported discussing their concerns, praying, information seeking, reading, relaxation, and exercise as common coping mechanisms (Agazio, Ephraim, Flaherty, et al., 2003). Additional common sources of support include friends and relatives, as well as chaplain and social or child life workers.

Examine how the family has dealt with the health needs of the child if the child has been hospitalized or required home care in the past. (See Developing Cultural Competence: Supporting Alternative Health Practices.) Determine the family members' level of understanding related to the child's hospitalization and anticipated therapy. Collaborate with family members to determine their desired role in the child's care. Assess the family's needs for referral to family service agencies or other community organizations which may be required. Evaluate the need for support groups or agencies that provide medical equipment or other assistance.

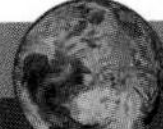

DEVELOPING CULTURAL COMPETENCE
Supporting Alternative Health Practices

Many cultural groups, such as Chinese Americans and Mexican Americans, use a combination of Western medicine and traditional therapies such as home treatments or a traditional healer or curandismo. This information may not be shared with nurses or physicians, both out of respect for Western medicine and in fear that they will be told not to use traditional methods. Recognizing and supporting use of both Western and traditional practices can promote health and provide comfort for children and families. Ask the families about the use of traditional, complementary, or alternative therapies in an accepting and nonjudgmental manner.

Teaching the child and family, providing support, and referring them to community resources are key elements in providing family-centered care. Additional resources available for the child and family include social workers, child and family psychology professionals, and advanced practice nurses. Additionally, hospital programs and parent support groups are available to assist families in coping with a child's illness.

ADAPTATION TO HOSPITALIZATION

Hospitalization of the child may be planned or unexpected. A child may be hospitalized for any of the following reasons.

- The child develops an acute illness or exacerbation of chronic illness.
- The child requires diagnostic or treatment procedures or requires elective surgery.
- The child who was previously healthy suffers a serious injury, necessitating unexpected hospitalization.

Planned Hospitalization

When hospitalization is planned, children and their parents have time to prepare for the experience. (See Partnering with Families: Parental Preparation of Children for Hospitalization.) Through preadmission preparation, children and their families are introduced to the acute care setting. Assess the family's knowledge and expectations and provide information about likely experiences. A variety of approaches can be used to provide information and allay fears.

- Tours of the hospital unit or surgical area are helpful. This activity assists the child and family to become familiar with the environment they will encounter. During tours, preschoolers and school-age children are provided opportunities to see and handle items with which they will come in contact. The surgical team's attire is less frightening if the child has had a chance to try it on and engage in play while wearing the attire (Figure 17–1 ■). Medical equipment is not as frightening when the child learns what it does and observes how it is used, for example, through demonstration on a doll (Figure 17–2 ■).
- If a tour is not possible, photographs or a videotape can be used to demonstrate the medical setting and procedures.

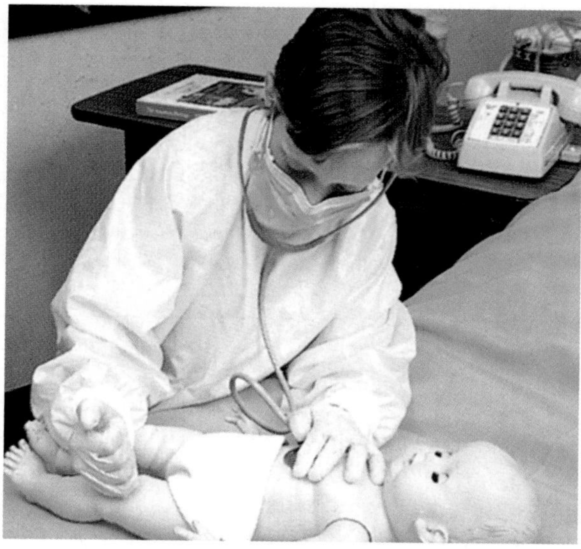

FIGURE 17–1 ■ Allowing the child to dress up as a doctor or a nurse helps prepare the child for the hospitalization experience. This helps the child adjust to treatment, care, and the recovery process. Why? What might the child's concerns be? Can you think of any concerns that might be related to cultural background?

- Puppets and skits are another effective method of explaining procedures to children.
- Many hospitals offer health fairs to explain health procedures to children. During a tour, while hospitalized, or at home, the child can be exposed to books or films that explain in age-appropriate terms what to expect during various procedures (Table 17–5). Coloring books or other methods can also be utilized to reinforce teaching.

Different approaches are useful when adolescents are being prepared for hospitalization. They learn not only from written materials, models, and videotapes, but also from talking with peers who have had similar experiences. To demonstrate respect of privacy, an opportunity for asking questions without parents present is also provided to the adolescent.

Include the family in preparing the child of any age for hospitalization (Figure 17–3 ■). Parents can be instrumental in preparing a child for hospitalization by reviewing material presented, being available to answer questions, and being truthful and supportive (Box 17–2). Determine the child's normal routine,

PARTNERING WITH FAMILIES

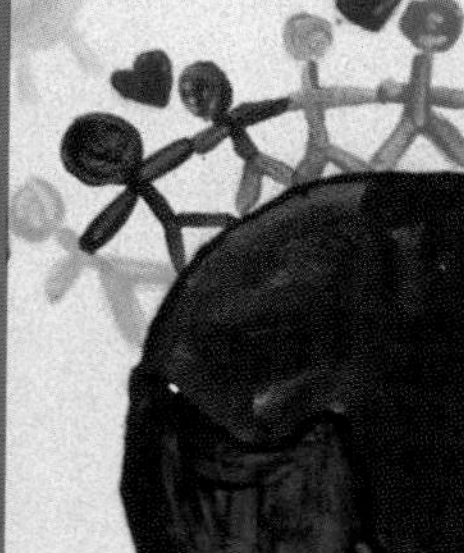

Parental Preparation of Children for Hospitalization

The nurse can assist the parents in preparing the child for hospitalization by suggesting the following interventions.

- Read stories to the child about the experience. Numerous books and pamphlets are available.
- Talk about going to the hospital, what it will be like. Talk about coming home.
- Encourage the child to ask questions.
- Encourage the child to draw pictures of what the hospital will be like.
- Visit the hospital unit before hospitalization if possible.
- Let the child touch or see equipment if possible.
- Plan for support via parents' presence, telephone calls, special items of the parents that the child can keep during the stay.
- Be honest.

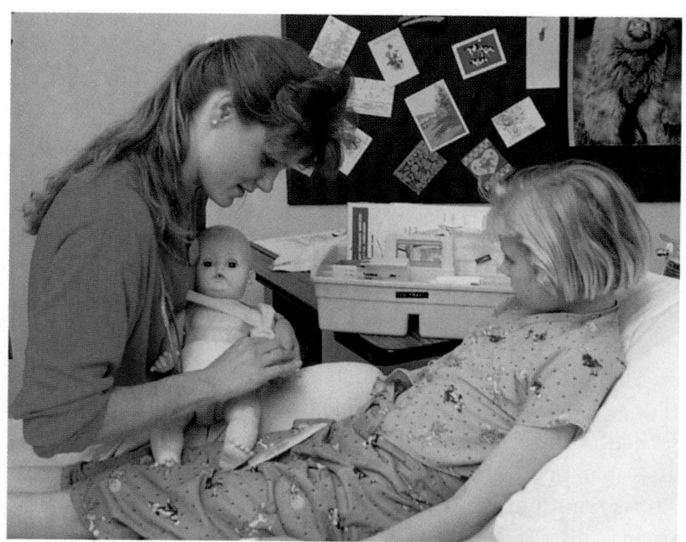

FIGURE 17–2 ■ The child's anxiety and fear often will be reduced if the nurse explains what is going to happen and demonstrates how the procedure will be done by using a doll. Based on your experience, can you list five actions you can take to prepare a school-age child for hospitalization?

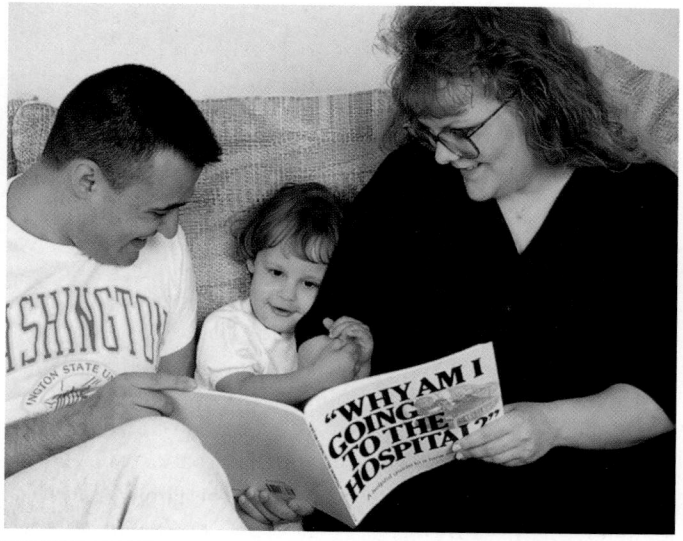

FIGURE 17–3 ■ Jasmine's parents are taking the time to prepare her for hospitalization by reading a book recommended by the nurse. Such material should be appropriate to the child's age and culture. Why do you think that having the parents read this material is valuable?

TABLE 17–5 Sample Teaching Materials for Children Regarding Hospitalization and Healthcare

VIDEOTAPES	PUBLISHERS
Clean Intermittent Catheterization	Learner Managed Designs, Inc.
I Have Epilepsy Too	Epilepsy Foundation
What Do I Tell My Children? How to Help a Child Cope with the Death of a Loved One	Life Cycle Productions
BOOKS	
Barney Is Best, by N. W. Carlstrom	HarperCollins
Barney and Baby Bop Go to the Doctor, by M. Larsen	Lyrick Publishers
The Berenstain Bears Go to the Doctor, by S. Berenstain & B. Berenstain	Random House
Chris Gets Ear Tubes, by B. Pace & K. Hutton	Kendall Green Publishers
Curious George Goes to the Hospital, by M. Rey & H. A. Rey	Houghton Mifflin Company
Cut, by P. McCormick & P. McCormick (Mental health hospitalization of a teen.)	Front Street Publishers
David's Story: A Book About Surgery, by B. Brink	Lerner Publications
Doctors and Nurses: What Do They Do? by C. Green	HarperCollins
The Fall of Freddie the Leaf, by L. Buscaglia	Henry Holt & Co.
Going to the Hospital, by F. Rogers & J. Judkis	Penguin Putnam Books
The Hospital Book, by J. Howe	Crown Publishers
Let's Talk About Going to the Hospital, by M. Johnston	Rosen Publishers
A Night Without Stars, by J. Howe	Avon
No Measles, No Mumps for Me, by P. Showers	Thomas Y. Crowell
Corduroy Goes to the Doctor, by D. Freeman & L. McCue	A Golden Book
Rita Goes to the Hospital, by M. Davison	Random Books
Tubes in My Ears: My Trip to the Hospital, by V. Dooley & M. Katon	Mondo Publishers
A Visit to the Sesame Street Hospital, by D. Hautzig	Random Books
When Molly Was in the Hospital: A Book for Brothers and Sisters of Hospitalized Children, by D. Duncan	Rayve Productions
Why Am I Going to the Hospital? by C. Cilliota & C. Livingston	Lyle Stuart

reactions to stressful situations, and prior experiences with hospitalization to assist in establishing a plan of care for the child.

Unexpected Hospitalization

An unanticipated admission places the child at emotional risk for several reasons, including the lack of preparation for the experience, the uncertainty and unpredictability of events that follow, the unfamiliarity of the environment, and the heightened anxiety of parents. An admission for exacerbation of a disease such as cystic fibrosis or leukemia can provoke feelings of depression or hopelessness.

Assist the child and family who are not prepared for hospital admission to adapt to the experience by orienting them to their immediate environment, providing an opportunity for questions, offering truthful responses, and explaining all procedures and expectations. Discuss the anticipated plan of care for the child and involve the family in the child's care. Provide the family an opportunity to express their fears and concerns. Refer to social services and/or parent support groups if additional support is needed.

BOX 17–2 Development: Providing Concrete Details

Children who focus on the specific details of a healthcare procedure are better able to cope emotionally and recover faster than those who worry about vague aspects of their condition or treatment. Researchers suggest that nurses communicate clearly and tell children about the concrete aspects of their treatment (LaMontagne, 2000). For example, tell them what stitches do for an incision and when they can be removed; explain how a piece of machinery works, and show them the display of their vital signs while they touch vital sign equipment.

NURSING CARE OF THE HOSPITALIZED CHILD

Nursing care of the hospitalized child focuses on providing family-centered care by promoting the child's and family's coping strategies to deal with the stressors of hospitalization, promoting optimal development and safety (Box 17–3), and minimizing disruption of the child's usual routine as much as possible.

Special Units and Types of Care

Children admitted to a hospital may be cared for in one or more of the following units: short-stay unit, outpatient unit, or ambulatory surgical units, general pediatric unit, emergency department, neonatal intensive care unit, or pediatric intensive care unit. Hospitalized children may require surgical treatment involving preoperative and postoperative care. Children with infectious diseases require isolation precautions. Other children may require rehabilitative care to achieve or restore maximum potential.

Short-Stay, Outpatient, and Ambulatory Surgical Units

Hospitalization stays for children have generally become short, with many procedures performed in outpatient units such as minor surgery (in ambulatory surgical centers), diagnostic tests such as cardiac catheterizations, radiology studies requiring sedation, and treatments such as chemotherapy. The child may be admitted in the morning and discharged later that same afternoon. In addition, children who have potentially serious illnesses may be placed on a short-stay or 23-hour observation unit for monitoring or limited treatment, after which a decision is made to either hospitalize the child for additional treatment or discharge the child home if improvement occurs.

These short stays are considered beneficial primarily because they cause minimal disruption of family patterns and are cost effective for the institution, insurance company, and family. Nurses assist parents to prepare the child properly for planned admissions, monitor the child during the procedures, encourage family participation in care, and keep families well informed (Box 17–4).

Nursing care of the child in short-stay, outpatient, and ambulatory surgical units is the same as for regular hospital admission (see following discussion); however, time for teaching is compressed, requiring the nurse to implement a variety of teaching methods in a minimal amount of time to ensure the

BOX 17–3 Safety Measures for the Hospitalized Child

NEWBORN AND INFANTS

- Use age-appropriate crib and bedding.
- Secure equipment cords under infant's gown or shirt.
- Do not allow infant to chew on cords.
- Properly dispose of syringe caps and other small items that may present a choking hazard.
- Establish with parents a list of persons that may visit the child.

TODDLERS AND PRESCHOOLERS

- Maintain bed in low position.
- Do not allow children to chew on cords.
- Keep room clutter free.
- Remove all unnecessary equipment from child's room.
- Properly dispose of medical equipment.
- If toddlers and preschoolers are curious about hospital equipment, provide them the opportunity to explore the equipment safely and with guidance (e.g., syringes without equipment, blood pressure cuffs).
- Keep in mind that these children are naturally curious and explorative.
- Instruct family members to inform staff when they are leaving the room to ensure that the toddler or preschooler is being observed.

SCHOOL-AGE CHILD

- Instruct children to avoid manipulating hospital equipment such as intravenous fluid pumps, PCA pumps, and oxygen masks.
- Allow the child the opportunity to explore hospital surroundings and equipment with guidance.
- Instruct family members to inform staff when they are leaving the room to ensure that the child is being observed.

ADOLESCENT

- Address issues such as smoking in the room and consuming alcohol since friends could possibly bring cigarettes or alcohol to the hospitalized adolescent.

family understands discharge instructions. Effective teaching methods include demonstration, videos, pamphlets with verbal review, and informal teaching sessions.

General Pediatric Care Unit

General pediatric units may be subcategorized into medical and/or surgical units, orthopedic units, oncology units, mental health units, and units specific to developmental levels (e.g., adolescent unit). Whereas some facilities utilize one unit or area (depending on the size of the hospital) which incorporates all of these care specialties, larger medical centers and children's hospitals generally employ separated units for specific specialties.

Admission to these units may be the result of an acute condition, such as pneumonia or trauma, or as the result of an exacerbation of a chronic condition such as asthma. Other causes for admissions include surgical procedures requiring longer than 24-hour stays and the need for inpatient treatments and services.

Nursing care includes orienting the child and family to the unit and procedures, adhering to the child's normal routine as much as possible, including child and family in the decision-making process, promoting a safe environment for the child, and promoting the child's growth and developmental needs.

BOX 17–4 Nursing Considerations in Preparing Parents and Child for Planned Short-Stay Admission

- Are there special requirements, such as not being permitted food or drink or needing extra fluid intake?
- What time and where must the child appear?
- Are any special forms, insurance numbers, or previous records needed?
- How long will the child stay in the hospital?
- Are parents expected or encouraged to be with the child or stay in the health facility?
- Is there a chance the child may need to remain longer than expected?
- What will the child's condition be for transfer home?
- Will special equipment or care be needed?
- What symptoms can indicate problems?
- Where can the family go or whom can they call in case of problems or questions?

Emergency Care

When a child is brought to an emergency department, the parents are usually frightened and insecure and may even be in a state of shock. The fast pace and critical nature of the unit creates an atmosphere in which parents are hesitant to ask questions and are anxious about the outcome. Anxiety and stress are caused by uncertainties in a critical care environment and the necessity of quick decision making. Numerous procedures, tests, treatments, and fear of pain also lead to stress related to minimal preparation in emergency situations. (See Chapter 21∞.) The nurse keeps both the child and the family informed about what is being done and when more news may be available.

Parents and child are encouraged to remain together as much as possible. Parents who wish to remain with a child even during invasive procedures or resuscitation efforts should be allowed to do so. The Emergency Nurses Association (2001) supports the option of family presence during invasive procedures and resuscitation. The nurse collaborates with the family members to determine their desired presence in critical situations and keeps them informed about the healthcare provided.

Intensive Care Unit

Intensive care units provide specialized nursing care to neonates, infants, and children requiring advanced technical support and interventions and continuous monitoring. See Chapter 21∞ for further discussion of care of the family with a child in an intensive care unit.

Neonatal Intensive Care Unit. The neonatal intensive care unit (NICU) provides specialized care to the neonate. Preterm neonates with complications, those born with congenital defects affecting cardiovascular or respiratory function, and neonates in other life-threatening situations receive care in the neonatal intensive care unit.

Pediatric Intensive Care Unit. The pediatric intensive care unit (PICU) provides specialized nursing care to infants and children. The patient population includes children with trauma, life-threatening illnesses, acute exacerbations of chronic illness (such as status asthmaticus), or any other condition requiring advanced support and continuous monitoring.

Parents of a newborn in the neonatal intensive care unit or a child in a pediatric intensive care unit (PICU) are likely to be anxious, particularly since the child's illness may be severe and the prognosis may be guarded. The unfamiliar equipment may create an atmosphere of fear or anxiety. Sensory overload as well as sensory deprivation is a potential problem for the child in the NICU or PICU. Numerous healthcare professionals work in the intensive care environment, and without effective and open communication, parents may not know whom to question or even what questions to ask.

Nurses provide comprehensive care to the child, as well as emotional support, explain the purpose of treatments and machines, help parents to hold or touch their child, and provide referral to other services if appropriate. Partner with the family and encourage them to write down their questions and direct them to the appropriate source if unable to answer the question. See Chapter 21∞ for a discussion of stressors in parents and children in an intensive care unit and the nursing strategies intended to address these stressors.

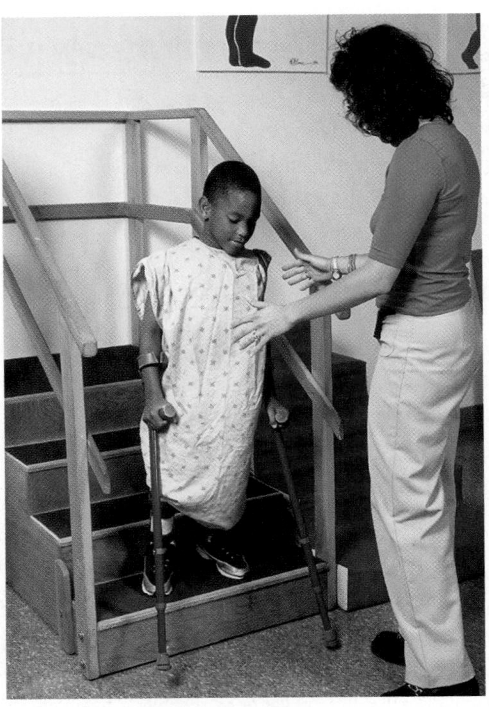

FIGURE 17–4 ■ Rehabilitation units provide an opportunity for the child to relearn such tasks as walking and climbing stairs. They provide an important transition from hospital to home and community.

Isolation

Children who require isolation to prevent spread of infection may experience lack of stimulation due to limited contact with other children and visitors. Frequent family visits are important and should be encouraged. Family members may be reluctant to wear protective garments either out of fear of using them incorrectly or a belief that they are unnecessary. The nurse ensures that the family understands the reason for isolation and any special procedures. Having contact with and holding the child are encouraged when possible. (Standard precautions are described in the Skills Manual.) Discussion of isolation techniques is found in Chapters 19 and 28∞.

Rehabilitation

Rehabilitation is the process of assisting a child with physical or mental challenges to reach full potential through therapy and education. Rehabilitation units provide children with ongoing care and support to continue recovery beyond the initial period of illness or injury (Figure 17–4 ■). These may be separate units within a hospital or independent centers. The rehabilitation may be on an inpatient or outpatient basis. Children who experience brain injury, spinal cord injury, near drowning, and burns commonly require extensive rehabilitation. The rehabilitation process can be lengthy; families may need support in adapting to changes in lifestyle, income, finances, and responsibilities.

The objective of rehabilitation is to assist the child with physical, psychosocial, or educational challenges to reach his or her fullest potential and to promote achievement of developmentally appropriate skills. Collaboration with a multidisciplinary team including parental involvement is essential.

Parental Involvement and Parental Presence

Family-centered care recognizes that families are essential to the child's care during illness. The nurse partners with the family and multidisciplinary team to involve the parents in the decision-making process and facilitate parental participation in the care of the child (Daneman, Macaluso, & Guzzetta, 2003).

Integrity of the family unit is fostered through parental involvement during the child's hospital stay. Additionally, parental participation prepares the family for care that will be required when the child goes home. The child benefits greatly from parental presence and participation. The child experiences reduced emotional distress and anxiety. Additionally parent–child attachment is uninterrupted, and the child experiences a decrease in behavioral maladjustments. Parental presence during painful procedures is particularly beneficial in reducing the child's anxiety and stress (Daneman et al., 2003).

Parental Reactions

Parents experience tremendous stress and anxiety when their child is hospitalized. Expressions of anger are not uncommon, particularly in high-stress situations such as having a child in the intensive care unit or not knowing or understanding the reason for the child's illness. Common sources of parental anger in the hospital setting include visiting restrictions, an unexpected change in the child's health status, confusion resulting from conflicting or insufficient information provided by the staff, and feeling undervalued in the care of their infant or child (Griffin, 2003b). The nurse implements a family-centered approach to develop strategies to reduce sources of parental anger and to handle these stressful situations in a professional and therapeutic manner.

Visiting Restrictions

Many hospitals maintain visitation policies which place limitations on who can visit, when they can visit, and the number of visitors allowed. Although many pediatric settings claim 24-hour visitation, families are often required to leave the child's bedside or unit during nursing report, medical rounds, admissions, and emergency situations. Parents may become upset when these restrictions deny them access and interfere with the amount of time they are able to spend with their hospitalized child (Griffin, 2003a).

Nurses are instrumental in assisting facilities to adapt policies which reflect a family-centered approach (Box 17–5). Partner with the family to provide them the opportunity to decide whose presence is most beneficial to the child and family.

Unexpected Change in the Child's Health Status

Nurses frequently experience changes in a child's condition; however, for parents this fluctuation in condition is an alarming event, particularly if the family was not provided anticipatory guidance that the event could occur, and if the family was not notified of the change in the child's condition. When parents are not informed in a timely manner of the change in condition, or they arrive on a unit and find their child in a different bed space, on another unit, or with a change in equipment, they may exhibit confusion and anger (Griffin, 2003b).

Nursing techniques include informing the family of potential changes in condition that may occur. If a change in condition occurs, make every effort to inform the family immediately. Partner with the family to identify methods of communication, such as a cellular telephone, pager, or alternate phone numbers and place these methods of contact on the child's chart. Determine in advance when parents would like to be notified of common procedures such as blood transfusions, radiologic examinations, and other procedures, to provide them a choice about whether to be present.

If parents are upset, nurses acknowledge understanding the situation the parents experienced and collaborate with the family to ensure trust is maintained (Griffin, 2003b). Encourage participation in parent-to-parent support groups where other parents of hospitalized children share their experiences and coping mechanisms.

Conflicting or Insufficient Information

Parents of hospitalized children may come in daily contact with numerous healthcare providers, leading to inconsistent or conflicting information. This causes anger and frustration, particularly where conflict in the diagnosis or discharge planning exists. The nurse acts as family advocate by collaborating with the multidisciplinary team and establishing a plan of care and communication sheet to ensure continuity of care and consistent communication.

Feeling Undervalued in the Care of Their Infant or Child

Parents may feel undervalued in the care of their infant or child, especially in high-technology intensive care units. Feeling unable to provide care to their child may lead the parents to express anger toward the staff. In applying a family-centered approach, nurses partner with the parents and include them in all aspects of the infant or child's care. Encourage the parent to ask questions. Collaborate with them to determine their desired level of involvement in the child's care. Simple tasks, such as weighing the child, feeding, holding, and providing hygiene care, provides the parent opportunities to participate in the care of the child (Griffin, 2003b).

Nurses need support when confronting challenging clinical situations such as angered parents. Nurses implement a variety of techniques to handle these challenges, including education such as inservice training on managing anger in the clinical setting, support through peers, mentoring, or debriefing opportunities. Additionally the nurses' own defensiveness and anger in response to parental anger can also be addressed by use of these techniques (Griffin, 2003b).

BOX 17–5 Taking "Visitation" Out of the Pediatric Care Setting

A family-centered approach to pediatric hospitalization recognizes that the family is an integral part of the child's life and care. Parents and family members should not be made to feel as though they are "visitors" to their child. A better approach to policy is to use terms such as "family time" rather than "visiting hours" or "visiting policy." Nurses can be the impetus for this movement by encouraging a change in policy and the language used.

CLINICAL TIP

When an angry parent becomes loud, the nurse acknowledges the anger and emphasizes his or her desire to help. Using a calm, supportive manner may diffuse parental anger and redirect the discussion to offering support to the parent. In situations where parents are disturbing other infants or children and their families, statements such as "I care about what is happening to your child and how you feel. Let's go someplace private where we can talk." If the situation becomes volatile and the parent becomes physically or verbally abusive, notify security immediately.

Preparation for Procedures

Numerous procedures may occur during hospitalization, from collection of urine or blood specimens to lumbar punctures and surgery. Special techniques can help the child to understand and cope with feelings about these procedures.

Psychological Preparation

Preparation may begin a few moments to several days before the procedure, depending on the child's age. In providing sensitive care to the child, nurses assume that a procedure can potentially be traumatic for the child. Even providing urine in a specimen cup or undergoing radiologic examination can be frightening if the child does not understand the reason for the procedure or what to expect. Administration of medication can also be frustrating or anxiety inducing for the child. The nurse prepares the child for medication administration and adapts techniques used with adults to ensure the correct medication is safely given (Table 17–6). A common procedure for which children need support is venipuncture.

TABLE 17–6 Variations in Medication Administration to Children

ROUTE	DEVELOPMENTAL CONSIDERATIONS	TECHNIQUES
Oral	Children under 5 years cannot generally swallow pills and capsules.	➤ Medications are usually given in liquid form (elixir, syrup, or suspension) ➤ Sometimes tablets are crushed or capsules are opened and mixed with one spoon of food. Check with pharmacy to be sure this does not inactivate the drug. Never crush enteric-coated or timed-release medicine. ➤ When choosing a vehicle for crushed tablets, use only one spoonful of applesauce, pudding, jelly, or similar food. ➤ Use TB syringe for amounts less that 1 mL to increase accuracy.
	Children may not want to take medicine.	➤ Position young children upright to avoid choking and aspiration. ➤ Give liquid medicines slowly by oral syringe (for infants) aimed at the inside of the cheek or by medicine cup (for toddler and preschooler) for drinking. ➤ Have the expectation that the medicine will be taken. Let children choose the type of fluid to drink after, but do not ask if they will take their medicine now.
Rectal	Colon is small in size.	➤ For children under 3 years, the nurse's gloved fifth finger is used for insertion. After this age, the index finger can usually be used. ➤ Lubricate the tip of the suppository.
Ophthalmic and otic	Young children may be fearful of medicines placed in the eyes or ears.	➤ Adequate restraint is needed to avoid injury. ➤ The nurse's hand can be stabilized by resting the wrist on the child's head. ➤ Explanations and therapeutic play can be used with children old enough to explain the process of administration. ➤ Have medication at room temperature.
Topical	Skin of infants is thin and fragile.	➤ Only prescribed doses and medicines appropriate for young children should be used on the skin. ➤ Covering the area or keeping the child's hands occupied may be necessary to ensure adequate contact of medication with the skin.
Intramuscular	Anatomy and physiology of children differ from that of adults.	➤ Gluteus maximus muscle (dorsal gluteal site) must not be used until the child has been walking for at least 1 year. ➤ Vastus lateralis site is preferred for young children. ➤ Amounts to be administered should be limited to no more than 1–2 mL for ventrogluteal site depending on muscle size. ➤ The deltoid muscle is rarely used in young children except for the small amounts injected in some vaccines.
Intravenous	Veins are small and fragile.	➤ Careful maintenance of sites is needed. ➤ Common infusion sites include hands and feet, although scalp veins are sometimes used in infants. ➤ Infusion pumps require frequent monitoring.
	Fluid balance is critical.	➤ Syringe pumps are often used when minimal fluid is to be given over an extended period of time. ➤ Central lines are commonly used for long-term intravenous medication therapy.

See Skills Manual for further medication administration techniques. Adapted from Bindler & Howry, 2005.

To assess the child's feelings about the procedure, ask the following questions.

- Does the child know the purpose of the procedure?
- Has the child experienced this procedure before? Was the experience painful, frightening, or reassuring?
- What does the child think will happen? Are the child's beliefs accurate?
- Is the procedure painful?
- What techniques does the child use to gain control in challenging situations?
- Will the parents or other caregiver be present to provide support?

When explaining, use words that the child understands to describe the procedure and its purpose (see Chapter 6). Older children require explanations geared to their cognitive level and previous experiences (Figure 17–5 ■). They will want to know

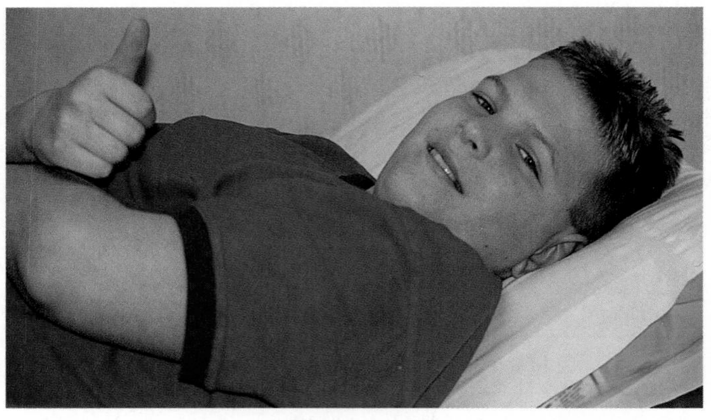

FIGURE 17–5 ■ This boy was formerly afraid of blood draws but with the aid of health professionals has overcome his fear and can now have the procedure done calmly. He shows his mastery over the situation. What can you do to help children afraid of procedures to develop coping mechanisms to assist them?

what is happening, why, and what they can do to cope during the procedure (Table 17–7).

Provide written information, videos, and other available media for adolescents and schedule time for questions and discussions. Adolescents can make many choices about their own healthcare. For example, they can be asked such questions as "Do you want your hand numbed for the intravenous start?" Some adolescents desire their parents to be involved in their care, while others prefer to minimize their parents' role. Maintain a positive attitude when preparing the child and reassure the child that it is normal to be frightened of unknown experiences. The nurse partners with the adolescent to ensure that the adolescent's wishes are known regarding parental presence. Parental presence can provide comfort and support to the child during procedures.

Physical Preparation

Preparation depends on the age of the child and the procedure. Preprocedural sedation may be required. Procedural checklists are often utilized.

> **CLINICAL TIP**
>
> When a potentially painful procedure will be occurring, an anesthetic cream such as EMLA, ELA-MAX, NUMBIES, or TAC is applied before the planned procedure. This can lessen discomfort and, therefore, fear in the child.

Performing the Procedure

Procedures on children are generally performed in a **treatment room** (a room designated for performing treatments such as intravenous starts, blood drawing, and lumbar punctures) to promote the child's sense of security that his or her own room is a "safe" and relatively pain-free site (Box 17–6). Infants may be provided sucrose for procedures (see Chapter 18∞ for pain management for all ages). After the procedure, the child is returned to his or her room for comfort and reassurance. A choice of reward often soothes the young child. Older children can be given the option of treatments in the treatment room or in their own hospital room. Older school-age children and adolescents may prefer to remain in their room rather than visit the treatment room.

> **BOX 17–6 Treatment Room**
>
> The treatment room is a special room utilized for the pediatric population for procedures such as intravenous starts, lumbar punctures, and blood draws. The treatment room is utilized rather than the child's own hospital room so that the child always has a "safe" environment and comfort zone by knowing that no unpleasant or painful procedures will occur in his or her room.
>
> Pediatric hospitals and large medical centers generally provide treatment rooms on each unit. Smaller hospitals and community hospitals may not provide a specific treatment room designated for pediatrics; however, any room other than the child's own room is an appropriate alternative. If smaller hospitals do not have a treatment room or provide an alternative, nurses acting as a child advocate should be vigilant in encouraging the establishment of such a room to minimize the stressors the hospitalized child experiences.

MediaLink Treatment Room Video

> **CLINICAL TIP**
>
> Procedures should never be performed in a playroom or during a play activity. The nurse acts as the child's advocate by ensuring that treatments by other healthcare professionals (such as blood draws or respiratory treatments) are not performed in the playroom. Assist the child to the treatment room and reassure the child that he or she may return to the playroom after the treatment is completed.

TABLE 17–7 Assisting Children Through Procedures

DEVELOPMENTAL STAGE	BEFORE PROCEDURE	DURING PROCEDURE
Infant	None for infant. Explain to parents the procedure, the reason for it, and their role.	Restrain infant securely and gently. Perform procedure quickly. Use touch, voice, pacifier, and bottle as distractions. Ask parent to hold, rock, and sing to infant after procedure.
Toddler	Give explanation just before procedure, since toddler's concept of time is limited. Explain that child did nothing wrong; the procedure is simply necessary.	Perform in treatment room. Give short explanations and directions in a positive manner. Avoid giving choices when none are available. For example, "We are going to do this now" is better than "Is it okay to do this now?" Allow child to cry or scream. Comfort child after procedure. Give child a choice of favorite drink or special sticker.
Preschool child	Give simple explanations of procedure. Basic drawings may be useful. While providing supervision, allow the child to touch and play with equipment to be used if possible. Since any entry into the body is viewed as a threat, state that the child's body will remain the same, and use adhesive bandages to reassure the child that the body is intact and parts will not "fall out."	Perform in treatment room. Restrain securely. Give short explanations and directions in a positive manner. Encourage control by having the child count to 10 or spell name. Allow child to cry. Give positive feedback for cooperation and getting through procedure. Encourage the child to draw afterward to explore the experience.
School-age child	Clear, thorough explanations are helpful. Use drawings, pictures, books, and contact with equipment. Teach stress-reduction techniques such as deep breathing, and visualization. Offer a choice of reward after procedure is completed.	Be ready to restrain child if needed. Allow child to remain in position by self if child is able to be still. Explain throughout procedure what is happening. Facilitate use of stress-control techniques. Praise cooperative efforts.
Adolescent	Give clear explanations orally and in writing. Teach stress-reduction techniques. Explore fear of certain procedures, such as staple removal or venipuncture.	Assist adolescent in self-control. Assist with use of stress control techniques. Explain expected outcome and tell when results of test will be completed.

The procedure is performed as quickly and efficiently as possible. The parents or nurse can be designated to support the child by way of a gentle touch, talking, singing, reassurance, or a stress-reduction technique. Refer to Chapter 18 for discussion of pain management.

Parents may wish to be involved or may prefer to be available afterward to comfort the child. If the parents wish to participate, teach comfort hold measures that the parent can utilize to provide comfort to the child while providing restraint for some procedures. Following the procedure, no matter how the child responded, the child should be praised.

Preparation for Surgery

A child's surgical experience may be elective, planned in advance, or a result of an emergency or trauma. How a child responds to the experience is related to the psychologic and physical preparation he or she receives. The accompanying nursing care plan, beginning on page 544, summarizes key elements of preoperative and postoperative care.

Preoperative Care

Preoperative care of the child includes both psychosocial and physical preparation for surgery. The goal of preoperative teaching is to reduce the fear associated with the unknown and decrease stress and anxiety associated with surgery.

Psychosocial Preparation

Preoperative teaching is geared to the child's developmental level. If child life specialists (discussed later in the chapter) are available, they can also play an important role in preparing the child for surgery. When the child will be transferred to an intensive care unit or recovery room after surgery, a visit to the area before surgery can reduce the fear and anxiety associated with waking up in a strange environment filled with frightening sights, sounds, and smells. The use of videotapes, anatomically correct puppets and dolls, drawings, and models is encouraged to teach the child about the surgical procedure. For example, a doll was used as a teaching aid in preparing Sabrina, the preschooler described in the opening vignette, for surgery. Playing with stethoscopes, gowns, masks, and syringes without needles also helps the child feel more in control (see discussion about therapeutic play later in this chapter). Children are reassured that their parents can accompany them to the operating room floor and will be waiting when they awaken from surgery.

Prepare family members for what to anticipate and what is expected of them. Special equipment such as intravenous setups and monitoring devices are explained. In some hospitals, only one or two immediate family members are allowed to visit the child at one time. Visitors may be required to wear special gowns, shoes, or hats, and they may be restricted to certain areas.

MediaLink Case Study: Preparing an Adolescent for Surgery

Physical Preparation

Preparation for surgery may occur in designated preoperative areas. Procedures generally conducted in preoperative areas include premedication, intravenous start (if not performed following general anesthesia), and preparation of the surgical site. If urinary catheterization is necessary, it is usually not performed until the child has been anesthetized.

Preoperative procedures and guidelines vary among hospitals and outpatient surgical centers. Preoperative checklists are used in ambulatory and acute care settings to ensure proper physical preparation of patients for surgery. A sample preoperative checklist is provided in Box 17–7. Weigh the preoperative child accurately, measure vital signs, and ask about last fluid intake amount and type. Monitor urinary output. Reinforce teaching regarding necessary NPO status.

Nursing management during the preoperative period includes establishing accurate baseline data, administering prescribed fluids, and performing assessments of fluid status. When an intravenous infusion is prescribed, start the infusion (see the Skills Manual), ensuring that the type of fluid and flow rate match those that are ordered and that would be expected for the weight of the child.

Of necessity, the young child who undergoes surgery usually is restricted from consuming oral foods and fluids just before, during, and for a period after surgery, thus creating a risk of fluid imbalance. The length of time the child is kept without oral intake is usually dependent on the child's age. Older children will have a longer time without intake, infants much shorter. This is due to anatomic development of the gastrointestinal tract, absorption, and standard diet for infants versus adolescents (American Society of Anesthesiologists, 2004.) Infants are especially unable to conserve fluids; therefore, even a short time of NPO status for a diagnostic test may lead to imbalance. Surgery often causes fluid loss from bleeding, which can further compromise fluid balance. In addition, the child may experience third spacing, a loss or pooling of fluid in a body space such as the abdomen, either in response to surgery or the child's condition.

BOX 17–7 Preoperative Checklist

- ___ Check that consent forms are witnessed and signed and in the patient's chart.
- ___ Be sure the child's name band is in place.
- ___ Be sure any allergies are prominently noted in the child's chart and on a special name band.
- ___ Remove any prosthetic devices, including orthodontic appliances and body piercings.
- ___ Check the child's mouth for loose teeth and tongue piercings.
- ___ Remove eyeglasses and jewelry.
- ___ Bathe and cleanse the operative site if ordered.
- ___ Put the child in an operating room gown, allowing the child to wear underwear.
- ___ Check that all special tests have been completed and the results are in the child's chart.
- ___ Have the child void before surgery.
- ___ Keep the child NPO before surgery.
- ___ Give the child prescribed medications.
- ___ Transport the child safely to the operating room.

While decisions about the total amount of fluid required is determined by anesthesiologists during the surgery, the nurse needs an understanding of the amount of fluid generally required during the perioperative period. Table 17–8 describes the amount of fluid needed on an hourly basis for maintenance of normal body requirements. In addition, losses from blood, third-space collection, or elevated temperature require replacement.

If a child is NPO prior to surgery and no intravenous line has been started, the fasting deficit is calculated using the formula in Table 17–8. Therefore a child who has fasted for 2 hours requires additional fluids during and after surgery to compensate for those not taken in during the period of fasting.

The decisions regarding the types of fluids administered before, during, and after surgery are determined based on the child's condition, length of surgery, and clinical condition. Generally, solutions with dextrose and saline are most common, such as $D_5$1/2NS or $D_5$1/4NS. Occasionally saline solutions are used in surgery rather than dextrose/saline combinations, since the stress of surgery induces the body to produce glucose. In addition, blood, plasma, albumin, balanced salt solution (lactated Ringer's), and nonprotein colloid solutions (hetastarch and dextran) may be administered when needed. During surgery, nurses continue to administer fluids and measure fluid losses, and assess the child continuously.

Parental Presence During Anesthesia Induction

Many hospitals now allow parents to be present with their child during anesthesia induction and again in the postanesthesia recovery area. Parents often want to support their child before and immediately after a surgical procedure, and their presence offers reassurance and comfort to the child. The nurse explains expectations such as surgical gown, cap, shoe covers, and the parent's role in presence during induction. The nurse offers the parents an opportunity to ask questions and voice concerns.

Postoperative Care

Postoperative area care units (PACU) or post-anesthesia recovery units (PAR) are the receiving areas for children following surgery. In the PACU or PAR, the child is recovered from anesthesia and is either discharged home or transferred to the unit specified.

Postoperative care of the child includes both physical and psychologic care. In the immediate postoperative period, perform baseline monitoring of vital signs; evaluate evidence of fluid loss via dressings, vomiting, or drainage tubes; and record hourly urinary output. Maintain effective airway clearance and monitor for evidence of respiratory depression or distress. Examine the postoperative orders and ensure that the child receives the type and amount of intravenous fluid indicated.

The child's level of consciousness is evaluated, and vital signs are assessed frequently according to protocol, generally every 15 minutes for 1 hour, then every 30 minutes for 1 hour, followed by hourly vital signs for 4 hours. The surgical site is observed for drainage, and dressings are monitored for bleeding. The nurse monitors the child's intake and output hourly and provides comfort and pain relief. See Chapter 18∞ for details concerning pain management. Resumption of oral intake is dependent on the surgical procedure, the child's condition, and surgeon protocol. Once oral fluids are resumed, monitor for emesis.

Parents are encouraged to visit with the child as soon after surgery as possible and culturally competent care is implemented (Figure 17–6 ■). The child may be discharged home directly from an outpatient surgical procedure, such as placement of pressure equalizing ear tubes (see Chapter 24∞), or, depending on the child's condition, may be transferred to a general pediatric unit or intensive care unit.

Postoperative Home Care Instructions

Routine postoperative instructions for the family of the child undergoing outpatient or 1-day-stay surgical procedures include monitoring for signs of infection such as drainage, redness, or swelling of the surgical incision, fever, and change in behavior. Instructions for follow-up visit, medications, other

TABLE 17–8 Calculation of Fluid Needs in Surgery

BODY WEIGHT	MAINTENANCE AMOUNT
Up to 10 kg	4 mL/kg/hr
11–20 kg	40 mL + (2 mL/kg/hr for weight above 10 kg)/hr
> 20 kg	60 mL + (1 mL/kg/hr for weight above 20 kg)/hr

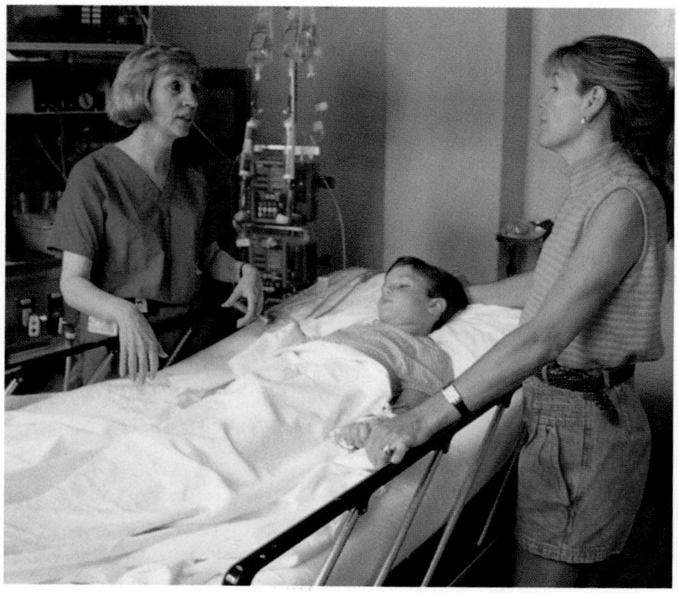

FIGURE 17–6 ■ This child has just undergone surgery and is in the post anesthesia care unit (PACU). Although the child's physical care is immediate and important, remember that both the child and the family have strong psychosocial needs that must be addressed concurrently. It is important to reunite the family as soon as possible after surgery.

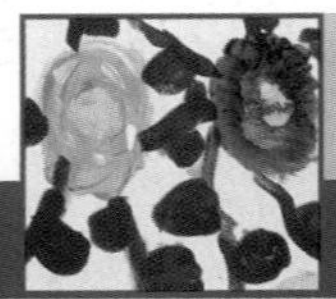

Nursing Care Plan

THE CHILD UNDERGOING SURGERY

GOAL	INTERVENTION	RATIONALE	EXPECTED OUTCOME
Preoperative Care			
1. Deficient Knowledge related to preoperative and postoperative events			
	NIC Priority Intervention—*Teaching, Preoperative:* Assisting a patient to understand and mentally prepare for surgery and postoperative recovery		**NOC Suggested Outcome—***Knowledge:* Extent of understanding conveyed about treatment regimen
The child and family will acquire knowledge related to the operation.	▪ Ask questions of the parent and child about surgery.	▪ Prior knowledge and understanding can be reinforced and used to guide your presentation.	The child and family are able to verbalize details about expected preoperative and postoperative events. They ask questions that demonstrate understanding.
	▪ Teach about preoperative and postoperative events using appropriate developmental methods such as dolls, drawings, stories, and tours.	▪ Developmental level determines the cognitive approach that works best for teaching.	The child demonstrates skills needed in the postoperative period.
	▪ Reinforce information the family has received about the purpose of surgery.	▪ The physician may have explained the operation.	
	▪ Have the child demonstrate post-operative events that pertain to his or her case such as deep breathing, putting bandage on doll, taping intravenous line on doll, and pressing patient-controlled analgesia button.	▪ Concrete experience promotes learning.	
	▪ Allow the parents and child to ask questions.	▪ Learners must have opportunity to ask questions.	
2. Anxiety related to change in health status			
	NIC Priority Intervention—*Anxiety Reduction:* Minimizing apprehension, dread, foreboding, or uneasiness related to an unidentified source of anticipated danger.		**NOC Suggested Outcome—***Coping:* Actions to manage stressors that tax an individual's resources.
The child and family will show decreased behavior indicating anxiety.	▪ Question the child about expectations of hospitalization and previous experiences.	▪ Previous experiences can influence present anxiety level.	The child and family demonstrate less anxiety. They verbalize understanding and comfort in hospital routines.
	▪ Orient the child to the hospital setting, routines, staff, and other patients.	▪ Familiarity with the setting and people can decrease anxiety by removing unknown factors.	Parents support the child for traumatic procedures.
	▪ Institute age-appropriate play and interactions with the child.	▪ Play can increase trust level and decrease anxiety.	
	▪ Explain procedures and prepare for those that might cause trauma. Encourage parents to support the child.	▪ The child is more likely to trust caregivers if they are truthful and if parents are present.	
	▪ Allow the parents and child to ask questions.	▪ Questioning provides an opportunity to explain the unknown, which decreases anxiety.	

MediaLink Care Plan: Preparing a School-Age Child for Surgery

Nursing Care Plan THE CHILD UNDERGOING SURGERY (continued)

GOAL	INTERVENTION	RATIONALE	EXPECTED OUTCOME
3. Risk for Infection and Injury related to exposure to nosocomial infection and use of preoperative medication			
	NIC Priority Intervention—*Infection Control and Fall Prevention:* Minimizing the acquisition and transmission of infectious agents, and instituting special precautions with patient at risk of falling.		**NOC Suggested Outcome**—*Risk Control:* Actions to eliminate or reduce actual, personal, and modifiable health risks.
The child will show no signs of infection.	■ Monitor vital signs at least every 4 hours. Inspect skin and respiratory status each shift.	■ Increase in vital sign levels, skin lesions, nasal drainage, or adventitious breath sounds can indicate signs of infection in the child.	The child's vital signs and assessment are within normal limits.
The child will remain free of injury.	■ Report any variations from expected vital signs.	■ Symptoms are reported so surgery can be canceled if necessary.	The child is transported safely to the operating room.
	■ Keep side rails up after preoperative medication is given. Maintain NPO status when ordered. Transport the child to the operating room safely secured.	■ Preoperative medication can alter level of consciousness. NPO status prevents aspiration.	
Postoperative Care			
4. Impaired skin integrity related to disruption of skin surface			
	NIC Priority Intervention—*Wound Care:* Prevention of wound complications and promotion of wound healing.		**NOC Suggested Outcome**—*Wound Healing:* The extent to which cells and tissues have regenerated following intentional closure.
The child will be free of infection.	■ Monitor vital signs per hospital routine. Record and report changes from baseline.	■ Changes in vital signs, especially increased temperature and pulse, can indicate infection.	The child shows no signs of infection.
	■ Monitor surgical dressing and drains every hour.	■ Excess drainage may indicate infection.	The surgical wound heals without infection.
	■ Change or reinforce dressings when wet.	■ Wet dressing can allow organisms to come into contact with surgical wound.	
	■ Check the intravenous site every 2 hours for redness, swelling, pain, or pallor.	■ Intravenous lines may become infiltrated or cause thrombophlebitis.	The intravenous line remains patent without signs of infection.
	■ Teach parents signs of infection before discharge. Teach parents aseptic technique for dressing change and wound care.	■ Parents report signs of infection and perform home care as needed.	The child continues to demonstrate no signs of infection at home.
5. Risk for Constipation related to surgical procedure and anesthetics			
	NIC Priority Intervention—*Constipation Management:* Establishment and maintenance of regular bowel elimination		**NOC Suggested Outcome**—*Bowel Elimination:* Ability of the gastrointestinal tract to form and evacuate stool effectively.
The child will achieve and maintain normal bowel functioning by the fourth postoperative day.	■ Auscultate bowel sounds every 4 hours. Offer liquids only when bowel sounds are present. Assess the abdomen for distention.	■ Restricting fluids avoids distention if peristalsis is not normal.	The child has bowel movement within 2 to 3 days after surgery with normal pattern by the fourth postoperative day.
	■ Document the character and frequency of bowel movements.	■ Knowledge of bowel status ensures early identification of constipation.	
	■ Advance the diet as tolerated.	■ Fluids and roughage promote normal bowel functioning.	
	■ Increase activity as ordered and tolerated.	■ Physical activity promotes peristalsis.	

(continued)

Nursing Care Plan THE CHILD UNDERGOING SURGERY (continued)

GOAL	INTERVENTION	RATIONALE	EXPECTED OUTCOME
6. Risk for Fluid Volume Imbalance related to intravenous infusion and NPO status			
	NIC Priority Intervention—*Fluid Management:* Promotion of fluid balance and prevention of imbalance complications.		**NOC Suggested Outcome—***Fluid Balance:* Balance of water in intracellular and extracellular components.
The child will achieve and maintain proper circulating volume. The child will tolerate oral intake when started, with no nausea, vomiting, or dehydration present.	■ Monitor vital signs per hospital routines.	■ Changes in vital signs, especially pulse or blood pressure, can indicate fluid imbalance.	The child remains in fluid balance with no vomiting in postoperative period.
	■ Record intake and output. Be alert for fluid loss via dressings or watery stools. Evaluate hydration status by skin turgor and mucous membranes.	■ Intake and output are roughly equivalent. Urinary retention sometimes occurs postoperatively as a result of anesthesia. Fluid status can be assessed by skin and mucous membrane hydration.	
	■ Monitor laboratory values of hematocrit and hemoglobin.	■ Increased hematocrit and hemoglobin can indicate hemoconcentration and underhydration. Decreased serum values can indicate hemodilution or overhydration.	
	■ Begin oral intake after assessment of bowel sounds. Record vomiting. Administer antiemetics if indicated.	■ Vomiting can cause fluid loss.	
7. Impaired Gas Exchange related to anesthetics and pain			
	NIC Priorty Intervention—*Airway Management:* Facilitation of patency of air passages.		**NOC Suggested Outcome—***Respiratory Status:* Ventilation: Movement of air in and out of lungs.
The child will maintain adequate ventilation with no respiratory impairment.	■ Auscultate lungs every 2 hours. Record rate, rhythm, and quality of respiration. Evaluate respiratory rate after analgesics.	■ Early identification of respiratory difficulty aids early treatment. Analgesics, especially morphine, may slow respiratory rate.	The child moves adequate air in and out of lungs.
	■ Administer oxygen if ordered.	■ Oxygen may facilitate breathing status postoperatively.	
	■ Reposition the child every 2 hours.	■ Repositioning ensures expansion of all lung fields.	
	■ Encourage deep breathing and coughing every 2 hours. Use incentive spirometer, pinwheels, or other blow toys appropriate for the development level of the child.	■ All areas of the lungs must be expanded. Mucus is expectorated.	
	■ Ensure proper intake and output.	■ Balanced fluid status ensures liquification of secretions and prevents excess fluid accumulation.	
8. Pain related to surgical procedure			
	NIC Priority Intervention—*Pain Management:* Alleviation of pain or a reduction in pain to a level of comfort that is acceptable to the patient.		**NOC Suggested Outcome—***Pain Control Behavior:* Personal actions to control pain
The child will maintain an adequate comfort level.	■ Assess behavioral cues (e.g., crying, movement, guarding).	■ Behavior of preverbal children provides clues to pain experience.	The child's pain is controlled as demonstrated by a low number on the pain control scale (behavioral or verbal).
	■ Use an appropriate pain scale with verbal children.	■ Pain scales allow children to quantify the amount of pain (see Chapter 18).	
	■ Administer prescribed pain medications on a regular basis.	■ Narcotics and nonnarcotic analgesics alter pain perception.	
	■ Use age-appropriate nonpharmacologic methods of pain control (e.g., distraction, repositioning).	■ Nonpharmacologic interventions interfere with pain perception.	

Nursing Care Plan THE CHILD UNDERGOING SURGERY (continued)

GOAL	INTERVENTION	RATIONALE	EXPECTED OUTCOME
9. Risk for Impaired Skin Integrity related to limited mobility after surgery			
	NIC Priority Intervention—*Skin Surveillance and Pressure Management:* Collection and analysis of patient data to maintain skin integrity and minimizing pressure to body parts.		**NOC Suggested Outcome—***Risk Control:* Actions to eliminate or reduce actual personal and modifiable health threats.
The child's skin will remain intact.	■ Turn and reposition the child every 2 hours. ■ Keep linens clean and dry. ■ Check pressure areas when turning and rub erythematous areas with lotion. ■ Get the child up and ambulating when ordered. ■ Check the incision for drainage, redness, and intactness of staples or stitches every 4–8 hours.	■ Repositioning takes pressure off the skin and allows increased circulation. ■ Clean linen decreases the chance of skin breakdown. ■ Rubbing increases circulation. ■ Movement decreases pressure on skin. ■ Early identification of infection or problems with wound healing can ensure fast treatment.	The child develops no pressure areas. The wound heals without complication.
10. Anxiety (child and family) related to change in health status and environments			
	NIC Priority Intervention—*Anxiety Reduction:* Minimizing apprehension, dread, foreboding, or uneasiness related to an unidentified source of danger.		**NOC Suggested Outcome—***Coping:* Actions to manage stressors that tax an individuals' resources.
The child and family will verbalize comfort with postoperative care and outcome.	■ Explain monitors, drainage dressings, intravenous lines, and procedures. ■ Reassure the child and family that anxiety is a normal response to the stressful event of surgery. ■ Encourage parental presence and care of the child. ■ Use touch and other nonverbal and verbal communication with the child and family	■ Knowledge of purpose decreases anxiety. ■ Knowledge of what is expected decreases anxiety. ■ The child's anxiety decreases with parental presence. ■ Effective communication reassures child and family.	The child and family demonstrate coping skills to deal with hospitalization.
11. Deficient Knowledge (child and family) related to lack of exposure to needed home care			
	NIC Priority Intervention—*Teaching, Postoperative:* Health System Guidance: Facilitating a patient's location and use of appropriate health services.		**NOC Suggested Outcome—***Knowledge:* Extent of understanding conveyed about home care.
The child and family will verbalize self-care required at home.	■ Provide oral and written home care instructions regarding surgical wound care, medications, activities, and diet. ■ Provide a number to call for questions or concerns. Instruct on follow-up visits.	■ Teaching regarding home care is necessary early in hospitalization. ■ Parents need to know emergency information and that follow-up care is required.	The child and family demonstrate skills needed for home care following discharge. They verbalize plans for future care.

treatments, and wound care, as well as signs and symptoms that require medical attention, are also provided. Additional instructions are tailored according to the surgical procedure and the child's condition. The nurse ensures the family understands home care instructions through their return demonstration and verbalization of understanding.

STRATEGIES TO PROMOTE COPING AND NORMAL DEVELOPMENT OF THE HOSPITALIZED CHILD

During hospitalization, care of the child focuses not only on meeting physiologic needs, but also on meeting psychosocial and developmental needs. Several strategies may be used to help children adapt to the hospital environment, promote effective coping, and provide developmentally appropriate activities (Figure 17–7 ■). These strategies include child life programs, rooming in, therapeutic play, and therapeutic recreation.

Rooming In

The practice of **rooming in** involves a parent staying in the child's hospital room during the course of the child's hospitalization. Some hospitals provide cots, while others have special built-in beds on pediatric units, and in some institutions a parent is provided a separate room on the unit. A parent who is rooming in may want to perform all of the child's basic care and to assist with some of the nursing care such as medication administration. Communication between nurse and family is important so that the parent's desire for involvement is understood and supported.

Rooming in provides the child with the comfort and security of parental presence. Parents may feel more comfortable staying with their child and participating in care, while others may experience more stress if they are missing work and are away from home and other children. Partner with the parent to assist them in establishing a rooming-in plan that is beneficial to both the child and family. For example, parents may alternate turns staying with the child, and even grandparents, aunts and uncles, and grown siblings may be included in the plan.

Some facilities offer free or reduced-cost meals to the parent rooming in. The parent who does not receive these meals may often skip many meals due to the financial impact on an already overburdened budget related to illness and hospitalization. Collaborate with the parent on cost-effective ways to ensure adequate nutrition for the parent. Emphasize the importance of the child's need for a healthy parent. Social services may be able to assist the family in obtaining meals while rooming in with the hospitalized child.

Parents rooming in with their child for an extended hospitalization can be encouraged to take advantage of the Ronald McDonald house, or other housing available for parents, at some point during the stay as a respite for a few days. This will provide them with an opportunity for needed rest and privacy.

Child Life Programs

Many hospitals have child life programs that focus on the psychosocial needs of hospitalized children. Professional child life specialists, paraprofessionals, and volunteers staff these departments. A **child life specialist** plans activities to provide age-appropriate playtime for children either in the child's room or in a specialized playroom. Some of the planned activities are designed to assist children in working through feelings about illness. Examples include playing with medical equipment, acting out procedures or treatments on dolls, using games to act out feelings, or drawing pictures about hospital treatments (Figure 17–8 ■). A trusted child life specialist may stay with a child dur-

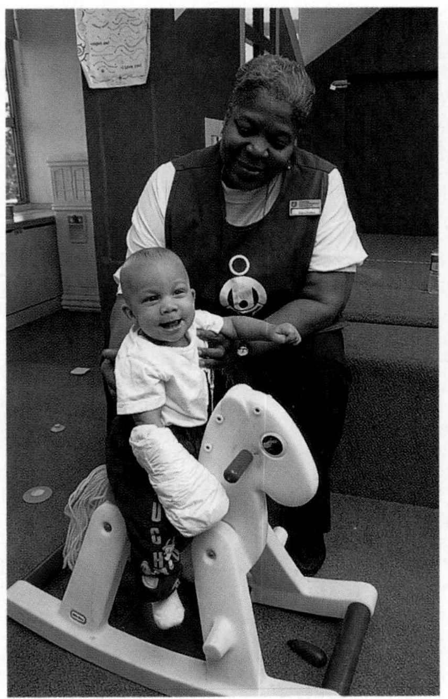

A

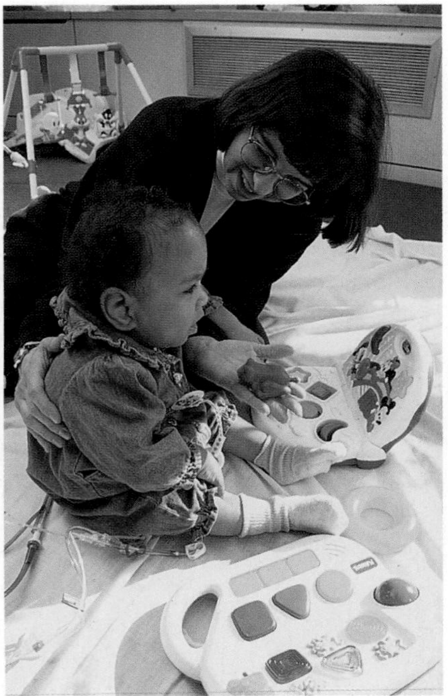

B

FIGURE 17–7 ■ *A,* Volunteers such as this foster grandmother can provide stimulation and nurturing to help young children adapt to lengthy hospitalizations. *B,* Child life specialists plan activities for young children in the hospital to facilitate play and stress reduction.

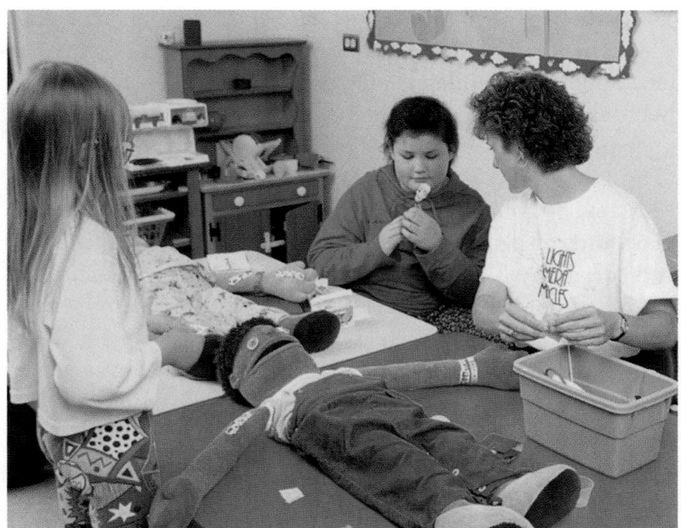

FIGURE 17–8 ■ A child life specialist works with children being treated for cancer. Special dolls are used to familiarize children with the procedures they undergo.

ing a particularly frightening procedure such as a venipuncture or bone marrow aspiration.

Both the child life department and the nursing staff focus on the emotional needs of hospitalized children. Child life specialists and nurses collaborate to formulate a plan together to assist children with particular needs. Before engaging in activities, attention is given to the child's level of mobility, fatigue, readiness to participate, and other barriers such as pain.

Therapeutic Play

Play is a significant component of childhood. The stress of illness and hospitalization increases the value of play. Not only is normal development facilitated by play, but also play sessions can provide a means for the child to learn about healthcare, to express anxieties, to work through feelings, and to achieve a sense of mastery or control over frightening or little-understood situations. In the present era of cost containment, play programs may be minimized in hospitals; therefore, nurses should document the need for and benefits of play.

Play that presents an opportunity to deal with the fears, concerns, and stressors of health experiences is called **therapeutic play.** Therapeutic play has many benefits for both the child and the health professional. It allows the child an opportunity to relive, understand, and integrate fearful healthcare experiences. Children can achieve a sense of mastery by being in control of the occurences during play. This helps lessen the child's stress and anxiety. In addition, the health professional can observe the child's play to learn what type of events are the subject of play and have been anxiety producing. The child's coping methods can be observed and additional techniques offered to the child. In contrast, *play therapy* is a mental health technique used to treat children with mental health problems, rather than normal life events that have caused anxiety. This technique is discussed in Chapter 34.

Through therapeutic play, the child's knowledge of his or her illness or injury can be assessed. A common technique involves using an outline drawing of the body (Figure 17–9 ■) or stories and asking the child to draw in or talk about what the illness or injury means to him or her (Ramsey, 2000). Alternatively, the child may be asked to draw a picture or make up a story, allowing the nurse to assess fears and other emotions. The Goodenough Draw-a-Person test helps to assess the cognitive level of children between 3 and 13 years of age (Box 17–8). The Gellert Index is another tool that helps to assess the child's knowledge of the body (Table 17–9). In addition to assessment, drawing can be used as a nursing intervention. Demonstrate to the child on a drawing what will occur during surgery or a treatment. The child's drawings of healthcare experiences allow him or her to express fears and gain mastery over the situation.

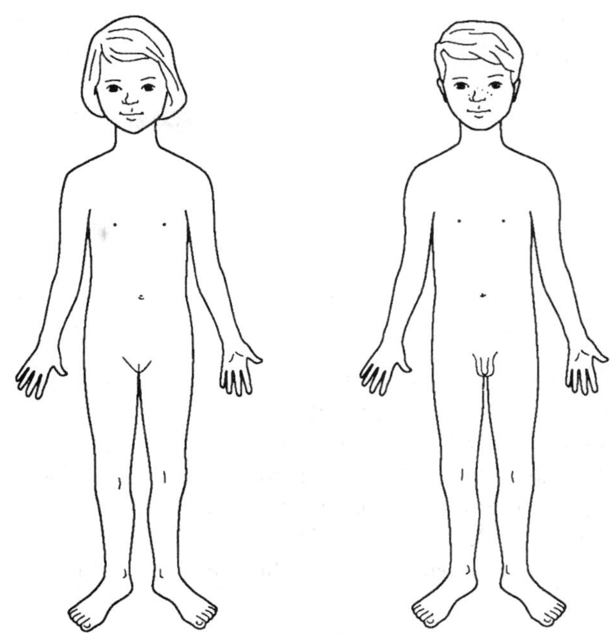

FIGURE 17–9 ■ The nurse can use a simple gender-specific outline drawing of a child's body to encourage children to draw what they think about their medical problem. Such drawings reveal a child's interpretation, which the nurse can work with to provide enhanced teaching.

BOX 17–8 Goodenough Draw-a-Person Test

- The child is asked to draw a picture of a person and to do so carefully and completely, taking his or her time. It is preferable to have the child take the test alone, away from parents.
- Points are assigned for specific details included in the drawing, for example, 1 point each for the presence of head, legs, arms, trunk, and eyes. Additional points are assigned depending on the complexity of details.
- For every 4 points assigned, another year is added to a baseline age of 3 years. For example, a child who scores 24 points (by including 24 details) would have a total score of 9 years (6 plus 3 baseline years). This number is compared to the child's chronologic age to determine his or her cognitive level.

The Goodenough Test may be obtained from the Psychological Corporation, 555 Academic Court, San Antonio, TX 78204; 1-800-872-1726; www.psychcorp.com.

TABLE 17–9 Gellert Index of Body Knowledge

Part A

What do you have inside you? Tell me as many things as you can think of that are inside you.

Part B

1. Show me the head. What is in the head? (Tell me all the things that are in the head.)
2. Make a circle showing where and about how big the heart is. What does the heart do? (What is it for?) What would happen if we didn't have a heart?
3. Show me some places where you have bones. (Try for a minimum of five locations.) What do we have bones for? What would happen if we didn't have bones?
4. Make a circle showing where and about how big the stomach is. What does the stomach do? Show me where the food goes after you swallow it. (Sketch in diagram.) And then? (If excretion is not mentioned spontaneously, ask: Does it ever come out anywhere? If the answer is affirmative, ask: Show me where it comes out.)
5. Make a circle showing about where and about how big the ribs are. Why do we have ribs? (What for?) What would happen if we didn't have ribs?
6. Make a circle showing about where and about how big the liver is. What does the liver do? What would happen if we didn't have a liver?
7. What do you think we have a skin for? What would happen if we didn't have a skin?
8. Make a circle showing where and about how big the lungs are. How many lungs are there? What do we have lungs for? What would happen if we didn't have lungs?
9. Do you have any nerves? (If no, ask: Does anybody else? If so, who?) What would happen if we didn't have any nerves?
10. Make a circle showing where and about how big the bladder is. What do we have a bladder for? What would happen if we didn't have a bladder?
11. How come we have bowel movements? (What for?) Where do bowel movements come from? (Probe for derivation from food, stomach, intestines.) Show me on the diagram. What would happen if we didn't have bowel movements? About how often (how many times) should people have bowel movements? About how often do you have bowel movements?

Part C

1. What do you think is the most important part of you? (If you picked one part of you as the most important, which one would you pick?)
2. Are there any parts of you that you could live (get along) without? Which ones?

From Gellert, E. (1962). Children's conceptions of the content and functions of the human body. Genetic Psychology Monographs, *65, 293–405. Reprinted with permission of the Helen Dwight Reid Education Foundation. Published by Heldref Publications, 1319 18th St NW, Washington, DC 20036-1802.*

Dramatic play, in which medical situations encountered are reenacted by the child, often assist the child to cope with painful treatments and intrusive procedures. The use of games, creation of art, and play with healthcare materials such as tongue depressors, syringes without needles, and other equipment is effective in encouraging dramatic play. These activities allow the child the opportunity to become familiar with the hospital environment and procedures allowing an outlet for anxiety in stressful and confusing situations. Observation of dramatic play offers insight into the child's concerns and level of understanding of the experiences, thus providing an opportunity to correct misconceptions.

A variety of techniques may be used to promote therapeutic and dramatic play (Table 17–10). Specific techniques are chosen to reflect the child's developmental stage. The nurse ensures that a variety of age-appropriate toys and distraction materials (stress balls, bubbles, music) are available (Box 17–9). Families are encouraged to bring the child's favorite age-appropriate toys from home.

Many hospitals, particularly children's hospitals, provide playrooms on each of the units to allow children a place to play and socialize with same-age peers. These rooms are generally brightly decorated in children's themes, and provide numerous opportunities for play, such as board games, video games, supplies for painting or drawing, and age-appropriate toys for each developmental level. Portable electronic play stations may be available to children in isolation or those unable to come to the playroom. Specific interventions according to developmental level are discussed later in this section.

Newborn and Infants

Newborns and infants require external stimuli for growth. The use of mobiles, music, mirrors, and other stimulation helps to promote stimulation and offer comfort to the newborn or infant. Parents and family are encouraged to cuddle or rock the infant and sing lullabies. Talking to the infant encourages interaction and play.

Toddler

Through play, toddlers explore the environment and learn to identify with significant people in their lives. Play is also an acceptable way for toddlers to release tensions caused by stress or aggressive impulses.

Toddlers are approached slowly, and the initial approach should be made in their parents' presence, if possible, to decrease feelings of stranger anxiety (wariness of strangers). Playing a variation of peek-a-boo or hide-and-seek using the curtain surrounding the toddler's crib or bed helps promote the realization that objects out of sight, such as parents, do return. The use of **transitional objects,** such as a familiar blanket or stuffed animal, can temporarily substitute for the security of parents. The toddler who is restrained can be read familiar stories. Repetition of stories promotes a sense of stability in the unfamiliar hospital environment.

A doll is a familiar toy that can be used to recreate a stressful environment, thereby providing an opportunity for the child to express and work through feelings. Other developmentally appropriate toys for toddlers include familiar objects from home such as measuring cups or spoons, wooden puzzles, building

BOX 17–9 Cheer or Surprise Basket

A "cheer" or "surprise" basket is an effective method of providing rewards and distraction to the toddler, preschooler, and even school-aged child. The basket contains age-appropriate toys, games, and items that the child may choose from as reward for participating in a procedure. For example, bubbles, stuffed animals, small dolls, coloring books, balls, and books are inexpensive or donated items from which the child can choose. Of importance, even if the child is uncooperative, once the procedure is completed the child should be praised and offered the opportunity to choose from the cheer basket.

TABLE 17–10 Therapeutic Play Techniques

TECHNIQUE	ASSESSMENT	INTERVENTIONS
Stories	Have the child make up a story about a picture. Analyze content and emotional clues in the story. Have children tell a story about an important experience in a group of other children.	Read or make up stories to explain illness, hospitalization, or other specific aspects of healthcare. Emotions such as fear can be included.
Drawings	Administer Goodenough Draw-a-Person test (see Table 17–10) to evaluate cognitive level. Consider subject matter, size and placement of items in drawings, colors used, presence or absence of physical barriers, and general emotional feeling. Administer Gellert Index (Table 17–11) to learn about the child's knowledge of the body and its functioning before planning teaching.	Use the child's drawings or outlines of the body to explain care, procedures, or conditions. Provide an opportunity for the child to draw pictures of his or her choice or directed topics such as a picture of the child's family or healthcare encounter. Ask the child: "Tell me about your picture." Be alert to the child's emotions: "This child must be frightened by the big x-ray machine."
Music	Observe types of music chosen and effects of played music on behavior.	Encourage parents and children to bring favorite tapes to the hospital for stress relief. Have tapes playing during tests and procedures. Parents can tape their voices to play for infants and young children during separations. During longer hospitalizations children can tape messages for siblings or classmates, who are then encouraged to retape their responses. Playtime can include the opportunity to play instruments and sing.
Puppets	The puppets can ask questions of young children, who are often more likely to answer the puppet than a person.	Perform short skits to teach children necessary healthcare information. Include emotional content when appropriate.
Dramatic play	Provide dolls and medical equipment, and analyze the roles assigned to dolls by the child, the behavior demonstrated by the dolls in the child's play, and the apparent emotions. Dolls with handicaps like those of the child are especially helpful (see Figure 17–10B).	Provide dolls and equipment for play sessions. To ensure safety, supervise closely when actual equipment is used. Respond to emotions and behavior shown. Use dolls and equipment such as casts, nebulizer, intravenous apparatus, and stethoscope to explain care. Use dolls with problems or handicaps similar to those of the child when available. Provide toys that foster expres sion of emotion, such as a pounding board and indoor darts.
Pets	Provide pet therapy. Watch the interaction between child and animal. (See Figure 17–11.)	Respond to emotions the child shows. Facilitate touch and stroking of animals.

Additional techniques, such as sand or water play or pet therapy, may be appropriate in specific situations.

blocks, and push-and-pull toys. Playing with safe hospital equipment (bandages, syringes without needles, and stethoscopes) helps toddlers to overcome the anxiety associated with these items. Supervise these play sessions and remove hospital equipment when you leave.

Preschooler

The nurse can intervene to reduce the stress produced by preschoolers' fears through the use of certain kinds of play. A simple outline of the body or a doll can be used to address the child's fantasies and fears of bodily harm. Playing with safe hospital equipment may help preschoolers to work through feelings such as aggression (Figure 17–10 ■).

Preschoolers prefer crayons and coloring books, puppets, felt and magnetic boards, play dough, books, and recorded stories. Preschoolers and older children often enjoy **pet therapy.** Children's hospitals and units can have visits from pets, most commonly dogs, to provide diversion and physical contact (Figure 17–11 ■). Both preschool and school-age children may enjoy playing with a toy hospital.

School-Age Child

Although play begins to lose its importance in the school-age years, the nurse can still use some techniques of therapeutic play to help the hospitalized child cope with stress. School-age children often regress developmentally during hospitalization, demonstrating behaviors characteristic of an earlier state, such as separation anxiety and fear of bodily injury. Age-appropriate crafts and activities provide diversion and a sense of accomplishment. Outlines of the body and, occasionally, dolls can be used to illustrate the cause and treatment of the child's illness. Terms for body parts that are suitable for older children are used. Drawings provide an outlet for expression of fear and anger.

School-age children enjoy collecting and organizing objects and often ask to keep disposable equipment that has been used in their care. They may use these items later to relive the experience with their friends. Games, books, school work, crafts, tape recordings, and computers, and video games provide an outlet for stress and increase self-esteem in the school-age child. The type of play used should promote a sense of mastery and achievement.

Adolescent

Many of the special play techniques used with younger children are not suitable for adolescents. However, adolescents do require a planned **therapeutic recreation** program to assist them in meeting developmental needs during hospitalization. Peers are very important to the adolescent, and the isolation of hospitalization can be difficult. Telephone contact with other teenagers and visits from friends should be encouraged. Interactions with other hospitalized teenagers at a pizza party, video game, movie night, or during other activities can help adolescents feel a sense of normalcy (Figure 17–12 ■). Physical activities that provide an outlet for stress are recommended. Even adolescents on bed rest or in wheelchairs can play a modified form of basketball.

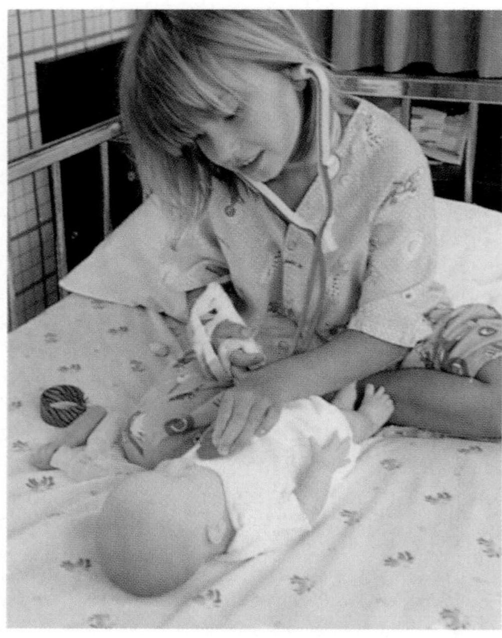

A

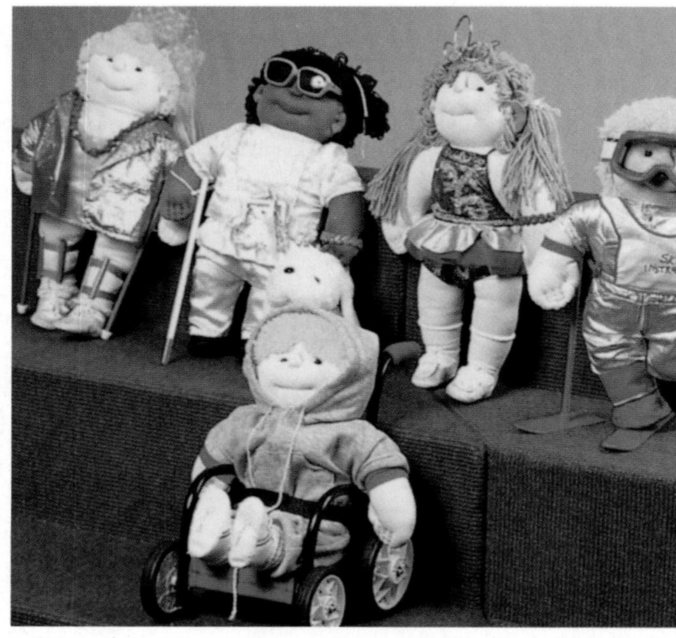

B

FIGURE 17–10 ■ A, Age-appropriate play will help the child adjust to hospitalization and care. B, Having the child play with dolls that have "conditions" similar to his or her own will help the child adjust. Such play helps the child realize what activities are possible.

The independence of adolescence is interrupted by illness. Nurses can provide choices for teenagers to assist them in regaining control. Providing the adolescents options and encouraging them to choose an evening recreational activity can promote their feelings of independence.

Adolescents and school-age children also prefer to wear their own clothing while hospitalized. Depending on the adolescent's condition, passes to leave the hospital for special activities and recreation may be possible.

Strategies to Meet Educational Needs

Some hospitalizations are so short that the absence of the child or adolescent from school and peers is of minimal concern.

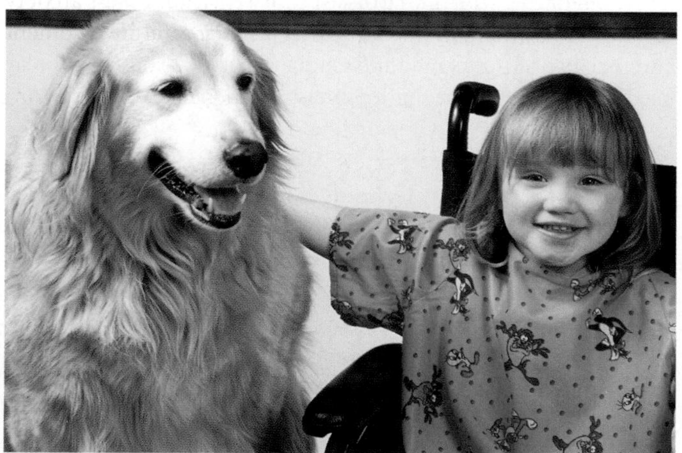

FIGURE 17–11 ■ Hospitals may have pet therapy from specially trained animals to provide comfort and distraction during healthcare. Both the child and the dog seem to be smiling!

However, if hospitalization is expected to last longer than a few days or if the child's condition will change, necessitating special school arrangements, the nurse assesses the effects of hospitalization on the child's education. The Commission on Accreditation of Healthcare Organizations (2004) mandates provision for schooling of the child in a healthcare facility for an extended period.

When an elective procedure occurs, partner with families to assist in the arrangement of the extended school absence with teachers. The child can then be provided with schoolwork to complete in the hospital or at home when capable. This minimizes educational deficits and future problems for the child. Pencils, paper, comfortable work areas, computers, and quiet work times are provided to meet the child's educational needs. Telephone calls, Internet connections, and live video conferencing with teachers can be arranged as needed. Pediatric hospitals generally provide in-house teachers to meet the child's educational needs. The hospital teachers collaborate with the child's school teachers to ensure the child is meeting the educational objectives to avoid deficits upon return to school.

The social aspects of school and peers are also considered. Peers are encouraged to visit a hospitalized classmate, send cards and letters, call on the telephone, or communicate via the Internet. Classmates may even want to videotape a class session, allowing everyone the opportunity to send a message to the child. When the child returns to school, the nurse can visit the classroom to provide classmates with information about the child's medical condition or assist the child in creating his or her own presentation about the hospital experience and medical condition.

The hospital nurse may contact the child's school nurse when special arrangements are necessary for situations such as mobil-

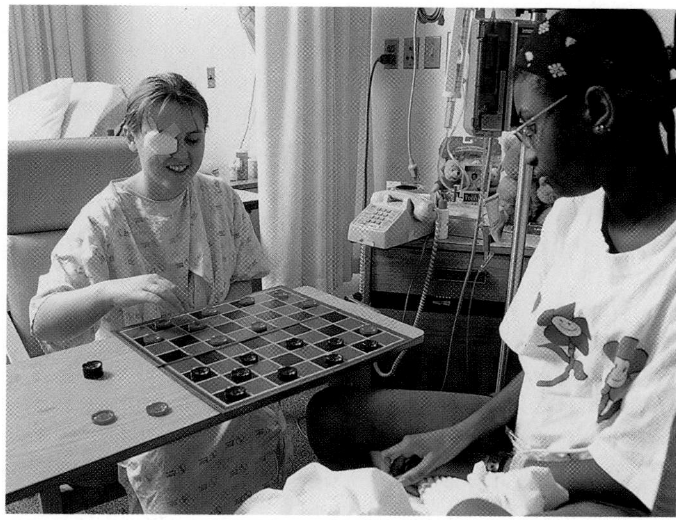

FIGURE 17–12 ■ Having interaction with other hospitalized adolescents and maintaining contact with friends outside the hospital are very important so that the teenager does not feel alone. A friendly yet competitive checkers game helps to stimulate these teenagers and allows for self-expression. What are the other benefits?

ity challenges. For example, the child who is wearing a large cast or who requires medications or other treatments, such as tracheostomy care, may offer challenges in a traditional school setting. Refer to Chapter 16∞ for further discussion of caring for the child in the community.

The child with chronic health problems or requiring long-term hospitalization has additional needs with regard to school. Hospitals or rehabilitation units may have classrooms, teachers, and facilities to promote learning (Figure 17–13 ■). Many school districts provide tutors or computer connections for students who are hospitalized or receiving home care for extended periods. Teachers can visit children at the hospital or at home. Parents are often pivotal in making arrangements to meet the child's educational needs, since they interact with the child, the school, and the healthcare team. Further discussion of meeting the educational needs of the child with a chronic condition is provided in Chapter 20∞.

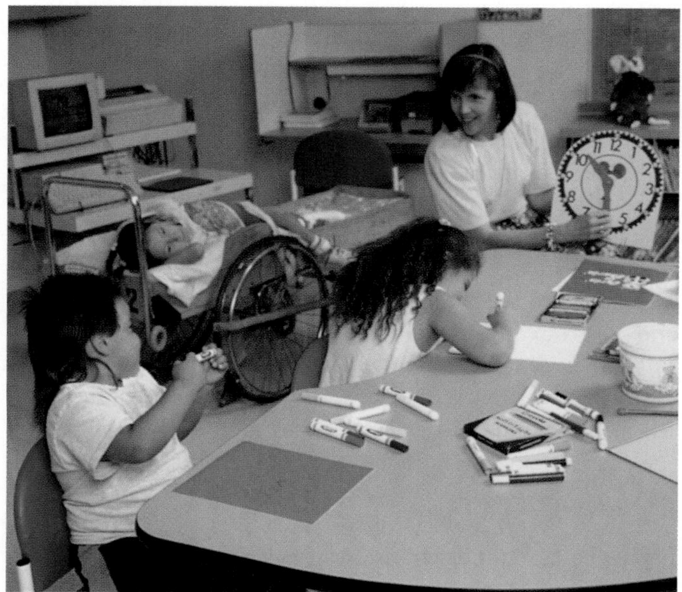

FIGURE 17–13 ■ Shriner's Hospital in Spokane, Washington, has a special classroom and teacher for children undergoing a lengthy hospital stay, enabling them to remain current with their school work. The child who falls behind other students might not fit in when he or she returns to school or might be required to repeat a grade. What are the potential consequences of these situations?

Child and Family Teaching

Teaching is an essential part of the nurse's role in care of hospitalized children and their families and begins with the initial contact of the family with healthcare providers. The American Nurses Association's and Society of Pediatric Nursing's statement on the scope and standards of pediatric clinical nursing practice mandates teaching as a component of pediatric nursing care (American Nurses Association & Society of Pediatric Nurses, 2003).

Teaching may be informal, as when the nurse integrates an explanation during routine care, or structured, as when the nurse plans and implements a formal teaching program. However, with shorter hospitalization stays few group interactions are possible, necessitating that most teaching be conducted during conversations and patient care (London, 2004).

Nurses inform the family that most teaching will occur in informal sessions rather than in formalized programs. The family should be aware of the teaching process to encourage active listening and participation. Essential to ensuring the family's understanding is to actively involve them in the learning process. The nurse and family partner together to identify the family's learning needs and appropriate teaching method to best convey the information. Recall that family members may be at various cognitive and anxiety levels and therefore have different teaching needs. Collaborate with both the family and other healthcare professionals to facilitate learning among the child and family members.

Teaching about the behaviors observed in hospitalized children and the strategies to deal with these behaviors is helpful for parents. For instance, providing information for parents of hospitalized toddlers on the typical behaviors of hospitalized children, and on the strategies to assist children, leads to less anxiety on the part of the parents and to greater parental involvement and support of the child during the hospitalization.

Teaching directed at children takes into account their developmental levels and cognitive abilities. Learning is achieved more successfully when teaching involves more than one sense (such as hearing, vision, and touch). Teaching directed at parents must be geared to their level of understanding. If English is not spoken or is the parents' second language, then a translator may be necessary. If translators are needed to facilitate understanding, be sure they are arranged and available for teaching sessions (see Chapters 3 and 6∞ for further discussion of the use of translators).

Timing is a critical factor in teaching. Parents and children are less receptive to teaching when they are preoccupied with stress or activities. Collaborating with the parents in scheduling specific times for teaching sessions may be helpful.

Depending on the information to be presented, teaching may use the cognitive, psychomotor, or affective domains of learning. Teaching that includes all three domains is more effective. Explanations or reading materials are tailored to a level the parent can understand. The choice of tools used varies depending on the child's diagnosis and available materials; included are pamphlets, booklets, videos, and models.

Teaching Plans

A teaching plan is a written document that includes goals and expected outcomes, interventions needed to achieve the specified goals and a method, and time for evaluation of the expected outcomes. The teaching plan may also specify teaching methods and types of materials to be used. Multidisciplinary teaching plans provide clear communication for all health team members in the teaching process. Documentation of teaching allows for continuity of care between nurses and other disciplines. Developing a teaching plan helps to ensure that all the necessary information is included and makes teaching more efficient.

The child's primary caretaker is an active participant in the development of the teaching plan as well as the implementation. The primary caretaker is most often a parent but may be a close family member (uncle, aunt, or grandparent). The first step in establishing a teaching plan is to assess the child's or parent's knowledge, skills, and feelings by asking the following questions.

- What does the parent/caretaker or child know about the health issue?
- What are the expectations of the child and family?
- What is the cognitive level or ability to learn?
- Is there a desire to learn?
- What previous experiences affect the learning experience, either positively or negatively?
- What previous interventions have been the most useful for the child and family?
- What resources are available to the parents, child, and nurse that enhance understanding of the health condition?
- Are there feelings or beliefs that might interfere with the learning process?
- What complementary care does the family use, and how does this relate to the teaching plan?

The second step involves deciding what knowledge, skill, or change in attitude is desired. Outcome criteria or objectives are established with the parent and child.

Possible teaching methods and a range of approaches are explored. A variety of sources, including written materials (books, pamphlets, handouts, and stories), computer software, audiovisual presentations, and others, are available to encourage interest from the child and family. Refer to Chapter 1∞ for information on reading level of patient education materials. In some settings, audiovisual and computer resources may be limited. Small group teaching sessions (e.g., for children with recently diagnosed diabetes or cystic fibrosis) may be another option and provide the child with an opportunity to interact and learn from peers experiencing the same condition. Gathering two or three parents or children together on a unit to learn and share experiences may also be helpful.

For children who can hear, touch, see a model or equipment, read, look at pictures, or even smell such items as alcohol swabs, learning is more complete. This basis is particularly important for the school-age child in the stage of concrete operational thought, who must be able to manipulate materials in order to learn. For some conditions, standardized teaching plans are available in books and from healthcare agencies (see Partnering with Families: Standardized Teaching Plan: Care During a Seizure for an example). These plans can serve as a guide in developing an individualized teaching plan.

Teaching for Children with Special Healthcare Needs

Children who have disabilities may have special learning needs. If the child has a visual impairment or perceptual difficulty, material is presented in auditory and tactile ways. Children who have hearing deficits require visual and tactile presentations. When psychomotor skill performance is needed, special aids and devices may be necessary for the child with neuromuscular conditions to allow the child to hold a syringe, draw up a liquid, or perform other tasks. Children who have learning disabilities may require more frequent reinforcement and shorter teaching sessions. These children are evaluated often for comprehension in order to adjust teaching as necessary.

Nurses individualize teaching plans and sessions according to the child's ability and needs. Adequate assessment of the child's strengths and abilities, along with collaboration with parents and other members of the multidisciplinary team, can assist the nurse to establish an individualized plan to establish the most effective teaching methods for the child.

Children who have chronic conditions or special healthcare needs may have been hospitalized numerous times and have received other healthcare at home and in the community. They usually have adapted coping mechanisms that help them deal with the chronic illness. Nurses can talk with the child to determine what has helped in the past, provide information about what to expect during the current hospitalization, assign staff members who are familiar when possible, and follow each child's lead in assisting his or her coping.

Nurses do not assume that the child with a history of numerous hospitalizations understands all activities since each hospitalization is different. Explain even the most routine activities. Regularly review the updated plan of care with parents and child. Provide the child with opportunities to ask questions and express concerns and fears. Assess the child's individual learning needs. Older children can be asked how they best like to learn. Determine the necessity for special equipment or teaching methods.

PREPARATION FOR HOME CARE

Nurses play an important role in preparing the child and family for discharge home; this preparation starts on admission to the hospital. Family-centered care includes keeping the family informed of discharge plans as families prefer being informed of the discharge date ahead of time so that they are able to plan in advance (Suderman, Deatrich, Johnson, et al., 2000).

PARTNERING WITH FAMILIES

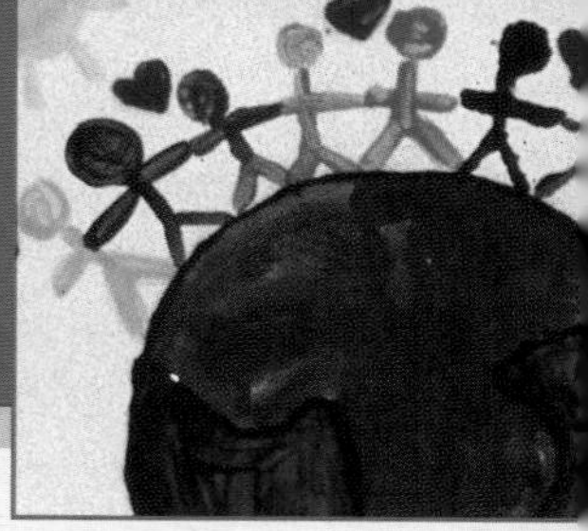

Standardized Teaching Plan: Care During a Seizure

Seizures are characterized as periods of involuntary muscle contractions and relaxations that the child has no control over. Seizures may be caused by high fever, head trauma, birth defects, and other neurologic problems. It is hard to predict when a seizure is going to occur. Some safety measures can help to prevent injuries to your child during a seizure.

What to do during a seizure

Seizure activity often means that the child is at risk for injury. Remember these safety guidelines when your child has a seizure.

- Remain calm and stay with your child.
- Protect your child from any injury.
- Place your child on the floor when the seizure occurs.
- Remove any dangerous objects from your child's reach, such as furniture, glass, or objects that can fall on the floor. Do not restrain or hold down your child during a seizure.
- If the floor is hard (tile, cement, uncarpeted), place a small pillow, sweater, or your hand under your child's head.
- Loosen your child's clothing if it is too tight.
- Turn your child's head to one side to prevent choking. Do not put anything into your child's mouth during a seizure.
- Provide time for your child to recover after the seizure stops. Reassure your child that he or she is okay. Speak softly. Explain what happened. Do not give food or drink until your child has fully recovered from the seizure.

When to call for emergency help

- If your child's seizure continues for more than 5 minutes.
- If your child has trouble breathing or does not breathe after the seizure.
- If your child has one seizure after another without waking up between them.

Everyday safety guidelines

- Have your child wear a safety helmet while riding a bike or skating to reduce the chances of a head injury.
- Keep bathroom and bedroom doors unlocked. It will be easier for you or other family members to get into a room to help.
- If the child prefers a bath rather than a shower, use just a few inches of water in the tub. Supervise the young child during the bath. Be sure someone is at home when a teenager is bathing.
- Your child should always swim with a buddy. If a seizure occurs, it is easier to rescue a child in a pool than a child in a pond or lake.
- Teach your child to hold onto the handrails when using stairs.
- Move glass, furniture, and extra pillows away from the child's bed to reduce the chance of injury during a seizure. Think about placing your child's mattress on the floor. This would keep the child from falling out of bed during a seizure.
- Give antiseizure medicines as prescribed to decrease the number of times your child has a seizure.
- Have your child wear a medical identification bracelet at all times.
- Inform relatives, babysitters, and teachers that your child has seizures. Tell them about any special care to be given during a seizure.

From Ball, J. (1998). Pediatric patient teaching guides *(pp. 1–4). St. Louis: Mosby–Year Book. Used with permission.*

Assessing the Child and Family in Preparation for Discharge

The discharge process is best started upon admission to the hospital. The healthcare team, including the primary healthcare provider, nurse, social worker, and discharge planner partner with the family to ensure a smooth transition. Assess the family's ability to manage the child's care and if any special adaptation to the home environment is necessary.

When a child who has been hospitalized for an extended time is to be discharged home, personnel contact the school district and make plans for education or reentry into school. This involves an assessment of the child by the school district and formulation of an individualized education plan (IEP). The IEP may include home tutors, specialized services from persons such as physical or speech therapists, or arrangements for transport of the child with a disability to the school and provisions for special medical care as needed. An individualized health plan (IHP) may also be required. See Chapters 16 and 20∞ for a detailed discussion on individualized education plans and individualized health plans.

Some common problems that interfere with successful discharge planning include financial concerns, the family's unavailability for teaching and planning, lack of equipment and lack of teamwork among involved healthcare disciplines. Nurses who assess for these potential problems from the initial contact with the child and family can intervene and assist the family to resolve these problems as soon as possible.

Preparing the Child and Family for Discharge

The family may need to learn physical and rehabilitative procedures for the child's care. Short-term care may be necessary until the child regains full function. In other situations, care may be required throughout the child's life. This may involve measuring vital signs or assessing blood glucose levels. For the child requiring complex long-term care, parents may need to learn about intravenous lines, medications, oxygen administration, or ventilators

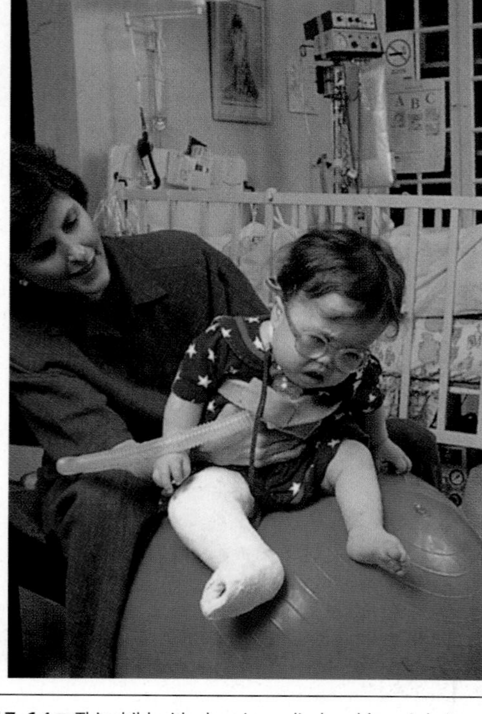

FIGURE 17–14 ■ This child with chronic medical problems is being cared for at home. Are there any legal implications for the hospital and the nurse associated with the preparation of the child and family for home care?

(Figure 17–14 ■). Some facilities provide families with the opportunity to provide 24-hour care to the child prior to discharge in order to help them gain confidence in providing care and allow the nurse to assess for areas requiring further teaching. See Chapter 20 for discussion of the child with a chronic condition.

Collaborate with the parents to teach them treatment procedures and proper equipment use as needed for the child's care. The goals of teaching include parents' ability to demonstrate care technique, their appropriate use of equipment, and their ability to identify symptoms requiring report to the healthcare provider.

Parents of children at risk for respiratory or cardiac arrest are encouraged to learn cardiopulmonary resuscitation (CPR) (refer to Skills Manual). Arrangements for individual sessions to teach the family CPR can be arranged. Some families require support and assistance to become providers of end-of-life care (see Chapter 22 for end-of-life care).

Not all children discharged after hospitalization will require additional care. However, these families still have need of support and education, as they may continue to be anxious or stressed over their child's hospitalization. Standard discharge plans for routine hospital discharge include the follow-up appointment date, phone number to call for questions, medication instructions, signs and symptoms to monitor for that are specific to the condition, and care at home. Ensure that the family understands these instructions and has ample time for questions before discharge home.

MediaLink Rehabilitation Resources and Support

Preparing the Child and Family for Home Healthcare

Children discharged from the hospital may require short- or long-term home healthcare. Children with multisystem conditions may require home care involving specialized equipment and personnel. Early planning provides the family time to investigate health insurance benefits, support services in the community, and other needs before discharge. The education provided and the parents' ability to perform care is discussed with a visiting nurse or individual who manages the home care program.

The nurse collaborates with the social service department, home care agencies, and the family to plan for equipment, procedures, and other home care needs. Home care nurses then assume the child's care and assist families to meet the child's healthcare needs. See Chapter 16 for further discussion of home healthcare.

Preparing the Child and Family for Long-term Care or Rehabilitation

When ill or injured children require long-term care, they are often transferred from an acute care hospital to a rehabilitation center or other long-term care facility. Like discharge planning, the rehabilitation phase of the treatment does not begin at the time of discharge from the acute care hospital but, instead, early in the hospitalization phase. The case team institutes the plan of care in the hospital, begins interventions and therapies, and makes plans for continued care. This multidisciplinary team, including the nurse, social worker, and case manager, coordinates the process and collaborates with the family to ensure a transition that causes the least disruption to the child and family. (See Chapter 1.)

When it becomes apparent that a child will require long-term care, the healthcare team explores with the family the options and resources available to provide the following care.

- Home care with support services such as visiting nurses and physical therapists
- A long-term care facility
- A specialized rehabilitation center that can provide care for an extended period

The nurse supports the family during the decision-making process about which option will be the most beneficial, considering the needs of the child, the financial implications, the roles and supports available to the family unit, and the resources available in the community. Guidelines to assist parents in evaluating rehabilitation centers are available from the Brain Injury Association of America (2004). Families can also be referred to the Commission on Accreditation of Rehabilitation Facilities.

Families often require assistance in determining the insurance coverage for long-term care or rehabilitation as coverage for these services may be limited. Social services can play an important role in assisting the family in identifying insurance resources. If a parent must take a leave of absence from work to provide care for the child, inform them about the coverage provided by Family Medical Leave Act (U.S. Department of Labor, 2004). Partner with social services to assist the family in completing the applications, if needed.

Nurses in acute care hospitals frequently coordinate services when transfer to another facility occurs. This involves providing information about the child's history, plan of care, and treatment and current status to the new facility. Forms are available to assist the person responsible for coordinating the transfer.

Copies of nursing and medical care plans are often provided to ensure continuity of care.

Families require support and assistance in dealing with the transfer from the acute care setting to another facility. The family may benefit from a visit to the facility before the child is transferred. Meeting the staff and becoming familiar with the environment can assist the family in preparing the child for a new environment. The family can then provide the child with brochures, pictures, and other materials from the facility and explain what the child can anticipate experiencing upon transfer. If possible, visits from rehabilitation center or long-term care facility nursing staff to the child before transfer can also be beneficial.

Regardless of the needs of the child after discharge, whether they are discharged home without need for further care or with the need for home healthcare or rehabilitative care, the nurse maintains a family-centered approach to provide the child and family with information and support during the discharge process. The nurse ensures that the family is prepared for the discharge and that any treatments and monitoring are understood by the family. Contact information is provided and any support services required are arranged before the child is discharged.

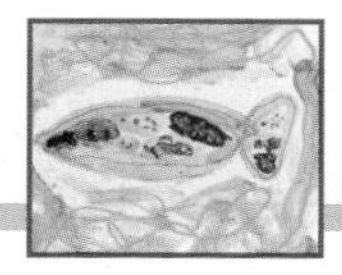

CHAPTER HIGHLIGHTS

- Hospitalization is a stressful event for all children and their families, especially when the hospitalization was unplanned and sudden.
- The understanding of children about their illnesses and hospitalizations is based on cognitive abilities at each developmental stage, and upon previous healthcare experiences.
- Nurses assess the impact of the child's illness or hospitalization on the family unit.
- Families are always disrupted by a child's hospitalization, and various approaches can help them to understand the process and cope more successfully with this challenge.
- When hospitalization is planned, both the child and parents can prepare for the experience. Nurses assist this process by teaching about what to expect.
- A teaching plan includes goals and expected outcomes, interventions needed to achieve the specified goals, and a method and time for evaluation of the expected outcomes.
- Strategies such as child life programs, rooming in, therapeutic play, and therapeutic recreation help meet the psychosocial needs of the hospitalized child.
- The nurse assists the family to plan for the child's long-term healthcare needs and home care issues. Culturally competent care is integrated throughout all provisions of care.

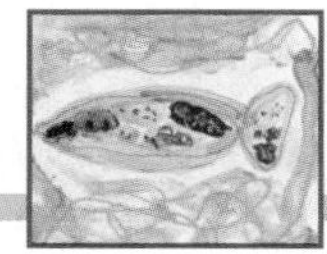

CRITICAL THINKING IN ACTION

INTRODUCTION

Recall Sabrina, the preschooler described in the chapter beginning. She is a 4-year-old living with both adoptive parents and her siblings, ages 9 and 7. She was diagnosed with coarctation of the aorta and is scheduled for a cardiac catheterization this week, followed by open heart surgery next week. Her family lives approximately 50 miles from the medical center where Sabrina is to receive her care.

DESCRIPTION

The parents and Sabrina discuss the upcoming catheterization and heart surgery with the nurse. During the family assessment, the nurse learns that the family has only been living in this area approximately 5 months and they have no relatives in the area but do feel they have established a good relationship with their "church family." Financially, the family reports they are stable but express concern about the extra costs of traveling and hotel expenses out of town during Sabrina's hospitalizations. Moving has depleted their savings and they are unprepared for these additional expenses.

The parents report that Sabrina has been anxious about her nosebleed episodes and she is difficult to calm down once she begins bleeding. Sabrina has not been told yet that she will be hospitalized for a cardiac catheterization and then for open heart surgery.

Sabrina's siblings are very concerned about the nosebleed episodes, but do not understand what is happening. The parents report that they have not explained to the other children Sabrina's heart condition and that she requires surgery.

DISCUSSION

1. Identify the stressors the family may experience as a result of Sabrina's illness and hospitalization. What interventions can you implement in response to those stressors? How will you evaluate the effectiveness of the interventions?
2. Based on Sabrina's age and psychosocial developmental stage, what are the most common fears and stressors caused by illness, hospitalization, and surgery that Sabrina will most likely experience? What interventions can you implement in response to those stressors?
3. Based on Sabrina's age and psychosocial development, what communication techniques would you employ? When should Sabrina be told about the cardiac catheterization? When should she be told about the open heart surgery? How will you explain each of these events?
4. Based on Sabrina's siblings' ages and psychosocial developmental stage, what should each of them be told regarding Sabrina's illness and need for surgery? What feelings and fears might each sibling be experiencing regarding Sabrina's illness? What measures can be implemented to reduce the siblings' stressors and fears? How should each child be included in the activities related to the hospitalization?

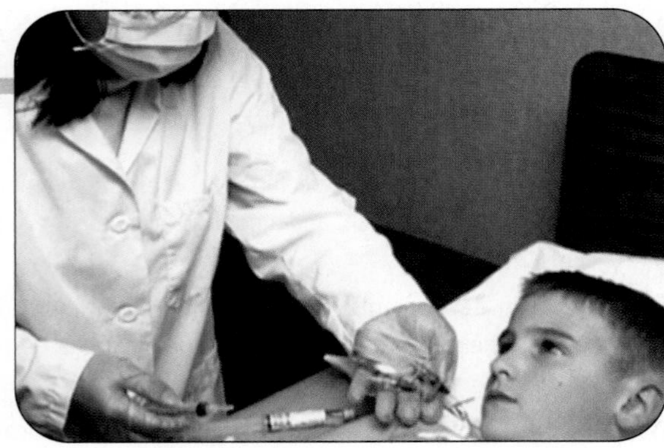

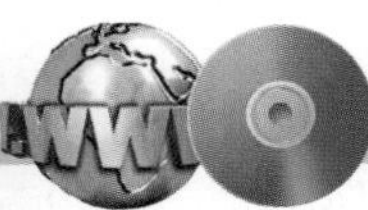

EXPLORE MediaLink

- NCLEX review, case studies, and other interactive resources for this chapter can be found on the Companion Website at **www.prenhall.com/ball**. Click on Chapter 17 to select the activities for this chapter.
- For animations, more NCLEX review questions, and an audio glossary, access the accompanying CD-ROM in this textbook.

http://www.prenhall.com/ball

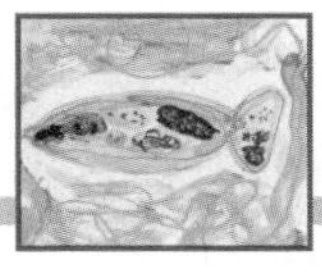

REFERENCES

Agazio, J. B., Ephraim, P., Flaherty, N. J., & Gurney, C. A. (2003). Effects of nonlocal geographically separated hospitalizations upon families. *Military Medicine, 168*, 778.

American Nurses Association & Society of Pediatric Nurses. (2003). *Scope and standards of pediatric nursing practice*. Washington, DC. Author. www.nursesbooks.org.

American Society of Anesthesiologists. (2004). Practice guidelines for fasting and the use of pharmacologic agents to reduce the risk of aspiration: Application to healthy patients undergoing elective procedures.www.asahq.org/publicationsAndServices/ NPO.pdf, accessed 12/15/04.

Bowlby, J. (1960). Separation anxiety. *International Journal of Psychoanalysis, 41*, 89–113.

Boyd, J. R., & Hunsberger, M. (1998). Chronically ill children coping with repeated hospitalizations: Their perceptions and suggested interventions. *Journal of Pediatric Nursing, 13*, 330–342.

Brain Injury Association of America. (2004). www.biausa.org/Pages/splash.html.

Bricher, G. (2000). Children in the hospital: Issues of power and vulnerability. *Pediatric Nursing, 26*, 277–282.

Commission on Accreditation of Rehabilitation Facilities. (2004). www.carf.org.

Daneman, S., Macaluso, J., & Guzzetta, C. (2003). Healthcare providers' attitudes toward parent participation in the care of the hospitalized child. *Journal for Specialists in Pediatric Nursing, 8*, 90–98.

Emergency Nurses Association. (2001). Position statement: Family presence at the bedside during invasive procedures and resuscitation. www.ena.org/about/position/familypresence.asp, accessed 7/15/2004.

Flores, G., Milagros, A., Chaisson, C. E., & Donglin, S. (2003). Keeping children out of hospitals: Parents' and physicians' perspectives on how pediatric hospitalization for ambulatory care-sensitive conditions can be avoided. *Pediatrics, 112*, 1021–1030.

Gellert, E. (1962). Children's conceptions of the content and functions of the human body. *Genetic Psychology Monographs, 65*, 293–405.

Gregor, F. M. (2001). Nurses' informal teaching practices: Their nature and impact on the production of patient care. *International Journal of Nursing Studies, 38*, 461–470.

Griffin, T. (2003a). Facing challenges to family-centered care I: Conflicts over visitation (family matters). *Pediatric Nursing, 29*, 135–137.

Griffin, T. (2003b). Facing challenges to family-centered care II: Anger in the clinical setting. *Pediatric Nursing, 29*, 212–214.

Huckabay, L. M. D., & Tilem-Kessler, D. (1999). Patterns of parental stress in PICU admission. *Dimensions of Critical Care Nursing, 18*(2), 36–42.

Hughes, C. K. (2003-April). Play therapy in an outpatient setting. *Advance for Nurse Practitioners*, 41–44.

Jackson, P. L., & Vessey, J. A. (2004). *Primary care of the child with a chronic condition* (4th ed.). St. Louis: Mosby.

Lau, W. K. (2002). Stress in children: Can nurses help? *Pediatric Nursing, 28*, 13–19.

LaMontagne, L. L. (2000). Effects of surgery type and attention focus on children's coping. *Nursing Research, 49*, 245–252.

London, F. (2004). How to prepare families for discharge in the limited time available. *Pediatric Nursing, 30*, 212–214, 227.

Marino, B. L., & Marino, E. K. (2000). Practice applications of research. Parents' report of children's hospital care: What it means for your practice. *Pediatric Nursing, 26*, 195–198.

Meleski, D. D. (2002). Families with chronically ill children. *American Journal of Nursing, 102*, 47–54.

Melnyk, B. M. (2000). Intervention studies involving parents of hospitalized young children: An analysis of the past and future recommendations. *Journal of Pediatric Nursing, 15*, 4–13.

Pinckney, R. B., & Stuart, G. W. (2004). Adjustment difficulties of adolescents with sickle cell disease. *Journal of Child and Adolescent Psychiatric Nursing, 17*, 5–12.

Proctor, E. K., Morrow-Howell, N., Kitchen, A., & Wang, Y. T. (1995). Pediatric discharge planning: Complications, efficiency, and adequacy. *Social Work in Health Care, 22*, 1–18.

Ramsey, C. A. (2000). Storytelling can be a valuable teaching aid. *Association of Operating Room Nurses Journal, 72*, 497–499.

Suderman, E. M., Deatrich, J. V., Johnson, L. S., & Sawatzky-Dickson, D. M. (2000). Action research sets the stage to improve discharge preparation. *Pediatric Nursing, 26*, 571–579.

United States Department of Labor. (2004). Family and Medical Leave Act. www.dol.gov/esa/whd/fmla/

Votroubek, W., & Townsend, J. L. (1997). *Pediatric home care*. Gaithersburg, MD: Aspen Publishers.

Chapter

18

Pain Assessment and Management

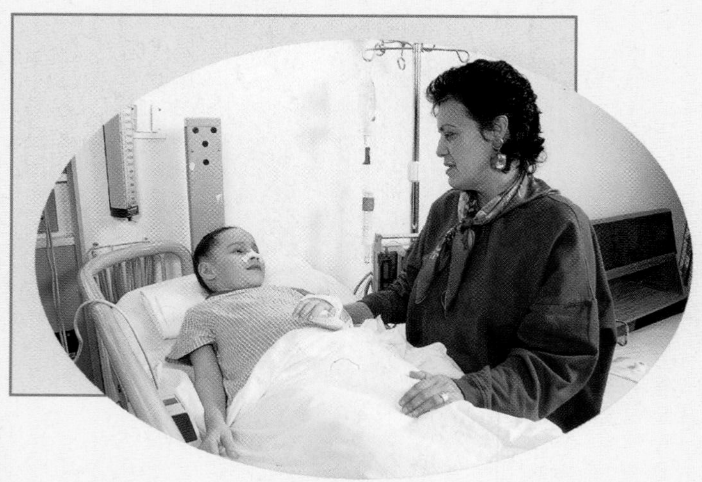

Felicia Alba, who is 5 years old, was struck by a car. Six hours ago she had surgery to repair a liver laceration. She also has numerous abrasions on her legs and arms. Fortunately she did not experience a traumatic brain injury. After spending 3 hours in the postanesthesia unit, she was moved to the pediatric inpatient unit. She has an intravenous line in place, as well as a nasogastric tube for suction. Her abdominal dressing is clean and dry. Felicia has orders for morphine IV every 3 hours around the clock for the first 24 hours.

Felicia's mother is rooming in with her during her hospital stay. Twelve hours after surgery Felicia is dozing but is responsive to verbal stimuli. Her most recent IV morphine was given 2 hours ago. The nurse attempts to determine how well Felicia's pain is managed. Her facial expression indicates that she is not in pain. Felicia's mother feels that she is resting fairly comfortably. The nurse asks Felicia to look at a copy of the faces on the Oucher Scale and to tell her which picture is the one most like how she feels. Felicia points to the second face for a score of 2 on the pain scale.

"I am really worried about Felicia. How do we know she is not in a lot of pain? She might be afraid to tell us she has pain because she has had so many things done to her already. She may be afraid of getting another needle."

—Maria, age 14

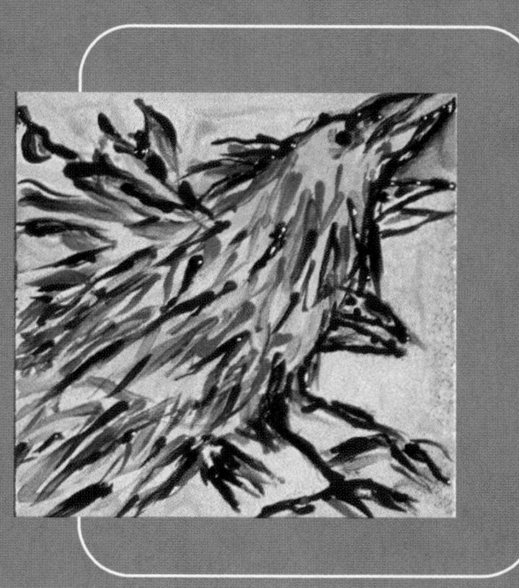

Learning Outcomes

After completing this chapter, you will be able to:

- Describe the pathophysiology of pain and rationales for effectiveness of nonpainful touch and massage in reducing pain.
- Describe the physiologic and behavioral consequences of pain in children.
- Assess the developmental abilities of children in different age groups to perform a self-assessment of pain intensity and select an appropriate tool to assess the pain of children in each age group.
- Assess children of different ages with acute pain and develop a nursing care plan that integrates pharmacologic interventions in addition to developmentally appropriate complementary and alternative therapies.
- Contrast the nursing care for children receiving an opioid analgesic and a nonsteroidal anti-inflammatory medication.
- Assess the child receiving sedation and analgesia for a medical procedure and develop a nursing care plan for monitoring the child throughout the procedure and during recovery.

MediaLink http://www.prenhall.com/ball

Resources for this chapter can be found on the CD-ROM accompanying this textbook, and on the Companion Website at www.prenhall.com/ball. Click on Chapter 18 to select the activities for this chapter.

CD-ROM

Animations/Videos

- *Morphine*
- *Pain Management Kit*
- *Pain Perception*

Nursing in Action

- *Administering Patient-Controlled Analgesia (PCA)*
- *Conscious Sedation Monitoring*

NCLEX Review

Audio Glossary

COMPANION WEBSITE

A & P Review

Clinical Manifestations Review

Medication Match-Up

NCLEX Review

MediaLink Applications

- *Calculating Opioid Dosage*
- *Managing Conscious Sedation*
- *Postoperative Pain Assessment*
- *Pain and Distraction Techniques*
- *Emergency Equipment and Sedation*
- *Teaching Plan: Managing Pain at Home*

Key Terms

acute pain/562
anxiolysis/586
chronic pain/562
deep sedation/586
distraction/579
electroanalgesia/579
equianalgesic dose/573
light sedation/586
nociception/562
nociceptors/562
NSAIDs/574
opioids/573
pain/562
pain threshold/564
patient-controlled analgesia (PCA)/576
reliability/568
sedation/586
tolerance/581
validity/568
withdrawal/577

ACUTE AND CHRONIC PAIN

Everyone has his or her own perception of pain. A neurologic response to tissue injury, **pain** is a highly personal and subjective unpleasant sensory and emotional experience associated with actual or potential tissue damage. Much of the acute pain infants and children feel associated with medical conditions and procedures can be prevented or greatly relieved. Effective pain management is every child's right.

Pain exists when the patient says it does (McCaffery & Pasero, 1999). Pain may be either acute or chronic. **Acute pain** is sudden pain of short duration that may be associated with a single event, such as surgery, or an acute exacerbation of a condition such as a sickle-cell crisis. There is an immediate pain response that occurs right at the time of tissue damage. The inflammatory response that follows causes an established or sustained pain response (Fuller, 2001). **Chronic pain** is persistent pain lasting longer than 6 months that is generally associated with a prolonged disease process such as juvenile rheumatoid arthritis.

Pathophysiology of Pain

Two fibers have the primary responsibility for the **nociception,** the transmission of pain impulses from the periphery to the dorsal horn of the spinal cord. The large, myelinated A-delta fibers quickly transmit sharp, well-localized pain. The small, unmyelinated C-polymodal fibers slowly transmit dull, burning, diffuse pain, as well as chronic pain (Figure 18–1 ■). **Nociceptors,** free nerve endings at the site of tissue damage with the capacity to distinguish painful stimuli, transmit information to these specialized nerve fibers. Nociceptors are stimulated by mechanical, thermal, and chemical injury. Various substances (bradykinin, prostaglandin, leukotrienes, serotonin, histamine, catecholamines, and substance P) are produced in response to tissue damage. These substances help move the pain impulse from the nerve endings to the spinal cord. Other neurons can be recruited to transmit pain impulses, increasing the pain perceived.

After the sensory information reaches the substantia gelatinosa in the dorsal horn of the spinal cord, the pain signal may be modified depending on the presence of other stimuli from either the brain or the periphery. The pain signal is then transmitted to the brain through the spinothalamic, reticulospinal, and spinomesoencephalic nerve pathways, where perception occurs. The descending tracts may alter or modulate pain perception through the release of inhibitory neurotransmitters. Once the pain sensation reaches the brain, emotional responses, past experiences with pain, and the nature of the painful event may increase or decrease the intensity of the pain perceived. The autonomic nervous system is activated in response to pain, producing tachycardia, peripheral vasoconstriction, diaphoresis, pupil dilation, and increased secretion of catecholamines and adrenocorticoid hormones.

MediaLink Pain Perception Video

The gate-control theory of pain helps explain how the pain impulses are allowed to proceed to the brain. Impulses are transmitted by the nociceptors through the large A-delta and small C fibers to terminate in the substantia gelatinosa in the dorsal horn of the spinal cord. The substantia gelatinosa serves as a gate and regulates the transmission of pain and other impulses to the central nervous system (Huether & Leo, 2002). Since pain and nonpain impulses are sent along the same pathways, nonpain impulses can compete with pain impulses for transmission. (See Complementary Therapy: Pain Control.)

Neonatal Pathophysiology

All of the necessary peripheral and central nervous system anatomical structures and functional ability to process pain are developed in the fetus by 20 weeks' gestation (Pasero, 2002). Additionally, the hypothalamic-pituitary-adrenal axes are well developed enabling the newborn to release catecholamines and cortisol in response to stress (Franck, Greenberg, & Stevens, 2000). However, there are some differences in the nociceptive processing between infants and adults due to neurophysiologic and cognitive immaturity. Since myelination of spinal fibers continues after birth, most pain impulses in newborns are transmitted along the nonmyelinated C fibers. The pain signal being transmitted is less precise. Even though the pain transmitted is along the slower C fibers, the distance from the site of pain to the brain is short. The descending neurotransmitters are underdeveloped, and newborns are less able to modulate the pain impulses (Anand & Hickey, 1987). Therefore preterm and full-term newborns may be more sensitive to pain stimuli than older infants and children because of the immaturity of the descending control mechanisms that enable older infants and children to reduce the transmission of pain. By 6 months of age, infants have a memory of pain and demonstrate anticipatory fear of pain when taken to a location where they once experienced it (McGrath & Craig, 1989).

Physiologic Consequences of Pain

Unrelieved pain is stressful and has many undesirable physiologic consequences on several body systems (Table 18–1). In addition to elevations in vital signs, there is an increased release of catecholamines, glucagon, and corticosteroids. This can result in a catabolic state that can have a serious effect on newborns and young infants with higher metabolic rates and fewer nutritional reserves.

Pain in the newborn and infant drains energy resources the infant needs for growth and healing. The autonomic nervous system becomes unstable, reflected in vital sign and oxygen saturation changes. Diaphragmatic splinting increases the intracranial blood volume and intracranial pressure, potentially leading to intraventricular hemorrhages. Repeated disruption of the sleep-awake cycle can affect the child's neurodevelopment,

> **COMPLEMENTARY THERAPY**
> **Pain Control**
>
> The gate-control theory helps explain why complementary pain management techniques are effective in helping to control pain. Stimulation of the larger A-delta fibers by nonpainful touch and pressure such as massage causes the substantia gelatinosa in the dorsal horn of the spinal cord to "close the gate" and decrease the transmission of pain impulses to the brain (Franck, Greenberg, & Stevens, 2000; Huether & Leo, 2002).

PATHOPHYSIOLOGY ILLUSTRATED

Acute Pain Perception

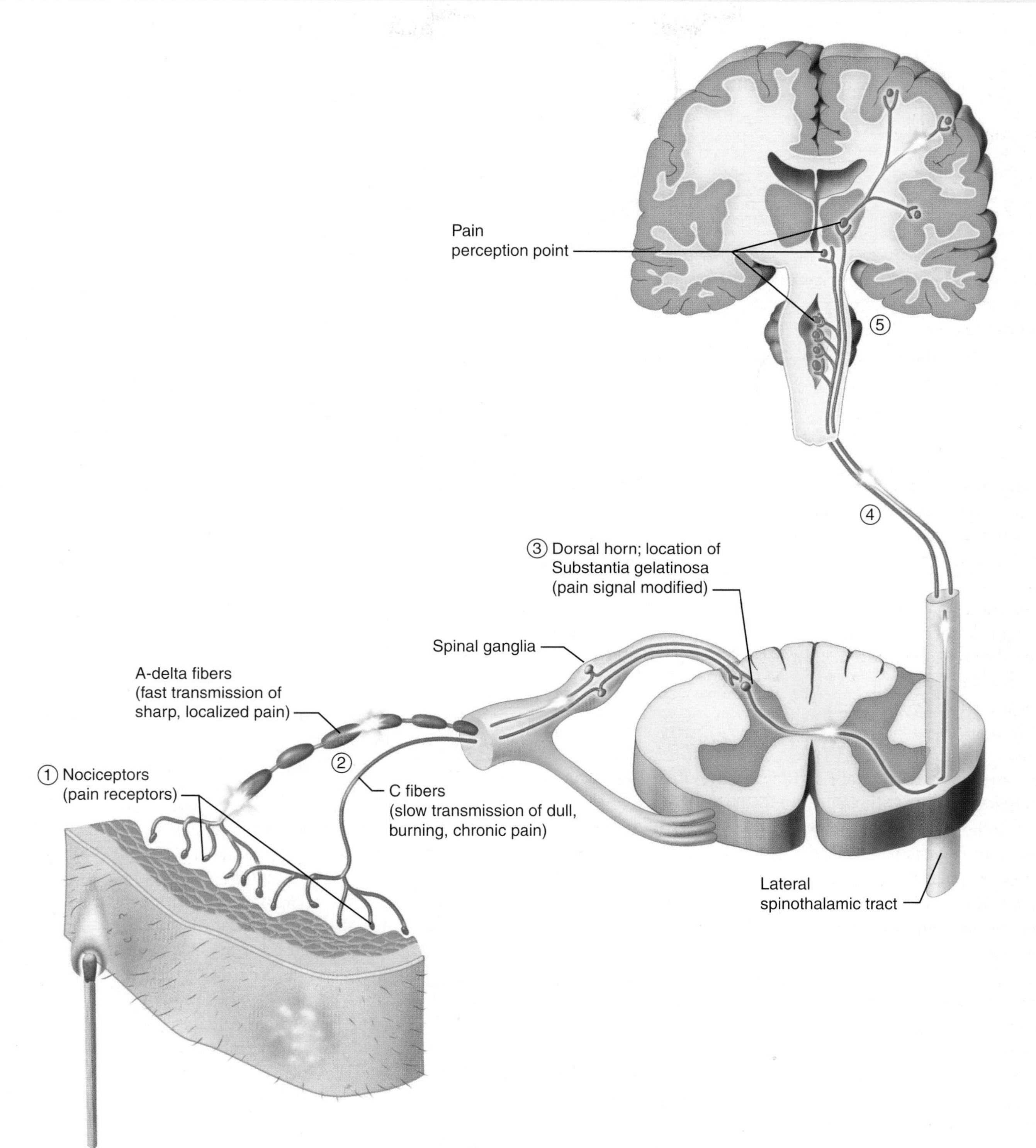

FIGURE 18–1 ■ Nociceptors transmit pain impulses along A-delta and C fibers to the dorsal horn of the spinal cord. After the sensory information reaches the dorsal horn of the spinal cord, the pain signal may be modified depending on the presence of other stimuli, from either the brain or the periphery. Along the nerve conduction pathways between the periphery, spinal cord, and the brain are "gates" that control the number of impulses sent to the brain. Nonpain impulses can compete with pain impulses for transmission along the spinal tracts to the brain. Once the impulse reaches the brain, the pain is perceived.

TABLE 18–1 Physiologic Consequences of Unrelieved Pain in Children

RESPONSES TO PAIN	POTENTIAL PHYSIOLOGIC CONSEQUENCES
Respiratory Changes	
Rapid shallow breathing	Alkalosis
Inadequate lung expansion	Decreased oxygen saturation, atelectasis
Inadequate cough	Retention of secretions
Neurologic Changes	
Increased sympathetic nervous system activity	Tachycardia, change in sleep patterns, increased blood glucose and cortisol levels
Diaphragmatic splinting in preterm infants increases intracranial blood volume	Increased intracranial pressure and potential for intraventricular hemorrhage
Metabolic Changes	
Increased metabolic rate with increased perspiration	Increased fluid and electrolyte losses
Immune System Changes	
Depression of immune response	Increased risk of infection
Gastrointestinal Changes	
Increased intestinal secretions and smooth muscle sphincter tone	Impaired gastrointestinal functioning Ileus

Data from Eland, J. M. (1990). Pain in children. Nursing Clinics of North America, *25, 871–884; Altimier, L., Norwood, S., Dick, M. J., et al. (1994). Postoperative pain management in preverbal children: The prescription and administration of analgesia with and without caudal analgesia.* Journal of Pediatric Nursing, *9(4), 226–232; McCaffrey, M., & Pasero, C. (1999).* Pain: Clinical manual *(2nd ed., pp. 24, 27). St. Louis: Mosby; Mitchell, A., & Boss, B. J. (2002). Adverse effects of pain on the nervous systems of newborns and young children: A review of the literature.* Journal of Neuroscience Nursing, *34(5), 228–236.*

which may put the child at risk for attention deficits and emotional disturbances (Mitchell & Boss, 2002).

Repeated pain experiences in newborns and infants are thought to cause changes in the **pain threshold** (the point at which the transmission of pain stimulus begins) and the perception and tolerance of pain throughout life. Because the pain pathways continue to develop during infancy and childhood, the painful experiences may have an impact on the development of the overall pain system. Repeated pain may lead to hypersensitivity and decrease the pain threshold, potentially leading to pain syndromes later in life, but research has not yet confirmed this (Mitchell & Boss, 2002).

The child with acute postoperative pain takes shallow breaths and suppresses coughing to avoid more pain. These self-protective actions increase the potential for respiratory complications. Unrelieved pain may delay the return of normal gastric and bowel functions and cause a stress ulcer. Anorexia associated with pain decreases nutritional intake and delays the healing process. The long-term effects of pain on the child's physical or psychologic condition are unknown. However, research has revealed that children who have intensely painful procedures report long-term sequelae that resemble posttraumatic stress disorder (Bowers, 2002).

Behavioral Consequences of Pain

Children learn about pain through the first experience. Newborn memory of pain has been reported to influence later behavior with increased behavioral responses to pain, altered temperament, infant distress behavior, and anxiety states (McCaffrey & Pasero, 1999). Short-term changes in behavior have been noted in infants after painful stimuli (McCaffrey & Pasero, 1999), such as the following:

- Changes in sleeping and wakefulness patterns
- Changes in parent-infant interaction
- Changes in feeding patterns
- Poor self-soothing abilities
- Greater motor activity for 24 hours after the stimuli

Children who are inadequately treated for procedural pain may have higher pain ratings during subsequent procedures, even when efficacious pain relief measures are used (Weissman, Bernstein, & Schecter, 1998).

Barriers to Pain Management in Children

In the past, infants and children did not receive adequate treatment for pain. Infants and children are at particular risk for undertreatment of pain because of an inability to describe their pain. Undertreatment still occurs, but much progress is being made due to the following:

- Research has revealed that infants and children feel pain just as adults do.
- Improved assessment tools have been developed for infants and children.
- Attitudes about pain management are changing.
- Teaching about pain includes a better understanding of the side effects of pain medications, such as respiratory depression.
- Standards of pain management are mandated in hospitals for all age groups (Box 18–1).

Healthcare professionals once believed that infants and children feel less pain than adults. In fact, most physicians did not prescribe pain medication for children or ordered it only as needed. This undertreatment was based on the attitudes of healthcare professionals about pain, the difficulty and complexity of pain assessment in infants and children, and inadequate research. For a review of past myths and the contrasting reality, see Table 18–2.

Research has shown that past beliefs about the ability of infants and children to perceive pain were incorrect. Even the smallest infants do feel and remember pain. Evidence-Based Practice: Challenges to Adequate Pain Management on page 566 explains how these outdated beliefs still result in undermedication of children for pain.

Developmental Aspects of Pain Perception and Memory

Although every infant and child perceives pain, their understanding, responses to pain, and memory of painful events change as they develop. See Table 18–3 for children's understanding of pain by developmental age.

BOX 18–1 JCAHO Pain Management Standards

In 2001, the Joint Commission on Accreditation of Healthcare Organizations (JCAHO) introduced standards for the assessment and management of pain in patients in accredited hospitals and other healthcare organizations.

- Standard RI.1.2.8: Patients have the right to appropriate assessment and management of pain.
- Standard PE 1.4: Pain is assessed in all patients.
- Standard PF.3.4: Patients are educated about pain and managing pain as part of treatment, as appropriate.

Additionally, these standards are applicable to the administration of pain and monitoring its effectiveness.

- Standard TX 3.3: Prescribing and ordering of medications follows established procedures.
- Standard TX 6.4: The patient is monitored during the post procedure period.
- Standard CC 6.1: The follow-up process provides for continuing care based on the patient's needs.

From Joint Commission on the Accreditation of Healthcare Organizations. (2001). Pain standards for 2001. *Oakbrook Terrace, IL: Author.* www.jcaho.org, *accessed 2/28/2003.*

With regard to painful events, even newborns appear to have a memory of them. When newborns who have experienced numerous heel sticks smell alcohol, they anticipate the heelstick and attempt to pull the foot away (Shah, Taddio, Bennett, et al., 1997). Newborns exposed to repeated painful experiences in the intensive care unit demonstrate memory of pain by holding their breath when approached by care providers (McGrath & Craig, 1989).

By 6 months, infants demonstrate fear of situations where pain was previously experienced, such as locations where immunizations were given. Infants experiencing circumcision without anesthesia demonstrate more exaggerated responses to painful immunizations (Taddio, Goldbach, Ipp, et al., 1995; Taddio, Katz, Ilersich, et al., 1997). Older children have no difficulty remembering a past painful experience. For example, preschool-age children make efforts to delay a painful procedure.

Cultural Influences on Pain

Culture and social learning have a tremendous influence on children's expression of pain. They are exposed to pain through their own direct experiences and through the observations of others suffering and attempting to cope with pain. These experiences enable the child to learn family and cultural traditions that provide guidance about self-control, coping, and enlisting the assistance of others (Huether & Leo, 2002). Some religious cultures rationalize pain and suffering as "bringing people closer to God" or a divine state of salvation. Sometimes pain is viewed as character building, as evidenced by a common phrase, "no pain, no gain." Some ethnic groups, such as Asian, Anglo-Saxon–Germanic, and Irish encourage a more stoic response in which expression of pain is diminished. People of Italian and Jewish descent are more likely to use both verbal and nonverbal methods to express pain freely.

TABLE 18–2 Misconceptions About Pain in Infants and Children

MYTH	REALITY
Neonates and infants are incapable of feeling pain. Children do not feel pain with the same intensity as adults because a child's nervous system is immature.	By 20 weeks' gestation, a fetus has most of the anatomic and functional requirements for pain processing. Term infants have the same level of sensitivity to pain as older infants and children. Preterm infants may actually have greater sensitivity.
Infants are incapable of expressing pain.	Infants express pain with both behavioral and physiologic cues that can be assessed.
Infants and children have no memory of pain.	Preterm infants have been noticed to associate the smell of alcohol with heel sticks and try to pull the foot away to avoid the pain. Infants cry in anticipation of immunizations.
Parents exaggerate or aggravate their child's pain.	Parents know their child and are able to identify when the child is in pain.
Children are not in pain if they can be distracted or they are sleeping.	Children use distraction to cope with pain, but they soon become exhausted when coping with pain and fall asleep.
Repeated experience with pain teaches the child to be more tolerant of pain and cope with it better.	Children who have more experience with pain respond more vigorously to pain. Experience with pain teaches how severe the pain can become.
Children tolerate discomfort well. They become accustomed to pain after having it for a while.	Children do not tolerate pain any better than adults, and may have less tolerance with prior painful experiences. They do not become accustomed to pain or cope with it better than adults.
Children recover more quickly than adults from painful experiences such as surgery.	Children heal quickly from surgery, but they have the same amount of pain from surgery as an adult.
Children tell you if they are in pain. They do not need medication unless they appear to be in pain.	Children may be too young to express pain or afraid to tell anyone other than a parent about the pain. The child fears the treatment for pain may be worse than the pain itself.
Children without obvious physical reasons for pain are not likely to have pain.	The cause of pain cannot always be determined. The feeling of pain is subjective and should be accepted by nurses.
Children run the risk of becoming addicted to pain medication when used for pain management.	Addiction is extremely rare when the child is treated for an acute condition.

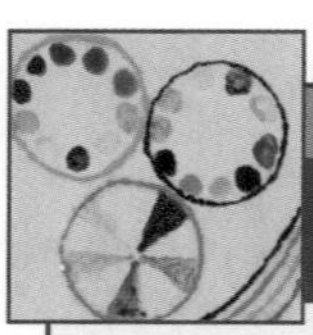

EVIDENCE-BASED PRACTICE
Challenges to Adequate Pain Management

PROBLEM

Adequate management of children with acute pain by health professionals continues to be a problem despite significant efforts over the last 20 years to increase knowledge about children's needs for pain relief.

EVIDENCE

In studies reported as recently as 1998 and 1999, researchers found that up to half of the children were undermedicated for pain and reported moderate to severe levels of pain (Tesler, Holzemer, & Savedra, 1998; Higgins, Turley, Harr, et al., 1999). In most cases physicians had ordered adequate pain medication, but it was the nurses who did not administer the pain medication around the clock on a fixed schedule as ordered, or they administered less than 40% of the amount of analgesia available to the child from the physician's order (Vincent, 2001).

A study conducted in 1999 and 2000 in a pediatric emergency department identified that 96 children between 6 and 24 months of age and 84 children between 6 to 10 years of age who had long bone fractures or burns were treated differently for pain management. Results revealed that the children between 6 and 24 months of age more often received no pain medication for fractures or burns in comparison with children 6 to 10 years of age. When the younger children were given pain medication, it was more likely to be an NSAID rather than an opioid medication while the older children were more likely to be given the opioid medication (Alexander & Manno, 2003).

IMPLICATIONS

Nurses have a responsibility to administer adequate pharmacologic treatment of pain when ordered and to advocate for adequate pain management when not ordered, regardless of the child's age.

CRITICAL THINKING APPLICATION

What could have been the reason for undermedication of children by nurses? Why would younger children be less likely to receive opioid analgesia for significant injuries? What is the role of the nurse to improve the pain management of children in all settings?

However, not everyone in a cultural group conforms to an expected response. Children will have individualized responses to pain based on past experiences, and younger children have had less time to acquire culturally learned behaviors.

Children learn directly and indirectly from their parents about how to respond to pain. By showing approval and disapproval, parents teach their children how to behave when in pain. For example, boys are usually encouraged to hide their pain by acting brave and not crying, but open expressions of pain are tolerated in girls (Abu-Saad, 1984). Types of feedback children obtain from family members about their pain experiences that help them learn socially and culturally acceptable pain responses include the following:

- How much discomfort justifies a complaint
- How to express the complaint
- How and when to stop complaining
- Whom to approach for pain relief

See Developing Cultural Competence: Examine Your Experience.

TABLE 18–3 Children's Understanding of Pain by Developmental Stage

DEVELOPMENTAL STAGE	UNDERSTANDING OF PAIN
Newborns and infants less than 6 months	No apparent understanding of pain Responsive to parental anxiety
Infants 6–12 months	Infants have memory of pain Responsive to parental anxiety
Toddlers 1–3 years	Lack understanding of what causes pain and why they might be experiencing it Demonstrate a fear of painful situations Use common words for pain such as *owie* and *boo-boo*
Preschoolers 3–6 years (preoperational)	Pain is a *hurt* Have language skills to express pain on a sensory level, and as the child grows older, provides more descriptive terms for the pain Do not relate pain to illness but may relate pain to an injury Often believe pain is punishment Not able to understand why a painful procedure will help them feel better or why an injection takes the pain away
School-age Children 7–9 years (concrete operations)	Can understand simple relationships between pain and disease but have no clear understanding of the cause of pain Can understand the need for painful procedures to monitor or treat disease May associate pain with feeling bad or angry May recognize psychologic pain related to grief and hurt feelings
10–12 years (transitional)	Have a more complex awareness of physical and psychologic pain, such as moral dilemmas and mental pain Better able to understand relationship between an event and pain
Adolescents 13–18 years (formal operations)	Have a capacity for sophisticated and complex understanding of the causes of physical and mental pain Can relate to the pain experienced by others Pain has both qualitative and quantitative characteristics

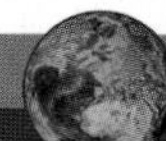

DEVELOPING CULTURAL COMPETENCE
Examine Your Experience

Think about your personal pain experiences during childhood and how your family members encouraged you to be stoic or to express pain. These types of experiences often contribute to a health professional's outdated attitudes about pain experienced by children. For example, some nurses and healthcare assistants (as well as parents) may believe that being in pain for a little while is not so bad, that pain helps build character, or that using pain medication is a sign of a weak character. Every nurse needs to acknowledge that the child has the right to have any level of pain managed, and it is a current standard of care.

Developmental Responses to Pain

A child's responses to and understanding of pain depend on age, stage of development, and other situational factors (McGrath, 1995). See Table 18–4 to learn more about the child's responses at each age. Young children are unable to give a detailed description of their pain because of limited vocabulary and pain experiences. Depending on their developmental stage, children use different coping strategies to deal with their pain (such as escape, postponement or avoidance, diversion, and imagery). Healthcare professionals now recognize that children do not complain of pain for several reasons.

- Some children believe they need to be brave.
- Preschoolers and adolescents may assume the nurse knows they have pain.
- Other children may be afraid that the injection to relieve pain will hurt more than the pain already does.

Clinical Manifestations of Pain

Physiologic Indicators

Acute pain stimulates the adrenergic nervous system and results in physiologic changes, including tachycardia, tachypnea, hypertension, pupil dilation, peripheral vasoconstriction, pallor, increased perspiration, and increased secretion of catecholamines and adrenocorticoid hormones. Changes in these signs demonstrate a complex stress response. These signs are not specific to pain, so they cannot be used for monitoring acute pain. These signs can be used in association with behavioral changes and self-reporting.

CLINICAL TIP

As the body adapts physiologically to acute pain, vital signs return to near normal and perspiration decreases after several minutes. Thus changes in vital signs are not a reliable indicator of pain in children because they last such a short time and they may also be an indication of anxiety or fear.

Chronic pain of long duration permits physiologic adaptation so normal heart rate, respiratory rate, and blood pressure levels are often seen (Huether & Leo, 2002).

Behavioral Indicators

Newborns and infants demonstrate a large number of behaviors when in acute pain. These behaviors include knitted brows, squinted eyes with cheeks raised, eyes closed, crying not oriented to a person or broadcast crying, crying around a pacifier, consoling intermittently, jerky or flailing movements, and stiff posture (Fuller, 2000). Many of these behaviors are the basis for the pain assessment tools developed for use in this age group. A sick newborn or infant will have a weaker cry, and not have the energy to make as many body movements as the well infant.

Preverbal infants and children may show conflicting signs of pain (increased or decreased vital signs, agitation or withdrawal, grimacing, crying, or anger), thus making assessment and monitoring of pain management more challenging.

Facial expression is a reliable and consistent indicator of pain. Facial characteristics with the eyes forcefully closed, brows lowered and furrowed, deepened nasolabial fold, a square

TABLE 18–4 Behavioral Responses and Verbal Descriptions of Pain by Children of Different Developmental Stages

AGE GROUP	BEHAVIORAL RESPONSE	VERBAL DESCRIPTION
Infants		
< 6 months	Generalized body movements, chin quivering, facial grimacing, poor feeding	Cries
6–12 months	Reflex withdrawal to stimulus, facial grimacing, disturbed sleep, irritability, restlessness	Cries
Toddlers 1–3 years	Localized withdrawal, resistance of entire body, aggressive behavior, disturbed sleep	Cries and screams, cannot describe intensity or type of pain
Preschoolers 3–6 years (preoperational)	Active physical resistance, directed aggressive behavior, strikes out physically and verbally when hurt, low frustration level	Can identify location and intensity of pain, denies pain, may believe pain is obvious to others
School-age Children 7–9 years (concrete operations)	Passive resistance, clenches fists, holds body rigidly still, suffers emotional withdrawal, engages in plea bargaining	Can specify location and intensity of pain and describe its physical characteristics in relation to body parts
10–12 years (transitional)	May pretend comfort to project bravery, may regress with stress and anxiety	Able to describe intensity and location with more characteristics, able to describe psychologic pain "Pain" and "hurt" mean greater pain than "ache" (LaFleur & Raway, 1999)
Adolescents 13–18 years (formal operations)	Want to behave in a socially acceptable manner (like adults), show controlled behavioral response	More sophisticated descriptions as experience is gained
	Pain causes conflict with their need for independence and bodily control	Use common meanings of words to describe pain (*pain, hurt, ache*) similar to adults
	May not complain about pain if they perceive that nurses and other healthcare providers believe it should be tolerated	May think nurses are attuned to their thoughts, so they do not need to tell them they are in pain

Adapted from Ball, J. W., & Bindler, R. C. (2003). Pediatric nursing: Caring for children, 3rd ed. *(p. 292) Upper Saddle River, NJ: Prentice Hall.*

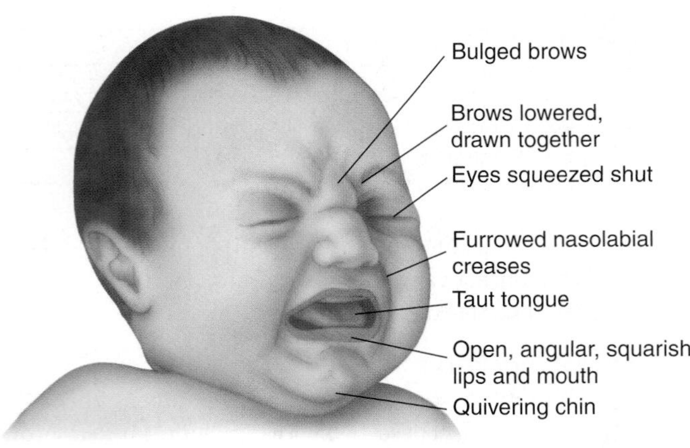

FIGURE 18–2 ■ Neonatal characteristic facial responses to pain include bulged brow; eyes squeezed shut; furrowed nasolabial creases; open angular, squarish lips and mouth; taut tongue, and a quivering chin. Redrawn from Carlson, K. L., Clement, B. A., & Nash, P. (1996). Neonatal pain: From concept to research questions and the role of the advanced practice nurse. *Journal of Perinatal Neonatal Nursing, 10*(1), 64–71.

mouth, and a taut, cupped tongue are associated with acute pain (Figure 18–2 ■). In older children facial characteristics indicative of acute pain include facial grimacing and biting or pursing lips. Children in acute pain behave in many of the same ways as children who show signs of fear and anxiety (Hazinski, 1999; Tesler, Holzemer, & Savedra, 1998). Exhibited behaviors that could indicate pain or anxiety in infants and toddlers include the following: restlessness or agitation, hyperalert and vigilant, sleep disturbances, and irritability or difficulty comforting the child. Preschoolers, school-age children, and adolescents may exhibit many of the following behaviors.

- Short attention span (child is difficult to distract)
- Posturing (guarding a painful joint by avoiding movement), remaining immobile, or protecting the painful area
- Drawing up knees, flexing limbs, massaging affected area
- Lethargy, remaining quiet, or withdrawal
- Sleep disturbances
- Depression and/or aggressive behavior, especially for those with emotional distress and fear that the discomfort will worsen

COLLABORATIVE CARE

Diagnostic Procedures

No laboratory tests are routinely used to assess pain. Prolonged, severe pain produces a physiologic stress response that includes the chemical release of catecholamines, cortisol, aldosterone, and other corticosteroids. Insulin secretion also decreases, leading to increased amounts of glucose and severe hyperglycemia (Hazinski, 1999). Existing conditions such as infection, trauma, and anemia or stress can cause the vital sign changes seen with sudden pain.

Pain Assessment Scales. Self-report assessment tools are considered to be the best method of assessing pain in children and adolescents who can provide such information (Box 18–2).

> **BOX 18–2 Research: Self-Reporting and Pain**
>
> School-age children and adolescents may not exhibit distress in direct proportion to their pain intensity. Thus, behavioral measures may not match the child's self-report of pain intensity. Older children often appear calm, expressionless, and limit movement following surgery, but report pain of moderate to severe levels (Tesler et al., 1999). Because children in these age groups can accurately report pain intensity, use the self-report as the valid pain assessment.

Assessment tools that combine behavioral and physiologic signs are the most valid for health professionals to use in rating the level of pain in infants and nonverbal children. Pain assessment tools for children have been developed and tested primarily to evaluate procedural or postsurgical pain. Many pain tools have been tested for **validity** (the extent to which an instrument or scale measures what it is supposed to measure) and **reliability** (the extent to which the same score is obtained when an instrument or scale is used either by different persons or by the same person at different times).

Newborn and Infant Pain Assessment. Knowing the diagnosis severity and associating it with pain helps nurses decide to use the behavioral and physiologic indicators of pain in newborns and infants. While numerous tools have been developed, three tools have validity and reliability, ease of use in the clinical setting, and wide acceptance.

- The CRIES scale was developed to evaluate postoperative pain in preterm and full-term neonates in the ICU (Table 18–5). The CRIES scale measures crying, oxygen saturation, heart rate, blood pressure, expression, and sleeplessness with scores of 0 to 2 for each. This tool has been demonstrated to have validity and good inter-rater reliability. Some facilities have established a score of 3 for the administration of analgesia with the CRIES scale (Pasero, 2002).
- The Neonatal Infant Pain Scale (NIPS) was developed to evaluate procedural pain in preterm and full-term neonates (Table 18–6). Facial expression, cry, breathing pattern, arms, legs, and state of arousal are assessed with a score from 0 to 1 or 0 to 2 for each. The tool has high inter-rater reliability and validity.
- The Premature Infant Pain Profile (PIPP) was developed to evaluate procedural pain in preterm and full-term neonates between 28 and 40 weeks' gestation. Gestational age, behavioral state, heart rate, oxygen saturation, brow bulge, eye squeeze, and nasolabial furrow are assessed with a score from 0 to 3 for each (Mitchell, Brooks, & Roane, 2000). The tool has been the most rigorously validated for use with procedural pain, and it has been additionally validated for postoperative pain. The tool also has good inter-rater and intra-rater reliability.

Infants and Young Children. The FLACC Behavioral Pain Assessment Scale is an easily administered tool to assess acute pain in infants and young children following surgery. This tool can be used until the child is able to self-report pain with another

TABLE 18–5 CRIES Neonatal Postoperative Pain Measurement Tool

	0	1	2
Crying	No	High-pitched	Inconsolable
Requires O_2 for oxygen saturation > 95%	No	< 30%	> 30%
Increased vital signs	HR and BP = or < preoperative value	HR or BP ↑ < 20% of preoperative value	HR or BP ↑ > 20% of preoperative value
Expression	None	Grimace	Grimace/grunt
Sleeplessness	No	The baby wakes at frequent intervals	The baby is awake continuously

Coding Tips for CRIES

Crying	The characteristic cry of pain is high-pitched If there is no crying or it is not high-pitched .... score **0** If crying is high-pitched but the baby is easily consoled .... score **1** If crying is high-pitched and the baby is inconsolable .... score **2**
Requires O_2 for oxygen saturation > 95% (Consider other causes of changes in oxygenation: atelectasis, pneumothorax, oversedation, etc.)	Look for changes in oxygenation. Babies experiencing pain manifest decreases in oxygenation as measured by TCO_2 or oxygen saturation. If no oxygen is required .... score **0** If < 30% O_2 is required .... score **1** If > 30% O_2 is required .... score **2**
Increased vital signs	Note: Take blood pressure last, as this may wake the baby, making other assessments difficult. Use baseline preoperative parameters from a period free of stress. Multiply baseline HR × 0.2, then add this total to the baseline value to determine whether the HR is 20% faster. Do likewise for BP, using the mean value. If HR and BP are both either unchanged or less than at baseline .... score **0** If either HR or BP is increased less than 20% of baseline .... score **1** If either one is increased more than 20% from baseline .... score **2**
Expression	The facial expression most often associated with pain is a grimace characterized by a lowered brow, the eyes squeezed shut, a deepening of the nasolabial furrow, and open lips and mouth. If no grimace is present .... score **0** If grimace alone is present .... score **1** If grimace and a vocalization without crying (grunt) are present .... score **2**
Sleeplessness	This parameter is scored according to the infant's state during the preceding hour. If the baby has been continuously asleep .... score **0** If the baby has awoken at frequent intervals .... score **1** If the baby has been awake continuously .... score **2**

HR = heart rate; BP = blood pressure; ↑ = increase; TCO_2 = transcutaneous CO_2

From Krechel, S. W., & Bildner, J. (1995). CRIES: A new neonatal postoperative pain measurement score. Initial testing of validity and reliability. Pediatric Anesthesia, *5(1), 53–61. This neonatal pain assessment tool was developed at the University of Missouri–Columbia. Copyright 1995 S. W. Krechel and Jo Bildner. Adapted with permission.*

pain scale (Table 18–7). FLACC is an acronym for the five assessment categories: face, legs, activity, cry, and consolability. To use the FLACC, observe the child during routine care for 1 to 5 minutes, and then select the score that most closely matches each behavior noted. The scores for the five categories are added together for the total score. The tool has validity and reliability for evaluation of postoperative pain (Manworren & Hynan, 2003; Willis, Merkel, Voepel-Lewis, et al., 2003).

Young children (3 years and older) can localize pain if given a body outline facing front and back (Figure 18–3 ■). The child can be asked to mark where the pain is located or to color the area of pain with crayons. Ask the child to use one color for the place where it hurts the most, and then to choose a different color for areas with less pain. Children often use red, black, or purple to indicate severe pain, however, it is important to ask the child about the colors selected and used to indicate different pain intensities.

Once the child has developed number concepts, a self-report tool to assess pain can be used. Follow the guidelines in Box 18–3 to assess the child's readiness for pain scales. Examples of self-report tools developed for children include the Faces Pain Rating Scale and the Oucher Scale. Young children who have not yet developed number concepts may select the extreme ends of a continuous or multiple-item scale and ignore the middle items on the scale (Champion, Goodenough, von Baeyer, et al., 1998).

The Faces Pain Rating Scale has a series of six cartoonlike faces with expressions from smiling to tearful (Figure 18–4 ■). Children from 3 years through adolescence can use it. After explanations about the meaning for each face, the child selects the face that is the closest match to the pain felt. The nurse should not use

TABLE 18–6 Neonatal Infant Pain Scale (NIPS)

CHARACTERISTIC	SCORING CRITERIA
Facial expression	
0 = Relaxed muscles	➤ Restful face with neutral expression
1 = Grimace	➤ Tight facial muscles; furrowed brow, chin, and jaw (Note: At low gestational ages, infants may have no facial expression.)
Cry	
0 = No cry	➤ Quiet, not crying
1 = Whimper	➤ Mild moaning, intermittent cry
2 = Vigorous cry	➤ Loud screaming, rising, shrill, and continuous (Note: Silent cry may be scored if infant is intubated, as indicated by obvious facial movements.)
Breathing patterns	
0 = Relaxed	➤ Relaxed, usual breathing pattern maintained
1 = Change in breathing	➤ Change in breathing, irregular, faster than usual, gagging, or holding breath
Arm movements	
0 = Relaxed/restrained (with soft restraints)	➤ Relaxed, no muscle rigidity, occasional random movements or arms
1 = Flexed/extended	➤ Tense, straight arms; rigid; or rapid extension and flexion
Leg movements	
0 = Relaxed/restrained (with soft restraints)	➤ Relaxed, no muscle rigidity, occasional random movements of legs
1 = Flexed/extended	➤ Tense, straight legs; rigid; or rapid extension and flexion
State of arousal	
0 = Sleeping/awake	➤ Quiet, peaceful, sleeping; or alert and settled
1 = Fussy	➤ Alert and restless or thrashing; fussy

From Lawrence, J., Alcock, D., McGrath, P., et al. (1993). The development of a tool to assess neonatal pain. Neonatal Network, *12(6), 61.*

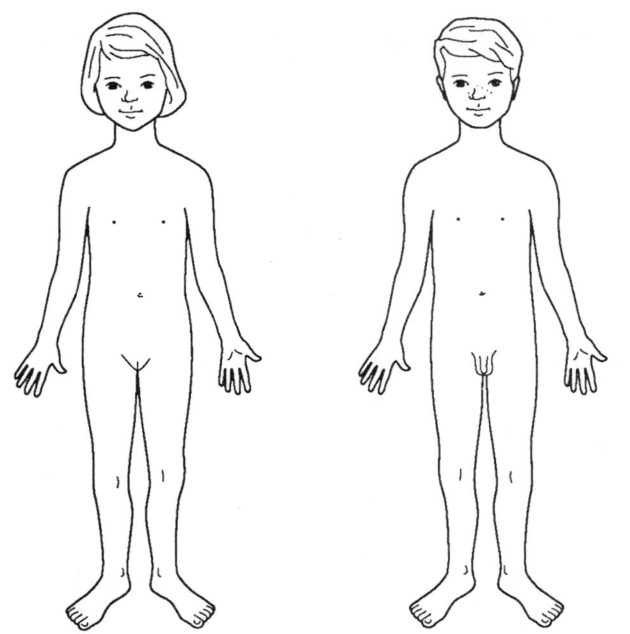

FIGURE 18–3 ■ Use a body outline for children to identify the location of pain either with a marker or crayon. Children have the opportunity to mark all the different locations of pain. Different color crayons can be used to identify different amounts of pain. This tool can be used independently or as part of the Adolescent Pediatric Pain Tool.

the tool to compare with the child's facial expression to determine pain level. Older children can use the words associated with the tool to provide a pain rating. When contrasted to other self-report pain assessment tools, the faces pain assessment tool was preferred by children and nurses (Keck, Gerkensmeyer, Joyce, et al., 1996). The Faces Pain Rating Scale has been studied for validity and reliability. A neutral face as the "no pain" anchor for the scale rather than a happy face may increase the tool's sensitivity in measuring pain rather than positive or negative emotion (Chambers & Craig, 1998).

MediaLink Pain Resources and Support

The Oucher Scale presents a series of six photographs of a child expressing increased intensity of pain in combination with a vertical Visual Analogue Scale (Figure 18–5 ■). The tool has been developed and tested in three cultural groups: Caucasian, African American, and Hispanic. The tools have validity and reliability for children between 3 and 12 years of age. Validity and reliability of the African American tool was confirmed by further testing (Luffy & Grove, 2003).

School-Age Children and Adolescents. All of the tools listed for infants and children may be used for school-age children; but with a better understanding of language and number concepts, additional tools can be used to assess pain. In each case, the child should be asked about the location of pain and descriptions about the type of pain. The ability to give a separate rating for the intensity of pain and to describe how unpleasant the pain is begins at about 8 years of age (Jedlinksy, McCarthy, & Michel, 1999).

- The Visual Analogue Scale (VAS) or numeric scale is a single horizontal or vertical line anchored with descriptors of

BOX 18–3 Assessing Readiness for Use of Pain Scales

Young children gradually develop the understanding of concepts important in being able to use pain scales. The child must understand the basic concept of a little or a lot of pain well enough to communicate about it. Assess the child's language skills—ability to use words in sequence, follow simple directions, and answer simple questions.

Children 2–3 years old are usually able to understand the concept of "more or less." With the development of this concept, the child cannot be given more than three choices on a pain scale (none, some, a lot) to assess the amount of pain.

Once the child can understand rank order and magnitude and be able to classify, match, and estimate, the child can use a numerical scale. Only 26% of 5-year-olds had the conceptual understanding to use a numerical scale (Fanurik, 1998). The correct response to either of the activities below indicates the child has the conceptual understanding to use a numerical scale (Merkel, 2002).

➤ Ask the child which number is larger, 5 or 9? Then ask which number is smaller, 7 or 4?

➤ Ask the child to place several blocks or pieces of paper of different sizes in a row from biggest to smallest.

TABLE 18–7 FLACC Behavioral Pain Assessment Scale

CATEGORIES	SCORING		
	0	1	2
Face	No particular expression or smile	Occasional grimace or frown; withdrawn, disinterested	Frequent to constant frown, clenched jaw, quivering chin
Legs	Normal position or relaxed	Uneasy, restless, tense	Kicking or legs drawn up
Activity	Lying quietly, normal position, moves easily	Squirming, shifting back and forth, tense	Arched, rigid, or jerking
Cry	No cry (awake or asleep)	Moans or whimpers, occasional complaint	Crying steadily, screams or sobs; frequent complaints
Consolability	Content, relaxed	Reassured by occasional touching, hugging, or being talked to; distractable	Difficult to console or comfort

How to Use the FLACC

In patients who are awake: observe for 1 to 5 minutes or longer. Observe legs and body uncovered. Reposition patient or observe activity. Assess body for tenseness and tone. Initiate consoling interventions if needed.

In patients who are asleep: observe for 5 minutes or longer. Observe body and legs uncovered. If possible, reposition the patient. Touch the body and assess for tenseness and tone.

Face

- Score 0 if the patient has a relaxed face, makes eye contact, shows interest in surroundings.
- Score 1 if the patient has a worried facial expression, with eyebrows lowered, eyes partially closed, cheeks raised, mouth pursed.
- Score 2 if the patient has deep furrows in the forehead, closed eyes, an open mouth, deep lines around nose and lips.

Legs

- Score 0 if the muscle tone and motion in the limbs are normal.
- Score 1 if patient has increased tone, rigidity, or tension; if there is intermittent flexion or extension of the limbs.
- Score 2 if patient has hypertonicity, the legs are pulled tight, there is exaggerated flexion or extension of the limbs, tremors.

Activity

- Score 0 if the patient moves easily and freely, normal activity or restrictions.
- Score 1 if the patient shifts positions, appears hesitant to move, demonstrates guarding, a tense torso, pressure on a body part.
- Score 2 if the patient is in a fixed position, rocking; demonstrates side-to-side head movement or rubbing of a body part.

Cry

- Score 0 if the patient has no cry or moan, awake or asleep.
- Score 1 if the patient has occasional moans, cries, whimpers, sighs.
- Score 2 if the patient has frequent or continuous moans, cries, grunts.

Consolability

- Score 0 if the patient is calm and does not require consoling.
- Score 1 if the patient responds to comfort by touching or talking in 30 seconds to 1 minute.
- Score 2 if the patient requires constant comforting or is inconsolable.

Whenever feasible, behavioral measurement of pain should be used in conjunction with self-report. When self-report is not possible, interpretation of pain behaviors and decisions regarding treatment of pain require careful consideration of the context in which the pain behaviors are observed.

Interpreting the Behavioral Score

Each category is scored on the 0–2 scale, which results in a total score of 0–10.

0 = Relaxed and comfortable
4–6 = Moderate pain
1–3 = Mild discomfort
7–10 = Severe discomfort or pain or both

From Merkel, S. I., Voepel-Lewis, T., Shayevitz, J. R., & Malviya, S. (1997). The FLACC: A behavioral scale for scoring postoperative pain in young children. Pediatric Nursing, 23(3), 293–297. The FLACC scale was developed by Sandra Merkel, MS, RN, Terri Voepel-Lewis, MS, RN, and Shobha Malviya, MD, at C. S. Mott Children's Hospital, University of Michigan Health System, Ann Arbor, MI. Used with permission.

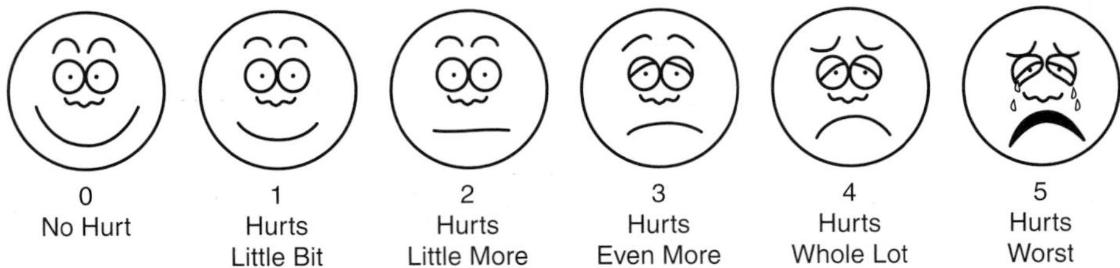

FIGURE 18–4 ■ The Faces Pain Rating Scale is valid and reliable in helping children to report their level of pain. After determining that the child has an understanding of number concepts, teach the child how to use the scale. Point to each face and use the words under the picture to describe the amount of pain the child feels. Then ask the child to select the face that comes closest to the amount of pain felt.

From Wong, D. L., Hockenberry, Eaton, M., Wilson, D., Winkelstein, M. L., Schwartz, P.: Wong's Essentials of Pediatric Nursing, 6/e, *St. Louis, 2001, P. 1301. Copyrighted by Mosby Inc. Reprinted by permission.*

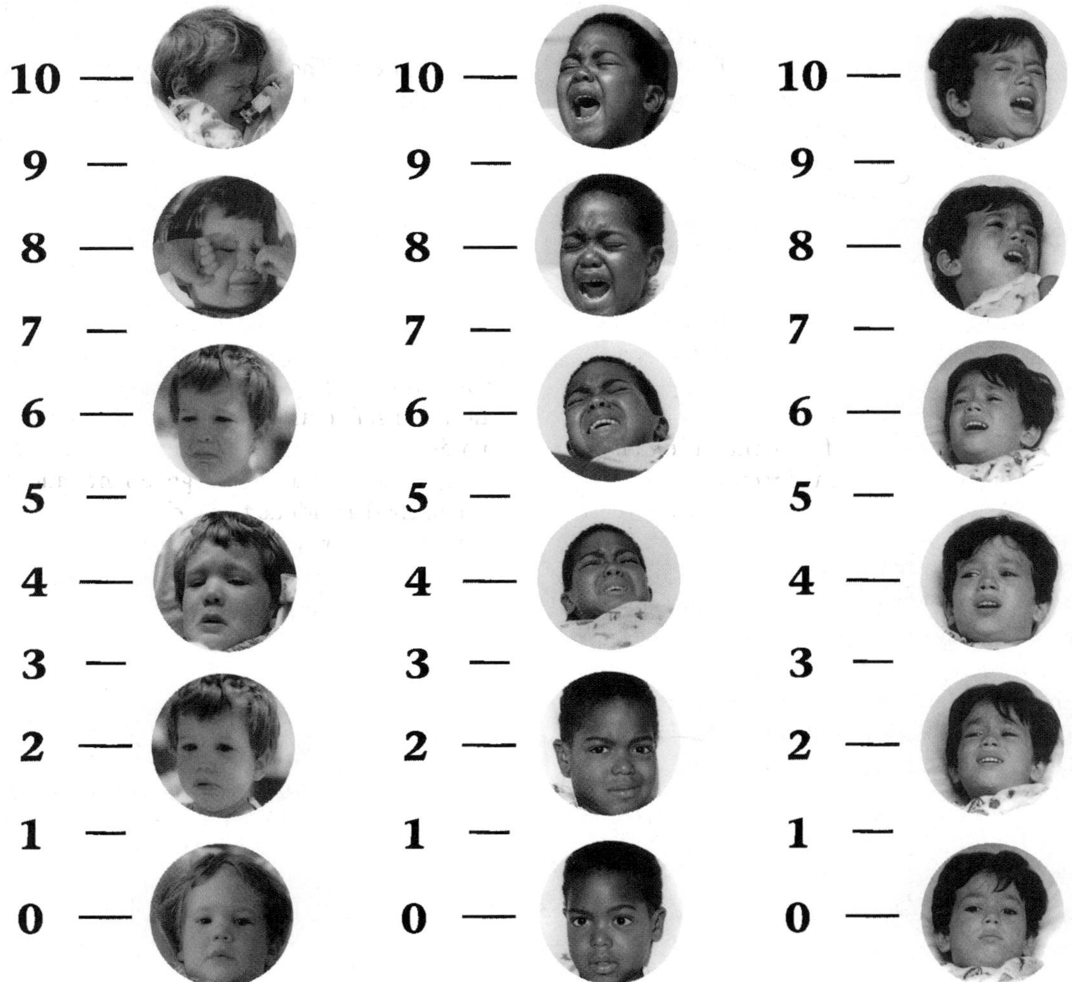

FIGURE 18–5 ■ Use the Oucher version that is the best match for the ethnicity of the child. After determining that the child has an understanding of number concepts, teach the child to use the Oucher. Point to each photo and explain that the bottom picture is "no hurt," the second photo is a "little hurt," the third photo is a "little more hurt," the fourth photo is "even more hurt," the fifth photo is "a lot of hurt," and the sixth photo is the "biggest or most hurt you could ever have." The numbers beside the photos can be used to score the amount of pain the child reports.

*In the form presented in this book, the Oucher is for educational purposes only and cannot be used for patient care.

[a]*Reliability is the extent to which the same score is obtained when an instrument or scale is used either by different persons or by the same person at different times. Validity is the extent to which an instrument or scale measures what it is supposed to measure.*

[b]*A, The Caucasian version of the Oucher, developed and copyrighted by Judith E. Beyer, RN, Ph.D., 1983. B, The African-American version of the Oucher, developed and copyrighted by Mary J. Denyes, RN, Ph.D., and Antonia M. Villarruel, RN, Ph.D., 1990. Cornelia P. Porter, RN, Ph.D. and Charlotta Marshall, RN, MSN, contributed to the development of the scale. C, The Hispanic version of the Oucher, developed and copyrighted by Antonio M. Villarruel, RN, Ph.D., and Mary J. Denyes, RN, Ph.D., 1990.* www.oucher.org.

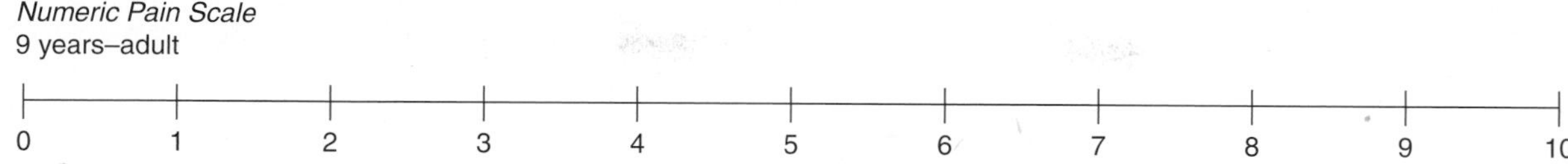

FIGURE 18–6 ■ The Numeric Pain Scale or Visual Analogue Scale is used for older school-age children and adolescents. Teach the child to use the scale by saying that 0 is no pain and 10 is the most pain ever felt. In between are numbers that can be used to report small or large amounts of pain. Ask the child to make a mark any place along the line that is the best match for the amount of pain felt.

From PAIN *28.27–38, Varni, J. W. et al. © 1987 International Association for the Study of Pain. Used with permission.*

pain at each end (Figure 18–6 ■). This tool sometimes has marks at equal intervals to provide a numeric dimension to the tool. A 10 cm line is usually the standard, with a mark and number at each cm. A VAS designed as a pain thermometer is appropriate for use in children. The child needs to have good cognitive ability and be 6 to 7 years of age to be successful in accurately reporting pain severity (Shields, Palermo, Powers, et al., 2003). See Partnering with Families: Assessing Pain in Children with Cognitive Impairments who Cannot Communicate.

- The Poker Chip Scale includes four checkers or poker chips to use to quantify pain (Figure 18–7 ■). The child is told one chip is a little pain or hurt and four chips is the most pain he or she could have. The child is asked to pick the number of chips that best match the pain felt. The tool has been validated, but is difficult to use in the postanesthesia care unit.
- The Word-Graphic Scale uses a horizontal line and has words at describing increasing pain intensity across the bottom (Figure 18–8 ■). The child is given instructions to mark the line that is closest to the pain felt. A millimeter ruler can then be used to quantify the pain and record the number as the pain score. This scale can be used to help children understand the concept of the increasing pain severity using the five-word anchors at specific points along the scale.
- The Adolescent Pediatric Pain Tool includes a human figure drawing, the Word-Graphic Rating Scale, and a choice of descriptive words. It can be used for children between 8 and 17 years. The human figure drawing can be used for the adolescent to indicate the location of all pain sites. The Word-Graphic Rating Scale is used as described, and the word choices help provide the adolescent with the different ways to characterize the pain felt. It provides various methods for adolescents to describe pain and its location.

Clinical Therapy

Pain management includes both pharmacologic and nonpharmacologic pain measures. While children need to be assured of adequate pharmacologic pain medication, nonpharmacologic measure can enhance the pain management and ultimately reduce the amount of pain medication needed.

Pharmacologic Pain Management. Pain medications include opioids, nonsteroidal anti-inflammatory drugs (NSAIDs), and nonnarcotic analgesics (acetaminophen).

Opioids. **Opioids** such as morphine and codeine may be administered by oral, subcutaneous, intramuscular, and intravenous routes. Opioids are commonly given for severe pain, particularly after surgery or for a significant injury. See the medication table on page 575 for opioids commonly used for children. Administration of opioids by an oral route is as effective as by intramuscular and intravenous routes when the drug is given in an **equianalgesic dose** (the amount of drug, whether given by oral or parenteral routes, needed to produce the same analgesic effect). The oral and intravenous routes are preferred since children often experience increased stress as well as pain when receiving intramuscular and subcutaneous injections. Rectal preparations of some opioids are also available. The optimal analgesic dose varies widely among patients in all age groups (American Pain Society, 1999).

Common side effects include sedation, nausea, vomiting, constipation, urinary retention, and itching. Potential complications of opioids include respiratory depression, cardiovascular collapse, and addiction. See the Practice Alert box for more information on respiratory depression. When the child's condition is unstable, as in trauma or critical illness, the dosage of opioids must be carefully calculated to match the child's cardiorespiratory status, although infants and children are no more likely than adults to develop respiratory depression following administration of a weight-specific dose of narcotics (Holder & Patt, 1995). Addiction is a rare complication in adults treated for painful conditions, and the same holds true for children.

PRACTICE ALERT

Respiratory depression (unresponsiveness and a respiratory rate less than 12 breaths/min in young children) may progress to respiratory arrest and is the major life-threatening complication of opioid administration. Respiratory depression is most likely to occur when the child is sleeping. This augments the depressant effect on the respiratory center and potential airway obstruction by the tongue (American Pain Society, 1999). Identify the time interval before drug-specific peak respiratory depression action occurs, and then carefully monitor the child's vital signs during that period to detect respiratory depression.

Clinical signs that predict the development of respiratory depression include sleepiness, small pupils, and shallow breathing. Children at particular risk for respiratory depression induced by an opioid are those with an altered level of consciousness, an unstable circulatory status, a history of apnea, or a known airway problem.

Avoid use of opioid agonists such as nalbuphine (Nubain), pentazocine (Talwin), and butorphanol (Stadol) as first-line drugs for pain. These drugs were developed to exert effects on

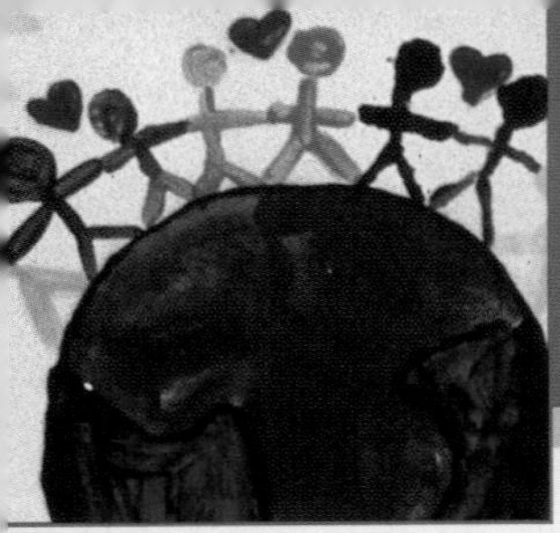

PARTNERING WITH FAMILIES

Assessing Pain in Children with Cognitive Impairments Who Cannot Communicate

For nonverbal children with cognitive impairments, parents may be coached to develop the Individualized Numeric Rating Scale (INRS). Categories of the FLACC Behavioral Pain Assessment Scale can be used to describe pain behaviors on a Visual Analogue Scale. Parents can be asked to recall a time when their child had a painful experience, and then to think about the behaviors the child demonstrated using the face, legs, activity, cry, and consolability characteristics. The parent can then write the pain behaviors on the line that corresponds to their interpretation of the child's pain intensity ranging from 0 (no pain) to 10 (worst possible pain). This tool has not been evaluated for validity and reliability, and accuracy is dependent upon the parent's ability to describe the child's pain behaviors on paper. However, this does provide a method to evaluate children who cannot communicate by other means (Solodiuk & Curley, 2003).

Directions:

1. Think about your child's past painful events. How does your child act when in mild pain, moderate pain, or severe pain?
2. In the diagram below, write in your child's typical pain behaviors on the line that corresponds to its pain intensity where 0 = no pain and 10 = worst possible pain.
3. When describing your child's pain, think about changes in:
   1. Facial expression
      Squinting eyes, frowning, distorted face, grinds teeth, thrusts tongue
   2. Leg or general body movements
      Tense, gestures (more or less) or touches part of body that hurts
   3. Activity, or social interaction
      Not cooperative, cranky, irritable, unhappy; Not moving, less active, quiet or more active, fidgety
   4. Cry or vocalization
      Moaning, whimpering, crying, yelling
   5. Consolability
      Less interaction, seeks comfort or physical closeness, difficult to distract/satisfy
   6. Other changes: Tears, sweating, holds breath, gasping

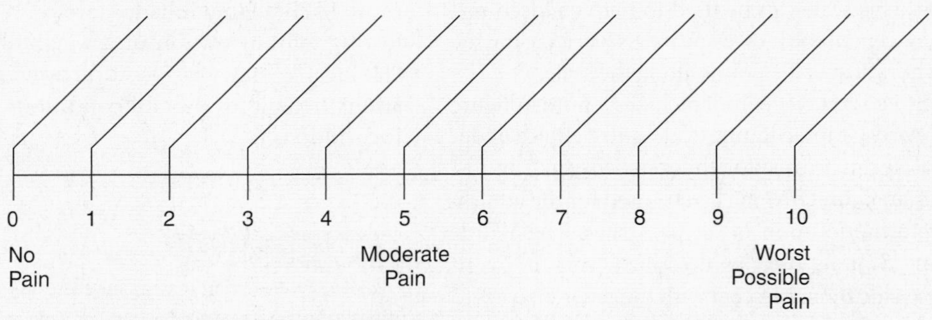

Individualized Numeric Rating Scale to assess pain in children with cognitive impairments who cannot communicate.

From Solodiuk, J., & Curley, M. A. Q. (2003). Pain assessment in nonverbal children with severe cognitive impairments: The individualized numeric rating scale. Journal of Pediatric Nursing, *18(4), 295–299. Used with permission from Elsevier.*

one opioid receptor and antagonize a second receptor. Although this mixed agonist-antagonist action may limit potential side effects such as respiratory depression, the drugs have a ceiling to analgesia. They are inappropriate for escalating pain (Hazinski, 1999). Naloxone is the drug used for reversal of opioid adverse effects that include respiratory depression, sedation, and hypotension.

Acetaminophen and Nonsteroidal Anti-inflammatory Drugs. **NSAIDs** such as aspirin, which are primarily given orally, are effective for the relief of mild to moderate pain and chronic pain. The medication table on page 576 presents recommended dosages of these drugs. They are most commonly used for bone, inflammatory, and connective tissue conditions. An NSAID may be prescribed in combination with an opioid to increase the

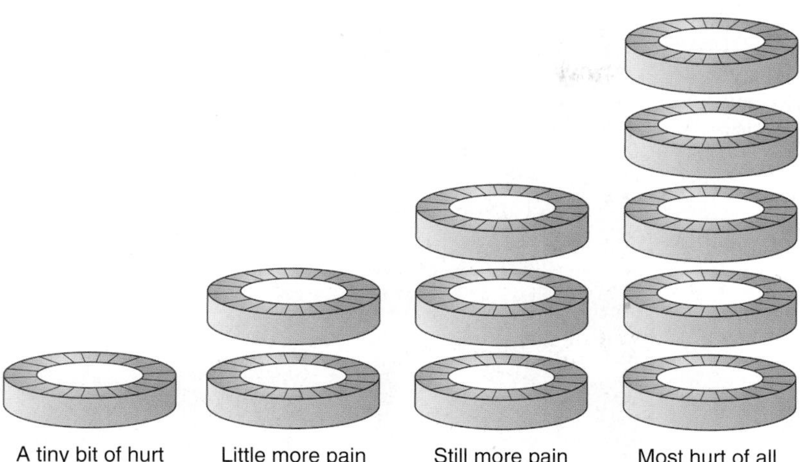

FIGURE 18–7 ■ The Poker Chip Scale uses four poker chips or checkers. Teach the child to use the number of chips to indicate the amount of pain felt. One chip is a tiny bit of hurt, two chips is a little more pain, three chips is more pain, and four chips is the most hurt of all.

From Hester, N., Foster, R., & Kristensen, K. (1990). Measurement of pain in children: Generalizability and validity of the pain ladder and poker chip tool. In D. C. Tyler & E. J. Krane (Eds.), Advances in pain research therapy *(Vol. 15, pp. 79–93). New York: Raven.*

effectiveness of the narcotic drug. This combination may ultimately reduce the amount of opioids needed for pain relief.

Acetaminophen is a nonnarcotic analgesic that is used like NSAIDs. It produces analgesia by raising the pain threshold and is equal to aspirin in analgesic properties.

Drug Administration. Pain from surgery, major trauma, or cancer will be present for predictable periods because of the effects of tissue damage. Pain relief should be provided around the clock. Every effort should be made to give the child analgesics without causing more pain. The preferred routes of administration are intravenous, local nerve block, and oral.

Continuous-infusion analgesia, which eliminates the peaks and valleys in pain control, is recommended to keep drug levels constant in children with continuous or persistent severe pain. Analgesics may also be given intravenously on a scheduled basis (e.g., every 3–4 hours). Delays in giving analgesics on a scheduled basis increase the chances of breakthrough pain and the

MEDICATIONS Opioid Analgesics and Recommended Doses for Children and Adolescents*

DRUG	APPROXIMATE EQUIANALGESIC ORAL DOSE	APPROXIMATE EQUIANALGESIC PARENTERAL DOSE	RECOMMENDED STARTING DOSE (ADULTS > 50 KG) ORAL	PARENTERAL	RECOMMENDED STARTING DOSE (CHILDREN & ADULTS < 50 KG) ORAL	PARENTERAL
Morphine	30 mg	10 mg	15–30 mg q 3–4 hr	10 mg q 3–4 hr	0.3 mg/kg q 3–4 hr	0.1 mg/kg q 3–4 hr
Codeine	130 mg	75 mg IM or subcutaneous	30–60 mg q 3–4 hr	60 mg q 2 hr	0.5–1 mg q 3–4 hr[a]	NR
Hydromorphone (Dilaudid)	7.5 mg	1.5 mg	4–8 mg q 3–4 hr	1.5 mg q 3–4 hr	0.06 mg/kg q 3–4 hr	0.015 mg/kg q 3–4 hr
Levorphanol (Levo-Dromoman)	4 mg (acute) 1 mg (chronic)	2 mg (acute) 1 mg (chronic)	2–4 mg q 6–8 hr	2 mg q 6–8 hr	0.04 mg/kg q 6–8 hr	0.02 mg/kg q 6–8 hr
Meperidine (Demerol)	300 mg	100 mg	NR	100 mg q 3 hr	NR	0.05–1.5 mg q 2–4 hr
Methadone (Dolophine, others)	20 mg (acute) 2–4 mg (chronic)	10 mg (acute) 2–4 mg (chronic)	5–10 mg q 6–8 hr	10 mg q 6–8 hr	0.2 mg/kg q 6–8 hr	0.1 mg/kg q 6–8 hr
Oxycodone	30 mg	NA	5–10 mg q 3–4 hr	NA	0.1-0.2mg/kg q 3–4 hr[a]	NA
Fentanyl	NA	0.01 mg	5 mcg/kg Lozenge	1 mcg/kg	5–15 mcg/kg Oralet[b]	1 mcg/kg

NR = Not recommended NA = Not available

**For all parenteral opioids, start with the low dose and titrate to effective pain control.*

[a]Caution: Doses of aspirin and acetaminophen in combination with opioid/NSAID preparation must also be adjusted to the patient's body weight.

[b]Oralet is not widely used because of nausea and vomiting side effects.

Resources: American Pain Society (1999). Principles of analgesic use in the treatment of acute pain and cancer pain, *4th ed., Glenview, IL: Author: pp. 6–8, 14–15, 20; Hazinski, M. F., (1999). Analgesia, sedation, and neuromuscular blockade in pediatric critical care. In Hazinski, M. F.* Manual of Pediatric Critical Care, *St. Louis: Mosby, pp. 44–72; and Acute Pain Management Guideline Panel (1992).* Acute pain management in infants, children, and adolescents: Operative and medical procedures. Quick reference guide for clinicians. *(AHCPR Pub. No. 92-0020). Rockville, MD: Agency for Healthcare Policy and Research, U.S. Public Health Service, Department of Health and Human Services.*

MediaLink Morphine Animation

MediaLink Nursing in Action: Administering Patient-Controlled Analgesia

No Pain	Little Pain	Moderate Pain	Large Pain	Worst Possible Pain

FIGURE 18–8 ■ The Word-Graphic Rating Scale can be used independently or as part of the Adolescent Pediatric Pain Tool. Words rather than numbers are under the line. Teach the child to use the scale by pointing to the side of the line that is no pain. Then run your finger along the line to the other side and tell the child that this location is the worst possible pain. Ask the child to make a mark along the line that is the best match for the amount of pain felt. Use a millimeter ruler to measure from the "no pain" end of the line to the marked location to identify the pain score. Make sure a line of the same length is used each time pain is assessed for comparison.

From Sinkin-Feldman, L., Tesler, M., & Savedra, M. (1997). Word placement on the word-graphic rating scale by pediatric patients. Pediatric Nursing, *23, 31–34.*

subsequent anticipation of pain. Giving analgesics on an as-needed basis for acute pain also results in the loss of pain control. More medications are often needed to restore pain control than would have been required for continuous-infusion analgesia.

Patient-Controlled Analgesia. **Patient-controlled analgesia (PCA)** is a method of administering an intravenous or epidural analgesic, such as morphine, using a computerized pump that is programmed by the healthcare professional and controlled by the child. After initial pain control has been achieved with a continuous IV infusion of morphine, the child presses a button to receive a smaller analgesic dose for episodic pain relief (Figure 18–9 ■). A continuous infusion prevents a recurrence of pain during long sleeping periods. This method of pain management is used in the immediate postoperative period, and for up to 48 hours after surgery when oral pain management is not possible.

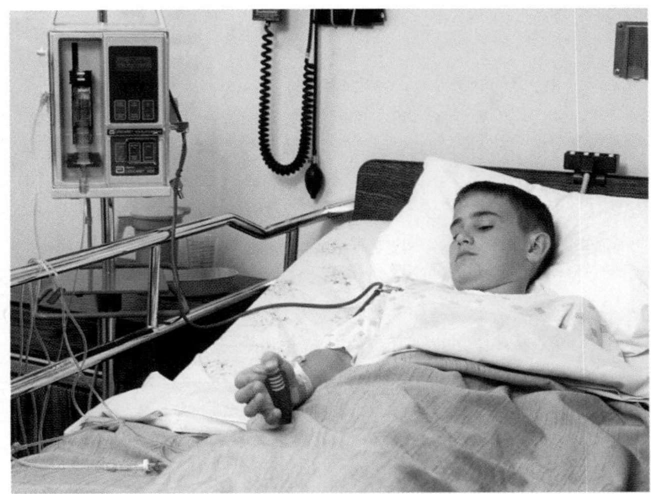

FIGURE 18–9 ■ By using patient-controlled analgesia, the older child is able to regulate the intake of an intravenous analgesic such as morphine.

PCA is prescribed mostly for children 5 years and older. Children selected for PCA should be able to push the injection button and should understand that pushing the button will give them medication to relieve pain. Parents are sometimes given responsibility for pushing the injection button for younger children or for those with disabilities. Additional pain medication is often ordered as needed to supplement the continuous and patient-administered infusion when pain control is not maintained. See Partnering with Families: Teaching About Patient-Controlled Analgesia and the Skills Manual).

Children and adolescents benefit from PCA by receiving continuous pain control and having the ability to control their com-

MEDICATIONS Recommended Doses of Acetaminophen and NSAIDs for Children and Adolescents

ORAL PEAK ACTION TIME	USUAL ADULT DOSE	USUAL PEDIATRIC DOSE	COMMENTS
Nonopioid Analgesic			
Acetaminophen 0.5–2 hr	500–1000 mg q 4–6 hr	10–15 mg/kg q 4–6 hr	Lacks the peripheral anti-inflammatory activity of other NSAIDs; rectal suppository available
NSAIDs			
Aspirin 1–2 hr	650–975 mg q 4–6 hr	10–15 mg/kg q 4 hr	Do not use in children under 12 years with possible viral illness; may cause gastric upset and bleeding; rectal suppository available
Choline magnesium trisalicylate (Trilisate) 2 hr	1000–1500 mg q 12 hr	25 mg/kg q 12 hr	Does not increase bleeding time like other NSAIDs; also available as oral liquid
Ibuprofen (Motrin, others) 0.5 hr	200–400 mg q 4–6 hr	10 mg/kg q 6–8 hr	Available as oral suspension
Naproxen (Naprosyn) 2–4 hr	500 mg initial dose followed by 250 mg q 6–8 hr	5 mg/kg q 12 hr	Available as oral liquid

Resources: American Pain Society (1999). Principles of analgesic use in the treatment of acute pain and cancer pain, *4th ed., Glenview, IL: Author; pp. 6–8, 14–15, 20; Hazinski, M. F., (1999). Analgesia, sedation, and neuromuscular blockade in pediatric critical care. In Hazinski, M. F.* Manual of Pediatric Critical Care, *St. Louis: Mosby, pp. 44–72; and Acute Pain Management Guideline Panel (1992).* Acute pain management in infants, children, and adolescents: Operative and medical procedures. Quick reference guide for clinicians *(AHCPR Pub. No. 92-0020). Rockville, MD: Agency for Healthcare Policy and Research, U.S. Public Health Service, Department of Health and Human Services.*

fort level with no trauma from injections. Once children can take oral analgesics, PCA is discontinued.

Children who have been given opioids over an extended period of time may experience **withdrawal,** the physical signs and symptoms that occur when a sedative or pain drug is stopped suddenly in a patient with physical dependence. An example would be a child in an intensive care setting who experienced life-threatening injuries and required multiple surgeries and invasive procedures for long-term treatment. If withdrawal signs and symptoms are anticipated or noticed in a child, slowly weaning the child off of the opioid over 2 to 4 weeks will prevent withdrawal symptoms. See Table 18–8 for signs and symptoms of withdrawal.

CLINICAL TIP

When withdrawal is anticipated, the plan for weaning the child off of the opioid is to give half of the previous day's total dose split into four doses a day for 2 days, followed by a 25% reduction of the previous day's total dose every 2 days thereafter, until a dose of 0.6 mg/kg/day is reached. This low dose is given for 2 days and the opioid is discontinued (American Pain Society, 1999).

Regional Pain Management. Epidural pain control provides selective analgesia and has become more common for postoperative pain management. A catheter is inserted into either the lumbar or the caudal space (Figure 18–10 ■). Continuous infusion with a small pump may be used to maintain pain control for the first 24 to 48 hours after surgery. Only minute doses of drugs are needed because of the high concentration achieved at the opioid receptors in the spinal cord's dorsal horn (Pasero, 2003).

Local nerve blocks, such as a popliteal block for anesthesia and analgesia of a lower extremity are used more frequently for pain control after surgery. A subcutaneous catheter is inserted into the local area for infusion of the analgesia. Pain control is achieved without systemic side effects from the anesthesia. Tingling felt in the fingers or toes of the affected limb is the first sign that the nerve block is receding.

TABLE 18–8 Signs and Symptoms of Opioid or Sedative Withdrawal

SYSTEM	SIGNS AND SYMPTOMS
Central nervous system	➤ Irritability, increased wakefulness, tremulousness, hyperactive deep tendon reflexes, clonus, inability to concentrate, frequent yawning, sneezing, delirium, hypertonicity, visual or auditory hallucinations
Gastrointestinal system	➤ Feeding intolerance with vomiting, diarrhea, nausea, uncoordinated suck and swallow
Sympathetic nervous system	➤ Tachycardia, tachypnea, increased blood pressure, nasal stuffiness, sweating, fever, chills, hot flashes

Data from Tobias, J. D. (2000). Tolerance, withdrawal, and physical dependency after long term sedation and analgesia of children in the pediatric intensive care unit. Critical Care Medicine, *28(6), 2122–2132.*

PARTNERING WITH FAMILIES

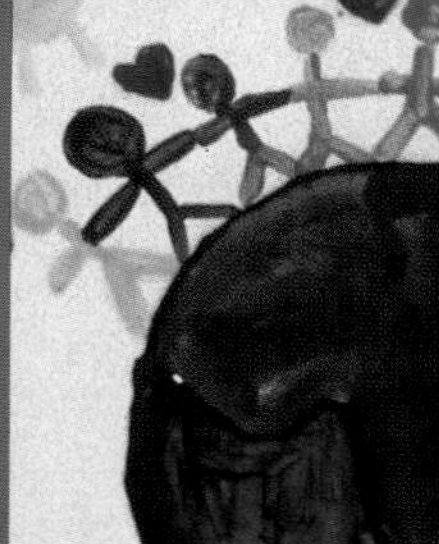

Teaching About Patient-Controlled Analgesia (PCA)

- ➤ What is PCA? Analgesia means pain relief: You get to control the amount of medicine you receive by using the machine.
- ➤ The machine gives the medicine by passing it through the tube that is connected to your intravenous line. When you push the button, the machine pumps pain medicine into the intravenous line to make you feel better.
- ➤ The machine limits the amount of medicine you can get, up to amount ordered by the physician. You can get any amount up to the maximum by pushing the button repeatedly. The push button will not let you make a mistake if you drop it or roll on it.
- ➤ Whenever you feel pain, hurt, or discomfort, push the button to get more medicine. You should be the only one to push the button.
- ➤ No needles for pain shots are needed as long as the intravenous line is in place.
- ➤ The PCA may not relieve all of your pain, but it should make you feel comfortable. Let the nurse know if you think your PCA is not working.
- ➤ The PCA will be used until you can take pills or drink liquid pain medicine.

Complementary and Alternative Therapies. Complementary pain control therapies are usually used with analgesics. These therapies may involve cognitive or behavioral methods; however, techniques such as touch, heat or cold applications, and a sugar-coated pacifier should not be overlooked for pain management.

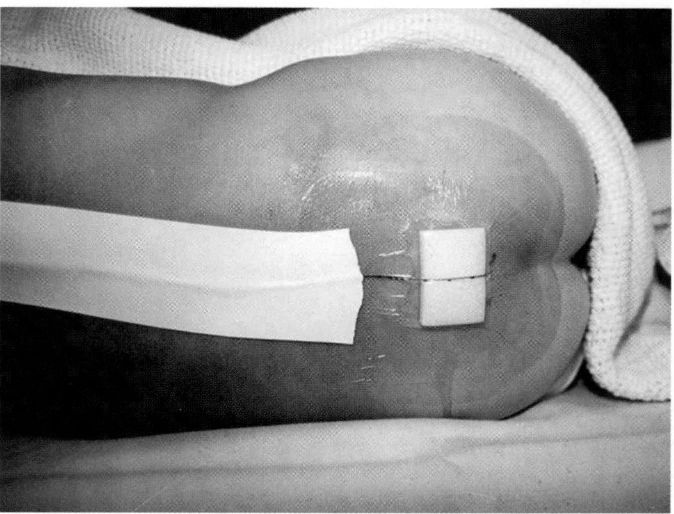

FIGURE 18–10 ■ An epidural pain block is one example of a regional analgesia used for postoperative pain management. Once the epidural catheter is placed, it is taped and wrapped securely; small doses of pain medication are then continuously infused by a pump.

Courtesy of Shriner's Hospital for Children, Spokane, WA.

See the range of complementary and alternative therapies that could be used for pain management on page 579. One or more of these methods may provide adequate pain relief when the child has low levels of pain. When used with analgesics, complementary therapies often enhance the effectiveness of the analgesic or reduce the dosage required. When used in association with a medical procedure, remember to use an intervention before, during, and after the procedure. This gives the child a chance to recover, feel mastery, and remember coping (Fanurik, Koh, Schitz, et al., 1997).

NURSING MANAGEMENT OF ACUTE PAIN

Nurses have an ethical obligation to relieve a child's suffering not only because of the consequences of unrelieved pain but also because appropriate pain management may have benefits such as earlier mobilization, shortened hospital stays, and reduced costs.

Nursing Assessment and Diagnosis

The goal of pain assessment is to provide accurate information about the location and intensity of pain and its effects on the child's functioning. A number of factors influence the pain perceived by the child, in addition to the maturation of the nervous system, the child's developmental stage, and previous pain experiences. See Box 18–4 for a listing of these factors. Because there are so many factors related to pain, the perception of pain and response to it are unique for each infant, child, and adolescent.

BOX 18–4 Situational Factors Influencing Pain in Children

COGNITIVE FACTORS

- Understanding of pain source
- Ability to control what will happen
- Expectations about the quality and strength of pain
- Whether attention is focused on painful event or distractor

BEHAVIORAL FACTORS

- Use of a pain control strategy
- Response of parents and healthcare personnel
- Whether or not restrained
- Ability to continue usual activities

EMOTIONAL FACTORS

- Fear
- Anxiety
- Frustration
- Anger
- Depression

Adapted from McGrath, P. A. (1995). Pain in the pediatric patient: Practical aspects of assessment. Pediatric Annals, *24(3), 126–138.*

When assessing pain in children, keep the following questions in mind.

- What is happening in tissues that might cause pain? Assume that children who have had surgery, an injury, a vaso-occlusive episode, or illness are experiencing pain, since these events also cause pain in adults. What external factors could be causing pain? For example, is the cast too tight or is the child poorly positioned in bed?
- Are there any indicators of pain, either physiologic or behavioral?
- How is the child responding emotionally?
- How does the child or parent rate the pain?

Partnering with families for pain assessment can provide a great deal of information about the child's response to pain that will be beneficial when planning nursing care, such as the following:

- How the child typically expresses pain, both verbally and behaviorally (Children and parents use similar terms to describe pain. Some examples of words used are a *hurt, owie, boo-boo, stinging, sore, cutting, burning, itching, hot,* and *tight.* Knowing the appropriate word to use makes communicating with the child easier.)
- The child's previous experiences with painful situations
- How the child copes with pain (The child with several past pain experiences may not exhibit the same types of stressful behaviors as the child with few pain experiences.)
- The parent's and child's preferences for analgesic use

See Developing Cultural Competence: Describing Pain.

Older children may be able to give a history of painful procedures. When attempting to obtain information about the child's pain experiences and present level of pain, ask the child and parent similar open-ended questions, such as those listed in Table 18–9. Many children modify their pain descriptions depending on the type of questions asked and what they expect will happen as a result of their response.

When working with an infant or child, determine which pain scale is most appropriate for the circumstance and developmental stage of the infant or child. When using a self-report assessment tool, use the same tool each time you assess for pain or for an evaluation of pain management. This makes comparison of assessment results possible. A chronological record of the child's pain assessments must be documented along with actions taken to relieve pain and follow-up assessment to determine the effectiveness of those actions. See

DEVELOPING CULTURAL COMPETENCE
Describing Pain

The terms *pain, hurt,* and *ache* have been found to describe pain intensity across cultures. Pain is most intense, hurt is less severe, and ache is least severe (Gaston-Johansson, Albert, Fagan, et al., 1990).

The terms *tender* and *tenderness* may be confusing for some families in which English is a second language. These terms are more commonly associated with caring, romance, or meat rather than soreness or pain.

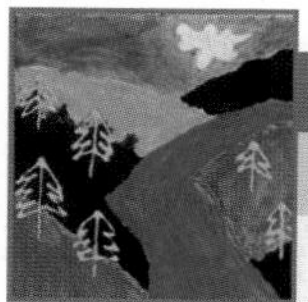

COMPLEMENTARY THERAPIES

Pain Control Methods

CUTANEOUS STIMULATION

Cutaneous stimulation involves gently rubbing the painful area, massaging the skin gently, and holding or rocking the child. Touching provides a stimulus to compete with the pain stimuli that are transmitted from the peripheral nerves to the spinal cord and brain. These actions may reduce the pain felt by the child. Swaddling and blanket rolls may calm a distressed neonate by decreasing tactile stimulation and containing gross motor behaviors (Lynn, Ulma, & Spreker, 1999).

SUCROSE SOLUTION

Concentrated sucrose solutions (12% or 24%) with a pacifier may be used as a pain relief measure in newborns. Sucrose may provide a natural pain relief by activating endogenous opioid systems in the body. The analgesic effect of sucrose lasts approximately 3 to 5 minutes, with a peak action in 2 minutes (Mitchell & Waltman, 2003). Sucking on a pacifier reduced pain behaviors in infants when the infant sucked at a rate more than 32 sucks per minute (Blass & Watt, 1999). A moistened pacifier dipped in a packet of sugar given to the infant during a painful procedure reduced pain behaviors such as duration of crying and vagal tone during a heel stick procedure (Greenberg, 2002).

DISTRACTION

Distraction involves engaging a child in a wide variety of activities that help focus attention on something other than pain and the anxiety associated with the procedure. Examples of distraction activities are listening to music, singing a song, blowing bubbles, playing a game, watching television or a video, and focusing on a picture while counting. Guided imagery and breathing techniques may be forms of distraction for school-age children and adolescents. Select activities that are developmentally appropriate for the child. Children in severe pain cannot be distracted; but do not assume the pain is gone if a child can be distracted.

GUIDED IMAGERY

Imagery is a cognitive process that encourages the child to relax and focus concentration on an event or place unrelated to the pain process. The focus can be on exploring a favorite place, doing a favorite activity, remembering a funny story, or being a superhero. This method is most effective in children over 6 years of age. Ask the child to think about all the sights, sounds, smells, tastes, and feelings that will help him or her to experience the favorite place, activity, or story. The purpose is to help the child feel good and be less afraid. Guided imagery is a form of self-hypnosis, and it is most effective when preceded by a progressive muscle relaxation exercise.

PROGRESSIVE MUSCLE RELAXATION TECHNIQUES

Relaxation techniques are used to reduce muscle tension because pain is often aggravated when muscles are tensed. Children can be taught to tense and relax different muscle groups, starting with the hands and feet, and then moving centrally. The child is asked to tense a muscle group for 10 seconds and notice how it feels. Then the child is asked to relax the muscle group for 10 seconds and compare it to how it felt when tensed. The exercise is best done in a quiet location with the child focusing on something pleasant. With practice, the child should be able to detect the difference between tense and relaxed muscles and then to reduce the tension. Relaxation methods include rhythmic breathing (repeatedly taking a deep breath and slowly releasing it), alternately tensing and relaxing selected muscle groups for 10 seconds each. Progressively move from specific muscle groups to more central muscles. Relaxation is enhanced if the child is encouraged to focus attention on something pleasant.

BREATHING TECHNIQUES

Various breathing techniques can be used for either distraction or muscle relaxation. One technique is rhythmic deep breaths. The child or adolescent is encouraged to take a deep breath, hold it for 5 seconds, and blow out through the mouth and push the tension out or the needle away. It can be used to promote relaxation and for distraction during a painful procedure, or as a mechanism to reduce stress. Patterned, shallow breathing is another technique. The child is encouraged to take shallow breaths in through the nose and blow out through the mouth while thinking of a particular image. The image could be a train and short breaths could be the "toot, toot" of the train engine. The child could also pretend to blow bubbles.

HYPNOSIS

Hypnosis is an altered state of consciousness in which the child's concentration is focused, narrowed, or absorbed, resulting in diminished peripheral awareness. Hypnosis is a tool that uses language for the purpose of establishing therapeutic rapport, comfort, awareness of self-control, and setting positive expectations. All hypnosis is self-hypnosis. Children more easily respond to hypnosis than adults because of their imaginative powers for fun and fantasy, and to cope with fears and challenges. Those who are successfully hypnotized respond to posthypnotic suggestions for the relief of anxiety, tension, and pain by achieving a progressively deeper level of relaxation and pain relief. Hypnosis has been successful in assisting children to control acute postoperative pain, procedural pain, and acute pain associated with conditions such as hemophilia and sickle-cell anemia. It is also useful for pain associated with chronic diseases. The precise physiologic mechanism for the success of hypnosis in pain control is not known; however, the gate-control theory may be a factor.

APPLICATION OF HEAT AND COLD

Heat application promotes dilation of blood vessels. The increased blood circulation permits the removal of cell breakdown debris from the site. Heat also promotes muscle relaxation, breaking the pain-spasm-pain cycle. To reduce edema, do not apply heat in the first 24 hours after an injury.

The application of cold is believed to slow the ability of pain fibers to transmit pain impulses. Cold also controls pain by decreasing edema and inflammation, and by causing partial or complete anesthesia or numbness of the skin. When cold is applied, assess the skin for redness or signs of irritation. Care should be taken to avoid causing thermal injury. Discontinue cold applications immediately if the skin alternately blanches and reddens afterwards or if blisters or redness do not subside between applications.

ELECTROANALGESIA

Also known as transcutaneous electrical nerve stimulation (TENS), **electroanalgesia** delivers small amounts of electrical stimulation to the skin by electrodes. This electronic stimulation is stronger than the pain impulses and, because of the gate-control theory, is thought to interfere with the transmission of pain impulses from the peripheral nerves to the spinal cord and brain. The alternative theory about why TENS is effective is that it may stimulate the body to produce endorphins or natural painkillers. The endorphins act at the pain receptors and block the perception of pain (Rusy & Weisman, 2000). TENS may be used for both acute and chronic pain management. The only known side effect is skin irritation at the electrode site.

BIOFEEDBACK

Instruments (α-electroencephalography, muscle electromyography, skin temperature, and temporal pulse feedback) can be used to raise the awareness of physical states in the body such as pain and stress. Through different biofeedback instruments, the child can learn voluntary control enabling the relaxation of specific muscles or to make changes in peripheral and cranial blood flow, thus helping to control pain. Because of the time needed to learn these techniques, they are best used for chronic pain management rather than acute postoperative pain.

ACUPUNCTURE

A traditional Chinese treatment for pain relief, acupuncture has been gaining greater acceptance in Western medicine. Acupuncture is based on the theory that energy or chi flows along channels through the body (meridians) that are connected by acupuncture points. Pain occurs with obstruction of the energy flow, and inserting needles at the appropriate acupuncture points restores the energy flow (Rusy & Weisman, 2000). Limited research has been conducted about the use and effectiveness of acupuncture use in children. Because of the use of needles, few children under 10 years will cooperate with the procedure.

TABLE 18–9 Pediatric Pain History for Children and Parents

QUESTIONS FOR CHILDREN	QUESTIONS FOR PARENTS
Past Pain Experiences	**Past Pain Experiences**
Tell me what pain is. Tell me about the hurt you have had before. Do you tell others when you hurt? Who? What do you do for yourself when you are hurting? What helps the most to take your hurt away? What do you want others to do for you when you hurt? What don't you want others to do for you when you hurt? Is there anything special you want me to know about when you hurt? What?	What word(s) does your child use to describe pain? Describe pain experiences your child has previously had. Does your child tell you or others when he or she is in pain? How do you know when your child is in pain? How does your child usually react to pain? What do you do for your child when he or she is in pain? What does your child do to manage pain? What works best to reduce or take away your child's pain? Is there anything special you would like me to know about your child and pain?
Present Pain Experiences	**Present Pain Experiences**
Where is the pain? What does it feel like? What do you think is causing the pain? What would you like me to do for you?	Tell me about the pain your child is having now. Where is it and what does it feel like? What would you like me to do for your child?

Adapted from Hester, N. O., & Barcus, C. S. (1986). Assessment and management of pain in children. Pediatrics: Nursing Update, 1, *2–8.*

Evidence-Based Practice: Selecting a Pain Scale for Use with Young Children.

Surgery and trauma can result in multiple sites of pain (e.g., incision or laceration, cut or bruised muscles, interrupted blood supply, nasogastric tube placement, insertion sites of intravenous lines). When using pain scales in the assessment of a verbal child, attempt to identify all sites of pain, and then identify the intensity of pain at each site. The presence of physiologic symptoms such as nausea, fatigue, dyspnea, bladder and bowel distention, and fever may also influence the intensity of pain felt by a child. The child's behavior or responses to pain stimuli may also be affected by fear, anxiety, separation from parents, anger, culture, age, or a previous pain experience (Figure 18–11 ■).

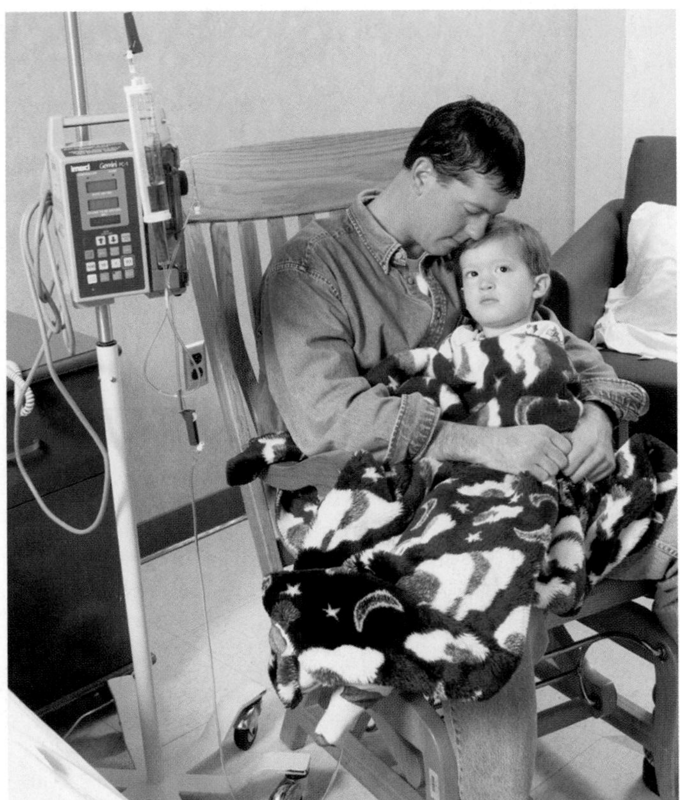

FIGURE 18–11 ■ The presence of the parent is an important part of pain management. Children often feel more secure telling parents about their pain and anxiety.

Examples of nursing diagnoses for children in pain include the following:

- Acute Pain (abdominal) related to injury and surgery
- Anxiety related to anticipation of pain from an invasive procedure
- Sleep Pattern Disturbed related to inadequate pain control
- Ineffective Therapeutic Regimen Management related to self-management of pain control, and use of nonpharmacologic pain control measures
- Ineffective Breathing Pattern related to opioid overdose

■ Planning and Implementation

Nursing management involves the following actions to increase and maintain patient comfort once the assessment is completed and nursing diagnoses are developed. Pain management involves the use of analgesic and anesthetic medications, as well as complementary and alternative therapies. The nurse must also monitor, evaluate, and document the effectiveness of pain control measures to provide optimal comfort. When physician orders for pain management are inadequate, the nurse is also responsible for advocating for improved pain control for the child.

Use the questions in Box 18–5 to assess the child's pain management. Many facilities have established a score of 3 for the administration of analgesia with the CRIES and FLACC scale (Merkel, Voepel-Lewis, & Malviya, 2002). Determine what guidelines exist for administration of analgesia in your healthcare facility when using one or more pain scales. The accompa-

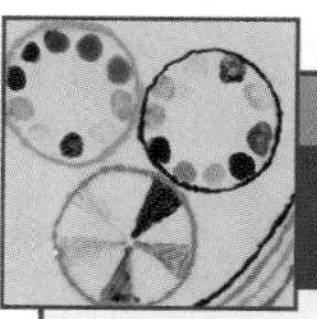

EVIDENCE-BASED PRACTICE

Selecting a Pain Scale for Use with Young Children

PROBLEM

Selecting an appropriate pain assessment tool to use for a specific child is important in ensuring that an accurate assessment of pain is made. Self-report of pain severity is considered the best method when the child is able to use a self-report scale. What pain assessment tool is the most appropriate to use in young children 3 to 7 years of age for self-reporting pain severity?

EVIDENCE

Children need to have several developmental skills before they can use a numerical scale to report pain severity. They must understand rank order and magnitude, and be able to classify, match, and estimate. Few children under 6 years of age have these skills (Fanurik, Koh, Harrison, et al., 1998; Shields et al., 2003). The selection of valid and reliable assessment tools is also important. The Wong-Baker Faces Pain Scale and the Oucher Pain Scale have both demonstrated good validity and reliability when used in children of this age group (Wong & Baker, 1988; Beyer & Wells, 1989; Beyer, Denyes, & Villarruel, 1992). The Faces Pain Scale was preferred by nurses and children when contrasted to other self-report pain assessment tools (Keck et al., 1996). However, the Oucher Pain Scale is specially developed for children in three cultural groups—Caucasian, African American, and Hispanic. Do children in different cultural groups have a different preference for a pain scale? A study recently conducted examined the validity, reliability, and preference of a pain assessment tool by 100 African American children with sickle-cell disease. Findings of this study replicated the validity and reliability of the Faces Pain Scale and Oucher African American Pain Scale of the original scale developers. Significantly more African American children under 7 years of age (56%) preferred the Faces Pain Scale to the Oucher Pain Scale (26%) (Luffy & Grove, 2003).

IMPLICATION

Studies continue to confirm that young children can describe their pain using special tools developed for them. With the evidence that children have preferences for the pain scale they use, nurses should consider giving children a choice of tools for self-reporting pain, helping them to feel that they have more control over their care.

CRITICAL THINKING APPLICATION

When planning pain assessment, think about how you can provide children a choice in pain self-report tools. Are a variety of tools available in the clinical setting? How can you ensure that the same tool is used each time to assess the child's pain so that pain ratings can be compared? How would this be documented in the child's record?

nying nursing care plan summarizes nursing care for the child with postoperative pain.

Pharmacologic Intervention

Give analgesics as ordered by the physician, ensuring that the dose is appropriate for the child's weight and medical situation. The goal is to control the pain as rapidly as possible, and the starting dose should be optimal, and further doses titrated depending upon the child's response. When administering an opioid by intravenous infusion or PCA, monitor the flow rate and the site for infiltration. Make sure analgesic antagonists such as naloxone are available should complications develop. The dose should be precalculated and the medication immediately available when an opioid is used. Consider using pulse oximetry or a cardiorespiratory monitor to continuously assess respiratory function when an opioid is used.

CLINICAL TIP

Naloxone may be used to treat respiratory depression caused by an opioid drug at a dose and slow infusion rate that does not reverse the pain control effects of the narcotic. A continuous infusion or repeated doses may be needed for severe overdoses.

Monitor the child's vital signs for complications related to opioids, such as respiratory depression. Other vital signs (heart rate and blood pressure) may not change in response to effective analgesia when infection, trauma, or other stressors keep them elevated. Check for the presence of other side effects of analgesics, such as sedation, nausea, vomiting, itching, urinary retention, and constipation.

Assess the child for the pain 15 to 30 minutes following IV pain medication and 1 hour after oral pain medication to determine if adequate pain control was achieved. Use information collected from the child and parent, as well as from an appropriate pain scale, as was done with Felicia in the chapter opener. Dramatic reductions in pain should occur, although all pain may not disappear. Evaluate the child's level of pain at regular intervals to detect an increase in pain intensity, and the need for more pain medication. Be certain to record results of pain control measures to guide future nursing actions. A flowsheet should be used to document assessments and medication administration during the postoperative period.

Many children sleep after receiving an analgesic. This sleep is not a side effect of the drug or a sign of an overdose, but the result of pain relief. Pain interrupts sleep, and once pain is relieved, the child can sleep comfortably. On the other hand, sleep does not always indicate pain control. A child in pain may fall asleep in exhaustion. Look for other symptoms of pain, such as excess movement or moaning.

Become an advocate for children when the dose or type of analgesic ordered is inadequate. **Tolerance** is a decrease in a drug's effect over time or the need for increasing amounts of the

BOX 18–5 Questions to Assess the Child's Pain Medication Management

- Is the child being assessed at appropriate intervals?
- Are analgesics ordered for prevention as well as relief of pain?
- Is the analgesic dose appropriate for the pain being experienced or expected?
- Is the timing of the medication administration appropriate?
- Is the route of administration appropriate?
- Is the child adequately monitored for the occurrence of side effects? Is the nurse appropriately prepared to manage side effects that occur?
- Has the analgesia provided adequate comfort to the child?

From Acute Pain Management Guideline Panel. (1992). Acute Pain Management in Infants, Children, and Adolescents: Operative and Medical Procedures: Quick Reference Guide for Clinicians (Publication No. 92-0020). Washington, DC: Public Health Service, U.S. Department of Health and Human Services.

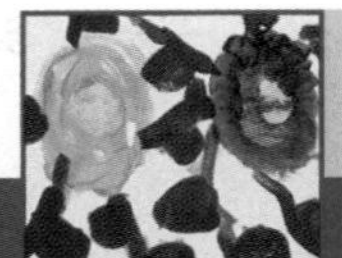

Nursing Care Plan

THE CHILD WITH POSTOPERATIVE PAIN

GOAL	INTERVENTION	RATIONALE	EXPECTED OUTCOME
1. Severe Abdominal Pain related to surgery and injury			
	NIC Priority Intervention—*Pain Management:* Alleviation of pain or a reduction in pain to a level of comfort that is acceptable to the patient.		**NOC Suggested Outcomes**—*Comfort Level:* Feelings of physical and psychologic ease.
The child will report pain relief (to a level acceptable to child on a pain scale).	■ Give analgesic by a pain-free method.	■ The child may deny pain to avoid analgesia by painful route.	The child reports pain relief after administration of analgesia.
	■ Have the child select a pain scale and rate the amount of pain perceived before and 30–60 minutes after analgesia is given to ensure pain relief.	■ The child's pain rating is the best indicator of pain. Maintenance of pain control requires less analgesia than treating each acute pain episode.	
	■ Assess pain control each hour to ensure that the child's pain is relieved.	■ Frequent monitoring identifies inadequate pain control before it becomes significant.	
	■ Reposition the child every 2 hr to maintain good body alignment.	■ New positions decrease muscle cramping and skin pressure.	
	■ Provide therapeutic touch or massage. Encourage the parents to read a story or play favorite music.	■ Complementary therapy reduces stress and enhances the analgesic action.	
2. Sleep Pattern Disturbance related to inadequate pain control			
	NIC Priority Intervention—*Sleep Enhancement:* Facilitation of regular sleep-awake cycles.		**NOC Suggested Outcome**—*Sleep:* Extent and pattern of sleep for mental and physical rejuvenation.
The child will experience fewer disruptions of sleep by pain.	■ Give analgesia by continuous infusion or every 3–4 hr around the clock.	■ Pain breakthrough occurs even during sleep and disturbs the healing effects of sleep.	The child's sleep is undisturbed by pain. Child sleeps for age-appropriate number of hours per day.
3. Ineffective Individual Therapeutic Regimen Management related to self-management of pain control and use of complementary therapy pain control measures			
	NIC Priority Intervention—*Self-Modification Assistance:* Reinforcement of self-directed change initiated by the patient to achieve personally important goals.		**NOC Suggested Outcome**—*Treatment Behavior Pain Control:* Personal actions to palliate or eliminate pain.
The child and family will effectively use patient-controlled analgesia (PCA) and complementary therapy pain control measures.	■ Teach the child how the PCA works and when to push the button.	■ The child must know that pushing the PCA button will keep pain under control.	The child's pain rating stays low.
	■ Teach the family and the child how to use age-appropriate imagery, distraction, relaxation techniques, and other complementary therapy pain relief measures.	■ Complementary therapy pain control measures reduce amount of analgesia needed.	The child and family independently use complementary therapies for pain control.
The child and family will use appropriate analgesia after discharge.	■ Discuss appropriate pain control to use at home after discharge.	■ The family and child may be anxious about pain management at home.	The family understands pain relief measures for use at home and knows where to call if help is needed.
4. Ineffective Breathing Pattern related to opioid overdose			
	NIC Priority Intervention—*Respiratory Monitoring:* Collection and analysis of patient data to ensure airway patency and adequate gas exchange.		**NOC Suggested Outcome**—*Vital Signs Status:* Temperature, pulse, respirations, and blood pressure within expected range for the individual.

Nursing Care Plan THE CHILD WITH POSTOPERATIVE PAIN (continued)

GOAL	INTERVENTION	RATIONALE	EXPECTED OUTCOME
4. Ineffective Breathing Pattern related to opioid overdose (continued)			
The child will maintain adequate ventilations.	■ Verify that the correct dose of opioid analgesia is given for the child's weight. ■ Monitor vital signs and depth of inspirations before analgesic is administered and at the time of peak drug action. ■ Calculate the agonist dose ordered by physician to be sure it will reverse respiratory depression, but not counteract the effect of analgesia.	■ Respiratory depression is a significant complication of opioid analgesia when too much analgesia is given. ■ Respiratory depression episode must be identified before progression to respiratory arrest occurs. All opioids act on the brainstem center that decreases responsiveness to CO_2 tension. ■ Valuable time will be saved if the agonist is needed for an episode of respiratory depression. Complete reversal of analgesia will cause the child to have significant pain.	There is no episode of respiratory depression associated with analgesia.
5. Constipation related to opioid administration and decreased motility of gastrointestinal tract.			
	NIC Priority Intervention—*Constipation Management:* Prevention and alleviation of constipation.		**NOC Suggested Outcome**—*Bowel Elimination:* Ability of gastrointestinal tract to form and evacuate stool effectively.
The child will have minimal constipation.	■ Palpate the abdomen, and assess bowel sounds and abdominal distention. ■ Request physician order for stimulating laxative and stool softener. ■ Provide fluids of choice to increase fluid intake when IV fluids are decreased. ■ Inform family and child that constipation is a possible side effect of pain medication.	■ Signs of constipation must be anticipated and identified. ■ Opioids increase the transit time of feces and interfere with bile enzymes needed for evacuation. ■ Extra fluids will counteract the opioid action of increasing the absorption of water from the large intestine. ■ Parents can become partners in managing fluid intake and monitoring bowel movements.	The child has bowel movements at least every 2 days while on opioid pain control.

drug to produce or maintain the same level of pain relief or sedation effect. This may occur when children with severe pain have been taking opioids or sedatives for several days. The first sign of tolerance may be a decrease in the duration of effective analgesia. Breakthrough pain occurs, and an increase in dosage is needed to achieve the previous level of pain relief. Tolerance can be delayed with effective use of pain scales to allow appropriate drug dosing, and often less analgesia is needed. Magnesium is being investigated as an agent to slow the development of tolerance (Tobias, 2000).

Analyze all of the information about the child's pain management before asking the physician to change the analgesia dosage. Review the child's record for documentation that the prescribed drug has been given at the appropriate dose and frequency and that the child's pain relief is ineffective despite the drug administration. After verifying the record, provide the physician with information about the characteristics of the child's pain and ask that the medication be changed.

Oral NSAIDs or acetaminophen are generally ordered for less severe pain or chronic pain. These medications may also be given with opioids to ensure effective analgesia in the child with tolerance and to avoid an immediate increase in opioid dose. NSAIDs and acetaminophen may mask fever. Be alert to the potential complication of gastrointestinal hemorrhage in critically ill children who have increased gastric acids as a physiologic stress response to pain.

When an epidural or regional nerve block is used, the analgesic effect does not recede for several hours after the catheter is removed, but the time of effectiveness varies by type of analgesia used. Since the epidural catheter may be maintained for a day or more, continuous infusion or patient-controlled epidural anesthesia may be used. Assess the child for pain and monitor the child for tingling of fingers or toes, an indication that the analgesic effect is receding at least every 2 hours. Assess motor function by asking children if they can move their legs, wiggle their toes, and lift their buttocks off the bed. Determine if there are any numb or tingling areas on the skin. Monitor voiding and catheterize the child as necessary for urinary retention (Pasero, 1999). Care must be taken to avoid injury to the limb that has the regional nerve block as the limb has a "dead" feeling, particularly if the child is being ambulated on an affected leg. The affected limb may be placed in a splint or sling while the nerve block is working, to protect it. Regular assessment for pain is still important as breakthrough pain can still occur with a nerve block. Effective oral analgesia should be initiated to maintain pain control.

Pain assessment and management of newborns in an intensive care nursery has different challenges. Adapt the assessment and management interventions described for infants in caring for these newborns. Guidelines for the assessment and management of newborns are listed in Box 18–6.

Partnering with Families

Parents are the single most powerful nonpharmacologic method of pain relief available to children. A parent's presence greatly reduces the anxiety associated with pain and hospitalization (Broome, 2000). Children often feel more secure telling parents about their pain and anxiety.

Educate school-age children and adolescents about pain that may occur with elective procedures, the use of pain scales, and the methods available for pain relief, both pharmacologic and nonpharmacologic. Parents can accurately rate their child's pain using a quantitative scale, so involve them in their child's pain management.

When parents are actively participating in the child's care during hospitalization, make sure they know the appropriate interventions for pain relief. Teach them about how complementary therapies can be used to enhance the child's pain management, and help the parent select the age-appropriate complementary therapies for the child as listed in Table 18–10. Encourage children and parents to use the techniques that work best for them.

BOX 18–6 Guidelines for the Prevention and Management of Pain in Newborns

ASSESSMENT

- Assess the neonate for pain every 4–6 hours, concomitantly with the vital signs, or as indicated by the pain scores or clinical condition of the infant. Document the findings.
- Use standardized pain assessment methods with evidence of validity, reliability, and clinical utility.
- Select the pain assessment tool sensitive and specific for the infant's gestational age and for the nature of the pain (acute, recurrent, or continuous).
- A comprehensive and multidimensional assessment process should be used.
- Perform the pain assessment after each potentially painful procedure and evaluate the effectiveness of all pain control methods (behavioral, environmental, and pharmacologic).

PAIN MANAGEMENT

- Prevent pain, and avoid recurrent painful stimuli.
- Use environmental interventions to reduce stress, such as minimizing noise and light levels and clustering care.
- Use behavioral methods of pain management, such as sucrose, nonnutritive sucking, swaddling, and holding and rocking.
- Use medications for preemptive analgesia and for ongoing pain.

Anand, K. J. S., & the International Evidence-Based Group for Neonatal Pain. (2001). Consensus statement for the prevention and management of pain in the newborn. Archives of Pediatric and Adolescent Medicine, *155(2), 173–180.*

TABLE 18–10 Complementary Therapies for Pain Management by Age Group

COMPLEMENTARY THERAPY	APPROPRIATE AGE FOR USE
Cutaneous stimulation	Newborns and infants
Pacifier	
Swaddling with limbs close to the trunk	
Nesting in blanket rolls with extremities flexed and hands near mouth	
Massage	All ages
Touch	
Comfort measures	Newborns and infants
Music (intrauterine sounds)	
Sucrose solution	
Distraction	
Stories	2–6 years
Bubbles	
Counting	
Video games	6–10 years
Suggestion	5–10 years
Magic glove	
Magic blanket	
Pain switch	
Breathing techniques	
Patterned	2–7 years
Shallow	7–18 years
Rhythmic	
Deep chest	
Guided imagery	4 years and older
Music	
Imagine being superhero	
Imagine special place	
Progressive muscle relaxation	6 years and older
Hypnosis	4 years and older

Adapted from Rusy, L. M., & Weisman, S. J. (2000). Complementary therapies for acute pediatric pain management. Pediatric Clinics of North America, *47(3), 591. Used with permission from Elsevier.*

Discharge Planning and Home Care Teaching

Children are frequently discharged from the hospital, emergency department, or healthcare center with oral analgesics following surgery, injury, or treatment of acute medical conditions. Teach parents and children about the dosage and frequency of administration and the side effects of the analgesic ordered. Make sure parents know that a sudden increase in pain intensity indicates the development of a complication requiring medical attention. Provide guidelines for follow-up care in the event of increasing pain.

Parents have the responsibility to provide adequate pain control for their child after day surgery. As the child leaves the surgical center pain free, the parents may not anticipate pain. Because of cultural values, certain parents may feel the child should learn to tolerate some amount of pain. Provide information about the child's need for pain medication around the clock for the first 1 to 2 days to prevent the child from feeling pain. Provide guidance to help parents assess their child's pain and directions for giving pain medications. Take the time to discuss the importance of pain management and its benefits in promoting the child's healing. (See Partnering with Families: Pain Management for the Child at Home.)

Remember that many common health problems (otitis media, pharyngitis, and urinary tract infection) have pain as one of their presenting symptoms. Often the only medication prescribed is an antibiotic to clear the infection. This may leave the child in pain for 48 to 72 hours until the antibiotic brings the infection under control. Give parents recommendations for pain control and comfort measures during this period.

Evaluation

Expected outcomes of nursing care include the following:

- Children at risk for pain are identified, assessed, and pain management is implemented.
- The child's pain level is assessed frequently and pain management is effective in improving the child's comfort.
- When the child's pain medication dosage is inadequate, advocacy for additional pain medication is successful.
- The child successfully uses a PCA pump to control acute pain.
- Age-appropriate complementary and alternative methods of pain management enhance the comfort provided by medications.
- Parents understand the importance of pain management and implement effective interventions for the child at home.

NURSING MANAGEMENT OF CHRONIC PAIN

Children do experience medical conditions that cause chronic pain and episodic acute pain, such as rheumatoid arthritis, cancer, headaches, recurrent abdominal pain, and HIV infection. Chronic pain does not arouse the sympathetic nervous system in the same way as acute pain does. Therefore, the child may not appear to be in pain but may still perceive pain. Ongoing stimulation of nociceptors can sensitize the peripheral and central nervous systems that lead to neuroanatomical, neurochemical, and neurophysiological changes. Physical and psychological signs and symptoms should be viewed together. Behavioral indicators of chronic pain and pain of long duration include posturing and inactivity to avoid pain, depression, difficulty sleeping, and an inability to concentrate (Shapiro, 1995).

No tools have been developed to assess chronic pain for any child age group. Assessment and evaluation of chronic pain in children should include the following aspects (American Pain Society, 2003).

PARTNERING WITH FAMILIES

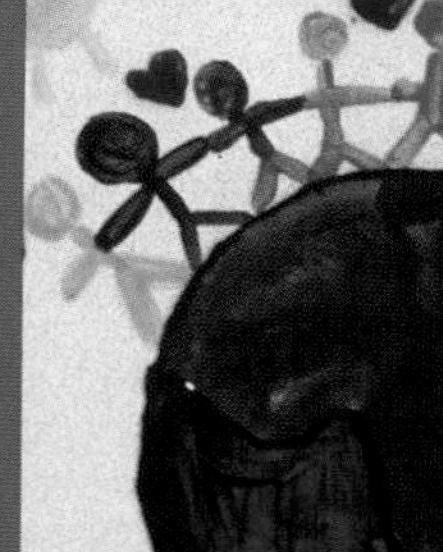

Pain Management for the Child at Home

- Review the child's pain behaviors and the fact that the child may still have pain even though watching television, playing, or sleeping.
- Discuss why pain management is important and how uncontrolled pain can slow recovery.
- Discuss the need for scheduled pain medication rather than waiting for the onset of pain to begin treatment.
- Review the child's pain management plan.
- Review the complementary therapies and the role they play in pain management.

- Approach pain as the present problem and obtain the history of pain onset, its development over time, intensity, duration, location, what makes it worse or relieves it, and its impact on daily life (sleeping, appetite, school, and social interactions).
- Determine the amount of distress the child and family experience with pain, including anxiety, depression, and hopelessness.
- Determine what the family and child believe causes the pain and their response to it.
- Identify past pain problems in the family and the current methods of treatment.
- Observe the child's appearance, posture, gait, emotional and cognitive state.
- Assess muscle spasms, trigger points, areas sensitive to light touch; perform a complete neurologic examination.

Older children with recurrent episodes of pain can be encouraged to keep a diary or log to describe the characteristics, timing, activities, and potential triggers of their pain, as well as their response to pain treatment measures. A pain assessment scale should be used to rate the pain intensity before and after medications and other pain control measures are used. See Figure 18–12 ■. This record can help improve pain management.

MediaLink Helping a Child Cope with Pain

Examples of nursing diagnoses for children with chronic pain include:

- Chronic (hand) Pain (moderate, dull) related to arthritic joint degeneration
- Sleep Pattern Disturbed related to inadequate pain control
- Risk for Constipation related to opioid pain medication and limited activity

Children with chronic conditions (arthritis, sickle-cell disease, hemophilia, cancer, recurrent headaches, etc.) often need long-term pain management. NSAIDs and acetaminophen are

FIGURE 18–12 ■ A pain diary is an important tool to help record the painful episodes experienced with chronic conditions such as rheumatoid arthritis or episodic conditions such as migraine headaches. A pain scale should be used to record pain intensity 1 hour after intervention.

Date	Time	Pain Intensity	Pain Medication Taken	How Much	Other Pain Relief Methods	Amount of Pain 1 Hour Later

often ordered for pain management. See Box 18–7 for strategies for chronic pain management. These children may also need additional pain medication for acute flare-ups of their condition. It is important to remember that they need effective preventive pain management for procedural pain, as many of these children have numerous medical procedures.

The parents must be actively engaged in pain control for the child. They are in the best position to assess the level of pain intensity. As for the child having acute pain, the parent needs to be taught about the importance of pain control. Teach parents how to use a variety of complementary therapies that can be used for the child to supplement the pain medications administered. Children with long-term pain should be referred to a pediatric pain program to be evaluated for customized strategies to manage pain.

SEDATION AND PAIN MANAGEMENT FOR MEDICAL PROCEDURES

MediaLink Nursing in Action: Conscious Sedation Monitoring

Children undergo a wide variety of painful diagnostic and treatment procedures in the hospital and in outpatient settings. Procedures such as chest tube insertion, arterial puncture, lumbar puncture, bone marrow aspiration, insertion of a central or peripheral intravenous line, fracture reduction, laceration repair, and burn debridement cause significant pain in children. The anticipation of these procedures causes anxiety and emotional distress that can lead to greater intensity of pain. Children who have experienced severe pain in the past associated with one of these procedures may be unwilling to cooperate with healthcare personnel.

BOX 18–7 Strategies for Chronic Pain Management

- Explain and validate the pain and its causes.
- Define treatment goals, including medications.
- Use distraction, relaxation, self-hypnosis, TENS, and exercise.
- Develop strategies for functional restoration.
- Give guidelines for a gradual increase in activity.
- Have a plan for sudden painful episodes.
- Explore stressors and potential pain triggers.
- Consider whether the child uses manipulative behaviors for attention or secondary gain.
- Refer to a mental health professional or pain management team as needed.

Adapted from Shapiro, B. S. (1995). Treatment of chronic pain in children and adolescents. Pediatric Annals, *24(3), 148–156.*

COLLABORATIVE CARE

Clinical Therapy for Minor Medical Procedures

Topical anesthetics can be used to reduce the pain associated with the first needle stick. Vapocoolant sprays can be used for injections. Eutetic mixture of local anesthetics (EMLA) cream, a mixture of 2.5% lidocaine and 2.5% prilocaine in an emulsion, is effective if applied 1 to 2 hours before a needle stick procedure on intact skin (Figure 18–13 ■). A new preparation, ELA-MAX, 4% liposomal lidocaine, is effective if applied 30 minutes before needle stick (Eichenfiled, Funk, Fallon-Friedlander, et al., 2002). Alternatively, Numby Stuff (2% lidocaine with 1:100,000 epinephrine) can be applied by iontophoresis, electric DC type current, to transport the ionizable drugs across intact skin in about 13 minutes (Squire, Kirchoff, & Hissong, 2000).

A local anesthetic such as lidocaine buffered by sodium bicarbonate is often injected to provide analgesia for emergent invasive procedures. Lidocaine can also be injected subcutaneously in a small area to reduce the pain of deeper needle insertion.

Sedation

Sedation is a medically controlled state of depressed consciousness (light to deep) used for painful diagnostic and therapeutic procedures and analgesia. Procedures such as burn debridement, laceration repair, bone marrow aspiration, and fracture reduction are associated with so much pain and anxiety that children need premedication with analgesia and **anxiolysis,** mild sedation. Sedation is often used to gain the cooperation of the child for the medical procedure. See the medication table on page 587 for medications used for sedation.

When given in lower doses **light sedation** occurs in which the child maintains protective reflexes, retains the ability to independently and continuously maintain a patent airway, and retains the ability to make an appropriate response to physical stimuli or verbal command. **Deep sedation** is a controlled state of depressed consciousness or unconsciousness in which protective airway reflexes are lost. See Table 18–11 for the signs of light and deep sedation.

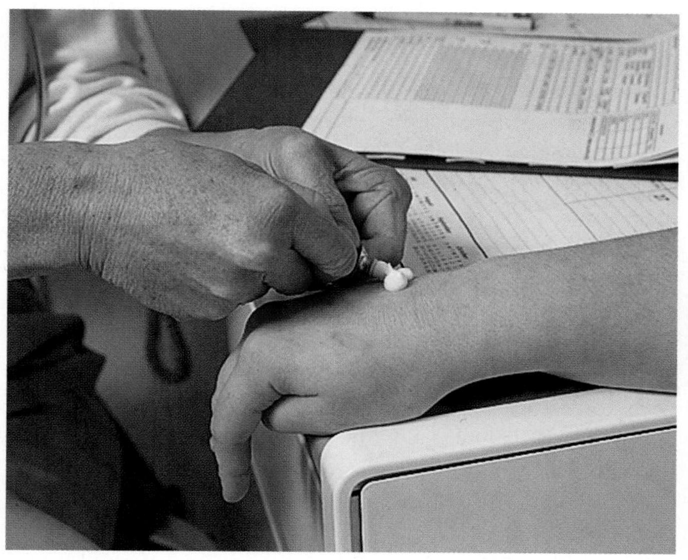
A

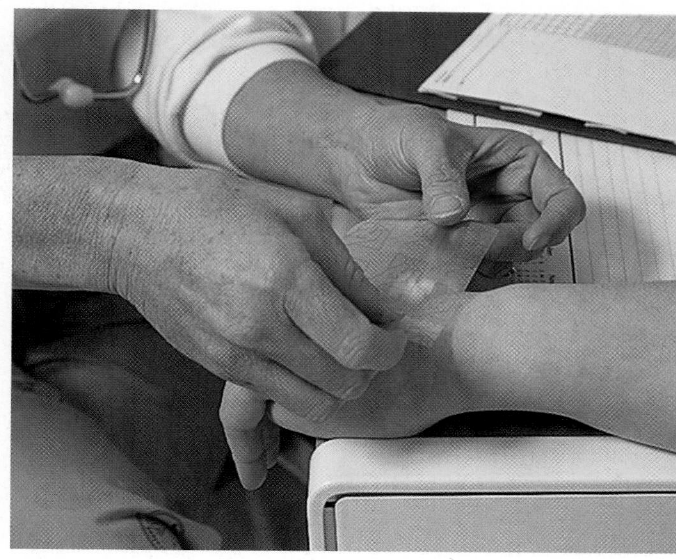
B

FIGURE 18–13 ■ When painful procedures are planned, use EMLA cream to anesthetize the skin where the painful stick will be made. A, Apply a thick layer of cream over intact skin (1/2 of a 5-g tube). B, Cover the cream with a transparent adhesive dressing, sealing all the sides. The cream anesthetizes the dermal surface in 45–60 minutes.

The goals of procedural sedation and analgesia are to prevent or relieve pain and anxiety, make it easier to do the medical procedures, and prevent complications such as respiratory distress, an obstructed airway, aspiration, or an adverse reaction to the medications used. Guidelines should exist in every healthcare facility where pediatric sedation is performed to ensure safe healthcare practices. Analgesia must be given in association with sedation as the sedated child can still feel pain but not communicate its

MEDICATIONS Used for Sedation

MEDICATION	ACTION	NURSING CONSIDERATIONS
Benzodiazepines Midazolam (Versed) Lorazepam (Ativan) Diazepam (Valium) May be reversed by flumazenil	Midazolam is preferred for its rapid and short action time. It produces skeletal muscle relaxation, amnesia, and anxiolysis. Pain is still perceived.	Analgesia should be co-administered to manage pain associated with the procedure. Simultaneous administration of potent opiates such as fentanyl increases the risk of hypoventilation and apnea. May cause paradoxical reaction in some children (hysteria, restlessness, inconsolability, and agitation).
Hypnotics (barbiturates) Thiopental Pentobarbital	Thiopental is preferred for its ultra-short action that produces hypnosis and sedation.	The drug has a histamine release and must be used with caution in asthmatics. Can cause significant hypotension.
Analgesics Fentanyl Alfentanil May be reversed by naloxone	Opioid with rapid and short duration of action. Children appear to be asleep, but may be able to maintain awareness.	Rapid administration may lead to rigidity of the chest wall, bradycardia, facial pruritis, nausea, and vomiting.
Ketamine	Has analgesic, sedative, and amnestic properties. Child appears awake with eyes open but does not respond behaviorally.	Airway reflexes and respirations are unimpaired. Upper airway secretions are increased. Up to 10% of children will vomit during recovery. Other signs seen during emergence from sedation include inconsolable crying, agitation, and restlessness. Should not be used in children with brain injury.
Propofol	Sedative, hypnotic, and muscle relaxant with rapid onset and quick return to baseline. Mild antiemetic.	May be combined with fentanyl. Contraindicated in children with allergies to soybean oil, egg yolk, glycerol, and EDTA (ethylenediamine-tetraacetic acid)

Data from Proudfoot, J. (2002). Pediatric procedural sedation and analgesia (PSA): Keeping it simple and safe. Pediatric Emergency Medicine Reports, *7(2), 16–18.*

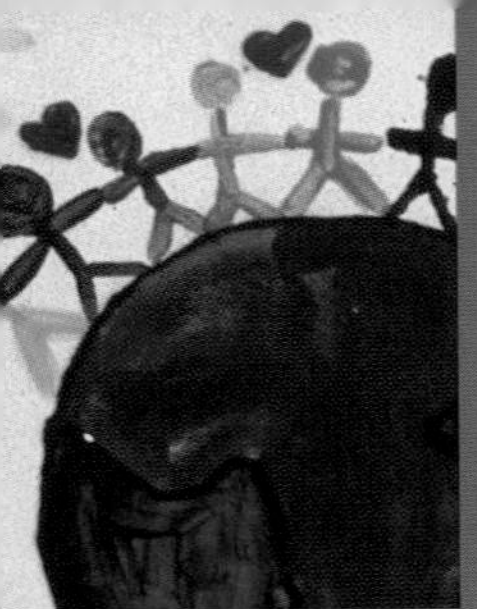

PARTNERING WITH FAMILIES

Placing EMLA Cream at Home

Teach parents to prepare the child for an immunization or venipuncture by placing EMLA cream on the skin before departing for the healthcare visit. Provide directions for the amount of cream that should be applied to the child's arm or leg, based on the child's age and weight (Bell, 2003).

- For infants under 3 months of age, use no more than 1 g, cover no more than a 10 cm^2 area.
- For infants 3 to 12 months of age, use no more than 2 g, cover no more than a 20 cm^2 area.
- For children 1 to 6 years of age, use up to 10 g, cover no more than a 100 cm^2 area.
- For children 7 to 12 years, use up to 20 g, cover no more than a 200 cm^2 area.

An occlusive dressing should be applied over the cream. If a dressing does not come with the cream, kitchen plastic wrap can be substituted.

presence. These guidelines often require health professionals monitoring the child to have specific qualifications, such as pediatric advanced life support training. The child must be carefully monitored for respiratory depression and signs of deep sedation as the child may become more deeply sedated when the stimulus of the procedure is discontinued (American Academy of Pediatrics Committee on Drugs, 2002). Antagonist agents are available for opioids and benzodiazepines when the effects of sedation and respiratory depression need to be reversed.

Nursing Management

Make every effort to increase the child's comfort during painful procedures. Help the child cope with a painful procedure by explaining what sensations to expect and what will happen during the procedure. This reduces stress more effectively than just providing information about the procedure. Chapter 17∞ gives methods for preparing children of different developmental ages for procedures.

The nurse has an important role in advocating for effective sedation and pain management for the child undergoing an invasive diagnostic or therapeutic procedure. Prevent anticipated procedure-related pain with an analgesic, and give time for the medication to become effective. Make sure that the child with preexisting pain, such as from a burn, has effective pain management prior to debridement of the burn. When possible, administer drugs by a nonpainful route (oral, transmucosal, or intravenous). Avoid intramuscular and subcutaneous injections. When procedures must be repeated (e.g., bone marrow aspirations for children with leukemia), give optimal sedation and analgesia for the first procedure to reduce anxiety about future procedures. To prevent increased anxiety, avoid delays in performing procedures. Make sure the results of pain management are documented.

When the child receives sedation, monitoring the child's status is important during the procedure and until the medication wears off. Nursing assessments include *visual* confirmation of respiratory effort, color, and vital signs. Pulse oximetry and other technology may also be used for monitoring, but this equipment must not replace visual assessment. Vital signs must be checked every 15 minutes until the child regains full consciousness and level of functioning. If light sedation progresses to deep sedation, airway management is essential, and vital signs should be checked every 5 minutes. Resuscitation equipment and antagonist agents must be precalculated and ready to administer.

PRACTICE ALERT

When light sedation is given, be sure to have the resources available to monitor the child's vital signs and to provide advanced life support if the child should progress to deep sedation. All healthcare facilities have special protocols for management of children receiving sedation.

If complications occur, the following equipment should be immediately available: suction apparatus, a bag-valve mask for assisted ventilation with capability of 90% to 100% oxygen delivery, an oxygen supply (5 L/min for more than 60 min), and antagonists to sedative medication.

Medications may not be used for quick procedures, such as a dressing change, or an unexpected intravenous insertion, injec-

TABLE 18–11 Characteristics of Light Sedation and Deep Sedation

ASSESSMENT FACTORS	LIGHT SEDATION	DEEP SEDATION
Airway	Able to maintain airway independently and continuously	Unable to maintain airway independently or continuously
Cough and gag reflexes	Reflexes intact	Partial or complete loss of reflexes
Level of consciousness	Easily aroused with verbal or gentle physical stimulation	Not easily aroused, may not respond purposefully to verbal or gentle physical stimulation

Data from Proudfoot, J. (2002). Pediatric procedural sedation and analgesia (PSA): Keeping it simple and safe. Pediatric Emergency Medicine Reports, *7(2), 1–2.*

tion, or venipuncture. For a planned quick procedure, such as an immunization, other injection, intravenous insertion, or venipuncture, use a topical anesthetic such as EMLA, ELA-MAX, or vapocoolant spray on the skin. (See Partnering with Families: Placing EMLA Cream at Home.) Complementary and alternative therapies, especially imagery, relaxation techniques, and distraction, may reduce the anxiety associated with the anticipation of the procedure. Teach parents and children to use these therapies before procedures. Help children to control their anxiety through therapeutic play as described in Chapter 17∞. See Complementary Therapy: A Pain Management Kit.

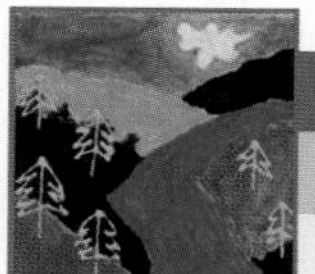

COMPLEMENTARY THERAPY

A Pain Management Kit

Assemble a pain management kit to promote distraction, imagery, and relaxation in children. Items that might be included are magic wands, pinwheels, bubble liquid, a slinky spring toy, a foam ball, party noisemakers, and pop-up books. It may also be helpful to include items for therapeutic play such as syringes, adhesive bandages, alcohol swabs, and other supplies from a medical kit. The pain management kit may be especially helpful for children who are being prepared for surgery or for painful procedures and need to be distracted. Parents can also help the child to cope with mild or moderate pain during a procedure by using items in this kit that match the child's developmental stage and individual interests.

MediaLink Pain Management Kit Video

Discharge Planning

Criteria for discharge after sedation includes the following (Bindler & Ball, 2003):

- Child shows satisfactory and stable cardiovascular function and airway patency.
- Child is easily arousable, with protective reflexes intact.
- Hydration is adequate.
- Infant is able to hold the head up and sit up unassisted if old enough to do so, or the child can stand and walk without assistance.
- Discharge status is the same as admission status.

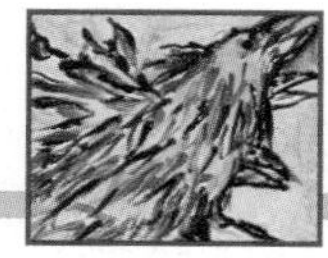

CHAPTER HIGHLIGHTS

- Pain is an unpleasant sensation that is either acute or chronic, perceived in response to tissue damage.
- Research has revealed that infants and children feel pain, like adults, despite past beliefs to the contrary.
- Pain behaviors in children are similar to the behaviors of fearful and anxious children.
- Every infant, child, and adolescent has the right to adequate pain control.
- The goal of pain assessment is to provide accurate information about the location and intensity of the child's pain and how the child responds to it.
- Learning how the child expresses pain, both verbally and behaviorally, will help the nurse make a better assessment.
- Children learn how and when to seek help for pain and how to cope with pain by observing other family members.
- Numerous tools have been developed and validated to assess pain in infants and children.
- Pharmacologic interventions for pain control include opioids, nonsteroidal anti-inflammatory drugs (NSAIDs), and acetaminophen.
- Opioids are equally as effective when given orally, intramuscularly, and intravenously when an equianalgesic dose is used.
- Analgesia for continuous or severe pain should be given around the clock to maintain pain control. Patient-controlled analgesia is one method of administering a continuous infusion of an opioid medication and allowing the child to infuse additional small doses for episodic pain.
- Epidural and regional nerve blocks are pain control methods gaining acceptance because they have many fewer side effects associated with systemic medications.
- Complementary and alternative therapies for pain management include the following: parental presence, distraction, cutaneous stimulation, sucrose solution, electroanalgesia, guided imagery, breathing techniques, progressive muscle relaxation techniques, hypnosis, application of heat and cold, biofeedback, and acupuncture.
- Parents need education and preparation to provide pain control for children who are discharged home following surgery and injuries. Children with chronic conditions often need long-term pain management.
- Many diagnostic and therapeutic procedures cause pain and anxiety in children. Provide optimal prophylactic pain management to reduce the anxiety associated with future procedures.
- Sedation is used to reduce the child's anxiety associated with painful procedures. Analgesia is usually given in association with sedation when the procedure would cause pain or discomfort in an alert child.

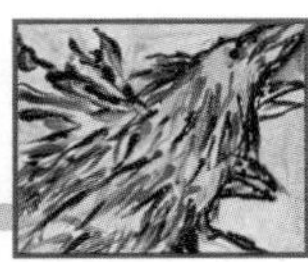

CRITICAL THINKING IN ACTION

INTRODUCTION

Consider Felicia in the opening scenario. Review the nursing care and pain management during the initial period following her injury and surgery. Her pain seems to be well managed at the moment. Both her mother and 14-year-old sister Maria are with her to provide comfort and security.

DESCRIPTION

As the next day begins, Felicia will be expected to get out of bed and perform coughing and deep breathing to aerate the lungs. Felicia's sister is asking how the nurses know if she is in pain because she has lots of reasons to be in pain. After all, she was struck by a car and has lots of bumps and bruises, she had surgery, and now she has an IV and nasogastric tube. Getting out of bed and taking deep breaths must hurt her. Consider how the nursing care plan will integrate considerations about pain assessment and management with regard to these activities.

DISCUSSION

1. How well is Felicia's pain being managed? Does Felicia need more pain medication than what has been ordered? How would you reassure her sister about her pain assessment and management plan?
2. Could Felicia's anxiety about being in the hospital have an impact on how much pain she feels? What other pain relief measures could reduce or help to control her pain?
3. As Felicia begins feeling better, taking fluids and foods, and visiting the playroom, she seems to have little pain. She has oral pain medication ordered as needed. What factors need to be considered in determining whether to give her pain medication?

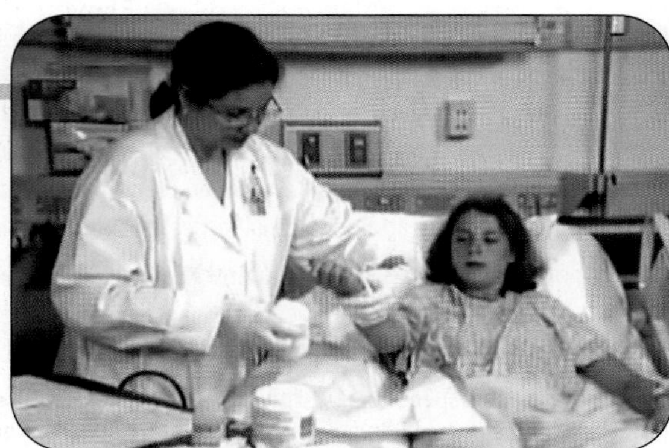

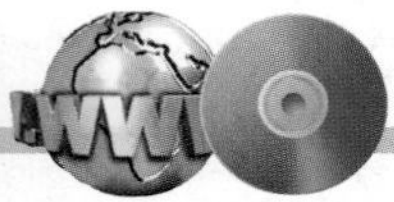

EXPLORE MediaLink

- NCLEX review, case studies, and other interactive resources for this chapter can be found on the Companion Website at **www.prenhall.com/ball**. Click on Chapter 18 to select the activities for this chapter.
- For animations, more NCLEX review questions, and an audio glossary, access the accompanying CD-ROM in this textbook.

http://www.prenhall.com/ball

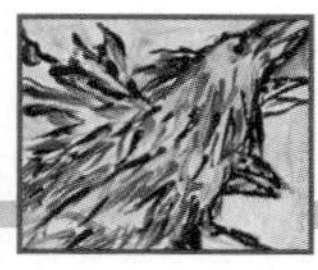

REFERENCES

Abu-Saad, H. (1984). Cultural components of pain: The Asian-American child. *Children's Health Care, 13,* 11–14.

Alexander, J., & Manno, M. (2003). Analgesia administration in the very young: The practice is uncommon. *Annals of Emergency Medicine, 41*(5), 617–622.

American Academy of Pediatrics Committee on Drugs. (2002). Guidelines for monitoring and management of pediatric patients during and after sedation for diagnostic and therapeutic procedures: Addendum. *Pediatrics, 110*(4), 836–838.

American Pain Society. (1999). *Principles of analgesic use in the treatment of acute pain and cancer pain* (4th ed.). Glenview, IL: Author.

American Pain Society. (2003). Pediatric chronic pain: A position statement from the American Pain Society. www.ampainsoc.org/cgi-bin/print/print/pl, accessed 10/22/2003.

Anand, K. J. S., & Hickey, P. R. (1987). Pain and its effects in the human neonate and fetus. *New England Journal of Medicine, 317,* 1321.

Anand, K. J. S., & the International Evidence-Based Group for Neonatal Pain. (2001). Consensus statement for the prevention and management of pain in the newborn. *Archives of Pediatric and Adolescent Medicine, 155*(2), 173–180.

Bell, E. A. (2003, March). Using topical anesthetics for common procedures in children. *Infectious Diseases in Children,* 7–8.

Beyer, J. E., & Wells, N. (1989). The assessment of pain in children. *Pediatric Clinics of North America, 36*(4), 837–854.

Beyer, J. E., Denyes, M. J., & Villarruel, A. M. (1992). The creation, validation and continuing development of the Oucher: A measure of pain intensity in children. *Journal of Pediatric Nursing, 7*(5), 335–346.

Bindler, R. C., & Ball, J. W. (2003). *Clinical skills manual for pediatric nursing: Caring for children,* (3rd ed.). Upper Saddle River, NJ: Prentice Hall.

Blass, E. M., & Watt, L. B. (1999). Sucrose as an analgesic for newborn infants. *Pediatrics, 87,* 215–218.

Bowers, P. (2002). Children in pain. *Nursing Spectrum, 15*(4), 22–24.

Broome, M. E. (2000). Helping parents support their child in pain. *Pediatric Nursing, 26*(3), 315–317.

Chambers, C., & Craig, K. D. (1998). An intrusive impact of anchors in children's faces pain scales. *Pain, 78,* 27.

Champion, G. D., Goodenough, B., von Baeyer, C. L., et al. (1998). Measurement of pain by self-report. *Progress in Pain Research and Management, 10,* 123–160.

Eichenfiled, L. F., Funk, A., Fallon-Friedlander, S., & Cunningham, B. B. (2002). A clinical study to evaluate ELA-MAX (4% liposomal lidocaine) as compared with eutectic mixture of local anesthetics cream for pain reduction of venipuncture in children. *Pediatrics, 109*(5), 1093–1099.

Fanurik, D., Koh, J., Schitz, M., & Brown, R. (1997). Pharmacobehavioral intervention: Integrating pharmacologic and behavioral techniques for pediatric procedures. *Children's Health Care, 26*(1), 1–13.

Fanurik, D., Koh, J. L., Harrison, R. D., Conrad, T. M., & Tomerlin, C. (1998). Pain assessment in children with cognitive impairment. *Clinical Nursing Research, 7*(2), 103–119.

Franck, L. S., Greenberg, C. S., & Stevens, B. (2000). Pain assessment in infants and children. *Pediatric Clinics of North America, 47*(3), 487–512.

Fuller, B. F. (2000). Fluctuations in established infant pain behaviors. *Clinical Nursing Research, 9*(3), 298–316.

Fuller, B. F. (2001). Infant behaviors as indicators of established acute pain. *Journal of Society of Pediatric Nurses, 6*(3), 109–115.

Gaston-Johansson, F., Albert, M., Fagan, E., & Zimmerman, L. (1990). Similarities in pain descriptions of four different ethnic-culture groups. *Journal of Pain and Symptom Management, 5*(2), 94–100.

Greenberg, C. S. (2002). A sugar-coated pacifier reduces procedural pain in newborns. *Pediatric Nursing,* 22(3), 271–277.

Hazinski, M. F. (1999). Analgesia, sedation, and neuromuscular blockade in pediatric critical care. In M. F. Hazinski, *Manual of pediatric critical care* (pp. 44–72) St. Louis: Mosby.

Higgins, S. S., Turley, K. M., Harr, J., & Turley, K. (1999). Prescription and administration of around the clock analgesics in postoperative pediatric cardiovascular surgery patients. *Progress in Cardiovascular Nursing, 14*(1), 19–24.

Holder, K. A., & Patt, R. B. (1995). Taming the pain monster: Pediatric postoperative pain management. *Pediatric Annals, 24*(3), 164–168.

Huether, S. E., & Leo, J. (2002). Pain, temperature regulation, sleep, and sensory function. In K. L. McCance & S. E. Huether (Eds.), *Pathophysiology: The biologic basis for disease in adults and children* (4th ed., pp. 401–410). St. Louis: Mosby.

Jedlinksy, B. P., McCarthy, C. F., & Michel, T. H. (1999). Validating pediatric pain measurement: Sensory and affective components. *Pediatric Physical Therapy, 11,* 368–374.

Joint Commission on the Accreditation of Health Care Organizations. (2001). Pain standards for 2001. Oakbrook Terrace, IL: Author. www.jcaho.org, accessed 2/28/2003.

Keck, J. F., Gerkensmeyer, J. E., Joyce, B. A., et al. (1996). Reliability and validity of the faces and word descriptor scales to measure procedural pain. *Journal of Pediatric Nursing, 11,* 368.

LaFleur, C. J., & Raway, B. (1999). School-age child and adolescent perception of pain intensity associated with three word descriptors. *Pediatric Nursing, 25*(1), 45–55.

Luffy, R., & Grove, S. K. (2003). Examining the validity, reliability, and preference of three pediatric pain measurement tools in African-American children. *Pediatric Nursing, 29*(1), 54–59.

Lynn, A. M., Ulma, G. A., & Spreker, M. (1999). Pain control in very young infants: An update. *Contemporary Pediatrics, 16*(11), 39–66.

Manworren, R. C. B., & Hynan, L. S. (2003). Clinical validation of FLACC: Preverbal patient pain scale. *Pediatric Nursing, 29*(2), 140–146.

McCaffery, M., & Pasero, C. (1999). *Pain: Clinical manual* (2nd ed.). St. Louis: Mosby.

McGrath, P. A. (1995). Pain in the pediatric patient: Practical aspects of assessment. *Pediatric Annals, 24*(3), 126–138.

McGrath, P. J., & Craig, K. D. (1989). Developmental and psychological factors in children's pain. *Pediatric Clinics of North America, 36*(4), 823–836.

Merkel, S. (2002). Pain assessment in infants and young children: The finger span scale. *American Journal of Nursing, 102*(11), 55–56.

Merkel, S., Voepel-Lewis, T., & Malviya, S. (2002). Pain assessment in infants and young children: The FLACC scale. *American Journal of Nursing, 102*(10), 55–57.

Merkel, S., Voepel-Lewis, T., Shayevitz, J. R., & Malviya, S. (1997). The FLACC: A behavioral scale for scoring postoperative pain in young children. *Pediatric Nursing, 23*(3), 293–297.

Mitchell, A., & Boss, B. J. (2002). Adverse effects of pain on the nervous systems of newborns and young children: A review of the literature. *Journal of Neuroscience Nursing, 34*(5), 228–236.

Mitchell, A., & Waltman, P. A. (2003). Oral sucrose and pain relief in preterm infants. *Pain Management Nursing, 4*(2), 62–69.

Mitchell, A., Brooks, S., & Roane, D. (2000). The premature infant and painful procedures. *Pain Management Nursing, 1*(2), 58–65.

Pasero, C. (1999). Epidural analgesia in children. *American Journal of Nursing, 99*(5), 20.

Pasero, C. (2002). Pain assessment in infants and young children: Neonates. *American Journal of Nursing, 102*(8), 61–65.

Pasero, C. (2003). Epidural analgesia for postoperative pain. *American Journal of Nursing, 103*(10), 62–64.

Proudfoot, J. (2002). Pediatric procedural sedation and analagesia (PSA): Keeping it simple and safe. *Pediatric Emergency Medicine Reports, 7*(2), 16–18.

Rusy, L. M., & Weisman, S. J. (2000). Complementary therapies for acute pediatric pain management. *Pediatric Clinics of North America, 47*(3), 589–598.

Shah, V. S., Taddio, A., Bennett, S., & Speidel, B. D. (1997). Neonatal pain response to heelstick vs. venipuncture for routine blood sampling. *Archives of Diseases in Childhood, 77,* F143–F144.

Shapiro, B. S. (1995). Treatment of chronic pain in children and adolescents. *Pediatric Annals, 24*(3), 148–156.

Shields, B. J., Palermo, T. M., Powers, J. D., Grewe, S. D., & Smith, G.A. (2003). Predictors of a child's ability to use a visual analog scale. *Child Care Health Development, 29*(4), 281–290.

Solodiuk, J., & Curley, M. A. Q. (2003). Pain assessment in nonverbal children with severe cognitive impairments: The individualized numeric rating scale. *Journal of Pediatric Nursing, 18*(4), 295–299.

Squire, S. J., Kirchoff, K. T., & Hissong, K. (2000). Comparing two methods of topical anesthesia used before intravenous cannulation in pediatric patients. *Journal of Pediatric Health Care, 14*(2), 68–72.

Taddio, A., Goldbach, M., Ipp, M., Stephens, B., & Koren, G. (1995, February). Effect of neonatal circumcision on pain responses during vaccination in boys. *The Lancet, 345,* 291–292.

Taddio, A., Katz, J., Ilersich, A., & Koren, G. (1997, March). Effect of neonatal circumcision on pain response during subsequent routine vaccinations. *The Lancet, 349,* 599–603.

Tesler, M. D., Holzemer, W. L., & Savedra, M. C. (1998). Pain behaviors: Postsurgical responses of children and adolescents. *Journal of Pediatric Nursing, 13,* 41–47.

Tobias, J. D. (2000). Tolerance, withdrawal, and physical dependency after long-term sedation and analgesia of children in the pediatric intensive care unit. *Critical Care Medicine, 28*(6), 2122–2132.

Vincent, C.V. (2001). Nurses' analgesic practices with hospitalized children. *Journal of Child and Family Nursing, 4*(2), 79–89.

Weissman, S.J., Bernstein, B., & Schecter, N.L. (1998). Consequences of inadequate analgesia during painful procedures in children. *Archives of Diseases in Pediatric and Adolescent Medicine, 152,* 147–149.

Willis, M. H. W., Merkel, S. I., Voepel-Lewis, T., & Malviya, S. (2003). FLACC behavioral pain assessment scale: A comparison with the child's self-report. *Pediatric Nursing, 29*(3), 195–198.

Wong, D. L., & Baker, C. M. (1988). Pain in children: Comparison of assessment scales. *Pediatric Nursing, 14,* 9–16.

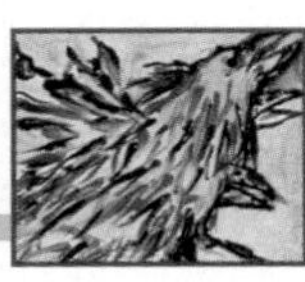

ADDITIONAL REFERENCES

American Academy of Pediatrics and Canadian Pediatric Society (2002). Prevention and management of pain and stress in the neonate. *Pediatrics, 105*(2), 454–461.

Buck, M. L. (2002). Naloxone for the reversal of opioids adverse effects. *Pediatric Pharmacology, 8*(8), http://www.medscape.com/viewarticle/441915_print, accessed 10/17/2002.

Chambers, C. T., Gresbrecht, K., Craig, K. D., Bennett, S. M., & Huntsman, E. (1999). A comparison of faces scales for the measurement of pediatric pain: Chidren's and parent's ratings. *Pain, 83*, 25–35.

Dresser, S., & Melnyk, B. M. (2003). The effectiveness of conscious sedation on anxiety, pain, and procedural complications in young children. *Pediatric Nursing, 29*(4), 320–323.

Haouari, N., Wood, G., Griffiths, G., & Levene, M. (1995). The analgesic effect of sucrose on full term infants: A randomized controlled trial. *British Medical Journal, 310*, 1498–1500.

Jonas, D. A. (2003). Parent's management of their child's pain in the home following day surgery. *Journal of Child Health Care, 7*(3), 150–162.

Merkel, S., & Malviya, S. (2000). Pediatric pain, tools, and assessment. *Journal of PeriAnesthesia Nursing, 15*(6), 408–414.

Pao, M. (2003). Managing pain: An exploration of psychotropic medications. *Contemporary Pediatrics, 20*(10), 43–63.

Pölkki, T., Pietilä, A., Vehviläïnen-Julkunen, K., Laukkala, H., & Ryhänen, P. (2002). Parental views on participation in their child's pain relief measures and recommendations to health care providers. *Journal of Pediatric Nursing, 17*(4), 270–278.

Porter, F. L., Wolf, C. M., & Miller, J. P. (1999). Procedural pain in newborn infants: The influence of intensity and development. *Pediatrics [serial on line], 104*(1), e13.

Sugarman, L. I. (1996). Hypnosis: Helping children help themselves. *Contemporary Pediatrics, 13*(11), 107–123.

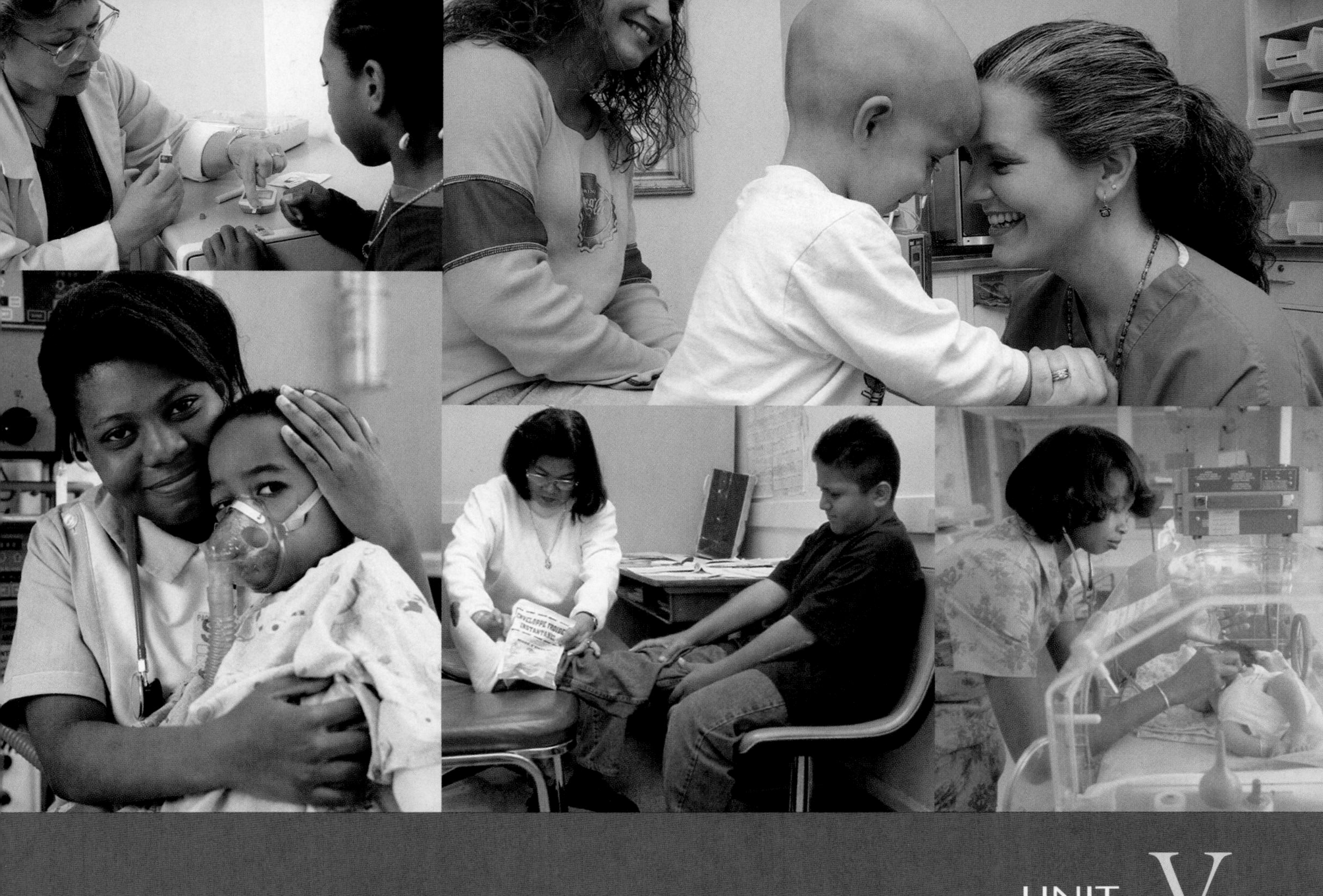

UNIT V

Health Conditions: Episodic to End-of-Life

Children experience a wide range of health conditions throughout childhood, from simple infectious or communicable diseases to life-threatening conditions. Pediatric nurses need to be prepared to work with children in any stage of acute or chronic illness, as well as provide effective end-of-life care. Essential to providing family-centered care is the nurse's understanding of the child and family responses to these conditions. The pediatric nurse partners with the family to individualize care for the child, and collaborates with other health professionals to ensure the child and family are adequately supported in both the hospital and community settings. The nurse applies knowledge of the child's developmental, cognitive, and psychosocial levels to address needs specific to children and their families in any setting.

Chapter

19

Infectious and Communicable Diseases

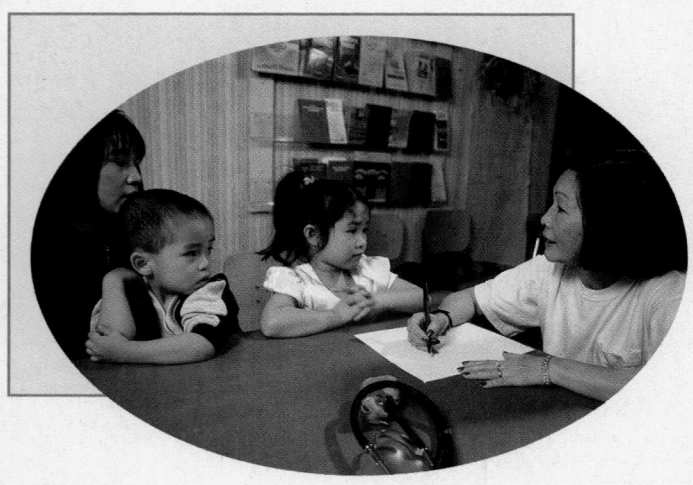

Lian Zhao, 5 years old, has accompanied her mother and 2-year-old brother, Chang, to the pediatric clinic. Her mother is concerned because Chang has had a fever of 38.3°C (101°F) for the past 3 days. Chang has been to this office several times in the past few months for illnesses, but this is the first time Lian has come along.

When the nurse asks about Lian's last visit to the doctor and the status of her immunizations, her mother says Lian has not been seen for about 2 years. She is not sure whether Lian has had all of her shots. In checking Lian's health records, the nurse notes that she is in need of several immunizations, including DTaP, polio, varicella, pneumococcal, and the hepatitis B series. Chang needs polio, Hib and hepatitis B boosters, and the MMR vaccine.

Should Lian be given any of these immunizations today, even though her brother is ill? Can immunizations be given at the same time? Should Chang also receive any immunizations today?

"Why do I have to get a shot? It hurts! I really don't like coming here."

—Lian, 5 years old

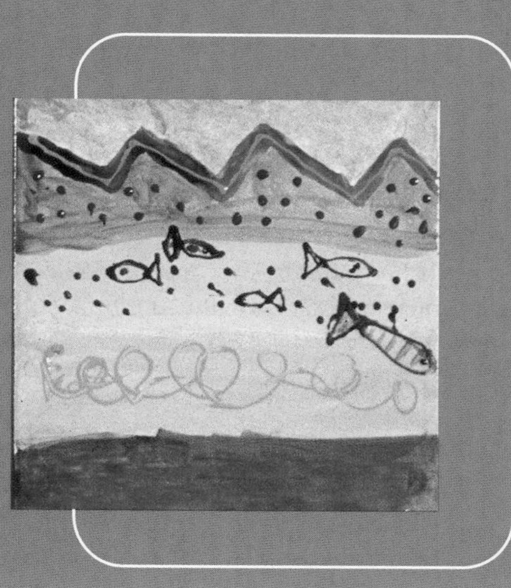

Learning Outcomes

After completing this chapter, you will be able to:

- Describe why children are more vulnerable than adults to infectious and communicable diseases.
- Describe the process of infection and modes of transmission.
- Understand the role that vaccines play in reduction and elimination of infectious and communicable diseases.
- Develop a nursing care plan for children of all ages needing immunizations.
- Recognize common infectious and communicable diseases.
- Describe the medical and nursing management of common infectious and communicable diseases.

MediaLink http://www.prenhall.com/ball

Resources for this chapter can be found on the CD-ROM accompanying this textbook, and on the Companion Website at www.prenhall.com/ball. Click on Chapter 19 to select the activities for this chapter.

CD-ROM

Animations
- *Inflammation with Phagocytosis*

NCLEX Review

Audio Glossary

COMPANION WEBSITE

Clinical Manifestations Review

Medication Match-Up

NCLEX Review

Case Study: Consequences of Vaccine Shortages

Case Study: Develop an Immunization Education Plan for a Reluctant Parent

Case Study: Reporting an Adverse Vaccine Event

Care Plan: Develop an Immunization Schedule
- *Healthy Infant*
- *Infant with HIV*
- *Preschooler*

MediaLink Applications
- *Bioterrorism Preparedness*
- *Develop an Infection Control Plan*
  - *Childcare Center*
  - *Health Clinic*
- *Immunization FAQ*
- *Immunizations and Older Children*
- *Storing Vaccines During a Disaster*
- *Vaccine Administration Records*

Key Terms

acellular vaccine/600
active immunity/599
antigen/599
communicable disease/596
conjugated vaccine/600
disease surveillance/598
endogenous pyrogens/618
indirect transmission/596
infectious disease/596
killed virus vaccine/600
live virus vaccine/600
nosocomial infection/637
opisthotonus/631
passive immunity/599
phagocytosis/617
prostration/625
recombinant vaccine/600
toxic appearance/636
toxoid/600
transplacental immunity/601
zoonosis/619

An **infectious disease** is any communicable disease caused by microorganisms that are commonly transmitted from one person to another or from an animal to a person. A **communicable disease** is an illness that is directly or indirectly transmitted from one person or animal to another by contact with body fluids, by contact with contaminated objects, or by vectors (ticks, mosquitoes, other insects). Infectious and communicable diseases are a major cause of morbidity in infants and children in the United States, and in some cases result in death.

For a communicable disease to occur, the following links need to be present (Figure 19–1 ■).

- An infectious agent, or pathogen
- An effective means of transmission
- A susceptible host

VULNERABILITY OF CHILDREN TO INFECTION

Infants and young children are often susceptible hosts. Their immune systems are not fully developed and they have not yet developed antibodies to many agents (see Chapter 26∞). Therefore, they cannot defend themselves against infectious and communicable diseases as well as older children and adults. Other characteristics, such as immunodeficiency and poor health, may increase a child's risk of contracting an infectious disease.

Young children such as Lian and Chang are particularly susceptible to illnesses that are transmitted among close contacts or through exposure to microorganisms in various settings. Children can develop complications or secondary infections resulting from the infectious disease that require healthcare intervention and may be an economic burden to families. Nurses have an important health promotion role in reducing the transmission of infectious diseases by immunization and in partnering with families to interrupt the transmission of infection in other ways, such as quarantine or handwashing.

Reducing the number of preventable childhood illnesses is a major national goal in *Healthy People 2010,* and nurses are important partners in this effort. Specific objectives are targeted at the reduction or elimination of the following infectious diseases (Department of Health and Human Services, 1999).

- *Elimination*—rubella and congenital rubella syndrome, diphtheria, Haemophilus influenza type b, measles, mumps, polio, and tetanus
- *Reduction*—pertussis, hepatitis B, varicella, food-borne pathogens, and HIV infection

The national objectives reflect the significance of these preventable diseases as a public health problem. When infectious diseases are not prevented, there is an impact on the family and the healthcare system. There is the cost to families and health insurance payors. Excessive healthcare resources are used when the infectious disease becomes widely transmitted and treatment is required by infected children and their families. Parents miss work while caring for the child and may become ill themselves, and children are directly impacted when they miss time from school and interrupt their learning.

PATHOPHYSIOLOGY ILLUSTRATED

The Chain of Infection

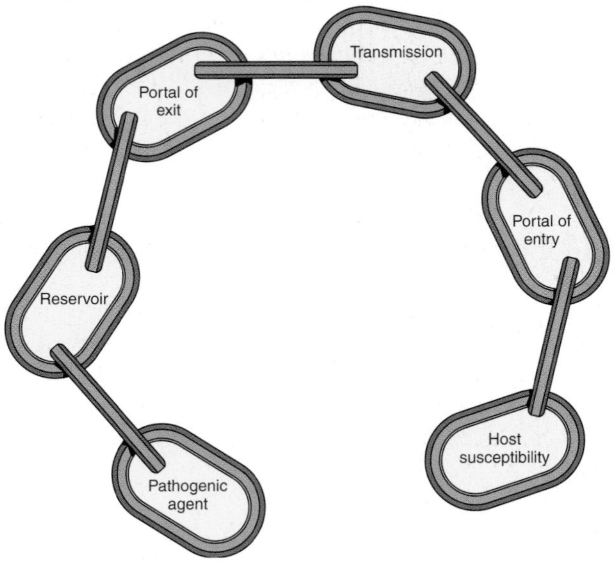

Transmission
Portal of exit
Portal of entry
Reservoir
Host susceptibility
Pathogenic agent

FIGURE 19–1 ■ An effective chain of transmission for infection requires a suitable habitat, or reservoir, for the pathogen. A reservoir may be living or nonliving. Transmission may be direct or indirect. Direct transmission involves physical contact between the source of the infection and the new host. **Indirect transmission** occurs when pathogens survive outside humans before causing infection and disease. To achieve infection control, one of the links in the chain must be broken.

Special Vulnerability of Newborns and Young Infants

The capability and function of the immune system of newborns and young infants is becoming more clearly understood. Infants are particularly vulnerable to infectious diseases for the following reasons.

- *The immune system is not fully mature at birth.* Synthesis of immunoglobulin M antibodies begins at birth in response to antigens in the environment, and adult levels are present by 1 year of age. Natural killer cells are present in adult levels at birth. Levels of complement (plasma proteins important in the inflammatory response that are defenders against bacterial infection) are only 50% to 75% of adult levels in full-term infants and even lower in preterm infants. While neutrophils are fairly numerous in both full-term and preterm infants, the storage pool in the bone marrow is only 20% to 30% of an adult level. This storage pool can be rapidly depleted when the newborn acquires an infection. Once the storage pool is depleted, it then takes 5 to 7 days for the bone marrow to produce a mature granulocyte from a stem cell (McKenney, 2001). See Chapter 27∞ for more information on the development of the immune system.

- *Passively acquired maternal antibodies provide limited protection.* Immunoglobulin G is transferred through the placenta so that full-term infants have levels comparable to their mother, but the half-life of IgG provided through the placenta is about 20 days. Placental transfer of antibodies for gram-negative organisms is minimal, and the newborn has protection only for viruses and gram-positive organisms to which the mother has been exposed. Other immunoglobulins (IgA, IgE, IgD, and IgM) do not transfer through the placenta. In addition, preterm infants may have fewer maternal antibodies as most of the placental transfer occurs after 31 weeks' gestation (McKenney, 2001). Breastfeeding provides some continuing passive protection, but many infants are not breastfed.
- *Disease protection through immunization is incomplete.* Newborns are at risk for infection before, during, and immediately after birth. See Table 19–1 for factors that increase their infection risk.

As children grow, they develop immunity through immunization or exposure to the natural disease. As children mature and become more active, they interact more frequently with other children and adults, which increases their exposure to infectious agents (Figure 19–2 ■). Young children in childcare, for example, are in close contact with other children who are susceptible to most infectious organisms. In some cases it is not possible to limit exposure to certain organisms as a child may be contagious before symptoms appear, such as with varicella (chickenpox) and parvovirus B-19 (Fifth disease). See Table 19–5 on page 620 for more information about these communicable diseases.

TABLE 19–1 Risk Factors for Infection in Newborns

TIME PERIOD	RISK FACTORS
Prenatal	Maternal infection Preterm labor Premature rupture of membranes Maternal substance abuse
Perinatal	Maternal infection in gastrointestinal and genitourinary tracts Internal fetal monitoring Assisted delivery resulting in skin lacerations Vaginal examinations of mother
Postnatal	Low birth weight, preterm, intrauterine growth restriction Skin breakdown Invasive catheters Endotracheal intubation Exposure to infections of other infants or healthcare personnel

Adapted from McKenney, W. M. (2001). Understanding the neonatal immune system: High risk for infection. Critical Care Nurse, *21(6), 38.*

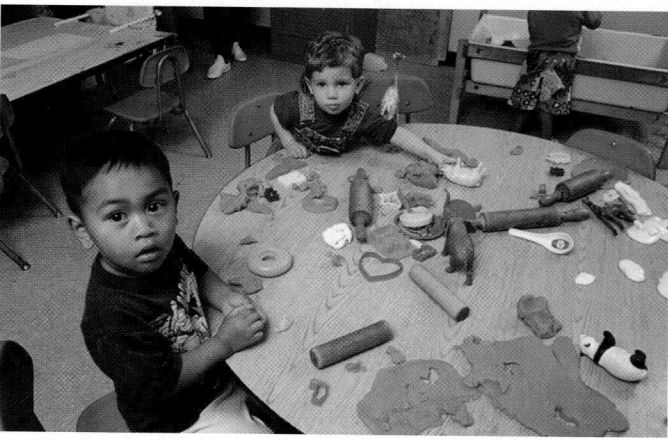

FIGURE 19–2 ■ Infectious diseases are easily transmitted in setting such as childcare centers where children handle common objects after coughing, sneezing, or drooling on them. The organisms survive to be picked up by another child handling the same object. The child then may rub the eyes, nose, or mouth and introduces the infection. Young children depend upon caregivers to help break the chain of infection.

As healthy children are exposed to more infections, they develop antibodies naturally. Thus, subsequent infections with the same type of organism may be less severe or avoided. (Refer to "Anatomy and Physiology of Pediatric Differences" in Chapter 27∞.) See Developing Cultural Competence: Disease Causation.

Infection Control

The poor hygiene behaviors of young children and their caregivers facilitate transmission of infectious diseases among young children in childcare settings and other environments such as hospitals, clinics, and physician offices. The fecal–oral and respiratory routes are the most common sources of transmission in children. Children usually do not wash their hands after toileting unless they are closely supervised. They put toys and their hands in their mouths, and then rub their nose and eyes. They often are unable to care for a runny nose without help. Diapers may leak stool and provide the fecal exposure to organisms. In addition, caregivers in childcare centers, other persons caring for children, and healthcare professionals may not use proper handwashing techniques (Figure 19–3 ■). All of these behaviors promote the transmission of infection. See Partnering with Families: Reducing the Transmission of Infection.

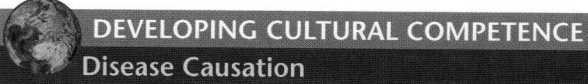

DEVELOPING CULTURAL COMPETENCE
Disease Causation

In some cultures infectious diseases are seen as punishment or the result of curses or evil spirits. For example, some Native Americans traditionally view illnesses as the result of disharmony or displeasing the spirits. They may not believe in the germ theory of disease causation.

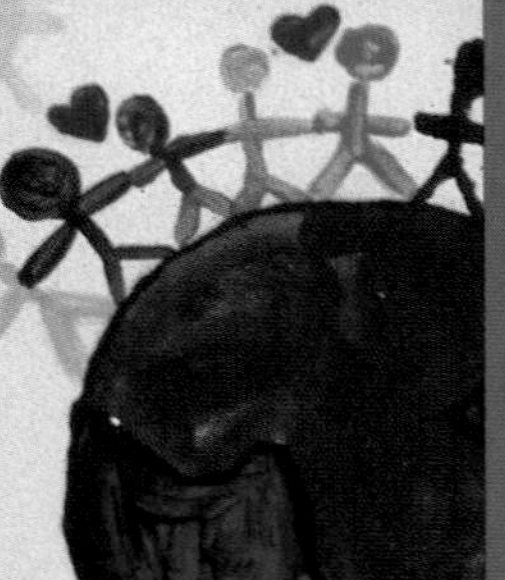

PARTNERING WITH FAMILIES

Reducing the Transmission of Infection

Teach families to reduce transmission of infection among family members with the following practices.

- Use disposable tissues and discard immediately after use.
- Wash hands thoroughly with soap and water or gels after all contact with the child's diaper, runny nose, and mucous membranes.
- Teach children to cough or sneeze into their elbow rather than into their hands.
- Teach children to wash their hands with soap and water after toileting and before eating.
- Do not allow children to share dishes and utensils.
- Wipe kitchen counters and surfaces where food is prepared and eaten with a disinfectant such as Lysol or a bleach solution. Wash hands well before preparing food. Follow guidelines for safe food preparation and storage.
- Wash dishes in warm soapy water or use the sanitizing cycle on the dishwasher.
- Wipe counters and surfaces that are used for diaper change or that the child touches with a disinfectant such as Lysol, a bleach solution, or isopropyl alcohol. Make sure the diaper changing area is well away from food preparation areas.
- Dispose of diapers in closed containers.

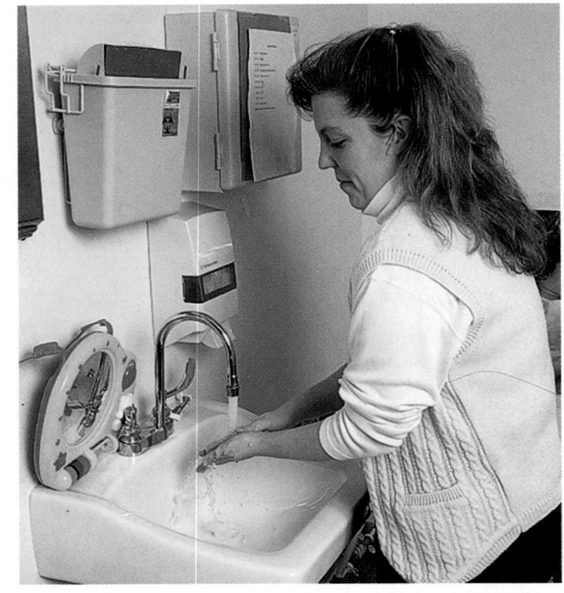

FIGURE 19–3 ■ Proper handwashing with soap and water for 1 to 2 minutes is one of the most effective measures in preventing transmission of microorganisms. Alcohol-based hand rubs which take less than 30 seconds to use are a good alternative to handwashing. Selecting a hand rub with an emollient may reduce dryness and cracking of the skin. Placing dispensers in convenient locations may increase the number of times the hands are cleaned.

Preventing the spread of infectious diseases is a process that involves several strategies that must be well coordinated. Proper handwashing is one of the most important health promotion strategies for all age groups of children as well as childcare providers (Box 19–1).

Nurses have a significant role in this process and are responsible for implementing several infection control strategies.

- Use standard precautions. See Box 19–2 for standard precautions and transmission-based precautions guidelines.
- Separate or quarantine ill children from well children. Perform triage of children frequently in clinics and physician offices to identify children who should not stay in the waiting room with other children. Similarly, separate hospitalized children with infections from those at great risk for infection, such as children with compromised immune systems.
- Promote and provide immunizations. See the immunization schedule on page 602.
- Eliminate the habitat or reservoir of the host (e.g., eliminate standing water where mosquitoes breed, killing mosquitoes that carry west Nile virus).
- Kill the pathogen (e.g., sanitize toys and contact surfaces).
- Educate parents and caregivers of children about the need for handwashing and standard precautions, safe food preparation and storage, taking action to avoid exposure to certain organisms (e.g., ticks that cause Lyme disease), and the importance of immunizations.

Public health authorities conduct **disease surveillance,** monitoring patterns of disease occurrence from the cases of infectious and communicable diseases reported by healthcare workers to state health officials. Outcomes of past disease surveillance efforts have resulted in major public health programs and scientific advances such as safer drinking water, better sanitation, improved standards of living, national immunization

BOX 19–1 Research: Handwashing in the Classroom

A study conducted in five school districts involving 16 schools and 6,000 children in four states evaluated the impact of a waterless alcohol gel hand sanitizer on elementary school absenteeism. Students and teachers in the study group classrooms were educated about the importance of handwashing, and dispensers with the hand sanitizing gel were placed in each classroom. Students were asked to use the hand gel upon entering and leaving the classroom, after using the restroom, and after they coughed or sneezed. Students in the control classrooms were asked to continue their usual procedure for handwashing in the restroom. Significant reductions in student absenteeism were found in three of five school districts; one school district had reduced student absenteeism but not at a statistically significant level. Additionally, a 10% reduction in teacher absenteeism was found in the largest school district. This study supports the earlier studies about the value of handwashing in controlling the transmission of infection (Hammond, Ali, Fendler, et al., 2000). This study reaffirms the value of handwashing, and the role of nurses in teaching parents and children the importance of frequent handwashing as a health promotion measure.

BOX 19–2 Infection Control Methods

STANDARD PRECAUTIONS

- Wash hands before and after patient contact and when needed during contact.
- Wear gloves when contact with blood, body fluids, secretions, excretions, nonintact skin, or mucous membranes might occur. Change gloves each time they are contaminated with these substances, washing hands before regloving.
- Wear additional protective equipment such as gown, mask, and goggles if body fluid splashes can occur.
- Wear the protective equipment to clean up body fluid spills. Discard waste in appropriate body substance waste containers. Clean the area with bleach or another acceptable cleaner. Bag contaminated laundry in secured and labeled bags.
- Discard needles, scalpels, and lancets in labeled sharps containers without recapping.
- Place patients who could contaminate the environment with airborne or droplet infection in private rooms.

TRANSMISSION-BASED PRECAUTIONS

- Use airborne precautions for diseases transported by the airborne route, such as measles, chickenpox, or tuberculosis. Care providers use high-efficiency particulate air filter respirators (or other respirators that filter inspired air) for protection. In addition, a negative airflow ventilation system room is needed for tuberculosis. The patient in airborne precautions must wear a surgical mask when leaving the room to filter expired air. Keep the patient's room door closed.
- Use droplet precautions for diseases transmitted by the droplet route, such as Haemophilus influenzae type b, pneumonia, rubella, and pertussis. A surgical mask is needed when coming within 3 feet of the patient. The patient wears a mask when leaving the room. The room door can remain open, and special respirators are not required.
- Use contact precautions for diseases, such as hepatitis A, E. coli, and gonorrhea, that spread by direct contact with the skin or by indirect contact with a contaminated object in the patient's environment. Apply gloves for all care. Use antimicrobial soap for handwashing after removing gloves, and do not touch potentially contaminated surfaces or items in the patient's room. Gowns are worn if the healthcare professional's clothing may come in contact with contaminated surfaces or the patient. Patients should be placed in a private room or with other patients with the same pathogen.

initiatives, and advanced medical treatment that have resulted in reduction or elimination of many infectious and communicable diseases over the past century. See Chapter 1∞. While many infectious and communicable diseases have decreased in occurrence, they remain a significant source of morbidity and mortality in infants and children, especially in developing countries.

IMMUNIZATION

The development and widespread availability of vaccines has been one of the great breakthroughs of modern medicine. The average infant born in 2004 receives 20 immunizations for 11 childhood diseases by the age of 6 years. The 11 childhood diseases for which vaccines are routinely recommended include the following: measles, mumps, rubella, polio, pertussis (whooping cough), diphtheria, tetanus, Haemophilus influenzae type b, hepatitis B, pneumococcus, and varicella (chickenpox). Beginning in 2004, the influenza vaccine is recommended for infants 6 months of age and older. Administering these vaccines greatly improves the health of children and reduces the parental burden of caring for ill children.

Before the 1950s, when infants and childhood immunization programs were initiated, the annual impact of infectious and communicable diseases in the United States was as follows (Children's Hospital of Philadelphia, 2003):

- Polio paralyzed 10,000 children.
- Rubella caused birth defects and mental retardation in up to 20,000 newborns.
- Measles infected 4 million children and caused 3,000 deaths.
- Diphtheria was one of the most common causes of death in school-age children.
- Haemophilus influenzae type b caused meningitis in 15,000 children, leaving many with permanent brain damage.
- Pertussis-related deaths occurred in thousands of infants.

MediaLink Infectious and Communicable Diseases Resources

Etiology and Pathophysiology

Immunization introduces an **antigen** (a foreign substance that triggers an immune system response) into the body, allowing immunity against a disease to develop naturally. The person produces antibodies, which are proteins capable of responding to specific antigens. In **active immunity** (in which antibody production is stimulated without causing clinical disease), an antigen is given in the form of a vaccine.

When a child needs antibodies faster than the body can develop them, **passive immunity** may be induced, with antibodies produced in another human or animal host and given to the child. This approach is also used with at-risk children after a single exposure to a disease to prevent the disease from occurring or to reduce its severity. For example, if a child who has never had a tetanus immunization steps on a rusty nail, the child needs immediate protection (passive immunity) from tetanus. Tetanus immune globulin injection is given to combat the tetanus toxin produced by the bacterial spores introduced by the nail. Because passive immunity does not confer lasting immunity, the process of antibody development (active immunity) is then initiated with the administration of a tetanus toxoid vaccine.

Since the first vaccines were developed in the late 1800s, many diseases have decreased dramatically in incidence. The introduction of vaccines against childhood diseases such as smallpox, polio, and measles either eradicated or virtually eliminated deaths due to the disease. Since the introduction of the pneumococcal conjugate vaccine in 2000 and the administration of 20 million doses of the vaccine in the United States, a 35% reduction of invasive disease (meningitis and pneumonia) caused by pneumococcal strains resistant to penicillin, and a 78% reduction in disease caused by strains targeted in the vaccine has been seen in children less than 2 years of age (Whitney, Farley, & Hadler, 2003; Peters & Edwards, 2002). See Box 19–3 for the impact of the Canadian childhood immunization program.

Improvements in vaccine technology continue to increase the safety and efficacy of immunization against an increasing number of diseases. Today's vaccines are often produced synthetically by

BOX 19–3 Impact of the Canadian Immunization Program

Vaccine-preventable illnesses were significantly reduced in Canada following the implementation of universal immunization programs for measles, rubella, poliomyelitis, and Haemophilus influenzae type b. The average rate of reported disease in the 5-year period after the implementation of the programs fell by 90% for Haemophilus influenzae type b, 93% for measles, 99% for rubella, and 100% for poliomyelitis. No significant changes in sanitation, water, nutrition, healthcare, or other socioeconomic factor occurred during the period of estimating the benefit of the immunization program that could be responsible for these reductions (Bigham & Hoefer, 2001).

means of recombinant DNA technology or genetic engineering. This technology offers the benefit of decreased side effects while providing immunity for diseases. Many other vaccines are in development, including meningococcal conjugate vaccine, group A streptococccal vaccine, respiratory syncytial virus vaccine, and a parainfluenza virus vaccine. See Box 19–4 for the various types of vaccines used in childhood immunization programs.

Clinical Manifestations

Children receiving vaccines can have a variety of responses as the body responds to the injected antigen stimulating the immune response. Depending on the specific immunization, up to 50% of vaccine recipients have a local reaction that includes erythema, swelling, pain, and induration at the site of the injection. Systemic reactions that often occur include fever, fussiness or irritability, malaise, and anorexia. With some vaccines other systemic reactions include a rash or arthralgia.

Allergic reactions to vaccines do occur; however, the rate is low, with only 2,281 allergic reactions in 1.9 billion doses in the United States between 1991 and 2001. This is in contrast to the incidence of allergic reactions to food (6% to 8%) and antibiotics (7.3%) in children (Schuval, 2003). Local allergic reactions, such as a wheal and urticaria, can occur in minutes to hours after the injection. A severe local allergic reaction is manifested by warmth, erythema, edema, petechiae, or ulceration occurring 2 to 8 hours after vaccination. A non-life-threatening systemic allergic reaction, such as generalized urticaria or transient petechiae, may occur within minutes. Anaphylaxis is a life-threatening reaction that is manifested by hypotension, generalized urticaria, angioedema, and laryngeal edema has occurred in rare cases with nearly every vaccine. The reactions to specific vaccines can be found on the medications table listing common pediatric immunizations on page 606.

Other serious reactions to vaccines occur in rare instances, for which the National Vaccine Injury Compensation Program was established. See Box 19–5 for more information. The range of illnesses and disabilities that may occur include the following: anaphylaxis, encephalopathy, bacterial neuritis, chronic arthritis, thrombocytopenia purpura, and death. The significant reactions eligible for compensation specific to each vaccine are listed in Table 19–2.

BOX 19–4 Types of Vaccines

- **Killed virus vaccine**—a vaccine that contains a microorganism that has been killed but is still capable of inducing the human body to produce antibodies (e.g., inactivated poliovirus vaccine)
- **Toxoid**—a toxin that has been treated (by heat or chemical, such as formaldehyde) to weaken its toxic effects but retain its antigenicity (e.g., tetanus toxoid)
- **Live virus vaccine**—a vaccine that contains a microorganism in live but attenuated, or weakened, form (e.g., measles and varicella vaccines)
- **Recombinant forms**—an organism that has been genetically altered for use in vaccines (e.g., hepatitis B and pertussis **acellular vaccine,** which is a vaccine that uses proteins from, say, pertussis rather than the whole cell to stimulate the process of active immunity)
- **Conjugated forms**—an altered organism that is joined with another substance to increase the immune response (e.g., the Pneumococcal Conjugate Vaccine and Haemophilus influenzae type b (Hib) vaccine are conjugated with a protein carrier such as tetanus toxoid or diphtheria toxoid; however, there is no immunity to tetanus or diphtheria conferred by these vaccines)

MediaLink Vaccine Schedule

COLLABORATIVE CARE

The recommended schedule for immunization is updated at least annually to reflect new vaccines and the need for repeat immunization. The Advisory Committee on Immunization Practices (ACIP) of the Centers for Disease Control, the American Academy of Pediatrics (AAP), and the American Academy of Family Practitioners (AAFP) collaborate to provide a uniform vaccination schedule. See Figure 19–4 ■ for the recommended schedule of immunizations in the United States; see Figure 19–5 ■ for the immunization schedule for Canadian infants and children. Because the vaccine schedule changes at least annually, visit the CDC website for the most current recommendations. This schedule applies to immunizations all children should receive, and schedules and recommendations vary for children who begin immunizations later in childhood or need catch-up doses. Other immunization recommendations are made for children who recently received blood products or immunosuppressive agents. Supplemental immunizations for meningococcal and pneumococcal infections are recommended for certain children, as noted in the table on page 609.

Pediatric healthcare providers—physicians, nurses, advance practice nurses, and physician associates—use the immunization

BOX 19–5 Vaccine Safety

The National Childhood Vaccine Injury Act of 1986 provides compensation if a link between immunization and a serious adverse effect is found. This act resulted after serious neurologic adverse reactions from pertussis immunizations were reported, creating significant liability concerns for healthcare professionals. The Vaccine Adverse Event Reporting System (VAERS) was established in 1988 to track serious vaccine reactions. Follow-up of the patient's condition occurs at 60 days and 1 year after the adverse event. Follow guidelines for reporting according to the Vaccine Adverse Event Reporting System detailed in Table 19–2.

TABLE 19–2 National Vaccine Injury Compensation Program—Vaccine Injury Table

VACCINE	ILLNESS, DISABILITY, INJURY, OR CONDITION COVERED	TIME PERIOD FOR FIRST SYMPTOM OR MANIFESTATION OF ONSET OR OF SIGNIFICANT AGGRAVATION AFTER VACCINE ADMINISTRATION—FOR COMPENSATION
Tetanus toxoid-containing vaccines (e.g., DTaP, DTP-Hib, DT, Td, or TT)	Anaphylaxis or anaphylactic shock	0–4 hours
	Bacterial neuritis	2–28 days
	Any acute complication or sequela (including death) of above events.	Not applicable
Pertussis antigen-containing vaccines (e.g., DTaP, DTP, P, DTP-Hib)	Anaphylaxis or anaphylactic shock	0–4 hours
	Encephalopathy (or encephalitis)	0–72 hours
	Any acute complication or sequela (including death) of above events.	Not applicable
Measles, mumps, rubella virus-containing vaccines in any combination (e.g., MMR, MR, M, R)	Anaphylaxis or anaphylactic shock	0–4 hours
	Encephalopathy (or encephalitis)	5–15 days
	Any acute complication or sequela (including death) of above events.	Not applicable
Rubella virus-containing vaccines (e.g., MMR, MR, R)	Chronic arthritis	7–42 days
	Any acute complication or sequela (including death) of above events.	Not applicable
Measles virus-containing vaccines	Thrombocytopenia purpura	7–30 days
	Vaccine strain measles viral infection in an immunodeficient recipient.	0–6 months
	Any acute complication or sequela (including death) of above events.	Not applicable
Polio inactivated virus-containing vaccines (e.g., IPV)	Anaphylaxis or anaphylactic shock	0–4 hours
	Any acute complication or sequela (including death) of above events.	No limit
Hepatitis B antigen-containing vaccines	Anaphylaxis or anaphylactic shock	0–4 hours
	Any acute complication or sequela (including death) of above events.	No limit
Haemophilus influenzae type B polysaccharide conjugate vaccines	No condition specified for compensation	Not applicable
Varicella vaccine	No condition specified for compensation	Not applicable
Rotavirus vaccine	No condition specified for compensation	Not applicable
Vaccines containing live, oral, rhesus-based rotavirus	Intussusception	0–30 days
	Any condition or sequela (including death) of above event	Not applicable
Pneumococcal conjugate vaccine	No condition specified for compensation	Not applicable

From: Health Resources and Services Administration Office of Special Programs. (2002). National Childhood Vaccine Injury Act Vaccine Injury Table, http://www.hrsa.gov/osp/ vicp/table.htm. *Accessed 9/30/2003. For aids to interpret defined conditions – go to the Vaccine Injury Table at the above website.*

schedules to ensure that infants and children become fully immunized. Vaccines should be administered at specific ages and intervals. Timing for first immunizations is determined by the age at which **transplacental immunity** (passive immunity transferred from mother to infant) decreases or disappears, and the infant or child develops the ability to make antibodies in response to the vaccine. Scientists continue to study the duration of protection from vaccines. Some vaccines do not confer lifelong immunity, and variable numbers of doses are required depending on vaccine and the age of the child to whom it is administered.

Vaccine ▼ / Age ▶	Birth	1 month	2 months	4 months	6 months	12 months	15 months	18 months	24 months	4–6 years	11–12 years	13–18 years
Hepatitis B[1]	HepB #1	HepB #2			HepB #3				HepB Series			
Diphtheria, Tetanus, Pertussis[2]			DTaP	DTaP	DTaP		DTaP			DTaP	Td	Td
Haemophilus influenzae type b[3]			Hib	Hib	Hib	Hib						
Inactivated Poliovirus			IPV	IPV	IPV					IPV		
Measles, Mumps, Rubella[4]						MMR #1				MMR #2	MMR #2	
Varicella[5]						Varicella			Varicella			
Pneumococcal[6]			PCV	PCV	PCV	PCV			PCV		PPV	
Influenza[7]					Influenza (Yearly)					Influenza (Yearly)		
Vaccines below red line are for selected populations												
Hepatitis A[8]										Hepatitis A Series		

This schedule indicates the recommended ages for routine administration of currently licensed childhood vaccines, as of December 1, 2004, for children through age 18 years. Any dose not given at the recommended age should be given at any subsequent visit when indicated and feasible.

▬ Indicates age groups that warrant special effort to administer those vaccines not previously given. Additional vaccines may be licensed and recommended during the year. Licensed combination vaccines may be used whenever any components of the combination are indicated and the vaccine's other components are not contraindicated. Providers should consult the manufacturers' package inserts for detailed recommendations. Clinically significant adverse events that follow immunization should be reported to the Vaccine Adverse Event Reporting System (VAERS). Guidance about how to obtain and complete a VAERS form can be found on the Internet: **www.vaers.org** or by calling **800-822-7967**.

Range of recommended ages | **Only if mother HBsAg(−)**

Preadolescent assessment | **Catch-up immunization**

1. **Hepatitis B (HepB) vaccine.** All infants should receive the first dose of hepatitis B vaccine soon after birth and before hospital discharge; the first dose may also be given by age 2 months if the infant's mother is hepatitis B surface antigen (HBsAg) negative. Only monovalent HepB can be used for the birth dose. Monovalent or combination vaccine containing HepB may be used to complete the series. Four doses of vaccine may be administered when a birth dose is given. The second dose should be given at least 4 weeks after the first dose, except for combination vaccines which cannot be administered before age 6 weeks. The third dose should be given at least 16 weeks after the first dose and at least 8 weeks after the second dose. The last dose in the vaccination series (third or fourth dose) should not be administered before age 24 weeks.

   Infants born to HBsAg-positive mothers should receive HepB and 0.5 mL of Hepatitis B Immune Globulin (HBIG) within 12 hours of birth at separate sites. The second dose is recommended at age 1–2 months. The last dose in the immunization series should not be administered before age 24 weeks. These infants should be tested for HBsAg and antibody to HBsAg (anti-HBs) at age 9–15 months.

   Infants born to mothers whose HBsAg status is unknown should receive the first dose of the HepB series within 12 hours of birth. Maternal blood should be drawn as soon as possible to determine the mother's HBsAg status; if the HBsAg test is positive, the infant should receive HBIG as soon as possible (no later than age 1 week). The second dose is recommended at age 1–2 months. The last dose in the immunization series should not be administered before age 24 weeks.

2. **Diphtheria and tetanus toxoids and acellular pertussis (DTaP) vaccine.** The fourth dose of DTaP may be administered as early as age 12 months, provided 6 months have elapsed since the third dose and the child is unlikely to return at age 15–18 months. The final dose in the series should be given at age ≥4 years. **Tetanus and diphtheria toxoids (Td)** is recommended at age 11–12 years if at least 5 years have elapsed since the last dose of tetanus and diphtheria toxoid-containing vaccine. Subsequent routine Td boosters are recommended every 10 years.

3. ***Haemophilus influenzae* type b (Hib) conjugate vaccine.** Three Hib conjugate vaccines are licensed for infant use. If PRP-OMP (PedvaxHIB or ComVax [Merck]) is administered at ages 2 and 4 months, a dose at age 6 months is not required. DTaP/Hib combination products should not be used for primary immunization in infants at ages 2, 4 or 6 months but can be used as boosters following any Hib vaccine. The final dose in the series should be given at age ≥12 months.

4. **Measles, mumps, and rubella vaccine (MMR).** The second dose of MMR is recommended routinely at age 4–6 years but may be administered during any visit, provided at least 4 weeks have elapsed since the first dose and both doses are administered beginning at or after age 12 months. Those who have not previously received the second dose should complete the schedule by the visit at age 11–12 years.

5. **Varicella vaccine.** Varicella vaccine is recommended at any visit at or after age 12 months for susceptible children (i.e., those who lack a reliable history of chickenpox). Susceptible persons aged ≥13 years should receive 2 doses, given at least 4 weeks apart.

6. **Pneumococcal vaccine.** The heptavalent **pneumococcal conjugate vaccine (PCV)** is recommended for all children aged 2–23 months. It is also recommended for certain children aged 24–59 months. The final dose in the series should be given at age ≥12 months. **Pneumococcal polysaccharide vaccine (PPV)** is recommended in addition to PCV for certain high-risk groups. See *MMWR* 2000;49(RR-9):1-35.

7. **Influenza vaccine.** Influenza vaccine is recommended annually for children aged ≥6 months with certain risk factors (including but not limited to asthma, cardiac disease, sickle cell disease, HIV, and diabetes), healthcare workers, and other persons (including household members) in close contact with persons in groups at high risk (see *MMWR* 2004;53[RR-6]:1-40) and can be administered to all others wishing to obtain immunity. In addition, healthy children aged 6–23 months and close contacts of healthy children aged 0–23 months are recommended to receive influenza vaccine, because children in this age group are at substantially increased risk for influenza-related hospitalizations. For healthy persons aged 5–49 years, the intranasally administered live, attenuated influenza vaccine (LAIV) is an acceptable alternative to the intramuscular trivalent inactivated influenza vaccine (TIV). See *MMWR* 2004;53(RR-6):1-40. Children receiving TIV should be administered a dosage appropriate for their age (0.25 mL if 6–35 months or 0.5 mL if ≥3 years). Children aged ≤8 years who are receiving influenza vaccine for the first time should receive 2 doses (separated by at least 4 weeks for TIV and at least 6 weeks for LAIV).

8. **Hepatitis A vaccine.** Hepatitis A vaccine is recommended for children and adolescents in selected states and regions and for certain high-risk groups; consult your local public health authority. Children and adolescents in these states, regions, and high-risk groups who have not been immunized against hepatitis A can begin the hepatitis A immunization series during any visit. The 2 doses in the series should be administered at least 6 months apart. See *MMWR* 1999;48(RR-12):1-37.

FIGURE 19–4A ■ Recommended immunization schedule for United States children and adolescents, United States, 2005. Department of Health and Human Services, Centers for Disease Control and Prevention.

The tables below give catch-up schedules and minimum intervals between doses for children who have delayed immunizations. There is no need to restart a vaccine series regardless of the time that has elapsed between doses. Use the chart appropriate for the child's age.

CATCH-UP SCHEDULE FOR CHILDREN AGED 4 MONTHS THROUGH 6 YEARS

Vaccine	Minimum Age for Dose 1	Minimum Interval Between Doses			
		Dose 1 to Dose 2	Dose 2 to Dose 3	Dose 3 to Dose 4	Dose 4 to Dose 5
Diphtheria, Tetanus, Pertussis	6 wks	4 weeks	4 weeks	6 months	6 months[1]
Inactivated Poliovirus	6 wks	4 weeks	4 weeks	4 weeks[2]	
Hepatitis B[3]	Birth	4 weeks	8 weeks (and 16 weeks after first dose)		
Measles, Mumps, Rubella	12 mo	4 weeks[4]			
Varicella	12 mo				
Haemophilus influenzae type b[5]	6 wks	**4 weeks** if first dose given at age <12 months **8 weeks (as final dose)** if first dose given at age 12-14 months **No further doses needed** if first dose given at age ≥15 months	**4 weeks[6]** if current age <12 months **8 weeks (as final dose)[6]** if current age ≥12 months and second dose given at age <15 months **No further doses needed** if previous dose given at age ≥15 mo	**8 weeks (as final dose)** This dose only necessary for children aged 12 months–5 years who received 3 doses before age 12 months	
Pneumococcal[7]	6 wks	**4 weeks** if first dose given at age <12 months and current age <24 months **8 weeks (as final dose)** if first dose given at age ≥12 months or current age 24–59 months **No further doses needed** for healthy children if first dose given at age ≥24 months	**4 weeks** if current age <12 months **8 weeks (as final dose)** if current age ≥12 months **No further doses needed** for healthy children if previous dose given at age ≥24 months	**8 weeks (as final dose)** This dose only necessary for children aged 12 months–5 years who received 3 doses before age 12 months	

CATCH-UP SCHEDULE FOR CHILDREN AGED 7 YEARS THROUGH 18 YEARS

Vaccine	Minimum Interval Between Doses		
	Dose 1 to Dose 2	Dose 2 to Dose 3	Dose 3 to Booster Dose
Tetanus, Diphtheria	4 weeks	6 months	**6 months[8]** if first dose given at age <12 months and current age <11 years **5 years[8]** if first dose given at age ≥12 months and third dose given at age <7 years and current age ≥11 years **10 years[8]** if third dose given at age ≥7 years
Inactivated Poliovirus[9]	4 weeks	4 weeks	IPV[2,9]
Hepatitis B	4 weeks	8 weeks (and 16 weeks after first dose)	
Measles, Mumps, Rubella	4 weeks		
Varicella[10]	4 weeks		

1. **DTaP.** The fifth dose is not necessary if the fourth dose was given after the fourth birthday.
2. **IPV.** For children who received an all-IPV or all-oral poliovirus (OPV) series, a fourth dose is not necessary if third dose was given at age ≥4 years. If both OPV and IPV were given as part of a series, a total of 4 doses should be given, regardless of the child's current age.
3. **HepB.** All children and adolescents who have not been immunized against hepatitis B should begin the HepB immunization series during any visit. Providers should make special efforts to immunize children who were born in, or whose parents were born in, areas of the world where hepatitis B virus infection is moderately or highly endemic.
4. **MMR.** The second dose of MMR is recommended routinely at age 4–6 years but may be given earlier if desired.
5. **Hib.** Vaccine is not generally recommended for children aged ≥5 years.
6. **Hib.** If current age <12 months and the first 2 doses were PRP-OMP (PedvaxHIB or ComVax [Merck]), the third (and final) dose should be given at age 12–15 months and at least 8 weeks after the second dose.
7. **PCV.** Vaccine is not generally recommended for children aged ≥5 years.
8. **Td.** For children aged 7–10 years, the interval between the third and booster dose is determined by the age when the first dose was given. For adolescents aged 11–18 years, the interval is determined by the age when the third dose was given.
9. **IPV.** Vaccine is not generally recommended for persons aged ≥18 years.
10. **Varicella.** Give 2-dose series to all susceptible adolescents aged ≥13 years.

FIGURE 19–4B ■ Recommended immunization schedule for children and adolescents who start late or who are more than 1 month behind, United States, 2005.

A. Routine Immunization Schedule for Infants and Children

Age at Vaccination	DtaP[1]	IPV	Hib[2]	MMR	Td[3] or dTap[10]	Hep B[4] (3 doses)	V	PC	MC
Birth									
2 months	X	X	X					X[8]	X[9]
4 months	X	X	X			Infancy		X	X
6 months	X	(X)[5]	X			or		X	X
12 months				X		preadolescence	X[7]	X	
18 months	X	X	X	(X)[6] or		(9-13 years)			or
4-6 years	X	X		(X)[6]					
14-16 years					X[10]				X[9]

DTaP Diphtheria, tetanus, pertussis (acellular) vaccine
IPV Inactivated poliovirus vaccine
Hib *Haemophilus influenzae* type b conjugate vaccine
MMR Measles, mumps, and rubella vaccine
Td Tetanus and diphtheria toxoid, adult type with reduced diphtheria toxoid
dTap Tetanus and diphtheria toxoid, acellular pertussis, adolescent/adult type with reduced diphtheria and pertussis components
Hep B Hepatitis B vaccine
V Varicella
PC Pneumoccoccal conjugate vaccine
MC Meningococcal C conjugate vaccine

B. Routine Immunization Schedule for Children < 7 Years of Age Not Immunized in Early Infancy

Timing	DTaP[1]	IPV	Hib	MMR	Td[3] or dTap[10]	Hep B[4] (3 doses)	V	P	M
First visit	X	X	X[11]	X[12]		X	X[7]	X[8]	X[9]
2 months later	X	X	X	(X)[6]		X		(X)	(X)
2 months later	X	(X)[5]						(X)	
6-12 months later	X	X	(X)[11]			X			
4-6 years of age[13]	X	X							
14-16 years of age					X				

P Pneumococcal vaccine
M Meningococcal vaccine

FIGURE 19–5 ■ Recommended immunization schedule for Canadian infants and children, Pediatric Clinical Guidelines, Table 10–7B. Immunization schedule, http:/www.phac-aspc.gc.ca/dird-dimr/is-cv/index.html. Accessed 9/27/2004. Health Canada, reproduced with the permission of the Minister of Public Works and Government Services Canada, 2004.

Efforts to increase the numbers of children protected from vaccine-preventable diseases and to monitor immunization status is a national public health initiative. *Healthy People 2010* states important goals for reduction of vaccine preventable diseases.

- Adequately immunize 90% of U.S. children by their second birthday.
- Adequately immunize 95% of children in kindergarten and first grade.
- Have 95% of children less than 6 years of age participating in a fully operational population-based immunization registry. Once fully operational, the registries should meet 13 functional standards that will enable states or managed care organizations to monitor the immunization status of their population (Department of Health and Human Services, 1999; Centers for Disease Control, 2002b).

Many missed opportunities to immunize children have been identified. Children (and siblings present) should have their immunization status assessed during all healthcare visits, hospitalizations, and in schools. Efforts to increase immunization levels among children are also supported by managed care organizations that require contracted healthcare providers to comply with the pediatric immunization standards, and patient records are audited to ensure compliance.

The reported level of full immunization for children between 19 and 35 months of age in 2002 was 65.5%. Full immunization was defined as four doses of DTP/DT/DTaP, three doses of poliovirus vaccine, one measles-containing vaccine,

C. Routine Immunization Schedule for Children > 7 Years of Age Not Immunized in Early Infancy

Timing	dTap[10]	IPV	MMR	Hep B[4] (3 doses)	V	M
First visit	X	X	X	X	X	X[9]
2 months later	X	X	X[6]	X	(X)[7]	
6-12 months later	X	X		X		
10 years later	X					
M Meningoccocal vaccine						

1. DTaP (diphtheria, tetanus, acellular or component pertussis) vaccine is the preferred vaccine for all doses in the vaccination series, including completion of the series in children who have received > 1 dose of DPT (whole cell) vaccine.
2. Hib schedule shown is for PRP-T or HbOC vaccine. If PRP-OMP is used, give at 2, 4 and 12 months of age.
3. Td (tetanus and diphtheria toxoid), a combined adsorbed "adult type" preparation for use in people > 7 years of age, contains less diphtheria toxoid than preparations given to younger children and is less likely to cause reactions in older people.
4. Hepatitis B vaccine can be routinely given to infants or preadolescents, depending on the provincial/territorial policy; three doses at 0, 1 and 6 month intervals are preferred. The second dose should be administered at least 1 month after the first dose, and the third at least 2 months after the second dose. A two-dose schedule for adolescents is also possible (see chapter on Hepatitis B Vaccine).
5. This dose is not needed routinely, but can be included for convenience.
6. A second dose of MMR is recommended, at least 1 month after the first dose for the purpose of better measles protection. For convenience, options include giving it with the next scheduled vaccination at 18 months of age or with school entry (4-6 years) vaccinations (depending on the provincial/territorial policy), or at any intervening age that is practicable. The need for a second dose of mumps and rubella vaccine is not established but may benefit (given for convenience as MMR). The second dose of MMR should be given at the same visit as DTaP IPV (+ Hib) to ensure high uptake rates.
7. Children aged 12 months to 12 years should receive one dose of varicella vaccine. Individuals > 13 years of age should receive two doses at least 28 days apart.
8. Recommended schedule, number of doses and subsequent use of 23 valent polysaccharide pneumococcal vaccine depend on the age of the child when vaccination is begun.
9. Recommended schedule and number of doses of meningococcal vaccine depends on the age of the child.
10. dTap adult formulation with reduced diphtheria toxoid and pertussis component.
11. Recommended schedule and number of doses depend on the product used and age of the child when vaccination is begun (see the 6th *Edition 2002 Canadian Immunization Guide* for specific recommendations). Not required past age 5.
12. Delay until subsequent visit if child is < 12 months of age.
13. Omit these doses if the previous doses of DTaP and polio were given after the fourth birthday.

FIGURE 19–5 ■ (Continued)

three doses of Hib vaccine, three doses of hepatitis B vaccine, and one dose of varicella vaccine. If varicella vaccine is not considered, the level of immunization is 74.8% (Barker, Darling, McCauley, et al., 2003). Very small gains in levels of vaccination have occurred over the past few years, but many children are not fully immunized and at risk for vaccine-preventable diseases. The reported level of full immunization (with the exception of hepatitis B) for children entering kindergarten and first grade, based on state requirements, was ≥ 95% in 29 states and ≥ 90% in 45 states (Centers for Disease Control, 2003a).

Immunization of Immigrants

Children less than 10 years of age who are internationally adopted are not required to have proof of immunizations prior to entry into the United States; however, adoptive parents are required to indicate their intent to have the child become fully immunized. For other child immigrants, such as refugees, vaccines should be administered according to a catch-up schedule when no record of immunizations is available. Alternatively, antibody titers can be measured for the various vaccines to determine the child's need for additional immunizations (American Academy of Pediatrics, 2003). Many vaccines on the U.S. recommended schedule may not be available in countries of the child's origin.

Challenges in Achieving Optimal Immunization Rates

Lower immunization rates of children are often associated with economic factors, limited access to healthcare, lack of primary care at hours convenient for working parents, inadequate education regarding the importance of immunization, and religious prohibitions. The federal Vaccine for Children program that provides free vaccines for qualified children and adolescents less than 19 years of age has resolved some of the economic factors associated with vaccine coverage. However, the cost of vaccines such as the pneumococcal conjugate vaccine (at about $75 per

MEDICATIONS Common Pediatric Immunizations

IMMUNIZATION TYPE	SIDE EFFECTS	CONTRAINDICATIONS	NURSING CONSIDERATIONS
Diphtheria and Pertussis Vaccines and Tetanus Toxiod (DTaP) *Type:* Inactivated *Route:* Intramuscular *Dosage:* 0.5 mL *Age(s) Given:* 2, 4, 6, 15–18 months; 4–6 years (five doses) May give at same time as all other vaccines, in a separate site. *Storage:* Store in body of refrigerator at 2–8°(35–46°F). Do not freeze. Tripedia and Infanrix are licensed for all 5 doses. Daptacel is licensed for the first 4 doses. Pediarix is composed of DTaP, Hep B, and IPV and can be given as the primary series. TriHiBit is composed of DTaP and Hib.	*Common:* Redness, pain, swelling, nodule at injection site; temperature up to 38.3°C (101°F); drowsiness, irritability, fussiness; anorexia within 2 days of injection. Increase in frequency and magnitude of local reactions with doses 4 and 5, e.g., entire limb swelling. *Serious:* Allergic reaction, anaphylaxis; shock or collapse (hypotonic-hyperresponsive episode— sudden loss of muscle tone, pallor, fever, and unresponsiveness), fever above 38.8°C (102°F); febrile seizure; persistent inconsolable crying; coma or permanent brain damage.	Gelatin allergy (do not use Tripedia) Occurrence of a serious side effect after previous administration of DTaP, such as anaphylaxis or encephalopathy within 7 days after DTP or DTaP. Precautions in additional doses should be considered in children with the following reactions within 48 hours of the previous dose: ➤ Fever ≥ 40.5°C (105°F) ➤ Continuous inconsolable crying lasting ≥ 3 hours ➤ Pale or limp episode or collapse Convulsion within 3 days of dose. Administration should be delayed for 1 month after immunosuppressive therapy and until moderate to severe febrile illnesses have resolved. Administration of immune serum globulin within last 90 days.	Use same brand for all doses where feasible. Prior to immunization, ask about previous reactions to immunization. DTaP may coincide with or hasten the recognition of a seizure disorder. In children with a history of seizures with or without fever, give acetaminophen at the time of vaccine and then every 4 hours for 24 hours. Shake vaccine before withdrawing. Solution will be cloudy. If it contains clumps that cannot be resuspended, do not use. Daptacel stopper vial contains latex. Pediarix stopper vial is latex free. When required, simultaneous administration of tetanus immune globulin or diphtheria antitoxin should be given in separate sites with a new needle and syringe. Inform parents of the chance of increased reaction to doses 4 and 5. Defer the vaccine when the child has a progressive neurologic problem until the child is stable. DT is given to children < 7 years of age who have had a serious reaction to the pertussis component of the DTP or DTaP vaccine. Td is given to children ≥ 7 years. The series does not need to be restarted, no matter how long since the previous dose was given.
Poliovirus Vaccine (IPV) *Type:* Inactivated *Route:* Subcutaneous or intramuscular depending upon vaccine used *Dosage:* 0.5 mL *Age(s) given:* 2, 4, 12–18 months; 4–6 years (four doses) May give at same time as all other vaccines in a separate site. *Storage:* Store in body of refrigerator at 2–8°C (35–46°F). Do not freeze. Pediarix includes IPV along with DTaP and HepB. IPV may be given as single vaccine preparation.	*Common:* Swelling and tenderness, irritability, tiredness *Serious:* Allergic reaction or anaphylaxis	Hypersensitivity to vaccine components: neomycin, streptomycin, polymyxin B. Anaphylactic response. Pregnancy.	Prior to immunization, ask if the child has an allergy to neomycin, streptomycin, or polymyxin B (whichever of these antibiotics the specific vaccine to be used contains). Clear, colorless suspension. Do not use if it contains particulate matter, becomes cloudy, or changes color. Recommended for use in all vaccine doses. All doses must be separated by at least 4 weeks. The series does not need to be restarted, no matter how long since the previous dose was given.
Measles, Mumps, Rubella Vaccines (MMR) *Type:* Live attenuated *Route:* Subcutaneous *Dosage:* 0.5 mL *Age(s) given:* 12–15 months; 4–6 years (2 doses) May give at same time as all other vaccines in a separate site. *Storage:* Store in body of refrigerator at 2–8°C (35–46°F). When reconstituted, keep refrigerated and away from light; discard if unused within 8 hours. Diluent is stored at room temperature or in refrigerator. Do not freeze.	*Common:* Elevated temperature 1–2 weeks after immunization; redness or pain at injection site; noncontagious rash; joint pain. *Serious:* Allergic reaction or anaphylaxis; febrile seizure; meningitis (usually mild); encephalopathy; thrombocytopenia purpura; and rare cases of coma and permanent brain damage.	Prior anaphylactic reaction to vaccine Allergy to neomycin or gelatin. Severely impaired immune system due to malignancy, immune deficiency disease, immunosuppressive therapy. Wait at least 3–11 months after administration of immune serum globulin or blood products (time determined by the type) before giving vaccine. Pregnancy or possibility of pregnancy within 4 weeks. Thrombocytopenia or history of thrombocytopenic purpura Tuberculosis or positive PPD	Prior to immunization, ask if child has allergy to neomycin or gelatin. Observe the child with an egg allergy for 90 minutes after injection. Inquire about immunosuppression. MMR vaccine is recommended for those infected with HIV. Instruct adolescent girls to childbearing age to avoid pregnancy for 3 months after immunization. Give tuberculosis (TB) test at same time as MMR or 4–6 weeks later. If MMR and Varivax are not given on the same day, space them ≥ 28 days apart. Reconstituted vaccine is a clear, yellow solution. Give entire contents of reconstituted vial even if more than 0.5 mL. As college students are at greater risk due to decreasing immunity, make sure they have received a second MMR dose.

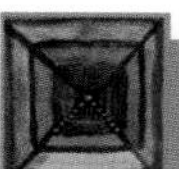

MEDICATIONS Common Pediatric Immunizations (continued)

IMMUNIZATION TYPE	SIDE EFFECTS	CONTRAINDICATIONS	NURSING CONSIDERATIONS
Hepatitis B Vaccine (HB) *Type:* Inactivated *Route:* Intramuscular *Dosage:* Engerix-B: 10 mcg or Recombivax HB: 5 mcg *Age(s) given:* Birth-2 months, 1 month after first dose; 6 months after first dose *or* Birth–2 months, 1–4 months, 6–18 months (3 doses) May give at same time as all other vaccines in a separate site. *Storage:* Store in body of refrigerator at 2–8°C (35–46°F). Do not freeze. Storage out of recommended temperature range decreases potency. Engerix-B and Recombivax HB are single vaccine preparations. Comvax is a combination of Hib and Hep B	*Common:* Pain or redness at injection site; headache; photophobia; altered liver enzymes. *Serious:* Allergic reaction or anaphylaxis; fever	Prior anaphylaxis, liver abnormalities. Serious allergic reaction to past dose. Yeast hypersensitivity	Prior to immunization, check status of mother's hepatitis B test and presence of other liver disease. Note: If mother has HbsAg+, vaccine must be given to infant within 12 hours of birth along with hepatitis B immune globulin at the same time in another site with new needle and syringe. Shake vaccine before withdrawing. Solution will appear cloudy. Various formulations (pediatric, adult, dialysis) are available in different strengths. Read package insert carefully to determine proper dosage for age for the particular formulation used. A 3-dose series can be started at any age. Minimum spacing for children and teens is 4 weeks between doses 1 and 2, and 8 weeks between doses 2 and 3. The last dose in an infant series should not be given before 6 months of age. Vaccine brands can be interchanged for 3-dose series. The series does not need to be restarted, no matter how long since the previous dose was given.
Haemophilus influenza Type B (Hib) *Type:* Inactivated *Route:* Intramuscular *Dosage:* 0.5 mL *Age(s) given:* 2, 4, 6, 12–15 months; (4 doses for HbOC[a] [HibTITER] and PRP-T[a] [ActHIB]) *or* 2, 4, 12–15 months (3 doses for PRP-OMP[a] [PedvaxHIB]) May give at same time as all other vaccines in a separate site. *Storage:* Store in body of refrigerator at 2–8°C (35–46°F). Do not freeze. Use or discard reconstituted ActHIB and OmniHIB within 30 minutes. Refrigerate reconstituted PedvaxHIB and discard within 24 hours. HibTITER, ActHib, OmniHib, and PedvaxHib are single vaccine preparations Comvax is a combination of PRP-OMP plus HB. TriHiBit is composed of DTaP and Hib	*Common:* Pain, redness, or swelling at site *Serious:* Allergic reaction of anaphylaxis (extremely rare); fever	Prior anaphylactic reaction to this vaccine.	Prior to immunizations, ask if child is immunosuppressed. Solution is clear and colorless. Since schedules for product preparations of different companies vary, it is important to read package inserts carefully. If the first dose is given between 7 and 11 months of age, 3 doses are needed. If the first dose was given at 12 to 14 months of age, give a booster dose in 8 weeks. If the first dose is given when the child is over 15 months or under 5 years, only 1 dose is needed. Second and third doses can be given 4 to 8 weeks after the first. Use the same vaccine preparation for all doses of the primary series if possible. The series does not need to be restarted, no matter how long since the previous dose was given.
Heptavalent Pneumococcal Conjugate Vaccine (PCV) *Type:* Inactivated *Route:* Intramuscular *Dosage:* 0.5 mL *Age(s) given:* 2, 4, 6, 12–15 months *Storage:* Store in body of refrigerator at 2–8°C (35–46°F). Do not freeze. Prevnar is a single vaccine preparation.	*Common:* Soreness, swelling, redness at injection site; mild to moderate fever; irritability, drowsiness, restless sleep, decreased appetite, vomiting and diarrhea, rash or hives. *Severe:* Allergic reaction or anaphylaxis	Hypersensitivity to diphtheria toxoid.	Clear, colorless, or slightly opalescent liquid. In addition to infants this vaccine is a priority for children 2-5 years with sickle cell disease, asplenia, HIV infection, or immunocompromised. The vaccine is also a priority for American Indian and Native Alaskan children 2-5 years because of their increased risk for pneumococcal disease. The series does not need to be restarted, no matter how long since the previous dose was given. (continued)

MEDICATIONS Common Pediatric Immunizations (continued)

IMMUNIZATION TYPE	SIDE EFFECTS	CONTRAINDICATIONS	NURSING CONSIDERATIONS
Varicella Virus Vaccine *Type:* Live attenuated *Route:* Subcutaneous *Dosage:* 0.5 mL *Age(s) given:* 12–18 months; or any time up to 12 years of age (one dose); 13 years or older (two doses 4–8 weeks apart) *Storage:* Frozen at 5°F or colder. May be stored in refrigerator at 2°–8°C (35°–46°F) up to 72 hours before reconstitution. Once reconstituted, vaccine must be used within 30 minutes or discarded. Do not refreeze. Diluent kept at room temperature. Varivax is a single vaccine preparation.	*Common:* Pain or redness at injection site; fever up to 38.8°C (102°F) in children or up to 37.7°C (100°F) in adults. Less commonly a vaccine-related rash (mild exanthem of 6 to 10 lesions that last for 2–3 days) may occur during first month after the injection. *Severe:* Allergic reaction or anaphylaxis; thrombocytopenia; febrile seizure; CNS manifestations.	Prior anaphylactic reaction to vaccine. Allergy to neomycin or gelatin. Immunodeficiency or receiving immunosuppression therapy. Administration of immune serum globulin or blood products in last 3–11 months. Active untreated TB. Pregnancy. Moderate or severe febrile illness.	Prior to immunization, ask if child is immunodeficient or on immunosuppression treatment or had an allergy to neomycin or gelatin. Determine if a family member is immunocompromised. Clear, colorless to pale yellow liquid when reconstituted. Give the entire contents of the vial even if more than 0.5 mL. Instruct adolescent girls of childbearing age to avoid pregnancy for 3 months after immunization. The vaccine is effective. Only very mild cases occurred in children who were immunized, primarily caused by wild type virus (Vazquez, LaRussa, Gershon, et al., 2001).
Hepatitis A *Type:* inactivated *Route:* intramuscular *Dosage:* 0.5 mL, 1 mL over 17 years for Vaqta[a], 1 mL over 18 years for Havrix[a] *Age(s) given:* 2–18 years, 6–12 months after first dose (2 doses) in areas with increased incidence. May give at same time as all other vaccines in a separate site. *Storage:* Store in body of refrigerator at 2–8°C (35–46°F). Do not freeze; do not use if frozen. Havrix and Vaqta are single vaccine preparations.	Rare reports of anaphylaxis/anaphylactoid reactions.	Known hypersensitivity to any component of vaccine. Prior hypersensitivity reaction to the vaccine.	Shake well, slightly opaque white suspension. Can be given for postexposure prophylaxis against Hepatitis A. Immune globulin and vaccine can be given at the same time in different sites. High incidence areas include the states of Alaska, Arkansas, Arizona, California, Colorado, Idaho, Missouri, Montana, New Mexico, Nevada, Oklahoma, Oregon, South Dakota, Texas, Utah, Washington, and Wyoming. Other high-risk populations to receive this vaccine include incarcerated youth, Native Alaskans, and American Indians. Do not restart the series, no matter how long since the previous dose. Vaccine brands can be interchanged.
Influenza *Type:* Inactivated (TIV), live attenuated for intranasal use (LAIV) *Route:* Intramuscular (all ages), intranasal (5 years and older) *Dosage:* 0.25 mL in infants 6–35 months, 0.5 mL beginning at 3 years May give at same time as all other vaccines in a separate site. *TIV Storage:* Store in body of refrigerator at 2–8°C (35–46°F). Do not freeze; do not use if frozen. *LAIV Storage:* Keep frozen. May be thawed and kept in refrigerator at 2–8°C (35–46°F) for no more than 24 hours before use. Flu Shield (Trivalent, inactivated vaccine) Flu Mist (LAIV)	*Common after TIV:* May have soreness or swelling at injection site, fever, aches. Life-threatening allergic reactions are rare. *Common after intranasal vaccine:* Runny nose or nasal congestion, fever, headache or muscle aches, abdominal pain and occasional vomiting. No life-threatening problems were detected during clinical trials.	Contraindicated in children with history of egg anaphylaxis, known sensitivity to gentamycin or other aminoglycosides. LAIV is contraindicated in children on long-term aspirin therapy; known or suspected immune deficiency disorders; immunosuppressed; or have an altered immune status due to various therapies. Should not be given within 3 days of pertussis vaccine (Mosby's Drug Consult, 2004) Postpone vaccine when child has acute febrile illness until symptoms abate, but may be given with minor illness, with or without fever.	Thawed intranasal vaccine is pale yellow, clear to slightly cloudy. Administered annually in autumn. Children with no history of influenza illness or vaccine need 2 doses 1 month apart. Intranasal dose is split (0.25 mL) with a dose divider clip. Administer in each nostril while child is sitting in an upright position. Insert the tip of the sprayer inside the nose and depress the plunger to spray. Children 8 years of age or younger who are receiving the influenza vaccine for the first time should get 2 doses separated by at least 4 weeks (injectable) and 6 weeks (intranasal). Must be reimmunized each year as immunity wanes.

[a]*Trade names*

Data from American Academy of Pediatrics. (2003). Red Book: Report of the Committee on Infectious Disease *(26th ed.). Elk Grove Village, IL: Author; Immunization Action Coalition; Mosby. (2004).* Mosby's drug consult 2004. *St. Louis: Mosby, Inc.; Bindler, R. M., & Howry, L. B. (1997).* Pediatric drugs and nursing implications *(2nd ed.). Stamford, CT: Appleton & Lange.*

MediaLink Case Study: Immunization Education Plan for the Reluctant Parent

MEDICATIONS Supplemental Immunizations

VACCINE	RECOMMENDATION
Meningococcal	For children older than 2 years of age with asplenia. Vaccine duration is 5 years or longer in children older than 4 years at the time of immunization. The vaccine is also recommended for college students residing in dormitories or other group living arrangements. The vaccine should be repeated after 1 year if the child is younger than 4 years at the time of initial immunization.
23-valent Pneumococcal	For children older than 2 years of age with sickle-cell disease, asplenia, chronic cardiovascular and pulmonary disorders, nephrotic syndrome, renal failure, HIV infection, cerebrospinal fluid leaks, or those undergoing immunosuppressive therapy. Repeat the immunization after 3–5 years if the child is younger than 10 years at the time of first immunization or at severe risk for pneumococcal infection.

Adapted from the American Academy of Pediatrics Committee on Infectious Disease. (2003). Red book: Report of the Committee on Infectious Disease *(25th ed.). Elk Grove Village, IL: Author.*

dose) is a barrier for children with private health insurance. This is particularly true in rural areas where private healthcare providers do not stock the vaccine due to cost. Children with health insurance are not eligible for the Vaccines for Children program; so local health departments do not provide the vaccine to these insured children (Bechtel, 2003). However, these children may not have access to a healthcare provider who stocks the vaccine or the ability to pay for the vaccine out of pocket. See Box 19–6.

However, an increasing number of parents are choosing not to immunize their children for philosophical reasons. Some of these reasons include the following (Coyer, 2002; Mera & Hackley, 2003):

- Vaccines are dangerous and may cause harm to their child, such as autism and sudden infant death syndrome. Additional concerns emerged when pressure was placed on vaccine manufacturers to remove thimerosal from vaccines (Box 19–7).
- Vaccines do not work—even some vaccinated children get the infectious disease, so the vaccines are not all that protective.
- There is disagreement with government regulation and monitoring of immunizations.
- The threat of the disease has diminished with vaccine success and improved sanitary conditions, and the need for immunization of their child is less important.
- The number of adverse events to vaccines now exceeds the number of cases of vaccine-preventable diseases, and the public has increased access to this information.
- Parents believe that they can control their child's susceptibility to disease and the outcome if they become infected.

See Table 19–3 for common misconceptions some parents have about vaccines and correct information. All healthcare providers should be consistent in their message about the value of vaccines and provide the following information to parents (Stinchfield, 2001).

- Immunization is one of the most important ways you can protect your child.
- Vaccines safety continues to improve because of advancements in medical research and review by public health professionals.

BOX 19–6 Vaccine Shortages

Vaccine shortages have occurred periodically since 2000 for 8 of the 11 vaccine-preventable diseases. Reasons for these shortages include:

- Manufacturers choose to stop producing a vaccine
- Manufacturers have production problems
- Efforts to remove thimerosal (a preservative) from vaccines
- Unanticipated demands for a new vaccine (Pneumococcal Conjugate Vaccine)
- The lengthy clinical testing and review for new vaccines required by the Food and Drug Administration

States have responded during times of vaccine shortage by loosening immunization requirements for childcare and school entry. As vaccines became available children were recalled for immunizations (Heinrich, 2002). The Centers for Disease Control and Prevention's Advisory Committee on Immunization Practices and the American Academy of Pediatrics have developed guidelines for immunizing children when there are vaccine shortages, ensuring that there is coverage for all children rather than have some children not be protected.

CRITICAL THINKING

What are potential consequences of vaccine shortages? What guidelines can be developed to ensure that children are recalled for immunizations when vaccine supplies are restored?

BOX 19–7 Thimerosal Use in Vaccines

Thimerosal, a bacteriostatic agent that contains ethyl mercury, was used to sterilize vaccines in multidose vials. Because of the possible association between mercury poisoning and nerve and brain damage, healthcare advocates called for the removal of thimerosal from vaccines. Vaccine manufacturers are working to eliminate the use of thimerosal from vaccines while maintaining their sterility. The cumulative mercury exposure in vaccines administered within the first 6 months has fallen from the 1999 level 187.5 mcg to 3 mcg in 2002 (Greene, 2002). Research conducted by the Immunizations Safety Review Committee of the Institute of Medicine also shows that it is not possible to declare a causal relationship between thimerosal exposures in childhood vaccines and subsequent development of autism, attention deficit hyperactivity disorder, and a speech and language delay (Institute of Medicine, 2001b). In contrast, a recent study reported that the number of autism cases rose after thimerosal was discontinued from vaccines in Denmark (Madsen, Lauritsen, Pedersen, et al., 2003).

MediaLink Case Study: Consequences of a Vaccine Shortage

TABLE 19–3 Vaccine Safety Information

MISINFORMATION	CORRECT INFORMATION
Vaccine-preventable diseases have been eliminated.	Even though the incidence of these vaccine-preventable diseases is low in the United States, most diseases are never completely eliminated. They still exist in other countries. Travelers may reintroduce the disease from a country or another community where the disease still exists. If numerous parents in one community decide not to immunize their children, the herd immunity level drops and the community's children are at higher risk of infection. For example, pertussis is now common in Boulder, Colorado, as many parents are refusing to have their children immunized (Allen, 2002).
Immunization weakens the immune system. Multiple vaccines overload the immune system and cause harmful effects.	Vaccination uses the body's immune system to prevent a future infection. A small amount of an inactivated or attenuated virus or bacteria is given to the child. The child's immune system recognizes the foreign substance and develops antibodies to protect against it. Science has revealed that infants are capable of generating protective immune responses to multiple vaccines given simultaneously. Even though infants are given more vaccines than in the 1980s, the vaccines contain fewer antigens (Humiston & Judelsohn, 2003).
It would be better to let the child get the disease than get immunized.	Many of the diseases preventable by vaccines can cause great suffering, permanent disability, and even death. Children who are not immunized are at a much greater risk of getting the disease. They also increase the risk that pregnant women and high-risk infants and children will get the disease.
Vaccines do not work. Children still get the disease.	The widespread use of vaccines has reduced the incidence of vaccine-preventable diseases by 95%. No vaccine is 100% effective, but most vaccines protect 90% or more of the children immunized. When vaccines are given widely in the community, they indirectly protect other persons, including young infants who are not yet fully immunized and those who have medical reasons to not be immunized (Evers, 2000).

- Infants and young children are vulnerable to infectious diseases, so they need protection by immunization.
- If your child is not immunized and gets sick, it increases the risk that other vulnerable children become exposed and get the infection.
- Although information about immunizations is available online and in the media, not all the information is correct. Provide the parents with recommendations for trustworthy information about immunizations.

NURSING MANAGEMENT

Nursing management focuses on the health promotion activities of immunization by teaching parents about vaccines and their possible side effects, addressing their fears about possible reactions, obtaining consent, administering vaccines, and reporting adverse reactions.

Nursing Assessment and Diagnosis

Nurses are responsible for reviewing a child's immunization record and determining whether the child needs immunization. Inquire about the child's preventive care as well as health problems. Record the child's history carefully, specifying any previous reactions to immunizations, allergies, and immune diseases (Box 19–8).

Make sure you use the most current guidelines for comparison with the child's record. If the child is behind in appropriate immunizations for age, determine the best combination of vaccines to give at this visit to better protect the child. Identify opportunities to give needed immunizations to siblings accompanying the family on the visit, such as Lian in the opening scenario. A minor illness should not deter the nurse from giving an immunization to a child, such as Lian's brother Chang.

To avoid missed opportunities in administering immunizations, be sure to evaluate the child's immunization record (as well as the record of siblings present) in all healthcare settings: on acute care units in the hospital, in the emergency department, and during well-child health or chronic condition care. To reduce the number of missed opportunities for full immunization of children, use the following guidelines (American Academy of Pediatrics, 2003).

- Immunizations can be given when the child has a minor illness with or without a low-grade fever, and with antibiotic treatment. Recent exposure to an infectious disease is not a reason to defer a vaccine.
- Several vaccines—diphtheria, tetanus, and acellular pertussis (DTaP); measles, mumps, and rubella (MMR); hepatitis B

BOX 19–8 Questions for Vaccine Screening

When talking with a parent to identify if an infant or child who needs an immunization has any contraindications to receiving a vaccine, the following questions can help.

- Is the child sick today?
- Does the child have allergies to medications (certain antibiotics), food (eggs or gelatin), or any vaccine?
- Has the child had a serious reaction to a vaccine in the past?
- Has the child had a seizure or brain condition?
- Does the child have cancer, leukemia, AIDS, or any other immune system problem?
- Has the child taken cortisone, prednisone, other steroids, or anticancer drugs or had radiograph treatments in the past 3 months?
- Has the child received a transfusion of blood or blood products, or been given a medicine called immune (gamma) globulin in the past year?
- Is the child/teen pregnant or is there a chance she could become pregnant in the next month?
- Has the child received any vaccinations in the past 4 weeks?

When the parent answers yes to any of the questions, refer to the contraindications for specific vaccines in Table 19–3 or the packet insert before administering a needed vaccine.

From Immunization Action Coalition. (2004). Screening questionnaire for child and teen immunization. Needle Tips and the Hepatitis B Coalition News, 14*(1), Item #P4060.*

(HBV); Haemophilus influenzae type b (Hib); inactivated polio (IPV); varicella; and heptavalent pneumococcal vaccines—can be given at the same visit.
- Combination vaccines, such as Pediarix (combining DTaP, HepB, and IPV) can reduce the overall number of injections needed in the first 2 years from 20 to 14.
- Two injections can be given in different sites on the same extremity.
- Premature and low-birth-weight infants have the same requirements for immunizations as full-term infants.

PRACTICE ALERT

Preterm and low-birth-weight infants are vulnerable to infection. The latest research regarding the ability of preterm and low-birth-weight infants to develop protection from vaccines has revealed that although their immune response may be somewhat decreased, they do respond adequately and develop full immunity by the end of the vaccination series. Therefore, preterm and low-birth-weight infants who are medically stable should receive all routinely recommended vaccines at the same chronologic age and in the same dosage as full-term infants.

The only difference in immunization recommendations is for a delay in initiation of Hepatitis B vaccine for infants weighing less than 2000 g whose mother is hepatitis B negative. The Hepatitis B vaccine should be given at 30 days of age or upon hospital discharge if the infant is consistently gaining weight (Saari & Committee on Infectious Diseases, 2003).

- Immunizations can be given when there was a local reaction to a prior vaccine or a family member had an adverse response.

True contraindications for a vaccine are an anaphylactic reaction to the vaccine or one of its components and a moderate to severe acute illness. Some additional contraindications for specific vaccines may also exist, such as pregnancy and allergy to some components of the vaccine (e.g., neomycin, gelatin, eggs) (see the table on page 606).

Assess the child for potential contraindications to vaccines. Inquire about past reactions to vaccines as well as allergy to key vaccine components such as eggs, gelatin, or neomycin. Determine whether female teens could be pregnant.

Inquire about recent administration of immune globulin or blood products. Antibody response to vaccines may be decreased. Follow guidelines for administration of specific live virus vaccines (e.g., measles, varicella).

PRACTICE ALERT

Health professionals need to know if a child has received immune globulin or blood products before the administration of vaccines to determine if the child will be able to develop immunity. Immune globulin inhibits the response to live virus vaccines such as measles, mumps, rubella, and varicella. Refer to the most current guidelines to identify the appropriate interval (3 or more months) between administration of immune globulin or blood products and live virus vaccine administration.

Similarly, if immune globulin or blood products must be given within 14 days after administration of a measles-containing vaccine or other live virus vaccine, these live virus vaccines should be administered again after the period specified in the most current guidelines, unless serologic testing determines that the child developed adequate serum antibodies (American Academy of Pediatrics, 2003).

The accompanying nursing care plan explores three potential nursing diagnoses that may apply to the child needing immunizations. Additional nursing diagnoses may include the following:

- Ineffective Airway Clearance related to an airway obstructed by swelling
- Risk for Impaired Skin Integrity related to vaccine response
- Ineffective Health Maintenance related to cultural beliefs regarding routine immunization

Planning and Implementation

Nurses should be strong advocates for immunization. Being well informed about immunizations, their potential side effects, and recommended schedules assists immunization efforts.

PRACTICE ALERT

Make every effort to stay current on immunization guidelines and information about vaccines, safe administration, adverse effects, etc. Two major resources provide more extensive information about immunization schedules and specific vaccines, as well as infectious and communicable diseases; they are the American Academy of Pediatrics and the Centers for Disease Control and Prevention. The American Academy of Pediatrics *Red Book: Report of the Committee of Infectious Diseases* is updated about every 3 years. The revised immunization schedule is published each January in the American Academy of Pediatrics newsletter and its journal, *Pediatrics*, as well as several pediatric nursing journals. The Centers for Disease Control and Prevention maintains a regularly updated website with detailed information about immunizations, the most recent vaccine schedule, and infectious and communicable diseases.

MediaLink Immunization and Vaccine Resources

Family Education and Informed Consent

Federal legislation requires consent to be obtained before administering a vaccine. In most healthcare settings, the nurse has the responsibility to inform the parents or the child's legal guardian, supply literature, and obtain written consent before the vaccine is administered. The nurse is required to record the (1) month, day, and year of administration, (2) vaccine given, (3) manufacturer, (4) lot number and expiration date of the immunization given, (5) site and route of administration, and (6) name, title, and address of the person who administers the vaccine. Obtain written consent to give the needed vaccines on the healthcare facility's standardized form from the parent or guardian. Provide parents with a record of the child's immunizations, and record the vaccines given in the healthcare agency's official records.

Discuss vaccine risks and benefits with parents. They have often heard sensational stories about the consequences of vaccines and correct information is needed to help them make informed decisions. See Box 19–9 for research findings indicating a lack of relationship between immunizations and various conditions. Provide the current Vaccine Information Statement (VIS) to parents for each vaccine the child will receive as required by the National Childhood Vaccine Injury Acts of 1986 and 1993. The information provided about the vaccine includes the following:

- Concise information about the vaccine
- Risks and benefits of the vaccine
- Recommended schedule
- What to do if adverse effects occur
- Description of the National Vaccine Injury Compensation Program

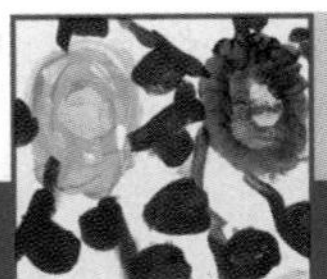

Nursing Care Plan

THE CHILD NEEDING IMMUNIZATIONS

GOAL	INTERVENTION	RATIONALE	EXPECTED OUTCOME
1. Risk for Infection related to incomplete immunization series			
	NIC Interventions: *Immunization Administration:* Provision of immunizations for prevention of communicable disease.		**NOC Outcome:** *Risk Control:* Actions to eliminate or reduce actual, personal, and modifiable health threats.
The child will become adequately protected from disease-preventable illnesses.	■ Review the child's immunization record for needed vaccines at each healthcare visit. ■ Identify all due vaccines that can be provided simultaneously. ■ Identify potential contraindications to needed vaccines. Review past reactions to vaccines.	■ Assessment identifies the children who have missed needed immunizations. ■ Many vaccines can be given at the same visit to more adequately protect the child. This also saves healthcare trips for families. ■ Reduces the risk for the child and other caretakers to have adverse reactions to vaccines.	The child is adequately protected from vaccine-preventable illnesses.
2. Knowledge Deficit (parent) related to potential side effects of vaccines			
	NIC Interventions: *Teaching, Prescribed Vaccines:* Preparing a patient to safely take prescribed vaccines and monitor their effects.		**NOC Outcome:** *Knowledge:* Vaccine reactions and comfort measures: Extent of understanding conveyed about treatment regimen.
Parents will sign consent for vaccines to be given.	■ Educate the parents about the need for specific vaccines and the risk if not given. Obtain signed consent before giving vaccines. ■ Review past reactions to vaccines and describe common potential reactions and why they occur.	■ Informed consent is required for all treatments. ■ Parents should expect common reactions and know they indicate the child's body is building protection to the illness.	The parent(s) complete(s) consent form, which is placed in the child's file.
Parents will state the side effects of vaccines given.	■ Describe serious side effects that should be reported to healthcare provider.	■ Parents need to be prepared for potential serious side effects so they can obtain care.	Parents report all serious side effects to the healthcare provider.
Parents will manage common side effects of vaccines.	■ Teach parents general comfort measures for children's common side effects, for example: ■ Cool pack to tender leg ■ Acetaminophen or ibuprofen for fever and discomfort ■ Rocking and holding the infant ■ Gentle movement of affected extremity	■ Parents will know how to make the child more comfortable during the 24–48 hours after the vaccine is given.	The child is given comfort measures after vaccine administration.
3. Acute Pain related to injection and associated anxiety			
	NIC Intervention: *Pain Managment:* Alleviation of pain or a reduction in pain to a level of comfort that is acceptable to the patient.		**NOC Outcome:** *Pain Level:* Amount of reported or demonstrated pain.
The child's anxiety and pain associated with immunizations is reduced.	■ Prepare all immunization injections and supplies enabling injections to be given quickly. ■ Provide guidelines for parents to hold child and provide distraction and reassurance during injections. ■ Right before giving injections, tell child what to expect, that it is okay to cry, and how to cooperate.	■ Shortening exposure to syringes and needles reduces period of anxiety. ■ Distraction and security of being held by parent provides comfort and reduces anxiety. ■ Information about what will happen and how to cooperate helps child manage anxiety.	The time the child cries during and after injections is brief. The child is easily comforted.

MediaLink Care Plan: Develop an Immunization Schedule

Nursing Care Plan THE CHILD NEEDING IMMUNIZATIONS (continued)

GOAL	INTERVENTION	RATIONALE	EXPECTED OUTCOME
3. Acute Pain related to injection and associated anxiety (continued)			
	■ Use vapocoolant spray on injection sites. ■ Inform the child when all injections have been completed and offer praise and comfort.	■ Spray will reduce pain due to needle stick. ■ Information and comfort lets child know when to relax.	
4. Risk for Injury related to vaccine reaction			
	NIC Intervention: *Vital Sign Monitoring:* Reducing the risk of a systemic reaction to vaccine.		**NOC Outcome**: *Risk Control:* Actions to eliminate or reduce actual, personal, and modifiable health threats.
The child's potential vaccine reactions will be safely managed.	■ Prepare for life-threatening reactions by having resuscitation drugs and equipment immediately available. ■ Monitor the child for 15 minutes after the vaccine is given before letting the child go home. ■ Assess the child for extreme anxiety and injection fearfulness. ■ Have the fearful child sit or lie down until symptoms of vasovagal response have disappeared. ■ Report all vaccine-related reactions to the appropriate agency using the standard form.	■ Anaphylactic reactions must be managed quickly and effectively. ■ A life-threatening response will usually become apparent within this time frame. ■ These are potential signs the child may have a vasovagal response to the injection. ■ The child who faints may sustain a head injury. ■ Legal requirements for all healthcare providers.	The child has no reaction or has a severe reaction to a vaccine that is managed effectively.

The VIS for each vaccine is updated by the Centers for Disease Control National Immunization Program and they are available through the program's website. It is the nurse's responsibility to make sure that the most current VIS is provided to the parents about the vaccines to be administered. When teaching about immunizations, make sure that the parents understand the information in the VIS and answer any questions the parents might have. Identify the vaccines due to be given at this visit and on the next visit so that the parents know their child's immunization status. It may save time to give the VIS for the next vaccines to the parents to take home and review prior to the next visit. See Developing Cultural Competence: Vaccine Information Statements.

Provide guidelines for managing expected mild reactions at home. (See Partnering with Families: Care of the Child after Immunizations.) See recommended acetaminophen doses for children of various ages in the medications table on page 576. Schedule the child's next appointment for a health supervision visit to complete needed immunizations for age.

Parents have the right to refuse immunizations, but they must be aware that if there is a disease outbreak, the nonimmunized child must be kept out of school. Local, city, or state courts decide how to settle any conflicts. If the parent chooses not to have the child receive a particular vaccine, document an informed refusal. This is one method to communicate the seriousness of not allowing the child to be protected by a vaccine-preventable disease. A form that can be used for documentation of informed refusal is available from the American Academy of Pediatrics.

DEVELOPING CULTURAL COMPETENCE
Vaccine Information Statements

Consider literacy and reading level when giving Vaccine Information Statements (VIS) to parents. While written at a sixth-grade reading level, they may be too difficult for some parents to read. It is acceptable to read the statement to the parents, but the nurse must make sure the parent understands the information. Supplement the VIS with other teaching materials such as videotapes when possible.

The VIS is also available in a number of languages from the National Immunization Program, and the Minnesota Department of Health has the statements available in 25 languages. Provide translators to provide verbal explanations and answer questions when necessary.

Reducing Pain and Anxiety

Prepare the parent to help reduce the anxiety and pain of the immunizations. Let them know it is okay to be anxious, but to try to stay calm for the child. See Evidence-Based Practice: Nursing Care During Immunizations.

CLINICAL TIP

Coach the parent to hold and talk with the child during the injections. Funny faces or a toy for distraction might also help. Then encourage the parent of an infant to breastfeed or bottle-feed after the injection. This will often help console the infant (Lugo, et al., 2003).

MediaLink Professional Resources

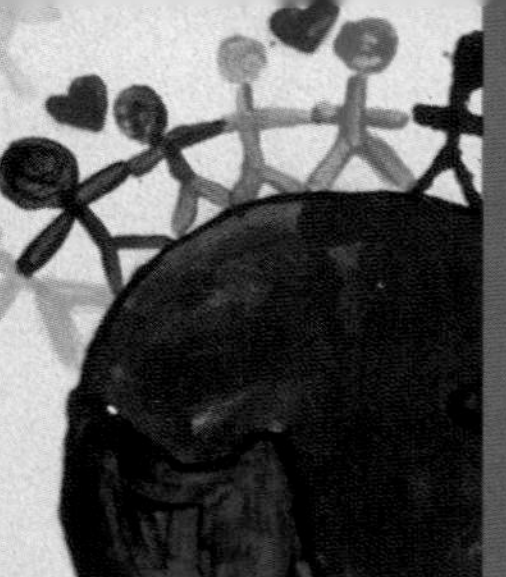

PARTNERING WITH FAMILIES

Care of the Child after Immunizations

After your child receives an immunization, observe for any reactions that might occur (Schuval, 2003).

- Check the injection site. Local pain, redness, and swelling are common. Ice can be put on the site to help reduce swelling and pain. Acetaminophen may be given to reduce a fever and pain. The symptoms disappear in 1–2 days.
- The child may have a fever, joint pain, muscle aches, or fatigue within hours to days after the vaccine is given. Give acetaminophen for pain, and call your healthcare provider if you are concerned about the symptoms.
- If your child has a mild allergic reaction to the vaccine, you might notice a few hives around the injection site.
- A severe allergic reaction is indicated by a flushed face; swelling of the face, mouth, or throat; wheezing or other difficulty breathing; shock (confusion, lack of movement or response, or unconsciousness). If these symptoms occur, call 9-1-1 or your emergency number so your child can be taken to the emergency department for treatment. While waiting for the ambulance to arrive lie the child down on his or her back and raise the legs to promote blood return to the vital organs.

Give the appropriate immunizations to the child as efficiently as possible, while providing support to the child (Figure 19–6 ■). Nurses should make efforts to reduce the pain associated with vaccine injections, especially since infants and children must return for more injections in the future. Reducing pain will also lessen the anxiety associated with future visits for healthcare. Suggestions for pain management include the following techniques.

- Give young infants 25% sucrose water to drink (mix 1 packet of table sugar with 10 mL of tap water) prior to the injection. Then allow the infant to suck on a pacifier or bottle of for-

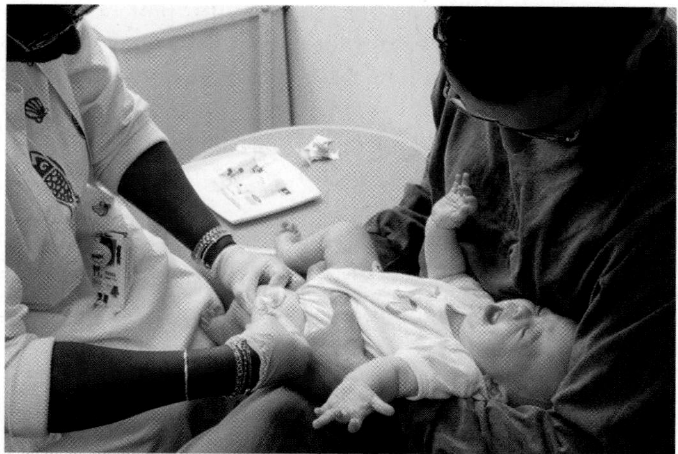

FIGURE 19–6 ■ Give immunizations quickly and efficiently. Do not prolong the wait and let fear grow. The child will be anxious, especially if more than one injection is to be given.

BOX 19–9 Research: Potential Adverse Effects of Vaccines

It is the nurse's responsibility to know the potential adverse consequences of vaccines and to be informed about the latest research regarding potential vaccine-related conditions. To provide informed consent, the nurse needs to respond to their questions and be able to correct any misinformation. This is especially important when parents with philosophical reasons for not immunizing their children could potentially see the value of getting some or all of the vaccines recommended. To respond to the concerns about the potential adverse effects of vaccines, numerous studies have been conducted, and continue to be conducted so that health professionals are fully informed about vaccine risks and vaccine safety.

Febrile seizures. MMR vaccine has been associated with an increased risk of febrile seizures in immunized children 8 to 14 days after vaccination. Diphtheria tetanus toxoids and whole pertussis (DTP) are associated with a febrile seizure on the day of administration. However, these children were not found to be at a higher risk for subsequent seizures or neurodevelopmental disabilities (Barlow, Davis, Glasser, et al., 2001).

Inflammatory bowel disease. No association has been found between MMR vaccine and the development of inflammatory bowel disease (Taylor, Miller, Lingram, et al., 2002).

Autism. No association has been found between the development of autism and the MMR vaccine (DeStefano, Bhasin, Thompson, et al., 2004; Institute of Medicine, 2001a; Madsen, et al., 2003; Taylor, Miller, Farrington, et al., 1999).

Multiple sclerosis. Hepatitis B vaccine has been found to have no association with the development of multiple sclerosis or to increase the risk of short-term relapse of multiple sclerosis (Ascherio, Zhang, Hernan, et al., 2001; Confavreux, Samy, Saddier, et al., 2001).

Sudden infant death syndrome. Inadequate evidence exists to accept or reject a causal relationship between sudden infant death syndrome and the following individual vaccines: Hepatitis B, DTaP, Hib, and oral polio. No association was found between exposure to multiple vaccines and sudden infant death syndrome (Institute of Medicine, 2003).

Asthma. No association has been found between the development of asthma and the following vaccines: DTP, oral polio, measles, mumps and rubella, Hib, and Hepatitis B (DeStefano, Gu, Kramarz, et al., 2002).

Diabetes type 1. No association was found between the risk for development of type 1 diabetes and multiple immunizations (Institute of Medicine, 2002; Hviid, Stellfeld, Wohlfahrt, et al., 2004).

The Vaccine Safety Datalink project continually evaluates vaccine safety on more than 6 million people. Studies in process are examining the association of immunizations with diabetes mellitus and of MMR vaccine with inflammatory bowel disease (American Academy of Pediatrics, 2003).

CRITICAL THINKING IN ACTION

How would you explain these research findings in a convincing manner to parents concerned about the potential linkage between vaccines and other health conditions?

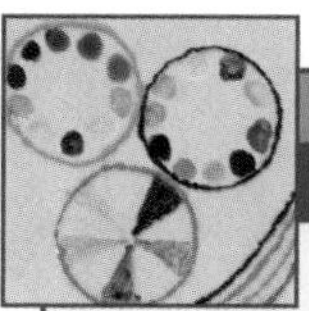

EVIDENCE-BASED PRACTICE
Nursing Care During Immunizations

PROBLEM

Young infants receive several injections for immunizations at health promotion visits. Parents are increasingly concerned about the number of immunizations given during the same visit (Gellin, Maibach, & Marcuse, 2000) and the pain associated with the injections. Some anti-immunization efforts could be influencing the attitudes of parents regarding immunization of their children.

EVIDENCE

A telephone survey of parents of young children was conducted to assess parents' knowledge and perceptions regarding current immunizations, and to evaluate parents' attitudes toward immunizations in general, and toward watching their children receive immunizations. A sample of 1,000 parents with children aged birth to 24 months was fairly representative of all U.S. households with children in this age group. Parents were supportive of immunizations: 98% agreed they were important to their child's health, 98% said if you can prevent a disease by immunization you should do so. However, many parents did not recognize most of the vaccine-preventable diseases, such as whooping cough, hepatitis, and polio. Most parents underestimated the number of injections needed to fully immunize the child. Most parents (84%) reported feeling sympathy pain for the child being immunized, regardless of the age of the child. Most parents (75%) wished to have the number of immunizations decreased without reducing their child's protection. Combination vaccines were desirable (Lugo, Montoya, & Petraco, 2003). A study of the use of distraction to reduce the distress of immunizations was conducted with 90 infants aged 2 months to 3 years in a rural health department. Nurses performing injections were trained in the use of appropriate behaviors and distraction techniques (age-appropriate toy and a popular cartoon movie) to use with the study children. Children in the control group could be provided with comfort, reassurance, and empathy, but no toy or movie. Interactions were videotaped and scored by researchers. Infants in the distraction group displayed less distress than the control group. In many cases the parents helped supplement the distraction provided by the nurse (Cohen, 2002). A recent study explored methods to reduce the pain stress associated with four immunization injections provided to 116 infants between 6 and 16 weeks of age. The intervention group received a bottle with 10 mL of 25% sucrose 2 minutes before the injections. They were then allowed to suck on a pacifier or bottle of formula throughout the injections and afterwards. Parents were asked to hold the infants on their lap with the upper bodies close to the parent, making the legs available for injection. The control group received immunizations on the examining table with no specific comfort measures provided. Infants in the intervention group cried less and parents expressed the desire for the same procedure to be used in future visits (Reis, Roth, Syphan, et al., 2003).

IMPLICATIONS

The vast majority of parents want their children to be fully immunized, but they are distressed by the number of injections and their associated pain. Simple comfort measures and distraction are effective in reducing pain and distress associated with immunizations when utilized.

CRITICAL THINKING IN ACTION

Review and identify the different methods for comforting infants receiving immunizations by the nurses in a busy clinical setting. Identify those that seem to be more effective at reducing the distress of infants. Make a personal comparison of the distress experienced by infants who have distraction or sucrose solution provided versus those without comfort measures.

mula during the injections. Sucrose has been found to have the ability to reduce the perception of pain in infants. See Chapter 18∞. Allowing the parent to hold the infant may also lessen the infant's distress with multiple injections.

- Instruct parent how to apply EMLA cream to the site 1 hour before the injection. A prescription can be given at the end of the visit for use prior to the next health visit when vaccines are given. See Chapter 18∞ for information regarding use of EMLA cream.
- Use vapocoolant spray immediately before the injection. Spray on the planned injection site for 3 to 7 seconds from a distance of 3 to 9 inches. It may also be sprayed on a cotton ball that is then held against the skin. Prepare the skin as usual for the injection. The child will not feel the initial needle stick, but may feel the medication being injected (Clark & Manworren, 2001).
- Apply pressure at the site for 10 seconds before the injection.
- Give two injections simultaneously in different extremities using two different providers.
- Use age-appropriate distraction techniques (see Chapter 18∞).
- Use of longer needles (25 mm rather than 16 mm) reduces the rate of local reactions and tenderness in infant immunizations (Table 19–4). This may ensure that the vaccine is given intramuscularly rather than subcutaneously (Diggle & Deek, 2000).
- Do not prolong the process of giving immunizations, and give the child honest answers that the needles will cause some pain.

TABLE 19–4 Recommended Length of 22 to 25 Gauge Needles for Intramuscular Immunization Administration

AGE AND INJECTION LOCATION	SUBCUTANEOUS NEEDLE SIZE	INTRAMUSCULAR NEEDLE SIZE
Newborns and preterm infants—anterolateral thigh	5/8th inch	5/8th inch
Infants 2 to 12 months—anterolateral thigh	5/8th to 3/4th inch	7/8th to 1 inch
Toddlers—anterolateral thigh	5/8th to 3/4th inch	7/8th to 1 inch
Toddlers and older children—deltoid	5/8th to 3/4th inch	7/8th inch
Adolescents—deltoid	5/8th to 3/4th inch	1 to 2 inches

From Immunization Action Coalition. (2004). How to administer subcutaneous injections and How to administer intramuscular injections. www.immunize.org/datg.d/p2020.pdf, *accessed 2/25/2004.*

- Let the child select the arm or leg for the injection and forms of distraction to promote coping. After the injections are completed, let the parent comfort the child.

Preparation for Emergencies

Be prepared for potential vaccine anaphylaxis. Keep epinephrine 1:1000 and resuscitation equipment immediately available. The dose for epinephrine (aqueous 1:1000) is 0.01 mL/kg per dose up to 0.5 mL intramuscularly. The dose can be repeated every 10 to 20 minutes for up to a total of three doses until symptoms subside or other emergency care interventions are initiated (American Academy of Pediatrics, 2003). Check the date of available epinephrine to be assured of its potency as it has a short shelf life. Ensure that specific serious reactions following immunization are reported to the U.S. Department of Health and Human Services, as required by law.

Vaccine Storage

Assure the effectiveness of the vaccines administered. An improperly stored or poorly administered vaccine may be rendered ineffective, thus preventing the child from developing immunity. Read the package inserts of vaccines to determine proper storage conditions. When reconstituting vaccines, it is important to use the solution provided or follow the manufacturer's directions. Write the date and time on the bottle if it is a multidose vial. Many reconstituted vaccines (e.g., varicella vaccine) have a very short shelf life. See vaccine-specific information in the table on page 606.

PRACTICE ALERT

Special care must be taken to assure the potency of the vaccines that are stored in the office, clinic, and hospital setting to ensure that they are effective in promoting immunity in the children to whom they are given. Read the package inserts of vaccines to determine proper storage conditions. Some vaccines are frozen; others are refrigerated.

Vaccines should be stored in a refrigerator that has separate doors for the refrigerator and freezer units. Check the temperature of the refrigerator and freezer units twice daily and record the temperatures on a log. Automatic temperature measurement systems are available that check and record temperatures at established times. The refrigerator should maintain a consistent temperature in the range of 35 to 46°F (2 to 8° C). The freezer should maintain a consistent temperature of 5°F (15°C) or lower. Keep jugs of water in the refrigerator and trays of ice in the freezer to help keep the temperature of the units consistent. Store the vaccines in the middle of the refrigerator and freezer, placing older vaccines in front, where the temperature is maintained in the desired range. Make sure the facility has an emergency plan for safe storage of vaccines in case of a power outage or natural disaster. Manufacturers of the vaccine and the CDC can be consulted for advice about how to handle vaccine that has been subjected to a power outage.

When accepting new shipments of vaccine, check for damage and identify if any delay in the shipment could have resulted in exposure to temperatures that could damage the vaccine potency.

When reconstituting vaccines, it is important to use the solution provided and follow the manufacturer's directions. Write the date and time on the bottle if it is a multidose vial. Many reconstituted vaccines (e.g., varicella vaccine and MMR) have a very short shelf life so they are only available in single-dose vials.

Critical Thinking Application Develop a plan to safely store and preserve vaccine potency for a health clinic when a power outage is threatened or occurs due to a natural disaster.

MediaLink Storing Vaccines During a Disaster

Evaluation

Expected nursing outcomes include the following:

- Parents are fully informed and give consent for immunizations.
- All age-appropriate immunizations are provided for the child at each health visit or catch-up immunizations are provided as needed.
- The parents are prepared to manage mild reactions to immunizations at home.
- Parents are able to identify and report serious reactions to immunizations.

INFECTIOUS AND COMMUNICABLE DISEASES IN INFANTS AND CHILDREN

Infectious and communicable diseases cause acute illnesses. These diseases are caused by bacterial, viral, protozoan, or fungal organisms. As noted earlier, infants and children develop infectious and communicable diseases more frequently than adults do. Active immunity to microorganisms does not occur until there is natural exposure that leads to the development of antibodies. Therefore, they are more susceptible to the large number of infectious organisms to which they have no resistance.

Epidemiology and Pathophysiology

Microorganisms use the human body to reproduce and in some cases have a mutually beneficial relationship, such as occurs with the bacteria in the gastrointestinal tract that help with digestion. Other microorganisms are pathogens that cause infectious and communicable diseases. They enter the body through direct contact with mucous membranes and injured skin, inhalation, and ingestion. Biting insects or animals (vectors) also inject organisms into the skin and blood. The microorganisms spread through the lymph and blood to other tissues and organs where they multiply.

Bacteria

Most bacteria have found ways to prevent destruction by the inflammatory and immune systems. Bacteria avoid destruction and cause disease in the following ways.

- By producing toxins that kill phagocytes and injure cells or tissues, as occurs with staphylococcus
- By producing a thick capsule of carbohydrate or protein that prevents efficient phagocytosis, as occurs with the polysaccharide covering of the pneumococcus

The initial response of the body to invasion by bacteria is inflammation. Endotoxins increase capillary permeability and trigger fever.

When antibodies have developed to a specific microorganism to which the child is exposed, they protect the child by:

- Neutralizing bacterial toxins by serving as an antitoxin, preventing the toxin from binding with the tissues
- Neutralizing viruses by preventing the initial attachment and entrance of viruses into the cells

- Producing a substance (opsonin) that makes the bacterial outer capsule susceptible to **phagocytosis** (the engulfment and destruction of microorganisms, dead cells, and foreign particles)
- Activating the inflammatory response

When a microorganism succeeds in invading the body through its defenses (such as the skin and mucous membranes), the inflammatory response is initiated (Figure 19–7 ■). Neutrophils are the predominant phagocytic cell in the early inflammatory response (removes debris in sterile lesions and

PATHOPHYSIOLOGY ILLUSTRATED

Inflammatory Response

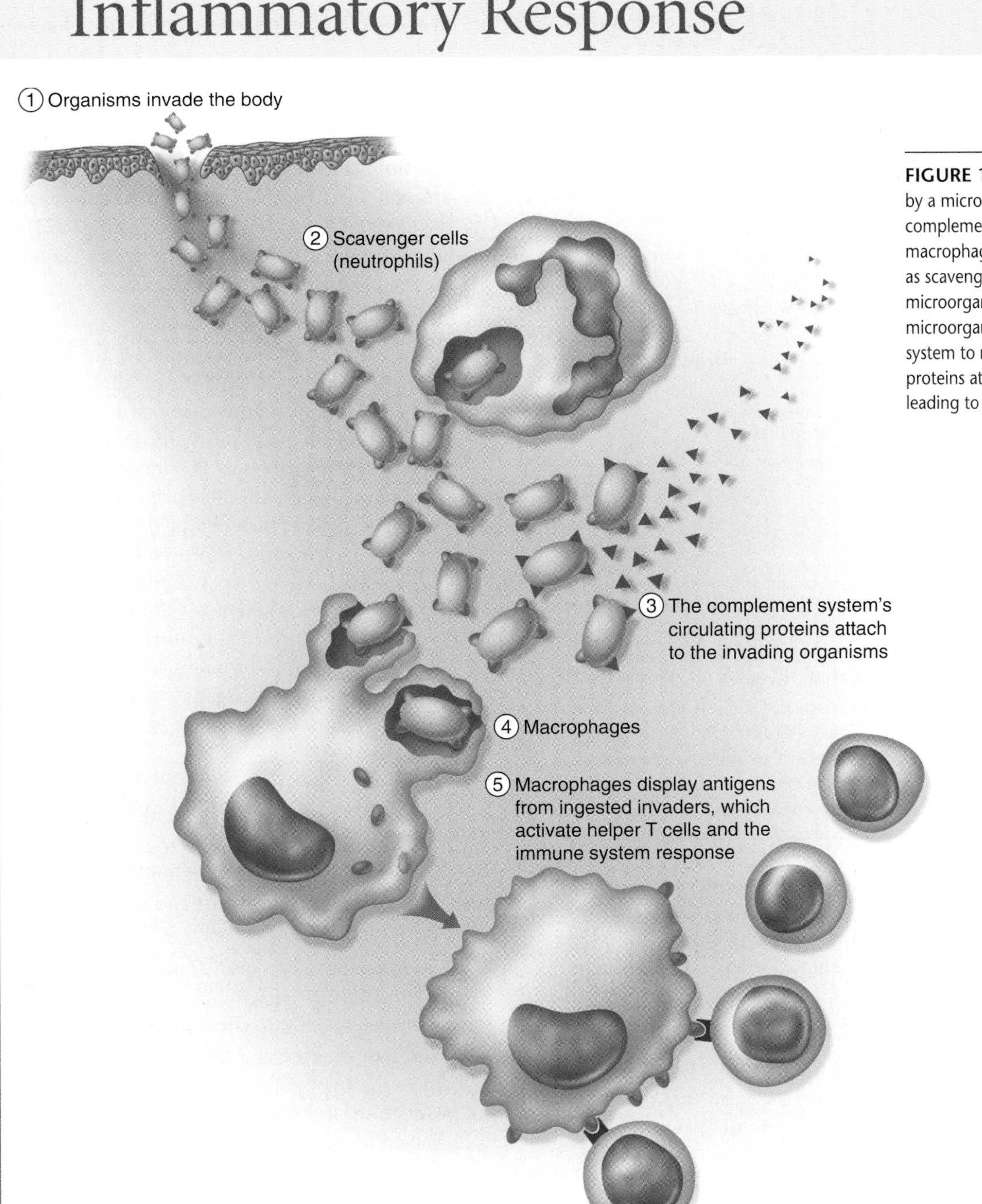

(1) Organisms invade the body
(2) Scavenger cells (neutrophils)
(3) The complement system's circulating proteins attach to the invading organisms
(4) Macrophages
(5) Macrophages display antigens from ingested invaders, which activate helper T cells and the immune system response

FIGURE 19–7 ■ After the body is invaded by a microorganism, neutrophils, the complement system proteins, and macrophages rush to the site. Neutrophils act as scavenger cells and engulf microorganisms. Macrophages also engulf microorganisms and trigger the immune system to respond. The complement system's proteins attach to the microorganisms leading to their death.

MediaLink Inflammation with Phagocytosis Animation

PATHOPHYSIOLOGY ILLUSTRATED
Fever

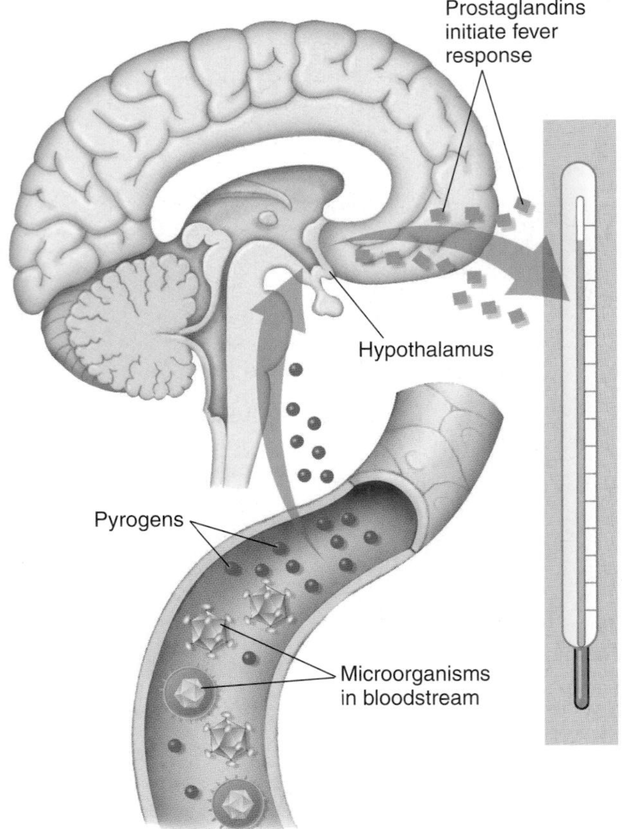

FIGURE 19–8 ■ The hypothalamus functions as the body's thermostat, directing the body to conserve or dissipate heat. When microorganisms invade the body, endogenous pyrogens are released into the bloodstream. These substances travel to the hypothalamus, where they trigger the production and release of prostaglandins, which initiate the fever response. Blood is diverted from the extremities to more central vessels. This helps increase the core body temperature by decreasing heat loss. Shivering, the rapid contraction and relaxation of the skeletal muscles, burns energy and produces heat until the blood is the temperature of the altered temperature set point in the hypothalamus. The body then maintains the temperature at the new set point until antipyretics are given or the organisms causing the fever are eliminated.

phagocytosis of bacteria in nonsterile lesions). Macrophages and monocytes also serve a role in phagocytosis. Cytokines, such as interleukins and interferons, enhance the inflammatory response. Interferons help prevent viruses from infecting healthy cells by attaching to neighboring cells of the virus-invaded cell, stimulating the healthy cells to produce an antiviral protein. Antimicrobials also prevent the growth of or destroy microorganisms that have not developed antibiotic resistance. See Chapter 27∞ for more information about the inflammatory and immune response.

Viruses

Viruses are the most common cause of infections in humans. They are parasitic organisms that invade the cells and take them over for their own survival and reproduction. The cell's protein synthesis is halted. Viruses usually hide in the cells and avoid the typical inflammatory and immune responses. They penetrate the cell and release the viral genetic material into the cytoplasm. The cell's lysosomal membrane is disrupted, releasing enzymes that can kill the cell. As they reproduce cell to cell, eventually the body's immune response to the virus overwhelms it and the infection is cured. In some cases the virus reproduces at such a slow rate that the infected person is asymptomatic and becomes a carrier of the virus. Secondary bacterial infection can occur in virus-damaged cells. See Chapter 27∞ for more information about the immune response and viral infections such as HIV.

Fever

In cases of infection, fever occurs in which the body temperature is regulated at a higher level. The hypothalamus is the control center for the regulation of body temperature and is frequently compared to a thermostat due to its regulatory function (Figure 19–8 ■). As blood circulates through the hypothalamus, this brain structure regulates body temperature by directing body systems to conserve or dissipate heat, depending on the temperature of the blood.

- If body temperature is lower than normal, vasoconstriction is initiated to conserve heat. The adrenal glands produce epinephrine and norepinephrine, which cause an increase in metabolism, more vasoconstriction, and more heat production.
- Shivering or chills may occur, which in turn may increase heat production.
- When excess heat is produced, the body responds with an increase in temperature. The heart rate and respiratory rate increase.

CLINICAL TIP

One degree of temperature elevation causes an increase in respiratory rate by four breaths per minute and increases oxygen need by 7%.

- Vasodilation occurs and the skin flushes, becoming warm to the touch. As the temperature decreases, the child may start to perspire, and the heart and respiratory rates return to normal.

Endogenous pyrogens (interleukins, interferons, and tumor necrosis factor) are released by macrophages in response to an invasive organism. These pyrogens travel through the circulatory system to the hypothalamus, where they trigger the production of prostaglandins. Prostaglandins are believed to raise the body's thermoregulatory set point, thus causing the fever to occur (Cimpella, Goldman, & Khine, 2000).

Infectious and communicable diseases differ in their epidemiology, transmission, and incubation period. Many infectious diseases are communicable between humans, but many are vaccine preventable. The epidemiology, clinical manifestations, treatment, prevention, and nursing care of selected infectious and communicable diseases of childhood are detailed in Table 19–5 starting on page 620. Some infectious diseases are transmitted by insects or animals (**zoonosis**) and are not communicable from person to person. See Table 19–6 on page 632. See Chapter 36∞ for information about impetigo, scabies, and lice; Chapter 24∞ for information about conjunctivitis; Chapter 31∞ for information on sexually transmitted infections; and Chapter 30∞ for information on hepatitis and parasites.

Clinical Manifestations

The child with an infectious or communicable disease has several symptoms. Initially there may be nonspecific symptoms such as fatigue, malaise, weakness, and decreased responsiveness or reduced ability to concentrate. Skin rash, poor appetite, malaise, vomiting and/or diarrhea, and body aches are common signs and symptoms. Fever is the most common sign of infectious disease in infants and children. Signs and symptoms of infection in newborns, infants, and children are associated with the system involved (see table below).

CLINICAL MANIFESTATIONS of Infection in Infants and Children by Age Group

SYSTEM	NEWBORNS	INFANTS	CHILDREN
Central nervous system	Lethargy Decreased responsiveness Seizures Subtle changes in muscle tone or hypotonia High-pitched cry	Irritable Decreased responsiveness Lethargy Bulging anterior fontanel High-pitched cry Muscle weakness	Irritable or combative Stiff neck Back pain Decreased responsiveness Photophobia Brudzinski sign Kernig sign Malaise
Cardiovascular	Hypotension Mottling, pallor Cyanosis Decreased perfusion Tachycardia or bradycardia Weak, thready pulse Delayed capillary refill time	Tachycardia Decreased perfusion Weak peripheral pulses Pallor or mottled skin Flushed, dry skin Delayed capillary refill time	Tachycardia Decreased perfusion Weak peripheral pulses Pallor or flushed, dry skin Delayed capillary refill time
Respiratory	Grunting, retractions, nasal flaring Tachypnea Crackles Decreased oxygen saturation Increased or new-onset oxygen requirement Apnea (new onset or increased episodes)	Tachypnea Increased work of breathing Retractions Nasal flaring Crackles Cough Stridor Decreased oxygen saturation Irregular breathing	Tachypnea Dyspnea Retractions Nasal flaring Crackles Cough Stridor Decreased oxygen saturation
Gastrointestinal	Abdominal distention Poor feeding or feeding intolerance Abdominal wall discoloration Hepatosplenomegaly Paralytic ileus Bloody stool Jaundice	Vomiting Diarrhea Abdominal distention Poor feeding	Nausea and vomiting Diarrhea Abdominal discomfort Abdominal distention Poor appetite
Renal	Decreased urine output Hematuria, proteinuria	WBCs and bacteria in urine	WBCs and bacteria in urine
Hematopoietic	Neutropenia Fraction of band cells > 0.20 Thrombocytopenia	Neutropenia Increased immature WBCs (bands) in bacterial infections Lymphocytosis in viral infections	Leukocytosis Increased immature WBCs (bands) in bacterial infections Lymphocytosis in viral infections
Metabolic	Hypoglycemia or hyperglycemia Temperature instability or hypothermia	Hyperthermia or hypothermia Hypoglycemia or hyperglycemia	Hyperthermia Chills Hypothermic in septic shock
Other	Petechiae Purpura	Rash Dry mucous membranes Poor skin turgor Sunken anterior fontanel	Rash Petechiae and/or purpura Dry mucous membranes Poor skin turgor

Newborn data adapted from McKenney, W.M. (2001). Understanding the neonatal immune system: High risk for infection. Critical Care Nurse, *21*(6), *40.*

TABLE 19–5 Selected Infectious and Communicable Diseases in Children

DISEASE	CLINICAL MANIFESTATIONS	CLINICAL THERAPY	NURSING MANAGEMENT
Chickenpox (Varicella)*+ *Causal agent:* Varicella-zoster, human herpesvirus 3. *Epidemiology:* Peak occurrence is in the late fall, winter, and spring. Maternal antibodies disappear 2–3 months after birth. *Transmission:* Direct contact of the virus to the mucous membranes or conjunctiva primarily through airborne spread of secretions and occasionally with lesion contact. It has an attack rate of nearly 90%. When introduced into a population who have not been vaccinated or have not had the disease, it spreads until most or all susceptible children and adults have been infected (Arvin, 2002). *Incubation period:* 14–21 days. *Period of communicability:* As long as 5 days before the onset of the rash to a maximum of 6 days after the appearance of the first group of vesicles, when all lesions have crusted over. This period may be prolonged after passive immunization or in immunodeficient children. 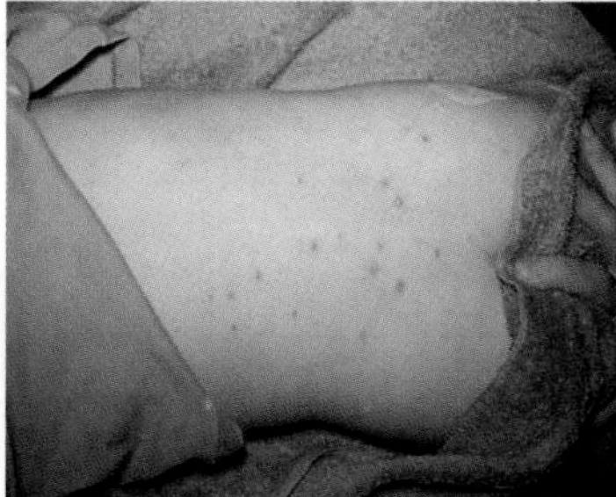 Chicken pox *Used with permission of the American Academy of Pediatrics, http://www.vaccineinformation.org/ photos/varlaap 002.jpg, accessed 6/20/2004.*	The onset of symptoms is acute. Mild fever, malaise, anorexia, headache, mild abdominal pain, and irritability occur before and with eruption. Itching is present once the rash appears. The rash begins as a macule on an erythematous base and progresses to a papule, then a clear, fluid-filled vesicle. Lesions are often described as a "teardrop on a rose petal" and may erupt for 1–5 days. Lesions of all stages may be present at any one time. Crusts may remain for 1–3 weeks. The lesions begin on the trunk, scalp, and face, and then spread to the rest of the body. Ulcerative lesions may be seen in the oropharyngeal, conjunctival, and vaginal mucosa. Lesions in the mouth may lead to decreased fluid intake and dehydration. *Complications:* Complications are rare but can include secondary infection, cellulitis, lymphadenitis, local abscesses, sepsis, encephalitis, varicella pneumonia, thrombocytopenia, hepatitis, glomerulonephritis, arthritis, meningitis, and Reye syndrome. Varicella may cause significant illness or death. Chickenpox can be fatal in immunocompromised children. Children who are undergoing chemotherapy, steroid treatment, or transplant therapy should be carefully monitored after exposure to the disease. Varicella-zoster immune globulin is usually administered as soon as possible after exposure.	Diagnostic tests include tissue culture from vesicle fluid. There is no cure for chickenpox. Medical management is supportive. Oral and IV acyclovir is used for immunocompromised patients, adolescents, children with chronic cutaneous and pulmonary diseases treated with chronic salicylate therapy, and oral or aerosol corticosteroids. If acyclovir is started within 24 hours of first lesions, it will decrease new lesion formation, the total number of lesions, and prevent life-threatening illness. It is not recommended for healthy children or adolescents with uncomplicated chickenpox (American Academy of Pediatrics, 2003). *Prognosis:* Most children recover fully. Children who are immunocompromised must be treated aggressively. This includes children with conditions listed above plus those on chemotherapy. The disease is more severe when steroids have been given during the incubation period (Arvin, 2002). *Prevention:* Chickenpox is a vaccine-preventable disease. The immunization may be given to susceptible children at any time after 12 months of age. The vaccine may be given within 72 hours after exposure to prevent or significantly modify the disease. Varicella-zoster immune globulin may be given to newborns of infected mothers and to exposed immunocompromised children with no history of chickenpox or immunization up to 4 days after exposure. Wild virus cases and breakthrough cases occur in vaccinated children.	➤ Use airborne and contact precautions for children in the hospital or agencies providing sick childcare while they are contagious. ➤ Obtain a history of varicella immunization and recent exposure in susceptible children upon admission to the hospital. Place all children exposed to varicella in isolation as a means of protecting newborns and immunocompromised patients. Nurses caring for the child should have a varicella titer to be certain of their immune status if they have not had a documented case of chickenpox. ➤ Most children are treated at home. While contagious, isolate them from all susceptible individuals, especially children and adults who are medically fragile and immunocompromised, and women early in pregnancy. Notify the school or childcare facility of the child's illness. ➤ Secondary cases in the home are often more severe than the primary case. ➤ Skin damage from eczema or sunburn may result in a more severe rash. ➤ Give nonaspirin antipyretics to control fever. ➤ Give oral antihistamines for relief of itching. Oatmeal and Aveeno baths are soothing. Caladryl lotion applied in moderation to lesions may also provide relief. ➤ Keep the child's fingernails short and clean. Young children may need to wear soft cotton mittens to prevent infections when itching cannot be controlled. ➤ Change bed linens frequently. Linen should be washed in mild soap and rinsed well. Reassure the child that the lesions are temporary and will go away. ➤ Observe the child closely for symptoms of complications such as drowsiness, meningeal signs, respiratory distress, and dehydration. Disorientation and restlessness may indicate viral encephalitis. ➤ Monitor for acyclovir side effects: nausea, vomiting, diarrhea, abdominal pain, as well as allergic skin reactions or headache. Monitor renal function if the child has renal insufficiency.

**Indicates that a vaccine or antitoxin is available for use in high-risk or as-needed situations.*

+Indicates that the disease has a safe and effective vaccine.

TABLE 19–5 Selected Infectious and Communicable Diseases in Children (continued)

DISEASE	CLINICAL MANIFESTATIONS	CLINICAL THERAPY	NURSING MANAGEMENT
Coxsackievirus *Causal Agent:* Coxsackievirus A16 and Enterovirus 71 cause a wide group of acute diseases that ranges from minor and self-limiting to potentially fatal. *Epidemiology:* Occurs worldwide, most commonly in summer and early fall. Sporadic outbreaks are seen, especially among children in out-of-home settings. Illnesses include the common cold; pharyngitis; pneumonia; hand, foot, and mouth disease; and herpangina. Immunity probably occurs after clinical or subclinical infection, but duration of the immunity is unknown. *Transmission:* Fecal–oral and respiratory routes. *Incubation period:* 3–6 days. *Period of communicability:* 2 days before rash to 2 days after it disappears.	Each of the coxsackieviruses is responsible for a different set of manifestations. Herpangina is an acute, self-limiting viral disease characterized by the sudden onset of fever, sore throat, and small, discrete grayish papulovesicular ulcerative pharyngeal lesions that gradually increase in size. In hand, foot, and mouth disease the lesions are more diffuse and may occur on the buccal surfaces of the cheeks, gums, and sides of the tongue. Papulovesicular lesions occur on the hands and feet and last for 7–10 days. Children may be irritable and have a fever, anorexia, dysphagia, malaise, and a sore throat. *Complications:* Enterovirus 71 caused a fatal epidemic in Taiwan in 1998. 78 deaths resulted from 90,000 cases of hand, foot, and mouth disease (Chang, Lin, Hsu, et al., 1999).	Diagnostic tests include a cell culture to detect the virus. There is no specific treatment. An antiviral medication, pleconaril, is being evaluated for use in immunodeficient children (American Academy of Pediatrics, 2003). *Prognosis:* Recovery is generally good with supportive care. *Prevention:* Avoid contact with infected persons early in the disease.	➤ Isolate the child while contagious. Use standard and contact precautions if the child is hospitalized. ➤ Apply topical lotions and give systemic medications as ordered to lessen the pain and relieve the irritation. ➤ Offer cool drinks and soft, bland foods (no citrus, salty, or spicy foods). Swallowing may be painful. ➤ Offer warm saline mouth rinses. ➤ Observe for dehydration. ➤ Provide reassurance and support to parents. ➤ Give nonaspirin antipyretics for fever. Keep the child out of school or childcare while febrile.
Diphtheria*+ *Causal agent: Corynebacterium diphtheriae,* a bacterium. *Epidemiology:* Occurs mostly during colder months in temperate zones in unimmunized, partially immunized, and immunized children with waning immunity. In tropical areas, cases of cutaneous and wound diphtheria occur sporadically. Maternal immunity lasts as long as 6 months after birth. While there are less than five cases annually in the United States, the disease is endemic in areas where immunization is no longer routine, such as Russia. *Transmission:* By contact with an infectious patient or carrier's nasal or eye discharge, or skin lesion; or less commonly, indirectly by contact with contaminated articles. Unpasteurized milk has also served as a vehicle. *Incubation period:* 2–7 days, sometimes longer. *Period of communicability:* Varies but is usually 2–4 weeks or until 4 days after antibiotics were initiated.	Symptoms can be mild or severe with a gradual onset over 1–2 days. Low-grade fever, anorexia, malaise, rhinorrhea with a foul odor, cough, sore throat, hoarseness, stridor or noisy breathing, cervical lymphadenitis, and pharyngitis may be present. In more severe cases the membranes of the tonsils, pharynx, and larynx are affected. The characteristic membranous lesion is a thick, bluish white to grayish black patch that covers the tonsils. It can spread to cover the soft and hard palates and the posterior portion of the pharynx. Attempts to remove the membrane result in bleeding. *Complications:* Produces an endotoxin that causes myocarditis and peripheral neuropathy (diplopia, slurred speech, difficulty swallowing, or paralysis of the palate) or ascending paralysis similar to Guillain-Barré syndrome.	Diagnostic tests include a culture from the nose or throat or any mucosal or cutaneous lesion. Administration of IV antitoxin and antibiotics within 3 days of onset of symptoms. The child must be tested for sensitivity to horse serum before giving the antitoxin. When diphtheria is suspected, antibiotic therapy (penicillin G or erythromycin) should be initiated without waiting for laboratory results. Removal of membrane may be needed to treat airway obstruction. *Prognosis:* With treatment, prognosis is good. If untreated, diphtheria can cause death from airway obstruction. *Prevention:* Diphtheria is a vaccine-preventable disease. The immunization series is initiated at 2 months of age and is usually given in combination with tetanus and pertussis. Diphtheria-tetanus (Td) is administered to children over 7 years. *This is a reportable disease.*	➤ Use droplet precautions for pharyngeal disease and contact precautions for cutaneous disease. ➤ Monitor closely for signs of increasing respiratory distress, as well as cardiac and neurologic complications. Provide humidified oxygen as necessary. ➤ Have emergency airway equipment available. ➤ Administer antibiotics. Give no medications containing caffeine or other stimulants. ➤ Use oral suction gently as necessary. ➤ Allow children to use mouthwash if desired. Gargling is not permitted because it can irritate the back of the throat. ➤ Encourage liquids as tolerated. Intravenous fluids may be necessary. ➤ Provide emotional support to the family. ➤ Initiate the trace for contacts with the patient to give antibiotics and immunization boosters.

(continued)

TABLE 19–5 Selected Infectious and Communicable Diseases in Children (continued)

DISEASE	CLINICAL MANIFESTATIONS	CLINICAL THERAPY	NURSING MANAGEMENT
Erythema Infectiosum (Fifth Disease) *Causal agent:* Human parvovirus B-19. *Epidemiology:* Occurs worldwide, most often in winter and spring. The disease also occurs in epidemics, with peak activity every 6 years. The incidence is highest in children between the ages of 5 and 14 years. *Transmission:* Respiratory secretions and blood. *Incubation period:* 6–14 days. *Period of communicability:* Believed to be the highest before the onset of the disease. 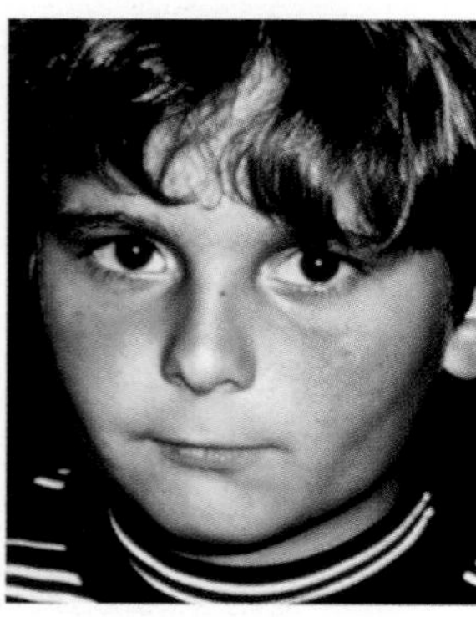 Erythema infectiosum *Courtesy of Centers for Disease Control and Prevention.*	The child first manifests a flulike illness (headache, chills, malaise, nausea, body ache) that lasts 2–3 days; 1 week later, a fiery-red rash appears on the cheeks giving a "slapped face" appearance. The rash is accompanied by circumoral pallor. In 1–4 days a lacelike symmetric, erythematous, maculopapular rash appears on the trunk and limbs, spreading proximal to distal. The palms and soles are spared. During the third stage, lasting 1–3 weeks, the rash fades but can reappear if the skin is irritated or exposed to sunlight. The rash may be mildly pruritic. *Complications:* Children with hemolytic conditions may have transient aplastic crisis.	Diagnostic testing includes determining if parvovirus B-19-specific immunoglobulin (Ig) M antibody is present. There is no specific treatment, and recovery is usually spontaneous. Children with hemolytic conditions may need blood transfusions if an aplastic crisis occurs. Immunodeficient patients may develop a chronic infection for which IV immune globulin therapy is often effective (American Academy of Pediatrics, 2003). *Prognosis:* Fetal infection may occur resulting in fetal hydrops or spontaneous abortion. *Prevention:* Avoid contact with infected persons early in the disease.	➤ Children with aplastic crisis are often hospitalized. ➤ Isolation is needed only for children with aplastic crisis or when immunosuppressed. Use standard and droplet precautions. ➤ Nonaspirin antipyretics may be given to control fever. ➤ Use soothing oatmeal or Aveeno baths if the rash is pruritic. Antipruritics may also help to relieve itching. ➤ Encourage rest and offer frequent fluids. ➤ Keep children out of direct sunlight if possible. ➤ Provide protective, light, loose clothing if exposure to sunlight cannot be avoided. ➤ Provide quiet diversionary activity. There is no reason to keep the immune competent child out of school or childcare. ➤ Explain the three stages of rash development to parents.
Haemophilus Influenzae Type B⁺ (H.Influenzae Type B) *Causal agent:* Coccobacilli *H. influenzae* bacteria, which has several serotypes and can be encapsulated or nonencapsulated. *Epidemiology:* Occurs most often in the spring and summer. Most commonly affected are infants and young children in childcare centers. Low-birth-weight children and children with chronic illnesses also have an increased susceptibility. Invasive disease has decreased significantly since introduction of the vaccine. *Transmission:* Direct person-to-person contact or droplet inhalation. The organism is frequently asymptomatically colonized in the respiratory tract. Incubation period: Unknown. *Period of communicability:* 3 days from onset of symptoms.	*H. influenzae* type B starts with a viral upper respiratory infection. The organism passes through the mucosal barrier to directly invade the bloodstream. It can cause several severe invasive illnesses, including meningitis, epiglottitis, pneumonia, septic arthritis, and cellulitis. It is also a cause of sepsis in infants. Other illnesses include sinusitis, otitis media, bronchitis, and pericarditis. Each disease has very specific clinical manifestations. *Complications:* Illness caused by *H. influenzae* type B responds to antibiotic therapy. Left untreated, severe sequelae and death, especially in young infants, can occur from conditions such as meningitis, epiglottitis, sinusitis, pneumonitis, and cellulitis.	Treatment consists of antibiotic therapy; however, one third of strains are resistant to ampicillin. Rifampin may be given to unprotected household contacts (not pregnant women), if another child has not completed immunizations, within 1 week after diagnosis. In this case, the infected child also gets rifampin to eliminate nasopharyngeal colonization. *Prognosis:* With rapid diagnosis and treatment, the outlook for recovery is good but highly dependent on the disease the organism has caused. When treatment has been delayed, the prognosis for full recovery becomes much more guarded. *Prevention:* Immunization is now available for *H. influenzae* type B as part of the recommended childhood immunization series beginning at 2 months of age. Other types of *H. influenzae* are not vaccine preventable.	➤ Use droplet precautions until 24 hours after the initiation of antibiotics. ➤ Antibiotic therapy is administered intravenously for severe infections. Infections such as otitis media can be managed at home with oral antibiotics. ➤ Children under the age of 4 years who have not been immunized are at increased risk for developing disease from *H. influenzae.* Specific prophylactic measures for susceptible children may be ordered by the physician. ➤ Administer antipyretics to help the child feel more comfortable. ➤ Closely monitor IV sites for patency and infiltration. ➤ Perform nursing care measures specific to the illness. ➤ Inform family members that rifampin turns urine and other body fluids orange, and it will cause stains.

**Indicates that a vaccine or antitoxin is available for use in high-risk or as-needed situations. +Indicates that the disease has a safe and effective vaccine.*
Hepatitis A, Hepatitis B, and Hepatitis C, see Chapter 30.

TABLE 19–5 Selected Infectious and Communicable Diseases in Children (continued)

DISEASE	CLINICAL MANIFESTATIONS	CLINICAL THERAPY	NURSING MANAGEMENT
Herpetic Gingivostomatitis *Causal agent:* Herpes simplex, type 1 (HSV-1). *Epidemiology:* Worldwide distribution with an infection rate of approximately 70% in the United States. Infants and young children 2 to 4 years are at increased risk as maternal antibodies decrease. Exposure occurs primarily between children in childcare settings. The virus is transported to the trigeminal ganglia and becomes dormant. Illness, stress, sun exposure, menses, fever, or immune suppression reactivates the virus. *Transmission:* The virus is shed by infected individuals and when direct contact is made with mucous membranes or broken skin of an uninfected individual, it invades the epithelial cells. *Incubation period:* 3–7 days. *Period of communicability:* The virus is usually shed for a week or longer.	Mild cases may be asymptomatic. Primary sign with an initial infection is blistering oral lesions, but it can occur on any skin surface. Herpetic gingivostomatitis syndrome signs include fever (up to 103° F), malaise, irritability, and bilateral cervical, submental, and submaxillary lymphadenopathy. Fragile vesicles appear on the mucosa inside the upper lip, but may also appear on the gingivae, buccal mucosa, tongue, and hard palate. Vesicles progress to ulcers that are painful. Mouth odor is present. The child may have too much pain to swallow saliva, resulting in drooling. Symptoms may last 1–2 weeks. Herpetic whitlow, an inflamed finger with a single or multiple vesicles can occur if the infected child sucks a thumb or finger and spreads the infection to that location, or potentially another location where there is broken skin. Cold sores (fever blisters) appear at the border of the lip when the virus is reactivated. Neonatal infection signs can include disseminated disease involving multiple organs, most prominently liver and lungs or localized central nervous system disease. *Complications:* Immunocompromised children are at increased risk for secondary infection. Central nervous system complications include Bell's palsy, atypical pain syndromes, trigeminal neuralgia, ascending myelitis, and postinfectious encephalomyelitis (American Academy of Pediatrics, 2003).	If diagnostic testing is required, cell cultures of HSV-1 can be grown. Direct fluorescent antibody stain of infected cells scraped from lesions may be positive for lesions that are healing. An enzyme immunoassay can be used to diagnose HSV-1. Oral acyclovir is used to treat herpetic gingivostomatitis. It reduces viral shedding and shortens the healing time. Acyclovir also shortens the duration of lesions during a recurrence. Viscous lidocaine, a local anesthetic, can be prescribed for topical application to lesions, providing relief for 10–15 minutes. *Prognosis:* In children this is a self-limiting primary infection with reactivation of the latent virus. In neonates significant neurologic sequelae occur, and up to 25% of neonates with disseminated infection die, even with acyclovir treatment (American Academy of Pediatrics, 2003). *Prevention:* There is no vaccine for this infection; however, vaccine research is being conducted.	➤ Use contact precautions with gloves to avoid direct contact with mucous membranes, lesions, and saliva. Gowns may be needed to avoid contact when the child is drooling. ➤ Children will usually be cared for at home. Teach parents about the transmission of the virus and how to protect themselves and other family members from infection. ➤ Encourage the use of acetaminophen or ibuprofen for fever and mild pain management. Teach parents how to apply viscous lidocaine to oral lesions before encouraging the child to drink fluids. ➤ Encourage the child to eat cold soft foods and cool liquids that have low acidity (avoid orange and pineapple juice). Higher acidity liquids will irritate the lesions and cause pain. Foods and liquids that should be encouraged: jello, applesauce, pudding, popsicles, white grape or apple juice. Help parents set goals for fluid intake so that dehydration is avoided. ➤ Provide oral care with glyoxide (glycerine and peroxide) to help sooth the mucous membranes. ➤ Teach the parents to monitor the child for dehydration (see Chapter 23∞) and to contact the health professional if the child does not drink enough fluids or has less frequent voiding than normal with dark and strong-smelling urine. ➤ Monitor the child for side effects of acyclovir. ➤ If dehydration occurs, the child is likely to be hospitalized for IV fluids. ➤ If an infant who is breastfeeding becomes infected, encourage the mother to pump her breasts and use a bottle to feed the breast milk until the lesions have disappeared. This will help prevent transmission of the virus to her breasts. ➤ Do not allow the child to return to childcare until active lesions are healed and drooling has stopped.
Influenza[+] *Causal agent: Orthomyxoviridae,* types A and B. *Epidemiology:* Spreads by aerosolized particles and direct contact with respiratory secretions. Prevalent in the United States from October to March, but the virus is active in other parts of the world year-round. During annual epidemics, 10% to 40% of healthy children are infected, and 1% are hospitalized (Cheung, & Lieberman, 2002).	Abrupt onset of fever (38–40°C), chills, cough, runny nose, sore throat, malaise, aches, headache, and anorexia. Children may have nausea and vomiting, diarrhea, and abdominal pain. Children may also present with croup, bronchiolitis, conjunctivitis, or other nonspecific febrile illness. *Complications:* Otitis media, exacerbations of chronic lung conditions such as asthma and cystic	Diagnostic tests may include rapid test for influenza from a nasopharyngeal swab, throat swab, or nasal washing (Directigen Flu A+B, FluOIA, QuickVue), and viral culture. Treatment is usually supportive with nonaspirin antipyretics for fever. Antiviral therapy (amantadine, rimantadine, oseltamivir, and zanamivir) is indicated for children 1 year of age or older at high risk of complications, those with severe influenza, and patients in contact	➤ Use droplet and contact precautions for hospitalized infants and children. ➤ The child is usually cared for at home. Encourage parents to wash hands frequently and to reduce exposure of other family members to the infected child. ➤ Provide fluids to keep nasal secretions moist and to prevent dehydration. ➤ Provide acetaminophen or ibuprofen for fever management and mild pain. ➤ Provide rest and quiet diversional activities. ➤ Teach parents to be alert to signs of complications from the viral infection.

(continued)

TABLE 19–5 Selected Infectious and Communicable Diseases in Children (continued)

DISEASE	CLINICAL MANIFESTATIONS	CLINICAL THERAPY	NURSING MANAGEMENT
Influenza (continued) *Incubation period:* 1–4 days. *Period of communicability:* One day before symptoms until 5 days after onset of illness.	fibrosis. Lower respiratory infections such as pneumonia, croup, bronchiolitis, and wheezing may occur in up to 25% of children. Myositis, myocarditis, encephalitis, transverse myelitis, Reye syndrome, and Guillain-Barré syndrome are all potential complications.	with high-risk individuals in an effort to reduce transmission of the virus (Cheung & Lieberman, 2002). When antiviral medication is initiated within 2 days of symptoms the duration of symptoms may be reduced by 1–2 days. *Prevention:* Influenza vaccine is now recommended for infants and children over 6 months of age.	
Measles (Rubeola)*+ *Causal agent:* Mobillivirus, a member of the paramyxovirus group. *Epidemiology:* Occurrence peaks in the late winter and early spring. In developed countries, measles occurs mostly in outbreaks among children, which are largely the result of lack of immunization or possibly declining immunity. Many cases are imported from countries without routine immunization. Maternal immunity is active in the infant until the age of approximately 12–15 months. Vaccination induces lifelong immunity. In developing countries, measles remains largely an endemic problem and is a significant cause of infant and child morbidity and mortality. *Transmission:* Airborne, respiratory droplets, and contact with infected persons. *Incubation period:* About 8–12 days. *Period of communicability:* Begins during the prodromal phase and ends about 2–4 days after the rash appears. Measles *Courtesy of Centers for Disease Control and Prevention.*	Children are quite ill in the 3–5 day prodromal phase, with symptoms including high fever, conjunctivitis, coryza, cough, anorexia, and malaise. Small, irregular, bluish white spots on a red background, called Koplik spots, appear on the buccal mucosa about 2 days before and after the onset of the rash. The characteristic red, blotchy, maculopapular rash that becomes confluent usually appears 2–4 days after onset of prodromal phase. The rash begins on the face and spreads to the trunk and extremities. Symptoms gradually subside in 4–7 days. Other symptoms include anorexia, malaise, fatigue, and generalized lymphadenopathy. *Complications:* Diarrhea, otitis media, bronchopneumonia, bronchitis, laryngotracheobronchitis, and encephalitis. Complications and sequelae occur most often in children who are malnourished, medically fragile, and immunosuppressed. The younger the child, the greater the risk for complications.	Diagnosis can be made by a serologic test result for immunoglobulin (Ig) M measles antibody. There is no cure for measles. Treatment is supportive. Antibiotics are used for bacterial secondary infections. *Prognosis:* Recovery is generally good with supportive care. *Prevention:* Measles is a vaccine-preventable disease. The measles vaccine is available alone (M), in combination with the rubella vaccine (MR), or in combination with the rubella and mumps vaccines (MMR). Immune globulin, administered up to 6 days after exposure, may be helpful in preventing the disease in susceptible persons (immunocompromised children, infants less than 1 year of age, pregnant women). All healthcare workers should have documented immunity. *This is a reportable disease.*	➤ If the child is hospitalized, maintain airborne precautions during the contagious period (5 days after the rash appears). ➤ Use a cool-mist vaporizer to help clear respiratory passages. ➤ Suction nose and oral cavity gently as necessary. ➤ Give nonaspirin antipyretics for fever and antipruritics for itching. ➤ Assess lungs carefully, especially in young children, in whom pneumonias are a common complication. ➤ Antitussives may be ordered to control coughing. ➤ Keep lights dim, and cover windows if the child has photophobia. ➤ Elevate the head of the bed. Keep the room cool with good air circulation. Provide light, nonirritating blankets. ➤ Keep skin clean and dry. No soaps should be used. ➤ Maintain fluid intake. Offer cool liquids frequently in small amounts. Blended, pureed, and mashed foods are most easily tolerated. ➤ Maintain bed rest. Visitors should be immune to measles. ➤ Provide diversions such as music, stories, and favorite toys.

**Indicates that a vaccine or antitoxin is available for use in high-risk or as-needed situations.*
+Indicates that the disease has a safe and effective vaccine.

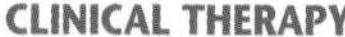

TABLE 19–5 Selected Infectious and Communicable Diseases in Children (continued)

DISEASE	CLINICAL MANIFESTATIONS	CLINICAL THERAPY	NURSING MANAGEMENT
Meningococcus* *Causal agent: Neisseria meningitidis.* *Epidemiology:* Most often in winter or early spring. Spread by respiratory droplets from human carriers. Majority of infections are caused by serogroups B and C in the United States. Highest rates are in children under 5 years of age, with a peak attack rate in 3 to 5 months old. Outbreaks have occurred in childcare centers, college dormitories, and military recruit camps. *Incubation period:* 1–10 days. *Period of communicability:* Until 24 hours after antibiotics is started. 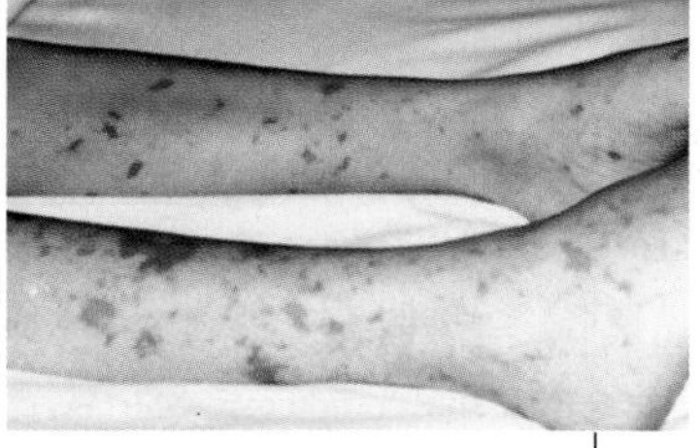 Purpura *Used with permission of the American Academy of Pediatrics, http://www.vaccineinformation.org/photos/variaapoo3.jpg, accessed 6/20/04.*	Abrupt onset of flulike symptoms of fever, chills, malaise, vomiting, and **prostration** (extreme exhaustion). Meningitis has the neurologic signs including drowsiness, disorientation, hallucinations, and convulsions. Meningococcemia: An urticarial, maculopapular, or petechial rash also appears that may progress to purpura. The condition may further deteriorate to shock, hypotension, disseminated intravascular coagulation, and coma. *Complications:* Loss of limbs due to necrosis, hearing loss, arthritis, myocarditis, pericarditis, ataxia, seizures, hemiparesis, cranial nerve palsies, and obstructive hydrocephalus. *Prognosis:* Up to 15% of children with invasive meningococcal disease die (Ferguson, Hormann, Parks, et al., 2002).	Diagnostic tests include, complete blood count and a blood culture. Lumbar puncture for culture of cerebrospinal fluid is performed when the child is hemodynamically stable and has no increased intracranial pressure. Cultures from petechial scrapings may also be done. *Treatment:* Penicillin G is given IV (cefotaxime, ceftriaxone, and ampicillin are alternate antibiotics), and choloramphenicol is used for children allergic to penicillin. Use of steroids is controversial. The child is managed aggressively in the intensive care unit to maintain the airway, assisted ventilation, management of shock with IV fluids and vasopressers when needed to maintain the blood pressure. Plasma, blood, or platelets are used to treat the disseminated intravascular coagulation. *Prevention:* A vaccine available for children > 2 years with chronic conditions or asplenia, and students living in school or college dormitories. Immunization of freshman college students living in dormitories available at the student's or family's request. Close contacts are given medication (rifampin, ceftriaxone, or ciprofloxacin) for prophylaxis. Only health professionals with unprotected direct contact with oral secretions need prophylaxis (American Academy of Pediatrics, 2003). *This is a reportable disease.*	➤ The child will be hospitalized. Use standard precautions and droplet precautions until antibiotic has been administered for 24 hours. ➤ Disease onset is abrupt and rapidly progresses to life threatening. Be alert for development of shock and respiratory compromise. Have emergency equipment available and be prepared to perform resuscitation. ➤ When giving IV fluids and blood products, make sure the child does not get overloaded with fluids, and monitor for evidence of increased intracranial pressure. ➤ Keep the family informed of the child's status and treatment as the disease progresses. Help the family identify and mobilize its support system. ➤ The surviving child will likely need rehabilitation. Work with the social worker or case manager to transition the child to long-term care. ➤ Help identify close contacts that should receive prophylactic antibiotics and educate them about the expected side effects (i.e., orange urine with rifampin). ➤ Teach close contacts to be observant for signs of illness and to seek healthcare promptly if they occur.
Mononucleosis *Causal agent:* Epstein-Barr virus (EBV), a member of the herpes-virus group. *Epidemiology:* Occurs worldwide. In developing countries, the disease occurs in young children and may be asymptomatic or mild. In developed countries, the disease is more common in older children and adolescents. *Transmission:* Direct contact with infected oropharyngeal and genital tract secretions. EBV can survive for several hours outside the body. EBV can also be transmitted by blood transfusion. Approximately 85% of adults have antibody to EBV.	In very young children mononucleosis may cause irritability, but be otherwise asymptomatic. A maculopapular rash may be seen in a few cases. In other children, the disease is characterized by malaise, headache, anorexia, abdominal pain, fatigue, and fever for 2–3 days, followed by lymphadenopathy and a sore throat. Hepatosplenomegaly may occur. Pain from swelling of the tonsils and lymph nodes may be significant. The syndrome typically lasts 2–3 weeks and is self-limited. Weakness and lethargy may continue for several months. *Complications:* Rare side effects include central nervous system	Diagnostic tests include the serologic monospot test or testing EBV antibodies by immunofluorescence. Abnormal liver enzymes are often found with a chemistry panel. On a blood smear, lymphocytes are enlarged with atypical nuclei (Downey cells). There is no specific treatment as this is a viral illness. Corticosteroids may be used to control tonsillar swelling and pain when there is impending airway obstruction, massive splenomegaly, myocarditis or hemolytic anemia. Antibiotics (ampicillin and amoxicillin) should be avoided as a nonallergic rash often develops (American Academy of Pediatrics, 2003).	➤ Children are usually treated at home. Standard precautions should be used. ➤ Give antipyretics and analgesics for fever and sore throat. Offer warm salt water for gargling. Offer soft foods and encourage fluids. ➤ Maintain bed rest. ➤ Give adolescents a sense of responsibility by involving them in decisions about care when possible. Be sure to include parents and adolescents in discussions. ➤ Reassure adolescents who may be worried about keeping up with schoolwork that they can return to school when the fever is gone and swallowing is normal. ➤ Teens should avoid kissing until the fever has been gone several days. ➤ Contact sports should be avoided until the liver and spleen are normal, usually in about 4 weeks.

(continued)

TABLE 19–5 Selected Infectious and Communicable Diseases in Children (continued)

DISEASE	CLINICAL MANIFESTATIONS	CLINICAL THERAPY	NURSING MANAGEMENT
Mononucleosis (continued)			
Incubation period: 10–50 days. *Period of communicability:* Virus is shed for up to 18 months after the clinical course of the disease. The infected individual becomes a lifelong carrier (American Academy of Pediatrics, 2003).	symptoms such as encephalitis, aseptic meningitis, and Guillain-Barré syndrome. Splenic rupture, respiratory failure, and hematologic complications such as thrombocytopenia can also occur. In immunodeficient children, fatal infections or lymphomas can develop.	*Prognosis:* After recovery, the virus remains latent in the lymphoid system. It can be reactivated during periods of immunosuppression. *Prevention:* No known prevention.	
Mumps (Parotitis)[+] *Causal agent:* Rubulavirus in the paramyxovirus family. *Epidemiology:* Occurs worldwide in unvaccinated children, most often in winter and spring. Infection and vaccination induce lifelong immunity. Maternal antibodies begin to disappear in infants at the age of 12–15 months. *Transmission:* Contact with respiratory tract secretions. *Incubation period:* 12–25 days. *Period of communicability:* 7 days before parotid swelling until 9 days after swelling subsides. 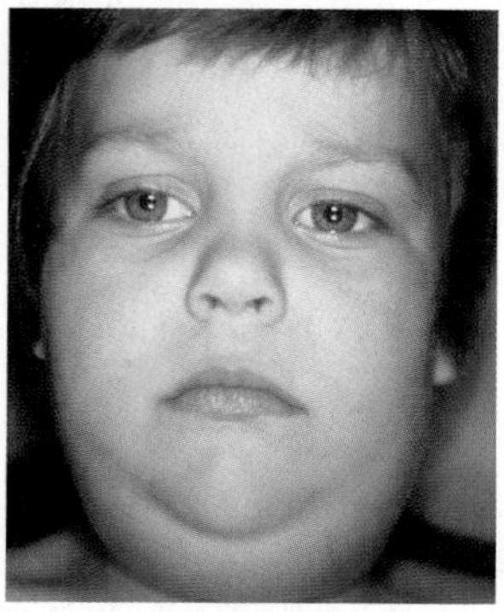 Mumps *Courtesy of Centers for Disease Control and Prevention.*	Malaise; low-grade fever; and earache, headache, malaise, pain with chewing, decreased appetite and activity; followed by bilateral or unilateral parotid gland swelling. Swelling peaks around the third day. Meningeal signs (stiff neck, headache, and photophobia) occur in about 15% of patients. *Complications:* Orchitis (inflammation of the epididymis, pain on testicular palpation, and scrotal swelling—most often unilateral) may occur in postpubertal males; sterility is relatively rare (American Academy of Pediatrics, 2003). Oophoritis, pancreatitis, aseptic meningoencephalitis, and unilateral permanent deafness are sometimes seen.	Diagnostic tests include a viral culture from a throat washing, urine, or cerebrospinal fluid. Serum mumps immunoglobulin (Ig) G antibody titer may also be performed. There is no specific treatment. Therapy is supportive, focused on symptom relief. *Prognosis:* Mumps is usually self-limiting. *Prevention:* Mumps is a vaccine-preventable disease. The vaccine is usually administered in combination with measles and rubella vaccines (MMR) at 12–15 months of age and again at either 4–6 years or 11–12 years. *This is a reportable disease.*	➤ Children are generally uncomfortable but are rarely very ill. They are usually cared for at home. ➤ Use standard and droplet precautions for hospitalized children while contagious. Avoid exposure to immunocompromised individuals or susceptible persons. ➤ Keep children out of school or childcare until 9 days after parotid swelling occurs. Encourage diversional activities. ➤ Give nonaspirin analgesics and antipyretics to control fever and pain. Give steroids if ordered. Encourage fluid intake. Swallowing and chewing may be painful. Offer soft and blended foods. Avoid foods and beverages that increase salivary flow (citrus, spices, and candies) because they cause pain. ➤ Talking may be painful. Provide a bell or other attention-getting device. ➤ Apply warm or cool compresses, whichever is preferred, to the parotid area. ➤ Be alert for signs of complications. Headache, stiff neck, vomiting, and photophobia may indicate meningeal irritation. ➤ Provide scrotal supports if testicular swelling occurs. ➤ Reassure children who may be upset about the facial swelling that it will go away.
Pertussis (Whooping Cough)[+] *Causal agent: Bordetella pertussis.* Occurs worldwide. Predominantly a childhood disease that is most common in children under 6 months of age. Epidemic cycles occur every 3–4 years. Pertussis also occurs in healthcare workers or adults who may have weakened or incomplete immunity. Adults may become only mildly ill but can	The onset is insidious. Catarrhal stage: The disease begins with nasal congestion, a runny nose, low-grade fever, and a mild nonproductive cough, lasting about 2 weeks. Paroxysmal stage: The cough becomes more severe at night and changes into spasms of paroxysmal coughing when the child attempts to expel a thick mucoid plug. This is followed by inspiration, stridor, or "whooping." (Young infants do not	Diagnostic tests include culture and polymerase chain reaction (PCR) testing. Treatment consists of antibiotics (erythromycin and other macrolides), corticosteroids, if ordered, and supportive care. *Prognosis:* The disease is most severe in infants under 1 year of age, and most deaths occur in this age group. *Prevention:* Pertussis is a vaccine-preventable disease. Active	➤ Use droplet precautions until 5–7 days after the initiation of antibiotics. Most hospitalized cases occur in children under the age of 5 years. ➤ Closely monitor respirations and oxygen saturation. The smaller the child, the greater the risk for respiratory distress and apnea. ➤ Remain with the child during coughing spells, when hypoxic and apneic episodes are most likely. Give oxygen if ordered. Have emergency equipment available. ➤ Provide humidification. Gentle suctioning may be necessary.

**Indicates that a vaccine or antitoxin is available for use in high-risk or as-needed situations.*
+Indicates that the disease has a safe and effective vaccine.
Parasites, see Chapter 30∞.

TABLE 19–5 Selected Infectious and Communicable Diseases in Children (continued)

DISEASE	CLINICAL MANIFESTATIONS	CLINICAL THERAPY	NURSING MANAGEMENT
Pertussis (Whooping Cough) (continued)			
spread the disease to unimmunized children. Approximately 20 to 40 million cases occur annually in the world (World Health Organization, 1999). *Transmission:* Respiratory droplets and direct contact with discharge from the respiratory membranes. *Incubation period:* 7–21 days (commonly 7–10 days). *Period of communicability:* Begins approximately 1 week after exposure. Pertussis is communicable for 5–7 days after the initiation of antibiotic therapy. The disease is most contagious before the paroxysmal cough stage.	manifest the "whooping." Rather they present with frequent apnea.) The whoop sound results from forceful inhalation and a narrowed glottis. Sucking on a bottle may trigger the coughing spell. May be accompanied by flushing, cyanosis, vomiting, profuse drainage from the nose, eyes, and mouth. Dehydration may result from decreased oral intake. Paroxysmal coughing may last 1–4 weeks or more. Convalescent stage: up to 6 weeks when paroxysms gradually subside. *Complications:* Pneumonia, atelectasis, otitis media, encephalopathy, seizures, and death. Highest mortality rate and complication rate is in infants under 1 year. In 2000, 17 infants under 4 months of age died due to pertussis (Centers for Disease Control, 2002a).	immunization should be given in early infancy. During the 1990s the incidence of pertussis has increased in infants less than 6 months of age, adolescents and adults, but remained stable in children 6 months to 4 years of age, indicating effectiveness of the acellular pertussis vaccine (Centers for Disease Control, 2002c). Healthcare professionals who are in close contact with infected children before diagnosis may need antibiotics to prevent transmission. Vaccine protection wanes after 5 to 10 years allowing adolescents and adults to become infected and transmit the infection to susceptible infants. *This is a reportable disease.*	➤ Give nonaspirin antipyretics as needed for fever. ➤ Encourage frequent rest periods. ➤ Allow the child to eat desired foods in small frequent feedings. ➤ Encourage the child to take fluids. The child may need IV hydration if oral intake is not tolerated. ➤ Provide emotional support to parents. ➤ Teach parents to watch for signs of respiratory failure and dehydration if the child is managed at home.
Pneumococcal infection*⁺ *Causative agent: Streptococcus pneumoniae,* a gram-positive diplococcus. *Epidemiology:* The organism is found in the pharynx of healthy people. Outbreaks occur in the winter and spring when people are more crowded in physical settings. In temperate climates, of 90 serotypes, 8 account for most of the invasive pediatric infections. The disease is more common in African Americans, American Indians, and Alaskan Natives. It occurs most commonly in the 6-month to 2-year age group, and among children in childcare settings. Of particular concern is the development of penicillin and multiantibiotic-resistant strains. *Transmission:* Respiratory secretions and droplets. Upper respiratory infections help the spread. *Incubation period:* 1–3 days. *Period of communicability:* Unknown. Probably less than 24 hours after initiation of effective antibiotic therapy.	The signs and symptoms are related to the focal area of infection. The organism causes otitis media, sinusitis, pharyngitis, laryngotracheobronchitis, pneumonia, meningitis, and bacteremia. In otitis media, upper respiratory infection, fever, ear pain, and decreased appetite are seen. In bacteremia, there is unexplained fever and no localized infection site. In pneumonia, fever, chills, chest pain, dyspnea, malaise, and a productive cough are seen. In meningitis, inconsolable crying, increased irritability, lethargy, refusal to eat, nausea, vomiting, diarrhea, myalgia, photophobia, and seizures are seen. *Complications:* This organism is one of the leading causes of morbidity and mortality. It is the leading cause of acute otitis media, and a major cause of meningitis, bacteremia, and pneumonia (Tan, 2002). Other complications include septic arthritis, osteomyelitis, endocarditis, and brain abscess.	Penicillin is given for penicillin-sensitive strains, but up to 48% of infections are penicillin resistant. Macrolide antibiotics are used for mild disease if the child is allergic to penicillin. Penicillin-resistant strains are treated with third-generation cephalosporins (cefotaxime or ceftriaxone). Vancomycin and rifampen are used in combination when strains are resistant to antibiotics listed above (American Academy of Pediatrics, 2003). Symptomatic care is also provided. *Prevention:* Many serotypes are preventable with immunization. Active immunization should begin in infancy with the 7-valent vaccine (Prevnar). Significant reduction in pneumonia, meningitis, bacteremia, and otitis media have occurred with the vaccine. No increase of invasive pneuomoccal disease with nonvaccine serotypes has been detected (Keyserling, 2002). A 23-valent vaccine is available for older children at high risk of pneumococcal disease.	➤ If the child is hospitalized, maintain standard precautions. ➤ Provide nonaspirin antipyretics for control of fever and comfort. ➤ Encourage fluids, and monitor intake and output. ➤ Monitor vital signs and consciousness level to identify signs of worsening condition. ➤ Educate parents about the need for the vaccine, as the unimmunized child could become infected repeatedly with different serotypes. ➤ Many children with mild disease will be treated at home. Educate parents about signs indicating a need to seek additional medical care, the need for proper medication administration, and comfort measures for the child. ➤ Individuals with congenital asplenia or traumatic splenectomy, malignancy, sickle-cell disease, and nephrotic syndrome are at higher risk for invasive disease with this organism. ➤ Additional factors that increase risk of pneumococcal disease include poverty, crowded housing, homelessness, and exposure to tobacco smoke.

(continued)

TABLE 19–5 Selected Infectious and Communicable Diseases in Children (continued)

DISEASE	CLINICAL MANIFESTATIONS	CLINICAL THERAPY	NURSING MANAGEMENT
Poliomyelitis+ *Causal agent:* Poliovirus is an enterovirus with three serotypes. *Epidemiology:* Occurs worldwide. Polio primarily affects children, although some of the cases involve transmission to immunocompromised or non-polio-protected adults caring for infants who had received live poliovirus vaccine. The disease can be mild or severe. The vaccine induces lifelong immunity. With the discontinuation of the live poliovirus vaccine in the United States, no cases of wild poliomyelitis have occurred since 2000. *Transmission:* Primarily by the fecal-oral route, but also the respiratory route. *Incubation period:* Usually 7–10 days (range 3–36 days). *Period of communicability:* Greatest shortly before and right after clinical symptoms develop when the virus is in the throat. Excreted in the feces for several weeks.	Affects the central nervous system. Less severe infections may be limited to fever and stiffness in the neck and back, headache, vomiting, and sore throat. In other cases, fever, headache, stiff neck, Kernig or Brudzinski sign, decreased deep tendon reflexes, and progressive weakness occur. With cranial nerve involvement there may be respiratory difficulties. An increased respiratory rate may interfere with the ability to talk because frequent pauses are needed. Onset of paralysis may be sudden, in hours, or gradual over 3–5 days. Paralysis results from damage to motor neurons. *Complications:* Permanent motor paralysis, respiratory arrest, myocardial failure, aseptic meningitis, and postpolio syndrome.	Diagnosis is made by cell culture from stool or throat swabs. Treatment is supportive. No chemotherapeutic agents that directly kill the poliovirus are available. *Prognosis:* Respiratory complication is life threatening and involves 5%–10% of all cases. Respiratory paralysis may lead to death. Motor paralysis may result in long-term disability. *Prevention:* Poliomyelitis is a vaccine-preventable disease. Children should be immunized with the inactivated poliovirus vaccine (IPV) according to the recommended schedule. *This is a reportable disease.*	➤ Use standard and droplet precautions in the hospital and keep the child on strict bed rest. ➤ Observe closely for respiratory paralysis (ineffective cough, talking with frequent pauses, shallow and rapid respiratory rate). Have emergency equipment at bedside. Assist ventilations as needed until mechanical ventilation is set up. ➤ Administer sedatives and nonaspirin analgesics as ordered to allow for rest and comfort. Moist hot packs may relieve discomfort. ➤ Encourage fluids. ➤ Position the child to promote body alignment. ➤ Perform range-of-motion exercises to prevent contractures after the acute phase. ➤ Provide emotional support. ➤ Patients are alert and aware. Tell them what is happening to them. ➤ Long-term orthopedic (physical therapy) support may be needed by some children.
Roseola (Exanthem Subitum, Sixth Disease) *Causal agent:* Herpesvirus type 6. *Epidemiology:* Occurs worldwide, primarily in children 6–24 months of age (after maternal antibodies decline). No seasonal pattern. *Transmission:* Likely to be from respiratory secretions of healthy individuals. *Incubation period:* Appears to be 5–15 days. *Period of communicability:* Lifelong persistent infection and virus shedding in healthy individuals (American Academy of Pediatrics, 2003).	Sudden, high fever up to 40.5°C (105°F) for 3–8 days, during which the child does not appear toxic (normal appetite and behavior). The fever phase is followed by a characteristic pale pink, discrete, maculopapular rash, which starts on the trunk and spreads to the face, neck, and extremities. The rash can last for 1–2 days. The child's appetite is normal. *Complications:* Children may have febrile seizures during high fever stage. Encephalopathy may develop in rare cases.	Roseola is self-limiting, and there is no treatment other than supportive care. *Prognosis:* Roseola is benign in most cases.	➤ Children are rarely hospitalized, but if they are, use standard precautions. ➤ Give nonaspirin antipyretics to control fever. ➤ Observe closely for any seizure activity, especially during the acute febrile periods. ➤ Encourage fluids. ➤ Reassure parents that the rash will disappear in a few days.
Rubella (German Measles)+ *Causal agent:* An RNA virus, member of the family Togaviridae, genus Rubivirus. *Epidemiology:* Occurs worldwide and is most prevalent in the winter and spring. Children are susceptible after loss of transplacentally acquired maternal antibodies about 6–9 months after birth. Natural infection or	Rubella is generally a mild disease with a characteristic pink, nonconfluent, maculopapular rash. The rash appears on the face, progresses to the neck, trunk, and legs, and disappears in the same order. Prodromal symptoms occur 1–5 days before the rash and include low-grade fever, headache, malaise, coryza, sore	Diagnostic tests include cell culture from a nasal swab, and detection of IgM or IgG antibodies. Treatment is supportive. Rubella is generally self-limiting in children. *Prognosis:* Disease is usually mild and benign. Major risk is for fetus if the mother is infected in the first trimester. Abortion, stillbirth, or fetal death is common (10% die after	➤ Children are usually treated at home and rarely require hospitalization. They should not attend school or childcare while contagious, and they should be isolated from pregnant women. School and childcare facilities should be notified of the child's illness. ➤ Maintain standard and droplet precautions for contagious children. Maintain contact precautions for infants with congenital rubella syndrome until 1 year of age unless

**Indicates that a vaccine or antitoxin is available for use in high-risk or as-needed situations.*

+Indicates that the disease has a safe and effective vaccine.

TABLE 19–5 Selected Infectious and Communicable Diseases in Children (continued)

DISEASE	CLINICAL MANIFESTATIONS	CLINICAL THERAPY	NURSING MANAGEMENT
Rubella (continued) vaccination induces lifelong immunity. Most cases occur in the adults 20–29 years of age. Most cases in the United States occur among foreign-born Hispanic adults who are from countries that do not have rubella vaccination programs. Congenital rubella syndrome is most likely the result of lack of immunization rather than vaccine failure. Each year an average of 6 infants are born with congenital rubella syndrome (Reef, Frey, Theall, et al., 2002). *Transmission:* Droplet spread, direct contact with infected persons, or contact with articles soiled by nasal secretions. *Incubation period:* 14–21 days (most commonly 16–18 days). *Period of communicability:* From about 7 days before until about 4 days after the onset of the rash. Infants with congenital rubella may shed the virus for months after birth and should not be exposed or cared for by persons who are not immune to the disease.	throat, and anorexia. Forschheimer spots (discrete, erythematous pinpoint or larger lesions on the soft palate) are seen during the prodromal phase. Generalized lymphadenopathy involving the postauricular, suboccipital, and posterior cervical areas is common up to 7 days before the rash. Many cases are asymptomatic. Signs of congenital rubella syndrome include growth retardation, radiolucent bone disease, hepatosplenomegaly, thrombocytopenia, and purpuric skin lesions (giving a "blueberry muffin" appearance). No obvious signs may be found with mild forms of the disease at birth. *Complications:* Complications are rare, but include arthritis in adolescents, encephalitis, and congenital rubella syndrome.	birth). Many other anomalies may be present, such as intrauterine growth retardation, cardiac, ear, and eye anomalies. *Prevention:* Rubella is a vaccine-preventable disease. It is important to immunize females of childbearing age because of the severe complications rubella poses to the fetus during the first trimester. All healthcare workers should have documented immunity. Of the 47 countries in North, Central, and South America 44 have initiated rubella vaccination programs in the past 3 years (Reef et al., 2002). It is hoped that this will reduce the incidence of rubella and congenital rubella syndrome in the United States.	nasopharyngeal and urine cultures are repeatedly negative after 3 months of age (American Academy of Pediatrics, 2003). ➤ Give nonaspirin analgesics and antipyretics for any pain and fever. ➤ Allow children to choose what they would like to eat and drink. Encourage fluids. ➤ Provide quiet activities. ➤ Exclude children from childcare or school for 7 days after onset of rash. 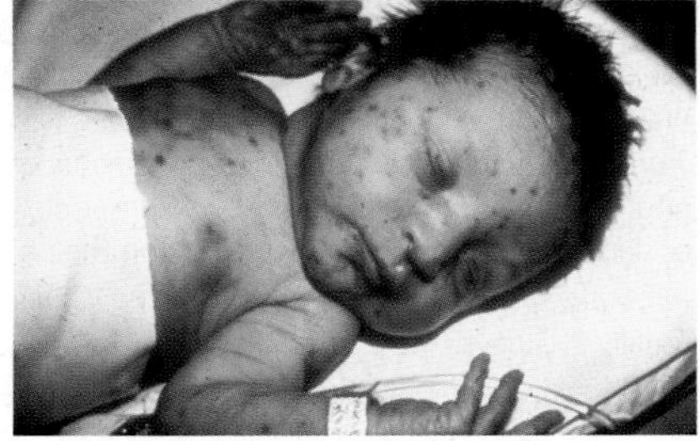 Congenital rubella syndrome *Courtesy of Centers for Disease Control and Prevention*
Severe Acute Respiratory Syndrome (SARS) *Causative agent:* A coronavirus. *Epidemiology:* Emerging infection believed to be animal to human transmission initially. Then transmission occurs by close contact, potentially spread through the airborne route. Transmission is primarily thought to be associated with travel within 10 days of onset of symptoms to an area with documented or suspected community transmission of SARS or close contact within 10 days of onset of symptoms with a person known or suspected to have SARS. *Incubation period:* 2–7 days, up to 10 days.	Onset with a 1–2 day fever over 38.0°C (100.4°F), chills, headache, malaise, and myalgia. Asymptomatic or mild respiratory illness with symptoms such as rhinorrhea and a dry cough that may progress to dyspnea. Diarrhea or a rash may be present in rare cases. The lower respiratory phase begins after 3 to 7 days with a dry cough, shortness of breath, or dyspnea that may progress to pneumonia, respiratory distress syndrome, or hypoxemia. The disease severity ranges from mild to severe. The clinical course in young children has been less severe than in adults and adolescents. Recovery occurs in about a week. *Complications:* Mortality of 6%–7% in adults, rare pediatric deaths.	Diagnostic tests include reverse transcriptase-polymerase chain reaction performed on a nasopharyngeal specimen or cell culture. Supportive care. Antiviral drugs do not appear to be effective. Antibiotics providing broad coverage may be prescribed for pneumonia or other respiratory organisms. *Prevention:* There is no vaccine. *This is a reportable disease.*	➤ Use airborne precautions and place the child in a negative pressure room. If this is not available, place the child in a private room and keep the door closed. Wear gown, gloves, and mask. ➤ Minimize patient transport and restrict visitors. ➤ Keep the child comfortable and use distraction to reduce the child's anxiety. ➤ Monitor respiratory symptoms for progression in severity and prepare to move to intensive care if condition worsens. ➤ Keep the child hydrated. ➤ Provide information and support to family members. ➤ If children have been exposed, they should be monitored for fever and respiratory symptoms over the 10 days following exposure. Children do not need to limit their activities or school attendance when symptom free (Centers for Disease Control 2003b).

(continued)

TABLE 19–5 Selected Infectious and Communicable Diseases in Children (continued)

DISEASE	CLINICAL MANIFESTATIONS	CLINICAL THERAPY	NURSING MANAGEMENT
Streptococcus A *Causal agent:* Group A streptococci (GAS). *Epidemiology:* The illness is caused by various M-protein groups of group A alpha- and beta-hemolytic streptococci. In recent years severe infections have appeared, in some cases threatening life and limb. Different strains are associated with pharyngeal and pyodermal infections. Pharyngeal infections tend to occur more in late fall, winter, and spring. Pyodermal infections tend to occur in warmer seasons because of the association with minor skin trauma and insect bites. *Transmission:* Contact with respiratory secretions for pharyngitis or skin lesions for pyoderma. *Incubation period:* Pharyngeal: usually 2–5 days. Pyodermal: usually 7–10 days. *Period of communicability:* For weeks in untreated pharyngeal infections. The child is most contagious during the acute stage of the illness.	*Pharyngeal:* Onset is abrupt, with a sore throat, dysphagia, malaise, high fever, chills, headache, abdominal pain, anorexia, and vomiting. A beefy red pharynx with exudate (strep throat) and tender cervical nodes is seen. Palatal petechiae may be seen. *GAS respiratory tract infection:* Toddlers may develop serous rhinitis and a respiratory illness with moderate fever, irritability, and anorexia rather than pharyngitis. *Scarlet fever:* A characteristic erythematous, sandpaper rash associated with scarlet fever appears in some cases 12–48 hours after onset of symptoms, starting on the neck and spreading to the trunk and extremities. In 3–4 days, the rash begins to fade and the tips of the toes and fingers begin to peel. The classic strawberry tongue is seen on day 4- 5. *Pyodermal:* Lesions (impetigo) are honey-colored crusts at the site of open lesions. *Complications:* If untreated, acute otitis media, sinusitis, peritonsillar or retropharyngeal abscess, cervical lymphadenitis, acute rheumatic fever, acute glomerulonephritis, toxic shock syndrome, bacteremia, and necrotizing fasciitis or myositis can occur.	Diagnosis can be made by a rapid strep test or a culture of secretions from the pharynx and tonsils. Cultures of skin lesions are not indicated (American Academy of Pediatrics, 2003). Prompt antibiotic treatment is effective. Penicillin is the drug of choice. Erythromycin is used if the child is allergic to penicillin. The fever decreases after treatment is begun. Uncomplicated impetigo is treated with mupirocin ointment. Invasive strains causing necrotizing fasciitis or myositis need surgical intervention (exploration and debridement of dead tissue). *Prognosis:* Recovery is usually good with antibiotic therapy. Ten to 20% of school-age children become chronic carriers. *Prevention:* None. 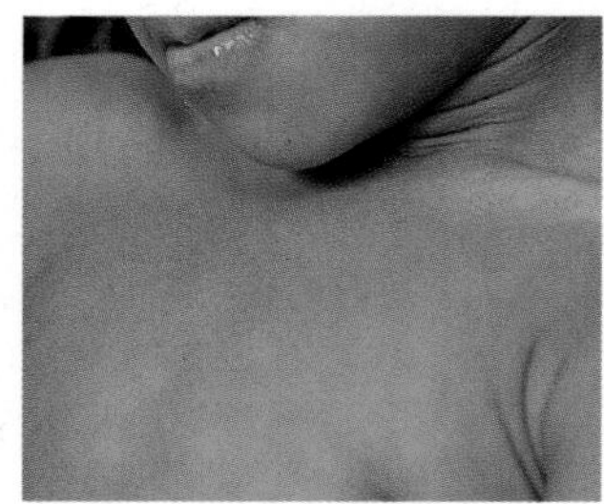 Scarlet fever from group A beta-hemolytic streptococcus *Courtesy of Centers for Disease Control and Prevention*	➤ Children with uncomplicated streptoccocal infections are usually cared for at home. Promote bedrest during the febrile stage. Give nonaspirin antipyretics to control fever. Teach parents important signs of a worsening condition. ➤ For pharyngeal infections, offer warm saltwater for gargling; a soft diet and nonacidic beverages. Encourage fluids. Provide cool, clear liquids. Swallowing may be difficult. ➤ Explain to parents the importance of the child taking antibiotics for the full number of days prescribed. ➤ Encourage other family members with sore throats to have throat cultures taken. ➤ For impetigo, teach the parents to wash the skin, remove crusts, and apply antibiotic ointment. ➤ If the child is hospitalized, maintain droplet precautions for pharyngeal infections and contact precautions for skin lesions for 24 hours after beginning antibiotics. Monitor vital signs, especially temperature. Administer antibiotics as ordered. ➤ If the child develops invasive streptococcal infection, use standard precautions. The child with toxic shock syndrome will need intensive care to manage shock and fluid and electrolyte imbalances.
Streptococcus B *Causal agent:* Group B streptococci (GBS), a gram-positive, aerobic diplococcus. *Epidemiology:* The gastrointestinal tract is the natural reservoir for GBS and is the likely source for vaginal colonization. Rates of colonization during pregnancy are between 15% to 40% (American Academy of Pediatrics, 2003). The woman is usually asymptomatic. Increased risk of infection occurs in cases of preterm infants (< 37 weeks of gestation), prolonged rupture of membranes	Early onset: Newborn becomes acutely ill, often within 24 hours of birth, with signs of systemic infection, respiratory distress, apnea, and shock caused by sepsis, pneumonia, meningitis, osteomyelitis, or septic arthritis. Late onset: Newborn between 1 and 4 weeks of age may develop signs of bacteremia or meningitis. *Complications:* Death, brain injury that could result in cognitive and motor disabilities, hearing loss.	*Diagnostic tests:* Complete blood count, chest radiograph, cultures of body fluids, including blood, urine, cerebrospinal fluid, and breaks in the skin or open lesions. Antibiotics are initiated when GBS infection is suspected and before culture results are known. Ampicillin and gentamycin are used in newborns. Penicillin G and aminoglycosides are also used. Duration of treatment is dependent upon focus of infection.	➤ Use standard precautions for infected newborns. Wash hands after each contact with the infant. Adhere to all infection control guidelines to reduce the risk of transmitting the infection to other newborns. ➤ Ensure that the appropriate IV antibiotic dosage is administered at the correct rate and on time to maintain optimal blood levels. ➤ Monitor the newborn for side effects and toxicity associated with the antibiotic. ➤ Maintain a neutral thermoregulatory environment.

**Indicates that a vaccine or antitoxin is available for use in high-risk or as-needed situations.*
+Indicates that the disease has a safe and effective vaccine.

TABLE 19–5 Selected Infectious and Communicable Diseases in Children (continued)

DISEASE	CLINICAL MANIFESTATIONS	CLINICAL THERAPY	NURSING MANAGEMENT
Streptococcus B (continued) (≥18 hours), positive vaginorectal culture in mother, young maternal age intrapartum fever, chorioamnionitis, or GBS bacteriuria during the pregnancy. *Transmission:* Not sexually transmitted. Intrauterine infection of fetus can occur from ascending GBS; however, early onset GBS usually occurs from mother to infant after onset of labor or membrane rupture. Late onset GBS may be transmitted person to person after delivery. *Incubation period:* Fewer than 7 days. *Period of communicability:* Unknown.		*Prognosis:* Case-fatality ratios range from 5% to 8% but are higher in preterm neonates (American Academy of Pediatrics, 2003). *Prevention:* Current guidelines recommend screening all pregnant women by vaginal and rectal cultures between 35 and 37 weeks' gestation to identify GBS carriers who should then receive IV antibiotics during labor to protect the newborn. Infants born of these mothers are carefully monitored for signs of infection (Centers for Disease Control, 2002e). Prenatal vaginorectal cultures and intrapartum antibiotics are not effective strategies for late-onset GBS.	➤ Monitor vital signs, and observe for signs indicating progression or resolution of the infection. Monitor for development of complications such as septic shock, seizures, renal failure, hypoglycemia, hyperglycemia, acidosis, hyponatremia, and hypocalcemia. ➤ Provide adequate fluid and caloric intake. Monitor weight, urine output, and urine specific gravity. ➤ Provide respiratory support as needed with oxygen and assisted ventilation if needed. ➤ Provide honest information and support the parents. Permit parents to touch the baby and participate in care as much as the newborn's condition permits.
Tetanus[+*] *Causal agent: Clostridium tetani* or tetanus bacillus. *Epidemiology:* The bacillus is common and exists as a spore in soil, dust, and animal excretions. The organism produces an endotoxin that affects the central nervous system. *Transmission:* The organism is transmitted to humans through puncture wounds or broken skin exposed to contaminated soil, manure, or implements. Newborns can acquire tetanus via the umbilical cord if they are born in an unclean area, a contaminated implement is used to cut the cord, or clay is applied to the umbilical cord as a ritual in some Middle Eastern cultures. *Incubation period:* 3 days–3 weeks (average 8 days). *Period of communicability:* Not communicable to other individuals except through skin wounds.	Stiffness of the neck and jaw, with painful facial spasms and difficulty chewing and swallowing over a few days, and headache. Noise or sudden movement may stimulate spasms. Spasms of facial muscles may produce a grinning expression (risus sardonicus). Localized prolonged and painful muscle contraction may occur at the site of the wound. Eventually rigidity of the abdomen and trunk produce **opisthotonus** (rigid hypertextension of the entire body), spasms, and fever occur along with difficulty swallowing the increased oral secretions. Respiratory muscles can be affected and cause airway obstruction and suffocation. Newborns have difficulty with sucking, progressing to an inability to suck, irritability, and nuchal rigidity. *Complications:* Laryngospasm, respiratory distress, death.	Tetanus immune globulin is given to unimmunized persons as soon as possible. Tetanus toxoid is given at the same time in a separate site. Medications are provided to treat muscle spasms. Intensive care is provided with cardiorespiratory monitoring, assisted ventilation, IV metronidazole or penicillin G, nutrition, and supportive care. Wound cleansing and debriding is performed. Survival beyond 4 days indicates an increased chance of recovery. Paroxysms become less frequent and complete recovery may take weeks. *Prognosis:* 30% mortality; much higher in newborns. Intensive care has improved mortality. *Prevention:* Tetanus immunizations are routinely given. They must be updated every 10 years, or, if a potentially contaminated wound occurs, in 5 years. Proper surgical debridement of wounds decreases the chance of infection.	➤ Prevent disease by checking immunization records and administering immunizations as necessary. ➤ Give immune globulin to unimmunized persons. ➤ Assist with wound debridement. ➤ The child with tetanus is hospitalized. Use standard precautions. ➤ Monitor the child's condition. Handle as little as possible. Reduce stimulation by placing child in a quiet, darkened room. ➤ Offer skin and respiratory care. The child may need an endotracheal tube, suctioning, and supplemental oxygen for airway support. ➤ Provide feedings via total parenteral nutrition or feeding tube. ➤ Maintain hydration with IV fluids and electrolytes. ➤ Try to reduce the child's anxiety, as mental status may be unaffected. ➤ Prepare the family for a possible poor prognosis.

Tuberculosis, see Chapter 25∞.

TABLE 19–6 Selected Infectious Diseases Transmitted Insect or Animal Hosts (Zoonosis)

DISEASE	CLINICAL MANIFESTATIONS	CLINICAL THERAPY	NURSING MANAGEMENT
Lyme Disease* *Causal agent:* Borrelia *burgdorferi,* a spirochete, which is transmitted by ixodid ticks. *Epidemiology:* Distribution in the United States correlates highly with the distribution of various tick carriers (vectors). It occurs in 49 states and the District of Columbia. 80% of cases occur in the Northeastern, Mid-Atlantic, and North Central states (Centers for Disease Control, 2002d). Exposure occurs in any outdoor setting where ticks are endemic. Animals such as dogs and cats can also have the disease. Lyme disease occurs year round, with the highest risk of infection in the summer. Children between 5 and 14 years are at highest risk because of outdoor activities. Infection does not induce immunity. *Transmission:* Tick bite. The tick transmits the infected spirochete when it draws blood. The tick must feed for 36 hours to transmit the disease. Lyme disease is the most common vector-borne illness in North America. *Incubation period:* 3–32 days after an infected tick bite. A rash in 48 hours is an allergic reaction or infection, not Lyme disease. *Period of communicability:* The infection is not contagious from person to person. 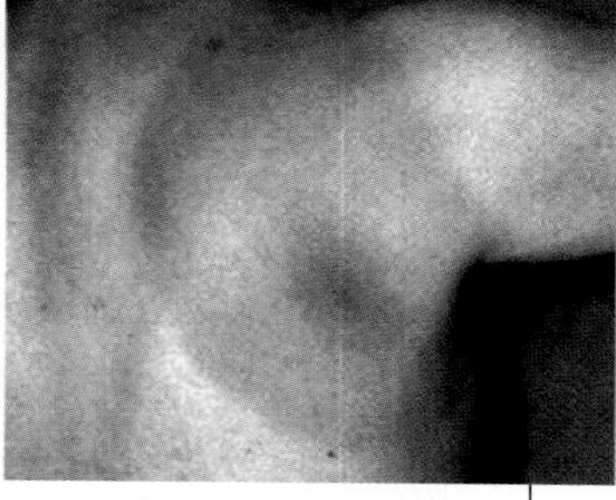 Lyme Disease	The most typical early symptom is a slowly expanding red rash that develops a bull's-eye appearance called erythema migrans at the site of the bite. The bite is often found on the groin, axilla, or thigh. The rash starts as a flat or raised red area and may progress to partial clearing; develop blisters or scabs in the center. It is usually at least 5 cm in diameter. The rash may look like a bruise in dark-skinned patients. It resolves spontaneously within 4 weeks. Only 50%–75% of patients have the rash (Wade, 2000). Stage 1 symptoms, lasting 5–21 days, include malaise, fatigue, headache, stiff neck, mild fever, and muscle and joint aches. Stage 2 (early disseminated) occurs 1–4 months after the bite. The most common symptoms of untreated disease are pain and swelling of the joints, most commonly the knee (Lyme arthritis), facial palsy, meningitis, AV block. Stage 3 (late disseminated) occurs months later and includes problems such as Lyme arthritis and central nervous system changes. These may become chronic problems. *Complications:* Left untreated, Lyme disease can cause significant neurologic deficits, including arm and leg weakness, Bell's palsy, encephalopathy, optic neuropathy, meningitis, severe headaches, and cognitive and behavioral changes as well as chronic arthritis, and disorders of the peripheral nerves. The sproichete can cross the placental barrier and infect the fetus (Wade, 2000).	Diagnostic tests include the enzyme-linked immunosorbent assay (ELISA) plus the Western blot test. Antibiotics are the treatment of choice. Amoxicillin or cefuroxime axetil are most often used in children 8 years of age or younger. Doxycycline or tetracycline is given to children over the age of 8 years. A 2-week course of oral medication is given. If recurrent arthritis, central nervous system difficulty, or carditis occurs, treat for 4 weeks with IV ceftriaxone, cefotaxime, or penicillin G. Relapse can occur. *Prognosis:* Lyme disease does not cause acute life-threatening illness, but it may result in significant morbidity, especially when chronic. *Prevention:* ➤ A vaccine, LYMErix, is approved for high-risk patients 15–70 years. Some clinical trials in younger children appear promising. ➤ Avoid areas that are heavily tick infested, and wear protective clothing. Check for ticks (especially hidden in hair) after every outing. Check pets because they can carry home ticks that are then transferred to the child. Remove ticks as soon as possible. There is no acquired immunity.	➤ Children with early disease are usually treated at home. Children with progressive symptoms may be hospitalized. Use standard precautions. ➤ Educate parents about the need for the long course of medications, informing them that the spirochete can go dormant. ➤ Tell parents to have the child avoid sun exposure when taking doxycycline. Nonaspirin analgesics and antipyretics may provide relief of mild fevers, headaches, and muscle and joint aches. ➤ Children with Lyme disease may tire easily. Promote rest and avoid vigorous activities that may be difficult. ➤ Educate parents and children about the disease and early recognition of the symptoms. ➤ Teach parents to safely remove ticks. To remove a tick, grasp it gently but firmly with fine-point tweezers where the mouthparts are attached. Pull gently—avoid squeezing of the tick's body—until it releases. Clean the area with soap and water (American Academy of Pediatrics, 2003). ➤ Tell parents to mark the date of tick bite on the calendar and monitor the child's health for flulike symptoms over the next 30 days. Encourage them to seek medical attention promptly if symptoms develop. ➤ Provide emotional support.

** Indicates that a vaccine or antitoxin is available for use in high-risk or as-needed situations*

TABLE 19–6 Selected Infectious Diseases Transmitted Insect or Animal Hosts (Zoonosis) (continued)

DISEASE	CLINICAL MANIFESTATIONS	CLINICAL THERAPY	NURSING MANAGEMENT
Malaria *Causal agent: Plasmodium,* four species (*P. falciparum,* P. vivax, P. ovale, P. malariae) *Epidemiology:* Occurs in tropical and subtropical regions on four continents (Africa, Americas, Asia, and Oceana). The highest mortality is in children 6 months to 3 years of age. The disease is acquired during travel to an endemic area. P. falciparum causes the most serious disease. *Transmission:* The bite of an infected female Anopheles mosquito during a nocturnal blood meal permits the parasite to enter the human bloodstream. The parasite passes to the liver and infects hepatic cells. During an asymptomatic 5–16 day cycle, the parasite transforms to become a merozoite that can reproduce asexually. The merozoites are released as parasites that infect the red blood cells. Transmission can also occur by blood transfusion. *Incubation period:* Varies by type. P. falciparum in 7–10 days, for the other types it can remain dormant for a year or longer. *Period of communicability:* Not communicable except by blood or blood product transfusion, or the transplantation of organs from an infected person.	Nonspecific signs such as myalgia, malaise, headache, abdominal pain, back pain, pallor, diarrhea, nausea and vomiting are common. Spiking fever > 40°C occurs at the time red blood cells rupture, becoming a classical cyclic pattern every 48–72 hours. Periods of symptomatic improvement are sometimes seen between spells. Seizures and altered consciousness indicate the development of cerebral malaria. Hepatosplenomegaly and jaundice from hemolysis are often seen. Attacks may recur over the course of the year after infection, but the parasites die out gradually if reinfection does not occur. Children who live in endemic areas and survive the first 5 years of life develop immunity to the severe effects of the disease as long as they have frequent reexposure to the infection. *Complications:* When more than 5% of red blood cells are infected, severe anemia is seen; cerebral malaria with seizures, increased intracranial pressure, confusion, stupor, coma, and frequently death are most common in children. Pulmonary edema, respiratory failure, renal failure, spontaneous bleeding, and shock are seen in older children and adolescents. Children with asplenia are at high risk for death. Causes 1–2 million deaths worldwide annually. Risks are higher during pregnancy and the fetus may become infected. If the fetus survives, intrauterine growth retardation is common (Howell, 2001).	Malaria can be diagnosed by examining blood smears for parasites, or with a plasmodium HRP2 antigen enzyme-linked immunosorbent assay (ELISA). Laboratory tests often reveal anemia (Hgb <12 gm/dl) and thrombocytopenia (<150,000/mm^3). The patient is hospitalized to receive fluid replacement, antipyretics, and anemia management. The blood is regularly monitored for parasite density. In severe disease with greater than 5% parasitemia, intensive care and IV treatment is needed. Careful monitoring is needed to detect mental status changes, severe anemia, renal failure, and pulmonary edema. Exchange transfusion may be used in some children with greater than 5% parasitemia (Shingadia, & Shulman, 2000). Oral chloroquine is the treatment of choice for all species except P. faciparum. Quinine sulfate and tetracycline are used for therapy in children over 8 years for chloroquine-resistant P. falciparum. Atovaquone-proguanil was recently approved by the FDA to treat malaria and for prophylaxis. Hypoglycemia may result from quinine treatment. Primaquine (sometimes used along with chloroquine to prevent relapses) will cause severe anemia if given to individuals with G6PD disorder. *Prevention:* Minimize contact with mosquitoes, use DEET insect repellent, screened rooms, DEET-treated mosquito netting, and cover the body with light-colored clothing when traveling in endemic regions. Antimalarial chemoprophylaxis (mefloquine) should be used 1 week before arrival, weekly during travel, and 4 weeks after leaving the risk area. Doxycycline may be used as an alternate chemoprophylaxis in children over 8 years, but must be taken daily.	➤ Use standard precautions for the hospitalized patient. ➤ Maintain fluid intake. Monitor intake and output. ➤ Monitor blood glucose level and be prepared to respond to sudden hypoglycemia. ➤ Observe for signs of increasing illness severity such as confusion, seizures, and shock. Be prepared to protect the patient from injury and provide emergency support with airways and oxygen supplementation until the child can be transferred to intensive care. ➤ Monitor the hematocrit and hemoglobin levels. ➤ Administer antipyretics to control the fever and promote comfort. ➤ Provide education and emotional support to parents of children with severe malarial symptoms. ➤ Educate families traveling to endemic areas about the importance of antimalarial chemoprophylaxis. Explain the need to take the medication correctly despite the common side effects of nausea and vomiting. Discuss the need to protect children during nocturnal feeding times of mosquitoes with protective clothing, mosquito repellent, and mosquito netting around the bed.

(continued)

TABLE 19–6 Selected Infectious Diseases Transmitted Insect or Animal Hosts (Zoonosis) (continued)

DISEASE	CLINICAL MANIFESTATIONS	CLINICAL THERAPY	NURSING MANAGEMENT
Rabies (Hydrophobia)* *Causal agent: Rhabdoviridae,* two types (urban, in dogs; wild, in wildlife). *Epidemiology:* Occurs worldwide. Urban rabies is generally controlled by vaccination of domestic animals susceptible to the infection, especially dogs and cats. Rabies can occur in many wild animals, particularly bats, foxes, skunks, and raccoons. *Transmission:* Infected saliva from bite of rabid animal. Virus enters the wound and travels along the nerves from point of entry to the brain where it multiplies and migrates along the efferent nerves to the salivary glands. *Incubation period:* Highly variable (3–7 weeks); average 6 weeks. This period depends on the amount of virus in the saliva, how close to the brain or major nerves the bite occurred, and how deeply the saliva penetrated the skin.	Children may be free of symptoms during the long incubation period. Initial acute symptoms include pain or paresthesia at the site of exposure along with headache, fever, loss of appetite, and malaise. Painful contractures in the muscles used for swallowing lead to hydrophobia (50% of patients), a reflex contraction at the sight of liquid. Neurologic symptoms such as hallucinations, disorientation, periods of excitability (mania) and quiet, and seizures later occur. Some patients may have confusion with or without agitation with progression to stupor and coma. Symptoms last about 2 weeks. *Complications:* Usually results in death.	Diagnosis is made on the basis of history and clinical symptoms. The diagnosis is usually confirmed by fluorescent antibody staining of the dead animal's brain tissue. Diagnostic tests performed on the victim include fluorescent microscopy of skin biopsy from the nape of the neck, from the saliva, from antibody in the cerebrospinal fluid or by detection of viral nucleic acid in infected tissues (American Academy of Pediatrics, 2003). Immediately wash animal bites thoroughly with soap and water and irrigate well. Suturing should be avoided if possible. Human rabies immune globulin (HRIG) and human diploid cell rabies vaccine (HDCV) should be given to all persons bitten by animals that may be rabid. Half of the HRIG is infiltrated around the wound and the remainder is given IM. Follow local guidelines for delay in HRIG and HDCV if testing of the animal's brain is done. The vaccine is of no value once rabies symptoms are present. *Prognosis:* If symptoms develop, no drug improves the prognosis. *Prevention:* Postexposure prophylaxis with HRIG and HDCV should be given as soon as possible after exposure. HDCV is repeated on days 3, 7, 14, and 28 after the bite (five doses). The HDCV series may be stopped if the animal is found free of rabies. Expert advice on the administration of these vaccines is available from state and local health officials. Prevention also includes immunizing all domestic animals against rabies.	➤ Work with family members and local animal control to have any animal suspected of having rabies quarantined, if possible. ➤ Administer HRIG and HDCV as ordered. Assist family with obtaining help to find and quarantine the animal for observation. ➤ Provide emotional support to the family while reinforcing the urgency for the vaccine and the need for a series of injections. ➤ Inform parents and the child about the side effects of the vaccine — irritation at the injection site, itching, headache, muscle aches, nausea, and dizziness. ➤ If the child acquires rabies, he or she will be hospitalized. ➤ Institute standard and contact precautions. The virus is transmitted primarily in the saliva and cerebrospinal fluid. ➤ Make the child as comfortable as possible. ➤ Keep liquids out of sight of the hydrophobic child. ➤ Use caution in the late stages of the disease when children are usually combative. Various medications, paralyzing agents, and sedatives may be used to provide relief. Coma and death occur after an exhaustive period of excitement and agitation that may last for days. ➤ Provide emotional support to the family of the dying child. ➤ Participate in local education about rabies and safe interactions with dogs. See Chapter 36. ➤ Teach children to avoid contact with all unknown animals, dead or alive.
Rocky Mountain Spotted Fever (Tickborne Typhus Fever, Sao Paulo Typhus) *Causal agent: Rickettsia rickettsii,* a bacterium that is transmitted by infected ticks. *Epidemiology:* Rocky Mountain spotted fever (RMSF) occurs in most of the United States, southwestern Canada, and Mexico. Nearly half of all U.S. cases occur in Oklahoma, North Carolina, South Carolina, and Tennessee. Generally occurs between April and September. Most infections occur in children who are less	RMSF is a multisystem disease that can be mild, moderate, or severe. Onset may be gradual or rapid. Children may be very ill. Sudden onset is characterized by a moderate to high fever (40°C) that ordinarily lasts for 2–3 weeks, significant malaise, abdominal pain, nausea, vomiting, deep muscle pain, persistent headache, chills, and conjunctival injection. The characteristic rash, which usually appears between	Diagnostic tests include the indirect immunofluorescent antibody assay, enzyme immunoassay, or indirect hemagglutination test. Treatment of choice is doxycycline, regardless of the patient's age (Jacobs, Ogborn, & Tunnessen, 2001). *Prognosis:* Without early recognition and treatment, morbidity is significant and mortality in children is 2%–3% in children under 10 years (Centers for Disease	➤ Use standard precautions. ➤ Children may require prolonged hospitalization, including monitoring in the intensive care unit. ➤ Have hemodynamic monitoring equipment and emergency supplies readily available. ➤ Administer antibiotics as ordered. ➤ Observe for any abnormal bleeding. ➤ Make the child as comfortable as possible. If the child is unconscious, support the extremities and keep the eyes closed and lubricated.

* *Indicates that a vaccine or antitoxin is available for use in high-risk or as-needed situations*

TABLE 19–6 Selected Infectious Diseases Transmitted Insect or Animal Hosts (Zoonosis) (continued)

DISEASE	CLINICAL MANIFESTATIONS	CLINICAL THERAPY	NURSING MANAGEMENT
Rocky Mountain Spotted Fever (continued) than 15 years of age. Infection induces immunity. *Transmission:* Transmitted by bites of ticks, principally dog and wood ticks. *Incubation period:* 2–12 days (most commonly 7 days) after bite of an infected tick. *Period of communicability:* There is no evidence of person-to-person transmission.	the third and fifth days, starts on the extremities, including the palms and soles, and moves to the trunk. Initially the rash is maculopapular and blanches with pressure. It later becomes petechial and more defined; it is rarely pruritic. Up to 25% of children do not develop a rash. The child may have splenomegaly, hepatomegaly, and jaundice. *Complications:* In severe cases bleeding from the gastrointestinal tract and from disseminated intravascular coagulation (DIC) can be significant. Pulmonary complications, especially pneumonitis, pulmonary edema, and respiratory distress syndrome are common and can become life threatening. Central nervous system involvement can cause significant encephalitis and overall severe neurologic dysfunction. Cardiac and renal complications can also occur, leading to shock in severe cases.	Control 2000). Mortality in untreated cases is 20%–25% (Jacobs, et al., 2001). *Prevention:* Avoid areas that are heavily tick infested, and wear protective clothing. Check for ticks and if found remove promptly. Infected ticks must be attached and feeding for 4–6 hours to transmit the disease. Seek medical attention promptly for a child who has been bitten and becomes symptomatic.	➤ Provide quiet diversion activities. ➤ Provide emotional support, and keep parents informed about the child's condition. Rocky Mountain Spotted Fever
West Nile Virus *Causative agent:* An arbovirus, genus Flavivirus. *Epidemiology:* Infected wild birds (crow family) and the mosquitoes that feed on them carry the illness. The infection has occurred in 44 of the U.S. states and several Canadian provinces. The majority of the cases occur during summer months. Transmission may also occur by blood transfusion or organ transplant from an infected donor. The elderly and those with weak immune systems are at greatest risk. *Incubation period:* 2–14 days. *Period of communicability:* This infection is not transmitted from person to person.	Most people are asymptomatic, but about 20% of infected individuals develop flulike symptoms including fever, body aches, skin rashes, and lymphadenopathy. Symptoms may last 3–6 days. About 1% of infected individuals develop severe neurologic illness, with symptoms that include fever, headache, and altered mental status. Risk of illness is substantially lower in children under 19 years than in the elderly. *Complications:* Encephalitis, meningitis, or both. Death may occur.	Diagnostic tests include testing the serum or cerebrospinal fluid for IgG and IgM antibodies against West Nile Virus. No established treatment exists for West Nile Virus, so treatment is supportive. For severe cases the patient will be in intensive care and supported with IV fluids, airway management, respiratory support, management of cerebral edema, and management of secondary infections. *Prevention:* There is no vaccine. Blood collection centers should check donor blood for West Nile Virus. Reduce or eliminate potential breeding locations for mosquitoes by dumping out standing water in tires, flowerpots, puddles, etc. Change the water in birdbaths, pet water bowls, and wading pools at least weekly. Stock ponds and fountains with fish that eat mosquito larvae. Wear insect repellent and long-sleeved clothing, especially in the dawn and twilight hours when mosquitoes bite. *This is a reportable disease.*	➤ Use standard precautions. ➤ Provide supportive care for those with encephalitis and meningitis. ➤ Be prepared to provide emergency airway and respiratory support. ➤ Teach families to control mosquito breeding and to protect children and adults from mosquito bites.

COLLABORATIVE CARE

For many infectious and communicable diseases, management is supportive. In addition to diagnostic tests, collaborative care includes fever management, promoting the child's comfort, antibiotic administration for bacterial infections, and in some cases antiviral agents for specific viral illnesses.

Diagnostic Procedures

Diagnostic tests include cultures from sites where the infection may potentially be located, such as the skin, pharynx, blood, urine, feces, and cerebrospinal fluid. See the Skills Manual for guidelines related to collection of specimens. In some cases, radiographs or special imaging may be used to identify localized infection in an organ such as the lungs.

Clinical Therapy

An elevated temperature can be a beneficial physiologic response, helping to eradicate organisms that thrive at lower body temperatures, and mobilizing the immune response. It may also enhance the effect of antibiotics. In addition, fever decreases the plasma iron concentration, which may limit the growth of microorganisms (Cimpella et al., 2000). Fever is not inherently harmful until it reaches 41°C (105.9°F). For this reason, medical management may include postponing treatment of low-grade fevers under 38.9°C (102°F) to promote the body's natural defenses against an infection. If not managed, elevated temperatures can result in febrile seizures, which usually have no long-term sequelae. Thus, fevers greater than 38.9°C (102°F) should be treated, especially if associated with discomfort. Persistent temperatures of 38.3 to 38.5°C (101 to 101.5°F) may also benefit from antipyretic treatment. Acetaminophen and ibuprofen are the preferred antipyretics for children. See Complementary therapy: Hot and Cold. Antipyretics reduce fever by inhibiting prostaglandin synthesis, which results in lowering of the body's temperature set point. Aspirin is no longer recommended for children because of its association with Reye syndrome. See Chapter 33.

Administration of antibiotics is often another component of clinical therapy for infectious diseases. Before the introduction of antibiotics, children were often unable to fight infection and died as the result of overwhelming sepsis. Antibiotics have been responsible for decreases in morbidity and mortality from infections among children. However, strains of bacteria have developed resistance to many antibiotics. Children with chronic illnesses such as cystic fibrosis, sickle-cell disease, and acquired immunodeficiency syndrome (AIDS) are particularly susceptible to infection by drug-resistant pathogens.

Antiviral medications, such as acyclovir, may be ordered for certain types of viral infections, such as chickenpox, herpes simplex virus type I, influenza, and others. In cases when the child is immunocompromised, the antiviral medication needs to be provided very early in the infectious period to minimize the potentially life-threatening consequences of the infection.

Often cases of an infectious or communicable disease must be reported to the state health department. Cases can be reported on standardized state forms or on designated websites. This enables disease surveillance and a measure of how effective preventative measures such as immunizations are. For example, data about immunization rates in a community or state can be matched with reported cases of disease to evaluate public health and health promotion interventions.

> **COMPLEMENTARY THERAPY**
>
> **Hot and Cold**
>
> Many Latino and Asian cultures subscribe to the hot and cold theory of disease causation. "Hot" and "cold" do not refer to temperature but to categories. Fever, a hot condition, is treated by giving the patient cold substances (foods or medicines). Cold foods include vegetables, fruits, and fish. Cold medicines include orange flower water, linden, and sage. Ask parents how they think the illness should be treated. Encourage them to use that treatment as long as it is not known to cause harm. Check current literature for guidance when needed. Teach such clients additional Western medicine treatments they can use. (See Chapter 3.)

NURSING MANAGEMENT

The goal of nursing management is to assess the child for initial symptoms and potential progression in severity of the infection. Nursing care is focused on managing the child's symptoms, promoting the child's hydration, and preventing the spread of infection.

■ Nursing Assessment and Diagnosis

Assess the child's hydration status and fluid intake, vital signs, comfort level, and appetite and observe for seizures and for a **toxic appearance** (lethargy, poor perfusion, hypoventilation or hyperventilation, and cyanosis). The child with a fever may be irritable and restless, sleep fitfully, and have nonspecific muscular pain. Identify those children who may be at higher risk for a serious illness in association with a fever, in particular:

- Infants and children having a toxic appearance
- Neonates less than 28 days of age with a temperature over 38°C (100.4°F)
- Children less than 4 years of age with a temperature over 41°C (105.8°F)
- Children with conditions such as a ventriculoperitoneal shunt, congenital heart disease, asplenia, and sickle-cell anemia

Observe the child for other signs of infection, such as a rash, nausea and vomiting, and/or diarrhea, as well as generalized symptoms of a poor appetite and malaise.

Examples of nursing diagnoses that may be appropriate for children with infectious and communicable diseases are as follows:

- Hyperthermia related to infectious disease process
- Risk for Deficient Fluid Volume related to hypermetabolic state

- Impaired Skin Integrity related to hyperthermia and self-mutilation of skin lesions
- Impaired Oral Mucous Membrane related to infectious disease process
- Deficient Fluid Volume related to repeated episodes of vomiting and diarrhea
- Ineffective Therapeutic Regimen Management (family) related to complexity of care required by the child

Planning and Implementation

Most children with infectious diseases are cared for at home; however, children may be evaluated in various healthcare settings.

Assist with the collection of cultures. Be sure that infants and children have pain management for painful diagnostic procedures such as lumbar punctures.

Nursing care of children with infectious diseases in healthcare settings focuses on preventing the spread of infection. Children with suspicious rashes should be isolated from other children. When possible, hard surfaces and toys in the waiting and examining rooms where the child was seen should be wiped down with antiseptic solution before another child uses the room. Linens are disposed of in appropriately marked linen bags.

Children are often admitted to the hospital for treatment of severe infections. In addition, countless numbers of **nosocomial** (hospital-acquired) **infections** occur each year. The fecal–oral and respiratory routes are the most common sources of infections in children. For the preterm infant, a break in the skin for catheters or chest tubes may increase the risk of nosocomial infections. All items with which the infected child comes into contact are considered contaminated (e.g., linens, toys, medical equipment). Transmission-based precautions, including isolation, must be implemented to reduce exposure of other children and staff to the infectious agent. Follow the facility's standard precautions and transmission-based precautions to reduce the spread of infectious diseases to staff and other patients. Bring any questions and concerns to the hospital's infection control nurse. (Refer to the Skills Manual for more detailed information.)

Nursing care for treatment of fever includes administering antipyretics, removing unnecessary clothing, and careful continued monitoring of temperature progression. Identify clear fluids the child prefers to drink, and encourage the intake of extra fluids.

CLINICAL TIP

The practice of alternating acetaminophen with ibuprofen in the care of children with fever is not based on scientific evidence. Each medication is effective in managing fever. However, because the medications have different durations of action (4 hours for acetaminophen and 6 hours for ibuprofen) and many different preparations, there is risk for overdosing the child if the administration schedule is not strictly followed. In addition there are potentially synergistic effects on the kidneys by the two medications when given in an alternating schedule that can cause renal tubular toxicity. An important patient safety initiative is to use only one antipyretic for fever management of children (Carson, 2003).

PRACTICE ALERT

A study comparing methods of fever reduction in febrile children aged 5 to 68 months with temperatures of more than 38.9°C (102°F) found no significant differences in temperature reduction over a 2-hour period when the child was given acetaminophen alone or with a 15-minute tepid sponge bath. However, the children who were given sponge baths had significantly higher discomfort scores (Sharber, 1997).

Encourage parents to assist with their child's care. Nursing care also includes treating infection, administering antibiotics on schedule, monitoring antibiotic blood levels if indicated to ensure appropriate results, monitoring the child's response to therapy, staying alert for signs that the infection is worsening, and educating parents.

Care in the Community

Teach parents to care for their child at home, including how and when to give antipyretics, over-the-counter medications, and antibiotics if ordered; what foods and beverages are appropriate; and how to care for rashes and other topical symptoms. Provide guidelines about the types of fluids to encourage. Parents often fear a fever, believing it is a disease rather than a symptom of an illness. Their greatest fears about the harmful effects of fever include seizure, brain damage, and death (Crocetti, Moghbeli, & Serwint, 2001). Provide information and reassurance. Help them to recognize signs of the child's worsening condition in association with the child's specific disease. See Partnering with Families: Guidelines for Evaluating and Treating Fever in Children.

Teach parents the importance of proper use of antibiotics when ordered to help reduce the development of antibiotic-resistant bacteria (Larrabee, 2002).

- Give all the antibiotic dosages as prescribed for the full number of days ordered. Spread the doses around the clock to keep blood levels constant, as much as possible. This will help ensure that the bacteria causing the infection are eradicated, rather than having some bacteria left alive to mutate and resist the antibiotic in the future.
- Make sure parents know to give the antibiotic with food or without food to promote optimal absorption.
- Discard the antibiotic when all doses have been given. Antibiotics have an expiration date and lose potency after that date.
- Do not share the antibiotic with any other family member. If that family member is ill, there will not be enough antibiotic to fully treat the infection, even if the same bacteria is causing the infection.

Educate parents about methods to reduce disease transmission in the home. Encourage parents to limit the exposure of elderly family members and infants to the ill child. Make sure that the ill child's dishes and utensils are washed in hot soapy water or sanitized in a dishwasher. Encourage handwashing when the caregiver is in contact with body fluids.

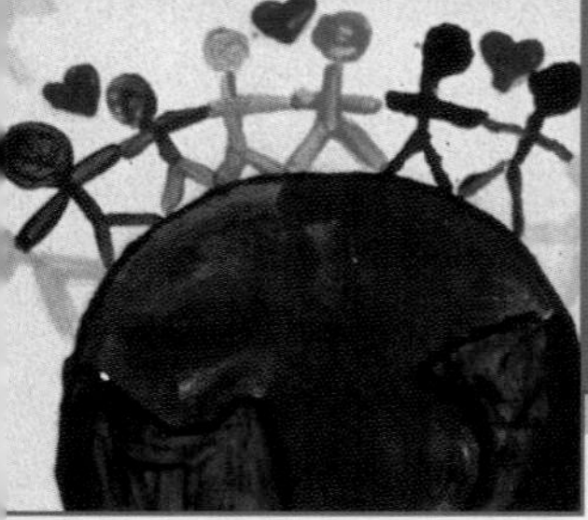

PARTNERING WITH FAMILIES

Guidelines for Evaluating and Treating Fever in Children

About fevers

- A fever is not a disease; it is the body's physiologic response to an infection. A fever means the child's body is using natural defenses to fight an infection and kill viruses and bacteria.
- If the child has a fever and does not look sick, it may be better to let the child use the natural defenses to fight off the virus or bacteria causing the fever.

Care for a fever

- Use a thermometer to check the child's temperature. See Skills Manual.
- Assess the child for other symptoms.
- Lower the temperature with acetaminophen or ibuprofen (do not use aspirin) using the correct dose for the child's weight. Do not alternate the medications. Alternating the medications increases the risk that the infant or child will get an overdose that could cause harm. There is no evidence that alternating the medications improves the treatment of the fever (Mayoral, Marino, Rosenfeld, et al., 2000).
- Use the correct dose of the medication—drops and syrups do not have the same concentration.
- Remove all but a light layer of the child's clothing to help lower the temperature.
- Monitor the child's behavior and response to the fever medication. The main goal of fever medication is improving the child's comfort.
- Provide generous amounts of fluids for the child to drink and allow the child to rest.
- The temperature may rise again 4 hours after giving acetaminophen or 6 hours after ibuprofen. Check the temperature and give another dose of fever medication. Check recommendations on the bottle for the maximum number of doses allowed per day.

Call your healthcare provider immediately if:

- The child is under 3 months old and has a fever higher than 38.0°C (100.4°F)
- The child has a fever over 40.1°C (104.2°F), and symptoms below are present.
- The child is crying inconsolably or whimpering. The child cries when moved or otherwise touched by the parent or other family members.
- The child is difficult to awaken.
- The child's neck is stiff.
- There are any purple spots present on the skin.
- Breathing is difficult and no better after the nose is cleared.
- The child is drooling saliva and is unable to swallow anything.
- The child has a convulsion.
- The child acts or looks very sick.

Call your healthcare provider within 24 hours if:

- The child is 2–4 months old (unless fever occurs within 48 hours of a DTP shot and the infant has no other serious symptoms).
- The fever is higher than 40.1°C (104.2°F) (especially if the child is under 3 years old).
- The child complains of burning or pain with urination.
- The fever has been present more than 24 hours without an obvious cause or location of infection.
- The fever went away for more than 24 hours and then returned.
- The fever has been present for more than 72 hours.

Correct any misconceptions parents and childcare workers may have about the occurrence or cause of the infectious disease in their child. The parents and other providers may believe that they have exposed the child to certain germs or bacteria. Teach them that infection control will reduce exposure of other children and family members to the infectious disease.

Evaluation

Expected outcomes of nursing care include the following:

- Opportunities for spread of infection are minimized between patients and family members.
- The child's fever is effectively managed with antipyretics.
- The full treatment with antibiotics, if ordered, is completed.

SEPSIS

Sepsis is a significant infection in which bacteria invade the bloodstream followed by a systemic inflammatory response. Infants in the first year of life are at a high risk for developing sepsis, especially those with low birth weight. The incidence of sepsis in newborns is 0.3 per 100 live births (Watson, Carcillo, Linde-Zwirble, et al., 2003).

Epidemiology and Pathophysiology

Newborns can acquire infections during the prenatal and perinatal periods, as well as during the first weeks of life. During the prenatal and perinatal periods, microorganisms can be transmitted through ingestion or aspiration of infected amniotic fluid during labor; transfer of microorganisms from the mother to the fetus during prolonged rupture of the membranes; and transplacental transfer of viruses and other organisms. Low-birth-weight infants often have invasive procedures performed that increase their risk for infections. Refer to Table 19–1 for newborns at risk for infection. Common microorganisms associated with sepsis include group B streptococcus, *E. coli, Haemophilus influenzae,* and staphylococcus. Because the newborn has inadequately developed inflammatory and immune system responses, the microorganisms can rapidly invade, spread, and multiply (see page 596).

Clinical Manifestations

Symptoms of sepsis in newborns are often nonspecific, such as subtle changes in appearance and behavior. Rather than a fever, newborns often have hypothermia. Subtle changes in color, tone, and activity provide clues that the newborn is ill. Feeding problems such as decreased intake, poor sucking, lack of interest in feeding, abdominal distension, vomiting, or diarrhea may be noted. Nonspecific respiratory distress or apnea may be noted, especially if group B streptococcus is the causative organism. See the clinical manifestations table on page 619 for signs of infection in newborns by body system.

COLLABORATIVE CARE

Care focuses on diagnosis of sepsis and aggressive therapy to promote the infant's survival and to reduce the potential consequences such as neurologic damage.

Diagnostic Procedures

Diagnosis is often suspected from clinical signs and symptoms. Because a focal site of infection is usually not apparent, culture specimens are obtained from the blood, urine, cerebrospinal fluid, and skin lesions. Radiographs of the lungs and other potential sites may reveal signs of infection. Blood is obtained for a complete blood count and white blood cell differential. A low neutrophil count and a high band (immature white blood cell) count indicate the presence of an infection. A C-reactive protein level may or may not be elevated.

Clinical Therapy

To reduce the risk for development of neurologic sequelae and progression to severe sepsis or septic shock, aggressive therapy is initiated with antibiotics before culture and sensitivity results are known. Two broad-spectrum antibiotics are often given in large doses initially in an effort to make sure the microorganism is treated. Once the culture and sensitivities are known, the antibiotic is changed if necessary to target the specific microorganism causing the infection. Additional therapy includes oxygen, intravenous fluids, and management of acid-base and electrolyte imbalances. Cardiorespiratory monitoring and temperature regulation of the environment are performed. Nutritional support is provided. See Chapter 26∞ for clinical therapy associated with septic shock.

NURSING MANAGEMENT

Nursing care is focused on identifying the infant with signs of infection, monitoring the newborn's status during clinical therapy, and preventing the development of sepsis in low-birthweight newborns.

■ Nursing Assessment and Diagnoses

Maintain a high level of suspicion for the development of sepsis in high-risk newborns. Monitor the newborn's condition for signs and symptoms of infection and sepsis, especially high-risk newborns that have invasive procedures performed or are treated with various types of technology.

Assess and monitor the vital signs and temperature of newborns with sepsis. Monitor hydration, intake and output, and weight. Ensure that the cardiorespiratory monitor leads are attached so that episodes of apnea are detected. Observe the newborn for signs that the condition is worsening or resolving. Monitor the newborn for side effects of various antibiotics used, especially when they may cause renal or other organ system damage.

Examples of nursing diagnoses may include the following:

- Ineffective Thermoregulation related to illness affecting temperature regulation and immaturity of newborn's temperature-regulating mechanism
- Interrupted Breastfeeding related to infant illness
- Ineffective Protection related to prematurity and inadequately developed inflammatory and immune system response
- Risk for Delayed Development related to neonatal infection

■ Planning and Implementation

Ensure that antibiotics are administered appropriately. Make sure that the newborn's environmental temperature and oxygen level are maintained. Carefully manage the IV fluid volume administered to ensure that the newborn is adequately hydrated.

Assist in the care of newborns during diagnostic procedures. Ensure the provision pain management, and soothe the infant afterwards with positioning, a pacifier, low lighting, and swaddling.

Provide support to parents who are stressed, because the newborn has the potential for development of disabilities or progression of the condition to severe sepsis or septic shock. Provide information about the newborn's illness and treatment plan. Encourage the parents to participate in the newborn's care as much as possible.

Prevention of infection is a significant role of the nurse and includes frequent and thorough handwashing with soap and water or gels by all persons touching the newborn, use of aseptic technique for all procedures, and limiting exposure to individuals with infections. Feeding preterm infants with human milk is associated with a reduction in the number of nosocomial infections (Hylander, Strobino, & Dhanireddy, 1998). Other measures to reduce the risk of infection in neonates include skin care with barriers that maintain skin integrity.

Discharge planning includes educating parents about the need to administer antibiotics until the full course is completed. Teach parents to identify signs and symptoms that the infection is not resolving as expected. Encourage the parents to keep healthcare appointments so that the infant can be monitored for signs of neurologic impairment.

Evaluation

Expected outcomes of nursing care include:

- Early recognition of the signs of sepsis permit rapid initiation of treatment that minimizes potential sequelae.
- The newborn's temperature-regulation mechanism stabilizes.
- The parents complete the newborn's antibiotic medications and keep healthcare follow-up visits so the newborn can be monitored for neurologic sequelae.

EMERGING INFECTION CONTROL THREATS

Special attention is now directed at disease surveillance associated with infectious agents. Weapons of terrorists (anthrax, smallpox, plague, botulism, hemorrhagic fever, or tularemia) or the emergence of rare infectious diseases, such as severe acute respiratory syndrome (SARS), need to be identified as early as possible so that public health measures can be initiated.

Due to differences in physical characteristics and physiologic responses, infants and children have unique problems when exposed to various biologic and chemical agents that could be used by terrorists. See Table 19–7.

TABLE 19–7 Problems Specific to Children Exposed to Biologic and Chemical Terrorism

ANATOMY AND PHYSIOLOGY	RESULTING PROBLEM
Increased body surface area	More surface area to absorb toxins
Smaller blood volume	More susceptible to fluid volume losses associated with vomiting and diarrhea
Thinner, under-keratinized epidermis	Skin is more permeable to toxins Increased absorption of toxins
Faster respiratory rate	Greater contact with aerosol biologic or chemical agents
Shorter, closer to the ground	Chemical biologic agents are heavier than air, and being closer to the ground increases exposure
Immature immune system Immature blood-brain barrier	More susceptible to certain biologic agents

Data From Cieslak, T. J., & Henretig, F. M. (2003). Ring-a-ring-a-roses: Bioterrorism and its peculiar relevance to pediatrics. Current Opinion in Pediatrics, *19, 107–111.*

MediaLink Bioterrorism Preparedness Resources

BOX 19–10 The Public Health Response to Bioterrorism

The United States and Canada are on high alert for outbreaks of infection that could potentially be related to a bioterrorism event or to the emergence of a new or rare infectious disease, such as occurred with severe acute respiratory syndrome (SARS). (See Table 19–5 on page 629 for more information about this disease.) This level of alertness is important to identify the infection early, as well as potential sources and contacts. Then infection control procedures are implemented to minimize the number of persons who contract the illness. Once an infectious disease outbreak is identified, health professionals are notified through the national Health Alert Network (HAN) and educated about the signs and symptoms to be alert for, to isolate the infected, and to refer those most seriously ill to designated hospitals or centers of care. State health departments have developed guidelines for infection control management and are partnering with hospitals and local health providers to prepare them to manage hundreds of ill patients in an epidemic. This international public health response was successful in containing the SARS epidemic in 2003.

Specific biologic agents that could potentially be used for terrorism, signs and symptoms, and clinical therapy are described in the table on page 641. The state public health system is activated to identify cases, to control the spread of infection, and to prepare the mass casualty response to care for the potential large numbers of ill adults and children. See Box 19–10.

NURSING MANAGEMENT

Nurses have responsibility for maintaining a high level of suspicion when numerous individuals with similar signs and symptoms seek care in any healthcare facility. Initiating infection control measures such as airborne and contact precautions may help reduce the transmission of infection. Instituting isolation before a definitive diagnosis is appropriate when the level of suspicion is high. Assess children and provide supportive nursing care for the identified infection.

Nurses should regularly review guidelines posted by the Centers for Disease Control and Prevention about the management of specific health threats. They should also participate in planning for the healthcare facility's preparedness to respond to potential epidemics as a partner in the state and local emergency preparedness planning. See Chapter 16∞.

CLINICAL MANIFESTATIONS of Aerosolized Organisms that Are Potential Biological Weapons of Terrorists

ORGANISMS	AEROSOL TRANSMISSION CLINICAL MANIFESTATIONS	CLINICAL THERAPY
Anthrax *Causal agent:* *Bacillis anthracis* Cutaneous anthrax	■ Cutaneous—papule that progresses to a vesicle that develops into a skin ulcer with a depressed black scab area in the center. Not painful. Child may have fever, malaise, headache, and regional lymphadenopathy. ■ Gastrointestinal—nausea, loss of appetite, bloody diarrhea, hematemesis, fever, stomach pain, severe abdominal pain followed by fever and septicemia. ■ Inhalation—brief prodrome with respiratory symptoms like a sore throat, mild fever, malaise, muscle aches followed by development of dyspnea, cough, chest pain, shortness of breath, and systemic symptoms. Shock, pleural effusion, and meningitis may develop without treatment.	■ IV ciprofloxacin or doxycycline for patients over 12 years. For children under 12 years, IV ciprofloxacin plus clindamycin. ■ For postexposure prophylaxis: oral ciprofloxacin or amoxicillin for 60 days.
Botulism *Causal agent:* *Clostridium botulinum*	■ Ptosis, diplopia, blurred vision. Sluggishly reactive pupils. ■ Speech and swallowing problems, dysarthria, dysphonia, dysphagia, and loss of gag reflex. ■ Acute, afebrile symmetric descending flaccid paralysis, progressing to loss of head control, hypotonia, generalized weakness, deep tendon reflexes diminish or disappear. Constipation. ■ May be preceded by abdominal cramps, nausea, vomiting, or diarrhea. ■ May become confused or obtunded.	■ Slow IV infusion of equine antitoxin diluted in normal saline. ■ Epinephrine and diphenhydramine for serum sickness or urticaria.
Hemorrhagic Fever *Causal agent:* Ebola or Marburg virus	■ Abrupt onset of fever, myalgia, headache, nausea, vomiting, abdominal pain, photophobia, diarrhea, chest pain, cough, pharyngitis. ■ Maculopapular rash prominent on trunk soon after fever, bleeding into skin (petechiae, ecchymosis, subconjunctival hemorrhages), shock and circulatory collapse in short period. ■ Ghostlike appearance, looks critically ill.	■ Management of hypotension and shock and maintenance of fluid and electrolyte balance. ■ Replacement of blood, platelets, and plasma for severe hemorrhage.
Plague *Causal agent:* *Yersinia pestis* Pneumonic plague with aerosol route of transmission	■ Severe respiratory illness with high fever, chills, headache, cough, breathing difficulty ■ Rapidly developing pneumonia, bloody or watery sputum. ■ May lead to respiratory failure and shock.	■ Streptomycin IM or gentamycin IV. Alternate antibiotics include IV chloramphenicol or doxycycline.
Smallpox *Causal agent:* Variola major virus Smallpox	■ Prodrome 2 to 4 days before rash: abrupt onset with fever (101°F or higher), malaise, headache, muscle pain, prostration, nausea and vomiting, and backache. ■ Rash begins with red spots in mouth and on tongue that develop sores and break open. Then a few macules known as herald spots appear on the forehead, face, and extremities. Over the next few days a generalized rash develops, progressing from macules to papules, to tense vesicles, to tense deep pustules with an umbilicated appearance. Most cases have discrete, semiconfluent to confluent vesicles. Lesions are firm, all in same stage of development, more concentrated on the extremities than the trunk. The temperature usually falls and the patient feels better. ■ The pustules form scabs by the end of the second week, and the scabs fall off after 3–4 weeks.	■ Supportive care. ■ Antibiotics for secondary infection.
Tularemia *Causal agent:* *Francisella tularensis*	■ Febrile illness, fatigue, chills, headache, malaise, dyspnea, chest pain. ■ May develop hemorrhagic inflammation of airways that progresses to pneumonia, pleuritis, and hilar lymphadenopathy. ■ May also have pharyngitis, bronchiolitis, and pneumonia with systemic symptoms.	■ Supportive care in the intensive care unit. ■ Streptomycin IM or gentamycin IV, alternate drug is IV ciprofloxacin. For children use gentamycin IV, alternate drugs are doxycycline and chloramphenicol. ■ Postexposure prophylaxis for 14 days with ciprofloxacin, for children use doxycycline.

Data from Yetman, R. J., Parks, D., & Taft, E. (2002). Management of patients exposed to biologic weapons. Journal of Pediatric Health Care, 16*(5), 256–261; Centers for Disease Control and Prevention. (2003).* www.bt.cdc.gov*, accessed 9/24/2003. Photos courtesy of the Centers for Disease Control and Prevention.*

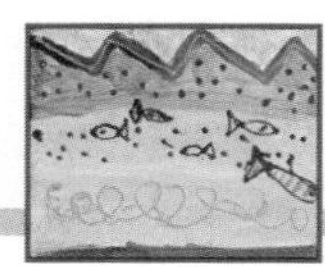

CHAPTER HIGHLIGHTS

- Reducing the number of preventable childhood illnesses is a major national public health goal.
- An infectious disease is an illness caused by microorganisms that are commonly communicated from one host (animal or human) to another.
- Newborns and infants are especially vulnerable to infectious diseases because their immune systems are immature, their passively acquired maternal antibodies provide limited protection, and disease protection through immunization is not yet complete.
- For a child to acquire a communicable disease, an infectious agent or pathogen, an effective means of transmission, and a susceptible host need to be present.
- Infection control measures caregivers can take include the following: using good handwashing techniques, disinfecting hard surfaces touched by the child, telling children not to kiss pets, disinfecting toys the child has mouthed before letting other children play with them, and making sure all children are fully immunized.
- Major public health efforts that have decreased the occurrence of infectious and communicable diseases include safer drinking water, better sanitation, improved standards of living, and increased immunization.
- The public health system is conducting disease surveillence to detect the emergence of rare infections or the presence of infectious disease potentially caused by terrorists.
- The average infant born in 2003 received 20 immunizations for 11 childhood diseases by 6 years of age. In the United States, immunizations protect children from diphtheria, tetanus, pertussis, polio, hepatitis B, Haemophilus influenza type b, measles, mumps, rubella, varicella, and pneumococcus. Influenza vaccine was added to the recommended list for infants and children over 6 months of age in 2004.
- Vaccines must be given at specific ages and intervals. Immunization timing is related to decreasing maternal antibody protection, to the child's developing ability to make antibodies in response to a vaccine, and whether the vaccine provides lifelong immunity.
- The Vaccines for Children program provides free immunizations for low-income children to assure that finances are not a barrier to full immunization of those children.
- Increasing numbers of parents are choosing not to immunize their children for religious and philosophical reasons. The nurse's role is to provide these parents with accurate information and to recognize that their child may be at a significant risk for infection with potential serious consequences without immunization.
- Vaccines must be stored properly and administered appropriately to ensure their effectiveness.
- The National Vaccine Injury Acts of 1986 and 1993 provides compensation if a link between immunization and a serious adverse effect is found. The Vaccine Adverse Event Reporting System has been established to track serious vaccine reactions.
- Immunization information is updated frequently. It is the nurse's responsibility to regularly check credible sources for the latest information about vaccines, immunization schedule, and important information for parents.
- Infectious and communicable diseases are caused by bacterial, viral, protozoan, or fungal organisms.
- Fever is often a sign of infectious disease in children. The hypothalamus functions as the body's thermostat, directing the body to conserve or dissipate heat. When microorganisms invade the body, endogenous pyrogens are released into the bloodstream. These substances travel to the hypothalamus, where they trigger the production and release of prostaglandins, which initiate the fever response.
- The child with a toxic or septic appearance has the following signs: lethargy, poor perfusion, tachypnea or bradypnea, and pallor or cyanosis.
- The appropriate use and administration of antibiotics to help reduce the development of antibiotic-resistant bacteria includes the following: Give antibiotic dosages as prescribed for the full number of days ordered, do not share with other family members who might be ill, and discard when all doses have been given.
- Signs and symptoms of sepsis in newborns are often nonspecific, including subtle changes in appearance and behavior such as feeding problems and changes in color, tone, and activity.
- Children need special care when exposed to biologic and chemical agents that could be used by terrorists because of their smaller anatomy and physiologic responses. Work to ensure that children's special needs are integrated into local healthcare facility planning for epidemics.

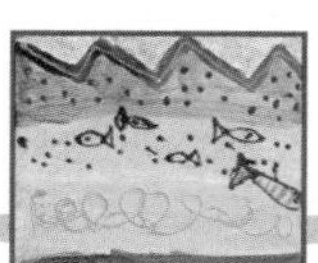

CRITICAL THINKING IN ACTION

INTRODUCTION

Recall the scenario at the beginning of the chapter involving 5-year-old Lian and 2-year-old Chang. This pediatric clinic has recently increased its efforts to improve the number of children fully immunized because quality improvement initiatives detected several deficiencies. New guidelines have been developed that encourage nurses to look for opportunities to review immunization records for all children coming to the clinic.

DESCRIPTION

Because Lian will be starting school in the fall, she will need to have the complete series of immunizations over the next 5 months. Chang needs to complete his immunization series for his age.

DISCUSSION

1. List the vaccines that should be given to Lian and Chang at today's visit. Identify when Lian and Chang should return to the clinic for their next immunizations. What vaccines are appropriate to give each child at the next visit?
2. Identify nursing interventions to reduce the anxiety and pain associated with the injections for each age child.
3. Develop the teaching plan for the care of each child at home following the immunizations.

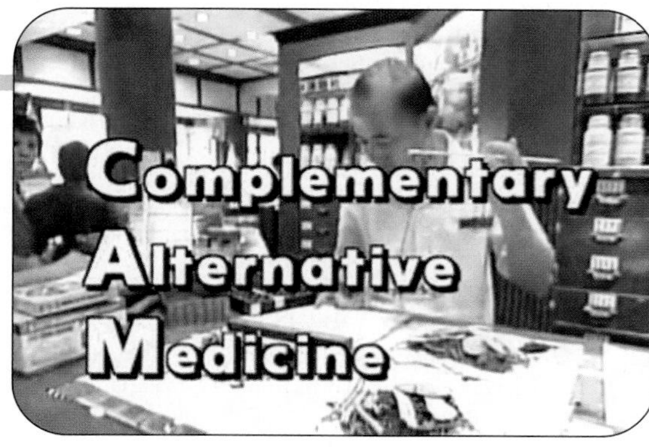

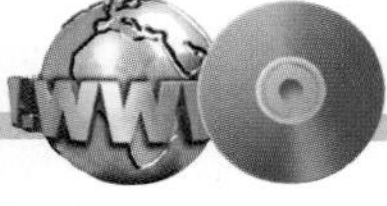

EXPLORE MediaLink

- NCLEX review, case studies, and other interactive resources for this chapter can be found on the Companion Website at **www.prenhall.com/ball**. Click on Chapter 19 to select the activities for this chapter.
- For animations, more NCLEX review questions, and an audio glossary, access the accompanying CD-ROM in this textbook.

http://www.prenhall.com/ball

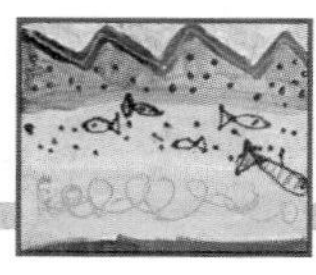

REFERENCES

Allen, A. (2002, September). Bucking the herd. *Atlantic Monthly.* www.immunize.org/exemptions/allen.htm, accessed 10/10/2002.

American Academy of Pediatrics Committee on Infectious Disease. (2003). *Red book: Report of the Committee on Infectious Disease* (26th ed.). Elk Grove Village, IL: Author.

Arvin, A. M. (2002). Antiviral therapy for varicella and herpes zoster. *Seminars in Pediatric Infectious Diseases, 13*(1), 12–21.

Ascherio, A., Zhang, S., Hernan, M., Olek, M., Copeland, P., Brodovicz, K., & Walker, A. (2001). Hepatitis B vaccination and the risk of multiple sclerosis. *New England Journal of Medicine, 344,* 327–332.

Barker, L., Darling, N., McCauley, M., & Santoli, J. (2003). National, state, and urban area vaccination levels among children aged 19–35 months, United States, 2002. *MMWR, 52*(31), 728–732.

Barlow, W. E., Davis, R. L., Glasser, J. W., Rhodes, P. H., Thompson, R. S., Mullooly, J. P., et al. (2001). The risk of seizures after receipt of whole-cell pertussis or measles, mumps, and rubella vaccine. *New England Journal of Medicine, 345*(6), 656–661.

Bechtel, B. (2003, February). Insured children in rural areas having a hard time getting PCV7. *Infectious Diseases in Children,* 18, 21.

Bigham, M., & Hoefer, M. (2001). Comparing benefits and risks of immunizations. *Canadian Journal of Public Health, 92*(3), 173–177.

Carson, S. M. (2003). Alternating acetaminophen and ibuprofen in the febrile child: Examining the evidence regarding efficacy and safety. *Pediatric Nursing, 29*(5), 379–382.

Centers for Disease Control and Prevention. (2000). Consequences of delayed diagnosis of Rocky Mountain spotted fever in children—West Virginia, Michigan, Tennessee, and Oklahoma, May–July 2000. *Morbidity and Mortality Weekly Report, 49*(39), 885–888.

Centers for Disease Control and Prevention. (2002a). Pertussis deaths—United States, 2000. *Morbidity and Mortality Weekly Report, 51*(28), 616–618.

Centers for Disease Control and Prevention. (2002b). Immunization registry use and progress—United States, 2001. *Morbidity and Mortality Weekly Report, 51*(3), 53–56.

Centers for Disease Control and Prevention. (2002c). Pertussis—United States, 1997–2000. *Morbidity and Mortality Weekly Report, 51*(4), 73–76.

Centers for Disease Control and Prevention. (2002d). Lyme disease—United States, 2000. *Morbidity and Mortality Weekly Report, 51*(2), 29–31.

Centers for Disease Control and Prevention. (2002e). Prevention of perinatal group B streptococcus disease: Revised guidelines from CDC. www.cdc.gov/mmwr/pdf/rr/rr5111/pdf, accessed 5/25/2004.

Centers for Disease Control and Prevention. (2003a). Vaccination coverage among children entering school—United States, 2002–2003 school year. *Morbidity and Mortality Weekly Report, 52*(33), 791–793.

Centers for Disease Control and Prevention. (2003b). Interim domestic guidance for health departments in the management of school students exposed to severe acute respiratory syndrome (SARS). www.cdc.gov/ncidod/sars, accessed 9/30/2003.

Centers for Disease Control Advisory Committee on Immunization Practices. (2005). Recommended childhood and adolescent immunization schedule—United States, 2005. www.cdc.gov/ nip/recs/child-schedule-fourpages.pdf, accessed 02/27/2005.

Chang, L. Y., Lin, T. Y., Hsu, K. H., Huang, Y. C., Lin, K. L., et al. (1999). Clinical features and risk factors of pulmonary edema after Enterovirus 71–related hand, foot, and mouth disease. *Lancet, 354*(9191), 1682–1686.

Cheung, M., & Lieberman, J. M. (2002). Influenza: Update on strategies for management. *Contemporary Pediatrics, 19*(10), 82–94.

Children's Hospital of Philadelphia. (2003). Vaccine education. www.chop.edu/consumer/jsp/microsite/microsite.jsp?id=75918, accessed 8/12/2003.

Cimpella, L. B., Goldman, D. L., & Khine, H. (2000). Fever pathophysiology. *Clinical Pediatric Emergency Medicine, 1*(2), 84–93.

Clark, L. M., & Manworren, R. C. B. (2001). Immunizations: Could they hurt less? *Journal of Pediatric Health Care, 15*(6), 322–323.

Cohen, L. L. (2002). Reducing infant immunization distress through distraction. *Health Psychology, 21*(2), 207–211.

Confavreux, C., Samy, S., Saddier, P., Bourdes, V., & Vukusic, S. (2001). Vaccinations and the risk of relapse in multiple sclerosis. *New England Journal of Medicine, 344*, 319–326.

Coyer, S. M. (2002). Understanding parental concerns about immunizations. *Journal of Pediatric Health Care, 16*(4), 193–196.

Crocetti, M., Moghbeli, N., & Serwint, J. (2001). Fever phobia: Have parent misconceptions about fever changed in 20 years? *Pediatrics, 107*(6), 1241–1246.

Department of Health and Human Services, Office of Disease Prevention and Promotion. (1999). *Healthy People 2010.* Washington, DC: Author.

DeStefano, F., Bhasin, T. K., Thompson, W. W., Yeargin-Allsopp, M., & Boyle, C. (2004). Age at first measles-mumps-rubella vaccination in children with autism and school-matched control subjects: A population-based study in metropolitan Atlanta. *Pediatrics, 113*(2), 259–266.

DeStefano, F., Gu, D., Kramarz, P., Truman, B. I., Iademarco, M. F., Mullooly, J. P., et al. (2002). Childhood vaccinations and risk of asthma. *Pediatric Infectious Disease Journal, 21*(6), 498–504.

Diggle, L., & Deek, J. (2000). Effect of needle length on incidence of local reactions to routine immunizations in infants aged 4 months: Randomized control trial. *British Medical Journal, 321*(7266), 931–933.

Evers, D. B. (2000). Childhood immunizations: Policies, problems, and remedies. *JONA's Healthcare Law, Ethics, and Regulation, 2*(2), 67–72.

Ferguson, L. E., Hormann, M. D., Parks, D. K., & Yetman, R. J. (2002). Neisseria meningitidis: Presentation, treatment, and prevention. *Journal of Pediatric Health Care, 16*(3), 119–124.

Gellin, B. G., Maibach, E. W., Marcuse, E. K. (2000). Do parents understand immunizations? A national telephone survey, *Pediatrics, 106*(5), 1097–1102.

Greene, A. (2002, October). Vaccination fears: What the school nurse can do. *Journal of School Nursing* (Supplement), 31–35.

Hammond, B., Ali, Y., Fendler, E., Dolan, M., & Donovan, S. (2000). Effect of hand sanitizer use on elementary school absenteeism. *American Journal of Infection Control, 28*(5), 340–346.

Healy, T. L. (2000). The impact of Lyme disease on school children. *Journal of School Nursing, 16*(2), 12–18.

Heinrich, J. (2002). *Childhood vaccines: Challenges in preventing future shortages.* Washington, DC: United States General Accounting Office, GAO-02–1105T.

Howell, K. (2001). Malaria: Part 2. *Practice Nursing, 12*(11), 464–466.

Humiston, S. G., & Judelsohn, R. G. (2003). A practical guide to using the new combination vaccines. *Contemporary Pediatrics, 20*(2), 36–53.

Hviid, A., Stellfeld, M., Wohlfahrt, J., & Melbye, M. (2004). Childhood vaccination and type 1 diabetes. *New England Journal of Medicine, 350*(14), 1398–1404.

Hylander, M. A., Strobino, D. M., & Dhanireddy, R. (1998). Human milk feedings and infection among very low birth weight infants. *Pediatrics, 102*(3), e38.

Immunization Action Coalition. (2004). Screening questionnaire for child and teen immunization. *Needle Tips and the Hepatitis B Coalition News, 14*(1), Item #P4060.

Institute of Medicine Board of Health Promotion and Disease Prevention. (2001a). *Immunization safety review: Measles-mumps-rubella vaccine and autism.* Washington, DC: National Academy Press.

Institute of Medicine Board of Health Promotion and Disease Prevention. (2001b). *Immunization safety review: Thimerosal-containing vaccines and neurodevelopmental disorders.* Washington, DC: National Academy Press.

Institute of Medicine Board of Health Promotion and Disease Prevention. (2002). *Immunization safety review: Multiple immunizations and immune dysfunction.* Washington, DC: National Academy Press.

Institute of Medicine Board of Health Promotion and Disease Prevention. (2003). *Immunization safety review: Vaccinations and sudden unexpected death in infancy.* Washington, DC: National Academy Press. http://books.nap.edu/books/0309088860/html/1.html, accessed 9/25/2003

Jacobs, E. S., Ogborn, J., & Tunnessen, W. W. (2001). Fever and abdominal pain in a 13-year-old: Time for rash decisions. *Contemporary Pediatrics, 18*(10), 20–26.

Keyserling, H. L. (2002). Prevention of pneumococcal disease in children. *Medscape.* www.medscape.com/viewprogram/1807_pnt, accessed 12/20/2002.

Larrabee, T. (2002). Prescribing practices that promote antibiotic resistance: Strategies for change. *Journal of Pediatric Nursing, 17*(2), 126–132.

Lugo, N. R., Montoya, C., & Petraco, M. B. K. (2003). Parents' perspectives on immunizations: A survey. *American Journal for Nurse Practitioners, 7*(11), 8–20.

Madsen, K. M., Lauritsen, M. B., Pedersen, C. B., Thorsen, P., Plesner, A. M., Anderson, P. H., & Mortensen, P. B. (2003). Thimerosal and the occurrence of autism: Negative ecological evidence from Danish population-based data. *Pediatrics, 112*(3, Part 1), 604–606.

Mayoral, C. E., Marino, R. V., Rosenfeld, W., & Greensher, J. (2000). Alternating antipyretics: Is this an alternative? *Pediatrics, 105*(5), 1009–1012.

McKenney, W. M. (2001). Understanding the neonatal immune system: High risk for infection. *Critical Care Nurse, 21*(6), 35–47.

Mera, K. E., & Hackley, B. (2003). Childhood vaccines: How safe are they? *American Journal of Nursing, 103*(2), 79–88.

Mosby. (2004). Mosby's drug consult 2004, St. Louis: Mosby. Inc.

Peters, T. R., & Edwards, K. M. (2002). Pneumococcal vaccines: Present and future. *Pediatric Annals, 31*(4), 261–268.

Reef, S. E., Frey, T. K., Theall, K., et al. (2002). The changing epidemiology of rubella in the 1990s: On the verge of elimination and new challenges for control and prevention. *Journal of the American Medical Association, 287*(4), 464–472.

Reis, E. C., Roth, E. K., Syphan, J. L., Tarbell, S. E., & Holubkov, R. (2003). Effective pain reduction for multiple immunization injections in young infants. *Archives of Pediatrics & Adolescent Medicine, 57*, 1115–1120.

Rennels, M. B., Edwards, K. M., & Keyserling, H. L. (1998). Safety and immunogenicity of heptavalent pneumococcal vaccine conjugated to CRM in United States infants. *Pediatrics, 101*(4), 604–611.

Saari, T. N., & Committee on Infectious Diseases. (2003). Immunization of preterm and low-birthweight infants. *Pediatrics, 112*(1), 193–198.

Schuval, S. (2003). Avoiding allergic reactions to childhood vaccines and what to do if they occur. *Contemporary Pediatrics, 20*(4), 29–53.

Sharber, J. (1997). The efficacy of tepid sponge bathing to reduce fever in young children. *American Journal of Emergency Medicine, 15*(2), 211–213.

Shingadia, D., & Shulman, S. T. (2000). Recognition and management of imported malaria in children. *Seminars in Pediatric Infectious Diseases, 11*(3), 172–177.

Stinchfield, P. K. (2001). Vaccine safety communication: The role of the pediatric nurse. *Journal of the Society of Pediatric Nurses, 6*(3), 143–146.

Tan, T. Q. (2002). Pneumococcal infections in children. *Pediatric Annals, 31*(4), 241–247.

Taylor, B., Miller, E., Farrington, C. P., Petropoulos, M. C., Favot-Mayaud, I., Li, J., & Wright, P. A. (1999). Autism and measles, mumps, and rubella vaccine: No epidemiologic evidence for a causal relationship. *Lancet, 353*(9169), 2026–2029.

Taylor, B., Miller, E., Lingram, R., et al. (2002). Measles, mumps, and rubella vaccination and bowel problems or developmental regression in children with autism: Population study. *British Medical Journal, 324*, 393.

Vazquez, M., LaRussa, P. S., Gershon, A. A., Steinberg, S. P., Freudigman, K., & Shapiro, E.D. (2001). The effectiveness of the varicella vaccine in clinical practice. *New England Journal of Medicine, 344*(13), 955–960.

Wade, C. F. (2000). Keeping Lyme disease at bay: An integrated approach to prevention. *American Journal of Nursing, 100*(7), 26–31.

Whitney, C. G., Farley, M. M., & Hadler, J. (2003). Decline in invasive pneumococcal disease after introduction of protein-polysaccharide conjugate vaccine. *New England Journal of Medicine, 348*(18), 1737–1746.

World Health Organization. (1999). Pertussis vaccines WHO position paper. *Weekly Epidemiological Record, 74*, 137–144.

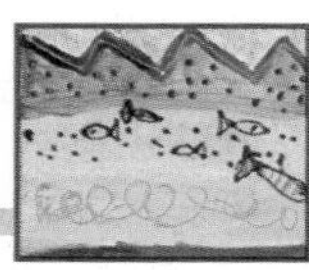

ADDITIONAL REFERENCES

Andreae, M. (2004). How to recognize and manage herpes simplex virus type 1 infections. *Contemporary Pediatrics, 27*(2), 41–59.

Baltimore, R. S. (2003). Smallpox: Preparing for an old (but no longer familiar) threat. *Contemporary Pediatrics, 20*(5), 42–60.

Blevins, J. Y. (2003). Primary herpetic gingivostomatitis in young children. *Pediatric Nursing, 29*(3), 199–202.

CDC. (2003). Guidelines for maintaining and managing the vaccine cold chain. *Morbidity and Mortality Weekly Report, 52*(42), 1023–1025.

Coleman, E. A., & Yegler, M. E. (2002). Botulism. *American Journal of Nursing, 102*(9), 44–47.

Easter, A. (2002). Ebola. *American Journal of Nursing, 102*(12), 49–52.

Foster, J. A., & Chen, J. S. (2002). General principles of disease transmission. *Pediatric Annals, 31*(5), 293–298.

Gerber, M. A., & Shapiro, E. D. (2001). Late Lyme disease: Clearing up the confusion. *Contemporary Pediatrics, 18*(7), 46–56.

National Vaccine Advisory Committee (2003). Standards for child and adolescent immunization practices. *Pediatrics, 112*(4), 958–963.

Raucci, J., Whitehill, J., & Sandritter, T. (2004). Childhood immunizations (Part one). *Journal of Pediatric Health Care, 18*(2), 95–99.

Reilly, C. M., & Deason, D. (2002). Plague. *American Journal of Nursing, 102*(11), 47–50.

Reilly, C.M., & Deason, D. (2002). Smallpox. *American Journal of Nursing, 102*(2), 51–55.

Rideout, M. E., & First, L. R. (2001). Fever: Measuring and managing a sizzling symptom. *Contemporary Pediatrics, 18*(5), 42–50.

Watson, R. S., Carcillo, J. A., Linde-Zwirble, W. T., et al. (2003). The epidemiology of severe sepsis in children in the United States. *American Journal of Respiratory and Critical Care Medicine, 167,* 695–701.

Yetman, R. J., Parks, D., & Taft, E. (2002). Management of patients exposed to biologic weapons. *Journal of Pediatric Health Care, 16*(5), 256–261.

Chapter

20 Nursing Care of the Child with a Chronic Condition

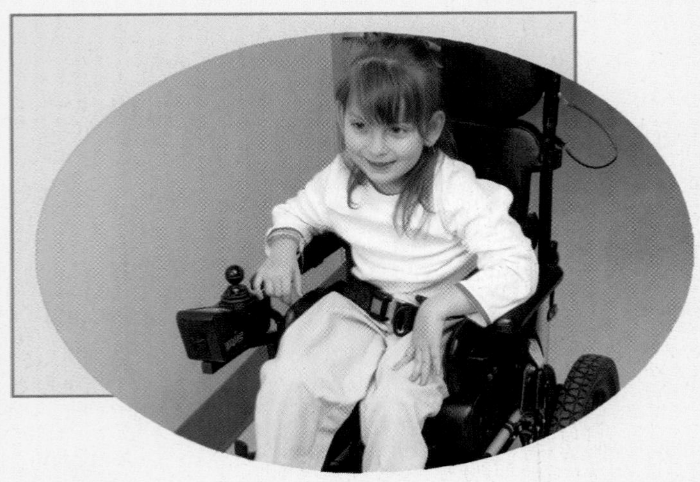

Haley Leftwich is an 8-year-old girl with cerebral palsy. She had an intraventricular hemorrhage during her neonatal intensive care unit (NICU) hospitalization for very low birth weight. Haley lives with her mother and two older siblings, ages 10 and 13. Her parents divorced when Haley was 3 years old. She has frequent contact with her father, who she visits on weekends. Her father is supportive emotionally, physically, and financially in the care of Haley and her siblings.

Haley's mother is the full-time primary care provider. Routine care includes hygiene, supplemental enteral tube feedings to promote adequate nutrition in between oral feedings, range of motion (ROM) exercises, and home schooling. Haley uses her motorized wheelchair without difficulty, and her mother has decided that she would benefit from social interaction and a structured educational environment at the local public school. Her family asks the clinic nurse and case manager at the cerebral palsy clinic for assistance in helping with planning Haley's entry into school.

How can the clinic nurse and case manager assist Haley and her family in this transition? What special arrangements are needed to permit a child to receive care for a chronic condition while at school? What measures can be taken to ensure an effective transition between home and school?

"I am excited to finally be going to school, but I am afraid too. What if the other kids don't like me? Is my mommy going to be okay while I am gone?"

—Haley, 8 years old

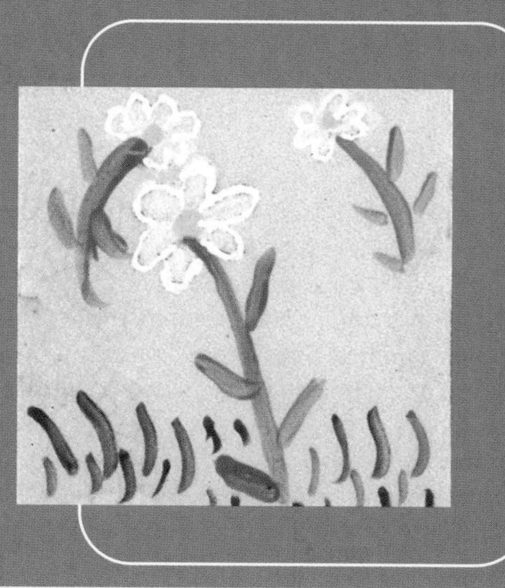

Learning Outcomes

After completing this chapter, you will be able to:

- Discuss the various categories of chronic conditions and their etiology.
- Assess the child with a chronic condition and identify specific nursing interventions for the child at different ages.
- Assess the family of a child with a chronic condition and discuss the impact of the child's condition on the family.
- Describe family-centered nursing interventions to assist the family of the child with a chronic condition to effectively care for the child in the home.
- Describe nursing management for the child with a chronic condition to support transition to school and adult living.
- Discuss the family's role in care coordination and case management.

Key Terms

MediaLink http://www.prenhall.com/ball

Resources for this chapter can be found on the CD-ROM accompanying this textbook and on the Companion Website at www.prenhall.com/ball. Click on Chapter 20 to select the activities for this chapter.

CD-ROM

Videos

- *Caregiver Burden*
- *Complementary and Alternative Modalities*
- *School Reentry*

NCLEX Review

Audio Glossary

COMPANION WEBSITE

NCLEX Review

Case Studies:

- *Preschool Entry for a 3-year-old with Asthma*
- *School Reentry for an Adolescent with a Chronic Condition*

Care Plan: The Adolescent Preparing for Transition

Teaching Plan: Educating Classmates

MediaLink Applications

- *Develop an Individualized Education Plan (IEP)*
- *Assisting Parents in Case Management*

GENERAL CONCEPTS IN THE CARE OF CHILDREN WITH CHRONIC CONDITIONS

While specific chronic conditions are discussed in detail in the chapters addressing body systems, this chapter focuses on general care concepts for the child requiring additional care coordination for a chronic condition. Nurses are essential in providing family-centered care to children with a chronic condition and their families. Nurses may assume many roles in this process, including direct care in the hospital, community setting, home, or school. Nurses often assume the role of care coordinator or case manager to help the family link with appropriate resources, plan care while wisely using health insurance resources, and integrate services needed to promote the best care for the child and family.

The following skills and abilities have been identified as essential to nurses providing care to children with specific chronic conditions (Allen, 2004).

- Knowledge of the pathophysiology of the chronic condition and anticipated disease trajectory
- Understanding of child and family reactions to the stress of the chronic condition
- An ability to work with family members in their efforts to manage the child's normal growth and development
- An ability to provide culturally sensitive care to the child and family experiencing a chronic health condition
- Assessment skills to identify changes in the child's condition requiring referral or consultation
- The ability to communicate effectively with other healthcare providers regarding any changes in the child's physical or psychosocial health
- The ability to work collaboratively with other healthcare providers
- Knowledge of resources (community agencies, tertiary care centers, specialty professionals) appropriate for the child and family with a chronic condition
- The ability to identify a family needing intervention

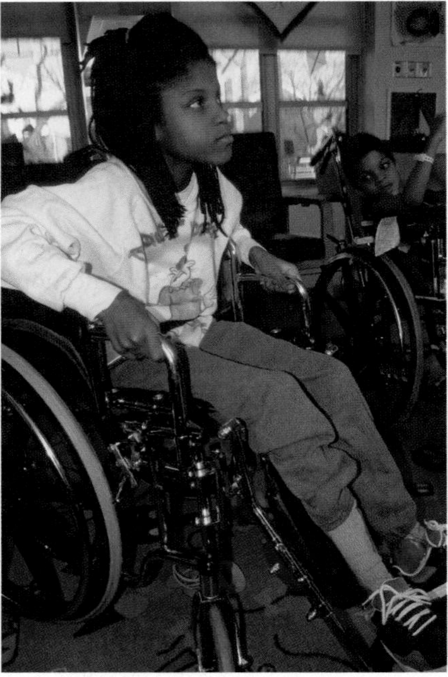

A

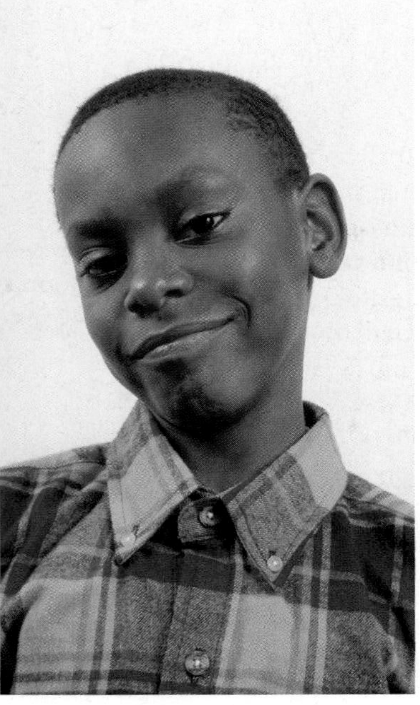

B

FIGURE 20–1 ■ Children with chronic conditions may have a visible or nonvisible health condition, or nonvisible until an acute episode of their condition makes the condition visible. *A,* The child in a wheelchair has a visible disability. *B,* The child with a seizure may have no visible signs of the condition unless a seizure is witnessed.

A **chronic condition** is a health problem that at the time of diagnosis is expected to last longer than 3 months (Perrin, 2002). The wide variety of chronic health conditions experienced by children and the different nature of these conditions impact the child's growth and development and health status in unique ways (Figure 20–1 ■). Chronic conditions have often been defined by diagnostic categories or by functional or social limitations. Examples of categories of chronic conditions include the following (Allen, 2004):

- Limitations in function that would typically be expected for the child's age and development
- Disfigurement
- Dependency on medications or a special diet for control of the condition
- Dependency on medical technology for functioning
- Need for more medical care and related services than typically used by a healthy child of the same age
- Special ongoing treatments at home or school

Children with chronic conditions that fall under these categories may require specialized healthcare: The term **children with special healthcare needs (CSHCN)** is applied to this set of children by the Maternal and Child Health Bureau of the U.S. Department of Health and Human Services, Health Resources and Services Administration. Children with special healthcare needs are those who have or are at risk for a chronic physical, developmental, behavioral, or emotional condition and who also require health and related services of a type or amount beyond that required by children generally (McPherson, Arango, Fox, et al., 1998). This definition focuses on the criteria of the need for additional health services rather than categories of limitations of diagnoses.

Using this definition, a national survey conducted by the Maternal and Child Health Bureau and the National Center for Health Statistics revealed that 12.8% (9.3 million) of children in the United States under the age of 18 years have special healthcare needs (van Dyck, Kogan, McPherson, et al., 2004). Findings revealed that the **prevalence** (the number of new and existing cases of a chronic condition during a particular period of time in the population) of special healthcare conditions increased with age, most likely because some children acquire conditions at later ages and other children with special health conditions are identified over time. For example, many children with special healthcare needs are identified upon school entry, due to conditions that require special education services or limit school participation.

Special healthcare needs for this population can be narrowed to three categories:

- Dependency on prescription medications or special diet
- Use of health services beyond what is considered usual or routine
- Functional limitations

See Table 20–1 for examples of chronic conditions that fall into these categories. Some children with chronic conditions have special healthcare needs that fall into two or all three categories. In the majority of cases, the more severe the chronic condition, the greater the number of categories of special healthcare needs. Many of these children have a **disability,** a limitation that interferes with a child's ability to fully participate in society, which can be related to one of the following (Msall, Avery, Tremont, et al., 2003):

- *Medical impairment*—chronic health condition
- *Functional limitation*—a mobility, self-care, communication (hearing or speaking), or learning behavior impairment
- *Difficulty maintaining a social role* in school or play

A **handicap** is the term applied by society to the individual with a functional limitation that creates barriers to full participation in society. The individual with a functional limitation may also self-impose barriers to societal participation.

With improved healthcare and technology, approximately 90% of children with chronic conditions will reach their 20th birthday and most of these individuals will live on into adulthood (Lindeke, Leonard, Presler, et al., 2002).

Healthcare Finance Considerations

Children with chronic conditions average medical charges from 4 to 20 times greater than healthy children. They account for 60% of all inpatient charges and 75% of all durable medical equipment, nursing, and home care charges (Neff, 2002). The 12.8% of children with special healthcare needs consume an estimated 45% of pediatric healthcare costs, demonstrating their need for increased health services (Allen, 2004). Efforts by health insurance providers and Medicaid to reduce healthcare costs have shifted the care of children with chronic conditions from hospitalization to primary healthcare providers and families. Considerable coordination of care among families and healthcare providers is essential to ensure that children have access to needed care as changes to the healthcare system continue.

Efforts to improve the health status and healthcare delivery to children with chronic conditions are a continuing public health focus. For example, *Healthy People 2010* includes objectives focused on children with special healthcare needs (Box 20–1). To help states develop strategies to achieve these objectives, the Maternal and Child Health Bureau of the U.S. Department of Health and Human Services, Health Resources and Services Administration administers Title V of the Social Security Act. This federal program provides block grants to states for the purpose of improving the health of children and their families. States are required by law to spend at least 30% of their federal block grant funds on children with special healthcare needs (CSHCN) (Maternal and Child Health Bureau, 2002). Some states use the funds to coordinate and provide direct care to children through specialty clinics, while other state programs are consultative and focus on policy development and research, providing families with referral information and resources. Table 20–2 provides a discussion of these needs and the nursing implications related to planning health service delivery to children and their families.

Overview of Chronic Conditions

Chronic conditions vary in etiology, manifestations, and their effect on the child's physical, psychosocial, and cognitive development. Chronic conditions develop from multiple causes.

- Genetic or inheritable conditions may be manifest as a chronic condition. Examples include muscular dystrophy, hemophilia, sickle cell disease, and cystic fibrosis.
- Conditions may result from congenital defect or insult to the infant during fetal development, such as neural tube defect, maternal substance abuse, cleft palate, and cerebral palsy.
- Insult or injury may be associated with birth and care following birth (sepsis, prematurity, intraventricular hemorrhage) that lead to conditions such as bronchopulmonary dysplasia, attention deficit disorder, and vision or hearing impairment.
- Conditions can be acquired through injury or acute medical condition such as brain injury, cancer, HIV infection, near drowning, and mental health problems.

TABLE 20–1 Examples of Conditions by Special Healthcare Need Category

SPECIAL HEALTHCARE NEED CATEGORY	CHRONIC HEALTH CONDITION EXAMPLES
Dependent on prescription medications or special diet	Diabetes mellitus, asthma, seizures, phenylketonuria, organ transplantation
Increased use of healthcare services	Cancer, bronchopulmonary dysplasia, renal failure, sickle cell disease, cystic fibrosis
Functional limitations	Down syndrome, brain injury, autism, myelodysplasia, cerebral palsy

BOX 20–1 *Healthy People 2010* Objectives for Children with Special Healthcare Needs

- ➤ All CSHCN will receive regular ongoing comprehensive care within a medical home.
- ➤ All families with CSHCN will have adequate private and/or public insurance to pay for the services they need.
- ➤ Services for CSHCN and their families will be organized in ways that families can use them easily.
- ➤ Families of CSHCN will participate in decision making at all levels and will be satisfied with the services they receive.

Source: U.S. Department of Health and Human Services. (2000). Healthy People 2010 *(2nd ed.). Washington, DC: U.S. Government Printing Office.*

TABLE 20–2 Healthcare Needs of Children with Chronic Disorders

HEALTHCARE NEED	DEFINITION	NURSING ACTIONS
Access to care	Availability and accessibility to providers with knowledge as well as ancillary services needed by children and their families	Assist the family in identifying local and specialized healthcare providers Assist the family in obtaining transportation assistance if required
Appropriateness of care	Services and care delivered by individuals with expertise and experience that are developmentally and culturally appropriate for the child and family	Assist the family in identifying healthcare providers that provide health promotion and other services to address the child's specific healthcare needs
Comprehensiveness	Coverage of the preventive, primary, and tertiary care needs of children, and linkages with other service systems, such as education, social services, and family support systems	Support the family by outlining educational and health services needed when developing an individualized education plan (IEP) and individualized health plan (IHP) Provide the family with resource contacts such as social services, family support groups, and other systems to help the family manage the child's condition
Coordination	Families linked to medical care, financial health resources, educational and community-based services; information is centralized	Assist the family in identifying a care coordinator Provide guidance and resources if the family decides to assume the role of care coordinator
Continuity	Through a medical home or healthcare home; linkages between primary, specialty, therapeutic, and home care exist throughout childhood	Encourage the family to collaborate with the healthcare team to ensure continuity of care Facilitate communication between all the child's healthcare providers
Degree to which services and the service system are family centered	Importance of the family reflected in the way services are planned and delivered, building on individual and family strengths, and respecting the diversity of each family	Include the family and older child in all decision making Determine the family and child's needs to ensure they are being addressed Recognize and respect the culture of the child and family

In most cases, these chronic conditions become lifelong disorders, but the impact on the affected child is variable according to the severity of the condition, the stage of growth and development when the condition occurs, and the child's and family's responses to the condition. While some conditions require intense monitoring and technological support for survival, other conditions cause few limitations and minimal effect on quality of life.

Technological advancements have improved the survival rate of children with conditions that previously were associated with high mortality rates, such as very low birth weight, complex cardiac defects, and serious brain injury. Thousands of very-low-birth-weight infants and other sick newborns are admitted to neonatal intensive care units (NICUs) each year with dependency on technology for survival. These infants have increased long-term healthcare needs after experiencing respiratory or cardiovascular disorders, hypoxia, congenital infection, brain injury, prematurity, or intrauterine drug exposure, and they may spend weeks to months in the NICU in order to receive specialized care (Kessenich, 2003).

Many of these infants and children become **medically fragile,** dependent on a medical device for survival or prevention of further disability (Figure 20–2 ■). **Technology dependence** can be categorized into four aspects of care (Haffner & Schurman, 2001).

- Respiratory support through ventilator, oxygen, and/or tracheostomy
- Intravenous medications
- Nutritional support (parenteral and enteral)
- Other medical services (such as peritoneal or hemodialysis)

Children assisted by technology can be cared for at home because equipment has been made small enough to be portable. Equipment used in the home for the child with a chronic condition may include ventilators, enteral feeding tubes, intravenous catheters, infusion pumps, dialysis equipment, and oxygen.

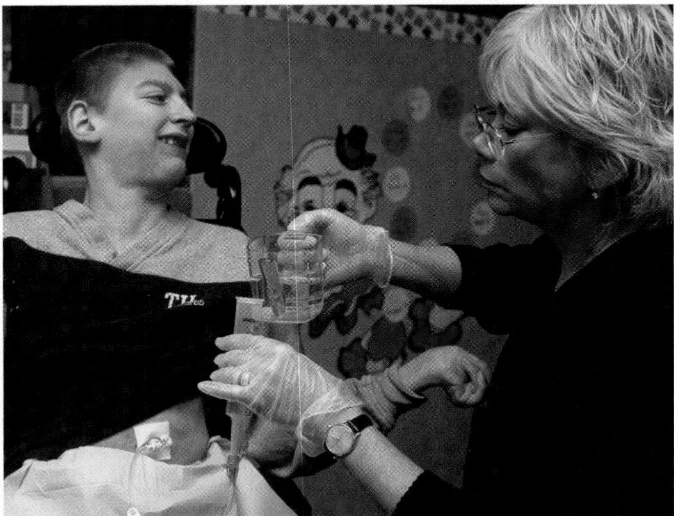

FIGURE 20–2 ■ This child needs a gastrostomy tube to ensure adequate nutrition is obtained to support growth and promote resistance to infection.

With the support of home health services, parents can learn to manage the child's care. The benefit to the child is support of physical, emotional, and cognitive growth and development within the home care setting. The child who is technology dependent may, however, be hindered in the ability to participate in normal childhood activities due to the presence of technological equipment (O'Brien & Wegner, 2002). Required treatments may also prohibit normal activities. For example, the child required to visit a dialysis center three times a week may miss school if the dialysis sessions are not planned according to the child's education program.

All families with children experiencing a chronic condition need to make some lifestyle adjustments, ensuring a baseline of care that helps maintain the child's health status and promotes growth and development. In many cases, the child has a baseline level of home management with episodic exacerbations that require the family to make sudden adjustments in family routines, such as may occur with the child who has seizures, asthma, or juvenile rheumatoid arthritis. These exacerbations often cause stress and disrupt family routines. In other cases, the chronic condition requires the family to learn and provide care that is complex and time-intensive, such as cystic fibrosis, diabetes mellitus, bronchopulmonary dysplasia, and significant cognitive impairment. These more severe chronic conditions often impact the child's physical and psychologic development.

Developmental Considerations of a Chronic Condition on the Child

The child with a chronic condition has the same developmental and emotional needs as the healthy child and should be encouraged to achieve the same developmental milestones as a child without a chronic condition. However, the impact of the chronic condition on the child's cognitive, physical, and emotional health may lead to altered developmental achievement expectations. A **developmental delay** results when there is failure to achieve anticipated developmental milestones during specific developmental stages.

Newborn and Infant

Medically fragile newborns and infants are at risk for chronic conditions related to brain injury, oxygen deprivation, and respiratory problems (Figure 20–3 ■). Newborns cared for in the NICU are exposed to a negative environment of bright lights, loud noises, frequent handling, and painful procedures, all which may adversely affect their neuropsychological development (Kessenich, 2003).

Nursing actions to promote development include encouraging the parents to spend time with the infant and engage in face-to-face interaction, touching, soothing, and caring for the infant. Provide sensory stimuli such as mobiles, soft music, and different textures for the infant to touch.

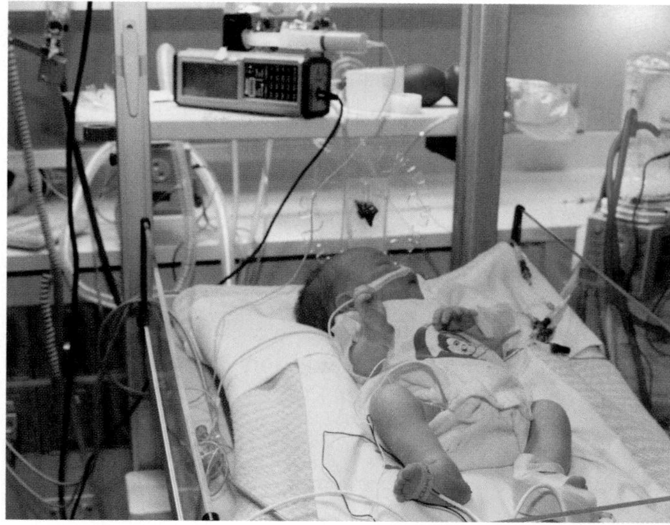

FIGURE 20–3 ■ Development of trust may be disrupted for the infant in the NICU or hospital unit when there are multiple caregivers and experiences of painful stimuli. When parents are overwhelmed by the infant's health condition or when frequent hospitalizations prolong separation, parent–infant bonding may be impaired. The infant who experiences a lack of attachment behaviors (cuddling, holding, talking) may become withdrawn (Murray, 2000).

Toddler

When the toddler has a chronic condition, parents may need to control and set limits on movement, play, behavior, or social interactions, which interferes with the achievement of autonomy and development of self-control (Figure 20–4 ■). Some parents desire to protect the child or assist with tasks they feel the child is incapable of accomplishing, rather than encouraging the child to explore. The child ultimately loses independence and lacks

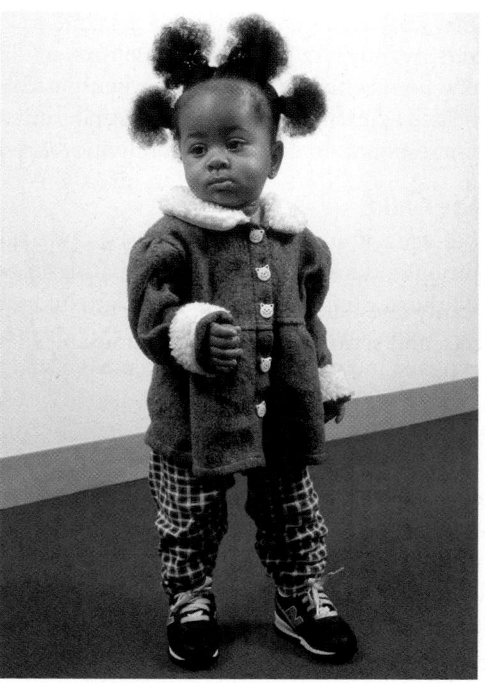

FIGURE 20–4 ■ Toddlers may experience difficulty in adapting to constraints of the condition and treatments related to their disorder. Depending on the condition, toddlers may be unable to achieve developmental milestones such as walking, toilet training, and feeding self. Delays in speech also become apparent during this stage.

opportunities for meeting developmental tasks. The parents may become overprotective and lead to vulnerable child syndrome in which the child becomes demanding, dependent, and has disturbed interactions with the parents (Melnyk, Feinstein, Moldenhouer, et al., 2001).

Nursing actions to promote development of toddlers with chronic conditions include offering the child choices when possible, such as which color gown to wear or which food to eat first. Help parents recognize the toddler's capabilities and to let the child take the time to practice and learn a skill. Identify the next most appropriate developmental accomplishments parents should help the child achieve and some strategies to support those developmental milestones.

Preschooler

Preschool children recognize the association between body parts and problems associated with the chronic condition. The preschooler engages in magical thinking during this stage, and the child may believe that his or her thoughts or behaviors cause the condition or feel that the condition is a form of punishment.

Limitations of the condition, such as decreased energy, may interfere with the preschooler's ability to learn about the environment, develop social relationships, gain a sense of self-confidence, and learn a sense of purpose (Vessey & Rumsey, 2004). The developing self-concept may be strongly influenced by the disability and discomfort experienced.

Nursing actions to promote development include explaining the purpose of treatments and procedures in terms the preschooler can understand, and emphasizing that treatments and procedures are not punishment for any wrongdoing. Through play, look for opportunities for the child to learn, perform an activity, and feel a sense of accomplishment. Encourage social interactions with other children when possible. Simple concepts related to learning about self-care can be initiated. Provide positive feedback for all successful activities and self-care.

School-Age Child

Early school-age children have an increased understanding of their condition and are capable of participating in certain aspects of monitoring and care. Late school-age children begin to understand the long-term needs associated with their condition. They also understand more about management of the condition and are capable of assuming more responsibility of their care such as serum glucose sampling, monitoring the condition of skin under braces, or intermittent self-catheterization. When some children with chronic conditions enter school, they are found to have learning difficulties and other limitations that interfere with education and social competence.

Gaining social skills, peer interaction, mastering new information, learning to cope with stress, and acquiring skills that lead to self-sufficiency are all important for the development of a sense of industry. Depending on the type of chronic condition, the child may have functional limitations (self-care, communication, mobility, stamina, and learning) that interfere with participation in school activities and thus interfere with gaining a sense of industry (Msall et al., 2003). The impact of a chronic condition may result in feelings of inferiority and a low self-concept as children recognize differences between themselves and peers.

Nursing actions to promote the development of the school-age child include encouraging the child to interact with children in the same age group and, when possible, with children experiencing the same condition. Link the child to a peer support group to promote social interaction and to help the child recognize that others also have the same condition. Encourage contact from school peers and friends through letters, cards, computer messages, as well as video and tape recordings. Encourage the child to complete school assignments when possible. Begin to identify aspects of the child's care that the child can begin to assume under supervision of the parents. When available, families may be encouraged to permit the child to attend a special camp for children with the chronic condition to promote recreation, social interaction, and learning skills of self-care.

Adolescent

Adolescence presents numerous challenges due to rapid changes in growth and sexual maturation; ongoing development of identity, body image, and self-concept; and the need to plan for vocational and healthcare transitions. This stage is normally a time of profound physical, psychological, and physiological changes. The adolescent may experience heightened awareness of differences between self and peers. For example, puberty may be delayed in some chronic conditions. Cognitive development and abstract thinking skills are achieved during this stage, allowing the adolescent to develop an understanding of the short-term and long-term consequences related to the condition (Figure 20–5 ■).

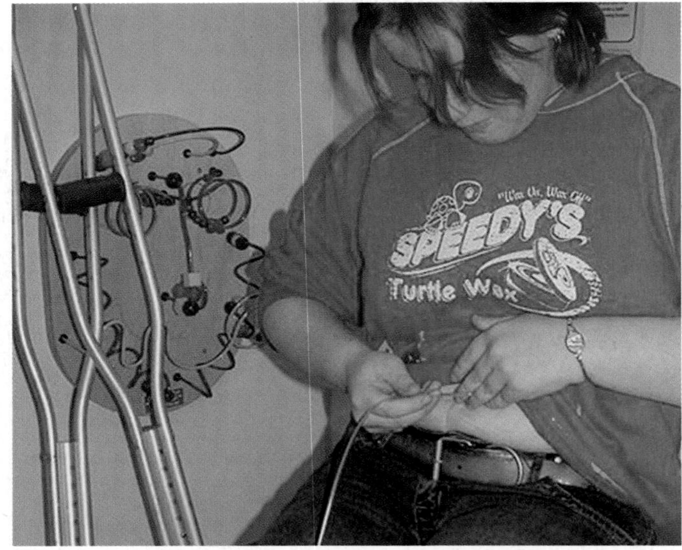

FIGURE 20–5 ■ All adolescents need to learn how to assume responsibility for their personal care and to make good decisions about future life plans. The adolescent with a chronic condition must also learn to independently manage the health condition (such as this girl performing self-catheterization) and to take that condition into consideration when making future life plans. This may be more challenging for adolescents who have a limited life expectancy or when parents are unable to relinquish their control and thus fail to encourage the child to assume more responsibility for self-care.

Some adolescents are unable to cope with the recognizable differences between themselves and healthy peers, and they withdraw from social activities and relationships. Others may engage in risky behavior that may be harmful to themselves or to management of their condition, just to be accepted by peers.

Nursing actions to promote development of the adolescent include the provision of patient education to help the adolescent learn about the chronic condition, care needed to manage or control the condition, and problem solving and specific skills for self-care so they can integrate the care management into their daily lives. Parents need to be coached to transition care over to the adolescent and to support the adolescent to make healthy decisions regarding care. Encourage the adolescent to build a safety net of friends who know enough about the chronic condition to assist if a problem occurs, such as a seizure, asthma episode, or insulin reaction. Discuss sexual maturation and the importance of protected sexual activity and discourage risky behaviors by the adolescent. Provide the adolescent an opportunity to express concerns regarding self-management, vocational planning, and future independent living.

THE FAMILY OF A CHILD WITH A CHRONIC CONDITION

Informing the Parents

The path to parents becoming aware of and informed about their child's chronic condition is as variable as the presentation of the condition.

- Some chronic conditions are apparent at birth, such as a neural tube defect.
- The child's condition may be detected as the result of a routine screening test, such as newborn screening tests for hypothyroidism or phenylketonuria.
- The infant may develop a chronic condition as a result of complications of care provided in the NICU, such as an intraventricular hemorrhage or bronchopulmonary dysplasia.
- Parents may suspect that the infant or child has a problem and seek a diagnosis, such as when the infant does not achieve motor developmental milestones as in cerebral palsy.
- Episodic illnesses may develop in a pattern and lead to the diagnosis of a chronic condition such as asthma.
- Some children do not have their chronic condition recognized until they begin school, when learning and behavior problems are identified.
- In other cases, parents wait anxiously following a child's serious illness or injury (sepsis, meningitis, near drowning, brain injury) to learn if the child will make a full recovery or have disabilities.

Parents in all cases must patiently wait for information as diagnostic procedures are performed, historical information is obtained, and the child is examined. During the period of diagnostic studies and medical evaluation, the parents face uncertainty, anxiety, and stress. If the condition is potentially life threatening, the parents' uncertainty and stress will be increased. Studies conducted among parents of children with chronic conditions have revealed that the time of diagnosis is one of the most stressful times for families (Meleski, 2002). This begins the initial transition to becoming a family with a child having special healthcare needs.

CLINICAL TIP

When discussing a child's chronic condition with family, use the child's name. Avoid labeling the child with a condition, such as "diabetic child"; instead refer to the situation as "the child with diabetes." This places the emphasis on the *child* rather than the *condition.*

The manner in which parents are informed of their child's condition influences their ability to cope (Figure 20–6 ■). Nurses should ensure that families understand all information presented to them regarding their child's health. A heightened anxiety level may reduce the comprehension of information heard. Each communication approach should be individualized according to the family's level of understanding and communication techniques (Swallow & Jacoby, 2001). See Developing Cultural Competence: Communication.

The following guidelines may be considered when informing parents of the diagnosis of a chronic illness or disability in their child (Ahmann, 1998).

1. Inform parents of their child's diagnosis in person, in a private setting, and free from interruptions. Tell both parents together. In a single-parent family, the parent should be offered the opportunity to have a relative or friend as a support person when informed of the diagnosis.
2. Inform parents of the diagnosis early on. As part of informing families, consideration should be given to the whole child and to pointing out strengths and positive attributes, as well as limitations and characteristics related to the illness or disability.
3. Use simple, direct language without medical jargon. Individualize the pace of the interview and approaches taken to

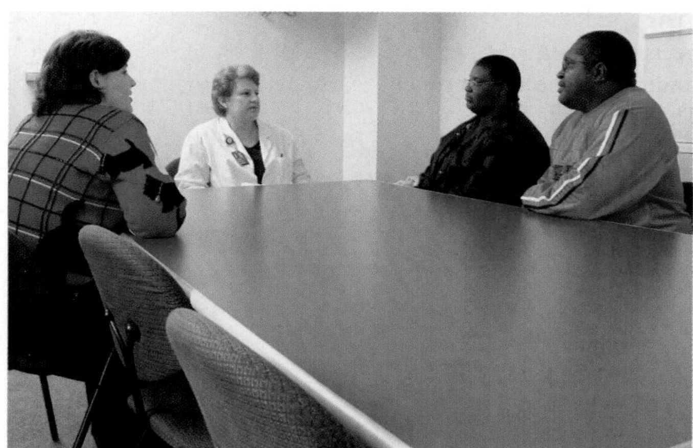

FIGURE 20–6 ■ Inform the family about the child's chronic condition in an area with privacy, and be sure to provide adequate time for the family to initially absorb the information and then to ask questions. Offer to meet the next day to review the information and respond to additional questions.

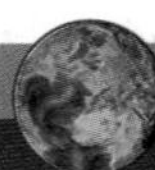

DEVELOPING CULTURAL COMPETENCE
Communication

The family who speaks English as a second language may experience difficulty in communicating and understanding information presented in English during stressful situations. A translator should be used during these times. Until a translator is available, support the family and promote a calm environment to assist in reducing the family's stress.

English-speaking Mexican American families of children with chronic conditions have reported that they recognize some advantages over Mexican American families who could not communicate easily with nursing staff. Conversely, they also indicated that their lack of Spanish fluency served as a barrier to support from parents of their cultural group that predominantly spoke Spanish (Rehm, 2003).

present the explanation. The specific diagnosis may affect the types of information parents need and want initially. For example, the parents of a child diagnosed with diabetes require immediate information related to glucose monitoring, insulin administration, and signs and symptoms of hypo- and hyperglycemia. Long-term care and management of a child with diabetes is best discussed in stages.

4. Share accurate, up-to-date information about the diagnosis, treatment options, specialty referrals, and community resources.
5. Evaluate the discussion to assess whether the family's affective and information needs were met and to provide support and/or additional or more accurate information as necessary. An evaluation can also be used to determine the family's unique and/or culturally based understanding of the condition and preferences regarding treatment.

Informing the Child

Informing the child of a newly acquired chronic condition is individualized and is based on the child's developmental level and age. Questions the child may ask vary, but often focus on the cause of the condition, how to make it better, and how it will affect daily life. Provide information tailored to the child's level of understanding and answer questions honestly. (See Chapter 6∞).

Parental Reactions

It is not possible for the parents to comprehend the diagnosis and its impact on their lives at the time of the initial discussion. A wide range of responses is a normal part of the process of adapting to the news. In some cases, the parents will feel a sense of relief that there is finally a diagnosis after all the concern, diagnostic testing, and uncertainty. In other cases, the information is a shock or very distressing news that is further compounded by the need to understand medical information and rapidly make decisions about treatment (Meleski, 2002). Responses of parents are the same as when a child has a life-threatening illness—shock, disbelief, denial, and anger (see Chapter 22∞ for a discussion of grief). Other emotions experienced by parents include despair, depression, frustration, and confusion (Melnyk et al., 2001). The specific diagnosis may also have an effect on the parents' initial response. For example, parental reaction to the diagnosis of asthma should vary significantly from the parental reaction to the diagnosis of leukemia. The nurse should be empathetic and supportive of parental emotional expression.

Parents go through a grieving process for the many losses that the child's chronic illness may bring, such as the following:

- Loss of family routines and goals
- Siblings' loss of normal childhood
- Loss of expectations for the development and life expectancy of the child with the chronic condition
- The child's loss of a normal childhood

Parents often experience sorrow and helplessness as they mourn the loss of the "perfect child." Parents may also feel the need to blame someone or something for their child's condition. They may blame themselves or their spouse if the condition is genetic.

Some parents have difficulty becoming involved with or bonding with the affected infant due to feelings of guilt, disappointment, fearing that the infant will not survive, or recognizing how differently the infant looks or behaves. The enforced separation imposed by a prolonged hospitalization after birth may contribute to difficulty with bonding (Noyes, 2000). Parents of the child with a chronic condition, particularly one that results in significant disability, have a daily reminder of their losses and differences from other families.

Parents learn to adapt to the changes imposed by the child's chronic condition; however, they may never fully accept the child's illness or disability or reach closure. Parents of children with a chronic disorder have reported episodes of recurrent sorrow, particularly at times of important transitions in the child's life that remind parents that their children are different from healthy children. At other times, the same parents deny having sorrow. This pattern of periodic grieving interspersed by periods of denial, called **chronic sorrow,** is believed to be a coping mechanism that permits parents to carry on with responsibilities at other intervals (Melnyk et al., 2001). The periods of denial prevent progression through the full stages of grieving, allowing parents to hope so that they can function (Meleski, 2002).

Siblings' Reactions

Siblings of children with a chronic condition may be affected in a variety of ways. Their self-esteem, social support, mood, understanding of the illness, and attitude toward the child's illness are interrelated (Williams, Williams, Graff, et al., 2002). They may experience feelings of jealousy, embarrassment, resentment, and a sense of loneliness and isolation (Beckman, 2002). Some siblings may fear that they themselves will have the same disease or condition as the affected child. Younger siblings may believe, because of magical thinking, that they caused the child's disability (Beckman, 2002). Some siblings may experience behavioral problems because of the disruption in family life or the lack of attention and guidance received from parents. However, some siblings have positive responses and demonstrate increased responsibility, independence, maturity, and a tolerance for differences in other. See Chapter 17∞ for siblings' responses to the child experiencing an illness.

A significant nursing action to help promote improved adjustment for the sibling of a child with a chronic condition is to help parents recognize the need to spend individual time with the sibling. Maintenance of family routines is helpful in promoting a sense of the normal. Help the family with selection of appropriate ways the sibling can help with the care of the child with a chronic condition while recognizing that the sibling needs a childhood with peer interactions, physical exercise, and recreation.

Nurse's Reactions to Care of Children with a Chronic Condition

Nurses and other healthcare professionals generally describe their role in caring for families and children with chronic conditions as very rewarding. However, over time these nurses may experience conflicting feelings, including grief, fatigue, and burnout, particularly if the needs of families and children served are difficult to meet (Maytum, Heiman, & Garwick, 2004). Nurses need to recognize signs of **compassion fatigue,** an emotion that comes from understanding the traumatic events experienced by families and the stress from helping or wanting to help the families. The weariness and lack of energy associated with compassion fatigue may become severe and affect the ability to function at work or home if the nurse's coping mechanisms are not effective.

Self-care activities such as exercise, meditation, recreation, maintaining a sense of humor, and social nonwork relationships are beneficial short-term personal coping strategies. Taking vacations to rest and reenergize, changing patient assignments, or transferring to a new work area are other strategies that can help the nurse balance personal mental health with the compassion needed for ongoing work with these families.

STRESSORS ON THE FAMILY

Having a child with a chronic condition places great demands on parents. Numerous stressors have been identified, and the following are commonly reported by families.

- Learning as much as possible about the child's condition and expected progression in severity
- Learning how to provide care to the child and integrate care into family routines
- Identifying ways that each family member can contribute to the child's care
- Communicating with health professionals about the child's care, attempting to serve as a full partner in the child's care, and identifying the most appropriate resources for the child
- Determining how to integrate employment responsibilities into the care routine
- Managing a family budget that is drained by expenses for care not covered by health insurance plans and other financial resources
- Attempting to provide siblings as normal a life as possible
- Opening the home to strangers that provide home care to the child
- Coping with episodes when the child's condition worsens and fearing that the child will die
- Working with the child to gradually assume more responsibility for self-care

Certain transitions or events are more stressful for the family, as they disrupt family routines or require adaptation by the family. As mentioned earlier, the time of diagnosis is the initial transition or event that results in changes in a family's expectations. Other times of transition that cause stress or trigger more intense feelings of sorrow include (Melnyk et al., 2001):

- When development milestones do not occur as expected, such as walking at 12 to 15 months and speech delays at 24 to 30 months
- If younger siblings surpass the affected child in developmental milestone achievement
- School entry, when differences (physical appearance, cognitive ability, or social skills) between the affected child and other children the same age become apparent to parents
- Onset of adolescence
- During transition to adult roles and health services (21 years)
- When parents must seriously plan for guardianship of the child
- When the family considers institutionalizing the child

The marriage relationship is at risk for breakdown if the couple is not able to communicate, share in the care of the child and other family members, and have common expectations for the child's condition and abilities to perform self-care. Marital and role strain as well as high levels of psychologic distress are experienced more often by parents of chronically ill children than parents of healthy children (Melnyk et al., 2001). This may be compounded by concurrent family illnesses, a death in the family, or the presence of a family conflict. However, recent studies on divorce rates have revealed that this population does not have rates that exceed that of the general population (Eddy & Walker, 1999).

Caregiver Burden

Caregiver burden, the unrelenting pressure and anxiety related to providing daily care to a child with disabilities while meeting other family obligations, is a major stressor for families of the child with a chronic condition (Figure 20–7 ■). For parents of the medically fragile child, technical skills and complicated procedures may cause the caregiver's burden to be even greater. Greater personal strain and caregiver distress are found when the child has poor functional status, needs extensive care, and a financial burden exists (Kuster, Badr, Chang, et al., 2004). The parents must perform technical care, keep records, be vigilant in monitoring symptoms, and make clinical decisions about symptoms detected based on what is best for the child and family. Additional demands include scheduling and logistics, and attending appointments to meet the therapy, medical, and educational needs of the child (Beckman, 2002).

The complexity of scheduled care combined with family responsibilities such as shopping, preparing meals, doing laundry, cleaning, ensuring that the affected child and other family members get to all appointments, paying bills, spending time with

MediaLink Caregiver Burden Video

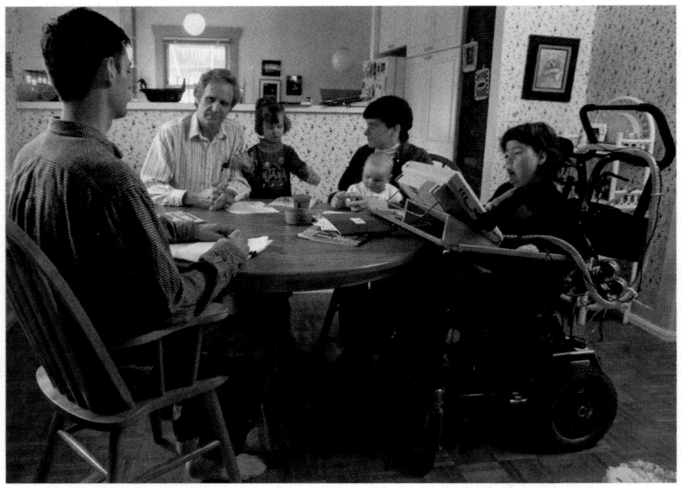

FIGURE 20–7 ■ Daily caregiving demands of the child who is medically fragile continue 24 hours a day, 7 days a week. Parents need to identify ways to share the care of the child and other family care management. When the child lives with a single parent, additional healthcare resources are needed so the parent can sleep.

other children, and managing to find personal time for a brief break can be challenging even when a family support infrastructure exists (Box 20–2). A constant struggle exists in keeping the child's needs and the family's needs in balance. Social isolation may be experienced by the parent who remains in the home providing care to the chronically ill child. Spousal support is essential to manage all the family and childcare requirements. Employment responsibilities also must be integrated into the schedule, and often hours of work must be negotiated to ensure parental health insurance coverage for the child's care.

BOX 20–2 Research: Coping and Health Promotion Participation

A study of 38 mothers of children who were technology assisted by a ventilator revealed that they rarely participated in personal health behaviors (planned exercise, balanced nutrition, adequate sleep). Those who were able to participate had children functioning at a higher level and the impact of the child's condition on the family was lower. When mothers perceived that the impact of the child's illness on the family was greater, participation in fewer health promotion activities was reported (Kuster et al., 2004).

Healthy behaviors are one form of coping and can help with the stress associated with managing the child's care. Encouraging the use of social supports or respite may enable the mother and other family members to participate in health promotion activities and could improve the mother's overall health.

Even when parents develop the capacity and skills in care coordination of the child's medical care, advocacy on behalf of the child remains intensive. Administrative work such as scheduling appointments, keeping records, developing and maintaining lists, completing health insurance claim forms, and appealing denied payments is ongoing. Seeking resources and opportunities for the affected child continues and changes with the child's condition and developmental status.

This type of workload is demanding and must be sustained long term. Parents need to learn to pace themselves, as there are limits on how much they can do and continue long term. Despite the challenges described, some families of children with chronic conditions do lead constructive lives with periods of joy and hope (Kearney & Griffin, 2001). See Table 20–3 for nursing actions to assist families with significant stressors.

TABLE 20–3 Common Stressors for Families of a Child with a Chronic Condition

STRESSORS	NURSING IMPLICATIONS
Uncertainty	Be honest in responding to the parents' questions. Serve as an advocate to ensure information from primary healthcare provider or specialists is being relayed to family.
Fear of potential loss of the child	If the death of the child is likely or uncertain, support the family and refer to social services or other support to assist the family in anticipatory grieving. Ensure that the family is kept informed about all changes in the child's condition.
High-technology environment of the neonatal or pediatric intensive care unit	Orient the parents to the child's environment. Explain all equipment and procedures. Encourage them to be an active participant in the child's care.
Communication with healthcare providers	Partner with the family and serve as their advocate to ensure communication is shared between the multidisciplinary team. Ensure the family understands all communication, and offer clarification if required. Ensure that the parents are fully informed and participate in all decision making regarding the child's care.
Deciding whom to inform about the chronic condition	Assist the family in identifying all individuals who need to know about the child's condition. Extended family members and friends can offer support and may provide assistance with care. Recommend that childcare or school officials (if school age) be informed since the child is in their care for a majority of time.
Increased out-of-pocket expenses	Partner with the family to identify cost-effective measures to reduce expenses. Refer the family to social services to determine any available assistance for healthcare, respite care, meals, or other expenses.
Social isolation and role strain	Encourage the family to participate in support groups. Parent-to-parent support groups can offer support and guidance. Encourage family to take respite time from care of child. Assist the family in determining satisfactory arrangements for respite care (e.g., family member, healthcare or respite provider).
Dividing time between well children and child with chronic condition	Encourage parents to take "special time" with siblings of child with chronic condition. Also encourage family to include all members in planning family activities and to ensure that each child has an opportunity to plan activities. Identify social supports to help provide transportation and enable participation in recreational or peer group activities.

The stressors for parents of a child who is technology dependent vary according to the child's functional status, the extent of care needed, and the financial burden (Box 20–3). Additional stressors include giving up privacy to have a home health worker provide some of the child's care, conflicts over authority and control, and child rearing decisions (O'Brien & Wegner, 2002). This burden may be compounded by the family's lack of trust in care professionals, unreliable or unskilled care, and the need to supervise the care professional in the home (Ratliffe, Harrigan, Haley, et al., 2002). Responses to these stressors are dependent upon the family's strengths, resiliency, and resources available. See Chapter 2∞ for family assessment and nursing interventions for family support.

Stressors on families directly influence the adjustment of the child with a chronic condition. In impoverished families, mothers of children with a disability report that the disability caused them to experience sleep deprivation, or have work and financial burdens. These children are approximately twice as likely to have poor psychosocial adjustment as other children with disabilities from families above poverty level. Additionally, mothers with poor health are 70% more likely to have a child who is maladjusted, and mothers with distress or depression are 90% more likely to have a child who is maladjusted (Witt, Riley, & Coiro, 2003).

Maltreatment of the Child with a Chronic Condition

Child maltreatment is reported to occur more frequently among children who are chronically ill or disabled. Causal factors contributing to the abuse and neglect of children with chronic conditions are generally the same as those for all children (see Chapter 7∞). Other factors that increase the risk of abuse in children with chronic conditions include the following (American Academy of Pediatrics, 2001b):

- Higher emotional, physical, economic, and social demands on the family
- Limited social and community support and the inability of parents to cope with the care and supervision responsibilities
- Failure of child to receive medications, appropriate educational placement, adequate medical care
- Increased stress related to the child's behavioral characteristics (e.g., communication problems, aggressiveness)

Risks for sexual abuse of the child with chronic conditions include the following:

- Infrequent contact with others can decrease opportunities to develop trusting relationships with someone to whom the child may disclose the abuse.
- The child dependent on caregivers for physical needs may become accustomed to having his or her body routinely touched by adults.

Assess the family for ineffective coping and the potential for abuse of the child with a chronic condition. Assist the family in dealing with the demands and pressure of caring for a child with a chronic condition by making appropriate referrals to support services such as mental health counseling and social services. Provide the family with a local hotline number that provides immediate support for parents experiencing stress or ineffective coping.

MediaLink Family Support Resources

BOX 20–3 Research: Parental Perceptions of Rearing a Technology-Dependent Child

A qualitative nursing study of 16 parents with a child with technology dependence and 15 registered nurses who provided home care revealed that parent perceptions of rearing a technology-dependent child were similar but different to that of raising other children. Differences noted were primarily due to the presence of technology (O'Brien & Wegner, 2002).

This finding illustrates the parents' efforts to normalize the child with a chronic condition. Home health nurses perceived that parents treated technology-dependent children differently than other children, either by not using normal behavioral expectations for the child or by denying the child's problems. Parents and home health nurses reported conflict with each other related to child rearing approaches and styles. Both parents and nurses felt that equipment interfered with the ability of the child to participate in normal childhood and family activities.

Parents also revealed difficulty in obtaining child rearing information specific to the technology-dependent child. Nurses should make efforts to support parents who wish to integrate the child with a chronic condition into normal activities. The findings suggest that improved collaboration and communication between parents and nurses may reduce parental stress and enhance development for children who are dependent on technology.

Family Financial Issues

The economic impact of caring for a child with a chronic condition is significant. Even with good insurance coverage, the family still incurs a major financial burden (Ratliffe et al., 2002). The family faces issues with insurance and provider services such as coverage limitations, inadequate service coverage, establishing medical necessity per insurer protocol, policies on providing for generic versus brand-name medications, inadequate reimbursement, and other policies affecting the care delivery for the child with a chronic condition (Newacheck, McManus, Fox, et al., 2000). Examples of additional expenses that families pay out of pocket may include special diets, durable equipment and supplies, transportation to healthcare visits, respite care, and copayment for health services. Despite these issues, the child with health insurance is more likely to have a usual source of care and a regular healthcare provider (Newacheck et al., 2000). Underinsured children with chronic illnesses are significantly more likely to go without needed care (Wood, Smith, Romero, et al., 2002).

Although health insurance payers view the limitation of services as a means to save money, this may not be an effective plan when caring for medically fragile children (Ratliffe et al., 2002). Because of the rapidly rising cost of healthcare, all health insurance plans are implementing additional controls to slow the increase in the cost of care. Depending on the type of health insurance, children with significant and expensive health conditions may reach their maximum coverage level after only a few years. Case management, supported by health insurance payers, is one mechanism used by health plans to contain costs while improving the utilization and distribution of limited resources (Lindeke et al., 2002).

Another financial concern for the family and child with a chronic condition in the home is the high incidence of job instability that can occur as a direct result of the child's condition. Parents may lose their employment due to excessive absences to provide care for the child or be required to reduce hours worked to make sure the child receives adequate care. Such job instability further threatens the family's access to health insurance for the remainder of the family as well as the child with a chronic condition.

Promoting Healthy Family Coping

A key role for nurses is to assess the family for its strengths and coping mechanisms. (See Chapter 2∞.) To cope effectively with all the stressors associated with caring for a child with a chronic condition, families have identified supports that are essential or important to them (National Resource Center for Community Based Family Resource and Support, 2002). These supports include:

- Basic needs (food, clothing, housing)
- Financial assistance
- Medical/health-related supports (home health aides, special equipment)
- Parent-to-parent support
- Recreation
- Respite care
- Technology and services that assist in tempering limitations
- Transportation

Many families identify unmet needs that interfere with effective coping. See Evidence-Based Practice: Identifying and Responding to Unmet Needs for additional information.

Families often engage in a coping strategy called **normalization.** Through normalization, the family views the care of the child with a chronic condition as a "normal" part of life, rather than an inconvenience or something outside of routine. The family continues to recognize the serious nature of the child's condition. However, the family redefines what is considered "normal" for them by adopting a "normalcy lens," enabling them to see that the family follows some normal routines like all other families. With normalization, the parents may be able to move the child's condition to the subconscious, so that it does not take a dominant place in the family's life and thoughts. They choose to focus on the normal aspects of the child and the family's life. Through normalization, the family perceives success in meeting the needs of the family (Rehm & Rohr, 2002).

The following defining attributes are exhibited by families that experience normalization (Knafl & Deatrick, 2002).

- They acknowledge the child's condition and know that it has the potential to threaten the family's lifestyle.
- They adopt a normalcy lens for defining child and family; the child and family are not changed in important ways.
- Their parenting behaviors and family routines are consistent with the normalcy lens.
- The child's treatment regimen is integrated into the usual routines of the family and child, being consistent with the normalcy lens.

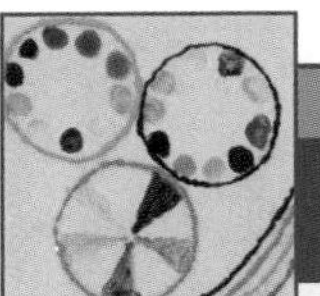

EVIDENCE-BASED PRACTICE
Identifying and Responding to Unmet Needs

PROBLEM

Parents having a child with complex healthcare conditions have reported difficulties in obtaining the supports needed to manage the child's care. What are the specific unmet needs reported by families, and do these unmet needs differ by family characteristics or the functional level of the child?

EVIDENCE

A study of the mothers, fathers, and pediatricians of 123 children with chronic conditions surveyed all three study participants per child about which of 23 items or services would benefit the child (Perrin, Lewkowicz, & Young, 2000). The majority of parent respondents were of middle income status. Information about the child's condition and services was identified by more than 65% of respondents. More than 50% identified needs associated with arranging for school programs, finding social activities for the child, and educating the child about the specific condition and treatments; further unmet needs were identified when the child had a severe or multiple conditions. The physicians consistently underestimated needs of the child and family when compared to the parents. A more recent study of lower income mothers of 83 children with complex health problems treated in primary care offices revealed similar needs (Farmer, Marien, Clark, et al., 2004). The most frequently identified need was about services for the child and ways to promote the child's growth and development. More than 50% of parents also reported a need for caregiver supports, community services, help with family relationships, and financial costs. A greater number of unmet needs were reported when the child functioned at a lower level and mothers expressed more caregiver burden. Interviews with 30 families (30 mothers and 13 fathers) having one or more children with special healthcare needs helped describe the wide range of responsibilities that parents have in managing their children's healthcare (Ray, 2002). Findings revealed that parents spent a large amount of time searching for information, people who could be relied upon for information, and services.

IMPLICATIONS

All studies revealed that families with children having special healthcare needs seek information, but the type of information sought varies by the type of condition or special healthcare need. However, ways to promote the child's growth and development and community services that match the child's needs are desired by nearly all families. Nurses are in a position to assist families by seeking information about their needs and then attempting to provide the information, and by maintaining current listings of community services for these families.

CRITICAL THINKING APPLICATION

Select a specific pediatric chronic condition that usually requires parents to follow a complex routine to care for the child. Construct a series of questions to ask the family in order to learn about their perceived needs. Consider the potential supports and services such a family might need and compile a list of local resources that could be recommended to the family.

- The parents interact with others based on their view of the child and family as normal.

Some families are unable to achieve or sustain the sense of normalization; however, they often view it as a desired goal. In many cases, these families are still adjusting to their child's condition, the child's condition may have recently changed, or another family stressor is present. These families view their life and their child as different from other families because of the child's condition. The following examples may occur (Knafl & Deatrick, 2002).

- The child's condition is a major focus of family life.
- The child's condition is a source of conflict in the family.
- The child is viewed as different from peers, and the parents have modified their parenting style to accommodate their dramatically changed view of the child.
- The child's treatment regimen is viewed as a significant burden in ways that make the family different from other families.

There are several threats to sustaining normalization. The child's health status may worsen and make the parents more aware of the child's serious condition. Management routines that previously were effective may need to be modified to integrate developmental transitions, new additions to the family, or other family situational changes. Nurses can be effective in working with families by listening to the issues and offering suggestions. Often the opportunity to talk through the child's management plan will help the family consider different strategies that may be effective. The nurse may also provide linkages to community resources that may help the family.

EDUCATION/SCHOOLING

Many children have school activity limitations that can range from an inability to attend school, or limited school attendance, to receiving or needing special education services. The majority of children with a functional disability need special education services (Msall et al., 2003). Chronic health impairments by themselves or in combination with other functional disabilities also cause school activity limitations.

All children, including those with chronic conditions and special healthcare needs, are entitled to a free education that is matched to their developmental and functional capabilities by federal law. The age range for educational services includes infants and toddlers, with the hope that early intervention in provision of educational services will lower the total cost of educational services for these children. Provisions for transitional planning for adult living, including vocational training and independent living, are also included in the Individuals with Disabilities Education Act. See Box 20–4 for federal laws that provide assurances for educational services.

Attending school is an important transition for children with special healthcare needs and their families. Sending the child to school has several benefits for the child and family. Children have an opportunity for socialization with children and adults beyond the immediate family. Parents gain a sense of normalization as the child attends school like all other children. Parents also benefit by respite from the child's care during the school day (Rehm & Rohr, 2002). Haley, the child in the opening vignette, looks forward to attending school, but also expresses fears. Her integration into the school system will require the collaboration of her family, school personnel, the nurse, and other members of the healthcare team.

Careful planning is needed when a child with special needs attends school or receives other education services.

BOX 20–4 Federal Laws for Providing Education Services for Children with Special Healthcare Needs

- Rehabilitation Act, PL 93-112 of 1973 prohibited discrimination against people with a disability. Section 504 specifies that each student who has a disability is entitled to accommodations needed to attend school and participate as fully as possible in school activities (Betz, 2001).
- The Education for All Handicapped Children Act, PL 94-142 of 1975 mandated that all children, even those with handicaps, be provided with public education and related services.
- Education for All Handicapped Children Amendments, PL 99-457 of 1986 expanded the scope of PL 94-142 to include appropriate services for infants and toddlers with disabilities and their families.
- Individuals with Disabilities Education Act (IDEA), PL 105-17 of 1997 ensures that all children with disabilities have available to them a free appropriate public education that emphasizes special education and related services designed to meet their unique needs and prepare them for employment and independent living. Every child with a disability must have a written individualized education plan, and parents have the right to question placement decisions and to due process when settling differences.

- An **individualized family service plan** (**IFSP**) is developed for the early intervention process for infants with special healthcare needs and their families. The IFSP contains information about the services required to support a child's development and enhance the family's capacity to facilitate the child's development. The family and education service providers work as a team to plan, implement, and evaluate services specific to the family's unique concerns, priorities, and resources.
- An **individualized education plan** (**IEP**) is developed for the child in the school setting with cognitive, motor, social, and communication impairments who needs special education services. The IEP is jointly planned with the school administrator, teacher, parents, and other special support professionals as appropriate for the child's condition. The child is also included in the process when possible. The plan is developed after an assessment of the child's abilities and specific functional limitations. See Box 20–5 for the elements of an IEP.
- An **individualized health plan** (**IHP**) is developed for the child with medical conditions that need to be managed within the school setting. An IHP may be developed simultaneously with the IEP for the child with a health problem and a coexisting functional impairment. Some children only need an IHP for management of their chronic medical condition at school, such as daily medication administration or for glucose monitoring and insulin injection. Learning may be challenged when the child has frequent exacerbations of the illness that result in missed days of school, and the IHP often integrates methods to prevent the child from being penalized for those absences.
- An **individualized transition plan** (**ITP**) is included in the development of an IEP for each child with a chronic disability who is 14 years or older. The ITP focuses on assisting the individual to receive vocational training and in

MediaLink Case Studies: School Reentry

BOX 20–5 Elements of an IEP

- Student's name
- Date of meeting to develop or review the IEP
- Statement of transition service needs of student beginning at age 14 years
- Present level of assessments and education performance, including how the child's disability affects the child's involvement and progress in a general curriculum or participation in appropriate activities
- Measurable annual goals that include benchmarks or short-term objectives in meeting the child's needs that enable the child to be involved in or progress in the general curriculum or participate in appropriate activities
- Special education and related services, supplementary aids and services, and program modifications or supports for school personnel needed to enable the child to make advancements toward attaining annual goals
- Explanation to the extent that the child will or will not participate with nondisabled children
- Any specific modification in the administration of state or district-wide assessments of achievement that are needed for the child to participate in the assessment, or reasons for excluding the child from assessment
- How the child's progress toward annual goals will be measured
- How the child's parents will be regularly informed of the child's progress toward annual goals and the extent to which the child's progress is sufficient to meet goals by the end of the year

Data from U.S. Department of Education. (2004). A guide to the individualized education program. http://www.ed.gov/parents/needs/speced/iepguide/index.htm, *accessed 10/14/2004.*

moving successfully from the home into other community living settings as they grow older.

During school entry, parents may experience judgmental attitudes of school professionals. The child's deficits, rather than abilities, may be the focus of school professionals (Beckman, 2002). Special education is provided in the "least restrictive environment," meaning that where possible, the child should be able to participate in as many school activities as possible. Ongoing debate in education exists regarding full inclusion or "least restrictive environment," in which the child with a chronic condition is placed in general educational settings, versus optimal or partial inclusion, in which the child is placed in a general classroom for part of the school day and in a special resource room at other times for education tailored to the child's abilities and educational goals (Rehm & Rohr, 2002).

MediaLink Develop an IEP

Parents have an important role in advocating for their child to ensure that the child receives the most appropriate educational services. School systems must provide a full range of educational services for the children with special healthcare needs, including services that support cognitive development, self-care skills, mobility, improved communication, and social skills. Because each child's severity and combination of impairments is unique, identifying and matching the specific services for each child requires discussion and negotiation. Parents should make an effort to learn about the different types of educational services that address a child's specific disability in preparation for the IEP meeting (Figure 20–8 ■). In this way, the parents are better prepared to participate in the educational planning and development of the child's IEP. See Partnering with Families: Preparing for an IEP Meeting.

Many children have chronic medical conditions that require management during the day in the school environment, such as asthma, diabetes, and attention deficit disorder. Medications may need to be administered regularly or episodically to the child. Additional aspects of care may also be integrated into the school day, such as blood glucose monitoring or intermittent self-catheterization. The education system is obligated to provide reasonable accommodations to ensure that the child's medical needs are met during the school day.

As with the IEP, the development of an IHP is a joint activity of the child's teacher, school administrator, school nurse, parents, and the child. The child's healthcare provider will provide information about the child's condition and special health condition management that must be integrated into the child's school day. When medications and special treatments are needed, a physician order for those aspects of the child's care is required. In discussing the IHP and management plan, efforts must be made to reduce barriers to the care needed (Box 20–6).

Teachers will need to learn to identify specific health problems, such as increased respiratory effort in a child with asthma or sweating, and pallor and loss of concentration in a child with diabetes. The child's teachers become part of the child's safety net for rapid access to needed healthcare intervention. With support from the school administration and school nurse, teachers can learn about the child's condition and special care that may be needed during the school day, such as a snack for the child with diabetes, management of the child who has a seizure, and ways to reduce the spread of infection within the classroom.

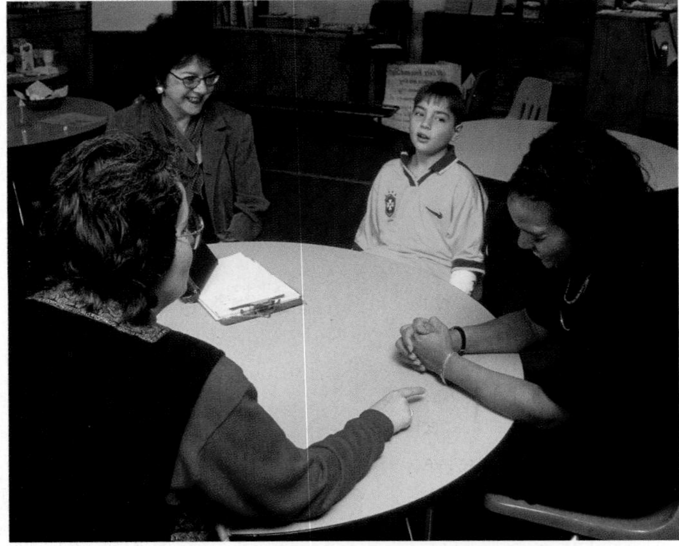

FIGURE 20–8 ■ An annual meeting of the school administrator, teacher, school nurse, and other school personnel, as well as the parents and child, is important in identifying the educational goals for the child and the special education resources to help meet those goals.

PARTNERING WITH FAMILIES

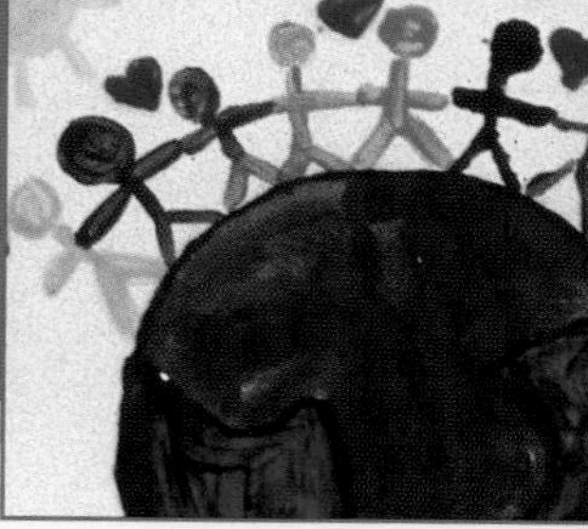

Preparing for an IEP Meeting

Parents need to be prepared to meet with the school administrator, teacher, and other health professionals when the child's IEP will be developed so they can be effective advocates. Provide parents with the following suggestions.

- Talk with another parent who has experienced the IEP process to help prepare for the meeting. Inquire about what information should be shared about the child and what types of requests for services are appropriate. Parent support groups are a good place to talk with other parents who have gone through the process. Parent information and training programs often have parents who can provide support and mentoring for parents participating in the IEP process the first time. The National Information Center for Children and Youth with Disabilities website has a state-by-state directory of resources.
- Learn about the range of special education services available. Discussions with parent mentors can provide information about the special education services available for a child with specific disabilities.
- The child must be evaluated prior to the development of the IEP. Provide parental consent for the evaluation and carefully review the result of the evaluation. Ask for assistance in interpreting evaluation results if they are unclear.
- Attend the IEP planning meeting in person, and when appropriate bring the child to the meeting.
- Be prepared to provide a summary of the child's strengths and parental concerns about enhancing the child's education.
- During discussions about potential educational strategies for the child, parents should listen carefully and ask questions to be fully informed about the special education service options.
- Listen to the educational goals and objectives as well as how evaluation of the child's progress in meeting those goals and objectives will be accomplished. Parents should ask questions or raise issues if they disagree with the IEP goals and objectives.
- Review the written plan to ensure that it matches the discussion during the IEP meeting. If the plan does not seem to match the child's needs, parents have the right to ask for revisions of the IEP. If the parents feel that special education is not being provided as outlined in the child's IEP or a good faith effort is not being made to assist the child to achieve the goals and objectives in the IEP, due process can be initiated.
- Request a new IEP planning meeting if the child appears to have made substantial progress in meeting goals and objectives during the school year. More frequent revisions to the IEP with new goals and objectives may be needed to support the child's progress.

BOX 20–6 School Reentry Planning for the Child with a Chronic Illness

A study was conducted to identify and describe specific concerns and educational needs of parents and school personnel for school reentry for the child with a chronic illness. Data were collected by telephone interviews of 21 parents of children with chronic conditions and with questionnaires answered by 24 school personnel, that included social workers, principals, psychologists, teachers, and school nurses (Kliebenstein & Broome, 2000). The survey results revealed five areas of concern.

- How parents informed the school about the child's illness (*breaking the news*)
- The processes related to the child's reentry into the school (*making the transition*)
- Ongoing monitoring of the child's health status both parents and teachers felt necessary (*watching the child*)
- The need to educate school personnel about unexpected health problems (*teaching the teachers*)
- School personnel's expectations for the child (*working with the child*)

Nurses can use these five areas of concern as an outline to help the family plan for sharing information with the school system about the child's new or changed condition. Nurses in hospital or clinic settings caring for the child can help assemble information about the child's condition and physician orders for medical care at school, and serve as a liaison with the school nurse to help parents provide information to school administrators and teachers.

The Child's Response to Entering School

Children with chronic conditions—whether they cause minimal interference in the child's daily life or are dependent on technology—face certain challenges in the school setting. School-age children with special healthcare needs may for the first time recognize differences between themselves and other children, such as appearance, abilities, social skills, or special treatment needs. They also may experience social stigma for the first time, experience teasing, or have difficulties forming friendships (Melnyk et al., 2001). Some children, particularly adolescents, may attempt to hide their condition or fail to adhere to necessary recommendations, such as dietary restrictions, to appear like their peers.

Education for Children Who Are Medically Fragile

MediaLink School Reentry Video

Children who are medically fragile or dependent on technology are also entitled to a free and appropriate education and education services in the school setting. In some cases, the education of these children is provided through a home schooling program. However, other families prefer that their child attend school. The child's need for skilled supportive care for management of medical needs must be carefully considered by both the parents and the school system. Parents often have anxiety and concerns about how well the child will be cared for as they relinquish the child's care to others during the school day. The school administration is obligated to plan for and ensure that the personnel resources and equipment needed to provide care are consistently available. The school and classroom setting may need modifications to accommodate the child, such as wheelchair ramps or an elevator.

In some cases the child is placed in a classroom with healthy children, and the teacher is expected to monitor the child's health status and provide care as needed. Examples of care include suctioning a tracheostomy, feeding the child with a gastrostomy tube, and changing diapers. Health aides are sometimes assigned to provide care for one or more children, and school nurses supervise or assist with care provided. Some children are placed in classes for children with special healthcare needs, where health aides are more readily available to provide needed healthcare.

Risks in the school setting for the child who is medically fragile or dependent on technology include safety issues related to ventilators, tracheostomy, and medication therapy. These children may also have less resistance to infections than healthier school-age children. Proper emergency resuscitative equipment must be available for certain children, and teachers and school personnel need to be instructed in resuscitative procedures. Some families request a Do Not Resuscitate (DNR) order for the child at school. The school personnel may challenge this request on the basis of legal concerns, personal beliefs, and educational considerations (American Academy of Pediatrics, 2000a). See Chapter 22∞ for more information about issues related to DNR orders.

Teachers often feel conflicted because their primary role is to educate children, and they are increasingly being required to provide skilled supportive care as well. They often feel overwhelmed by the responsibility of providing skilled supportive care, just as parents did when they first were learning to provide the care. Teachers are also fearful of their own liability in providing the care. Because they do not have training in special supportive medical skills, teachers rely on parents and school nurses to provide the preparation needed to provide care for these children. School nurses are often on-call in schools that have children who are medically fragile or dependent on technology.

Nurses play a key role in assisting the family to understand that a teacher's primary responsibility is to teach, not to provide healthcare. The teacher is responsible for the health and safety of all children in the classroom. Parents need to be realistic in their expectations about the level of skilled support services that can be provided in a classroom. Teachers and education leaders are often challenged as they attempt to meet the obligations for the child's special education services in balance with the needs of all the other children in the classroom.

MediaLink Care Plan: The Adolescent Preparing for Transition

Home Schooling

The family of a child who is medically fragile or technology dependent may choose the option of home schooling the child, with resources provided through the school system. Home schooling may be used for all of the child's education or for periods when the child is experiencing exacerbations or more complications from the condition. The benefits of home schooling include continuity of education when the child would otherwise be unable to attend school and reducing the child's stress and fatigue. Potential negative effects of home schooling include lack of peer and social interaction and decreased opportunity to develop social skills. The family that chooses home schooling needs to establish a routine for the education process with limited interruptions.

Transition to Adulthood

Adulthood is considered the time when children move into their own home and begin to financially support themselves. Depending on the adolescent's chronic condition and abilities, customized **transition** planning is needed for self-determination. An ITP is developed through the IEP process, using a multidisciplinary approach in collaboration with the family to assist in identifying appropriate support programs, living arrangements, and employment (Beckman, 2002). Transition planning should focus on the following areas (American Academy of Pediatrics, 2000b).

- Identifying and transitioning the adolescent or young adult to adult-oriented healthcare services
- Identifying and selecting an alternate living arrangement so the child can leave home and live in the community
- Helping the adolescent learn work skills and apply them in the workplace in preparation for leaving the school environment

Healthy Ready to Work services may be particularly helpful to adolescents and families in planning for the transition to adulthood. For adolescents with chronic conditions who have the ability to seek higher education, parents may need assistance in visiting the program or school and seeking information about support services that are available. Campus disability support programs can provide information on the school's view of students with disabilities and their accommodations.

COLLABORATIVE CARE

Care of the child with a chronic condition generally requires a multidisciplinary health professional approach, including physicians, nurse practitioners, nurses, nutritionists, social workers, case workers, physical therapists, occupational therapists, and a case manager.

Hospitalization

Children with chronic disorders are more likely to be hospitalized than children without chronic disorders. Depending on the severity of the condition, long-term hospitalization for months or years may be required for the child with a chronic condition. The family is an integral part of the plan of care for an ill or hospitalized child. Acute hospitalization resulting from exacerbation of the child's disorder places increased demands and stressors on the child and family. The child and parent may fear worsening of the condition or even death. Refer to Chapter 17∞ for a discussion of nursing care of the hospitalized child.

Ethical Issues

Ethical issues often arise for children with chronic conditions or disabilities since they may be unable to make autonomous choices or give informed consent for research or medical procedures. Who ultimately makes the decisions—parents or the primary healthcare providers—about withholding treatments, implementing treatments, and other medical care issues is an ongoing debate. Issues regarding clinical ethics related to children with chronic conditions or disabilities include the following:

- Withholding and refusal of treatment
- Advanced directives (Do Not Resuscitate orders) (see Chapter 1 and Chapter 22∞ for further discussion)
- Genetic testing and screening programs
- Prenatal diagnosis, therapeutic abortion, and fetal therapy
- Sexual and reproductive rights
- Sterilization of adolescents with mental retardation
- Organ donation and rationing of care
- Research involving individuals with disabilities

Additional ethical issues arise from rationing of care, or withholding treatment on the basis of outcome and cost. For example, a child born with a severe congenital malformation may be denied surgical intervention due to increased likelihood of poor outcomes and the cost of treatment. These situations present a challenge to the family and healthcare providers. Most healthcare facilities have an ethics committee with established procedures and guidelines for addressing issues for the child with a chronic disorder or disability.

Transition Between Hospital and Home

Many families become the primary caregiver for the child with a chronic condition, assuming responsibility for assessment and treatment despite the level of skill and complexity involved in that care. Numerous benefits to home care include the promotion of normalcy and development for the child, fewer hospitalization days, and decreased financial costs to health insurance providers (Balinsky, 1999). However, many question the true financial savings, since many families of medically fragile children report limited access to healthcare services and limited insurance to meet their child's needs (Newacheck, McManas, Fox, et al., 2000). Because of the burden of care, parent caregivers may experience depression, social isolation, poor physical health, and a high degree of stress associated with caring for the medically fragile child.

The family faces numerous challenges for home care, including modification of the home. Management of the condition involves technological support, medications, and treatment regimens, all potential necessities to maintain the child in the home. Family members must decide who has responsibility for different aspects of the child's care. Many families must also decide whether both spouses will continue to work or if one parent will stay home to care for the child. Home health nursing care may be needed if both parents continue to work or to cover the night shift so parents can sleep.

Moving the child who is chronically ill or technology dependent to the home setting is a life-changing decision for the family, and it must be done with collaboration between the family and the healthcare team. Preparation for the transition of the child with a chronic condition or technology dependence requires that the family receive extensive training and instructions on the care of the child. This transition is often challenging and intimidating for the family who now must assume the role of independent caregiver. Family members often feel unprepared to handle the complex situation of chronic condition and/or technological supports. The family may be assuming care of a child that has been hospitalized for months or even years before being discharged home (Harrigan, Ratliffe, Patrinos, et al., 2002).

Several factors have been identified as necessary for a successful transition from the hospital to home. First, the family must be motivated to provide care for the child at home. If the family's motivation is substantial, if they possess strength and resiliency factors, they are more likely to overcome the difficulties and obstacles that arise. Adequate health insurance and financial resources are also needed. Lastly, the family must be connected to available community services (Harrigan et al., 2002). In some cases, if the appropriate level of home care cannot be achieved, the child may be placed in a care facility outside of the home.

Barriers to Family Support Services. Parents of children with disabilities often identify barriers that prevent them from receiving adequate family support services. The family of the child with a chronic condition may not initially recognize the barriers that interfere with receiving adequate social support. The nurse assists the family in first recognizing any barriers. Once barriers are identified, appropriate referral (e.g., financial assistance, healthcare providers) and other resources can be recommended. See Table 20–4 for potential barriers and nursing implications.

Health Promotion and Health Maintenance of Children with Chronic Conditions

Most children with chronic conditions are cared for at home with or without home nursing or other healthcare services, and they may rely solely on the family for their support and care. Children with chronic health conditions require regular health promotion, health screening, and health maintenance care, as well as specialized health services to assist the child and family in the management of the condition. Many children with chronic conditions require additional health supervision visits for additional immunizations, such as the meningococcal, pneumococcal 24-valent, and respiratory syncytial virus vaccines.

The child's chronic condition may predispose a higher risk for other complications, such as infectious diseases, injury, or developmental delay. Parents require education and guidance to reduce risks for further illness and injury and to foster the child's development. The goal is to promote the child's growth and development and permit the child to have as normal a childhood as possible. See the Health Promotion and Maintenance Overview on page 665.

The child with a chronic condition needs a medical or healthcare home to ensure that all the child's healthcare needs are met. Ideally this healthcare provider is located in the community where the family resides, making it more convenient for the family to obtain healthcare as well as care for episodic illnesses. Having a regular healthcare provider has many advantages for the family.

TABLE 20–4 Barriers to Family Support Services

BARRIER	NURSING IMPLICATIONS
Attitudes and beliefs of healthcare providers	Evaluate personal biases and beliefs regarding working with children with special healthcare needs
Family's awareness of condition and treatment	Assess the family's level of understanding of the child's condition and treatment Offer careful explanation over multiple visits to provide the family opportunities for questions and to develop an understanding Encourage the family to discuss their fears and concerns
Collaboration and respect between healthcare providers and family members	Be familiar with program policies and standards of practice Encourage a family-centered care team approach between the family and healthcare provider team Demonstrate respect for the family's decisions Demonstrate respect for the family's culture Assist the family in choosing a case manager or in assuming the role of case manager themselves
Cost of care	Provide the family with information regarding healthcare insurance or health reimbursement options, such as Medicaid, Title V, or social security income.
Resources	Assist the family to identify appropriate healthcare providers to meet the child's special healthcare needs Refer family to child and parent advocacy groups Provide families with names, telephone numbers, and addresses of other significant resources Assist the family in identifying local services that are appropriate to meet the child's healthcare needs Refer the family to counseling if appropriate

Data from National Resource Center for the Community-Based Family Resource and Support (CBFRS) Program. (2002, August). http://www.friendsnrc.org/, *accessed 2/11/2004.*

- Because the child and family are seen more frequently, a trusting relationship can develop. The relationship may enable a more family-centered approach to care, providing important information to the family and supporting the family to make decisions regarding proposed interventions.
- The healthcare provider sees the child and family when things are going well and during exacerbations, and thus develops a more global view of the family and potential needs. This may enable the provider to identify strategies that may help the family to better coordinate the child's care.
- When the provider is based in the same community as the child there is a better chance that knowledge about community resources will already be assembled and can be shared with the family. This information can significantly reduce the effort families often make to identify and match appropriate resources to the child's needs.

An optimal healthcare arrangement for the child with a chronic condition exists when the medical or healthcare home provider collaborates with a pediatric team specializing in the care of children with a specific chronic condition. Pediatric specialists, advanced practice nurses, and other healthcare providers (e.g., physical therapists, occupational therapists, social workers, and nutritionists) often function as a team, providing coordinated care to the family and child with a chronic condition such as spina bifida, cystic fibrosis, or cerebral palsy. In this way, the child benefits from the most current healthcare guidelines and expertise for a specific condition. These specialty teams are often found in major medical centers, requiring travel to the facility. The team approach often makes it possible to have a coordinated visit with all specialists on the same day. Communication between the child's healthcare provider and the specialty team helps ensure that families have a healthcare provider to monitor new treatments and to seek further consultation if a change in the child's status occurs. The primary healthcare provider serves as the child's advocate in the larger healthcare system.

Alternate patterns of care are also seen.

- A pediatric specialist may serve as the child's medical or healthcare home. Although this may seem like a good strategy for care, there are some risks that health promotion services will be minimized. It is important to ensure that regular health promotion and health maintenance services, such as immunizations, are not overlooked during the care of acute exacerbations of the chronic condition.
- The child may be cared for by a generalist physician or pediatrician and be referred to a pediatric specialist on an episodic basis to review the child's health status and management plan. Recommendations for diagnostic procedures and condition management are provided to the child's primary healthcare provider. The child's healthcare provider assists the family in making decisions to implement the recommendations.

One innovative model of healthcare delivery has been successful in helping families of children with chronic conditions. Pediatric nurse practitioners in pediatric office settings help families by obtaining letters of medical necessity, getting referrals, arranging early medical care when the child was ill, setting goals for the child, helping to develop IEPs and IHPs, and providing the families with one nurse for consistent communication. This healthcare delivery system has improved the parents' satisfaction with healthcare delivery, reduced the number of lost work days of parents, and reduced hospitalizations for the child (Palfrey, Sofis, Davidson, et al., 2004).

Health Promotion & Maintenance Overview

The Child with a Chronic Condition

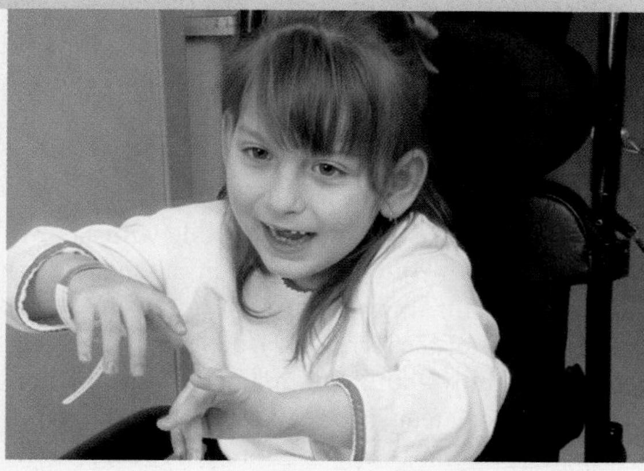

The child with a chronic condition requires monitoring and intervention in order to foster growth and development. The nurse can help promote and maintain health in the following ways.

Growth and Development Surveillance

- Monitor the child's growth and developmental patterns.
- Monitor for developmental delays.
- Explain to parents that regression following rehospitalization or exacerbation of condition in the toddler or older child is normal. Be patient and work with the child to regain developmentally acquired skills.
- Ask the family about financial resources to pay for physical therapy, occupational therapy, speech therapy, and other services that promote the acquisition of developmentally appropriate skills. Financial constraints can impede adherence with recommended therapies; refer the family to resources.

Nutrition

- Refer the family to a nutritionist and to resources for nutritional supplements or special dietary food, as well as for enteral or parenteral nutrition equipment.
- Assist mother in learning how to breastfeed the infant if desired

Physical Activity/Recreation

- Encourage the parents to promote physical activities within the child's ability.
- Assist the family in identifying appropriate activities for the child, such as swimming classes for children with disabilities.
- Encourage the child to participate in a camp for children with similar chronic conditions.

Oral Health

- Encourage regular dental visits for dental caries screening and other oral health issues such as grinding the teeth.
- Teach the parents to provide and promote good dental hygiene.

Mental and Spiritual Health

- Assess the child for self-esteem status related to body image if the condition affects physical appearance. Help the child and family identify strengths that can help enhance self-esteem.
- Ask the older child about experiences with any teasing associated with the condition or physical appearance. Discuss possible responses when teasing occurs.
- Refer the child for counseling if indicated.

Relationships

- Evaluate the parents for parental–infant bonding.
- Encourage peer interaction.
- Encourage participation in social activities within the child's ability.

Disease Prevention Strategies

- Teach the family to maintain a record of the child's immunizations, illnesses, and treatments. Ensure that the child obtains additional immunizations appropriate for higher risk status for infection, such as the pneumococcal 24-valent vaccine, meningococcal vaccine, and Palizumab for RSV.
- Ask school personnel to provide information when an increase in acute infectious diseases among classmates is noticed so parents can decide if child should remain home from school for a few days.
- Encourage consistent handwashing before and after providing care to the child.

Injury Prevention Strategies (Safety)

- Assist parents to establish a safe home environment for children with visual or motor difficulties.
- Ensure that parents obtain injury prevention guidance offered to families with healthy children, such as use of car safety seats and seating the child in the back seat of the car.
- Customize injury prevention guidance to the special needs of the child, such as testing bath water temperature for children with reduced sensation in the lower extremities.

NURSING MANAGEMENT

In collaboration with the family and a multidisciplinary healthcare team, the nurse assists the family to manage the child's care at home, provides guidelines to promote the child's health and growth and development, and supports the family by facilitating psychosocial adaptation.

The role of the nurse in caring for the chronically ill child includes the following: providing health supervision from infancy to transition into adulthood, collaborating with the multidisciplinary healthcare team, partnering with parents or caregivers to manage the child's care at home, referring the family to appropriate community services, assisting with planning for education services, promoting positive parenting behaviors and psychosocial adaptation and well-being of the child and family, and promoting growth and development of siblings.

Nursing Assessment and Diagnosis

Physiologic and Developmental Assessment

Conduct a physical assessment of the child, noting general health and also specifically focusing on systems affected by the chronic condition. Perform a developmental assessment to help identify future developmental goals and offer anticipatory guidance.

FAMILY ASSESSMENT

Assess individual family members' level of understanding of the condition, treatment, and anticipated outcome of the condition. Determine the family's stage of acceptance of the child's chronic illness, and how well the child's care is integrated into family routines. Evaluate the child's home care environment to determine the potential for abuse, lack of adequate care, or neglect. Assess the family's strengths, stressors, risk factors, and coping strategies.

Nursing diagnoses that may apply to the family of a child with a chronic condition include:

- Compromised Family Coping related to prolonged condition management and inadequate financial resources
- Fatigue related to excessive role demands in caring for the child with chronic condition and other family members
- Anticipatory Grieving related to child's deteriorating health status
- Deficient Knowledge related to complex condition management plan
- Risk for Impaired Parenting related to stress with caring for child with chronic condition and lack of social support system
- Caregiver Role Strain related to child's illness chronicity and 24-hour care responsibility

Nursing diagnoses that may apply to the child are provided in the nursing care plan on page 668. Additional nursing diagnoses may be found in the nursing care plans for children with specific chronic conditions in systems chapters.

Planning and Implementation

Newborn Care

Promote parent–newborn attachment by demonstrating to parent how to hold (if possible), stroke, touch, rub, and talk to the newborn attached to technology. Explain the purpose of all technology, the sights and sounds, and what they indicate to help reduce anxiety in handling the newborn. Reduce environmental noise and bright lights, but provide developmentally appropriate visual stimulation for the newborn, such as pictures of a face or a patterned design. When possible, provide continuity of nursing staff for the newborn to help parents bond with the newborn, to educate the parents about the child's condition, and to begin preparing for home care. Ensure adequate pain management for procedures performed. See Chapter 18∞.

The Child with a Newly Diagnosed Chronic Condition

Just as with the newborn's family, it is equally important to address the fears and concerns of the family of a child with a newly diagnosed chronic condition. Provide the condition-specific education to help prepare the family for care at home and begin discharge planning. Care of the technology-dependent child includes educating the family about equipment use and maintenance, specific tasks associated with treatment, and monitoring of the child. Ongoing assistance may be required to help families deal with financial issues, time management, and other challenges. See the systems chapters later in this textbook for condition-specific family education and discharge planning.

Discharge Planning and Home Care Teaching

As the newborn or child with a newly diagnosed chronic condition transitions to the home, parents often feel overwhelmed with preparations for home care, the anxiety of caring for a newborn with special healthcare needs, grief for the loss of their expectations for a healthy baby, and supporting the child's growth and development needs. Partner with the parents to ensure a smooth transition from hospital to the home environment. Assist the family in the initial discussions with the multidisciplinary team that participates in developing the child's care plan. Ensure that the family understands the role of each care provider.

Education to provide care of the child at home may be initiated by the hospital nursing staff, and then transitioned to special nurse educators or the home health nurses. Care is taken to ensure that all aspects of management are discussed with the family and that they demonstrate an understanding and ability to perform the care required.

Collaborate with the family and healthcare team to ensure that the child has a medical or healthcare home in the local community to provide health promotion and maintenance and to assist with the coordination of local community resources. Promote communication and joint planning of care between the specialty care provider and local healthcare provider. Nurses working in hospital specialty clinics and other community settings can help ensure that children with chronic conditions receive multidisciplinary referrals and have appointments scheduled. Social services may be called to assist the family with identifying financial resources and other community resources for home management.

Coordination of Care

Care coordination involves promoting timely access to services, continuity of care, and enhancing the family's well-being (Lindeke et al., 2002). The nurse partners with the family and healthcare team to coordinate care and services to meet the individualized needs of the child and family. Care coordination also involves matching the family's needs for services based on assessment findings.

The goals of care coordination include (American Academy of Pediatrics, 1999):

- Gaining access to and integrating services and resources on behalf of the child
- Linking service systems with the family
- Preventing duplication of services and unnecessary cost
- Advocating for improved individual outcomes

Care coordination may also include assisting the family to adapt the home to support required technology, such as mechanical ventilation. Assistance may be required in purchasing or leasing specialized equipment such as ventilators, infusion pumps, and wheelchairs. The coordination plan also includes determining the responsibility for caregiver tasks and the potential need for home health nursing or other home health services, such as physical therapy.

Because numerous healthcare providers and healthcare agencies are often involved in the care of the child with a chronic illness or an injury requiring long-term care, coordination of health services is important to prevent gaps and overlaps. A **case manager,** often a nurse or social worker, may be given responsibility to help the family with care coordination. The role includes coordinating the healthcare team, determining family needs, identifying resources, and arranging for healthcare needs. In some hospitals, nurses act as case managers. (See Chapter 1∞ for more on the role of the nurse as case manager.)

Once management goals are set by the multidisciplinary team, the case manager partners with the family to assist in decision making about which healthcare provider or agency is responsible for assisting the child to meet each goal. An important role is helping the family to determine cost-effective strategies to meet healthcare goals, to prevent the child from reaching the cap on health insurance benefits for as long as possible.

Often families will assume the role of care coordinator for their child. It is essential for the family to understand that care coordination is time consuming and requires ongoing assessment and evaluation of the child's status and anticipated outcomes. Support family members in their decision to lead the care coordination process by helping the parents to become knowledgeable about the child's condition and treatment regimen. Support the parents to take an active role in the treatment planning and decision-making process so that they gain confidence in their abilities. Many hospitals have workshops for parents who are managing the complex care of their children. Additionally, parent-to-parent support groups can be valuable to the family by providing advice, support, and suggestions for referrals. Review the care coordination to ensure that the child has access to the most appropriate care and resources. Provide positive feedback to the parents as their advocacy skills increase.

Suggest that the family maintain a log of the healthcare team members, their roles, when the child was seen and any interventions, the results of interventions, and future planned interventions or treatments. The family can use this information when communicating with the healthcare providers, particularly in an emergency, and it may also help eliminate unnecessary duplication of procedures.

Respite Care

Respite care is an important support service for families to help them keep the child with a chronic condition in the home. Respite care and other support services (home health services and parent support groups) may also reduce the risk of abuse. Assist the family in identifying respite care that meets the individual family's needs from the services available in the community. Many states have passed legislation for in-home family support services that include respite care. Because many respite services charge for their assistance, the family may require help in identifying respite waiver subsidies available to them. Reliable childcare and enrollment in school are other mechanisms for families to obtain respite care.

MediaLink Respite Resources

Support for the Child with a Chronic Condition

Provide the child with opportunities to express concerns about the condition and the effect the condition has on quality of life. The child who has had the chronic condition since birth or early childhood requires assistance in understanding more about the condition as cognitive development and understanding increase. As the child grows, collaborate with the child and family to include the child in self-care management according to cognitive and developmental level, and to participate in decision-making process. Encourage the child to assume a role in care and management of the condition. This may include maintaining a journal, self-administering medications, or monitoring glucose levels. See Partnering with Families: Developmental Strategies for Promoting the Child's Self-Care for more information.

Health Promotion

Review the next stage of expected development with parents and provide suggestions and strategies to help the child with a chronic condition achieve developmental milestones. Partner with the family to ensure that other children in the family are also receiving appropriate care and stimulation to promote their growth and development. Discuss with parents routine health promotion and maintenance needs of all children in the family such as immunizations, dental hygiene, and any screening tests. See Chapters 11 through 15∞.

Discuss parenting approaches for the child with a chronic condition. Encourage a structured environment with limitations as developmentally appropriate for the child. Assist the family as needed in providing a nurturing environment and offering praise for achievement of tasks.

Support the transition of adolescents to adult health services by introducing the adolescent to members of the healthcare team that will eventually assume a role in providing care.

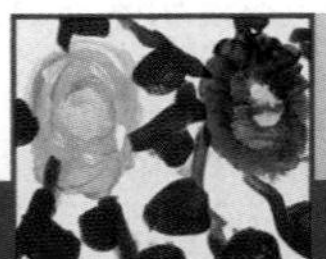

Nursing Care Plan

THE CHILD WITH A CHRONIC CONDITION

GOAL	INTERVENTION	RATIONALE	EXPECTED OUTCOME
1. Deficient Knowledge (child) related to learning self-care skills			
	NIC Priority Intervention— *Individual Teaching:* Planning, implementation, and evaluating a teaching program designed to address a patient's particular need.		**NOC Suggested Outcomes—** *Knowledge:* Extent of understanding conveyed about treatment regimen.
The child will acquire self-care skills for lifetime management	▪ Assess the child's developmental level and select an educational approach and self-care activities to match. ▪ Review with the child all steps involved in the self-care skill and how to perform the skill. ▪ Use demonstration/return demonstration until the child is comfortable with procedures. ▪ Help parents develop a planned sequence of self-care skills to teach the child. ▪ Discuss a plan for increased responsibility for self-care with the child and parents.	▪ Learning goals for the child must match knowledge and skill expectations appropriate for developmental stage. ▪ The child may have watched the routine used by parents many times, and asking the child to list each step helps the nurse identify extra training needed. ▪ Evaluation permits positive reinforcement and guidance for modification of techniques. ▪ Parents need guidance to identify appropriate self-care skills that the child is developmentally ready to learn. ▪ Parents often need encouragement to transition responsibility to the child, becoming a supervisor rather than the person controlling care.	The child demonstrates the proper technique in the self-care skill and is able to assume responsibility for that skill with supervision by the parent. Responsibility for self-care increases as new skills are learned.
2. Interrupted Family Processes related to management of a chronic disease			
	NIC Priority Intervention— *Normalization Promotion:* Assisting parents and other family members of children with chronic illnesses or disabilities in providing normal life experiences for their children and families.		**NOC Suggested Outcomes—** *Family Health Status:* Overall health status and social competence of family unit.
The child and family will manage the required treatments, monitoring, and medication regimen for the child's condition while maintaining family routines and functioning.	▪ Assess the child's and family's lifestyle and attempt to fit the child's care needs into those schedules. ▪ Discuss the family's routines for special occasions and vacations and any activities important to the child. Identify ways to modify the child's management for these occasions and activities.	▪ Fitting the child's care to the child's and family's lifestyle promotes adherence to regimen and healthier family processes. ▪ It is important for the child to participate in special events with the family and peers as a normal child to promote psychological development.	The child and family maintain important family routines and successfully manage the child's condition.
3. Individual Readiness for Enhanced Family Coping related to self-care management of chronic condition			
	NIC Priority Intervention—*Decision-Making Support:* Providing information and support for a patient who is making a decision regarding healthcare.		**NOC Suggested Outcomes—** *Decision Making:* Ability to choose between two or more options.
The child will develop a support system network.	▪ Talk with the child about how to tell friends, teachers, and other important persons about the chronic condition.	▪ These important persons can assist the child in an emergency if they have enough information to assess the problem.	The child identifies the friends, teachers, and other important persons informed about the chronic condition who can provide support when needed.

Nursing Care Plan THE CHILD WITH A CHRONIC CONDITION (continued)

GOAL	INTERVENTION	RATIONALE	EXPECTED OUTCOME
3. Individualized Readiness for Enhanced Family Coping related to self-care management of chronic condition (continued)			
	■ Discuss ways to explain the condition to important persons and how to answer questions. Role-play ways to talk about the condition with friends and teachers. ■ Encourage the child to attend peer support groups or camps specific to the child's condition.	■ Having an opportunity to plan and role-play the conversation will reduce the child's anxiety about condition disclosure. Sharing information about the condition helps others understand changes in lifestyle needed by the child. ■ Learning and support networks developed at camp can promote development of problem-solving skills that increase coping abilities.	
4. Health-Seeking Behaviors (Child) related to learning self-management of chronic disorder			
	NIC Priority Intervention— *Self-Modification Assistance:* Reinforcement of self-directed change initiated by the patient to achieve personally important goals.		**NOC Suggested Outcomes—** *Health Promotion:* Actions to sustain or increase wellness.
The child will develop independent ability to manage condition.	■ Allow the child to perform as many self-care procedures as possible at each developmental stage. ■ Encourage the child to problem solve and make decisions regarding care. Review decisions and provide feedback or appropriate guidance. ■ Encourage parents to stay involved even when the adolescent takes primary responsibility for care. ■ Encourage the child to discuss the condition and care directly with the healthcare provider.	■ Gradually learning self-care skills helps make this seem a regular expected behavior. ■ Problem-solving skills and competence in self-care management develop with positive feedback or corrective guidance. ■ The child is likely to adhere to treatment plan when the parents continue to show interest and supervise care. ■ The child begins to learn the process for seeking healthcare and becoming an advocate for own care.	The child performs appropriate daily management of self-care and seeks help to appropriately manage episodic acute problems.

Encourage the adolescent to take a more assertive role in healthcare visits with the pediatric healthcare team in preparation for working with a new healthcare team. Ensure that the adolescent understands the role each new member of the team will assume.

Facilitate Education Service Planning

Assist the family with school entry of the child with a chronic condition. Discussions with the family can help them in defining appropriate expectations and goals. The nurse can also take a role in communicating with school personnel about any classroom modifications required by the child, and in educating teachers and other school personnel about the medical or assistive equipment used by the child. This information is then integrated into the child's IHP, which may be a stand-alone plan or tied to an IEP. Encourage the family to establish regular communication with the school personnel and school nurse.

The school nurse can also play a key role in assisting the family with Section 504 planning activities by serving as a liaison between the school and the child's healthcare team. Key health records that are needed for the planning of the IHP should be assembled after the family provides informed consent. Inform the family that special accommodations for the child with disabilities may include extending test-taking times, tutors, note takers, and the use of technological equipment to assist in the learning environment. Encourage parents to ask questions regarding computer accessibility, arrangements for tutors or note takers, private study areas, and individualized attention. Partner with the child and family to determine the appropriate level of participation in school activities, including after-school activities.

In the case of a Do Not Resuscitate (DNR) request for the child at school, encourage collaboration with school personnel, teachers, and other members of the healthcare team as necessary to facilitate an agreement between the school and family. Many school systems do not have a policy that permits honoring a DNR request, and the school nurse is an important liaison in the

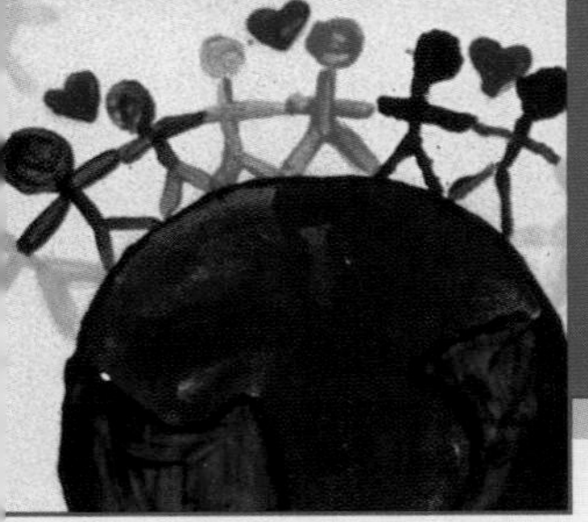

PARTNERING WITH FAMILIES

Developmental Strategies for Promoting the Child's Self-Care

When the child is cognitively able to learn about the chronic condition and begin to take some responsibility for self-care, knowledge of cognitive and psychomotor development helps in developing strategies to teach the child about self-care. Ideally such learning should begin early in life, but even when the condition develops at a later age, educating the child can still be based on knowledge of the child's development. Education and assumption of self-care responsibility should be appropriately matched to the child's developmental abilities. The ultimate goal is to transition all self-care responsibility to an adolescent who has learned all important aspects of the condition, who can manage daily routines and problem solve when an issue with care occurs, and who knows when and how to seek healthcare (Kieckhefer & Trahms, 2000).

- Toddlers (1 to 3 years) can cooperate with the daily routines of care and assist in simple ways, such as holding an item. The toddler can also learn simple concepts such as foods allowed or not allowed. When a routine is established, the toddler learns what to expect through daily repetition.
- Preschoolers (4 to 5 years) are able to imitate some of the parent's behaviors regarding care, and they can learn simple terms that describe their condition and how they feel when the condition is not well controlled (e.g., weak and dizzy with diabetes, difficulty breathing with asthma).

  Parents can help teach the child the simple terms about the condition and having the child practice telling the information to other family members. Help the parent identify a simple task that is part of the management care routine that the child can do to help (e.g., holding the spacer during the asthma treatment, washing the hands, taking supplies out of a bag or box).
- Early school-age children (6 to 9 years) are more aware of physical feelings associated with when the condition is and is not well controlled. The child is also capable of performing some aspects of care (e.g., finger stick for glucose monitoring, writing the glucose reading in a log, controlling inhalation to use aerosol medication, selecting appropriate foods for a meal or snack), having seen it performed by parents repeatedly or after being taught and coached to do it well.

  The parent can support the child's learning by increasing the information provided about the condition and need for treatment. Give the child an option about which self-care skill to learn first, next, and so on. The parent is then able to select skills appropriate to the child's developmental ability and teach the child to perform them. As the child demonstrates proficiency with a skill, a new skill can be added. The child can take responsibility for learned self-care skills with supervision, and the parent performs other unlearned skills.
- Late school-age children (10 to 12 years) have a greater understanding of how the body works and the impact of the chronic condition. They have the capability of discussing some aspects of care directly with the healthcare provider. By 12 years of age, the child can learn to perform all the psychomotor skills associated with the condition.

  Parents can support the child in assuming more responsibility for self-care by initially providing a list of all steps in the management plan or other tools that will help with decision making (e.g., dose of insulin, adding food to diet on days with soccer practice). Provide corrective feedback as necessary. Continue to be present to answer questions, particularly when problem solving and decisions need to be made about care. Encourage the child to talk independently with the healthcare provider rather than control the discussion.
- Adolescents can, with the prior steps of preparation, become the primary managers of their daily care. They usually have the cognitive ability to problem solve and make adjustments in the care routine for special occasions or illness and to ask for help when a complex care situation develops. The adolescent should have a network of friends and family who are informed about the condition and able to assist in an emergency.

  Parents should monitor the self-care provided without interfering in the adolescent's care routine unless corrective feedback is needed. Encourage the adolescent to take full responsibility for self-care management, but encourage open communication about the condition and other healthcare concerns. Discuss risky behaviors and the potential impact on general health and the condition specifically. Provide support and assistance during the time the adolescent transitions to adult healthcare providers.

---

discussion and development of the policy. Refer to Chapter 22∞ for further discussion of DNR requests in school.

Support Family's Psychosocial Adjustment

Collaborate with the child and parents and provide them the opportunity to discuss how the experience of a chronic illness affects their daily lives (Jacobs, 2002). Well siblings may feel neglected by parents as a result of the time-consuming care process for the child with a chronic condition. Listening and offering strategies to improve the organization of care, as well as the use of community and family supports, can help enhance the family's coping. The family's social network—extended family, neighbors, and friends—are also beneficial to coping with stressors (Beckman, 2002). Help the family see that simple chores performed by the social network can reduce stress especially during times when the child is hospitalized, such as meals cooked for the family, transportation for well siblings to recreational events, or picking up needed supplies at the supermarket. Partner with the family to identify support systems and to encourage open communication with those systems to maintain adequate support. Referral to a support group for parents, as well as siblings, may assist the family with information, encouragement, and care suggestions (Keefe, 2003). Counseling may be helpful to parents experiencing marital stress.

Identify ways to improve accessibility of services to children with chronic conditions and their families. For example, arranging transportation, finding resources closer to home, and arranging for home visits may improve accessibility.

Assist the family to provide information to the siblings about the child's disability at the appropriate developmental level so that the information is tailored specifically to the siblings' level of understanding. Provide instructional materials, videos, books, pamphlets, and other information when available.

Inform the parents that siblings of the child with a chronic condition may experience an array of feelings including anger, jealousy, grief, denial, and aggression. Encourage the parents to permit the siblings to express their feelings and concerns. Conflicts or resentment may arise when older siblings are requested to assume increasing responsibility in the care of the child, especially when it interferes with social and recreational activities. Discuss ways of determining the appropriate balance of responsibilities for each family member. If available, referral to support groups for siblings may be beneficial.

CLINICAL TIP

Siblings of children with chronic conditions may feel overwhelmingly guilty about their feelings of jealousy, shame, and anger. Inform the siblings that these feelings are normal and that they are not "bad" for having them.

Evaluation

Expected outcomes for care of the family of a child with a chronic condition may include:

- The child and family establish effective coping mechanisms.
- The child and family experience reduced anxiety.
- The child and family demonstrate understanding and management of condition.
- Parenting patterns are appropriate and supportive of the child's growth and development.
- Role conflict and caregiver strain are minimized.
- Caregivers achieve adequate rest, sleep, and socialization.
- The child and family adjust to the child's chronic condition.
- The adolescent successfully transitions to adult health services and living arrangements.

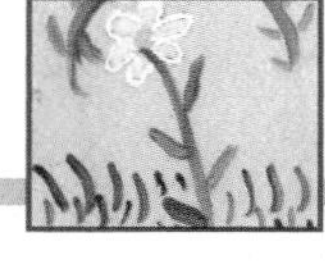

CHAPTER HIGHLIGHTS

- A chronic condition lasts or is expected to last 3 months or more and may involve any of the following alone or in combination: functional limitations, disfigurement, dependence on technology, medications, special diet for management of the condition, and requiring more healthcare services than a healthy child.
- Children with special healthcare needs represent approximately 12.8% (9.3 million) of the U.S. children less than 18 years of age. Approximately 45% of all pediatric healthcare costs are related to healthcare services used by this group of children.
- Chronic conditions can occur as a result of a genetic condition, congenital anomaly, injury during fetal development or at birth, complication of care after birth, serious infection, or significant injury.
- Children who are medically fragile are those dependent on a medical device for survival or prevention of further disability.
- A developmental delay results when there is failure to achieve anticipated developmental milestones during specific developmental stages.
- Parents may experience many of the same responses to the diagnosis of a child's chronic condition as if they had experienced the child's death, including shock, disbelief, anger, denial, and despair. Siblings of the child with a chronic illness may have feelings of jealousy, embarrassment, resentment, and a sense of loneliness and isolation.
- Nurses who specialize in caring for children with complex chronic conditions may experience compassion fatigue as they continue their efforts to meet the ongoing needs of these families.
- The time of diagnosis is one of the most stressful times for families of children with chronic conditions as the parents wait anxiously for the outcome of diagnostic procedures. Other times associated with significant stressors for the family include developmental milestones, school entry, adolescence, planning for the transition to adult health and vocational services, and planning for long-term guardianship.
- Caregiver burden, the ongoing pressure of caring for children with special healthcare needs, causes fatigue and makes it difficult for the parents to meet other family obligations.
- The financial burden of caring for a child with special healthcare needs is significant even when the family has health insurance.
- In an effort to cope and feel a sense of control of the family's life, the parents may use normalization, a process of focusing on those aspects of family life and routine that are similar to other families while integrating the needs of the child with a chronic condition.
- Sending the child to school has several benefits for the child and family including the following: socialization for the child beyond the immediate family, respite for parents, and promotion of a sense of normalization in the family.

- An individualized education plan (IEP) is developed for the child in the school setting for a child with cognitive, motor, social, and communication impairments who needs special education services. An individualized health plan (IHP) is developed for the child with medical conditions that need to be managed within the school setting.
- Children who are medically fragile or dependent on technology are entitled to a free and appropriate education and education services in the school setting. The school administration is obligated to plan for and ensure that the personnel resources and equipment needed to provide care are consistently available.
- An individualized transition plan (ITP) is developed for adolescents with a chronic condition in collaboration with the family to assist in identifying appropriate support programs, living arrangements, and employment for adult life.
- The child with a chronic condition is more likely to be hospitalized than the child without a chronic condition. Sudden hospitalization resulting from exacerbation of the child's disorder places increased demands and stressors on the child and family.
- Moving the chronically ill child or technology-dependent child to the home setting is a life-changing decision for the family, and it must be done with collaboration between the family and the healthcare team.
- Children with chronic health conditions require regular health promotion, health screening, and health maintenance care, as well as specialized health services to assist the child and family in the management of the condition.
- The role of the nurse in caring for the child with a chronic condition includes providing health supervision from infancy to transition into adulthood, collaborating with the multidisciplinary healthcare team, and partnering with the family to manage the child's care at home.

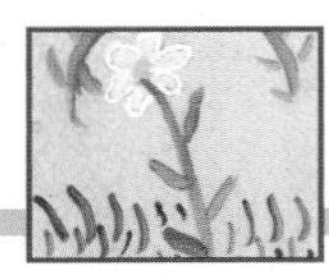

CRITICAL THINKING IN ACTION

INTRODUCTION

Recall Haley, the child with cerebral palsy who will be attending school for the first time. Her mother had initially preferred home schooling for Haley, and now wants to support her social development with other children. Haley's sister is in the local elementary school and, if possible, her mother would like Haley to attend the same school. A case manager is asked to assist with facilitating Haley's entry into school.

DESCRIPTION

The case manager coordinates a multidisciplinary meeting of the clinic nurse, physical therapist, physician, and Haley's family to review her health status and to discuss the transition to school. They also discuss potential accommodations needed for Haley's mobility limitations. A full educational evaluation has not yet been performed, and the family is encouraged to talk with the school system to initiate that process. The multidisciplinary team assists the parents in developing a plan for Haley's transition to school. Once her mother has signed consent, the case worker will ensure that needed medical records are transferred to the school for development of the IEP and IHP.

DISCUSSION

1. What role will the clinic nurse and case manager have in helping develop Haley's IEP and IHP?
2. What role will the school nurse have with the child, caregivers, teacher, and classmates during the facilitation of school entry?
3. Based on Haley's age and developmental stage, what feelings, fears, and concerns might she be expected to experience related to entry into school? What interventions would be beneficial to Haley?
4. What actions will the mother need to take in preparing the school personnel for Haley's health needs?
5. Haley's 10-year-old sister attends the same school. What effects of Haley's entry into school might the sibling experience?

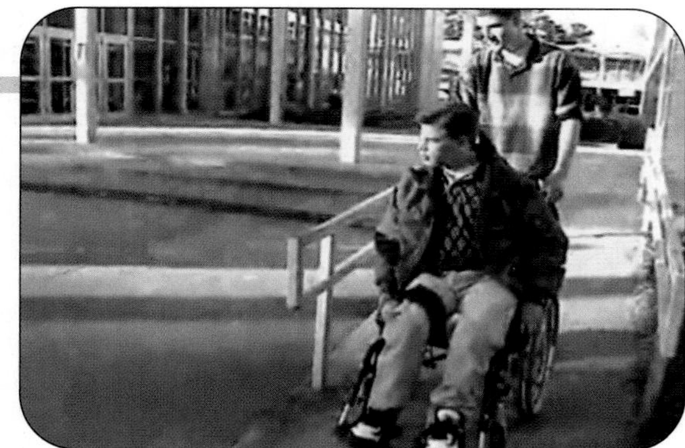

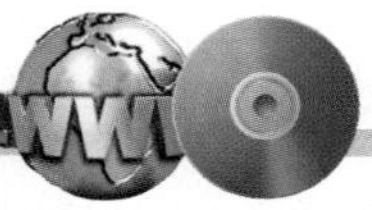

EXPLORE MediaLink

- NCLEX review, case studies, and other interactive resources for this chapter can be found on the Companion Website at **www.prenhall.com/ball**. Click on Chapter 20 to select the activities for this chapter.
- For animations, more NCLEX review questions, and an audio glossary, access the accompanying CD-ROM in this book.

http://www.prenhall.com/ball

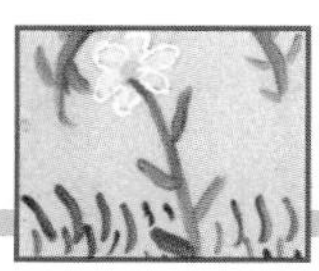

REFERENCES

Ahmann, E. (1998). Review and commentary: Two studies regarding giving "bad news." *Pediatric Nursing, 24*(6), 554–556.

Allen, P. J. (2004). The primary care provider and children with chronic conditions. In P. J. Allen & J. A. Vessey, *Primary care of the child with a chronic condition* (4th ed., pp. 3–22). St. Louis: Mosby.

American Academy of Pediatrics. (1999). Committee on children with disabilities. Care coordination: Integrating health and related systems of care for children with special health care needs. *Pediatrics, 104,* 978–981.

American Academy of Pediatrics. (2000a). Do not resuscitate orders in schools (RE9842). *Pediatrics, 105*(4), 878–879.

American Academy of Pediatrics. (2000b). The role of the pediatrician in transitioning children and adolescents with developmental disabilities and chronic illness from school to work or college. *Pediatrics, 106*(4), 854–856.

American Academy of Pediatrics. (2001a). Counseling families who choose complementary and alternative medicine for their child with chronic illness or disability. *Pediatrics, 107*(3), 598–601.

American Academy of Pediatrics. (2001b). Policy statement: Assessment of maltreatment of children with disabilities. *Pediatrics, 108*(2), 508–512.

Balinsky, W. (1999). Pediatric home care: Reimbursement and cost benefit analysis. *Journal of Pediatric Health Care, 13*(6), 288–294.

Beckman, P. J. (2002). Providing family-centered services. In M. L. Batshaw (Ed.), *Children with disabilities* (5th ed., pp. 683–691). Baltimore: Paul H. Brookes Publishing Co.

Betz, C. L. (2001). Use of 504 plans for children and youth with disabilities: Nursing application. *Pediatric Nursing, 27*(4), 347–352.

Dokken, D., & Sydnor-Greenberg, N. (2000). Exploring complementary and alternative medicine in pediatrics: Parents and professionals working together for new understanding. *Pediatric Nursing, 26*(4), 383–396.

Eddy, L. L., & Walker, A. J. (1999). The impact of children with chronic health problems on marriage. *Journal of Family Nursing, 5,* 10–33.

Farmer, J. E., Marien, W. E., Clark, M. J., Sherman, A., & Selva, T. J. (2004). Primary care supports for children with chronic health conditions: Identifying and predicting unmet family needs. *Journal of Pediatric Psychology, 29*(5), 355–367.

Haffner, J. C., & Schurman, S. J. (2001). The technology-dependent child. *Pediatric Clinics of North America, 48*(3), 751–761.

Harrigan, R. C., Ratliffe, C., Patrinos, M. E., & Alice, T. (2002). Medically fragile children: An integrative review of the literature and recommendations on future research. *Issues in Comprehensive Pediatric Nursing, 25,* 1–20.

Jacobs, L. A. (2002). Living with a chronically ill child. *American Journal of Nursing, 102*(5), 24A-24C.

Kearney, P. M., & Griffin, T. (2001). Between joy and sorrow: Being a parent of a child with a developmental disability. *Journal of Advanced Nursing, 34*(5), 582–592.

Keefe, S. (2003). Parenting a child with special needs. *Advance for Nurse Practitioners, 11*(10), 73–80.

Kessenich, M. (2003). Developmental outcomes of premature, low birth weight, and medically fragile infants. *Newborn and Infant Nursing, 3*(3), 80–87.

Kieckhefer, G. M., & Trahms, C. M. (2000). Supporting development of children with chronic conditions: From compliance toward shared management. *Pediatric Nursing, 26*(4), 354–364.

Kliebenstein, M. A., & Broome, M. E. (2000). School re-entry for the child with chronic illness: Parent and school personnel perceptions. *Pediatric Nursing, 26*(6), 579–594.

Knafl, K. A., & Deatrick, J. A. (2002). The challenge of normalization for families of children with chronic conditions. *Pediatric Nursing, 28*(1), 49–54.

Kuster, P. A., Badr, L. K., Chang, B. L., Wuerker, A. K., & Benjamin, A. E. (2004). Factors influencing health promoting activities of mothers caring for ventilator-assisted children. *Journal of Pediatric Nursing, 19*(4), 276–287.

Lindeke, L. L., Leonard, B. J., Presler, B., & Garwick, A. (2002). Family-centered care coordination for children with special needs across multiple settings. *Journal of Pediatric Health Care, 16*(6), 290–297.

Little, L. (2002). Differences in stress and coping for mothers and fathers of children with Asperger's syndrome and nonverbal learning disorders. *Pediatric Nursing, 28*(6), 565–570.

Maternal and Child Health Bureau. (2002). *Understanding the Title V of the Social Security Act.* Rockville, MD: Department of Health and Human Services, Health Resources and Services Administration, Maternal and Child Health Bureau.

Maytum, J. C., Heiman, M. B., & Garwick, A. W. (2004). Compassion fatigue and burnout in nurses who work with children with chronic conditions and their families. *Journal of Pediatric Health Care, 18*(4), 171–179.

McPherson, M., Arango, P., Fox, H., Lauver, C., McManus, M., et al. (1998). A new definition of children with special health care needs. *Pediatrics, 102*(1), 137–140.

Meleski, D. D. (2002). Families with chronically ill children. *American Journal of Nursing, 102*(5), 47–54.

Melnyk, B. M., Feinstein, N. F., Moldenhouer, Z., & Small, L. (2001). Coping in parents of children who are chronically ill: Strategies for assessment and intervention. *Pediatric Nursing, 27*(6), 548–558.

Msall, M. E., Avery, R. C., Tremont, M. R., Lima, J. C., Rogers, M. L., & Hogan, D. P. (2003). Functional disability and school activity limitations in 41,300 school age children: Relationship to medical impairments. *Pediatrics, 111*(3), 548–553.

Murray, J. S. (2000). Understanding sibling adaptations to childhood cancer. *Issues in Comprehensive Pediatric Nursing, 23*, 39–47.

National Resource Center for Community Based Family Resource and Support (CBFRS) Program. (2002, August). http://www.friendsnrc.org/, accessed 2/11/2004.

Neff, J. M. (2002, Fall). Chronic conditions in children: A decade of change. *Children's Hospitals Today, 10*, 14–16.

Newacheck, P. W., McManus, M., Fox, H. B., Hung, Y. Y., & Halfon, N. (2000). Access to health care for children with special health care needs. *Pediatrics, 105*(4), 760–766.

Noyes, J. (2000). Ventilator-dependent children who spend prolonged periods of time in intensive care units when they no longer have a medical need or want to be there. *Journal of Clinical Nursing, 9*, 774–783.

O'Brien, M. E., & Wegner, C. B. (2002). Rearing the child who is technology dependent: Perceptions of parents and home care nurses. *Journal of Society of Pediatric Nursing, 7*(1), 7–15.

Palfrey, J. S., Sofis, L. A., Davidson, E. J., Liu, J., Freeman, L., & Ganz, M. L. (2004). The pediatric alliance for coordinated care: Evaluation of a medical home model. *Pediatrics, 113*(5), 1507–1516.

Perrin, E. C., Lewkowicz, C., & Young, M. H. (2000). Shared vision: Concordance among fathers, mothers, and pediatricians about unmet needs of children with chronic health conditions. *Pediatrics, 105*(1, Pt 3), 277–285.

Perrin, J. M. (2002). Health services research for children with disabilities. *Milbank Quarterly, 80*(2), 303–324.

Ratliffe, C. E., Harrigan, R. C., Haley, J., Tse, A., & Olson, T. (2002). Stress in families with medically fragile children. *Issues in Comprehensive Pediatric Nursing, 25*, 167–188.

Ray, L. D. (2002). Parenting and childhood chronicity: Making visible the invisible work. *Journal of Pediatric Nursing, 17*(6), 424–438.

Rehm, R. S., (2003). Cultural intersections in the care of Mexican American children with chronic conditions. *Pediatric Nursing, 29*(6), 434–439.

Rehm, R. S., & Rohr, J. A. (2002). Parents', nurses', and educators' perceptions of risks and benefits of school attendance by children who are medically fragile/-technology-dependent. *Journal of Pediatric Nursing, 17*(5), 345–354.

Swallow, V. M., & Jacoby, A. (2001). Mothers' coping in chronic childhood illness: The effect of presymptomatic diagnosis of vesicoureteric reflux. *Journal of Advanced Nursing, 33*(1), 69–78.

U.S. Department of Education. (2004). *A guide to the individualized education program.* http://www.ed.gov/parents/needs/speced/iepguide/index.htm, accessed 10/14/2004.

U.S. Department of Health and Human Services. (2000). *Healthy People 2010* (2nd ed.). Washington, DC: U.S. Government Printing Office.

Van Dyck, P. C., Kogan, M. D., McPherson, M. G., Weissman, G. R., & Newcheck, P. W. (2004). Prevalence and characteristics of children with special health care needs. *Archives of Pediatric and Adolescent Medicine, 158*(9), 884–490.

Van Dyck, P. C., McPherson, M., Strickland, B. B., Nesseler, K., Blumberg, S. J., Cynamon, M. L., & Newacheck, P. W. (2002). The national survey of children with special health care needs. *Ambulatory Pediatrics, 2*(1), 29–37.

Vessey, J. A., & Rumsey, M. (2004). Chronic conditions and child development. In P. J. Allen & J. A. Vessey, *Primary care of the child with a chronic condition* (4th ed., pp. 23–43). St. Louis: Mosby.

Williams, P. D., Williams, A. R., Graff, J. C., Hanson, S., Stanton, A., Hafeman, C., Liebergen, A., Leuenberg, K., Setter, R. K., Ridder, L., Curry, H., Barnard, M., & Sanders, S. (2002). Interrelationships among variables affecting well siblings and mothers in families of children with a chronic illness or disability. *Journal of Behavioral Medicine, 25*(5), 411–424.

Witt, W., Riley, A. W., & Coiro, M. J. (2003). Childhood functional status, family stressors, and psychosocial adjustment among school-aged children with disabilities in the United States. *Archives of Pediatric and Adolescent Medicine, 157*, 687–695.

Wood, P. R., Smith, L. A., Romero, D., Bradshaw, P., Wise, P. H., & Chavkin, W. (2002). Relationships between welfare status, health insurance status, and health and medical care among children with asthma. *American Journal of Public Health, 92*(9), 1446–1452.

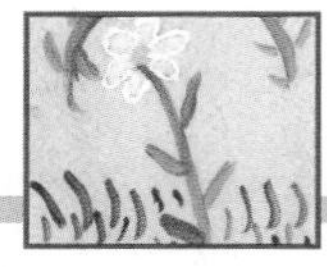

ADDITIONAL REFERENCES

American Academy of Pediatrics, American Academy of Family Physicians, American College of Physicians—American Society of Internal Medicine. (2002). A consensus statement on health care transitions for young adults with special health care needs. *Pediatrics, 110*(6, Suppl), 1304–1306.

American Academy of Pediatrics Committee on Children with Disabilities. (1999). The pediatrician's role in development and implementation of an individual education plan (IEP) and/or an individual family service plan (IFSP). *Pediatrics, 104*(1), 124–127.

American Academy of Pediatrics Committee on Children with Disabilities. (2000). Provision of educationally-related services for children and adolescents with chronic diseases and disabling conditions. *Pediatrics, 105*(2), 448–451.

Betz, C. L., & Redcay, G. (2003). Creating healthy futures: An innovative nurse-managed transition clinic for adolescents and young adults with special health care needs. *Pediatric Nursing, 29*(1), 25–30.

Reiss, J., & Gibson, R. (2002). Health care transition: Destination unknown. *Pediatrics, 110*(6, Suppl), 1307–1314.

Smith, P. J., Mathews, K. S., Hehir, T., & Palfrey, J. S. (2002). Educating children with disabilities: How pediatricians can help. *Contemporary Pediatrics, 19*(9), 102–127.

The Child with a Life-Threatening Illness or Injury

Chapter

21

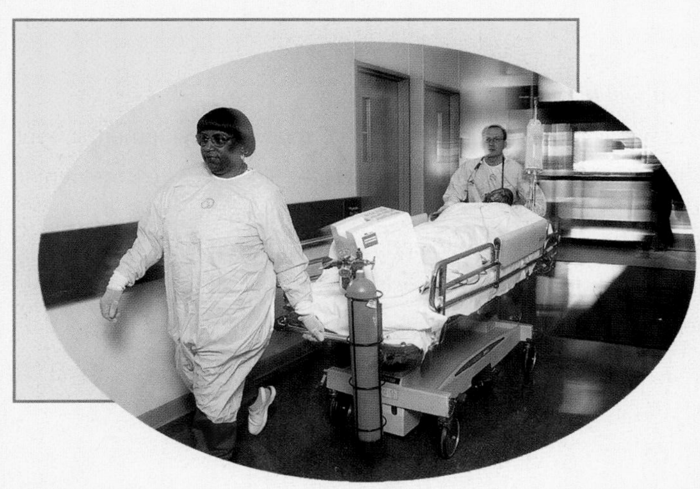

The telephone in the pediatric intensive care unit (PICU) at a large medical center rings at 8:30 A.M. A referring hospital is calling to request the transport of an unstable 12-year-old boy, Jeremy Dees, who is in status epilepticus. Jeremy has a seizure disorder that is usually controlled with medications, but several days ago he abruptly stopped taking the medication. After aggressive treatment by the emergency department at the referring hospital to try to end the seizures, Jeremy is now unconscious and must be intubated until he can maintain his airway.

The transport team is in the air within minutes and arrives at the rural community hospital 25 minutes later. After stabilizing Jeremy and receiving reports from the medical and nursing teams, the transport team meets briefly with his parents, answers their immediate questions, and secures Jeremy in the helicopter in preparation for the return flight to the medical center.

Jeremy is admitted directly to the PICU, where the unit team has been preparing for his arrival. He is connected to cardiorespiratory and noninvasive blood pressure monitors, while his existing intravenous lines and endotracheal tube are evaluated for patency. Team members quickly complete a head-to-toe assessment. The unit clerk enters Jeremy's room to inform the staff that his parents have arrived in the emergency department and are being escorted to the PICU.

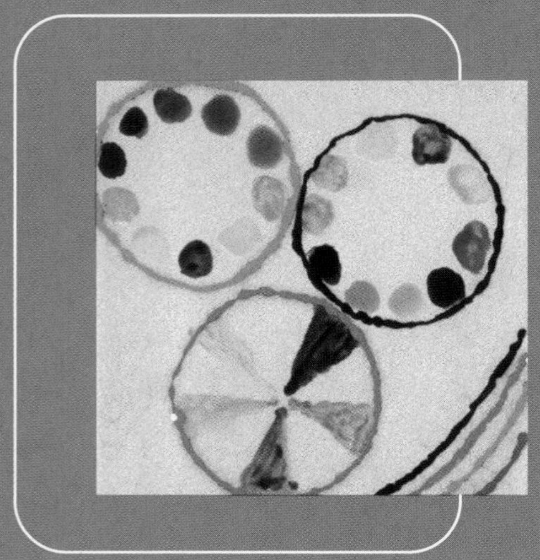

"I was so scared when I woke up and had tubes in my mouth, arms, and everywhere else and I couldn't move. The noise was terrible—every machine in there made weird noises. Then, all these strangers were talking to me and I realized that I didn't know where I was. I just wanted to see my mom and dad and go home. I never want to go back there again."

—Jeremy, age 12

Key Terms

coping/680
family crisis/680
neonatal intensive care unit (NICU)/678
pediatric intensive care unit (PICU)/677
regression/680
repression/680
support systems/690
treatment interference/679

Learning Outcomes

After completing this chapter, you will be able to

- Describe the child's experiences with life-threatening illness according to developmental level.
- Discuss the variety of settings in which the nurse may encounter a child with a life-threatening condition.
- Describe the coping mechanisms utilized by the child and family in response to stress.
- Discuss the family's experience and reactions to having a child with a life-threatening illness.
- Develop a plan of care for the child with a life-threatening illness and the family.

MediaLink 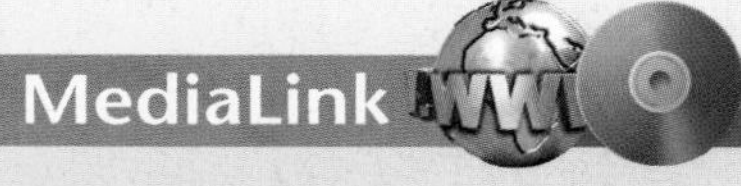 http://www.prenhall.com/ball

Resources for this chapter can be found on the CD-ROM accompanying this textbook and on the Companion Website at www.prenhall.com/ball. Click on Chapter 21 to select the activities for this chapter.

CD-ROM

Videos

Involving Family in NICU Setting
Presenting Bad News to Families

NCLEX Review

Audio Glossary

COMPANION WEBSITE

NCLEX Review

Case Study: Neonate in NICU with Bronchopulmonary Dysplasia

Care Plan: Adolescent in PICU with Brain Injury

Care Plan: Toddler in ED for Near-Drowning Episode

What experiences do children like Jeremy face after admission to the pediatric intensive care unit (PICU)? What strategies can you use to help such critically ill or injured children cope with the experience? What stressors will parents face during the initial period when you work with them? How can you intervene to help them in this crisis? What strategies should be used to help siblings understand what has happened to their brother or sister? This chapter will enable you to answer these questions and will assist you in providing supportive care to critically ill and injured children like Jeremy and to their families.

The intense emotional and physical demands placed on the critically ill or injured child present a challenge to nurses' attempts to provide developmentally appropriate care. The child's parents and siblings are confronted with a stressful situation. Family-centered care offers a framework for performing nursing interventions that help to minimize stress and enhance coping by parents, siblings, and the ill or injured child.

LIFE-THREATENING ILLNESS OR INJURY

A threat to a child's life may be expected, as in a progressive chronic condition or disabling disease, or unexpected, as in an unintentional injury or acute illness. How children, parents, siblings, and other family members cope with the threat will depend upon the nature of the event, the conditions surrounding the child's admission to the hospital, and the support system of the family. Some potential life-threatening situations that may occur in children include: trauma, septic shock, meningitis, status asthmaticus, status epilepticus, and diabetic ketoacidosis. (See Chapter 1∞ for specific information related to causes of death and hospitalization of children.)

When death results from a chronic condition or terminal illness, the child and family have time to adjust to episodes of life-threatening crisis and impending death. Parents of children with chronic or terminal illness are encouraged to become involved in the child's therapy as integral members of the treatment team. Emergency admission for an acute illness or unintentional injury, on the other hand, brings with it sudden stressors as the child and family are thrust into an unfamiliar environment, confronted with frightening or invasive procedures, and faced with an uncertain outcome.

Nursing care of children and families coping with specific chronic conditions or terminal illnesses such as cancer, cystic fibrosis, or muscular dystrophy, as well as care of the dying child, is discussed in other chapters throughout the textbook. The following discussion focuses on general concepts of care for children with acute life-threatening illnesses or injuries.

SETTINGS ENCOUNTERED BY CHILDREN WITH A LIFE-THREATENING CONDITION

Children with a life-threatening condition may experience admission to a variety of healthcare settings. Included are emergency departments, pediatric intensive care units, and neonatal intensive care units. These departments are staffed with nurses who specialize in the care of children with life-threatening conditions.

Emergency Department

Trauma is the leading cause of death in children ages 1–19. Approximately 43% of all pediatric deaths are a result of unintentional injury (White & Dalton, 2002). Leading causes of childhood mortality and morbidity are related to injury from motor vehicle crashes, falls, burns, and drowning. Over four million emergency department visits annually for children younger than age 18 years are the result of home environment injuries (Posner, Hawkins, Garcia-Espana, et al., 2004). While most emergency department visits are not life-threatening, the nurse must be prepared to respond to critical pediatric emergencies. The American Heart Association offers courses in pediatric advanced life support, in which nurses and other healthcare providers learn the emergency protocols for life-threatening events such as respiratory arrest and hypovolemic shock. See Appendix E∞ and the Skills Manual.

The role of the emergency department nurse includes triaging the child, initiating lifesaving measures (e.g., pediatric advance life support), collaborating with the multidisciplinary emergency department team, and providing support to the family.

Children and their families may encounter a fast-paced environment in the emergency department, with the child receiving simultaneous care from multiple healthcare providers. The unfamiliar, hectic environment compounded with the uncertainty of the child's life-threatening condition, can be a frightening experience and a significant source of stress for the family. Each emergency department develops its own set of unique requirements and protocols, which may limit the number of family members who can accompany the child. Family members who are asked to remain in the waiting room while the child receives treatment may experience additional stress and anxiety.

The nurse, in addition to other healthcare professionals, should keep family informed of the care provided and the child's status. Many facilities provide a social worker in the emergency department to coordinate the flow of information and support the families of critically ill children. Other emergency departments have limited personnel, and a nurse may take a leadership role to ensure the family receives adequate support.

CLINICAL TIP

In addition to the stressors experienced due to life-threatening injury or illness in their child, parents may also suddenly be faced with the dilemma of arranging for the care of other children. For example, the sibling may be at band practice and need to be picked up by a certain time. Parents may need assistance to make these arrangements when they are in a state of crisis. Collaboration among health team members is essential to ensure adequate support.

Pediatric Intensive Care Unit

The **pediatric intensive care unit (PICU)** is a highly specialized care unit for children with life-threatening illness or injury. Children undergoing procedures such as thoracic,

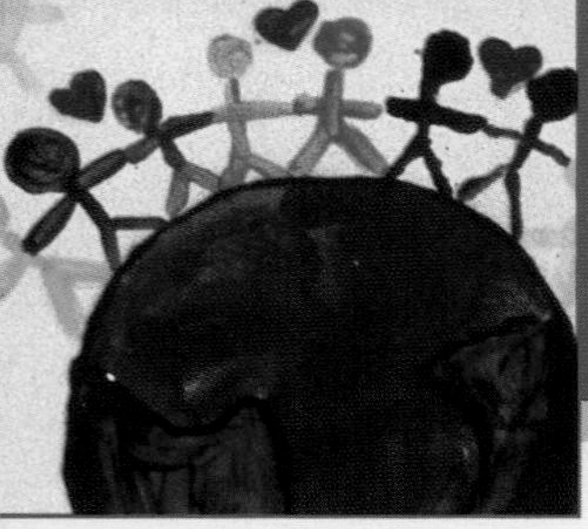

PARTNERING WITH FAMILIES

Terms Commonly Used in Pediatric Intensive Care Units

Families are often overwhelmed with the terminology used in the neonatal or pediatric intensive care unit. What is everyday language to the healthcare team may be foreign to family members. The nurse can provide the family with a list of terms clarifying their meaning, and encourage family members to ask questions if they do not understand. Understanding the terminology may help to reduce the family's stress. Common terms in the PICU include:

- **Arterial blood gases (ABGs):** A sample of blood from an artery that helps to identify the level of oxygenation and provides a guide for changes necessary in treatment. The blood sample may be obtained through an arterial line.
- **Arterial line:** A catheter inserted into an artery, which allows for continuous monitoring of blood pressure and for the blood sampling for arterial blood gases.
- **ET tube (endotracheal tube):** The plastic tube that is placed into the child's trachea or airway, either through the nose or mouth. The tube is usually connected to a ventilator (breathing machine) to help the child breathe.
- **Isolation:** A method used to prevent the transfer of infections to the child or visitors. Gowns, gloves, mask, and a special isolation room may be included in the isolation guidelines.
- **IV (intravenous) line:** A catheter inserted into a blood vessel. The catheter provides a method to administer fluids, nutrition, and medications. IVs may be inserted into the veins in the hand, arm, or foot, or into the neck, head (in infants), chest, or groin area.
- **Monitor:** A screen that shows your child's heart rhythm and rate, blood pressure, and oxygen level.
- **NG tube (nasogastric tube):** A tube that is inserted in the child's nose and into the stomach. The tube can be used to drain stomach fluids or to administer feedings.
- **Oxygen saturation:** A measure of the amount of oxygen in the blood.
- **Pulse ox (pulse oximeter):** A probe that is taped to the child's finger or toe. You will note a red light on the probe. This measures the oxygen saturation in the child's blood.
- **Restraint:** Soft wraps that may be secured around the child's hands to keep them from pulling out tubes.
- **Ventilator:** A machine that is connected to an endotracheal tube (or tracheostomy) that assists the child to breathe.

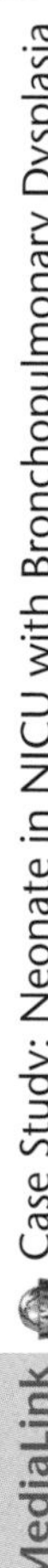

cardiovascular, airway, craniofacial, and abdominal surgeries, and organ transplants, are often admitted to the PICU postoperatively as well. While the number of pediatric beds for general care has decreased in hospitals throughout the country, the number of PICU beds has increased (Melnyk, Small, & Carno, 2004).

Not all hospitals are equipped with pediatric intensive care units; therefore, the child and family may experience a transfer from one facility to another that provides specialized care for critically ill children. The child admitted to the pediatric intensive care unit experiences multiple sensory stimuli, ranging from constant sounds of monitor alarms and supportive equipment to bright lights, and interventions from multiple healthcare professionals.

The role of the nurse in the pediatric intensive care unit includes maintaining life support measures such as ventilatory support and vasoactive medications. The nurse explains the environment and equipment, which may include ventilators, dialysis machines, arterial lines, central venous pressure lines, intracranial pressure lines, and warming/cooling blankets. Families are often overwhelmed by the presence of so much equipment attached to the child, in addition to the altered appearance of their child requiring these supportive devices. Before the family visits the child for the first time, the nurse prepares the family for visual, auditory, and olfactory experiences they may have in the intensive care unit. It is especially important that the nurse explain any difference in appearance the child may have. For example, the nurse might say, "Danny will not look like himself because his face is swollen and bruised. He has a tube in his mouth to help him breathe." See Partnering with Families: Terms Commonly Used in Pediatric Intensive Care Units.

Families of children in the intensive care unit may also experience hospital rules regarding visitation. Many children's hospitals support open visitation by parents and siblings and encourage parents to spend as much time as possible with their critically ill child. Other intensive care units may restrict such visitations, limiting the specific hours and length of visits. The number of people who can visit at a time may also be limited. These restrictions are often a source of frustration for families, especially when the child's outcome is uncertain. Nurses can be instrumental in supporting family-centered care by encouraging their hospitals and specialized units to reduce or remove restrictive visitation policies (Box 21–1).

Neonatal Intensive Care Unit

Newborns with life-threatening conditions are admitted to the **neonatal intensive care unit (NICU).** Common reasons for NICU admission include prematurity (Jones, 2004), congenital heart defects, congenital diaphragmatic hernia, bronchopulmonary dysplasia, necrotizing enterocolitis, infection, meconium aspiration syndrome, and neural tube defects. Approximately 320,000 preterm infants are discharged from the NICU every year (Verma, Sridhar, & Spizer, 2003).

BOX 21–1 Visitation Rules

Intensive care settings generally have policies on how many people can visit at a time. There are times when flexibility is essential. For example, a family of four, with one member being the ill or injured child, needs to be together at times. In addition, extended family members visiting from out of town may want to spend time not only with the hospitalized child, but with the parents of the child as well. When a child is critically ill, the presence of several family members at the bedside when updates are being given not only ensures that everyone hears the same information, but also serves as a means of support for each other (Griffin, 2003a).

The role of the nurse in the neonatal intensive care unit is similar to that of the nurse in the pediatric intensive care unit, though there are distinct differences. The NICU nurse deals primarily with premature newborns and those with congenital defects that are life threatening.

The family of the newborn in neonatal intensive care experiences a unique situation since the newborn is admitted to a critical care unit rather than being sent home with the parents as anticipated. When an infant is admitted to the NICU shortly after birth, the family is in a state of crisis. The family is separated from the newborn and experiences feelings of anxiety and loss of control (Loo, Espinosa, Tyler, & Howard (2003). Families may experience the same visitation issues as families of children in the pediatric intensive care unit. For the neonate admitted to the neonatal intensive care unit the potential for impaired parental-newborn attachment exists. Parents may also experience grief over loss of the "perfect child."

CHILD'S EXPERIENCE OF A LIFE-THREATENING ILLNESS OR INJURY

Admission to the hospital, emergency department, or pediatric intensive care unit (PICU) is one of the most frightening occurences a child can experience. The critically ill child may appear extremely anxious and fearful, or withdrawn, solemn, and preoccupied with his or her physical condition. The illness or injury often brings pain, decreased energy, and changes to the child's level of consciousness.

Young children admitted to the PICU may be unable to understand what is happening to them. The environment appears overwhelming, fast paced, and frightening. Equipment that hisses, blinks, beeps, and alarms may be seen as a monster or alive to a preschooler. The child's normal sleep patterns can be disrupted due to the lack of day–night patterns in many intensive care units. Being cared for by strangers produces anxiety in the child. Procedures are performed despite the child's protests and sometimes pain results. The child's limited ability to move intensifies feelings of powerlessness and vulnerability. Children admitted to an intensive care setting are at risk for psychological trauma (Melnyk, Small, & Carno, 2004). An increased incidence of posttraumatic stress disorder (PTSD) has been noted in children with life-threatening illnesses and injuries (Box 21–2) (see Chapter 34∞ for a discussion of posttraumatic stress disorder).

Children's responses to stress are influenced by their developmental levels, past experiences, types of illness, coping mechanisms, and available emotional support. (See page 529 for a discussion of stressors based on developmental level.) Nurses must consider how the child's developmental level and coping skills will influence his or her ability to deal with the emergency department or PICU experience. Successful coping can provide the child with the skills to handle difficult situations in the future.

The four most significant stressors for hospitalized children of all ages are as follows:

1. Separation from parents or the primary caretaker
2. Loss of self-control, autonomy, and privacy
3. Being subjected to multiple painful and invasive procedures
4. Fear of bodily injury and disfigurement

In addition to dealing with these stressors, the critically ill child experiences an intense emotional and physical threat to his or her well-being. An unanticipated admission places the child at emotional risk for several reasons, including the lack of preparation for the experience, the uncertainty and unpredictability of events that follow, the unfamiliarity of the environment, and the heightened anxiety of parents. An admission for an acute exacerbation of a disease such as cystic fibrosis or leukemia can provoke feelings of depression or hopelessness.

In the critical care environment, children often self-remove or threaten to self-remove technological equipment or devices employed in their care. For example, the child may engage in self-removal of an endotracheal tube, peripheral intravenous line or central line, nasogastric tube, or arterial line. The child's actions are often referred to as **treatment interference.** Treatment interference may be conscious or unconscious. Parents and nurses can partner to prevent treatment interference. Intervention strategies by parents include supervision, simple instructions, a calm approach, setting limits, a sense of security, and repositioning. Suggested nursing interventions include distraction, supporting family-centered care, and providing adequate instruction. It is also important that the nurse position devices in a way that maintain comfort as much as possible (Snyder, 2004). Physical restraints are frequently used in children with an altered level of consciousness to prevent unintentional removal of technological devices or equipment. The use of physical restraint should be limited and only used when absolutely necessary. The Joint Commission on Accreditation of Healthcare Organizations (JCAHO) requires that hospitals have policies and procedures in place for the use of restraints.

BOX 21–2 Research: PTSD

Injured children requiring hospitalization for injury are at risk for posttraumatic stress disorder (PTSD). Variables predictive of PTSD include child acute stress, parental stress, and the degree of the psychological trauma exposure. One study reported 12.5% of injured children met diagnostic criteria for PTSD at 1 month after the injury (Daviss, Mooney, Racusin, et al., 2000). Refer to Chapter 34∞ for detailed discussion on PTSD.

Coping Mechanisms

Coping refers to the cognitive and behavioral responses that help a person to manage specific internal and external demands that exceed personal resources, thus enabling the person to solve problems and to respond appropriately. The child may mirror the parents' behaviors and responses, which may help or hinder the child's response to stress. The child's temperament, previous coping experiences, and availability of support systems all combine to influence his or her ability to cope with the current experience.

The nature and severity of the illness and an emergency admission to the hospital stress a child's coping capabilities. Defense mechanisms displayed by children in these situations include **regression,** or return to an earlier behavior (a common reaction to stress), denial, **repression** (involuntary forgetting), postponement, and bargaining. The nurse can encourage the child and family to utilize positive coping mechanisms that have worked for them in the past. See Chapter 17∞ for detailed discussion on coping mechanisms for hospitalized children.

PARENTS' EXPERIENCE OF A CHILD'S LIFE-THREATENING ILLNESS OR INJURY

The uncertainty and unpredictability of a child's life-threatening illness challenge a family's coping and stability (Figure 21–1 ■). Families have different reactions and coping mechanisms when challenged. Children who are hospitalized for a critical illness cannot be adequately cared for if their families' needs are not met. Not only will parents find it difficult to support the child if their own needs are not met, but they also can transmit their anxiety to the child, who then becomes even more anxious. The nurse recognizes that parents may exhibit a variety of emotions and behavior including irritability, crying, hostility toward staff, and withdrawal. Discuss with the parent that these symptoms are stress related and are common experiences of parents of the child with a life-threatening illness. (See Chapter 17∞ for a discussion on dealing with hostile family members.)

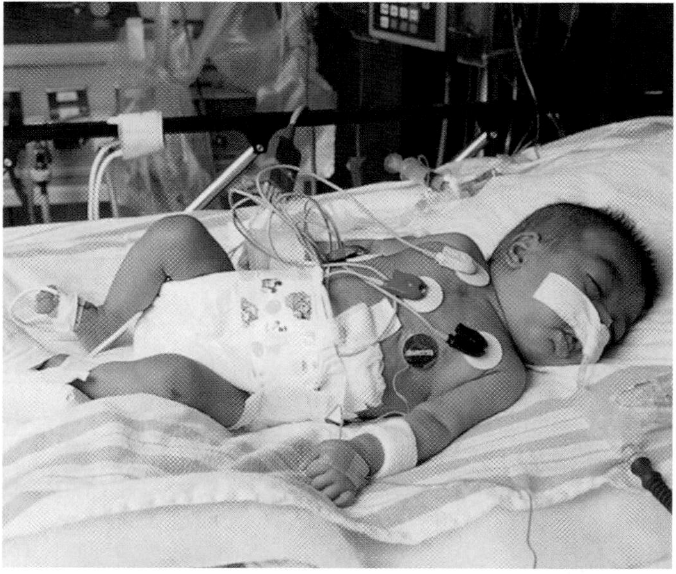

FIGURE 21–1 ■ Jooti feels pain, hears noises, has her sleep disrupted, and has limited mobility because of all the equipment attached to her. What care and comfort can you offer parents who see their child like this?

Situations that lead to increased stress in a critical care environment are as follows: "(a) uncertainty about the child's conditions and prognosis, (b) not knowing how to best care for the child's emotional and physical needs during hospitalization, and (c) the child's emotional and behavioral responses" (Melnyk, Small & Carno, 2004). In addition, factors related to the environment itself such as alarms, equipment and constant activity have also been identified as stressors for parents. See Evidence-Based Practice: Parental Stressors When the Child is in the PICU.

CLINICAL TIP

Explain to the child and parents, in easy-to-understand terms, the purpose of equipment that is being used. Answer alarms quickly. Follow with an explanation of why alarms sound including the fact that many times monitor alarms will sound when the child moves, if the monitor becomes disconnected, or if the monitor patches are loose.

Nurses implementing a family-centered approach recognize that the reactions and actions of family members to a child's life-threatening situation are influenced by a variety of factors, and unique to the person experiencing the crisis (Sydnor-Greenberg & Dokken, 2000). Effective communication with family members is essential to effective family-centered care (Griffin, May/June, 2003).

The Family in Crisis

The critical care environment and the implications of a life-threatening illness or injury of a child are far removed from the everyday experiences of most families. The family in this situation may experience a **family crisis,** which occurs when the family encounters a problem that seems insurmountable and with which they cannot cope in its usual ways. The unfamiliar environment and the uncertainty and seriousness of the illness or injury create a crisis for the family. Box 21–3 lists the primary needs of parents during a child's critical illness or injury.

The interruption of the unique parent–child relationship can be more stressful to parents than the physical PICU environment. Siblings are also affected; see Partnering with Families: Strategies for Working with Siblings of an Ill or Injured Child. (See Chapter 17∞ for further discussion on interventions for siblings of hospitalized child.) Extended family members such as grandparents are affected as well. Grandparents have concern for both their critically ill grandchild and their child, one of the parents of the ill child (Hall, 2004). Grandparents' should be included in family-centered care of the critically ill child unless a situation exists contraindicating their involvement.

Stresses are intensified when divorce, separation, and step-parenting are involved. Other family stresses such as financial problems, long distance from home to hospital, or another fam-

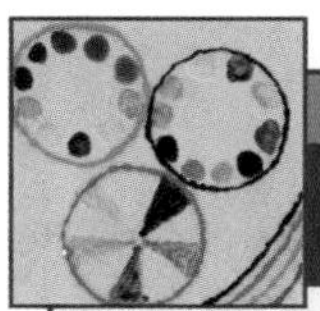

EVIDENCE-BASED PRACTICE

Parental Stressors When the Child is in the PICU

PROBLEM

Nurses expect parents to experience stress when their child has a life-threatening condition, but what causes the most stress? Do mothers and fathers experience the same stressors?

EVIDENCE

In a recent nursing study, responses of parents (31 mothers and 15 fathers) with a child in the intensive care unit to a self-administered questionnaire, Parental Stressor Scale: PICU, were compared to the responses of parents (32 mothers and 10 fathers) with a child admitted to the general care unit. Nurse researchers identified the greatest sources of stress reported by 90% or more of the mothers with children in the PICU included "total experience is stressful," "injections/shots," "sudden sounds of monitor alarms," "seeing heart rate on monitor," "sound of monitors and equipment," "putting needles in the child," "too many people talking to me," and "tubes in my child." Mothers (90% or more) of children cared for on the general care unit were stressed by "putting needles in the child," "child acting or looking like in pain," and "child crying or whining" (Board & Ryan-Wenger, 2003). The greatest sources of stress for the 90% or more of the fathers with child in the PICU were "tubes in my child," "putting needles in my child for fluids, procedures or tests," and "not knowing how best to help my child during the crisis." Other high ranking stressors for 80% or more of fathers included "total ICU experience," "injections/shots," "sudden sounds of monitor alarms," and "having machine breathe for my child" (Board, 2004). The most significant stressors for fathers of children on the general care unit included "putting needles in my child for fluids, procedures or tests," and "not knowing how best to help my child during this crisis" (Board, 2004). Parents with children in the PICU have more stressors, and seem to be more stressed by the physical aspects of the critical care environment rather than issues such as communication. Efforts of PICU nurses and physicians to involve parents in care decisions may help explain why communication was less of a stressor for parents.

IMPLICATIONS

Many PICUs have open visiting hours for parents, so they witness many of the procedures performed on the child, such as suctioning, starting IVs and central lines, and obtaining blood. The illness acuity of children in PICUs is often quite high, and the number of invasive devices and machines contributes to the stress perceived by parents. Making an effort to reduce the stressors of parents is a significant nursing role. Explaining the changes that will be noted in the child's appearance, the purpose for all the tubes and devices used is important after the child is admitted. Identifying ways that the parents can participate in the child's care, such as mouth care, cleaning the diaper area, is important so that a sense of the parental role is maintained.

CRITICAL THINKING IN ACTION

Consider what your response would be if it were your child in the PICU. Would your stressors be different than these parents reported because of your nursing education? How would you want the nurse caring for your child to support you? After considering your personal responses, does it help you identify nursing care strategies for working with parents of a child with a life threatening condition?

ily member with an illness can add to the state of crisis. (Refer to Chapter 2∞ for discussion of family assessment and family resiliency.) In addition, the outcome of the admission may not be positive, and nurses need to be equipped to support families in this situation (Box 21–4).

BOX 21–3 Parental Needs During Hospitalization of a Critically Ill or Injured Child

INFORMATION (THE MOST IMPORTANT IDENTIFIED NEED)

- Information and frequent updates about the child's condition. Repeat the information and provide other materials frequently as parents forget or cannot concentrate on details due to stress
- Explanations they can understand about the child's condition, equipment being used, and procedures of care
- Discussion with a physician or care coordinator daily
- General information about unit policies, team members, and phone numbers

PROXIMITY

- Permission to remain at the bedside
- Permission to touch and speak with the child
- Open, flexible visiting hours

REESTABLISHMENT OF THE PARENTAL CONTROL

- Recognition as important to the child's recovery
- Recognition as the decision maker regarding the child's treatment options

PARTICIPATION IN THE CHILD'S CARE

- Performance of care (e.g., bathing, diaper changes, feeding, range of motion exercises, massages, hair care)
- Provision of comfort measures (e.g., reading, singing, telling stories, touching, talking)
- Explanation of equipment and procedures to the child to decrease the child's fears

CONFIDENCE IN THE TREATMENT PLAN AND CAREGIVERS

- Continuity in staffing and healthcare contacts
- Evidence that staff care about the child
- Assurance that the child is receiving appropriate treatment and pain management

PSYCHOLOGIC SUPPORT

- Acknowledgment that the situation is difficult
- Help to focus on the positive or unchanged aspects of the child's appearance
- Rest and nutrition to maintain physical resources necessary for coping
- Space and privacy as needed
- Hope—an essential component of coping
- Choice of other family members to be present
- Preparation for responses of siblings and the long-term emotional responses of the pediatric patient

Parental Reactions to Life-threatening Illness or Injury

How do parents react to a threat to their child's life? What parental behaviors might nurses observe when a child is critically ill or injured? Parents typically progress through stages that may include shock and disbelief; anger and guilt; deprivation and loss; anticipatory waiting; and readjustment or mourning.

Shock and Disbelief

The universal reaction to a child's life-threatening condition is shock and disbelief. As the familiar is disrupted, parents experience a loss of control, an inability to regain their bearings, and

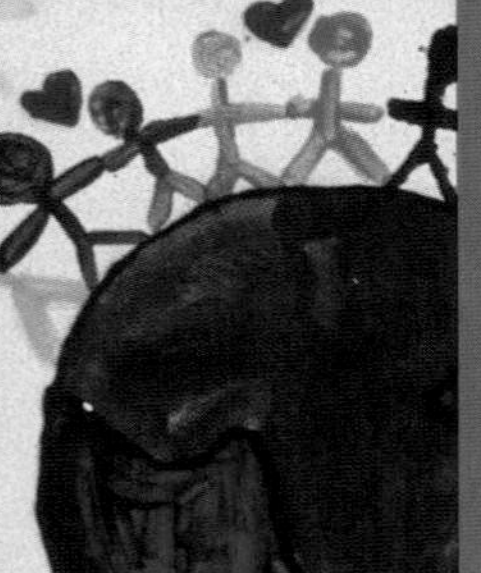

PARTNERING WITH FAMILIES

Strategies for Working with Siblings of an Ill or Injured Child

Sibling visitation is beneficial to both the ill or injured child and the sibling. Before siblings visit the child, however, the nurse should prepare them for expected sights, sounds, smells, and the appearance of their brother or sister. The nurse working with siblings of an ill or injured child can promote the sibling's understanding and coping by utilizing the following strategies.

- Be truthful. Explain why the child is hospitalized, what the treatment involves, and how long the hospitalization is expected to last.
- Assure siblings that they did not cause the illness and that the ill child did nothing wrong. If a sibling had some involvement in or responsibility for the health crisis, referral for psychological counseling is needed.
- Allow siblings to ask questions and state fears and other feelings.
- Encourage siblings to express their feelings related to the disruptive effect of the child's hospitalization on family life.
- Allow siblings to visit if possible. Cover tubes and wires with a sheet. Wash off blood or cover bloody bandages if possible. Prepare them for any equipment, dressing, and procedures they might see.
- Warn siblings if the ill child is not speaking. Say something like, "John can't talk now. He seems to be sleeping deeply. He may be able to hear, though, so you can touch him and talk to him."

feelings of immobility. The hospital environment, emergency department, or PICU may seem unreal. The emotions parents experience initially are intensified by the physical appearance of their child, particularly after a significant injury; the presence of monitors, tubing, and equipment; and the actual injury or illness (Figure 21–2 ■). As the mother of a 5-year-old trauma patient said, "I felt distanced, in a daze, in and out of it that first day after the accident."

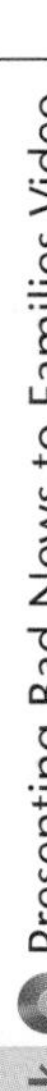

Shock and disbelief set in in the first few moments after hearing the "news" and can last for days. The shock helps postpone the full impact of the crisis. For most parents, however, the overwhelming sense of shock passes during the first 24 hours. During this period, parents grope for answers and explanations about the illness or injury. Information may need to be repeated many times to parents, since in this stage they are often unable to assimilate information easily.

Anger and Guilt

Anger and guilt surface as parents become more aware of their child's illness or injury. Their anger may be directed toward themselves, each other, healthcare providers, or other children or parents, as in the case of a motor vehicle crash involving a group of teenagers. Parents may also be angry with their child.

BOX 21–4 Presenting Bad News to Families

The nurse and other members of the healthcare team can use the following tips for presenting information concerning a child's life-threatening condition to family members.

PREPARATION

- Respectful and clear communication is an essential professional obligation.
- Plan for the delivery of bad news, including the words, tone, time, and place. Have information that is as complete as possible.
- Be prepared to deal with shock, grief, anger, panic, and other strong emotions.
- Have someone trained to respond to the family's emotional and practical needs and who will be able to stay with the family.
- Try to have both parents present, if clinical and family circumstances permit; ask if they would like their child or others to be present. If the answer is yes, plan for someone to accompany the child if he or she chooses to leave.
- Deliver the news in a private, quiet place where everyone can be seated comfortably and you can make eye contact with the family members and touch them if that seems supportive.
- Have a trained translator present if necessary.

CONVERSATION

- Indicate at the start that the news is not good.
- Show your concern, empathy, and respect for the child and family. Listen carefully.
- Adjust the style and content of communication—including the use of physical contact—according to the family's needs.
- Use the everyday language of the family except when clinical terms are likely to be helpful.
- Consider using sketches and diagrams to support explanations of the diagnosis and prognosis.
- Allow time for families to absorb and process information.
- Assess (if the child's condition permits) whether discussion of options, goals, and plans should be initiated or postponed to a defined later time.
- Assess family members' understanding of the information.
- Reassure families that it is normal to be emotional, confused, or overwhelmed.
- Provide written information and suggest other information resources.
- Offer to help parents prepare for talking with their child if the child is not present.
- Encourage parents to write down questions so that they can be discussed later.
- Respect parents' need for hope and reassurance but avoid evasions or deceits that may undermine trust and prevent preparation for what lies ahead.

FOLLOW-UP

- Arrange for further discussions as appropriate, including with the child (if he or she was absent), siblings, and others.
- Document the conversation (in addition to documenting diagnosis and prognosis) as a guide for future discussions.
- Reflect on the conversation and what might be done better in the future.

Adapted from Field, M. J., & Behrman, R. E. (2003) When children die: Improving palliative and end-of-life care for children and their families. *National Academies Press: Washington, D.C. pp. 116–117.*

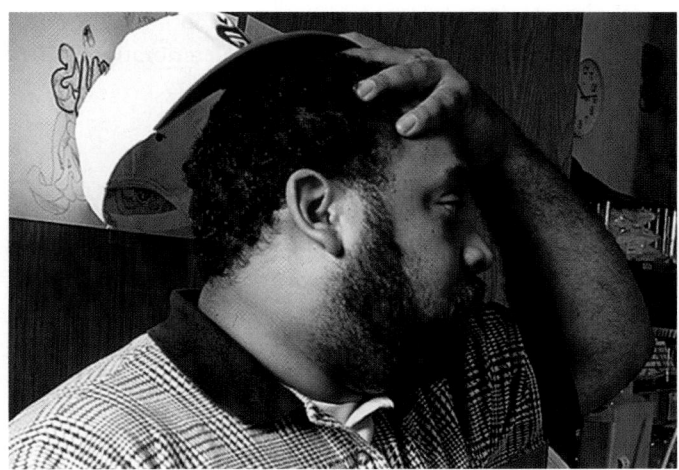

FIGURE 21–2 ■ This father is in a state of shock following his child's injury. He is unable to pay attention to information being provided, so repeat important information until it is understood.

This anger may be a result of injuries the child sustained when breaking known rules such as drinking and driving, playing with matches, or riding a bicycle without a helmet. Lastly, the anger may not be directed at anyone specifically. Injuries caused by natural disasters such as an earthquake, flood, or hurricane provoke as much anger as those that result from the actions of people. Situations such as natural disasters may also create a challenge to the parents' spiritual beliefs.

Parents typically react to their child's illness or injury with some degree of guilt. This reaction may be magnified in the intensive care environment. The fact that the guilt usually has no basis in real events does not lessen the feeling. A question parents frequently ask at this stage is, "Why not me instead of my child?" Parents' feelings of guilt may have one of two causes.

1. They may feel responsible for causing the illness or injury. Statements such as, "If only I hadn't sent him to the store on his bike, this wouldn't have happened," or, from the father of a 2-year-old who nearly drowned, "Maybe if I hadn't been working, he would have been in my care and this wouldn't have happened," reflect feelings of guilt for causing or failing to prevent the injury.
2. They may feel guilty about not noticing the onset of an illness or disregarding earlier symptoms of an illness. For example, the mother of a 1-year-old with meningitis repeatedly said, "I shouldn't have waited so long to take her to the doctor!"

Deprivation and Loss

As the shock slowly recedes, parents enter a stage of deprivation and loss related to their parental role. Within minutes or hours, parents have gone from the familiar role of being a parent of a healthy child to the unexpected and unfamiliar role of being a parent of a critically ill child (Figure 21–3 ■). Parents have compared this deprivation and loss to that experienced when a family member dies.

Parents' difficulties and ambivalence in releasing to strangers a part of their responsibility as the child's primary caretakers can threaten their self-esteem and self-control. Moreover, if parents cannot participate in the child's care, they may feel helpless or worthless.

Anticipatory Waiting

Once the child's condition is stabilized and survival seems likely, parents often move into a period of anticipatory waiting. This stage is characterized as "life suspended in time." Parents spend a great deal of time waiting: for test results, for explanations, for their child to become conscious, or for surgery to be over. Parents may fear leaving the area because they may miss an important procedure, physician visit, or decisions or changes in treatment. Lack of mobility decreases the parents' use of typical coping mechanisms, therefore anxiety and the sense of powerlessness may increase. A pager system has been adopted in some facilities to allow parents freedom to take breaks away from the child's bedside, knowing they will be alerted to important events. Pagers provided to family members of critically ill patients have been shown to decrease overall stress. Family members also revealed a higher level of satisfaction because the healthcare team could easily be in contact with them (Gavaghan, S. R. & Carroll, D. L., 2002). Use of pagers or cellular phones can also decrease feelings of frustration and anger associated with arriving at the beside to find that there has been a change in their child's condition (Griffin, 2003b).

Parents may have a preoccupation with medical details. During this period, parents may ask questions about the long-term

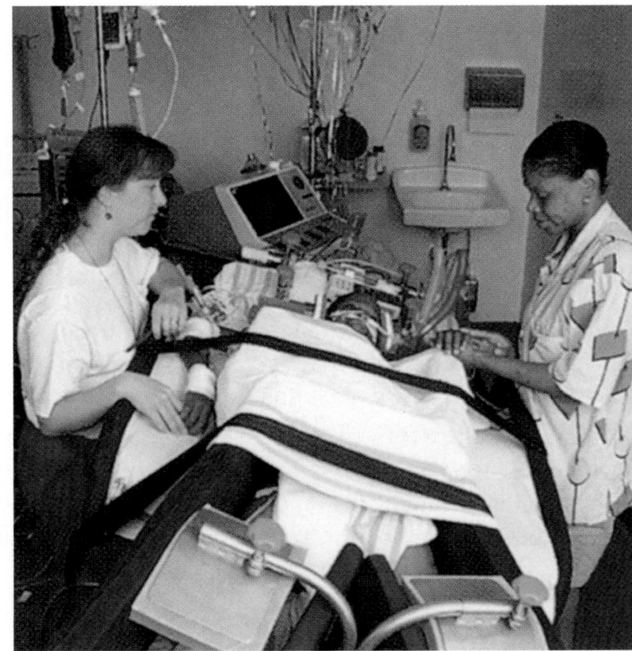

FIGURE 21–3 ■ By their very nature, PICUs are ominous and sterile. To lessen this effect, it can help to personalize the child's space. Being there with the child and parent, answering questions, or just talking can be a comfort to both.

effects of the illness or injury on the child, about the potential for brain damage, or about the need for additional surgeries. Parents may place demands on staff and become frustrated when the child's progress is slow.

Readjustment or Mourning

The last stage that parents experience is readjustment or mourning. Readjustment is experienced as the child recovers, improves steadily, and prepares for transfer and discharge. In contrast, parents of the child who dies reenter the cycle of emotions characteristic of grief (see Chapter 22 for further discussion of end-of-life issues). Mourning also occurs when the child remains seriously ill or unresponsive, when the outcome remains uncertain for an extended period, or when long-term care is required.

NURSING MANAGEMENT

Nursing care of the child with a life-threatening illness and his or her family includes assessing the child's physical and psychosocial needs, assessing the family's psychosocial needs, providing physical and psychosocial care for the child, and providing support for parental physical and emotional needs.

Nursing Assessment and Diagnosis

Nursing assessment of the child involves, in addition to physiologic parameters, skilled observation of the child's psychosocial and emotional needs. The nurse utilizes knowledge of normal psychosocial and cognitive development to plan developmentally appropriate interventions.

Physical Assessment

MediaLink Care Plan: Adolescent in PICU for Brain Injury

Nurses in the emergency department initially conduct a rapid head-to-toe assessment with focus on airway, breathing, and circulation. After the child's condition has been stabilized, the nurse conducts a thorough assessment of the child. (See Appendix E and the Skills Manual for triage assessment and subsequent procedures performed in the emergency department).

Nurses in the neonatal or pediatric intensive care unit are continuously assessing the child for changes in physiologic status and for responses to interventions. Physiologic monitoring in the neonatal intensive care unit (NICU) and pediatric intensive care unit (PICU) may include:

- Cardiac monitoring
- Respiratory monitoring
- Blood pressure monitoring via arterial line or noninvasive measurements
- Intracranial pressure (ICP) monitoring
- Central venous pressure (CVP)
- Hemodynamic monitoring
- Neurological checks

Careful attention to lung sound changes in children who are mechanically ventilated is essential to detect dislodged endotracheal tube, esophageal intubation, and pneumothorax. Frequent neurological checks are essential to detect deterioration in neurological status following traumatic brain injury.

Psychosocial Assessment

The challenge to nurses in critical care environments is to blend and balance technology with caring. Assessment of the child's psychosocial status includes the child's response to illness, the environment, coping strategies, and the need for information and support.

Nurses who work with families of critically ill children have a unique opportunity to help them adapt and to promote family functioning. Begin by assessing the family's reaction to the illness, their coping skills, and risk factors. This initial assessment provides a baseline of information to develop a care plan and strategies that meet the psychosocial and physiologic needs of the family. Ongoing reassessment provides a measure with which to evaluate the family's ability to manage the crisis. (See Chapter 2 for family assessment tools.) Use a family-centered approach to meet the needs of families, minimize stress, and enhance family coping.

The accompanying nursing care plan includes common nursing diagnoses for the child with a life-threatening illness or injury. The following additional nursing diagnoses may apply to parents who are dealing with their child's critical illness or injury.

- Parental Role Conflict related to the child's critical illness or injury and PICU policies
- Fatigue related to extreme stress, sleep deprivation, and crisis
- Hopelessness related to the child's deteriorating physiologic condition
- Anticipatory Grieving related to potential death of the child or loss of body functions
- Family Coping: Compromised related to the critical illness of the child
- Sleep Pattern Disturbance related to circadian asynchrony, excessive stimulation, pain, and anxiety caused by the critical care unit environment

Planning and Implementation

Nursing care focuses on promoting a sense of trust, providing physical and psychosocial care for the child and family, providing education about the illness or injury, preparing the child for procedures, facilitating the use of play, facilitating positive relationships, and promoting a sense of control.

Provide Physical and Psychosocial Care for the Child

Children admitted to a pediatric intensive care unit (PICU) are often presented with a traumatic experience for which they require support when they are alert. Nurses play a key role in providing developmentally appropriate support to the child. Nursing interventions are directed at building a trusting relationship, minimizing the stressors experienced by the child, and promoting

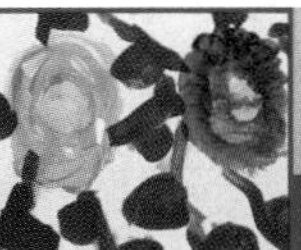

Nursing Care Plan

THE CHILD COPING WITH A LIFE-THREATENING ILLNESS OR INJURY

GOAL	INTERVENTION	RATIONALE	EXPECTED OUTCOME
1. Anxiety (child) related to separation from parents, foreign environment, strangers as caretakers, invasive procedures			
	NIC Priority Intervention—*Anxiety Reduction:* Minimizing apprehension, dread, or uneasiness related to an unidentified source of anticipated danger.		**NOC Suggested Outcome—***Anxiety Control:* Ability to eliminate or reduce feelings of apprehension and tension from unidentified source.
The child will exhibit or express an increased sense of security.	▪ Encourage parents to remain at bedside (open visitation) and to participate in the child's care by touching, talking to, reading to, and singing to the child. ▪ Talk with the child. Avoid discussions at bedside that the child should not overhear. ▪ Offer to arrange a visit from the chaplain or other spiritual support. ▪ Provide the child with developmentally appropriate explanations when possible; encourage the child to ask questions, and express concerns. ▪ Prepare child in advance for procedures using developmentally appropriate techniques. ▪ Make the child's bedside more personal and familiar by encouraging parents to bring in security objects, family photos, and favorite toys from home. ▪ Involve the child in play appropriate to developmental age (see Chapter 5∞). ▪ Provide care using a primary nursing care model.	▪ Presence of parents is comforting to the child. ▪ The child may overhear and remember, even if unconscious. ▪ Spiritual support often provides comfort and sustenance in a time of crisis. ▪ Information reduces anxiety and builds trust. ▪ Preparation decreases anxiety related to the unknown. ▪ Security objects decrease unfamiliarity of hospital environment. The child derives comfort from presence of personal items. ▪ Play provides familiarity, decreases fantasy, and provides motor activity. ▪ Consistency in caregivers helps to build the child's trust. Caregiver learns child's cues.	The child appears more relaxed, acknowledges parents' presence, and behavioral manifestations of anxiety are absent. Restful periods of sleep are noted. Vital signs are within normal limits.
2. Powerlessness (moderate) related to inability to communicate, and control relinquished to the healthcare team			
	NIC Priority Intervention—*Self-Esteem Facilitation:* Encouraging a patient to assume more responsibility for own behavior.		**NOC Suggested Outcome—***Health Beliefs: Perceived Control:* Personal conviction that one can influence an outcome.
The child or adolescent will have an increased sense of control over the situation.	▪ Provide opportunities for choices when possible. Encourage participation in self-care. ▪ Prepare the child or adolescent in advance (timing dependent on developmental level) for procedures. Describe the sensations that will be experienced. Allow some choice in timing or method of pain relief. ▪ Provide routines for the child both within a 24-hour period and for scheduled care. Tell the child before the procedure (timing is dependent upon developmental level), repeat explanation of why procedure is necessary, complete procedure in a consistent manner, and offer praise	▪ Such opportunities provide sense of control and autonomy through decision making. ▪ Information provides anticipatory guidance and a sense of involvement and value to the child. ▪ Self-control is maintained through routines.	The child or adolescent expresses satisfaction over ability to control some elements of situation. The child or adolescent participates in self-care and decision making.

(continued)

Nursing Care Plan THE CHILD COPING WITH A LIFE-THREATENING ILLNESS OR INJURY (continued)

GOAL	INTERVENTION	RATIONALE	EXPECTED OUTCOME
2. Powerlessness (moderate related to inability to communicate, and control relinquished to the health care team (continued)			
	or a special story when completed. When possible, incorporate routines from home.		
	■ Encourage play as a means of expressing feelings.	■ Play is a normal activity for children and provides freedom of expression.	
	■ Provide other means of communication to the intubated child (e.g., a word board or finger board).	■ Maintaining communication provides autonomy and independence for the child.	
	■ For the child requiring restraints, use as seldom as possible, provide appropriate explanations, and release at regular intervals. Wrapping IV lines well and using armboards can help maintain lines and avoid restraints.	■ Release from restraints helps diminish the sense of powerlessness that accompanies their use.	
3. Acute pain related to injuries, invasive procedures, surgery			
	NIC Priority Intervention—*Pain Management:* Alleviation of pain or a reduction in pain to a level of comfort that is acceptable to the patient.		**NOC Suggested Outcome**—*Comfort Level:* Feelings of physical and psychologic ease.
The child will experience reduced pain and improved comfort.	■ Assess the child's pain: location, intensity, what makes it better or worse.	■ Assessment provides baseline information from which a plan of care can be developed.	The child experiences a perceived or actual improvement in comfort level.
	■ If appropriate age, use self-report pain assessment scale (see Chapter 18∞). Use appropriate pain scale for nonverbal children.	■ Use of scale provides continuity and consistency in monitoring of the child's pain.	
	■ Prepare the child for procedures using developmentally appropriate language and format. Describe the sensations that the child will feel, smell, taste, or see. Comfort the child after the procedures. Provide rest periods between procedures.	■ Information reduces anxiety and fear associated with the unknown and helps the child maintain self-control.	
	■ Provide topical anesthetic as prescribed for painful procedures.	■ Reduces pain associated with needle sticks.	
	■ Provide optimal pain relief with prescribed analgesics. Provide comfort measures—position changes, backrubs, etc. Provide diversional activities as appropriate or possible. Incorporate the family in pain relief modality.	■ Physiologic and psychologic methods of pain control can be used in combination to maximally improve outcomes.	

MediaLink Care Plan: Toddler in ER for Near-Drowning Episode

coping. Ongoing reassessment of progress in meeting the child's needs is critical.

General care for the child in a critical care unit may include the following:

- Pain management
- Maintenance of mechanical ventilation
- Nutritional support
- Maintenance of hemodynamic monitoring equipment
- Use of sedating and paralytic agents
- Maintenance of life support such as extracorporeal membranous oxygenation (ECMO). See Chapter 25∞.
- Maintenance of intravenous medications such as vasopressors and insulin
- Wound care

For the child who is unconscious or sedated, additional care may include eye care, oral care, range of motion exercises, and skin care to prevent breakdown.

Implement the following to promote psychosocial care.

- Provide a thorough explanation of all environmental sights, sounds, sensations, and smells.
- Explain all procedures and their purposes.

- Keep child and family informed of any status changes.
- Provide the child an opportunity to ask questions and express fears and anxieties.
- Decrease excess environmental stimuli as much as possible (e.g., bright lights and loud alarms).
- Encourage parental visitation and participation in child's care as frequently as possible.
- Cluster nursing care to allow for periods of rest.
- Maintain honesty in all responses.

Provide for Parental Physical and Emotional Needs

The experience of having a child with a critical illness drains parents' physical and emotional reserves. Parents often need encouragement to take care of themselves. A statement such as, "It is important for you to eat and rest because Jeremy is really going to need you when he wakes up," helps parents to realize that becoming exhausted benefits neither them nor the child.

CLINICAL TIP

Encourage parents to take time for themselves to be alone, alternating times to be away for a short break. Suggest places they can go such as a lounge, chapel, or courtyard. There are times when both parents may need to get away together. Provide parents with a beeper, if possible, to reduce anxiety when they are away from the unit. In addition, if parents are hesitant to leave the child alone, ask if another family member or friend might be able to stay with the child for short periods. Hospitals generally have volunteers that can sit with children for a while to allow parents to feel comfortable leaving the child.

Orienting parents to the hospital, as well as to the unit routines, helps them to adapt to their surroundings. Many communities now have Ronald McDonald houses, an inexpensive but warm and supportive environment for parents of ill children (Figure 21–4 ■). Computer resources at Ronald McDonald houses may make it possible to keep in contact with family and concerned friends and provide updates. When financial burdens are a consideration, family and social service referrals may be needed.

Parents are often at different levels of coping during a crisis. The child's critical illness may foster cohesion between the couple and build a stronger relationship. Unfortunately, the reverse may also be true—differences in styles or levels of coping may foster a sense of isolation, placing a strain on the couple's relationship. Nurses should be alert to family dynamics and risk factors, and refer the family for counseling or therapy, if indicated.

Promote Parental Involvement

An important nursing role is to encourage and support parents in their parenting role. The parents' place when possible is at the bedside—their very presence can comfort the child, minimize fears, and reduce the child's experiences with pain during invasive procedures. They provide continuity and may notice subtle changes that a newly assigned nurse may miss. Participation in the care of their child helps parents to cope with the child's life-threatening illness (Katz, 2002).

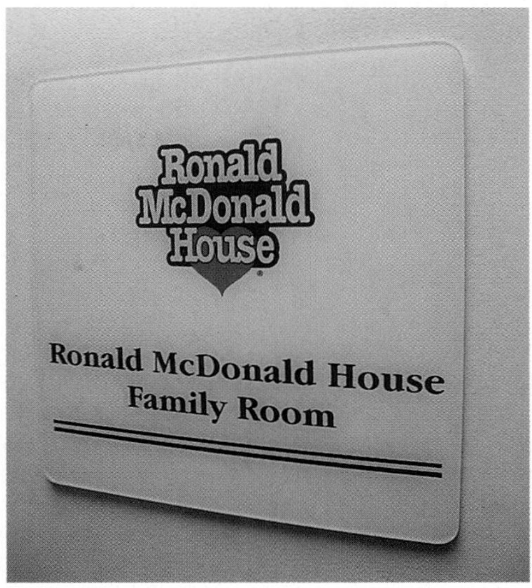

FIGURE 21–4 ■ A Ronald McDonald family room in a large metropolitan hospital provides a comfortable setting where families of seriously ill children can go to get away from the high-tech hospital atmosphere while remaining near the ill child.

Encourage parental and other family member involvement in the care of the neonate or infant. This provides the family with a sense of control over the situation and instills a feeling of empowerment (Sydnor-Greenberg & Dokken, 2000). Parents who are not allowed to remain at the bedside with their child may feel undervalued. (Griffin, 2003a). Giving parents a role at the child's bedside, such as providing personal care, is one example of encouraging parental involvement. See Partnering with Families: Involving Family Members in NICU/PICU Settings.

If the child is in the NICU or PICU, parents and siblings are prepared by the nurse before they see their child for the first time. Explain to them what tubes and monitors are present and how their child will look and react. Throughout the child's hospitalization, parents will continue to require reassurance and encouragement. Open visitation by parents is important to maintain their parenting role.

FAMILY PRESENCE DURING RESUSCITATION OR INVASIVE PROCEDURES

Although controversial, more families are witnessing the resuscitation of their loved ones. For healthcare providers, many issues arise with the parental presence during a child's resuscitation, including parental understanding of potentially disturbing resuscitative activities (e.g., open cardiac massage), potential for parental interference with resuscitative efforts, and the potential for a negative psychosocial impact of witnessing a child's resuscitation (Table 21–1).

However, for many parents, witnessing resuscitation is important for them to feel that everything possible has been performed to help their child. (See Partnering with Families: Presence During Resuscitation.) To make the opportunity for

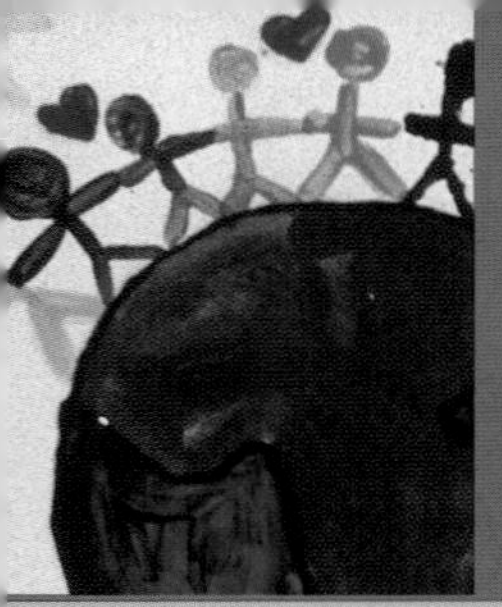

PARTNERING WITH FAMILIES

Involving Family Members in NICU/PICU Settings

Family participation in the care of the child in the pediatric or neonatal intensive care unit can be extremely beneficial to both the child and family. The child benefits from parental presence and continuity of care, while parents benefit from having some sense of control over their child's situation. Nurses can encourage family members to become involved in their child's care by suggesting the following:

- Talking to the NICU or PICU staff by telephone about the infant or child's condition and progress (if unable to visit)
- Sending photos, audiotapes, toys, or clothes for the baby or child
- Being present in the NICU or PICU, sitting with the baby or child
- Providing hands-on care (e.g., feeding, diapering, bathing)
- Doing research about the baby or child's medical condition, gathering information about resources, requesting conferences with staff
- Bringing other family members to the NICU or PICU
- Interacting with staff and establishing connections
- Interacting with other NICU or PICU parents and establishing connections
- Learning special caretaking skills from nurses and other staff (e.g., administering medication, physical therapy)
- Planning/organizing (e.g., active role in discharge planning)
- Establishing communication with a veteran NICU or PICU parent and/or family and/or joining an appropriate support group

Adapted from Sydnor-Greenberg, N., & Dokken, D. (2000). Coping and caring in different ways: Understanding and meaningful involvement. Pediatric Nursing, *26(2), 185–190.*

parental presence more acceptable to all involved, see the following steps (Levetown, 2004, p. 38).

1. Prior to entering the room where the child is being resuscitated, the nurse informs the parents about the environment—the equipment they will see in, on, and near their child and its purpose—and tells them who is in the room (she is a doctor, he is a nurse, she is a respiratory therapist) working on the child.
2. The nurse informs the parents that if they feel uncomfortable or if they get in the way of the resuscitation team's work, they will be escorted out.
3. Have the parents sit so that they are able to look at the child's face, holding his or her hand. The parents can be given duties (e.g., "Sit near Jeff s face, and let him know how much you love him").
4. If the parents are looking around, explain what is being done for the child and why. Parents need to know that their child did not endure unnecessary suffering. Attention to procedure-related pain management is important.
5. If the child is declared dead in the ED, reassure the parents that they were there at the last moment and that their child (use the child's name) felt loved.

CLINICAL TIP

If parents choose not to witness the resuscitation efforts, regular updates (15-minute intervals or more often is suggested) should be provided to the parents as they wait in a private area. The hospital chaplain or other family support team member should be notified so that support can be provided to parents while they wait.

Promote a Sense of Security

For children of all ages, feeling secure depends on a sense of physical and psychologic safety. A sense of physical security is difficult to attain within the PICU due to the constant barrage

MediaLink Involving Family in NICU Setting Video

TABLE 21–1 Perceptions of Health Professionals About Family Presence During Resuscitation

ADVANTAGES	DISADVANTAGES
Bonding between patients, patients' family members, and caregivers is facilitated	Child's family members may disrupt resuscitation efforts
Family members can observe the efforts of the healthcare team	Healthcare staff may not be able to control their emotions
Family members can provide comfort to their child, and speak words of encouragement	The child's family may be offended and potentially engage in negative behavior
Family's ability to obtain closure and accept outcome is facilitated	Fear of litigation might inhibit staff from performing necessary tasks well
Families perceive that they are actively participating in the resuscitation	Potential exists for emotional scarring of family or staff, with violent emotional memories of event
Family members can touch the child while the child is still warm	Long-term effects on family's emotional status are unknown
Staff may view the child as part of a loving family	Stress for staff involved may be increased
The mystery of activities behind closed doors of resuscitation room is reduced	The child's privacy may be violated
Being present during the resuscitation, rather than hearing only a verbal accounting, may dispel family members' doubts about the course of events	The child's family might not understand the tasks and procedures performed
Holistic approach with acknowledgement of family as part of the child is fostered	Having the child's family present might influence the decision about the duration of the resuscitation effort

Adapted from McGahey, P. R. (2002). Family presence during pediatric resuscitation: A focus on staff. Critical Care Nurse, *22(6), 29.*

of procedures that are part of the child's treatment plan. A sense of psychologic safety is best achieved through the presence of parents. An open visitation policy that enables parents to be at the bedside is optimal. Including parents as partners in the child's care provides comfort and reassurance to the child. Children whose parents have high anxiety levels pick up their parents' emotional cues and become more anxious. Interventions to lower the parents' anxiety may benefit the child. Consistency of staff is invaluable in developing familiarity and a trusting relationship with the child.

Personalizing the child's bedside and room can promote comfort and a sense of security for the child. Pictures from home, a favorite blanket or toy, music tapes, or posters can make the environment friendlier and more familiar to the child (Figure 21–5 ■). Religious or spiritual icons may also provide psychological support.

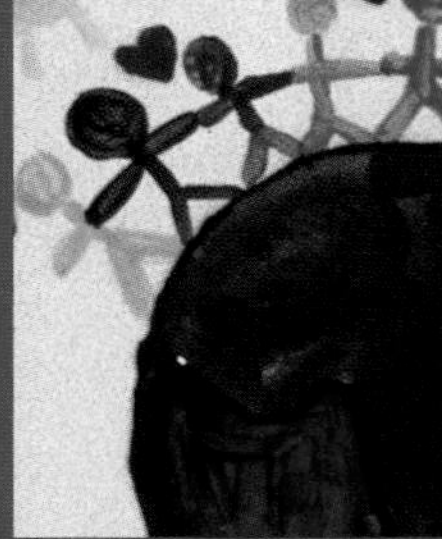

PARTNERING WITH FAMILIES

Presence During Resuscitation

The Emergency Nurses Association (2004) supports the option of family presence during invasive procedures and resuscitation. Parents and other family members (e.g., grandparents) may wish to be present during invasive procedures (such as lumbar puncture) or resuscitation of the child. The nurse partners with the family to determine their needs at the time. To better facilitate the needs of the family, the following is determined:

- Who desires to be present during resuscitation or invasive procedures?
- What role will they play during the procedure (e.g., snuggle child for comfort)?

Healthcare agencies should have established protocols for family presence during invasive procedures or resuscitation (Emergency Nurses Association, 2001). The nurse providing family-centered care recognizes that each situation is individualized according to the child's and family's needs. The nurse ensures that a support person from the multidisciplinary team (e.g., another nurse, social worker) is available to stay with the family members during resuscitation.

Provide Education About the Illness or Injury and Prepare the Child for Procedures

Children's understanding of the cause of the illness and its therapy depends on their cognitive abilities. Explain to younger children that illness and hospitalization are not punishments.

Preparation for procedures is important at all ages, even for the unconscious or sedated child. The timing of this preparation depends on the child's cognitive level. Generally, the younger the child, the shorter the interval should be between the time of the teaching and the actual procedure.

Children often are able to feel and hear even when unconscious, so touch and verbal interchanges are important. Toddlers will benefit from being talked to, soothed, and touched during and after the procedure. Provide preschoolers, school-age children, and adolescents with an explanation of the sensations they can expect to experience (temperature, vibrations, sounds, smells, tastes, sight). In any explanations to the child, avoid medical jargon; use simple language appropriate to the child's developmental level. See Chapter 17∞ for further discussion of educating and preparing the hospitalized child for procedures.

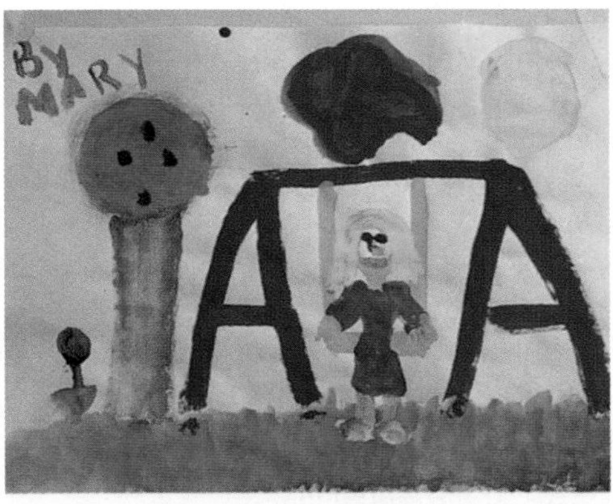

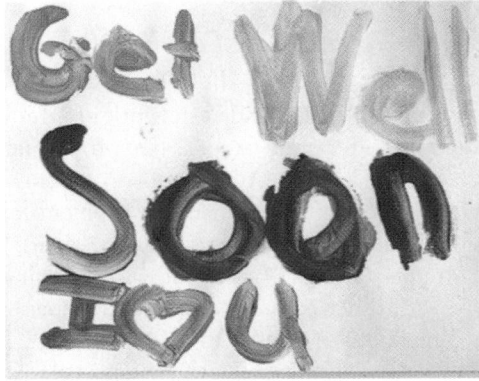

FIGURE 21–5 ■ It is important that parents and siblings feel comfortable communicating with the seriously ill child. If siblings cannot visit, they should be encouraged to paint or record messages. They need to be able to express themselves and to feel that they are helping.

Facilitate the Use of Play

The use of play is important in alleviating stress and helping children to prepare for procedures. It is also another way for the nurse to assess the child's developmental level. Therapeutic play adds familiarity, diminishes negative fantasies, provides motor activity, and helps the child develop a sense of mastery (see Chapter 5∞). Children who are immobilized by tubes and restraints can still feel a sense of accomplishment, for example, by completing a puzzle, even if the nurse points to each piece and, through nods and gestures, indicates where it should be placed. Play can help children work through a painful situation, making it more tolerable. See Chapter 17∞ for further discussion of the use of play in the hospitalized child.

Promote a Sense of Control

Children between toddlerhood and adolescence experience a loss of control during a life-threatening illness. This loss of control may be related to the body, emotions, normal routines, or privacy. Nursing interventions should promote a sense of control over these areas.

Allow the child choices when possible. Even the simple choice of choosing a gown color can help the child feel in control. Scheduling routine activities and treatments at the same time each day adds predictability and lessens anxiety. Limited mobility and the use of restraints, although sometimes necessary, contribute to the child's sense of powerlessness. Review the hospital's policies and procedures for the use of restraints. If restraints must be used, plan to release them regularly for short periods of time. Restrain children as little as possible, and when they are necessary, explain the rationale for restraints, emphasizing that they are not a punishment. Provide diversional activities for the child, for example, by reading stories, playing music, or watching videotapes (see Chapter 17∞).

Enhance the child's coping skills by teaching the child and family a combination of relaxation, visual imagery, or distraction techniques, and comforting self-talk phrases such as, "This will be over soon. If I stay calm, it will be all right. It will be over faster and then I can do something fun." Help the parents become the child's coping coaches.

Facilitate Positive Staff–Parent Relationships and Communication

The information given to parents must be accurate, and provided frequently. Information on the child's illness, condition, and plan of care should be delivered in a manner and language readily understandable to parents. Upon admission, parents need to be given an idea of what to expect in the days ahead and be prepared for special procedures or major changes in therapy that may become necessary. The parents are also provided with updates at least daily, and more often if the child's status changes. Inform the parents of the planned procedures for the day.

Given the intensity of the parents' experience when their child is critically ill, it is understandable that problems can arise between staff and parents. Each healthcare team member must be aware of the child's current status so that parents receive the same information from all staff. Consistency in the message can instill confidence. Provide explanations geared to the parents' level of understanding, using language the parents can understand.

Parents need to know who has the overall responsibility for the care of their child. They should be introduced to the nurse and physician who are responsible for the child's care. This is especially important in teaching hospitals that have rotating staff. The staff physician with the overall responsibility should meet with parents as often as necessary to talk about changes in the child's condition or treatment plan and to allow time for parents to ask questions (Figure 21–6 ■). Encourage parents to keep a daily log or notebook to record information on the child's care, progress, and needs. Parents should also be encouraged to write questions down in order to help them remember what they want to discuss with physicians, nursing staff, and other healthcare team members. Family care conferences can be helpful when a large number of team members provide care. Honesty in discussions with parents is extremely important. If parents feel misled or that information is being withheld, a trusting relationship will be impossible. Trust is facilitated when parents believe that the staff truly cares about the child and sees him or her as an individual, special child.

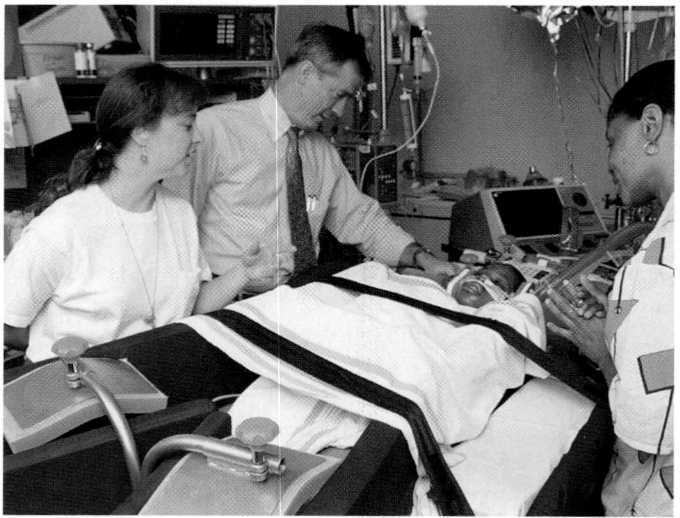

FIGURE 21–6 ■ In times of crisis, everyone likes to know that someone is in charge and who that person is. The parents should meet and talk with the staff physician in charge and the nurses as often as possible. Parents need to know that someone is responsible, even if different people are providing care.

Nurses collaborate with the multidisciplinary team to ensure that parents are informed and encouraged by each team member to be active participants in decision making. Parents also need a sense of hope regarding their child's illness to help them cope. Focus on the positives as the child progresses through the different phases of the critical illness.

Maintain or Strengthen Family Support Systems

Support systems are the extended network of family, friends, and religious and community contacts that provide nurturance, emotional support, and direct assistance to parents, thus enabling them to cope with overwhelming problems and crises. Most parents indicate that having family or friends nearby is crucial as a support system. Parents may also benefit from support groups with other parents who are also experiencing the life-threatening illness of a child.

Parents may require reassurance that it is acceptable to ask for help from family, friends, or community services. They may be uncomfortable asking for help, instead attempting to handle multiple responsibilities themselves, often to the point of exhaustion. Some parents are unable to respond to offers of help because it requires too great a mental effort on their part.

Nurses may be required to intervene on parents' behalf when they are overwhelmed with numerous people offering support. Parents may be frustrated by people who visit unannounced, stay too long, or visit too often. They may also find it difficult to tell well-meaning friends and family that they cannot deal with visitors at the moment. In these situations, offering to serve as a gatekeeper may be helpful. Partnering with the family to establish suggested "visiting times" for friends and extending family members may help to alleviate some of the parents' frustration and fatigue. The nurse can suggest to the parents that they inform friends and family of the most comfortable time for visits. See Partnering with Families: Lessening the Burden.

Families of critically ill or dying children often have emotional needs beyond the support capabilities of the nurse caring for the child. Referrals to family and professionally led support services or pastoral care may be beneficial in these instances. Refer to Chapter 22∞ for a discussion of nursing care of the family experiencing the death of a child.

Evaluation

Expected outcomes of nursing care include the following:

- The nurse establishes a trusting relationship and effective communication with the family.
- Parents participate in their child's care as much as desired.
- Family members receive emotional support and nurturance needed to sustain them through the child's illness.
- The child's social interactions, coping, and growth and development are promoted through diversional activities.
- The child's and family's coping is promoted through education and preparation for procedures.

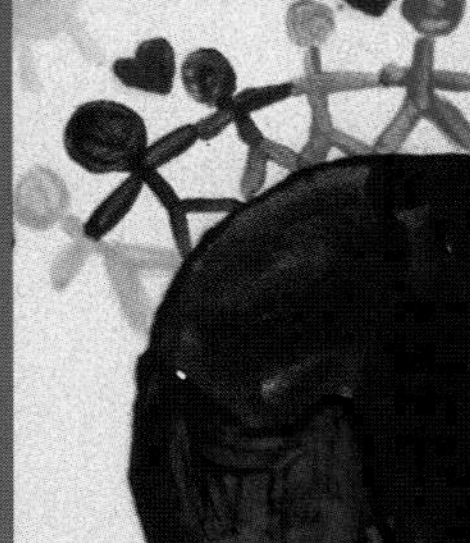

PARTNERING WITH FAMILIES

Lessening the Burden

Families of critically ill children are often overwhelmed and burdened with well-meaning inquiries from friends, co-workers, and extended family members. Parents are often required to repeat the same information numerous times to those inquiring about the child's condition, and this can be exhausting for the parents. Partner with the family to identify some effective methods of communicating the child's status while reducing the burden on the family. Suggestions can include:

- Designating a family member or another person to be responsible for relaying information to others
- Identifying a specific time period for calls and visits to allow for rest (e.g., between 10 A.M. and 12 noon and 6 P.M. and 8 P.M.)
- For prolonged hospitalizations, suggest the family create a website to post updates about the child's condition and treatments. The site can also be used to allow friends and family to provide responses and words of encouragement.
- Develop an email list and send updated messages periodically.

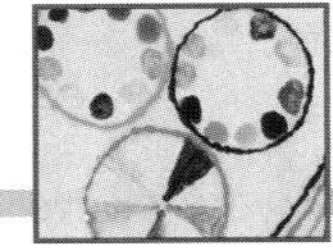

CHAPTER HIGHLIGHTS

- A life-threatening illness or injury places intense emotional and physical demands on the child and family due to the unfamiliar environment of the PICU, frightening or invasive procedures, and an uncertain outcome.
- The four most significant stressors for hospitalized children are separation from parents or the primary caretaker; loss of self-control, autonomy, and privacy; being subjected to multiple painful and invasive procedures; and fear of bodily injury and disfigurement.
- The child's developmental stage, temperament, previous coping experiences, and support system influence how he or she will cope with the current experience.
- When the child is hospitalized, work to meet the family members' needs so they can manage their anxiety and support the child.
- Parents typically progress through the stages of shock and disbelief; anger and guilt; deprivation and loss; anticipatory waiting; and readjustment or mourning when their child has a life-threatening illness or injury.
- For many parents, witnessing the resuscitation is important for them to feel sure that everything that could have been done has been tried.
- General care for the child in a critical care unit may include pain management, maintenance of mechanical ventilation, nutritional support, maintenance of hemodynamic monitoring equipment, use of sedating and paralytic agents, and maintenance of life support such as ECMO.

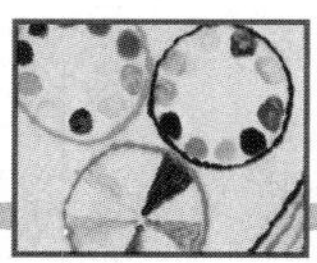

CRITICAL THINKING IN ACTION

INTRODUCTION

Recall Jeremy, the 12-year-old described in the chapter opener. After self-discontinuation of his seizure medications, Jeremy experienced status epilepticus and was transferred via helicopter from the local hospital to a medical center pediatric intensive care unit (PICU). He is intubated, unconscious, and has several intravenous lines. He has been placed on cardiorespiratory and noninvasive blood pressure monitors. His parents have arrived and are being escorted to the PICU.

DESCRIPTION

The PICU nurse assigned to the care of Jeremy has conducted a complete assessment, and his vital signs at the moment are stable. However, Jeremy remains unconscious, intubated, and is receiving mechanical ventilation.

Jeremy's parents are in the waiting room and are anxious to hear about their child's condition. The unit clerk informs the staff that the parents state Jeremy is the youngest of three children. His siblings are ages 14 and 15. The clerk also states that Jeremy's maternal and paternal grandparents are enroute to the hospital and they are bringing Jeremy's siblings with them.

DISCUSSION

1. What will the parents, siblings, and grandparents likely be experiencing as a result of Jeremy's life-threatening condition?
2. What measures will you implement to assist the family in dealing with the stressors of Jeremy's condition? How do you determine their coping mechanisms and support structure?
3. What will you explain to the parents and how will you prepare them before they visit Jeremy in the PICU for the first time?
4. Should Jeremy's siblings be allowed to visit him in the PICU while he is still unconscious? If so, how will you prepare Jeremy's siblings before they visit him in the PICU for the first time?
5. Jeremy demonstrates consciousness the following evening. Given the PICU environment, and Jeremy's developmental stage, what stressors will he likely experience at this time? What strategies will you implement to help Jeremy cope with the stressors?
6. The family remains together in the waiting room. Jeremy's father states, "This is all Jeremy's fault because he stopped taking his medicine." Jeremy's mother becomes very angry and begins to shout at the father. The siblings are present during this argument and begin to cry. What interventions can you implement in this situation?

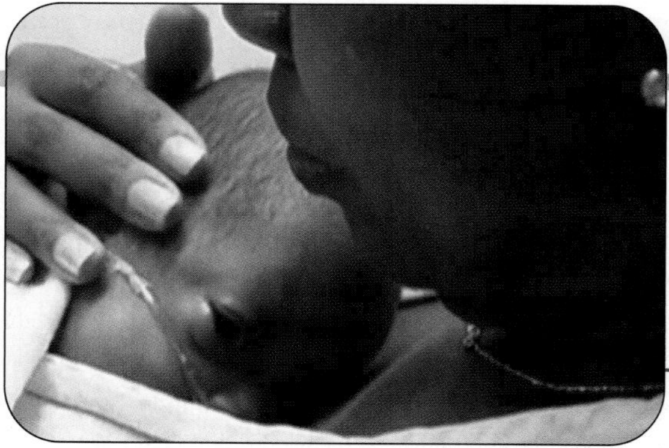

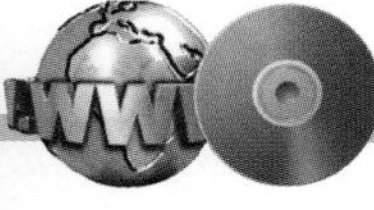

EXPLORE MediaLink

- NCLEX review, case studies, and other interactive resources for this chapter can be found on the Companion Website at **www.prenhall.com/ball**. Click on Chapter 21 to select the activities for this chapter.
- For animations, more NCLEX review questions, and an audio glossary, access the accompanying CD-ROM in this book.

http://www.prenhall.com/ball

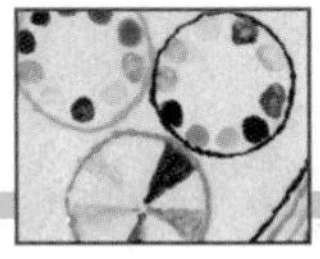

REFERENCES

Board, R. (2004). Father stress during a child's critical care hospitalization. *Journal of Pediatric Health Care, 18*(5), 244–249.

Board, R., & Ryan-Wenger, N. (2003). Stressors and stress symptoms of mothers with children in the PICU. *Journal of Pediatric Nursing, 18*(3), 195–202.

Daviss, W. B., Mooney, D., Racusin, R., Ford, J. D., Fleischer, A., & McHugo, G. J. (2000). Predicting posttraumatic stress after hospitalization for pediatric injury. *Journal of American Academy of Child and Adolescent Psychiatry, 39*(5), 576–583.

Emergency Nurses Association. (2004). Position statement: Family presence at the bedside during invasive procedures and resuscitation. www.ena.org/about/position/familypresence.asp, accessed 8/6/2004.

Field, M. J., & Behrman, R. E. (2003). *When children die: Improving palliative and end-of-life-care for children and their families.* National Academies Press: Washington, D. C. pp. 116–117.

Gavaghan, S. R., & Carroll, D. L. (2002). Families of critically ill patients and the effect of nursing interventions. *Dimensions of Critical Care Nursing, 21*(2), 64–71.

Griffin, T. (2003a). Facing challenges to family-centered care I: Conflicts over visitation. *Pediatric Nursing, 29*(2), 135–137.

Griffin, T. (2003b). Facing challenges to family-centered care II: Anger in the clinical setting. *Pediatric Nursing, 29*(3), 212–214.

Hall, E. O. C. (2004). A double concern: Grandmothers' experiences when a small grandchild is critically ill. *Journal of Pediatric Nursing, 19*(1), 61–69.

Jones, J. (2004, February). Neonatal nursing: The first six weeks. *Critical Care Nurse,* Suppl, 6-8.

Katz, S. (2002). When the child's illness is life-threatening: Impact on parents. *Pediatric Nursing, 28*(5), 453–464.

Levetown, M. (2004). Breaking bad news in the emergency department: When seconds count. *Topics in Emergency Medicine, 26*(1), 35–43.

Loo, K. K., Espinosa, M., Tyler, R., & Howard, J. (2003). Using Knowledge to Cope with Stress in the NICU: How parents integrate learning to read the physiologic and behavioral cues of the infant. *Neonatal Network, 22*(1), 31–37.

McGahey, P. R. (2002). Family presence during pediatric resuscitation: A focus on staff. *Critical Care Nurse, 22*(6), 29.

Melnyk, B. M., Small, L., & Carno, M. (2004). The effectiveness of parent-focused interventions in improving coping/mental health outcomes of critically ill children and their parents: an evidence base to guide clinical practice. *Pediatric Nursing, 30*(2), 143–148.

Posner, J. C., Hawkins, L. A., Garcia-Espana, F., & Durbin, D. R. (2004). A randomized, clinical trial of a home safety intervention based in an emergency department setting. *Pediatrics, 113*(6), 1603–1608.

Small, L. (2002). Early predictors of poor coping outcomes in children following intensive care hospitalization and stressful medical encounters. *Pediatric Nursing, 26*(4), 393–398, 401.

Snyder, B. S. (2004). Preventing treatment interference: Nurses' and parents' intervention strategies. *Pediatric Nursing, 30*(1), 31–40.

Stephenson, J. (2000). Palliative and hospice care needed for children with life-threatening conditions. *Journal of the American Medical Association, 284*(19), 2437–2438.

Sydnor-Greenberg, N., & Dokken, D. (2000). Coping and caring in different ways: Understanding and meaningful involvement. *Pediatric Nursing, 26*(2), 185–190.

Verma, R. P., Sridhar, S., & Spitzer, A. R. (2003). Continuing care of NICU graduates. *Clinical Pediatrics, 42*(4), 299–315.

White, J. R. M., & Dalton, H. J. (2002). Pediatric trauma: Postinjury care in the pediatric intensive care unit. *Critical Care Medicine, 30*(11) S478–S488.

Chapter 22

End-of-Life Care and Bereavement

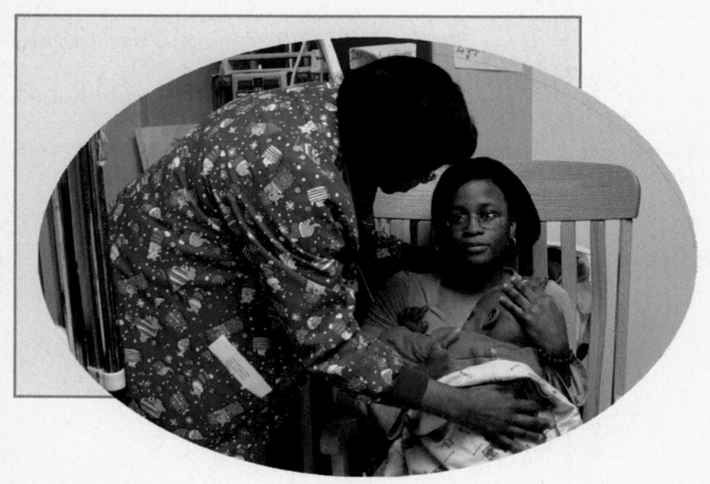

Zachary Conway is a 3 1/2-year-old who began experiencing motor difficulties and demonstrating bizarre emotional behavior a few months ago. After a series of diagnostic studies, he was diagnosed with an inoperable, rapidly progressing brain tumor. Zachary underwent radiation and chemotherapy to reduce the size of the tumor. He is currently hospitalized after experiencing grand mal seizures and dehydration from poor nutritional intake.

Zachary's condition has deteriorated and his death is expected within two to three days. Emphasis is now on promoting his comfort and supporting his family during the death vigil. Zachary is awake but appears lethargic. He now receives enteral feedings via a nasogastric tube. He interacts very little with anyone other than his mother.

Zachary's mother remains with him at all times during hospitalization while other family members visit. His father spends several hours each day at the hospital. Zachary's sister, Marilee, attends school in the second grade. She is being cared for by grandparents after school when her mother and father are with Zachary.

What is the role of the nurse in caring for Zachary and his family? What nursing interventions address the physiologic and psychologic needs of the child who is dying? How can you provide family-centered care?

"My daddy told me my baby brother Zach wasn't coming home because he is going to die. Mommy stays with Zach in the hospital all of the time. I just wish everyone would come home. Why does Zach have to die anyway?"

—Marilee, age 7

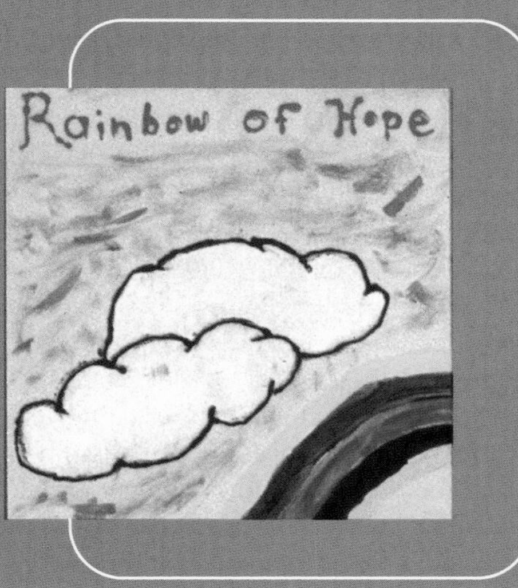

Learning Objectives

After completing this chapter, you will be able to:

- Describe the development of the child's concept of death, loss, and grief.
- Describe the child's responses to death, loss, and grief.
- Identify the causes of loss and grief for the child by developmental level.
- Identify the cultural and spiritual influences on the child and family's responses to death, loss, and grief.
- Identify the physiologic and psychologic changes that occur in the dying child.
- Develop a nursing care plan to provide family-centered care for the dying child and family.
- Implement strategies to assist the family in coping with the death of a child.

MediaLink http://www.prenhall.com/ball

Resources for this chapter can be found on the CD-ROM accompanying this textbook and on the Companion Website at www.prenhall.com/ball. Click on Chapter 22 to select the activities for this chapter.

CD-ROM

Video

Parental Reactions to Death of a Child

NCLEX Review

Audio Glossary

COMPANION WEBSITE

NCLEX Review

Case Study: Loss of a Schoolmate

Family-Centered Care Plan: Death of a Child at Various Ages

MediaLink Applications

Helping Families Grieve

Preparing the Family for Hospice

Key Terms

In the United States, approximately 55,000 children up to age 19 die annually, with infants accounting for nearly half of those deaths. Childhood death may be the result of a chronic condition, sudden illness, or injury (Institute of Medicine [IOM], 2003). Refer to Tables 1–4 through 1–14 in Chapter 1∞ for a thorough discussion of the neonatal, postnatal, age-specific death rates, and the leading causes of injury deaths in children of all ages.

The death of a child is a devastating, life-altering experience for the parents, siblings, and other family members. The nurse caring for the child and family experiencing death, loss, and grief must consider the personal, ethical, legal, spiritual, cultural, and biologic influences on these individuals. This enables the nurse to provide supportive and sensitive care to the dying child and family and assist them through the grieving process (Box 22–1).

When the family is faced with end-of-life care of a child, the process leading up to this may involve a chronic condition or multiple acute care episodes (Figure 22–1 ■). However, some deaths occur suddenly, which does not allow the opportunity for such planned care. Whether the child's death is the result of a chronic condition or an acute circumstance, the nurse is pivotal in providing valuable care and support to the child and family.

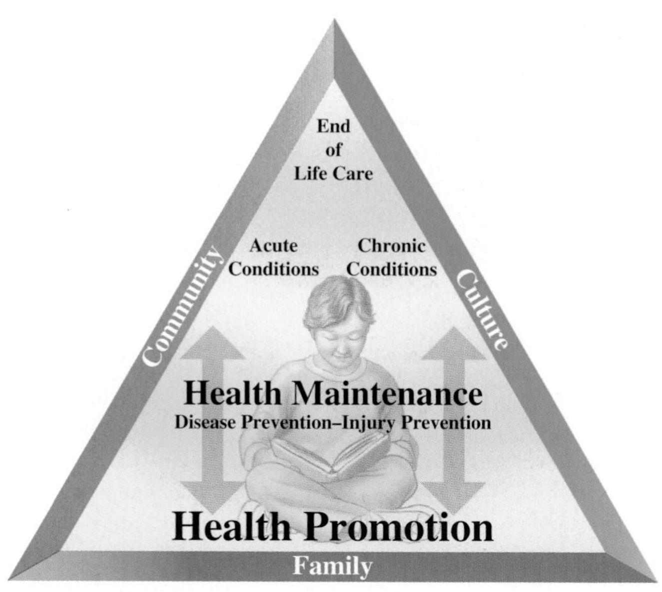

FIGURE 22–1 ■ The Bindler-Ball Child Health Continuum illustrates the paths that may lead to a child's death. In many cases, the child's death is associated with a chronic condition such as cancer or congenital anomalies, but it is important to remember that more than 40% of child deaths between 1 and 19 years of age are caused by unexpected injury (Health Resources and Services Administration, 2002).

CONCEPTS OF LOSS, DEATH, AND GRIEF

Loss, death, and grief are experienced by everyone at some point in life. Children may suffer loss as a result of a changed relationship through death of a parent, separation or divorce of parents, or death of a grandparent.

BOX 22–1 Nursing Roles in Improving Pediatric Palliative, End-of-life, and Bereavement Care

The nurse and other members of the healthcare team work collaboratively to improve end-of-life care for children and their families through the following actions.

1. Plan nursing care for children with life-threatening medical conditions and their families that matches the child's physical, cognitive, emotional, and spiritual level of development.
2. Implement family-centered care, ensuring that families are part of the care team and their beliefs, feelings, and desires are respected.
3. Plan and provide compassionate care for children with life-threatening conditions and for their families beginning at the time of diagnosis through death and bereavement.
4. Seek information, education, and mentoring to gain proficiency and skill in working effectively with children who are dying and their families.
5. Work within the healthcare facility to promote needed changes that will improve the palliative, end-of-life, and bereavement care for children and their families.
6. Participate in research designed to increase healthcare professional understanding of clinical, cultural, organizational, and other practices or perspectives that can improve palliative, end-of-life, and bereavement care for children and their families.

Adapted from Institute of Medicine. (2003). When children die: Improving palliative and end-of-life care for children and their families. *Washington, DC: National Academies Press, p. 7.*

Loss

Loss is an actual or potential change in status of something valued, so that it is no longer available to be experienced. An **actual loss** is one that is recognized by others. A **perceived loss** is experienced by an individual but cannot be confirmed by others. **Anticipatory loss** is experienced before the loss actually transpires. Sources of loss for children may include:

- Loss of a loved one (e.g., parent, sibling, grandparent, friend, childcare provider)
- Loss of an aspect of oneself, such as a body part or function (e.g., amputation, organ failure, hearing or vision loss)
- Loss of an object (e.g., pet or favorite toy)
- Separation from an accustomed environment (e.g., relocation to new neighborhood or new school)

Death

A lack of consensus has led to various definitions of death. Traditionally, death has been defined as the irreversible cessation of circulatory and respiratory functions, also referred to as **heart-lung death.** However, death has become more difficult to define since the inception of technology to support blood circulation and respirations. Another commonly accepted definition of death is **cerebral death** (also called brain death), or the irreversible cessation of all functions of the brain, including the cerebral cortex and brainstem (Box 22–2). Special guidelines are applied in determining brain death in children of different ages.

Depending on the institution and practice guidelines, additional confirmatory tests may be conducted in some circumstances. Currently, there are no clinically applicable criteria for brain death in infants less than 1 week of age due to the unique physiologic changes of brain blood flow during the transition period from fetus to newborn infant (IOM, 2003).

Grief and Bereavement

Grief describes an individual's feelings and behaviors in response to death. Sadness, anger, fatigue, inability to concentrate, numbness, and sleep disturbances are normal responses to a loved one's death (IOM, 2003). Additional symptoms that may accompany grief include anxiety, blurred vision, chest pain, depression, difficulty swallowing, dizziness, dyspnea, excessive sweating, headaches, menstrual disturbances, palpitations, skin rashes, syncope, vomiting, and weight loss.

Anticipatory grief occurs before an expected loss, in anticipation of that loss. This may occur before an expected death or following the diagnosis of a child's serious condition. Parents may express strong feelings of sadness, regret, loss, and possibly guilt and anger (IOM, 2003). Children with life-threatening illnesses may also experience anticipatory grief, exhibiting sadness and anger.

Disenfranchised grief occurs when the individual is unable to acknowledge the loss to others. **Dysfunctional grief** is an unhealthy grief that may be unresolved or inhibited. Unresolved grief is extended in severity and length. With inhibited grief, the individual suppresses many of the normal symptoms of grief, but may experience somatic symptoms. Signs of dysfunctional grief after a death may include the following:

- Persistent guilt and lowered self-esteem
- Failure to grieve (does not cry, does not attend funeral)
- Inability to discuss the deceased even after a period of time
- Declining relationships with family and friends
- Refusal to participate in memorial services or visit the grave
- Thoughts of suicide to reunite with the deceased

Factors contributing to unresolved grief after a death include a highly emotional attachment to the dead person (failure to grieve helps to avoid the reality of loss), a perceived need to be in control, and the lack of support systems.

Bereavement describes experiencing loss through the death of a loved one, but not the emotional aspect of the loss. **Mourning** is the social ritual and expression of loss, as well as the behavioral and psychological process of adapting to the loss. Mourning is often influenced by custom, spiritual beliefs, and culture.

Stages of Grieving

Though many theorists have described phases or stages of grieving, the most well known is Kübler-Ross's five stages of grieving (1969): denial, anger, bargaining, depression, and acceptance. According to Kübler-Ross, not everyone dealing with a loss will experience all of these stages and individuals who do experience all stages may not experience them in the sequence described. This process is not linear, and individuals may experience some or all of the stages at varying times. See Table 22–1 for a description of stages of grieving and pediatric implications.

BOX 22–2 Brain Death Criteria

Coma—totally nonresponsive, no vocalization, no purposeful activity

Absent brainstem function

- Pupils fully dilated or midposition, nonreactive to light
- No spontaneous eye movements induced by oculocephalic or oculovestibular testing
- Absence of bulbar musculature—no facial or oropharyngeal muscle movements; absent corneal, gag, cough, sucking, and rooting reflexes
- Apnea when removed from ventilator

Flaccid tone, no spontaneous movements

Required observation period by age of child prior to declaration of brain death is as follows:

- 7 days to 2 months—2 examinations and 2 EEGs, separated by at least 48 hours
- 2 months to 1 year—2 examinations and 2 EEGs, separated by at least 24 hours
- Over 1 year—observation period of at least 12 hours. No EEG or laboratory testing is needed if irreversible cause is known

Adapted from Task Force for the Determination of Brain Death in Children (1987). Guidelines for the determination of brain death in children. Neurology, *37, 1077–1078.*

FACTORS INFLUENCING RESPONSES TO DEATH AND LOSS

Cultural beliefs, spiritual beliefs, and social support systems are central factors influencing a child and family's response to death and loss. Other factors specifically influencing the child's response, including their developmental level, are discussed in the following section.

Culture

Recognizing and understanding a family's cultural traditions and practices when they are experiencing the death of a child helps nurses to provide individualized care to the dying child and family. Each culture has its own way of defining, addressing, and acknowledging death. Customs, ceremonies, religious laws, and beliefs are strongly connected with such events. Culture influences the individual's reaction to loss, and the expression of grief is often determined by the customs of the culture. Some families may believe that grief is a private matter, and they may internalize and repress their feelings. Others may believe that outward demonstration of the expression of grief is acceptable and is even encouraged. See Developing Cultural Competence: Assessing Cultural Differences in Dealing with Death.

TABLE 22–1 Stages of Grieving and Pediatric Implications

STAGE	BEHAVIORAL RESPONSES	NURSING IMPLICATIONS
Denial	Refuses to believe that loss is happening Is not prepared to deal with practical problems, such as funeral arrangements following child's unexpected death May assume artificial cheerfulness to prolong denial May make statements such as "This can't be happening" or "This can't be true" "I know she is not dead—she is just hiding"	Be verbally supportive but refrain from reinforcing denial Examine your own behavior to ensure that you do not share in person's denial Don't argue—allow the child or parents to come to terms in their own time
Anger	Child or family may direct anger at nurse or staff about matters that normally would not bother them	Emphasize that anger is a normal response to feelings of loss and powerlessness Avoid withdrawal or retaliation; do not take anger personally—remain with the child or parents even though they express anger. Silence and presence indicate understanding Address any issues associated with underlying anger (e.g., parents not being informed of how their child died)
Bargaining	Seeks to bargain to avoid loss May express feelings of guilt or fear of punishment for past sins, real or imagined	Be supportive and listen to expressions of guilt or fear Offer spiritual support if appropriate
Depression	Grieves for events that will not happen (e.g., graduation, wedding) May talk freely (e.g., reviewing child's life) or may withdraw	Communicate nonverbally by remaining quiet and allowing the opportunity for expression Encourage expression of sadness and other feelings Convey caring by touch if appropriate
Acceptance	Comes to terms with loss May have decreased interest in surroundings and support people May wish to begin making plans for the future	Assist family and friends to understand the individual's decreased need to socialize Encourage participation in making plans

Data from Kübler-Ross, On Death and Dying *(1969);* On Children and Death. *1983, New York: Macmillan.*

Religion and Spirituality

In providing family-centered care, it is essential for the nurse to examine human spirituality when facing issues related to dying and death. The impact of religion and spirituality on the practices related to death and dying is especially significant given that religious beliefs can influence treatment decisions (Hickman, Tilden, & Tolle, 2004).

Spirituality is derived from unique experience. The quality of the child and family's spirituality determines the sense of depth with which they will comprehend their own death as well as the deaths of those they love. The spiritual needs of dying children are as important as those of dying adults (Davies, Brenner, Orloff, et al., 2002).

When dealing with death and dying, religion and spirituality may be a fundamental coping mechanism (Flannelly, Weaver, & Costa, 2004). Most religious groups have specific practices related to death, which may be expressed through prayer, meditation, rituals, worship, music, art, and dance. See Table 22–2 for an overview of religious traditions in mourning and after-death rites. Religious practices are also significant as a means of coping with grief (Figure 22–2 ■). An individual's spiritual beliefs and practices considerably influence his or her reactions to loss and subsequent behavior. In order for the nurse to provide care to the dying child, the family's religious needs must be assessed. However, it important to note that not all families observe traditional rites and rituals. (See Complementary Therapy: Prayer.)

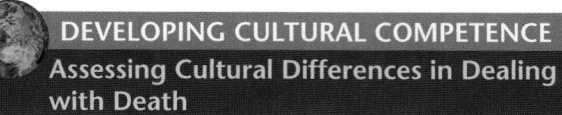

Consider the customs and attitudes that might reflect the family's cultural heritage and affect their response to death. Information about these customs will help plan nursing care to families. For example try to learn about the following:

- How much to reveal to a child about the diagnosis and prognosis
- How much the child and family want to participate in medical decision making
- The degree of trust in the medical system
- The amount of emotional display that is appropriate
- The role of children, women, and the elderly
- The concept of an afterlife and how it is prepared for (e.g., special ceremonies)
- Whether death should take place alone, with the family, or with an extended group
- Whether death should take place in the home or in the hospital
- Funeral and burial customs
- The length of the mourning period

From Lewis, L., Brecher, M., Reaman, G. H., & Sahler, O. J. (2002). How can you help meet the needs of dying children? Contemporary Pediatrics, *19(4), 147–159.*

Social Support System

Those closest to the grieving child and family can be a great source of physical, emotional, and functional support which

TABLE 22–2 Spiritual Traditions in Mourning and After-Death Rites

RELIGIOUS GROUP	POSSIBLE RITUALS	ORGAN DONATION OR AUTOPSY BELIEFS
American Indians	Beliefs and practices vary widely Navajo do not touch the deceased or their belongings Mourning is done in private	Varies among tribes
Buddhism	Last-rite chanting at bedside Cremation common	Organ donation considered act of mercy, autopsy individual choice
Catholicism	Sacrament of the sick Obligated to take ordinary but not extraordinary means to prolong life Burial	Autopsy, organ donation acceptable
Christian Science	Unlikely to seek medical help to prolong life Disposal of body and parts decided by family	Individual decides about organ donation
Hinduism	No restrictions to right-to-die issue Religious prayers chanted before and after death Cremation common Men and women display outward grief Thread tied around wrist signifies a blessing, do not remove	Autopsy, organ donation acceptable
Islam	Attempts to shorten life prohibited Body is washed only by Muslim of same gender	Organ donation acceptable Autopsy only for medical or legal reasons
Jehovah's Witness	Use of extraordinary means to prolong life is individual choice Burial determined by family preference	Autopsy if required by law Organ donation forbidden
Judaism	If death is inevitable, no new procedures needed, but must continue those ongoing Body ritually washed Burial as soon as possible, all body parts must be buried together Seven-day mourning period	Autopsy permitted in certain circumstances, organ donation is a complex issue
Mennonite	Do not believe life must be continued at all cost	Autopsy and organ donation acceptable
Mormonism	If death inevitable, promote a peaceful and dignified death Burial in temple clothes	Autopsy permitted with permission of next of kin, organ donation is permitted
Protestantism	Burial or cremation is individual decision	Organ donation and autopsy are individual decisions
Seventh-Day Adventist	Follow ethic of prolonging life Disposal of body and burial are individual decisions	Autopsy, organ donation acceptable

Adapted from Spector, R. E. (2000). Cultural diversity in health and illness *(5th ed., pp. 137–138, 144–149). Upper Saddle River, NJ: Prentice Hall Health.*

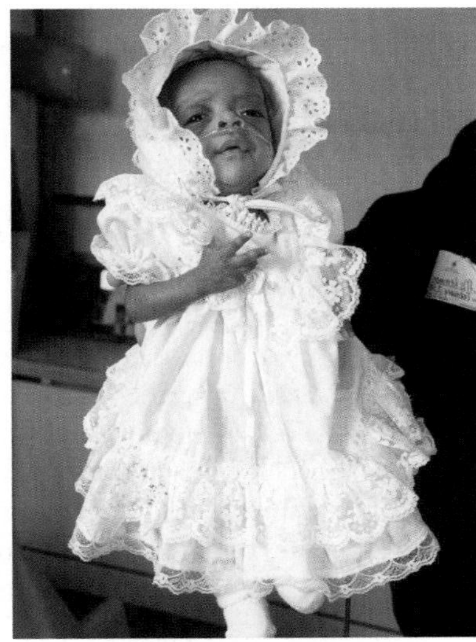

FIGURE 22–2 ■ Religious rituals, such as baptism and blessing of an ill infant, may provide great comfort to the family. When the infant is stable, a traditional baptism may be performed in the home or church with family and friends present. When the infant has a life-threatening illness, baptism may be performed in the hospital by a chaplain or health professional.

can positively influence the successful resolution of grief. However, some people are uncomfortable or lack experience in dealing with death, and rather than offering support in the time of need, they may withdraw from the grieving person or family. Others may offer support initially, but as they return to their usual activities, they may cease to provide ongoing support for those still grieving. Another consideration is that the

COMPLEMENTARY THERAPY

Prayer

In the United States, religious practices such as prayer represent the most prevalent complementary and alternative therapies. A study revealed that 82% of Americans believe in the healing power of prayer, 73% believe that praying for others can help cure them, and 77% believe that God sometimes intervenes to cure people (Barnes, Plotnikoff, Fox, et al., 2000). A national telephone survey of 2,055 households explored the use of prayer and other complementary therapies. Results revealed that 35% of respondents used prayer for health concerns. Prayer was often directed toward wellness, but it was also used in conjunction with conventional medical care (McCaffrey, Eisenberg, Legedza, et al., 2004).

grieving individual may be unable or unwilling to accept support when it is offered. Social factors that can interfere with grieving include a lack of social recognition of the loss, perceived inability to share the loss, and traumatic circumstances of the loss.

THE CHILD'S UNDERSTANDING OF LOSS AND DEATH

Children differ from adults in their understanding of loss and death. Their understanding and behavioral responses vary according to their developmental level, and their previous experience with loss and death. Table 22–3 provides a summary of the child's understanding of death and lists some possible behavioral responses to death.

Communicating with children about death is often a difficult task for parents. Parents and other adults should avoid euphemisms such as "she has gone to sleep" or "he passed away," since this may confuse children and hinder their understanding of the finality of death. Parents and healthcare providers should not be afraid to use the word *death* or *dead* when explaining these concepts to children. After discussing death with children, provide them with the opportunity to ask questions and express their feelings.

For children, major losses associated with death include the death of a parent, death of a grandparent, death of a sibling, and death of a friend. The death of a sibling is discussed later in this chapter. Children also experience loss through a myriad of circumstances not related to the death of a person, including parental separation or divorce, loss of a pet, loss of a possession, and relocation. The significance of the loss to the child determines the amount and type of grieving the child experiences.

Death of a Parent

In the United States, more than 2 million children and adolescents younger than 18 years have experienced the death of a parent (Christ, Siegel, & Christ, 2002). The death of a parent is an extremely traumatic event for the child and can seriously disrupt the child's psychosocial development. For example, if the mother or primary caregiver dies during a child's early years of life, the child may experience significant lifelong psychosocial problems such as enduring stress. Preschoolers experiencing the death of a parent may also have significant psychosocial problems as a result. Children in this age group engage in magical thinking and may believe the death of the parent is their fault, punishment for an actual or imagined wrongdoing. School-age children may experience a sense of responsibility and guilt for the death of the parent. Adolescents may experience difficulty in mastery of the developmental task of establishing an intimate relationship with members of the opposite sex.

MediaLink Case Study: Loss of a Schoolmate

The child's reaction to the death of a parent is greatly influenced by the manner the surviving parent reacts to the death and the manner in which the child is supported by the surviving parent. Children can become angry and may focus their anger on the surviving parent, especially when that parent moves into a new relationship.

CLINICAL TIP

Encourage adults to help children deal with the loss of a parent by keeping memories alive with pictures, stories about the parent, and letting children know that they too feel sad. Provide honest answers to questions and return to normal routines. Older children and adolescents may benefit from a support group and counseling (Menke, 2002).

Additional losses for the child may occur as the result of a parent's death. The death may bring about relocation or a change in living arrangements. For example, the child may have to live with a noncustodial parent, grandparent, or other extended family member. The family's financial status may change as a result of the loss of a wage earner. Older children may be expected to assume more responsibility for the home or younger siblings, allowing them less time with peers and recreational activities. See Partnering with Families: Leaving Memories for Children.

Death of a Grandparent

The death of a grandparent is often the first experience a child has with death of a significant individual. The child's grandparent may have been essential in the development of the child's sense of trust, love, and belonging. With an understanding of a grandparent's death, the child may also come to the realization that their parents will die also.

The child's reaction to the loss of a grandparent is dependent on the significance of the grandparent to the child. In many families and cultures, grandparents are important influences in the child's life. Children may be raised by a grandparent, they may be cared for by a grandparent while the parents work, or they may reside in the same household with the grandparent. Grandparents are often a child's link to his or her heritage through the grandparent's storytelling and sharing family history. The influence of the grandparent on the child may therefore have considerable meaning to the child and the impact of a grandparent's death may be as significant as the death of a parent. See Partnering with Families: Assisting Children with Grieving.

Death of a Friend

Children may experience the death of a friend due to a chronic condition, acute illness, or an injury. Since children with chronic and life-threatening conditions are living longer and are able to attend school and engage in social activities, they are likely to have developed close friendships with other children. The childhood friends and schoolmates of chronically ill children should be prepared for the potential death according to their developmental level. When a friend dies suddenly, there is no time for preparation. Whether the death of a friend was anticipated or sudden, the child experiences the same stages of grief as with other losses. The death of a peer may bring about the first realization that the elderly are not the only ones who die. The adolescent's sense of invulnerability may be shaken.

TABLE 22–3 Children's Understanding of Death and Possible Behavioral Responses

UNDERSTANDING OF DEATH	POSSIBLE BEHAVIORAL RESPONSES
Infant	
Cognitive Stage: Sensorimotor Lacks understanding of concept of death May sense caregivers are tense, routines are altered Senses separation	May show sadness by turning away from the gaze of others Resists cuddling and eats less Clinging more than usual Crying excessively Sleeps more than usual Regression
Toddler	
Cognitive Stage: Preoperational Unable to distinguish fact from fantasy No understanding of true concept of death Aware someone is missing—separation anxiety Unable to distinguish death from temporary separation or abandonment	Clingy, refuses to let parent out of sight Stops walking and talking Shows distress by biting, hitting, tears Fearful Problems eating and sleeping Sleep disturbances Reacts to others around them Regression from previously achieved milestones (such as bowel and/or bladder training)
Preschooler	
Cognitive Stage: Preoperational Believes death is temporary and that the dead person will return Believes bad thoughts cause death Magical thinking (believes the dead person can be brought back to life or is the cause of death) Has beginning experience with death of animals and plants	May fear going to sleep, has nightmares, afraid of dark Out-of-control behavior, hyperactivity, tantrums, regression Problems with bowel and bladder control Crying spells Seems morbidly fascinated with death Asks a lot of questions Displays anger at failure to keep person "alive," breaks toys, is aggressive to friends Regression to baby talk or thumb sucking Complaints of abdominal pain
School-Age Child	
Cognitive Stage: Concrete Operations Acquires more realistic understanding of death By 8–10 years, understands that death is permanent and irreversible, and that people die from internal and external causes Believes that death is universal and will happen to him or her May have exaggerated concerns about death	May deny sadness by hiding tears and acting more like adults Difficulty concentrating on school work Psychosomatic complaints—stomachache or headache Acting-out behavior, anger at being abandoned May try to comfort parents by taking over tasks May display aggression May fear someone else they love will die May have nightmares May display feelings of guilt
Adolescent	
Cognitive Stage: Formal Operations Intellectually capable of understanding death Has a better grasp of association between illness and death Sense of invincibility conflicts with fear of death Able to recognize effect of death on others	Same as school-age child May have severe depression May feel angry or guilty Acting-out behavior—risk-taking behavior, delinquency, suicide attempts, promiscuity, pseudo indifference Difficulties eating and sleeping

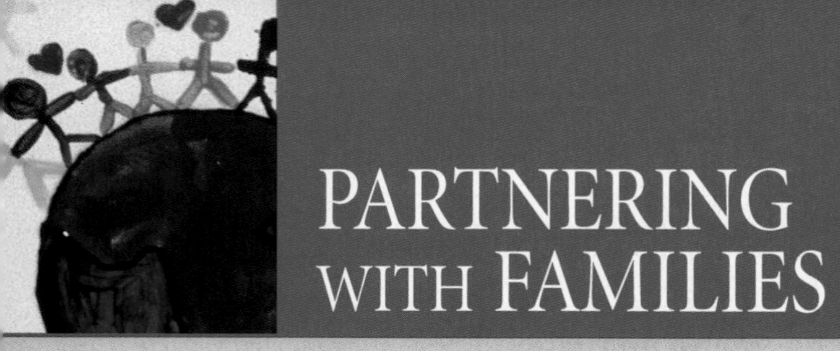

PARTNERING WITH FAMILIES

Leaving Memories for Children

Dying parents may ask the nurse about leaving memories for their child. Suggestions that the nurse could offer include the following:

- Making video recordings and dating them according to when they wish the child to view them (e.g., special occasions such as birthdays and graduation)
- Journaling or writing to the child about their love for the child and their experience of being a parent to them
- Writing out birthday cards and providing special gifts for each of the child's birthdays and having family members give to the child at the appropriate time
- Writing letters and asking family members to mail them to the child at the designated time
- Making a "memory book" of the parent's life from birth
- Sharing special moments (e.g., "I remember the first time you smiled at me," or "I remember the first day you said 'mama') either in writing or on videotape

Some schools offer grief support and counseling to provide opportunities for the children's expressions of grief and sadness. The development of a memorial is often helpful for children. Planting a tree, hanging a plaque, or creating a play area at school in memory of the deceased child helps the children to express their grief. (See Table 22–4 for further resources.)

Other Potentially Significant Losses

Crime, school shootings, homicide, natural or man-made disasters, and terror attacks such as the events of September 11, 2001, are types of trauma to which children in the United States are exposed. Children are the population most vulnerable to the negative effects of trauma (Meier, 2002). After hearing about incidents on television, children may have questions for parents.

- As the preschooler is still egocentric, when concerns about death are voiced it is to determine how the death may impact the child. For example, the 5-year-old who asks about the children or families of victims and how they will be cared for may actually be seeking reassurance that his or her parents will continue to be there to provide care (Goldman, 2004).
- The school-age child who asks for many details about the incident may be using intellectualization as a coping mechanism. School-age children think logically and are able to conceptualize their thoughts and fears. They can understand causality and see the link between a terrorist with a weapon who causes a plane to crash and the resultant death of many people. Children at this developmental level may wonder about an afterlife and voice concerns about where a loved one has gone.

The effects of the traumatic event are greater if the child directly experiences the event, sustains loss, is separated from parents, or observes parents in distress (Meier, 2002). Children may experience posttraumatic stress syndrome (PTSD) following ex-

TABLE 22–4 Books for Children Who Experience a Friend's Death

BOOK	PUBLISHER	AGE/DEVELOPMENTAL STAGE
A Separate Peace, by John Knowles	New York: MacMillan	12 and up
A Taste of Blackberries, by Doris Buchanan Smith	New York: Harper Collins	8–12
A Time for Dancing, by Davida Wills Hurwin	Boston: Little, Brown	12 and up
Blackwater, by Eve Bunting	New York: Harper Collins	12 and up
Blow Me a Kiss, Miss Lilly, by Nancy White Carlstrom	New York: Harper and Row	4–8
Bridge to Terabithia, by Katherine Paterson	New York: Harper Collins	10–14
Bye, Mis' Lela, by Dorothy Carter	New York: Farrar, Straus and Giroux	4–8
Charlotte's Web, by E. B. White	New York: Harper and Row	4–8
Dinah Forever, by Claudia Mills	New York: Farrar	9–12
Dorothy's Darkest Days, by Judith Casely	New York: Greenwillow	7–10
Flying Solo, by Ralph Fletcher	New York: Clarion	8–12
Forever Friends, by Candy Boyd	New York: Puffin Books	10–14
I Had a Friend Named Peter, by Janice Cohn	New York: William Morrow and Co	5–10
The Kids' Book About Death and Dying, E. E. Ropes, Editor	Toronto: Little Brown and Company	4–8
Love Ya Like a Sister, by Katie Ouriou	Toronto: Tundra Books	12 and up
On My Honor, by Marion Dane Bauer	New York: Bantam Doubleday Dell Publishing	8–12
Phoenix Rising, by Karen Hesse	New York: Henry Holt and Co.	12 and up
Rudi's Pond, by Eve Bunting	New York: Clarion	5–8
Secret Friends, by Elizabeth Laird	New York: G.P. Putnam's Sons	10–14
When a Friend Dies: A Book for Teens and Grieving and Healing, by Marilyn E. Gootman	Minneapolis: Free Spirit Press	12 and up

Data from Rivlin, D. (2001). Books for children when a friend dies. Contemporary Pediatrics, 18*(10), 134–138.*

posure to a traumatic event or disaster. Refer to Chapter 34∞ for further discussion of PTSD.

For many children, the first significant loss is that of a pet. A pet is often viewed by the child as a source of unconditional love and acceptance. The child typically views a pet as a friend, companion, and member of the family. The child may experience a pet's loss through death (anticipated or unexpected), or because the pet ran away or was stolen. How the parents and other adults support the child and handle the loss can impact the manner in which children learn to cope with loss and death later in life.

Parents should offer honest, simple, and developmentally appropriate explanations to help the child understand what happened. Telling a child that the dog was old and sick, so it had to be "put to sleep" may cause anxiety in the 4-year-old about what will happen when he or she sleeps at night. The 8-year-old who is told "God was lonely, so he took Cocoa to live with him," may become concerned about what other possessions God may desire.

Suggestions for helping the child cope with the loss of a pet include having a memorial service for the pet, creating a scrapbook, and planting a tree or small garden in memory of the pet (Clements, Benasutti, & Carmone, 2003).

PARTNERING WITH FAMILIES

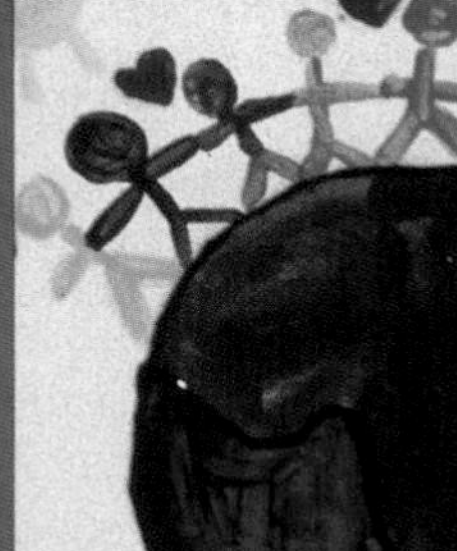

Assisting Children with Grieving

Families can help the child express feelings about the loss of a grandparent in a variety of ways. Some examples include the following:

- Write a good-bye letter or draw a picture.
- Draw a picture of each family member and show how each person is grieving. An older child could write about how each person is grieving.
- Make a paper boat. Help the child write or draw his or her thoughts and feelings on the paper before folding it. Release the boat to sail away on a lake or pond.
- Allow children to play with toys and act out their feelings.

Adapted from Busch, T., & Kimble, C. S. (2001). Grieving children: Are we meeting the challenge? Pediatric Nursing, *27(4), 414–418.*

THE DYING CHILD'S EXPERIENCE

A child's understanding of and responses to death varies according to developmental stages as previously described in Table 22–3. Children as young as 5 years of age can sense when they are seriously ill. A child's awareness of death develops more rapidly when he or she is experiencing the progression of a disease and related medical treatment. Children with life-threatening illnesses often learn about death and their own illness from exposure to other seriously ill and dying children when they are receiving treatment during hospitalization or clinic visits. Parents may prefer not to talk with the child about the seriousness of the illness and potential death out of a desire to protect the child from bad news, and a fear that the child will lose hope (Mazanec & Tyler, 2003). Major considerations in planning care for the dying child are that the child does not want to experience pain or to be left alone. Kübler-Ross (1983) notes that children are more fearful of abandonment than death.

Infants and Toddlers

Although infants and toddlers are not actually aware of death, they are aware of and react to changes in normal routines and parental nonverbal communication (Figure 22–3 ■). Toddlers may know they "feel bad" but do not understand their physical symptoms are associated with impending death.

Toddlers may sense a difference in the way parents interact with them. The parent who inspired trust through providing predictable and consistent care may become less predictable. Whereas the parent once met all the child's needs, now he or she may feel helpless in meeting needs such as freedom from pain.

Preschooler

Preschool children can see their body deteriorate and feel the toxic effects of endogenous chemicals during disease progression and treatment. Changes in self-concept occur as they perceive these body changes. The preschool child often describes illness in terms of mutilation to the body. The child may realize that he or she is dying because of these physical changes.

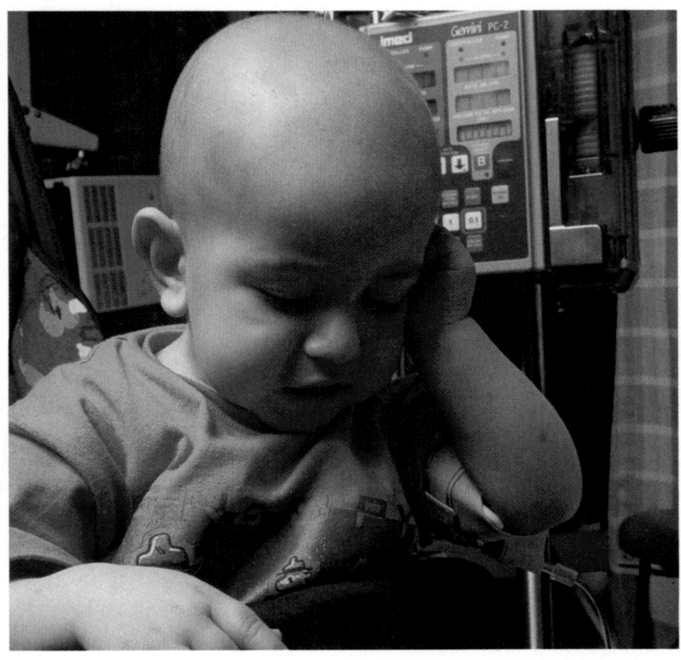

FIGURE 22–3 ■ The toddler with a life-threatening disorder recognizes that he feels bad and that routines are different. His anxiety may increase due to the concern and feelings of sadness exhibited by his parents.

When parents instruct the healthcare team to avoid any mention of death, the intent is usually to protect the child from an unpleasant truth. The child may have some realization about impending death, and a "conspiracy of silence" may lead the child to avoid the subject in an attempt to protect the parents from the truth. The child may believe that expressing an awareness of death and related fears will place added emotional burdens on family members. The result is that both parent and child miss the opportunity to share the comfort and love that could make the death more peaceful for the child and family survivors.

School-Age Child

School-age children also have subtle fears about body integrity and anxieties related to the serious nature of their illness. This greater preoccupation with illness is considered by many professionals as the child's version of **death anxiety,** a feeling of apprehension or fear of death. Children may express death anxiety as a concern with treatments that invade the body or interfere with normal body functions.

While the child at this developmental stage can conceptualize concrete facts, such as death occurring when the body stops working, abstract concepts such as the existence of an afterlife are harder to understand. The child may feel a loneliness associated with separation from family and the world as he or she knows it.

Kübler-Ross (1969) identifies anger as a stage of grief experienced by both the dying person and loved ones. When parents refuse to acknowledge the child's impending death, or when they acknowledge it to themselves but are determined to shield the child from the inevitable, they are denying the child the opportunity to resolve anger and move on in the grieving process. The message sent to the child is that the topic of death is taboo. The child may fear being emotionally abandoned by family members, so displays of anger are often avoided because the child fears desertion more than death.

Waechter's (1987) classic study of hospitalized and fatally ill children revealed that children who were given an opportunity to discuss issues related to death openly did not experience greater anxiety about death. The permission to discuss any aspect of the illness made the child feel less isolated and alienated from the parents. The child also felt that the illness was not too terrible to discuss.

Adolescents

Adolescents have a mature understanding of death, but the normal developmental milestones of adolescence add to their challenges in facing a terminal illness. They are struggling to establish their own identity and plans for the future. At a time when body image is extremely important, they may be faced with the possibility of mutilation and disfigurement. Dying adolescents are often isolated from their peers during a period when peers are the most essential social group. Adolescents with terminal illnesses may be angry because they recognize their loss at a time when the whole world is opening up to them.

Adolescents should not be expected to handle feelings in the same way as adults. They often avoid expressing anger against the family, seeking to control and direct these feelings elsewhere. Adolescents often become angry at changes in treatment procedures, lack of explanations, and threats to their independence. As death nears, the adolescent may permit comforting and support and may accept care from warm and loving family members, as long as he or she is not treated condescendingly. Talking about death with a friend or a nurse with whom there is a close relationship may be easier than talking with the parents. Some dying adolescents will attempt to control the situation by planning their funeral in detail and identifying who should receive specific possessions (Klopfenstein & Young-Saleme, 2002).

End-of-life care for the adolescent is particularly challenging due to relevant developmental, legal, and ethical considerations specific to this age group. (See Chapter 1∞ for more information on ethical issues.) The adolescent may express a desire to refuse treatment or request withdrawal of treatment. Open and honest discussion with the adolescent can help parents and the healthcare team to determine if he or she fully understands the implications of terminating curative therapy. If the intent is to avoid more painful procedures, then the adolescent needs to be informed about options for pain relief. Because of the adolescent's desire for autonomy, information about all choices should be provided, including but not limited to withdrawal of treatment. However, the adolescent may have reached the acceptance stage in the grieving process and is ready for death to occur. Once parents are satisfied that the adolescent has reached a resolution based on facts, it may be easier for the parents to support and respect the adolescent's wishes. The nurse who has established a trusting relationship with the adolescent may be able to help him or her recognize the parents' wishes to continue nurturing and protecting their child.

CLINICAL TIP

The Patient Self-Determination Act of 1990 (PSDA) supports the rights of persons 18 years of age or older to make decisions about their medical care. Although many adolescents younger than 18 have the cognitive skills necessary for decision making and are involved in decisions concerning their care, the PSDA limits their legal rights. Creative strategies are needed to develop a model of decision-making rights and responsibilities for adolescents that is built on the PSDA and shared with parents who ultimately will be responsible for decisions on care.

END-OF-LIFE CONSIDERATIONS AND DECISION-MAKING ISSUES

The family of the dying child is faced with numerous decisions; the end-of-life decision-making process is extremely difficult. During this time, the family relies on the primary healthcare providers, nursing staff, and other members of the healthcare team to provide them with honest information including various treatment options and potential outcomes. The family in stress may need additional time to make informed decisions. The degree of a child's participation in the decision-making process depends on the child's cognitive abilities, developmental stage, physical and mental status, as well as prior experience with healthcare (Haddad, 2000).

Communication between family and healthcare professionals is essential in assisting the family with decisions on end-of-life care. Issues concerning end-of-life care that the families may consider include palliative care, hospice care, do-not-resuscitate requests, continuation of schooling, discontinuation of treatments, organ/tissue donation, and autopsy. The ethical principles of beneficence and nonmaleficence and the child's quality of life can provide a framework for the family and healthcare team during the decision-making process (Stutts & Schloemann, 2002). See Chapter 1∞.

Families have different beliefs about full disclosure of information about the illness and prognosis based on their culture. Most Western cultures are accepting of sharing information about a serious illness and death with the patient. Families from non-Western cultures may choose not to disclose all information to the patient (Mazanec & Tyler, 2003). Talk with the family to learn about cultural values regarding sharing information with the child.

At the proper time, assist the parents in planning the developmentally appropriate way of sharing the truth with their child, or as much information as the family is ready to share. Collaborate with the healthcare team and family to discuss the family's fears and concerns about telling the child the truth. Explain that the child needs to trust in his or her parents and healthcare providers. Even when the family is unwilling to talk with the child about death, some information should be provided to the child about the ongoing need for treatment and procedures. If they are performed without explanation, the child may experience increased anxiety and accompanying symptoms. Be available to offer support and answer questions.

When the family is ready, assist them in role-playing or possible words to use when informing the child that he or she is dying. Emphasize to the parents that the child may actually need to hear the word *dying* in order to understand.

Palliative Care and Hospice Care

The World Health Organization defines **palliative care** as the active total care of patients whose disease is not responsive to curative treatment (Ferrell & Coyle, 2002). It combines active and compassionate therapies intended to comfort, soothe, and relieve persons with a life-limiting condition (IOM, 2003). It may be combined with therapies aimed at reducing or curing the illness and treating symptoms more aggressively than hospice care. Palliative care focuses on the child and family by addressing their physical, psychologic, social, and spiritual issues. The goal of palliative care is the achievement of the best quality of life for the child and the family. Palliative care may occur in the home, hospital, or other facility.

According to the World Health Organization (2001), palliative care:

- Provides relief from pain and other distressing symptoms
- Affirms life and regards dying as a normal process
- Intends neither to hasten nor postpone death
- Integrates the psychologic and spiritual aspects of patient care
- Offers a support system to help patients live as actively as possible until death
- Offers a support system to help the family cope during the patient's illness and in their own bereavement
- Uses a team approach to address the needs of patients and their families, including bereavement counseling, if indicated
- Will enhance quality of life, and may also positively influence the course of illness

It is estimated that approximately 5,000 children die each year from life-limiting illnesses such as cancer, congenital anomalies, neurogenerative disorders, cystic fibrosis, and HIV infection who could potentially benefit from palliative care (Chaffee, 2001). Barriers to providing good pediatric palliative care include attitudinal, educational, institutional, regulatory, and financial. A significant barrier is the cultural denial of the fact that children actually die (Rushton & Catlin, 2002). Therefore, children may live for many years with a life-limiting condition without the family and healthcare supports and services that could improve quality of life. Improvements in palliative care services can be performed by assessing the needs of children and families for such services (Box 22–3).

Hospice care helps those with short life expectancies to live their remaining time to the fullest—alert, without pain, and with choices and dignity. Hospice care does not seek to prolong life, but rather regards dying as a normal part of life and provides support for a dignified and peaceful death. Hospice approaches end-of-life care through emotional, psychologic, spiritual, and medical support of the child and family. It is estimated that less than 1% of dying children receive hospice services (American Academy of Pediatrics, 2000b).

For hospice care to be successful, the child and family must perceive hospice as a desirable choice (Vickers & Carlisle, 2000). Some families may not find the hospice approach as an acceptable alternative because it requires them to accept the impending death of the child, and may imply that they are giving up hope (Klopfenstein & Young-Saleme, 2002). The family may require assistance to view hospice care as an opportunity to focus on the time left with the child. Other families may view hospice as the child and family's choice in determining where the child dies (Vickers & Carlisle, 2000). In pediatric hospice, the family learns to focus on the quality of life by keeping communication open between the child and family members.

For the child who will receive palliative and/or hospice care, the family and healthcare providers collaborate to determine which treatments are appropriate to continue with the child's end-of-life care. These treatments may include total parenteral nutrition (TPN), intravenous fluids, gastric or nasogastric tube feedings, and certain medications.

Nurses collaborate with a multidisciplinary healthcare team which includes the primary care provider, social workers, pastoral or other spiritual counselors, and volunteers to provide comprehensive care to the dying child and family. Financial concerns should be addressed. Social workers can assist the family's

MediaLink Hospice and Palliative Care Resources

BOX 22–3 Assessments Needed in Devising and Revising a Palliative Care Plan

The nurse assisting in devising or revising a palliative care plan should first collect and consider information related to the child's disease status, family and child's preferences and goals, and the child's functional status. Then information about available therapies and the family's resources can be assessed.

DISEASE STATUS AND SYMPTOMS ASSESSMENT

- The child's diagnosis and prognosis and uncertainty about the child's future course
- When death is expected, potentially within a few months or sooner
- Symptoms present and those likely to emerge
- Effect of the disease on the child's physical, intellectual, and emotional functioning

FAMILY PREFERENCES AND GOALS

- Parents' understanding of their child's medical condition and care options, need for more information or assistance in understanding the information provided, including palliative care and end-of-life resources
- Child's understanding of his or her medical condition and care options, his or her competence and interest in being involved in care decisions
- Assessment of the agreement of the child's and parents' preferences
- Explanation of benefits and burdens of therapy options; discussion of end-of-life issues and plans for the child's condition
- Documentation of DNR or allow natural death orders in the medical record as appropriate for the child's medical status; copies also available for home and school

PSYCHOSOCIAL AND SPIRITUAL ASSESSMENT

- Child's hopes and fears for the present and future
- Child assured of care, not abandonment
- Family (parents and siblings) coping, hopes and fears for the present and future
- Support by a counselor or chaplain offered and arranged as appropriate

CHILD'S FUNCTIONAL STATUS

- Child's self-care abilities, assistance required at home or school
- Help needed by family and teachers

THERAPY REVIEW AND EVALUATION

- Assessment of pain and other symptoms, monitor for side effects
- Palliative interventions in use or being considered; results to date; benefits and burdens of therapies for child, family, and caregivers
- Availability of reliable assistance 24 hours a day, 7 days a week

RESOURCE AND LOGISTICS REVIEW AND EVALUATION

- Need for additional professional and nonprofessional personnel; their availability in the community
- Preference of child and family for primary location of care, including at the time when death is expected; potential barriers to accommodating these preferences
- Adequacy of home physical facilities (e.g., accessible bathroom), transportation, economic, and other relevant resources
- Financial burden on the family, availability of other resources; potential that existing resources be used more effectively or efficiently

Data from Institute of Medicine. (2003). When children die: Improving palliative and end-of-life care for children and their families. *Washington, DC: National Academies Press, pp. 136–137.*

communication with insurance providers to determine the benefits covered. For the uninsured, community programs may be available to assist families with the expenses associated with hospice and other care of dying children. Refer the family to appropriate community resources.

The hospice nurse discusses signs and symptoms of impending death, such as nausea and respiratory difficulty, and develops a plan to alleviate them. Hospice provides anticipatory guidance to the child and family so they are not alarmed by the child's unexpected distress (Klopfenstein & Young-Saleme, 2002). If the child is in pain, the family is instructed on appropriate pain management to ensure the promotion of comfort. Hospice also offers assurance that following the death of their child, parents will not have to face their grief alone as counseling and support are provided for 1 year following the death of the child.

Parents may choose hospice home care for their terminal newborn or infant. This provides the infant and family the opportunity to spend time together unencumbered by technical equipment and the presence of strangers. Nurses can encourage the bonding process by allowing the parents to dress the infant, introduce the infant to siblings, and take photographs with the infant as part of the family unit. Special considerations for this family are necessary since they are experiencing the child's entire life cycle in a short duration (Box 22–4).

Withdrawal or Withholding Treatment

The decision to withdraw or withhold life-sustaining treatments from the dying child is extremely difficult and highly emotional for the parents. The decision to withhold nutrition and hydration is particularly difficult for parents because they often associate the provision of food with nurturing and love. Common reasons cited for ordering intravenous fluids at the end of life include the fear of hastening death or causing starvation (Ramer-Chrastek, Brunnquell, & Hasse, 2002). Other treatments, including certain

BOX 22–4 Research: Dying at Home

Nursing research has explored parental perspectives on caring for a dying child at home (Vickers & Carlisle, 2000). The qualitative study revealed a common theme—choice and control—which linked all other concepts. The main findings are as follows:

- Home is viewed by parents as the place of choice for terminal care of the child.
- Choice and control are fundamental to parents' coping strategies.
- Parents desire to care for their terminally ill child at home, but the responsibility entails concerns and fears.
- Decision making at the transition from curative to palliative care is crucial for parents.
- The hospital environment is perceived as stressful and lacking privacy.
- Philosophy of hospice care can be adapted to whatever setting a family chooses.
- Sense of normalcy and balance of control are important factors in choosing to care for the child at home.

From Vickers, J. L. & Carlisle, C. (2000). Choices and control: Parental experiences in pediatric terminal home care. Journal of Pediatric Oncology Nursing, 17*(1), 12–21.*

medications, mechanical ventilation, and dialysis, may also be withdrawn in the event the outcome of the child is inevitable death and continuation of the treatment inflicts more suffering than benefit for the child. See Evidence-Based Practice: Improving the Quality of Pediatric End-of-life Care in the PICU.

Conflicts Regarding Parental Refusal of Treatment

Conflicts may arise between parents and the healthcare providers when there is disagreement over what, if any, medical interventions should be provided. Parents may refuse treatments based on religious convictions or because they wish to avoid prolonging the child's life in order to provide a peaceful death (IOM, 2003). Initiating highly technical, but possibly futile, interventions may cause emotional and financial stress that can overwhelm young parents.

In certain situations in which recommended care is refused, court intervention may be initiated by the healthcare team to have a surrogate legal guardian appointed. This intervention is based on the legal principle that failing to obtain adequate medical care for a child violates the state child neglect laws (IOM, 2003). Consultation by the hospital's ethics committee is often a first step in clarifying the issues involved and it helps reduce the emotion associated with the conflict. An unbiased professional can collect facts about the child's condition and beliefs and values of parents and health professionals, and can improve communication while investigating options for compromise (Rushton, 2004). The nurse may be put in the uncomfortable position of trying to provide care to the infant or child while an adversarial rather than a supportive relationship exists with the parents. See Box 22–5.

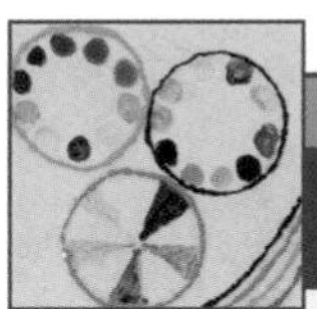

EVIDENCE-BASED PRACTICE
Improving the Quality of Pediatric End-of-life Care in the PICU

PROBLEM

The majority of children who die due to life-limiting conditions die in the hospital setting, and many times in the pediatric intensive care unit (PICU). What are the parents' perspectives with regard to improving their child's quality of care?

EVIDENCE

A study involving parents of 56 children who had died in the PICU focused on care provided to the child and parental end-of-life decision making. Parents struggled with issues such as adequacy of information about particular aspects of the child's care and loss of control. The results of the study indicated that when parents were considering withdrawal of life support, they placed the highest priorities on quality of life, likelihood of improvement, and their perception of the child's pain and discomfort (Meyer, Burns, Griffith, et al., 2002). Another study was conducted by interviewing parents of 44 children who had died at one children's hospital. Themes emerging from the interviews included the following: parents appreciated being highly involved in decision making, difficult news should be delivered by a familiar person, one caregiver should be in charge throughout all phases of treatment, improved services for siblings are needed, and pain management is critical. Effective caregivers were described as those who were honest, clinically accurate, compassionate, and available. Language barriers with Spanish-speaking families compromised the ability of these families to fully understand the child's care and to feel isolated (Contro, Larson, Scofield, et al., 2002).

IMPLICATIONS

Identifying the specific care valued by parents during this time is important for planning nursing care and multidisciplinary palliative care. Nurses can assist the family through the decision-making process by providing honest, factual responses to the family's questions. Planning of care and communication should ensure that family-centered care is integrating values important to the family.

CRITICAL THINKING APPLICATION

Consider the special needs of the parents of a newborn with a cardiac congenital anomaly that cannot be corrected by surgery. Identify a family-centered care plan of palliative care for the infant who is expected to die within the next few days.

Do-Not-Resuscitate Orders

Parents faced with a child's inevitable death as a result of a terminal illness or condition may be asked to consider a **do-not-resuscitate (DNR) or do-not-intubate (DNI) order.** For children with end-stage, irreversible life-limiting conditions, the family and healthcare providers must decide if a resuscitation attempt would be in the child's best interest. Factors influencing the decision for a DNR or DNI status include allowing the child to die with dignity and the possibility of causing more harm and suffering if resuscitative measures are implemented.

The decision is emotionally challenging for the family as well as healthcare providers. Parents require ongoing support as they may feel they are "giving up" on their child. When faced with the decision of requesting a DNR or DNI for their child, the family requires honest information. It is essential that the family understand compliance with a DNR or DNI order does not mean the child will no longer receive further care or interventions. Oxygen, suctioning, and control of pain, as well as other comfort measures and supportive nursing care, continue in the presence of a DNR order (Box 22–6).

School Considerations

The American Disabilities Act of 1990 and the Education for All Handicapped Children Act mandate that all disabled children—including those with terminal illnesses—are entitled to the same education as other students. Policy challenges in the school setting related to hospice care and do-not-resuscitate orders have resulted in some school systems (Ramer-Chrastek, 2000). Additional issues requiring consideration of the dying child at school include

BOX 22–5 Critical Thinking: Effective Communication

A family refuses to consent to medical care that the healthcare team believes will improve and prolong the dying child's life. You do not agree with the family's decision. How will disagreeing with the family's decision affect your communication with the family? Your care of the child? Your support of the family? How can you ensure that personal views do not interfere with the nurse–child–family relationship? What resources exist to help the family and healthcare team reach agreement with regard to care of the dying child?

BOX 22-6 DNR and AND

Some institutions are now replacing the phrase do not resuscitate (DNR) with the phrase "allow natural death" (AND). This provides the family with a point of view that may make the decision more acceptable. To the families, rather than requesting intervention to be withheld (DNR), they are requesting that the child be allowed to die peacefully. This helps them to consider the choice as being in the child's best interest, rather than "giving up" (Ramer-Chrastek et al., 2002).

the effects on the well children at school who may witness a child's physical deterioration and potentially the child's death.

Do-Not-Resuscitate Orders in Schools

Children with chronic or terminal illnesses may be at high risk of dying while in school. The issue of a do-not-resuscitate (DNR) order in the school leads to various concerns for the school officials. Concerns include the effect of a death of a student on classmates. Parents may not want their healthy children exposed to death in a classroom or other school setting. Other concerns include the potential for misinterpretation of the DNR order, in which the child may not receive emergency attention for life-threatening events such as choking, and the legal issues of liability for the school if a child dies while in attendance (American Academy of Pediatrics [AAP], 2000a). Some school districts refuse to honor DNR orders (Ramer-Chrastek, 2000).

The best approach for handling DNR requests at school is collaboration between the child, family, nurse and other healthcare providers, school officials, and social workers or other personnel with knowledge or expertise in DNR requests at school. This partnership will facilitate the development of an understanding of the positions of all parties involved and subsequently enable them to reach agreement regarding the handling of the DNR request that respects the rights and interests of dying children.

Euthanasia

The American Academy of Pediatrics does not support the practice of physician-assisted suicide or euthanasia for children. The American Nurses Association (ANA) holds that nurses should not participate in active euthanasia or to participate in assisted suicide because the act is in direct violation of the Code for Nurses, the ethical traditions and goals of the profession, and its covenant with society (American Nurses Association, 2003a; American Nurses Association, 2003b). The ANA emphasizes the nurse's obligation to provide timely, humane, comprehensive, and compassionate end-of-life care. However, honoring the refusal of treatments is considered ethically and legally permissible.

If a child or adolescent requests euthanasia, the healthcare team responds with compassion and emphasizes the focus of alleviating sources of distress (AAP, 2000b). Once the child receives support in alleviating distress, the requests for euthanasia usually cease.

Tissue and/or Organ Donation

In many states, healthcare workers are required to provide the family of the deceased with the option of making an anatomical gift. Nurses can best serve the family of the dying child and potential organ donor recipients by becoming familiar with the state's legal aspects of organ donation and their institution's criteria for establishing the procurement of organs or tissue.

Information about organ and tissue donation is discussed in a sensitive manner with the family. The appropriate time to approach the family concerning organ donation may be difficult to determine for nurses not accustomed to discussing these difficult circumstances with families. To maintain the rights and dignity of the dying child and family, a person with experience in communicating with families during times of crises, such as with a dying child, would be ideal for this situation. Most facilities have personnel trained in identifying and coordinating the appropriate time to discuss organ and tissue donation. Generally, an organ procurement organization (OPO) coordinator will work in collaboration with the nurses and other members of the healthcare team (Smith, 2003).

Autopsy

When the exact cause of death is not clear, an autopsy may be suggested. Parents may be hesitant to consent to an autopsy because they are uneasy with the prospect of their child's body being further invaded. The family is informed that the autopsy will likely reveal the cause of death, which is especially important if the cause of death is related to a genetic disorder and may affect future child-bearing decisions. The family is supported during this decision-making process.

In the event of an unnatural death, such as suicide or murder, an autopsy is required by state law. Other situations requiring an autopsy may include the sudden death of an infant or child previously considered healthy, an acute illness resulting in death, and cases of suspected abuse. Because the decision to conduct an autopsy in these situations is not a choice made by parents, the family requires support as they may feel they have relinquished control over their child's body.

THE DEATH OF A CHILD

Informing Parents of Child's Serious Illness or Death

Research indicates that the manner in which parents receive bad news regarding their child's illness or death may influence their ability to cope with the situation, and can have lasting effects. Parents find certain approaches more helpful when hearing difficult news (Serwint & Rutherford, 2000). The death of a child should be disclosed in a sensitive manner with compassion and sympathy. Refer to Chapter 21∞ for a discussion of communicating bad news to families.

The location and environment for the communication of bad news is important. A private room used for the meeting is ideal as it provides the opportunity to present the news without interruptions or distractions, and provides the parents privacy to express their emotions. The person or persons most able to provide answers to the parents' questions are generally the best choice for who will deliver the news.

Awareness of body language is important for healthcare professionals during the disclosure of bad news. Eye contact, sitting rather than standing, and providing touch, such as holding a hand or touching an arm, provides the parents with assurance that the focus is on them and their child.

When possible, both parents should be present during the explanation. If only one parent is available, try to have another family member or support person available. It is important to begin to set the stage for the information to come with a phrase such as, "I am sorry, but I have bad news for you." Avoid the use of medical jargon; use terms that the family members understand. Frequently evaluate the parents' understanding of what they have been told. Truthfulness is essential during this period. Parents should be told everything possible, and uncertainties should be acknowledged.

Younger children should not be present initially when parents are being told of their illness or condition. Parents need an opportunity to process the information, express their emotions, and ask questions before revealing the news to the child.

Once parents receive their child's prognosis, they should be allowed time to process the information before sharing with others. Repeat information as necessary. Allow parents to set the pace of the interaction. They will make eye contact and ask questions when they are ready to continue. Care is taken to avoid the sense of being rushed. Acknowledge emotions and responses as being a normal reaction to receiving bad news (Serwint & Rutherford, 2000).

CLINICAL TIP

Questions such as "Who can I call for you right now?" and "What can I do for you and your family right now?" provide a sense of caring and acknowledge your willingness to assist the family during a difficult time.

Parents' Reactions to a Child's Death

The death of one's child is likely the most traumatic event a parent will experience. When the loss is sudden and unexpected, the abruptness adds a dimension of shock that may last for 4 to 5 weeks. When a child dies suddenly, the parents have no time to prepare themselves emotionally. The shock that accompanies the death of a child may be manifested by shortness of breath, a choking sensation, hyperventilation, loss of strength, and crying.

Grief is painful, individualized, and exhausting. Many factors influence the parents' grief responses, including their perception of the preventability of the illness or injury, the suddenness and circumstances of the death, the nature of their attachment to the child, previous losses, spiritual or religious orientation, and culture.

Although parents progress through distinct stages of grief, the timeline and nature of the grief process differ for each individual. The intense pain and shock initially felt by parents gradually give way to feelings of anger, guilt, depression, and loneliness. Very slowly, and with much support, energy returns and parents again begin to enjoy life experiences. Parents may process grief on different timelines. Spouses experiencing stages of grief at different levels may need additional support to prevent a sense of loneliness or isolation. Insomnia, fatigue, preoccupation with sleep, and decreased or increased activity level may also be experienced during the grieving process.

MediaLink Parental Reactions to Death of a Child Video

The Unexpected Death of a Child

The experience of a child's unexpected death is different from that of a death that was anticipated. A sudden or unexpected death that results from sudden infant death syndrome, injury, illness, suicide, or violence can lead to more intense grief, and take longer to resolve than grief experienced after an expected death (Menke, 2002). Parents and other family members have not had the opportunity to prepare for the child's death, and are not able to engage in anticipatory grieving and psychologic preparation. A child's suicide produces agonizing anger, guilt, and confusion: The fact that the child ended his or her own life compounds the feelings of guilt because parents may think they missed signs of the child's intentions. Parents need support to deal with the death of their child and to deal with their surviving children. Parents are often unavailable emotionally to the living children, requiring additional family members or close friends to offer support to those children. See Partnering with Families: Strategies for Working with Parents Whose Child Dies Suddenly.

The Death of a Newborn or Young Infant

Approximately 15,000 children are born each year who are dying at birth or who have conditions that are incompatible with prolonged life beyond the first year (Catlin & Carter, 2002). The death of a newborn forces the parents to experience their child's entire life cycle in a short period of time, and they are faced with overwhelming grief at a time when they anticipated the experience of joy. The death of a newborn may occur shortly after birth, in the hospital as a result of congenital anomalies, or at home as a result of sudden infant death syndrome (SIDS) (refer to Chapter 25∞ for further discussion of SIDS).

Unique situations arise when a multiple birth results in the death of one or more of the infants. The death of one twin, while the other twin lives, leads to conflicting emotions for parents. While they mourn the loss of one child, they must parent and bond with the survivor. Concerns arise as the parents may fear losing the other twin (Lundqvist, Nilstun, & Dykes, 2002).

The family experiencing the death of a newborn may appreciate an offer to take pictures of the baby and family together, if picture-taking is not prohibited by religious or cultural traditions. Some families may feel uncomfortable taking pictures with their dead baby and refuse the offer.

Wrap the baby in a blanket and offer the mother and other family members the opportunity to hold the baby. Offer the parents the opportunity to bathe and dress the infant. If the baby is disfigured, clothe or wrap the baby in a manner that optimizes his or her best physical characteristics. Some mothers may avoid a mother–child relationship and refuse to provide care or hold their dead or dying newborn.

The infant's blanket, hat, or lock of hair may be given to the parents as a keepsake. Handprints and footprints may be captured using ink pads or clay, and can be given to the parents.

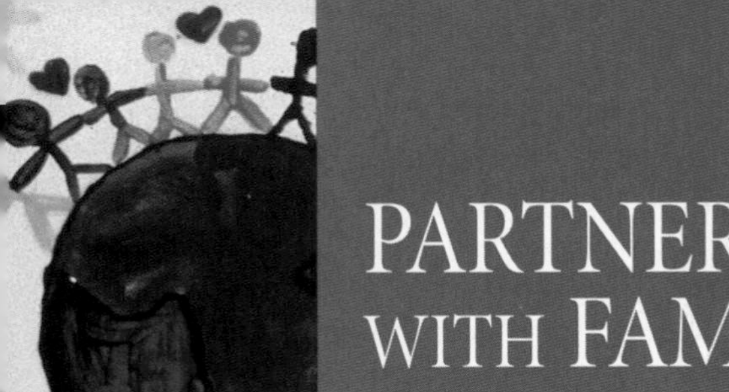

PARTNERING WITH FAMILIES

Strategies for Working with Parents Whose Child Dies Suddenly

The following strategies can assist the nurse in working with parents whose child dies suddenly.

- Identify a spokesperson for the medical team to keep the family informed during resuscitation efforts. Have both parents present if possible.
- Provide private space with telephone access.
- Create time for families to assimilate the child's worsening status by providing several updates during the resuscitation. Prepare them for what is to come.
- Offer to telephone clergy, family, and friends.
- After the death, prepare the body for viewing.
- Provide time and a place for the family to say good-bye.
- Sit close, make eye contact. Share your emotions with the family. Accept whatever emotions family members express.
- Convey information to the family about the cause of death, autopsy, funeral preparations, and the normal grief process.
- Arrange for family follow-up to see how they are responding to the child's loss and to review autopsy findings.

Data from Lipton, H., & Coleman, M. (1999). Bereavement practice guidelines for healthcare professionals in the emergency department. *Washington, DC: National Association of Social Workers.*

Some parents may initially refuse to take any of the baby's personal items or pictures. These items should be stored to allow the parents the opportunity to obtain them at a later date.

The nurse should question the family about baptism or other ritual requests for the newborn, and facilitate arrangements for a priest or pastor at the family's request. Another consideration is lactation; the mother experiencing the death of a newborn requires instructions on lactation suppression or milk donation options if she has been breastfeeding or pumping the breasts (Moore & Catlin, 2003).

Referral to a perinatal bereavement program or support group may help parents through the grieving process. Some facilities offer parental follow-up programs to assist with bereavement related to the death of an infant. Siblings anticipating the addition of a new baby to the family will also feel the loss. Children should be provided with information as they would for an older sibling's death.

Siblings' Reactions to a Child's Death

Siblings who experience the death of a brother or sister require supportive and compassionate care. In the course of the child's illness, the siblings may have received less attention from parents. Depending on their developmental level, they may fear that they caused their brother or sister to be injured or become ill, or worry that bad thoughts on their part brought on the illness. It is also not uncommon for the sibling to worry that he or she may also die. The nurse and other support personnel assist the child in adapting to their parents' grief, distraction, and increased protectiveness of them. Siblings need to understand that their parents' grief in no way diminishes the love they have for them.

When talking with the siblings of a dying child, honesty is most important (Figure 22–4 ■). Provide explanations in language that is developmentally appropriate. Reassure siblings that they did not cause their brother or sister to die and that death was not a punishment for wrongdoing. Allow the siblings to ask questions. Acknowledge the emotions they are feeling and emphasize that it is all right for them to be sad, angry, frightened, or tearful. Ask how they feel about saying good-bye to the dying child, and provide physical and emotional support. Prepare the siblings before they see the dying child by briefly explaining what they may see, feel, hear, and smell. Answer questions truthfully. The nurse may need to repeat information and offer explanations several times.

As appropriate and comfortable for the family, siblings should be permitted to participate in planning the child's memorial or funeral service; this provides them a sense of connection to the parents during a difficult time. Children should be allowed, but not forced, to attend the funeral. Prepare them for what to expect and provide a support person, a close family member or friend who can monitor the siblings' needs while the parents attend to other matters. Children may ask what happens to their sibling's soul or spirit and the response to the child is dependent on the family's spiritual and cultural beliefs. Prepare the sibling for "open-casket" visitation. Some families practice the ritual of kissing the deceased as a final farewell. Children should not be forced to kiss their dead sibling, and if they choose to do so, they should be informed that their brother or sister will "feel" cold.

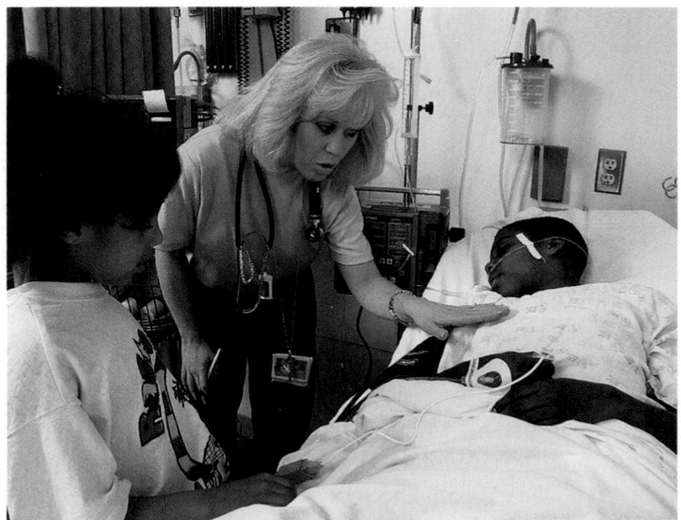

FIGURE 22–4 ■ During the sibling's visit with the dying child, it is important to talk with the sibling and answer any questions asked in an honest manner at a level the child can understand.

PARTNERING WITH FAMILIES

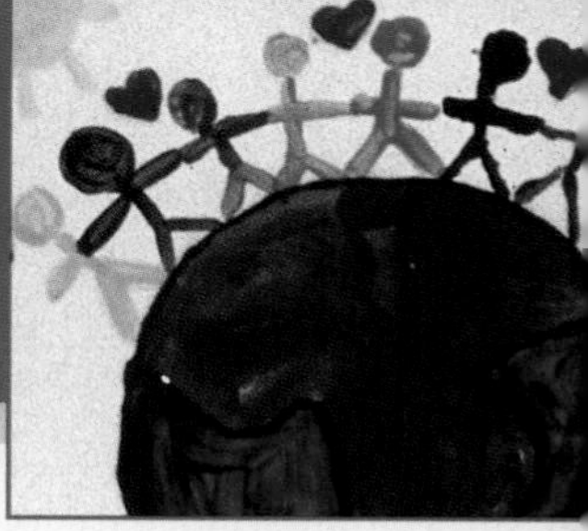

Strategies to Help Children and Adolescents Handle Grief

Nurses can share the following information with families when a child has died. Suggested strategies are provided according to developmental level.

Infants to age 3 years

- Provide a sense of security by being with the infant or child and by holding and hugging him or her.
- Verbally tell the infant or child you will be there to provide care.
- Try to return to usual routines.
- Be tolerant of regressive behaviors.
- Talk and answer questions.

Preschoolers

- Listen to the child and answer questions honestly.
- Try to return to usual routines and provide reassurance that you will be with the child.
- Be tolerant of regressive behaviors.
- Keep memories alive with pictures and other things that remind the child of the loved one.
- Participate in rituals such as going to the cemetery, releasing helium balloons, and planting flowers.
- Provide play activities.

School-Age children

- Listen to the child and answer questions honestly.
- Return to usual routines and activities.
- Keep memories alive through activities such as art, music, creating a memory book, sewing a quilt, and planting a garden.
- Share Internet resources.
- Use coping support groups.

Adolescents

- Be available and foster open communication.
- Share your own grief and feelings with the adolescent.
- Keep memories alive with pictures and other things that remind the child of the loved one.
- Access counseling and support groups.
- Share Internet resources.

Adapted from Menke, E. M. (2002). Handling children's grief at the first anniversary. Journal of Pediatric Health Care, 16*(5), 267–270.*

As with their parents, sibling bereavement is a lifelong process. Let children express all feelings, including sadness, guilt, and anger. When they perceive the level of parental distress, children may conceal feelings and suppress questions as a method of protecting their parents. Encourage siblings to express grief through art, stories, and writing.

Ensure that other caregivers and teachers are aware of and acknowledge a sibling's loss. The nurse can be instrumental in assisting an understanding of the child's death through a discussion with classmates, close friends, and other children affected by the death of the child. Children can be encouraged to celebrate their sibling's life by preparing collages of photographs, collecting the child's favorite toys and making a keepsake box, or even making a video about their sibling's life. See Partnering with Families: Strategies to Help Children and Adolescents Handle Grief.

Grandparents' Reactions to Death of Child

Grandparents grieve not only for the loss of their grandchild, but also for their bereaved adult children (Moffitt, 2001). Grandparents may experience uncertainty whether to openly share their grief with their bereaved children. They may feel they are adding further burden to their bereaved children by openly expressing their grief. On the other hand, some grandparents may feel the need to avoid expressing grief in the attempt to demonstrate that they are in control. The grandparents may wish to be included in the final arrangements, and some grandparents may assume the responsibility entirely to relieve some of their adult child's burden.

END-OF-LIFE NURSING CARE FOR THE DYING CHILD

Care of the dying child and family presents one of the greatest challenges to the nurse, requiring the utmost sensitivity and compassion. An understanding of the dying child's experiences during each developmental stage can assist the nurse in delivering individualized care to the child. See Box 22–7.

BOX 22–7 Research: Hospital Staff and Its Ability to Support Families

Nurse researchers conducted a questionnaire with 45 parents of children who died during a 2-year period at a regional children's hospital (Davies & Connaughty, 2002). Results revealed that only 14% of parents felt they had received adequate information regarding their child's deteriorating physical condition as death neared. Parents suggested that staff anticipate their needs and offer information accordingly, because parents do not know what to expect or ask. Additionally, the results indicated that staff should assess the parents' desire to discuss sensitive topics such as the child's impending death, funeral arrangements, and bereavement issues.

MediaLink Family-Centered Care Plan: The Death of a Child

NURSING MANAGEMENT

Nursing care of the dying child and family focuses on providing family-centered support for the physical and psychosocial needs of the child and family members.

Nursing Assessment and Diagnosis

Nursing assessment of the dying child and family includes a physiologic assessment of the child and a psychosocial assessment of all family members, assessment of cultural and spiritual influences of the child and individual family members, and an assessment of the child and family's social support system.

Physiologic Assessment of the Dying Child

Physiologic changes in the dying child are individualized according to the child's disease process or injury. However, certain basic processes are universal as death draws near (Box 22–8). The signs and symptoms of approaching death are discussed in the clinical manifestations table on the next page.

Psychosocial Assessment of the Dying Child

The dying child is usually aware of impending death even before being told. Parents may feel incapable of dealing directly with the child's questions about dying. They may feel that talking about the impending death takes away the child's hope. They may fear that they will be unable to cope with their own feelings during a frank discussion of the possibility of the child's imminent death. The types of questions that children may ask include the following:

- What will death be like?
- What will happen to me when I die? What happens after I die?
- Will I be punished for the bad things I have done?
- When will I be with [person(s) closest to child] again?
- Will my parents be all right?
- Will I experience much pain?
- What does heaven look like?
- Can you come with me?
- Will you remember me?

BOX 22–8 Manifestations of Death

- Absences of pulse and respirations
- Flat encephalogram
- Absence of reflexes
- Fixed and dilated pupils
- Release of urine and stool
- Pallor as blood settles to dependent areas
- Drop in body temperature

Some parents require help in understanding and answering the child's questions at a developmentally appropriate level for the child.

Psychosocial Assessment of the Dying Child's Family

Assessment of the family includes assisting family members to openly express their fears and concerns and to cope with the realization that the child is going to die. The nurse should be aware of the altered sensorium that individuals may experience during shock and disbelief. Parents may express feelings of numbness, helplessness, loneliness, and unreality.

Conduct an assessment of personal coping skills. Questions regarding previous and current losses, the nature of the loss, and the significance of the loss are explored to evaluate the individual's ability to cope. Information to discuss in the assessment includes general health status, cultural and spiritual traditions, rituals, beliefs related to loss and grieving, other stressors, and social support.

Assessing the spiritual needs of the child and family may include asking the following questions.

- Which spiritual rituals and resources have significance to the child and family?
- What is the child's understanding of the spiritual aspects surrounding life and death?

Assessing the cultural needs of the child and family may include asking the following questions.

- What are the cultural influences which have significance to the dying child and family?
- What are the cultural practices, rites, and rituals related to the dying child and family?

Examples of nursing diagnoses that apply to the dying child and family include the following:

- Fear (child) related to own impending death and unanswered questions
- Hopelessness (parental) related to the child's impending death
- Risk for Caregiver Role Strain related to parental care of dying child
- Disabled Family Coping related to sudden death of child
- Anticipatory Grieving related to imminent death of child

Planning and Implementation

Nursing care for the dying child and the family includes maintaining physiologic and psychologic comfort, assisting the child in a peaceful death, assisting the family and child with coping strategies, and facilitating grief (Figure 22–5 ■). Goals for the nurse providing palliative care for a dying child and the family are provided in Table 22–5 and in the nursing care plan on page 717.

Meet the Physiologic Needs of the Child

Pain during end of life is one of the greatest fears of the dying child and the family. A major goal of care of the dying child is to promote comfort and keep the child pain free. Narcotic anal-

CLINICAL MANIFESTATIONS of the Dying Child

SYSTEM	CLINICAL MANIFESTATIONS
Cardiovascular system	The heart rate may initially increase in an attempt for compensation, but as hypoxia develops, the heart rate and blood pressure decrease, resulting in decreased cardiac output. A change in pulse pressure and a decrease in the volume of Korotkoff's sounds is a predictive indicator of imminent death. Peripheral circulation decreases, leading to diaphoresis, clammy skin, and changes in skin coloring, which varies from mottled to cyanosis. The skin feels cool to touch. Blood begins pooling in the sacrum and lower back as a result of compromised perfusion. Mottling is considered a cardinal sign of imminent death.
Respiratory system	Impaired cardiac function and lymphatic congestion (due to the decreased protein levels in the blood) lead to pulmonary congestion and hypoxia. The child may exhibit diminished breath sounds, adventitious breath sounds, or both. Dyspnea (shortness of breath) is commonly reported in dying patients. **Air hunger,** the most severe form of dyspnea, may be manifested by a look of panic, gasping for breath, and sitting upright. Tachypnea may occur in combination with dyspnea. **Cheyne-Stokes respirations,** in which breathing becomes irregular with periods of shallow breathing alternating with periods of apnea, is a sign of imminent death. As the muscles relax, secretions accumulate in the oropharynx and bronchi. As air passes through these secretions a loud gurgling sound, known as the "death rattle," can be heard. This causes extreme distress in family members as they associate the sound with impending death. The child near death may moan or grunt when breathing. This is not uncommon and families should be assured that pain assessment and management are a continuous part of the child's care.
Neurologic system	Decreased cerebral perfusion, hypoxemia, metabolic acidosis, the influences of disease-related factors, and an accumulation of toxins from renal and liver failure can contribute to neurologic dysfunction in the dying child. The child may exhibit agitation during the final hours. Other signs may include withdrawal, increasing drowsiness, restlessness, confusion, and incontinence of bowel and bladder. The child may speak of visions of persons or objects not visible to others. Hearing and vision acuity may deteriorate, though it is important to remember that hearing is considered to be the last of the senses to diminish during death. The child may be unconscious during the final hours of death. Pain or discomfort may be increased, decreased, or remain the same for the child.
Musculoskeletal system	A decrease in muscular function leads to extreme muscle weakness and fatigue. Sensations and reflexes diminish. The child may be unable to reposition self, toilet self, or effectively expectorate accumulated respiratory secretions. Difficulty with swallowing also becomes apparent.
Renal system	Decreased kidney function and urine production results from the altered cardiac function. With altered cardiac output, intravascular blood volume diminishes, resulting in decreased renal perfusion. The kidneys will cease to function in response to decreased renal perfusion. Anuria occurs as a result of renal shutdown. Sphincters relax during the dying process and incontinence can occur.
Altered nutritional intake and fluid and electrolyte imbalances	Decreased oral fluid intake is normal during the dying process. Depending on the primary care provider, parenteral fluids may or may not be indicated as they may cause increased edema and increased respiratory secretions leading to shortness of breath and cough. The child may experience "third spacing," where fluids move into the extracellular spaces, causing edema and ascites. Anorexia and a decreased food intake are normal in the dying child. Parents are often distressed by the inability of their child to drink water or eat, since in most cultures food and drink are associated with comfort and health.

gesics may be prescribed and are administered routinely to promote optimal pain relief. For the child who remains alert, delivery of opioids via patient-controlled analgesia (PCA) pump is an option, as this provides the child with some sense of control. Oral or rectal pain medications are available for families who choose to withhold intravenous fluids. Nurses may also implement nonpharmacotherapeutic approaches to pain management such as distraction and guided imagery to children who are able to participate. Refer to Chapter 18∞ for detailed discussion of pain management of the child.

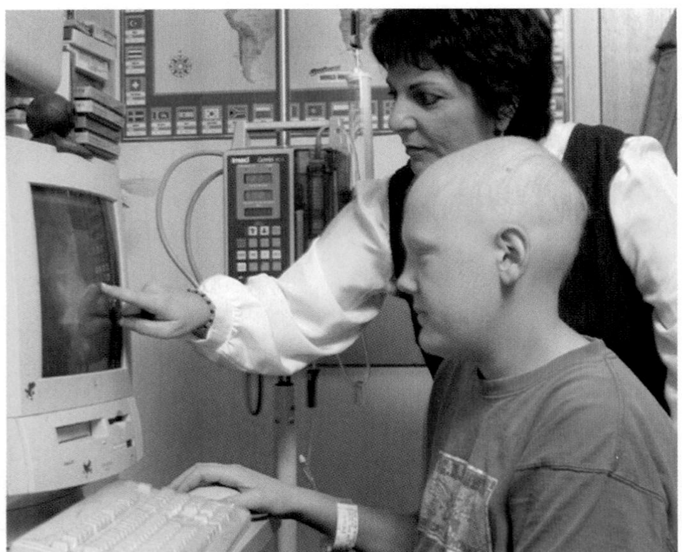

FIGURE 22–5 ■ A child and his mother explore chat rooms for terminally ill children receiving palliative care.

Morphine or another opioid may be prescribed for air hunger or tachypnea. Morphine dilates the pulmonary vessels, reduces oxygen consumption, and decreases pulmonary congestion. Elevate the head of the bed, open a window, or use a circulating fan if the child is experiencing air hunger. Table 22–6 provides additional information on meeting the physiologic needs of the dying child.

Meet the Psychologic Needs of the Dying Child and Family

The ability of the nurse to communicate and offer support will depend on the child and family's awareness of the impending death. The child and family may share one of three types of awareness.

- In **closed awareness,** the child is unaware of impending death. The child and family may not understand why the child is ill, and they may believe the child's condition will improve.
- **Mutual pretense** exists when the child, family, and healthcare personnel know that the outcome is terminal but do not discuss the subject. Mutual pretense leaves the dying child with no one in whom to confide.
- With **open awareness,** the child and family, as well as other members of the healthcare team, are aware of the impending death and are comfortable with discussing the situation, even though this may prove difficult for them.

Promote a trusting nurse–child–family relationship. Be honest in responses to the child and family. Allow opportunities for communication by listening and being present (Box 22–9). The nurse's acceptance of the child's and family's feelings and attitudes helps to promote trust. Demonstrate respect for the child's and family's religion, culture, and values.

Provide the child with opportunities for fantasy play, drawings, and storytelling, without emphasizing or reinforcing death themes. Listen to what children tell you about themselves and their lives. **Death imagery,** references to death or death-related topics (going away, separation, and funerals), or anticipated experiences with treatment may be themes of their stories. These themes are expected and do not reflect repression or other pathology.

CLINICAL TIP

Provide children an opportunity to tell you about themselves. For example, sitting with a child and reviewing family photos provides the child an opportunity to share as well as providing them time to discuss their feelings.

TABLE 22–5 Common Family Goals and Nursing Interventions for Palliative Care

GOAL	NURSING INTERVENTIONS
Physical comfort	Prevent or relieve a child's pain fatigue or other symptoms through the use of medication and behavioral interventions. Support improved function and pain relief with physical therapy.
Emotional comfort	Use various techniques to provide comfort, such as psychotherapy, play, art, music, and other expressive therapies. Encourage visits from family and friends.
Normal life	Promote maintenance of normal routines as long as possible. Involve the child in decision making (consistent with intellectual and emotional maturity). Plan for the child's return to school in collaboration with teachers and school administrators. Organize travel or camp experiences. Refer family to organizations such as Make a Wish Foundation and Starlight Foundation.
Family functioning	Help parents make special time for siblings. Support and encourage the parents to use respite care and assist the family in making arrangements.
Cultural or spiritual values	Accommodate religious rituals and traditional customs. Encourage families to continue or adapt family holiday traditions.
Preparing for death	Talk with families about their preferences for who will be present at the time of the child's death. Help families develop remembrances or legacies of the child's life including pictures, videos, locks of hair, and handprints or handmolds.

Adapted from Institute of Medicine (2003). When children die: Improving palliative and end-of-life care for children and their families. *Washington, DC: National Academies Press, p. 128.*

TABLE 22–6 Nursing Care for the Child at End-of-Life

PHYSIOLOGIC NEED	NURSING INTERVENTIONS
Airway clearance	Place the conscious child in Fowler's position to promote effective airway clearance. Place the unconscious child in lateral position to promote effective airway clearance. Suction oral and throat secretions as needed. Maintain oxygen as indicated for hypoxia.
Bathing/hygiene	To maintain dry and intact skin: Maintain dry bed linens and bathe diaphoretic child frequently. Provide frequent oral care as needed for dry mouth. Apply lotions and creams for dry skin (encourage parents to participate in this activity). Apply moisture barrier skin preparations for incontinence.
Elimination	Encourage dietary fiber intake as tolerated to avoid constipation. Administer stool softeners or laxatives as indicated. Provide call light within reach for assistance onto bedpan or commode. Ensure that bedpan, urinal, or commode chair are within easy access. Place absorbent pads under incontinent child; change linen as often as indicated. Perform catheterization if necessary. Maintain clean and odor-free room.
Nutrition	Administer antiemetics for vomiting. Encourage liquid foods as tolerated. Provide the child with preferred foods—family may bring the child's favorite foods from home. Encourage family participation at meal time.
Physical mobility	Reposition the bedridden child at frequent intervals (every 2 hours or as indicated). Support the child's position with pillows, blanket rolls, or towels as needed. Use pressure-relieving surfaces as indicated. If the child is able to sit in chair, assist the child out of bed periodically.
Sensory/perceptual changes	Monitor child's blood pressure, heart rate, and tolerance to activity when sitting up. Ask the child's (if alert) preference for light in room. When addressing the child or other individuals in the room, speak clearly and do not whisper (recall that hearing is not diminished). Maintain wrinkle-free linens. Implement pain management protocol if indicated.

Collaborate with the parents and provide guidance about appropriate methods and words to use that will support the child (Box 22–10). Some parents may prefer that the child's questions be answered honestly by another professional. A professional who has special training in bereavement counseling can assist children and families with discussions.

When caring for adolescents, remember that outbursts of anger are common but not personally directed at the nurse. Provide activities to help adolescents channel their feelings. Continue providing support despite their behavior. This approach may encourage adolescents to accept comforting without losing face. Be available to listen when the adolescent wants to talk and express feelings and frustrations. Promote friendships with other adolescents having similar interests or problems. Provide adolescents with as much independence and control over their situation as possible. Include the adolescent in the decision-making process

BOX 22–9 Communicating with the Family

- Be honest and truthful. Encourage and respond to questions.
- Do not abandon the patient/family.
- Elicit and request the family's values and goals and provide as much help as possible to achieve them.
- Help patients explore their realistic options.
- Take the time to listen.
- Be supportive, but avoid offering unrealistic hope.

BOX 22–10 Strategies for Talking with a Dying Child

- Be flexible.
- Recognize that some children communicate best through nonverbal means (e.g., art or music). The child may be willing to talk through a puppet or a stuffed animal.
- Respect the child's need to be alone and his or her desire to share. Allow communication, but do not force it.
- Be receptive when children initiate a conversation.
- Be specific and literal in explanation of death.
- Acknowledge that a child's life can be complete, even if it is brief. Let dying children know they will always be loved and remembered. Help them find a sense of accomplishment and purpose in the lives they have led.
- Empower children as much as possible in circumstances concerning their deaths. Reassure them of continued love and physical closeness.

From Faulkner, K. W. (1997). Talking about death with a dying child. American Journal of Nursing, *97(6), 64–69.*

and provide them the opportunity to express their feelings, concerns, and wishes. Answer questions honestly without using a condescending tone.

Work closely with the family when the child's death is imminent, because they will remember the experience and words spoken for the rest of their lives. Prepare the family for changes in the child's appearance and behavior. Providing parents with a room in which to be alone with the child ensures privacy at this extremely personal time. Ask the family in a nonjudgmental, supportive manner what is important to them in the last moments or hours of their child's life and what will be important to them in the grief process.

Holding the child is a universal request and is always permitted. Many families find that saying good-bye as a group is helpful. Families need the opportunity to cry together and to tell each other how much they will miss the child. They also should be assured that the death vigil is important, so the child does not feel isolated or abandoned as death approaches. The dying child should never be left alone when death is imminent.

CLINICAL TIP

When the child's death is imminent and parents are incapable of remaining with the child due to emotional distress, arrange for another family member or close person to remain with the child. If no one is available, a nurse (or other member of the healthcare team with whom the child is familiar) should remain present to ensure that the child does not die alone.

Encourage the parents to communicate with the dying child. Let them know that they can hold, stroke, kiss, and talk soothingly to the child, which may offer comfort to both child and parents and facilitate their grieving. The family can also be encouraged to lie in the bed and "snuggle" with the dying child. This offers support and comfort to both the child and family. Encourage parents to maintain their parental role by continuing with caregiving activities such as bathing or dressing the child for the last time.

Some parents may feel they need to give the child "permission" to die by telling the child "mommy and daddy are going to be alright," or some other phrase that communicates this message to the child.

Promote Spiritual and Cultural Needs

The nurse discusses the family's spiritual needs and arranges access to those individuals who can provide spiritual care. (See Developing Cultural Competence: Spiritual Assistance.) To provide family-centered care, nurses must be aware of their own spiritual issues and avoid imposing their own religious or spiritual beliefs on the family. Interventions may include locating appropriate clergy or spiritual leaders for the family and facilitating the establishment of an environment in which the family may pray, meditate, or engage in other spiritual practices.

The nurse partners with the family to determine their spiritual and cultural preferences related to death rituals. It is important for the nurse to determine who will be responsible for carrying out the activities. For example, cultural rituals may include special procedures for washing, dressing, shrouding, and positioning the dead. Identify which family member will perform the cultural rituals. Refer to Chapter 3 for further discussion of cultural influences on the child and family.

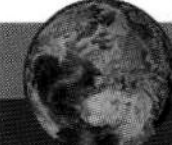

DEVELOPING CULTURAL COMPETENCE
Spiritual Assistance

Depending on the family's cultural and religious beliefs, a chaplain or other healthcare professional specializing in the care of terminally ill children and families may help reduce a child's spiritual fears and promote peace and comfort among family members. The nurse asks the family about specific cultural and religious needs and facilitates arranging for chaplains, priests, or other religious or cultural representatives. Special rites or ceremonies may be requested and should be accommodated when possible.

Promote Social Support System

Help the child maintain contact with peers on the hospital unit as long as the child has energy to benefit from the companionship. Interaction with peers reduces the child's feelings of isolation.

Support from others facilitates grief work and decreases feelings of loneliness and isolation. Assist family members in identifying their social support systems and refer them to sources such as social services, religious leaders, and bereavement groups to assist them during the child's impending death.

Facilitating Grief

The nurse collaborates with the family and other support persons, including grief counselors, to assist the family in understanding what to expect during the grief process. Include the family's cultural, religious, and personal values when encouraging the child and family to express grief. Encourage the child and family to express their grief as appropriate to their cultural customs. Inform the child and family that certain emotions such as fear, sadness, guilt, and anger are normal responses to grief. Informing the family of the stages of grief and what to expect reassures them that their reactions are a normal response to grief and loss.

Care in the Community

The family may choose hospice or home health care for the dying child. The nurse collaborates with home healthcare agencies, a hospice care agency, support groups, and other resources to facilitate the child and family's transition to home care or hospice care. Refer to previous discussion in this chapter regarding hospice or home health care.

■ Evaluation

Expected outcomes of caring for the dying child and family may include the following:

- The child is pain free and comfortable, and physiologic needs are met.

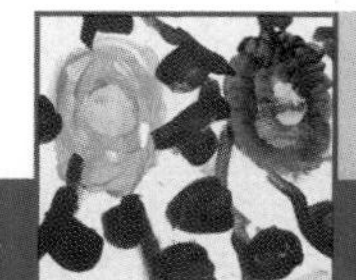

Nursing Care Plan

THE DYING CHILD

GOAL	INTERVENTION	RATIONALE	EXPECTED OUTCOME
1. Fear (parents) related to being alone and separated from support system at the time of the child's death			
	NIC Priority Intervention—*Coping Enhancement:* Assisting a parent to adapt to perceived stressors, changes, or threats which interfere with meeting life demands and roles		**NOC Suggested Outcome**—*Fear Control:* Ability to eliminate or reduce disabling feelings of alarm aroused by an identifiable source
The parents will have reduced fears related to remaining with the dying child during the death vigil.	▪ Provide information to the family about the signs and symptoms of approaching death.	▪ Information about expected changes in breathing patterns, consciousness level, agitation, ability to swallow, and cool skin reduce anxiety in parents when these changes occur.	Parents will take an active role in caring for the dying child. Parents seek support of family members or friends during the death vigil.
	▪ Encourage parents to invite close family members or friends to share the death vigil.	▪ Presence of supportive family and friends reduces parents' feeling of isolation.	
	▪ Ask the family if they would like to have a spiritual leader notified or present.	▪ A spiritual leader often provides comfort and enables the family to cope with the death.	
	▪ Provide information about the nursing interventions and medications used to keep the child comfortable and that regular assessments of the child's comfort are performed.	▪ Parents often fear that the child will have a painful death or that giving the pain medication will cause the child's death.	
	▪ Provide information about comfort measures parents can provide to the child, such as singing, massage, providing warm blankets, a cool cloth to the head, praying, or reading.	▪ Providing comfort gives the parents an active role in the child's care and a sense of purpose.	
	▪ Educate the parents about the signs and symptoms of death and what to do if they suspect the child has died.	▪ Parents often fear being alone when the child dies and not knowing how to react or what to do.	
2. Impaired Adjustment (parents) related to intense emotional state following the child's death			
	NIC Priority Intervention—*Coping Enhancement:* Assisting a patient to adapt to perceived stressors, changes, or threats which interfere with meeting life demands and roles		**NOC Suggested Outcome**—*Psychosocial Adjustment: Life Change:* Psychosocial adaptation of an individual to a life change
The parents will adjust to the immediate loss of the child and begin to make funeral or memorial service plans.	▪ Remove medical supplies, equipment, and tubing from the room. Cover leaking wounds and use a diaper as needed for incontinence.	▪ Removing medical supplies helps the family see the dead child as a loved family member rather than as a patient.	The parents say good-bye to the child and take the next steps in planning a funeral or memorial service.
	▪ Ask the family if they have preferences for the bathing or care of the body or for dressing the dead child.	▪ This honors cultural practices and shows respect for the child and family.	
	▪ Encourage parents to hold the child, and provide as much time as needed to say good-bye.	▪ Providing time will facilitate closure. Time may be needed for other family members to arrive and say good-bye.	
	▪ Offer to assist with phone calls to family, friends, spiritual leaders.	▪ Some parents are unable to make needed phone calls immediately and may appreciate assistance.	
	▪ Assist with decision making for the funeral or memorial service arrangements as needed.	▪ Providing options helps promote family choice.	
	▪ Provide follow-up bereavement support with phone calls and cards. Refer the family to community bereavement resources.	▪ Follow-up contact lets the family know that they and the child are not forgotten. An assessment of the need for ongoing bereavement support can be made.	

- The child's other physiologic needs are met.
- The cultural and spiritual needs of the dying child and family are met.
- The dying child and family receive support during the dying process.
- The family receives continued support after the child's death.

NURSING CARE FOLLOWING THE DEATH OF A CHILD

After the child's death, allow the family to spend as much time as they need with the child's body. Never rush family members who are saying good-bye to the child. Save all of the child's personal items—especially in the case of an infant, whose parents may have few mementos. A lock of hair, hand or foot prints, the infant's identification band, the child's weight and height, the last clothes or patient gown worn by the child sealed in a plastic bag to retain the child's scent, or a picture of the infant can be sources of comfort and remembrance for families. Always ask the parents before cutting a lock of the child's hair. Some cultures and religions forbid the cutting of hair.

CLINICAL TIP

It may be traumatic for parents to receive the child's possessions, and placing them in a plastic garbage bag is insensitive. When possible, a special container should be used for this purpose.

Postmortem Care

Nursing personnel are responsible for conducting or supervising the care of the body after death. Follow the policy of the institution for postmortem care. Religious or cultural practices may influence the manner in which the care of the body is delivered. The nurse determines the family's wishes for postmortem care before performing any care. Ask family members before removing any jewelry or other item from the child because cultural or spiritual practices may specify that the jewelry or article remain on the child after death.

The child is positioned according to protocol or cultural/religious practices, the room is cleaned, and all medical equipment (e.g., tubes, suction equipment) should be removed to provide a clean environment before the family views the child's body. Do not remove the body from the room until the family acknowledges they are ready. They may be waiting on other family members or friends to view the body. Parents may require direction about resources available to help with a memorial service or funeral. Refer them to support personnel who can assist them in making these arrangements.

MediaLink Resources and Support for Families

Psychosocial Support

Advise parents that certain dates—such as the day of the week the child died, the child's birthday, or family holidays—may be difficult and possibly trigger intense sadness. Parents may benefit from keeping a journal of their thoughts and memories, or writing letters or poems to or about their child.

Emphasize to parents that although the period surrounding their child's death is difficult, caring for themselves physically and mentally is important. Parents may experience friction because each may move through the stages of grief at different rates and with different intensity. For example, a father in denial may be unable to offer support to a mother experiencing anger or depression. The family is supported in order to achieve a positive resolution of the grieving process. It is important to inform grieving parents that although their pain may diminish as time passes, they will revisit their loss for the remainder of their lives (Box 22–11).

A list of appropriate support groups, books, and articles can be given to parents for later use. Parents can be referred to national organizations, such as the Candlelighters Foundation or Compassionate Friends, and to local support groups for bereaved parents or siblings who may feel isolated and alone. Some institutions have formal follow-up programs for bereaved parents to encourage a healthy progression through the grieving process.

Care in the Community

Following the death of a child, parents and families may require ongoing care to assist them in adapting to the loss of a child. Home care follow-up serves as a bridge between the support the family received at the time of death and their need for continued support in adapting to life at home following the death of their child.

BOX 22–11 Suggestions for a Healthy Grieving Process

Nurses can assist families toward a healthy grieving process after a child's death with the following information.

- Explain that grief exerts tremendous stress on even the most loving relationships.
- Encourage parents to show their emotions so youngsters will learn and understand appropriate grieving behavior.
- Alert parents to the special needs of young children, who may feel guilty about the death due to unresolved sibling rivalries.
- Advise parents to be watchful for their adolescents' responses to the death through withdrawal or the use of alcohol, drugs, or sexual activity.
- Recommend open lines of communication between parents and bereaved siblings.
- Explain that many family members and friends may distance themselves because they are uneasy with death and grief.
- Caution families to expect especially difficult emotional times during major holidays and anniversary dates of the child's birth and death.

Adapted from Moffitt, P. (2001). The impact of the child's death on the extended family. Journal of Child and Family Nursing, *4(2), 152–155.*

Family follow-up support is essential to facilitating the family's grief. Especially in the case of an unexpected death, the family may not have understood all of the information provided to them at the time of their child's death. A follow-up visit provides parents the opportunity to ask questions at a later time. If an autopsy has been performed, explaining the results may clarify uncertainties and assist the parents through their grieving process.

NURSES' REACTIONS TO CARING FOR THE DYING CHILD

Children are highly valued by society because of their potential future contributions. Children are expected to have a normal life span, and the death of a child is often viewed as a tragedy. Caring for dying children is especially stressful and demanding for healthcare professionals. Nurses involved in long-term relationships with children experience severe grief when these children die. Some nurses may cope by distancing themselves socially from the dying child and family to maintain composure and a professional demeanor and to protect themselves from the pain of repeated loss. Caring for the dying child may be especially difficult for nurses with young children of their own. They tend to identify with the child, making it more likely that they will have difficulty dealing with the death in a professional manner.

CLINICAL TIP

Although crying with families was once considered unprofessional to some, it is now recognized as an expression of caring and empathy. Nurses should feel free to express their sorrow and grief for the child and family.

Nurses may feel unable to adequately intervene with the anxiety and fears experienced by the dying child and family due to their own personal defenses against their sense of helplessness to alter the course of the child's disease. Nurses who work with children who are terminally ill and their families require special preparation to meet the needs of these individuals and to manage personal stress simultaneously. Mentorship with experienced hospice nurses, as well as additional educational experiences, may help promote professional nursing care. Nurses who work with dying children and families must learn to cope effectively with grief and to develop empathy, competence, and confidence in their ability to provide more humane and effective nursing care. Sharing grief with the family after a child's death assists both the nurse and family to cope with their feelings about the loss. Nurses should also understand that experiencing a child's death and the family's grief may reactivate feelings about unresolved grief in their own lives.

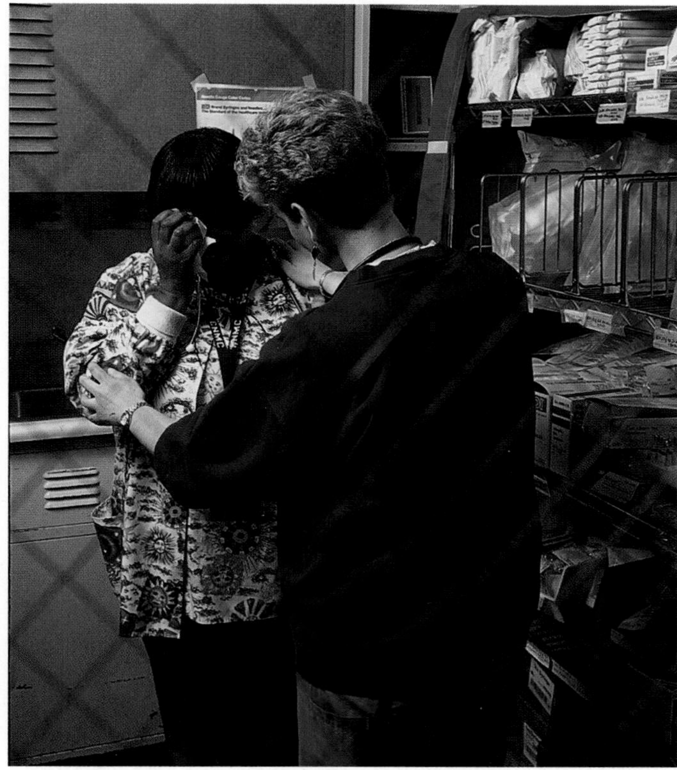

FIGURE 22–6 ■ Nurses need to express their own grief in a supportive environment after a child's death. Nurses who do not share the sadness and grief or futility of resuscitation efforts with colleagues may be unable to continue to provide supportive care to the next families who need compassionate care.

Nurses who work in emergency departments caring for children who die suddenly, or in hospice settings and hospital units caring for terminally ill children, need support systems to help balance the stresses of working with dying children. The workplace should acknowledge the stress and overwhelming feelings nurses experience when working with terminally ill children or those who die unexpectedly. Support systems may include discussions with peers or debriefing group sessions with mental health professionals that provide an opportunity to discuss their feelings and concerns (Figure 22–6 ■). Participating in team decisions regarding the dying child's plan of care (palliative rather than curative) helps many nurses manage their distress.

Nurses may be requested by the family to attend the child's funeral services, or they may personally desire to attend the funeral. Attending the services may assist the nurses with their own grieving and promote closure. Additionally, the presence of nurses who provided care to the child may offer the family continued support as this displays a meaningful way of demonstrating their care for the deceased child and the family.

MediaLink Grief Resources for Nurses

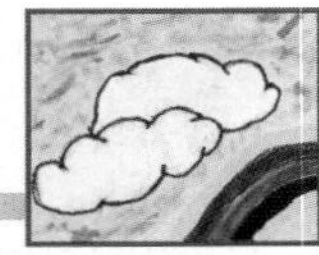

CHAPTER HIGHLIGHTS

- The child's developmental level, culture, spirituality, and parental support directly affect the child's response to loss, death, and grief.
- Children may experience loss through death of a parent, grandparent, pet, or friend, and through losses associated with relocation, trauma, and loss of an object.
- It is essential to work closely with the family when a child's death is imminent, helping to provide the support and services most important to them in the last moments or hours of their child's life.
- Children with life-threatening illnesses often learn about death and their own illness through exposure to other ill and dying children. Even if they have not been told they are dying, they will know their condition is worsening with extra treatments, feeling ill, and cues from their parents.
- The families of dying children are faced with many decision-making issues such as do-not-resuscitate requests, palliative and/or hospice care, the withholding or withdrawing of treatments, and organ and tissue donation.
- Palliative care combines therapies to comfort and support persons with a short life expectancy, by providing therapies to improve the quality of remaining life.
- The nurse caring for the dying child and family offers physiologic and psychosocial support during end-of-life care.
- Caring for a dying child is difficult, and nurses need special preparation to meet the needs of the child and family while managing their own personal stress.

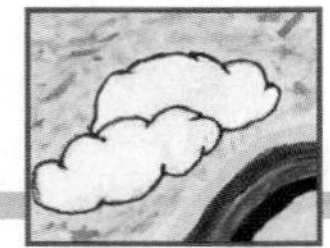

CRITICAL THINKING IN ACTION

INTRODUCTION

Recall Zachary, the 3-year-old child with an inoperable brain tumor hospitalized and near death. His seizures and dehydration are being treated. He is also receiving morphine for pain. His mother remains at his bedside while his father and other family members visit.

DESCRIPTION

Despite aggressive therapy, Zachary's condition has continued to deteriorate. After consulting with Zachary's healthcare team, the parents agree to discontinue the radiation and aggressive treatment. He will continue to receive antiseizure medications, pain medication, and nutrition. They have requested a do-not-resuscitate order and the family wishes to have time with Zachary to say goodbye. The parents want guidance to help Marilee say goodbye.

DISCUSSION

1. What role does the hospital nurse play in facilitating hospice care for Zachary?
2. What other decisions should be made regarding Zachary's continued treatment and care?
3. Based on Marilee's developmental level, what is her understanding of Zachary's imminent death? What nursing interventions should be offered?
4. Identify at least three priority nursing diagnoses for Zachary's family during the transition from hospitalized care to hospice care.
5. Develop a family-centered nursing care plan for Zachary's hospice care.

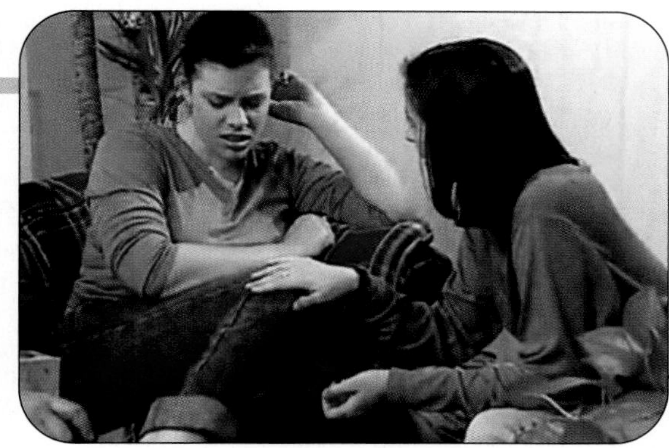

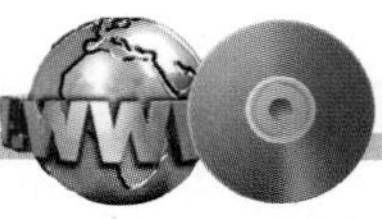

EXPLORE MediaLink

- NCLEX review, case studies, and other interactive resources for this chapter can be found on the Companion Website at **www.prenhall.com/ball**. Click on Chapter 22 to select the activities for this chapter.
- For animations, more NCLEX review questions, and an audio glossary, access the accompanying CD-ROM in this book.

http://www.prenhall.com/ball

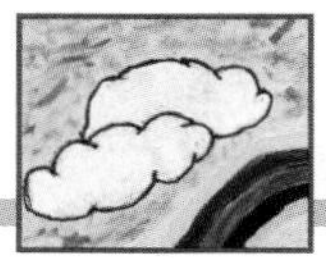

REFERENCES

American Academy of Pediatrics. (2000a). Policy statement: Do not resuscitate orders in schools. *Pediatrics, 105*(4), 878–879.

American Academy of Pediatrics. Committee on Bioethics and Committee on Hospital Care. (2000b). Palliative care for children. *Pediatrics, 106*(2), 351–357.

American Academy of Pediatrics. (2000b). Palliative care for children. *Pediatrics, 106*(2), 351–357.

American Association of Colleges of Nursing. (1999). *Peaceful death: Recommended competencies and curricular guidelines for end-of-life nursing care.* Washington, DC: AACN.

American Nurses Association. (2003a). Position statement: Active euthanasia. www.nursingworld.org/readroom/position/ethics/eteuth.htm, accessed 7/20/2004.

American Nurses Association. (2003b). Position statement: Assisted suicide. www.nursingworld.org/readroom/position/ethics/etsuic.htm, accessed 7/20/2004.

Barnes, L. L., Plotnikoff, G. A., Fox, K., & Pendleton, S. (2000). Spirituality, religion, and pediatrics: Intersecting worlds of healing (Part 2). *Pediatrics, 106*(4), 899–909.

Busch, T., & Kimble, C. S. (2001). Grieving children. Are we meeting the challenge? *Pediatric Nursing, 27*(4), 414–418.

Catlin, A., & Carter, B. (2002). Creation of a neonatal end-of-life palliative care protocol. *Neonatal Network, 21*(4), 37–49.

Chaffee, S. (2001). Pediatric palliative care. *Primary Care: Clinics in Office Practice, 28*(2), 365–390.

Christ, G. H., Siegel, K., & Christ, A. E. (2002). Adolescent grief: "It never really hit me . . . until it actually happened." *JAMA, 288*(10), 1269–1278.

Clements, P. T., Benasutti, K. M., & Carmone, A. (2003). Support for bereaved owners of pets. *Perspectives in Psychiatric Care, 39*(2), 49.

Cole, L. (2003). Say when . . . end-of-life decisions in PICU. *Pediatric Nursing, 29*(2), 138–139.

Contro, N., Larson, J., Scofield, S., Sourkes, B., & Cohen, H. (2002). Family perspectives on the quality of pediatric palliative care. *Archives of Pediatric and Adolescent Medicine, 156*(1), 14–19.

Davies, B., Brenner, P., Orloff, S., Sumner, L., & Worden, W. (2002). Addressing spirituality in pediatric hospice and palliative care. *Journal of Palliative Care, 18*(1), 59–68.

Davies, B., & Connaughty, S. (2002). Pediatric end-of-life care: Lessons learned from parents. *The Journal of Nursing Administration, 32*(1), 5–6.

Davies, B., Cook, K., O'Loane, M., Clarke, D., MacKenzie, B., Stutzer, C., Connaughty, S., & McCormick, J. (1996). Caring for dying children: Nurses' experiences. *Pediatric Nursing, 22*(6), 500–507.

Faulkner, K. W. (1997). Talking about death with a dying child. *American Journal of Nursing, 97*(6), 64–69.

Ferrell, B. R., & Coyle, N. (2002). An overview of palliative care. *American Journal of Nursing, 102*(5), 26–31.

Ferri, R. S., & Safer, D. (2002). Grieving mothers of stillborn infants. *American Journal of Nursing, 102*(10), 18.

Flannelly, K. J., Weaver, A. J., & Costa, K. G. (2004). A systematic review of religion and spirituality in three palliative care journals, 1990–1999. *Journal of Palliative Care, 20*(1), 50–56.

Goldman, L. (2004). Counseling with children in contemporary society. *Journal of Mental Health Counseling, 26*(2), 168–187.

Haddad, A. (2000). Ethics in action. *RN, 63*(11), 21–23.

Health Resources and Services Administration, Maternal and Child Health Bureau. (2002). *Child health USA, 2002.* Rockville, MD: U.S. Department of Health and Human Services.

Heilferty, C. M. (2004). Spiritual development and the dying child: The pediatric nurse practitioner's role. *Journal of Pediatric Health Care, 18*(6), 271–275.

Hickman, S. E., Tilden, V. P., & Tolle, S. W. (2004). Family perceptions of worry, symptoms, and suffering in the dying. *Journal of Palliative Care, 20*(1), 20–27.

Institute of Medicine. (2003). Patterns of childhood death in America. In *When children die: Improving palliative and end-of-life care for children and their families* (pp. 41–71). Washington, DC: National Academy Press.

Klopfenstein, K. J., & Young-Saleme, T. (2002). Your role in the spectrum of adolescent cancer: Diagnosis through treatment to care at life's end. *Contemporary Pediatrics, 19*(8), 105–127.

Kübler-Ross, E. (1969). *On death and dying.* New York: Macmillan.

Kübler-Ross, E. (1983). *On children and death.* New York: Macmillan.

Lewis, L., Brecher, M., Reaman, G. H., & Sahler, O. J. (2002). How you can help meet the needs of dying children. *Contemporary Pediatrics, 19*(4), 147–159.

Lipton, H., & Coleman, M. (1999). *Bereavement practice guidelines for health care professionals in the emergency department.* Washington, DC: National Association of Social Workers.

Lundqvist, A., Nilstun, T., & Dykes, A. (2002). Experiencing neonatal death: An ambivalent transition into motherhood. *Pediatric Nursing, 28*(6), 621–626.

Mazanec, P., & Tyler, M. K. (2003). Cultural considerations in end-of-life care. *American Journal of Nursing, 103*(3), 50–58.

McCaffrey, A. M., Eisenberg, D. M., Legedza, A. T. R., Davis, R. B., & Phillips, R. S. (2004, April 26). Prayer for health concerns: Results of a national survey on prevalence and patterns of use. *Archives of Internal Medicine, 164,* 858–862.

Meier, E. (2002). Effects of trauma and war on children. *Pediatric Nursing, 28*(6), 626–629.

Menke, E. M. (2002). Handling children's grief at the first anniversary. *Journal of Pediatric Health Care, 16*(5), 267–270.

Meyer, E. C., Burns, J. P., Griffith, J. L., & Truog, R. D. (2002). Parental perspectives on end-of-life care in the pediatric intensive care unit. *Critical Care Medicine, 30*(1), 226–231.

Moffit, P. (2001). The impact of a child's death on the extended family. In D. Dokken & N. Syndnor-Greenberg (Eds.), *Journal of Child and Family Nursing, 4*(2), 152–155.

Moore, D. B., & Catlin, A. (2003). Lactation suppression: Forgotten aspect of care for the mother of a dying child. *Pediatric Nursing, 29*(5), 383–384.

Nelson, L. (1995). When a child dies: Practical, sensitive advice for helping parents through their worst nightmare. *American Journal of Nursing, 95*(3), 61–64.

Ramer-Chrastek, J. (2000). Hospice care for a terminally-ill child in the school setting. *Journal of School Nursing, 16*(2), 52–56.

Ramer-Chrastek, J., Brunnquell, D., & Hasse, S. (2002). Letting nature take its course. *American Journal of Nursing, 102*(10), 24CC–24JJ.

Rivlin, D. (2001). Books for children when a friend dies. *Contemporary Pediatrics, 18*(10), 134–138.

Rushton, C. H. (2004). Ethics and palliative care in pediatrics. *American Journal of Nursing, 104*(4), 54–63.

Rushton, C. H., & Catlin, A. (2002). Pediatric palliative care: The time is now! *Pediatric Nursing, 28*(1), 57–70.

Serwint, J. R., & Rutherford, L. (2000). Sharing bad news with parents. *Contemporary Pediatrics, 17*(3), 45–66.

Smith, S. (2003). Organ and tissue donation and recovery. Organ Transplant. www.medscape.com/viewarticle/451208, accessed 4/9/2003.

Stephenson, J. (2000). Palliative and hospice care needed for children with life-threatening conditions. *Journal of the American Medical Association, 284*(19), 2437–2438.

Stutts, A., & Schloemann, J. (2002). Life-sustaining support: Ethical, cultural, and spiritual conflicts. Part I: Family support—a neonatal case study. *Neonatal Network, 21*(3) 23–36.

Task Force for the Determination of Brain Death in Children. (1987). Guidelines for the determination of brain death in children. *Neurology, 37*, 1077–1078.

Vickers, J. L., & Carlisle, C. (2000). Choice and control: Parental experiences in pediatric terminal home care. *Journal of Pediatric Oncology Nursing, 17*(1), 12–21.

Waechter, E. H. (1987). Children's reactions to fatal illness. In T. Krulik, B. Holaday, & I. M. Martinson (Eds.), *The child and family facing life-threatening illness.* Philadelphia: Lippincott.

World Health Organization. (2001). Palliative care. www.who.int/hiv/topics/palliative/PalliativeCare/en/print.html, accessed 7/11/203.

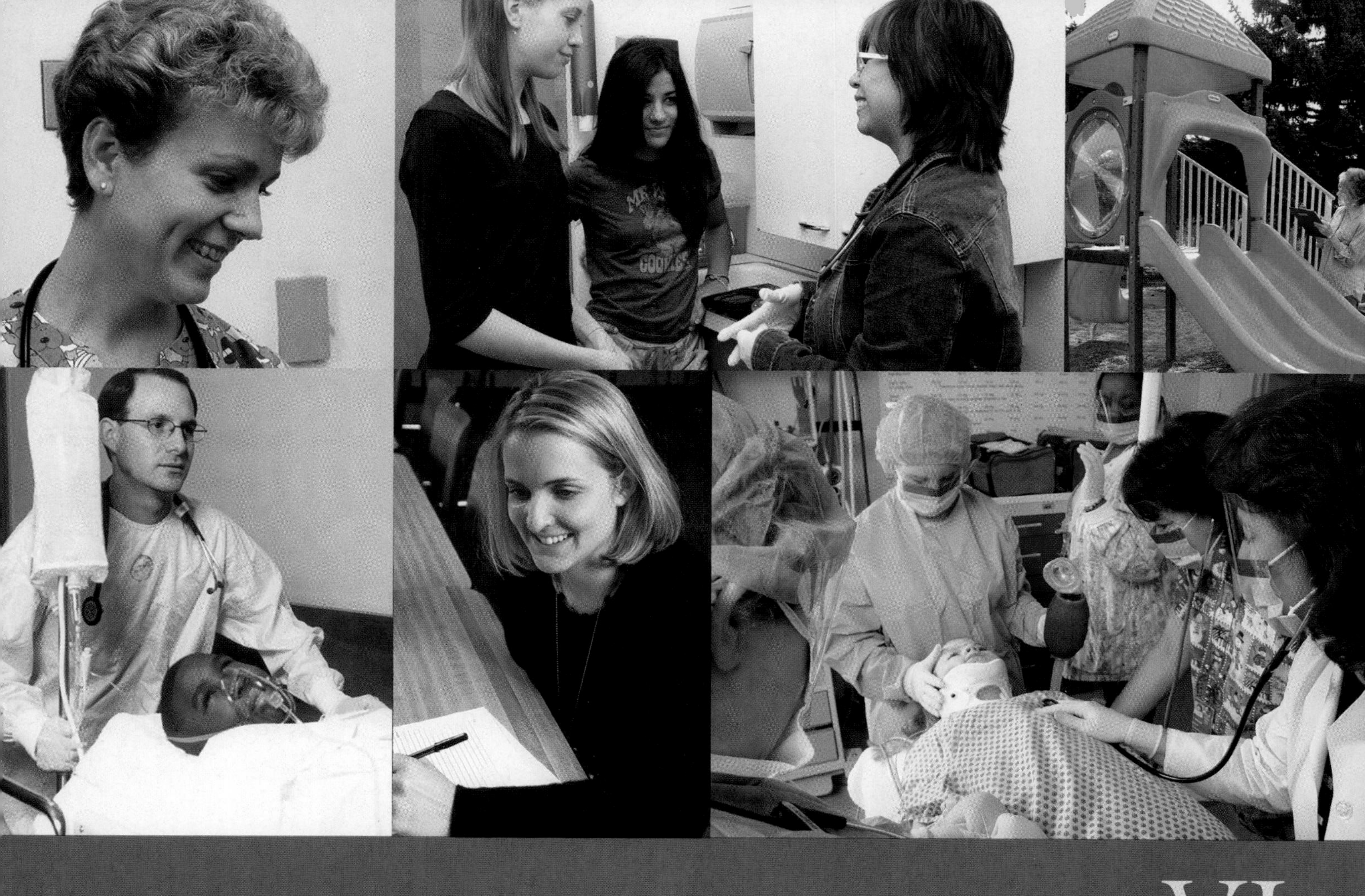

UNIT VI

Nursing Care of Specific Health Conditions

A child's healthcare needs are determined by the developmental level and specific health condition. The child may experience a health alteration related to any one body system, or may experience health alterations to several body systems simultaneously. The nurse applies knowledge of growth and development, anatomy, and pathophysiology in assessing the child with an altered health status. The nurse partners with the family in establishing a plan of care that will promote optimal achievement of growth and development, which may be affected by specific health conditions. The nurse also collaborates with other health professionals to provide individualized healthcare to the child and family.

Chapter

23

Alterations in Fluid, Electrolyte, and Acid–Base Balance

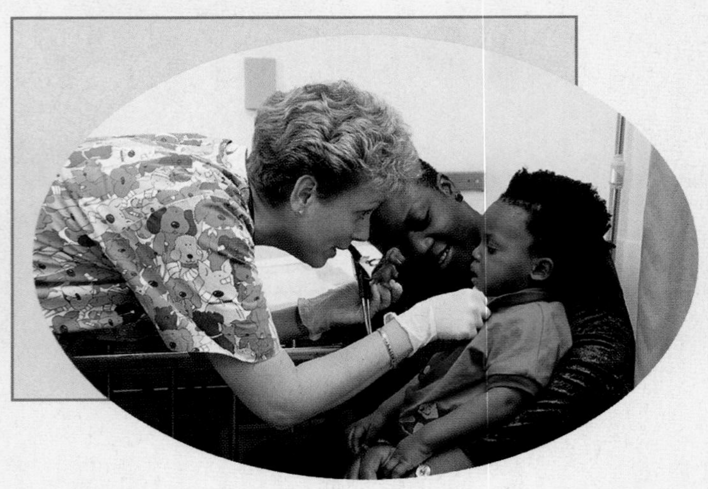

Vernon Smith is 18 months old. Several days ago he developed vomiting and diarrhea. His parents tried to get him to eat, but he had little appetite. He drank a few sips of water and juice, but the next morning he was listless and would not drink anything. The diarrhea continued.

His mother brought him to the urgent care center. Vernon is irritable on arrival, and his mother reports that he has been alternately irritable and lethargic. His mucous membranes and tongue appear dry, and skin turgor over the abdomen is slightly decreased. His mother notes that Vernon has had only two wet diapers today and says the urine in his diapers was dark in color. She also reports that he weighed 12 kg (26 lb) at the clinic last week. However, when the nurse weighs him, the scale reads only 11 kg (24.5 lb). Vernon is moderately dehydrated and needs rapid replacement of the proper type of fluids. He is started on oral replacement therapy at the urgent care center and is kept for monitoring. His mother makes arrangements for someone to care for her 4-year-old daughter, Shawna, at home for the day.

What happens inside the body when dehydration occurs? How can a nurse recognize dehydration? What laboratory studies provide clues to the degree of Vernon's dehydration? What types of fluid does Vernon need? What nursing management is important for his recovery? Why are young children at greater risk for dehydration than adults? What do parents need to be taught to prevent and manage dehydration? This chapter presents information that will enable you to answer these questions.

"Vernon didn't want to play. Grandma says Mommy took him to the clinic so they can make him better."

—Shawna, age 4

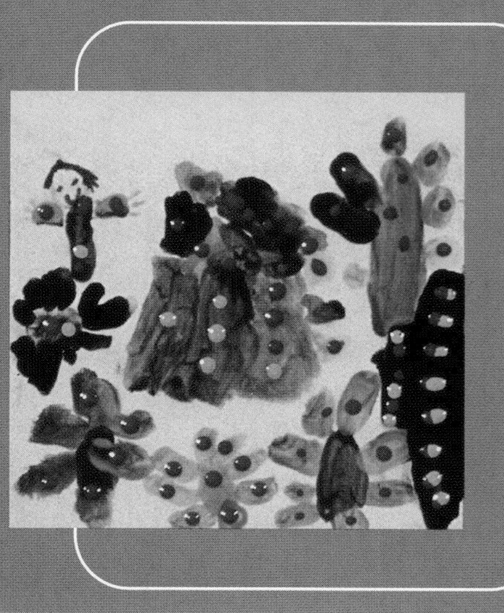

Learning Outcomes

After completing this chapter, you will be able to:

- Describe normal fluid and electrolyte status for children at various ages.
- Identify regulatory mechanisms for fluid and electrolyte balance.
- Recognize threats to fluid and electrolyte balance in children.
- Analyze assessment findings to recognize fluid-electrolyte problems and acid–base imbalance in children.
- Describe appropriate interventions for children experiencing fluid-electrolyte problems and acid–base imbalance.

MediaLink http://www.prenhall.com/ball

Resources for this chapter can be found on the CD-ROM accompanying this textbook, and on the Companion Website at www.prenhall.com/ball. Click on Chapter 23 to select the activities for this chapter.

CD-ROM

Animations/Videos

Acid–Base Balance

NCLEX Review

Audio Glossary

COMPANION WEBSITE

A & P Review

Clinical Manifestations Review

NCLEX Review

Case Study: Dehydration and Fluid Calculation

Care Plan: Infant Feeding

Care Plan: Hyponatremic Dehydration in Breastfeeding

MediaLink Applications

Formula Preparation at a Home Visit
Identifying Intravenous Fluids
Interpreting Blood Gases
Understanding School-Age Athletes and Fluid Needs

Key Terms

Key Terms *(continued)*

isotonic fluid/744
Kussmaul respirations /765
oncotic pressure/741
osmolality/743
osmosis/726
Pco_2/759
Po_2/759
pH/758
saline/738
sensible/726
third-spacing/729

A thorough understanding of fluid, electrolyte, and acid–base homeostasis and imbalances is essential when providing nursing care to pediatric patients like Vernon, in the preceding scenario. This chapter presents information about the processes that maintain fluid and electrolyte balance, and describes the common imbalances that may occur in children. It also describes how the body regulates acid–base status and explains the management of acid–base imbalances.

Many health conditions cause changes in body fluids and electrolytes, or alter acid–base balance, requiring regulation and management. Gastroenteritis, burns, respiratory problems, and kidney disorders are examples of such conditions. Sometimes management of fluid status in the home or in a short-term ambulatory facility can prevent more serious illness or hospitalization. Children who cannot take in normal fluids by mouth due to surgery need short-term management of fluid by intravenous route. When children with a chronic condition cannot ingest adequate fluids due to neuromuscular conditions, measures such as gastrostomy feeding tubes can ensure balanced intake. Athletes and those exercising in hot weather need management of intake to promote fluid and electrolyte balance. In all of these cases, nursing care is needed to evaluate intake, assess the child, and plan and implement appropriate interventions.

ANATOMY AND PHYSIOLOGY OF PEDIATRIC DIFFERENCES

Much of the human body is composed of water. Water provides important functions in the body such as aiding in metabolism, excretion of waste products, and temperature regulation, and it serves as a main component of blood and lymphatic fluid. **Body fluid** is body water that has solutes dissolved in it. Some of the solutes are **electrolytes,** or charged particles (ions). Electrolytes such as sodium (Na^+), potassium (K^+), calcium (Ca^{++}), magnesium (Mg^{++}), chloride (Cl^-), and inorganic phosphorus (Pi) ions must be present in the proper concentrations for cells to function effectively.

Fluid in the body is in a dynamic state. In persons of all ages, fluid continuously leaves the body through the skin, in feces and urine, and during respiration. **Sensible** water loss is that which is measurable and observable, such as in urine or through drainage tubes. **Insensible** water loss cannot be directly measured or observed, such as that lost through the skin and respirations. For adults and children, intake of oral fluid is approximately equivalent to urinary output in normal circumstances. Likewise, water provided in food and by the body's metabolic processes is approximately the same as insensible loss from feces, skin, and respirations.

In persons of all ages, body fluid is located in several compartments. The two major fluid compartments contain the **intracellular fluid** (fluid inside the cells) and the **extracellular fluid** (fluid outside the cells). The extracellular fluid is made up of **intravascular fluid** (the fluid within the blood vessels) and **interstitial fluid** (the fluid between the cells and outside the blood and lymphatic vessels). The concentrations of electrolytes in the fluid differ depending on the fluid compartment. For example, extracellular fluid is rich in sodium ions; intracellular fluid, by contrast, is low in sodium ions but rich in potassium ions (Table 23–1). In addition, the percentage of the fluid that is located in each compartment varies during development, as discussed below.

Fluid moves between the intravascular and interstitial compartments by a process called **filtration.** Water moves into and out of the cells by the process of **osmosis.** These processes are discussed later in the chapter. Electrolytes move over cell membranes both by **diffusion** of particles from a location of greater to less concentration and by active transport that is effective even against the concentration gradient.

Infants and young children differ physiologically from adults in ways that make them vulnerable to fluid, electrolyte, and acid–base imbalances. The percentage of body weight that is composed of water varies with age. The percentage is highest at birth (and higher in premature than in full-term infants) and decreases with age (Figure 23–1 ■). In addition to variations in total body water, the proportion in the various compartments differs with age. Neonates and young infants have a proportionately larger extracellular fluid volume than older children and adults because their brain and skin (both rich in interstitial fluid) occupy a greater proportion of their body weight. Much of the body's extracellular fluid is exchanged each day. During infancy, there is a high daily fluid requirement with little fluid volume reserve in the intracellular compartment; this makes the infant vulnerable to dehydration. As an infant grows, the proportion of water in-

TABLE 23–1 Electrolyte Concentrations in Body Fluid Compartments

	EXTRACELLULAR FLUID (ECF)		INTRACELLULAR FLUID (ICF)
COMPONENTS	***VASCULAR***	***INTERSTITIAL***	
$Na+$	High	High	Low
K^{+}	Low	Low	High
Ca^{++}	Low	Low	Low (higher than ECF)
Mg^{++}	Low	Low	High
Pi	Low	Low	High
Cl^{-}	High	High	Low
Proteins	High	Low	High

side the cells increases, extracellular amount decreases in comparison, and the risk of fluid imbalance begins to decrease (Figure 23–2 ■).

The normal newborn has the most striking differences in fluid status from older infants. These include:

- Basal metabolic rate double that of children
- Approximately 4 to 5 times greater water intake needs/kg of body weight
- Only 10% of the ability to excrete sodium (Merenstein & Gardner, 2003)

The newborn adapts to extrauterine life in the first few days, showing variations in fluid status. In the first day of life, urine output is limited and body weight is stable. Newborns experience a diuresis in the first 3 to 5 days of life, causing a weight loss of about 10% (Cloherty, Stark, & Eichenwald, 2003). Near the end of the first week, urine output and fluid intake become approximately equal in amount. Prematurity (born before 37 weeks' gestation) delays the ability to manage fluid and electrolyte balance (Cote, Todres, Goudsouzian et al., 2001). Thus, the newborn, particularly when premature, who requires surgery or other treatment, requires the expertise of a neonatologist and neonatal nurse practitioner to manage fluid needs. The very-low-birth-weight baby (< 1500 g) has an even greater than normal loss of body fluid in the period after birth, and often requires greater intake of fluids to maintain balance.

Infants and children under 2 years of age lose a greater proportion of fluid each day than older children and adults and are thus more dependent on adequate intake. They have a greater proportion of skin surface or **body surface area (BSA)** and thus have greater insensible water losses through the skin. Because of this large BSA, they are also at greater risk for dehydration and electrolyte imbalance when burned.

CLINICAL TIP

BSA is a relationship between height and weight measured in squared meters. BSA in m^2 = the square root of [height in cm × weight in kg]/3600.

See the Skills Manual for further description of BSA, which is often considered when determining fluid needs of infants and children over 10 kg in weight, and can be used to calculate medication dosages for children.

In addition, respiratory and metabolic rates are high during early childhood. These factors lead to greater water loss from the lungs and greater water demand to fuel the body's metabolic processes (Figure 23–3 ■). Due to these factors, the exercising child dehydrates easily and must consume more fluid during physical activity, particularly during hot weather (Committee on Sports Medicine and Fitness, 2000). Recommendations for fluids during exercise will be found later in the chapter.

When fluid status is compromised, a number of body mechanisms are activated to help restore balance. Several of these mechanisms occur in the kidney. The kidneys conserve water and needed electrolytes while excreting waste products and drug metabolites. In children under 2 years of age, however, the glomeruli, tubules, and nephrons of the kidneys are immature.

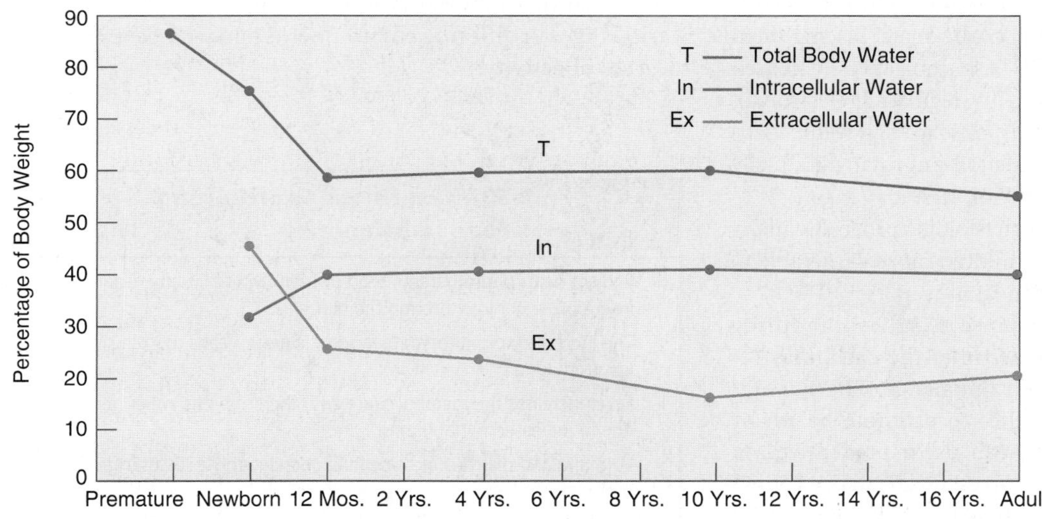

FIGURE 23–1 ■ The major body fluid compartments at various ages. *Extracellular* fluid is composed mainly of intravascular fluid (fluid in blood vessels) and interstitial fluid (fluid between the cells and outside the blood and lymphatic vessels). *Intracellular* fluid is that within cells.

From Bindler, R., & Howry, L. (2005). Pediatric Drug Guide. *Upper Saddle River, NJ: Prentice Hall.*

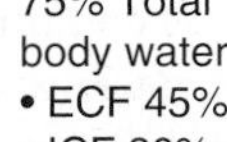

AS THEY GROW

Fluid and Electrolyte Differences

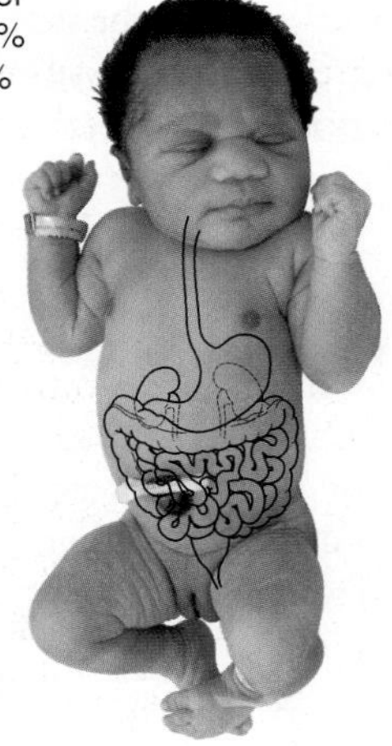
Newborn
75% Total
body water
• ECF 45%
• ICF 30%
Brain and skin occupy
a greater proportion of
body weight and are
high in interstitial fluid

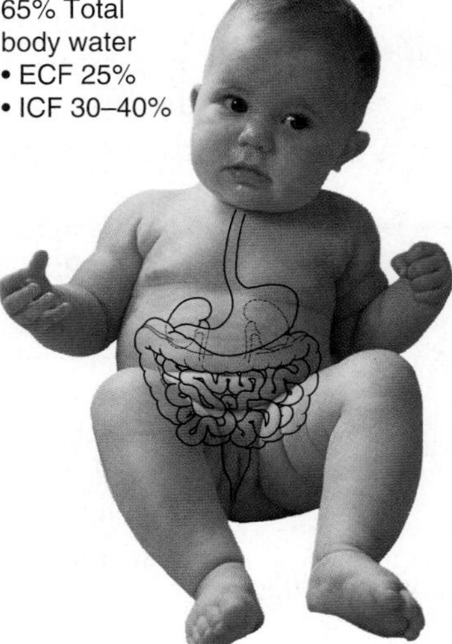

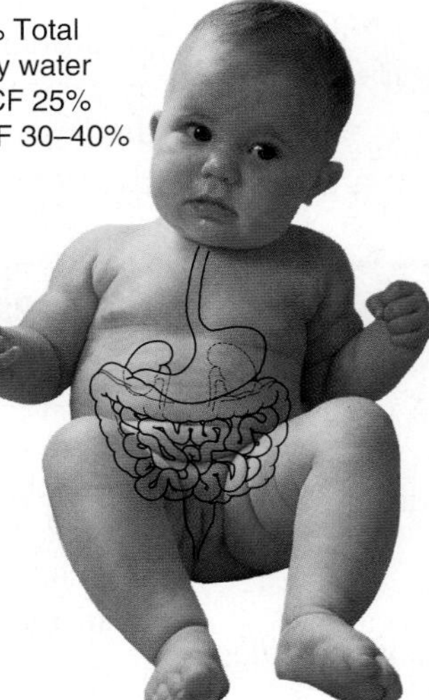
Infant
65% Total
body water
• ECF 25%
• ICF 30–40%
High BSA
promotes fluid loss
5–6x greater fluid
exchange daily
Little fluid reserve
in intracellular fluid
High metabolic rate requires
generous fluid intake

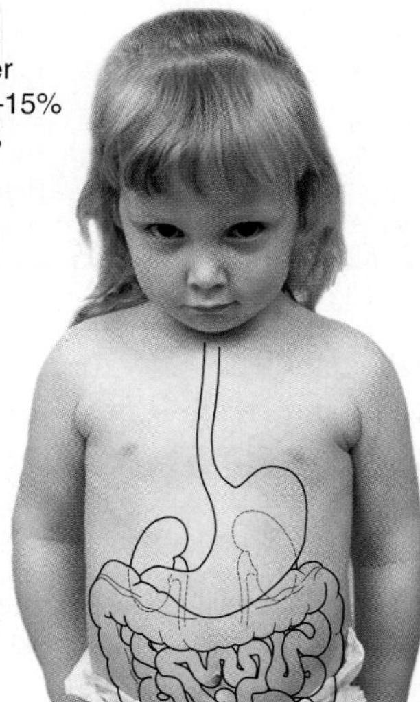
Child/Adolescent
50% Total
body water
• ECF 10–15%
• ICF 40%
Kidneys are immature
until 2 years and unable
to conserve water and
electrolytes or fully assist
in acid–base balance

FIGURE 23–2 ■ The newborn and infant have a high percentage of body weight comprised of water, especially extracellular fluid, which is lost from the body easily. Note the small stomach size which limits ability to rehydrate quickly.

They are thus unable to conserve or excrete water and solutes effectively (see Chapter 31∞). Because more water is generally excreted, the infant and young child can become dehydrated quickly or develop electrolyte imbalances. In addition, infants have a weaker transport system for ions and bicarbonate, placing them at greater risk for acidosis and acid–base imbalances. Children under 2 years of age also have difficulty regulating electrolytes such as sodium and calcium. Renal response to high solute loads is slower and less developed, with function improving gradually during the first year of life (Hewitt-Taylor, 1999).

In addition to the immaturity of physiologic processes, many health conditions also make young children more vulnerable to fluid deficit. Examples are listed in Box 23–1.

Although disruptions in fluid balance usually occur during an illness, at other more predictable times the child may require management to prevent fluid imbalance. The nurse is well positioned to work with families to promote health by maintenance of fluid balance and can use a preventive approach to ensure fluid balance. Nurses in specialized areas such as newborn and pediatric intensive care units, emergency rooms, and operative suites provide intensive and careful management of fluids. See Chapter 17∞ for a discussion of fluid needs during the perioperative period. Nurses also partner with childcare centers and schools to plan for appropriate fluid for children; partner with parents in all clinical settings so that they are aware of fluid needs for children of various ages in differing environments and who have different degrees of activity.

BOX 23–1 Health Conditions Contributing to Fluid Imbalance

- Radiant heat (phototherapy) used to treat hyperbilirubinemia increases insensible water loss through the skin.
- The increased respiratory rate in some illnesses leads to excessive water loss from lungs.
- Fever increases the metabolic rate and, therefore, the water demands due to increased metabolism.
- Vomiting and diarrhea increase fluid and electrolyte losses from the gastrointestinal system.
- Fistulas, blood loss, and drainage tubes contribute to fluid deficits.
- Renal disease can influence rates of fluid excretion.

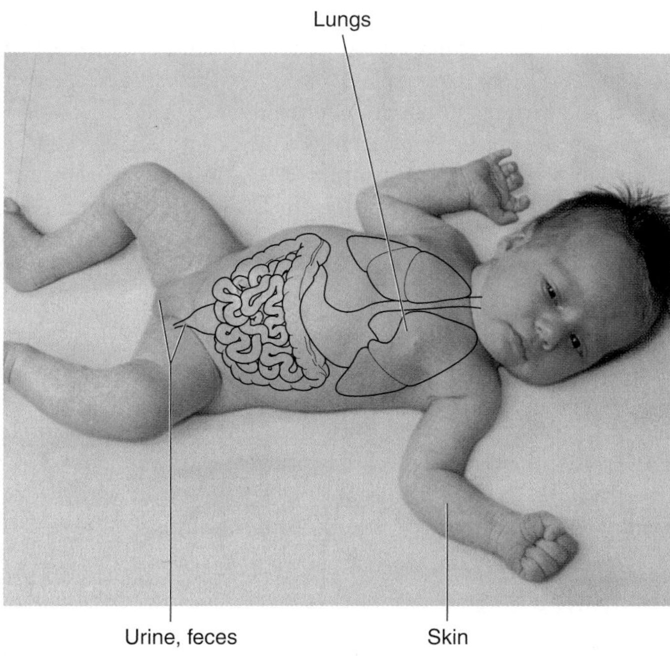

FIGURE 23–3 ■ Normal routes of fluid excretion from infants and children.

FLUID VOLUME IMBALANCES

When fluid excretion and losses are balanced by the proper volume and type of fluid intake, fluid balance will be maintained. If, however, fluid output and intake are not matched, fluid imbalance may occur rapidly. The major types of fluid imbalances are extracellular fluid volume deficit (**dehydration**), extracellular fluid volume excess, and interstitial fluid volume excess (**edema**).

Extracellular Fluid Volume Imbalances

Extracellular Fluid Volume Deficit (Dehydration)

Extracellular fluid volume deficit occurs when there is not enough fluid in the extracellular compartment (intravascular and interstitial). Depending on the cause of dehydration, sodium may be at a normal, low, or elevated level. (Hyponatremia and hypernatremia are described later in the chapter, on pages 743 and 745.) The state of body water deficit is called dehydration. The three major types of dehydration are as follows:

- **Isotonic dehydration** (or **isonatremic dehydration**) occurs when fluid loss is not balanced by intake and the loss of water and sodium are in proportion. The serum sodium is therefore within normal limits even though the circulating blood volume is lowered. Most of the fluid lost is from the extracellular component. This type of dehydration is commonly manifested in the illnesses of young children such as vomiting and diarrhea.
- **Hypotonic dehydration** (or **hyponatremic dehydration**) occurs when fluid loss is characterized by a proportionately greater loss of sodium than water. Serum sodium is below normal levels. Compensatory fluid shifts occur from the extracellular to intracellular components in an attempt to establish normal proportions, thus leading to even greater extracellular dehydration. Severe and prolonged vomiting and diarrhea, burns, and renal disease can lead to this condition, as well as administration of intravenous fluid without electrolytes in treatment of dehydration.
- **Hypertonic dehydration** (or **hypernatremic dehydration**) occurs when sodium loss is proportionately less than water loss. Serum sodium is above normal levels. Compensatory fluid shifts occur from the intracellular to extracellular components in an attempt to establish normal proportions. The extracellular component therefore remains fairly normal, delaying the onset of signs and symptoms of dehydration until the condition is quite serious. Neurologic symptoms reflecting intracellular imbalance may occur simultaneously with more common symptoms of dehydration. The condition may be caused by health problems such as diabetes insipidus or administration of intravenous fluid or tube feedings with high electrolyte levels.

The body continuously attempts to compensate for fluid and electrolyte imbalance by shifting fluid and electrolytes from one component to another. Therefore, it is rare for only one type of dehydration to occur; the child's fluid and electrolyte status and symptoms are constantly changing. Ongoing assessment and management will be needed.

Etiology and Pathophysiology. Extracellular fluid volume deficit is usually caused by the loss of sodium-containing fluid from the body. The situations that most often cause loss of fluid containing sodium are vomiting, diarrhea, nasogastric suction, hemorrhage, and burns. Vomiting and diarrhea are common manifestations of disease in children throughout the world, and each year up to 5 million children die from dehydration related to diarrhea. About 300 to 500 die annually in the United States from this problem; about 220,000 are hospitalized (accounting for 9% of pediatric hospitalizations); and many more receive care on an outpatient basis (Shamir, Zahavi, Abramowich, et al., 1998; Nager & Wang, 2002).

Another cause of extracellular fluid volume deficit in infants is increased water loss in low-birth-weight infants who are kept under radiant warmers to maintain heat (Figure 23–4 ■). Remember that their high BSA puts them at risk of dehydration due to insensible fluid loss through the skin. Less frequently, adrenal insufficiency, accumulation of extracellular fluid in a third space such as the peritoneal cavity (**third-spacing**), or overuse of diuretics may be the cause. The latter etiology is most often seen in bulimic adolescents for weight control (see Chapter 9∞). In general, newborns and infants are at highest risk to develop dehydration because of their physiologic differences and poorly developed compensatory mechanisms.

Excessive exercise during very hot weather without sufficient fluid replacement can lead to fluid and electrolyte imbalance. Children are more prone than adults to imbalance from exercise, for several of the physiologic differences described earlier in the chapter. Because children have a greater BSA, they can gain more heat from the environment when it is hot, and lose more when it is cold (Binkley, Beckett, Casa, et al., 2002). In addition,

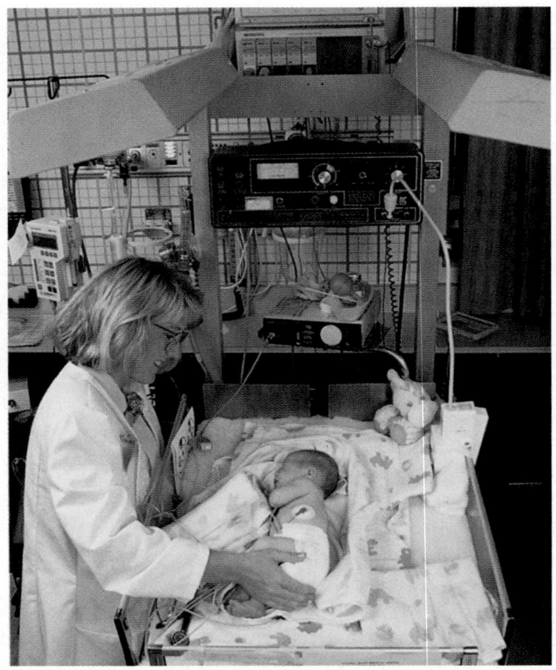

FIGURE 23–4 ■ Use of an overhead warmer or phototherapy increases insensible fluid excretion through the skin, thus increasing the fluid intake needed.

the high metabolic rate of children is further increased during exercise so that fluid lost in metabolism is significant. Young children do not sweat effectively and may be unable to eliminate heat by this method. Children may not feel thirsty and so fail to drink even when dehydrated (Committee on Sports Medicine and Fitness, 2000). Several types of heat illness are possible; see the clinical manifestations table on page 731.

Burns involve complex health problems that are described in Chapter 36∞. Burns of the skin usually involve huge loss of body fluids, including water and electrolytes, particularly sodium. Hypotonic dehydration is the type most commonly seen in the initial period after a burn. Serum proteins are also lost so body fluid is more likely to leak into interstitial spaces, causing edema and further contributing to the fluid deficit. The kidneys decrease urine production because of their decreased blood flow leading to decreased urinary output. While the fluid imbalance of burns is therefore complicated, the first imbalance encountered is often that of dehydration with accompanying hyponatremia.

For burns, gastroenteritis, and other illness, initial dehydration in the first 3 days reflects a high loss of extracellular fluid. About 80% of the fluid loss is extracellular; about 20% is intracellular. With time, however, the relationship begins to change so that in illnesses over 3 days, about 60% of fluid loss is extracellular while 40% is intracellular (Johns Hopkins Hospital, 2003). Since the electrolyte composition of extracellular and intracellular fluids differs (see Table 23–1), electrolyte management will need to change for long-term conditions.

CLINICAL TIP

Many conditions that cause dehydration are accompanied by fever which produces additional demands for fluid. For each degree of Celsius increase above 37°, 0.42 mL/kg/hr of additional fluid is needed.

Clinical Manifestations. The signs of dehydration relate to the severity or degree of the body water deficit (Table 23–2). They are a result of both the decreased fluid (e.g., diminished turgor and mucous membrane moisture) and the body's response to the fluid deficit (e.g., pulse and blood pressure changes). See page 731 for clinical manifestations of extracellular fluid volume deficit.

Mild dehydration is hard to detect, because children appear alert and have moist mucous membranes. Infants may be irritable and older children are thirsty. In moderate dehydration, the child is often lethargic and sleepy, but may have periods of rest-

TABLE 23–2 Severity of Clinical Dehydration

CLINICAL ASSESSMENT	MILD	MODERATE	SEVERE
Percent of body weight lost	Up to 5% (40–50 mL/kg)	6%–9% (60–90 mL/kg)	10% or more (100 + mL/kg)
Level of consciousness	Alert, restless, thirsty	Irritable or lethargic (infants and very young children); alert, thirsty, restless (older children and adolescents)	Lethargic to comatose (infants and young children); often conscious, apprehensive (older children and adolescents)
Blood pressure	Normal	Normal or low; postural hypotension (older children and adolescents)	Low to undetectable
Pulse	Normal	Rapid	Rapid, weak to nonpalpable
Skin turgor	Normal	Poor	Very poor
Mucous membranes	Moist	Dry	Parched
Urine	May appear normal	Decreased output (< 1 mL/kg/hr) dark color; increased specific gravity	Very decreased or absent output
Thirst	Slightly increased	Moderately increased	Greatly increased unless lethargic
Fontanel	Normal	Sunken	Sunken
Extremities	Warm; normal capillary refill	Delayed capillary refill (>2 sec)	Cool, discolored; delayed capillary refill. (> 3–4 sec)
Respirations	Normal	Normal or rapid	Changing rate and pattern

CLINICAL MANIFESTATIONS of Exertional Heat Illness

CONDITION	ETIOLOGY	SIGNS AND SYMPTOMS
Heat cramps	Dehydration Electrolyte imbalance Neuromuscular fatigue	Acute, painful muscle cramps Thirst Fatigue
Heat syncope	Peripheral vasodilation Reduced cardiac output Cerebral ischemia	Tunnel vision Pale, sweaty skin Decreased pulse Dizziness, faintness
Heat exhaustion	Elevated core body temperature Sodium loss	Sweating, pallor Dehydration Muscle cramps Nausea, anorexia, diarrhea Decreased urinary output Weakness, fainting, dizziness
Heat stroke	Elevated core temperature (> 104°F) Temperature regulation overwhelmed by heat production or absence of adequate heat loss Organ system failure from overheating	Tachycardia Hypotension Sweating Hyperventilation Altered mental status, seizures, coma Vomiting, diarrhea Death can occur from severe acidosis, hyperkalemia, renal failure, and disseminated intravascular coagulation
Exertional hyponatremia	Serum sodium < 130 mmol/L Exercise over 4 hours with water or other low-solute fluids for replenishment	Disorientation, headache, lethargy Swollen extremities Vomiting Pulmonary or cerebral edema Death can occur from sodium imbalance

Adapted from Binkley et al., (2002). National Athletic Trainers' Association Position Statement: Exertional heat illnesses. Journal of Athletic Training, *37, 329–343.*

lessness and irritability, especially if an infant. Skin turgor is diminished, mucous membranes appear dry, and urine is dark in color and diminished in amount. Pulse rate is usually increased and blood pressure can be normal or low. Vernon, described at the beginning of this chapter, was displaying symptoms of moderate dehydration. His urine output was decreased, and he had lost about 8% of his body weight (Box 23–2). What other signs and symptoms of moderate dehydration can you identify in the opening scenario? What additional assessments would you want to perform on Vernon?

Severe dehydration is manifested by increasing lethargy or nonresponsiveness, low to markedly decreased blood pressure, rapid pulse, poor skin turgor, dry mucous membranes, and markedly decreased (oliguria) or absent (anuria) urinary output.

CLINICAL MANIFESTATIONS of Extracellular Fluid Volume Deficit

ETIOLOGY	CLINICAL MANIFESTATIONS
Decreased fluid volume	Weight loss Sunken fontanel (infant)
Inadequate circulating blood volume to offset the force of gravity when in upright position	Postural blood pressure drop (older children) Dizziness
Decreased intravascular volume	Increased small-vein filling time Delayed capillary refill time Flat neck veins when supine (older children)
Inadequate circulation to the brain	Dizziness, syncope
Inadequate circulation to the kidneys	Oliguria
Cardiac reflex response to decreased intravascular volume	Thready, rapid pulse
Decreased interstitial fluid volume	Decreased skin turgor

CLINICAL TIP

Normal urinary output is 1–2 mL/kg/hour.

BOX 23–2 Calculation of Percentage of Weight Loss

To calculate percent of weight loss:

- Subtract the child's present weight from the original weight to find the loss.
- Divide the loss by the child's original weight.

Example: In the opening scenario, Vernon weighed 12 kg (26 lb) at the clinic last week. However, when he is weighed today, the scale reads only 11 kg (24.5 lb). In this case, subtracting 11 kg from 12 kg yields 1 kg of weight loss. Dividing 1 kg by his original weight of 12 kg reveals that he has lost approximately 8% of his body weight, which indicates moderate dehydration.

Recall that in hypertonic dehydration, the more common symptoms of mild and moderate dehydration may be delayed since fluid is being moved from the intracellular to the extracellular component. Some of the first manifestations of dehydration may therefore indicate severe dehydration as compensatory mechanisms fail. Level of consciousness, seizures, or profoundly decreased urinary output may seem to quickly be manifested.

COLLABORATIVE CARE

Nurses work with other healthcare providers to provide care for the child with dehydration. Physicians, nurse practitioners, and physician assistants often provide primary care in hospitals, urgent care centers, and clinics during extracellular fluid volume deficit. You will provide ongoing assessments, administer intravenous and oral fluids, and collect necessary laboratory specimens. Nurses also partner with parents to instruct them about prevention, recognition, and treatment of dehydration.

Diagnostic Tests

The diagnosis of dehydration is best accomplished by clinical observations as described in Table 23–2. In isotonic dehydration, the amount of fluid lost is in direct relationship with the loss of sodium, so serum sodium levels will appear within normal limits (see sections on hyponatremia and hypernatremia later in this chapter). The major observation that provides clues about the degree of dehydration is percent of weight loss. Selected laboratory tests may be helpful in severe and continuing dehydration that is complicated by electrolyte imbalance or acidosis. The tests include serum electrolytes, creatinine, and glucose (Liebelt, 1998). Elevated blood urea nitrogen (> 25 mg/dL) and serum bicarbonate (> 17 mEq/L) are useful to identify moderate and severe diarrhea (Eliason & Lewan, 1998). The results can be used to target the fluid type and amount to best meet the imbalances identified.

Clinical Therapy

Medical management depends on accurate identification of the degree of dehydration. The treatment of extracellular fluid volume deficit is administration of fluid containing sodium. This may be accomplished by oral rehydration therapy or by intravenous fluids.

Oral rehydration therapy has been used for a number of years in developing countries without an accessible supply of intravenous fluids. More recently, the benefits of using this therapy early to prevent severe dehydration and to treat mild and moderate dehydration in children in developed countries has been recognized. The therapy is successful in treating the dehydration caused by many gastrointestinal illnesses and prevents hospitalization for many infants and young children (Armon, Stephenson, MacFaul, et al., 2001). It is the treatment of choice for children with diarrhea who have mild to moderate dehydration (King, Glass, Bresee, et al., 2003). Solutions are available commercially that contain water, carbohydrate (sugar), sodium, potassium, chloride, and lactate. Some clinicians allow lactose-free milk, breast milk, or half-strength milk to be given in addition to oral rehydration therapy solution. The WHO/UNICEF solution was developed for use with cholera and is not generally used for diarrhea treatment in the United States, as its sodium and chloride loads are higher than that of other commercial solutions (Box 23–3). When the child is severely dehydrated, intravenous fluid is administered, often accompanied with oral rehydration. The intravenous fluid is often Ringer's lactate or 0.9% normal saline, followed by or accompanied with dilute saline, such as one half or one quarter normal saline (Aker & O'Sullivan, 1998). The fluid combination replenishes the extracellular fluid volume and adds solutes to return the body fluid to normal. See Table 23–3 for a description of the most common types of intravenous fluids. The child may be hospitalized or treated with intravenous fluids in a short-stay unit until the dehydration is controlled. Once hydration is completed, the child may resume an age-appropriate diet (Burkhart, 1999).

In developing countries with a high rate of diarrheal diseases in childhood, supplementation with zinc has been associated with less persistent and severe disease. In these countries the diet may be deficient in this mineral, which is commonly found in meats, liver, eggs, and seafood. In addition, certain functional

BOX 23–3 Research: Use of Oral Rehydration Therapy

Despite the recommendation of the American Academy of Pediatrics (Provisional Committee on Quality Improvement, 1996) and other groups to use outpatient oral rehydration therapy (ORT) for mild and moderate dehydration, many healthcare providers continue to hospitalize these children and administer intravenous therapy (Nager & Wang, 2002). Hospitalization is expensive and disrupting for families, while care providers state that it seems easier than keeping a child in an outpatient setting for several hours to institute ORT.

Several analyses of studies performed with children have demonstrated the success and efficacy of ORT (Larson, 2000). In order to study the possibility of decreased treatment time, 96 children from 3 to 36 months of age were randomly assigned as moderately dehydrated children to receive either rapid nasogastric hydration or rapid intravenous (IV) hydration, both accomplished within 3 hours in an emergency department. Both techniques were effective in treating children for dehydration, while the nasogastric rehydration was significantly less expensive. The authors offer the possibility of rapid rehydration as a cost-effective management technique for moderately dehydrated children (Nager & Wang, 2002). In another study of 18 moderately dehydrated children with gastroenteritis, half were given ORT and half were started on intravenous therapy. The length of treatment in the emergency department was significantly lower for the ORT group than the IV group, and ORT required significantly less staff time. Parents reported greater satisfaction with ORT, and the outcomes for the children were comparable (Atherly-John, Cunningham, & Crain, 2002).

Nurses can support ORT for children with mild or moderate dehydration. Teach parents to keep appropriate fluids at home and to institute the therapy early during vomiting and diarrhea episodes. Monitor children receiving the therapy in outpatient settings, whether by traditional oral therapy or rapid nasogastric hydration.

Critical Thinking Application: Why do you think physicians and nurses might resist applying findings related to the efficacy of ORT and continue to hospitalize and use intravenous therapy for mild or moderate dehydration? How could knowledge of the benefits of ORT change the care provided in emergency departments and other outpatient settings? (See Ozuah, Avner, & Stein, 2002 for ideas.) What are some of the risks of hospitalization and intravenous use?

TABLE 23–3 Common Intravenous Solutions, Uses, and Components

IV SOLUTION	USES	COMPONENTS							
		CHO (g/100 mL)	Protein (g/100 mL)	Cal/L	NA^+ (mEq/L)	K^+ (mEq/L)	Cl^- (mEq/L)	HCO_3 (mEq/L)	Ca^{++} (mEq/L)
D_5W	Restores water loss, plasma volume, and calories; lowers sodium levels	5	—	170	—	—	—	—	—
Normal saline (0.9% NaCl)	Restores water and sodium loss; maintains sodium and chloride at present levels	—	—	—	154	—	154	—	—
Ringer's solution	Expands intracellular fluid; replaces extracellular losses	0–10	—	0–340	147	4	155.5	—	4
Lactated Ringer's solution	Replaces fluid loss from burns, bleeding, and severe diarrhea	0–10	—	0–340	130	4	109	28	3
Albumin 25% (salt poor albumin)	Restores major plasma protein in blood loss that has been treated with NS (plasma expander)	—	25	1000	100–160	—	< 120	—	—

Note: Variations and combinations are available to tailor intake to needs of the child. For example, ½ NS (0.45% NaCl) or ¼ NS (0.225% NaCl) are often used in young children; the lower sodium content helps to avoid inadvertent hypernatremia. D_5W ½ NS and D_5W ¼ NS are combinations of D_5W and NS; they provide both carbohydrate and sodium. Amino acid 8.5% is an additional plasma expander to restore loss of plasma proteins.

Information adapted from Nechyba, C., and Gunn, V. (eds.) (2003). The Harriet Lane handbook *(16th ed.). Johns Hopkins University Press; and LeMone, P., & Burke, K. M. (2004).* Medical surgical nursing *(3rd ed.). Upper Saddle River, NJ: Prentice Hall Health.*

foods that contain normal intestinal bacterial flora, or substances that promote normal flora, are under investigation for preventing diarrhea in children at risk (King et al., 2003).

NURSING MANAGEMENT

Nurses assess children of all ages for signs of fluid imbalance. Partnering with parents to prevent fluid imbalance is important. Nurses provide information on normal needs of infants and children and special needs during exercise or illness, and help parents to recognize imbalances. Nurses collaborate with other healthcare providers to perform and analyze laboratory tests for diagnosis, administer intravenous and oral fluids as needed, and provide comfort measures for the child experiencing imbalance.

■ Nursing Assessment and Diagnosis

Prevention of dehydration is the major aim. Teach parents of all newborns and infants how to identify the problem. This age group is most at risk for dehydration and the signs are hardest to detect. When the child is admitted to a facility, weigh the child without clothing and with the same scale as used for previous weights. If hospitalized, continue with daily weights.

CLINICAL TIP

1 L of fluid weighs about 1 kg. The approximate amount of fluid deficit can be calculated using this formula.

Compare to past weights and calculate weight loss. Carefully measure intake and output, urine specific gravity, level of consciousness, pulse rate and quality, skin turgor, mucous membrane moisture, quality and rate of respirations, and blood pressure (Figure 23–5 ■). Urine specific gravity may increase in older children who are dehydrated; but due to the inability of the child under 2 years of age to concentrate urine effectively, a rising specific gravity may not be seen in the younger dehydrated child. The child with renal disease may also not show increased urine specific gravity due to the kidney's inability to concentrate urine.

CLINICAL TIP

To obtain urine from an infant for testing specific gravity, place two cotton balls in the diaper. When they are wet, put on gloves, push them into a 10 mL syringe, and squeeze out the urine with the plunger.

Compare the blood pressure when the child is supine with the pressure when the child is sitting with legs hanging down or standing. If the child is dehydrated, the sitting or standing blood pressure will be lower than the supine blood pressure, because blood accumulates in the dependent legs. The nurse will obtain samples of urine and blood as needed for laboratory tests.

The nursing diagnosis, Deficient Fluid Volume, applies to all children who have an extracellular fluid volume deficit. Other diagnoses depend on the severity of the condition and the age of the child. Several nursing diagnoses that might be appropriate for the mildly to severely dehydrated child are included in the accompanying nursing care plans. Additional care of the child with dehydration from gastroenteritis can be found in Chapter 30∞. Specific examples of nursing diagnoses include the following:

- Fluid Volume, Deficient related to active fluid volume loss or failure of regulatory mechanisms

MediaLink Case Study: Dehydration and Fluid Calculation

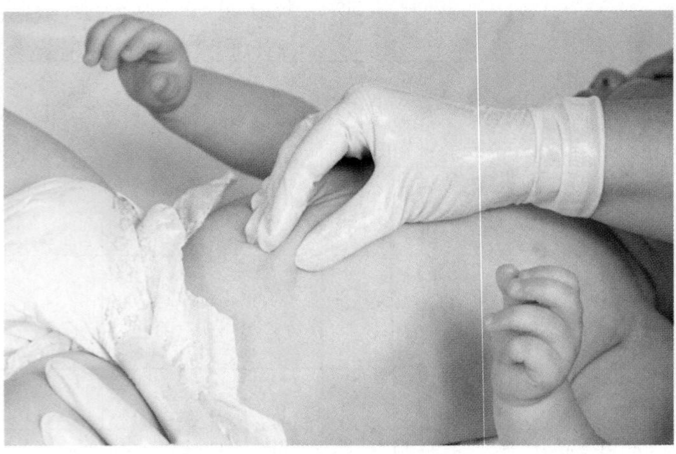
A

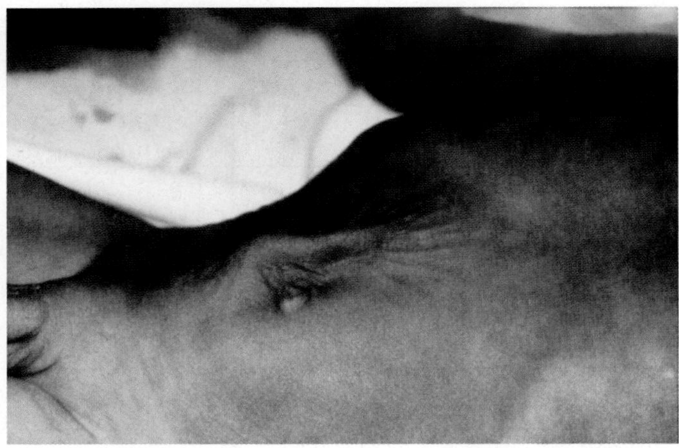
B

FIGURE 23–5 ■ Assessing skin turgor takes skill and practice. A, In moderate dehydration the skin may have a doughy texture and appearance. B, Later, in severe dehydration, the more typical "tenting" of skin is observed. Diminished turgor is most easily assessed in infants or children with little subcutaneous fat; it is more difficult to assess in those with larger amounts of fat. The chest, abdomen, and upper thighs are locations to measure turgor.

- Risk for Ineffective Peripheral Tissue Perfusion related to hypovolemia
- Risk for Injury related to postural hypotension

Planning and Implementation

Nursing care of the dehydrated child focuses on preventing dehydration when possible, providing oral rehydration fluids, teaching parents oral rehydration methods, and, if necessary, administering intravenous fluids to restore fluid balance. The accompanying nursing care plans on pages 736 and 737 summarize care of the child with mild to severe dehydration. Daily weights, frequent vital signs, neurologic assessments, and intake and output measures are important components of care that provide data needed for care management. Document findings and report changes in condition. Take measures to ensure the child's safety such as keeping side rails up and providing assistance when out of bed. Administer fluids and electrolyte solutions by intravenous and oral routes as prescribed.

MediaLink Care Plan: Hyponatremic Dehydration in Breastfeeding

Prevent Dehydration

Nursing care can often prevent dehydration. Carefully monitor temperature probes in radiant warmers and isolettes for newborns to prevent overheating and resulting dehydration. Teach parents proper clothing for infants to prevent overheating. Nurses play an important role in educating parents, youth, school personnel, and coaches about the dangers of heat-related illness. Prevention is key, so that children can exercise safely. Prior to a new exercise regime, assessment for risk factors is performed. This includes medical conditions that put the child at high risk, such as cystic fibrosis, diabetes, obesity, or mental retardation. Prior history of heat-related illness or recent change from a cooler to hotter environment increases risk. Long exercise periods increase the stress upon the body. Major nursing interventions involve partnering with families and athletic coaches to prevent problems and to recognize and treat them promptly. See Partnering with Families: Preventing Heat-Related Illness. Recognize that heat syndromes can result in death so that prevention and prompt recognition and treatment are essential.

Provide Oral Rehydration Fluids

In mild or moderate dehydration, oral rehydration fluid is the first intervention (Box 23–4). It is given in frequent small amounts; for example, 1 to 3 teaspoons of fluid every 10 to 15 minutes is a useful guideline for starting oral rehydration. For the first 2 to 4 hours of treatment, 50 mL of fluid for each kilogram of the child's weight should be the target intake (Endsley & Galbraith, 1998; Larson, 2000). Instruct parents to continue to administer the 1 teaspoon every 2 to 3 minutes even if the child vomits, as small amounts of the fluid may still be absorbed. See Partnering with Families: Oral Rehydration Therapy Guidelines on page 738.

PRACTICE ALERT

Sugar facilitates the absorption of sodium in oral rehydration fluids. Tell parents not to give diet beverages for oral rehydration, because they contain no sugar and will not be effectively absorbed. On the other hand, if an oral rehydration solution is too concentrated, it can worsen diarrhea. Juice and cola are highly concentrated and should be diluted to half strength when given to a child with diarrhea. Encourage parents to keep an oral rehydration solution in liquid or powder form on hand at all times and to use these solutions rather than juice or soda when the child first develops diarrhea.

BOX 23–4 Oral Rehydration and Maintenance Fluids for Mild and Moderate Dehydration

- Pedialyte
- Infalyte
- Rehydralyte
- Resol
- Lytren
- Nutralyte
- Ricelyte
- Hydralyte
- Cerealyte
- ReVital
- KaoLectrolyte
- Equalyte
- Pediatric Oral Maintenance Solution ORS
- WHO/UNICEF oral rehydration solution

PARTNERING WITH FAMILIES

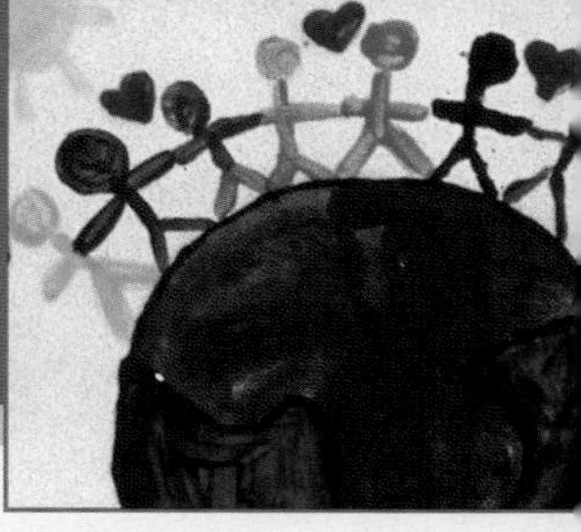

Preventing Heat-Related Illness

Teach parents, coaches, and youth the following preventive techniques.

- Precede exercise programs with physical examination designed to identify risks.
- Reduce intensity of activity when temperature or humidity are high.
- Allow a 10–14 day period of acclimation to higher temperatures before reaching usual exercise level.
- Ensure hydration before activity begins.
- During activity, stop for fluids every 15–20 minutes. Children up to 90 lb should drink 150 mL (5 oz) and those over 90 lb should drink 250 mL (9 oz). A combination of water and sports drink is best.
- Recognize low urine volume or dark color as a sign of dehydration.
- Wear light-colored, light clothing. Never use rubber clothing designed to promote weight loss through sweating.
- Maintain adequate sleep and nutritional status.

Additional tips for coaches:

- Weigh all children before and after events to evaluate if weight and therefore fluids are maintained.
- Be familiar with signs of heat-related illness.
- Have cell phones or other mechanisms available to call for emergency assistance.
- At least two adults should always be present at exercise sessions.
- Keep adequate fluids and sports drinks readily available.
- During all-day practices, allow 2–3 hours rest during the middle of the day with fluids and food provided.
- Practice in shade or use fans if possible.
- Obtain and use a wet-bulb globe temperature (WBGT) risk measurement that considers humidity (70% of heat stress), radiation (20% of heat stress), and temperature (10% of heat stress). For WBGT < 75°F activities are allowed with monitoring for heat-related problems, for 75–79°F enforce longer rest periods in the shade every 15 minutes, for 79–84°F limit activities for all children and eliminate activity for those not acclimated, and > 85° cancel all athletic activity.
- Understand symptoms for recognition of all heat-related problems.
- Obtain prompt first-aid treatment for any heat-related problems.

Data from Binkley et al., 2002; Committee on Sports Medicine and Fitness, 2000.

Teach Parents Oral Rehydration Methods

Instruct parents about the types of fluids and amounts to be given. Begin teaching with parents of all newborns and reinforce teaching at each well-child visit. Advise parents to continue the child's normal diet in addition to providing the rehydration solution. Cereals, starches, soups, fruits, and vegetables are allowed. Tell parents to avoid simple sugars, which can worsen diarrhea because of osmotic effects, including soft drinks (if used, soft drinks should be diluted with equal parts of water), undiluted juice, Jell-O, and sweetened cereal.

Repeated vomiting of large volumes of fluid or a worsening of the child's condition can indicate the need for intravenous therapy. Teach parents when to seek further medical care. If the child's condition worsens or does not improve after 4 hours of oral rehydration therapy, parents should contact a healthcare professional.

Monitor Intravenous Fluid Administration

Ill neonates usually receive all fluids intravenously, and many babies and children in intensive care units receive most fluids intravenously. The child hospitalized for dehydration usually requires administration of intravenous fluids. Be sure that the amount of fluid administered to all infants and children corresponds with the diagnosed dehydration state and maintenance fluid needs of the child (Box 23–5). Usually, about half of the 24-hour total maintenance and replacement needs will be given to a dehydrated child in the first 6 to 8 hours, with a slower rate infused for the remainder of the 24 hours. During the first 1 to 3 hours, the infusion rate may be highest to rapidly expand the vascular space. Rapid infusion of 20 to 30 mL/kg over 1 to 2 hours is sometimes used in outpatient settings, followed by oral fluids. When oral fluids are maintained, the decision for discharge can be made and hospitalization avoided. Maintain the intravenous line carefully so fluid infusion can be kept on schedule (refer to the Skills Manual). See Evidence-Based Practice: Intravenous Starts on page 739. Use a pump to prevent inadvertent, rapid infusion, which can lead to fluid overload and electrolyte imbalance (Figure 23–6 ■). Play with the toddler and preschool child

BOX 23–5 Calculation of Intravenous Fluid Needs

1. First, calculate the maintenance fluid needs of the child, according to the following guideline.

Usual Weight	Maintenance Amount
Up to 10 kg	100 mL/kg/24 hr
11–20 kg	1000 mL + (50 mL/kg for weight above 10 kg)/ 24 hr
> 20 kg	1500 mL + (20 mL/kg for weight above 20 kg)/ 24 hr

   Example: *Vernon's weight is 12 kg. He needs 1000 mL + (50 × 2), or 1100 mL/24 hr for maintenance fluid.*
2. Next, calculate replacement fluid for that loss.
   Example: *Vernon has lost 1 kg (8%) of his body weight. Multiplying the percentage of body weight × 10 yields the mL/kg/24 hr required:*
   $$8 \times 10 = 80 \text{ mL/kg/24 hr}$$
   $$80 \text{ mL/kg} \times 12 \text{ kg} = 960 \text{ mL}$$
   Thus, Vernon's replacement fluid needs are 960 mL/24 hr.
3. Finally, calculate continued losses and add to the total maintenance and replacement needs.

Note: These fluid needs are for normal children who have a problem causing dehydration. In special circumstances, such as very-low-birth-weight infants, or children with problems such as renal disease, the maintenance amounts need to be adjusted. Consult with specialists treating the child and specialized references to learn about fluid needs in these situations.

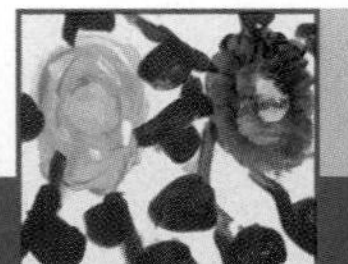

Nursing Care Plan

THE CHILD WITH MILD OR MODERATE DEHYDRATION

GOAL	INTERVENTION	RATIONALE	EXPECTED OUTCOME
1. Ineffective Management of Therapeutic Regimen related to family knowledge deficit about diarrhea and vomiting			
	NIC Priority Intervention: *Family Involvement:* Facilitate family participation in care of the child.		**NOC Suggested Outcome:** *Participation: Healthcare Decisions:* Personal involvement in selecting healthcare options.
Parents will describe appropriate home management of fluid replacement for diarrhea and vomiting.	■ Explain how to replace body fluid with an oral rehydration solution. Encourage parents to keep the solution at home and begin use with the first sign of diarrhea. ■ Teach parents to continue the child's normal diet in addition to providing replacement fluids for diarrhea. ■ Provide verbal and written instructions to parents at each well-child visit.	■ Use of an oral rehydration solution can enable successful treatment of vomiting and diarrhea at home. ■ Diet plus fluid supplementation leads to faster recovery. ■ Parents are provided with a reference for later use.	Parents are successfully able to treat the child's diarrhea and vomiting at home. Child is adequately hydrated.
2. Knowldege, Deficient (parent) related to causes of dehydration			
	NIC Priority Intervention: *Teaching:* Teach causes of dehydration.		**NOC Suggested Outcome:** *Knowledge:* Extent of understanding conveyed about treatment regimen
Parents will state common causes of childhood dehydration.	■ Teach parents childhood conditions that commonly lead to dehydration.	■ If parents recognize situations that can lead to dehydration, they will be more alert to its appearance.	Parents recognize conditions of risk for dehydration in children.
3. Risk for Fluid Volume, Deficient related to worsening of child's condition			
	NIC Priority Intervention: *Fluid Management:* Promote fluid balance.		**NOC Suggested Outcome:** *Fluid Balance:* Balance of water in extra- and intracellular compartments of body.
Parents will seek healthcare for the child's worsening condition.	■ Teach parents to seek care when the child's vomiting or diarrhea worsens, or the child's mental alertness changes.	■ Severe dehydration may occur if milder forms are not successfully treated.	Parents seek prompt attention for the child's worsening condition, preventing the development of severe dehydration.

frequently and use diversionary methods, as necessary, to distract the child from the intravenous line. Monitor the child carefully and implement safety precautions as necessary. Once the child begins to tolerate some oral fluids, oral rehydration therapy is substituted for intravenous fluid administration, and frequent administration of appropriate fluids is needed.

■ Discharge Planning and Home Care Teaching

Prevention of dehydration is the best approach when possible. Encourage breastfeeding because it is associated with a decreased incidence of gastroenteritis. During health promotion and health maintenance visits, encourage all parents to keep oral rehydration fluids at home in case they are needed at some time; they are available in most grocery stores and pharmacies (Box 23–6). Address the need for increasing fluids in hot weather and when the child is exercising. Reinforce safety teaching to decrease incidence of burns, an important cause of dehydration. Teach the signs and symptoms of vomiting and diarrhea so parents recognize these

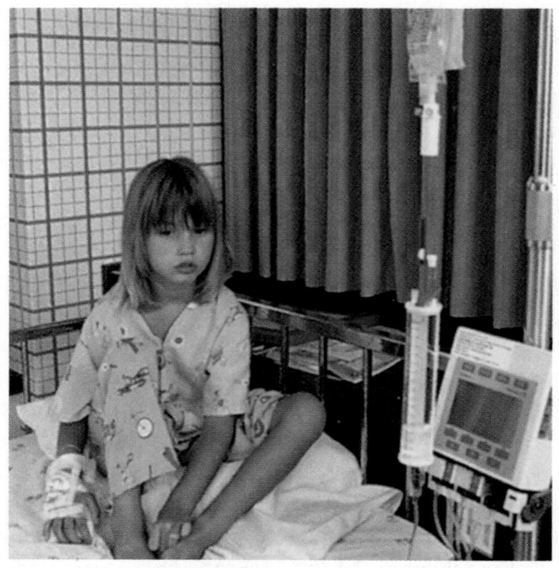

FIGURE 23–6 ■ The use of a volume control device with an intravenous saline infusion is important to prevent a sudden extracellular fluid volume overload.

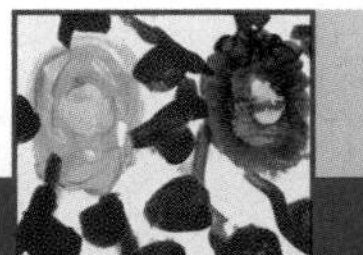

Nursing Care Plan

THE CHILD WITH SEVERE DEHYDRATION

GOAL	INTERVENTION	RATIONALE	EXPECTED OUTCOME
1. Fluid Volume, Deficient related to excess losses and inadequate intake			
	NIC Priority Intervention: *Fluid Management:* Promote fluid balance.		**NOC Suggested Outcome:** *Fluid Balance:* Balance of water in extra- and intracellular components of the body.
The child will return to normal hydration status and will not develop hypovolemic shock.	■ Monitor weight daily. Assess intake and output every shift. Assess heart rate, postural blood pressure, skin turgor, small-vein filling time, capillary refill time, fontanel (infant), and urine specific gravity every 4 hours or more frequently as indicated. ■ Administer intravenous fluids as ordered. Monitor for crackles in dependent portions of the lungs.	■ Frequent assessment of hydration status facilitates rapid intervention and evaluation of the effectiveness of fluid replacement. ■ Replace fluid lost from the body. Excessive replacement of sodium-containing fluids could cause extracellular fluid volume excess.	The child has signs of normal hydration.
2. Risk for Injury related to decreased level of consciousness			
	NIC Priority Intervention: *Fall Prevention:* Institute special precautions.		**NOC Suggested Outcome.** *Fall Prevention:* Minimize risk factors that precipitate falls.
The child will not experience injury.	■ Raise the side rails of the bed. Ensure that a small child does not become tangled in bed covers. ■ Monitor level of consciousness every 2–4 hours or more often as indicated. ■ Monitor serum sodium concentration daily or more often. ■ Have the child sit before rising from bed and assist to stand slowly.	■ Safety measures protect the child. ■ Frequent assessment provides evidence of the need for safety interventions and of the effectiveness of therapy. ■ Elevated serum sodium concentration causes brain cell shrinkage and decreased level of consciousness. ■ Slow adjustment to upright posture reduces light-headedness from decreased blood volume.	The child does not fall or suffer other injury.
3. Activity Intolerance related to bed rest/immobility			
	NIC Priority Intervention: *Activity Therapy:* Plan activities to meet child's developmental needs.		**NOC Suggested Outcome:** *Energy Conservation:* Manage energy to sustain activity.
The child will engage in normal activity for age.	■ Plan activities appropriate for the age of the child that can be done in bed. ■ Group nursing interventions to provide time for the child to rest. ■ Provide assistance during meals and other activities as needed.	■ Activities will provide distraction and promote recovery. ■ The child will require more rest than usual. ■ Prevention of overexertion will conserve body fluid and promote healing.	The child engages in normal developmental activities and receives adequate rest.

problems accurately. Prior to discharge from the hospital or outpatient facility after dehydration treatment, parents need instructions about types of fluids and amounts to encourage. Teach the signs of dehydration that parents can recognize such as increasing lethargy, dry mucous membranes, decreased urine output, and either increased thirst or anorexia. Parents should seek help immediately when these symptoms occur. Emphasize that the newborn and infant are at highest risk and that prompt care is needed if dehydration persists. After treatment, instruct parents to begin the child's normal diet once hydration is complete, determined by adequate urinary output and normal behaviors. Review methods of minimizing the child's chance of acquiring gastrointestinal infections (e.g., avoiding contact with other children who are infected; using careful handwashing and dishwashing procedures when a child in the home is affected). Most gastroenteritis is viral in origin and the child can return to school or childcare once the symptoms

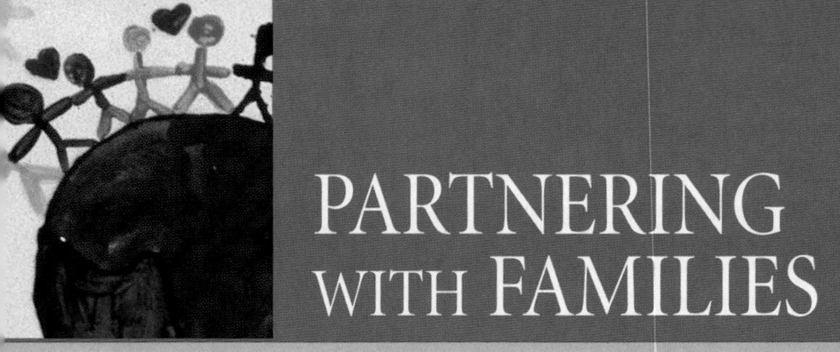

Oral Rehydration Therapy Guidelines

Calculate the specific amounts required for individual children based on the following guidelines and instruct parents in terminology they understand. Provide measuring devices with proper amounts marked.

- Children with diarrhea and no dehydration should be continued on age-appropriate diets.
- For mild dehydration, give 50 mL/kg oral rehydration therapy in first 4 hours in addition to replacing fluids lost in stool and emesis. (Measure emesis and give 10 mL/kg of fluid for each diarrheal stool.)
  - Start slowly, administering 3–5 mL in a small cup or spoon every few minutes. Increase amounts gradually if no vomiting occurs.
  - Recommend or provide samples of ORT solutions. Suggest ready-to-feed or powdered forms for choice by parents.
- For moderate dehydration, give 100 mL/kg oral rehydration therapy in first 4 hours in addition to replacing fluids lost as described above.
- For severe dehydration, the child is hospitalized and treated with intravenous fluids. When hydrated adequately or concurrently with intravenous rehydration, begin oral rehydration therapy with 50–100 mL/kg of fluid in 4 hours and stool replacement as described above.
- Recalculate fluid needs after first 4 hours and adjust as needed. If the child is not taking increased fluids and otherwise improving by this time, contact healthcare provider.
- When rehydration is complete, resume normal diet.

Data from Provisional Committee on Quality Improvement, Subcommittee on Acute Gastroenteritis. (1996). Practice parameter: The management of acute gastroenteritis in young children. Pediatrics, *97, 424–436.*

of vomiting and diarrhea have disappeared. However, in bacterial cases, such as those caused by *E. coli* or *Shigella*, negative stool cultures may be needed prior to exposure to other children and stool cultures may be recommended for close contacts in the family or school (Committee on Infectious Diseases, 2003). See Chapter 30∞ for further discussion of gastrointestinal illness and Chapter 19∞ for infectious and communicable diseases.

■ Evaluation

Expected outcomes of nursing care for the child with dehydration include the following:

- Balance of water and electrolytes in intracellular and extracellular compartments
- Normal urinary output
- Adequate fluid intake for maintenance needs
- Vital signs within normal limits

Extracellular Fluid Volume Excess

Extracellular fluid volume excess occurs when there is too much fluid in the extracellular compartment (intravascular and interstitial). This imbalance may also be called saline excess or extracellular volume overload. If this disorder occurs by itself (without saline disturbance), the serum sodium concentration is normal. There is simply too much extracellular fluid, even though it has a normal concentration.

Infants and children who develop an extracellular fluid volume excess have a condition that causes them to retain **saline** (sodium and water) or they have been given an overload of sodium-containing isotonic intravenous fluid (Figure 23–7 ■).

CLINICAL TIP

A normal saline solution is a salt solution that has the same percentage of salt as the human body. This is a 0.9% solution of sodium chloride. The term *normal* indicates that there is the same weight, in grams, of sodium and chloride in the solution. There are 154 mEq/L of sodium and 154 mEq/L of chloride in normal saline.

What conditions cause retention of saline? The hormone aldosterone is secreted by the adrenal cortex. One of its normal functions is to cause the kidneys to retain saline in the body (Figure 23–8 ■). Saline excess can be caused by any condition that results in excessive aldosterone secretion, such as adrenal tumors that secrete aldosterone, congestive heart failure, liver cirrhosis, and chronic renal failure (Figure 23–9 ■). Most glucocorticoid medications (such as prednisone) have a mild saline-retaining effect when taken long term.

Because fluid has weight, extracellular fluid volume excess is characterized by weight gain.

CLINICAL TIP

You can tell if a child's weight gain is due to normal growth or to the development of extracellular fluid volume excess by looking at the speed with which the increase develops. Sudden weight gain (e.g., 0.5 kg [approximately 1 lb] in 1 day) is due to the accumulation of fluid. Gain of 0.5 kg overnight is due to retention of about 500 mL of saline.

BOX 23–6 Research: Knowledge of Diarrhea

In a study with ethnically diverse and medically underserved parents, 229 families completed questionnaires related to knowledge of diarrhea among young children. More highly educated parents had greater knowledge about diarrhea and its treatment. Many parents did not start oral rehydration therapy early in a diarrheal illness, citing cost, taste, and availability as problems. In addition, parents often restricted food, fluids, and even breastfeeding during diarrhea. Parents were receptive to teaching and most indicated that information from a health professional was important to them (Anidi, Bazargan, & James, 2002). Nurses should not assume parents know how to recognize and treat common illnesses leading to dehydration. Integrate such teaching into each health promotion/health maintenance visit. Emphasize the benefits of oral rehydration for treatment of mild diarrhea and provide clear guidelines for parents regarding types and amounts of feedings to use.

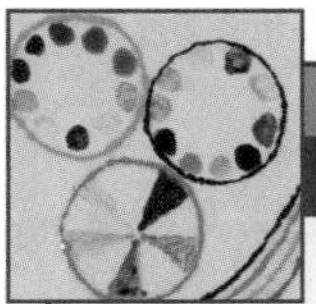

EVIDENCE-BASED PRACTICE
Intravenous Starts

PROBLEM

Parents often voice dissatisfaction with the number of intravenous starts to which their young hospitalized children are subjected, as children experience pain and anxiety when intravenous lines are initiated.

EVIDENCE

The Children's Hospital of Denver created a task force to address problems of venous access. Co-chairs in this collaborative project included a nurse from the neonatal intensive care unit, a general surgeon, and a radiologist. Additional nurses from units using peripheral intravenous lines served as committee members. A tracking tool was developed to collect information on intravenous placements for a 1-month period. Other children's hospitals were also surveyed for their practices regarding venous access policies and procedures. (The Venous Access Task Force, 2002).

IMPLICATIONS

Based on the analysis of internal and external data, the task force developed recommendations to (1) develop a group of specially trained nurses to act as resources for other staff nurses, (2) create an algorithm to provide guidelines for decisions about peripheral versus peripherally inserted central venous catheter versus central venous catheter insertion, (3) use the specially trained nurses to educate staff members about the new algorithm, and (4) develop a tracking/evaluation mechanism for the new algorithm and trained nurse group.

CRITICAL THINKING APPLICATION

This clinical situation is an example of partnership among healthcare specialists to improve care for hospitalized children. What were the benefits of having an interdisciplinary group to examine the topic of intravenous starts? How would you suggest that parent satisfaction before and after a program like this be measured? What could be the benefits of having a nursing resource group and an intravenous start guideline to positively influence the hospitalization of young children requiring intravenous infusion for dehydration?

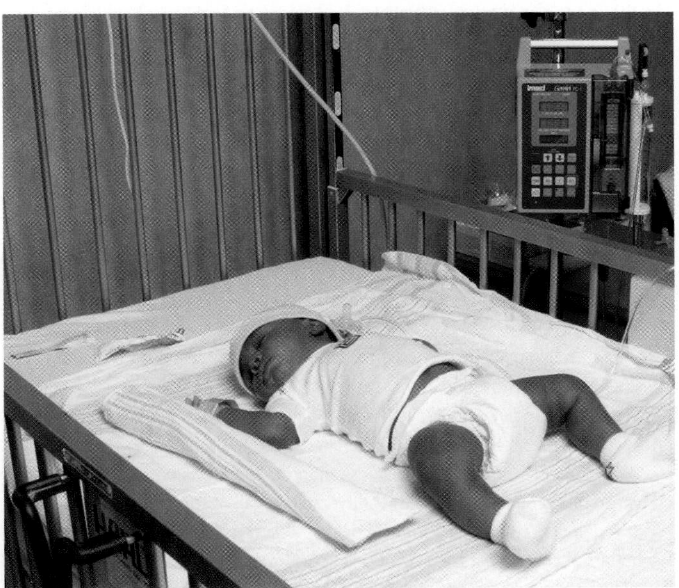

FIGURE 23–7 ■ If isotonic fluid containing sodium is given too rapidly or in too great an amount, an extracellular fluid volume excess will develop. Carefully monitor fluid intake, excretion, and retention in infants and children.

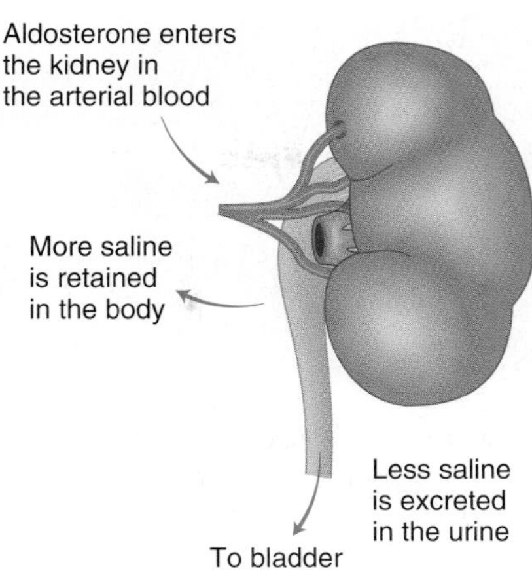
Aldosterone enters
the kidney in
the arterial blood
More saline
is retained
in the body
Less saline
is excreted
in the urine
To bladder

FIGURE 23–8 ■ Aldosterone has a saline-retaining effect. Increased aldosterone secretion can be caused by adrenal tumors or congestive heart failure.

An overload of fluid in the blood vessels and interstitial spaces can cause clinical manifestations such as bounding pulse, distended neck veins in children (not usually evident in infants), hepatomegaly, dyspnea, orthopnea, and lung crackles. Edema is the sign of overload of the interstitial fluid compartment (see description later in the chapter). In an infant, edema is often generalized. Edema in children with extracellular fluid volume excess occurs in the dependent parts of the body, that is, in the parts closest to the ground. Thus, edema is evident in sacral areas in a child supine in bed. Edema that develops from other causes is described in the next section of this chapter.

Intravenous fluid volume regulation is important, especially in young children. Inaccurate calculation of needed fluid or inadvertent infusion of excess fluids can cause overload.

Clinical therapy for extracellular fluid volume excess focuses on treating the underlying cause of the disorder. For example, a child who has congestive heart failure is given medications to strengthen the heart's ability to contract (see Chapter 26∞ for further discussion of management of fluid volume excess in congenital heart disease). In addition, diuretics may be given to remove fluid from the body, thus reducing the extracellular fluid volume directly.

NURSING MANAGEMENT

Rapid weight gain is the most sensitive index of extracellular fluid volume excess. Therefore, daily weighing is an important nursing assessment. Measure the child's intake and output. When treatment is successful, output is greater than intake.

CLINICAL TIP

The infant's urine output is important to monitor both dehydration and edema. Weigh the diaper before and after use. A 1 g weight increase in the diaper equals 1 mL of urine volume. Change the diaper frequently to minimize urine loss from evaporation.

Assess the character of the pulse and observe for neck vein distention when the child is sitting (usually visible only in older children). Monitor for signs of pulmonary edema (an indication

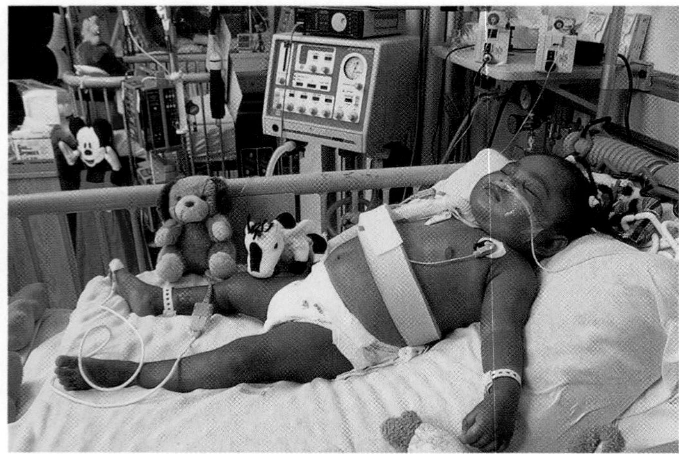

FIGURE 23–9 ■ This infant with congenital heart disease has signs of generalized edema. Note the fluid retention in the face and abdomen.

of severe imbalance) by listening to lung sounds in the dependent lung fields (crackles) and assessing for respiratory distress (rapid respiratory rate, use of accessory muscles of respiration). Observe for edema.

The potential for a child to develop a fluid overload is present whenever an isotonic intravenous solution containing sodium is being administered. Examples include normal saline (0.9% NaCl), Ringer's solution, and lactated Ringer's solution. In such cases, monitor the infusion rate frequently and carefully and use a pump when possible to aid in accurate administration.

PRACTICE ALERT

Occasionally intravenous fluid is infused too rapidly, causing extracellular fluid volume excess and endangering the fluid and electrolyte status of a young child. The nurse can take the following measures to minimize this risk.

- Use small bags of fluid, so if the fluid were to infuse quickly, the amount infused would be limited.
- Always use infusion pumps when available so that the rate is programmed and monitored.
- Check and double-check the machine after setting to be sure it was properly programmed.
- Have another nurse check your calculation of rates and total fluid to be infused until you are certain of your skill in this area.
- Finally, remember that even mechanical pumps can have faulty performance so check the intravenous line, bag, and rate frequently.

If an excess of fluid has already developed, administer the medical therapy as prescribed and monitor for any complications of the therapy. For example, many diuretics increase potassium excretion in the urine, an increase that may lead to an abnormally low plasma potassium concentration unless potassium intake is increased. (Refer to the discussion of hypokalemia later in this chapter.) It is also important to monitor for the development of extracellular fluid volume deficit as a result of diuretic therapy.

If edema is present, provide careful skin care and protection for edematous areas. Teach parents how to provide skin care and perform position changes at home. See the following section for additional interventions related to edema.

If a child has a long-term condition such as chronic renal failure that predisposes to extracellular fluid volume excess, a dietary sodium restriction may be prescribed (see Chapter 31 ∞ for further detail). Teach parents how to manage sodium restriction. See Developing Cultural Competence: Low-Sodium Diets. Plan low-sodium meals that fit the family's cultural practices. If the child is old enough to participate, incorporate games into the teaching. If a scale is available, teach parents to take and record an accurate daily weight.

Expected outcomes include electrolyte balance, maintenance of intact skin, and dietary intake as prescribed.

Interstitial Fluid Volume Excess (Edema)

Edema is an abnormal increase in the volume of interstitial fluid. It may be caused by an extracellular fluid volume excess or it may be due to other causes.

The causes of edema are best understood in the context of normal capillary dynamics. Fluid moves between the vascular and interstitial compartments by the process of filtration. Filtration is the net result of forces that tend to move fluid in opposing directions. The strongest forces will determine the direction of fluid movement.

At the capillary level, two forces (blood hydrostatic pressure and interstitial osmotic pressure) tend to move fluid from the capillaries into the interstitial fluid, while two other forces (blood colloid osmotic pressure and interstitial fluid hydrostatic pressure) tend to move fluid in the opposite direction (from the interstitial fluid into the capillaries). The net result of these forces usually moves fluid from the capillaries into the interstitial compartment at the arterial end of the capillaries and fluid from the interstitial compartment back into the capillaries at the venous end of the capillaries. This process brings oxygen and nutrients to the cells and removes carbon dioxide and other waste products.

Edema occurs if the balance of these four forces is altered so that excess fluid either enters or leaves the interstitial compartment (Figure 23–10 ■). This may occur through (1) increased blood hydrostatic pressure, (2) decreased blood colloid osmotic pressure, (3) increased interstitial fluid osmotic pressure, or (4) blocked lymphatic drainage. Various clinical conditions are associated with these altered forces (Table 23–4), as described here.

DEVELOPING CULTURAL COMPETENCE
Low-Sodium Diets

To adapt teaching about low-sodium diets to the cultural practices of a family, ask clients what types of food they usually eat. Help them to choose low-sodium foods from their diets and to avoid high-sodium foods. This approach is more effective than giving the same list of restricted foods to each family.

For example, some Asians may use monosodium glutamate to flavor foods and can be encouraged to add this at the table for family members who can have extra sodium rather than during cooking. Many Hispanic groups use large amounts of cheese that can provide significant sodium. Encourage them to look for low sodium cheese and substitute cottage cheese for other types since it is lower in sodium. Canned foods tend to have high sodium so teach all families to use fresh produce rather than canned when possible. Low-sodium milk is available and a good option for young children.

PATHOPHYSIOLOGY ILLUSTRATED

Capillary Dynamics and Edema

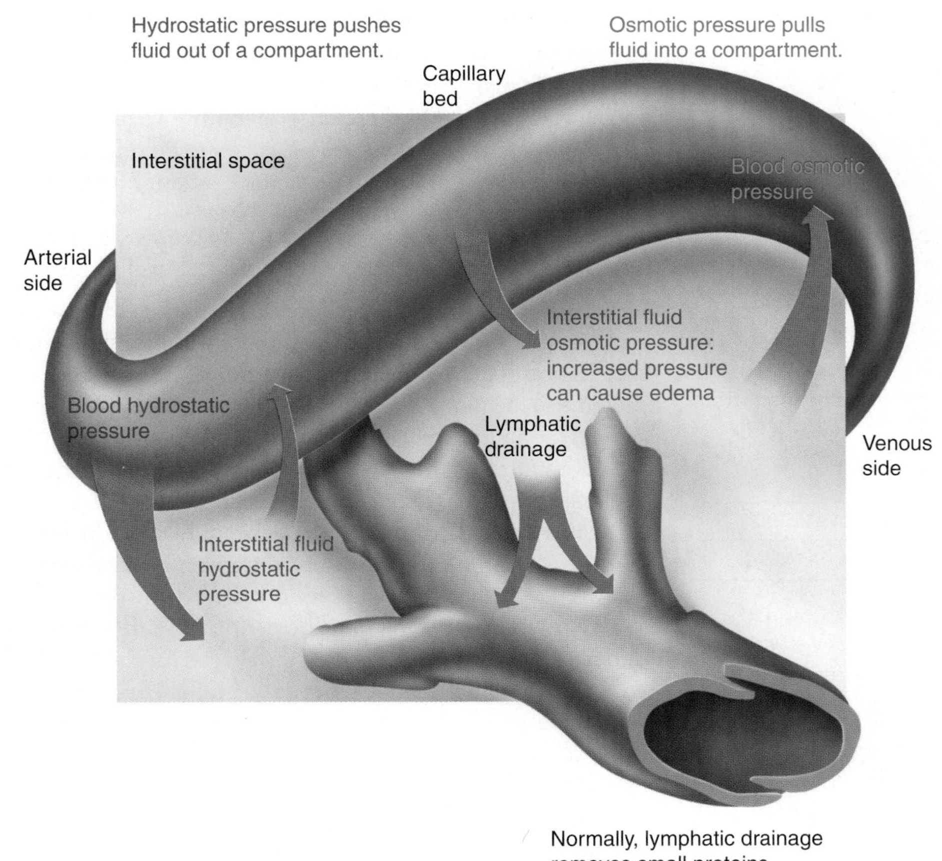
Hydrostatic pressure pushes fluid out of a compartment.
Osmotic pressure pulls fluid into a compartment.
Capillary bed
Interstitial space
Blood osmotic pressure
Arterial side
Interstitial fluid osmotic pressure: increased pressure can cause edema
Blood hydrostatic pressure
Lymphatic drainage
Venous side
Interstitial fluid hydrostatic pressure
Normally, lymphatic drainage removes small proteins and excess interstitial fluid. Blocked lymphatic drainage can cause edema.

FIGURE 23–10 ■ With normal capillary dynamics, fluid moves out of the compartment by the force of hydrostatic pressure in the blood vessel and is pulled out by interstitial osmotic pressure. Fluid is forced into the compartment by interstitial hydrostatic pressure and pulled in by compartment osmotic pressure. Abnormal capillary dynamics can cause edema.

1. **Increased blood hydrostatic pressure.** When extracellular fluid volume excess occurs, the increased fluid volume in the vascular compartment congests the veins. The pressure against the sides of the capillary is increased and more fluid then enters the interstitial compartment.
2. **Decreased blood colloid osmotic pressure.** Much of the osmotic pressure that pulls fluid into the capillaries is due to the presence of albumin and other plasma proteins made by the liver. The part of the blood osmotic pressure that is due to plasma proteins is often called **oncotic pressure** or blood colloid osmotic pressure. Any condition that decreases plasma proteins will decrease blood colloid osmotic pressure and cause edema. For example, if a clinical condition causes large amounts of albumin to leak into the urine, the liver will not be able to make albumin fast enough to replace it. As a result, the plasma protein level will fall, decreasing the blood osmotic pressure. Without this pulling force to return fluid to the capillaries, edema will occur. This is the cause of the edema that occurs in children who have nephrotic syndrome (see Chapter 31∞). Another cause in children is prolonged surgical procedures with significant blood loss. Intravenous fluids and blood may be infused during surgery to replace those losses, but plasma proteins are lost and not fully restored by infusion. Edema may be seen in the postoperative period.
3. **Increased interstitial fluid osmotic pressure.** Ordinarily, only a few small proteins enter the interstitial fluid, and the interstitial fluid osmotic pressure is small. If the capillary becomes abnormally permeable to proteins, however, the influx of large amounts of proteins into the interstitial fluid causes a dramatic increase in interstitial fluid osmotic pressure. This increased pulling force keeps an abnormal amount of fluid in the interstitial compartment. This mechanism plays an important part in the edema caused by a bee sting or a sprained

MediaLink Edema Animation

TABLE 23–4 Clinical Conditions That Cause Edema

EDEMA DUE TO INCREASED BLOOD HYDROSTATIC PRESSURE
Increased Capillary Blood Flow
Inflammation Local infection
Venous Congestion
Extracellular fluid volume excess Right heart failure Venous thrombosis External pressure on vein Muscle paralysis
EDEMA DUE TO DECREASED BLOOD OSMOTIC PRESSURE
Increased Albumin Excretion
Nephrotic syndrome (albumin leaks into urine) Protein-losing enteropathies (excess albumin in feces)
Decreased Albumin Synthesis
Kwashiorkor (low-protein, high-carbohydrate starvation diet provides too few amino acids for liver to make albumin) Liver cirrhosis (diseased liver unable to make enough albumin)
EDEMA DUE TO INCREASED INTERSTITIAL FLUID OSMOTIC PRESSURE
Increased Capillary Permeability
Inflammation Toxins Hypersensitivity reactions Burns
EDEMA DUE TO BLOCKED LYMPHATIC DRAINAGE
Tumors Goiter Parasites that obstruct lymph nodes Surgery that removes lymph nodes

ankle. It occurs to a greater extent in burns, leading to swelling at the same time that there is a great loss of fluid volume through the burned skin (see Chapter 36∞).

4. **Blocked lymphatic drainage.** The lymph vessels normally drain small proteins and excess fluid from the interstitial compartment and return them to the blood vessels. If this process is blocked, fluid accumulates in the interstitial compartment. This may occur when a tumor blocks lymphatic drainage.

Edema causes swelling, which may be localized or generalized. The swelling of tissue may cause pain and restrict motion. Edema that is due to extracellular fluid volume excess or right-sided heart failure usually occurs in the dependent portion of the body. In a child who is walking, dependent edema is observed in the ankles; in a bedfast supine child, it is seen in the sacral area. The skin over an edematous area often appears thin and shiny.

The main focus of clinical therapy for edema is to treat the underlying condition that caused the edema. Such conditions are discussed throughout this book. The edema from inflammation of an injury is initially treated with cold to reduce capillary blood flow and thus reduce blood hydrostatic pressure.

NURSING MANAGEMENT

A child or parent may make comments that alert the nurse to the development of edema. Shoes may become tight by the end of the day (dependent edema); the waistband of pants or a skirt may be "outgrown" suddenly (generalized edema or ascites, which is accumulation of fluid in the peritoneal cavity); the eyes may be puffy (periorbital edema); a ring may be too tight; fingers may "feel like sausages." In many cases visual inspection is sufficient to recognize edema. Observe for the presence of pitting edema. To detect changes in the amount of swelling, measure around the edematous part (Figure 23–11 ■). See Chapter 8∞ for further description of assessment of edema. If the edema is caused by extracellular fluid volume excess, daily measurements of weight and intake and output are a necessary part of the daily assessment. Carefully perform such assessments in all children at risk such as those who had recent surgery with blood loss and those with health conditions such as heart failure or nephrotic syndrome. Nursing assessment should also focus on the integrity of the skin, presence of pain, restricted motion, and alterations in the child's body image.

Elevation of an area of localized edema helps to reduce the swelling. The skin over an edematous area needs extra care because it is fragile (Figure 23–12 ■). Carefully position an infant or child who is on bed rest and turn frequently to prevent pressure sores. Use sheepskin and special mattresses to decrease pressure on the skin. Turning must be performed carefully to avoid skin abrasion by rubbing against the sheets. Pat the skin dry after cleansing rather than rubbing it. Trim the child's fingernails smooth to prevent scratching. Teach parents skin care for the child at home and recommend checking for redness or skin breakdown several times daily. Teach older children to inspect their skin carefully to identify areas needing special care. Prevention and care of pressure ulcers is described in Chapter 36∞.

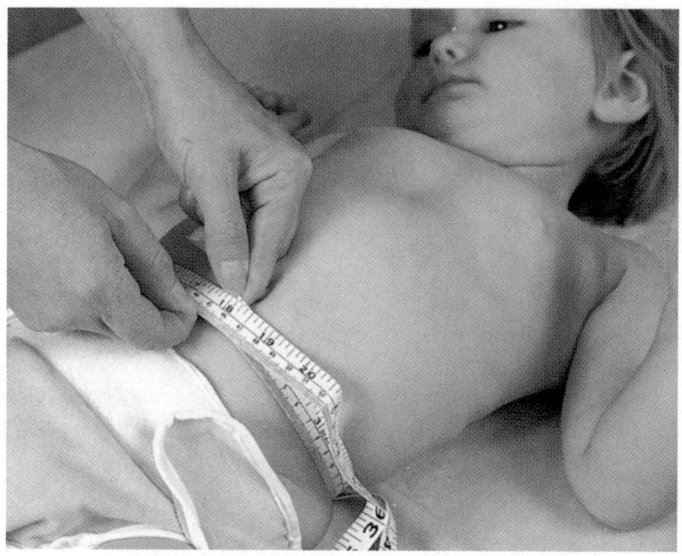

FIGURE 23–11 ■ Finding the same location each day for measuring circumference to assess edema can be accomplished by use of a reference point. An indelible marker may be used to mark the measurement location on the skin, if this is acceptable to the child and parents.

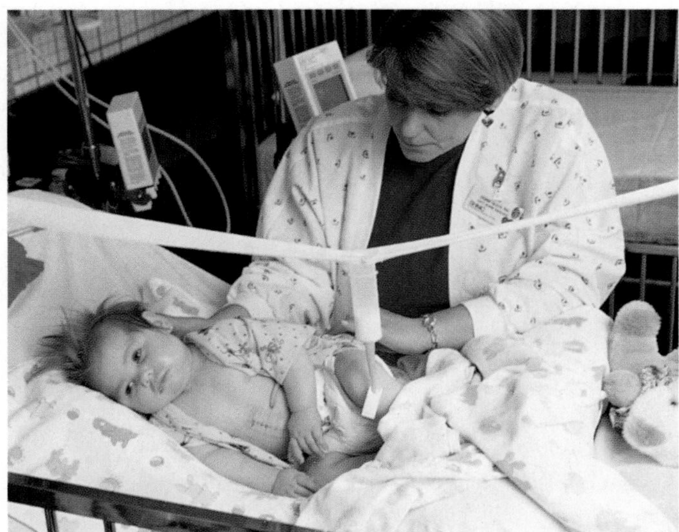

FIGURE 23–12 ■ Edematous tissue is easily damaged. It must be kept clean and dry and free of pressure.

If restricted mobility is a problem, specific plans to help the child manage activities are needed. For example, if an edematous finger restricts hand movement, food can be cut into bite-size portions before the meal is served, so that the child can still eat independently.

Discomfort from edema may require creative interventions by the nurse. Distraction with toys or activities appropriate to the child's developmental level can be useful. Interventions to treat the underlying problem can also reduce the edema and its accompanying discomfort. Interventions for edema should be added to the nursing management of the underlying condition that causes the edema. Administration of the prescribed medical therapy and observation for the complications of therapy are nursing responsibilities.

Discuss with school-age children and adolescents feelings of embarrassment about the edematous appearance. They need to understand the reason for edema and be able to explain it to peers. Arrange for the child to meet other children with similar concerns.

Desired outcomes of care include maintenance of intact skin, normal respiratory sounds and effort, normal weight patterns, and maintenance of fluid and electrolyte balance.

ELECTROLYTE IMBALANCES

All body fluids contain electrolytes, although the concentration of those electrolytes varies, depending on the type and location of the fluid. When a serum electrolyte value is reported from the laboratory, it provides information about the concentration of that electrolyte in the blood. It may not necessarily reflect the concentration of the electrolyte in other body compartments. Each laboratory has standard values based on the machines and assay techniques used. Refer to local laboratory norms and realize that levels in references are general or average levels that may differ slightly from a specific laboratory standard. Refer to Table 23–1 to see which electrolytes are highest and lowest concentration in the blood and other fluid compartments.

Electrolytes are normally gained and lost in relatively equal amounts so the body remains in balance. However, when a child has an abnormal route of loss, such as vomiting, wound drainage, or nasogastric suction, electrolyte balance can be disturbed. In addition, supplementation with electrolytes via IV fluids in proportion different than body fluids can also cause electrolyte imbalance. Children with disease states that interfere with normal mechanisms of electrolyte regulation, such as renal disease, also have disturbance in electrolyte levels. Monitoring for signs of imbalance becomes important in all of these cases.

Sodium Imbalances

The serum sodium concentration reflects the **osmolality** of body fluids, that is, their degree of concentration or dilution. It refers to the number of moles of the substance per kilogram of water in the solution. Serum sodium concentration reflects the proportion of water and sodium in the extracellular compartment. When the osmolality of body fluids becomes abnormal, the cells swell or shrink. These cell size changes are due to osmosis, the movement of water across a semipermeable membrane into an area of higher particle concentration (Figure 23–13 ■). Sodium levels are maintained at high extracellular and low intracellular levels by the sodium-potassium pump, which moves these electrolytes against their expected concentration gradients.

Sodium plays several important roles in the body and is an important **cation** (positively charged particle). It is important in blood pressure regulation and maintenance of fluid volume.

Hypernatremia

Hypernatremia is a condition of increased osmolality of the blood. The body fluids are too concentrated, containing excess sodium relative to water. A serum sodium level above 148 mmol/L in children (146 mmol/L in newborns) is diagnostic of hypernatremia.

Etiology and Pathophysiology. Hypernatremia results from conditions that cause the body to lose relatively more water than sodium or to gain relatively more sodium than water (Table 23–5). Examples include children who do not have access to adequate water or are developmentally delayed and do not perceive thirst. Special circumstances in which a high solute intake may occur without adequate water include an infant formula that is too concentrated or one that is prepared with salt instead of sugar. A breast-fed baby not receiving adequate breast milk who has normal water loss may develop hypernatremic dehydration (Livingstone, Willis, Abdel-Wareth, et al., 2000.) See Box 23–7. Newborns in the neonatal intensive care unit usually do not require sodium in intravenous infusions until about day 3 of life, when newborn diuresis occurs; earlier administration of sodium may lead to hypernatremia.

Clinical Manifestations. An infant or child who has hypernatremia is generally thirsty. The urine output is low unless the hypernatremia is caused by diabetes insipidus. A decreased level of consciousness manifested by confusion, lethargy, or coma

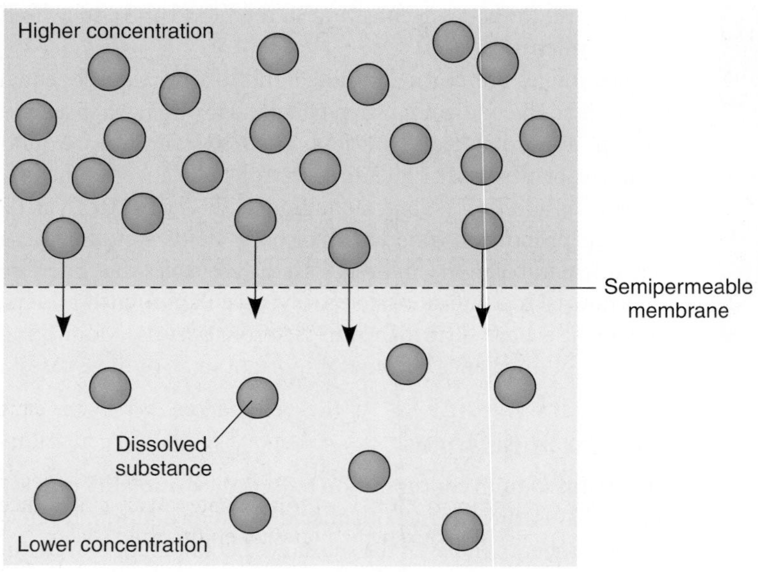

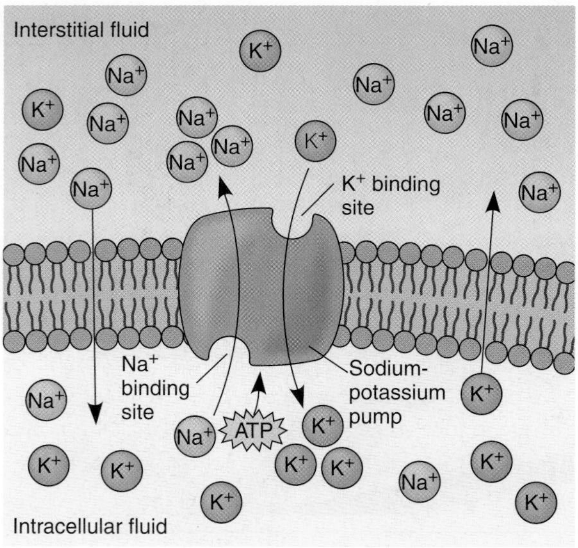

FIGURE 23–13 ■ *A,* Water balance is maintained by the simple passage of molecules from greater to lesser concentration across cell membranes. *B,* Sodium levels are maintained by an active transport system, the sodium-potassium pump, which moves these electrolytes across cell membranes in spite of their concentrations.

results from shrinking of the brain cells. Seizures can occur when hypernatremia occurs rapidly or is severe. Severe hypernatremia can be fatal.

COLLABORATIVE CARE

The major laboratory test that is diagnostic of sodium imbalance is serum sodium. Normal level for newborns is 133 to 146 mmol/L and for children 135 to 148 mmol/L. See Table 23–6 for normally acceptable laboratory values for electrolytes. Specific gravity of urine is concentrated in hypernatremia and dilute in hyponatremia. The normal levels are 1.001 to 1.015 in infants to 2 years of age, and 1.010 to 1.030 for children over 2 years.

TABLE 23–5 Causes of Hypernatremia

LOSS OF RELATIVELY MORE WATER THAN SODIUM	GAIN OF RELATIVELY MORE SODIUM THAN WATER
Inadequate intake from breastfeeding with normal output	Inability to communicate thirst
Diabetes insipidus (not enough antidiuretic hormone)	Limited or no access to water
Diarrhea or vomiting without fluid replacement	High solute intake without adequate water (e.g., tube feedings)
Excessive sweating without fluid replacement	Improper formula preparation leading to excessive concentration.
High solute intake without adequate water (causes kidneys to excrete water)	Intravenous hypertonic saline
Increased aldosterone	

CLINICAL TIP

Specific gravity compares the density of urine with the density of water (water density is 1.000). The infant's kidney is less able to concentrate urine so the specific gravity indicates dilution of urine.

Hypernatremia is treated by intravenous administration of **hypotonic fluid,** or fluid that is more dilute than normal body fluid. This therapy dilutes the body fluids back to normal concentration. If a child is dehydrated, **isotonic fluids** (those with the osmolality of body fluids) may be ordered first to replenish

BOX 23–7 Research: Causes of Hypernatremia

In recent years, the major causes of hypernatremia in infants have changed. Formerly, untreated diarrhea was a common cause. Presently, there has been an increase in the number of breastfed babies diagnosed with hypernatremia in the newborn period. When babies have the normal diuresis at 2–3 days of age but are not able to feed well or the mother does not have adequate breast milk, hypernatremia can occur. Decrease in activity and alertness, seizures, and excessive weight loss (≥ 10% of birth weight) in the first few days are symptoms in the neonate (Manganaro, Mami, Marrone, et al., 2001). Nurses teach mothers of newborns how to evaluate the feeding behaviors of their babies, weigh babies especially when early discharge after delivery occurs, and perform careful physical assessments to find infants with decreased neurologic response.

Another important cause of hypernatremia at present is inadequate provision or offering of water to hospitalized children (Blonshine, 2000; Moritz & Ayus, 1999). Nurses should ensure that children, especially those with developmental delays or who are unable to care for themselves, be offered adequate amounts of fluid. Assess intake and output and be alert for signs of neurologic change.

TABLE 23–6 Normal Serum Values for Electrolytes in Infants and Youth

	NEWBORN	INFANT AND CHILD
Sodium	131–144 mmol/L	132–141 mmol/L
Potassium	Premature 4.5–7.2 mmol/L Term 3.2–5.7 mmol/L	3.3–4.7 mmol/L
Calcium	Premature 3.5–4.5 mEq/L (1.7–2.3 mmol/L) Term 4–5 mEq/L (2–2.5 mmol/L or 8.5–10.6 mg/dL)	4.4–5.3 mEq/L (2.2–2.7 mmol/L or 8.7–10.7 mg/dL)
Magnesium	1.3–2.7 mg/dL (0.5–1.1 mmol/L)	1.6–2.7 mg/dL (0.7–1.1 mmol/L)

** Laboratories may have slightly different levels of normal depending on assays performed. Always consult the normal values for your particular laboratory.*

the volume, followed by hypotonic fluid to correct the osmolality. The underlying cause of the disorder is also treated.

NURSING MANAGEMENT

Teaching can prevent many cases of hypernatremia. Be sure the breastfeeding mother has instruction and resources about lactation before discharge after delivery. If discharged soon after birth, be sure the infant has an appointment to have weight checked within the first few days, and alert the parents to expected output of four to six wet diapers daily. By about 10 days, infants should have regained the birth weight. Assess the infant's alertness and general neurologic status (see Chapter 8∞).

When an infant is sick or developing slowly, parents sometimes want to feed the infant more concentrated formula to build the child's strength. Parents and caregivers of bottle-fed babies should be taught never to give undiluted formula concentrate or evaporated milk due to the high sodium content.

CLINICAL TIP

Careful teaching about how to mix powdered formula so that it is not too concentrated can help prevent hypernatremia. Pictures are an important teaching tool if the parents are not able to read labels or instructions. Ask for return demonstration to evaluate ability to mix formula accurately.

Children with delayed development are at risk for hypernatremia since they may not be able to recognize thirst or obtain fluids when dehydrated. Teach parents about the child's fluid requirements (use Box 23–5 to calculate) and offer adequate fluids when the child is hospitalized.

Parents should be cautioned to keep salt out of reach, because eating handfuls of salt has caused hypernatremia. Teach parents to offer extra fluids during hot weather. See Partnering with Families: Preventing Heat-Related Illness on page 735. Teach oral rehydration therapy for use at home during mild vomiting and diarrhea (see page 738).

When a child is hospitalized for hypernatremia, monitor serum sodium level and measure intake and output and urine specific gravity. Specific gravity changes toward normal levels as therapy progresses. Frequently assess responsiveness to monitor the effect of hypernatremia on brain cells. As the concentration of body fluids returns to normal, the child will become more alert and responsive. Watch for rebound hyponatremia while monitoring the fluid replacement. Implement safety interventions such as raised bed rails for protection. Ensure adequate rest and introduce developmentally appropriate activities when the child is alert.

Water deprivation is a form of child neglect or abuse. In neglect, the parents simply do not provide adequate water for the child. A form of child abuse that sometimes includes water deprivation is Munchausen syndrome by proxy (see Chapter 7∞). A small child who is hospitalized with hypernatremia that does not have a detectable cause may be subject to water deprivation. Assess the child's general condition, developmental tasks, the family dynamics, and parent's understanding of formula preparation and the child's fluid intake needs.

Nurses can prevent hypernatremia in hospitalized infants and children by administering water between tube feedings, keeping water available, and offering it frequently. Offering frequent small amounts and using popsicles and other creative interventions can increase children's intake.

Desired outcomes of treatment for hypernatremia include balance of electrolytes and fluid in the intracellular and extracellular compartments, and alert level of consciousness.

Hyponatremia

In hyponatremia, the osmolality of the blood is decreased. The body fluids are too dilute, containing excess water relative to sodium. Hyponatremia is the most common sodium imbalance in children (Behrman, Kliegman, & Jenson, 2004). A serum sodium level below 135 mmol/L in children (133 mmol/L in newborns) is diagnostic of hyponatremia.

Etiology and Pathophysiology. Hyponatremia results from conditions that cause gain of relatively more water than sodium or loss of relatively more sodium than water (Table 23–7). Intake of excessive water is called water intoxication. As an example, oral intake of water causes hyponatremia in unusual conditions such as forced fluid intake. More commonly, parents feed an infant only water or dilute formula to save money instead of regular-strength formula or breast milk. Excessive swallowing of swimming pool water by an infant can have the same effect. Infants are vulnerable to the type of hyponatremia caused by water intoxication, because they have a poorly developed thirst mechanism and may continue to drink, and then are unable to

TABLE 23–7 Causes of Hyponatremia

GAIN OF RELATIVELY MORE WATER THAN SODIUM	LOSS OF RELATIVELY MORE SODIUM THAN WATER
Excessive intravenous D_5W (5% dextrose in water)	Diarrhea or vomiting with replacement by tap water only instead of fluid containing sodium
Excessive tap water enemas	Excessive sweating such as in cystic fibrosis
Irrigation of body cavities with distilled water	Diuretics, especially thiazides
Excessive antidiuretic hormone	
Forced excessive oral intake of tap water	
Congestive heart failure	

excrete excess water quickly due to immature kidney function (Behrman et al., 2004).

Clinical Manifestations. The child with hyponatremia has a decreased level of consciousness, which results from swelling of brain cells. This can be manifested as anorexia, headache, muscle weakness, decreased deep tendon reflexes, lethargy, confusion, or coma. If hyponatremia arises rapidly or is extreme, seizures may occur. Hyponatremia is a frequent cause of seizures in infants under 6 months of age. Nausea and vomiting also occur in some children. Severe hyponatremia can be fatal.

COLLABORATIVE CARE

Nurses partner with other healthcare providers to gather laboratory specimens helpful in assessing for sodium imbalance. Careful correction of fluid and electrolyte balance is managed by the nurse, physician, neonatal nurse practitioner, pediatric nurse practitioner, and other care providers. Serum sodium is the major diagnostic test. Antidiuretic hormone (ADH) levels and 24-hour urinary output are helpful in diagnosing diabetes insipidus as the cause of hyponatremia. In most cases, hyponatremia is treated by restricting the intake of water. This therapy allows the kidneys to correct the imbalance by excreting excess water from the body. If a child is having seizures from hyponatremia, intravenous **hypertonic fluid** (more concentrated than body fluid) may be administered. Use of this concentrated saline is a way to rapidly increase body fluid concentration, but it must be monitored carefully because it can easily cause rebound hypernatremia.

NURSING MANAGEMENT

Nurses carefully assess all infants and children who are at risk for hyponatremia and promptly report symptoms to the primary care provider. Appropriate fluids with electrolytes are administered and monitored closely.

Nursing Assessment and Diagnosis

Monitor serum sodium level and measure intake and output. If an infant with hyponatremia has normal antidiuretic hormone (ADH) levels, and other causes have been ruled out, careful questioning about proper preparation of formula and feeding practices is needed. A toddler or school-age child may be subjected to forced fluid intake as a form of child abuse. Sensitive interviewing and a caring manner on the part of the nurse can help identify such problems in a family.

Because hyponatremia is characterized by decreased level of consciousness, frequent assessment of responsiveness will be necessary to monitor the response to therapy. The child will become more alert and responsive as the concentration of body fluids returns to normal.

The highest priority nursing diagnosis for hyponatremia addresses the risk for injury related to the child's decreased level of consciousness. The following diagnoses might also apply.

- Self-care Deficit related to weakness and tiredness
- Ineffective Health Maintenance related to parental information misinterpretation about infant formula
- Ineffective Breastfeeding related to inadequate sucking by infant or inadequate milk production

Planning and Implementation

Nurses can prevent hyponatremia in hospitalized children by using normal saline instead of distilled water for irrigations and by avoiding tap water enemas. It is important to help the child comply with prescribed fluid restrictions and teach the parents how to do this at home. See Partnering with Families: Interventions for a Child Who Has a Fluid Restriction. Allow the child to choose favorite fluids to drink. Teach parents to replace body fluids lost through diarrhea or vomiting with oral electrolyte solutions (see page 738). The child with diseases such as cystic fibrosis or taking thiazide diuretics needs intake above that recommended for maintenance fluids.

Evaluation

Expected outcomes of nursing care for hyponatremia include the following:

- Avoidance of injury
- Balance of fluid and electrolytes
- Establishment of adequate intake of formula and/or breast milk

---

Potassium Imbalances

Potassium is an essential **anion** (negatively charged particle) that performs many necessary functions in the body. It is present in high levels in intracellular fluids and is active in enzyme performance in cells. It is needed for contractility of heart and skeletal muscle. Potassium intake in healthy children comes from potassium-rich foods such as fruits and vegetables. Potassium is absorbed easily from the intestine. A potassium imbalance arises when the serum potassium concentration rises or falls outside the normal range. Potassium imbalances are caused by alterations in potassium intake, distribution, or excretion; or by loss of potassium through an abnormal route such as burns, emesis, or renal failure.

Most of the potassium ions in the body are found inside the cells. The sodium-potassium pump in cell membranes moves potassium ions into cells to maintain the high intracellular potassium concentration (see Figure 23–13). Potassium ions can be shifted into or out of cells by various physiologic factors (Figure 23–14 ■). Potassium is excreted from the body through urine, feces, and sweat. The hormone aldosterone increases potassium excretion in the urine.

Hyperkalemia

Hyperkalemia is an excess of potassium in the blood. It is reflected by a level above 5.8 mmol/L in children or above 5.2 mmol/L in newborns.

Etiology and Pathophysiology. Hyperkalemia is caused by conditions that involve increased potassium intake, shift of potassium from cells into the extracellular fluid, and decreased potassium excretion. Indeed, renal insufficiency is a primary cause of hyperkalemia (Blonshine, 2000). Premature infants commonly have low systemic blood flow and resultant poor renal function, leading to hyperkalemia (Kluckow & Evans, 2001). Increased potassium intake is usually due to intravenous potassium overload. Excessive or too rapid intravenous administration of potassium-containing solutions can occur if potassium requirement is overestimated or if the intravenous infusion infuses too quickly.

Blood transfusion is another source of potassium intake that may cause hyperkalemia. Potassium ions leak out of red blood cells that are stored in a blood bank. The longer the blood is stored, the more potassium leaks out of cells and accumulates in the fluid portion of the transfusion. Hyperkalemia from administration of stored blood arises when multiple units are transfused, as when infants receive exchange transfusions or children receive multiple blood transfusions after a serious injury or in surgery.

Shift of potassium from cells into the extracellular fluid occurs when there is massive cell death, as with a crush injury, in sickle cell anemia (hemolytic crisis), in severe acidosis causing respiratory failure and organ failure, or when chemotherapy for a malignancy is rapidly effective. In these situations, the dead cells release their high-potassium contents into the extracellular fluid. Potassium ions also shift out of cells in metabolic acidosis caused by diarrhea and in diabetes mellitus when insulin levels are low.

Decreased potassium excretion occurs with acute or chronic oliguria during renal failure, prematurity, severe hypovolemia,

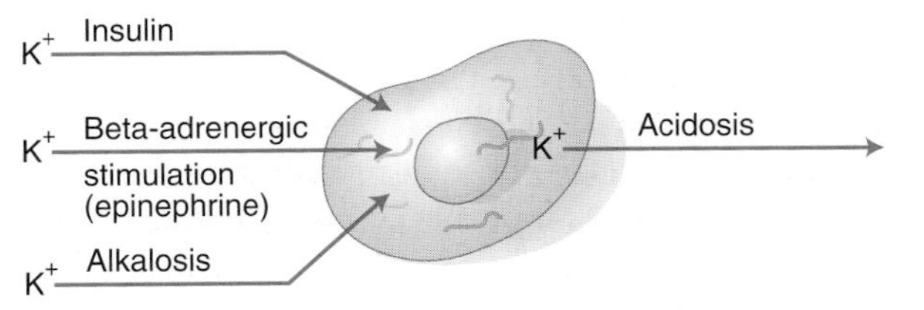

FIGURE 23–14 ■ Factors that shift potassium ions into or out of cells.

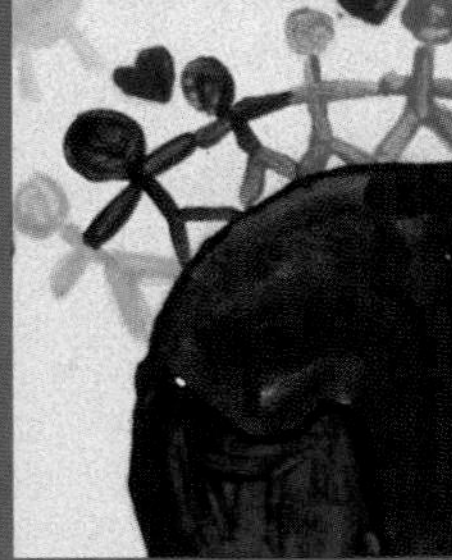

PARTNERING WITH FAMILIES

Interventions for a Child Who Has a Fluid Restriction

- Give cold rather than lukewarm fluids.
- Use an insulated glass that looks bigger than it is. This works well with preschoolers and school-age children.
- Be sure that extra fluids are removed from meal trays before the child sees them.
- Have the child swish fluids around in the mouth before swallowing to relieve thirst. School-age children and adolescents can often use this intervention.
- Provide frequent oral care on all children.
- Suggest eating meals dry and drinking between meals.
- Provide a chart so an older child can keep intake records.

and conditions that decrease the secretion of aldosterone by the adrenal cortex (lead poisoning, Addison's disease, hypoaldosteronism). The following medications can cause hyperkalemia.

- Potassium-containing preparations
- Cytotoxic agents
- Potassium-sparing diuretics
- Angiotensin-converting enzyme inhibitors
- Nonsteroidal anti-inflammatory analgesics

Clinical Manifestations. All clinical manifestations of hyperkalemia are related to muscle dysfunction because potassium plays a vital role in muscle activity. Hyperactivity of gastrointestinal smooth muscle causes intestinal cramping and diarrhea in some children. The skeletal muscles become weak, beginning typically with leg weakness and ascending. Weakness can progress to flaccid paralysis. The child is often lethargic. Dysfunction of cardiac muscle causes cardiac arrhythmias such as tachycardia and may result in heart failure and cardiac arrest. Abnormalities in the electrocardiogram include a prolonged QRS complex, a peak in T waves, AV block, and ventricular tachycardia (Nechyba & Gunn, 2003).

COLLABORATIVE CARE

Nurses collaborate with other healthcare providers to perform accurate diagnosis of hyperkalemia, to treat the underlying conditions that cause the imbalance, and to restore electrolyte balance.

Diagnostic Tests

The major diagnostic test is serum potassium. Normal levels for premature infants are 4.5 to 7.2 mmol/L. Full-term newborns have levels from 3.7 to 5.2 mmol/L, and children have levels from 3.5 to 5.8 mmol/L.

CLINICAL TIP

If an infant's hyperkalemia was diagnosed using blood obtained from a heel stick, intracellular fluid may have contaminated the sample. Intracellular fluid has a higher level of potassium which may leak into the extracellular fluid if cells are damaged during the draw. A venous sample should be obtained to verify the potassium level.

Clinical Therapy

Hyperkalemia is treated by management of the underlying condition that caused the imbalance. If the serum potassium concentration is very high or is causing dangerous cardiac arrhythmias, treatment to decrease the serum potassium level may be ordered. These treatments may remove potassium from the body or drive it from the extracellular fluid into the cells. Potassium is removed from the body by peritoneal dialysis or hemodialysis, by potassium-wasting diuretics, or with a cation exchange resin (Kayexalate) that is administered orally or rectally. Medical treatments that drive potassium ions into cells are intravenous calcium and bicarbonate, intravenous insulin, and glucose.

NURSING MANAGEMENT

Nursing management for the child with hyperkalemia is focused on restoring electrolyte balance and maintaining safety and health until normal potassium levels return.

Nursing Assessment and Diagnosis

Monitor serum potassium levels. Ongoing assessment of muscle strength is important, because the muscle weakness may progress to flaccid paralysis. (This paralysis is reversible on correction of the potassium imbalance.) Diarrhea can occur in infants and children. An older child may complain of intestinal cramping. Monitor the pulse rate carefully. Monitor urinary output in those with renal disease and in all infants, especially premature babies.

Nursing diagnoses for a child who has hyperkalemia depend on the severity of the clinical manifestations. The cause of the imbalance may also lead to useful diagnoses that guide teaching for the child and the parents regarding safety measures and accurate medication administration. The following nursing diagnoses may apply.

- Activity Intolerance related to decreased cardiac output secondary to cardiac arrhythmias
- Risk for Injury related to muscle weakness
- Self-care Deficit: Hygiene and Dressing related to neuromuscular impairment
- Anxiety related to change in health status
- Ineffective Health Maintenance related to parental lack of knowledge of sources of potassium intake in children with chronic renal failure
- Ineffective Management of Therapeutic Regimen by Family related to complexity of therapy

Planning and Implementation

Nursing care includes measures to prevent hyperkalemia from developing in hospitalized children. If hyperkalemia does develop, care shifts to administering intravenous solutions, continuous monitoring of cardiopulmonary status, ensuring safety, promoting adequate nutrition, and preparing the child and family for discharge. Provide for easy bathroom access for older children and frequently check diapers for younger children. For the child in the community, potassium levels are monitored when the child is taking a drug such as those for cancer treatment that cause hyperkalemia.

Prevent Hyperkalemia

Any child who is receiving an intravenous infusion that contains potassium is at risk for hyperkalemia. Check that urine output is normal before administering intravenous potassium solutions. Intravenous solutions to which potassium has been added should be mixed thoroughly by gentle turning of the solutions before they are connected to the infusion tubing.

Be sure blood or packed red blood cells are fresh, especially for the child receiving multiple transfusions, and for all neonates. Use a cardiac monitor during infusion of these products to watch for arrhythmias.

Administer Intravenous Solutions

Once a child is diagnosed as hyperkalemic, ensure that any infusions with added potassium are stopped. Several infusions may need to be managed, including glucose, bicarbonate, and calcium gluconate. Maintain the infusion at the ordered rate and monitor the child's condition frequently.

Monitor Cardiopulmonary Status

Upon diagnosis of hyperkalemia, an electrocardiogram is performed and a cardiac monitor applied. Monitor for any changes in cardiac status and for cardiac arrhythmias. Report abnormal rate and character of pulse as well as shortness of breath.

Ensure Safety

Since the child is weak, side rails should be raised. Position the child carefully. Assist the child with activities requiring leg muscle strength, such as climbing into bed or pushing up in bed. Encourage quiet activities with frequent rest periods, considering both the child's developmental level and the degree of muscle involvement. Document and report any change in muscle weakness.

Promote Adequate Nutritional Intake

Adequate caloric intake is necessary to prevent tissue breakdown and the resultant potassium release from cells. Offer the child nourishing snacks if his or her appetite is decreased. Restrict potassium-rich foods. See Partnering with Families: Potassium-Rich Foods.

Discharge Planning and Home Care Teaching

If the child has chronic renal failure or another condition that decreases aldosterone secretion, parents and the child need to be taught to restrict foods that are high in potassium. Most oral rehydration solutions, including Pedialyte, contain potassium and should not be used to provide fluid for the child. Likewise, cola drinks contain potassium and should be avoided. Instruct the family not to use salt substitutes, which commonly contain potassium. Parents should check with the care provider and pharmacist before giving even over-the-counter products to the child, as some of these medications contain potassium. Management of renal failure at home with frequent visits for dialysis and other treatments can be challenging. Refer to Chapter 31∞ for further suggestions to help parents handle this condition.

Evaluation

Expected outcomes of nursing care for hyperkalemia include the following:

- Return to a state of fluid and electrolyte balance
- Maintenance of safety
- Adequate nutritional intake to provide essential potassium
- Normal cardiac rate and rhythm

Hypokalemia

Hypokalemia occurs when the serum potassium concentration is too low. Total body potassium may be decreased, normal, or even increased when the serum level is low, depending on the cause of the imbalance. Serum potassium levels below 3.5 mmol/L in children (3.7 mmol/L for newborns) are diagnostic of hypokalemia.

Etiology and Pathophysiology

Hypokalemia is caused by conditions that involve increased potassium excretion, decreased potassium intake, shift of potassium from the extracellular fluid into cells, and loss of potassium by an abnormal route.

Increased potassium excretion is a major cause of hypokalemia in children. In addition to diuretics and other medications, causes of increased urinary potassium excretion are osmotic diuresis (glucose present in urine), hypomagnesemia, increased aldosterone (hyperaldosteronism, congestive heart failure, nephrotic syndrome, cirrhosis), and increased cortisol (Cushing's disease and syndrome). Eating large amounts of black licorice increases renal excretion of potassium. Diarrhea causes potassium to be excreted in the feces and is a major cause of the imbalance in developing countries. In the chapter opening vignette, Vernon had increased potassium excretion due to diarrhea.

Decreased potassium intake will lead to hypokalemia slowly, or more rapidly if combined with increased excretion or loss of potassium. Hospitalized children may be placed on NPO status and receive prolonged intravenous therapy without potassium. Adolescents concerned about weight loss or those with anorexia nervosa may embark on diets low in potassium and may take medications that induce diuresis or diarrhea.

PARTNERING WITH FAMILIES

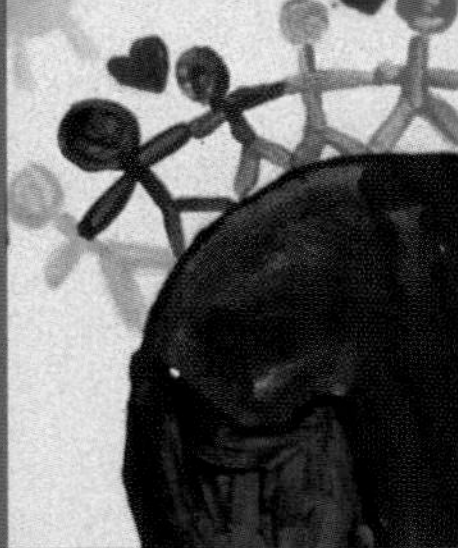

Potassium-Rich Foods

When the child is hyperkalemic, teach the parents about some common foods that contain high amounts of potassium so that they can be avoided. Likewise, when the child is hypokalemic, have the family choose at least two of the foods that could be inserted into the daily diet.

Apricots	Orange juice
Bananas	Peaches
Cantaloupe	Potatoes
Cherries	Prunes
Dates	Raisins
Figs	Strawberries
Molasses	Tomato juice

Shift of potassium from the extracellular fluid into cells occurs in alkalosis and hypothermia (unintentional or induced for surgery). Hyperalimentation often causes hypersecretion of insulin, which also shifts potassium into cells.

Loss of potassium by an abnormal route occurs through vomiting. Self-induced vomiting in bulimia is an example of this cause. Nasogastric suctioning (Figure 23–15 ■) and intestinal decompression can cause potassium loss. Hypokalemia can also be caused by several medications. Common examples are as follows:

- Beta-adrenergic agonists
- Insulin
- Potassium-wasting diuretics
- Parenteral penicillins

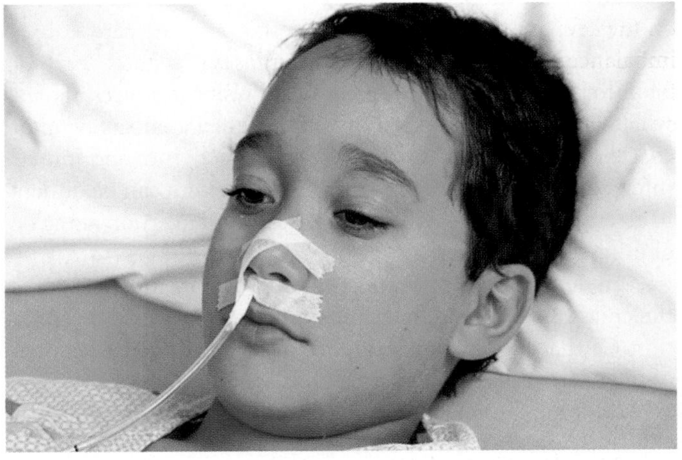

FIGURE 23–15 ■ Because this child has a nasogastric tube in place that requires suctioning, it is important to monitor his potassium levels.

- Glucocorticoids
- Aminoglycoside antimicrobials
- Systemic antifungals
- Antineoplastics
- Laxatives

Clinical Manifestations

Since the ratio of intracellular to extracellular potassium determines the responsiveness of muscle cells to neural stimuli, it is not surprising that the clinical manifestations of hypokalemia involve muscle dysfunction. Gastrointestinal smooth muscle activity is slowed, leading to abdominal distention, constipation, or paralytic ileus. Skeletal muscles are weak and unresponsive to stimuli, and weakness may progress to flaccid paralysis. The respiratory muscles may be impaired. Cardiac arrhythmias can occur. Polyuria results from changes in the kidney caused by hypokalemia. Symptoms may range from mild fatigue with potassium levels less than 3.5 mmol/L, to muscle necrosis at less than 2.5 mmol/L, and flaccidity and respiratory problems at less than 2 mmol/L (English, 2002).

COLLABORATIVE CARE

Nurses and other healthcare professionals collaborate to perform accurate laboratory tests to identify hypokalemia and to treat the causes in order to restore normal balance.

Serum measurement of potassium is the major laboratory test. See normal values in the previous section on hyperkalemia. Medical management of hypokalemia focuses on replacement of potassium while treating the cause of the imbalance. Potassium replacement may be given intravenously or orally.

NURSING MANAGEMENT

Nurses collect serum specimens for analysis, monitor for signs and symptoms of the imbalance, and intervene to ensure the child's safety and restore potassium balance.

Nursing Assessment and Diagnosis

Monitor serum potassium levels. Observe for muscle weakness, which is frequently detected first in the legs. Parents may report that muscle weakness restricts the child's activities and impairs interactions with peers. Skeletal muscle strength can be difficult to assess if the child is lethargic, as shown with Vernon at the beginning of the chapter.

Muscle weakness may affect the respiratory muscles. Assess the child frequently to determine the need for assisted ventilation. Cardiac monitoring is important for continued assessment of hypokalemia-associated arrhythmias.

Assess for diminished bowel sounds. Ask the parents if the child has recently been awakening to use the toilet at night or has begun bedwetting after previously being dry at night. These may be symptoms of polyuria associated with underlying disease, which has led to hypokalemia.

The most important nursing diagnoses in the child with severe hypokalemia relate to cardiac arrhythmias and respiratory muscle weakness. The following nursing diagnoses may apply.

- Risk for Activity Intolerance related to decreased cardiac output secondary to cardiac arrhythmia
- Ineffective Breathing Pattern related to respiratory musculoskeletal impairment
- Risk for Injury related to muscle weakness
- Self-care Deficit: Hygiene and Dressing related to neuromuscular impairment
- Constipation related to decreased motility
- Anxiety related to change in health status
- Ineffective Health Maintenance related to management of potassium supplements or high-potassium diet
- Ineffective Management of Therapeutic Regimen related to complexity of potassium therapy
- Imbalanced Nutrition: Less than Body Requirements related to lack of basic nutritional knowledge regarding safe weight-loss diet

Planning and Implementation

Nursing care of the child with hypokalemia focuses on ensuring adequate potassium intake, monitoring cardiopulmonary status, promoting normal bowel function, ensuring safety, providing dietary counseling, and preparing the child and family for discharge.

Ensure Adequate Potassium Intake

Since potassium is excreted from the body every day, daily potassium intake is necessary to prevent hypokalemia. A hypokalemic child who is able to eat should be given a high-potassium diet. Teach parents (and the child if old enough) which foods are high in potassium and how to incorporate them into the daily diet (see Partnering with Families on page 749).

Children who have no oral intake for a period of time should receive intravenous fluids that contain potassium. Calculate the dosage to ensure accuracy, and be sure that the infusion runs on schedule. Sometimes the child will complain of burning along the vein when potassium is infused. The infusion may need to be slowed temporarily to alleviate pain and maintain the intravenous line. Remain vigilant to maintain patency of the vein in order to avoid infiltration which can cause painful tissues. Consult the hospital formulary for dilution and administration guidelines. Check serum potassium for high or low potassium levels. Monitor urine output. An oliguric child can develop hyperkalemia when receiving supplements.

Monitor Cardiopulmonary Status

Hypokalemia potentiates digitalis toxicity. A hypokalemic child who is receiving digitalis needs careful surveillance for digitalis toxicity, which is manifested as anorexia, nausea, vomiting, and bradycardia. Observe for these effects. Take the pulse rate and rhythm regularly. Monitor respirations and ease of breathing to watch for decreased respiratory muscle activity.

PRACTICE ALERT

Bradycardia occurs at different levels for children of various ages. For infants, a pulse rate below 100 beats per minute (bpm) is considered bradycardia. For young children, 80 bpm may be the identified number, whereas for adolescents, a pulse below 60 bpm is bradycardia. Look at the child's age and normal pulse range to find changes that indicate bradycardia.

Promote Normal Bowel Function

Ensure adequate fluids and fiber in the diet. Monitor and record the number of stools and report inadequate stools.

Ensure Safety

Keep side rails up. Assist the child as needed to move into and out of bed. Reposition the child frequently to preserve skin integrity of limbs that are not moved regularly. Perform passive range of motion if the child is not moving. Use supportive pillows to position the child properly.

Provide Dietary Counseling

The adolescent who is trying to lose weight and not consuming a nutritious diet needs dietary teaching. More intensive treatment will be needed for teens who are anorexic or bulimic (see Chapter 9∞ for interventions in these cases).

Discharge Planning and Home Care Teaching

Teach parents how to give potassium supplements, if prescribed. Liquid or powdered potassium supplements can be mixed with juice or sherbet to improve the bitter taste. The parent should call the mixture "medicine" so that the child does not learn to dislike all juices. Teach the parents signs of both hypokalemia and hyperkalemia and whom to call to report these symptoms. The signs must be reported promptly so medications can be adjusted.

■ Evaluation

Expected outcomes of nursing care during hypokalemia include the following:

- Normal rate and rhythm of heart and respiratory system
- Regular bowel movements
- Maintenance of safety
- Knowledge of child and family regarding food sources of potassium

Calcium Imbalances

A normal serum calcium concentration is important for many physiologic functions, including muscle and nerve function, secretion of hormones, bone formation and strength, and clotting of the blood. Calcium is the most abundant mineral in the body, with about 98% of it being present in bones (Umpaichitra, Bastian, & Castells, 2001). A discussion of dietary calcium intake and its importance in bone formation can be found in Chapter 9∞. See Developing Cultural Competence: Calcium Intake and Osteoporosis.

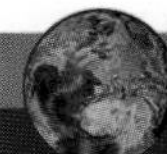

DEVELOPING CULTURAL COMPETENCE
Calcium Intake and Osteoporosis

Ingestion and absorption of calcium is important in the growing child to ensure formation of strong bones. Adolescents who ingest more calcium have less risk of osteoporosis later in life. It has been noted that Black women have less bone loss and fewer fractures than White women. A study with Black and White adolescent girls showed that the Blacks absorbed more calcium from the diet, and lost less in their urine, leading to increased bone density (Bryant et al., 2003). Nurses should recognize this difference and monitor intake of all adolescents. Recognize the high risk of developing osteoporosis in those who are White and consuming little calcium. Interventions should focus on ways of increasing intake.

Calcium imbalances are caused by alterations in calcium intake, absorption, distribution, or excretion. Calcium absorption requires vitamin D for maximum efficiency and is greatest in the duodenum. Calcium distribution involves calcium entry into and exit from bones and the distribution of different forms of calcium in the plasma. Excretion of calcium occurs in urine, feces, and sweat (Figure 23–16 ■). The three forms of calcium in plasma are either bound to protein, bound to small organic ions (e.g., citrate), or are free ionized calcium (Ca^{++}), the only physiologically active form.

Parathyroid hormone is the major regulator of the plasma calcium concentration. It increases this concentration by increasing calcium absorption, increasing calcium withdrawal from bones, and decreasing calcium excretion in the urine. The plasma calcium concentration has an important influence on cell membrane permeability and influences the threshold potential of excitable cells. For this reason, calcium imbalances alter neuromuscular irritability.

Hypercalcemia

Hypercalcemia refers to a plasma excess of calcium (above 5.3 mEq/L [2.7 mmol/L] in children or 5 mEq/L [2.5 mmol/L] in newborns). Because so much calcium is stored in the bones, however, the serum levels of calcium may not reflect body stores.

Etiology and Pathophysiology. Hypercalcemia is caused by conditions that involve increased calcium intake or absorption, shift of calcium from bones into the extracellular fluid, and decreased calcium excretion. Hypercalcemia due to increased calcium intake or absorption may occur if an infant is fed large amounts of chicken liver (source of vitamin A) or is given megadoses of vitamin D or vitamin A, or if a child or adolescent consumes large amounts of calcium-rich foods concurrently with antacids (milk-alkali syndrome). Infants with very low birth weight can develop hypercalcemia if they have inadequate phosphorus intake, as bone phosphorus and calcium will be resorbed. Hypercalcemia may also occur when children receiving total parenteral nutrition are given doses of calcium that are too high.

Most cases of hypercalcemia in children are due to a shift of calcium from bones into the extracellular fluid. The excessive

PATHOPHYSIOLOGY ILLUSTRATED

Calcium Imbalance

Some causes of excess calcium in the blood (hypercalcemia)

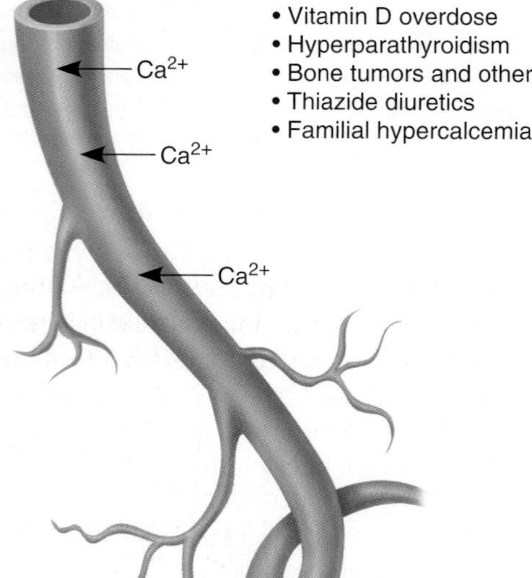

Some causes of decreased calcium in the blood (hypocalcemia)

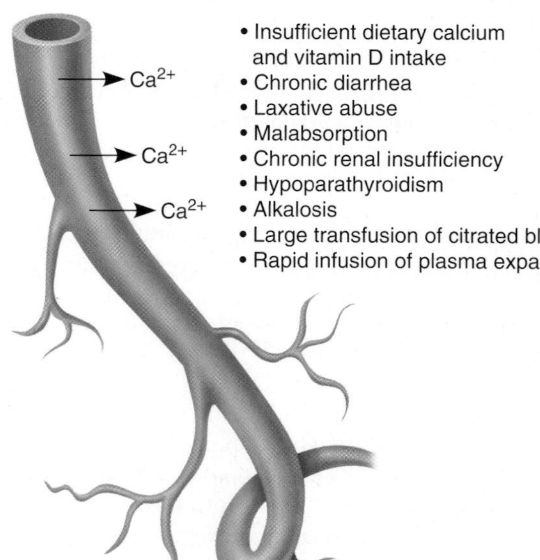

FIGURE 26-16 ■ A variety of conditions can lead to hypercalcemia and hypocalcemia.

amounts of parathyroid hormone produced in hyperparathyroidism cause calcium withdrawal from bones. Prolonged immobilization also causes withdrawal of calcium from bones. Often, the excess calcium ions are excreted in the urine. However, if calcium is withdrawn from bones faster than the kidneys can excrete it, hypercalcemia results. Hypercalcemia also occurs with many types of malignancies such as leukemias. The malignant cells produce substances that circulate in the blood to the bones and cause bone resorption. The calcium from the bones then enters the extracellular fluid, causing hypercalcemia. Bone tumors and chemotherapy destroy bone directly, leading to the release of calcium. In spite of high calcium in the blood, the levels in bone are low and the child is prone to fractures. Familial hypercalcemia and infantile hypercalcemia are rare congenital disorders.

Thiazide diuretics (e.g., thiazide and hydrochlorthiazide) decrease calcium excretion in the urine and may contribute to development of hypercalcemia.

Clinical Manifestations. Hypercalcemia may have nonspecific symptoms, making diagnosis difficult. Many of the signs and symptoms of hypercalcemia are manifestations of decreased neuromuscular excitability. Constipation, anorexia, nausea, and vomiting can occur. Fatigue and skeletal muscle weakness predominate. Confusion, lethargy, and decreased attention span are common, and polyuria develops. Renal calculi may form due to the high calcium levels. Severe hypercalcemia may cause cardiac arrhythmias and arrest. Neonates with hypercalcemia have flaccid muscles and exhibit failure to thrive. Hypercalcemia increases sodium and potassium excretion by the kidneys and can lead to polyuria and polydipsia.

COLLABORATIVE CARE

Nurses collaborate with other healthcare providers to assess for hypercalcemia. Treatments focus on medications and care during dialysis when this treatment is needed.

Normal laboratory values for calcium in serum are 3.5 to 4.5 mEq/L for premature infants, 4 to 5 mEq/L for normal newborns, and 4.4 to 5.3 mEq/L for children. Remember that much of the calcium is stored in bone so that serum values may not fully reflect the body's state of balance.

Hypercalcemia is treated by increasing fluids and administering the diuretic furosemide (Lasix) to increase excretion of calcium in the urine. Treatment to decrease intestinal absorption of calcium involves effective use of glucocorticoids. Bone resorption can be decreased by administration of glucocorticoids and calcitonin. Phosphate is sometimes given to treat hypercalcemia, but it may cause dangerous precipitation of calcium phosphate salts in body tissues. Dialysis may be used, if necessary.

NURSING MANAGEMENT

The nurse assesses calcium status and plans nursing care to help in establishing normal calcium balance.

Nursing Assessment and Diagnosis

Nursing assessment of a child with hypercalcemia includes monitoring serum calcium levels, level of consciousness, gastrointestinal function, urine volume, specific gravity, cardiac rhythm, and pH. With chronic hypercalcemia, assessment of activity tolerance and developmental level becomes important.

Many nursing diagnoses are appropriate for children who have hypercalcemia. Diagnoses that address cardiac and neuromuscular manifestation are especially important. The following nursing diagnoses may apply.

- Risk for Activity Intolerance related to decreased cardiac output secondary to cardiac arrhythmia
- Risk for Injury related to decreased level of response
- Risk for Injury related to neuromuscular impairment
- Risk for Injury related to possibility of spontaneous fractures
- Self-care Deficit: Hygiene and Dressing related to neuromuscular impairment
- Anxiety related to change in health status
- Constipation related to decreased motility
- Risk for Imbalanced Nutrition: Less than Body Requirements related to anorexia and nausea
- Risk for Impaired Urinary Elimination related to renal calculi

Planning and Intervention

Carefully calculate calcium in total parenteral nutrition and other solutions, administer these solutions with caution, and use cardiac monitoring to prevent hypercalcemia in hospitalized children.

Interventions to increase fluid intake are important for children with hypercalcemia or those who are immobilized. A generous fluid intake, appropriate to the child's age, is necessary to keep the urine dilute and to help reduce constipation (a common symptom of hypercalcemia). An acidic urine helps to keep calcium from forming stones. Because urinary tract infections may cause the urine to be alkaline, nursing interventions to prevent urinary tract infection are necessary. Thiazide diuretics, which decrease calcium excretion, should not be given to the hypercalcemic child. Provide a high-fiber diet to help reduce constipation.

Increasing mobility through assisted weight bearing helps to decrease the withdrawal of calcium from bones that is caused by immobility. If the hypercalcemia is caused by withdrawal of calcium from bones, the child is at risk for fractures with minor trauma and must be handled with special care. See Chapter 35∞ for further discussion of care following fractures and prolonged casting. A further description of metabolic emergency with hypercalcemia during cancer treatment can be found in Chapter 29∞.

Teach parents to avoid giving calcium-rich foods and calcium antacids (e.g., Tums) to children with hypercalcemia. Suggest juices and frozen fruit desserts as an alternate to milk and ice cream. Vitamin D supplements should be avoided as they increase calcium absorption from the gastrointestinal tract.

Evaluation

Expected outcomes of nursing care include the following:

- Cardiac pump effectiveness with absence of arrhythmias
- Safety to ensure prevention of fractures
- Normal bowel excretion
- Adequate nutritional status

Hypocalcemia

Hypocalcemia is a serum deficit of calcium (below 4.4 mEq/L [2.2 mmol/L] in children, 4 mEq/L [2 mmol/L] in newborns, or 3.4 mEq/L [1.7 mmol/L] in premature infants) (Umpaichitra et al., 2001). Serum calcium levels may not reflect body stores of this mineral, as most of the body's calcium is stored in bone.

Etiology and Pathophysiology. Hypocalcemia is caused by conditions that involve decreased calcium intake or absorption, shift of calcium to a physiologically unavailable form, increased calcium excretion, and loss of calcium by an abnormal route.

Decreased calcium intake or absorption causes hypocalcemia in children with chronic generalized malnutrition, or with a diet that is low in vitamin D and calcium. Female adolescents trying to lose or maintain a low weight often decrease foods that contain calcium and may develop chronic hypocalcemia. In these cases, premature bone loss and inadequate bone formation occur. (See Chapter 9∞ for further discussion of calcium intake during adolescence.) This deficit cannot be made up later in life, thus increasing the risk of osteoporosis.

Even with a normal calcium intake, hypocalcemia occurs if the mineral is not absorbed. If a child does not have enough vitamin D, calcium is not absorbed efficiently from the duodenum. Sunlight speeds formation of vitamin D in the skin. Children who are institutionalized without access to sunlight (e.g., severely developmentally delayed children), those with very dark skin, or children kept well covered when outside may become hypocalcemic due to lack of vitamin D (see Chapter 9∞). Uremic syndrome is another cause of vitamin D deficiency. It interferes with the kidney's ability to activate vitamin D. High phosphate intake can cause hypocalcemia. Chronic diarrhea and steatorrhea (fatty stools) also reduce calcium absorption from the gastrointestinal tract.

About 40% of calcium is bound to proteins and is not available for interactions, 10% is bound to small organic ions such as citrate, and about 50% is ionized and physiologically active. The shift of calcium into a physiologically unavailable form occurs when calcium shifts into bone or free ionized calcium in plasma binds to proteins or small organic ions in the plasma. Too much calcium shifts into bones in various types of hypoparathyroidism, including DiGeorge syndrome (congenital absence of the parathyroid glands; see Chapter 27∞ for further description of this syndrome). Alkalosis causes more calcium to bind to plasma proteins and become physiologically inactive. Citrate, found in transfused blood, can bind to body calcium. Hypomagnesemia impairs parathyroid hormone function and may cause hypocalcemia. Some types of neonatal hypocalcemia are associated with delayed parathyroid hormone function or hypomagnesemia. A genetic abnormality can result in calcium-sensing receptor defect. Infants of diabetic mothers may have hypocalcemia in response to glycosuria that leads to hypomagnesemia. Very-low-birth-weight babies and newborns with respiratory impairment are prone to develop hypocalcemia. Calcium shifts rapidly into bone when rickets is treated. A high plasma phosphate concentration causes plasma calcium to decrease. Ionized hypocalcemia, which is due to an increased binding of plasma ionized calcium, occurs rapidly. The ionized hypocalcemia persists until the alkalosis resolves or the citrate is metabolized by the liver. Children who receive liver transplants are hypocalcemic for several days due to impaired citrate metabolism.

Increased calcium excretion occurs in steatorrhea, when calcium secreted into the gastrointestinal fluid binds to the fecal fat in addition to the dietary calcium bound in the feces. A similar situation occurs in acute pancreatitis.

Loss of calcium by an abnormal route may contribute to hypocalcemia as calcium is lost from the body through burn or wound drainage or sequestered in acute pancreatitis. Many different medications can cause hypocalcemia, including:

- Antacids (if overused)
- Laxatives (if overused)
- Oil-based bowel lubricants
- Anticonvulsants
- Phosphate-containing preparations
- Protein-type plasma expanders during rapid infusion
- Antineoplastics

Clinical Manifestations. The signs and symptoms of hypocalcemia are manifestations of increased muscular excitability (tetany). In children they include twitching and cramping, tingling around the mouth or in the fingers, carpal spasm, and pedal spasm. Infants may demonstrate tremors, muscle twitches, and brief tonic-clonic seizures. Laryngospasm, seizures, and cardiac arrhythmias are more severe manifestations of hypocalcemia and may be fatal. Hypocalcemia may cause congestive heart failure, especially in neonates.

Although these symptoms are diagnostic of acute calcium deficiency, a more common state in children and adolescents is chronic low intake of calcium. This may be manifested by spontaneous fractures in infants and in adolescents who exercise excessively.

COLLABORATIVE CARE

Laboratory measurements of serum calcium can be helpful.

CLINICAL TIP

Clinical conditions can alter calcium levels and interfere with their interpretation. For example, each 0.1 decrease in pH increases measured ionized calcium by 0.2 mg/dL (Umpaichitra et al., 2001).

Hypocalcemia is treated by oral or intravenous administration of calcium. See the medication table below. The original cause of the imbalance is also treated. If the hypocalcemia is due to hypomagnesemia, the magnesium must be replenished before the calcium replacement can be successful. When the cause is chronic low dietary intake, counseling is needed about high-calcium foods, and perhaps the necessity for vitamin D intake or supplements.

NURSING MANAGEMENT

Nurses assess diets and partner with families to ensure adequate calcium intake by children and adolescents. Careful assessments of the child with hypocalcemia are ongoing. Acute hypocalcemia is treated, associated problems monitored, and medications administered to restore calcium balance.

■ Nursing Assessment and Diagnosis

Carefully assess growth in the young female who is trying to diet. When an adolescent female is very thin, be sure to ask about excessive sports and other activities, and about regularity of menstrual periods. If periods are irregular or not occurring, collect additional dietary information to help determine whether the

MEDICATION Used to Treat Acute Hypocalcemia

MEDICATION	ACTION	NURSING IMPLICATIONS
10% calcium gluconate IV	Calcium is a normal body electrolyte and may need to be infused in infants or young children with health problems leading to low calcium. It is also used during exchange transfusion in neonates since citrate in the blood transfusion can bind body calcium. In the form of CaCl, calcium may be used during resuscitation. Calcium regulates excitability of muscles and nerves, and therefore affects cardiac function (inotropic effect); is necessary for blood clotting; plays a role in storage and release of neurotransmitters, in renal function, and in maintaining cell membranes; antidote to excessive magnesium infusion.	Verify dose carefully with the prescriber and another nurse. Monitor heart rate and rhythm—hypotension and bradycardia can occur. Use extreme caution if given in cardiac or renal disease. Maintain IV carefully to avoid extravasation; do *not* administer by peripheral infusion, scalp vein, IM, or SC. Precipitates when given in infusion with bicarbonate.

girl is lacking in intake of calcium, calories, and other nutrients. These assessments are needed even if serum calcium values are normal. Look for signs of inadequate nutrition such as fat and muscle wasting, dry hair, and cold hands and feet.

In those who may have acute hypocalcemia, assess for muscle cramps, stiffness, and clumsiness; grimacing caused by spasms of facial muscles and twitching of arm muscles; and laryngospasm. Increased neuromuscular excitability may be detected by testing for Trousseau's sign or Chvostek's sign. Many healthy newborns have a positive Chvostek's sign; however, this assessment should be reserved for children over several months of age (Box 23–8). Monitor serum calcium levels and perform continuous cardiac monitoring to observe for cardiac arrhythmias.

The effects of increased neuromuscular excitability in the child with hypocalcemia are the basis for the following nursing diagnoses.

- Risk for Injury related to potential for fractures
- Risk for Ineffective Breathing Pattern related to laryngospasm
- Activity Intolerance related to decreased cardiac output secondary to cardiac arrhythmias
- Disturbed Sensory Perception related to electrolyte imbalance
- Imbalanced Nutrition: Less than Body Requirement related to lack of basic nutritional knowledge of sources and recommended amounts of calcium intake

Planning and Implementation

To correct calcium deficiency in the hospitalized child, give oral or intravenous calcium as ordered. Monitor for complications of calcium supplementation (Box 23–9). A 10% IV calcium gluconate solution should be readily available for emergency use in severe hypocalcemia. Calcium is never given intramuscularly because it causes tissue necrosis.

Take measures to ensure safety for the child who is hospitalized with hypocalcemia. Seizure precautions may be necessary. Explain the cause of muscle cramps to parents and older children.

Counsel the family about dairy products and nondairy foods rich in calcium (Box 23–10). For the adolescent female whose weight is low and menstrual patterns show irregularities, total calories and calcium intake should be increased. Teaching may also be needed about proper calcium intake and its importance both to athletic performance and to prevention of osteoporosis. Encourage three glasses of nonfat milk per day. Teach ways to use milk in the diet. For example, sprinkle nonfat dry milk on cereal and other foods. If the child is lactose intolerant, emphasize nondairy sources of calcium and advise parents to purchase special milk treated with lactase. This milk is more costly, and inadequate family finances may be an impediment to its use. If a child has a health condition leading to chronic diarrhea, encourage increased intake of calcium-rich foods. Calcium supplements in the form of calcium carbonate tablets may be used.

Evaluation

Expected outcomes of nursing care for hypocalcemia include the following:

- Ingestion of recommended dietary allowances for calcium
- Absence of discomfort from muscle spasms related to calcium imbalance
- Freedom from injury due to fractures

BOX 23–9 Medications: Calcium Supplements

ORAL CALCIUM

Calcium tablets and powders are available for relief of acid indigestion and to increase calcium intake when it is deficient. Popular products contain calcium carbonate (e.g., Tums), calcium acetate, calcium citrate, tricalcium phosphate, calcium lactate, calcium gluconate, and calcium polycarbophil. Since so many forms exist, be sure that chewable tablets are chewed, sustained release tablets are swallowed whole, and powders mixed and administered as recommended. The most common side effect is constipation; other side effects are hypercalcemia and renal calculi.

INTRAVENOUS CALCIUM

Intravenous calcium is administered to treat severe hypocalcemia such as in tetany due to parathyroid disease, in cardiac resuscitation, during exchange transfusions in newborns, and to relieve muscle cramps caused by insect bites. Intravenous calcium has several serious potential side effects, so nursing care centers on maintaining an intact intravenous line, continuous cardiorespiratory monitoring, and monitoring calcium and phosphate levels.

BOX 23–8 Physical Assessment: Trousseau's and Chvostek's Signs

To test for Trousseau's sign, apply a blood pressure cuff to the arm and leave inflated for 3 minutes. If a carpal spasm occurs, the Trousseau's sign is positive. To test for Chvostek's sign, tap the skin lightly just in front of the ear (over the facial nerve). If the corner of the mouth draws up because of muscle contraction, the Chvostek's sign is positive. These findings may be indicative of hypocalcemia and/or hypomagnesemia.

BOX 23–10 High-Calcium Foods

- Milk
- Cheese
- Yogurt
- Pudding
- Egg yolks
- Legumes
- Nuts
- Figs
- Chicken
- Salmon (canned with bones)
- Grains (Cream of Wheat, farina, bran muffins)
- Sardines (canned)
- Tofu
- Fruit drinks with added calcium

Magnesium Imbalances

Magnesium is necessary for enzyme function in cells, acetylcholine release, glycolysis, stimulation of ATPases, and bone formation. Magnesium is a component of chlorophyll; thus, magnesium intake is aided by eating dark green leafy vegetables. Nuts and grains are also good sources of this mineral. Magnesium is absorbed primarily from the terminal ileum. It is distributed among the extracellular fluid (small amounts), the cells (larger amounts), and the bones (largest amounts). Magnesium excretion occurs in urine, feces, and sweat.

Magnesium imbalances are caused by alterations in magnesium intake, distribution, or excretion; by loss through an abnormal route; or by a combination of these factors. The plasma magnesium concentration influences the release of acetylcholine at neuromuscular junctions. Thus, magnesium imbalances are characterized by alterations in neuromuscular irritability.

Hypermagnesemia

Hypermagnesemia occurs when the plasma magnesium concentration is too high (above 2.4 mg/dL [0.99 mmol/L]). Keep in mind that the serum levels measured in the laboratory may not reflect body magnesium stores, because most of the magnesium in the body is located in the bones and inside the cells.

Hypermagnesemia is caused by conditions that involve increased magnesium intake and decreased magnesium excretion. Impaired renal function leading to decreased magnesium excretion is the most common cause of hypermagnesemia in children. In both oliguric renal failure and adrenal insufficiency, magnesium ions that cannot be excreted in the urine accumulate in the extracellular fluid.

Less frequently, increased magnesium intake may cause hypermagnesemia. Magnesium sulfate given to treat eclampsia in the mother before delivery causes hypermagnesemia in the newborn. Abnormally high amounts may also be taken in magnesium-containing enemas, laxatives, antacids, and intravenous fluids. Aspiration of seawater, as in near-drowning, is an uncommon but potentially serious source of excessive magnesium intake. Children with Addison's disease can have abnormally high magnesium levels.

Normal serum concentration of magnesium during infancy and childhood is 1.6 to 2.4 mg/dL (0.66 to 0.99 mmol/L). Clinical manifestations of hypermagnesemia include decreased muscle irritability, hypotension, bradycardia, drowsiness, lethargy, and weak or absent deep tendon reflexes. In severe hypermagnesemia, flaccid muscle paralysis, fatal respiratory depression, cardiac arrhythmias, and cardiac arrest occur.

Hypermagnesemia is managed primarily by increasing the urinary excretion of magnesium. This is usually accomplished by increasing fluid intake (except in oliguric renal failure) and by the administration of diuretics. Dialysis may sometimes be necessary.

NURSING MANAGEMENT

The goal of nursing management is to provide assessment of magnesium status in infants and children at risk of imbalance, and to intervene to restore balance when necessary. Monitor serum magnesium levels. Take the child's blood pressure (to watch for hypotension), heart rate and rhythm (to monitor for bradycardia and cardiac arrhythmias), respiratory rate and depth (to watch for respiratory depression), and deep tendon reflexes (to check muscle tone and paralysis or movement). Keep the side rails of the bed raised. Children with hypermagnesemia or oliguria should not be given magnesium-containing medications or sea salt.

Teach parents of children with chronic renal failure that these children should never be given milk of magnesia, antacids that contain magnesium, or other sources of magnesium. Parents should learn to read labels carefully to look for products that contain magnesium. When hypermagnesemia is treated with diuretics, monitor potassium levels to watch for hypokalemia.

Expected outcomes of nursing care include maintenance of electrolyte balance, normal neuromuscular tone, safety, and regular heart rate and rhythm.

Hypomagnesemia

Hypomagnesemia refers to a plasma magnesium concentration that is too low (below 1.5 to 1.7 mg/dL [0.62 to 0.70 mmol/L]). Remember that the serum levels of magnesium may not reflect body stores, as most of the magnesium in the body is found in cells and bones.

Hypomagnesemia is caused by conditions that involve decreased magnesium intake or absorption, shift of magnesium to a physiologically unavailable form, increased magnesium excretion, and loss of magnesium by an abnormal route. Hypocalcemia often accompanies and contributes to hypomagnesemia.

Neonates whose mothers are diabetic sometimes develop hypomagnesemia in the newborn period. Decreased magnesium intake or absorption can occur if a child who is not eating has prolonged intravenous therapy without magnesium. Chronic malnutrition is another cause of decreased magnesium intake. Magnesium absorption is decreased in chronic diarrhea, short bowel syndrome, malabsorption syndromes, and steatorrhea.

A shift of magnesium to a physiologically unavailable form may occur after transfusion of many units of citrated blood products, because magnesium bound to the citrate is not physiologically active. Such transfusions cause prolonged hypomagnesemia in liver transplant patients who have impaired citrate metabolism. Magnesium shifts rapidly into bones that have been deprived of adequate stores.

Increased magnesium excretion in the urine occurs with diuretic therapy, the diuretic phase of acute renal failure, diabetic ketoacidosis, and hyperaldosteronism. Chronic alcoholism, occasionally seen in adolescents, increases urinary magnesium excretion. Magnesium contained in gastrointestinal secretions is bound to fat and excreted in the stool.

Loss of magnesium by an abnormal route occurs with prolonged nasogastric suction and through sequestration of magnesium in acute pancreatitis. Several medications may cause hypomagnesemia, such as magnesium-wasting diuretics, some antineoplastic agents, systemic antifungals, aminoglycoside antibiotics, and laxatives.

Hypomagnesemia is characterized by increased neuromuscular excitability (tetany). The clinical manifestations are hyperactive reflexes, skeletal muscle cramps, twitching, tremors, and cardiac arrhythmias. Seizures can occur with severe hypomagnesemia. Hypomagnesemia is associated with high mortality for children in the pediatric intensive care unit (Singhi, Singh, & Prasad, 2003).

Magnesium serum levels are measured, along with serum calcium and potassium, since these electrolyte disturbances often occur together. See the normal level for serum magnesium in the previous section. Hypomagnesemia is managed by administering magnesium and treating the underlying cause of the imbalance.

NURSING MANAGEMENT

In addition to monitoring serum magnesium levels, nursing assessment of hypomagnesemia includes monitoring deep tendon reflexes, testing for Trousseau's and Chvostek's signs, monitoring cardiac function, and observing for muscle twitching. Children who are able to talk will report muscle cramping. Because magnesium levels are not routinely measured in many settings, request the test for any child who has risk factors and early manifestations of hypomagnesemia. When intramuscular or intravenous magnesium is ordered, administer carefully as directed and monitor vital signs. Electrocardiogram and renal studies may precede drug administration. Have resuscitative drugs and equipment readily available during drug administration.

Teach parents of a child with hypomagnesemia or continuing risk factors such as chronic diarrhea to include magnesium-rich foods in the diet (Box 23–11). Before administering magnesium supplements, verify that the child's urine output is adequate. Monitor deep tendon reflexes if intravenous magnesium is given, and observe for complications of magnesium supplementation (Box 23–12).

Expected outcomes for nursing care include restoration and maintenance of electrolyte balance.

Critical Thinking: Clinical Evaluation of Fluid and Electrolyte Imbalance

How can you evaluate children appropriately for fluid and electrolyte imbalance without thinking through the clinical manifestations of every possible disorder one after the other? First, perform a rapid risk factor assessment on each child to see which factors are present (Tables 23–8 and 23–9). Remember that most imbalances influence other factors so it is common to find more than one type of fluid and electrolyte problem. Examining several body systems such as cardiovascular, respiratory, and neurologic will be necessary to get a comprehensive picture of the child.

BOX 23–11 Magnesium-Rich Foods

- Whole-grain cereal
- Dark green vegetables
- Soy
- Almonds
- Peanut butter
- Bananas
- Egg yolk

BOX 23–12 Medications: Magnesium Supplements

ORAL MAGNESIUM

Magnesium tablets, capsules, solution, and suspension are available for relief of acid indigestion and to stimulate peristalsis. Popular products contain magnesium citrate, magnesium hydroxide, magnesium oxide, and magnesium salicylate. When used as a cathartic, administer the recommended amount of water to ensure bowel evacuation. The most common side effect is abdominal cramping accompanied by diarrhea; other side effects are dehydration, respiratory depression, and electrolyte imbalance.

INTRAVENOUS MAGNESIUM

Intravenous magnesium is administered in the form of magnesium sulfate to treat severe hypomagnesemia, refractory hypocalcemia, and intractable seizures. Intravenous magnesium has side effects of hypermagnesemia, respiratory depression, hypotension, and CNS depression. This form of therapy requires close monitoring of body systems and electrolyte status.

A risk factor assessment may be performed mentally during routine tasks. Look for factors that alter the intake, retention, and loss of isotonic fluid and water. This information is used to evaluate which fluid imbalance is most likely to occur in a particular child. Next, look for factors that alter electrolyte intake and absorption, distribution between plasma and other electrolyte pools, excretion, and abnormal routes of electrolyte loss. This information is used to evaluate which electrolyte imbalances are most likely to occur in the child. A review of pathophysiology is important to understand the role of the other electrolytes and substances, such as phosphorus, in the body. Apply growth and development to realize what types of problems might be most common in various age groups. For example, the newborn is more likely to be dehydrated due to lack of adequate intake, while the toddler more commonly suffers fluid loss from nausea and vomiting.

After evaluating possible imbalances for the child, perform a clinical assessment. Assessment of fluid imbalances is performed by assessing weight changes, vascular volume, interstitial volume, and cerebral function (Table 23–10). Assessment of electrolyte imbalances is performed by assessing serum electrolyte levels, skeletal muscle strength, neuromuscular excitability, gastrointestinal tract function, and cardiac rhythm (Table 23–11). Next, check for other manifestations that are specific to a particular high-risk imbalance (e.g., polyuria in hypokalemia). Evaluate any serum laboratory values available. This method of risk factor assessment followed by clinical assessment provides a rapid yet thorough approach to assessment for fluid and electrolyte imbalances.

TABLE 23–8 Risk Factor Assessment for Fluid Imbalances

ISOTONIC FLUID (EXTRACELLULAR FLUID VOLUME IMBALANCES)	WATER
Source of increased intake?	Source of increased intake?
Aldosterone secretion increased or decreased?	Antidiuretic hormone secretion increased or decreased?
Source of loss from the body?	Source of unusual loss from the body?

TABLE 23–9 Risk Factor Assessment for Electrolyte Imbalances

ELECTROLYTE INTAKE AND ABSORPTION	ELECTROLYTE SHIFTS	ELECTROLYTE EXCRETION	ELECTROLYTE LOSS BY ABNORMAL ROUTE
Increased? Decreased?	From electrolyte pool to plasma? From plasma to electrolyte pool?	Increased? Decreased?	Vomiting? Diarrhea? Nasogastric suction? Wound? Burn? Excessive sweating?

PHYSIOLOGY OF ACID–BASE BALANCE

Normal acid–base balance is necessary for proper function of the cells and the body. The number of hydrogen ions (H^+) present in a fluid determines its acidity. Increasing the hydrogen ion concentration makes a solution more acidic. Because the hydrogen ion concentration in body fluids is very low, acidity is expressed as **pH** (the negative logarithm of the hydrogen ion concentration) rather than as the hydrogen ion concentration itself. The range of possible pH values is 1 to 14. A pH of 7 is neutral. The lower the pH, the more acidic the solution. A pH above 7 is basic. The higher the pH, the more basic the solution. Body fluids are normally slightly basic as the normal range is 7.35 to 7.45. A pH above 7.454 indicates excess base and below 7.34 indicates excess acid in the human body (Table 23–12).

The pH of body fluids is regulated carefully to provide a suitable environment for cell function. The pH of the blood influences the pH inside the cells. **Acidemia** is a term that refers to a decreased blood pH below normal levels, whereas **alkalemia** is an increased blood pH. For the enzymes outside the cells to function optimally, the pH must be in the normal range. If the pH inside the cells becomes too high or too low, then the speed of chemical reactions becomes inappropriate for proper cell function. Cell protein function relies on the correct level of hydrogen ions. Thus, acid–base imbalances result in clinical signs and symptoms, and, in severe cases, may cause death.

In the course of their normal function, all cells in the body produce acids. Cells produce two kinds of acids: carbonic acid (H_2CO_3) and metabolic (noncarbonic) acids. Examples of common metabolic acids are pyruvic acid, sulfuric acid, acetoacetic acid, lactic acid, hydrochloric acid, and beta-hydroxybutyric acid. These acids are released into the extracellular fluid and must be neutralized or excreted from the body to prevent dangerous accumulation. They can be neutralized to some degree by the buffers in body fluids. Metabolic acids are excreted by the kidneys. Carbonic acid is excreted by the lungs in the form of carbon dioxide and water (as shown by the formula $H_2CO_3 = CO_2 + H_2O$). It is also part of the carbonic acid–bicarbonate buffer system and can be converted to bicarbonate (HCO_3) when needed to restore acid–base balance.

Buffers

The maintenance of hydrogen ions within normal range relies heavily on buffers. A **buffer** is a compound that binds hydrogen ions when their concentration rises and releases them when the concentration falls (Figure 23–17 ■). Several kinds of buffers

TABLE 23–10 Summary of Clinical Assessment of Fluid Imbalances

ASSESSMENT CATEGORY	SPECIFIC ASSESSMENTS	CHANGES WITH FLUID IMBALANCES
Rapid changes in weight	Daily weights	Weight gain—extracellular volumes excess Weight loss—extracellular volume deficit; clinical dehydration
Vascular volume	Small-vein filling time	Increased—extracellular volume deficit, clinical dehydration
	Capillary refill time	Increased—extracellular volume deficit; clinical dehydration
	Character of pluse	Bounding—extracellular volume excess Thready—extracellular volume deficit; clinical dehydration
	Postural blood pressure meaurements	Postural drop—extracellular volume deficit; clinical dehydration
	Lung sounds in dependent portions	Crackles—extracellular volumes excess
	Central venous pressure	Increased—extracellular volume excess Decreased—extracellular volume deficit; clinical dehydration
	Tenseness of fontanel (infants)	Bulging—extracellular volume excess Sunken—extracellular volume deficit; clinical dehydration
	Neck vein filling (older children)	Full when upright—extracellular volumes excess Flat when supine—extracellular volume deficit; clinical dehydration
Interstitial volume	Skin turgor	Skin tents—extracellular volume deficit; clinical dehydration
	Presence or absence of edema	Edema—extracellular volume excess
Cerebral function	Level of consciousness	Decreased—clinical dehydration

TABLE 23–11 Summary of Clinical Assessment of Electrolyte Imbalances

ASSESSMENT CATEGORY	SPECIFIC ASSESSMENTS	CHANGES WITH ELECTROLYTE IMBALANCES
Skeletal muscle function	Muscle strength	Weakness, flaccid paralysis—hyperkalemia; hypokalemia
Neuromuscular excitability	Deep tendon reflexes	Depressed—hypercalcemia; hypermagnesemia Hyperactive—hypocalcemia; hypomagnesemia
	Chvostek's sign (except in infants)	Positive—hypocalcemia; hypomagnesemia
	Trousseau's sign	Positive—hypocalcemia; hypomagnesemia
	Paresthesias	Digital or perioral—hypocalcemia
	Muscle cramping or twitching	Present—hypocalcemia; hypomagnesemia
Gastrointestinal tract function	Bowel sounds	Decreased or absent—hypokalemia
	Elimination pattern	Constipation—hypokalemia; hypercalcemia Diarrhea—hyperkalemia
Cardiac rhythm	Arrhythmia	Irregular—hyperkalemia; hypokalemia; hypercalcemia; hypocalcemia; hypermagnesemia; hypomagnesemia
	Electrocardiogram	Abnormal—hyperkalemia; hypokalemia; hypercalcemia; hypocalcemia; hypermagnesemia; hypomagnesemia
Cerebral function	Level of consciousness	Decreased—hyponatremia; hypernatremia

are present in the body (Table 23–13). Various body fluids have buffers to meet their special needs. For example, the bicarbonate buffer system neutralizes metabolic acids (Figure 23–18 ■).

All buffer systems have limits. For example, if there are too many metabolic acids, the bicarbonate buffers become depleted. The acids then accumulate in the body until they are excreted by the kidneys. Clinically, this is seen as a decreased serum bicarbonate concentration and decreased blood pH.

Role of the Lungs

The lungs are responsible for excreting excess carbonic acid from the body. A child breathes out carbon dioxide and water, the components of carbonic acid, with each breath. With faster and deeper breaths, more carbonic acid is excreted. Since carbonic acid is converted in the body to carbon dioxide and water by the enzyme carbonic anhydrase, an indirect laboratory measurement of carbonic acid is **PCO_2**, the partial pressure of carbon dioxide in arterial blood.

Although a child can voluntarily increase or decrease the rate and depth of respirations, they are usually involuntarily controlled. The **PO_2** (partial pressure of oxygen in arterial blood), PCO_2, and pH of the blood are monitored by chemoreceptors in the hypothalamus of the brain and in the aorta and carotid arteries. The input from the chemoreceptors is combined with other neural input to change breathing according to needs. Rate and depth increase or decrease according to the amount of carbonic acid that needs to be excreted.

If a child has a condition that decreases the excretion of carbonic acid or causes breathing to be too slow or shallow (such as overmedication following surgery), carbonic acid accumulates in the blood. Clinically, this is seen as an increased blood PCO_2 and is a form of respiratory acidosis. The reverse will also be true in the child breathing excessively or deeply. This leads to decreased PCO_2 and respiratory alkalosis.

Role of the Kidneys

The kidneys excrete metabolic acids from the body in two ways. They reabsorb filtered bicarbonate and form bicarbonate when needed to restore balance. Bicarbonate is formed when acids and ammonium combine with extra ions. The blood bicarbonate concentration is an indicator of the amount of metabolic acids present, because bicarbonate is used in buffering the acids. When the concentration is normal, metabolic acids are present in usual amounts (Figure 23–19 ■).

In a healthy child, the result of these renal processes is excretion of metabolic acids and maintenance of blood bicarbonate concentration within normal limits. These processes may take several hours to days to be effective in restoring balance when acidosis occurs. In the child whose kidneys are not producing enough urine, metabolic acids may not be effectively excreted. Accumulation of these acids uses up many of the available bicarbonate buffers, resulting in a decreased serum bicarbonate concentration and metabolic acidosis.

TABLE 23–12 Normal Blood pH and Gases

	INFANTS	CHILDREN	ADOLESCENTS
Arterial blood pH	7.18–7.5	7.27–7.49	7.35–7.41
Arterial blood PO_2	60–70 mm Hg (8–9.3 pKa)	80–108 mm Hg (10.7–14.4 pKa)	80–100 mm Hg (10.7–13.3 pKa)
Arterial blood PCO_2	27–41 mm Hg (3.6–5.5 pKa)	32–48 mm Hg (4.3–6.4 pKa)	32–48 mm Hg (4.3–6.4 pKa)
Arterial blood HCO_3^- (bicarbonate)	19–24 mmol/L	18–25 mmol/L	20–29 mmol/L

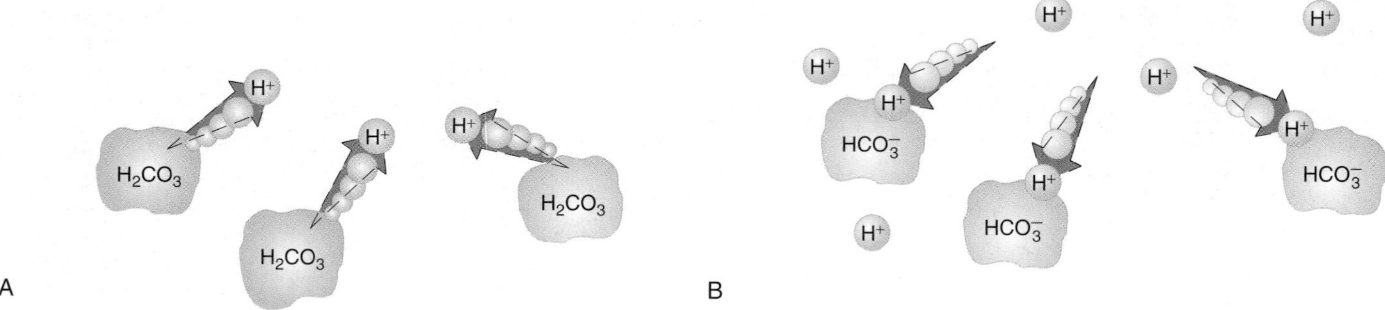

H+
H_2CO_3
H+
H_2CO_3
H+
H_2CO_3
A
H+
H+
HCO_3^-
H+
H+
H+
HCO_3^-
H+
H+
HCO_3^-
H+
B

FIGURE 23–17 ■ *A,* How buffers respond to an excess of base. If the blood has too much base, the acid portion of a buffer pair (e.g., H_2CO_3 of the bicarbonate buffer system) releases hydrogen ions (H^+) to help return the pH to normal. *B,* How buffers respond to an excess of acid. If the blood has too much acid, the base portion of a buffer pair (e.g., HCO_3^-) of the bicarbonate buffer system) takes up hydrogen ions (H^+) to help return the pH to normal.

Role of the Liver

The liver also plays a role in maintaining acid–base balance by metabolizing protein, which produces hydrogen ions. In addition, it synthesizes proteins needed to maintain osmotic pressures in the fluid compartments.

ACID–BASE IMBALANCES

Of the four acid–base imbalances, two are the result of processes that cause too much acid in the body and are referred to as **acidosis.** The other two imbalances are the result of processes that cause too little acid in the body and are called **alkalosis** (Noble, 1999). An acid–base disorder caused by too much or too little carbonic acid is called a respiratory acid–base imbalance. A disorder caused by too much or too little metabolic acid is called a metabolic acid–base imbalance (Box 23–13). Mixed imbalances are possible as well.

Arterial blood gas measurements (ABGs) provide a laboratory evaluation of a child's current acid–base status. See Table 23–12 for normal values for each measurement and Box 23–14 for a method that can help to interpret the pH, PCO_2, and bicarbonate concentrations, which are the most important acid–base measures. Capillary blood gases are commonly used with neonates and infants to decrease amount of blood used for samples. End-tidal CO_2 can provide a continuous noninvasive measurement. (Remember that PCO_2 reflects carbonic acid status and bicarbonate concentration reflects the metabolic acid status.)

MediaLink Acid–Base Balance Animation

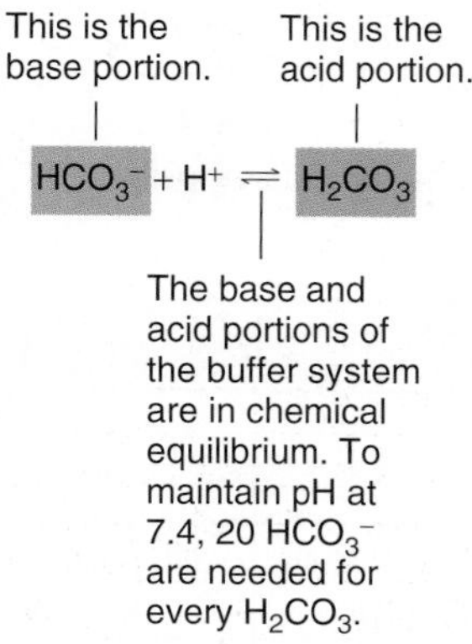

This is the base portion.
This is the acid portion.
$HCO_3^- + H^+ \rightleftharpoons H_2CO_3$
The base and acid portions of the buffer system are in chemical equilibrium. To maintain pH at 7.4, 20 HCO_3^- are needed for every H_2CO_3.

FIGURE 23–18 ■ The bicarbonate buffer system.

BOX 23–13 Acid–Base Imbalances

Acidosis: Relatively too much acid in the body
- *Respiratory acidosis:* Relatively too much carbonic acid
- *Metabolic acidosis:* Relatively too much metabolic acid

Alkalosis: Relatively too little acid in the body
- *Respiratory alkalosis:* Relatively too little carbonic acid
- *Metabolic alkalosis:* Relatively too little metabolic acid

Respiratory Acidosis

Respiratory acidosis is caused by the accumulation of carbon dioxide in the blood. Since carbon dioxide and water can be combined into carbonic acid, respiratory acidosis is sometimes called carbonic acid excess. The condition can be acute or chronic. It is controlled by the lungs.

Etiology and Pathophysiology

Any factor that interferes with the ability of the lungs to excrete carbon dioxide can cause respiratory acidosis. These factors may interfere with the gaseous exchange within the lungs, may impair the neuromuscular pump that moves air in and out of the lungs, or may depress the respiratory rate (Table 23–14; Figure 23–20 ■).

As the PCO_2 begins to increase, the pH of the blood begins to decrease. Compensatory mechanisms begin to act in the

TABLE 23–13 Important Buffers

BUFFER	MAJOR LOCATIONS IN THE BODY
Bicarbonate	Plasma; interstitial fluid
Protein	Plasma; inside cells
Hemoglobin	Inside red blood cells
Phosphate	Inside cells; urine

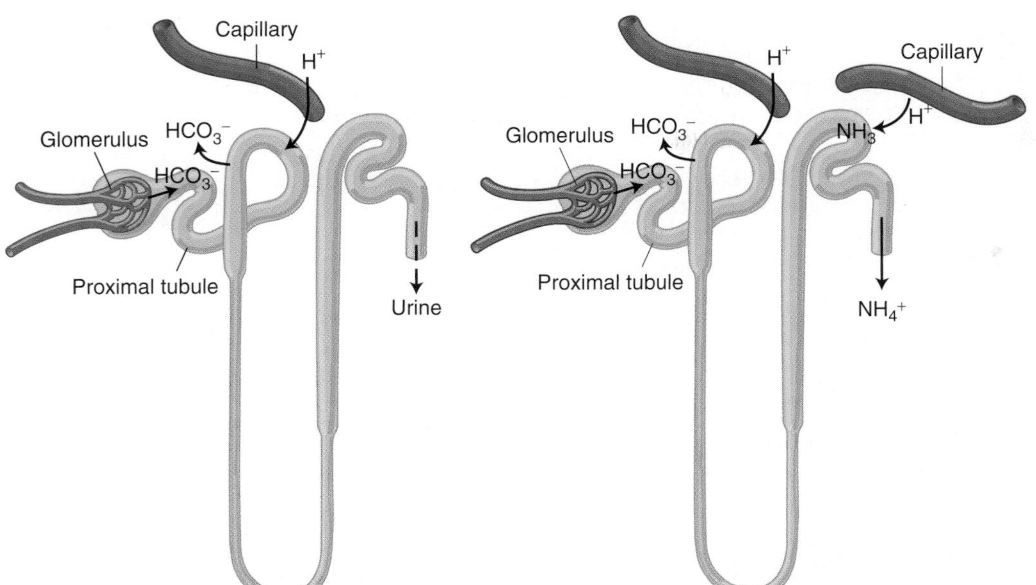

FIGURE 23–19 ■ The kidneys and metabolic acids. *A,* Recycling of bicarbonate by the kidneys. Bicarbonate ions that are in the blood are filtered into the renal tubules at the glomerulus. In the proximal tubules, bicarbonate ions are reabsorbed into the blood at the same time that hydrogen ions are transported from the blood into the renal tubular fluid. *B,* Secretion and buffering of hydrogen ions in the kidneys. If the urine is too acidic, the cells that line the urinary tract could be damaged. To prevent this problem, hydrogen ions secreted into the distal tubules are neutralized by phosphate buffers or bound to ammonia and excreted in the form of ammonium ions.

form of nonbicarbonate buffers, additional hydrogen ion excretion by the kidneys, and formation and decreased bicarbonate excretion by the kidneys. These compensatory mechanisms may take several days to become clinically evident in most situations, depending on the underlying cause and the amount of compensation occurring.

BOX 23–14 Critical Thinking: How to Interpret Arterial Blood Gas Measurements

Ask the following questions to analyze blood gas results.

1. What is the pH? If the pH is normal, the child has no imbalance or has compensated for an imbalance. If the pH is below normal, the child has acidosis. If the pH is above normal, the child has alkalosis.
2. What is the P_{CO_2}? If the P_{CO_2} is normal, the child does not have a respiratory acid–base imbalance. If the P_{CO_2} is above normal, the child has respiratory acidosis. This may be the primary disorder or may be a compensatory response to metabolic alkalosis. Looking at the bicarbonate concentration helps you decide. If the P_{CO_2} is below normal, the child has respiratory alkalosis. Again, this can be the primary disorder or may be a compensatory response to metabolic acidosis.
3. What is the bicarbonate concentration? If the bicarbonate concentration is within normal range, the child does not have a metabolic acid–base imbalance. If the bicarbonate is above normal, the child has metabolic alkalosis. This can be a primary disorder or can be compensatory in respiratory acidosis. When bicarbonate is below normal, the child has metabolic acidosis, either as a direct disorder or as a compensatory response to respiratory alkalosis.
4. What do the results together tell you? If the pH is abnormal and either the P_{CO_2} or bicarbonate concentration is normal, there is an uncompensated acid–base disorder. If all three values are abnormal, the child has a partially compensated disorder and the pH will provide the definitive answer. If P_{CO_2}, pH, and bicarbonate are all decreased, then partially compensated metabolic acidosis is most likely. If pH is normal and P_{CO_2} and bicarbonate are abnormal, there is a fully compensated acid–base disorder.
5. What are the child's history and clinical signs? Does your interpretation fit with what you know about the child's medical condition and with assessments you are making? This last step helps you to integrate laboratory data with the clinical picture to strengthen your nursing care of the child with an acid–base imbalance.

Clinical Manifestations

Acidosis in the brain cells causes central nervous system depression, manifested by confusion, lethargy, headache, increased intracranial pressure, and even coma. Acute respiratory acidosis can lead to tachycardia and cardiac arrhythmias. The child's arterial blood gases always show an increased P_{CO_2}, the laboratory sign of increased carbonic acid. Serum pH can be decreased or normal.

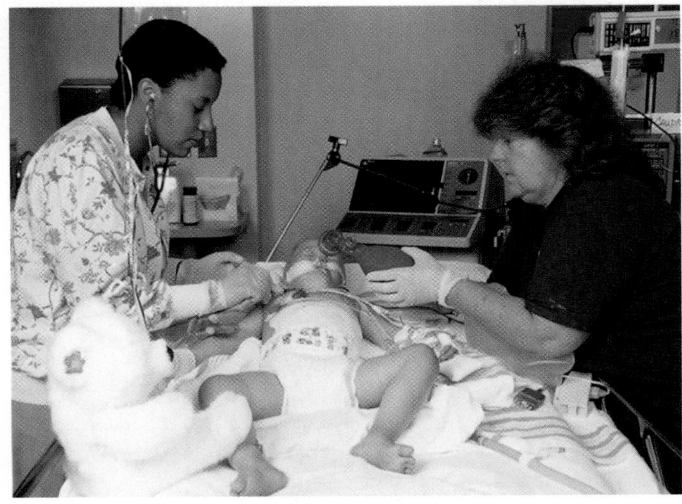

FIGURE 23–20 ■ This child may develop respiratory acidosis or respiratory alkalosis. If the tidal volume is set too low during mechanical ventilation, carbon dioxide (carbonic acid) will accumulate in the body (respiratory acidosis) because it is not being excreted by the lungs. If the tidal volume is set too high, carbon dioxide will be depleted in the body (respiratory alkalosis) because it is being excreted in great quantities.

TABLE 23–14 Causes of Respiratory Acidosis

FACTORS AFFECTING THE LUNGS	FACTORS AFFECTING THE NEUROMUSCULAR PUMP	FACTORS AFFECTING CENTRAL CONTROL OF RESPIRATION
Aspiration	Flail chest	Sedative overdose
Spasm of the airways	Pneumothorax or hemothorax	General anesthesia
Laryngeal edema	Mechanical underventilation	Head injury
Epiglottitis	Hypokalemic muscle weakness	Brain tumor
Croup	High cervical spinal cord injury	Central sleep apnea
Pulmonary edema	Botulism	
Atelectasis	Tetanus	
Severe pneumonia	Kyphoscoliosis	
Cystic fibrosis	Poliomyelitis	
Bronchopulmonary dysplasia	Muscular dystrophy	
Pulmonary embolism	Congenital diaphragmatic hernia	
	Guillain-Barré syndrome	

COLLABORATIVE CARE

Laboratory tests involve arterial blood gases as described previously. Treatment of respiratory acidosis requires correction of the underlying cause. For example, treatment may include bronchodilators for bronchospasm, mechanical ventilation for neuromuscular defects, decreasing sedative use, or surgery for kyphoscoliosis (Table 23–15).

NURSING MANAGEMENT

The nurse assumes an important role in assessment of the child with an acid–base problem. Early identification of increasing imbalance is key to early therapeutic interventions. Nursing interventions focus on keeping the child safe, monitoring effects of treatment, and ensuring management of respiratory, cardiovascular, renal, and other body systems.

Nursing Assessment and Diagnosis

Nursing assessment plays a pivotal role in decisions about interventions for respiratory acidosis, especially in chronic conditions such as cystic fibrosis and kyphoscoliosis. Assess respiratory rate, rhythm, and depth carefully. Take the apical pulse and be alert for tachycardia or arrhythmia. A cardiac monitor may be used. Obtain serial arterial blood gas measurements in acute conditions to evaluate changing status. Assess the level of consciousness and energy. Observe for chronic fatigue, headache, or decreased level of consciousness.

Several nursing diagnoses may apply to the child with respiratory acidosis. The most important of these addresses the child's

TABLE 23–15 Laboratory Values in Acid–Base Imbalance

IMBALANCE	Pco_2	pH	HCO_3^-
Respiratory Acidosis			
Uncompensated	Increased	Decreased	Normal
Partially compensated	Increased	Decreased but moving toward normal	Increasing
Fully compensated	Increased	Normal	Increased
Respiratory Alkalosis			
Uncompensated	Decreased	Increased	Normal
Partially compensated	Decreased	Increased but moving toward normal	Decreasing
Fully compensated	Decreased	Normal	Decreased
Metabolic Acidosis			
Uncompensated	Normal	Decreased	Decreased
Partially compensated	Decreasing	Decreased but moving toward normal	Decreased
Fully compensated	Decreased	Normal	Decreased
Metabolic Alkalosis			
Acute condition; uncompensated	Normal	Increased	Increased
Partially compensated	Increasing	Increased but moving toward normal	Increased
Fully compensated	Full compensation limited by the need for oxygen	Full compensation limited by the need for oxygen	Full compensation limited by the need for oxygen

risk for injury. Other nursing diagnoses depend on the specific clinical manifestation and the particular cause of the acidosis. Examples include:

- Risk for Injury related to decreased level of consciousness
- Activity Intolerance related to decreased cardiac output secondary to cardiac dysrhythmias
- Ineffective Breathing Pattern (hypoventilation) related to neuromuscular impairment
- Acute Pain (headache) related to cerebral vasodilation
- Ineffective Family Management of Therapeutic Regimen related to complexity of bronchodilator therapy

■ Planning and Intervention

Prevention is a major focus of nursing care for the child at risk of respiratory acidosis. When the condition has developed, the nurse engages in measures to correct the acidosis and maintain safety for the child.

Care in the Community

Teach children at risk for respiratory acidosis and their parents preventive measures to use at home. For the child with a chronic condition such as cystic fibrosis, muscular dystrophy, or kyphoscoliosis, demonstrate deep breathing and encourage its use several times each day. Teach the family signs of infection—including fever, increased respiratory secretions, and discomfort with breathing—so the problems can be treated promptly to prevent further respiratory involvement. Position the child to facilitate chest expansion (Figure 23–21 ■). Teach parents about proper administration of any necessary medications. For example, the child with cystic fibrosis may receive antibiotics to prevent respiratory infections. Teach parents and older children about home respirator use (Figure 23–22 ■).

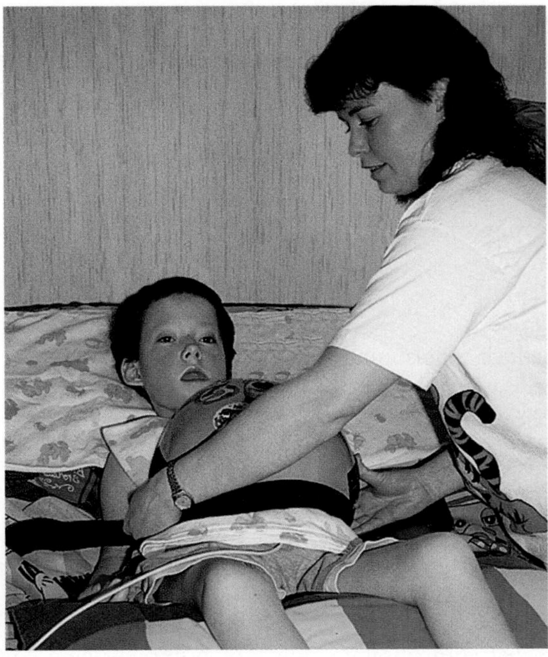

FIGURE 23–22 ■ This child, who has muscular dystrophy, uses a "turtle" respirator at home to assist with breathing. His parents required instructions from the nurse on use of the respirator. The family has a generator to provide electricity for the respirator during power outages.

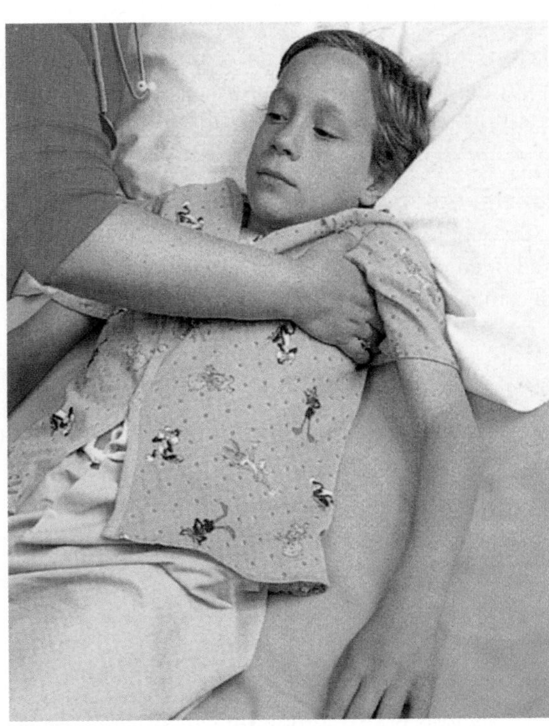

FIGURE 23–21 ■ Positioning to facilitate chest expansion. If the child is positioned to avoid chest compression or slumping to the side, this will help correct respiratory acidosis.

Hospital-based Care

For the hospitalized child, the focus is on ensuring safety. Keep side rails raised, and turn and position the child frequently. Evaluate mental status and document and report any changes in alertness. When laboratory values of blood pH and P_{CO_2} are available, evaluate them promptly and report any changes or abnormalities. Administer medications as ordered. Carefully watch the doses of sedatives to avoid further respiratory depression. Provide suctioning as needed and encourage deep breathing. It is usually difficult to get a young child to do deep breathing or to use the "blow bottle" that is often given to older children and adults. To make deep breathing fun, use a pinwheel and have the child turn it during play. Alternatively, give a child a straw and have him or her blow bubbles in a glass of water, or have the child use the straw to blow scraps of paper across the bedside table.

■ Evaluation

Expected outcomes of nursing care for the child with respiratory acidosis include the following:

- Maintenance of safety
- Adequate rate and rhythm of respirations
- Management of causative disorders

Respiratory Alkalosis

Respiratory alkalosis occurs when the blood contains too little carbon dioxide. It is sometimes called carbonic acid deficit.

Excess carbon dioxide loss is caused by hyperventilation, in which more air than normal is moved into and out of the lungs. Common causes of hyperventilation include:

- Hypoxemia
- Anxiety
- Pain
- Fever
- Salicylate poisoning
- Meningitis
- Encephalitis
- Septicemia caused by gram-negative bacteria
- Mechanical overventilation

Some of the most common causes in young children are hypoxia such as that from severe asthma, salicylate poisoning, and sepsis (Foster, Vaziri, & Sassoon, 2001).

In many cases, respiratory alkalosis lasts for several hours only. Renal compensation does not occur, as these compensatory mechanisms take several days to begin action. An example is the hyperventilation that occurs with acute anxiety. If the condition persists, however, the kidneys will begin to retain more acid and excrete more bicarbonate. Hydrogen ions will be released from body buffers to decrease plasma bicarbonate. While the imbalance continues, cellular function is thus protected by returning pH to normal levels.

Arterial blood gas measurements show a decreased P_{CO_2} in respiratory alkalosis. Blood pH is generally elevated. The lack of carbon dioxide causes neuromuscular irritability and paresthesias in the extremities and around the mouth. Muscle cramping and carpal or pedal spasms can occur. The child may be dizzy or confused.

Clinical therapy focuses on correcting the condition that caused the hyperventilation, sepsis, hypoxia, or other condition so that the body's compensatory mechanisms can return carbon dioxide levels to normal. Oxygen therapy may be helpful in some cases of hypoxia, salicylates are removed from the body (see Chapter 30∞ for treatment during poisoning), drugs that have interfered with breathing are stopped, and sepsis is treated with effective medications. Anxiolytic medications may also be prescribed in severe situations.

NURSING MANAGEMENT

Assess the child's level of consciousness and ask if the child feels light headed or has tingling sensations or numbness in the fingers, toes, or around the mouth. Assess the rate and depth of respirations. Monitor the hospitalized child's P_{O_2} with serial arterial blood gas measurements to evaluate changes in status. A careful assessment is needed regarding the cause of hyperventilation. Did an occurrence cause anxiety for the child? Is pain present (see Chapter 18∞)? Has the child received salicylates in any form? Is the child mechanically ventilated? Is there a central nervous system infection such as meningitis?

Nursing care for the child with respiratory alkalosis centers on teaching stress management techniques, maintaining pain control, promoting respiratory function, ensuring safety, maintaining fluid status, and providing health supervision and home care.

PRACTICE ALERT

The P_{O_2} must be checked before any therapy for respiratory alkalosis is started, because it is dangerous to stop hyperventilation if oxygenation is poor. When P_{O_2} is low, the child's hyperventilation may be a protective mechanism to increase blood oxygenation. Other measures such as oxygen therapy or mechanical ventilation may need to start first, followed by treatment for the cause of respiratory alkalosis.

Teach Stress Management Techniques. When anxiety is the cause of respiratory alkalosis, instruct the child to breathe slowly, in rhythm with your own breathing. Teach stress control techniques such as relaxation or imagery, and use other developmentally appropriate interventions for situations that cause anxiety in children and adolescents (Table 23–16).

Maintain Pain Control. Use medications, imagery, distraction, positioning, massage, and other techniques to decrease pain and maintain pain management. Chapter 18∞ describes these and other measures to assist with pain control.

Promote Respiratory Function. Have the child cough, or suction as needed. Be certain that mechanical ventilation systems are working properly.

Ensure Safety. Provide a safe environment for the child who has a decreased level of consciousness. Be sure the child is supervised when sitting or standing up. Keep bed rails raised.

Regulate Fluid Status. Renal compensation to manage ongoing respiratory alkalosis requires adequate urinary output. Regulate fluid intake to ensure urine output unless fluids are restricted due to medical condition.

Care in the Community. Teach parents to keep aspirin and other salicylate products out of reach of children, preferably in a locked medicine box. Instruct parents to call the poison control center immediately in case of poison ingestion.

■ Evaluation

Expected outcomes of nursing care for the child with respiratory alkalosis include the following:

- Normal respiratory rate and rhythm
- Maintenance of safety
- Regulation of fluid status

Metabolic Acidosis

Metabolic acidosis is a condition in which there is an excess of any acid other than carbonic acid. For this reason, it is sometimes called noncarbonic acid excess.

TABLE 23–16 Techniques for Reducing Anxiety in Children with Parethesias

INFANT	TODDLER OR PRESCHOOLER	YOUNG SCHOOL-AGE CHILD	OLDER SCHOOL-AGE CHILD OR ADOLESCENT
Calming touch Quiet voice Swaddling Holding quietly	Stuffed toy to hug Singing familiar quiet nursery songs Acknowledging the child's feelings Holding calmly	Talking quietly about a happy event Telling a familiar story Reading a familiar book together Explaining that the tingling will go away Use of simple guided imagery supportive listening	Explaining the reason for the tingling and that it will go away Use of guided imagery Familiar music on tape or radio Asking what the child does when anxious or scared Talking about coping strategies

Etiology and Pathophysiology

Metabolic acidosis is caused by an imbalance in production and excretion of acid or by excess loss of bicarbonate (Table 23–17). Excess accumulation occurs by one of two mechanisms. First, a child can eat or drink acids or substances that are converted to acid in the body. Examples include aspirin, boric acid, and antifreeze. Second, cells can make abnormally high amounts of acid that cannot be excreted. This is the case in ketoacidosis of untreated diabetes mellitus, untreated growth hormone deficiency (Glaser, Shirali, Styne, et al., 1998), in children with bladder construction that uses part of the bowel (Mundy, 1999), or the starvation that can occur in anorexia or bulimia. A disorder of excretion occurs in conditions such as oliguric renal failure (Figure 23–23 ■).

Bicarbonate can be lost from the body through the urine or through excessive loss of intestinal fluid. Diarrhea, fistulas, and ileal drainage are all possible sources. Carbonic anhydrase inhibitors can cause loss of excess bicarbonate in the urine.

When the pH of the blood decreases below normal, the chemoreceptors in the brain and arteries are stimulated and respiratory compensation begins. The child's rate and depth of breathing increase and carbonic acid is removed from the body. The blood pH shifts to a more normal range even though the cause is not corrected. The underlying condition and the degree of compensation will alter the clinical laboratory values observed.

Clinical Manifestations

Laboratory values show decreased blood pH and decreased HCO_3- and Pco_2. An attempt at respiratory compensation causes one of the most important signs of metabolic acidosis, increased rate and depth of respirations (hyperventilation) or **Kussmaul respirations.** Severe acidosis can cause decreased peripheral vascular resistance and resultant cardiac arrhythmias, hypotension, pulmonary edema, and tissue hypoxia. Confusion or drowsiness may result, as well as headache or abdominal pain.

TABLE 23–17 Causes of Metabolic Acidosis

GAIN OF METABOLIC ACID	LOSS OF BICARBONATE
Ingestion of acids (e.g., aspirin) Ingestion of acid precursors (e.g., antifreeze) Oliguria (e.g., renal failure) Distal renal tubular acidosis Hyperalimentation Diabetic ketoacidosis Starvation ketoacidosis Some inborn errors of metabolism (e.g., maple syrup urine disease) Tissue hypoxia (lactic acidosis) Loss of bicarbonate	Diarrhea Intestinal or pancreatic fistula Proximal renal tubular acidosis

COLLABORATIVE CARE

Laboratory tests include blood pH and blood gases, as described in the clinical manifestation section. Treatment of metabolic acidosis depends on identification and treatment of the underlying cause. For example, renal failure is treated with medications or dialysis, an intestinal fistula is repaired, and hyperalimentation formula is regulated to decrease acidosis. In severe metabolic acidosis, intravenous sodium bicarbonate may be used to increase the pH and to prevent cardiac arrhythmias. This treatment is

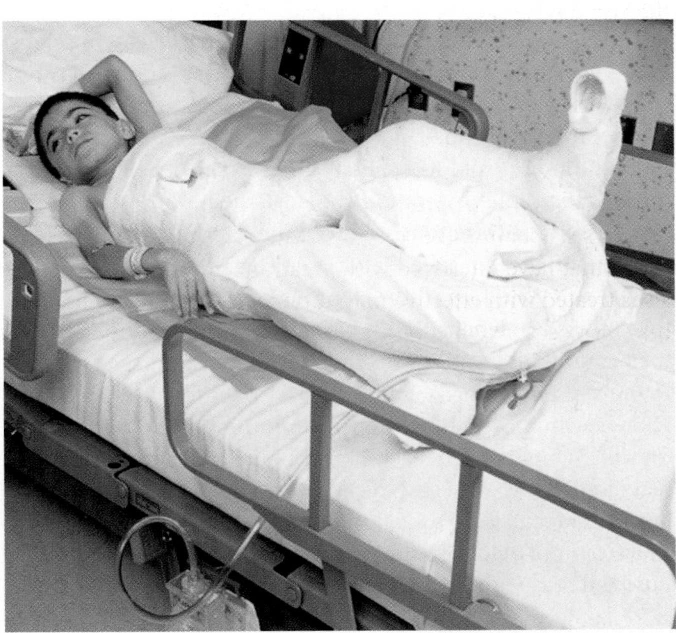

FIGURE 23–23 ■ With any postoperative or immobilized child, it is important to monitor urine output to detect oliguria. If the kidneys do not produce very much urine, the metabolic acids accumulate in the body and cause metabolic acidosis. Inadequate fluid intake in the postoperative or immobilized child can lead to oliguria and, potentially, metabolic acidosis. Note this child's urine collection device.

difficult to manage, because renal excretion can cause excess retention of bicarbonate; therefore, intravenous sodium bicarbonate is used only in severe situations, such as prolonged cardiac arrest.

NURSING MANAGEMENT

Nurses seek to prevent metabolic acidosis by partnering with families to avoid accidental ingestion of harmful substances by young children and to avoid complications of diabetes when possible. Nursing interventions seek to restore balance, and include monitoring of arterial blood gases and body systems.

Nursing Assessment and Diagnosis

Assess the rate and depth of respirations. Evaluate the child's level of consciousness frequently. Be alert for signs or complaints of headache and abdominal pain. Serial arterial blood gas measurements will usually be obtained to evaluate changes in status.

The following nursing diagnoses can apply to the child with metabolic acidosis.

- Risk for Injury related to confusion/drowsiness or decreased responsiveness
- Risk for Decreased Cardiac Output related to cardiac dysrhythmias
- Ineffective Tissue Perfusion: Cerebral related to tissue hypoxia
- Ineffective Family Management of Therapeutic Regimen related to complexity of management of diabetes mellitus

Planning and Implementation

Ensure safety, taking into account the child's level of consciousness and alertness. Turn the child and change his or her position to prevent pressure on the skin. Limit the child's activities to decrease cardiac workload.

Position the child to facilitate chest expansion. Provide oral care during rapid respirations because the mouth may become dry. Monitor intravenous solutions and laboratory values indicating acid–base balance. Report changes promptly.

Once the child is stabilized, provide teaching to compensate for knowledge deficits. Teach parents of young children to keep medications and acids locked in a secure place and out of reach to prevent poisoning (Figure 23–24 ■). This includes medicines with aspirin as well as substances commonly kept in the garage for car maintenance. Teach about home management of diabetes and about early identification and treatment to avoid diabetic ketoacidosis. Expected outcomes of nursing care relate to prevention of acidosis and restoration of normal body balance during disease processes.

Metabolic Alkalosis

Metabolic alkalosis occurs when there are too few metabolic acids. It is sometimes called noncarbonic acid deficit.

A gain in bicarbonate or a loss of metabolic acid can cause metabolic alkalosis (Table 23–18). Bicarbonate is gained through excessive intake of bicarbonate antacids or baking soda or through metabolism of bicarbonate precursors such as the citrate contained in blood transfusions. Increased renal absorption of bicarbonate can occur with diuretic use, in profound hypokalemia, primary hyperaldosteronism, or extreme deficit in extracellular fluid volume. Acid can be lost through severe vomiting, such as that seen in infants with pyloric stenosis and in continued removal of gastric contents through suction.

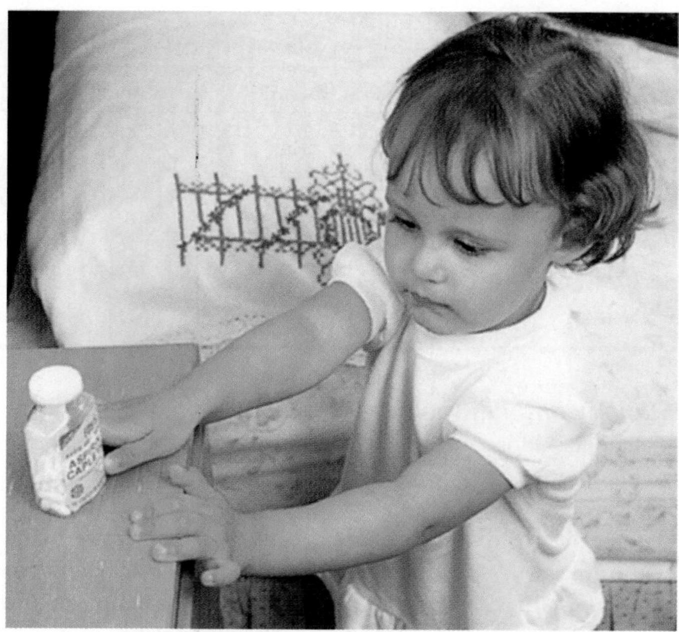

FIGURE 23–24 ■ Teaching parents to use safety latches on cabinets to keep aspirin away from small children can prevent one cause of metabolic acidosis.

When the chemoreceptors in the brain and arteries detect the rising pH of metabolic alkalosis and respirations decrease, carbonic acid is retained in the body. This carbonic acid can neutralize the bicarbonate and return pH toward normal.

Blood pH, bicarbonate, and P_{CO_2} are usually elevated in metabolic alkalosis. Hypokalemia often occurs simultaneously (refer to page 749 to review signs of hypokalemia). Respiratory rate and depth usually decrease. Increased neuromuscular irritability, cramping, paresthesia, tetany, seizures, and excitation

TABLE 23–18 Causes of Metabolic Alkalosis

GAIN OF BICARBONATE	LOSS OF METABOLIC ACID
Ingestion of baking soda Ingestion of large quantities of bicarbonate antacids Exchange transfusion or massive transfusion (citrate is metabolized to bicarbonate) Increased renal absorption of bicarbonate	Prolonged vomiting (e.g., pyloric stenosis) Nasogastric suction Cystic fibrosis Hypokalemia Diuretic therapy Hyperaldosteronism Adrenogenital syndrome Cushing's syndrome

can occur. Finally, this state can progress to weakness, confusion, lethargy, and coma.

See Table 23–15 for laboratory findings. Clinical therapy is directed at treating the underlying cause of the condition. Increasing the extracellular fluid volume with intravenous normal saline is used to facilitate renal excretion of bicarbonate. Medications such as acetazolamide increase renal excretion of bicarbonate as well.

NURSING MANAGEMENT

Assess the child's level of consciousness frequently. Alertness may decrease after an initial period of excitement, so regular assessments are needed. Monitor neuromuscular irritability. Observe for nausea and vomiting. Assess the rate and depth of respirations carefully. Obtain serial arterial blood gas measurements as ordered.

Facilitate ease of respirations. Ensure safety by keeping bed rails elevated and by turning the child frequently. Position the child on the side to avoid aspiration of vomitus.

If antacids were the cause of the alkalosis, teach the child and parents about correct use of these medications.

Mixed Acid–Base Imbalances

It is possible for two acid–base imbalances to occur simultaneously. For example, a child with cystic fibrosis can develop respiratory acidosis from lung problems and concurrent metabolic alkalosis from vomiting during an illness. Treatment with diuretics may cause concurrent metabolic alkalosis resulting from extracellular volume depletion and hypokalemia in a child with congestive heart failure and chronic respiratory acidosis. In these cases, all underlying causes must be identified and treated. Care of children with mixed acid–base imbalances is often complicated, requiring hospitalization and careful management. Upon discharge, the nurse can teach parents about signs of imbalance that need to be reported and treated to prevent further complications. Evaluation of care is based on outcomes of adequate respiratory ventilation and metabolic balance.

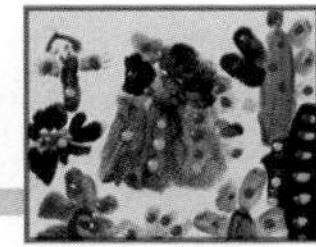

CHAPTER HIGHLIGHTS

- Young children are at risk for fluid and electrolyte imbalance due to differences in body fluid compartments and regulation systems.
- Nurses institute health promotion and health maintenance measures to maintain normal body fluids for children who exercise in hot weather and those undergoing surgery.
- Extracellular fluid volume deficit manifests as dehydration.
- Extracellular fluid volume excess is due to an excess of saline in the body.
- Interstitial fluid volume excess manifests as edema and weight gain.
- Nurses carefully manage fluid status of young children and teach parents prevention and treatment of fluid imbalances caused by gastroenteritis and other disease states.
- The most common electrolyte imbalances are hypernatremia and hypokalemia, and thus involve sodium and potassium.
- Normal acid–base balance is necessary for proper function of cells in the body.
- The lungs, kidneys, and liver play a role in maintaining acid–base balance.
- Acid–base imbalance can involve alkalosis or acidosis; either can have a respiratory or metabolic origin.

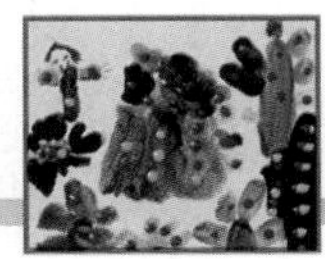

CRITICAL THINKING IN ACTION

INTRODUCTION

Consider the scenario involving 18-month-old Vernon at the chapter beginning. He has had vomiting and diarrhea for several days. Assessment of body weight loss, skin turgor, and level of activity suggests moderate dehydration. His mother has arranged child care for today for her 4-year-old daughter.

DESCRIPTION

Vernon refuses attempts at feeding him orally and his pulse becomes rapid and blood pressure decreases. After several hours in the monitoring unit, he has not voided and has a capillary refill of about 4 seconds.

DISCUSSION

1. What type of dehydration is Vernon likely experiencing now?
2. Has he lost both water and sodium in proportion (isotonic dehydration), or relatively more water (hypotonic dehydration) or sodium (hypertonic dehydration)?
3. What type of intravenous fluid might be ordered for Vernon if intravenous therapy is started?
4. What is his needed maintenance fluid? His replacement fluid?
5. What amount of oral rehydration therapy (ORT) is recommended as therapy begins?
6. Consider Vernon's age and developmental stage. How will you promote intake of oral fluid?
7. Vernon improves and is sent home tonight. Instruct his mother about how to continue the ORT.
8. Since Vernon has gastroenteritis, what precautions do you suggest to prevent other family members from becoming affected?
9. How will you assist Vernon's mother to plan care for him as well as her 4-year-old daughter?

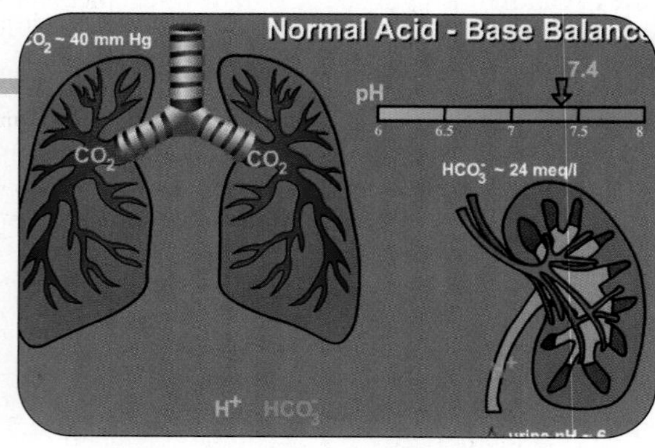

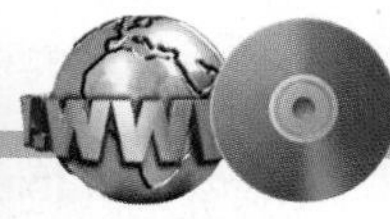

EXPLORE MediaLink

- NCLEX review, case studies, and other interactive resources for this chapter can be found on the Companion Website at **www.prenhall.com/ball**. Click on Chapter 23 to select the activities for this chapter.
- For animations, more NCLEX review questions, and an audio glossary, access the accompanying CD-ROM in this book.

http://www.prenhall.com/ball

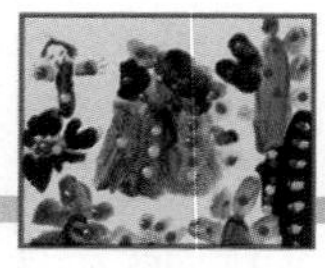

REFERENCES

Aker, J., & O'Sullivan, C. (1998). The selection and administration of perioperative intravenous fluids for the pediatric patient. *Journal of PeriAnesthesia Nursing, 13,* 172–181.

Anidi, I., Bazargan, M., & James, F. W. (2002). Knowledge and management of diarrhea among underserved minority parents/caregivers. *Ambulatory Pediatrics, 2,* 201–206.

Armon, K., Stephenson, T., MacFaul, R., Eccleston, P., & Werneke, U. (2001). An evidence and consensus based guideline for acute diarrhoea management. *Archives of Diseases in Children, 85,* 132–142.

Atherly-John, Y. C., Cunningham, S. J., & Crain, E. F. (2002). A randomized trial of oral vs. intravenous rehydration in a pediatric emergency department. *Archives of Pediatric and Adolescent Medicine, 156,* 1240–1243.

Behrman, R. E., Kliegman, R., & Jenson, H. B. (2004). *Nelson textbook of pediatrics* (17th ed.). Philadelphia: Saunders.

Bindler, R., & Howry, L. (2005). *Pediatric Drug Guide.* Upper Saddle River, NJ: Prentice Hall.

Binkley, H. M., Beckett, J., Casa, D. J., Kleiner, D. M., & Plummer, P. E. (2002). National Athletic Trainers' Association position statement: Exertional heat illnesses. *Journal of Athletic Training, 37,* 329–343.

Blonshine, S. (2000). Sodium, potassium, and ionized calcium. *AARC Times, 24*(4), 46–48.

Bryant, R. J., Wastney, M. E., Martin, B. R., Wood, O., McCabe, G. P., Morshidi. M., Smith, D. L., Peacock, M., & Weaver, C. M. (2003). Racial differences in bone turnover and calcium metabolism in adolescent females. *Journal of Clinical Endocrinology and Metabolism, 88,* 1043–1047.

Burkhart, D. M. (1999). Management of acute gastroenteritis in children. *American Family Physician, 60,* 2555–2563.

Cloherty, J. P., Stark, A. R. & Eichenwald, E. (Eds.). (2003). *Manual of neonatal care* (5th ed.). Philadelphia: Lippincott, Williams & Wilkins.

Committee on Infectious Diseases (2003). *Redbook: Report of the Committee on Infectious Diseases* 26th ed. Elk Grove Village, IL: American Academy of Pediatrics.

Committee on Sports Medicine and Fitness. (2000). Climatic heat stress and the exercising child and adolescent. *Pediatrics, 106,* 158–159.

Cote, C. J., Todres, I. D., Goudsouzian, N. G., Todres, I. D., & Ryan, J. F. (2001). *Practice of anesthesia for infants and chidren* (3rd ed.). Philadelphia: Saunders.

Dabbagh, S., Ellis, D., & Grus Kin, A. B. (1996). In E. K. Motoyama & P. J. Davis (Eds.), *Smith's anesthesia for infants and children* (6th ed., pp. 105–137). St. Louis: Mosby-Year Book.

Eliason, B. C., & Lewan, R. B. (1998). Gastroenteritis in children: Principles of diagnosis and treatment. *American Family Physician, 58,* 1769–1776.

Endsley, S., & Galbraith, A. (1998). Are you overlooking oral rehydration therapy in childhood diarrhea? *Postgraduate Medicine, 104,* 159–166, 171.

English, M. (2002). Challenges in managing profound hypokalemia. *British Medical Journal, 324,* 269–270.

Foster, G. T., Vaziri, N. D. & Sassoon, C. S. H. (2001). Respiratory alkalosis. *Respiratory Care, 46,* 384–391.

Glaser, N. S., Shirali, A. C., Styne, D. M., & Jones, K. L. (1998). Acid–base homeostasis in children with growth hormone deficiency. *Pediatrics, 102,* 1407–1414.

Hanna, J. D., Scheinman, J. I., & Chan, J. C. M. (1995). The kidney in acid–base balance. *Pediatric Clinics of North America, 42,* 1365–1396.

Hewitt-Taylor, J. (1999). Children in intensive care: Physiological considerations. *Nursing in Critical Care, 4,* 40–45.

King, C. K., Glass, R., Bresee, J. S., & Duggan, C. (2003). Managing acute gastroenteritis among children. *MMWR, 52*(RR16), 1–16.

Kluckow, M., & Evans, N. (2001). Low systemic blood flow and hyperkalemia in preterm infants. *Journal of Pediatrics, 139,* 227–232.

Larson, C. E. (2000). Safety and efficacy of oral rehydration therapy for the treatment of diarrhea and gastroenteritis in pediatrics. *Pediatric Nursing, 26,* 177–179.

Lasche, J., & Duggan, C. (1999). Managing acute diarrhea: What every pediatrician needs to know. *Contemporary Pediatrics, 16,* 74–83.

Leelanukrom, R., & Cunliffe, M. (2000). Intraoperative fluid and glucose management in children. *Paediatric Anaesthesia, 10,* 353–359.

Liebelt, E. L. (1998). Clinical and laboratory evaluation and management of children with vomiting, diarrhea, and dehydration. *Current Opinion in Pediatrics, 10,* 461–469.

Lipp, J., Lord, L. M., & Scholer, L. H. (1999). Fluid management and enteral nutrition. *Nutrition in Clinical Practice, 14,* 232–237.

Livingstone, V. H., Willis, C. E., Abdel-Wareth, L. O., Thiessen, P., & Lockitch, G. (2000). Neonatal hypernatremic dehydration associated with breast-feeding malnutrition: A retrospective survey. *Canadian Medical Association Journal, 162,* 647–652.

Manganaro, R., Mami, C., Marrone, T., Marseglia, L., & Gemelli, M. (2001). Incidence of dehydration and hypernatremia in exclusively breast-fed infants. *Journal of Pediatrics, 139,* 673–675.

Merenstein, G. B., & Gardner, S. L. (2003). *Handbook of neonatal intensive care* (5th ed.). St. Louis: Elsevier.

Moritz, M., & Ayus, J. C. (1999). The changing pattern of hypernatremia in hospitalized children. *Pediatrics, 104,* 435–439.

Mundy, A. R. (1999). Metabolic complications of urinary diversion. *Lancet, 353,* 1813–1814.

Nager, A. L., & Wang, V. J. (2002). Comparison of nasogastric and intravenous methods of rehydration in pediatric patients with acute dehydration. *Pediatrics, 109,* 566–572.

Nechyba, C., & Gunn, V. (eds). (2003). *The Harriet Lane handbook* (16th ed.). St Louis: Mosby.

Noble, K. A. (1999, June 28). Putting the puzzle together: Arterial blood gas interpretation. *Advance for Nurses,* 19–22.

Ozuah, P., Avner, J. R., & Stein, R. E. K. (2002). Oral rehyrdration, emergency physicians, and practice parameters: A national survey. *Pediatrics, 109,* 259–261.

Provisional Committee on Quality Improvement, Subcommittee on Acute Gastroenteritis. (1996). Practice parameter: The management of acute gastroenteritis in young children. *Pediatrics, 97,* 424–436.

Shamir, R., Zahavi, I., Abramowich, T., Poraz, I., Tal, D., Pollak, S., & Dinari, G. (1998). Management of acute gastroenteritis in children in Israel. *Pediatrics, 101,* 892–894.

Singhi, S. C., Singh, J., & Prasad, R. (2003). Hypo- and hypermagnesemia in an Indian pediatric intensive care unit. *Journal of Tropical Pediatrics, 49,* 99–103.

Umpaichitra, V., Bastian, W., & Castells, S. (2001). Hypocalcemia in children: Pathogenesis and management. *Clinical Pediatrics, 40,* 305–312.

Vega, R., & Avner, J. R. (1997). A prospective study of the usefulness of clinical and laboratory parameters for predicting percentage of dehydration in children. *Pediatric Emergency Care, 13,* 179–182.

The Venous Access Task Force (2002). Using evidence-based practice to create a venous access team. *Journal of Pediatric Nursing, 17,* 450–454.

Weaver, C. M. (2003). Racial differences in calcium metabolism. *Journal of Clinical Endocrinology and Metabolism, 88,* 1043–1047.

White, V. M. (1997). Hyperkalemia. *American Journal of Nursing, 97*(6), 35.

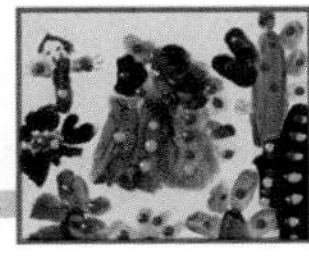

ADDITIONAL REFERENCES

Askin, D. F. (1997a). Interpretation of neonatal blood gases, Part I: Physiology and acid–base homeostasis. *Neonatal Network, 16,* 17–21.

Askin, D. F. (1997b). Interpretation of neonatal blood gases, Part II: Disorders of acid–base balance. *Neonatal Network, 16,* 23–29.

Barber, C., & Masiello, M. (1996). Oral rehydration therapy. *Topics in Emergency Medicine, 18*(3), 21–26.

Bar-Or, O. (1996). Water and electrolyte replenishment in the exercising child. *International Journal of Sport Nutrition, 6,* 93–99.

Clark, S. L. (1999). Arterial lines: An analysis of good practice. *Journal of Child Healthcare, 3,* 23–27.

Escalente-Kanashiro, R., & Tantalean-Da-Fieno, J. (2000). Capillary blood gases in a pediatric intensive care unit. *Critical Care Medicine, 28,* 224–226.

Ferry, R. J., Kesavula, V., Kelly, A., Katz, L. E. L., & Mosbang, T. (2001). Hyponatremia and polyuria in children with central diabetes insipidus: Challences in diagnosis and management. *Journal of Pediatrics, 138,* 744–747.

Johnson, M. D. (1994). Disordered eating in active and athletic women. *Clinics in Sports Medicine, 13,* 355–369.

Jones, P. M. (2001). Case studies: Electrolytes, blood gases, and acid-base balance. *Laboratory Medicine, 9,* 537–540.

Jospe, N., & Forbes, G. (1996). Fluids and electrolytes— clinical aspects. *Pediatrics in Review, 17,* 395–404.

Khan, N., Licata, A., & Rogers, D. (2001). Intravenous bisphosphonate for hypercalcemia accompanying subcutaneous fat necrosis: A novel treatment approach. *Clinical Pediatrics, 40,* 217–219.

Lain, I. A., & Wong, C. M. (2002). Hypernatraemia in the first few days: Is the incidence rising? *Archives of Disease in Childhood, 87,* 158–162.

McGillivray, C., Ducharme, F. M., Charron, Y., Mattimoe, C., & Treherne, S. (1999). Clinical decision-making based on venous versus capillary blood gas values in the well-perfused child. *Annals of Emergency Medicine, 34,* 58–63.

Mizock, B. A., & Hathiwala, S. C. (1998). Using the sodium-chloride difference to diagnose acid-base disorders. *Journal of Critical Illness, 13,* 701–704.

Oddie, S., Richmond, S., & Coulthard, M. (2001). Hypernatraemic dehydration and breast feeding: A population study. *Archives of Disease in Childhood, 85,* 318–320.

Santosham, M. (2002). Oral rehydration therapy. *Archives of Pediatric and Adolescent Medicine, 156,* 1177–1179.

Sarker, S. A., Mahalanabix, D., Lam, N. H., Sharmin, S., Khan, A. M., & Fuchs, G. J. (2001). Reduced osmolarity oral rehydration solution for persistent diarrhea in infants: A randomized controlled clinical trial. *Journal of Pediatrics, 138,* 532–538.

Straughn, A., & English, B. (1996). Oral rehydration therapy. *American Journal of Maternal-Child Nursing (MCN), 21,* 144–147.

Tanzi, M., Gardner, M., Megellas, M., Lucio, S., & Restino, M. (2003). Evaluation of the appropriate use of albumin in adult and pediatric patients. *American Journal of Health-System Pharmacy, 60,* 1330–1335.

Chapter 24

Alterations in Eye, Ear, Nose, and Throat Function

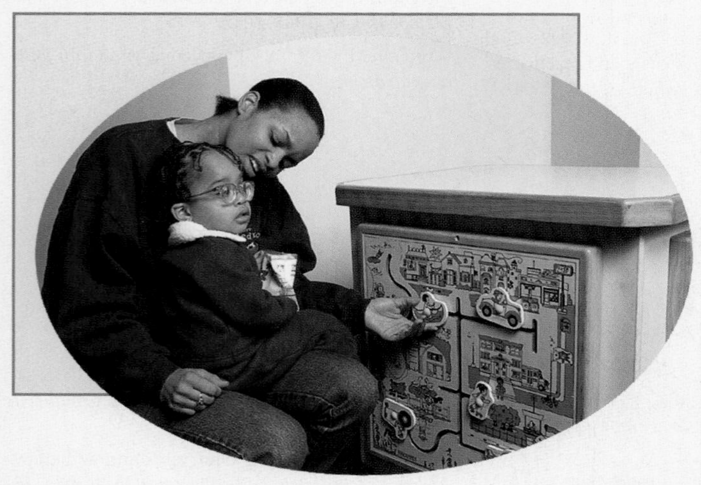

Raeanne Cross, 3 years old, has a severe visual impairment. Born prematurely at 25 weeks' gestation, she received oxygen therapy, and had damage to her retinal blood vessels. As a result, Raeanne developed retinopathy of prematurity. While in the hospital, Raeanne was given frequent ophthalmoscopic examinations. She received cryotherapy to the retinal vessels—a treatment designed to prevent detached retinae and the resulting total vision loss. Although this treatment halted progression of the disorder, Raeanne was left severely myopic (nearsighted).

For the first 3 years of life, Raeanne and her mother attended an early intervention program, which provided stimulation for Raeanne and helped teach her mother techniques for enhancing her developmental progress. Raeanne will soon begin attending preschool. Her speech is well developed for a 3-year-old; she is socially mature, converses readily, and shows no developmental delays. However, she has had little contact with other children.

As the nurse in the preschool Raeanne will be attending, how will you partner with both her parents and the preschool staff in facilitating Raeanne's adaptation to the preschool experience? Your role includes helping her parents to prepare her for this new experience. You also provide information to the other preschool staff members to help them ensure a safe environment for Raeanne, assist her in adjustment to working and playing in a group of children, and foster her development.

"Why can't my Mommy be here with me? I have a friend; her name is Kiley."

—Raeanne, age 3

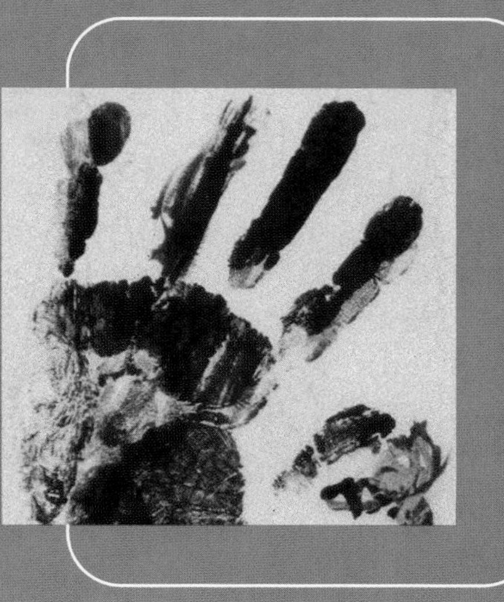

Learning Outcomes

After completing this chapter, you will be able to:

- Describe abnormalities of the eyes, ears, nose, throat, and mouth in children.
- Plan for screening programs and identification of children with vision and hearing abnormalities.
- Plan nursing care for children with vision or hearing impairments.
- Use current recommendations when implementing care and teaching for children with abnormalities of eyes, ears, nose, throat, and mouth.
- Integrate preventive and treatment principles when implementing care for children related to eyes, ears, nose, and throat.

Key Terms

amblyopia/777
audiography/798
binocularity/777
conductive hearing loss/797
decibels/795
esotropia/772
exotropia/779
mixed hearing loss/798
myringotomy/792
nystagmus/772
sensorineural hearing loss/797
strabismus/777
tinnitus/795
tympanogram/798
tympanostomy tubes/792
vision/772
visual acuity/772

MediaLink http://www.prenhall.com/ball

Resources for this chapter can be found on the CD-ROM accompanying this textbook and on the Companion Website at www.prenhall.com/ball. Click on Chapter 24 to select the activities for this chapter.

CD-ROM

Animations/Videos

- *3D Ear/Ear Anatomy*
- *3D Eye/Eye Anatomy*
- *Ear Abnormalities*
- *Middle Ear Dynamics*
- *Otitis Media*
- *The Child's Ear*

Nursing in Action

- *Eye, Ear, and Nose Medication Administration*
- *Obtaining a Sample for Throat Culture*

NCLEX Review

Audio Glossary

COMPANION WEBSITE

A & P Review

Clinical Manifestations Review

Medication Match-Up

NCLEX Review

Case Study: Otitis Media

MediaLink Applications

- *Early Identification and Intervention for Hearing Loss*
- *Neonate Screening and the Law*
- *Plan a Vision Screening Program*
- *Plan Interventions for Visual Disorders*

How are conditions of the eye, ear, nose, and throat or mouth related? Which conditions have the potential to affect a child's growth, development, and behavior? What important testing during the newborn period can help to identify and intervene early with children who may have an abnormality in this system? In what settings do children with eye, ear, nose, throat, and mouth conditions receive care?

Because the eye, ear, nose, throat, and mouth are connected, a malformation, infection, or other condition in one of these structures may affect them all. Intact sensory structures are necessary for attainment of developmental milestones; thus alterations, especially to the eye and ear, may delay a child's development. In the preceding scenario, Raeanne's condition was diagnosed when she was very young, and she was enrolled in a program to help her develop normally. Although Raeanne received her initial diagnosis and treatment in the hospital, most children with eye, ear, nose, and throat disorders are treated at home or in the community rather than in the hospital. Most screening for disorders occurs in newborn nurseries, clinics, and schools. This chapter will explore the screening guidelines for hearing, vision, and speech; the treatment for common disorders of the eye, ear, nose, throat, and mouth (including upper respiratory infections); nursing interventions that can prevent problems; and methods of partnering with parents and other health professionals to foster development of children with alterations in this body system.

ANATOMY AND PHYSIOLOGY OF PEDIATRIC DIFFERENCES

Eye

How are the eyes of children different from those of adults? Chapter 8 provides a detailed discussion of the assessment of the eyes and **visual acuity,** the ability to discriminate letters or other objects. The eyes of neonates differ from the eyes of adults in several ways. Visual acuity in neonates ranges between 20/100 and 20/400, making them hyperopic or farsighted. The lens is more spherical and cannot accommodate to both near and far objects, which means that the neonate sees best at a distance of about 20 cm (8 in.). Because the optic nerve is not yet completely myelinated, the ability to distinguish color and other details is decreased. If the infant is preterm, especially less than 32 weeks' gestation, retinal vascularization, particularly in the periphery of the retina, may be incomplete. Pupillary reflex reaction is detected by about 28 to 30 weeks' gestation and so may be sluggish in preterms. The rectus muscles that control binocular vision may be somewhat uncoordinated at birth. The eyes should be aligned and movement coordinated by the age of 3 months. Transient **nystagmus** (involuntary rapid eye movement) and **esotropia** (momentary turning inward of eyes) are common in neonates, but decrease in incidence during the first few months of life. Conjunctival and retinal hemorrhages may be observed in the newborn as a result of the trauma of birth; they usually gradually improve and have no lasting effects. The red reflex should always be examined in children because it is a key abnormality in retinoblastoma (see Chapter 8 for the method to evaluate red reflex and Chapter 29 for a description of retinoblastoma).

MediaLink A & P Review

CLINICAL TIP

To examine the eye of a newborn who has eyes tightly closed, instead of prying the eyelid open, it is easier and less traumatic to encourage the baby to open the eyes normally. Most newborns will open the eyes if held securely and tipped up and down several times, especially when accompanied by dim lighting and soft talking. Parents may also hold them upright over their shoulder to encourage eye opening.

The cornea of the infant and young child occupies a larger portion of the orbit than in the adult. Because the eyeball is relatively unprotected laterally, it is more easily injured. The sclera of the neonate is thin and translucent with a bluish tinge, and the iris is blue or gray. Eye color changes during the first 6 months of life, until reaching the child's natural color. Infants produce tears to nourish and oxygenate the outer layers of the cornea. Parents do not see tears when a young infant cries because the infant's lacrimal system drains them efficiently into the nasal cavity. However, the amount of tears is less in preterm infants, which can lead to dry corneas and concentration of medications administered into the eye (Behrman, Kliegman, & Jenson, 2004). See Figure 24–1 ■ for the parts of the normal eye.

As infants grow, their eyes mature and their vision improves. By the age of 2 or 3 years, most children have a visual acuity of 20/50, and by the age of 6 or 7 years, it is 20/20. Visual acuity is measured using standardized letter or picture charts (see Chapter 8 and the Skills Manual). **Vision** refers to the complex process of acquiring meaning from what is seen, involving the eye, brain, and related neurologic and physiologic structures. Cognitive development interacts with a child's maturing physiologic system to bring increasing meaning to objects in sight (Table 24–1). The first few years of life are considered crit-

TABLE 24–1 Visually Related Developmental Milestones

AGE	MILESTONE
Term neonate	Demonstrates alertness to visual stimulus presented 8–12 in. (20–30 cm) from eyes
1 month	Follows an object 60 degrees horizontally and 30 degrees vertically; blinks at an approaching object
2 months	Follows a person from 6 ft (2 m) away; smiles in response to a face; raises head 30 degrees from prone
3 months	Tracks an object through 180 degrees; inspects own hand; begins visual-motor coordination
4–5 months	Social smile; reaches for a cube 12 in. (30 cm) away; notices a raisin 12 in. (30 cm) away
7–8 months	Picks up a raisin by raking
8–9 months	Pokes at holes in a peg board; neat pincer grasp; crawling
12–14 months	Stacks blocks; places a peg in a round hole; stands and walks

From Scheiner, A. P. (1996). Vision problems: Impairment to blindness. In A. M. Rudolph, J. I. E. Hoffman, & C. D. Rudolph (Eds.), Rudolph's pediatrics *(20th ed., p. 167). Stamford, CT: Appleton & Lange.*

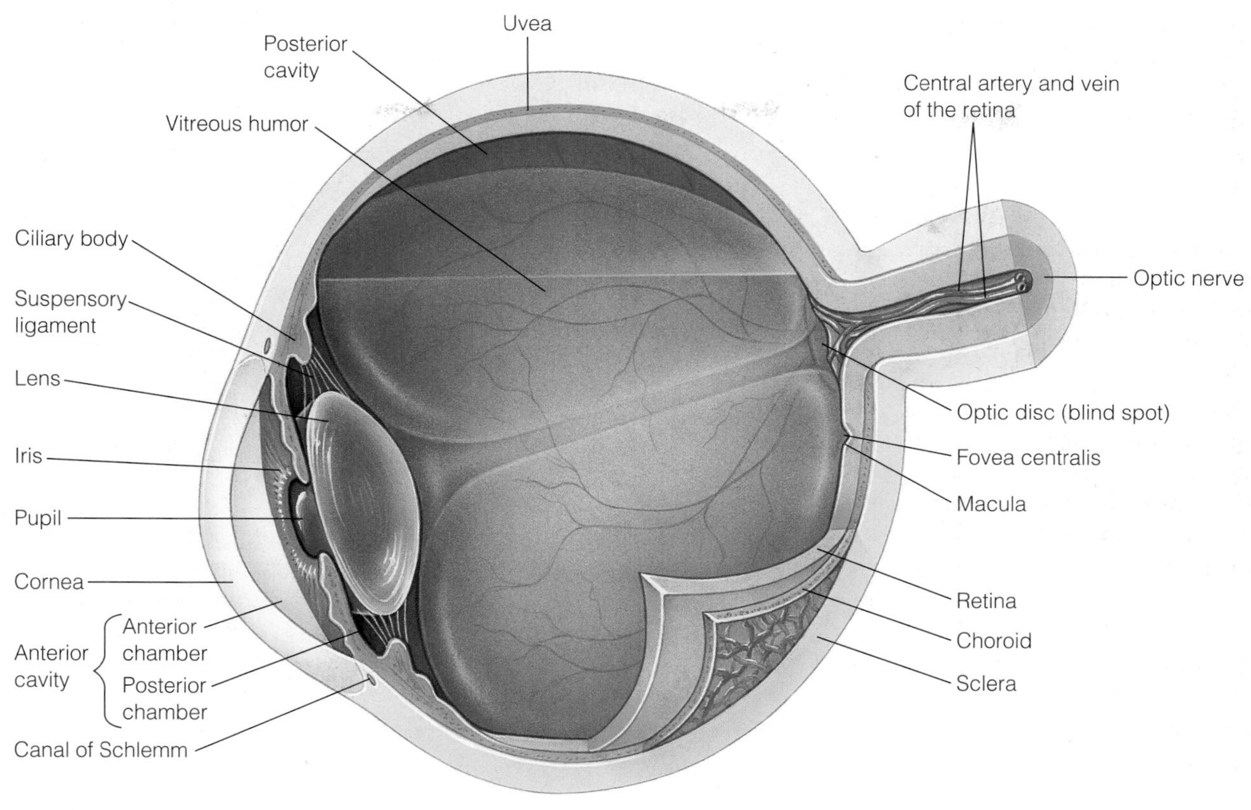

FIGURE 24–1 ■ Parts of the normal eye.

ical for the formation of normal vision. As acuity improves, the brain learns to interpret messages received from the eyes. Disturbances in vision, even in one eye, can affect the retinal nerve function, muscle function in the eye, or the brain's ability to interpret visual input.

Ear

Why do infants and young children have more ear problems than adults? The eustachian tube, which connects the nasopharynx to the middle ear, is proportionately shorter, wider, and more horizontal in infants than in older children or adults (Figure 24–2 ■). During sucking, yawning, and other movements, the tube opens for milliseconds, allowing free passage of air between the nasopharynx and the middle ear. This predisposes young children to development of otitis media or middle ear infection.

The external ear canal is small at birth, although the internal ear and middle ear are relatively large. As a result, the tympanic membrane is close to the surface and can be easily injured.

Babies can hear at about 20 weeks' gestation while the auditory nerve function is mature at about 5 months of age in the infant. Before 34 weeks' gestation, the exterior ear is soft with little cartilage apparent. When the ear of a preterm is folded forward and released, its recoil is slow, while with term neonates the recoil is strong and fast. (See Figure 8-67 for normal newborn ear recoil.)

Nose, Throat, and Mouth

Up to the age of 6 months, infants are primarily nasal breathers. Edema and nasal discharge may interfere with adequate air intake and feeding. Newborns may need bulb suctioning of the nose occasionally at feeding time to remove mucus so that breathing is facilitated (see Skills Manual for bulb suctioning procedure). Mucosal swelling and exudate may block the small nasal passages of infants and toddlers during respiratory infections (see discussion later in this chapter of upper respiratory infection and Chapter 25 for description of lower respiratory infection in children).

The palatine tonsils, which are visible on oral examination, are located on each side of the oropharynx. The method for examining a child's throat is discussed in Chapter 8. Although tonsils vary in size considerably during childhood, they are normally large, especially in school-age children. Lymph tissue decreases in size by about 10 years, so its appearance after this age can indicate abnormality. The nasopharyngeal tonsils (adenoids) lie in the posterior wall of the nasopharynx, just above the oropharynx. In children, the adenoids may become enlarged, harboring bacteria and interfering with breathing.

The mucosal membranes of the mouth are expected to be intact and without lesions at all ages. The first teeth commonly erupt at about 6 months of age, and the first loss of teeth begins at about 6 years. See Chapter 8 for thorough descriptions of assessment of the oral cavity in infants and children.

MediaLink 3D Eye/Eye Anatomy Video

AS THEY GROW

Eustachian Tube

FIGURE 24–2 ■ Of the three anatomical differences in the eustachian tube between adults and small children (shorter, wider, more horizontal), which do you think could cause more problems for the child and why? Answer: More horizontal. Small children who are bottle fed in a supine position have a greater probability of developing otitis media because the eustachian tube opens when the child sucks and the horizontal angle provides easy access to the middle ear. In older children the greater angle helps keep foreign substances and germs away from the middle ear.

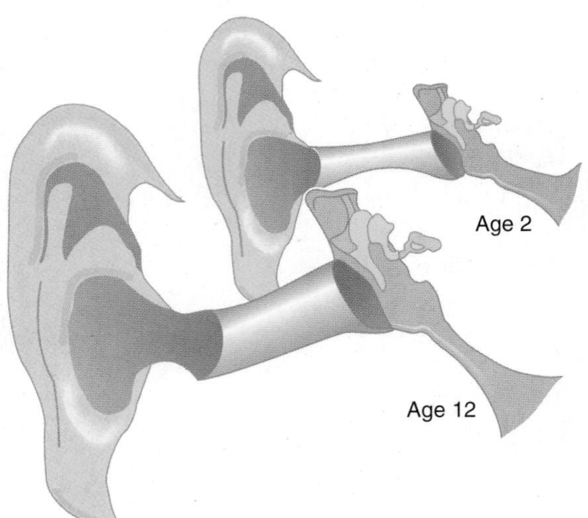

Position of eustachian tube is at less of an angle (more horizontal) in the young child, resulting in decreased drainage.

End of eustachian tube in nasal pharynx opens during sucking.

Eustachian tube equalizes air pressure between the middle ear and the outside environment and allows for drainage of secretions from middle ear mucosa.

DISORDERS OF THE EYE

Infectious Conjunctivitis

Conjunctivitis is an inflammation of the conjunctiva, the clear membrane that lines the inside of the lid and sclera. There are several types of conjunctivitis, depending on the cause of inflammation. Bacteria, viruses, allergies, trauma, or irritants cause the conjunctiva to become swollen and red with a clear, yellow, or white discharge (Figure 24–3 ■). Some additional less common causes of conjunctivitis include inflammation of eyelash follicle, tumor, or uveitis (Gross, 2002). Parents commonly refer to all conjunctivitis as "pink eye."

Swollen eyelid

Purulent discharge

Inflamed conjunctiva

FIGURE 24–3 ■ Acute conjunctivitis. The major difference between bacterial and viral conjunctivitis is that bacterial conjunctivitis has a purulent discharge that may result in crusting whereas the discharge from viral conjunctivitis is serous (watery). Allergic conjunctivitis produces watery to thick drainage and is characterized by itching. Which type of conjunctivitis is seen in this picture?

Reprinted from Newell, F.W. (1996). Ophthalmology: Principles and concepts *(8th ed.). St Louis: Mosby Year-Book. Used with permission from Elsevier.*

MediaLink 3D Ear/Ear Anatomy Video

Ophthalmia Neonatorum

Conjunctivitis in an infant under 30 days of age is called ophthalmia neonatorum. These infections are usually acquired from the mother during vaginal delivery as a result of contact with infected vaginal discharge containing organisms such as *Chlamydia trachomatis* and *Neisseria gonorrhoeae.* Such infections can cause serious damage to the eye and lead to permanent corneal damage. Antibiotics are instilled into the eyes of newborns soon after birth as a prophylactic measure against ophthalmia neonatorum. Chemical conjunctivitis occasionally occurs in newborns (Alcorn, 2001) as a reaction to the prophylactic medication. It is considered as a possible cause when conjunctivitis develops within 24 to 48 hours after instillation of the medication.

PRACTICE ALERT

By federal law, all infants born in the United States are given prophylactic eye treatment soon after delivery to help prevent ophthalmia neonatorum. The nurse is responsible for administering this eye ointment. Penicillin, tetracycline, erthromycin, or povidone-iodine ointments are most commonly used.

Bacterial Conjunctivitis

Bacterial conjunctivitis can occur in older children as well. It is characterized by edema of the eyelid, red conjunctiva, and enlarged preauricular lymph glands. There is usually mucopurulent exudate that causes matting, making the eyes difficult to open upon awakening. Older children with conjunctivitis complain of itching or burning, mild photophobia, and a feeling of scratching under the lids.

CLINICAL TIP

Place a gloved index finger on the child's nose next to the inner corner of the eye and apply gentle pressure for several seconds. If mucopurulent drainage is discharged from the eye, bacterial conjunctivitis may be present.

Some common organisms include *Haemophilus influenzae, Streptococcus pneumoniae, Moraxella catarrhalis,* and *Escherichia coli.* Most cases are caused by hand-to-eye contact and the disease can rapidly spread when groups of youth spend time together, such as among young children and adolescents in schools and childcare centers, and even among college students in dormitories, sororities, fraternities, and on sports teams (Stephenson, 2003; Gross, 2002). Although bacterial conjunctivitis can be bilateral, it is more commonly unilateral.

PRACTICE ALERT

Some youth are using decorative contact lenses and some even "trade" such lenses with other youth. Contact lenses should only be prescribed and fitted by a qualified eye professional. There have been reports of bacterial conjunctivitis, corneal damage, and allergic reactions to these cosmetic lenses. The U.S. Food and Drug Administration (FDA) has issued a press release about the dangers of improperly obtained lenses (www.fda.gov/bbs/topics/news/2002/new00846.html)

Viral Conjunctivitis

Other infections in newborns and older children can be caused by viruses. Viral conjunctivitis is commonly bilateral. Adenovirus is a common cause and spreads from respiratory adenovirus infection in a hand-to-eye manner. Herpes simplex virus (HSV) can also cause infection, either by transfer from a herpes-infected mother to a neonate during birth or by contact with an infected person in infants or children of any age. Ophthalmic herpes infection is often accompanied by characteristic vesicular lesions on the skin of the face. A culture of the lesions is performed for diagnosis and any accompanying conjunctivitis is assumed to be caused by herpes virus. For the infection caused by HSV, prompt and vigorous treatment is needed to prevent eye injury or blindness, which can occur in children with recurrent herpes virus infections as a result of antibody reaction to the viral antigen. Herpes virus infections commonly recur so periodic treatment and sometimes prophylaxis may be needed.

In infants who have frequent tearing and mattering (eyelid discharge that has formed a crust) on awakening, a plugged lacrimal duct may mimic conjunctivitis. Treatment involves massaging the tear duct several times toward the direction of the nose every 4 hours when the infant is awake. Lacrimal ducts that remain plugged after the age of 1 year may have to be opened surgically.

Allergic Conjunctivitis

When conjunctivitis is caused by an allergy, the child complains of intense itching. Examination reveals red eyes with watery discharge and the conjunctivae have a "cobblestone" appearance. The eyes may also appear puffy and swollen.

COLLABORATIVE CARE

The goal of collaborative care is prompt diagnosis and treatment of any conjunctivitis to prevent both continued discomfort for the baby or child and any long-term damage to the eye.

In most cases, a diagnosis of the cause of conjunctivitis is made based on the history and symptoms. Cultures can be taken, especially in infants or in cases suspected of being unusual bacterial illness or herpes viruses. A Gram stain of discharge and conjunctival scraping for potential Chlamydia or herpes is performed. Infants and children must be promptly referred to primary care providers or eye specialists for treatment of possible eye infections. When diagnosed in an infant in the neonatal intensive care unit, the infant is isolated to prevent spread to other infants.

Antibiotic eye medication is prescribed in droplet or ointment form if a bacterial infection is suspected. Treatment may be started after a laboratory sample is obtained but before the results are known. Fluoroquinolones are now frequently used to treat bacterial conjunctivitis; drops or ointment can be used. When gonococcal conjunctivitis occurs in newborns, ceftriaxone is recommended; the disease is resistant to penicillin. Chlamydial infections are treated with oral erythromycin or tetracycline. Careful total evaluation of the newborn with any conjunctivitis is also performed to watch for other signs of infection. Instructions for instilling eye medications are given in the Skills Manual.

Viral conjunctivitis may be treated with comfort measures such as cleaning drainage away with a warm clean cloth, avoiding bright lights, and avoiding reading. Ophthalmic antibiotics are sometimes given to prevent bacterial invasion due to frequent rubbing of the eyes. Herpes simplex virus infections of the eye are treated promptly by an ophthalmologist, neonatologist, or other professional trained in this serious disease. Topical drugs are used, and often are combined with a systemic antiviral agent such as acyclovir (Alcorn, 2001; Gross, 2002). Neonatal herpes simplex virus is treated vigorously with parenteral acyclovir for 14 days (or longer if central nervous system involvement is found upon lumbar puncture), and with topical ophthalmic medication (trifluridine, iododeoxyuridine, or vidarabine). Recurrent lesions may necessitate suppressive or prophylactic treatment with oral acyclovir (Committee on Infectious Diseases, 2003).

If an allergen is diagnosed as the cause of conjunctivitis, systemic or topical antihistamines may be prescribed. Decongestants can be combined with systemic antihistamines for short-term therapy. More current treatment involves use of mast-cell stabilizers to decrease the activation of mast cells that accompanies allergic reactions. Most mast-cell stabilizers have been tested and found to be safe in children 3 years of age and older (Alexander, 2003). See the medication table on page 776.

PRACTICE ALERT

Topical steroids can be used to treat allergic conjunctivitis. However, these drugs could mask the symptoms of an infection with herpes virus, leading to serious eye damage. Any red eye should be diagnosed by an ophthalmologist or well-trained pediatric care provider so that viral infections are ruled out before use of steroids. *How do steroids work? Why could masking a herpes infection have important implications?*

MEDICATIONS Used to Treat Conjunctivitis

MEDICATION	ACTION/INDICATION	NURSING IMPLICATIONS
Fluoroquinolones (e.g., norfloxacin, ciprofloxacin, ofloxacin, levofloxacin, sparfloxacin)	Antibiotic effective against a broad spectrum of gram-positive and gram-negative organisms; generally interfere with enzymes needed for DNA replication in bacteria causing eye infections	If a culture and sensitivity test is ordered, perform the test before beginning the antibiotic. Teach parents correct administration of drops or ointment. Be alert for signs of reactivity to medication which might be manifested as local burning, crusting, itching, and edema.
Acyclovir	Anitviral drug effective against herpes simplex virus (HSV).	Most viral conjunctivitis infections are not treated; good hygiene practices are followed and the infection clears without treatment by medication. However, herpes simplex virus infections must be treated because they can harm vision. Acyclovir is administered intravenously to neonates and some children with HSV; ongoing suppressive oral therapy is used for recurrent infections. Teach family to recognize characteristic herpes skin lesions and report them and all eye redness immediately. Ensure that family and other care providers understand the possible chronic nature of HSV and engage in careful hygiene to prevent spread when infections are active. Prepare and administer IV form as ordered, over at least 1 hour. Shake oral suspension when that form is used for children.
Mast-cell stabilizers (e.g., cromolyn, nedocromil, olopatadine)	Inhibit release of histamine from mast cells, thereby decreasing allergic response. Used to treat itching and other symptoms of allergic conjunctivitis.	Teach family the correct installation of medication. Encourage other methods to decrease itching such as cool compresses several times daily to the eyes. Avoid rubbing eyes which can introduce bacteria or virus to the already inflamed eyes. If medication does not provide relief or additional eye symptoms appear, consult again with healthcare provider.

NURSING MANAGEMENT

Nurses routinely instill prophylactic antibiotics into the eyes of newborns after birth. A careful examination should occur so that any cases of ophthalmia neonatorum are referred promptly to an ophthalmologist. Women infected with gonococcus or chlamydia should be identified so their babies can receive attention and medication at birth to prevent infection (Brocklehurst & Rooney, 2000). Babies born at home should have ocular examinations soon after birth.

Because bacterial conjunctivitis is contagious, advise parents that children should not return to childcare or school until they have been using an antibiotic for 24 hours. For all types of conjunctivitis, teach parents the importance of careful handwashing and the avoidance of shared towels. Inform parents that children should not rub their eyes; soft cotton mittens may help prevent infants from doing so. Toddlers may be distracted by activities that keep their hands busy. Teach parents the proper techniques for instilling eye medications. Answer questions about types of infections; some parents do not understand that most viral infections are not treated with antibiotics. For children with allergies, alert parents to signs of infection such as increased redness and thickness of discharge, so if the child gets an eye infection, prompt treatment will be obtained. For the child at the appropriate developmental level, the itching of allergic conjunctivitis may be relieved by lying clean washcloths with very cold water over the eyes for several minutes two to three times daily. It is best not to use contact lenses during periods of allergic conjunctivitis since they can further exacerbate the condition. See Partnering with Families: Instilling Eye Medications.

Periorbital Cellulitis

Periorbital cellulitis is an infection of the eyelid and surrounding tissues that is usually caused by bacteria. Children present with swollen, tender, red or purple eyelids; restricted, painful movement of the area around the eye; and fever. Periorbital cellulitis should be treated promptly to prevent the spread of the infection to the posterior orbit. Orbital cellulitis is a serious outcome that can lead to bacterial meningitis and all of its possible sequallae (see Chapter 33∞). Clinical therapy includes hospitalization for intravenous administration of antibiotics and the application of hot packs. Children usually respond favorably within 48 to 72 hours.

Nursing management of periorbital cellulitis begins with identification of potential cases and prompt referral for treatment. When the child is hospitalized, the nurse administers antibiotics, provides supportive care, monitors vital signs, and teaches the family about the infection. Desired outcomes are rapid resolution of the infection and return to normal daily activity with no impairment in eye function. See Chapter 26∞ for additional information about cellulitis in other body parts.

Visual Disorders

Vision, the complex process of acquiring meaning from what is seen, depends on many factors. The eyes must move quickly and in a coordinated manner (see Chapter 8∞ for discussion of eye movement assessment). They must function together for clear, single vision to occur. If this ability, called **binocularity,** is not present (perhaps due to strabismus or amblyopia), the child cannot make sense of the images the brain receives. Normally, the objects seen are integrated with other senses through eye–hand coordination, and with the brain through visual imagery and discrimination of objects seen. Although visual acuity is essential, the child's movements, mental processes, and other senses all interact to give meaning to objects that are viewed. Vision therefore influences learning and school performance.

Etiology and Pathophysiology

Several of the common visual disorders involve errors of refraction (Figure 24–4 ■). As light enters the eye, it is bent or refracted to fall on the retina. Variations in shape of the eyeball are often genetic in nature and can cause light rays to fall in another area of the eye, where they cannot be interpreted. Common refractive errors include:

- ***Hyperopia* (farsightedness).** Light rays focus posterior to the retina, resulting in an inability to focus on nearby objects. All children have some degree of hyperopia until 9 to 10 years of age. However, their eyes can accommodate sufficiently to enable them to see near objects clearly. Blurring of vision occurs only in children with excessive hyperopia, or a difference in accommodation between the two eyes. Amblyopia, or weakened vision of the poorer eye, can occur in these children if treatment is not obtained.
- ***Myopia* (nearsightedness).** Light rays focus anterior to the retina, resulting in an inability to see far-off objects. Although children of any age can manifest myopia, it most commonly develops at about 8 years of age. The child may complain of headaches and often squints to improve distance vision.
- **Astigmatism.** Light rays are refracted differently depending on their place of entry to the eye. The curvature of the cornea or lens is not uniformly spherical, causing blurred images. The child with astigmatism often holds pages very close to the face to obtain the best visual image (DeRespinis, 2001).

Other common visual disorders in children are characterized by abnormal musculature that causes asymmetric eye movement and by other anatomic abnormalities. They include:

- **Strabismus**—abnormal turning of the eye, usually inward or outward. The eyes are misaligned so that symmetric vision, or binocularity, is not possible. The condition is usually present at birth and up to approximately 6 months of age, but can develop as a result of amblyopia, described next. When strabismus is the primary disorder, it may also lead to amblyopia since the eye with abnormal musculature may lose its ability to see normally.
- **Amblyopia**—reduced vision of the eye. Generally one eye has much poorer vision than the other, resulting in loss of binocularity. As noted, the child's muscle in the poorer eye may fail to function normally over time, resulting in strabismus. Amblyopia is usually genetic and appears at birth. At times it is the result of another eye abnormality such as glaucoma, cataract, or even eye injury.
- **Cataracts**—lens opacity. Some cataracts are present at birth while others are acquired during childhood. Some of the causes of acquired cataracts include retinopathy of prematurity (described later in this chapter), metabolic diseases such as galactosemia, diabetes mellitus, and long-term use of corticosteroids. A major cause of congenital cataracts in the past was congenital rubella syndrome, the mother's infection with rubella during gestation. Since children and women now receive rubella vaccine, there are very few cases of rubella in pregnant women and consequently few cases of cataracts from the syndrome.
- **Glaucoma**—refers to increased intraocular pressure. Some infants have congenital glaucoma present at birth and other children manifest a genetically caused glaucoma sometime during childhood. Secondary or acquired glaucoma can result from eye injury or prolonged steroid use. The pressure can alter structures of the eye when left untreated, leading to permanent visual impairment.
- **Retinoblastoma**—tumor of the retina, described in Chapter 29∞. Other cancers that may affect the eye include optic nerve glioma, optic nerve meningioma, and rhabdomyosarcoma.

Clinical Manifestations

Children with eye abnormalities may show a variety of behaviors. An infant who notices objects only on one side or consistently holds the head more to one side may have a decrease

PARTNERING WITH FAMILIES

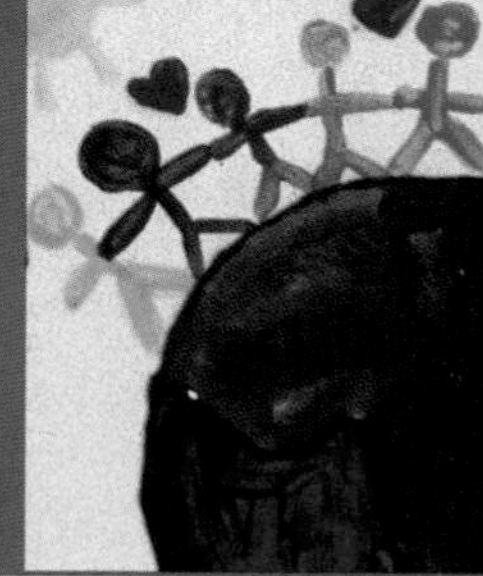

Instilling Eye Medications

It can be challenging to safely instill eye medication into young children. Give parents the following suggestions.

- Wash hands well.
- Be sure the medicine is warmed at least to room temperature.
- Remove any drainage from the eye with a clean or sterile moist, warm cloth or gauze.
- Wash hands again.
- Have the child lie on the back with eyes closed.
- Gently pull the lower lid down to form a small pocket.
- Apply a thin string (for ointment) or drops (for liquid) of the medicine.
- Allow the eyelid to return to normal position.
- Have the child keep the eye closed for several seconds.
- Help prevent spread of the infection by keeping the child's hands clean.
- Enhance comfort by keeping the head elevated to decrease swelling and by avoiding exposure to bright light.

PATHOPHYSIOLOGY ILLUSTRATED

Visual Abnormalities

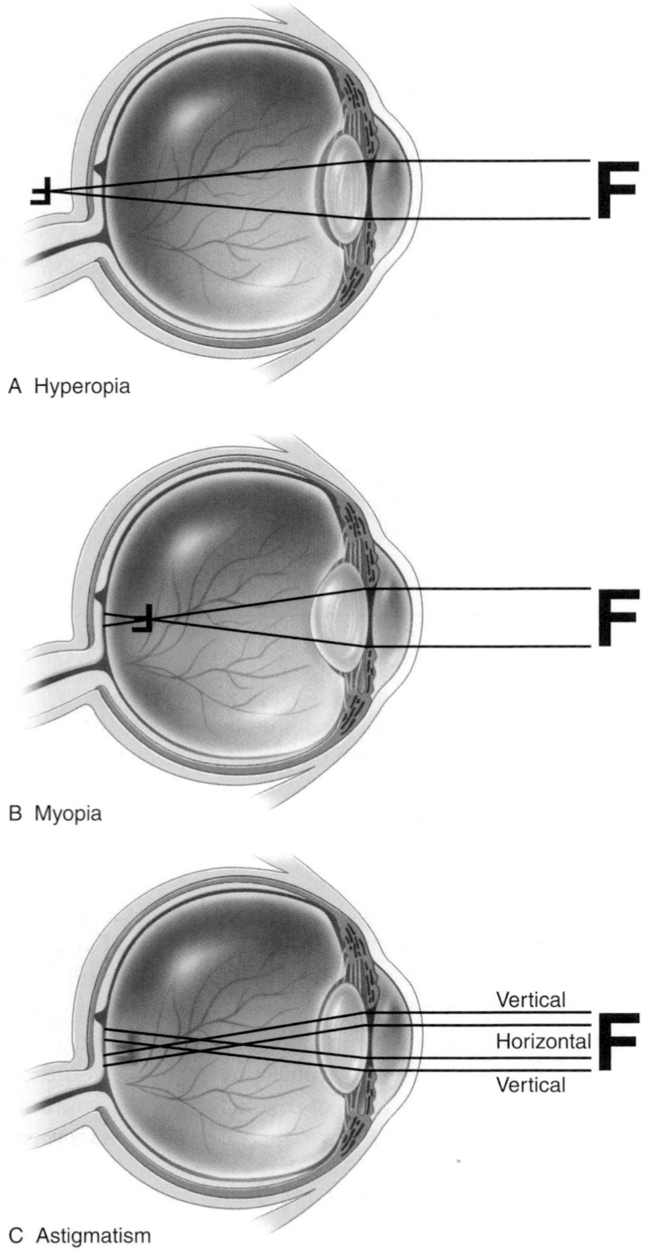

A Hyperopia

B Myopia

C Astigmatism

Vertical

Horizontal

Vertical

FIGURE 24–4 ■ In hyperopia light rays focus behind the retina, making it difficult to focus on objects at close range. In myopia light rays focus in front of the retina, making it difficult to focus on objects that are far away. In astigmatism light rays do not uniformly focus on the eye due to abnormal curvature of cornea or lens.

in vision in the other eye. Cataracts may be visualized as the lens appears cloudy. Muscular problems may be evident when the eyes do not move symmetrically or one eye deviates inward or outward. Some children squint, cover one eye, hold toys or books close to the face, or have watering eyes. For further detail on clinical manifestations of specific eye conditions, see the clinical manifestations table on page 779.

COLLABORATIVE CARE

The goal of collaborative care for visual disorders is early detection of abnormalities and prompt treatment. Since vision is developing in early childhood, a problem with one eye can affect permanent visual acuity if not detected and treated.

Diagnostic Tests

Visual disturbances must be diagnosed and treated promptly to prevent impairment or loss of visual acuity (Altemeier, 2000; *Healthy People 2010,* 2000). Most children undergo a simple test for visual acuity during healthcare visits as soon as they can cooperate with the examiner. Once in school, children's visual acuity is screened every 2 to 3 years during the elementary years. Table 24–2 provides a series of questions that can be asked to identify visual disturbances in children. A child who does not pass vision screening is referred to an ophthalmologist or optometrist for more detailed examination of near and far vision, eye structure and movement, and color discrimination. During health promotion visits, infants and young children should be examined by using the cover–uncover test and the red reflex should be examined with an ophthalmoscope. See Chapter 8∞ for thorough descriptions of both of these tests.

Clinical Therapy

Compensatory lenses are prescribed for many visual disorders, particularly refractive disorders. A significant difference in visual acuity between the eyes is often a result of amblyopia or strabismus, and further treatment by patching or surgery may be needed. The visual acuity of a child with compensatory lenses should be reevaluated every 1 to 2 years. More frequent visits to an eye specialist are needed when a child is being treated for amblyopia or strabismus.

Cataracts are generally treated surgically with removal of the lens, placement of lens transplant, or use of corrective contact lenses. Glaucoma frequently requires surgery in children to provide outflow for fluid and resultant decrease in intraocular pressure. The variety of cancers are treated with surgery and chemotherapy.

CLINICAL MANIFESTATIONS of Visual Disorders

ETIOLOGY	CLINICAL MANIFESTATIONS	CLINICAL THERAPY
Strabismus Can be congenital or acquired. Seen in 5% of all children Most common types: **Esotropia:** inward deviation of eyes ("crossed eyes") **Exotropia:** outward deviation of eyes ("wall- eyes") Strabismus *Reprinted from* Paediatrics, *2e, Thomas & Harvey, p. 130, 1997, by permission of the publisher Churchill Livingstone.*	Eyes appear misaligned to observer. May occur only when child is tired. Symptoms include squinting and frowning when reading; closing one eye to see; having trouble picking up objects; dizziness and headache. Corneal light reflex and cover–uncover tests confirm diagnosis. Child may have no other abnormalities but certain conditions such as cerebral palsy, hydrocephalus, Down syndrome, and seizure disorder are more commonly accompanied by strabismus.	Occlusion therapy (patching the fixating or good eye to force use of the weak eye) Compensatory lenses Surgery of the rectus muscles to correct muscle imbalance Eye drops to cause blurring of the good eye Prisms Vision therapy (eye exercises) If treatment is begun before 24 months of age, amblyopia (reduced vision in one or both eyes) may be prevented.
Amblyopia ("lazy eye") Reduced vision in one or both eyes; affects 7% of children. Amblyopia can result from anything which causes visual deprivation to one eye. The most common causes are untreated strabismus, with the child "tuning out" the image in deviating eye, congenital cataract, or visual differences between eyes.	Symptoms are the same as for strabismus. Vision testing can be used to diagnose condition.	Compensatory lenses Occlusion therapy for 2–6 hours daily Occasionally vision therapy (eye exercises) is used in an attempt to improve the weaker eye. Atropine 1% 1 gtt/day in unaffected eye. Treatment is discontinued when visual faculty no longer improves; 20/20 acuity rarely attained. Treatment is most successful if received by 5–6 years of age.
Cataracts Occur when all or part of lens of eye becomes opaque, which prevents refraction of light rays onto retina Seen in 1 of every 250 newborns Congenital cataract. *From Vaughan, D., Asbury, T., & Riordan-Eva, P. (1992)* General ophthalmology *(13th ed., p. 172). New York: McGraw-Hill Companies.*	Can affect one or both eyes and may be congenital or acquired. Clouding of lens indicates presence of cataract, however, cataracts are not always visible to naked eye. Symptoms included distorted red reflex, symptoms of vision loss (see strabismus), white pupil. May be present alone but sometimes associated with fetal alcohol syndrome and Down syndrome.	Must be diagnosed at a young age for successful treatment; many cases are missed. Specific treatment depends on whether one or both eyes are affected, extent of clouding and presence of other ocular abnormalities. Surgical removal of lens and corrective lenses; contact lenses frequently used; results of surgery are good; surgery before the age of 2 months is associated with the best results; visual acuity in 55% of children is 20/40 or better. Lens implant may be used. Eye protectors and restraints are used postoperatively to prevent injury; antibiotic or steroid drops may be used for several weeks; treatment for amblyopia may be necessary.

(continued)

CLINICAL MANIFESTATIONS of Visual Disorders (continued)

ETIOLOGY	CLINICAL MANIFESTATIONS	CLINICAL THERAPY
Glaucoma Increased intraocular pressure damages eye and impairs visual function; ciliary body of eye produces aqueous fluid that flows between iris and lens into anterior chamber; if enough fluid accumulates, blindness results; affects 1 in 100,000 newborns. May be congenital (primary) or acquired (secondary) and affect one or both eyes. Congenital glaucoma. *From Vaughan, D., Asbury, T. & Riordan-Eva, P. (1992)* General ophthalmology. *(13th ed., p. 172). New York: McGraw-Hill Companies.*	Symptoms of congenital glaucoma include tearing, blinking, corneal clouding, eyelid spasms, and progressive enlargement of eye; photophobia (extreme sensitivity to light). Symptoms of acquired glaucoma include constant bumping into objects in child's periphery (painless visual field loss); seeing halos around objects. Diagnosis is made using tonometer, which measures intraocular pressure.	Surgery to reduce intraocular pressure is treatment of choice, since medications used to combat glaucoma in adults are not as effective in children. Compensatory lenses used following surgery. Treatment is not always successful, especially if the child has congenital glaucoma, so parents' feelings regarding care of a visually handicapped child should be explored.

Data from Alterneier, W. A. (2000). Preschool vision screening: The importance of the two-line difference. Pediatric Annals, 29, 264–267; Bacal, D. A., & Wilson, M. C. (2000). *Strabismus: Getting it straight.* Contemporary Pediatrics, 17, *49–60; Starr, N. B. (2000). Vision therapy for learning disabilities and dyslexia.* Journal of Pediatric Health Care, 14, *32–33.*

NURSING MANAGEMENT

The nurse focuses activities on identification of children with eye problems, and on partnering with parents and other professionals to provide care for the child with a visual disorder.

■ Nursing Assessment and Diagnosis

The nurse plays an important role in identifying eye disorders in children. You will perform careful eye examinations of newborns and children. Observe for symmetry of placement and movement, ability to follow objects with each eye, and any abnormalities in appearance. The light reflex test, cover–uncover test, and visual acuity testing are essential for every child. See Chapter 8∞ for a description of eye examination and the Skills Manual for visual acuity tests.

Nurses in schools plan and carry out visual acuity screening on children. Generally certain grades (such as kindergarten, 2, 5, and 8) are screened annually along with any children new to a district. The nurse performs and records the screening results,

TABLE 24–2 Assessment Questions for Identifying Visual Disturbances in Children

INFANT	YOUNG CHILD	SCHOOL-AGE CHILD
Ask the parents:	Ask the parents:	Ask the parents:
Does your baby follow an object from one side to the other?	Does your child follow you with his or her eyes as you come into a room?	Does your child like to look at pictures and read?
What is your baby's reaction when you are directly in front and close?	Are other objects followed with ease?	Does your child hold toys or books close, or sit very close to the television?
Does the baby seem to notice an object to the right and left sides?	Do both eyes work together or does one seem to wander off?	Does your child squint or rub the eyes?
Do your baby's eyes ever appear to move asymmetrically?	At what age did your baby sit, stand, walk?	Is he or she performing at grade level in all subjects?
What is your baby learning to do right now?	Does your child have any difficulty picking up objects?	Has your child demonstrated any learning difficulties?
		Does he or she use a computer, watch television, or play computer games?
		Does your child play sports and games at the same level of ability as peers?

and informs the school and families of any children with abnormal results who are referred to an eye specialist for care. An important part of the screening process is following up on referrals to be certain that children receive the diagnostic care they need.

Potential diagnoses related to visual problems are as follows:

- Disturbed Sensory Perception related to error of refraction
- Delayed Growth and Development related to effects of visual impairment
- Situational Low Self-esteem related to poor school performance resulting from visual impairment

Planning and Implementation

When abnormalities are found on screening, nurses refer families to the care of an eye specialist. When prescriptive lenses are used, the nurse instructs the parent and child on correct wear practices and care. See the Skills Manual for information about contact lens care. Sometimes nurses partner with community resources to provide financial assistance to provide for care. The Lions Club and other groups may be able to provide glasses for children if the family cannot afford them.

Provide explanations for parents who are confused about the diagnosis or treatment. Instruct parents in patching for the recommended period of time daily (usually 2 to 6 hours) for the child with amblyopia.

If surgery is needed, surgical and postoperative follow-up are needed. This will include pain control, observing for signs of infection (ophthalmic or systemic), and administering needed eye medications. Sterile technique is used postoperatively to provide eye care. Promptly report deviations from normal such as increased pain, redness, discharge, or edema of the eye; increased temperature or pulse, which may indicate infection; increased sensitivity to light; or other abnormalities. Children are usually discharged home with instructions to minimize vigorous activities for a certain period of time. Perform postoperative and discharge teaching and emphasize the importance of follow-up visits.

Evaluation

The nurse evaluates the effectiveness of vision screening and treatment for individuals and groups of children. Use the *Healthy People 2010* (2000) objectives related to vision as a guide to evaluation of programs (Table 24–3). See the section on visual impairment later in the chapter for information on the child with a diagnosed decrease in vision.

Color Blindness

Color blindness is an X-linked recessive disorder found in 8% of White and 4% of Black males and very rarely in females. The most common form affects the ability to distinguish between the colors red and green. Preschool boys are tested for color blindness in some clinics to identify those with the disorder. The Ishihara color blindness test is often used and consists of

TABLE 24–3 *Healthy People 2010* Objectives Related to Vision in Children

OBJECTIVE	NURSING IMPLEMENTATION
28–2 Increase the proportion of preschool children aged 5 years and under who receive vision screening.	➤ Establish programs to screen preschoolers in childcare centers for visual acuity, symmetry of eye movement, and ability to focus ➤ Sponsor programs at schools, clinics, vans, religious organizations, and other settings to screen vision of young children
28–3 Reduce uncorrected visual impairment due to refractive errors.	➤ Establish a referral and follow-up plan for children who do not pass screening ➤ Post resources on bulletin boards, online websites, and other places where parents look for health information
28–4 Reduce blindness and visual impairment in children and adolescents aged 17 years and under.	➤ Ensure that pregnant women obtain recommended prenatal care in order to reduce prematurity which is a risk factor for visual impairment ➤ Perform screening for visual impairment during each health encounter ➤ Refer children to eye specialists when parents are concerned about a child's vision or any abnormalities are noted
28–9 Increase the use of appropriate personal eyewear in recreational activities and hazardous situations around the home.	➤ Assist families to understand that most eye injuries are preventable ➤ Partner with families to plan for protection during sports such as hockey and racquetball, as well as yard work ➤ Include teaching about emergency care for eye injuries to teachers, coaches, and parents
28–10 Increase the use of vision rehabilitation services and adaptive devices by people with visual impairments.	➤ Screen children with glasses or contact lenses in place ➤ Check for fit of glasses; strap to keep glasses on toddler ➤ Encourage annual visits to eye specialist for child with visual impairment ➤ Assist families and school personnel to provide safe and stimulating environments for children with visual impairment

Adapted from U. S. Department of Health and Human Services. (2000). Healthy People 2010 *(2nd ed.). Washington, DC: U.S. Government Printing Office.* www.healthypeople.gov

MediaLink Vision Impairment Resources

numbers embedded in a background that are difficult for persons with color blindness to see. Color blindness is not treatable and management focuses on issues of safety (e.g., problems in distinguishing red–green traffic signals) and techniques to improve discrimination of colors in the affected color groups.

Retinopathy of Prematurity

Retinopathy of prematurity (ROP) occurs when immature blood vessels in the retina constrict and become necrotic. This condition, which may occur in infants of low birth weight or of short gestation, can heal completely or lead to mild myopia or retinal detachment and blindness.

Etiology and Pathophysiology

Retinopathy of prematurity results from injury to the developing capillaries of the retina. Oxygen therapy is associated with the development of ROP (Figure 24–5 ■), but other factors such as respiratory distress, assisted ventilation, apnea, bradycardia, heart disease, multiple blood transfusions, infection, hypoxia, hypercarbia, acidosis, shock, and sepsis have been linked with the disorder. Cerebral palsy is sometimes an associated factor and more cases are seen in multiple births. It is most common in infants born before 28 weeks' gestation and weighing under 1,600 g (3 lb, 8 oz) at birth. A genetic link may be present as White infants are more commonly affected than those of African heritage, and Alaskan natives have a high rate of the disorder. In developed countries ROP is the second most common cause of blindness, occurring in 12.5% of infants born from 23 to 26 weeks' gestation (Wheatley, Dickinson, Mackey, et al., 2002).

The retina is normally vascularized by about 8 months' gestation. For the premature infant, however, this process must continue after birth and the environmental and other conditions listed in the preceding paragraph appear to affect its course. Arteriole constriction, followed by vascular proliferation of abnormal vessels, occurs. In most cases, the abnormal vessels gradually regress and normal vascularization occurs. Sometimes, however, the abnormal vascularization continues into the vitreous cavity, causing abnormalities of the retina, optic disc, and macula. It is not known why the disease progresses in some cases, but progression is directly linked to lower birth weight, greater prematurity, and duration (not necessarily concentration) of oxygen therapy. Raeanne, the child described in the scenario at the beginning of this chapter, developed retinopathy of prematurity after assisted ventilation and other treatments for her prematurity (Box 24–1).

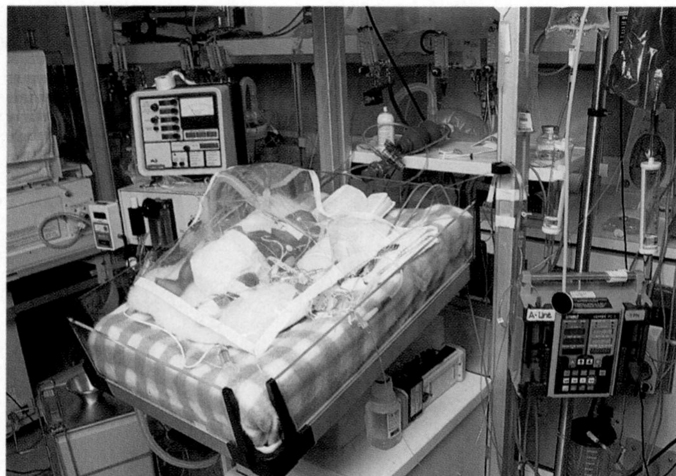

FIGURE 24–5 ■ This premature infant in the neonatal intensive care unit is receiving artificial ventilation—a risk factor for retinopathy of prematurity. The infant will need careful management of oxygen as well as periodic eye examinations.

Although the developing capillaries are lost, in up to 90% of cases some degree of revascularization occurs later. The degree of visual loss, varying from slight to total, is determined by the degree of revascularization that occurs.

Clinical Manifestations

Retinopathy of prematurity is characterized by progressive changes in the retinal blood vessels, and in severe disease, by retinal detachment. Premature and low-birth-weight infants at risk for the disease are given frequent ocular examinations to ensure early detection of these changes. For infants who do not receive ophthalmologic examinations, resulting visual impairment may be detected only later in infancy when the child progresses slowly in meeting developmental milestones, fails to reach for objects, and does not follow objects or faces with the eyes. When visual impairment is present, the child usually manifests myopia. Total loss of vision can occur in the child who suffers a retinal detachment.

COLLABORATIVE CARE

The goal of collaborative care is to provide ongoing evaluation of infants at risk for retinopathy of prematurity, to provide care for the disorder to minimize effects, and to support the child who has visual impairment due to the disorder.

Diagnostic Tests

Diagnosis is made by ophthalmologic examination. A classification system is used to describe the location, extent, and severity of the disease (American Academy of Pediatrics, Section on Ophthalmology, 2001). All infants at risk, particularly those under 2,000 g (4 lb, 3 oz) at birth or born before 33 weeks' gestation are assessed frequently by an ophthalmologist who is experienced with the condition. The disease does not manifest itself before 4 to 6 weeks after birth, so it is important that the infant receive

BOX 24–1 Retinopathy of Prematurity and Reduction of Light Exposure

Several groups have studied whether retinopathy of prematurity is associated with exposure to bright lights in neonatal intensive care units. It has been hypothesized that since babies would normally be in a dark womb and their retinal vessels are still developing, damage might be done by environmental light. In a meta-analysis of five studies, pooled data provided no support for the hypothesis. Placing premature infants in goggles or other eye covers does not appear to lower the incidence of retinopathy of prematurity (Phelps & Watts, 2003).

regular eye examinations until the risk is discounted. If the infant shows signs of disease, eye examinations continue every 1 to 2 weeks. Involvement of blood vessels in the periphery of the retina rarely leads to visual impairment. With involvement in other areas of the retina, risk of visual problems is more common.

Clinical Therapy

Treatment of infants with severe retinopathy of prematurity involves using cryotherapy or laser therapy to stop progression of the disease process. Other surgical procedures such as a scleral buckle procedure and vitrectomy have been used in retinal detachments. For children like Raeanne who have resulting visual impairment, it is important to treat problems such as strabismus, amblyopia, and myopia to promote maximal development (see previous section).

NURSING MANAGEMENT

Nursing management focuses on referring the infant at risk for retinopathy of prematurity for ophthalmoscopic evaluation and for assisting the family in coping with visual impairment when that is a result of the disorder.

Nursing Assessment and Diagnosis

Assessment of the infant at risk for retinopathy of prematurity begins at birth by identifying infants who may require oxygen therapy. Look for risk factors such as prematurity and low birth weight. Assess the infant's breathing efforts and report any changes. Be certain the ventilation equipment is properly set to deliver the correct amount of oxygen. Ventilatory equipment is meticulously monitored. The nurse weans the infant from oxygen as indicated by oxygen saturation reading in concordance with standing orders in the neonatal intensive care unit. Note the cumulative risks in a particular case (longer exposure to oxygen increases risk) and suggest the need for a referral to an ophthalmologist, as necessary. See Tables 24–4 and 24–5 for referral criteria for assessment and classification of cases.

The accompanying nursing care plan outlines several nursing diagnoses for a child such as Raeanne with a visual impairment secondary to retinopathy of prematurity. Following are other nursing diagnoses that may be appropriate for an infant with the potential to develop ROP or a child with resulting visual impairment.

- Sensory/Perceptual Alteration (visual) related to altered transmission of impulses
- Potential Impaired Gas Exchange related to ventilation-perfusion imbalance
- Alteration in Growth and Development related to effects of visual impairment
- Altered Family Processes related to a child with a visual impairment

Planning and Implementation

The nurse plays an important role in preventing retinopathy of prematurity. Encourage early and regular prenatal care to prevent unnecessary premature births. Administer oxygen only to newborns who need it, and in the amount specified by the physician. Ensure that the proper ventilatory settings are used. Be alert for infants with multiple risk factors and refer them, when appropriate, for ophthalmologic examination. Parents of infants at risk for ROP require information about the disorder, as well as support, as the long-term effects on the child's vision are often identified only after subsequent examinations as the child grows. Families may be frustrated that a prognosis cannot be made at the time of the first eye examination. Explanations and consistent updates on the infant's condition can be reassuring.

The accompanying nursing care plan summarizes care for the child with a visual impairment resulting from retinopathy of prematurity. The nurse is instrumental in case management for such children. Reinforce to parents the importance of follow-up eye examinations. Teach methods of stimulating development for the visually impaired child (refer to the next section in this chapter).

TABLE 24–4 Diagnosis of Retinopathy of Prematurity

ZONE (AREA OF RETINA INVOLVED WITH ABNORMAL VASCULATURE)	STAGE (SEVERITY OF ROP WHEREVER IT IS PRESENT)	PLUS DISEASE (VASCULAR DILATION AND TORTUOSITY IS NOTED IN POSTERIOR POLE IN AREA NEAR OPTIC NERVE)	THRESHOLD (MEASURE OF SEVERITY OF DISEASE; USED TO JUDGE WHEN TREATMENT IS NEEDED)
Zone I (most posterior and near optic nerve head)	Stage 1 (line divides vascular and avascular retina)	Presence	Threshold I (stage 3 ROP in Zone I or II and five continuous or eight cumulative "clock hour" areas with plus disease; treatment is required)
Zone II (outside or area anterior to Zone I)	Stage 2 (line of demarcation is elevated)	Absence	
Zone III (only present on temporal side of eye; nasal quadrants are adequately vascularized)	Stage 3 (New vascularization is present in the demarcation area)		

Data from Good, W. V., & Gendron, R. L. (2001). Retinopathy of prematurity. Ophthalmology Clinics of North America, 14, *513–519.*

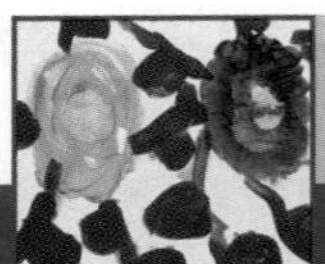

Nursing Care Plan

THE CHILD WITH A VISUAL IMPAIRMENT SECONDARY TO RETINOPATHY OF PREMATURITY

GOAL	INTERVENTION	RATIONALE	EXPECTED OUTCOME
1. Disturbed Visual Sensory Perception related to altered reception, transmission, and integration resulting from retinopathy of prematurity			
	NIC Priority Intervention: *Visual Deficit Enhancement:* Assistance in accepting and learning alternate methods for living with diminished vision.		**NOC Suggested Outcome:** *Developmental Progression:* Compensate for sensory deficits by maximizing use of impaired senses.
The child will receive adequate sensory input	■ Provide kinesthetic, tactile, and auditory stimulation during play and in daily care (e.g., talking and playing). Provide music while bathing an infant using bells and other noises on each side of infant. Verbally describe to a child all actions being carried out by adult.	■ Because visual sensory input is not present, the child needs input from all other senses to compensate and provide adequate sensory stimulation.	The child demonstrates minimal signs of sensory deprivation.
2. Risk for Injury related to impaired vision			
	NIC Priority Intervention: *Fall Prevention:* Instituting special precautions with patients at risk for injury.		**NOC Suggested Outcome:** *Risk Control:* Actions to eliminate or reduce modifiable health threats.
The child will be protected from safety hazards that can lead to injury.	■ Evaluate environment for potential safety hazards based on age of child and degree of impairment. Be particularly alert to objects that give visual cues to their dangers (e.g., stoves, fireplaces, candles). Eliminate safety hazards and protect the child from exposure. Take the child on a tour of new rooms (e.g., schools, hotel room, hospital room).	■ The child may be at risk for injury related both to developmental stage and inability to visualize hazards.	The child will experience no injuries.
3. Risk for Altered Growth and Development related to Impaired vision			
	NIC Priority Intervention: *Developmental Enhancement:* Facilitating or teaching parents and caregivers to facilitate optional growth and development of children.		**NOC Suggested Outcome:** *Child Growth and Development*: Milestones of developmental progression.
The child has experiences necessary to foster normal growth and development.	■ Help parents plan early, regular social activities with other children. ■ Provide opportunities and encourage self-feeding activities. ■ Provide an environment rich in sensory input. ■ Assess growth and development during regular examinations to identify the child's strengths and needs.	■ The visually impaired child benefits developmentally from contact with other children. ■ To obtain adequate nutrients, the child needs to feel comfortable feeding self. ■ Sensory input is needed for normal development to occur. ■ Regular examinations aid in early identification of growth problems or developmental delays, so that appropriate interventions can be planned.	The child demonstrates normal growth and development milestones.

Nursing Care Plan THE CHILD WITH A VISUAL IMPAIRMENT SECONDARY TO RETINOPATHY OF PREMATURITY (continued)

GOAL	INTERVENTION	RATIONALE	EXPECTED OUTCOME
4. Risk for Compromised Family Coping related to child's prolonged disability from sensory impairment			
	NIC Priority Intervention: *Family Mobilization:* Utilization of family strengths to influence child's health positively.		**NOC Suggested Outcome:** *Positive Coping:* Extent to which family can mobilize resources to deal with the child's needs.
The family identifies methods for coping with their visually impaired child.	■ Provide explanation of visual impairment as appropriate.	■ The parents may feel guilt about the child's visual impairment, which can be allayed by knowledge of the cause.	The family successfully copes with the experience of having a visually impaired child.
	■ Refer parents to organizations, early intervention programs, and other parents of visually impaired children.	■ The parents will receive needed information and support from others.	
	■ Assist parents to plan for meeting developmental, educational, and safety needs of their visually impaired child. Offer resources for changing home environment to assist visually impaired child.	■ The child may require an enhanced environment in order to foster developmental progress.	

Evaluation

Expected outcomes of nursing care for the child with retinopathy of prematurity include:

- Early identification of visual impairment
- Normal developmental milestone achievement
- Positive management of child's visual condition by the family

Visual Impairment

Visual impairment accounts for 11% of chronic medical conditions in children. Legal blindness (defined as visual acuity of 20/200 or worse in the corrected eye or significantly reduced visual fields) occurs in 1 per 35,000 children. About 1 in 500 children have partial vision. About half of the children who are blind or have partial vision have other disabilities as well. Between 5% and 10% of preschoolers and 20% to 30% of school-age children have some type of vision problem (Burns, Brady, Dunn, et al., 2000; Halle, 2002).

Many conditions discussed earlier in this chapter lead to temporary or permanent visual impairment. Infants who are premature; whose mothers were infected prenatally with rubella, toxoplasmosis, or other viruses; and who have certain congenital and hereditary conditions have a high risk of visual problems (Table 24–6). Fetal alcohol syndrome (FAS) is a major cause of visual disturbance; 90% of children with FAS have eye abnormalities (see Chapter 34∞ for further description of FAS).

TABLE 24–5 Assessment and Treatment for Retinopathy of Prematurity

INITIAL ASSESSMENT	FOLLOW-UP ASSESSMENT	TREATMENT
Who? All infants less than 1,500 g or less than 28 weeks' gestation; babies from 1,500–2,000 g who have other risk factors	Every 2–3 weeks if vasculature is immature and extends to Zone II but no retinopathy is present; continue until normal vascularization is seen in Zone III	Ablative therapy with laser or cryotherapy for infants reaching threshold disease; treatment needed within 72 hours of diagnosis to minimize chance of retinal detachment
When? 4–6 weeks postnatal age or 31–33 weeks of postconceptual age	Every 2 weeks if ROP is in Zone II but is not severe	
What? At least two funduscopic examinations with pupil dilation using binocular indirect ophthalmoscopy by an ophthalmologist; one examination is satisfactory if full retinal vascularization is seen bilaterally	Every 1–2 weeks if no ROP but having incomplete vasculature in Zone I	
	Every week for infants with ROP in Zone II, stage 3 ROP without plus disease, or stage 2 ROP with plus disease, or stage 3 ROP with plus disease not severe enough for surgery	

Data from American Academy of Pediatrics Section on Ophthalmology. (2001). Screening examination of premature infants for retinopathy of prematurity. Pediatrics, 108, *809–811.*

TABLE 24–6 Common Causes of Visual Impairment in Children

Congenital or Hereditary	Acquired
Cataracts	Injury to eye or head
Glaucoma	Infections
Tay-Sachs disease	Rubella
Marfan syndrome	Measles
Down syndrome	Chickenpox
Fetal alcohol syndrome	Brain tumor
Prenatal infections (maternal infection)	Retinopathy of prematurity
Rubella	Cerebral palsy
Toxoplasmosis	
Herpes simplex	
Retinoblastoma	

The signs of visual impairment depend on the cause and degree of the problem and the age of the child (Table 24–7). The child's eyes may appear crossed or watery, and the lids may be crusty. Verbal children may complain of itching; dizziness; headache; or blurred, double, or poor vision.

COLLABORATIVE CARE

Diagnostic tests include vision screening, followed by referral to an eye specialist for full examination. Responses to visual stimuli, symmetry of eye movements, location of corneal light reflex, cover–uncover testing, visual field testing, and fundoscopic examination of retina are commonly performed. The American Optometric Association and American Public Health Association recommend comprehensive vision examination starting at 6 months of age, while the American Academy of Ophthalmology and American Academy of Pediatrics recommend screening by 3 years of age (Center for Health and Health Care in Schools, 2004). The United States Preventive Services Task Force (USPSTF) recommends screening to detect amblyopia, strabismus, and defects in visual acuity in children younger than 5 years (USPSTF, 2004). In spite of the differences in timing, it is clear that all young children should have vision examinations to identify vision problems early in life.

Clinical therapy depends on the child's condition and may include surgery, medication, and supportive aids. In the case of a disorder that results in permanent visual impairment, an interdisciplinary team of specialists works with the child and family. Nurses have an important role in this team, as evidenced by the care provided to Raeanne.

TABLE 24–7 Signs of Visual Impairment

INFANTS	TODDLERS AND OLDER CHILDREN
May be unable to follow lights or objects	May rub, shut, or cover eyes
Do not make eye contact	Tilt or thrust head forward
Have a dull, vacant stare	Blink frequently
Do not imitate facial expressions	Hold objects close
	Bump into objects
	Squint

NURSING MANAGEMENT

The nurse plays a key role in identifying children with visual impairment and in partnering with families to provide an environment for the child with visual impairment that fosters normal growth and development.

Nursing Assessment and Diagnosis

Vision screening facilitates early detection and treatment of conditions that can lead to vision loss. Visual testing can be done at any age, including immediately after birth. By 3 years of age, it should be performed at each health promotion/health maintenance visit. Developmental milestones that require vision, such as following bright lights, reaching for objects, or looking at pictures in a book, can be used to assess vision. For children over the age of 3 years, visual acuity is most frequently measured by means of an age-appropriate acuity test (see Chapter 8 and the Skills Manual). The photo screener is a device that can be used to take a photo of the child's eyes and is useful for infants, toddlers, and preschoolers. The photo can be used to diagnose refraction errors, eye opacities, and misalignment (Gomez & Davis, 2001). Visual fields and the ability to discriminate colors are tested at school age, when children can cooperate.

Children who are visually impaired may lag in development of cognitive and other skills. Sighted children learn the word *cup* using four senses—sight, touch, hearing, and taste—to obtain the information necessary to connect the word with the object it represents. In contrast, children with visual impairments rely on only three senses—touch, hearing, and taste. They learn concepts through differences in sounds, textures, and shapes. Vision affects both fine and gross motor development, so skills such as hand-to-mouth coordination and walking may be delayed in children with visual impairment.

In addition, many visual disorders are linked with other conditions that influence development. Thus, a child with cerebral palsy or fetal alcohol syndrome should be assessed frequently to identify a visual disorder, as well as to evaluate normal developmental milestones.

Nursing diagnoses for the child with impaired vision may include the following:

- Disturbed Sensory Alteration (visual) related to altered sensory perception
- Risk for Injury related to poor vision
- Risk for Delayed Growth and Development related to visual impairment
- Risk for Ineffective Family Coping related to demands of a child with a sensory impairment

Planning and Implementation

The first intervention used by nurses in all settings is prevention of visual impairment when possible, both in children with normal sight and those with some visual impairment in order to prevent further damage. Prevent visual deficits by teaching safety in activities that can injure the eye. Encourage protective eyewear in sports such as hockey, handball, and football. Work with school personnel to establish guidelines for protective eye wear for chemistry or other science or industrial education courses that may present a risk to eyes. Keep laser pointers away from children since they can cause retinal damage, especially when stared at for 10 seconds. Young children do not blink as often as adults or older children and so are at greater risk of retinal damage.

Several strategies can be used by nurses who work with children who are visually impaired (Box 24–2). Nursing care focuses on encouraging the child's use of all senses, promoting socialization, helping parents to meet the child's developmental and educational needs, and providing emotional support to parents. Refer the parents to an early intervention program upon diagnosis. Be sure that a regular series of developmental screening is performed either in the early intervention program or during healthcare visits. Developmental screening should be done about every 2 months during infancy, and every 6 months from 1 to 5 years. As the child grows, assess for physical activity, since visually impaired children are less likely than sighted children to pass activity criteria such a 1-mile walk/run, arm strength tests, and curl ups (Lieberman & McHugh, 2001). Nearly all care will occur in community and home settings.

Encourage Use of All Senses

Children who are partially sighted or blind use other senses to a great extent. Encouraging the use of the eyes as much as possible is important even if a child has poor vision (Figure 24–6 ■). See Partnering with Families: Enhancing Development of the Child Who is Visually Impaired.

Promote Socialization

The child's interactions and socializations should be as normal as possible (i.e., similar to those of sighted children of the same age and development).

- Stroke, rock, and hug infants and children who are visually impaired. Sing and talk to them. Infants with visual impairment appreciate and use touch and verbal interactions more, both in interactions with others and when exploring new objects. These infants do not make eye contact and have rather blank expressions. Encourage parents to plan for interactions between the child and a variety of other children.
- Teach parents to read body language and vocalization as expressions of emotion. Facial expressions give a great deal of information, but infants and children with poor vision do not have the ability to learn by visual imitation. Show parents how to use tactile means to teach appropriate facial expressions. For example, a touch on the arm can be soft and stroking to indicate a smile, but firmer to indicate dismay or frown.
- Explain to parents that discipline and rewards for children with poor vision should be the same as those for other children in the family. The child should be given age-appropriate tasks.

BOX 24–2 Strategies for Nurses Working with the Child Who is Visually Impaired

- Call the child's name and speak before touching the child.
- Tell the child when you are leaving the room.
- Describe what each procedure will feel like (e.g., blood pressure cuff, otoscope).
- Let the child touch the equipment to establish familiarity.
- Describe what foods are present and their locations on the food tray.

PARTNERING WITH FAMILIES

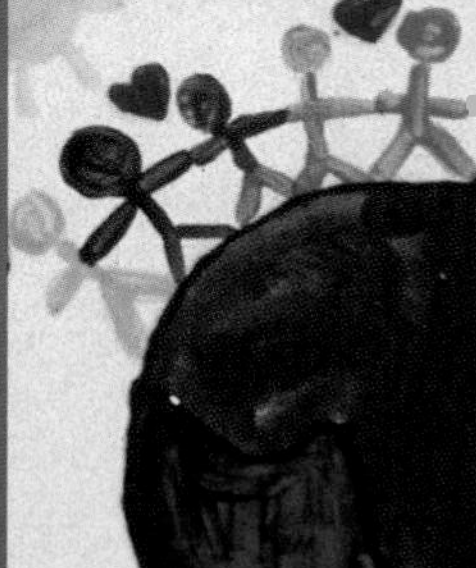

Enhancing Development of the Child Who is Visually Impaired

- Encourage a toddler or preschooler who is visually impaired to look at pictures in well-lit settings. Have a school-age child read large-print books. Computers designed for the visually impaired are also available. The Optacon (a device that raises print so it can be felt by the child) and View Scan (which magnifies print) are instruments that improve the ability to read.
- Expose the infant and child to everyday sounds.
- Encourage the infant to use the sense of touch to explore people and objects. Have the parents purchase toys with sound and texture in mind. Directional concepts can be taught using games. Responding to the infant's and child's vocalizations encourages the use of speech.
- Teach specific techniques for toileting, dressing, bathing, eating, and safety.
- When the child becomes mobile, furniture and other objects in the environment should be kept in the same positions so the child can safely move around independently. Extra care must be taken to prevent injuries when a child does not see.
- Emphasize the child's abilities. Adolescents can use seeing-eye dogs or a white cane to function independently.
- Encourage the child to function independently within normal developmental parameters.
- If in the hospital or another strange environment, orient the child to the placement of objects and do not rearrange them.
- Teach those around the child to:
  - Announce their presence to the child when approaching.
  - When walking with a blind child, walk slightly ahead of the child so he or she can sense your movements.
  - Let the child hold the seeing person's arm rather than the reverse.
  - Identify the contents of meals and encourage the child to feed self.

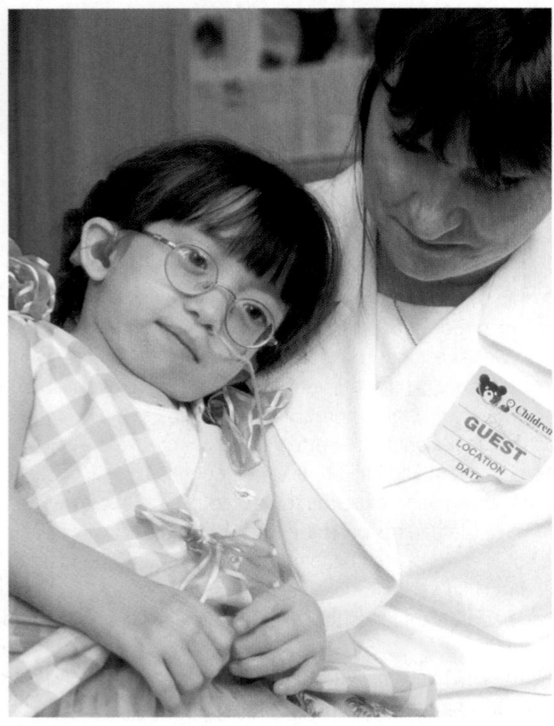

FIGURE 24–6 ■ This child with a visual impairment needs ongoing developmental assessments and a comprehensive individual education plan. Note that she is receiving tube feedings and therefore has other healthcare needs.

- Encourage contact with peers as the child grows older. Teach the child to look directly at persons who are talking to him or her. Play, sports, and other activities can be modified to give the visually impaired child the same social experiences as a sighted child.
- Foster physical activity for visually impaired children by encouraging involvement in early intervention programs; recommending programs that increase cardiovascular strength, endurance, upper body strength and flexibility; facilitating participation in and reward for sports and athletics (Lieberman & McHugh, 2001).

Care in the Community

Public laws require that each state provide educational and related services for children with disabilities (see Chapter 1∞). Parents and professionals should develop an individualized education plan (as discussed in Chapter 16∞) that maximizes the child's learning ability. If possible, the child with a vision problem should attend childcare and preschool with children who have normal visual acuity. While some developmental skills such as feeding and dressing may be slower to develop than in sighted children, plans for encouraging development tailored to the child's needs can assist in learning skills. What nursing actions are needed to help a child such as Raeanne, introduced at the beginning of this chapter, in adjusting to childcare or school?

- Provide parents with information about educational options before their child reaches school age. Education should take place in a setting that allows the child to have contact with other children and to participate in social activities. As the child enters middle and high school, it may be challenging to move to new schools or communities unfamiliar to the child. Help the parents to plan activities that will enable the youth to meet new friends.
- The child may be mainstreamed with a tutor, be partially mainstreamed in a resource room, attend special classes, or be tutored at home. If the child is to attend public school, suggest to parents that they contact the school well before enrollment to ensure that school personnel understand the child's disability.
- Make sure that items such as large-print books, braille materials, audio equipment, or an Optacon (described earlier) is available. Ensure that frequent eye examinations are performed and assist with proper use and care of prescribed glasses or contact lenses, as necessary.
- Familiarize the child with the new environment.

Provide Emotional Support

Family members often need help to understand the child's abilities and disabilities. Having a child with visual impairment can be a challenge for parents, causing anxiety about the child's future, worry about ability to meet the child's needs, financial concerns, and having insufficient time for the marital partner and other family members (Troster, 2001). Support them as they learn about the child's visual problems, tell friends and family, and then adjust to supporting the child. Assist them in explaining the child's visual impairment to school personnel or other children in a classroom.

- Encourage habilitation as soon as realistically possible. Make the adjustment easier by providing information about the child's specific type of visual impairment, available community services, and groups or associations for children with similar vision conditions. Suggest resources to families of children with visual disorders.
- Be supportive and listen to the family's concerns regarding the child's visual deficit.
- Ensure that parents meet their own physical and emotional needs so they are better able to care for and provide support to their child. Support groups, respite care, and financial resources in the community may all lower stress for parents.

■ Evaluation

Expected outcomes of nursing care for the child with a visual impairment include:

- Prevention of injury
- Growth and development to maximum potential
- Establishment of successful individualized education plan
- Adequate stress management by family members

Injuries of the Eye

In the United States, eye injuries are common in boys 11 to 15 years of age and in all children aged 9 to 11 years. Boys from 11 to 15 years have four times more eye injuries than girls. About 42,000 sports injuries occur annually with about half of these in children (Committee on Sports Medicine and Fitness, 2004). Sports, darts, fireworks, air-powered BB guns, blunt and sharp objects, chemical and thermal burns, physical irritants, and abuse may cause eye trauma (Behrman et al., 2004). Recreational activities such as sports and projectile toys are common causes. Older children may be injured by chemicals in school science laboratories.

Prevention is an important part of health promotion. Protective eyewear should be used by participants in all sports with a risk of eye injury. The most common injuries occur in baseball, basketball, swimming, bicycling, and football (Center for Health and Health Care in Schools, 2004). The best lenses for most sports are polycarbonate. Sports requiring eye protection include:

- Badminton
- Baseball
- Basketball
- Bicycling
- Fencing (face cage)
- Hockey (field, ice, roller, street)
- Handball
- Lacrosse
- Racquetball
- Soccer
- Squash
- Swimming (swim goggles)
- Tennis
- Track and field
- Water polo

(American Academy of Pediatrics, 2001)

When athletes have the best-corrected visual acuity of worse than 20/40 in the lowest vision eye, they should wear eye protection during all sports (Committee on Sports Medicine and Fitness, 2004). Some injuries can be treated at home, but many necessitate a trip to the emergency department or require hospitalization. Personnel take careful history of the injury, perform assessment of the eye, and measure visual acuity. See the table below for a summary of clinical manifestations and emergency treatment of common eye injuries.

PRACTICE ALERT

Be sure to check the immunization status of the child with an eye injury. If the child has not had a tetanus booster within 5 years, this immunization should be given. A Td or tetanus-diphtheria booster should be administered in most cases.

NURSING MANAGEMENT

The nurse's role in eye injuries has two main components. First, perform teaching at each health promotion examination about ways to avoid eye injuries in children. Second, be well informed

CLINICAL MANIFESTATIONS and Emergency Treatment of Eye Injuries

CONDITION AND ETIOLOGY	CLINICAL MANIFESTATIONS	CLINICAL THERAPY
Subconjunctival hemorrhage (caused by coughing, mild trauma, or increased physical activity)	Reddened area in conjunctiva	Usually heals spontaneously; child should see ophthalmologist if most of sclera is covered or if condition does not clear up in 1–2 weeks
Periorbital ecchymosis	"Black eye" or bruising of the skin around the eye	Apply ice to eye area (both eyes) for 5–15 minutes every hour for the first 1–2 days after injury (even if only one eye is affected, both eyes may discolor); then apply warm compresses beginning the second day after injury
Foreign body on conjunctiva	Intense pain or feeling of something in the eye	Do not let child rub eye; remove material on surface of eye by closing upper lid over lower lid, irrigating or everting upper lid, visualizing material, and removing it with a slightly damp handkerchief; patch eye and transport child to emergency department if foreign body cannot be removed
Corneal abrasion	Intense pain and redness	Superficial corneal abrasions are diagnosed by touching a sterile fluorescein strip to lower conjunctiva; dye remains where corneal epithelial cells are disrupted; most corneal abrasions heal spontaneously or antibiotic ointment may be prescribed and eyes patched in some children
Burns (alkaline burns readily penetrate cornea and are more serious than acid burns)	Pain and/or complaints of "blindness" or vision loss	For child with chemical burn, irrigate eye for 15–30 minutes; transport child to emergency department, where irrigation should continue (see Skills Manual); pupils are dilated to reduce pain and prevent adhesions; after irrigation is complete, eyes are patched and antibiotics are prescribed
Penetrating and perforating injuries	Pain	Obtain medical assistance immediately; never try to remove an object that has penetrated the child's eye; such objects should be removed by an ophthalmologist; prevent the child from rubbing injured eye; cover both eyes with shield before transportation to emergency department
Eye injuries caused by severe blows to head and eye (blunt trauma can seriously injure all eye structures, including orbit, which can be fractured)	Pain and redness	Transport immediately to ophthalmologist's office or emergency department for evaluation and treatment. Personnel should be aware that retinal hemorrhage is a common presentation of the type of child abuse called "shaken child syndrome" (see Chapter 7 for further discussion of child abuse)

about emergency treatment of eye injuries and provide necessary information to school personnel and families. This information is important for all children, but is especially vital for those with impaired vision already or with only one functional eye. When the extent of injury is not clear, always recommend that the child be evaluated in an emergency care facility.

Recognize that visual impairment caused by trauma is largely preventable. Scissors, knives, and other sharp objects should be out of the reach of young children. They should be supervised when using scissors, pencils, and other sharp objects. Parents should be aware of sharp and exploding parts of toys and purchase those only intended for the age of the child. All children should be encouraged to wear protective eyewear during sports that most commonly lead to eye injury. School nurses can ensure that students use protective eye gear in chemistry classes and that emergency treatment for injury is posted in classrooms. When eye injury does occur, the nurse may care for the child at home and in the community. The permanent loss of vision from an injury can cause feelings of guilt and anger in the child and family and the nurse may need to provide emotional support.

DISORDERS OF THE EAR

Otitis Media

MediaLink Middle Ear Dynamics Animation

Otitis media, or inflammation of the middle ear, is sometimes accompanied by infection. This condition is one of the most common childhood illnesses. About 70% of infants have at least one case of acute otitis media during the first year of life, and 93% have been diagnosed with the problem by age 7 years. Peak incidence is in the first 2 years of life, particularly from 6 to 12 months of age (Hoberman, Marchant, Kaplan, et al., 2002). Otitis media occurs more frequently among boys and in children who attend childcare centers, in those with allergies, children exposed to tobacco smoke, and those who use pacifiers several hours daily. It is most common during the winter months. Children with conditions such as cleft lip and palate or Down syndrome more often experience otitis media. Breastfeeding appears to be protective against otitis media. In the past decade, an increased number of cases have been observed, and recent changes have been made in recommendations for treatment (Sagraves, 2002; American Academy of Pediatrics 2004).

Etiology and Pathophysiology

The specific cause of otitis media is unknown, but it appears to be related to eustachian tube dysfunction. Often an upper respiratory infection precedes the development of otitis media. This infection causes the mucous membranes of the eustachian tube to become edematous. As a result, air that normally flows to the middle ear is blocked, and the air in the middle ear is reabsorbed into the bloodstream. Fluid is pulled from the mucosal lining into the former air space, providing a medium for the rapid growth of pathogens. The tympanic membrane and fluid behind it become infected. The most common causative organisms are *Streptococcus pneumoniae, Haemophilus influenzae,* and *Moraxella catarrhalis* (Hoberman et al., 2002).

Conditions such as enlarged adenoids or edema from allergic rhinitis can also obstruct the eustachian tube and lead to otitis media. Pacifier use raises the soft palate and thus alters dynamics in the eustachian tube, providing for entry of microorganisms from the nasopharynx (Garrelts & Melnyk, 2001). See Developing Cultural Competence: Otitis Media.

Clinical Manifestations

Otitis media is the general term for inflammation of the middle ear. *Acute otitis media* (AOM) is diagnosed when the child has acute onset of ear pain, marked redness of the tympanic membrane upon otoscopy, and middle ear effusion (Figure 24–7 ■). Recurrent acute otitis media indicates repeated bouts of AOM, such as three in 6 months, or four in 12 months. *Otitis media with effusion* (OME) is evidence of fluid in the middle ear without inflammation (Figure 24–8 ■). OME sometimes becomes chronic in nature (continuing more than 3 months) and is more commonly associated with hearing loss. See the clinical manifestations table on page 791.

Infants and young children have characteristic behaviors that can indicate otitis media may be present. Pulling at the ear is a sign of ear pain (Figure 24–9 ■). Diarrhea, vomiting, and fever are typical of otitis media. Irritability and "acting out" may be signs of a related hearing impairment. The child with otitis media often has night awakenings with crying due to increased pressure when prone or supine.

COLLABORATIVE CARE

Health professionals collaborate in care for children to accurately diagnose children with otitis media and to implement current guidelines for treatment.

Diagnostic Tests

Diagnosis of otitis media is based on otoscopic examination. Acute otitis media is diagnosed with certainty when there is a history of acute onset, presence of middle ear effusion (bulging or decreased mobility of the tympanic membrane, air fluid behind the membrane or otorrhea or discharge), and signs and symptoms of inflammation (erythema of tympanic membrane or discomfort that makes sleep and other activities difficult for the child) (Subcommittee on Management of Acute Otitis Media, 2004). Otoscopic examination includes visualization and pneumatic otoscopy. The trained clinician can perform pneumatic otoscopy in which positive air pressure in the external canal is

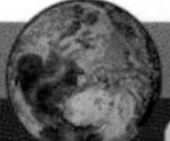

DEVELOPING CULTURAL COMPETENCE
Otitis Media

American Indian and Alaska Native (AI/AN) children have a very high rate of otitis media, perhaps due to culturally related bony structure of the ear, nose, and mouth. A recent study found that AI/AN children are seen about 3 times more frequently in outpatient clinics for otitis media than are other U.S. children (Curns, Holman, Shay, et al., 2002). Be alert for the common incidence in these population groups, plan prevention programs, and ensure prompt care and teaching about treatments for families of children affected. *What prevention measures would you emphasize with these families?* See the nursing management section in otitis media for suggestions of preventive approaches.

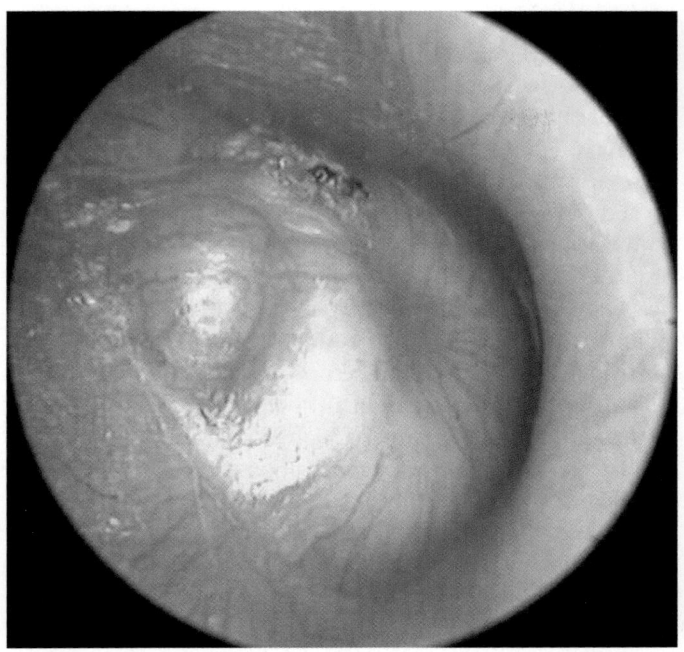

FIGURE 24–7 ■ Acute otitis media is characterized by abrupt onset, pain, middle ear effusion, and inflammation. Note the injected vessels and altered shape of cone of light. See Chapter 8 for a normal tympanic membrane.

Courtesy of Kevin Kavanagh, MD, FACS.

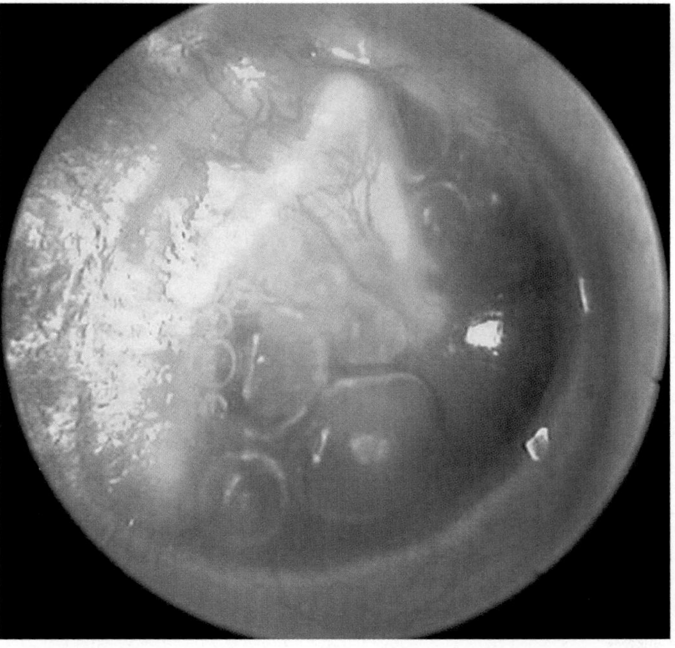

FIGURE 24–8 ■ Otitis media with effusion is noted on otoscopy by fluid line or air bubbles. Pneumatic otoscopy or tympanometry shows a nonmobile tympanic membrane. Note that the light reflex is not in the expected position due to a change in tympanic membrane shape from air bubbles. Where would you expect to see the light reflex? (See Chapter 8 for a description of normal findings.)

Courtesy of Kevin Kavanagh, MD, FACS.

used to measure the movement of the tympanic membrane. This is commonly done by blowing a puff of air into the ear canal using a pneumatic otoscope. Special gradient acoustic reflectometry (SGAR) measures the condition of the middle ear by introducing a sound and measuring the tympanic membrane response (Hoberman & Paradise, 2000). A flat tympanogram is also suggestive of otitis media. (The tympanogram is described in the section on hearing impairment later in this chapter.)

Occasionally, the middle ear fluid is cultured so that the causative organism can be identified. If the tympanic membrane is not intact, the culture is easy to obtain; in cases with repeated antibiotic treatment failure, a tympanocentesis may be done to aspirate some fluid from the middle ear through the tympanic membrane. See the clinical manifestations table below for additional detail concerning manifestations of otitis media.

Since otitis media with effusion may only involve fluid in the middle ear, it is best diagnosed by pneumatic otoscopy and tympanometry. Since this type of otitis media is most commonly associated with hearing loss, audiological testing should be performed in the pediatric healthcare home (medical home) if

CLINICAL MANIFESTATIONS of Acute Otitis Media and Otitis Media with Effusion

ETIOLOGY	CLINICAL MANIFESTATIONS	CLINICAL THERAPY
Acute otitis media—bacterial infection in the middle ear from pathogens transferred from the nasopharynx; most common infectious agents are *S. pneumoniae, H. influenzae, M. catarrhalis*	*Behavioral*—ear pain, pulling at ear, rapid onset, irritability, malaise, poor feeding *Examination*—bulging tympanic membrane, air or fluid bubbles present behind tympanic membrane; immobile or poorly mobile tympanic membrane, red (or other color change such as white, gray, or yellow as long as bulging is present) tympanic membrane, reduced visibility of tympanic membrane landmarks with displaced light reflex	Treat ear pain with local anesthetic, local herbal pain products, or systemic acetaminophen or ibuprofen Observe child's condition for 48–72 hours and if not improved, treat with course of antibiotics
Otitis media with effusion—collection of fluid in the middle ear behind the tympanic membrane which is not infected with bacteria	*Behavioral*—difficulty hearing or responding as expected to sounds *Examination*—signs of acute inflammation are NOT present; tympanic membrane is retracted or neutral; immobile or partly mobile tympanic membrane; yellow or gray tympanic membrane; opaque or thickened tympanic membrane with visibility of landmarks reduced	Symptomatic treatment or pain Careful observation of hearing acuity over several months Speech assessment if loss of hearing acuity occurs Developmental assessment

MediaLink Otitis Media Video

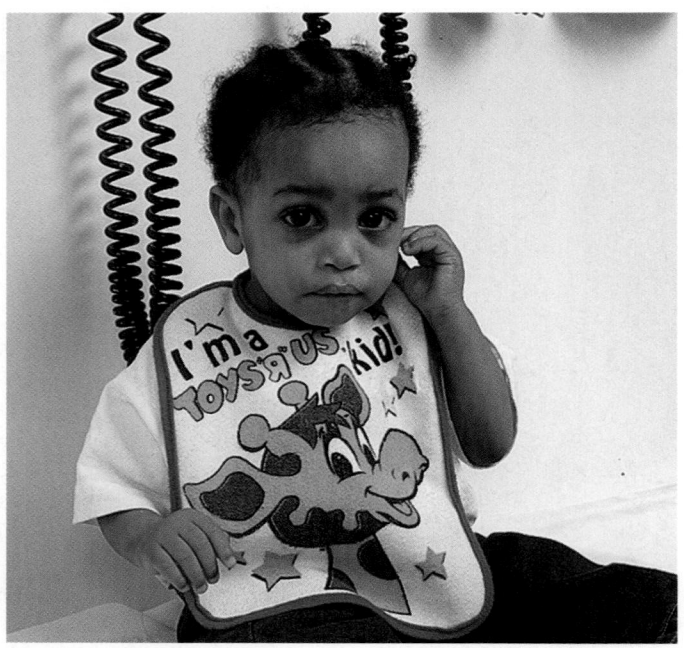

FIGURE 24–9 ■ This young child is pulling at the ear and acting fussy, two important signs of otitis media. Ask the parents about the presence of fever and night awakenings, additional signs that are often observed in children with this condition.

the effusion persists for 3 months or longer. A referral to audiologist should be made for children who fail testing in the office or are less than 4 years of age (Otitis Media with Effusion, 2004).

Clinical Therapy

Concern has developed about the increasing appearance of drug-resistant antimicrobials as causative agents in otitis media. These organisms may explain the increase in otitis media observed in the last decade. Based on current knowledge, the American Academy of Pediatrics and the American Academy of Family Physicians joined to establish recommendations in 2004 (Subcommittee on Management of Acute Otitis Media, 2004). Acute otitis media is now treated with antibiotic therapy for 10 days in children under 6 years, and 5 to 7 days for children 6 years and over. Consistent with current guidelines, acute otitis media treatment is delayed for 48 to 72 hours after diagnosis in children 6 months to 2 years with nonsevere illness at presentation AND uncertain diagnosis, or in children 2 years and older without severe symptoms OR with uncertain diagnosis.

When prescribed, the choice of antibiotic depends on the probable organism, ease of administration, cost, previous effectiveness, and any history of allergies. First-line therapy is amoxicillin at a dose of 80 to 90 mg/kg/day. Amoxicillin with clavulanate or cefuroxime are second-line drugs. If an intramuscular drug is preferred, cefdinir at 14 mg/kg/day, cefpodoxime at 10 mg/kg/day, or cefuroxime at 30 mg/kg/day can be prescribed (Zacharyczuk, 2004). See the medication table below.

When antibiotic therapy is not prescribed initially, the child can be given ibuprofen or acetaminophen for pain relief and returns for further treatment if symptoms continue. Sometimes topical anesthetic ear drops are used to provide comfort for several days. (See Complementary Therapy: Naturopathic Extract for Ear Pain in Otitis Media.)

OME is not treated with antibiotics but is evaluated periodically to be sure there is not an additional AOM that needs treatment. Children with OME generally improve within 3 months. Since this type of otitis is more commonly associated with hearing loss and cochlear damage, follow-up with audiology is essential. If hearing is abnormal, speech testing should be performed (Otitis Media with Effusion, 2004).

Neither decongestants nor antihistamines have been shown to be effective in the treatment of otitis media with or without effusion. Steroids also do not appear to have any long-term beneficial effect. If infection recurs despite antibiotic treatment for acute otitis media or if OME continues 4 months or more with persistent hearing loss present, **myringotomy** (surgical incision of the tympanic membrane) may be performed and **tympanostomy tubes** (pressure-equalizing tubes) may be inserted to drain fluid from the middle ear. In one study, children with otitis media with effusion were followed for 4 years. They did have greater hearing loss and

MEDICATIONS Used to Treat Acute Otitis Media

MEDICATION	ACTION/INDICATION	NURSING IMPLICATIONS
Amoxicillin	Broad-spectrum antibiotic which inhibits mucoprotein synthesis in cell wall of bacteria; used to treat some gram-positive and gram-negative infections	Assess for previous allergy to drug, penicillins, cephalosporins Take as instructed for entire period prescribed If oral suspension is given, refrigerate and shake well before administration Teach parents how to administer drug to the child Have family report side effects such as rash and diarrhea
Amoxicillin and clavulanate potassium	Action and use are similar to amoxicillin. However, clavulanate is a β-lactamase inhibitor that enhances effect of amoxicillin	See amoxicillin
Cefuroxime	A second generation cephalosporin that binds to one or more of the penicillin-binding proteins in cell walls of bacteria; useful in treatment of most gram-negative and some gram-positive infections	Assess for previous allergy to drug, penicillins, cephalosporins Take as instructed for entire period prescribed If oral suspension is given, refrigerate and shake well before administration Teach parents how to administer drug to the child Have family report side effects such as rash and diarrhea

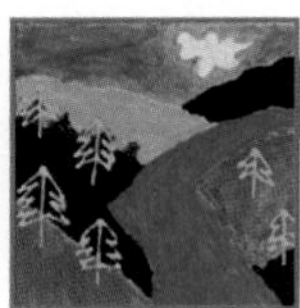

COMPLEMENTARY THERAPY

Naturopathic Extract for Ear Pain in Otitis Media

Since many children with otitis media experience ear pain that can disrupt their sleep and that of family members, anesthetic ear drops have been used for their analgesic effect on the tympanic membrane. Since some families might prefer use of natural remedies for ear pain, a study comparing Otikon (a naturopathic herbal extract of *Allium sativum, Verbascum thapsus, Calendula flores,* and *Hypericum peroforatum*) with a local anesthetic of ametocaine and phenazone was conducted. About half of the total 103 children received each of the pain treatments and parents rated the children after training with a pain tool. Both treatments were effective in decreasing ear pain over the 3 days of the study. There was no significant difference in success rates of local anesthetic and naturopathic agent; in fact, the naturopathic agent was as effective or more effective than anesthetic at each measurement period. It is concluded that herbal pain control may be beneficial for treatment of ear pain, and can help to decrease the need for antibiotic treatment for every case of otitis media (Sarrell, Mandelberg, & Cohen, 2001).

lower verbal and math scores than peers in early grades. However, they caught up with peers by school entry or by second grade (Roberts, Burchinal, & Zeisel, 2002). More studies are needed to determine whether tube placement is helpful for some children with otitis media with effusion or if school performance is affected.

NURSING MANAGEMENT

Nursing management in the child with otitis media focuses on prevention of infection when possible, prompt identification of treatment, and teaching for the family so that the child is successfully treated.

Nursing Assessment and Diagnosis

The tympanic membrane is assessed at each health promotion visit and during examinations for illness. Examine the color, transparency, mobility, presence of landmarks, and light reflex. Ask the parents if the child has had a fever, been fussy, or been pulling at the ears. Observe for signs of impaired hearing, observing for the child's ability to hear whispered or soft sounds.

Several nursing diagnoses that may apply to the child with otitis media are included in the accompanying nursing care plan on pages 796–797. Additional nursing diagnoses may include the following:

- Risk for Imbalanced Body Temperature: Hyperthermia related to infectious process
- Fatigue (child and parent) related to sleep deprivation
- Disturbed Sensory Perception (auditory) related to chronic ear infections and altered sensory reception

Planning and Implementation

Most children with otitis media are not hospitalized; therefore, nursing management centers on care of the child in the home. Parents may not understand why the child with a possible infection is not given antibiotics. Explain to them the problem of developing resistant strains of bacteria, and new research that indicates most children improve after 48 to 72 hours even without antibiotics (Box 24–3). Encourage them to bring the child back for care if the condition worsens or has not improved in the recommended time.

Likewise, parents of children with OME need explanations about why there is a waiting period of about 3 months with no medications or other medical care. Explain that antibiotics, steroids, and antihistamines/decongestants have not been effective treatment and that most children improve in 3 months. Assure them that if the effusion continues beyond that time, the child will be tested for hearing acuity, and if indicated, for speech development.

MediaLink Case Study: Otitis Media

The child who is having tympanostomy tubes inserted is generally treated in a day surgery setting. Occasionally, children admitted to the hospital for other problems have a concurrent ear infection. The accompanying nursing care plan summarizes nursing care for the child with otitis media.

Preventive measures should be emphasized. Exposure to secondhand smoke in the home increases the incidence of otitis media in children; therefore, parents who smoke should be encouraged to avoid smoking near the child or in the home. If young children are in childcare with fewer than 10 children, incidence decreases. Breastfeeding provides some protection from the disease. Placing babies to sleep with a pacifier may increase incidence and should be avoided in the infant with prior infections (Niemela, Pihakari, Pokka, et al., 2000). See Evidence-based Practice: Otitis Media.

CLINICAL TIP

Many cases of otitis media are related to microbes such as *Haemophilus influenzae* and *Pneumococcal pneumoniae,* so immunization against these pathogens (see Chapter 19) can be effective preventive measures. Hib vaccine is effective against *H. influenzae* type B and pneumococcal vaccine is effective against several strains of *P. pneumoniae.*

BOX 24–3 Research: Mechanisms of Bacterial Resistance

Drug resistance to antibiotics has developed as some organisms evolve to interfere with the actions of medications. Some organisms inactivate antibiotics by producing beta-lactamase, an enzyme that breaks through the beta-lactam ring of penicillin and related drugs. A common infectious agent in otitis media, *Streptococcus pneumoniae,* has been affective in inactivating common antibiotics; it has also been able to reduce permeability of cells to some antibiotics and increase production of penicillin-binding proteins that decrease drug action. The Centers for Disease Control and Prevention currently use surveillance techniques to track penicillin-resistant *S. pneumoniae* (PRSP) and it is believed that about 30% of the organisms are now resistant to penicillin-type drugs (Sagraves, 2002). Study of drug resistance has led to recent changes in recommendations for treatment of otitis media. Some resistance may develop because antibiotics have been used too freely to treat all cases of otitis media, rather than only those that are clearly caused by bacterial infection. In addition, parents may have failed to give entire courses or accurate doses of medication, allowing the bacteria to continue to grow and then evolve into a drug-resistant strain. Research knowledge has assisted in clarifying treatment for various types of otitis media. Nurses play a major role in being sure that parents understand why an antibiotic might not always be ordered, and to ensure proper measurement and administration of antibiotics that are prescribed.

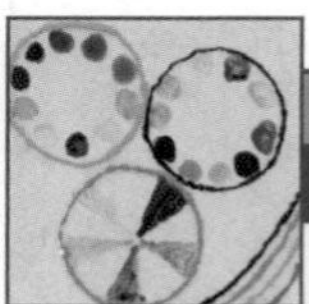

EVIDENCE-BASED PRACTICE
Otitis Media

PROBLEM

Sometimes rather simple interventions can positively influence a healthcare issue. Research can assist in identifying interventions that have an effect on common problems. Acute otitis media is an important pediatric issue since it affects about 70% of all children by the time of their third birthday. Nurses may be able to identify the problem but until recently have had little to offer to families to help prevent otitis media.

EVIDENCE

In a type of research called systematic review, or summary of studies on a topic, two nurses described the collective results of research that examined relationships between incidence of otitis media and pacifier use (Garrelts & Melnyck, 2001). One study enrolled nearly 500 infants and divided them into control and intervention groups (Niemela et al., 2000). Parents in the control group received usual instructions during healthcare visits, while the intervention group parents were instructed to limit pacifier use after 6 months of age, and to discontinue the pacifier after 10 months when the baby's sucking need was lessened. Incidence of otitis media was recorded and parents reported on pacifier use. Although the intervention group did not show decreased incidence of pacifier use, the babies in that group were using the pacifier significantly less daily than the control group babies. The occurrence of acute otitis media was 29% less in the intervention group than the control group.

In a second study, researchers followed over 800 children for an average of 10 months (Niemela, Uhari, & Mottonen, 1995). Parents completed questionnaires about their children's health and answered questions about pacifier use. About 29.5% of the children younger than 2 years who used pacifiers had three or more episodes of acute otitis media, while 20.6% of those who did not use pacifiers had the history of otitis media. For children from 2–3 years acute otitis incidence was 30.6% in pacifier users and 13.2% in nonusers.

In another study of 200 children, charts were reviewed for incidence of otitis media and parents completed questionnaires about pacifier use (Jackson & Mourino, 1999). Prevalence of otitis media was 36% for pacifier users and 23% for nonusers.

IMPLICATIONS

Many children use pacifiers and parents are often not aware that this practice can influence incidence of otitis media. The common nature of ear infections makes it important to apply knowledge to decrease its incidence among young children. In addition, some children have hearing loss or need surgery due to the disorder. Parents can be informed that babies over 6 months of age do not have the same need for sucking as younger babies (Garrelts & Melnyk, 2001). This would be a good age to decrease pacifier use. Perhaps parents will be receptive to offering a pacifier when the baby goes to sleep but not using it during waking hours.

CRITICAL THINKING APPLICATION

How will you phrase questions to ask in a sensitive manner about pacifier use by young children? How can you approach a parent during a well-child visit with a 2-year-old if you notice the child still using a pacifier? If a parent is interested in decreasing pacifier use for a baby, what strategies can you suggest to lessen the number of hours of daily use gradually? Develop an information sheet that can be used in a clinic to teach parents about the connection between pacifier use and acute otitis media.

The chronic nature of otitis media in some children can create many problems for the family. The child's waking at night with ear pain results in lack of sleep and parental fatigue. Parents often become frustrated and disillusioned because of the inability of the healthcare system to cure the child and may fear a permanent hearing impairment. Reassure parents that as the child grows older, the recurrent infections eventually cease. Teach them that asking for courses of antibiotics for every infection may not be the treatment of choice. Provide pain relief techniques such as teaching correct administration of ear drops, oral administration of acetaminophen, and positioning the baby with the head slightly elevated. Provide hearing and language examinations at regular intervals, inform parents of results, and refer to an audiology specialist if hearing problems are identified. Parents of children with tympanostomy tubes need to be taught how to care for the child and what symptoms to report. (See Partnering with Families: Care of the Child with Tympanostomy Tubes.) For the child with some hearing loss due to otitis media with effusion, a home environment that fosters math, reading, and verbal skills can overcome the effects of lowered hearing during the time of infection (Roberts et al., 2002). Nurses should focus interventions on helping parents to read and talk with children frequently who have otitis media with effusion.

Evaluation

Expected outcomes of nursing care for the child with otitis media include:

- Return to normal sleep and feeding patterns
- Maintenance of normal hearing and speech development
- Effective pain and temperature management
- Understanding of treatment regimen by parents

Otitis Externa

Otitis externa is an inflammation of the skin and surrounding soft tissue of the ear canal. It is sometimes called "swimmer's ear" because it is common in children who swim frequently, especially during hot and humid weather. The ear canal can also be injured by use of cotton-tipped applicators, foreign objects, or sprays used near the face. If the tympanic membrane is not intact because of tympanostomy tubes or breakage of the membrane, there may be drainage visible in the canal; this drainage may irritate the canal and lead to otitis externa. Any irritation of the canal can become infected with bacteria, virus, or fungi; sometimes it represents an allergic reaction. The child usually complains of pain and itching, and may have intense pain when the examiner presses on the tragus, or skin tab in front of the ear. Sometimes the ear appears swollen and redness or drainage of the canal may be seen upon otoscopic examination.

Treatment of otitis externa requires removing the dried and flaking epithelium and cerumen. Burrows solutions or normal saline are used to irrigate and clean the canal. Steroid eardrops are used to decrease inflammation and antibiotic drops are also used if a bacterial infection is suspected. Ibuprofen or acetaminophen may be helpful for pain control. The ear canal should then be kept dry by using ear plugs or a swim cap for swimming and gently blow drying the canal after bathing. The child should not return to swimming for about 5 days. Cotton-tipped applicators or other objects should not be placed in the ear canal so that the skin in the canal can heal. If hair sprays or other solutions are irritating, they should not be used by the child or adolescent.

Nurses should be aware of the signs of otitis externa such as a painful ear, drainage, and irritated canal. Verify that the tympanic membrane is intact during otoscopic examination. Teach families to avoid the irritants identified such as cotton-tipped applicators, sprays, and frequent swimming. Demonstrate proper instillation of drops (see Skills Manual) and give instructions for use of acetaminophen for pain relief in the acute period.

Hearing Impairment

Approximately 1 million children in the United States have some form of hearing impairment. These hearing impairments are expressed in terms of **decibels (dB),** which are units of loudness, and rated according to severity (Table 24–8). Children who have only a mild hearing loss (35 to 40 dB) may miss 50% of everyday conversation and are considered at high risk for school failure. Children with a hearing loss of more than 90 dB are considered legally deaf. From 2 to 6 children per 1,000 have a hearing loss (Bachman & Arvedson, 1998).

Etiology and Pathophysiology

About 50% of hearing loss is genetically caused, usually with a recessive inheritance pattern. Another 25% is due to environmental causes around the time of birth; the remainder is due to unknown causes. Hearing loss is present in about 1 to 2 infants per 1,000 births (Walter et al., 2000). Newborns at risk for hearing loss include those with:

- A family history of congenital hearing loss
- Positive titer for TORCH infections (toxoplasmosis, rubella, cytomegalovirus, syphilis, herpes)
- Craniofacial abnormalities
- Very low birth weight (< 1,500 g)
- Bilirubin > 16 mg/dL
- Aminoglycoside medication administration > 5 days
- Low Apgar score at 1 or 5 minutes
- Bacterial meningitis
- Mechanical ventilation > 5 days
- Presence of syndromes associated with hearing loss (Down syndrome, Pierre Robin syndrome, Arnold-Chiari malformation)

(Vohr, Widen, Cone-Wesson, et al., 2000)

TABLE 24–8 Severity of Hearing Loss

TYPE OF LOSS	DECIBEL LEVEL (dB)	HEARING ABILITY
Slight/mild	26–40	Some speech sounds are difficult to perceive, particularly unvoiced consonant sounds
Moderate	41–60	Most normal conversational speech sounds are missed
Severe	61–80	Speech sounds cannot be heard at a normal conversational level
Profound	81–90	No speech sounds can be heard
Deaf	> 90	No sound at all can be heard

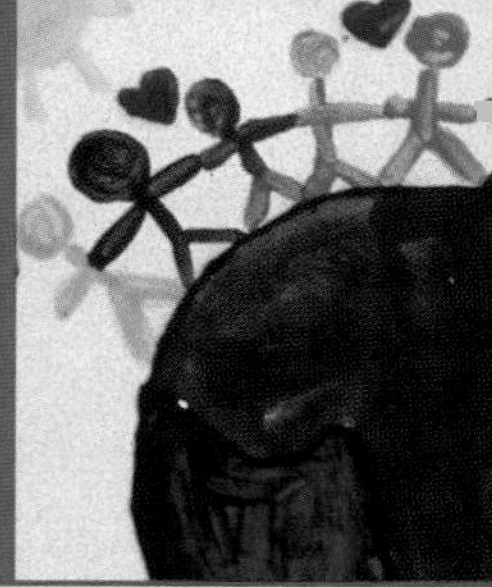

PARTNERING WITH FAMILIES

Care of the Child with Tympanostomy Tubes

After surgery

- Encourage the child to drink generous amounts of fluids.
- Reestablish a regular diet as tolerated.
- Give pain medication (acetaminophen) as ordered for discomfort and at bedtime.
- Place drops in child's ears if instructed.
- Restrict the child to quiet activities.

Following postoperative period

- Follow the physician's instructions regarding swimming and water (some caution against swimming and other activities that might get water in ears; others do not).
- Ear plugs can be used to prevent water from getting into ears.
- Be alert for tubes becoming dislodged and falling out and alert physician (they usually fall out within 1 year).
- Report purulent discharge from the ear, which may indicate a new ear infection. Contact the care provider.

Common causes of conductive hearing loss include impacted cerumen, the most frequent reason for conductive loss; outer ear infection ("swimmer's ear"); trauma; or a foreign body. Conductive loss also occurs if the tympanic membrane does not fully vibrate, as in otitis media. In these cases loss may be restored after the infection clears. Chronic and untreated ear infections may lead to ear structural changes and permanent hearing impairment. The loss of acuity may be gradual or rapid and results in diminished hearing in all ranges.

Conditions leading to sensorineural hearing loss may be congenital (maternal rubella), genetic (Tay-Sachs disease), or acquired (such as from ototoxic drugs, bacterial meningitis, or loud noise). In sensorineural hearing loss, high-frequency sounds are most affected. Such hearing loss may be preceeded by **tinnitus** or ringing in the ears. Teenagers who use earphones at high volumes or attend many rock concerts are at risk for hearing loss (Figure 24–10 ■). Other noise hazards include firecrackers, guns, and power and farm equipment (Box 24–4).

MediaLink Ear Abnormalities Animation

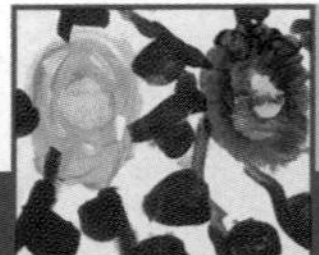

Nursing Care Plan

THE CHILD WITH OTITIS MEDIA

GOAL	INTERVENTION	RATIONALE	EXPECTED OUTCOME
1. Acute Pain related to inflammation and pressure on tympanic membrane			
	NIC Priority Intervention: *Pain Management:* Alleviation or reduction in pain to a level of comfort acceptable to patient and family.		**NOC Suggested Outcome:** *Pain Level:* Amount of reported or demonstrated pain.
The child or parent will indicate absence of pain.	▪ Give analgesic such as acetaminophen. Use analgesic eardrops. ▪ Have the child sit up, raise head on pillows, or lie on unaffected ear. ▪ Apply heating pad or warm hot water bottle. ▪ Have the child chew gum or blow on balloon to relieve pressure in ear.	▪ Analgesics after perception or response to pain. ▪ Elevation decreases pressure from fluid. ▪ Heat increases blood supply and reduces discomfort. ▪ Attempts to open the eustachian tube may help aerate the middle ear.	Verbal child states that pain is relieved. Nonverbal child has improved disposition and comfort.
2. Infection related to presence of pathogens			
	NIC Priority Intervention: *Infection Control:* Minimizing the acquisition and transmission of infectious agents.		**NOC Suggested Outcome:** *Risk Control:* Actions to eliminate or reduce health threats.
The child will be free of infection	▪ Encourage breastfeeding of infants. ▪ Instruct the parents to administer antibiotics exactly as directed and to complete prescribed course of medication. ▪ Telephone the parents 2–3 days after initial examination. ▪ Examine ear 3–4 days after completion of antibiotic treatment, symptomatic treatment.	▪ Breastfeeding affords natural immunity to infectious agents. ▪ Taking antibiotics as prescribed minimizes chance for overgrowth of pathogens. ▪ If symptoms have not improved in 36 hours, treatment should be evaluated. ▪ Check-up determines if treatment is effective.	The child's temperature is normal, symptoms have disappeared, and tympanic membrane shows no signs of infection.
3. Risk for Caregiver Role Strain related to chronic disease			
	NIC Priority Intervention: *Caregiver Support:* Provision of necessary support, information, and advocacy to facilitate care by parents.		**NOC Suggested Outcome:** *Caregiver Performance:* Provision by family care provider of healthcare for child.
The parents will manage the child's condition with minimal stress.	▪ Determine the parents' ability to manage condition. Provide frequent information and feedback. ▪ Encourage parental input in managing care. ▪ Listen carefully to parental expressions of frustration and fatigue and try to understand parents' feelings.	▪ Many parents can treat children at home. Knowledge of condition allows parents to make informed decisions and to manage condition effectively. ▪ Active participation increases confidence and ability to manage condition. ▪ Reacting empathically encourages parents to communicate.	The parents express confidence about treating the child and state that stress is reduced.

Nursing Care Plan THE CHILD WITH OTITIS MEDIA (continued)

GOAL	INTERVENTION	RATIONALE	EXPECTED OUTCOME
4. Risk for Infection related to knowledge deficit about infection in children			
	NIC Priority Intervention: *Infection Control:* Minimizing the acquisition and transmission of infectious agents.		**NOC Suggested Outcome:** *Knowledge:* Extent of understanding conveyed about infectious disease prevention.
The parents will state understanding of preventive measures.	■ Teach family members to cover mouths and noses when sneezing or coughing and to wash hands frequently. Have parents isolate sick children.	■ Good hygiene prevents spread of pathogens.	Parents express understanding of measures to lead to fewer infections.
	■ Encourage optimal nutrition, rest, and exercise.	■ Physical well-being helps the body fight disease.	
	■ Position bottle-fed infants upright when feeding. Do not prop bottles.	■ Elevated position prevents passage of milk and pathogens into the eustachian tube.	
	■ Eliminate allergens and upper respiratory irritants such as tobacco, smoke, and dust.	■ Fewer irritants and allergens may decrease susceptibility to respiratory infections. Secondhand smoke contributes to higher incidence of otitis media.	
5. Risk for Delayed Growth and Development related to hearing loss			
	NIC Priority Intervention: *Developmental Enhancement:* Facilitating optimal growth and development of the child.		**NOC Suggested Outcome:** *Growth and Development:* Milestones of developmental progression.
The child will have normal hearing.	■ Assess hearing ability frequently.	■ Monitoring detects hearing loss early.	The child's general health and hearing improve, and incidence of condition decreases.
The child will have normal motor and language development.	■ Assess motor and language development at each healthcare visit.	■ Early detection of developmental delays can lead to appropriate intervention.	The child has language and motor development within norms for age group.

Clinical Manifestations

Hearing is both an innate and a learned behavior. Infants and children who are hearing impaired exhibit a range of behaviors, depending on the child's age and the severity of the deficit. Infants who hear normally respond to sound in both obvious and subtle ways that do not occur in those who are hearing impaired (Table 24–9). As children with hearing impairments mature, language skills are affected. Hearing loss is often manifested as a cognitive deficit, a behavioral problem, or both.

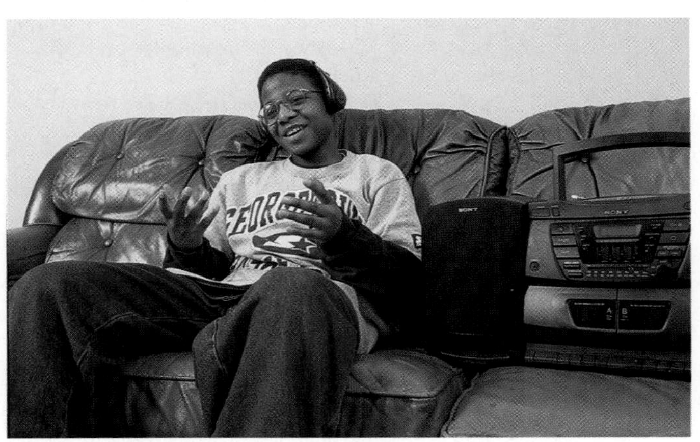

FIGURE 24–10 ■ Listening to loud music with headphones or at rock concerts is a frequent cause of hearing loss among teenagers and young adults. This adolescent needs to be informed about the possible outcomes of this activity.

Hearing disorders can be classified according to the location of the deficit. **Conductive hearing loss** occurs when conditions in the external auditory canal or tympanic membrane prevent sound from reaching the middle ear. **Sensorineural hearing loss** occurs when the hair cells in the cochlea or along the auditory nerve (cranial nerve VIII) are damaged. This leads to permanent

BOX 24–4 Research: Noise-Induced Hearing Loss

Current research shows that 12% of school-age children may have hearing impairments due to noise-induced hearing loss (NIHL), often in ranges not screened during school auditory testing. Hearing loss is even more common among teens. Preventing these hearing losses is possible, so nurses should identify and find sources of noise in the child's environment. They may include stereos, airplanes, firearms, power tools, machinery, and toys. Encourage use of earplugs during hazardous activities (Niskar, Kieszak, & Holmes, et al., 2001).

TABLE 24–9 Behaviors Suggestive of Hearing Impairment

AGE	BEHAVIOR
Infant	Has a diminished or absent startle reflex to loud sound Does not awaken when environment is very noisy Awakens only to touch Does not turn head to sound at 3–4 months Does not localize sound at 6–10 months Babbles little or not at all
Toddler and preschooler	Speaks unintelligibly, in a monotone, or not at all Communicates needs through gestures Appears developmentally delayed Appears emotionally immature, yells inappropriately Does not respond to doorbell or telephone Appears more interested in objects than people and prefers to play alone Focuses on facial expressions rather than verbal communications
School-age child and adolescent	Asks to have statements repeated Answers questions inappropriately, except when able to view speaker's face Daydreams and is inattentive Performs poorly at school or is truant Has speech abnormalities or speaks in a monotone Sits close to or turns television or radio up loudly Prefers to play alone

hearing loss. A **mixed hearing loss** indicates a hearing loss having a combination of conductive and sensorineural causes.

COLLABORATIVE CARE

Care focuses on preventing hearing impairment when possible and providing an environment that supports development for the child with a hearing impairment.

Diagnostic Tests

Early identification of hearing loss is a key element in successful treatment. Normal hearing is indicated when infants and young children respond automatically with a blink or the startle reflex to unexpected or loud noises. As they mature, they localize the sound source and look in its direction, then understand speech sounds, and finally, by about 1 year of age, begin to communicate verbally. Detection of hearing loss in infants is important to ensure optimal development. Universal screening of all infants is recommended before 1 month of age, with diagnostic audiologic evaluation before 3 months, and beginning of early intervention programs by 6 months of age for those with hearing impairment (Walter et al., 2000). Many state laws now mandate screening of newborns. Observations of response to noise in all newborns should be accompanied by more sophisticated testing such as auditory brainstem response or transient evoked otoacoustic emissions especially in those at high risk of deficits (Figure 24–11 ■). See Table 24–10.

An otoscopic examination and a tympanogram can be performed on an older infant to determine conductive hearing loss. The **tympanogram** is a test performed with a machine called a tympanometer that provides a graph of the ability of the middle ear to transmit sound. An airtight probe is inserted into the external ear canal and a tone is emitted. The pressure is measured by the probe and plotted on a graph. A flat tympanogram suggests that the tympanic membrane cannot move normally due to fluid behind it and is therefore indicative of conductive hearing loss (Figure 24–12 ■). **Audiography** can be used with cooperative children over 3 years of age. Sounds of various frequencies and intensities are presented to the child through earphones with a machine called an audiometer, and the child is instructed to raise a hand upon hearing the sound. Audiography cannot detect hearing loss caused by middle ear effusion but can indicate sensorineural loss. The hearing of preschool and school-age children is tested by asking them to repeat whispered

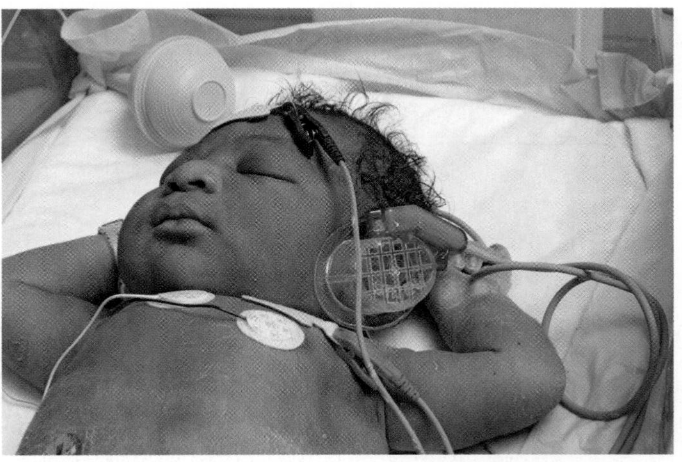

FIGURE 24–11 ■ Newborn hearing screening is an effective tool in diagnosing some cases of hearing impairment very early in life.

TABLE 24–10 Screening Tests for Newborn Hearing

TEST	MECHANISM OF ACTION
Otoacoustive emission (OAE) (either transient-evoked [TEOAE] or distortion-product [DPOAE])	A measure of low-intensity sounds from the cochlear hair cells in response to clicks clicks from a probe placed in the ear canal Sensitive in frequency range above 1,500 Hz May show false negative for loss below 1,000–1,500 Hz Detects inner ear hearing loss by evaluating cochlear and hair cell function Does not detect neural damage to 8th cranial nerve Can be sensitive to outer ear canal obstruction or middle ear effusion, leading to false positive result
Auditory brainstem response (ABR)	Electrical response to auditory stimuli from three surface scalp electrodes Reflects activity of cochlea, cranial nerve 8, and auditory brainstem pathways Detects hearing loss from 1,000–8,000 Hz May show false negative results for losses in the 500–2,000 Hz levels Will give a positive result even if cochlear loss is not present

words. Hearing of school-age children and adolescents also is assessed with the Weber and Rinne tests (see Chapter 8∞).

Clinical Therapy

If a hearing loss is permanent, a multidisciplinary team of pediatrician, audiologist, otolaryngologist, speech-language pathologist, nurse, teacher, and social worker should assist the child and family with adaptation to the disability (Brookhouse, Beauchaine, & Osberger, 1999). If the deficit is due to recurrent otitis media with effusion, tympanostomy tube insertion may improve hearing. Extra verbal stimulation by parents and care providers may help the child with otitis media with effusion to have normal cognitive and verbal performance.

A hearing aid may be prescribed for a conductive loss. It collects and magnifies the sound that is presented to the auditory nerve. A sensorineural loss is more difficult to treat, but cochlear implants and bone conduction hearing aids have been used in some children. Cochlear implants are increasingly being used in children and have restored hearing in some who are profoundly deaf (Cheng, Rubin, Powe, et al., 2000) (Box 24–5).

For children with uncorrectable hearing loss, several approaches are used to enhance communication (Table 24–11). Children with hearing impairment may receive speech therapy and instructions in lipreading, signing, cuing, and fingerspelling.

NURSING MANAGEMENT

Nursing roles include partnering with families to prevent hearing loss when possible, administering diagnostic tests and assessing development to identify hearing loss, and supporting the family of a child with impairment to maximize communication skills and developmental progression.

■ Nursing Assessment and Diagnosis

Nurses conduct newborn hearing tests soon after birth and make observations of the infant's responses to sound. As the child grows, hearing should be assessed at every well-child visit. The best judges of hearing are parents; ask them if they have concerns about their child's hearing. Be alert for parents who believe their children do not have normal hearing, since they are often the first to diagnose a hearing impairment. An infant's reaction to rattles, bells, or handclapping

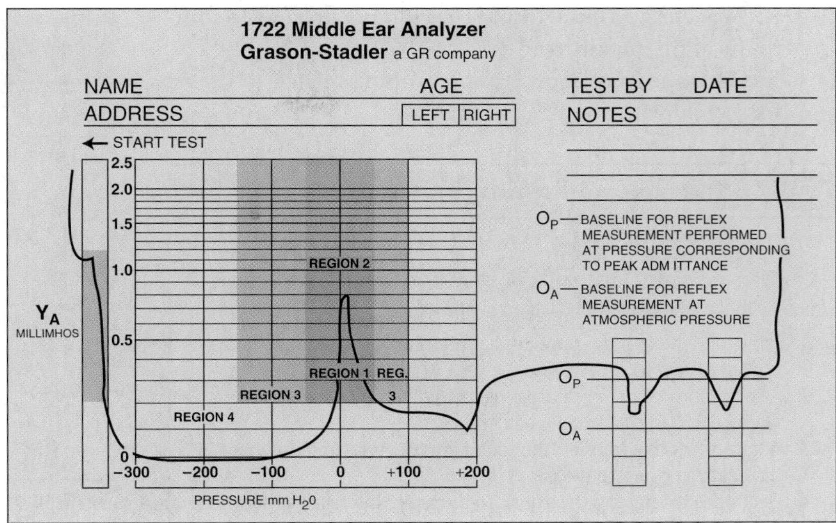

A

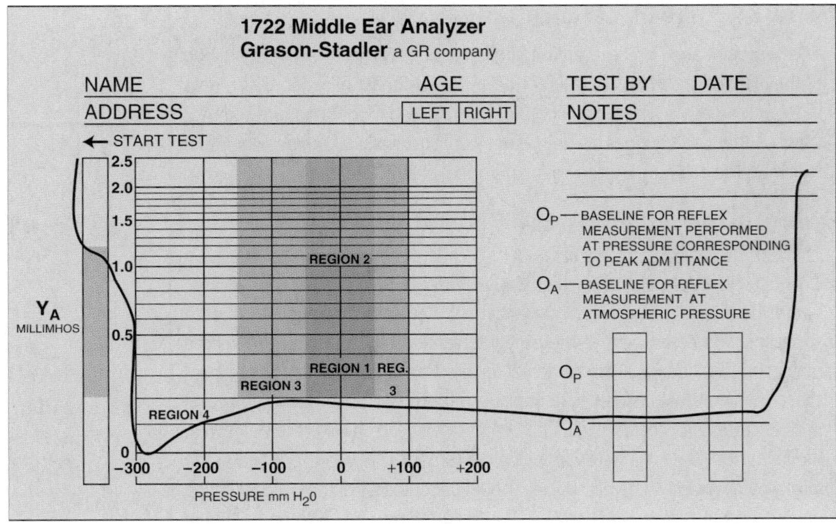

B

FIGURE 24–12 ■ *A,* This tympanogram demonstrates normal hearing as evidenced by the curve showing the tympanic membrane's movement when a sound wave is emitted into the ear canal. Mobility is between 0.2 mL and 1 mL, the normal range. *B,* In contrast, note the flat pattern in the second tympanogram, which shows very restricted mobility of the tympanic membrane in response to sound.

30 cm (12 in.) from the ear is an important observation. Language milestones should be evaluated when the older infant and child are examined. Language development is a major area of focus in deaf children. Deaf infants begin to babble at about 5 to 6 months of age, the same age as hearing infants. However, this babbling decreases and then ceases several months later in the child with a hearing impairment.

School nurses use audiometers to evaluate hearing during screening programs in schools, and refer children who do not pass the screening test. See the Skills Manual for techniques in performing hearing screening. Nurses in offices often use tympanometers to evaluate ear function.

Following are common nursing diagnoses for the child with impaired hearing.

- Risk for Impaired Verbal Communication related to hearing loss
- Disturbed Sensory Perception related to sound transmission

- Risk for Delayed Growth and Development related to communication impairment
- Readiness for Enhanced Family Coping related to caring for a child with a hearing impairment

BOX 24–5 Cochlear Implants

WHAT IS A COCHLEAR IMPLANT?

A cochlear implant is a small electronic device that helps to provide sound for those who are deaf or profoundly hard of hearing. It consists of the following:

1. A microphone to pick up sound that is located outside of the body; it is worn as a headpiece behind the ear
2. A speech processor which organizes sound from the microphone; worn behind the ear or on a belt
3. A transmitter that transfers the sound into electrical impulses; part of the headpiece behind the ear
4. Electrodes which send the signals to the brain; this receiver is implanted in the skin behind the ear with a wire leading to the cochelar fluid in the middle ear

WHEN CAN CHILDREN GET COCHLEAR IMPLANTS?

The minimum age to receive an implant is 12 months, upon recommendation of the National Institutes of Health (1995). The reason for allowing the surgery at this young age is the recognition that most speech foundations are laid by 2 years of age, and younger children have more success in language acquisition following the implant (Ertmer, Young, Grohne, et al., 2002).

WHAT FOLLOW-UP IS NEEDED FOR CHILDREN AFTER COCHLEAR IMPLANT?

Children with implants receive carefully planned speech therapy and families are taught how to promote speech development. Regular assessments by speech specialists with adjustment of the early intervention program are needed. The major complication following surgery is an infection of the insertion site or associated meningitis. All children with implants must receive pneumococcal vaccine prior to surgery for the implant. Children under 2 years should receive Prevnar, the pneumococcal conjugate vaccine before surgery. Children over 2 years who have already received Prevnar vaccine should get one dose of the polysaccharide pneumococcal vaccine (Pneumovax 23). Children from 24–50 months should receive two doses of Prevnar 2 or more months apart, followed by Pneumovax 23 at least 2 months later. Children 5 years and older should receive one dose of Pneumovax 23. Consult the Centers for Disease Control and Prevention (CDC) and Canadian Health Network for updates on immunization recommendations.

MediaLink Immunization Resources

WHY IS THERE SOME CONTROVERSY ABOUT COCHLEAR IMPLANTS?

Many people who are deaf consider deafness a culture, similar to an ethnic group, or group with other common traits and experiences. They believe they are fully functional, communicate and socialize with others satisfactorily, and do not view deafness as a defect. They believe that it is an affront to their culture to consider that someone should try to change from being deaf to hearing. Others note that only a select few can obtain cochlear implants due to their cost and the fact that health insurance may not cover the surgery or instrumentation or speech therapy. Other people are opposed to use of cochlear implants for children because of the surgical risk involved and the fact that children are not old enough to make their own decision about choosing the surgery. On the other hand, the earlier the child has the surgery and hears sounds, the more likely speech is to develop. Read about the controversy in resources such as Christiansen, J.B., & Leigh, I.W. (2001). *Cochlear implants in children: Ethics and choices.* Washington, DC: Gallaudet University Press. Imagine the difficulty parents have as they try to make the choice about treatment for the child who is hearing impaired.

TABLE 24–11 Communication Techniques for Children Who Are Hearing Impaired

TECHNIQUE	DESCRIPTION
Cued speech	Supplement to lipreading; eight hand shapes represent groups of consonant sounds and four positions about the face represent groups of vowel sounds; based on the sounds the letters make, not the letters themselves; child can "see-hear" every spoken syllable a hearing person hears
Oral approach	Uses only spoken language for face-to-face communication; avoids use of formal signs; uses hearing aids and residual hearing
Total communication	Uses speech and sign, fingerspelling, lipreading, and residual hearing simultaneously; child selects communication technique depending on the situation
Sign language	A separate or foreign language that allows the user to communicate quickly and accurately with others who understand signs. The signs or hand movements represent words or concepts. When a sign is not available, the word can be spelled out using signs. American Sign Language (ASL) is most often used; British Sign Language (BSL) is common in Europe.

Planning and Implementation

The goals of *Healthy People 2010* (2000) can guide nurses in planning assessments and interventions (Table 24–12).

Early Identification

Early identification of hearing loss in infants and children is facilitated by newborn screening, developmental assessment, and childhood screening programs. Infants should be tested for hearing loss by 3 months of age and in cases of loss, intervention should begin before 6 months of age (Joint Committee on Infant Hearing, 2000). Be alert for expected language milestones during early childhood as this can be a clue to hearing impairment (see Table 24–9).

Care in the Community

Most of the care for children with hearing impairment takes place in the community. Nurses in a variety of settings can encourage prevention of hearing loss from exposure to loud noises such as from music and power and farm equipment. Music should be turned down and ear protection worn for other activities. School nurses should be active in hearing conservation education programs in school (Folmer, 2003). Several programs are available to assist the school nurse in teaching school children at targeted ages about noise-induced hearing loss. The nurse should develop and deliver hearing conservation curricula to children at elementary, middle, and high school levels; inform teachers and other professionals about noise-induced hearing loss; and train volunteers to assist with school programs.

Nurses may be active in the community to encourage access for those with hearing impairment. This may include attending

TABLE 24–12 *Healthy People 2010* Objectives Related to Hearing in Children

OBJECTIVE	NURSING IMPLEMENTATION
28–11 Increase the proportion of newborns who are screened for hearing loss by age 1 month, have audiologic evaluation by age 3 months, and are enrolled in appropriate intervention services by age 6 months.	Perform screening of newborns in nurseries. Evaluate results of hearing tests during health promotion visits and home visits to families with infants. Refer newborns with abnormal results for further screening. Refer babies with diagnosed impaired hearing to early intervention programs before they are 6 months of age.
29–12 Reduce otitis media in children and adolescents.	Partner with families to provide treatment as prescribed for otitis media. Provide teaching on correct administration of medications, need for immunizations that prevent against types of otitis media, and comfort measures for children with ear pain.
29–13 Increase access by persons who have hearing impairments to hearing rehabilitation services and adaptive devices, including hearing aids, cochlear implants, or tactile or other assistive or augmentative devices.	Refer families to audiologic counseling to receive overview of services helpful to the child. Explain and interpret services available. Assist the family in identifying useful services and the financial resources to assist in their use. Partner with families to liaison with schools to explain the adaptive devices used by the child and to form an individualized education plan.
28–14 Increase the proportion of persons who have had a hearing examination on schedule.	Perform screening in newborn nurseries, and at each health promotion or home visit for infants. Organize school screening programs to screen children at least at each age prescribed by state laws (often K, 2, 5, 8 grades and for new children to the district).
28–16 Increase the use of appropriate ear protection devices, equipment, and practices.	Teach all children about ear protection. Be alert for signs of hearing loss such as tinnitis. For those at risk of hearing loss, ensure regular audiometric testing.
28–17 Reduce noise-induced hearing loss in children and adolescents under 17 years.	Integrate hearing conservation instruction into each health maintenance visit. Ask about use of ear phones, participation in rock bands, and attendance at rock concerts. Assist schools to establish regular curricula related to hearing conservation.

Adapted from U.S. Department of Health and Human Services. (2000). Healthy People 2010 *(2nd ed.). Washington, DC: U.S. Government Printing Office.* www.healthypeople.gov

and requesting classes in American Sign Language at local community colleges and schools, or arranging for sign language interpretation at public events.

Nursing care of the child with a hearing impairment also takes place in the community and focuses on facilitating the child's ability to receive spoken language and to send information, on helping parents to meet the child's schooling needs, and on providing emotional support to parents. Refer the parents to an early intervention program as soon as the diagnosis of hearing impairment is made, in order to foster the child's development. If a cochlear implant is planned, the child needs surgical care and follow-up to monitor results and integrate sound gradually into the child's life (Slattery & Fayad, 1999) See the Photo Story on pages 802–803. Parents often need help to decide on the best method for hearing and language enhancement for the child. You may need to interpret information, refer to Internet and other resources, and help parents partner with parents who have chosen various approaches for their own children. The nurse integrates special care into the health promotion and health maintenance visits of children with hearing impairments (Figure 24–13 ■). See the Health Promotion and Maintenance Overview on page 804.

Facilitate Ability to Receive Spoken Language

Be aware of how the child compensates for hearing loss and use the following strategies in communication.

- If hearing loss is mild or temporary or if the child reads lips, first obtain the child's visual attention by lightly touching the child or saying the child's name.
- Position your face 1 to 2 m (3 to 6 ft) from the child's face and make sure that the child's eyes are focused on your face and

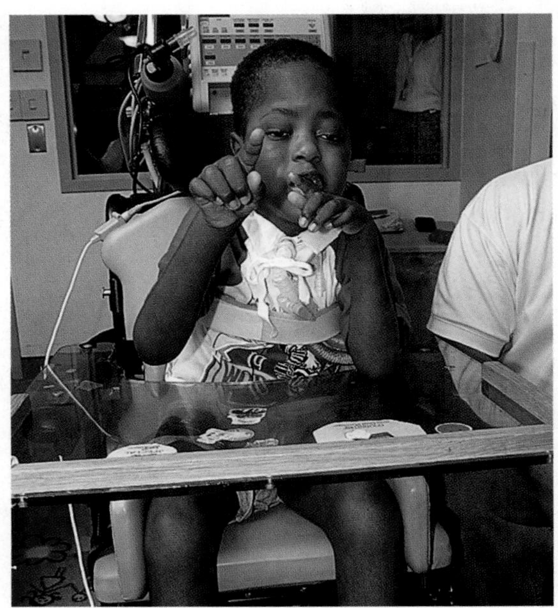

FIGURE 24–13 ■ This child with a hearing impairment and tracheostomy is communicating by means of American Sign Language.

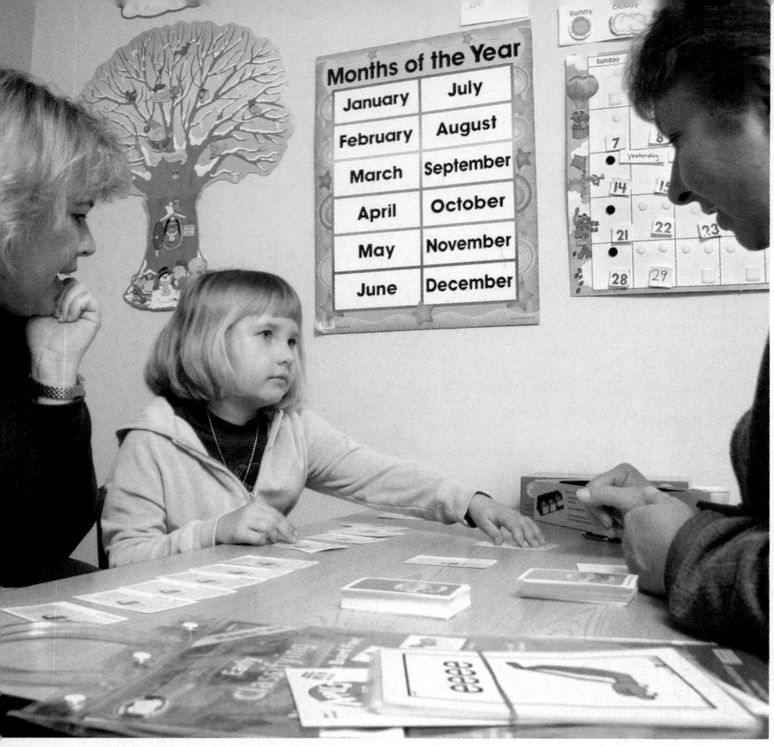

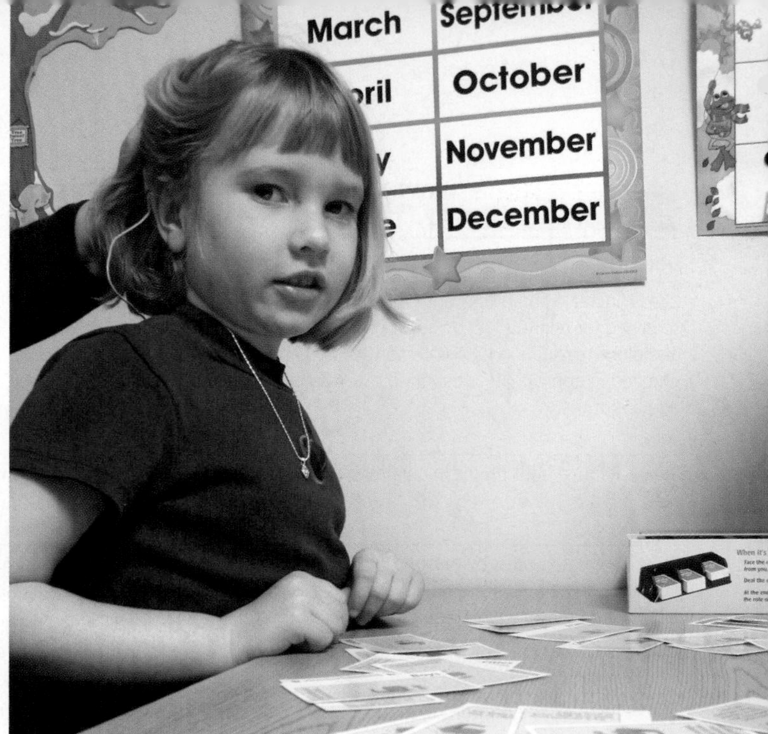

Kate is playing a card game with the speech therapist while her mother sits next to her. Notice her visual attention to the therapist which enhances her interpretation of speech. ***(left)***

Kate is learning to integrate vision, hearing, and cognition before she speaks. ***(right)***

PHOTOStory...

Communicating with a cochlear implant

Kate is 5 years old and has had decreased hearing ability from birth. She was born at term and had no other risk factors for hearing loss. When she was several months old, Kate's parents suspected that she was hard of hearing. Her father designed an experiment: He crashed pans together behind her and found no response. The family was devastated but sought care and explored options to assist Kate with communication. They decided on a cochlear implant in her inner ear when Kate was 2 years of age. The implant connects to a microphone that is placed outside her head. She wears a sound processor on her belt that codes signals so that she can receive them in the implant. Kate communicates verbally now and visits a speech therapist each week who helps her to learn how to listen for sounds, solve problems, and respond verbally. The therapist, Kate, and her mother work in these photos on a card game that combines problem solving, visual recognition, and verbal skills.

Kate's father attends most of the speech therapy visits also and appreciates the therapist's willingness to periodically review with him the anatomy of the ear so that he can better understand his daughter's impairment and surgery. Recall that teaching needs to be repeated and enlarged upon as the family is able to understand the condition more fully. Kate will attend kindergarten next year and continue to receive speech therapy to enhance her ability to listen, comprehend, and verbalize.

The experience of Kate's family is quite typical. Although there are risk factors for development of hearing impairment such as an infant who is premature or has a family history of impairment, the majority of children with a hearing impairment do not have any known risk factors. Because of this, healthcare providers are often not proficient at identifying the impairment during infancy, when institution of sign language and other methods of communication are most effective. Nurses are instrumental in performing hearing testing on all newborns, on carefully monitoring developmental progression, and testing response to sounds during all healthcare visits. Parents are usually the first to notice the child's inability to hear normally, as demonstrated by the case of Kate's father. Ask them about their perceptions of the child's hearing ability.

What other healthcare needs can you identify for Kate now that she is five years old? Recall that she is at risk for infection and so immunizations such as pneumoccocal vaccine, and Haemophilus influenzae type b, need to be up-to-date. As Kate begins kindergarten, what do her teachers and classmates need to know? How can the family and school nurse partner to establish an individualized education plan to enhance Kate's learning? ■

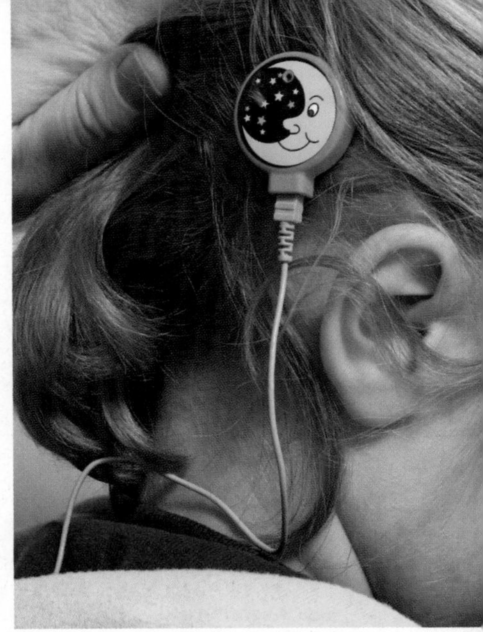

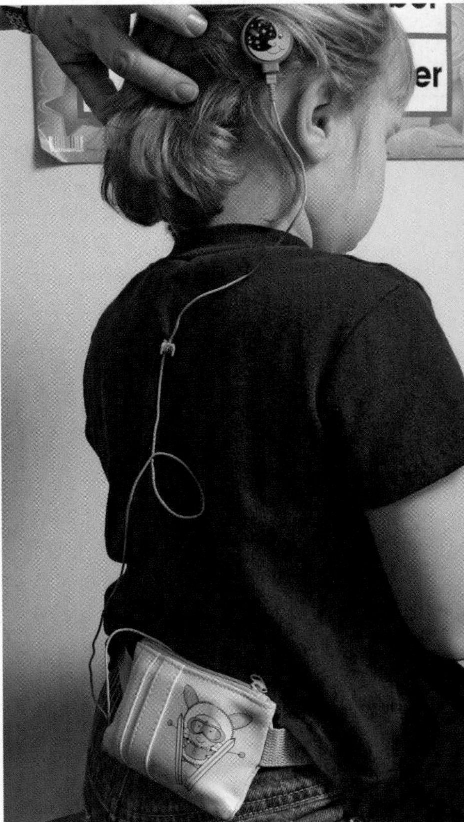

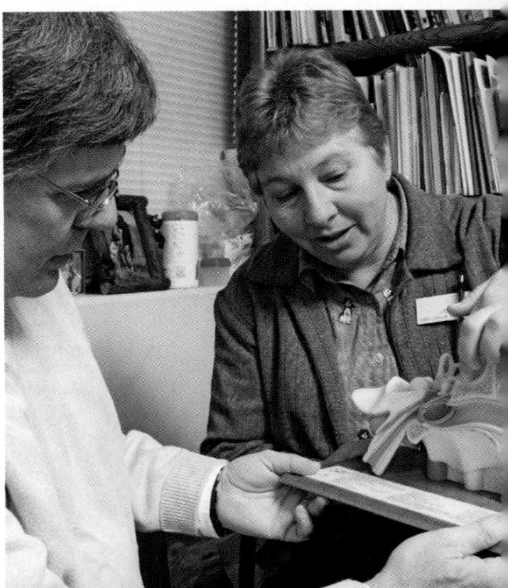

The cochlear implant is connected to this microphone which Kate wears under her hair. ***(top)***

Notice the belt pack that Kate is wearing. Her microphone connects to the sound processor which enables her to hear and make sense of sounds. ***(middle)***

The speech therapist reinforces prior teaching about cochlear implants with Kate's father. ***(bottom)***

Health Promotion & Maintenance Overview

The Child with a Hearing Impairment

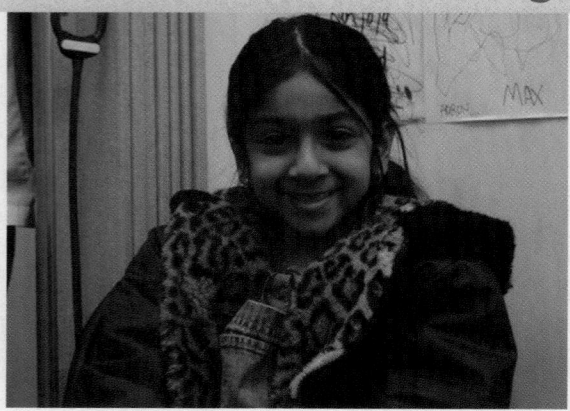

Growth and Developmental Surveillance

- Ensure that the child receives all immunizations at scheduled times. All children with cochlear implants should have pneumococcal vaccine (PCV7 for under 5 years or PPV23 for over 5 years). The immunization should be completed 2 weeks before surgery for cochlear implant. Children should be up to date on all immunizations, but rubella, mumps, and measles are especially important since infections with the diseases could cause further hearing loss.
- Complete developmental assessment, including receptive and expressive verbal skills at each visit.
- Teach about safety precautions for those with hearing impairment, such as inability to hear announcements at school, fire alarms at home, or sirens when in travel. Assist the family to install visual stimuli for fire alarms and other safety needs.

Communication

- Review the type of communication used by the child and the family's satisfaction.
- Ask about relationships with other children, both hearing impaired and those with normal hearing.
- Review discipline techniques used by the parents and consistency of limit setting.

Nutrition and Physical Activity

- Complete 24-hour diet recall and be sure the child receives adequate nutrition appropriate in energy for activities.
- Review the child's exercise patterns since some children with hearing impairment may avoid interactions with other children in sports.
- Refer the family to community activity programs as needed.

Mental Health

- Find out stressors parents may feel.
- Locate community resources for early intervention and ongoing programs.
- Assist the youth and family to plan for moves to new schools and communities, and for plans related to transition to young adulthood, including college, trade schools, or work in the community.

Disease Prevention Strategies

- Be sure signs of ear infection such as fever, irritability, disturbed sleep, rubbing ear, or ear drainage are promptly evaluated in the pediatric healthcare home.
- Teach parents to administer antibiotics for ear infections exactly as prescribed.
- Encourage breastfeeding of infants and avoiding smoking to minimize incidence of ear infections.
- Be sure the child has all recommended immunizations.

Injury Prevention Strategies

- Encourage family to preserve any hearing the child may have by avoiding exposure to loud sounds; when children are old enough to understand be sure they safeguard against exposure to loud music, guns, and other risks.
- Teach the child and family to plan for safety when crossing streets, driving cars, escaping house fires, and other situations that normally rely on hearing.

lips. Make sure the room is well lit, with no backlighting. Speak at a normal rate and tone, and use facial expressions that show caring or concern. If the child does not understand, rephrase the information in shorter, simpler sentences. Use specific, concrete explanations, and give the child time to comprehend. Watch for subtle signs of misinterpretations and give consistent and immediate feedback because only 30% of the English language is visible on the lips.

- Be familiar with the different types of hearing aids. Hearing aids, which are microphones that amplify all sounds, can be worn in or behind the ear, in the frame of glasses, or on the body with a wire attached to the ear. When talking to a child with a hearing aid, speak slowly and be positioned 15 to 45 cm (6 to 18 in.) from the microphone using a normal conversational tone. Talk to the child even if the child is not looking at you. Make sure the batteries are fresh for the best reception. All sound is amplified, so reduce background noise as much as possible. (See Partnering with Families: Care of the Hearing Aid.)
- Acoustic feedback, an audible whistling sound that cannot always be heard by the child, is a common problem with hearing aids. To eliminate this sound, readjust the hearing aid to ensure that it is inserted properly and that no hair or ear wax is caught between the ear mold and canal. Turning down the volume may also help.
- A remote microphone system is another type of device designed to improve hearing. This is often used in the classroom situation because it eliminates background noise. The speaker wears a transmitter that picks up the voice and transmits it to a receiver worn by the child.

Facilitate Ability to Send Information

Maintain the child's hearing aid in proper condition. Many children with impaired hearing communicate using speech, which is enhanced through speech therapy. In addition, they are taught to sign, fingerspell, or use cued speech (Figure 24–14 ■). Articulation may be difficult, and understanding what the child is trying to say may be frustrating for both the nurse and the child. Taking time to listen carefully is important.

Measures to promote speech and communication development as well as safety are implemented. Ask the parents to explain the child's communication techniques and to help interpret words. Have younger children point to pictures. Use assisted technologies such as a computer or picture board, as well as drawings or gestures if necessary. This technique is especially helpful for communicating feelings of pain and hunger during hospitalization. If the child signs or fingerspells, be sure you understand the signs for important functions. Give older children paper and pencil to write requests. People other than parents should be able to understand what the child is trying to communicate. Have an interpreter available if the child uses American Sign Language. Learn some common signs yourself to communicate simple words or phrases. Orient the child carefully to new settings such as the hospital room or a new school.

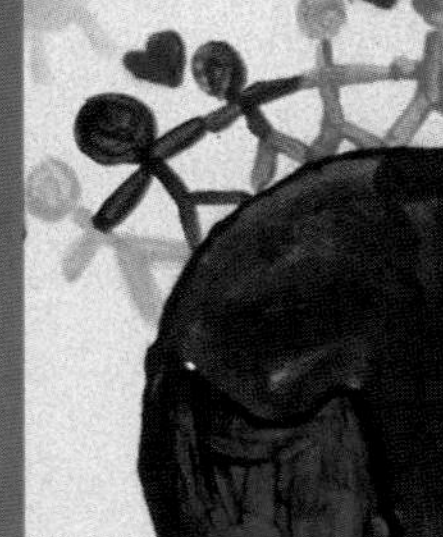

PARTNERING WITH FAMILIES

Care of the Hearing Aid

Families need to know how to maintain the child's hearing aid in proper condition to ensure its function. They can be taught when the child receives the first hearing aid, with at least annual updates to check on knowledge and questions. Items to include in teaching are as follows:

- The three types of hearing aid are those that fit totally in the ear canal, those that fit in the external ear canal, and those that fit behind the ear.
- The hearing aid should be cleaned each day with a damp cloth. Change the batteries as needed, usually about once a week. Disconnect the battery when not in use.
- Place the hearing aid in the ear with the volume off, then slowly turn up to half volume. Adjust as needed.
- Be sure the hearing aid fit is checked yearly, as the child's growth may necessitate a new fitting.

Help Parents to Meet Child's Educational Needs

Public laws apply to the education of children who are hearing impaired (see Chapter 1∞). After diagnosis, the parents and professionals together agree on an individualized education plan (see discussion in Chapter 16∞). Childcare and preschool are recommended for children with hearing problems in order to foster socialization skills and increase time for communicating with others. Some parents may choose to send the child to a separate program or school for the deaf and may need assistance to find such resources.

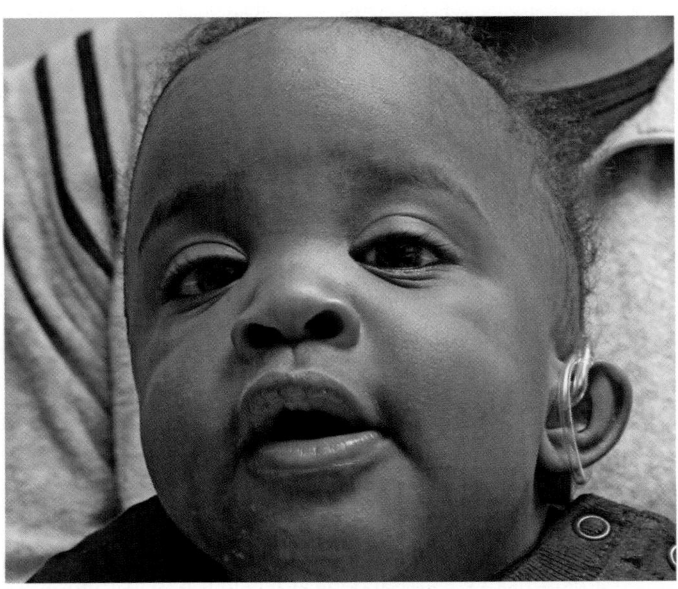

FIGURE 24–14 ■ This child with a hearing impairment has been fitted with a hearing aid and hears and responds to sounds in the environment.

- Provide parents with information about adjustments that may have to be made for the child with a hearing impairment who attends public school. By sitting at the front of the classroom, the child can hear and see more clearly. The teacher should always face the child when speaking, and background noise should be reduced.
- Tell parents that children who are hearing impaired have the same intelligence quotient (IQ) distribution as children without hearing impairment. However, communication and learning can be difficult, and extra support is needed.
- Children with hearing impairment should reach their intellectual potential, although development in certain areas may take place more slowly than it does in children with no hearing impairment.

Provide Emotional Support

By recognizing the effects of the diagnosis on the family, the nurse can help family members deal with their reactions to the child's hearing loss. Supporting healthy coping is an important intervention to help the parents carry on with their lives.

- Help the parents understand the child's hearing ability and its effect on speech and language development. Provide accurate information about their concerns. Work jointly with other healthcare professionals and social service workers if necessary.
- Tell the family about the community services available for medical, nursing, psychologic, and financial assistance. Link the family with the deaf or hearing-impaired community and resources.

MediaLink Hearing Impairment Resources

Evaluation

Expected outcomes of nursing care for a child with hearing impairment include the following:

- Successful establishment of communication method
- Growth and development to maximum potential
- Establishment of successful individualized education plan
- Positive family coping

Injuries of the Ear

Ear injuries of many types commonly occur in children. Lacerations, infections, and hematomas may occur in the external ear structures, especially the pinna. Children may place foreign objects in the ear, and insects may enter the ear canal.

PRACTICE ALERT

If an alkaline button battery (like those found in many toys or watches) is inserted in a child's ear, it can rapidly destroy tissue, causing perforation of the tympanic membrane, destruction of the ossicles, and local tissue ulceration. Removal should be performed with the child under sedation or general anesthesia.

Rupture of the tympanic membrane may result from head injuries, blows to the ear, or insertion of objects into the ear canal. Serous drainage from the ear can indicate a basilar skull fracture. Be alert for ruptured tympanic membranes in combination with conjuntival hemorrhage and other signs of shaken child syndrome (see Chapter 7 for further discussion of this type of child abuse).

See Table 24–13 for information on the emergency treatment of ear injuries. Any injury resulting in earache, decreased hearing, imbalance problems, persistent bleeding, or other discharge should be seen by a physician.

TABLE 24–13 Emergency Treatment of Ear Injuries

INJURY	TREATMENT
Pinna	
Minor cuts or abrasions	Wash thoroughly with soap and water and rinse well; leave exposed to air if possible or apply adhesive bandage, monitor for infection.
Hematomas	Needle aspiration should be performed and pressure dressing applied; undrained hematomas may become fibrotic; "cauliflower ear" deformity may develop.
Cellulitis or abscesses	Apply moist heat intermittently; make sure that prescribed antibiotic is taken; minor surgery may be performed for an abscess.
Deep lacerations	Apply pressure to stop bleeding; transport to physician's office or emergency department for suturing.
Ear Canal	
Foreign bodies	Have child lie on back and turn head over edge of bed, with affected side down; wiggle earlobe and have child shake head; foreign object may fall out as result of gravity; if object remains in ear, call physician; do not try to remove foreign body with tweezers since this may push the object further into the ear.
Insects	Shine flashlights into ear to try to attract insect; instilling a few drops of mineral oil, olive oil, or alcohol kills insect, and irrigating ear canal gently may remove dead insect (see Skills Manual).
Tympanic Membrane	
Ruptures	Call physician if child has persistent ear pain after blow, blast injury, or insertion of foreign object; cover external ear loosely with piece of sterile cotton or gauze; if tympanic membrane has been ruptured, systemic antibiotics are prescribed.

DISORDERS OF THE NOSE, THROAT, AND MOUTH

A variety of disorders affect the nose, throat, and mouth of children. They commonly relate to infection or trauma. The areas are anatomically connected, and with the upper bronchi they comprise the upper respiratory system. Several of the disorders of the upper respiratory system are discussed in the following section.

Epistaxis

Epistaxis, or nosebleed, is common in school-age children, especially boys. Kiesselbach's plexus, an area of plentiful veins located in the anterior nares, is a usual source of bleeding, commonly caused by irritation from nosepicking, foreign bodies, or low humidity. Other causes include forceful coughing, allergies, or infections resulting in congestion of the nasal mucosa. Bleeding from the posterior septum is more serious and may be life threatening. Hospitalization may be necessary. Posterior nosebleeds have a variety of causes, some of which may indicate systemic disease (i.e., bleeding disorder) or injury.

Children with nosebleeds are sometimes brought to the emergency department by a parent who has been unable to stop the flow of blood within a few minutes. Both parent and child may be frightened. Ask the parent briefly about any history of nosebleeds and other contributing factors, including medications. Take the child's pulse and blood pressure to monitor for hypovolemia when there is excessive blood loss. Carefully examine the nasal mucosa by asking the child to blow any clots out gently, if possible. Suctioning may be necessary.

Observing the flow may help determine if the blood is coming from an anterior or a posterior location. A nosebleed confined to one side of the nose is almost always anterior, but posterior bleeding can flow on one or both sides. If blood cannot be seen, the child may be swallowing it and may become nauseated. Suspect posterior bleeding in children who have sustained blunt trauma to the head.

The child with anterior bleeding should sit upright quietly. The head should be tilted forward to prevent blood from trickling down the throat, which can lead to vomiting. The nares should be squeezed just below the nasal bone and held for 10 to 15 minutes while the child breathes through the mouth. An ice bag can be applied to the nose or back of the neck. If the bleeding does not stop, a cotton ball or swab soaked with Neo-Synephrine, epinephrine, thrombin, or lidocaine may be inserted into the affected nostril to promote topical vasoconstriction or anesthesia. Once the bleeding has stopped, the nostril may have to be cauterized with silver nitrate or electrocautery. If the bleeding cannot be stopped, absorbable packing may be used.

Posterior bleeding must also be stopped by packing, and the child must be monitored carefully. Arterial ligation is occasionally needed. Repeated or severe nosebleeds need further evaluation.

Nursing Management

Assess the child's hematocrit or hemoglobin if significant bleeding has occurred. Report abnormal results to the primary care provider. Children with frequent epistaxis should have a complete history taken and physical examination performed to rule out systemic disease.

After the nosebleed has stopped, the child is more vulnerable to recurrent bleeding and should avoid bending over, stooping, strenuous exercise, hot drinks, and hot baths or showers for the next 3 to 4 days. Sleeping with the head elevated on two or three pillows and humidifying the air with a vaporizer may also prevent a recurrence. Provide parents with suggestions for prevention and home management of epistaxis. See Partnering with Families: Prevention and Home Management of Epistaxis.

Nasopharyngitis

Nasopharyngitis, also known as upper respiratory infection (URI) or the common cold, causes inflammation and infection of the nose and throat and is probably the most common illness of infancy and childhood. More than 200 viruses and numerous bacteria can cause this condition. The most common viruses include rhinovirus and coronavirus, and the most frequently occurring bacterium is group A streptococcus. The organisms incubate in 1 to 3 days, and the infection is communicable several hours before symptoms develop and for 1 to 2 days after they begin. Symptoms may last 4 to 10 days or longer. The pathogens are believed to spread when the infected person touches the hand of an uninfected person, who then touches his or her mouth or nose, resulting in self-inoculation.

A red nasal mucosa with clear nasal discharge and an infected throat with enlarged tonsils may be apparent in children with nasopharyngitis. Vesicles may be present on the soft palate and in the pharynx. Accompanying symptoms may vary, depending on the child's age (Table 24–14).

Between episodes of nasopharyngitis, the child should be asymptomatic. If a child continues to have upper respiratory infections or a chronic cough, the presence of an underlying condition such as allergy, asthma, or polyps should be ruled out.

Nursing Management

For infants who cannot breathe through the mouth, normal saline nose drops can be administered every 3 to 4 hours, especially before feeding. (Refer to the Skills Manual for instructions on how to administer nose drops.) For infants over 9 months of age, nasal stuffiness can be treated with either normal saline nose drops or a decongestant such as phenylephrine (0.125% to 0.25%, depending on the child's age). Older children can use nasal sprays.

Although decongestant nose drops and sprays are more effective than systemic decongestants, they should not be used for more than 4 or 5 days or more often than recommended. Antihistamines may be helpful for children with allergic rhinitis or profuse nasal drainage. Long-acting nasal sprays and medications with several ingredients are not recommended. See Partnering with

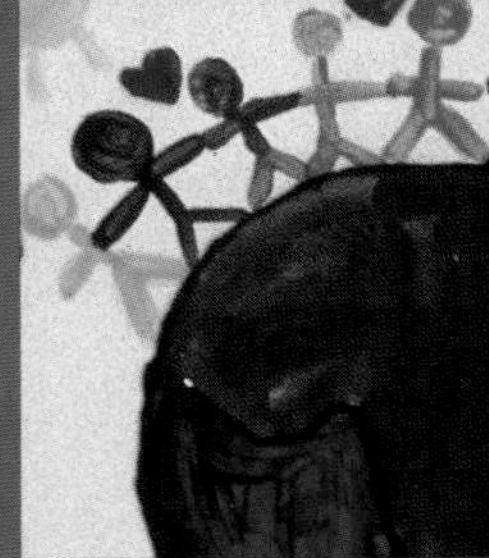

PARTNERING WITH FAMILIES

Prevention and Home Management of Epistaxis

Prevention

- Humidify the child's room, especially during the winter.
- Discourage the child from picking or rubbing the nose or inserting foreign objects in the nose.
- Instruct the child to blow the nose gently and release sneezes through the mouth.

Home management

- Keep the child calm.
- Sit the child upright with head tilted slightly forward so blood does not run down the nasopharynx.
- Press a roll of cotton under the upper lip to compress the labial artery.
- Apply steady pressure to both nostrils just below the nasal bone with the thumb and forefinger for 15–20 minutes. Time by the clock.
- Apply an ice pack or cold compress to the bridge of the nose or the back of the neck.
- Call healthcare provider if the bleeding does not stop.
- Avoid further bleeds by sleeping with the head elevated on pillows, avoiding hot showers and drinks, and avoiding aspirin or other noncoagulant drugs during the first few days after a nosebleed.

Adapted from Newland, J. A., & Rich, E. (1998). Epistaxis. American Journal of Nursing, 98, *16HHH.*

TABLE 24–14 Symptoms of Nasopharyngitis

INFANTS YOUNGER THAN 3 MONTHS OF AGE	INFANTS 3 MONTHS OF AGE OR OLDER	OLDER CHILDREN
Lethargy Irritability Feeding poorly Fever (may be absent)	Fever Vomiting Diarrhea Sneezing Anorexia Irritability Restlessness	Dry, irritated nose and throat Chills, fever Generalized muscle aches Headache Malaise Anorexia Post-nasal drip Thin nasal discharge, which may later become thick and purulent Sneezing

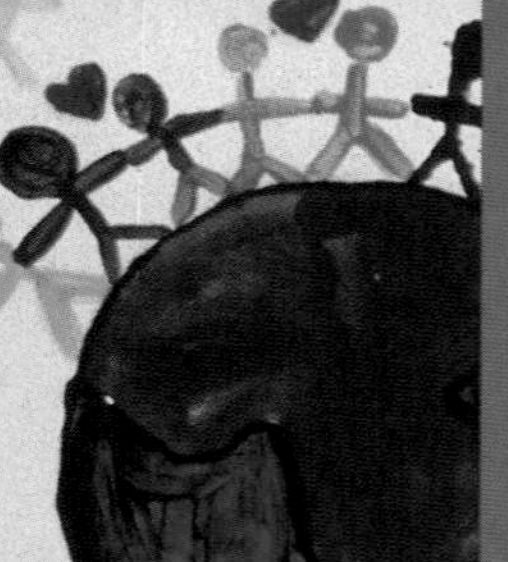

PARTNERING WITH FAMILIES

Teaching about Over-the-Counter Cough and Cold Medications

Parents may try to treat children who have upper respiratory infections with the same medications they are accustomed to taking for a cold. Prepare them during a health promotion visit and help them plan for how to handle medications for the child. Guidelines are as follows:

- Read the label to be sure the medication is recommended for the child's age and condition. Give only the dose recommended for the age and weight of the child.
- Be sure you know how to measure the medication. Tablespoon and teaspoon are *not* the same. Use the measuring device that is provided with some liquids for greatest accuracy.
- Consult the pharmacist, nurse, or doctor if you have questions, if the medication is not recommended for the age of your child, if the child's condition does not improve, or if other symptoms appear.
- Use the child-resistant cap after each opening of the bottle. Store the medication out of reach of all children, preferably in a locked location.
- If you use home remedies or other herbal products to treat colds, be sure to check on their safety with your healthcare provider first.

Adapted from U.S. Food and Drug Administration. Got a sick kid? www.fda.gov/cder/consumerinfo/sickkids.htm, accessed 1/1/2004.

Families: Teaching about Over-the-Counter Cough and Cold Medications and Complementary Therapy: Cold Treatments.

Room humidification may help prevent drying of nasal secretions. Antipyretics such as acetaminophen or ibuprofen reduce fever and make the child more comfortable. Aspirin is not recommended because of its association with Reye syndrome (refer to Chapter 33∞).

Children should avoid strenuous physical activity and engage in quiet play such as reading, listening to music or stories, or watching television or videotapes. Children should not be forced to eat, but the intake of favorite fluids to liquify secretions should be encouraged. (See Developing Cultural Competence: Hot and Cold Disease Theory.) Parents should be told that no medicine or vaccine can prevent the common cold, but eliminating contact with infected persons can reduce the spread of infection. Proper handwashing and disposal of tissues help to decrease the spread of the infection.

Sinusitis

Sinusitis is an inflammation of one or more of the paranasal sinuses. These sinuses, which have respiratory epithelium and are continuous with the respiratory tract, are air-filled hollow cavities and include the maxillary, ethmoid, frontal, and sphenoid sinuses (Box 24–6). The sinuses may become infected with

COMPLEMENTARY THERAPY

Cold Treatments

Many families use home and herbal remedies for treatment of colds. Although some of these are harmless and may actually increase the child's comfort, some may not help. For example, Echinacea is a product derived from a plant that has been used as an immune stimulant; it is available in capsules, juice, tea, and other preparations. A recent study funded by the National Center for Complementary and Alternative Medicine did not find Echinacea effective in treating upper respiratory tract infections in children from 2 to 11 years of age. While the treatment was generally found to be safe, there was an increased risk of rash in treated children (Taylor, Weber, Standish, et al., 2003).

Some products designed for colds may actually be harmful. Herbal products that contain aristolochic acid, a substance that can cause cancer and kidney disease, can be found on numerous Internet sites, and several are marketed as cold remedies (Gold & Slone, 2003).

Be sure to ask families if they use any home or herbal remedies to treat a child's upper respiratory infection, and check to be sure these products are safe for use in children. Refer to Chapter 3∞ for further information on helping families evaluate safety of products used.

bacteria following a viral upper respiratory infection; sinusitis occurs in 5% to 10% of children following upper respiratory infections (Duchene, 2000). In most cases, the child's history reveals a cold for several days, followed by improvement in the cold symptoms, but with an increase in purulent nasal drainage or other symptoms. There is often accompanying facial pain, headache, and fever. The most common infectious agents are the same as those for otitis media, namely *Streptococcus pneumoniae, Haemophilus influenzae,* and *Moraxella catarrhalis* (Subcommittee on Management of Sinusitis and Committee on Quality Improvement, 2001). Chronic sinusitis may occur in children with uncontrolled allergies and asthma.

Signs and symptoms of sinusitis in children are sometimes nonspecific. A history of recent upper respiratory infection is common, persistent cough from postnasal drip can occur, and nasal discharge or swelling can be apparent. Malodorous breath, fever, mouth breathing, hyponasal speech, and cervical lymphadenopathy may be present (Duchene, 2000; Hayes, 2001; Leung & Kellner, 2004). Young children may be anorexic or have difficulty feeding while older children may complain of headache.

Diagnosis of sinusitis is usually based on history and physical examination findings. Percussion and illumination of sinuses are not generally useful in children. Computed tomography (CT), magnetic resonance imaging (MRI), and radiographs may be done, but they can be costly and require sedation of young chil-

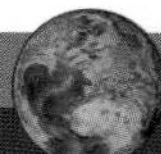

DEVELOPING CULTURAL COMPETENCE

Hot and Cold Disease Theory

Many Hispanic and Asian cultural groups believe in the "hot and cold theory" of disease, in which health problems are viewed as the result of imbalance. For example, some Mexican Americans traditionally treat a "cold disease" such as an earache or common cold with "hot" substances. Ask families if they prefer to eat certain foods during an illness. Incorporating such preferences may help the child and increase the confidence of the family in healthcare providers.

BOX 24–6 Growth and Development

The ethmoid and maxillary sinuses form during gestation by about month 3–4. Sphenoid sinuses begin developing by 1–2 years and are formed by 5 years of age; frontal sinuses form from 5–8 years of age but are not complete until adolescence (Subcommittee on Management of Sinusitis and Committee on Quality Improvement, 2001). Children over 1 year of age commonly experience sinusitis following upper respiratory infections.

dren and results may not be conclusive. For the child with repeated sinusitis or who appears toxic, aspiration of sinus aspirate may be performed for culture by an otolaryngologist.

Although most primary care providers treat suspected sinusitis with antibiotics, many cases will clear spontaneously without treatment. Amoxicillin is the first choice for therapy; amoxicillin/clavulanate and cephalosporins are also sometimes used (Sinus and Allergy Health Partnership, 2000; Kakish, Mahafza, Batieha, et al., 2000). Children with recurrent sinusitis should be referred for further care by an otolaryngologist and allergy specialist.

Parents whose child has persistent and purulent nasal drainage should be told to see a healthcare provider, particularly if the drainage is accompanied by facial pain, headache, and fever. Teach parents to correctly administer antibiotics (e.g., to take medications for the full course) if prescribed, and to use saline nose drops if needed for comfort. Infants may need their nose cleared with nose drops and a bulb syringe prior to feedings. (Refer to the Skills Manual for correct use of a bulb syringe.) Antipyretics can be given for fever and to relieve pain.

Pharyngitis

Acute pharyngitis is an infection that primarily affects the pharynx, including the tonsils. It is seen most frequently in children 4 to 7 years and is rare in children less than 1 year. Approximately 80% of these infections are caused by viruses; the rest are caused by bacteria. Bacterial pharyngitis is commonly known as strep throat, because it is most often caused by group A beta-hemolytic streptococcus (GABHS). About 20% to 40% of pharyngitis is GABHS. Viral pharyngitis is caused by a large number of enteroviruses.

The major complaint is a sore throat. See the clinical manifestations table on this page for manifestations of viral pharyngitis and strep throat. Children with symptoms of strep throat who have minimal throat redness and pain, exudate, mild lymphadenopathy, and a low-grade fever, and who have been exposed to someone who has pharyngitis, should have a throat culture. The classic signs of purulent drainage and white patches are not present in all cases of strep throat. A child who finds swallowing difficult or extremely painful, who drools, or who exhibits signs of dehydration or respiratory distress should be seen by a physician immediately. These signs could be indicators of serious conditions such as epiglottitis (see Chapter 25) or diphtheria (see Chapter 19). Peritonsillar abscess (a tonsil infection that spreads into surrounding tissues and causes cellulites) or retropharyngeal abscess (an infection of the lymph nodes that drain the adenoids, nasopharynx, and paranasal sinuses) are other serious conditions.

CLINICAL MANIFESTATIONS of Viral Pharyngitis and Strep Throat (Group A Beta-hemolytic Streptococcus [GABHS])[a]

VIRAL PHARYNGITIS	STREP THROAT
Nasal congestion	Abrupt onset
Mild sore throat	Tonsillar exudate[b]
Conjunctivitis	Painful cervical lymphadenopathy[b]
Cough	Anorexia, nausea, vomiting, abdominal pain
Hoarseness	Severe sore throat
Mild pharyngeal redness	Headache, malaise
Minimal tonsillar exudate	Fever > 38.3°C (101°F)
Mildly tender anterior cervical lymphadenopathy	Petechial mottling of soft palate
Fever < 38.3°C (101°F)	

[a]Children 6 months to 3 years of age may have streptococcus with symptoms that resemble those of viral pharyngitis. Children with scarlet fever have the symptoms of strep throat plus a sandpaper-textured erythematous generalized rash and pallor around the lips.

[b]Classic signs of strep throat.

Collaborative Care

The diagnosis of strep throat is made by throat culture, using the rapid or traditional strep tests. Results of the rapid strep test may be available within minutes; those for the traditional test are available in 24 to 48 hours.

CLINICAL TIP

Throat cultures must be properly performed for accurate diagnosis. A sterile cotton-tip applicator is swabbed across the tonsils, posterior edge of the soft palate, and uvula. Cooperative children can be asked to put their hands under their buttocks, open their mouth, and laugh or pant like a dog. The throat is quickly swabbed. Uncooperative and young children are placed on their back with their hands next to their head and held by a parent or an assistant. The tongue is gently depressed with a tongue blade and the throat is swabbed. Be sure to swab both tonsils.

Early signs of strep throat should be treated with oral penicillin for 10 days or by long-acting penicillin given in one injection. If the child is allergic to penicillin, erythromycin is given. Acute symptoms should resolve within 24 hours of therapy, at which time the child is no longer contagious. For pharyngitis that is caused by a virus, symptomatic treatment alone is used (Feder, 2001).

Nursing Management

Nursing care focuses on symptomatic relief. Acetaminophen reduces throat pain and generalized fever. Cool, nonacidic fluids and soft foods, ice chips, or frozen juice pops given frequently in small amounts facilitate swallowing and prevent dehydration. Humidification, chewing gum, and gargling with warm salt water (5 g to 250 mL water; 1/4 teaspoon to 8 oz water) soothe an irritated throat.

MediaLink Nursing in Action: Obtaining a Sample for Throat Culture

CLINICAL TIP

Children may be more willing to gargle with salt water if the mixture is placed in a spray bottle and sprayed gently toward the throat. Do you know why? The salt water bypasses the salt sensation on the outer part of the tongue and is not as distasteful. The gentle spray does not stimulate a gag reflex; it delivers the salt solution directly to the throat area where it can be gargled and then spit out.

Commercial throat sprays or throat lozenges are not generally more effective than these home remedies. Encourage the child to rest, to conserve energy and promote recovery.

Teach parents the importance of completing the entire course of antibiotics if prescribed for bacterial pharyngitis. After about 2 days on the medication, have the parents replace the child's toothbrush with a new one to avoid reinfection by bacteria that can survive on the moist brush. Reinforce to parents the importance of treating streptococcal infections, as untreated infections may lead to rheumatic fever, cervical adenitis, sinusitis, glomerulonephritis, or meningitis.

Tonsillitis

Tonsillitis is an infection or inflammation (hypertrophy) of the palatine tonsils. Although most children with pharyngitis have infected tonsils, they do not necessarily have inflammation that indicates tonsillitis.

Etiology and Pathophysiology

Like pharyngitis, tonsillitis may be caused by a virus or bacterium. The primary site of infection is the tonsils. The condition tends to recur several times in certain children.

Clinical Manifestations

Symptoms suggestive of tonsillitis include frequent throat infections with breathing and swallowing difficulties; persistent redness of the anterior pillars; and enlargement of the cervical lymph nodes. If children breathe through their mouths continuously, the mucous membranes may become dry and irritated.

COLLABORATIVE CARE

The goal of treatment is relief from discomfort for the child. Symptomatic treatment, antibiotics, and occasionally surgery are used.

Diagnostic Tests

Diagnosis is made on the basis of visual inspection and clinical manifestations. Tonsils appear large and inflamed. During normal development children often have a growth of tonsillar tissue in childhood so the tonsils normally appear large. A diagnosis of tonsillitis requires enlarged tonsils with pain and inflammation.

Clinical Therapy

Symptomatic treatment for tonsillitis is the same as for pharyngitis. Surgical removal of tonsils (tonsillectomy) is often recommended when children have recurrent throat infections (about three per year for 3 years), chronic tonsillitis, obstructive sleep apnea, or malformations causing nasal speech or a facial growth abnormality. If the child is under 3 years of age, the surgery is postponed if possible because it may stimulate growth of other lymphoid tissue in the nasopharynx. If the pharyngeal tonsils (adenoids) are enlarged, as suggested by mouth breathing, cough, impaired taste and smell, a muffled quality to the voice, and chronic otitis media, then they may be removed at the same time. Surgical tonsillectomy is a common operation in children with most cases involving both tonsillectomy and adenoidectomy (Paradise, Bluestone, Colborn, et al., 2002). A newer technique is under study for use with children who have sleep obstruction due to large tonsillar size. Temperature-controlled radiofrequency (TCRF) has been used to decrease the size of tonsils in children from 4 to 13 years. Children had increased comfort, decreased snoring and other sleep problems, and very quick recovery from the procedure (Nelson, 2003).

NURSING MANAGEMENT

The goal of nursing care in tonsillitis is promotion of comfort for the child and successful treatment of infection. If surgical removal is indicated, the nurse prepares the family and child for the surgery, provides postoperative care, and teaches information needed for postsurgical home care.

■ Nursing Assessment and Diagnosis

Assess the throat carefully during each physical examination. Observe for tonsils that are simply large (a common finding in childhood) and those that are inflamed. Look for the degree of redness and presence of any exudate. Ask if the child has pain or difficulty swallowing. Ask about the history of past tonsillar infections and the length of time of the present discomfort. Collect information about snoring, restlessness, or repeated night wakenings.

If surgery is indicated, take a complete history of the child preoperatively. Remember to evaluate for loose teeth and report them to the surgeon since they are common in children of this age. Monitor vital signs and observe for respiratory distress, hemorrhage, and dehydration postoperatively. Ask about medication usage.

The following nursing diagnoses may apply to the child with tonsillitis:

- Acute Pain related to inflammation of the pharynx
- Risk for Deficient Fluid Volume related to inadequate intake
- Risk for Ineffective Breathing Pattern related to obstruction by enlarged tonsils
- Impaired Swallowing related to inflammation and pain
- Deficient Knowledge (parents) related to home care following discharge

Planning and Implementation

The nurse provides general supportive care and, if medication is prescribed, encourages completion of the full course of treatment. The nursing management of children with tonsillitis is similar to that of children with pharyngitis (see earlier discussion).

If surgery is indicated, the nurse helps parents prepare their child for a short-term surgical procedure with a possible overnight stay in the hospital (see Chapter 17∞). Children should be free of sore throat, fever, or upper respiratory infection for at least 1 week before surgery. Any medications, such as ibuprofen, that alter bleeding time should not be given within the 2 weeks prior to surgery. Although not usually recommended for children, aspirin alters bleeding time, so specifically teach parents to avoid that analgesic. See Chapter 33∞ for further description of reasons to avoid aspirin use in children. Check if any herbal medications are taken and report them to the physician and anesthesiologist, because some may interfere with anesthetic drugs used in surgery or interfere with normal blood clotting.

Discharge Planning and Home Care Teaching

Discharge planning includes teaching parents about pain management, fluid and nutrition intake, activity restrictions, and possible complications in the postoperative period. Most children will have a sore throat for 7 to 10 days after tonsillectomy. Advise parents how to relieve the child's throat pain.

Children may experience ear pain, especially when swallowing, between 4 and 8 days after tonsillectomy. Advise parents that this pain is the result of referred pain from the tonsillar area and does not indicate an ear infection.

Emphasize to parents the importance of adequate fluid intake. Children should be given any liquid they prefer for the first week, except citrus juices, which may produce a burning sensation in the throat. Soft foods such as gelatin, applesauce, frozen juice pops, and mashed potatoes can be added as tolerated.

Children do not need to be confined to bed, but vigorous exercise should be avoided for the first week after surgery. Advise parents that the child may return to school approximately 10 days after tonsillectomy.

Any surgery carries with it the risk of postoperative complications. Teach parents the normal signs of healing in the postoperative period, as well as signs of complications. (See Partnering with Families: Care after Tonsillectomy and Complications of Tonsillectomy and Adenoidectomy.)

Evaluation

Expected outcomes of nursing care for the child with tonsillitis include:

- Adequate intake of food and fluids
- Management of pain and fever
- Absence of postoperative complications such as bleeding, hemorrhage, dehydration
- Healing without impairment following tonsillectomy

PARTNERING WITH FAMILIES

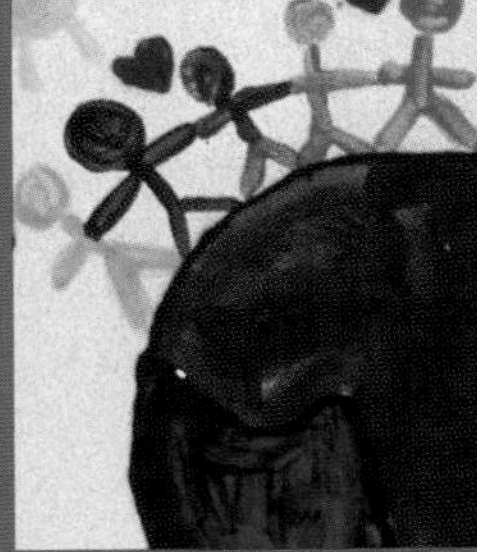

Care after Tonsillectomy

After a child's tonsillectomy, the parent can institute measures to increase the child's comfort.

- Have the child drink adequate cool fluids or chew gum, as this reduces spasms in the muscles surrounding the throat.
- Give acetaminophen elixir, as ordered.
- Apply an ice collar around the child's neck.
- Have the child gargle with a solution of 2.5 g (0.5 teaspoon) each of baking soda and salt in 8 oz of water.
- Have the child rinse the mouth well with viscous lidocaine, if prescribed by the surgeon, and then swallow the solution.

Mouth Disorders

The mouth is an important structure that is directly linked to both the gastrointestinal and respiratory systems. Structural problems can occur in the mouth, often in conjunction with other defects. See Chapter 30∞ for a description of tracheoesophageal fistula and cleft lip and palate. Both of these defects are commonly connected with structural defects of the mouth, most notably a cleft or opening in the palate. See Chapter 8∞ for a description of examination of the mouth and tongue in neonates and older children in order to identify structural problems.

Another type of mouth disorder in children is ulceration. Children sometimes have changes in the mucous membranes of the mouth, associated with illnesses, infections, or as a side effect of drug treatments. These disorders are discussed later in the chapter.

Trauma is a third cause for mouth disorders in children. Accidents can cause fractures of the jaw or other trauma. Fractures are discussed in Chapter 35∞, while trauma that leads to dental emergencies is discussed later in the chapter.

Mouth Ulcers

A variety of conditions can cause mouth ulcers in children. They commonly occur in conjunction with certain medications or diseases. Oral mucosa has a fast rate of growth so that conditions that impair cell synthesis will cause breakdown in the mucosa with lack of new tissue growth. The growth of mucosal tissue requires adequate moisture so dehydration is a risk factor for development of oral ulcers.

Trauma is another cause of oral ulcers. See the clinical manifestations table on page 813 for the etiology, clinical manifestations, and clinical therapy for conditions leading to oral ulcers in children.

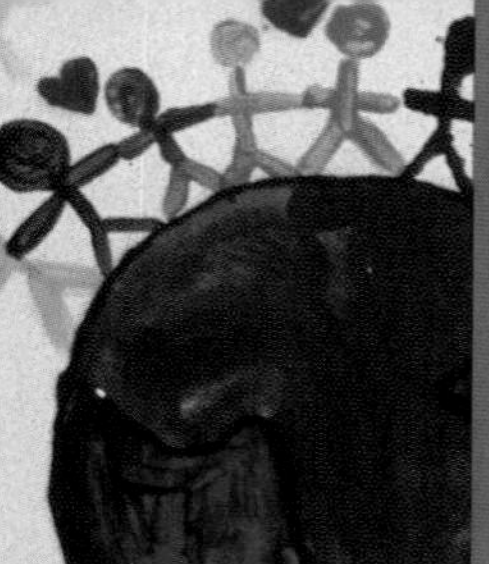

PARTNERING WITH FAMILIES

Complications of Tonsillectomy and Adenoidectomy

Bleeding

- To prevent bleeding, ibuprofen or other drugs that alter bleeding should not be given for pain for the first postoperative week. Use acetaminophen instead.
- Bleeding is most likely to occur within the first 24 hours or 7–10 days after the tonsillectomy, when the scar is forming. Report any trickle of bright red blood to the physician immediately.

Infection

- The back of the throat will look white and have an odor for the first 7–8 days after the surgery. The child may also have a low-grade fever. These are not signs of infection.
- For temperatures over 38.3°C (101°F), acetaminophen may be used.
- Call the physician if the child develops a fever above 38.8°C (102°F).

Pain

- Administer acetaminophen as ordered.
- Offer frequent small amounts of cool liquids. Avoid citrus juice.
- Provide for rest and quiet activities for several days.

COLLABORATIVE CARE

The goals of collaborative care are relief from pain and promotion of ulcer healing.

Diagnostic Tests

Most mouth ulcers and other oral lesions are diagnosed by history and appearance. Culture of exudate may be helpful in identifying an infective cause. Biopsy may be performed if the cause is not clear or a mouth cancer is possible. Occasionally laboratory blood analysis is done and may show leukocytosis in infectious cases and Stevens-Johnson syndrome.

Clinical Therapy

Most mouth ulcers are treated symptomatically. Since the oral mucosa is fast growing, the cells can rapidly heal. Keeping the mouth clean and administering systemic or topical analgesics can assist with comfort. Foods should be mild and nonirritating. Acyclovir may be administered for treatment of herpes infections. Antibiotics are needed for bacterial infection of oral lesions. Stevens-Johnson syndrome necessitates removing the drug that causes the reaction, and treating the child with oral antihistamines and supportive therapy.

NURSING MANAGEMENT

Nurses assess oral mucosa and implement treatments for oral ulcers.

Nursing Assessment and Diagnosis

Nurses assess the oral cavity of all children beginning in the neonatal period. Structural abnormalities are promptly referred for further diagnostic work. Mouth ulcers are examined for size, location, drainage, and pain. For those at risk, such as children on chemotherapy, regular careful examinations of the oral mucosa is an important part of care. Some of the appropriate nursing diagnoses for children with oral ulcers include:

- Pain related to injury of oral cavity
- Impaired Oral Mucous Membrane related to chemotherapy or infection
- Imbalanced Nutrition: Less than Body Requirements related to inability to ingest adequate foods

Planning and Implementation

Nurses play an important role in treatment of oral ulcers. Most ulcers are treated symptomatically and will heal rapidly. Ensure that children have good oral care, including brushing teeth with a soft bristle brush or by use of mouth sponges. Rinse the mouth after all meals and snacks. Teach the family correct administration of oral medications and topical preparations designed to treat infection or provide comfort. When oral mucosa ulcers are predicted, such as with chemotherapy or in AIDS, begin oral protocols before lesions occur to decrease their appearance and severity (Cheng, Molassiotis, Chang, et al., 2001; Gibson & Nelson, 2000). Encourage a diet that has only mild foods, avoiding spices and very sweet, sour, and acidic items. Cold foods may be better accepted. Monitor hydration status to ensure adequate fluid intake. Teach parents correct administration of acetaminophen or other analgesic treatment. Use standard precautions to protect the child from infections and prevent their flora from being transferred to other children or family members. Encourage parents to keep children with herpes gingivostomatitis out of contact with other children if active lesions or drooling are present (Blevins, 2003).

Evaluation

Desired outcomes of nursing care for children with oral problems include:

- Decreased reports of oral pain or disruptive effects on dietary intake

CLINICAL MANIFESTATIONS of Mouth Ulcers in Children

DISORDER	ETIOLOGY	CLINICAL MANIFESTATIONS
Chemotherapy-related oral mucositis	Many chemotherapy drugs used to treat cancer attack all rapidly growing cells in the body. Lack of intake of sufficient fluids to provide adequate hydration exacerbates the development of mucositis.	The oral mucosa may have painful ulcers that bleed, become infected, or interfere with food intake.
AIDS-related oral mucositis	Some of the drugs used to treat HIV infections and the poor nutritional state of children with AIDS can promote the development of oral ulcers.	Painful oral ulcers further interfere with adequate food intake.
Stevens-Johnson syndrome (see Chapter 36∞)	Erythema multiforme is a rare mucocutaneous disease and erythema multiforme major is also known as Stevens-Johnson syndrome. After a prodromal period with fever, malaise, fatigue, and sore throat, the characteristic lesions of the disease erupt. Stevens-Johnson syndrome may occur with recurrent herpes virus infection, *Mycoplasma pneumoniae,* or as a reaction to drugs such as nonsteroidal anti-inflammatories, anticonvulsants, and sulfonamides.	Endothelial cells, epithelial cells, and mucosal cells are affected, causing blisters and erosion of conjunctiva, oral cavity, and genital mucosa. A bullous erythematous rash also is common and pneumonia can result.
Aphthous ulcers	These lesions are commonly called "canker sores." An allergic or autoimmune cause is suspected, but herpes gingivitis should be ruled out.	They often recur in the same child over time. Ulcers are on the inside of the lips or throughout the mouth; about 1–3 ulcers occur at a time.
Herpes simplex gingivostomatitis (see Chapter 19∞)	Herpes virus is the causative organism. Herpes simplex infections of the face and nose are referred to as "cold sores."	Multiple ulcers and vesicles of the gingiva, palate, buccal mucosa, lips, and tongue appear. They may be accompanied by skin vesicular lesions characteristic of herpes on the face.
Traumatic ulcers	Trauma to the oral mucosa can lead to ulcers. Children may bite the side of the mouth, may poke a pencil or other object into the mucosa, or can have burns from hot liquids or acidic substances.	One or more ulcerations are visible and may become infected due to source of trauma.

- Structural intactness and normal function of oral mucosal membranes
- Adequate fluids and nutrients ingested

Mouth and Dental Emergencies

Children may have trauma to the mouth and teeth during sporting activities and during other injuries. About 10% of children experience some dental trauma (Diangelis & Bakland, 1998). Nurses inform parents of proper treatment for injuries and may provide emergency treatment in schools and other community settings. Injury prevention is encouraged through use of protective gear during sports. See Chapter 7∞ for a discussion of protective sporting gear and of body piercing which may include the oral cavity. Mouth guards can be helpful to prevent dental damage. The best guards are custom made by dentists because they fit the mouth well and are more likely worn because of their comfort.

Because the mouth has a profuse blood supply, bleeding may be extensive for even minor injuries. It is best to use clean cloths to absorb the blood and prevent choking on it, and get the child to an emergency facility to have the lesion carefully examined.

Dental injuries may involve fracture of a tooth, luxation (partial extrusion), or avulsion (complete removal). The child should be transported immediately to an emergency facility or dentist. If otherwise stable, an emergency dental visit is the best choice. When avulsion has occurred, fast care improves the chance that a permanent tooth can be reimplanted and kept alive. When reimplanted within 30 minutes, the chances of survival of tooth are best (Rudy, 2001). Nurses can perform care or teach parents what to do in case of dental emergency. Referral to dental resources may be needed. See Chapters 10 to 15 for specific dental care needs for health promotion and health maintenance at each age during childhood and adolescence. See Partnering with Families: Care of a Tooth Avulsion.

PRACTICE ALERT

For families with financial constraints, dental care is often delayed or not available. Dental caries is the most common cause of chronic disease in childhood. The highest rates of caries occur in Asian and Pacific Islanders, then Hispanics, followed by African Americans and Whites (Children's Oral Health, 2003). Ask families about what they do for dental care, and how they would seek care if the child has a dental emergency. Many communities have an association of dentists and dental workers who provide care at clinics and other facilities for children without dental insurance. Nurses can help the families to find resources in their communities to provide regular dental visits and care for dental emergencies.

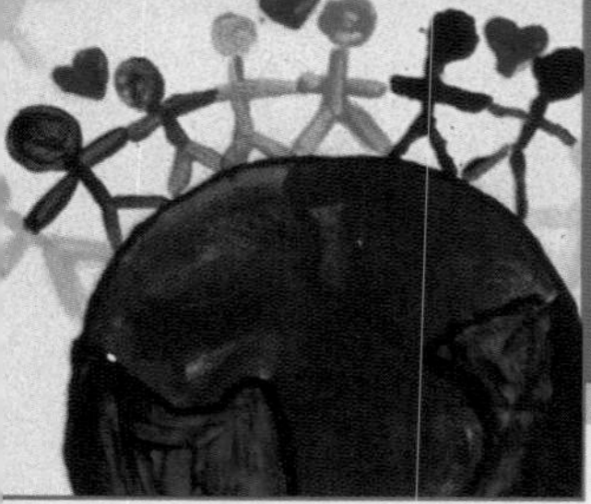

PARTNERING WITH FAMILIES

Care of a Tooth Avulsion

When a tooth is removed during an injury, prompt treatment may influence the chance that it can be reimplanted. If the child's condition is stable, try to reimplant the tooth and then transfer the child to an emergency dental facility.

- Handle the tooth only by the crown (its top).
- Gently rinse the tooth in a bowl of tap water. Do not place it under running water.
- Insert into the socket.
- Have the child provide gentle pressure by biting a piece of gauze or a tea bag.

If child is unstable or has other injuries, enlist emergency medical transportation (call 9–1–1). In this case, the tooth is transported with the child.

- Place the tooth in milk, saline, saliva, or water. If a dental aid kit is available, it may contain a transport liquid called Hank's Balanced Salt Solution.

Adapted from Rudy, C. A. (2001). Dental trauma. School Nurse News, 18*(1), 33–35.*

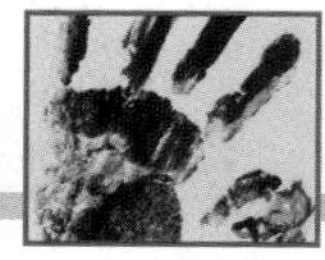

CHAPTER HIGHLIGHTS

- Health conditions affecting the eyes and ears are common in childhood, partially due to anatomical differences in structure.
- Disorders of the eye and ear can lead to developmental and communication delays.
- Conjunctivitis can occur throughout childhood, and can be caused by bacteria, viruses, and allergy.
- Conjunctivitis in the newborn, ophthalmia neonatorum, can be acquired during birth from the mother, and can provide a serious health threat.
- Children manifest a wide array of visual disorders such as hyperopia, myopia, and astigmatism.
- Conditions that can seriously affect vision are strabismus, amblyopia, cataracts, and glaucoma.
- An iatrogenically caused visual disorder is retinopathy of prematurity.
- Nurses commonly screen vision of children in schools and health facilities to identify those with visual impairment.
- Interventions for the child with visual impairment center on providing input through other senses to maximize child development.
- Otitis media is the most common childhood health condition, and has increased in incidence in the past decade.
- Overgrowth of resistant organisms has made treatment of otitis media difficult.
- Treatment of otitis media may begin with up to 3 days of monitoring, followed by antibiotic therapy if the child's condition worsens.
- Newborns should be screened for response to sounds; those at high risk of hearing impairment should be carefully monitored in early childhood.
- Hearing loss may be conductive, sensorineural, or mixed.
- Nursing plan interventions maximize development and communication in the child with a hearing impairment.
- Common disorders of the nose and throat in children include epistaxis, nasopharyngitis, pharyngitis, and tonsillitis.
- Common disorders of the mouth in children are structural abnormalities and oral ulcers.
- Nurses are influential in providing care in dental emergencies and referring families for adequate dental care.

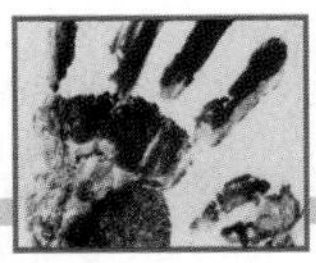

CRITICAL THINKING IN ACTION

INTRODUCTION

Consider the opening scenario with Raeanne, who is visually impaired due to retinopathy of prematurity in the newborn period. Raeanne and her family have had several major challenges in her short life, and they appear to be adapting well.

DESCRIPTION

Raeanne is about to begin preschool after having an early intervention program with her mother for the first 3 years of her life. Raeanne's mother has been considering the possibility of a part-time job to help with expenses; Raeanne's father has been working long hours and is able to spend very little time with his daughter.

DISCUSSION

As Raeanne begins attendance at a preschool, what new challenges will her family face? How can you help them to learn about and become oriented to this new facility? What help might Raeanne's mother need as she makes a possible transition to a part-time job?

Use Bronfenbrenner's ecological theory (Chapter 5∞) to develop questions about Raeanne's microsystem, mesosystem, exosystem, and macrosystem that will influence her healthcare and support.

1. In about 2 more years, as Raeanne begins school, how could you intervene to assist the family in that important transition?
2. What have you learned about individualized education programs, and how can they help Raeanne?
3. If Raeanne's parents decide to have another child, what help will they need to prevent premature birth?

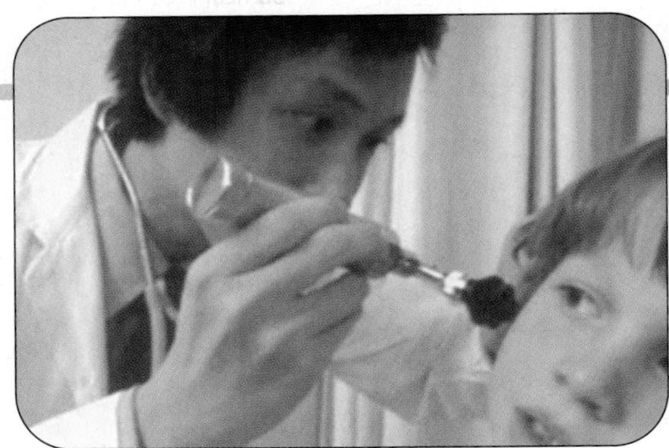

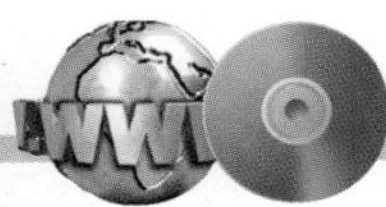

EXPLORE MediaLink

- NCLEX review, case studies, and other interactive resources for this chapter can be found on the Companion Website at **www.prenhall.com/ball**. Click on Chapter 24 to select the activities for this chapter.
- For animations, more NCLEX review questions, and an audio glossary, access the accompanying CD-ROM in this book.

http://www.prenhall.com/ball

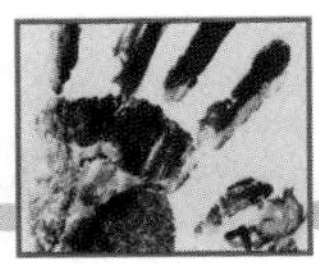

REFERENCES

Alcorn, D. M. (2001, March). Red eye: When to treat and when to refer. *Infectious Diseases in Children*, 3–8.

Alexander, M. (2003). Ocular allergy: Treatment options for children. *Contemporary Pediatrics*, Supplement, 3–6.

Altemeier, W. A. (2000). Preschool vision screening: The importance of the two-line difference. *Pediatric Annals, 29*, 264–267.

American Academy of Pediatrics. (2001). Sports with high risk of eye injury with appropriate eye protectors. www.aaporg/policy/01497t2.htm, accessed 7/16/2004.

American Academy of Pediatrics, Section on Ophthalmology. (2001). Screening examination of premature infants for retinopathy of prematurity. *Pediatrics, 108*, 809–811.

American Academy of Pediatrics, Subcommitte on management of acute otitis media (2004). Diagnosis and management of acute otitis media. *Pediatrics* 113, 1451–1465.

American Academy of Pediatrics. (2001). Subcommittee on Management of Sinusitis and Committee on Quality Improvement. Clinical practice guideline: Management of sinusitis. *Pediatrics, 108*, 798–808.

Bacal, D. A., & Wilson, M. C. (2000). Strabismus: Getting it straight. *Contemporary Pediatrics, 17,* 49–60.

Bachman, K. R., & Arvedson, J. C. (1998). Early identification and intervention for children who are hearing impaired. *Pediatrics in Review, 19,* 155–165.

Behrman, R. E., Kliegman, R. M., & Jenson, H. B. (2004). *Nelson textbook of pediatrics* (17th ed.). Philadelphia: Saunders.

Blevins, J. Y. (2003). Primary herpetic gingivostomatitis in young children. *Pediatric Nursing, 29,* 199–202.

Brocklehurst, P., & Rooney, G. (2000). Interventions for treating genital Chlamydia trachomatis infection in pregnancy. *Cochrane Database Systematic Review 2000, 2,* CD000054.

Brookhouse, P. E., Beauchaine, K. L., & Osberger, M. J. (1999). Management of the child with sensorineural hearing loss: Medical, surgical, hearing aids, cochlear implants. *Pediatric Clinics of North America, 46,* 121–142.

Burns, C. E., Brady, M. A., Dunn, A. M., & Starr, N. B. (2000). *Pediatric primary care* (2nd ed.). Philadelphia: Saunders.

Center for Health and Health Care in Schools. (2004). Childhood vision: What the research tells us. www.healthinschools.org, accessed 6/15/2004.

Cheng, K. K., Molassiotis, A., Chang, A. M., Wai, W. C., & Cheung, S. S. (2001). Evaluation of an oral care protocol intervention in the prevention of chemotherapy-induced oral mucositis in paediatric cancer patients. *European Journal of Cancer, 37,* 2056–2063.

Cheng, A. K., Rubin, H. R., Powe, N. R., Mellon, N. K., Francis, H. W., & Niparko, J. K. (2000). Cost-utility of the cochlear implant in children. *Journal of the American Medical Association, 284,* 850–856.

Children's oral health national facts. (2003). Washington, DC: Children's Dental Health Project.

Committee on Infectious Diseases. (2003). *Red book* (26th ed.). Elk Grove Village, IL: American Academy of Pediatrics.

Committee on Sports Medicine and Fitness. (2004). Protective eyewear for young athletes. *Pediatrics, 113,* 619–622.

Coody, D., Banks, J. M., Yetman, R. J., & Musgrove, K. (1997). Eye trauma in children: Epidemiology, management, and prevention. *Journal of Pediatric Health Care,* 11, 182–188.

Curns, A. T., Holman, R. C., Shay, D. K., Cheek, J. E., Kaufman, S. F., Singleton, R. J., & Anderson, L. J. (2002). Outpatient and hospital visits associated with otitis media among American Indian and Alaska Native children younger than 5 years. *Pediatrics, 109*(3). www.pediatrics.org/cgi/content/full/109/3/e41

DeRespinis, P. A. (2001). Eyeglasses: Why and when do children need them? *Pediatric Annals, 30,* 455–461.

Diangelis, A. J., & Bakland, L. K. (1998). Traumatic dental injuries: Current treatment concepts. *Journal of the American Dental Association, 129,* 1401–1414.

Duchene, T. M. (2000). Managing sinusitis in children. *Nurse Practitioner, 25*(9), 42–55.

Ertmer, D. J., Young, N., Grohne, K., Mellon, J. A., Johnson, C., Corbett, K., & Saindon, K. (2002). Vocal development in young children with cochlear implants: Profiles and implications for intervention. *Language, Speech & Hearing Services in Schools, 33,* 184–195.

Feder, H. M. (2001). Acute pharyngitis: Fitting the drug to the bug. *Contemporary Pediatrics, 8,* 41–59.

Folmer, R. L. (2003). The importance of hearing conservation instruction. *Journal of School Nursing, 19,* 140–148.

Garrelts, L., & Melnyk, B. M. (2001). Pacifier usage and acute otitis media in infants and young children. *Pediatric Nursing,* 27, 516–518.

Gibson, F. & Nelson, N. (2000). Mouthcare for children with cancer. *Paediatric Nursing, 12,* 18–22.

Gold, L. S., & Slone, T. H. (2003). Aristolochic acid, an herbal carcinogen, sold on the Web after FDA alert. *New England Journal of Medicine, 349,* 1576–1577.

Gomez, S., & Davis, R. L. (2001). Photoscreening—A viable method for referral. *School Nurse News, 18*(1), 18–20.

Good, W. V., & Gendron, R. L. (2001). Retinopathy of prematurity. *Ophthalmology Clinics of North America, 14,* 513–519.

Gross, R. D. (2002). Understanding ocular infections and strategies for management. *Contemporary Pediatrics,* Supplement, 4–7, 10–12.

Halle, C. (2002). Achieve new vision screening objectives. *Nurse Practitioner, 27*(3), 15–37.

Hayes, D. (1999). State programs for universal newborn hearing screening. *Pediatric Clinics of North America, 46,* 89–94.

Hayes, R. O. (2001). Pediatric sinusitis. *Clinician Reviews* 11(10), 53–58.

Hoberman, A., & Paradise, J. L. (2000). Acute otitis media: Diagnosis and management in the year 2000. *Pediatric Annals, 29,* 609–620.

Hoberman, A., Marchant, C. D., Kaplan, S. L., & Feldman, S. (2002). Treatment of acute otitis media consensus recommendations. *Clinical Pediatrics, 41,* 373–390.

Jackson, J. M., & Mourino, A. P. (1999). Pacifier use and otitis media in infants twelve months of age and younger. *Pediatric Dentistry, 21,* 256–260.

Joint Committee on Infant Hearing. (2000). Joint Committee on Infant Hearing 2000 Position Statement: Principles and guidelines for early hearing detection and intervention programs. *Pediatrics, 106,* 798–817.

Kakish, K. S., Mahafza, T., Batieha, A., Ekteish, F., & Daoud, A. (2000). Clinical sinusitis in children attending primary care centers. *Pediatric Infectious Disease Journal, 19,* 1071–1074.

Leung, A. K. C., & Kellner, J. D. (2004). Acute sinusitis in children: Diagnosis and management. *Journal of Pediatric Health Care, 18,* 72–76.

Lieberman, L. J., & McHugh, E. (2001). Health-related fitness of children who are visually impaired. *Journal of Visual Impairment & Blindness, 5,* 272–287.

Mills, M. D. (1998). Perianesthesia care of adult and pediatric strabismus surgery patients. *Journal of PeriAnesthesia Nursing, 13,* 16–25.

Nance, W. E., Cunningham, G. C., Davis, J. G., Morton, C. C., Elsas, L. J., Finitzo, T., Falk, R. E., Ing, P. S., Pandya, A., McCabe, E. R. B., & Smith, R. J. H. (2000). Statement of the American College of Medical Genetics on Universal Newborn Hearing Screening. *Genetics in Medicine, 2,* 149–150.

National Institutes of Health (1995). Consensus statement: Cochlear implants. Accessed 9/20/04 from http://consensus.nih.gov/cons/100/100—intro.htm.

Nelson, L. M. (2003). Temperature-controlled radiofrequency tonsil reduction in children. *Archives of Otolaryngology—Head & Neck Surgery, 129,* 533–537.

Newland, J. A., & Rich, E. (1998). Epistaxis. *American Journal of Nursing, 98,* 16HHH.

Niemela, M., Pihakari, O., Pokka, T., Uhari, M. S., & Uhari, M. S. (2000). Pacifier as a risk factor for acute otitis media: A randomized, controlled trial of parental counseling. *Pediatrics, 106,* 483–488.

Niemela, M., Uhari, M., & Mottonen, M. (1995). A pacifier increases the risk of recurrent acute otitis media in children in day-care centers. *Pediatrics, 96,* 884–888.

Niskar, A. S., Kieszak, S. M., Holmes, A. E., Esteban, E., Rubin, C., & Brody, D. J. (2001). Estimated prevalence of noise-induced hearing threshold shifts among children 6 to 19 years of age: The third national health and nutrition examination survey, 1988–1994, United States. *Pediatrics, 108,* 40–43.

Otitis media with effusion, clinical practice guideline. (2004). *Pediatrics, 113,* 1412–1429.

Paradise, J. L., Bluestone, C. D., Colborn, K., Bernard, B. S., Rockette, H. E., & Kurs-Lasky, M. (2002). Tonsillectomy and adenotonsillectomy for recurrent throat infection in moderately affected children. *Pediatrics, 110,* 7–15.

Phelps, D. L., & Watts, J. L. (2003). Early light reduction for preventing retinopathy of prematurity in very low birth weight infants. *Cochrane Library, 2,* 1–15.

Roberts, J. E., Burchinal, M. R., & Zeisel, S. A. (2002). Otitis media in early childhood in relation to children's school-age language and academic skills. *Pediatrics, 110,* 696–706.

Rudy, C. A. (2001). Dental trauma. *School Nurse News, 18*(1), 33–35.

Sagraves, R. (2002). Increasing antibiotic resistance: its effect on the therapy for otitis media. *Journal of Pediatric Health Care, 16,* 79–87.

Sarrell, E. M., Mandelberg, A., & Cohen, H. A. (2001). Efficacy of naturopathic extracts in the management of ear pain associated with acute otitis media. *Archives of Pediatric and Adolescent Medicine, 155,* 796–799.

Sinus and Allergy Health Partnership. (2000). Antimicrobial treatment guidelines for acute bacterial rhinosinusitis. *Otolaryngology and Head and Neck Surgery, 123,* 5–31.

Slattery, W. H., & Fayad, J. N. (1999). Cochlear implants in children with sensorineural inner ear hearing loss. *Pediatric Annals, 28,* 359–363.

Starr, N. B. (2000). Vision therapy for learning disabilities and dyslexia. *Journal of Pediatric Health Care, 14,* 32–33.

Stephenson, M. (2003). Mucopurulent discharge is good sign conjunctivitis is bacterial. *Infectious Diseases in Children, 3,* 32–33.

Taylor, J. A., Weber, W., Standish, L., Quinn, H., Goesling, J., McGann, J., & Calabrese, C. (2003). Efficacy and safety of Echinacea in treating upper respiratory tract infections in children: A randomized controlled trial. *Journal of the American Medical Association, 290,* 2824–2830.

Troster, H. (2001). Sources of stress in mothers of young children with visual impairments. *Journal of Visual Impairment & Blindness, 10,* 623–637.

U.S. Department of Health and Human Services. (2000). *Healthy People 2010* (2nd ed.). Washington, DC: U.S. Government Printing Office. www.healthypeople.gov.

United States Preventive Services Task Force. (2004). Screening for visual impairment in children younger than age 5 years. www/ahrq.gov/clinic/3rduspstf.visionscr/sicshrs.htm, accessed 6/1/2004.

Vohr, B. R., Widen, J. E., Cone-Wesson, B., Sininger, Y. S., Gorga, M. P., Folsom, R. C., & Norton, S. J. (2000). Identification of neonatal hearing impairment: Characteristics of infants in the neonatial intensive care unit and well-baby nursery. *Ear & Hearing, 21,* 373–382.

Walter, W. E., Cunningham, G. C., Davis, J. G., Morton, C. C., Elsas, L. J., Finitzo, T., Fack, R. E., Ing, P. S., Pandya, A., McCabe, E. R.B., & Smith, R. J.H. (2000). Statement of the American College of Medical Genetics on universal newborn hearing screening *Genetics in Medicine* 2, 149–150.

Wheatley, C. M., Dickinson, J. L., Mackey, D. A., Craing, J. E., & Sale, M. M. (2002). Retinopathy of prematurity: Recent advances in our understanding. *Archives of Disease in Childhood, 87,* F78-F82.

Zacharyczuk, C. (2004, April). New guidelines outline AOM management options. *Infectious Diseases in Children,* 24.

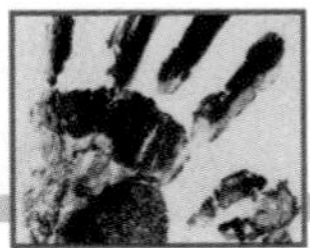

ADDITIONAL REFERENCES

Agency for Healthcare Research and Quality. (2001). Management of acute otitis media (AHRQ Publication No. 00-E010). Rockville, MD: Author.

Bacal, D. A., & Wilson, M. C. (2000). Strabismus: Getting it straight. *Contemporary Pediatrics, 2,* 49–60.

Beck, A. D. (2001). Diagnosis and management of pediatric glaucoma. *Ophthalmology Clinics of North America, 14,* 501–512.

Butler, C. C., & van der Voort, J. H. (2001). Steroids for otitis media with effusion. *Archives of Pediatric and Adolescent Medicine, 155,* 641–647.

Chan, L. S., Takata, G. S., Shekelle, P., Morton, S. C., Mason, W., & Marcy, S. M. (2001). Evidence assessment of management of acute otitis media: Research gaps and priorities for future research. *Pediatrics, 108,* 248–254.

Clarkson, L. J. (2002). Retinopathy of prematurity: Current treatment options. *Journal of Neonntal Nursing 8,* 7–10.

Clinical treatment guideline: Retropharyngeal & parapharyngeal abscess. http://chwebapps. Tch. harvard.edu/cpg/rpa_cov.html, accessed 5/19/2003.

Hall, J. W. (2000). Infant hearing impairment and universal hearing screening. *Journal of Perinatology, 20,* S113-S121.

Leibovitz, E., Greenberg, D., Piglansky, L., Raiz, S., Porat, N., Press, J., Leiberman, A., & Dagan, R. (2003). Recurrent acute otitis media occurring within one month from completion of antibiotic therapy: Relationship to the original pathogen. *Pediatric Infectious Disease Journal, 22,* 209–216.

Little, P., Gould, C., Williamson, I., Moore, M., Warner, G., & Dunleavey, J. (2001). Pragmatic randomized controlled trial of two prescribing strategies for childhood acute otitis media. *British Medical Journal, 322,* 336–342.

Magnuson, M., & Hergils, L. (2000). Late diagnosis of congential hearing impariment in children: The parents' experiences and opinions. *Patient Education and Counseling, 41,* 285–294.

Mandel, E. M., Casselbrant, M. L., Rockette, H. E., Fireman, P., Kurs-Lasky, M., & Bluestone, C. D. (2002). Systemic steroid for chronic otitis media with effusion in children. *Pediatrics, 110,* 1071–1080.

McCracken, G. H. (2002). Diagnosis and management of acute otitis media in the urgent care setting. *Annals of Emergency Medicine, 39,* 413–421.

MMWR. (2003). Infants tested for hearing loss—United States, 1999–2001. *Morbidity and Mortality Weekly Report, 52,* 981–984.

Nickerson, B. (2002). Nursing care of the pediatric patient following strabismus repair surgery. *Insight, 27,* 64–65.

Norton, S. J., Gorga, M. P., Widen, J. E., Folsom, R. C., Sininger, Y., Cone-Wesson, B., Vohr, B. R., & Fletcher, K. A. (2000). Identification of neonatal hearing impairment: Summary and recommendations. *Ear & Hearing, 21,* 529–535.

Paradise, J. L., Feldman, H. M., Campbell, T. F., Dollaghan, C. A., Colburn, D. K., Bernard, B. S., Rockette, H. E., Janosky, J. E., Pitcairn, D. L., Sabo, D. L., Kurs-Lasky, M., & Smith, C. G. (2001). Effect of early or delayed insertion of tympanostomy tubes for persistent otitis media on developmental outcome at the age of 3 years. *New England Journal of Medicine, 344,* 1170–1187.

Ramsey, A. M. (2002). Diagnosis and treatment of the child with a draining ear. *Journal of Pediatric Health Care, 16,* 161–169.

Roberts, G., Scully, C., & Shotts, R. (2000). ABC of oral health: Dental emergencies. *British Medical Journal, 321,* 559–562.

Siegel, R. M., Kiely, M., & Bien, J. P. (2003). Treatment of otitis media with observation and a safety-net antibiotic prescription. *Pediatrics, 112,* 527–531.

Takata, G. S., Chan, L. S., Shekelle, P., Morton, S. C., Mason, W., & Marcy, S. M. (2001). Evidence assessment of management of acute otitis media: The role of antibiotics in treatment of uncomplicated acute otitis media. *Pediatrics, 108,* 239–247.

Waldman, H. B., Periman, S. P., & Swerdloff, M. (2000). Orthodontics and the population with special needs. *American Journal of Dentofacial Orthoptics, 118,* 14–17.

Chapter

25 Alterations in Respiratory Function

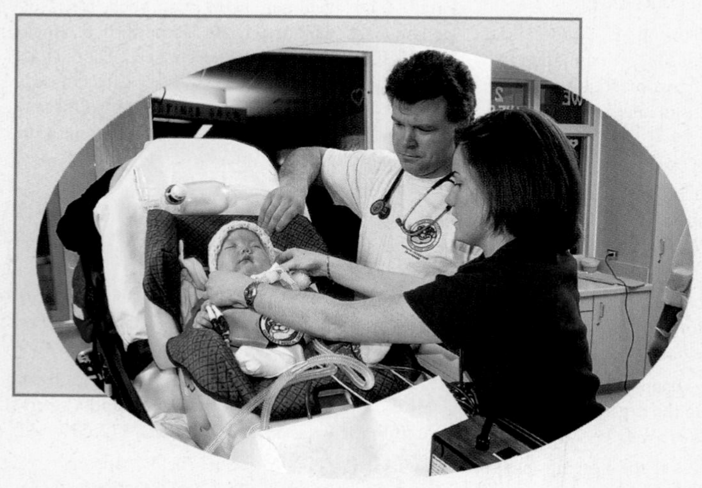

Emily Chow, a 6-month-old infant with bronchopulmonary dysplasia, lives at home with her mother and two siblings who are 4 and 8 years old. Emily has a tracheostomy and receives humidified oxygen. When Emily developed a fever, labored breathing, and more secretions than usual in the tracheostomy, her mother called for an urgent care visit with Emily's healthcare provider.

When Emily is initially seen by the office nurse, her temperature is 38.8°C (102°F), her respiratory rate is 50, and her heart rate is 130. Intercostal and substernal retractions are visible, and crackles can be heard over the lower right lobe. The nurse assists Emily's mother in suctioning her tracheostomy as the secretions seem to be excessive. Because of her respiratory signs, the nurse moves Emily ahead of other children waiting to be seen by the physician. After assessing Emily, the physician believes that her respiratory distress may worsen. She may need oxygen supplementation as well as IV fluids and medication that cannot be provided in the office setting. A chest radiograph is also needed for diagnosis. While the physician coordinates Emily's transfer to the hospital's short-stay unit for observation and treatment, the office nurse talks with Emily's mother, who has become increasingly anxious. The nurse listens to her concerns, provides support, and makes sure she understands the reason for the planned transfer. The nurse also obtains consent to provide all documentation from this visit and important historical information to the pediatric transport team that transfers Emily to the hospital.

"Mom spends a lot of time taking care of Emily. I try to help as much as I can. I help to listen and make sure she does not have trouble breathing when she takes a nap. Then I try to play with her when she is awake."

—Isabel, age 8

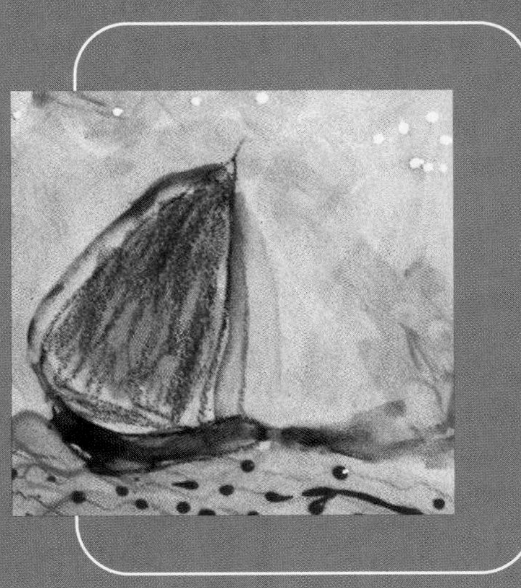

Learning Outcomes

After completing this chapter, you will be able to:

- Describe unique characteristics of the pediatric respiratory system anatomy and physiology and apply that information to the care of children with respiratory conditions.
- Define the different respiratory conditions and injuries that can cause respiratory distress in infants and children.
- Assess the child's respiratory signs and symptoms to distinguish between mild, moderate, and severe respiratory distress and describe the appropriate nursing care for each level of severity.
- Describe different methods to evaluate the infant and child with a respiratory condition.
- Synthesize information and develop a nursing care plan in partnership with the family for a child with common acute respiratory conditions.
- Synthesize information and develop a nursing care plan in partnership with the family for a child with a chronic respiratory condition.

Key Terms

adventitious sounds/825
airway remodeling/859
airway resistance/821
alveolar hypoventilation/826
apnea/829
atelectasis/842
bronchiolitis obliterans/876
cor pulmonale/833
dysphagia/840
dysphonia/840
dyspnea/823
grunting/829
hypercapnia/826
hypoxemia/826
hypoxia/827
laryngospasm/837
paradoxical breathing/825
periodic breathing/829
polysomnography/834
pulsus paradoxus/859
retractions/822
stridor/836
tachypnea/823
tidal volume/832
tracheostomy/828
trigger/859

MediaLink http://www.prenhall.com/ball

Resources for this chapter can be found on the CD-ROM accompanying this textbook, and on the Companion Website at www.prenhall.com/ball. Click on Chapter 25 to select the activities for this chapter.

CD-ROM

Animations/Videos

- *Alternative Asthma Treatments*
- *Asthma*
- *Carbon Dioxide Transport*
- *Cystic Fibrosis*
- *Gas Exchange in the Lung*
- *Lung Sounds*
- *Passive Smoke Exposure*
- *Pediatric Respiratory Emergency Management*
- *SIDS*

Nursing in Action

- *Apnea Monitor*
- *Endotracheal Tube Suctioning*
- *Pulse Oximetry and Oxygen Delivery Systems*
- *Using a Metered Dose Inhaler*

NCLEX Review

Audio Glossary

COMPANION WEBSITE

A & P Review

Clinical Manifestations Review

Medication Match-Up

NCLEX Review

Care Plan: The Child with Bronchopulmonary Dysplasia

Care Plan: The Child with Cystic Fibrosis

MediaLink Applications

- *Determine the Respiratory Risks in a Childcare Setting*
- *Teaching Plan: Dust Mites*
- *Teaching Plan: Educating Asthmatics Based on Severity*
- *Teaching Plan: Metered-Dose Inhaler*

This chapter explores several special factors in the child's respiratory system that create ongoing threats to respiratory function and overall health. Most respiratory problems in children produce mild symptoms, last a short time, and can be managed at home. Other respiratory conditions are chronic and have a significant impact on the child's growth and development. Pediatric respiratory conditions may occur as a primary problem or as a complication of nonrespiratory conditions. They may be life threatening or have long-term implications. Acute respiratory problems are the most common cause of illness requiring hospitalization in infants and children under 10 years of age and a leading cause of hospitalization in children between 10 and 15 years of age (Health Resources and Services Administration, 2002).

Respiratory conditions may be a result of structural problems, functional problems, or a combination of both. Structural problems involve alterations in the size and shape of parts of the respiratory tract. Functional problems involve alterations in gas exchange and threats to this normal process from irritants (such as large particles and chemicals) or invaders (such as viruses or bacteria). Alterations in other organ systems, especially the immune and neurologic systems, may also threaten respiratory function. Nurses must learn to assess the child's current respiratory status quickly, monitor progress, and anticipate potential complications. When reading this chapter, keep in mind the distinction between structural and functional problems to help you understand what is normal and what is abnormal about the child's maturing respiratory system. Refer to Chapter 24 ∞ for information on upper respiratory conditions such as colds, otitis media, sinusitis, and pharyngitis.

ANATOMY AND PHYSIOLOGY OF PEDIATRIC DIFFERENCES

The child's respiratory tract constantly grows and changes until about 12 years of age. The young child's neck is shorter than an adult's, resulting in airway structures that are closer together.

AS THEY GROW

Comparison of Airway Structures

Smaller nasopharynx, easily occluded during infection.
Lymph tissue (tonsils, adenoids) grows rapidly in early childhood; atrophies after age 12.
Smaller nares, easily occluded.
Small oral cavity and large tongue increase risk of obstruction.
Long, floppy epiglottis vulnerable to swelling with resulting obstruction.
Larynx and glottis are higher in neck, increasing risk of aspiration.
Because thyroid, cricoid, and tracheal cartilages are immature, they may easily collapse when neck is flexed.
Because fewer muscles are functional in airway, it is less able to compensate for edema, spasm, and trauma.
The large amounts of soft tissue and loosely anchored mucous membranes lining the airway increase risk of edema and obstruction.

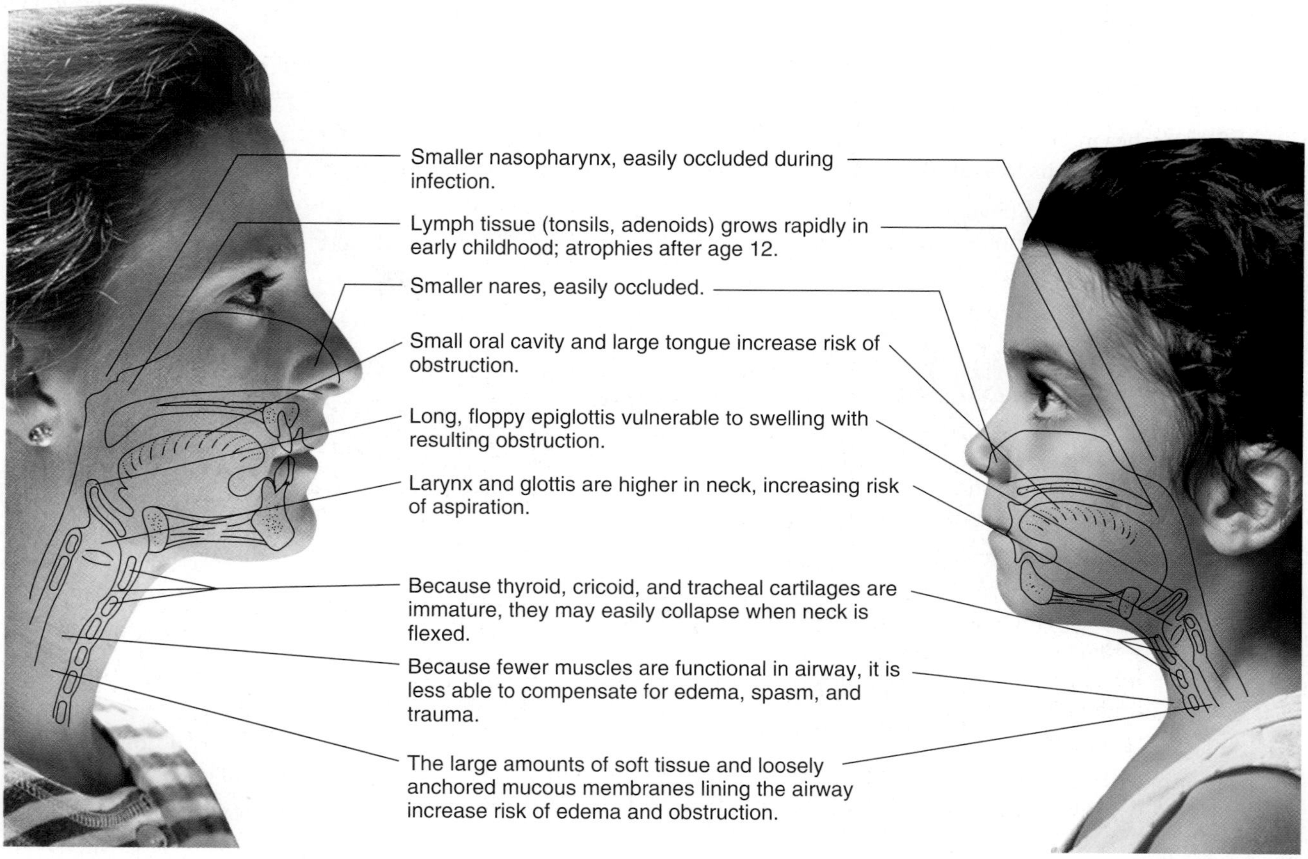

FIGURE 25–1 ■ It is easy to see that a child's airway is smaller and less developed than an adult's airway, but why is this important? The infant and child are more vulnerable to the consequences of an upper respiratory tract infection, enlarged tonsils and adenoids, an allergic reaction, positioning of the head and neck during sleep, and small objects that can be aspirated. All can cause an airway obstruction that results in respiratory distress.

TABLE 25–1 Summary of Upper Airway Differences Between Children and Adults

DIFFERENCE IN CHILDREN	SIGNIFICANCE
Small oral cavity and large tongue	Increases risk of obstruction; nasal patency is critical in infants
Newborns and young infants are nose breathers	Will not automatically open mouth to breathe if nose is obstructed. Nasal passages must be kept patent.
Rapid growth of lymph tissue (tonsils and adenoids) during early childhood, atrophy after age 12	Larger tissues in smaller pharyngeal structures; infection can easily cause obstruction of upper airway as lymph tissues swell in response
Larynx and glottis high in neck	Increases chance of aspiration
Thyroid, cricoid, and tracheal cartilages immature and incomplete	Easily collapse when neck is flexed, further narrowing airway; less protective of glottis
Large amount of soft tissue and loosely anchored mucous membranes lining length of airway	Increases likelihood of airway edema and obstruction
Long, floppy epiglottis	Vulnerable to swelling with resultant obstruction
Fewer functional muscles in the airways	Less able to compensate for edema, spasm, and trauma; may swallow more mucus than able to sneeze or cough out

Upper Airway Differences

The child's tracheal airway is shorter and narrower than an adult's airway. These differences create a greater potential for obstruction (Figure 25–1 ■ and Table 25–1). The infant's airway is approximately 4 mm in diameter, about the width of a drinking straw or the diameter of the infant's little finger, in contrast to the adult's airway diameter of 20 mm. The upper airway increases in length rather than diameter during the first 5 years of life. The trachea in a child is higher and at a different angle than the adult's (Figure 25–2 ■).

The **airway resistance,** the effort or force needed to move oxygen through the trachea to the lungs, is greater in the child's narrower airway than in an adult (Figure 25–3 ■). As air moves from the child's nares down the trachea to the distal airways (alveoli), it must flow through a relatively small area. Friction and increasing resistance are generated as air passes through the airway. When edema and swelling of the trachea occur in response to a virus, bacterium, or other irritant, the airway is further narrowed, and air is inspired more quickly to maintain oxygenation status. The resulting negative pressure in the airway draws tissues closer together, further narrowing the airway and increasing airway resistance.

Physiologically the upper airway is the port for inspiration of oxygen and expiration of carbon dioxide. Infants, children, and adults can breathe through either the nose or the mouth. Until at least 4 weeks of age, newborns are obligatory nose breathers. The coordination of mouth breathing is controlled by maturing neurologic pathways; thus, young infants do not automatically open the mouth to breathe when the nose is obstructed. The only time newborns breathe through the mouth is when they cry. Nasal patency in newborns is therefore essential for activities such as breathing and eating.

Lower Airway Differences

While the tracheobronchial tree is complete at birth, the child's lower airway is also constantly growing. At birth, the lung tissue contains only 25 million alveoli, which are not fully developed. The number of alveoli increases to 300 million by

AS THEY GROW

Trachea Position

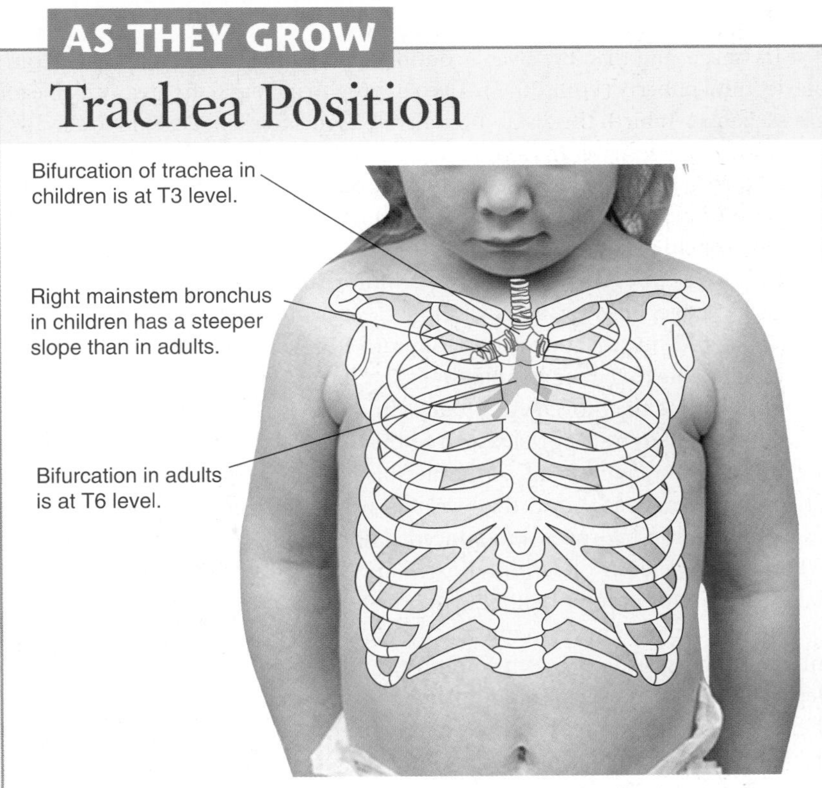
Bifurcation of trachea in children is at T3 level.
Right mainstem bronchus in children has a steeper slope than in adults.
Bifurcation in adults is at T6 level.

FIGURE 25–2 ■ In children, the trachea is shorter and the angle of the right bronchus at bifurcation is more acute than in the adult. Where is an aspirated foreign body likely to land? When you are resuscitating or suctioning, you must allow for the differences in the length of the trachea as it is easier to slip into the right bronchus with an endotracheal tube or suction catheter.

MediaLink A & P Review

PATHOPHYSIOLOGY ILLUSTRATED
Airway Diameter

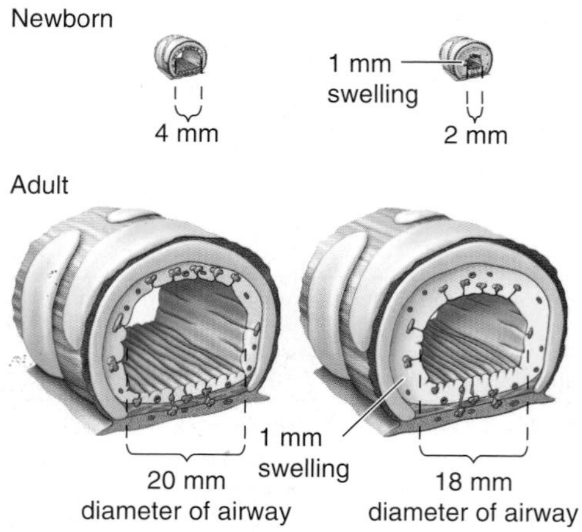

FIGURE 25–3 ■ The diameter of an infant's airway is approximately 4 mm, in contrast to an adult's airway diameter of 20 mm. An inflammatory process in the airway causes swelling that narrows the airway, and airway resistance increases. Note that swelling of 1 mm reduces the infant's airway diameter to 2 mm, but the adult's airway diameter is only narrowed to 18 mm. Air must move more quickly in the infant's narrowed airway to get the same amount of air to the lungs. The friction of the quickly moving air against the side of the airway increases airway resistance. The infant must use more effort to breathe and breathe faster to get adequate oxygen.

8 years of age, and then the alveoli continue developing in size, shape, and complexity until puberty (Froh, 2002). Alveolar growth increases the area available for gas exchange. At birth the distal (peripheral) bronchioles that extend to the alveoli are narrow and fewer in number than in an adult. The child's overall growth can be correlated to the increased branching of the peripheral bronchioles as the alveoli continue to multiply. The taller the child, the greater the lung surface area.

The bronchi and bronchioles are lined with smooth muscle. The newborn does not have enough smooth muscle bundles to help trap airway invaders. By 5 months of age, however, sufficient muscles exist to react to irritants by bronchospasm and muscle contraction. Smooth muscle development is complete and comparable to that of an adult by 1 year of age (Webster & Huether, 1998).

Ventilation is the movement of air in and out of the lungs and alveoli. The circulatory system transports oxygen to the tissues and carbon dioxide back to the lungs for the gas exchange at the alveolar-pulmonary capillary membranes. Chemoreceptors respond to the levels of arterial oxygen and carbon dioxide levels and to the hydrogen ion concentration in the blood and spinal fluid. When excessive levels of carbon dioxide are detected, the chemoreceptors signal the respiratory center that regulates the respiratory muscles.

The lungs, which have no muscles of their own, rely on the diaphragm and intercostal muscles to power respiration. Children up to 6 years are primarily dependent upon the diaphragm to breathe. The negative pressure caused by the downward movement of the diaphragm draws in air, and the abdomen rises as the abdominal contents are slightly compressed. The intercostal muscles increase the chest diameter. As the ribs are primarily cartilage and very flexible, and the intercostal muscles are less strong, their efficiency in assisting ventilation is reduced. In cases of respiratory distress the increased effort to move air through a narrower airway with increased airway resistance causes **retractions,** seen as indentations between the ribs during inspiration. See Figure 25–4 ■ for sites of retractions associated with respiratory distress.

MediaLink CO_2 and O_2 Transport Animation

From the moment a child is born, airway integrity is vulnerable because of the immaturity of the respiratory muscles and neurologic system. For example, preterm and full-term infants respond differently to hypoxia and elevated P_{CO_2} levels than adults. Preterm infants' response to hypoxia is blunted, further depressing the respiratory center's sensitivity to an elevated carbon dioxide level. As a consequence, these infants have a diminished rather than an increased inspiratory effort (Head & Bhatia, 2000).

RESPIRATORY DISTRESS AND RESPIRATORY FAILURE

Many conditions associated with the respiratory system progress from difficulty breathing to respiratory distress, and if the condition is not managed, it progresses to respiratory failure. Recognition of the child's respiratory signs and symptoms is critical in ensuring that appropriate care is provided to prevent the progression to respiratory failure. Foreign-body aspiration is a common cause of respiratory distress.

Foreign-Body Aspiration

Airway obstruction exists when air passage in the respiratory tract and lungs is slowed or blocked. Foreign-body aspiration is the inhalation of any object (solid or liquid, food or nonfood) into the respiratory tract. It is a major health problem for infants and young toddlers due to their increasing mobility and tendency to place small objects in the mouth. In young children aspiration occurs most often during feeding and reaching activities, while crawling, or during playtime. However, aspiration may occur in children of any age.

In 2001, 17,537 children 14 years of age and younger were treated in an emergency department for a choking-related episode. Rates were highest for infants less than 1 year of age and rates decreased with advancing age (Centers for Disease Control and Prevention [CDC], 2002). Foreign-body aspirations result in approximately 300 childhood deaths annually in the United States, and they are a common cause of unintentional injury death in the home among children under 6 years of age (Muniz & Joffe, 1999).

Etiology and Pathophysiology

In infants over 6 months of age and in children, aspiration may be caused by small objects that

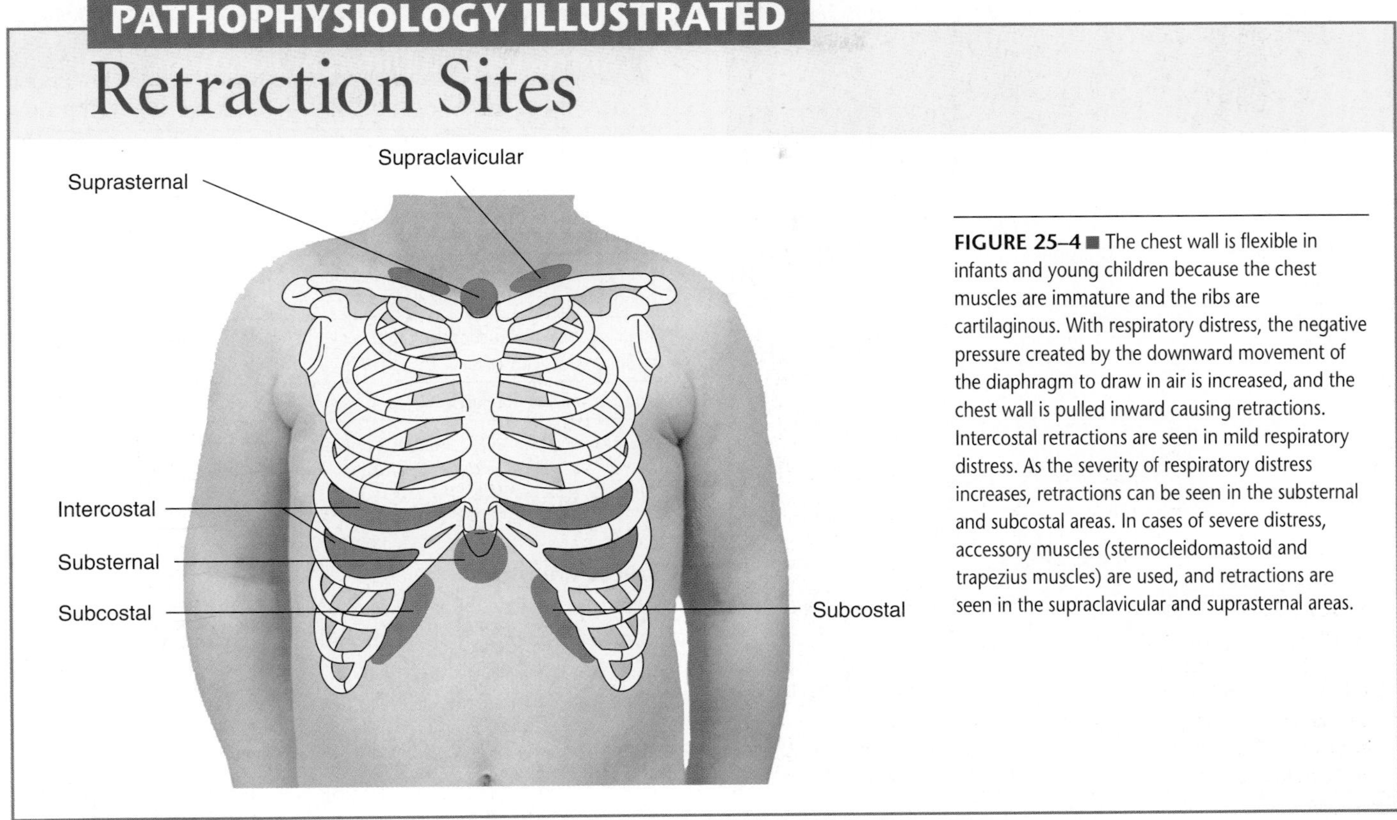

FIGURE 25–4 ■ The chest wall is flexible in infants and young children because the chest muscles are immature and the ribs are cartilaginous. With respiratory distress, the negative pressure created by the downward movement of the diaphragm to draw in air is increased, and the chest wall is pulled inward causing retractions. Intercostal retractions are seen in mild respiratory distress. As the severity of respiratory distress increases, retractions can be seen in the substernal and subcostal areas. In cases of severe distress, accessory muscles (sternocleidomastoid and trapezius muscles) are used, and retractions are seen in the supraclavicular and suprasternal areas.

enter the child's mouth. Common aspirated items include the following:

- Foods such as nuts, popcorn, hard candy, or small pieces of raw vegetables or hot dog
- Small, loose toy parts such as wheels and bells
- Household objects and substances such as beads, safety pins, coins, buttons, balloon pieces, colorful liquids (mouthwash, perfume), and enticing packages (small screw bottle tops)

Many aspirations occur when the young child who has something in the mouth takes a deep and rapid inspiration after bumping the head or falling. Partial and sometimes complete airway obstruction may occur.

The severity of the obstruction depends on the size and composition of the object or substance and its location within the respiratory tract. The majority of aspirated foreign bodies (AFBs) usually cause bronchial, not tracheal, obstruction. An object lodged high in the airway above the vocal cords is frequently coughed out easily or with some assistance (such as use of chest thrusts and back blows or the abdominal thrust). The right lung is the more common site of lower airway aspiration because of the sloped angle of its bronchus (see Figure 25–2 ■). Objects may migrate from higher to lower airway locations. An object may also move back up to the trachea, creating extreme respiratory difficulty. An object lodged in the trachea is a life-threatening situation. If oxygen is depleted for an extended time, brain damage may occur.

Clinical Manifestations

The child may initially have spasmodic coughing, or gagging without fever or other symptoms of illness. The child may have signs of increased respiratory effort such as **dyspnea** (difficulty breathing), **tachypnea** (increased respiratory rate), nasal flaring, and retractions (a visible drawing in of the skin of the neck and between the ribs of the chest, which occurs on inspiration in infants and young children in respiratory distress). As respiratory distress progresses, the child may have a concentrated focus on breathing, have an anxious expression, and sit in a forward position with the neck extended, as if to straighten out the airway. Retractions may not be present if air movement is diminished. As the child becomes increasingly hypoxic, behavior changes such as irritability and decreased responsiveness will be seen.

The older child who aspirates and has an airway obstruction may clutch the neck—the universal sign for choking (Figure 25–5 ■). In some cases, the child becomes asymptomatic after coughing for 15 to 30 minutes as the airway adapts to the foreign body. Coughing, choking, gagging, dysphonia, and wheezing may be brief or may persist for several hours if the object drops below the trachea into one of the mainstem bronchi. See the clinical manifestations table on page 824 for signs associated with obstructions in various locations of the airway. If the foreign body drops into the lower airway and is not removed, the child may present weeks later with complications of the aspiration such as a chronic cough, persistent or recurrent pneumonia, or a lung abscess.

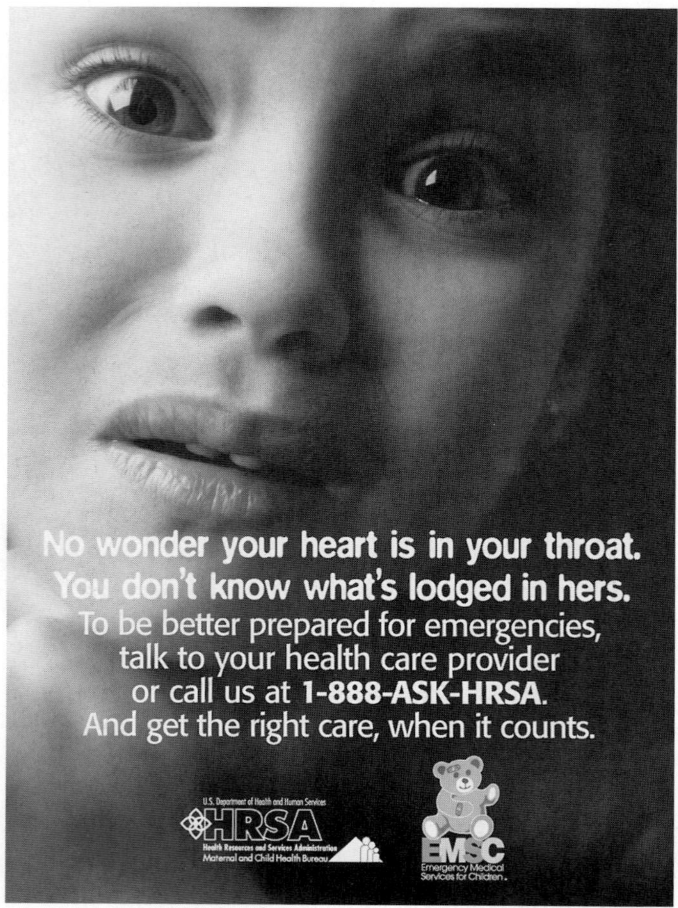

FIGURE 25–5 ■ The universal sign of choking is grabbing the neck. The individual who is choking is usually panicky because of the inability to breathe.
Courtesy of Health Resources and Services Administration, Maternal and Child Health Bureau, Emergency Medical Services for Children.

COLLABORATIVE CARE

Initial management is focused on maintaining a patent airway and relieving the airway obstruction.

Diagnostic Tests

Children are usually brought to the hospital after a sudden episode of coughing. Discovery of an open container with small objects may prompt parents to seek medical assistance for the child. Clinical therapy focuses on taking a careful history to determine whether aspiration has actually occurred. Choking associated with feeding or crawling on the floor is usually a confirming event. The physical examination often reveals decreased breath sounds, stridor, and respiratory distress in the child without a witnessed aspiration.

A chest radiograph is performed. When the object aspirated is radiopaque, it can be seen on the radiograph (Figure 25–6 ■). A special chest radiograph, called a forced expiratory film, may also be ordered. This shows abnormalities caused by the foreign body, such as local hyperinflation (air trapping) and a mediastinal shift away from the affected side (Hazinski, 1999).

CLINICAL MANIFESTATIONS of Airway Obstructions in Different Locations

LOCATION OF AIRWAY OBSTRUCTION	CLINICAL MANIFESTATION
Nasopharyngeal obstruction, enlarged tonsils or adenoids	Sonorous snoring
Partially obstructed upper airway (in the larynx, subglottic space, and upper trachea)	Inspiratory stridor
Obstruction of the mid to lower trachea and central bronchus	Expiratory stridor or wheeze
Supralaryngeal obstruction, epiglottitis or retropharyngeal abscess	Muffled voice
Croup or tracheal foreign body	Harsh, barking cough

Data from Froh, D.K. (2002). Alterations in pulmonary function in children. In McCance, K. L. & Huether, S. E., Pathophysiology: The Biological Basis for Disease in Adults and Children, *(4th ed.) St. Louis: Mosby, p. 1149.*

Clinical Therapy

When total airway obstruction occurs, efforts to clear the obstruction include back blows and chest thrusts in an infant. Abdominal thrusts are used on older children. In the emergency department, oxygen is administered. Efforts are made to visualize the foreign

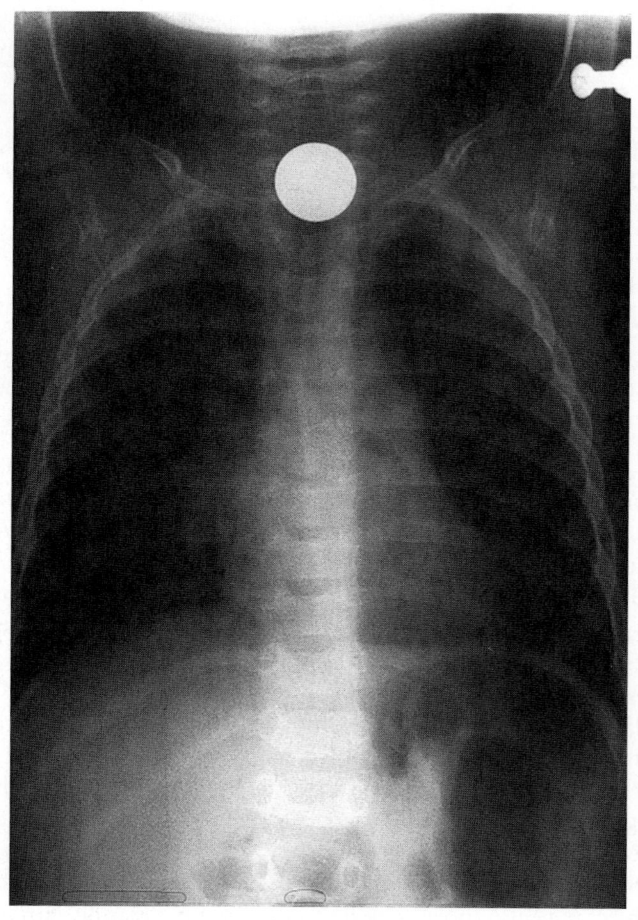

FIGURE 25–6 ■ An aspirated foreign body (coin) is clearly visible in the child's trachea on this chest radiograph.
Courtesy of Rockwood Clinic, Spokane, WA.

body with a laryngoscope and remove it with Magill forceps. When possible, the child is taken to the operating room so that optimal conditions exist to protect and maintain the child's airway during removal of the foreign body. When a partial airway obstruction exists, fluoroscopy and fiber-optic bronchoscopy may be used to identify, locate, and extract the foreign body.

Following removal of the foreign body, the child is stabilized and observed for a few hours in a short-stay unit. Depending on the type of object, location of the object, and degree of obstruction, surgical removal and hospitalization may be required. See the section on pneumonia, page 850, for clinical therapy for the child with complications due to aspiration.

NURSING MANAGEMENT

Nursing management is focused on assessment and monitoring the child until the obstruction can be removed, supporting the child and family during the crisis, and preventing future airway obstructions.

Nursing Assessment and Diagnosis

Physiologic Assessment

The child will be in respiratory distress. Perform the respiratory assessment following guidelines in Box 25–1 and Table 25–2. If the object remains lodged in the airway, observe the child for increasing signs of respiratory distress, especially vital signs and audible wheezing on auscultation. Identify the types of retractions present to help determine the severity of respiratory distress. If the obstruction occurs above the trachea, inspiration is more affected. If the obstruction occurs below the trachea, expiration is more affected.

CLINICAL TIP

If the child cannot say "P" in words like *Pluto* or *Peter Pan,* the expiratory effort is noticeably diminished as a result of the foreign body.

Changes in breath sounds, from noisy to decreasing to absent, on the affected side are noted. This can indicate that the object is moving and blocking a mainstem bronchus.

PRACTICE ALERT

The depth and location of retractions is associated with the severity of respiratory distress. Isolated intercostal retractions indicate mild distress. Subcostal, suprasternal, and supraclavicular retractions indicate moderate distress. These retractions accompanied by use of accessory muscles in the neck indicate severe distress.

Attach the child to a cardiorespiratory monitor and pulse oximeter to assess the child for subtle signs of increasing hypoxia associated with the obstruction. See Box 25–2 for guidelines to increase the accuracy of pulse oximeter readings. Constant assessment is performed as the child may develop a complete obstruction.

PRACTICE ALERT

The following signs and symptoms signal the body's response to increased metabolic demands for oxygenation as a result of stress or impending illness.

- Increasing restlessness, irritability, unexplained sudden confusion
- Rapid heart rate accompanied by a rapid respiratory rate

Psychosocial Assessment

The unexpected and acute nature of the event creates anxiety for parents and child. The child will be anxious and fearful because

BOX 25–1 Assessment Guidelines for a Child in Respiratory Distress[a]

QUALITY OF RESPIRATIONS

- Inspect the rate, depth, and respiratory effort. (See Table 25–2 for expected respiratory rate ranges by age.)
- Identify the signs of respiratory distress: tachypnea (abnormally rapid rate of respirations), retractions, nasal flaring, inspiratory stridor, expiratory grunting.
- Note lack of simultaneous chest and abdominal rise with inspiration **(paradoxical breathing)**.
- Auscultate breath sounds. Note if they are bilateral, diminished or absent, if **adventitious sounds** are present (wheezes, crackles, rhonchi).
- Assess nasal patency in newborn.

QUALITY OF PULSE

- Assess the rate and rhythm. *Tachycardia may indicate hypoxia.*
- Compare pulse sites (apical to brachial) for strength and rate.

COLOR

- Observe overall color. With respiratory distress, color progresses from pallor to mottled to cyanosis. *Central cyanosis is a late sign of respiratory distress.*
- Compare peripheral and central color. Assess capillary refill and nailbed color and inspect mucous membranes. *Central cyanosis in mucous membranes is more ominous.*
- Note whether crying improves or worsens color.

COUGH

- Quality: note whether dry (nonproductive), wet (productive, mucousy), brassy (noisy, musical), croupy (barking, seal-like).
- Effort: note whether forceful or weak. *Weak cough may indicate an airway obstruction or fatigue from prolonged respiratory effort (not valid in newborns).*

BEHAVIOR CHANGE

- Note level of consciousness. *Lethargy may indicate hypoxia.*
- Restlessness and irritability are associated with hypoxia.
- Watch for abrupt behavior changes. *Restlessness, irritability, and lowered level of consciousness may indicate increasing hypoxia.*

SIGNS OF DEHYDRATION

- Inspect for dry mucous membranes, lack of tears, poor skin turgor, sunken fontanel in an infant, and decreased urine output, which indicate that fluid needs are not being met.

[a]Refer to Chapter 8 for the actual assessment techniques mentioned in this table.

MediaLink Pediatric Respiratory Emergency Management Video

TABLE 25–2 Normal Respiratory Rate Ranges by Age

AGE	RESPIRATORY RATE PER MINUTE
Newborn	30–60
1 year	20–40
3 years	20–30
6 years	16–22
10 years	16–20
17 years	12–20

of the difficulty breathing. Parents may be experiencing a variety of other emotions such as fear, anger, or guilt. Assess the family's level of distress and coping ability.

Developmental Assessment

As the child's condition stabilizes, observe how well the child's developmental abilities match the parents' understanding of age-appropriate behaviors. See Chapters 12 and 13∞.

Common nursing diagnoses for a child with an aspirated foreign body include the following:

- Ineffective Airway Clearance related to foreign-body aspiration
- Impaired Spontaneous Ventilation related to foreign-body aspiration and respiratory muscle fatigue
- Fear (parent or child) related to uncertainty of prognosis, unfamiliar surroundings, and procedures

■ Planning and Implementation

The period immediately after aspiration until the foreign body can be removed is critical, and subtle changes in the child's respiratory status during this period must be documented and reported promptly. A nurse must remain with the child who has significant airway obstruction, and emergency resuscitation equipment must be immediately accessible.

Allow the child to select the position of comfort. In many cases this will be sitting upright or a semi-Fowler's position. Avoid performing any procedures that will increase the child's anxiety or stress. Sudden movements or increased respiratory efforts may cause the obstruction to move and potentially completely obstruct the airway.

BOX 25–2 Guidelines for Increasing the Accuracy of Pulse Oximetry Readings

- Place the sensor probe over clean and dry skin that is exposed to minimal movement. Avoid sites with nail polish as this can interfere with the sensor.
- Avoid exposing the sensor probe to bright light or sunshine as this may falsely increase the reading.
- Make sure the heart rate detected by the pulse oximeter matches the child's heart rate by direct assessment for accuracy. The oximeter may be unable to accurately detect pulsatile blood flow if the extremity used is cool with vasoconstriction present, or if peripheral blood flow is decreased due to dysrhythmias or shock.

Note: Data from Popovich, D. M, Richiuso, N., & Danek, G. (2004). Pediatric health care providers' knowledge of pulse oximetry. Pediatric Nursing, *30(1), 14–20.*

MediaLink Nursing in Action: Pulse Oximetry and Oxygen Delivery Systems

Keep the child and family informed about planned procedures and provide them with emotional support. Provide a quiet environment and encourage the presence of the parents to help reduce the child's fear and anxiety.

Discharge Planning and Home Care Teaching

Prevention of future foreign-body aspirations is a major focus for nursing care. Provide education or reinforcing information about developmental characteristics of the child and potential safety hazards in the environment. Encourage the parents to learn CPR, choking-prevention techniques, and back blows, chest thrusts, or abdominal thrusts.

■ Evaluation

Expected outcomes of nursing care include the following:

- The child regains the ability to ventilate spontaneously after removal of the foreign body.
- Parents complete a safety check of the home environment to prevent future aspiration incidents.

Respiratory Failure and Acute Respiratory Distress Syndrome

Respiratory failure occurs when the body can no longer maintain effective gas exchange. The physiologic process that ends in respiratory failure begins with hypoventilation of the alveoli.

Etiology and Pathophysiology

Alveolar hypoventilation occurs when any of the following factors exist.

- The body's need for oxygen exceeds actual oxygen intake.
- The airway is partially occluded.
- The transfer of oxygen and carbon dioxide in the alveoli is disrupted. This disruption may occur either because of a malfunction of respiratory center stimulation (the alveoli do not receive the message to diffuse) or because the alveolar membrane is defective (a structural problem).

Gas exchange is optimal in children when there is an equal match between ventilation and pulmonary blood flow. The usual ratio between ventilation and perfusion is 0.8 to 0.9 because perfusion (circulation) is somewhat greater than ventilation in the lung bases (less inspired air reaches the lowest levels of the lungs). A mismatch between ventilation and perfusion can occur because airflow is inadequate to well-perfused areas of the lungs, such as occurs with constriction of the bronchi or when alveoli are obstructed or collapsed. In this case the blood flowing through pulmonary capillaries receives less oxygen than normal and thus causes hypoxemia. Supplemental oxygen does not effectively treat the condition because the blood flowing through the affected capillary beds never gets exposed to the oxygen. Poor perfusion with well-ventilated lungs may also result in a ventilation-perfusion mismatch, such as occurs with hypovolemia (Froh, 2002). See Figure 25–7 ■.

Alveolar hypoventilation results in **hypoxemia** (lower than normal blood oxygen level) and **hypercapnia** (greater than normal amount of carbon dioxide in the blood). When the blood

PATHOPHYSIOLOGY ILLUSTRATED

Ventilation-Perfusion Ratio

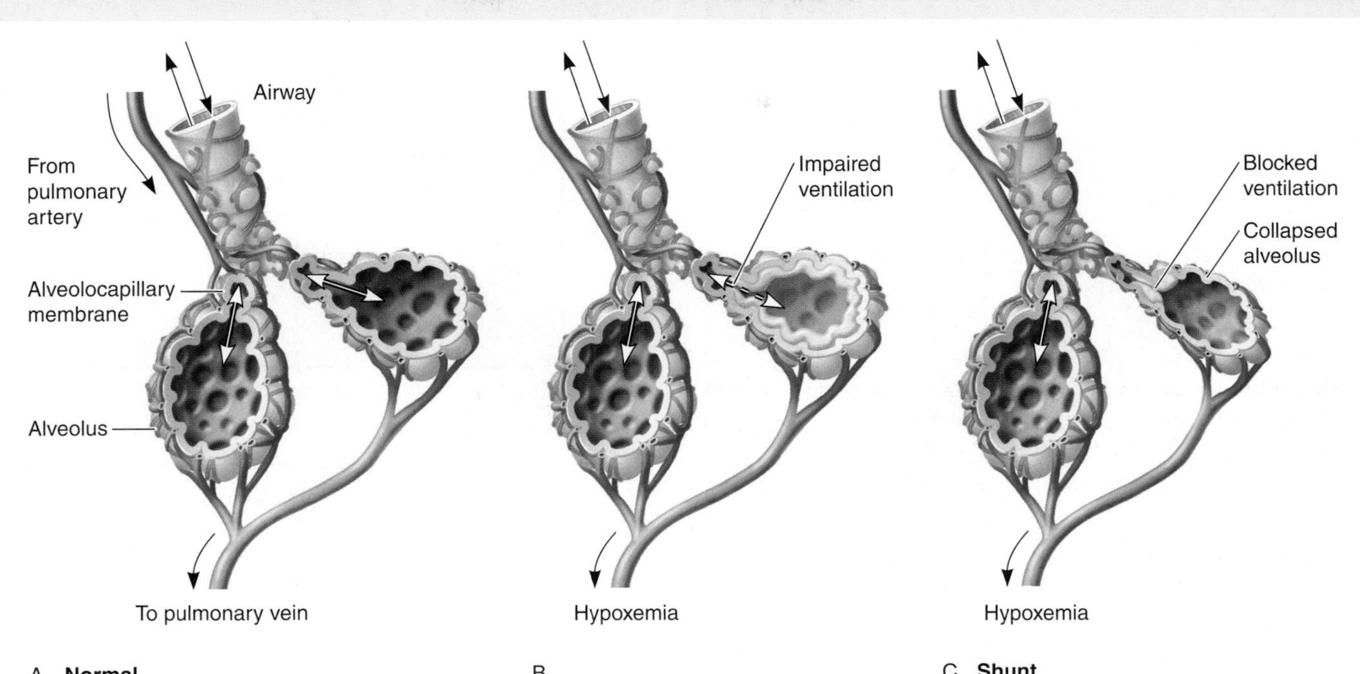

FIGURE 25–7 ■ A ventilation-perfusion mismatch can occur when an infant or child has an abnormal distribution of ventilation or perfusion. *A,* Children with normal lung function and circulation have a ventilation-perfusion ratio of 0.8 to 0.9 because perfusion is greater than ventilation (air exchange) in the lung bases. *B,* When ventilation is inadequate to well-perfused areas of the lungs, the ventilation-perfusion ratio is low or mismatched, resulting in shunting. Blood passing through the pulmonary capillaries gets less oxygen exchange than normal and hypoxemia occurs. This is the case in asthma due to bronchoconstriction and in pneumonia because alveoli are filled with fluid. *C,* In the case of neonatal hyaline membrane disease the alveoli are collapsed, so blood passes through the alveolar capillaries and no oxygenation occurs. The ventilation-perfusion ratio is very low with significant shunting that does not respond to oxygen therapy because the capillary bed never gets exposed to the supplemental oxygen.

levels of oxygen and carbon dioxide reach abnormal levels, **hypoxia** (lower than normal oxygen level in the tissues) occurs and respiratory failure begins.

Children may develop respiratory failure and acute respiratory distress syndrome (ARDS). An acute lung injury causes an inflammatory-immune response and alveolar capillary membrane damage. Examples of conditions that injure the lungs include sepsis, pneumonia, meconium aspiration, aspiration of stomach contents, smoke inhalation, and near drowning. Information on most of these conditions occurs later in the chapter. (See Chapter 33∞ for information on near drowning.)

The increased permeability of the damaged alveolar-capillary membrane allows fluid and protein to accumulate in the alveoli. This in turn results in decreased lung compliance and functional residual capacity, reducing airflow and causing a ventilation-perfusion mismatch and hypoxemia (Moloney-Harmon, 1999). Other body systems may also contribute directly or indirectly to an increased workload, causing the respiratory system to fail.

Clinical Manifestations

Signs of respiratory distress worsen with impending respiratory failure and include irritability, lethargy, cyanosis, diaphoresis, and increased respiratory effort such as dyspnea (difficulty breathing), tachypnea (increased respiratory rate), nasal flaring, and retractions.

CLINICAL TIP

As the child tires from the prolonged effort of breathing, the respiratory rate may begin to decrease. This is an ominous sign and may progress to respiratory arrest without intervention.

See the table on page 828 for clinical manifestations of respiratory failure and imminent respiratory arrest. Hypoxemia is unresponsive to increased oxygen administration due to a ventilation-perfusion mismatch.

PRACTICE ALERT

When the child has a chronic respiratory condition, development of respiratory failure may be gradual. Signs will be subtle. Be particularly alert to behavior changes in addition to respiratory signs. Pulse oximetry and serial blood gases may be needed to monitor the child.

COLLABORATIVE CARE

Physicians, nurses, and respiratory therapists collaborate on treating the respiratory failure and its cause in an effort to prevent its progression to death.

MediaLink Gas Exchange Animation

CLINICAL MANIFESTATIONS of Respiratory Failure and Imminent Respiratory Arrest

PHYSIOLOGIC CAUSE	CLINICAL MANIFESTATIONS
These signs occur because the child is attempting to compensate for oxygen deficit and airway blockage. Oxygen supply is inadequate; behavior and vital signs reflect compensation and beginning hypoxia.	***Respiratory failure*** *Initial signs* Restlessness Tachypnea Tachycardia Diaphoresis
The child attempts to use accessory muscles to assist oxygen intake; hypoxia persists and efforts now waste more oxygen than is obtained.	*Early decompensation* Nasal flaring Retractions Grunting Wheezing Anxiety and irritability Mood changes Headache Hypertension Confusion
These signs occur because oxygen deficit is overwhelming and beyond spontaneous recovery. Cerebral oxygenation is dramatically affected; central nervous system changes are ominous.	***Imminent respiratory arrest*** *Severe hypoxia* Dyspnea Bradycardia Cyanosis Stupor and coma

Diagnostic Tests

The child's history, vital signs, and respiratory signs provide important clues about the progression from respiratory distress to respiratory failure. Pulse oximetry and arterial blood gases are used to assess respiratory failure. Pulse oximetry provides an estimate of the hemoglobin saturated by oxygen (Spo_2) and it is expressed as the percentage of hemoglobin capable of transporting oxygen. See Figure 25–8 ■ for guidelines to interpret pulse oximetry readings. See Table 25–3 for normal ranges of arterial blood gases. Refer to Chapter 23∞ for interpretation of acidosis and alkalosis that must be considered simultaneously with assessment of oxygenation status. Hypercarbia in the presence of acidosis is a sign of respiratory failure. Hypoxemia even when supplemental oxygen is given is also a sign of respiratory failure.

Clinical Therapy

Medical management is focused on treating the cause of respiratory failure and reversing the severe hypoxemia with oxygen, mechanical ventilation, and positive end-expiratory pressure (PEEP) to increase functional residual capacity. As the child becomes more hypoxic, the level of responsiveness deteriorates and the child's ability to keep the airway patent decreases. Respiratory problems that do not respond to oxygen therapy or medications require the insertion of an endotracheal tube to stabilize the airway. Assisted ventilation must be provided until the child breathes spontaneously or until a ventilator is hooked up. Oxygen saturation and end-tidal CO_2 monitoring are helpful to assure appropriate positioning of the endotracheal tube. A **tracheostomy,** the creation of a surgical opening into the trachea through the anterior neck at the cricoid cartilage, is often performed if long-term airway management is

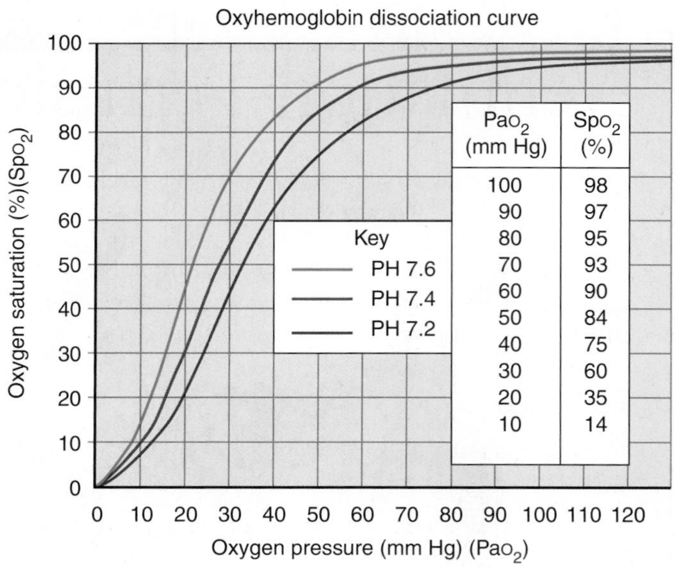

FIGURE 25–8 ■ Oxyhemoglobin Dissociation Curve. The relationship between the partial pressure of oxygen in arterial blood (Pao_2) and pulse oximetry reading (Spo_2) is not linear. When hypoxia exists, the hemoglobin releases oxygen in the body tissues. When hypoxia does not exist, oxygen remains bound to the hemoglobin. A fall in pulse oximetry reading is associated with a more dramatic reduction in Pao_2. The oxyhemoglobin dissociation curve demonstrates the relationship between Spo_2 and Pao_2 and is important in correctly interpreting the pulse oximetry reading. For example,

- When cardiac output is normal, the hemoglobin concentration is adequate, and the pH is normal (7.4), a Spo_2 above 93% to 95% is associated with a Pao_2 of 90 mm Hg or adequate oxygen delivery.
- A Spo_2 of 90% or less indicates hypoxemia with a Pao_2 of ≤ 60 mm Hg.
- A Spo_2 of 60% or less indicates severe hypoxemia with a Pao_2 of < 30 mm Hg.
- If anemia or low cardiac output is present, a $Spo_2 > 95\%$ can indicate inadequate oxygen delivery.
- If the child has a higher pH, the hemoglobin does not as easily release the oxygen to the tissues. In this case the oxyhemoglobin dissociation curve shifts to the left, and the Spo_2 of 90% is associated with a Pao_2 of 50 mm Hg.
- If the child has a lower pH, the hemoglobin more readily releases oxygen to the tissues. In this case the oxyhemoglobin dissociation curve shifts to the right, and the Spo_2 of 90% is associated with a Pao_2 of > 70 mm Hg.

needed. Children are often sedated to optimize ventilation. Continuous positive airway pressure (CPAP) is one form of PEEP used to improve oxygenation and lung compliance. Nitric oxide administered by inhalation is used in some cases to promote vasodilation and increase blood flow in the alveoli that are well ventilated. When respiratory failure becomes life threatening, extracorporeal membrane oxygenation (ECMO)

TABLE 25–3 Normal Ranges of Arterial Blood Gases

Partial Pressure of Oxygen (Pao_2)	
All children:	83–108 mm Hg
Partial Pressure of Carbon Dioxide ($Paco_2$)	
Infant:	27–41 mm Hg
Children:	32–48 mm Hg

Note: From Soldin, S. J., Brugnara, C., & Wong, E. C. (2003). Pediatric reference ranges *(4th ed.). Washington, DC: AACC Press. Used with permission.*

may be initiated. ECMO is a highly invasive cardiopulmonary bypass system with external oxygenation and a pump mechanism that can be used to provide respiratory and hemodynamic support while the lungs heal. It also reduces mechanical ventilation time and associated complications; however, several significant complications may occur in the child placed on ECMO. This complex and expensive treatment is available in special neonatal and pediatric intensive care centers, so the child may have to be transferred to another hospital to receive this therapy. Survival rates are influenced by the severity of the condition causing the respiratory failure (Morris, Gonzalez, Stewart, et al., 2000).

NURSING MANAGEMENT

Nursing care is focused on the recognition of progression from respiratory distress to respiratory failure and supportive care to the child and family.

Nursing Assessment and Diagnosis

Early recognition of impending respiratory failure is the most important aspect of care for a child with any signs of respiratory compromise. Perform the respiratory assessment using guidelines in Box 25–1. **Grunting,** a physiologic mechanism that slows the expiratory flow to increase the lung volume and alveolar pressure, is a sign associated with the onset of respiratory failure in newborns and infants. Attach a cardiorespiratory monitor and pulse oximeter. Monitor the child for changes in vital signs, respiratory status, and level of responsiveness.

If the child has an endotracheal or a tracheostomy tube, assess for secretions that may further obstruct the airway.

Examples of nursing diagnoses associated with respiratory failure include:

- Ineffective Breathing Pattern associated with prolonged tachypnea and muscle fatigue
- Ineffective Airway Clearance related to sedation and loss of protective cough reflex
- Impaired Gas Exchange related to structural injury to the alveolar membrane
- Compromised Family Coping related to child's life-threatening illness

Planning and Implementation

Place the child in an upright position (by elevating the head of the bed) and the head in midline to help maintain the airway. Administer oxygen as ordered. See the Skills Manual for a review of oxygen delivery systems and amount of oxygen delivered by each. Keep a bag-valve mask and emergency equipment readily available at the bedside to assist ventilations if respiratory status deteriorates.

Because endotracheal and tracheostomy tubes prevent vocal cord vibration, intubated children cannot cry or talk. Once infants and young children who are intubated recover from the sedation or anesthesia, they often express initial frustration and fear when they cannot communicate verbally. Explain the reasons for the inability to cry and talk to the child and parents. When the child is alert, give suggestions for ways to make noise and gain attention when needed, such as striking the mattress. For older children obtain and demonstrate the use of a communication board.

Suction airway secretions as needed, and provide tracheostomy care if present. See Skills Manual for tracheostomy care procedures. Provide good skin care around the endotracheal tube or tracheostomy to prevent breakdown over pressure points.

Provide support to parents and children. The parents will be stressed because of the life-threatening nature of the disorder. Help the family identify resources and support to care for other children so parents may spend more time with the child who is critically ill. Provide age-appropriate information to the child once sedation wears off to reduce fear, and permit the parents to be with the child as much as possible.

Once the child begins responding to clinical therapy, the child is weaned from the ventilator and the endotracheal tube is removed. The child will be moved to the pediatric nursing unit for the remainder of treatment for the condition causing respiratory failure.

Discharge Planning and Home Care Teaching

Many children are discharged from the hospital and cared for at home for an extended period with a tracheostomy tube in place. It is essential to teach parents how to maintain and suction the airway, clean the tracheostomy site, and change the tube. They must demonstrate competence in all aspects of tracheostomy care, as well as emergency resuscitation skills adapted to the tracheostomy. Make a referral to a home health agency and supply company. A home health care nurse can provide follow-up care and support for the child and family. See Skills Manual for management of the tracheostomy tube.

Evaluation

Expected outcomes of nursing care include the following:

- The child's airway and ventilation are supported until the respiratory failure is reversed.
- The child is provided with a method of communication when alert but unable to talk.
- Skin integrity is maintained around the artificial airway and pressure surfaces of the body.
- The family is educated to provide tracheostomy care at home and referrals are made to provide family support.

APNEA

Newborns normally have **periodic breathing**, an irregular rhythm with occasional pauses of up to 20 seconds between breaths. This breathing pattern is not apnea. **Apnea** is the cessation of respiration lasting longer than 20 seconds, or any pause in respiration associated with cyanosis, marked pallor, hypotonia, or bradycardia. Apnea can be characterized in the following ways.

- Central apnea—complete cessation of breathing effort
- Obstructive apnea—absence of nasal airflow when respiratory efforts are present (remember that newborns are nasal breathers and thus do not open the mouth to breathe.)
- Mixed apnea—central respiratory pause that either precedes or follows airway obstruction

Apnea may be the first major sign of respiratory dysfunction in the neonate. Two types of apnea occur during infancy, but they are different conditions. Apnea of prematurity (AOP) occurs in preterm infants, usually as a result of immaturity. An apparent life-threatening event (ALTE), sometimes referred to as apnea of infancy, occurs in near-term or term infants. In the past, both AOP and ALTE were often called "near-miss sudden infant death" or "aborted crib death." These terms erroneously implied a close association between such episodes and sudden infant death syndrome (SIDS). SIDS should not be confused with apnea and is discussed later in this chapter. Obstructive sleep apnea occurs in children.

Apnea of Prematurity

AOP is a pathologic apnea with no definable cause in infants less than 37 weeks gestational age. It usually presents between 2 and 7 days of life, and its incidence increases with lower gestational age. It resolves in most infants by 40 weeks postconceptional age (Theobald, Botwinski, Albanna, et al., 2000).

AOP may be caused by neurologic and immunologic immaturity, or immature muscle development and coordination. The primary sign of AOP is one or more episodes of cessation of breathing for 20 seconds or longer associated with bradycardia and color change. The clinical manifestations of AOP are associated with the potential cause of the condition. See clinical manifestation below for signs and symptoms associated with AOP.

Collaborative Care

Diagnostic procedures performed include a pneumogram and other tests to identify potential underlying conditions contributing to the AOP. These include gastroesophageal reflux, sepsis, metabolic errors or electrolyte abnormalities, poor thermoregulation, seizures, and anatomic abnormalities. See the clinical manifestations table below for specific tests performed.

Therapy is initiated to prevent irreversible neurologic damage that could result from repeated or prolonged episodes. Any infant considered to be at high risk for apnea will have cardiorespiratory monitors set to detect prolonged pauses in breathing. Medications are given orally or intravenously to stimulate breathing. See the medication table on page 831. CPAP may also be used when obstructive apnea is suspected.

Nursing Management

Nurses play an important role in evaluating signs and symptoms associated with potential contributing factors. Monitor the infant for apnea episodes.

CAUSES AND CLINICAL MANIFESTATIONS of Apnea of Prematurity and Apparent Life-Threatening Event

ETIOLOGY	CLINICAL MANIFESTATIONS	DIAGNOSTIC PROCEDURES
Functional or structural airway problem or immaturity	Apnea of 20 sec or longer; accompanied by bradycardia or cyanosis	Cardiorespiratory monitoring, sleep study, pneumogram, sepsis workup
Aspiration as a result of dysfunctional swallowing or gastroesophageal reflux	Choking, coughing, cyanosis, vomiting	Barium swallow, esophageal pH probe
Cardiac problems	Tachycardia, tachypnea, dyspnea	Cardiorespiratory monitoring, electrocardiogram, echocardiogram, arterial blood gases
Drug toxicity or poisoning; maternal history of ingestion	Central nervous system depression, hypotonia	Serum magnesium level, toxicity screen
Environmental, thermoregulation problem	Lethargy, tachypnea, hypothermia or hyperthermia	Cardiorespiratory and temperature monitoring, environmental temperature level (ambient air temperature)
Impaired oxygenation, respiratory disease (pulmonary edema, atelectasis, pneumonia)	Cyanosis, tachypnea, respiratory distress, anemia, choking, coughing	Oximetry, chest radiograph, arterial blood gases, complete blood count, upper airway evaluation, sleep study, serum electrolytes
Acute infection (sepsis, meningitis, necrotizing enterocolitis)	Feeding intolerance, lethargy, temperature instability	Complete blood count, cultures when appropriate, C-reactive protein, chest and abdominal radiographs
Intracranial pathology (intraventricular hemorrhage, ventricular dilation, CNS anomalies, meningitis)	Abnormal neurologic examination, seizures	Cranial ultrasound, computed tomography scan, electroencephalogram, magnetic resonance imaging, cerebrospinal fluid evaluation
Metabolic disorders	Jitteriness, poor feeding, lethargy, central nervous system depression or irritability, hypotonia	Serum electrolytes (potassium, sodium, chloride), glucose, calcium, arterial blood gases

Note: Data from Theobald, K., Botwinski, C., Albanna, S., & McWilliam, P. (2000). Apnea of prematurity: Diagnosis, implications for care, and pharmacologic management. Neonatal Network, *19(6), 17–24; and Eichenwald, E., & Stark, A. (1992). Apnea of prematurity: Etiology and management.* Tufts University School of Medicine Reports on Neonatal Respiratory Diseases, *2(1), 1–11.*

MEDICATIONS Used to Treat Apnea of Prematurity

MEDICATION	ACTION	NURSING CONSIDERATIONS
Methylxanthines aminophylline, caffeine	Stimulates the respiratory center in the brain, stimulates diaphragmatic contractility and prevents diaphragmatic fatigue. Caffeine is preferred because it enhances diaphragmatic contraction, has a longer action time, fewer side effects, and a more stable plasma concentration. The drug is discontinued once the infant is past 37 weeks postconceptional age.	Monitor vital signs and clinical response. Monitor the serum drug level because the metabolism and elimination rates of the drug can be unpredictable. Because of the delayed elimination of the medications, the infant should be carefully monitored for apneic episodes for 7 to 10 days after discontinuation to ensure that the condition has resolved.
Doxapram	Respiratory and CNS stimulant used only when apnea of prematurity is not responsive to methylxanthines.	IV formulation has benzyl alcohol and must be used with caution. Oral formulation is poorly absorbed by preterm infants.

Supportive care for AOP includes placing the neonate with the head at midline and the neck in the neutral position or slightly extended to minimize upper airway obstruction. Tactile stimulation, such as rubbing the infant's back or feet, often is enough to halt an apneic episode.

The medication dosage administered is small and must be carefully titrated. Observe the neonate for the drug's side effects. Monitor the neonate for apneic episodes until the drug is completely eliminated from the body. Prolonged follow-up provides assurance that the respiratory system has matured adequately, and further apneic spells should not occur.

Apparent Life-threatening Event (ALTE)

ALTE is defined as an episode of central or obstructive apnea occurring in a near-term or term infant who is greater than 37 weeks' gestation. The majority of these events occur in infants under 4 months of age, with a peak incidence between 1 week and 2 months (Davies & Gupta, 2002).

Etiology and Pathophysiology

Potential causes of ALTE include infection, gastrointestinal reflux, seizures or breath-holding spells, cardiac arrhythmias, respiratory center dysfunction, obstructive sleep apnea, and metabolic and endocrine problems. In the case of repeated episodes without identifiable cause, ALTE may be the result of intentional suffocation or Munchausen syndrome by proxy, both a form of child abuse (see Chapter 7∞).

Clinical Manifestations

Clinical manifestations include apnea (central or obstructive) accompanied by a color change (cyanosis, pallor, or occasionally ruddiness), limp muscle tone, choking, or gagging. These episodes may occur during sleep, wakefulness, or feeding.

COLLABORATIVE CARE

After an ALTE, the infant is usually admitted to the hospital for evaluation and cardiorespiratory monitoring. See the clinical manifestations table on page 830 for potential causes and tests used for diagnosis. In 50% of cases, however, no cause is identified (Loughlin & Carroll, 1999). Physical stimulation or emergency resuscitation is usually required to revive the infant.

NURSING MANAGEMENT

Nursing care includes collecting a detailed history of the event, observing and monitoring cardiorespiratory status, providing supportive care to the infant and family, facilitating the diagnostic process, and anticipating the need for emergency resuscitation and for the diagnostic process.

■ Nursing Assessment and Diagnosis

Establish rapport with the parents to create a sense of trust. Do not give parents the impression that their parenting skills are being judged or questioned. Collect historical information that includes the infant's color, tone, apnea, rescue breaths or CPR, state of arousal, and duration of the episode. Seek information about the potential relationship between the event and feeding. Additional information about any past episodes, recent infections, medications, seizure activity, birth history or perinatal insults, family history of infant deaths, apnea, or cardiac problems should also be collected. Ask family members about how they responded to the event (CPR, bulb suctioning, and repositioning) and the infant's response.

Attach a cardiorespiratory monitor to continuously assess the heart rate and respiratory rate while the infant is awake and asleep (Figure 25–9 ■). Pulse oximetry provides continuous evaluation of the infant's oxygenation status.

Examples of nursing diagnoses associated with ALTE include:

- Ineffective Breathing Pattern related to airway obstruction or metabolic disorder
- Caregiver Role Strain associated with need for continuous respiratory monitoring and fear of future apneic episodes
- Interrupted Breastfeeding related to infant's hospitalization and change in established routines
- Interrupted Family Processes related to increased monitoring of infant and change in family routines

■ Planning and Implementation

ALTE can frighten the parent or observer, who often fears the infant has died. Parents experience fear and anxiety about the infant's prognosis. Explanations of tests and treatment help to

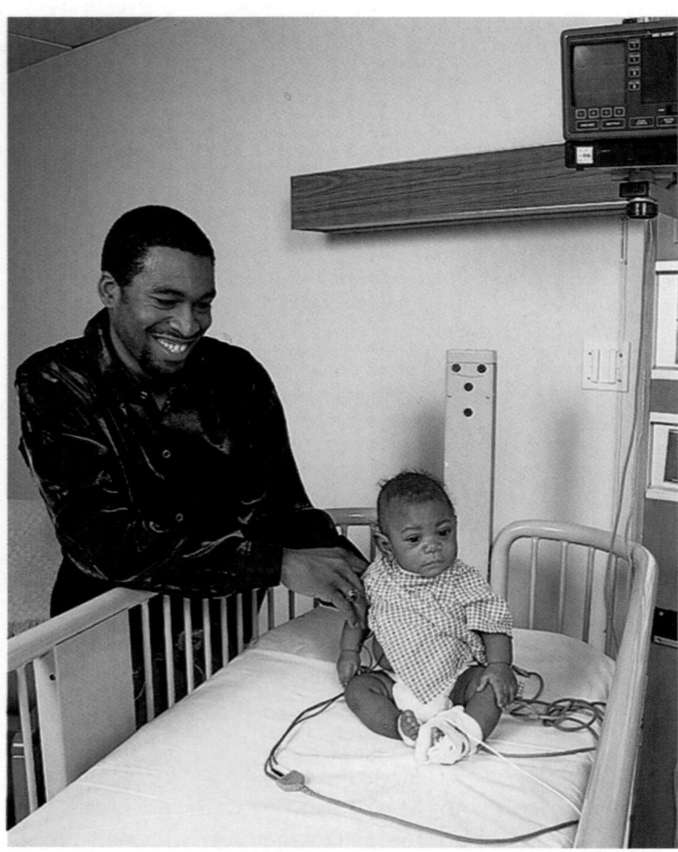

FIGURE 25–9 ■ Infants who experience an episode of apnea or apparent life-threatening event are usually admitted to the hospital for cardiorespiratory monitoring.

decrease parental anxiety and increase their understanding of the situation.

During hospitalization the infant should be held and cuddled to provide a sense of security and well-being. Encouraging parents' participation in the infant's care helps to meet these needs and promotes family bonding. Often parents are afraid they might disconnect the monitoring cable if they handle the infant. Wrapping the cable inside the infant's blanket helps secure the wires, thus increasing parents' feelings of confidence when handling the infant.

Assist the mother to continue breastfeeding and maintaining the supply of breast milk by pumping if necessary. Support the mother's desire to continue breastfeeding by ensuring that she gets adequate fluids and nutrition. Provide privacy for breast pumping, and store breast milk for future feedings.

Because the infant who has had an ALTE continues to be at risk for cardiopulmonary arrest, emergency resuscitation equipment and drugs should be readily accessible at all times.

Discharge Planning and Home Care Teaching

Home care needs should be identified and addressed early during the hospitalization. Some infants will be sent home with an apnea monitor, and parents need to be taught how to operate it. See Partnering with Families: Home Care Instructions for the Infant Requiring Apnea Monitoring. Teach parents what to do when the infant has an apneic episode and techniques for choking intervention. Encourage parents to attend a cardiopulmonary resuscitation (CPR) class. Talk with parents about how to manage this new family stressor and still meet needs of other family members.

■ Evaluation

Expected outcomes of nursing care include the following:

- The child's apneic episode is managed promptly and respirations are restored.
- Parents learn to identify and manage future apneic episodes.
- The mother continues to breastfeed the infant.
- The infant's sense of security and development is promoted.

Obstructive Sleep Apnea

Obstructive sleep apnea (OSA) syndrome is a disorder of breathing during sleep that is characterized by prolonged partial upper airway obstruction and/or intermittent complete obstruction (obstructive apnea) that disrupts normal ventilation during sleep and normal sleep patterns (American Academy of Pediatrics, 2002). When the child tries to move air past the obstruction, the breathing becomes labored, and snoring or noisy breathing is heard. Snoring is noticed in 7% to 12% of children; however, not all children who snore have OSA syndrome (Perkin, Downey, & MacQuarrie, 1999). The severe obstruction and resulting impact on the child's health occurs in about 2% of children of all ages, including newborns. Its incidence peaks between 2 and 6 years of age when tonsils and adenoids are at their largest in relation to the size of the airway; however, it is also a relatively common condition in children up to 11 years of age. Black children are at higher risk than White children, and former preterm infants are at higher risk than full-term infants (Rosen, Larkin, Kirchner, et al., 2003).

Etiology and Pathophysiology

The upper airway contains about 30 muscles that permit the pharynx to collapse enabling the child to talk and swallow, but also maintain airway patency. When the child is awake, muscle tone is maintained and the airway remains patent even when obstructions such as enlarged adenoids and tonsils, craniofacial anomalies, or obesity are present. During sleep, the airway muscles relax and the pharynx becomes obstructed. Breathing during sleep is also less deep as the ventilatory drive decreases. During nonrapid eye movement sleep, the **tidal volume** (the amount of air inhaled and exhaled during a normal breath) and respiratory rate are lower, resulting in a lower volume breathed each minute (minute ventilation). When the airway muscles are relaxed, airway resistance is increased. During rapid eye movement sleep, the skeletal muscles relax and the respiratory rate is irregular. The combination of decreased intercostal muscle activity, a variable respiratory rate, and tidal volume predisposes the child to hypoxemia. Reduced upper airway tone and obstruction then result in apnea episodes.

PARTNERING WITH FAMILIES

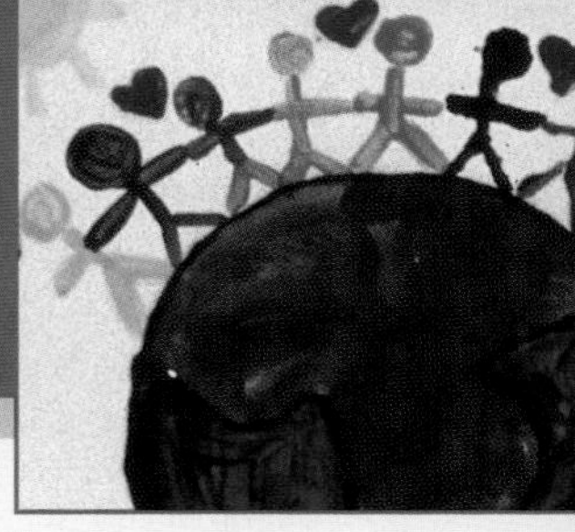

Home Care Instructions for the Infant Requiring Apnea Monitoring

Apnea equipment

- Understand monitor type, lead wires, placement of skin electrodes or chest belt, battery power, manual for troubleshooting.

Emergency preparation

- Notify telephone company, electric company, local rescue squad, local emergency department (establishes priority status).
- Post phone numbers of rescue squad, physician, equipment company, power company, emergency number, cardiopulmonary resuscitation (CPR) guidelines, other important numbers (neighbor, parents' work numbers) in at least two places in the home; have at least one added extension phone.
- Keep the apnea monitor battery fully charged.

Safety precautions

- Place monitor on firm surface; keep away from other appliances (television, microwave oven) and water.
- Ensure that alarms are audible from all locations.
- Double-check that monitor is on before going to bed.
- Thread cable and wires through lower end of infant's clothes.
- Ensure integrity of leads, monitor cable, power cord (replace if frayed).

Routine care

- Understand reasons for apnea monitor and frequency of use.
- Be able to attach and detach infant chest leads and belt.
- Evaluate skin for irritation or breakdown from electrode placement and give skin care (no oils or lotion; move patches correctly).

Emergency care

- Develop plan for respiratory failure and power failure.
- Demonstrate CPR and back blows and chest thrusts for airway obstruction.
- Understand how to respond to alarms for apnea, bradycardia, or loose lead.

Apnea alarm

- First observe infant's respiratory movement to determine if the alarm is for a real event.
- If respiration is absent or infant is lethargic, stimulate by calling name and gently touching, proceeding to vigorous touch if needed.
- If no response, proceed with CPR.

Bradycardia alarm

- Stimulate infant; infant should respond quickly.

Loose lead

- Check electrode patch. Is it loose? Dirty? Belt loose?
- Check wires from electrode or monitor cable.
- Check power supply. Is battery low? Power failure? Monitor malfunctioning?

Severity of this condition may range from a continuous partial airway obstruction to episodes of no air movement despite breathing effort. Many children arouse frequently and repeatedly from sleep to increase airway muscle tone so that they can breathe. Other children do not arouse from sleep easily and sleep with obstructive hypoventilation, a partial airway obstruction that lasts for several hours without interruption (Marcus, 1998). In both cases, the child experiences hypoxemia, hypercapnia, acidemia, and hemodynamic alterations, such as elevated blood pressure and increased pulmonary arterial pressure in association with apnea episodes. Cerebral blood flow is also decreased during sleep.

Hypertrophy of the adenoids and tonsils is the most common cause of OSA. Other children at risk for OSA include those with craniofacial anomalies (e.g., Apert syndrome, Pierre Robin syndrome, Treacher Collins syndrome, Crouzon syndrome), Down syndrome, obesity, neuromuscular disorders (e.g., cerebral palsy, muscular dystrophy), macroglossia, Prader Willi syndrome, and mucopolysaccharidoses.

Clinical Manifestations

Children with OSA snore and have signs of labored breathing during sleep such as retractions and paradoxical breathing. After pauses in snoring or lack of airflow, the child may be noted to snort, gasp, choke, move, or arouse to take a breath. Sleep is restless and the child may sleep in unusual positions to hyperextend the neck and airway. Daytime sleepiness and other symptoms of sleep deprivation (poor attention, increased activity, aggression, acting out behavior, poor school performance) may be noted. The child may also have enuresis and report a morning headache resulting from carbon dioxide retention.

On physical examination, findings may be normal but mouth breathing and enlarged tonsils and adenoids may be seen. Failure to thrive may be present, potentially because the airway obstruction makes eating difficult or because of increased energy expenditure due to the work of breathing. Without treatment, complications develop that can include failure to thrive, pulmonary hypertension, **cor pulmonale** (obstruction of pulmonary blood flow that leads to right ventricular hypertrophy and heart failure), systemic hypertension, and cognitive impairment.

COLLABORATIVE CARE

Clinical management is focused on diagnosing children with OSA and selecting the appropriate therapy for the child.

MediaLink Nursing in Action: Apnea Monitor

BOX 25–3 History Questions for Assessment for Obstructive Sleep Apnea

- Does your child snore? If so how often, and how loudly?
- Do you ever see your child stop breathing during sleep?
- Is your child restless during sleep or assume unusual sleep positions?
- Does your child wet the bed?
- Does your child exhibit signs of being excessively sleepy during the day?
- Does your child complain of headaches in the morning?
- Does your child often breathe with the mouth open?
- Is your child having difficulty with schoolwork or relationships?
- Does your child have any signs of hyperactivity or aggressiveness?

Note: Reprinted from Yantis, M. A. (1999). Assessing children for obstructive sleep apnea. Journal of Pediatric Health Care, *13(3), 99–104, with permission from Elsevier.*

Diagnostic Tests

Health professionals must be proactive in inquiring about snoring and its characteristics during examinations. See Box 25–3 for screening questions to use for OSA and associated problems. Diagnosis is made by **polysomnography,** a sleep study that simultaneously records brain activity, eye movement, and respiration. The number of hypopnea and apnea episodes and associated oxygen desaturation and sleep disturbances are measured.

Clinical Therapy

Adenotonsillectomy is the most common treatment for OSA and resolution of the condition occurs in the majority of children. (See Box 25–4 for children at higher risk for respiratory complications in the immediate postoperative period.) Weight-loss strategies may be implemented for children with obesity. Continuous positive airway pressure (CPAP) is used for children with surgical contraindications or those with persistent OSA (craniofacial anomalies, Down syndrome, or neuromuscular disorders) after adenotonsillectomy. CPAP levels are set at the pressure that eliminates apneic episodes, sleep arousals, and hypoxemia. Pressure levels may need to be changed as the child grows. Craniofacial surgery or even tracheostomy may be treatment options in some cases. Oxygen is not usually prescribed as it decreases the ventilatory drive. Polysomnography is usually repeated about 6 to 8 weeks after surgery to determine if any residual OSA remains.

BOX 25–4 Children with Severe OSA at Risk for Respiratory Complications after Adenotonsillectomy

- Younger than 3 years of age
- Severe OSA on polysomnography
- Cardiac complications of OSA (e.g., right ventricular hypertrophy)
- Failure to thrive
- Obesity
- Prematurity
- Recent respiratory infection
- Craniofacial anomalies
- Neuromuscular disorders

Note: Adapted from American Academy of Pediatrics Section on Pediatric Pulmonology, Subcommittee on Obstructive Sleep Apnea Syndrome. (2002). Clinical practice guideline: Diagnosis and management of childhood obstructive sleep apnea syndrome. Pediatrics, *109(4), 704–712. Used with permission.*

NURSING MANAGEMENT

The goal of nursing care is to identify children at risk for OSA and to support the family during surgery or other therapies.

Nursing Assessment and Diagnoses

In the community setting, all children should be screened for snoring as part of their routine healthcare. Assess the child for signs of nasal obstruction, mouth breathing, and enlarged tonsils. Determine if the child has symptoms of sleep deprivation or a condition is present that places the child at high risk for OSA. Coordinate referral to a sleep center for polysomnogram evaluation.

Following adenotonsillectomy, the child is usually hospitalized overnight to monitor for development of complications. Carefully assess the child for bleeding and respiratory complications.

The following nursing diagnoses might be appropriate for the child with OSA

- Impaired Gas Exchange related to airway obstruction associated with enlarged tonsils and adenoids
- Ineffective Tissue Perfusion (cerebral) related to hypoventilation
- Ineffective Therapeutic Regimen Management (child and family) related to nonadherence in use of continuous positive airway pressure

Planning and Implementation

Nursing care in the community is initially focused on educating the parents about the potential serious complications associated with OSA and the interventions that can resolve or control the condition. Explain the purpose of polysomnography evaluation and how to prepare the child for the strange setting and wires that will be attached during the sleep study. Most pediatric centers will allow the parent to stay with the child during the study. Encourage the family to return for a follow-up sleep study after adenotonsillectomy to determine if the condition is resolved or if additional intervention is needed. Ongoing growth and development is monitored to observe for improved growth patterns and behavior after intervention begins.

Following adenotonsillectomy, the hospital nurse monitors the child for bleeding and respiratory distress, such as obstructive sleep apnea and pulmonary edema. Continuous pulse oximetry is used to detect oxygen desaturation. See Chapter 24∞ for additional nursing care, family education, and home care following adenotonsillectomy.

Sleep center nurses provide education and support to families of children who need to use CPAP to treat the OSA. The nurse helps identify the best fitting mask or nasal prong system for CPAP delivery. Parents may need guidance about helping children to go to sleep wearing the mask until they are accustomed to it.

Evaluation

Expected outcomes of nursing care include the following:

- The child has minimal snoring and sleep is no longer disturbed by apnea episodes.
- Catch-up growth for children with failure to thrive is noted.
- Behavior and school performance improve.

SUDDEN INFANT DEATH SYNDROME

Sudden infant death syndrome (SIDS) has been defined as the sudden death of an infant under 1 year of age that remains unexplained after a complete autopsy, a death scene investigation, and review of the history. It remains a leading cause of death in infants between 1 month and 1 year of age, with 90% of cases occurring before 6 months of age (American Academy of Pediatrics Committee on Child Abuse and Neglect, 2001). SIDS occurs rarely in infants less than 2 weeks. It is unpredictable and in some cases unpreventable.

Etiology and Pathophysiology

The current evidence suggests a genetic susceptibility to SIDS, and no relationship exists between apnea and SIDS (American Academy of Pediatrics Committee on Fetus and Newborn, 2003). One theory regarding the etiology of SIDS is that an abnormality in the arcuate nucleus of the brainstem causes a delayed development of arousal, cardiorespiratory control, or cardiovascular control (Parnighrahy, Filiano, Sleeper, et al., 1997). Sleep studies conducted on infants who later died due to SIDS revealed less frequent cortical arousal during sleep (Kato, Franco, Groswasser, et al., 2003). Other proposed causes include *H. pylori* gastrointestinal infection and a cardiac dysrhythmia called long QT syndrome. See Box 25–5 for the infant, maternal, and familial factors that appear to place infants at risk for SIDS. SIDS has not been found to be associated with newborn apnea or immunizations for diphtheria, tetanus, and pertussis (DTP). Child abuse or homicide may be associated with 1% to 5% of suspected SIDS cases (American Academy of Pediatrics Committee on Child Abuse and Neglect, 2001).

SIDS is referred to as a "syndrome" because of the many and varied autopsy and clinical findings that characterize most infants who die from the disorder. The autopsy typically does not identify a disease process that caused the death.

Clinical Manifestations

The first symptom is cardiopulmonary arrest. Clinical findings include evidence of a struggle or change in position and the presence of frothy, blood-tinged secretions from the mouth and nares. SIDS occurs more often in the fall and winter and during periods of sleep. Most deaths are unobserved. Typically parents find the infant dead in the crib in the morning and report having heard no cries or disturbances during the night.

BOX 25–5 Risk Factors for Sudden Infant Death Syndrome

INFANT

- Prematurity, gestational age < 28 weeks
- Low birth weight
- Multiple birth
- Race (in decreasing order of frequency): most common in Native American infants, followed by African American, Hispanic, White, and Asian infants
- Gender: more common in males than females
- Age: most common in infants between 2 and 4 months of age
- Time of year: more prevalent in winter months
- Exposure to passive smoke
- History of cyanosis, respiratory distress, irritability, and poor feeding in the nursery
- Sleeping in bed with others, particularly siblings
- Use of pillows and quilts with bedding
- Sleeping prone or sleeping on side and turning to prone position

MATERNAL AND FAMILIAL

- Maternal age less than 20 years
- Prenatal smoking, binge alcohol use, and illicit drug use (increases incidence 10 times)
- Anemia
- Multiple pregnancies, with short intervals between births
- History of sibling with SIDS (increases incidence 4 to 5 times)
- Low socioeconomic status; crowding
- No or late prenatal care, low weight gain

COLLABORATIVE CARE

The Back to Sleep Campaign, which encourages the placement of infants in supine position for sleeping, was initiated in 1992. The SIDS postneonatal mortality rate declined 38.9% between 1991 and 1997 presumably as a result of this changed sleeping position. Fears of aspiration in infants associated with supine sleep position have not been noted, as the mortality rate for aspiration-related deaths also declined in the same time period (Malloy, 2002).

PRACTICE ALERT

The American Academy of Pediatrics recommends that infants be placed on their back to sleep (American Academy of Pediatrics Committee on Fetus and Newborn, 2003). The dramatic decrease in SIDS deaths, from 67% of postneonatal deaths in 1993 to 28% in 1998, is believed to be related to the success of educational campaigns about infant sleep position. Recent findings indicate that infants who are placed to sleep on the stomach have a 13.1 times greater risk for SIDS while those placed to sleep on the side who then turn to the stomach have a 45.4 times greater risk for SIDS. This is believed to be a factor in the rising incidence of SIDS found in childcare settings (Cote, Gerez, Brouillette, et al., 2000; Moon, Patel, & Shaefer, 2000).

MediaLink SIDS Video

NURSING MANAGEMENT

The sudden, unexpected nature of the infant's death is confirmed in the emergency department. The nurse's role is to be empathetic and provide support during one of the greatest crises a family must face. The focus is on supporting the family during the acute grieving period (Table 25–4). Guidelines for the support of families experiencing SIDS should include baptism services, religious support, grief counseling, assistance with funeral arrangements, and counseling on cessation of breastfeeding when appropriate. Giving parents information about the potential reactions of siblings can help them address their needs. See Chapter 22∞.

Reassure the parents that they are not responsible for the infant's death and assist them in contacting other family members and mobilizing support. Older children may need reassurance that SIDS will not happen to them. They may also believe that bad thoughts or wishes about their baby brother or sister caused the death. Support groups can help parents, siblings, and other family members express these fears and work through their feelings about the infant's death. The SIDS Alliance and SHARE organizations can help families locate a support group in their geographic area. Parents may need extra support with the birth of a subsequent newborn.

Nurses can play an important role in educating the public about the link between SIDS and infant positioning during sleep. Educate all parents of neonates and infants about the recommended sleep position for their infants at home and ask them to make sure this sleep position is used when the infant is cared for by another family member, babysitter, or childcare center (Moon et al., 2000). In addition to sleep position, parents and care providers should place the infant on a firm mattress and avoid the use of loose bedding, toys, and pillows. Avoid overheating the infant with too many clothes and blankets. Parents should stop smoking. Hospitalized infants should be placed to sleep in *supine position* rather than side-lying or prone.

CROUP SYNDROMES

Croup is a term applied to a broad classification of upper airway illnesses that result from swelling of the epiglottis and larynx. The swelling usually extends into the trachea and bronchi. Included under the classification of croup syndromes are virus-caused syndromes such as spasmodic laryngitis (spasmodic croup), laryngotracheitis, and laryngotracheobronchitis (LTB) as well as bacterial-caused syndromes such as bacterial tracheitis and epiglottitis (Figure 25–10 ■ and Table 25–5).

LTB, epiglottitis, and bacterial tracheitis are referred to as the "big three" of pediatric respiratory illness because they affect the greatest number of children across all age groups in both sexes. LTB is the most common disorder, but epiglottitis and bacterial tracheitis are more serious. The initial symptoms of all three conditions include inspiratory **stridor** (a high-pitched, musical sound that is created by narrowing of the airway), a seal-like barking cough, and hoarseness. See the following sections for differences between these conditions. Laryngitis and laryngotracheitis are mild illnesses that can be managed at home. LTB is the most serious type of viral croup, frequently necessitating an emergency department visit for infants and children under 6 years of age. Epiglottitis is a life-threatening illness.

Laryngotracheobronchitis

Although the term *croup* is applied to several viral and bacterial syndromes, it most often refers to LTB, a viral invasion of

TABLE 25–4 Supportive Care for the Family of an Infant with SIDS

NURSING INTERVENTION	RATIONALE
Provide parents with a private area and a support person who reinforces that the infant's death was not their fault.	Parents need to be able to express their grief in their own way and be told that they are not being blamed for the infant's death.
Prepare the family for the viewing of the infant. Describe how the infant will look and feel.	You can say "Paul's (use the infant's name) skin will feel cool. He will be very still and his eyes will be closed." They probably know this, but a gentle explanation demonstrates empathy. Explain that pooling of blood on the dependent areas will look like bruises.
Allow parents to hold, touch, and rock the infant if desired.	Viewing the infant allows parents a chance to say good-bye. Before bringing the infant to parents, wrap in a clean blanket, comb the hair, wash the face, swab the mouth clean, and apply petroleum jelly to lips.
Reinforce the physician's explanation about the need for an autopsy.	An autopsy is required for all unexplained deaths. You can say to parents, "It is the only way we can be sure of what caused your baby's death."
Answer parents' questions and provide them with sources for further information. Provide literature and a name of the local contact for a SIDS support group, as well as for the national foundation.	Parents may not be able to take in all of your answers. Many emergency departments and pediatric units have a social worker who provides ongoing contact with the family. Provide names of resource persons and phone numbers for SIDS support groups.
Advise parents that surviving siblings may benefit from psychologic support.	Siblings often require emotional support in the weeks and months after the death. Social workers can help the family obtain counseling and support for all members.
Provide parents with a lock of hair, footprints, and handprints, if they desire.	Personal items can be placed in a memory book. This reaffirms the child's existence for many parents.

PATHOPHYSIOLOGY ILLUSTRATED

Airway Changes with Croup

Epiglottis swells
occluding airway
Cricoid
cartilage
Trachea swells against
cricoid cartilage
resulting in restriction

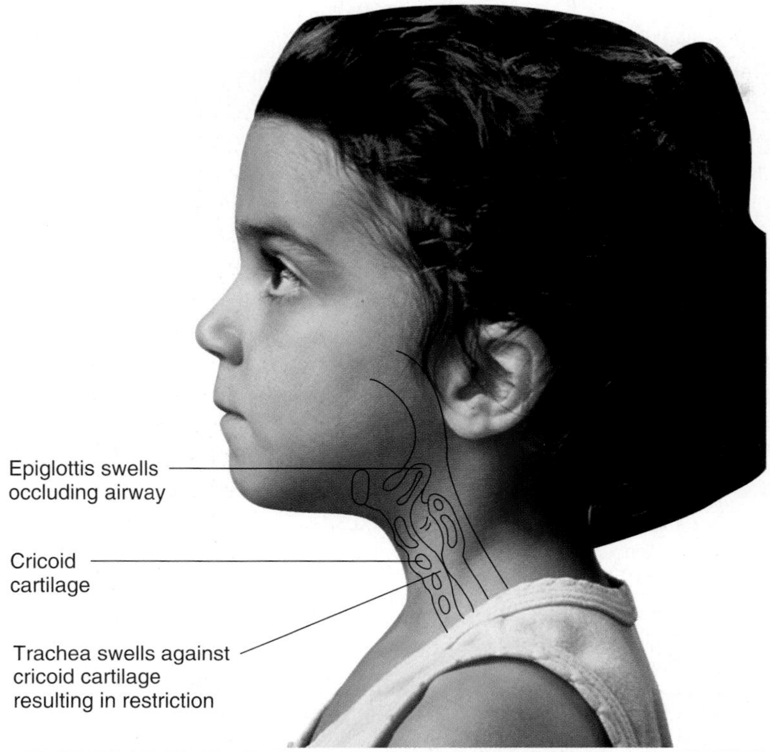

FIGURE 25–10 ■ There are two important changes in the upper airway in croup: the epiglottis swells, thereby occluding the airway, and the trachea swells against the cricoid cartilage, causing restriction.

the upper airway that extends throughout the larynx, trachea, and bronchi. Table 25–5 compares LTB and other croup syndromes.

Etiology and Pathophysiology

Acute viral LTB is most common in children 3 months to 4 years of age but can occur up to 8 years of age. Males are affected more often than females. LTB is of greatest concern in infants and children under the age of 6 years, due to potential airway obstruction. The causative organism is usually parainfluenza virus type I, II, or III, which appears during winter months in clustered outbreaks. Other viruses causing this disorder include influenza A and B, adenovirus, respiratory syncytial virus, and measles (Perkin & Swift, 2002).

The tracheal and laryngeal airway tissues respond to the invading virus with inflammation and edema. Copious, tenacious secretions further increase the child's respiratory distress. The laryngeal inflammation causes the airway diameter to narrow in the subglottic area, the narrowest part of the airway. Even small amounts of mucus or edema can quickly obstruct the airway (see Figure 25–10 ■). Both the large and small airways can be affected.

Clinical Manifestations

Most children brought to the emergency department with LTB have been ill for a couple of days with upper respiratory symptoms. These symptoms progress to a cough and hoarseness. Low-grade fever and an inflamed pharynx may or may not be present. Common presenting signs are runny nose, tachypnea, inspiratory stridor, and a seal-like barking cough. The presence of expiratory stridor, severe tachypnea, retractions, and oxygen desaturation are associated with a more serious illness. Table 25–6 can be used to assess the severity of stridor.

COLLABORATIVE CARE

Diagnostic Procedures

Diagnosis is often made by history and clinical signs. Pulse oximetry is used to detect hypoxemia. If the diagnosis of LTB is in question, anteroposterior (AP) and lateral radiographs of the upper airway are taken; these may show a tapered symmetric subglottic narrowing called a "steeple sign" in about 50% of children. Another rationale for the radiograph is to rule out the presence of a foreign body that could be causing symptoms.

> **PRACTICE ALERT**
>
> Throat cultures and visual inspection of the inner mouth and throat are contraindicated in children with LTB and epiglottitis. These procedures can cause **laryngospasms** (spasmodic vibrations that close the larynx) to occur as a result of the child's anxiety or of probing this reactive and already compromised area.

Clinical Therapy

Management consists of maintaining and improving respiratory effort with humidification, medications, and supplemental oxygen when the saturated oxygen level is less than 92%. Nebulized epinephrine constricts the capillary arterioles and reduces laryngeal mucosal edema with improvement in symptoms occurring in less than 30 minutes. Dexamethosone is given orally or intramuscularly to reduce inflammation until the child recovers from the virus. See medications used to treat laryngotracheobronchitis on page 839.

Children with a positive response to medications are often sent home from the emergency department after a 3- to 4-hour observation period. Children with persistence of moderate to severe symptoms after medication administration are admitted for further observation and treatment. Heliox, a mixture of 60% to 80% helium and 20% to 40% oxygen, may be used to manage severe LTB. It decreases the density of the gas and work of breathing by reducing the airway resistance. Heliox treatment is used to support the child until other therapeutic agents work effectively. Airway obstruction is a potential complication of severe LTB. The child may require intubation and transfer to the PICU to maintain airway patency

TABLE 25–5 Summary of Croup Syndromes

	VIRAL SYNDROMES			BACTERIAL SYNDROMES	
	ACUTE SPASMODIC LARYNGITIS (SPASMODIC CROUP)	**LARYNGOTRACHEO-BRONCHITIS**	**LARYNGOTRACHEITIS**	**BACTERIAL TRACHEITIS**	**EPIGLOTTITIS (SUPRAGLOTTITIS)**
Severity	Least serious	Most common[a]	Most serious; progresses if untreated	Guarded; requires close observation	Most life threatening (medical emergency)[a]
Age affected	3 months to 3 years	3 months to 8 years	3 months to 8 years	1 month to 13 years[a]	2 years to 8 years
Onset	Abrupt onset; peaks at night, resolves by morning (recurs)[a]	Gradual onset; starts as URI, progresses to moderate respiratory difficulty	Gradual onset; starts as URI, progresses to symptoms of respiratory distress	Progressive from URI (1–2 days)	Progresses rapidly (hours)[a]
Clinical manifestations	Afebrile; mild respiratory distress; barking-seal cough	*Early:* mild fever [<39.0°C (102.2°F)]; hoarseness; barking-seal, brassy, croupy cough; rhinorrhea; sore throat; stridor; apprehension (inspiratory) *Progressing to* labored respirations	*Early:* mild fever [<39.0°C (102.2°F)]; barking-seal, brassy, croupy cough; rhinorrhea; sore throat; stridor (inspiratory); apprehension; restless/irritable *Progressing to* retractions (progressive); increasing stridor; cyanosis	High fever [>39.0°C (102.2°F)]; URI appears as viral croupy cough; croup initially; stridor (tracheal); purulent secretions	High fever [>39.0°C (102.2°F)]; URI; intense sore throat; dysphagia[a], drooling[a]; increased pulse and respiratory rate; prefers upright position (tripod position with chin thrust)[a]
Etiology	Unknown; suspect viral with allergic/emotional influences	Parainfluenza, types I and II, RSV, or influenza	Parainfluenza, types I and II, RSV, or influenza	*Staphylococcus*	*Haemophilus influenzae*

[a] Classic parameter or key point (distinguishes condition).

if total obstruction is imminent. Most children, however, respond positively to the medications and oxygen therapy and are discharged within 48 to 72 hours.

NURSING MANAGEMENT

Nursing Assessment and Diagnosis

The initial and ongoing physical assessment of the child with LTB focuses on adequacy of respiratory functioning. Table 25–7 provides guidelines for assessment and rationale for actions. Close monitoring is required to identify changes in airway patency. The child should be continuously monitored in the emergency department, short-stay observation area, or the PICU. Infants and preverbal toddlers require constant supervision to monitor respiratory status. A means of communication (sign language or simple word cues) must be established to enable the older child to alert nursing staff about respiratory difficulty.

Particular attention should be paid to the child's respiratory effort, breath sounds, and responsiveness. Physical exhaustion can diminish the intensity of retractions and stridor. As the child uses the remaining energy reserve to maintain ventilation, breath sounds may actually diminish. Noisy breathing (audible airway congestion, coarse breath sounds) in this situation verifies adequate energy stores. Responsiveness will decrease as hypoxemia increases.

The following nursing diagnoses might be appropriate for the child with acute LTB:

- Ineffective Breathing Pattern related to tracheobronchial obstruction, decreased energy, and fatigue
- Ineffective Airway Clearance (copious secretions)
- Risk for Fluid Volume Deficit related to inadequate fluid intake
- Fear (child) related to dyspnea, unfamiliar surroundings, procedures, and separation from support system

TABLE 25–6 Clinical Scoring System for Assessing Children with Stridor

SIGN	0	1	2	3
Stridor	None	With agitation	Mild at rest	Severe at rest
Retraction	None	Mild	Moderate	Severe
Air entry	Normal	Normal	Decreased	Severe decrease
Color	Normal	Normal	Cyanotic with agitation	Cyanotic with rest
Level of consciousness	Normal	Restless if disturbed	Restless if undisturbed	Lethargic

Scoring: To quantifiy the severity of stridor, add the individual scores for each of the sign categories. A score between 0 and 15 is possible. A rating of severity based on total score is as follows: < 6 is mild, 7–8 is moderate, > 8 is severe.

Note: From Perkin, R. M., & Swift, J. D. (2002). Infectious causes of upper airway obstruction in children. Pediatric Emergency Medicine Reports, *7(11), 120.*

MEDICATIONS Used for Symptomatic Treatment of Laryngotracheobronchitis

MEDICATION	ACTION/INDICATION	NURSING CONSIDERATIONS
Beta-agonists and beta-adrenergics (e.g., albuterol, racemic epinephrine): aerosolized through face mask	Rapid-acting bronchodilator, decreases bronchial and tracheal secretions and mucosal edema, used to decrease symptoms of moderate to severe respiratory distress; and constriction of subglottic mucosa and submucosal capillaries. Used until dexamethasone begins working.	Provides only temporary relief; improvement in 30 minutes which lasts about 2 hours, it gives time for the steroid to work; the child may experience tachycardia (160–200 beats/min) and hypertension; dizziness, headache, and nausea may necessitate stopping medication; reduces the need for artifical airway.
Corticosteroids (e.g., dexamethasone): IM, PO Nebulized budesonide	Anti-inflammatory, used to decrease edema; has a long half-life of 36–54 hours.	The child may experience cardiovascular symptoms (hypertension): requires close observation for individual response; children less frequently need emergency airways; stridor resolves faster.

Planning and Implementation

Skillful nursing care can greatly assist children with LTB and their families to cope with the symptoms of the illness. Nursing care focuses on maintaining airway patency, promoting fluid balance, reducing stress, and teaching the family how to care for the child at home.

Maintain Airway Patency

Supplemental oxygen with humidity may be needed for hypoxemia. Allow the child to assume a position of comfort, which will most likely be sitting or lying with the head elevated. Administer medications. Cool mist is presumed to moisten airway secretions and soothe the inflamed mucosa; however, research has not revealed a significant benefit to this treatment (Perkin & Swift, 2002).

An important developmental consideration is the child's ability to communicate reliably. The nurse must be immediately available to attend to the child's respiratory needs during emergency department or outpatient care. If hospitalization is needed, place the child in a room near the nurses' station and maintain emergency resuscitation equipment at the bedside. Parents are helpful in providing support to the child and alerting the nurse when the respiratory symptoms worsen.

Meet Fluid and Nutritional Needs

The illness preceding the emergency department visit may have compromised the child's fluid status. Recognizing fluid deficit and monitoring the child's hydration and nutritional status are essential. Respiratory distress can compromise the child's ability and desire to drink fluids. Fluids promote liquification of secretions and provide calories for energy and metabolism. Children with LTB usually prefer cool, noncarbonated, nonacidic drinks such as apple juice or fruit-flavored drinks. Remember that gelatin, ice, and fruit-flavored ice pops are also fluids. Oral rehydration fluids may also be used. Parents can be encouraged to participate in gaining the child's cooperation in taking oral fluids. An intravenous infusion may be necessary to rehydrate the child, maintain fluid balance, or provide emergency medication access. The child should be observed closely for difficulty in swallowing or drooling, which may be an early sign of epiglottitis or bacterial tracheitis.

Discharge Planning and Home Care Teaching

During the child's observation period, the nurse should take every opportunity to assess the parents' knowledge of symptoms of LTB and discuss actions to take if symptoms recur. For example, instruct parents to call the child's healthcare provider if the following occurs.

- Mild symptoms do not improve after 1 hour of humidity and cool air treatment.
- The child's breathing is rapid and labored.
- The child does not drink adequate liquids, and urine output is reduced

TABLE 25–7 Nursing Assessment of Child with Respiratory Difficulty

NURSING ACTION	RATIONALE
Assess heart rate and respiratory rate.	Tachypnea and tachycardia indicate increasing respiratory effort.
What is the child's position (sitting, prone, or supine)?	Upright or semi-Fowler's promotes airway patency; the child's change to a more upright position may signal increased distress.
Assess overall quality of respiratory effort. Determine inspiratory and expiratory breath sounds, ability to speak, and presence of stridor, cough, retractions, nasal flaring, cyanosis.	Reflects overall adequacy of airway and respiratory function.
Initiate stridor severity assessment (Table 25–6), continue scoring every 30 minutes or more frequently if distress increases; initiate nursing actions appropriate for croup score.	Provides consistent and objective assessment data with score for future comparison.
Attach cardiorespiratory monitor and pulse oximeter.	Provides continuous assessment data as part of ongoing physiologic monitoring.

Evaluation

Expected outcomes of nursing care include the following:

- The child responds to medications with decreased respiratory distress.
- The child's fear and anxiety are managed with family support and explanations about care.

Epiglottitis (Supraglottitis)

Epiglottitis (also known as supraglottitis) is an inflammation of the tissues surrounding the epiglottis, the long, narrow structure that closes off the glottis during swallowing. Because edema in this area can rapidly (within minutes or hours) obstruct the airway by occluding the trachea, epiglottitis is considered a potentially life-threatening condition. (Table 25–5 compares epiglottitis and other croup syndromes.)

Etiology and Pathophysiology

Epiglottitis is caused by bacterial invasion of the soft tissue of the supraglottic area by streptococcus, staphylococcus, or by Haemophilus influenzae type B (Hib) in unimmunized children. The resulting cellulitis causes swelling in the tissues surrounding the epiglottis leading to airway obstruction. Since use of the Hib vaccine has become widespread, there has been a 10-fold decrease in the incidence of epiglottitis (Isaacson & Isaacson, 2003).

Clinical Manifestations

Characteristically, a previously healthy child suddenly becomes very ill. The child initially develops a high fever (greater than 39°C [102.2°F]), with a severe sore throat. The four classic signs of epiglottitis, in order of their appearance, are as follows:

- **Dysphonia,** muffled, hoarse, or absent voice sounds
- **Dysphagia,** difficulty in swallowing
- Drooling, the child refuses fluids or resists swallowing due to intense throat pain
- Distressed respiratory effort with inspiratory stridor

To fully open the airway and improve air intake, the child sits up and leans forward with the jaw thrust forward in the classic "sniffing" or tripod posture and refuses to lie down. The child's anxiety increases as respiratory distress progresses.

COLLABORATIVE CARE

Care of the child with suspected epiglottitis is focused on rapid diagnosis and assuring an emergency airway.

Diagnostic Procedures

Diagnosis is often based on a lateral neck radiograph (Figure 25–11 ■), which reveals a narrowed airway and an enlarged, rounded epiglottis, seen as a mass at the base of the tongue. Laryngospasm and airway obstruction can occur as a result of the severe irritation and hypersensitivity of the airway muscles. For this reason, visual inspection of the mouth and throat is contraindicated in children with suspected epiglottitis. A culture of the epiglottis is performed after an endotracheal tube has been inserted and the child is stabilized.

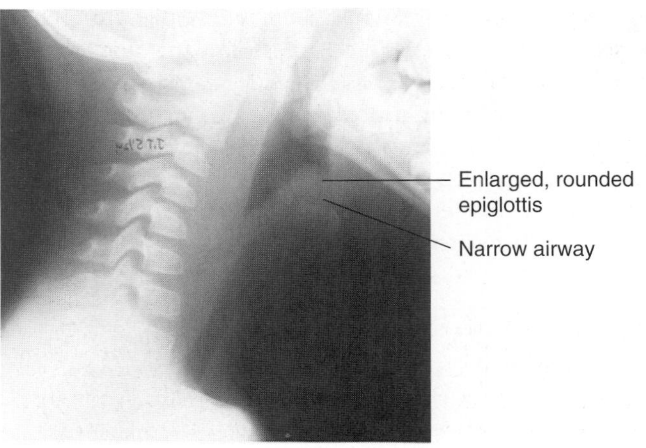

FIGURE 25–11 ■ The phrase "thumb sign" has been used to describe this enlargement of the epiglottis. Recall the trachea's usual "little finger" size. Do you see the stiff, enlarged "thumb" above it in this lateral neck radiograph?

Clinical Therapy

Immediate clinical therapy usually involves insertion of an endotracheal tube to maintain the airway, usually in the operating room. At the same time, the airway is inspected and a direct culture of the supraglottic tissue is taken. Antibiotics effective for gram-positive organisms and *H. influenzae* (second- or third-generation cephalosporin) are given until blood culture sensitivities are available when the antibiotic may be changed to one that is more specific for the organism. No evidence exists that corticosteroids are beneficial.

NURSING MANAGEMENT

Nursing management consists of airway management, drug therapy, hydration, and emotional and psychosocial support of the child and parents.

Nursing Assessment and Diagnosis

The child's respiratory and airway status should be observed closely and often. The child often breathes slowly and with great concentration as the airway obstruction increases. Note any change in the child's level of consciousness—from anxiety to lethargy to stupor as hypoxia increases.

Examples of nursing diagnoses include the following:

- Ineffective Airway Clearance related to increased swelling of the epiglottis and drooling
- Anxiety (child) related to increasing difficulty breathing
- Anxiety (parents) related to sudden onset of life-threatening illness

Planning and Implementation

Until intubated, the child is never left unattended or transported away from equipment or from personnel who can perform emergency airway interventions. Allow the child to sit upright or assume a position of comfort to maintain the airway patency and breathe more easily. Supplemental humidified oxygen may be used initially to reverse hypoxemia. Provide a quiet environment with as little stress as possible to decrease anxiety and crying. Anxiety-provoking procedures, such as venipuncture, are postponed until the airway is secure. Crying stimulates the airway, increases oxygen consumption, and can precipitate laryngospasm; the calmer the child, the better the respiratory function (Eichelberger, Ball, Pratsch, et al., 1998).

PRACTICE ALERT

Observe the child continuously for absence of voice sounds, increasing degree of respiratory distress, inability to swallow, and acute onset of drooling (an ominous sign of supraglottic obstruction). If any of these signs occur, get medical assistance immediately. The quieter the child, the greater the cause for concern.

Provide support to parents as they cope with the sudden onset of a life-threatening illness. Identify ways to help parents notify family members and ensure that other children are cared for during the crisis. Keep parents informed about the child's status and permit them to stay with the child to help keep the child calm.

The child is often cared for in an intensive care unit after the airway has been stabilized. Administer prescribed antibiotics to treat the infection and IV fluids to provide hydration. Because the child was febrile with a sore throat before admission, fluid intake may have been compromised. Most children show rapid improvement once cool mist and oxygen, antibiotics, and fluid therapy are started. The endotracheal tube can usually be removed within 24 to 36 hours once the child is afebrile and swallowing comfortably (Hazinski, 1999).

The dyspnea and loss of voice, or even the inability to create sounds, can be frightening to a child. The unfamiliar hospital environment and strange equipment can create stress for child and parent alike. It is important to reassure the parents that the child's voice loss is temporary and to explain the need for the various pieces of equipment. Home care may involve completing the course of antibiotics. Parents need instructions on proper administration and potential side effects of drug therapy.

■ Evaluation

Expected outcomes of nursing care include the following:

- The child's acute infection resolves, the endotracheal tube is removed, and the voice returns.
- The parents cope effectively during the child's illness and provide support to the child.

Bacterial Tracheitis

Bacterial tracheitis occurs as a secondary infection of the upper trachea following an initial viral laryngotracheitis. The secondary infection may be caused by *Staphylococcus aureus, alpha-hemolytic Streptococcus, group A Streptococcus, Moraxella catarrhalis,* or *Haemophilus influenzae.* The disorder starts with a viral upper respiratory infection, croupy cough, and stridor but progresses to include a high fever greater than 39°C (102.2°F), respiratory distress, and a toxic appearance (Stroud & Friedman, 2001). No drooling is present. Table 25–5 compares bacterial tracheitis and other croup syndromes.

Diagnosis is often made by blood cultures after the child is found unresponsive to usual LTB management. Endoscopic examination may be performed on children with minimal airway symptoms. The subglottis is edematous with ulceration, and thick mucopurulent exudate may obstruct the trachea and main bronchi. Culture and sensitivities are obtained.

Due to the similarity of symptoms, bacterial tracheitis is often misdiagnosed initially as LTB. Instead of improving with nebulized epinephrine, the child's condition worsens. Antibiotics are given for 10 to 14 days. Most children are intubated for 3 to 11 days. Frequent suctioning, humidification, and monitoring for patency of the endotracheal tube are required.

Nursing Management

The child with bacterial tracheitis is frequently cared for in the intensive care unit after intubation. The child must have airway patency assessed frequently. Airway maintenance is often required because of the thick tracheal secretions that pool high in the upper airway. Since most children need to be intubated for 3 to 11 days, monitor the patency of the endotracheal tube, suction as needed, and provide humidified air or oxygen. Mechanical suctioning helps remove the thick secretions to help maintain the airway. Children generally prefer lying flat to sitting up. This seems to be a position of comfort that allows the child to conserve energy. Antibiotics are administrated as ordered.

The earlier section on epiglottitis discusses other nursing care interventions that may also be appropriate for the child with bacterial tracheitis.

LOWER AIRWAY DISORDERS

The lower airway, or bronchial tree, lies below the trachea and includes the bronchi, bronchioles, and alveoli. Lower airway disorders occur because a structural or functional problem interferes with the lungs' ability to complete the respiratory cycle. Lower airway disorders include neonatal respiratory distress syndrome, meconium aspiration, transient tachypnea of the newborn, bronchitis, bronchiolitis, pneumonia, and tuberculosis.

Neonatal Respiratory Distress Syndrome

Neonatal respiratory distress syndrome (RDS), also known as hyaline membrane disease, manifests during the first hours of life in preterm newborns with surfactant deficiency. RDS is the most common cause of respiratory failure and death in the newborn, accounting for 20% to 30% of preterm newborn deaths (Froh, 2002). RDS is more common in Whites and males.

Etiology and Pathophysiology

In utero, the fetal lungs are filled with fluid. When the infant takes the first breath after birth, this fluid is expelled from the alveoli. Most of the fetal lung fluid is moved to the interstitial spaces and absorbed. A small amount is expelled in a term birth, but less is expelled by preterm newborns because of the lack of mechanical forces during passage through the birth canal. With the onset of breathing, inspiration and negative thoracic pressures fill the alveoli with air. When the surface tension of the lung tissue is high, the alveoli are difficult to inflate.

Surfactant is a substance that lowers the surface tension of the alveoli and prevents the interior walls of the alveoli from adhering. Pulmonary surfactant consists of 90% lipid and 10% protein. It plays a major role in development of the normal surface lining layer of the lung (Krauss, 2003). Without sufficient surfactant, fluid droplets remaining in the alveoli cause the surface tension to increase and the sides of the alveoli collapse or stick together on expiration. Significant negative pressure is needed for the newborn to breathe and reopen the alveoli. This is difficult due to the compliant chest wall and stiff lungs, leading to **atelectasis** (collapse of a portion of the lung). Atelectasis actually results because of surfactant depletion. As a consequence the newborn uses more energy to exert this negative pressure and becomes exhausted and is unable to sustain the work of breathing. Fatigue associated with respiratory effort results in decreased air movement and hypoxia. The hypoxia and atelectasis lead to vasoconstriction of the pulmonary vascular beds, increased pulmonary vascular resistance, respiratory acidosis, and partial return to fetal circulation. (See information on fetal circulation in Chapter 26∞.) Metabolic acidosis develops following a prolonged lack of oxygen at the cellular level. Several factors are associated with the development of chronic lung disease following RDS such as long-term ventilatory support, oxygen administration, and infections.

Clinical Manifestations

Signs and symptoms become apparent shortly after birth. They include tachypnea (at rates greater than 60 breaths/min), nasal flaring, intercostal and subcostal retractions, expiratory grunting, crackles, cyanosis, slow capillary refill, paradoxical breathing (in which the chest falls and the abdomen rises on inspiration), decreased breath sounds, and labored breathing. Apnea and irregular breathing are seen as the newborn tires.

COLLABORATIVE CARE

Care focuses on identifying the newborn with potential for respiratory distress and providing surfactant and ventilatory support.

Diagnostic Procedures

Diagnosis is often made within minutes of birth when resuscitation is needed for severe respiratory distress. Prior knowledge of the history and anticipated gestational age are also part of the diagnostic picture. A chest radiograph may show diffuse fine granular densities with portions of an air-filled tracheobronchial tree as early as 6 hours after birth. An echocardiogram is used to assess for a vascular shunt (patent ductus arteriosis) that enables blood to bypass the lungs.

Clinical Therapy

Management focuses on emergency intervention at birth, temperature control, and assisted ventilation to expand the alveoli and preserve respiratory function. Surfactant is instilled down an endotracheal tube shortly after birth to decrease the alveolar surface tension. Repeated doses may be given every 12 hours for about 48 hours, depending upon the newborn's need. Supplemental oxygen may be provided through ventilatory support from CPAP and PEEP, or various devices such as high-frequency oscillation or jet ventilation. Careful monitoring is needed to reduce the risk of adverse effects of hyperoxia, such as bronchopulmonary dysplasia and retinopathy of prematurity. Intravenous fluid therapy and medications are administered to support function of the respiratory and other body systems. Blood products may be administered to expand blood volume, thus increasing oxygen capacity.

NURSING MANAGEMENT

The newborn is cared for in a neonatal intensive care nursery. The respiratory status of the infant with RDS is closely monitored. Nursing assessment focuses on identifying changes in respiratory status such as quality of respirations and pulse, grunting respirations, nasal flaring, retractions, apnea, overall color, signs of dehydration, and changes in the infant's behavior. Pulse oximetry and blood gases are monitored to aid in assessment. Care of the infant is organized to eliminate unnecessary physical stimulation, as this additional stress contributes to respiratory compromise. The infant is usually placed in a warmer to stabilize the temperature and to reduce metabolic demands. Fluid management is critical as excess fluids can lead to pulmonary edema. Provide fluids and nutrition to help meet energy needs. Position the infant to facilitate breathing. Parents need clear explanations about the infant's health status and planned interventions. By remaining available to parents and answering their questions, the nurse establishes a positive relationship and facilitates essential communication.

Due to the potential for respiratory distress and chronic lung disease after discharge, parents should be taught CPR and oxygen administration if ordered. The infant also has apnea or if supplemental oxygen is ordered, a home apnea monitor may be used. Some monitors permit data to be downloaded enabling the healthcare provider to evaluate the frequency and length of apnea spells that occur at home. Home care nursing may be needed to provide follow-up support. Parents may benefit from a referral to a support group.

Meconium Aspiration Syndrome

Meconium is the greenish-black, sticky material present in the bowels of the fetus. It consists of amniotic fluid, mucus, lanugo, bile, exfoliated cells, glycoproteins, various enzymes, minerals, and lipids. In cases of fetal distress, the meconium may be released into the amniotic fluid and then aspirated in utero, during labor, or during delivery. Amniotic fluid is stained by meconium in 8% to 19% of term deliveries, and the risk increases with advancing gestational age. Thicker meconium-stained amniotic fluid and a longer duration of exposure to it increase the risk for developing meconium aspiration syndrome. As many as 33% of infants born with meconium-stained amniotic fluid may develop meconium aspiration syndrome (Fuloria & Wiswell, 2000).

Etiology and Pathophysiology

Meconium aspiration can lead to partial or complete airway obstruction, atelectasis, air trapping with increased functional residual capacity, and air leaks. Meconium causes a chemical inflammation of the airway leading to pulmonary edema, and cellular necrosis. Meconium interferes with the production of surfactant and its ability to reduce the surface tension of pulmonary fluids. Air can be inhaled but not exhaled, leading to distention and rupture of the alveoli. This can cause air leaks, pneumomediastinum, or a pneumothorax. Nearly one third of infants with meconium aspiration syndrome develop persistent pulmonary hypertension with persistent fetal circulation. See Chapter 26∞ for more information. All of these pathophysiologic changes lead to hypoxia, hypercapnia, and respiratory and metabolic acidosis.

Clinical Manifestations

Newborns have respiratory distress with tachypnea, grunting, flaring, retractions, and cyanosis. Yellowish staining of the skin, nails, and umbilical cord is usually present because of meconium in the amniotic fluid. Typical findings on chest radiograph are patchy infiltrates, areas of consolidation, and hyperinflation. Signs of neurologic depression are also apparent. Grunting slows the expiratory flow and increases the lung volume and alveolar pressures. This sign of severe disease suggests the onset of respiratory failure (Margolis & Gadomski, 1998).

COLLABORATIVE CARE

A chest radiograph will be obtained to identify if a pneumothorax or air leak is present. An umbilical arterial line is inserted to monitor the arterial blood pressures, blood pH, and blood gases as needed.

Newborns with meconium-stained amniotic fluid must have the nasal and oral pharyngeal airways suctioned as soon as the baby's head is delivered in an effort to reduce aspiration. Newborns with depressed respiratory or neurologic function are aggressively resuscitated after thorough suctioning is completed. Immediate tracheal suctioning and intubation of infants born through meconium-stained amniotic fluid is performed when the newborn has depressed respirations or requires positive pressure ventilation soon after birth. IV fluids, blood, and medications are infused through an umbilical arterial line. Surfactant replacement therapy may be used. Other therapies are under investigation, such as bronchoalveolar lavage, glucocorticoids, and nitrous oxide. If the newborn progresses to respiratory failure and is not responding to other therapies, transfer to a neonatal intensive care unit for nitric oxide or extracorporeal membranous oxygenation (ECMO) therapy may be necessary.

NURSING MANAGEMENT

The newborn with meconium aspiration syndrome is cared for in a neonatal intensive care nursery. Nursing management follows guidelines previously described for RDS. Actions involve carefully assessing and monitoring the newborn for hypoglycemia, signs of complications, and response to treatment. Regulation of the environmental temperature and maintenance of adequate oxygenation and ventilation are essential. Caloric requirements, IV fluids, and medication administration are priorities of nursing care.

Provide support to families who must cope with suddenly changed expectations about having a healthy baby. Help them understand the infant's health problems and rationale for the treatment provided.

Transient Tachypnea of the Newborn

Transient tachypnea of the newborn is a progressive respiratory distress disorder that commonly develops in near-term infants that is sometimes difficult to distinguish from RDS. The disorder often follows a preterm or term newborn delivery that was uneventful.

Etiology and Pathophysiology

The primary cause of this disorder is failure to clear the airway of fetal lung fluid, mucus, or other debris. Alternatively excess fluid may be in the lungs because amniotic fluid or tracheal fluid is aspirated. The lung fluid is believed to decrease pulmonary compliance (increased lung stiffness) and tidal volume while increasing dead space. Vaginal-birth newborns less commonly develop the disorder because their thorax is compressed during delivery, forcing out some of the lung fluids. Other newborns at risk include those with intrauterine asphyxia due to maternal oversedation, maternal bleeding, prolapsed cord, breech birth, or maternal diabetes (Ladewig, London, Moberly, et al., 2002).

Clinical Manifestations

The newborn has no initial breathing difficulties at birth. Shortly after birth respiratory distress develops with signs including expiratory grunting, nasal flaring, retractions, and mild cyanosis when on room air. Tachypnea with rates up to 100 to 140 breaths per minute develops within 6 hours of birth. No crackles or rhonchi are heard on auscultation. These infants often do not appear to be severely ill. Condition improvement begins by 8 to 24 hours of age. Recovery is usually sudden within 72 hours of age.

COLLABORATIVE CARE

Diagnosis is based on absence of adventitious breath sounds and chest radiograph. Blood gas and electrolyte levels may be obtained. Radiograph findings reveal prominent vascular markings, hyperaeration of the alveoli, and a flattened diaphragm contour. The chest radiograph findings clear within 48 to 72 hours. Clinical therapy sometimes involves supplemental oxygen (usually less than 40% concentration), fluids, and electrolytes.

NURSING MANAGEMENT

Nursing assessment and management for transient tachypnea of the newborn is the same as for RDS during the acute care phase. Monitor and identify changes in newborn's respiratory status, as well as fluid and electrolyte levels. Attach a cardiorespiratory monitor and pulse oximeter. Monitor oxygen delivery and infant's response to supplemental oxygen.

Organize care to the infant to eliminate unnecessary physical stimulation. The infant is usually placed in a warmer to stabilize the temperature and to reduce metabolic demands. Feedings may be postponed because of the rapid respiratory rate. Support the mother's effort to breastfeed as soon as the infant's condition allows it. Parents need clear explanations about the infant's health status and planned interventions. Help parents to identify changes in the infant's condition indicating recovery.

Bronchitis

Acute bronchitis, inflammation of the trachea and bronchi, rarely occurs in childhood as an isolated problem. The bronchi can be affected simultaneously with adjacent respiratory structures during a respiratory illness. Bronchitis occurs most often in children under 4 years of age, usually following a mild upper respiratory tract problem, but it can occur at any age (D'Auria, 1997). Bronchitis is caused most often by a virus but may also result from invasion of bacteria or in response to an allergen or irritant.

The classic symptom of bronchitis is a coarse, hacking cough, which increases in severity at night. Children with bronchitis look tired. The chest and ribs may be painful due to deep and frequent coughing. There is often a deep, rattling quality to breathing. Some children have audible wheezing that can be heard without a stethoscope. Treatment is palliative unless a secondary bacterial infection occurs.

Nursing Management

Nursing management includes supporting respiratory function through rest, humidification, hydration, and symptomatic treatment. Refer to the sections on asthma and pneumonia for detailed information on treatment measures.

Home care should emphasize the self-limiting nature of the disorder. Parents who smoke should be advised that quitting or refraining from smoking in the child's presence may benefit the child.

Bronchiolitis

Bronchiolitis is a lower respiratory tract illness that occurs when an infecting agent (virus or bacterium) causes inflammation and obstruction of the small airways, the bronchioles. The peak age for bronchiolitis is 2 to 6 months (Cooper, Banasiak, & Allen, 2003). Infection is most severe in infants under 6 months of age and in children with lung or heart disease. Bronchiolitis accounts for 90,000 hospital admissions and 4,500 deaths per year, mostly among infants under 6 months of age (Agency for Healthcare Research and Quality, 2003).

Etiology and Pathophysiology

Respiratory syncytial virus (RSV) is the most common cause of bronchiolitis, but bacteria, mycoplasms, and other viruses can be causative organisms. RSV occurs in annual epidemics from October to March. It is transmitted through direct contact with respiratory secretions or indirectly through contaminated surfaces. Nearly all children have been infected with RSV by 2 years of age, and reinfection (via siblings or close family contacts) throughout life is common (National Respiratory and Enteric Virus Surveillance System, 2000). RSV is the most common cause of lower respiratory tract infections in infants and children. RSV causes severe or fatal illness in infants with conditions such as congenital heart disease, bronchopulmonary dysplasia (BPD), prematurity, and immunosuppression.

Viruses are able to invade the mucosal cells that line the small bronchi and bronchioles. The invaded cells die when the virus bursts from inside the cell to invade adjacent cells. The membranes of the infected cells fuse with adjacent cells creating large masses of cells or "syncytia." The resulting cell debris clogs and obstructs the bronchioles and irritates the airway. In response, the airway lining swells and produces excessive mucus. Despite this protective response by the bronchioles, the actual effect is partial airway obstruction during expiration and bronchospasms.

The cycle is repeated throughout both lungs as the airway cells are invaded by the virus. The partially obstructed airways allow air in, but the mucus and airway swelling block expulsion of the air. This creates the wheezing and crackles in the airways. Atelectasis occurs in some areas and air trapping and hyperinflation in others. Hypoxemia results because of the ventilation-perfusion mismatch. See page 827. The child with RSV is therefore at risk for respiratory failure as the oxygen level decreases and the carbon dioxide level increases. Apnea and pulmonary edema may occur.

Clinical Manifestations

The infant or child with bronchiolitis may have been ill with upper respiratory symptoms such as nasal stuffiness, cough (not usually noted in infants), and fever (less than 39°C [102.2°F]) for a few days. As the illness progresses and the lower respiratory tract becomes involved, symptoms increase and include rhinitis, low-grade fever, inspiratory and expiratory wheezing; a deeper, more frequent cough; tachypnea; retractions; and more labored breathing. In severe cases, signs and symptoms include rapid, shallow respirations, nasal flaring and marked retractions, crackles, cyanosis, and decreased breath sounds. As the airflow continues to decrease, breath sounds diminish. Thus the noisier the lungs, the better, as this indicates that the child is still able to move air in and out of the lungs.

Dehydration may be present if the child has been sick for several days. Abdominal distention may occur due to air swallowing. Parents report that the infant or child is acting more ill—appearing sicker, less playful, and less interested in eating. Infants especially may refuse to feed or may spit up what they eat along with thick, clear mucus. Airway hyperresponsiveness may persist for weeks after the virus has resolved.

COLLABORATIVE CARE

Care is focused on providing oxygen, fluids, and medications to support the infant and young child until the infection resolves.

Diagnostic Procedures

The history and physical examination provide the data needed to diagnose bronchiolitis. Laboratory tests that are used to identify the virus causing bronchiolitis include enzyme-linked immunosorbent assay (ELISA) or direct fluorescent assay that can provide information in a few hours. The assays are performed on nasal wash specimens placed in viral transport medium. Chest radiographs show hyperinflation, patchy atelectasis, and other signs of inflammation.

Clinical Therapy

Children who test positive for RSV are isolated, roomed together, or placed on the same unit to minimize the spread of the virus to other hospitalized children. Oxygen administration and supportive care are provided, especially when the causative agent is unknown and the condition is mild to moderate in severity. See Table 25–8 for additional clinical therapies.

Various medications may be prescribed for RSV and bronchiolitis in an effort to treat symptoms and shorten the course of the infection. Bronchodilators, nebulized epinephrine, and corticosteroids are occasionally used, but effectiveness has not been documented by studies (Figure 25–12 ■). Research continues to be conducted to identify medications that might be effective in treating bronchiolitis, such as oral dexamethasone and montelukast. Antibiotics are not used routinely unless the child also has a bacterial infection.

The child with apnea or respiratory failure will be cared for in the critical care unit and may be intubated and ventilated. Ribavirin is an antiviral drug specifically available for RSV treatment, and acts to slow viral replication. Because studies have not confirmed its effectiveness, it is reserved for life-threatening cases, such as infants with complicated congenital heart disease, BPD, cystic fibrosis, or other chronic lung disease (Wright, Pomerantz, & Luria, 2002).

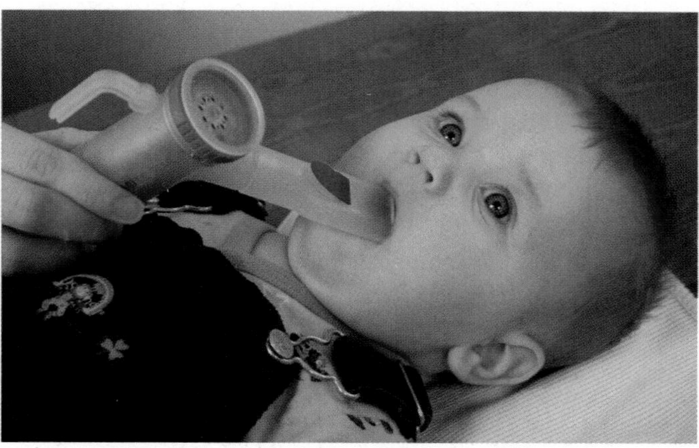

FIGURE 25–12 ■ Nebulized epinephrine administration for bronchiolitis. Parents can hold the nebulizer and reduce the infant's fear.

While RSV bronchiolitis resolves in 5 to 7 days, increased airway resistance and airway hypersensitivity may persist for weeks or even months. Some evidence suggests that bronchiolitis in infancy may increase the risk for childhood wheezing and asthma. It also may be a major risk factor for chronic obstructive pulmonary disease later in life (Webster & Huether, 1998).

Prevention of RSV is a focus for children under 2 years of age at high risk for severe bronchiolitis caused by RSV. The characteristics of children who fall into this high-risk category are the following (American Academy of Pediatrics Committee on Infectious Diseases and Committee on Fetus and Newborn, 2003a):

- Prematurity—born at 32 week's gestation or earlier, particularly if less than 6 months of age at the start of the RSV season

TABLE 25–8 Clinical Therapy for Bronchiolitis

COLLABORATIVE CARE	RATIONALE
Cardiorespiratory monitor and pulse oximeter	Enable provider to follow course and assess need for specific therapies.
Humidified oxygen therapy by hood or face tent, mask or nasal cannula	Delivery method chosen based on desired concentration of oxygen, degree of humidity, and child's response.
Intubation and assisted ventilation (PEEP/CPAP)	Used when the child becomes too fatigued to breathe effectively.
Hydration with intravenous or oral fluids	Provider must consider insensible fluid loss, decreased intake, the child's current electrolyte and hydration status, and risk for pulmonary edema.
Postural drainage and chest physiotherapy	Helps to further loosen and mobilize trapped mucus.
Systemic medications	Symptomatic treatment may include antipyretics (acetaminophen or ibuprofen preferred; no antibiotics are given unless evidence of secondary bacterial infection [e.g., otitis media] is present). Bronchodilators, nebulized epinephrine, and corticosteroids are occasionally used.
High-Risk Infant or Child[a]	
RSV immune globulin (Respigam) IV Palivizumab (Synargis) IM	Give for 5 consecutive months during RSV season to high-risk children. May prevent RSV bronchiolitis or reduce severity of disease. Both are very expensive, but less than hospitalization.

[a]Defined as a child with congenital heart disease, bronchopulmonary dysplasia, chronic lung problems, cystic fibrosis, or an infant who is premature or severely ill and less than 6 weeks old.

- Chronic lung disease such as BPD who have required supplemental oxygen, bronchodilator, diuretic or corticosteroid therapy within 6 months of the start of RSV season
- Complicated congenital heart disease, particularly those on medication to control congestive heart failure, with cyanosis, and with moderate to severe pulmonary hypertension
- Immunocompromised infants and children

Intravenous RSV immune globulin (Respigam) or intramuscular palivizumab (Synagis) may be used for prophylaxis for the above group of children under 2 years of age. Prophylactic treatment is expensive, so it is limited to high-risk children. Monthly treatment for 5 months beginning in October or November is initiated at the onset of the RSV season and terminated at the end of the RSV season. Monthly treatment has been associated with reduced hospitalization of high-risk infants. Palivizumab is preferred treatment because it is easier to administer and has fewer side effects. Palivizumab does not interfere with vaccine administration, but children receiving RSV immune globulin should wait 9 months before receiving the live virus vaccines (MMR and varicella). Children under 2 years of age with complicated cyanotic or congenital heart disease should only receive palivizumab. Children with severe immunodeficiencies receiving immune globulin monthly could have RSV immune globulin substituted during RSV season (American Academy of Pediatrics Committee on Infectious Diseases and Committee on Fetus and Newborn, 2003a).

NURSING MANAGEMENT

An important nursing role is prevention of RSV by educating parents and caregivers about methods to reduce exposure and transmission of the disease by frequent handwashing, eliminating exposure to crowds and other children, as well as cigarette smoke.

Nursing Assessment and Diagnosis

Physiologic Assessment

Assess airway and respiratory function carefully. Good observation skills are important to ensure timely interventions for worsening respiratory symptoms and prevention of respiratory distress (see Box 25–1 and the clinical manifestations table on page 828). A decreased oxygen saturation level below 90% is the best indicator of the severity of the disease.

PRACTICE ALERT

Signs of life-threatening illness in the infant with bronchiolitis include central cyanosis, respiratory rate greater than 70 breaths per minute, listlessness, and apneic spells. The chest is hyperinflated and air exchange is so poor that breath sounds are very diminished on auscultation.

The nurse may be asked to obtain the nasal wash specimen. Use standard precautions. Instill 1 to 2 drops of sterile saline without preservative into each naris. Then gently suction nasal contents using an 8 French catheter attached to a suction trap. Follow hospital guidelines for adding viral transport medium and transport to the laboratory. The child may have increased coughing and nasal secretions after the procedure.

Psychosocial Assessment

Children and their parents should be observed for signs of fear and anxiety (Box 25–6). The unfamiliar hospital environment and procedures can increase stress. Parents' questions, as well as their nonverbal cues, help direct nursing interventions during admission and throughout hospitalization.

The accompanying nursing care plan lists common nursing diagnoses for the child with bronchiolitis. The following diagnoses might also be appropriate.

- Ineffective Airway Clearance related to increased airway secretions, fatigue from coughing and dyspnea, and air trapping
- Activity Intolerance related to imbalance between oxygen supply and demand
- Risk for Deficient Fluid Volume related to inability to meet fluid needs and increased metabolic demands (insensible loss, fever, thickened or increased respiratory secretions)

Planning and Implementation

Nursing management focuses on maintaining respiratory function, supporting overall physiologic function and hydration, reducing the child's and family's anxiety, and preparing the family for home care. Refer to the accompanying nursing care plan, which summarizes nursing care for the child with bronchiolitis.

Maintain Respiratory Function

Close monitoring is essential to evaluate the child's improvement or to spot early signs of deterioration. Oxygen and pulmonary care therapies are administered. High humidity and supplemental oxygen may be provided with a mist tent if the child requires only moisture and minimal oxygen. If more concentrated oxygen is required, it can be given via nasal cannula, hood, or tent. Pulse oximetry is used to evaluate oxygenation.

BOX 25–6 Psychosocial Assessment of the Child with an Acute Respiratory Illness

CHILD

- Assess for indications of anxiety or fear that may have an impact on respiratory status.
- For young children, inquire about security objects (such as a blanket or doll), the child's reaction to strangers, and reaction to absence of parents.
- For older children, ask whether this is the first hospital stay and what previous illness and hospital experiences have meant to the child.

PARENTS

- Assess parents' reactions: Are they anxious? Fearful? Verbal or quiet? Asking appropriate questions?
- Observe for nonverbal cues. Often parents have financial worries (cost of hospital stay, lost work and wages) and personal worries (siblings at home who are ill) that they may not readily share with staff.

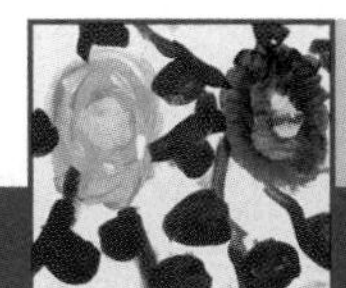

Nursing Care Plan

THE CHILD WITH BRONCHIOLITIS

GOAL	INTERVENTION	RATIONALE	EXPECTED OUTCOME
1. Ineffective Breathing Pattern related to increased work of breathing and decreased energy (fatigue)			
	NIC Priority Intervention—*Respiratory Monitoring*: Collection and analysis of patient data to ensure airway patency and adequate gas exchange.		**NOC Suggested Outcome**—*Vital Signs Status*: Temperature, pulse, respiration, and blood pressure within expected range for the child's age.
The child will return to respiratory baseline. The child will not experience respiratory failure.	■ Assess respiratory status (Box 25–1) when child is calm and not crying a minimum of every 2–4 hours, or more often as indicated for an increasing or decreasing respiratory rate and episodes of apnea. Cardiorespiratory monitor and pulse oximeter attached with alarms set. Record and report changes promptly to physician.	■ Changes in breathing pattern may occur quickly as the child's energy reserves are depleted. Assessment and monitoring baseline reveal rate and quality of air exchange. Frequent assessment and monitoring provides objective evidence of changes in the quality of respiratory effort, enabling prompt and effective intervention.	■ The child returns to respiratory baseline within 48–72 hours.
The child's oxygenation status will return to baseline.	■ Administer humidified oxygen via mask, nasal cannula, hood, or tent.	■ Humidified oxygen loosens secretions and helps maintain oxygenation status and ease respiratory distress.	■ The child's respiratory effort eases. Pulse oximetry reading remains ≥ 95% oxygen saturation during treatment.
	■ Assess pulse oximetry on room air and compare to reading when child is on oxygen.	■ Comparison of pulse oximetry readings provides information about improvement status.	
	■ Note child's response to ordered medications.	■ Medications act systemically to improve oxygenation and decrease inflammation.	■ The child tolerates therapeutic measures with no adverse effects.
	■ Position head of bed up or place child in position of comfort on parent's lap, if crying or struggling in crib or bed.	■ Position facilitates improved aeration and promotes decrease in anxiety (especially in toddlers) and energy expenditure.	■ The child rests quietly in position of comfort.
	■ Assess tolerance to feeding and activities.	■ Provides an assessment of condition improvement.	
2. Risk for Imbalanced Fluid Volume related to inability to meet body requirements and increased metabolic demand			
	NIC Priority Intervention—*Fluid Management*: Promotion of fluid balance and prevention of complications resulting from abnormal or undesired fluid levels.		**NOC Suggested Outcome**—*Hydration*: Amount of water in intracellular and extracellular compartments of body.
Child's immediate fluid deficit is corrected.	■ Evaluate need for intravenous fluids. Maintain IV, if ordered.	■ Previous fluid loss may require immediate replacement.	■ Child's hydration status is maintained during acute phase of illness.
	■ Calculate maintenance fluid requirements and give oral and/or IV fluids.	■ Assessment ensures child receives appropriate fluids to maintain hydration while transitioning to oral fluids.	
Child will be adequately hydrated, be able to tolerate oral fluids, and progress to normal diet.	■ Maintain strict intake and output monitoring and evaluate specific gravity at least every 8 hours.	■ Monitoring provides objective evidence of fluid loss and ongoing hydration status.	■ Child takes adequate oral fluids after 24–48 hours to maintain hydration.
	■ Perform daily weight measurement on the same scale at the same time of day. Evaluate skin turgor.	■ Further evidence of improvement of hydration status.	■ Child's weight stabilizes after 24–48 hours; skin turgor is supple.
	■ Assess mucous membranes and presence of tears. Report changes promptly to physician.	■ Moist mucous membranes and tears provide observable evidence of hydration.	■ Child shows evidence of improved hydration.
	■ Offer clear fluids and incorporate parent in care. Offer fluid choice when tolerated.	■ Choice of fluid offered by parent gains the child's cooperation.	■ The child accepts beverage of choice from parent or nursing staff.

(continued)

Nursing Care Plan THE CHILD WITH BRONCHIOLITIS (continued)

GOAL	INTERVENTION	RATIONALE	EXPECTED OUTCOME
3. Anxiety (child and parent) related to acute illness, hospitalization, uncertain course of illness and treatment, and home care needs			
	NIC Priority Intervention—*Anxiety Reduction*: Minimizing apprehension, dread, foreboding, or uneasiness related to an unidentified source of anticipated danger.		**NOC Suggested Outcome**—*Anxiety Control*: Ability to eliminate or reduce feelings of apprehension and tension from an unidentifiable source.
Child and parents will demonstrate behaviors that indicate decrease in anxiety.	■ Encourage parents to express fears and ask questions; provide direct answers and discuss care, procedures, and condition changes. ■ Incorporate parents in the child's care. Encourage parents to bring familiar objects from home. Ask about and incorporate in care plan the home routines for feeding and sleeping.	■ Provides opportunity to vent feelings and receive timely, relevant information. Helps reduce parents' anxiety and increase trust in nursing staff. ■ Familiar people, routines, and objects decrease the child's anxiety and increase parents' sense of control over unexpected, uncertain situation.	■ Parents and child show decreasing anxiety and fear as symptoms improve and as child and parents feel more secure in hospital environment. *Parent* freely asks questions and participates in the child's care. The *child* cries less and allows staff to hold and/or touch him or her.
Parents will verbalize knowledge of bronchiolitis symptoms and use of home care methods before the child's discharge from the hospital.	■ Explain symptoms, treatment, and home care of bronchiolitis. ■ Provide written instructions for follow-up care arrangements, as needed.	■ Anticipate potential for recurrence. Assist family to be prepared should respiratory symptoms recur after discharge. ■ Written and oral instructions reinforce knowledge. Parents may not "hear" and remember the particulars of home care if presented only orally.	■ Parent accurately describes respiratory symptoms and initial home care actions.

Patent nares are important to promote oxygen intake. A bulb syringe and saline nose drops can be used to quickly and easily clear the nasal passages. The head of the bed should be elevated to ease the work of breathing and drain mucus from the upper airways. Chest physiotherapy is often administered by a respiratory therapist.

Support Nutrition

Infants may have feeding difficulties and are at risk for aspiration. Smaller volumes and more frequent feedings will help conserve energy for infants with bronchiolitis who are formula and breastfed. Thickened formula may improve swallowing and prevent aspiration in infants with RSV bronchiolitis (Gadomski, 2002).

Support Physiologic Function

The grouping of nursing tasks promotes the child's physiologic function by decreasing stress and promoting rest. Rest is a key component in improving the child's breathing and overall health. Medications may be administered to control fever and promote comfort as needed. An intravenous infusion may be ordered to rehydrate and maintain fluid balance until the child is capable of taking sufficient oral fluids.

Reduce Anxiety

The need for hospitalization and assistive therapies creates anxiety and fear in the child and parents. The parents may be frightened by the child's continued respiratory difficulty and the presence of assistive equipment at bedside. An important part of nursing care is anticipating, recognizing, and acting to decrease the child's and parents' anxiety. Provide parents with regular updates and explanations, and answer questions they may have about planned care.

Partner with parents to care for the child in the hospital. Their presence and ability to calm the infant or child can be helpful in the child's recovery. They should be reassured that holding or touching the child will not dislodge wires or tubing. If the child has been ill for a few days before admission, the parents are likely to be tired. Acknowledging parents' physical and emotional needs facilitates a spirit of caring and enhances communication between staff and family. Encourage the parents to take turns at the child's bedside and to take breaks for meals and rest.

Discharge Planning and Home Care Teaching

Children are discharged once they show sufficient stability in maintaining adequate oxygenation (as evidenced by easing of respiratory effort and decreased mucous production). In most children, symptoms decrease within 24 to 72 hours; however, resolution of all symptoms may take weeks. Coughing may continue for a few weeks postdischarge. The same supportive therapies implemented in the hospital may be needed at home.

- Use of the bulb syringe to suction the nares of an infant under 1 year of age

- Fluid intake to thin respiratory secretions (making them easier to clear) and provide sucrose in water for energy (since the child's appetite may not return to normal for several days)
- Rest

Children are usually capable of recognizing their own activity limits. However, parents should encourage active toddlers to nap and take rest periods. Teach the parents proper administration of medications. Acetaminophen may be prescribed for persistent low-grade fevers and general discomfort. Advise parents that RSV infection can recur; therefore, they need to know how to recognize symptoms and when to call the physician. See Partnering with Families: Recognizing Worsening Condition in the Child with Bronchiolitis.

Evaluation

Expected outcomes of nursing care are provided on the accompanying nursing care plan.

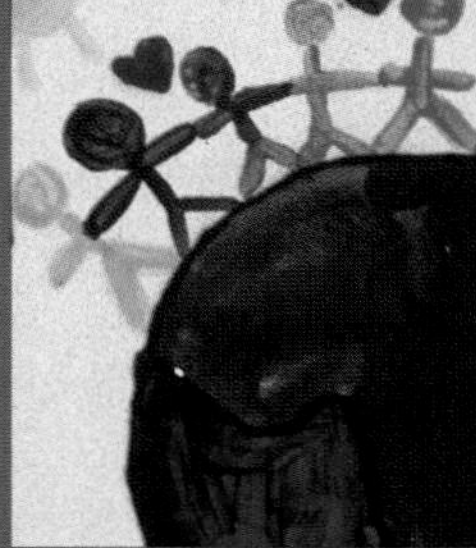

PARTNERING WITH FAMILIES

Recognizing Worsening Condition in the Child with Bronchiolitis

Advise parents to call the healthcare provider if:

- Respiratory symptoms interfere with sleep or eating
- Breathing is rapid or difficult
- Symptoms persist in a child who is less than 1 year old, has heart or lung disease, or was premature and had lung disease after birth
- The child acts sicker—appears tired, less playful, less interested in food (parents just "feel" the child is not improving)

Pneumonia

Pneumonia is an inflammation or infection of the bronchioles and alveolar spaces of the lungs. It occurs most often in infants and young children. The incidence of pneumonia in the United States is 35 to 40 cases for every 1,000 children younger than 5 years of age, and 16 to 22 years for every 1,000 children older than 5 years of age (Patel & Turcios, 2003). Pneumonia in children often resolves much sooner than in adults. The key is early recognition, enabling most children to be managed at home rather than in the hospital. Risk factors for developing pneumonia include chronic lung disease, anatomic problems, gastroesophageal reflux with aspiration, neurologic disorders that compromise the airway, and altered immune status (Sectish & Prober, 2004).

Etiology and Pathophysiology

Infectious organisms that can cause pneumonia are viral, bacterial, mycoplasmal, and fungal. In children under 5 years, pneumonia is most often caused by viruses such as RSV, influenza, parainfluenza virus, adenovirus, rhinovirus, and enterovirus. Bacteria more commonly cause pneumonia in children over 5 years of age. Common bacterial organisms include the following:

- *Staphylococcus aureus* is a common complication of viral pneumonia.
- *Streptococcus pneumoniae* is a common bacterial cause of pneumonia in all age groups, but it is anticipated that a decline in incidence should occur as more children are immunized.
- *Group B streptococci* and *Chlamydia trachomatis* are common causes of pneumonia in newborns.
- *Haemophilus influenza type b* is now an uncommon cause in immunized children.

Mycoplasma pneumoniae is a common cause of pneumonia in school-age children. Children with an underlying illness such as cystic fibrosis or immunosuppression are susceptible to many other bacterial, parasitic, or fungal infections.

Bacterial Pathophysiology. Bacterial invaders circulate through the bloodstream to the lungs, where they damage cells. An inflammatory response and edema usually result. Cellular debris and mucus cause airway obstruction. This leads to the proliferation of organisms that spread to nearby areas. Bacteria tend to be distributed evenly throughout one or more lobes of a single lung, a pattern termed unilateral lobar pneumonia.

Viral Pathophysiology. Viruses frequently enter from the upper respiratory tract, infiltrating the alveoli nearest the bronchi of one or both lungs. There they invade the cells, replicate, and burst out forcefully, killing the cells and sending out cell debris. Airway obstruction occurs due to swelling and cellular debris. The viral cells rapidly invade adjacent areas, distributing themselves in a scattered, patchy pattern, often referred to as bronchopneumonia. The small airway in infants increases the risk for progression to atelectasis, edema, and a ventilation-perfusion mismatch. The resulting lung injury makes the child susceptible to secondary bacterial pneumonia.

Aspiration Physiology. Aspiration of materials, such as foods, emesis, gastric reflux, or hydrocarbons, causes a chemical lung injury and resulting inflammatory response. Often the pH of the material is related to the severity of the chemical injury and pneumonitis, with a lower pH (acidic) causing greater irritation. Newborns may aspirate amniotic fluid and debris during birth, and develop pneumonia as a secondary infection. Hypoxemia, atelectasis, hemorrhagic pneumonitis, necrosis of damaged airway tissues, intravascular fluid shifts, and pulmonary edema may result. The stage is then set for a secondary bacterial invasion.

Clinical Manifestations

Pneumonia is often preceded by an upper respiratory tract infection including rhinitis and a cough. Regardless of the causative agent, symptoms include fever (usually a lower temperature is associated with viral pneumonia), crackles, wheezes, cough, dyspnea, tachypnea, restlessness, and decreased breath sounds if consolidation exists. Newborns and infants may have grunting, nasal flaring, irritability, lethargy, and a diminished appetite. Diminished breath sounds may be noted. Children with bacterial pneumonia may have chest pain and try to splint the chest when coughing. As the condition increases in severity, the infant or child will have increased work of breathing, cyanosis, retractions, and use of accessory muscles. See the clinical manifestations table below.

COLLABORATIVE CARE

Diagnostic Procedures

Diagnosis is made based on history, physical signs and symptoms. Chest radiography helps distinguish the type of pneumonia present. See the clinical manifestations below for characteristic findings. The child's age, severity of symptoms, and presence of an underlying lung, cardiac, or immunodeficiency disease may result in some children having variations from classical clinical findings. Children with recurrent pneumonia (two or more episodes in a year or a lifetime total of three or more episodes) need to be evaluated for immunodeficiency syndromes, foreign-body aspiration, obstruction or compression of the airway, structural abnormality, cystic fibrosis, and asthma.

Clinical Therapy

Clinical management for all types of pneumonia includes symptomatic therapy (pain and fever control) and supportive care through airway management, fluids, fever management, and rest. Mycoplasma and bacterial pneumonias are treated with organism-sensitive antibiotics; viral pneumonias usually improve without antibiotics, but antibiotics may be ordered if secondary bacterial invasion is suspected. Infants and children with severe infections will be hospitalized to monitor the condition and observe for increased respiratory distress. Some children need oxygen and IV fluids to maintain hydration.

NURSING MANAGEMENT

Most children with pneumonia are cared for at home. For those infants and children who are hospitalized, the goal of nursing care is to monitor the child's condition for increasing respiratory distress and to restore optimal respiratory function.

Nursing Assessment and Diagnosis

Assess the infant's or child's condition, paying particular attention to respiratory rate, heart rate, and temperature, and observe color for pallor or cyanosis. Attach a pulse oximeter to monitor the Spo_2 level. Assess hydration status. Assess for the presence of pain with coughing.

Examples of nursing diagnoses include the following:

- Fatigue related to respiratory distress and coughing
- Ineffective Breathing Pattern related to constant coughing and inability to clear airways
- Risk for Deficient Fluid Volume related to increased metabolic rate, fever, and anorexia

Planning and Implementation

Assist the child to take deep breaths to fully aerate the lungs and to promote coughing to clear secretions and cellular debris. Teach the child and parent how to splint the chest, by hugging a small pillow, teddy bear, or doll, to make coughing less painful. Pain medication (acetaminophen or ibuprofen) can provide the added benefits of temperature control and may aid in sleep.

Maintain hydration by offering preferred clear fluids. Administer IV fluids when the infant or child is unable to maintain an adequate fluid intake. Encourage small amounts of soft foods when tolerated. Give medications as prescribed.

Discharge Planning and Home Care Teaching

Discharge planning should be addressed early in the hospital stay. Medications, especially antibiotics, must be taken at pre-

CLINICAL MANIFESTATIONS of Pneumonia by Causative Organism

ETIOLOGY	CLINICAL MANIFESTATIONS	CHEST RADIOGRAPH FINDINGS
Mycoplasma pneumoniae	Insidious onset, malaise, muscle aches, headache, fever, sore throat, rhinorrhea, dry hacking cough that becomes productive, fine crackles, anorexia.	Patchy infiltrates and mild pleural effusions
Viral pneumonia	Sudden or insidious onset, rhinitis, slight cough that may become productive, fever and chills, crackles, and wheezes.	Hyperinflation and diffuse, patchy infiltrates
Streptococcus pneumoniae	Sudden onset, high fever, cough, shaking, chills, chest pain, nasal flaring, retractions, fine crackles, dullness on percussion, fremitus.	Lobar consolidation
Staphylococcus aureus	Upper respiratory infection and abrupt change in condition, high fever, cough, shaking, chills, lethargy, chest pain, nasal flaring, retractions, fine crackles, dullness on percussion, fremitus.	Limited patchy infiltrate, usually only right lung involved.
Chlamydia pneumoniae	Insidious onset, minimal or absent fever, tachypnea, malaise, persistent cough, pharyngitis.	Pleural effusions and lobar infiltrates

scribed intervals and for the full course. Make sure parents learn the proper administration of drugs and any side effects. Inform parents of signs indicating the infant's or child's condition may be worsening that need immediate care, such as increased difficulty breathing and refusal to take fluids. A chest radiograph may be obtained during a follow-up visit to see if the lungs are clear. Symptoms of pneumonia usually disappear long before the lungs are completely healed. Some children continue to have worsening reactive airway problems or abnormal results on pulmonary function tests. Most children, however, recover uneventfully.

Preventive measures against pneumonia are limited; however, the Hemophilus influenza b vaccine has dramatically reduced the incidence of pneumonia due to that organism. The pneumococcal conjugate vaccine, now regularly administered to infants, may help reduce the incidence of pneumonia caused by *Streptococcus pneumoniae.* The 23-valent pneumococcal vaccine is recommended for children over 2 years of age who are immunosuppressed or have chronic diseases (sickle-cell disease, other types of functional or anatomic asplenia, human immunodeficiency virus [HIV] infection, or primary immunodeficiency and children who are receiving immunosuppressive therapy). See Chapter 19∞ for information about immunization schedules and a discussion on pertussis.

Tuberculosis

Tuberculosis (TB) is caused by the organism *Mycobacterium tuberculosis,* which is transmitted through the air via droplets. It is estimated that approximately 32% of the world's population is infected (Dye, Scheele, Doulin, et al., 1999). Children less than 15 years are a major group infected, and Southeast Asia and Africa are locations with high rates in this age group. The epidemic of acquired immunodeficiency syndrome is largely responsible for the increase in TB infections and deaths. Even though the incidence has decreased 50.5% since 1992, the overall incidence of TB in the United States is 5.2 cases per 100,000 people. In 2002, rates were highest among foreign-born individuals and U.S.-born non-Hispanic Blacks (Centers for Disease Control and Prevention, 2003). Incidence rates in Canada are similar to the United States (Dye et al., 1999).

The risk of transitioning from latent TB to an active infection is greatest during the first 2 years of life and during adolescence. Adolescents are more likely to develop active TB due to hormonal changes and metabolic changes associated with growth spurts (Morisky, Malotte, Ebin, et al., 2001). Other children at risk are those with altered immune status. Foreign-born children have accounted for more than one third of newly diagnosed cases in children 14 years of age or younger in recent years (American Academy of Pediatrics, 2003b).

Adults with active laryngeal or pulmonary TB may transmit the disease to children. Children under 12 years of age with active pulmonary tuberculosis are rarely contagious, because they have small pulmonary lesions, an unproductive cough, and inadequate force to expel bacilli (American Academy of Pediatrics, 2003b).

Etiology and Pathophysiology

By coughing, sneezing, speaking, or singing, a person with active TB sends out tiny droplets of moisture that remain in the air. If these droplets are inhaled, the bacillus is small enough to travel directly to the alveoli where the organism replicates. Frequently, however, the organism is trapped in the upper airway, preventing infection. Pulmonary infection occurs only when the bacillus reaches the alveoli. Four factors are associated with the transmission of TB.

- Number of organisms disseminated by the infected individual
- Concentration of the organisms in the air (a small space and poor ventilation will increase the concentration)
- Length of time the exposed person breathes the contaminated air
- Immune status of the exposed person (a person with a compromised immune status or HIV infection is more likely to develop active TB if infected)

Once the bacillus reaches the alveoli, an immune response is initiated and macrophages are sent to kill it. If the bacillus survives, it begins to multiply within the macrophage that has surrounded it and walled it off in small hard capsules, called tubercles. The tubercle bacillus grows slowly, dividing every 25 to 32 hours within the macrophage. The organisms grow for 2 to 12 weeks until they number 1,000 to 10,000. At this point, the cellular immune response to TB can be elicited by a response to the TB skin test. However, before the development of cellular immunity, the tubercle bacilli may spread by the lymphatic system to the hilar lymph nodes and then to the bloodstream and to other sites. Children have a greater risk for developing extrapulmonary TB, such as TB meningitis and miliary (disseminated) TB (Maltezou, Spyridis, & Kafetzis, 2000).

In persons with intact cell-mediated immunity, activated T cells and macrophages form granulomas that limit multiplication and spread of the organism. Proliferation of TB is arrested once cell-mediated immunity develops, but small numbers of viable bacilli may remain in the granuloma. These individuals have latent tuberculosis infection rather than active disease, and thus are not infectious and cannot transmit the disease.

In young children, the disease develops as an immediate complication of the primary infection. Children with HIV infection or immunosuppression may have more rapidly progressive disease. If the tubercle extends into a blood vessel, the bacillus may spread through the bloodstream to affect the liver, spleen, kidney, bone marrow, or meninges (tubercular meningitis). This systemic form of TB (meningeal or miliary tuberculosis) may lead to serious illness or death.

Clinical Manifestations

Infants, children, and adolescents with latent TB (exposed and infected) are asymptomatic. If the disease develops, signs and symptoms may appear between 1 and 6 months after becoming infected. Infants with TB may have a persistent cough, weight loss or failure to gain weight, and fever. Wheezing, crackles, and decreased breath sounds may be present. Children with active

TB may have fatigue, cough, anorexia, weight loss or growth delay, night sweats, chills, and a low-grade fever.

COLLABORATIVE CARE

Diagnostic Procedures

Tuberculosis is diagnosed by a positive tuberculin skin test (5 tuberculin units of purified protein derivative [PPD]) that is injected intradermally. See Box 25–7 for interpretation of PPD tests. A positive test indicates that the child has been exposed to and infected with TB, and antibodies have been produced against the bacillus. See Table 25–9 for current recommendations for PPD skin testing in children. Only those children at high risk of exposure or at high risk for acquiring the infection because of immune status are routinely tested.

See Table 25–10 for other diagnostic procedures that may be required to confirm the diagnosis. Acid-fast stains of blood, gastric aspirate, and sputum cultures reveal the bacillus. Chest radiographic findings vary depending on the child's condition, and may include a granuloma, calcification, adenopathy, atelectasis, or infiltrate of a segment or lobe; pleural effusion; cavitary lesions; or miliary (disseminated) disease. For infants, children, and adolescents with active TB, a chest radiograph should be obtained after 2 to 3 months of therapy to evaluate response.

Clinical Therapy

Management focuses on diagnosis and treatment of active and latent TB with antitubercular drug therapy. See the medications used to treat TB on page 854. Drug resistance to these medications has occurred because infected individuals did not complete courses of medications, permitting the TB bacillus to develop resistance. Therapy for active, drug-susceptible TB usually involves a 6-month regimen consisting of isoniazid, rifampin, and pyrazinamide for the first 2 months and isoniazid and rifampin for the remaining 4 months. Direct observed drug therapy is recommended for treatment of children and adolescents with active TB in the United States to reduce treatment failure and development of drug-resistant organisms.

For infants, children, and adolescents with latent TB, a single daily dose of isoniazid is given for 9 months, as only one drug is

BOX 25–7 Interpreting Tuberculin Skin Test Results in Infants, Children, and Adolescents*

INDURATION > 5 MM

- Children in close contact with known or suspected contagious cases of tuberculosis disease
- Children suspected to have tuberculosis disease: with findings on chest radiograph consistent with active or previously active tuberculosis or clinical evidence of potential tuberculosis disease (i.e., meningitis)
- Children receiving immunosuppressive doses of corticosteroids or having immunosuppressive conditions, including HIV infection

INDURATION > 10 MM

- Children at increased risk of disseminated disease: younger than 4 years of age; with other medical conditions, including Hodgkin disease, lymphoma, diabetes mellitus, chronic renal failure, or malnutrition
- Children with increased exposure to tuberculosis disease: born in (or parents born in) high-prevalence regions of the world; frequently exposed to adults who are HIV infected, homeless, users of illicit drugs, residents of nursing homes, incarcerated or institutionalized, or migrant farm workers; or travel to high-prevalence regions of the world

INDURATION > 15 MM

- Children 4 years of age or older with no risk factors

*These definitions apply regardless of previous bacille Calmette-Guérin (BCG) immunization

Note: From American Academy of Pediatrics. (2003b). Red book: 2003 Report of the Committee on Infectious Diseases *(26th ed.). Elk Grove Village, IL: Author.*

TABLE 25–9 Recommendations for Tuberculin Skin Testing in Children

CLASSIFICATION OF CHILDREN	FREQUENCY OF TESTING
Contact with persons confirmed or suspected infectious TB	Immediate and 10–12 weeks later
Children with radiologic or clinical findings suggesting TB	Immediate
Children emigrating from countries with high rates of TB (Asia, Middle East, Africa, Latin America)	Immediate and 10–12 weeks later
Children with travel history to countries with high rates of TB or contact with indigenous persons in those countries	Immediate and 10–12 weeks later
Infected with HIV	Annual
Incarcerated adolescent	Annual
Exposed to the following individuals: HIV infected, homeless, nursing home residents, institutionalized adolescents or adults, users of illicit drugs, incarcerated adolescents or adults, migrant farm workers; foster children with exposure to persons in these high-risk groups	Every 2–3 years
Parents immigrated from region of the world with high prevalence of TB; continued potential exposure by travel to the endemic areas and/or household contact with people from the endemic areas (with unknown TST status)	Once at 4–6 years Once at 11–16 years
Children beginning immunosuppressive therapy, including prolonged steroid administration, for any child with an underlying condition that necessitates immunosuppressive therapy	Once prior to beginning therapy
Children without a specific risk factor who reside in a high-risk neighborhood or community within a large city	Once at 4–6 years Once at 11–16 years

Note: Used with permission of the American Academy of Pediatrics. (2003b). Red book: 2003 Report of the Committee on Infectious Diseases *(26th ed.). Elk Grove Village, IL: Author.*

TABLE 25–10 Diagnostic Procedures for Tuberculosis

DIAGNOSTIC TEST	INDICATION AND RATIONALE
Intradermal injection of purified protein derivative (PPD)	Confirms infection (latent or active) with the TB organism (3–12 weeks after exposure)
Chest radiograph (anteroposterior and lateral views)	Confirms presence of pulmonary TB (small, seedlike opacities may be visible); however, radiologic changes may look like other chronic lung conditions
Blood cultures for Mycobacterium tuberculosis	Proves diagnosis; defines specific drug sensitivity
Gastric washings (aspirates), performed in early morning after overnight fast on 3 consecutive days	Confirms active pulmonary TB. Used in children under 12 years as they do not produce sputum
Sputum cultures (expectorated or from bronchoscopic examination)	Confirms active pulmonary TB
Pleural biopsy for culture and tissue examination	Taken when pleural effusion is present
Lumbar puncture	Confirms meningeal TB

used. When adherence with daily therapy with isoniazid cannot be ensured, twice-a-week direct observed drug therapy can be considered.

NURSING MANAGEMENT

Nursing Assessment and Diagnosis

Assessment focuses on retaining a heightened awareness that certain children are at higher risk for exposure to TB and for developing the infection, such as recent contact with a case of tuberculosis, family history of tuberculosis, positive tuberculin skin test reactions in other current household members, and foreign birth or prolonged travel to a country with high tuberculosis rates (American Academy of Pediatrics, 2003b). Additionally consider the child's immigration status, immunosuppression status, and exposure to individuals with HIV infection. Follow guidelines for tuberculin skin testing in these children presented in Table 25–9.

Carefully evaluate infants and young children who have a tuberculin skin test conversion as they are at greater risk to develop active TB over the next few months. When the ill child presents for healthcare, perform a complete physical assessment, but carefully assess for weight loss, fever, fatigue, coughing, and respiratory status. If TB is suspected, implement standard precautions until the infection status is known. The nurse assists with the collection of blood, sputum, and gastric aspirate cultures so that drug sensitivity can be identified.

Examples of nursing diagnoses that might be appropriate include the following:

- Imbalanced Nutrition: Less than Body Requirements related to anorexia and active infection
- Activity Intolerance related to active infectious process
- Ineffective Therapeutic Regimen Management related to nonadherence to daily medication regimen

Planning and Implementation

Nursing care centers on administering medications, education, and providing supportive care. Parents and children need to be taught about the disease process, medications, strategies for medication administration to infants and toddlers, possible side effects, the importance of long-term therapy (e.g., that drug therapy may last for 6 to 9 months), and the need for frequent follow-up.

Children with active TB should receive "directly observed drug therapy" by a nurse or other healthcare provider to ensure that the drug is being taken. Direct observation should be done daily for at least 2 weeks and then decreased to twice a week if the patient is responding to treatment and is compliant with the treatment regimen (Stowe & Jacobs, 1999). Children with latent TB should receive "directly observed drug therapy" twice a week (American Academy of Pediatrics, 2003b).

The nurse works with the families of children and adolescents with latent TB infections to encourage completion of therapy. Help the family to develop a strategy that enables them to remember to give the medication. In the case of an adolescent, the nurse encourages increased responsibility for healthcare. Although parents need to be involved, the adolescent can make choices about the time of day to take the medication and to set up a reminder system to take it. Parents can support the adolescent by establishing a contract with incentives when the adolescent takes all medications in the established time period.

Unless the child is seriously ill, hospitalization is not needed. In most cases when the child is hospitalized, standard precautions are maintained as the child is not infectious. If the child or adolescent has extensive pulmonary infection, positive sputum cultures, or suspected congenital tuberculosis airborne precautions are used, including room isolation and a "fitted" and "sealed" particulate respirator for all patient contacts. Airborne precautions are used until culture smears indicate a diminishing number of organisms and the child's cough is improving (American Academy of Pediatrics, 2003b). Family members should use masks (reverse airborne precautions) when visiting the child in the hospital until it is determined that they are not infectious, to reduce the risk of infection to other children and hospital staff. Facilitate tuberculin skin testing of family members and close contacts followed by chest radiographs as necessary.

The family needs information and education to care for the child at home. Emphasize the importance of taking medications as prescribed on an empty stomach, and ensuring proper

MEDICATIONS Used to Treat Latent and Active TB in Infants, Children, and Adolescents

MEDICATION	NURSING CONSIDERATIONS
Isoniazid bactericidal	• Obtain baseline bilirubin and liver function studies as hepatotoxicity can occur. • Obtain a baseline weight. • Assess ophthalmologic and hematopoietic status studies. • Give 1 hour before or 2 hours after meals unless GI irritation occurs, then give with food. Tablets can be crushed. • Interferes with hepatic metabolism of phenytoin, may cause toxicity. • Monitor for symptoms of hypersensitivity, signs of hepatotoxicity (anorexia, fever, malaise, nausea, vomiting, diarrhea, weight loss), dark urine, jaundice. • Adolescent should avoid alcohol. • Pyridoxine supplementation (vitamin B_6) is recommended for children and adolescents with meat- and milk-deficient diets, with nutritional deficiencies, and those who are pregnant or HIV infected to prevent peripheral neuritis and seizures.
Rifampin bactericidal	• Obtain baseline bilirubin and liver function studies as this drug can alter the pharmacokinetics and serum concentrations of other drugs. • Assess renal and hematopoietic status studies. • Give 1 hour before or 2 hours after meals unless GI irritation occurs, then give with food. Capsule contents can be sprinkled on applesauce or suspended in flavored syrup. • Monitor for symptoms of jaundice and other side effects. • Assess medications taken for interaction with rifampin (i.e., diazepam, beta-adrenergics, barbiturates, analgesics, corticosteroids, oral contraceptives, digitalis, and others). • Inform parents and child about orange body fluids. • Contact lenses will become permanently discolored if used. • Sexually active adolescent females should not use oral contraceptives as rifampin makes them ineffective.
Pyrazinamide	• Obtain baseline liver function studies, and renal and hematopoietic status studies. Monitor for symptoms of hepatotoxicity. • Monitor blood glucose level in children with diabetes as glycemic control may be affected. • When used in combination with isoniazid and rifampin, a 6-month course of therapy is possible.
Ethambutol bacteriostatic or bactericidal, depending on dosage used	• Obtain baseline liver function studies, and renal and hematopoietic status studies. • Perform a baseline and monthly ophthalmologic test of visual acuity, visual fields, and color discrimination as the drug may cause reversible or irreversible optic neuritis, particularly in children with impaired renal function. • Give with meals if gastrointestinal irritation occurs. • Inform parents and child to report any vision changes.
Streptomycin may occasionally be used for initial 4–8 weeks of treatment for active TB	• IM injections are painful so provide guidance for pain management. • Monitor for ototoxicity, assess hearing acuity regularly. • Monitor intake and output, looking for signs of reduced kidney function. • Educate parents to immediately report these symptoms: nausea, vomiting, incoordination, dizziness, impaired hearing, fullness in ears.

nutrition and rest to promote normal growth and development. The child can return to school or childcare when effective therapy has been instituted, adherence to therapy has been documented, and clinical symptoms have diminished substantially (American Academy of Pediatrics, 2003b). Most children who have been successfully treated for TB are able to lead essentially normal lives.

By law, cases of active TB must be reported immediately to the public health department so that disease contacts can be traced to help prevent the further spread of TB. Public health nurses have a significant role in tracking close contacts, arranging tuberculin skin testing, and encouraging treatment or supervising "directly observed drug therapy."

■ Evaluation

Expected outcomes of nursing care include the following:

- The child completes the full course of preventive TB medications.
- The child recovering from active TB regains energy and appetite, and catch-up growth is documented.
- Family members and close contacts are tested for TB and have treatment initiated as appropriate.

CHRONIC LUNG DISEASES

Bronchopulmonary Dysplasia (Chronic Lung Disease)

Bronchopulmonary dysplasia (BPD), also called chronic lung disease (CLD), results from an acute respiratory disease during the neonatal period. It is the most prevalent and serious chronic respiratory disorder that begins during infancy. Premature infants are affected more often than full-term infants, and morbidity is greater in males than in females. Risk factors for developing BPD include prematurity, lung immaturity, RDS in the neonatal period, high inspired oxygen concentrations, positive pressure ventilation, patent ductus arteriosis, and vitamin A deficiency (Froh, 2002). The incidence is increasing due to advances in medical technology that permit very-low-birth-weight infants to survive (Daigle & Cloutier, 1997). It is estimated that 10% to 35% of very-low-birth-weight infants develop BPD (Froh, 2002).

Etiology and Pathophysiology

BPD results from positive pressure ventilation and oxygen treatment for RDS and inflammatory changes in the airways. The sequence of events is as follows: an interruption in alveolar development that occurs when preterm infants need mechanical ventilation and supplemental oxygen. Inflammation and persistent hypoxia also contribute to the development of the chronic lung disease. Other disorders that contribute to the development of BPD include neonatal pneumonia, meconium aspiration syndrome, patent ductus arteriosis, fluid overload, and lung hypoplasia (Capper-Michel, 2004).

Clinical Manifestations

The infant with BPD has persistent signs of respiratory distress: tachypnea, wheezing, crackles, irritability, nasal flaring, grunting, retractions, pulmonary edema, and failure to thrive. The severity of the condition varies in infants. The infant has intermittent bronchospasms and mucous plugging. Air trapping persists and in time the chest assumes a barrel shape (Figure 25–13 ■). The infant may seem stable and improving, and then has a BPD episode that consists of sudden respiratory deterioration associated with an expiratory airflow limitation due to tracheobronchial narrowing. The child becomes dusky or cyanotic and agitated. The episodes may be caused by a sudden increase in pulmonary vascular resistance. Normal activities, such as feeding, can create increased oxygen demands that are difficult for the compromised infant to meet.

COLLABORATIVE CARE

Care is focused on supporting the infant's lung function and providing care for episodes of respiratory compromise until lung healing and development occur.

Diagnostic Procedures

The chest radiograph is the best indicator of lung changes and is the key to medical diagnosis. The radiograph often shows hyperexpansion, atelectasis, and interstitial thickening (Capper-Michel, 2004).

Clinical Therapy

Management focuses initially on prevention of BPD with gentle ventilation techniques, shortened intubation time, early treatment of a patent ductus arteriosis, infections, and nutritional support. Once BPD has occurred, clinical therapy focuses on symptomatic treatment that supports respiratory function and good nutrition, which helps to accelerate lung maturity. Infants with severe BPD must be cautiously weaned off assisted ventilation. Supplemental oxygen with humidity is used to keep the SaO_2 more than 90% to 92% even during sleep and feeding. A tracheostomy may be performed for long-term airway management.

Increased calories are provided to support growth, but fluids are restricted to prevent pulmonary edema. Some children require gastrostomy or nasogastric feeding to get adequate calories. Chest physiotherapy and medications (diuretics, bronchodilators, anti-inflammatories, and inhaled corticosteroids) are also used. See the medications table on page 856 for specific medications and their action.

With improvement and adequate weight gain, the child is weaned off of oxygen, diuretics, and bronchodilators. Long-term sequelae include asthma and respiratory infections with frequent rehospitalization. Potential long-term outcomes for the child with BPD include developmental delays, growth retardation, continuing airway obstruction, and persistent airway hypersensitivity.

NURSING MANAGEMENT

The goal of nursing management is to assess and manage the infant's acute episodes, assuring adequate nutritional support and thus promoting the infant's growth and development.

PATHOPHYSIOLOGY ILLUSTRATED

Barrel Chest

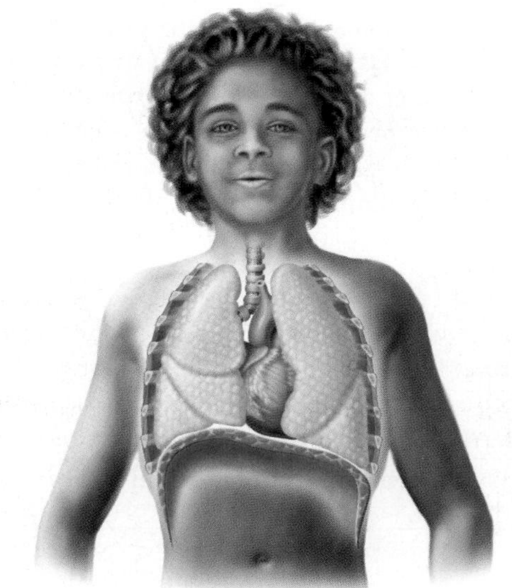

FIGURE 25–13 ■ A barrel chest may result from chronic respiratory conditions such as asthma or bronchopulmonary dysplasia, in which air trapping or hyperinflation of the alveoli occur.

Nursing Assessment and Diagnosis

The infant with chronic BPD may become acutely ill at any time, as occurred with Emily in the opening scenario. Observe for signs of infection that can be a threat because of a compromised immune system. During hospitalizations for acute infections, a cardiorespiratory monitor and pulse oximeter will be used. Assess airway and respiratory function, vital signs, color, and behavior changes to identify signs of worsening respiratory symptoms even when oxygen is provided. Observe for airway obstruction when the infant has a tracheostomy and suction as needed. See the Skills Manual for tracheostomy care.

Monitor growth as the infant often experiences poor weight gain. Evaluate development regularly as the infant may develop motor, language, and cognitive delays. Coordinate a periodic assessment of hearing and vision.

Nursing diagnoses that may be appropriate include:

- Dysfunctional Ventilatory Weaning Response related to inappropriate pacing of diminished ventilator support and BPD
- Risk for Caregiver Role Strain related to 24-hour responsibility for infant with BPD
- Delayed Growth and Development related to inadequate calories to support physical growth and energy needed for respiratory functions
- Ineffective Infant Feeding Pattern related to oral hypersensitivity resulting from long-term orogastric feeding

Planning and Implementation

Care of the hospitalized infant is organized to eliminate unnecessary physical stimulation, as this additional stress contributes to respiratory compromise. Position the infant to facilitate breathing and provide tracheostomy care when present. Provide humidified oxygen if ordered.

Provide fluids and nutrition to help meet energy needs. Fluid management is critical as excess fluids can lead to pulmonary edema. Support the mother who desires to breastfeed. Caloric supplementation may be needed for either the breastfed or formula-fed infant. Administer medications as ordered. Management of fever will help minimize energy needs.

Provide toys and mobiles that are age appropriate but do not encourage excessive activity so that growth and development is promoted. Support the parents with clear explanations about the infant's health status and planned interventions to reduce anxiety.

Discharge Planning and Home Care

Plans for care at home must be carefully planned and coordinated early in the child's hospitalization. Including parents in the infant's care early on promotes bonding and prepares them for home care responsibilities. Make referrals for needed oxygen, respiratory supplies, medications, an early intervention program, and follow-up care. Some families require home health nursing assistance, especially during the initial transition period. Help families identify additional family members who might be willing to learn how to care for the infant so that the parent can have a few hours of respite during the week. Families may need assistance in planning a schedule that the infant receives needed care and leaves some time free for other children and family activities. Inform families of the need for RSV prophylaxis and provide the first injection prior to discharge if during RSV season.

Once home, many infants need assisted ventilation therapy, supplemental oxygen, and medications (Figure 25–14 ■). Electrolytes may be monitored monthly. It is important to provide for the infant's normal development through rest, nutrition, stimulation, and family support. Frequent rehospitalization may occur. While the lungs may function adequately, they remain vulnerable throughout childhood to common respiratory illnesses. Infants with BPD do not have the same respiratory reserve as healthy infants, and can become very ill rapidly.

Teach parents to identify signs of respiratory compromise indicating a need for rapid intervention. Such planning was done with Emily's parents, and the healthcare providers were called before a crisis developed. However, an emergency care plan should also be developed for the parents in those cases when the infant becomes suddenly ill and emergency care is needed. A model emergency information form for emergency care providers is available on page 516.

Nutritional requirements to support growth must be balanced with fluid restrictions to prevent the development of pulmonary edema. A formula supplemented with carbohydrates and medium chain triglycerides may be given to promote weight

MEDICATIONS Used to Treat Bronchopulmonary Dysplasia

MEDICATION	ACTION/INDICATION
Bronchodilators (β_2-adrenergics, anticholinergics, theophylline, albuterol nebulizer)	Decreases airway resistance, increases expiratory flow in small airways, stimulates mucus clearance; different drugs work together for best response
Anti-inflammatory agents (corticosteroids, inhaled cromolyn, beclomethasone)	Reduces pulmonary edema and inflammation in small airways, enhances effect of bronchodilators; helps decrease the need for other drugs and oxygen; for moderate disease only
Diuretics (furosemide, chlorothiazide, spironolactone)	Helps remove excess fluid from lungs, decreases pulmonary resistance and increases pulmonary compliance; may cause electrolyte imbalances
Potassium chloride	Prevents electrolyte imbalances associated with diuretics
Antibiotics	Specific treatment for identified organisms
Vitamin A	Plays a role in normal lung development
Palivizumab (Synargis)	Protects infant from respiratory syncytial virus

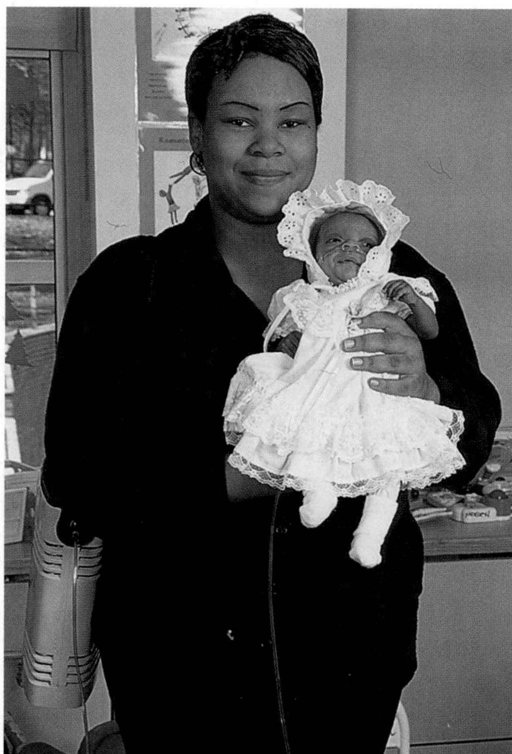

FIGURE 25–14 ■ Many children with BPD are cared for at home, with the support of a home care program to monitor the family's ability to provide airway management, oxygen, and support. This premature infant girl, who is now 4 months old but weighs only about 5 pounds, requires respiratory support with oxygen.

gain. Some children need nasogastric or gastrostomy tube feedings to get adequate nutrition when cyanosis is noted with feeding. Oral tactile hypersensitivity that interferes with feeding may be a problem in these children because of the long term use of nasogastric, orogastric, and endotracheal tubes. See Chapter 9∞. All infants with BPD need more frequent health promotion visits and immunizations.

Evaluation

Expected outcomes of nursing care may include:

- The infant receives adequate calories to sustain growth in length and weight. Introduction of oral foods is tolerated.
- Acute illness episodes are rapidly identified by the family and emergency care is provided to prevent and/or manage the infant's respiratory decompensation.
- The infant receives attention and exposure to developmentally appropriate toys and activities to promote development.

Health Promotion & Maintenance Overview

The Child with Bronchopulmonary Dysplasia

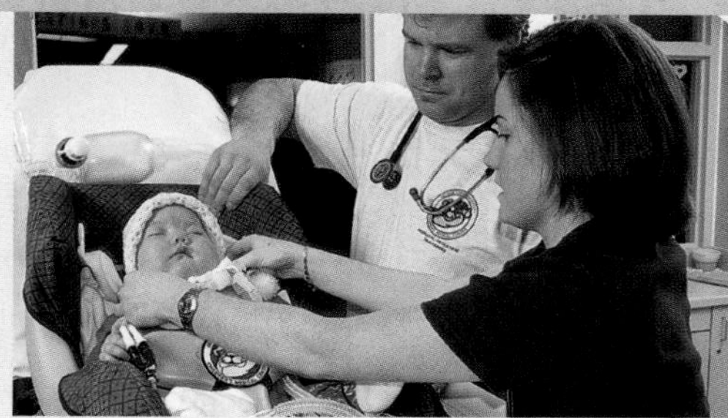

Health Supervision

- Assess blood pressure to detect abnormal findings associated with pulmonary hypertension.
- Perform hematocrit frequently during the first year of life to assess for anemia.
- Perform a chest radiograph and pulmonary function tests annually or as needed for clinical condition.
- Perform routine hearing assessment at each visit.
- Coordinate vision screening by an ophthalmologist every 2–3 months during the first year of life. Myopia and strabismus are common.
- Coordinate pulmonary function tests annually or as needed for clinical condition.
- Perform other screening tests as recommended for age.

Growth and Developmental Surveillance

- Assess growth and plot measurements on a growth chart corrected for gestational age. Even if length and weight are lower than normal, monitor for continued growth following the growth curves.
- Perform the Denver II and record the developmental assessment corrected for gestational age.

Nutrition

- Review caloric intake and ensure that intake is optimal for growth. Assess difficulties with feeding related to oral motor function. Refer to a nutitionist as necessary.

Physical Activity

- Organize care so that child has periods of time to rest during the day.

Relationships

- Identify ways to coordinate care during the night to reduce number of times child and family have sleep disturbed.
- Provide discipline appropriate for developmental age.
- Encourage development. Provide developmentally appropriate toys and activities.

Disease Prevention Strategies

- Reduce exposure to infections. If out-of-home childcare is used, select a provider caring for a small number of children. If possible, avoid the use of childcare centers during RSV season.
- Immunize the child with the routine schedule based on chronological age.
- Give the influenza vaccine annually and 23-valent pneumococcal vaccine at 2 years of age.
- Provide monthly injections of palivizumab throughout the RSV season to protect the child from respiratory syncytial virus.

Condition-Specific Guidance

- Develop an emergency care plan for times when the infant's condition rapidly worsens.

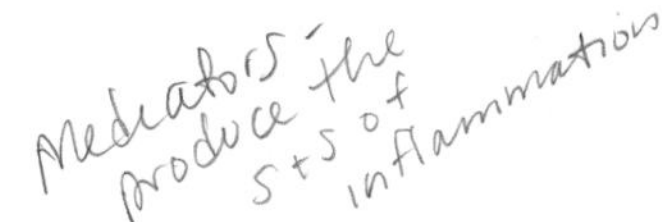

Asthma

Asthma (also called bronchial asthma) is a chronic inflammatory disorder of the airway with airway obstruction that can be partially or completely reversed and increased airway responsiveness to stimuli (Kieckhefer & Ratcliffe, 2004). It affects about 5 million children in the United States. Nearly 3.8 million children (a rate of 54 per 1,000 children) between 0 and 17 years had an asthma attack in the previous year (Centers for Disease Control and Prevention, 2001). See Figure 25–15 ■ for the change in age-specific asthma prevalence in children. Canada estimates that 12.2% of its children and youth under 20 years of age have asthma, and it is one of the country's most prevalent chronic conditions (Health Canada, 1999).

In the United States, the greatest increase in asthma prevalence has been noted in children 0 to 4 years of age, at a rate of 160% between 1980 and 1994 (Foley, 2002). Affected children have about 10 days of school absenteeism and 20 days of restricted activity per year (Sydnor-Greenberg & Dokken, 2000). Most children with asthma experience their first symptoms before the age of 5 years.

Asthma is a chronic condition with acute exacerbations or persistent symptoms. Children require continuous coordinated care to control sudden symptoms and minimize long-term airway changes. Although unusual in the past, severe persistent asthma is more common now. Hospitalizations for asthma have increased from 21.6 per 10,000 children in 1980–1981 to 26.9 per 10,000 children in 1998–1999, with the highest hospitalization rates found in children between 0 to 4 years of age. In the same time period, asthma mortality increased from 1.8 to 3.3 per 1 million children, with the highest mortality found in non-Hispanic Black children (10.1 per million) and in children between 11 and 17 years (4.4 per million) (Akinbami & Schoendorf, 2002). Risk factors for death from asthma include (American Academy of Allergy, Asthma, and Immunology, 1999):

- Past history of sudden exacerbation of asthma
- Prior intubation for asthma
- Prior admission to an intensive care unit for asthma
- Three or more emergency care visits for asthma in the past 12 months
- Hospitalization or emergency care visit for asthma in the past month
- Use of more than one canister per month of inhaled short-acting $beta_2$-agonist
- Current and long-term (chronic) use of oral corticosteroids
- Lack of accurate self-perception of symptom severity
- Low socioeconomic status and urban residence
- Illicit drug use
- Serious psychiatric disease or psychosocial problems

The significance of asthma and the increased prevalence of the condition in children has focused attention on the need for a national public health response. See Table 25–11 for national recommendations to address the management of asthma in children.

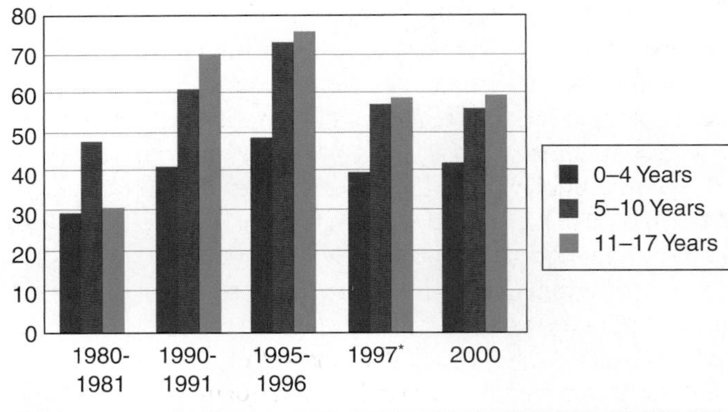

FIGURE 25–15 ■ Age-Specific Prevalence of Asthma by Selected Years

* In 1997, the definition of asthma prevalence (asthmatic episode confirmed by a health professional in the last 12 months) was changed for the National Health Information Survey from which prevalence estimates are made. This makes it difficult to compare the current prevalence of asthma with the rates in earlier years; however, the prevalence of asthma has increased dramatically since 1980.

Note: Data from Akinbami, L. J., & Schoendorf, K. C. (2002). Trends in childhood asthma: Prevalence, health care utilization, and mortality. Pediatrics, *110(2), 317.*

TABLE 25–11 Public Health Policy Recommendations for Improving Childhood Asthma Outcomes

For Promoting Quality of Care for Key Childhood Asthma Services

- Develop and implement primary care performance measures for childhood asthma care.
- Teach all children with persistent asthma and their families a specific set of self-management skills.
- Provide case management to high-risk children.

For Expanding Coverage and Improving Benefits Design

- Extend continuous health insurance coverage to all uninsured children.
- Develop model benefit packages for essential childhood asthma services.
- Educate healthcare purchasers about asthma benefits.

Public Health Funding of Asthma-Related Community and Health Services Not Currently Funded by Insurance System

- Establish public health grants to foster asthma-friendly communities and home environments.
- Promote asthma-friendly schools and school-based asthma programs.

Increasing Public Awareness and Knowledge of Asthma

- Develop a national asthma surveillance system.
- Develop and implement a national agenda for asthma prevention research.

Note: Reproduced with permission from Lara, M., Rosenbaum, S., Rachelefsky, G., et al. (2002). Improving childhood asthma outcomes in the United States: A blueprint for policy action. Pediatrics, *109(5), 919–930.*

Etiology and Pathophysiology

Asthma is a chronic inflammatory disease of the lungs that is caused by multiple factors, including environmental exposures, viral illnesses, allergens, and a genetic predisposition. It is thought that several chromosomal regions may be the site of genes leading to asthma susceptibility, including chromosomes 5q, 6p, 11q, 12q, and 13q (Foley, 2002). Exposure to environmental factors early in life or in utero is thought to stimulate the onset of asthma. For the development of asthma, a recent report found strong evidence that house dust mites and environmental tobacco smoke, and suggestive evidence that cockroaches, infections with respiratory syncytial virus, and mold resulting from indoor home dampness contributed to the development of asthma (Institute of Medicine, 2000).

The respiratory difficulties of an asthmatic episode result from inflammation that contributes to airway obstruction. The inflammation causes the normal protective mechanisms of the lungs (mucous formation, mucosal swelling, and airway muscle contraction) to react excessively in response to a stimulus. Asthma is a progressive disease. Chronic inflammatory changes result in airway remodeling that includes thickening of the basement membrane, airway smooth muscle hypertrophy, and mucus gland hypertrophy (Froh, 2002).

The stimulus, more correctly termed a **trigger,** that initiates an asthmatic episode can be inflammatory or noninflammatory. Triggers increase the frequency and severity of smooth muscle contraction, and airway responsiveness is enhanced through inflammatory mechanisms. Asthmatic triggers include exercise, viral or bacterial agents, allergens (mold, dust, pollen, furry pets, birds), fragrances, food additives, pollutants, weather changes (humidity and temperature), and emotions. See Box 25–8 for more information on the link between passive smoke exposure and asthma. Exercise is also a trigger in some children and adolescents. The lungs lose heat and water during exercise. A bronchospasm is triggered by rapidly breathing air that is cooler and dryer than the air in the respiratory tract, occurring during or shortly after vigorous physical activity (Baker, Friedman, & Schmitt, 2002a).

During the acute allergic reaction, an antigen binds to the specific immunoglobulin E surface on the mucosal mast cells, and histamine is released along with intercellular chemical mediators (leukotrienes, prostaglandin platelet-activating factor, and certain cytokines) resulting in bronchospasm, mucosal edema, and mucous secretion. The late allergic response starts 6 to 9 hours later when inflammatory cells respond and another wave of mediator release occurs. This stimulates more airway inflammation and bronchospasm (Kieckhefer & Ratcliffe, 2004). The reactive airway responses to stimuli are present before the trigger initiates the physiologic sequence that results in an asthmatic episode.

Airway narrowing results from bronchial constriction, airway swelling, and production of copious amounts of mucus. Mucus clogs small airways, trapping air below the plugs (Figure 25–16 ■). The airways swell, creating muscle spasms that often become uncontrolled in the large airways. Decreased perfusion of the alveolar capillaries results from hypoxic vasoconstriction and increased pressure due to hyperinflation of the alveoli. Hypoxemia leads to an increased respiratory rate with a reduced minute volume (air breathed per minute) because of airway resistance. With time, repeated episodes of bronchospasm, mucosal edema, and mucous plugging can damage the respiratory cells that line the airway. This is referred to as **airway remodeling,** an irreversible thickening of the subepithelial basement membrane and proliferation of smooth muscle cells in size and number. This results in decreased airway elasticity and decreased lung function.

MediaLink Asthma Animation

The psychologic sequence of events during an asthmatic episode starts with moderate anxiety as the episode begins. The anxiety becomes severe as the episode intensifies. Severe anxiety, in turn, intensifies physical responses and symptoms. Recognizing and addressing the child's fear and panic are essential for reestablishing normal respirations.

BOX 25–8 Research: Passive Smoke Exposure

Research has confirmed that passive smoke exposure (secondhand smoke) contributes significantly to the development of respiratory problems in children. Passive smoke exposure has been linked specifically to an increase in asthma symptoms, emergency department visits, and hospital admissions in children of parents who smoke. It is believed to be responsible for thousands of new cases of asthma in children each year. In addition, children exposed to tobacco smoke in utero have a higher rate of asthma. It is thought that the increased number of women smokers may have contributed to the increased rates of asthma (Gilliland, Yu-Fen, & Peters, 2001). Asthmatic children with high levels of smoke exposure were also found more likely to have moderate and severe asthma and decreased lung function than those with low levels of smoke exposure (Mannino, Homa, & Redd, 2002).

Clinical Manifestations

Asthma is characterized by airway inflammation, airway obstruction or narrowing, and airway hyperreactivity. The sudden appearance of breathing difficulty (cough, wheeze, or shortness of breath) is often referred to as an asthmatic episode, or "asthma attack."

During an acute episode, respirations are rapid and labored and the child often appears tired because of the ongoing effort required to breathe. Nasal flaring and intercostal retractions may be visible. The child exhibits a productive cough and expiratory wheezing, prolonged expiratory phase, decreased air movement, and respiratory fatigue. The child may complain of chest tightness. In cases of severe obstruction, wheezing may not be heard because of the lack of airflow. Head bobbing may be seen in young children with the use of accessory muscles (sternocleidomastoids) to breathe. **Pulsus paradoxus,** when the arterial blood pressure during expiration exceeds the arterial pressure during inspiration by 10 mm Hg, may be present. The resulting hypoxia, as well as the cumulative effect of previously administered medications, contributes to behaviors ranging from wide-eyed agitation to lethargic irritability. See clinical manifestations by exacerbation severity below. In children who have repeated acute episodes, a barrel chest (hyperinflation of the thorax) and the use of accessory muscles of respiration are common findings (see Figure 25–13 ■).

COLLABORATIVE CARE

Diagnostic Procedures

Preliminary diagnosis is initially based on physical signs and symptoms of airway constriction. A spirometer tests how effectively the

PATHOPHYSIOLOGY ILLUSTRATED

Asthmatic Episode

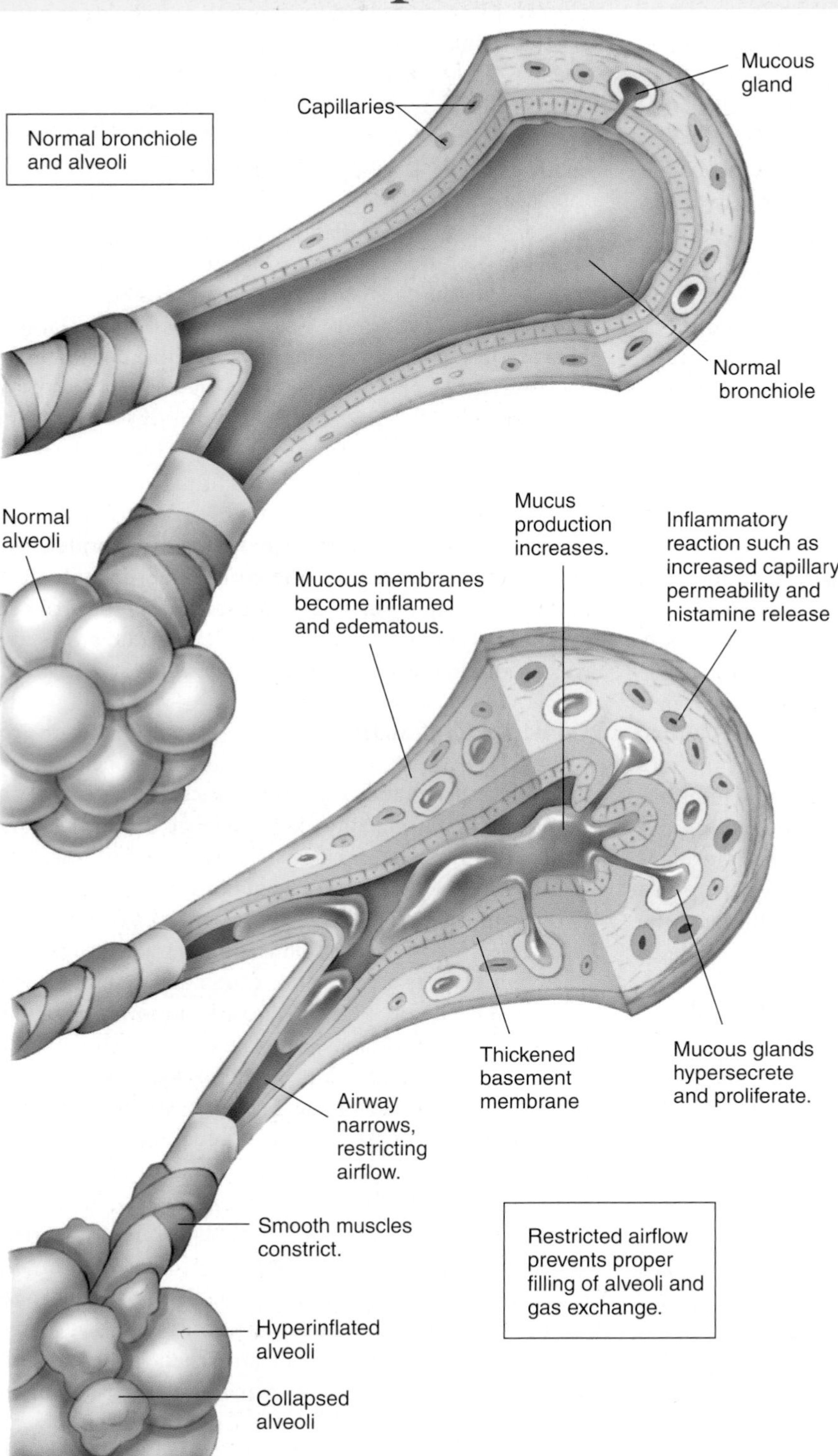

Normal bronchiole and alveoli
Capillaries
Mucous gland
Normal bronchiole
Normal alveoli
Mucous membranes become inflamed and edematous.
Mucus production increases.
Inflammatory reaction such as increased capillary permeability and histamine release
Thickened basement membrane
Mucous glands hypersecrete and proliferate.
Airway narrows, restricting airflow.
Smooth muscles constrict.
Hyperinflated alveoli
Collapsed alveoli
Restricted airflow prevents proper filling of alveoli and gas exchange.

FIGURE 25–16 ■ What can cause an asthmatic episode? Some asthma triggers are exercise, infection, and allergies. This illustration shows how asthma obstructs airflow through bronchoconstriction and inflammatory changes, narrowing the airway and thus increasing production of mucus.

lungs work by measuring the volume of air the child can expel from the lungs after a maximal inspiration. Both a forced vital capacity (FVC) and a forced expiratory volume in 1 second (FEV_1) readings are taken. Three readings are taken to compare with predicted normal values. Because the test requires children to cooperate and follow instructions, it is usually administered to children over 4 or 5 years of age.

CLINICAL TIP

Coach the child to give the best effort each time. Encourage the child to seal the lips tightly around the mouthpiece. The child is then instructed to breathe out as hard as possible, and then to breathe in deeply.

The spirometer helps to assess the severity of airway obstruction. A chest radiograph may be taken if other causes of the respiratory difficulty are suspected, such as a foreign body. Skin testing may be used to identify allergens (asthma triggers). The final diagnosis of asthma has four key elements: symptoms of episodic airflow obstruction; partial reversibility of bronchospasm with bronchodilator treatment; exclusion of alternate diagnosis; and confirmation by spirometry of measurement of forced expiratory flow variability.

Clinical Therapy

Management includes medications, hydration, education, and support of parents and child. See Box 25–9 on page 865 for an explanation of good asthma control. See Developing Cultural Competence: Asthma Management. Pharmacologic therapies

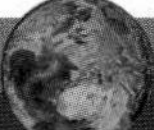

DEVELOPING CULTURAL COMPETENCE
Asthma Management

Asthma attack prevalence (having at least one asthma attack in the past 12 months) varies greatly among children under 18 years by race/ethnicity. In 1998, non-Hispanic Black children had the highest prevalence at 68.1% per 1,000 children, non-Hispanic White children had a prevalence of 52.1%, and Hispanic children had a prevalence of 47.4% (Centers for Disease Control and Prevention, 2000). A recent study investigating these disparities compared children in the above race/ethnicity groups and found a difference in the use of preventive medications for asthma. Among variables studied, specialist use, preventive visits, pets, and smoking in the home were found to be equal among the study population, indicating that these differences did not account for the asthma prevalence. Findings also revealed that Black and Hispanic children with similar insurance and sociodemographic characteristics to White children were 31% and 42%, respectively, less likely to be using inhaled anti-inflammatory medications to prevent the beginning or worsening of an asthma episode. This study suggests that factors such as differences in health beliefs, fear of steroids, or communication issues, rather than financial barriers, may play a role in the use of preventive medications (Lieu, Lozano, Finkelstein, et al., 2002).

are matched to the severity of asthma for long-term control and for management of acute episodes. See Table 25–12 and Table 25–13 on pages 862–863 for nationally recommended guidelines for the treatment of children under 5 years of age and children 5 years of age and older with acute and chronic asthma. See the medications used to treat asthma box on pages 864–865. Control of asthma symptoms is the goal, and

CLINICAL MANIFESTATIONS of Asthma in Children by Severity of Acute Exacerbations

ASSESSMENT CRITERIA	MILD	MODERATE	SEVERE
PEFR[a]	70–90% predicted or personal best	50–70% predicted or personal best	< 50% predicted or personal best
Respiratory rate, resting or sleeping	Normal to 30% increase above the mean	30–50% increase above mean	Increase over 50% above mean
Alertness	Normal	Normal	May be decreased
Dyspnea[b]	Absent or mild; speaks in complete sentences	Moderate; speaks in phrases or partial sentences; infant's cry softer and shorter; has difficulty sucking and feeding	Severe; speaks only in single words or short phrases; infant's cry softer and shorter; stops sucking and feeding
Pulsus paradoxus[c]	< 10 mm Hg	10–20 mm Hg	20–40 mm Hg
Accessory muscle use	No intercostal to mild retractions	Moderate intercostal retractions with tracheostemal retractions; use of sternocleidomastoid muscles; chest hyperinflation	Severe intercostal retractions, tracheosternal retractions with nasal flaring during inspiration; chest hyperinflation
Color	Good	Pale	Possibly cyanotic
Auscultation	End-expiratory wheeze only	Wheeze during entire expiration and inspiration	Breath sounds becoming inaudible
Oxygen saturation	> 95%	90–95%	< 90%
Pco_2	< 35	< 40	> 40

Note: Within each category, the presence of several parameters, but not necessarily all, indicate the general classification of the exacerbation.
[a]For children 5 years of age or older.
[b]Parents or physicians' impressions of degree of children's breathlessness.
[c]Pulsus paradoxus does not correlate with phase of respiration in small children.
Note: From National Asthma Education and Prevention Program. (1994). Acute exacerbations of asthma; Care in a hospital-based emergency department *(p. 13). Bethesdo, MD: National Heart, Lung, and Blood Institute, National Institutes of Health.*

TABLE 25–12 Asthma Severity Classification and Preferred Clinical Therapy for Children Younger than 5 Years of Age

CLASSIFICATION (STEPS)	DESCRIPTION	MEDICATIONS FOR LONG-TERM CONTROL
Step 1: Mild intermittent	Brief exacerbations with symptoms no more often than twice a week. Nighttime symptoms no more than twice a week.	No daily medications needed.
Step 2: Mild persistent	Exacerbations more than twice a week, but less than once a day. Nighttime symptoms more than twice a month.	Preferred treatment ➤ Low-dose inhaled corticosteroid (with nebulizer or MDI with hold ing chamber with or without face mask or DPI). Alternate treatment ➤ Cromolyn (nebulizer is preferred or MDI with holding chamber). OR ➤ Leukotriene receptor antagonist.
Step 3: Moderate persistent	Daily symptoms of coughing and wheezing. Nighttime symptoms more than once per week.	Preferred treatment ➤ Low-dose inhaled corticosteroids and long-acting B_2-agonists. OR ➤ Medium-dose inhaled corticosteroids. Alternate treatment ➤ Low-dose inhaled corticosteroids and either leukotriene receptor antagonist or theophylline. If needed (particularly in children and adolescents with recurring severe exacerbations) Preferred treatment ➤ Medium-dose inhaled corticosteroids and long-acting inhaled B_2-agonists. Alternative treatment ➤ Medium-dose inhaled corticosteroids and either leukotriene receptor antagonist or theophylline.
Step 4: Severe persistent	Continuous daytime symptoms, limited physical activity. Frequent nighttime symptoms.	Preferred treatment ➤ High-dose inhaled corticosteroids. Plus ➤ Long-acting inhaled B_2-agonists. And if needed, ➤ Oral corticosteroids at 2 mg/kg/day (not to exceed 60 mg per day). Repeated efforts should be made to reduce systemic corticosteroids and maintain control with high-dose inhaled corticosteroids.
Quick relief	Bronchodilator as needed for symptoms. Intensity of treatment will depend on severity of exacerbation. ➤ Preferred treatment: Short-acting inhaled β_2-agonists by nebulizer, face mask, and space/holding chamber. ➤ Alternative treatment: oral β_2-agonist. With viral respiratory infection ➤ Bronchodilator every 4 to 6 hours up to 24 hours (longer with physician counsel); in general, repeat no more than once every 6 weeks. ➤ Consider systemic corticosteroids if exacerbation is severe or patient has a history of previous severe exacerbations. Use of short-acting β_2-agonists > 2 times a week in intermittent asthma (daily, or increasing use in persistent asthma) may indicate the need to initiate (increase) long-term control therapy.	

Note: Adapted from National Asthma Education and Prevention Program. (2002). Expert Panel Report II: Guidelines for the diagnosis and management of asthma—Update on selected topics 2002 *(NIH Publication No. 02-5075). Bethesda, MD: NHLBI, NIH.*

TABLE 25–13 Asthma Severity Classification and Preferred Clinical Therapy for Children Older than 5 Years of Age

CLASSIFICATION (STEPS)	DESCRIPTION	MEDICATIONS FOR LONG-TERM CONTROL
Step 1: Mild intermittent	Brief exacerbations with symptoms no more often than twice a week. Nighttime symptoms no more than twice a week. Asymptomatic and normal PEFR between exacerbations. No emergent visits and no asthma-related absences from school. PEFR ≥ 80% of predicted with variability < 20%.	No daily medications needed. Severe exacerbation may occur, separated by long periods of normal lung function and no symptoms. A course of systemic corticosteroids is recommended.
Step 2: Mild persistent	Exacerbations more than twice a week, but less than once a day. Nighttime symptoms more than twice a month. Exacerbations may affect activity and cause absences from school. PEFR ≥ 80% of predicted with variability of 20% to 30%.	Preferred treatment ➤ Low-dose inhaled steroid. Alternate treatment ➤ Cromolyn, leukotriene modifier, or nedocromil. OR ➤ Sustained-release theophylline to serum concentration of 5–15 mcg/mL.
Step 3: Moderate persistent	Daily symptoms of coughing and wheezing. Exacerbations at least twice a week that may last for days. Nighttime symptoms more than once per week. Exacerbations affect activity and several school absences occur. PEF or FEV_1 > 60% but < 80% of predicted with variability > 30%	Preferred treatment ➤ Low-to medium-dose inhaled corticosteroid. Plus Long-acting β_2-agonists Alternate treatment ➤ Increase inhaled corticosteroids to within medium-dose range OR ➤ Low-dose inhaled steroid and either leukotriene modifier or theophylline. If needed (particularly in children and adolescents with recurring severe exacerbations) Preferred treatment ➤ Increase inhaled corticosteroids within medium-dose range and add long-acting inhaled β_2-agonists. Alternative treatment ➤ Increase inhaled corticosteroids within medium-dose range and add either leukotriene modifier or theophylline.
Step 4: Severe persistent	Continuous daytime symptoms, limited physical activity. Frequent exacerbations. Frequent nighttime symptoms. Limited physical activity. Hospitalizations are frequent with PICU admissions for severe exacerbations. PEF or FEV_1 ≤ 60% of predicted, with variability > 30%	Preferred treatment ➤ High-dose inhaled corticosteroids. Plus ➤ Long-acting inhaled β_2-agonists. And if needed, ➤ Oral corticosteroids at 2 mg/kg/day (not to exceed 60 mg per day). Repeated efforts should be made to reduce systemic corticosteroids and maintain control with high-dose inhaled corticosteroids.
Quick relief	Bronchodilator as needed for symptoms. Intensity of treatment will depend on severity of exacerbation. ➤ Preferred treatment: Short-acting inhaled β_2-agonists by nebulizer, face mask, and space/holding chamber. ➤ Alternative treatment: oral β_2-agonist. With viral respiratory infection ➤ Bronchodilator every 4–6 hours up to 24 hours (longer with physician counsel); in general, repeat no more than once every 6 weeks. ➤ Consider systemic corticosteroids if exacerbation is severe or patient has a history of previous severe exacerbations. ➤ Use of short-acting β_2-agonists > 2 times a week in intermittent asthma (daily or increasing use in persistent asthma) may indicate the need to initiate (increase) long-term control therapy.	

Note: Adapted from National Asthma Education and Prevention Program. (2002). Expert Panel Report II: Guidelines for the diagnosis and management of asthma—Update on selected topics 2002 *(NIH Publication No. 02-5075). Bethesda, MD: NHLBI, NIH.*

MEDICATIONS Used to Treat Asthma

RESCUE MEDICATION	ACTION/INDICATION	NURSING CONSIDERATIONS
Beta$_2$-agonists (short-acting) Albuterol, metaproterenol, terbutaline, levalbuterol: inhalation, PO	Relax smooth muscle in airway, increase water content in bronchial mucus to promote muciliary clearance resulting in rapid bronchodilation within 5–10 minutes. Drug of choice for acute therapy (MDI or nebulizer).	• Use this rescue medication before inhaled steroid, wait 1–2 minutes between puffs, wait 15 minutes to give inhaled steroid. Child should hold breath 10 seconds after inspiring. Then rinse mouth and avoid swallowing medication. Use spacer. • Some side effects (tachycardia, nervousness, nausea and vomiting, headaches), but these are usually dose related. • Repetitive or excessive use can mask increasing airway inflammation and hyperresponsiveness and increase need for higher dosage to get same effect. • Use of more than 1 canister a month indicates inadequate control.
Corticosteroids Methylprednisolone: IV Prednisone Prednisolone: PO	Diminish airway inflammation and obstruction, enhance bronchodilating effect of β_2-agonists. Used for moderate to severe acute exacerbations when single β^2-agonist dose given in emergency department does not resolve symptoms.	• Not used as primary treatment. • Onset of action is 4–6 hours. • Short-term therapy for 3–10 days until symptoms resolve or child achieves 80% peak expiratory flow personal best. • Give with food. • Give daily oral dose in early morning to mimic normal peak corticosteroid blood level. • Assess for potential adverse effects of long-term therapy: decreased growth, unstable blood sugar, immunosuppression.
Anticholinergic Ipratropium: inhalation	Inhibits bronchoconstriction and decreases mucus production. Provides additive effects to short-acting β_2-agonists during acute exacerbation.	• Not for primary treatment. • Side effects include increased wheezing, cough, nervousness, dry mouth, tachycardia, dizziness, headache, palpitations. • Avoid eye contact.
CONTROLLER MEDICATION	**ACTION/INDICATION**	**NURSING CONSIDERATIONS**
Beta$_2$-agonists (long acting) Salmeterol Formoterol: inhalation	Relax smooth muscle in airway, used for nocturnal symptoms and prevention of exercise-induced bronchospasm.	• Should not be used for acute asthma attack. • Should not be used in place of inhaled corticosteroids. • Caution against overdosage as side effects such as tachycardia, tremor, irritability, insomnia will last 8–12 hours. • Report use of more than 4 puffs a day as this may indicate need for stepped-up therapy.
Methylxanthines Theophylline: PO Aminophylline: IV	Relax muscle bundles that constrict airways; dilate airway; provide continuous airway relaxation; sustained release for prevention of nocturnal symptoms. Aminophylline may be used for emergency adjunct therapy in ICU, but use is controversial.	• Tablet should not be crushed or chewed. • Used for long-term control, so continuous administration is needed; works best when a specific amount is maintained in the bloodstream (therapeutic serum level, 10–20 mcg/L). • Requires serum level checks and dose adjustment. • Side effects include tachycardia, dysrhythmias, restlessness, tremors, seizures, insomnia, hypotension, severe headaches, vomiting, and diarrhea.
Mast Cell Inhibitors Cromolyn sodium Nedocromil: aerosol	Anti-inflammatory, inhibit early- and late-phase asthma response to allergens and exercise-induced bronchospasm; may be used for unavoidable allergen exposure	• Not used at time of symptom development or acute exacerbation. • Must be used up to 4 times a day to be effective. • Therapeutic response seen in 2 weeks, maximum benefit may not be seen for 4–6 weeks. • Adverse reactions include wheezing, bronchospasm, throat irritation, nasal congestion, anaphylaxis.

MediaLink Nursing in Action: Using a Metered Dose Inhaler

MEDICATIONS Used to Treat Asthma (continued)

CONTROLLER MEDICATION	ACTION/INDICATION	NURSING CONSIDERATIONS
Corticosteroids Beclomethasone Budesonide Fluticasone Triamcinolone: aerosol	Anti-inflammatory, controls seasonal, allergic, and exercise-induced asthma. Effectively reduces mucosal edema in airways; usually combined with other asthma medications for control. First-line therapy in asthma management.	• Administer with spacer or holding chamber. • Rinse mouth following treatment to reduce chance of thrush and dysphonia. • Monitor growth. • Monitor for headache, gastrointestinal upset, dizziness, infection. • Use exactly as prescribed.
Leukotriene Modifiers Montelukast: PO Zafirlukast: PO	Reduces inflammation cascade responsible for airway inflammation. Improves lung function and diminishes symptoms and need for rescue medications. Adjunct to inhaled corticosteroids in moderate to severe asthma or substitute for inhaled corticosteroids in mild asthma.	• Administer montelukast in evening; may be given with or without food. • Administer zafirlukast 1 hour before or 2 hours after meal. • Family needs to report fever, acute asthma attacks, flu-like symptoms, severe headaches, or lethargy. • Take as prescribed, do not withdraw abruptly.
Other Hyposensitization (allergy shots), subcutaneous	Series of injections that can reduce sensitivity to unavoidable allergens (e.g., environmental organisms—mold, pollen); gradual dose increase over time (buildup) increases the child's tolerance to allergic substances; has been of help in some children.	• Use is controversial; some question about actual effect.

Note: Data from Baker, V. O., Friedman, J., & Schmitt, R. (2002b). Asthma management, part II: Pharmacologic management. Journal of School Nursing, 18*(5), 257–269; Belcher, D. (2002, November). Breathing easier with pediatric asthma: Pharmacologic management.* Advance for Nurse Practitioners, *37–38, 79; Baren, J. M., & Puchalski, A. (2002). Current concepts in the ED treatment of pediatric asthma.* Pediatric Emergency Medicine Reports, *7(10), 105–115.*

BOX 25–9 Markers of Good Asthma Control

- Minimal or no chronic symptoms day or night
- Minimal or no exacerbations
- No limitations on activities, no school missed, parents do not miss work
- Minimal use of short-acting β_2-agonists (< 1 time a day or < 1 canister a month)
- Minimal or no adverse effects from medications

Note: From National Asthma Education and Prevention Program. (2002). NAEPP Expert Panel Report: Guidelines for the diagnosis and management of asthma—Update on selected topics 2002 *(NIH Publication No. 02-5075). Bethesda, MD: National Institutes of Health, NHLBI.*

if control is not achieved with the regimen prescribed, then the regimen should be changed to correspond to the next step of asthma severity. Once control of asthma symptoms is achieved, the treatment plan can be reviewed in 1 to 6 months to determine if a reduction in asthma severity is appropriate (Hogan & Wilson, 2003). See Box 25–10.

The use of a peak expiratory flow (PEF) meter can assist in the management of asthma by helping to identify when obstruction occurs. This device measures the maximum flow of air that the child can push forcefully out of the lungs when cooperating. See Table 25–14 on page 866 for interpretation of peak expiratory flow meter readings. Medication administration can be based on peak expiratory flow rate (PEFR) readings and the effectiveness of treatment confirmed by improved PEFR numbers.

Most children with acute exacerbations respond to aggressive management in the emergency department. Children who do not respond or who are already being managed at home on corticosteroids have a greater chance of being admitted. Some children will need mechanical ventilation.

BOX 25–10 Research: Inhaled Corticosteroids

The use of inhaled corticosteroids as a first-line therapy for young children is of concern to many professionals and families despite their effectiveness in controlling symptoms and postponing irreversible damage to the lungs. Some studies have found associations between corticosteroid use and complications such as declines in growth, and the potential for brittle bones, glaucoma, and cataract development. The Steroid Therapy as Regular Therapy (START) study, a randomized control trial involving 1,974 children between 5 and 10 years and 1,221 children between 11 and 17 years, as well as 3,970 adults, compared the use of once daily low-dose budesonide with a placebo. All children were allowed to take their regular asthma medication in addition to the budesonide or placebo. Findings revealed that budesonide significantly reduced the risk of first severe asthma-related event for all age groups, and this group had more symptom-free days during the entire study period. Growth of enrolled children was measured and the overall reduction in growth for the children taking budesonide was 1.34 cm over 3 years; however, children attained normal adult height while continuing treatment on budesonide. New evidence for the regular use of inhaled steroids for control of mild persistent asthma has been provided (Pauwels, Pedersen, Busse, et al., 2003).

TABLE 25–14 Assessing Peak Expiratory Flow Rate (PEFR)

ZONE	PEFR (BEST AND PREDICTED FOR AGE)	ACTION
Green	80–100%	Good control. No asthma symptoms. Take medications as usual.
Yellow	50–80%	Caution! An acute episode may be present. Use action plan provided by healthcare provider. Inform healthcare provider if the child stays in this zone after giving medications listed in action plan.
Red	< 50%	Medical alert! Severe asthma episode. Use action plan provided by healthcare provider. Call healthcare provider or go to emergency department if PEFR does not return to yellow or green zone.

The child's personal best is determined after reviewing the recorded PEFRs measured two to four times a day for 2 to 3 weeks. The child should be optimally treated with medications during the day so the best reading is obtained (Richman, 1997). These zones are guidelines only. Specific zones and management should be individualized for each child.

Note: Adapted from American Academy of Allergy, Asthma, and Immunology (AAAAI). (1999). Pediatric asthma: Promoting best practice. Guide for managing asthma in children. *Milwaukee, WI: Author.*

NURSING MANAGEMENT

The goal of nursing management is to perform assessments and interventions to support the child during acute asthmatic episodes and to assist the child and family to control asthma symptoms.

Nursing Assessment and Diagnosis

Hospital-Based Care

The nurse usually encounters the child and family in the emergency department, nursing unit, or health center. Acute care has become necessary because the child's level of respiratory compromise cannot be managed at home.

PHYSIOLOGIC ASSESSMENT

Identify the child's current respiratory status first by assessing the ABCs—airway, breathing, and circulation—to make sure that the child's condition is not life threatening. If the child is moving air or talking, assess the quality of breathing. Assess the respiratory rate. Inspect the chest for retractions to assess the severity of respiratory distress. Auscultate the lungs for the quality of breath sounds and for the presence or absence of wheezing. Note whether a cough or stridor is present. Observe the child's color and assess the heart rate. Determine the severity of symptoms from the clinical manifestations table on page 861. Only after no life-threatening respiratory distress is found should the assessment move on to other systems.

Attach a pulse oximeter to monitor oxygen saturation. Assess peak expiratory flow rate, skin turgor, intake and output, and urine specific gravity. Because asthma can be a symptom of another illness, a head-to-toe assessment should be performed to identify other associated problems. See Box 25–1 and Table 25–7 for assessment guidelines.

The infant or child who has had episodes of frequent coughing or frequent respiratory infections (especially pneumonia or bronchitis) should also be evaluated for asthma. The cough is the warning signal that the child's airway is very sensitive to stimuli; it may be the only sign in "silent" asthma.

PSYCHOSOCIAL ASSESSMENT

Assess the child's anxiety. (Refer to Box 25–6 for guidelines.) The child and parents may be frustrated because another asthma episode has occurred. Assess whether the child thinks this episode could have been avoided if medications had been taken. The nurse should look for clues to hidden stress and self-blaming.

Common nursing diagnoses for the child experiencing an acute asthmatic episode include the following:

- Ineffective Airway Clearance related to airway compromise, copious mucous secretions, and coughing
- Impaired Gas Exchange related to airway obstruction, possible additional respiratory illness, and poor response to medication
- Risk for Deficient Fluid Volume related to difficulty in taking adequate fluids with respiratory distress
- Anxiety/Fear (child and parents) related to difficulty breathing and change in health status
- Ineffective Therapeutic Regimen Management (family) related to inadequate education on daily management of a chronic disease

Planning and Implementation

Pharmacologic and supportive therapies are used to reverse the airway obstruction and promote respiratory function. Nursing interventions focus on maintaining airway patency, meeting fluid needs, promoting rest and stress reduction for the child and parents, supporting the family's participation in care, and providing the child and family with information to enable them to manage the child's disease and ongoing developmental needs.

Maintain Airway Patency

If the child is exhibiting breathing difficulty, supplemental oxygen is required. Oxygen is best administered by nasal cannula or face mask. Humidified oxygen should be used to prevent drying and thickening of mucous secretions. The child should be placed in a sitting (semi-Fowler's) or upright position to promote and ease respiratory effort. The effectiveness of positioning, response to medications, and oxygen administration is evaluated by pulse oximeter and by observing for improved respiratory status.

The respiratory distress and need for supplemental oxygen can be stressful for parents and child alike (Figure 25–17 ■). Encouraging the parents' presence can be reassuring for the child. The parents should be kept informed of procedures and results, and their input should be obtained in developing the treatment plan.

Many medications are given by inhalation route (Figure 25–18 ■). The advantages of inhalation are that the medication acts quickly, enabling the pulmonary blood vessels to absorb the medication; systemic effects are minimized; and the inhaled droplets provide the added benefit of moisture. Continuous aerosol treatments may be implemented in some children with severe exacerbations. Monitor the child for medication side effects. The frequency of vital sign assessment is determined by the severity of symptoms. See Box 25–11 on page 868 .

Meet Fluid Needs

Fluid therapy is often necessary to restore and maintain adequate fluid balance. Adequate hydration is essential to thin and break up trapped mucous plugs in the narrowed airways. An adequate oral intake may not be possible with the child's compromised respiratory status. An intravenous infusion may be needed, and this route also may be used for administering medications and providing glucose. Overhydration must be avoided to prevent pulmonary edema in severe asthma attacks.

As respiratory difficulty diminishes, oral fluids can be offered slowly. Continue to monitor the child's hydration status. Involving parents in feeding can help gain the child's cooperation in taking oral fluids. The child's fluid preferences should be determined and choices provided when possible.

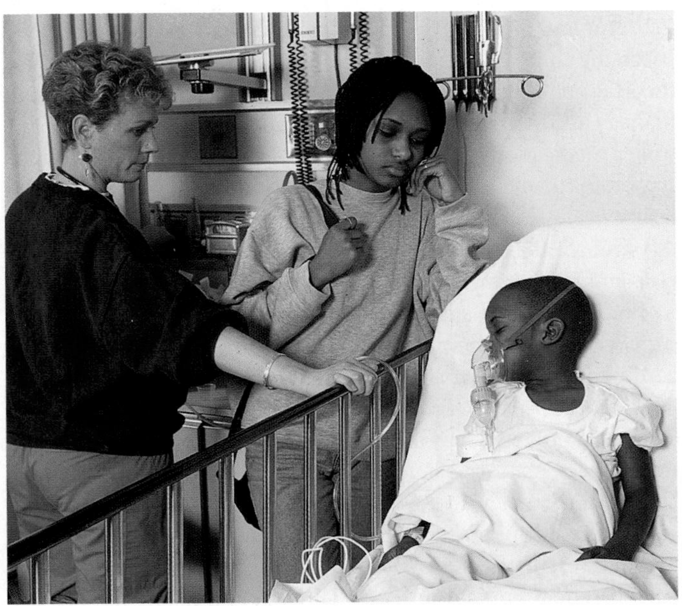

FIGURE 25–17 ■ Acute exacerbations of asthma may require management in the emergency department. The child is placed in a semisitting position to facilitate respiratory effort. Providing support to both the child and parent is an important part of nursing care during these acute episodes. The mother is exhausted after a sleepless night of caring for her son.

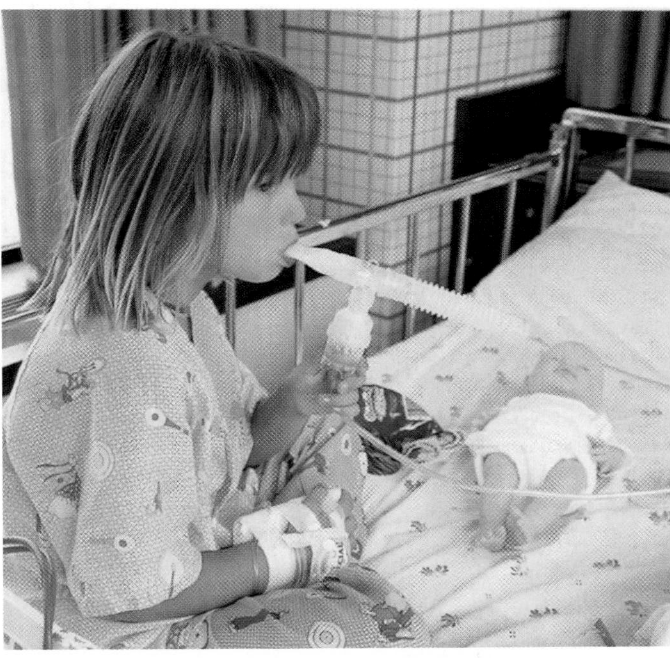

FIGURE 25–18 ■ Medications given by aerosol therapy allow children to get optimal therapy without injections and their associated pain and stress.

CLINICAL TIP

Iced beverages precipitate bronchospasms in some children with asthma. It is safest to offer the child room temperature or slightly cooled fluids without ice.

Promote Rest and Stress Reduction

The child who has had an acute asthmatic episode is usually very tired when admitted to the nursing unit. Labored breathing and low oxygenation may leave the child exhausted. Place the child in a quiet, private room if possible, to promote relaxation and rest. By grouping tasks, nurses can avoid repeatedly disturbing the child.

Support Family Participation

The parents may stay with the child, but may be exhausted after hours of their child's respiratory distress. Give parents the option of assisting with the child's treatments, rather than expecting them to do the care in addition to comforting the child. Provide frequent updates about the child's condition and encourage the parents to take breaks as needed.

Length of hospitalization depends on the child's response to therapy. Any underlying or accompanying health problem, such as preexisting lung disease or pneumonia, can complicate and extend the child's hospital stay. Communicate with the family of the hospitalized child frequently about the child's condition.

Discharge Planning and Home Care Teaching

Parents need a thorough understanding of asthma—how to prevent acute episodes and how to use treatment to maintain the child's health and avoid unnecessary hospitalization. When possible, educate parents when they are rested, but refer the parents

BOX 25–11 Medication Administration: Growth and Development Considerations

Inhalation is the preferred method of asthma medication administration. Metered-dose inhalers, nebulizers, and dry powder inhalers are devices used for this route of medication administration. Inhalation rapidly delivers the medication to the lungs for prompt onset of action. Other benefits are reduced risk of adverse effects and lower dosing compared to the oral route. However, inhalers are relatively inefficient and have special challenges for infants and young children. Effective medication delivery to the lung is affected by respiratory rate, degree of airflow obstruction, the medication, and the device used. Many devices require cooperation, coordination, and appropriate technique (Pongracic, 2003).

- Children over 6 years usually have the ability to use a metered-dose inhaler, coordinating medication release and inspiration; however, they may prefer to use a holding chamber or spacer with a valve.
- Spacers help increase the proportion of particles in the range that can reach the lungs. They also trap larger particles preventing them from reaching the mouth and being swallowed, which can cause local and systemic side effects. Valves prevent the escape of medication during use. With proper technique 12% to 15% of the dose may reach the lower airways.
- Spacers have a mouthpiece or mask attachment. When selecting a spacer for infants and young children, choose one with a mask because these children tend to be nasal breathers. Choose a mask size that fits the child's face and that has a flexible seal to prevent an air leak around the facial features. When the young child is uncooperative, it may still be difficult to maintain a seal. Work with young children to improve cooperation for medication delivery with play and distraction. Crying leads to prolonged exhalation and short inspiratory efforts which reduces lung deposition.
- Some inhaler and spacer brands have a whistle on inhalation that indicates that a breath is too fast or too shallow, but in others it indicates an adequate breath has been taken. When teaching the child and family about inhaler use, make sure you know what the whistle indicates.
- Nebulizers do not require coordination, making them easier for young children to use. A mask or mouthpiece must be used. They provide increased humidification during treatment. When the nebulizer mouthpiece is held 1 cm from the mouth, lung deposition of the medication is reduced by 50%. When it is held 2 cm from the mouth, up to 80% of the medication does not reach the lungs (Marshik, 2004). Nebulizers are inefficient, expensive, and take 8 to 10 minutes for the treatment. Infants and young children may have difficulty cooperating for the duration of the nebulizer treatment. Crying and a face mask that is too large for the child's face can further decrease the delivery of the medication to the lower airways.
- Dry powder inhalers are activated when the patient takes a breath, so puffs do not need to be coordinated with inhalation. No spacer is required, so it is more convenient to carry. No propellant is used. Delivery to the lower airway varies between 15% and 30% depending upon the type of inhaler. Children under 6 years of age who are wheezing may not be able to inspire at a rate fast enough to obtain the optimal amount of medication.

and child to a healthcare provider who can provide more comprehensive education. Support of the parents and child should focus on helping them to understand and cope with the diagnosis and the need for daily management to promote near-normal respiratory function while the child continues to grow and develop normally.

Discharge planning for the asthmatic child focuses on increasing the family's knowledge about the disease, medication therapy, and the need for follow-up care according to guidelines of the National Asthma Education and Prevention Program. The required lifestyle changes may be difficult for the child and parents. The need to modify the home by removing a loved pet or by having family members stop smoking in the home may create stress and resistance.

The nurse can play a role in keeping lines of communication open and can facilitate discussion and clarification of ways to prevent asthmatic episodes. Teach the family how to measure and interpret peak expiratory flow rate readings. Discuss the rescue medications used to manage asthma episodes, as well as controller medications for daily management. Begin encouraging school-age children to assume more responsibility for care, including avoidance of known triggers, early symptom recognition, relaxation breathing, and the proper use of inhaled medications. The family should be reassured that most children with asthma can lead a normal life with some modifications. See Partnering with Families: Home Care for the Child with Asthma on page 870.

Care in the Community

Nurses provide care to children with asthma in pediatricians' offices, specialty asthma clinics, schools, and summer camps. Once the stress of the acute episode has passed, take advantage of opportunities to provide more extensive education at each health visit.

Teach children how the lung works and what happens when an asthmatic episode occurs. Special summer camps are available that help children with asthma learn to manage their disease.

Make sure the parents and the child understand that asthma is a chronic and progressive condition rather than an episodic illness. Teach the child and family about the importance of the controller medication program and develop a written plan to help the family manage asthma. The plan should include not only the daily controller medications, but also the rescue medications to take once symptoms of an asthma episode are identified and when to call the health professional. Determine if the family uses any complementary and alternative therapies for asthma management. See Complementary Therapy: Alternative Asthma Treatments on page 871.

Provide printed educational materials and referral to a local support group to help parents gain additional knowledge and confidence that will enable them to help their child lead a normal life (Figure 25–19 ■). *Pediatric Asthma: Promoting Best Practice* is a good resource for families and is available from the American Academy of Asthma, Allergy, and Immunology.

Regularly review the child's technique for using an inhaler to ensure that proper technique is used. Assess how often the child uses the rescue inhaler by how frequently a new inhaler is purchased. There are 200 puffs per inhaler, and if one inhaler per month (or 6 to 7 puffs per day) is used, further investigation is needed. This could reflect poor asthma control or poor technique in using the inhaler so that full benefit of the medication is not gained.

Review the family's daily plan for monitoring the child's respiratory status. Evaluate the child's technique for PEFR and the parent's ability to identify the timing and type of stepped-up care needed to manage worsening symptoms. The goal is to bring asthma episodes under control with stepped-up care before a significant episode occurs. This can be achieved only with daily monitoring.

Environmental control is an important part of asthma management. When possible, pets and plants should not be kept in the home (and never in the child's bedroom). Active dust mite control should be attempted, but is challenging as mites live in the carpets, mattresses, upholstered furniture, bedcovers, soft toys, and clothes. Particular attention should be directed at controlling dust mites in the child's bed and bedroom. The child's mattress and pillow should be encased in plastic covers. Cockroach eradication should be initiated. Smoke from cigarettes, wood stoves, and fireplaces should be eliminated.

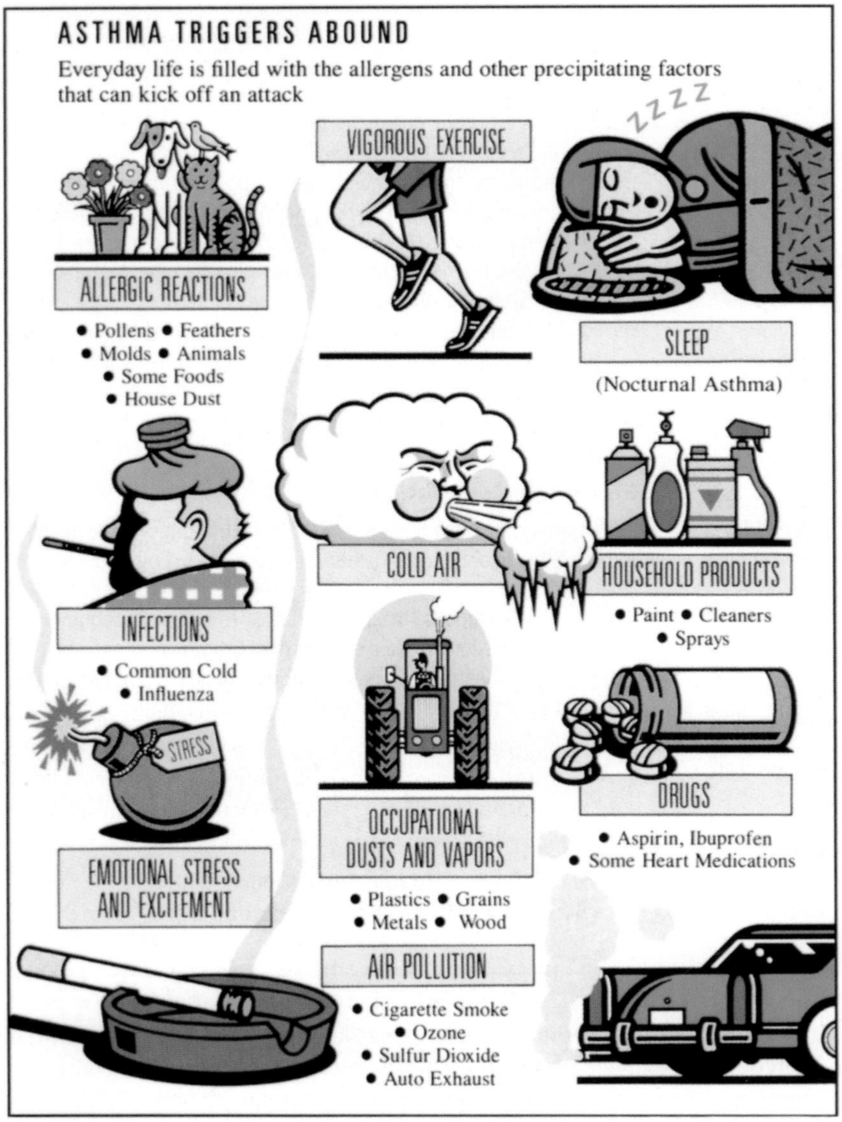

Help the child learn the signs of early respiratory distress so that treatment can be obtained before signs become more serious. Help parents to communicate with school personnel regarding the child's condition, and to have an individual school health plan developed so that medications are given as needed, even in preparation for exercise. For young school-age children, make sure their teachers can help recognize respiratory distress and can reduce their fear of going to the nurse for rescue medications. Make sure the child has a supply of medications at school or childcare as well as at home.

Encourage the school-age child or parent of younger children to use a symptom diary to note the daytime and nighttime symptoms, including peak flow measurements for 2 weeks prior to the next health visit.

Assess family support systems and family response to the chronic illness. Work to establish a partnership with the child and family that supports their ability to perform and maintain controller medication regimens. Reasons for nonadherence include the following:

- Improper use of delivery devices
- Inconvenient or frequent dosing regimens
- Lag time for medications to suppress inflammation
- Length of time for reappearance of symptoms following discontinuation of medications
- Fear of side effects
- Lack of support from family

See Evidence-Based Practice: Effective Asthma Management on page 871.

Ensure that the child gets regular health promotion and maintenance care, including routine and supplemental immunizations (influenza). If the child has severe asthma and uses high doses of aerosol or oral glucocorticoids to control asthma episodes, monitor the child's growth every 6 months as the disease and these medications may affect overall growth. Recent studies have revealed that inhaled corticosteroids may reduce the growth of prepubescent children, but the effect diminishes with chronic treatments, and final adult height is not affected. However, untreated asthma may reduce growth velocity in a child by nearly 0.9 cm per year (Stempel, Pedersen, & Blaiss, 2002).

Exercise is important for all children for physical fitness and to maintain appropriate body weight. Assess the amount of exercise children

FIGURE 25–19 ■ This educational piece from the American Lung Association explains what triggers an asthmatic episode. The required lifestyle changes for the child and family will be significant, so be sensitive to the family's situation and needs. Culture sometimes plays a significant part in exposure to lifestyle triggers.

Reprinted with permission ©2004 American Lung Association. For more information on how you can support to fight lung disease, the third leading cause of death in the United States, please contact the American Lung Association at 1-800-LUNG-USA (1-800-586-4872) or log on to the website at www.lungusa.org.

MediaLink Asthma Resources and Support

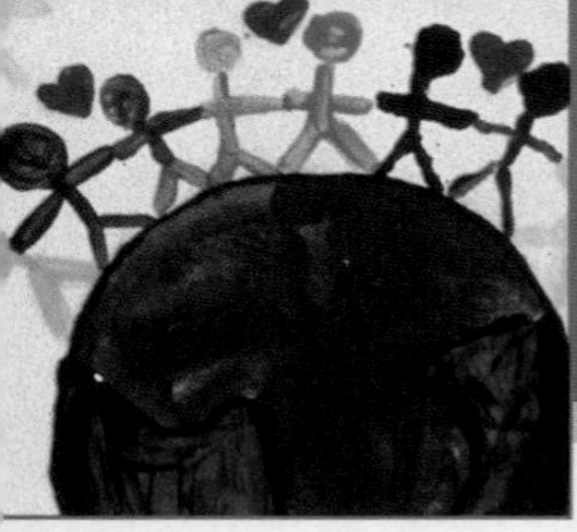

PARTNERING WITH FAMILIES

Home Care for the Child with Asthma

Identify parents' knowledge about the condition

- Review why asthma occurs and assess parents' understanding of the physiologic process. Ask:
  - What happens in your child's lungs during an asthma attack?
  - What are the early warning signs of an asthma episode in your child?
  - What are your child's symptoms and how does he or she respond to them? Does your child use the peak expiratory flow meter to evaluate symptoms?
  - To help toddlers learn how to use a peak flow meter, have them practice by blowing into party favors (i.e., noisemakers).
  - Determine if the parents or child understands that asthma is a chronic condition that needs daily medication and environmental management to be controlled.
- Help parents explore and understand how asthma affects their child.
  - Does the child wake up at night?
  - Does the child cough a lot? When?
  - Does the child avoid sports practice? What physical activities does the child like to do? If none, why?
  - Does asthma interfere with social activities or activities with friends?
- Identify asthma triggers and assess parents' understanding of how to prevent, avoid, or minimize their effect in a timely manner. Ask:
  - Do you know your child's personal asthma triggers? (Suggest that the parents and child keep a notebook to track episodes so they can learn more about these triggers.) Where do most episodes begin—home, school, outdoors, with exercise?
  - What steps can you take to minimize or eliminate your child's exposure to indoor pollutants (cigarette smoke, molds, dust mites, allergens, furry animals, etc.)?

Set up a schedule for parents to learn asthma management

- Make sure the parents understand the need for daily management and how that enables the family and child to have control over asthma.
- Ensure that the family knows when and where to seek emergency medical help? Describe actions the family can take before seeking medical assistance.

Review parents' understanding of medication therapy

- Provide information about medications: name, type of drug, dose, method of administration, expected effect, possible side effects. Make sure the parent knows the difference between controller medications to be used every day and rescue medications to be used during an episode.
  - Color labels to match the peak flow meter zones can be used to help children and parents tell the difference between their medications. A green label can be used on controller medications, to be used every day. Yellow and red labels can be used on the rescue medications with the number of puffs to use when the childs's peak flow meter reading is in either color zone.
- Evaluate the child's technique for the use of an inhaler. To help children use a metered-dose inhaler, let them practice breathing in slowly through a straw. To help children use a dry powder inhaler, obtain a practice inhaler from the pharmaceutical representative so the child learns to listen for the whistle corresponding to correct use for that inhaler. (Some inhalers have a whistle when the inspiration is too fast or when the inspiration is the correct rate.)
  - To help parents provide a nebulizer treatment to the infant or young child, suggest different types of diversion that might be used to help the child cooperate during the 8- to 10-minute treatment.
- Make sure the parent and child have a written action plan that includes daily management and steps to take when an episode begins.

Address associated issues

- Do parents know how to store and properly transport medications?
- What are the financial considerations of medication cost and lifestyle changes?
- Has the child's school or teacher been notified? What arrangements have been made for the child's use of medications at school?
- Has a medical identification bracelet or medallion been obtained for the child to facilitate assistance when away from home?

Identify need for follow-up care

- Do parents know when to see a physician? When drug levels need to be checked?
- Does child need to see an allergist?
- Do the child and parents have special emotional needs?
- Would a self-help group or camp experience be helpful for the child?

---

with asthma are getting and any symptoms they experience such as chest tightening, wheezing, or shortness of breath. Exercise-induced asthma typically occurs 5 to 10 minutes after stopping the activity and resolves in another 20 to 30 minutes. In the infant and toddler, excitement, giggling, and crying are exercise equivalents (Strunk, 2002). Avoid asking questions such as, "Do you have asthma symptoms when exercising?" or "Do you use your rescue inhaler for exercise?" without first determining that the child gets some exercise. Determine how frequently the child has symptoms of asthma and compare that to the classification of asthma severity in Table 25–13. For example, exercise-induced asthma symptoms that occur daily would put the child in the *moderate persistent* category. Ensure the appropriate controller and rescue medication treatment plan is used by the child.

Refer to the nursing care plan for the child with asthma in the community setting.

■ Evaluation

Expected outcomes of nursing care include the following:

- The child recognizes early asthma symptoms and uses rescue medications, hydration, and relaxation breathing before severe respiratory distress occurs.

- The child learns to avoid asthma triggers.
- The child and family implement a daily treatment plan for asthma and reduce the number of asthmatic episodes the child has.
- The child with a serious asthmatic episode responds to oxygen, fluids, and medication therapy, avoiding hospital admission.

Status Asthmaticus

Status asthmaticus is unrelenting, severe respiratory distress and bronchospasm in an asthmatic child, which persists despite pharmacologic and supportive interventions. These children are in acute respiratory distress and use many accessory muscles, appear restless and anxious, have altered mental status, cannot say more than a word or two without gasping for a breath, are diaphoretic, and are dusky or cyanotic. The child may have diminished or absent breath sounds and pulsus paradoxus. Laboratory findings for the child who needs admission to an intensive care unit may include:

- Significant hypoxemia (arterial oxygen saturation < 90% when on oxygen)
- Hypercarbia
- Peak expiratory flow rate < 25% predicted

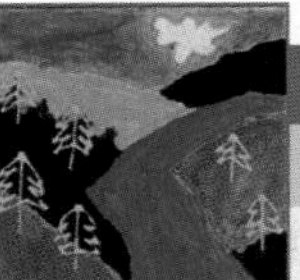

COMPLEMENTARY THERAPY
Alternative Asthma Treatments

Parents of children from different cultures may have concerns about daily medication regimens. Some prefer to use folk medicines such as rubbing oils or camphor (Vicks VapoRub) preparations on the child's chest. Learn about the family's cultural beliefs and practices (Sydnor-Greenberg & Dokken, 2000). Up to 80% of Hispanic, African American, and immigrant adolescents attending an inner-city high school reported the use of complementary therapies for the treatment of asthma that included rubs, teas (chamomile, ginger, wild root, and eucalyptus), prayer, and massage. There was no association between complementary therapy use and ethnicity or immigrant status. Nearly all adolescents indicated that they would repeat the use of the complementary therapy. It is important to ask about complementary therapy use by children and adolescents with asthma, and how it is used in conjunction with traditional therapy (Reznik, Ozuah, Franco, et al., 2002).

MediaLink Alternative Asthma Treatments Video

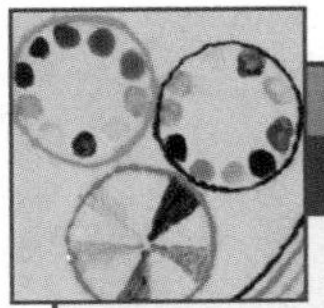

EVIDENCE-BASED PRACTICE
Effective Asthma Management

BACKGROUND

Adherence to recommended controller asthma medications is important to help manage asthma symptoms so the child has as normal a life as possible. Many children with asthma have less than optimal medication management to control symptoms. As a result many children have increased asthmatic episodes and suboptimal asthma control. What information about the knowledge and perceptions about managing the child with asthma is available to help nurses improve their communication and partnership with families for effective asthma management?

EVIDENCE

A study of children with persistent asthma symptoms in East Harlem revealed that anti-inflammatory medications were underused (Diaz, Sturm, Matte, et al., 2000). Parental concerns specific to long-term medication use were identified as a barrier to effective asthma management in another study (Mansour, Lamphear, & DeWitt, 2000). Recent research on parental beliefs, knowledge, experience of living with a child who has asthma, and attitudes about controller medication was conducted through interviews with 18 mothers of children and adolescents with asthma. Parents expressed that they learned to manage the child's asthma through "trial and error." Even though they had been taught about medications at one time, they had significant gaps in current knowledge with regard to medication actions. Parents expressed the desire to have health professionals (particularly those providing episodic and emergency care) listen to them regarding their child's healthcare needs. These same parents reported that taking medications on a daily basis was the most difficult aspect of asthma care; however, when they did use them they saw a good response in the child (Peterson-Sweeney, McMullen, Yoos, et al., 2003). A questionnaire was administered to parents of 109 children with asthma to explore their attitudes and understanding of asthma. Findings revealed that 31 children had mild intermittent asthma, and only 27 of the 78 children with persistent asthma had an appropriate medication regimen. Seventeen parents reported no anti-inflammatory medication use even when the child had moderate to severe asthma. Parents in this study had various beliefs about inhaled steroids, such as they should be a last-resort therapy and after they are taken for a while they will fail to work when needed. These parents also anticipated that their children would have activity limitations and episodic emergency department visits (Yoos, Kitzman, & McMullen, 2003).

IMPLICATIONS

The expressed desire for parents to be respected by health professionals for their knowledge about their children and daily management of asthma is important to acknowledge. Such respect for the parent's knowledge of the child's health status and response to asthma management is essential for an effective partnership with the parent. It is important to talk with parents about their beliefs about inhaled steroids to make sure appropriate information is provided. The following screening statements may be useful in identifying parents and children with a suboptimal asthma regimen (Yoos et al., 2003).

- There is little I can do to control my child's symptoms.
- Using inhaled steroids should be a last resort in treating asthma.
- After a child has taken inhaled steroids for a while, the steroids won't work when they are really needed.
- My child thinks that taking daily medicine is a hassle.
- I believe that my child can be symptom free most of the time.
- I expect that asthma will not affect my child's school attendance.
- I expect that my child can fully participate in gym and normal physical activity.
- I expect that my child will have no emergency room visits or hospitalizations because of asthma.

CRITICAL THINKING APPLICATION

Consider the possible perceptions and beliefs of parents and children with asthma in your practice setting. Use these statements to survey parents of children with moderate to severe persistent asthma to identify their beliefs about asthma and medication management. Then develop an education program that integrates these beliefs and perceptions to help improve their understanding of medication actions, the differences between inhaled and oral corticosteroids, and collaboration with health professionals to improve the control of their child's asthma.

Note: From Yoos, H. L., Kitzman, H., & McMullen, A. (2003, July). Barriers to anti-inflammatory medication use in childhood asthma. Ambulatory Pediatrics, *3, 181–190.*

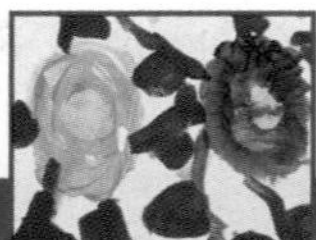

Nursing Care Plan

THE CHILD WITH ASTHMA IN THE COMMUNITY SETTING

GOAL	INTERVENTION	RATIONALE	EXPECTED OUTCOME
1. Readiness for Enhanced Family Coping related to increased control of asthma with daily therapeutic care			
	NIC Priority Intervention—*Family Support*: Promotion of family interests and goals.		**NOC Suggested Outcome—***Coping:* Actions to manage stressors that tax the family's resources.
The child and parents will work in partnership with the nurse to improve the child's asthma management.	■ Listen to the family's concerns about asthma management and respond with information to correct any misconceptions.	■ The parents' concerns may not be the same as the nurse's. If the parents' concerns are not addressed, the parents may not comply with recommended care.	■ The parents express greater confidence in averting and managing their child's asthma attacks.
	■ Teach the family skills (assessment, use of equipment, and giving medications) for managing the child's asthma.	■ Proper use of equipment and appropriate medication dosage will help alleviate asthma symptoms.	
	■ Provide telephone consultation to the parents during management of the first few asthma attacks.	■ Support and reinforcement of learning during an asthma attack will increase the parents' confidence in managing future attacks.	
	■ Educate the parents about when to call for future medical advice or to seek emergency treatment.	■ Parents need guidelines for judging the severity of asthma attacks.	
2. Ineffective Family Therapeutic Regimen Management related to knowledge deficit			
	NIC Priority Intervention—*Family Involvement*: Facilitating family participation in the emotional and physical care of the patient.		**NOC Suggested Outcome—** *Knowledge:* Treatment Regimen: Extent of understanding conveyed about a specific treatment regimen.
The child and parents will recognize early signs of an asthma episode and begin appropriate treatment.	■ Teach the child and parents to use a peak flow meter.	■ The peak flow meter helps quantify changes in respiratory status before symptoms are detected.	■ The number of asthma attacks requiring medical intervention is reduced.
	■ Help the child recognize his or her personal best peak flow and range indicating development of asthma symptoms.	■ Identifying a personal best peak flow helps establish the ranges to be used for future symptom identification.	
	■ Teach the family and child to give medications when the peak flow falls to the yellow range.	■ Giving medications before an asthma attack becomes established may help avert the actual attack.	
	■ Teach the child and family to monitor the child's response to medications with the peak flow meter.	■ Monitoring the response gives the family information to determine when home care is inadequate and medical intervention is needed.	

Without aggressive and immediate intervention the child with status asthmaticus may progress to respiratory failure and die. The child is placed on a cardiorespiratory monitor and pulse oximetry. Aggressive treatment with continuous nebulized albuterol and intravenous medications such as corticosteroids and aminophylline are implemented.

Heliox may be used to improve oxygenation and reduce the work of breathing. If improvement is not noted with these interventions, the child may ultimately require endotracheal intubation and mechanical ventilation. The section on respiratory failure earlier in the chapter gives additional information on the nurse's role in providing respiratory care for the child who is critically ill.

Cystic Fibrosis

Cystic fibrosis is a common inherited autosomal recessive disorder of the exocrine glands that results in physiologic alterations in the respiratory, gastrointestinal, and reproductive systems. The incidence of cystic fibrosis varies by race—1:3,300 in Caucasians, 1:17,000 in African Americans, 1:8,000 in Hispanics, and 1:32,000 in Asian Americans (McMullen & Bryson, 2004). Gender is not a factor in incidence (Figure 25–20 ■). Approximately 30,000 children and adults have cystic fibrosis in the United States, and approximately one third of these individuals are adults (Cystic Fibrosis Foundation, 2004). The mean age at diagnosis is 4.8 years; however, some children with a milder form of the disease may be adolescents or young adults before symp-

Nursing Care Plan THE CHILD WITH ASTHMA IN THE COMMUNITY SETTING (continued)

GOAL	INTERVENTION	RATIONALE	EXPECTED OUTCOME
3. Ineffective Health Maintenance related to lack of school asthma management plan			
	NIC Priority Intervention—*Health System Guidance*: Facilitating a patient's location and use of appropriate health services.		**NOC Suggested Outcome**—*Health-Promoting Behavior*: Actions to sustain or promote optimal wellness, recovery, and rehabilitation.
An Individual Health Plan (IHP) will be developed to help control and manage the child's asthma symptoms at school.	■ Provide the family with educational materials to give to the school nurse and school administrators.	■ School personnel need the latest information about effective asthma management in school settings.	■ Implementation of the school health plan reduces the number of school absences for asthma attacks that occur during school hours and increases participation in school activities.
	■ Advocate for all children to have an asthma management plan developed.	■ Establishing a school policy will help all children with asthma receive appropriate care.	
	■ Support the family to have a school health plan that includes the healthcare provider's written orders customized for the child.	■ The child with asthma needs a personalized care plan to be most successful in controlling asthma attacks.	
	■ Include in the IHP participation in regular school/class activities such as field trips and physical education, and what to do if asthma symptoms occur at school.	■ Participation, even with modification or premedication, prior to activities promotes self-esteem and peer relationships.	
	■ Help the family to obtain extra equipment and medications that can be provided to the school.	■ Schools will provide care, but the families must provide all supplies, equipment, and medications.	
	■ Work with the parents and school nurse to teach the specific asthma interventions to a designated person in the school nurse's absence.	■ School nurses often travel between several schools. The school administrator or secretary often serves as the backup care provider.	
4. Risk for Situational Low Self-Esteem (child) related to need to seek special care during school hours			
	NIC Priority Intervention—*Self-Esteem Enhancement*: Assisting a patient to increase his or her personal judgment of self-worth.		**NOC Suggested Outcome**—*Child Development, Middle Childhood*: Milestones of physical, cognitive, and psychosocial progression by 8 years of age.
The child's improved control over asthma will increase his or her self-esteem and peer relationships.	■ Assess the child's peer relationships and opportunities for age-appropriate interactions.	■ Assessment is important to identify the best strategies to support the child and family.	■ The child establishes friendships and engages in activities with peers.
	■ Motivate the child and family to gain increased control of asthma so the child can participate in normal childhood activities.	■ Motivation may increase adherence to recommended daily asthma control interventions.	
	■ Identify types of conflict and teasing the child experiences with peers, and teach the child defense tactics to deal with them.	■ If the child is able to gain some control over these situations, his or her self-esteem will be improved.	

toms appear (Farrell, Kosorok, Rock, et al., 2001). The median life span for individuals with cystic fibrosis in the United States is 32 years, but it is even higher in Canada (Orenstein, Winnie, & Altman, 2002).

Etiology and Pathophysiology

A gene isolated on the long arm of chromosome 7 directs the function of the cystic fibrosis transmembrane conductance regulator (CFTR). There are nearly 1,000 mutations of the CFTR gene that can cause cystic fibrosis (Orenstein, et. al., 2002). Approximately 1 in 29 individuals in the United States is a carrier of a defective CFTR gene (Parad & Comeau, 2003).

With a defective CFTR, there is defective chloride-ion transport across the exocrine and epithelial cells that causes decreased chloride secretion and increased sodium absorption. Decreased water flows across cell membranes, resulting in an abnormal accumulation of viscous, dehydrated mucus that affects the respiratory, gastrointestinal, and reproductive systems. Inflammation and lung changes are present as early as 4 weeks of age. Ultimately, all body organs with mucous ducts become

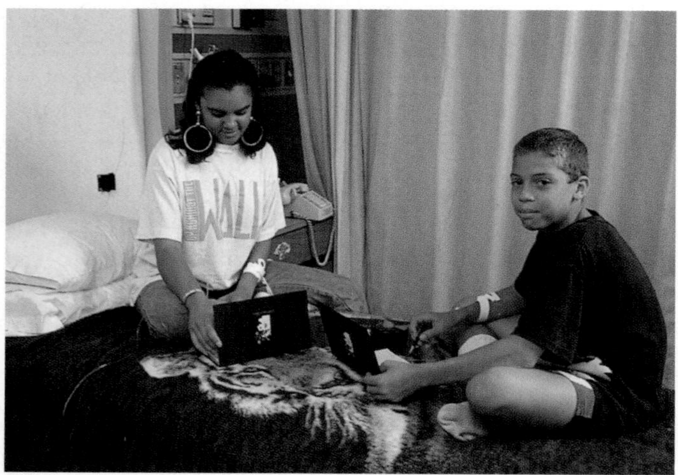

FIGURE 25–20 ■ Cystic fibrosis is an inherited autosomal recessive disorder of the exocrine glands, so it is not uncommon to see siblings with it such as this brother and sister.

obstructed and damaged (McMullen & Bryson, 2004). The rate of progression is variable among affected children.

Because of the blocked pancreatic ducts and resulting pancreatic damage, the natural enzymes necessary to digest fats and proteins are not secreted. Food is poorly digested and thick mucus is also found in the intestines. This results in poor digestion and malabsorption in 90% of children with cystic fibrosis by 1 year of age, resulting in failure to thrive in many children. In some children the pancreas may stop producing sufficient insulin and the body may fail to utilize insulin normally, resulting in the development of diabetes mellitus.

Children have a classic cough because the lungs are filled with thick mucus, which the respiratory cilia cannot clear. This causes air to become trapped in the small airways, resulting in hyperinflation and atelectasis. Secondary respiratory infections and chronic bacterial colonization occur because the thick secretions provide an environment conducive to bacterial growth. Pneumothorax and hemothorax may occur in older children. Respiratory failure is the major leading cause of mortality.

Nearly all males who have cystic fibrosis are sterile because of blockage or absence of the vas deferens. Females have difficulty conceiving because of chronic illness and thickened mucous secretions in the reproductive tract that interfere with the passage of sperm (McMullen & Bryson, 2004).

Metabolic function is altered as a result of the imbalances created by excessive electrolyte loss through perspiration, saliva, and mucous secretion. These children are at risk for dehydration secondary to electrolyte imbalance. The "salty taste" of the skin is the result of sodium chloride that makes its way through skin pores to the skin surface.

MediaLink Cystic Fibrosis Video

Clinical Manifestations

The primary symptom of cystic fibrosis is the production of thick, sticky mucus. Up to 10% of newborns with cystic fibrosis present in the first 48 hours with meconium ileus, a small bowel obstruction (McMullen & Bryson, 2004). Stools of the child with cystic fibrosis may have the following characteristics: steatorrhea (fatty or greasy), frothy (bulky and large quantity), foul smelling, and floating. Constipation is common and intestinal obstruction may occur in older children. Rectal prolapse, resulting from the large, bulky, difficult-to-pass stools, may occur (Figure 25–21 ■).

Respiratory signs and symptoms include a chronic moist, productive cough and frequent infections. Frontal headaches, facial tenderness, purulent nasal discharge, and postnasal discharge are associated with chronic sinus infections. Nasal polyps are found in 10% of children with cystic fibrosis (McMullen & Bryson, 2004). Most children have a voracious appetite, but have difficulty maintaining and gaining weight because of malabsorption of food and an increased metabolic rate associated with frequent infections. Clubbing, an enlargement of the distal phalanges of the fingers and toes, occurs as the disease progresses due to chronic fibrotic changes within the lungs (Figure 25–22 ■). Children with a milder form of the disease may reach the teenage or young adult years before symptoms appear.

Various disorders develop in the older child with more advanced cystic fibrosis. Unilateral chest pain of sudden onset associated with shortness of breath is an indication of pneumothorax. Minor hemoptysis (blood streaking the expectorated mucus) is common; however, massive hemoptysis (240 mL in 24 hours) is a serious complication and much less common (McMullen & Bryson, 2004). Distal intestinal obstruction syndrome, presenting as crampy abdominal pain and decreased stooling, occurs in about 10% of adolescents and adults.

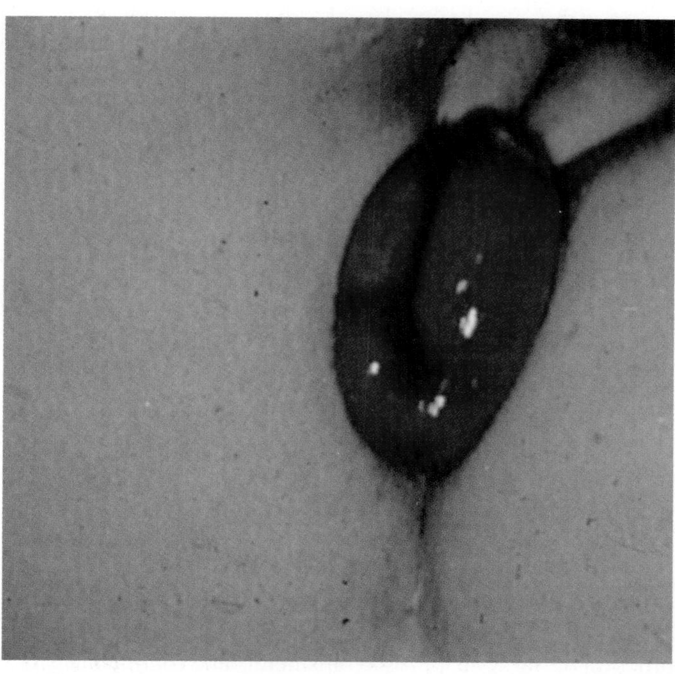

FIGURE 25–21 ■ Rectal prolapse.

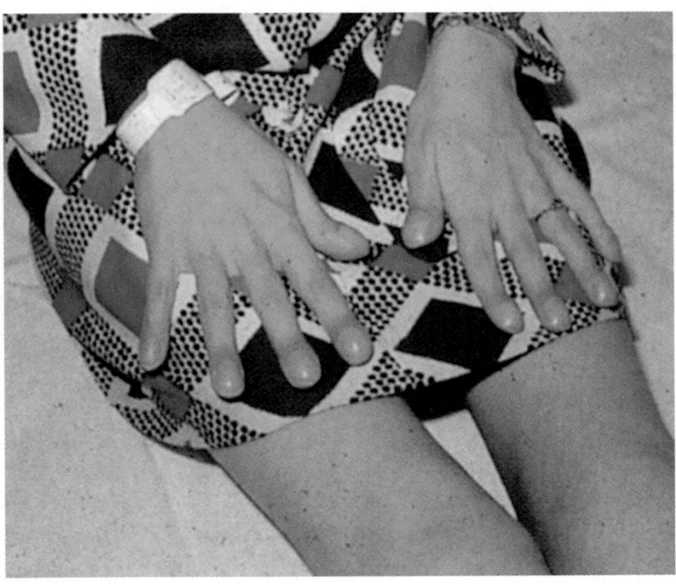

FIGURE 25–22 ■ Digital clubbing.

COLLABORATIVE CARE

Diagnostic Procedures

Cystic fibrosis is usually diagnosed in infancy or early childhood following one of three major presentations: newborn meconium ileus, malabsorption or failure to thrive, or chronic recurrent respiratory infections. In infants and toddlers, fecal impaction and intussusception ("telescoping" of the bowel) may be the first signs of cystic fibrosis (see Chapter 29∞).

Genetic testing is available for adults with a positive family history, partners of individuals with cystic fibrosis, and couples seeking prenatal testing to detect the majority of CF gene alterations. Rare CF gene alterations are not always detected in genetic testing (Cystic Fibrosis Foundation, 2004).

Newborns with CF have an elevated serum level of the pancreatic enzyme trypsinogen. Newborn screening can be performed on dried blood samples to detect immunoreactive trypsinogen, although this test has high false-positive and false-negative rates. Therefore genetic testing of the child's DNA is performed on the positive immunoreactive trysinogen tests. Approximately 10% of newborns are screened in the United States. Newborn screening for CF is mandated in Wisconsin, Colorado, Wyoming, Mississippi, New Jersey, and New York, and offered as an option in several other states (Parad & Comeau, 2003).

A sweat chloride test by pilocarpine iontophoresis is considered the gold standard for diagnosis of cystic fibrosis. The majority of children with cystic fibrosis are diagnosed by a positive sweat chloride test and the presence of classic symptoms or a positive family history (McMullen & Bryson, 2004) (Table 25–15). Sweat chloride tests can be performed on infants who are only a few days old; however, inadequate sweat samples may not be collected until the infant is more than 4 weeks (Orenstein et al., 2002; McMullen & Bryson, 2004). Two tests are performed to confirm the diagnosis (Figure 25–23 ■).

A spirometer is used on children older than 6 years to monitor pulmonary function. Forced vital capacity (FVC) and forced expiratory volume in 1 second (FEV_1) readings are taken. Sputum specimens are obtained to test for culture and sensitivity for treatment.

Clinical Therapy

Clinical therapy focuses on maintaining respiratory function, managing infection, promoting optimal nutrition and exercise, and preventing intestinal obstruction. See Table 25–16. Newly diagnosed children who begin treatment before the onset of symptomatic lung disease are aggressively treated to improve their outcome and maintain near-normal lung function as long as possible. The goal of therapy is to prevent or slow the progression of airway damage. Pulmonary function declines 2% to 4% per year even with aggressive treatment (Varlotta, 1998).

Treatment is focused on controlling infection and inflammation, and on reducing mucus accumulation. Various forms of bronchial hygiene therapy, such as manual chest physiotherapy, are used regularly to reduce the accumulation of mucus in the lungs. See Box 25–12 for the various types of chest physiotherapy used by children with cystic fibrosis.

Frequent prolonged courses of antibiotics for infections may be prescribed to improve pulmonary function, exercise tolerance, and quality of life. Infection management directed at *Haemophilus influenzae*, Staphylococcus, and *Pseudomonas aeruginosa* are important for children with mild disease; however, sputum culture results and sensitivities are also important in selection of the specific antibiotics used. Children who have evidence of *Pseudomonas aeruginosa* or *Burkholderia cepacia* infections have a poorer outcome. The Cystic Fibrosis Foundation has a policy stating that individuals infected with *Burkholderia*

TABLE 25–15 Diagnostic Test for Cystic Fibrosis (Sweat Test)

TEST	PURPOSE	NORMAL VALUES	DIAGNOSTIC VALUES
Sweat test (pilocarpine iontophoresis)	Analysis of sodium and chloride content in sweat	Sodium: 10–30 mEq/L Chloride: 10–35 mEq/L	Chloride: 50–60 mEq/L—suspicious; > 60 mEq/L—diagnostic with other clinical signs

To collect the sweat, pilocarpine is applied to a small area on the arm or leg. An electrode with weak electrical current is placed on the area to stimulate the child to sweat. The area is cleaned and a piece of filter paper is placed over the area and covered in plastic. The filter paper is removed after 30 minutes and the sweat content is analyzed.

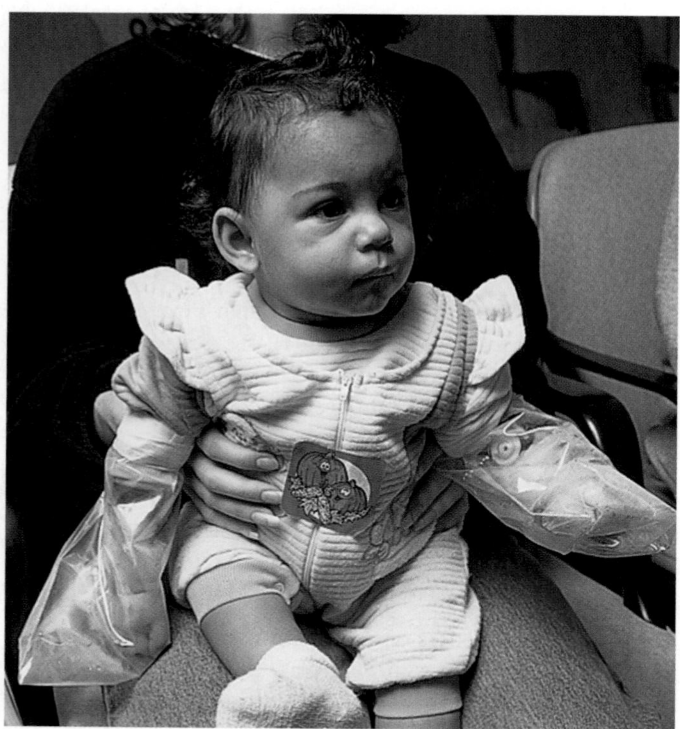

FIGURE 25–23 ■ The parent may hold and reassure the infant or small child being evaluated for cystic fibrosis with a sweat chloride test. Sweat is being collected under the wrappings for later analysis of the amount of sodium and chloride.

cepacia may not attend foundation-sponsored events in an effort to reduce the cross infection to uninfected children (Cystic Fibrosis Foundation, 2000).

Medications are used to reduce sputum viscosity and to dilate the airways. Anti-inflammatory treatment is sometimes prescribed. Vitamins and pancreatic enzymes are also provided to improve the child's nutritional status. See the table of medications used to treat cystic fibrosis on page 878.

Improvements in medical management and optimal nutrition now enable many children with cystic fibrosis to survive into adulthood. As more adolescents survive into adulthood, new complications are becoming apparent and need carefully coordinated management along with cystic fibrosis. Cystic fibrosis–related diabetes is challenging to manage, because the large caloric intake needed for these adolescents needs to be balanced by insulin dosage.

Cystic fibrosis is ultimately terminal, however, because of the progressive multisystem changes and the difficulty of long-term infection management. Double-lung transplantation is occasionally performed when the patient is in the disease's end stages to temporarily halt the disease progression, and approximately 50% of cases survive for the first 5 years (McMullen & Bryson, 2004). The posttransplant course can be complicated by infection and rejection of the grafted lungs. Acute rejection can be managed by immunologic medications. Chronic rejection, also known as **bronchiolitis obliterans,** involves irreversible changes to the lung tissue that are unresponsive to immunologic med-

TABLE 25–16 Clinical Therapy for Cystic Fibrosis

CLINICAL THERAPY	RATIONALE
Respiratory Therapy	
Exercise and physical fitness	Promotes maintenance of lung function
Chest physiotherapy for all lung segments (bilateral percussion or vibration while the patient is in a position to promote sputum drainage)	In association with coughing and breathing techniques secretions move to bronchi from lung areas, performed twice a day
Antibiotics (oral, IV, inhalation)	Treats infection
Immunizations	Prevention of viral and some bacterial infections
Chest tube drainage of air leaks	Resolves pneumothorax
Thorocoscopy to sew over ruptured alveoli	Repairs area of recurrent pneumothorax and prevents future episode in same location
Hospitalization for intense airway clearance	Promotes resolution of pulmonary exacerbations
Lung transplantation	Reversal of respiratory failure
Gastrointestinal Tract Therapy	
Acid suppression preparation	Gastric acid hypersecretion may cause gastroesophageal reflux that worsens lung function; enteric coating of enzyme supplements is reduced with high acid levels in duodenum
Hyperosmolar enemas	Relieves meconium ileus in most infants
Isotonic fluid lavage of the intestines orally or by nasogastric tube	Reduces partial obstruction caused by distal intestinal obstruction syndrome (DIOS)
Nutrition	
Well-balanced diet with 120–150% of RDA calories and 200% of RDA protein and moderate fat	Promotes essential nutrient balance for health, growth, and weight maintenance; nutritional counseling to support high-caloric intake; cultural-socioeconomic issues important
Pancreatic enzyme supplements	Assists in digestion of nutrients and decreasing fat and bulk

BOX 25–12 Bronchial Hygiene Therapy

Various methods of bronchial hygiene therapy have evolved over time to treat patients needing extra support to clear mucus and secretions from the lungs. Limited research comparing the various methods has revealed that their effectiveness is fairly comparable in clearing secretions from the airway. A more definitive long-term study to compare the efficacy of chest physiotherapy, the high-frequency chest wall oscillation vest, and the flutter device is currently being conducted by the Cystic Fibrosis Foundation.

For the child with cystic fibrosis, chest physiotherapy is time consuming and unpleasant, so adherence is often less than optimal. Finding a method that the family and child will use is important in disease management. Use the following information to assist families to select the method of bronchial hygiene therapy that has a better chance of fitting into their lives.

- **Chest physiotherapy.** Considered the gold standard in bronchial hygiene therapy. A parent or therapist percusses or applies vibration over each lung segment for 3 to 5 minutes while the child is maintained in the different positions that promote drainage of the secretions loosened by percussion or vibration. This method is preferred for infants and toddlers. See the skills manual for correct techniques.
- **Positive expiratory pressure (PEP).** The patient breathes in and out about 15 times through a mouthpiece attached to a breathing device with a special expiratory valve that creates a positive pressure in the airways during exhalation. The child then removes the mouthpiece and performs two to three forced exhalations followed by a cough (huff cough technique). This method creates a back pressure in the lungs and stabilizes the smaller airways. It improves aeration to the alveoli by prolonging exhalation against positive pressure. The technique has been mastered by children as young as 3 years, but is more commonly used by school-age and older children. Studies have reported that it is comparable to manual chest physiotherapy for mucus clearance in children with cystic fibrosis (McIlwaine, Wong, Peacock, et al., 1997).
- **Flutter valve.** This form of PEP uses deep breathing and forced exhalation to promote airway clearance. The patient breathes through a mouthpiece attached to a handheld device that has a steel ball inside. The patient controls exhalations through the device and the weight of the steel ball (flutter) provides intermittent positive expiratory pressure that vibrates the airway walls to loosen secretions. Deep breathing and breath holding allow the air to get behind the mucus and the positive expiratory pressure created helps move the mucus to the larger airways. School-age and older children can use this method. A study comparing the flutter valve to conventional chest physiotherapy revealed that each therapy was effective (Homnick, Anderson, & Marks, 1998).
- **High-frequency chest wall oscillation.** The patient puts on an inflatable vest that creates an oscillating motion against the chest wall by an air pulse generator that rapidly inflates and deflates the vest. Deep breathing and coughing help mobilize secretions loosened. Children older than 4 years can use this method. One study found no statistical difference between this device and others when studying patient satisfaction and efficacy (Oermann, Accurso, Castile, et al., 1997).

ication management. The presence of bronchiolitis obliterans is a sign of impending patient death unless another lung transplant is performed.

NURSING MANAGEMENT

The goal of nursing management is to partner with families to manage the disease by promoting optimal nutrition and in reducing the incidence of infection.

Nursing Assessment and Diagnosis

Physiologic Assessment

Assess the child's respiratory status. Respiratory function tests are usually performed every 6 months during cystic fibrosis center visits. Inquire about the frequency and character of the child's cough and characteristics of the sputum. Compare this information with the child's baseline. Changes in the cough may be more important than its presence or absence related to the development of a new infection. Auscultate the chest for breath sounds, crackles, and wheezes. Note any cyanosis or clubbing of the extremities. Obtain oxygen saturation and spirometry readings if changes in respiratory status are suspected.

Evaluate the child's growth, plotting the weight and height on a growth curve. Determine whether the child is maintaining an appropriate growth pattern. Children with significantly lower percentiles for height and weight on the growth curve should be considered malnourished. Inquire about the child's appetite and dietary intake. How are nutritional supplements, pancreatic enzymes, and vitamins used?

Assess the child's stooling pattern. Identify whether the child has problems with abdominal pain or bloating, and whether these problems can be related to eating, stooling, or other activities. Palpate the abdomen for liver size, fecal masses, and evidence of pain.

Assess hearing acuity on a regular basis, especially if the antibiotic tobramycin is used as this medication has been associated with hearing loss.

Psychosocial Assessment

Inquire about the family's and child's emotional and psychosocial responses to managing the illness. The emotional stress of this chronic disease may not be readily apparent on admission, or in clinic settings particularly if the child's symptoms are mild and not imminently life threatening. These issues are important when the child is going through major developmental stages. Ongoing observation of the child's and parents' behavior helps direct nursing interventions. See Box 25–6 on page 846 for guidelines. Parents may feel guilt as carriers of the disease. Siblings may also show signs of difficulty in dealing with the illness, particularly if not affected by the disease. Siblings may also be affected if the child is showing signs of significant deterioration, being forced to acknowledge their own future course with the disease.

The nurse should ask parents how the child's illness has affected day-to-day functioning, potential conflicts with family activities, and how they have adapted to the child's plan of care. Identify what parents of young children have told the child and siblings about the disease. What kind of questions have the child and siblings asked about cystic fibrosis, and how have parents answered them? Has the child ever asked about his or her life expectancy? If not, what would parents say if asked?

Developmental Assessment

Growth and development may be altered by the chronic nature of the disease. Children with cystic fibrosis may be growth delayed. Compare the child's height and weight to age norms and observe the adolescent for the appearance of secondary sex

MEDICATIONS Used to Treat Cystic Fibrosis

MEDICATIONS	ACTIONS
Aerosol bronchodilators	Opens large and small airways; use before chest physiotherapy and with symptoms; few studies exist to demonstrate their effectiveness.
Aerosol DNAse	Loosens, liquefies, and thins pulmonary secretions; decreases risk of developing pulmonary infections requiring parenteral treatment in some patients (McMullen & Bryson 2004).
Corticosteroids and high-dose ibuprofen on alternate days	Anti-inflammatory agents: reduces inflammatory response to infection; alternate day use to decrease side effects of steroids; decreases progression of lung damage in preadolescents with mild disease.
Antibiotics (oral, IV, and inhalation)	Treats infections. Higher doses than normal and prolonged courses may be needed. Antibiotic selection should be based on culture sensitivities. Intermittent administration of tobramycin by inhalation improves pulmonary function.
Pancreatic enzyme supplements (Cotazym-S, Pancrease, Viokase)	Assists in digestion of nutrients decreasing fat and bulk; given prior to food ingestion, taken with meals and snacks.
Multivitamins and vitamin E in water-soluble form; vitamins A, D, and K given when deficient; iron supplementation	Cystic fibrosis interferes with vitamin production; supplements are required in water-soluble form for better absorption (vitamins A, D, E, and K are naturally fat soluble); iron deficiency results from malabsorption syndrome.
Ursodeoxycholate	May slow progression of hepatic lesion in CF. Given when patient has elevated liver enzymes or evidence of portal hypertension.
Lactulose	May abort early distal intestinal obstruction syndrome and prevent recurrences.

characteristics, which are often delayed due to nutrition status. School-age children and adolescents often are embarrassed at being viewed as different from playmates and peers. Ask how the child or adolescent feels about the need for a special diet, medications, and the daily routine of respiratory management.

Common nursing diagnoses for the child with cystic fibrosis include the following:

- Ineffective Airway Clearance related to thick mucus in lungs
- Ineffective Breathing Pattern related to thick tracheobronchial secretions and airway obstruction
- Risk for Infection related to the presence of mucous secretions conducive to bacterial growth
- Imbalanced Nutrition: Less than Body Requirements related to inability to digest nutrients
- Parental Role Conflict related to interruptions in family life due to the home care regimen and child's frequent exacerbations

■ Planning and Implementation

Nursing management involves supporting the child and family initially, when the diagnosis is made, during subsequent hospitalizations, and during visits to specialty and primary healthcare providers. The nurse's role begins with implementing specific medical therapies and providing nursing care to meet the child's physiologic and psychosocial needs. Respiratory therapy, medications, and diet must be coordinated to promote optimal body function. Psychosocial support and reinforcement of the child's daily care needs are important in preparation for home care.

Children with cystic fibrosis require periodic hospitalization when a severe infection occurs or for a pulmonary and nutritional "tune-up." Respect the parents' experiences as the child's primary care provider and include them in the child's routine care as much as possible. However, parents may view the hospital stay as a break from the rigorous daily pulmonary routine at home and need support to take advantage of the respite. The family often becomes proficient at providing physical care to the child, but the nurse should take the opportunity provided during rehospitalization to review basic and new information about respiratory care, medications, and nutrition. Keeping lines of communication open and validating parents' understanding of their child's disease and care needs are important steps in preparing the family to cope with this chronic health challenge.

The hospitalized child is usually placed in a single room with standard precautions to reduce spread of infectious organisms. Children with cystic fibrosis are not co-roomed to reduce risk for transfer of Pseudomonas aeruginosa and Burkeholderia cepacia.

Provide Respiratory Therapy

Chest physiotherapy is usually performed one to three times per day before meals to facilitate the removal of secretions from the lungs (Figure 25–24 ■). DNAse is given by nebulizer to help thin respiratory secretions. Respiratory therapists and nurses often collaborate in teaching parents and other family members the skills for these necessary treatments. Pulmonary care may involve aerosol treatments and antibiotics when indicated. Some children use an oscillating vest for 30 minutes twice a day rather than chest physiotherapy. Exercise therapy is often utilized to increase endurance.

Administer Medications and Meet Nutritional Needs

Antibiotics for an acute exacerbation are provided by oral, inhalation, and intravenous routes. They are continued until the child achieves the best possible lung function, often for at least 14

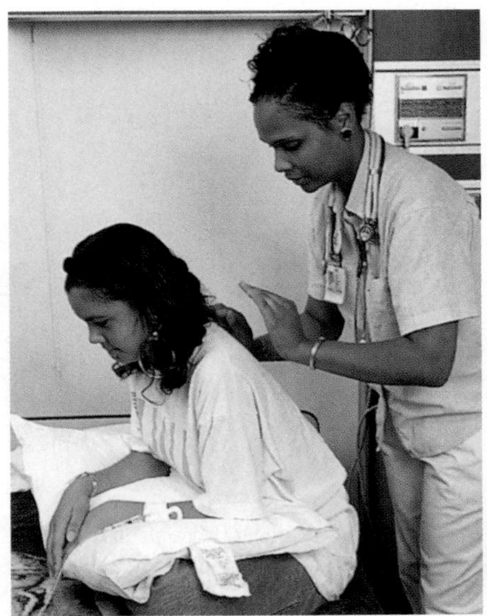

A

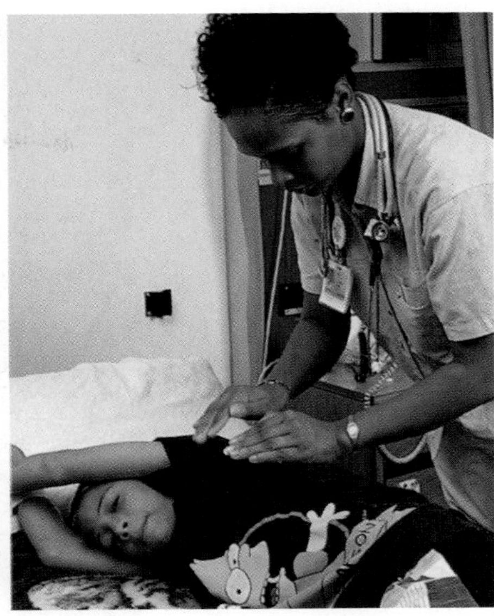

B

FIGURE 25–24 ■ Postural drainage can be achieved by clapping with a cupped hand on the chest wall over the segment to be drained. This action creates vibrations that are transmitted to the bronchi so that secretions are loosened and drain by gravity to the bronchi. *A,* If the obstruction is in the posterior apical segment of the lung, the nurse can do this with the child sitting up. *B,* If the obstruction is in the left posterior segment, the child should be lying on the right side. Several other positions can be used depending on the location of the obstruction. See the Skills Manual.

days. Children with cystic fibrosis have an increased clearance of nearly all antibiotics, and therefore they need higher dosages and longer treatment courses than other children. Due to the higher antibiotic dosages, renal function needs to be monitored. Serum drug levels of antibiotics may be ordered to ensure therapeutic dosing. In some cases, IV antibiotics may be given at home to enable an earlier discharge. A portacath or peripherally inserted central catheters (PICC lines) are often placed for home IV therapy.

Digestive problems can be eased with pancreatic enzymes and dietary modification. Pancreatic enzyme supplements come in powder sprinkles and capsule form and are taken orally with all meals and large snacks. The amount needed is individualized based on the child's nutritional needs and digestive response to these supplements. Parents need to learn what foods if any should be avoided or eliminated because of the child's gastrointestinal problems. Referral should be made to a nutritionist before the time of discharge. The goal is to achieve near-normal, well-formed stools and adequate weight gain.

Fat-soluble vitamins (A, D, E, and K) are not completely absorbed from food; therefore, they must be taken in water-soluble form. Multivitamins taken twice daily usually are sufficient to prevent vitamin deficiency.

Respiratory complications necessitate additional energy expenditure, and some children require nutritional supplements or, supplemental nasogastric or gastrostomy feedings, to gain and maintain weight. The diet should be well balanced, with an emphasis on high caloric value. Children with CF may require 1.5 times the daily caloric requirements. Fats and salt are both necessary in the diet. Balanced with pancreatic enzyme supplements, moderate fat intake adds an important source of calories.

Psychosocial Support

The nurse should assist the parents and child to learn ways to promote health after discharge. Emotional support is essential because the diagnosis of this disorder creates anxiety and fear in both the parents and the child. The child and parents need assistance with emotional and psychosocial issues relating to discipline, body image (stooling and odor, clubbing, barrel chest), frequent rehospitalization, the potential fatal nature of the illness, the child's feeling of being different from friends, and overall financial, social, and family concerns. Because the disorder is inherited, families may have more than one child with cystic fibrosis. Parents may have unspoken feelings of anger and guilt, blaming themselves for their children's condition. Refer families to genetic counseling.

Discharge Planning and Home Care Teaching

The financial burden of medications, supplies, and medical follow-up may not be recognized immediately by a family overwhelmed by the diagnosis. Initially, parents need assistance in obtaining necessary equipment. If the family requires financial assistance, they should be referred to the appropriate social services. Home care of the child with cystic fibrosis is expensive and can be draining on the family's finances. The cost of care varies by the severity of the child's condition, so annual costs increase as the child ages, and may range from $5,600 to $60,700 (Balinsky & Zhu, 2004).

The chest physiotherapy regimen of three or four times a day has a significant impact on family time. See Photo Story: Managing Cystic Fibrosis on page 880. Alternate bronchial hygiene therapy techniques, such as a vest, may be more easily accepted by the family, especially if the parent does not have to physically perform the percussion and vibration. A regular vigorous exercise regimen is also beneficial in improving lung function, respiratory muscle strength, endurance, and airway clearance. Aerobic fitness is a significant factor in longer survival and quality of life for patients with cystic fibrosis.

Managing the child's nutritional needs is important and takes time and energy. Parents often have a difficult time encouraging the child with cystic fibrosis to eat the extra calories needed for optimal nutrition, setting the stage for a potential mealtime battleground. To be successful, parents need guidance about managing negative mealtime behaviors, in addition to guidelines for preparing nutritional calorie-dense foods. Increase calorie intake by offering high-calorie snacks between meals and before bed.

CLINICAL TIP

Use of cream or half and half added to soups, casseroles, and puddings; cream cheese spread on breads, muffins, and crackers; sour cream added to casseroles, and powdered milk added to regular milk, meatloaf, and custards are all ways to increase the calories in food eaten.

Have the family work with a nutritionist to plan high-calorie meals and snacks that will meet the child's calorie needs. Recipes for children with cystic fibrosis are available online. Children with adequate nutrition have a longer life expectancy. Extra intervention, such as a gastrostomy tube for nighttime feedings, may be needed when the child's weight is 85% to 90% of ideal weight for height.

Children with cystic fibrosis lose more than normal amounts of salt in their sweat. This loss can become intensified during hot weather, strenuous exercise, and fever. During periods of exercise and increased sweating, the child should be encouraged to drink more fluids and increase salt intake. Parents should allow the child to add extra salt to food and should permit some salty snacks (pretzels with salt, pickles, carbonated soda). Teach parents to recognize early symptoms of salt depletion, including fatigue, weakness, abdominal pain, and vomiting, and to contact the child's health-care provider if these symptoms occur.

At follow-up visits review the child's use of bronchodilators and airway clearance techniques. To prevent a change in pulmonary status from progressing, short-term changes in care may be recommended. These may include intravenous and aerosol medications and antibiotics, an increase in the number of times chest physiotherapy is performed daily, and changes in dietary management. Help the family select the best time to fit the additional treatment into the schedule.

Adolescents have special developmental issues and needs that must be addressed since the median survival rate has increased

PHOTO Story...

Managing cystic fibrosis

Shaun, a 13-year-old with cystic fibrosis, has a challenging time managing all the aspects of his disease management. Shaun has an older sister who does not have cystic fibrosis. He lives with his mother and sister in a town about 50 miles from the cystic fibrosis center at the university medical center. He is in the 7th grade at a local middle school. He plays on a little league baseball team and enjoys riding his bicycle. He manages to keep his grades at a "C" level despite occasional school absences because of infection flare ups. He usually spends a few days in the hospital each year for intensive therapy sessions to clear his lungs.

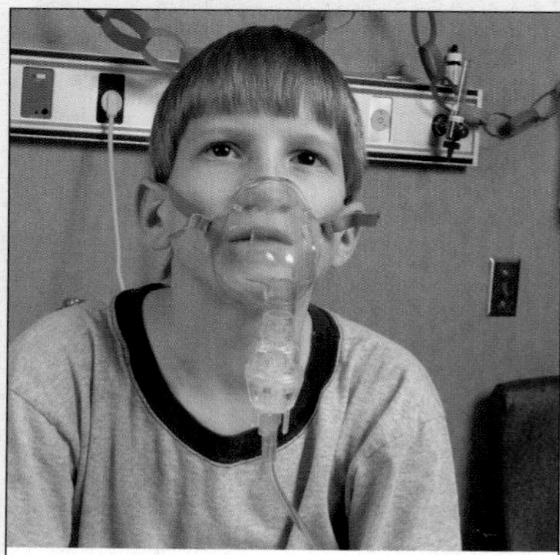

Shaun takes his nebulizer treatment with DNAse prior to chest physiotherapy to increase moisture of mucous secretions.

Management of cystic fibrosis takes a lot of time each day, whether at home or in the hospital. All of his care must be scheduled around school and recreation. In most cases, the treatments cut in to his recreational time. Shaun has learned to manage many aspects of his care, relieving his mother of some responsibilities. For example, Shaun can set up his nebulizer treatment and even measure the amount of DNAse to use. After the nebulizer treatment, he uses an oscillating vest for chest physiotherapy for about 20 minutes per treatment. Coughing up sputum during and after the treatment is very tiring.

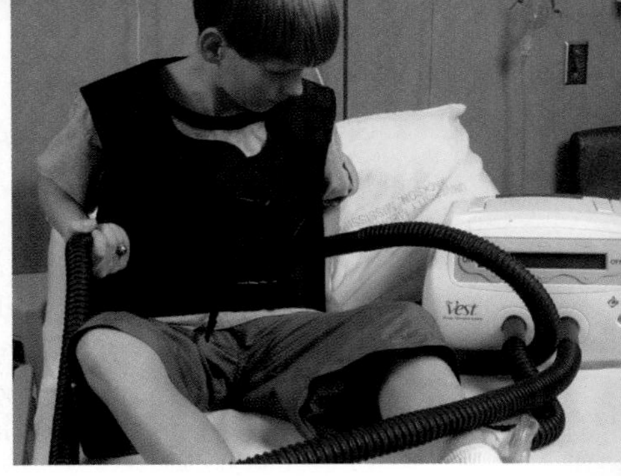

Shaun needs many extra calories to grow as well as to meet metabolic demands. His mother works hard to prepare and provide the extra calories he needs throughout the day. He must take pancreatic enzymes to help him digest the foods. Because Shaun sometimes has difficulty getting enough calories, he has a gastrostomy tube for nighttime feedings. This has made it possible to get enough calories to help support his adolescent growth spurt. ■

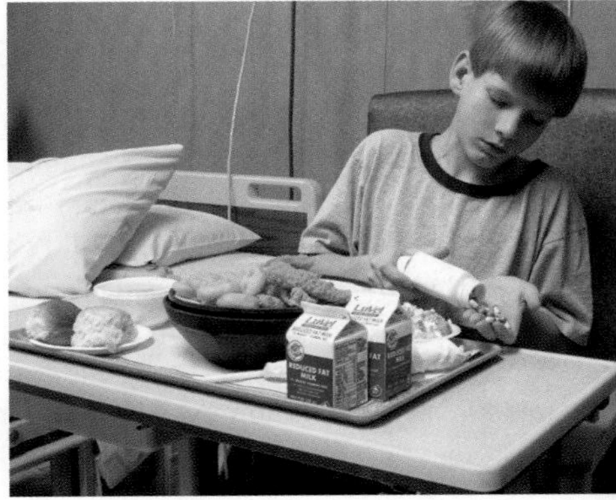

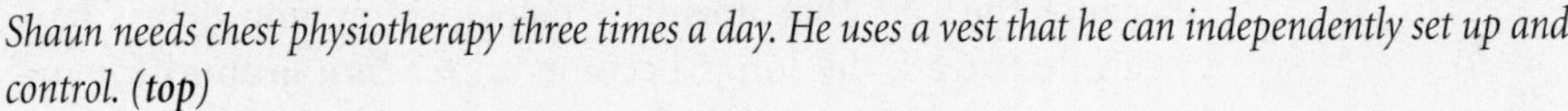

Shaun needs chest physiotherapy three times a day. He uses a vest that he can independently set up and control. ***(top)***

Shaun needs lots of calories and takes his pancreatic enzymes prior to eating lunch which is composed of double portions and high-calorie foods. ***(middle)***

Shaun and his mother take time for recreation with a game to break the monotony of his time in the hospital. ***(bottom)***

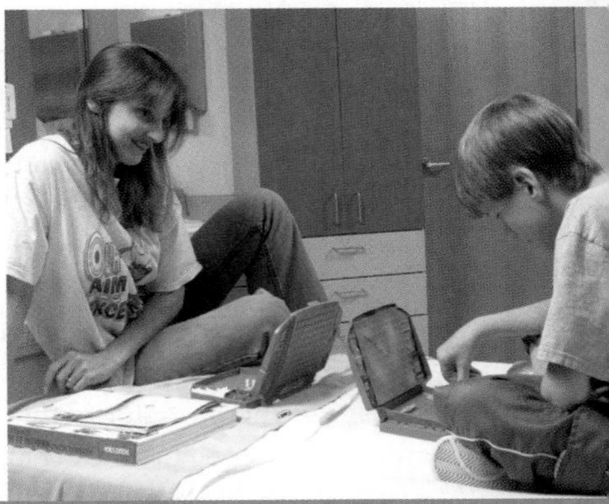

to more than 30 years of age. Gradual assumption of responsibility for daily disease management is necessary, and may be challenging when there is rebellion and defiance to treatment. Individualized planning to achieve their daily care regimen may be helpful to these adolescents and still enable them to interact with peers at school.

Adolescents with cystic fibrosis know they are different from their peers, and must learn how to cope with that difference. They also need to develop normal relationships and establish intimacy with a partner. Information about potential infertility must be provided along with the guidelines for safe sexual practices to reduce the risk for sexually transmitted diseases. Females may potentially be able to conceive and should be given contraception.

Adolescents must deal with the fact that they have a terminal condition, and they often need help to establish appropriate educational and occupational goals for their future. Transitioning to adult health-care services and planning for independent life with a chronic disease requires support and planning. Palliative care planning should be initiated in adolescents and young adults as the disease progresses to respiratory failure. Discussions about options, such as a double lung transplant, may be initiated with those considered to be candidates for the surgery. The patients who receive a transplant are not cured, but trade the problems of end-stage cystic fibrosis with lifelong immunosuppression and the resulting complications.

Cystic fibrosis affects all family members and disrupts activities of daily living for everyone. It is important to refer families to counseling and group therapy with families of other children with cystic fibrosis if indicated. The Cystic Fibrosis Foundation is a source for information on current advances in the disorder. Local chapter activities also provide emotional support for parents and children.

■ Evaluation

Expected outcomes of nursing care include the following:

- The child and family develop proficiency in providing the daily pulmonary care and reducing the incidence of respiratory infections.

MediaLink Cystic Fibrosis Resources and Support

- The child and family cope effectively with the child's disease and develop a schedule and routine for daily pulmonary care that fits into family and school activities.
- The child consumes adequate calories and pancreatic enzymes to support growth and to stay within desirable weight ranges.

INJURIES OF THE RESPIRATORY SYSTEM

Airway compromise after an unintentional injury can cause death if not managed quickly and effectively. Children are vulnerable to changes in respiratory function after accidental injury because the small size of the child's airway makes it vulnerable to obstruction. The tongue, small amounts of blood, mucus, or foreign debris or swelling in the respiratory tract or adjacent neck tissue may block the airway and lead to hypoxia and respiratory failure. If the child's neck is flexed or hyperextended, the soft laryngeal cartilage may compress and obstruct the airway.

PRACTICE ALERT

Never allow a child's neck to hyperextend (bend completely backward) or hyperflex (bend completely forward). Hyperextension flattens the trachea because there is no firm cartilage to provide structural support. Hyperflexion can kink and compress the trachea. Both maneuvers obstruct rather than open the airway.

Smoke Inhalation Injury

Exposure of the child's face and airway to fire or thermal conditions leads to dramatic responses in the child's respiratory tract. In every age group, inhalation injury from smoke and heat significantly increases the child's chance of death by 20%, and it also increases the likelihood that the burned child will develop pneumonia (Kim, 2001). Children are more vulnerable to smoke inhalation injury because their smaller airway diameter can be obstructed by edema and a higher respiratory rate increases their exposure to noxious chemicals.

Etiology and Pathophysiology

The severity of a smoke inhalation injury is influenced by the type of material burned and whether the child was exposed in an open or closed space. The composition of materials determines how easily it ignites, how fast it burns, and how much heat is released. These factors influence the production of smoke and toxic gases. Smoke, a product of the burning process that is composed of gases and particles, is generated in varying volumes and density. Chemicals and irritants from the gases result in mucosal airway damage, bronchospasm, depletion of alveolar surfactant, and mucous plugging from soot and sloughed airway mucosa. The type and concentration of invisible toxic gases affect the severity of pulmonary damage. The duration of exposure to the smoke produced and any toxic gases contribute significantly to the child's prognosis.

Exposure to extreme heat, common in house fires, leads to surface injury and upper airway damage. The upper airway normally removes heat from inhaled gases, sparing the lower airway from thermal damage when the patient is conscious. This thermal injury results in marked edema of the upper airway, placing the small child at risk for airway obstruction.

Carbon monoxide (CO) is a clear, colorless, odorless gas that is present in all fire conditions as the fire consumes oxygen. This is a significant concern when the child is trapped in a closed-space fire, when the concentration of oxygen is decreased by up to 50%. The CO molecule binds more firmly to hemoglobin than does oxygen. As a result, it replaces oxygen in circulation and rapidly produces hypoxia in the child. The longer the exposure to CO, the greater the hypoxia. The brain and heart receive inadequate oxygen, resulting in confusion, myocardial depression, and ventricular arrhythmias.

Damage to the lower airway most often results from chemicals or toxic gas inhalation. Soot is carried deep into the lungs, where it combines with water in the lungs to deposit acid-producing chemicals on the lung tissue. These acids burn the tissue, causing loss of cilia, loss of surfactant, and edema. Tissue destruction, edema, and disruption of gas exchange produce the initial insult to the lungs and potential airway obstruction. Days later, the damaged tissue sloughs off, obstructing the airways. Because the cilia that normally help in removing debris have been destroyed, the lungs become a breeding ground for microorganisms. Pneumonia becomes a major health concern. The damaged alveoli heal by scar tissue formation. This can greatly reduce the future functioning of the lungs.

Clinical Manifestations

Burns of the face and neck, singed nasal hairs, soot around the mouth or nose, and hoarseness with stridor or voice change all indicate inhalation injury, even when the child initially has no respiratory distress. Edema develops rapidly over a few hours and may lead to airway obstruction with signs such as tachypnea, stridor, coughing, and wheezing. Respiratory distress develops and can lead to respiratory failure. If carbon monoxide poisoning is present the child will be confused or unconscious, and have cardiac arrhythmias.

COLLABORATIVE CARE

Diagnosis is based on history of the child being exposed to smoke in a closed area, as well as signs of soot around the nose and mouth. If the child has minimal signs and symptoms when seen in the emergency department, admission for close observation and monitoring for progression of respiratory distress is often indicated. Initial treatment is 100% humidified oxygen administered through a nonrebreather mask. With the development of respiratory distress, aggressive airway management with endotracheal tube insertion, mechanical ventilation, and monitoring are provided in the intensive care unit. Bronchodilators by inhalation may be prescribed. Pulmonary physiotherapy may be provided. All other injuries sustained in the fire are treated.

NURSING MANAGEMENT

Nursing assessment for respiratory distress is a key initial role. Check vital signs frequently. Attach a pulse oximeter to monitor the oxygen saturation. Auscultate the lungs for crackles, wheezes, and decreased breath sounds. Assess for level of consciousness and behavior changes that could indicate increasing hypoxia. Assess the family's response to the life-threatening crisis and offer support with information about the child's condition.

Provide oxygen as ordered. Position the child to promote respiratory function. If the child's condition deteriorates, assist with procedures to secure the child's airway and prepare the child for transfer to the intensive care unit.

Blunt Chest Trauma

Blunt trauma is a common injury in children, especially associated with motor vehicle crashes (Pieper, 2000). Chest injuries may not be obvious and can be extremely difficult to evaluate.

Most children who die after sustaining severe blunt trauma were hypoxic due to poor airway and ventilatory control. A child's elastic, pliable chest wall and thin abdominal muscles provide minimal protection to underlying organs. This elasticity often spares bone but not the underlying organs. The presence of a rib fracture in children under 12 years indicates trauma of significant force. The energy from blunt trauma is transferred directly from an external force to the internal organs, often causing a pulmonary contusion or pneumothorax.

Pulmonary Contusion

A pulmonary contusion is defined as bruising damage to the tissues of the lung that often occurs without bony injury to the thorax. This causes bleeding from the capillaries into the alveoli, which may lead to capillary rupture in the air sacs. Pulmonary edema develops in the lower airways as blood and fluid from damaged tissues accumulate. Lower airway obstruction and atelectasis may result in impaired gas exchange, acute respiratory distress, and respiratory failure (Hazinski, 1999).

Pulmonary contusion occurs in up to 76% of children with blunt or nonpenetrating chest trauma. Initially the child may appear asymptomatic. Signs of respiratory distress often develop over several hours, and include wheezing, hemoptysis, fever, crackles, and evidence of hypoxemia. Careful observation is required during the first 12 hours after the injury to detect decreased perfusion related to ventilatory impairment.

Nursing Management

The child's level of consciousness is an excellent indicator of respiratory function. Agitation and lethargy can signal increasing hypoxia. When monitoring the status of a child who has a pulmonary contusion, do not rely on the child's color as an indicator of adequate oxygenation. Cyanosis in children is often a late indicator of respiratory distress. Observe for hemoptysis (fresh blood in the sputum), dyspnea, decreased breath sounds, wheezes, crackles, and a transient temperature elevation. The thorax should be inspected for symmetric chest wall movement and equal presence of breath sounds in both lungs. The child may initially appear stable but requires careful and thorough monitoring to detect signs of deterioration.

Nursing care focuses on providing necessary physiologic support, such as oxygen therapy, pulmonary management, positioning, ventilatory support to provide positive end-expiratory pressure, and comfort measures.

Children with significant injuries are cared for in the intensive care unit. Some children require ventilator support as the pulmonary tissues heal. Fluids are carefully managed to prevent large increases in pulmonary edema. With severe pulmonary contusion intubation and mechanical ventilation are needed. Diuretics may be given to decrease edema in the interstitial pulmonary tissue. The child is at risk for development of acute respiratory distress syndrome. See page 826.

Pneumothorax

A pneumothorax occurs when air enters the pleural space because of tears in the tracheobronchial tree, the esophagus, or the chest wall. If blood collects in the pleural space, it is called a hemothorax, and if blood and air collect, it is called a pneumohemothorax.

Etiology and Pathophysiology

Pneumothorax may develop as a complication of mechanical ventilation or high peak inspiratory or end-expiratory pressure used to achieve adequate oxygenation and ventilation. It may also occur in chronic lung conditions such as neonatal respiratory distress syndrome, status asthmaticus, and cystic fibrosis in which there is gas trapping and alveolar hyperinflation. A pneumothorax is one of the more common thoracic injuries in pediatric trauma patients.

The three types of pneumothorax are open, closed, and tension. An open pneumothorax, sometimes referred to as a sucking chest wound, results from any penetrating injury that exposes the pleural space to atmospheric pressure. Air is able to move freely in and out of the chest wall, collapsing the lung.

A closed pneumothorax is sometimes caused by blunt chest trauma with no evidence of rib fracture (Figure 25–25 ■). The chest may be compressed against a closed glottis, causing a sudden increase in pressure within the thoracic cavity. The child spontaneously holds his or her breath when the thorax is struck, accounting for the involuntary closing of the glottis. The pressure increase is transferred to the alveoli, causing them to burst. A single burst alveolus may be able to seal itself off, but with the destruction of many alveoli the lung collapses.

A tension pneumothorax is a life-threatening emergency that results when the air leaked on inhalation cannot be vented to escape during exhalation. Internal pressure builds, compressing the chest contents and collapsing the lung. A mediastinal shift occurs when venous return to the heart is impaired as the trachea, heart, vena cava, and esophagus are compressed toward the unaffected lung, leading to decreased cardiac output.

Clinical Manifestations

With an open pneumothorax, a sucking sound may be heard as the air moves through the opening on the chest wall. The child may show signs of restlessness, cyanosis, and subcutaneous emphysema (air leakage in the tissue). The child with a closed pneumothorax may have breath sounds decreased or absent on the injured side, and the child may be in respiratory distress. Signs of tension pneumothorax include increasing respiratory distress, absent breath sounds, cardiovascular instability, and a tracheal shift to the unaffected side.

PATHOPHYSIOLOGY ILLUSTRATED

Pneumothorax

Parenial pleura (outer lining)
Air in pleural space
Visceral pleura (inner lining)
Partially collapsed lung

A

B

FIGURE 25–25 ■ *A,* A pneumothorax is air in the pleural space that causes a lung to collapse. Whether the air results from an open injury or from bursting of alveoli due to a blunt injury or hyperinflation, it is important to focus on airway management and maintain lung inflation. *B,* Pneumothorax, note the collapsed lung on the patient's right side. *Courtesy of Dorothy Bulas, M.D., Children's National Medical Center, Washington, DC.*

COLLABORATIVE CARE

Immediate treatment for an open pneumothorax is covering the wound with an airtight seal, however, a gloved hand can be used until a bandage is prepared. With a closed pneumothorax, a thoracostomy is performed and a chest tube inserted. A closed drainage system is attached to help remove the air and reinflate the lung by reestablishing negative pressure. Immediate care for a tension pneumothorax is a needle thoracentesis to allow air to escape and relieve the tension. A chest tube is then inserted and attached to a closed drainage system.

NURSING MANAGEMENT

Nursing care focuses on airway management and maintaining lung inflation. The child usually arrives on the nursing unit with a chest tube and drainage system in place. Continued close observation for respiratory distress is essential. Vital signs are carefully monitored. When the chest tube is removed, the site is covered with an occlusive dressing and the child's respiratory status is carefully monitored for signs of respiratory distress.

Complications of chest tube placement include hemothorax (if the thoracostomy and chest tube are improperly placed), lung tissue injury, and scarring from poor tube placement (especially if the tube is placed too near the breast in girls).

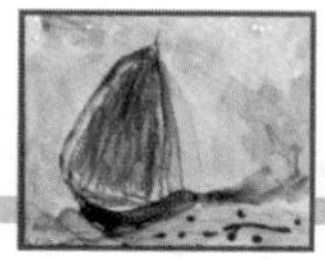

CHAPTER HIGHLIGHTS

- Acute respiratory problems are the most common cause of illness requiring hospitalization in infants and children under 10 years of age and a leading cause of hospitalization in children between 10 and 15 years of age.
- The child's airway is shorter and narrower than an adult's. These differences create a greater potential for obstruction. The lungs have no muscles of their own, so respiration is powered by the diaphragm and intercostal muscles.
- Foreign-body aspiration is most often caused by small objects that make their way into the child's mouth, such as foods, small toy parts, or household objects like beads, safety pins, coins, or buttons.

- Signs of impending respiratory failure in infants and children include worsening respiratory distress, irritability, lethargy, cyanosis, and increased respiratory effort such as dyspnea (difficulty breathing), tachypnea (increased respiratory rate), nasal flaring, and retractions.
- Apnea, by definition, is cessation of respiration lasting longer than 20 seconds, or any pause in respiration associated with cyanosis, marked pallor, hypotonia, or bradycardia.
- Three types of apnea are noted in neonates: central apnea in which there is complete cessation of breathing; obstructive apnea in which there is an absence of nasal airflow when respiratory efforts are present; and mixed apnea in which a central respiratory pause either preceeds or follows airway obstruction.
- Obstructive sleep apnea syndrome is a disorder of breathing during sleep that in children is commonly caused by enlarged tonsils and adenoids. Children have symptoms of sleep deprivation such as daytime sleepiness, poor attention, increased activity, aggression or acting-out behavior, and poor school performance.
- Sudden infant death syndrome (SIDS), a leading cause of death in infants, is the sudden death of an infant under 1 year of age that remains unexplained after a complete autopsy, a death scene investigation, and review of the history.
- Laryngotracheobronchitis (LTB) is a viral croup syndrome with signs of an upper respiratory illness, hoarseness, tachypnea, inspiratory stridor, and a seal-like barking cough. Fever may or may not be present.
- Epiglottitis is caused by bacterial invasion of the soft tissue of the larynx causing inflammation and edema of the tissues and the epiglottis that can result in life-threatening airway obstruction. Classic signs of epiglottitis include dysphonia, dysphagia, drooling, and distressed respiratory effort. Fortunately, the number of cases of epiglottitis has decreased significantly because of the Hib vaccine.
- Neonatal respiratory distress syndrome is the most common cause of respiratory failure and death in newborns, accounting for 20% to 30% of preterm newborn deaths.
- Meconium aspiration syndrome occurs in 33% of newborns born with meconium-stained amniotic fluid. The meconium causes a chemical inflammation of the airway that results in pulmonary edema and cellular death. Some newborns progress to develop pulmonary hypertension with persistent fetal circulation.
- Although many bacterial and mycoplasmal organisms may cause bronchiolitis, infection with respiratory syncytial virus (RSV) is the most common cause. Bronchiolitis is a major cause of hospitalization in infants under 6 months of age.
- Symptoms of pneumonia in infants and children include elevated temperature, rales, crackles, wheezes, cough, dyspnea, tachypnea, restlessness, and decreased breath sounds if consolidation occurs.
- In children, the risk of developing tuberculosis is increased in those under 2 years of age. Clinical manifestations of tuberculosis in infants include a persistent cough, fever, and weight loss or failure to gain weight. Wheezing and decreased breath sounds may be present. Older children may be asymptomatic.
- Bronchopulmonary dysplasia (BPD) is often a consequence of neonatal respiratory distress syndrome and inflammatory changes in the airway. Treatment with mechanical ventilation causes further inflammation and damage to the bronchioles, resulting in fibrosis and edema of the bronchioles and smooth muscle hypertrophy.
- Asthma affects about 5 million children in the United States and, for those children, results in about 10 days of school absenteeism and 20 days of restricted activity per year. Asthma mortality in children has increased from 1.8 to 3.3 per 1 million children between 1980–1981 and 1998–1999.
- Status asthmaticus is persistent severe respiratory distress and bronchospasm in an asthmatic child that persists despite medications and supportive interventions. Without aggressive and immediate intervention the child may progress to respiratory failure and die.
- In cystic fibrosis, defective chloride-ion transport across the exocrine and epithelial cells results in an abnormal accumulation of viscous, dehydrated mucus that affects the respiratory, gastrointestinal, and reproductive systems.
- Signs of smoke inhalation injury in children include burns of the face and neck, singed nasal hairs, soot around the mouth or nose, and hoarseness with stridor or voice change.
- Pulmonary contusion occurs in the majority of children with nonpenetrating chest trauma. Although the child may appear initially asymptomatic, respiratory distress often develops within a few hours.
- A pneumothorax may become life threatening if internal pressure from a closed pneumothorax is not vented. Air leaking into the chest cavity during inspiration cannot escape during expiration, increasing compression. Venous blood return to the heart is impaired as the mediastinum shifts toward the unaffected lung.

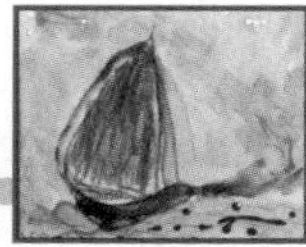

CRITICAL THINKING IN ACTION

INTRODUCTION

Return to the scenario at the beginning of the chapter. Once Emily and her mother arrive at the emergency department, she is assessed for current respiratory status and moved into one of the short-stay unit rooms.

DESCRIPTION

Emily's respiratory signs and symptoms have not changed substantially from those present in the primary care provider's office. Suctioning is needed to clear secretions from the airway. Secretions are sent for a culture and sensitivity. The pulmonary specialist orders a chest radiograph. Nebulizer treatments via the tracheostomy tube will begin as soon as Emily returns from the diagnostic imaging department.

DISCUSSION

1. Describe the signs that would indicate Emily's respiratory status is worsening. Consider the information the mother might be able to contribute. What laboratory studies will contribute to the assessment? Develop a nursing care plan to respond to those worsening conditions.
2. Identify historical information that should be obtained about the mother's home management plan for Emily's care. Describe how this information can be used to partner with the family and integrate needed changes into the home care plan as a result of this episode.
3. Identify Emily's stage of development and recommend appropriate toys or activities that the mother may use to promote Emily's development.
4. Emily's chest radiograph reveals pneumonia and hospitalization is planned. Develop the nursing care plan for Emily's hospital care.

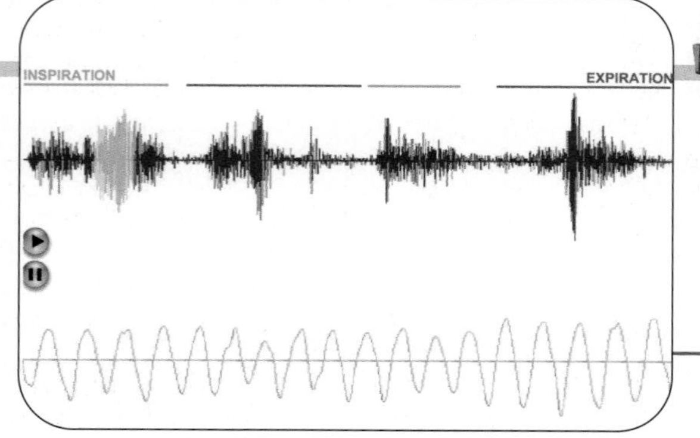

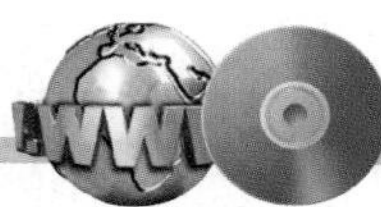

EXPLORE MediaLink

- NCLEX review, case studies, and other interactive resources for this chapter can be found on the Companion Website at **http://www.prenhall.com/ball**. Click on Chapter 25 to select the activities for this chapter.
- For animations, more NCLEX review questions, and an audio glossary, access the accompanying CD-ROM in this book.

http://www.prenhall.com/ball

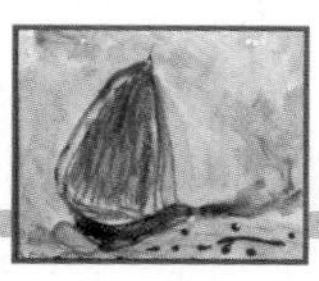

REFERENCES

Agency for Healthcare Research and Quality. (2003). *Management of bronchiolitis in infants and children, summary*. Evidence Report/Technology Assessment: Number 69, AHRQ Publication Number 03-E009. Rockville, MD: Author. www.ahrq.gov/clinic/epcsums/broncsom.htm, accessed 3-29-2004.

Akinbami, L. J., & Schoendorf, K. C., (2002). Trends in childhood asthma: Prevalence, health care utilization, and mortality. *Pediatrics, 110*(2), 315–322.

American Academy of Allergy, Asthma, and Immunology. (1999). *Pediatric asthma: Promoting best practice, guide for managing asthma in children*. Milwaukee, WI: Author.

American Academy of Pediatrics Committee on Infectious Diseases and Committee on Fetus and Newborn. (2003a). Revised indications for the use of palivizumab and respiratory syncytial virus immune globulin intravenous for the prevention of respiratory syncytial virus. *Pediatrics, 112*(6), 1442–1446.

American Academy of Pediatrics. (2003b). *Red book: 2003 Report of the Committee on Infectious Diseases* (26th ed.). Elk Grove Village, IL: Author.

American Academy of Pediatrics Committee on Child Abuse and Neglect. (2001). Distinguishing sudden infant death syndrome from child abuse fatalities. *Pediatrics, 107*(2), 437–441.

American Academy of Pediatrics Committee on Fetus and Newborn. (2003). Apnea, sudden infant death syndrome, and home monitoring. *Pediatrics, 111*(4), 914–917.

American Academy of Pediatrics Section on Pediatric Pulmonology, Subcommittee on Obstructive Sleep Apnea Syndrome. (2002). Clinical practice guideline: Diagnosis and management of childhood obstructive sleep apnea syndrome. *Pediatrics, 109*(4), 704–712.

American Thoracic Society and Centers for Disease Control and Prevention. (2000). Diagnostic standards and classification of tuberculosis in adults and children. *American Journal of Respiratory and Critical Care Medicine, 161*, 1376–1395.

Baker, V. O., Friedman, J., & Schmitt, R. (2002a). Asthma management, part I: An overview of the problem and current trends. *Journal of School Nursing, 18*(3), 128–137.

Baker, V. O., Friedman, J., & Schmitt, R. (2002b). Asthma management, part II: Pharmacologic management. *Journal of School Nursing, 18*(5), 257–269.

Balinsky, W., & Zhy, C. W. (2004). Pediatric cystic fibrosis: Evaluating costs and genetic testing. *Journal of Pediatric Health Care, 18*(1), 30–34.

Baren, J. M., & Puchalski, A. (2002). Current concepts in the ED treatment of pediatric asthma. *Pediatric Emergency Medicine Reports, 7*(10), 105–115.

Belcher, D. (2002, November). Breathing easier with pediatric asthma: Pharmacologic management. *Advance for Nurse Practitioners*, 37–38, 79.

Capper-Michel, B. (2004). Bronchopulmonary dysplasia. In P. J. Allen, & J. A. Vessey, (Eds.), *Primary care of the child with a chronic condition* (4th ed., pp. 282–298). St. Louis: Mosby.

Centers for Disease Control and Prevention (2000). Measuring childhood asthma prevalence before and after the 1997 redesign of the National Health Interview Survey. *Morbidity and Mortality Weekly Report, 49*(40), 908–911.

Centers for Disease Control and Prevention, National Center for Health Statistics (2001, October). New estimates for asthma tracked. Accessed January 23, 2003 from www.cdc.gov/nchs/releases/01facts/asthma.htm.

Centers for Disease Control and Prevention (CDC). (2002). Nonfatal choking-related episodes among children—United States, 2001. *Morbidity and Mortality Weekly Report, 51*(42), 945–948.

Centers for Disease Control and Prevention (CDC). (2003). Trends in tuberculosis morbidity—United States, 1999–2002. *Monthly Morbidity and Mortality Report, 52*(11), 217–222.

Cooper, A. C., Banasiak, N. C., & Allen, P. J. (2003). Management and prevention strategies for respiratory syncytial virus (RSV) bronchiolitis in infants and young children: A review of evidence-based practice interventions. *Pediatric Nursing, 29*(6), 452–456.

Cote, A., Gerez, T., Brouillette, R. T., & Laplante, S. (2000). Circumstances leading to a change to prone sleeping in sudden infant death syndrome victims. *Pediatrics, 106*(6), 1–5.

Cystic Fibrosis Foundation. (2000). B. cepacia policy. Accessed March 17, 2004, from www.cff.org/living_with_cf/B_cepacia_policy.cfm.

Cystic Fibrosis Foundation. (2004). Genetic carrier testing for CF. Accessed March 10, 2004, from www.cff.org.

Daigle, K. L., & Cloutier, M. M. (1997). Office management of bronchopulmonary dysplasia. *Comprehensive Therapy, 23*(10), 656–663.

D'Auria, J. P. (1997). Respiratory system. In J. A. Fox (Ed.), *Primary health care of children* (pp. 415–418). St. Louis: Mosby.

Davies, F., & Gupta, R. (2002). Apparent life threatening events in infants presenting to an emergency department. *Emergency Medicine Journal, 19*, 11–16.

Dickinson-Herbst, D. (2001). Cystic fibrosis and lung transplantation: Ethical concerns. *Pediatric Nursing, 27*(1), 87–92.

Diaz, T., Sturm, T., Matte, T., Bindra, M., Lawler, K., Findley, S., et al. (2000). Medication use among children with asthma in East Harlem: Are national guidelines followed? *Pediatrics, 106*, 886–896.

Dye, C., Scheele, S., Dolin, P., Pathania, N., Raviglione, M. C., for the WHO Global Surveillance and Monitoring Project. (1999). Global burden of tuberculosis: Estimated incidence, prevalence, and mortality by country. *JAMA, 282*(7), 677–686.

Eichelberger, M. R., Ball, J. W., Pratsch, G. S., & Clark, J. R. (1998). *Pediatric emergencies* (2nd ed.). Englewood Cliffs, NJ: Brady.

Farrell, P. M., Kosorok, M. R., Rock, M. J., Laxova, A., & Zeng, L., et al. (2001). Early diagnosis of cystic fibrosis through neonatal screening prevents severe malnutrition and improves long-term growth. *Pediatrics, 107*(1), 1–13.

Foley, S. M. (2002). Infant asthma: Genetic predisposition and environmental influences. *Newborn and Infant Nursing Reviews, 2*(4), 200–206.

Froh, D. K. (2002). Alterations in pulmonary function in children. In K. L. McCance & S. E. Huether (Eds.), *Pathophysiology: The biologic basis for disease in adults and children* (4th ed., pp. 1145–1169). St. Louis: Mosby.

Fuloria, M., & Wiswell, T. E. (2000). Managing meconium aspiration. *Contemporary Pediatrics, 17*(4), 125–136.

Gadomski, A. (2002). Bronchiolitis dilemma: A happy wheezer and his unhappy parent. *Contemporary Pediatrics, 19*(11), 40–59.

Gilliland, F. D., Yu-Fen, L., & Peters, J. M. (2001). Effects of maternal smoking during pregnancy and environmental tobacco smoke on asthmatic and wheezing in children. *American Journal of Respiratory and Critical Care Medicine, 163*, 429–436.

Hazinski, M. F. (1999). *Manual of pediatric critical care*. St. Louis: Mosby.

Head, G., & Bhatia, J. (2000). Current options in the management of apnea of prematurity. *Clinical Pediatrics, 39*(6), 327–336.

Health Canada. (1999). Asthma prevalence. *Measuring Up: A Health Surveillance Update on Canadian Children and Youth*. Accessed July 2, 2003, from www.hc-sc.gc.ca/pphb-dgspsp/ publicat/meas-haut/mu_r_e.html.

Health Resources and Services Administration, Maternal and Child Health Bureau. (2002). *Child health USA 2002*. Rockville, MD: U.S. Department of Health and Human Services.

Hogan, M. B., & Wilson, N. W. (2003). Asthma in the school-aged child. *Pediatric Annals, 32*(1), 20–25.

Homnick, D. N., Anderson, K., & Marks, J. H. (1998). Comparison of flutter device to standard chest physiotherapy in hospitalized patients with cystic fibrosis: A pilot study. *Chest, 114*, 993–997.

Institute of Medicine. (2000). *Clearing the air: Asthma and indoor air exposures*. Washington, DC: National Academy of Sciences.

Isaacson, G., & Isaacson, D. M. (2003). Pediatric epiglottitis caused by group G beta-hemolytic streptococcus. *Pediatric Infectious Disease Journal, 22*(9), 846–847.

Kato, I., Franco, P., Groswasser, J., Scaillet, S., Kelmanson, I., & Kahn, A. (2003). Incomplete arousal processes in infants who were victims of sudden death. *American Journal of Respiratory and Critical Care Medicine, 168*(1), 1298–1303.

Kieckhefer, G., & Ratcliffe, M. (2004). Asthma. In P. J. Allen & J. A. Vessey (Eds.), *Primary care of the child with a chronic condition* (4th ed., pp. 174–197). St. Louis: Mosby.

Kim, Y. (2001). Smoke inhalation injury in children. *Office and Emergency Pediatrics, 14*(1), 27–30.

Krauss, A. N. (2003). New methods advance treatment for respiratory distress syndrome. *Pediatric Annals, 32*(9), 585–591.

Ladewig, P. W., London, M. L., Moberly, S. M., & Olds, S. B. (2002). *Contemporary maternal-newborn nursing care* (5th ed., p. 690). Upper Saddle River, NJ: Prentice Hall Health.

Lara, M., Rosenbaum, S., Rachelefsky, G., Nicholas, W., Morton, S. C., et. al. (2002). Improving childhood asthma outcomes in the United States: A blueprint for policy action. *Pediatrics, 109*(5), 919–930.

Lassieur, S. M., & Jacobs, R. F. (1999). Pediatric pneumonia: Recognizing usual—and unusual—causes. *Journal of Respiratory Diseases, 20*(2), 126–143.

Lieu, T. A., Lozano, P., Finkelstein, J. A., Chi, F. W., Jensvold, N. G., et al. (2002). Racial/ethnic variations in asthma status and management practices among children in managed Medicaid. *Pediatrics, 109*(5), 857–865.

Loughlin, G. M., & Carroll, J. L. (1999). Apparent life-threatening events. In J. A. McMillan, C. D. DeAngelis, R. D. Feigin, & J. B. Warshaw (Eds.), *Oski's pediatrics: Principles and practice* (3rd ed., pp. 589–596). Philadelphia: Lippincott, Williams & Wilkins.

Malloy, M. H. (2002). Trends in postneonatal aspiration deaths and reclassification of sudden infant death syndrome: Impact on the "Back to Sleep" program. *Pediatrics, 109*(4), 661–665.

Mansour, M., Lamphear, B., & DeWitt, T. (2000). Barriers to asthma care in urban children: Parent perspectives. *Pediatrics, 106*, 512–519.

Maltezou, H. C., Spyridis, P., & Kafetzis, D. A. (2000). Extra-pulmonary tuberculosis in children. *Archives of Disease in Childhood, 83*(4), 342–346.

Mannino, D. M., Homa, D. M., & Redd, S. C. (2002). Involuntary smoking and asthma severity in children: Data from the Third National Health and Nutrition Examination Survey. *Chest 122*(2), 409–415.

Marcus, C. L. (1998). Does your child snore? *Contemporary Pediatrics, 15*(2), 101–115.

Margolis, P., & Gadomski, A. (1998). Does this infant have pneumonia? *Journal of the American Medical Association, 279*(4), 308–313.

Marshik, P. L. (2004). Pharmacologic treatment of pediatric asthma. *Advance for Nurse Practitioners, 12*(3), 35–36, 41–46.

McGrath, N. E., DeMasi, J., & DeMasi, M. (2002). Infants with an apparent life-threatening event (ALTE): Recognizing the symptoms, the seriousness. *Journal of Emergency Nursing, 28*(3), 255–258.

McIlwaine, P. M., Wong, L. T., Peacock, D., & Davidson, A. G. F. (1997). Long-term comparative trial of conventional postural drainage and percussion versus positive expiratory pressure physiotherapy in the treatment of cystic fibrosis. *Journal of Pediatrics, 131*, 570–574.

McMullen, A. H., & Bryson, E. A. (2004). Cystic fibrosis. In P. J. Allen, & J. A. Vessey, *Primary care of the child with a chronic condition* (4th ed., pp. 404–425). St. Louis, Mosby.

Moloney-Harmon, P. A. (1999). When the lung fails: Acute respiratory distress syndrome in children. *Critical Care Clinics of North America, 11*(4), 519–528.

Moon, R. Y., Patel, K. M., & Shaefer, S. J. M. (2000). Sudden infant death syndrome in child care settings. *Pediatrics, 106*(2), 295–300.

Morisky, D. E., Malotte, C. K., Ebin, V., Davidson, P., Cabrera, D., et al. (2001). Behavioral interventions for the control of tuberculosis in adolescents. *Public Health Reports, 116*(6), 568–574.

Morris, D. S., Gonzalez, L. S., Stewart, S. R., & Sampers, J. (2000). Extracorporeal membrane oxygenation (ECMO): A treatment for neonates in respiratory failure. Infant-Toddler Intervention. *The Transdisciplinary Journal, 10*(4), 215–238.

Muniz, A. E., & Joffe, M. D. (1999). Foreign bodies, ingested and inhaled. *JAAPA, 12*(6), 23–46.

National Asthma Education and Prevention Program. (2002). *NAEPP Expert Panel Report: Guidelines for the diagnosis and management of asthma—Update on selected topics 2002* (NIH Publication No. 02–5075). Bethesda, MD: National Institutes of Health, NHLBI.

National Respiratory and Enteric Virus Surveillance System. (2000). Respiratory syncytial virus activity—US, 1999–2000 season. *MMWR Weekly, 49*(48), 1091–1093.

Oermann, C., Accurso, F., Castile, R., & Sockridder, M. (1997). Evaluation of the safety, efficacy, and impact on the quality of life of the ThAIRpy Vest and Flutter compared to conventional chest physical therapy in patients with cystic fibrosis. *American Journal of Respiratory and Critical Care Medicine, 155*, A638.

Orenstein, D. M., Winnie, G. B., & Altman, H. (2002). Cystic fibrosis: A 2002 update. *Journal of Pediatrics, 140*(2), 156–164.

Parad, R. B., & Comeau, A. M. (2003). Newborn screening for cystic fibrosis. *Pediatric Annals, 32*(8), 528–535.

Park, J. W., & Barnett, D. W. (2002). Respiratory syncytial virus infection and the primary care physician. *Southern Medical Journal, 95*(3), 353–359.

Patel, P. B., & Turcios, N. L. (2003). Pneumonia that recurs: Your diagnostic challenge. *Contemporary Pediatrics, 20*(3), 82–106.

Pauwels, R., Pedersen, S., Busse, W., Tan, W. C., Chen, Y., et al., on behalf of the START Investigators Group. (2003, March 29). Early intervention with budesonide in mild persistent asthma: A randomised, double-blind trial. *Lancet, 361* 1071–1076.

Perkin, R. M., Downey, R., & Macquarrie, J. (1999). Sleep disordered breathing in infants and children. *Respiratory Care Clinics of North America, 5*(3), 395–426.

Perkin, R. M., & Swift, J. D. (2002). Infectious causes of upper airway obstruction in children. *Pediatric Emergency Medicine Reports, 7*(11), 117–128.

79. Peterson-Sweeney, K., McMullen, A., Yoos, H. L., & Kitzman, H. (2003). Parental perceptions of their child's asthma: Management and medication use. *Journal of Pediatric Nursing, 17*(3), 118–125.

Pieper, P. (2000). Pediatric trauma. In B. V. Wise, C. McKenna, G. Garvin, & B. J. Harmon (Eds.), *Nursing care of the general pediatric surgical patient* (pp. 459–479). Gaithersburg, MD: Aspen.

Pongracic, J. A. (2003). Asthma delivery devices: Age-appropriate use. *Pediatric Annals, 32*(1), 50–54.

Popovich, D. M., Richiuso, N., & Danek, G. (2004). Pediatric health care providers' knowledge of pulse oximetry. *Pediatric Nursing, 30*(1), 14–20.

Reznik, M., Ozuah, P. O., Franco, K., Cohen, R., & Motlow, F. (2002, October). Use of complementary therapy by adolescents with asthma. *Archive of Pediatric and Adolescent Medicine, 156*, 1042–1044.

Richman, E. (1997). Asthma diagnosis and management: New severity classifications and therapy alternatives. *Clinician Reviews, 7*(8), 76–112.

Rosen, C. L., Larkin, E. K., Kirchner, L., Emancipator, J. L., Bivens, S. F., et. al. (2003). Prevalence and risk factors for sleep-disordered breathing in 8 to 11 year old children: Association with race and prematurity. *Journal of Pediatrics, 142*(4), 383–389.

Sectish, T. C., & Prober, C. G. (2004). Pneumonia. In R. E. Behrman, R. M. Kliegman, & H. B. Jenson, *Nelson textbook of pediatrics* (17th ed., pp. 1432–1435). Philadelphia: Saunders.

Stempel, D. A., Pedersen, S., & Blaiss, M. S. (2002). Inhaled corticosteroids and growth: How big a dose of caution? *Contemporary Pediatrics, 19*(3), 49–64.

Stowe, C. D., & Jacobs, R. F. (1999). Treatment of tuberculosis infection and disease in children: The North American perspective. *Pediatric Drugs, 1*(4), 299–312.

Stroud, R. H., & Friedman, N. R. (2001). An update on inflammatory disorders of the pediatric airway: Epiglottitis, croup, and tracheitis. *American Journal of Otolaryngology, 22*(4), 268–275.

Strunk, R. C. (2002). Defining asthma in the preschool-aged child. *Pediatrics, 109*(2), 357–361.

Sydnor-Greenberg, N., & Dokken, D. (2000). Communicating information at diagnosis: Helping families and children manage asthma. *Journal of Child and Family Nursing, 3*(4), 290–295.

Tan, T. Q., Mason, E. O., Wald, E. R., Barson, W. J., Schutz, G. E., et al. (2002). Clinical characteristics of children with complicated pneumonia caused by Streptococcus pneumoniae. *Pediatrics, 110*(1), 1–6.

Theobald, K., Botwinski, C., Albanna, S., & McWilliam, P. (2000). Apnea of prematurity: Diagnosis, implications for care, and pharmacologic management. *Neonatal Network, 19*(6), 17–24.

Varlotta, L. (1998). Management and care of the newly diagnosed patient with cystic fibrosis. *Current Opinion in Pulmonary Medicine, 4*, 311–318.

Webster, H., & Huether, S.E. (1998). Alterations in pulmonary function in children. In K.L. McCance & S.E. Huether (Eds.), *Pathophysiology: The biologic basis of disease in adults and children* (3rd ed., pp. 1201–1220). St. Louis: Mosby.

Wright, R. B., Pomerantz, W. J., & Luria, J. W. (2002). New approaches to respiratory infections in children. *Emergency Medicine Clinics of North America, 20*(1), 93–114.

Yantis, M. A. (1999). Assessing children for obstructive sleep apnea. *Journal of Pediatric Health Care, 13*(1), 99–104.

Yoos, H. L., Kitzman, H., & McMullen, A. (2003, July). Barriers to anti-inflammatory medication use in childhood asthma. *Ambulatory Pediatrics, 3*, 181–190.

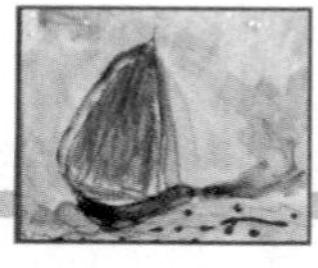

ADDITIONAL REFERENCES

National Education and Prevention Program. (1997). *Expert panel report II: Guidelines for diagnosis and management of asthma* (NIH Publication No. 97–4051). Bethesda, MD: National Institutes of Health.

Ozuah, P. O., Ozuah, T. P., Stein, R. E. K., Burton, W., & Mulvihill, M. (2001). Evaluation of risk assessment questionnaire used to target tuberculin skin testing in children. *JAMA, 285*(4), 451–453.

Robinson, W. (2000). Palliative care in cystic fibrosis. *Journal of Palliative Medicine, 3*(2), 187–192.

Stubblefield, C., & Murray, R. (2000). Making the transition: Pediatric lung transplantation. *Journal of Pediatric Health Care, 14*(6), 280–287.

Teets, J. M., & Borisuk, M. J. (2004). Pediatric thoracic organ transplants: Challenges in primary care. *Pediatric Nursing, 30*(1), 23–30.

Weiland, J., Schoettker, P. J., Byczkowski, T., Britto, M. T., Pandzik, G., & Kotagal, U. R. (2003). Individualized schedules for hospitalized adolescents with cystic fibrosis. *Journal of Pediatric Health Care, 17*(6), 284–289.

Chapter 26

Alterations in Cardiovascular Function

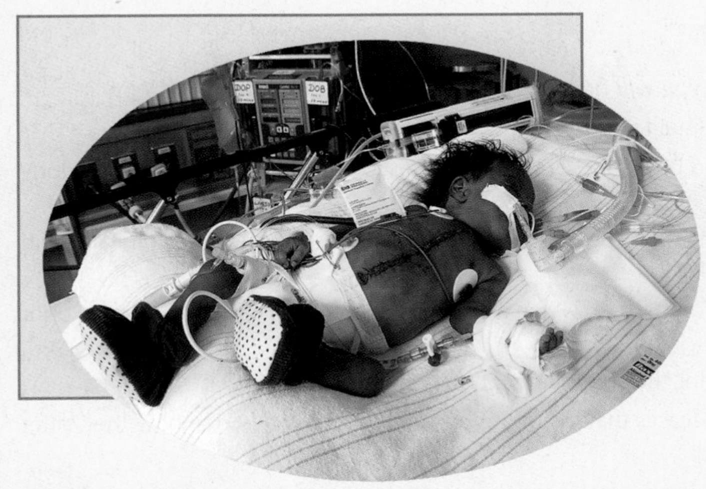

Brandy DeVries, who is 1 month old, was diagnosed with a ventricular septal defect (VSD) at birth. Her parents were just beginning to accept that she had a heart defect that might require surgical repair when signs of respiratory distress and difficulty in feeding developed.

Brandy's mother had been alerted to watch for these signs as a possible indication of congestive heart failure. Brandy was quickly hospitalized so her condition could be treated with digoxin, furosemide (Lasix), and potassium. Over the next 2 days she lost the weight she had gained due to fluid retention.

Because Brandy developed problems so soon after birth, it was decided that she should undergo surgical correction of her heart defect. A cardiac catheterization was performed prior to surgery to make sure no other congenital defects were present. Corrective surgery was performed to place a patch over the septal opening. Brandy is being cared for in the intensive care unit before being transferred to another unit.

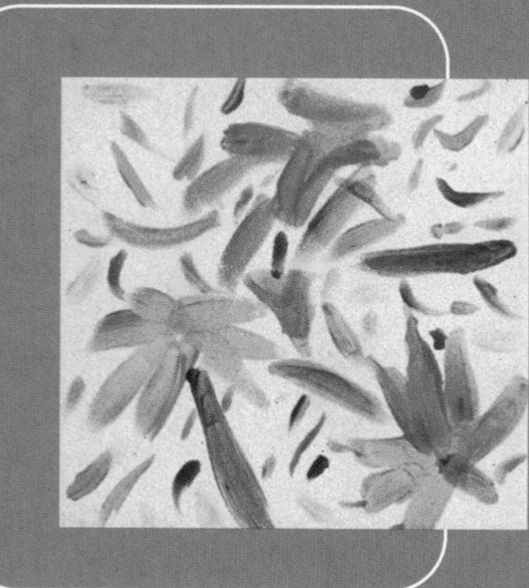

"Where's the baby? Daddy, bring home Mommy and baby."

—Ben, age 3

Key Terms

afterload/894
arrhythmias/935
cardiac output/894
cardiomegaly/896
compliance/893
contractility/894
desaturated blood/893
digitalization/896
ductus arteriosus/891
ductus venosus/891
endocardial cushions/912
foramen ovale/891
gallop/895
heaving/897
hemodynamics/891
hypoplastic/905
hypoxemia/893
normalization/924
oxygen saturation/893
palliative procedure/905
polycythemia/917
preload/894
radiofrequency ablation/939
shock/944
shunt/904
stenosis/stenotic/905
synchronized cardioversion/938
syncope/919
valvuloplasty/905

Learning Outcomes

After completing this chapter, you will be able to:

- Describe the transition from fetal to pulmonary circulation.
- Understand the anatomy and physiology of the cardiovascular system and pathophysiology associated with increased pulmonary circulation and decreased pulmonary circulation.
- Perform a nursing assessment and recognize the signs of congestive heart failure in infants and children, and develop a nursing care plan.
- Develop a nursing care plan for the child with a congenital heart defect cared for at home prior to corrective surgery.
- Develop a nursing care plan for the child undergoing open heart surgery.
- Identify the acquired heart diseases that occur during childhood and describe how they differ from congenital heart defects.
- Describe the development of hypovolemic shock and nursing management of the condition.

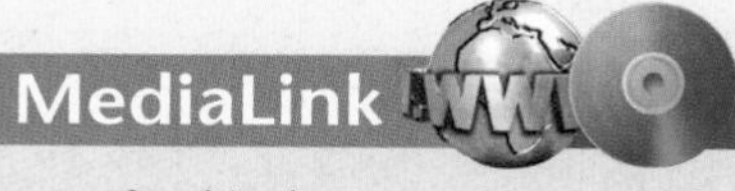

MediaLink http://www.prenhall.com/ball

Resources for this chapter can be found on the CD-ROM accompanying this textbook and on the Companion Website at www.prenhall.com/ball. Click on Chapter 26 to select the activities for this chapter.

CD-ROM

Animations/Videos
- *Blood Pressure*
- *Congenital Heart Defects*
- *Digoxin*
- *Heart Sounds*

NCLEX Review

Audio Glossary

COMPANION WEBSITE

A & P Review

NCLEX Review

Case Study: Newborn after Heart Surgery

Care Plan: Pediatric Heart Transplant

MediaLink Applications
- *Ethical Dilemma*
- *Exercise: Hematocrit*
- *Teaching Plan: Infective Endocarditis Prophylaxis*
- *Teaching Plan: Healthy Heart Curricula*

Alterations in cardiovascular function may be the result of a congenital defect, acquired infection, or injury. Congenital heart disease is the leading cause of death, excluding prematurity, during the first year of life. It is estimated that about one third of children born with congenital heart disease die as a result of their cardiac disease and about a third of those deaths occur in the first year of life (Connor, 2002). More than 35 types of heart defects have been documented. The frequency of occurrence is increasing, possibly due to improved detection. Congenital heart defects, like Brandy's ventricular septal defect, occur in approximately 1 in 170 live births and often require surgical correction (Neilson & Robin, 2002). Rapid advances in the treatment of congenital heart defects allow children to have surgery at younger ages. As a result, nursing care required to identify and manage responses of infants and children with heart disease has become more challenging.

ANATOMY AND PHYSIOLOGY OF PEDIATRIC DIFFERENCES

Fetal Circulation

Blood flows from the placenta to the fetus through the umbilical vein. Blood flow through the **ductus venosus** (the fetal vascular channel between the umbilical vein and the inferior vena cava) permits the blood to enter the right atrium of the heart. The **foramen ovale,** an opening between the atria in the fetal heart, allows blood to flow from the right to the left atrium. From here the blood travels to the left ventricle and is pumped to the aorta and the systemic circulation. Some blood returns from the head and upper extremities to the superior vena cava and right atrium. It flows to the right ventricle where it is pumped to the pulmonary artery. The majority of the blood passes through the **ductus arteriosus,** the fetal vascular channel between the pulmonary artery and the descending aorta, to enter the systemic circulation. A small amount of the blood from the pulmonary artery goes to the lungs. Blood eventually returns to the placenta by way of the umbilical arteries. See Figure 26–1 ■.

During fetal circulation, the blood with the highest oxygen content goes to the heart and the brain. The constricted pulmonary vessels limit blood flow to the lungs (high pulmonary vascular resistance). Blood, however, flows easily to the extremities because systemic vascular resistance is low. After the umbilical cord has been cut, the newborn must quickly adapt to receiving oxygen from the lungs.

Transition from Fetal to Pulmonary Circulation

The transition from fetal to pulmonary circulation occurs within just a few hours after birth. The first breath expands the lungs and blood that previously passed through the ductus arteriosus begins flowing to the lungs. Increased pulmonary blood flow and decreased pulmonary vascular resistance results. Pressure in the left atrium increases as increased blood flow is returned from the lungs through the pulmonary veins.

Systemic vascular resistance increases and right atrial pressure falls after the umbilical cord is cut. Increased pressure in the left atrium stimulates closure of the foramen ovale. The flaps of the foramen ovale close and fibrin deposits permanently seal the opening unless there is excess pressure on the right side of the heart. Table 26–1 provides a comparison of fetal and neonatal circulation and Figure 26–2 ■ illustrates the differences.

The ductus arteriosus, responding to higher oxygen saturation, normally constricts and closes within 10 to 15 hours after birth. Permanent closure usually occurs by 10 to 21 days after birth. If the infant's oxygen saturation remains low, the ductus arteriosis closure may be delayed or prevented. Fetal tissues are accustomed to low oxygen saturation. This may explain why newborns with cyanotic heart disease appear relatively comfortable even when the arterial partial pressure of oxygen (PaO_2) is 20 to 25 mm Hg. Older children and adults would rapidly develop acidosis and cerebral anoxia with such a low PaO_2.

Heart Hemodynamics

Once the transition to extrauterine life is complete, the blood travels through the heart and lungs with each side of the heart working in parallel. Review the normal heart **hemodynamics,** the pathways blood takes through the heart and pulmonary system as well as the pressures generated by blood against the chamber

TABLE 26–1 Comparison of Fetal and Neonatal Circulation

BLOOD VESSELS AND CHANNELS	FETAL	NEONATAL
Pulmonary blood vessels	Constricted, with very little blood flow; lungs not expanded	Vasodilation and increased blood flow; lungs expanded; increased oxygen stimulates vasodilation
Systemic blood vessels	Dilated, with low resistance; blood mostly in placenta	Arterial pressure rises due to loss of placenta; increased systemic blood volume and resistance
Ductus arteriosus	Large, with no tone; blood flow from pulmonary artery to aorta	Reversal of blood flow; now from aorta to pulmonary artery because of increased left atrial pressure. Ductus arteriosus is sensitive to increased oxygen and body chemicals and begins to constrict
Foramen ovale	Patent, with increased blood flow from right atrium to left atrium	Increased pressure in left atrium attempts to reverse blood flow and shuts one-way valve
Ductus venosus	Patent, blood flow from placenta to liver and inferior vena cava	Blood flow stops when umbilical cord is cut, ductus venosus begins to constrict

Adapted from Ladewig, P. W., London, M. L., Moberly, S., & Olds, S. B. (2002). Contemporary maternal-newborn nursing care *(5th ed., p. 521). Upper Saddle River, NJ: Prentice Hall.*

MediaLink A & P Review

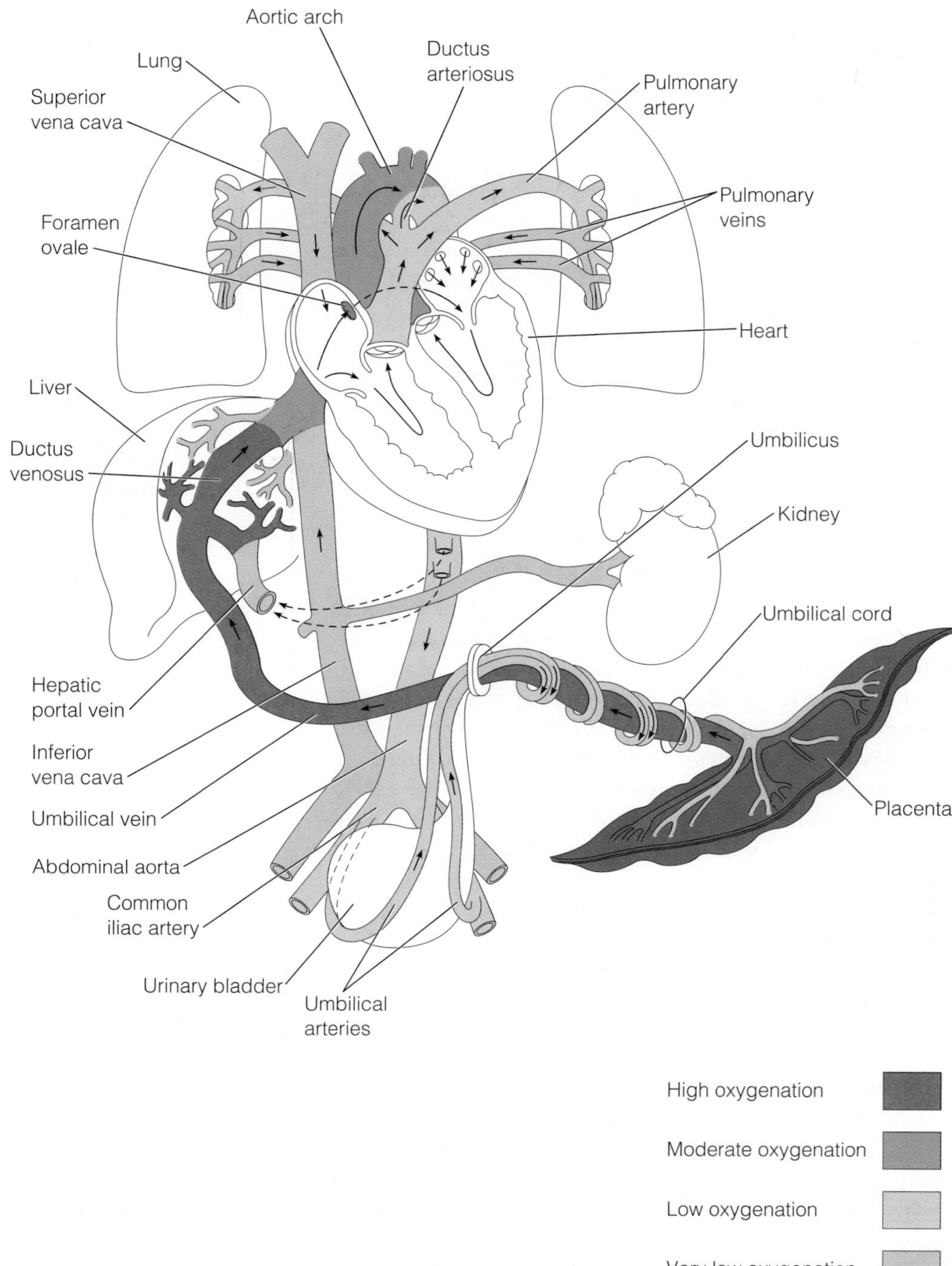

FIGURE 26–1 ■ Fetal circulation. Blood leaves the placenta and enters the fetus through the umbilical vein. The ductus venosus, the foramen ovale, and the ductus arteriosus allow the blood to bypass the fetal liver and lungs. After circulating through the fetus, the blood returns to the placenta through the umbilical arteries.

From Ladewig, P. W., London, M. L., Moberly, S., & Olds, S. B. (2002). Contemporary Maternal-Child Nursing Care *(8th ed,. p. 51). Upper Saddle River, NJ: Prentice Hall.*

walls, to understand the pathophysiology of various heart conditions. See Figure 26–3 ■ for an illustration of the heart chambers and vessels, and their associated oxygen saturation and pressure gradients. (Refer to Figure 26–2B for the normal flow of blood through the heart.) See Table 26–2 for a description of the coordinated blood flow through the heart chambers and valves.

Cardiovascular Changes as the Child Grows

The infant's cardiovascular system is proportionately larger in relation to body size than an adult's. The right ventricle is larger than the left at birth because the high pulmonary resistance during fetal life forced the right ventricle to be as thick and strong as the left ventricle. As the pulmonary resistance drops, the right ventricle thins out, and by 2 months of age the left ventricle is twice as large as the right ventricle. The higher systemic vascular pressures force the left ventricle to develop quickly.

The decreasing pulmonary vascular resistance at birth leads to thinning of the small pulmonary arteriole lining, leading to an increased diameter in these blood vessels. The pulmonary bed also develops in response to lung growth. Both changes result in development of pulmonary resistance of adult levels by 2 months of age. However, the neonate who experiences condi-

AS THEY GROW

Transition of Fetal Circulation to Postnatal Pulmonary Circulation

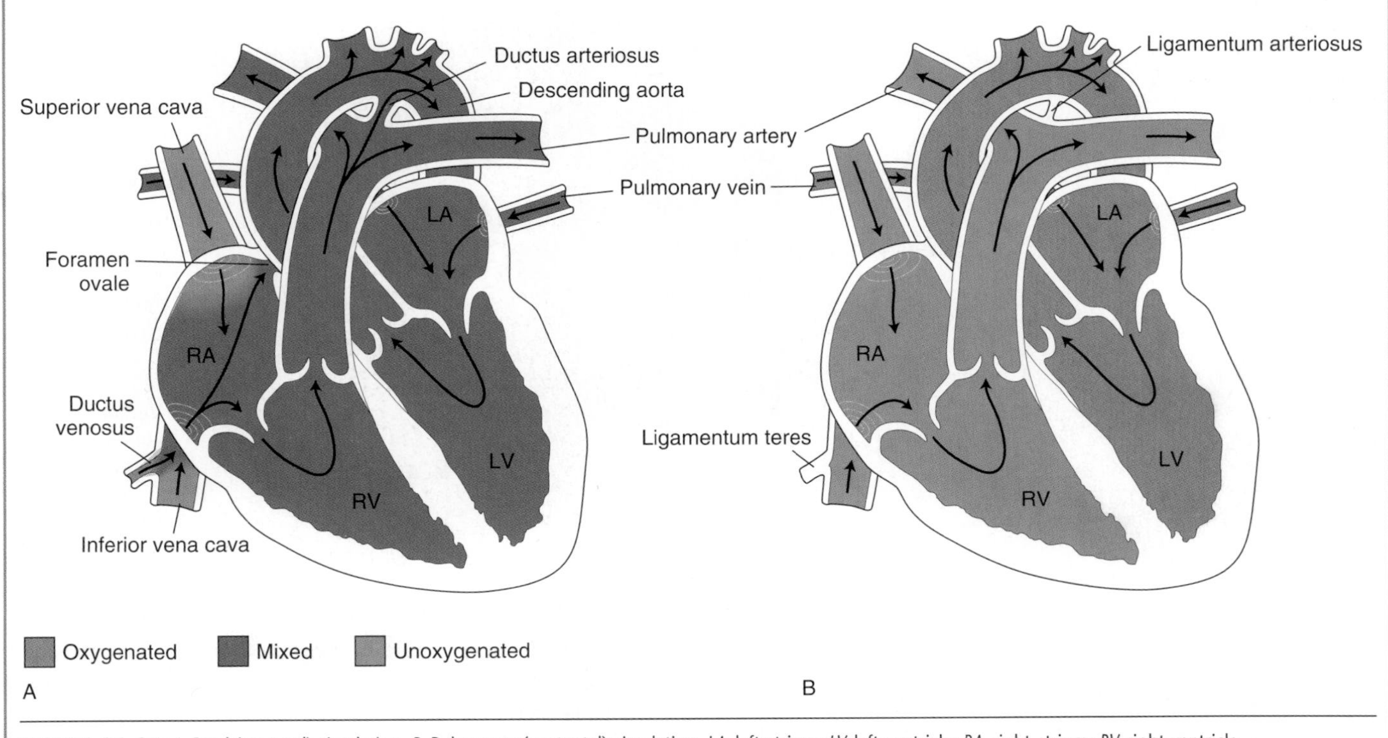

FIGURE 26–2 ■ *A*, Fetal (prenatal) circulation. *B*, Pulmonary (postnatal) circulation. *LA*, left atrium; *LV*, left ventricle; *RA*, right atrium; *RV*, right ventricle.

tions such as alveolar hypoxia, acidosis, and hypothermia may develop prolonged pulmonary vasoconstriction that results in pulmonary hypertension (Connor, 2002).

Infants have a greater risk of heart failure than older children because the immature heart is more sensitive to volume or pressure overload. During infancy, the muscle fibers of the heart are less developed and less organized, resulting in limited functional capacity. The decreased left ventricular strength is one reason for the neonate's low systolic blood pressure (approximately 39 to 59 mm Hg). Less **compliance** (amount of distention or expansion the ventricles can achieve to increase stroke volume) of the heart muscle means that stroke volume cannot increase substantially. The heart muscle fibers develop during early childhood and by 9 years of age, the weight of the heart has increased by six times (Kohr & Sims, 1998). As the child's heart grows and develops, the systolic blood pressure rises, reaching adult levels by puberty.

Oxygenation

Oxygen bound to hemoglobin is transported to the tissues by the systemic circulation. Hematocrit and hemoglobin concentrations appropriate for the child's age are necessary for adequate oxygen transport (see Chapter 27∞). The arterial **oxygen saturation** is the amount of oxygen that can potentially be delivered to the tissues. **Desaturated blood** results when oxygenated and unoxygenated blood mix due to a congenital heart defect. Cyanosis, which indicates **hypoxemia** (lower than normal amounts of oxygen in the blood), results from a concentration of 5 or more grams of deoxygenated hemoglobin per 100 mL of blood or from arterial saturations less than 85%. An anemic infant or child with congenital heart disease may be hypoxic but not have evidence of cyanosis because of less circulating hemoglobin. Refer to Box 25–2∞ and Figure 25–8∞ for a review of pulse oximetry use and interpretation (Box 26–1).

The child's bone marrow responds to chronic hypoxemia by producing more red blood cells to increase the amount of hemoglobin available to carry oxygen to the tissues. This occurs when the increase in red blood cells is greater than normal. A hematocrit value of 50% or higher is common in children with cyanotic heart defects because their bodies attempt to increase available oxygen by increasing red blood cell production. Extreme polycythemia is determined by a hemoglobin concentration greater than 20 g/dL. A hematocrit greater than 55% to 60% is dangerous. Blood viscosity is increased, and the child is at risk for a thromboembolism.

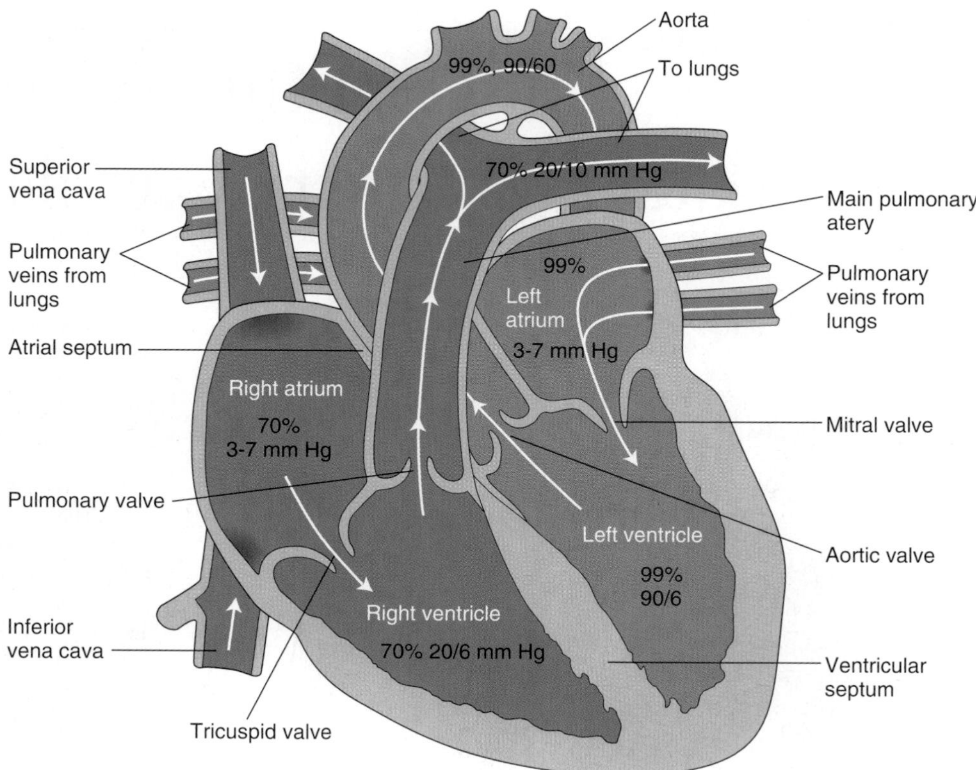

FIGURE 26–3 ■ Normal pressure gradients and oxygen saturation levels in the heart chambers and great vessels. The ventricle on the right side of the heart has a lower pressure during systole than the left ventricle because less pressure is needed to pump blood to the lungs than to the rest of the body.

The child's metabolic rate and oxygen consumption doubles at birth so the heart must maintain a high cardiac output. This is primarily accomplished with a higher heart rate, between 100 and 180 beats per minute. With the limited functional capacity of the heart, this results in minimal cardiac reserves for managing physiologic stresses until oxygen requirements decrease. By 2 months of age the oxygen consumption reduces by half (Connor, 2002).

TABLE 26–2 Hemodynamics of the Normal Heart

ACTION	RIGHT SIDE OF HEART	LEFT SIDE OF HEART
Blood return to heart	Systemic circulation by way of the superior vena cava and inferior vena cava	Lungs by way of the left and right pulmonary veins
Diastolic phase	Pulmonary valve closes, tricuspid valve opens Blood flows through the right atrium, through the tricuspid valve into the right ventricle	Aortic valve closes and the mitral valve opens Blood flows through the left atrium, through the mitral valve and into the left ventricle
Systolic phase	Tricuspid valve closes and pulmonary valve opens Blood is pumped from the right ventricle into the pulmonary artery where it passes to the right and left pulmonary arteries and lungs	Mitral valve closes and aortic valve opens Blood is pumped from the left ventricle into the aorta where it enters the systemic circulation

Cardiac Functioning

Cardiac systolic functioning or **cardiac output,** volume of blood ejected from the left ventricle each minute, is controlled by four interrelated actions.

- Heart rate.
- **Preload,** the volume of blood in the ventricle at the end of diastole that stretches the heart muscle before contraction.
- **Contractility,** the ability of the heart muscle fibers to contract forcefully
- **Afterload,** the systemic resistance to the ventricular ejection of blood

Cardiac output in newborns and young children depends primarily on heart rate until the heart muscle is fully developed at 5 years of age. The undeveloped muscle fibers in the myocardium are unable to expand their stretch to increase the ventricular volume. Weight-specific cardiac output decreases during childhood. During stress, exercise, fever, or respiratory

BOX 26–1 Lab Values

Pulse oximetry can be used to measure arterial oxygen saturation. A reading of 95%–98% is normal in children. The following values indicate hypoxemia.

- Mild hypoxemia: 90%–95%
- Moderate hypoxemia: 85%–90%
- Severe hypoxemia: 85%

A lower pulse oximetry reading level may be appropriate in some children before corrective cardiac surgery.

distress, infants and children become tachycardic, which increases their cardiac output.

PRACTICE ALERT

Children respond to severe hypoxemia with bradycardia. Cardiac arrest in children generally results from prolonged hypoxemia related to respiratory failure or shock rather than from a primary cardiac insult as in adults. Bradycardia is therefore a significant warning sign that cardiac arrest is imminent. Management of hypoxemia with assisted ventilation and 100% oxygen often reverses bradycardia and prevents cardiac arrest.

CONGESTIVE HEART FAILURE

Congestive heart failure is a disorder of circulation in which cardiac output is inadequate to support the body's circulatory and metabolic needs. It may result from a congenital heart defect that causes increased pulmonary blood flow or obstruction to the systemic outflow tract, from problems with heart contractility, or from pathologic conditions that require high cardiac output, such as severe anemia, acidosis, or respiratory disease. Congestive heart failure also results from acquired heart disease, such as cardiomyopathy, rheumatic heart disease, and Kawasaki syndrome.

Etiology and Pathophysiology

Heart chamber and vessel pressures as well as blood volume overloads associated with congenital heart defects are the most common cause of congestive heart failure in infants. Up to 90% of these children develop congestive heart failure within the first 6 to 12 months of life (Connor, 2002). Brandy, described at the beginning of this chapter, developed congestive heart failure as a result of one such defect. Some defects allow blood to flow from the left side of the heart to the right so that extra blood must be pumped to the pulmonary system rather than through the aorta when the left ventricle contracts. This overloads the pulmonary system, and if prolonged can lead to pulmonary artery hypertension, an often irreversible condition leading to life-threatening pulmonary vascular resistance (see page 930). Obstructive congenital defects (i.e., abnormally small pulmonary vessels) restrict the flow of blood so the heart hypertrophies to work harder to force blood through these structures. This increases cardiac output initially, but eventually the hypertrophied muscle becomes ineffective (Balaguru, Artman, & Auslender, 2000). Initially the right or left side of the heart may fail, but eventually failure is bilateral. See Table 26–3 for the types of congenital defects that cause congestive heart failure during the first months of life.

When cardiac output remains insufficient, the body's organs and tissues do not receive adequate oxygen. The decrease in blood pressure stimulates a sympathetic nervous system response that releases catecholamines and stimulates beta receptors, resulting in an increased rate and force of myocardial contraction, and peripheral vascular resistance. More blood is returned from the extremities as the venous smooth muscle tone increases. Blood flow to the skin, spleen, and kidneys is decreased so that blood flows to the vital organs. The kidneys respond to the lowered circulating volume by activating the renin-angiotensin

TABLE 26–3 Congenital Heart Defects that Cause Congestive Heart Failure in the First Months of Life

TIMING	DEFECT
At birth	Hypoplastic left heart syndrome Arterial venous fistula Tricuspid regurgitation and resulting volume overload
In first week of life	Hypoplastic left heart syndrome Aortic atresia Transposition of great vessels Coarctation of aorta Patent ductus arteriosus in preterm infants
In first month of life	Coarctation of aorta Total anomalous pulmonary venous connection with obstruction Ventricular septal defect with large left to right shunt Tricuspid atresia All previously mentioned defects
After 4 weeks of age	Transposition of great vessels Endocardial cushion defect with large left to right shunt Ventricular septal defect Endocardial fibroelastosis Persistent truncus arteriosus with large left to right shunt

From Connor, J. A. (2002). Alterations in cardiovascular function in children. In K. L. McCance & S. E. Huether, Pathophysiology: The biologic basis for disease in adults and children *(4th ed., p. 1055). St. Louis: Mosby.*

MediaLink Congenital Heart Defects Animation

mechanism to retain salt and water which then increases volume in the circulatory system. The heart muscle fibers stretch to accommodate the increased blood volume and the myocardium hypertrophies to manage the increased ventricular pressure. Without intervention, the compensatory mechanisms increase their intensity, demanding more effort from the compromised heart. Ultimately, the heart muscle cannot stretch the fibers any further to accommodate increased volume in the ventricles and the force of contractions is decreased. This results in progressive systemic edema and pulmonary congestion.

Clinical Manifestations

Congestive heart failure often develops subtly, and symptoms may not be recognized at first (see clinical manifestations on page 896). The infant tires easily, especially during feeding. Weight loss or lack of normal weight gain, diaphoresis, irritability, and frequent infections may be evident. Older children may have exercise intolerance, dyspnea, abdominal pain or distention, and peripheral edema. Skin color changes such as mottling or pallor are seen.

As the disease progresses, symptoms such as tachypnea, tachycardia, pallor or cyanosis, nasal flaring, grunting, retractions, cough, or crackles may occur. An S_3 **gallop** (a third heart sound that produces a rhythm like the gait of a horse) may be auscultated. Generalized fluid volume overload is seen more commonly in toddlers and older children. Periorbital and facial edema, jugular vein distention, and hepatomegaly are signs of fluid volume excess. See the clinical manifestations table for more detail.

CLINICAL MANIFESTATIONS in Congestive Heart Failure

ETIOLOGY	CLINICAL MANIFESTATIONS
Pulmonary venous congestion	Tachypnea, wheezing, crackles, retractions, cough, dyspnea on exertion, grunting, nasal flaring, cyanosis, feeding difficulties, irritability, tiring with play
Systemic venous congestion	Hepatomegaly, ascites, periorbital edema, peripheral edema, weight gain from retained fluids, neck vein distention in children
Impaired cardiac output	Tachycardia, weak thready pulses, hypotension, gallop rhythm, capillary refill time > 2 sec, pallor, cool extremities, oliguria, fatigue, restlessness, enlarged heart
High metabolic rate	Failure to thrive or slow weight gain, perspiration

Cardiomegaly, enlargement of the heart by hypertrophy of its walls, occurs as the heart attempts to maintain cardiac output. Cyanosis, weak peripheral pulses, cool extremities, hypotension, and heart murmur are precursors of cardiogenic shock, which can occur if congestive heart failure is not adequately treated. (Cardiogenic shock is discussed on page 949.)

COLLABORATIVE CARE

The goals of medical management are to make the heart work more efficiently and to remove excess fluid. This decreases the cardiac workload and improves systemic circulation without flooding the pulmonary system.

Diagnostic Procedures

Diagnosis is based primarily on clinical manifestations such as tachycardia, respiratory distress, and crackles. A chest radiograph reveals cardiac enlargement and venous congestion or signs of pulmonary edema. Echocardiography may be performed to diagnose specific cardiac defects or ventricular dysfunction. An electrocardiogram may show arrhythmias or ventricular hypertrophy. See Table 26–6 on page 906 for more information about diagnostic procedures.

Clinical Therapy

Diuretics, such as furosemide, chlorothiazide, and spironolactone, are given to promote fluid excretion. Because most diuretics (except for spironolactone) cause potassium loss, serum potassium levels are monitored and potassium supplements may be ordered.

Inotropic medicines and afterload-reducing agents (such as angiotensin-converting enzyme inhibitors) are sometimes used to lessen the workload of the heart and help it to work more efficiently. Digoxin is the drug most commonly used to improve the heart's ability to contract and therefore increase its output. Occasionally a higher than normal dose is given initially, followed by a lower maintenance dose. This process, called **digitalization,** speeds the child's response to the drug to achieve therapeutic blood levels more quickly. Beta-blockers, such as propanolol and carvediol, have been used successfully in cases of chronic heart failure (Azeka, Ramires, Valler, et al., 2002). Long-term changes in clinical manifestations include improved contractility, improved left ventricular ejection, reduced ventricular volumes, and improved blood pressures after treatment with beta-blockers (Balaguru, et al., 2000).

Surgery or interventional catheterization to correct a congenital heart defect may become the treatment of choice when congestive heart failure is difficult to manage, as occurred with Brandy (see pages 905–908). Cardiac transplantation may be performed for children with end-stage cardiomyopathy or complex congenital heart defects such as hypoplastic left heart syndrome (see page 928).

Other medical therapy is supportive. Airway management, ventilatory support, rest, and fluid and dietary management are also part of the treatment plan. Oxygen may be ordered (Figure 26–4 ■). Most children improve rapidly after medication is administered.

MEDICATIONS Used to Treat Congestive Heart Failure

DRUG	ACTION
Digoxin	Increases myocardial contractility improving systemic circulation
Furosemide	Rapid diuresis; blocks reabsorption of sodium and water in renal tubules
Thiazides: Chlorothiazide (suspension) Hydrochlorothiazide (tablets)	Maintenance diuresis, decreases absorption of sodium, water, potassium, chloride, and bicarbonate in renal tubules
Spironolactone	Maintenance diuresis (potassium sparing)
ACEi (angiotensin-converting enzyme inhibitor)	Promotes vascular relaxation and reduced peripheral vascular resistance, reduces afterload
Propranolol	Increases contractility
Carvedilol	Improves left ventricular function, promotes vasodilation of systemic circulation for chronic heart failure and dilated cardiomyopathy

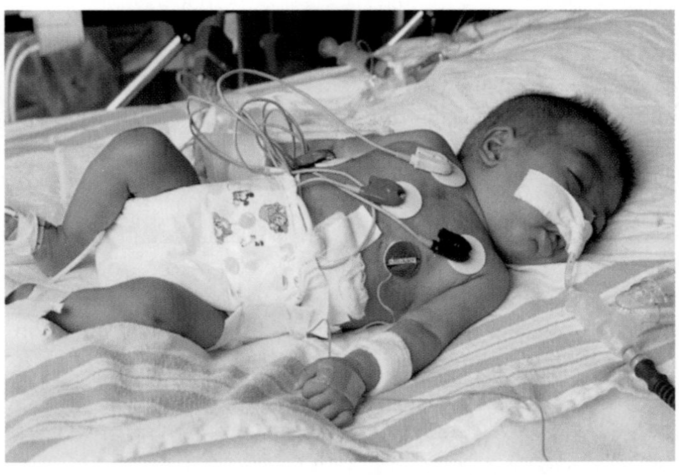

FIGURE 26–4 ■ Jooti is receiving intravenous fluids and oxygen. Her condition is being continuously monitored for congestive heart failure.

NURSING MANAGEMENT

The focus of nursing care is careful assessment of the child and family, promoting oxygenation and cardiovascular functioning, safely administering medications, fostering growth and development, and helping the family plan to care for the child at home.

■ Nursing Assessment and Diagnosis

Physiologic Assessment

As diagnosis of congestive heart failure depends primarily on physical symptoms, nursing observations are important. Assess the child's behavioral patterns, cardiac function, respiratory function, and fluid status as described in Box 26–2. Obtain a detailed history of the onset of symptoms from the parents, as congestive heart failure often develops slowly. Be suspicious of

BOX 26–2 Assessment Guidelines for a Child in Cardiac Condition[a]

QUALITY OF RESPIRATIONS

- Inspect the rate, depth, and respiratory effort.
- Is a cough present?
- Identify the signs of increased respiratory effort: tachypnea (abnormally rapid rate of respirations), dyspnea, retractions, nasal flaring, expiratory grunting.
- Auscultate breath sounds: Note if adventitious sounds are present (wheezes, crackles).

QUALITY OF PULSE

- Assess the rate, rhythm, and quality.
- Compare pulse sites (apical to brachial or radial) for strength and rate.
- Compare strength of pulse between upper and lower extremities (brachial to femoral). *A weaker femoral pulse is associated with coarctation of aorta.*

EVALUATE THE BLOOD PRESSURE

- Compare the blood pressure to expected value for age, sex, and height percentile. (See Table 8–16∞.)
- Compare blood pressure values between upper and lower extremities. *A lower systolic blood pressure in the legs in comparison to the arms is associated with coarctation of aorta.*

COLOR

- Observe overall color: Note pallor, dusky color, or cyanosis.
- Compare peripheral and central color: assess capillary refill and nailbed color and inspect mucous membranes. *Central cyanosis in mucous membranes is seen in cyanotic heart conditions.*
- Note whether crying improves or worsens color. *In cyanotic conditions crying worsens the cyanosis.*

ASSESS THE HEART

- Inspect the anterior chest. *Bulging on the left side or* **heaving** *(lifting of the chest wall during contraction) may indicate an enlarged heart.*
- Palpate the chest wall over the heart for any pulsations, heaves, or vibrations. *A thrill is caused by turbulent blood flow from a defective heart valve and a heart murmur.*
- Locate the point of maximum intensity using topographical landmarks.
- Auscultate the heart for the heart sounds and their quality (loud versus weak, distinct versus muffled). *Muffled or indistinct sounds are associated with congestive heart failure or a heart defect.*
- Determine if any extra heart sounds are present (a third or fourth heart sound, murmurs). See Table 8–15∞ for information on grading the loudness of murmurs. *Extra heart sounds and murmurs are associated with various cardiac conditions.*
  - Describe murmurs present by intensity, location, radiation, timing, and quality.
- Auscultate the heart with the child in sitting and reclining positions to detect differences in heart sounds.

SIGNS OF FLUID STATUS

- Observe for signs of periorbital, facial, or peripheral edema.
- Observe for abdominal distention.
- Palpate the liver to detect hepatomegaly.
- Observe for signs of dehydration with acute illnesses. *Dehydration is especially dangerous in children with polycythemia.*

ACTIVITY AND BEHAVIOR

- Determine if exercise intolerance is present or if the child tires with feeding.
- Identify changes in activity level. *Reduction in usual activity level may indicate increased hypoxia.*
- Watch for abrupt behavior changes. *Restlessness, irritability, and lowered level of consciousness may indicate increasing hypoxia.*

GENERAL

- Assess pattern of growth.
- Note presence of diaphoresis and when it occurs.

[a] Refer to Chapter 8∞ for the actual assessment techniques mentioned in this table.

developing congestive heart failure if feedings take 30 minutes or longer.

Measure intake and output carefully. Weigh the infant's diapers before use and after changing. The difference in weight provides information about output (1 g = 1 mL urine). Weigh the child at the same time each day because fluid volume varies throughout the day. If ascites is present, take serial abdominal measurements to monitor changes (see the Skills Manual for guidelines).

Observe for changes in peripheral edema and circulation. (See Figure 23–9). Turn the child frequently to assess the skin for redness and breakdown. Assessment of weight and weight gain is important to determine the child's response to treatment and need for surgical intervention. Some children have difficulty gaining weight as inadequate calories are consumed for the energy expended feeding. In other children weight gain may be noticed, and it is important to determine if it is fluid or growth accounting for the weight gain.

Family Assessment

Take a history of the child's previous hospitalizations and assess the family's knowledge about the child's condition. Families of children with congestive heart failure are anxious and fear the potential serious outcome of the problem and the need to provide ongoing care. Assess the family's anxiety level and coping strategies. Evaluate the family's economic status. Medication is crucial to treatment, and a family's inability to afford or obtain the necessary medications jeopardizes the child's ability to survive.

Assess the parents' understanding of the child's condition and ability to provide the necessary care at home. Correct medication dosage is critical. Extensive time is needed to feed the infant so that adequate nutrition is obtained. Identify their ability to make the observations of change in the child's condition as well as provide needed care. Find out if another family member is available who could support young parents to ensure that the child's needs are met or to provide respite care.

Developmental Assessment

Because fatigue limits the activities of the child with congestive heart failure, he or she does not have the opportunity to practice the skills needed to attain normal developmental milestones. Perform developmental assessment with a tool such as the Denver II (see Chapter 10). In addition, parents can provide information about the attainment of expected developmental milestones such as sitting, manipulating objects, standing, or walking. When congestive heart failure is well controlled, the child's energy level increases and developmental skills often improve. In infants and toddlers, assessments every 2 to 3 months are useful to observe development and evaluate disease management.

Parents may limit the child's contact with other children because of frequent infections and exercise intolerance. Ask parents about contact and play with other children and a typical day's activity schedule.

Several nursing diagnoses that may apply to the child with congestive heart failure are given in the accompanying nursing care plans. The primary nursing diagnosis is Decreased Cardiac Output related to cardiac anomaly.

■ Planning and Implementation

Nursing care for the child with congestive heart failure focuses on administering and monitoring effects of medications, maintaining adequate oxygenation and myocardial function, promoting rest, fostering development, providing adequate nutrition, and providing emotional support to the child and family.

Administer and Monitor Prescribed Medications

Children with congestive heart failure usually receive digoxin and diuretics. These medications are potent and must be administered correctly. Provide frequent skin care when edema is present.

PRACTICE ALERT

Digoxin and digitoxin are both digitalis preparations but they are not the same drug. Digoxin is the drug of choice in pediatrics. Digitoxin is 10 times more powerful than digoxin, and is rarely used in children. Read labels carefully and double-check doses to ensure that the child receives the right dose of the right drug. Give digoxin at the same times daily with or without food to ensure equal bioavailability. Food slows absorption, but it does not decrease total absorption.

Check the child's apical heart rate for a full minute before giving any dose to determine if bradycardia is present. If the heart rate is below the guideline noted in a physician's order, call for advice before giving the drug. Check the child's serum potassium level if diuretics are also ordered as a low potassium level increases the risk for digoxin overdose.

Observe the child carefully for digoxin toxicity. Early signs include tachycardia in young children or bradycardia in older children, nausea, vomiting, anorexia, dizziness, headache, weakness, fatigue, and arrhythmia. Serum digoxin levels are usually taken 6 to 8 hours after a dose. The therapeutic serum level ranges from 1.1 to 1.7 ng/mL.

Certain antibiotics increase digoxin serum concentration. It is believed that alteration in the normal gastrointestinal flora that metabolizes digoxin can lead to digoxin toxicity. The antibiotics reported to be associated with this antibiotic-digoxin interation include the following: macrolides (clarithromycin, roxithyromycin, erythromycin), azithromycin, tetracyclines, and beta-lactams (Ten Eick & Reed, 2000).

Maintain Oxygenation and Myocardial Function

Oxygen therapy may be ordered. Ensure that tubing is patent, the oxygen flow rate is correct, the oxygen delivery device is working properly, and humidification is provided. Keep the child calm and quiet. Place the child in a semi-Fowler's or 45-degree angle position to promote maximum oxygenation.

Promote Rest

Group assessments and interventions together to ensure that the child has some uninterrupted rest each hour. Feedings should last no more than 20 to 30 minutes. Frequent small feedings generally work best, with burping after every 0.5 oz of intake to minimize vomiting. Rocking is restful and comforting for infants. Encourage older children to engage in quiet activities such as playing board or computer games or watching television and reading.

Foster Development

Encourage parents to play with the child, using toys to stimulate eye–hand coordination and fine motor movements. Such toys include rattles, blocks, and stuffed animals for infants and books, paper and pencil, and dolls for older children. Encourage sitting, standing, or walking for short periods with adequate rest afterward to promote the development of large muscles. Singing, talking, and playing music encourage the development of cognitive and language skills.

Provide Adequate Nutrition

Teach parents about feeding techniques. The mother who chooses to breastfeed the infant should not be discouraged. The antibodies contained in breast milk reduce infections, and the milk is naturally low in sodium. However, the sucking involved in feeding may cause dyspnea and force the infant to rest frequently during feeding. Infants should be burped frequently to permit rest and prevent vomiting. They may need small frequent feedings and longer feeding periods.

CLINICAL TIP

Ways to decrease the work of feeding, either with breast or bottle, include the following (Cook & Higgins, 2004):

- Hold the infant at a 45-degree angle. If the parent gets fatigued due to the long feeding time the infant can be shifted to an infant seat at a 45-degree angle. This position helps to decrease venous return to the heart and reduce metabolic demand.
- Limit feeding time to 40 minutes so the infant does not get overtired.
- Permit the infant to set rhythm for feeding and resting.
- Follow the infant's cues for hunger, satiety, and tiring.

Attempting to have the infant eat adequate calories to satisfy hunger and to support growth puts a lot of pressure on the parents. Encourage parents to use the feeding time for nurturing and bonding with the infant, as they learn the infant's cues for hunger and satiety.

Make sure parents understand that changes in feeding habits (decreased intake, vomiting, sleeping through feedings, and increased perspiration with feedings) may indicate deteriorating cardiac status. The American Heart Association publishes a helpful booklet, *Feeding Infants with Congenital Heart Disease,* for parents.

Adequate nutrition is needed to support the infant's growth. These infants often require up to 150 kcal/kg or more per day for their increased metabolic rate and to sustain weight gain. Some infants need a higher caloric formula (24 to 30 cal/oz) to obtain adequate nutrition or to meet fluid restrictions. It is not unusual for infants with heart problems to develop failure to thrive as the result of feeding difficulties (see Chapter 9∞). When infants have significant dyspnea with

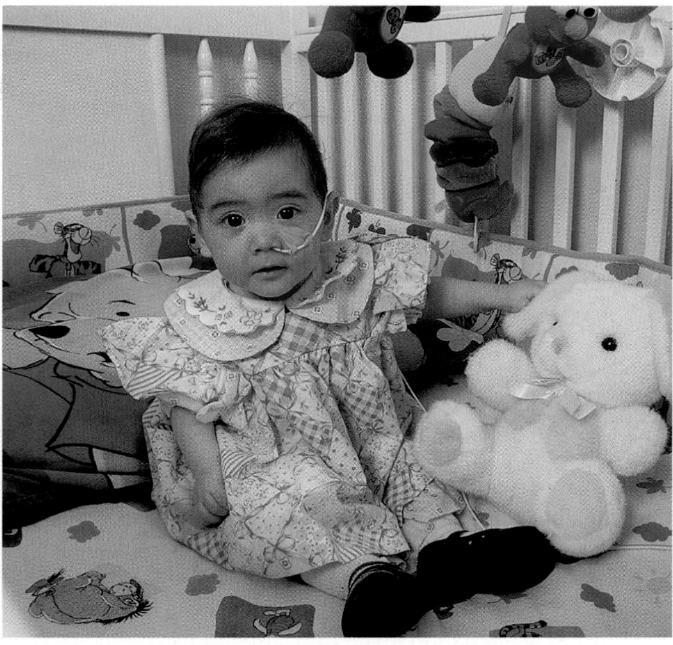

FIGURE 26–5 ■ Infants with cardiac conditions often require supplemental feedings to provide sufficient calories for growth and development. The parents of this infant girl have been taught how to give her nasogastric feedings at home.

feeding, special feeding techniques are needed. Other infants require nutritional supplementation by nasogastric or gastrostomy tube (Figure 26–5 ■). Parents are often advised to give the infant a chance to feed normally for a specific period. The remainder of the formula is then given by nasogastric or gastrostomy tube.

Provide Emotional Support

When a child is hospitalized with congestive heart failure, the family is often anxious about his or her condition. Give parents an opportunity to express concerns about their child's condition. Explain the child's treatment regimen, and make sure family members understand the child's need for nutrition and rest. Answering questions about the child's prognosis and the ultimate outcome can be reassuring. Provide family members with information, and relay questions to the physician. Talking to other parents of children with cardiac conditions may be a source of emotional support. Refer parents to the appropriate support groups.

Discharge Planning and Home Care Teaching

Home care needs should be identified and addressed as early as possible before discharge. While the child is hospitalized, teach the family about the administration of medications and signs of a worsening condition. Arrange for home care nursing visits to reinforce the education provided for home care management and to monitor the child's condition. Ensure that the family has a phone contact for emergency assistance if they live a distance from the healthcare provider.

MediaLink Congenital Heart Disease Resources for Families

Medication Administration

Demonstrate administration of drugs, and then supervise while the parents measure and administer medications. Make sure parents have oral syringes or other appropriate measuring devices to ensure that the infant receives the correct dose. Teach parents about the toxic effects of digoxin and other drugs and provide an information sheet for home reference. Advise them to notify the physician immediately if any of these side effects occur. Digitalis is a very dangerous drug. Encourage parents to keep it locked up at home and away from children. In case of accidental ingestion, immediate medical care is needed. Make sure the parents have the poison control number posted on every phone.

Educate parents about signs and symptoms of dehydration when the child is managed on diuretics. An acute illness could lead to dehydration more quickly because of those medications.

Assessment for Worsening Condition

Show parents how to feed the child to maximize nutritional intake. Tell them to watch for symptoms such as increased feeding difficulty, irritability, lethargy, breathing difficulty, and puffiness around the eyes or extremities, which indicate that congestive heart failure is worsening. Parents are frequently taught to take the child's pulse and to report any significant change to the physician. An increase in pulse rate can signal congestive heart failure, and a decrease in pulse rate can indicate digoxin toxicity.

Care in the Community

The second of the two accompanying nursing care plans outlines home care of the child with congestive heart failure. Parents play a critical role in the care of the child with heart disease by facilitating normal development and limiting the development or consequences of congestive heart failure. Home care nurses often collaborate with cardiac specialists and advance practice nurses in the hospital outpatient setting to support the family and child so that the child's condition is appropriately managed in the home. These children are evaluated frequently for progression in signs and symptoms, appropriate weight gain, and developmental progress. Families are evaluated for their ongoing ability to manage the child's condition and coping with the stress of caring for a sick child. Additional needs for psychosocial support or for financial resources are monitored. Daily care of these children is taxing, and usually requires that a parent or caregiver be present 24 hours a day. Identify how the family is managing the needs of other children.

Parents are educated about the potential interaction between digoxin and certain antibiotics so that they can more carefully monitor the child if a primary care provider orders these antibiotics for an infection.

Evaluate family resources so that adequate child or respite care can be arranged if needed. Periodically review how the family assesses the child's energy level, physical condition for progressively worsening signs, and feeding problems. Observe medication administration and correct any errors. Watch the child feeding and provide suggestions as necessary. Reinforce any education or guidance that will help the family in the daily plan of care for the child.

■ Evaluation

Expected outcomes of nursing care can be found on the nursing care plans.

CONGENITAL HEART DISEASE

Congenital heart disease refers to a defect in the heart or great vessels, or persistence of a fetal structure after birth. Congenital heart defects are estimated to occur in 1% of all pregnancies and 1 of every 170 live births (Neilson & Robin, 2002). They are the second most common birth defect after developmental disabilities.

Individuals with congenital heart disease are living longer than those born in past decades. Between 1979 and 1997, deaths from heart defects declined by 39.4% (Boneva, Botto, & Moore, et al., 2001). This is attributed to diagnostic advances, surgical technique refinements, and intensive care.

Etiology and Pathophysiology

The heart develops during the fourth and seventh weeks of gestation, the time when it is most susceptible to teratogens. Therefore, most congenital heart defects develop during the first 8 weeks of gestation. They are usually the result of a combined or interactive effect of genetic and environmental factors, as follows:

- Fetal exposure to drugs such as phenytoin and lithium
- Fetal exposure to alcohol (tetralogy of Fallot, atrial septal defect, ventriculoseptal defect)
- Maternal systemic viral infections such as rubella (patent ductus arteriosis, pulmonic stenosis, coarctation of aorta) or coxsackie B5 (endocardial fibroelastosis)
- Increased maternal age (ventriculoseptal defect, tetralogy of Fallot)
- Maternal metabolic disorders such as phenylketonuria (coarctation of aorta and patent ductus arteriosis), diabetes mellitus (ventricular septal defects, cardiomegaly, transposition of great arteries), and hypercalcemia (aortic stenosis, pulmonic stenosis, aortic hyperplasia)
- High altitude (patent ductus arteriosis, atrial septal defect)
- Maternal complications of pregnancy such as increased age and antepartal bleeding
- Genetic factors (family recurrence patterns)
- Prematurity (patent ductus arteriosis, ventricular septal defect)
- Chromosomal abnormalities such as Turner syndrome, Noonan syndrome, Marfan syndrome, DiGeorge syndrome, cri du chat syndrome, Down syndrome, and trisomy syndromes 13, 15, 18, and 21 (Kohr & Sims, 1998); the prevalence of heart defects in children with Down syndrome is about 12% to 44%, and in children with trisomies 13 and 18, the incidence increases to 80% and higher (Connor, 2002)

text continues on page 904

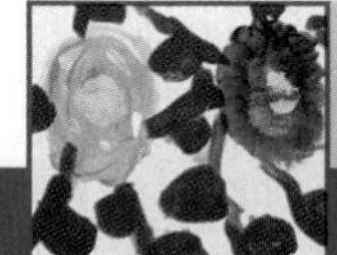

Nursing Care Plan

THE CHILD HOSPITALIZED WITH CONGESTIVE HEART FAILURE

GOAL	INTERVENTION	RATIONALE	EXPECTED OUTCOME
1. Decreased Cardiac Output related to cardiac anomaly (VSD)			
	NIC Priority Intervention—*Hemodynamic Regulation:* Optimization of heart rate, preload, afterload, and contractility		**NOC Suggested Outcome**—*Cardiac Pump Effectiveness:* Extent to which blood is ejected from the left ventricle per minute to support systemic perfusion pressure
The child's cardiac output will be sufficient to meet the body's metabolic demands.	▪ Administer digoxin as ordered.	▪ Digoxin increases contractility of the heart and force of contraction.	The child's cardiac output is sufficient as indicated by increased energy, adequate feeding intake, and decreased edema.
	▪ Take apical pulse and listen to heart sounds regularly, especially before each dose of digoxin. Record apical pulse with each recorded dose of digoxin.	▪ Digoxin toxicity may cause bradycardia. Pulse and heart sounds provide information about heart functioning.	
	▪ Use cardiac monitor if ordered.	▪ Monitor identifies tachycardia and arrhythmias.	
	▪ Prevent injury by monitoring for digoxin side effects and serum potassium level.	▪ Digoxin is a potent drug with serious side effects. Hypokalemia increases risk of digoxin toxicity.	The child maintains normal serum levels of potassium and therapeutic levels of digoxin.
	▪ Provide for rest periods each hour.	▪ Rest decreases need for high cardiac output.	The child rests hourly and has adequate energy to eat and play.
The child will manifest adequate oxygenation.	▪ Place child in semi-Fowler's position.	▪ Position facilitates lung expansion.	The child has normal respiratory rate for age with no evidence of adventitious sounds or diaphoresis.
	▪ Evaluate respiratory rate and sounds. Take pulse oximetry readings to determine oxygen saturation.	▪ Absence of tachypnea and adventitious sounds and oxygen saturation above 95% (or appropriate baseline for specific heart defect) indicate ease of respiration.	
	▪ Provide oxygen and humidification if ordered. Observe for diaphoresis, a sign of increased respiratory effort.	▪ Supplemental oxygen decreases tachypnea, and humidification moistens secretions to keep airway clear.	
2. Fluid Volume Excess related to heart failure			
	NIC Priority Intervention—*Fluid Management:* Promotion of fluid balance and prevention of complications resulting from abnormal or undesired fluid levels		**NOC Suggested Outcomes**—*Fluid Balance:* Balance of water in the intracellular and extracellular compartments of the body
The child's peripheral and central edema will decrease. Intake and output will be balanced once excess fluid is excreted.	▪ Administer diuretics as ordered.	▪ Diuretics mobilize fluids and facilitate excretion.	The child's edema is reduced, intake and output are proportional, and electrolyte levels remain within normal ranges.
	▪ Weigh daily. ▪ Measure abdominal girth daily if ascites is present. Observe for peripheral edema.	▪ Assessments demonstrate effectiveness of treatment.	
	▪ Measure intake and output carefully. Weigh diapers to obtain output of young child.	▪ Adequate output is a good indicator of renal perfusion.	
	▪ Maintain fluid-restricted diet if ordered.	▪ Fluid restriction is sometimes used to decrease cardiac load.	
	▪ Monitor electrolytes.	▪ Electrolyte imbalance is common when fluids are restricted and diuretics are given.	

(continued)

Nursing Care Plan THE CHILD HOSPITALIZED WITH CONGESTIVE HEART FAILURE (continued)

GOAL	INTERVENTION	RATIONALE	EXPECTED OUTCOME
3. Risk for Impaired Skin Integrity related to altered fluid status			
	NIC Priority Intervention—*Pressure Management:* Minimizing pressure to body parts		**NOC Suggested Outcomes**—*Risk Control:* Actions to eliminate or reduce actual, personal, and modifiable health threats
The child will have no skin breakdown associated with peripheral edema.	■ Provide frequent skin care for edematous body parts and elevate extremities. ■ Change child's position frequently. ■ Inspect skin frequently for redness and skin breakdown over pressure points.	■ Edematous skin injures easily. Elevation promotes return of fluid from extremities. ■ Position change promotes circulation to skin over pressure points. ■ Inspection identifies earliest stages of skin breakdown.	The child has no skin breakdown after edema resolves.
4. Altered Nutrition: Less than Body Requirements related to high metabolic needs and rapid tiring while feeding			
	NIC Priority Intervention—*Nutrition Management:* Assistance with or provision of a balanced dietary intake of food and fluids		**NOC Suggested Outcome**—*Nutrition Status:* Extent to which nutrients are available to meet metabolic needs.
The infant or child will demonstrate normal weight gain for age.	■ Hold infant at 45-degree angle for feeding. ■ Record intake carefully. ■ Weigh child daily. ■ Give frequent small meals with rest periods in between. ■ Use high-calorie formula or give high-calorie snacks as ordered. ■ Use soothing approaches such as holding infants for feeding and having parents eat with older child. ■ Transition to supplemental nasogastric feeding if infant is not able to gain weight.	■ Position facilitates breathing while eating. ■ Evaluation of intake indicates whether caloric and other nutritional needs are met. ■ Weight indicates growth (in absence of fluid retention with congestive heart failure). ■ Digesting small meals requires less energy. ■ High-calorie formulas and snacks provide calories efficiently. ■ Restful approach facilitates intake with minimum cardiac work. ■ Nasogastric feeds provide added calories but do not force infant to use energy to eat.	The infant or child gains recommended weight according to growth grids. All dietary requirements are met, and mealtimes are pleasant.
5. Ineffective Family Coping, Compromised related to unknown nature of child's disease			
	NIC Priority Intervention—*Family Involvement:* Facilitating family participation in the emotional and physical care of the patient.		**NOC Suggested Outcome**—*Coping:* Actions to manage stressors that tax an individual's resources
Parents will express lessened anxiety as hospitalization proceeds.	■ Encourage parents to room in or stay with child. Explain procedures and treatment. Involve parents in care as much as possible. Have parents plan child's play periods. ■ At discharge, provide clear instructions and information about what to do in an emergency, and whom and where to call with questions. ■ Allow parents to verbalize questions, concerns, and feelings. Refer parents to support groups or other resources as needed.	■ Involvement in child's care lessens parental anxiety and fear of unknown. ■ Having resources available provides feelings of security. ■ Emotional support is needed to lessen anxiety.	Parents participate in developing and implementing the treatment plan and providing care to the child.

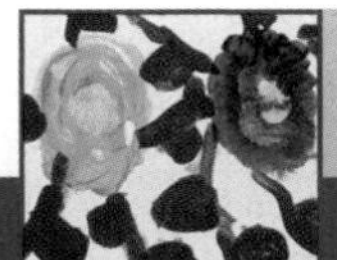

Nursing Care Plan

THE CHILD WITH CONGESTIVE HEART FAILURE BEING CARED FOR AT HOME

GOAL	INTERVENTION	RATIONALE	EXPECTED OUTCOME
1. Altered Growth and Development related to effects of physical disability			
	NIC Priority Intervention—*Developmental Enhancement:* Teaching parents to facilitate optimal gross motor, fine motor, language, cognitive, social, and emotional growth of preschool children		**NOC Suggested Outcome**—*Child Development* (2 years): Milestones of physical, cognitive, and psychosocial progression by 2 years of age
The child will meet developmental milestones for age group.	▪ Perform baseline developmental assessment.	▪ Assessment provides comparison for later assessments and basis for planning specific games, toys, and activities to promote developmental skills.	The child displays normal language, fine motor, and gross motor activity.
	▪ Plan for short play periods after rest.	▪ Short play periods maintain energy and facilitate play.	
	▪ Introduce age-appropriate toys and activities such as rattles and blocks for infants and art projects for older children.	▪ Play activities facilitate learning and mastery of developmental tasks.	
	▪ Plan for interactions with healthy children.	▪ Social skills are learned through contact with others.	
2. Ineffective Therapeutic Regimen Management (family) related to complexity of therapeutic regimen			
	NIC Priority Intervention—*Family Involvement:* Facilitating family participation in the emotional and physical care of the patient		**NOC Suggested Outcome**—*Coping:* Actions to manage stressors that tax an individual's resources.
Parents will demonstrate correct administration of medications.	▪ Have parents prepare the medication dosages and administer the digoxin, diuretics, and other medications to the child under the supervision of a home health nurse.	▪ Demonstration of techniques used to administer medications provides opportunities to identify dosage errors and to suggest methods to help ensure that the child gets all of needed medications.	Parents report that child continues to demonstrate improvement and adequate cardiac output with absence of congestive heart failure.
Parents will state side effects of medications and symptoms of congestive heart failure.	▪ Describe side effects of medications. Give parents handouts with telephone number to call to ask questions or report side effects.	▪ If side effects are recognized, the child will get care earlier, and serious complications can be avoided.	
	▪ Describe subtle onset of congestive heart failure and its symptoms (increasing weakness, exhaustion, irritability, feeding difficulty, cough, difficult respirations, edema).	▪ Parents can evaluate child regularly and note subtle changes requiring medical management.	
3. Altered Nutrition: Less than Body Requirements related to chronic illness and tiring while feeding			
	NIC Priority Intervention—*Weight Gain Assistance:* Facilitation of body weight gain		**NOC Suggested Outcome**—*Nutritional Status: Food and fluid intake:* Amount of food and fluid taken into the body over a 24-hour period
The infant or child will demonstrate normal weight gain for age.	▪ Teach parents methods to promote food intake related to positioning, size of feedings, food choices.	▪ Positioning, frequency of feedings, size of feedings, and use of high-caloric formulas or foods can enhance nutritional intake.	The infant or child shows normal weight gain.
	▪ Observe feeding during home visit.	▪ Feedback can assist parents in integrating positive feeding techniques.	Parents report and demonstrate successful feedings of child.

(continued)

Nursing Care Plan THE CHILD WITH CONGESTIVE HEART FAILURE BEING CARED FOR AT HOME (continued)

GOAL	INTERVENTION	RATIONALE	EXPECTED OUTCOME
4. Activity Intolerance (child) related to poor cardiac output			
	NIC Priority Intervention—*Energy Management:* Regulating energy use to treat or prevent fatigue and optimize function		**NOC Suggested Outcome**—*Energy Conservation:* Extent of active management of energy to initiate or sustain activity
The child will perform all necessary activities of daily living without undue tiring.	■ Help parents alternate activities and rest throughout the child's day. ■ Have parents limit child's exposure to persons with contagious disease. ■ Help family plan quiet surroundings to provide for child's rest.	■ Activities to promote development must be alternated with rest due to decreased cardiac output. ■ When the child is ill and tired, the immune system can be compromised. ■ Home setting may need to be altered to promote rest.	The child performs necessary activities and rests frequently each day.
5. Caregiver Role Strain (parent) related to 24-hour responsibility for child's care			
	NIC Priority Intervention—*Caregiver Support:* Provision of the necessary information, advocacy, and support to facilitate primary patient care by someone other than a healthcare professional		**NOC Suggested Outcome**—*Caregiver Endurance Potential:* Factors that promote family care provider continuance over an extended period of time
Parents will express ability to meet own needs.	■ Assess family and community supports. Provide information related to respite care. ■ Encourage parents to seek activities to meet personal needs.	■ Variable family and community supports are available. ■ Parents need time to meet own personal needs in order to successfully care for child.	Parents report some time away from the child and report renewal in caring for the child.

Evidence shows that the use of multivitamins by women at the time of conception may reduce the risk of certain defects (transposition of the great vessels, tetralogy of Fallot, and truncus arteriosis) (Botto, Khoury, Mulinare, et al., 1996).

Congenital heart defects can occur as an isolated defect or as a malformation associated with a genetic syndrome. Chromosome 22q11 is one of the most frequent genetic sites associated with development of cardiovascular defects such as truncus arteriosus, tetralogy of Fallot, and pulmonary atresia (Lewin, 2000). Other known chromosomes with associated cardiovascular defects include chromosome 7q11.23 deletion, chromosome 20p12 region deletions, and TBX5 gene mutation on chromosome 12q24. While some conditions develop due to mutations of genes, others are transmitted in an autosomal dominant or autosomal recessive pattern. See Chapter 4∞ for more information on genetic transmission. Because of this genetic component, the incidence of congenital heart defects is expected to slowly rise as persons with some of these defects survive and have children of their own (Table 26–4). There is an increased incidence of congenital heart defect in families as shown in Table 26–5.

Congenital heart defects are generally categorized by the pathophysiology and hemodynamics. An understanding of the normal heart hemodynamics is important to understand the pathophysiology associated with different heart defects.

Clinical Manifestations

The presence of a heart murmur is often the first indication of a congenital heart defect. A loud murmur indicates blood is flowing with higher pressure than normal to get through a narrowed valve or vessel, or through a **shunt** (movement of blood between the systemic and pulmonary circulation through an abnormal anatomic opening). The other clinical manifestations and the timing of their appearance vary by the pathophysiology and severity of the defect (see clinical manifestations on page 906). Newborns may be initially asymptomatic but develop symptoms in the first few days of life. Other newborns are symptomatic as soon as the umbilical cord is cut. Infants and children may be asymptomatic except for a heart murmur, such as with a small atrial septal defect. See Chapter 8∞ for assessment of murmurs. Signs and symptoms of congenital heart disease in older children include exercise intolerance, chest pain, arrhythmias, syncope, and sudden death.

COLLABORATIVE CARE

Diagnostic Procedures

Multiple tests are used to diagnose cardiac defects. See Table 26–6 for the diagnostic procedures commonly used. Blood tests include hematocrit and hemoglobin. Arterial blood gases may

TABLE 26–4 Congenital Heart Defects Commonly Associated with Genetic Disorders

GENETIC DISORDER	ASSOCIATED CONGENITAL HEART DEFECTS
Trisomy 13	Ventriculoseptal defect, atrial septal defect, patent ductus arteriosus, anomalous pulmonary venous connection, bicuspid aorta, and overriding aorta
Trisomy 18	Ventriculoseptal defect, patent ductus arteriosus, patent foramen ovale, bicuspid aorta, dextrocardia
Down syndrome (trisomy 21)	Endocardial cushion defect, ventriculoseptal defect, patent ductus arteriosus, atrial septal defect, transposition of great arteries, tetralogy of Fallot, truncus arteriosus, coarctation of aorta, endocardial fibroelastosis
Cri du chat	Patent ductus arteriosus, mixed defects
Turner syndrome (monosomy 23)	Coarctation of aorta, peripheral pulmonic stenosis, aortic stenosis, patent ductus arteriosus, septal defects
Neurofibromatosis	Pulmonic stenosis
Williams syndrome (chromosome 7q11.23 deletion)	Supravalvular aortic stenosis, atrial septal defect, peripheral pulmonic stenosis, aortic hypoplasia
DiGeorge syndrome, velocardiofacial syndrome (chromosome 22q11 microdeletion)	Interrupted aortic arch, tetralogy of Fallot, pulmonic stenosis, septal defects, truncus arteriosus
Marfan syndrome (defect in fibrillin 1 gene on chromosome 15)	Aortic or mitral valve abnormalities, dissecting aortic aneurysms, myocardial disease
Alagille syndrome (chromosome 20p12 region deletions)	Peripheral pulmonic stenosis, tetralogy of Fallot, ventricular septal defect, atrial septal defect, aortic stenosis, coarctation of aorta
Holt-Oram syndrome (TBX5 gene mutation on chromosome 12q24)	Ventricular septal defect, atrial septal defect, mitral valve prolapse, hypoplastic left heart syndrome, coarctation of aorta, tetralogy of Fallot, aortic stenosis, pulmonic stenosis, patent ductus arteriosus, dextrocardia

Adapted from Connor, J. A. (2002). Alterations in cardiovascular function in children. In K. L. McCance & S. E. Huether, Pathophysiology: The biologic basis for disease in adults and children *(4th ed., pp. 1048–1081). St. Louis: Mosby; Neilson, D. E., & Robin, N. H. (2002). Advances in the genetics of pediatric heart disease.* Contemporary Pediatrics, *19(1), 85–100.*

be obtained for some children, especially when cyanosis or a complex heart defect is suspected.

Clinical Therapy

Genetic testing should be provided to patients and their families so they have accurate information and receive counseling about the cause of and risks for recurrence in subsequent pregnancies.

Surgical Intervention. One third of infants born with congenital heart defects develop life-threatening symptoms in the first few days of life. Treatment for congenital heart defects depends on the severity of symptoms and whether the condition is imminently life threatening. Surgical correction is the treatment of choice for many defects. Many heart defects can be completely repaired with restoration of normal hemodynamics and physiology. For complex heart defects, treatment may only be **palliative,** a surgical procedure that does not create normal anatomical or hemodynamic results that are used for children with a potentially fatal or lethal condition. In some cases a palliative procedure is used initially while the infant is small, with definitive corrective surgery performed after some growth has been achieved. Table 26–7 lists the types of surgical procedures performed on children with congenital heart defects.

Interventional Catheterization. Interventional cardiac catheterization is performed to correct some congenital heart defects as described below (Vincent, & Diehl, 2002; Uzark, 2001).

Opening Narrowed Passages. A balloon is used during cardiac catheterization to create a larger opening in the atrial septum, perform a **valvuloplasty** (dilating a **stenotic** [narrowed or small] pulmonic or aortic valve), and to expand a coarctation of the aorta. See Figure 26–6 ■ on page 908. Another intervention involves inserting a stent into a patent ductus arteriosis to maintain patency as an alternative to long-term prostaglandin E_1 (PGE_1) infusion. Insertion of a stent may also be used to treat a stenotic **hypoplastic** (underdeveloped structure) pulmonary artery. Balloon dilation techniques have also been used to improve stenosis of prosthetic conduits and systemic venous stenosis following surgery for complex heart defects. Aortic regurgitation is a potential complication of aortic valvuloplasty. Development of an aortic aneurysm is a potential complication of balloon dilation of aortic coarctation. Anticoagulant therapy is needed for children with stents placed in pulmonary arteries, as thrombus formation is a significant risk.

TABLE 26–5 Increased Frequency of Congenital Heart Defects in Families

FAMILIAL RELATIONSHIP	INCIDENCE OR RISK OF RECURRENCE
Unaffected parents	Incidence of 2% to 6%
One parent has congenital heart defect	Incidence of 5% to 15%
Two siblings have congenital heart defect	Recurrence risk of 9% in next child
Three siblings have congenital heart defect	Recurrence risk of 50% in next child

Data from Connor, J. A. (2002). Alterations in cardiovascular function in children. In K. L. McCance & S. E. Huether, Pathophysiology: The biologic basis for disease in adults and children *(4th ed., pp. 1053–1054). St. Louis: Mosby.*

CLINICAL MANIFESTATIONS of Heart Defects by Pathophysiology

ETIOLOGY	TYPES OF DEFECTS	CLINICAL MANIFESTATIONS
Increased pulmonary blood flow	Patent ductus arteriosus, atrial septal defect, ventricular septal defect, atrioventricular canal defect (endocardial cushion defect), truncus arteriosus, total anomalous pulmonary venous return	Tachypnea, tachycardia, murmur, congestive heart failure, poor weight gain, diaphoresis, periorbital edema, frequent respiratory infections
Decreased pulmonary blood flow	Pulmonic stenosis, tetralogy of Fallot, pulmonary atresia, tricuspid atresia, transposition of the great arteries	Cyanosis, hypercyanotic spells, poor weight gain, polycythemia
Obstruction to systemic blood flow	Coarctation of aorta, aortic stenosis, hypoplastic left heart syndrome, mitral stenosis, interrupted aortic arch	Diminished pulses, poor color, delayed capillary refill time, decreased urine output, congestive heart failure with pulmonary edema
Mixed defects—postnatal survival is dependent upon mixing of systemic and pulmonary blood	Transposition of great arteries, total anomalous pulmonary venous, connection, truncus arteriosus, double outlet right ventricle	Cyanosis, poor weight gain, pulmonary congestion, congestive heart failure may occur with increased shunting

Closing Openings. A coil can be used to occlude a patent ductus arteriosis, atrial septal defect, and occasionally for a ventricular septal defect. A surgically created Blalock-Taussig shunt may be occluded with a coil when no longer needed after corrective surgery (Figure 26–7 ■). A small persistent shunt may remain in about 5% of cases following patent ductus arteriosus closure (Uzark, 2001). In some cases hemolysis occurs with the residual shunt and requires placement of additional coils until the shunting is stopped. Embolization of the coil to the pulmonary artery may necessitate repeat catheterization and retrieval of the coil. Complications are rare following the septal closure of an atrial septal defect, and they are primarily associated with thrombus formation and potential pulmonary or cerebral embolism. Anticoagulant therapy is often ordered during the procedure and for several months following the placement of the occlusion device.

Outcomes and Prognosis. Lifelong assessment and medical care will be required for children with complex congenital heart defects following palliative or corrective heart surgery. Some will require multiple stages of surgery to provide improved quality of life. Others will need valve replacements and revisions of previous

TABLE 26–6 Diagnostic Procedures for Diagnosing and Evaluating Congenital Heart Defects

DIAGNOSTIC PROCEDURE	PURPOSE
Chest radiograph	Assess the size and contour of the heart and the great arteries. Characteristics of pulmonary blood flow are assessed through the vascular markings.
Electrocardiogram (ECG)	Records the quality of major electrical activity in the heart. Information about the heart rate and conduction patterns, muscular damage, hypertrophy, electrolyte imbalance, and influence of various drugs can be obtained. See Figure 26–6.
Ambulatory ECG (Holter monitor)	Permits a 24–48-hour ECG recording so that conduction pattern changes during a day's activities can be identified.
Exercise testing	Records an ECG with a controlled increase in activity to identify significant cardiac compensation or inadequate cardiac output.
Cardiac monitoring	Performed on hospitalized children to monitor the heart rate and rhythm through a digital display or by printed tracings as needed.
Two-dimensional echocardiogram	Identifies the heart structures and their size; the pattern of the heart's movement; the presence, position, and function of the valves; the hemodynamics and velocity of blood flow; and the presence of defects. Fetal echocardiography can often reveal congenital heart disease prenatally.
Transesophageal echocardiogram	A transducer is passed into the esophagus to an area behind the atria to provide two-dimensional images of the heart from a posterior view. This view often provides better imaging of the left atrium and left ventricle structures. This procedure requires general anesthesia or sedation.
Cardiac catheterization—An invasive procedure that passes a radiopaque catheter through a large vein to the heart	Enables precise measurement of oxygen saturation within the heart's chambers and great arteries, and pressure gradients in each of these structures. Contrast material is used to identify the anatomy and blood flow patterns. In some cases a biopsy of the heart muscle may also be obtained to evaluate muscle function problems, inflammation, or heart transplant rejection. Potential complications include arrhythmias during the procedure due to catheter manipulation; perforation of a blood vessel; allergic reaction to the contrast media; hypotension; stroke; vascular injury or thrombus formation at the large vein access site; vascular compromise in the leg, and bleeding.
Magnetic resonance imaging	Evaluates the great arteries outside the heart, such as for coarctation of the aorta. The ventricles can also be evaluated for size and volume.
Hyperoxia test	Measures differences in arterial blood gas level when child is on room air and on 100% oxygen. In children with defects causing cyanosis, the oxygen saturation will only increase to 80%–85% with 100% oxygen, whereas those children with pulmonary conditions will have an increase in oxygenation saturation to 95% (Saenz, Beebe, & Triplett, 1999).

TABLE 26–7 Clinical Interventions for Congenital Heart Defects

CARDIAC CATHETERIZATION PROCEDURES	PURPOSE	THERAPEUTIC USE
Angioplasty	Dilatation of coarctation of aorta or a stenotic vessel during cardiac catheterization	Palliative or Corrective COA
Balloon valvuloplasty	A deflated balloon is inserted into the opening of a narrowed valve and inflated to stretch the valve open during cardiac catheterization	Corrective or Palliative PS, AS
Patent ductus arteriosus closure	Closure of ductus arteriosus by surgery or an umbrella or coil device during cardiac catheterization.	Corrective PDA
Rashkind—Balloon atrial septostomy	Creation of larger defect (at the foramen ovale) between atria to increase blood mixing, performed during cardiac catheterization.	Palliative TGA
Transcatheter closure	Closure of a septal defect by a septal occluder during cardiac catheterization.	Corrective ASD, PDA, VSD
SURGICAL PROCEDURES	**PURPOSE**	**THERAPEUTIC USE**
Aorta end-to-end anastomosis	Resection of the narrowed section of the aorta and connecting the proximal and distal sections	Corrective COA
Blalock-Taussig shunt, modified	Creation of aorto-pulmonary conduit (from the subclavian artery to pulmonary artery) to increase pulmonary blood flow	Palliative TOF, other defects of decreased pulmonary blood flow
Brock	Blind incision of pulmonary valve	Corrective PS
Damus-Kaye-Stansel	Pulmonary artery is cut in two with the proximal section attached to the ascending aorta and the distal section to the right ventricle	Corrective TGA, complex single ventricle defects
Fontan	Creation of conduit between inferior vena cava and pulmonary artery to increase pulmonary blood flow—total right heart bypass. This permits the right ventricle to assume the responsibility for the systemic circulation and eject blood into the aorta	Palliative HLHS, single ventricle defects
Glenn	Superior vena cava connected to right pulmonary artery along with closure of aorto-pulmonary shunt. Systemic venous blood from the head is sent to the lungs directly without ventricular pumping	Palliative HLHS, single ventricle defects
Jatene (arterial switch)	Aorta and pulmonary arteries are transected and re-anastomosed to opposite stumps, coronary arteries are moved to new aorta area	Corrective TGA
Mustard or Senning (venous switch or intra-atrial baffle)	Baffling blood in atria to reestablish a proper blood flow in transposition of great vessels	Palliative TGA
Norwood	Atrial septectomy, anastomosis of the main pulmonary artery to the aorta, and an arterial-pulmonary shunt	Palliative HLHS
Norwood with Sano modification	Creation of a right ventricle to pulmonary artery conduit so that the direct pulmonary and aorta blood flow originates in the right ventricle	Palliative HLHS
Patch aortoplasty	Insertion of a Dacron patch to expand the lumen of the aorta	Corrective COA
Pulmonary artery banding	Placement of constricting band around pulmonary artery to reduce pulmonary blood flow	Palliative VSD, single ventricle defects
Rastelli	Creation of a conduit between the right ventricle to pulmonary artery with closure of the ventricular septal defect. In the case of truncus arteriosus, the pulmonary arteries are removed from the truncus	Corrective TGA with pulmonic stenosis, TOF, tricuspid atresia, truncus arteriosus
Ross	The diseased aortic valve is replaced with the patient's pulmonic valve (pulmonary autograft), and a homograft (valve from a human donor) replaces the pulmonic valve	Corrective AS
Subclavian flap aortoplasty	Division of the distal subclavian artery and inserting a flap into the aorta through the coarcted segment	Corrective COA
Transplant	Replacement of diseased heart with donor heart	Corrective HLHS, complex defects, cardiomyopathies

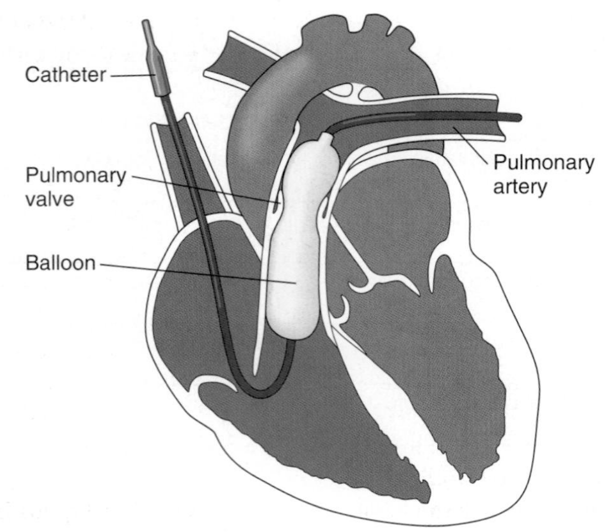

FIGURE 26–6 ■ Interventional catheterization, balloon valvuloplasty to open the pulmonary valve.

surgeries or interventional catheterization to reopen valves or vessels that have become stenotic. Some children have recurrent arrhythmias that require implantation of a pacemaker. Arrhythmias may be associated with congenital anomalies of the conduction system or unavoidable surgical incisions in areas of the sinoatrial node, sinoventricular node, and tissues around these nodes. The Mustard and Senning procedures for transposition of the great arteries (TGA), the Fontan procedure for hypoplastic left heart syndrome (HLHS), truncus arteriosus, tricuspid atresia, and repair of tetralogy of Fallot (TOF) are associated with increased risk of postsurgical arrhythmius. See page 935. An implantable cardioverter-defibrillator may be used in older children with life-threatening ventricular arrhythmias (LeRoy, 2001).

Infants with complex congenital heart defects are at risk for preoperative neurologic insult. Conditions such as congestive heart failure, prolonged hypoxemia, profound acidosis, or low cardiac output place the infant at risk for long-term neurologic sequelae. Inadequate nutrition to support growth during the first year of life when the brain is rapidly developing also places the infant at greater risk. In addition, intraventricular hemorrhage has been documented in nearly 25% of neonates with congenital heart defects. An ultrasound of the brain may be performed to identify preexisting intraventricular hemorrhage prior to surgery. Cardiopulmonary bypass and deep hypothermic circulatory arrest used in most surgery for congenital heart disease has the potential to insult the neurologic system. Seizures have been noted in the immediate postoperative period (Mahle & Wernovsky, 2001). See Chapter 33∞ for more information about seizures.

In general, studies have demonstrated that preschool and school-age survivors of congenital heart disease have normal IQ scores. Some children with complex defects such as TGA and HLHS are at an increased risk for neurodevelopmental problems. Visuospatial, visual motor, and speech deficits have been identified in children with TGA even when IQ scores have been within normal ranges. Children with HLHS are at higher risk for neurocognitive impairment than many other children with congenital heart defects. Reasons include a higher incidence of congenital brain abnormalities, ductal-dependent systemic blood flow, severe acidosis at time of diagnosis, duration of deep hypothermic cardiac arrest for the stage 1 Norwood procedure, and the challenge of maintaining adequate systemic blood flow and cerebral perfusion in the immediate postoperative period. Many children evaluated in the past decade have been found to have mental retardation or a significantly lower IQ than the general population (Mahle & Wernovsky, 2001). Improvements in earlier recognition of neonates with HLHS as well as in operative and postoperative care are expected to improve the neurodevelopmental outcomes of these children.

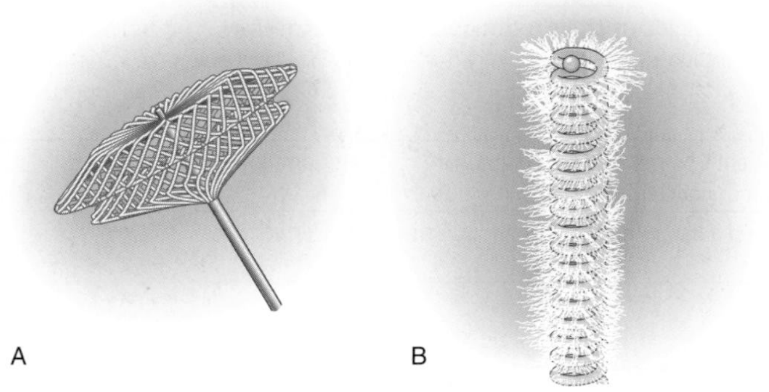

FIGURE 26–7 ■ *A*, Septal occluder used to close an atrial septal defect (ASD) and less commonly to close a ventricular septal defect (VSD). *B*, Coil used to close a patent ductus arteriosus (PDA). The coil of wire covered with tiny fibers occludes the ductus arteriosis when a thrombus forms in the mass of fabric and wire.

NURSING MANAGEMENT OF THE CHILD UNDERGOING A CARDIAC CATHETERIZATION

Cardiac catheterization is often an outpatient procedure, but some children will be admitted for observation. Various diagnostic tests may be performed before the procedure, such as a chest radiograph, ECG, complete blood count, and electrolytes. The child is NPO for several hours, except for medications, and arrives at the catheterization laboratory 1 to 2 hours before the procedure. Before entering the laboratory, the child is asked to void and is given an oral sedative. Infants and young children usually need deeper sedation to keep them still during the procedure.

■ Nursing Assessment and Diagnosis

Physiologic Assessment

Before the procedure, assess the child's vital signs, hematocrit and hemoglobin concentrations, and capillary refill, skin temperature and color, and strength of the pedal and popliteal pulses for comparison with postcatheterization assessments.

For several hours after the procedure, monitor the child for potential complications such as arrhythmia, bleeding, hematoma development, thrombus formation, and infection. No bleeding should occur at the catheterization site. Assess vital signs, perfusion of the lower extremities (pedal and popliteal pulses, skin temperature, color, capillary refill, and sensation), and the pressure dressing over the catheterization site every 15 minutes for 1 hour and then every 30 minutes for 1 hour. Pedal pulses, capillary refill, sensation, warmth, and color of the lower extremities should match the precatheterization assessment. The child's temperature, heart rate, respiratory rate, and blood pressure should remain stable. Monitor intake and output because the contrast medium may cause diuresis. The child's intake and output should be balanced. Infants and children treated with diuretics have a greater potential for dehydration, and excessive urinary excretion is important to identify so that additional fluids can be provided.

PRACTICE ALERT

Ileofemoral artery injury associated with cardiac catheterization is more common in newborns and young infants. Reduced limb warmth and decreased pedal perfusion in the extremity following transfemoral cardiac catheterization is an indication of potential arterial occlusion and limb ischemia. Immediate medical intervention is needed to prevent permanent neurovascular damage to the extremity.

Psychosocial Assessment

Assess the parents' need for emotional support. This is often the first invasive procedure performed on a newborn with a congenital heart defect. The parents have had little time to understand and cope with the infant's condition. Older children may have fears about all the equipment and people that will be performing invasive procedures while he or she is awake.

The following nursing diagnoses may apply to the child who undergoes cardiac catheterization.

- Fear related to separation from support system in a stressful situation
- Anxiety (family) related to potential for serious diagnosis
- Risk for Imbalanced Fluid Volume related to inadequate fluid intake due to NPO status, diuretic therapy, and diuretic effect of contrast medium
- Impaired Tissue Perfusion (cardiopulmonary) related to mechanical reduction of arterial and venous blood flow
- Decreased Cardiac Output related to ventricular restriction (obstruction by balloon catheter)

■ Planning and Implementation

Prepare the child for cardiac catheterization with age-appropriate information. A tour of the catheterization laboratory for a preschooler or school-age child may reduce the child's fears about the large equipment. Because the child will be sedated but arousable for the procedure, explain the sensations that he or she will experience.

Nursing care during a cardiac catheterization focuses on monitoring the child's vital signs, reassuring the child, and providing emergency care if necessary. After the catheters and guide wires are removed at the end of the procedure, direct pressure must be applied for 15 minutes. A pressure dressing is then placed over the site for 6 hours. Regular assessment of the site of catheterization and distal extremity is performed for several hours after the procedure.

CLINICAL TIP

The catheterization site is initially checked every 15 minutes and then every 30 minutes. Be sure to check under the buttocks to make sure that blood does not ooze out and run under the child.

The child is kept on bed rest for 6 hours with an effort to keep the leg straight for several hours. Avoid elevating the head of the bed as flexion of the hips is not permitted during this period. Activity is then limited for 24 hours. Provide quiet diversional activities to keep the child occupied.

Encourage the intake of small amounts of clear liquids initially, and then progress to other fluids and food as the child tolerates them. Maintaining hydration is important because the contrast medium used during the procedure has a diuretic effect. Monitor intake and output.

CLINICAL TIP

If the child has been treated with diuretics, careful monitoring of intake and output is even more important because the child could become dehydrated.

Discharge Planning and Home Care Teaching

Children are usually discharged several hours after the cardiac catheterization. Teach the parents to watch the child for signs of complications and make sure they know when to notify the physician. See Partnering with Families: Home Care after Cardiac Catheterization.

Children whose heart defect is corrected by cardiac catheterization have the same risks for infective endocarditis as children with surgical correction. Use the information provided later in this chapter to teach parents about infective endocarditis prophylaxis.

■ Evaluation

Expected outcomes of nursing care include the following:

- Any potential complications (thrombosis or hemorrhage) following cardiac catheterization are rapidly identified.
- No permanent injury to the limb occurs.
- The child maintains fluid balance.

Congenital Heart Defects that Increase Pulmonary Blood Flow

Etiology and Pathophysiology

The most common congenital heart defects result from a connection between the left and right side of the heart (septal defect) or between the great arteries (patent ductus arteriosus) that allows blood to flow between the left and right side of the heart. Because the pressures on the left side of the heart are

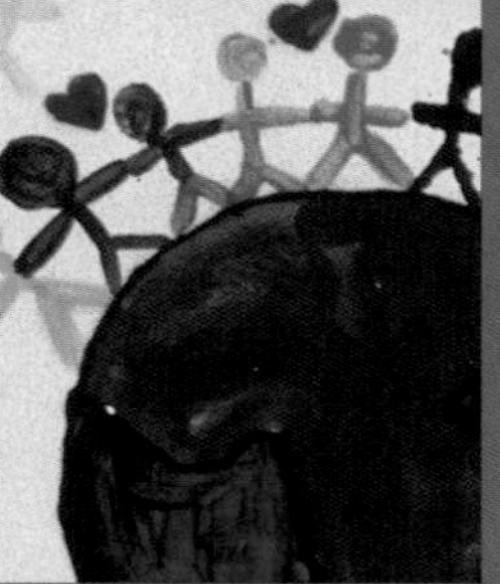

PARTNERING WITH FAMILIES

Home Care After Cardiac Catheterization

Check for signs of complications several times in the first 24 hours after catheterization.

- Fever
- Bleeding at the catheterization site
- A bruise increasing in size at the catheterization site
- Foot on side of catheterization site is cooler than other foot
- Loss of feeling in foot on side of catheterization

If the child is treated with diuretics, observe for signs of dehydration.

- Dry mucous membranes
- No tears
- Sunken fontanel

Notify physician immediately if any of these signs are noted within the first 24 hours after the catheterization.

Encourage fluids to help flush the dye out of the body and to prevent dehydration. Permit quiet play such as crayons or markers, board games, puzzles, books, music, and videos for 24 hours.

higher than on the right side, blood will shunt from the left side of the heart to the right side and increase the amount of blood that needs to be pumped to the lungs. The size of the connection and how much blood passes through it determine if or how quickly the child will develop signs associated with congestive heart failure. The increased pulmonary blood flow causes increased pulmonary vascular resistance, or constriction of the pulmonary vascular bed in an effort to reduce the blood flow, and pulmonary hypertension. Right ventricular hypertrophy develops to counteract the increasing pulmonary vascular resistance and deliver the increased volume of blood to the lungs.

Clinical Manifestations

As the lungs attempt to accommodate the increased pulmonary blood flow, the infant heart rate and respiratory rate are increased, as is the metabolic rate. Sucking takes energy and diaphoresis may be noted with feeding. Often the infant is unable to take in enough calories to support the metabolic rate and growth, so poor weight gain is noted. Congestive heart failure may develop if the amount of blood passing from the left to the right side of the heart overloads the pulmonary system. If this occurs, the child has dyspnea, tachypnea, intercostal retractions, and periorbital edema. Frequent respiratory infections occur as the wet environment in the lungs supports bacterial growth. The symptoms of congestive heart failure appear earlier when the heart defect is more severe and complex. See Table 26–8 for the pathophysiology, clinical manifestations, and clinical therapy for the congenital heart defects that increase pulmonary blood flow.

COLLABORATIVE CARE

Diagnostic Procedures

See Table 26–8 for tests used to diagnose the condition. Prior to surgery a complete blood count and urinalysis are collected, along with a chest radiograph. Coagulation studies, platelet counts, and serum electrolytes are commonly obtained for children having open heart surgery.

Clinical Therapy

Surgery to correct or manage defects that cause significant increased pulmonary blood flow is performed early in infancy to prevent irreversible pulmonary vascular disease, such as with a patent ductus arteriosis or large ventricular septal defect. Unless complications develop before surgery, the child should make a complete recovery without limitations. The major complication of these defects is pulmonary hypertension. See Table 26–8 for clinical therapy for the specific congenital heart defects.

Conservative treatment, such as waiting until the child is symptomatic or older, may be selected initially for some children with increased pulmonary blood flow defects. For example, a small ventricular septal defect may close spontaneously, and often repair of an atrial septal defect is postponed until preschool or early school-age years. Indomethacin may be given to preterm infants with a patent ductus arteriosis when immediate closure of the ductus is needed.

Cardiac catheterization, an invasive procedure used for diagnosis of some congenital heart defects, is also performed as a therapeutic procedure for some conditions. Recently developed techniques using transcatheter devices permit treatment of some heart defects causing increased pulmonary blood flow during cardiac catheterization, such as patent ductus arteriosis and atrial septal defects.

A potential complication of surgery is postpericardiotomy syndrome when surgery involved a pericardiotomy (incision through the pericardium), leading to pericardial and pleual inflammation. Children over 2 years of age have a higher rate of occurrence than infants. The specific etiology is not known, but it may result from a viral infection, an autoimmune response, or a reaction to blood in the pericardium. The syndrome generally develops within a few weeks to a few months after surgery. It is characterized by a high fever up to 40°C (104°F) and severe chest pain that worsens with deep inspiration and in supine position. The median duration of the condition is 2 to 3 weeks. Mild cases are treated with bed rest and NSAIDs. Severe cases may need hospitalization and more aggressive treatment with pericardiocentesis, diuretics, and corticosteroids (Park, 2002).

TABLE 26–8 Pathophysiology, Clinical Manifestations, and Clinical Therapy for Heart Defects that Increase Pulmonary Blood Flow

DEFECT PATHOPHYSIOLOGY | **CLINICAL MANIFESTATIONS AND CLINICAL THERAPY**

Patent Ductus Arteriosus (PDA)

Common congenital defect caused by persistent fetal circulation that accounts for 9%–12% of all congenital heart defects (Driscoll, 1999). When pulmonary circulation is established and systemic vascular resistance increases at birth, pressures in the aorta become greater than in the pulmonary arteries. Blood is then shunted from the aorta to the pulmonary arteries, increasing circulation to the pulmonary system. It is a common problem of preterm infants, and is present in nearly all preterm infants less than 27 weeks' gestation (Tran, 2002). The ductus arteriosus in the preterm newborn is not as responsive to the increased oxygen content with the conversion to pulmonary circulation, and it is less likely to close.

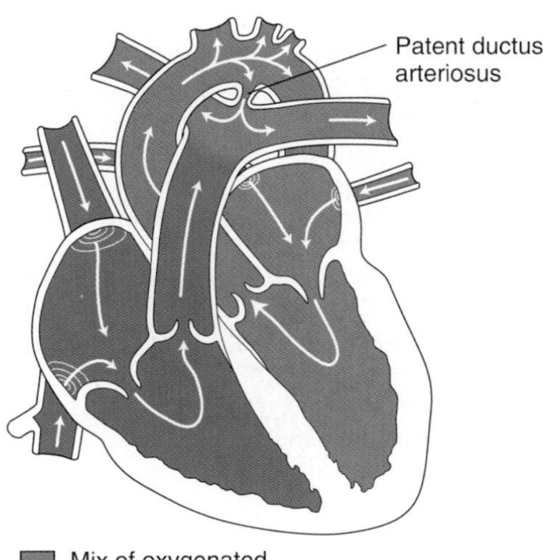

Clinical Manifestations

Dyspnea; tachypnea; tachycardia; full, bounding pulses; widened pulse pressure; hypotension may be noted when cardiac output is low.

Poor development

A continuous "machinery" murmur is auscultated during both systole and diastole, and a thrill may be palpated in the pulmonic area.

The infant is at risk for frequent respiratory infections, pneumonia, and infective endocarditis.

When a large PDA exists, congestive heart failure, intercostal retractions, hepatomegaly, and growth failure are also seen.

Diagnostic Procedures

The chest radiograph and ECG show left ventricular hypertrophy.

The PDA can be visualized, and left to right shunt can be measured on echocardiogram.

Clinical Therapy

Surgical ligation of PDA is the treatment of choice.

Intravenous indomethacin often stimulates closure of the ductus arteriosus in premature infants. Intravenous ibuprofen holds promise as another medication to stimulate closure of the ductus arteriosus once further research is conducted (Tran, 2002).

Transcatheter closure by obstructive device is sometimes attempted in children over 18 months of age. Prophylaxis for infective endocarditis is required until the PDA is closed.

Prognosis: No long-term sequelae occur if treated before pulmonary vascular disease develops. If PDA is not treated, child's life span is shortened because pulmonary hypertension and pulmonary vascular obstructive disease develop.

Atrial Septal Defect (ASD)

The opening in the atrial septum permits left to right shunting of blood. Three types of ASDs occur: ostium secundum, ostium primum that is an endocardial cushion defect with anomalies of one or both of the tricuspid and mitral valves, and sinus venosus that is associated with partial anomalous pulmonary venous connection. The opening may be small, as when the foramen ovale fails to close, or large, as when the septum may be completely absent. Of children with congenital heart defects, 6%–10% have an ASD (Driscoll, 1999).

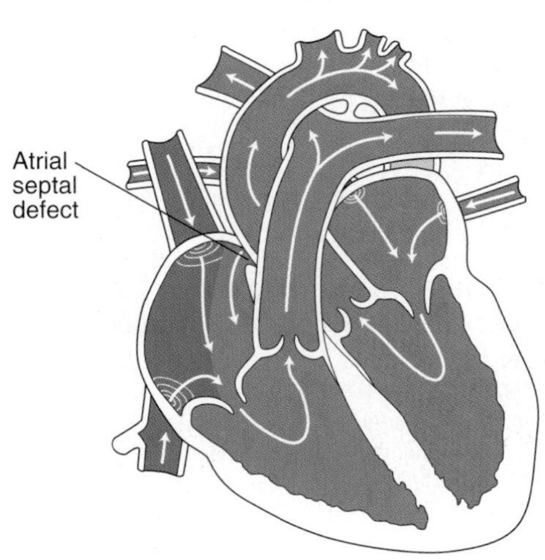

Clinical Manifestations

Infants and young children usually have no symptoms.

Small and midsize ASDs are usually not diagnosed until preschool years or later.

Congestive heart failure, easy tiring, and poor growth occur with a large ASD.

A soft systolic ejection murmur is usually heard in the pulmonic area with wide splitting of S_2. The split second sound remains the same regardless of the phase of respiration.

Diagnostic Procedures

Diagnosis is made by echocardiogram that identifies a dilated right ventricule due to blood overload and the shunt size.

The chest radiograph and ECG reveal little information unless the ASD is large, or excessive shunting and right ventricular hypertrophy is present.

Clinical Therapy

Spontaneous closure of some types of ASDs occurs within the first 4 years of life. Those larger than 8 mm rarely close spontaneously. No activity limitations are needed.

Surgery to close or patch the ASD is performed when significant increased pulmonary blood flow causes congestive heart failure, or when an ASD has not closed spontaneously by 4 years of age.

Secundum ASDs may be closed by a transcatheter device (septal occluder) during cardiac catheterization.

Prognosis: Many persons with uncorrected small and midsize ASDs have lived to middle age without symptoms, however, congestive heart failure and pulmonary hypertension may develop in untreated adults. Atrial arrhythmias may also occur in adults regardless of the type of treatment provided.

(continued)

TABLE 26–8 Pathophysiology, Clinical Manifestations, and Clinical Therapy for Heart Defects that Increase Pulmonary Blood Flow (continued)

DEFECT PATHOPHYSIOLOGY	CLINICAL MANIFESTATIONS AND CLINICAL THERAPY
Ventricular Septal Defect (VSD) An opening in the ventricular septum results in increased pulmonary blood flow. Blood is shunted from the left ventricle directly across the open septum into the pulmonary artery. This most common congenital heart defect occurs in approximately 20% of all children with congenital heart disease (Driscoll, 1999). It can occur in any area of the septum. 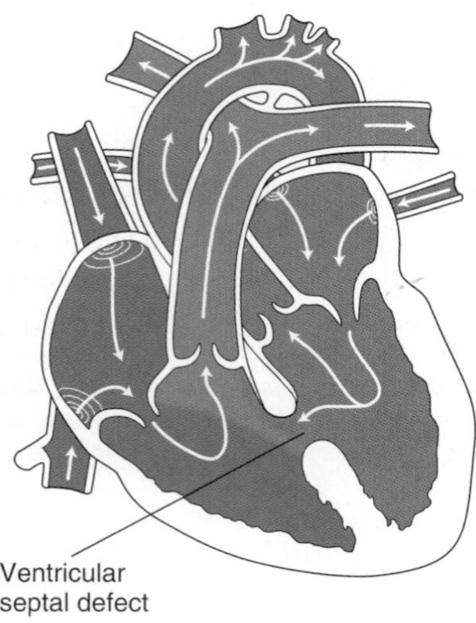 	**Clinical Manifestations** Only 15% of VSDs are large enough to cause symptoms, such as tachypnea, dyspnea, poor growth, reduced fluid intake, congestive heart failure, increased number of pulmonary infections, and pulmonary hypertension. A systolic murmur is auscultated at the third or fourth left intercostal space at the sternal border. **Diagnostic Procedures** A chest radiograph and ECG reveal few findings in cases of small VSDs. Larger VSDs with shunting are associated with enlarged heart and pulmonary vascular markings on chest radiograph. On ECG right and left ventricular hypertrophy may be seen. Echocardiogram establishes the diagnosis if shunting is present. Cardiac catheterization is used only in preparation for surgery. Increased oxygen is noted in the right ventricle and increased systolic pressure is found in the right ventricle and pulmonary artery. **Clinical Therapy** Most small VSDs close spontaneously within the first 6 months of life. Treatment is conservative when no signs of congestive heart failure or pulmonary hypertension are present. Surgical patching of VSD during infancy is performed when poor growth is evident. Closure of VSD by transcatheter device (i.e., Rashkind device) during cardiac catheterization may be attempted for some defects. Prophylaxis for infective endocarditis is required. *Prognosis:* Highest risk associated with surgical repair is in the first few months of life. Children respond well to surgery and experience substantial catch-up growth. Malignant tachyarrhythmias and right bundle branch block are possible complications.
Atrioventricular Canal (Endocardial Cushion Defect) Atrioventricular (AV) canal refers to a combination of defects in the atrial and ventricular septa and portions of tricuspid and mitral valves. Of children with congenital heart defects, 4%–5% have a total or partial AV canal (Driscoll, 1999). This defect is associated with Down syndrome. **Endocardial cushions** are fetal growth centers for mitral and tricuspid valves and AV septum. The most complex AV canal malformation results in one AV valve and large septal defects between both atria and ventricles. 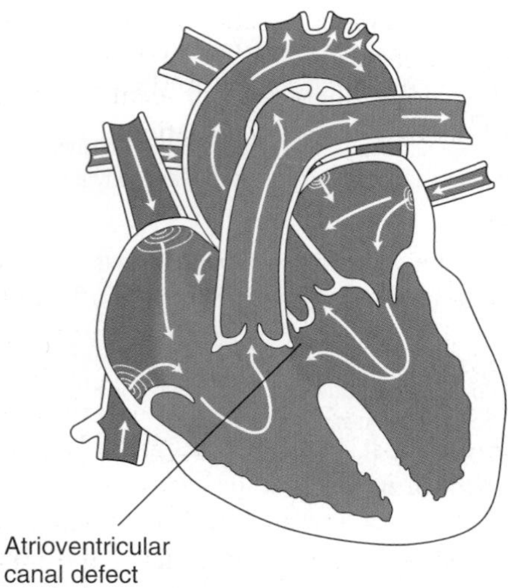 	**Clinical Manifestations** Severity of symptoms depends on amount of mitral regurgitation and the left to right shunting of blood across the septum. Infants have congestive heart failure, tachypnea, tachycardia, poor growth, recurrent respiratory infections, and repeated respiratory failure. A holosystolic murmur is loudest at left lower sternal border, and the intensity reflects the amount of mitral regurgitation. S_1 is accentuated and S_2 is split. **Diagnostic Procedures** On chest radiograph, cardiomegaly and pulmonary vascular markings are present. On ECG, atrial enlargement, right ventricular hypertrophy, and an incomplete right bundle branch block are noted. Echocardiogram reveals presence of dilation of the ventricles, septal defects, and details of valvular malformation. Cardiac catheterization reveals increased oxygen in the right atrium, increased right ventricle and/or pulmonary artery pressure. **Clinical Therapy** Surgery is performed during infancy to prevent pulmonary vascular disease. Palliative pulmonary artery banding may be performed to reduce blood flow to the lungs and congestive heart failure in an effort to let the infant grow before corrective surgery is performed. Patches are placed over septal defects, and valve tissue is used to form functioning valves. Occasionally the mitral valve is replaced. Oxygen may be required until surgery, but oxygen may also increase the pulmonary blood flow and worsen congestive heart failure. Prophylaxis for infective endocarditis is required. *Prognosis:* Information on long-term survival following successful surgery is lacking. Arrhythmias and mitral valve insufficiency occur postoperatively. There is no difference in short-term survival rates between infants with and without Down syndrome.

NURSING MANAGEMENT PRIOR TO SURGERY

Nursing Assessment and Diagnosis

Physiologic Assessment

Prior to surgery the infant or child is seen regularly to assess growth, and for progression of signs of congestive heart failure. Many infants will have no problems growing because their defect is small, such as those infants and children with an atrial septal defect or small ventricular septal defect. Failure to gain weight is an indication of an increased metabolic rate and inability to consume adequate calories for both metabolic function and growth. Assessment of length and head circumference growth is also important to determine the full impact of the condition on growth.

Psychosocial Assessment

Assess the ability of the parents to cope with the diagnosis of their infant's congenital heart defect. Initially parents may be in shock and feel guilty and anxious. The newborn often looks healthy and has few symptoms. Parents need an opportunity to express their feelings and to begin learning to cope with their child's illness. The initial period of diagnosis, hospitalization, and early care of the infant at home is very stressful. Parents need special support if their infant has a life-threatening heart defect.

Following are examples of nursing diagnoses associated with heart defects having increased pulmonary blood flow and their complications.

- Excess Fluid Volume related to heart failure and pulmonary vasculature overload
- Ineffective Infant Feeding Pattern related to shortness of breath and fatigue
- Risk for Infection related to pulmonary vascular congestion and chronic illness
- Interrupted Family Processes related to crisis of child's serious illness

Planning and Implementation

Nursing management is similar to the care provided to the child with congestive heart failure. See page 898 for specific nursing interventions.

Family Education

Participate with members of the cardiology team to provide information and education to the family about the child's condition. Information may include the following:

- General information about the congenital heart disease, including a description of the heart's anatomy and physiology and the defect (Box 26–3)
- Specific information about the multiple interactive factors associated with congenital heart disease; this information can often help reduce parents' guilt about the child's defect
- Sample case histories with good and poor prognoses
- Overview of the child's prognosis and timing of medical and surgical interventions

BOX 26–3 Resources for Parents and Children with Congenital Heart Defects

MediaLink: Support for Families

For Parents

If Your Child Has a Congenital Heart Defect by the American Heart Association

The Parent's Guide to Children's Congenital Heart Defects by Gerri Freid Kramer and Shari Maurer, Three Rivers Press

King of Hearts: The True Story of the Maverick Who Pioneered Open Heart Surgery by G. Wayne Miller.

For Children and Teens

Pump the Bear by Gisella Olivo Whittington, Brown Books (Young Children)

Overcoming Challenges! Congenital Heart Defects: Life After Heart Surgery by Melissa Curnel, Gorham Printing (Children and Teens)

A Night Without Stars by James Howe, Camelot (Older Children, Teens and Adults)

Psychosocial Support

Parents may need support for their anxiety regarding an uncertain outcome of surgery. Determine if parents have a support system as they learn about the infant's diagnosis and make difficult decisions about the child's surgery. Identify some resources for support, such as social services or pastoral services, if the parents do not have adequate support systems. Some parents may be concerned that signing consent for surgery places the child in even more danger of illness or even death. Consider identifying a parent whose child has a similar heart defect to provide support and information.

Parents should be offered genetic counseling if planning a future pregnancy. Parents may need support and care during pregnancy as fetal echocardiography can identify structural heart defects as early as 18 to 20 weeks' gestation.

Home Care

Children are often managed at home until surgery is scheduled. The initial important focus is on growth, so the parents should encourage feeding, but allow the infant to nurse or take formula for up to 30 minutes. Breastfeeding is encouraged because of its beneficial effects for the infant. If the infant has difficulty gaining weight, high caloric formula may be used. Feedings through a nasogastric or gastrostomy tube may also be given at night or 24 hours a day. Even when nasogastric or gastrostomy feedings are used, encourage the infant to take some formula orally to provide positive oral stimulation. See page 897 regarding nursing management of congestive heart failure.

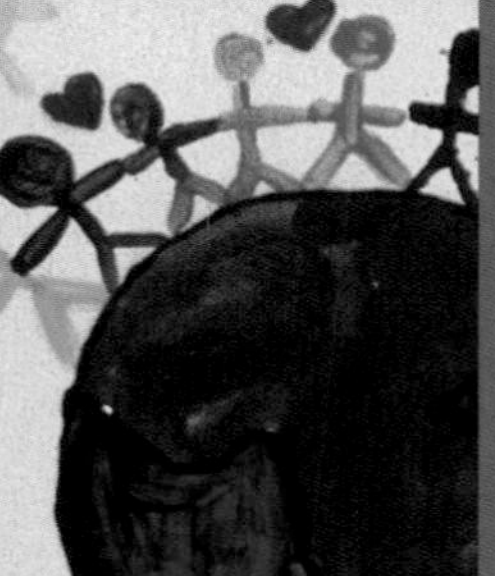

PARTNERING WITH FAMILIES

Home Care of Children with Congenital Heart Defects Before Surgery

Routine healthcare

- Wash hands frequently to prevent transmission of infections to the infant.
- Provide well-child care and all immunizations, including influenza vaccine and monthly injections of Palivizumab for respiratory syncytial virus during the fall and winter. Live virus vaccines may need to be postponed for 3 months if surgery is scheduled and blood products will be used.
- Brush the teeth twice a day and provide fluoride treatment if the water is not fluoridated. Have the child visit the dentist beginning at 2 to 3 years of age for preventive dental care.

Administration of medications

- Give medications safely with a dosage schedule that fits the family's routine.
- Keep digoxin locked up to prevent ingestion by the patient or other children in the family.

Signs of illness

- Notify physician if the child has the following signs: fever, vomiting, or diarrhea. It is important to maintain adequate hydration.
- Notify the physician if the infant or child begins feeding poorly. This may be the initial sign of congestive heart failure.

Activity

- Allow the child to set his or her own activity level. Children with congenital heart defects usually do not overexert themselves.

Efforts should be made to reduce the infant's exposure to infectious diseases as the illness can further increase the stress on the child's cardiac system.

PRACTICE ALERT

Children with complex congenital heart defects have a greater risk for developing infections, and for experiencing special problems when ill. Examples of problems causing extra concern include the following:

- Severe respiratory infections make hypoxemia worse in children with cyanosis.
- Fever increases the metabolic rate and oxygen demands which can further stress the heart.
- If the child has polycythemia, dehydration can lead to thrombus formation.
- If the child has vomiting and diarrhea leading to electrolyte disturbances, the heart function can be affected and digoxin toxicity can develop if the child takes digoxin.

Adapted from Cook, E. H., & Higgins, S. S. (2004). Congenital heart disease. In P. Jackson Allen & J. A. Vessey, Primary care of the child with a chronic condition *(4th ed., p. 389), St. Louis: Mosby.*

Regular well-child visits should be made and all immunizations provided according to the recommended schedule. Monthly prophylaxis for respiratory syncytial virus with Palivizumab should be provided during the peak season. See Chapter 25∞. See Partnering with Families: Home Care of Children with Congenital Heart Defects Before Surgery.

Preparation for Surgery

When preschool age or older, prepare the child for the settings, equipment, and experiences to expect during anesthesia induction and in the postoperative period. Pictures or a visit to the intensive care unit will be helpful. Follow guidelines for preoperative treatment described in Chapter 17∞. If an infant or toddler is having surgery, provide parents with information about how the child will look, equipment that will be used, and what care will be provided in the immediate postoperative period.

Evaluation

- Adequate nutritional intake is by oral feeds and supplemental nasogastric feeding as necessary.
- The child maintains a growth pattern that follows the established growth curve percentile.
- The child receives all immunizations and RSV prophylaxis to reduce the potential for acute illnesses.

NURSING MANAGEMENT AT THE TIME OF SURGERY

Children with these heart defects are hospitalized either because of complications, such as congestive heart failure, or for surgery. The goal of nursing management is to perform assessments, provide supportive care to the family, and meet the child's nursing care needs before and after surgery.

Nursing Assessment and Diagnosis

At the time of surgery, the child needs a careful history and physical examination to detect the presence or potential development of any acute illnesses. Assess the child's behavioral patterns, cardiac function, respiratory function, weight, and fluid status. Refer to the earlier discussion of nursing assessment for children with congestive heart failure on page 897 for additional assessment guidelines for the child with a congenital heart defect of increased pulmonary blood flow.

Critical Care

In the immediate postoperative period the child will be cared for in the intensive care unit (Figure 26–8 ■). The child's arterial and venous pressures, vital signs, oxygen saturation, core temperature (as hypothermia is commonly used during surgical procedures), and level of consciousness are frequently assessed to assure adequate tissue perfusion and to detect arrhythmias. The heart is auscultated for clarity of heart sounds, and lungs are

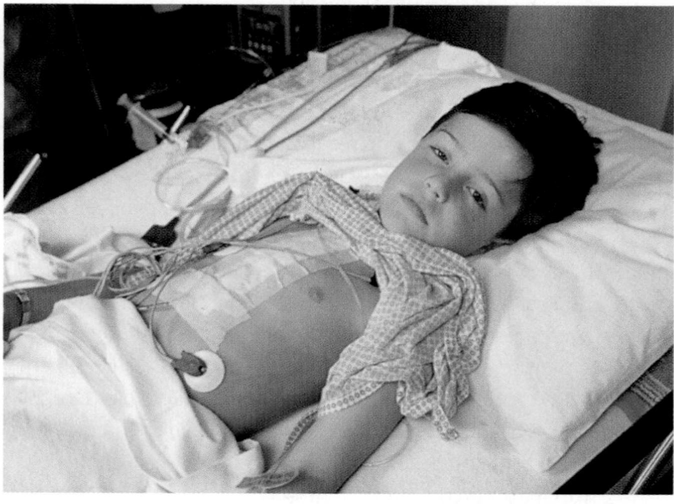

FIGURE 26–8 ■ A child with atrial septal defect repair. Surgery is performed with this type of defect to prevent pulmonary vascular obstructive disease as an adult.

auscultated to assess breath sounds. Assess for arrhythmias. Supraventricular arrhythmias are the most common in the early postoperative period for most surgeries. Postoperative junctional ectopic tachycardia is seen most often following repair of complex defects (LeRoy, 2001). Monitoring cardiac output is especially important as the child's history of increased pulmonary blood flow can result in increased pulmonary vascular reactivity. Monitor fluid intake and output. Monitor for chest tube drainage and bleeding, acid–base and electrolyte imbalances, and the child's pain level.

General Nursing Unit

After the child's return to the general nursing unit, assessment focuses on signs of surgical complications such as infection, arrhythmias, and impaired tissue perfusion. Monitor the child's temperature and inspect the surgical incision site. Fever, excessive incisional pain, spreading erythema around the incision, and wound drainage beginning 3 to 4 days postoperatively may be early signs of infection. Assess the respiratory system for breath sounds, respiratory effort, and signs of distress that may indicate pneumonia or fluid in the pleural space. Monitor the vital signs, including blood pressure.

Because the child may no longer be on a cardiac monitor, auscultation of the apical pulse to detect an irregular heart rate or bradycardia is essential. Either condition is an indication of reduced cardiac output that requires immediate intervention. To assess for impaired tissue perfusion, check pulse oximetry, capillary refill, extremity warmth, pedal pulses, level of consciousness, and urine output. Reduced urine output is a sign of decreased cardiac output. Continue to assess the child's pain.

Examples of nursing diagnoses following cardiac surgery include the following:

- Ineffective Breathing Pattern related to respiratory muscle fatigue
- Acute Pain related to surgical incision and expansion of chest with coughing and deep breathing exercises
- Risk for Imbalanced Fluid Volume related to impact of surgery on heart's pumping action
- Impaired Spontaneous Ventilation related to sedation and pain management

■ Planning and Implementation

Critical Care Unit

Nursing care following surgery focuses on promoting the child's recuperation. Following surgical correction of the heart defect, the child is usually cared for in an ICU until stable. Depending upon the complexity of surgery and potential complications, the ICU stay may be 1 or more days. The child will be initially intubated and on a ventilator, and when the child is stable and able to breathe independently, the ventilator will be turned off and the endotracheal tube will be removed. Suctioning is performed as needed until the child can handle secretions. Several intravenous lines will be placed after the child is under anesthesia to monitor arterial and venous pressures, and to infuse fluids. Blood samples may be obtained from the arterial line. Chest tubes will be placed to drain air, fluids and blood from around the heart and lungs. Radiant heat warmers may be used to help maintain the child's temperature or to rewarm a child when hypothermia has been used during surgery.

Pain Management

Pain management with 24-hour intravenous opioids should be provided for several days postoperatively until the child is taking fluids. Once the child is taking oral fluids and foods, oral analgesics may be provided, but these should also be provided around the clock. Follow the guidelines for pain management provided in Chapter 18∞. Make sure parents and caregivers know how to lift and move the child in a manner that reduces stress on the incision and potential pain.

Promoting Respiratory Function

Encourage the child to take deep breaths and cough or to perform spirometry exercises regularly to promote full lung expansion. Provide tips for splinting the chest (a pillow or stuffed animal) to reduce the pain associated with coughing and deep breathing. Chest physiotherapy may be performed in children under 3 years of age. Inspect the child's incision regularly for signs of infection.

Manage Fluids and Nutrition

Encourage the infant or child to begin oral fluids and nutrition when permitted. Although oral fluids are rarely limited, intake and output should be assessed carefully. Parents may be encouraged to bring in favorite foods to encourage the child when they can be tolerated. Administer antibiotics as ordered. If intravenous antibiotics are continued after the child's oral intake is normal, the intravenous line can be converted to a heparin or saline lock.

Encourage the child to increase activity gradually with longer periods out of bed every day. However, assure adequate

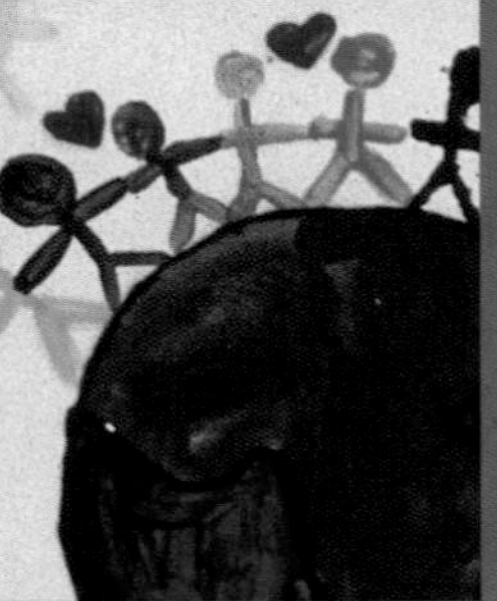

PARTNERING WITH FAMILIES

Home Care of the Child After Cardiac Surgery

- Sponge bathe the infant or use a tub bath with low water level to bathe the child. Avoid soaking the incision for a prolonged period of time until sutures are out and the incision is healed. Clean the incision daily with gentle baby or pH-balanced soap. Do not use oils, creams, lotions, or ointments on the incision. Cover the incision with a clean shirt or bib to keep it clean and dry. In infants, make a special effort to keep the area under the chin clean and dry to reduce the risk of infection in this area of the incision.
- Avoid picking the child up with hands placed under the arms as this will put stress on the incision and cause pain. Pick infants and young children up by placing one hand under the head and the other hand under the hips.
- Allow the child to increase activity gradually as tolerated. Report increased fatigue or decreased activity tolerance to the physician.
- Call the healthcare provider about any concerns regarding the child's health and recovery.
  - Report any signs of wound infection (redness, swelling, tenderness, or drainage around the incision), fever over 40.3°C (101°F), flulike symptoms, a change in appetite or activity level, irritability, or an increased respiratory rate.
  - High fever, chest pain, increased respiratory and heart rates occurring within a few weeks of surgery may indicate postpericardiotomy syndrome. The child needs to be evaluated for severity of the condition.
- Acetaminophen or ibuprofen can be given for pain control. Use the dose appropriate for the weight of the infant or child.
- Place infants in car safety seats for travel home from the hospital. Place a small blanket over the incision to prevent the straps from rubbing the incision area.
- Allow the child to gradually increase activity. Physical activities such as rough play, bike riding, or climbing should be postponed for 6 weeks until the sternum incision has healed completely. The child should return to school in approximately 3 weeks, but this varies by type of surgery performed.
- Antibiotics should be given for dental and surgical procedures as directed (some children need for several months and some need for the rest of their lives). Report any unexplained fever or illness during the first 2 months following surgery. The child is at higher risk for infective endocarditis during this period.

rest periods to promote healing. Provide diversional activities and opportunities for therapeutic play so the child can better manage the stresses associated with pain and frightening procedures.

Discharge Planning and Home Care Teaching

Infants and children may be discharged from the hospital within a few days of surgery. Parents need information spread over several days rather than at one session to prepare for continuing care of the child at home. This enables the parents to hear information more than once and to identify questions and concerns. Encourage a nutritious diet and snacks so the infant or child has an opportunity to catch up for previous growth deficits. Acetaminophen or ibuprofen may be used for pain management after discharge. See Partnering with Families: Care of the Child After Cardiac Surgery.

Prepare parents for potential behavior problems of young children that may result from the stressful experience of the hospitalization. It is not unusual for children to experience nightmares, separation anxiety, and overdependence on parents. Encourage parents to reassure children about their security, to promote play and other means to deal with their feelings. When the child's symptoms continue for several weeks, referral for psychological assessment and support may be needed for posttraumatic stress disorder. See Chapter 34∞.

Reassure parents by telling them that the child with a complete correction of the cardiac defect should have no further cardiovascular problems. Provide parents with full information about the child's defect and the surgery performed, so parents are able to share with the child's current and future healthcare providers. Encourage parents to allow the child to live a normal and active life. The normalization of the child's life should be reinforced at the surgical follow-up visits.

Children are at risk for infective endocarditis, especially within the first 6 months after surgery. The child should receive prophylactic antibiotics according to the American Heart Association recommendations in the medication box on page 917. Any unexplained fever or malaise seen in the 2 months following surgical repair or after dental work may be a sign of infection. The child should be examined for petechiae and spleenomegaly. Blood cultures, blood cell count, and urinalysis should be performed to assist in the diagnosis. Children with positive cultures are referred for immediate treatment.

■ Evaluation

Examples of expected outcomes of nursing care include the following:

- The child's pain is effectively managed.
- Full lung expansion is maintained with spirometry exercises or chest physiotherapy.
- The child's incision heals without infection.
- Catch-up growth occurs over the next few months to years.

Defects Causing Decreased Pulmonary Blood Flow and Mixed Defects

Etiology and Pathophysiology

Defects Causing Decreased Pulmonary Blood Flow. Defects that obstruct the pulmonary blood flow to the lungs or an embryologic failure that permits no connection of the right-sided blood flow to the lungs decrease pulmonary blood flow. This results in little or no blood reaching the lungs to get oxygenated. If an atrial or ventricular septal opening exists between the left and right side of the heart, right-sided pressures

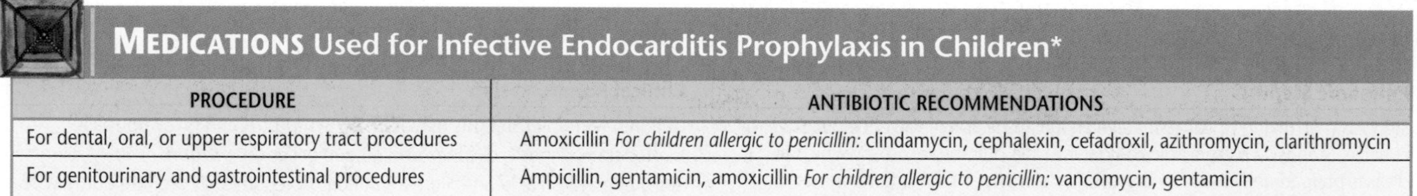

MEDICATIONS Used for Infective Endocarditis Prophylaxis in Children*

PROCEDURE	ANTIBIOTIC RECOMMENDATIONS
For dental, oral, or upper respiratory tract procedures	Amoxicillin *For children allergic to penicillin:* clindamycin, cephalexin, cefadroxil, azithromycin, clarithromycin
For genitourinary and gastrointestinal procedures	Ampicillin, gentamicin, amoxicillin *For children allergic to penicillin:* vancomycin, gentamicin

**One large dose is given 1 hour before the procedures. In high-risk patients, a smaller dose may be given 6 hours after the procedure.*

Modified from Dajani, A. S., Taubert, K. A., Wilson, W., Bolger, A. F., & Bayer, A., et al. (1997). Prevention of bacterial endocarditis: Recommendations of the American Heart Association. Journal of the American Medical Association, *277*(22), 1794–1801.

exceed those on the left, resulting in right to left shunting. Evidence of cyanosis that does not respond as expected to oxygen is a classic sign of decreased pulmonary blood flow related to congenital heart disease (Figure 26–9 ■).

The kidneys produce the erythropoietin hormone that stimulates the bone marrow to produce more red blood cells, resulting in **polycythemia,** an above-normal increase in the number of red cells in the blood to increase the amount of hemoglobin available to carry oxygen. Over time the survival time of platelets is reduced, and there is impaired synthesis of vitamin K–dependent clotting factors. These factors increase the infant's risk of bleeding with surgery.

Chronic polycythemia can result in sluggish blood flow through the small vessels placing infants and children at increased risk for thromboembolism in the cerebral and pulmonary vessels. Brain abscesses are more common in children with cyanotic heart defects. The capillaries in the lungs usually filter out bacteria in the blood returning from the systemic circulation. However, when unoxygenated blood enters the systemic circulation through the right to left shunt, bacteria can travel directly to the brain.

When infants and children with cyanosis rise in the morning, they may experience an abrupt decrease in systemic resistance and pulmonary blood flow. This physiologic change can trigger a hypercyanotic (hypoxic or "tet") episode when combined with a sudden increase in cardiac output and venous return associated with such activities as crying, feeding, exercise, warm bath, and straining with defecation. The partial pressure of oxygen (PO_2) is lowered, and the partial pressure of carbon dioxide (PCO_2) rises. In this severe decompensation the hypoxemia becomes progressively worse as the respiratory center in the brain overreacts, increasing the respiratory effort. The additional respiratory effort further increases the cardiac output and contributes to a life-threatening decline unless rapid intervention is successful.

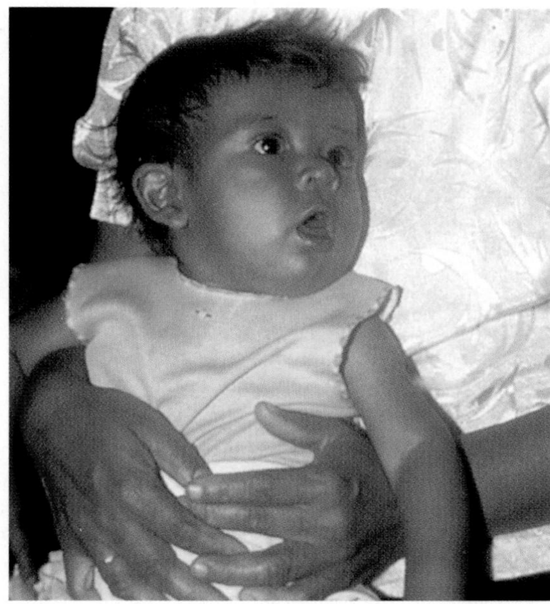

FIGURE 26–9 ■ This infant has a congenital heart defect with decreased blood flow. What is the prognosis for an infant who has either of the most common malformations—tetralogy of Fallot or transposition of the great vessels?

Mixed Defects. Many complex congenital heart defects involve a combination of defects that fall into one of the previous three categories. What is unique about them is that the newborn is dependent upon the mixing of the pulmonary and systemic circulations for survival during the postnatal period. This mixing of saturated and desaturated blood results in a general desaturated systemic blood flow and cyanosis. Pulmonary congestion occurs because of increased pulmonary blood flow and obstruction of systemic flow.

Clinical Manifestations

Defects Causing Decreased Pulmonary Blood Flow. Clinical manifestations in infants initially include cyanosis, dyspnea, and a loud murmur. Cyanosis often occurs when the ductus arteriosus closes, causing hypoxemia. The skin may initially be ruddy or mottled before cyanosis is observed. Signs and symptoms of chronic hypoxemia include fatigue, clubbing of the fingers and toes, exertional dyspnea, and delayed developmental milestones. The infants may need to stop sucking periodically during feedings to breathe, and diaphoresis may be seen with the increased work of eating. These infants have a higher metabolic rate, and inadequate calories may be consumed resulting in poor weight gain. See Table 26–9 for the pathophysiology, clinical manifestations, and clinical therapy for the congenital heart defects that decrease pulmonary blood flow.

PRACTICE ALERT

Cyanosis is typically observed when the amount of reduced hemoglobin in the veins reaches a level of about 5 g/100 mL, usually because of desaturation of arterial blood in children with congenital heart defects (Park, 2002). When the child is anemic, the oxygen saturation must be very low before cyanosis is observed because there is less overall circulating hemoglobin. In cases of polycythemia, there is much greater circulating hemoglobin, so cyanosis becomes apparent at a higher oxygen saturation level.

TABLE 26–9	Pathophysiology, Clinical Manifestations, and Clinical Therapy for Heart Defects with Decreased Pulmonary Blood Flow

DEFECT PATHOPHYSIOLOGY	CLINICAL MANIFESTATIONS AND CLINICAL THERAPY
Pulmonic Stenosis Stenosis (narrowing of valve or valve area) can be above valve, below valve, or at valve. Stenosis obstructs blood flow into the pulmonary artery, which increases preload and results in right ventricular hypertrophy. Pulmonic stenosis is the second most frequent congenital heart defect, accounting for 8%–12% of all cases (Park, 2002). Stenosis may progress as the heart muscle grows and develops in the subvalvular area. 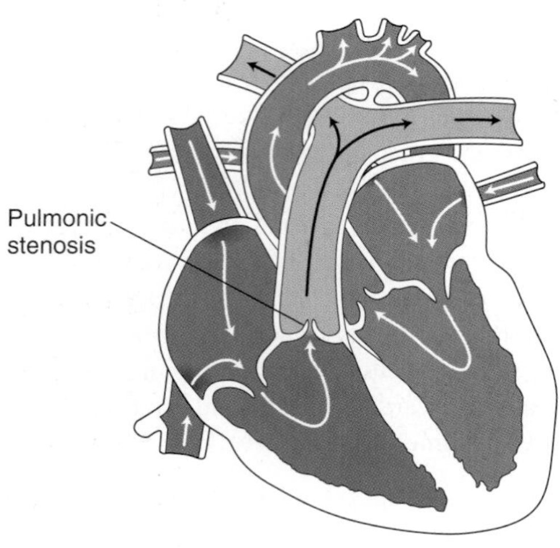 	**Clinical Manifestation** Children with mild stenosis may have no symptoms and grow normally. In moderate stenosis, dyspnea and fatigue occur on exertion. Signs of congestive heart failure and hepatosplenomegaly are rare but may result from chronic pressure overload. Heart failure and chest pain on exertion may occur in severe cases. A loud systolic ejection murmur with a widely split S_2 and thrill may be found in the pulmonic listening area. **Diagnostic Procedures** Diagnosis is usually made at birth after auscultation of murmur. The chest radiograph may show an enlarged pulmonary artery with normal heart size and normal pulmonary vascularity. The ECG may demonstrate right atrial enlargement and right ventricular hypertrophy. Echocardiogram provides information about pressure gradient across valve and size of valve ring. Cardiac catheterization findings include increased right ventricular pressure and a normal or slightly lowered pulmonary artery pressure. **Clinical Therapy** Dilation by balloon valvuloplasty, performed during cardiac catheterization, has been widely successful for treatment of simple pulmonic stenosis. Surgical valvotomy may still be used, especially when other defects such as VSD are present. Surgical resection may be needed for narrowing above the valve area. Pulmonary regurgitation may result, but is not a significant problem. *Prognosis:* Pulmonic stenosis does not typically increase in severity. Lifelong infective endocarditis prophylaxis is necessary.
Tetralogy of Fallot A combination of four defects: pulmonic stenosis, right ventricular hypertrophy, ventricular septal defect (VSD), and overriding of aorta make up the condition. Some children have a fifth defect: open foramen ovale or atrial septal defect (ASD). About 10% of children with congenital heart defects have tetralogy of Fallot (Park, 2002). Elevated pressures in right side of heart, causing right to left shunt, characterize this defect. 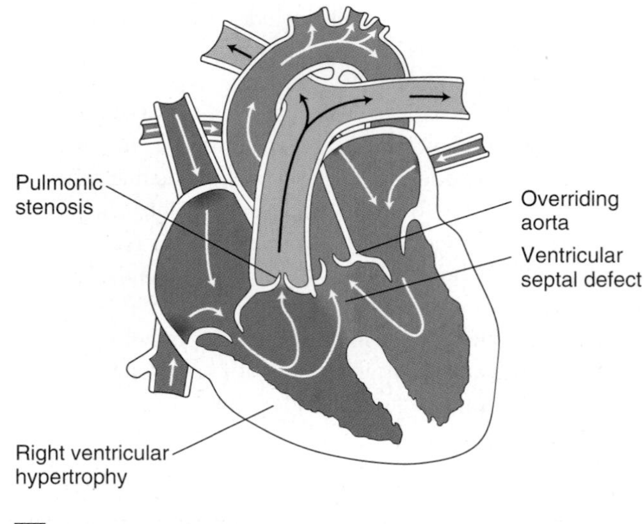 	**Clinical Manifestations** As ductus arteriosus closes, infant becomes hypoxic and cyanotic. The degree of pulmonary stenosis determines severity of symptoms. Infants have a systolic murmur heard in pulmonic area that is transmitted to suprasternal notch. A thrill may also be palpated in the pulmonic area. Polycythemia, hypoxic spells, metabolic acidosis, poor growth, clubbing, and exercise intolerance may develop. Toddlers instinctively squat (assume a knee–chest position) to decrease the return of systemic venous blood to the heart. **Diagnostic Procedures** A chest radiograph shows the boot-shaped heart due to the large right ventricle, decreased pulmonary vascular markings, and a prominent aorta. Electrocardiogram (ECG) shows right ventricular hypertrophy. Echocardiogram demonstrates VSD, obstruction of pulmonary outflow, an overriding aorta, and the size of the pulmonary arteries. Cardiac catheterization provides details about the anatomy of the right ventricular outflow region, the location of all anatomic structures, and any additional defects. Blood laboratory tests reveal increased hematocrit and hemoglobin levels and an increased clotting time. **Clinical Therapy** Management of hypercyanotic episodes includes placing the infant in knee–chest position, calming the child, giving oxygen, and administering morphine and propranolol intravenously. Monitoring the child for metabolic acidosis or prolonged unconsciousness is critical. A total repair is often performed before 6 months of age when the infant has a hypercyanotic episode. Corrective surgery may be attempted in asymptomatic children by 6 months of age. *Prognosis:* Not all children are cured by surgery, but most have improved quality of life and improved longevity. Arrhythmias and right ventricular dysfunction may be residual problems (Waldman & Wernly, 1999). Lifelong infective endocarditis prophylaxis is required.

TABLE 26–9 Pathophysiology, Clinical Manifestations, and Clinical Therapy for Heart Defects with Decreased Pulmonary Blood Flow (continued)

DEFECT PATHOPHYSIOLOGY	CLINICAL MANIFESTATIONS AND CLINICAL THERAPY
Pulmonary Atresia Pulmonary atresia is the absence of communication between the right ventricle and the pulmonary artery, either at the site of the pulmonary valve or in the main pulmonary artery. The right ventricle pushes blood back through the tricuspid valve for passage through the foramen ovale. The PDA provides the only flow of blood to the pulmonary arteries. A ventricular septal defect (VSD) or transposition of the great arteries (TGA) is also often present. 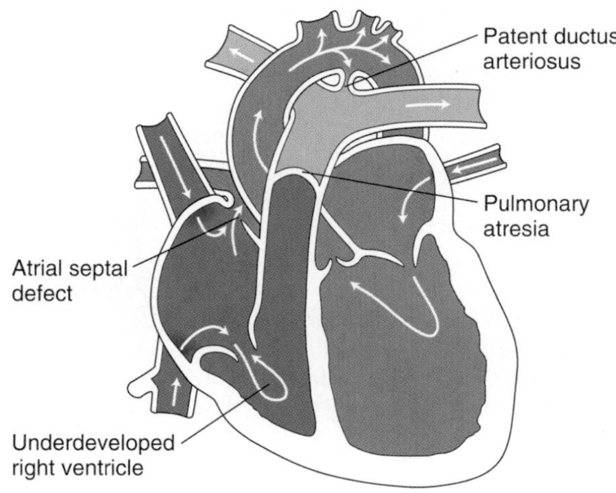 	**Clinical Manifestations** Cyanosis is present at birth. Tachypnea, congestive heart failure, pulmonary edema, hepatomegaly, acidosis, hypoxic spells, clubbing, polycythemia, and growth delays occur. A continuous murmur from the PDA is heard in pulmonic area. A single S_2 is heard in the aortic area, and a harsh systolic murmur may be heard in the tricuspid area. **Diagnostic Procedures** The chest radiograph may reveal a normal-size heart or one slightly enlarged. The ECG may reveal right atrial hypertrophy. The echocardiogram shows a small hypoplastic right ventricular cavity and tricuspid valve, the absence of the right ventricular outflow tract, a dilated right atrium, and right to left shunting across the atrial septum. If a VSD is present, right to left shunting will be detected with the possibility of a normal-size right ventricle. **Clinical Therapy** Prostaglandin E_1 is given immediately to maintain a patent ductus arteriosus. Digoxin and diuretics are also used. The Rastelli balloon atrial septostomy is performed to increase the atrial opening. A Rastelli or modified Fontan procedure results in improved survival. *Prognosis:* Outcome depends upon the size of the pulmonary outflow tract developed by surgery and the fibrosis in the right ventricle. The child is at increased risk for arrhythmia and right ventricular dysfunction.

When the infant or child has severe obstruction to pulmonary blood flow, hypercyanotic episodes can occur suddenly. Toddlers with uncorrected cyanotic heart disease often squat to relieve dyspnea (Figure 26–10 ■). The knee–chest position reduces the cardiac output by decreasing the venous return from the lower extremities and by increasing the systemic vascular resistance. Hypercyanotic episodes usually appear between 2 months and 2 years of age. Signs include:

- Increased rate and depth of respirations
- Increased cyanosis, pallor, and poor tissue perfusion
- Increased heart rate
- Diaphoresis
- Irritability and crying
- Seizures and loss of consciousness

Older children with a diagnosis of congenital heart disease may have additional symptoms. Exercise-induced dizziness and **syncope** (transient loss of consciousness and muscle tone) are serious signs indicating a need for medical evaluation.

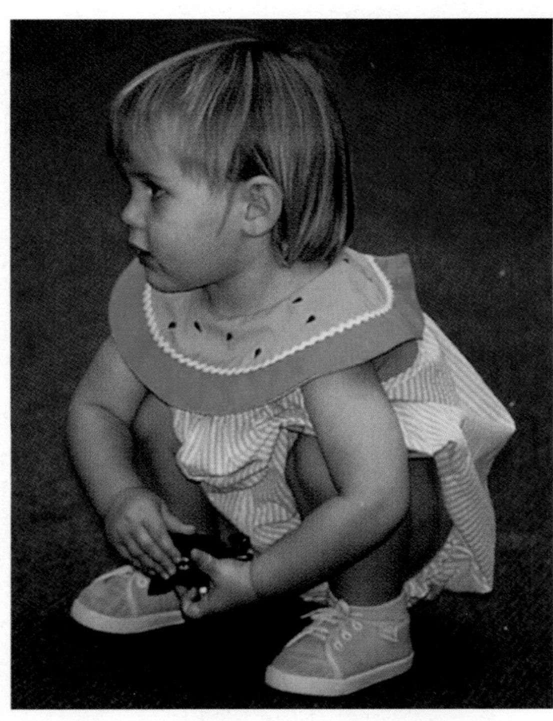

FIGURE 26–10 ■ A child with a cyanotic heart defect squats (assumes a knee–chest position) to relieve cyanotic spells.

Mixed Defects. Infants with these complex congenital heart defects have varying degrees of cyanosis and congestive heart failure. In cases when the pulmonary vascular resistance is lower than the systemic resistance, pulmonary congestion develops, followed by congestive heart failure. In cases when the pulmonary blood flow is decreased, the infant will have more severe cyanosis and polycythemia (Suddaby, 2001). See Table 26–10 for the pathophysiology, clinical manifestations, and clinical therapy for these complex mixed defects.

TABLE 26–10 Pathophysiology, Clinical Manifestations, and Clinical Therapy for Mixed Defects

DEFECT PATHOPHYSIOLOGY	CLINICAL MANIFESTATIONS AND CLINICAL THERAPY
Transposition of the Great Arteries (TGA) In this disorder the pulmonary artery is the outflow tract for left ventricle, and the aorta is the outflow tract for the right ventricle, creating parallel circulations. This condition is life threatening at birth, and survival initially depends on an open ductus arteriosus and foramen ovale. This condition occurs in about 5% of children with congenital heart disease (Grifka, 1999). An ASD or VSD may also be present with TGA. 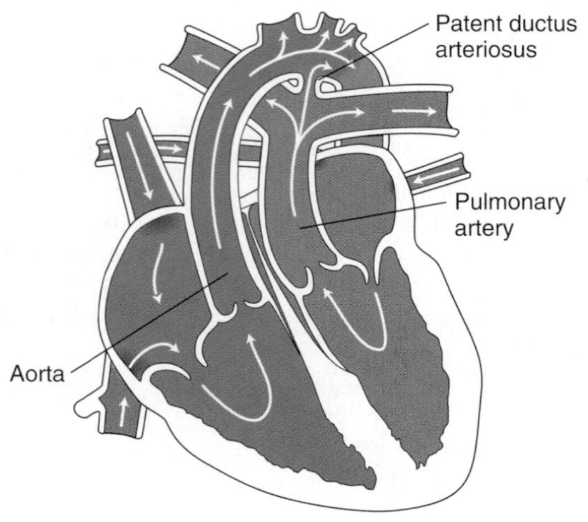 	**Clinical Manifestations** Cyanosis, apparent soon after birth, progresses to hypoxia and acidosis. Cyanosis does not improve with oxygen administration. However, cyanosis may be less apparent when a large VSD is also present. Congestive heart failure may develop immediately or over days or weeks. Tachypnea (60 respirations/min) is often present without retractions or other signs of dyspnea. A systolic murmur is auscultated if a VSD is present; otherwise no murmur is generally heard. S_2 is loud. Infants take a long time to feed and need frequent rest periods because of rapid respiratory rate and fatigue. Growth failure may be evident as early as 2 weeks of age if corrective surgery is not performed. **Diagnostic Procedures** A chest radiograph may reveal a classic egg-shaped heart on a string (narrow superior mediastinum) with enlarged ventricles and increased pulmonary vascular markings. The ECG reveals right ventricular hypertrophy. The echocardiogram reveals the abnormal positioning of the great arteries when the position of arteries arising from ventricles is visible. Cardiac catheterization shows increased right ventricular pressure, and the catheter can enter the aorta through the right ventricle. Blood laboratory tests reveal increased hematocrit and hemoglobin levels or polycythemia. **Clinical Therapy** Prostaglandin E_1 is initially ordered to maintain a patent ductus arteriosus until a palliative procedure can be performed. Corrective surgery (arterial switch) is usually performed before 1 week of age. Balloon atrial septostomy may be performed during cardiac catheterization in newborns as a first stage. This may also be corrected surgically. Other defects may be repaired in stages as the infant grows. *Prognosis:* Survival without surgery is impossible. The 5-year survival following an arterial switch is 82%. Arrhythmias, right ventricular failure, and sudden death are long-term complications (8–15 years) after the Mustard procedure, so the Mustard or Rastelli procedure is performed only when significant pulmonary valve stenosis is present (Grifka, 1999). Other complications of surgical repair include pulmonic or aortic stenosis, coronary artery obstruction, and mitral regurgitation. Infective endocarditis prophylaxis may be necessary.
Truncus Arteriosus A single large vessel empties both ventricles and provides circulation for the pulmonary, systemic, and coronary circulations. A VSD is usually present. This occurs in less than 1% of congenital heart defects. 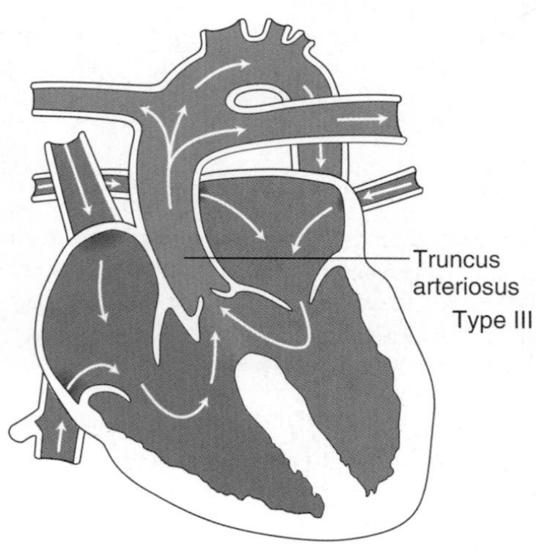 	**Clinical Manifestations** Cyanosis develops soon after birth, however, this is also a condition of increased pulmonary blood flow. Severe congestive heart failure, dyspnea, retractions, fatigue, poor feeding, poor growth, polycythemia, clubbing, increased pulse pressure, bounding peripheral pulses, frequent respiratory infections, and cardiomegaly also occur. The VSD produces a harsh systolic murmur in the lower sternal border. A systolic click may be auscultated in the apex and pulmonic area. Bounding pulses and a widened pulse pressure may also be present. **Diagnostic Procedures** The chest radiograph shows cardiomegaly, a large aorta, and increased pulmonary vascular markings. The ECG reveals right and left ventricular hypertrophy. The echocardiogram shows the absence of two semilunar valves. Cardiac catheterization documents a left to right shunt at the level of the ventricle, equal pressure in the ventricles, the truncus, and pulmonary arteries. **Clinical Therapy** Rastelli procedure is performed to close the VSD and create a passage to pulmonary arteries. Digoxin and diuretics are given. Repeated surgery is necessary to enlarge pulmonary artery conduit. *Prognosis:* Survival is improved, but truncal valve stenosis and regurgitation result. The long-term prognosis is unknown.

TABLE 26–10 Pathophysiology, Clinical Manifestations, and Clinical Therapy for Mixed Defects (continued)

DEFECT PATHOPHYSIOLOGY	CLINICAL MANIFESTATIONS AND CLINICAL THERAPY
Total Anomalous Pulmonary Venous Return The pulmonary veins empty into right atrium or veins leading to the right atrium rather than into the left atrium. The foramen ovale must remain patent for mixed blood from the right atrium to pass to the systemic circulation. Any obstruction of the pulmonary veins increases severity of the condition. 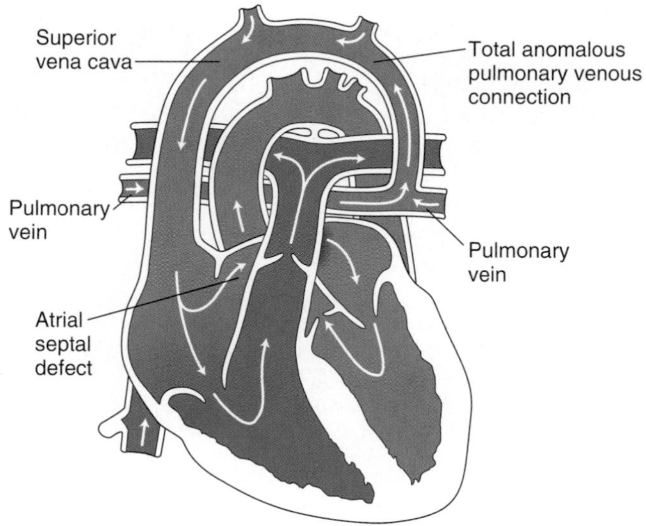 	**Clinical Manifestations** The infant may have mild cyanosis and frequent respiratory infections. If the pulmonary veins are obstructed in any way, cyanosis will be increased and there will be increased pulmonary blood flow resulting in tachycardia, dyspnea, pulmonary edema, retractions, crackles, hepatomegaly, poor feedings, irritability, and failure to thrive. Increased cyanosis may occur with feedings as the filled esophagus compresses the common pulmonary vein. A precordial bulge may be palpated. On auscultation S_2 has a wide, fixed split when there is no pulmonary vein obstruction. An ejection murmur may be auscultated in the pulmonic area, along with a gallop rhythm. If the pulmonary veins are obstructed, S_2 will be loud and single, along with a gallop rhythm. An ejection murmur may or may not be auscultated. **Diagnostic Procedures** The chest radiograph shows cardiac enlargement, a large pulmonary artery, and increased pulmonary blood flow. The ECG reveals right ventricular hypertrophy, and right atrial hypertrophy after 1 month of age. The echocardiogram shows enlargement of the right atrium, a patent foramen ovale, and the lack of continuity between the pulmonary veins and the left atrium. Cardiac catheterization shows higher oxygen level in the right atrium and the abnormal circulation. **Clinical Therapy** Prostaglandin E_1 is given to maintain patent ductus arteriosus. Hypoxemia and congestive heart failure are treated. Balloon atrial septostomy may be performed to promote better mixing of blood to enable surgery to be delayed until the infant is stabilized. Surgery to reconnect or baffle the pulmonary veins to the left atrium is performed. *Prognosis:* Survivors have lived more than 20 years after correction.
Double Outlet Right Ventricle Both of the great arteries leave the right ventricle causing increased pulmonary blood flow and reduced systemic blood flow. The only outlet for the left ventricle is a large ventricular septal defect. This occurs in < 1% of all congenital heart defects.	**Clinical Manifestations** Growth retardation, tachypnea, signs of congestive heart failure, cyanosis, clubbing Loud S_2 and a systolic murmur at the upper left sternal border, with or without a systolic thrill. **Diagnostic Procedures** Chest radiography shows cardiomegaly with increased vascular markings and a prominent pulmonary artery segment. The ECG shows right axis deviation, atrial hypertrophy, and right ventricular hypertrophy, and right bundle branch block. First degree AV block may be present. The echocardiogram shows the origin of both great arteries from the anterior right ventricle, the absence of the left ventricle outflow, and the ventricular septal defect. **Clinical Therapy** Digoxin and diuretics for treatment of congestive heart failure. Pulmonary artery banding may be performed in some infants with symptomatic increased blood flow while balloon atrial septostomy is performed in others. An arterial switch or Senning procedure with an intraventricular tunnel is created between the VSD and the pulmonary artery is used for some types. Alternatively an intraventricular tunnel between the VSD and the subaortic outflow tract with a Dacron patch is used. Infective endocarditis prophylaxis is required. *Prognosis:* About 20% of patients require additional surgery on the intraventricular tunnel (Park, 2002). Ventricular arrhythmia may cause sudden death.

COLLABORATIVE CARE

Early management of these defects is important to prevent secondary damage to the heart, lungs, and brain, including the adverse effects of hypoxemia on the child's cognitive and psychomotor development. For this reason, corrective surgery is being performed at younger ages, often in infancy. A palliative procedure may be performed first to preserve life in children with potentially lethal heart defects and complications (see Table 26–7). With some defects, corrective surgery can be postponed with a palliative procedure. This gives the infant an opportunity to grow and improve the success of corrective surgery. See Figure 26–11 ■ for various palliative shunts (surgically created channels for blood flow) that may be performed. See Tables 26–9 and 26–10 for clinical therapy for specific congenital heart defects.

Antibiotic prophylaxis for infective endocarditis is needed before and after surgical correction for many congenital heart defects. See the medications box on page 917 for a list of recommended antibiotics. Antibiotic prophylaxis for specific heart defects is provided with clinical therapy descriptions for each.

If closure of the ductus arteriosus causes life-threatening cyanosis in newborns, such as those with tricuspid atresia, pulmonary atresia, transposition of great arteries, and truncus arteriosis, prostaglandin E_1 (PGE_1) is prescribed to reopen the ductus arteriosus. These infants depend on a patent ductus arteriosus for survival or improvement in pulmonary or systemic blood flow. Treatment with PGE_1 provides time for the newborn to be transferred to a cardiac center for diagnostic evaluation and surgical intervention. Response time to PGE_1 varies depending on the type of defect. Some infants being treated with PGE_1 develop apnea that has been responsive to aminophylline. The child's hemoglobin level and hematocrit values must be monitored to ensure that the blood does not become too viscous. Polycythemia may be managed by red blood cell pheresis if the blood viscosity becomes too high. These children are also monitored for anemia, as they do not tolerate the lower hemoglobin and oxygen-carrying capacity.

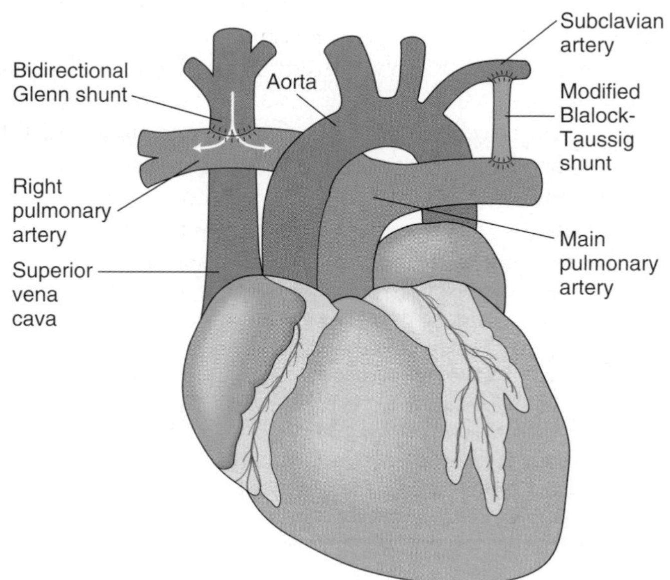

FIGURE 26–11 ■ Anatomic location of the modified Blalock-Taussig and Glenn shunts for palliative procedures.

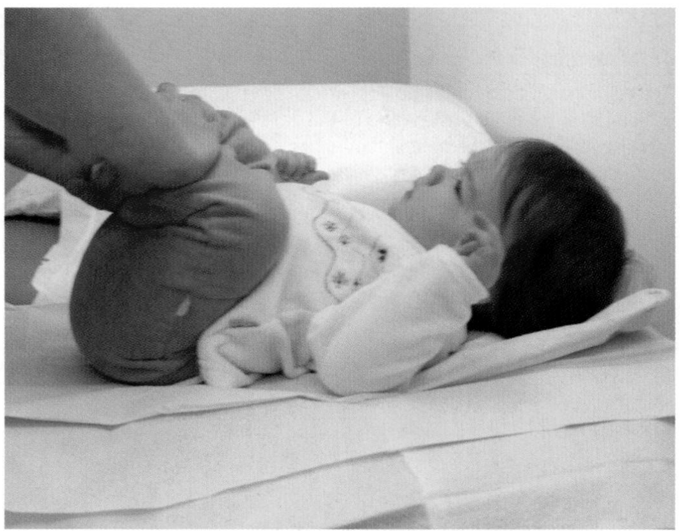

FIGURE 26–12 ■ Place the infant who has a hypercyanotic spell in the knee–chest position. This position increases systemic vascular resistance in the lower extremities.

Hypercyanotic Episodes

Hypercyanotic episodes are treated aggressively. To decrease the pulmonary vascular resistance, the initial treatment involves calming the child, giving oxygen, and administering morphine and propranolol intravenously. Packed red blood cells may be administered to improve oxygen delivery to the tissues when the child is anemic. Postpone all unpleasant procedures. To increase the systemic vascular resistance, the child is placed in the knee–chest position (Figure 26–12 ■) and given intravenous fluids to expand circulatory volume. Dopamine or phenylephrine (Neosynephrine) is also given. Once a hypercyanotic episode has occurred, immediate palliative or corrective surgery is often scheduled. Oral propranolol is administered to decrease the frequency of hypercyanotic episodes because of its action to minimize spasms of the pulmonary outflow tract (DeBoer, 1996).

NURSING MANAGEMENT

Nursing management of the hospitalized child focuses on monitoring PGE_1 therapy (for newborns only; used until palliative surgery is performed), treating hypercyanotic episodes, and providing postsurgical care. Nursing management involves supporting parents to care for the child at home until surgery is performed by reducing parental anxiety, providing adequate nutrition, helping parents recognize signs of illness or progression of the child's condition, and formulating a plan for emergency treatment.

■ Nursing Assessment and Diagnosis

Physiologic Assessment Prior to Surgery

The cardiovascular status of infants receiving PGE_1 therapy needs to be closely monitored. Assess vital signs, heart rhythm, skin color, peripheral pulses, and capillary refill time. Observe for signs of improvement in vital signs and color as the oxygen saturation increases and acidosis decreases following the initial treatment. In addition, watch for tachycardia, tachypnea, crackles, frothy secretions, low urine output, and edema, because these infants are at risk for congestive heart failure.

Prior to or between stages of surgery the infant or child is seen regularly to assess growth, and for signs of progressive deterioration in cardiac status. These children are at risk for growth problems that affect height and weight, and potentially the head circumference. The child's weight and length measurements are plotted on a growth curve to monitor the significance of the growth problems.

The child needs careful observation for signs of increased cyanosis in the morning or at other high-risk times. Observe for neurologic signs of thromboembolitic complications from polycythemia such as headache, dizziness, excessive irritability, and paralysis. Older children with cyanotic defects may have clubbing of the fingers and toes (Figure 26–13 ■).

Assessment Following Surgery

Children are admitted to the ICU following surgery. Refer to the section on nursing assessment of the child with increased pulmonary blood flow on page 914 for nursing care guidelines. Once the child returns to the general nursing unit, monitor the child's heart functioning. Assess vital signs, pulse oximetry, skin color, perfusion of the skin by capillary refill, and distal pulses. A sudden sustained increase in pulse and respirations and a decrease in peripheral perfusion may be early signs of hemorrhage. Monitoring fluid intake and output following surgery is critical. Note any signs of respiratory distress that may indicate the development of a pneumothorax or congestive heart failure.

Psychosocial Assessment

Assess the parents' need for information and emotional support. In many cases, the infant's condition is first identified at birth; however, a defect could have been identified by sonogram prenatally. The parents will be grieving the loss of a perfect newborn and be extremely anxious about the infant's condition and prognosis.

Following are nursing diagnoses that may apply to a child with cyanotic heart disease.

- Decreased Cardiac Output related to ventricular restriction and an obstructed outflow tract
- Risk for Infection related to unfiltered bacteria in the blood and sites of blood shunting that promote bacterial growth'
- Acute Pain related to palliative or corrective surgery
- Caregiver Role Strain related to care of a child with chronic illness
- Activity Intolerance related to cyanosis and dyspnea on exertion
- Delayed Growth and Development related to congenital anomaly and hypoxemia
- Ineffective Family Therapeutic Regimen Management related to complexity of therapeutic regimen: assessment and management of cyanotic spells, which are unpredictable events

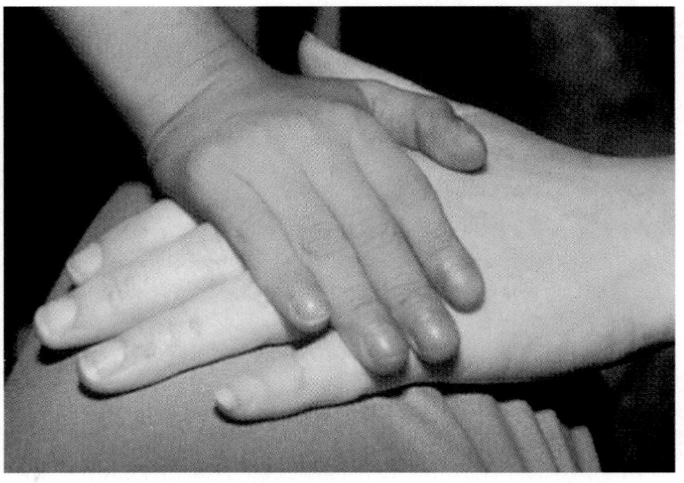

FIGURE 26–13 ■ Clubbing of the fingers is one manifestation of a cyanotic defect in an older child. What neurologic signs may be associated with such a defect?

■ Planning and Implementation

Home Care of the Child Before Surgery

Infants with tetralogy of Fallot and other defects are often managed at home initially as they grow and potentially improve surgical outcome. Parents are usually anxious because of the need to wait before surgery can be performed. They often fear that the infant will not survive until surgery or that they will be unable to manage any problems the infant may have. Provide parents with information and teach them how to care for the child at home. Some infants have such special home care needs that home health nursing and other community services are required. Many of these children require supplemental nutrition and oxygen for emergencies. These children maintain a low oxygen saturation rate because unoxygenated blood mixes with oxygenated blood, and oxygen has no effect on improving the oxygen saturation level. See Evidence-Based Practice: Parental Stress Associated with Having a Child with a Congenital Heart Defect.

Cyanosis with or without congestive heart failure often results in delayed gross motor skills. Parents become concerned that the level of cyanosis will damage the brain. Developmental specialists can help parents set realistic developmental goals for the child. Make referrals to community-based early-intervention programs to promote the child's development. Provide information about the long-term developmental outcomes of children with periods of cyanosis and subsequent surgery to help reduce their anxiety.

Encourage parents to treat the infant as normally as possible. Children with mild cyanotic lesions do not need to adjust activity. The child with moderate to severe disease should be able to tolerate crying for a few minutes without difficulty.

CLINICAL TIP

Crying may improve cyanosis caused by lung disease or disorders of the central nervous system. In children with cyanotic heart disease, crying usually makes cyanosis worse. Prolonged crying should not be permitted because it causes fatigue and further hypoxia.

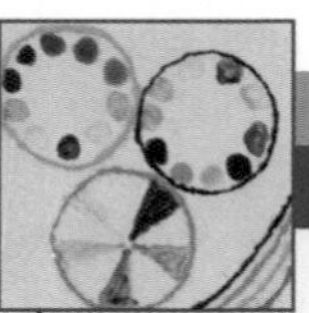

EVIDENCE-BASED PRACTICE
Parental Stress Associated with Having a Child with a Congenital Heart Defect

PROBLEM

Because the heart is known to be an organ essential for survival, it is appropriate to anticipate that parents of children will have stress and concern for their child's well-being and ability to be a normal child. Do parents of a child with a congenital heart defect have any more or less stress than parents with children having other chronic conditions?

EVIDENCE

Interest in the subject of how much stress these parents perceive was stimulated by findings that parents of infants with congenital heart disease reported higher stress than parents of children with cystic fibrosis, specifically in the sense of parental competence and acceptability of the child (Goldberg, Morris, Simmons, et al., 1990). More recently, parents of a child with congenital heart disease or Down syndrome were found to report more stress and distress than control parents or parents of a child with cleft lip and/or cleft palate (Pelchat, Ricard, Bouchard, et al., 1999). The Parenting Stress Index (PSI), a 36-item self-report measure of the amount of stress experienced by parents of young children, was used in several recent studies to further describe the nature of parenting stress. It is composed of three subscales:

- *Parental Distress*—amount of distress a parent is experiencing in his or her role as a parent, or as a function of personal factors related to parenting
- *Parent-Child Dysfunctional Interaction*—parent's perception that his or her child does not meet the parent's expectations and the interactions with his or her child are not reinforcing
- *Difficult Child*—basic behavioral characteristics of children that make them either easy or difficult to manage

A recent study reported that 80 parents of children with congenital heart disease reported significantly greater stress than the parent population in whom the PSI had been normalized; and 17.5% reported a total stress score at or above the 90th percentile. The parents also had significantly higher stress scores for the Difficult Child subscale. Parenting stress was not related to the severity of the child's heart disease (Uzark & Jones, 2003). In a study using the Swedish version of the PSI, parents of 26 children with a complex heart defect requiring multiple surgeries and 32 children with a simple defect (ventricular septal defect) requiring a single surgery were compared. No significant differences were found in parental stress (even when scores of mothers and fathers were analyzed separately) by the type of their child's congenital heart defect (Mörelius, Lundh, & Nelson, 2002). These findings were consistent with those of a study that included children with 11 different types of congenital heart defects (Davis, Brown, Bakeman, et al., 1998). One study did reveal no significant differences in PSI total and subscale scores between 30 mothers of children with moderate to severe congenital heart defects and 30 mothers of matched control healthy children. However, scores on the Parent Behavior Checklist revealed that mothers of the children with heart defects had significantly lower developmental expectations of their children than mothers of the healthy controls (Carey, Nicholson, & Fox, 2002).

IMPLICATIONS

Since the studies do not demonstrate significant differences in stress level between parents by the severity of their child's heart defect, it is important to consider the factors that could contribute to the parent's stress and help them find coping mechanisms. Nursing interventions to help parents manage their anxiety and promote healthy lives for their children and the entire family should be part of every health visit for these children (Carey et al., 2002).

- Perform a family assessment to address social supports, strengths, and resources available to the family (see Chapter 2∞).
- Provide initial education and reinforce the education provided about the child's diagnosis and treatment.
- Promote **normalization,** a philosophy of raising children as close to normal as possible, with anticipatory guidance about age-appropriate expectations about development and activity, nurturing, and strategies for discipline.
- Allow parents the time to tell stories about living with their child to help understand their stresses and strengths. This will provide valuable information to help parents develop strategies to manage their stress and to correct any misunderstandings they may have about their child's condition.

CRITICAL THINKING APPLICATION

Refer back to Brandy's situation at the beginning of the chapter. What stresses do you believe her parents are experiencing? How would you assess their anxiety and coping mechanisms? Identify two nursing interventions to help this family cope with their stress.

Teach parents to observe for signs of worsening cyanosis, particularly in the morning that could signal the beginning of a hypercyanotic episode. Provide guidelines for the initial management of the hypercyanotic episode. The parents should call for an ambulance and try to calm and reassure the infant. The infant should be placed in knee–chest position by holding the infant facing the chest, placing one arm under the knees, and folding the legs upward toward the infant's chest. Use the other arm to support the infant's back. If oxygen is available, provide it in a manner that does not further upset the infant. If none is available in the home the emergency medical technicians will administer it during transport to the emergency department.

PRACTICE ALERT

Cyanotic spells become life threatening if not treated immediately. The child becomes progressively more hypoxic and limp, loses consciousness, is likely to have a seizure or cerebrovascular accident, and may die. If they occur when the infant is at home, parents should begin recommended treatment and call 9–1–1 or their emergency number.

Vomiting and diarrhea may lead to dehydration, and parents must notify the physician when the infant or child has these symptoms. Dehydration is a particular risk in children with polycythemia because the blood can become even more viscous. Fever increases the metabolic rate and causes further stress on the heart. In dehydration, the systemic vascular resistance is decreased, resulting in a further decrease in blood flow to the pulmonary system. Aggressive management with antipyretic medication and fluid volume replacement is necessary. (See Developing Cultural Competence: Medication Interactions.)

Teach parents to observe the child for signs of infective endocarditis, including low-grade fever, fatigue, and malaise. They need to notify the physician if these symptoms occur within 2 months of surgery or a high-risk procedure. Educate parents about the need to request antibiotic prophylaxis for the child.

Assist parents to formulate an emergency plan in case the infant develops acute problems such as a hypercyanotic episode or respiratory distress. Cardiopulmonary resuscitation should be taught to the parents. Ask parents to notify the local rescue squad about the infant's problem. Prepare a card or brief history form with information about the child's condition, medications, and necessary emergency care and the physician's name for parents to keep at home (American Academy of Pediatrics Committee on Pediatric Emergency Medicine, 1999). When an acute problem occurs, this form gives important information to the emergency medical technicians and emergency department staff.

Although parents may travel with cyanotic children, they should not take them to areas of high altitude without first consulting with the physician. Supplemental oxygen when traveling on an airplane may be necessary.

Hospital-Based Care of Infant and Child

CARE OF THE NEWBORN

Monitor and carefully maintain the central, umbilical, or peripheral intravenous lines in the newborn receiving continuous infusion of PGE_1. Observe the infant for side effects of prostaglandin treatment. Common side effects of PGE_1 therapy include cutaneous vasodilation, bradycardia, tachycardia, hypotension, seizure activity, fever, and apnea. Have intubation equipment and a resuscitation bag and mask at bedside in case of apnea. Have intravenous fluids available to control hypotension.

INFANTS AND TODDLERS PRIOR TO SURGERY

If a hypercyanotic episode occurs, immediately place the child in the knee–chest position and administer oxygen. Administer morphine as ordered. Immediately notify the physician for further orders if these procedures are ineffective and the episode continues. Avoid any unpleasant or anxiety-provoking procedures.

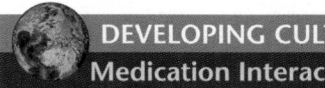

DEVELOPING CULTURAL COMPETENCE
Medication Interactions

Caution parents of children with congenital heart defects to avoid using complementary therapies such as herbal products as they may interfere with the medications being used to manage the child's heart condition. Products containing ginkgo are known to interact with warfarin, of particular concern for any child on anticoagulant therapy. Full research on many of these herbal remedies has not been conducted, so the potential side effects and interactions with prescribed medications is not known (Cook & Higgins, 2004).

FOLLOWING SURGERY

The child is initially cared for in the intensive care unit as described on page 914. Postoperative bleeding is a potential risk in children with polycythemia, because bleeding times are prolonged and platelet counts are low. Chest tube output is monitored carefully for bright red blood or excessive volume. Bright red blood in the chest tube is a significant sign of hemorrhage. Fluids and diuretics are used to maintain preload (the volume of blood in the ventricle at the end of diastole that stretches the heart muscle before contraction) in the right ventricle whereas inotropic drugs are used to support cardiac output. Children are transferred to the general nursing unit once heart function has stabilized.

Once the child returns to the general nursing unit, nursing care is the same as described for the child having surgery for increased pulmonary blood flow.

Evaluation

Examples of expected nursing care outcomes include the following:

- The parents recognize a hypercyanotic episode, initiate emergency treatment, and seek emergency care for the child.
- The parents manage fever and medical illnesses to prevent dehydration and potential hypercyanotic episodes.
- The child becomes stable following surgery and has no complications.
- The child attains expected developmental progress in gross motor, fine motor, and language skills following surgical repair of the congenital heart defect.

See the Health Promotion and Maintenenance Overview on page 926.

Defects Obstructing Systemic Blood Flow

Etiology and Pathophysiology

An anatomic **stenosis** (narrowing of a valve, area around the valve, or in the great artery above the valve) causes obstruction to blood flow and results in a pressure load on the ventricle and decreased cardiac output. The greater the narrowing, the more obstructed the blood flow is to the pulmonic or systemic circulation. This results in a higher-pressure gradient in the ventricle, increased afterload on the ventricle, and decreased cardiac output.

Clinical Manifestations

Clinical manifestations of these congenital heart defects are those associated with a low cardiac output: diminished pulses, poor color, delayed capillary refill time, and decreased urinary output. The blood cannot move past the obstruction, so it backs up into the left atrium and then into the lungs, causing congestive heart failure and pulmonary edema. With mild obstructions, the child may have leg cramps, cooler feet than hands, and stronger pulses in the upper extremities than the lower extremities. The blood pressure which is usually 10 to 15 mm Hg higher in the legs than the arms may be lower than the reading in the arms. Decreased blood supply to the gastrointestinal tract may result in necrotizing enterocolitis. See Chapter 30∞. See Table 26–11 for the

Health Promotion & Maintenance Overview

The Adolescent with Congenital Heart Disease

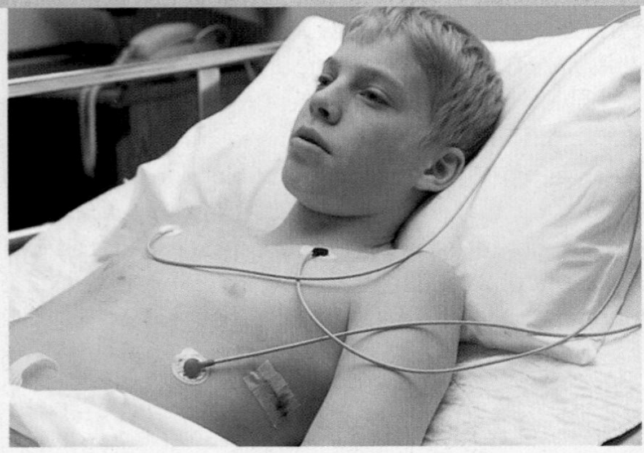

Disease Prevention Strategies

- Ensure that the adolescent completes all immunizations and adolescents with a significant congenital heart disease should get the influenza vaccine annually.
- Encourage visits to the dentist twice a year for cleaning and restoration of decayed teeth as needed. Make sure the adolescent knows this is one way to reduce endocarditis risk.
- Encourage regular visits to the primary care provider for general health and illness care.
- Provide appropriate health screening according to recommended schedules (see Chapter 15∞).
- Encourage female adolescents to initiate gynecologic care to ensure that appropriate contraception and other gynecologic care needs are addressed. Ensure that the adolescent understands risks associated with pregnancy and the potential need for special care during pregnancy.
- Provide counseling about health risks associated with tobacco use, alcohol and drug use, and unprotected sex.

Nutrition and Physical Activity

- Inquire about the adolescent's preferred exercise and activity level. An individualized assessment with graded exercise testing on a treadmill or bicycle should be performed to determine specific exercise and activity limitations for the adolescent's condition. Depending on the significance of the congenital heart disease, participation in competitive sports and strenuous work may be limited. Adolescents who have had a complete repair can participate in team sports. Adolescents taking anticoagulants may have other activity limitations.
- Encourage the adolescent to participate in normal gym activities and other recreational and sports activities to the best of their physical abilities.
- Encourage the adolescent to eat nutritious meals and snacks, and to avoid excess weight gain that could stress the heart function.

Endocarditis Risk and Prophylaxis

- Discuss situations that place the adolescent at risk for endocarditis: body piercing, tattooing, acupuncture, electrolysis, dental care, intrauterine device for contraception, and various diagnostic and surgical procedures (Alderman, 2000).
- Provide education about the need for antibiotic prophylaxis and the need to inform all healthcare providers about the defect and need for prophylaxis. Provide the adolescent with the guidelines for endocarditis prophylaxis published by the American Heart Association. See page 917.

Mental and Spiritual Health

- Discuss the adolescent's concerns for the future, as there may be significant uncertainty about the disease course and outcome.
- Identify and refer adolescents as needed for counseling or to a support group of adolescents of similar age with congenital heart disease.
- Begin the process of transitioning the adolescent to adult healthcare in which full responsibility for ongoing healthcare will become the role of the individual rather than the parents.

Patient Education

- Provide education directed to the adolescent about the specific nature of the congenital heart defect, surgeries that have been performed, and the types of symptoms resulting. Remember that previous education has been targeted to the parents.
- Provide a written succinct summary of the key points regarding medical management of the adolescent's condition that can be used when visiting other health professionals. This summary should include the following: diagnosis, operations, medications and their side effects, contraception, exercise prescription, endocarditis prophylaxis, and frequency of medical follow-up (Higgins & Tong, 2003).
- Discuss the medications needed and why, and develop plans for the adolescent to assume responsibility for self-administration.
- Discuss the future treatment needed for the condition and frequency of cardiac evaluations. Make sure the adolescent understands the need for preventive healthcare and finding a primary care provider.
- Discuss the genetic aspects of the condition and provide resources for genetic counseling if desired.
- Discuss any activity or other limitations, such as strenuous work.
- Discuss the danger signs of the condition (such as arrhythmias, or the potential of dehydration in an adolescent with cyanosis) and how to seek urgent or emergency care. Role-play may help the adolescent gain confidence in seeking advice from health professionals.

Vocational Education

- Reassure the adolescents who have had complete repairs of the congenital heart defect and have no disabilities that they have no limitations in their career or vocational selection.
- Provide career and vocational counseling to adolescents with cardiac disabilities that match their interests and clinical limitations. If a job application asks about disabilities, the adolescent does not need to disclose the heart problem if it will not interfere with the job being sought.
- Inform adolescents with congenital heart disease–related disabilities about their rights under the Americans with Disabilities Act of 1990.
- Families and patients should be informed to identify health insurance options, and to identify those policies that have fewer restrictions. Adolescents need to be informed about carefully investigating healthcare coverage when considering a job change so that healthcare coverage is not lost (Canobbio, 2001).

TABLE 26–11 Pathophysiology, Clinical Manifestations, and Clinical Therapy for Heart Defects that Obstruct the Systemic Blood Flow

DEFECT PATHOPHYSIOLOGY | **CLINICAL MANIFESTATIONS AND CLINICAL THERAPY**

Aortic Stenosis

Narrowing of the aortic valve obstructs blood flow to systemic circulation. The narrowing may be subvalvular, at the valve, or supravalvular. Aortic stenosis accounts for 3%–6% of all cases of congenital heart defects (Fedderly, 1999). This defect is often associated with bicuspid rather than normal tricuspid valve. The pressure gradient across the valve usually increases as the child grows and cardiac output increases.

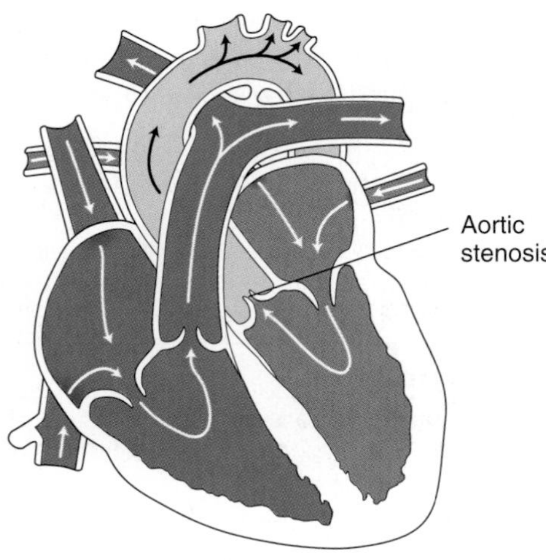

Clinical Manifestations

A majority of infants and young children are asymptomatic and grow and develop normally.

Some newborns have life-threatening aortic stenosis noted at birth.

The blood pressure is normal, but there is often a narrow pulse pressure.

Occasionally the child complains of chest pain after exercise, but exercise intolerance is uncommon.

Peripheral pulses may be weak.

Fainting and dizziness are serious signs that require intervention.

Congestive heart failure develops in infants with significant stenosis.

A systolic heart murmur and thrill in the aortic or pulmonic listening areas with transmission to the neck are usually detected in routine physical examination in the school-age child or adolescent. An ejection click may be heard. With severe aortic stenosis splitting of the S_2 may be noted. Aortic insufficiency may result from interventions, causing a high-pitched diastolic decrescendo murmur along the left sternal border near the mitral area.

Diagnostic Procedures

The chest radiograph is usually normal, but may reveal a slight prominence of the left ventricle and aorta with increased severity.

The ECG is usually normal in mild cases, but may show mild left ventricular hypertrophy and inverted T waves with increased severity.

An echocardiogram reveals the number of the valve cusps, pressure gradient across valve, and size of aorta.

Stress testing may be used in asymptomatic children to determine amount of obstruction present with exercise.

Clinical Therapy

Newborns with life-threatening aortic stenosis need PGE_1 to maintain a patent ductus arteriosis until the aortic valve can be dilated.

The aortic valve may be successfully dilated by balloon valvuloplasty.

Surgical treatment is palliative rather than curative.

Surgical valvuloplasty may also be performed.

Aortic valve replacement is performed when stenosis is severe or if significant regurgitation results from other interventions.

Prognosis: Chest pain, syncope, and sudden death can occur in symptomatic children, particularly during vigorous exercise. Stenosis is usually progressive during childhood as the valve calcifies. Valve replacement may ultimately be necessary, once the child reaches adulthood, at which time lifelong anticoagulant therapy will be needed. Lifelong infective endocarditis prophylaxis is required.

Coarctation of the Aorta

Narrowing in the descending aorta near the ductus arteriosus or left subclavian artery obstructs systemic blood outflow. This defect is common, occurring in 5%–8% of all children with congenital heart disease (Fedderly, 1999).

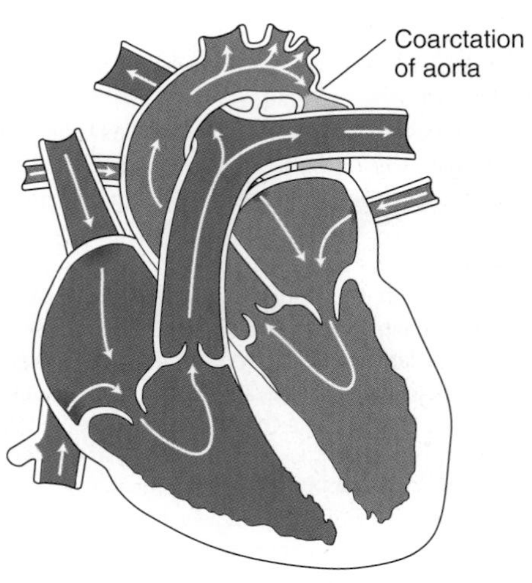

Clinical Manifestations

Many children are asymptomatic and grow normally, but constriction is progressive.

Up to 20%–30% of infants develop congestive heart failure by 3 months of age.

Reduction in blood flow through the descending aorta causes lower blood pressure in legs and higher blood pressure in arms, neck, and head. In cases when significant reductions in systemic circulation occur, renal failure and necrotizing enterocolitis may develop.

Brachial and radial pulses are typically bounding, but femoral pulses are weak or absent.

Older children may complain of weakness and pain in the legs after exercise.

S_2 is loud and single on auscultation. A systolic ejection murmur may be heard at the upper right and middle or lower left sternal border. A thrill may be palpated in the suprasternal notch.

Diagnostic Procedures

The chest radiograph may reveal cardiomegaly, pulmonary venous congestion, and indentation of descending aorta. Rib notching (change in the smooth contour of the rib apparent on radiograph) from collateral vessels is rarely seen before 10 years of age.

ECG shows left ventricular hypertrophy, and right ventricular hypertrophy may be seen in severe cases.

(continued)

TABLE 26–11	**Pathophysiology, Clinical Manifestations, and Clinical Therapy for Heart Defects that Obstruct the Systemic Blood Flow (continued)**

DEFECT PATHOPHYSIOLOGY	CLINICAL MANIFESTATIONS AND CLINICAL THERAPY
	Diagnostic Procedures (continued) Echocardiogram permits measurement of the size of the aorta, imaging of the actual coarctation, and functioning of the aortic valve and left ventricle. Both cardiac catheterization and magnetic resonance imaging show the site of coarctation. **Clinical Therapy** Balloon dilation may be performed during cardiac catheterization for both initial relief and recoarctation. Some centers are performing balloon dilation on infants under 3 months of age through the umbilical artery to avoid injury to the femoral artery (Rao, Jureidini, Balfour, et al., 2003). Balloon dilation and surgical resection and anastomosis are palliative, as coarctation may recur. Surgical resection can be performed with the subclavian artery used as a patch in the infant. Repair in the first year of life is preferred to decrease exposure to hypertention. *Prognosis:* Postcoarctectomy syndrome (abdominal pain and distention) occurs in 20% of patients (Walters, 2000). Persistent hypertension in adulthood is common. Infective endocarditis prophylaxis is needed.
Hypoplastic Left Heart Syndrome Absence or stenosis of mitral and aortic valves associated with an abnormally small left ventricle, a small aorta, and aortic or mitral stenosis or atresia. As one of the most severe congenital heart defects, it is the largest contributor of infant deaths due to congenital heart disease (Cook & Higgins, 2004). 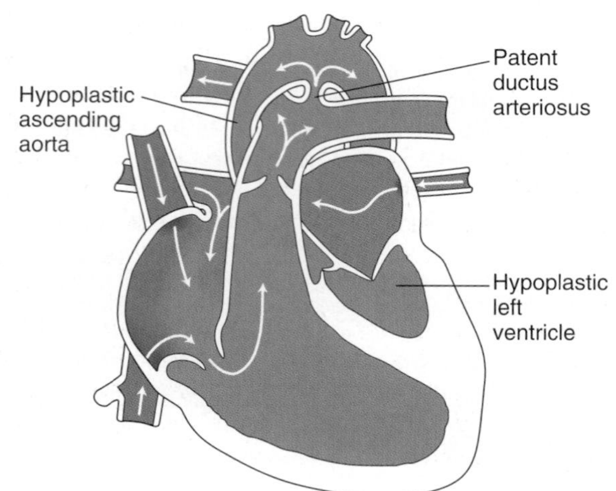	**Clinical Manifestations** Signs are initiated with closure of ductus arteriosus and include progressive cyanosis, tachycardia, tachypnea, dyspnea, retractions and decreased peripheral pulses. A systolic murmur may be present or absent. Poor peripheral perfusion, pulmonary edema, and congestive heart failure eventually lead to shock, acidosis, and death. **Diagnostic Procedures** The chest radiograph shows cardiomegaly and increased pulmonary vascularity. The echocardiogram shows the small left ventricle. This condition may be diagnosed prenatally, as early as the first trimester. Cardiac catheterization may be performed in preparation of surgical intervention. **Clinical Therapy** Prostaglandin E_1 is given to maintain a patent ductus arteriosus. Supplemental oxygen avoided. Three treatment options are currently available for these infants: comfort or palliative care, the Norwood procedure, and heart transplantation. See page 929 for care associated with heart transplantation. Over the past 10 years, surgery has been offered more frequently, and by 2004 it is anticipated the Norwood procedure will be offered as the first intervention to 50% of these infants in the United States. Surgery is performed in three stages. The Norwood procedure is performed in the first week of life, and it carries the highest risk of mortality. The Glenn procedure is performed at about 3 to 8 months of age, and the Fontan procedure is performed between 18 months and 3 years of age. The surgical palliative procedures give the child a chance to reach adolescence before the heart fails and a heart transplant is needed. See Table 26–6 for more information about these procedures. Up to 63% of infants waiting for a heart transplant die waiting for a donor heart (Jenkins, Flanagan, Jenkins, et al., 2000). In Canada, approximately 50% of parents choose comfort care (Osiovich, Phillipos, Byrne, et al., 2000). *Prognosis:* Without surgery, the median survival time is 3 days, and only a few survive longer than 1 month. Mortality rates in infants having a first-stage Norwood procedure are approximately 10%–20% in the first year of life (Cook & Higgins, 2004). Some large centers have achieved a 70% 5-year survival rate with the Norwood procedure, but mortality remains high in many centers (Chang, Chen, & Klitzner, 2002). The child will have some limitations in physical activity because of a single ventricle. Additionally, many of these children have significant neurocognitive and neurodevelopmental impairment (Mahle, Clancy, Moss, et al, 2000). Failure of the single ventricle occurs over time, and these children may require a heart transplant during adolescence or adulthood.

pathophysiology, clinical manifestations, and clinical therapy for the congenital heart defects that obstruct systemic blood flow.

Collaborative Care

Neonates with critical left outflow obstruction or left ventricular dysfunction may develop decreased cardiac output and shock. PGE_1 and inotropes may be required to support the systemic circulation until the obstruction is relieved or ventricular function improves.

Nursing Management

Children with aortic stenosis and coarctation of the aorta should have nursing care as described in the nursing management sections in "Congenital Heart Defects that Increase Pulmonary Blood Flow." Infants with hypoplastic left heart syndrome should have nursing care as described in the nursing management sections in "Defects Causing Decreased Pulmonary Blood Flow and Mixed Defects."

Parents of children with life-threatening defects such as hypoplastic left heart syndrome are put in the position of making quick decisions about the best treatment for their child. For this condition there is no cure, and a decision must be made that is best for their individual situation. Parents have not yet had the opportunity to grieve the loss of a normal infant or cope with their emotions before being faced with the potential death of the newborn. Parents do not have the time to carefully weigh the information about the various treatment options; however, it is important to try to support parents through this difficult decision-making period. Share the following information with parents so they are fully informed for decision making: treatment options and their associated mortality, the intense care that the surviving child will need, potential neurocognitive and neurodevelopmental outcomes, and unknown long-term survival. If parents choose comfort or palliative care, interventions such as PGE_1 are discontinued and the infant is given appropriate pain medication and comfort. Seek the support of clergy, social workers, or other supportive individuals in the family's life to assist them through this period. (See Chapter 22∞.)

Cardiomyopathy

Cardiomyopathy is a serious disorder of the heart's muscle. An annual incidence of 1.13 to 1.24 per 100,000 children has been estimated (Lipshultz, Sleeper, Towbin, et al., 2003; Nugent, Daubeney, Chondros, et al., 2003). It occurs most often in infancy. The population at higher risk for the condition includes Hispanics and African Americans; a strong familial or genetic influence is also apparent (Lipshultz, et al., 2003). Cardiomyopathy may be primary, or not due to a specific cause. The highest incidence of cardiomyopathy in the pediatric population occurs during the first year of life, and the second peak incidence is during adolescence. Males have a higher incidence than females. Almost 40% of children with symptoms of cardiomyopathy die of the condition within 2 years or receive a heart transplant (Strauss & Lock, 2003).

Dilated Cardiomyopathy

Dilated cardiomyopathy accounts for about 51% of cases. Neuromuscular disorders, such as muscular dystrophy, and viral myocarditis were the most common identified causes of this type of cardiomyopathy (Lipshultz et al., 2003). Barth syndrome is a genetically linked cardiac disease that primarily targets males. Most cases have an unknown cause. It is often diagnosed in the first year of life and can cause dilated cardiomyopathy. This form may develop as the ventricles stretch or dilate to accommodate increased blood volume. However, the heart muscle does not contract and pump blood effectively. The blood flows more slowly through the heart and clots may form. This places the child at risk for emboli to the lungs and the brain. The child usually presents in congestive heart failure with tachypnea, wheezing, and poor cardiac output. Arrhythmias may develop that can cause cardiac arrest. Treatment involves anticoagulants, vasodilators, antiarrhythmics, diuretics and digoxin, and ultimately a heart transplant may be considered. An implantable cardioyerter-defibrillator may be used for the child who survives cardiac arrest or for the child who has evidence of ventricular arrhythmias.

Hypertrophic Cardiomyopathy

Hypertrophic cardiomyopathy accounts for about 42% of cases. Approximately 30% to 60% of cases appear to be genetically transmitted as an autosomal dominant trait (Park, 2002). This form is associated with the enlargement or hypertrophy of the ventricular muscles or enlargement of the ventricular septum makes the ventricular walls rigid. The resulting reduced size of the ventricular chamber causes obstruction of blood flow and does not allow the heart to relax appropriately. Symptoms include exertional dyspnea, fatigue, dizziness, fainting, palpitations, and chest pain. Digoxin is contraindicated and diuretics may worsen symptoms (Park, 2002). Surgery for subaortic stenosis may be performed if this is the cause of left ventricular outflow obstruction. Antiarrhythmic medications may be used based on findings of ambulatory ECG monitoring. An implantable cardioverter-defibrillator may be used when the child with this condition has unexplained syncope. Abnormal heart rhythms may lead to sudden death. Recent studies show that 36% of young athletes who die suddenly have hypertrophic cardiomyopathy (American Heart Association, 2003).

Nursing Management

Nursing management for dilated cardiomyopathy is the same as for children with congestive heart failure unless or until a heart transplant is performed. Nursing management for hypertrophic cardiomyopathy involves frequent visits to assess the child's condition and to review progress with antiarrhythmic medications. See page 938.

Heart Transplantation

Approximately 375 pediatric heart transplants are performed annually. The indications for heart transplant vary by age (Odim, Laks, Burch, et al., 2000).

- Infants—primarily congenital heart disease, such as hypoplastic left heart syndrome and other complex defects
- Children 1 to 10 years—cardiomyopathy (50%), congenital heart disease (40%)
- Adolescents—cardiomyopathy (65%), congenital heart disease (25%)

MediaLink Care Plan: Pediatric Heart Transplant

In the cases of children and adolescents with congenital heart disease, the cause is often associated with acquired myopathy associated with past reconstructive and palliative procedures. Contraindications for heart transplantation include significant pulmonary vascular resistance, severe metabolic disease, severe hepatic dysfunction, multiple congenital anomalies, and advanced multiple organ failure.

With improved immunosuppressive protocols and surgical techniques, patient survival rates are increasing (89% at 1 year and 65% at 5 years) (Boucek, 2000; Luikart, 2001). The use of ventricular assist devices and extracorporeal membrane oxygenation (ECMO) prior to transplantation has been found to improve the child's recovery from end-organ failure and enhance transplantation outcome (Luikart, 2003).

Rejection and infection are the major causes of mortality and morbidity, particularly in the first year following the transplant. The triple immunosuppression regimen often includes tacrolimus or cyclosporin A, azathioprine, and corticosteroids. Tacrolimus is now preferred for immunosuppression rather than cyclosporin in many centers (Buck, 2003). High dose intravenous steroids are used to treat episodes of acute rejection.

Endomyocardial biopsy, performed during a cardiac catheterization, is used to detect rejection in the early postoperative period. Echocardiograms are also used to assess cardiac function, cardiac wall motion, and wall thickness. Signs of organ rejection include the following (Duitsman, Suddaby, & Masterson, 1999):

- Increasing resting heart rate, arrhythmias, bradycardia
- Presence of a third heart sound
- Cool and mottled extremities
- Inspiratory crackles, diaphoresis, tachypnea, pulmonary edema
- Hepatosplenomegaly
- Oliguria

Bacterial, fungal, and viral (i.e., cytomegalovirus, herpes viruses, varicella zoster) infections cause the most problems; however, some common childhood illnesses (acute otitis, colds) may be well tolerated. Many children who survive the initial year after transplant may survive to reach adulthood; however, hypercholesterolemia and graft coronary artery disease then become causes of late transplant failure. Medications, such as lovastatin, to reduce the serum cholesterol level may be given. Calcium channel blockers may be used to treat hypertension. Some children have received a second heart transplant for graft coronary artery disease, although morbidity and mortality are greater with the retransplantation.

Nursing Management

After recovery from surgery, children may have near-normal exercise capabilities and normal heart function, and return to school and other activities. Immunosuppressive medications will be continued long term and can cause a variety of physical side effects such as the following: hair growth, gum hyperplasia, weight gain, short stature, moon facies, acne, and rashes. Children and adolescents may need support to develop positive self-esteem due to their appearance.

Depending on the age at time of transplant, the child may not have had all immunizations. Live virus vaccines are often not given to immunosuppressed children (see Chapter 19∞). Help parents arrange for schools and childcare centers to provide early notification of cases of measles, mumps, rubella, and chickenpox. Preventive treatment for the child can be provided as necessary. Handwashing and other methods to reduce the spread of infection should be encouraged both at home and at school.

Organ rejection is a major concern of families. Provide education for the parents and child to carefully follow the immunosuppression regimen, to recognize the signs of rejection, and to seek treatment promptly. Adolescents may be at particular risk of nonadherence to their immunosuppression regimen and risk rejection (Ringewald, Gidding, Crawford, et al., 2001). Osteoporosis and obesity may occur as a result of corticosteroid treatment. Families need to encourage a diet and exercise program to reduce the child's risk for obesity and osteoporosis.

Pulmonary Artery Hypertension

Pulmonary artery hypertension is a complication of many congenital heart defects, as well as pulmonary conditions and congenital diaphragmatic hernia.

Etiology and Pathophysiology

In children with congenital heart defects that increase pulmonary blood flow, pulmonary vascular resistance develops. The pulmonary vascular bed compensates to reduce this excessive pulmonary blood flow by vasoconstriction. Over time the smooth muscle in the small pulmonary arteries increases to sustain the vasoconstriction if the increased pulmonary blood flow is not controlled. If the child has left ventricular dysfunction, pressures in the pulmonary venous system increase. The pulmonary artery pressure must then increase to push blood across the vascular bed. Inflammation, hypertrophy of pulmonary vessels, and fibrosis develop. The increased pressure leads to a right to left shunt, and right heart function is impaired. The condition may become life threatening (Barst, 1999).

Clinical Manifestations

Hypoxemia and acidosis result from pulmonary hypertension and help maintain the vasoconstriction. The infant displays tachypnea, cyanosis, retractions, and fatigue. Feeding is difficult, and weight loss with fluid and electrolyte imbalance is likely. Older children will have exertional dypsnea, chest pain, and syncope.

Collaborative Care

Clinical therapy involves surgery to correct an obstructive lesion or close a defect. Therapy for pulmonary artery hypertension related to noncardiac conditions involves bronchodilators, antibiotics, corticosteroids, and low flow oxygen. No cure is available, but life can be prolonged with these measures (Barst, 1999). Short-term nitric oxide therapy has been effective in reducing pulmonary vascular resistance through vasodilation, and has been found to shorten the duration of mechanical ventilator support (Kinsella, Parker, Ivy, et al., 2003).

Nursing Management

Nursing care focuses on promoting rest for oxygen conservation, monitoring fluid intake and output carefully, and administering medications and oxygen. Airplane travel may be possible with supplemental oxygen. Exercise should be tailored to avoid dyspnea. Give parents needed support and information about their child.

ACQUIRED HEART DISEASES

Infective Endocarditis

Infective endocarditis is an inflammation of the lining, valves, and arterial vessels of the heart caused by bacterial, enterococci, and fungal infections. It is not preventable in all cases. The frequency of infective endocarditis appears to have increased in recent years due to the following:

- Improved survival of children with complex congenital heart disease
- Increased numbers of children and newborns with multiple complex medical problems treated in critical care units with indwelling venous catheters

Etiology and Pathophysiology

An increasing number of children with infective endocarditis have had corrective or palliative surgery with or without implanted vascular grafts, patches, or prosthetic valves. The highest risk for infective endocarditis appears to be in children who had surgery for obstruction to pulmonary blood flow or aortic valve replacement (Ferrieri, Gewitz, Gerber, et al., 2002).

Infections may occur after the causal organism enters the bloodstream during dental work or surgery and lodges on damaged or abnormal endocardial tissue. In children with congenital heart disease, a high velocity or turbulent blood flow can injure the endocardium. Indwelling catheters positioned in the right side of the heart also damage the endocardium or valve endothelium.

Clinical Manifestations

Symptoms can be mild and develop slowly, or they can be severe and develop rapidly. The child may have a prolonged low-grade fever and other symptoms such as fatigue, weakness, weight loss, joint and muscle aches, and diaphoresis. Signs may include a new or changing murmur, congestive heart failure, decreased oxygen saturation levels, dyspnea, hematuria, petechiae, and splenomegaly (Brook, 1999). Children with indwelling catheters may initially have pulmonary symptoms or signs related to septic pulmonary embolism. Newborns have variable and nonspecific signs such as feeding difficulties, respiratory distress, and tachycardia, which are difficult to distinguish from congestive heart failure and septicemia (Ferrieri et al., 2002).

COLLABORATIVE CARE

Diagnostic Procedures

The Duke Criteria are used for the diagnosis of infective endocarditis (Box 26–4). Infective endocarditis is diagnosed primarily by blood culture; however, urine and cerebrospinal fluid also may be cultured. Elevated erythrocyte sedimentation rate, anemia, elevated C-reactive protein level, increased white blood cell count, alterations in the electrocardiogram, and changes in heart sounds and murmurs are indicators of the condition. Two-dimensional echocardiography is the main method to detect the presence of vegetation or infective lesions in the heart, extent of valve damage, and cardiac function. Color doppler is used to detect valve insufficiency and valve flow disturbances.

BOX 26–4 Duke Criteria for Diagnosis of Infective Endocarditis

MAJOR CRITERIA

1. Positive blood culture from two or more separate blood cultures
2. Evidence of endocardial involvement noted on echocardiogram of an intracardiac mass on a valve or supporting structure, abscess, or new partial dehiscence of a prosthetic valve; alternatively new valvular regurgitation is discovered

MINOR CRITERIA

1. Predisposing heart condition or IV drug use
2. Temperature ≥ 38.0°C (100.4°F).
3. Vascular phenomena such as major arterial emboli, septic pulmonary infarcts, mycotic aneurysm, intracranial hemorrhage, conjunctival hemorrhages, and Janeway lesions
4. Immunologic phenomena such as glomerulonephritis, Osler nodes, Roth's spots, and rheumatoid factor
5. Microbiologic evidence of positive blood culture but does not meet major criteria or serologic evidence of active infection with organism consistent with infectious endocarditis
6. Echocardiograph findings consistent with infectious endocarditis but do not meet the major criterion above

The infectious endocarditis diagnosis is definitive when specific pathologic criteria related to a vegetation or intracardiac abscess are met as well as the following clinical criteria:

- 2 major criteria, or
- 1 major criterion and 3 minor criteria, or
- 5 minor criteria

Adapted from Durack, D. T., Lukes, A. S., & Bright, D. K. (1994). New criteria for diagnosis of infective endocarditis: Utilization of specific echocardiographic findings. American Journal of Medicine, *96, 200–209.*

MediaLink Infective Endocarditis Resources

Clinical Therapy

Clinical therapy consists of administering antibiotics such as penicillin G, ampicillin, vancomycin, nafcillin, or gentamicin. Intravenous administration is preferred, with therapy continuing for 2 to 8 weeks until the infective organism is eradicated. Serum levels of antibiotics are monitored to maintain a therapeutic range. Surgery is often necessary to replace a heart valve or because of the risk of embolism. If congestive heart failure occurs because of damage to a heart valve, bed rest and medications such as digoxin and furosemide are prescribed initially until it is determined whether medical therapy is adequate or if surgery will be required.

NURSING MANAGEMENT

■ Nursing Assessment and Diagnoses

Assessment focuses on the child's respiratory and cardiovascular status. Pay careful attention to the vital signs, oxygen saturation, and level of consciousness as congestive heart failure and embolism may occur. The child will be on a cardiac monitor and pulse oximeter. Monitor the child's temperature, intake and output, and level of comfort. The parents will be very anxious about the child's condition, especially if this occurs following surgery for a congenital heart defect or in a critically ill child or newborn. Monitor the parents' coping skills and need for information.

Nursing diagnoses that may be associated with infective endocarditis include the following:

- Effective Therapeutic Regimen Management related to appropriate requests for antibiotic prophylaxis
- Risk for Infection related to congenital heart disease
- Risk for Caregiver Role Strain related to child's increasing care needs
- Risk for Spiritual Distress (parents) related to child's deteriorating health status and challenge to their belief and values system

Planning and Intervention

Nursing care focuses on preventing infective endocarditis for those cases when it is preventable. See guidelines on page 917. Parents of children and adolescents need to tell every healthcare provider about the risk for infective endocarditis. They need to become advocates and ask for prophylaxis, specifically prior to procedures such as professional teeth cleaning, other dental procedures, tonsillectomy or adenoidectomy, bronchoscopy, and surgery on the respiratory, gastrointestinal, and genitourinary systems. Make sure the family has copies of the wallet card produced by the American Heart Association that can be shared with healthcare providers.

Children at moderate to high risk for infective endocarditis should be discouraged from body piercing and tattoos as endocarditis may occur despite prophylaxis. Reports have indicated increased incidence of endocarditis with piercings of the nose, tongue, and nipple (Goldrick, 2003).

When the child has infective endocarditis, nursing care focuses on assessing the child's condition, administering medications, and teaching the parents about the child's care. Take the child's vital signs and assess gastrointestinal discomfort. Administer medications as ordered and monitor serum antibiotic levels. Monitor for side effects of antibiotics and for infiltration or extravasation at the infusion site. Keep invasive procedures to a minimum. Use careful aseptic technique in performing venipunctures, urinary catheterizations, and other procedures.

Make sure the parents are fully informed about the child's care and potential for complications. Permit time for them to express their feelings and frustrations over the development of this infection. Identify ways that parents can contribute to the care of the child and plan appropriate activities as the child is often lethargic and on bed rest.

Discharge Planning and Home Care Teaching

Begin discharge planning and education for the care of the child at home as soon as possible. Home infusion antibiotic therapy may be ordered so that care can be provided on an outpatient basis. At discharge, arrange home health nursing and instruct parents about care needed for the child's recuperation. Home schooling will be needed during the recovery period. Help parents to maintain contact with the child's friends and encourage social interactions. Reinforce the need for follow-up visits. Explain the importance of informing physicians and dentists about the child's history of endocarditis so that care is taken to prevent infection before invasive procedures.

Evaluation

- The child with a complex congenital heart disease does not develop infectious endocarditis.
- The child with infective endocarditis is monitored for complications and these are identified rapidly during the course of hospitalization.

Rheumatic Fever

Rheumatic fever is an inflammatory connective tissue disorder that follows an initial infection by some strains of group A beta-hemolytic streptococci. This disorder affects the heart, joints, brain, and skin tissues. Rheumatic fever causes significant morbidity, and even with modern antibiotic therapy some mortality from rheumatic heart disease still occurs in the United States. Although not common, the disorder has occurred more frequently since the 1980s, probably due to a virulent strain of group A streptococcal infections (Steeg, Walsh, & Glickstein, 2000). The exact cause of the disorder is unknown, but one possible cause is an autoimmune response in a genetically predisposed child (Steeg et al., 2000).

Clinical Manifestations

One to 3 weeks after an untreated streptococcal infection, the hallmark signs of rheumatic fever may occur. Major manifestations include the following:

- Carditis is found in 50% to 75% of cases and it varies in severity. Aschoff bodies (hemorrhagic bullous lesions) develop in the connective tissue of the heart. Endocarditis may involve the mitral and aortic valves, myocardium, and pericardium. Murmurs of mitral and aortic insufficiency must be heard to fulfill this manifestation criterion.
- Arthritis in which the child's joints become inflamed and painful occurs in about 70% of patients. The large joints are more commonly affected with pain, swelling, tenderness, erythema, and heat. The condition may migrate from joint to joint (migratory polyarthritis).
- Subcutaneous nodules may be palpable near joints in about 5% of patients.
- A skin rash called erythema marginatum, with pink macules and blanching in the middle of the lesions, is infrequently seen. The nonpruritic rash is seen on the trunk and proximal extremities, but not on the face.
- Sydenham chorea (St. Vitus dance), which is characterized by aimless movements of the extremities and facial grimacing, may be seen in about 10% of cases if the central nervous system is involved.

COLLABORATIVE CARE

Diagnostic Procedures

Diagnosis is based on clinical signs (Jones criteria; Table 26–12) and conclusive evidence of a preceding streptococcal infection. Laboratory testing for antistreptococcal antibodies is performed. Antistreptolysin-O (ASLO) titers of 320 Todd units are an indication of a recent streptococcal infection (Steeg et al., 2000). If a low titer is found and some major and minor criteria have been met, other streptococcal antibody titers should be performed.

Clinical Therapy

Clinical therapy includes antibiotics (penicillin, sulfadiazine or erythromycin) to eradicate the streptococcal infection. Aspirin is the traditional anti-inflammatory medication prescribed for 3 to 4 weeks, or longer if carditis is present. Serum salicylate levels are monitored. Aspirin works effectively to relieve joint pain and inflammation and to reduce fever, although it does not prevent the development of long-term cardiac complications. Other nonsteroidal anti-inflammatories are sometimes used, such as naproxen. Children should be monitored carefully for residual heart involvement by echocardiogram. Steroids may be used for severe carditis with congestive heart failure. Most children recover fully, but they are at risk for subsequent episodes of rheumatic fever. Recommendations for long-term antibiotic prophylaxis to reduce the risk of recurrent attacks are as follows (Dajani, Taubert, Ferrieri, et al., 1995):

- Rheumatic fever without carditis—5 years or until 21 years old, whichever is longer
- Rheumatic fever with carditis, but no residual heart disease—10 years or well into adulthood, whichever is longer
- Rheumatic fever with carditis and residual heart disease—≥ 10 years since last episode and until ≥ 40 years, whichever is longer, or lifelong

Children with cardiac valve damage from rheumatic fever need antibiotic prophylaxis to prevent infectious endocarditis. See the medication box on page 917.

TABLE 26–12 Guidelines for Diagnosis of Initial Attack of Rheumatic Fever (Jones Criteria, updated 1992)

MAJOR MANIFESTATIONS	MINOR MANIFESTATIONS
Carditis	*Clinical findings*
Polyarthritis	Arthralgia
Chorea	Fever
Erythema marginatum	*Laboratory findings*
Subcutaneous nodules	Elevated acute-phase reactants
	Erythrocyte sedimentation rate
	C-reactive protein
	Prolonged PR interval

Supporting evidence of antecedent group A streptococcal infection: (1) positive throat culture or rapid streptococcal antigen test; (2) elevated or rising streptococcal antibody titer.

** If supported by evidence of preceding group A streptococcal infection, the presence of two major manifestations or one major and two minor manifestations indicates a high probability of acute rheumatic fever.*

Data from Special Writing Group of the Committee on Rheumatic Fever, Endocarditis, and Kawasaki Disease of the Council on Cardiovascular Disease in the Young of the American Heart Association. (1992). Guidelines for the diagnosis of rheumatic fever. Jones Criteria, 1992 update. Journal of the American Medical Association, 268*(15), 2069–2073.*

NURSING MANAGEMENT

The most important role of the nurse is prevention of rheumatic fever. Nurses in clinics, offices, and schools need to ensure that all children with possible streptococcal infections have a throat culture taken. Even if the sore throat is mild, a culture is needed if family members or other contacts have had a streptococcal infection. Emphasize to the family the importance of giving the entire 10-day course of antibiotics when a culture is positive.

In a case of severe rheumatic fever, the child will be hospitalized for a period of time. Nursing care focuses on assessing the child's condition, promoting recovery, and ensuring adherence to the treatment regimen.

During the acute inflammatory phase, take the child's temperature at least every 4 hours and monitor vital signs. The child is on bed rest while monitoring for the onset of carditis, and for 4 weeks if carditis develops. Auscultate the child's heart and note any unusual sounds. Observe the child for changes in skin, joints, or behavior. Family members should have throat cultures done to identify possible asymptomatic streptococcal carriers.

Administer antibiotic and aspirin as ordered. The child is usually lethargic and often has joint pain. Aspirin often relieves pain dramatically after a few doses. Place the child's joints in neutral position and handle them carefully. Provide quiet activities, as the child is often confined to bed. Encourage visits or telephone calls from family members and friends. For the child with chorea, provide emotional support because the purposeless involuntary movements that can last for 5 to 15 weeks can be disturbing. Encourage the family to participate in the child's hospital care.

During the recovery phase, the child will generally be cared for at home. Activities may be limited, especially if heart damage is suspected. Help parents plan quiet activities, such as playing board games, working with computers, or reading, and arrange rest periods after the child returns to school. Reassure the child and parents that the effects of chorea will eventually subside.

On discharge, a daily oral low-dose antibiotic is prescribed or monthly long-acting antibiotic injection is given. Make sure the child and parents understand the importance of taking prescribed medication until adulthood to prevent future infection and possible heart damage from recurrent rheumatic fever. Stress the importance of telling future healthcare providers, including dentists and surgeons, about the child's rheumatic fever history so prophylactic antibiotics can be given to prevent infective endocarditis during invasive procedures.

Make sure the parents understand that the child's future sore throats may be streptococcal and that a throat culture should be taken even when the child is taking daily antibiotics. The child may need additional antibiotics for the infection. Emphasize the importance of follow-up care to prevent new infections and to monitor heart function.

Kawasaki Syndrome

Kawasaki syndrome is an acute febrile, systemic inflammatory illness of unknown cause. It is the leading cause of acquired heart disease in children in North America and most developed countries. The annual incidence of the disease in the United States increased from 8.1 to 18.5 cases per 100,000 children between 1988 and 1997. Hawaiian children have a significantly higher incidence at 47.7 cases per 100,000. Children under 5 years account for 75% of the cases, and nearly half of those cases occurred in children under 2 years. Significantly more males than females develop the disease. Although this disorder is most commonly found in Asian children, it is seen in all races. The increasing incidence of this disease may possibly be associated with improved diagnosis and because the Asian American population in the United States increased by more than 50% between 1990 and 2000. Mortality has decreased significantly with current treatment (Chang, 2002).

Etiology and Pathophysiology

The etiology of Kawasaki syndrome is unknown, but the primary cause is theorized to be infectious in genetically predisposed children. A seasonal distribution of cases occurs with the greatest incidence occurring in the winter and spring and the lowest incidence in the summer. It does not appear to be spread by person-to-person contact, but frequently is preceded by an upper respiratory tract infection. This multisystem inflammatory disease involves the small and midsize arteries, including the coronary arteries. Coronary artery damage may result in aneurysms, ischemic heart disease, and potentially infarcts.

Clinical Manifestations

The three stages of the disease are acute, subacute, and convalescent. The acute stage of Kawasaki syndrome is characterized by irritability, fever, conjunctival hyperemia, red throat, swollen hands and feet, rash on the trunk and perineal area, unilateral enlargement of the anterior cervical lymph nodes, diarrhea, and hepatic dysfunction (Figure 26–14 ■). The subacute stage is characterized by cracking lips and fissures, desquamation of the skin on the tips of the fingers and toes starting at about 10 days after the fever begins, joint pain, cardiac disease, and thrombocytosis. In the convalescent stage, 6 to 8 weeks after disease onset, the child appears normal but lingering signs of inflammation may be present. Some cases have an atypical presentation. Other clinical manifestations may include abdominal pain, paralytic ileus, diarrhea and vomiting, hydrops of the gallbladder, uveitis, meatitis, dysuria, aseptic meningitis, pneumonitis, and arthritis.

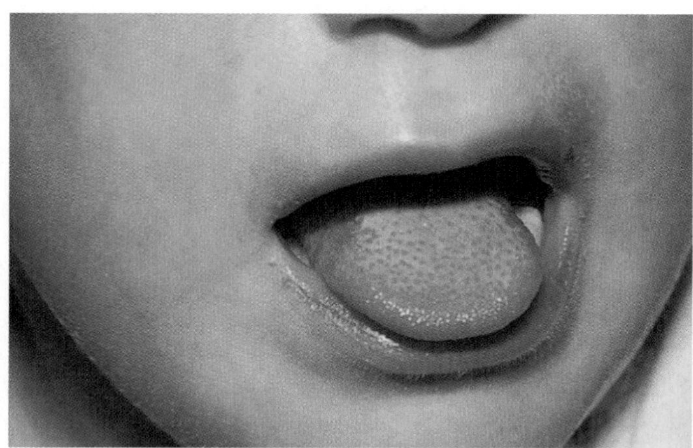

FIGURE 26–14 ■ This child shows many of the signs of the acute stage of Kawasaki syndrome.

COLLABORATIVE CARE

Diagnostic Procedures

Diagnosis is based on clinical signs using the criteria given in Box 26–5, as there is no specific diagnostic test. Blood studies show some abnormalities such as elevated erythrocyte sedimentation rate, elevated white blood cell count, mild anemia, thrombocytosis, elevated platelet count, an elevated C-reactive protein level, moderately elevated transaminase levels, and hypoalbuminemia. A two-dimensional echocardiogram is used to identify specific vascular changes in the heart and coronary arteries such as the following: diffuse dilation of the coronary arteries, coronary aneurysms, myocarditis, and aortic and mitral regurgitation. Repeat echocardiograms are performed frequently to monitor the development of coronary lesions during the acute phases of the disease, and then periodically during recovery and long-term follow-up to observe for resolution of coronary artery lesions.

Clinical Therapy

Kawasaki syndrome is treated with intravenous immunoglobulin (2 g/kg given in a single infusion) and oral aspirin. High doses of aspirin (80 to 100 mg/kg/day in four divided doses) are given while the fever is high. The dose is decreased to 3 to 5 mg/kg/day once the fever has dropped for about 6 to 8 weeks. Aspirin is taken until the platelet count is normal and may be continued on a long-term basis if cardiac abnormalities occur. High doses of immune globulin and aspirin given before the 10th day of fever have been shown to reduce the incidence of

BOX 26–5 Diagnostic Criteria for Kawasaki Disease

Kawasaki disease is diagnosed when a high spiking fever over 39°C (102.2°F) for 5 days or longer is present along with four of the following five criteria not explained by another disease process.

- Bilateral conjunctivitis without exudate, typically with distinctly visible vessels early in the disease
- Intense erythema of the buccal and pharyngeal surfaces with dry, swollen, cracked, and fissuring lips and a strawberry tongue
- Dermatitis of the extremities, intense palmar and plantar erythema, induration of the hands and feet, and then desquamation after 2 or more weeks of symptoms
- Dermatitis of the trunk with an erythematous maculopapular rash
- Acute cervical lymphadenopathy, frequently unilateral, with a node over 1.5 cm in diameter found early in the disease

Modified from Rowley, A. H., & Shulman, S. T. (1999). Kawasaki syndrome. Pediatric Clinics of North America, *46(2), 313–329.*

coronary artery lesions and aneurysms, and to decrease fever and inflammatory signs (Rowley & Shulman, 1999). When the fever persists after the first administration of immune globulin, a second dose may be given. When the second dose of immune globulin is ineffective, corticosteroids may be administered.

Children are usually hospitalized for 3 or more days, depending on the presence of cardiac lesions and persistence of the fever. Most children recover fully. Careful monitoring for cardiac disease continues for several weeks or months. Coronary aneurysms and coronary artery stenosis with a risk of thrombosis are the most serious complications. Some children with stenosed coronary arteries may need angioplasty or coronary artery bypass grafts.

NURSING MANAGEMENT

Nursing care focuses on promoting comfort, monitoring for early signs of complications or disease progression, and supporting the family.

■ Nursing Assessment and Diagnoses

Assessment is important in identifying signs of Kawasaki syndrome, as the acute phase of this disorder is commonly confused with other diseases. The nurse in the community must be alert to early signs and symptoms. When the child is hospitalized, take the temperature every 4 hours and before each dose of aspirin. Carefully assess the extremities for edema, redness, and desquamation every 8 hours. Examine the eyes for conjunctivitis and the mucous membranes for inflammation. Monitor the child's dietary and fluid intake and weigh the child daily. Carefully assess heart sounds and rhythm.

Nursing diagnoses that may be appropriate for the child with Kawasaki disease include:

- Impaired Oral Mucous Membrane related to infection
- Impaired Skin Integrity related to hyperthermia and disease state
- Hyperthermia related to illness

■ Planning and Implementation

Administer aspirin and immune globulin as ordered. Monitor for side effects of aspirin such as bleeding and gastrointestinal upset. Administer intravenous immune globulin as a blood product, carefully regulating the infusion rate to run slowly according to the physician's orders, and watching for any reactions to the infusion. The infusion rate should not be over 1 mL/min. If symptoms of reaction are noted, stop the infusion immediately (see Chapter 27∞).

Promote the child's comfort. Keep the child's skin clean and dry, and lubricate the lips. Use cool compresses and tepid sponges to make the feverish child more comfortable. Change the child's clothes and bed linens frequently. Give frequent small feedings of soft foods and liquids that are neither too hot nor too cold.

Use passive range of motion exercises to facilitate joint movement. Because the child with Kawasaki syndrome is frequently lethargic and irritable, plan rest periods and quiet, age-appropriate activities. Encourage the parents to participate in their child's care to promote comfort and reassurance for the child. Provide the parents with information about the disease and the child's treatment.

Discharge Planning and Home Care Teaching

Before the child is discharged, teach the parents to administer aspirin as ordered and to watch for side effects. Advise the parents that the child may need to avoid contact sports or other activities that could cause bleeding. Limitation of strenuous activity is recommended for all children with coronary aneurysms or stenoses. Have them take the child's temperature daily and report any fever above 37.8°C (100°F) to the physician. Emphasize the need for follow-up care to monitor for cardiac complications (Figure 26–15 ■).

Inform the parents of a child with Kawasaki syndrome to postpone measles and varicella immunizations for 11 months after immune globulin administration, but other immunizations may be given on schedule. Influenza vaccine should be administered, particularly for those children on long-term aspirin therapy, because of the risk for Reye syndrome (American Academy of Pediatrics, 2003).

■ Evaluation

Examples of expected nursing care outcomes include the following:

- Nursing care of the child's acute symptoms or rash, fever, and irritability promote comfort.
- The child has balanced periods of rest and quiet activity that promote recovery.

CARDIAC ARRHYTHMIAS

Cardiac **arrhythmias** (abnormal rhythms or dysrhythmias) occur frequently in children, but not as commonly as in adults. Arrhythmias must be recognized because they can cause decreased cardiac

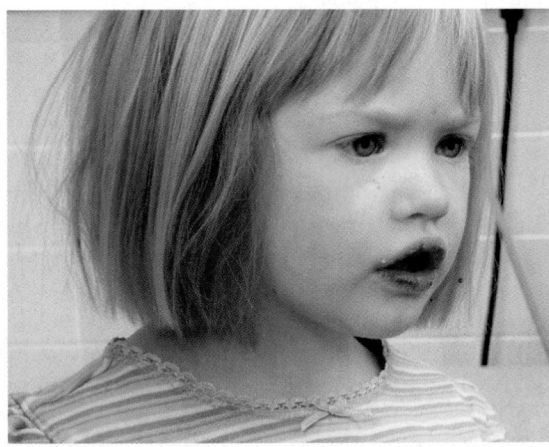

FIGURE 26–15 ■ This child has returned for one of her frequent follow-up visits to assess her cardiac status after treatment for Kawasaki syndrome. Notice the lips that show the inflammation and cracking.

output and congestive heart failure or further progress to an even more serious arrhythmia that could result in sudden death.

Etiology and Pathophysiology

Tachyarrhythmias (sinus tachycardia) and bradyarrhythmias (sinus bradycardia) occur with acute conditions, such as hypoxia, acidosis, increased intracranial pressure, abdominal distention, hypothermia, and hypoglycemia. These types of arrhythmias generally resolve once the underlying condition is treated. Sinus tachycardias may result from drug or stimulant use by adolescents. Some arrhythmias result from genetic conditions, such as forms of supraventricular tachycardia (SVT) and long QT syndrome. Other arrhythmias have a congenital cause, such as the newborn of a mother with an autoimmune condition like systemic lupus erythethematosis (Starr & Freitas-Nichols, 2000). Less common arrhythmias are often associated with congenital heart disease, especially as many more children are surviving surgeries for complex defects. Review Figure 26–16 ■ for the normal electrical conduction system to determine where specific stimulation or interruption occurs in association with various arrhythmias.

Newborns and young children may be predisposed to SVT due to a congenital heart defect or Wolff-Parkinson-White syndrome. Short periods of arrhythmia (several seconds), which may be caused by paroxysmal atrial tachycardia, are rarely dangerous; however, prolonged episodes (> 24 hours) of continuous SVT may lead to congestive heart failure. Cardiac output is affected because diastolic filling cannot occur with such a rapid heart rate.

Clinical Manifestations

Bradycardias

Bradycardia and the various degrees of heart block are characterized by general symptoms such as fatigue, exercise intolerance, dizziness, and syncope. Criteria for bradycardia by age group are as follows (Hanish, 2001):

- Infants to 3 years — < 100 beats per minute
- Children 3 to 9 years — < 60 beats per minute
- Children 9 to 16 years — < 50 beats per minute
- Adolescents over 16 years — < 40 beats per minute

Refer to Chapter 8∞ for normal heart rate ranges by age.

Tachycardias

Supraventricular tachycardia (SVT), the most common pathologic tachycardia, is the abrupt onset of a rapid, regular heart rate, often too fast to count. The presenting heart rate in infants with SVT may be up to 260 beats/min. In older children, a heart rate between 150 and 240 beats/min may be seen. For SVT early signs in infants include poor feeding, irritability, and pallor. Older children may have episodes of altered consciousness (dizziness or syncope). Recurrent attacks are common. Prolonged episodes of SVT are life threatening and can progress to congestive heart failure or cardiogenic shock if untreated. Signs and symptoms of different classifications of arrhythmias can be found in the clinical manifestations table on page 937.

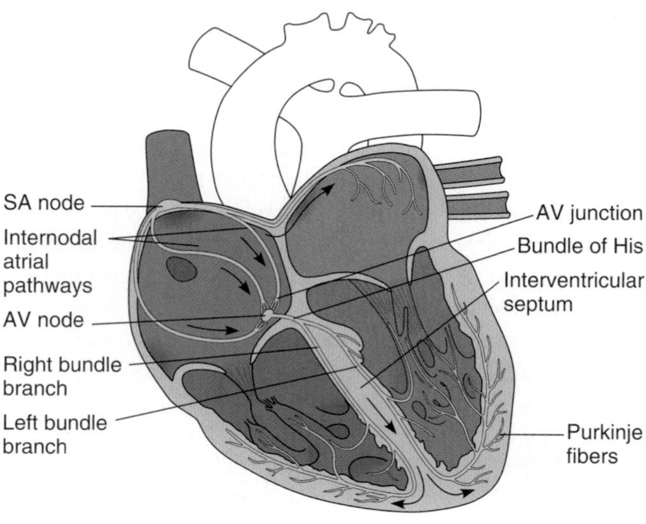

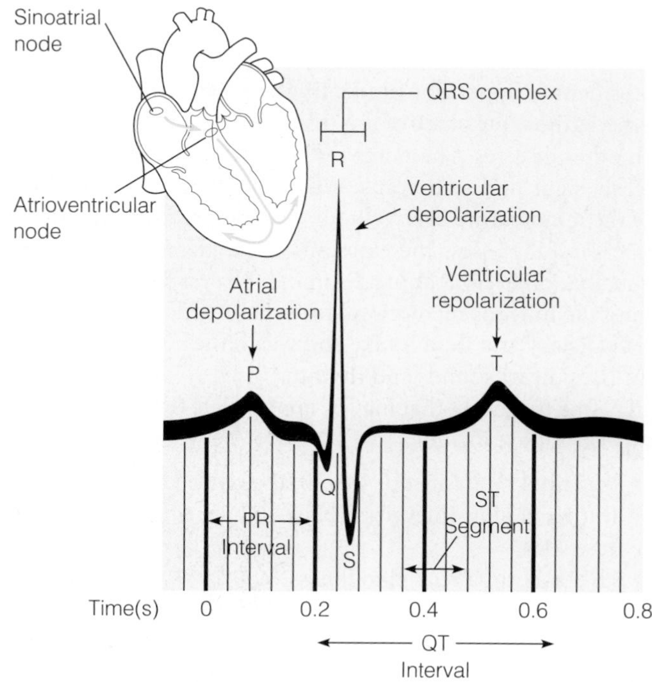

FIGURE 26–16 ■ *A,* Electrical conduction system of the heart. Depolarization normally follows a sequence that begins in the sinoatrial (SA) node and travels through the atrial muscle to the atrioventricular (AV) junction, and then through the AV node to the ventricular muscles. The pathway in the ventricles begins in the bundle of His and divides into the right and left bundle branches. The pathway terminates in the Purkinje system so that the impulse spreads across the myocardium. *B,* Normal electrocardiogram pattern.

P wave—atrial depolarization

P-R interval—time between the beginning of atrial depolarization to beginning of ventricular depolarization

QRS complex—ventricular depolarization

T wave—ventricular repolarization

ST segment—period between ventricular depolarization and repolarization

CLINICAL MANIFESTATIONS of Arrhythmias

ETIOLOGY	CLINICAL MANIFESTATION	CLINICAL THERAPY
Sinus node dysfunction—surgical injury to the sinoatrial node or its arterial supply, right atrial dilatation, myocarditis, antiarrhythmic medications.	Bradycardia, fatigue, exercise intolerance, dizziness, syncope	Adequate ventilation, oxygenation, Medications: epinephrine, atropine, Temporary or permanent pacing
Incomplete conduction of impulses through the atrioventricular node, surgery for transposition of great arteries, tetralogy of Fallot, endocardial cushion defect, ventricular septal defect, subaortic resection, aortic valve replacement, inflammation due to myocarditis, Lyme disease, rheumatic fever	Heart block (first, second, or third degree), slow ventricular heart rates Congestive heart failure, fatigue, exercise intolerance, dizziness, syncope	Temporary or permanent pacemaker
Reentrant circuit with or without an accessory conduction pathway, or an ectopic focus; Wolff-Parkinson-White syndrome	Sustained tachyarrhythmia of 130–300 beats per minute depending on age and etiology, supraventricular tachycardia, atrial flutter in some cases Infants: irritability, lethargy, poor feeding, signs of congestive heart failure Older children: palpitations, chest discomfort, dizziness, syncope, cardiac arrest	Vagal maneuvers Medications: adenosine, amiodarone, digoxin, or propanolol Synchronized cardioversion Radiofrequency catheter ablation Implantation of an anti-tachycardia pacemaker or cardioverter-defibrillator
Severe electrolyte or metabolic abnormalities, hypoxia, hypothermia, drug toxicity, cardiomyopathy, ventriculotomy for congenital heart defect, long QT syndome	Ventricular tachycardia with abrupt onset, torsade de pointes, heart rate > 220 beats per minute, cardiac arrest Infants: lethargy, tachypnea, poor feeding, pallor or cyanosis, diaphoresis Older children: palpitations, chest discomfort, dizziness, nausea, syncope, sudden cardiac death	Amiodarone, beta-blocker medications Synchronized cardioversion, implantable pacemaker, or cardioverter-defibrillator Radiofrequency ablation in a few cases Surgical intervention (revision of previous heart surgery, cryoablation, transplant)
Hypovolemia, febrile illness, drugs or stimulant medications	Sinus tachycardia, gradual onset, heart rate < 200 beats per minute	Fluids or blood replacement Antipyretic
Inheritance of one or more genes associated with long QT syndrome	A prolongation of the QT interval on ECG, torsade de pointes, syncope, palpitations, seizure, cardiac arrest	Medications: beta-blocker (propanolol, atenolol), sodium channel blockers Pacemaker or cardioverter-defibrillator Avoid triggers and drugs that cause QT interval to be prolonged

Data from Hanish, D. (2001). Pediatric arrhythmia. Journal of Pediatric Nursing, 16*(5), 351–362; LeMone, P., & Burke, K. (2004)* Medical-Surgical Nursing: Critical Thinking in Client Care *(3e). Upper Saddle River, NJ: Prentice Hall.*

COLLABORATIVE CARE

Diagnostic Procedures

An electrocardiogram is initially used to diagnose an arrhythmia. If symptoms are episodic, a 24-hour Holter monitor or an event monitor may be used to capture the arrhythmia. With an event monitor, the patient can push a button on the monitor to activate the mark of the ECG tracing at the time of the symptoms. The event monitor retains the ECG tracing immediately before and during the episode. The ECG record can then be transmitted by telephone for immediate interpretation. Stress testing may also be performed when exercise either triggers or is associated with the symptoms.

Invasive procedures may be needed to diagnose some arrhythmias.

- Electrophysiologic cardiac catheterization allows electrode catheters to be placed in the right side of the heart. Areas of the heart can be selectively stimulated to trigger the arrhythmia. Medications can then be given intravenously to identify which medication can be used to effectively treat the arrhythmia.
- Transesophageal recording involves passing an electrode catheter into the lower esophagus to stimulate and record the arrhythmia.

Clinical Therapy

Treatment for arrhythmias depends upon the type and severity.

Bradycardias. For sinus bradycardia due to an acute condition, oxygen, ventilation, and medications such as epinephrine or atropine are used until the condition resolves. Other chronic bradycardias due to heart block often require a pacemaker. The criterion for implanting a pacemaker is the concurrent observation of a symptom such as syncope with bradycardia or asystole longer than 3 seconds (Gregoratos, Abrams, Epstein, et al., 2002).

Tachycardias. Supraventricular tachycardia episodes are initially treated with vagal maneuvers to slow the heart rate when the infant or child is stable. In infants the application of ice or iced saline solution to the face or rectal stimulation with a thermometer may reduce the heart rate. An older child can perform the Valsalva maneuver (holding the breath and bearing down as if to have a bowel movement, inducing the gag reflex, or blowing forcefully on the thumb) to increase intrathoracic and venous pressures, and thus slow the heart rate. Adenosine may be given intravenously when the vagal maneuvers are unsuccessful. Digoxin, amiodarone, or propanolol may also be used during acute episodes if more aggressive therapy is needed. See medications used to treat arrhythmias below. In life-threatening situations the child is sedated and invasive maneuvers are used to convert the tachycardia to sinus rhythm.

- In **synchronized cardioversion**, the timed administration of a calibrated electrical charge by a defibrillator is used in an effort to convert the arrhythmia to a sinus rhythm.
- With esophageal overdrive pacing, an electrode is inserted into the esophagus and positioned behind the left atrium. The heart is stimulated at a very rapid rate to interrupt the tachycardia.

Recurrent episodes of SVT are common, and long-term digoxin and propranolol may be given to reduce the frequency

MEDICATIONS Commonly Used for the Treatment of Arrhythmias

MEDICATION	USE AND ACTION
Epinephrine Alpha- and beta-adrenergic agonist	Used for bradycardia Strengthens myocardial contraction, restores cardiac rhythm
Atropine Anticholinergic	Used for sinus bradycardia or asystole Decreases AV conduction time, shortens PR interval, increases heart rate
Adenosine Class IA antiarrhythmic	Used for supraventricular tachycardia, atrial flutter Slows conduction through the AV and SA nodes, interrupts reentry pathways through the AV node
Amiodarone Class III antiarrhythmic	Used for life-threatening ventricular tachycardia, supraventricular tachycardia, and ventricular fibrillation Acts directly on cardiac tissue, decreases AV and SA node conduction and prolongs the refractory period
Propranolol Class II antiarrhythmic	Used for supraventricular tachycardia, Wolf-Parkinson-White syndrome, and ventricular tachycardia Reduces myocardial irritability, depresses automaticity of sinus node, decreases AV and intraventricular conduction velocity
Digoxin	Used for supraventricular tachycardia and atrial flutter Decreases conduction velocity through the AV node
Verapamil Class IV antiarrhythmic	Used for refractory supraventricular tachycardia and ventricular tachycardia. Not used in infants under 1 year of age Decreases and slows SA and AV node conduction
Procainamide Class IA antiarrhythmic	Used for supraventricular tachycardia, ventricular tachycardias, and atrial tachycardias Decreases myocardial excitability and conduction velocity, increases duration of refractory period
Lidocaine Class IB antiarrhythmic	Used for ventricular arrhythmias Suppresses automaticity of His-Purkinje conduction system, increases electrical stimulation threshold of the ventricles during diastole

Data from Miller-Hoover, S. R. (2003). Pediatric and cardiovascular pharmacology. Pediatric Nursing, *29(2),109; Wilson, B. A., Shannon, M. T., & Stang, C. L. (2003).* Nurse's drug guide 2003. *Upper Saddle River, NJ: Prentice Hall; Atkins, D. L., Dorian, P., Gonzalez, E. R., et al. (2001). Treatment of tachyarrhythmias.* Annals of Emergency Medicine, *37(4), S91-S109.*

MediaLink Digoxin Animation

of episodes (Starr & Freitas-Nichols, 2000). **Radiofrequency ablation**, the use of radio energy to destroy a very small section of the myocardium through which an accessory conduction pathway passes, may be performed in the cardiac catheterization laboratory with specialized electrophysiology equipment. A catheter is guided to the site of the accessory conduction system pathway triggering the tachycardia. Radiofrequency energy is transmitted to the muscle cells through which the accessory conduction system passes. The muscle cells in that small area die and block the transmission of the extra impulses triggering the tachycardia. This procedure is frequently successful and medications to control the tachycardia can be discontinued. The Cox-Maze procedure, in which surgical and cryoablation lesions are strategically placed to interrupt specific conduction pathways, may also be used for the surgical treatment of atrial flutter and atrial fibrillation (LeRoy, 2001). In some cases, however, a cardioverter-defibrillator may need to be implanted.

NURSING MANAGEMENT

The focus of nursing care is assessment of the child, preparing the child and family for diagnostic procedures, and educating the parents about medications and other interventions for the specific rhythm problem.

Nursing Assessment and Diagnoses

The child suspected of having an arrhythmia should have the heart rate and other vital signs monitored. A cardiorespiratory monitor and pulse oximetry should be used to identify deterioration of the child's condition. Carefully observe and record changes in level of consciousness, color, weakness, irritability, and feeding pattern as hypoxia may develop.

PRACTICE ALERT

When the heart rate reaches 180 beats/min in a child (220 beats/min in an infant), the time needed for blood to fill the ventricles during diastole is too short. As a result, the cardiac output and stroke volume fall. Life-threatening shock may develop if corrective action is not taken to reduce the heart rate (Eichelberger, Ball, Pratsch, et al., 1998).

Any child in the community found to have an abnormal ECG finding, unusual heart rhythm, syncope (especially with exercise), or dizziness with palpitations should be referred to a pediatric cardiologist for evaluation.

Nursing diagnoses that may be considered for the child with arrhythmias include:

- Decreased Cardiac Output related to dysfunctional electrical conduction
- Compromised Family Coping related to recurrent life-threatening arrhythmia in infant
- Risk for Disorganized Infant Behavior related to repeated illness episodes
- Impaired Social Interaction related to ban from team sports

Planning and Implementation

The child will be treated in the emergency department or intensive care unit, depending upon the type of arrhythmia and how stable the child is while being treated. Attach the cardiorespiratory monitor or external pacing leads and equipment as ordered. Assist with vagal maneuvers if ordered for SVT and monitor for recurrence of the arrhythmia. Administer medications as ordered and monitor for response. Provide for rest and adequate nutrition.

Prepare the child and family for procedures. When sedation is ordered for invasive procedures such as synchronized cardioversion, follow the institution's guidelines for frequent assessment and intervention. Have emergency drugs and resuscitation equipment available at bedside.

Episodes of arrhythmia are frightening for both the child and parents. Carefully explain the treatment plan and home care. Teach parents to take the child's apical pulse. Make sure parents are trained in cardiopulmonary resuscitation. Provide telephone numbers of emergency medical facilities and help parents plan how to seek emergency care. Emphasize that medications help prevent or reduce episode frequency.

Discharge Planning and Home Care Teaching

Teach the parents about the condition and how to take the child's pulse for a full minute. Parents and other family members should learn to perform CPR. Make sure the parents and child with supraventricular tachycardia (SVT) understand the need to avoid using cardiac stimulant drugs such as decongestants as these drugs might trigger another episode of SVT. Describe and provide written instructions about the danger signs indicating a recurrence of the acute condition and how to seek emergency care. Provide preparation for the child and family for procedures such as radiofrequency ablation, or pacemaker or cardioverter-defibrillator implantation.

Evaluation

Expected outcomes of nursing care include the following:

- The child reduces the frequency of arrhythmia episodes by adherence to prescribed medications.
- Parents respond to an episode by appropriately seeking emergency care and notifying the cardiologist or designated healthcare provider.

Long QT Syndrome

Long QT syndrome is a rhythm disturbance of autosomal dominant and autosomal recessive inheritance that places children at risk for ventricular fibrillation and sudden death. It may also result from electrolyte abnormalities, malnutrition associated with anorexia and bulimia, myocarditis, and central nervous system trauma (Berul, 2000). It is thought to be associated with some cases of sudden infant death syndrome.

The arrhythmia commonly occurs without warning and often results in death. Syncopal episodes and sudden cardiac death may be triggered by extreme emotion, a loud noise, or demanding physical activity. Swimming is a specific trigger in approximately 15% of patients (Hampton, 2003). Others have episodes at rest or during sleep. Early signs include a fast heart rate (too fast to count), irritability, lethargy, poor feeding, poor perfusion (cool pale skin, increased capillary refill time), decreased responsiveness, and decreased blood pressure.

If the child is resuscitated or evaluated because of early signs, the arrhythmia is commonly detected by electrocardiogram. The disorder is treated by beta-adrenergic blockade, and often a pacemaker (Lewin, 2000).

Nursing Management

Nursing care is as described for other arrhythmias. Parents and children need to avoid triggers that cause arrhythmia episodes such as competitive athletics, swimming, loud noises, and hypokalemia. These children should not receive anti-arrhythmic medications and the potential adverse effects of other medications (e.g. antihistamines, macrolide antibiotics) should be reviewed by the healthcare provider as many of these medications can trigger episodes (Erickson & Jones, 2000). Teach the parents and adolescents to remind the primary care provider about prescription medications that should be avoided; an updated list of these medications can be found online.

Commotio Cordis

Commotio cordis, also known as a cardiac concussion, is a blunt, nonpenetrating blow to the precordium that causes ventricular fibrillation and sudden death. The majority of victims are healthy children and youth participating in sports such as baseball, softball, ice hockey, and lacrosse. In some cases the event is triggered by physical contact with another person, such as a fist, elbow, knee, or head. The timing of the impact on the precordium is believed to coincide with the period of vulnerable cardiac repolarization, in the terminal 15 to 30 mseconds before the peak of the T wave. The narrower anteroposterior diameter of the chest and increased compliance of the chest wall in children and youth may contribute to the transfer of more energy from the chest wall to the heart. Currently designed chest protective gear may reduce risk, but does not fully protect the wearer (Maron, Gohman, Kyle, et al., 2002).

The most common arrhythmias recorded after the victim's collapse include ventricular fibrillation and ventricular tachycardia. Prompt cardiopulmonary resuscitation or defibrillation is the only treatment. The majority of victims do not survive.

DYSLIPIDEMIA

Dyslipidemia is a condition in which one or more lipids have an abnormal level in the blood that causes the following:

- Increased total cholesterol
- Increased low-density lipoproteins
- Increased triglycerides
- Decreased high-density lipoprotein level

Although children do not usually die of atherosclerotic heart disease, its development begins during childhood and progresses through the adult years leading to coronary heart disease, the major cause of death in the United States. It is important to identify children who have a genetic history or lifestyle that makes them more susceptible to future coronary heart disease and implement preventive health measures to reduce their risk of disease and premature death as adults. In young adults who were monitored from the age of 4 years, the following factors were found to increase risk for the presence of coronary artery calcium, including obesity and increased body mass index, elevated blood pressure in childhood, and dyslipidemia (Kavey, Daniels, Lauer, et al., 2003).

Epidemiology and Pathophysiology

Cholesterol and triglycerides are the major lipids transported in the blood as lipoproteins to the sites where they are used. Lipids serve many important functions, such as biosynthesis of hormones, synthesis of bile acids needed to absorb fats from the small intestine, and energy storage and production. The lipoproteins vary by size, density, and lipid composition. Low-density lipoproteins (LDLs) carry the majority of cholesterol to the cells where it is used for cell membrane structure and the production of hormones. These lipoproteins (LDLs) are associated with increased cardiovascular risk if high levels are present in the blood. High-density lipoproteins (HDLs) attract free cholesterol and support the transfer of cholesterol from the lower density lipoproteins and peripheral tissues to the liver. These lipoproteins (HDLs) are associated with a reduced cardiovascular risk. Abnormalities in the lipid levels may be the result of excessive production, lack of clearance of the lipoprotein particles, a genetic defect in lipid metabolism, or other defects such as enzyme deficiencies.

Some children have primary dyslipidemia due to familial hypercholesterolemia in which they may have cholesterol levels as high as 600 to 1,000 mg/dL and lipid deposits in their corneas and tendons. As the excessive fat circulates, it causes changes in blood vessels. Children may also have secondary dyslipidemia that can result from a diet rich in saturated fat and too little exercise, diseases such as diabetes, and certain drugs such as anabolic steroids (Kingsbury, 2003). Most commonly, children have milder lipid abnormalities that arise from a combination of heredity and lifestyle factors. The fatty streaks that appear in childhood become fibrous plaques in adolescence. These atherosclerotic plaques continue to grow in adulthood and may cause hemorrhage, thrombi, and occlusion of vessels.

Clinical Manifestations

Children and adolescents rarely have signs or symptoms of dyslipidemia, and the condition is usually only discovered during blood screening tests.

COLLABORATIVE CARE

Diagnostic Tests

Dyslipidemia is identified by a blood test. Cholesterol, including total cholesterol (TC), high-density lipoprotein cholesterol (HDL-C), and triglycerides are measured. The low-density lipoprotein cholesterol (LDL-C) level is calculated using an equation based on the triglyceride, HDL, and total cholesterol levels. See Table 26–13 for recommended, borderline, and high values for each lipid.

Because primary prevention of atherosclerosis should begin during childhood, the American Heart Association and the National Cholesterol Education Program's Expert Panel on Blood Cholesterol in Children and Adolescents recommends that all children over 2 years of age who have the following risk factors be screened with a fasting lipid panel (Kavey et al., 2003).

- Family history of cardiovascular disease before age 55 years (parents or grandparents), a parent has an elevated total serum cholesterol (240 mg/dL), or when family history is unknown
- Blood pressure > 90th percentile for age, sex, and height
- Overweight, BMI > 85th percentile
- Other risk factors such as smoking and diabetes

Children without the previous risk factors should be evaluated at each health visit to identify the development of potential risk factors that would become an indication for fasting lipid testing. At each visit, assess the child's height, weight, and BMI as well as diet and physical activity. Starting at age 3 years assess the blood pressure and compare to norms for age, sex, and height. At about 9 to 10 years inquire about cigarette smoking. The family history should be updated regularly with regard to obesity, hypertension, dyslipidemia, diabetes, cigarette smoking, and cardiovascular disease before 55 in men and 65 in women (Kavey et al., 2003).

Clinical Therapy

The primary management of dyslipidemia in most children includes dietary modifications, exercise, and other changes in lifestyle. The child's diet is carefully analyzed and changes are made to satisfy the dietary guidelines given in Table 26–14.

If the child continues to have high serum lipid levels, a lipid specialist should be consulted. Cholestyramine or colestipol, which bind bile acid in the intestine, and niacin, are occasionally prescribed for children over 10 years of age. Lovastatin received FDA approval in 2002 for use in adolescent boys and girls who are 1 year past menarche for treatment of familial hypercholesterolemia. Criteria for its use include the following (Buck, 2002):

- An LDL-C > 189 mg/dL despite diet therapy
- An LDL-C > 160 mg/dL in adolescents with a family history of premature cardiovascular disease or two or more risk factors for cardiovascular disease

A new long-term randomized control clinical trial has been initiated to test the efficacy, safety, and tolerability of simvastatin in the treatment of children with familial hypercholesterolemia. Study results will hopefully provide guidelines for future therapy (de Jongh, Stalenhoef, Tuohy, et al., 2002).

Other studies of the long-term effects of high lipid levels and different management strategies implemented during childhood continue. It is hoped that careful monitoring and management of lipid levels in childhood will decrease the incidence of cardiovascular disease.

TABLE 26–13 Laboratory Values for Assessment of Dyslipidemia in Children Between 2 and 19 years old

TEST	RECOMMENDED LEVEL	LEVELS OF HIGHER RISK
Total cholesterol	< 170 mg/dL	Borderline: 170–199 mg/dL High: ≥ 200 mg/dL
LDL-C	< 110 mg/dL	Borderline: 110–129 mg/dL High: ≥ 130 mg/dL
Triglyceride	100 mg/dL	Borderline: 100–150 mg/dL High: > 150 mg/dL
HDL-C	≥ 35 mg/dL	< 35 mg/dL

From National Cholesterol Education Program. (1993). Expert panel on blood cholesterol in children and adolescents, NIH parent's guide (NIH Publication No. 93-3102). Washington, DC: National Institute of Health, NHLBI. www.americanheart.org/presenter.jhtml?identifier=4499, *accessed 8/4/2003.*

TABLE 26–14 Recommended Nutrient Intake in Children and Adolescents with Dyslipidemia

NUTRIENT	RECOMMENDED INTAKE
Saturated fatty acid	Less than 10% of calories
Total fat	No more than 30% of calories
Polyunsaturated fat	Up to 10% of calories
Monounsaturated fat	10%–15% of calories
Cholesterol	Less than 300 mg/day

Data from the National Cholesterol Education Program Coordinating Committee. (1991). Report of the expert panel on blood cholesterol levels in children and adolescents. Washington, DC: U.S. Department of Health and Human Services; Krauss, R. M., Eckel, R. H., Howard, B., et al. (2001). AHA scientific statement: AHA dietary guidelines. Journal of Nutrition, 131, *132–146.*

NURSING MANAGEMENT

Nursing care focuses on identifying children at risk for dyslipidemia, providing education about diet and exercise, and monitoring eating patterns. Identification and management of dyslipidemia takes place in a variety of community agencies. Office and clinic nurses identify children who need to have serum lipids measured. Nurses in schools provide education on ways to reduce risk factors. The child's history of exercise patterns, weight and BMI percentiles, and dietary intake provides important information. Obtain data on familial heart disease, hypertension, diabetes, and smoking to determine risk factors. Total cholesterol level screening does not require fasting, but the child will need to fast for 12 hours before blood is drawn for a complete lipid evaluation.

Work with nutritionists to provide dietary teaching and monitor family eating patterns. Emphasize the importance of teaching and modeling food choices that help reduce lipid levels. For children with familial hypercholesterolemia, lifelong dietary control is essential (Box 26–6). Emphasize the importance of exercise in keeping the heart and blood vessels free from atherosclerotic changes. Encourage parents to promote physical

BOX 26–6 Research: Dietary Fat

A long-term study evaluating the safety and efficacy of a diet to lower total fat and saturated fat to very low levels in children with elevated LDL-C revealed that dietary fat modification can be achieved and sustained in actively growing children. Improvements in LDL-C levels can be made without adverse effects on the child's growth and maturational development (Obarzanek, Kimm, Barton, et al., 2001).

activity, limit sedentary time for their children, and serve as role models. Help the child select an enjoyable moderate to intense activity to participate in every day, and then to participate in 30 minutes of vigorous, aerobic activities at least 3 to 4 times a week to promote cardiovascular fitness. Aerobic exercise includes running or jogging, aerobic dancing, swimming, fast walking, hiking, biking, rollerblading, and soccer. When 30 minutes is not possible, encourage two 15-minute exercise periods. The exercise will help control the child's weight and blood pressure, reduce the risk of diabetes, and help raise the HDL cholesterol level.

Smoking by the child or the parents should be discouraged. Secondhand smoke may affect blood pressure and plaque formation, and thus increase the risk for the development of cardiovascular disease (Giddings, 1999).

Since many affected children have family members with dyslipidemia, it is important to include the entire family in the treatment plan. Lifestyle changes such as diet and exercise are difficult for a single family member to implement. The family of a child with dyslipidemia requires continual teaching and reinforcement. Nutrition assessments and evaluation of family diet should be performed periodically.

HYPERTENSION

Hypertension is present in 0.8% to 5% of the pediatric population, meaning that 350,000 children and adolescents potentially have elevated blood pressures (Peters & Flack, 2003). Mildly elevated blood pressure in children and adolescents may precede adult hypertension (National High Blood Pressure Education Program, 1996). This becomes a significant concern as hypertension becomes a major risk factor for heart disease and stroke during adulthood.

MediaLink Blood Pressure Animation

Etiology and Pathophysiology

Hypertension in infants and prepubescent children is often associated with underlying conditions such as kidney disease or heart defects, and is considered secondary hypertension. In children under 13 years, kidney disease, including glomerulonephritis, renal stenosis, and reflux nephropathy, is responsible for 70% to 80% of secondary hypertension (Peters & Flack 2003). Other causes of secondary hypertension include coarctation of the aorta, endocrinopathies (hyperthyroidism, adrenal cortical hyperplasia, or pheochromocytoma), increased intracranial pressure, and ingestion of agents such as cocaine or amphetamines. See Table 26–15 for medications and other agents that can cause an elevated blood pressure.

TABLE 26–15 Medications and Other Agents that Elevate the Blood Pressure

CLASSIFICATION OF AGENT	SPECIFIC MEDICATIONS AND AGENTS
Over-the-counter medications	Caffeine Ephedrine Pseudoephedrine Nonsteroidal anti-inflammatory drugs
Prescription medications	Cyclosporin, tacrolimus Dexedrine Erythropoietin Glucocorticoids Methylphenidate Oral contraceptives Phenylpropanolamine Pseudoephedrine Tricyclice antidepressants
Other agents	Cocaine Ethanol Heavy metals (lead, mercury) Ecstasy (MDMA) Tobacco

From Flynn, J. T. (2003). Recognizing and managing the hypertensive child. Contemporary Pediatrics, *20(8), 48.*

Primary or essential hypertension may be associated with a genetic or familial predisposition and obesity. All children with blood pressures in the 90th percentile for age and height are significantly more likely to develop hypertension as adults (Bartosh & Aronson, 1999). See Developing Cultural Competence: Blood Pressure.

Clinical Manifestations

Children rarely have symptoms of hypertension and the condition is usually detected during a health examination. Symptoms of severe hypertension may include headaches, dizziness, and visual changes. The child may also present with symptoms of the underlying condition, such as growth failure. In the case of hypertensive encephalopathy, the child may have vomiting, ataxia, and seizures.

COLLABORATIVE CARE

Diagnostic Procedures

The diagnosis of hypertension is based on three separate readings of an elevated blood pressure. The child with an elevated blood

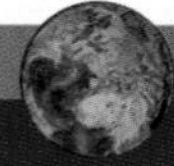

DEVELOPING CULTURAL COMPETENCE
Blood Pressure

A recent study contrasting the blood pressure of African American and Caucasian children and adolescents found no significant differences in blood pressure by ethnicity alone. Differences found were most often attributable to body mass index (BMI). African American children were more likely to have higher blood pressure and more hypertension at lower levels of BMI. Hypertension in Caucasian children was more likely to occur with higher BMIs (Rosner, Prineas, Daniels, et al., 2000).

pressure should have blood chemistry (BUN, creatinine, glucose, and electrolytes), a complete blood count with differential and platelet count, urinalysis and culture (to test for hematuria, proteinuria, and infection), and a lipid panel to detect secondary causes of hypertension. Depending upon the findings and the symptoms of other conditions that could cause hypertension, additional laboratory tests may be ordered. Renal ultrasonography, a 24-hour urine creatinine clearance and protein excretion, and urine and serum catecholamines may also be ordered if kidney disease is suspected. See Chapter 31∞ for more information about assessment of kidney functioning. Thyroid and adrenal hormone levels may be obtained. Fasting insulin and glucose tests may also be ordered (Flynn, 2003). Echocardiogram can be performed to assess for coarctation of the aorta and to begin monitoring for left ventricular hypertrophy which develops in many children with primary hypertension (Daniels, Witt, Glascock, et al., 2002). Ambulatory blood pressure monitoring—obtaining automated and multiple blood pressure readings over a 24-hour period—is used in some centers to determine the significance of elevated blood pressure readings. This may become a more useful diagnostic tool in the future, when standards for interpretation of 24-hour readings are developed for children.

Clinical Therapy

Nonpharmacologic measures for reduction of blood pressure focus on lifestyle changes that include weight reduction, increased exercise, and dietary modification to reduce sodium, provision of three to five fruit servings daily, and adequate intake of calcium and dietary fiber. Less than 10% of calories should come from saturated fats. The Dietary Approaches to Stop Hypertension (DASH) diet that is low in sodium and enriched in calcium and potassium has helped reduce the blood pressure in adults, and may well work with children. Smoking, alcohol, and drugs should be strongly discouraged.

Medications are used for children with persistent, severe hypertension that is not resolved with nonpharmacologic therapies. End organ damage (left ventricular hypertrophy, retinopathy, or microalbuminuria) is another indication for pharmacologic therapy. The goal of therapy is to reduce the blood pressure to less than the 95% for age, sex, and height. Angiotensin-converting enzyme (ACE) inhibitors, angiotensin-receptor blockers, calcium channel blockers, and beta-agonists are approved for the treatment of childhood hypertension (Flynn, 2003).

NURSING MANAGEMENT

Nursing care focuses on detecting the child with hypertension and helping the child and family make lifestyle changes that help prevent hypertension or control the blood pressure when hypertension occurs.

■ Nursing Assessment and Diagnosis

Take a complete history for the child with borderline hypertension and other associated diseases. Are parents or siblings hypertensive? Is the child obese? How many servings of fruit does the child eat daily? What is the number of servings of dairy products? What is the child's daily salt intake? What are the child's daily exercise routines?

When assessing the child for hypertension, make sure the appropriate size cuff is used and take readings at different times of day. Have the child sit quietly for 5 minutes before taking the blood pressure. Attempt to have another healthcare provider, such as a school nurse, take one or more readings. This might help determine if the higher systolic reading is associated with stress of a visit to the physician. Make sure at least one blood pressure reading is made using the leg, to assess for coarctation of the aorta. The systolic reading in the leg is normally at least 10 to 20 mm Hg higher than the arm reading (Flynn, 2003).

Monitor the blood pressure of the child with borderline hypertension every 3 to 6 months. Be sure that the correct size cuff and the appropriate technique are used to assess the blood pressure. Take at least two readings during the visit and average them if they differ. Compare readings to normal blood pressure for age and gender and plot them on a graph (see Table 8–16∞).

Examples of nursing diagnoses for the child with hypertension include the following:

- Health-Seeking Behavior (hypertension) related to family history and risk
- Risk for Disproportionate Growth related to low activity level and excess calories
- Readiness for Enhanced Nutrition related to plans for reduction of fats and sodium from the diet

MediaLink Hypertension Resources

■ Planning and Implementation

Teach the child and parents the importance of weight reduction and dietary changes. Provide suggestions about substitute seasonings for salt and lists of salty foods to avoid. Children of African American descent may be particularly susceptible to increased blood pressure caused by dietary intake of sodium. Encouraging these children to follow a low-salt diet is important. Increasing intake of low-fat dairy products and fruits can contribute to blood pressure control.

Discuss ways to increase activity and reduce time watching television or playing computer games. Provide suggestions for the management of stress and stressful situations (See Complementary Therapy: Transcendental Meditation). See Chapter 7∞. Emphasize the importance of avoiding smoking, alcohol, and drugs. Teaching that involves the entire family is usually the most effective. Instruct the family on correct administration of prescribed medications when used.

■ Evaluation

Expected outcomes of nursing care include the following:

- The child eats a diet low in fat and maintains an appropriate weight for age and height.
- Foods high in sodium can be listed by the child and family.
- Regular follow-up visits are kept for hypertension evaluation.

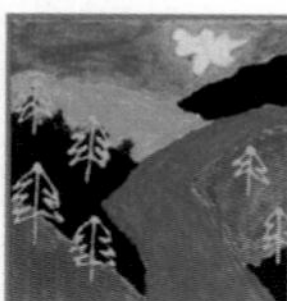

COMPLEMENTARY THERAPY

Transcendental Meditation for Stress Management and Blood Pressure Control

The relationship between stress and cardiovascular reactivity and subsequent development of primary hypertension in adults has been documented. African American adolescents have been found to exhibit greater blood pressure reactivity to stress than Caucasian adolescents. A randomized clinical trial with 35 adolescents 15 to 18 years of age with high normal resting blood pressure (between 85th and 95th percentiles) compared the impact of a 2-month transcendental meditation program with a control group that received lifestyle education sessions. Each group had similar numbers of males and females, but 34 of the participants were African American and 1 was Caucasian. Participants in the transcendental meditation group practiced two 15-minute sessions while sitting comfortably with eyes closed to obtain a deeply restful state of wakefulness. Participants in the control group attended seven weekly 1-hour health education sessions. The study was conducted in collaboration with the public school system. Anthropometric measurements, heart rate, blood pressure, cardiac output, and total peripheral resistance were evaluated at the beginning of the study and during exposure to stressful experiences (a car-driving simulation and a social situation interview). Study results revealed that the transcendental meditation group had greater decreases in resting systolic blood pressure and a trend toward greater decreases in diastolic blood pressure than the control group, particularly with the car-driving simulation. Transcendental meditation shows promise as a potential complementary therapy to help control blood pressure in adolescents. Further study is needed to determine if the blood pressure reductions are sustained long term with this intervention (Barnes, Treiber, & Davis, 2001).

INJURIES OF THE CARDIOVASCULAR SYSTEM

Hypovolemic Shock

Shock is an acute, complex state of circulatory dysfunction resulting in failure to deliver sufficient oxygen and other nutrients to meet cell and tissue demands. It can be caused by a variety of conditions such as hemorrhage, dehydration, sepsis, obstruction of blood flow, and cardiac pump failure. Hypovolemic shock is a clinical state of inadequate tissue and organ perfusion resulting from the movement of blood or plasma out of the intravascular compartment, leading to an inadequate intravascular volume (Figure 26–17 ■). The blood or plasma in the vascular space may be decreased because of hemorrhage or fluid movement into the interstitial spaces.

Etiology and Pathophysiology

Major causes of decreased intravascular blood volume include the following:

- Hemorrhage from significant injury
- Redistribution of blood volume or increased capillary permeability that may result from burns, nephrotic syndrome, and sepsis (In some cases the fluids move to a location that is neither intravascular nor intracellular and cause edema, a mechanism known as "third spacing" of fluids.)
- Fluid and electrolyte loss associated with dehydration, diabetic ketoacidosis, and diabetes insipidus

Shock results in inadequate delivery of oxygen and nutrients to cells and accumulation of toxic wastes in the capillaries. This reduction in circulating blood volume causes a decrease in cardiac output and mean arterial pressure. Cellular hypoxia and acidosis develop simultaneously. The accumulation of toxins and inadequate tissue oxygenation cause cellular damage.

The child's body attempts to compensate with adrenergic and renal mechanisms.

- When perfusion of the kidneys is reduced, the renin-angiotensin-aldosterone system is stimulated to begin sodium and water retention.
- Reduced blood volume to the atria stimulates secretion of antidiuretic hormone leading to free water retention by the kidneys.
- The heart rate and myocardial contractility increase to improve cardiac output.
- The respiratory rate increases to improve oxygenation and decrease waste accumulation in the cells.
- The hydrostatic pressure falls, permitting fluid to shift into the vascular space and increasing the circulating blood volume.
- The peripheral vasculature constricts to maintain the systemic vascular resistance to increase left ventricular afterload and provide perfusion of the brain, heart, and lungs as long as possible.

The compensatory efforts increase the myocardium's consumption of oxygen and tachycardia may impair coronary blood flow that may lead to myocardial ischemia if rapid intervention does not occur. The child is able to compensate until 20% to 25% of volume loss occurs, and then life-threatening hypotension and hypoxemia result, leading to potential end-organ failure.

Clinical Manifestations

Signs of early hypovolemic shock in children are nonspecific, but they need to be recognized before hypotension occurs. Signs indicating that the child is compensating for a decreased blood volume are persistent tachycardia, usually sustained at a rate greater than 130 beats/min, increased respiratory effort, prolonged capillary refill time (> 2 sec), weak peripheral pulses, pallor or mottled color, and cold extremities (signs of decreased perfusion). The blood pressure is often within normal values for age until compensatory mechanisms are exhausted. The infant and child may be irritable and anxious and then become progressively less responsive as hypovolemia increases. Urine output decreases due to the decreased renal blood flow. Low urine output is < 1 to 2 mL/kg/hr in newborns and < 0.5 to 1 mL/kg/hr in infants and children. In cases of dehydration, dry mucous membranes and poor skin turgor are also present.

If treatment is not initiated in the early stages of hypovolemic shock, the condition progresses until the child can no longer compensate. At that time, the systolic blood pressure drops and the pulse pressure decreases. A decreased level of consciousness ultimately results from reduced cerebral blood flow. If shock is not reversed, the condition progresses to cardiopulmonary failure. The clinical manifestations table on page 946 compares the signs associated with early, uncompensated, and profound shock.

PATHOPHYSIOLOGY ILLUSTRATED

Hypovolemic Shock

1. Blood loss from hemorrhage occurs or continues.
2. Signs and symptoms include altered responsiveness and cool extremities.
3. Blood pressure falls; if uncorrected, circulatory collapse results.
4. Tachycardia and vasoconstriction occur as the body attempts to compensate for falling blood pressure and flow.
5. Blood is shunted to vital organs in an attempt to maintain perfusion.

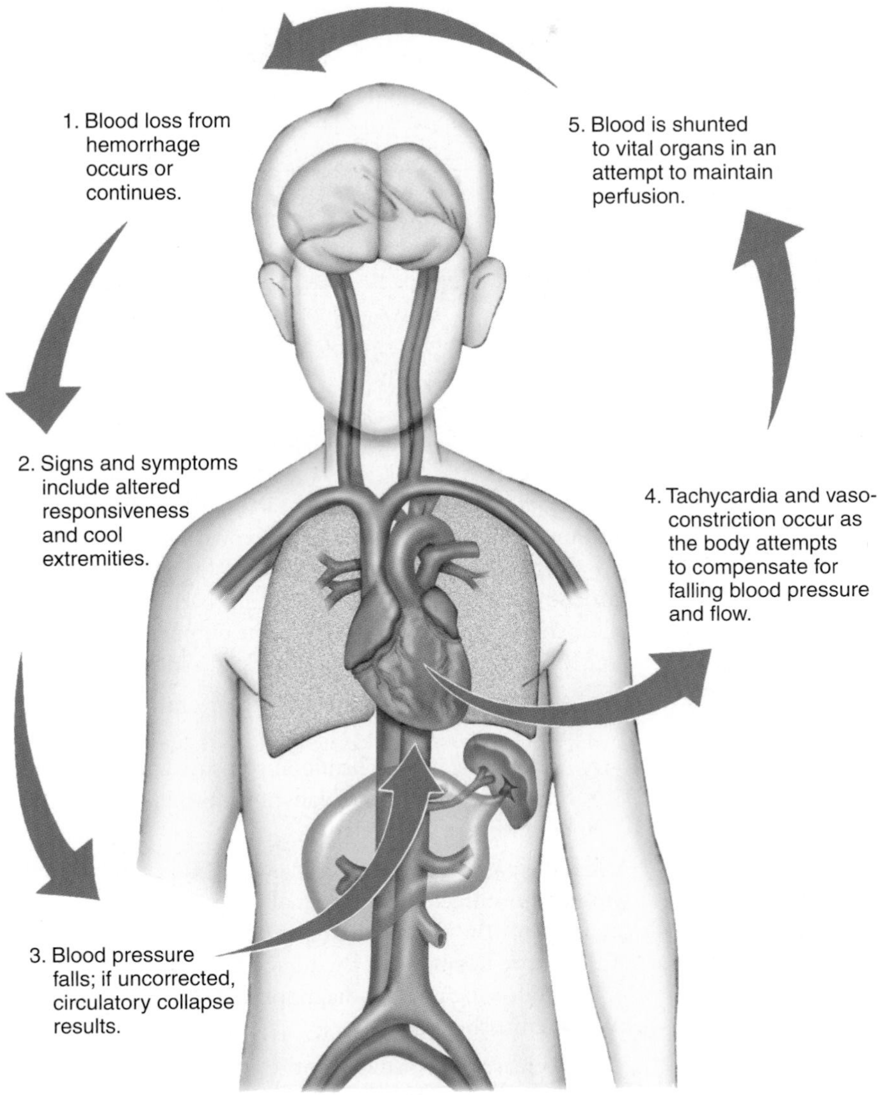

FIGURE 26–17 ■ If hemorrhage reduces the circulating blood volume sufficiently then vasoconstriction occurs, shifting blood to maintain the perfusion of vital organs. When the blood loss exceeds 20%–25%, the child's body can no longer compensate and hypovolemic shock ensues.

COLLABORATIVE CARE

Diagnostic Procedures

No laboratory values can be used to evaluate the volume deficit rapidly enough to diagnose hypovolemic shock. The child is examined for characteristic signs to confirm the diagnosis. Laboratory tests commonly performed after hypovolemic shock is diagnosed include hematocrit and hemoglobin, arterial blood gases, serum electrolytes, glucose, osmolality, blood urea nitrogen (BUN), and urinalysis. The BUN and specific gravity are usually elevated when dehydration is the cause of hypovolemia. The type and severity of dehydration present influence the serum sodium and osmolality levels (see Chapter 23∞ for more information about dehydration and electrolyte levels.

Clinical Therapy

Emergency care focuses on improving tissue perfusion by correcting the intravascular volume deficit and providing supplemental oxygen. An open airway is established, oxygen is administered, and ventilation is assisted if necessary. Bleeding is controlled, and an intravenous or intraosseous line is started to provide large volumes of crystalloid fluids (Ringer's lactate or normal saline).

Ringer's lactate solution is the preferred fluid for initial resuscitation. A fluid volume of 20 mL/kg is administered rapidly over 5 minutes. The same amount of fluid is given in 5 minutes if the

CLINICAL MANIFESTATIONS of Hypovolemic Shock

SYSTEM	EARLY SHOCK	UNCOMPENSATED SHOCK	PROFOUND SHOCK
Cardiac	Tachycardia, weak distal pulses	Tachycardia, absent distal pulses, decreasing systolic blood pressure	Frank hypotension, bradycardia, weak central pulses
Neurologic	Normal, anxious, irritable, or combative behavior	Confusion, lethargy, decreased pain response	Comatose state
Skin	Mottled appearance; capillary refill time > 2 sec; cool, clammy extremities	Cyanosis, capillary refill time > 3 sec, cold extremities	Pale, cold skin
Renal	Decreased urine output, increased specific gravity in older infants and children (newborns cannot concentrate urine)	Oliguria, increased specific gravity	No urine output

Modified from Waisman, H., & Eichelberger, M. R. (1993). Hypovolemic shock. In M. R. Eichelberger (Ed.), Pediatric trauma: Prevention, acute care, rehabilitation *(p. 182). St. Louis: Mosby-Yearbook.*

child's physiologic condition does not improve after fluid is first administered. Clinical signs indicating that a child is responding to fluid resuscitation include improved color, improved responsiveness, lower heart rate, and faster capillary refill time. If no improvement is seen after the second fluid bolus, blood or albumin is usually ordered. Some children need inotropic medications provided in intravenous drips to sustain cardiac output and increase renal perfusion as the cause of hypovolemic shock is identified and treated. Once the child's physiologic condition is stabilized, the cause of the hypovolemic shock becomes the focus of examination and treatment.

When an injured child is admitted to the hospital for a problem such as a liver or spleen laceration, assess the child's circulatory status frequently. Current medical treatment for these injuries is conservative. Surgeons give the liver or spleen a chance to heal spontaneously rather than perform immediate surgery to control bleeding and repair the laceration. Even if the child's circulatory condition was stabilized during emergency care, shock can develop again if bleeding continues.

NURSING MANAGEMENT

Nursing care is focused on early detection of hypovolemic shock so that intervention is initiated before the blood pressure falls.

■ Nursing Assessment and Diagnosis

Ask the parent (or child, if appropriate) about possible injuries or the duration and severity of acute illnesses. If no external bleeding is evident, determine whether an injury may be causing internal bleeding. For example, the liver and spleen are highly vascular organs that have little protection from direct blunt forces. Significant bleeding from injury to one of these organs can cause hypovolemic shock without evidence of bleeding. An acute illness such as gastroenteritis with prolonged vomiting and diarrhea can also result in dehydration and hypovolemic shock.

If external bleeding is apparent, determine the amount of blood lost. Although children lose the same amount of blood from a laceration as adults, the total volume of blood lost is proportional to their weight.

CLINICAL TIP

The child has approximately 80 mL of blood for every kilogram of body weight.

- Newborn: 3 kg × 80 mL = 240 mL (1 cup)
- 5-year-old child: 25 kg × 80 mL = 2,000 mL (2 quarts)
- 13-year-old child: 50 kg × 80 mL = 4,000 mL (1 gallon)

Frequently assess the child's heart rate, respiratory rate, blood pressure, capillary refill time, level of consciousness with the Glasgow Coma Scale (see Chapter 33∞), color, and skin temperature to identify any changes that indicate improvement or deterioration in the child's condition. Monitor urine output and specific gravity hourly. Signs of the child's improved status include the following:

- A decrease in heart rate, respiratory rate, and capillary refill time
- An increase in systolic blood pressure and urine output
- Improved color, level of consciousness, and skin temperature
- Regaining of lost weight

Assess the parents' response and coping mechanisms to the potentially life-threatening injury of their child. Families are unprepared for the abrupt change in the child's condition because of the unpredictability of the injury. See Chapter 21∞.

The following nursing diagnoses may apply to the child with hypovolemic shock.

- Decreased Cardiac Output related to hypovolemia
- Deficient Fluid Volume related to active fluid volume loss
- Ineffective Tissue Perfusion (cardiopulmonary, renal, and cerebral) related to impaired transport of oxygen across alveolar and capillary membrane
- Ineffective Airway Clearance related to altered level of consciousness
- Compromised Family Coping related to life-threatening condition of the child

■ Planning and Implementation

Nurses in the emergency department and intensive care unit participate in the resuscitation of the child in hypovolemic shock. See the Photo Story on pages 948–949. Assist with the child's assessment and the establishment of intravenous access.

Calculate and prepare the amount of intravenous fluid needed for administration according to the child's weight (20 mL/kg). Ensure rapid fluid administration by intravenous push or pressure bag. Monitor the child's physiologic response to the fluid bolus within 5 minutes. Prepare a second and third fluid bolus.

Use warmed intravenous fluids for resuscitation because hypothermia may interfere with the child's response to treatment. Keep the child covered or use heat lamps to reduce body heat loss.

When packed red blood cells are administered, verify that the correct blood has been obtained for the child. Change the intravenous fluid to normal saline solution to prevent clotting during blood administration. Assess the child carefully for a transfusion reaction (see Chapter 28∞). Monitor the child's physiologic circulatory responses for improvement or deterioration in status. Notify the physician of any deterioration.

Provide support to the child and family during the acute phase of treatment. Parents and children with hypovolemic shock resulting from injury or severe dehydration are usually apprehensive. The child may be fearful because of the sudden hospitalization or may be agitated because of an altered level of consciousness. Determine the causes of the child's anxiety. The parents often fear for the child's life in cases of severe injury. In cases when the parent is present during the resuscitation, ensure that a healthcare provider is assigned to give information and support during the emergency care provided. Update the parents about the child's condition frequently if the parent is in the waiting area. Explain the care being provided and how it helps the child. Listen to their concerns and correct any misconceptions.

■ Evaluation

Examples of expected nursing care outcomes include the following:

- The child receives adequate fluid resuscitation to prevent progression to uncompensated shock.
- The family copes with the stress of the child's injury.

Maldistributive Shock

Maldistributive shock is an abnormal distribution of blood volume usually resulting from a decrease in systemic vascular resistance. The blood accumulates in the extremities because of vasodilation and capillary permeability. Less blood is returned to the heart, so preload drops and cardiac output falls.

PATHOPHYSIOLOGY ILLUSTRATED

Maldistributive Shock

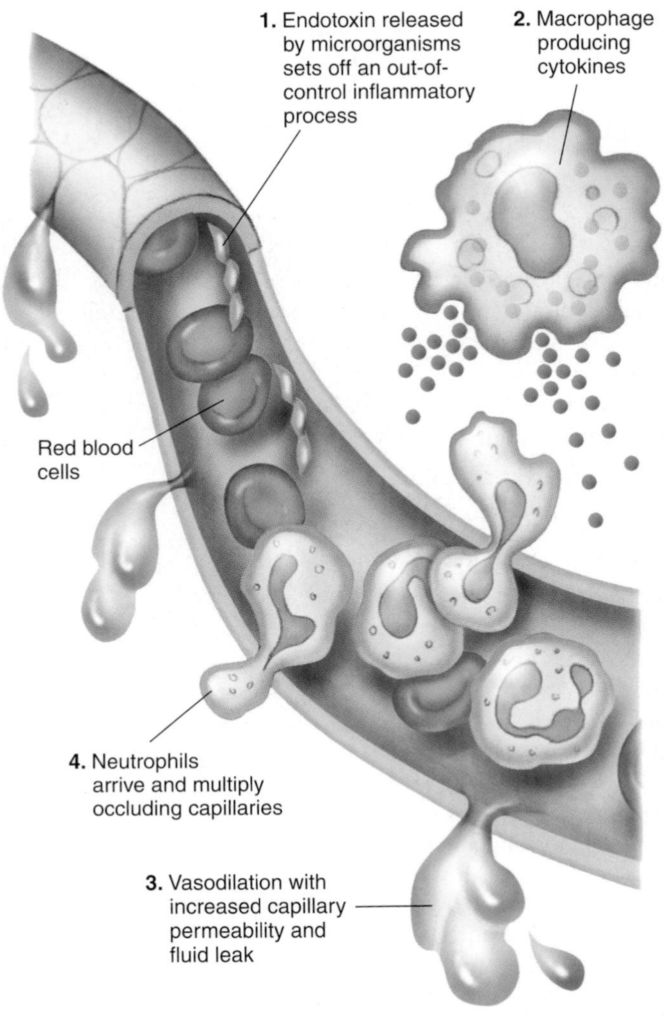

FIGURE 26–18 ■ In septic shock, blood pools in the extremities. Blood flow is sluggish and the tissues receive amounts of oxygen inadequate for cell metabolism.

Causes of maldistributive shock include the following:

- Neurogenic in which vasodilation occurs with loss of vasomotor tone, such as occurs with a spinal cord injury or various medications (morphine, beta-blockers, barbiturates, antihypertensives, anesthetic agents) (Figure 26–18 ■).
- Anaphylaxis with profound vasodilation and capillary leak resulting from the release of mediators from the tissue mast cells in an immediate hypersensitivity reaction. See Chapter 27∞.
- Sepsis that may result from these organisms: beta-hemolytic streptococcus, *Haemophilus influenza type B, Neisseria meningitidis, Streptococcus*

PHOTO Story...

Managing hypovolemic shock

Seven-year-old Sandy was seated in the back seat of her parents' car wearing a regular lapbelt and no shoulder harness. When the car crashed, the lapbelt caused injury to her abdomen, but protected her from a brain injury. She was also holding a book that left a bruise on her left upper abdomen. She has just arrived in the emergency department and her airway, breathing, and circulation are being quickly evaluated. An IV is started because hypovolemia could develop. A liver laceration is suspected based on the mechanism of the injury. The nurse is an important member of the trauma team and takes vital signs and talks with the child to assess pain and level of consciousness.

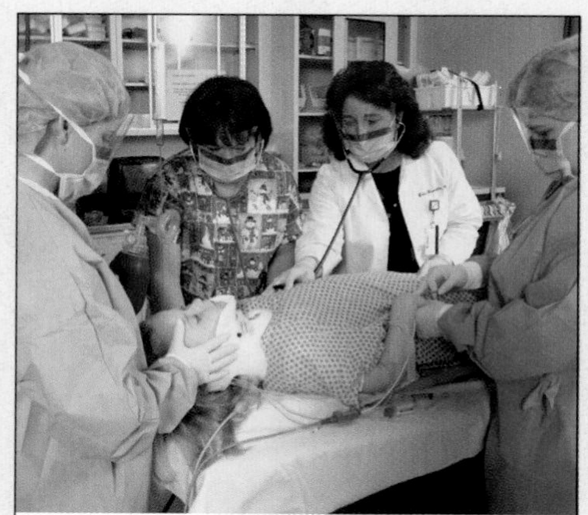

The initial emergency assessment and management of Sandy's condition.

pneumoniae, Staphylococcus aureus, Staphylococcus epidermidis, Pseudomonas, and *Candida*

Immunodeficient children are at high risk for septic shock. Septic shock begins as an infection that progresses to sepsis with a bacterial toxin. Once the toxin enters the circulatory system, the body's inflammatory processes go out of control. White blood cells multiply throughout the body and macrophages produce cytokines, which dilate the blood vessels and increase permeability. Congestion occurs in some tissue beds reducing delivery of oxygen and nutrients to the cells, and bacteria may be trapped and multiply unchecked. Systemic and pulmonary edema develops as organ ischemia occurs (Hazinski, 1999). The metabolism is altered, and cardiac dysfunction may ultimately occur. The progression of this form of shock can be very rapid with death occurring in hours. Toxic shock syndrome is one form of septic shock that results from toxin-producing strains of *Staphylococcus aureus.*

Septic shock has three phases: compensated, uncompensated and refractory. During the compensated phase the child has tachycardia and tachypnea. A fever (> 38°C or 100.4°F) or hypothermia (< 36°C or 96.8°F) may be present. Because of decreased systemic vascular resistance and increased blood flow to the extremities, warm dry extremities, a bounding pulse, and a brisk capillary refill time will be seen. Urine output may be normal. Level of responsiveness may be diminished. The body attempts to maintain vital signs and vital organ perfusion. Perfusion appears adequate; however, because of infection and fever, oxygen demand in the tissues is much higher and perfusion is actually inadequate.

Cardiac output is high, but systemic vascular resistance is low, leading to an uneven blood flow and pooling in the extremities. Blood moves sluggishly, and anaerobic metabolism and lactic acidosis occur in some tissue beds where oxygen no longer circulates. Microvascular thrombi may develop causing further obstruction to blood flow.

In the second phase, the child's compensatory mechanisms begin to fail resulting in hypotension and inadequate oxygen and nutrient delivery to the tissues. Cellular damage from the infection may be so significant that the metabolic processes cannot be supported, even when adequate fluids have been administered to maintain intravascular volume. Poor tissue perfusion of the vital organs becomes apparent and multiple organ failure begins.

In the refractory or third phase, the shock becomes irreversible with significant damage to the vital organs. Cardiac output falls as the myocardium becomes unresponsive.

Sandy is now on the general pediatric floor following surgery after it was determined that she had an injury to the bowel that needed to be repaired. Her liver laceration is expected to heal on its own, but careful monitoring is needed for several days to make sure that any subsequent bleeding from the liver is identified and treated. She receives general postoperative nursing care, including assessment of pain.

Sandy has been discharged. Her parents want to make sure this type of injury is not repeated in the future. They visit a car seat inspection station to make sure she has the appropriate booster seat and that it is installed properly for use with the shoulder and lap belt. ■

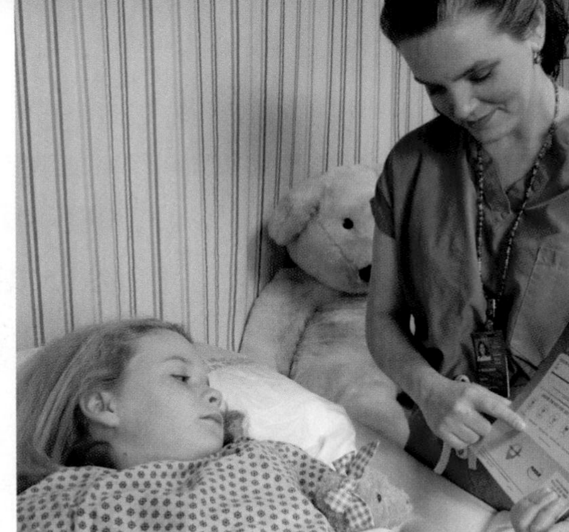

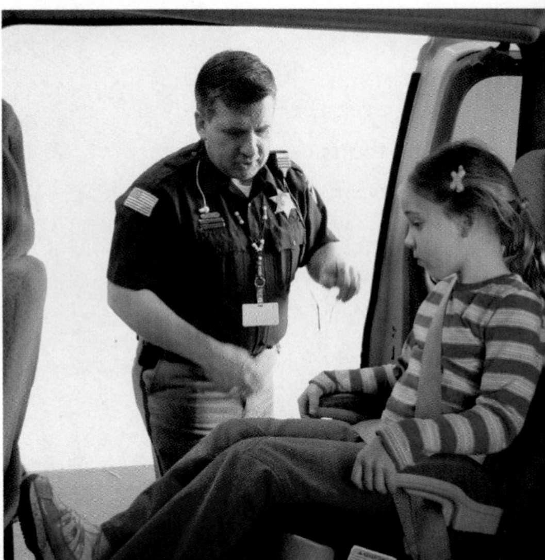

The nurse administers a pain assessment tool after Sandy's surgery. **(top)**

Sandy's parents take their van to a safety seat inspection station. **(bottom)**

Treatment for septic shock is actually initiated with the treatment of sepsis, with appropriate antibiotics effective for the suspected or confirmed organisms. As signs of septic shock develop, aggressive fluid administration is used to stabilize the circulation and ensure adequate tissue perfusion (Figure 26–19 ■). Hemodynamic monitoring is performed in the intensive care unit. Vasopressors are given to maintain the blood pressure. Metabolic acidosis is treated. Morbidity and mortality are high even when treatment is initiated early. Complications include disseminated intravascular coagulation and adult respiratory distress syndrome.

Obstructive Shock

Obstructive shock occurs when a blockage of the main bloodstream interferes with tissue perfusion (Figure 26–20 ■). Causes in children include compression of the vena cava, pericardial tamponade, pulmonary embolism, tension pneumothorax, pleural effusion, and congenital heart defects with outflow obstruction (e.g., coarctation of the aorta). Management is focused on treatment of the underlying condition.

Cardiogenic Shock

Cardiogenic shock is an abnormality of myocardial function in which the heart fails to maintain adequate cardiac output and

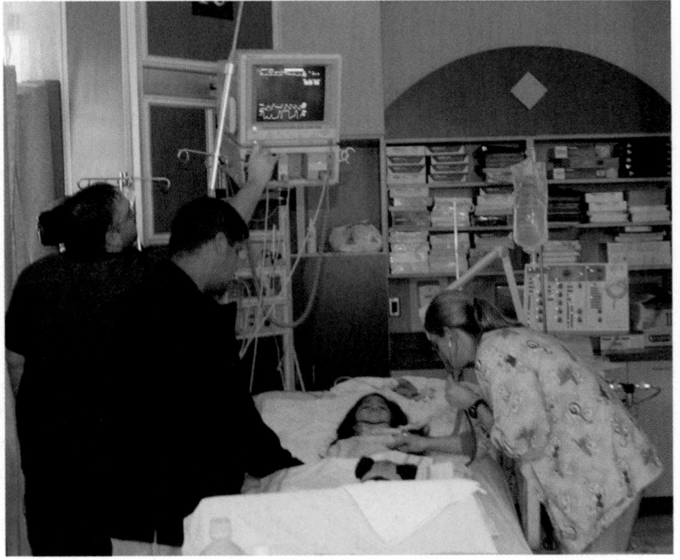

FIGURE 26–19 ■ Tina was involved in a motor vehicle crash that resulted in a cervical spine injury. She is on a ventilator and she has experienced spinal shock, a maldistributive shock syndrome due to the cervical spine injury. The intensive care unit nurses carefully monitor her status and manage her condition with IV fluids and medications.

PATHOPHYSIOLOGY ILLUSTRATED

Obstructive Shock

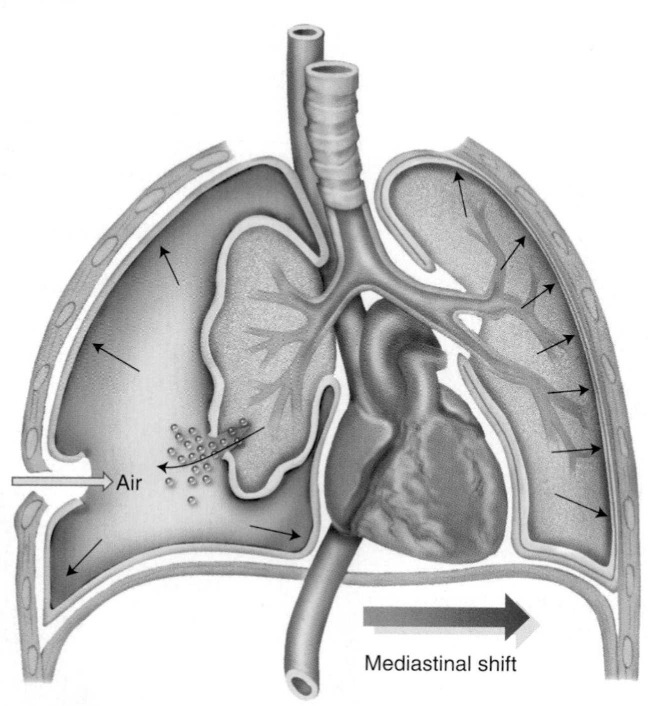

FIGURE 26–20 ■ Mediastinal shift can occur when a tension pneumothorax obstructs blood flow to and from the heart. Here, the great vessels are compressed during the mediastinal shift leading to obstructive shock.

tissue perfusion (Figure 26–21 ■). Causes of cardiogenic shock in children may include congestive heart failure, cardiovascular surgery, severe obstructive congenital heart disease such as coarctation of the aorta and hypoplastic left heart syndrome, cardiomyopathy, and arrhythmias such as bradycardia and supraventricular tachycardia. Cardiogenic shock may also be an end stage for other acute and chronic conditions such as sepsis, prolonged shock, asphyxia, hypoglycemia, and muscular dystrophy.

Clinically, cardiogenic shock resembles hypovolemic shock with low cardiac output. Tachycardia, tachypnea, decreased oxygen saturation, hypotension, diminished peripheral pulses, and cool, pale extremities are common signs. Disorientation and restlessness occur as the compensatory mechanisms fail. Compensatory responses divert blood to the heart and brain; however, reduced blood flow to the kidneys, liver, and intestines can lead to ischemia and end-organ failure. Increased systemic vascular resistance puts more stress on the failing heart. Each contraction causes more blood to accumulate in the heart and pulmonary vessels, eventually leading to congestive heart failure, reduced perfusion of the coronary arteries, metabolic acidosis, and circulatory collapse. Signs of respiratory distress will be seen when congestive heart failure develops. The cardiac output and blood pressure fall resulting in myocardial ischemia and progressive myocardial dysfunction. Multisystem organ failure can occur from persistent ischemia.

An enlarged heart and pulmonary congestions may be seen on a chest radiograph. The goal of medical treatment is rapid restoration of myocardial function with adequate ventilation, resolution of the initial metabolic insult, correction of arrhythmias, fluid management, and administration of diuretics and inotropic drugs.

Myocardial Contusion

Myocardial contusion, a rare injury in children, results from a strong, blunt force against the chest wall that injures the heart muscle. Blood flow to areas of the heart muscle is disrupted, or myocardial cells are directly destroyed. This potentially life-threatening condition is often associated with a motor vehicle–related injury. It most often occurs in adolescents who have struck the steering wheel of a motor vehicle during a crash or children who have been struck in the chest with a baseball.

A myocardial contusion should be suspected in cases of injury to the anterior chest. The child has chest discomfort because of fractured ribs or chest wall contusion. An electrocardiogram reveals arrhythmias or signs of myocardial infarct. A two-dimensional echocardiogram may show an abnormality in heart wall movement. Cardiac troponin I levels may be useful as this is a specific biochemical marker for myocardial injury. Levels greater than 0.15 ng/mL indicate cardiac injury. Cardiac isoenzyme concentrations may also be monitored for elevation. Because of the risk of sudden arrhythmias, the child is admitted to the intensive care unit for cardiac monitoring. Long-term sequelae are unknown, but could potentially include aneurysm, myocardial rupture, and postcontusion pericarditis.

PATHOPHYSIOLOGY ILLUSTRATED

Cardiogenic Shock

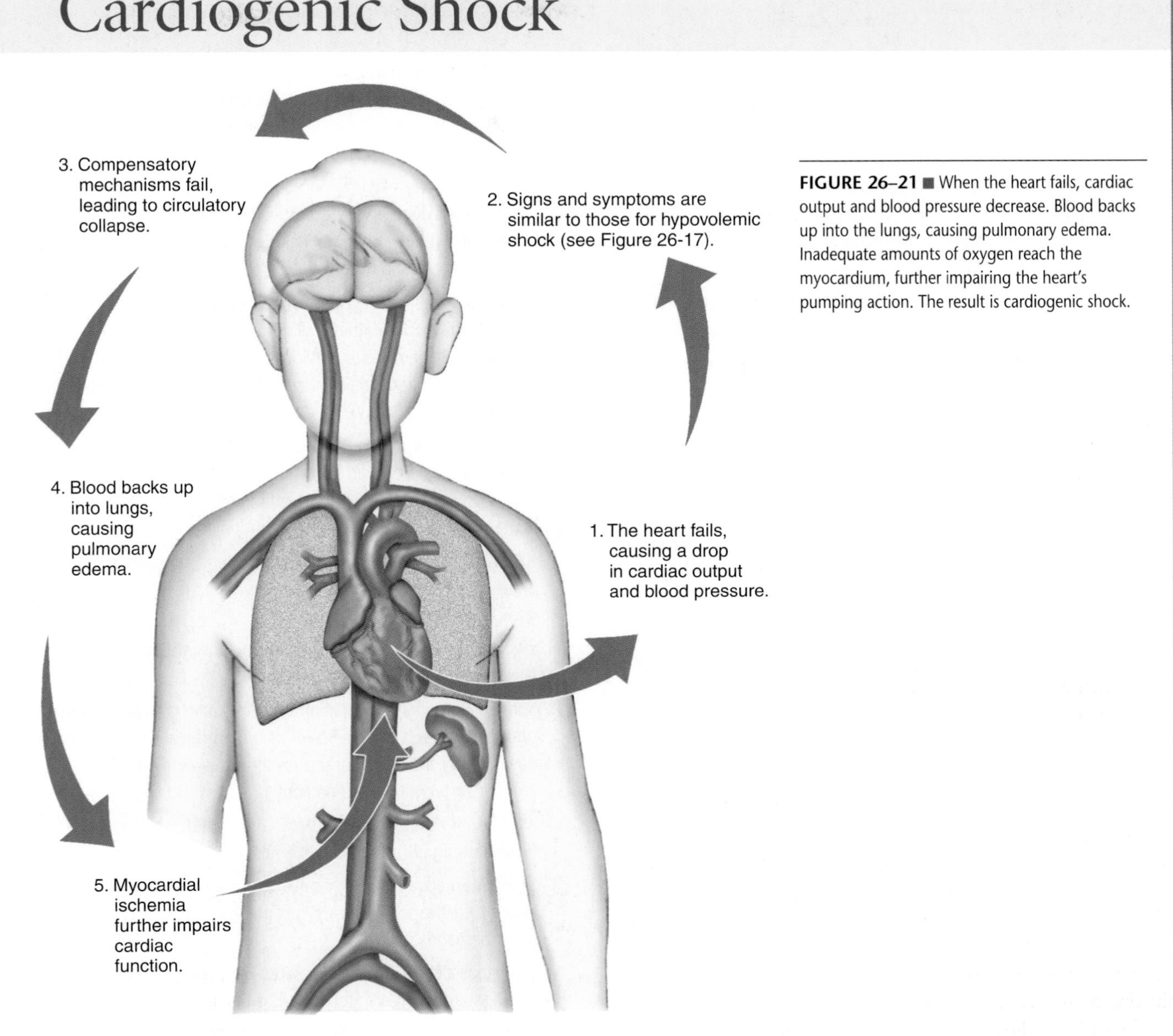
3. Compensatory mechanisms fail, leading to circulatory collapse.
2. Signs and symptoms are similar to those for hypovolemic shock (see Figure 26-17).
4. Blood backs up into lungs, causing pulmonary edema.
1. The heart fails, causing a drop in cardiac output and blood pressure.
5. Myocardial ischemia further impairs cardiac function.

FIGURE 26–21 ■ When the heart fails, cardiac output and blood pressure decrease. Blood backs up into the lungs, causing pulmonary edema. Inadequate amounts of oxygen reach the myocardium, further impairing the heart's pumping action. The result is cardiogenic shock.

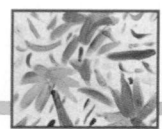

CHAPTER HIGHLIGHTS

- Infants are at risk of heart failure because their immature heart is more sensitive to volume or pressure overload. The heart muscle fibers are less developed and the ventricles have less compliance so that stroke volume cannot increase substantially.
- Increasing cardiac output is primarily heart rate dependent in infants and children under 5 years of age. After that age, the muscle fibers in the myocardium are developed enough to stretch and increase ventricular volume.
- Pressure and blood volume overloads associated with congenital heart defects are the most common causes of congestive heart failure in infants.
- Signs of congestive heart failure may include tachypnea, tachycardia, pallor or cyanosis, nasal flaring, grunting, retractions, cough, crackles, periorbital and facial edema, jugular vein distention, and hepatomegaly.
- Most congenital heart defects develop during the first 8 weeks of pregnancy, and they are usually the result of a combined or interactive effect of genetic and environmental factors.
- Congenital heart defects are categorized by pathophysiology and hemodynamics: increased pulmonary blood flow, decreased pulmonary blood flow, and decreased systemic blood flow.
- An obstructive defect (i.e., aortic or pulmonic stenosis) causes pressure overload and hypertrophy of the closest ventricle.
- Cardiac catheterization provides a means for the evaluation of the anatomy, as well as the hemodynamics and pressure gradients within the heart. Cardiac catheterization also provides a mechanism to correct certain congenital defects without surgery.
- Some children have complex congenital heart defects that require multiple stages of surgery to improve the quality of life. Many of these children are surviving to adulthood and careful planning is needed to prepare them for a vocation and transition to adult health services.
- Infants with congenital heart defects that increase pulmonary blood flow are at high risk for development of congestive heart failure. Pulmonary artery hypertension can develop if the defect is not corrected at an early age.
- The child with the congenital heart defect tetralogy of Fallot that decreases pulmonary blood flow may have life-threatening hypercyanotic spells requiring emergency treatment. Palliative or corrective surgery is often performed soon afterwards to prevent other life-threatening attacks.
- Congenital heart defects that obstruct systemic blood flow cause signs and symptoms associated with low cardiac output: diminished pulses, poor color, prolonged capillary refill time, and decreased urinary output.
- Cardiomyopathy during childhood occurs most often in infancy and adolescence.
- Heart transplantation is performed in infants and children for complex heart defects or cardiomyopathy. Rejection and infection are the major causes of mortality and morbidity during the first year following the transplant.
- Pulmonary artery hypertension is a life-threatening complication of congenital heart disease with excessive pulmonary blood flow. Irreversible pulmonary vascular changes include inflammation, hypertrophy of pulmonary vessels, and fibrosis.
- Children who have a congenital heart defect, rheumatic heart disease, or a central venous catheter or who have had heart surgery are at risk for infective endocarditis. Children at high risk should be discouraged from body piercing because infections have occurred despite antibiotic prophylaxis.
- Rheumatic fever is an inflammatory connective tissue disease following a streptococcal infection that may affect the heart, joints, skin, or central nervous system. Long-term antibiotic therapy is prescribed after the acute phase of the illness to prevent repeated infections.
- Kawasaki disease is an acute febrile, systemic inflammatory illness with an unknown etiology. Coronary artery damage is a potential significant complication.
- Two potentially life-threatening cardiac arrhythmias are supraventricular tachycardia and long QT syndrome.
- Some children have familial or lifestyle-related dyslipidemia that causes undesirable levels of cholesterol or triglycerides. These children should have dietary intervention and exercise regimens to reduce the risk of coronary artery disease as an adult.
- All children with blood pressures in the 90th percentile for age, sex, and height are significantly more likely to develop hypertension as adults.
- Shock is an acute, complex state of circulatory dysfunction resulting in failure to deliver sufficient oxygen and other nutrients to meet cell and tissue demands.
- Signs that a child is in compensated hypovolemic shock include tachycardia, increased respiratory effort, prolonged capillary refill time, weak peripheral pulses, pallor, and cold extremities.
- Maldistributive shock is an abnormal distribution of the blood volume that results from a decrease in vascular resistance. It may be caused by anaphylaxis, sepsis, or spinal cord injury.
- Myocardial contusion results from a strong, blunt force against the chest wall that injures the heart muscle. Blood flow to areas of the heart muscle may be disrupted or myocardial cells may be directly destroyed.

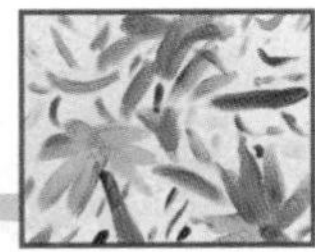

CRITICAL THINKING IN ACTION

INTRODUCTION

Return to the scenario at the beginning of the chapter. One-month old Brandy is recuperating from corrective surgery to repair her ventricular septal defect after developing congestive heart failure.

DESCRIPTION

Brandy's parents have had little time to adjust to the new baby in the family, dealing with the fact that she had a heart defect and the special care needed, and now are coping with the emergency corrective surgery. While they are thrilled that Brandy is making good progress following surgery and that she will be moved to the general care unit later in the day, they are exhausted by the emotional stressors. They have begun asking about the special care Brandy will need when she returns home. The parents have a toddler named Ben at home who is bewildered by all the changes in his life. One of his grandmothers is caring for him, and his parents have had little time to spend with Ben except to talk with him on the phone and tuck him in to bed at night.

DISCUSSION

1. Outline the nursing care that Brandy will need on the general care unit and describe how Brandy's parents can play an active role in her care.
2. Describe the care that Brandy will need in the first couple of weeks at home and develop a discharge plan. Identify the signs that might indicate an urgent need to return for medical evaluation.
3. Talk with the parents about their toddler's potential responses to all the changes in the family over the past month. Collaborate with the parents to outline strategies to meet Ben's developmental needs for attention, comfort, and security once Brandy returns home.
4. What information can you share with Brandy's parents to help them understand her prognosis so they begin to see her as a healthy child rather than a vulnerable child with a chronic condition?

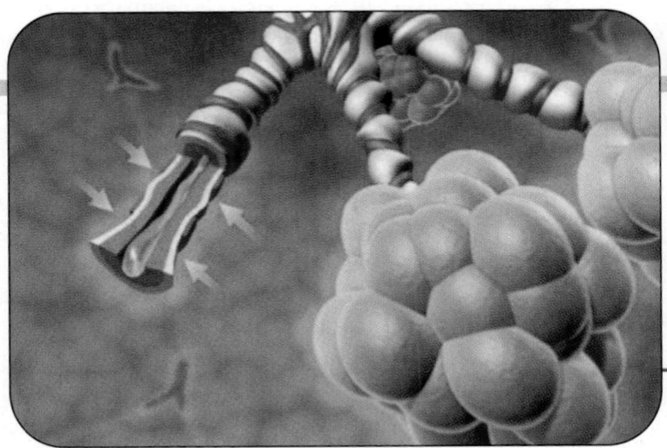

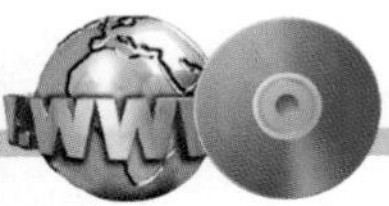

EXPLORE MediaLink

- NCLEX review, case studies, and other interactive resources for this chapter can be found on the Companion Website at **www.prenhall.com/ball**. Click on Chapter 26 to select the activities for this chapter.
- For animations, more NCLEX review questions, and an audio glossary, access the accompanying CD-ROM in this book.

http://www.prenhall.com/ball

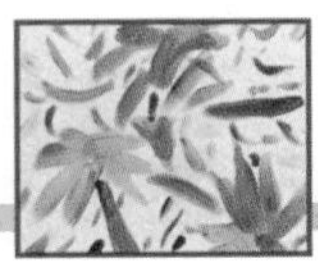

REFERENCES

Alderman, L. M. (2000). At risk: Adolescents and adults with congenital heart disease. *Dimension of Critical Care Nursing, 19*(1), 2.

American Academy of Pediatrics Committee on Infectious Disease. (2003). *Red book: Report of the Committee on Infectious Disease* (26th ed.). Elk Grove Village, IL: Author.

American Academy of Pediatrics Committee on Pediatric Emergency Medicine. (1999). Emergency preparedness of children with special health care needs. *Pediatrics, 104*(4), e53.

American Heart Association. (2003). Youth and cardiovascular diseases—Statistics. www.americanheart.org, accessed 8/4/2003.

Atkins, D. L., Dorian, P., Gonzalez, E. R., Gorgels, A. P. M., Kudenchuk, P. J., Lurie, K. G., et. al. (2001).

Treatment of tachyarrhythmias. *Annals of Emergency Medicine, 37*(4), S91-S109.

Azeka, E., Ramires, J. A. F, Valler, C., & Bocchi, E. A. (2002). Delisting of infants and children from the heart transplantation waiting list after carvedilol treatment. *Journal of the American College of Cardiology, 40*(11), 2034–2038.

Balaguru, D., Artman, M., & Auslender, M. (2000). Management of heart failure in children. *Current Problems in Pediatrics, 30*(1), 1–36.

Barnes, V. A., Treiber, F. A., & Davis, H. (2001). Impact of transcendental meditation on cardiovascular function at rest and during acute stress in adolescents with high normal blood pressure. *Journal of Psychosomatic Research, 51,* 597–605.

Barst, R. J. (1999). Recent advances in the treatment of pediatric pulmonary artery hypertension. *Pediatric Clinics of North America, 46*(2), 331–345.

Bartosh, S. M., & Aronson, A. J. (1999). Childhood hypertension: An update on etiology, diagnosis, and treatment. *Pediatric Clinics of North America, 46*(2), 235–252.

Berul, C. I. (2000). Cardiac evaluation in the young athlete. *Pediatric Annals, 29*(3), 162–165.

Boneva, R. S., Botto, L. D., Moore, C. A., Yang, O., Correa, A., & Erickson, J. D. (2001). Mortality associated with congenital heart defects in the United States: Trends and racial disparities, 1979–1997. *Circulation, 103*(19), 2376–2381.

Botto, L. D., Khoury, M. J., Mulinare, J., & Erickson, J. D. (1996). Periconceptional multivitamin use and the occurrence of contruncal heart defects: Results from a population-based, case-control study. *Pediatrics, 98*(5), 911–917.

Boucek, M. M. (2000). Issues in pediatric heart transplantation.http://transplantation.medscape.com/Medscape/transplantation/Clinical Mgmt/CM.v08/index-CM.v08.html

Brook, M. M. (1999). Pediatric bacterial endocarditis: Treatment and prophylaxis. *Pediatric Clinics of North America, 46*(2), 275–287.

Buck, M. L. (2002). HMG-CoA reductase inhibitors for the treatment of hypercholesterolemia in children and adolescents. *Pediatric Pharmacology, 8*(9). www.medscape.com/viewarticle/442460_print, accessed 10/17/2002.

Buck, M. L. (2003). Immunosuppression with tacrolimus after solid organ transplantation in children. *Pediatric Pharmacology, 9*(5). www.medscape.com/viewarticle/457649_print

Canobbio, M. M. (2001). Health care issues facing adolescents with congenital heart disease. *Journal of Pediatric Nursing, 16*(5), 363–370.

Carey, L. K., Nicholson, B. C., & Fox, R. A. (2002). Maternal factors related to parenting young children with congenital heart disease. *Journal of Pediatric Nursing, 17*(3), 174–183.

Chang, R. R. (2002). Hospitalizations for Kawasaki disease among children in the United States, 1988, 1997, *Pediatrics, 109*(6) e87 www.pediatries.org/cgi/content/full/109/6/e87.

Chang, R. R., Chen, A. Y., & Klitzner, T. S. (2002). Clinical management of infants with hypoplastic left heart syndrome in the United States, 1988–1997. *Pediatrics, 110*(2), 292–298.

Connor, J. A. (2002). Alterations in cardiovascular function in children. In K. L. McCance & S. E. Huether, *Pathophysiology: The biologic basis for disease in adults and children* (4th ed., pp. 1048–1081). St. Louis: Mosby.

Cook, E. H., & Higgins, S. S. (2004). Congenital heart disease. In P. Jackson Allen & J. A. Vessey, *Primary care of the child with a chronic condition* (4th ed., 382–403). St. Louis: Mosby.

Dajani, A., Taubert, K., Ferrieri, P. et al. (1995). Treatment of acute streptococcal pharyngitis and prevention of rheumatic fever: A statement for health professionals. *Pediatrics, 96,* 758.

Dajani, A. S., Taubert, K. A., Wilson, W., Bolger, A. F., & Bayer, A., et al. (1997). Prevention of bacterial endocarditis: Recommendations of the American Heart Association. *Journal of the American Medical Association, 277*(22), 1794–1801.

Daniels, S. R., Witt, S. A., Glascock, B., Khoury, P. R., & Kimball, T. R., (2002). Left atrial size in children with hypertension: The influence of obesity, blood pressure, and left ventricular mass. *Journal of Pediatrics, 141*(2), 186–190.

Davis, C. C., Brown, R. T., Bakeman, R., & Campbell, R. (1998). Psychological adaptation and adjustment of mothers of children with congenital heart disease: Stress, coping, and family functioning. *Journal of Pediatric Psychology, 23*(4), 219–228.

DeBoer, S. (1996). The care of the blue baby: Emergency department management of tetralogy of Fallot. *Journal of Emergency Nursing, 22*(2), 73–76.

de Jongh, S., Stalenhoef, A. F. H., Tuohy, M. B., Mercuri, M., Bakker, H. D., Kastelein, J. J. P. (2002). Efficacy, safety, and tolerability of simvastatin in children with familial hypercholesterolemia. *Clinical Drug Investigation, 22*(8), 533–540.

Driscoll, D. J. (1999). Left-to-right shunt lesions. *Pediatric Clinics of North America, 46*(2), 355–368.

Duitsman, D. M., Suddaby, E. C., & Masterson, G. (1999). Unique considerations for the pediatric heart transplant recipient: The role of the school nurse. *Journal of School Nursing, 15*(3), 10–13.

Durack, D. T., Lukes, A. S., & Bright, D. K. (1994). New criteria for diagnosis of infective endocarditis: Utilization of specific echocardographic findings. *American Journal of Medicine, 96,* 200–209.

Eichelberger, M. R., Ball, J. W., Pratsch, G. S. & Clark, J. R. (1998) *Pediatric emergencies* (2nd ed.). Englewood Cliffs, NJ: Brady.

Erickson, C. C., & Jones, C. S. (2000). Pediatric sudden cardiac death: What the pediatrician needs to know. *Pediatric Annals, 29*(8), 509–518.

Fedderly, R. T. (1999). Left verticular outflow obstruction. *Pediatric Clinics of North America,* 46(2), 369–384.

Ferrieri, P., Gewitz, M. H., Gerber, M. A., Newburger, J. W., Dajani, A. S., Shulman, S. T., et al. (2002). Unique features of infective endocarditis in children. *Pediatrics, 109*(5), 931–943.

Flynn, J. T. (2003). Recognizing and managing the hypertensive child. *Contemporary Pediatrics, 20*(8), 38–60.

Giddings, S. (1999). Preventive pediatric cardiology: Tobacco, cholesterol, obesity, and physical activity. *Pediatric Clinics of North America, 46*(2), 253–262.

Goldberg, S., Morris, P., Simmons, R. J., Fowler, R. S., & Levinson, H. (1990). Chronic illness in infancy and parenting stress: A comparison of three groups of parents. *Journal of Pediatric Psychology, 15,* 347–358.

Goldrick, B. A. (2003). Endocarditis associated with body piercing. *American Journal of Nursing, 103*(1), 26–27.

Gregoratos, G., Abrams, J., Epstein, A. E., Freedman, R. A., Hayes, D. L., Hlatky, M. A., et al. (2002). ACC/AHA/NASPE 2002 guideline update for implantation of cardiac pacemakers and antiarrhythmia devices: A report of the American College of Cardiology/American Heart Association Task Force on Practice Guidelines. www.acc.org/clinical/guidelines/pacemaker/pacemaker.pdf, accessed 8/8/2003.

Grifka, R. G. (1999). Cyanotic congenital heart disease with increased blood flow. *Pediatric Clinics of North America, 46*(2), 405–425.

Hampton, C. T. (2003). Long QT syndrome. *Clinician Reviews, 13*(1), 40–46.

Hanish, D. (2001). Pediatric arrhythmia. *Journal of Pediatric Nursing, 16*(5), 351–362.

Hazinski, M. F. (1999). *Manual of pediatric critical care* (pp. 130–160). St. Louis: Mosby.

Higgins, S. S., & Tong, E. (2003). Transitioning adolescents with congenital heart disease to adult health care. *Progressive Cardiovascular Nursing, 18*(2), 93–98.

Jenkins, P. C., Flanagan, M. F., Jenkins, K. J., Sargent, J. D., Canter, C. E., Chinnock, R. E., et al. (2000). Survival analysis and risk factors for mortality in transplantation and staged surgery in hypoplastic left heart syndrome. *Journal of American College of Cardiology, 36,* 1178–1185.

Kavey, R. E. W., Daniels, S. R., Lauer, R. M., Atkins, D. L., Hayman, L. L., & Taubert, K. (2003). American Heart Association guidelines for primary prevention of atherosclerotic cardiovascular disease beginnings in childhod. *Journal of Pediatrics, 142*(4), 368–372.

Kingsbury, K. J. (2003). Understanding the essentials of blood lipid metabolism. *Progressive Cardiovascular Nursing, 18*(1), 13–18.

Kinsella, J. P., Parker, T. A., Ivy, D., & Abman, S. H. (2003). Noninvasive delivery of inhaled nitric oxide therapy for late pulmonary hypertension in newborn infants with congenital diaphragmatic hernia. *Journal of Pediatrics, 142,* 397–401.

Kohr, L. M., & Sims, S. L. (1998). Alterations in cardiovascular function in children. In K. L. McCance & S. E. Huether, *Pathophysiology: The biologic basis for disease in adults and children* (3rd ed., pp. 1093–1130). St. Louis: Mosby.

Ladewig, P. W., London, M. L., Moberly, S., & Olds, S. B. (2002). *Contemporary maternal-newborn nursing care* (5th ed., p. 521). Upper Saddle River, NJ: Prentice Hall.

LeRoy, S. S. (2001). Clinical dysrhythmias after surgical repair of congenital heart disease. *AACN Clinical Issues, 12*(1), 87–99.

Lewin, M. B. (2000). The genetic basis of congenital heart disease. *Pediatric Annals, 29*(8), 469–480.

Lipshultz, S. E., Sleeper, L. A., Towbin, J. A., Lowe, A. M., Orav, E. J., Cox, G. F., et. al. (2003, April 24). The incidence of pediatric cardiomyopathy in two regions of the United States. *New England Journal of Medicine, 348,* 1647–1655.

Luikart, H. (2001). Pediatric cardiac transplantation: Management issues. *Journal of Pediatric Nursing, 16*(5), 320–331.

Mahle, W. T., Clancy, R. R., Moss, E. M., Gerdes, M., Jobes, D. R., & Wernovsky, G. (2000). Neurodevelopmental outcome and lifestyle adjustment in school-aged and adolescent children with hypoplastic left heart syndrome. *Pediatrics, 105,* 1082–1089.

Mahle, W. T., & Wernovsky, G. (2001). Long-term developmental outcome of children with complex congenital heart disease. *Clinics in Perinatology, 28*(1), 235–247.

Maron, B. J., Gohman, T. E., Kyle, S. B., Estes, N. A. M., Link, M. S. (2002). Clinical profile and spectrum of commotio cordis. *Journal of American Medical Association, 287*(9), 1142–1146.

Miller-Hoover, S. R. (2003). Pediatric and cardiovascular pharmacology. *Pediatric Nursing, 29*(2), 105–113.

Mörelius, E., Lundh, U., & Nelson, N. (2002). Parental stress in relation to the severity of congenital heart disease in the offspring. *Pediatric Nursing, 28*(1), 28–32.

National High Blood Pressure Education Program, Working Group on Hypertension Control in Children and Adolescents. (1996). Update on the 1987 task force report on high blood pressure in children and adolescents: A working group report from the National High Blood Pressure Education Program. *Pediatrics,* 98(4), 649–658.

Neilson, D. E., & Robin, N. H. (2002). Advances in the genetics of pediatric heart disease. *Contemporary Pediatrics, 19*(1), 85–100.

Nugent, A. W., Daubeney, P. E. F., Chondros, P., Carlin, J. B., Cheung, M., Wilkinson, L. C., et al. (2003, April 24). The epidemiology of childhood cardiomyopathy in Australia. *New England Journal of Medicine, 348,* 1639–1646.

Obarzanek, E., Kimm, S. Y. S., Barton, B. A., Van Horn, L., Kwiterovich, P. O., & Simons-Morton, D. G., et al. (2001). Long-term safety and efficacy of a cholesterol-lowering diet in children with elevated low-density lipoprotein cholesterol: Seven-year results of the dietary intervention study in children (DISC). *Pediatrics, 107*(2), 256–264.

Odim, J., Laks, H., Burch, C., Komanapalli, C., & Alejos, J. C. (2000). Transplantation for congenital heart disease. *Advances in Cardiac Surgery, 12,* 59–76.

Osiovich, H., Phillipos, E., Byrne, P., & Robertson, M. (2000). Hypoplastic left heart syndrome: "To treat or not to treat." *Journal of Perinatology, 20,* 363–365.

Park, M. K. (2002). *Pediatric cardiology for practitioners* (4th ed.). St. Louis: Mosby.

Pelchat, D., Ricard, N., Bouchard, J. M., Perreault, M., Saucier, J. F., Berrthiaume, M., et al. (1999). Adaptation of parents in relation to their 6-month-old infant's type of disability. *Child: Care, Health and Development, 25,* 377–397.

Peters, R. M., & Flack, J. M. (2003). Diagnosis and treatment of hypertension in children and adolescents. *Journal of the American Academy of Nurse Practitioners, 15*(2), 56–63.

Poustie, V. J., & Rutherford, P. (2001). Dietary treatment for familial hypercholesterolemia. *Cochrane Database System Review,* 2001(2):CD001918.

Rao, P. S., Jureidini, S. B., Balfour, I. C., Singh, G. K., & Chen, S. (2003). Severe aortic coarctation in infants less than three months: Successful palliation by balloon angioplasty. *Journal of Invasive Cardiology, 15*(4), 202–208.

Ringewald, J. M., Gidding, S. S., Crawford, S. E., Backer, C. L., Mavroudis, C., & Pahl, E. (2001). Nonadherence is associated with late rejection in pediatric heart transplant recipients. *Journal of Pediatrics, 139*(1), 75–78.

Rosner, B., Prineas, R., Daniels, S. R., & Loggie, J. (2000). Blood pressure differences between Blacks and Whites in relation to body size among US children and adolescents. *American Journal of Epidemiology, 151*(10), 1007–1019.

Rowley, A. H., & Shulman, S. T. (1999). Kawasaki syndrome. *Pediatric Clinics of North America, 46*(2), 313–329.

Saenz, R. B., Beebe, D. K., & Triplett, L. C. (1999). Caring for infants with congenital heart disease and their families. *American Family Physician, 59*(7), 1857–1866.

Starr, N. B., & Freitas-Nichols, J. (2000). Cardiac arrythmias in children. *Journal of Pediatric Health Care, 14*(3), 127–129.

Steeg, C. N., Walsh, C. A., & Glickstein, J. S. (2000). Rheumatic fever: No cause for complaisance. *Contemporary Pediatrics, 17*(1), 128–141.

Stinson, J., & McKeever, P. (1995). Mother's information needs related to caring for infants at home following cardiac surgery. *Journal of Pediatric Nursing, 10*(1), 48–57.

Strauss, A., & Lock, J. E. (2003, April 24). Pediatric cardiomyopathy—A long way to go. *New England Journal of Medicine, 348,* 1703–1705.

Suddaby, E. C. (2001). Contemporary thinking for congenital heart disease. *Pediatric Nursing, 27*(3), 233–238, 270.

Ten Eick, A. P., & Reed, M. D. (2000). Hidden dangers of coadministration of antibiotics and digoxin in children: Focus on azithromycin. *Current Therapeutic Research, 61*(3), 148–160.

Tran, J. (2002). Current treatment strategies of symptomatic patent ductus arteriosus. *Journal of Pediatric Health Care, 16*(6), 306–310.

Uzark, K. (2001). Therapeutic cardiac catheterization for congenital heart disease—A new era in pediatric care. *Journal of Pediatric Nursing, 16*(5), 300–307.

Uzark, K., & Jones, K. (2003). Parenting stress and children with heart disease. *Journal of Pediatric Health Care, 17*(4), 163–168.

Vincent, R. N., & Diehl, H. J. (2002). Interventions in pediatric cardiac catheterization. *Critical Care Nursing Quarterly, 25*(3), 37–47.

Waldman, J. D., & Wernly, J. A. (1999). Cyanotic congenital heart disease with decreased pulmonary blood flow in children. *Pediatric Clinics of North America, 46*(2), 385–404.

Walters, H. L. (2000). Congenital cardiac surgical strategies and outcomes: HEARTS. *Pediatric Annals 29*(8), 489–498.

Wilson, B. A., Shannon, M. T., & Stang, C. L. (2003). *Nurse's drug guide 2003.* Upper Saddle River, NJ: Prentice Hall.

Chapter 27

Alterations in Immune Function

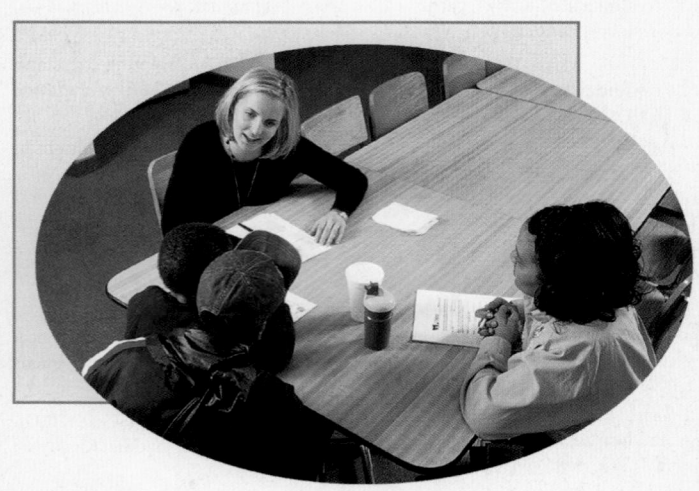

Raymond Estment, a 2-year-old child, has had recurrent infections since he was born. In the last 3 months he has experienced bronchitis twice, otitis media three times, and several colds. Raymond has had a fever, vomiting, and diarrhea for several days, and does not appear to be improving. His mother brings him to an ambulatory clinic for evaluation. His 5-year-old sister, Rachel, expresses her concerns for Raymond's well-being after repeated visits to the clinic.

After a thorough history and physical assessment, serum laboratory tests are performed to assess Raymond's immune function. On the basis of an evaluation of Raymond's clinical symptoms and the results of the laboratory tests, which revealed altered immunity, he is referred to a specialist and is subsequently diagnosed with acquired immunodeficiency syndrome (AIDS). Raymond is admitted to a special unit of the hospital for children with AIDS so that his treatment can begin.

Raymond is often irritable and difficult to console. He is diagnosed as having failure to thrive, a common sequelae of AIDS. Broad-spectrum antibiotics are given, and he is assessed frequently for the development of new infections. Pharmacologic therapy for the treatment of human immunodeficiency virus (HIV) is initiated.

Based on Raymond's diagnosis, the healthcare team recommends that his mother obtain testing for HIV. Diagnostic studies confirm that she is positive for HIV. Raymond's sister, Rachel, is also tested, and the results are negative for HIV infection. The nurse collaborates with a multidisciplinary team, including physicians, nutritionists, child life specialists, and social services professionals, in planning Raymond's care and assisting his family to cope with the diagnoses of Raymond and his mother.

"Why do we always have to take Raymond to the doctor? I don't like it here because it makes him cry."

—Raymond's sister Rachel, age 5

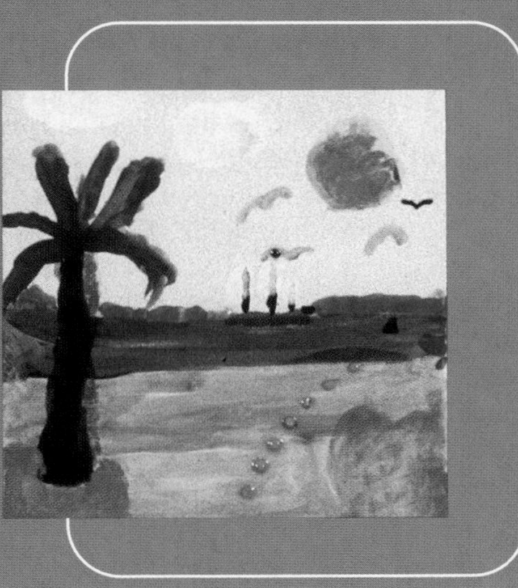

Learning Outcomes

After completing this chapter, you will be able to:

- Describe the structure and function of the immune system and apply that knowledge to the care of children with immunological disorders.
- Explain the differences between active and passive immunity.
- Identify infection control measures to prevent the spread of infection in children with an immunodeficiency.
- Develop a nursing care plan in partnership with the family for a child with human immunodeficiency virus (HIV).
- Describe nursing management for the child with systemic lupus erythematosus.
- Describe exposure prevention measures for the child with latex allergy.
- Apply nursing interventions and prevention measures for the child experiencing hypersensitivity reactions.

Key Terms

MediaLink http://www.prenhall.com/ball

Resources for this chapter can be found on the CD-ROM accompanying this textbook, and on the Companion Website at www.prenhall.com/ball. Click on Chapter 27 to select the activities for this chapter.

CD-ROM
Animations/Videos
AIDS/HIV
HIV Infection/Transmission
NCLEX Review
Audio Glossary

COMPANION WEBSITE
A & P Review
NCLEX Review
Case Study: Postexposure Management of Needlestick Injuries
Case Study: Toddler with HIV

Signs and symptoms of immunological disorders in children are often nonspecific. Raymond's admitting signs and symptoms, described in the opening scenario, are characteristic of several different immunodeficiency disorders. The immune system is one of the few body systems that regulate, either directly or indirectly, all other body functions. Thus, a problem with the immune system can result in multisystem consequences since the conditions may be mild to severe to life threatening. This chapter will examine the more common disorders of immune function and discuss nursing care of immunodeficient children and their families.

ANATOMY AND PHYSIOLOGY OF PEDIATRIC DIFFERENCES

The function of the immune system is to recognize any foreign substances within the body—in simple terms, to distinguish "nonself" from "self"—and to eliminate foreign substances as efficiently as possible. When the body recognizes the presence of a substance that it cannot identify as part of itself, the body protects itself through the immune response. Normally, the immune system responds to an invasion of foreign substances, or antigens, in numerous ways (Table 27–1). The immune system produces **antibodies,** or proteins that work against **antigens,** the foreign substances that trigger the immune response. There are many types of antibodies, which are described later in this section. The immune system also produces other types of cells, such as T lymphocytes and natural killer (NK) cells.

Immunity is either natural or acquired. **Natural immunity** is comprised of the defenses present at birth, such as intact skin, body pH, natural antibodies from the mother, and inflammatory and phagocytic properties. **Acquired immunity** consists of humoral (antibody-mediated) and cell-mediated immunity and is not fully developed until a child is about 6 years of age.

Humoral immunity is responsible for destroying bacterial antigens. B lymphocytes, produced in the bone marrow, develop into plasma cells that produce antibodies. Antibodies are a type of protein called **immunoglobulins,** of which there are five types: IgM, IgG, IgA, IgD, and IgE (Table 27–2). IgM, IgG, and IgA act to control a number of body infections and are the most important to the neonate, whereas IgE is useful in combating parasitic infections and is part of the allergic response. The role of IgD is unknown. Humoral immunity antibodies are found in serum, body fluids, and certain tissues. When a child is first exposed to an antigen, the B lymphocyte system begins to produce antibodies that react specifically to that antigen, known as **primary immune response,** in approximately 3 days (Figure 27–1 ■). Subsequent encounters with the antigen trigger memory cells, resulting in a **secondary immune response** within 24 hours.

Infants and children have differing amounts of some immunoglobulins. IgG is the only immunoglobulin that crosses the placenta; as a result, a newborn's levels are similar to those of the mother's. This maternal IgG disappears by 6 to 8 months of age. The infant's IgG then increases gradually until mature levels are reached at 7 to 8 years. IgM levels are low at birth, rise markedly at 1 week of age, and continue to increase until adult levels are reached at about 1 year. IgA and IgE are not present at birth. Manufacture of these immunoglobulins begins by 2 weeks of age; however, normal values are not achieved until 6 to 7 years. It is thus easy to understand why children under 6 years of

TABLE 27–1 Cells and Tissues of the Immune System

COMPONENT	LOCATION	FUNCTION
Leukocytes		
Granulocytes		
Neutrophils	Circulation	Phagocytosis and chemotaxis
Eosinophils	Circulation, respiratory tract, and gastrointestinal tract	Phagocytosis Protection against parasites Involved in allergic response
Basophils	Circulation	Release of chemotactic substances
Monocytes and macrophages	Circulation (monocytes) and body tissue, such as skin (histocytes), liver (Kupffer's cells), alveoli, spleen, tonsils, lymph nodes, bone marrow, brain	Trapping and phagocytizing of foreign substances and cellular debris Secretion of interleukin-1 to stimulate lymphocyte growth
Lymphocytes		
T Cells (mature in thymus gland)	Circulation, lymph system, tissues	Activation of T and B cells Control of viral infections and destruction of cancer cells Involved in hypersensitivity reactions and graft tissue rejection
B Cells (mature in bone marrow)	Circulation, spleen	Production of antibodies (immunoglobulins) to specific antigens
NK (natural killer) cells	Circulation	Cytotoxic; killing of tumor cells, fungi, viral-infected cells, and foreign tissue
Lymphoid Tissues		
Primary or central lymphoid structures	Bone marrow and thymus gland	Production of immune cells; sites for cell maturation
Secondary or peripheral lymphoid structures	Lymph nodes, spleen, tonsils, intestinal lymphoid tissue, lymphoid tissue in other organs	Sites for activation of immune cells by antigens

From LeMone P. and Burke, K. (2004) Medical-Surgical Nursing: Critical Thinking in Client Care (3rd ed.) *Upper Saddle River: Prentice Hall Health.*

MediaLink A & P Review

TABLE 27–2 Classes of Immunoglobulins

IMMUNOGLOBULIN	LOCATION	ACTION
IgM	Present in intravascular spaces (blood and lymph)	Mediates cytotoxic response and activates complement First antibody produced with primary immune response
IgG	Present in all body fluids	Active against bacteria, bacterial toxins, and viruses Activates complement The only immunoglobulin to cross the placenta
IgA	Present in secretions of gastrointestinal, respiratory, and genitourinary tracts	Prevents binding of viruses to cells of the respiratory and gastrointestinal tracts
IgD	Present in blood, lymph, and surfaces of B cells	Function is not fully understood
IgE	Present in internal and external body fluids	Releases chemical mediators responsible for immediate hypersensitivity response

age become ill so often—they do not have a full complement of immunoglobulins.

In contrast, cell-mediated immunity achieves full function early in life. T lymphocytes, produced in the thymus, provide cellular immunity and protect against most viruses, fungi, slowly developing bacterial infections such as tuberculosis, and tumors. In addition, T lymphocytes control the timing of the response in delayed hypersensitivity reactions, such as the purified

PATHOPHYSIOLOGY ILLUSTRATED

Primary Immune Response

Antigen presenting cell
Macrophage ingests antigens and signals helper T cells that antigens are present. B cells also signal T cells.
Message sent
Helper T cells
Helper T cells stimulate rapid cell division in B cells and killer T cells.
Humoral immunity (in body fluids)
Stimulates division
Cellular immunity (in body cells)
Stimulates division
B cells produce plasma cells.
B cells
Killer T cells
Killer T cells directly attack and destroy body cells infected with antigen.
Plasma cells produce antibodies.
Plasma cells
Memory T cells
Memory B cells and T cells remember how to identify the antigen and will reactivate at future time if same type of antigen is present.
Memory B cells
Antibodies directly attack and destroy antigens either before or after antigens invade body cells.

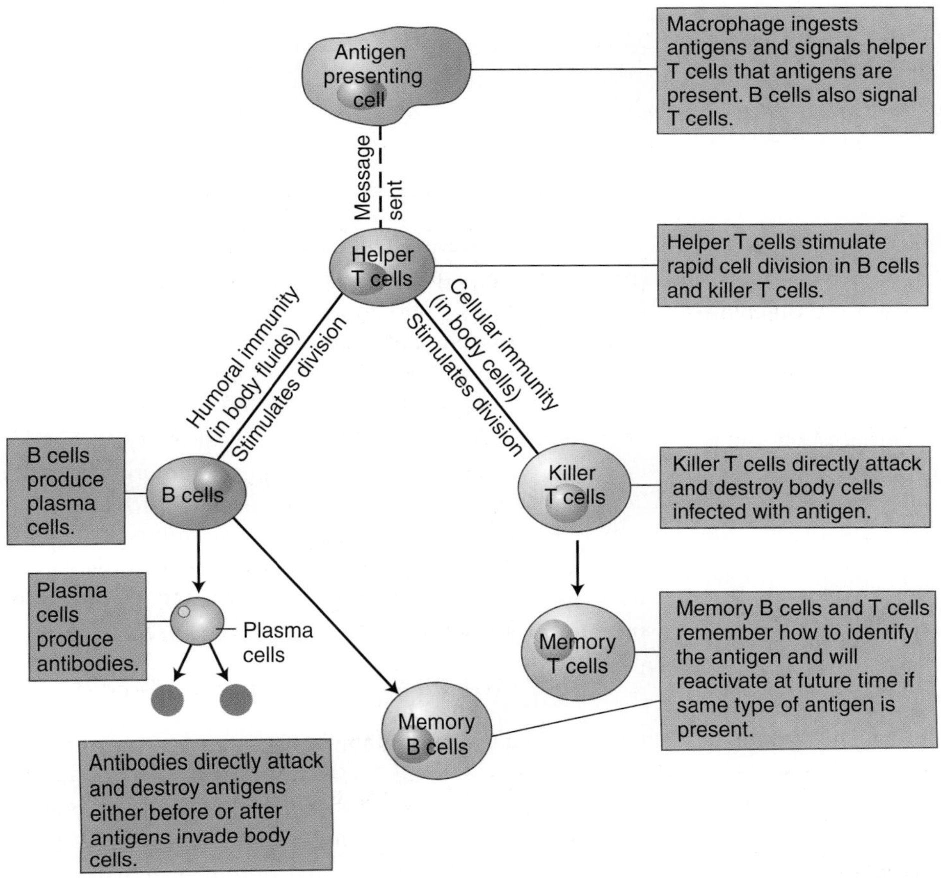

FIGURE 27–1 ■ The primary immune response encompasses a cascade of events that involve humoral and cellular immunity. What part of the response enables the body to react quickly the next time a specific antigen is sensed in the body?

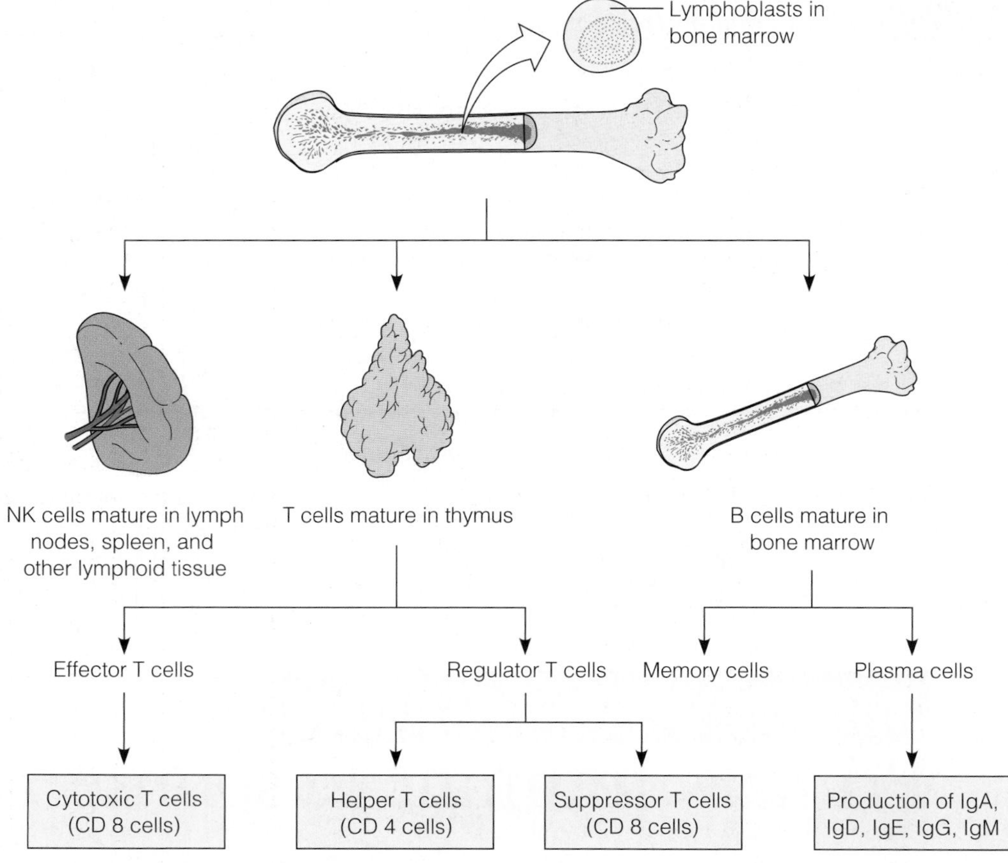

FIGURE 27–2 ■ Development and differentiation of lymphocytes from the lymphoid stem cell (lymphoblasts). The cells circulate, mature in lymph tissue, and are activated to their specific functions when exposed to antigens.

protein derivative (PPD) test, and they are responsible for the rejection of foreign grafts, such as transplants. For this reason, the blood infused into newborns is generally irradiated to prevent **graft-versus-host disease** (a series of immunologic reactions in response to transplanted cells, discussed later in the chapter) from transfused lymphocytes.

Specialized types of T lymphocytes include killer T cells, suppressor T cells, and helper T cells.

- Suppressor T cells inhibit B lymphocytes from differentiating into plasma cells.
- Helper T cells aid in the proliferation and immunologic function of other cells.
- T lymphocytes have proteins on their surfaces that can be used to measure the immune activity of these cells. For example, common proteins are CD2, CD3, CD4, CD5, CD7, and CD8.

Natural killer (NK) cells (also known as non-B/non-T lymphocytes) originate in the bone marrow and thymus and migrate to the blood and spleen. They play a role in control of viral infection, tumors, and autoimmune disease. Newborns have somewhat lower numbers of NK cells than older children and adults, decreasing their ability to respond to certain antigens. See Figure 27–2 ■ for the differentiation between B and T lymphocytes and NK cells.

Complement is a component of blood serum consisting of 11 protein compounds. It is an inactive enzyme that activates in response to antigen–antibody functions, resulting in a generalized inflammatory reaction that kills foreign cells. Complement also plays a role in causing some autoimmune diseases. The levels of some complement proteins are lower in newborns than in older children and adults, thus delaying and hampering response to certain infections.

IMMUNODEFICIENCY DISORDERS

Immunodeficiency, a state of decreased responsiveness of the immune system, can occur to varying degrees in response to any number of events. Children with congenital immunodeficiency, or **primary immunodeficiency,** are born with a failure of humoral antibody formation (B-cell disorder), a deficient cellular immune system (T-cell disorder), or a combination of both defects. Approximately 50,000 new cases of primary immunodeficiency are diagnosed each year (Cooper, Pommering, & Koranyi, 2003). In congenital disorders, the immune deficiency is not caused by another condition. However, immunodeficiency may also be acquired, as in human immunodeficiency virus (HIV) infection. Acquired immunodeficiency is also called **secondary immunodeficiency.**

B-cell and T-cell Disorders

In B-cell disorders, immunoglobulins may be present in inadequate numbers or nearly absent. X-linked hypogammaglobulinemia, selective IgA deficiency, and common variable immunodeficiency are examples of such disorders. Because newborns are protected from infection by maternal antibodies in the first months after birth, symptoms of B-cell disorders usually become apparent after 3 months of age once the infant loses maternal antibodies. Infants with these disorders have frequent recurrent bacterial infections and failure to thrive. With treatment, consisting of intravenous immunoglobulins and antibiotics, most children survive into adulthood. Prognosis depends on the degree of antibody deficiency.

T-cell disorders are characterized by inadequate numbers of T lymphocytes or absence of T-cell functions. Isolated T-cell disorders are rare, usually accompanied by a B-cell disorder, and may be associated with congenital abnormalities (as in DiGeorge syndrome, described below) or of unknown cause. Table 27–3 compares laboratory values for selected congenital immunodeficiency disorders.

DiGeorge syndrome is most often accompanied by abnormalities in chromosome 22, and is usually diagnosed soon after birth. The syndrome is characterized by the absence of parathyroid or thymus glands, resultant hypocalcemia, cardiac defects, low-set ears, hypertelorism (widely set eyes), tetany 48 hours after birth, and viral and fungal infections in the neonatal period. Pneumonia and failure to thrive are common, and T-lymphocyte counts are often < 1,500/mm^3 for CD3 (low for age) and < 1,000/mm^3 for CD4 cells (Elder, 2000) (normal to low for age since CD4 counts of 650 to 1,200 cells/mm^3 represents normal levels). Children diagnosed with the disorder are treated with antibiotics for prophylaxis against pneumonia from *Pneumocystis carinii*, oral calcium, thymus transplantation, and HLA-identical bone marrow transplantation. Without thymus transplantation, few children survive beyond 5 years.

Immunodeficiency with hyper-IgM is a T-cell disorder that affects mainly males and causes decreased T-cell function, variable abnormal levels of immunoglobulins, and high titers of some antibodies. It is usually X linked, but may be autosomal in some cases. Pulmonary and sinus bacterial infections generally occur in the first 2 years of life (Koleilat, Williams, & Ryan, 2003). Treatment with intravenous immune globulin (IVIG) therapy is helpful although later malignancies and liver disease can occur.

TABLE 27–3 Laboratory Findings for Selected Congenital Immunodeficiency Disorders

DISORDERS	LABORATORY FINDINGS
B Cell	
X-linked hypogammaglobulinemia	Reduced IgA, IgM, IgE, IgG (< 100 mg/dL), absence of B cells in peripheral blood, normal T cells
Selective IgA deficiency	IgA < 10 mg/dL
Common variable immunodeficiency	IgA, IgM reduced; IgG < 250 mg/dL
T Cell	
DiGeorge syndrome	Lymphopenia; absent T-cell functions, decreased T cells, normal B cells
Immunodeficiency with hyper-IgM	Reduced IgG, IgA; elevated IgM; mutations in T-cell surface proteins
Combined	
Severe combined immunodeficiency syndrome (SCID)	Complete absence of T- and B-cell and NK immunity
Wiskott-Aldrich syndrome	Thrombocytopenia, low platelet volume, nonfunctional B cells, normal IgG, decreased IgM, increased IgA,increased IgE; inability to respond to polysaccharide antigens

Severe Combined Immunodeficiency Disease

Severe combined immunodeficiency disease (SCID), the most severe form of primary immunodeficiency, is a congenital condition characterized by absence of both humoral and cellular immunity, which is manifested by lack of functioning T cells and B cells. Severe combined immunodeficiency disease occurs in X-linked recessive, autosomal recessive, and sporadic forms. The disorder is more common in males than females (Cooper et al., 2003). Without appropriate treatment children born with severe combined immunodeficiency disease usually die within the first 2 years of life.

Etiology and Pathophysiology

Severe combined immunodeficiency disease is caused by genetic mutations of cellular receptors to interleukin. The mutations lead to impaired lymphoid development in children with low T and NK cells. The B lymphocytes present may appear normal in number but are defective in performance (Candotti, 2000).

Clinical Manifestations

Symptoms in a child born with severe combined immunodeficiency disease develop early in life. The neonate often demonstrates a susceptibility to infection by 3 months of age, after loss of maternal immunity. Manifestations include oral candidiasis, failure to thrive, chronic diarrhea, sepsis, and chronic infections such as otitis media or pneumonia. Additionally, failure to completely recover from infection, frequent reinfection, and infection with viruses such as cytomegalovirus and the bacterium *P. carinii* are common to the child with severe combined immunodeficiency disease. Often the first infection observed is a resistant oral candidiasis. Children with severe combined immunodeficiency disease are also highly susceptible to serious infections such as meningitis, skin or organ infection, osteomyelitis, or sepsis. Failure to thrive is a consequence of persistent illness.

Some infants experience graft-versus-host disease (see section later in this chapter) as a result of placental transfer of maternal T lymphocytes. The reaction may be manifested by a perinatal rash which resembles measles or atopic dermatitis (Koleilat et al., 2003). If the child receives foreign tissue, for example, in a blood transfusion, signs such as skin rash, fever, hepatosplenomegaly, and diarrhea may occur.

COLLABORATIVE CARE

The goal of clinical therapy is to restore immune function. In addition to diagnostic studies, collaborative care includes prevention and treatment of systemic infection, promotion of skin integrity, managing medication therapy, and providing parental support. The family of the child undergoing hematopoietic stem cell transplantation will require additional education and support.

Diagnostic Tests

A marked reduction in lymphocyte counts is indicative of severe combined immunodeficiency disease. B and T lymphocytes are generally few in number or absent from the peripheral blood and lymphoid tissues. In some cases, the B-lymphocyte count may be elevated, although these cells do not function normally. Natural killer (NK) cells are few in number. Immunoglobulin levels are significantly reduced. See Table 27–3 for laboratory findings in severe combined immunodeficiency disease. Diagnosis is usually made after confirmation of absent proliferative response of lymphocytes, confirming the depressed T- and B-cell function (Koleilat et al., 2003). In addition to a complete blood count, erythrocyte sedimentation rate, and B- and T-cell lymphocyte counts, other studies including IgA, IgG, and IgM antibody titers to immunizations received, and neutrophil count, may be performed (Table 27–4). A chest radiograph is conducted to assess thymus size.

Clinical Therapy

The standard therapy for severe combined immunodeficiency disease is the administration of intravenous immune globulin (IVIG), which is administered to provide protection until humoral immunity is established. Hematopoietic stem cell transplantation (see Chapter 28∞) can be curative for the child with severe combined immunodeficiency. However, the donor must be histocompatible. T-cell function is corrected with the stem cell transplantation, and new cells appear 3 to 4 months after infusion of the donor stem cell. Prognosis for the child is poor without aggressive therapy.

With the identification of the genetic defect for severe combined immunodeficiency disease in recent years, gene therapy has been successfully attempted to treat a small number of children. This experimental therapy is expected to be used more often in the future (Champi, 2002). Enzyme replacement therapy may be implemented in certain forms of autosomal recessive severe combined immunodeficiency disease caused by adenosine deaminase deficiency.

For children with primary immunodeficiencies, prevention of infection is essential. Antibiotic therapy should be targeted at infectious agents affecting the child. Prompt treatment with effective drugs and doses is needed (Koleilat et al., 2003). Additional management consists of antibiotic prophylaxis and immunizations for encapsulated bacteria (e.g., heptovalent pneumococcal vaccine, Haemophilus b conjugate vaccine, meningococcal polysaccharide vaccine). Children with T-cell deficiencies should receive cytomegalovirus-negative irradiated blood products due to the risk of infection and graft-versus-host disease from lymphocytes in the donor blood (Cooper et al., 2003).

NURSING MANAGEMENT

Nursing care is focused on preventing the spread of infection, promoting proper nutrition and skin care, supporting the family, and promoting growth and development.

■ Nursing Assessment and Diagnosis

Obtain a thorough history of infections, including age of onset, type of causal organism, frequency, and severity. Assess family history and determine if the child has had any unusual reactions to vaccines, medications, or foods. Measure the child's height and weight accurately to identify failure to thrive. Assess the child's nutritional intake and fluid and electrolyte balance. Assess for evidence of infections involving the skin, subcutaneous tissues, respiratory system, and mucous membranes. Palpate the abdomen for hepatomegaly and the lymph nodes for lymphadenopathy. Perform a developmental assessment and assess for delays in achievement of developmental milestones. Assess family support systems and coping mechanisms when a child is diagnosed with the disorder.

The primary nursing diagnosis for a child with severe combined immunodeficiency disease is risk for infection related to immunodeficiency. Other nursing diagnoses may include the following:

- Imbalanced Nutrition: Less than Body Requirements
- Risk for Impaired Skin Integrity related to immunologic deficit
- Risk for Caregiver Role Strain related to a child with a chronic, life-threatening illness
- Risk for Delayed Growth and Development related to physical disability and chronic illness

TABLE 27–4 Cells Evaluated in Laboratory Studies for Immune Conditions

TEST AND TYPE OF CELL EVALUATED/ NORMAL VALUES	ACTION	IMPLICATION OF INCREASED OR DECREASED LEVELS
White Blood Cell (WBC) Count		
Neutrophil (polys) (54%–62%)	Phagocytic cell that defends against bacteria	Increased in bacterial infection, inflammatory processes, and some malignancies
Eosinophil (1%–3%)	Associated with antigen–antibody reaction	Increased in allergic reaction; decreased in children receiving corticosteroids
Lymphocytes (T, B, non-B/non-T [NK]) (25%–33%)	Major components of immune system	Increased in many infections; decreased in children with immune deficiency
Immunoglobulins		
IgM, IgG, IgA, IgD, IgE (See Appendix C∞ for age-specific values)	Many roles in a number of immunologic reactions	Increased in presence of infection or allergic response; decreased in children with immune deficiency

Planning and Implementation

Nursing care of the immunodeficient child focuses on preventing infection. However, even with the use of environmental controls, such as maintaining children inside special units (negative pressure rooms) to maintain a sterile environment, these children are prone to opportunistic infections (those caused by normally nonpathogenic organisms in persons who lack normal immunity).

Prevent Systemic Infection

Frequent and thorough handwashing is essential. Standard precautions are always maintained and transmission-based precautions are established when required. Implement sterile aseptic technique when caring for all sites where needles, catheters, central lines, endotracheal tubes, pressure-monitoring lines, peripheral intravenous lines, or other invasive equipment enters the child's body. Food and other items entering the hospital room may require special treatment. The child should be placed in a negative pressure room, and contact with infectious individuals should be avoided. Inform parents that because of the risk of infection to the child, live vaccines are avoided for the child as well as siblings, parents, and other household members (Champi, 2002). Refer to the current recommendations for immunizations for the immunocompromised child. (See Chapter 19∞).

Promote Skin Integrity

The skin is the only intact defense that many immunodeficient children have. Provide good skin care, and observe all possible pressure areas closely for signs of breakdown or infection. Implement measures to avoid skin trauma. Reposition the child frequently and encourage range of motion exercises.

Promote Nutritional Balance

Encourage adequate fluid and nutritional intake. Provide foods that the child prefers. For children with evidence of failure to thrive, offer small frequent feedings of high-calorie, protein-rich foods. Protein intake can be increased by adding dried milk powder to foods. This increases the calorie content of the food without increasing the volume, which is important to maximize nutrient intake. Energy intake can be increased by adding small amounts of cooking oil, margarine, or butter. Foods that are soft and moist are easier to chew for those with mouth ulcers. Yogurt can help reduce diarrhea which often accompanies various drug regimes; only pasteurized milk products should be used to avoid chance of infection. Pay close attention to growth patterns and developmental achievements since they may reflect nutritional status. Lastly, a referral or consultation with a dietitian will aid parents in customizing a diet plan to their child's individual needs.

Manage Medication Therapy

Many of the medications used in the long-term treatment of children with severe combined immunodeficiency disease have numerous side effects. Monitor closely for side effects of antibiotics, such as overgrowth of resistant organisms (e.g., thrush infections in the mouth, *Clostridium difficile* infections of the gastrointestinal tract) and administer IVIG safely (Table 27–5).

Provide Emotional Support and Referrals

Severe combined immunodeficiency disease is a life-threatening and devastating disease and requires the collaboration of a multidisciplinary team approach. Even with aggressive therapy, the prognosis is poor for children who do not receive hematopoietic stem cell transplantation. Evaluate the family's knowledge about the disease and educate them on infection control measures and signs of infection. Involve the parents by encouraging them to assist in the care of their child. The parents may be experiencing guilt because of the genetic nature of the disease and the difficulties of treatment. Partner with the family and provide them the opportunity to discuss their feelings and concerns. Listen closely to their concerns and encourage them to discuss their fears.

Assist the family to plan care for the child at home. Offer referrals to an appropriate support group or counselor if needed. The family should be referred for genetic counseling (see Chapter 4∞). See Chapter 21∞ for more information on life-threatening illnesses.

The family of a child who undergoes hematopoietic stem cell transplantation requires additional information, support and

TABLE 27–5 Nursing Considerations in the Administration of Intravenous Immune Globulin (IVIG)

USE	SIDE EFFECTS	NURSING IMPLICATIONS
Intravenous globulin is prepared from pools of multiple samples of human plasma and contains globulin (primarily IgG). It is used after exposure to diseases such as hepatitis B, in idiopathic thrombocytopic purpura, in Kawasaki disease, AIDS, and other disorders. Specific types of immune globulin are effective against specific diseases. For example, RespiGam helps to decrease incidence of respiratory syncytial virus, and HBIG is effective to prevent infection after exposure to hepatitis B.	Local inflammatory reaction, malaise, fever, nausea, vomiting, arthralgia; hypersensitivity reaction with fever, chills, anaphylactic shock; infusion reaction with nausea, flushing, chills, headache, difficulty breathing, pain in back or abdomen.	Have emergency drugs and equipment readily available to treat hypersensitivity reaction or infusion reaction. Child may be treated with antipyretic or antihistamine before the infusion. Follow manufacturer directions for reconstitution, dilution, and intravenous infusion rates. Do not mix with other medications for infusion. Monitor vital signs throughout infusion. Stop infusion immediately and notify physician for any signs of hypersensitivity. Activate emergency system as needed. Have family instruct healthcare providers about IVIG therapy as immunization recommendations will be altered.

Data from Bindler, R.M. & Howry, L.B. (2005). Pediatric Drug Guide with Nursing Implications. *Upper Saddle River, NJ: Prentice Hall.*

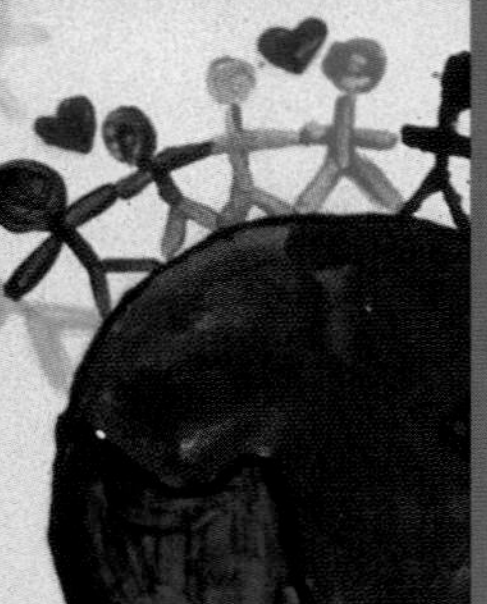

PARTNERING WITH FAMILIES

Reducing Risk of Infection

Teach family members the following practices to reduce the risk of transmission of infection:

- Wash all bottles, nipples, and pacifiers with hot water and soap, or in the dishwasher.
- Do not allow child to share utensils, cups, bottles, or pacifiers.
- Use safe food preparation practices such as peeling fruit and vegetables and using different surfaces and utensils for preparing meats vs. other foods.
- Change diapers frequently and cleanse skin with mild soap and dry thoroughly.
- Wash hands before handling child, after changing diapers, and before feeding child.
- Maintain clean pets and keep the pet's environment clean.
- Avoid exposing the child to other family members' illnesses, such as colds.

referrals. The transplantation procedure involves surgery for both the ill child and the donor, which is often another child in the family. After the infusion of the donor marrow, the ill child will be hospitalized for several months until T-lymphocyte levels are sufficient to provide resistance to infection. During this period, parents may need to rely on social services to help manage the family situation, particularly if the child is hospitalized at a medical center far from the family's home. Assess the family's situation and make appropriate referrals to social service and to support groups. Introduce parents to other families undergoing hematopoietic stem cell transplantation. (See Chapter 28∞ for discussion of hematopoietic stem cell transplantation.) See Partnering with Families: Reducing Risk of Infection.

Evaluation

Expected outcomes of nursing care include the following:

- The child is free from infection.
- The child receives adequate nutritional status as determined by normal growth patterns.
- The child's skin remains intact.
- The family adapts to demands of a chronic illness.
- The child achieves developmental milestones appropriate for age.

Wiskott-Aldrich Syndrome

A combined congenital immunodeficiency syndrome, Wiskott-Aldrich syndrome (WAS) is an X-linked recessive disorder that occurs in males and causes mutation in the WAS gene and changes in the WAS protein (Elder, 2000). The gene resides on Xp11.22–23. The incidence is 4 in 1 million live male births (Dibbern & Routes, 2004). The IgG levels are normal or elevated, IgM levels are decreased, and IgA and IgE levels are increased. Wiskott-Aldrich syndrome is characterized by thrombocytopenia, eczema, hemorrhagic tendencies, and recurrent infections (Champi, 2002). Thrombocytopenia with bleeding tendencies appears during the neonatal period. Eczema appears by 1 year of age. Infections involve the middle ear and often lead to chronic otitis media. Meningitis is caused by organisms such as *H. influenzae, P. carinii, S. pneumoniae*, and varicella. Children are particularly susceptible to infections from herpes viruses and lymphoreticular malignancies, especially of the lymphatic system.

The diagnosis is made in the early neonatal period on the basis of the thrombocytopenia, which leads to bleeding as evidenced by petechiae, hematuria, bloody diarrhea, and hematemesis (see Table 27–3).

Manifestations of Wiskott-Aldrich syndrome vary and some children maintain normal lymphocyte levels for years. Treatment is supportive, which includes antibiotic prophylaxis with platelet infusions, and monthly intravenous immune globulin infusions. Hypersplenism is a complication that may necessitate a splenectomy. However, this is done sparingly due to the risk of life-threatening infection following the procedure (El-Alfy & El-Sayed, 2004; Conley, Saragoussi, & Notarangelo, et al., 2003). Hematopoietic stem cell transplantation corrects the inherent genetic defect found in Wiskott-Aldrich patients and is generally performed in younger children before the toll of repeated infections has further weakened the immune system (Ochs, 1998). Without hematopoietic stem cell transplantation most children die within the first 5 years of life. Infection, bleeding, or malignancy (leukemia or lymphoma) may be the cause of death (Elder, 2000).

Nursing Management

Nursing care is similar to that for the child with severe combined immunodeficiency. In addition to this care, assess for splenomegaly, cervical lymphadenopathy, and hepatomegaly. Observe for excessive bleeding following circumcision and for bloody diarrhea. Refer the parents for genetic counseling to help them understand the transmission of the disease and the probability of having another child with the same disorder (see Chapter 4∞). Arrange for psychologic support for those parents who may be overwhelmed with guilt from learning that the illness is inherited.

Partner with the family and assist them with establishing coping skills to deal with the knowledge that the child has a chronic and potentially fatal illness. Referral to family counseling may be appropriate. Expected outcomes are the child's return to normal immunologic function, absence of hemorrhage, and successful coping with a life-threatening illness.

Human Immunodeficiency Virus and Acquired Immunodeficiency Syndrome

Acquired immunodeficiency syndrome (AIDS) is caused by the human immunodeficiency virus (HIV-1). As HIV destroys the body's ability to fight infection, opportunistic infections that would normally not affect healthy people begin to attack the HIV-infected individual and AIDS, the advanced stages of HIV infection, is subsequently diagnosed.

Soon after HIV and AIDS were recognized in homosexual adults and intravenous drug abusers, cases of AIDS were seen in children. Increasing numbers of children infected with the human immunodeficiency virus have been diagnosed, making HIV infection a leading cause of immune disease in infants and children and AIDS a major cause of death in children. As of December 2003, there were an estimated 9,419 children with AIDS under age 13 years in the United States (Box 27–1). Additionally for the same time period, the estimated number of deaths related to AIDS was 5,315 for children under age 15 (CDC, 2005). Canadian numbers are much lower for the 10–19 year age group, which comprises less than 1% of the total 18,929 AIDS cases reported as of June 2003 (Health Canada, 2004).

Of the children infected with HIV at birth, 10% to 20% are likely to die by 4 years of age and the remaining 80% to 90% will have a median survival expected to exceed 9 years of age. HIV is found in varying concentrations in blood, semen, vaginal fluids, breast milk, saliva, and tears; however, contact with saliva, tears, or sweat has not been shown to result in transmission of HIV (CDC, 2003a).

Most cases of HIV in children—and virtually all new cases—are the result of **perinatal transmission.** The Centers for Disease Control and Prevention estimates that approximately 300 infants are born with HIV infection each year in the United States (MMWR, 2003). These numbers are down from the previously reported estimates of 1,000 to 2,000 infants born annually with HIV infection during the early 1990s.

According to the American Academy of Pediatrics (2001), half of all new human immunodeficiency virus (HIV) infections in the United States occur among young people between the ages of 13 and 24. Most cases of HIV during adolescence are acquired through sexual transmission.

BOX 27–1 Pediatric AIDS Statistics

As of December 2003, 9,419 cases of AIDS were reported in U.S. children under 13 years of age, 891 additional cases had occurred in children from 13 to 14 years of age, with an additional 37,599 cases in individuals from 15 to 24 years of age. These numbers integrated the new cases reported for 2003 which included 59 cases in children under 13 years, 59 additional cases in children from 13 to 14 years, and 1,991 cases in persons from 15 to 24 years.

The cumulative U.S. deaths from AIDS by the end of 2003 represented 5,492 children under 13 years and 518,568 deaths in adolescents and adults; of these numbers 83 children under 13 years died in 2003 and 17,934 adolescents and adults died of AIDS in 2003.

The primary cause of pediatric AIDS in the U.S. is shown by 2003 data that demonstrated 58 cases with perinatal transmission, and 1 case of another cause, while cumulative data on children has described 8,749 cases of perinatal transmission, and 670 cases in children with hemophilia, blood transfusions, and other causes.

Health Canada, as of 2003, reported 18,929 AIDS cases. Only 93 cases (0.49%) were from the 10 to 19 year age group.

Worldwide, an estimated 2.5 million children under age 15 are living with HIV or AIDS. During 2003, AIDS caused the death of approximately 500,000 children under age 15 years.

Data from Centers for Disease Control and Prevention (CDC). www.cdc.gov/hiv/stats.htm, *accessed 3/16/05; Public Health Agency of Canada.* www.hc.sc.ga.ca/englis/diseases/aids.html, accessed 12/03/04.

The virus affects multiple systems and eventually destroys the child's immune system. An understanding of the natural history of HIV disease is still evolving, as there are several important differences in the disease progression and clinical manifestations of pediatric and adult HIV infection.

MediaLink AIDS/HIV Video

Etiology and Pathophysiology

Because HIV kills or damages the cells of the body's immune system, it eventually destroys the body's ability to fight infection. HIV destroys the CD4 T cells (helper cells), which are crucial to the normal function of the human immune system. HIV selectively targets and destroys the T cells, thereby decreasing and eventually eliminating cellular immunity and affecting humoral immunity. This process results in major effects on the viral load and the death of the CD4 cells (Figure 27–3 ■).

- A T4 (CD4) count of 500 to 1,500 cells/mm^3 represents no suppression.
- A T4 count of 200 to 499 cells/mm^3 indicates a moderate suppression
- A T4 count of less than 200 cells/mm^3 is an AIDS indicator of severe suppression. (Aids info, 2004)

Once the death of the CD4 cells occur, the child is left unprotected against a myriad of bacterial, viral, fungal, and opportunistic infections, which are ultimately fatal. Every organ system can be affected.

Most children acquire HIV in a form of perinatal transmission from their mothers transplacentally or during delivery. Transmission can occur during birth from blood, amniotic fluid, and exposure to genital tract secretions, and after birth through breast milk from HIV-positive mothers. However, risk for perinatal transmission has been significantly reduced since mothers identified as infected are delivered by cesarean section, and receive zidovudine (AZT) during pregnancy and delivery as does the newborn after birth (Ramstead, 2003). Due to the high rate of transmission from mother to infant, HIV counseling and voluntary testing are encouraged for all pregnant women (Box 27–2).

Before mandatory screening of blood and blood products was instituted in 1985, HIV was also transmitted to children through transfusions of infected blood. Most children were infected during treatment for hemophilia. Before adequate screening of blood, 30% of adolescents with AIDS also had hemophilia, with infected blood the expected etiology of AIDS. Adolescents now most commonly acquire the virus through intravenous drug abuse or unprotected sexual activities.

Sexual exploration can occur at early ages and may include bisexual experimentation and practices which put youth at risk for

BOX 27–2 HIV Screening in Prenatal Care

The 2001 CDC recommendations for pregnant women include HIV screening as a routine part of prenatal care. Informed consent is required. If the woman refuses HIV screening, explore the reasons for refusal (e.g., fear of diagnosis, fear of not receiving proper prenatal care) and provide counseling to the woman. The opportunity to receive HIV screening at a later time during the pregnancy should be offered (CDC, 2001).

PATHOPHYSIOLOGY ILLUSTRATED

Human Immunodeficiency Virus

(1) HIV uses the CD4 antigen to bind to the surface of the target cell

Helper T cell (target cell)

Nucleus with DNA

CD4 antigen

HIV

(2) Virus sheds protein coat

(3) Viral RNA is converted with reverse transcriptase into viral DNA

(4) Viral DNA integrates with host cell DNA

Virus remains latent

Virus infects daughter cells during host replication

Viral proliferation results in the lysis of the infected cell

(5) The net result of an HIV infection is decreased cellular immunity

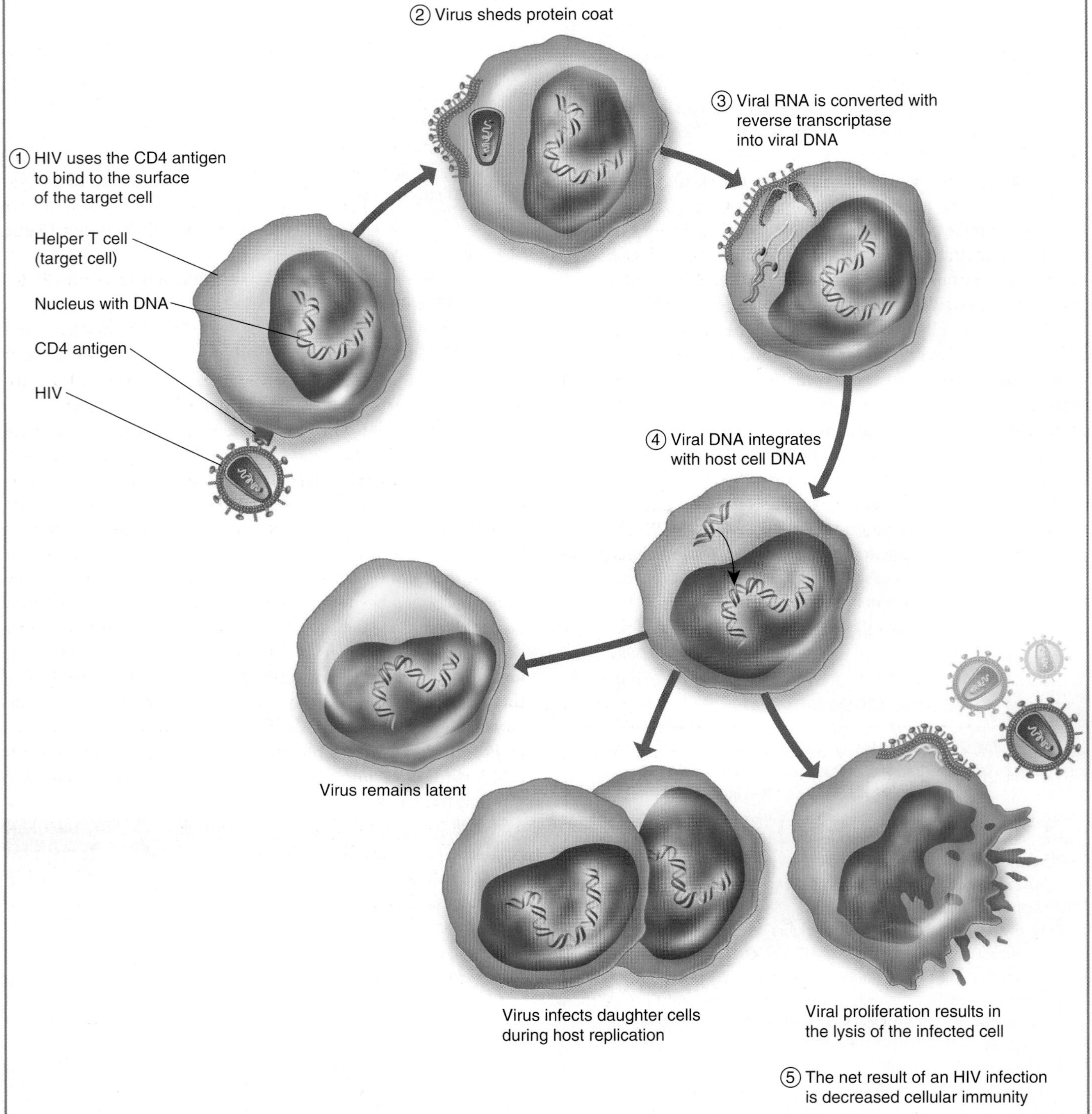

FIGURE 27–3 ■ The human immunodeficiency virus gains entry into helper T cells, uses the cell DNA to replicate, interferes with normal function of the T cells, and destroys the normal cells.

HIV and other sexually transmitted infections. Comprehensive school- and community-based programs that focus on delaying sexual behavior and provide information on how sexually active youth can protect themselves from infection have shown success in reducing risk-taking behavior.

Clinical Manifestations

The neonate is asymptomatic at birth. The time period for the development of opportunistic infections varies; however, the interval from HIV infection to the onset of overt AIDS is shorter in children than in adults, and shorter in children infected perinatally than in those infected through transfusion. See the table below for clinical manifestations of human immunodeficiency virus in children.

Most children with AIDS have nonspecific findings, including lymphadenopathy, hepatosplenomegaly, nephropathy, oral candidiasis, failure to thrive and weight loss, delayed development, chronic diarrhea, chronic eczema and dermatitis, and fever. Severe or persistent symptoms usually appear within 2 years in children born with HIV infection. These children also may have frequent infections, and severe forms of bacterial infections, such as conjunctivitis (pink eye), ear infections, and tonsillitis, may be present. Raymond, described at the beginning of this chapter, had several of these findings, manifested by a history of recurrent, acute infections (bronchitis, otitis media, and colds). Bacterial and **opportunistic infections,** such as *Streptococcus, Haemophilus influenzae*, Salmonella, and *Pneumocystis carinii* pneumonia (PCP), and malignancies such as lymphomas, frequently occur as the disease progresses.

Children infected with HIV at birth have a higher cancer risk than other children, with the average age of cancer diagnosis at 5 to 6 years (Caselli, 2000). Lymphocytic interstitial pneumonitis is a common manifestation of pediatric AIDS. Frequently children develop encephalopathy resulting in developmental delay or a deterioration of motor skills and intellectual functioning. Adolescents with HIV infection often are also infected with hepatitis B virus (Rogers, 2000).

COLLABORATIVE CARE

There is no cure for HIV or AIDS. Care focuses on the prevention of HIV transmission, the detection of the presence of HIV, aggressive therapy to reduce progression to AIDS, and promoting the infant or child's growth and development and survival.

Diagnostic Tests

Most children with HIV are diagnosed early in life. Serologic tests for detection of the virus are monitored in infants born to HIV-positive mothers. These tests are performed within 48 hours of birth (as many as 40% of infected infants can be identified at this time). Infants with initially negative virologic tests should be retested at age 1 to 2 months. Those who had negative virologic assays at birth and age 1 to 2 months should have the test repeated at 3 and 6 months, then again between 15 and 18 months.

The preferred test is the polymerase chain reaction (PCR); other tests include p24 antigen, or HIV culture (which is not universally available). Any positive result is confirmed by retesting. HIV infection is confirmed by two positive assays (PCR or viral culture) on two separate specimens. A positive HIV antibody test at > 18 months of age indicates HIV infection.

In March 2004, the Federal Drug Administration (FDA) approved the OraQuick Advance HIV½ Antibody Test™ for use with oral fluids as well as on plasma specimens. The oral method of testing is not considered a saliva test as it requires collection of oral fluids which differ from saliva. Oral fluids are obtained by gently swabbing both the upper and lower outer gums of the mouth. Test results are available in approximately 20 minutes. The testing process for using plasma is the same for a whole blood specimen and also yields results in 20 minutes. Both oral and plasma versions of the test have been shown to correctly identify individuals who are positive for the HIV virus 99% of the time. Accuracy in detecting those negative for the virus was also in the 99% range (CDC, 2003, 2004a). Individuals who test positive using the OraQuick test should be counseled that the result is only preliminary and referral for further testing is

MediaLink HIV Infection/Transmission Animation

CLINICAL MANIFESTATIONS of Human Immunodeficiency Virus in Children

ETIOLOGY	CLINICAL MANIFESTATIONS	CLINICAL THERAPY
Frequent, chronic, or unusual infections due to poor immune response	Chronic bilateral otitis media Oral candidiasis *Pneumocystis carinii* pneumonia (PCP) Skin disorders Fever	Vigorous antimicrobial therapy for treatment of infections Limit exposure to groups of people Obtain recommended immunizations
Poor nutritional intake due to lack of appetite caused by disease and medications	Failure to thrive (eating disorder of childhood) Weight and body mass index below 10th percentile Chronic diarrhea Skin irritation	Monitor growth Supplemental intake such as enteral feedings at night, and TPN if needed Meticulous skin care to prevent breakdown
Immune system overgrowth to compensate for lack of proper immune response	Hepatosplenomegaly and lymphadenopathy	Assess abdomen frequently Teach about safe transport to avoid injury to liver and spleen

Note: Be alert for the possibility of HIV infection in infants with combinations of listed clinical manifestations, especially in infants known to be at risk.

needed. Those testing negative but having a known exposure risk for HIV should be encouraged to repeat testing in 3 months (CDC, 2003).

The Centers for Disease Control and Prevention (CDC) considers children under 13 years of age to be infected if their symptoms meet the CDC criteria for AIDS, if they have HIV in the blood or tissues, or if they have antibodies to HIV. The CDC criteria address two issues: the diagnosis of HIV and the clinical classification of children infected with HIV (Table 27–6).

CLINICAL TIP

Two types of tests are commonly used to test for HIV infection. One is ELISA, or enzyme-linked immunosorbent assay, and the other is PCR, or polymerase chain reaction. Although the PCR has the greatest sensitivity, it is costly (about $175) and identifies some false positive results. ELISA is less expensive (about $50) but not as sensitive, especially for children under 18 months. For this reason, repeated tests are recommended, especially in the infant who may become HIV positive after birth to an infected mother. In developing countries where expense prohibits repeated tests, the ELISA is often used with astute clinical observations of the child at risk.

TABLE 27–6 Clinical Staging of Pediatric HIV Infection

Diagnosis of HIV Infection in Children

- HIV infected (two or more positive tests for HIV or demonstrates AIDS)
- Perinatally exposed (born to a mother known to be infected with HIV)
- Seroconverter (born to a mother known to be infected with HIV but has had two negative HIV tests)

When Infected, the Child with HIV is Classified as

- Category N (not symptomatic)
- Category A (mildly symptomatic)
- Category B (moderately symptomatic)
- Category C (severely symptomatic; multiple, recurrent infection)

From Guidelines for the use of antiretroviral agents in pediatric HIV infection. (1998). MMWR *(RR-4), 1–43.*

Clinical Therapy

Medical management begins with prevention of the spread of HIV from mother to newborn. Due to the rapidity of disease progression in perinatally transmitted HIV infection, early identification of infected infants is important to ensure the most effective treatment. HIV-infected mothers should be identified during pregnancy, and their infants should undergo periodic laboratory testing, as described earlier. Pregnant women infected with HIV who are treated with zidovudine (AZT) and deliver their babies by cesarean section reduce the chance of transmission of the virus to the baby down to a rate of 1%. The neonate is also treated prophylactically with AZT.

Medication Therapy

There are currently 12 antiretroviral agents approved for pediatric use, in children as young as 3 months of age (Aidsinfo, 2004). Treatment with highly active antiretroviral therapy (HAART), a drug regime aimed at maximizing the effect of viral load suppression, has had a dramatic impact on the health of HIV-infected children. Combination therapy is recommended for all infants, children, and adolescents who are treated with antiretroviral agents including nucleoside reverse transcriptase inhibitors (NRTIs) such as zidovudine (AZT), didanosine (DDI), zalcitabine (DDC), lamivudine (3TC), and stavudine (D4T) (Edmunds & Mayhew, 2004).

The protease inhibitors (PIs) ritonavir, nelfinavir, amprenavir, and lopinavir/ritonavir have now been approved for use in children over 2 years, and other PIs are now under investigation (Temple, Koranyi, & Nahata, 2001; Edmunds & Mayhew, 2004). Protease inhibitors are most effective when used in combination with nucleoside reverse transcriptase inhibitors, which slow replication of the virus. Recent drug trials have demonstrated reduction of serum viral HIV load in infants who acquired the infection from their mothers and were treated with a combination of several antiviral drugs. The antineoplastic drug hydroxyurea can be used in combination with nucleoside reverse transcriptase inhibitors (Kline, Calles, Simon, et al., 2000). Use of AZT as a single agent is appropriate only when used in infants of indeterminate HIV status during the first 6 weeks of life to prevent perinatal HIV transmission. A CBC with differential is performed at birth, 4 to 6 weeks, and 12 weeks to monitor for drug side effects. See the medication table on page 969.

Regardless of the results of diagnostic tests, all infants born to infected mothers should begin prophylaxis against *P. carinii* pneumonia (a commonly serious or fatal outcome in infants) by the age of 4 to 6 weeks and continue to 12 months, or until two negative HIV tests have been documented. Intravenous immune globulin (IVIG; see Table 27–5) has been used to prevent bacterial infections in children under the age of 2 years. Treatment involves prompt therapy for bacterial and opportunistic infections.

Medications used for *P. carinii* pneumonia (PCP) prophylaxis include trimethoprim-sulfamethoxazole (Bactrim or Septra), dapsone, or aerosolized pentamidine. In addition, all infected mothers should receive oral zidovudine (AZT) after the first trimester of pregnancy and intravenous AZT during labor and delivery.

The earlier the child develops AIDS, the poorer the prognosis. However, as treatment protocols improve, more children are living longer with the disease. Younger children are more likely to die of pulmonary diseases or infection, while those who survive past 10 years of age are more likely to die of cardiac disease, protein-energy malnutrition, encephalopathy, and infection with Mycobacterium avium complex. The average age for survival of a child after diagnosis of HIV infection is 8 years (Langston, Cooper, Goldfarb, et al., 2001).

NURSING MANAGEMENT

The initial goal of nursing management is to implement health promotion measures to reduce the risk of transmission of HIV to newborns, infants, children, and adolescents. Once a child with HIV or AIDS is identified, nursing care is focused on managing the child's symptoms, promoting growth and development, reducing the child's exposure to infectious organisms, and preventing further transmission of HIV.

MEDICATIONS Used to Treat Human Immunodeficiency Virus

MEDICATION	ACTION	NURSING IMPLICATIONS
Nucleoside Analogs or Nucleoside Reverse Transcriptase Inhibitors (NRTIs)		
Examples: Zidovudine (AZT) Didanosine Zalcitabine Stavudine Lamivudine Abacavir	Inhibits action of viral reverse transcriptase, an enzyme in the conversion of RNA to DNA	Baseline data include physical assessment, laboratory studies (especially measurement of white and red blood cell counts); monitored at least monthly for changes Common side effects include fever, headache, insomnia, myalgia, nausea, vomiting, diarrhea, anorexia, bone marrow suppression with resulting granulocytopenia and anemia, dyspnea, cough, skin rash. Teach signs and symptoms of infection. Be sure family realizes that the drug neither cures HIV nor prevents transfer from the person infected to others.
Protease Inhibitors		
Examples: Saquinavir Ritonavir Indinavir Nelfinavir Kaletra (lopinavir/ritonavir combination) Fosamprenavir	Blocks the function of the enzyme protease needed for viral formation and growth	Baseline data include physical assessment and laboratory studies (such as serum electrolytes, CBC, liver function studies, blood glucose, hemoglobin A_{1c}, serum amylase, CPK); monitored at least monthly for changes. Side effects include CNS, CV changes, life-threatening hematologic changes, respiratory distress, and allergy; monitor for specific side effects of the particular drug administered. Oral forms taken within 2 hours of a full meal. Be sure family realizes that the drug neither cures HIV nor prevents transfer from the person infected to others.
Nonnucleoside Reverse Transcriptase Inhibitors		
Examples: nevirapine, delavirdine	Bind to viral reverse transcriptase and disrupt the conversion of RNA to DNA	Baseline data include physical assessment and laboratory studies (such as liver and kidney function tests, CBC and differential); monitored at least monthly for changes Side effects include fever, headache, nausea, diarrhea, hepatitis, altered liver function, anemia, neutropenia, drowsiness and fatigue, rash, Stevens-Johnson syndrome. Be sure family realizes that the drug neither cures HIV nor prevents transfer from the person infected to others. Teach the family to: Notify healthcare provider immediately if rash appears. Use caution in driving or other hazardous activity due to fatigue. Avoid St. John's wort which may decrease the medication's activity.

Note: The average cost of annual therapy with a combination of drugs as recommended is about $10,000 (Burpo, 2000). What special financial needs will families have when someone is treated for HIV?

Nursing Assessment and Diagnosis

For infants at risk of HIV infection, obtain the HIV test results of the mother if available. When the results are positive, the infant should be screened for HIV infection according to the CDC guidelines as described in the previous section. Facilitate the screening and explain the necessity to the family.

Physiologic Assessment

Assessment centers on observation and evaluation of potential sites of infection. Assess breath sounds, respiratory status, arterial blood gases, level of consciousness, and mental status. Any evidence of lymphocytic interstitial pneumonitis or neurologic abnormalities are reported for immediate evaluation. Assess the child's height and weight frequently. Observe for signs of failure to thrive and assess for anemia. Assess for Candida infections in the mouth and the diaper area. Note any developmental delays in motor skills or intellectual functioning, which could result from encephalopathy and poor nutrition, and can signal the progression from HIV infection into AIDS (Pearson, McGrath, Nozyce, et al., 2000). These findings should be reported immediately so that further medical evaluation can be implemented.

Psychosocial Assessment

Assess family support systems and coping mechanisms, as the stressors of caring for a child with HIV or AIDS may overwhelm parents. Assess the family's ability to care for the child. If the mother is infected, inquire about the extended family's ability to provide daily care as well as emotional support. Support the family when they decide to inform a school-age child or adolescent of the diagnosis. When assessing an adolescent with AIDS, evaluate the teen's understanding of how AIDS is transmitted and the response to the diagnosis. See Partnering with Families: Informing the Child of HIV Status.

The accompanying nursing care plan includes common nursing diagnoses that may apply to a child hospitalized with AIDS. Other nursing diagnoses may include the following:

- Diarrhea related to gastrointestinal infection, malignancy, or drug reactions
- Impaired Gas Exchange related to pulmonary disease

MediaLink Case Study: Toddler with HIV

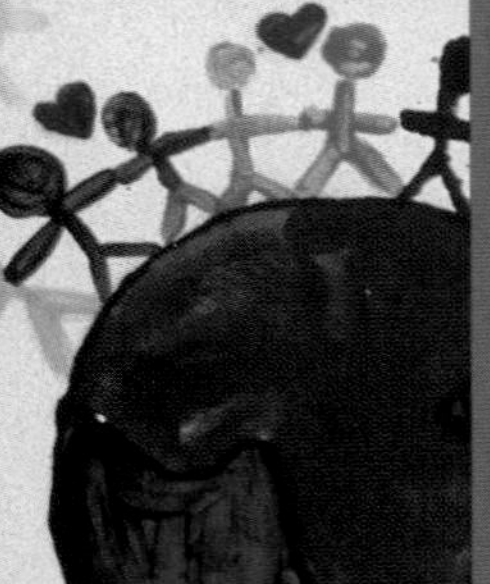

PARTNERING WITH FAMILIES

Informing the Child of HIV Status

The American Academy of Pediatric Committee on Pediatric AIDS recommends that school children and adolescents with HIV be informed of their diagnosis. Telling the child is difficult for parents and they often avoid doing so. Because parents usually want to be the ones to tell the child, they need help to plan how to discuss the issue and ongoing support in the process of communication (Instone, 2000). Nurses can assist in the following ways.

- Help parents understand the need to discuss the diagnosis with the child.
- Provide information about how to tell the child. Role play with the parents how to tell the child; assist parents to be honest.
- Provide sources of hope—the success of treatment, children living with HIV, and maintaining an active life.
- Assist the family to join support groups or web-based groups.
- Help the family plan for respite care as needed.
- Provide emotional support for this difficult task and allow for ongoing opportunities to express concerns, fears, and anxieties.

- Delayed Growth and Development related to chronic infection and poor nutrition
- Risk for Compromised Family Coping related to child's life-threatening illness

Planning and Implementation

Nursing care centers on preventing infection and providing emotional support and developmentally appropriate health promotion and health maintenance. The first step in managing HIV infection is prevention. Nurses must be active in evaluating test results and instituting measures to prevent perinatal transmission of HIV to the infants of infected mothers. Adequate testing, prophylaxis for HIV and PCP, and follow-up visits for evaluation of general health and development for all infants at risk of the disease is advised.

Guidelines from the American Academy of Pediatrics recommend that pediatricians offer HIV testing and counseling to adolescents who are sexually active or involved in substance abuse (Committee on Pediatric AIDS, 2001). There are also recommendations for inclusion of HIV and AIDS education into comprehensive health education for students from kindergarten through 12th grade (Committee on Pediatric AIDS, 1998) (Box 27–3). Nurses can implement these policies and counsel teens about the dangers and prevention measures for HIV.

If the child is diagnosed with HIV, close health supervision is needed to ensure medications are given and examinations are carried out. When HIV progresses to AIDS, nursing care is similar to that of a child with any serious chronic, life-threatening disease. The accompanying nursing care plan summarizes nursing care for the child hospitalized with acquired immunodeficiency syndrome.

BOX 27–3 Teaching about AIDS

The American Academy of Pediatrics recommends that HIV and AIDS education be part of health education in kindergarten through 12th grade. School nurses should be educated about HIV/AIDS, ethics, testing, and counseling. The particular roles defined for nurses in school settings include:

1. Participate in education programs for teachers.
2. Assist schools and other organizations to develop education programs.
3. Review, adapt, and develop educational materials.
4. Participate in public discussions about HIV/AIDS.
5. Take part in meetings with school administrators, staff, and parents.
6. Facilitate networking among parents and AIDS community groups.

Adapted from Committee on Pediatric AIDS. (1998). Human immunodeficiency virus/acquired immunodeficiency syndrome education in schools. Pediatrics, 101, 933–935.

Prevent Infection

Protection of the neonate from HIV-infected maternal secretions is essential. Measures to implement include avoidance of the use of fetal scalp electrodes and other invasive devices during labor. Bathe the newborn as soon as possible after delivery and wash the eyes and face before administration of prophylactic eye drops or ointment. Heel sticks and newborn injections should be delayed until after the newborn has been bathed. To avoid transmission of HIV through breast milk, encourage the mother to formula-feed the baby instead of breastfeeding (Luxner, 2003). (See Developing Cultural Competence: Breastfeeding and HIV/AIDS.)

Properly dispose of needles and contaminated materials to reduce the transmission of HIV (Figure 27-4 ■). Standard precautions (see Chapter 19∞) are implemented to prevent exposure to HIV. See the Skills Manual.

Immunosuppressed children become infected with bacteria as well as other organisms that are common in the environment. Frequent handwashing and prevention of exposure of the child to individuals with upper respiratory or other infections are the best interventions to protect the child with HIV from acquiring other infections. See Partnering with Families: Childcare Center Safety Precautions.

A modified immunization schedule that avoids exposure to varicella vaccine should be followed. See Chapter 19∞ for the CDC's recommended guidelines for immunization schedules. Because the risk of serious outcomes for measles disease is great, a live measles-mumps-rubella vaccine is used unless the child is severely affected with AIDS. Tuberculosis is more common in children with AIDS; therefore, annual skin tests that are performed

DEVELOPING CULTURAL COMPETENCE
Breastfeeding and HIV/AIDS

In countries such as the United States, where artificial formula is readily available, infant survival is greatest if the HIV-positive mother does not breastfeed her infant. In developing countries where artificial formula is not available or in areas where hygiene and sanitation conditions are poor and access to clean water is not available to reconstitute the formula, breastfeeding should be used as the primary source of nutrition.

Data from Linkages Project. (2004). www.linkagesproject.org, *accessed 12/7/2004.*

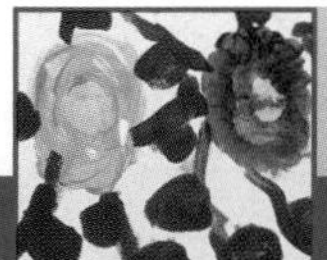

Nursing Care Plan

THE CHILD WITH ACQUIRED IMMUNODEFICIENCY SYNDROME

GOAL	INTERVENTION	RATIONALE	EXPECTED OUTCOME
1. Risk for Infection related to immunosuppression			
	NIC Priority Intervention—*Infection Control:* Minimizing the acquisition and transmission of infectious agents		**NOC Suggested Outcome—***Risk Control:* Actions to eliminate or reduce actual, personal, and modifiable health threats
Risk factors for infection will be eliminated as evidenced by infection control.	■ Assess the child every 2–4 hours for fever; lesions in the mouth; redness, inflammation, soreness, and lesions on the skin or around intravenous lines.	■ Fever is one of the few signs of infections in the immunosuppressed child who does not have a sufficient number of white blood cells.	The child has no fever and shows no other signs of infection.
	■ Auscultate for changes in breath sounds every 2 hours. Perform pulmonary toilet (coughing, deep breathing, incentive spirometry) every 2–4 hours.	■ Pneumonia is a likely infection in the child with AIDS.	
	■ Enforce strict handwashing. Allow no fresh flowers, fruits, or vegetables in child's room. Screen visitors for colds or recent exposure to varicella. Use blood and body fluid precautions (refer to the Skills Manual). Practice strict asepsis for dressing changes and suctioning.	■ Control of environmental factors helps prevent infection.	
	■ Coordinate patient care assignments to avoid exposing the child to individuals with recent infections or immunizations.	■ Planning minimizes chances for infection.	
	■ Organize patient care activities to allow for adequate period of rest.	■ Rest periods allow the child to regain energy.	
	■ Follow recommendations of CDC and AAP for immunizing immunosuppressed children. Avoid varicella vaccine. Perform annual TB testing.	■ Special recommendations consider the child's decreased immune response and the danger of acquiring disease from certain live virus vaccines.	
2. Imbalanced Nutrition: Less Than Body Requirements related to loss of appetite and decreased absorption of nutrients			
	NIC Priority Intervention—*Nutrition Management:* Assistance with or provision of a balanced dietary intake of food and fluids		**NOC Suggested Outcome—** *Nutritional Status:* Nutrient value: adequacy of nutrients taken into the body
The child will demonstrate adequate nutritional status to meet metabolic needs.	■ Encourage frequent small meals to promote nutritional and fluid intake.	■ Additional nutrition is required to rebuild the immune system.	The child eats frequent meals of adequate nutritional content.
	■ Maintain nasogastric tube feeding, if ordered. Hyperalimentation may be necessary to ensure adequate nutrition.		
	■ Eliminate unpleasant stimuli and odors from the environment during meals.	■ Unpleasant stimuli decrease the desire for food.	
	■ Monitor skin turgor every shift.	■ Skin turgor reflects hydration status.	
	■ Involve a nutritionist in planning a diet for the child that includes favorite foods.	■ Including favorite foods encourages intake.	

(continued)

Nursing Care Plan THE CHILD WITH ACQUIRED IMMUNODEFICIENCY SYNDROME (continued)

GOAL	INTERVENTION	RATIONALE	EXPECTED OUTCOME
3. Risk for Impaired Skin Integrity related to skin infection, immobility, or diarrhea			
	NIC Priority Intervention—*Skin Surveillance:* Collection and analysis of patient data to maintain skin integrity		**NOC Suggested Outcome—***Risk Control:* Actions to eliminate or reduce actual, personal, and modifiable health threats
The child will have structural intactness and normal physiologic function of skin.	■ Observe all pressure areas closely for signs of infection or breakdown. ■ Keep skin clean and dry. Provide perineal care to minimize irritation from diarrhea.	■ Skin care is important in the immunocompromised child. The skin may be the only intact defense the child has. ■ Prevents breaking or cracking of skin.	The child is free of preventable skin breakdown.
4. Risk for Impaired Oral Mucous Membrane related to infection			
	NIC Priority Intervention—*Oral Health Restoration:* Promotion of healing for a patient who has an oral mucosal lesion		**NOC Suggested Outcome—***Tissue Integrity:* Structural integrity and normal physiologic function of mucous membranes
The child will have intact oral mucous membranes.	■ Inspect mouth for sign of blistering or lesions. ■ Provide mouth care with normal saline solution or lemon-glycerine swabs every 2–4 hours.	■ Candidal infection is frequently associated with immunodeficiency. ■ Provides comfort and promotes healing.	The child has intact oral mucous membranes.
5. Pain related to infections			
	NIC Priority Intervention—*Pain Management:* Alleviation of pain or a reduction in pain to level of comfort that is acceptable to the patient		**NOC Suggested Outcome—***Comfort Level:* Feelings of physical and psychologic ease
The child will be free of pain or experience only mild pain/discomfort.	■ Observe for signs of pain and discomfort. ■ Medicate for pain as ordered, monitor and document results. ■ Implement general comfort measures (e.g., holding, rocking).	■ Pain relief adds to comfort of the child and family.	The child demonstrates evidence of pain relief.
6. Deficient Knowledge (parent) related to home care of child with AIDS			
	NIC Priority Intervention— *Teaching, Treatment:* Preparing a patient and family to understand and mentally prepare for a treatment		**NOC Suggested Outcome—** *Knowledge, Treatment Regimen:* Extent of understanding conveyed about AIDS treatment
The parent(s) will demonstrate knowledge about home care, measures to prevent infection, and signs and symptoms to report to healthcare providers.	■ Explain the importance of optimizing the child's health status and reducing risk of complications through diet, rest, and meticulous personal hygiene. Be sure that parents and other family members understand how AIDS is spread and appropriate precautions. ■ Discuss with parents and child reasons for protective measures. ■ Inform family about signs and symptoms of infection that should be reported promptly to the physician or nurse (fever, chills, cough, mild erythema).	■ Knowledge about the disorder and preventive measures is necessary to provide safe and effective home care for the child. ■ Knowledge of rationale increases compliance. ■ Prompt treatment improves outcome.	The parent describes appropriate home care and preventive measures for a child with AIDS.

Nursing Care Plan THE CHILD WITH ACQUIRED IMMUNODEFICIENCY SYNDROME (continued)

GOAL	INTERVENTION	RATIONALE	EXPECTED OUTCOME
7. Caregiver Role Strain related to anxiety about child's condition and demands of providing care			
	NIC Priority Intervention—*Caregiver Support:* Provision of the necessary information, advocacy, and support to facilitate primary patient care by someone other than a health professional		**NOC Suggested Outcome—** *Caregiver Emotional Health:* Feelings, attitudes, and emotions of a family care provider while caring for the child over an extended period of time
The parent(s) will demonstrate emotional health as evidenced by decreased anxiety related to the child's condition and care.	■ Encourage family members to express fears and concerns regarding the child's prognosis. ■ Advise family about support services or other resources available in the community.	■ Expression of fears helps to decrease anxiety. ■ Provides additional support to help family cope with the child's illness and the dying process, when needed.	The parent states decreased anxiety.

and read by health professionals are recommended (Cohen, Chen, Sunkle, et al., 2000). Educate sexually active adolescents on the importance of practicing safe sex and the ramifications of high-risk sexual behaviors and intravenous drug abuse (see Chapter 15∞). See Developing Cultural Competence: HIV/AIDS and Hispanics.

Promote Medication Regimen Adherence

A treatment regimen including antiretroviral therapies for the child with HIV or AIDS may be complex, time consuming, and costly, presenting an overwhelming challenge to the child and family. Nonadherence to the prescribed antiretroviral treatment regimen will likely result in increased morbidity and mortality. Some common reasons for nonadherence include frequent dosing, child's displeasure with medication (large pills, gritty powders, bitter taste), and associated side effects including nausea and rashes (Brackis-Cott, Mellins, Abrams, et al., 2003). Strategies for achieving optimal management of the treatment regimen include educating the parent or care provider, and child when developmentally appropriate, about the purpose of the medication, the benefits of adhering to the regimen, and the potential consequences of failure to adhere to the regimen. Behavior modification techniques, using positive reinforcement, can be very effective in promoting the child's adherence. Provide support to the family and tailor the medication regimen to the family's routine when possible. Praise should be offered to the child and parent for adhering to the regimen. If problems exist in the management of the treatment regimen, carefully listen to the family to help determine the cause. Collaborate with the family in establishing goals to help meet the prescribed treatment regimen. If further intervention is required, options include direct observational therapy or home visits. See Evidence-based Practice: Adolescents with HIV Infection and Medication Regimen Adherence.

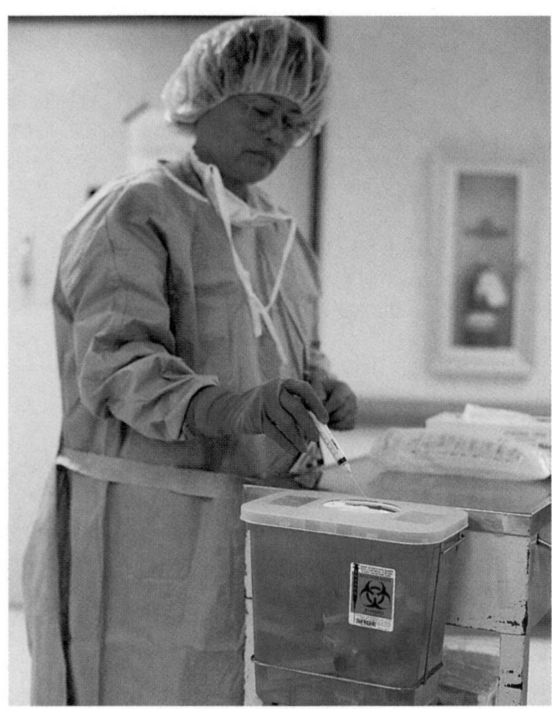

FIGURE 27–4 ■ This nurse is disposing of a needle and syringe in a biohazard container, a necessary practice to avoid the transmission of HIV through needle sticks with contaminated needles.

Promote Respiratory Function

Because many children with AIDS develop pneumonia, encourage the child to cough and deep breathe every 2 to 4 hours. Blowing cotton balls with a straw, blowing bubbles, or other games may engage the interest of a younger child. Reposition infants frequently so all areas of the lungs can fully expand. Rest

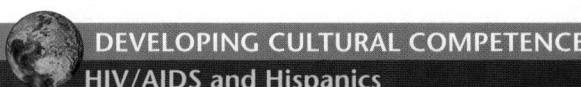

DEVELOPING CULTURAL COMPETENCE
HIV/AIDS and Hispanics

Hispanics account for approximately 14% of the total U.S. population; however, they account for a disproportionate 18% of the total AIDS cases diagnosed due primarily to poverty and inadequate access to quality healthcare. Additionally, women may be reluctant to ask male partners to wear a condom due to machismo behavior displayed by some Hispanic males; this can increase the risk of heterosexual spread of disease. Nurses need to be aware of these cultural concerns in the Hispanic population and provide them an opportunity to discuss concerns about HIV/AIDS. CDC-funded programs are now providing community-based free health clinics and other bilingual services (CDC, 2004b).

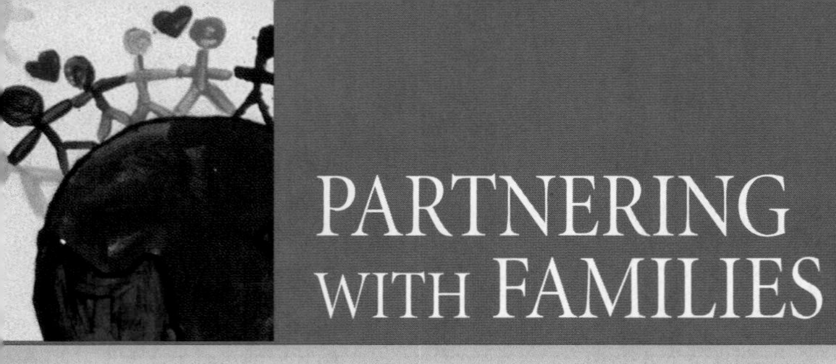

PARTNERING WITH FAMILIES

Childcare Center Safety Precautions

Because children with HIV or other bloodborne infections may be enrolled in childcare centers, staff in these centers should use standard precautions in handling blood and body fluids. Partner with the family and childcare centers to provide instructions to childcare center personnel in use of these precautions. Assist childcare centers in establishing procedures to notify all parents when a child with an infectious disease has been at the center. Encourage parents of immunocompromised children to take any necessary precautions to minimize the chances of their children becoming ill. Parents of HIV-infected children must be very cautious to limit the exposure of their children to infectious diseases.

periods to conserve energy and lower the body's demand for oxygen should be included in the plan of care.

Promote Adequate Nutritional Intake

Because many children with AIDS have failure to thrive, nutrition is an important part of their care. (See Chapter 9 for information to include in a detailed nutritional assessment.) A nutritionist should be involved in planning an appropriate diet for the child that provides necessary calories, protein, and other nutrients. Vitamins may be especially lacking in the diets of infected children. Antioxidants (vitamin A, vitamin E, zinc, and selenium) are known to enhance general immune system function and should be consumed at recommended levels. Periodic dietary analysis and teaching are needed. Adequate nutrition is sometimes provided by hyperalimentation, nasogastric, or gavage feeding.

Diarrhea resulting from gastrointestinal infection and lactose intolerance is a common finding in these children and complicates other nutritional disturbances. Antidiarrheal medications or alternative formulas may be prescribed. Carefully monitor hydration status, skin turgor, and urine output. Provide careful perineal skin care to prevent infection.

The frequency of Candida infections leads to blisters, cracking, and discharge involving the oral mucous membranes. Mouth care with a nonalcohol-based solution such as normal saline or lemon-glycerine swabs to keep the child's lips and mouth moist should be performed every 2 to 4 hours. Precautions to guard against foodborne illness are particularly important for the HIV-infected child. See Partnering with Families: Food Safety and HIV.

Provide Emotional Support

The family of the child with HIV or AIDS is under emotional stress; this is compounded if others in the family are infected. Integrate social services and support groups into the care of the child as soon as the diagnosis is made. Spend time with the family to provide them an opportunity to discuss their fears and feelings. In many parts of the United States, HIV and AIDS still carry a tremendous stigma, and the family may not be able to discuss their feelings outside of the healthcare environment. Safeguard the wishes of the family regarding the privacy of the diagnosis (Box 27–4).

Clarify any misconceptions the older child with HIV or AIDS may have about the transmission of the disease (Box 27–5). Routes of transmission and the need for safe sexual practices must be clearly discussed with adolescents. Providing support for adolescents is particularly important, as the dependence that this chronic and terminal disease brings can make it difficult to meet the developmental task of independence. Adolescents may benefit from contact with other infected peers. See Partnering with Families: Supporting the Family of a Child with HIV/AIDS.

Discharge Planning

The diagnosis of HIV or AIDS is surrounded by strong emotions and fears. Be honest and direct. Education is essential and

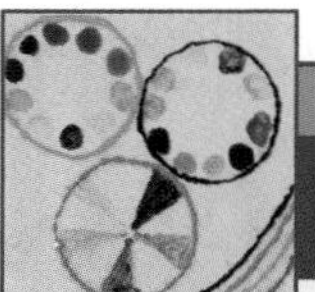

EVIDENCE-BASED PRACTICE
Adolescents with HIV Infection and Medication Regimen Adherence

PROBLEM

Medication adherence is a major problem in the HIV-infected adolescent.

EVIDENCE

There has been an increase in incidence of human immunodeficiency virus in the United States, particularly among young people ages 13–19 years. Adherence to highly active antiretroviral therapy (HAART) has been shown to decrease morbidity and mortality; however, medication adherence in this age group is often poor. The Reaching for Excellence in Adolescent Care (REACH) project has conducted studies evaluating medication adherence in the HIV-positive adolescent.

In face-to-face interviews of HIV-infected adolescents enrolled in REACH from several U.S. cities, only 41% (n = 161) reported consistently taking their medication as prescribed (Murphy, Wilson, Durako, et al., 2001). Depressed mood was a major factor in nonadherence.

Another REACH study involved 114 HIV-positive adolescents prescribed HAART who were interviewed regarding barriers associated with medication adherence (Murphy, Sarr, Durako, et al., 2003). Participants reported simply forgetting to take their medication, not having medication available to take (e.g., left medication at home), and variations in their daily routine as key reasons for not taking the prescribed medications as directed.

NURSING IMPLICATIONS

In these studies, adherence to medication regimens was noted to be closely tied to depressed mood, lack of understanding of the importance of strictly following medication directions, and daily routine. This suggests that improving organizational skills and providing better education and treatment for depression could have a positive impact on medication adherence.

CRITICAL THINKING APPLICATION

What barriers may lead to medication nonadherence in the HIV-positive adolescent? What support does the adolescent need to improve medication adherence? What measures can the nurse take to improve medication adherence in the adolescent?

BOX 27–4 Confidentiality

Disclosure of patient information is a breach of confidentiality that may subject a nurse to legal action. Disclosure of confidential information occurs when a patient's condition—for example, a diagnosis of AIDS—is discussed inappropriately with any third party. In addition, privacy must be provided when calling individuals in for office visits and in all provisions of care.

begins at the time of admission or diagnosis. Explain that there is no evidence that casual contact among family members can spread the infection. For the child who has been hospitalized, home care needs should be identified in advance of discharge.

Discuss the family's finances as well as health insurance coverage for the child's care. Assess the family's ability to provide nutritious food, required medications, and a supportive environment. Refer to services as needed to ensure provision of quality care for the child after discharge.

Support groups, home healthcare nursing services, financial assistance, and psychological counseling are usually needed at some point during the child's illness, and the family should be aware of the availability of such services. Assist the family with coping mechanisms to deal with feelings of guilt about the child's condition.

PARTNERING WITH FAMILIES

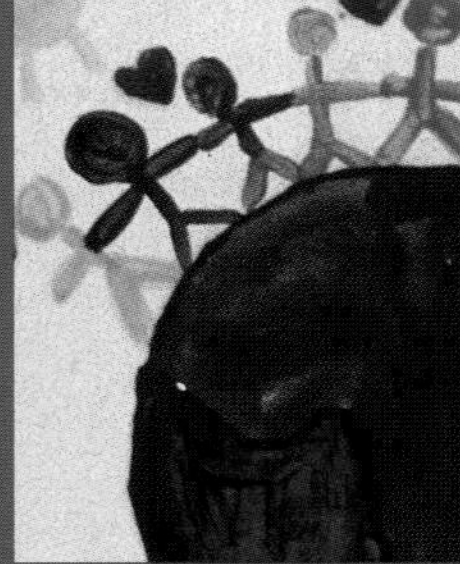

Food Safety and HIV

The child with HIV infection is more prone to foodborne disease. Instruct parents to practice the following:

- Use a separate cutting board for meats, and wash it with hot soapy water after use.
- Wash all utensils with hot soapy water between any uses.
- Wash and peel fresh fruits and vegetables. Consider use of canned varieties to limit exposure to microorganisms.
- Use a disposable cloth or cloth that is washed after each meal to clean dishes. A sponge can harbor organisms and should not be used.
- Have well water checked for contaminants regularly if that is the source of drinking water.
- Do not allow the child to eat raw or undercooked meats, fish, eggs, or cookie dough. Avoid natural honey.
- Bleach solution (2 tablespoons liquid chlorine bleach added to 1 quart cold water) is the best product for cleaning surfaces in the kitchen.

Care in the Community

Much of the care of the child with HIV infection or AIDS takes place in the community. With the continued success of aggressive therapy, the majority of HIV-infected children can be expected to attend childcare and school. Additionally, a substantial number of these children will reach adolescence, and some will reach adulthood. Evaluate the family and community support systems and provide resources and referrals as needed. Many children with HIV infection are placed in foster homes, and these families require careful instruction to manage this multifaceted illness.

School attendance guidelines for children with HIV or AIDS by the American Academy of Pediatrics (AAP) and the CDC recommend unrestricted school attendance and/or childcare center attendance for children with AIDS or AIDS-related complex with physician approval. In addition, children should be allowed to participate in all activities to the extent that their health and other recommendations for management of contagious diseases permit. Contraindications to school attendance include lack of control over body secretions, biting, and open wounds that cannot be covered. Since it is not required that the school or childcare center be notified of a child's HIV status, the nurse should prepare the school personnel with training related to care for children with known and unknown cases of HIV. The nurse also may be responsible for providing medicines or other care for the HIV-infected child at school. CDC guidelines for standard precautions should always be followed in the school, childcare, and home settings.

Even though the child's HIV status is confidential, in certain instances the HIV status of a child attending childcare or school is known. Parents of other children, school teachers, other school personnel, classmates, as well as others in the community may express concerns regarding the school attendance of a child infected with HIV. The child infected with HIV may face social stigma and fear associated with the disease. An important role for the nurse is to educate individuals about the disease and its transmission, dispeling myths regarding the disease (Box 27–5). Factual information presented in a professional manner and the opportunity to ask questions may reduce the potential for ostracizing the child in this situation.

Assist the family in altering the home environment to provide standard precautions during care. See Partnering with Families: Preventing HIV Transmission.

Parents will also require instruction on correct administration and side effects of any medications the child is taking. Giving a child a complicated combination of drugs can be challenging for

BOX 27–5 Dispelling Myths about HIV Transmission

- Although HIV has been found in saliva and tears, it does not necessarily mean that HIV can be transmitted by that body fluid. HIV has not been recovered in the sweat of HIV-infected individuals. Contact with saliva, tears, or sweat has never been shown to result in the transmission of HIV.
- Casual, closed-mouth or "social" kissing is not a risk for transmission of HIV. The risk of open-mouth kissing is believed to be very low (only one documented case of HIV infection may have been attributed to contact with blood during open-mouth kissing).
- Human biting is not a common method of transmitting HIV. In cases of HIV transmission by a bite, severe trauma with extensive tissue tearing and damage and the presence of blood were documented.
- There is no evidence that HIV is transmitted through insect bites.

Adapted from the Centers for Disease Control and Prevention (2003). www.cdc.gov, accessed 12/24/04.

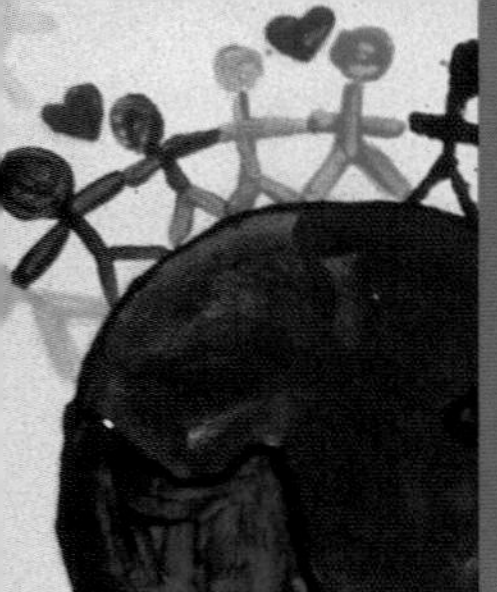

PARTNERING WITH FAMILIES

Supporting the Family of a Child with HIV/AIDS

The majority of children infected with HIV received the infection as a result of perinatal transmission. This presents a challenge for the family because not only is the child infected but also the mother. The mother may be burdened with strong emotional and physical barriers that could prevent the ability to provide the appropriate care to the child. An essential role of the nurse is collaboration with the family to determine support systems, available assistance, needs of the child, and needs of the mother. Referrals to social services as well as other services may assist the family in obtaining the needed support for providing care to both the mother and the child. The child may require foster care if the mother is too ill or has died as a result of the HIV infection.

all families; therefore, teaching is tailored to the particular family and is followed by repeated evaluation of the family's success with medication administration.

Emphasize the importance of promoting the child's development. Periodic screening should be performed to assess for delays in growth and development. Provide the parents with information on how to support the child in achieving developmental milestones. Encourage contact with other children and adults, provide for appropriate toys, teach parents how to encourage the child's communication, and praise the family for what the child has already accomplished. Children who manifest decreasing developmental milestones or other neurologic symptoms should be referred immediately to the primary healthcare provider to be assessed for signs of HIV-induced encephalopathy. The nurse's record of the child's development will be of great importance in this situation. The child must receive regular health maintenance care, such as child health supervision visits, immunizations, and care for any other health conditions. See the health promotion and maintenance overview on page 978.

PRACTICE ALERT

Childhood Infections

When a child has been diagnosed with HIV, even common childhood infections are a cause for concern. Conditions such as respiratory infection, fever, chickenpox, or gastrointestinal illness can progress rapidly to a life-threatening stage. Teach families to seek prompt treatment at the first sign of illness. Realize also that the typical signs of infection may be weakened or not present. The parent's close observation and feeling that something is not right should be cause for concern and medical evaluation.

The nurse plays a key role in identifying the adolescent population at risk for HIV infection. Box 27–6 provides sample questions that the nurse can ask the adolescent to screen for the risk of HIV.

BOX 27–6 Questions to Screen the Adolescent at Risk for HIV

1. Do you inject drugs and/or share needles, syringes, or other equipment?
2. Have you engaged in unprotected vaginal, anal, or oral sex with anyone who might be infected with HIV (e.g., someone with multiple or anonymous sexual partners, men who have had sex with other men, a partner who injects drugs, someone who has been treated for sexually transmitted infections)?
3. Have you engaged in unprotected sex with more than one partner?
4. Have you been diagnosed or treated for a sexually transmitted infection?
5. Have you ever experienced a fever or illness of unknown cause?

Data from Centers for Disease Control and Prevention. (2001). Revised guidelines for HIV counseling, testing, and referral and revised recommendations for HIV screening of pregnant women. MMWR, 50 *(RR-19), 1–58. www.cdc.gov/mmwr/preview/mmwrhtml/rr5019a1.htm*

Evaluation

There are many desired outcomes of care for the child with HIV infection or AIDS. Expected outcomes of nursing care include the following:

- The child experiences a decreased number of diarrhea stools.
- The child exhibits adequate respiratory function, perfusion, and gas exchange.
- The child achieves growth and developmental milestones appropriate for age.
- The family demonstrates successful coping with the stress of chronic disease.

AUTOIMMUNE DISORDERS

In an immune system damaged by pathologic changes, an immune response may occur to some of the body's own proteins, resulting in the production of autoantibodies. These pathologic conditions in which the body directs the immune response against itself—identifying "self" as "nonself"—are called **autoimmune disorders.**

The primary feature of autoimmune disorders is tissue injury caused by a probable immunologic reaction of the host with its own tissues. Structural or functional changes occur as immune cells attack other cells in the body. Autoimmune disorders are grouped into systemic and organ-specific diseases. Systemic diseases, which generally involve more than one organ, include systemic lupus erythematosus and juvenile rheumatoid arthritis, which are discussed in this chapter. Organ-specific diseases, which primarily affect a single organ, include insulin-dependent diabetes mellitus (discussed in Chapter 32∞) and thyroiditis. Idiopathic (or immune) thrombocytic purpura is an immune disease affecting blood platelets and clotting, as discussed in Chapter 28∞.

Systemic Lupus Erythematosus

Systemic lupus erythematosus (SLE), is a chronic inflammatory, autoimmune disease of unknown origin that involves many organ systems. The disease is characterized by remissions and exacerbations. Systemic lupus erythematosus affects 7 per 100,000 individuals and is more common in Blacks, Hispanics, and Asians than in Caucasians. Females are affected more than males with a 9:1 ratio (Stichweh, Aree, & Paseual, 2004; Pullen, Cannon, & Rushing, 2003). The majority of cases are diagnosed during the teenage and early adult years.

The five classifications of systemic lupus erythematosus are as follows (Lupus Foundation of America, 2004):

- *Systemic lupus*—involves one or more of the following systems: cardiovascular, central nervous system, hematological, kidneys, lungs, musculoskeletal.
- *Drug-induced lupus*—associated with some antineoplastic drugs, isoniazid (INH), hydralazine (Apresoline), and others. Symptoms generally subside after the drugs are discontinued.
- *Discoid/Cutaneous lupus*—involvement of the disorder is limited to the skin.
- *Overlap*—several autoimmune disorders overlap with lupus including rheumatoid arthritis, scleroderma, and Sjögren's syndrome.
- *Neonatal lupus*—occurs when maternal autoantibodies are acquired by the infant during delivery. Symptoms affecting the skin, heart, and blood of the newborn may develop.

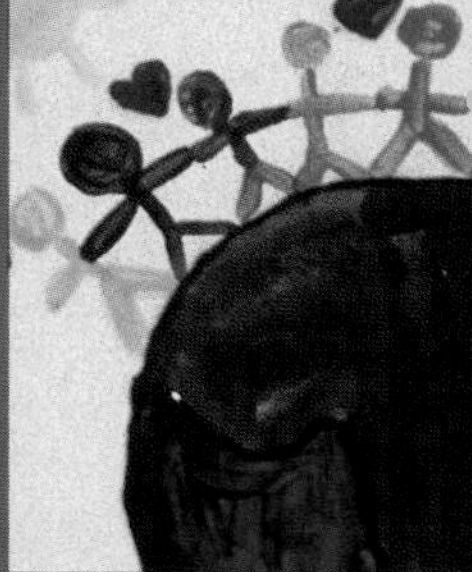

PARTNERING WITH FAMILIES

Preventing HIV Transmission

Ensure that the child and family understand that HIV is transmitted through blood, urine, stool, and other body secretions. Educate family members on the importance of careful hygiene. Encourage careful handwashing and instruct parents to use precautions when handling body fluids. Explain that they should wear gloves when changing diapers; disposing of urine, stool, and emesis; or treating the child's cuts and scrapes. Wash hands immediately after contact with blood or other body fluids. Instruct parents to use a bleach solution for disinfection of objects when necessary and to avoid contact with persons with infectious illnesses. The sharing of razors and toothbrushes should be avoided. Use only appropriate puncture-proof containers for the disposal of needles and other sharp instruments used in the child's care. Do not recap needles by hand or remove needles from syringes (CDC, 2003).

Etiology and Pathophysiology

The exact etiology of systemic lupus erythematosus is unknown. It is believed that an outside environmental agent causes the body to initiate an abnormal immune system response to its own tissues. A genetic component is clear as the disease is common when familial autoimmunity is present. Diet, hormones, sunlight, stress, and infections have been linked to systemic lupus erythematosus (Stichweh, et al., 2004). Cardiac, antihypertensive, and neuropsychiatric drugs have also been associated with drug-induced lupus (Lupus Foundation of America, 2004). Approximately 5% of the children born to individuals with lupus will develop the illness (Lupus Foundation of America, 2004).

The body produces autoantibodies and combines with antigens to form immune complexes. These antigen–antibody complexes are deposited in the connective tissue, triggering an inflammatory response. The chronic inflammation then destroys connective tissue. The tissue damage varies according to the organ involvement, though the tissues most likely to be affected are the small blood vessels, glomeruli, joints, spleen, and heart valves. Because many systems can be affected simultaneously, organ damage with subsequent multisystem failure may occur.

Clinical Manifestations

Manifestations of systemic lupus erythematosus may be acute, with onset of nephritis, arthritis, or vasculitis; or may be noted as a gradual onset with nonspecific symptoms. Symptoms vary and depend on the organ involved and the amount of tissue damage that has occurred. Initial symptoms include fever, chills, fatigue, oral ulcers, malaise, and weight loss. The most common symptoms are joint pain, occurring in about 80% to 90% of patients with systemic lupus erythematosus and skin rash. A butterfly rash on the face, consisting of a pink or red rash over the bridge of the nose extending to the cheeks, is a characteristic finding (Figure 27–5 ■). See the table on page 979 for additional manifestations of systemic lupus erythematosus.

Approximately 80% of children affected with systemic lupus erythematosus experience renal involvement since autoantibodies commonly attack the body's kidney cells. Inflammation of the kidneys, called lupus nephritis, occurs when the inflammatory process damages the capillaries of the kidneys. This disorder varies widely in severity, from mild to fatal end-stage renal disease.

Systemic lupus erythematosus is characterized by periods of remission and exacerbation (flares). Flares are triggered by a variety of causes including sun exposure, a cold or other infection, and stress. Family stressors include divorce, death, changes in schools, moving, and other life-altering events. The child or family may be able to identify other triggers to flares, such as particular events, activities, or situations. Infections and renal failure are the most common cause of death for those with systemic lupus erythematosus.

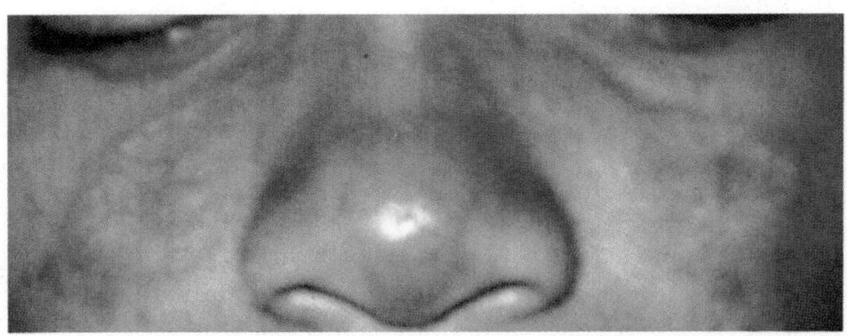

FIGURE 27–5 ■ This child displays a "butterfly" rash across the cheeks and bridge of the nose. It is often seen in the child with SLE.

From Zitelli, B. J., & Davis, H. W. (Eds.). (1997). Atlas of pediatric physical diagnosis *(3rd ed., p. 192). St. Louis: Mosby.*

Health Promotion & Maintenance Overview

The Child with HIV or AIDS

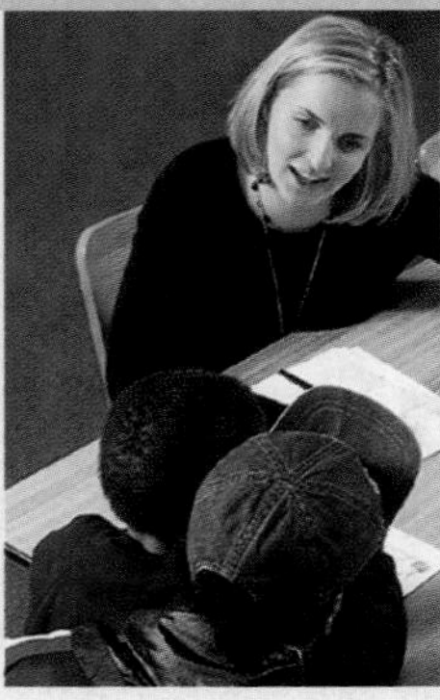

Growth and Development Surveillance

- Monitor and record growth, including head circumference, monthly.
- Assess for developmental delay using the Denver Developmental Screening Test.
- Monitor BMI.
- Teach the family techniques to encourage development.
- Refer the family to a local early intervention program.
- Refer the family to special services if required (e.g., speech or physical therapy).
- Assist the family in establishing a homecare and childcare plan for the infant, toddler, and preschooler, and individualized education plan for the school-age child.
- Emphasize the need for routine vision and hearing examinations.
- Refer the adolescent to appropriate sources to assist with transition into adulthood.

Nutrition

- Monitor for failure to thrive.
- Encourage the use of dietary supplements if needed.
- Teach the family proper care of enteral or tube feedings.
- Monitor the child for diarrhea, vomiting, and weight loss.
- Develop strategies to foster a well-balanced diet.

Physical Activity

- Encourage the child to engage in physical activity appropriate for age. Ensure precautionary measures if the child is thrombocytopenic.

Oral Health

- Teach the family that dental caries are a source of infection, and that the child should be screened beginning at age 2 to 3 years, and every 6 months thereafter.
- Teach the family how to provide proper oral care to child.

Mental and Spiritual Health

- Ask the child or adolescent to describe feelings related to having a chronic disease.
- Refer the child to counseling if appropriate.
- Encourage the child to participate in peer support groups.
- Ask the child and family to identify sources of spiritual strength.

Relationships

- Discuss the transmission of HIV through sexual contact.
- Ask the sexually active adolescent to identify his or her methods of safe sex.
- Refer the adolescent to counseling if required since adolescence is the period of sexual identity and a time for sexual experimentation.

Disease Prevention Strategies

- Refer to the current CDC recommendations for immunizations in children with HIV/AIDS.
- Teach the family about standard blood and fluid precautions.
- Instruct the family to avoid exposing the child to persons with infections.

Injury Prevention Strategies

- Teach the family how to properly and safely store medications.
- Encourage frequent handwashing by all family members. Suggest placing small bottles of antibacterial hand sanitizer throughout the house.
- Monitor the child's platelet count.
- Encourage the use of car seats, seat belts, and bicycle helmets as indicated.

COLLABORATIVE CARE

The goals of clinical therapy are to create a remission of symptoms, to prevent exacerbations of the disease, and to prevent complications.

Diagnostic Tests

Crucial to preventing organ damage is early diagnosis of systemic lupus erythematosus. Blood studies including C3, C4, ESR, CRP, and immune complexes are performed. Radiologic examinations included chest radiographs and CT scans; MRI of affected joints may also be conducted. A 24-hour urine collection, imaging studies, and renal biopsies may be performed to evaluate lupus nephritis. When four of the main symptoms of the disease are present (Table 27–7), a diagnosis of SLE is made.

Clinical Therapy

See the medication table on page 981 for pharmacologic therapy for systemic lupus erythematosus. Diet may be restricted if the child has excessive weight gain or fluid retention from steroids and renal damage. See Partnering with Families: Side Effects of Corticosteroids.

Prognosis depends on the severity of the internal organ involvement; however, where systemic lupus erythematosus was once considered a fatal disease the survival rate now is more than 97% with 5-year survival rate for children of 78–92% (American College of Rheumatology, 2003; Stichweh, et al., 2004). Kidney failure is managed by hemodialysis or peritoneal dialysis. Renal transplantation has been very successful for treatment of renal failure secondary to lupus nephritis. See Chapter 31 ∞ for a discussion of renal failure.

CLINICAL MANIFESTATIONS of System Lupus Erythematosus

SYSTEM	CLINICAL MANIFESTATIONS
Integumentary	A butterfly rash on the face, consisting of a pink or red rash over the bridge of the nose extending to the cheeks, is a characteristic finding Photosensitivity Alopecia Mouth or nose ulcers
Hematologic	Hemolytic anemia Leukopenia (low white blood cells) Thrombocytopenia (low platelet count) Bleeding disorders
Musculoskeletal	Joint pain Raynaud's phenomenon (fingers turning white and/or blue in the cold) Arthritis Arthralgia
Neurological	Headache Chorea Dizziness Seizures Cerebral vascular accident (CVA) and resultant quadriplegia
Pulmonary	Pleural effusions Pleuritis Pulmonary hemorrhage
Cardiac	Pericarditis Vasculitis Hypertension
Renal	Glomerulonephritis Renal failure Lupus nephritis
Other	Hypergammaglobulinemia Extreme fatigue Neuropsychiatric syndrome

NURSING MANAGEMENT

Nursing management focuses on identifying triggers, reducing exacerbations (flares), minimizing complications associated with the disease process, and promoting optimal growth and development.

Nursing Assessment and Diagnosis

Since systemic lupus erythematosus generally consists of multiorgan involvement, careful assessment of each of the systems is essential to detect any complications as early as possible. A thorough physiological assessment as well as a thorough psychosocial assessment is essential.

Physiologic Assessment

A thorough assessment is needed, as symptoms are widespread. Assess the child's nutritional status including baseline weight and history of recent weight loss or weight gain. Observe the skin for rashes, ulcers, photosensitivity, ecchymosis, petechiae, cyanosis, and hair loss. Auscultate breath sounds and respiratory rate, and assess for pleural effusion or pleuritis. Assess vital signs, and heart tones for symptoms of pericarditis or friction rub. Musculoskeletal assessment includes joint pain, joint deformity, weakness, and ability to perform activities of daily living. Neurologic assessment includes changes in affect or cognitive abilities and seizure activity. Gastrointestinal assessment includes splenomegaly, abdominal pain, and anorexia. Measure intake, output, and weight.

PARTNERING WITH FAMILIES

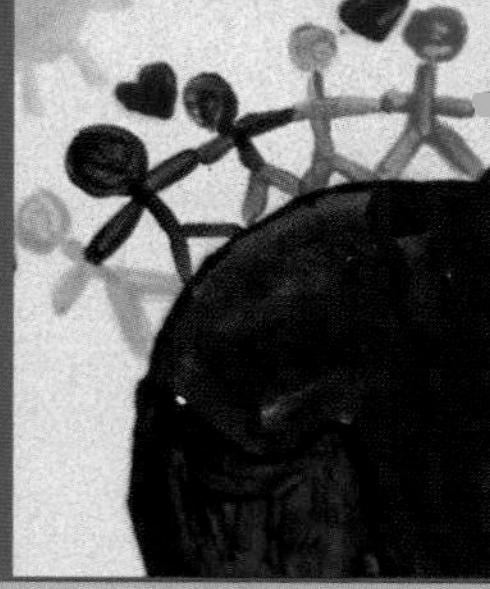

Side Effects of Corticosteroids

The side effects of the corticosteroids, immunosuppressants, and antimalarial drugs used in the treatment of children with systemic lupus erythematosus are significant and include hair loss, susceptibility to infection, "moon face," retinal damage, and bone loss. These are significant side effects for the adolescent who is commonly concerned about appearance. Special teaching, guidance, and support may be needed for teens with systemic lupus erythematosus. The adolescent may benefit from peer interaction with others who have the same experiences. Encourage the adolescent to find methods to explain the side effects and appearance. For example, a science teacher or health teacher may allow the adolescent the opportunity to present information about the disease and treatment.

Psychosocial Assessment

Because systemic lupus erythematosus is a chronic disease that affects primarily adolescents, psychosocial assessment is indicated. Assess family interactions, exploring stressful situations such as divorce or trauma. Treatment-related restrictions associated with medications, and changes in appearance such as weight gain, cushingoid appearance, and skin rashes can lead to withdrawal, depression, and suicidal tendencies. Perform psychological assessments periodically as the child grows and adapts to the disorder or faces new developmental challenges with a chronic disease. Evaluate school performance.

The following nursing diagnoses may apply to the child with systemic lupus erythematosus.

- Pain related to joint inflammation and injury
- Risk for Infection related to immunosuppressive medications
- Risk for Ineffective Tissue Perfusion (renal) related to interrupted blood flow in kidneys
- Risk for Impaired Skin Integrity related to immunologic deficit
- Risk for Activity Intolerance related to chronic disease and joint involvement
- Risk for Disturbed Body Image related to side effects of medications and skin alterations

TABLE 27–7 Diagnostic Criteria for Systemic Lupus Erythematosus

CRITERION	DEFINITION
Malar rash	Fixed erythema, flat or raised, over the facial cheeks, tending to spare the nasolabial folds
Discoid rash	Erythematous raised patches with adherent keratotic scaling and follicular plugging; atrophic scarring may occur in older lesions
Photosensitivity	Skin rash as a result of unusual reaction to sunlight
Oral ulcers	Oral or nasopharyngeal ulceration, usually painless, observed on examination
Arthritis	Arthritis involving two or more peripheral joints, characterized by tenderness, swelling, or effusion
Serositis	Pleuritis—history of pleuritic pain or rubbing or evidence of pleural effusion OR Pericarditis—documented by ECG or rub or evidence of pericardial effusion
Renal disorder	Persistent proteinuria greater than 0.5 g per day OR Cellular casts—may be red cell, hemoglobin, granular, tubular, or mixed
Neurologic disorder	Seizures—in the absence of causative drugs or known metabolic illness, e.g., uremia, ketoacidosis, or electrolyte imbalance OR Psychosis—in the absence of causative drugs or known metabolic illness, e.g., uremia, ketoacidosis, or electrolyte imbalance
Hematologic disorder	Hemolytic anemia—with reticulocytosis OR Leukopenia—less than 4,000/mm^3 total on two or more occasions OR Lymphopenia—less than 1,500/mm^3 on two or more occasions OR Thrombocytopenia—less than 100,000/mm^3 in the absence of causative drugs
Immunologic disorder	Positive LE cell preparation OR Anti-DNA: antibody to native DNA in abnormal titer OR Anti-Sm: presence of antibody to Sm nuclear antigen OR False positive serologic test for syphilis known to be positive for at least 6 months and confirmed by *Treponema pallidum* immobilization or fluorescent treponemal antibody absorption test
Positive antinuclear antibody	An abnormal titer of antinuclear antibody by immunofluorescence or an equivalent assay at any point in time and in the absence of drugs known to be associated with "drug-induced lupus" syndrome

Note: An individual should have four or more of these symptoms to suspect lupus. All symptoms do not have to occur simultaneously.

Adapted from Tan, E. M., Cohen, A. S., Fries, J. F., Masi, A. T., McShane, D. J., & Rothfield, N. F., et al. (1982). The 1982 revised criteria for the classification of systemic lupus erythematosus. Arthritis Rheum, 25, *1271–1277.*

Planning and Implementation

The goals of nursing care are to assist the child to manage and cope with a chronic disease, prevent infection, promote adequate nutrition, and assist the child in avoiding triggers.

Maintain Fluid Balance

Because most children with systemic lupus erythematosus have renal involvement, nursing care includes maintaining accurate intake and output measurements and frequent evaluation of the child's fluid and electrolyte status. Renal dysfunction may be manifested by edema, muscle cramps, diarrhea, tetany, and seizures.

Promote Adequate Nutrition

Currently, there are no specific dietary plans for the child with systemic lupus erythematosus; however, the diet may be restricted dependent on renal involvement, weight gain, weight loss, or other complications. The child is at risk for weight gain associated with treatment with steroids and a decreased activity level during exacerbations of this disease. A well-balanced, nutritious diet with calcium and Vitamin D supplements as well as appropriate fluid intake for age should be encouraged.

Promote Skin Integrity

Presence of the ulcers on mucous membranes can cause weakening of the tissues, placing the child at increased risk for infection. Encourage the use of good hygienic measures and a mild soap. Recommend that adolescents limit their use of cosmetics. Reinforce the importance of avoiding sunlight as much as possible and the use of sun protection factor (SPF) of 30 or higher at all times when in the sun. Encourage the child to wear protective clothing to limit exposure to sunlight (see Chapter 36 for discussion of sun exposure). Additionally, avoidance of unprotected fluorescent lighting should be included since exacerbations of systemic lupus erythematosus have been reported following this exposure. Encourage the adolescent to avoid the use of tanning beds. Provide instructions on oral care to maintain intact oral mucosa. Provide instructions on the care of the head if alopecia occurs.

MediaLink Animation: Methotrexate

MEDICATIONS Used to Treat Systemic Lupus Erythematosus

MEDICATION	ACTION/INDICATION	NURSING IMPLICATIONS
Corticosteroids prednisone	To control inflammation	Monitor for side effects including weight gain, mood changes, insomnia, and elevated serum glucose Caution must be taken with corticosteroids as they may interfere with normal growth and increase susceptibility to infection
Topical steroids fluocinonide cream (Lidex)	To treat dermatologic symptoms	Apply to clean, dry skin Apply thin layer
Antimalarial preparations hydroxychloroquine (Plaquenil) chloroquine	To treat symptoms associated with skin lesions and renal and arthritic pain. Although the exact action of these drugs on SLE is not known, they often permit continued remission with a lowered dose of steroids.	Administer with milk or meals to reduce gastric irritation Teach family to report the following serious side effects: Weakness Visual symptoms Hearing loss Bruising Unusual bleeding Skin eruptions
Nonsteroidal anti-inflammatories (NSAIDs) aspirin ibuprofen naproxen	To relieve muscle and joint pain	Monitor for side effects including abdominal pain, bleeding, and gastrointestinal complications Teach family to monitor for side effects and to avoid administration of additional NSAIDs
Immunosuppressants cyclosporine methotrexate	To help control systemic lupus erythematosus during acute exacerbations	Monitor for infection Implement measures to reduce risk of infection Monitor for thrombocytopenia Teach family that child should avoid exposure to sunlight; wear sunscreen and sunglasses

Promote Rest and Comfort

The child with systemic lupus erythematosus experiences fatigue and joint pain, leaving little energy reserve during acute episodes of the disease. Encourage frequent rest periods and a nutritious diet to maximize energy stores. A physical therapist can plan a therapeutic exercise program to encourage mobility and increase muscle strength. Implement measures such as application of heat to painful areas. See Complementary Therapy: SLE and Stress.

Avoidance of Flare Triggers

Many children and their parents can recognize the signs of an impending flare and the triggers that precede them. Partner with the parents and child to implement measures to avoid these triggers. Discuss such preventive behaviors as avoiding sun exposure and stressors. Adolescents should be warned that alcohol, smoking, and drugs also pose an increased risk due to the potential to stimulate flares. Female adolescents who are sexually active should avoid birth control pills which contain the hormone estrogen, because the extra estrogen may exacerbate symptoms. Alternate birth control methods should be discussed with the adolescent. See Partnering with Families: SLE and Fertility.

COMPLEMENTARY THERAPY
SLE and Stress

Systemic lupus erythematosus exacerbations have been linked to stress. Stress-reducing techniques such as guided imagery, reading, yoga, and quiet games can benefit the child or adolescent and reduce exacerbations of systemic lupus erythematosus. The nurse can review the child's activities and partner with the child and family to evaluate the need for stress reduction. It may be necessary to discontinue a sport or music lesson temporarily to provide a chance for the child to relax each day. *What stressors are common to children, and how can they be reduced in the child with SLE?*

Prevent Infection

Infections are a leading cause of death for patients with systemic lupus erythematosus. Prophylactic antibiotics may be required for dental work and surgical procedures. Instruct the patient and family to inform all healthcare providers of the disease in order to plan for prophylactic measures. Educate the patient and family on the importance of adhering to the immunization schedule, and to obtain a yearly influenza vaccine to prevent infection. Instruct the family on handwashing and infection control measures in the home. Warn adolescents about the dangers of tattooing and body piercing due to risk of infection.

Manage Side Effects of Medications

Observe for side effects of medications used for treatment, and teach the child and family about these effects. For example, immunosuppressant drugs can promote infection anywhere in the body; and nonsteroidal anti-inflammatory drugs commonly cause gastric distress and bleeding of the gastrointestinal tract.

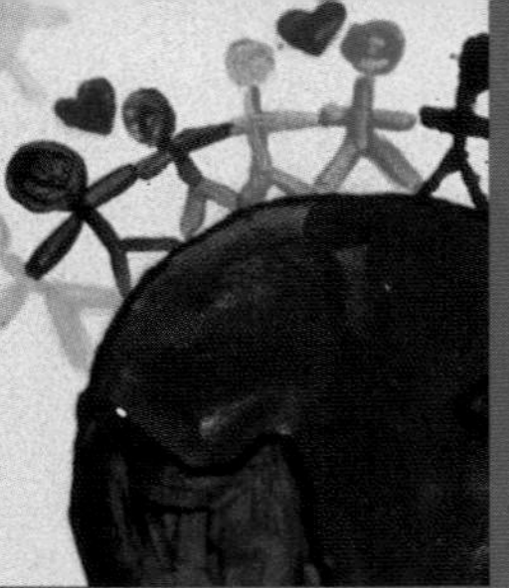

PARTNERING WITH FAMILIES

SLE and Fertility

The female adolescent with systemic lupus erythematosus may express concern about her future ability to have children. Explain that there is no reason that a female with lupus should not get pregnant, unless she has moderate to severe organ involvement (e.g., central nervous system, kidney, or heart and lungs) which would place her (the mother) at risk. However, because of the increased risk of disease activity during or immediately after (3 to 4 weeks) pregnancy, those who are pregnant and have systemic lupus erythematosus should be carefully monitored by their healthcare provider.

MediaLink Lupus Resources and Support

The antimalarial drug hydroxychloroquine increases the risk of retinopathy and blindness; therefore, eye examinations should be performed every 6 months. Corticosteroid side effects include cushingoid effects, weight gain, and hypertension. Sulfa drugs should be avoided because they increase photosensitivity.

Provide Emotional Support

Adolescents may have an altered body image as a result of rash, alopecia, arthritic changes in the joints, and chronic disease. Referral to a lupus support group, social services, or counseling may be helpful. The American Lupus Society and the Lupus Foundation of America can provide information to help parents and children adjust to the disease. The Arthritis Foundation also publishes a useful pamphlet, "Meeting the Challenge: A Young Person's Guide to Living with Lupus." Numerous Internet support groups are also available for those with systemic lupus erythematosus.

Care in the Community

Care of the child with systemic lupus erythematosus occurs primarily in the community since the child is generally only hospitalized for acute exacerbations or a coexisting health condition. The parents and child should be taught the avoidance of triggers and stressors and the signs and symptoms of impending flares. Teach parents the importance of infection control measures in the home and environment. Partner with the parents to promote the child's growth and development and to establish an individualized education plan if needed. Encourage the parents to allow the child to participate in activities as long as the child is physically capable and measures to prevent sun exposure are implemented (e.g., wide-brim hats, long sleeves, sunscreen). Instruct the parent to notify the primary healthcare provider of any of the following symptoms: bloody stools, easy bruising (with or without nosebleeds), seizures, new or high fever, and chest or abdominal pain. Refer the adolescent and family to appropriate sources for vocational counseling. Refer the family to the Lupus Foundation of America, Inc. and other resources.

Evaluation

Successful outcomes of nursing care involve management of this chronic disease. Expected outcomes of nursing care include the following:

- The child is free from pain.
- The child is free from infection.
- The child maintains adequate intake and output levels, with demonstrated fluid and electrolyte balance and renal function.
- The child's skin remains intact.
- The child maintains a balance of rest and activity adequate to promote development.
- The child demonstrates a positive body image.

Juvenile Rheumatoid Arthritis

Juvenile rheumatoid arthritis (JRA) is a chronic autoimmune inflammatory disease characterized by joint inflammation resulting in decreased mobility, swelling, and pain that occurs slightly more often in girls than in boys. Juvenile rheumatoid arthritis is the most common type of arthritis in children and adolescents, and usually occurs in children between 2 and 5 or between 9 and 12 years of age. Children may enter remission or manifest continued symptoms of a chronic disease. Approximately 5 to 18 of every 100,000 children develop juvenile rheumatoid arthritis each year (Ilowite, 2002).

Juvenile rheumatoid arthritis affects joints and surrounding tissues in addition to potential effects on other organs such as the heart, lungs, liver, and eyes. During its course, the child may experience pain, impaired mobility, and interference with normal growth and development. Of children with juvenile rheumatoid arthritis, 70% experience permanent remission of the disease by adulthood. Rarely, the disease is unresponsive to treatment or the child may suffer lasting impairment such as bone and joint changes. Children with early onset have a better prognosis for complete recovery.

Etiology and Pathophysiology

The cause of juvenile rheumatoid arthritis is unknown, but it is thought to have an autoimmune basis. Inflammation begins in the joint and leads to pain and swelling (Figure 27–6 ■). Scar tissue eventually develops, resulting in limited range of motion. The three major types of juvenile rheumatoid arthritis are pauciarticular arthritis, systemic arthritis, and polyarticular arthritis (Ilowite, 2002).

- *Pauciarticular arthritis* primarily affects the knees, ankles, and elbows, and occurs more frequently in females. Approximately 50% of children with juvenile rheumatoid arthritis have pauciarticular arthritis. It generally manifests between infancy and age 5 years. Four or fewer joints are affected in this type of JRA.
- *Systemic arthritis* affects males and females equally and is characteristically manifested by high fever, polyarthritis, and rheumatoid rash. Systemic arthritis affects internal or-

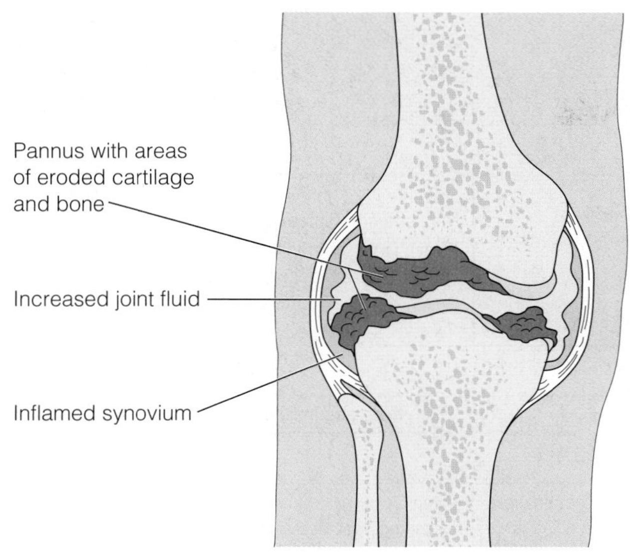

FIGURE 27–6 ■ Joint inflammation and destruction in rheumatoid arthritis.

gans and joints. Approximately 15% of children with juvenile rheumatoid arthritis have systemic arthritis.

- *Polyarticular arthritis* involves many joints (five or more), particularly the small joints of the hands and fingers. It may also affect the hips, knees, feet, ankles, and neck. This type of arthritis affects approximately 35% of the children with juvenile rheumatoid arthritis.

Clinical Manifestations

Juvenile rheumatoid arthritis may be restricted to a few joints or be systemic with involvement of multiple joints. One of the most common complaints is morning joint stiffness accompanied by joint swelling. This commonly affects the knees and the joints in the hands and feet. Characteristic signs of juvenile rheumatoid arthritis are fever and a rash.

Symptoms may also include lymphadenopathy, splenomegaly, and hepatomegaly, which mainly occur with the systemic and polyarticular forms of juvenile rheumatoid arthritis. The child may develop a limp or obviously favor one extremity over the other. Older children may develop symmetric involvement of the small joints of the hand. Just as with systemic lupus erythematosus, another autoimmune disorder, juvenile rheumatoid arthritis is characterized by periods of remission and exacerbation. Remission may last for months, years, or for a lifetime. A slow rate of growth or uneven growth of extremities may also be noted.

COLLABORATIVE CARE

Diagnosis is made primarily on the basis of the history and assessment findings, in particular, arthritis having an onset before 16 years of age and persisting for at least 6 weeks, with no other identifiable cause (Gottlieb & Ilowite, 2000). Multidisciplinary care involves drug therapy, physical therapy, and, when necessary, surgery.

Diagnostic Tests

Although there are no specific laboratory tests for the disease, in some children, rheumatoid factor, human leukocyte antigen (HLA) B27, and antinuclear antibody (ANA) tests are positive, and the erythrocyte sedimentation rate (ESR) may be elevated. Radiographs are generally performed to exclude other causes, such as fractures, rather than as a definitive diagnosis, though the radiographs are useful in monitoring for joint damage and bone development. See Box 27–7 for the criteria for classification of juvenile rheumatoid arthritis.

Clinical Therapy

The goals of treatment are to relieve pain, suppress the inflammatory process, prevent contractures, preserve joint function, and promote normal growth and development. Pharmacological management of juvenile rheumatoid arthritis is provided in the table on page 984.

In addition to medication therapy, physical and/or occupational therapy are performed to increase strength and mobility of joints while protecting them from injury. The physical therapist and/or occupational therapist tailors an exercise regimen specifically to the child. Range of motion exercises are essential to maintain joint mobility. The therapist may recommend the use of splints or other special equipment. Exercise such as swimming is encouraged because it involves a majority of the muscles and joints with minimal impact and stress on joints. Surgery is occasionally performed to relieve pain and maintain or improve joint function in children with joint contractures.

Complications such as chronic uveitis, which results from chronic inflammation, may occur in children with juvenile rheumatoid arthritis, especially those with pauciarticular arthritis. Children with polyarticular and systemic juvenile rheumatoid arthritis should be examined by an ophthalmologist for eye inflammation every 6 months and children with pauciarticular arthritis should be examined every 3 months.

Growth interference for the child with juvenile rheumatoid arthritis is a potential complication. The specific disorder may result in bone growth disturbance such as contractures or effusions, and the administration of corticosteroids can also inhibit growth.

BOX 27–7 Criteria for the Classification of Juvenile Rheumatoid Arthritis

1. Age of onset < 16 years
2. Arthritis (e.g., swelling or effusion or presence of two or more of the following signs: limitation of range of motion, tenderness or pain on motion, increased heat) in one or more joints
3. Duration of disease > 6 weeks
4. Type of onset defined by type of disease in first 6 months:
   a. Polyarthritis: ≥ inflamed joints
   b. Oligoarthritis: < five inflamed joints
   c. Systemic: arthritis with characteristic fever
5. Exclusion of other forms of juvenile arthritis

Adapted from Cassidy, J. T., & Petty, P. E. (2001). Textbook of pediatric rheumatology *(4th ed.). Philadelphia: W.B. Saunders.*

MEDICATIONS Used to Treat Juvenile Rheumatoid Arthritis

MEDICATION	ACTION/INDICATION	NURSING IMPLICATIONS
Nonsteroidal Anti-inflammatory Drugs (NSAIDs)		
aspirin tolmetin sodium choline magnesium trisalicylate naproxen diclofenac ibuprofen	To reduce inflammation and pain	Monitor for side effects including abdominal pain, bleeding, and gastrointestinal complications Teach family to monitor for side effects and to avoid administration of additional NSAIDs
Cox-2 Inhibitors		
celecoxib (Celebrex)	To reduce inflammation and pain	Side effects are similar to traditional NSAIDs
Disease-modifying Antirheumatic Drugs (DMARDs)		
The most commonly used DMARD for children is methotrexate (Rheumatrex) Other DMARDs include gold compounds such as auranofin (Ridaura) and aurothioglucose (Solganal) sulfasalazine (Azulfidine, Azaline) hydroxychloroquine (Plaquenil, Quineprox)	DMARDs may be prescribed in combination with NSAIDs or used alone when NSAIDS are ineffective in relieving symptoms of joint pain and swelling	Monitor for gastrointestinal side effects—nausea, vomiting, oral ulcers, diarrhea Monitor liver enzymes Live virus vaccines should not generally be administered to the child receiving methotrexate or etanercept; consult the CDC for immunization recommendations
Corticosteroids		
prednisone (Deltasone, Orasone)	These medications are generally prescribed to children with the more severe forms of JRA to control symptoms until a DMARD takes effect	May be administered by mouth or by injection Side effects include weight gain, mood changes, insomnia, and elevated serum glucose Caution must be taken with corticosteroids as they may interfere with normal growth and increase susceptibility to infection
Biologic Response Modifiers		
etanercept (Enbrel) infliximab (Remicade)	Tumor necrosis factor (TNF) inhibitor	Enbrel: Administered subcutaneously twice weekly Monitor for side effects of itching, redness, or swelling at injection site Do not administer live vaccines Do not administer medication during active infection Remicade: Administered intravenously Monitor for side effects including chest pain, headache, upper respiratory infection

NURSING MANAGEMENT

Nursing care focuses on pain relief, maintaining joint mobility, preventing deformities, promoting self-care, and promoting growth and development.

Nursing Assessment and Diagnosis

A careful history is important, as it is sometimes the primary mode of diagnosis. Assess for joint swelling and deformities, pain, decreased mobility, morning stiffness, fever, nodules under the skin, delayed growth, and enlarged lymph nodes.

The following nursing diagnoses may apply to the child with juvenile rheumatoid arthritis.

- Activity Intolerance related to chronic pain
- Impaired Physical Mobility related to joint stiffness and inflammation
- Anxiety related to stress of chronic illness
- Pain related to joint inflammation
- Disturbed Body Image related to illness and physical appearance

Planning and Implementation

Nursing care focuses on promoting mobility, encouraging adequate nutrition, and teaching the parents and child about the disease and its management. Most care will occur in the community, including physical therapy, with only occasional hospitalizations at the time of an exacerbation of the disease or in the presence of a coexisting condition.

Promote Improved Mobility

The goals of physical therapy are to maintain joint function, strengthen muscles, increase tone, maintain body alignment, and prevent permanent deformities such as contractures. The nurse supports the physical and occupational therapy program goals by encouraging range of motion exercises, stretching, hydrotherapy, and swimming to help prevent deformities (Figures 27–7 ■ and 27–8 ■). Encourage the child to perform activities of daily living. Exercise may be painful or even difficult for the child; however, it strengthens and stretches the muscles and prevents potential bone deformities (contractures). Emphasize the importance of establishing a regular exercise and activity routine. Encourage periods of rest during exacerbations, as the child fatigues more easily.

During exacerbations, the activities will be modified and individualized according to the child's ability and comfort level. Teach the child methods to reduce stress on joints, such as using wrist splints when lifting. If the child requires splints, a schedule for removal should be established. See Partnering with Families: Reducing Joint Stiffness.

PARTNERING WITH FAMILIES

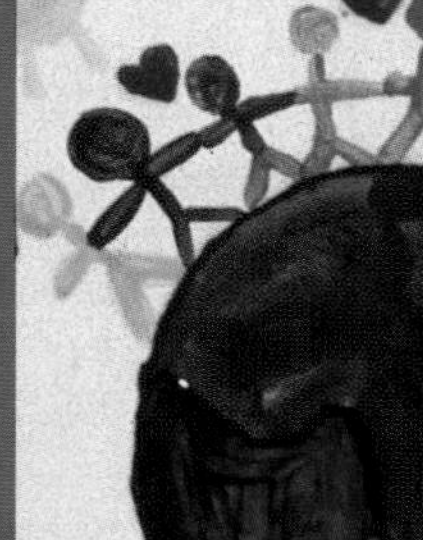

Reducing Joint Stiffness

The child with juvenile rheumatoid arthritis experiences joint stiffness which is generally more severe in the mornings upon awakening. Teach the child and family the following steps to help reduce joint stiffness.

- Maintain proper body alignment while in bed to promote pain relief and prevention of contractures.
- Medications may be given to reduce joint swelling and inflammation.
- Warm compresses to the involved joints and warm baths or showers each morning are soothing since heat promotes relief of pain and joint stiffness.
- Moist heat may also include the use of whirlpools, hot tubs, or heated paraffin baths.
- Some children may prefer cold packs applied to joints rather than heat packs.

Encourage Adequate Nutrition

Promote general health by encouraging a well-balanced diet. Children with decreased mobility may have reduced metabolic needs, and excess weight causes additional muscle strain. Pain may also reduce the child's appetite. The child's emotional status may affect nutritional intake. Observe for irritability, apathy, or depression. Encourage adequate hydration to reduce risk of constipation associated with immobility. Dietary consultation will help ensure that the child receives adequate calories and a well-balanced diet. Monitor the child's food and liquid intake and output.

Manage Side Effects of Medication

Aspirin and corticosteroids may lead to gastric irritation. To decrease the risk of stomach irritation or pain, aspirin should be administered with food, milk, or a prescribed antacid. Since high doses of aspirin are given, monitor for signs and symptoms

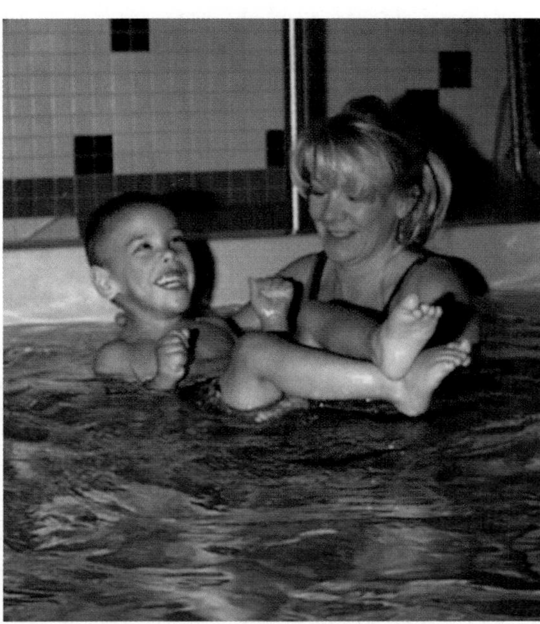

FIGURE 27–7 ■ The physical therapist uses hydrotherapy to maintain joint function in a child who has juvenile rheumatoid arthritis.

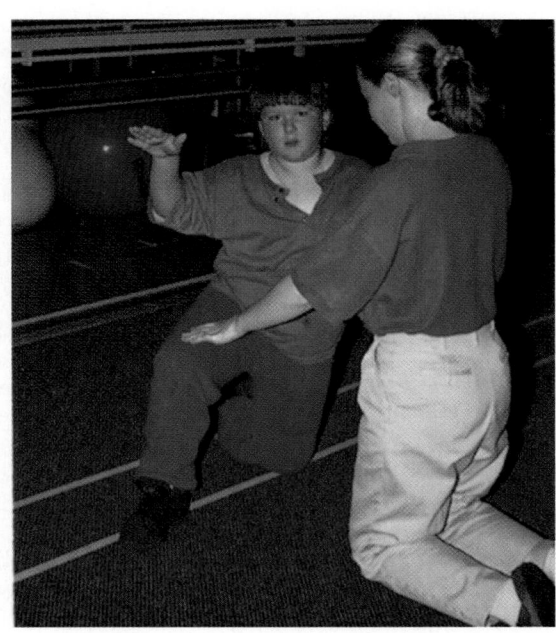

FIGURE 27–8 ■ Stretching exercises are an important part of physical therapy for a child who has juvenile rheumatoid arthritis.

MediaLink JRA Resources and Support

of aspirin toxicity, including tinnitus, decreased hearing, nausea, vomiting, drowsiness, irritability, and rapid, deep breathing. The family is cautioned against simultaneous use of other NSAIDs.

PRACTICE ALERT

Infants and children with juvenile rheumatoid arthritis who are receiving aspirin therapy are at risk of developing Reye syndrome if they contract influenza or varicella. For unknown reasons children with influenza or chickenpox who are treated with aspirin have a higher incidence of Reye. Since that connection was observed and children are generally treated with acetaminophen or ibuprofen for viral illness, incidence of Reye has drastically dropped. However, because many children with juvenile rheumatoid arthritis receive aspirin for treatment, they have a higher risk of Reye syndrome if they have influenza or varicella. These children should be immunized with influenza vaccine in the fall of each year and should meet current recommendations for varicella vaccine.

Care in the Community

The child with juvenile rheumatoid arthritis may never, or rarely, be hospitalized. Most care takes place during visits to healthcare offices, clinics, and physical therapy. Educate parents on the child's condition and prognosis, and answer their questions about the child's treatment. The child may need support to adjust to the diagnosis of a chronic illness. Allow the child to express anger about the diagnosis of juvenile rheumatoid arthritis. Allow the opportunity for the child and parents to express feelings regarding the crippling effects of the disease. Social services, a child life specialist, or a psychologist is consulted as needed.

Encourage the child to maintain contact with peers and to attend school when possible. Partner with the child and family to assist in identifying activities of interest for the child to engage in and provide them with opportunities for social contacts. Arts and science clubs, choir, scouts, and other similar organizations can provide the child social activities. Encourage parents to allow the child to participate in activities as the child desires as long as the child is following the recommendations of the primary healthcare provider and/or physical or occupational therapist. Explain to the child and parents that overexertion may lead to exacerbation of the disease. Inform parents about possible complications of juvenile rheumatoid arthritis, such as altered growth related to early closure of epiphyseal plates, small joint contractures, and synovitis. Refer the family to the American Juvenile Arthritis Organization and other organizations.

Partner with the family and school officials to meet the child's needs (Table 27–8). Accommodations at school may include providing a set of books for the home so that the child is not required to carry the books home daily. Additional time may be required for the child to move from class to class. Parents and children can be referred to the Arthritis Foundation and the American Juvenile

TABLE 27–8 Mobility Issues for the Child and Adolescent with Rheumatoid Arthritis

NURSING DIAGNOSIS	NURSING INTERVENTIONS
Impaired Physical Mobility related to inability to walk hallways, climb stairs, open locker, obtain lunch, carry books	➤ Work with the school to identify methods of transport such as wheelchair access, use of elevators, and placement/opening of locker ➤ Identify methods of carrying items such as lunch and books ➤ Consider having two sets of books and other items—one at home and one at school, to eliminate need to carry these items ➤ Explore with the child access to supportive shoes to facilitate adequate support when walking ➤ If arthritic symptoms worsen upon inactivity, arrange for the child to rise, walk, or exercise on a schedule that facilitates movement
Impaired Communication related to inability to raise hand or write	➤ Partner with school personnel to establish an individualized education plan for the child that includes methods of communication appropriate to condition ➤ Evaluate the child for use of computer or tape recorder at home and school and ensure access to these resources if needed ➤ Refer to occupational therapy specialist if special pens or pencils could enhance writing ability ➤ Consider the use of a cell phone or other device that the child can manipulate and use to call identified persons for help if needed
Risk for Self-Care Deficit: Dressing/Grooming and Toileting related to weakness and inability to manipulate clothing	➤ Partner with occupational therapy to plan clothing and fasteners that the child can manipulate ➤ Locate toilet in the school that provides room, adequate space, and privacy for the child who needs extra time to toileting activities ➤ Identify a member of the school staff who the child can turn to for assistance in completing dressing or other activities
Activity Intolerance related to insufficient energy to complete daily activities	➤ Determine activities that create fatigue ➤ Provide place for rest during school hours if needed ➤ Consider partial days of school attendance if the child is receptive
Risk of Delayed Growth and Development related to effects of physical condition	➤ Encourage the child to maintain contact with friends and usual activities, such as attending sports practice and assisting the coach if unable to play ➤ Enlist help of peers to assist the child with mobility in school and transferring items as needed ➤ Refer children to others who have had arthritis as a source of support ➤ Refer to summer camps and other special programs for children with arthritis ➤ Plan methods to help the child maintain independence and meet developmental milestones

Data from Rettig, P. A., Merhar, S. L., & Cron, R. Q. (2004). Juvenile rheumatoid arthritis and juvenile spondifoarthropathy. In P. J. Allen & J. A. Vessey. Primary care of the child with a chronic condition. *St. Louis: Mosby.*

Arthritis Foundation for further information and support. Refer the adolescent for vocational counseling and offer support for transition into adult services.

Evaluation

Expected outcomes of nursing care for the child with juvenile rheumatoid arthritis include the following:

- The child participates in desired activities and tolerates without difficulties.
- The child maintains joint mobility and experiences no joint deformity.
- The child is free from anxiety.
- The child is free from pain.
- The child demonstrates a positive body image.

ALLERGIC REACTIONS

For unclear reasons, there continues to be a rise in the number of children diagnosed with some type of allergy, such as allergic rhinitis and asthma. Why are some children allergic to cats, for instance, although no one else in the family has allergies? To answer this question, the nurse requires a basic understanding of the mechanisms of allergy. An overview of allergic reactions, anaphylaxis, and latex allergies are discussed in this section. Other allergic reactions, including atopic dermatitis, contact dermatitis, erythema multiforme, and Stevens-Johnson syndrome are discussed in Chapter 36∞.

Allergy is an abnormal or altered reaction to an antigen. Antigens responsible for clinical manifestations of allergy are called **allergens.** Allergens can be ingested in food or drugs or injected or absorbed through contact with unbroken skin, and inhaled (Box 27–8). An allergic reaction is an antigen–antibody reaction and can manifest itself as anaphylaxis, atopic disease, serum sickness, or contact dermatitis.

Therefore, the symptoms can be mild to severe or life threatening and they can be localized or systemic. Characteristic findings in children with allergies are summarized in the clinical manifestations table on this page.

The **hypersensitivity response,** an overreaction of the immune system, is responsible for allergic reactions. Hypersensitivity reactions have been classified into four types (Table 27–9).

BOX 27–8 Common Childhood Allergens

Common childhood allergens include:

- Animal dander
- Cockroaches
- Cow milk
- Dust
- Egg whites
- Medications (e.g., penicillin)
- Mites
- Mold
- Plant pollens
- Peanuts
- Seafood
- Shellfish
- Soy
- Tree nuts
- Wheat

CLINICAL MANIFESTATIONS of Allergic Reactions in Children

SYSTEM	CLINICAL MANIFESTATIONS
Respiratory system	Asthma Rhinitis (seasonal and perennial) Serous otitis media Cough Pneumonia Croup Edema of glottis Nasal congestion or discharge
Gastrointestinal system	Abdominal pain and colic Stomatitis Constipation Diarrhea Bloody stools Geographic tongue Vomiting
Skin	Angioedema Urticaria Eczema Atopic dermatitis Erythema multiforme Purpura Drug and food rashes Contact dermatitis
Nervous system	Headache Tension Fatigue Seizures Ménière syndrome Tremors Irritability Sleep disorders Decreased concentration
Eyes	Conjunctivitis Cataract Ciliary spasm Iritis Itching of eyes Tearing
Hematologic	Thrombocytopenic purpura Hemolytic anemia Leukopenia Agranulocytosis
Musculoskeletal system	Arthralgia Myalgia Rheumatoid arthritis Torticollis
Genitourinary system	Dysuria Vulvovaginitis Enuresis
Miscellaneous	Anaphylactic shock Serum sickness Autoimmune diseases

TABLE 27–9 Types of Hypersensitivity Reactions

TYPE	MECHANISM OF ACTION	CLINICAL MANIFESTATIONS	EXAMPLES
Type I Localized or systemic reactions (anaphylaxis)	Antibodies bind to certain cells, causing release of chemical substances that produce an inflammatory reaction.	Hypotension, wheezing, gastrointestinal spasm, uterine spasm; stridor, urticaria	Extrinsic asthma Hay fever
Type II Tissue-specific reactions	Antibodies cause activation of complement system, which leads to tissue damage.	Variable; may include dyspnea or fever	Transfusion reaction ABO incompatibility Hemolytic disease of the newborn
Type III Immune-complex reactions	Immune complexes are deposited in tissues, where they activate complement, which results in a generalized inflammatory reaction.	Urticaria, fever, joint pain	Acute glomerulonephritis Serum sickness
Type IV Delayed reactions	Antigens stimulate T cells that release lymphokines, which cause inflammation and tissue damage.	Variable; may include fever, erythema, pruritus	Contact dermatitis Tuberculin skin test Graft-versus-host disease Allograft rejection

Type I hypersensitivity reactions, the most common allergic reactions, are immediate reactions that occur within seconds or minutes of exposure to the antigen. Symptoms can include a wheal and flare in the skin, edema, spasm of smooth muscle, wheezing, vomiting, diarrhea, or anaphylaxis. The release of chemical substances such as histamine is responsible for the signs and symptoms exhibited.

Type II sensitivity reaction is immediate, within 15 to 30 minutes after exposure to the antigen. Symptoms vary and may include fever and dyspnea. Type III hypersensitivity reaction may be difficult to distinguish from type II reaction. Hypersensitivity reactions generally peak within 6 hours.

Type IV reactions are delayed responses that do not appear until several hours after exposure and require 24 to 72 hours to fully develop. A type IV reaction, which is not confined to any specific tissue, is elicited by relatively complex antigens such as those of bacteria and viruses and by simple antigens such as drugs and metals. Symptoms include contact dermatitis, itching, and blistering.

The first time a child is exposed to the allergen, there is no reaction. With every exposure thereafter, however, the allergic child may have a reaction to the allergen.

Collaborative Care

Assessment of the child with allergy includes a complete physical examination; laboratory, radiograph, and pulmonary function studies; tests of nasal function; and skin testing. Food removal trials or oral food challenges can identify sources of food allergens (Bacharier, 2004). Treatment generally involves avoidance of the allergen, such as substitution of a different drug when the child has a drug allergy. Desensitization may sometimes be used with increasing doses of the allergen administered intradermally in an office where resuscitation is readily available. This treatment is useful for allergy to bees or some pollen. For skin allergies, the allergen is avoided, skin is kept well lubricated, and topical steroids may be used. Oral antihistamines are sometimes used to treat allergy. When exposure to an allergen occurs, medical care may require treatment of anaphylaxis.

Nursing Management

The child with allergies requires a thorough assessment, including a complete past medical history, family history, personal and social history, and review of symptoms. The history focuses on the following areas.

- What symptoms does the child experience? Encourage the child to describe the difficulty in his or her own words.
- Are the symptoms continuous or intermittent? What are the frequency and duration of episodes?
- When did the child first begin to experience symptoms? Did the child have eczema or a feeding problem in infancy or childhood? Did the infant have frequent bouts of colic or skin problems when new foods were introduced? Was there a change in symptoms at puberty? Are the symptoms becoming worse or spontaneously improving?
- What known agents in the environment cause difficulties?
- Are there seasonal variations in symptoms? At what time of the day or night do symptoms usually occur?

The nurse may be responsible for performing intradermal skin tests for allergies (Figure 27–9 ■). Nursing care focuses on

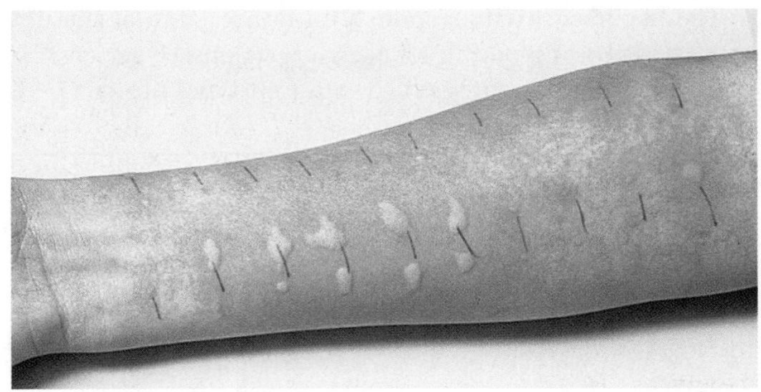

FIGURE 27–9 ■ Results of intradermal skin testing on the forearm. Injections are given on each side of the markings. Note the positive results marked by induration and erythema in response to certain antigens.

From VU/Southern Illinois University/Visuals Unlimited.

treating the symptoms, alleviating the anxiety of the child and parents, and identifying the allergens. Educating the child and family on methods to minimize or avoid exposure to allergens is important. Parents of children who have had severe reactions to bee or wasp stings should be taught how to take precautions and how to provide emergency treatment if the child is stung. An EpiPen® may be prescribed, and the parents and child will require instructions on its proper use. (See Partnering with Families: Using an EpiPen®.)

Partner with the family to determine effective measures to allergy-proof the home. Pets, dust, carpets, fabrics, feather pillows and bedding, and cigarette smoke can all cause allergic reactions. If families are reluctant to give up pets, frequent baths can reduce dander, which is the usual allergen. (See Partnering with Families: Removing Common Allergens from the Home.) When the child has type I reactions to an environmental substance, avoidance of the allergen is most critical. In addition, care providers, families, and school personnel must be able to treat anaphylaxis if exposure to the allergen occurs. School nurses keep records regarding children's allergies and inform school personnel about the allergies and cautions that should be followed. Be sure to label the child's chart, bed, and apply a red armband to alert others to allergies when the child is hospitalized. See Chapter 9 for more information about food allergies. Nurses must be aware of the resuscitation procedures and equipment in all facilities such as hospital units, offices, childcare centers, and schools. See Chapter 25 for airway maintenance and refer to the Skills Manual for resuscitation procedures.

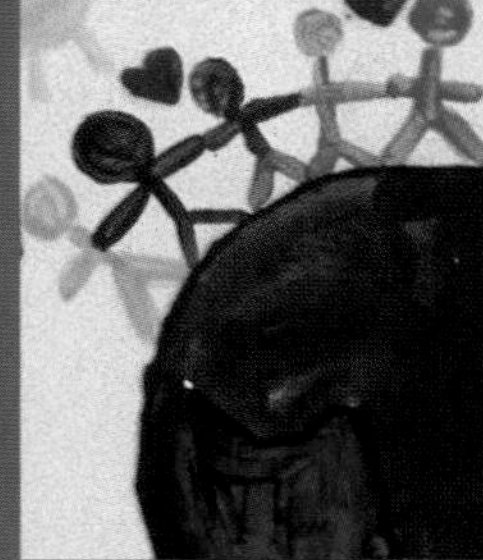

PARTNERING WITH FAMILIES

Using an EpiPen®

If the child has had a severe or systemic reaction in the past, ensure that the parents know how to handle an anaphylactic reaction if the child experiences another reaction.

- Kits with syringes of premeasured epinephrine are available by prescription.
- Ensure that family members understand how to use the kit.
- Instruct the family on proper storage of the kit and to avoid exposing the kit to sun or high temperature.
- Instruct the family to frequently check the expiration date of the adrenaline.
- Encourage the child to wear a medical alert bracelet.
- Emphasize to the family that a kit should be readily available at school, camp, childcare, or other settings, with someone instructed in its use.

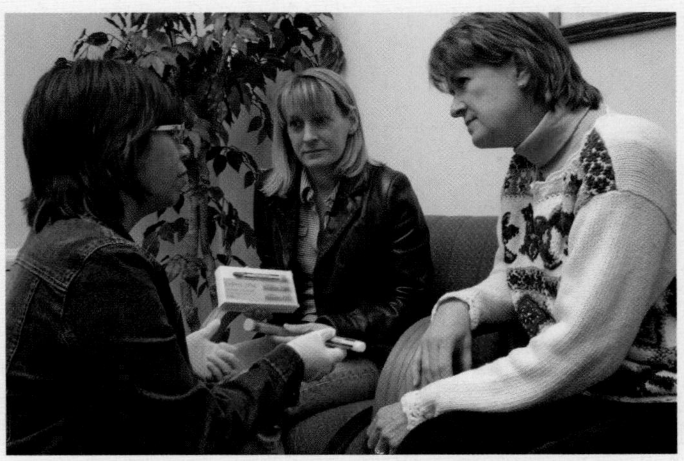

Anaphylaxis

Anaphylaxis, also called anaphylactic shock, is a potentially life-threatening systemic reaction to an allergen. Symptoms can occur within minutes or up to 2 hours after exposure to an allergy-causing substance. The disorder is rare in children, and annual incidence of anaphylactic reactions is approximately 30 per 100,000 individuals (including adults). Those with asthma, eczema, or hay fever are at greater relative risk of experiencing anaphylaxis (The Food Allergy and Anaphylaxis Network, 2004).

Etiology and Pathophysiology

Peanut allergy is the leading cause of fatal and near-fatal food anaphylaxis in the United States, and each year approximately 50 to 100 individuals die from accidental ingestion of peanuts (American Academy of Allergy, Asthma, & Immunology, 2003). Anaphylaxis from other sources causes approximately 1,500 deaths in the United States annually (Tang, 2003). Other causes of anaphylaxis include latex, medications, insect stings, and foods such as milk, eggs, and shellfish.

The child does not experience anaphylaxis with the first exposure to an allergen, but rather produces immunoglobulin E (IgE) antibodies against the antigen. Following a subsequent exposure, the antigen reacts with the IgE antibodies, causing a disruption in cellular integrity. Histamine in large quantities is released, causing increased capillary permeability and massive vasodilation, resulting in hypotension and eventual vascular collapse. Respiratory distress occurs as histamine causes constriction of the bronchioles. As serotonin is released, the capillary permeability in the lungs is increased, leading to plasma leakage into the alveoli, resulting in pulmonary edema. Death can occur within minutes if severe anaphylaxis is not treated immediately.

Clinical Manifestations

Anaphylaxis is an exaggerated hypersensitivity reaction that may manifest with itching; localized or generalized hives on the hands, feet, or mucosa; soft-tissue swelling; cough; dyspnea; pallor; sweating; and tachycardia. Severe reactions may lead to respiratory distress or death. See page 990 for clinical manifestations of anaphylaxis.

COLLABORATIVE CARE

Essential to preservation of life is the immediate recognition and treatment of anaphylactic reaction. Procurement of a stable airway and intravenous access are established. Epinephrine is the medication of choice for treating an anaphylactic reaction

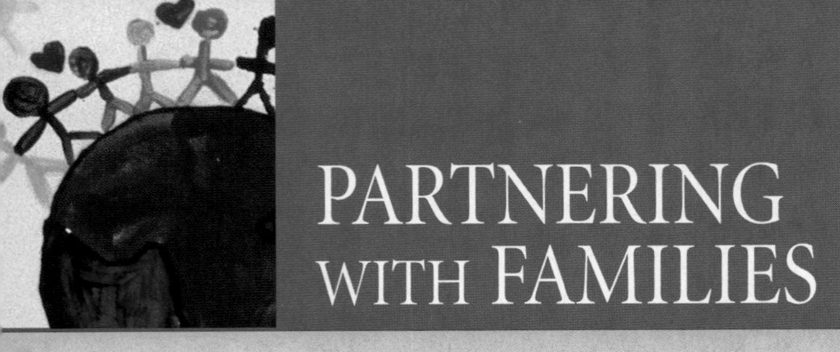

Removing Common Allergens from the Home

Exposure to the known allergens in the home setting is important. Several measures the nurse can instruct the families to take in order to minimize contact with allergens are as follows:

- Remove household pets.
- Control dust by frequent cleaning.
- Clean with moist cloths and mops to remove dust.
- Use plastic covers on mattresses and pillows.
- Avoid carpeting when possible.
- Avoid toys that collect dust (plastic and wood toys are better alternatives than stuffed fabric toys).
- Use high-efficiency air filters.
- Repair homes to prevent entry of water and subsequent molds.
- Consider dehumidification in moist climates.

(Tang, 2003). Epinephrine may be administered subcutaneously, intramuscularly, or via endotracheal tube. Epinephrine reverses the symptoms of an anaphylactic reaction by causing vasoconstriction and reversing airway constriction.

Antihistamines, such as Benadryl, and steroids are often administered to the child experiencing an anaphylactic reaction. Though antihistamines and steroids may be administered with epinephrine, they are never prescribed as a substitute for epinephrine since they cannot reverse many of the symptoms of anaphylaxis (Food Allergy and Anaphylaxis Network, 2004). The child is placed in supine position with legs elevated to increase venous return.

PRACTICE ALERT

The Trendelenburg position is no longer recommended for the treatment of shock. The position causes abdominal organs to press against the diaphragm, which impedes respirations, and decreases coronary artery filling.

Intravenous access is obtained for fluid resuscitation, because large volumes of fluids may be required to treat hypotension caused by increased vascular permeability and vasodilation. Oxygen is administered. The child may require endotracheal intubation and mechanical ventilation (see Chapter 25∞). The child is monitored for an observation period of 2 to 6 hours after mild episodes, and 24 hours after more severe episodes (Tang, 2003).

Prevention of reexposure to the allergen is essential. Determining the cause of anaphylaxis, if uncertain, may require numerous diagnostic studies. Previous tolerance of a substance does not rule it out as the trigger. Direct skin testing and radioallergosorbent testing (RAST) are available for some antigens.

CLINICAL MANIFESTATIONS of Anaphylactic Shock

SYSTEM	CLINICAL MANIFESTATIONS	CLINICAL THERAPY
Respiratory	Wheezing Stridor Dyspnea Laryngospasm Bronchospasm Pulmonary edema Cyanosis	Monitor respiratory status Monitor breath sounds Monitor arterial blood gases Administer epinephrine, oxygen, and fluids (protocol for anaphylactic shock) Ventilatory support as needed
Cardiovascular	Profound hypotension Tachycardia Dysrhythmias Decreased central venous pressure	Monitor heart rate, blood pressure, cardiac rhythm Monitor peripheral pulses Manage fluid intake and output
Neurological	Anxiety Restlessness Lethargy Progression to coma	Conduct neurological assessment at regular intervals Assess for changes in level of consciousness Assess for changes in anxiety level
Gastrointestinal	Vomiting Diarrhea Abdominal pain	Assess for vomiting or diarrhea Assess for abdominal pain Assess bowel sounds and limit intake when not present
Integumentary	Edematous face, lips, tongue, hands, feet Skin warm	Assess for edema, rashes Assess skin temperature Ensure comfort measures
Renal	Oliguria progressing to anuria	Monitor intake hourly Adjust intake and medications to maintain normal urinary output Monitor serum BUN and creatinine

NURSING MANAGEMENT

The goal of nursing care is to recognize and immediately treat anaphylaxis and educate the child and family to avoid exposure to allergens.

Nursing Assessment and Diagnosis

Assess the child for respiratory distress, hypotension, tachycardia, and edema. Assess breath sounds for wheezing, and monitor oxygen saturation. Assess all vital signs including peripheral pulses. Monitor urine output hourly. Assess skin temperature, color, and moisture.

Nursing diagnoses that apply to the child with anaphylaxis include:

- Decreased Cardiac Output related to profound hypotension and shock
- Ineffective Tissue Perfusion (all systems) related to decreased blood flow, hypotension, and shock
- Deficient Fluid Balance related to shock
- Anxiety (parental and child) related to life-threatening emergent condition

Planning and Implementation

Nursing roles involve preventing anaphylactic reactions by partnering with families to minimize exposure to allergens and by alerting all healthcare personnel in hospitals and clinics to the child's allergy. In addition, knowledge of emergency procedures is important in all facilities such as schools, homes, and hospitals.

Emergency management of anaphylaxis consists of administration of epinephrine, oxygen, and fluids. Maintain the child on bed rest immediately following anaphylaxis until the observation period has concluded. Provide the child and family the opportunity to express anxiety and concerns.

For home care, partner with the family to ensure that the child and family members can properly administer epinephrine. Emphasize to the family that the child should always wear a medical identification tag and have an EpiPen® available for emergencies. Ensure that the childcare providers or school officials can recognize the signs and symptoms of anaphylaxis and can appropriately administer epinephrine. Instruct the child and family to activate the emergency medical system (EMS) (9-1-1) after epinephrine is administered.

Evaluation

Expected outcomes of nursing care of the child with anaphylaxis include:

- Cardiac output is stabilized and vital signs are within baseline limits.
- Tissue perfusion to all organs is stabilized.
- Fluid balance is restored.
- The child and family express anxiety and utilize effective coping mechanism.

Latex Allergy

Latex allergy is a common finding among certain occupations, including healthcare workers, and in specific types of patients. For example, about 10% of healthcare workers, 50% of children with neural tube defects, and 34% of children with three or more surgeries are sensitive to latex (Brehler & Kutting, 2001). Healthcare products such as gloves, drains, catheters, and intravenous ports, contain latex, which is a sap from the rubber tree. Latex allergy is caused by an IgE-mediated response that develops after repeated exposure to latex. In some cases, intraoperative deaths have occurred when allergic individuals were exposed to latex products during surgery. A reaction to latex products can be manifested as irritant reaction of the skin; type IV of delayed hypersensitivity, with redness, inflammation, and blisters on the skin; or type I hypersensitivity which is immediate and often has systemic manifestations (itchy eyes, asthma, or anaphylaxis).

PRACTICE ALERT

Starting in September 1998, the Food and Drug Administration ordered that medical products with latex carry the warning: "Caution: This product contains natural rubber latex, which may cause allergic reactions." Check product labels in your healthcare facility for this warning. *What products do you expect to need the label?*

Children most at risk for latex allergy include those with myelodysplasia and congenital urinary tract anomalies. Up to 70% of children with neural tube defects have immunoglobulin E (IgE) antibodies to latex, and other at risk groups include children with bladder exstrophy (Houribane, Allard, Wade, et al., 2002). Persons who have had repeated surgeries are also at higher risk due to high exposure to latex during surgery. Healthcare personnel are also at risk for latex allergy due to exposure in the workplace (Box 27–9).

Collaborative Care

Children and adolescents at high risk should receive allergy testing for latex; the radioallergosorbent test (RAST) is most often

BOX 27–9 Measures to Protect Against Latex Allergy

Healthcare personnel are at high risk of developing latex allergy because of intense exposure to products containing latex. An estimated 8% to 12% of healthcare workers are latex sensitive. You can protect yourself by using the following measures.

- Decrease exposure by choosing alternative products when available (use synthetic rubbers, polyethylene, nitrile, neoprene, vinyl gloves).
- Use powder-free gloves if using latex gloves (the powder has high amounts of latex, which can be inhaled).
- Avoid use of oil-based hand creams and lotions before putting on latex gloves, as these preparations break down the latex.
- When symptoms of sensitivity to latex occur on exposure (rash, hives, nasal congestion, conjunctivitis, cough, or wheeze), contact the employee health department of your facility.
- If diagnosed as latex allergic, avoid all contact and wear a medical alert bracelet.

used. Healthcare personnel should use alternative products when caring for those persons at risk (Box 27–10).

When a positive skin test has occurred or when the child has had a reaction to latex, all latex products must be removed from the allergic individual's environment.

Nursing Management

Assess the child for the potential for latex allergy (Box 27–11). Alternative products, such as nonlatex gloves and catheters, must be used when providing healthcare. Emphasize to the family that the child with latex allergy should wear a medical alert identification bracelet at all times, and should have an epinephrine kit readily available at home and school.

Be alert for any signs of hypersensitivity when the child is receiving healthcare, and be prepared with drugs and equipment to treat anaphylaxis. This is especially important in operative settings when acute anaphylaxis is often life threatening. Emphasize to parents and children that many everyday products contain latex, including latex balloons and condoms (Table 27–10).

BOX 27–11 Latex Allergy Questionnaire

1. Has the child ever had allergies, asthma, hay fever, eczema, or problems with rashes?
2. Has the child ever had respiratory distress, rapid heart rate, or swelling?
3. Has the child ever had swelling, itching, hives, or other symptoms after contact with a balloon?
4. Has the child ever had swelling, itching, hives, or other symptoms after a dental examination or procedure?
5. Has the child/adolescent ever had swelling, itching, hives, or other symptoms following a vaginal or rectal examination or after contact with a diaphragm or condom?
6. Has the child ever had swelling, itching, or hives during or within 1 hour after wearing rubber gloves or a bandage with latex?
7. Has the child ever had a rash on his or her hands that lasted over 1 week?
8. Has the child ever had swelling, itching, hives, runny nose, eye irritation, wheezing, or asthma after contact with any latex or rubber product?
9. Has the child ever had swelling, itching, or hives after being examined by someone wearing rubber or latex gloves?
10. Has a physician ever informed the parent that the child has a rubber or latex allergy?
11. Is the child allergic to bananas, papaya, avocado, kiwi fruits, other stone fruits, tomatoes, raw potatoes, or chestnuts?
12. Has the child ever had an unexplained anaphylactic episode? If so, please describe.

Data from Association of Operating Room Nurses. (2004). AORN latex guideline. AORN Journal, 79(3), 653–678.

GRAFT-VERSUS-HOST DISEASE

Most of us are quite familiar with the fact that transplantation of organs can lead to an immune reaction that results in rejection by the recipient. Blood and HLA tissue typing minimize the incidence of rejection. Immunosuppressant drugs are given, usually for life, to further decrease incidence of organ rejection. Many people are less aware that blood acts as a body organ as well. While reaction to a blood transfusion has already been discussed, another type of reaction can occur when bone marrow cells or stem cells are transfused into a recipient. Typically, bone marrow or stem cells are transplanted into a child with diseased blood cells such as in leukemia, or into a child with severe combined immunodeficiency disease (see a discussion of that disease earlier in this chapter and a discussion of leukemia in Chapter 29∞).

Etiology and Pathophysiology

In a child with severe immunodeficiency disease, lymphocyte production does not occur or is impaired. For a child with leukemia, the child's lymphocyte production is blocked by irradiation or chemotherapy that purposefully destroys bone marrow function. The child then receives donor bone marrow or stem cells by intravenous infusion. After a period of time in isolation to prevent infection, the new cells attach to the child's bone marrow and begin production. The child's lymphocyte production increases and immune response develops. (See further description of this treatment's use for cancer in Chapter 29∞.) However, despite blood and tissue typing, sometimes the donor cells are incompatible with the recipient cells and the new cells begin to mount an immunologic response in the child who has received the transplant. The incidence of the disease is less in matched siblings than in matched nonsibling transplants.

In graft-versus-host disease, the host is immunocompromised while the donor tissue is immunologically competent. The host, or recipient, cannot raise a defense to the infused and incompatible cells; however, the donor cells release cytokines and become enlarged or inflamed, leading to tissue damage in many body organs such as the gastrointestinal system and the skin. The process is further worsened by the recipient's general tissue condition. The preparatory irradiation or chemotherapy has already caused tissue damage and release of the child's own inflammatory cytokines in these tissues (Behrman, Kliegman, & Jenson, 2004; Vogelsang, Lee, & Bensen-Kennedy, 2003).

BOX 27–10 RAST

RAST is a common laboratory test used to detect IgE antibodies. It measures circulating IgE antibodies to many allergens and generally correlates well with skin test results. It is not as sensitive as skin tests, however, so those tests are generally preferred when available for specific allergens.

Clinical Manifestations

Graft-versus-host disease may be either acute or chronic. Acute disease occurs in the first 100 days after transplant. The skin is most commonly affected and manifests a rash that is pruritic and macular/popular. It generally begins on the extremities and progresses to the trunk. Blistering and a burning sensation may occur. Gastrointestinal effects of graft-versus-host disease may include nausea, vomiting, anorexia, diarrhea, cramping, and abdominal pain. Impaired liver function is evident from jaundice and abnormal liver function tests.

Chronic graft-versus-host disease generally occurs after 100 days posttransplant. This reaction is similar to an autoimmune reaction in the recipient's body. Recurrent infections, skin reactions, and thrombocytopenia are frequent occurrences. Mouth, throat, and esophageal ulcers; gastrointestinal disorders; cholestasis; and dry, irritated eyes can occur (Behrman et al., 2004; Higman & Vogelsang, 2004).

TABLE 27–10 Sources of Possible Latex Contact

FREQUENTLY CONTAIN LATEX	EXAMPLES OF LATEX-SAFE ALTERNATIVES/BARRIERS
Adhesives, skin (Smith + Nephew)	Mastisol (Ferndale)
Anesthesia circuits, bags, oxygen masks	Neoprene (Anesthesia Associates, Ohmeda adult), *some* Vital Signs
Bandaids	Active Strip (3M), CURAD Neon, Readi-Bandages, NHP, *some* Airstrip
Blood pressure cuff, tubing (J&J)	Cleen Cuff (Vital Signs), nylon (*some* Trimline) *selected* Davol, Medline, Rusch, Premium, Baxter
Bulb syringe	
Casts: Delta-Lite Podiatry, Orthoflex (J&J)	Scotchcast soft, Delta-Lites, *recent* Conformable (J&J), Caraglas Ultra, liners (Gore)
Catheters, condom	Clear Advantage, ProSys NL, *selected* Coloplast, Rochester, PolyTech (Hollister)
Catheters, indwelling & systems, UDS	*some* Am BioMed, Argyle, Bard, Cook, Dale, Kendall, Lifetech, Mentor, Rochester, Rusch, Vitaid. Adapters & plug (Addto)
Catheters, cardiac, vascular, pulmonary	*some* World Medical, Am BioMed
Catheters, straight, coude	Mentor, RobNel (Sherwood), Coloplast, *selected* Bard, Rusch catheters
Catheters, feeding	Accumark feeding catheter (Sims Portex)
CPR manikins & Medical training aids	*most* Laerdal products
Dressings: Dyna-flex, butterfly closures (J&J) BDF Elastroplast, Action Wrap, Coban (3M) Lyofoam (Acme), Spandage (Medi-tech), Telfa	Duoderm, Reston foam (3M), Opsite, Venigard, Comfeel, Sorbaview, Telfa (some) Xeroform, PinCare, Bioclusive, Montg'ry strap (J&J), Webril, Metalline, Selopor, Opraflex, Centurion brief, *some* Airstrips, Rainbow Net (Surgilast), VAC
Note: Latex in package only: Steri-strip wound closure system, Tegaderm, Active Strips (3M), Nu-Derm (J&J), CURAD	
Ear plugs	Grainger (5F767)
Elastic wrap: ACE, Esmarch, Zimmer Dyna-flex, Elastikon (J&J)	E-Cotton, CEB elastic (coNco), Champ (Carolon), Adban Adhesive, X-Mark (Avcor) Co-Flex, PowerFlex (Andover), Comprilan (Jobst), Esmark (DeRoyal, NHP)
Electrode bulbs, pads, grounding	*some* Baxter, Dantec EMG, Conmed, ValleyLab, Vermont Med, Staodyn, Neotrode
Endotracheal tubes, airways	*selected* Berman, Mallinckrodt, Polamedco, Portex, Rusch, Sheridan, Shiley
Enemas	BabyLax, Bowel Man't Tube (MIC), Pharmaseal set, all Fleet Ready-to-use, cone irrigation set (Convatec), silicone retention cuff tip (Lafayette)
G-tubes, buttons	Silicone (Bard, Flexiflo, MIC, Rusch, Stomate)
Gloves: sterile, clean, surgical, orthodontic	Allergard (J&J), dermaprene (Ansell), N-DEX (Best), Safeskin Nitrile, Neolon, SensiCare, Tru-touch (Maxxim), Nitrex, Tactyl 1,2 (SmartPractice), Duraprene (Allegiance Healthcare), Elastyren (Hermal, Center Labs), Boston Medical, Masel, Neotech
Incentive deep breathing exerciser	Voldyne 5000 (Sherwood David & Geck), Triflo II
IV access: injection ports, Y-sites, bags, pumps, buretrol ports, PRN adapters, needless systems	**Cover Y-sites and bag ports—do not puncture. Use stopcocks for meds.** Polymer injection caps + burettes + Safsite (Braun), Abbot systems, Walrus, Gemini (IMED), *selected* Baxter (InterLink), Statlock, Ready Med, ConMed, Clave, Alaris, Hudson, *select* Sims, IV boards (Avcor), Terumo Pumps: Mach II, ADS 100; Clic-Open (vial top remover—Sepha Pharm.)
OR/Infection Control masks, hats, shoe covers	*some* by Kimberly Clark, TECNOL; OR & sterile packs (CML, DeRoyal) twill ties
Medication vial stoppers	*some* AmRegent, Astra, Bedford Labs, Fujisawa, Gensia, Glaxo, Lilly, Roche
Miscellaneous items	Soft-Grip fabric clamp covers (Scanlan), Precision Dynamics I.D. bracelets
Ostomy supplies	Check with individual companies regarding latex content of products
Penrose drains	Jackson-Pratt, Zimmer Hemovac
Pulse oximeters, thermometer probes	Nonin oximeters, *selected* Nellcor sensors, Diatec probe covers
Reflex hammers	Cover with plastic bag
Respirators	Advantage (MSA), HEPA-Tech (Uvex), PFR 95 (Tecnol), 3M 1860
Resuscitators, manual	*certain* Ambu, Armstrong, Laerdal, Puriton Bennett, Vital Blue, Respironics, Rusch
Spacer (for metered-dose inhaler)	ACE spacer (Center Labs), OptiHaler (HealthScan)
Stethoscope tubing	PVC (*some* Littman) cover with ScopeCoat or latex-free stockinette (Albahealth)
Suction tubing	PVC (Davol, Laerdal, Mallinckrodt, Superior, Yankauer) Medline, Ballard
Syringes, disposable	Terumo Medical, Abbott PCA Abboject, Norm-Ject (Air-Tite), EpiPen, *selected* BD syringes, AdvantaJet (Activa)
Tapes: pink, Waterproof (3M), Zonas, Moleskin, cloth, Waterproof (J&J), adhesive felt (Acme)	Dermicel (J&J), Durapore, Microfoam, Micropore, Transpore (3M) Cath-Strip (Genetic Labs), Ice Tape (P.O.Pak), All-Felt (Universal Foot Care), Hypafix
Tonopen disposable covers (glaucoma tester)	
Tourniquets	Children's Medical, Grafco, VelcroPedic, X-Tourn straps (Avcor), Free-Band (Kent)
Theraband (also strip, tube), other OT supplies	REP Bands & Cords (OPTP), Exercise putty (Rolyan), new Thera-Band Exercisers plastic tubing-Tygon LR-40 (Norton), elastic thread, sheets (JPS Elastomerics)
Tubing, sheeting	
Vascular stockings	Compriform Custom (Jobst)

(continued)

TABLE 27–10 Sources of Possible Latex Contact (continued)

FREQUENTLY CONTAIN LATEX	EXAMPLES OF LATEX-SAFE ALTERNATIVES/BARRIERS
Latex in the Home and Community	
Art supplies: paints, glue, erasers, fabric paints	Elmers (School Glue, Glue-All, GluColors, Carpenters Wood Glue, Sno-Drift paste) FaberCastel erasers, Crayola (**except** stamps, erasers), Liquitex paints, DickBlick Tempera & acrylic paints & soap erasers, Play-Doh
Balloons Balls: Koosh balls, tennis balls, bowling balls	Mylar balloons, self-sealing *Myloons* PVC (Headstrom Sports Ball), Nerf Foam Balls
Carpet backing, gym floor, basement sealant Chewing gum Clothes: applique on Tees, elastic on socks, underwear, sneakers, sandals Condoms, contraceptive sponges, diaphragm Crutches: tips, axillary pads, hand grips	Provide barrier—cloth or mat Bubblicious, Trident (Warner-Lambert), Wrigley gums (check new products) Cloth-covered elastic, neoprene (Decent Exposures, NOLATEX Industries) Buster Brown elastic-free socks (Vermont Country Store) Polyurethane (Avanti), female condom (Reality), Wideseal Silicone Diaphragms (Milex), Trojan Supra Condom Cover with cloth, tape
Dental dams, cups, bands, root canal material, orthodontic rubber bands Diapers, incontinence pads, rubber pants	PURO/M27 intraoral elastics (Midwest Orthodontic), wire springs, sealant (Delton), dams (Meer Dental, Hygenic Corp), John O Butler, Earloop masks (Richmond) Huggies, First Quality, Gold Seal, Tranquility, Always, *some* Attends, Drypers Diapers (not training pants), Confidence (Paper-Pak), Pampers, Luvs
Feeding nipples Food handled with latex gloves	Silicone, vinyl (*selected* Gerber, Evenflo, MAM, Ross, Mead Johnson) Synthetic gloves for food handling
Note: Associated allergies are reported to banana, avocado, chestnut, kiwi, and other fruits.	
Handles on racquets, tools, bicycles	Vinyl, leather handles, or cover with cloth or tape
Infant toothbrush-massager	Soft bristle brush or cloth, Gerber/NUK
Kitchen cleaning gloves	PVC MYPLEX (Magla), cotton liners (Allerderm)
Latex paints, sealants, stains	There is no natural rubber in latex paint; it may be present in some waterproof paints and sealants
Miscellaneous items	Some medical stickers by MediBadge, UAL, Cushie Tushie Potty Seat
Newsprint, ads, coupons, lottery scratch tickets	
Pacifiers Play pits, playground surfaces	Soothies (Children's Med Ventures), *selected* Binky, Gerber, Infa, Kip, MAM Natural rubber latex may be a component
Rubber bands, bungee cords	Plasti bands
Toys—Stretch Armstrong, old Barbies	Jurassic Park figures (Kenner), 1993 Barbie, Disney dolls (Mattel), many toys by Fisher Price, Little Tikes, Playschool, Discovery, Trolls (Norfin), Silly-putty
Water toys & equipment: beach thongs, masks, bathing suits, caps, scuba gear, goggles Wheelchair cushions, tires	PVC, plastic, nylon, Suits Me Swimwear Jay, ROHO cushions, use leather gloves, Sof Care bed/chair cushions (Gaymar)
Zippered plastic storage bags	Waxed paper, plain plastic bags, Ziploc bags

Adapted from the Spina Bifida Association of America. www.sbaa.org. 4590 MacArthur Blvd NW, Suite 250, Washington, DC 20001-4226. Used with permission.

COLLABORATIVE CARE

The aim of collaborative care is to prevent graft-versus-host disease when possible—to identify it early and to intervene to decrease the immune response in the recipient.

Diagnostic Tests

Careful physical examination of all systems and laboratory tests assist in determining presence of the disease and stage of reaction. Clinical staging ranges from stage 1 for mild disease to stage IV for severe disease. Mild skin involvement includes presence of rash on about 25% of skin surface, while severe involvement is indicated when much of the body is affected with blisters and desquamation. Mild liver involvement is evident with a bilirubin of 2–3 mg/dL, while severe disease is indicated with a bilirubin of > 15mg/dL (see Appendix C∞ for additional expected liver function test results in children). Mild diarrhea indicates some gastrointestinal involvement, whereas severe diarrhea and abdominal pain indicate advanced disease. Total blood counts and immunoglobulins are measured regularly to monitor for disease occurrence.

Clinical Therapy

The first therapy is prevention of the disease by tissue typing. Studies are being conducted to identify further differentiation of tissue types that may be helpful in preventing disease. Early identification is key to beginning therapy and stopping progression of the disease. Several immunosuppressant drugs are used in treatment, commonly cyclosporine and prednisone administered on alternating days. See the medication table on page 995 for common drugs used to treat graft-versus-host disease. When

MEDICATIONS Used to Treat Graft-Versus-Host Disease

MEDICATION	ACTION/INDICATION	NURSING IMPLICATIONS
Corticosteroids *Prednisone*	Suppress inflammatory cytokines; decrease inflammation and immune response	Monitor for adverse effects such as hyperglycemia (check blood glucose), confusion and psychosis, muscle weakness, delayed healing, gastrointestinal distress. Perform regular weight and height measurements and report changes in percentiles; record blood pressure. Perform serum electrolytes and routine laboratory studies frequently.
Antimetabolite *Methotrexate (MTX)*	Folic acid antagonist that decreases proliferation of T lymphocytes; interferes with immune response to hematopoietic stem cell transplant	Obtain baseline liver and kidney function tests, CBC, and chest radiographs. Monitor for renal, hepatic, and gastrointestinal toxicity. Encourage generous fluid intake for age of child. Prevent exposure to infectious agents and have families report signs of infection. Teach families to perform thorough and gentle mouth care to prevent oral problems.
Interleukin-2 suppressors *Cyclosporine and tacrolimus*	Blocks calcium-dependent signal transduction to T-cell receptor, thereby interfering with antibody production	Observe carefully during and after administration for signs of transfusion reaction. Monitor intake and output, vital signs, neurologic function. Obtain liver and kidney function tests. Take oral form of cyclosporine with meals to decrease gastrointestinal effects; oral tacrolimus should be taken on an empty stomach. Oral cyclosporine can be mixed with small amount of milk or juice just before giving as long as child can drink the entire amount.

Adapted from Bindler, R. M., & Howry, L. B. (2005). Prentice Hall pediatric drug guide with nursing implications. *Upper Saddle River, NJ: Prentice Hall Health; Vogelsang, G. B., Lee, L., & Benserr-Kennedy, D. M. (2003). Pathogenesis and treatment of graft-versus-host disease after bone marrow transplant.* Annual Review of Medicine, *54, 29–54.*

these drugs are not successful in treating the disease, antithymocyte globulin, anti-CD33 (gemtuzumab ozogamicin), anti-CD20 (rituximab), and mycophenolate mofetil may be used.

NURSING MANAGEMENT

Nursing management focuses on careful physical assessment to assist in early identification of the disease process, and partnering with other health professionals and families to ensure treatment for the child. All body systems can be involved, especially in chronic disease, so frequent and thorough assessments are needed. Place particular emphasis on skin examination and reporting rashes that occur. Monitor gastrointestinal functioning by asking about nausea, vomiting, diarrhea, abdominal pain, bloody stools, and dietary intake. Weigh and measure the child and compare to earlier findings. Auscultate the lungs and be alert for signs of infection. Inquire about pain in joints or other body parts. Perform regular eye examinations and ask about burning or itching of eyes. Perform prescribed blood tests to monitor for liver and bone marrow function.

Nursing care for the child who has had a bone marrow or stem cell transplant is complex. Emphasize the need for regular examinations to identify any signs of disease. Provide resources if the family needs transportation or financial assistance to obtain these examinations. Teach the family the importance of obtaining immunizations as recommended; children with immunosuppression may require special additional immunizations and may require prophylaxis to infections such as pneumonia. Instruct the family on administration of medications if the child receives immunosuppressants. Have the family report fever, change in behavior or neurological functioning, dietary intake changes, gastrointestinal symptoms, or other concerns. Have the child avoid contact with infectious individuals and settings such as shopping malls. Help the family arrange for a home tutor and an individualized education plan if the child must remain out of school for a period of time.

Medications used to treat graft-versus-host disease have many side effects. Assist families to administer them properly, become familiar with side effects, and perform monitoring such as blood tests, height and weight, developmental, and other necessary evaluations. See the medications box above for information about some of the most commonly used medications.

The desired outcomes for care of the child with a hematopoietic stem cell transplant include adequate blood cell production and healthy immune response, prevention and early treatment of graft-versus-host disease, and normal growth and development without sequellae of disease.

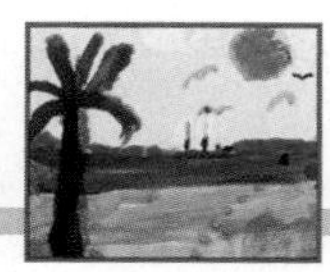

CHAPTER HIGHLIGHTS

- The infant is born with natural immunity from the mother, and develops acquired immunity gradually in the first 6 years of life.
- Acquired immunity is humoral (antibody mediated) and cell mediated.
- B cells, T cells, natural killer (NK) cells, and complement proteins are the major components of a healthy immune system.
- Disorders of the immune system can be due to genetic causes (primary immunodeficiency), or can be acquired (secondary immunodeficiency).
- Severe combined immunodeficiency disease (SCID) is life threatening and requires careful medical and nursing management.
- Human immunodeficiency virus (HIV) can lead to acquired immunodeficiency syndrome (AIDS); care focuses on prevention of this major viral infection.
- When the child is infected with HIV, support for nutrition, infection control, and developmental stimulation is needed.
- Nurses provide support for families of children with severe immune deficiency with a focus on finances, provision of complex medical care, and emotional support.
- Autoimmune disorders such as eczema, juvenile rheumatoid arthritis, and systemic lupus erythematosis occur when the body perceives its own tissue as foreign and mounts a defense against it.
- Systemic lupus erythematosus (SLE), a generalized disorder mainly occurring in females, is a chronic inflammatory, autoimmune disease of unknown origin that involves many organ systems.
- Juvenile rheumatoid arthritis (JRA) is a chronic autoimmune inflammatory disease characterized by joint inflammation resulting in decreased mobility, swelling, and pain that occurs slightly more often in girls than in boys.
- Although progress is slow, the body may return to normal after manifestation of autoimmune disorder.
- Approximately 2 million children have some type of allergy, making this one of the major chronic illnesses of children today.
- Peanut allergy is the leading cause of fatal and near-fatal food anaphylaxis in the United States, and each year approximately 50 to 100 individuals die from accidental ingestion of peanuts.
- A thorough assessment and careful teaching can help the child with allergies to successfully manage reactions.
- Allergy to latex products is commonly seen in children, healthcare workers, and the general population.
- Children most at risk for latex allergy include those with myelodysplasia and congenital urinary tract anomalies.
- Graft-versus-host disease (GVHD) is a type IV hypersensitivity reaction in which the donor T lymphocytes are stimulated by the recipient's antigen-presenting cells.

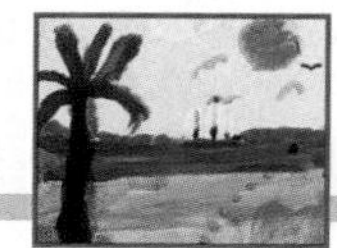

CRITICAL THINKING IN ACTION

INTRODUCTION

Recall Raymond, the 2-year-old who, after repeated infections, was diagnosed with AIDS. Because Raymond had no other risk factors for HIV and AIDS, the healthcare team recommended that Raymond's mother also be tested for the infection since Raymond could have received the infection as a result of maternal–fetus infection. Raymond's mother was subsequently diagnosed with HIV. Raymond's 5-year-old sister, Rachel, tested negative for HIV.

DESCRIPTION

Raymond begins pharmacologic treatment with HAART. Raymond's mother also begins pharmacologic treatment for HIV. Raymond's current viral load is 170,000 and his CD4 count is less than 200 cells/mm^3. He is 2 standard deviations below his expected growth curve.

DISCUSSION

1. Based on Raymond's diagnosis and physical condition, what is the immediate plan of care for Raymond?
2. What are the primary teaching goals for Raymond's mother?
3. Based on Raymond's developmental stage, identify appropriate interventions for medication administration and other nursing interventions during hospitalization.

4. Based on Rachel's developmental stage, what should she be told about her brother's illness? Her mother's diagnosis? How can the nurse assist Raymond's mother to explain these issues to Rachel?
5. What critical issues will Raymond and his family face based on his diagnosis of AIDS and his mother's diagnosis of HIV?
6. What home and community care must be established before Raymond's discharge from the hospital? What are the short-term goals for home management? What are the long-term goals for home management?

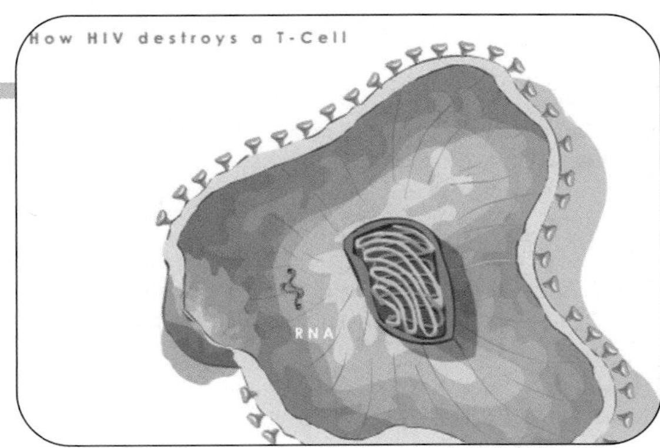

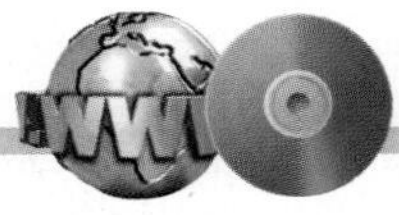

EXPLORE MediaLink

- NCLEX review, case studies, and other interactive resources for this chapter can be found on the Companion Website at **www.prenhall.com/ball**. Click on Chapter 27 to select the activities for this chapter.
- For animation, more NCLEX review questions, and an audio glossary, access the accompanying CD-ROM in this textbook.

http://www.prenhall.com/ball

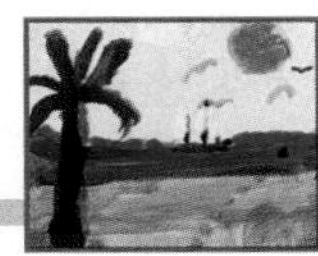

REFERENCES

Aidsinfo. (2004). Guidelines for the use of antiviral agents in pediatric HIV infection. aidsinfo.nih.gov, accessed 12/5/2004.

American Academy of Allergy, Asthma, & Immunology. (2003, July 10). New research on peanut allergies. www.aaaai.org/media/news_releases/2-003/07/071003.stm, accessed 6/22/2004.

American Academy of Pediatrics, Committee on Pediatric AIDS and Committee on Adolescence. (2001). Adolescents and human immunodeficiency virus infection: The role of the pediatrician in prevention and intervention (RE0031). *Pediatrics, 107*(1), 188–190.

American College of Rheumatology. (2003). http://rarediseases.about.com/gi/dynamic/offsite.htm?site=http%3A%2F%2Fwww.rheumatology.org%2Fpatients%2Ffactsheet%2Fsle.html, accessed 12/22/2003.

Bacharier, L. B. (2004). Are the results of oral food challenges predictable? *Annals of Allergy, Asthma, and Immunology, 92*(2), 195–197.

Behrman, R. E., Kliegman, R. M., & Jenson, H. B. (2004). *Nelson textbook of pediatrics* (17th ed., pp. 738–741). Philadelphia: Saunders.

Bindler, R. M., & Howry, L. B. (2005). *Prentice Hall pediatric drug guide with nursing implications.* Upper Saddle River, NJ: Prentice Hall Health.

Brackis-Cott, E., Mellins, C. A., Abrams, E., Reval, T., & Dolezal, C. (2003). Pediatric HIV medication adherence: The views of medical providers from two primary care programs. *Journal of Pediatric Health Care, 17,* 252–260.

Brehler, R., & Kutting, B. (2001). Natural rubber latex allergy. *Archives of Internal Medicine, 161,* 1057–1064.

Burpo, R. H. (2000). Common antiviral agents used in women's and children's care. *Journal of Obstetric, Gynecologic and Neonatal Nursing, 29,* 181–200.

Candotti, F. (2000). The potential for therapy of immune disorders with gene therapy. *Pediatric Clinics of North America, 47,* 1389–1408.

Caselli, D. (2000). Human immunodeficiency virus–related cancer in children: Incidence and treatment outcome—Report of the Italian Register. *Journal of Clinical Oncology, 18,* 3854–3861.

Cassidy, J. T., & Petty, P. E. (2001). *Textbook of pediatric rheumatology* (4th ed.). Philadelphia: W.B. Saunders.

Centers for Disease Control and Prevention. (2003). OraQuick rapid HIV-1 antibody test. www.cdc.gov, accessed 12/4/2004.

Centers for Disease Control and Prevention. (2004a). OraQuick rapid HIV test for oral fluid. Frequently asked questions. www.cdc.gov, accessed 12/4/2004.

Centers for Disease Control and Prevention. (2004b). HIV/AIDS among Hispanics. www.cdc.gov/hiv/pubs/facts/hispanic.htm, accessed 12/5/2004.

Centers for Poison Control and Prevention. (2005).

Champi, C. (2002). Primary immunodeficiency disorders in children: Prompt diagnosis can lead to lifesaving treatment. *Journal of Pediatric Health, 16*(1), 16–21.

Cohen, H., Chen, X. C., Sunkle, S., Davis, L., Geromanos, K., Xanthos, G., & Shearer, W. (2000). Ability of caregivers to read delayed hypersensitivity skin tests in children exposed to and infected by HIV. *Journal of Pediatric Health Care, 14,* 50–55.

Committee on Pediatric AIDS. (1998). Human immunodeficiency virus/acquired immunodeficiency syndrome education in schools. *Pediatrics, 101,* 933–935.

Committee on Pediatric AIDS and Committee on Adolescence. (2001). Adolescents and human immunodeficiency virus infections: The role of the pediatrician in prevention and intervention. *Pediatrics, 107,* 188–190.

Conley, M. E., Saragoussi, D., Notarangelo, L., Elzioni, A., & Casanova, J. L. (2003). An international study examining therapeutic options used in treatment of Wiskott-Aldrich syndrome. *Clinical Immunology 109,* 272–277.

Cooper, M. A., Pommering, T. L., & Koranyi, K. (2003). Primary immunodeficiencies. *American Family Physician, 68,* 2001-2008.

Copstead, L. C., & Banasik, J. L. (2005). *Pathophysiology: Biological and behavioral perspectives* (3rd ed.). St. Louis: Elsevier Saunders.

Dibbern, D. A., & Routes, J. M. (2004). Wiskott-Aldrich syndrome. www.emedicine.com/med/topic1162.htm, accessed 6/20/2004.

Drug Digest. (2004). www.drugdigest.org/DD/HC/treatment/0,4047,550408,00.html, accessed 12/5/2004.

Edmunds, M. W., & Mayhew, M. S. (2004). *Pharmacology for the primary care provider* (2nd ed.). Philadelphia: Elsevier Mosby.

El-Alfy, M. S., & El-Sayed, M. H. (2004). Overwhelming postsplenectomy infection: Is quality of patient knowledge enough for prevention? *Hematology Journal, 5,* 77–88.

Elder, M. E. (2000). T-cell immunodeficiencies. *Pediatric Clinics of North America, 47,* 1253–1274.

Food Allergy & Anaphylaxis Network www.foodallergy.org, accessed 2004.

Giarelli, E., & Jacobs, L. A. (2003). Traditional healing and HIV-AIDS in KwaZula-Natal, South Africa. *American Journal of Nursing, 103*(10), 36–47.

Gottlieb, B. S., & Ilowite, N. T. (2000). Meeting the challenge of rheumatologic diseases in teens. *Contemporary Pediatrics, 17,* 61–98.

Grosch-Worner, I. (2000). An effective and safe protocol involving zidovudine and caesarean section to reduce vertical transmission on HIV-1 infection. *AIDS, 14,* 2903–2911.

Higman, M. A., & Vogelsang, G. B. (2004). Chronic graft-versus-host disease. *British Journal of Haematology, 125,* 435–454.

Houribane, J. O., Allard, J. M., Wade, A. M., & McEwan, A. I. (2002). Impact of repeated surgical procedures on the incidence and prevalence of latex allergy: A prospective study of 1263 children. *Journal of Pediatrics, 140,* 479–482.

Ilowite, N. T. (2002). Current treatment of juvenile rheumatoid arthritis. *Pediatrics, 109,* 109–115.

Instone, S. L. (2000). Perceptions of children with HIV infection when not told for so long: Implications for diagnosis disclosure. *Journal of Pediatric Health Care, 14,* 235–243.

Kaiser, H. B. (2004). Risk factors in allergy and asthma. *Allergy and Asthma Proceeding, 25,* 7–10.

Kline, M. W., Calles, N. R., Simon, C., & Schwarzwald, H. (2000). Pilot study of hydroxyurea in human immunodeficiency virus–infected children receiving didanasine and/or stavudine. *Pediatric Infectious Disease Journal, 19,* 1083–1086.

Koleilat, M. A., Williams, L. W., & Ryan, M. E. (2003). Read the warning signs of primary immunodeficiency. *Contemporary Pediatrics, 20*(6), 65– 81.

Langston, C., Cooper, E. R., Goldfarb, J., Easley, K. A., Husak, S., Sunkle, S., Starc, T. J., & Colin, A. A. (2001). Human immunodeficiency virus–related mortality in infants and children: Data from the pediatric pulmonary and cardiovascular complications of vertically transmitted HIV study. *Pediatrics, 107,* 328–338.

Lee, M. H., & Kim, K. T. (1998). Latex allergy: A relevant issue in the general pediatric population. *Journal of Pediatric Health Care, 12,* 242–246.

Lindegren, M. L., Steinberg, S., & Byers, R. H. (2000). Epidemiology of HIV/AIDS in children. *Pediatric Clinics of North America, 47,* 1–20.

Linkages Project. (2004). Breastfeeding and HIV/AIDS—Frequently asked questions. www.linkagesproject.org, accessed 12/7/2004.

Lupus Foundation of America. (2004). www.lupus.org/education/types/html, accessed 12/4/2004.

Luxner, K. L. (2003). The complicated prenatal experience. In M. H. Hogan & R. S. Glazebrook (Eds.), *Maternal-newborn nursing.* Upper Saddle River, NJ: Prentice Hall.

Mariani, S. M. (2003). Conference report: Severe immunodeficiencies: Bone marrow transplantation or gene therapy? Highlights from the 90th meeting of the American Association of Immunologists, May 6–10, Denver, Colorado. www.medscape.com/viewarticle/455460

Morbidity and Mortality Weekly Report. (2003). Advancing HIV prevention: New strategies for a changing epidemic—United States. *MMWR, 52,* 329–332.

Murphy, D. A., Wilson, C. M., Durako, S. J., Muenz, L. R., & Belzer, M. (2001). Antiretroviral medication adherence among the REACH HIV-infected adolescent cohort in the USA. *AIDS Care, 13*(1), 27–41.

Murphy, D. A., Sarr, M., Durako, S. J., Moscicki, A. B., Wilson, C. M., & Muenz, L. R. (2003). Barriers to HAART adherence among human immunodeficiency virus-infected adolescents. *Archives of Pediatric Adolescent Medicine, 157,* 249–255.

National Institute of Health. (2004). Guidelines for the use of antiretroviral agents in pediatric HIV infection. www.aidsinfo.nih.gov/guidelines/pediatric/PED_012004.html#stratad

Nielsen, K., & Bryson, Y. J. (2000). Diagnosis of HIV infection in children. *Pediatric Clinics of North America, 47,* 39–64.

Ochs, H. D. (1998). The Wiskott-Aldrich syndrome. *Seminars in Hematology, 35,* 332–345.

Parkman, R. (2004). Getting a handle on graft-versus-host disease. *The New England Journal of Medicine, 350,* 614–615.

Pearson, D. A., McGrath, N. M., Nozyce, M., Nichols, S. L., Raskino, C., Brouwers, P., Lifschitz, M. C., Baker, C. J., & Englund, J. A. (2000). Predicting HIV progression in children using measures of neuropsychological and neurological functioning. *Pediatrics, 106*(6). www.pediatrics.org/cgi/content/full/106/6/e76, accessed 1/15/2002.

Pugatch, D., Bennett, L., & Patterson, D. (2002). HIV medication adherence in adolescents: A qualitative study. *Journal of HIV/AIDS Prevention & Education for Adolescents & Children, 5*(1/2), 9–28.

Pullen, R. L., Cannon, J. D., & Rushing, J. D., (2003). Managing organ-threatening systemic lupus erythematosus. *Medsurg Nursing 12,* 368–379.

Ramstead, C. (2003). HIV counseling, testing, and referral: Putting revised guidelines to use. *Clinician Reviews, 13*(11), 58–64.

Rettig, P. A., Merhar, S. L., & Cron, R. Q. (2004). Juvenile rheumatoid arthritis and juvenile spondifoarthropathy. In P. J. Allen & J. A. Vessey. *Primary care of the child with a chronic condition* (pp. 582–600). St. Louis: Mosby.

Rogers, A. S. (2000). Serologic examination of hepatitis B infection and immunization in HIV-positive youth and associated risks. *AIDS Patient Care and STDs, 14,* 651–657.

Sack, K. E., & Fye, K. H. (1997). Rheumatic diseases. In D. P. Stites, A. T. Terr, & T. G. Parslow (Eds.), *Medical immunology* (pp. 456–479). Stamford, CT: Appleton & Lange.

Santhanam, H., & Goins, M. (2004). Antiretroviral update. *Advance for Nurse Practitioners, 12*(11), 53–56.

Schwartz, S. A. (2000). Intravenous immunoglobulin treatment of immunodeficiency disorders. *Pediatric Clinics of North America, 47,* 1355–1370.

Stichweh, D., Arce, E., & Pascual, V. (2004). Update on pediatric systemic lupus erythematosus. *Current Opinion in Rheumatology 16,* 577–587.

Tang, A. W. (2003). Practical guide to anaphylaxis. *American Family Physician, 68,* 1325.

Temple, M. E., Koranyi, K., & Nahata, M. C. (2001). The safety and antiviral effect of protease inhibitors in children. *Pharmacotherapy, 21,* 287–294.

Vogelsang, G. B., Lee, L., & Bensen-Kennedy, D. M. (2003). Pathogenesis and treatment of graft-versus-host disease after bone marrow transplant. *Annual Review of Medicine, 54,* 29–54.

Chapter 28

Alterations in Hematologic Function

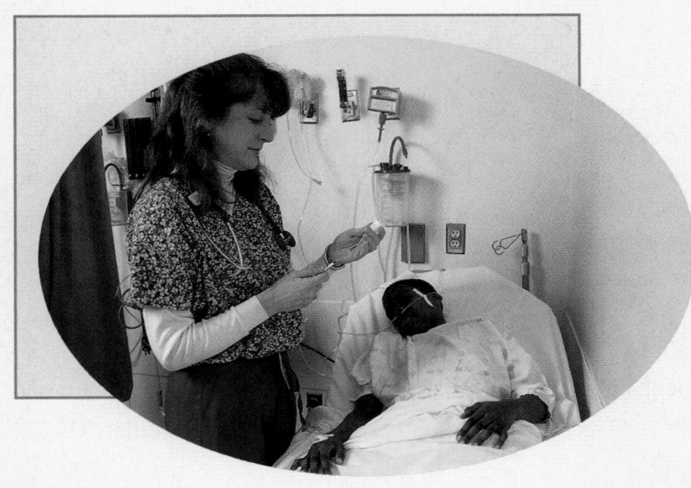

Michael Draper is a 12-year-old African American boy who is admitted to the hospital with severe abdominal pain. He was diagnosed with sickle cell anemia at 1 year of age. Although Michael is in relatively good health he was hospitalized on two previous occasions related to complications of the disease. Recently, Michael has had several viral illnesses, leading his primary care provider to suspect that his spleen is filled with abnormal cells (a complication associated with sickle cell anemia), which leads to impairment of his immune function. Michael complains of abdominal pain and large joint pain. He is admitted to the hospital for treatment.

Upon physical examination, the nurse notes that Michael is small for his age and has several ecchymotic areas on his lower legs. Michael has tachypnea, tachycardia, and has a temperature of 101.6°F. He appears anxious and complains of pain in his abdomen and knees. Michael's parents are knowledgeable about sickle cell anemia. They understand that Michael is experiencing an episode of sickle cell crisis.

An intravenous infusion is immediately started and Michael's pain is aggressively managed with fluids and opioid pain medication via a patient-controlled analgesia (PCA) pump. Michael receives oxygen by nasal cannula to increase his oxygen saturation to normal levels. The nurse clusters the care and performs multiple tests and procedures together to allow Michael time to have regular rest periods. Additionally, the nurse collaborates with the multidisciplinary team and the family to establish an individualized plan of care for Michael.

Michael's hospitalization experience is similar to that of other children with sickle cell anemia. It represents the wide variety of conditions that effect the hematologic system, ranging from mild to life-threatening. This chapter will assist the nurse in planning care for children like Michael who have disorders of the hematologic system.

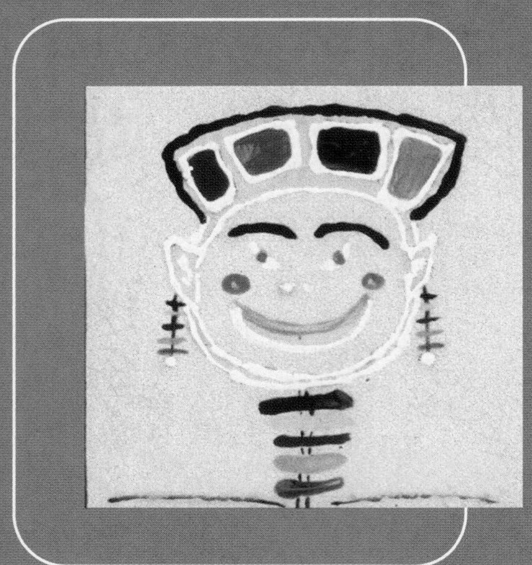

"I am fine most of the time, I feel just like a normal kid until I get sick. Then the pain reminds me that I am not a normal kid, I have a disease and it hurts—a lot."

—Michael, age 12

Key Terms

- allogeneic transplantation/1031
- anemia/1001
- anemia of prematurity/1004
- autologous transplantation/1031
- ecchymosis/1024
- erythrocytes/1001
- erythropoiesis/1001
- erythropoietin/1001
- hemarthrosis/1023
- hematopoiesis/1001
- hemochromatosis/1019
- hemosiderin/1019
- hemosiderosis/1012
- hypersplenism/1002
- isogeneic transplantation/1031
- leukocytes/1001
- leukopenia/1002
- menorrhagia/1004
- pancytopenia/1022
- petechiae/1022
- physiologic anemia of infancy/1004
- polycythemia/1001
- purpura/1022
- reticulocyte/1001
- thrombocytes/1001
- thrombocytopenia/1002
- vaso-occlusion/1008

Learning Outcomes

After completing this chapter, you will be able to:

- Describe the function of red blood cells, white blood cells, and platelets.
- Discuss the pathophysiology and clinical manifestations of the major disorders of red blood cells affecting the pediatric population.
- Discuss the pathophysiology and clinical manifestations of the major disorders of white blood cells affecting the pediatric population.
- Discuss the pathophysiology and clinical manifestations of the major disorders of platelets affecting the pediatric population.
- Describe the nursing management and collaborative care of a child with a hematologic disorder.
- Discuss nursing implications for a child receiving hematopoietic stem cell transplantation (HSCT).

MediaLink 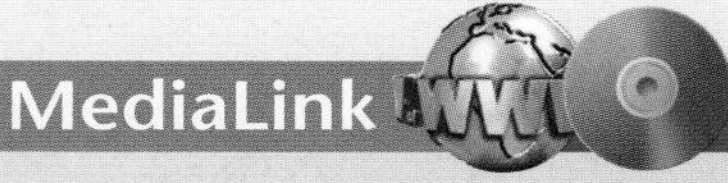 **http://www.prenhall.com/ball**

Resources for this chapter can be found on the CD-ROM accompanying this textbook and on the Companion Website at www.prenhall.com/ball. Click on Chapter 28 to select the activities for this chapter.

CD-ROM

Animations/Videos

- *Circulatory System*
- *Types of Blood Cells*
- *Sickle Cell Anemia*

Nursing in Action: Administering Blood or Blood Products

NCLEX Review

Audio Glossary

COMPANION WEBSITE

A & P Review

Clinical Manifestations Review

Medication Match-Up

NCLEX Review

Case Study: An Adolescent in Sickle Cell Crisis

Care Plan: A School-Age Child with Hemophilia

MediaLink Applications

- *Ethical Considerations: Hemophilia*
- *Hematopoietic Stem Cell Transplantation (HSCT)*

The hematologic system is one of the few body systems that directly or indirectly regulates all other body functions. The functions of blood include transport of hormones and oxygen, regulation of body temperature, and maintenance of acid–base balance, cellular nutrition, and defense against foreign antigens. Because blood is involved in the function of all tissues and organs, changes in the blood may result in altered functioning of many body organs and structures.

This chapter provides a discussion of the most common disorders of the blood and blood-forming organs in children. (Refer to Chapter 29∞ for a discussion of leukemia, a white blood cell cancer.)

ANATOMY AND PHYSIOLOGY OF PEDIATRIC DIFFERENCES

Blood has two components: a fluid portion called plasma and a cellular portion known as the formed elements of the blood. Plasma contains proteins, electrolytes, clotting factors, antibodies, and anticoagulants. The cellular elements are red blood cells (**erythrocytes**), white blood cells (**leukocytes**), and platelets (**thrombocytes**) (Figure 28–1 ■). A summary of normal values for these and other blood components in children is provided in Table 28–1.

Production of red blood cells occurs in the fetus by the second week of gestation, with white blood cell and platelet production beginning at 8 weeks. Most of this early production occurs in the liver and spleen; however, by 20 to 24 weeks' gestation, liver production decreases as bone marrow production begins to predominate (Ohls & Christensen, 2004).

At birth, **hematopoiesis,** or blood cell production, occurs in the marrow of almost every bone. The flat bones such as the sternum, ribs, pelvic and shoulder girdles, vertebrae, and hips retain most of their hematopoietic activity throughout life.

Red Blood Cells

Red blood cells (RBC), or erythrocytes, are the most abundant of the cellular elements of blood. The RBCs are formed through a process called **erythropoiesis.** The primary function of red blood cells is to transport oxygen from the lungs to the tissues. These cells also help to carry carbon dioxide from the tissues back to the lungs. Hemoglobin, a red pigment of protein and iron, is essential to this function because it is the iron-containing pigment in the red blood cell and is responsible for carrying oxygen to the tissues. **Reticulocytes** are precursors to mature RBCs. The normal lifespan of the RBC is 120 days. Upon destruction of the RBC by the spleen, most of the iron from the cell is stored for later use in development of new red blood cells. **Erythropoietin,** which is produced by the kidney in response to hypoxia, stimulates RBC production (Figure 28–2 ■).

Anemia is a reduction in the number of red blood cells. The various types of anemia are discussed in the following section.

Polycythemia is an above-average increase in the number of red cells in the blood. Any condition that causes the quantity of oxygen transported to the tissues to decrease ordinarily increases the rate of red blood cell production and polycythemia may result. When a child becomes anemic secondary to hemorrhage, for instance, the bone marrow immediately begins to produce large quantities of red cells. Children with cyanotic heart defects experience polycythemia in an attempt to compensate for the chronic deoxygenated state. Polycythemia

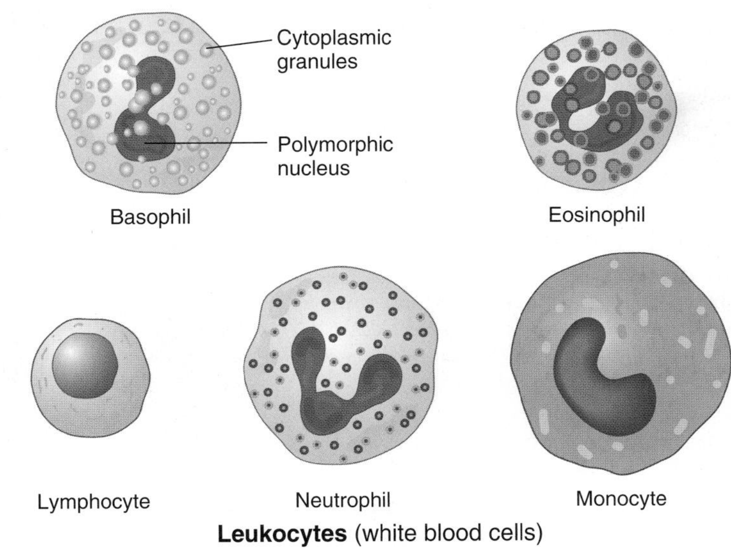

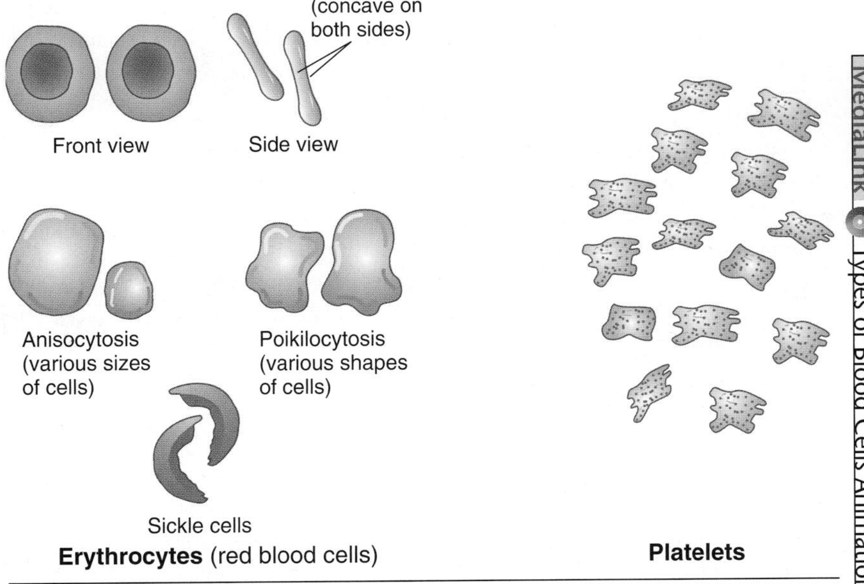

FIGURE 28–1 ■ Types of blood cells.

MediaLink Types of Blood Cells Animation

TABLE 28–1 Normal Blood Values in Children

TEST*	NORMAL VALUE
Red blood cell (RBC)	$3.90–5.03 \times 10^6/\mu L$
Hemoglobin (Hb)	10.5–13.3 g/dL
Hematocrit (HCT)	31.7–39.6%
Mean corpuscular volume (MCV)	$72.7–86.5\ \mu m^3$
Mean corpuscular hemoglobin (MCH)	24.1–29.4 pg
Mean corpuscular hemoglobin concentration (MCHC)	32.4–35.3%
Reticulocyte count	0.8–2.2%
White blood cell (WBC)	$5.3–11.5 \times 10^3/\mu L$
Platelets	$202–403 \times 10^3/\mu L$
Differential	
Neutrophils	34.3–72.9%
Eosinophils	2.4–4.8%
Basophils	1%
Lymphocyte	13.5–52.8%
Atypical lymphocytes	2.6–5.6%
Monocytes	3.5–13.4%

From Soldin, S. J., Brugnara, C., & Wong, E. C. (2003). Pediatric reference ranges *(4th ed.). Washington, DC: AACC Press.*

**Note all values are for the 2- to 12-year-old child. Laboratory values vary according to the procedures and type of testing used. Values listed are only approximate for common methods of measurement. Consult the normative values for the laboratories used by your healthcare facilities to evaluate whether a specific child's values are normal or abnormal.*

can also occur in the newborn with delayed clamping of the umbilical cord. The major complication associated with polycythemia is increased blood viscosity, which can lead to complications such as cerebral vascular accident.

CLINICAL TIP

Be aware that a heelstick sample in the newborn may reveal a falsely elevated red blood cell count. If an abnormal result is suspected, another sample should be obtained.

At birth, the newborn has a naturally occurring elevation in red blood cells due to a high level of erythropoietin, which stimulates red cell production. Once the newborn begins breathing air and the oxygen level in the blood increases, this production slows. Levels of RBCs fall until about 2 to 3 months of age, and then begin increasing. Adult levels are reached during adolescence and males have red blood cell levels slightly higher than females (see Appendix C∞).

White Blood Cells

White blood cells, or leukocytes, are the mobile units of the body's protective system. They are formed in bone marrow and lymph tissue. The white blood cell count is highest at birth, although levels vary greatly among infants. By 1 week of age, white blood cell values stabilize. Throughout childhood, there is a very slow decrease in white blood cell count (Boxer, 2004).

As a protective response, white blood cells normally elevate in the presence of infection. Other physiologic stressors causing an elevated white blood cell count include anesthesia, pain, some medications such as steroids, and surgery.

The five types of white blood cells each have a distinct function (Table 28–2). A differential blood count indicates the percentages of the different types of white cells present in the blood and is sometimes useful in identifying the cause of an illness. For example, infections cause an increase in neutrophils; and allergies produce an increase in eosinophils. The function of lymphocytes is discussed with acquired immunodeficiency syndrome in Chapter 27∞.

A decrease in the number of white blood cells is called **leukopenia,** and can be caused by immune or bone marrow disorders. It may also be seen in viral infection.

Platelets

Platelets, or thrombocytes, are cell fragments that can form hemostatic plugs to contribute to the coagulation process. The function of platelets is primary coagulation and capillary hemostasis. Platelets are synthesized from components in the red bone marrow and are stored in the spleen. Platelet levels in newborns are lower than in older children and adults. Levels of many clotting factors, particularly those requiring vitamin K for activation (factors II, VII, IX, X and anticoagulant factors—proteins C and S), are also lower in infants. For this reason, all newborns receive a prophylactic injection of vitamin K at birth. Values of platelets and other coagulation products soon reach normal childhood levels (Montgomery & Scott, 2004). A deficiency of platelets, termed **thrombocytopenia,** can lead to bleeding disorders.

ANEMIA

Anemia is defined as a reduction in the number of red blood cells, the quantity of hemoglobin, and the volume of packed red cells to below-normal levels. This condition can be caused by increased loss or destruction of existing red blood cells or by an impaired or decreased rate of red cell production. Anemia also can be a clinical manifestation of an underlying disorder, such as lead poisoning or **hypersplenism** (a syndrome characterized by splenomegaly and blood cell deficiencies). The types of anemia in children discussed in this chapter are iron deficiency anemia, normocytic anemia, sickle cell anemia, hereditary spherocytosis, the thalassemias, and aplastic anemia.

TABLE 28–2 White Blood Cells and Their Functions

CELL TYPE	FUNCTION
Neutrophils	Phagocytosis
Eosinophils	Allergic reactions
Basophils	Inflammatory reactions
Monocytes (macrophages)	Phagocytosis, antigen processing
Lymphocytes	Humoral immunity (B cell), cellular immunity (T cell)

PATHOPHYSIOLOGY ILLUSTRATED

Erythropoietin Feedback Mechanism

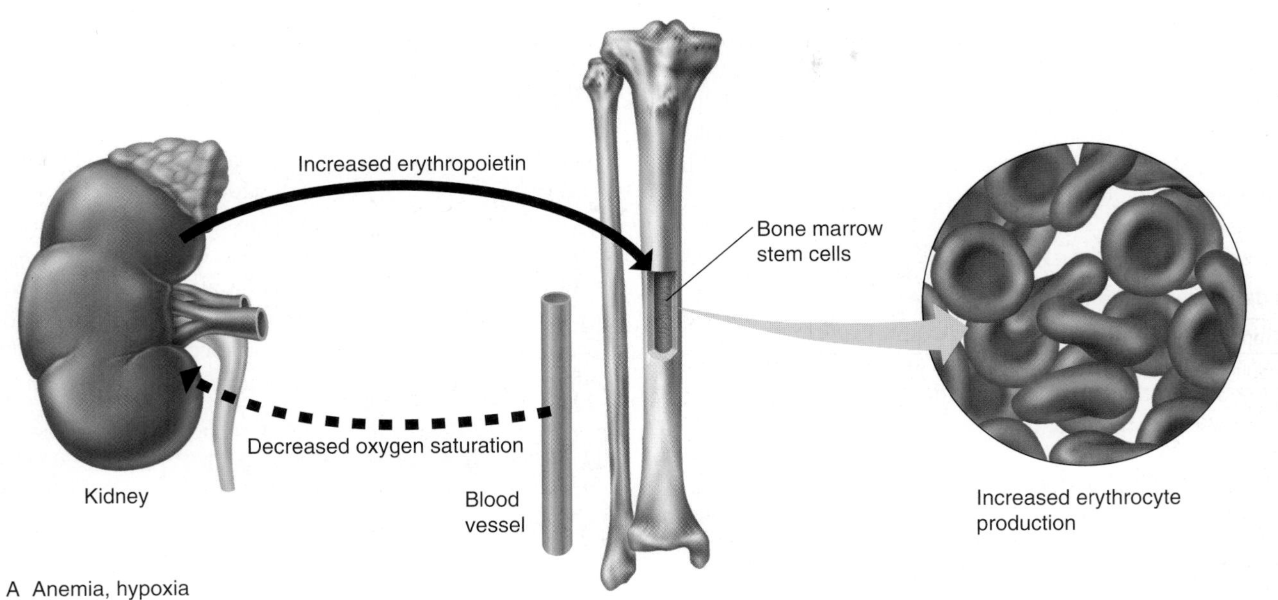

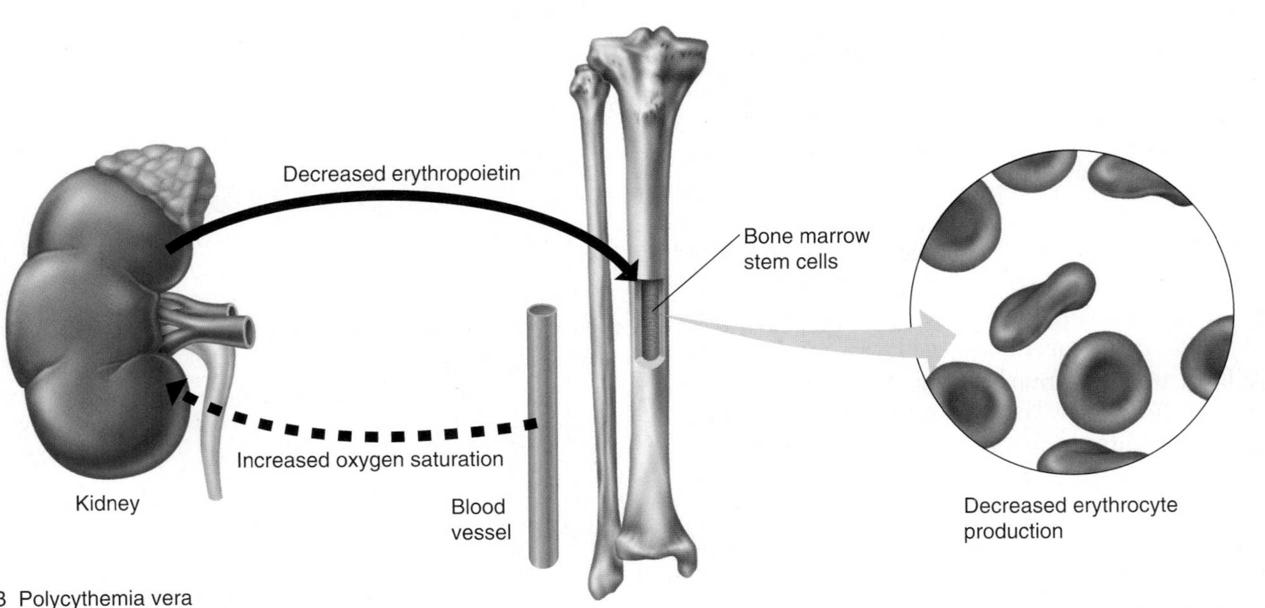

FIGURE 28–2 ■ The kidneys respond to altered oxygen delivery by increasing or decreasing erythropoietin, which stimulates red blood cell production. *A,* As a compensatory mechanism, alterations such as anemia and hypoxia prompt the kidneys to increase erythropoietin, which in turn stimulates the bone marrow to increase red blood cell production. *B,* For conditions in which there is an excess production of red blood cells, such as in polycythemia vera, the kidneys decrease erythropoietin release, which in turn stimulates the bone marrow to decrease red blood cell production.

Physiologic anemia of infancy is a normal occurrence. After birth, erythropoietin synthesis, and therefore production of red blood cells, abruptly decreases in response to the higher oxygenation of tissues. In the following 6 to 12 weeks, the hemoglobin reaches a low level of 9 to 11 g/dL in term infants and 7 to 9 g/dL in premature infants. The erythropoietin production is again naturally stimulated, red blood cell production increases, and the hemoglobin level is returned to normal. No management is necessary for physiologic anemia except when it falls below normal newborn levels or when folic acid intake is inadequate, such as in the premature infant with feeding difficulties (Irwin & Kirchner, 2001).

Iron Deficiency Anemia

Iron deficiency anemia is the most common type of anemia and the most common nutritional deficiency in children. Three percent of children younger than 2 years of age, 9 to 11% of adolescent females, and less than 1% of adolescent males are affected by iron deficiency anemia (Carley, 2003).

Etiology and Pathophysiology

The body requires iron for the production of hemoglobin. Insufficient quantities of iron limit hemoglobin production. This in turn affects the production of red blood cells. Because red blood cells are required to carry oxygen throughout the body, anemia results in less oxygen reaching the cells and tissues, thereby affecting their function.

Iron deficiency anemia can result from a variety of causes. Included is anemia secondary to blood loss, malabsorption, or poor nutritional intake. Increased internal demands (such as rapid growth periods) for blood production can also lead to anemia. Rapidly growing adolescents whose diets are high in fat and low in vitamins and minerals are particularly susceptible to iron deficiency anemia since rapid growth increases iron requirements.

The term newborn receives iron stores from the mother during pregnancy; this generally provides sufficient iron for the infant for about 4 to 6 months after birth. Premature infants do not have as much time in utero; therefore, they do not have as extensive iron stores, and may become iron depleted earlier in postnatal life. This is sometimes called **anemia of prematurity.** In addition, when mothers have inadequate nutritional status during pregnancy, or give birth to two or more babies in a pregnancy, or have had several pregnancies in close succession, their babies may not have iron stores that last the usual 4 to 6 months after birth.

Infants who do not consume adequate solid foods after 6 months of age and are fed only breast milk or formula that is not fortified with iron are also at risk because neonatal iron stores have been depleted by this time and their iron needs are not being met. Feeding regular cow milk before one year of age can cause gastrointestinal bleeding and resultant anemia. The child over 1 year of age who consumes greater than 24 oz of cow milk in a day is also at risk for iron deficiency anemia (Lesperance et al., 2002).

Chronic blood loss is also a potential cause of iron deficiency anemia. The infant who has had bleeding in the neonatal period; the child who loses blood as a result of conditions such as hemophilia, gastrointestinal ulcers, or bleeding from a parasitic gastrointestinal illness; and the adolescent female who has **menorrhagia** (heavy menstrual bleeding) may all be at risk of anemia. As a result of an inadequate supply of iron, the RBCs are smaller, the number of RBCs is reduced, the quantity of hemoglobin is reduced, and oxygen-carrying capacity of the blood is decreased.

Clinical Manifestations

Clinical manifestations and severity of symptoms are directly related to the amount of iron deficiency anemia. Pallor, fatigue, and irritability are characteristic findings. With chronic anemia, nailbed deformities, growth retardation, developmental delay, muscle weakness, tachycardia, headache, and systolic heart murmur can occur. A behavior that may also be associated with iron deficiency anemia is pica, the consumption of nonfood items. Lead poisoning (plumbism) may occur with iron deficiency anemia since lead absorption is increased with anemia.

COLLABORATIVE CARE

Care for the child with iron deficiency anemia focuses on identifying the anemia, correcting the cause, and treating with medications and/or dietary management until a normal RBC count is achieved.

Diagnostic Tests

Diagnosis is made on the basis of clinical presentation and laboratory studies, including hematocrit, hemoglobin level, mean corpuscular hemoglobin volume, red blood cell distribution width, microscopic analysis (Figure 28–3 ■), serum ferritin, and serum iron-binding capacity.

The degree of anemia is related to the value of hemoglobin (Carley, 2003), as follows:

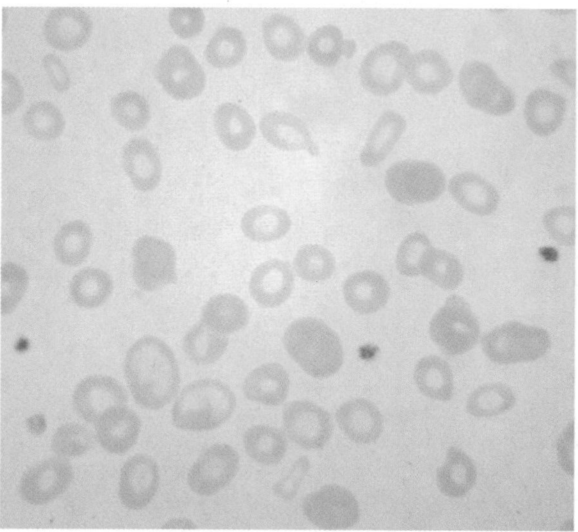

FIGURE 28–3 ■ In iron deficiency anemia, red blood cells appear hypochromic as a result of decreased hemoglobin synthesis.

Courtesy of Dr. Ed Wong, Laboratory Medicine, Children's National Medical Center, Washington, DC.

- Hemoglobin 9.5–11 g/dL — mild iron deficiency anemia
- Hemoglobin 8–9.4 g/dL — moderate iron deficiency anemia
- Hemoglobin < 8 g/dL — severe iron deficiency anemia

Reticulocyte counts reveal the bone marrow's response to anemia (Box 28–1). For children consuming cow milk, the stool is tested for occult blood. Serum lead levels may be conducted to rule out plumbism, also known as lead poisoning. (See Chapter 30∞ for a full description of lead poisoning.)

On microscopic examination, the red blood cells are microcytic (small) in size and hypochromic (pale) in appearance (Cook, 2000). Anemia is a common symptom associated with a variety of diseases, disorders, and dietary deficiencies. A review of hemoglobin and hematocrit levels may not be sufficient to determine the severity of the underlying problem. Hemoglobin, hematocrit, reticulocyte count, and serum iron concentration are decreased. RBC count and total iron-binding capacity are elevated. Serum ferritin is low (< 15 µg/L or < 15 ng/mL).

Clinical Therapy

Treatment of iron deficiency anemia centers on correction of the iron deficiency with supplemental oral elemental iron preparations, such as oral ferrous sulfate, and a diet high in food with iron. Anemia is treated with 3 to 6 mg/kg/day of iron for about 4 weeks. If the hemoglobin has increased by more than 1 g/dL or if hematocrit has increased by more than 3%, a diagnosis of anemia is confirmed. Treatment continues for 2 months, and blood values are reevaluated. Once normal values are reached and iron supplementation is tapered off, blood values should be measured after about 6 months to be sure food intake is meeting the requirement (Carley, 2003; Committee on Nutrition, 2004).

If the anemia is not improved by iron intake and is a result of bleeding, the cause is identified and treated to prevent future excess blood loss. Other causes such as myelosuppresion or genetic diseases are treated as appropriate. If lead poisoning has occured, removal from the source and chelation therapy are needed (See Chapter 30∞).

NURSING MANAGEMENT

Nursing care focuses on screening for the disorder and educating the parents and children about the causes of iron deficiency anemia, dietary management, and the importance of complying with the medication regimen.

BOX 28–1 Reticulocyte Counts

Reticulocytes are immature or newly released red blood cells. Elevated reticulocyte counts indicate the bone marrow is responding to anemia by releasing new RBCs into the circulation. A low reticulocyte count in the presence of anemia indicates that the bone marrow is not responding appropriately to anemia. Further testing is needed to find the cause of decreased red blood cell production.

Nursing Assessment and Diagnosis

Children with iron deficiency anemia are usually identified and treated in community settings. Screening for anemia is performed between 9 months and 1 year for most infants, with a second screening at 15 to 18 months. Premature infants are generally screened at 4 months and then periodically during infancy and toddlerhood. Follow-up screening for all children at 2 and 3 years of age may decrease the risk of developmental complications related to iron deficiency anemia (Segal, Hirsh, & Feig, 2002; Committee on Nutrition, 2004). Screening during adolescence is also recommended (American Academy of Pediatrics, 2000).

For screening, a hematocrit or hemoglobin level is obtained. More detailed tests, such as those identified in the diagnostic tests section, are performed if the blood test is abnormal. Children at high risk for nutritional deficiencies, such as those in low-income groups and Women, Infants, and Children (WIC) programs, may require more frequent screenings. Most children in Head Start are screened annually by nurses. In addition, children demonstrating signs of anemia should be screened. Height and weight measurements are obtained at each healthcare visit, plotted on growth charts, and compared with percentiles obtained at previous visits. Slow downward trends in percentiles are of concern and require further nutritional analysis. Developmental screening tests are performed to assess for developmental delays (refer to Chapter 5∞). A diet history and analysis can provide information related to food intake (refer to Chapter 9∞ for guidelines about diet history).

Nursing diagnoses that may apply to the child with iron deficiency anemia include:

- Imbalanced Nutrition, Less than Body Requirements related to dietary intake
- Ineffective Tissue Perfusion (all organ systems) related to anemia
- Activity Intolerance related to decreased oxygen-carrying capacity
- Risk for Delayed Growth and Development related to decreased tissue perfusion
- Deficient Knowledge related to management of iron deficiency anemia

Planning and Implementation

The goal of nursing care is centered on educating the family on dietary management, medication therapy, and prevention.

Dietary Management

Dietary management is the preferred long-term treatment for iron deficiency anemia. Teach the child and family to plan for foods that are rich in iron (Table 28–3). Iron-fortified formula and baby cereals are used in the diet of the infant. For the infant who consumes large quantities of milk and refuses to eat solid food, restrictions on milk intake may be required. Older infants and toddlers are provided with finger foods such as thinly sliced

TABLE 28–3 Food Sources of Iron and Vitamin C

IRON-RICH FOODS	FOOD SOURCES OF VITAMIN C
Meats, fish, poultry	Orange juice
Vegetables	Citrus fruits
Dried fruits	Strawberries
Legumes	Tomatoes
Enriched grain products	Broccoli and other green leafy vegetables
Whole-grain cereals	Potatoes
Iron-fortified dry cereals	Some dry cereals

meats. Adolescents are encouraged to eat foods with high iron content and vitamin C, such as hamburgers and dried fruits. Protein and vitamin C are necessary to produce new blood cells and folic acid helps to convert iron from ferritin to hemoglobin. Vitamin C also enhances the absorption of iron when the two nutrients are taken in at the same time.

Medication Therapy

Oral iron preparations are often administered to correct anemia. Teach the family techniques for proper medication administration.

> **CLINICAL TIP**
>
> Liquid iron preparation should be taken through a straw and the mouth rinsed after administration to avoid staining the teeth. For infants, the iron preparation is administered into the back of the mouth.

Ferrous sulfate should be administered on an empty stomach, and given with a vitamin C source such as orange juice or apple juice to promote iron absorption. Milk and other dairy products containing calcium, whole-grain products, and antacids should not be administered at the same time as the iron preparation since these products may inhibit iron absorption. Iron preparations can cause gastrointestinal upset. Although administration on an empty stomach increases absorption, some children do not tolerate this method and need to take the medication with a small amount of food.

Instruct the family about side effects of iron preparations such as black stools, constipation, gastrointestinal discomfort, and a foul aftertaste. Emphasize the importance of drinking fluids and eating foods high in dietary fiber to minimize these side effects.

Teach the family to monitor for evidence of iron overload. Signs and symptoms of iron overdose include abdominal pain, vomiting, and bloody diarrhea. Severe overdose leads to shortness of breath and shock. Immediate emergency treatment is required as death may result from iron overdose. Safety precautions to prevent accidental iron ingestion and overdose are reviewed with parents. These precautions include keeping the iron preparation out of the reach of children and administering only the prescribed amount.

Screening and Prevention

Universal screening for anemia in areas with high prevalence rates is recommended by the American Academy of Pediatrics (AAP). As discussed, routine screenings and assessment for children and adolescents at risk of iron deficiency anemia should be performed (Carley, 2003). Refer to Chapter 10 for more information regarding health maintenance recommendations for children.

Prevention measures include encouraging breastfeeding mothers to introduce iron-containing foods after 6 months. Iron-fortified formulas should be consumed by the formula-fed infant, and iron-rich foods should be introduced at 6 months. Inform the parents that although cow milk is a good source of calcium, it is low in iron. Additionally, cow milk should be avoided in the first year since it can cause bleeding from the gastrointestinal tract, leading to anemia. Vitamin C–containing foods should be introduced and encouraged because vitamin C enhances iron absorption.

■ Evaluation

Expected outcomes for nursing care of the child with iron deficiency anemia include:

- A normal red blood cell level is attained.
- The family verbalizes an understanding of treatment.
- The child consumes recommended dietary foods.
- The child is free from side effects of the medication such as constipation.
- The child is active and does not demonstrate fatigue.
- Appropriate developmental and growth expectations are achieved.

Normocytic Anemia

In normocytic anemia, the red blood cells, although decreased in number, are of normal size with a pale center (Cook, 2000). This type of anemia may occur as a result of hemorrhage, disease-induced inflammation, disseminated intravascular coagulation (DIC; refer to the discussion later in this chapter), G6PD (glucose-6-phosphate dehydrogenase) deficiency (Chapter 32), hemolytic-uremic syndrome (refer to Chapter 31), or several other conditions. The anemia will often resolve itself once the cause is corrected. Some infectious and inflammatory etiologies of anemia are listed in Table 28–4.

The etiology of normocytic anemia associated with chronic inflammation or infection is related to increased red blood cell destruction, decreased iron release from storage sites, and ineffective bone marrow response (Irwin & Kirchner, 2001). In hemorrhage, anemia is a direct result of loss of blood.

TABLE 28–4 Infectious and Inflammatory Causes of Anemia

INFECTIONS	INFLAMMATIONS
Haemophilus influenzae type b	Arthritis
HIV/AIDS	Cancers
Orbital cellulitis	Chronic heart or liver disease
Meningitis	
Septic arthritis	

Clinical manifestations are similar to those seen in iron deficiency anemia, with the possible occurrence of hepatomegaly and splenomegaly as well.

Collaborative Care

Microscopic examination of red blood cells confirms diagnosis. Treatment of normocytic anemia depends on the underlying cause. When one of the aforementioned conditions exists in a child diagnosed with anemia, an infectious or inflammatory condition should be suspected as the cause of the identified anemia and treated first. For anemia caused by renal failure, recombinant human erythropoietin is administered. When hemorrhage is the underlying cause, the source of the bleeding is identified and treated. In hypovolemia in acute emergencies, blood products are infused to make up for some of the losses. When G6PD deficiency is the cause, infections are treated vigorously and blood cells are managed to reflect normal levels.

Nursing Management

Nursing management of normocytic anemia is dependent on the cause of the decreased red blood cells. Children with inflammatory or infectious diseases require careful assessment and management of medication and other treatment regimens. Administer blood products and other intravenous fluids as ordered to restore blood volume (refer to section later in chapter on administration of blood products). Follow-up and home visits are conducted to assess hematocrit, hemoglobin, and dietary intake. (Refer to the discussion later in this chapter for management of DIC; to Chapter 30∞ for management of intestinal infections; and to Chapter 31∞ for management of hemolytic-uremic syndrome.)

Sickle Cell Disease

Sickle cell disease is a genetic condition affecting the hemoglobin of red blood cells. Sickle cell anemia (SS) is the most common type of sickle cell disease. Sickle cell disease is an autosomal recessive disorder and is one of the most common genetic diseases in the United States. If both parents have the sickle cell gene, for each pregnancy the risk of having a child with the disease is 25%, the risk of having a child with the trait (carries only one gene for the disease) is 50%; and the odds of having a nonaffected child is 25%. The disease occurs primarily in African Americans and other people of African descent, although occasionally it affects people of Mediterranean descent. Sickle cell anemia occurs in approximately 1 in 375 African American infants born in the United States; and 1 in 12 African American infants born will have sickle cell trait (Jakubik & Thompson, 2000). (Refer to Chapter 4∞ for a discussion of recessive gene transmission.)

Prognosis depends on the severity of the child's disease; children with more frequent exacerbations and hospitalization have poorer prognosis. Approximately one third of deaths associated with sickle cell occur during an acute crisis (Ogedegbe, 2002). Neonatal screening, early intervention, prophylactic antibiotics, and parent education have allowed children with sickle cell disease to live into adulthood.

Etiology and Pathophysiology

Sickle cell anemia is characterized by the partial or complete replacement of normal hemoglobin with abnormal hemoglobin S (Hb S) (Table 28–5). The hemoglobin S forms by a genetic mutation in which the amino acid valine replaces the amino acid glutamic acid. The hallmark features of this disease are vaso-occlusion resulting in ischemic tissue injury to organs, and chronic hemolytic anemia.

Those with the sickle cell trait, in which the child inherits the Hb S from one parent and normal hemoglobin (Hb A) from the other, generally do not manifest symptoms or may have mild symptoms. The sickle cell trait is revealed upon screening.

The process of sickle cell anemia is as follows:

1. Deoxygenation occurs (can result from causes such as dehydration, or being at high altitude).
2. Instead of the normal smooth, flexible, doughnut-shaped cell, the hemoglobin in the red blood cell acquires an elongated crescent or sickle shape (Figure 28–4 ■).
3. The sickled cells are rigid, causing clumping of red blood cells, which leads to obstruction of capillary blood flow (Figure 28–5 ■).
4. Microscopic obstructions lead to engorgement and tissue ischemia. This causes intense pain and organ infarction.
5. Because the sickled cell is rigid, it becomes fragile and is easily hemolyzed, leading to destruction of red blood cells.
6. Sickled cells are hemolyzed or sequestered in the spleen, causing blood pooling and infarction of splenic vessels.
7. The local tissue hypoxia causes further sickling and ultimately large infarctions.
8. Damaged tissues in organs throughout the body become scarred, resulting in impaired function.
9. Acidosis occurs as a result of tissue hypoxia.
10. Anemia triggers erythropoiesis.

TABLE 28–5 Sickle Cell Disorders

DISORDER	CHARACTERISTICS
Sickle Cell Trait (Hb SA)	Most common form of sickle cell disease in the United States Heterozygous condition (child has one sickle cell hemoglobin gene and one normal hemoglobin gene) Child is carrier of sickle cell anemia and has no symptoms or mild symptoms of the disease
Sickle Cell Anemia (Hb SS)	Homozygous condition (child has two sickle hemoglobin genes) Child is subject to sickle cell crises
Sickle Cell Syndromes	*Sickle cell Hb C disease (Hb SC)* Second most frequent form of sickle cell disease in African Americans and other individuals of African descent Different from sickle cell anemia only in that the sickle cell assumes a C shape instead of an S shape
Rare Syndromes	Combination of sickle cell trait and thalassemia trait most often seen in people of Mediterranean descent Sickle cell beta-thalassemia disease (Hb SB)

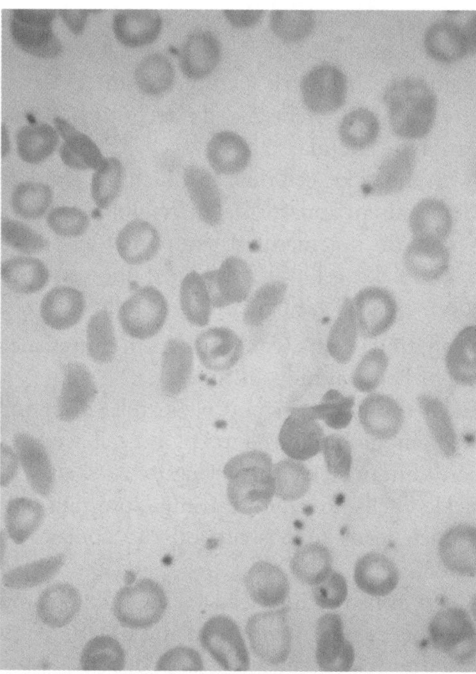

FIGURE 28–4 ■ Many of these red blood cells show an elongated crescent shape characteristic of sickle cell anemia.

Courtesy of Dr. Ed Wong, Laboratory Medicine, Children's National Medical Center, Washington, DC.

Sickling may be triggered by fever and emotional or physical stress. Potential causes of hypoxia or low oxygen tension include high altitudes, poorly pressurized airplanes, hypoventilation, vasoconstriction when cold, dehydration, acidosis, or an emotionally stressful event. Any condition that increases the body's need for oxygen or alters the transport of oxygen (such as infection, trauma, or dehydration) may result in sickling of the cells.

Sickled cells can resume a normal shape when rehydrated and reoxygenated. Because the membrane of these cells is more fragile, the cell life is shortened to 10 to 20 days rather than the usual 120 days. In response, bone marrow spaces enlarge to produce more red blood cells. Continuous formation and destruction of the child's red blood cells contributes to the severe hemolytic anemia that is characteristic of sickle cell anemia (Tanyi, 2003).

MediaLink Sickle Cell Anemia Animation

Children with sickle cell anemia can also suffer from splenic sequestration when blood is trapped in the spleen, a life-threatening complication resulting in cardiovascular collapse (refer to the following discussion on splenic sequestration). Many children must undergo splenectomy in early childhood, leading to severely compromised immunity. Infection rate is high due to impaired immunity, and bacterial infections are the leading cause of death in young children with sickle cell disease.

The outcome and complications of sickle cell disease vary according to the individual, the incidence of sickle cell crisis, and management of complications. Stroke is a significant risk to children with sickle cell anemia and can lead to developmental delay, mental retardation, and other neurologic outcomes (National Heart, Lung, and Blood Institute, 2002). With advances in treatment and newborn diagnosis and intervention, those affected with sickle cell disease are living longer, at least until middle age.

Clinical Manifestations

The manifestations of sickle cell disease range over nearly all of the organ systems (Ogedegbe, 2002). Pathologic changes occur in most body systems and result in multiple signs and symptoms.

Affected children are usually asymptomatic until 4 to 6 months of age because sickling is inhibited by high levels of fetal hemoglobin. Clinical manifestations are directly related to the shortened life span of blood cells (hemolytic anemia) and tissue destruction resulting from **vaso-occlusion** (blockage of a blood vessel).

Pain is the most common complaint of children with sickle cell disease. Hospitalization of the child with sickle cell anemia is commonly associated with acute complications including pain, splenic sequestrations, and febrile illness. Less common complications include cerebral vascular accident (stroke), aplastic crisis, and priapism. Chronic complications associated with sickle cell include anemia, delayed growth and development, jaundice, cholithiasis, hepatobiliary disease, renal dysfunction, retinopathy, and avascular necrosis of the hips and shoulders (Jakubik & Thompson, 2000). These and other complications associated with sickle cell anemia are discussed in Table 28–6.

Because children with sickle cell trait have some abnormal hemoglobin, they may develop symptoms of the disease under conditions of abnormally low oxygen such as flying in an inadequately pressurized airplane over 7,000 feet or during anesthesia. The most common symptoms experienced by those with sickle cell trait are splenic infarction and hematuria. However, most persons who carry the trait never have symptoms, even with low oxygen concentrations.

Sickle Cell Crisis. Sickle cell crises are acute exacerbations of the disease that vary markedly in severity and frequency. Precipitating factors for sickle cell crisis include increased blood viscosity (such as from dehydration or fever) and hypoxia or low oxygen tension (Box 28–2). Michael, the child described at the beginning of this chapter, was experiencing sickle cell crisis.

The most common types of crises affecting children with sickle cell disease—vaso-occlusive crisis, splenic sequestration, and aplastic crisis—are described below. These crises may occur individually or in combination.

- Vaso-occlusive crisis (thrombotic crisis)
  - Most common type of crisis
  - Precipitated by dehydration, exposure to cold, acidosis, or localized hypoxemia

(continued on page 1011)

BOX 28–2 Precipitating Factors Contributing to Sickle Cell Crisis

- Fever
- Dehydration
- Altitude
- Extremes in temperature
- Vomiting
- Emotional distress
- Fatigue
- Alcohol consumption
- Pregnancy
- Elevated hemoglobin levels
- Elevated reticulocyte counts
- Excessive exercise or physical activity
- Acidosis

PATHOPHYSIOLOGY ILLUSTRATED

Sickle Cell Anemia

Hemoglobin S and Red Blood Cell Sickling

Sickle cell anemia is caused by an inherited autosomal recessive defect in Hb synthesis. Sickle cell hemoglobin (HbS) differs from normal hemoglobin only in the substitution of the amino acid valine for glutamine in both beta chains of the hemoglobin molecule.

When HbS is oxygenated, it has the same globular shape as normal hemoglobin. However, when HbS loses its oxygen, it becomes insoluble in intracellular fluid and crystallizes into rodlike structures. Clusters of rods form polymers (long chains) that bend the erythrocyte into the characteristic crescent shape of the sickle cell.

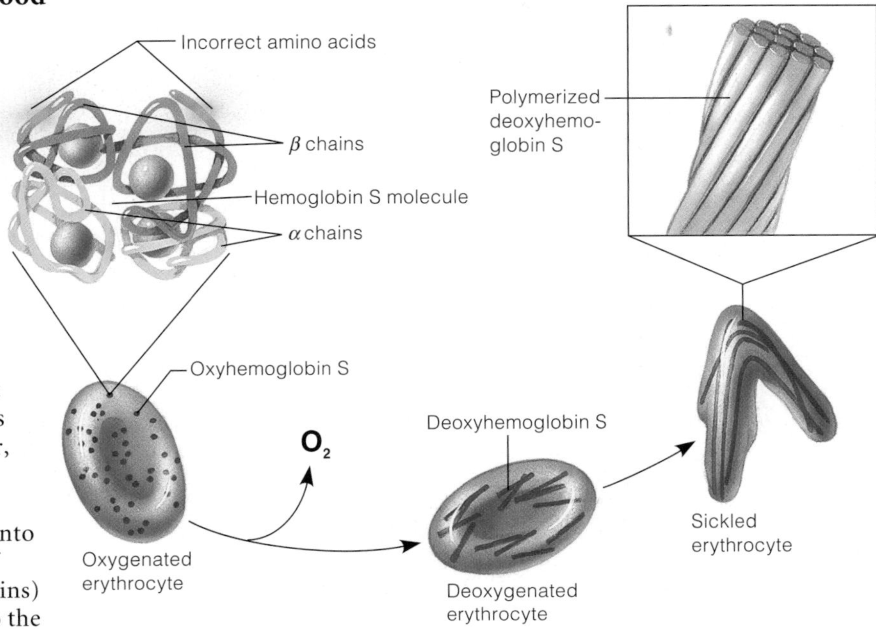

The Sickle Cell Disease Process

Sickle cell disease is characterized by episodes of acute painful crises. Sickling crises are triggered by conditions causing high tissue oxygen demands or that affect cellular pH. As the crisis begins, sickled erythrocytes adhere to capillary walls and to each other, obstructing blood flow and causing cellular hypoxia. The crisis accelerates as tissue hypoxia and acidic metabolic waste products cause further sickling and cell damage.

Sickle cell crises cause microinfarcts in joints and organs, and repeated crises slowly destroy organs and tissues. The spleen and kidneys are especially prone to sickling damage.

Microinfarct
Necrotic tissue
Damaged tissue
Inflamed tissue
Hypoxic cells
Mass of sickled cells obstructing capillary lumen
Capillary

FIGURE 28–5 ■ The clinical manifestations of sickle cell anemia result from pathologic changes to structures and systems throughout the body.

TABLE 28–6 Complications Associated with Sickle Cell Anemia

COMPLICATION	CLINICAL MANIFESTATIONS	CLINICAL THERAPY
Infection, sepsis, and meningitis	➤ Bacterial infections are a major cause of morbidity and mortality for the child with sickle cell disease ➤ *S. pneumoniae* septicemia/meningitis is the most common cause of death during early childhood ➤ Fever in a child younger than 5 years of age with SS often indicates a life-threatening bacterial infection	➤ Routine immunization schedule ➤ Pneumococcal vaccine ➤ Prophylactic penicillin ➤ Aggressive treatment of infection
Limp	➤ Gait abnormality ➤ Often the presenting symptom in a child, especially the preverbal child ➤ Consider septic arthritis or other bone or joint infections ➤ Consider bone infarct or osteomyelitis	➤ Depends on underlying cause ➤ Refer to orthopedic or neurologic consults
Osteomyelitis	➤ Increased incidence of infections of the bones and joints in SS ➤ Tenderness, swelling, warmth, erythema, or other signs of infection may indicate osteomyelitis ➤ Systemic symptoms include fever, weight loss, recurrent pain ➤ Leukocytosis and elevated ESR	➤ Bone biopsy or aspiration to identify organism ➤ Aggressive intravenous antibiotic therapy lasting approximately 6–8 weeks
Acute anemia	➤ Usually triggered by suppression of the bone marrow from viral or other infections, pooling of blood in the spleen or liver, or increased intravascular hemolysis ➤ Usually presents with acute onset of weakness, lethargy, pallor, breathlessness, palpitations, abdominal pain, and occasionally increased jaundice ➤ Other manifestations include tachycardia, tachypnea, pallor, jaundice, suddenly enlarged spleen/liver, S_3 gallop, and/or congestive heart failure	➤ Compare hemoglobin, hematocrit, reticulocyte count, and bilirubin with baseline values ➤ Treatment is individualized according to degree of anemia and clinical status
Chest pain and acute chest syndrome	➤ Acute chest syndrome describes new pulmonary findings on radiograph; a leading cause of death and morbidity and mortality ➤ Common causes are infarction of bones of the thoracic cage and/or acute pulmonary disease ➤ Common symptoms include pain, cough, fever, and occasional, abdominal pain ➤ Signs include tachypnea and shallow respirations ➤ Lungs may be clear to auscultation or rales may be present ➤ Palpate chest to identify swelling, warmth, and erythema, which may indicate rib and/or vertebral infarction	➤ Hematology referral ➤ Analgesics ➤ Hydration ➤ Incentive spirometry ➤ Pulse oximetry ➤ Oxygen ➤ Antibiotics ➤ Transfusion for severe anemia or hypoxemia
Cerebrovascular accident (CVA)	➤ Ischemic strokes are more common in children with SS ➤ Transient ischemic attacks (TIAs) may occur ➤ Mortality is unusual from a first ischemic stroke; however, morbidity may be substantial with severe motor and neuropsychologic deficits ➤ Intracranial hemorrhage in sickle cell patients has a 25% mortality rate ➤ Approximately 15% of children with SS have "silent infarcts" in which an MRI is suggestive of infarction but there are no overt neurologic deficits ➤ Ischemic stroke most commonly presents with sudden onset of numbness or weakness of an arm and or leg on one side of the body ➤ Children are most susceptible to stroke between the ages of 2 and 10 years	➤ CT scan or MRI should be performed immediately upon suspicion of CVA ➤ Rule out meningitis ➤ Neurosurgical consultation ➤ Chronic transfusions are generally prescribed
Transfusion therapy	➤ Alloimmunization ➤ Transmission of infectious diseases such as hepatitis and HIV	➤ Phenotyping ➤ Monitor transfusion history ➤ Use sickle cell negative blood for transfusion
Surgery and anesthesia	➤ Increased risk of perioperative complications ➤ Surgical procedures that have an increased probability of ischemia or hypoxia deserve special attention (cardiothoracic surgery, techniques associated with hypotension, hypothermia, hyperventilation, and vascular surgery) ➤ Laparoscopic surgery appears to lower the postoperative complications of SS and should be used when available	➤ Evaluation by anesthesiologist ➤ Maintenance fluids at least 12 hours before surgery ➤ Transfusion if necessary ➤ Monitor pulmonary function tests and oxygen saturation measured by pulse oximetry ➤ Echocardiogram ➤ Renal and liver function ➤ Incentive spirometry preoperatively and postoperatively

TABLE 28–6 Complications Associated with Sickle Cell Anemia (continued)

COMPLICATION	CLINICAL MANIFESTATIONS	CLINICAL THERAPY
Heart disease	➤ Caused by chronic anemia, pulmonary arterial occlusion leading to cor pulmonale and myocardial damage resulting from small infarcts and iron deposition ➤ Cardiomegaly is seen in most children with SS by the age of 5 ➤ Signs and symptoms include exercise intolerance, cardiomegaly, pulmonary hypertension and cor pulmonale after recurrent acute chest syndrome	➤ Baseline cardiac screening ➤ Treat hypertension, valvular disease, mitral valve prolapse, and cor pulmonale ➤ Limits on activity are generally set by the child
Ocular involvement	➤ Red blood sickling can occur in the microvascular of the eye ➤ Signs may be demonstrated in the conjunctiva, uvea, retina, and optic nerve ➤ Proliferative sickle cell retinopathy may cause vitreous hemorrhage and retinal detachment with loss of vision	➤ Regular ophthalmologic evaluations starting at age 10 years ➤ Small lesions can be treated to avoid large lesions ➤ Laser therapy to obliterate aberrant vessels so as to prevent retinal hemorrhage and to treat detached retina
Priapism	➤ Persistent painful erection of the penis ➤ Common in SS ➤ Can occur at any age ➤ May persist for hours, days, or even weeks ➤ Episodes often begin during sleep ➤ May be associated with dehydration, hypoventilation, and/or a full bladder ➤ Major episodes can last several days and are associated with a high risk of erectile dysfunction	➤ Males should seek medical attention if episodes exceed 3 hours in length or are recurrent ➤ Priapism should be managed by a urologist and hematologist familiar with sickle cell disease ➤ Management of prolonged episode includes hospitalization, hydration, analgesia, and often transfusions
Avascular necrosis (AVN)	➤ Avascular necrosis of the humeral and femoral heads is accompanied by varying degrees of pain and disability ➤ AVN of the humeral head is usually less disabling than femoral head AVN as the shoulder is a non-weight-bearing joint ➤ May also be seen in other bones such as the knees and spine ➤ Symptoms include acute pain in the hips, buttocks, or shoulders with motion limitation because of pain ➤ Pain is intermittent or persistent	➤ Analgesics (NSAID or narcotic), local heat, and restriction of weight bearing ➤ Healing has been reported in children and teenagers ➤ Hip fusion or reconstruction may be required
Liver/hyperbilirubinemia	➤ Chronic hemolysis leads to icteric sclera, production of gallstones ➤ Acute attacks with pain in right upper quadrant or diffuse abdominal pain, nausea, vomiting, icteric sclera, fever, leukocytosis ➤ Acute hepatomegaly may occur during a painful crisis ➤ Note: hepatomegaly is present in 40%–80% of patients with SS	➤ Management is indicated by symptomology and will include intravenous fluids/NPO, analgesics, intravenous antibiotics, and transfusions ➤ Elective cholecystectomy within 6 weeks after attacks subside
Kidney/urinary tract	➤ Renal intravascular sickling is common in SS ➤ Occurs early in life and continues throughout the life of the patient ➤ Chronic renal failure may occur ➤ Renal disease is frequently asymptomatic	➤ Regular urinalysis monitoring for proteinuria and/or microscopic hematuria ➤ Urine cultures ➤ Treat urinary tract infections with vigorous antibiotic therapy

Adapted from the Sickle Cell Advisory Committee of The Genetic Network of New York, Puerto Rico, and the Virgin Islands. (March, 2002). Guidelines for the treatment of people with sickle cell disease.

(continued from page 1008)

- Extremely painful
- Caused by stasis of blood with clumping of cells in the microcirculation, ischemia, and infarction
- Thrombosis and infarction of local tissue may occur if the crisis is not reversed
- Clinical manifestations include fever, pain, tissue engorgement, painful swelling of joints in hands and feet, priapism, severe abdominal pain
- Cerebral occlusion results in stroke, manifested by paralysis and/or other central nervous system complications
- May last for days or weeks

- Splenic sequestration
  - Life-threatening crisis; death can occur within hours; high mortality (as much as 50%)
  - Caused by pooling of blood in the spleen
  - The spleen is capable of holding as much as one fifth of the body's blood supply at one time—leading to cardiovascular collapse
  - Clinical manifestations include profound anemia, hypovolemia, and shock
- Aplastic crisis
  - Diminished erythropoiesis and increased destruction of red blood cells
  - Triggered by viral infection or depletion of folic acid
  - Clinical manifestations include profound anemia, pallor, fatigue

Pain. The most common reason for hospitalization of the child with sickle cell is acute painful episodes. The sickled RBCs cause vaso-occlusion, microinfarction, and ischemia. Pain results from avascular necrosis of the bone marrow. Pain is typically experienced in the back, abdomen, chest, and joints (Jacob, 2001). Children may also experience chest tightness and shortness of breath.

Pain intensity and duration vary depending on the individual and the location. Pain may be transient in a localized area, such as the wrist, to severe, generalized pain that lasts for several days or weeks and may require hospitalization (Jacob, 2001). The pain is often severe enough to require opioid analgesics and the use of a patient-controlled analgesic (PCA) pump. See Complementary Therapy: Pain and Sickle Cell Anemia.

COLLABORATIVE CARE

No cure for sickle cell anemia exists. Supportive care is aimed at the prevention and treatment of sickling episodes and management of pain. Preventing exposure to infections, preventing exposure to cold, preventing acidosis, and maintaining normal hydration are important steps in avoiding crises.

Diagnostic Tests

The initial diagnosis of sickle cell anemia in newborns is often made by testing cord blood using hemoglobin electrophoresis. The sickle turbidity test (Sickledex) may be used for quick screening purposes in children over 6 months of age, once the fetal hemoglobin levels have fallen. Hemoglobin electrophoresis is performed to verify positive Sickledex test results. Newborn screening of infants for hemoglobinopathies now occurs in most states. A complete blood cell count will reveal decreased hemoglobin and an increased reticulocyte count.

It is recommended that all newborns be screened, as sickle cell disease can occur in several groups in addition to African Americans, such as those of Mediterranean, South American, Arabian, and East Indian descent. A child's heritage cannot be predicted from appearance or name alone. Individuals with a family history are at greatest risk of this genetic disease. Prenatal testing is recommended if it has not been routinely done in that state.

During therapy, the reticulocyte count is monitored regularly to ensure that the bone marrow is still functioning.

Clinical Therapy

Management focuses on pain control, hydration, oxygenation, prevention of infection, and prevention of associated complications. Treatment of crises involves aggressive hydration, oxygen, pain management, and bed rest to reduce energy expenditure.

Pain Control, Hydration, and Oxygenation. Parenteral analgesics, such as morphine, are generally administered around the clock or via patient-controlled analgesia. Pain medications should not be ordered solely on a prn basis, as this increases the child's anxiety and delays medication administration. Oral and intravenous fluid replacement also promotes pain relief since dehydration is often a cause of crisis. Fluids also reduce the viscosity of the blood. Oxygen is usually administered although the best method of promoting oxygenation is the reversal of sickling.

> **COMPLEMENTARY THERAPY**
> **Pain and Sickle Cell Anemia**
>
> Pain management for children with sickle cell disease is a major challenge, both for healthcare providers and families. A nursing study that determined effectiveness of pain control and types of comfort measures used by families provides information that can be applied in caring for children with sickle cell disease in the hospital and home (Beyer, J. E. & Simmons, L. E., 2004). The mothers in this study described a combination of traditional medicine and complementary approaches. They emphasized the importance of keeping the child healthy, in order to avoid crisis, by avoiding overheating or chilling. Regular medical checkups, adequate hydration, and immunizations were considered important. Being alert to early signs of pain was important so that the families could begin pharmacological treatment as well as complementary therapies such as applying heat via baths and hot towels to decrease pain and increase relaxation; touching, holding, and massaging the extremities or chest and back; praying together; distraction and diversionary activities such as playing games and taking drives. Nurses can learn from and apply these approaches with families. Ask them what they do to identify pain early and alleviate it. Add to the list of interventions the family can try and then partner with them to evaluate results. Continue to emphasize medical care while integrating the other comfort measures the family and child find helpful into nursing care plans.

Prevention and Treatment of Infection. Children who are functionally asplenic or have had a splenectomy have a resultant decreased capability to fight infection. For this reason, infection is a serious condition regarding immediate attention. Daily prophylactic penicillin VK 125 mg twice daily is recommended for children from 2 months to 3 years. From 3 to 5 years of age the recommended dosage is 250 mg twice daily. Amoxicillin or injections of Bicillin every 3 weeks can be substituted. If the child is allergic to penicillin, erythromycin ethyl succinate (20 mg/kg divided into two doses) can be used for prophylaxis (Wilson, Krishnamurti, & Kamat, 2003).

When an infection is suspected, cultures (blood, urine, and throat) are obtained to identify source of infection and the offending organism. Aggressive antibiotic therapy is implemented immediately.

It is recommended that the pneumococcal vaccine (PCV 7 for infants and toddlers or 23 valent for children over 2 years of age) is administered for all infants and children with sickle cell disease (National Institutes of Health, 2002). The *Haemophilus influenzae* type b (Hib) vaccine series should be started at 2 months of age and continued at recommended ages to prevent infection with Hib. Other vaccines such as the influenza and meningococcal vaccines may also be administered.

Transfusion of Red Blood Cells. Other therapeutic measures include transfusions of red blood cells. See Table 28–7 for blood products used in sickle cell disease and other hematologic conditions. The benefits of transfusions include improved blood and tissue oxygenation, a reduction in sickling, and a temporary suppression of the production of RBCs containing the Hb S (Ogedegbe, 2002).

A complication associated with frequent transfusions is an overload of iron in the body. The iron is stored in tissues and organs (**hemosiderosis**), due to the body's limited ability to excrete

TABLE 28–7 Type of Blood and Blood Products for Administration

TYPE OF BLOOD OR BLOOD PRODUCT	INDICATION FOR USE
Whole blood	To replace blood volume Generally given in hemorrhagic emergencies and shock
Packed red blood cells	To increase oxygen-carrying capacity in anemia and some leukemias
Fresh frozen plasma	To expand blood volume
Cryoprecipitate	To replace factor VIII, factor XIII, von Willebrand factor, and fibrinogen
Clotting factors	
Factor VIII	To treat factor VIII deficiency (hemophilia A) and von Willebrand disease
Factor IX	To treat factor IX deficiency (hemophilia B)
Albumin	To expand blood volume in shock and trauma

iron. For this reason, an iron-chelating drug such as deferoxamine may be given with vitamin C to promote iron excretion. Another complication of multiple transfusions is the development of alloimmunization to red cell and platelet antigens (Ogedegbe, 2002). Alloimmunization occurs when the child's immune system reacts against antigens on the donated tissues (e.g., blood and stem cells) (See Chapter 27∞).

Additionally, chronic transfusions have proven to be an effective treatment of stroke complications related to sickle cell disease. In children who have had strokes from the disease, periodic transfusions (about every 3 to 4 weeks) can reduce the incidence of future strokes (National Heart, Lung, and Blood Institute, 2002). If administered early in the crisis, blood transfusions may relieve the ischemia caused by vaso-occlusion in major organs and body parts such as the spleen, lung, kidney, brain, and penis. Exchange transfusion is preferred in order to reduce the potential of fluid volume excess. (See Developing Cultural Competence: Blood Products.)

Other Therapies. Treatment with hydroxyurea has been helpful in adults, and is now being used more frequently in children. This cytotoxic medication decreases production of abnormal blood cells and leads to a lesser amount of pain being experienced (Day & Wynn, 2000). Side effects of hydroxyurea include bone marrow suppression, headaches, dizziness, nausea, and vomiting.

Hematopoietic stem cell transplantation (HSCT) may be considered; however, a recurrence of the disease is demonstrated in approximately 10% of recipients. Refer to later discussion regarding HSCT.

DEVELOPING CULTURAL COMPETENCE
Blood Products

For the Jehovah's Witness, receiving blood and blood products is forbidden. For a child who is critically ill and requires blood or blood product transfusions for survival, collaboration with the family and healthcare team is essential. Healthcare providers are often challenged with ethical decisions regarding refusal of treatments for children. Depending on the state and the circumstances, healthcare providers or medical facilities may seek legal intervention on the child's behalf.

NURSING MANAGEMENT

Nursing care is focused on identifying children at risk for sickle cell disease, recognition and management of sickle cell crisis, promoting growth and development, prevention of complications associated with the disease, and supporting the child and family.

Nursing Assessment and Diagnosis

Once a child is diagnosed with the disease, a comprehensive physical assessment is essential considering sickle cell anemia can affect any body system.

Physiologic Assessment

In children who are known to have sickle cell anemia, obtain a detailed history from the parents or child about past crises, precipitating events, medical treatment, and home management. Measure the child's height and weight accurately and compare with past measurements, since failure to thrive is common. Assess achievement of developmental milestones. Ask about chronic or acute pain that the child is experiencing. Pain may occur in nearly any body part, but most commonly manifests as headache, extremity pain, or abdominal discomfort. Use a pain scale and identify pain perception in each body part where pain exists (See Chapter 18∞). Assess the pain management protocols the family has used and what has been most successful. Palpate the spleen and assess for tenderness. Assess for complications associated with sickle cell disease (see Table 28–6 on pages 1010–1011).

The ill child with sickle cell disease should receive a careful multisystem assessment. Fever is an emergency that necessitates prompt treatment. When the child is in crisis, assess pain and note the presence of any signs of inflammation or infection. Carefully monitor the child for signs of shock (refer to Chapter 26∞).

Psychosocial Assessment

The child who experiences frequent painful crises may exhibit problems with low self-esteem and self-concept, anxiety, dissatisfaction with body image, depression, social isolation, poor peer and family relationships, and decreased participation in normal activities of daily living (Jacob, 2001). Assess the child for development of psychosocial problems.

The family of a child with sickle cell disease requires a thorough psychosocial assessment. If the child is newly diagnosed with the disorder, the family will require assistance to deal with feelings related to the serious, life-threatening nature of the disease. Assess parents' understanding of the disease transmission and ask whether genetic counseling has been obtained.

PRACTICE ALERT

Information about genetic testing is confidential and must not be shared with persons other than those tested. In the 1970s, when genetic testing for sickle cell disease and trait first became available, discrimination in jobs and insurance occurred against Blacks who had the trait for sickle cell disease.

MediaLink Case Study: An Adolescent in Sickle Cell Crisis

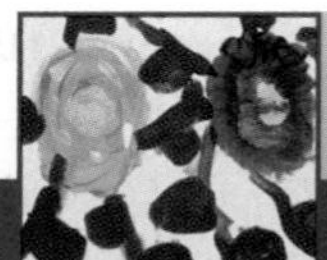

Nursing Care Plan

THE CHILD WITH SICKLE CELL ANEMIA

GOAL	INTERVENTION	RATIONALE	EXPECTED OUTCOME
1. Ineffective Tissue Perfusion (all systems) related to affinity of hemoglobin for oxygen			
	NIC Priority Intervention—*Circulatory Care:* Promotion of arterial and venous circulation		**NOC Outcome**—*Tissue Perfusion:* Extent to which blood flows through the vessels of the body vasculature and maintains tissue function
The child will show few signs and symptoms of tissue hypoxia.	■ Instruct child to avoid physical exertion, emotional stress, low oxygen environments (e.g., airplanes, high altitudes), and known sources of infection.	■ Decreased activity and exposure reduce body's need for oxygen.	The child has no shortness of breath and shows no signs of hypoxia.
	■ Administer blood transfusions as ordered.	■ Packed cells increase number of red blood cells available to carry oxygen to tissue cells. Transfusions promote circulation.	
	■ Perform several caregiving activities together when possible.	■ Grouping activities allows for optimum rest.	
	■ Give oxygen as ordered.	■ High concentration of oxygen in alveoli increases diffusion of gas across membranes.	
Repeated cerebrovascular accidents will be avoided.	■ Administer and teach the family to administer prophylactic transfusions for the child who has had a cerebrovascular accident.	■ Lowers potential for a future cerebrovascular accident.	The child does not suffer a cerebrovascular accident.
2. Risk for Deficient Fluid Volume related to inadequate fluid intake and dehydration			
	NIC Priority Intervention—*Fluid Management:* Promotion of electrolyte balance and prevention of complications resulting from abnormal or undesired fluid levels		**NOC Suggested Outcome**—*Hydration:* Amount of water in the intracellular and extracellular compartments of the body
The child will maintain or be restored to adequate hydration.	■ Calculate the child's daily fluid requirements. Monitor the child's usual fluid consumption and make necessary adjustments. Encourage the child to take fluids. Observe for signs of dehydration.	■ Optimizing fluid intake ensures that the child gets needed fluid. Dehydration exacerbates crises.	The child shows signs of adequate hydration.
	■ Record intake and output.	■ Early intervention can be effective in minimizing complications from dehydration. Child may need oral or intravenous rehydration therapy.	
	■ Instruct family to report fever, vomiting, diarrhea, or other signs of fluid imbalance immediately.	■ Recording enables you to monitor daily fluid intake and spacing throughout the day.	
3. Pain related to chronic physical disability and clustering of sickled cells			
	NIC Priority Intervention—*Pain Management:* Alleviation of pain or a reduction in pain to a level of comfort acceptable to the patient		**NOC Suggested Outcome**—*Comfort Level:* Feelings of physical and psychologic ease
The child will verbalize that pain is controlled.	■ Administer analgesics, such as morphine or hydromorphine (Dilaudid), as ordered. Continuous intravenous infusion is used for the duration of a painful crisis.	■ Pain of sickle cell crises is excruciating.	The child is pain free, or pain control is significantly improved.
	■ Position carefully.	■ Joints and extremities can be extremely painful.	

Nursing Care Plan THE CHILD WITH SICKLE CELL ANEMIA (continued)

GOAL	INTERVENTION	RATIONALE	EXPECTED OUTCOME
3. Pain related to chronic physical disability and clustering of sickled cells (continued)			
	■ Ask family what pain relief measures are helpful and integrate them into care for the child.	■ Complementary therapy such as holding the child, massage, warmth, distraction, and other measures may be instrumental in managing the child's pain.	
4. Risk for Infection related to chronic disease and splenic malfunction			
	NIC Intervention—*Infection Control:* Minimizing the acquisition and transmission of infectious agents		**NOC Suggested Outcome**—*Risk Control:* Actions to eliminate or reduce actual, personal, and modifiable health threats
The child will not develop infection.	■ Ensure adequate nutrition by providing high-calorie high-protein diet. Ensure that the child's immunizations are up to date. Report any signs of infection to physician immediately. ■ Isolate the child from possible sources of infection. Instruct parents about signs of infection and encourage them to seek prompt healthcare.	■ Chronically ill children are at greater risk of infection. ■ Restriction of persons with infection decreases the child's contact with infectious agents. Prompt care for infection reduces the chance of sickle cell crisis.	The child is free of infection.
5. Deficient Knowledge (child and parents) related to lack of exposure about cause and treatment of sickle cell anemia			
	NIC Intervention— *Teaching Disease Process:* Assisting the patient to understand information related to a specific disease process		**NOC Suggested Outcome**—*Knowledge:* Extent of understanding conveyed about sickle cell disease
The child and family will verbalize understanding of risk factors for sickle cell crises and how to minimize them.	■ Review basics of sickle cell disease. Teach the child and family about signs and symptoms of crises. ■ Arrange for genetic counseling and testing for sickle cell trait for family members if desired.	■ Knowledge of disease helps ensure compliance with treatment regimen and adherence to preventive measures. ■ Questions and concerns regarding future pregnancies can be allayed through knowledge of disease and transmission.	The child and parent can verbalize precipitating events of crises.

Assist the family with resources for the child's long-term medical expenses. The nurse assesses the older child's knowledge about the disease and explores the child's feelings related to the management of a chronic condition. When siblings or other family members are carriers, counseling is needed periodically during the life span so that implications for dating, marriage, and having children are understood.

Several nursing diagnoses that may apply to the child with sickle cell anemia are presented in the accompanying nursing care plan.

Other nursing diagnoses may include the following:

- Risk for Impaired Tissue Perfusion (cerebral) related to interrupted blood flow
- Delayed Growth and Development related to effects of physical disability
- Caregiver Role Strain related to child's chronic illness
- Risk for Impaired Parenting related to having a child with a chronic illness
- Impaired Physical Mobility related to pain

Planning and Implementation

The accompanying nursing care plan summarizes nursing care for the child with sickle cell anemia. Nursing management for the child in crisis, such as Michael in the chapter's opening scenario, focuses on promoting increased tissue perfusion, promoting hydration, controlling pain, preventing infection, ensuring adequate nutrition, preventing complications related to the disease, and providing emotional support to the child and family.

Promote Increased Tissue Perfusion

Administer blood transfusions and oxygen as ordered (Box 28–3). To prevent hemolysis, the intravenous fluid used before and after a blood transfusion must be saline rather than D_5W. It is important for all health facilities to have current guidelines for transfusion protocols. Become familiar with the policies and procedures where you work. For example, two nurses should check the child's blood type and patient identification before starting the infusion. Refer to the Skills Manual for further discussion of blood transfusions.

BOX 28–3 Principles of Blood and Blood Product Administration

Nurses should consider the following principles when administering blood and blood products.

- Verify the blood type, patient number, donor number, and Rh factor with another RN.
- Check the blood for sediment, or any nonuniform or unusual characteristics.
- Assess the child's history for previous transfusion reactions.
- Assess the child's vital signs before transfusion and every 15-30 minutes throughout transfusion.
- Remain with the child during the first 20 minutes of the transfusion to monitor for undesirable reaction.
- If transfusion reaction occurs, immediately discontinue the transfusion, change the IV to normal saline, and notify the primary healthcare provider.

(Refer to Skills Manual for administering blood or blood products procedure.)

CLINICAL TIP

When administering a transfusion, never infuse cold blood because it may increase sickling. Use a blood-warming coil to bring blood to room temperature.

For small children, blood is usually infused without saline because they cannot manage the extra volume. Monitor for transfusion reactions; see clinical manifestations below. Work with the child and family to assist with support for emotional stress. Any activities that increase cellular metabolism also result in tissue hypoxia. Schedule caregiving activities and play periods to allow the child the opportunity to obtain optimal rest.

PRACTICE ALERT

Blood reactions can occur as soon as the blood transfusion begins. Administer the first 20 mL of blood slowly and observe the child carefully for a reaction. Repeatedly assess the child according to agency policy.

MediaLink Nursing in Action: Administering Blood or Blood Products

Promote Hydration

The child with sickle cell anemia is adversely affected by dehydration since higher blood viscosity and further sickling is a consequence of dehydration. Calculate the child's fluid maintenance requirements (minimum daily fluid intake) (see Chapter 23) and monitor the child's oral fluid intake. The dehydrated child generally requires a fluid bolus intravenously, followed by an intravenous fluid maintenance. Adjust oral intake as necessary to keep the child well hydrated. See Partnering with Families: Fluid Intake.

Pain Management

Administer prescribed analgesics around the clock during crises. If patient-controlled analgesia (PCA) is used, ensure that the constant infusions run as ordered and that the parent or child understands the use of bolus infusions, when needed (refer to Chapter 18 for additional information on pain management). Assist the child to assume a comfortable position. Avoid putting stress on painful joints. The small child or infant should be handled carefully and repositioned with care, supporting the joints and extremities during repositioning. See Evidence-Based Practice: Sickle Cell Anemia and Pain Management.

PRACTICE ALERT

Neither hot nor cold compresses should be used for pain management in the child who has sickle cell anemia. Ischemic tissue is fragile and has reduced sensation, increasing the risk of burn injury. Cold compresses promote sickling. However, many children find that warmth, such as a warm bath, helps to increase comfort and alleviate pain.

Prevent Infection

Infection makes the child more susceptible to a crisis, and the crisis, in turn, increases susceptibility to infection. Teach the parents how to administer antibiotics for prophylaxis or treatment of infection. Partner with the parents to ensure that they have the necessary resources to obtain and give daily antibiotics. Because infections can be particularly virulent and can cause death in these children, parents should be instructed to obtain immediate

CLINICAL MANIFESTATIONS of Blood Transfusion Reactions

TYPE OF REACTION	CLINICAL MANIFESTATION	ETIOLOGY	CLINICAL THERAPY
Allergic reaction	Urticaria, itching, respiratory distress	Immune response to protein in the blood	Stop the transfusion; call physician; administer antihistamines as ordered; monitor vital signs; maintain intravenous infusion of normal saline; keep intravenous line open; check urine for hematuria
Hemolytic reaction	Fever, chills, hematuria, headache, chest pain; can progress to shock	Mismatched blood, history of multiple transfusions, or infusion with a solution containing dextrose or other additives	
Febrile or septic	Chills, fever, headache, decreased blood pressure, nausea and/or vomiting, and leg and back pain	Usually a result of contamination of blood; may also be caused by idiopathic conditions	Inform primary healthcare provider. Diuretics may be ordered
Circulatory overload	Labored breathing, chest or lower back pain, productive cough with rales heard on auscultation, and distended neck veins; central venous pressure may increase	Results from infusion of excessive amounts of fluid or too rapid administration	

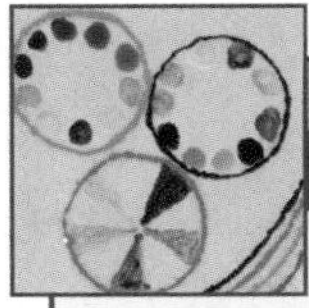

EVIDENCE-BASED PRACTICE

Sickle Cell Anemia and Pain Management

PROBLEM

Severe episodes of sickle cell crises require hospitalization for pain management. Relief of pain is the primary goal for healthcare providers and is most significant to the child experiencing pain. However, different pain management regimens may be used during each hospitalization and effective regimens are not well documented. Studies are needed to identify effective pain management strategies for children with sickle cell disease. In addition, parents use a variety of pain relief measures at home but these may not be integrated into care when the child becomes hospitalized, leading to poor pain management.

EVIDENCE

Nurse researchers conducted a descriptive longitudinal study with 27 children to evaluate the pain management strategies used in sickle cell disease when they experienced pain during a vaso-occlusive episode. The children ranged in age from 5 to 19 years; there were 40 hospital admissions during the 9-month study. The researchers noted several surprising findings from the study. First, they found that children on average self-administered only 35% of the pain medication that was prescribed. The second finding was that the children did not report significant pain relief. It is surmised that adequate pain relief was not achieved during hospitalization because the dose of analgesics administered was too low. In another study in which 21 female caretakers of children with sickle cell disease were interviewed, a variety of techniques were used to manage pain at home. Oral medications, massage, warmth to painful body parts, and other techniques were considered helpful (Jacob et al., 2003; Beyer & Simmons, 2004).

IMPLICATIONS

Hospitalized children who self-administered their medication consistently undermedicated themselves and failed to achieve pain relief. Children may not be taught how to use the PCA device properly and may interpret that they use it as little as possible. Thus, healthcare provider practices influence the child's pain management. In addition, children and families have developed many effective pain relief measures at home that may not be included in hospital care. More information is needed about methods of integrating these techniques into hospital care.

Recommendations include the need to evaluate whether increasing analgesic use to at least the amount prescribed would increase the amount of pain relief. Additional research is needed to determine the effectiveness of different PCA regimens and to evaluate the effectiveness of pain management algorithms. Effective evaluation tools are needed to measure effectiveness of the child self medication by patient controlled analgesia. Tools for evaluating home care pain management are needed. Nurses must be willing to integrate the family's measures into care while the child is hospitalized.

CRITICAL THINKING APPLICATION

How will you determine if the child in sickle cell crisis is obtaining adequate pain relief? What personal beliefs of healthcare providers may influence effective pain management? How can these beliefs be addressed? If the primary healthcare provider has prescribed a subtherapeutic dosage of pain medication for a child in sickle cell crisis, what action could you take?

care when the child is ill or has a fever. Evaluate the child's immunization schedule and provide needed immunizations.

Ensure Adequate Nutrition

Emphasize the importance of adequate nutrition to promote growth. Encourage the child to eat a high-protein, high-calorie diet. Emphasize the importance of folic acid supplements and vitamin C as ordered. Perform regular growth measurements and if slow growth is apparent, perform 24-hour recalls and other nutritional assessments.

PARTNERING WITH FAMILIES

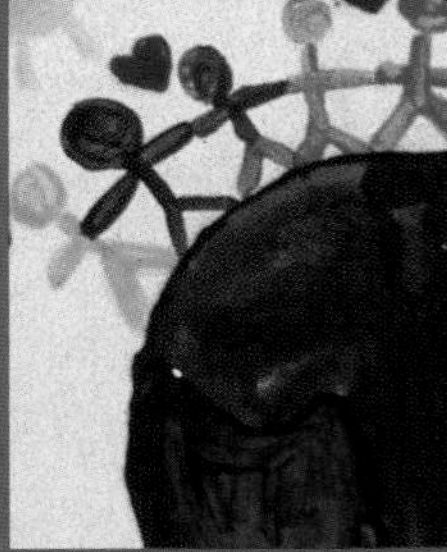

Fluid Intake

Parents often claim they have difficulty in getting their child with sickle cell anemia to consume adequate fluids. Provide the family with these tips on encouraging fluid intake in a small child.

- Use a favorite cup or glass.
- Use a straw.
- Take advantage of times the child is thirsty such as on awakening or after play.
- Leave a cup within easy reach of the child.
- Offer frozen juice pops, crushed ice drinks, and flavored ice chips.
- Make "games" out of drinking fluids such as a contest to see at what time a child can finish a drink.

Prevent Complications of Crises

Observe the child for signs of increasing anemia and shock (mental status change, pallor, vital sign changes). Maintain ongoing monitoring of the child's neurologic status for evidence of altered cerebral function. Administer blood transfusions and observe the child for any adverse reaction.

Provide Emotional Support

Sickle cell anemia is a chronic disease that is accompanied by life-threatening episodic crises. Family members often need support to help them deal with their feelings about the diagnosis and its implications. For example, consider the effects of sickle cell anemia on Michael (the child in the opening scenario) and his family. Parents may experience guilt because the disease is genetically transmitted. Referrals to support groups and contact with others with the disease can be helpful.

Collaborate care with family members and provide them with ongoing support to deal with the stress of having a child with a chronic condition. (See Partnering with Families: Home Care Considerations for the Child with Sickle Cell Anemia.) Provide resources, respite care for parents, and information as needed for siblings. Sickle cell disease and some other hematologic disorders of childhood require that parents provide ongoing monitoring and care for their children with chronic conditions. Nurse researchers have found that parents describe a sense of chronic sorrow and eventual adjustment to the uncertainty of the condition. The nurse should realize that parents are constantly changing in their understanding and coping mechanisms. Periodic evaluations of their coping skills and needs are

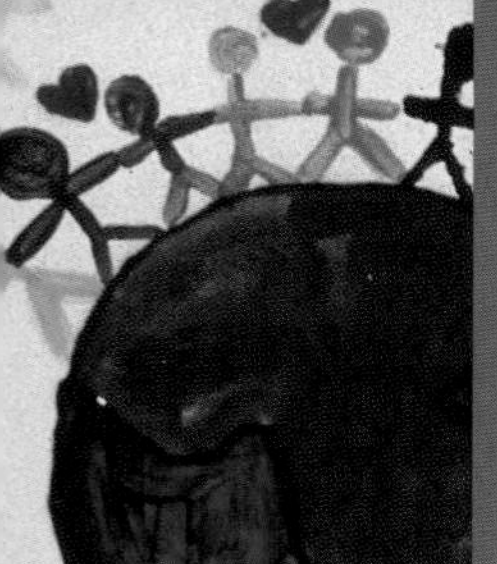

PARTNERING WITH FAMILIES

Home Care Considerations for the Child with Sickle Cell Anemia

- Follow recommended schedules for well-child care visits.
- Be sure the child is up to date with immunizations, including hepatitis B, annual influenza, pneumococcal vaccine, and tuberculosis skin test.
- Special testing, such as heart and eye examinations, may be needed periodically to check for any sequelae of the disease.
- Special medications, such as antibiotics, may be needed; pain relief medicine and blood transfusions may be administered.
- Dehydration is dangerous. Be sure the child gets extra fluids in hot weather, when ill, during physical activity, and during travel.
- As the child develops, provide information about the disease and encourage self-care. Be sure the school personnel understand the child's diagnosis and any care required during school hours.
- Contact your healthcare provider if the child has a high fever, a common illness that lasts more than a day, seizures, change in behavior, severe pain, abnormal skin color or breathing pattern, or any other symptoms of concern.

helpful in adapting teaching and resource recommendations to them (Northington, 2000). Refer to Chapter 20∞ for a discussion regarding transition of a child with a chronic disorder into adulthood. Refer parents to support groups such as the National Association of Sickle Cell Disease for further information.

Discharge Planning and Home Care Teaching

Partner with the family to identify and address home care needs well in advance of discharge. Provide parents with information about sickle cell disease and the child's treatment. Even parents of a child previously diagnosed with the disorder may benefit from information about the disease process and its management. Explain the basic effect of tissue hypoxia and the effects of sickling on circulation. Partner with the family to explore resources in the home and community and determine if parents will be able to administer medications and fluids and to provide adequate nutrition. Assess their knowledge of signs of infection and of sickle cell crisis and when to seek medical care for the child. Refer the parents for genetic counseling, particularly if they plan to have more children. Encourage adolescents and young adults in the family to receive genetic counseling and testing as well.

MediaLink Sickle Cell Resources and Support

Partner with the family to be sure they understand the importance of monitoring for signs of dehydration, such as dry mucous membranes, weight loss, and sunken fontanels in infants. Provide specific instructions regarding how many ounces of liquid the child needs to drink each day. Emphasize that increased fluid intake is needed to replace the fluids lost from overheating or exposure to hot weather. Make sure both the child and family understand the triggers and precipitating factors for sickle cell crises. Encourage the avoidance of situations that cause crises. Instruct the child and parents about signs and symptoms of crises and that these signs should be reported to their healthcare provider.

Provide the family with careful instructions about infusion therapy. When regular blood infusions are required, the resulting iron overload is damaging to body organs. These children will likely receive deferoxamine (Desferal) for iron overload. The medication is usually given by subcutaneous or intravenous routes over 8 to 10 hours. Prompt recognition of side effects and careful management of the lengthy infusion process are important. The child should be monitored for skin reactions and allergic responses. Have parents demonstrate the infusion technique and state what to do in case of reactions. Pain management may be required during infusion as the site may be tender and uncomfortable.

Instruct parents that it is important to inform all treating physicians and dentists of the child's medical condition. Special precautions are necessary when the child undergoes surgery of any kind, as hypoxia resulting from anesthesia is a major surgical risk. The child should also wear a medical identification tag or medical alert bracelet.

Encourage older children with sickle cell anemia to participate in activities with other children between crises, but to avoid strenuous physical exertion and contact sports. Play and social interactions that promote learning and development are important. Monitor the child's growth and development, as delays in sexual maturation and growth are common.

Situations such as flying at high altitudes may result in sickling. The child and family should be aware of this risk. Recommend discussing flights with the primary healthcare provider before any plans are made.

Care in the Community

The child may receive home care nursing for transfusion therapy. The nurse partners with the child and family to establish a plan of care. An individualized school health plan will need to be established. The nurse can assist the family and school with establishing this plan.

School personnel must be aware of the child's disease, as prompt care if the child exhibits any sign of sickle cell crisis is essential. The nurse can identify key staff members in the school and partner with them to ensure that essential management actions are understood by all staff members. Members of the school staff should be instructed in management of emergencies and contact numbers for parents should be readily available. Assist the family and school to plan an appropriate schedule of activities without overprotecting the child. An individualized education plan and ongoing cognitive evaluations are needed. Children with sickle cell disease should not engage in activities, such as running and heavy exercise, which may increase oxygen demand resulting in sickling.

■ Evaluation

Expected outcomes of nursing care for the child with sickle cell anemia include the following:

- The child is free from pain.
- Adequate hydration is achieved.
- The child is free from infection.
- Complications are promptly treated.
- Normal growth and development are achieved.
- Family and child demonstrate understanding of disease and treatment regimen.

Hereditary Spherocytosis

Hereditary spherocytosis (HS), also known as congenital hemolytic anemia, is a hemolytic disorder in which there is no abnormality of hemoglobin. HS is an autosomal dominant disorder caused by an abnormality of proteins by an unknown cause. The cells are disproportionately permeable to sodium, leading to an usual characteristic cell structure. The blood cells are sequestered and hemolyzed in the spleen.

Clinical manifestations appear in the neonatal period or during early infancy. Severity of the anemia varies, but mild jaundice is usually evident. Aplastic crisis (discussed in sickle cell section) is the most serious complication the child experiences. Gallstones are a complication associated with hereditary spherocytosis. No single test confirms hereditary spherocytosis; however, complete blood count reveals anemia and microscopic examination reveals the abnormally shaped cells.

Anemia and hyperbilirubinemia require phototherapy or exchange transfusions. Surgical removal of the spleen, generally around the age of 5 years, produces a clinical cure by eliminating hemolysis; however it does not correct the red blood cell defect. Removal of the spleen increases the risk of infection and sepsis. The prognosis after splenectomy is favorable; the child is generally able to lead a normal life. Nursing care for the child with hereditary spherocytosis is the same as care for the child with anemia.

Thalassemias

The thalassemias are a group of inherited blood disorders of hemoglobin synthesis characterized by anemia that can be mild to severe. The three types of beta-thalassemias (sometimes identified as β-thalassemia) are discussed in this chapter. β-thalassemia major, also known as Cooley anemia, is the most common type. Alpha-thalassemias (sometimes identified as A-thalassemia) vary from only having the recessive trait to the fatal disorder alpha-thalassemia major, in which all four alpha-forming genes are defective. Beta-thalassemia occurs more commonly than alpha-thalassemia.

These disorders most often occur in people of Mediterranean descent but are also found among Middle Eastern, Asian, and African populations (Cook, 2000). β-thalassemia is an autosomal recessive disorder; therefore, if both parents carry the abnormal gene, with each pregnancy there is a 25% chance of passing the disorder on to the child.

Etiology and Pathophysiology

Beta-thalassemia. In β-thalassemia, defective hemoglobin is synthesized as a result of impaired production of the beta chain of hemoglobin A (Hb A). To compensate for decreased Hb A, production of Hb F (fetal hemoglobin) increases. The RBCs are fragile and are easily destroyed, shortening their lifespan. As hemolysis increased, **hemosiderin** (iron-containing pigment accumulated from hemoglobin as the red blood cells are destroyed) is deposited in the skin, causing a bronze appearance. Chronic anemia leads to hyperplasia of the bone marrow cavity and thinning of the bone marrow cortex as the bone marrow attempts to compensate for the anemia. Pathologic fractures and skeletal deformities may occur as a result of these bone marrow changes. Splenomegaly results from hyperactivity of the spleen and from pooling of cells.

The three types of β-thalassemia are as follows:

- Thalassemia minor, or thalassemia trait (produces mild anemia)
- Thalassemia intermedia (produces moderate anemia)
- Thalassemia major (produces anemia requiring transfusion)

Long-term complications related to **hemochromatosis** (excessive absorption and accumulation of iron in the body) include gallbladder disease, liver enlargement and cirrhosis, growth retardation, endocrine complications, jaundice, and cardiac complications including heart failure. Skeletal changes include pathologic fractures and skeletal deformities such as an enlarged head and thickened cranial bones. Death is generally the result of heart failure resulting from severe anemia or iron overload. Other causes of death include liver disease and infection. However, with improved treatment, survival is now possible to age 20 to 30 years.

Alpha-thalassemia. In alpha-thalassemia, the defect occurs on the alpha chain of adult hemoglobin. As with beta-thalassemia, the severity of the disorder is dependent on the number of genes that are defective.

The four types of alpha-thalassemia are as follows:

- Alpha trait—defect in a single alpha chain–forming gene
- Alpha-thalassemia minor—defect in two genes
- Hemoglobin H disease—defect in three genes
- Alpha-thalassemia major—defect in all four alpha-forming genes

Clinical Manifestations

Beta-thalassemia. Clinical manifestations of β-thalassemia are caused by the defective synthesis of hemoglobin, structurally impaired red blood cells (Figure 28–6 ■), and the shortened life span of the red blood cells. The infant with β-thalassemia manifests pallor, failure to thrive, hepatosplenomegaly, and severe anemia (hemoglobin < 6 g/dL) that leads to chronic hypoxemia. See clinical manifestations of β-thalassemia on page 1021. Hemochromatosis may result as the body conserves iron from the destructed red cells as well as from the transfused

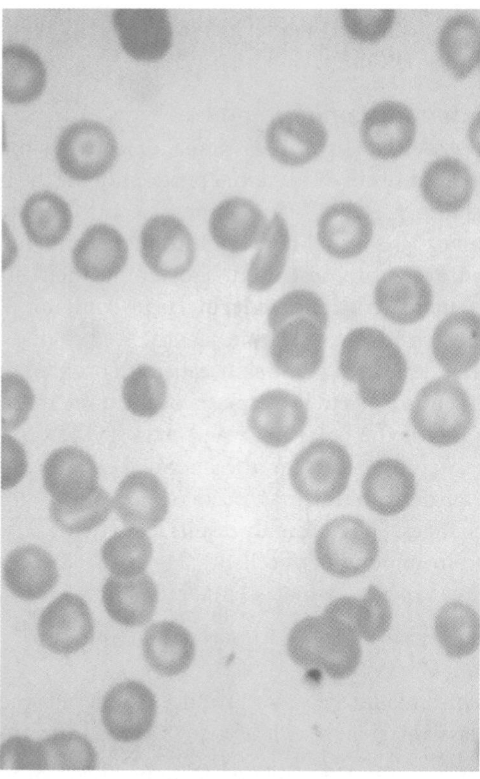

FIGURE 28–6 ■ Red blood cell appearance in β-thalassemia. What characteristic abnormalities can be seen on this microscopic view?

Courtesy of Dr. Ed Wong, Laboratory Medicine, Children's National Medical Center, Washington, DC.

cells. Manifestations of chronic hypoxia include lethargy, exercise intolerance, anorexia, headache, and bone pain. The liver enlarges as a result of hemosiderosis, and the spleen enlarges as a result of extramedullary hematopoiesis and increased hemolysis of red blood cells.

Alpha-thalassemia. The child with alpha trait is generally symptom free. Clinical manifestations of alpha-thalassemia minor are similar to those of beta-thalassemia minor. Manifestations of hemoglobin H disease are similar, though they tend to be milder, to those of beta-thalassemia major. Alpha-thalassemia major results in hydrops fetalis, intrauterine congestive heart failure (the oxygen is unable to be related to the tissues due to defective alpha chains), cardiomegaly, and hepatomegaly.

COLLABORATIVE CARE

The goal of collaborative care is to maintain normal hemoglobin levels and to prevent long-term complications associated with the disorder.

Diagnostic Tests

Diagnosis is made by hemoglobin electrophoresis, which reveals a decreased production of one of the globin chains in hemoglobin and an elevated F and A hemoglobin. A complete blood count (CBC) reveals a decreased hemoglobin, hematocrit, and reticulocyte count. Thalassemia can be detected early in infancy as characteristic erythrocyte cell changes are often recognized in infants by 6 weeks of age. Prenatal testing using chorionic villus sampling (CVS) or amniocentesis can detect or rule out thalassemia in the fetus.

A chest radiograph may be performed to evaluate heart size. MRI and CT scans may be performed to evaluate the liver. A liver biopsy may be performed to evaluate the degree of hemochromatosis.

Clinical Therapy

Treatment for thalassemia is supportive. A hypertransfusion program, in which blood transfusions are administered every 2 to 4 weeks, is the conventional therapy used to treat children with severe disease. Since iron overload is a side effect of this treatment, children may be required to receive an iron-chelating drug such as deferoxamine (Desferal), which binds excess iron so it can be excreted by the kidneys. Deferoxamine 30 to 40 mg/kg/day is infused over 8 to 12 hours during the child's sleep for 5 days each week by a mechanical pump. The medication may be administered subcutaneously or intravenously. A port provides ease of intravenous access and reduced irritation for the child. Pain, induration, and erythema are common side effects with subcutaneous infusions.

Other potential complications of long-term transfusion therapy are transfusion reactions and alloimmunization (antibody formation). A splenectomy may be required for the child with splenomegaly. Hematopoietic stem cell transplantation (HSCT) may be offered as an alternative therapy for children newly diagnosed with the disorder (Box 28–4).

Diet is normal for age and should include folic acid and ascorbic acid (vitamin C). Iron should not be administered and foods rich in iron should be avoided.

NURSING MANAGEMENT

Nursing care focuses on observing for complications of transfusion therapy, supporting the child and family in dealing with a chronic life-threatening illness, and referring the family for genetic counseling.

■ Nursing Assessment and Diagnoses

Assess for the classic manifestations which are pallor, failure to thrive, severe anemia, skin discoloration, and hepatosplenomegaly.

BOX 28–4 β-Thalassemia and Transplantation

The results of treating children with β-thalassemia by transplantation with bone marrow stem cells from family members have been successful. In a study at the University of California, San Francisco, overall survival with this treatment was 94%; those surviving without complications was 71% (Mentzer & Cowan, 2000). It is expected that collection of cord blood from siblings of affected children will increasingly be the treatment of choice (Reed, Walters, & Lubin, 2000).

CLINICAL MANIFESTATIONS of β-Thalassemia

BODY ORGANS	CLINICAL MANIFESTATIONS	CLINICAL THERAPY
Red blood cells (anemia)	Hypochromic and microcytic changes Folic acid deficiency Frequent epistaxis	Hypertransfusion program Administer folic acid and increase dietary consumption of folic acid and vitamin C
Skeletal changes	Osteoporosis Delayed growth Susceptibility to pathologic fractures Facial deformities: enlarged head, prominent forehead due to frontal and parietal bossing, prominent cheek bones, broadened and depressed bridge of nose, enlarged maxilla with protruding front teeth, eyes with mongolian slant and epicanthal fold	Assess growth and plot on chart—monitor for delays in growth Teach safety precautions to avoid fractures
Heart	Chronic congestive heart failure Myocardial fibrosis Murmurs	Monitor for signs of congestive heart failure EKG and echocardiogram may be conducted to assess heart function
Liver/gallbladder	Hepatomegaly Hepatic insufficiency	MRI or CT scans may be conducted to evaluate liver and gallbladder Liver biopsy may be performed
Spleen	Splenomegaly	MRI or CT scans may be conducted to evaluate spleen
Endocrine system	Delayed sexual maturation Fibrotic pancreas, resulting in diabetes mellitus	Assess sexual maturation using the Tanner staging
Skin	Darkening of skin	Assess for skin changes

Assess heart sounds, breath sounds, and respiratory effort. Assess for signs of infection. Assessment also includes monitoring for signs of iron overload, including abdominal pain, vomiting, bloody diarrhea, leading to shortness of breath and shock. As previously mentioned, immediate emergency treatment is required as death may result from iron overdose.

Nursing diagnoses for the child with thalassemia may include:

- Risk for Infection related to splenectomy
- Deficient Knowledge related to disease process and management
- Activity Intolerance related to anemia
- Disturbed Body Image related to discoloration of skin
- Ineffective Tissue Perfusion (all systems) related to anemia

Planning and Implementation

Care for the child with thalassemia is generally managed at home unless the child has a coexisting complication. Transfusions of packed cells are often given. Partner with the family to teach parents techniques for infusing packed cells and administration of deferoxamine to prevent iron overload.

Home care nurses may provide care to the child receiving intravenous infusions. Needles and tubing should be discarded after use and should not be reused..

Deferoxamine may be given by IV, IM, or subcutaneous routes so teaching about administration will be needed when the family administers the drug. Chronic toxicity may result from usually high doses of deferoxamine, and resulting complications include hearing loss and renal calcium loss. Blurred vision, decreased visual acuity, and night blindness may occur. Blurred vision should be immediately reported. Periodic ophthalmologic examinations are recommended. Inform parents and child that deferoxamine discolors urine to a reddish color.

If the child has undergone a splenectomy, the risk for infection is increased. Teach the parents and child infection control measures, including proper handwashing and aseptic technique for infusion. Long-term prophylactic antibiotics are generally prescribed.

Provide parents information about thalassemia and its treatment, and encourage them to obtain genetic counseling. The nurse provides emotional support to the child and parents and implement measures to assist them in coping with a chronic life-threatening illness (see Chapters 20 and 21∞).

Encourage parents to take an active role in the child's treatment regimen. Partner with the parents and child to provide opportunities for physical activities, such as swimming, that do not increase the risk of fractures. Collaborate with the family and school to establish individualized health and education plans. Discuss potential body image changes with the child and provide an opportunity for them to express their concerns. The child may require referral for counseling in helping to cope with the body image changes.

Compliance with transfusion therapy often becomes an issue as children reach adolescence. Offering the adolescent a choice regarding treatment options, such as when to undergo transfusion, can help to improve compliance. Adolescents with β-thalassemia and parents of newly diagnosed children can be referred to the Thalassemia Action Group, a national organization for patients, or to the Cooley's Anemia Foundation.

MediaLink Thalassemia Resources

Evaluation

Expected outcomes of nursing care for the child with thalassemia include:

- The child is free from infection.
- The child and family demonstrate understanding of treatment regimen and signs of potential complications.
- The child participates in age-appropriate, safe activities without experiencing fatigue.
- The child demonstrates positive body image.
- Evidence of effective tissue perfusion demonstrated.

Aplastic Anemia

Aplastic anemia is a deficiency of the blood cells that results from failure of the bone marrow to produce adequate numbers of circulating blood cells. The condition may be congenital or acquired. Aplastic anemia is more common between the ages of 15 and 25 years and is more common in the Asian population (Derivan & Ferrante, 2002).

Etiology and Pathophysiology

Bone marrow hematopoiesis failure leads to **pancytopenia** (decreased number of all blood cell components) as a result of alterations from infection, congenital condition, or toxin. The cause is unknown in 50% of all diagnosed cases (Derivan & Ferrante, 2002). The syndrome is manifested by a marked reduction in stem cells and the replacement of red bone marrow by fat.

Cogenital aplastic anemia (Fanconi anemia) is a rare autosomal recessive syndrome consisting of multiple congenital anomalies. Children with congenital aplastic anemia are at risk for developing malignancies such as acute nonlymphocytic leukemia (D'Andrea & Hord, 2004).

Acquired aplastic anemia in children can be idiopathic or occur after ingestion of medications such as sulfonamides, chloramphenicol, quinacrine, penicillamine, chemotherapeutic agents, and nonsteroidal anti-inflammatory drugs. Aplastic anemia can also develop after exposure to ionizing radiation or insecticides, benzene solvents in model airplane glue, and lead. This type of anemia can also be a result of an infectious process such as viral hepatitis, mononucleosis, cytomegalovirus, military tuberculosis, and human immunodeficiency virus.

Clinical Manifestations

Regardless of the etiology, manifestations vary depending on the degree of thrombocytopenia, anemia, and neutropenia. The most common symptom is bleeding secondary to thrombocytopenia. Platelet counts may be as low as 20,000/mm^3. Other symptoms related to thrombocytopenia include **petechiae** (pinpoint hemorrhages), **purpura** (bleeding into the tissues) (Figure 28–7 ■), weakness, bloody stools, epistaxis, retinal bleeding, and tachycardia. Symptoms associated with anemia include pallor, fatigue, tachycardia, and congestive heart failure. Symptoms related to neutropenia include fever and bacterial infections. Death can result from complications associated with hemorrhage, sepsis, and malignancy.

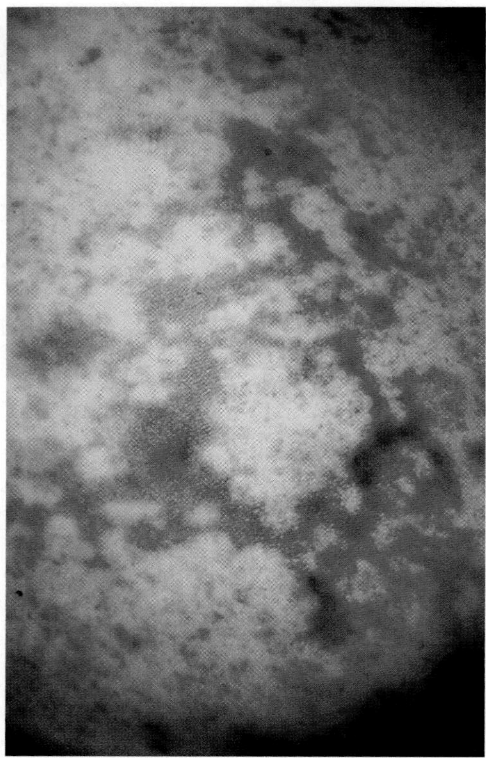

FIGURE 28–7 ■ Nonpalpable purpura with bleeding into the tissues below the skin.

Courtesy of the Department of Hematology/Oncology, Children's National Medical Center, Washington, DC.

COLLABORATIVE CARE

Management includes identifying the child with aplastic anemia; removing any causal agents and treating underlying disorder or infection; preventing complications associated with neutropenia, thrombocytopenia, and anemia; and supporting the family and child with a life-threatening illness.

Diagnostic Tests

Diagnosis is made by complete blood count studies, which reveal anemia, leukopenia with marked neutropenia, thrombocytopenia, and pancytopenia. Serum iron is elevated. Bone marrow aspiration reveals yellow, fatty bone marrow instead of red bone marrow.

Clinical Therapy

For acquired aplastic anemia, determine risk factors such as exposure to toxin or chemical, current medications, or previous viral infection, and prevent further exposure to the causal agent. Supportive treatment may include transfusions of packed cells, platelets, and granulocytes.

Because it is believed the child's immune system is reacting against the bone marrow, immunosuppressive therapy is administered to reduce the immune response, allowing the bone marrow to produce blood cells again. Immunosuppressive agents include antithymocyte globulin (ATG) and cyclosporine.

Cyclosporine may be given in combination with androgens to stimulate blood cell production (Aplastic Anemia and MDS International Foundation, 2003). Antibiotics are administered if infection is confirmed. Chelation therapy should be considered in cases of elevated iron levels. The treatment of choice is hematopoietic stem cell transplantation (HSCT) from a compatible sibling or family member donor; and survival rate is up to 90% in children.

NURSING MANAGEMENT

Nursing care is similar to care provided for the child with leukemia (see Chapter 29∞). Nursing actions focus on preventing bleeding, administering and monitoring blood transfusions, preventing infection, encouraging mobility as tolerated, educating the parents and child about the disorder, and providing emotional support. Monitor for signs and symptoms of bleeding and implement measures to protect against bleeding, such as avoiding invasive procedures and trauma. Standard precautions and transmission-based precautions are implemented for the child in the hospital setting to prevent exposure to infection.

The nurse partners with the child and family to assist the child with activities of daily living and cluster patient care to conserve energy since fatigue, poor tissue oxygenation, and weakness may be experienced. Observe for complications associated with administration of blood products, including transfusion reaction and fluid overload. For the child receiving hematopoietic stem cell transplantation, refer to the section discussing HSCT later in this chapter.

Families require support in dealing with a child who has a life-threatening disease. A collaborative approach including social services, spiritual care, and other support services offers comfort and education to families with these special needs. Assistance with both personal and social resources can help families to cope with these trying circumstances (Pelchat and Lefebvre, 2004). Expected outcomes of nursing care include maintenance of normal levels of white and red blood cells and platelets to support body functions.

CLOTTING DISORDERS

Clotting disorders, depending on the type, result in various bleeding tendencies. Some disorders are hereditary, such as hemophilia and von Willebrand disease, while others such as disseminated intravascular coagulation and idiopathic thrombocytopenic purpura, are acquired. These clotting disorders are discussed in the following section.

Hemophilia

Hemophilia refers to a group of hereditary bleeding disorders that result from a deficiency in specific clotting factors. The most common type, factor VIII deficiency (also known as hemophilia A or classic hemophilia), is caused by a deficiency of clotting factor VIII in the blood and accounts for 80% of persons with hemophilia. About 1 in 5,000 male births are affected by factor VIII deficiency (hemophilia A). Hemophilia B, also known as Christmas disease or factor IX deficiency, is caused by a deficiency of clotting factor IX. Of persons with hemophilia, 15% have hemophilia B. The severity of the disease may range from mild to severe bleeding tendencies. Hemophilia C, a deficiency in factor XI, is an autosomal recessive disease, occurring equally in males and females. The bleeding in factor XI deficiency is generally less severe than in factors VIII and IX deficiencies (Curry, 2004; Nechyba & Gunn, 2002). See Table 28–8.

Etiology and Pathophysiology

Genes for clotting factors VIII and IX are located near the terminal long arm of the X chromosome (Montgomery & Scott, 2004). Hemophilia A and B are X-linked recessive traits, which manifests almost exclusively as affected males and carrier females. A daughter who inherits the trait from her father has a 50% chance at each pregnancy of transmitting it to her sons (refer to Chapter 4∞ for a description of genetic transmission). However, as many as one third of the children affected by hemophilia do not have a family member with a history of a clotting disorder. In these cases, the disorder is caused by a new mutation.

The degree of bleeding is related to the amount of clotting factor, which is dependent upon the phase of coagulation affected, and the severity of the injury. Potential complications of hemophilia include internal hemorrhaging, transfusion reactions, shock, and death.

Clinical Manifestations

Hemophilia is manifested in different children by bleeding tendencies that range from mild to moderate or severe. Children with hemophilia often do not manifest symptoms until after 6 months of age as they become more mobile and incur injuries and bleeding from falls or from tooth eruption. Spontaneous bleeding, **hemarthrosis** (bleeding into a joint space), and deep tissue hemorrhage occur. Affected children frequently experience bleeding into the joint spaces of the knees, ankles, and elbows. Bleeding into joint spaces or bursae causes the child to have limited motion because of pain, tenderness, and swelling. Bone

TABLE 28–8 Coagulation Factors

FACTOR	SYNONYM
I	Fibrinogen
II	Prothrombin
V	AC-Globulin
VII	Prothrombin conversion accelerator
VIII	Antihemophiliac factor
IX	Christmas factor
XI	Plasma thromboplastin antecedent (PTA)
XII	Hageman factor
XIII	Fibrin-stabilizing factor (FSF)

changes, contractures, and disabling deformities can result from immobility and from the effects of blood in the joint structures.

The male infant may have excessive bleeding after circumcision. Other signs or symptoms include easy bruising (**ecchymosis**), nosebleeds, hematuria, spontaneous bleeding, and bleeding after tooth extraction, minor trauma, or minor surgical procedures. Large subcutaneous and intramuscular hemorrhages sometimes occur. Bleeding into the tissues of the neck, mouth, or chest is particularly serious because of the potential for airway obstruction. Retroperitoneal and intracranial bleeding may also occur and can be life threatening (Stover, 2000). Bleeding for these children is a lifelong problem.

Females who carry the trait for hemophilia do not usually manifest symptoms of the disease. However, they may have prolonged bleeding during dental work, surgery, or trauma.

COLLABORATIVE CARE

The goal of medical management is to control bleeding by replacing the missing clotting factor and to prevent complications associated with bleeding.

Diagnostic Tests

Diagnosis of affected children and carriers can be done before birth through chorionic villus sampling or amniocentesis. Genetic testing of family members is increasingly being used to identify carriers. Diagnosis can also be made on the basis of the history, physical examination, and laboratory data. Laboratory tests will show low levels of factor VIII or IX, and prolonged activated partial prothrombin time (APPT). Prothrombin time (PT), thrombin time (TT), fibrinogen, and platelet count are normal. See Table 28–9.

Clinical Therapy

Factor replacement therapy with cryoprecipitate is indicated when the child experiences a mild or major hemorrhage or faces a life-threatening situation. The factor replacements are cryoprecipitate, which is rich in factor VIII, and Christmas disease concentrate for factor IX deficiency. Prompt and adequate treatment is needed to prevent serious bleeding episodes and their sequelae (Stover, 2000). A synthetic drug that is effective for mild hemophilia is desmopressin acetate (DDAVP). An analog of vasopressin, DDAVP is administered intravenously and causes a two- to fourfold increase in factor VIII activity. The outlook for children with hemophilia has been greatly improved by the availability of factor (cryoprecipitate) transfusion therapy.

Transfusions started at home and early interventions prevent many disease complications. In the past, many children with factor VIII deficiency died in the first 5 years of life. Today, children with moderate or mild hemophilia can lead normal lives.

Gene therapy is being explored for treatment of hemophilia. One approach is to infuse carrier organisms into the body where they would act on target cells to promote manufacture of deficient clotting factor. These research approaches offer the promise of new treatment options in the future (White, 2001).

TABLE 28–9 Diagnostic Tests for Clotting Disorders

TEST	NORMAL VALUE	
Bleeding time	2–9 minutes	
Fibrinogen	200–500 mg/dL (5.9–14.7 μmol/L)	
Partial thromboplastin time (PTT)	42–54 seconds	
Platelet count ($\times 10^3/\mu l$)	Males	Females
Newborns	164–351	234–346
1–2 months	275–567	295–615
2–6 months	275–566	288–598
6 months–2 years	219–452	229–465
2–6 years	204–405	204–402
6–12 years	194–364	183–369
12–18 years	165–332	185–335
> 18 years	143–320	171–326
Prothrombin time (PT)	11–15 seconds	
Thrombin time (π)	12–16 seconds	

From Soldin, S. J., Brugnara, C., & Wong, E. C. (2003). Pediatric reference ranges *(4th ed.). Washington, DC: AACC Press.*

NURSING MANAGEMENT

Nursing care focuses on identifying the child with hemophilia, implementing measures to prevent or control bleeding and collaborating with child and family to reduce risk of complications associated with the disorder.

■ Nursing Assessment and Diagnosis

Nursing assessment centers on signs and symptoms that indicate bleeding, achievement of expected growth and development stages, and the child and family's coping strategies.

Physiologic Assessment

Obtain a complete medical history from the parents or child. In particular, inquire about previous episodes of bleeding and the occurrence of hemophilia or any other bleeding disorders in family members. The history of bleeding will vary depending on the severity of the disease.

PRACTICE ALERT

Take the following precautions when caring for children with bleeding disorders.

- Avoid taking temperatures rectally or giving suppositories.
- Check blood pressure by cuff as infrequently as possible.
- Avoid intramuscular or subcutaneous injections.
- Use only paper or silk tape for dressings.
- When indicated, perform mouth care every 3 hours with a glycerin swab.
- Except for factor replacement therapy, avoid all venipunctures.
- Use a peripheral fingerstick to obtain blood samples.
- Do not give aspirin.

Assess the child for any joint pain, swelling, or permanent deformity, particularly around the knees, elbows, ankles, and shoulders. Assess for pain. Note the presence of hematuria and mild flank pain. Assess skin for evidence of ecchymosis or petechia. Note that nosebleeds and oozing from intravenous access sites also indicate clotting disorders. A neurologic assessment is conducted, as the risk for intracranial hemorrhage and bleeding can lead to peripheral neuropathies.

Psychologic Assessment

It is difficult for families to manage care of the child with hemophilia, especially if the disease is severe. Assess the family's coping mechanisms and support systems. Determine the family's resources to manage procedures and treatments for the chronically ill child; the factor concentrates and infusion equipment are costly. Determine if the parents have respite care that enables them to take time for themselves while knowing that the child is cared for safely. Assess older children's understanding of the disease, limitations, and their adaptation to the disease.

Developmental Assessment

Because the child with hemophilia may have physical activity restrictions, physical skills may be delayed. Perform frequent developmental assessments, being particularly attentive to fine and gross motor skills.

The most important nursing diagnosis for the child with hemophilia is Risk for Injury related to bleeding disorder. Following are other nursing diagnoses that may apply.

- Pain related to bleeding episodes
- Risk for Injury related to excessive bleeding
- Impaired Physical Mobility related to joint stiffness or contractures
- Deficient Knowledge (child and parent) related to disease and management
- Interrupted Family Processes related to family role shift required to care for a child with a chronic illness
- Delayed Growth and Development related to effects of physical disability

■ Planning and Implementation

The goals of nursing care include preventing and controlling bleeding episodes, limiting joint involvement and managing pain, and providing emotional support to the child and family. Both short-term interventions and long-term management are necessary.

Prevent and Control Bleeding Episodes

CARE IN THE COMMUNITY

Bleeding problems are rare in infants with hemophilia. As children learn to walk and develop other motor skills, however, they often fall and suffer cuts and bruises. The risk of injury can be reduced by emphasizing to parents the need for close supervision and a safe environment. Parents should encourage children to play with toys that are safe and age appropriate. For the child learning to walk, a helmet is recommended to protect the head from injuries due to frequent falls. The home environment should be adapted to promote safety (e.g., remove rugs the child could trip over, remove or pad sharp-edged furniture).

If dental surgery or tooth extraction is necessary, it is performed in a controlled environment by experienced staff. Use of a dental irrigation device is often recommended if the child has excess bleeding from gums. Advise adolescents to shave only with an electric razor to avoid cuts.

If the child experiences a bleeding episode, control any superficial bleeding by applying pressure to the area for at least 15 minutes. Immobilize and elevate the affected area, and apply ice packs to promote vasoconstriction. If the child sustains a head, abdominal, or other major injury, immediate medical attention is required.

HOSPITAL-BASED CARE

Make the hospital environment safe for children by orienting them to the room and keeping room and floor clear. Avoid injections and monitor intravenous site for bleeding. Apply pressure for 15 minutes to lab puncture sites. A saline lock (*without* heparin flush) may be inserted to provide access for blood drawing rather than the child receiving repeated venous draws.

If significant bleeding does occur, offer supportive measures and assist with factor replacement therapy. Carefully monitor the child's condition for any side effects when factor replacement therapy is administered.

Limit Joint Involvement and Manage Pain

During bleeding episodes, hemarthrosis is managed by elevating and immobilizing the joint and applying ice packs. Analgesics are administered to promote pain relief. Once bleeding has been controlled, range of motion exercises are performed to strengthen muscles and joints and to prevent flexion contractures. Outpatient physical therapy may be required. Because excessive weight can place an added stress on joints, encourage the child to maintain an appropriate weight. Oral opioids may be required for pain relief. Refer to nursing management of sickle cell anemia pain for more information.

Provide Emotional Support

The needs of families with hemophiliac children are best met through a comprehensive partnership approach. Refer the parents for genetic counseling as soon as possible after diagnosis. Emphasize the importance to identify family members who are carriers of the trait, as they may suffer excessive bleeding during surgery.

Encourage parents to verbalize their feelings. Be understanding and sensitive to their needs. Mothers may feel guilty about having transferred the disease to the child and may require assistance in dealing with these feelings. Refer to counseling as appropriate. Partner with the family and teach the parents about hemophilia and explain how the disorder affects both the child and other family members. Refer the parents and child to organizations such as the National Hemophilia Foundation for further information. The family should also be referred for genetic counseling.

MediaLink Care Plan: A School-Age Child with Hemophilia

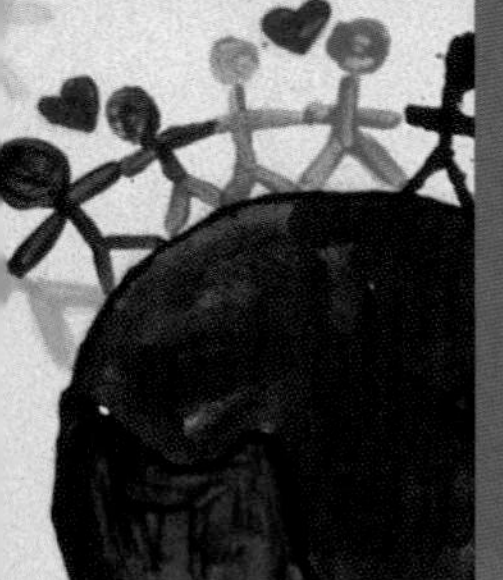

PARTNERING WITH FAMILIES

Activities and Safety

Parents of children with hemophilia may be hesitant to allow their child to participate in activities for fear of a bleeding episode. Partner with the family to assist in identifying safe activities in which the child and adolescent can participate. Encourage children with hemophilia to participate in leisure activities such as computer games, reading clubs, crafts, and social clubs such as Boy Scouts. Swimming, bicycle riding, and other noncontact sports are excellent options for the child. Knee pads, elbow pads, and helmets should always be used when participating in any physical sports. Activities important to development can be encouraged when coaches, teachers, and others know how to treat bleeding episodes.

MediaLink Hemophilia Resources

Discharge Planning and Home Care Teaching

The child may be hospitalized briefly during the first manifestation of bleeding for diagnosis and management. Most care will subsequently take place in the home. Home care needs are identified and addressed well in advance of discharge. Explain how the parents can partner with a number of health professionals to coordinate the child's care. Provide ongoing case management, assisting the family to take on this task if able.

Partner with parents and child to plan safe activities for the child to promote growth and development (see Partnering with Families: Activities and Safety). Advise parents to have the child wear a medical identification tag. Explain the cause of bleeding so both the child and parents understand the disease process. Teach the child and family how to identify internal bleeding. Signs and symptoms such as joint pain, abdominal pain, and obvious bleeding are indicators for immediate factor infusion. Make sure the child and parents know what situations could cause bleeding to occur. Head trauma can be life threatening. Review mental status changes with parents and inform them to seek immediate care for the child sustaining a head injury. Teach parents to give acetaminophen to relieve pain instead of aspirin or other nonsteroidal anti-inflammatory agents that can alter platelet activity.

Instruct the parents and the child, when appropriate, in the preparation and administration of factor concentrate (cryoprecipitate). If infusion of the missing factor is scheduled on a regular basis, bleeding episodes can be controlled or avoided. Have the parents demonstrate the procedure and make sure they can administer the product correctly. The parents need to be familiar with properties of the factor concentrate to prepare the mixture correctly. As the child advances in age, he or she can assume some of the management responsibilities of care. Partner with the child and family to assist in determining the roles the child will assume.

The child will require an individual school health plan (refer to Chapters 16 and 20∞). School personnel must be able to care for the hemophiliac child when bleeding occurs as prompt care is essential. The nurse can identify key staff members in the school and partner with them to ensure essential management actions are understood by all staff members. Members of the school staff should be instructed in management of emergencies and contact numbers for parents should be readily available. Assist the family and school to plan an appropriate schedule of activities without overprotecting the child. Children with hemophilia should not engage in contact sports such as football and soccer, which may result in injury and trauma. Instead, sports such as swimming, hiking, and bicycling are encouraged.

Hemophilia is not only a debilitating disorder for the child, but also a financial and emotional drain for the family. Frequent outpatient visits, emergency department visits, hospital admissions, and the cost of factor concentrate can exhaust a family's resources. If indicated, referral should be made to appropriate social services (e.g., the state's maternal and child health program for children with special health care needs) and organizations such as the National Hemophilia Foundation. Sharing experiences with other families of children with hemophilia can provide support.

■ Evaluation

Expected outcomes of nursing care may include the following:

- The child is free from pain.
- The child is free from injury.
- The child exhibits full joint mobility.
- The child and family demonstrate understanding of disease process and management.
- The family demonstrates positive adaptation to role of caring for chronically ill child.
- The child achieves growth and development milestones appropriate for age.

Von Willebrand Disease

Like hemophilia, von Willebrand disease is a hereditary bleeding disorder. There are approximately 20 different disorders involving a deficiency of von Willebrand factor (vWF), which is a plasma protein and the carrier for clotting factor VIII, thereby playing a necessary role in platelet adhesion (McDaniel, 2000). The most common form of the disorder is transmitted as an autosomal dominant trait, and the disease can occur in both males and females. The gene for the disease is located on chromosome 12.

Normally, vWF concentration increases in the area of an injury and binds to platelets to facilitate their binding to the damaged vessel wall. With von Willebrand disease, the vWF is not sufficient in quantity or is dysfunctional, therefore clot forming and bleeding control is impaired.

The three types of von Willebrand disease and their characteristics are as follows:

• Type I	Decreased amount of normal vWF
• Type II	Presence of abnormal vWF
• Type III	Near complete absence of vWF

The characteristic manifestations are easy bruising and epistaxis. Children with von Willebrand disease frequently have gingival bleeding, epistaxis, ecchymosis, and increased bleeding with lacerations or during surgery and dental extractions. Fortunately, children with von Willebrand disease usually do not experience spontaneous hemarthrosis as experienced by children with hemophilia. Affected teenage girls may have menorrhagia (increased menstrual bleeding). Gastrointestinal bleeding may also occur.

Because the manifestations are generally mild, children with this disorder remain undiagnosed until an excessive bleeding episode occurs, such as following dental procedures or surgery.

Collaborative Care

Management focuses on identifying the child with von Willebrand disease, restoring clotting function, and preventing complications associated with bleeding.

Diagnosis of von Willebrand disease is made after laboratory studies reveal decreased von Willebrand factor levels, von Willebrand factor antigen levels, and factor VIII activity; reduced platelet agglutination; prolonged bleeding time; and prolonged or normal activated partial thromboplastin time (APPT).

Treatment is similar to that for the child with hemophilia and involves infusion of von Willebrand protein concentrate. Desmopressin (DDAVP) is administered to promote release of stored vWF (see DDAVP administration as discussed in hemophilia section) and to prevent bleeding associated with dental or surgical procedures. Locally administered medications such as aminocaproic acid are sometimes used to manage bleeding in the mucous membranes.

Nursing Management

Nursing care is the same for a child with hemophilia (refer to previous discussion). Teach parents about the disorder and instruct them not to give the child aspirin or other drugs that can cause bleeding or inhibit platelet function. Teach management of bleeding episodes and intravenous infusion techniques which are the same as for hemophilia. The prognosis is good, and children with von Willebrand disease usually have a normal life expectancy. Expected outcomes of nursing care include prompt management of bleeding and prevention of disease complications.

Disseminated Intravascular Coagulation

Disseminated intravascular coagulation (DIC) is a life-threatening process which occurs as complication of other serious illnesses in infants and children, such as hypoxia, shock, trauma, burns, liver disease, necrotizing enterocolitis, cancer, and viruses.

Etiology and Pathophysiology

The most common cause of DIC is infection. Other causes include trauma, burns, hemolysis, fat embolism, hemolytic uremic syndrome, and blood transfusions. DIC is an acquired pathologic process in which the clotting system is abnormally activated, resulting in widespread clot formation in the small vessels throughout the body. The disorder results from increased protease activity which is caused by unregulated release of thrombin. Excess thrombin is generated, followed by deposition of fibrin strands in body tissues. These changes slow the circulating blood and cause tissue hypoxia, resulting in eventual tissue necrosis. The circulating fibrin fragments later begin to interfere with platelet aggregation and other aspects of the clotting mechanism, resulting in bleeding or hemorrhage.

The sequence of events for DIC is as follows (LeMone & Burke, 2004):

1. Widespread formation of tiny blood clots occurs within the microcirculation of all body organs.
2. The fibrinolytic pathway is activated, promoting the dissolution of the clots that have been formed.
3. The amount of thrombin that enters the systemic circulation greatly exceeds that of clotting inhibitors to regulate it.
4. The deposit of thrombin decreases blood flow to organs, which may eventually cause tissue ischemia, infarction, and necrosis.
5. The excessive amounts of thrombin also activate platelet aggregation—causing thrombocytopenia with an increased risk of bleeding—and the fibrinolytic pathway (causing bleeding).
6. Plasma begins to break down fibrin before a stable clot is formed.
7. Fibrin degradation products, which are potent anticoagulants, are released and further increase bleeding.
8. Clotting factors are depleted, the ability to form clots is lost, and hemorrhage occurs.

Clinical Manifestations

The clinical manifestations of DIC result from bleeding and clotting disorders. The manifestations range from minor oozing to hemorrhage (see page 1028).

COLLABORATIVE CARE

Treatment of DIC focuses on controlling bleeding, identifying and correcting the primary cause of the disorder, and preventing further activation of clotting mechanisms.

Diagnostic Tests

The prothrombin time and partial thromboplastin time are prolonged, platelet count and fibrinogen levels are decreased, and levels of fibrin–fibrinogen split products are high.

Clinical Therapy

Management is supportive and includes identification and treatment of the underlying disorder; administering fluids, replacement of depleted coagulation factors by administering fresh frozen plasma, fibrinogen, and platelets. Heparin, although controversial since there are no documented clinical research studies utilizing heparin as a treatment modality for DIC, may be used in some cases to interrupt the clotting cascade and stop the cycle. Oxygen should be administered, and pulse oximetry oxygen saturation and arterial blood gases are monitored.

CLINICAL MANIFESTATIONS of Disseminated Intravascular Coagulation

ETIOLOGY	CLINICAL MANIFESTATIONS	CLINICAL THERAPY
Cardiovascular System Tachycardia Hypotension Circulatory collapse Major vessel thrombosis	Decreased perfusion, shock Inappropriate clotting	Administer fluids as ordered; monitor intake and output Monitor vital signs
Respiratory System Tachypnea Decreased breath sounds	Impaired gas exchange due to microclots in the pulmonary vasculature	Monitor respiratory status Maintain ventilatory support if required
Central Nervous System Confusion Coma Seizures	Impaired cerebral perfusion	Conduct neurologic assessment every 2 hours during critical period, then every 4 hours until stabilized
Urinary System Oliguria Anuria Renal failure Hematuria	Impaired renal perfusion Impaired clotting mechanisms lead to bleeding	Monitor urine output hourly Maintain patent urinary catheter Monitor urine for blood
Gastrointestinal System Gastrointestinal bleeding Abdominal distention Bleeding from mucous membranes Occult blood in stool or emesis	Impaired clotting mechanisms lead to bleeding	Monitor for occult blood in stools and emesis Monitor for overt signs of bleeding from gums Measure abdominal girth every 4 hours
Integumentary System Petechiae Purpura Ecchymosis Bleeding or oozing from wounds or intravenous access site Pallor Cool extremities Cyanosis of extremities Gangrene	Impaired clotting mechanism leads to bleeding Impaired tissue perfusion	Monitor skin for evidence of bleeding Protect from injury Monitor distal pulses, temperature, and capillary refill
General: weakness, malaise Oozing from body orifices	Shock, decreased perfusion Impaired clotting mechanism lead to bleeding	Cluster care to allow for rest periods Maintain bed rest

NURSING MANAGEMENT

DIC is a complex disorder that is managed by a critical care team. Nursing care focuses on assessing for bleeding, preventing further injury, and administering prescribed therapies.

Nursing Assessment and Diagnosis

Because all body systems can be involved, careful assessment of all systems is needed on a continual basis. Observe for petechiae, ecchymoses, and oozing every 1 to 2 hours. Careful monitoring of dependent areas is essential, as blood will pool in these locations. Intravenous sites are particularly prone to oozing and should be assessed every 15 minutes. Examine stool for the presence of blood, and measure blood loss as accurately as possible. Assess extremities for capillary refill, warmth, and pulses. Frequently assess vital signs and level of consciousness. Assess intake and output. Monitor urine for presence of blood. BUN and creatinine are monitored to assess renal function.

Nursing diagnoses for the child with disseminated intravascular coagulation may include:

- Ineffective Tissue Perfusion to all body systems
- Impaired Gas Exchange related to decreased perfusion
- Impaired Skin Integrity related to bleeding
- Fear (parental) related to critically ill child

Planning and Implementation

The child with DIC requires critical care nursing. Institute bleeding control precautions and monitor for signs of bleeding (oozing from intravenous sites, orifices). Administer replacement therapy of blood products as prescribed. Monitor vital signs frequently and report any signs of complications. Monitor for signs of shock.

Monitor oxygen saturations and arterial blood gases. The child may require mechanical ventilation. Maintain patency of airway and implement safety measures to preserve endotracheal tube position.

Implement measures to maintain skin integrity, such as repositioning gently and avoiding the use of adhesive tape. Implement feeding plan as prescribed (tube feedings, TPN). Identify the family's coping strategies and support system to facilitate their ability to manage this crisis.

■ Evaluation

Expected outcomes of nursing care for the child with DIC may include:

- The child demonstrates adequate functioning and perfusion of all body systems.
- The child demonstrates adequate gas exchange.
- The child's skin integrity remains intact.
- The family effectively copes with the child's life-threatening illness and fear is reduced.

Idiopathic Thrombocytopenic Purpura

Idiopathic thrombocytopenic purpura (ITP), also known as autoimmune thrombocytopenic purpura, is a disorder characterized by increased destruction of platelets in the spleen, even though platelet production in the bone marrow is normal.

Platelets are destroyed as a result of the binding of autoantibodies to platelet antigens. When the rate of platelet destruction exceeds the rate of platelet production, the number of circulating platelets decreases and blood clotting slows.

ITP is the most common bleeding disorder in children. It occurs most frequently in children 2 to 10 years of age, with peaks between ages 2 and 5 years of age. The disorder occurs equally in males and females, and is seen more often in Caucasian children than other races. The disorder usually follows a viral infection such as measles, chickenpox, or rubella, as part of an inappropriate immune response (Bolton-Maggs, 2000). Symptoms include multiple ecchymoses, petechiae, and purpura (purplish areas where blood has collected due to bleeding from blood vessels); bleeding from gums, nosebleeds, blood in urine, and blood in stools. At least half of the children affected will have complete remission (Jayabose, Levendoglu-Tugal, & Ozkaynkak, et al., 2004).

Collaborative Care

Management of idiopathic thrombocytopenic purpura focuses on identifying the disorder, preventing bleeding and associated complications, and restoring platelet count.

Diagnosis is made by history and through physical and laboratory findings, which reveal a decreased platelet count (< 20,000–30,000 mm^3/dL) and antiplatelet antibodies in the peripheral blood. Antinuclear antibodies may be present, and direct and indirect Coombs' test may be performed to detect the presence of antibodies. Bone marrow aspiration may be considered to rule out leukemia (Yetman, 2003; Kuhne, Buchanan, & Zimmerman et al., 2003). Red and white blood cell counts are normal in ITP.

Treatment is dependent on the platelet count and clinical presentation. Corticosteroids, generally prednisone or methylprednisolone, are administered for platelet counts less than 50,000 mm^3/dL. Children presenting with platelet counts less than 20,000 mm^3/dL and present with minor purpura are administered intravenous immune globulin (IVIG) (Fischer, 2003). Platelet administration is not usually indicated unless hemorrhaging occurs. For those children who do not respond to drug therapy over a period of 6 months to 1 year, splenectomy may be the treatment of choice since the platelets are destroyed in the spleen. Spontaneous remission is seen in 90% of children with ITP.

Nursing Management

Nursing care focuses on controlling and reducing the number of bleeding episodes. Assess vital sign and level of consciousness. Assess for evidence of bleeding, including petechiae and purpura. The abdomen is assessed for hepatosplenomegaly. Monitor for nosebleeds, oozing at intravenous sites, gastrointestinal bleeding, and indications of intracranial bleeding. Signs of intracranial bleeding include vomiting and seizures.

Preventive measures are similar to those for the child with hemophilia. Teach parents to use acetaminophen, rather than aspirin or other drugs that influence bleeding times, to control pain. The child should avoid contact sports and other activities that may increase risk of injury. Ensure that the family and child are aware of the signs and symptoms indicating bleeding, including signs of intracranial bleeding. Refer to Table 33–1∞ for signs of intracranial bleeding.

Expected outcomes of nursing care are prevention or control of bleeding and restoration of normal coagulation patterns.

Meningococcemia

Meningococcemia is the most severe disease process that follows infection with *Neisseria meningitidis*. This infection is thought to be an immune response to the endotoxins of the organism. Approximately 60% to 90% of the cases of meningococcemia occur in children, and most are less than 4 months old. The disease is particularly devastating due to its rapid progression. Mortality rates for this disease are 17% to 60% and are almost 100% in children who have shock and are comatose (Smillova & Walker, 2000).

Etiology and Pathophysiology

N. meningitidis is transmitted through airborne droplets and close contact. The incubation period is less than 10 days from initial contact to dissemination into the bloodstream (Smillova & Walker, 2000). In meningococcemia, the bacteria are located primarily in the systemic circulation. This gram-negative sepsis leads to clinical shock. The bacteria multiply and release an endotoxin (lipopolysaccharide), and this endotoxin triggers other events such as altered immune response, DIC, and circulatory collapse (Smillova & Walker, 2000). Endotoxins from the bacteria are thought to impair protein C, which causes thrombosis formation.

Clinical Manifestations

Onset of manifestations is sudden. Often, a respiratory infection is followed by high fever, petechial rash, massive skin and mucosal hemorrhage, hypotension, disseminated intravascular coagulation, and shock. Vomiting, abdominal pain, headache, lethargy, and myalgia may also be noted (Smillova & Walker, 2000). The child, usually under 2 years of age, is critically ill and demonstrates multisystem disease. Symptoms can progress to a critical level within 12 to 48 hours of onset. Coagulopathy, microvascular thrombosis, and secondary hemorrhages may occur. Pulmonary edema occurs secondary to capillary leakage, therefore respiratory effort is increased. Ischemia of the digits and limbs may occur secondary to decreased cardiac output, microthrombi, vasoconstriction, and DIC. Impaired circulation to the limbs may result in gangrene and amputation.

COLLABORATIVE CARE

Care is focused on identifying the disease without delay in order to improve outcome since the mortality rate for meningococcemia is high, particularly when there is a delay in treatment. Treatment includes antibiotics, fluid volume replacement, and management of complications such as DIC and shock.

Diagnostic Tests

Blood cultures reveal *N. meningitidis*, a gram-negative organism. The bacteria or antigens may also be found in cerebrospinal fluid, urine, scrapings from nodular lesions, and joints (Smillova & Walker, 2000). Other findings may include the presence of other pathogens and idiopathic thrombocytopenia. A lumbar puncture is performed to determine the presence of organisms in the cerebrospinal fluid.

Clinical Therapy

Respiratory isolation is implemented to prevent spread of infection. Treatment consists of antibiotics such as penicillin or third-generation cephalosporin, removal from sources of infection, and multisystem shock management. (See Chapter 26∞ for a description of distributive shock.) Prompt administration of antibiotics to the child who manifests fever with purpura can decrease the severity of outcome. Fluid volume replacement is essential to support blood pressure and correct hypovolemic shock. For the child in septic shock, an arterial catheter is inserted for constant monitoring of blood pressure, and a pulmonary artery catheter may be considered to monitor fluid volume status. Inotropic agents are administered for hypotension and to decrease vascular resistance in vital organs (Smillova & Walker, 2000).

DIC is managed with cryoprecipitate, fresh frozen plasma, platelets, and vitamin K (refer to previous section on DIC management). Depending on the child's condition, total parenteral nutrition, sedation and pain relief, dialysis, or amputation may be required. Close contacts of the child should receive prophylactic antibiotics immediately and should be monitored closely for fever or other signs and symptoms of developing infection. Children may receive high-pressure oxygen therapy via hyperbaric chamber to assist in perfusion of affected tissues.

NURSING MANAGEMENT

Nursing care of the child with meningococcemia is complex. Treatment must begin quickly and the child generally has a lengthy hospitalization in a pediatric intensive care unit followed by years of care that may involve plastic surgery or prosthetic adaptation.

■ Nursing Assessment and Diagnosis

Thorough assessments of all body systems are performed. Ongoing assessment of vital signs is essential. Continually assess for changes in level of consciousness. Urinary output is measured to evaluate renal function. Assess for alterations in tissue perfusion by noting cold extremities and circumoral cyanosis. Assess oxygen saturation levels and arterial blood gas values as performed. Assess for indications of seizure activity.

Appropriate diagnoses for the child with meningococcemia may include:

- Ineffective Tissue Perfusion (all systems) related to shock
- Deficient Fluid Volume related to hypovolemia
- Parental Anxiety related to critically ill child
- Risk for Injury related to seizures
- Disturbed Body Image (if amputation is required)

■ Planning and Implementation

Meningococcal vaccine can prevent some cases of the disease. The vaccine is recommended for college students and other select groups (see Chapter 19∞) Nursing care centers on managing fluids, maintaining respiratory support, administration of medications, and monitoring for complications associated with meningococcemia. Intravenous infusions must be administered when ordered to ensure correct and timely administration of fluids, antibiotics, and other therapies such as vasopressive agents. Meticulous skin care is necessary to preserve the integrity of tissues. Implement measures to prevent further infections. Nutritional support in the form of total parenteral nutrition is common. Maintain ventilatory support and arterial lines if they are present. Implement safety precautions for seizures (refer to nursing care of seizures in Chapter 33∞), include padding on crib or side rails and suction equipment at bedside. Assist with wound care debridement as required. Maintain sterile technique.

The nurse offers the family support to deal with the changing critical nature of the child's illness and the possibility that death or permanent, severe deformities will result. When the child improves, continuing comprehensive care in the hospital and then in the community is needed to manage complex issues related growth, development, nutrition, amputations, and prosthetics. Refer to Chapter 33∞ for nursing care of the child with meningitis.

■ Evaluation

Expected outcomes of nursing care for the child with meningococcemia include:

- The child demonstrates adequate tissue perfusion to all systems.
- Fluid balance is restored.
- The family verbalizes fear and anxiety and receives appropriate support.
- The child is free from injury.
- The child demonstrates a positive body image.

HEMATOPOIETIC STEM CELL TRANSPLANTATION (HSCT)

Hematopoietic stem cell transplantation (previously referred to as bone marrow transplantation) is a treatment used for diseases such as severe combined immunodeficiency disease, severe and unresponsive aplastic anemia, and leukemia (refer to Chapters 27 and 29∞). Sources of stem cells now include bone marrow, peripheral blood, and cord blood. Hematopoietic stem cells exist primarily in the bone marrow but also circulate in the peripheral blood. These cells can grow into new body cells, and have become useful in treatment of immune and hematologic diseases when restoration of normal cells is needed. Stem cells can be obtained from bone marrow, cord blood, or peripheral blood and frozen for later use (Trigg, 2004).

COLLABORATIVE CARE

The three types of hematopoietic stem cell transplants are autologous, isogeneic (or syngeneic), and allogeneic. In **autologous transplantation,** the child's own marrow is taken, treated, stored, and reinfused after the child has received chemotherapy. In **isogeneic transplantation,** the marrow is taken from a genetically identical twin. In **allogeneic transplantation,** the donor, often a sibling, has a compatible human leukocyte antigen (HLA). Human leukocyte antigens are proteins found on the surface of nearly all nucleated cells within the body, and they are responsible for regulating the immune response. When no relative is found to match the child, a histocompatible donor may be sought from the National Marrow Donor Program. With the development of this registry, bone marrow transplantation from HLA-matched unrelated donors has become possible for some children.

Clinical Therapy

Pretransplant Phase. After a thorough evaluation of the child, including HLA typing, evaluation of organ functions, and laboratory studies, the child will begin receiving high doses of chemotherapy and, sometimes, total body irradiation directed at destroying circulating blood cells and the diseased bone marrow in the ill child. Common chemotherapeutic agents used include cyclophosphamide, busulfan, cytarabine, carmustine, iotepa, and lomustine (Ryan, Kristovich, & Haugen, et al. 2002). The chemotherapy program for destruction of bone marrow ranges from 4 to 12 days. During this time, the child is cared for in strict isolation in a special unit that provides a negative pressure environment (Figure 28–8 ■). Side effects of chemotherapy provide challenges for care in addition to those of preventing infection (refer to Chapter 29∞). The child is without immunity for a minimum of 10 days after transplantation. It is of critical importance that the immunocompromised child be placed in protective isolation and strict measures implemented to prevent transmission of infection. Precautionary measures may include irradiating food and sterilizing utensils and other items the child uses.

MediaLink National Marrow Donor Program

Transplant Phase. Following the immunosuppression procedure, the child receives an intravenous transfusion with the donor stem cells. This procedure is similar to administration of a blood product. The healthy stem cells migrate to the bone marrow. Healthy bone marrow, capable of making blood cells, is the anticipated result. If the transplantation is successful, the cells implant in the bone and begin to grow. The transplanted and implanted cells in the marrow start producing hematopoietic blood cells in approximately 2 to 4 weeks.

Posttransplant Phase. Pancytopenia (marked decrease in RBCs, WBCs, and platelets) lasts for several weeks following the transplantation. The major risks during this period are infection, anemia, and bleeding. Transfusion of red blood cells

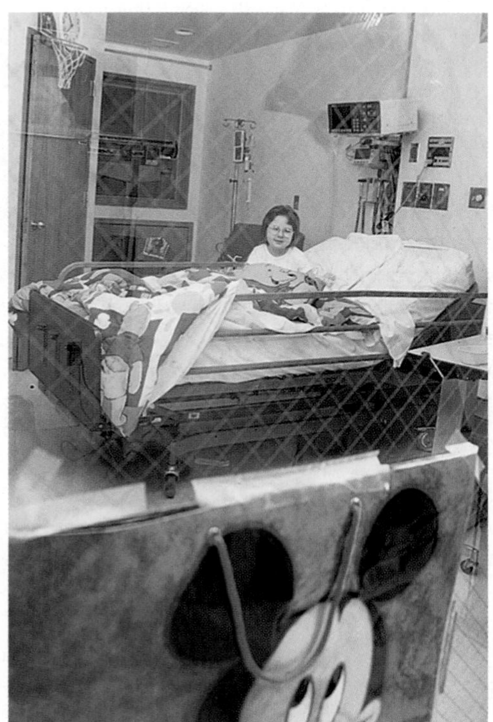

FIGURE 28–8 ■ The child undergoing bone marrow transplantation is hospitalized in a special sterile unit while receiving chemotherapy before the transfusion. The child remains in the unit for several weeks afterward until the new marrow produces enough cells to maintain health.

Health Promotion & Maintenance Overview

The Child with Hematopoietic Stem Cell Transplantation (HSCT)

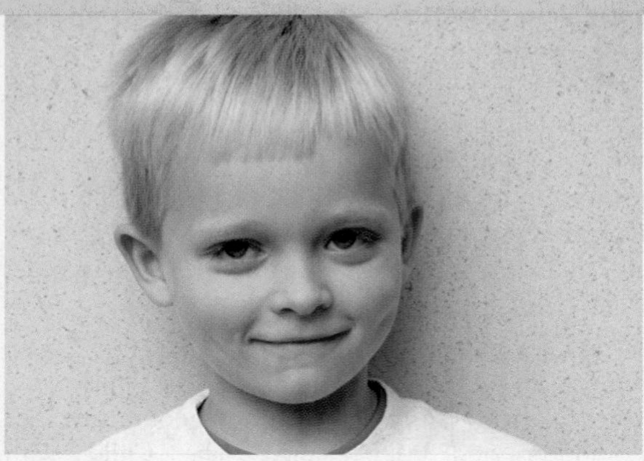

Growth and Development

- Measure and plot height and weight at each visit using standard growth curve charts.
- Measure onset and progression of puberty using Tanner staging.
- An individualized education plan (IEP) should be performed yearly to identify learning problems.
- Routine hearing screening is advised since hearing loss may occur as a result of ototoxic drug therapy.
- Vision should be screened at each primary care visit since corticosteroid use can cause cataracts, cGVHD can result in keratoconjunctivitis, and cytomegalovirus (CMV) can cause retinitis.
- Blood pressure should be monitored each visit since children are commonly placed on medication for hypertension after HSCT because of nephrotoxic medications.
- Instruct parents to record blood pressure at home if necessary.

Nutrition

- Teach family to avoid foods with potential vectors for infection, such as unpasteurized products and undercooked meats.
- A low-sodium diet may be required if the child has hypertension.
- Calcium supplements may be administered to reduce the risk of osteopenia.

Physical Activity

- If the child has thrombocytopenia, physical activity may be restricted.
- The child may experience fatigue. Ask about activity tolerance.

Oral Health

- Dental screening and any required restorative care should be done before transplant to reduce potential sources of infection.
- Routine dental care is resumed once the child's immune system is restored. Ask the family about the child's routine dental care.

Mental and Spiritual Health

- Apply developmental approaches to assess the child's feelings after a HSCT.
- Ask the child about coping with being in the hospital and at home rather than attending school.
- Many physical changes occur with treatment that may interfere with body image. Assess the child's or adolescent's body image in a manner appropriate to age.

Relationships

- In-hospital or in-home schooling is required after HSCT for 6 to 12 months until immune function has been obtained to reduce the risk of infection.
- Encourage peer contact, telephone calls, e-mail, and letters to reduce the child's feelings of isolation.
- On returning to school, the child is encouraged to participate fully in school activities.
- For the adolescent, sex education is important, especially to avoid sexually transmitted infections.

Disease Prevention Strategies

- Teach the family that handwashing is essential to prevent the spread of infection.
- The child should have his or her own eating utensils. Teach safe food preparation techniques.
- In-home childcare is recommended because of the risk of infection in other childcare settings.
- Teach the family that the child should have minimal direct contact with animals to avoid infections.
- Determine the child's immunization schedule and the need for immunizations.
- Encourage the family to obtain an influenza vaccine annually for the child and all household or close contacts.
- Teach signs and symptoms of infection and stress the importance of prompt reporting.

Injury Prevention Strategies

- Ask the family how they store medications.
- Ask the family how they dispose of used needles and syringes.

and platelets may be required. The child's illness and the side effects related to the chemotherapy may alter nutritional status. Total parenteral nutrition (TPN) may be implemented to meet the child's nutritional needs during this period.

Except for children receiving syngeneic transplants, immunosuppressive agents are administered to prevent graft-versus-host disease. Once the bone marrow begins to produce new cells, graft-versus-host disease (rejection) is the major threat. Refer to Chapter 27∞ for a discussion of this disease.

NURSING MANAGEMENT

Supportive care after the transplantation procedure focuses on preventing infection, controlling bleeding, maintaining adequate nutrition and hydration, monitoring for signs of rejection, and providing psychosocial support.

Nursing Assessment and Diagnosis

Monitor for this multisystem disorder by assessing the skin, mucous membranes, gastrointestinal function, respiratory function, cardiac function, and hydration status. Because graft-versus-host disease may occur at any time, even after the child returns home, frequent thorough assessments are necessary after discharge. Refer to Chapter 27∞ for a discussion of graft-versus-host disease.

Nursing diagnoses that apply to the child undergoing HSCT include:

- Risk for Infection related to immunocompromised state
- Anxiety (parental and child) related to procedures
- Risk for Delayed Growth and Development related to lengthy hospitalization and illness
- Social Isolation related to isolation procedures

Planning and Implementation

The treatment is lengthy, the child is often critically ill, and parents may have traveled to a medical center many miles from home for the procedure. Ask parents about other family members and how they are managing. Provide information about inexpensive housing available near the medical center, such as in a Ronald McDonald house. Encourage parents to discuss their feelings with other parents of children receiving bone marrow transplantation. Organizations such as the Bone Marrow Transplant Family Support Network can serve as resources for families.

Because hospitalizations of children undergoing bone marrow transplantation are usually lengthy, the child experience interruptions in developmental achievements. Evaluate the child's age and developmental stage and establish developmental goals to be met during the hospitalization. Implement nursing plans to meet the child's developmental needs and encourage further growth. When the child is ready for discharge, be sure the family is prepared to administer medications, recognize signs of graft-versus-host disease, provide adequate nutrition for the child, and perform other necessary care. Partner with the family to arrange for follow-up visits and provide the names of local healthcare contact persons who can offer support and provide information. Homebound schooling, if available, should be recommended since the child may be unable to return to school for several months following the transplant. The child may require assistance to promote integration back into the school setting. See Health Promotion and Maintenance: The Child with Hematopoietic Stem Cell Transplantation on page 1032.

Evaluation

The major expected outcome of nursing care is that the child remains free from infection.

Other desired outcomes include:

- The family and child verbalize their anxiety and receive adequate support.
- The child achieves growth and development milestones appropriate for age.
- The child does not experience social isolation and has appropriate interaction and contact with family and peers.

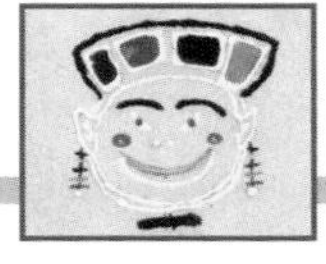

CHAPTER HIGHLIGHTS

- Erythrocytes (red cells) are a major component of the blood and transport oxygen from the lungs to body tissues.
- Polycythemia is an increase in the number of red blood cells and anemia characterized by a decrease in red blood cell number. Leukocytes (white cells) are important in the cell's defenses against disease.
- Thrombocytes (platelets) are necessary for normal clotting of blood.
- The major anemias of childhood include iron deficiency anemia, thalassemia, aplastic anemia, normocytic anemia, and sickle cell anemia.
- Sickle cell anemia is a genetic disease in which an abnormal shape, or sickling of red blood cells, prevents the normal flow of blood.
- Major complications of sickle cell anemia include pain, strokes, retinopathy, enlarged liver and spleen, urinary complications, poor peripheral blood flow, and osteoporosis.
- Nurses assist families in dealing with chronic diseases such as sickle cell anemia by providing information about the disorder and resources that can provide assistance, monitoring child growth and development, instituting preventive care, and managing exacerbations of the disease.
- Hereditary spherocytosis, also known as congenital hemolytic anemia, is an autosomal dominant disorder caused by an abnormality of proteins by an unknown cause. The cells have an usual characteristic cell structure and become sequestered and hemolyzed in the spleen.
- The thalassemias are a group of genetic diseases of red blood cells, which cause defective synthesis of hemoglobin.
- Aplastic anemia is a deficiency of all blood cells related to poor bone marrow function; it can be congenital or acquired after exposure to certain drugs or harmful environmental toxins.
- Hemophilia is a bleeding disorder transmitted by genes; hemophilia A is most common and results in a decrease in clotting factor VIII.
- The goal of treatment for hemophilia is to control bleeding by preventive care and replacement of the missing factor.
- Major nursing concerns for the child with hemophilia include managing bleeding episodes, controlling pain during bleeds, minimizing physical immobility, supporting the family in learning management of this chronic disease, and explaining genetic implications of the disease.

- Disseminated intravascular coagulation is a serious condition in which clotting mechanisms are disturbed, leading to extensive clotting and tissue damage.
- Idiopathic thrombocytopenic purpura causes destruction of platelets and most frequently follows a childhood viral disease.
- Management of idiopathic thrombocytopenic purpura includes corticosteroids and immunoglobulins since the disease is considered to be autoimmune in nature.
- Occasionally, infection with organisms such as *Neisseria meningitidis* or *Streptococcus pneumoniae* is followed by a severe systemic disease known as meningococcemia.
- Meningococcemia is manifested by sudden high fever, rash, skin and mucosal hemorrhage, and shock; prompt treatment with antibiotics is needed.
- Hematopoietic stem cell transplant (HSCT) is a useful treatment in some diseases of the hematologic system and some cancers; it involves infusion of bone marrow, peripheral stem cells, or neonatal stem cells from a donor into the blood of the recipient where it circulates, implants into the bone marrow, and begins making new blood cells.
- Nursing care before and after HSCT includes infection prevention, careful physical assessment, administration of medications, and support for the family.

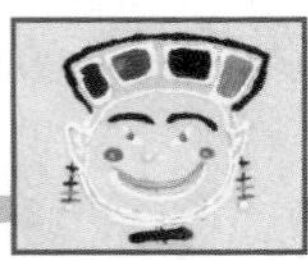

CRITICAL THINKING IN ACTION

INTRODUCTION

Recall Michael, the child in the opening scenario who is admitted with sickle cell crisis. Michael is receiving intravenous and oral fluids, oxygen, and opioids via a patient-controlled analgesia (PCA) pump. His hemoglobin on admit was 7.7 g/dL, hematocrit was 22%. His WBC on admit was elevated at 22,000. Michael's father has returned to work and he visits in the evenings. Michael's mother remains at the hospital with her son.

DESCRIPTION

Two days after Michael's admission, he requires less pain medication and has longer periods of time between doses. He acknowledges achieving adequate pain relief, though he still "aches" all over. His respirations, heart rate, and blood pressure are all within Michael's normal baseline. Michael's WBC count is dropping after receiving intravenous antibiotics.

DISCUSSION

1. Considering Michael's diagnosis, what immediate care does he require while hospitalized? What additional immediate care will Michael require at home?
2. What long-term care will Michael require at home? What considerations are necessary for school?
3. As Michael approaches adolescence, what developmental issues will he face with this disease? What issues may Michael face regarding body image, self-esteem, and sexuality? What health promotion strategies should be implemented to assist Michael through adolescence?
4. Considering Michaels's age and developmental stage, what specific communication techniques will the nurse implement when teaching him about this disease?
5. What are the expected outcomes related to the teaching plan for Michael and his family?

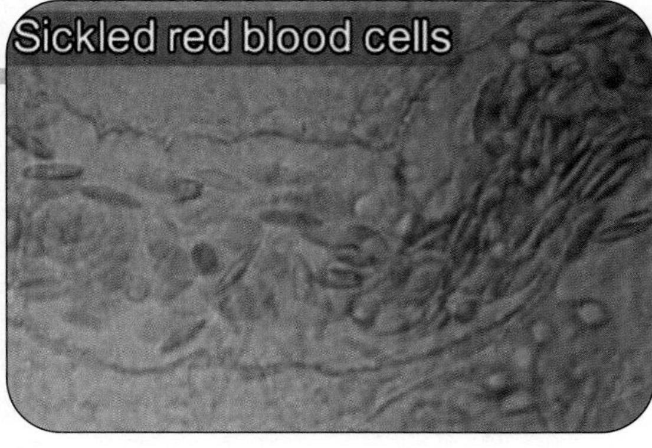

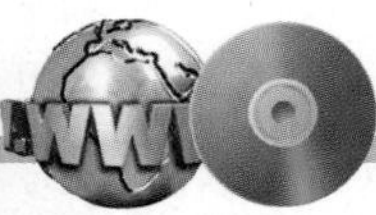

EXPLORE MediaLink

- NCLEX review, case studies, and other interactive resources for this chapter can be found on the Companion Website at **www.prenhall.com/ball**. Click on Chapter 28 to select the activities for this chapter.
- For animations, more NCLEX review questions, and an audio glossary, access the accompanying CD-ROM in this book.

http://www.prenhall.com/ball

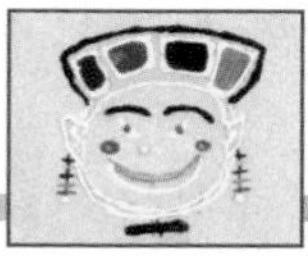

REFERENCES

American Academy of Pediatrics. (2000). *Guidelines for health supervision III.* Elk Grove Village, IL: American Academy of Pediatrics.

American Academy of Pediatrics. (2004). Clinical Practice Guidelines. Management of hyperbilirubinemia in the newborn infant 35 or more weeks of gestation Subcommittee on Hyperbilirubinemia. *Pediatrics, 114,* 297–316.

Aplastic Anemia and MDS International Foundation. 2003. www.aplastic.org/pdfs/ACQUIRED-APLASTIC-ANEMIA-BASIC-EXPLANATIONS.pdf, accessed 6/1/2004.

Beyer, J. E., & Simmons, L. E. (2004). Home treatment of pain for children and adolescents with sickle cell disease. *Pain Management Nursing 5,* 126–135.

Bhutani, V. K., & Johnson, L. H. (2004). Urgent clinical need for accurate and precise bilirubin measurements in the United States to prevent kernicterus. *Clinical Chemistry, 50,* 477–480.

Blackwell, J. T. (2003). Management of hyperbilirubinemia in the healthy term newborn. *Journal of American Academy of Nurse Practitioners, 15,* 194–198.

Bolton-Maggs, P. H. B. (2004). Idiopathic thrombocytopenic purpura. *Archives of Disease in Childhood, 83,* 220–223.

Boxer, L. A. (2004). Leukopenia. In R. E. Behrman, R. M. Kliegman, & H. B. Jenson (Eds.), *Nelson textbook of pediatrics* (17th ed., pp. 717–723). Philadelphia: WB Saunders.

Carley, A. (2003). Anemia: When is it iron deficiency? *Pediatric Nursing, 29,* 128–133.

Committee on Nutrition, American Academy of Pediatrics. (2004). *Pediatric nutrition handbook* (5th ed.). Elk Grove Village, IL: American Academy of Pediatrics.

Cook, L. S. (2000). A simple case of anemia: Pathophysiology of a common symptom. *Journal of Intravenous Nursing, 23,* 271–281.

Curry, Heather. (2004). Bleeding disorder basics. *Pediatric Nursing, 30,* 402–429.

D'Andrea, A. D., & Hord, J. D. (2004). The pancytopenias. In R. E. Behrman, R. M. Kliegman, & H. B. Jenson (Eds.), *Nelson textbook of pediatrics* (17th ed., pp. 1642–1646). Philadelphia: WB Saunders.

Day, S. W., & Wynn, L. W. (2000). Sickle cell pain & hydroxyurea. *American Journal of Nursing 100,* 32–38.

Derivan, M., & Ferrante, C. (2000). Aplastic anemia. *Clinical Journal of Oncology Nursing, 5,* 228–229.

Fischer, D. (2003, August 4). Thrombocytopenia. *Advance for Nurses,* 17–20.

Irwin, J. J., & Kirchner, J. T. (2001). Anemia in children. *American Family Physician, 64,* 1379–1386.

Jacob, E. (2001). The pain experience of patients with sickle cell anemia. *Pain Management Nursing, 2,* 74–83.

Jacob, E., Miaskowski, C., Savedra, M., Beyer, J. E., Treadwell, M. & Styles, L. (2003). Management of vaso-occlusive pain in children with sickle cell disease. *Journal of Pediatric Hematology/Oncology 25,* 307–311.

Jacob, E., Miaskowski, C., Savedra, M., Beyer, J. E., Treadwell, M., & Styles, L. (2003). Management of vaso-occlusive pain in children with sickle cell disease. *Journal of Pediatric Hematology/Oncology, 25,* 307–311.

Jakubik, L. D., & Thompson, M. (2000). Care of the child with sickle cell disease: Acute complications. *Pediatric Nursing, 26,* 373–380.

Jayabose, S., Levendoglu-Tugal, O., Ozkaynkak, J. F., Visintainer, P. & Sandor, C. (2004). Long-term outcome of chronic idiopathic thrombocytopenic purpura in children. *Journal of Pediatric Hematology and Oncology 26,* 724–726.

Kaplan, M., Herschel, M., Hammerman, C., Hoyer, J. D., & Stevenson, D. K. (2004). Hyperbilirubinemia among African American, Glucose-6-phosphate dehydrogenase-deficient neonates. *Pediatrics, 114,* 483–484.

Kristovich, K. M. (2004). Bone marrow transplantation. In P. J. Allen, & J. A.Vessey, (Eds.), *Primary care of the child with a chronic condition.* St. Louis: Mosby.

Kuhne, T., Buchanan, G. R., Zimmerman, S., Michaels, L. A., Kohan, R., Berchtold, W., & Imbach, P. (2003). A prospective comparative study of 2540 infants and children with newly diagnosed idiopathic thrombocytopenic purpura (ITP) from the intercontinental childhood ITP study group. *Journal of Pediatrics.* 143, 605–608.

LeMone, P., & Burke, K. M. (2004). *Medical surgical nursing: Critical thinking in client care* (3rd ed.). Upper Saddle River, NJ: Prentice Hall.

Lesperance, L., Wu, A. C., & Bernstein, H. (2002). Putting a dent in iron deficiency. *Contemporary Pediatrics, 19*(7), 60–79.

McDaniel, P. (2000). Focus on factors. *Journal of Intravenous Nursing, 23,* 282–289.

Mentzer, W. C., & Cowan, M. J. (2000). Bone marrow transplantation for beta-thalassemia: The University of California San Francisco experience. *Journal of Pediatric Hematology and Oncology, 22,* 598–601.

Montgomery, R. R., & Scott, J. P. (2004). Hemorrhagic and thrombotic diseases. In R. E. Behrman, R. M. Kliegman, & H. B. Jenson (Eds.), *Nelson textbook of pediatrics* (17th ed., pp. 1651–1674). Philadelphia: WB Saunders.

National Heart, Lung, and Blood Institute. (2002). The management of sickle cell disease. www.nhilbi.nih.gov/health/prof/blood/sickle/sc_mngt.pdf, accessed 6/1/2004.

National Institute of Health (2002). The management of sickle cell disease. www.nhlbi.nih.gov/health/prof/blood/sickle/sc_mngt.pdf

Nechyba, C., & Gunn V. L. (Eds.). (2002). *The Harriet Lane handbook* (16th ed., pp. 283–306). Philadelphia: Elsevier Science.

Northington, L. (2000). Chronic sorrow in caregivers of school age children with sickle cell disease: A grounded theory approach. *Issues in Comprehensive Pediatric Nursing, 23,* 141–154.

Odesina, V. (2001). Intravenous support for the patient in sickle cell crisis. *Journal of Intravenous Nursing, 24,* 32–37.

Ogedegbe, H.O. (2002). Sickle cell disease: An overview. *Laboratory Medicine, 7,* 515–543.

Ohls, R. K., & Christensen, R. D. (2004). The hematopoietic system. In R. E. Behrman, R. M. Kliegman, & H. B. Jenson (Eds.), *Nelson textbook of pediatrics* (17th ed., pp. 1599–1604). Philadelphia: WB Saunders.

Palmer, R. H., Clanton, M., Ezhuthachan, S., Newman, C., et al. (2003). Applying the "10 simple rules" of the Institute of Medicine to management of hyperbilirubinemia in newborns. *Pediatrics, 112.* 1388–1393.

Pelchat, D., & Lefebvre H. (2004). A holistic intervention programme for families with a child with a disability. *Journal of Advanced Nursing 48,* 124–131.

Porter, M. L., & Dennis, B. L., (2002). Hyperbilirubinemia in the term newborn. *American Family Physician, 65,* 599–606.

Reed, W., Walters, M., & Lubin, B. H. (2000). Collection of sibling donor cord blood for children with thalassemia. *Journal of Pediatric Hematology and Oncology, 22,* 602–604.

Ryan, L. G., Kristovich, K. M., Haugen, M. S., Coyne, K. D. & Hubbell, M. M. (2002). Hematopoietic stem cell transplantation. In C. R. Baggott, K. P. Kelly, D. Fochtman, & G. V. Foley (Eds.). *Nursing care of children and adolescents with cancer* (3rd ed., pp. 212–255). Philadelphia: Saunders.

Segal, G. B., Hirsh, M. G., & Feig, S. A. (2002). Managing anemia in pediatric office practice: Part 1. *Pediatrics in Review, 23,* 75–83.

Sickle Cell Information Center. (1997). The Georgia Comprehensive Sickle Cell Center at Grady Health System. www.emory.edu/PEDS/SICKLE/prod05.htm, accessed 6/1/2004.

Smillova, A., & Walker, E. (2000). Meningococcemia: A critical care emergency. *Critical Care Nurse, 20*(5), 28–38.

Stover, B. (2000). Training the client in self-management of hemophilia. *Journal of Intravenous Nursing, 23,* 304–309.

Tanyi, R. A. (2003). Sickle cell disease: Health promotion and maintenance and the role of primary care nurse practitioners. *Journal of the American Academy of Nursing Practitioners, 15,* 389–397.

Trigg, M. E. (2004). Hematopoietic stem cells. *Pediatrics, 13,* 1051–1057.

White, G. C. (2001). Gene therapy in hemophilia: Clinical trials update. *Thrombosis and Haemostasis, 86,* 172–177.

Wilson, R. E., Krishnamurti, L., & Kamat, D. (2003). Management of sickle cell disease in primary care. *Clinical Pediatrics, 42,* 753–761.

Yetman, R. J. (2003, September/October). Evaluation and management of childhood idiopathic (immune) thrombocytopenia. *Journal of Pediatric Health Care,* 261–263.

Chapter

29 Alterations in Cellular Growth

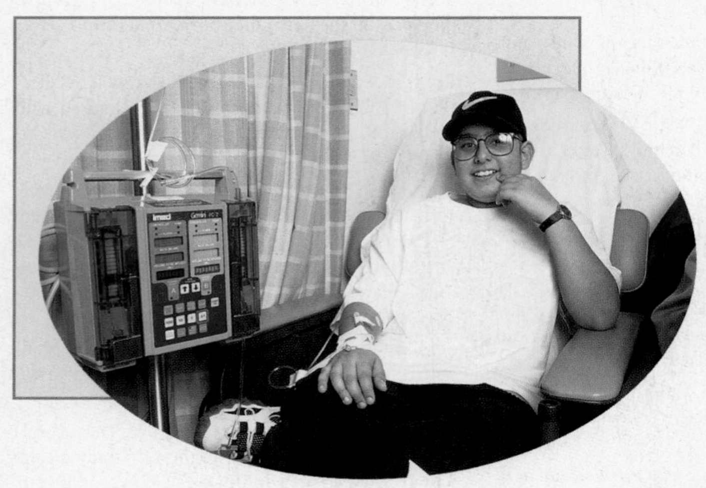

Twelve-year-old Rasheed Harper is admitted to the hospital with fever and explosive diarrhea. He is diagnosed with enterocolitis, an invasive infection of the small intestine and colon that has occurred several months into his therapy for acute lymphoblastic leukemia (ALL). As Rasheed's condition worsens day by day, his anxiety grows. His mother, who took a 3-month leave from work during the early phases of his treatment, is unable to take additional time off from work to be with him. At last, with aggressive antibiotic therapy and supportive nursing care, Rasheed conquers the complication and returns home. Rasheed and his parents feel they have met another challenge in his treatment for leukemia. When he was first diagnosed 7 months earlier, Rasheed was severely anemic and bruised easily. He was hospitalized for a short time after diagnosis for implantation of a central line for medication and began the first chemotherapy treatments. Soon, however, he was discharged home, returning for outpatient visits to receive chemotherapy and monitor his condition.

Rasheed has maintained a positive attitude throughout his treatment. He studied at home for a while, but has now returned to school. Keeping up with his schoolwork has been made easier by the gift of a computer from the Make-a-Wish Foundation. Partnerships between Rasheed's family, the oncology nurses in the hospital and outpatient clinic, and the school nurse and teachers have ensured that Rasheed has the support he needs during treatment.

"I can't figure out why I got so sick and had to come to the hospital. I did everything they told me to do. I'm kind of upset because I missed our field trip at school. Everyone went to see a play downtown that we had been reading about and then they ate at a pizza place."

—Rasheed, age 12

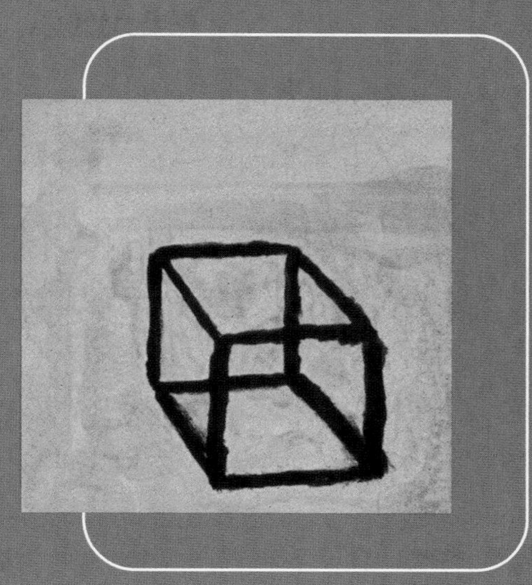

Learning Outcomes

After completing this chapter, you will be able to:

- Describe the incidence, known etiologies, and common clinical manifestations of cancer.
- Synthesize information about diagnostic tests and clinical therapy for cancer to plan comprehensive care for children undergoing these procedures.
- Integrate information about oncologic emergencies into plans for monitoring all children with cancer.
- Recognize the most common solid tumors in children, describe their treatment, and plan comprehensive nursing care.
- Plan care for children and adolescents of all ages who have a diagnosis of leukemia.
- Recognize the most common soft tissue tumors in children, describe their treatment, and plan comprehensive care.
- Describe the impact of cancer survival on children and use this information to plan for ongoing physiological and psychosocial care.
- Develop methods for an oncology team including nurses, social workers, psychologists, and child life therapists to partner with school personnel, children and adolescents, families, and others to meet the needs of children with cancer.

MediaLink http://www.prenhall.com/ball

Resources for this chapter can be found on the CD-ROM accompanying this textbook and on the Companion Website at www.prenhall.com/ball. Click on Chapter 29 to select the activities for this chapter.

CD-ROM

Animations/Videos

- *Cancer*
- *Cell Division*
- *Leukemia*

NCLEX Review

Audio Glossary

COMPANION WEBSITE

A & P Review

Clinical Manifestations Review

NCLEX Review

Case Study: Teen with Ewing's Sarcoma

MediaLink Applications

- *Exploring the Controversy: Stem Cell Transplantation*
- *Life with Leukemia: A Teen in Transition*

Key Terms

apoptosis/1038
benign/1038
biotherapy/1045
cachexia/1041
carcinogens/1039
chemotherapy/1043
complementary therapy/1048
debulk/1068
extravasation/1056
leukocytosis/1070
leukopenia/1070
malignant/1038
metastasis/1038
myelosuppression/1058
neoplasms/1038
neutropenia/1058
oncogene/1040
pancytopenia/1070
phantom pain/1075
polypharmacy/1056
protocol/1043
protooncogene/1040
radiation/1044
secondary cancers/1053
staging/1043
thrombocytopenia/1050
tumor suppressor genes/1040

Why do children like Rasheed develop different types of cancers than adults? Cancer in adults is often the result of dietary practices or habits such as smoking. Some adult-onset cancers are the result of oncogenic responses to stimuli, that is, responses that stimulate cancerous changes in cells. Other cancers that occur in adults result from prolonged exposure to toxins such as coal dust and asbestos. Some cancers are known to be related to genetic causes. In adults, prevention through general lifestyle changes is a major focus of interventions. In children, however, cancer is usually embryonic (occuring during development of the fetus) or oncogenic in origin (see description of oncogenes on page 1040). Thus, lifestyle changes that begin in childhood have little effect on the incidence of childhood cancer, although they may have a positive influence on the incidence of later cancer or other diseases. Occasionally, an environmental exposure is linked to the incidence of cancer in children.

Abnormal cellular growth can occur in any area of the body. Why are some growths called cancer and others not? Changes in cellular growth within the body are called **neoplasms** (meaning new growth). A neoplasm is further classified as benign or malignant. **Benign** means that a growth does not endanger life or health; it tends to not recur after treatment. **Malignant** means that if not treated, a growth will recur and continue to grow, and will result in spread to other sites in the body (**metastasis**), ending in death. The common term for this type of cellular growth is *cancer*.

ANATOMY AND PHYSIOLOGY OF PEDIATRIC DIFFERENCES

Cancers in children often have different etiology than those in adults. Most adult cancers are epithelial in origin, whereas in children, nonepithelial or embryonal cell types predominate. They often occur in deep body tissues and therefore may not be visible or palpable until quite large (Baggott, Kelly, Fochtman, et al., 2002).

Although not common, some neonates have cancer that is diagnosed soon after birth. The types of cancers most common in this age group include brain tumors, neuroblastoma, leukemia, retinoblastoma, and teratomas (arising from primary germ layers). While treatments are usually as effective in neonates as in older children, the rapid growth of this age makes side effects of therapy more serious (Askin, 2000).

A major physiologic difference between adults and children that affects cellular growth involves the immune system and how well it functions in the defense of the body. The rate of cell growth in children also can play a role in the rapidity with which some childhood cancers progress.

MediaLink A & P Review

The immune system defends the body against foreign organisms and substances through two responses: nonspecific and specific. In a nonspecific response, the components of the immune system attack a variety of targets. Nonspecific components include phagocytic (cell destroying) cells such as mononuclear leukocytes, polymorphonuclear (PMN) leukocytes, natural killer (NK) cells, and complements (noncellular proteins) that work together to destroy invading cells and substances. During the first month of a child's life, the nonspecific response is immature, so phagocytic cells have little ability to move toward cancer cells and fulfill their function. The nonspecific response is also impaired in premature and small-for-gestational-age (SGA) infants.

In a specific response, T lymphocytes and immunoglobulin (Ig) attack only one type of invader. The specific response capability is also immature in infants. B-cell production of various proteins called immunoglobins (IgM, IgG, and IgA) is below adult levels, so the infant is vulnerable to bacterial and viral infections. (For a detailed discussion of immune function, see Chapter 27∞.)

In children, fast cellular growth can lead to the proliferation of both cancerous and normal cells. Cell division that is out of control may normally trigger a mechanism called **apoptosis,** whereby the cell "realizes" something is wrong and destroys itself. The process of apoptosis or physiologic cell death may not be well developed in young children.

CHILDHOOD CANCER

The care of children who have cancer is a challenging specialty in pediatric nursing. For several years, the child undergoes aggressive treatments that may be life threatening and cause serious illness. Often the prognosis is quite hopeful; at other times, a terminal prognosis is expected. For some types of cancer, the child is cared for at home with outpatient visits for treatment and occasional hospitalization when needed for conditions such as fever and neutropenia. The periods of hospitalization are times of intense physical vulnerability for the child and intense emotional vulnerability for both the child and the family. For other cancers, multiple hospitalizations are needed to carry out therapy. To monitor the child closely, nurses need a sound knowledge of physiologic and psychologic responses, medical interventions, and nursing care. Effective communication skills are necessary to partner with the child and family and promote realistic hope.

During 2003, in the United States, cancer was diagnosed in approximately 9,000 children. In children under 15 years of age, cancer is the leading cause of disease-related death. In 2003, about 1,500 U.S. children died of cancer, one third of these from leukemia (American Cancer Society, 2004). However, mortality rates have declined by about 47% since 1975, and the rates continue to improve. Overall survival rate is 80% for childhood cancer (Baggott et al., 2002). Children treated in the 1980s and 1990s had significantly lower mortality rates than those treated in the 1960s and 1970s due to multimodal therapies including multiagent chemotherapy, surgery, and radiation therapy. There is a difference in survival rates for different types of cancer ranging from 69% for neuroblastoma to 94% for Hodgkin disease (American Cancer Society, 2004). Mortality rates are higher for females than males, for those diagnosed before 5 years of age, and for children with a central nervous system tumor or leukemia. The cause of death for most children is recurrence of the primary cancer (Moller, Garwicz, Barlow, et al., 2001). The most common forms of childhood cancers among children in different age groups are shown in Figure 29–1 ■.

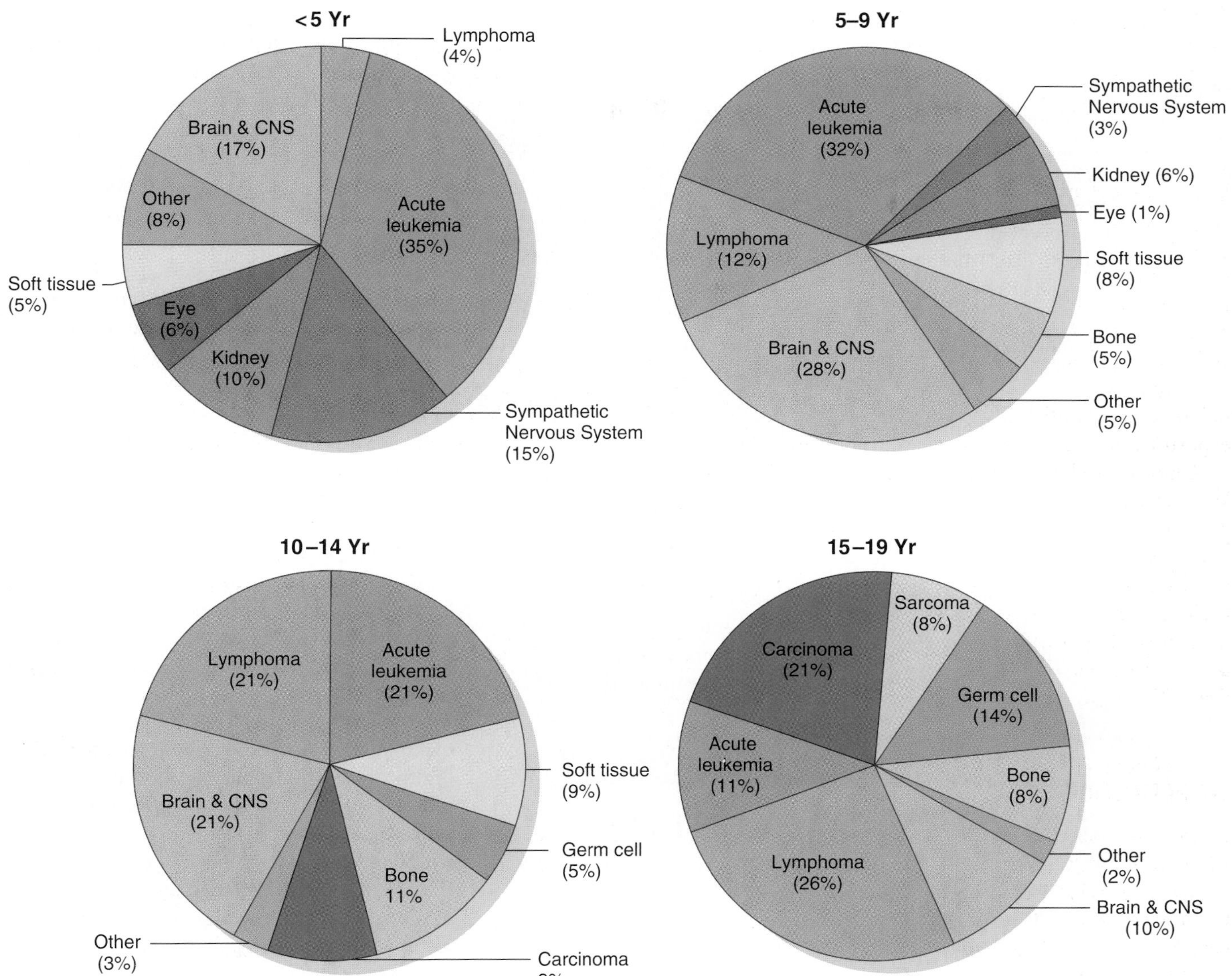

FIGURE 29–1 ■ Percentage of primary tumors by site of origin for different age groups. Notice that in the early years of life, in addition to leukemia, cancers that derive from embryonic cells such as sympathetic nervous system (neuroblastoma) and eye (retinoblastoma) are common. As the child grows, lymphoma becomes more common in school years, and germ cell cancers of ovary and testes emerge as more common causes in teens.

Data from Gurney, J. G., & Bondy, M. L. (2004). Cancer and benign tumors. In R. E. Behrman, R. M. Kliegman, & H. B. Jenson (Eds.), Nelson textbook of pediatrics *(17th ed., p. 1680). Philadelphia: Saunders.*

Etiology and Pathophysiology

Alterations in cellular growth occur in response to external and internal stimuli. Neoplasms are caused by one or a combination of three factors: (1) external stimuli that cause genetic mutations, (2) innate immune system and gene abnormalities, and (3) chromosomal abnormalities.

External Stimuli

External stimuli may affect the child's general health and cause mutations in body cells. **Carcinogens** are chemicals or industrial processes that, when combined with genetic traits and in interaction with one another, result in cancer. Several carcinogens cause cancers that are diagnosed during childhood. Others cause cancers that begin in childhood but are not identified until adulthood. Some chemicals suspected of causing childhood cancer include diethylstilbestrol or DES (maternal use of therapeutic estrogen hormones), anabolic androgenic steroids, alkylating chemotherapy agents, and immunosuppressants used for organ transplantation. Radiation exposure has been known to cause cancers such as leukemia and thyroid tumors in children exposed to nuclear fallout from atomic bombs, other nuclear accidents, and other excessive radiation sources.

External stimuli may also lead to secondary cancers in children, or those occurring after treatment for a primary cancer, and of a different cellular type than the primary cancer. Secondary cancers can result when the child is treated for a primary cancer with high doses of radiation. Excessive exposure to

MediaLink Cancer Overview Video

ultraviolet radiation from the sun predisposes children to development of skin cancer in adulthood.

Immune System and Gene Abnormalities

One critical function of a normal immune system is immune surveillance, in which phagocytic cells circulate throughout the body, detecting and destroying abnormal and cancerous cells. Children with congenital immune deficiencies, such as Wiskott-Aldrich syndrome, in which immune surveillance may fail, are at high risk for cancer. A form of non-Hodgkin lymphoma develops in some children treated with drugs that suppress the immune system. Children with acquired immunodeficiency syndrome (AIDS) may be at higher risk of certain types of cancer, such as Hodgkin disease, non-Hodgkin lymphoma, leiomyosarcoma, and Kaposi sarcoma (Biggar, Frisch, & Goedert, 2000).

Viruses and other substances may act in the body to alter the immune system, thereby allowing cancer to occur (Figure 29–2 ■). Their action is based on changing certain genes that normally regulate cellular growth and development (called **protooncogenes**) to related genes that allow unregulated cell division and cancerous growth (called **oncogenes**). Among the cancers thought to be linked to virus action and the change of protooncogenes to oncogenes are certain leukemias, rhabdomyosarcoma, Burkitt's lymphoma, and some forms of Hodgkin disease.

Sometimes a genetic change that occurs is passed on to future generations. Genetic changes can include autosomal dominant, autosomal recessive, and X-linked transfer. In these cases, the resulting cancers often occur relatively early in life. Cancers of these types are typically aggressive since the child has inherited the abnormal gene so it is within each cell, rather than a single mutation of one gene in a specific cell. Due to progress made in the Human Genome Project (see Chapter 4∞), there is increasing ability to perform genetic testing for certain familial cancers. Examples of cancers that are sometimes caused by genetic abnormalities within families include retinoblastoma (described later in this chapter), multiple endocrine neoplasia, type 2 (thyroid cancer), and familial adenomatous polyposis (invasive colon cancer). Not all cases of these cancers are familial, but their incidence suggests the needs for careful history taking to identify any other cases in the family. See Table 29–1 for several examples of cancers that are sometimes genetically linked within families.

When genetic testing is available, nurses with a specialty in genetics are often called on to support the family. For some parents it may be a relief to know whether the child has inherited the cancer gene, and in others it may lead to increased anxiety. If parents choose to have children genetically tested, the children will not have the option later in life to choose whether they want to be tested. This takes away their ability to make their own decision about this important healthcare decision. On the other hand, for some cancers, early testing may help to increase surveillance and early treatment. Nurses partner with families to advocate for both the child and the parents. Providing recommendations for referral to genetic counseling services and following up with further education and psychological support are important nursing roles (MacDonald & Lessick, 2000).

Tumor suppressor genes counteract the effect of oncogenes, keeping cellular growth within normal limits. When tumor suppressor genes are missing, unregulated cellular growth can occur. These genes are commonly missing in children with retinoblastoma and Wilms' tumor.

PATHOPHYSIOLOGY ILLUSTRATED

Protooncogene Alteration

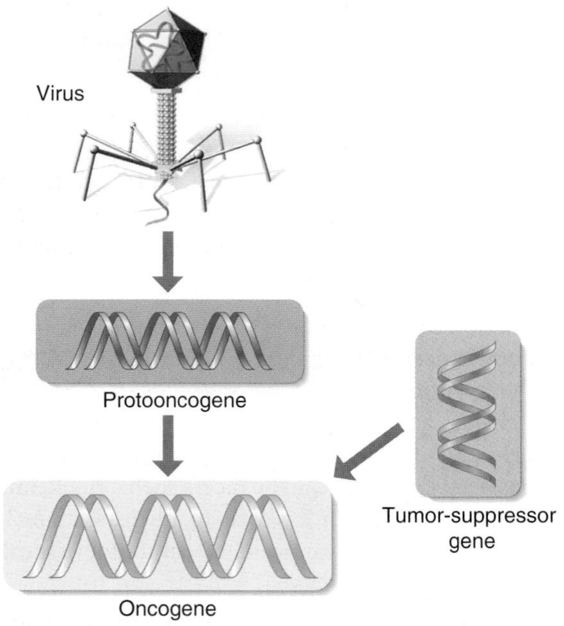

FIGURE 29–2 ■ A protooncogene normally regulates cellular growth and development. When altered by a virus or other external cause, it can change to an oncogene, which allows unregulated genetic activity and tumor growth. Tumor-suppressor genes regulate the effects of oncogenes to decrease wildly proliferating cellular growth.

Chromosomal Abnormalities

Normal chromosomes undergo change as a part of the genetic process. Most of the changes are not harmful, although some result in chromosomal abnormalities such as hyperploidy (more than the normal number of chromosomes), deletion, translocation, and breakage.

Some of these chromosomal abnormalities have been linked to an increased incidence of cancer. Children with the chromosomal disorder of Down syndrome have a 200 times higher incidence of leukemia than children without the syndrome. Children who are missing a band of

TABLE 29–1 Types of Familial Cancers

TYPE OF CANCER	GENETIC LOCATION	DESCRIPTION
Retinoblastoma	RB1 gene	Tumor of the eye retina
Wilms' tumor	Chromosomal band 11p13 WT1 gene	Tumor of the kidney
Beckwith-Wiedemann syndrome	Chromosome 11p15 Specific gene unknown	Multiple abnormalities including tumors of kidney, liver, and adrenals; oomphalocele, macroglossia
Multiple endocrine neoplasia, type 2	Protooncogene RET mutation	Medullary thyroid cancer
Familial adenomatous polyposis	APC tumor suppressor gene mutation on chromosome 5q21	Invasive widespread colon polyps
Li-Fraumeni syndrome	Germline TP53	Early onset breast and other soft tissue cancers
Von Hippel–Lindau disease	VHL gene on chromosome 3925-26	Hemangioblastoma of retina, cerebellum or spinal cord; renal cell carcinoma; pheochromocytoma

Data from Pakakasama, S., & Tomlinson, G. E. (2002). Genetic predisposition and screening in pediatric cancer. Pediatric Clinics of North America, *49, 1393–1413; MacDonald, D. J., & Lessick, M. (2000). Hereditary cancers in children and ethical and psychosocial implications.* Journal of Pediatric Nursing, *15, 217–225.*

genetic material on chromosome 13 often have retinoblastoma. Similarly, a Wilms' tumor often develops in children missing part of the genetic material from chromosome 11. Regardless of the location of abnormal cellular growth, the pathophysiologic process is similar. The altered cell begins to multiply as directed by the altered genetic structure of its DNA and the absence or inactivation of tumor suppressor genes. Each new cell transmits the altered pattern to the next generation. As the abnormal cells replicate, they form a growing neoplastic mass. Normal cells usually die as the increased metabolic rate of the neoplastic cells depletes available nutrition. The altered DNA in the tumor cells may also cause the abnormal cells to invade adjoining tissue. Through continued growth, the mass invades, disrupting a major vessel or a vital organ.

Clinical Manifestations

Each type of childhood cancer signals its presence differently. Because many of the presenting signs and symptoms of cancer are typical of common childhood illnesses, a delay in diagnosis can occur. In some cases, no symptoms are noted until the cancer is advanced. Children more commonly present with metastases (spread of the cancer to a site other than its origin) at time of diagnosis than do adults due to this difficulty in recognition of the disease. Common presenting symptoms of cancer are as follows:

- *Pain* may be the result of a neoplasm either directly or indirectly affecting nerve receptors through obstruction, inflammation, tissue damage, stretching of visceral tissue, or invasion of susceptible tissue.
- ***Cachexia*** is a syndrome characterized by anorexia, weight loss, anemia, asthenia (weakness), and early satiety (feeling of being full).
- *Anemia* may be experienced during times of chronic bleeding or iron deficiency. In chronic illness the body uses iron poorly. Anemia is also present in cancers of the bone marrow when the number of red blood cells (RBCs) is reduced, in part because of the presence of large numbers of other bone marrow products. Treatment of cancer often promotes further anemia.
- *Infection* is usually a result of an altered or immature immune system. In addition, infection occurs when bone marrow cancers inhibit maturation of normal immune system cells. Infection may also occur in children who are treated with corticosteroids. Because their immune response is altered, the normal signs of infection may not appear.
- *Bruising* can occur if the bone marrow cannot produce enough platelets; bleeding after even minor trauma can then lead to ecchymosis.
- *Neurologic symptoms* may result from impingement on the brain or nervous system. Signs of increased intracranial pressure, decreased or altered consciousness, eye abnormalities, or other neurologic or behavior changes may be evident.
- *A palpable mass* may be present for certain cancers. This is most commonly abdominal but may be mediastinal, in the neck, or other sites.

A variety of other symptoms can occur depending on the location of the cancer. Subctaneous nodules may appear if leukocytosis is present, superior vena cava syndrome or respiratory difficulty can occur with mediastinal tumors (such as neuroblastoma), and enlarged lymph nodes are common with lymphomas (Bleyer, 2004).

COLLABORATIVE CARE

Many health professionals work together with children and families in diagnosis and treatment of cancer. The goals of care are early diagnosis and development of an effective treatment plan, combined with psychosocial support to enhance coping.

Diagnostic Tests

The most common diagnostic tests performed on children with cancer are complete blood count with differential, bone marrow aspiration (BMA) and bone marrow biopsy (BMBX), lumbar puncture (LP) (Table 29–2), radiographic examination, magnetic resonance imaging (MRI), computed tomography (Figure 29–3 ■), ultrasound, and biopsy of tumor.

> **CLINICAL TIP**
>
> A child who has an implanted metallic object in the body should not undergo MRI scanning because of the strong magnetic field generated. Metallic objects include orthodontic braces, metal dental bridgework, surgical clips or plates, and orthopedic rods. Remove all jewelry and clothes with metal snaps from the child before the test. Ask about and remove body piercings; they may not always be visible.

Additional tests of serum may be helpful in diagnosis. Studies useful for certain cancers include nuclear medicine scans with radioactive isotopes such as gallium or iodine, bone scan with technetium 99m, or positron emission tomography (PET) and single photon emission computed tomography (SPECT) that combine nuclear medicine with CT (Leonard, 2002). Specific tests such as pulmonary function tests and echocardiograms may be used in certain situations.

The blood work is detailed and includes the following:

- RBC, WBC, platelets (CBC with differential)
- Hemoglobin and hematocrit
- RBC indices such as mean corpuscular volume (MCV), mean corpuscular hemoglobin concentration (MCHC), and mean corpuscular hemoglobin (MCH)
- WBC indices (manual differential) which include the percent of all five types (basophils, eosinophils, monocytes, lymphocytes, neutrophils; neutrophils are further divided into segmented and banded)
- Absolute neutrophil count (ANC) using both the segmented (mature) and band (immature) neutrophils as a measure of the body's infection-fighting capability, calculated by adding % of segmented neutrophils to % of bands, and then multiplying this % by the WBC count
- Serum chemistry which includes electrolytes, including sodium, potassium, chloride, calcium, magnesium, phosphorus, and carbon dioxide
- Additional studies that provide important diagnostic clues in some cases, for example, renal function studies such as blood urea nitrogen (BUN) and creatinine; liver studies such as total bilirubin, alanine aminotransferase (ALT), aspirate aminotransferase (AST), lactic dehydrogenase (LDH), and blood urea nitrogen (BUN); alkaline phosphatase may be elevated; uric acid is commonly elevated in leukemia
- Certain substances, or markers, that are elevated with some specific tumors, for example, α-fetoprotein may be elevated in liver tumors, vanillylmandelic acid (VMA) and homovanillic acid (HVA) may be elevated in adrenal tumors, and elevated catecholamines are found in neuroblastoma.

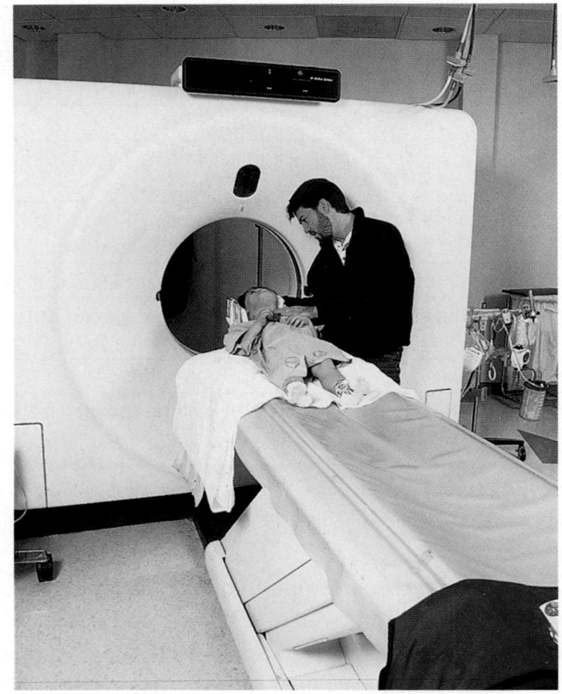

FIGURE 29–3 ■ Computed tomography (CT) can be a frightening procedure for children. This 2-year-old boy is comforted by his father before the procedure.

Urinalysis is performed. It may show abnormal cells such as RBCs (hematuria) that may assist in diagnosis of kidney tumors. Histological or laboratory analysis of tumor cells is often critical in diagnosis. A needle biopsy or endoscopic procedures of some tumors can be performed to obtain tumor cells. If the tumor is

TABLE 29–2 Selected Diagnostic Tests for Childhood Cancer

TEST	PURPOSE	NORMAL LABORATORY VALUES	DIAGNOSTIC VALUES
Bone marrow aspiration	Examines bone marrow	<5% blast cells (immature)	>25% blast cells in acute lymphoblastic leukemia, most with hypercellular marrow
Lumbar puncture	Examines cerebrospinal fluid	Cell count (μL) Polymorphonuclear leukocytes 0 Monocytes 0–5 RBCs 0–5	Presence of malignant cells indicates central nervous system involvement
Complete blood count and differential	Examines cellular components of blood	WBC <10,000/μL Platelets 150,000–400,000/μL Hemoglobin 12–16 g/dL	WBC <10,000/μL Platelets 20,000–100,000/μL Hemoglobin 7–10 g/dL
Absolute Neutrophil Count (ANC)	Blood component ratio: % of segmental neutrophils plus % of bands (immature neutrophils) times WBC count	ANC > 1000	ANC < 500 Risk of infection

removed during surgery, the entire tumor is available for study. The borders are examined to be certain it has been totally removed, and lymph nodes may also be removed to analyze possible spread via lymph system.

The tests are aimed at identifying the source of the cancer and any metastases to additional sites. This enables the physician to stage the cancer. **Staging** refers to the process of labeling the type of cancer cells, severity, and spread, to determine the recommended treatment. Stage 1 indicates less severe cancer without spread to other parts of the body, and higher numbers indicate greater severity and spread to other sites.

Clinical Therapy

Clinical therapy for cancer is extermely complex and is managed by a specialist in pediatric oncology. The cancer itself must be treated in order to cure the child or at least to lessen the effects of the cancer. Cancer has many effects on the body and all of those must be addressed. For example, they involve altered nutritional status from anorexia due to the cancer diverting nutrients to itself; decreased immune response from impaired manufacture of white blood cells and other immune components; and a variety of symptoms as a tumor presses on vital organs. In addition, cancer treatment itself has many potential side effects which require constant monitoring and adjustments in treatment.

Cancer is treated with one or a combination of several therapies including surgery, chemotherapy, radiation, biotherapy, and hematopoietic stem cell transplantation. Many families also choose some type of complementary therapy, in addition to traditional medical approaches. The treatment plan is determined by the type of cancer, site of primary tumor, and sites of metastasis (spread to other sites in the body).

The goal of treatment may be curative or palliative. See Box 29–1 for recommendations of the National Action Plan for Childhood Cancer (American Cancer Society, 2003). Curative treatment rids the child's body of the cancer. Almost 80% of childhood cancers are successfully treated, leading to at least a 5-year survival rate. Palliative treatment is designed to make the child as comfortable as possible when no curative treatment is possible (see Chapter 22∞ for a detailed discussion of palliative care for children). Supportive treatment for both curative and palliative approaches includes transfusions, pain management, antibiotics, and other interventions to assist the body's defenses and increase the child's comfort. Whatever combination of treatment is used, families will have questions and need resources for information.

BOX 29–1 Recommendations from the National Action Plan for Childhood Cancer

- Ensure that all children and adolescents suspected of having cancer are referred initially to a pediatric cancer center and have their care coordinated by the center.
- Establish national standards of quality care for children and adolescents with cancer, both medical and psychosocial, as defined by healthcare professionals and patient advocates.
- Quantify current patterns, quality, and outcomes of all phases of childhood and adolescent cancer care.
- Increase participation of children and adolescents in all phases of approved clinical trials.

(American Cancer Society, 2003).

Surgery. Surgery is used to remove or debulk (reduce the size of) a solid tumor. An example of a cancer that is commonly treated with surgery is a Wilms' tumor. Surgery is also used to determine the stage and type of cancer since the tumor cells can be examined microscopically once removed, and various body organs can be inspected for signs of cancer during the surgery.

Chemotherapy. Chemotherapy is the administration of specific drugs that kill both normal and cancerous cells. The administration of various chemotherapeutic drugs is timed to achieve the greatest cellular destruction. The schedule is determined by the cell's cycle of replication (Figure 29–4 ■). Several chemotherapeutic drugs are administered simultaneously to maximize their lethal impact on cells at all stages of activity. See the medications table on page 1046. Table 29–3 provides examples of common chemotherapy drug combinations.

Whereas DNA in a normal cell can repair itself after chemotherapy, the DNA in a neoplastic cell cannot. The particular chemotherapy treatment protocol used is based on research into different types of cancer cells. A **protocol** is a plan of action for chemotherapy that is based on the results of staging: type of cancer, its location, the particular cell type, and its degree of spread (Figure 29–5 ■).

Other drugs used in the treatment of children with cancer include colony-stimulating factors, antiemetics, and nutritional supplements. Colony-stimulating factors are hormone-like glycoproteins that enhance blood cell production and counteract the myelosuppressive effects of chemotherapy drugs. (See the medications table on page 1048.) For example, erythropoietin is produced in the kidney, and a recombinant form (epoietin) is available which can be used to treat anemia of cancer, thereby decreasing the number of transfusions needed (Agency for Healthcare Research and Quality, 2001a). Filgrastim (Neupogen) increases production of neutrophils by the bone marrow. Antiemetics, such as ondansetron (Zofran), can be used to treat the nausea and vomiting that are common side effects of therapy. Nutritional supplements can be given to maintain nutritional status. Some children may need periodic treatment with antibiotics or antiviral drugs to treat infections that occur as a result of decreased immune response.

Cancer chemotherapy is complex and requires care by specialists in oncology. Many drugs have severe side effects during the administration period. These side effects may require administration of other drugs for their treatment. Other drugs may have late side effects that occur after therapy is completed, while others are associated with different cancers in the future. The chemotherapeutic regimen often becomes even more complicated with very young children due to their inability to metabolize and excrete certain drugs. Administration of chemotherapy drugs requires specialized knowledge by the nurse. Guidelines for handling of substances posing occupational hazard from the Occupation Safety and Health Administration (OSHA) should be followed.

MediaLink OSHA Guidelines

PATHOPHYSIOLOGY ILLUSTRATED

Chemotherapy Drug Action

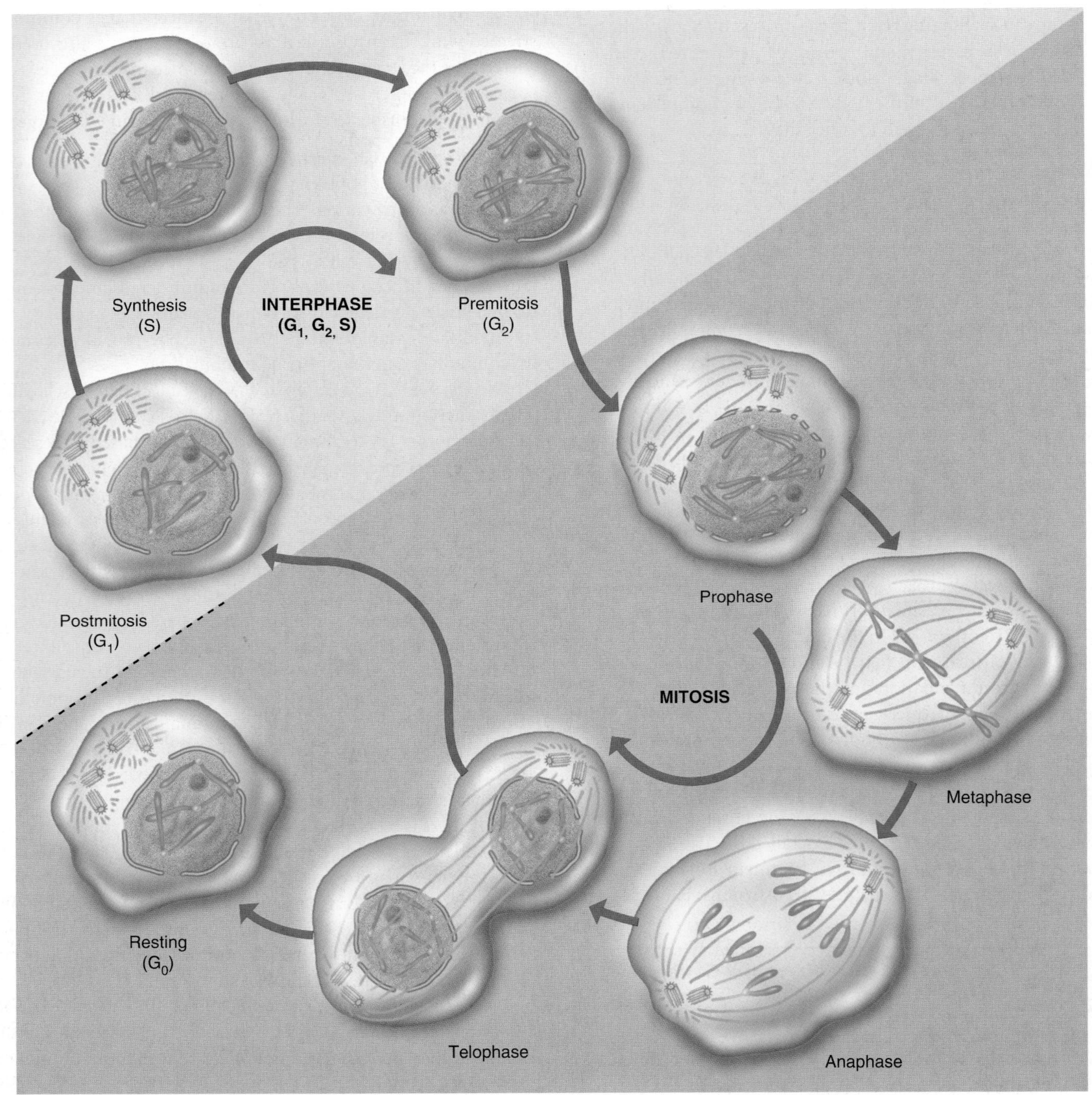

FIGURE 29–4 ■ Chemotherapy drugs either act at specific parts of the cell cycle or are nonspecific for action (act throughout all cell phases).

Radiation. **Radiation** therapy involves the use of unstable isotopes that release varying levels of energy to cause breaks in the DNA molecule and thereby destroy cells. Radiation has been used as a treatment method since the early 1900s, shortly after its discovery. It is often used for the local and regional control of cancer, and in combination with surgery and chemotherapy. It may be either curative or palliative.

The area to be irradiated (treatment field) includes the tumor site and sometimes other involved areas, such as lymph glands. The goal is to irradiate the tumor but not healthy adjacent tissue. The

TABLE 29–3 Commonly Used Chemotherapy Drug Combinations

ACRONYM	DRUG COMBINATION
A-COPP	Adriamycin (doxorubicin) + cyclophosphamide + vincristine (oncovin) + procarbazine + prednisone
ABVD	Adriamycin (doxorubicin) + bleomycin + vinblastine + dacarbazine
ABVE	Adriamycin (doxorubicin) + bleomycin + vincristine + etoposide
ABVE-PC	Adriamycin (doxorubicin) + bleomycin + vincristine + etoposide + prednisone + cyclophosphamide
ACE	Adriamycin (doxorubicin) + cyclophosphamide + etoposide
AOPE	Adriamycin (doxorubicin) + Oncovin (vincristine) + prednisone + etoposide
APE	Adriamycin (doxorubicin) + procarbazine + etoposide
BEACOPP	bleomycin + etoposide + adriamycin (doxorubicin) + cyclophosphamide + vincristine + procarbazine + prednisone
CAF	cyclophosphamide + doxorubicin + fluorouracil
CAMP	cyclophosphamide + doxorubicin + methotrexate + procarbazine
CAVe	lomustine + doxorubicin + vinblastine
CAVE or ECHO or CAPO or EVAC or VOCA	etoposide + cyclophosphamide + doxorubicin + vincristine
CHOP	cyclophosphamide + doxorubicin + vincristine + prednisone
CHOR	cyclophosphamide + doxorubicin + vincristine
CISCA	cisplatin + cyclophosphamide
CMF	cyclophosphamide + methotrexate + fluorouracil
COPP	cyclophosphamide + vincristine + procarbazine + prednisone
CY-VA-DIC	cyclophosphamide + vincristine + doxorubicin + dacarbazine
EBVP	etoposide + bleomycin + vinblastine + prednisone
FAC	fluorouracil + doxorubicin + cyclophosphamide
MACC	methotrexate + doxorubicin + cyclophosphamide + lomustine
MOPP	mechlorethamine + vincristine + procarbazine + prednisone
MTX + MP + CTX	methotrexate + mercaptopurine + cyclophosphamide
OEPA	vincristine + etoposide + prednisone + adriamycin (doxorubicin)
OPPA	vincristine + prednisone + procarbazine + adriamycin (doxorubicin)
PVB or VBP	vinblastine + bleomycin + cisplatin
T-2	dactinomycin + doxorubicin + vincristine + cyclophosphamide
VAMP	vinblastine + adriamycin (doxorubicin) + methotrexate + prednisone
VAP	vincristine + dactinomycin + cyclophosphamide
VEPA	vinblastine + etoposide + prednisone + adriamycin (doxorubicin)
VP-L-asparaginase	vincristine + prednisone + L-asparaginase

total dose of radiation is divided (or fractionated) and given over several weeks. A common course of radiation treatment might be once daily 4 or 5 days per week for a period of 2 to 7 weeks.

CLINICAL TIP

Nurses who care for a child receiving implant radiation or who work in a radiation department must wear a dosimeter film badge at all times to measure their exposure to radiation. If exposure exceeds limits, they will not be able to work in the setting for a period of time.

Examples of cancers treated with radiation include Hodgkin disease, stage III Wilms' tumor, brain tumors, rhabdomyosarcoma, and CNS disease in leukemia. Tumors that have a low sensitivity to radiation, such as osteosarcoma and soft tissue sarcomas, require higher doses of radiation, or may be treated by other therapies.

Biotherapy. **Biotherapy** is the use of biologic retooling and molecular intervention to produce targeted cancer therapy (Arceci & Cripe, 2002). Biologic retooling uses parts of the human body that are programmed to destroy cells, and applies them to the cancer cells. An example of this technique includes development of antibodies that are tumor specific to certain cancers. These antibodies promote apoptosis or death of the cancerous cells. Another example is the group of drugs that stimulate the body's own immune response. Cancer vaccines are under development that may work to help the body fight cancers. The actions of many of these agents are not completely understood, and some agents have more than one effect. For example, interferon has both antiviral and antiproliferative effects on some malignant cells. Interferon and tumor necrosis factor (TNF) are undergoing clinical trials to study their effectiveness and to develop protocols for their safe use against selected cancers. An additional type of biological therapy is

MEDICATIONS Used for Cancer Chemotherapy

MEDICATION	ACTION/INDICATION	NURSING IMPLICATIONS
Cell Cycle Specific Agents		
Antimetabolites ➤ 5-Azacytidine ➤ 5-Fluorouracil ➤ 6-Mercaptopurine ➤ 6-Thioguanine ➤ Cytosine arabinoside (cytarabine) ➤ Hydroxyurea ➤ Methotrexate	The antimetabolites work at synthesis phase of cell division; interfere with function of nucleic acid; inhibit DNA or RNA synthesis	Most common side effects are nausea and vomiting, myelosuppression, stomatitis. Specific agents such as methotrexate and cytarabine can cause neurologic toxicity with high doses. Consult drug books and package inserts for detailed list of side effects. Obtain baseline CBC, liver function, renal function. Monitor I&O and body weight. Ensure hydration and output levels ordered by oncologist. Monitor VS and cardiovascular and respiratory function. Watch for bleeding and signs of infection. Monitor carefully during administration for signs of anaphylaxis.
Vinca alkaloids ➤ Etoposide ➤ Teniposide ➤ Irinotecan ➤ Paclitaxel ➤ Vinblastine ➤ Vincristine	Act during mitosis; bind with cell proteins to inhibit nucleic acid and protein synthesis	Common side effects include nausea and vomiting, abdominal cramping and diarrhea, constipation, paralytic ileus, hair loss, hypotension or hypertension, peripheral neuropathy and neurological toxicity (latter especially with vinblastine and vincristine). Obtain baseline blood work. Consult specific drug information for period of maximum myelosuppressive effect. Be alert for bruising, infection, and other signs of myelosuppression. Monitor carefully during administration for signs of anaphylaxis.
Miscellaneous—G_1 phase activity ➤ L-asparaginase	Causes depletion of asparagine, needed by cancer cells; makes cell in G_1 phase vulnerable to other agents; interferes with prosynthesis. Used in combination with other agents in leukemia and other cancers.	Administered intravenously. Major side effects are severe nausea and vomiting, hypersensitivity, renal failure, myelosuppression, acid–base imbalance. CBC, serum amylase, glucose, coagulation factors, bone marrow function, liver function tests performed before therapy and twice weekly. Monitor I&O, neurologic status, gastrointestinal symptoms, abdominal pain.
Miscellaneous—G_2 phase activity ➤ Etoposide	Works at G_2 phase; binds cellular proteins to cause metaphase arrest; also acts on S phase of DNA synthesis. Used with other agents, particularly in recurrent disease.	Administered orally and intravenously. Common side effects are nausea and vomiting, myelosuppression, hair loss, diarrhea. Can cause anaphylaxis; hypotension and IV site pain with rapid infusion. Perform baseline CBC, liver and renal function tests. Check IV site frequently since extravasation can cause necrosis. Monitor VS during infusion and stop drug if hypotension occurs.
Cell Cycle Nonspecific Agents		
Alkylating agents ➤ Cyclophosphamide ➤ Carboplatin ➤ Cisplatin ➤ Busulfan ➤ Chlorambucil ➤ Ifosfamide ➤ Thiotepa ➤ Mechlorethamine ➤ Melphalan ➤ Procarbazine ➤ Dacarbazine	Substitute an alkyl group for a hydrogen atom, leading to blockage of DNA replication. Used for treatment of many cancers, either alone or in conjunction with other agents.	Most are administered orally and/or intravenously. Array of side effects depending on specific drug. Some common side effects are nausea and vomiting, diarrhea, myelosuppression, hair loss, neuropathies, pulmonary toxicity, renal damage; secondary tumors later in life associated with some agents. Obtain CBC and full blood work before and during treatment. Monitor for side effects of the specific agents administered. Ensure generous hydration and monitor I&O. Teach family the importance of long-term monitoring for secondary tumors.
Antibiotics ➤ Doxorubicin ➤ Mitomycin-C ➤ Dactinomycin ➤ Bleomycin ➤ Daunorubicin ➤ Idarubicin ➤ Mitoxantrone	Interfere with nucleic acid, inhibiting DNA or RNA synthesis. Used in combination with other agents to treat leukemia and other childhood cancers.	Most are administered intravenously. Common side effects include nausea and vomiting, myelosuppression, oral ulcers, skin and pulmonary toxicity. Several have cumulative dose toxicity, such as cardiac abnormalities (doxorubicin) and skin/pulmonary (bleomycin); total dose the child has received must be monitored. Obtain baseline CBC and other blood studies and monitor throughout therapy. Monitor VS, lung function, cardiac function, neurologic status throughout and following therapy. Be alert for signs of myelosuppression and mucosal ulcers.

MEDICATIONS Used for Cancer Chemotherapy (continued)

MEDICATION	ACTION/INDICATION	NURSING IMPLICATIONS
Cell Cycle Nonspecific Agents (continued)		
Nitrosoureas ➤ Carmustine ➤ Lomustine	Cross breakage in DNA strands so that DNA and RNA replication cannot occur. Used in lymphomas and other childhood cancers. Can cross blood-brain barrier.	Administered orally (lomustine) or intravenously (carmustine). Major side effect is myelosuppression. Others include pulmonary fibrosis, eye infarction, skin changes, hair loss, nausea, and vomiting. Obtain baseline and periodic CBC and other studies. Monitor pulmonary function, skin, and signs of infection or bleeding.
Hormones ➤ Prednisone ➤ Prednisolone ➤ Dexamethasone	Analog of hydrocortisone; anti-inflammatory; delayed and depressed immune response. Used in conjunction with other agents for many types of childhood cancer.	Often administered orally. Numerous side effects including edema, moon face, mood lability, increased appetite, disturbed sleep, immunosuppression, disturbed glucose control, osteoporosis. Teach child and family the effects of the drug. Minimize exposure to persons with infection. Monitor for infections in all systems. Monitor weight regularly. Take VS. Teach to take as directed. Drug must be tapered slowly at end of therapy.
Topoisomerase I inhibitor ➤ Irinotecan ➤ Mitoxantrone ➤ Topotecan	Inhibit the enzyme topoisomerase I in the cell nucleus, relaxing DNA and preventing its duplication. Used in conjunction with other agents to treat ALL and other childhood cancers.	Administered intravenously: topotecan can be given intrathecally. Common side effects include nausea and vomiting, diarrhea, fever, dehydration, myelosuppression. Can alter liver function and cause skin changes. Obtain baseline and periodic CBC and other studies, including liver function. Monitor for signs of myelosuppression, gastrointestinal distress, change in liver function.

gene therapy or attempting to replace a faulty gene with one that is normal.

Molecular targeting involves interference with metabolic pathways (for example, through enzyme disruption) in the tumor cells. It may also disturb the cell's growth and development and thereby depress proliferation.

Hematopoietic Stem Cell Transplantation. Hematopoietic stem cell transplantation (HSCT) is used to treat leukemia, neuroblastoma, and some noncancerous conditions such as aplastic anemia. The goal of therapy is to administer a lethal dose of chemotherapy and radiation that will kill the cancer, and then to resupply the body with stem cells either from the child's own bone marrow that was previously removed (autologous transplant) and stored or from a compatible donor (allogeneic transplant). Umbilical cord blood is another source of stem cells used for transplant. Peripheral blood stem cells are increasingly being used for transplant. The donor, whether autologous or allogeneic, can be given growth factors prior to donation to stimulate production of stem cells. An advantage of peripheral stem cells is that they can be easily collected rather than by the painful and invasive procedure of a bone marrow aspiration (Reiss & Bolotin, 2002).

HSCT has become the treatment of choice for some cancers when a relapse occurs while the child is receiving another form of cancer therapy and for primary treatment of certain cancers. First, a histocompatible donor must be located. The child then receives intensive chemotherapy, often followed by total body irradiation. Beginning 7 to 10 days before the transplant, this treatment kills all circulating blood cells and bone marrow contents (Alcoser & Burchett, 1999). Following this treatment, the child is intravenously transfused with the donor bone marrow or other source of stem cells. New blood cells usually form within 2 to 6 weeks (Alcoser & Rogers. 2003). (See Chapter 27∞ for a description of care for the child undergoing transplantation.)

Stem cells that become established in the host child's bone marrow can also be obtained from newborn umbilical cord blood. For some children this has become a better option than waiting for a matching bone marrow donor. Cord blood can be easily collected at birth from a sibling of the ill child, as histocompatible matches

Protocol = Map or plan of action

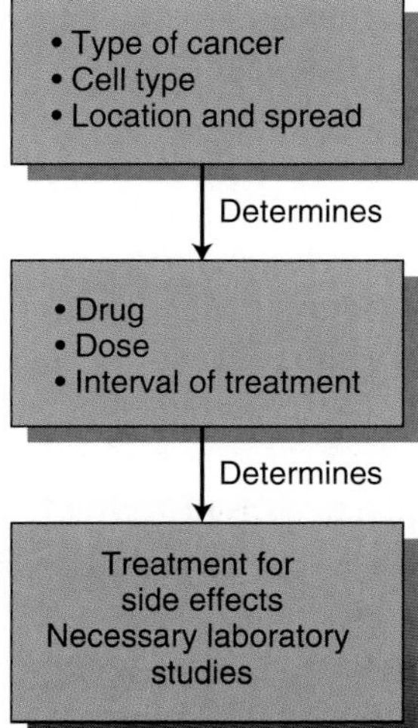

FIGURE 29–5 ■ Chemotherapy protocol. A protocol is a map or plan of action that directs therapy by identifying the drug and its accompanying treatment.

MEDICATIONS Used to Treat Cancer: Colony-Stimulating Factors

MEDICATION	ACTION/INDICATION	NURSING IMPLICATIONS
Epoetin alfa (human recombinant erythropoietin)	This glycoprotein stimulates the bone marrow in RBC formation; useful when numbers of RBCs are low due to chemotherapy effects	Give subcutaneously or intravenously. Do not shake and do not use if discolored or particles are present. Single-dose vials only so discard any solution that is not used. Obtain blood tests before therapy and periodically after; improvement in hematocrit should be seen in 7–14 days. Monitor blood pressure before and during therapy as hypertension can result. Monitor for change in neurologic response and headache; both seizures and strokes are possible side effects.
Filgrastim (Neupogen) and pegfilgrastim (Neulasta)	This human granulocyte colony-stimulating factor (G-CSF) increases production of neutrophils by the bone marrow	Administered subcutaneously and intravenously; prepare as directed for IV infusion to prevent its absorption by IV tubing. Single-dose vials only so discard any solution that is not used. Incompatible with many medications; check package insert; do not give within 24 hours before or after chemotherapy drugs or their effect may be decreased. Obtain baseline and twice weekly CBC. Monitor for side effects such as bone pain and heart arrhythmias; report fevers and be alert for other signs of infection when neutrophil count is low.
Oprelvekin (Neumega)	A hematopoietic growth factor, interleukin-11, that increases platelet count; useful in low platelet count due to chemotherapy effects on bone marrow	Administered subcutaneously. Single-dose vials only so discard any solution that is not used. Obtain baseline CBC and platelet count; monitor platelets throughout treatment. Monitor for side effects such as edema, fever, CNS changes, tachycardia, respiratory problems, and skin rash. Take daily weights and monitor for fluid retention.

often occur in siblings, or cord blood banks may offer a match. The umbilical cord blood is then infused into the child undergoing treatment and the same mechanism occurs as in transplantation of bone marrow—implantation of the stem cells into the child's bone marrow and production of normal blood cells over about 2 to 6 weeks. Advantages of umbilical cord blood are that, unlike bone marrow collection, it is not painful for the donor and does not require anesthesia; there is an opportunity to easily collect samples from many ethnic groups that are underrepresented in bone marrow donor registries; graft-versus-host disease after treatment is less prevalent; and storage of umbilical cord blood for use later in life is possible. A variety of federally funded and private blood banks are available to store and provide umbilical blood.

Complementary Therapies. Many families use **complementary therapies** in treatment of a child's cancer. These approaches to care are also referred to as alternative or unconventional, and may involve nutritional supplements, oral herbal supplements, touch therapy, and mind/body interventions. Little research has been done on complementary therapies, although up to 80% of children have used at least one such therapeutic approach (Kelly, Jacobsen, Kennedy, et al., 2000). Healthcare providers should be aware of these practices, inquire in a nonjudgmental manner about what therapies are used, and attempt to learn about specific therapies and practices. Although some herbal and nutritional products such as St. John's wort may decrease serum concentration of chemotherapeutic agents, or some may act as hormones in the body, most are not known to negatively impact contemporary medical treatment, and the families should be assisted in seeking information and supported in use of their chosen therapies (Dean, 2000; Chase, 2000). See Complementary Therapy: Cancer Prevention. Intake of fruits and vegetables is associated with lower cancer incidence in adults, and some foods such as garlic and oranges may slow cancer growth or enhance medical chemotherapy (Swerdlow, 2000). Some individuals use herbal supplements to treat cancer; these include cat's claw (bark of a tree root), mistletoe, and shark cartilage. The Food and Drug Administration has allowed testing of the efficacy of some herbal treatments for cancer (Kemper & Longwood Herbal Task Force, 1999). Several cancer drugs such as vincristine and paclitaxel are obtained from plant products. Some herbs are useful in treatment of nausea and vomiting, and others can boost the immune system's function (Kemper & Longwood Herbal Task Force, 1999).

Palliative Care. Despite modern medical practices and complementary therapies, some children do not survive childhood cancer. In these cases, the focus of healthcare is to provide comfort and emotional support for the child and family. Too often, healthcare providers feel uncomfortable when a child is expected to die and may withdraw from close contact with the child or family, fail to provide adequate comfort measures, and leave the family without access to needed resources. When delay in the recognition of prognosis occurs, children can experience

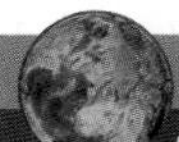

DEVELOPING CULTURAL COMPETENCE Cancer

Traditional Chinese view cancer as a result of weak or toxic blood, which allows pollutants to accumulate and become toxic. A variety of plant products and acupuncture are used to detoxify the blood, and good nutrition helps it to rebuild (Swerdlow, 2000). The nurse should ask what families think causes cancer and support their attempts to improve body functioning.

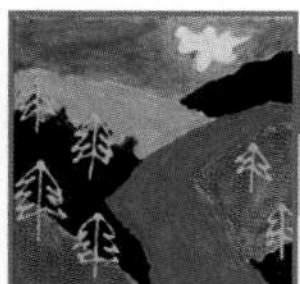

COMPLEMENTARY THERAPY
Cancer Prevention

Many parents ask what they can do to decrease the incidence of cancer in children as they grow into adulthood. The major teaching areas address complementary health practices. They are:

1. Have children increase intake of fruits and vegetables. Most children do not eat enough of these foods and increased intake is associated with lower rates of many cancers. Aim for a minimum of five servings daily.
2. Protect skin with sunscreen. Early excessive exposure to sun and having been sunburned increase chance of skin cancers in adulthood.
3. Discourage smoking among children and be sure children are not exposed to environmental tobacco smoke. This will decrease future chance of developing lung cancer.
4. Have homes tested for radon. Be alert for exposure to any potential hazardous substances in the home or on parents' clothes if they work in industries with chemicals or other harmful substances.

greater suffering and potentially less integration of palliative care (Wolfe, Klar, & Grier, et al., 2000). Some of the symptoms for which children are commonly undertreated include pain, dyspnea, nutrition, elimination, and fatigue (Wolfe, Klar, Grier, et al., 2000). See Chapter 22∞ for a detailed description of palliative care for children with terminal disease (Box 29–2).

BOX 29–2 Research: Preparation for Palliative Care

Healthcare providers often feel uncomfortable in treating children who are dying of cancer, and may not be adequately prepared for the task by their educational programs. The presence of a palliative care team and an integrated plan of care; collaboration between families, primary care provider, and other practitioners; and focus on the child's developmental level and the needs of the family can enhance the care provided for the dying child (Chaffee, 2001; Hilden, Emanuel, Fairclough, et al., 2001).

Special Issues in Childhood Cancer

Oncologic Emergencies. Oncologic emergencies result from the cancer itself or as a side effect of treatment. They can be organized into three groups: metabolic, hematologic, and those involving space-occupying lesions. Overall, the most common oncologic emergencies are tumor lysis syndrome, septic shock, brain herniation, spinal cord compression, and superior vena cava compression from a superior mediastinal mass.

Metabolic Emergencies. Metabolic emergencies result from the lysis (dissolving or decomposing) of tumor cells, a process called tumor lysis syndrome. This cell destruction releases high levels of uric acid, potassium, and phosphates into the blood. Low levels of sodium and calcium occur and metabolic acidosis results. This syndrome is seen most commonly in children with Burkitt's lymphoma and acute lymphocytic leukemia (Baggott et al., 2002). See the table below for laboratory findings and management of tumor lysis syndrome. The nurse collects laboratory studies, including CBC, absolute neutrophil count (ANF), serum electrolytes, bicarbonate, uric acid, BUN and creatinine; and urinalysis. The emergency can be life threatening and the family will need ongoing support and explanations about care.

A second type of metabolic emergency is septic shock. During periods of immune suppression the child is vulnerable to overwhelming infection, resulting in circulatory failure, hypothermia or hyperthermia, tachypnea, mental changes, inadequate tissue perfusion, and hypotension. Septic shock can be fatal (see Chapter 26∞ for a full description of septic shock). Factors contributing to massive infection include inadequate neutrophil production, abnormal granulocytes (not able to be actively phagocytic), erosions through normal barriers such as blood vessels and mucous membranes, and altered bone marrow production caused by chemotherapy and some forms of radiation. Such infections must be vigorously treated with antimicrobial therapy and hydration management.

A third type of metabolic emergency occurs when large amounts of bone are destroyed by treatment, resulting in hypercalcemia (elevated calcium in the serum). Hypercalcemia is most common in children with acute lymphocytic leukemia and rhabdomyosarcoma. Treatment includes hydration and adequate intake of phosphate by oral supplement.

CLINICAL MANIFESTATIONS and Management of Tumor Lysis Syndrome

ETIOLOGY	CLINICAL MANIFESTATIONS	CLINICAL THERAPY	NURSING IMPLICATIONS
Breakdown of malignant cells releases intracellular components into blood	Hyperuricemia Hyperkalemia Hyperphosphatemia Hypocalcemia	• Vigorous hydration with 2–4 times maintenance fluid • Correction of electrolyte imbalances • Administration of allopurinol or urate oxidase (Rasburicase) to reduce conversion of metabolic by-products to uric acid	• Administration of fluids, beginning before therapy • Careful intake and output measures • Daily weight • Urine specific gravity (should remain < 1.010) • Monitoring for desired and side effects of drug therapy
Electrolyte imbalance causes metabolic acidosis and serious abnormalities	Cardiac arrhythmias Impaired renal function Tetany, neurological and mental status changes	• ECG monitoring • Medications such as furosemide to facilitate potassium excretion • Dialysis may be needed	• Administration of electrolytes and medications • Urine pH (should remain 7.0 to 7.5) • Perform Trousseau's and Chvostek's signs for tetany monitoring and assess neurological function • Perform mental status examination • Obtain laboratory specimens as needed

Some children develop syndrome of inappropriate antidiuretic hormone (SIADH) and have excessive release of ADH. The resulting decreased urinary output leads to water intoxication. See Chapter 32∞ for a detailed description of SIADH.

Hematologic Emergencies. Hematologic emergencies result from bone marrow suppression or infiltration of brain and respiratory tissue with high numbers of leukemic blast cells (hyperleukocytosis). Bone marrow suppression results in anemia and **thrombocytopenia** (decreased platelets) with resultant coagulation disturbance and hemorrhage. Disseminated intravascular coagulation (DIC) occurs in some children and is a life-threatening complication. (See Chapter 28∞ for a thorough description of this condition.) Gastrointestinal and central nervous system bleeding (strokes) are common. Disruption of normal WBC production and resulting hyperleukocytosis can lead to obstruction of small blood vessels throughout the body.

Treatment involves infusion of packed red blood cells for anemia; and platelet transfusion, vitamin K, and fresh frozen plasma for thrombocytopenia and hemorrhage. Hyperleukocytosis is treated by hydration, bicarbonate infusion, and allopurinol (Baggott et al., 2002).

Space-Occupying Lesions. Extensive tumor growth may result in spinal cord compression, increased intracranial pressure, brain herniation, seizures, massive hepatomegaly, cardiac and respiratory complications, and superior vena cava syndrome (obstruction of the superior vena cava by tumor). These emergencies are often caused by neuroblastoma, medulloblastoma, astrocytoma, Hodgkin disease, or lymphoma. After biopsy of the mass, treatment involves radiation therapy, chemotherapy, and corticosteroids.

Psychosocial Needs. The diagnosis of cancer is devastating for families. They cannot believe that their vibrant, young child or adolescent has a potentially life-threatening disease. Families are in a state of crisis when the diagnosis is made, with the first response one of shock (Hendricks-Ferguson, 2000). At the same time that they are in a state of shock about the diagnosis, parents must gather resources to support the child, make treatment decisions, and adjust family life to integrate the needs of the child with cancer. Some families need to travel a great distance for the child's treatments and others may have financial constraints that make healthcare costs a major concern. For nearly everyone, parental work schedules and arrangements for other children must be adjusted. Most cancer treatment will last for a minimum of several months up to several years, necessitating nearly constant adaptation.

The child reacts to the diagnosis based on age. Infants and toddlers are unaware of the severity of the disease, while preschoolers are beginning to understand illness. However, they may think they caused their illness, and are confused about why the parent cannot make the illness go away. School-age children can understand a diagnosis of cancer and benefit from opportunities to talk about the experience. Adolescents find contact with others who have gone through their experience reassuring and supportive. A comprehensive review of studies on communicating with children and adolescents about their cancer did not find clear results and directions (Scott, Entwistle, Sowden, et al., 2003). Some programs such as group therapy sessions, computer programs about cancer and treatment, and school reintegration show potential for assisting youth who are adjusting to cancer. Children with cancer may have higher depression scores than healthy children, and therefore are at risk of disturbed mental health status (Cavusoglu, 2001).

NURSING MANAGEMENT

The complex nature of cancer is reflected in multifaceted nursing care. Oncology nursing is a specialty chosen by some nurses who manage the nursing care of children during the diagnostic and treatment phases. Other nurses such as those in schools, home healthcare, offices/clinics, and hospice care partner with oncology nurses to plan and provide for the child and family undergoing cancer treatment. Advanced practice nurses such as nurse practitioners often play key roles in both hospital and community management. Nursing interventions focus on preventive teaching for all families about risk factors for cancer, health promotion and health maintenance of the child undergoing cancer treatment, carrying out the treatment interventions, managing health problems related both to cancer and the side effects of treatment, and partnering with families to manage the challenging psychosocial needs that emerge when cancer is diagnosed.

■ Nursing Assessment and Diagnosis

History

During health promotion visits of all children, nurses are aware of the importance of a history of cancer in the family. Particularly when more than one person has had cancer, and when young children in the extended family have been affected, complete a pedigree to isolate cases in the family. (See Chapter 4∞.) A history of exposure to known carcinogens is also important. Does a parent work in an industry with chemicals or asbestos that might remain on clothing worn home? Was the child treated with radiation or chemotherapy for a previous cancer? Does the child have an identified condition such as Down syndrome? Does the child have any recognized congenital anomalies? A number of conditions are more commonly associated with certain types of cancer.

Physiologic Assessment

When performing any physiologic assessment on children, the nurse considers the possible signs and symptoms of cancer. These include anemia, frequent infections, bleeding disorders, loss of weight, fatigue, pain, and changes in mental health and neurological status. Assessment of children with the most significant types of childhood cancers is presented in separate sections throughout this chapter.

Once cancer has been diagnosed, a thorough physical assessment of all systems is needed to help in identifying the presence and extent of cancer (see Chapter 8∞). Systems needing particularly thorough assessments are neurologic, respiratory, cardiac, and gastrointestinal. Assess hydration status and the tumor site if it is visible. These assessments will be completed regularly at each treatment and monitoring visit. Height and weight should be carefully measured, and compared with prior findings for the child. Nutritional intake histories may be pertinent. Observe immunization status, developmental milestones gait and coordination, as well as any changes in mental status. Evaluate pain, fatigue, infections, bruising, shortness of breath, and elimination problems. Periodic laboratory studies will be performed.

Psychosocial Assessment

Assessment of stress and coping abilities, knowledge of the condition and cognitive level, support systems, developmental level, and body image provides data that help determine the appropriate nursing interventions for the child with cancer and the family.

STRESS AND COPING

The diagnosis of cancer is a major stressor for both the child and the family. Each child's prognosis and each family's coping mechanisms are unique, so begin by gathering information about the crisis from the perspective of the family (Hendricks-Ferguson, 2000). Assess the family (and child if old enough) for understanding and acceptance of the diagnosis. Evaluate if the family has told the child about the diagnosis and whether the family needs assistance in deciding how to do this (Ishibashi, 2001). Ask what they have told siblings, and if they need suggestions and support to decide how much and when to share information with the child's siblings.

Assess the level of anxiety during healthcare visits and scheduled treatments (Figure 29–6 ■). Evaluate the family's resilience and methods of coping, such as the ability to integrate relaxing and meaningful activities into family life, the use of support systems in the extended family and community, and the ability to alter expectations to take into account the child's health status. Concurrent stressors increase the family's difficulty in coping with childhood cancer. Evaluate the family for stressors such as illness or death of another family member, occupational changes, financial problems, relocation, and change in vacation plans. Evaluate the family's knowledge of the U.S. Family Leave Act, which provides for parental use of sick time to treat an ill family member.

KNOWLEDGE

People who are anxious tend to narrow their scope of attention and may read unintended messages into the behaviors of healthcare personnel. Anxiety also limits a person's ability to retain information.

The child's knowledge of cancer and its treatment should be assessed throughout the treatment period. As the child matures cognitively, new evaluations of knowledge are needed. Cancer and its treatment are complex topics and parents are exposed to information in various forms, including written material, news reports, discussions with others, and Internet websites and resources. Evaluate their knowledge and information sources, providing them with opportunities to ask questions. Evaluate the learning style of the child and family in order to adapt approaches to meet their needs.

SUPPORT SYSTEMS

Cancer treatment generally occurs over a long period of time. The extended family is crucial in providing necessary support to the child, parents, and siblings. Identify key persons in the family. They may be the parents, grandparents, or aunts and uncles. Thoroughly assess the coping strategies used by the family to meet the various challenges posed by the child's illness. This information helps to predict the success of interventions, such as home care with intravenous medications, and to decide when referrals for other supportive therapies are needed.

Assess family resources to identify support systems available to help the family during crises and if a child is expected to die. Extended supports include friends, jobs, insurance coverage, religious affiliations, cultural support systems, and the school system. Inquire if the insurance carrier provides for a case manager in

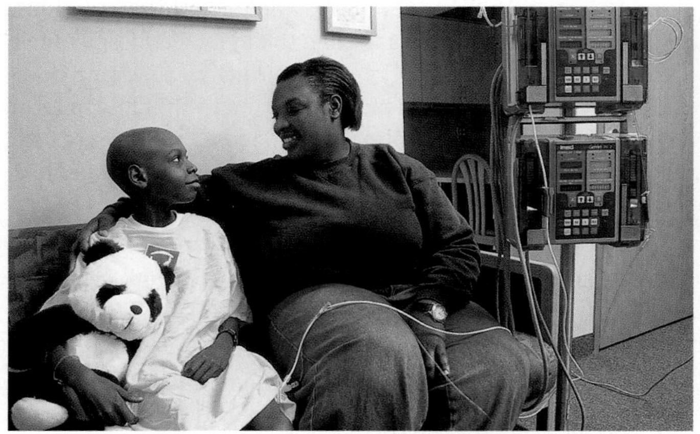

A

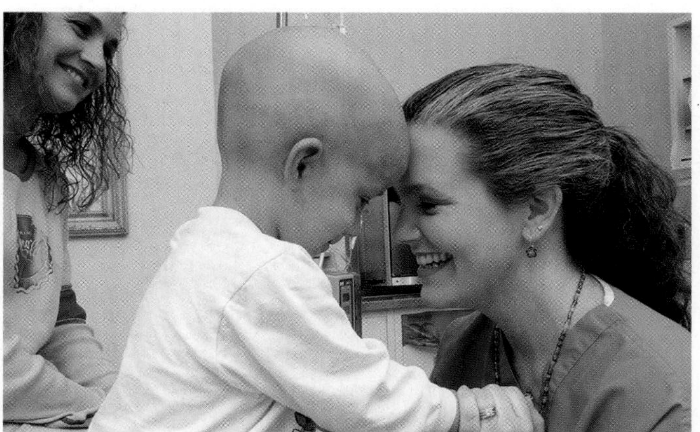

B

FIGURE 29–6 ■ *A,* The child with cancer depends on parents and family members to provide support. *B,* A special relationship often develops between the nurse and the child receiving treatment.

complex health needs such as cancer. Parents commonly lose contact with close friends following the diagnosis of cancer in a child. This is an additional stressor for the family. Jobs are often a source of support because coworkers may have gone through the same experience. It may also be comforting for parents to return to a job where they can feel a sense of security in tangible accomplishments. However, jobs can also be a source of stress if employers are unsympathetic to the demands of the child's hospitalization and clinic or office visits.

Faith-based affiliations can be an important source of support. Evaluate whether such affiliations are meaningful for the family and, if so, plan for visits from the appropriate clergy. In some cultures, spiritual leaders are an important part of the family's support. Enable a healer to visit the child and conduct a healing ceremony if that will be supportive to the family and child.

The return to school may pose difficulties for the child with cancer or it may be a source of support to be connected again to peers. The child is encouraged to go to school, even if only for half a day per week, to stay connected to peers. Evaluate the ability of the school to accept a medically vulnerable child into the classroom. Nurses who work in the oncology department of the hospital or clinic can ask if the family would give consent to visit the school, meet with the school nurse, and plan together to meet the child's educational needs. Assess whether the other children and teachers have been prepared for the appearance and needs of the child with cancer. Arrangements can be made for tutors to help the child keep up with schoolwork if he or she cannot attend school. An individualized education plan is needed. Parents need information about the legal right to this plan since the child is newly ill and they will likely not have been exposed to this in the past. See Chapter 20∞.

BODY IMAGE

Hair loss, surgical scars, and cushingoid changes are three common treatment-induced threats to body image. Most children being treated for cancer experience hair loss (Figure 29–7 ■). Children who have cranial surgery lose hair as part of the surgical preparation. Chemotherapy frequently results in some degree of hair loss. The speed of hair loss is unique to the child and can be as rapid as overnight or slower, evidenced by hair left on the pillow and in the hairbrush. Radiation may cause permanent hair loss or thinning.

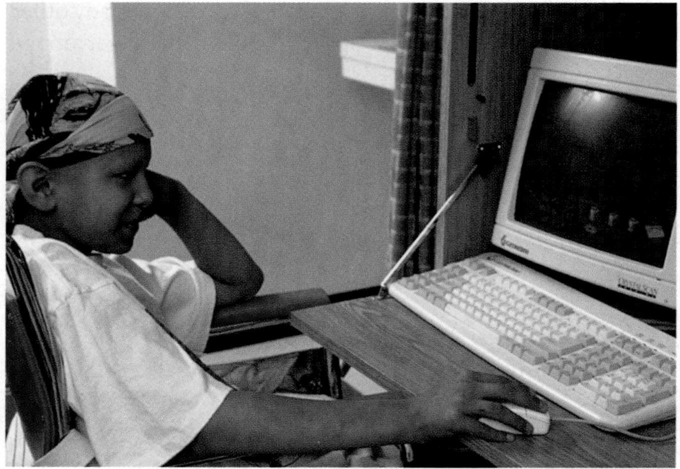

FIGURE 29–7 ■ One of the most common threats to a child's body image at any age is hair loss induced by chemotherapy. Use of hats can improve self-concept.

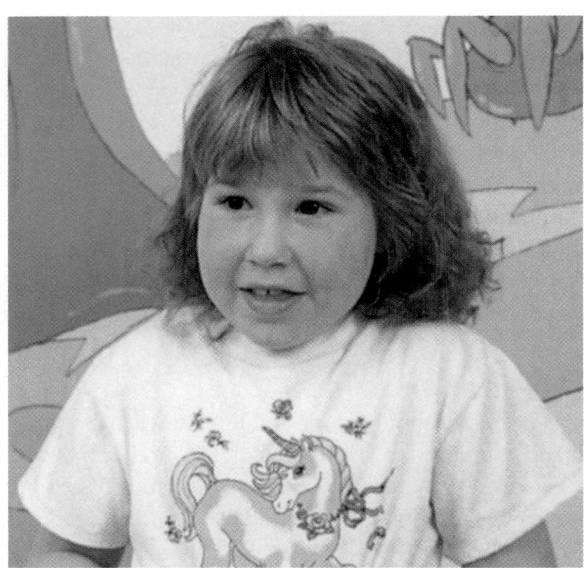

FIGURE 29–8 ■ The child with cushingoid features has a rounded face and prominent cheeks.

A second challenge to the child's body image is surgery. The scars of cranial and neck surgery are obvious, as are amputation and limb salvaging. Abdominal surgery for lymphoma is more easily concealed but is still a threat to the child's body image. A central line that is inserted for medications after surgery involves integration of this line to body image for a time.

A third source of altered body image is the cushingoid features such as round and flushed face, prominent cheeks, double chin, and generalized obesity (Figure 29–8 ■) that result from the use of corticosteroids. As the child's weight increases, stretch marks similar to those of pregnancy may occur. These stretch marks often remain after the corticosteroids are decreased.

Body image disturbances occur when a child cannot integrate changes and continues to cling to old images despite their inconsistency with reality. Common means for assessing body image are drawings, colored pictures cut out by the child to form a collage, discussion, and observation. See Chapter 17∞ for further discussion of these and other assessment techniques that can be used with children.

Developmental Assessment

Developmental assessment of children should be performed regularly during treatment for cancer, at times when the child feels well so that results are accurate. Children under 6 years of age who have cancer should receive regular developmental assessment with a standardized tool such as the Denver II Developmental Screening Test (see Chapter 10∞). A home healthcare nurse can perform such testing, or a nurse in the pediatric healthcare home (medical home) who sees the child for a general health supervision visit. Assessment of the child's physical and neurologic development helps in determining the progress made during treatment and provides a baseline for evaluating the long-term effects of treatment. Recommend referral to a neuropsychologist for testing early in treatment and if changes in developmental performance are noted. Observe developmental milestones at each contact with the child and refer for further assessment if regression has occurred. Performance in school and social activities with friends provides important information about expected developmental milestones in older children.

Assessment for Impact of Cancer Survival

Children with cancer have a variety of common psychologic and physiologic problems, regardless of their specific type of cancer. They and their families are dealing with a complex illness that influences their lives for years. The impact of this experience extends into all areas of function. Over the past 20 to 30 years, treatment for childhood cancers has been increasingly successful. About 1 in 1,000 young adults is a survivor of childhood cancer. The success of new modalities and treatment combinations has, however, created special healthcare needs for many survivors. See the Photo Story on pages 1054–1055.

Surgery can have many results. Body organs may be removed and manipulated, leading to adhesions, intestinal obstruction, visual impairment, neurologic disruption, and sterility. Removal of the spleen can lead to serious infections. Amputation necessitates the need for prosthetic devices and physical rehabilitation.

Radiation has several long-term effects. It can impair the growth of bones and teeth, leading to conditions such as scoliosis, leg length discrepancy, or poor dental health. Hypothyroidism can be observed in those who have had head and neck radiation (Castellino & Hudson, 2002). Cardiotoxicity and pulmonary toxicity can result from mediastinal radiation. Delayed puberty and sterility can result from radiation effects to the cranium and spinal regions. Impaired neurocognitive performance may occur as long-term effects of treatment, especially with higher doses of radiation. Some studies have found lower behavioral and social competence in treated children (Challinor, Miaskowski, Moore, et al., 2000). Secondary cancers, most commonly solid tumors, occur in some survivors. **Secondary cancers** are also called second malignant neoplasm (SMN) and are those that occur subsequent to the primary cancer and treatment but are of a different histologic type.

Chemotherapy can cause a wide variety of effects, both during its administration and for years afterward. See the clinical manifestations table on page 1056. Cardiomyopathy can occur with some drugs, especially the anthracyclines. Temporary and/or permanent pulmonary toxicity and renal complications can develop. Neurologic effects of some drugs can lead to hearing loss (e.g., cisplatin and ifosfamide), cataracts, and paraplegia (e.g., intrathecal methotrexate for leukemia). Learning disabilities and change in intelligence quotient (IQ) occur in some children. Infertility may result (Castellino & Hudson, 2002). Although radiation is responsible for most secondary tumors, some chemotherapy drugs have also been implicated.

The diagnosis and stress of treatment, along with the risk of recurrence, are significant stressors for the child with cancer. Families may find it difficult to obtain full insurance coverage for the child who has had a prior cancer. Employment can be a potential problem for cancer survivors if employers have concerns about the earlier cancer diagnosis. Most people with cancer report fear of recurrence of the disease, which is a stressor. Depression, suicidal thoughts, and concerns about appearance are more common in survivors of childhood cancer (Recklitis, O'Leary, & Diller, 2003). On the other hand, hopefulness and the sense of having an added purpose in life can be positive outcomes for many cancer survivors. Some meet with others who have a recent diagnosis, or work on fundraising events that financially support cancer research.

Nurses are involved with families when a diagnosis of cancer is made, during the therapy process, and in the years that follow. For a child who survives cancer, ongoing care is essential. Evaluate the child regularly with thorough physical, psychosocial, developmental, and cognitive assessments. Carefully monitor all body systems (e.g., cardiovascular; respiratory; musculoskeletal; eye, ear, nose, and throat; genitourinary). Record height and weight and general growth patterns. Ask about the child's interactions with peers and performance at school. Children who have received cranial radiation and intrathecal chemotherapy need regular scholastic evaluations. Impaired neurocognitive performance may occur as long-term effects of treatment, and appropriate interventions should be planned in these cases (Challinor et al., 2000). Be alert for signs and symptoms that could indicate a secondary tumor. Ask the parents about insurance coverage and other financial difficulties during ongoing care.

Plan care to assist the family to manage any long-term effects of cancer treatment. This may involve physical rehabilitation, support related to visual impairment, or treatment for cardiac or musculoskeletal abnormalities. Provide resources for information and support. Facilitate periodic evaluations in a healthcare agency so that serious outcomes of treatment can be identified early.

The accompanying nursing care plans include several diagnoses that may be appropriate for the child with cancer who is receiving care in the hospital or at home. Among the many other diagnoses that may be appropriate for a child with cancer are the following:

- Diarrhea related to radiation therapy and toxins
- Impaired Urinary Elimination related to chemotherapy
- Impaired Oral Mucous Membrane related to chemotherapy and radiation therapy
- Impaired Skin Integrity related to altered nutritional state, effects of medication, radiation, and immobilization
- Ineffective Individual Coping related to situational crises of chronic and acute illness
- Disturbed Sleep Pattern related to biochemical agents, anxiety, and unfamiliar surroundings
- Deficient Diversional Activity related to frequent lengthy treatments
- Disturbed Body Image related to chronic illness and treatments

PHOTOStory...

Survivors of childhood cancer

Most children survive the diagnosis and treatment of cancer. Each child and family has a unique way of coping with the challenges they face. The role of the nurse is to identify and draw upon the strengths of the family and provide resources to help increase coping skills. Three different families are shown in these photographs. Nicole, 11 years old, is undergoing chemotherapy for Ewing's sarcoma. Her mother emphasizes, "It's our faith that has gotten us through this. The hardest part is how busy you are coming to treatments all the time. Nicole's younger brother sometimes feels neglected." The family has learned to accept meals and other offers of help from friends. Nicole's teachers recently came to visit her at home when she was absent from school for several weeks due to treatment side effects. The nurse helps Nicole's mother to identify ways to include the brother in some trips to the hospital and other activities.

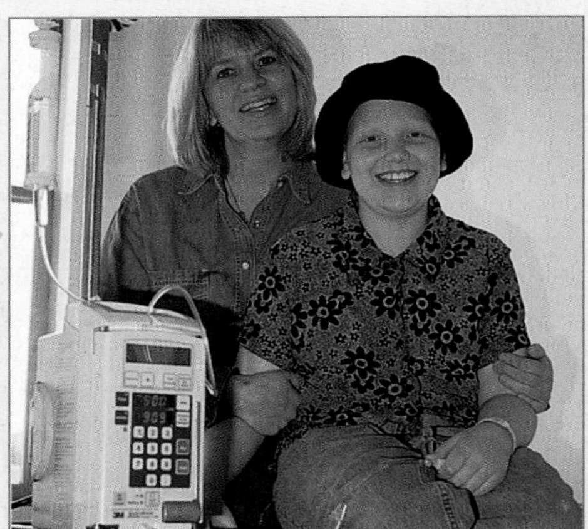

Nicole is receiving chemotherapy treatment for Ewing's sarcoma and a limb salvage surgical procedure is planned for her cancer site in the femur. What are the major psychosocial and physiological threats for the future surgery? How can Nicole be best prepared to meet these threats?

According to Jesse, who is 10 years old and waiting for a bone marrow transplant, "The thing that has helped me the most [in

- Deficient Knowledge (child or parents) related to lack of exposure to disease or treatments
- Anticipatory Grieving related to actual or potential loss of significant other

Planning and Implementation

The nursing care of children newly diagnosed with cancer and their families includes immediate physiologic and psychologic support, along with anticipatory guidance about imminent and future medical interventions. The family should be assisted and supported in making decisions about types of treatment that are appropriate for the child.

Nursing care of the hospitalized child with cancer and the child receiving ongoing therapy at home is summarized in the accompanying nursing care plans. These care plans are designed for the child who has progressed beyond the cancer diagnosis phase and is receiving chemotherapy.

Physiologic care of the hospitalized child focuses on providing support during treatment. This includes ensuring optimal nutritional intake, administering medications, managing the multiple side effects of chemotherapy and radiation, ensuring adequate hydration, preventing infection, and managing pain.

Ensure Optimal Nutritional Intake

Up to 30% of children with cancer are malnourished (Han-Markey, 2000). The high metabolic rate of cancer growth depletes the child's nutritional stores so that many children are cachectic at the time of diagnosis. Added to this is the catabolic effect of chemotherapy and radiation on normal cells, necessitating additional cellular replacement. The child needs increased nutritional intake at a time when nausea and vomiting are occurring as drug side effects, and when decreased activity and general health status result in diminished appetite. This often leads to extreme concern on the part of parents, and they may focus excessive attention on the child's intake.

Administer antiemetic drugs to lessen nausea from chemotherapy. Offer frequent, small meals. It may be helpful to offer the child's favorite foods at times when nausea and vomit-

dealing with acute lymphoblastic leukemia] is all the mail I got from my friends." His mother adds, "We're just really positive and believe that everything will turn out all right." Since contact with his peers is important, the nurse finds out his school and teacher's name so that when he has his transplant, which will be in a city about 300 miles from home, Jesse will again have cards from his friends. The nurse also helps the family plan for how they will manage when Jesse is hospitalized for several weeks for the transplant; options for housing near the hospital, access to food, and ways to ensure contact with the family at home are part of the nursing plan.

Cassie, 19 months old, has been diagnosed with neuroblastoma. At this age, it is hard for her to understand what is happening. Her mother has stayed with her each time she has come to the hospital, which has helped Cassie adjust to therapy. Her caregivers are confident that she will respond well to her treatment. The nurse encourages Cassie's mother to continue to spend time with her and also asks about the stress of leaving responsibilities at home behind. Developmental approaches appropriate to Cassie's age, including play therapy, are part of the nursing care plan. Survivors of childhood cancer need health promotion and health maintenance interventions throughout the treatment period and in the years following the initial diagnosis. ■

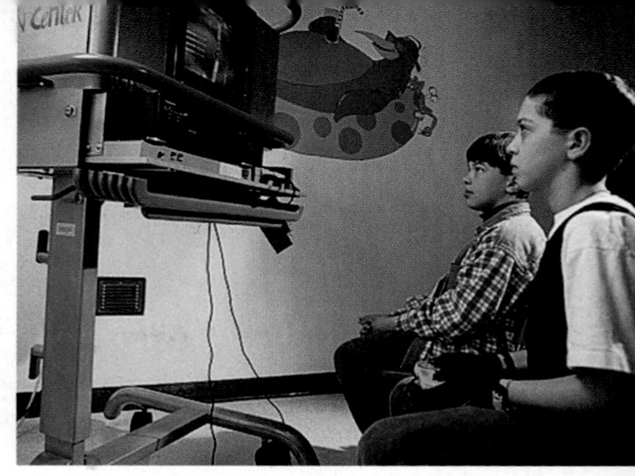

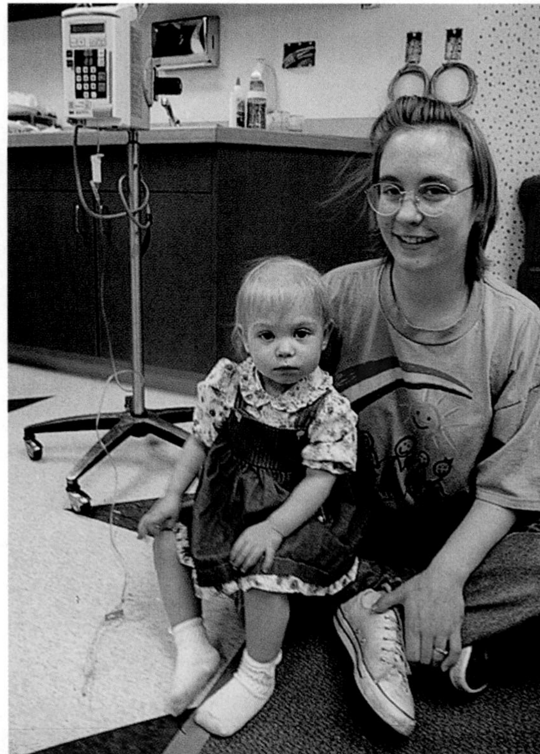

Jesse will be in an isolation room at the hospital when he gets his bone marrow transplant. What planning can you recommend now that might help him to plan for meeting school requirements? Once he is discharged and is going back to school, what teaching will you provide to minimize his chance of infection? ***(top right)***

Note that although Cassie is hospitalized she is wearing her own clothes. Why might this be important to children? What other interventions can promote a sense of comfort for a toddler who is hospitalized? ***(bottom right)***

ing are decreased. Ask the family what treatments they use to decrease the child's nausea and vomiting and inform them of techniques that may enhance intake. Perform 24-hour dietary recalls to assess the child's intake, and evaluate height and weight regularly. Special nutritional products may be given orally, nasogastric or nasoduodenal tube feedings may be given, or total parenteral nutrition may be necessary. When the child's nutritional status is deteriorating or parenteral nutrition is used, perform weekly studies of serum electrolytes, liver chemistry, glucose, and triglycerides. Partner with both the oncologist and the dietitian to plan interventions appropriate for meeting the needs of individual children.

Palliative care is administered when a child is not expected to live. Nutritional support becomes especially important during this time to improve quality of life, enhance comfort, and support the immune system. Children should be offered foods that they like and are easy to eat. Soft, nonspicy foods such as puddings, eggs, and purees provide high-energy density, ease in consumption, and digestibility. Ensure adequate fluids, and supplement fluids with powdered milk or energy supplements (Hill & Hart, 2001).

Administer Medications

One important intervention of the oncology nurse is administering medications safely. Most chemotherapeutic drugs are prescribed and calculated as dose per meter squared (dose/m^2), with m^2 calculated from the child's height and weight. (Refer to the section on administering medications in the Skills Manual.) Most often several chemotherapeutic drugs are used in combinations (see Table 29–3). Techniques such as generous hydration accompanying medications help to decrease side effects.

PRACTICE ALERT

A treatment known as *leucovorin rescue* is used in conjunction with high-dose methotrexate chemotherapy. Leucovorin (citorvorum factor) is a form of folic acid that helps to protect normal cells from the destructive action of methotrexate. It is started within 24 hours of methotrexate administration and is given along with hydration therapy. Usual administration is q 6 hours × 72 hours or until serum methotrexate is at the desired level.

Chemotherapy drugs are prepared with special techniques under laminar flow devices to minimize potential toxic effects

CLINICAL MANIFESTATIONS of Common Side Effects of Chemotherapy

SIDE EFFECT	CLINICAL MANIFESTATIONS	CLINICAL THERAPY
Bone marrow suppression	Evidence of suppression usually appears 7–10 days after administration of chemotherapy; recovery is usually complete within 3–4 weeks	Blood transfusions are administered when anemia is severe (Hgb < 7 g/dL) or platelets are very low Some institutions use a low-microbial diet to decrease the possibility that infectious organisms will colonize the intestine Septra is used for *Pneumocystis carinii* pneumonia prophylaxis; nystatin and oral vancomycin for antifungal and antibacterial prophylaxis Instruct the family and child about the importance of protecting the body from bruising during periods of mild to moderate thrombocytopenia (platelet count, < 5,000/mm^3) Careful handwashing is essential Encourage use of masks if family or staff have nasopharyngeal infections
Nausea and vomiting	Symptoms may occur immediately or 5–6 hours after administration of chemotherapy and may last 48 hours	Antiemetics, such as oldansetron, Kytril, Reglan, and Benadryl are used to treat this side effect Teach relaxation techniques, hypnosis, and systematic desensitization (a hypnotic process that progressively reduces reactions to objects that cause strong emotional or physical responses) to help to decrease the child's symptoms Encourage mild exercise and change of diet (eating only easily digestible foods) 12 hours before chemotherapy
Anorexia and weight loss	May occur at any time	Hyperalimentation is necessary if dietary changes are unsuccessful in halting the child's weight loss Pay careful attention to changes in taste that affect food preferences Referral to a dietician may be helpful to achieve successful modification of the child's diet
Mouth sores	The oral mucositis resulting from chemotherapy usually occurs within 3–4 days and is often a contributing factor in anorexia	Antifungal agents, such as nystatin or clotrimazole, lessen the possibility of candidal infection Promote good oral hygiene, use soft foam wand or water irrigation to clean teeth; commercial mouthwashes are not recommended because they contain alcohol and increase drying of the oral cavity
Constipation	Can occur at any time in treatment but becomes more common as therapy progresses and dietary intake and physical activity decrease	Stool softeners and laxatives are used to treat this side effect Advise parents to increase fluids and fibrous foods in the child's diet
Pain	Pain can occur at any time and is best understood by subjective explanations of the child.	Acetaminophen, morphine, steroids, nonsteroidal anti-inflammatory drugs, and antidepressants may be used to manage pain Careful pain assessment is important; the location of the pain may provide a clue to its cause, for example, metastasis to the skull, infiltration of joints, or damage to soft tissue; pain associated with chemotherapy may also be related to oral mucositis, myalgia, or tumor embolization; painful polyneuropathy can follow treatment with vincristine or cisplatin Acetaminophen for pain can mask the presence of fever, which signals infection; careful and complete physical assessment is needed to identify infection Pharmacologic, nonhypnotic (deep breathing, self-control), and hypnotic methods of pain control may be used; the nonpharmacologic methods often prove helpful to children with pain from multiple etiologies

on healthcare providers. Gloves and other hazardous drug protocols are used. Follow the guidelines of the Occupational Safety and Health Administration in "Controlling Occupational Exposure to Hazardous Drugs" (U.S. Department of Labor, 2003). Care must be taken to avoid **extravasation** of intravenous drugs (leakage into the soft tissue around the infusion site), as permanent tissue damage can result.

In addition to chemotherapy drugs, the nurse administers other medications, such as antiemetics to control nausea, vitamin supplements, and antibiotics. Antiemetics such as oldansetron are given prophylactically when a cancer agent is administered that has known emetic effects. Parents are asked about complementary therapy and medications they are obtaining from other sources and using at home. All medications must be safely administered and the child should be monitored for side effects. **Polypharmacy** (the use of several drugs at one time to treat multiple health conditions) can lead to multiple side effects and can challenge the body's ability to metabolize and excrete drugs.

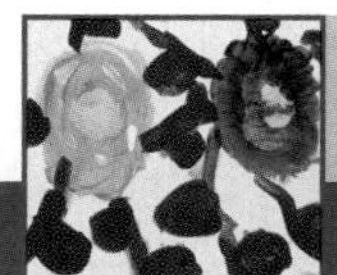

Nursing Care Plan

HOSPITAL CARE OF THE CHILD WITH CANCER

GOAL	INTERVENTION	RATIONALE	EXPECTED OUTCOME
1. Pain related to tissue injury			
	NIC Priority Intervention—*Pain Management:* Alleviation or reduction in pain to a level of comfort acceptable to patient.		**NOC Suggested Outcome**—*Comfort Level:* Feelings of physical and psychologic ease.
The child will report reduced pain that is manageable.	▪ Give analgesics as ordered. ▪ Teach relaxation techniques, deep breathing and distraction.	▪ Adequate medications can reduce pain. ▪ Nonpharmacologic methods work with the medication to reduce pain.	The child experiences pain reduced to the level that allows child to interact appropriately and gain rest.
2. Disturbed Sleep Pattern related to lack of sleep privacy/control			
	NIC Priority Intervention—*Sleep Enhancement:* Facilitation of regular sleep/wake cycles.		**NOC Suggested Outcome—***Rest:* Extent and pattern of diminished activity for mental and physical rejuvenation.
The child will sleep for hours appropriate to age. The child will report feeling rested.	▪ Alter the environment to allow designated rest periods. ▪ Plan care to reduce frequency of interruptions during normal rest and sleep times.	▪ A quiet environment encourages relaxation needed for resting. ▪ Reduced interruptions allow continuous sleep and rest.	The child rests and sleeps for an age-appropriate amount of time per day.
3. Imbalanced Nutrition: Less Than Body Requirements related to inability to ingest or digest food or absorb nutrients			
	NIC Priority Intervention—*Nutrition Management:* Assistance with and provision of a balanced dietary intake.		**NOC Suggested Outcome**—*Nutritional Status:* Extent to which nutrients are available to meet metabolic needs.
The child will maintain adequate nutritional intake.	▪ Offer small feedings. Encourage favorite foods. Refer to dietitian for special meals: Weight daily.	▪ Measures can increase caloric intake. Taste changes and mouth sores alter desire for food.	The child maintains admission weight.
The child will experience reduced effects of chemotherapy (i.e., nausea and vomiting)	▪ Teach the child distraction and relaxation techniques. Give antiemetics according to orders.	▪ Pharmacologic and nonpharmacologic methods are effective in helping to reduce nausea.	The child has minimal side effects of nausea and vomiting.
4. Risk for Constipation related to change in usual foods and eating patterns			
	NIC Priority Intervention—*Constipation Management:* Prevention and alleviation of constipation.		**NOC Suggested Outcome—***Bowel Elimination:* The ability of the gastrointestinal tract to form and evacuate stool effectively.
The child will reestablish normal bowel pattern.	▪ Record all output by size and description. Administer stool softeners. Test stool for guaiac. Report changes in stool to physician. Encourage adequate fluid intake.	▪ Chemotherapy or tumor may create constipation, diarrhea, or blood in stool.	The child has normal bowel pattern.
5. Fluid Volume Excess or Deficient related to medications.			
	NIC Priority Intervention—*Fluid Management:* Promotion of fluid balance and prevention of complications resulting from abnormal fluid levels.		**NOC Suggested Outcome—***Fluid Balance:* Balance of water in the intracellular and extracellular compartments of the body.
The child will be adequately hydrated.	▪ Record all intake. Monitor intravenous rate and solution as appropriate. ▪ Test specific gravity of urine daily.	▪ Some drugs (e.g., cyclophosphamide) necessitate a high level of fluid intake to prevent complications. ▪ Renal function may be affected by chemotherapy.	The child demonstrates adequate hydration. Mucous membranes are hydrated. Specific gravity remains within normal range.

(continued)

Nursing Care Plan HOSPITAL CARE OF THE CHILD WITH CANCER (continued)

GOAL	INTERVENTION	RATIONALE	EXPECTED OUTCOME
6. Risk for Infection related to immunosuppression, invasive procedures, malnutrition, or pharmaceutical agents			
	NIC Priority Intervention—*Infection Protection:* Prevention and early detection of infection in patient at risk.		**NOC Suggested Outcome—***Risk Control:* Actions to eliminate or reduce health threats.
The child will remain free of infection.	■ Wash hands often. Maintain in isolation if needed.	■ Handwashing is effective to reduce organisms. Transmission—based precautions may be needed to safeguard child.	The child remains infection free.
	■ Monitor temperature. Report elevation to physician.	■ Elevated temperature is a sign of infection.	
	■ Administer intravenous antibiotics as ordered. Monitor temperature. Use cooling mattress as ordered. Report elevations over 38°C (101°F) to physician.	■ Multiple antibiotics are needed to deal with bacterial and lung infections during neutropenia. Blood cultures may be taken to identify organism.	The child with an infection is effectively treated.
7. Ineffective Individual Coping related to situational crisis			
	NIC Priority Intervention—*Coping Enhancement:* Assisting a patient to adapt to stressors which interfere with meeting life demands and roles.		**NOC Suggested Outcome—***Coping:* Actions to manage stressors that tax an individual's resources.
The child will demonstrate normal adaptive coping methods.	■ Encourage drawings and other therapeutic play for expression of feelings. Allow for expression of angry feelings, such as hitting dolls and throwing sponge balls. Discuss how to behave during treatments.	■ Expression of feelings helps identify avoidance coping for further intervention. Play is a normal way for child to express self and ideas. Misinterpretations can be corrected. Knowledge of appropriate and helpful behaviors supports self-esteem.	The child continues to use usual coping strategies expected for developmental stage.
8. Ineffective Health Maintenance related to complex treatment, and lack of resources			
	NIC Priority Intervention—*Health System Guidance:* Facilitating use of health services.		**NOC Suggested Outcome—***Knowledge:* Health Behaviors: Extent of understanding conveyed about promotion and protection of health.
The child will state understanding of treatments and procedures.	■ Use age-appropriate teaching methods. Content areas include child's cancer, medications (actions and side effects), how to deal with body changes, and how to deal with response of others to those changes. Correct misinterpretations. Anticipate upcoming events and teach the child and family about them.	■ Education helps by increasing understanding, removing fantasy, and clarifying fears. Education promotes the use of new learning in all areas of life.	The child demonstrates age-appropriate knowledge of the cancer, its treatments, and medications. The child has age-appropriate understanding of how to deal with changes in the body.

When unapproved drugs are given investigationally in a clinical trial, consent by parents is mandatory. They should know the potential benefits and harm to the child. Children who are cognitively able should also give assent verbally or in writing. This assent can usually be obtained from children by the age of 7 to 9 years, depending on the child's level of understanding. Even when the family has given consent for a clinical trial they may have additional questions. Nurses can clarify information and refer the family to the research investigator for further explanations.

Many children will receive fluids and medications at home via central lines. Consider referral to home healthcare infusion agencies for monitoring of these treatments and provision of supplies for home use.

Manage Treatment Side Effects

All cancer treatments affect some normal body cells as well as cancer cells, causing a wide variety of side effects. A frequent occurrence is **myelosuppression,** or suppression of blood cell production in the bone marrow. Be alert for signs of a decreased white blood cell count, such as infections. **Neutropenia** is present when the absolute neutrophil count (ANC) is < 500 cells/mm^3 or if between 500 and 1,000 cells/mm^3 when chemotherapy is being given and falling levels are anticipated. At these levels, children will be given a broad-spectrum antibiotic; G-CSF may be given (see the medications table on page 1046) (Bryant, 2003). Take the child's temperature, isolate the child from others with infections, and perform serum laboratory studies as ordered. A colony-stimulating factor for white cell production may be administered, if necessary (see page 1048).

Protect the child from bruises and be alert for signs of bleeding such as petechiae, nosebleeds, dark colored or bloody stools, and presence of blood in vomit and urine; these are all effects of thrombocytopenia or decreased platelets. When thrombocytopenia occurs, minimize needle sticks and other intrusive procedures. Be ready to deal with nosebleeds and watch for bleeding gums. Report any bleeding episodes to the physician. Be sure parents know that the child should avoid contact sports or other rough activities and that any healthcare provider, such as a dentist, should be informed of the child's treatment and condition (Bryant, 2003). Infusions to increase platelets are sometimes administered.

Inadequate red blood cell production can result in anemia. Encourage the child to eat iron-rich foods and administer nutritional supplements, as needed. Blood transfusions are sometimes needed to treat severe anemia.

Chemotherapy affects all rapidly growing cells in the body, but especially those of the mucous membranes. Provide good oral hygiene with a soft toothbrush, foam wand, or water irrigation device. Report oral breakdown promptly. Partner with the oncologist, dentist, and nutritionist to plan treatment strategies to protect the oral health and erupting teeth of children. See Partnering with Families: Oral Care for common techniques to manage oral hygiene. Be alert for blood in vomitus and stool or dark colored stools, all of which can be indicators of bleeding in the gastrointestinal tract. Blood in the urine may also occur. Evaluate the effects of hair loss on the child. Know all side effects of specific drugs administered and monitor for them. Realize that some side effects are late and may be seen after therapy is completed. Emphasize importance of all follow-up visits scheduled in the future for monitoring of late effects.

Radiation can cause burns to the skin. Examine the skin daily during hospitalization or weekly when making home visits. Leave the marks on the skin that outline the radiation target area. Avoid use of lotions, powders, and soaps on the target skin area. Some children may need to be anesthetized to ensure correct positioning for radiation; postanesthesia care will then be needed.

Ensure Adequate Hydration

Hydration management can be a challenge as the child may not be thirsty but is excreting large numbers of cell fragments and other substances as a result of treatment. Offer frequent, small amounts of fluid. Include frozen ice pops or other fluid-containing foods such as Jell-O. Measure intake and output. To ensure adequate excretion, a number of chemotherapy drugs are given with intravenous fluids. It is important to administer fluids as ordered and ensure that the recommended urinary output excretion rate is maintained after drug administration.

Prevent and Treat Infection

Children with cancer have an altered immune system, both from the disease and from the effects of immunosuppressant drugs, and must be kept away from persons with known infections. Keep the child's immunization record so immunizations that have not been given yet can be administered in regular clinic visits after therapy is complete, using Centers for Disease Control and Prevention (CDC) recommendations for timing after treatment. Follow recommendations for the immunization of children with cancer as published by the Centers for Disease Control and Prevention and the American Academy of Pediatrics. Usually no immunizations are given to the child until 6 months after completing chemotherapy.

Teach parents to avoid taking the child to places that attract large gatherings of people, such as department stores, once the child returns home. Teach administration of any drugs being used to prevent infection such as pentamadine or sulfa preparations for pneumocystis pneumonia prophylaxis. Emphasize the need to report any exposure to contagious diseases, especially chickenpox. Signs of infection may be masked by some drugs, so be alert for any signs of mild infection. Fever, malaise, and mild respiratory infection must be reported promptly.

Management of infections is critical. Children are often hospitalized and central lines used for antibiotic administration. Blood cultures and cultures of infected body parts help to establish the causative organisms. Due to lowered immune status, unusual agents are sometimes identified. Administer medication treatment on time and as ordered. Ensure standard precautions and transmisson-based precautions are followed. Temperature, vital signs, and assessment of all body systems is performed at admission and at least every 4 hours.

PARTNERING WITH FAMILIES

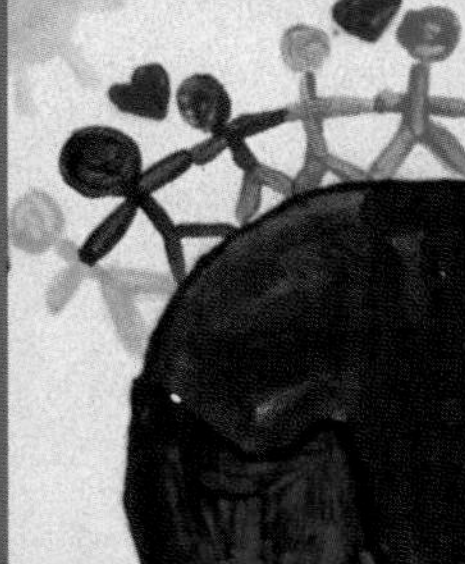

Oral Care

Since cancer treatment and poor nutritional status can adversely affect the oral status of children, families need help to plan and carry out prophylactic and treatment measures. Children continue to lose teeth, have new teeth erupt, and require nutrients to help in building teeth not yet erupted, even during cancer treatment. Some suggestions are:

- Provide a visit to the dentist early in treatment for assessment, treatment of dental disease, and to establish a prevention plan.
- Floss and brush teeth twice daily with a soft bristle brush and rinse with water.
- When granulocyte counts fall below 500/mm^3 or platelets fall below 40,000/mm^3, toothettes or gauze can be used to clean the teeth. Avoiding brushes will help to prevent bleeding and infection.
- Toothpaste can be used unless it causes discomfort.
- Medications may be used to prevent infection. They may include antibacterial mouthwash, nystatin, or fluconozole. Continue oral fluoride if it is not present in the drinking water.
- If bleeding, infection, or other oral care needs emerge, consult with the dentist and pediatric oncologist to develop a treatment plan.

(Chin, 1998; Gibson & Nelson, 2000)

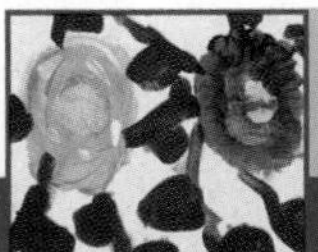

Nursing Care Plan

HOME CARE OF THE CHILD WITH CANCER

GOAL	INTERVENTION	RATIONALE	EXPECTED OUTCOME
1 Risk for Infection related to immunosuppression, chemotherapy, and presence of invasive lines			
	NIC Priority Intervention—*Infection Protection:* Prevention and early detection of infection in child at risk.		**NOC Suggested Outcome—***Risk Control:* Actions to eliminate or reduce health risks.
The child will remain infection free.	■ Educate the child and parents about meaning of blood counts. ■ Encourage parents/family members to use masks when they are ill. ■ Encourage good handwashing at all times. ■ Advise the child's teacher to tell parents if the child is exposed to communicable illness at school. ■ Clean vascular access site and inject heparin per protocol. Observe for signs of infection. Report infection to physician.	■ Knowledgeable parents and child can protect themselves. ■ Masks help decrease airborne infection if used properly. ■ Handwashing is best prevention. ■ Exposure can be reported to physician for possible use of antibiotic, antiviral drug, or admission for treatment. ■ Use of heparin maintains an open access route by preventing clotting.	The child remains infection free. All exposures are reported to physician immediately.
2. Imbalanced Nutrition: Less Than Body Requirements related to inability to ingest or digest adequate quantities of food or absorb adequate nutrients			
	NIC Priority Intervention—*Nutrition Management:* Assistance with and provision of a balanced dietary intake.		**NOC Suggested Outcome—***Nutritional Status:* Extent to which nutrients are available to meet metabolic needs.
The child will maintain adequate nutritional intake.	■ Encourage small and frequent high-calorie meals. Encourage small bites of a variety foods. ■ Promote good oral hygiene and use of nonalcohol mouthwashes. ■ Teach home enteral and parenteral nutrition if ordered.	■ Measures to increase caloric intake. Taste changes and favorite foods may no longer be preferred. ■ Mouth sores cause discomfort when eating, alcohol is painful on open sores. ■ Enternal or parenteral nutritional support may be used to enhance intake.	The child maintains normal weight for height.
3. Ineffective Management of Therapeutic Regimen related to complex therapy.			
	NIC Intervention—*Family Involvement:* Facilitating family participation in the emotional and physical care of the child.		**NOC Suggested Outcome—***Care Management:* Family ability to manage complex therapy.
The child will comply with oral medication regimen.	■ Educate parents and child about the importance of taking medication as prescribed. ■ Set up calender with dates, times, and medications clearly labeled. ■ Reward the child for taking medications.	■ Understanding can assist parents and child in placing importance on medication intake. ■ Visual reminders can help them recall instructions. ■ Reinforcing desired behaviors through rewards is effective with children.	The child takes all medications according to prescription.
4. Delayed Growth and Development related to serious illness			
	NIC Priority Intervention—*Developmental Enhancement:* Facilitating parents/caregivers to promote optimal/growth and development of child		**NOC Suggested Outcome—***Child Growth and Development:* Normal increase in body size and developmental skills.
The child will demonstrate normal physical, emotional, and cognitive development.	■ Encourage play appropriate to age. ■ Encourage the child to attend school.	■ Normal activities support self-esteem and self-knowledge. ■ School is the work of the child and promotes cognitive and social growth.	The child continues to develop physically, emotionally, and cognitively at a normal pace.

Nursing Care Plan HOME CARE OF THE CHILD WITH CANCER (continued)

GOAL	INTERVENTION	RATIONALE	EXPECTED OUTCOME
4. Delayed Growth and Development related to serious illness (continued)			
	■ Encourage communicating with peers when unable to attend school. ■ Work with teachers to support reentry to school. Use puppets, videotape, and discussion with classmates.	■ Peer contacts help the child in normal developmental tasks. ■ Classmates need to understand what has happened to their friend without asking the child directly.	
5. Fatigue related to disease state			
	NIC Priority Intervention—*Energy Management:* Regulating energy use to prevent fatigue and optimize function.		**NOC Suggested Outcome—***Energy Conservation:* Extent of management of energy to initiate and sustain activity.
The child will maintain energy levels necessary for normal activities.	■ Problem solve ways to save energy for play and school. ■ Plan with child for quiet activities during low-energy times.	■ The child and parents are assisted to see school and play as important. ■ Child is empowered to select and plan own activities.	The child plans use of time effectively to maintain energy for school and play. The child conserves energy during times of increased fatigue.
6. Interrupted Family Processes related to situational crisis			
	NIC Priority Intervention—*Family Process Maintenance:* Minimization of family process disruption events.		**NOC Suggested Outcome—***Family Process:* Extent of maintenance of family support system.
The child and family will demonstrate healthy adaptation.	■ Encourage open communication. ■ Suggest that all family members develop support networks. ■ Parents should be proactive with siblings about their feelings and needs. ■ Encourage attendance of all family members at oncology camps.	■ Open discussion allows problem solving and ego support. ■ Network expand support systems. ■ Siblings feel valued and problems are confronted early. ■ Oncology camps promote open discussion between peers for further support and fun.	Parents report better communication between themselves and the children. Family members report an increase in friends with whom they can share feelings. Family reports attending oncology camp and describe benefit of sharing with other families in same situation.

Manage Pain

The child with cancer may experience pain from the disease itself and from the medical interventions, such as lumbar puncture, bone marrow aspiration, and frequent intravenous infusions and blood draws. Use all possible pain management techniques to keep the child comfortable, as this will assist with comfort and encourage cooperation throughout the long treatment period. (See Chapter 18∞ for suggestions on methods of pain management.) See Complementary Therapy: Pain Management.

Management of cancer pain has been the subject of an evidence-based practice report by the Agency for Healthcare Research and Quality. The agency found a lack of adequate studies on pain management and a limited application of existing work. These factors limit effective pain management in many patients with cancer (Agency for Healthcare Research and Quality, 2001b). Nurses must examine research on effective pain management for children and integrate findings into practice.

Conscious sedation (see Chapter 18∞) may be used for some procedures. The American Academy of Pediatrics Subcommittee on Cancer Pain in Children recommends that children be given sedation before lumbar punctures are performed. Administer sedation as ordered for young children who are undergoing radiation. Coordinate other painful or intrusive tests so they can be done while the child is sedated for radiation.

Topical anesthetics such as EMLA cream may be used to numb the skin before a blood draw or an intravenous start.

CLINICAL TIP

EMLA cream, or eutectic mixture of local anesthetics, is a combination of lidocaine 2.5% and prilocaine 2.5% in an emulsion. Apply a thick layer of the cream to intact skin and cover with an occlusive dressing. Leave in place 1 hour for minor procedures and 2 hours for major procedures. Do not use EMLA on infants who are a gestational age of less than 37 weeks, under 20 kg, or in those under 12 months receiving treatment with methemoglobin-inducing agents. For all infants, be certain that parents realize the importance of limiting the area and duration as ordered and to keep the cream in a safe place to avoid ingestion by any children.

Another local anesthetic, Numby Stuff, uses lidocaine 2% and epinephrine 1:100,000 application followed by electrical current to produce local anesthesia. Some fast-acting sprays are available for even more minor anesthesia. Intradermal application of anesthesia with lidocaine is generally used for more painful and invasive procedures such as central line insertion. They may be combined with sedation to assist the child to relax.

When possible, include the parents in comforting the child after painful procedures.

Provide Psychosocial Support

A diagnosis of cancer brings with it many emotions for the family. Initially parents experience shock and anger. They need basic information about the disease and the purpose of the tests that will be performed. Instructions often need to be repeated as parents may not process information the first time it is presented due to their increased stress levels. Assist the parents to plan how and when to tell the child the diagnosis; what the child needs to know is based on his or her developmental level and understanding.

After progressing from the initial state of shock about the diagnosis, the family needs to learn more about the disease, including the pathophysiology, treatment, and expected outcome or the prognosis. Clarify the family's understanding of these areas and be ready to answer questions. Provide both verbal explanations and written material. Parents may talk with friends, purchase books, or search the Internet for information. Find out where they are getting information and provide additional resources when appropriate. Correct misconceptions and misinformation.

The family needs many strategies to deal with the challenge of long-term treatment for cancer. As the child experiences remissions and exacerbations or complications, the family feels alternately hopeful and discouraged. This was the case with Rasheed's family at the beginning of the chapter. Help the family to identify support systems, and intervene as needed to enhance these systems. Facilitate contact with extended family members who might be of help, religious or spiritual connections, social service agencies, and other resources such as Internet and parent support groups. Assist parents who are concerned about job obligations and financial concerns. Consider the impact on siblings when a child is being treated for cancer. They may alternately resent and feel guilty for the sibling's illness. They may not understand the treatments or disease. School progress may be slowed and teachers may not be aware of the sibling's stress. See Evidence-Based Practice: Cancer and Stress.

The child undergoing treatment for cancer needs support appropriate to his or her developmental stage and cognitive level (Figure 29–9 ■). (See Chapters 5 and 17∞ for developmental levels and effective support strategies for children of different ages.) Younger children primarily need support during painful procedures and separation from parents. Older children need intervention strategies to assist in working through feelings related to treatments (Figure 29–10 ■). A major developmental task of adolescence is to attain independence and control, but cancer often interferes with adolescents' ability to achieve this task. Therefore, plan nursing strategies that empower adolescents as much as possible. This might include asking them whether they prefer morning or afternoon appointments, being placed on a teen unit

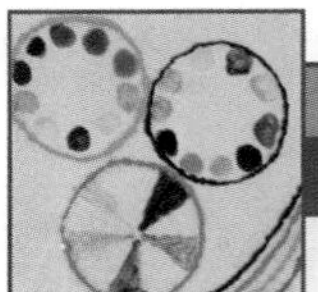

EVIDENCE-BASED PRACTICE
Cancer and Stress

PROBLEM

The family of a child with cancer experiences profound stress and all members of the family must adjust to their roles. The needs of family members are often overlooked as the ill child becomes the center of treatment and attention. Family members often provide care for the child, which can be emotionally and physically draining, and can deplete family financial resources.

EVIDENCE

In a study with 153 parents of children being treated at pediatric oncology facilities, nurses provided the Care of My Child with Cancer (CMCC) instrument. Six open-ended questions asked for information about the experience of caring for a child with cancer. Examples include: "How does the difficulty of caring for your ill child impact on your ability to care for yourself?" and "What things have helped the most in caring for your ill child?" Results indicated that parent caregivers commonly report lack of caring for self. They have reduced sleep, altered nutrition, and feelings of stress and anxiety. Helpful behaviors by health professionals included prompt and accurate information about the child, with support, understanding, and offers from others to care for other children or household responsibilities (James, Keegan-Wells, Hinds et al., 2002).

In another study, 50 siblings of children with cancer received the Nurse-Sibling Social Support Questionnaire. The tool asks siblings to write about things they wish nurses or parents would do to help them, and things that nurses or parents have done that were helpful. Siblings reported feeling left out and not being able to share feelings. They reported a need for emotional support and information, but also the need to be with other children like themselves who understand the situation (Murray, 2002).

IMPLICATIONS

Being a family member when a child has cancer is stressful. Both parents and siblings express a need for information about the ill child's condition and treatment. Nurses should provide information at each health encounter and frequently ask what questions the family members have. Ask about siblings and include them in visits when possible. In addition to information, support is vital. Ask who the parents and siblings have told about the ill child. Who can they turn to when they want to talk? Who can the parents call upon for help at home? Who can the siblings invite to school performances and other events if the parents are unable to attend?

CRITICAL THINKING APPLICATION

Refer back to Rasheed's situation at the chapter beginning. What information do you think his parents need, to understand the connection between his enterocolitis and leukemia? Explain the infection and its treatment in terms they will likely understand. What support will his mother need as she returns to work and cannot stay full time with Rasheed in the hospital during this hospitalization? Rasheed has a 7-year-old stepsister who comes to visit him in the hospital. She seems shy but interested in his care. How can you involve this younger sister in Rasheed's care and make her comfortable during her visit?

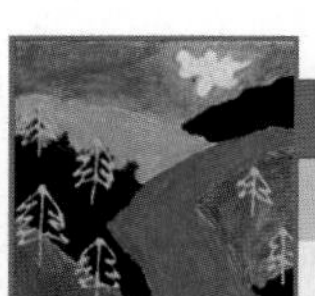

COMPLEMENTARY THERAPY
Pain Management

Children have many painful and invasive procedures during cancer treatment. In addition to use of medication they will be helped by the following pain management techniques.

- A parent can provide presence and support during procedures.
- Use distraction and relaxation techniques Either a parent or healthcare provider can work with the child and integrate techniques such as singing, counting, telling stories, and blowing bubbles. Children and teens can be taught to visualize positive scenes, use rhythmic breathing, or listen to music (Christensen & Fatchett, 2002).
- Hypnosis has been used successfully to manage both pain and nausea/vomiting during cancer treatment with children from 5–18 years (Liossi, 2000).

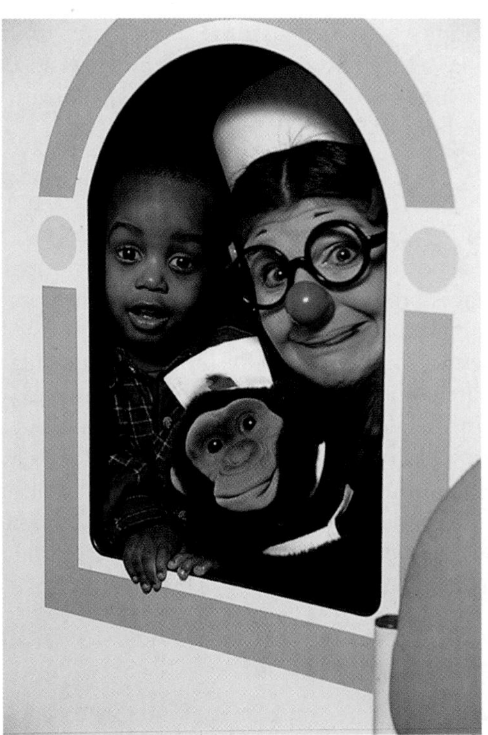

FIGURE 29–9 ■ Clowns from the Big Apple Clown Care Unit can help to ease the stress of hospitalization for seriously ill children and their families. Here, a clown doctor and her puppet distract a toddler who is waiting for his clinic appointment.

where they can receive treatments with other teens, and encouraging parents to allow them choices about issues at home.

For many parents, especially those with daughters, the loss of the child's hair during treatment can be devastating. Ask the parents and the child what this issue is like for them. Prepare them for the fact that it can be rapid or slow. Find out how they plan to cope. Some children want the hair cut very short so its loss will not be as traumatic. Offer resources for wigs, hats, or other ideas. Put them in touch with children who have lost hair and with those who have now regrown it.

CLINICAL TIP

Children with hair loss need to cover the head, wear sunscreen when outside, and avoid the sun when possible to minimize chance of burn to the head, which is prone to burning due to lack of prior sun exposure.

Talk with the child's teachers before the return to school after treatment to explain the child's condition and assist with plans to prepare the other children. Role-play with the child how to tell friends about any changes in appearance. A nurse or child life specialist could attend the class of a young child to explain what the child is experiencing. Arrange for tutors if necessary to assist the child with schoolwork during hospitalization and home care. Explore the option of summer camp for children with cancer. The Make-a-Wish Foundation strives to make dreams come true for ill children by sponsoring them for a desired activity or outing. Refer the child to this foundation if appropriate.

The siblings of a child who has cancer can be stressed by the changes in the family. They may grieve over the ill brother or sister and may feel sad and depressed. They also can experience anger, guilt, or resentment and may have a lack of knowledge about the disease and treatment. Inquire about siblings and ask what they know about the child's condition. Find out who is caring for siblings and whether their teachers have been informed about the family situation. Include siblings in care when possible. Invite them to visit and to participate both during hospitalization and at home care visits. They can be involved in play therapy sessions and recreational activities with the ill child. Ask the parents if the siblings are demonstrating symptoms such as depression, behavioral changes, or decrease in school performance and suggest interventions as appropriate. They may benefit from speaking with a school counselor or can be referred to a support group for siblings of children with cancer. Some cancer summer camps welcome siblings as well as children with cancer.

The family of a child with cancer is faced with a life-threatening illness. Refer to Chapter 21 ∞ for strategies to assist the family in coping with this stressor. For some types of cancer, the child may experience a remission with treatment, but then a recurrence of disease later as cancer cells grow again. The family may become angry or depressed about the relapse. Repeated treatments challenge the family's support systems. Waiting for the outcome of diagnostic tests can be an especially challenging time. Provide information as soon as possible. If the child's illness progresses, refer the family to hospice to assist them in caring for the terminally ill child and in working through the grieving process. Explore support groups and information related to cancer in order to share this information with families.

Care in the Community

Preparation for home care centers on creating a normal environment while supporting the child's physiologic and psychosocial responses to the cancer and treatments. Education is the primary focus of discharge planning. (See Partnering with Families: Cancer Therapy.) Teach the parents how to ensure adequate

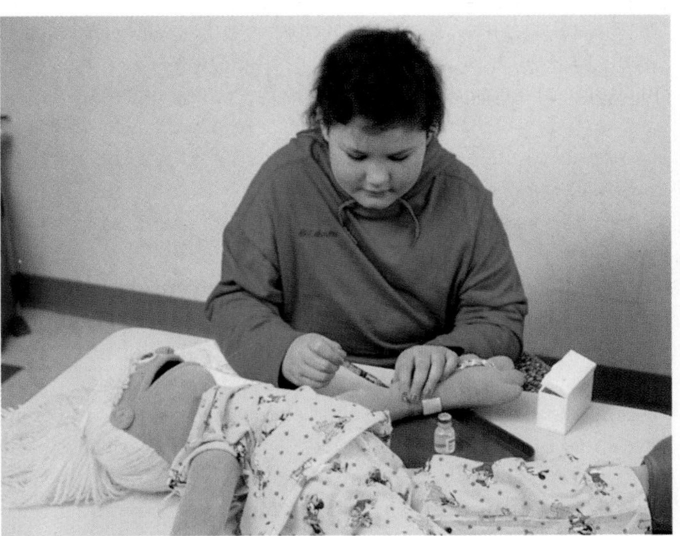

FIGURE 29–10 ■ A child in a pediatric oncology clinic giving injections to a doll. This type of play therapy helps the child deal with fear, thus lowering his or her stress level.

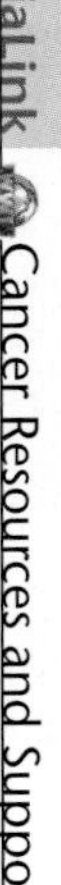

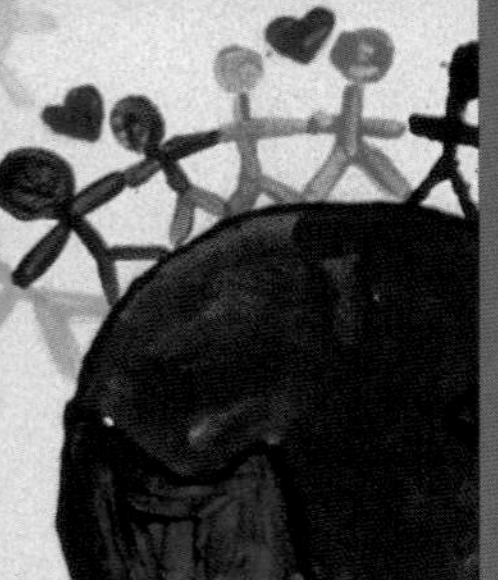

PARTNERING WITH FAMILIES

Cancer Therapy

Most parents are not aware of the effects of cancer treatment and how they can help children through this experience. Depending on the stage and type of treatment, the following suggestions are for parents.

- Children in radiation and chemotherapy are fatigued. Provide extra rest periods with shorter activity periods between them.
- Have an overnight bag ready in case the child develops a complication and needs to be taken to stay in the hospital for a few days. Several hospital stays of a few days are normal during treatment.
- When concerned about a symptom in the child, ask the care provider. Parents are often key in identifying problems early.
- Parents are usually concerned about central line care, but feel more comfortable after a few days of caring for the line.
- Children have poor appetites at times so nutritional intake is needed when they are hungry.
- Remember that children are still at the normal developmental age. Treat them as a reflection of their ages, not as if they are older or younger.
- Try to maintain contact with the child's peer group and family members.
- Seek information from other parents and resources on cancer care.
- Remind parents to get time away and relax so that parental energy remains high and they are better able to deal with the child's therapy.

nutritional intake, to be alert for signs of infection, to protect the child from exposure to communicable disease during times of neutropenia, to administer medications at home, and how to handle vomiting and pain. Assist the parents and child to deal with any obstacles to normal development and functioning. Teach the parents and family about symptoms that need to be treated immediately. (See Partnering with Families: Reportable Events for Children Receiving Chemotherapy.)

Home management of a vascular access device or central line, such as a Broviac catheter (refer to the Skills Manual), is an initial challenge for parents (Figure 29–11 ■). Alternatively, an implanted port may be used and allows the child freedom to swim and engage in other activities. Parents will need information about whatever device the child has received. Details about cleaning the site, instilling heparin in the line or reservoir, and other needed care should be demonstrated and reviewed prior to discharge to home. After teaching the parents, observe them performing the procedure before the child is discharged.

Emphasize the need for the child and family to have fun and engage in as many normal activities as possible. Play distracts the child and is essential in reducing fears. Children, parents, and siblings often benefit from participation in cancer support groups and cancer summer camps. These activities create additional support systems, build the child's self-esteem, and enhance coping skills through role modeling.

Make home visits to evaluate the family's strengths and needs in the home setting. Be sure that the family has adequate support from a hospice and other end-of-life services when the child's condition is terminal. See Chapter 22.

Health Promotion/Health Maintenance

Treatment for cancer is generally a long process. Most children are treated for a period of 2 to 3 years. Since normal developmental stages progress during this time, health promotion and health maintenance visits should still occur. Some usual care may have to be altered, but many of the same developmental concerns of all children should be addressed. Help parents to view the child as a "normal" child who is ill for a period of time, but still needs to have limits set on behavior, develop healthy lifestyles, have environmental stimulation to learn to talk, read, or perform motor and cognitive tasks. See the Health Promotion and Maintenance Overview on page 1065 for a summary of health promotion and health maintenance needs during cancer treatment.

■ Evaluation

The following expected outcomes of nursing care for the child with cancer relate to the specific disease, treatments, and responses.

- Adequate intake to promote normal growth
- Hydration that supports body processes and ensures drug and cancer cell product elimination
- Prompt identification and treatment to minimize treatment side effects

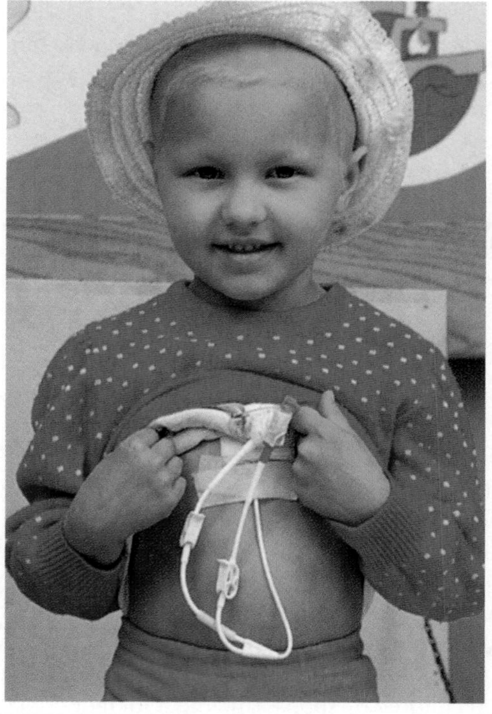

FIGURE 29–11 ■ A vascular access device allows chemotherapeutic agents to be administered without the need for repeated "sticks" to the child.

Health Promotion & Maintenance Overview

The Child Receiving Cancer Treatment

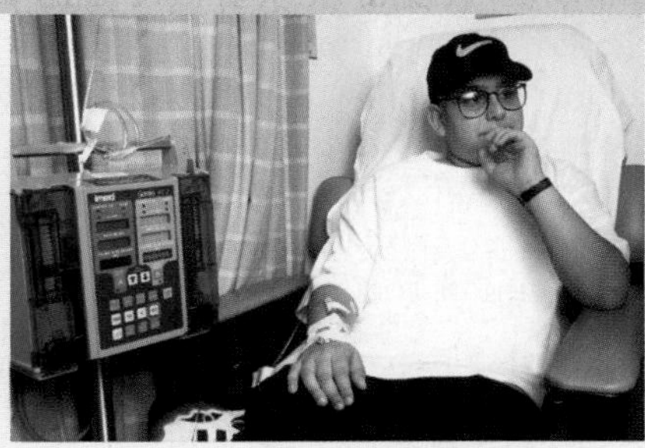

Cancer treatment often extends for several years, so the child needs to continue health promotion and health maintenance visits.

Growth and Development Surveillance

- The child is assessed for height, weight, and body mass index. This provides information about growth patterns which may be altered by cancer treatment. If indicated, 24-hour recalls and other assessments are performed.
- Teaching is provided about age-appropriate foods. Since appetite may be impaired during periods of treatment, the child may be lacking fruits, vegetables, or other foods, as well as the nutrients they include. Encourage parents to be sure the child has a well-balanced diet during periods of remission.
- Perform developmental screening of young children. Provide suggestions for parents about the stimulation that is appropriate for the child's age. Include quiet activities that can be used when the child is fatigued or receiving therapy. These might include reading books, listening to tapes and music, and working on a computer. Have the parent plan for these activities on days that the child goes for chemotherapy or other treatment.
- Ask about the school-age child's progress in school. Performance may be altered due to neurological effects of treatment as well as missing school. Plan for the family to partner with the school personnel for provision of tutors, computer programs, or other needed assistance.
- Encourage continued social contact with peers when blood counts are adequate to prevent infection.

Physical Assessment and Screening

- Careful physical assessments are performed to identify any abnormalities that may result from cancer or its treatment. Cardiopulmonary and neuromuscular assessments are particularly important. Vision and hearing should be assessed prior to treatment and periodically throughout. Include measurements of fine and gross motor activity.

Elimination

- Toddlers may have an interruption in toilet training during periods when they do not feel well. Help parents to understand this regression and encourage them to start again when the child is feeling better.
- Some medications cause diarrhea or constipation so evaluate bowel patterns and provide guidance as needed. Skin care instruction may be needed if the child has diarrhea and is relatively immobile. Increasing fluids and fiber foods may be needed for constipation.
- Evaluate urinary output since many medications have effects on kidney function. Encourage adequate fluids for age to ensure elimination of medications.

Sleep and Fatigue

- Children undergoing treatment often have disturbed sleep patterns. Parents of young children may become exhausted working all day, getting the child to treatments, and having disturbed sleep at night. Assess both the child's sleep patterns and the family's experiences. Encourage plans for respite care to enable rest periods. Provide cots, rocking chairs, and other comfortable settings for child and family members during treatments.
- Both child and parents may not expect or understand the profound fatigue that occurs during cancer treatment (Davies, Whitsett, Bruce, et al., 2002). They can be helped to plan for providing quiet times, and replenishing energy through naps, massage, relaxing baths, and spending time with family.

Physical Activity

- Since the child has periods of fatigue, patterns of physical activity may decrease. Emphasize the importance of integrating physical activity when the child feels well, since it is needed for learning gross motor skills, facilitating blood flow, improving mental status, and setting patterns for the future.

Disease and Injury Prevention Strategies

- The child with cancer has the same safety hazards as other children of the same age, and such topics as car safety seats, fire prevention, water safety, and violence prevention should be addressed.
- An important hazard for children with cancer is infection due to decreased immune response. Keep records of immunization status. Follow the recommendations of the CDC and AAP for other immunizations. Teach the hazards of large groups when the child's immune system is compromised. Teach care of central lines and other potential sources of infection. Have families report signs of infection and exposure to known illnesses promptly.

Mental and Spiritual Health

- Evaluate the child and family for signs of anxiety and depression. Ask how they are managing the cancer treatment and what poses the greatest challenges. Refer to other families with similar circumstances for support.
- Ensure that the child has contact with friends through childcare, school, or via phone, letters, and computer.
- Find out the impact of the child's cancer on the parent's jobs. Ask how the siblings have been coping, what changes there are in school performance, and whether teachers and others are aware of the stress the sibling may be experiencing.

Transitional Care

- As the child's treatment ends, instruct them about needed periodic follow-up with the oncologist. Continue to perform neurological examinations and ascertain school performance. Be alert for signs of secondary tumors.
- Ask about worries regarding the future. As teens grow older, have them take over more responsibility for informing care providers of their cancer history and assist them to transition to adult healthcare providers (Hobbie & Ogle, 2001).

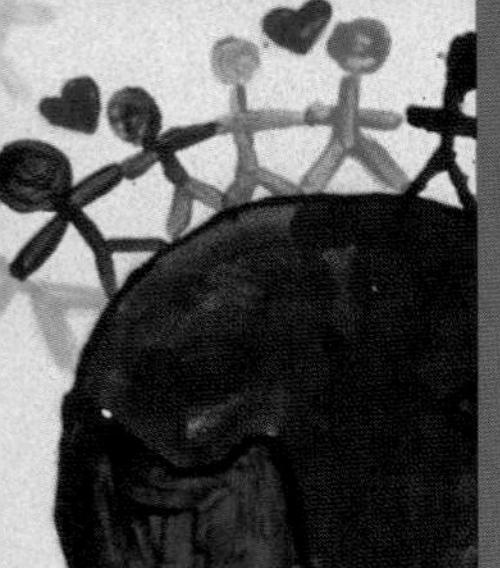

PARTNERING WITH FAMILIES

Reportable Events for Children Receiving Chemotherapy

Parents require verbal and written instructions about signs and symptoms to report to the child's oncologist while the child is receiving chemotherapy.

Have parents report the following events to the child's oncologist if they occur while the child is receiving chemotherapy:

- Temperature above 38°C (101°F)
- Any bleeding, such as nosebleeds, blood in stool or urine, petechiae, bruising
- Pain or discomfort with urination or defecation
- Sores in the mouth
- Vomiting or diarrhea
- Persistent pain anywhere, including headache
- Signs of infection, such as cough, fever, runny nose, tugging at ears
- Signs of infection in central lines, such as redness, drainage, or tenderness
- Exposure to communicable diseases, especially varicella (chickenpox)

Inform dentists and other healthcare providers that the child is receiving chemotherapy prior to procedures. Prophylactic antibiotics should be given before and after dental care.

Adapted from Bindler, R. M., & Howry, L. B. (2005). Pediatric drug guide. *Upper Saddle River, NJ: Prentice Hall Health.*

- Management of pain to a level of comfort satisfactory to child and family
- Family use of resources to provide necessary support during hospitalizations and treatments
- Knowledge of management of treatment regimens
- Acceptance of prognosis and support of all family members

Brain Tumors

Central nervous system or brain tumors are the most commonly occurring solid tumors in children and the second most common malignancy, after leukemia. Each year nearly 3,000 children and adolescents are diagnosed with tumors of the brain and central nervous system, accounting for one in five childhood cancers (Ryan-Murray & Petriccione, 2002).

Etiology and Pathophysiology

While a few cases are associated with other diseases, the cause of most brain tumors is unknown. There may be an association between parental work in aircraft or agricultural industry, paints, solvents, radiation, and electromagnetic fields and higher incidence of brain tumors in children (Ryan-Murray & Petriccione, 2002).

Brain tumors in children usually occur below the roof of the cerebellum and involve the cerebellum, midbrain, and brainstem (Figure 29–12 ■). In contrast, brain tumors in adults are usually located above the areas between the cerebrum and cerebellum.

The most common brain tumors in children are medulloblastoma, cerebral and cerebellar astrocytoma, ependymoma (from ependymal cells lining the brain ventricles and spinal cord canal), and gliomas of the cerebrum or brainstem. Less common are supratentorial embryonal tumors and craniopharyngioma.

Clinical Manifestations

Children with brain tumors can manifest behavioral and neurologic changes; these may occur rapidly or slowly and subtly. Some common symptoms include headache, nausea, vomiting, dizziness, change in vision or hearing, fatigue, and mental status changes.

CLINICAL TIP

Some children with brain tumors have nonspecific signs. They may have a subtle behavior change, perform poorly at school, or show some incoordination. Be alert to such signs and to the parents' statement that they notice a change in the child. Report such findings so appropriate assessments can be made.

Brainstem tumors can present with weight deficits, and may be mistakenly diagnosed as an eating disorder of infancy and childhood (failure to thrive). This may delay proper treatment (Lehman, Krishnamurthy, & Berlin, 2002). See the clinical manifestations table on page 1066 for common manifestations of certain types of tumors.

Medulloblastomas are brain tumors in the external layer of the cerebellum. They account for 20% of childhood brain tumors, and commonly occur in children age 5 to 6 years. They are fast growing and therefore often present with fast onset of symptoms such as increased intracranial pressure, manifested by increased head circumference in infants, vomiting, headache, ataxia, and vision changes. Astrocytomas arise from glial cells and can be either above or below the area between the cerebrum and cerebellum. They comprise 40% of childhood brain tumors, and vary from low-grade cerebellar to low-grade cerebral to high-grade tumors. The presenting symptoms vary depending on the location of the tumor. Endocrine, vision, and behavioral changes are all possible, as well as increased intracranial pressure and seizures (Ryan-Murray & Petriccione, 2002). Ependymomas commonly occur in the fourth ventricle of the posterior fossa and comprise 10% of childhood brain tumors. Impaired growth, hydrocephalus, seizures, and cranial nerve impairments are the most common manifestations. Brainstem gliomas are located in the pons and typically spread into the surrounding tissue. They account for 15% of childhood brain tumors (Conway, Asuncion, & DaRossa, 1999). Cranial nerve impairments, mental status changes, and motor symptoms occur.

COLLABORATIVE CARE

Collaborative care is needed to identify children with brain tumors and provide for them the comprehensive treatment required.

PATHOPHYSIOLOGY ILLUSTRATED

Sites of Brain Tumors in Children

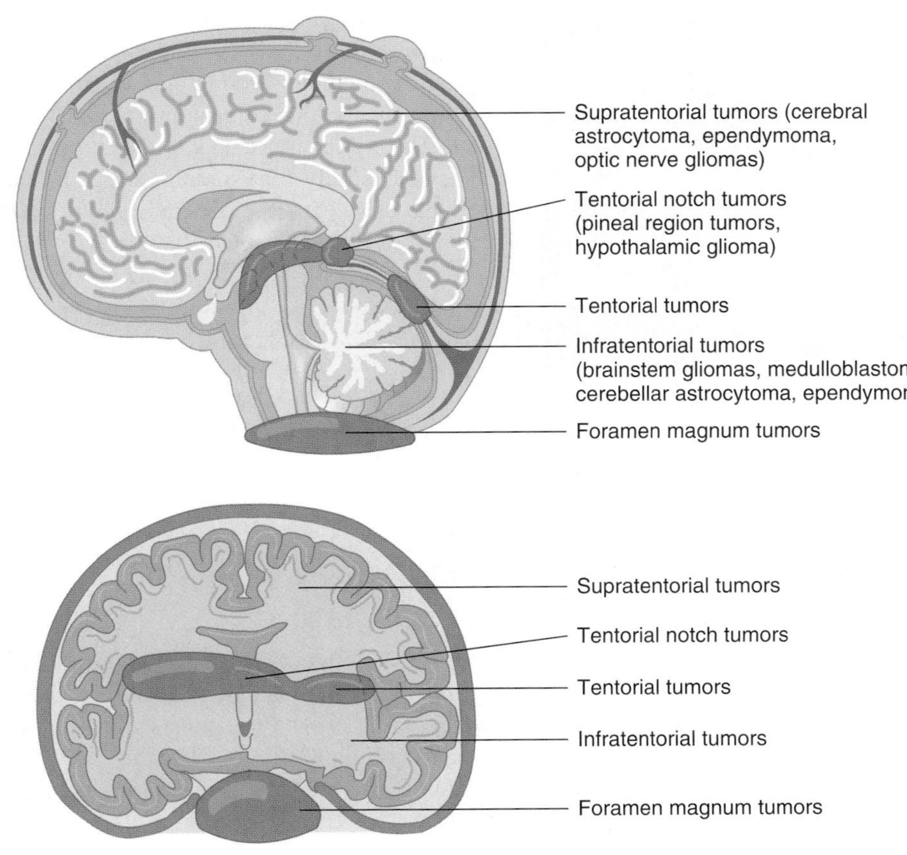

FIGURE 29–12 ■ Approximately 1,500 children under the age of 15 years are diagnosed annually as having tumors of the brain and central nervous system. The four most common brain tumors in children are medulloblastoma, cerebral astrocytoma, ependymoma, and brainstem glioma.

Diagnostic Tests

The first step in diagnosing brain tumors is a detailed health history and physical examination. Onset of symptoms, severity, and presentation of neurological symptoms is recorded. Brain tumors are then definitively diagnosed by means of computed tomography (CT; Figure 29–13A ■), magnetic resonance imaging (MRI; Figure 29–13B ■), positron emission tomography (PET), single-photon emission computed tomography (SPECT), myelography, and angiography. Neurophysiologic tests (electroencephalography and brainstem evoked potentials) are used to assess sensory pathway integrity and disease- or drug-related sensory dysfunction. Other tests that may be performed are examination for serum tumor markers such as α-fetaprotein and human chorionic gonadotropin. Lumbar puncture is used to identify abnormal cells

CLINICAL MANIFESTATIONS of Brain Tumors

TUMOR	ETIOLOGY	CLINICAL MANIFESTATIONS	CLINICAL THERAPY
Medulloblastoma	External layer of cerebellum	Headache, vomiting, ataxia	Surgery; chemotherapy with lomustine, vincristine, cisplatin, radiation
Astrocytomas	Glial cells, supratentorial or infratentorial	Seizures, visual disturbances, increased intracranial pressure, vomiting	Surgery; chemotherapy with vincristine, dactinomycin; radiation
Ependymoma	Fourth ventricle, posterior tossa	Hydrocephalus	Surgery, radiation
Brainstem gliomas	Pons	Cranial nerve (VI + VII) tract signs, nystagmus, ataxia, motor symptoms	Surgery, radiation

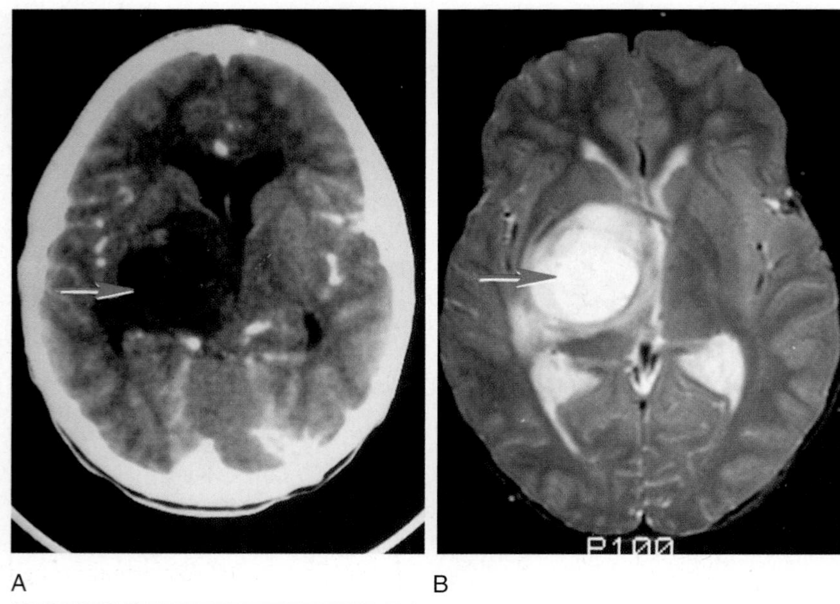

FIGURE 29–13 ■ Radiologic imaging of a child with a brain tumor. *A,* CT scan. *B,* MRI.

Courtesy of Carlos Sivit, M. D., Children's National Medical Center, Washington, DC.

in the cerebrospinal fluid. Bone marrow aspiration and bone scans identify any extracranial primary neoplastic growth, as cancers in other sites can metastasize to or from the brain.

Clinical Therapy

Treatment depends on the type of brain tumor. Surgery is a common treatment, and may be performed to obtain a biopsy specimen, to **debulk** (reduce the tumor size by partial removal) or excise the tumor, or to treat any hydrocephalus that may be present. During surgery, radiology images allow the neurosurgeon to see computerized images of the brain while at the same time stimulating nerves to determine their functioning. These techniques provide rapid feedback to the neurosurgeon. Laser surgery, which has delicate, precise control and accuracy, is used when tumors are close to sensitive neural or vascular structures.

Radiation is commonly used in treatment of brain tumors. Use of radiation following surgery and chemotherapy has improved the survival of children with medulloblastoma and ependymoma. Radiation has traditionally not been used in children under 3 years because of resultant damage to brain cells. However, newer and safer techniques of administration are being used with younger children. High-dose chemotherapy is often used, and this modality has improved the survival of children with central nervous system tumors (Conway et al., 1999). Low-dose chemotherapy can shrink and help manage some tumors. Intrathecal administration of chemotherapy is useful in some cases. However, the blood-brain barrier is a factor in the effectiveness of chemotherapy for children with brain tumors. For example, when methotrexate is administered intrathecally (in the spinal canal), only a small amount crosses normal brain capillaries. HSCT is an increasingly used treatment option.

Complications of treatment for children with brain tumors are significant. They include severe infections (commonly associated with high-dose chemotherapy), seizure activity, sensorimotor defects, hydrocephalus, and growth problems. Care is taken to treat infections early and aggressively. If a cerebrospinal shunt is used, infection or blockage can occur (see Chapter 33∞ for further discussion of cerbrospinal shunts in children). Anticonvulsants are commonly given prophylactically following surgery. Endocrine problems, such as growth hormone changes, hypothyroidism, and panhypopituitarism, may occur when the tumor is in the hyphothalamic-pituitary area. Treatment may also lead to impaired cognitive function and emotional or behavioral problems in some children. Memory deficits and selective attention deficits are the most common problems.

Diabetes insipidus is a special consideration in children with midline brain tumors, such as those that compress the hypothalamus, pituitary stalk, or posterior pituitary gland. Manifestations of diabetes insipidus include voiding of large amounts of dilute urine with a specific gravity of less than 1.005 to 1.010 (see Chapter 31∞).

NURSING MANAGEMENT

The goals of nursing management are to administer treatment, monitor for side effects, and support the child and family when a brain tumor occurs.

■ Nursing Assessment and Diagnosis

The focus of physiologic assessment of the child with a brain tumor is determined by its presentation (Table 29–4). Presenting signs can be categorized as follows:

- Nonspecific signs related to increasing intracranial pressure
- Secondary signs related to displacement of intracranial structures
- Focal signs suggesting direct involvement of the brain and cranial nerves

Thorough neurologic examination before surgery is essential to provide a record of baseline functioning and allow the evaluation of the child's changing physiologic status before surgery. Ask if the child has manifested slow changes over time or has had quickly developing symptoms. Measurement of head circumference and assessment of the anterior fontanel are necessary in children under the age of 18 months.

Perform developmental screening on young children using the Denver II or other developmental test (see Chapter 10∞). Ask about the child's social interactions, school performance, and any behavior changes that have occurred.

The following nursing diagnoses may be identified for the child with a brain tumor, depending on the type and location of the tumor.

- Imbalanced Nutrition: Less than Body Requirements related to loss of appetite

TABLE 29–4 Physiologic Assessment of Brain Tumors

CLINICAL MANIFESTATIONS	ASSESSMENT
Nonspecific signs: headache, morning vomiting, somnolence, irritability	Level of consciousness, pupil response, pupil shape and size
Secondary signs: disturbances of cranial nerves; other signs depend on site of tumor	All cranial nerves
Focal signs: truncal ataxia (midline brain tumors), general nystagmus, head tilting	Motor ability, head positions when watching television or looking at people (double vision, sixth cranial nerve involvement)

- Impaired Physical Mobility related to tumor pressure on coordination centers
- Delayed Growth and Development related to effects of disability
- Impaired Memory related to neurologic disturbance
- Acute Pain related to diagnostic tests and treatment

Planning and Implementation

The child with a brain tumor requires multidisciplinary care with partnerships among a neurologist, neurosurgeon, pediatrician, dietician, social worker, other specialists, and the family. The nurse can act as a case manager to coordinate the complex care needed by the child and help the family to understand the treatment.

For the nursing care of children immediately following surgery, refer to Chapter 17∞. In addition, close monitoring of neurologic status is needed postoperatively (refer to Chapter 33∞). Be especially alert for signs of increased intracranial pressure and infection. Subtle alterations such as visual differences, behavior or alertness variations, and gait changes can herald serious problems from the tumor or pressure in the brain. Many children return from surgery with a ventricular-peritoneal shunt. Observe for seizure activity. Administer drugs such as antibiotics, steroids, and anticonvulsants as ordered.

Signs and symptoms of diabetes insipidus may occur following brain surgery (see Chapter 18∞ for a description of diabetes insipidus). Nursing care includes hourly measurement of intake and output, measurement of serum sodium levels every 4 to 6 hours, accurate fluid replacement, and frequent assessment of neurologic status. An indwelling urinary catheter is useful for accurate measurement of urinary output.

Having a child with a diagnosis of brain tumor can be devastating to family members. While some tumors have a good prognosis, others do not. Whatever the prognosis, the surgery and other treatment protocols will be frightening to parents. Explain procedures, the purpose of lines, and the use of sedation to keep the child restful, and answer any questions. Ask parents about resources such as other family members, available sick leave from work, and places to stay if they live far from the hospital. Suggest periods of napping and rest, use of facilities to stay near the hospital, and other resources.

Care in the Community

Teach the parents to watch for an increase in voiding of dilute urine. Be sure they can recognize the signs of infection and changes in the child's neurologic status. Once the child is ready for discharge, chemotherapy or radiation may begin; inform parents of the reason and potential side effects of these treatments. Assist the family in obtaining any special equipment they may need to care for the child at home, such as a wheelchair, bed rails, or dressings. The American Cancer Society is a potential resource for assistance with these needs.

Children with brain tumors, especially those who have received radiation, often have some permanent sequelae. They may have slowed development, incoordination, learning disabilities, or other effects. These sequelae are most common in children who are 3 years of age or younger at the time of radiation therapy. Perform accurate height and weight measures at each healthcare visit. Assess developmental milestones. Ask about progress in school and any special services that might be needed. Perform thorough neurologic assessments. Support the family as they learn to deal with unknown or changed expectations for the child's performance (Freeman, O'Dell, & Meola, 2000). (Box 29–3.)

Evaluation

Expected outcomes of nursing care for the child with a brain tumor depend on the site of tumor, clinical therapy, and medical outcome. Possible outcomes include the following:

- Adequate nutritional intake to support growth and prevent malnutrition
- Maintenance of a safe environment

BOX 29–3 Research: Concerns of Children with Brain Tumors and Their Siblings

In a study with 87 families, children with a brain tumor and their siblings were asked to identify their concerns. Main concerns of children with a tumor included:

- Keeping up with school work and special needs at school
- Changes in physical activity level
- Changes in appearance
- Mood variations
- Getting together with friends

Concerns of siblings included:

- Worry about what might happen to the ill sibling
- Keeping up with schoolwork
- Information about cause of the tumor
- Help in dealing with the ill sibling regarding activity, mood, appearance, pain

For both groups information by healthcare providers and support by family, friends, and clergy were identified as the most helpful factors (Freeman, O'Dell, & Meola, 2003). Nurses can ask both affected children and their siblings what their concerns are throughout the treatment. Provide information that they desire and facilitate supportive contact with friends and clergy.

- Physical mobility allowed by developmental level and alterations of disease
- Provision of an environment to meet normal developmental milestones within capability of the child
- Management of pain of comfort level
- Parental understanding of diagnosis and treatment plan

Neuroblastoma

Neuroblastoma is the solid tumor most commonly occurring outside the cranium of children. It is responsible for 8% to 10% of childhood cancers and 15% of cancer deaths in children. The average age at onset is 22 months; it is the most common tumor in infants during the first year of life. Prognosis varies, depending on the staging of the tumor (Table 29–5) and the age of the child, with more favorable outcomes in infants under 1 year of age, and in presenting sites in the pelvis or thorax. Less favorable outcomes are associated with presence of N-myc oncogen amplification. Survival rates are 98% for stages 1 and 2, but drop to 22% for stage 4 (Dadd, 2002).

Neuroblastoma is commonly a smooth, hard, nontender mass that can occur anywhere along the sympathetic nervous system chain. A frequent location is the abdomen, although other sites are the adrenal, thoracic, and cervical areas. It is nearly unheard of after 10 years of age, is usually diagnosed in children under 5 years, and the median age at diagnosis is 2 years (McManus & Gilchrist, 2000).

Etiology and Pathophysiology

Neuroblastoma originates in primitive neurocrest cells that form the adrenal medulla, paraganglia, and sympathetic nervous system of the cervical sympathetic chain and the thoracic chain. Fifty percent of neuroblastomas develop in the adrenal medulla, 20% develop in the thorax, and the remaining 30% are elsewhere along the sympathetic chain (McManus & Gilchrist, 2000). Lymph node metastasis is common.

The cause of neuroblastoma is unknown. Theories that have been proposed center on the possible effects of environmental factors such as prenatal drug exposure from the mother and disturbed cellular nerve growth factors. Canada has recently noted a drop in neuroblastoma rates commensurate with fortification of flour with folate (French, Grant, Weitzman, et al., 2003). A genetic defect found in many cases of neuroblastoma is a deletion of the short arm of chromosome 1 (1p del). Oncogenes are commonly present in neuroblastoma cells in a DNA sequence known as N-myc, located on chromosome 2. High levels of the N-myc oncogene are associated with rapid disease progression and a poorer prognosis (Dadd, 2002).

TABLE 29–5 International Neuroblastoma Staging System

STAGE	DESCRIPTION
1	Localized tumor confined to the area of origin; complete gross excision, with or without microscopic residual disease; identifiable ipsilateral and contralateral lymph nodes negative microscopically
2A	Unilateral tumor with incomplete gross excision; identifiable ipsilateral and contralateral lymph nodes negative microscopically
2B	Unilateral tumor with complete or incomplete gross excision; with positive ipsilateral regional lymph nodes; identifiable contralateral lymph nodes negative microscopically
3	Tumor infiltrating across the midline with or without regional lymph node involvement; or unilateral tumor with contralateral regional lymph node involvement; or midline tumor with bilateral regional lymph node involvement
4	Dissemination of tumor to distant lymph nodes, bone, bone marrow, liver, and/or other organs (except as defined in stage 4S)
4S	Localized primary tumor as defined for stage 1 or 2 with dissemination limited to liver, skin, and/or bone marrow

Adapted from Castleberry, R. P. (1997). Biology and treatment of neuroblastoma. Pediatric Clinics of North America, *44, 919–938.*

Clinical Manifestations

The location of the mass determines the symptoms. Altered bowel and bladder function occur when the mass is retroperitoneal; characteristic signs are weight loss, abdominal distension, enlarged liver, irritability, fatigue, and fever. Dyspnea or infection may occur when the tumor is mediastinal. Neck and facial edema may result from vena cava syndrome if the tumor is mediastinal and large. Intracranial lesions may be present with periorbital ecchymosis. Malaise, fever, and a limp can occur if there has been metastasis to the bone. Bone marrow disease can manifest as **pancytopenia** (abnormal depression of all cellular blood components) with neutropenia (causing infections) and anemia (causing fatigue). Metastatic spread can result in an array of symptoms affecting multiple organs.

COLLABORATIVE CARE

The goal of care in neuroblastoma is early identification of disease so that it can be treated in its beginning stages. Support for the family during treatment is a focus of the entire care management team.

Diagnostic Tests

Diagnosis of neuroblastoma begins with a careful history and physical examination to identify changes in behaviors of the young child. The International Neuroblastoma Staging System (INSS) recommends different diagnostic and laboratory evaluations for diagnosis of the primary disease and of metastases (Table 29–6). Routine blood cell counts are needed, including CBC with differential. The test may reveal anemia and thrombocytopenia. There is no classic WBC response, although thrombocytopenia may occur in association with disseminated intravascular coagulation. **Leukocytosis** (higher than normal leukocyte count) and **leukopenia** (lower than normal leukocyte count) have been observed with bone marrow involvement. Serum electrolytes, liver function studies, LDH, coagulation studies, and urinalysis are performed. Baseline cardiac function is evaluated if doxorubicin will be used in treatment.

Tumor markers include VMA, HVA, dopamine, ferritin, NSE, LDH, and a ganglioside GD2. Vanillylmandelic acid (VMA) and homovanillic acid (HVA) are by-products of adrenal hormones and their levels are usually elevated in the urine and blood (see

TABLE 29–6 Diagnostic Tests for Neuroblastoma

TESTS FOR INITIAL DIAGNOSIS	TESTS FOR METASTASES
Tumor tissue diagnosis by light microscopy, or Biopsy of tumor cells plus laboratory evaluation showing increased urine or serum catecholamines (two separate measures each more than 3 standard deviations above the norm for age)	Bone marrow aspirate and biopsy Radiolabeled scanning with metaiodobenzylguanidine (MIBG) Bone scan Skeletal radiograph CT or MRI of abdomen, liver, brain, eye orbits MRI of spine Chest radiograph, with added CT or MRI if radiograph shows lesions

Appendix C∞ for normal values). Urinary catecholoamines are increased. Elevations in dopamine, ferritin, NSE (an enzyme in neural tissue), LDH, and GD2 (a sugar and lipid molecule on the surface of neural cells) are seen. All of these laboratory findings are used initially to diagnose the disease and later to follow its progress. A biopsy or surgical removal of the tumor will be followed by analysis of its type and genetic abnormalities. Areas of necrosis and calcification in major organs are readily identifiable with radiologic tests and MRIs. These tests also help in the staging of the disease by identifying metastases.

Clinical Therapy

The stage of the tumor (see Table 29–5) determines the treatment protocol. Surgical excision of the mass is performed and may be the only treatment in low-risk stages. With higher risk, surgery is followed by chemotherapy with a combination of drugs. Several courses of chemotherapy may be needed prior to surgery when the mass is large or wrapped around major blood vessels. Chemotherapy may include:

- Cyclophosphamide
- Ifosfamide
- Doxorubicin
- Cisplatin
- Carboplatin
- Teniposide
- Etoposide

Radiation is often used, especially in disseminated disease. HSCT may be performed for advanced disease, sometimes followed by the biological modifier *cis*-retinoic acid and fenretinide (to promote apoptosis). Studies are being conducted involving GD2, natural killer cells and other treatments, as well as gene therapy to interrupt growth of abnormal cells (Dadd, 2002). Neuroblastoma is most responsive to treatment in children under 1 year of age.

NURSING MANAGEMENT

Nursing management focuses on careful assessment of symptoms in this potentially multisystem disease. Physiological and psychological support during treatment are complex for the young child and family.

Nursing Assessment and Diagnosis

The presenting site of the tumor, such as the neck or abdomen, is assessed by observation and inspection. Palpation is contraindicated. Carefully document related functioning, such as bowel and bladder function. Take vital signs to watch for elevated temperature and vital sign changes caused by a thoracic mass. Observe gait and coordination. Take weight and height (or length for infant) and compare with earlier percentiles for the child. Specific assessments during treatment will depend on the treatment methods used (refer to the earlier discussions of chemotherapy and radiation treatment). Psychosocial assessment and emotional assessment of the family are needed.

The following nursing diagnoses may be appropriate for the child with neuroblastoma, depending on the location and extent of the presenting disease.

- Impaired Gas Exchange related to ventilation-perfusion imbalance
- Impaired Physical Mobility related to neuromuscular impairment
- Disturbed Sensory Perception (visual) related to altered sensory perception
- Pain related to tumor pressure and injury
- Anticipatory Grieving (family) related to potential loss of significant person

Planning and Implementation

The nursing management of the child with neuroblastoma can encompass the three phases of medical treatment: chemotherapy, surgery, and radiation. Specific postsurgical care depends on the size and site of the tumor. Normal postoperative care includes providing fluid support and respiratory care and preventing infection.

Nursing care during the chemotherapy phase includes minimizing side effects, preventing infection, teaching parents about the medications their child is receiving, and monitoring physical and emotional growth and development of the young child. When radiation is part of the treatment, use common nursing measures described earlier in the chapter. Topics for parent and family teaching and discharge planning are presented in Partnering with Families: The Child with Neuroblastoma.

Ongoing support and connection to resources to assist in management of the child's treatment at home will be needed. Longterm sequelae following surgery and other treatments require ongoing care. When the prognosis is poor, parents may appreciate referrals to hospice, to other parents who have experienced similar child illnesses, and to other community resources. See Chapter 22∞ for additional nursing care for end of life.

Evaluation

Expected outcomes of nursing care for the child with neuroblastoma include the following:

- Respiratory exchange to support daily activities
- Physical mobility to level possible considering developmental age

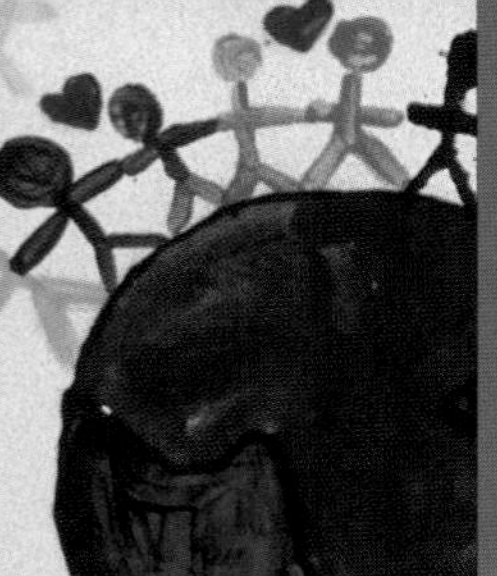

PARTNERING WITH FAMILIES

The Child with Neuroblastoma

Surgery phase

- Teach the parents to observe for signs of infection at the wound site and to take the child's temperature, if necessary.
- Assist the family to provide pain management including medication administration and various comfort measures.
- Teach the parents the importance of keeping accurate record of urine output and bowel movements and to notify physician if child does not have a bowel movement at least every 3 days.
- Continue with progression to a regular diet.

Chemotherapy phase

- The child frequently has a central line placed early in the chemotherapy phase. The central line greatly reduces the emotional trauma associated with chemotherapy and blood tests.
  - Teach the child how to help the parents with cleaning of the central line.
  - Teach the child how to protect the central line.
  - Teach the parents how to clean and dress the site of the central line.
  - Have the parents practice central line care with a model and then on the child before discharge to increase the parents' confidence.
  - Give the parents written and illustrated information about care of a central line.
  - Arrange for home care dressing supplies before discharge.
- Give the parents detailed chemotherapy information.
- Teach administration of any medications that the parent will perform via central line or other routes.
- Refer the family to the American Cancer Society for coloring books and other resources for children receiving chemotherapy

- Management of sensory/perceptual alterations to provide for safety and sensory input
- Management of pain to level of comfort
- Acceptance and integration of diagnosis into lives of family members

Wilms' Tumor (Nephroblastoma)

Nephroblastoma, an intrarenal tumor called Wilms' tumor, is a common abdominal tumor of childhood and accounts for 6% to 7% of all childhood tumors (Jaffe & Huff, 2004). The incidence of nephroblastoma is approximately 8.1 cases per 1 million children annually. Wilms' tumor occurs most frequently between 2 and 3 years of age, but may also occur in adolescents and adults (Drigan & Androkites, 2002).

Etiology and Pathophysiology

Wilms' tumor is associated with several congenital anomalies: aniridia (absence of the iris), hemihypertrophy (abnormal growth of half of the body or a body structure), genitourinary anomalies, nevi, and hamartomas (benign, nodulelike growths). This connection suggests a genetic link; chromosome deletions at 11p13 and 11p15 (locations for WT1 and WT2 genes) have been associated with Wilms' tumor (Kline & Sevier, 2003). It has a high incidence in Beckwith-Wiedemann syndrome which is characterized by macroglossia and hypoglycemia (McLorie, 2001). However, most children with Wilms' tumor have no other abnormalities. Only about 1-2% of children have a family history of Wilms'. In these cases a *WT 1* gene mutation occurs (Jaffe & Huff, 2004). Wilms' tumor grows very quickly, doubling its size in 11 to 13 days. Such fast growth generally contributes to a large tumor by the time of diagnosis. However, there is usually good response to chemotherapy drugs (Scott, Britt, Juneau, et al., 2001). Tissue type is associated with outcome, with anaplastic tumors having less favorable prognosis.

Clinical Manifestations

Wilms' tumor is usually an asymptomatic, firm, lobulated mass located to one side of the midline in the abdomen. Often a parent discovers the mass during the child's bath. Hypertension caused by increased renin activity related to renal damage is reported in 25% of cases. Hematuria or abdominal pain are sometimes present. Bilateral Wilms' tumors occur in 5% to 10% of cases (Anderson, 2000).

COLLABORATIVE CARE

Care by many professionals is needed for prompt diagnosis and treatment of Wilms' tumor.

Diagnostic Tests

The diagnosis of Wilms' tumor is based on an ultrasound study of the abdomen and an intravenous pyelogram. CT scanning or MRI of the lungs, liver, spleen, and brain may be performed to identify any metastases. This information is used in staging the tumor (Table 29–7). A complete blood count is obtained, as well as BUN and creatinine levels. Liver function tests are performed. Histologic examination is performed for tissue typing once the tumor is removed.

Clinical Therapy

Treatment is multifaceted and increasingly successful. About 90% of early stages and 70% of metastic cases have long-term survival (Pritchard-Jones, 2002). Surgery is performed to remove the affected kidney, to examine the opposite kidney, remove lymph nodes for examination, and to look for other sites of metastases. The total tumor is removed, taking care not to rupture the tumor capsule. Generally the entire kidney is removed, but when the disease is bilateral, a kidney-sparing procedure is needed. Such procedures are being examined for their success in treating unilateral disease as well. Chemotherapy or radiation therapy, alone or in combination, is sometimes used before surgery to reduce the size of the tumor. Children with stage III and IV disease often receive vincristine, dactinomycin, and doxorubicin; cyclophosphamide is sometimes added. Radiation may also follow surgery, especially in disseminated disease. Children whose tumors are almost com-

TABLE 29–7 National Wilms' Tumor Study Staging System

STAGE	DESCRIPTION
I	The tumor is limited to the kidney and completely excised.
	The surface of the renal capsule is intact. The tumor is not ruptured before or during removal. No residual tumor is apparent beyond the margins of the excision.
II	The tumor extends beyond the kidney but is completely excised. Regional extension of the tumor is present, i.e., penetration through the outer surface of the renal capsule into the perirenal soft tissues. Vessels outside the kidney substance are infiltrated or contain tumor thrombus. Biopsy may have been performed on the tumor, or local spillage of tumor confined to the flank has occurred. No residual tumor is apparent at or beyond the margin of excision.
III	Residual nonhematogenous tumor is confined to the abdomen. Any of the following may occur: ➤ Lymph nodes on biopsy are found to be involved in the hilus, the periaortic chains, or beyond. ➤ Diffuse peritoneal contamination by the tumor has occurred, such as by spillage of tumor beyond the flank before or during surgery, or by tumor growth that has penetrated through the peritoneal surface. ➤ Implants are found on peritoneal surfaces. ➤ The tumor extends beyond the surgical margins either microscopically or grossly. ➤ The tumor is not completely resectable because of local infiltration into vital structures.
IV	Hematogenous metastasis: deposits are present beyond stage III (e.g., lung, liver, bone, and/or brain).
V	Bilateral renal involvement is present at diagnosis. An attempt should be made to stage each side according to the above criteria on the basis of extent of disease before biopsy.

Adapted from Green, D. M., Grigoriev, Y. A., Nan, B., Takashima, J. R., Norkool, P. A., D'Angio, G. J., & Breslow, N. E. (2001). Congestive heart failure after treatment for Wilms' tumor: A report from the National Wilms' Tumor study group. Journal of Clinical Oncology, *19, 1926–1934.*

pletely excised and who have a favorable prognosis do not require irradiation of the tumor bed.

Long-term complications of treatment include liver damage, portal hypertension, and mild cirrhosis, which may occur in children treated for right-sided Wilms' tumor. Radiation damage (such as thinning or weakening) of the skeleton, pelvis, and thorax has been reported. Kyphosis and scoliosis may occur from irradiation of vertebral bodies and the pelvis. Glomerular damage to the remaining kidney may also occur. Second malignancies in the original radiation field have occurred with orthovoltage radiation, but recent changes in radiation therapy have reduced this risk.

NURSING MANAGEMENT

Nursing management focuses on referring the child with abdominal mass or other symptoms for prompt evaluation, supporting the child and family during therapy, and being alert for any further signs of cancer.

Nursing Assessment and Diagnosis

Perform a thorough baseline assessment of the child. Do not palpate the abdomen because of the potential for spreading the cancerous cells. Monitor the child's blood pressure carefully as hypertension is a common finding that may require treatment.

PRACTICE ALERT

If a mass is felt during palpation of a child's abdomen, **stop palpating immediately** and report the finding to the physician. Never palpate the liver or abdomen of a child with Wilms' tumor as this could cause a piece of the tumor to dislodge. Place a sign on the child's bed and in the chart alerting health providers not to palpate the child's abdomen.

Nursing diagnoses for a child with Wilms' tumor will differ depending on the phase of treatment. Common nursing diagnoses may include the following:

- Risk for Infection related to inadequate defenses
- Impaired Urinary Elimination related to anatomic obstruction
- Ineffective Cardiopulmonary Tissue Perfusion related to hypertension caused by mechanical reduction of blood flow
- Risk for Caregiver Role Strain related to child's illness severity
- Risk for Impaired Home Maintenance related to child's disease

Planning and Implementation

Nursing management can be divided into two phases: the postrenal surgery phase and the chemotherapy phase. (See Chapter 17∞ for general care of the child after surgery.) Drawings and special teaching dolls with removable kidneys can be used to teach young children about the surgery. Although chemotherapy may occur at two different times, before and after surgery, nursing management considerations remain the same.

Nursing care during the postrenal surgery phase focuses on pain management and close monitoring of fluid levels. A large incision is necessary to remove the kidney, and the resultant postoperative shift of organs and fluid in the abdominal cavity may create discomfort for the child. Frequently reposition the child and use noninvasive and pharmacologic pain interventions to improve the child's comfort. Gentle handling is important. Monitor fluids closely following surgery to prevent hypovolemia and to assess the shift of fluids out of the third space and out of the body. Assess daily weight, intake and output (I&O), and urine specific gravity. Monitor the function of the remaining kidney. Take blood pressure measurements frequently to watch for signs of shock and to assess the functioning of the remaining kidney.

During the chemotherapy phase, monitor the child for side effects of drugs, the potential for infection from the central line site, and the function of the remaining kidney. Advise parents about home care needs, administration of medications, and monitoring for drug side effects and ongoing needs for health monitoring. Be sure care is well coordinated among all healthcare providers.

Evaluation

Desired outcomes for nursing care of the child with nephroblastoma include balanced intake and output, normal vital signs, recovery from surgery, and successful family management of postsurgical care and ongoing treatments.

Bone Tumors

Osteosarcoma (or Osteogenic Sarcoma)

Osteosarcoma is a rare, malignant bone tumor that occurs predominantly in adolescent boys. Its peak incidence is during the rapid growth years. The tumor is usually located at the metaphysis of the distal femur, proximal tibia, or proximal humerus (Betcher, Simon, & McHard, 2002).

Etiology and Pathophysiology. Osteosarcoma occurs during growth spurts and is more common in tall youth. Bone tissue produced by osteosarcoma never matures into normal compact bone. Although the cause of osteosarcoma is unknown, radiation exposure (either environmental or treatment related) is associated with its development. Survivors of retinoblastoma have a greatly increased incidence of osteosarcoma. An abnormality of gene p53 has been noted in some cases of this cancer, leading to oncogene malformations and possibly to an absence of tumor suppressor genes (Betcher et al., 2002).

Clinical Manifestations. The common initial symptoms of osteosarcoma are pain, swelling or mass, and limp or decreased motion. The pain can be referred to the hip or back, which can delay diagnosis. Pulmonary metastasis occurs in up to 20% of cases. Other metastatic sites include kidney, adrenals, brain, and pericardium. When lung metastasis is the only site, lung resection may be successful for treatment. Disseminated metastases and bone lesions have poorer prognosis.

COLLABORATIVE CARE

Partnerships among professionals will enable the child with a bone tumor to obtain accurate diagnosis, treatment, and necessary rehabilitation.

Diagnostic Tests

Diagnosis of osteosarcoma is made through radiographic studies of the affected area and bone scan. CT or MRI scans of involved bone and other potential sites are performed. A complete blood count, liver studies, and renal studies are performed for clues to potential metastases. A blood test is included for serum alkaline phosphatase (level may be elevated), and tumor biopsy is performed to confirm the diagnosis. Arteriography may be performed if limb-sparing surgery is contemplated. Cardiac assessments are performed to establish baseline function prior to treatment with doxorubicin.

Clinical Therapy

Treatment involves both surgery and chemotherapy. The surgery is either a limb-salvage procedure or limb amputation. In limb-salvage procedures the tumor is removed and an internal prosthesis is inserted. A limb-salvage procedure is possible if bone growth has taken place and a neurobundle (area where several nerves converge) is not involved in the tumor. If these two criteria are not met, limb amputation is necessary. Physical rehabilitation will be needed after either amputation or limb-salvage procedure. Aggressive chemotherapy following surgery has improved the survival rate. At the time of diagnosis, most children have metastases (even though they may not be identifiable), so chemotherapy is needed. Chemotherapy is started before surgery to shrink the tumor, especially in cases where limb-salvage surgery is performed. It is also given postoperatively to treat and prevent metastasis. Drugs commonly used for osteosarcoma include:

- Doxorubicin
- Cisplatin
- Ifosfamide with mesna
- Methotrexate with leucovorin rescue

Radiation is generally not effective in treating osteosarcoma although it may be used with chemotherapy for recurrence at other sites.

Ewing's Sarcoma

Ewing's sarcoma is a malignant, small, round cell tumor usually involving the diaphyseal (shaft) portion of the long bones. The most common sites are the femur, pelvis, tibia, fibula, ribs, humerus, scapula, and clavicle, but any bone may be involved. Ewing's sarcoma occurs in two children per million, is most common in Whites and Hispanics, and is rare in Black and Asian children. The incidence is highest in children between the ages of 10 and 20 years (Betcher et al., 2002).

Translocations on chromosomes 11 and 22 have been identified in children with Ewing's sarcoma; these are t(11;22)(q24;q12). In addition, these tumors express a protooncogene, c-myc.

The symptoms are similar to those of osteosarcoma and may include pain, swelling, fever, an elevated WBC count, elevated erythrocyte sedimentation rate, and elevated C-reactive protein. Some children present with a fracture of the affected bone. A tumor biopsy is necessary for diagnosis. Diagnostic tests are the same as those for osteosarcoma.

Initial treatment for Ewing's sarcoma is chemotherapy to reduce the tumor, followed by surgical removal of the entire bone or intensive high-dose irradiation of the entire bone. Limb-salvage procedures are now commonly performed rather than amputation. Surgery is preferred because of the possibility of a secondary cancer from radiation. Chemotherapy is always used following initial treatment, as undetectable metastases are commonly present. Medications used to treat Ewing's sarcoma include:

- Vincristine
- Doxorubicin
- Cyclophosphamide
- Dactinomycin
- Etoposide
- Ifosfamide

NURSING MANAGEMENT

The goals of nursing management for bone tumors are to provide support during treatment and help the child adjust to any changes in body function.

Nursing Assessment and Diagnosis

Physiologic assessment of the child with a bone tumor includes assessment of the site before surgery. Assess the child's pain or discomfort, mobility, and gait. Take careful vital signs, especially noting temperature and respirations. Psychologic assessment of the child and family are needed, especially if amputation is planned. Body image disturbances occur when a limb is lost, particularly with school-age children and adolescents. Assess the child's understanding of the treatment and of care after surgery. Find out what support systems are available for assistance.

Observe the wound postoperatively for infection and hemorrhage. Assess circulation above and below the operative site. If edema is found, elevate the limb. If a limb-salvage procedure is performed, the child's extremity will be intact but it will not function as before, because muscle insertion sites and mass have been removed with the tumor during surgery. Detailed charting of the condition of the surgical site and limb function is important.

If the limb has been amputated, assess the child for the following signs indicating a disturbed body image.

- Refusal to look at or touch the altered or missing body part
- Preoccupation with loss or change
- Feelings of shame or embarrassment, either verbalized or demonstrated
- Distorted perception of normal body (easily seen in the child's drawings of the body)
- Fears of rejection or unwanted attention from others
- Overexposure or hiding of the affected body part
- Actual or perceived change in the structure and function of the body or body parts

Psychosocial assessment of the child and family is discussed in more detail earlier in the general section on childhood cancer (see page 1051).

Appropriate nursing diagnoses for the child with a bone tumor are based on the treatment and needs of each child.

- Risk for Infection related to amputation or limb-salvage procedure
- Impaired Skin Integrity related to mechanical forces of prosthesis
- Impaired Physical Mobility related to musculoskeletal impairment
- Impaired Adjustment related to disability and lifestyle change
- Disturbed Body Image related to treatment and injury
- Pain related to physical injury of tissues

Planning and Implementation

Care of the child after surgery involves general postoperative care (see Chapter 17∞). The child who has had an amputation has special needs regarding skin care and rehabilitation. Inspect the dressing for intactness and bleeding. When the dressing is changed (usually several days after surgery) inspect tissue at the surgical site, using sterile technique. Turn the child at least every 2 hours. The site needs to heal completely before chemotherapy can begin and a prosthesis can be made. Pain management is a major nursing care need. When amputation has occurred, the adolescent will often experience **phantom pain.** This is pain that feels as if it is in the amputated extremity and is caused by trauma to the nerves in the area of the amputation. Acknowledge the pain as real since the nerve endings are intact and the patient is perceiving real discomfort. Medicate adequately and use additional pain control measures such as repositioning the limb using gentle movement, supporting the limb, and using distraction or deep breathing (Gilger, Groben, & Hinds, 2002).

MediaLink Case Study: Teen with Ewing's Sarcoma

Discuss insurance and other financial arrangements with the parents, as prosthetics can be expensive. Physical therapy will be needed as well. Referral to a Shriners Hospital is an option for some families.

Implement plans to help the child deal with body image disturbance. Plan for a visit from another child who is well adjusted to a prosthesis. Help the child to gradually learn how to care for the stump. Slow progress may be made as the child first looks briefly, then for longer periods, and finally is willing to touch the stump. Show the child how it is possible to continue with sports such as baseball, skiing, or biking with a prosthesis. A discussion group with others can be very useful for adolescents. Plan with the child how to tell friends about the surgery and what issues he or she may face upon return to school. Make plans for elevator access if needed and emergency evacuation procedures. Some children or adolescents may need referral for counseling to assist in dealing with body image disturbance.

The child will be receiving physical rehabilitation while hospitalized and after discharge. When the child is discharged, explain to the family the importance of bringing the child for outpatient chemotherapy and physical rehabilitation visits. Special arrangements may be needed at the child's school to facilitate a wheelchair, crutches, or ambulation with a new prosthesis. Coordinate with the school nurse about the evaluation of the presence of buttons to open doors, wide doorways to facilitate passage, and any limitations of the building. Contact the school nurse or other school personnel to plan the child's return. The child will need careful management of a schedule that permits both healing of the surgical site with rehabilitation and then the demands of chemotherapy.

Follow-up care is needed to monitor for progress and to be alert for signs of metastases. Fracture may be a sign of recurrent tumor. All body systems such as lungs, heart, kidneys, and liver are monitored for signs of recurrence.

Evaluation

The following expected outcomes of nursing care for the child with a bone tumor focus on the treatments required and adaptation to changes in lifestyle:

- Healed surgical site with no signs of infection
- Adaptation to changes in mobility status
- Successful adjustment to changes required in school settings

- Maintenance of healthy skin
- Positive body image
- Management of pain to comfort level
- Successful integration of continuing medical therapy

Leukemia

Leukemia is the most commonly diagnosed pediatric malignancy in children under 14 years of age. A cancer of the blood-forming organs, leukemia is characterized by a proliferation of abnormal white blood cells in the body. Several types of leukemia are differentiated, depending on the blood cells affected. The main types are acute lymphoblastic leukemia, acute nonlymphocytic leukemia (acute myelogenous leukemia), and the rare chronic leukemias of childhood.

The most common type of childhood leukemia is acute lymphoblastic leukemia (ALL), which accounts for 25% of all childhood cancer and 75% of leukemias in children. The peak age at onset is 2 to 4 years (Landier, 2001). ALL is more common in Whites and in boys (Figure 29–14 ■) (Westlake & Bertolone, 2002). Subtypes of ALL are based on the French-American-British (FAB) system of classification. The three types of ALL in the FAB system are L1, L2, and L3. Rasheed, who is described in the opening scenario, has ALL.

Acute nonlymphocytic leukemia (ANLL) refers to all leukemias from myeloid cells. About 17% of childhood leukemias are ANLL. ANLL is most common in children younger than 2 years of age and in adolescents. It is more common in males than females, and in Asians/Pacific Islanders, Hispanics, and Whites than in Blacks (Landier, 2002; Reynolds, Von Behren, & Elkin, 2002). Following are subtypes of ANLL in the FAB classification.

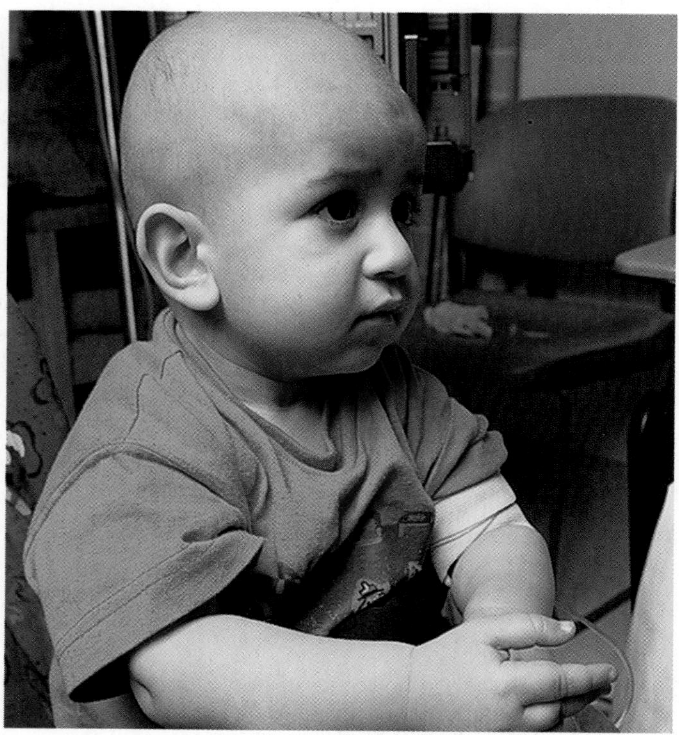

FIGURE 29–14 ■ Acute lymphoblastic leukemia is the most common type of leukemia in children and the most common cancer affecting children under 5 years of age.

- M0 = acute nonlymphocytic leukemia without maturation
- M1 = acute nonlymphocytic leukemia with poor maturation
- M2 = acute nonlymphocytic leukemia with maturation
- M3 = acute promyelocytic leukemia
- M4 = acute myelomonocytic leukemia
- M5 = actue monocytic leukemia
- M6 = erythroleukemia
- M7 = acute megakaryocytic leukemia

Because chronic leukemias such as chronic myelocytic, chronic myelomonocytic, and chronic lymphocytic leukemia are rare in children, the following discussion will focus on ALL and ANLL.

Etiology and Pathophysiology

The causes of leukemia are not well understood. Some investigators theorize that exposure to infectious agents can predispose children to leukemia (Kinlen & Balkwill, 2001). Genetic factors are believed to play a role in some types of the disease. For instance, children with chromosomal defects such as Down syndrome, neurofibromatosis type I, Bloom syndrome, and Shwachman syndrome have an increased incidence of ALL, and chromosomal abnormalities such as hyperploidy, hypodiploidy, tranlocations, and deletions are present in most children with ALL (Westlake & Bertolone, 2002). Children with immune deficiency states, such as ataxia-telangiectasia, congenital hypogammaglobulinemia, and Wiskott-Aldrich syndrome, have an increased risk of ALL.

Ionizing radiation exposure when in utero, and chemical agents such as treatment of an earlier cancer with chemotherapy (alkylating agents and topoisomerase II inhibitors) are thought to play a role in the development of ANLL. There are several chromosomal and genetic abnormalities associated with ANLL. For example, trisomy 8 is associated with all subtypes of the disease (Landier, 2002).

Leukemia occurs when the stem cells in the bone marrow produce immature WBCs that cannot function normally. These cells proliferate rapidly by cloning instead of normal mitosis, causing the bone marrow to fill with abnormal WBCs. The abnormal cells then spill out into the circulatory system where they steadily replace the normally functioning WBCs. As this occurs, the protective lymphocytic functions such as cellular and humeral immunity are reduced, leaving the body vulnerable to infections. The malignant WBCs rapidly fill the bone marrow, replacing stem cells that produce erythrocytes (red blood cells) and other blood products such as platelets, thereby decreasing the amount of these products in circulation. The stem cells are replaced by leukemic clones, eventually resulting in anemia. Children with leukemia commonly experience abnormal bleeding because of the reduced platelet amounts.

Clinical Manifestations

Children with ALL and ANLL usually have fever, pallor, overt signs of bleeding, lethargy, malaise, anorexia, and large joint or bone pain. Petechiae, frank bleeding, and joint pain are cardinal signs of bone marrow failure. Enlargement of the liver and spleen (hepatosplenomegaly) and changes in the lymph nodes (lymphadenopathy) are common. If the leukemia has infiltrated the central nervous system (entered it by means of the circulatory or lymphoid system), the child may exhibit signs such as headache, vomiting, papilledema, and sixth cranial nerve palsy (inability to move the eye laterally). These findings are caused by the leukemic cells massing and putting pressure on nerves. The testicles, spinal cord, and bone marrow are common sites for infiltration. The leukemic cells in the testicle become a mass that causes the testicle to enlarge, often painlessly.

COLLABORATIVE CARE

Many care providers join together as leukemia is diagnosed and treated. Periodic exacerbations or side effects from treatment require intensification in care. Partnerships with families are needed to provide the lengthy care required.

Diagnostic Tests

Diagnosis is based initially on blood counts and bone marrow aspiration. Blood counts reveal anemia, thrombocytopenia, and neutropenia. Bone marrow aspiration reveals immature and abnormal lymphoblasts and hypercellular marrow and is the differential test. Percent of blast cells in marrow is measured and 25% lymphoblasts is definitive of disease (Westlake & Bertolone, 2002). Neutropenia, thrombocytopenia, and anemia are commonly noted (Box 29–4). Other abnormal laboratory findings include elevated serum uric acid and elevated calcium, potassium, and phosphorus levels. New laboratory studies such as rapid flow cytometric assay are making the presence of even very small numbers of leukemic cells possible, so that treatment can be used to improve prognosis in children with minimal residual disease (Coustan-Smith, Sancho, Hancock, et al., 2000). Leukemic cells are examined and classified by FAB type, and DNA analysis may provide clues about genetic changes; all of these considerations are used to establish the protocol for treatment. Cells of children with ALL are B cell or T cell; these classifications are also used to establish treatment protocols.

Clinical Therapy

Treatment of ALL involves radiation and chemotherapy. Radiation is used for central nervous system disease, in T-cell leukemia, and for testicular involvement. Chemotherapy is organized into four phases:

1. Induction
   - Prednisone
   - Vincristine
   - L-asparaginase
   - Daunorubicin
2. Consolidation
   - L-asparaginase
   - Doxorubicin
3. Delayed intensification
   - Vincristine
   - ARA-C
   - Cyclophosphamide
4. Maintenance of remission
   - 6-mercaptopurine
   - 6-thioguanine
   - Methotrexate

An additional drug used for treatment of central nervous system disease or prophylaxis is intrathecal methotrexate. Maintenance therapy may continue for 2 to 3 years, causing decreased resistance to infection for this prolonged period of time.

Treatment of ANLL involves use of the following drugs during the induction and consolidation phases.

1. Induction phase
   - Daunorubicin
   - Coxorubicin
   - Mitoxantrone
   - Cytarabin
2. Consolidation phase
   - etoposide
   - teniposide

Maximum cell death occurs during the induction phase. The cells that remain after this period are more resistant to treatment. After 3 to 4 weeks, when a remission has occurred, central nervous system prophylaxis begins. Drugs are used in combination with cranial irradiation. During the consolidation phase, chemotherapy with L-asparaginase and doxorubicin is administered. Delayed intensification uses additional drugs to target the leukemic cells that have survived. Treatment during the maintenance phase is aimed at destroying the remaining leukemic cells. Combinations of active drugs are used to prevent resistance. Many complications can occur with such high doses and combinations of drugs, so much of the clinical therapy is aimed at managing these effects. In addition, long-term complications such as central nervous system toxicity; damage to pituitary, liver, kidneys, gastrointestinal tract, heart, lungs, gonads, blood and immune system; and secondary malignancies can occur.

The prognosis for children with leukemia is much improved with current therapy. However, several risk factors affect the long-term outcome. The most favorable findings are as follows:

- Age at onset between 2 and 10 years
- Initial hemoglobin level less than 10 g/dL
- Low initial WBC count
- Lack of B- or T-cell antigens
- Absence of extramedullary (outside bone marrow or spinal cord) involvement
- Rapid response to chemotherapy

The most important factor is the initial leukocyte count. The higher the leukocyte count (over 50,000/mm^3) at diagnosis, the

BOX 29–4 Laboratory Values in Leukemia

	Normal	Common Values in Leukemia
Leukocytes	< 10,000/μL	> 10,000/μL
Platelets	150,000–400,000/μL	20,000–100,000/μL
Hemoglobin	12–16 g/dL	7–11 g/dL

worse the prognosis. For children in the low-risk group, the probability of prolonged survival is as high as 90%. Infants under 12 months of age have a poor prognosis. Treatment methods and duration are adjusted for each child, depending on that child's risk factors. More aggressive treatment is undertaken for those in the higher risk groups.

Approximately 10% of children have a relapse within a year after completing treatment. Treatment for relapse consists of additional chemotherapy drugs. The prognosis is best if the relapse occurs late after the initial diagnosis and after the initial treatment is completed. HSCT is a treatment option for the child who has a relapse with ALL who then achieves a second remission; the transplant is given when the child is in remission. Transplant is also used for children with ANLL; they do not need to be in remission for the transplant to be performed. Chemotherapy itself can create numerous complications, affecting all body organs. Secondary malignancies sometimes occur later in life.

NURSING MANAGEMENT

Nursing management for the child with leukemia is complex due to the multisystem effects of the disease, and the long period of time required for therapy. Normal growth and development and prevention of sequelae from treatment are major goals.

Nursing Assessment and Diagnosis

A thorough physical assessment is important to ensure prompt identification of problems without injuring the child who has deficient coagulation and immune function. Perform assessments every 8 hours or more often depending on the chemotherapy regimen. Observe carefully for bruising and other new sites of bleeding, and fever or other signs of infection. Once chemotherapy has begun, closely monitor renal functioning through specific gravity, intake and output (I&O), and daily weight measurement. Monitor dietary intake, nausea, vomiting, and constipation. Observe for mucosal sores in the mouth. A central line is usually in place for intravenous infusion of medications, so careful assessment of the line for proper functioning and for signs of infection is needed. Ask the parents about any behavioral changes. Central nervous system infiltration can affect the child's level of consciousness, causing irritability, vomiting, and lethargy. However, these nonspecific signs can also be induced by chemotherapeutic drugs and antiemetics. Frequent venipunctures, bone marrow aspirations, and lumbar punctures require pain assessment and an evaluation of the level of knowledge and coping skills of child and family.

MediaLink Leukemia Video

Leukemia causes many changes in the body and confirmation of the disease is difficult for families to face. Among the many nursing diagnoses that might be appropriate for the child with leukemia are the following:

- Imbalanced Nutrition: Less than Body Requirements related to inability to ingest food
- Risk for Infection related to altered immune system functioning
- Risk for Injury related to bleeding
- Activity Intolerance related to generalized weakness
- Pain related to chemotherapy and disease process
- Disturbed Sleep Pattern related to chemotherapy drugs and disease process
- Anxiety (child and parent) related to change in health status

Planning and Implementation

Bone marrow suppression may necessitate transmission-based precautions (refer to the Skills Manual). Instruct parents in the prevention of infection and use nursing care measures to prevent infection also. Perform careful handwashing; take temperature frequently; give mouth care with antibacterial mouth washes; inspect skin, mouth, rectal area, and central line site for any signs of infection. Care of mouth sores and other side effects of chemotherapy is presented in the nursing care plan, earlier in this chapter.

Special attention to renal function is needed when the child receives cyclophosphamide. Gross hematuria is a side effect of this drug. Hydration with intravenous fluids to attain a specific gravity of less than 1.010 prevents or reduces the severity of hematuria. It also prepares the kidneys to manage products of tumor cell breakdown. To achieve the desired specific gravity, the child receives intravenous fluids at 1.5 times maintenance volume for at least 6 to 8 hours before and at least 1.5 hours after administration of the drug. Other chemotherapy drugs have different infusion times while some do not require hydration prior to infusion. Check drug references carefully for recommendations with each drug. Evaluate the infusion site before and frequently during infusion. Although extravasation is not as common with central lines used in cancer treatment as in peripheral lines, it still can occur. Many chemotherapy agents are extremely toxic to tissues. In addition, lysis of the cancer cells can produce toxic side effects (see oncologic emergencies described earlier in the chapter). Careful monitoring of I&O is required to record the intravenous fluids, assess kidney functioning, and monitor excretion of by-products from destroyed tumor cells. Monitor specific gravity every 8 hours, as well as before and during administration of the drug, and when the intravenous fluids are reduced to maintenance volume levels. Daily weight measurements are important to assist in planning adequate hydration during chemotherapy, as well as to measure nutritional status.

Drug side effects may necessitate infusion of platelets or packed red blood cells. See the Skills Manual for techniques to be used in these situations.

Many children are treated in an oncology clinic, staying in the hospital only on the day of intravenous drug administration, and receiving oral medications at home. The time at the hospital is used to assess how the family is managing issues such as nutrition, sleep, medication administration, and obtaining psychosocial support. Careful teaching for the family is needed to ensure safe drug adminstration and identification of issues requiring further care.

Nurses play a key role in the long-term multidisciplinary treatment of children with leukemia. The impact of a diagnosis of leukemia and the long-term nature of treatment can severely stress the coping abilities of both the child and the family. Ongoing psychosocial assessment and emotional support are essential (see the general discussion of psychosocial assessment in the Childhood Cancer section beginning on page 1038). Referral to support groups and social services may be beneficial. Assist the family in exploration of alternative therapies such as relaxation, imagery, and nutritional support that may aid the child. Be alert for any interactions that could occur between alternative therapies and the medical regimen. (See Partnering with Families: Chemotherapy for Leukemia and Complementary Therapy: Enhancing Chemotherapy Effectiveness.)

Evaluation

Following are expected outcomes for nursing care of the child with leukemia.

- Prevention of infection and other secondary complications of chemotherapy
- Adequate hydration
- Normal urinary output
- Blood values within normal limits
- Successful family adaptation to parenting a child with chronic illness
- Adequate parental knowledge related to disease process

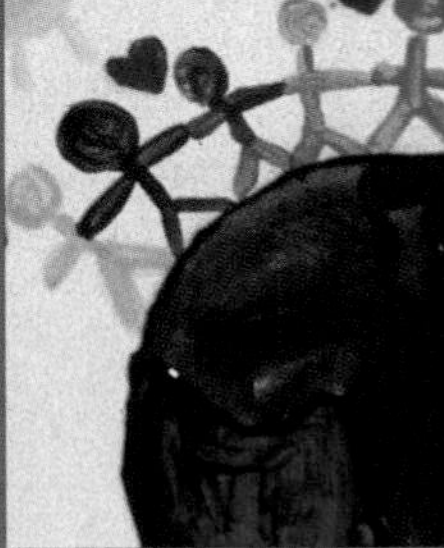

PARTNERING WITH FAMILIES

Chemotherapy for Leukemia

Physical care

- Schedule rest periods each day.
- Avoid areas of exposure to people with illnesses.
- Drink generous amounts of water.
- Eat a healthy diet, using frequent, small, and nutritious meals to obtain enough nutrients.
- Take medicines prescribed to decrease nausea.
- Maintain good oral hygiene with soft toothbrush and water pik.
- Avoid sun exposure and check skin each day for any signs of bruises, pressure areas, cuts, or scratches.
- Promote bowel elimination through regular dietary and toileting practices.
- Report any signs of infection, changes in condition, or other concerns.

Emotional care

- Prepare for loss of hair with plans for hats, wigs, or other alternatives.
- Continue contact with friends via phone, Internet, and in person when possible.
- Try relaxation techniques to aid in sleep and management of treatments.
- Talk with clergy, teachers, parents, counselors, friends, or other supportive people about the experience of having leukemia.
- Keep a journal to record feelings and experiences.

Soft Tissue Tumors

Hodgkin Disease

Hodgkin disease is a disorder of the lymphoid system. It usually arises in a single lymph node or an anatomic group of lymph nodes (Figure 29–15 ■). There are approximately 3 cases per 100,000 people, with the peak occurrence in adolescent boys. Hodgkin disease has a childhood form but is rare in those under 14 years. Most cases involve a young adult form that affects those between 15 and 35 years, and an older adult form, usually seen in persons over 55 years (Thompson, 1999).

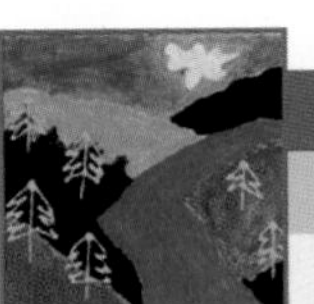

COMPLEMENTARY THERAPY

Enhancing Chemotherapy Effectiveness

Complementary medicine practices can often be easily integrated with and enhance effectiveness of chemotherapy. In a study of 20 children undergoing treatment for leukemia, parents were instructed to provide massage daily for 30 days. The children had an average age of 7 years. Parents and children completed anxiety and mood inventories and children had blood studies as well. Those in the massage groups had lower anxiety scores and higher mood scores after the intervention. In addition the children had improved white blood cell and neutrophil counts. Massage therapy may be a useful addition to treatment regimens of young children for leukemia (Field, Cullen, Diego, et al., 2001). Nurses can suggest this intervention to families and arrange for them to obtain massage therapy training if they are interested.

Etiology and Pathophysiology

Hodgkin disease occurs in clusters and has been reported in families. This suggests a possible genetic link as well as an infectious agent or environmental hazard.

Clinical Manifestations

The main symptom of Hodgkin disease is nontender, firm lymphadenopathy, usually in the supraclavicular and cervical nodes but occasionally in the mediastinal area. A mediastinal growth can cause respiratory difficulty because of pressure on the trachea or bronchi. Fever, night sweats, and weight loss occur in one third of children with Hodgkin disease and are associated with a more aggressive form of the disease. The leukocyte count and erythrocyte sedimentation rate (ESR) may be elevated.

COLLABORATIVE CARE

Primary care providers, diagnostic services, and oncologists work together when lymphoma occurs. Nurses provide ongoing care and monitoring for the child.

Diagnostic Tests

Diagnosis is based on lymph node biopsy; Reed-Stemberg cells (large cells with two nucleoli) are present. A staging classification

PATHOPHYSIOLOGY ILLUSTRATED

Hodgkin Disease

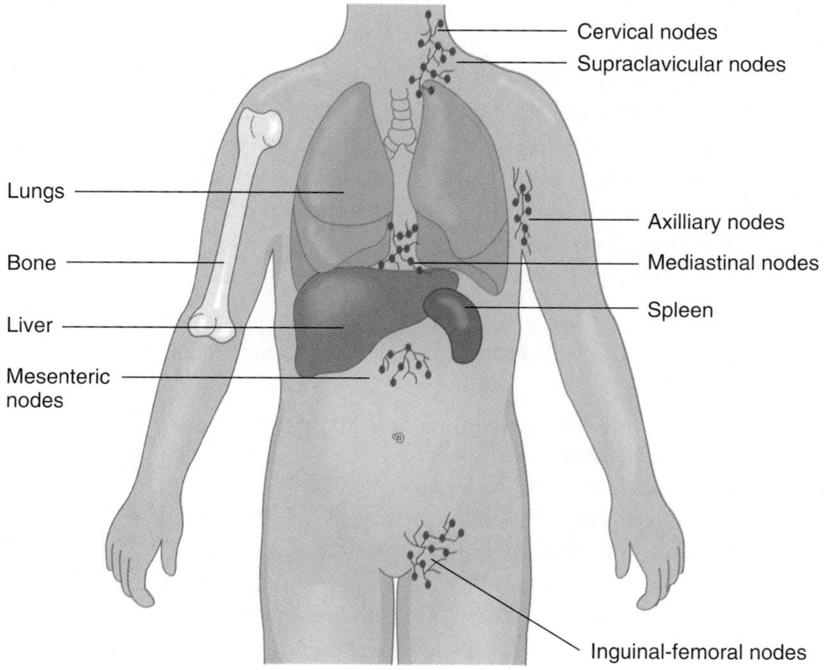

FIGURE 29–15 ■ Lymph nodes and organs affected in Hodgkin disease in children.

is used to determine disease severity (Table 29–8). The basis for staging is data obtained from the history, physical examination, radiographic study (for metastasis), chest CT scan, CT or MRI scans of the retroperitoneal nodes, lymphangiogram if there is retroperitoneal involvement, laboratory studies (complete blood count, erythrocyte sedimentation rate, serum copper level, liver function tests), PET, bone scans, and a radionuclide scan with gallium. Bone marrow biopsy, bone scan, or a staging laparotomy may be performed in certain situations when advanced disease is suspected.

TABLE 29–8 Staging System for Hodgkin Disease

STAGE	DESCRIPTION
I	Disease within a single lymph node region
IE	Disease within a single extralymphatic organ
II	Disease within two or more lymph node regions on same side of diaphragm
IIE	Disease within extralymphatic organ, and of one or more lymph node regions on same side of diaphragm
III	Disease of lymph node regions on both sides of diaphragm
IIIE	Disease of lymph node regions on both sides of the diaphragm with involvement of extralymphatic organ
IIIS	As in III, plus disease within spleen
IIISE	As in III, plus disease in extralymphatic organs and spleen
IV	Disseminated disease within one or more lymphatic organs with or without lymph node involvement

Clinical Therapy

Treatment is commonly performed in outpatient settings unless complications develop that require hospitalization. Chemotherapy using a four-drug combination has been found to be the most effective drug treatment. Drugs commonly used include:

- Adriamycin
- Bleomycin
- Vinblastine
- Dacarbazine
- Etoposide
- Prednisone
- Cyclophosphamide
- Procarbazine
- Methotrexate
- Mechlorethamine

Common drug combinations are:

- ABVD
- ABVE
- ABVE-PC
- AOPE

- BEACOPP
- COPP
- EBVP
- MOPP
- OEPA
- OPPA
- VAMP
- VEPA

(See Table 29–3 for description of these drug combinations.)

Radiation is commonly added, with low doses for children who are still growing, and larger doses for those who are physically mature or those whose disease is more advanced at diagnosis. The 5-year survival rate is approximately 90%, depending on the stage of the disease at diagnosis. Bone marrow transplantation is a treatment option in children with advanced disease or relapse.

Non-Hodgkin Lymphoma

About 12% of pediatric cancers are lymphoma and of these 40% to 45% are Hodgkin and 55% to 60% are non-Hodgkin. The three types of pediatric non-Hodgkin lymphoma are (1) lymphoblastic lymphoma (30% to 40%), (2) small noncleaved cell (Burkitt's) lymphoma (40% to 50%), and (3) large cell lymphoma (15%) (Hussong, 2002). Lymphomas of all types are the third most common group of malignancies in children, following leukemia and brain tumors (see Figure 29–1). Non-Hodgkin lymphomas are malignant tumors of lymphoreticular (internal framework of the lymph system) origin. The peak incidence for lymphomas occurs between the ages of 7 and 11 years, and is 3 times more common in boys than in girls.

Etiology and Pathophysiology

Lymphoblastic non-Hodgkin lymphomas are caused by T-cell abnormalities. These abnormal T cells are diffuse, highly malignant and aggressive, and do not mature. T-cell lymphomas produced by these cells often occur in children with congenital or acquired immunodeficiency states, chronic immune stimulation, or autoimmune disease. Some lymphomas have B-cell abnormalities, most specifically Burkitt's lymphoma; 8q24 chromosomal translocation may be found in these cases. Large cell lymphomas are variable in cell type affected and may also manifest chromosomal translocations (Hussong, 2002).

The incidence of lymphomas shows geographic variability. For example, a high incidence of Burkitt's lymphoma is found in equatorial Africa, where it causes 50% of childhood cancer. Incidence in Hispanic children is higher than in Whites, and Blacks have the lowest incidence (Wilkinson, Fleming, MacKinnon, et al., 2001). Males are affected more than females and children with immune system compromise are most commonly affected. Epstein-Barr virus has been associated with Burkitt's lymphoma (Hussong, 2002).

Clinical Manifestations

Children with non-Hodgkin lymphoma present with fever, weight loss, and night sweats less often than those with Hodgkin disease. The lymph glands are usually enlarged or nodular, with the most frequent sites being the cervical, axillary, inguinal, and femoral nodes. However, the disease may be diffuse, without nodular glands. The anterior mediastinum is the primary site for T-cell lymphomas. Tumors that occur in this area may compress the airway (causing breathing difficulty) or superior vena cava (leading to swelling of the face, neck, or arms), and can cause pain. Jaw involvement is common in Burkitt's lymphoma. An abdominal mass may cause pain, nausea, and vomiting.

COLLABORATIVE CARE

Comprehensive care to treat the illness and prevent complications are goals of collaborative care.

Diagnostic Tests

The symptoms of lymphoma are often nonspecific and treatments may already have been tried with antibiotics, if a mass is thought to be an infection, or other medication. A careful history will help determine the progression and possible location of disease. CBC is performed; additional blood tests include renal and liver function, electrolytes, uric acid, and LDH. Bone marrow aspiration and lumbar puncture are performed. Chest radiograph, bone scan, gallium scan, CT, and MRI can help to isolate affected body organs. Diagnosis is confirmed by tissue biopsy.

Clinical Therapy

A staging system is used to describe the tumor mass and extension to other body areas (Table 29–9). Treatment is tailored to the type of cancer and its stage. Stages I and II may be treated with drugs such as vincristine, cyclophosphamide, prednisone, and methotrexate for several months. Intrathecal medication is added if head and neck cancers are present. Stages III and IV are treated with additional drugs (up to nine total) for longer periods of time (1 to 2 years). Radiation is uncommonly used and may be helpful to treat a tumor that is impinging on a body part. Surgery is used to biopsy the tumor mass and treat any complications caused by the cancer. HSCT is used for children with recurrent disease.

TABLE 29–9 St. Jude Children's Research Hospital Staging Classification for Non-Hodgkin Lymphoma

STAGE	DESCRIPTION
I	Single tumor or node area involved; no tumor in abdomen or mediastinum
II	Single tumor with lymph node involvement; or two node areas or tumor on same side of diagphragm; or GI tumor in one site
III	Two tumors or node areas on different sides of diaphragm; or a primary mediastinal, intraabdominal, or epidural tumor
IV	Any involvement with CNS or bone marrow metastases

Adapted from Hussong, M. R. Non-Hodgkin's lymphoma. In C. R. Baggott, K. P. Kelly, D. Fochtman, & G. V. Foley, Nursing care of children and adolescents with cancer *(2002) (3rd ed., p. 539). Philadelphia: WB Saunders.*

Rhabdomyosarcoma

Rhabdomyosarcoma is a soft tissue cancer that is common in children. It occurs most often in the muscles around the eyes (extraorbital), in the neck, and less commonly in the abdomen, genitourinary tract, and the extremities. Genitourinary, bladder, and prostate cancers are more common in children under 5 years, while paratesticular and extremity cancer is more common among adolescents. Rhabdomyosarcoma occurs more often in Whites than in Blacks or Asians; it usually occurs in children under 5 years of age (Kotsubo, 2002). However, it is uncommon in newborns and if it presents in this age group, abdominal or pelvic sites are most common.

Etiology and Pathophysiology

The cause of rhabdomyosarcoma is unknown. It is more common in children with neurofibromatosis and Li-Fraumeni syndrome. Mutations in a tumor suppressor gene p53 are sometimes seen. Mothers of children with rhabdomyosarcoma are more likely to develop early breast cancer than other women (Ruymann & Grovas, 2000). The abnormal cells arise from mesenchyme which normally grows into muscle, fat, and bone (Kotsubo, 2002).

Clinical Manifestations

Tumors occurring close to the eye produce swelling, ptosis, visual disturbances, and eye movement abnormalities (Figure 29–16 ■). When the tumor occurs in the genitourinary tract, the result can be urinary obstruction, hematuria, dysuria, vaginal discharge, and a protruding vaginal mass. Rhabdomyosarcoma occurring in the abdomen may be asymptomatic. There is rapid metastasis to the lungs, bones, bone marrow, and distant lymph nodes.

COLLABORATIVE CARE

Soft tissue tumors that occur in young children require astute observations for early diagnosis. Providers then partner with parents to ensure both treatment and fostering of the young child's development.

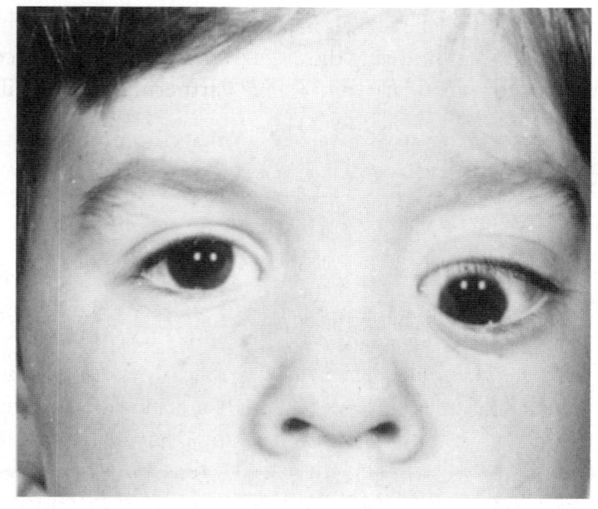

FIGURE 29–16 ■ Rhabdomyosarcoma is characterized by ptosis and swelling.
From Vaughn, D., Asbury, T., & Riordan-Eva, P. (1995). General opthalmology *(14th ed.). Norwalk, CT: Appleton & Lange.*

Diagnostic Tests

Diagnosis of the nonpainful mass is confirmed by CT, MRI, PET, bone marrow aspiration, and biopsy. CBC, renal and liver studies, and urinalysis are performed. Lumbar puncture may be used in head and neck tumors. A useful biologic marker, Desmin, allows differentiation of rhabdomyosarcoma from other round cell tumors. Because 20% of children have metastatic disease at the time of diagnosis, chest and lung CT scans are performed.

Clinical Therapy

Treatment includes surgical removal of the tumor when possible. However, if the tumor involves other structures removal may not be possible. Many children have metastasis at time of diagnosis so the primary tumor is removed. Surgery is followed by wide-field radiation and chemotherapy with a combination of drugs. Common drugs include:

- Vincristine
- Actinomycin
- Cyclophosphamide
  (VAC therapy)

Prognosis depends on the site, staging (Table 29–10), and histologic findings, with about 70% of children now surviving (Kotsubo, 2002).

Retinoblastoma

Retinoblastoma is an intraocular malignancy of the retina. It may be bilateral (20% to 30%) or unilateral. In 40% of children, the disease is inherited by an autosomal dominant gene (Dulczak & Frothingham, 2002). Family history is therefore important to collect, although many cases occur with no family history of the cancer.

Etiology and Pathophysiology

The tumor arises from embryonic retinal cells. It may be a new mutation or may be passed on to offspring of affected individuals. The retinoblastoma gene, RB1, is on chromosome 13q.

Clinical Manifestations

The first sign of retinoblastoma is a white pupil, termed leukokoria or cat's-eye reflex (Figure 29–17 ■). The red reflex is absent, asymmetrical, or of a differing color in the affected eye. Other symptoms may include a fixed strabismus (a constant de-

TABLE 29–10 Classification of Rhabdomyosarcoma

GROUP	DESCRIPTION
I	Localized, completely resected disease
II	Total gross resection with regional microscopic spread
III	Incomplete gross resection of biopsy
IV	Distant metastatic disease present

Note: From Wexler, L. H., & Helman, L. J. (1997). Rhabdomyosarcoma and the undifferentiated sarcomas. In P. A. Pizzo & D. G. Poplack (Eds.), Principles and practices of pediatric oncology *(3rd ed., p. 808). Philadelphia: Lippincott-Raven.*

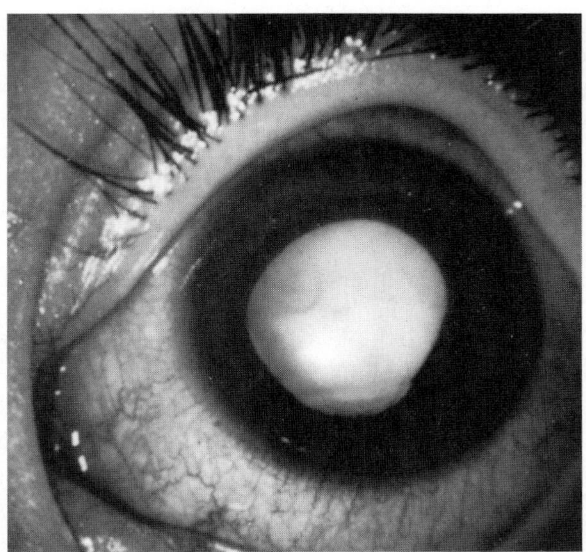

FIGURE 29–17 ■ Retinoblastoma is characterized by leukocoria, a white reflection in the pupil.

From Hathaway, W. E., Hay, W. W., Jr., Groothuis, J. R., & Paisley, J. W. (1993). Current pediatric diagnosis and treatment *(11th ed.). Norwalk, CT: Appleton & Lange.*

viation of one eye from the other), orbital inflammation, glaucoma, and heterochromia (irises of different colors).

Retinoblastoma is usually diagnosed when the child is between 1 and 2 years of age. A family history should alert healthcare providers so that regular ophthalmologic examinations can be performed frequently on infants and young children in the family. The appearance of a unilateral tumor demands regular examinations of the healthy eye since bilateral disease can develop. In some children a pineal gland tumor can also develop, causing central nervous system symptoms. The overall tumor-free survival rate is 90%, 5 to 10 years after diagnosis.

COLLABORATIVE CARE

Families work with healthcare professionals to identify and treat the disease, as well as support the child after treatment.

Diagnostic Tests

Children at risk for retinoblastoma due to family history can be tested for the RB1 gene. Diagnostic tests for the cancer include full ocular examination and CT or MRI scans of the eye orbit. All children with a history of retinoblastoma in the family should be examined by an ophthalmologist after birth, at 6 weeks, every 2 to 3 months until 2 years, then every 4 months until 3 years, and then annually (Dulczak & Frothingham, 2002; Pakakasama & Tomlinson, 2002) to aid in early diagnosis. Tumors are classified according to a staging system, from a very small, localized tumor (group I) to tumors involving more than half the retina and with seeding into the vitreous (group V).

Clinical Therapy

Treatment for retinblastoma may include removal of the eye (enucleation) when there is permanent retinal damage or failure to respond to other treatment. Other surgical treatments involve cryotherapy or photocoagulation (argon laser therapy). Radiation is nearly always used, either as the sole treatment or before surgery to shrink the tumor. Chemotherapy is sometimes used but is often ineffective as the drugs often fail to penetrate sufficiently into the eye. Chemotherapy drugs include carboplatin, etoposide, vincristine, and cyclosporine. Multiple therapies are more commonly used in children with bilateral retinoblastoma. Children with retinoblastoma are at increased risk of developing a secondary tumor, including another retinoblastoma or a sarcoma, most commonly osteogenic sarcoma. However, most young children who have been treated for the disease have good health and normal mental abilities several years after treatment. The most common sequella of retinoblastoma is decrease in visual acuity (Ross, Lipper, Abramson, et al., 2001).

PARTNERING WITH FAMILIES

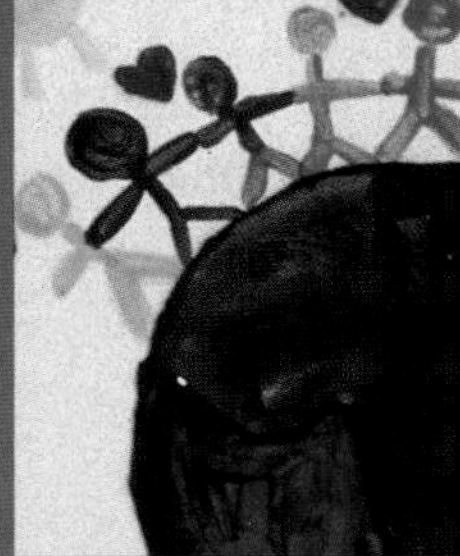

Care of the Child with a Soft Tissue Tumor

- ➤ Teach the family about the chemotherapy drugs and their side effects.
- ➤ Teach about the care of surgically placed venous access devices.
- ➤ Provide written and illustrated information about the chemotherapy protocol(s).
- ➤ Provide the family with radiation and surgery education specific to the tumor treatment.
- ➤ Refer the family to nutrition resources such as dietitians for ways to promote the child's adequate intake of food and fluid.

NURSING MANAGEMENT

Nursing management of the child with a soft tissue tumor involves supporting the child and family through the treatment for disease, and monitoring the child over time for recurrence of primary or for secondary tumor. (See Partnering with Families: The Child with a Soft Tissue Tumor.)

■ Nursing Assessment and Diagnosis

Physiologic Assessment

Careful family histories can sometimes identify children at risk who need frequent physical examinations. For example, if a family history of retinoblastoma is present, the child should receive frequent eye examinations. Physiologic assessment of the child with a soft tissue tumor, such as Hodgkin disease, non-Hodgkin lymphoma, rhabdomyosarcoma, and retinoblastoma, focuses on the child's general condition. Accurate height and weight measurements are essential to provide a baseline against which to measure the child's growth during treatment, as well as for calculation of chemotherapeutic drug dosages.

Observe the area of the tumor, such as the face, neck, and abdomen, and describe any changes. Monitor respiratory status if the tumor is on the face or neck. Report any changes in respiratory pattern to the physician. Avoid palpation of any tumor site or enlarged area; metastasis can be influenced by injudicious palpation and manipulation of a tumor site. Notify the physician of a change in any lymph node or any other area of the body.

Gastrointestinal and genitourinary function can be altered by the presence of a tumor and by treatment such as chemotherapy and radiation. Careful monitoring of the child's intake and output measurement is essential. Abdominal and pelvic tumors may affect defecation, so charting of all bowel movements is important. Explain to the family and child why keeping accurate records is necessary.

Observe wounds closely for lack of healing as a result of chemotherapy or radiation. Examine the mouth and extremities for wounds or ulcers. Nutritional changes caused by treatment will affect the body's ability to support healthy cells and heal wounds.

A thorough eye examination is warranted for any child who has a family history of retinoblastoma or has undergone treatment for a prior tumor. Assess color and position of the iris, eye movements, cover–uncover test, and other eye tests are described in Chapter 8. Be sure that the child has recommended evaluations by an ophthalmologist.

Psychosocial Assessment

Assessment of the family's psychosocial status and coping mechanisms is an essential component of nursing care. Refer to the general discussion of psychosocial assessment on page 1051. Assessment of body image is needed when the child has a soft tissue tumor affecting appearance of the head and neck. Even after treatment is successfully completed, lasting mental health changes can be apparent. Survivors of childhood lymphoma more commonly report depression and somatic distress (symptoms such as pain in the heart or chest, dizziness, weakness) than other individuals (Zebrack, Zeltzer, Whitton, et al., 2002). Ask about symptoms of depression such as loneliness, lack of interest, anxiety, suicidal thoughts.

The location and type of soft tissue tumor determine the specific nursing diagnoses for a particular child. Common nursing diagnoses may include the following:

- Impaired Tissue Perfusion (peripheral) related to interruption of blood flow
- Ineffective Breathing Pattern related to effect of tumor deformity on neck or chest wall
- Impaired Swallowing related to acquired anatomic defect
- Delayed Growth and Development related to effects of treatment
- Disturbed Body Image related to illness and treatment
- Disturbed Sensory Perception (visual) related to illness

■ Planning and Implementation

Nursing management of children with soft tissue tumors varies depending on the specific tumor. Children with lymphoma affecting the mediastinum may need respiratory support. Position the child so that the head is elevated. Administer chemotherapy drugs as ordered, maintaining adequate fluids to facilitate excretion of the resultant breakdown products. Monitor the central line used for chemotherapy administration, and teach parents care of the central line when the child is at home.

For the child with a rhabdomyosarcoma involving the bladder, monitor urinary output carefully. Report hematuria and painful urination. Monitor the changes that occur during therapy. For example, in children with eye tumors, observe for a decrease in ptosis, which may indicate successful treatment. Administer pain medications as needed and use distraction and other techniques to decrease the child's discomfort. Emphasize to parents the need for follow-up CT and MRI scans after completion of treatment.

When the child with retinoblastoma undergoes removal of the eye, the parents and child will need detailed instructions on postsurgical care. Demonstrate to the parents care of the socket and use of a conformer to maintain the eye socket shape. When healing is complete and the child receives a prosthetic eye, instruct parents about its insertion and care. The child can gradually be taught to take over this care when old enough. Encourage periodic healthcare visits to monitor for signs of a tumor in the other eye. It may be necessary to adapt developmental interventions to accommodate for sensory alterations. Attention is directed at the body changes of the cancer and its treatment. Children and adolescents may need suggestions to deal with hair loss, disfigurement, and living with serious illness. Referral to other children and teens with similar concerns may be helpful. Parents of all children need help to encourage normal development in the child with cancer.

The child with a soft tissue tumor often receives chemotherapy or radiation, or sometimes both modalities. Nursing management during chemotherapy and radiation is discussed earlier in this chapter in the general sections on these treatment measures (see pages 1054–1064) and in the Nursing Care Plan for Hospital Care of the Child with Cancer. Generally, the family will need help to adjust to the diagnosis of a life-threatening disease and to the care of the ill child. Refer to Chapter 17 for a description of postsurgical care. Consult Chapter 24 for strategies to assist the child and family if the child has a visual impairment resulting from a retinoblastoma. Topics for parent and family teaching and discharge planning are similar to those previously presented. Referral resources to support the families of children with these types of cancer can be found at our Companion Website.

Care in the Community

Reinforce with families the importance of long-term follow-up after treatment for a soft tissue tumor. Increased risk for secondary cancers for 20 to 30 years is possible, and early identification can help with prompt diagnosis (Metayer, Lynch, Clarke, et al., 2000). Partner with other healthcare providers to provide instructions to families as the child transitions from oncology treatment back to the pediatrician so they understand the importance of telling all care providers about the cancer and treatment. Establish oncology clinics to track and examine survivors. As children grow into teen and young adult years, help them to take over this important task in their care. Recommended annual examinations include:

- CBC
- Physical examination with special attention to skin, abdomen, and thyroid
- Monitoring for signs of hypo- and hyperthyroidism
- Neurological and developmental examinations; monitoring of school performance
- First mammogram at 25 years in those with chest radiation
- Pap and pelvic exams for teen and young adult women
- Mental status assessment

(Smith, 2003)

Evaluation

The following expected outcomes of nursing care for the child with a soft tissue tumor are examples that illustrate the varied tumor presentations.

- Successful management of treatment side effects
- Healed surgical site with no signs of infection
- Adaptation to sensory loss
- Adaptation to altered self-image
- Growth and development to maximum potential
- Anticipatory grieving by parents in cases of terminal disease

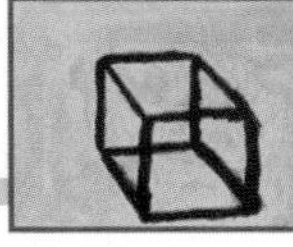

CHAPTER HIGHLIGHTS

- Cancer is a leading cause of illness and death among children.
- Cancer may be influenced by chromosomal or genetic messages, environmental carcinogens, or infectious processes. Often a combination of factors seems to be present.
- Cancer treatments include surgery, chemotherapy, radiation, biotherapy, and alternative therapies. Palliative care is needed when disease has relapsed and cure is no longer possible.
- Oncologic emergencies are life-threatening conditions caused by cancer or its treatment.
- Main types of oncologic emergencies are metabolic, hematologic, or space occupying.
- Key signs of childhood cancer are pain, cachexia, anemia, infection, bruising, and neurological symptoms.
- A protocol is a plan of action for chemotherapy that is based on the type of cancer, its stage, and the particular cell type.
- Nursing assessment for children with cancer involves detailed physical data, as well as psychological factors and developmental achievements.
- Common physical nursing interventions for children with cancer involve nutrition, medication adminstration, hydration, infection prevention, pain management, and measures to decrease side effects of treatment. Families require ongoing psychosocial support, information, and referral to diverse resources when caring for a child with cancer.
- While the number of children who are long-term survivors continues to grow, it is known that some of these children experience lasting effects such as cognitive or behavioral problems, recurrent or secondary cancers, or discrimination.
- Nursing care after cancer treatment is completed includes monitoring for any long-term physiological or psychosocial sequelae.
- Common brain tumors in children include medulloblastoma, astrocytoma, ependymoma, and gliomas.
- Headache, vomiting, ataxia, seizures, increased intracranial pressure, hydrocephalus, and sensory disturbances are the major clinical manifestations of brain tumors.
- Neuroblastoma is a tumor that is located along the sympathetic nervous system chain.
- Nephroblastoma (Wilms' tumor) is an intrarenal tumor; when suspected, the abdomen should not be palpated.
- Common bone tumors in childhood are osteosarcoma and Ewing's sarcoma; both are most common among adolescents.
- Leukemia is a common childhood malignancy, with the major types being acute lymphoblastic leukemia (ALL) and acute nonlymphocytic leukemia (ANLL).
- A variety of soft tissue tumors are seen in children and adolescents; they include Hodgkin disease, non-Hodgkin lymphoma, rhabdomyosarcoma, and retinoblastoma.
- Nurses are in a key position to assist families during a diagnosis for cancer, while therapy is carried out, in adjustment to school and other life tasks, and in providing palliative care for children who do not survive.

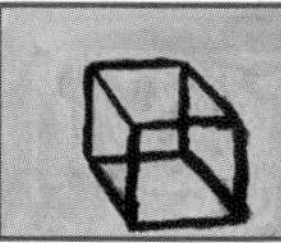

CRITICAL THINKING IN ACTION

INTRODUCTION

Recall 12-year-old Rasheed who is described at the chapter beginning. He has been admitted for treatment of enterocolitis secondary to his diagnosis of ALL. His parents are concerned about his illness, and his mother is upset that she cannot stay with him all the time in the hospital because of her job responsibilities. Rasheed was admitted with severe vomiting and diarrhea and was moderately dehydrated. He has been managed well with medications and intravenous infusions and is beginning to take fluids and food by mouth. His vital signs are temperature 100.6°F, pulse 100, respirations 22, blood pressure 104/56.

DESCRIPTION

The nurse learns that Rasheed's father had recently left the family, but has returned now that Rasheed is ill. While Rasheed is happy about this, his mother finds the situation stressful at times. Rasheed's parents have been taking turns bringing him to the oncology clinic for treatments. His blood values have improved and the oncologist is hopeful that he will recover. Rasheed's 7-year-old sister, Shanna, has not been to the hospital to visit, since the family lives about 70 miles away. The mother has told her only that Rasheed needs special care for a while because he is ill. Shanna's behavior at school was recently disruptive in the classroom and her mother is concerned that she cannot manage all of these problems. Rasheed is feeling better than he was upon admission, and is ready to get back to school. He is concerned about missing any more field trips or other activities.

DISCUSSION

1. Rasheed's family provides both stress and support for him as he goes through cancer treatment. List the risk factors in the family as well as the protective factors, or strengths.
2. Based on the risk and protective factors identified, list two or three nursing diagnoses related to the family. What nursing interventions will assist in dealing with these diagnoses? What is the highest priority nursing diagnosis? Why?
3. Rasheed seems very interested in his relationships at school. What psychosocial developmental stage is he in, according to Erikson? How will you integrate this knowledge into his plan of care?
4. Why was Rasheed anemic and manifesting bruises when he was first diagnosed? Describe what you would expect the laboratory values for RBC, WBC, hematocrit, hemoglobin, and platelets to be for Rasheed and why? See Appendix C∞ and Box 29–4.
5. Consider the ages of Rasheed and his sister, Shanna. Describe the cognitive level for each, according to Piaget. Based on that knowledge, construct two different teaching plans to teach important facts about leukemia to Rasheed and Shanna. How will the plans differ because of their cognitive abilities? What teaching aides will be most appropriate for each age?

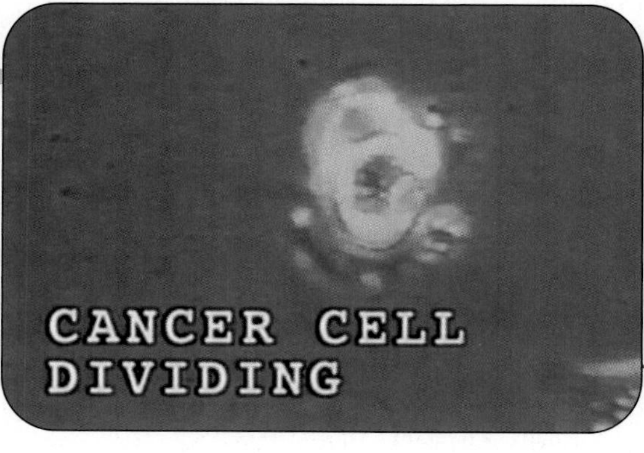

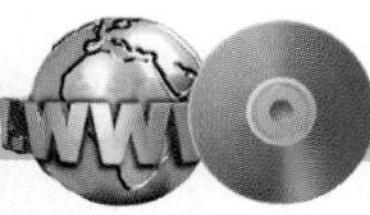

EXPLORE MediaLink

- NCLEX review, case studies, and other interactive resources for this chapter can be found on the Companion Website at **www.prenhall.com/ball**. Click on Chapter 29 to select the activities for this chapter.
- For animations, more NCLEX review questions, and an audio glossary, access the accompanying CD-ROM in this book.

http://www.prenhall.com/ball

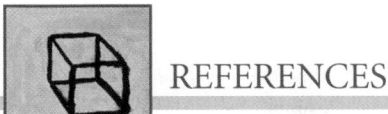

REFERENCES

Agency for Healthcare Research and Quality. (2001a). *Uses of epoetin for anemia in oncology.* Washington, DC: U.S. Department of Health and Human Services (Evidence Report/Technology Assessment No. 30).

Agency for Healthcare Research and Quality. (2001b). *Management of cancer pain.* Washington, DC: U.S. Department of Health and Human Services (Evidence Report/Technology Assessment No. 35).

Alcoser, P. W., & Burchett, S. (1999). Bone marrow transplantation. *American Journal of Nursing, 99,* 26–31.

Alcoser, P. W., & Rogers, C. (2003). Treatment strategies in childhood cancer. *Journal of Pediatric Nursing, 18,* 103–112.

American Cancer Society. (2003). National Action Plan for Childhood Cancer. www.cancer.org, accessed 2/16/2004.

American Cancer Society. (2004). Statistics. www.cancer.org.

Arceci, R. J., & Cripe, T. P. (2002). Emerging cancer-targeted therapies. *Pediatric Clinics of North America, 49,* 1339–1368.

Askin, D. F. (2000). Neonatal cancer: A clinical perspective. *Journal of Obstetrics and Gynecologic Nursing, 29,* 423–431.

Baggott, C. R., Kelly, K. P., Fochtman, D., & Foley, G. V. (2002). *Nursing care of children and adolescents with cancer* (3rd ed.). Philadelphia: WB Saunders.

Betcher, D. L., Simon, P. J., & McHard, K. M. (2002). Bone tumors. In C. R. Baggott, K. P. Kelly, & D. Fochtman, *Nursing care of children and adolescents with cancer* (3rd ed., pp. 575–588). Philadelphia: WB Saunders.

Biggar, R. J., Frisch, M., & Goedert, J. J. (2000). Risk of cancer in children with AIDS. *Journal of the American Medical Association, 284,* 205–209.

Bindler, R. M., & Howry, L. B. (2005). *Pediatric drug guide.* Upper Saddle River, NJ: Prentice Hall Health.

Bleyer, A. (2004). Principles of diagnosis; Principles of treatment. In R. E. Behrman, R. M. Kliegman, & H. B. Jenson, *Nelson textbook of pediatrics* (17th ed., pp. 1684–1693). Philadelphia: WB Saunders.

Bryant, R. (2003). Managing side effects of childhood cancer treatment. *Journal of Pediatric Nursing, 18,* 113–125.

Castellino, S., & Hudson, M. M. (2002). Health issues in survivors of childhood cancer. *Southern Medical Journal, 95,* 977–984.

Castleberry, R. P. (1997). Biology and treatment of neuroblastoma. *Pediatric Clinics of North America, 44,* 919–938.

Cavusoglu, H. (2001). Depression in children with cancer. *Journal of Pediatric Nursing, 16,* 380–385.

Chaffee, S. (2001). Pediatric palliative care. *Primary Care, 28,* 365–370.

Challinor, J., Miaskowski, C., Moore, I., Slaughter, R., & Franck, L. (2000). Review of research studies that evaluated the impact of treatment for childhood cancers on neurorecognition and behavioral and social competence: Nursing implications. *Journal for Specialists in Pediatric Nursing, 5,* 57–74.

Chase, S. (2000). St. John's wort: Not so safe. *RN, 63,* 114.

Chin, E. A. (1998, November/December). A brief overview of the oral complications in pediatric oncology patients and suggested management strategies. *Journal of Dentistry for Children,* 468–473.

Christensen, J., & Fatchett, D. (2002). Promoting parental use of distraction and relaxation in pediatric oncology patients during invasive procedures. *Journal of Pediatric Oncology Nursing, 19,* 127–132.

Conway, E. E., Asuncion, A., & DaRosso, R. (1999). Diagnosing and managing brain tumors: The pediatrician's role. *Contemporary Pediatrics, 16,* 84–97.

Coustan-Smith, E., Sancho, J., Hancock, M. L., Boyett, J. M., Behm, F. G., Raimondi, S. C., Sandlund, J. T., Rivera, G. K., Rubnitz, J. E., Ribeiro, R. C., Piu, C. H., & Campana, D. (2000). Clinical importance of minimal residual disease in childhood acute lymphoblastic leukemia. *Blood, 96,* 2691–2696.

Dadd, G. (2002). Neuroblastoma. In C. R. Baggott, K. P. Kelly, D. Fochtman, & G. V. Foley. *Nursing care of children and adolescents with cancer* (3rd ed., pp. 545–554). Philadelphia: WB Saunders.

Davies, B., Whitsett, S. F., Bruce, A., & McCarthy, P. (2002). A typology of fatigue in children with cancer. *Journal of Pediatric Oncology Nursing, 19,* 12–21.

Dean, R. (2000, September). Alternative therapies may cause interactions in oncology patients. American College of Clinical Pharmacology meeting. Reported by Reuters. http://pediatrics.medscape.com/reuters/prof/2000/09/09.19/2000091prof003.html, accessed 9/25/2000.

Derengowski, S. (1999, June 14). Pediatric non-Hodgkin's lymphoma. *Advance for Nurses,* 26–28.

Donaldson, S. S., Egbert, P. R., Newsham, I., & Cavenee, W. K. (1997). Retinoblastoma. In P. A. Pizzo & D. G. Poplack (Eds.), *Principles and practice of pediatric oncology* (3rd ed., pp. 699–716). Philadelphia: Lippincott-Raven.

Drigan, R., & Androkites, A. L. (2002). Wilms tumor. In C. R. Baggott, K. P. Kelly, D. Fochtman, & G. V. Foley. *Nursing care of children and adolescents with cancer* (3rd ed., pp. 568–574). Philadelphia: WB Saunders.

Dulczak, S., & Frothingham, B. (2002). Retinoblastoma. In C. R. Baggott, K. P. Kelly, D. Fochtman, & G. V. Foley. *Nursing care of children and adolescents with cancer* (3rd ed., pp. 589–597). Philadelphia: WB Saunders.

Field, T., Cullen, C., Diego, M., Hernandez-Feir, M., Sprinz, P., Beebe, K., Kissell, B., & Bango-Sanchez, V. (2001). Leukemia immune changes following massage therapy. *Journal of Bodywork and Movement Therapies, 5,* 271–274.

Freeman, K., O'Dell, C., & Meola, C. (2000). Issues in families of children with brain tumors. *Oncology Nursing Forum, 27,* 843–848.

Freeman, K., O'Dell, C., & Meola, C. (2003). Childhood brain tumors: Children's and siblings' concerns regarding the diagnosis and phase of illness. *Journal of Pediatric Oncology Nursing, 20,* 133–140.

French, A. E., Grant, R., Weitzman, S., Ray, J. G., Vermeulen, M. J., Sung, L., Greenberg, M., & Koren, G. (2003). Folic acid food fortification is associated with a decline in neuroblastoma. *Clinical Pharmacology Therapy, 74,* 288–294.

Gibson, F., & Nelson, W. (2000). Mouth care for children with cancer. *Paediatric Nursing, 12,* 18–22.

Gilger, E. A., Groben, V. J., & Hinds, P. S. (2002). Osteosarcoma nursing care guidelines: A tool to enhance the nursing care of children and adolescents enrolled on a medical research protocol. *Journal of Pediatric Oncology Nursing, 19,* 172–181.

Green, D. M., Grigoriev, Y. A., Nan, B., Takashima, J. R., Norkool, P. A., D'Angio, G. J., & Breslow, N. E. (2001). Congestive heart failure after treatment for Wilms' tumor: A report from the National Wilms' Tumor study group. *Journal of Clinical Oncology, 19,* 1926–1934.

Han-Markey, T. (2000). Nutritional considerations in pediatric oncology. *Seminars in Oncology Nursing, 16,* 146–151.

Hendricks-Ferguson, V. L. (2000). Crisis intervention strategies when caring for families of children with cancer. *Journal of Pediatric Oncology Nursing, 17,* 3–11.

Hilden, J. M., Emanuel, E. J., Fairclough, D. L., Link, M. P., Foley, K. M., Clarridge, B. C., Schnipper, L. E., & Mayer, R. J. (2001). Attitudes and practices among pediatric oncologists regarding end-of-life care: Results of the 1998 American Society of Clinical Oncology Survey. *Journal of Clinical Oncology, 19,* 205–212.

Hill, D., & Hart, K. (2001). A practical approach to nutritional support for patients with advanced cancer. *International Journal of Palliative Nursing, 7,* 317–321.

Hobbie, W. L., & Ogle, S. (2001). Transitional care for young adult survivors of childhood cancer. *Seminars in Oncology Nursing, 17,* 268–273.

Hussong, M. R. (2002). Non-Hodgkin's lymphoma. In C. R. Baggott, K. P. Kelly, D. Fochtman, & G. V. Foley, *Nursing care of children and adolescents with cancer* (3rd ed., pp. 536–544). Philadelphia: WB Saunders.

Ishibashi, A. (2001). The needs of children and adolescents with cancer for information and social support. *Cancer Nursing, 24,* 61–67.

Jaffe, N. & Huff, V. (2004). Neoplasms of the kidney. In R. E. Behrman, R. M. Kliegman, & H. B. Jenson (Eds.), *Nelson textbook of pediatrics* (17th ed., pp. 1711–1714). Philadelphia: WB Saunders.

James, K., Keegan-Wells, D., Hinds, P. S., Kelly, K. P., Bond, D., Hall, B., Mahan, R., Moore, I. M., Roll, L., & Speckhart, B. (2002). The care of my child with cancer: Parents' perceptions of caregiving demands. *Journal of Pediatric Oncology Nursing, 19,* 218–228.

Kelly, K. M., Jacobsen, J. S., Kennedy, D. D., Braudt, S. M., Mallick, M., & Weiner, M. A. (2000). Use of unconventional therapies by children at an urban medical center. *Journal of Pediatric Hematology/Oncology, 22,* 412–416.

Kemper, K. J., & Longwood Herbal Task Force. (1999). Shark cartilage, cat's claw, and other complementary cancer therapies. *Contemporary Pediatrics, 16,* 101–102, 105–106, 112, 115, 117–118, 121, 125–126.

Kinlen, L. J., & Balkwill, A. (2001). Infective cause of childhood leukemia and wartime population mixing in Orkney and Shetland, UK. *Lancet, 357*, 858.

Kleinhaus, S., & Boley, S. J. (1999). The latest news about minimally invasive surgery. *Contemporary Pediatrics, 16*, 125–134.

Kline, N. E., & Sevier, N. (2003). Solid tumors in children. *Journal of Pediatric Nursing, 18*, 96–102.

Kotsubo, C. Z. (2002). Rhabdomyosarcoma. In C. R. Baggott, K. P. Kelly, D. Fochtman, & G. V. Foley, *Nursing care of children and adolescents with cancer* (3rd ed., pp. 555–567). Philadelphia: WB Saunders.

Landier, W. (2001). Childhood acute lymphoblastic leukemia: Current perspectives. *Oncology Nursing Forum, 28*, 823–833.

Landier, W. (2002). Myeloid diseases. In C. R. Baggott, K. P. Kelly, D. Fochtman, & G. V. Foley, *Nursing care of children and adolescents with cancer* (3rd ed., pp. 491–502). Philadelphia: WB Saunders.

Lehman, R. A., Krishnamurthy, S., & Berlin, C. M. (2002). Weight and height deficits in children with brain stem tumors. *Clinical Pediatrics, 41*, 315–321.

Leonard, M. (2002). Diagnostic evaluations and staging procedures. In C. R. Baggott, K. P. Kelly, D. Fochtman, & G. V. Foley, *Nursing care of children and adolescents with cancer* (3rd ed., pp. 66–89). Philadelphia: WB Saunders.

Liossi, C. (2000). Clinical hypnosis in paediatric oncology: A critical review of the literature. *Sleep and Hypnosis, 5*, 268–274.

MacDonald, D. J., & Lessick, M. (2000). Hereditary cancers in children and ethical and psychosocial implications. *Journal of Pediatric Nursing, 15*, 217–225.

McLorie, G. A. (2001). Wilms' tumor (nephroblastoma). *Current Opinion in Urology, 11*, 567–570.

McManus, J., & Gilchrist, G. S. (2000). Neuroblastoma. In R. E. Behrman, R. M. Kliegman, & H. B. Jenson (Eds.), *Nelson textbook of pediatrics* (16th ed., pp. 1552–1554). Philadelphia: WB Saunders.

Metayer, C., Lynch, C. F., Clarke, E. A., Glimelius, B., Storm, H., Pukkala, E., Joensuu, T., van Leeuwen, F. E., et al. (2000). Second cancers among long-term survivors of Hodgkin's disease diagnosed in childhood and adolescence. *Journal of Clinical Oncology, 18*, 2435–2443.

Moller, T. R., Garwicz, S., Barlow, L., Falck Winther, J., Glattre, E., Olafsdotti, G., Olsen, J. H., Perfekt, R., Ritvanen, A., Sankila, R., & Tulinius, H. (2001). Decreasing late mortality among five-year survivors of cancer in childhood and adolescence: A population-based study in the Nordic countries. *Journal of Clinical Oncology, 19*, 3161–3181.

Murray, J. S. (2002). A qualitative exploration of psychosocial support for siblings of children with cancer. *Journal of Pediatric Nursing, 17*, 327–337.

Pakakasama, S., & Tomlinson, G. E. (2002). Genetic predisposition and screening in pediatric cancer. *Pediatric Clinics of North America, 49*, 1393–1413.

Pritchard-Jones, K. (2002). Controversies and advances in the management of Wilms' tumor. *Archives of Disease in Childhood, 87*, 241–244.

Recklitis, C., O'Leary, T., & Diller, L. (2003). Utility of routine psychological screening in the childhood cancer survivor clinic. *Journal of Clinical Oncology, 231*, 787–792.

Reiss, U., & Bolotin, E. (2002). New approaches to hematopoietic cell transplantation in oncology. *Pediatric Clinics of North America, 49*, 1437–1466.

Reynolds, P., Von Behren, J., & Elkin, E. P. (2002). Birth characteristics and leukemia in young children. *American Journal of Epidemiology, 155*, 603–613.

Ross, G., Lipper, E. G., Abramson, D., & Preiser, L. (2001). The development of young children with retinoblastoma. *Archives of Pediatric and Adolescent Medicine, 155*, 80–83.

Ruymann, F. B., & Grovas, A. C. (2000). Progress in the diagnosis and treatment of rhabdomyosarcomas and related soft tissue sarcomas. *Cancer Investigation, 18*, 223–241.

Ryan-Murray, J., & Petriccione, M. M. (2002). Central nervous system tumors. In C. R. Baggott, K. P. Kelly, D. Fochtman, & G. V. Foley, *Nursing care of children and adolescents with cancer* (3rd ed., pp. 503–523). Philadelphia: WB Saunders.

Schwartz, C. L. (2003). The management of Hodgkin disease in the young child. *Current Opinions in Pediatrics, 15*, 10–16.

Scott, C. M., Britt, R. B., Juneau, C., & McKracken, K. (2001). Wilms' tumor: A primary care case study and differential diagnosis. *Internet Journal of Advanced Nursing, 5*. www.ispub.com, accessed 1/20/2004.

Scott, J. T., Entwistle, V. A., Sowden, A. J., & Watt, I. (2003). Communicating with children and adolescents about their cancer. *Cochrane Library Issue, 2*. Oxford: Update Software.

Smith, P. C. K. (2002). The role of the primary care advanced practice nurse in evaluating and monitoring childhood cancer survivors for a second malignant neoplasm. *Journal of Pediatric Oncology Nursing, 19*, 84–96.

Swerdlow, J. L. (2000). *Nature's medicine: Plants that heal.* Washington, DC: National Geographic Society.

Thompson, K. A. (1999). Detecting Hodgkin's disease. *American Journal of Nursing, 99*, 61–64.

U.S. Department of Labor. (2003). *OSHA technical manual.* www.osha.gov, accessed 2/19/2004.

Westlake, S. K., & Bertolone, K. L. (2002). Acute lymphoblastic leukemia. In C. R. Baggott, K. P. Kelly, D. Fochtman, & G. V. Foley, *Nursing care of children and adolescents with cancer* (3rd ed., pp. 466–490). Philadelphia: WB Saunders.

Wilkinson, J. D., Fleming, L. E., MacKinnon, J., Voti, L., Wohler-Torres, B., Peace, S., & Trapido, E. (2001). Lymphoma and lymphoid leukemia incidence in Florida children: Ethnic and racial distribution. *Cancer, 91*, 1402–1408.

Wolfe, J., Grier, H. E., & Klar, N. (2000). Symptoms and suffering at the end of life in children with cancer. *New England Journal of Medicine, 342*, 326–333.

Wolfe, J., Klar, N., Grier, H. E., Duncan, J., Salem-Schatz, S., Emanuel, E. J., & Weeks, J. C. (2000). Understanding of prognosis among parents of children who died of cancer. *Journal of the American Medical Association, 284*, 2469–2475.

Zebrack, B. J., Zeltzer, L. K., Whitton, J., Mertens, A. C., Odom, L., Berkow, R., & Robison, L. L. (2002). Psychological outcomes in long-term survivors of childhood leukemia, Hodgkin's disease, and non-Hodgkin's lymphoma: A report from the Childhood Cancer Survivor Study. *Pediatrics, 110*, 42–52.

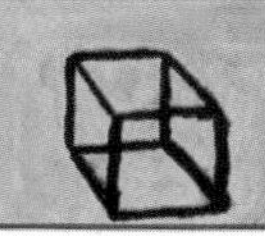

ADDITIONAL REFERENCES

Allen, P. J., & Vessey, J. A. (2004). *Primary care of the child with a chronic condition* (4th ed.). St. Louis: Mosby.

Auger, M., Kelly, K. P., Bayles, A., Bradlyn, A. S., Byron, P. J., Kinahan, K., Lafond, D., Moore, I. M., & Roy, S. C. (2000). Investigating cognitive consequences of treatment for childhood acute lymphoblastic leukemia. *Seminars in Oncology Nursing, 16*, 298–299.

Bleyer, A. (2002). Older adolescents with cancer in North America: Deficits in outcome and research. *Pediatric Clinics of North America, 49*, 1027–1042.

Dome, J. S., & Coppes, M. J. (2002). Recent advances in Wilms tumor genetics. *Current Opinion in Pediatrics, 14*, 5–11.

Halonen, P., Salo, J. K., & Makipernaa, A. (2001). Fasting hypoglycemia is common during maintenance therapy for childhood acute lymphoblastic leukemia. *Journal of Pediatrics, 138*, 428–431.

Hockenberry, M. J., Hinds, P. S., Barrera, P., Billups, C., Rodriguez-Galindo, C., Tan, M., Kline, M., & Razzouk, B. (2002). Incidence of anemia in children with solid tumors or Hodgkin disease. *Journal of Pediatric Hematology/Oncology, 24*, 35–37.

Hogan, D. K., & Rosenthal, L. D. (1998). Oncologic emergencies in the patient with lymphoma. *Seminars in Oncology Nursing, 14*, 312–320.

Hudson, M. M. (2002). Pediatric Hodgkin's therapy: Time for a paradigm shift. *Journal of Clinical Oncology, 21*, 3755–3757.

Kadan-Lottick, N. S., Robison, L. L., Gurney, J. G., Neglia, J. P., Yasui, Y., Hayashi, R., Hudson, M., Greenberg, J., & Mertens, A. C. (2002). Childhood cancer survivors' knowledge about their post diagnoses and treatment: Childhood Cancer Survivor Study. *JAMA, 287*, 1832–1839.

Kebudi, R., Bilgic, B., Gorgun, O., Ayan, I., & Demiryont, M. (2003). Is the Epstein Barr virus implicated in Ewing sarcoma? *Medical Pediatric Oncology, 40,* 256–257.

Kingma, A., van Commelen, R. I., Mooyaart, E. L., Wilmink, J. T., Deelman, B. G., & Kamps, W. A. (2001). Slight cognitive impairment and magnetic resonance imaging abnormalities but normal school levels in children treated for acute lymphoblastic leukemia with chemotherapy only. *Journal of Pediatrics, 139,* 413–420.

Louw, G., & Pinkerton, C. R. (2003). Interventions for early stage Hodgkin's disease in children. *Cochrane Review, 2.*

Nagarajan, R., Neglia, J. P., Clohisy, D. R., Yasui, Y., Greenberg, M., Hudson, J., Zevon, J. A., Tersak, J. M., Ablin, A., & Robison, L. L. (2003). Education, employment, insurance, and marital status among 694 survivors of pediatric lower extremity bone tumors. *Cancer, 97,* 2554–2564.

Pietsch, J. B., & Ford, C. (2000). Children with cancer: Measurements of nutritional status at diagnosis. *Nutrition in Clinical Practice, 15,* 185–188.

Ruble, K., & Kelly, K. P. (1999). Radiation therapy in childhood cancer. *Seminars in Oncology Nursing, 15,* 292–302.

Uusitalo, M., Wheeler, S., & O'Brien, J. M. (1999). New approaches in the clinical management of retinoblastoma. *Ophthalmology Clinics of North America, 12,* 255–264.

Van der Sluis, I. M., van den Heuvel-Eibrink, M. M., Hablen, K., Krenning, E. P., & Keizer-Schrama, S. M. (2002). Altered bone mineral density and body composition, and increased fracture risk in childhood acute lymphoblastic leukemia. *Journal of Pediatrics, 141,* 204–210.

Wagner, L. M., Neel, M. D., Pappo, A. S., Merchant, T. E., Poquette, C. A., Rao, B. N., & Rodriguez-Galindo, C. (2001). Fractures in pediatric Ewing sarcoma. *Journal of Pediatric Hematology/Oncology, 23,* 568–571.

Chapter

30

Alterations in Gastrointestinal Function

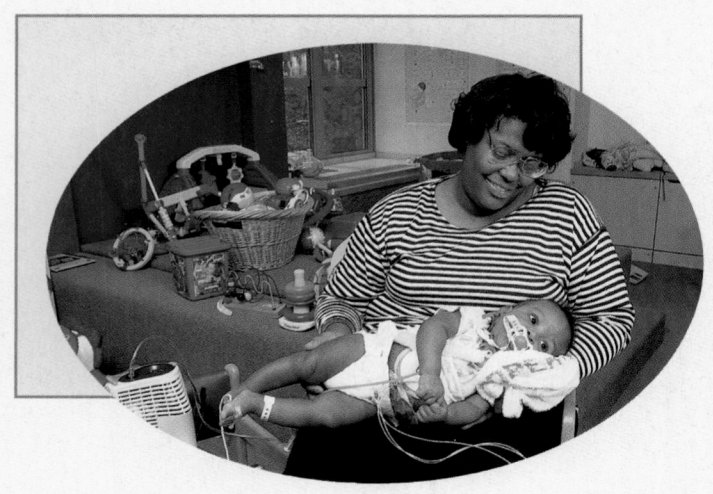

Jerome Sherlock was born 2 weeks prematurely after a normal pregnancy. Soon after birth, he was diagnosed with multiple gastrointestinal anomalies, the most severe of which were an imperforate anus and esophageal atresia (an incomplete esophagus leading to a blind pouch). He underwent two major surgeries in the immediate newborn period and has been hospitalized several times since birth to treat infections and electrolyte imbalance, provide nutritional support, and evaluate his condition.

Jerome is now 8 months old and weighs 15 pounds. Although he still receives most of his nutrition through enteral tube feedings, he is learning to suck more vigorously and is given a bottle every few hours. The muscle development facilitated by sucking will promote his intake of foods and formation of speech later.

Jerome has a colostomy that was placed during surgery for his imperforate anus. The plan is for closure of the colostomy at about 2 years of age, and it is anticipated that he will be able to develop normal bowel function. An ostomy nurse visits Jerome at home and when he is in the hospital to evaluate his care.

Jerome's mother has been devoted to his care, providing nearly all of his tube feedings and other care at home. A home health nurse visits frequently and helps arrange occasional respite care for the mother. Jerome's mother has received materials and talks on the phone with members of an ostomy support group. She finds this contact very helpful in providing additional ideas about colostomy care and the opportunity to discuss her feelings and concerns about Jerome.

"I hope that my baby brother can eat without that tube one day . . . I don't like that bag on his stomach either. Mommy is letting me hold him, so I think he is getting better."

—Amanda, age 6

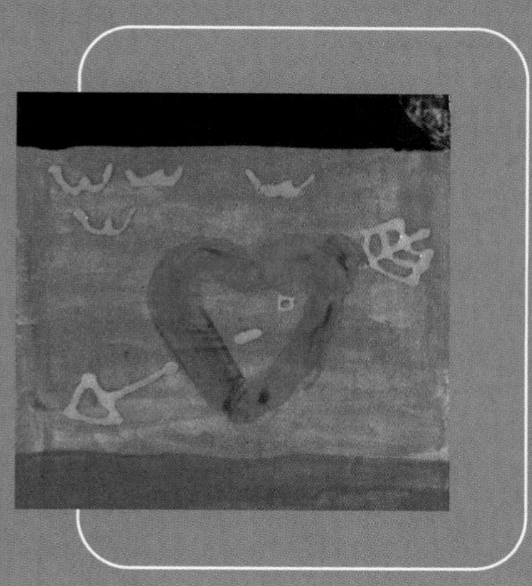

Learning Outcomes

After completing this chapter, you will be able to:

- Describe the general function of the gastrointestinal system.
- Discuss the pathophysiological processes associated with specific gastrointestinal disorders in the pediatric population.
- Identify signs and symptoms that may indicate a disorder of the gastrointestinal system.
- Describe nursing management and plan care for disorders of the gastrointestinal system.
- Analyze developmentally appropriate approaches for nursing management of gastrointestinal disorders in the pediatric population.
- Discuss nursing management of the child with an injury (trauma or ingestion of injurious agent) to the gastrointestinal system.

Key Terms

atresia/1092
bilirubin/1148
cholestasis/1138
chronic vomiting/1118
constipation/1121
cyclic vomiting/1118
diarrhea/1118
gastroesophageal reflux (GER)/1118
gastroesophageal reflux disease (GERD)/1118
gastroschisis/1109
gluconeogenesis/1092
hepatitis/1156
hernia/1114
hyperbilirubinemia/1148
intussusception/1107
occult blood/1140
omphalocele/1110
ostomy/1113
peristalsis/1092
projectile vomiting/1104
stoma/1113

MediaLink http://www.prenhall.com/ball

Resources for this chapter can be found on the CD-ROM accompanying this textbook and on the Companion Website at www.prenhall.com/ball. Click on Chapter 30 to select the activities for this chapter.

CD-ROM

Animations/Videos

- *Activated Charcoal*
- *Digestive System*
- *Lead Poisoning*
- *Stool Toileting: Refusals and Rewards*

Nursing in Action: Changing an Ostomy Pouch

NCLEX Review

Audio Glossary

COMPANION WEBSITE

A & P Review

Clinical Manifestations Review

Medication Match-Up

NCLEX Review

Case Study: The Child with a Cleft Palate

Care Plan: Managing Emesis in Pediatric Conditions

MediaLink Applications

- *Evaluating the Home for Poisons*

What causes structural defects such as esophageal atresia and imperforate anus? What special care will Jerome require to promote his growth and development while he undergoes treatment for his anomalies? The nurse providing care to the child with a gastrointestinal disorder will consider the causes and subsequent effects of these disorders. The nurse also collaborates with the other healthcare team members and the child's family to promote the child's growth and development. This chapter provides a discussion of the care of infants and children, like Jerome, who have structural defects and those with other common disorders of gastrointestinal functioning.

Through the gastrointestinal (GI) tract, a child ingests and absorbs the foods and fluids necessary to sustain life and promote growth. Most gastrointestinal disturbances produce symptoms that are short term and interfere with nutrition and fluid balance for only a brief period. Some disorders or severe defects lead to complications that prevent optimal nutrition and adequate growth. (See Chapter 23∞ for a discussion of specific fluid imbalances that may accompany gastrointestinal infections.)

Gastrointestinal disorders can result from a congenital defect, acquired disease, infection, or injury. Structural problems may occur when development is altered or ceases in the first trimester of gestation. Because various parts of the gastrointestinal system are developing at this point in gestation, it is not unusual for infants to have more than one structural defect of the gastrointestinal system. This was the case with Jerome in the opening vignette. Infections can cause an increase or decrease in motility and prevent proper absorption of nutrients. Interruption or destruction of the gastrointestinal system can also result from trauma or ingestion of caustic substances. As you read this chapter, remember that any interruption or alteration in the gastrointestinal system will decrease the body's ability to obtain nutrients, thus impairing growth.

ANATOMY AND PHYSIOLOGY OF PEDIATRIC DIFFERENCES

Although the fetus makes sucking and swallowing movements in utero and ingests amniotic fluid, the gastrointestinal system is immature at birth. The processes of absorption and excretion do not begin until after birth, because the placenta is responsible for providing nutrients and removing waste. Sucking is a primitive reflex that occurs when the lips or cheeks are stroked. The infant does not have voluntary control over swallowing until about 6 weeks of age.

MediaLink Digestive System Animation

The stomach capacity of the newborn is quite small, and intestinal motility (**peristalsis**) is greater than in older children (Box 30–1). These characteristics explain the newborn's need for small, frequent feedings and the increased frequency and liquid consistency of bowel movements. Because of the relaxed cardiac sphincter, infants frequently regurgitate small amounts of feedings. See page 277 for abdominal quadrants and associated organs.

Digestion takes place in the duodenum. Infants normally have a deficiency of the following enzymes: amylase (which digests carbohydrates), lipase (which enhances fat absorption), and trypsin (which catabolizes protein into polypeptides and some amino acids). Enzymes are usually not present in sufficient quantities to aid digestion until 4 to 6 months of age. Thus, abdominal distention from gas is common.

BOX 30–1 Stomach Capacity Increase Throughout Early Childhood

Age	Capacity (mL)
Newborn	10–20
1 week	30–90
2–3 weeks	75–100
1 month	90–150
3 months	150–200
1 year	210–360
2 years	500

Liver function is also immature at birth. After the first few weeks of life, the liver is able to conjugate bilirubin and excrete bile; until that age the liver is slow and immature in these functions. The processes of **gluconeogenesis** (formation of glycogen from noncarbohydrates), plasma protein and ketone formation, vitamin storage, and deamination (removal of amino group from amino compound) remain immature during the first year of life.

By the second year of life, gastrointestinal structures and digestive processes are fairly mature (Figure 30–1 ■). Stomach capacity increases and accommodates a three-meals-per-day feeding schedule. At about the same time, myelination of the spinal cord becomes complete and voluntary control over excretory functions can be achieved.

STRUCTURAL DEFECTS

Structural defects can involve one or more areas of the gastrointestinal tract. These defects occur when growth and development of fetal structures are interrupted during the first trimester. This can leave the structure incomplete, resulting in **atresia** (absence or closure of a normal body orifice), malposition, nonclosure, or other abnormalities. The structural defects

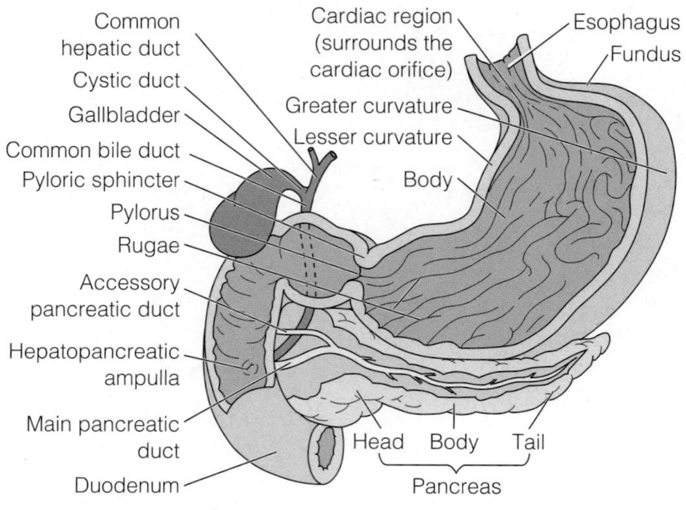

FIGURE 30–1 ■ The internal anatomic structures of the stomach, including the pancreatic, cystic, and hepatic ducts; the pancreas; and the gallbladder.

discussed in this section are cleft lip and cleft palate, esophageal atresia and tracheoesophageal fistula, pyloric stenosis, intussception, abdominal wall defects, and anorectal malformations. Ostomies are discussed in the next section of the chapter because they are a common surgical intervention during correction of structural defects.

Cleft Lip and Cleft Palate

Cleft lip and cleft palate are two distinct facial defects that can occur singly or in combination (Figure 30–2 ■). Cleft lip and palate are the most common congenital craniofacial deformities and the fourth most common birth defects overall in the United States (Cleft Palate Foundation, 2004). Incomplete fusion of the lip (cleft lip) with or without cleft palate occurs in approximately 1 in 700 births, and occurs approximately twice as often in males than females and occurs with greater severity (Mitchell & Wood, 2000). Cleft lip is more common in Native Americans and Asians with decreasing incidence in Whites and least common occurence in Blacks. Incomplete fusion of the palate (cleft palate) occurs in approximately 1 in 2,000 births. Each defect involves varying degrees of severity.

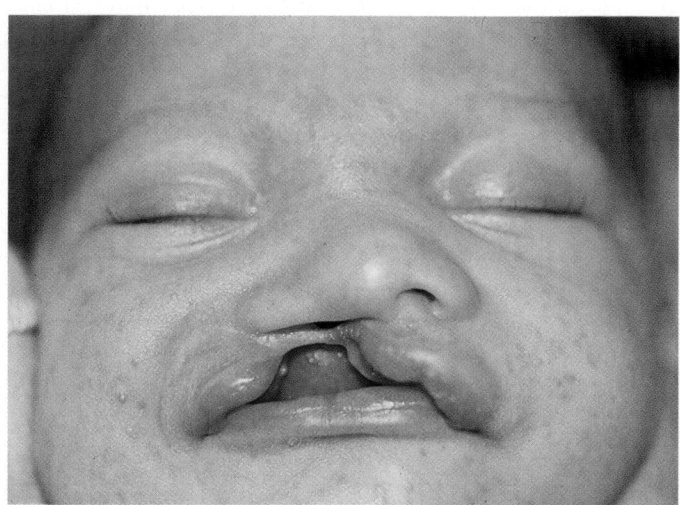

A

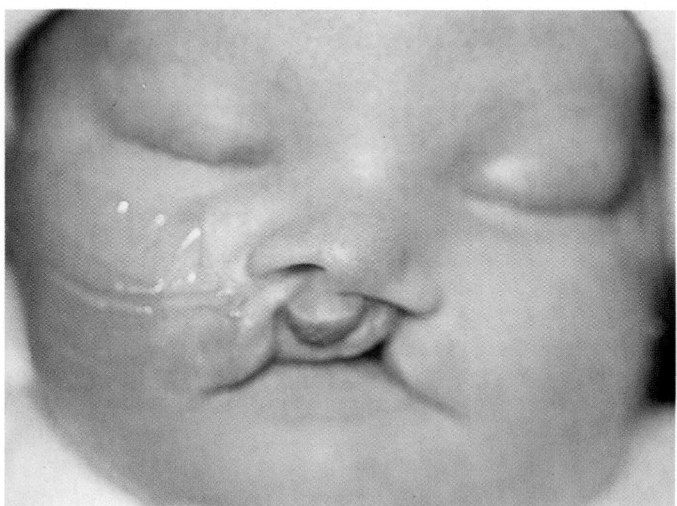

B

FIGURE 30–2 ■ *A,* Unilateral cleft lip. *B,* Bilateral cleft lip.

Courtesy of Dr. Elizabeth Peterson, Spokane, WA.

Etiology and Pathophysiology

Cleft lip with or without cleft palate results from a failure of the maxillary processes to fuse with the elevations on the frontal prominence during the sixth week of gestation. Normally union of the upper lip is complete by the seventh week (Mitchell & Wood, 2000). Fusion of the secondary palate occurs between 5 and 12 weeks of gestation. Failure of the tongue to move downward at the correct time will prevent the palatine processes from fusing.

The intrauterine development of the hard and soft palates is completed in the first trimester. It is during this time that other major organ systems develop. Congenital defects such as tracheoesophageal fistula, omphalocele, trisomy 13, and skeletal dysplasias are associated with cleft lip and palate defects in 20% to 30% of cases. There is an increased incidence in families with a prior history of cleft lip or palate. The cause is believed to be multifactorial, involving a combination of environmental and genetic influences. When fortification of cereals and breads with folate began in the United States in 1996 as a measure to decrease neural tube defects, it was found that the incidence of orofacial clefts also decreased. This may suggest a role for folate in formation of maxillary processes in the fetus (van Rooij, Vermeij-Keers, Kluijtmans, et al., 2003).

Additional etiologic factors include maternal use of tobacco, parental age, the use of anticonvulsants or steroids during pregnancy, and infections during pregnancy. Other medications that interfere with growth factors and enzymes crucial to cell differentiation and division include vitamin A, lithium, retinoids, and phenytoin (Mitchell & Wood, 2000).

Clinical Manifestations

Cleft lip may be detected during pregnancy on prenatal ultrasound by 13 to 16 weeks' gestation (Mitchell & Wood, 2000). A cleft that involves the lip is readily apparent at birth. The defect may be a simple dimple in the vermilion border of the lip or a complete separation extending to the floor of the nose. The defect may be unilateral or bilateral and may occur alone or in combination with a cleft palate defect. See the clinical manifestations table below. Varying degrees of nasal deformity may also be present.

CLINICAL MANIFESTATIONS of Cleft Lip and Cleft Palate

CLASSIFICATION	CLINICAL MANIFESTATIONS
Cleft lip	Unilateral or bilateral May or may not be associated with cleft palate Complete cleft lip extends into the nostril floor Incomplete cleft lip has a bridge of tissue connecting the central and lateral lip
Cleft palate	Occurs anywhere from the incisor foramen to the uvula Incomplete cleft palates involve mainly the soft palate

Cleft palate defects are less obvious when they occur without a cleft lip and may not be detected at birth unless a thorough examination of the oral cavity is performed. Clefts of the hard palate form a continuous opening between the mouth and nasal cavity and may be unilateral or bilateral, involving just the soft palate or both the soft and hard palates.

COLLABORATIVE CARE

Collaborative care focuses on identifying the defect, restoring lip and nasal form, promoting achievement of normal speech development, preventing hearing complications, and promoting normal dentition.

Cleft lip and cleft palate are generally diagnosed prenatally, at birth, or during the newborn assessment. Management requires the combined efforts of a multidisciplinary team. Because speech, hearing, and dentition may be affected, coordinated care by specialists in plastic and oral surgery, audiology, speech, otolaryngology, and orthodontics is necessary (Table 30–1).

Diagnostic Tests

Cleft lip and cleft palate are diagnosed by characteristic physical findings. Visual examination of the entire palate back to the tip of the uvula is performed. Palpation with a finger may reveal a notch in the posterior border of the hard palate (Mitchell & Wood, 2000).

Because clefts may be involved in many life-threatening malformations, immediate diagnostic studies to detect ear deformities, skeletal deformities, heart defects, and genitourinary defects are conducted.

Clinical Therapy

The cleft lip is usually repaired after 10 weeks of age (Figure 30–3 ■). The standard has traditionally been the "rule of tens"—weight greater than 10 pounds, age greater than 10 weeks, and hemoglobin greater than 10 mg/dL—when planning cleft lip repair (Mitchell & Wood, 2000). However, with advances in neonatology and pediatric anesthesia, it is now possible to perform cleft repair surgery for some infants during the neonatal period (Sandberg, Magee, & Denk, 2002).

The lip is sutured together, and a Logan bow or other stabilizing device or dressing is put in place to prevent tension on the suture line. After surgery, the infant's elbows may be restrained to prevent flexion, avoiding trauma to the facial suture lines (refer to the Skills Manual). To prevent injury to the suture line, crying is minimized by use of pain medication and physical comforting.

Early closure of the lip enables the infant to form a better seal around the nipple for feeding. The sucking motion strengthens the muscles necessary for speech. Special feeding devices such as longer nipples with enlarged holes are available to help meet the infant's nutritional needs before surgical correction.

Timing of the cleft palate repair varies among surgeons and depends on the size and severity of the cleft defect. Most surgeons perform closure operations when the infant is between 6 and 18 months old. This protects the formation of tooth buds and allows the infant to develop more normal speech patterns, since speech is adversely affected if the closure is delayed past the age of 2 years (Mitchell & Wood, 2000). Repair of cleft palate may require additional staged reconstructions if the cleft was severe.

Both surgical procedures require the use of general anesthesia, and the hospital stay is dependent upon the child's postoperative progress. Postoperative feeding protocols vary from the use of special nipples or syringes to breastfeeding. Infants with cleft lip and cleft palate are prone to recurrent otitis media, which can lead to hearing problems. Ear infections should be promptly evaluated by a health professional with expertise in ear

TABLE 30–1 Complications Associated with Cleft Lip or Cleft Palate

COMPLICATION	ETIOLOGY	CLINICAL THERAPY
Feeding problems	Inability to suck successfully Excess air intake and resultant gastrointestinal distress	Referral to feeding specialist for evaluation of need for special nipples and nursing routines Teaching for parents to encourage slow feeding with baby in upright position, frequent burping Frequent measurement to evaluate adequacy of growth
Speech development	Persistent structural abnormalities, dental problems, and hearing problems associated with cleft lip/cleft palate	Speech and language development are evaluated on a regular basis
Otologic	High risk for otitis media since the abnormal structure impairs the ventilatory function of the eustachian tubes Conductive hearing loss may occur as a result of ear effusions	Monitoring for ear infections Measures to prevent infections are taught to family and antibiotics are used to treat ear infections Audiology screening is conducted 1–2 times annually
Dental and orthodontic	Children with clefts have a higher prevalence of dental caries Teeth may be impacted, hypoplastic, or congenitally missing Higher risk for gingivitis, crowding, and crossbite	Promote good oral hygiene and regular dental visits Fluoride supplements if needed Palatal expansion may be required to correct crossbite Dental alignment with appliances
Developmental	Parent/infant attachment may be affected Older child may experience poor self-esteem if cosmetic correction was not performed (e.g., child is from a developing country) Reading complications may result from impaired hearing and speech	Support parent/infant attachment Refer child and family to counseling if required Screen for learning disabilities

Data from Mitchell, J. C., & Wood, R. J. (2000). Management of cleft lip and palate in primary care. Journal of Pediatric Health Care, 14, 13–19.

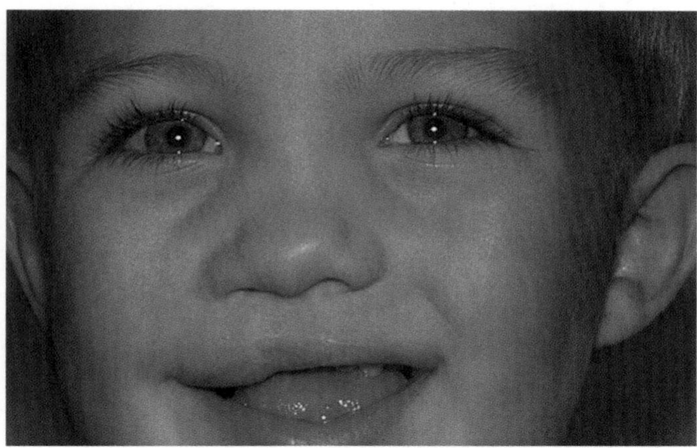

A

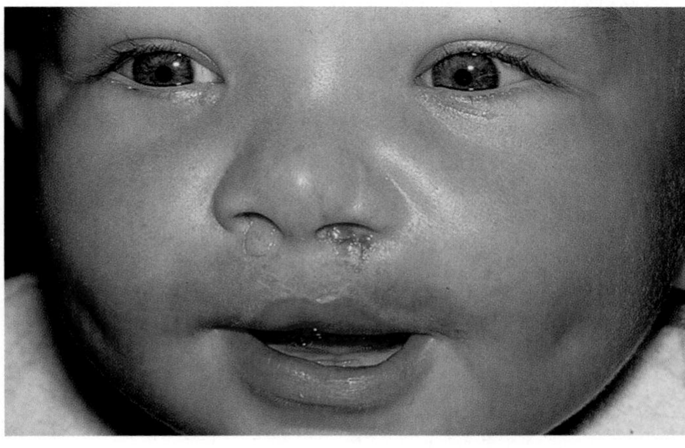

B

FIGURE 30–3 ■ *A,* Repaired unilateral cleft lip (see Figure 30–2A). *B,* Repaired bilateral cleft lip (see Figure 30–2B).

Courtesy of Dr. Elizabeth Peterson, Spokane, WA.

care and treatment. (Refer to Chapter 24∞ for care of the child with otitis media.) The child who has had cleft palate repair will require orthodontic care. Early visits will permit assessment of tooth eruption and the need for future orthodontic work.

NURSING MANAGEMENT

Nursing care involves facilitating feeding, providing emotional support, performing preoperative and postoperative care, assisting parents to coordinate care and maintain a healthy home environment, and making appropriate referrals.

■ Nursing Assessment and Diagnosis

Physiologic Assessment

A cleft lip defect is observable at birth. A cleft palate defect is usually noted during the newborn assessment by palpation of the hard palate with the finger. A description of the location and extent of the defect will assist the nurse in determining the correct method of feeding. A thorough and complete physical assessment is required since additional defects sometimes accompany cleft lip or cleft palate.

Psychosocial Assessment

Assessment of the family's reactions is an integral part of the overall nursing assessment. Physical deformities, especially of the face, can be devastating to parents. A poorly corrected defect can lead to the development of low self-esteem in the older child. Assess the child's developmental level and social interactions with peers.

The accompanying nursing care plan lists common nursing diagnoses for the infant with a cleft lip and/or palate. Additional diagnoses that may be appropriate include the following:

- Risk for Impaired Parent/Infant Attachment related to newborn's structural defect
- Acute Pain related to surgical repair of defect
- Risk for Delayed Growth and Development related to structural defect and altered nutritional intake

■ Planning and Implementation

The accompanying nursing care plan summarizes nursing care for the infant with a cleft lip and/or cleft palate. Additional nursing care includes facilitating feeding, providing emotional support, and providing preoperative and postoperative care.

Facilitate Feeding

Feeding problems for the infant with cleft lip or cleft palate depend on the severity of the anatomic defect. Infants with cleft lip without cleft palate, and those infants with isolated cleft of the soft palate generally are able to breast or bottle feed (Mitchell & Wood, 2000).

The infant with cleft palate may be able to breastfeed since the breast may fill the defect, allowing the development of negative intraoral pressure required to feed (Mitchell & Wood, 2000). The mother is generally assisted by a lactation specialist. If breastfeeding is not possible, the mother can be assisted to pump her breasts in order for the milk to be fed by a special nurser.

For infants requiring assistance to feed, several wide-based nipples, squeezable bottles, and other special bottles are available. Some infants may require a device placed in the mouth to enable them to establish suction. Several companies provide special nursers that may be helpful for children with cleft lip or palate. See Partnering with Families: Feeding the Infant with Cleft Lip or Cleft Palate.

Provide Emotional Support

Parents may require assistance to view their infant as a whole person, rather than focusing solely on the physical defect. Nurses can promote parent–infant bonding by explaining the nature of the structural defect and the procedure for correction. Interact and speak to the infant in the parents' presence and point out the infant's positive attributes such as alertness, soft skin, or active movements.

MediaLink Case Study: The Child with a Cleft Palate

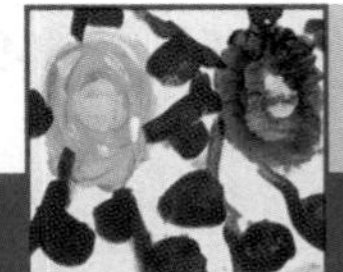

Nursing Care Plan

THE INFANT WITH A CLEFT LIP AND/OR PALATE

GOAL	INTERVENTION	RATIONALE	EXPECTED OUTCOME
Preoperative Care			
1. Risk for Aspiration (breast milk, formula, or mucus) related to anatomic defect			
	NIC Priority Intervention— *Aspiration Precautions:* Prevention or minimization of risk factors in the patient at risk of aspiration.		**NOC Suggested Outcome**—*Airway Maintenance:* Toleration of enteral feedings without aspiration.
The infant will have no episodes of gagging or aspiration.	▪ Assess respiratory status and monitor vital signs at least every 2 hours. ▪ Position on side after feedings. ▪ Feed slowly and use adaptive equipment as needed. ▪ Burp frequently (after every 15–30 mL of fluid). ▪ Position upright for feedings. ▪ Keep suction equipment and bulb syringe at bedside.	▪ Allows for early identification of problems. ▪ Prevents aspiration of feedings. ▪ Facilitates intake while minimizing risk of aspiration. ▪ Helps to prevent regurgitation and aspiration. ▪ Minimizes passage of feedings through cleft. ▪ Suctioning may be necessary to remove milk or mucus.	The infant exhibits no signs of respiratory distress.
2. Ineffective Family Coping related to situational crisis of birth of a child with a defect			
	NIC Priority Intervention—*Family Involvement:* Facilitating family participation in the emotional and physical care of the child.		**NOC Suggested Outcome**—*Positive Coping:* Extent of coping mechanisms and ability to perform child's physical and emotional care.
Parents will begin bonding process with the infant.	▪ Help parents to hold the infant and facilitate feeding process. ▪ Point out positive attributes of infant (e.g., hair, eyes, alertness). ▪ Explain surgical procedure and expected outcome. Show pictures of other children's cleft lip repair.	▪ Contact is essential for bonding. ▪ Helps parents see the child as a whole, rather than concentrating on the defect. ▪ Eliminating unknown factors helps to decrease anxiety.	Parents hold, comfort, and show concern for the infant.
The family's coping ability will be maximized. Parents will verbalize the nature and sequelae of the defect.	▪ Assess parents knowledge of the defect, their degree of anxiety and level of discomfort, and the interpersonal relationships among family members. ▪ Explore the reactions of extended family members. ▪ Support open visitation. ▪ Encourage parents to participate in caretaking activities (holding, diapering, feeding). ▪ Provide information about the etiology of cleft lip and palate defects and the special needs of these infants. Encourage questions. ▪ Refer to parent support groups.	▪ Helps to determine the appropriate timing and amount of information to be given regarding the child's defect. ▪ Extended family is an important source of support for most parents of a newborn. Family members can often help promote acceptance and compliance with the treatment plan. ▪ Allows parents to continue the bonding process. ▪ Participation in infant care decreases anxiety and provides parents with a sense of purpose. ▪ Concrete information allows parents time to understand the defect and reduces guilt. ▪ Support groups allow parents to express their feelings and concerns, to find people with concerns similar to their own, and to seek additional information.	The family demonstrates improved coping ability before discharge. Parents receive necessary support to care for their infant.

Nursing Care Plan THE INFANT WITH A CLEFT LIP AND/OR PALATE (continued)

GOAL	INTERVENTION	RATIONALE	EXPECTED OUTCOME
3. Imbalanced Nutrition: Less than Body Requirements related to the infant's inability to ingest nutrients			
	NIC Priority Intervention—*Nutrition Management:* Provision of a balanced dietary intake of foods and fluids.		**NOC Suggested Outcome**—*Nutrition Status:* Amount of food and fluid taken into the body over a 24-hour period.
The infant will gain weight steadily.	■ Assess fluid and calorie intake daily. Assess weight daily (same scale, same time, with infant completely undressed).	■ Provides an objective measurement of whether the infant is receiving sufficient caloric intake to promote growth. Using the same scale and procedure when weighing the infant provides for comparability between daily weights.	The infant maintains adequate nutritional intake and gains weight appropriately.
	■ Observe for any respiratory impairment.	■ Any symptoms of respiratory compromise will interfere with the infant's ability to suck. Feedings should be initiated only if there are no signs of respiratory distress.	
	■ Provide 100–150 cal/kg/day and 100–130 mL/kg/day of feedings and fluid. If the infant needs an increased number of calories to grow, referral to a nutritionist should be made. Formulas with higher calorie concentrations per ounce are available without increasing total fluids.	■ Provides optimal calories and fluids for growth and hydration.	
	■ Facilitate breastfeeding.	■ Breast milk is recommended as the best food for an infant. The process of breastfeeding helps to promote bonding between mother and infant.	Successful breastfeeding is achieved if desired.
	■ Hold the infant in a semisitting position.	■ Makes swallowing easier and reduces the amount of fluid return from the nose.	
	■ Give the mother information on breastfeeding the infant with a cleft lip and/or palate such as plugging the cleft lip and eliciting a letdown reflex before nursing.	■ Information and specific suggestions may encourage the mother to persist with breastfeeding.	
	■ Contact the LaLeche League for the name of a support person.	■ The LaLeche League promotes breastfeeding for all infants. It can provide support people with experience who will aid the mother.	
	■ If the mother is unable to breastfeed (or prefers not to), initiate bottle feeding.		
	■ Hold infant in an upright or semisitting position for feeding.	■ Facilitates swallowing and minimizes the amount of fluid return from the nose.	Feeding provides necessary nutrients and is a positive experience for parents and infant.
	■ Place nipple against the inside cheek toward the back of the tongue. May need to use a premature nipple (slightly longer and softer than regular nipple with a larger opening) or a Brecht feeder (an oval bottle with a long, soft nipple).	■ Use of longer, softer nipples makes it easier for the infant to suck. A Brecht feeder decreases the amount of pressure in the bottle and makes the formula flow more easily.	
	■ Feed small amounts slowly.	■ Small amounts and slow feeding do not tire the infant as quickly as do larger amounts given at a faster rate. They also decrease the energy used during feeding.	

(continued)

Nursing Care Plan THE INFANT WITH A CLEFT LIP AND/OR PALATE (continued)			
GOAL	INTERVENTION	RATIONALE	EXPECTED OUTCOME
Preoperative Care (continued)			
3. Imbalanced Nutrition: Less than Body Requirements related to the infant's inability to ingest nutrients (continued)			
	■ Burp frequently, after 15–30 mL of formula has been given. ■ Initiate nasogastric feedings if the infant is unable to ingest sufficient calories by mouth.	■ Frequent burping prevents the accumulation of air in stomach, which can cause regurgitation or vomiting. ■ Adequate nutrition must be maintained. Use of a feeding tube allows the infant who has difficulty with oral feeding to receive adequate nutrition for growth.	
Postoperative Care			
1. Risk for Infection related to location of surgical procedure			
	NIC Priority Intervention—*Infection Control:* Minimizing the acquisition and transmission of infectious agents.		**NOC Suggested Outcome**—*Risk Control:* Actions to eliminate or reduce actual, personal, or modifiable health risks.
The infant's mucosal tissue will heal without infection.	■ Assess vital signs every 2 hours. ■ Assess oral cavity every 2 hours or as needed for tenderness, reddened areas, lesions, or presence of secretions. ■ Cleanse suture line with normal saline or sterile water if ordered. ■ Cleanse the cleft areas by giving 5–15 mL of water after each feeding. ■ If a crust has formed, use a cotton swab to apply a half-strength peroxide solution or solution ordered by physician. ■ Apply antibiotic cream to suture line as ordered. ■ Use careful handwashing and sterile technique when working with suture line.	■ Elevated temperature may indicate infection. ■ Aids in identifying infection. ■ Helps decrease the presence of bacteria. ■ Prevents accumulation of carbohydrates, which encourage bacterial growth. ■ Helps loosen the crust, aiding in removal. ■ Counteracts the growth of bacteria.	The infant remains free of infection in the oral cavity. Tissues remain intact and pink. Healing process progresses without adverse events in postoperative period.
2. Ineffective Breathing Pattern related to surgical correction of defect			
	NIC Priority Intervention—*Airway Management:* Facilitation of patency of air passages.		**NOC Suggested Outcome**—*Vital Signs Status:* Temperature, pulse, respiration, and blood pressure within expected range for the infant/child.
The infant will maintain an effective breathing pattern.	■ Assess respiratory status and monitor vital signs at least every 2 hours. ■ Apply a cardiorespiratory monitor. ■ Keep suction equipment and bulb syringe at bedside. Gently suction oropharynx and nasopharynx as needed. ■ Provide cool mist for first 24 hours postoperatively if ordered. ■ Reposition every 2 hours.	■ Allows for early identification of problems. ■ Enables early detection of abnormal respirations, facilitating prompt intervention. ■ Gentle suctioning will keep the airway clear. Suctioning that is too vigorous can irritate the mucosa. ■ Moisturizes secretions to reduce pooling in lungs. Moisturizes oral cavity. ■ Ensures expansion of all lung fields.	The infant shows no signs of respiratory infection or compromise.

Nursing Care Plan THE INFANT WITH A CLEFT LIP AND/OR PALATE (continued)

GOAL	INTERVENTION	RATIONALE	EXPECTED OUTCOME
3. Impaired Tissue Integrity related to mechanical factors			
	NIC Priority Intervention—*Wound Care:* Prevention of wound complications and promotion of wound healing.		**NOC Suggested Outcome—***Wound Healing:* The extent to which cells and tissues have regenerated following intentional closure.
Lip and/or palate will heal with minimal scarring or disruption.	■ Position the infant with cleft lip repair on side or back only. ■ Use soft elbow restraints. Remove every 2 hours and replace. Do not leave the infant unattended when restraints are removed. ■ Maintain metal bar or Steri-Strips placed for stabilization over cleft lip repair. ■ Avoid metal utensils or straws after cleft palate repair. ■ Keep the infant well medicated for pain in initial postoperative period. Have parents hold and comfort the infant. ■ Provide developmentally appropriate activities (e.g., mobiles, music).	■ Prone position could cause rubbing on suture line. ■ Prevents the infant's hands from rubbing surgical site. Regular removal allows for skin and neurovascular checks. ■ Maintaining suture line will minimize scarring. ■ These devices may disrupt suture line. ■ Good pain management minimizes crying, which can cause stress on suture line. Increases bonding and soothes the child to decrease crying. ■ Soothes and keeps the infant calm.	Lip/palate heals without complications.
4. Deficient Knowledge (parent) related to lack of exposure and unfamiliarity with resources			
	NIC Priority Intervention—*Teaching, Disease Process:* Assisting the patient to understand information related to cleft lip/palate.		**NOC Suggested Outcome—***Knowledge:* Extent of understanding conveyed about cleft lip/palate treatment.
Before discharge, parents will verbalize home care methods for care of the infant with cleft lip and palate defect.	■ Explain care and treatment (both short term and long term). Discuss potential complications. ■ Demonstrate feeding techniques and alternatives. Allow parents to demonstrate before discharge. ■ Provide written instructions for follow-up care arrangements. ■ Introduce the parents (if possible) to a primary care provider in the setting where the infant will receive follow-up care after discharge.	■ Assists the family to deal with the physical and psychosocial aspects of a child with a congenital defect. ■ Provides visual instructions. Redemonstration confirms learning. ■ Written instructions reinforce verbal instruction and provide a reference after discharge. ■ Continuity of care is important. Since the infant will require long-term follow-up, a contact with the new provider is helpful.	Parents accurately describe and demonstrate feeding techniques to facilitate optimal growth of the infant; describe interventions if respiratory distress occurs; and take the written instructions home with them on discharge.
5. Imbalanced Nutrition: Less Than Body Requirements related to inability to ingest nutrients			
	NIC Priority Intervention—*Nutrition Management:* Promotion of a balanced dietary intake of foods and fluids.		**NOC Suggested Outcome—***Nutritional Status:* Extent to which nutrients are available to meet metabolic needs.
The infant will receive adequate nutritional intake.	■ Maintain intravenous infusion as ordered. ■ Begin with clear liquids, then give half-strength breast milk or formula as ordered. ■ Use Asepto syringe or dropper in side of mouth. ■ Do not allow pacifiers. ■ Give high-calorie soft foods after cleft palate repair.	■ Provides fluid when NPO. ■ Ensures adequate fluids and nutrients. ■ Avoids suture line and resultant accumulation of milk or formula in that area. ■ Sucking can disrupt suture line. ■ Rough foods, utensils, and straws could disrupt the surgical site.	The infant receives adequate nutritional intake. Infant resumes usual feeding patterns and gains weight appropriately.

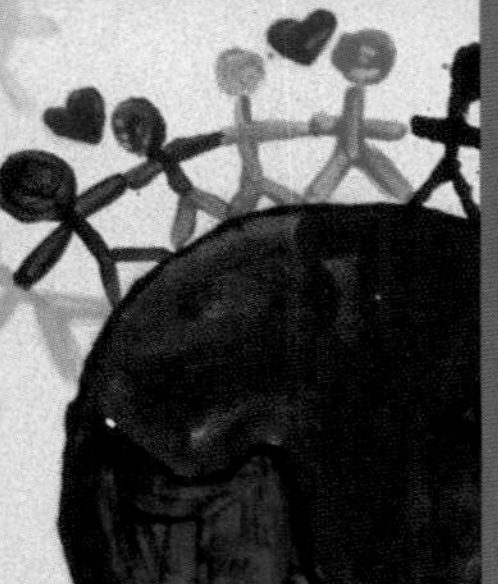

PARTNERING WITH FAMILIES

Feeding the Infant with Cleft Lip or Cleft Palate

The nurse assists the family to maintain feeding methods to promote the infant's growth and development. Inform parents of the following:

- The infant with a cleft may require additional time to feed, which may produce fatigue. Allow the child additional time to eat and provide opportunities for rest after feeding.
- Feed the infant with the head and chest elevated since gravity helps to prevent milk from coming through the baby's nose.
- Breastfeeding is encouraged if possible; special techniques can help to achieve success.
- Burp the baby frequently because infants with cleft palate tend to swallow air during feedings.
- A feeding specialist is available to assist, and can suggest specially designed bottles and other feeding techniques to facilitate feeding the baby.
- Maintain follow-up appointments so that infant is weighed and evaluated for growth and development.
- Inform primary care provider if the infant has difficulty feeding or develops a problem such as vomiting or respiratory difficulty.

CLINICAL TIP

Nurses can provide compassionate care to the family of the child born with cleft lip or cleft palate by pointing out the infant's positive aspects rather than focusing on the cleft. Examples include, "Congratulations on the birth of your new son. He has beautiful hair and long eyelashes. The cleft lip/palate is correctable. We will refer you to a team of professionals who will work together to correct the opening."

MediaLink Cleft Lip/Palate Resources and Support

Self-blame is common among parents. Provide them with opportunities to express fears and concerns. Refer parents to the American Cleft Palate–Craniofacial Association for information about the disorder. Some plastic surgeons have photos of children before and after correction to reassure parents that their child can have a "normal" appearance (Uhrich & Mackin, 2001). Introduce them to other families who have had a child with cleft lip or palate and can discuss treatments and offer support.

Parental anxiety is usual when children undergo surgery. This anxiety is heightened when the surgery involves an infant. To minimize anxiety, keep explanations to parents clear and concise. Allow sufficient time for parents to ask questions. Encourage parents to hold and cuddle the infant before surgery.

Provide Postoperative Care

Provide general postoperative care for the infant. (See the accompanying nursing care plan for the infant with a cleft lip and/or palate and also the nursing care plan for the child undergoing surgery in Chapter 17∞.)

Assess vital signs frequently and maintain the infant's airway. Assess respiratory status during feedings. Measure intake and output. Generally, the infant is allowed to begin feeding by bottle or breast immediately. Position the infant in a sitting position for the feedings to avoid aspiration. Frequently burp the infant during feedings. The infant then progresses to half-strength breast milk or formula. After each feeding, cleanse the suture line with water or normal saline to avoid accumulation of feedings. Provide routine administration of analgesics for pain relief.

Integrity of the suture line is essential to ensure healing. Place the infant in a supine or a side-lying position to avoid rubbing the suture line on the bedding. Avoid the prone position. Maintain appropriate measures to prevent infant from touching sutures (mummy wrap, soft elbow restraints). Maintain the protective device or Steri-Strips placed over the incision. If prescribed, apply antibiotic cream on the incision site. An infant who has had a cleft lip repair requires interventions to provide distraction in order to minimize crying, which can damage the suture line. Soft colorful toys, mobiles, and other visual objects are helpful. Music also can be used to soothe the infant.

Frequently monitor for signs and symptoms of pain and routinely provide postoperative analgesia to the infant to control pain and to minimize crying and stress on the suture line. After cleft palate surgery, avoid the use of metal utensils or straws, which may disrupt the surgical site.

Care in the Community

Home care needs are identified and addressed well in advance of discharge. Partner with the family and discuss all aspects of the infant's care with the parents throughout hospitalization and after surgery. Involve parents in the infant's care to increase their comfort level before discharge and to promote bonding. Collaborate care with the parents and teach proper feeding techniques, how to recognize signs of infection (redness or drainage at the incision site, fever, or increased crying or fussiness), proper positioning of the infant, and care for the suture line.

Management, especially in the first few months of life, involves many different healthcare professionals. In addition to hospital, clinic, and home health nurses, members of the healthcare team often include specialists such as the surgeon, speech therapist, geneticist, dentist, prosthodontist, audiologist, social worker, and pediatrician. The parents are the best coordinators of the child's care. Encourage them to keep a diary listing the professionals with whom they talk and the content of the discussions. The family may also implement complementary or alternative therapies for the child. Ask them about the use of these practices. See Complementary Therapy: Children with Special Needs Survey.

Discuss with the parents the financial implications of long-term care. Private insurance does not always cover all the costs of care necessary for the child. Refer parents to social services familiar with programs and financial aid for which the parents and child may be eligible. Relief of financial worries enables par-

COMPLEMENTARY THERAPY

Children with Special Needs Survey

A recent study assessed the frequency and type of complementary and alternative medicine (CAM) therapies used by families of children with special healthcare needs (Sanders, Davis, Duncan, et al., 2003). In this small sample study of families of 376 children, researchers found that 64% of the children were recipients of at least one of the listed CAM therapies (oral and topical herbs, megavitamins, massage, acupuncture, osteopathic manipulation, chiropractic manipulation, prayers/blessing/spiritual healing, self-hypnosis, special diets, homeopathy, hippotherapy, and "other") and almost 50% of the children had used CAM therapies within 6 months before completing the survey. Researchers also found that chiropractic and osteopathic manipulations, prayer, and spiritual blessings were used for children with cleft lip and cleft palate. Another finding was the use of CAM for the child strongly correlated with the use of CAM in the past by the family member who responded to the survey.

The nurse providing care to a child with cleft lip and/or palate should ask the family about any complementary or alternative treatments used for the child. Recall that treatment may last for several years as the child receives care for monitoring of feeding, and then for otologic or orthodontic complications. Ask regularly during the child's early childhood care about CAM treatments. Provide information that will help parents evaluate planned CAM, and reassure them when no harmful effects are known for the treatments they are using. Ask them what the outcomes have been for the child.

ents to concentrate on caring for the child. See Developing Cultural Competence: Surgical Correction.

Collaborate with parents on care needed for the child after discharge. If the child has siblings, emphasize that they will need preparation to enhance understanding and acceptance of the child. Sibling rivalry can be heightened when one child receives more attention within the home. Remind parents of the importance of setting limits and spending time with each child. Determine whether additional family supports are necessary. Provide parents with information on support groups, physicians, social workers, Internet resources, and local services that can help maintain family continuity.

Discuss ways to prevent the infant from touching the suture line. Teach parents how to bundle an infant in a blanket with arms tucked inside the blanket. A front-sling baby carrier may also be used to immobilize the arms. Front-sling carriers provide the additional benefits of comforting the infant through contact with the parent and of holding the infant upright, which aids in optimal positioning after feedings.

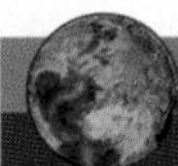

DEVELOPING CULTURAL COMPETENCE

Surgical Correction

Unlike the United States and Canada, in many developing countries infants do not have access to surgery for correction of cleft lip and palate. They may grow into childhood and adulthood with these abnormalities. Medical teams from the United States, Canada, and other countries sometimes travel to developing nations for short medical missions, performing surgery on the children and teaching local doctors surgical techniques. In some cases the children are brought to the sponsor country for a time to receive the needed surgery and care.

After surgical repair, teach parents how to feed the infant and identify signs of complications (fever, vomiting, respiratory distress). Referral to a home healthcare agency for support may be helpful. Encourage follow-up visits with healthcare professionals. The child may need further evaluation of speech development, ear infections, or a recommendation for plastic surgery. See the Health Promotion and Maintenance Overview for the child with cleft lip or palate on page 1102.

■ Evaluation

Following are expected outcomes of nursing care in the preoperative period.

- The child demonstrates absence of respiratory distress and maintenance of normal respirations.
- Parents and infant demonstrate positive bonding.
- Parents express support and comfort by family and community.
- Infant maintains normal weight.
- Parents display knowledge of defect, its correction, and infant needs.

Following are expected outcomes of postoperative nursing care.

- The child is free from infection.
- Anticipated healing stages of surgical area are achieved.
- The child demonstrates normal respiratory pattern and absence of respiratory distress.
- The child demonstrates relief of pain.
- Fluid and electrolyte balance is achieved.
- Anticipated weight gain appropriate for child's age is achieved.
- Parents properly demonstrate appropriate infant care and feeding.

Esophageal Atresia and Tracheoesophageal Fistula

Esophageal atresia is a malformation that results from failure of the esophagus to develop as a continuous tube during the fourth and fifth weeks of gestation. The defect affects approximately 1 in 4,000 neonates annually (Adzick & Nance, 2000). Approximately 30% of the infants are premature (Wyllie, 2004)

Etiology and Pathophysiology

In esophageal atresia, the foregut fails to lengthen, separate, and fuse into two parallel tubes (the esophagus and trachea) during fetal development. Instead the esophagus may end in a blind pouch or develop as a pouch connected to the trachea by a fistula (tracheoesophageal fistula) (Figure 30–4 ■).

Esophageal atresia is often associated with a maternal history of polyhydramnios. Associated anomalies may occur, including congenital heart defects, gastrointestinal or urinary tract anomalies, and musculoskeletal abnormalities. Jerome, described at the beginning of the chapter, had esophageal atresia as well as an imperforate anus.

Infants weighing less than 1,500 g at the time of birth and those with associated cardiac or chromosomal anomalies have

Health Promotion & Maintenance Overview

The Child with Cleft Lip or Cleft Palate

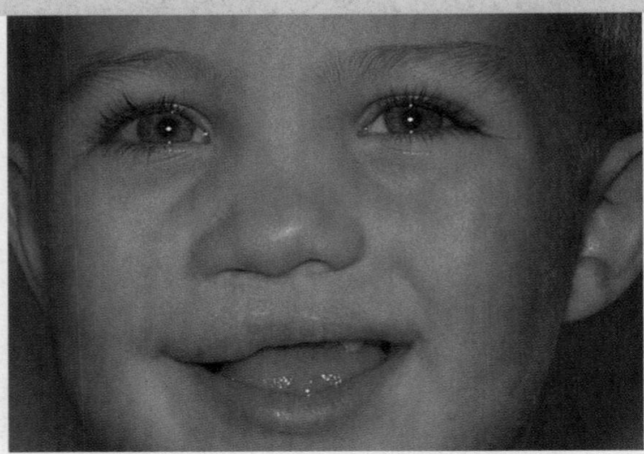

The child with cleft lip or cleft palate requires close monitoring and intervention to foster growth and development. The nurse can assist the child and family in many ways.

Growth and Development Surveillance

- Monitor the child's growth and developmental patterns.
- Monitor for developmental delays.
- Explain to parents that regression following surgery in the toddler or older child is normal.
- Ask the family about financial ability regarding speech therapy, dental care, and other services that may be required. Financial constraints can impede compliance to recommended therapies.

Nutrition

- Refer family to sources for nipples, nursers, and other special feeding devices.
- Assist mother with learning how to express breast milk and facilitate breast feeding.
- Teach parents to avoid foods that can pose a choking hazard to the child.
- Teach parents to avoid straws, metal spoons, and other sharp utensils that may damage palate.
- Teach parents to feed the infant in an upright position and to burp the child frequently during feedings.

Physical Activity

- Activity for the child having surgical procedures to correct cleft palate is generally restricted for approximately 2 to 3 weeks to allow for healing.
- After healing has occured, encourage the parents to promote the child's activities as they would any child without cleft lip or cleft palate.

Oral Health

- The child should be routinely screened for dental caries. Ask family about dental visits.
- Teach the parents to provide good dental hygiene to the child.
- Routine dental/orthodontic evaluation is necessary for the child with cleft palate.

Mental and Spiritual Health

- For uncorrected or poorly corrected cleft lip or palate, the child may experience poor self-esteem related to body image.
- Encourage family to adhere to treatment and surgical correction plan, including staged surgical corrections, dental care, and speech pathology assistance.
- Be alert for the child who has had experiences with teasing associated with articulation or physical appearance.
- Refer parents to websites such as Project Smile and other resources.
- Refer the child for counseling if indicated.

Relationships

- Evaluate the parents for parent–infant bonding.
- Promote bonding by encouraging the parents to participate in the infant's care, to hold the infant, and to recognize the infant's positive attributes.

Disease Prevention Strategies

- Teach family to recognize signs and symptoms of ear or other infections and to seek immediate evaluation. Treatment of acute otitis media by a specialist is necessary to prevent long-term effects of repeated infections.
- Emphasize to the parents the importance of audiology screening for children with cleft lip and palate to evaluate conductive hearing loss.

Injury Prevention Strategies (Safety)

- Assist parents to properly apply elbow restraints or to wrap child in mummy blanket to protect suture line in the postoperative period.
- Ask the parents about eating utensils the child uses.

the highest mortality rate. Early mortality is the result of cardiac or chromosomal abnormalities, whereas later mortality results from respiratory complications (Adzick & Nance, 2000).

Clinical Manifestations

Symptoms in the newborn include excessive salivation and drooling, often accompanied by the three classic signs—cyanosis, choking, and coughing. Sneezing may also be manifested.

During feeding, the infant returns fluid through the nose and mouth. Aspiration places the infant at risk for pneumonia. The abdomen may become distended secondary to air trapping.

COLLABORATIVE CARE

Collaborative care includes immediate identification of the defect, prevention of complications such as aspiration, respiratory and nutritional support as needed, and surgical intervention to correct the defect.

Diagnostic Tests

Diagnosis is usually confirmed by attempting to pass a 5 or 8 French nasogastric tube into the stomach. In most cases, the tube meets resistance and can be advanced only minimally. Specific defects and associated anomalies are determined by radiologic examination. Echocardiogram and abdominal ultrasound are performed. Careful examination of the lungs is needed. A delay in diagnosis can be fatal since ingested fluid or secretions may enter the lungs and lead to pneumonia.

Clinical Therapy

A nasogastric tube is inserted to suction the upper pouch. When using a small-bore nasogastric tube, gurgling can occur when the tube is in the esophagus or lung. Aspirate of contents confirms placement.

Begin intravenous antibiotics and fluids. Surgery is performed as soon as the infant is stable. Surgical correction may be accomplished in several stages (Adzick & Nance, 2000). The first stage usually involves ligation of the fistula and insertion of a gastrostomy tube. In the second stage, the two ends of the esophagus are reconnected, if possible. When surgical closure (anastomosis) is not initially possible, a gastrostomy tube must remain in place for use in feeding until surgery can be performed. Potential postoperative complications include gastroesophageal reflux, aspiration, and stricture formation. Generally, a simple repair results in a speedy recovery, though some conditions are complicated, requiring repeated surgeries and long-term management.

NURSING MANAGEMENT

Nursing care consists of collaborative identification of the defect in the immediate newborn period, preventing complications such as aspiration, providing preoperative and postoperative care, teaching family about the disorder and its treatment, and providing emotional support to the family. Ongoing care is also required to facilitate feeding and promote development.

■ Nursing Assessment and Diagnosis

The nurse may recognize the signs and symptoms in the immediate newborn period. Assess for difficulty feeding and excessive drooling. Assess for the classic signs of choking, coughing, and cyanosis. Assess for respiratory distress and assess the lung sounds carefully.

Esophageal atresia is a surgical emergency. Preoperatively the infant requires close observation and intervention to maintain a patent airway.

Diagnoses that may be appropriate for the infant with esophageal atresia or tracheoesophageal fistula include:

PATHOPHYSIOLOGY ILLUSTRATED

Esophageal Atresia and Tracheoesophageal Fistula

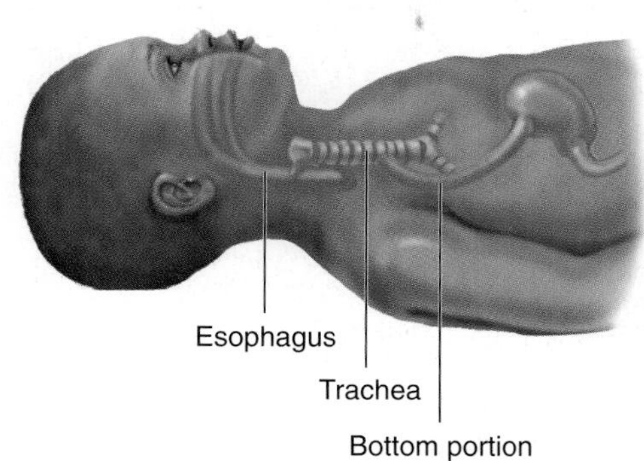

FIGURE 30–4 ■ In the most common type of esophageal atresia and tracheoesophageal fistula, the upper segment of the esophagus ends in a blind pouch connected to the trachea; the fistula connects the lower segment to the trachea.

- Risk for Aspiration related to regurgitation
- Deficient Fluid Volume related to NPO status
- Imbalanced Nutrition: Less than Body Requirements related to NPO status
- Risk for Infection (pulmonary) related to aspiration
- Risk for Impaired Parent/Infant Attachment related to emergency surgical intervention in the neonate

■ Planning and Implementation

Surgical intervention for a newborn is a stressful situation for the parents and family. The parents require emotional support throughout the infant's hospitalization. All procedures should be clearly explained. Partner with parents and encourage them to bond with the infant by stroking and talking to the child. Eliciting questions and allowing parents to participate in the infant's care, especially feeding (when permitted), can facilitate bonding and help to prepare parents for care of the infant after discharge.

Preoperative Nursing Care

Suction is readily available to remove any secretions that accumulate in the nasopharyngeal airway. Place the infant with the head of the bed slightly elevated to minimize aspiration of secretions into the trachea. Continuous or low intermittent suction via nasogastric tube is used to remove secretions from the blind pouch. Oral fluids are withheld, and the infant is maintained with fluids administered intravenously or through an umbilical artery catheter.

Postoperative Nursing Care

After surgery, gastrostomy drainage is maintained, and intravenous fluids and antibiotics are administered. Total parenteral nutrition may be required until gastrostomy or oral feedings are tolerated. Monitoring and assessment of feeding tolerance is ongoing. Feedings are introduced slowly and in small amounts. Assess for respiratory difficulty during reintroduction of feedings. Monitor weight and growth and developmental achievements.

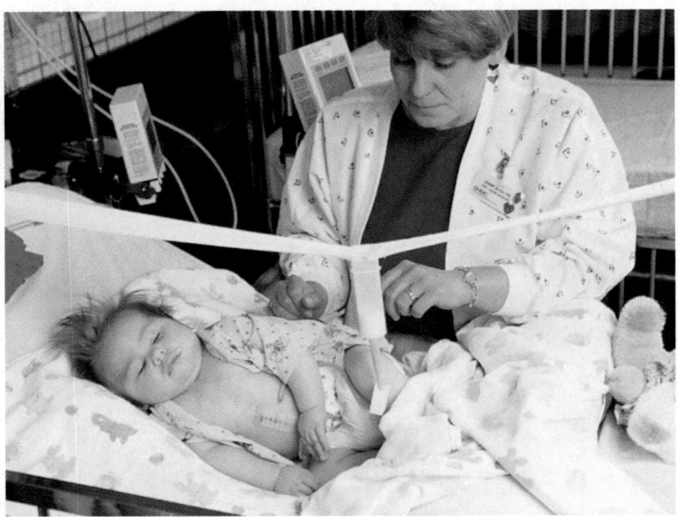

FIGURE 30–5 ■ Children with esophageal atresia and other gastrointestinal disorders often require a gastrostomy tube for feedings.

Some infants may have one surgery and progress without further complications, whereas others may require several surgical procedures and long-term intervention to ensure adequate nutrition, growth, and development.

Care in the Community

Once enteral feedings have been established, the infant may be discharged from the hospital with a gastrostomy tube in place (Figure 30–5 ■). (Refer to the Skills Manual for care of the child with a gastrostomy tube.) Collaborate with the parents regarding home care needs and teach them about gastrostomy tube care and feeding, signs of infection, and how to prevent postoperative complications. The family of an infant requiring multiple surgical procedures requires ongoing support. The infant is evaluated frequently for adequate nutrition, and growth and development patterns. See Partnering with Families: Home Care Instructions for the Child Requiring Gastrostomy Tube Feedings and Care.

■ Evaluation

Outcomes of nursing care depend on the extent of the defect and correction. Examples include the following:

- The infant demonstrates absence of respiratory distress.
- The infant achieves adequate intake of fluids to promote hydration and growth.
- The infant's nutritional intake is sufficient to meet growth and development needs.
- The infant is free from infection.
- Positive parent–infant bonding is demonstrated.

Pyloric Stenosis

Pyloric stenosis (also called hypertrophic pyloric stenosis) is a hypertrophy of the circular muscle of the pyloric canal causing obstruction. The disorder is common and most often affects first-born male infants. Pyloric stenosis occurs in approximately 1 to 4 cases per 1,000 live births and occurs 2 to 5 times more often in males than females, and is seen more in White children than in other races (Letton, 2001). Pyloric stenosis is a common cause of abdominal surgery in the first 6 months of life.

Etiology and Pathophysiology

The exact cause of pyloric stenosis is unknown although immature function or absence of pyloric ganglion cells has been suggested (Letton, 2001). Frequently there is a family history of the disorder.

Hypertrophy of the circular pylorus muscle results in stenosis of the passage between the stomach and the duodenum, partially obstructing the lumen of the stomach (Figure 30–6 ■). The lumen becomes inflamed and edematous, which narrows the gastric outlet opening until the obstruction becomes complete. At this time, vomiting becomes more forceful. As the obstruction progresses, the infant becomes dehydrated and electrolytes are depleted, resulting in metabolic imbalances.

Clinical Manifestations

Clinical manifestations usually become evident 2 to 8 weeks after birth, with peak incidence at 3 to 5 weeks (Letton, 2001), although onset may vary. Initially the infant appears well or regurgitates slightly after feedings. The parents may describe the infant as a "good eater" who vomits occasionally. The symptoms in the early stages may be erroneously attributed to overfeeding, milk allergy, feeding intolerance, or gastroesophageal reflux (Morash, 2002). As the obstruction progresses, the vomiting becomes projectile. In **projectile vomiting,** the contents of the stomach may be ejected up to 3 feet from the infant. The vomitus is nonbilious and may become blood tinged secondary to repeated irritation of the esophagus.

The infant generally appears hungry, especially after emesis, irritable, lethargic, fails to gain weight, and has fewer and smaller stools. Premature infants usually present symptoms sooner than term infants; however, their emesis is less projectile, resulting in delayed diagnosis (Letton, 2001). Loss of gastric secretions results in dehydration. On physical examination, visible peristaltic waves across the abdomen and an olive-sized mass in the right upper quadrant may be evident. Some infants have bloody gastric vomitus related to the mucosal erosion caused by gastritis or esophagitis.

COLLABORATIVE CARE

Collaborative care includes restoring fluid and electrolyte balance, correcting the defect, and preventing complications associated with the disorder.

Diagnostic Tests

An abdominal ultrasound is the most common study performed to confirm the diagnosis of pyloric stenosis, as the diameter and length of the pyloric muscle can be accurately measured. A thickened pylorus of >4 mm in diameter and length of >18 mm for the pyloric channel are diagnostic of pyloric stenosis (Blumer, Zucconi, Cohen, et al., 2004). An upper gastrointestinal (UGI) study may be performed. The UGI reveals a narrowing of the pyloric channel, preventing the passage of the contrast medium.

PARTNERING WITH FAMILIES

Home Care Instructions for the Child Requiring Gastrostomy Tube Feedings and Care

The nurse assists the family in learning care of gastrostomy tube and feedings. Provide the following information.

Equipment

- Prepared, prescribed feeding; enteral feeding pump; long-nosed syringe

Procedure

1. Wash hands.
2. Warm prescribed formula to room temperature.
3. Pour formula to run through the feeding bag.
4. Allow formula to run through the tubing to remove air. Close clamp.
5. Attach syringe to the end of the gastrostomy tube. Unclamp the gastrostomy tube.
6. Pull plunger back until resistance is felt. Check amount of formula in syringe. If more than half of the prescribed amount is withdrawn, refer to the section on problem solving. If less than the prescribed amount is withdrawn, push the formula gently back through the syringe.
7. Instill water through the tube.
8. Attach the feeding bag to the gastrostomy tube. Infuse at the prescribed rate.
9. Burp or bubble the infant throughout the feeding.
10. After feeding, flush the gastrostomy tube with water and clamp the tube.
11. Hold the infant or position the infant side lying with head elevated (NOT in sitting position) for 30 to 60 minutes after feedings.

Psychosocial needs

- Hold and rock the infant or child during feedings.
- Give a pacifier to an infant or a bottle or cup to a child to meet developmental needs.

Medication administration

- Use liquid medication when possible.
- Crush only uncoated tablets.
- Crush tablets to a fine powder and mix with water or juice.
- Flush tubing before and after medication administration.

Stoma care

- Wash the area around the stoma twice a day with soap and water.
- Use warm water and gentle washing to remove any crusting—do not scrub the area.
- Observe for signs of infection, such as redness, swelling, and discharge.
- Notify the primary care provider if any signs of infection or leakage are present.

Problem Solving

Problem	Cause	Action
Formula will not flow	Blocked tube (clamped, foreign material, viscous formula)	Check clamp Reposition Pull back on syringe Instill water Milk tube Notify primary care provider if actions do not resolve problem
	Pump malfunction	Check pump Call company if pump not working Administer feeding by gravity
Large volume of undigested formula removed before feeding	Delayed absorption	Reinfuse remaining formula If more than half of feeding, subtract from the next feeding Do not discard residual, but reinsert it
	Constipation	Check for last bowel movement Notify primary care provider
Constipation	Decreased free fluids	Give water and juice between feedings as tolerated Report bowel problems or hard stools to primary care provider
Diarrhea	Hyperosmolar formula Rapid rate of flow Cold formula	Dilute formula Feed at a slower rate Warm formula to room temperature before feeding
	Bacterial contamination	Treat with antibiotics
Dislodged tube	Inadequate stabilization	Bring child for emergency care
Skin irritation	Formula leakage	Provide skin care; barrier if needed

Data from Borkowski, S. (1998). Pediatric stomas, tubes, and appliances. Pediatric Clinics of North America, *45, 1419–1435; Young, C., & White, S. (1992). Preparing patients for tube feeding at home.* AJN, *92, 46–53.*

PATHOPHYSIOLOGY ILLUSTRATED

Pyloric Stenosis

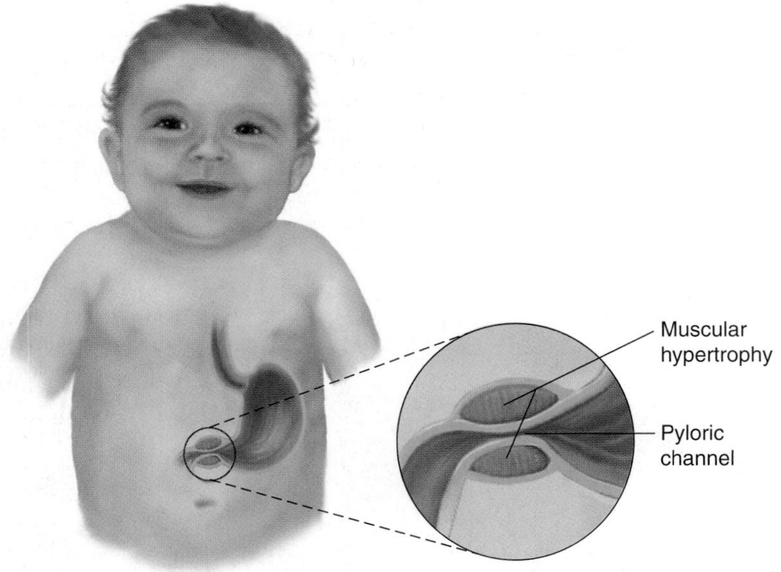

Muscular hypertrophy

Pyloric channel

FIGURE 30–6 ■ In pyloric stenosis, the hypertrophied pyloric muscle causes symptoms of projectile vomiting and visible peristalsis.

Due to the potential risk of vomiting and aspiration of barium following an UGI, the barium that is introduced is subsequently aspirated following the procedure (Morash, 2002). Serum electrolyte and acid-base measurements are used to determine the degree of dehydration, electrolyte imbalance, and anemia (see Chapter 23). Serum studies reveal hypochloremia, metabolic alkalosis, and hyperbilirubinemia.

Clinical Therapy

Preoperatively the infant's condition is stabilized with intravenous fluids and electrolytes. Antibiotics may be administered prophylactically. A nasogastric tube is inserted for gastric decompression if emesis is excessive.

Surgical correction (pyloromyotomy) is the treatment of choice. The surgery is performed as soon as possible after the infant's fluid and electrolyte balance is restored. Open pyloromyotomy is performed through a periumbilical incision or a small, transverse upper abdominal incision. Laparoscopic pyloromyotomy is now used, and patients undergoing this surgical method reach full feeding sooner, have less emesis, and require a shorter hospital stay than those having open procedure (Zitsman, 2003). With both procedures, the circular muscle fibers are released to allow the passage of food and fluid.

The prognosis postoperatively is good. Rare complications include infection and gastric or duodenal perforation (Morash, 2002). Although postoperative feeding schedules vary according to the surgeon, the infant is usually able to consume fluids within 6 hours following the procedure, and feedings are advanced according to protocol until full feedings are achieved. The infant is generally discharged the day following surgery.

In some countries, treatment of pyloric stenosis with intravenous atropine rather than surgery is showing promising results; further study is needed to learn if the treatment is safe and effective (Corner, 2003).

NURSING MANAGEMENT

Nursing care focuses on collaborative identification of the infant with pyloric stenosis, preventing complications such as dehydration, and preoperative and postoperative management.

Nursing Assessment and Diagnosis

Assess for signs and symptoms that may indicate the disorder. Observe the infant's abdomen for the presence of peristaltic waves. Bowel sounds are hyperactive on auscultation. Remember to auscultate for bowel sounds before palpating the abdomen because bowel patterns may change in response to the examiner's touch. Palpation reveals an olive-shaped mass in the right upper quadrant of the abdomen, especially when the stomach is empty such as following a vomiting episode.

Assess the infant's history of vomiting, vital signs, weight, and nutritional status. Assess skin turgor, fontanels, urinary output (weigh diapers), capillary refill, and mucous membranes to determine whether hydration is adequate. Measure vomitus and describe vomiting episodes. Be alert for signs of an electrolyte imbalance, particularly low levels of serum chloride, sodium, and potassium, and an elevated pH. (See Chapter 23 for a discussion of these electrolyte imbalances.) Assess parental anxiety related to the child's condition. The child is usually hungry and tries to feed. Crying and general discomfort are frequently observed.

Following are nursing diagnoses that may be appropriate for the child with pyloric stenosis.

- Deficient Fluid Volume related to active fluid volume loss
- Imbalanced Nutrition: Less than Body Requirements related to vomiting and inability to ingest nutrients
- Sleep Pattern Disturbed related to discomfort
- Pain related to surgical incision

Planning and Implementation

Nursing care centers on meeting the infant's fluid and electrolyte needs, minimizing weight loss, promoting rest and comfort, preventing infection, and providing supportive care for parents.

Meet Fluid and Electrolyte Needs

Oral feedings are withheld because they lead to projectile vomiting. Emphasize to the parents the importance of maintaining an NPO status preoperatively. Intravenous fluid therapy is administered to correct fluid and electrolyte imbalances and to maintain adequate hydration. Because gastric fluid is high in potassium, hypokalemia can result (see Chapter 23∞ for a discussion of this electrolyte imbalance and the signs of its occurrence). Monitor intake and output (including vomitus), blood urea nitrogen (BUN), creatinine, and urine specific gravity. Maintain patency of nasogastric tube and measure aspirated contents. Inform parents that all diapers will be weighed to measure the infant's output of urine and stool.

Postoperative reintroduction to fluids depends on the practitioner's preference. The traditional practice has been the slow reintroduction of feedings to prevent emesis. However, recent studies indicate that ad lib feedings once the infant has recovered from anesthesia are beneficial and do not result in more episodes of emesis (Morash, 2002). The infant is usually discharged after tolerating two feedings without emesis. See Evidence-Based Practice: Postoperative Feeding Methods Following Pyloromyotomy in Infants.

Minimize Weight Loss

The infant loses weight secondary to frequent vomiting. Monitor weight daily preoperatively and postoperatively. Begin formula or breast feedings according to protocol.

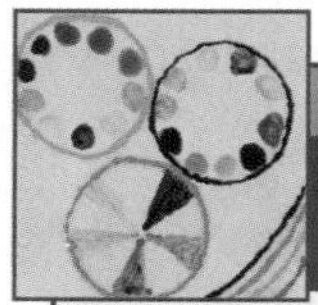

EVIDENCE-BASED PRACTICE

Postoperative Feeding Methods Following Pyloromyotomy in Infants

PROBLEM

Postoperative feeding methods for infants following surgical correction (pyloromyotomy) of pyloric stenosis have remained unchanged for several decades. Conventional feeding methods include a prolonged NPO period following pyloromyotomy, with slow, incremental increases in volume and strength of feedings once feeding has resumed. Recent evidence indicates that a more liberal feeding method may prove beneficial, rather than harmful, to the infant.

EVIDENCE

Nurse researchers, in collaboration with a pediatric surgeon, conducted a 6-month retrospective study of 36 hypertrophic pyloric stenosis patients to compare conventional regimen feeds to ad lib feeds according to surgeon preference (Morash, 2002). The study revealed that the interval from the operating room to toleration of full feedings was less with the ad lib group as compared to the conventional regimen group. Additionally, discharges occurred sooner in the ad lib group.

IMPLICATIONS

The interval from the operating room to toleration of full feeds was significantly less with the ad lib–fed infants compared to the conventionally fed infants. Significant decrease in length of stay was also noted. These findings led to practice changes at the hospital where the study was conducted.

CRITICAL THINKING APPLICATION

How is feeding tolerance determined in the post-pyloromyotomy infant? If a surgeon prescribes conventional regimen feeding for post-pyloromyotomy infants, what collaborative approach could the nurse take to improve the feeding approach?

Promote Rest and Comfort

During the preoperative period the infant is hungry and cries often. The infant is swaddled to maintain warmth and provide comfort. Encourage the parents to hold and cuddle the infant. Provide a pacifier to meet the infant's need to suck.

Postoperatively the infant is uncomfortable due to the surgical incision. Analgesics are administered routinely to relieve discomfort as ordered. (See Chapter 18∞ for a discussion of pain management.) Partner with the family and instruct parents to avoid pressure on the incision. Teach them when diapering the infant to slide the diaper gently under the buttocks rather than lifting the legs. Swaddling, rocking, and use of a pacifier provide comfort to the infant.

Prevent Infection

Postoperatively the incision is covered with collodion or Steri-Strips and should be kept clean and dry. Inspect the incision site for redness, swelling, or discharge. Monitor the infant's temperature every 4 hours. Auscultate lungs to assess for any adventitious breath sounds.

Provide Supportive Care

The need for hospitalization and surgery creates anxiety for parents. Collaborate care with the parents and encourage them to participate in the infant's care preoperatively and postoperatively. Encourage the parents to discuss their fears and concerns. Provide simple and clear explanations about the infant's condition and care. Advise parents that occasional vomiting after surgery may occur and the infant should continue to receive feedings.

Discharge Planning and Home Care Teaching

Instruct parents to observe the incision for redness, swelling, or discharge and to notify the physician immediately if these occur or if the infant's temperature is higher than 38.5°C (101°F). Continued vomiting and dehydration should be reported. To reduce the possibility of infection, advise parents to fold the infant's diaper so that it does not touch the incision. See Partnering with Families: Home Care Instructions Following Pyloromyotomy.

■ Evaluation

Expected outcomes of nursing care of the infant with pyloric stenosis include:

- The infant's fluid and electrolyte balance is restored.
- The infant achieves intake of recommended fluid and food with absence of vomiting.
- The infant experiences periods of rest and the family demonstrates implementation of comfort measures.
- The infant obtains relief of pain.

Intussusception

Intussusception occurs when one portion of the intestine prolapses and then invaginates or telescopes into another. This disorder is a frequent cause of intestinal obstruction during

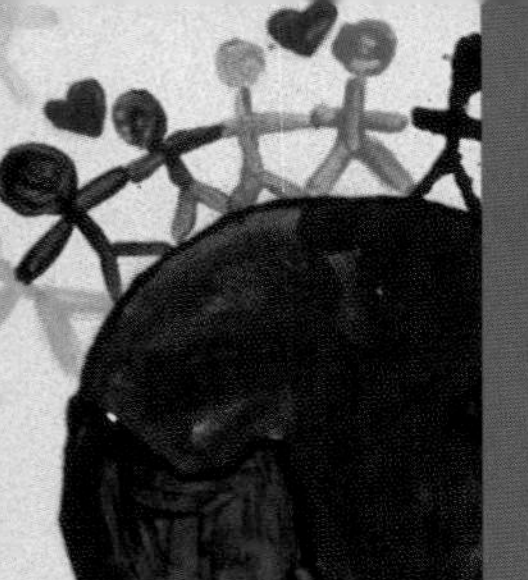

PARTNERING WITH FAMILIES

Home Care Instructions Following Pyloromyotomy

The infant is generally discharged home the day following surgery. Partner with the family to provide home feeding and care instructions. The following information is provided.

- The infant may bottle feed or breastfeed.
- An infant will sometimes vomit after feedings following surgery—this does not indicate the surgical correction was unsuccessful.
- If the infant vomits, offer breast or bottle as soon as interest in feeding resumes.
- The infant should be burped after every 1 to 2 ounces during feeding. If breastfeeding, burp the infant every 5 to 10 minutes.
- After feeding, place the baby in an upright position, holding for approximately 30 minutes, or position the infant on the right side with the head and upper body slightly elevated.
- The infant should not play or be rocked for 30 minutes following feedings.
- Administer analgesics as prescribed. Inform the healthcare provider if infant is not obtaining adequate pain relief.
- Keep the surgical wound area clean and dry. The bandage or strips may fall off, which is normal. If not, they will be removed at the follow-up visit.
- The infant should be sponge bathed only. Tub baths are avoided until the wound has healed or as instructed by the healthcare provider.
- Notify the healthcare provider if the infant demonstrates any of the following:
  - Redness, drainage, bleeding, or swelling at the surgical site
  - Fever of 100.5°F or higher
  - Inconsolable behavior
  - Vomiting the majority of two consecutive feedings

infancy, with an incidence of 1 to 4 in 1,000 births. Most cases occur in males between the ages of 3 months and 6 years (Wylie, 2004). Intussusception is more commonly observed in children with cystic fibrosis, celiac disease, and gastroenteritis.

Etiology and Pathophysiology

The etiology of intussusception is multifactorial and direct causes cannot always be identified. Virus infection, use of medications that influence gut motility, and the body's inflammatory mediators such as cytokine, nitric oxide, and prostaglandins are associated with increased rates of intussusception (Spiro, Arnold, & Barbone, 2003). Whatever the cause, decreased intestinal motility results, followed by impaired blood circulation to the intestinal tract involved. A proximal portion of the intestine invaginates into another portion of the intestine, typically in the direction of peristalsis. The walls of the intestine rub together, and the mesentery becomes compressed, resulting in inflammation, edema, obstruction, and decreased blood flow. Telescoping of the intestine obstructs the passage of stool. If uncorrected, intussusception can lead to life-threatening complications associated with necrosis, perforation, hemorrhage, and peritonitis. The most common site of intussusception is the ileocecal valve (Figure 30–7 ■).

Clinical Manifestations

The onset of intussusception is usually abrupt. A previously healthy infant or child suddenly experiences acute abdominal pain with vomiting and passage of brown stool. The infant may experience periods of comfort between acute episodes of pain. As the condition worsens, painful episodes increase. The stools become red and resemble currant jelly because of the mixture of blood and mucus. A long, cylindrical palpable mass may be present in the upper right quadrant or mid-upper abdomen. Rectal bleeding may also occur (Klein, Kapoor, & Shugerman, 2004).

COLLABORATIVE CARE

Collaborative care focuses on reducing the bowel compression and restoring fluid and electrolyte balance.

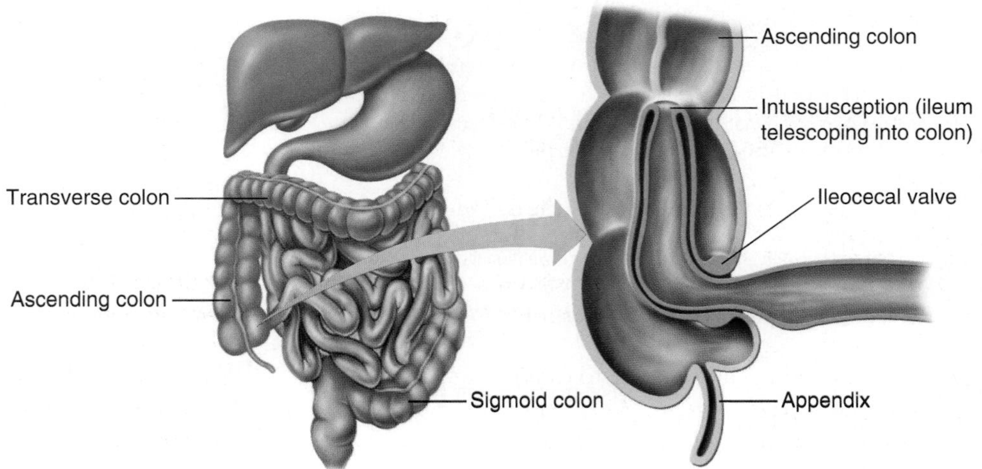

FIGURE 30–7 ■ In infants, intussusception is commonly associated with measles, viral disease, and gastroenteritis syndromes.

Diagnostic Tests

Diagnosis is made on the basis of the history and confirmed by radiographs and ultrasound of the abdomen (Orenstein, 2000). A contrast enema, which may utilize barium, or air, or a combination of both, is a common diagnostic study. Stool is tested for gross or occult blood (Klein et al., 2004). Hemoglobin and hematocrit are tested to assess for blood anemia from blood loss. Electrolytes are assessed before surgical intervention.

Clinical Therapy

In some cases, the hydrostatic pressure from the barium moves the bowel back into place. Oxygen, saline, and aqueous contrast material may also be used to reduce the intussusception. A nasogastric tube is inserted for gastric decompression. If reduction of the intussusception does not occur with these methods, surgical intervention to reduce the invaginated bowel and remove any necrotic tissue is necessary. Surgery is generally successful in correcting the problem; however, intussusception can recur after hydrostatic reduction or surgical correction.

NURSING MANAGEMENT

Nursing management focuses on maintaining or restoring fluid and electrolyte balance. Intravenous fluids are initiated immediately.

■ Nursing Assessment and Diagnosis

Preoperative assessment includes vital signs, monitoring for abdominal distention, and auscultating for bowel sounds every 4 hours. Monitor intravenous intake. Monitor urine output and measure any vomitus. Assess for number and characteristics of stools. Assess the infant or child for guarding of the abdomen. Monitor serum electrolytes.

> **PRACTICE ALERT**
>
> The passage of a normal brown stool may indicate that an intussusception has been reduced. Report this finding to the primary care provider immediately, as the course of treatment may be altered, especially in the case of a planned surgical reduction.

Postoperative assessment includes vital signs, bowel sounds, and intake and output. Assess surgical incision site. Assess for evidence of pain.

Nursing diagnoses that may apply to the child with intussusception include:

- Acute Pain related to bowel compression
- Ineffective Tissue Perfusion (gastrointestinal) related to bowel compression
- Deficient Fluid Volume related to vomiting and inability to consume foods/fluids with painful episodes
- Anxiety (parental and child) related to child's emergency condition

■ Planning and Implementation

Preoperative care focuses on relieving the child's pain and preparing the child and family for the surgical procedure. Maintain patent nasogastric tube.

Postoperative care focuses on monitoring for early signs of infection, managing the child's pain, and maintaining nasogastric tube patency. Feeding protocols vary among practitioners. Generally, after normal bowel function returns, clear liquid feeding or breastfeeding is begun. Feedings are then advanced to half-strength milk and other foods as the infant or child tolerates them.

Discharge occurs shortly after the infant or child begins taking full feedings. Partner with the family to ensure parents understand how to monitor the child for signs of infection, such as fever, wound drainage, and fussiness, and the importance of notifying the primary healthcare provider if symptoms recur or appetite decreases.

■ Evaluation

Expected outcomes for nursing care of the child with intussusception include the following:

- The child obtains pain relief.
- The child demonstrates patent bowel function, with relief of intussusception through reduction.
- The child achieves fluid and electrolyte balance.
- The parents and child express their fears and concerns and receive adequate emotional support.

Abdominal Wall Defects

In early fetal life, the intestines are extraabdominal, and move intraabdominally by about 11 weeks of gestation. The two most common congenital defects of the anterior abdominal wall are gastroschisis and omphalocele, which are discussed in this section.

Gastroschisis

Gastroschisis is a congenital defect of the ventral abdominal wall, characterized by herniation of abdominal viscera outside the abdominal cavity through a defect in the abdominal wall to the side (most often to the right) of the umbilicus. The most common abdominal organs involved are the small intestine and ascending colon, and no membrane covers the organs (Figure 30–8 ■). The umbilical cord is usually intact. The defect occurs in approximately 1 in 10,000 births, with incidence increasing in developed countries over the last decade. The disorder has an 8% mortality rate (Weir, 2003). Associated anomalies, other than cryptorchidism and intestinal atresia, are rare. Prognosis is determined primarily by the neurologic and vascular condition of the exposed bowel.

The cause of gastroschisis is multifactorial and involves vascular disruption of the fetal mesenteric vessels. Gastroschisis is more common in young mothers, particularly with a history of low socioeconomic status, smoking, and poor nutritional status.

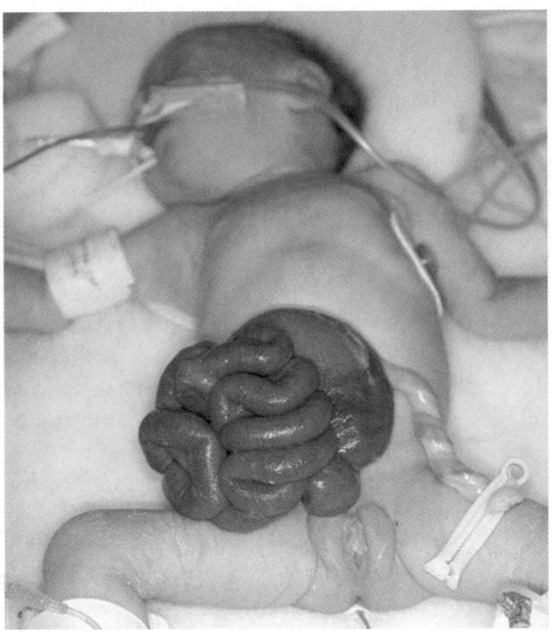

FIGURE 30–8 ■ The newborn with gastroschisis has abdominal contents located outside the abdominal wall.

Copyright protected material used with permission of the authors and the University of Iowa's Virtual Hospital®, www.vh.org.

Some over-the-counter medications, including ephedrine, and phenylpropanolamine, have also been implicated (Weir, 2003; Salihu, Boos, & Schmidt, 2002).

Omphalocele

Omphalocele is a congenital malformation in which intraabdominal contents herniate through the umbilical cord (Figure 30–9 ■). The defect results from failure of the abdominal contents, such as intestines and liver, to return to the abdomen when the abdominal wall begins to close by the eleventh week of gestation. Unlike gastroschisis, the tissues are covered by a translucent sac (peritoneum) into which the umbilical cord inserts. The size of the sac varies depending on the extent of the protrusion. Rupture of the sac results in evisceration of the abdominal contents. The defect can involve any abdominal organ; however, the large or small intestine, stomach, liver, gallbladder, pancreas, spleen, urinary bladder, or internal genitalia are most common.

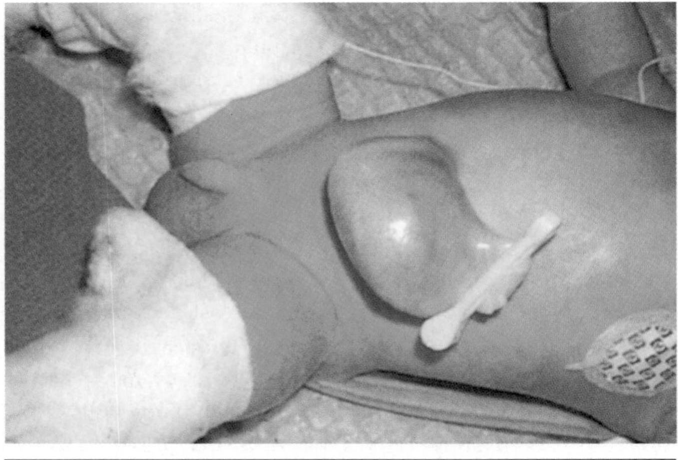

FIGURE 30–9 ■ In omphalocele, the size of the sack depends on the extent of the protrusion of abdominal contents through the umbilical cord.

From Rudolph, A. M., Hoffman, J. I. E., & Rudolph, C. D. (Eds). (1991). Rudolph's pediatrics *(19th ed., p. 1040). Stamford, CT: Appleton & Lange.*

Omphalocele is often associated with other congenital anomalies such as cardiac defects; genitourinary anomalies; trisomy 13, 18, or 21; craniofacial abnormalities; and diaphragmatic abnormalities (Weir, 2003). One example of a combination of anomalies is the chromosomal condition Beckwith-Weideman syndrome, characterized by omphalocele, macrosomia, macroglossia, ear fissures, facial hemangioma, and mental retardation. Omphalocele with intestinal contents in the sac occurs in 1.25 in 5,000 births, while those involving liver and intestines occur less often (Weir, 2003). The prognosis for a child with omphalocele is related to the presence of associated chromosomal and structural anomalies. The mortality rate is approximately 80% for cases with associated cardiac defects (Weir, 2003); without associated anomalies, the condition is usually successfully treated.

COLLABORATIVE CARE

Care of the child with gastroschisis or omphalocele centers on protecting the protruding abdominal organs, correcting the defect, and preventing complications such as hypothermia, infection, and injury to involved organs.

Diagnostic Tests

Diagnosis of both defects is confirmed by prenatal ultrasound or at birth. Since the intestines are normally extraabdominal until the eleventh week of gestation, diagnosis of abdominal wall defect is delayed until the fourteenth week of gestation to avoid an inaccurate diagnosis (Weir, 2003). Amniocentesis for karyotype analysis may be performed since some conditions are associated with chromosomal abnormalities.

Both gastroschisis and omphalocele are associated with elevation of maternal serum alpha-fetoprotein (MSAFP). Routine prenatal ultrasonography and determination of MSAFP levels permit early diagnosis and mobilization of the multidisciplinary team of obstetricians, geneticists, neonatologists, and pediatric surgeons needed to manage these congenital anomalies.

Clinical Therapy

The immediate action upon birth is to protect the sac (in omphalocele) or exposed abdominal contents (in gastroschisis) from injury by applying warm, sterile, saline-soaked dressings over defect. Temperature regulation is needed for the newborn due to heat loss through exposed viscera. Fluids are required to replace those lost through viscera. Blood cultures are performed before administering antibiotics. Orogastric or nasogastric tube may be inserted to prevent distention. A thorough examination is performed to rule out cardiac and other abnormalities.

In omphalocele, unlike gastroschisis, the extruded abdominal contents are covered by a two-layer membrane, making management of fluid losses and electrolyte stability less complicated than with gastroschisis.

Clinical therapy has usually consisted of urgent surgical reduction; however, aggressive attempts at primary closure can greatly increase abdominal pressure, resulting in impaired ventilation and vascular compromise and leading to bowel perforation and necrotizing enterocolitis. Current trends are to suture a prosthetic silo around the defect. The silo permits gradual return of the intestines to the abdominal cavity over 5 to 10 days as the cavity slowly enlarges (Weir, 2003). After the return of the intestines into the abdominal cavity, primary closure of epidermal and subdermal tissue is performed. Attainment of bowel motility and function varies and is often delayed for weeks after surgery. Parenteral nutrition for the infant is used during this period (Ashburn, Pranikoff, & Turner, 2002).

NURSING MANAGEMENT

Nursing care of the newborn with omphalocele or gastroschisis centers on protecting the sac or protruding organs, preventing hypothermia, preventing and identifying infection, providing preoperative and postoperative care, and supporting the family.

Nursing Assessment and Diagnosis

Assess for signs of associated congenital anomalies. (Refer to the discussions of tracheoesophageal fistula earlier in this chapter, to genitourinary anomalies in Chapter 31∞, and to congenital heart defects in Chapter 26∞.) Assess the integrity of the sac in omphalocele. Assess vital signs at least every hour.

Nursing diagnoses that apply to the newborn with omphalocele or gastroschisis include:

- Deficient Fluid Volume related to fluid loss through exposed abdominal organs
- Risk for Infection related to exposed abdominal organs
- Hypothermia related to heat loss through exposed abdominal organs
- Pain related to surgical incision
- Risk for Impaired Parent/Infant Attachment related to congenital defect, emergent surgery, and potential loss of neonate
- Anxiety (parental) related to threat to infant's health status

Planning and Implementation

During hospitalization of their child, parents require clear, accurate explanations about the infant's condition. Partner with the family to help the parents deal with the crisis of an acutely ill newborn, provide emotional support, and encourage parents to express their feelings. When the child has multiple anomalies, parents require ongoing support for the lengthy treatment, numerous hospitalizations, and management of nutritional intake. Referral to counselor or social services may be helpful to the family. In addition, the nurse provides intensive care to the infant before and after correction of the defect. Monitoring of health status, as well as providing comfort measures and nutritional support, are important nursing actions.

Preoperative Nursing Care

Immediately after birth, the omphalocele sac is covered with sterile gauze soaked in normal saline solution to prevent drying of the abdominal contents. A layer of sterile plastic wrap is placed over the gauze to provide additional protection against infection and loss of heat and moisture. Closely monitor temperature, as the infant can lose heat through the sac. The infant is placed in a warmer or isolette for maintenance of temperature control. Inspect the infant carefully for signs of infection. Because the infant is NPO preoperatively, fluid and electrolyte balance is maintained by administering intravenous fluids. Maintain orogastric or nasogastric tube patency. When the contents are reduced through a silo, intense monitoring of vital signs, sterile management to prevent infection, and supervision of fluid and electrolytes are needed.

Postoperative Nursing Care

Postoperative care includes measures to control pain, prevent infection, maintain fluid and electrolyte balance, and ensure adequate parenteral nutritional intake until oral intake is achieved. Administer pain medication routinely. Monitor vital signs several times hourly until stable, then according to protocol of the unit. Maintain parenteral nutrition as ordered. Promote parent–infant attachment by encouraging parents to participate in infant's care when feasible. Encourage touching, stroking, and soft talking to the infant. Ask about the family's distance from the hospital and ability to manage the child's condition once discharged. Refer to social services and other resources as needed.

Evaluation

Expected outcomes of nursing care of the neonate with gastroschisis or omphalocele may include the following:

- The neonate achieves fluid volume balance.
- The neonate is free from infection.
- The neonate maintains stable thermoregulatory function.
- The neonate obtains pain relief.
- Parents and infant demonstrate bonding and attachment.

Anorectal Malformations

Malformations of the anus and rectum are common congenital anomalies, occurring in approximately 1 in 5,000 live births (Gereige & Frias, 2002). They are often associated with anomalies of the genitourinary tract, esophagus, duodenum, musculoskeletal system, craniofacial area, cardiovascular system, and chromosomal abnormalities (Cho, Moore, & Fangman, 2001). The etiology of these malformations is not totally described, although a failure occurs in embryologic developmental sequences involving structures forming the normal rectum and lower urinary tract.

Associated anomalies are present in a majority of newborns with anorectal malformation. Approximately 30% of neonates demonstrate urinary abnormalities (commonly hydronephrosis), 38% have vertebral problems such as spina bifida, while other abnormalities include cardiac defect, tracheoesophageal fistula, and gastrointestinal and genital disruptions (Ratan, Ratan, Pandey, et al., 2004). Chromosomal abnormalities such as trisomy 13, 18, or 21 may coexist, and some babies have VACTERL conditions. VACTERL refers to three or more anomalies of vertebral formation, anal atresia, congenital heart disease, tracheoesophageal fistula, renourinary anomalies, and radial limb defects (Davies, Creighton, & Wilcox, 2004).

Anal Stenosis

Anal stenosis, a thickened and constricted anal wall, accounts for approximately 20% of anorectal malformations. Anal dilatation is the usual treatment for anal stenosis and may need to be continued for several months. Ribbonlike stools are characteristic until the anus is dilated.

Anal Atresia

Anal atresia affects males and females equally. Perineal inspection at birth reveals the absent anal opening. Failure to pass meconium is diagnostic for the condition. Stool in the urine usually indicates the presence of a fistula between the colon and urinary tract. Cloacal malformations in females, in which the urinary tract, vagina, and rectum drain through a common channel, may occur (Adzik & Nance, 2000).

Anal atresia is characterized as high or low, depending on where the rectum ends, either above the levator muscle or partially descending through this muscle and ending near the perineal floor. Often, the rectum ends in a fistula. In high anal atresia, the fistula often ends in the prostatic urethra in males and in the vagina in females.

Neonates with a low type of anal atresia usually have a well-formed sacrum, a prominent midline groove, and a prominent anal dimple. Low lesions are associated with a cutaneous fistula to the perineum. The orifice is usually located in the perineum anterior to the center of the external anal sphincter, close to the scrotum in the male and the vulva in the female. The abnormal anterior position of the fistula opening may be mistaken for the anus.

Anal atresia requires surgical correction to preserve bowel, urinary, and sexual function. A colostomy is initially performed in neonates with high anal atresia. Low lesions, including those with perineal fistulas, are corrected electively when the infant's condition is stable.

COLLABORATIVE CARE

Collaborative care focuses on preservation of bowel, urinary, and sexual function, as well as treatment of any associated abnormalities.

Diagnostic Tests

Diagnosis for both defects is usually made at birth or during the newborn assessment of anorectal structures and rectal patency. Ultrasound and lower gastrointestinal radiographic studies are used to confirm the diagnosis and demonstrate the extent of the anomaly. Anorectal manometry may be performed. Careful physical examination of all body systems is performed to identify any associated abnormalities.

Clinical Therapy

Management depends on the extent of the malformation and presence of associated conditions. Some anal stenosis can usually be treated with dilation alone. An imperforate anal membrane (Figure 30–10 ■) is excised surgically, followed by daily manual dilations.

Anal atresia requires reconstructive surgery. A temporary colostomy is frequently performed after reconstruction or for a high anal atresia. Closure of the colostomy is generally performed between the age of 6 months and 1 year.

NURSING MANAGEMENT

Nursing care focuses on newborn assessment of anal patency, preoperative and postoperative care, and family support.

■ Nursing Assessment and Diagnosis

During the initial newborn assessment, the perineal area is inspected for a poorly developed anal dimple or sacral anomalies. Observe and record passage of meconium. Carefully assess all body systems and promptly report abnormal findings. Be particularly alert for cardiac, respiratory, and urinary output problems.

CLINICAL TIP

Rectal thermometers are no longer recommended for use in determining rectal patency. Passage of stool is observed or elicitation of the anal wink reflex for appropriate anatomical position of the anus is used instead.

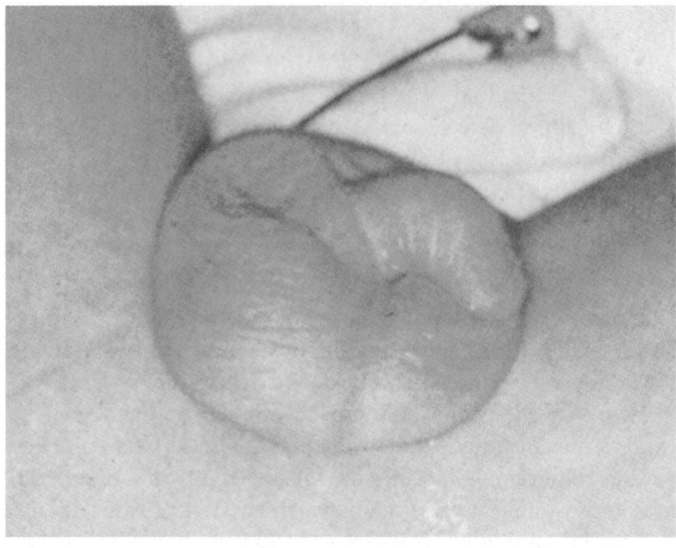

FIGURE 30–10 ■ Imperforate anus, which is often obvious at birth, can range from mild stenosis to a complex syndrome that includes associated congenital anomalies.

Nursing diagnoses that may apply to the infant with anorectal malformation include:

- Acute Pain related to surgical incision
- Anxiety (parental) related to infant's health status
- Risk for Infection related to impaired skin integrity (surgical incision)
- Risk for Deficient Fluid Volume related to NPO status
- Deficient Knowledge (parental) related to care of stoma

Planning and Implementation

Once the diagnosis of anorectal malformation has been made, intravenous fluids are initiated and a nasogastric tube is inserted to decompress the stomach. Monitor the child's intake and output and cardiorespiratory functioning. Provide emotional support to the parents and information about the planned treatments and surgery.

Postoperative care centers on preventing infection and respiratory complications from surgery, as well as maintaining hydration. Observe the incision for signs of infection, and provide careful wound care. Assess vital signs at least every 15 to 60 minutes after surgery.

Once the child's condition is stable, clear fluid oral intake or breast milk is allowed, advancing to half- and full-strength formula as tolerated.

The infant with a colostomy after surgery requires careful skin care around the stoma to prevent breakdown of the fragile area. Colostomy care is discussed in this chapter in the following section.

Discharge Planning and Home Care Teaching

All newborns are increasingly discharged from maternal-newborn units shortly after birth. Therefore, all parents require clear instructions about normal newborn stools and what abnormalities to report so that anorectal defects not obvious at birth are identified early.

For infants with a diagnosed abnormality, partner with the family to teach parents how to monitor the infant's temperature using the axillary route (see the Skills Manual). Have them demonstrate the proper technique before discharge. Explain the signs and symptoms of infection. Discuss feeding regimens and bowel habits necessary to maintain adequate nutrition for growth and development.

If a colostomy is performed, teach parents how to care for the ostomy site. Reassure parents that the colostomy will be closed in the future, and assist them in planning for that hospitalization. Discuss follow-up care and long-term management. Arrange follow-up and home care visits to evaluate the child's ostomy site and monitor growth. At later visits, advise parents that children with anorectal malformations may have difficulty achieving bowel control. Emphasize to parents that patience in toilet training is important and that some use of enemas may be needed to evacuate the bowel and achieve control. When the child reaches an age that is appropriate for toilet training, encourage the family to speak with a healthcare provider to discuss a plan for establishing continence and to monitor the child's progress.

The child with associated abnormalities may need several surgeries and interventions to treat all of the conditions present. Partnering with families and the healthcare team will assist in case management that facilitates the child's health and development. Health promotion and maintenance in regard to support of family members, ensuring immunizations, and monitoring developmental status is important.

Evaluation

Expected outcomes of nursing care include:

- The infant obtains pain relief.
- Parents express fears and concerns and receive adequate emotional support.
- The child is free from infection.
- The child maintains fluid and electrolyte balance.
- Parents demonstrate understanding of ostomy care and other treatment protocols.

OSTOMY

An intestinal **ostomy** is an opening, or **stoma**, into the small or large intestine that diverts fecal matter, to provide an outlet when a distal surgical anastomosis, obstruction, or nonfunctioning structures prevent normal elimination (Figure 30–11 ■). Depending on the integrity and function of anatomic structures, the ostomy may be temporary or permanent. Infants and small children with imperforate anus, necrotizing enterocolitis, Hirschsprung disease, volvulus, or intussusception may require a temporary or permanent colostomy or ileostomy. Ostomies may also be indicated for children with inflammatory bowel disease, intestinal tumors, or abdominal trauma.

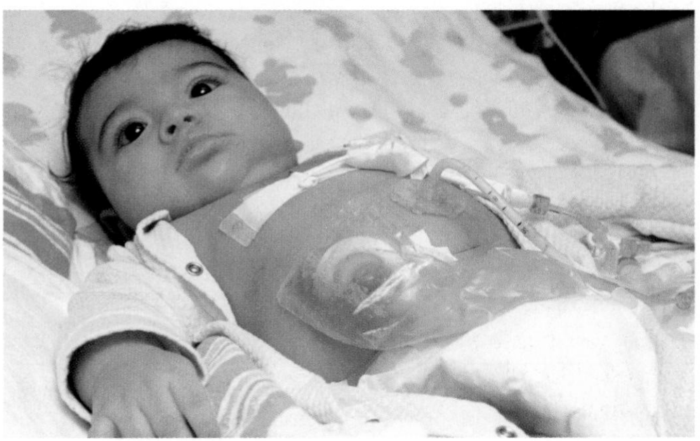

FIGURE 30–11 ■ This infant has several gastrointestinal problems and requires ostomies both for gastric feedings and for drainage of fecal material. Note the appearance of a healthy stoma.

An ostomy may be elective or a surgical emergency. In all cases it affects a child's lifestyle, alters body image, causes anxiety, and increases the risk for alterations in physiologic processes (electrolyte imbalance, increased nutritional requirements). For adolescents, it may also result in dependence at a time when autonomy is a major developmental need (Figure 30–12 ■).

When assessing the family and child approaching ostomy surgery, it is important to determine their ability to understand and accept the physical changes that will occur. Parents may feel guilt and anger about the ostomy surgery when the child has a genetically transmitted disease, has sustained an injury, or has developed an obstruction from necrosis of the bowel. Encourage parents and child to express their feelings, and correct any misunderstandings. Parents and older children may be referred for counseling and to support groups to help them deal with their feelings. Adolescents often benefit from a visit with an adolescent ostomate (someone who has an ostomy) who can answer questions about living with an ostomy.

Nursing Management

Nursing care focuses on preoperative teaching of the child and family and postoperative care of the child.

Preoperative Care

Preoperative education focuses on educating the child and family and preparing them for postoperative management. Discuss how the appliance will look, and explain the purpose of the pouch in developmentally appropriate terms. Provide examples of pouches and other stoma equipment. Encourage parents and child to touch and manipulate all equipment. A younger child can be shown how to place a pouch on a doll. Older children can practice placing a pouch on their skin. These measures help relieve anxiety by providing information and increasing familiarity with the appliance.

In addition to discussion of the appliance, preoperative education includes discussion of pain management (see Chapter 18) and measures that will be used to prevent postoperative complications. Instructions are geared to the child's developmental level. Encourage parental participation to promote compliance.

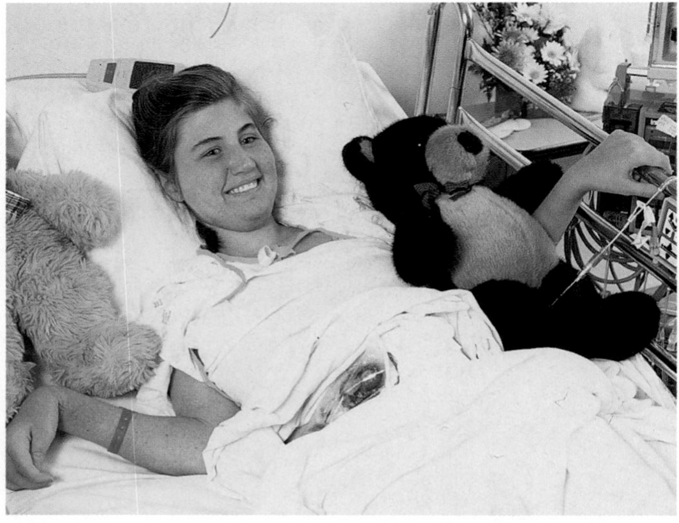

MediaLink Ostomy Resources and Support

FIGURE 30–12 ■ Nursing strategies to address altered perception of body image and increased feelings of dependence are important when working with adolescents who have ostomies. Support groups or a visit from another teenager who has had an ostomy can facilitate positive coping, as demonstrated by this adolescent female.

Postoperative Care

Postoperative care of a child with an ostomy is similar to that for any child who undergoes abdominal surgery. (See the earlier discussion in this chapter for the child having abdominal surgery and the nursing care plan for the child undergoing surgery in Chapter 17.) Management of the stoma may be coordinated by an ostomy nurse or other nurses. Major interventions involve ensuring proper function of the stoma, identifying complications, and instituting daily stoma care. See Table 30–2.

Assess the stoma, quality and amount of fecal matter, skin condition, and adherence of the pouch. Evaluate the understanding and ability of the family to care for the ostomy.

Care in the Community

Home care needs are identified and addressed well in advance of discharge. Instructions include skin and stoma care, appliance removal and application, and frequency of appliance changes.

CLINICAL TIP

Avoid adhesive enhancers on the skin of newborns and premature infants. Their skin layers are so thin that removal of the appliance can strip off the skin. Remember also that adhesive contains latex and its constant use is not advised due to risk of latex allergy development (see Chapter 27).

Teaching begins immediately after surgery with responsibility for care transferred gradually to the parents and child. See Partnering with Families: Assisting Families to Encourage Child's Participation in Stoma Care. (For information on caring for an ostomy, refer to the Skills Manual.) Discuss diet, activity level, hygiene, clothing, equipment, and financial considerations. Arrange for home visits to check periodically on the home management program.

Parents and children can be referred to the United Ostomy Association or a local ostomy group for information and support. Referrals should be made to social service, counseling, and a home health agency, if appropriate.

Expected outcomes of nursing care include the child's successful adjustment to the ostomy, thorough evacuation of the bowel, absence of infection and other complications, intact skin, and formation of a positive self-image in the child.

HERNIAS

A **hernia** is the protrusion or projection of an organ or a part of an organ through the muscle wall of the cavity that normally contains it. This protrusion may result from the failure of normal openings to close during fetal development or from weakness in

TABLE 30–2 Common Complications in Children with Stomas

COMPLICATION	CLINICAL THERAPY	NURSING IMPLICATIONS
Bowel prolapse through the stoma	If not engorged, prolapses can reduce spontaneously or be rolled back using a cold pack Surgical repair required if there is danger of bowel ischemia	Assess for bowel prolapse Teach family to assess for bowel prolapse
Stenosis of stoma	Pain and cramping associated with stenosis can be treated with manual dilatation, stool softeners, or surgery	Assess for pain and cramping
Parastomal hernia	Abdominal support garments may be helpful Hernias can be a source of embarrassment for the child because of fear the colostomy may be visible Approximately 10% of those developing parastomal hernias will require surgical intervention	Assess for difficulty in appliance adherence since this may be a problem associated with herniation Encourage child to verbalize feelings
Pain	Phantom pain or rectal fullness may be experienced, particularly after abdominoperineal resection These sensations often do not respond well to analgesics	Encourage use of nonpharmacologic methods for pain relief Suggest methods such as guided imagery and drawing
Flatus	Filters can be incorporated to prevent distension of the bag with flatus	Teach child and family that a well-balanced diet is essential to growth and development Teach the child and family about gas-causing foods: beans, leeks, excessive fiber, onions
Constipation	Moderate fiber intake with appropriate water consumption for age can help avoid constipation	Teach child and family that high-fiber foods (nuts, popcorn, dried fruits) can cause bolus obstruction
Diarrhea	Diarrhea is commonly seen in children with ileostomies and proximal colostomies because fluid outputs are normal in these situations due to loss of water absorption from the colon	Teach the child and family about appropriate fluid replacement according to age
Leakage and odor	Sigmoid or descending colon ostomies create solid intermittent output and require a closed bag that can be changed one to three times daily Ileostomies and colostomies that drain the proximal colon create frequent liquid or semisolid outputs and require a bag that can be drained and resealed several times per day Leakage, commonly caused by skin irregularities around the stoma, may require fillers of paste or wafers to provide a smooth surface for attachment	Assist the child and family with determining appropriate interventions for leakage Assist the child and family to choose from drops, powders, and sprays that are used to absorb odors
Skin problems	If the affected area of skin is close to the stoma, the flange opening may be too large, which allows bowel products to be in prolonged contact with skin	Assess for appropriate sizing of flange Teach child and family that bleeding usually is attributable to excessive cleaning Skin irritation and maceration often indicate leakage Teach the child and family that physical or chemical skin irritation may occur if the appliance is changed too frequently
Psychosocial issues (body image and social acceptance)	Child is evaluated for psychosocial issues	Recommend support groups and organizations to assist the child with self-esteem and social isolation issues Nurses specializing in stoma care can also assist the child and family Recommend counseling for the child who demonstrates depression or difficulty coping

Data from Walling, A. D. (2004). Multidimensional care of patients with colostomy. American Family Physician, *69(1), 193.*

MediaLink Nursing in Action: Changing an Ostomy Pouch

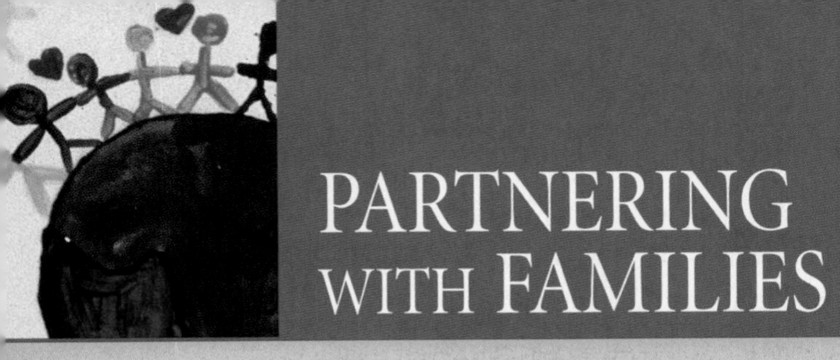

PARTNERING WITH FAMILIES

Assisting Families to Encourage Child's Participation in Stoma Care

Partner with parents to assist in understanding the abilities of the child at various developmental stages when planning the promotion of self-care.

- The preschooler has some manual dexterity and can help with parts of the procedure for changing an ostomy appliance and cleaning the stoma. The child should be taught using a doll or stuffed animal.
- Many school-age children are able to care for their ostomy independently. They should be taught how to avoid leakage around the bag, which could be embarrassing.
- Adolescents are generally totally independent in their self-care of ostomies; however, they may need support to deal with the fact that they are different from their peers.

the supporting musculature. When intraabdominal pressure increases (as when the infant cries or strains to pass stool), the weakened area separates, causing a protrusion of underlying organs. Inguinal hernias are the most common type of hernia occurring in children (see Chapter 31∞). Other hernias occurring frequently in children are congenital diaphragmatic hernias and umbilical hernias, which are discussed in this section.

Congenital Diaphragmatic Hernia

In a diaphragmatic hernia, abdominal contents protrude into the thoracic cavity through an opening in the diaphragm. Sites of herniation include the substernal space, posterolateral region, and the esophageal hiatus. The posterolateral site (foramen of Bochdalek) is the most common location.

Etiology and Pathophysiology

The cause of diaphragmatic hernia is a delay or failure in closure of the pleuroperitoneal musculature which forms the diaphragm. The diaphragm, which divides the thoracic and abdominal components, develops between 8 and 10 weeks' gestation.

Intestines and other abdominal structures enter the thoracic cavity through the opening in the diaphragm. The overall incidence of diaphragmatic hernia is 1 in 2,500 live births (Singh, Bhende, & Kinnane, 2001). Associated anomalies, particularly cardiac defects, occur in some infants. Pulmonary hypoplasia occurs secondary to intrauterine compression of the developing lungs by the herniated viscera (Adzik & Nance, 2000).

Clinical Manifestations

A diaphragmatic hernia is a life-threatening condition. Severe respiratory distress occurs shortly after birth. As the infant cries, abdominal organs extend into the thorax, decreasing the size of the thoracic cavity. The infant becomes dyspneic, with nasal flaring, tachypnea, and retractions. Cyanosis is also present. Characteristic findings include a barrel-shaped chest and sunken abdomen. Diminished or absent breath sounds are noted on the affected side. Bowel sounds may be auscultated over the chest. Heart tones may be auscultated on the right side of the chest. Pneumothorax may be an associated complication.

Rarely, diaphragmatic hernias may present after the neonatal period (Singh et al., 2001). The most common symptoms associated with delayed presentation of diaphragmatic hernia include respiratory distress and pneumonia.

COLLABORATIVE CARE

Collaborative care centers on immediate preservation of life, establishing ventilatory support, supporting fluid balance, and surgical correction of defect.

Diagnostic Tests

Congenital diaphragmatic hernia may be diagnosed in utero by ultrasound. If not identified prenatally, the condition is first identified postnatally by physical signs and symptoms; confirmation is made by chest radiologic examination. MRI is helpful in confirming the diagnosis and in determining the position of organs in the chest and abdomen (Hedrick, Crombleholme, Flake, et al., 2004).

Clinical Therapy

When a diaphragmatic hernia is diagnosed in utero, close prenatal observation and delivery at a facility with the capability of extracorporeal membrane oxygenation (ECMO) is recommended (Hedrick et al., 2004).

At the time of delivery, immediate respiratory support is essential. The infant is positioned with the head and thorax higher than the abdomen to facilitate downward movement of abdominal organs. Endotracheal intubation and ventilator support is necessary to manage respiratory compromise. A nasogastric tube is inserted to decompress the stomach. Intravenous fluids are administered through an umbilical artery catheter.

Once the infant's condition is stabilized, surgery is performed to correct the defect. ECMO may be used to provide cardiopulmonary bypass to rest the lungs (refer to Chapter 26∞ for discussion of ECMO).

Recent studies suggest the use of inhaled nitric oxide (iNO) and high-frequency oxygen ventilation (HFVO) preoperatively instead of ECMO improve survival outcomes and decrease concomitant morbidity (Bagolan, Casaccia, Crescenzi, et al., 2004).

The prognosis for the neonate is poor. Only 50% of infants survive, with death usually resulting from pulmonary hypoplasia. Even after surgery, the infant may do well initially and then manifest severe respiratory decompensation. Concomitant morbidity associated with diaphragmatic hernia includes pulmonary hypertension, hearing loss, tracheostomy, and neurologic impairment.

NURSING MANAGEMENT

Nursing care centers on maintaining ventilatory support of the infant, preoperative preparation, postoperative care, and supporting the family during this life-threatening event.

Nursing Assessment and Diagnosis

Assess the infant's vital signs and respiratory status by continuous monitoring. Assess for worsening of respiratory compromise. Assess cardiac rhythm by physical assessment and the cardiorespiratory monitor. Assess breath sounds—note presence of bowel sounds in thoracic cavity, and note presence of heart tones on right side of chest. Assess for cyanosis.

Nursing diagnoses that may apply to the infant with diaphragmatic hernia include the following:

- Ineffective Breathing Pattern related to presence of intraabdominal organs in thoracic cavity
- Risk for Deficient Fluid Volume related to NPO status
- Anxiety (parental) related to life-threatening condition of neonate
- Risk for Impaired Parent/Infant Attachment related to infant's life-threatening condition, surgery

Planning and Implementation

The infant with a diaphragmatic hernia is admitted to the neonatal intensive care unit (NICU) and requires continuous monitoring. The critical need for emergency surgical intervention and the poor survival rate place great stress on parents and family. Offer support and refer family to appropriate resources for stress management and support.

Preoperative Care

Preoperative management centers on providing supportive care to the infant and parents. Maintain intravenous fluid administration. Promote decreased stimulation to keep the infant calm and thus maintain low abdominal pressure. Keep parents informed about the infant's condition and provide emotional support both before and after surgery. Allow them to see and touch the infant if possible. Consult Chapter 25∞ for further detail regarding monitoring of respiratory status.

Postoperative Care

Postoperative care includes positioning the infant on the affected side to facilitate expansion of the lung on the unaffected side, observing closely for signs of infection, maintaining respiratory support, and carefully monitoring fluid and electrolyte balance. Cluster nursing care of infant to minimize exertion. Partner with parents to encourage participation in the infant's care to promote parent–infant attachment. Before discharge, instruct parents in wound care (see previous discussion in this chapter for abdominal wound care), prevention of infection, and feeding techniques.

Evaluation

Expected outcomes for nursing care of the infant with diaphragmatic hernia include:

- The infant establishes effective breathing pattern following surgical intervention.
- The infant achieves fluid balance appropriate for age.
- Family members verbalize fears and concerns and receive adequate emotional support.
- Parents and infant demonstrate bonding and attachment.

Umbilical Hernia

An umbilical hernia results from imperfect closure or weakness of the umbilical muscle ring (Figure 30–13 ■). The condition is often associated with diastasis recti (lateral separation of the abdominal muscles). Umbilical hernia occurs in one of every six children (Katz, 2001), and is nearly 10 times more common in African American children than White children. Umbilical hernias are also observed more frequently in females, infants with low birth weight, children with Down syndrome, and children with hypothyroidism. It is unknown why there is a higher incidence of umbilical hernias in these populations (Katz, 2001).

Closure of the umbilical ring normally begins at the end of the first trimester of gestation and follows the return of the intestines into the abdominal cavity at the eleventh week. As the rectus muscles and fascia migrate, the obliterated umbilical vessels occupy the defect in the umbilical ring and help to obliterate the space. There is no clear explanation why the umbilical ring closes incompletely (Katz, 2001).

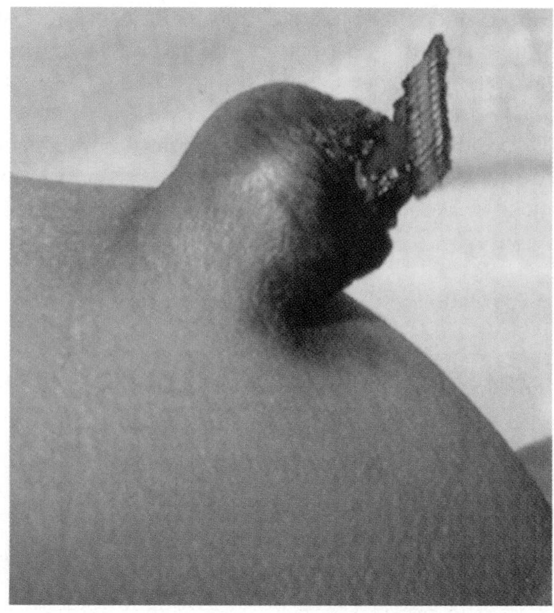

FIGURE 30–13 ■ The umbilical hernia of the newborn usually closes as the muscles strengthen in later infancy and childhood.

From Zitelli, B., & Davis, H. (Eds.) (1994). Atlas of pediatric physical diagnosis. *(2nd ed.). London: Mosby-Wolfe Publishing.*

The hernia appears as a soft swelling covered by skin. The size of the defect may vary among individuals. The herniated area protrudes with coughing, crying, or straining during a bowel movement. Contents of the hernia include omentum or portions of the small intestine.

The hernia is easily reduced by pushing the bowel back through the fibrous ring. Most defects resolve spontaneously by 3 to 4 years of age as the muscular ring closes. Surgery is indicated in cases of strangulation (closure of the umbilical ring around a portion of the bowel, preventing it from moving back into the abdomen), increased protrusion of the hernia after the age of 2 years, or little or no improvement in a large defect after the age of 4 years. Surgery is performed either laparoscopically or by open repair.

Nursing management is generally supportive. Instruct parents not to apply tape, straps, or coins to reduce the hernia. This can cause strangulation of the hernia, necessitating immediate surgery. If surgery is required, it is usually performed in a short-stay unit. Nursing care is similar to that of any child having abdominal surgery (see previous discussions). Postoperatively, teach parents how to care for the surgical site, to monitor for bleeding, and to recognize signs of infection. Reinforce the importance of returning for follow-up evaluation.

DISORDERS OF MOTILITY

Fluids are produced in large quantities as part of normal gastrointestinal functioning. As food passes through the intestines, fluids are reabsorbed and moderately soft stool is formed and evacuated. In disorders such as **diarrhea** (frequent, watery stools) and constipation, fluid production is altered, causing either more or less fluid to be reabsorbed. This can severely alter the characteristics of the stool.

Reabsorption of too little water produces diarrhea and can lead to fluid and electrolyte alterations. Reabsorption of too much fluid can cause constipation, which if untreated can lead to bowel obstruction.

Vomiting and gastroesophageal reflux are associated with return of gastric contents from the stomach. Disorders such as constipation, encopresis, Hirschsprung disease, and gastroenteritis affect bowel elimination. These disorders are discussed in this section.

MediaLink Care Plan: Managing Emesis in Pediatric Conditions

Vomiting

Vomiting is forceful regurgitation of gastric contents upward into the esophagus, mouth, and out of the body. Vomiting can occur with structural defects such as pyloric stenosis and tracheoesophageal fistula, which have already been described in this chapter. Vomiting often occurs when a child has a viral or bacterial gastrointestinal illness. See the section on gastroenteritis in this chapter and the discussion of fluid and electrolyte complications from gastroenteritis in Chapter 23∞. Vomiting and feeding disorders can occur throughout childhood as well as in infancy. In older children, a pattern of **chronic vomiting** (low-grade nearly daily emesis) or **cyclic vomiting** (repeated severe vomiting of an episodic nature) can occur. These patterns differ from vomiting seen in colic or gastroesophageal reflux. Chronic vomiting is most often associated with peptic ulcer or irritable bowel, and cyclic vomiting is indicative of a syndrome known as abdominal migraine when children have periodic bouts of abdominal pain and vomiting (headache does not usually occur with this condition). Continuous vomiting of any nature should be evaluated. Inquire about amount, quality, quantity, color, and odor of emesis. Ask about frequency of vomiting episodes and any distress that the child has prior to or following the episodes. Perform a diet recall as well as detailed nutritional and developmental assessments (see Chapter 9∞). Instruct parents on any treatments ordered, such as a change in formula or positioning after feeding. See the section later in this chapter on nursing interventions in gastrointestinal infections.

Gastroesophageal Reflux and Gastroesophageal Reflux Disease

Gastroesophageal reflux (GER) is the return of gastric contents into the esophagus, as the result of relaxation of the lower esophageal sphincter. GER is a common gastrointestinal disorder in children, affecting approximately 50% of healthy, full-term newborns (Jadcherla & Shaker, 2001). There is a higher incidence in premature infants, and males are affected 3 times more often than females. Children with neurologic impairments, such as cerebral palsy, more commonly experience GER. The peak age of onset is 1 to 4 months.

Gastroesophageal reflux disease (GERD) is a more serious manifestation of GER; it is a pathological process in infants manifested by poor weight gain, esophagitis, neurobehavioral changes, and persistent respiratory symptoms or complications (Arguin & Swartz, 2004). GERD is diagnosed in approximately 1 in 300 infants. Children most at risk include those with esophageal atresia repair, neurologic disorders, hiatal hernia, bronchopulmonary dysplasia, asthma, and cystic fibrosis (Jung, 2001).

Etiology and Pathophysiology

In the gastrointestinal tract, the lower esophageal sphincter is located at the distal end of the esophagus and is controlled by tonic smooth muscle (Jung, 2001). Three mechanisms allow reflux of the gastric contents across the esophagogastric junction and into the esophagus:

- Transient lower esophageal sphincter relaxations
- Hypotensive or incompetent lower esophageal sphincter
- Anatomic disruption of the esophagogastric junction

First, transient lower esophageal sphincter relaxations occur after postprandial gastric distention (Orlando, 2001). This vagal reflex accounts for most reflux episodes in healthy individuals and the majority of reflux episodes (50%–88%) in those with gastroesophageal reflux disease. Children with GERD have more transient sphincter relaxations than normal. Second, in some individuals, an incompetent lower esophageal sphincter allows for regurgitation of gastric contents with any increase in intraabdominal pressure such as coughing, crying, or straining. Infants are more predisposed to regurgitation than adolescents and adults due to the smaller reservoir of their esophagus and its limited ability to contain gastric fluids (Wylie, 2004). Lastly, in some children there is an anatomic variation that exerts pressure on the esophagogastric junction and allows regurgitation. This anatomic variation is called a hiatal hernia.

With repeated reflux of gastric contents, the acidity damages the esophageal mucosa. Aspiration of emesis may occur. The disorder may be self-limiting, resolving by 1 year of age. For cases that do not resolve, surgical intervention may be required.

Reflux of stomach contents can lead to aspiration, resulting in frequent bouts of pneumonia, reactive airway disease, color changes during feeding, apnea, or hematemesis (vomiting of blood) (Levy, 2001).

Clinical Manifestations

Manifestations vary from an occasional burp to persistent emesis and failure to thrive. Some "spitting up" after feedings is considered normal in newborns due to the weak cardiac sphincter of the stomach. It often resolves without surgical intervention by 6 to 12 months of age (Jung, 2001). Postprandial regurgitation is the most common sign of GER in infants. The regurgitation ranges from spitting to forceful vomiting (Sondheimer, 2003). Lasting or severe spitting up or emesis should be evaluated by a healthcare professional. See the clinical manifestations table below for clinical therapy and nursing implications.

Children with GER are frequently hungry and irritable. Although the infants are consuming nutrition, they continue to lose weight and experience failure to thrive. They have a history of vomiting and frequent upper respiratory infections. Apparent life-threatening events and cyanotic episodes may be reported (see Chapter 25).

Manifestations of respiratory problems associated with gastroesophageal reflux include cyanosis, wheezing, stridor, chronic cough, and recurrent croup.

COLLABORATIVE CARE

Collaborative care includes identifying gastroesophageal reflux, preventing complications associated with the disorder, and treatment through dietary and pharmacological management or surgical intervention.

Diagnostic Tests

Diagnosis is confirmed by a thorough history of the child's feeding patterns and by diagnostic evaluation using contrast upper gastrointestinal series (barium fluoroscopy), upper gastrointestinal endoscopy with esophageal biopsy, pH probe monitoring (insertion of a small catheter into the esophagus through the nose that is left in place for 18 to 24 hours to measure pH and thus determine number of reflux episodes), or gastroesophageal scintigraphy (radionuclide scanning to evaluate gastric emptying) (Murray & Christie, 2000; Jung, 2001). Laboratory studies may reveal anemia secondary to blood loss. There is no single definitive study to diagnose gastroesophageal reflux disease (Jung, 2001).

Testing for cow milk protein allergy—including cutaneous tests, eosinophil smears of the nasal mucosa, IgG antilactoglobulin levels, and intestinal biopsy—are generally performed due to the high association between GER and cow milk allergy (Arguin & Swartz, 2004). See Table 30–3.

CLINICAL MANIFESTATIONS of Gastroesophageal Reflux and Gastroesophageal Reflux Disease

CLINICAL MANIFESTATIONS	CLINICAL THERAPY	NURSING IMPLICATIONS
Gastroesophageal Reflux Regurgitation with normal weight gain No signs and symptoms of esophagitis, respiratory infection, excessive crying	Thicken formula with up to 1 tablespoon of rice cereal per 2–4 ounces of liquid or use specially thickened formula Consider change to hypoallergenic formula if condition persists	Teach parents recommended feeding techniques Monitor weight gain Monitor growth and development Assess for feeding difficulties
Gastroesophageal Reflux Disease Regurgitation with poor weight gain Persistent irritability due to pain Respiratory symptoms such as apnea, cyanosis, wheezing, pneumonia, cough Gastrointestinal symptoms such as hematemesis and iron deficiency anemia	Thicken formula as noted above or change type of formula for a trial period Treatment with antacids, histamine H_2 receptor blockers, or proton pump inhibitors (see medications table on page 1121)	Teach parents of infants: • Burp infant every 1–2 ounces of formula or after breastfeeding on each side • Avoid overfeeding • Hold infant upright for 30 minutes after feeding; avoid use of infant seat • Raise the head of the crib about 30 degrees so that the head is higher than the stomach Teach parents of older child: • Avoid foods that may cause reflux: caffeine, chocolate, spicy foods • Serve smaller, more frequent meals and snacks • The child should avoid eating 2–3 hours before bedtime • Encourage weight reduction if the child is overweight • Raise the head of the bed by about 6 inches

Data from Jung, A. D. (2001). Gastroesophageal reflux in infants and children. American Family Physician, *64, 1853–1860.*

TABLE 30–3 Diagnostic Tests for Gastroesophageal Reflux Disease

DIAGNOSTIC TEST	INDICATION	NURSING IMPLICATIONS
Gastroesophageal scintigraphy	Allows evaluation of gastric emptying or aspiration Scans the stomach, esophagus, and lungs	Oral ingestion or nasogastric tube instillation of radionuclide formula or food Administer radionuclide formula or food
Upper gastrointestinal (GI) examination	Identifies anatomic abnormalities such as pyloric stenosis, hiatal hernia, malrotation Identifies delayed gastric emptying and presence of reflux	No invasive procedure Explain procedure to child to alleviate fears
Intraesophageal pH probe monitoring	Considered the "gold standard" test for diagnosing GERD and for evaluating atypical symptoms such as apnea, stridor, or cough Placed in the distal esophagus to detect pH changes below 4.0 pH is measured and recorded every 4–8 seconds Acid reflux is defined by a pH of <4 for at least 15–30 seconds	Ensure pH probe is secured Prevent infant or child from inadvertent removal of probe Probe is left in place to measure pH for 24 hours Monitor and record pH measurements per protocol
Endoscopy with biopsy	Allows visualization and biopsy of the esophageal epithelium Endoscopy is useful in evaluating symptoms of pain, dysphagia, and hematemesis; and to differentiate GERD from peptic ulcer disease, *H. pylori* infection, gastritis, and duodenitis Histopathologic assessment of esophageal mucosa may be performed to grade the severity of esophagitis and detect early Barrett's esophagus	Administer sedation as prescribed Maintain NPO status preprocedure Explain procedure to parents and child Postoperatively monitor vital signs per protocol; resume oral feedings as prescribed

Data from Jung, A. D. (2001). Gastroesophageal reflux in infants and children. American Family Physician, *64, 1853–1860.*

Clinical Therapy

Treatment of GER and GERD depends on the severity of the condition. Generally, feeding modification, thickened feeds, and positioning are effective management for milder cases.

A smaller feeding volume may prove beneficial to avoid overdistention of the abdomen and subsequent reflux. The infant should be burped after every 1 to 2 ounces (Arguin & Swartz, 2004).

Rice cereal is sometimes placed in the infant's bottle to thicken feedings to a consistency similar to nectar (about 1 to 2 teaspoons per 4 ounce bottle). Note that breast milk will not readily thicken with addition of cereal. In addition, recent recommendations suggest caution when using thickened formula with rice cereal as it increases carbohydrate intake and decreases protein and minerals contained in the infant formula. Prethickened formulas are commercially available. For example, Enfamil AR contains added rice and is nutritionally balanced. These formulas can be administered without enlarging the nipple hole. Formula change to a protein hydrolysate or elemental formula, such as Pregestimil®, Nutramigen®, or Alimentum®, may be recommended (Arguin & Swartz, 2004). Fatty foods and citrus juices are avoided.

The best position in which to place the postprandial infant with GERD is the prone position with the head elevated. However, the prone position should not be used in the sleeping child due to the increased incidence of sudden infant death syndrome with this position. Caution parents to use the prone position only while the infant is awake and while being continuously observed by the parent (Arguin & Swartz, 2004). Other recommendations include positioning the infant with the head slightly elevated or in the left-lateral position. Parents are encouraged to hold their infant in an upright position for 20 to 30 minutes following feedings. Minimize seated positioning such as in an infant seat because this increases intraabdominal pressure and promotes reflux.

Medications (cholinergics, antacids, and histamine antagonists) may be prescribed to reduce the amount of stomach acid and lessen the child's discomfort. See the table on page 1121.

Treatment for severe cases of GERD such as those with persistent vomiting with failure to thrive, chronic esophagitis, esophageal strictures, or chronic pulmonary disease (Sondheimer, 2003), may include surgery to create a valve mechanism by wrapping the greater curvature of the stomach (fundus) around the distal esophagus (Nissen fundoplication). A gastrostomy tube is usually inserted during surgery and left in place for 6 weeks.

NURSING MANAGEMENT

Nursing management of the infant or child with gastroesophageal reflux or gastroesophageal reflux disease focuses on supporting the infant's or child's nutritional intake, promoting interventions to reduce associated complications, and supporting the family.

■ Nursing Assessment and Diagnosis

Obtain a thorough history of the child's feeding patterns. Table 30–4 on page 1122 provides history and assessment questions. Observe vomiting episodes and document amount, color, and consistency of emesis.

Monitor the infant's weight and plot progress on a growth chart. Observe for any signs of respiratory distress and keep the infant's nose and mouth clear of vomitus.

Nursing diagnoses that may apply to the infant with gastroesophageal reflux include:

- Risk for Aspiration related to reflux
- Fluid Volume, Deficient related to reflux
- Imbalanced Nutrition, Less than Body Requirements related to reflux and NPO status

MEDICATIONS Used to Treat Gastroesophageal Reflux Disease

MEDICATION	ACTION/INDICATION	NURSING IMPLICATIONS
Histamine H_2 receptor antagonists		
Zantac (ranitidine) Pepcid (famotidine)	Decreases acid secretion by inhibition of the histamine H_2 receptor on the gastric parietal cell	May be administered with or without food If antacids are prescribed, administer 2 hours before or after H_2 antagonists Teach parents to avoid OTC medications without checking with healthcare provider Monitor for side effects: Bradycardia, Constipation, Elevated serum creatinine, Fatigue, Headache, Irritability, Rash, Sedation, Thrombocytopenia
Proton-pump inhibitors		
Prevacid (lansoprazole) Prilosec (omeprazole)	These powerful inhibitors of acid secretion alleviate symptoms and help to heal esophagitis Blocks the final common pathway of acid production by inhibiting activated proton pumps in the gastric parietal cell canaliculus	Administer in the morning on an empty stomach Antacids may be administered with omeprazole Monitor for side effects: Abdominal pain, Diarrhea, Dizziness, Fatigue, Headache, Hematuria, Nausea, Proteinuria, Rash Teach family to inform primary healthcare provider if severe diarrhea occurs Teach family to inform primary healthcare provider if changes in urinary elimination, such as pain or discomfort associated with urination, occur.
Antacids		
Gaviscon	Antacids neutralize gastric acid by buffering the gastric fluid.	Not commonly used in infants and young children due to aluminum content Teach family to monitor for side effects: Osteopenia Neurotoxicity

Data from Gremse, D. A. (2002). Gastroesophageal reflux: Life-threatening disease or laundry problem? Clinical Pediatrics, 41*, 369–372; Hall, G. C., & Jacoby, H. I. (2002). Gastroesophageal reflux disease.* American Journal of Pharmaceutical Education, 66*, 148–152.*

- Risk for Infection (pulmonary) related to reflux
- Deficient Knowledge (parental) related to feeding techniques

Planning and Implementation

Adequate nutrition must be maintained in order for the child to achieve normal growth and development. Infants receiving oral feedings are administered smaller feedings. Elevate the head of the bed to prevent aspiration if vomiting should occur. If the child has difficulty maintaining this position, a Tracy harness or reflux board may be used. The harness, which is pinned to the mattress, supports the infant in an upright position. If the child has a gastrostomy tube, maintain skin integrity around the stoma site. Secure the tube so the infant cannot dislodge or pull on it.

CLINICAL TIP

Measure and record length of the gastrostomy tube daily to ensure it remains in proper position. Coil the tube that is outside the body, tape in place, and put a shirt on the infant to cover it. Frequently clean drainage around the tube as the acidic gastric contents are harmful to the skin.

Discharge planning focuses on instructing parents in how to feed and position the infant, as well as providing comfort and emotional support. Partner with parents and encourage them to hold and cuddle the infant during all feedings. Show them how to keep the upper body elevated and discourage use of infant seats. Caution the family that an enlarged nipple has the capacity to deliver too much formula too fast for the infant and may produce a choking hazard. Providing the infant with a pacifier helps to meet nonnutritive sucking needs. Teach parents how to suction the nose and mouth if vomiting occurs.

Evaluation

Expected outcomes of nursing care of the child with gastroesophageal reflux include:

- The infant is free from respiratory distress and other evidence of aspiration.
- The infant/child maintains balanced fluid and electrolyte status.
- The infant tolerates feeding and gains weight sufficient to meet growth and developmental needs.
- The infant remains free from infection.
- Parents demonstrate proper feeding techniques.

Constipation

Constipation is a common complaint in the pediatric population and accounts for one quarter of all pediatric gastroenterology referrals (Coughlin, 2003). Stools are hard but there is an absence of structural, endocrine, or metabolic conditions that

TABLE 30–4 History and Assessment Questions for Assessment of the Infant/Child with Gastroesophageal Reflux

Feeding practices/elimination	Do you breastfeed? How often and for how long? How frequently do you burp the baby? Show me how you burp the baby. Do you feed formula? What type? How many ounces does your baby consume with each feeding? How frequently do you burp the baby? Show me how you burp the baby. Have you introduced cereal and other foods? Which ones? When? How much and how often are the foods eaten? Does your infant seem hungry? Drink or eat very fast? Does the baby refuse food? In what position is the infant held during feedings? What position do you use after feedings? Describe the "spitting up," burping, or vomiting of the baby. How often do these occur? What type of fluid? How much? Color, odor? Is there ever blood? When does this occur—during, after, or between feedings? How often does the baby have bowel movements? Do they appear painful? Is there excessive passing of gas? Describe the consistency, color, odor. How often in a day does the baby have wet diapers?
Respiratory	Do you notice that your baby has a cough, hoarseness, or makes sounds when breathing? Is there choking, gagging, or a struggle to breathe during or between feedings? Has the baby had pneumonia? Has your baby had any episodes of apnea, or stopping breathing? Describe them. Describe the baby's sleep and awakening patterns.
Environment	Describe how and when the baby is usually fed. What activities are going on? Who feeds the baby? Is the baby held, fed lying down, or other? Is the infant/child exposed to tobacco smoke?

Adapted from Arguin, A. L., & Swartz, M. K. (2004). Gastroesophageal reflux in infants: A primary care perspective. Pediatric Nursing, 30, *45–52.*

could cause hard stools. For infants and children, the criteria for constipation (Lembo & Camilleri, 2003) include:

- Pebblelike, hard stools for a majority of bowel movements for at least 2 weeks
- Firm stools more than twice per week for at least 2 weeks

Constipation affects 3% of preschool-age children and 1% to 2% of school-age children. Constipation is more common in school-age males than females but at other ages is more common in females. Constipation leads to nearly 5% of outpatient visits to pediatric clinics and more than 25% of referrals to pediatric gastroenterologists (Arce, Ermocilla, & Costa, 2002; Lembo & Canilleri, 2003).

Because stool patterns vary among children, identification of an abnormal pattern is sometimes difficult. Infants usually have several bowel movements a day. For a young child, one bowel movement a day may be normal. As the child grows, however, three to four bowel movements in a week may be a normal pattern. The hardness of the stool rather than frequency is important to consider.

Breastfed infants may have bowel movements as frequently as with every feeding or just one bowel movement every several days. Because of differences in fat digestion and absorption, bottle-fed infants are more prone to hard stools (Coughlin, 2003).

Etiology and Pathophysiology

Constipation may be caused by an underlying disease, diet, or psychologic factor (Table 30–5). Constipation may result from defects in filling, or more commonly emptying, of the rectum. Pathologic causes of defective filling include ineffective colonic propulsive activity, caused by hypothyroidism or use of med-

TABLE 30–5 Factors Influential in Childhood Constipation

PHYSICAL FACTORS IN INFANCY	PHYSICAL FACTORS IN CHILDREN	PSYCHOLOGICAL FACTORS IN CHILDREN
Familial stool patterns High milk and low fiber intake Cow milk allergy Hard stools Dehydration Group A streptococcal infection of perianul area Medications such as diuretics, some anticonvulsants, analgesia Intestinal or anal conditions such as Hirschprung disease, cystic fibrosis, anorectal malformations	Hypertrophied rectum Residual stool blockage (fecalith) Overflow fecal soiling around a solid stool Poor rectal sensation Diseases that influence gastrointestinal or neurologic systems such as celiac disease, cerebral palsy Decreased mobility/activity	Embarrassment/shame related to soiling due to early or coercive toilet training or lack of privacy Fear of pain from hard stool Being too busy to use the bathroom Parental blame/anger related to soiling and toileting refusal Teasing and bullying related to incontinence

Adapted from Clayden, G., & Keshtgar, A. S. (2003). Management of childhood constipation. Postgraduate Medical Journal, *79, 616–621.*

ication, and obstruction; a structural anomaly (stricture or stenosis); or an aganglionic segment (Hirschsprung disease).

If the rectum fails to fill, stasis leads to excessive drying of the stools. Emptying of the rectum depends on the defecation reflex. Lesions of the spinal cord, weakness of the abdominal muscles, local lesions blocking sphincter relaxation, and a desire to avoid painful stools all may impede attempts to defecate (Box 30–2).

The three types of constipation are normal-transit constipation, defecation disorders, and slow-transit constipation.

1. **Normal-transit constipation,** also called functional constipation, is the most common form of constipation. With normal-transit constipation, stool traverses at a normal rate through the colon and the stool frequency is normal, yet individuals believe they are constipated. Normal-transit constipation is likely due to a perceived difficulty with evacuation or the presence of hard stools. Bloating and abdominal pain or discomfort may be experienced (Lembo & Camilleri, 2003).
2. **Defecation disorders** are commonly due to dysfunction of the pelvic floor or anal sphincter such as in children with anorectal malformations (see discussion in this chapter). Structural abnormalities such as intussusception, rectocele, and Hirschsprung disease are also causes. A desire to avoid pain associated with passing of a large, hard stool can result in defecation disorders. Ignoring or suppressing the urge to defecate can contribute to the development of mild constipation before the disorder becomes severe. Sexual or physical abuse or an eating disorder may be associated with defecation disorders (Lembo & Camilleri, 2003).
3. **Slow-transit constipation** occurs most commonly in young females who have infrequent bowel movements (once a week or fewer); the condition often begins at puberty. Associated symptoms are an infrequent urge to defecate, bloating, and abdominal pain or discomfort (Lembo & Camilleri, 2003).

Clinical Manifestations

Constipation is characterized by a decrease in the frequency of stool passage; the formation of hard, dry stools; or the oozing of liquid stool past a collection of hard, dry stool.

Constipation in the newborn should raise the suspicion of an obstructed large bowel such as that due to Hirschsprung disease or anorectal anomaly with anal stenosis (Clayden & Keshtgar, 2003).

BOX 30–2 Research: Stool Toileting Refusal

A recent study was conducted to determine whether constipation and painful bowel elimination occur as a result of stool toileting refusal (STR) or occur before STR. This prospective longitudinal study of toilet training followed 380 children between the ages of 17 and 19 months. Conclusions of the study are as follows: When hard bowel movements or painful bowel elimination is associated with stool toileting refusal, the first episode of constipation usually occurs *before* the STR. This suggests that for many children, constipation is a chronic problem that is not being treated effectively. Therefore, hard bowel movements and painful bowel elimination are factors that potentially contribute to the STR and for the majority of children are not caused solely by the STR behavior (Blum, Taubman, & Nemeth, 2004).

Constipation during infancy is commonly seen as a result of mismanagement of diet, although the disorder is generally easily managed with dietary changes. The transition from formula to cow milk may cause a transient constipation, since the bowel must adjust to the increased protein content of cow milk. Children who are difficult to feed because of prematurity or associated pathology such as gastroesophageal reflux disease, cleft palate, cerebral palsy, multiple operations, or even those intolerant to cow milk protein or gluten may present with difficulty in passing stools (Clayden & Keshtgar, 2003).

Constipation occurs most frequently in the toddler and preschool age groups. This increased incidence is often associated with learning to control bodily functions. Many children do not like the sensations of a bowel movement and may begin withholding stool, which accumulates in and dilates the rectum until the next urge to defecate. The increasingly hard and painful bowel movement reinforces the child's behavior, and a pattern develops (Castiglia, 2001).

Constipation in the school-age child, older child, and adolescent usually results in overflow fecal incontinence. Some children with constipation are discovered during their school years after being evaluated for recurrent urinary tract infections or enuresis (Clayden & Keshtgar, 2003).

COLLABORATIVE CARE

Collaborative care focuses on determining the underlying pathologic cause of constipation, correcting any structural defect or obstruction, eliminating contributing factors, and assisting the child to establish routine bowel elimination habits.

Diagnostic Tests

Diagnosis is based on a thorough history and physical examination. When constipation occurs along with growth failure, vomiting, or abdominal pain, further investigation is necessary to rule out other disorders. Tests may include abdominal radiographs; thyroid function tests; measurements of calcium, glucose, and electrolytes; a complete blood count; and urinalysis.

Anorectal manometry provides the pressure of the anal sphincter at rest and the maximal voluntary contract of the external sphincter, the presence or absence of relaxation of the internal anal sphincter during balloon distention (the anorectal inhibitory reflex), rectal sensation, and the ability of the anal sphincters to relax during straining (Lembo & Camilleri, 2003). Stool for occult blood may be conducted.

Clinical Therapy

Dietary and fluid management is the treatment of choice for constipation that has no underlying pathologic cause. Constipation in young infants can usually be corrected by increasing the amount of fluids or adding 2 ounces of pear or apple juice to daily intake. Increasing physical activity and fluid intake may be effective for some children.

Removing constipating foods (e.g., bananas, rice, and cheese) from the child's diet often decreases constipation. Increasing the child's intake of high-fiber foods (e.g., whole-grain breads, raw fruits and vegetables) and fluids also promotes bowel elimination.

In older infants, increasing the intake of fluids, cereals, fruits, and vegetables in the diet should correct the problem. A single glycerin suppository or enema may be required to remove hard stool.

In the school-age child, constipation may occur due to limited time for toileting. Busy school-age children may delay toileting. Children may also be hesitant to use an unfamiliar bathroom. Encouragement from parents and relaxation of bathroom privileges at school promote regularity and return of usual bowel patterns within a short time. Children may need to get up earlier to have breakfast and time for toileting before going to school.

Constipation may follow surgery, especially in children who are immobilized, such as by traction or a body cast. Stool softeners and a diet high in fiber and fluids are given to prevent and treat constipation.

Pharmacologic management of severe constipation usually occurs in two stages. The first stage involves softening the stool with medications such as lactulose, and the second stage involves evacuation of stool with a laxative (Clayden & Keshtgar, 2003). The evacuation phase is the most difficult for the child and those who are managing the child's constipation.

Once a stool softener is administered, consider the most effective means to evacuate the stool while causing the least amount of stress and anxiety to the child. Suppositories and enemas can cause fear in children. Golytely, Klean-prep, or Movicol can be administered orally or instilled via a nasogastric tube to promote stool evacuation (Clayden & Keshtgar, 2003). Once the stool has been evacuated, a routine stimulant laxative is given to prevent reaccumulation of stool in the bowel. Senokot or sodium picosulphate is usually the stimulant laxative of choice.

Behavior Management. Behavior modification may prove beneficial to managing constipation. For younger children, providing rewards for either overcoming the fear of toilets or toileting at routinely scheduled times is effective. Older children also respond to rewards (Clayden & Keshtgar, 2003), which can be simple items such as an afternoon spent with the parent playing a game. For children with psychological issues, child and family psychotherapy may be necessary. In these cases, the family is referred to a child and family counselor.

MediaLink Stool Toileting: Refusals and Rewards Video

NURSING MANAGEMENT

Nursing care focuses on teaching parents what constitutes normal bowel patterns in children and the importance of diet in maintaining such patterns.

Nursing Assessment and Diagnosis

Assess the child's diet history and obtain a description of bowel patterns and habits from parents. When was the child toilet trained and have those patterns changed? Has there been incontinence in the toilet-trained child? Ask what the family does to treat constipation. Ask about frequency, consistency, and the presence of blood in the stools. Ask the child or parents about pain upon passing of stool. Assessment of the child's food likes and dislikes may provide a clue to the cause of constipation. Assess fluid intake and level of activity. Assess for previous history of gastrointestinal complications or surgery, as well as present medications. Ask parents when the newborn passed meconium.

Physical Assessment

Palpate and assess the child's abdomen for firmness or tenderness and the presence of palpable mass (retained stool). Assess for bowel sounds. If a digital rectal examination is performed, assess for presence of stool in rectum. Assess for hemorrhoids, anal fissures, or other abnormalities of the abdomen or perineum.

Nursing diagnoses that may apply to the child with constipation include:

- Constipation related to dietary, nutritional, and/or elimination habits
- Bowel Incontinence related to leakage around formed stool

Planning and Implementation

Regular bowel habits are encouraged by placing the child on the toilet 30 minutes after a meal or around the time bowel elimination usually occurs. Providing positive reinforcement during toilet training helps to prevent a withholding pattern.

Partner with the family and teach parents dietary measures to promote regularity of bowel movements. Children can be given a high-fiber diet that includes fruits and vegetables. Offer cut fresh fruits, dried fruits, and fruit juice as snacks. A glycerin suppository can be used periodically if needed, as a natural stimulant and lubricant of the bowel.

Caution parents to avoid frequent use of laxatives, stool softeners, and enemas, because overuse can cause bowel dependency. Herbal stimulant laxatives are discouraged for children less than 12 years, although other intestinal motility aids are not generally harmful. Ask the family about any herbs they may commonly use. See Complementary Therapy: Children and Herbal Laxatives.

COMPLEMENTARY THERAPY
Children and Herbal Laxatives

Herbal stimulant laxatives are used by some families as complementary therapies. The following are not recommended for use in children under 12 years.

- Aloe
- Buckthorn bark
- Cascara sagrada bark
- Senna leaf or pod
- Coffee
- Tea
- Cola nut
- Mate
- Ma huang

Question parents about the use of complementary therapy for their child's constipation. Educate them regarding avoiding the use of any therapies that are not recommended for children.

Evaluation

Expected outcomes of nursing care for the child with constipation include:

- The child establishes a routine bowel elimination pattern.
- The child is free from constipation and diarrhea.

Encopresis

Encopresis is an abnormal elimination pattern characterized by the recurrent soiling or passage of stool at inappropriate times by a child who should have achieved bowel continence. It occurs in approximately 1% of school-age children. Children with primary encopresis have never achieved bowel control. Children with secondary encopresis have been continent of stool for several months.

Encopresis is usually associated with voluntary or involuntary retention of stool in the lower bowel and rectum, leading to constipation, dilation of the lower bowel, and incompetence of the inner sphincter. The retention of stool is usually a result of being "too busy"; the child puts off going to the bathroom because of the inconvenience of leaving an activity. The retention of stool leads to constipation that is untreated and chronic. Loose stool leaks around the hard feces, and the child becomes unaware of a need to eliminate. Soiling may occur during the day or night. Bowel movements are irregular, painful, small, and hard. The child may be ridiculed by peers because of offensive body odor. This rejection leads to withdrawal and behavioral problems, often resulting in altered school performance and attendance. The child continues to hold stool because the passage has become painful. Parents commonly seek healthcare, believing that the child has diarrhea or constipation.

The underlying constipation that leads to encopresis may be caused by the stress of environmental changes (e.g., birth of a sibling, moving to a new house, attending a new school), issues of anger and control related to bowel training, diet, a full schedule of activities, or a genetic predisposition.

A thorough history, physical examination, and diagnostic studies (possibly including barium enema) are necessary to rule out organic causes and anatomic abnormalities. Examination of mental health and cognitive functioning may be indicated. Information about the child's toilet training habits and parents' attitudes concerning those habits is obtained. A dietary history, including eating habits and types of foods eaten, is often helpful. Physical examination sometimes reveals a nontender mass in the lower abdomen.

Treatment may include behavior modification techniques, dietary changes, use of lubricants to clear the bowel of impacted stool and encourage normal defecation, and psychotherapy. Behavior modification programs that reward and reinforce appropriate toileting habits can be successful. Dietary changes include incorporating high-fiber foods such as fruits, vegetables, and whole-grain cereals into the diet. Limiting intake of refined and highly processed foods and dairy products also may be helpful. Drugs such as mineral oil, bulk-forming laxatives, and stool softeners are used temporarily to empty the bowel. The child should sit on the toilet for several minutes after morning and evening meals. It takes several months for the bowel to be retrained to respond to sphincter stimulation. Psychotherapy involving the child and family may be indicated in instances of dysfunctional parent–child relationships.

Nursing Management

Prevention of encopresis is the nursing goal. Partner with parents to teach toilet training techniques, emphasizing the child's developmental readiness (see Chapter 5∞). Parents are encouraged to praise the child for successes and to avoid punishment and power struggles. Encourage high-fiber diets and regular times for elimination.

Nursing care centers on educating the child and parents about the disorder and its treatment and on providing emotional support. Explain the treatment plan, including dietary changes and use of laxatives or stool softeners. Reassure the child that he or she has a healthy body and, with treatment, will achieve normal functioning. The child is monitored by the nurse for at least 6 months to be certain new patterns have been established.

Hirschsprung Disease

Hirschsprung disease, also known as congenital aganglionic megacolon, is a congenital anomaly in which inadequate motility causes mechanical obstruction of the intestine. The disease occurs in approximately 1 in 5,000 live births, and the incidence of transmitting this disease to offspring is approximately 3% (Swenson, 2002). Males are affected more commonly than females (Thompson, 2001). Hirschsprung disease may be either acute or chronic.

Hirschsprung disease occurs as an isolated trait in 70% of patients, is associated with a chromosomal abnormality in 12% of cases (trisomy 21 being the most frequent), and is associated with congenital anomalies, such as gastrointestinal malformation, cleft palate, polydactyly, cardiac septal defects, and craniofacial anomalies, in 18% of cases (Amiel & Lyonnet, 2001).

Etiology and Pathophysiology

Hirschsprung disease is the congenital absence of ganglion cells in the wall of a variable segment of rectum and colon. It is now known that the RET protooncogene is a major gene for the disease (Howard, 2001).

The pathogenesis of Hirschsprung disease is not well understood; however, in addition to genetic factors, a failure of the migration of neural crest cells (from which cells forming ganglia arise) during the embryonic stage has been implicated (Thompson, 2001).

The absence of autonomic parasympathetic ganglion cells in the colon prevents peristalsis at that portion of the intestine, resulting in the accumulation of intestinal contents and abdominal distention. The presence of trapped stool in the colon continues to build up, causing expansion of the colon to larger than normal, hence the name *megacolon*. See Box 30–3.

BOX 30–3 Chronic Intestinal Pseudo-Obstruction (Pseudo-Hirschsprung Disease)

Chronic intestinal pseudo-obstruction (pseudo-Hirschsprung disease) is a rare condition of small bowel dysmotility, and should be differentiated from the presence of Hirschsprung disease. It results from disorders of the smooth muscle of the bowel (myopathic type) or of the neurological network of the bowel (neuropathic type). Treatment includes drugs to increase intestinal motility and generally total parenteral nutrition (Barr, 2000).

Clinical Manifestations

Clinical manifestations vary depending on the child's age at onset. In newborns, symptoms include failure to pass meconium, refusal to suck, abdominal distention, and bile-stained emesis.

In the older child, symptoms may include failure to gain weight and delayed growth. The child may have a history of abdominal distention, severe constipation alternating with diarrhea (frequent, watery stools), and vomiting. The stool may be normal size or have a ribbonlike appearance.

COLLABORATIVE CARE

Collaborative care focuses on identifying Hirschsprung disease, surgical removal of the aganglionic section, promotion nutrition for growth and development, and achievement of normal bowel elimination patterns.

Diagnostic Tests

Diagnosis is made on the basis of the clinical criteria and history, bowel patterns, anorectal manometry, radiographic contrast studies such as barium enema, and rectal biopsy for presence or absence of ganglion cells (Swenson, 2002). The rectum is small in size on palpation and does not contain stool.

Abdominal radiograph and barium contrasts reveal a distended small bowel and proximal colon with an empty rectum. Rectal biopsy reveals the presence of aganglionic cells.

Anorectal manometry demonstrates absence of relaxation of the internal sphincter in response to rectal distension. Normally, distension of the rectum produces relaxation of the internal sphincter.

Clinical Therapy

If not treated, Hirschsprung disease can lead to complete obstruction, respiratory distress, and shock. Treatment in infancy involves surgical removal of the aganglionic bowel with end-to-end anastomosis to the anal canal (Thompson, 2001). Laparoscopic surgery may be considered versus the traditional open resection (Swensen, 2002).

In severe cases or in ill infants, a temporary colostomy is created. Closure of the colostomy and reanastomosis are performed approximately 3 to 6 months following the initial surgery (Rogers, 2001). A nasogastric tube is generally inserted preoperatively to relieve distention and is left in place approximately 24 hours after surgery.

For the child with a milder defect, management may involve dietary modification, stool softeners, and isotonic irrigations to prevent impaction until the child is toilet trained.

The return of normal bowel function depends on the amount of bowel involved. The majority of children achieve fecal continence; however, some fecal incontinence and constipation may persist following surgery and into adulthood (Thompson, 2001).

A serious complication of Hirschsprung disease is enterocolitis (inflammation of the intestines), which occurs in 20% to 60% of children after surgery. Symptoms of enterocolitis include gastrointestinal bleeding and diarrhea. Enterocolitis can occur before or after surgery, resulting in ischemia and ulceration of the bowel wall. Treatment may include total parenteral nutrition and a lactose-free diet.

NURSING MANAGEMENT

Nursing care focuses on collaborative identification of Hirschsprung disease, preoperative and postoperative nursing care, including nutritional support, and supporting the family.

■ Nursing Assessment and Diagnosis

Nursing assessment in the newborn period includes careful observation for the passage of meconium. Assess the newborn for refusal to suck, abdominal distention, and bile-stained emesis.

When the disease is diagnosed later in infancy or in childhood, obtain a thorough history of weight gain, nutritional intake, and bowel elimination habits. Assess the child's growth and developmental achievements. Assess the child for abdominal distention, severe constipation alternating with diarrhea (frequent, watery stools), and vomiting. Assess the stool appearance.

Nursing diagnoses that may apply to the child with Hirschsprung disease include:

- Risk for Deficient Fluid Balance related to ineffective bowel function, NPO status, and surgical intervention
- Risk for Imbalanced Nutrition, Less than Body Requirements related to ineffective bowel function, NPO status, and surgical intervention
- Acute Pain related to surgical incision
- Anxiety (parental) related to child's illness and required surgical intervention

■ Planning and Implementation

Nursing management consists of carefully monitoring fluid and electrolyte balance, maintaining nutrition, preoperative and postoperative care, providing pain relief, and promoting bowel elimination.

Nonsurgical Intervention Nursing Care

Newborns are often discharged within 24 hours of birth, so parents need to understand characteristics of normal early bowel movements, and should contact the healthcare professional if no stool is passed or if the abdomen becomes distended. If Hirschsprung disease is diagnosed, the family requires education about the disease. Teach parents the need for chronic care over time. Regular bowel movements are important to promote adequate elimination and prevent obstruction. Daily rectal irrigations of normal saline solution may be necessary. Teach parents how to prevent skin breakdown in the rectal area by changing diapers frequently, cleansing the area carefully, and applying protective ointment at each diaper change.

Preoperative Nursing Care

If surgical correction is necessary, nursing care includes monitoring for infection, managing pain, maintaining hydration, measuring abdominal circumference to detect any distention, and providing support to the child and family. Preoperative oral intake varies depending on the surgeon; however, intake is generally restricted to clear fluids the day before surgery. Normal saline enema may be performed to evacuate bowel.

Parents require instruction in ostomy care in those cases when the child has a colostomy (refer to the earlier discussion of colostomy care in this chapter). Provide appropriate referrals to an ostomy support group and enterostomal nurse specialist when indicated. Teach parents to be alert for and immediately report signs of complications. These complications include diarrhea and pelvic abscess from leakage of intestinal contents at the surgical site, characterized by fever and pain.

Children occasionally develop constipation, and parents may need guidance to adapt the diet and fluid intake to manage this complication. Because some children develop malabsorption, be alert for signs of poor growth or malnutrition.

Postoperative Nursing Care

Initial postoperative nursing care is the same for any other infant or child having abdominal surgery. Maintain intravenous fluids and nasogastric tube, and monitor intake and output. The colostomy is covered with sterile gauze initially. Once the colostomy is functional, approximately 24 to 48 hours postoperatively, apply a stoma pouch (Rogers, 2001). Administer pain medications routinely and assess at least every hour for evidence of pain utilizing a pain scale and documenting assessment.

Once bowel elimination is established, the child is feeding well without complications, and the family can manage pouch changes, the child is discharged home (Rogers, 2001). Home health nurse visits may be required to assist the family in managing the colostomy and in promoting the child's growth and development.

■ Evaluation

Expected outcomes of nursing care of the child with Hirschsprung disease may include the following:

- The child maintains fluid and electrolyte balance.
- The child's nutritional intake is adequate to promote growth and development.
- The child achieves relief from pain.
- The parents express their anxiety and concerns, and acknowledge receiving adequate support.

Gastroenteritis

Gastroenteritis is an inflammation of the stomach and intestines that may be accompanied by vomiting and diarrhea. Gastroenteritis can affect any part of the gastrointestinal tract. It may be an acute problem, caused by viral, bacterial, or parasitic infections, or a chronic problem. Acute gastroenteritis affects approximately 30 million children per year in the United States (Reeves, Shannon, & Fleisher, 2002). Children under age 5 years have an average of approximately two episodes of gastroenteritis each year. Infants and small children with gastroenteritis accompanied by diarrhea can quickly become dehydrated and are at risk for hypovolemic shock if fluid and electrolyte losses are not replaced (see Chapter 23∞).

Etiology and Pathophysiology

Gastroenteritis is commonly manifested in children by diarrhea. Diarrhea in children is related to many different causes (Table 30–6). The specific etiology is not always identified. The common mechanism is a decrease in the absorptive capacity of the bowel through inflammation, decrease in surface area for absorption, or alteration of parasympathetic innervation. Children in childcare centers and those living in substandard housing with improper sanitation are at increased risk.

TABLE 30–6 Causes of Diarrhea in Children

ETIOLOGY	BOWEL MANIFESTATIONS
Emotional stress (anxiety, fatigue)	Increased motility
Intestinal infection Bacteria *E. coli* *Salmonella* *Shigella* Viral Human rotavirus Enteric Adenovirus fungal overgrowth	Inflammation of mucosa Increased mucous secretion in colon
Food sensitivity Gluten Cow milk	Decreased digestion of food
Food intolerance Lactose Introduction of new foods Overfeeding	Increased motility Increased mucous secretion in colon Increased air trapping
Medications Iron Antibiotics	Irritation and superinfection
Colon disease Colitis Necrotizing enterocolitis Enterocolitis	Inflammation and ulceration of intestinal walls Reduced absorption of fluid Increased intestinal motility
Surgical alterations (short bowel syndrome)	Reduced size of colon Decreased absorption surface

Clinical Manifestations

Diarrhea may be mild, moderate, or severe.

- In mild diarrhea, stools are slightly increased in number and have a more liquid consistency.
- In moderate diarrhea, the child has several loose or watery stools. Other symptoms include irritability, anorexia, nausea, and vomiting. Moderate diarrhea is usually self-limiting, resolving without treatment within 1 or 2 days.
- In severe diarrhea, watery stools are continuous. The child exhibits symptoms of fluid and electrolyte imbalance (see Chapter 23∞), has cramping, and is extremely irritable and difficult to console.

COLLABORATIVE CARE

Collaborative care focuses on correcting fluid and electrolyte imbalance and restoring normal bowel elimination.

Diagnostic Tests

Diagnosis is based on the history, physical examination, and laboratory findings. A thorough history may help in identifying the causative factor. Stool cultures or other fecal testing, such as for pus and blood, may be conducted.

Physical examination provides a guide to the severity of dehydration. The stool can be examined for the presence of ova, parasites, infectious organisms, viruses, fat, and undigested sugars. Laboratory evaluation of serum electrolytes and urine helps in identification of electrolyte imbalances and other deficiencies.

Clinical Therapy

Management depends on the severity of the diarrhea and fluid and electrolyte imbalances. The goal of treatment is to correct the fluid and electrolyte imbalances. For mild to moderate dehydration, the child is rehydrated by means of oral rehydration therapy (see Chapter 23∞). This may be accomplished at home or in the short-stay observation unit in a hospital with solutions such as Pedialyte, Ricelyte, or Lytren. Carbonated beverages and those containing high amounts of sugar should not be given. Fermentation of sugar in the gastrointestinal tract causes increased gas, abdominal distention, and an increased frequency of diarrhea.

For severe dehydration, rehydration is accomplished by intravenous infusion with a solution chosen to correct the specific imbalances. Isotonic fluid such as normal saline with glucose or Ringer's lactate is commonly used (see Chapter 23∞ for further information about solutions to correct dehydration). As soon as possible, clear liquids or breast milk are introduced and then the child progresses to a regular diet. Foods generally are not withheld for more than 1 or 2 days. Refer to Chapter 23∞ for discussion of fluid replacement therapy.

If the diarrhea is caused by bacteria or parasites, antimicrobial therapy may be prescribed. Antiemetic and antidiarrheal medications such as Donnagel and Kaopectate are generally discouraged for infants and young children because they do not reduce actual fluid loss and can mask the signs and symptoms of more serious illnesses (Thielman & Guerrant, 2004).

NURSING MANAGEMENT

The focus of nursing is to prevent complications associated with diarrhea, maintain fluid and electrolyte balance, and promote comfort.

Nursing Assessment and Diagnosis

The nurse may encounter the child and family in the emergency department, urgent care center, clinic, or office. The child may be cared for over several hours at a clinic or urgent care center so that dehydration is treated with intravenous infusion and/or oral rehydration, and then sent home with instructions for parents to care for the child.

Ask parents about recent exposure to illnesses, use of antibiotics, travel, food and formula preparation, food sensitivities or allergies, and whether the child attends daycare.

If the child is hospitalized, assess onset, frequency, color, amount, and consistency of stools. If the child is also vomiting, monitor the amount and type of vomitus. Initial and ongoing physical assessment of the child focuses on observing for signs and symptoms of dehydration, which reflect underlying fluid and electrolyte status. Evaluate urinary output and specific gravity. Weigh the infant or child on admission and daily thereafter. Monitor vital signs every 2 to 4 hours. If the child is febrile, water loss will be increased, contributing to the dehydration. Assess skin integrity, especially in the perineal and rectal areas, and note any breakdown or rashes.

The accompanying nursing care plan lists common nursing diagnoses for a child with gastroenteritis. The following diagnoses may also be appropriate.

- Anxiety (child and parent) related to change in health status
- Sleep Pattern Disturbed related to pain
- Imbalanced Nutrition: Less than Body Requirements related to inability to ingest sufficient nutrients

Planning and Implementation

Nursing care focuses on providing emotional support, promoting rest and comfort, and ensuring adequate nutrition. The accompanying nursing care plan summarizes nursing care for the child with gastroenteritis.

Provide Emotional Support

The child may have been ill for several days or become suddenly ill a short time before seeking healthcare. The child and parents are usually anxious, so it is important to allow them to talk and ask questions. The child may require blood tests to help direct rehydration therapy. Most children are cared for at home, although care in a 24-hour monitoring unit may occur. For hospitalization

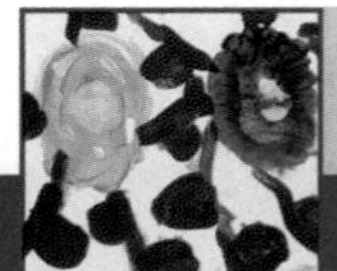

Nursing Care Plan

THE CHILD WITH GASTROENTERITIS

GOAL	INTERVENTION	RATIONALE	EXPECTED OUTCOME
1. Diarrhea related to infectious process			
	NIC Priority Intervention—*Diarrhea Management:* Prevention and alleviation of diarrhea.		**NOC Suggested Outcome—***Fluid and Electrolyte Balance:* Balance of water and electrolytes in the intracellular and extracellular compartments of the body.
The child's bowel function will be restored to normal.	▪ Obtain baseline vital signs and monitor every 2–4 hours.	▪ Fluid and electrolyte imbalances can alter vital body functions.	The child's bowel function returns to normal.
	▪ Observe stools for amount, color, consistency, odor, and frequency.	▪ Aids in the diagnosis and in monitoring the child's status.	
	▪ Test stools for occult blood.	▪ Frequent defecation and some infectious organisms can cause bleeding.	
	▪ Monitor results of stool culture and sample for ova and parasites.	▪ Rapid notification of the physician will facilitate treatment.	
	▪ Wash hands well before and after contact with the child.	▪ Helps prevent transmission of microorganisms.	
	▪ Isolate the child until the cause of the diarrhea is determined.	▪ Prevents exposure of other patients and staff to pathogens.	
	▪ Assist the child with toileting and hygiene.	▪ The child may be weak, incontinent, physically impaired, or anxious and require assistance to use the bathroom.	
	▪ Administer prescribed oral rehydration and intravenous solutions.	▪ Provides necessary fluids and nutrients.	
	▪ Notify the physician if diarrhea persists, stool characteristics change, or other symptoms of dehydration/electrolyte imbalance occur.	▪ Ensures early intervention.	
2. Deficient Fluid Volume related to active fluid volume loss			
	NIC Priority Intervention—*Fluid Monitoring:* Collection and analysis of patient data to regulate fluid balance.		**NOC Suggested Outcome—***Fluid and Electrolyte Balance:* Balance of water and electrolytes in the intracellular and extracellular compartments of the body.
The child will remain hydrated and will begin to drink fluids within 24 hours of admission.	▪ Monitor intake and output. Be sure to document time of each voiding.	▪ Will determine if output exceeds input. Long periods of time without urine output can be an early indicator of poor renal function. A child should produce 1 mL of urine/kg/hr.	The child has normal fluid and electrolyte balance as indicated by laboratory evaluation and physical examination.
	▪ Compare admission weight to preadmission weight. Assess weight daily.	▪ The degree of dehydration can be determined by the percentage of weight loss. Daily weights aid in determining progress toward rehydration.	
	▪ Assess level of consciousness, skin turgor, mucous membranes, skin color and temperature, capillary refill, eyes, and fontanels every 4 hours.	▪ Will determine degree of hydration and adequacy of interventions.	
	▪ Assess for vomiting.	▪ Vomiting frequently accompanies diarrhea and contributes to the child's fluid loss.	
	▪ Provide oral fluid and electrolyte replacement solution if able to tolerate.	▪ Less invasive than IV fluids. Provides for replacement of essential fluids and electrolytes.	
	▪ Provide and maintain IV replacement therapy, as ordered.	▪ Use of IV replacement is based on the degree of dehydration, ongoing losses, insensible water losses, and electrolyte results.	

(continued)

Nursing Care Plan THE CHILD WITH GASTROENTERITIS (continued)

GOAL	INTERVENTION	RATIONALE	EXPECTED OUTCOME
3. Risk for Impaired Skin Integrity related to altered fluid status			
	NIC Suggested Intervention—*Skin Surveillance:* Collection and analysis of patient data to maintain skin integrity.		**NOC Priority Outcome**—*Tissue Integrity:* Structural intactness and normal physiologic function of skin.
The child will remain free of skin breakdown and rashes.	■ Assess skin of perineum and rectum for signs of skin breakdown or irritation. ■ Provide prevention or restorative care for infants as follows:	■ Early assessment and intervention can prevent worsening of the condition.	The child's perianal and rectal tissue remains pink and intact.
Preventive Care			
	■ Change diapers every 2 hours or as needed. ■ Use cloth diapers rather than disposable. ■ Wash diaper area after each soiling. ■ Apply A & D ointment.	■ Minimizes skin contact with chemical irritants from stool and urine. ■ Minimizes the mechanical and chemical irritation from disposables. ■ Removes traces of stool if present. ■ Provides a barrier and protects intact or reddened skin from becoming excoriated.	
Restorative Care			
	■ Place the infant prone and leave the buttocks open to air. ■ Notify the physician if the skin is severely broken or peeling or if a rash is present. ■ For toddlers and older children: ■ Tub bathe at least daily (if condition allows) in tepid water. Pat the area dry. ■ Discourage the wearing of underwear if possible. ■ Apply A & D ointment at least four times daily	■ Promotes air circulation to the area. ■ Helps loosen any fecal matter without scrubbing, which can cause additional irritation to the skin. ■ Allows air to circulate and prevents accumulation of moisture. ■ Provides a barrier and protects intact or reddened skin from becoming excoriated	

or monitoring units, use therapeutic play techniques, such as allowing the child to manipulate equipment, to reduce anxiety (see Chapter 17∞). To promote a trusting relationship, be honest if a procedure will hurt. Encourage the child to express anger, fear, and pain.

Promote Rest and Comfort

Children with gastroenteritis may awaken frequently with periods of vomiting and diarrhea. Provide a quiet, restful environment and cluster nursing care to allow for periods of uninterrupted rest. Darken the room and keep interruptions to a minimum.

To reduce the child's anxiety, encourage parents to room-in. Place the child's favorite toys and comfort objects within reach. Keep the child's mouth moistened with a glycerine swab, a wet washcloth, or an occasional ice chip. Provide anal care after each diarrheal episode to maintain skin integrity. Avoid using commercial baby wipes when changing the diaper of an infant with diarrhea. Chemicals in the wipes may cause additional irritation and skin breakdown.

Ensure Adequate Nutrition

Liquids are offered throughout the illness, even if an intravenous infusion is in place. (Follow guidelines for oral rehydration therapy in Chapter 23∞.) Small amounts of normal diet for age are provided. Infants are breastfed or given formula. The child's diet progresses according to protocol or the child's tolerance for feedings.

Discharge Planning and Care in the Community

Discharge teaching begins on arrival at the healthcare facility. Partner with parents and teach them about the symptoms of dehydration and what actions to take if diarrhea recurs. Ensure that parents understand the recommended diet progression. Emphasize the necessity of good hygiene practices to prevent the spread of microorganisms that can cause gastroenteritis. If the child attends childcare, ask the parent to alert the care center about the gastroenteritis so the staff can monitor for other cases and take steps to prevent the spread of infection.

PRACTICE ALERT

Handwashing is the most important health maintenance measure that can be taken to prevent the spread of gastroenteritis. Wash hands often, particularly before and after care of each child. Instruct parents in the importance of handwashing, especially when caring for the child with gastroenteritis. Teach children in childcare centers and school how to wash their hands effectively to prevent spread of infectious diseases.

■ Evaluation

Expected outcomes of nursing care for the child with gastroenteritis include the following:

- The child's fluid and electrolyte balance are restored.
- The child achieves adequate nutritional intake to support growth and development.
- The child achieves adequate rest and sleep.
- Normal bowel function for the child is achieved.
- Family verbalizes description of signs of dehydration and appropriate interventions.
- Parents verbalize knowledge of importance of handwashing in decreasing transmission of infectious agents.

INTESTINAL PARASITIC DISORDERS

Intestinal parasitic disorders occur most frequently in tropical regions. Outbreaks take place in areas where water is not treated, food is incorrectly prepared, and people live in crowded conditions with poor sanitation. In the United States, outbreaks of diseases caused by protozoa or helminths (worms) are increasing. Young children, especially those in childcare centers, are most at risk of infection. They often lack good hygiene practices and are more likely to put objects and their hands into their mouths. The most common intestinal parasitic disorders are summarized in the clinical manifestations table on pages 1132–1133.

In addition, parasites are emerging in the United States that previously were not commonly seen. Included are *Cryptosporidium parvum, Dientamoeba fragilis, Blastocystis hominis,* and *Entamoeba coli.* The possibility of enteric infection should always be considered in children with continuing diarrhea or other intestinal symptoms (Cowden & Hotez, 2001).

Another common cause of young childhood infection is exposure to pets and wildlife. Pets should be checked for parasites and dewormed regularly. Public policies for cleanup of pet fecal material in parks can also decrease contamination. Some pets such as geckos and turtles may carry disease to young children.

Laboratory examination of stool specimens identifies the causative organism (protozoa, worms, larvae, or ova). Treatment usually involves an anthelmintic. See the medications table on page 1134.

Nursing Management

Nursing care centers on preventive teaching. Emphasize the importance of good hygiene practices, especially careful handwashing, after toileting and when handling food. Ensure the family understands proper medication administration. Instruct parents to administer prescribed medications as directed even if the child's condition seems to be improved.

Teach the family that sand and play boxes should be kept covered when not in use. Children should be taught good handwashing after exposure to their pets and not to approach or touch unfamiliar or wild animals (Kazacos, 2000).

INFLAMMATORY DISORDERS

Inflammatory disorders are reactions of specific tissues of the gastrointestinal tract to trauma caused by injuries, foreign bodies, chemicals, microorganisms, or surgery. These disorders may be acute or chronic and may involve various segments of the gastrointestinal tract. Peptic ulcer disease occurs in the esophagus, stomach, and/or duodenum. Appendicitis (the most common cause for emergency abdominal surgery in children), necrotizing enterocolitis (the most common gastrointestinal emergency occurring during the neonatal period), Meckel's diverticulum, recurrent abdominal pain, Crohn's disease, and ulcerative colitis are discussed in this section.

Peptic Ulcer

A peptic ulcer is an erosion of the mucosal tissue in the lower end of the esophagus, in the stomach (usually along the lesser curvature), or in the duodenum. Males are more likely to have peptic ulcers than females; however, peptic ulcers are much less common in children than in adults. African American and Hispanic children are at greater risk for peptic ulcers (Simpson & Ivey, 2003).

Etiology and Pathophysiology

Ulcers are classified as primary or secondary, depending on their etiology.

- *Primary peptic ulcers* occur in healthy children.
- *Secondary (stress) ulcers* occur in children with a preexisting illness or injury such as a burn, cancer, or HIV infection, and in children receiving medications such as salicylates, corticosteroids, and nonsteroidal anti-inflammatory drugs.

Diet usually is not a major factor in the development of peptic ulcers in children, although caffeine and alcohol consumption in adolescents may exacerbate the disease. It is now known that many cases of ulcer, in both adults and children, are caused by *Helicobacter pylori,* a gram-negative rod. This organism is transmitted by the fecal–oral or oral–oral route. Infections often occur in several members of a family, especially when the family's water supply is contaminated.

Clinical Manifestations

Clinical manifestations vary according to the age of the child and location of the ulcer. The most common symptom is abdominal pain

CLINICAL MANIFESTATIONS of Common Intestinal Parasitic Disorders

PARASITIC INFECTION	TRANSMISSION, LIFE CYCLE, PATHOGENESIS	CLINICAL MANIFESTATIONS	CLINICAL THERAPY	COMMENTS
Giardiasis Organism: protozoan *Giardia lamblia* Giardia lamblia	Transmission is through person-to-person contact, unfiltered water, improperly prepared infected food, and contact with animals. Cysts are ingested and passed into the duodenum and proximal jejunum, where they begin actively feeding. They are excreted in the stool.	May be asymptomatic. *Infants:* diarrhea, vomiting, anorexia, failure to thrive *Older children:* abdominal cramps; intermittent loose, foul-smelling, watery, pale, and greasy stools	Available medications include furazolidone and quinacrine. Furazolidone has fewer side effects than quinacrine but is more expensive. Metronidazole is also effective but is not licensed in the United States for treatment of giardiasis.	Most common intestinal parasitic organism in the United States. Infection may resolve spontaneously in 4–6 weeks without treatment. Parents or caregivers should wear gloves when handling diapers or stool of parasite-infected infant or child.
Enterobiasis (Pinworm) Organism: nematode *Enterobius vermicularis* Pinworm	Transmission is from discharged eggs inhaled or carried from hand to mouth. Eggs hatch in the upper intestine and mature in 15–28 days. Larvae then migrate to the cecum. After mating, the female migrates out of the anus and lays up to 17,000 eggs. Movement of worms causes intense itching. Scratching deposits eggs on the hands and under the nails.	Intense perianal itching, irritability, restlessness, and short attention span; in females, can migrate to the vagina and urethra to cause infection. Itching intensifies at night when the female comes to the anal opening to lay eggs.	Available medications include mebendazole, pyrantel pamoate, and piperazine citrate. The child and all household members should be treated at the same time. Treatment may be repeated in 2–3 weeks.	Most common helminthic infection in United States. Transmission is increased in crowded conditions such as housing developments, schools, and childcare centers.
Ascariasis (Roundworm) Organism: nematode *Ascaris lumbricoides* Roundworm	Transmission is from discharged eggs carried from hand to mouth. Adult lays eggs in small intestine. Eggs are excreted in stool, where they incubate for 2–3 weeks. Swallowed eggs hatch in the small intestine. Larvae may penetrate intestinal villi, entering the portal vein and liver, then moving to the lung. Larvae that ascend to upper respiratory tract are swallowed and proceed to the small intestine, where they repeat the cycle.	Mild infection may be asymptomatic. Severe infection may result in intestinal obstruction, peritonitis, obstructive jaundice, and lung involvement.	Available anthelmintic medications include mebendazole, pyrantel pamoate, or piperazine citrate. Stools should be examined 2 weeks after treatment and monthly for 3 months. Family members and contacts of the child should be treated if indicated. If the child has intestinal obstruction, treatment may include administering piperazine through a nasogastric tube and duodenal suction. Obstructing worms sometimes have to be surgically removed.	Most common in warm climates. Primarily affects children 1–4 years of age.

CLINICAL MANIFESTATIONS of Common Intestinal Parasitic Disorders (continued)

PARASITIC INFECTION	TRANSMISSION, LIFE CYCLE, PATHOGENESIS	CLINICAL MANIFESTATIONS	CLINICAL THERAPY	COMMENTS
Hookworm disease Organism: nematode *Necator americanus* Hookworm	Transmission is through direct contact with infected soil containing larvae. Worms live in the small intestine and feed on villi, causing bleeding. Eggs are deposited in the bowel and excreted in feces. Eggs hatch in damp shaded soil. Larvae attach to and penetrate the skin then enter the bloodstream, migrating to the lungs. Larvae then migrate to the upper respiratory passages and are swallowed.	In healthy individuals mild infection seldom causes problems. More severe infection may result in anemia and malnutrition. Presence of larvae on the skin may cause burning and itching, followed by redness and papular eruption.	Available medications include mebendazole and pyrantel pamoate. Stools should be examined 2 weeks after treatment and monthly for 3 months. Family members and contacts of the child should be treated if indicated.	Children should wear shoes when outdoors, although other unprotected areas of the skin may still come in contact with larvae.
Strongyloidiasis (Threadworm) Organism: nematode *Strongyloides stercoralis*	Transmission is from the ingestion of discharged larvae in the soil. Life cycle is similar to that of the hookworm, except the threadworm does not attach to the intestinal mucosa and feeding larvae (rather than eggs) may be deposited in the soil. Threadworm	Mild infection may be asymptomatic. Severe infection may result in abdominal pain and distention, nausea, vomiting, and diarrhea. Stools may be large and pale, with mucus. Severe infection may lead to a nutritional deficiency.	Available medications include thiabendazole or mebendazole. Treatment may need to be repeated if symptoms recur after treatment. Family members and contacts of the child should be examined and treated if indicated.	Most common in older children and adolescents.
Visceral larva migrans (Toxocarlasis) Organism: nematode *Toxocara canis* or *T. catis,* commonly found in dogs and cats	Transmission is through the ingestion of eggs in the soil. Ingested eggs hatch in the intestine. Mobile larvae then migrate to the liver and eventually to all major organs (including the brain). Once migration is complete, they encapsulate in dense fibrous tissue.	Most cases are asymptomatic. Affected children may have a low-grade fever and recurrent upper airway diseases. Severe symptoms include hepatomegaly, pulmonary infiltration, and neurologic disturbances. In all cases there is a hypereosinophilia of the blood.	There is no specific treatment. Corticosteroids have been used in severe cases. Thiabendazole has been recommended but efficacy is not established (infection usually resolves spontaneously).	Most common in toddlers. Deworm household pets monthly if indicated. Keep children away from areas contaminated with animal droppings.

Note: Giardia lamblia courtesy of the Centers for Disease Control and Prevention, Atlanta, GA; pinworm (p. 718), roundworm (p. 714), hookworm (p. 719), and threadworm (p. 721) from Rudolph, A. M., Hoffman, J. I. E., Rudolph, C. D. (1996). Rudolph's pediatrics *(20th ed.). Stamford, CT: Appleton & Lange.*

MEDICATIONS Used to Treat Intestinal Parasitic Infections

MEDICATION	INDICATION	NURSING IMPLICATIONS
Furazolidone	Used in treatment of: Giardiasis Enterobacter aerogenes Escherichia coli Proteus Salmonella Shigella Staphylococcus Vibrio cholerae	Protect medication from heat and light exposure Monitor for side effects: Abdominal pain Nausea, vomiting Diarrhea Fever Hypotension Headache Dizziness Hypoglycemia
Mebendazole	Used in treatment of: Pinworms Roundworm Hookworm Threadworm Whipworm	Tablets may be chewed and swallowed or crushed and mixed with food Monitor for side effects: Abdominal pain Diarrhea Fever
Pyrantel pamoate	Used in treatment of: Pinworms Roundworm Hookworm	Oral suspension should be shaken well before administration Administer with milk or fruit juices Monitor for side effects: Headache Anorexia Nausea Vomiting Diarrhea
Thiabendazole	Used in treatment of: Threadworm Pinworm Roundworm Hookworm	Administer after meals Chewable tablets must be chewed thoroughly Shake suspension well Monitor for side effects: Dizziness Anorexia Nausea Vomiting Diarrhea Pruritis Hematuria

Data from Bindler, R. M. & Howry, L. B. (2005). Pediatric Drugs & Nursing Implications. (3e). *Upper Saddle River, NJ: Prentice Hall Health.*

(burning) associated with an empty stomach, which may awaken the child at night. Vomiting and pain after meals, anemia, occult blood in stools, and abdominal distention may also be present.

COLLABORATIVE CARE

The goals of collaborative care are to relieve discomfort and promote healing.

Diagnostic Tests

Diagnosis is based on the history and radiologic studies. *H. pylori* can be diagnosed by culture of the organism taken via gastroscopy or measurement of *H. pylori* antigens in stool specimens. Urea breath test is effective (Kirschner, 2001), since the organism hydrolyzes urea.

Clinical Therapy

When *H. pylori* is the causative agent, antimicrobial agents such as bismuth salts, tetracycline, and metronidazole combination are given. Other drug combinations such as antacids in liquid form (Maalox, Mylanta) and histamine antagonists (ranitidine, cimetidine, and famotidine) are also used. Antibody titers are measured several times over 6 months to evaluate the effectiveness of therapy. The prognosis is usually good with early intervention.

NURSING MANAGEMENT

Nursing Assessment and Diagnosis

Assess the child for abdominal pain, vomiting, and abdominal distention. Monitor red blood cell (RBC) count and hemoglobin and hematocrit. Assess for family history of *H. pylori* infection.

Nursing diagnoses that may apply to the child with peptic ulcer include:

- Pain, Acute or Chronic related to erosion of gastric mucosal tissue
- Risk for Imbalanced Nutrition: Less than Body Requirements related to decreased food consumption, vomiting, and nausea
- Risk for Ineffective Coping (child) related to perceived stressful situations

Planning and Implementation

Nursing care centers on interventions to promote adequate nutritional intake, promote healing, and prevent recurrences. A nutritionally sound, age-appropriate diet is provided. Foods should be omitted only if they exacerbate the disorder.

Partner with the family and explain that antibiotics must be administered as scheduled. Emphasize the importance of continuing drug therapy. Encourage the family to continue the medications as ordered and to return for follow-up visits. Children who attend school may prefer to take antacids in the form of tablets, which are easier to carry than liquid preparations. A permission form to take medications at school will need to be filled out by the prescriber. Parents should discuss any additional medications with the primary healthcare provider before administering to the child.

Caution parents to avoid aspirin products, which irritate the gastric mucosa. If an antipyretic or pain medication is needed, administer acetaminophen. Advise parents to read medication labels if they are unsure of product contents.

Because psychologic stress can contribute to peptic ulcer disease, parents and child should be assisted to identify sources of stress in the child's life. Assess coping mechanisms and provide referral for psychologic counseling, if appropriate. Teach relaxation techniques and recommend community classes on yoga or other stress reduction.

■ Evaluation

Expected outcomes of nursing care of the child with peptic ulcer include:

- The child obtains pain relief and experiences decreased episodes of pain.
- The child consumes adequate nutrition to meet growth and development needs.
- The child engages in stress-reducing activities and acknowledges effectiveness of interventions.

PATHOPHYSIOLOGY ILLUSTRATED

Appendicitis

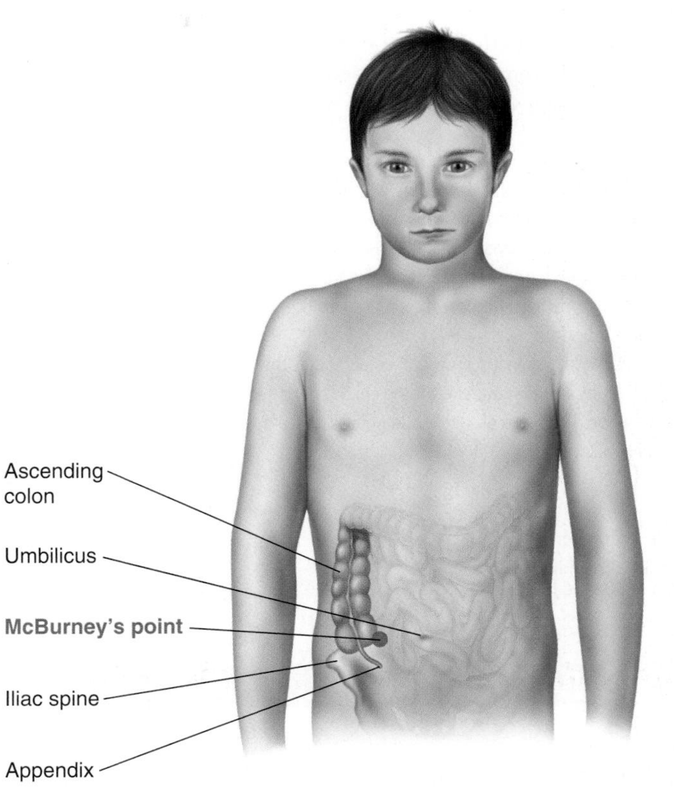

Ascending colon

Umbilicus

McBurney's point

Iliac spine

Appendix

FIGURE 30–14 ■ McBurney's point is the common location of pain in children and adolescents with appendicitis.

Appendicitis

Appendicitis is an inflammation of the vermiform appendix, the small sac near the end of the cecum. The condition occurs most often in adolescent males (10 to 19 years of age). It is rarely observed before 2 years of age. Appendicitis is the most common cause for emergency abdominal surgery in children and adolescents in the United States (Kosloske, Love, Rohrer, et al., 2004). Children account for 62,000 to 82,000 of the appendectomies performed every year in more than 250,000 Americans (Ziegler, 2004).

Etiology and Pathophysiology

Appendicitis almost always results from an obstruction in the appendiceal lumen, causing edema. Obstructions include fecalith (hard fecal mass), parasitic infestations, stenosis, hyperplasia of lymphoid tissue, or a tumor.

Continued secretion of mucus following acute obstruction of the lumen increases pressure, causing ischemia, cellular death, necrosis, and ulceration. As edema increases, the vascular supply to the appendix is compromised, increasing the permeability of the appendix. Bacteria then invade the appendix, causing further inflammation.

If untreated, appendicitis progresses to a life-threatening condition, as perforation or rupture of the appendix may occur, resulting in fecal and bacterial contamination of the peritoneum. Peritonitis spreads quickly and if untreated can result in small bowel obstruction, electrolyte imbalances, septicemia, hypovolemic shock, and death.

Clinical Manifestations

At onset, symptoms include periumbilical cramps, abdominal tenderness, and fever. Pain may be described throughout the abdomen with periumbilical pain common. In adolescent and young adult females, symptoms must be differentiated from those associated with ovulation (mittelschmerz), ruptured ectopic pregnancy, and pelvic inflammatory disease.

As the inflammation progresses, pain in the right lower abdomen becomes constant. Pain is often most intense at McBurney's point, halfway between the anterior superior iliac crest and the umbilicus (Figure 30–14 ■). In

30% of children, however, the appendix is in a different location, so the pain may occur elsewhere. Symptoms progress to include guarding, rigidity, nausea, vomiting, onset of pain before vomiting, anorexia, and rebound tenderness following palpation over the right lower quadrant. Rovsing's sign (indirect tenderness) and psoas sign (pain induced by flexion of the hip) may also be observed (Paulson, Kalady, & Pappas, 2003).

Diarrhea or constipation may be present. As appendicitis progresses, the child remains motionless, usually in a side-lying position with knees flexed.

PRACTICE ALERT

The most predictive signs and symptoms of acute appendicitis are pain in the right lower quadrant, abdominal rigidity, and migration of pain from the periumbilical region to the right lower quadrant. The nurse assessing these signs or symptoms should immediately report the findings to the primary care provider for urgent interventions.

Sudden relief of abdominal pain usually means that the appendix has ruptured. Notify the physician immediately if the child reports sudden relief of pain. Assess vital signs for indications of shock. Additional signs and symptoms of a ruptured appendix include:

- Fever
- Guarding
- Abdominal distention
- Rapid shallow breathing
- Pallor
- Chills
- Irritability or restlessness

COLLABORATIVE CARE

The focus of collaborative care includes early identification of appendicitis, pain management, surgical removal of the appendix, and prevention of complications.

Diagnostic Tests

Appendicitis should be suspected in any child with pain in the right lower quadrant. Diagnosis of appendicitis in young children can be difficult because their pain may be less localized and their symptoms more diffuse than in the older child. Continuing evaluations over several hours are often needed to establish diagnosis.

Numerous conditions mimic appendicitis and should be considered during the process of diagnosis. Such conditions include cholecystitis, sickle cell crisis, constipation, gastroenteritis, ectopic pregnancy, pelvic inflammatory disease, intestinal obstruction, inguinal hernia, testicular torsion, and urinary tract infection.

An elevated white blood cell count (above 15,000/mm^3) may occur. This leukocytosis occurs less often in young children than in teenagers. It is not uncommon, however, for the white blood cell count to be within normal limits with a nonperforated appendix; therefore, diagnosis is not dependent on this laboratory finding.

A history of abdominal pain, rebound tenderness, presence of a fecalith in the right lower abdomen on abdominal radiograph and abdominal ultrasound help to confirm or rule out the diagnosis. CT with contrast is rapidly becoming the diagnostic tool of choice. Urinalysis is performed to rule out other pathology, such as urinary tract infection. Serum C-reactive protein (CRP) may be evaluated. This measurement is elevated in appendicitis, although any infectious process also causes an elevated CRP.

Clinical Therapy

Treatment of acute appendicitis involves immediate surgical removal (appendectomy), either through laparoscopic or open method (Vegunta, Ali, Wallace, et al., 2004).

Preoperatively the child is kept NPO. Intravenous fluids and electrolytes are administered. Antibiotics are administered if the appendix is ruptured or the child is at high risk for infection. A nasogastric tube may be inserted before or after surgery.

Postoperatively intravenous fluids and antibiotics (if prescribed) are continued. If the appendix has ruptured before surgery, a Penrose drain is inserted and the wound may not be completely sutured. Wound irrigations may be required to assist with cleansing of the peritoneum. Recovery is usually complete following uncomplicated removal of the appendix.

NURSING MANAGEMENT

Nursing management includes collaborative identification of the child with appendicitis, preoperative and postoperative care, and preventing complications.

■ Nursing Assessment and Diagnosis

Physiologic Assessment

A detailed assessment of the child's pain is necessary to differentiate appendicitis from other illnesses (see Chapter 18∞).

Ask the child to point to the painful area and describe the pain. Utilize a pain scale to assess severity of pain. Recognize that localizing the pain may be difficult for young children. Note onset, location, and intensity of pain; precipitating factors; and relief measures tried. During abdominal assessment, perform palpation last to avoid causing additional pain. Deep palpation of the left side of the abdomen followed by removing the hand quickly can lead to pain in the area of the appendix (rebound tenderness). However, once appendicitis is suspected or verified, avoid abdominal palpation in order to minimize pain to the child.

Assess vital signs to determine baseline values and monitor every 2 hours thereafter. Ask about the last food and fluid intake and any vomiting that has occurred. Assess history of previous surgeries or abdominal conditions.

Psychosocial Assessment

Because appendicitis usually occurs in school-age children and adolescents, assessment of the child's coping skills is important. Adolescents, because of their preoccupation with body image, may be concerned about the surgical incision scar if open appendectomy is performed. Assess the parents' and child's anxiety about the sudden hospitalization and need for emergency surgery.

Following are nursing diagnoses that may be appropriate for the child with appendicitis.

- Acute Pain related to inflammation and surgery
- Risk for Deficient Fluid Volume related to fluid volume loss and inadequate fluid volume intake
- Anxiety (parental and child) related to acute physical condition and need for surgery
- Risk for Infection related to bowel trauma

■ Planning and Intervention

Nursing care focuses on promoting comfort, maintaining hydration, providing emotional support, supporting respiratory function, providing care of the surgical site, and monitoring for symptoms of infection.

Promote Comfort

Preoperatively, a side-lying position with knees bent is usually the most comfortable. Allow the child to assume any position that promotes comfort. Administer analgesics routinely as ordered, and note results of medications. Ask the family what might be comforting for the child such as music, gently stroking the back, or having family present.

Postoperative pain is managed similarly. The child is placed in a semi-Fowler's or side-lying position on the right side. If the appendix has ruptured, lying on the right side facilitates drainage from the peritoneal cavity. Administer pain medication routinely as prescribed. Avoid the use of a heating pad since it is contraindicated in children with appendicitis. Heat will only increase the inflammation and may contribute to rupture of the appendix if used preoperatively.

Maintain Hydration

Assess fluid volume status every 2 hours. Assess skin turgor, eyes, and mucous membranes for signs of dehydration. Monitor intake and output and assess vital signs. An intravenous infusion is initiated preoperatively and continued until bowel function returns after surgery. Once bowel sounds return, offer water in small amounts followed by other clear fluids, and advance to regular diet as tolerated. Listen for bowel tones postoperatively and be sure they are present before beginning oral fluids.

Provide Emotional Support

For many children, appendicitis may be the reason for their first hospitalization and only experience with healthcare personnel beyond their usual provider. The nurse must elicit a history, perform a physical examination, coordinate diagnostic tests, and prepare the child for surgery in a short period of time. Emotional support is essential for both child and parents. Good preoperative education can reduce anxiety. Answer any questions the child or parents may have. In the postoperative period, phone calls and visits from friends or family members may be helpful.

Support Respiratory Function

General anesthesia during surgery compromises respiratory function. Encourage the child to deep breathe by blowing bubbles or use incentive spirometry. Be alert for the child with asthma or other respiratory illness that will place the child at higher risk of respiratory complications

Recognize Symptoms of Infection

Assess vital signs and observe the abdominal incision every 4 hours for redness, edema, or drainage. If a drain is present, assess drainage for color, consistency, and amount. After the initial dressing has been changed, perform dressing changes routinely as indicated by agency protocol, and as necessary to keep the incision area clean and dry. Administer antibiotics as prescribed.

Discharge Planning and Home Care Teaching

The child is discharged once bowel function returns and he or she is taking fluids adequately. Give parents instructions on reestablishing a nutritious diet as recommended. Partner with parents to ensure that they are able to recognize the signs and symptoms of infection and understand the importance of seeking early treatment. Have them be alert for the child's first bowel movement and contact the care provider if constipation is a problem.

Normal activities can be resumed fairly quickly, but strenuous activities and contact sports should be avoided 6 weeks postoperatively or as indicated by the surgeon. Parents should check with the child's physician before allowing the child to resume sports activities. Generally the child is able to return to school soon after discharge if the surgery was noneventful and the appendix was not ruptured. In cases of complications or ruptured appendix, a longer hospitalization and longer home recovery are required. Home tutoring may be required for a short time so the child can remain current with school work.

■ Evaluation

Expected outcomes of nursing care include the following:

- The child obtains pain relief.
- The child maintains fluid balance.
- Parents and child express understanding of the condition and treatment, verbalize their fears and concerns, and receive adequate support.
- The child is free from infection.

Necrotizing Enterocolitis

Necrotizing enterocolitis (NEC) is a potentially life-threatening inflammatory disease of the intestinal tract that occurs primarily in premature infants. Necrotizing enterocolitis is the most common gastrointestinal emergency occurring during the neonatal period. The disorder affects from 4% to 13% of very-low-birth-weight infants and has up to a 40% mortality rate (Bell, 2005). Preterm infants are at greatest risk since maternal transport of immunoglobulins to the fetus occurs predominantly after 32 week's gestation, putting the premature infant at greatest risk for infectious processes.

Etiology and Pathophysiology

The etiology of necrotizing enterocolitis is multifactorial. Included are intestinal ischemia, bacterial or viral infection (a result of the premature infant's decreased immune response and greater risk for infection), and immaturity of the gastrointestinal mucosa (a result of the premature infant's decreased amount of gastric acid and proteolytic enzymes and underdeveloped protective intestinal mucin layer) (Kliegman & Willoughby, 2005). The disease occurs most often in the terminal ileum and colon.

Vascular compromise, leading to hypoxia and ischemia, causes a reduced blood flow to the bowel, leading to necrosis of the bowel mucosa. The damaged bowel stops secreting protective enzymes, allowing gas-forming bacteria to invade the necrotic tissue. This bacterial invasion further damages the intestinal mucosa by releasing bacterial toxins and gas, causing abdominal distention. Necrosis of the bowel can lead to intestinal perforation and general sepsis, making this a life-threatening condition.

Clinical Manifestations

Manifestations generally occur between 3 and 14 days of age, but can occur as early as the first day of life and as late as 3 months of age. The infant may initially show signs of feeding intolerance (increased gastric residuals, vomiting, irritability, and abdominal distention). The abdomen is initially mildly distended, progressing to severe distention. These signs are caused by inflammation and dilation of the bowel and accumulation of gas in the intestine. Bloody diarrhea may be present because of the hemorrhagic bowel. Urine output is decreased. Emesis may be bile stained. The clinical triad of abdominal distention, bilious vomiting, and bloody stools is characteristic of the infection. Signs of sepsis (e.g., hypothermia, hypotension, bradycardia, lethargy, apnea) usually follow, and the infant's condition rapidly deteriorates.

PRACTICE ALERT

Signs of sepsis in the newborn include:

- Hypothermia or hyperthermia
- Jaundice
- Respiratory distress
- Hepatomegaly
- Abdominal distention
- Anorexia
- Vomiting
- Lethargy

Report these symptoms to the primary healthcare provider immediately.

COLLABORATIVE CARE

The goal of collaborative care is to identify and reduce risk factors that lead to necrotizing enterocolitis, immediate identification and aggressive management of the disorder, and prevention of complications.

Diagnostic Tests

Diagnosis is made on the basis of characteristic clinical findings and the presence of free peritoneal gas, dilated bowel loops, bowel distention, and bowel wall thickening on abdominal radiographs. Stools and emesis are monitored for occult blood. Laboratory data reveal anemia, leukopenia, leukocytosis, thrombocytopenia, electrolyte imbalance, and metabolic or respiratory acidosis. Blood cultures are positive for organism present.

Clinical Therapy

Early aggressive enteral formula feeding of premature infants is avoided because of the increased incidence of the disease in these cases. Human milk has been shown to be protective against the disease; thus, breastfeeding or feeding the mother's expressed milk is the feeding method of choice for premature infants. Once diagnosed, necrotizing enterocolitis requires prompt intervention. Management begins with discontinuation of all enteral feedings. A naso-orogastric tube is inserted and maintained on low suction to prevent gastric distention, and intravenous fluids are started. Total parenteral nutrition may be initiated through a central line.

All cases of necrotizing enterocolitis are treated with strict enteric precautions to prevent the spread of infection to other premature infants on the unit. Antibiotics are administered prophylactically or to treat sepsis. Perforation or necrosis of the bowel necessitates surgical resection of the bowel. An ileostomy or colostomy may be performed in some cases.

Because the mortality rate associated with laparotomy for perforated necrotizing enterocolitis is significantly higher among neonates weighing less than 1,000 g than for larger neonates, peritoneal drains may be used initially instead of laparotomy for the management of perforation in these small neonates. The drains create a fistula, allowing drainage of the peritoneum.

New treatments are being attempted with probiotics, live and beneficial microorganisms that promote normal gut flora. *Lactobacillus acidophilus* and *Bifidobacterium infantis* are examples of organisms that can be administered by special formula.

Long-term complications of necrotizing enterocolitis include short bowel syndrome (discussed below), strictures, and cholestasis. Impaired nutrition may require total parenteral nutrition (TPN) therapy. **Cholestasis** is a disruption of bile flow, the most common problem in survivors of necrotizing enterocolitis. It is a complication of TPN and commonly occurs 2 weeks after TPN therapy has been initiated. Cholestasis is characterized by an elevated bilirubin (>0.2 mg/dL), hepatomegaly, and elevated serum transaminase. Abdominal perforation can lead to sepsis, shock, and death. The infant frequently has impaired growth and delayed developmental performance.

NURSING MANAGEMENT

Nursing care centers on prevention and early detection of necrotizing enterocolitis to minimize bowel loss, postoperative care, and family support.

■ Nursing Assessment and Diagnosis

Observe for feeding intolerance by aspirating gastric residual (if the infant is receiving enteral feedings). Measure abdominal circumference and assess bowel sounds in the premature or high-risk infant every 4 to 8 hours. Even minimal changes in circumference can indicate necrotizing enterocolitis and should be reported to the primary care provider. Careful monitoring of vital signs and intake and output is essential to detect complications.

Nursing diagnoses that apply to the infant with necrotizing enterocolitis may include:

- Risk for Infection related to presence of organisms
- Risk for Deficient Fluid Volume related to NPO status
- Ineffective Tissue Perfusion (gastrointestinal) related to vascular compromise
- Imbalanced Nutrition: Less than Body Requirements related to disease process and NPO status
- Risk for Impaired Parent/Infant Attachment related to critically ill status of newborn

Planning and Implementation

Maintaining fluid and electrolyte balance is essential. Provide comfort by holding and cuddling an infant who is NPO, and offer a pacifier to meet nonnutritive sucking needs. Careful assessment for infection and maintenance of skin integrity are essential. Feedings are gradually reestablished once bowel function returns. Administration of probiotics may be part of therapy.

Parents require emotional support and reassurance and help in bonding with their infant. They are coping with the birth of an infant who is critically ill. Make appropriate referrals for support as indicated. Because the symptoms of necrotizing enterocolitis do not appear until approximately 5 to 7 days after feedings are begun, parents may not be prepared for the infant's decline. The recovery of a premature infant is slow and can be complicated. Give clear explanations and encourage parents to ask questions and express their fears and concerns. If the infant's condition worsens, support for the parents of a dying child should be offered (see Chapter 22∞).

Once the infant is discharged, frequent follow-up care is needed. Encourage regular healthcare visits for monitoring of growth and development, and to receive preventive care such as immunizations. Schedule home visits to assist the family in managing healthcare and normal developmental issues. Partner with the parents to establish home care routine. If TPN is administered at home, parents will need education regarding proper administration of TPN and how to care for the central line. Oral and enteral nutritional intake is carefully assessed. Several medications are likely to be used. The nurse ensures the family understands correct administration techniques. If the infant requires an ostomy, teach parents proper care of the stoma. Refer to previous discussion of stoma care in this chapter.

The infant requires regular and thorough physical assessments to identify any complications. Growth of the child is monitored and compared with previous findings. Developmental progress is assessed by regular administration of a developmental test such as the Denver II (see Chapter 10∞).

Evaluation

Expected outcomes of nursing care for the child with necrotizing enterocolitis include:

- The infant is free from infection.
- The infant achieves fluid and electrolyte balance.
- Tissue perfusion is maintained following surgical removal of necrosed bowel.
- The infant receives adequate nutrition to support growth and development needs.
- Parent–infant attachment becomes secure.

If surgery is performed, complete healing without infection or other complication is desired. If the infant is not successfully treated, support and comfort for the parents is necessary. When the child survives, desired long-term outcomes include normal developmental progression and nutrition to support growth.

Meckel's Diverticulum

Meckel's diverticulum is the most common congenital anomaly of the gastrointestinal tract, with a male to female ratio of 3:2 (Sadovsky, 2001). It is the most common cause of lower gastrointestinal bleeding in children; it occurs in 2% of the population, although many individuals are asymptomatic and do not know they have the disorder.

Meckel's diverticulum results when the omphalomesenteric duct, which connects the midgut to the yolk sac during embryonic development, fails to atrophy. Instead, an outpouching of the ileum remains, usually located near the ileocecal valve. The pouch contains gastric or pancreatic tissue, which secretes acid, causing irritation and ulceration.

Clinical manifestations usually appear by 2 years of age. Common complaints include abdominal pain, nausea and vomiting, rectal bleeding, abdominal distention, peritonitis, and diarrhea (Neidlinger, Madan, & Wright, 2001). The rectal bleeding is usually painless dark or bright red, and results from the obstruction or ulceration. Often blood is passed without stool.

The child may have symptoms of intussusception, incarcerated hernia, volvulus, or intestinal obstruction. If untreated, diverticulitis may progress to perforation and peritonitis.

Bowel obstruction is the most common complication associated with Meckel's diverticulm (Neidlinger et al., 2001). Additional complications associated with Meckel's diverticulum include bowel inflammation, bleeding, and tumors (Sadovsky, 2001).

COLLABORATIVE CARE

Diagnosis of Meckel's diverticulum is based on the history. Contrast studies are usually not helpful, because the diverticulum is often too small to visualize and may not fill with barium. Radionuclide imaging and scanning can usually detect the gastric tissue, confirming the diagnosis. Laparoscopy may be performed to confirm diagnosis.

Treatment is surgical excision of the diverticulum and removal of any involved bowel via resection using either open or laparoscopic techniques (Sadovsky, 2001). The prognosis is good following surgical excision.

NURSING MANAGEMENT

Preoperatively an intravenous infusion is initiated to correct fluid and electrolyte imbalances. Monitor intake and output. Observe for rectal bleeding and test stools for **occult blood** (blood that is present in small quantities and measurable only by laboratory testing). Maintain the child on bed rest. Assess vital signs every 2 hours, and monitor for signs of shock.

Postoperative care is similar to that for an infant or child undergoing abdominal surgery. (See the earlier discussion of postsurgical nursing management of appendicitis and the nursing care plan for the child undergoing surgery in Chapter 17∞).

At the time of discharge, parents need instructions on caring for the surgical site, preventing infection, reintroducing of fluids and food, providing an adequate diet, and administering prescribed medications.

Recurrent Abdominal Pain

Recurrent abdominal pain (RAP) is a frequent problem among young children and adolescents, particularly girls of school age. The disorder affects approximately 10% to 15% of school-age children in the United States (Kohli & Li, 2004). Although organic causes such as motility problems, constipation, or inflammatory bowel disease exist, in most cases one cannot be found. This disorder is associated with the high-stress lifestyles common in contemporary society and has a strong environmental component. However, parents and healthcare professionals should not dismiss the child's pain because the cause is unknown or unidentified.

The pain is generally located in the periumbilical area and occurs on a regular basis. A thorough history and physical examination are necessary to rule out organic causes. Children with recurrent abdominal pain may have little independence and feel controlled by their parents. The history should explore the pressures and stresses in the child's life, the child's temperament or methods of coping, bowel elimination patterns, and history of sexual abuse.

Laboratory studies such as a complete blood count may be ordered to rule out other illness. Gastrointestinal studies may be performed in an outpatient setting. Children are occasionally hospitalized when their condition is severe and not treatable at home.

When no organic cause can be identified, treatment of recurrent abdominal pain focuses on providing outlets for the release of stress within the family and in other settings in the child's life, enhancing the child's coping methods, and promoting dietary changes that encourage regular bowel movements. Cognitive behavioral therapies, such as relaxation techniques, have proven effective since they reduce autonomic arousal and muscle tension (Hyman & Danda, 2004).

Nursing Management

Nursing care includes supporting the child during assessment and diagnostic testing. The child can be taught relaxation techniques and methods for coping with stress. Identify what life events are stressors for the child and ask about specific worries. Ask about school and anxiety related to friendships, grades, and activities. Explore methods for giving more independence to the child in the family. Teach the importance of eating a high-fiber diet and maintaining a regular elimination pattern. The child and family may need explanations to understand the pain, which can be compared with neck pain or a headache as an outcome of stress. Children with continuing or recurrent abdominal pain are referred to a mental health professional.

Inflammatory Bowel Disease

Inflammatory bowel disease encompasses two distinct chronic disorders, Crohn's disease and ulcerative colitis, which have similar symptoms and treatment. Both diseases involve faulty regulation of the immune response of the intestinal mucosa in individuals who are genetically predisposed and have a genetic trigger (Gokhale, 2001). Inflammatory bowel disease differs from irritable bowel syndrome, which is discussed in the section on feeding and elimination disorders in Chapter 9∞.

Etiology and Pathophysiology

Crohn's Disease. Crohn's disease is a chronic, inflammatory process. The disorder can occur randomly throughout the GI tract, with the ileum, colon, and rectum the most common sites. A distinct feature of Crohn's disease is the development of enteric fistulas between loops of bowel or nearby organs. Mucosal ulcers begin in small locations, and then grow in size and depth into the mucosal wall. Submucosal inflammation can be severe. The etiology is unknown. There is strong evidence to support a genetic association. Crohn's disease is more common in Whites and 3 to 6 times more prevalent in individuals of Jewish descent. It most often develops between 15 and 25 years of age, and has been increasing in incidence (Gokhale, 2001). The prevalence of Crohn's disease is approximately 10 in 100,000 children younger than age 18 years (Baron, 2002).

Complications associated with Crohn's disease include perforation, hemorrhage, strictures, fistulas, liver disease, and toxic megacolon.

Ulcerative Colitis. Ulcerative colitis is a chronic recurrent disease primarily of the large intestine and rectal mucosa of unknown etiology. Inflammation is limited to the mucosa, as opposed to Crohn's disease, which extends deep into the bowel wall. Ulcerative colitis involves the entire length of the bowel with varying degrees of inflammation, ulceration, hemorrhage, and edema. Emotional and other psychosocial factors may influence the presentation and course of the disease. It is more prevalent among persons of Jewish heritage. The disease develops before 20 years of age with peak onset at about 12 years.

Complications associated with ulcerative colitis include hemorrhage, sepsis, toxic megacolon, and increased incidence of cancer.

Clinical Manifestations

The onset of Crohn's disease is subtle. Cramping abdominal pain is usually reported first, followed by diarrhea. Other symptoms include fever, anorexia, growth failure or weight loss, general malaise, and joint pain. Perianal disease and oral or anal lesions (or both) may be present. Extraintestinal manifestations include skin lesions, arthritis of the large peripheral joints, and uveitis (Baron, 2002).

The first symptom of ulcerative colitis is usually diarrhea progressing to bloody stools. Lower abdominal pain and cramping are present before and during a bowel movement and are relieved by the passage of stool and flatus. The stool is often mixed with blood and mucus. Rectal bleeding and flatulence are also noted. Weight loss or delayed growth, nutritional deficiencies, and arthralgias often occur as effects of the disease. See Table 30–7 for a comparison of ulcerative colitis and Crohn's disease.

COLLABORATIVE CARE

Collaborative care focuses on promoting remission of the disease, optimal nutritional intake, and optimal growth and development.

Diagnostic Tests

Diagnosis centers on evaluating the cause and identifying the extent of involved bowel and differentiating an infectious process (organisms such as Shigella and Salmonella) from inflammatory bowel disease. Laboratory studies help to identify related nutritional, electrolyte, and blood abnormalities.

Diagnosis of inflammatory bowel disease is based on laboratory evaluation: Anemia is common; an elevated erythrocyte sedimentation rate, elevated C-reactive protein, hypoalbuminemia, and thrombocytosis are other possible findings. Stools are positive for occult blood. Antineutrophil cytoplasmic antibodies (ANCA) may be detected in serum studies. Perinuclear highlighting of those autoantibodies (pANCA) is associated with ulcerative colitis and Crohn's disease. Of individuals with Crohn's disease, 15% are pANCA positive, and 60% to 70% of individuals with ulcerative colitis are pANCA positive. Radiologic studies such as upper gastrointestinal (UGI) series may reveal deep ulcerations in the terminal ileum, a cobblestone appearance, or a narrowing in the small bowel; and fistulas may also be detected.

TABLE 30–7 Comparison of Ulcerative Colitis and Crohn's Disease

	ULCERATIVE COLITIS	CROHN'S DISEASE
Type of lesions	Continuous, superficial involvement	Segmental, transmural (through the wall) involvement
Clinical manifestations		
Anal or perianal lesions	Rare	Common
Anorexia	Mild to moderate	Can be severe
Diarrhea	Often severe	Moderate
Growth retardation	Mild	Significant
Pain	Present	Common
Rectal bleeding	Present	Absent
Weight loss	Moderate	Severe
Risk of cancer	Slightly increased	Greatly increased

A colonoscopy allows for direct visualization of the gastrointestinal tract surface. A biopsy conducted at this time confirms diagnosis of inflammatory bowel disease and is useful in determining the extent and severity of inflammation (Baron, 2002).

Clinical Therapy

Crohn's disease and ulcerative colitis have periods of remission and exacerbation. There is no cure for the diseases. Treatment for both diseases is highly individualized and includes pharmacologic interventions (administration of antibiotic, anti-inflammatory, immunosuppressive, and antidiarrheal medications), nutrition therapy, and in severe cases, surgery.

Pharmacologic Management. First-line pharmacologic treatment of Crohn's disease involves aminosalicylates. Sulfasalazine inhibits prostaglandin synthesis, thereby decreasing inflammation. See the medications table on page 1142. Corticosteroids are given orally and in the form of enemas to children with more severe disease.

Nutritional Management. Because children with Crohn's disease are at risk for nutritional deficiencies, a nutritionist is included as part of the multidisciplinary team treating the child. The goal of nutrition therapy is to provide adequate caloric intake and nutrients necessary for growth. Vitamin, iron, zinc, and folic acid supplementation is frequently required. Total parenteral nutrition is often given to treat nutritional deficiencies and malnutrition, which accompany inflammatory bowel disease. A high-protein, high-carbohydrate, low-fiber diet with normal amounts of fat is recommended. Enteral feedings of partially digested formulas via nasogastric (NG) tube at night and an unrestricted diet during the day may support maximal growth and minimize disease activity (Baron, 2002). Nutritional supplements may include iron for the child with anemia.

Surgical Management. If other treatment measures fail to reduce inflammation, surgery may be indicated. Bowel obstruction, perianal disease, abdominal abscess, and strictures are the most common reasons for surgical intervention. A temporary colostomy or ileostomy is performed to allow the bowel to rest. In Crohn's disease, however, ulcerations tend to recur elsewhere in the GI tract. In ulcerative colitis, removal of the diseased bowel provides a permanent cure. Increased production of inflammatory cytokines in the intestine has been observed in patients with Crohn's disease. The intravenous infusion of antitumor necrosis factor antibody has therefore shown promise of treatment for the disorder, decreasing the symptoms and incidence of surgery (Gokhale, 2001).

NURSING MANAGEMENT

Nursing management occurs mainly in the community and home and focuses on helping the child and family adjust to the emotional impact of a chronic disease, administering medications and diet therapy, monitoring nutritional status, monitoring growth status, and providing appropriate referrals.

MEDICATIONS Used for Treatment of Inflammatory Bowel Disease

MEDICATION	INDICATION	NURSING IMPLICATIONS
Aminosalicylates Sulfasalazine Mesalamine Olsalazine Balsalazide	Used for anti-inflammatory effect Inhibition of prostaglandins known to cause diarrhea and affect mucosal transport	Administer after meals Do not crush or chew sustained-released tablets Monitor for side effects: Nausea Bloody diarrhea Vomiting Anorexia
Corticosteroids Prednisone Methylprednisone Hydrocortisone enema	Used for anti-inflammatory effect	Administer with meals to reduce gastric irritation Teach family to avoid abrupt discontinuation of medication Teach family to report delayed wound healing Monitor for side effects: Nausea Cushingoid appearance Vomiting Leukocytosis
Immunosuppressants 6-Mercaptopurine (6-MP) Azathioprine Cyclosporine Methotrexate Tacrolimus (FK-506)	Given for immunosuppressant and anti-inflammatory actions	Monitor for side effects: Nausea Anorexia Vomiting Diarrhea Bone marrow depression Thrombocytopenia Teach family to avoid exposing child to persons with infection Teach family the importance of good hygiene for child to avoid infection
Biologic therapies Tumor necrosis factor (TNFα) Infliximab (Remicade) Interleukin-10 Thalidomide	Prevents TNFα from binding to its receptors (TNFα have been found in stools of patients with Crohn's disease)	Reconstitute IV preparation according to manufacturer directions and administer according to agency protocol Monitor for side effects: Infusion reactions—fever, chills, chest pain, hypotension, dyspnea, urticaria Discontinue IV infusion if infusion reaction is evident
Antibacterial Metronidazole Ciprofloxacil	Antibacterial against anaerobic bacteria and some gram-negative bacteria	Extended-release form should not be chewed or crushed Administer with food or milk to reduce gastrointestinal distress Monitor for side effects: Fever Vomiting Headache Overgrowth of Candida Nausea

Data from Baron, M. L. (2002) Crohn's disease in children. American Journal of Nursing, 102, *26–34.*

MediaLink Inflammatory Bowel Disease Resources and Support

Nursing Assessment and Diagnosis

Assess for abdominal distention, tenderness, and pain. Monitor bowel sounds and stool pattern; measure abdominal girth.

Nursing diagnoses that apply to the child with inflammatory bowel disease may include:

- Diarrhea related to disease process
- Imbalanced Nutrition: Less than Body Requirements related to bowel inflammation and poor nutritional intake
- Pain, Acute or Chronic related to inflammatory disease process
- Risk for Deficient Fluid Volume related to loss of fluids through diarrhea
- Disturbed Body Image related to disease process, presence of stoma, and medication side effects

Planning and Implementation

Provide emotional support and counseling to help the child adjust to feeling "different" from peers. Inability to compete with peers and frequent absences from school can affect the child's self-esteem. Collaborate care with parents and assist them in contacting the school district to arrange for tutoring in case extended absences from school become necessary. Encourage the child who is not attending school regularly to maintain contact with friends through telephone calls, cards, and visits.

Body image is a major concern for children and adolescents with inflammatory bowel disease. Corticosteroid therapy causes growth retardation and delayed sexual maturation. Encourage the child to discuss feelings about these side effects. If a permanent colostomy or ileostomy is required, the nurse can assist the child and family to understand the need for surgical treatment. (See the discussion of ostomies earlier in this chapter.) Introduce the child and family to other children who have stomas.

Providing adequate stress reduction may be helpful in control of inflammatory bowel disease. Collaborate with the parents to teach young children relaxation techniques, such as deep breathing, progressive tensing and relaxing of muscles, and visualization of favorite places. Encourage busy school-age children and teens to have quiet and restful times each day, in addition to physical activity periods.

Teach parents about medication administration and diet therapy. Reinforce to both the parents and child the importance of adhering to a strict medication regimen. Emphasize that medications should be continued even when the child is asymptomatic. Discuss side effects of the drugs and what to do if any of these symptoms occur. See Partnering with Families: Dietary Instructions for Inflammatory Bowel Disease. Since immune status may be altered by steroid use, have families avoid contact with infectious diseases when the child is taking steroids. Instruct them to report any diseases and fevers the child experiences, and to report the use of steroids to all healthcare providers. Immunization schedules may need to be altered.

If the child is able to eat, parents require instructions about dietary needs. If the child is unable to eat or the intake of calories is insufficient to meet basic nutritional and metabolic needs, TPN will be ordered. Frequent growth measurements and nutritional evaluations must be performed.

Parents also will require instructions for TPN and care of a central venous catheter, including dressing changes, sterile and nonsterile techniques, signs of infection, how to handle infusion pumps and tubing, and how to measure the child's intake and output. Assist parents in obtaining equipment and supplies necessary for the child's care. Have parents demonstrate their mastery of care for the central venous catheter and their understanding of TPN techniques during home visits and appointments for healthcare.

Refer parents to social services, the visiting nurse association, and home healthcare agencies if they are not receiving any of these services. For information about inflammatory bowel disease, refer families to the Crohn Colitis Foundation.

Evaluation

Expected outcomes of nursing care for the child with inflammatory bowel disease include the following:

- The child achieves normal growth and development.
- The child demonstrates absence of gastrointestinal distress.
- The child and family demonstrate successful management of medications without demonstration of side effects.
- The child remains free from infection due to TPN line.
- The child demonstrates a positive body image.
- The child demonstrates integration of stress-lowering practices into daily life.

PARTNERING WITH FAMILIES

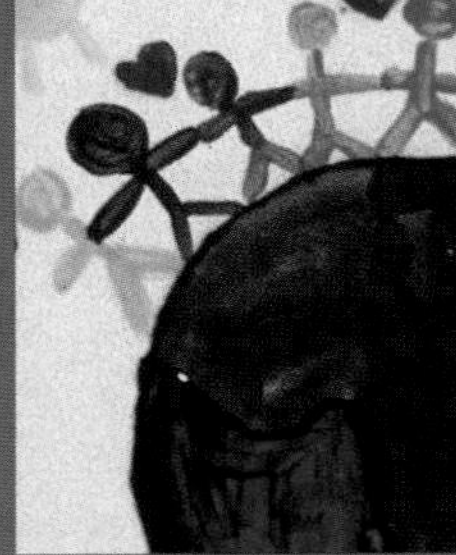

Dietary Instructions for Inflammatory Bowel Disease

Families require information regarding dietary accommodations for the child with inflammatory bowel disease. Provide families with the following information.

- Several small feedings are usually better tolerated than three meals daily.
- Limiting fiber intake can help to decrease intestine motility and inflammation. Peel fruits and avoid large quantities of whole grains and nuts.
- If the child is not eating well, offer high-calorie meals. If lactose intolerance is not a problem for the particular child, then cream soups, milkshakes, puddings, and custards can be offered.
- Liquid dietary supplements may be helpful to ensure that protein and caloric requirements are met.
- Watch for foods that cause intestinal problems for the individual child, and avoid them in the future.
- Avoid having mealtime become a reason for family strife. Seek help of nurses and dietitians if needed.

DISORDERS OF MALABSORPTION

Malabsorption occurs when a child is unable to digest or absorb nutrients in the diet. Disorders of malabsorption include short bowel syndrome, celiac disease, and lactose intolerance. Cystic fibrosis is a common cause of malabsorption and is discussed in Chapter 25.

Short Bowel Syndrome

Short bowel syndrome is a decreased ability to absorb and digest a regular diet due to a shortened intestine. Signs and symptoms of weight loss and malabsorption of fluids and micro- and macronutrients occur after surgical intestinal resection of a portion of the intestines (Scolapio, 2002). Loss of intestine may result from extensive bowel resection for treatment of necrotizing enterocolitis or inflammatory disorders or from a congenital bowel anomaly such as intestinal malrotation, gastroschisis, or atresia.

The extent and location of the involved bowel determine severity of the disorder. Because specific types of absorption occur primarily in certain parts of the bowel, the section lost determines the particular vitamins and other nutrients that are inadequate.

During the first 3 months after bowel resection, watery diarrhea is common. In the transition period, the remaining bowel usually increases its absorptive surface area and partially compensates for the absent intestine. The infant or young child requires nutritional support initially to provide sufficient nutrients for adequate growth and development. A combination of total parenteral nutrition via central line and oral fluids may be required. Once the bowel begins to recover, enteral feedings may be started. Enteral feedings include a high-fat, low-carbohydrate diet with added stimulants for mucosal growth hormones (gastrin, insulin, enteroglucagon, and growth hormone). Careful management of nucleotide, glutamine, polyamine, and fatty acid components in enteral feedings can also encourage growth of normal intestinal mucosa.

The section of the intestine that is resected will also determine the vitamin and nutrient deficiencies of the child with short bowel syndrome. When the ileum is resected, bile salts, fluids, and electrolyte absorption decrease so diarrhea can result. Loss of ileum also leads to steatorrhea and fat-soluble vitamins. When the colon is resected, fluid and electrolyte management is impaired. Resection of the jejunum is compensated for effectively by the remaining bowel (Jakubik, Colfer, & Grossman, 2000). Adaptation of the diet to facilitate absorption may include use of amino acids and peptides rather than protein, and use of medium-chain triglycerides rather than other sources of fat (American Academy of Pediatrics, 2004).

NURSING MANAGEMENT

Nursing care focuses on meeting the child's nutritional and fluid needs and teaching parents how to care for the child at home. Establishing an adequate nutritional intake and bowel pattern is a lengthy process. Total parenteral nutrition is provided initially until a feeding regimen can be established. Oral and enteral feedings are instituted gradually to allow the bowel time to compensate. Refer to Chapter 9 for nutritional assessment and detailed discussion regarding nutritional needs.

Partner with the family and child to provide support throughout this period. Teach parents how to prepare and administer parenteral feedings and care for the central line (see description in the Skills Manual). Once enteral or tube feedings are begun, teach management of the feeding pump and care of the feeding tube. Ensure regular bowel function and maintain skin integrity. Arrange home visits to monitor the child's growth and development, care of the central line and tube feeding site, and any side effects such as fluid and electrolyte imbalance and diarrhea.

Celiac Disease

Celiac disease, or gluten-sensitive enteropathy, is a chronic malabsorption syndrome that is more common in White European children than in African American or Asian children. It is also more common among members of the same family; therefore, a genetic factor may play a role in etiology. Approximately 1% to 4% of children with Down syndrome have celiac disease (Nehring, 2004). Current research is being directed at locating the potential genetic abnormalities that occur in celiac disease (Box 30–4).

BOX 30–4 Research: Genetics and Celiac Disease

By studying children at genetic risk of celiac disease, researchers have found that a transglutaminase antibody titer level identifies 70% to 85% of children who have intestinal changes on biopsy. The test may help in the future to identify and begin treatment for children with early nonsymptomatic celiac disease. Researchers also found that the consumption of 24 g of oat cereal daily did not worsen celiac disease, so once verified with further study, this may make management of the disease easier for children and families (Hoffenberg, Bao, & Eisenbarth, et al., 2000).

Etiology and Pathophysiology

Celiac disease is an immunologic disorder (Zelnik, Pacht, Obeid, et al., 2004) characterized by intolerance for gluten, a protein found in wheat, barley, rye, and oats (see Box 30–4). Inability to digest glutenin and gliadin (protein fractions) results in the accumulation of the amino acid glutamine, which is toxic to mucosal cells in the intestine. Damage to the villi ultimately impairs the absorptive process in the small intestine.

In the early stages, celiac disease affects fat absorption, resulting in excretion of large quantities of fat in the stools (steatorrhea). Stools are greasy, foul smelling, frothy, and excessive. As changes in the villi continue, absorption of protein, carbohydrates, calcium, iron, folate, and vitamins A, D, E, K, and B_{12} becomes impaired.

Clinical Manifestations

Symptoms usually occur when solid foods containing gluten are introduced to the child's diet (in the first 2 years of life), although celiac disease is sometimes first diagnosed in adulthood. The classic features of celiac disease in infancy include chronic diarrhea, malabsorption syndrome, failure to thrive, and abdominal pain (Zelnik et al., 2004). The child also exhibits vomiting, irritability, anemia, hypotonia, and ulcers of the mouth (Figure 30–15 ■). If diagnosis is delayed, the child begins to show evidence of protein deficiency (wasted musculature, abdominal distention), delayed dentition, and changes in bone density.

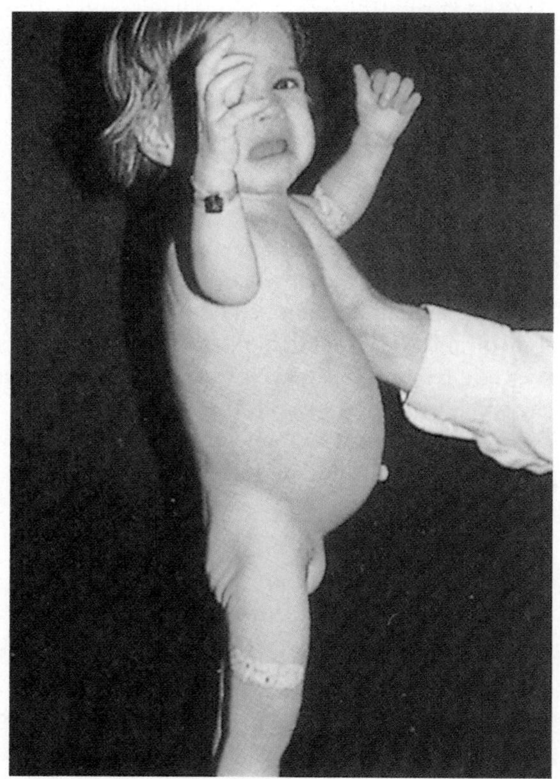

FIGURE 30–15 ■ The child with celiac disease commonly demonstrates failure to grow and wasting of extremities. The abdomen can appear large due to intestinal distension and malnutrition.

From Zitelli, B. J., & Davis, H. W. (Eds.). (1997). Atlas of pediatric physical diagnosis. *St. Louis: Mosby. Used with permission from Elsevier.*

Complications associated with the disorder include hypocalcemia, osteoporosis, osteomalacia, and rickets. Depression and anxiety are also associated with the disease. Malignancies such as lymphoma and carcinoma can result from undiagnosed and treated celiac disease.

COLLABORATIVE CARE

Collaborative care focuses on identifying the disorder, nutritional management, and promotion of growth and development.

Diagnostic Tests

Diagnosis is confirmed through measurement of fecal fat content, duodenal biopsy, and improvement with removal of gluten products from the diet. Serum screening tests for IgA antiendomysial antibodies and IgA antitissue transglutaminase antibodies are commonly used (Murdock & Johnston, 2005).

Clinical Therapy

Management of the disease is total exclusion of gluten from the diet. This gluten-free diet is a lifetime treatment. Barley, wheat, and rye are completely eliminated. Symptoms generally improve within a few days to weeks.

The intestinal villi return to normal in about 6 months. Growth should improve steadily, and height and weight should reach normal range within 1 year. Vitamin supplementation may be needed for a period of time if the child has become malnourished.

PARTNERING WITH FAMILIES

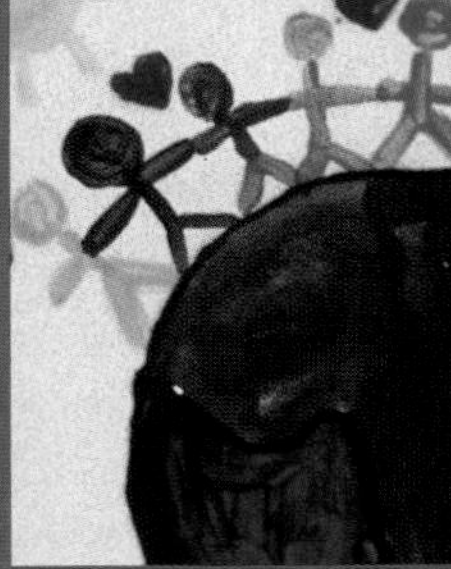

Hidden Sources of Gluten

Teach parents and older children to monitor for hidden sources of gluten. Many prepared foods contain hidden gluten. Examples include:

- Certain types of chocolate candy
- Some prepared hamburgers, hot dogs, luncheon meats
- Milk preparations such as malts and processed ice cream
- Canned soup
- Mayonnaise
- Catsup
- Malt flavoring
- Vinegar (except apple cider vinegar)
- Hydrolyzed vegetable protein
- Modified food starch

NURSING MANAGEMENT

Nursing care centers on teaching the family and older child appropriate nutritional guidelines and supporting the child's growth and development.

Nursing Assessment and Diagnosis

Assess the child for vomiting, irritability, anemia, hypotonia, and ulcers of the mouth. Assess growth pattern and developmental achievements. Ask family about the child's bowel elimination patterns. Observe stool patterns and characteristics.

Nursing diagnoses that apply to the child with celiac disease may include:

- Imbalanced Nutrition, Less than Body Requirements related to inability to digest gluten and diarrhea
- Risk for Delayed Growth and Development related to altered nutritional status
- Deficient Knowledge (parental and older child) related to dietary restrictions

Planning and Implementation

Nursing care focuses on supporting the parents in maintaining a gluten-free diet for the child. Partner with the parents to establish a nutritional plan for the child. Offer the parents a thorough explanation of the disease process. Emphasize the necessity of following a gluten-free diet.

Help parents to understand that celiac disease requires lifelong dietary modifications that should not be discontinued when the child is symptom free. Provide the parents and child with a list of foods that can be consumed (e.g., fruits, meats, rice, and vegetables). Discontinuation of the diet places the child at risk for growth retardation and the development of gastrointestinal cancers in adulthood. All children with celiac disease should be monitored by a dietitian several times during childhood, to assess nutrition and continue teaching to maintain a gluten-free diet.

Care in the Community

The diet of an infant or toddler is easily monitored at home. When the child enters school, however, ensuring adherence to dietary restrictions becomes more difficult. In addition to easily identified gluten-based foods such as bread, cake, doughnuts, cookies, and crackers, the child must also avoid processed foods that contain gluten as filler. See Partnering with Families: Hidden Sources of Gluten. School-age children and adolescents are often tempted to eat these foods, especially when among peers. Emphasize the need for compliance while meeting the child's developmental needs. Partner with the family to assist the child in establishing alternative choices during these periods of difficulty in adhering to dietary restrictions. Because adaptation to the diet must be made by the entire family, support and management skills are needed by parents and siblings.

The child's special dietary needs can place a financial burden on the family. Parents must purchase prepared rice or corn flour products or make their own bread and bakery products. Advise parents that obtaining a dietary prescription will enable them to deduct the cost of these ingredients and commercially prepared products as a medical expense.

MediaLink Celiac Disease Resources and Support

For information and support, refer parents and children to organizations including the American Celiac Society, the Celiac Sprue Association/United States of America, and the Gluten Intolerance Group. Written materials are also available from Children's Memorial Hospital in Chicago.

Evaluation

Expected outcomes of nursing care of the child with celiac disease include the following:

- The child achieves adequate nutrition to support growth and development needs.
- The child achieves growth and developmental milestones appropriate for age.
- The family (and older child) verbalize understanding of dietary restrictions and demonstrate appropriate meal planning.

Lactose Intolerance

Lactose intolerance is the inability to digest lactose, a disaccharide found in milk and other dairy products. It results from a congenital or acquired deficiency of the enzyme lactase. Congenital lactase deficiency of infancy is a rare disorder. Lactose intolerance is considered a biologic norm, occurring in approximately 70% of African Americans and Native Americans and >90% of Asian Americans (Barnard, 2003). See Chapter 9∞ for a general discussion of food intolerance.

Abdominal pain, flatulence, and diarrhea occur shortly after birth when the infant is unable to hydrolyze lactose. Diarrhea develops rapidly after the child ingests milk and milk products. Some children are able to tolerate small ingestions of lactose but have symptoms when larger amounts are consumed. Incidence of lactose intolerance increases with advancing age throughout childhood.

Diagnosis is based on a thorough history and a hydrogen breath test, which measures the amount of hydrogen left after fermentation of unabsorbed carbohydrates. Implementing a lactose-free diet for a period of time may eliminate the symptoms, thus confirming the diagnosis.

Treatment for infants includes switching to a soy-based formula. For older children, eliminating lactose-containing foods is recommended. Enzyme tablets such as LactAid can be added to milk or sprinkled on foods to aid digestion.

Nursing Management

Nursing care is primarily supportive. Carefully explain dietary modifications to parents and discuss alternate sources of calcium (see Chapter 9∞). Discuss the need for supplementation of calcium and vitamin D to prevent deficiencies. Suggest lactase tablets for children who want to have some dairy product intake. Caution parents to read food labels carefully to identify hidden sources of lactose. For example, milk solids are found in breads, cakes, some candies (e.g., milk chocolate, caramels, and toffee), some salad dressings, margarine, and various processed foods.

FEEDING DISORDERS

Feeding problems that interfere with a child's ability to ingest or tolerate certain forms of oral intake usually become apparent during the first year of life. To prevent complications of poor nutrition, feeding methods or diet may need to be altered. The following discussion focuses on the common disorders of colic and rumination. See Chapter 9∞ for a discussion of food allergy and sensitivity, feeding disorder of infancy and childhood (failure to thrive), and the eating disorders anorexia nervosa and bulimia.

Colic

Colic is a feeding disorder characterized by paroxysmal abdominal pain of intestinal origin and severe crying. Approximately 5% to 28% of infants have colic during the first few months of life. The onset of colic is usually between 2 and 6 weeks of life, and remission of symptoms generally occurs by 3 months of age (Miller, 2003).

Etiology and Pathophysiology

The etiology of colic is unknown. Proposed causes include feeding too rapidly and swallowing large amounts of air.

Clinical Manifestations

Colic is characterized by excessive and inconsolable crying, hypertonicity, and wakefulness (Miller, 2003). Episodes occur at the same time each day, usually in the late afternoon or early evening. Characteristically the infant cries loudly and continuously, often for several hours. The infant's face may become flushed. The abdomen is distended and tense. Often the infant draws up the legs toward the abdomen and clenches the hands. Abdominal distention and excessive flatus may also be noted (Garrison & Christakis, 2000). Crying may stop only when the child is completely exhausted or after passage of flatus or stool.

Clinical Therapy

The symptoms initially may resemble intestinal obstruction or peritoneal infection. These conditions must be ruled out along with sensitivity to formula. Treatment is supportive as there is currently no effective pharmacologic treatment for colic. Usually by 3 months of age the severity and frequency of symptoms decrease. There is currently no general medical consensus on effective treatments or interventions for colic. Carrying the child in the upright position is often helpful.

An important consideration is the significant impact of colic on families. Colic can place extreme stress and fatigue on the family. Recent studies indicate that aggressive thoughts and fantasies of infanticide were experienced by mothers in the study during their infant's colic episodes (Levitzky & Cooper, 2000). Active support and counseling for the mother and other family members is essential to reduce the risk of abuse to the infant.

NURSING MANAGEMENT

Nursing care focuses on supporting the infant and family during colic episodes.

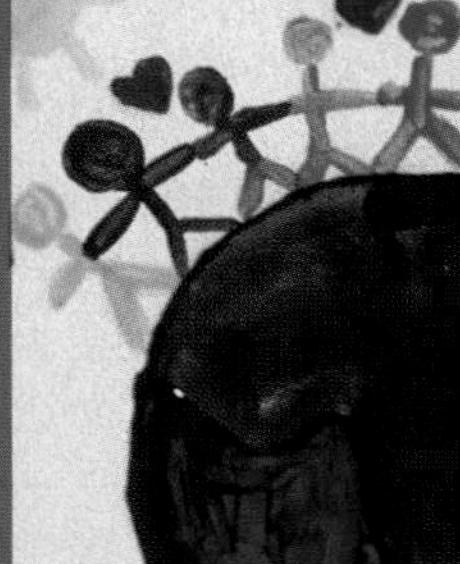

PARTNERING WITH FAMILIES

Suggestions for Alleviating Colic

Families of a child with colic require support and assistance. Offer the following suggestions to help alleviate colicky episodes.

- Provide rhythmic movement
  - Front-carrying sling carriers
  - Infant swing (battery-operated swing provides continuous motion)
  - Car ride
  - Ride in stroller
- Alternate positions
  - Swaddle infant in a soft, stretchy blanket with knees flexed up against abdomen or with legs straight
  - Place infant prone on parent's arm, supporting the body with one hand under the abdomen and cradling the head in the crook of the other arm
- Reduce environmental stimuli
  - Respond to crying
  - Provide quiet, soothing music
  - Prevent sudden loud noises
  - Avoid smoking
  - Dim lights
  - Play soft music
- Provide various tactile stimuli
  - Offer a pacifier
  - Provide a warm bath
  - Massage abdomen
- Alter intake
  - Feed smaller amount and burp frequently
  - Use a bottle with a collapsible bag in bottles to prevent sucking air
  - Hold upright for 30 minutes after feeding
  - Breastfeeding mothers: eliminate milk products and spicy or gas-producing foods from mother's diet

Nursing Assessment and Diagnosis

Nursing care requires a thorough history of the infant's diet and daily schedule and the events surrounding episodes of colicky behavior. Assessment of the infant's feeding patterns and diet includes type, frequency, and amount of feeding (if breastfeeding, maternal diet history) and frequency of burping. Episodes of colic are assessed for onset, duration, and characteristics of cry. Ask the parents what measures are used to relieve crying and their effectiveness. Assess parental response to infant behavior. Assess the family's mental health needs.

Nursing diagnoses that may apply to the infant with colic include:

- Pain related to colic episode
- Risk for Impaired Parent/Infant Attachment related to frequent crying episodes and parental fatigue
- Risk for Impaired Parenting related to parental inability to cope with frequent crying episodes

Planning and Implementation

If necessary, arrange a home visit during the reported time of the colicky episodes to ascertain feeding techniques and parental response (Belkengren & Sapala, 2002). Parents of infants with colic are often tired and frustrated. They require frequent reassurance that they are not to blame for the infant's condition. Suggest ways of alleviating some of the infant's symptoms and discomfort. (See Partnering with Families: Suggestions for Alleviating Colic.) See Chapter 11∞ for further interventions appropriate for colic.

Evaluation

Expected outcomes of nursing care for the infant with colic include:

- The infant experiences fewer colic episodes and receives support during painful episodes.
- Parents and infant demonstrate attachment.
- Parents respond appropriately to infant's needs. The infant is free from injury.

Rumination

Rumination is a rare and serious form of effortless chronic regurgitation of recently ingested food into the mouth, followed by rechewing and reswallowing or expulsion of the material (Chial, Camilleri, Williams, et al., 2003). The disorder may lead to malnutrition and growth failure in infancy. Chewing movements and mouthing of fingers often precede or accompany regurgitation. Close observation may reveal the infant actively initiating gagging with the tongue and fingers.

Rumination is commonly seen in infants and children with developmental delay, but occasionally occurs in older children, adolescents, and adults with normal intelligence (Chial et al., 2003). Rumination may be associated with poor maternal–infant bonding. This kind of behavior is seen in infants who are deprived of tactile, visual, or auditory stimuli for long periods. The infant substitutes repetitive self-stimulation for the lack of appropriate external stimulation. (See the discussion of failure to thrive in Chapter 9∞.) Complications of rumination syndrome include weight loss, malnutrition, halitosis, dental and esophageal erosions, and electrolyte abnormalities (Chial et al., 2003).

Diagnostic evaluation focuses on ruling out an organic cause and determining the degree and type of nutritional deficiencies. Treatment involves correcting the nutritional deficits and developing normal feeding patterns. A collaborative approach with a multidisciplinary team, including medical and nursing staff and social services, assists parents to meet the infant's nutritional and psychologic needs.

Nursing Management

Nursing care focuses on establishing a warm, caring relationship with the infant and the parents. Making eye contact with the infant, providing food regularly, and stimulating the infant through all the senses are ways to break the pattern of rumination.

Partner with parents and include them in the infant's care. Discuss proper nutrition and demonstrate feeding techniques and interactions that promote development. Determine parental support needs and make referrals to social service agencies as appropriate. A parent who is preoccupied with financial or other problems is less likely to attend to an infant's needs, resulting in continuation or recurrence of the pattern of rumination.

HEPATIC DISORDERS

The liver is one of the most vital organs in the body. Among its essential functions are blood storage and filtration; secretion of bile and bilirubin; metabolism of fat, protein, and carbohydrates; synthesis of blood-clotting components; detoxification of hormones, drugs, and other substances; and storage of glycogen, iron, fat-soluble vitamins, and vitamin B_{12}. Thus, any inflammatory, obstructive, or degenerative disorder that affects liver function can be life threatening. The following discussion focuses on four common liver disorders in children: hyperbilirubinemia in the newborn, biliary atresia, viral hepatitis, and cirrhosis.

Hyperbilirubinemia of the Newborn

Bilirubin is a yellow pigment produced from the breakdown of red blood cells (RBCs). Newborns have more RBCs per kilogram of weight than adults, and because the lifespan of the RBC is shorter in newborns than in adults, they are at risk for producing more bilirubin than their livers are capable of metabolizing. The preterm infant is especially prone to hyperbilirubinemia, due to an even shorter RBC lifespan than that of the term infant, and impaired bilirubin conjugation due to liver immaturity (Shaw, 2003).

Etiology and Pathophysiology

The majority of newborns experience some degree of jaundice in the first week of life (AAP, 2004), which is usually self-limiting and resolves quickly. The term newborn's bilirubin level usually peaks between the third and fifth day of life (Shaw, 2003). However, some newborns are at risk for **hyperbilirubinemia**, a level of bilirubin in the blood that requires timely assessment and appropriate intervention to prevent central nervous system injury (AAP, 2004).

The liver plays a major role in bilirubin metabolism. When the RBC deteriorates, unconjugated bilirubin, also called indirect bilirubin, attaches to circulating albumin in the bloodstream. However, as bilirubin production increases, albumin sites may be saturated, and the free indirect bilirubin moves into the fatty tissue where it causes jaundice, or in rare cases, into the brain, where it causes bilirubin encephalopathy. It is this free, unbound, and unconjugated bilirubin that causes complications in the newborn (Blackburn, 2003).

The unconjugated bilirubin that has attached to circulating albumin moves into the liver, where it is removed from the albumin and "conjugated" into direct bilirubin. The direct bilirubin, which is water soluble, is then excreted into the small intestine. At this point, it becomes urobilinogen, an orange product that gives stool its characteristic color. Most of the urobilinogen leaves the body through the stool. Some is reabsorbed in the colon and is then excreted in the urine (Blackburn, 2003). If delay occurs in intestinal movement, direct bilirubin can convert back to indirect bilirubin. Through a process called enterohepatic shunting, the indirect bilirubin is absorbed across the intestinal mucosa and reenters the circulation. This means the indirect bilirubin must reenter the liver and begin the process again (Blackburn, 2003).

Enzymes play an important part in the conjugation of bilirubin so that it can be excreted from the body. Glucuronyl transferase is needed for attaching unconjugated bilirubin to glucuronic acid in the liver, part of the process of changing unconjugated to conjugated bilirubin. On the other hand, the enzyme β-glucuronidase is present in the intestines and can split off bilirubin from the conjugated form to turn it back into unconjugated bilirubin; it will then be reabsorbed from the gut rather than excreted. High levels of that enzyme or delay in the passage of meconium facilitates this recycling of bilirubin to the unconjugated form, which can result in hyperbilirubinemia.

Two types of jaundice can occur in the newborn. Physiologic jaundice is normal and occurs in 50% to 60% of term newborns (Cash, 2004). Jaundice is usually visible 2 to 4 days after birth and lasts until day 6. Peak bilirubin concentration reaches 6–7 mg/dL; however, near-term newborns of 37 weeks' gestation may reach or exceed levels of 13 mg/dL. Preterm newborns are more susceptible to hyperbilirubinemia, with 63% reaching bilirubin levels of 10–19 mg/dL (Shaw, 2003).

Pathologic jaundice denotes a problem with the usual course of bilirubin metabolism (Blackburn, 2003). Pathologic jaundice can occur from conditions such as neonatal sepsis, intestinal obstruction, or polycythemia (Blackburn, 2003). More commonly, the problem originates from blood group incompatibility between the mother and the fetus, called ABO incompatibility. A second type of incompatibility is Rh sensitization, which is less common since the introduction of Rh immune globulin (RhIgG, RhIG, or RhoGAM) in 1964. Both ABO and Rh incompatibility can lead to pathologic jaundice in the newborn as a result of maternal response to a fetal antigen in her bloodstream.

ABO is the main blood group incompatibility between mother and fetus, and can occur when mother's blood type is O, and the fetal blood type is A or B (Shaw, 2003). ABO incompatibility occurs because human red blood cells contain antigens that mount an immune response to foreign bodies. Antigens in the plasma of one blood group produce agglutination (clumping) when mixed with antigens in a different blood group. In the ABO blood group system, anti-A and anti-B antibodies occur naturally (do not need exposure to an antigen in order to occur) in maternal type O blood. Maternal antibodies naturally cross the placenta and attach to the fetal RBCs, causing agglutination and hemolysis, releasing large amounts of bilirubin into fetal circulation. Fortunately, the undeveloped A and B antigens on the fetal and newborn RBC prevent a major immune response and less severe hemolysis occurs than with Rh sensitization. This is why only a small percentage of babies in an "ABO setup" become symptomatic. Of those who do become symptomatic, jaundice presents in the first 24 hours of life. Hemolysis and anemia are usually minimal; however, hepatosplenomegaly can be evident from fetal attempts to compensate for anemia by producing more RBCs. Problems with neonatal hyperbilirubinemia can result and phototherapy and exchange transfusion can become necessary (Shaw, 2003).

CLINICAL TIP

Remember which blood types are a setup for ABO incompatibility. In most cases, the mOm is blood type O and bABy is blood type A or B.

Rh incompatibility can cause hemolysis in the fetus, resulting in a serious condition called erythroblastosis fetalis (EBF). Rh incompatibility is potential when mother's blood type is Rh negative and fetal blood type is Rh positive (Shaw, 2003).

Fetal blood cells escape into maternal circulation through transplacental hemorrhage (TPH), which occurs spontaneously in 50% to 75% of all pregnancies (Shaw, 2003). Most TPH occurs during delivery; however, fetal RBCs can also pass into maternal circulation at any time during pregnancy through tiny breaks in the placenta, or during abortion, ectopic pregnancy, or amniocentesis. When the Rh-positive RBCs of the fetus contact maternal Rh-negative cells, a maternal antibody response occurs. An Rh-positive newborn is not usually affected in the first Rh incompatible pregnancy because initial sensitization most likely occurs during labor, and there is no time for maternal antibodies to develop and mount a response against the infant being born. The problem occurs in a subsequent pregnancy with an Rh-positive fetus, when previously formed maternal antibodies to Rh-positive blood cells enter the fetal circulation and destroy fetal RBCs. This can occur early in gestation and cause extensive damage in the developing fetus. In response to hemolysis, the fetus attempts to compensate by increasing erythropoiesis, and immature RBCs (erythroblasts) are released into the fetal circulation. In the worse case scenario, progressive hemolysis results in fetal hypoxia, cardiac failure, tissue edema, hydrops, and pericardial and pleural effusions. The fetus may be stillborn or born with acute respiratory and circulatory failure (Shaw, 2003).

All pregnant women receiving prenatal care have laboratory testing to determine their blood type and Rh status. Those women who are Rh negative and not yet sensitized (never before pregnant, or not sensitized as determined by laboratory testing) receive an intramuscular injection of Rh immune globulin (RhIgG, RhIG, or RhoGAM) within 72 hours after delivery or abortion of an Rh-positive infant or fetus. This prevents the development of maternal sensitization to the Rh factor. The anti-Rh antibodies in RhIG destroy fetal RBCs in the maternal circulation before they are recognized by the maternal immune system. This injection is necessary for each subsequent pregnancy, but is ineffective if Rh-positive antibodies are already present in maternal circulation from an earlier pregnancy. Administration of RhIG at 26 to 28 weeks' gestation further reduces the risk of Rh sensitization (Shaw, 2003).

The newborn with erythroblastosis fetalis can be seriously ill at birth. Bilirubin levels rise quickly and hepatosplenomegaly may be evident. If hydrops is severe, total body edema and pleural effusions necessitate resuscitation at birth and intensive care support. Congestive heart failure, severe anemia, low serum albumin levels, and blood clotting abnormalities may be problematic. Exchange transfusion is often required. Fortunately, antenatal screening and intervention can help safeguard the fetus and deliver the compromised newborn in the best possible condition (Shaw, 2003).

In both physiologic and pathologic jaundice, hyperbilirubinemia becomes dangerous when insufficient albumin binding sites result in indirect bilirubin leaving the circulation and entering the brain. In cases of severe and untreated hyperbilirubinemia, bilirubin encephalopathy can cause serious neurologic sequelae, including a severe form of athetoid cerebral palsy, auditory dysfunction, dental enamel dysplasia, paralysis of upward gaze, and intellectual and other handicaps (AAP, 2004). The term *acute bilirubin encephalopathy* is used to describe the effects of bilirubin toxicity in the first weeks of life. The term *kernicterus* is used when referring to the chronic and permanent clinical sequelae of bilirubin toxicity (AAP, 2004).

Clinical Manifestations

Newborn jaundice is first evident on the face, and then progresses to the trunk and finally to the extremities. Jaundice may be difficult to see in babies with dark skin color. Symptoms of hyperbilirubinemia include (AAP, 2004):

- Visible jaundice head to toe, including the sclerae
- Lethargy or irritability
- Poor breastfeeding or bottle feeding

Clinical manifestations of acute bilirubin encephalopathy include lethargy, hypotonia, and poor sucking ability (AAP, 2004). This progresses to irritability and hypertonia (backward arching of the neck and trunk), possibly accompanied by fever and high-pitched cry alternating with drowsiness and hypotonia. In the advanced phase, which probably denotes irreversible brain damage, the infant demonstrates pronounced hypertonia, shrill cry, no feeding, apnea, fever, coma, seizures, and ultimate death (AAP, 2004).

COLLABORATIVE CARE

Prevention of severe hyperbilirubinemia requires planned partnering among healthcare providers to establish and apply risk-reduction strategies. While rare, cases of kernicterus have been reported, including one registry that includes 90 cases in the United States from 1984 to 2001. Of these newborns, three died and all others sustained permanent damage to the central nervous system (Joint Commission on Accreditation of Healthcare Organizations [JCAHO], 2001).

The American Academy of Pediatrics recommends universal systematic risk assessment of all newborns, close follow-up after hospital discharge, and prompt intervention for newborns demonstrating signs of hyperbilirubinemia (AAP, 2004). The nurse's role is essential for identifying those newborns at risk, communicating risk and/or signs of developing jaundice to members of the newborn's healthcare team, promoting successful breastfeeding and making referrals for lactation support, teaching parents about newborn jaundice, and impressing upon parents the importance of timely follow-up after hospital discharge.

Diagnostic Tests

A blood test, performed by heelstick or venipuncture, measures total serum bilirubin (TSB) in the newborn. If phototherapy is already in progress, the TSB should be drawn with the phototherapy lights turned off because the lights can alter TSB results (Shaw, 2003). (See Developing Cultural Competence: G6PD Deficiency.)

A transcutaneous bilirubin (TcB) measurement device is recommended as a noninvasive way to estimate total serum bilirubin in babies whose TSB is less than 15 mg/dL. TcB generally provides measurements within 2–3 mg/dL of the TSB and can replace the blood test to measure TSB before phototherapy is initiated. Phototherapy "bleaches" the skin, making transcutaneous measurement unreliable after phototherapy is initiated (AAP, 2004).

A newborn undergoing phototherapy will have total serum bilirubin level checked periodically during treatment, and possibly 24 hours after discharge to check for rebound (rise in bilirubin after treatment is discontinued) (AAP, 2004).

Depending on risk factors and clinical history, additional laboratory tests may include blood typing and Rh factor, and Coombs' test. The Coombs' test looks for maternal antibodies coating the newborn's red blood cells. A direct positive Coombs' test indicates Rh incompatibility but not necessarily ABO incompatibility (Shaw, 2003). In addition, a complete blood count with differential and smear may be done to look for spherocytes (RBCs that are smaller and more fragile than normal RBCs) and to assess presence of infection. The presence of spherocytes occurs with ABO incompatibility, but not Rh incompatibility (Shaw, 2003). Urinalysis, urine culture, and cerebrospinal fluid are obtained if history or presentation suggests sepsis. If exchange transfusion is potential, a type and crossmatch is ordered (AAP, 2004).

Clinical Therapy

Phototherapy. Phototherapy most effectively reduces serum bilirubin in newborns with nonhemolytic jaundice. The aim of therapy is to keep the TSB below exchange transfusion level (AAP, 2004). Phototherapy is thought to reduce the amount of indirect, or unconjugated, bilirubin in the baby's bloodstream by promoting excretion via the intestines and kidneys. Phototherapy exposes the infant's skin to blue light at certain wavelengths, which changes bilirubin into water-soluble and excretable forms. Phototherapy also facilitates excretion of unconjugated bilirubin through the liver and speeds passage through the bowel (Shaw, 2003).

No standardized method exists for delivering phototherapy (AAP, 2004). Phototherapy may be delivered with fluorescent type lamps, halogen spotlights, and/or fiber-optic blankets or pads placed below or around the infant. Distance of the light from the infant influences the spectral irradiance, which is critical to the efficacy of the therapy (AAP, 2004). The adequacy of irradiance should be checked by nursing or bioengineering staff (Shaw, 2003) and documented in the newborn's record.

A sick term, premature, or low-birth-weight infant receives phototherapy in an open warmer or incubator to ensure temperature stability (Shaw, 2003). However, a large term infant can be placed nude in an open bassinet during phototherapy (AAP, 2004). The infant receives adequate phototherapy when the fluorescent tubes are placed within approximately 10 cm of the infant's body. However, halogen spotlights cannot be used in this manner due to risk of burns; follow manufacturer's recommendations. When bilirubin levels are extremely high, more of the newborn's surface area can be exposed to the light by lining the sides of the bassinet with aluminum foil or a white cloth (AAP, 2004). In most cases, the newborn's diaper can stay in place, which makes it easier to manage increased urine output and loose stools. However, if bilirubin levels are approaching exchange transfusion level, the diaper should be removed to expose more of the infant's skin surface to the effects of the phototherapy light (AAP, 2004). The infant's eyes are covered during phototherapy to prevent retinal damage, but eye protection should be removed during feeding and interaction with parents and caregivers (AAP, 2004). See Figure 30–16 ■.

Side effects of phototherapy may include skin rash, lethargy, abdominal distention, eye damage, and dehydration due to insensible water loss (Shaw, 2003). An uncommon complication, called "bronze infant" syndrome, may occur when a newborn with cholestatic jaundice, or a high direct (conjugated) bilirubin component, is exposed to phototherapy. These infants may develop a dark, grayish-brown color of the skin, serum, and urine, thought to occur when a photoproduct of bilirubin decomposition is deposited into the skin. This syndrome is not harmful, but can last several weeks to months and requires an explanation so that parents understand the condition (Shaw, 2003).

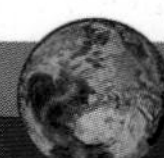

DEVELOPING CULTURAL COMPETENCE
G6PD Deficiency

Healthcare professionals should consider investigating an enzyme deficiency called glucose-6-phosphate dehydrogenase (G6PD) deficiency when a jaundiced infant's ethnicity is Mediterranean, Middle Eastern, Arabian peninsula, Southeast Asian, or African. G6PD deficiency is a global problem, and frequently goes unrecognized (AAP, 2004).

As a group, African American infants have much lower total serum bilirubin (TSB) levels than White or Asian infants; therefore, an African American infant with severe hyperbilirubinemia should be checked for G6PD. This condition occurs in 11% to 13% of African Americans (AAP, 2004).

Hydration. Many newborns with hyperbilirubinemia are also mildly dehydrated. Frequent breastfeeding (every 2 to 3 hours) is recommended; however, the interruption in phototherapy for feeding should be limited as much as possible. In some instances, supplemental fluid intake in the form of milk-based formula may be used to improve hydration and inhibit the enterohepatic circulation of bilirubin. Without evidence of dehydration, intravenous fluid or supplementation with

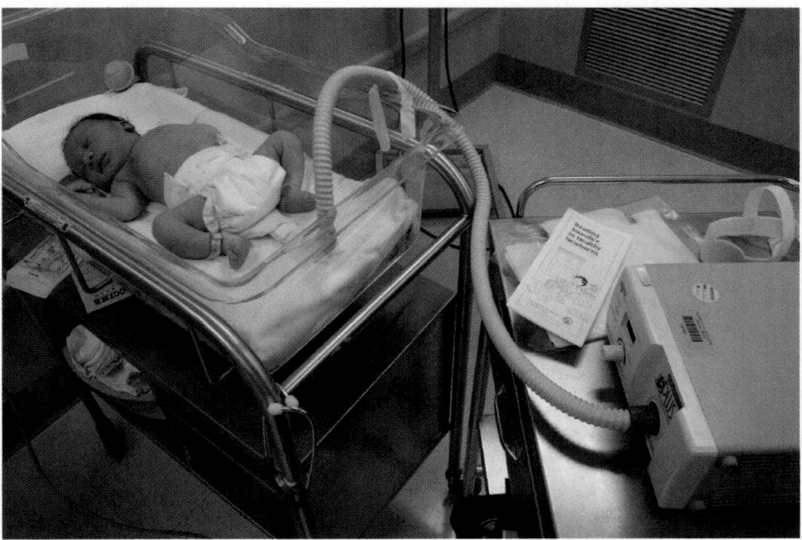

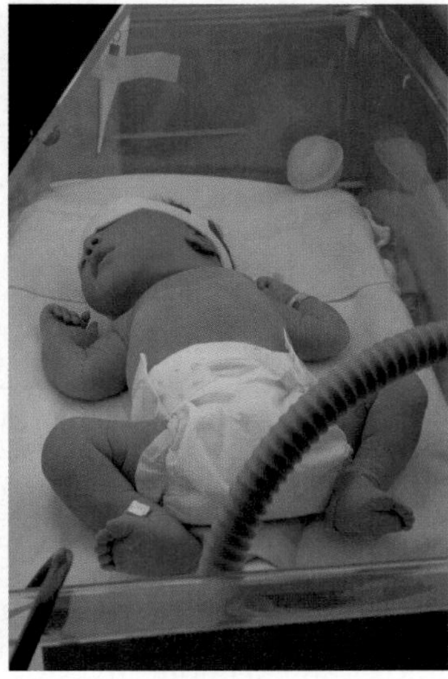

A B

FIGURE 30–16 ■ *A,* Infant receiving phototherapy on a phototherapy blanket. *B,* Infant receiving phototherapy in an incubator with overhead phototherapy lights.

dextrose water is not recommended for term and near-term infants receiving phototherapy (AAP, 2004).

Intravenous γ-Globulin. Administration of γ-globulin reduces the need for exchange transfusion in newborns with Rh and ABO hemolytic disease (AAP, 2004). This therapy may be indicated if bilirubin levels are rising despite intensive phototherapy and nearing exchange transfusion levels.

Exchange Transfusion. When intensive phototherapy fails to decrease the TSB and/or TSB rises to recommended levels for exchange, or if the newborn exhibits signs of intermediate to advanced stages of acute bilirubin encephalopathy, an exchange transfusion is indicated. This procedure should be conducted in a neonatal intensive care unit with full monitoring and resuscitation capabilities (AAP, 2004). Using catheters inserted into the newborn's umbilical vessels, aliquots of blood are drawn from the newborn and "exchanged" for the same amounts of fresh blood (Shaw, 2003).

Risks of exchange transfusion are difficult to estimate, due to the rarity of the procedure (AAP, 2004). Death occurs in approximately 3 in 1,000 procedures, although this may be an overestimation in well infants of more than 35 weeks' gestation. Other risks include apnea, bradycardia, cyanosis, vasospasm, thrombosis, necrotizing enterocolitis, and those usually associated with use of blood products. In addition, hypoxic-ischemic encephalopathy and acquired immunodeficiency syndrome have been reported in infants receiving exchange transfusions (AAP, 2004).

Tin-mesoporphyrin. Pharmacologic therapy with a drug called tin-mesoporphyrin may become more common in the future. This drug inhibits the production of heme oxygenase and can prevent or treat hyperbilirubinemia. If approved by the U.S. Food and Drug Administration, tin-mesoporphyrin may prevent the need for exchange transfusion in newborns with poor response to phototherapy (AAP, 2004).

NURSING MANAGEMENT

The nurse plays a critical role in identifying the newborn at risk, providing parent education and support, and providing nursing care to the newborn undergoing treatment for hyperbilirubinemia. The nurse coordinates communication among all members of the newborn's care team, including physicians, laboratory personnel, and parents.

■ Nursing Assessment and Diagnosis

The nurse should be aware of every infant's risk factors for developing hyperbilirubinemia (Box 30–5). Some clinical risk

BOX 30–5 Clinical Risk Factors for Development of Severe Hyperbilirubinemia

Important risk factors for severe hyperbilirubinemia in infants more than 35 weeks' gestation include breastfeeding, gestation less than 38 weeks, hyperbilirubinemia in a sibling, and visible jaundice prior to discharge (AAP, 2004, p. 301).

Additional risk factors for development of severe hyperbilirubinemia include:

- Bilirubin level higher than normal prior to hospital discharge
- Visible jaundice in the first 24 hours of life
- Blood group incompatibility or known hemolytic disease such as G6PD deficiency
- Significant bruising or cephalhematoma
- Problems with breastfeeding, especially if accompanied by excessive weight loss
- East Asian race

A term infant who is formula feeding is at very low risk of developing severe hyperbilirubinemia (AAP, 2004).

factors can be ascertained from the prenatal record or labor history, such as the newborn's gestational age and maternal blood type and Rh. Other clinical risk factors develop during the newborn's hospital stay, such as difficulties with breastfeeding or visible jaundice.

The nurse assesses the newborn for jaundice each time vital signs are assessed and no less than every 8 to 12 hours (AAP, 2004). To assess the presence of jaundice in the newborn, the nurse applies digital pressure to the newborn's skin, revealing the color of the subcutaneous tissue. Visual estimation of bililrubin levels can lead to errors, however, and is used only to assess the need for further investigation (AAP, 2004). If the nurse suspects the presence of jaundice, a TcB measurement or TSB level is indicated, reported to the newborn's primary care provider, and documented in the chart. Prior to discharge, the newborn's healthcare team follows a nursery protocol for assessing each newborn's risk of developing hyperbilirubinemia by using one or both of the following options.

- Assess risk of subsequent hyperbilirubinemia by obtaining a TcB level and/or a TSB level prior to discharge and plotting it on a nomogram (Figure 30–17 ■). A newborn whose predischarge TSB is in the low-risk zone is at very low risk of developing hyperbilirubinemia. If the predischarge TSB or TcB level places the newborn in a high-risk zone, decisions must be made regarding the advisability of discharge, initiation of phototherapy, or timing of follow-up to ensure prompt intervention if necessary.
- Assess clinical risk factors for development of hyperbilirubinemia, such as blood group incompatibility, prematurity, breastfeeding difficulties, or predischarge TSB or TcB level in the high-risk zone.

Assessment of Feeding

The breastfeeding mother should begin breastfeeding immediately after birth if possible (AAP, 2004; American Academy of Pediatrics and American College of Obstetricians and Gynecologists [ACOG], 2002) and nurse her infant at least 8 to 12 times per day for the first several days (AAP, 2004). The nurse should be alert to mother–infant pairs who are having difficulty and require lactation support during the hospital stay and following discharge. Supplemental formula or water is not recommended for the healthy term newborn and unsupplemented breastfeeding infants normally lose weight in the first days of life. Approximately 5% to 10% of fully breastfed infants experience a 10% weight loss by day 3 of life. If weight loss exceeds 10%, close monitoring of intake and weight loss is indicated, and the newborn is identified as being at risk for hyperbilirubinemia (AAP, 2004).

The breastfed newborn should have four to six thoroughly wet diapers and three to four stools per day by the fourth day of life. Meconium stool should have transitioned to mustard yellow, mushy stools by day 3 to 4 (AAP, 2004). If these parameters are not met, the infant may be at risk for dehydration due to inadequate intake, thus increasing the risk of hyperbilirubinemia (AAP, 2004). Because most mothers and term newborns are discharged before the fourth day, this is important information to teach parents prior to discharge.

Nursing diagnoses that may apply to the newborn with hyperbilirubinemia include:

- Imbalanced Nutrition: Less than Body Requirements related to inadequate nutritional intake
- Deficient Fluid Volume related to decreased oral intake
- Ineffective Breastfeeding related to prematurity
- Interrupted Breastfeeding related to newborn phototherapy treatment
- Risk for Impaired Parent/Newborn Attachment related to disruption of parental/newborn interaction due to hospitalization and treatment
- Risk for Imbalanced Body Temperature related to phototherapy
- Risk for Injury related to phototherapy

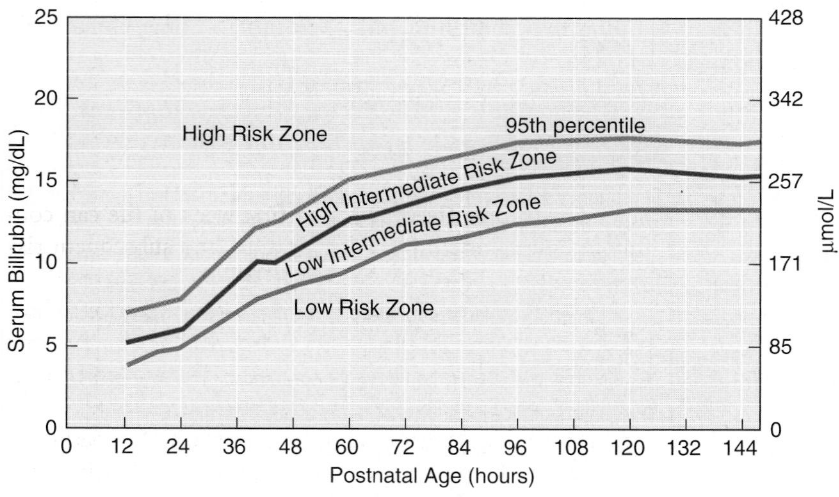

FIGURE 30–17 ■ This chart is recommended for use prior to infant discharge, to help assess the infant's risk of developing severe hyperbilirubinemia. For example, if a newborn is 48 hours old at discharge, and has a TSB or TcB of 12 mg/dL, the infant is in the high intermediate risk zone for developing severe hyperbilirubinemia. This assessment, in conjunction with other clinical factors, influences decisions regarding continued hospital care, or timing of postdischarge follow-up.

Redrawn from American Academy of Pediatrics. (2004.) http://aappolicy.aappublications.org/cgi/content/full/pediatrics;114/1/297.pdf, accessed 1/20/05.

■ Planning and Implementation

The role of the nurse is to identify the newborn at risk for hyperbilirubinemia, educate parents about newborn jaundice, and care for the newborn and family undergoing treatment for this condition. For the infant undergoing phototherapy, see the following guidelines.

Guidelines for Care of the Infant Receiving Phototherapy

- Draw TSB and other labs as ordered; report laboratory results to the newborn's care provider.
- Ensure that phototherapy lights are turned off while drawing blood for TSB.
- Measure glucose-6-phosphate dehydrogenase (G6PD) level in an infant whose family history or ethnic or geographic origin suggests the likelihood of this condition, or for an infant whose bilirubin level does not respond to phototherapy as expected.
- Monitor vital signs and continue to assess for concurrent problems, such as infection.
- Monitor feeding behavior and intake.
- Feed on demand if possible; attempt nursing every 2 to 3 hours.
- Provide lactation support and assistance as necessary.
- Monitor output: stool frequency and character, urine output.
- Monitor daily weight.
- Do not supplement feedings with water.
- Do not supplement breastfeedings with formula unless medically indicated.
- Observe skin color, note rashes or excoriation.
- Clean skin with warm water, especially diaper area.
- Reposition frequently to maintain skin integrity and maximize exposure to phototherapy.
- Perform periodic checks of phototherapy units to ensure adequate irradiance.
- Shield newborn's eyes from lights with opaque eye protection.
- Ensure that newborn's eyes are closed when applying eye protection to prevent corneal injury.
- Provide stable thermal environment and monitor newborn's temperature.
- Hold newborn during feedings as condition permits.
- Provide parents with ongoing education and information about newborn's condition.
- Provide parents with emotional support and allow frequent contact with newborn to reduce parental anxiety.
- Ensure plan for follow-up after discharge.

(Adapted from AAP, 2004; Shaw, 2003)

The following should help to prevent or manage hyperbilirubinemia in the term and near-term newborn.

- Provide support and advice to breastfeeding mothers. Initiate nursing as soon as possible after delivery if not medically contraindicated.
- Teach parents the importance of nursing the newborn at least 8 to 12 times per day for the first several days to reduce risk of poor caloric intake and dehydration.
- Notify the primary care provider of any infant who is visibly jaundiced in the first 24 hours of life and assess TSB or TcB.
- Encourage development of standing orders so that nurses can obtain a TcB level or order a TSB measurement on any infant when developing hyperbilirubinemia is suspected. Recognize that visual estimation of the degree of jaundice can lead to errors, particularly in darkly pigmented newborns.
- Interpret bilirubin levels according to the infant's age in hours.
- Develop and use a nursery protocol for assessing risk of hyperbilirubinemia in every infant prior to discharge, especially for infants discharged prior to 72 hours of age. Assessment of risk may use the predischarge measurement of TSB or TcB and/or assessment of clinical risk factors (see below).
- Provide written and verbal information to parents about jaundice and when to seek consultation after discharge. Ensure that education materials are culturally sensitive for the particular family.
- Ensure follow-up after hospital discharge by a licensed healthcare provider with competence in newborn assessment skills to assess overall infant status and presence of jaundice. This visit can take place in the hospital, outpatient clinic, or the family's home. Elements of assessment include weight, intake, pattern of voiding and stooling, and degree of jaundice. TSB or TcB level should be measured if there is any suspicion of jaundice. Timing of follow-up and number of follow-up visits depend on the clinical situation; however, general guidelines are as follows:
  - Infants discharged before age 24 hours of age should be seen by age 72 hours.
  - Infants discharged between 24 and 47.9 hours of age should be seen by age 96 hours.
  - Infants discharged between 48 and 72 hours of age should be seen by age 120 hours.
- Initiate phototherapy promptly when indicated (Figure 30–18 ■).

(Adapted from AAP, 2004; ACOG, 2002)

Care in the Community

Problems with breastfeeding in the first week of life can contribute to low caloric intake, dehydration, and subsequent risk of neonatal hyperbilirubinemia (AAP, 2004). The nurse plays a critical role in assessing adequacy of breastfeeding prior to hospital discharge and coordinating with the newborn's care provider in making appropriate referrals to lactation specialists and support groups in the community when necessary.

For term infants who develop uncomplicated hyperbilirubinemia, home phototherapy may be appropriate (AAP, 2004). Serum bilirubin levels must be monitored regularly at the physician's office, neighborhood laboratory, or by the home healthcare worker. A visiting or home healthcare nurse often visits the family to establish the phototherapy and inform parents about the care needed. The nurse partners with other professionals such as staff from a medical supply company to service equipment, lactation specialist, and pediatrician to coordinate services.

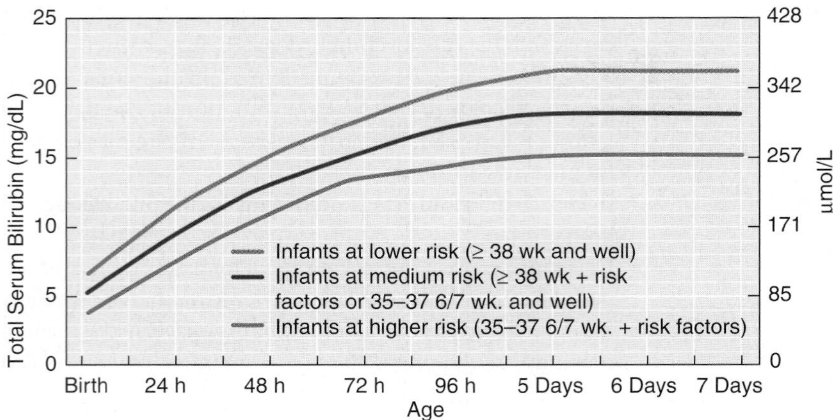

• Use total bilirubin. Do not subtract direct reacting or conjugated bilirubin.
• Risk factors = isoimmune hemolytic disease, G6PD deficiency, asphyxia, significant lethargy, temperature instability, sepsis, acidosis, or albumin < 3.0 g/dL (if measured)
• For well infants 35–37 6/7 wk can adjust TSB levels for intervention around the medium risk line. It is an option to intervene at lower TSB levels for infants closer to 35 wks and at higher TSB levels for those closer to 37 6/7 wk.
• It is an option to provide conventional phototherapy in hospital or at home at TSB levels 2–3 mg/dL (35–50 µmol/L) below those shown but home phototherapy should not be used in any infant with risk factors.

FIGURE 30–18 ■ This graph assists practitioners to decide when to initiate phototherapy in a newborn of 35+ weeks' gestation. First determine the infant's risk group (lower, medium, or higher) based on the graph's parameters. Then plot the infant's TSB and hours of age. If the TSB exceeds the line of the infant's risk category, the practitioner should initiate intensive phototherapy. For example, if a well newborn of 36 weeks' gestation has a TSB of 17 mg/dL at 84 hours of age, intensive phototherapy is advised.

Redrawn from American Academy of Pediatrics. (2004.) http://aappolicy.aappublications.org/cgi/content/full/pediatrics;114/1/297.pdf, accessed 1/20/05.

■ Evaluation

Expected outcomes of nursing interventions include:

- The term or near-term newborn at risk for hyperbilirubinemia is identified prior to discharge and receives appropriate and timely follow-up.
- The newborn's nutritional intake is adequate to meet growth and development requirements.
- The newborn's fluid intake is adequate for hydration and weight.
- Parents demonstrate appropriate attachment behaviors toward the newborn.
- The newborn's parents understand the basics of newborn jaundice and know who and when to call if they suspect development of hyperbilirubinemia.
- The newborn receives appropriate and timely intervention if hyperbilirubinemia occurs.
- The newborn is free of injury.

Biliary Atresia

Biliary atresia is the pathologic closure or absence of hepatic or common bile ducts at any point from the porta hepatic to the duodenum (Kotb, Kotb, Sheba, et al., 2001). The disorder leads to cholestasis, fibrosis, and cirrhosis (Kelly, 2002). It is the most common pediatric liver disease necessitating transplantation and the most common cause of infant jaundice.

Etiology and Pathophysiology

The cause of biliary atresia is unknown. Absence or blockage of the extrahepatic bile ducts results in blocked bile flow from the liver to the duodenum. This altered bile flow soon causes inflammation and fibrotic changes in the liver. In addition to blockage, the disease can also be caused by hepatocellular dysfunction. Lack of bile acids also interferes with digestion of fat and absorption of fat-soluble vitamins A, D, E, and K, resulting in steatorrhea and nutritional deficiencies. Without treatment the disease is fatal.

Clinical Manifestations

Initially the newborn is asymptomatic. Jaundice may not be detected until 2 or 3 weeks after birth. At that point, bilirubin levels increase, accompanied by abdominal distention and hepatomegaly (see Appendix C∞ for bilirubin levels and other liver function tests). As the disease progresses, splenomegaly occurs. The infant experiences easy bruising, prolonged bleeding time, and intense itching. Stools are puttylike in consistency and white or clay colored because of the absence of bile pigments. Excretion of bilirubin and bile salts results in tea-colored urine. Failure to thrive and malnutrition occur as the destructive changes of the disease progress.

COLLABORATIVE CARE

Collaborative care centers on immediate identification of the infant with biliary atresia, surgical correction of obstruction, and preparing the child and family for the necessity of liver transplantation.

Diagnostic Tests

Because liver damage develops rapidly in infants with biliary atresia, early diagnosis is essential. Diagnosis is based on the history, physical examination, and laboratory evaluation. Laboratory findings reveal elevated bilirubin levels, elevated serum aminotransferase and alkaline phosphatase values, prolonged prothrombin time, and increased ammonia levels. Abdominal ultrasound is used to rule out other causes. Percutaneous liver biopsy suggests biliary atresia, and an exploratory laparatomy confirms the diagnosis.

Ultrasonographic (US) triangular cord (TC) sign, which represents a cone-shaped fibrotic mass cranial to the bifurcation of the portal vein patients with biliary atresia, is useful in diagnosis of biliary atresia (Kotb et al., 2001).

Clinical Therapy

Treatment involves surgery to attempt correction of the obstruction (hepatoportoenterostomy) and supportive care. In the hepatoportoenterostomy

(Kasai procedure), a segment of the intestine is anastomosed to the porta hepatis. In most children this is a palliative treatment to promote bile drainage, maintain as much hepatic function as possible, and prevent the complications of liver failure.

Supportive treatment is directed at managing the bleeding tendencies by administering oral vitamin K, preventing rickets through vitamin D supplementation, controlling itching and irritability with cholestyramine and antihistamines, and promoting adequate nutrition. Low-dose oral antibiotics are administered to prevent cholangitis (Kelly, 2002).

Although the hepatoportoenterostomy improves the prognosis because it achieves biliary drainage in 60% of infants (Kelly, 2002), complications of liver disease continue to develop and eventually necessitate liver transplantation. In addition to biliary atresia, the most common reasons for liver transplants in children are metabolic liver disease, acute idiopathic hepatic necrosis, and cirrhosis.

Donor shortage is the major factor limiting the use of liver transplantation (Tran, Nissen, Poordad, et al., 2004). Advances in transplantation surgery now make it possible to perform partial liver transplants from living-donor resections. These advances, along with the development of cyclosporine and other immunosuppressants, have improved the first-year survival rate for children receiving liver transplantation to between 75% and 80% (Box 30–6).

Living-donor liver transplantation allows the opportunity for the procedure to be performed when the child is in optimal health, rather than waiting until an appropriate-size cadaver liver is available, and allows for donations from close family members who are often good tissue matches. The left lobe of the donor's liver is transplanted from the family member to the child. Excellent recipient and graft survival results are reported using this method (Tran et al., 2004). See Box 30–7.

NURSING MANAGEMENT

Nursing care in the initial stages of biliary atresia is the same as that for any healthy newborn. As symptoms develop, the focus of nursing care becomes long-term management and support.

Nursing Assessment and Diagnosis

Assess the abdomen for distention. Monitor stool pattern and assess for clay-colored, puttylike stools. Assess skin for jaundice and ecchymosis.

BOX 30–6 Pediatric Liver Transplantation

The Studies of Pediatric Liver Transplantation (SPLIT) had registered 1,144 child liver transplants in the United States and Canada by June 2000. Survival rate was 85% at 1 year and 77% at 2 years. Of the survivors, 89% of the school-age children attended school full time by 18 months after transplant (SPLIT Research Group, 2001).

BOX 30–7 Problems Encountered in Pediatric Liver Transplant

- **Lack of donors.** This problem is being solved by increasing use of split liver transplants when partial transplants are provided by a family member, alleviating the need to wait for cadaver donations.
- **Immunosuppression.** Immunosuppressive therapies have been tested less in children than in adults and increased research is needed.
- **Morbidity and mortality of treatment.** Many of the drugs used after transplant have side effects of renal toxicity, malignancy, and other serious sequellae. The effects can be magnified in children who have decades of exposure to these drugs.
- **Recurrent and new diseases.** Diseases that may be caused by immunosuppression can occur, such as those caused by infectious agents. Other liver diseases such as cirrhosis and nonspecific hepatitis are seen in some children.
- **Influences on growth and development.** Drugs, liver disease, emotional strain, and disturbed nutritional intake and metabolism may all influence the growth, cognitive function, and developmental variation of children. Attention and consistent screening of development and family adaptation are needed.

Note: From McDiarnid, S. V. (2000). Liver transplantation. The pediatric challenge. Clinical Liver Disease, *4, 879–927.*

Nursing diagnoses that apply to the infant with biliary atresia may include:

- Imbalanced Nutrition: Less than Body Requirements related to altered digestive processes
- Compromised Family Coping related to life-threatening illness of infant
- Anxiety related to life-threatening illness of infant
- Risk for Delayed Growth and Development related to nutritional deficiencies

Planning and Implementation

Nursing care includes preoperative and postoperative care, supporting the family, educating the family about home care, and preparing the family for organ transplantation.

Preoperative Nursing Care

Weight the infant daily. Administer TPN, intralipids, and fat-soluble vitamins A, D, E, and K as prescribed.

Diagnosis of this potentially fatal disorder can be devastating to parents. Provide emotional support and offer frequent explanations of tests during the initial diagnostic evaluation. As the disease progresses, the infant becomes irritable because of intense itching and the accumulation of toxins. Tepid baths may help to relieve itching and provide comfort. When drying the skin, pat the towel against the skin rather than rubbing which promotes vasodilation, and worsens the infant's itching and irritation. Promote rest by grouping nursing activities while the infant is awake.

Postoperative Nursing Care

Care following a hepatoportoenterostomy is similar to that for a child undergoing abdominal surgery. (See the earlier discussion of postsurgical nursing management for appendicitis and the nursing care plan for the child undergoing surgery in Chapter 17∞.)

Posttransplant care includes immunosuppressant drugs and close monitoring for vascular complications. For the child who has received a transplant, teach parents how to identify signs of rejection (nausea, vomiting, fever, jaundice), as well as the administration and side effects of immunosuppressant medications. Refer to Chapter 31∞ for further discussion of organ transplants.

Care in the Community

Discharge planning focuses on teaching parents how to care for the child's skin, provide for nutritional needs, administer medications, and monitor for increasing symptoms of liver disease.

Refer parents to support groups, clergy, or social services if indicated. They will require ongoing visits from a home healthcare nurse to help them in managing the complex care of the child.

Evaluation

Expected outcomes for nursing care of the child with biliary atresia are as follows:

- The child achieves adequate nutrition to support growth and development.
- The family utilizes effective coping skills.
- The family verbalizes anxiety and fears, and acknowledges receiving adequate support.
- The child achieves growth and developmental milestones expected for age.

Viral Hepatitis

Hepatitis is an inflammation of the liver caused by a viral infection. Hepatitis may occur as an acute or chronic disease. Acute hepatitis is rapid in onset and if untreated may develop into chronic hepatitis. The most frequently diagnosed causative organisms are hepatitis A virus (HAV), hepatitis B virus (HBV), hepatitis C virus (HCV), hepatitis D virus (HDV), and hepatitis E virus (HEV). Other types of non-A and non-B have been identified, such as hepatitis G. An estimated 136,000 cases of hepatitis occur annually in the United States, and one third of these are in children. Most cases are types A and B (Table 30–8).

Etiology and Pathophysiology

Hepatitis A is the most common form of acute viral hepatitis. Hepatitis A is highly contagious and traditionally has been referred to as infectious hepatitis. Infection occurs primarily through the fecal–oral route. Transmission is by direct person-to-person spread or through ingestion of contaminated water or food (particularly shellfish). Hepatitis A frequently occurs in children in childcare settings where hygiene practices are poor. Food handlers can spread hepatitis A if not aware of their infection; it is a common cause of foodborne illness. The virus can live on surfaces for 1 month. Because the virus is transmitted in the early stages of the disease when individuals are often asymptomatic or only mildly ill, large numbers of people may be exposed before the diagnosis is confirmed (Table 30–9). Although hepatitis A is a mild disease in many people, others may experience severe liver damage (Shovein, Damazo, & Hyams, 2000).

Hepatitis B, which has been known traditionally as serum hepatitis, is a serious disease. Transmission is usually by the parenteral route through the exchange of blood or any bodily secretion or fluid. Other common transmission routes include sexual activity and transmission from mother to fetus in utero. Adolescents who use intravenous drugs and have unprotected sexual intercourse are at risk for contracting hepatitis B. Major

TABLE 30–8 Comparison of Major Hepatitis Types

TYPE	INCUBATION	% ICTERIC	% WHO BECOME CHRONIC CARRIERS	CLINICAL FEATURES
Hepatitis A	4 weeks (10–50 days)			More acute onset; frequently subclinical in young children
Children <5 years		<5	0	
Adults		50–75	0	
Hepatitis B	1–6 months			Extrahepatic manifestations more common
Infants		<5	>90	
Adults		20–60	5–10	
Hepatitis C	6–7 weeks			Frequently manifests without jaundice; predisposes to hepatocellular carcinoma
All ages		20–30	≥60	
Hepatitis D	2–8 weeks			Most common viral cause of fulminant hepatitis
Coinfection with HBV		Not known	<5	
Superinfection of HBV carrier			>80	
Hepatitis E	2–9 weeks			Severe in pregnant women; high mortality and fetal loss
All ages		~10	0	

Adapted from Holst, B., & Ritter, D. (2001). Managing viral hepatitis. Clinician Reviews, 11, *51–62.*

TABLE 30–9 Transmission, Immunization, and Prophylaxis for Hepatitis

TYPE	PRIMARY TRANSMISSION	IMMUNIZATION AVAILABLE	PROPHYLAXIS
Hepatitis A	Fecal–oral	Yes	Immune serum globulin Hepatitis A vaccine
Hepatitis B	Blood products Intravenous drug use In utero Sexual activity	Yes	Hepatitis B immune globulin Hepatitis B vaccine
Hepatitis C	Blood products Sexual activity Intravenous drug use Body piercing	No	None
Hepatitis D	Blood products Intravenous drug use In utero Sexual activity	No	Hepatitis B vaccine
Hepatitis E	Fecal–oral	No	None

sources for the spread of HBV are healthy chronic carriers. All body fluids of infected individuals are potentially contaminated with the virus.

The hepatitis C virus (sometimes referred to as posttransfusion hepatitis) is transmitted primarily through blood and blood products, and blood banks now test for this virus. Infected children are commonly individuals who have had repeated transfusions (as in sickle cell disease or hemophilia). Intravenous drug use, body piercing, and multiple sexual partners are also risk factors. Infected mothers may infect their children before birth or during breastfeeding (Estrada, 2000; National Institutes of Health, 2000). Hepatitis C is the most common cause of chronic hepatitis.

Hepatitis D (delta virus) is a defective virus that can gain entry to a human only in connection with hepatitis B. This virus is suspected when someone who has been diagnosed with hepatitis B has diminishing liver function, increasing jaundice, and deteriorating mental status.

Hepatitis E infection is primarily transmitted through contaminated water and is most common in developing countries. Outbreaks may occur in flooding and rainy seasons. A related infection transferred primarily through blood transfusion is hepatitis G (Holst & Ritter, 2001).

Hepatitis G is transmitted through blood and is most commonly found in those who also have hepatitis C. More study is needed to establish the disease progression in individuals infected.

The liver's response to injury by the viruses that cause hepatitis is similar (Figure 30-19 ■). Initially, invasion of the parenchymal cells by the virus results in local degeneration and necrosis. Subsequent infiltration of the parenchyma by lymphocytes, macrophages, plasma cells, eosinophils, and neutrophils causes inflammation that blocks biliary drainage into the intestine. Impaired bile excretion causes a buildup of bile in the blood, urine, and skin (jaundice). Structural changes in the parenchymal cells account for other altered liver functions. Regeneration of parenchymal cells occurs within 3 months, and most children recover completely.

In some children, however, a progressive and total destruction of the hepatic parenchyma known as acute fulminating hepatitis develops. Children with this form of the disease usually die of liver failure within 2 weeks of onset unless they receive a liver transplant. Another complication, chronic active hepatitis, may lead to scarring of the liver and progressive deterioration of liver function. The prognosis depends on the degree of liver involvement. In some persons, especially those who develop chronic hepatitis, liver cancers and cirrhosis can develop.

Clinical Manifestations

Acute hepatitis infection is characterized by two phases:

- *Anicteric (absence of jaundice) phase.* This phase usually lasts 5 to 7 days. Signs and symptoms include nausea, vomiting, anorexia, malaise, fatigue, right upper quadrant pain, hepatosplenomegaly (Figure 30–20 ■), and fever. The child becomes irritable, looks ill, and requires rest.
- *Icteric (jaundice) phase.* In this phase, signs and symptoms include darkening of urine, clay-colored stools, and the characteristic yellowing of the skin and sclera.

In many cases of hepatitis in children, there is no jaundice (see Table 30–8), leading to delay in disease diagnosis and management. When jaundice does occur, it lasts approximately 4 weeks. Complete recovery with return of normal liver function and laboratory values may take 1 to 3 months.

In some cases hepatitis becomes chronic. The individual with chronic hepatitis carries the virus, can transfer it to others, and may develop serious liver disease after several years.

Manifestations of fulminating hepatitis include lethargy, restlessness, decreased level of consciousness, personality changes, and coma.

COLLABORATIVE CARE

The goals of collaborative care are early detection to prevent complications, support and monitoring during the acute phase of the disease, and prevention of the spread of the disease.

Diagnostic Tests

Diagnosis is often made on the basis of a thorough history and physical examination. A history of exposure to persons with the disease is significant. Physical examination reveals a tender, enlarged liver, abdominal pain, and flulike symptoms. Laboratory evaluation includes serologic testing to detect the presence of antigens and antibodies to HAV, HBV, HCV, or HDV, and liver function studies. Although a test for HEV has been developed, it is not available in developing countries, so diagnosis is usually based on the history. Serum glutamic-oxaloacetic transaminase (SGOT), serum glutamic pyruvic transaminase (SGPT), and bilirubin are elevated.

PATHOPHYSIOLOGY ILLUSTRATED

Viral Hepatitis

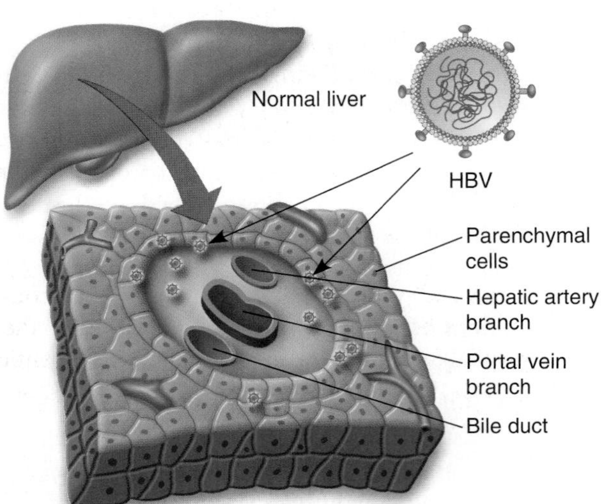

① Virus invades parechymal cells, causing local degeneration and necrosis

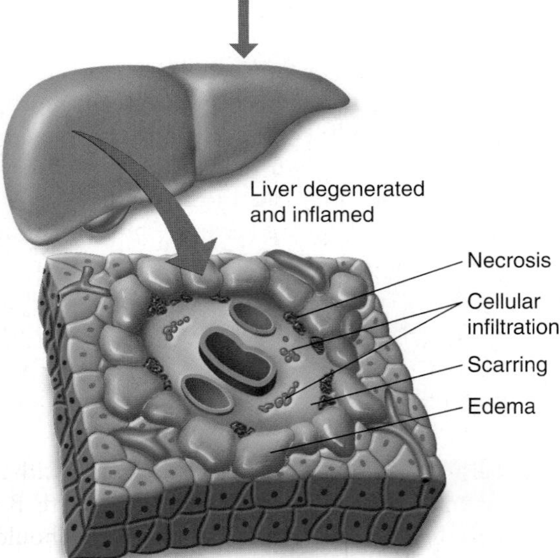

② Infiltration by lymphocytes, macrophages, and other white blood cells causes inflammation that blocks drainage

③ Structural changes occur in parenchymal cells, resulting in altered liver function:

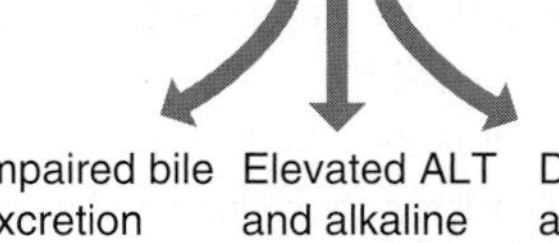

Impaired bile excretion

Elevated ALT and alkaline phosphatase levels

Decreased albumin synthesis

FIGURE 30–19 ■ The hepatitis virus causes degeneration and necrosis of the liver, which results in abnormal liver function and illness.

Clinical Therapy

Early diagnosis is essential to follow the course of the illness and identify potential complications. Management of the illness includes bed rest, hydration, and adequate nutrition during the flu-like phase. If prothrombin times are increased, vitamin K is administered.

The spread of viral infections can be interrupted by elimination of the virus from the infected population, institution of proper hygiene, and passive or active immunization. To date, no antiviral agent has been developed to combat the hepatitis viruses. Prevention depends on breaking the cycle of infection.

Active immunization for hepatitis A, a two-dose series, is recommended for all persons at risk of acquiring and transmitting the disease (e.g., men who have sex with men, international travelers) and for children and childcare workers in certain states with endemic disease (see Chapter 19∞). Individuals at risk include childcare staff and food handlers. Since childhood vaccination in high-risk areas was recommended, the overall hepatitis A rate has declined steadily, and in 2002, it was the lowest yet recorded (3.1 per 100,000) (Centers for Disease Control and Prevention [CDC], 2004). Passive immunity to HAV can be achieved with standard pooled immune globulin. It must be administered within 2 weeks of exposure.

Immunization for hepatitis B, a three-dose series, is recommended for all children and at-risk adults. The first dose is given within 12 hours of birth to the infant born to an infected mother or to a mother with unknown status (refer to the discussion of immunization in Chapter 19∞).

A total of 7,996 acute hepatitis B cases in the United States were reported in 2002, representing a >65% decrease since 1990 (21,102 cases). This decline in hepatitis B rates coincides with the implementation of a national strategy to achieve the elimination of hepatitis B virus (HBV) infection. The rate among children aged ≤18 years, the age group covered by the recommendation for routine childhood immunization, has declined by approximately 90% since 1990 (CDC, 2004).

Primary elements of this strategy to eliminate hepatitis B virus infection include:

- Screening of all pregnant women for HBV infection with provision of postexposure prophylaxis to infants born to infected women
- Routine vaccination of all infants and children aged ≤18 years

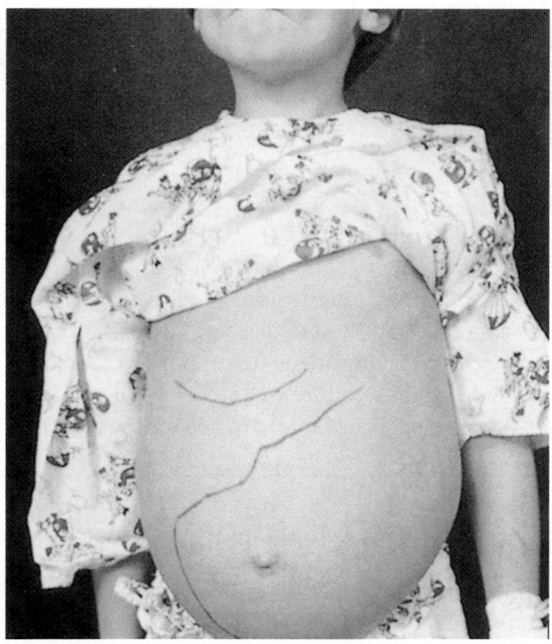

FIGURE 30–20 ■ Hepatosplenomegaly is a common finding in the child with hepatitis. Can you tell which organs are enlarged in this photo? Review methods for assessing for an enlarged spleen or liver in Chapter 8.

From Zitelli, B. J., & Davis, H. W. (Eds.). (1997). Atlas of pediatric physical diagnosis. *St. Louis: Mosby. Used with permission from Elsevier.*

- Vaccination of others at increased risk of acquiring hepatitis B (e.g., healthcare workers, injection drug users, and household and sex contacts of persons with chronic HBV infection)

Passive immunity to HBV can be achieved with hepatitis B immune globulin (HBIG). It is used for one-time exposure and for infants of infected mothers when it is given within 12 hours of birth.

NURSING MANAGEMENT

Nursing care focuses on preventing the spread of infection, providing fluid and nutritional support, promoting growth and development, reducing risk of complications, and supporting parents and child.

Nursing Assessment and Diagnosis

The nurse usually encounters the child and family in an outpatient setting. In addition to being observed for characteristic signs of hepatitis (jaundiced skin and sclera), the child is assessed for the presence of abdominal pain, anorexia, nausea and vomiting, malaise, and arthralgia. A history of the child's contacts over the past 45 days for HAV and up to 180 days for HBV is also obtained. For an infant, the hepatitis history of the mother and other family members is important.

Common nursing diagnoses for the child with acute hepatitis may include the following:

- Risk for Imbalanced Nutrition: Less than Body Requirements related to chronic illness
- Fatigue related to disease state
- Risk for Deficient Diversional Activity related to forced inactivity
- Risk for Body Image Disturbance (older child) related to jaundice
- Anxiety (parent and child) related to threat to health status
- Pain related to liver injury
- Risk for Infection related to potential spread of infection to child's contacts

Planning and Implementation

Nursing care involves home and community considerations, as children with hepatitis are seldom admitted to the hospital. The hospitalized child is placed in isolation. Prevention of the diseases is integrated into all healthcare by discussion of immunization and universal precautions.

When hepatitis cases have occurred in the family or community, parents require additional detailed information about health precautions and infection control measures. See Partnering with Families: Prevention of Hepatitis A Transmission. In addition, teach parents the importance of maintaining adequate nutrition, promoting rest and comfort, and providing diversional activities.

Prevent Spread of Infection

The practice of standard precautions is essential to prevent the transmission of hepatitis. Partner with parents (and child if old enough) to establish infection control measures to help prevent transmission of the virus. Good hygiene practices, such as washing hands before and after toileting and proper disposal of soiled diapers, are reinforced to parents. Siblings of a child with hepatitis B who have not already been immunized with the hepatitis B vaccine should be vaccinated immediately. Contacts of the child with hepatitis A should receive immune serum globulin and the first immunization in the hepatitis A series. Rifampin may be given in some cases.

Healthcare workers who come in contact with blood or other body fluids of children infected with hepatitis B are at risk for contracting the virus. Standard precautions should be used at all times and transmission-based precautions when appropriate (see the Skills Manual). Hepatitis B immunization (three doses) is recommended for nurses and other persons at high risk for exposure as well as all infants and previously nonimmunized children and adolescents.

Maintain Adequate Nutrition

Initially the child is encouraged to eat favorite foods. Once the anorexia and nausea have resolved, a high-protein, high-carbohydrate, low-fat diet is recommended. Increased protein helps to maintain protein stores and prevent muscle wasting. Increased carbohydrates ensure adequate caloric intake and prevent protein depletion. The use of low-fat foods lessens stomach distention. Offer the child small, frequent feedings.

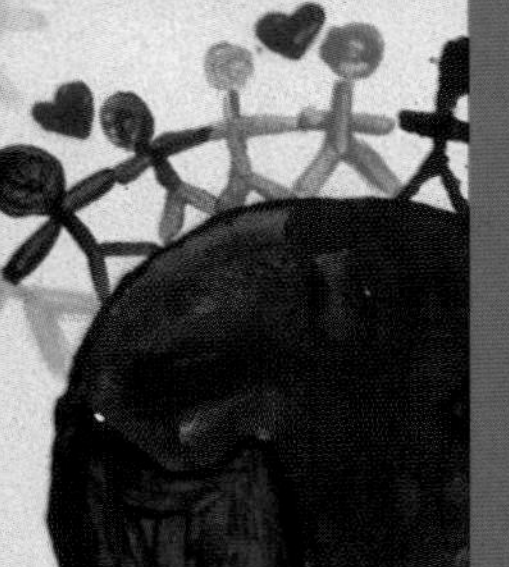

PARTNERING WITH FAMILIES

Prevention of Hepatitis A Transmission

Nurses can collaborate with the family and childcare center to provide assessment of the center's procedures and teaching to prevent hepatitis A transmission. Help the center to set standards related to the following areas if necessary.

- Handwashing after each diaper change
- Disposing of diapers properly
- Cleaning diaper-changing surfaces after each diaper change
- Never allowing food handlers to perform diaper changes
- Instructing parents to keep children at home for at least 2 weeks after a diagnosis of hepatitis A
- Informing parents of other children when there is a case of hepatitis A and teaching them the symptoms of the condition

Promote Rest and Comfort

Bed rest is necessary only if the child has severe fatigue and malaise. However, most children voluntarily limit their activities during the initial phase of the disease. Keep the child quiet and comfortable. Offer comfort items such as favorite toys, blankets, and pillows.

Medication Administration

Drug metabolism is altered during hepatitis since the liver cannot detoxify medications readily. As with all liver disorders, medications need to be administered carefully and the child's condition must be monitored for possible drug side effects. Caution parents to check with health professionals before giving any nonprescription medication. For example, acetaminophen is metabolized in the liver, and liver disease can interfere with its breakdown.

Provide Diversional Activities

Hospitalized children with hepatitis are kept in isolation. Nonhospitalized children with hepatitis do not require isolation but they should be kept at home for 2 weeks following the onset of symptoms. Young children can be provided with a new toy or favorite activities. Older children and adolescents can be provided with board games, puzzles, books or magazines, movies, or video games. Phone calls and short visits from friends help school-age children and adolescents maintain contact with peers.

Parents who cannot arrange to take time off from work may need to arrange for care at home. Refer the family to appropriate support services as indicated. Offer suggestions for diversional activities during this period.

Evaluation

Expected outcomes of nursing care for the child with hepatitis include the following:

- The child achieves adequate nutritional intake to meet growth and development needs.
- The child participates in self-care and other activities without experiencing fatigue.
- The child participates in quiet, non-fatiguing activities.
- The child demonstrates a positive body image.
- The child and family verbalize fears and concerns, and acknowledge receiving adequate support.
- The child obtains pain relief.
- There is no evidence of spread of hepatitis to child's contacts.

Cirrhosis (End-Stage Liver Failure)

Cirrhosis is a degenerative disease process that results in fibrotic changes and fatty infiltration in the liver. It can occur in children of any age as the end stage of several disorders, including biliary atresia (Kelly, 2002). The diffuse destruction and regeneration of the hepatic parenchymal cells result in an increase in fibrous connective tissue and disorganization of the liver structure. The balance between destruction and regeneration determines the specific clinical presentation.

Clinical manifestations of cirrhosis vary. When the disease process results from obstruction, as in biliary atresia, jaundice is an initial sign that intensifies with progression of the disease. In other diseases that cause cirrhosis, jaundice may be a late sign, intermittent, or absent. Steatorrhea is frequently present and can lead to rickets, hemorrhage, and failure to gain weight. Anemia can occur as a result of chronic blood loss from the gastrointestinal tract. Pruritus is common, particularly in children with biliary malformations. Clubbing of the digits and cyanosis are other common findings. Severe end-stage complications signaling hepatic failure can occur at any time and with little warning.

Diagnostic evaluation is based on the child's history of infection or disease with liver involvement. Physical examination may reveal jaundice, skin changes, ascites, and hemodynamic changes. Laboratory evaluation reveals abnormal liver function tests. A liver biopsy may help to determine the extent of the parenchymal damage.

Medical management focuses on treating the child's symptoms and achieving optimal nutritional status and growth. See the clinical manifestations table on page 1161 for a summary of treatment for complications of cirrhosis. Liver transplantation is the most common treatment for biliary atresia and metabolic disorders and is the only treatment for end-stage liver disease.

Nursing Management

Nursing care focuses on monitoring physiologic and psychosocial changes to identify early signs of end-stage hepatic failure. Monitor vital signs every 2 to 4 hours. Daily weight measure-

CLINICAL MANIFESTATIONS of Cirrhosis Complications

ETIOLOGY	CLINICAL MANIFESTATIONS	CLINICAL THERAPY
Fluid and electrolyte imbalance	Ascites	Restrict sodium, protein, and fluids Administer diuretics (e.g., furosemide [Lasix]) Administer intravenous albumin
Liver dysfunction	Hepatic encephalopathy	Restrict protein Administer lactulose (to control increased ammonia levels) Administer antibiotics Correct imbalances that can lead to coma (fluid and electrolyte imbalance)
Esophageal varices	Hemorrhage from esophageal varices	Administer blood and blood products Replace fluid and electrolytes Administer vitamin B complex and vitamin K Insertion of Sengstaken-Blakemore tube in cases of severe bleeding

ment is performed to assess for fluid retention. Close monitoring of electrolytes and liver function test results helps determine the need for fluid replacement therapy. Measure abdominal girth daily.

Careful administration of medications and monitoring for side effects are necessary because drug metabolism is altered in liver disorders. If ascites is present, provide a low-sodium, low-protein diet and restrict fluids. Remove all water pitchers, glasses, and straws to minimize the child's desire to drink.

Parents of a child with cirrhosis are coping with a life-threatening disorder, and their anxiety and stress levels are high. The child may be awaiting a liver transplantation that represents the only hope for recovery. Provide support to parents and encourage them to verbalize their fears and concerns (see Chapter 21∞). Encourage parents to participate in the child's care. Referral to a support group or counseling may be beneficial.

INJURIES TO THE GASTROINTESTINAL SYSTEM

Abdominal Trauma

Abdominal injuries may be caused by blunt or penetrating trauma. The kind of injury determines the extent of organ damage.

Etiology and Pathophysiology

Low-velocity trauma, for example, when a child strikes the handlebars of a bicycle, usually results in single-organ injury.

High-velocity blunt trauma, which may occur in motor vehicle crashes, usually involves multiple organs. Solid organs such as the liver and spleen are more vulnerable to injury than hollow organs such as the stomach, intestines, and bladder.

Motor vehicle crashes are the most common and also the most preventable unintentional injury in children (National Safety Council, 2003). On impact, small children who are held on a parent's lap or improperly restrained in a safety seat can easily become airborne, striking objects or being thrown from the car. When older children involved in severe crashes are wearing only lap belts, injury to the hollow organs may result. Bicycles are another cause of abdominal injuries in children. Bicycle accidents account for 5% to 14% of blunt abdominal trauma in children (Lam, Eunson, Munro, et al., 2001). Such injuries commonly occur when the child strikes the handlebars during a fall or sudden stop or is struck by a car. Child abuse is another major cause of abdominal trauma.

Injury to the abdominal organs can result in hemorrhage and organ necrosis. Digestive enzymes and/or bacterial contents of the bowel may be released into the peritoneum.

Clinical Manifestations

Clinical manifestations of abdominal injury include pain, abdominal distention, muscle guarding, decreased or absent bowel sounds, nausea and vomiting, hypotension, hypovolemia, and shock.

COLLABORATIVE CARE

Collaborative care focuses on identifying internal organ trauma, preventing blood and fluid loss, and surgical exploration or resection of damaged organs.

Diagnostic Tests

Suspected abdominal trauma in a child necessitates a thorough history and physical examination. The description of the event should be compared with the child's signs and symptoms. A CT scan is performed to assess for internal bleeding and air in the abdomen; however, CT scans may be unreliable in identifying mesenteric and hollow-organ injuries. Focused abdominal sonography for trauma (FAST) is more specific and can demonstrate the presence or absence of pericardial fluid, abdominal fluid, and some parenchymal injuries (Schulman, 2003).

Baseline laboratory studies, including blood type and cross-match, are done. Peritoneal lavage may be performed. A urinary catheter may be inserted to check for the presence of blood and bladder rupture.

During peritoneal lavage, a dialysis catheter is inserted into the abdominal cavity and normal saline or lactated Ringer's solution is instilled. The fluid is then drained and analyzed for the presence of red blood cells, amylase, and bacteria, which could indicate organ damage.

Clinical Therapy

Treatment of an abdominal, liver, or spleen injury takes place in the pediatric intensive care unit (PICU) and focuses on preventing or managing hemorrhage and monitoring for signs of shock. An intravenous infusion is initiated for fluid maintenance and to provide access for blood products. The child is kept NPO. A nasogastric tube is inserted. Blood transfusions and pharmacologic management are used to treat blood loss. Initially, the use of analgesics is minimized to avoid masking symptoms. Serial hematocrit levels are monitored during this period. Healing of the liver and spleen usually occurs without further intervention.

Exploratory laparatomy is performed to resect hollow organ injuries or to repair liver or spleen lacerations when bleeding is not controlled. The spleen is salvaged to help maintain the child's immune function. The child is usually discharged within 5 to 7 days following surgery. No strenuous activity is allowed for 6 to 8 weeks. The prognosis is generally good.

MediaLink Child Safety Resources

NURSING MANAGEMENT

Nursing care focuses on promoting hemodynamic stabilization through fluid and blood replacement therapy, preoperative and postoperative care, and supporting the child and family.

■ Nursing Assessment and Diagnosis

Nursing care includes initial and ongoing assessments of the child's condition. Initially, assess the abdomen for bruising, pain, guarding, rebound tenderness, distension, and absence of bowel sounds (Schulman, 2003). See Chapter 8∞ for techniques of abdominal assessment.

Monitor vital signs every hour or more frequently as warranted. Measurement of abdominal circumference (to detect distention), intake and output monitoring, serial hematocrit levels, and auscultation of bowel sounds are also performed hourly. Assess for increasing severity of pain, fever, and loss of bowel sounds, which may indicate a previously undiagnosed bowel or hollow-organ injury (Schulman, 2003). Back pain may indicate retroperitoneal bleeding. Monitor white blood cell (WBC) count, amylase, and alkaline phosphatase. Notify the primary healthcare provider of any changes.

Assess for increasing heart rate, hypotension, dyspnea, and other changes that may indicate shock.

PRACTICE ALERT

Trauma from bicycle handlebars is associated with severe abdominal injuries. The force of impact is applied via the small cross-sectional area of the end of the handlebars. Injuries to the spleen, liver, or kidneys are readily evident soon after the accident; however, injuries to the bowel and pancreas often present late and result in greater morbidity (Lam et al., 2001). The child sustaining impact from bicycle handlebars with no apparent injuries should be observed closely for vomiting, anorexia, weight loss, and increased epigastric pain. Instruct family that these symptoms should be reported immediately.

Nursing diagnoses for the child with abdominal trauma may include:

- Deficient Fluid Volume related to loss of blood from trauma
- Anxiety (parental and child) related to trauma and hospitalization
- Risk for Infection related to release of bacterial organisms from bowel into peritoneum

■ Planning and Implementation

The child and parents are usually fearful and anxious when the child is admitted to the hospital. If the injury was preventable, parents may have feelings of guilt or anger. Provide emotional support and avoid judgmental comments or statements that assign blame.

Administer fluids and blood products as prescribed. Maintain nasogastric tube if present. Prepare the child and parents for surgery if necessary. Refer to Chapter 17∞ for nursing care of the child undergoing surgery.

Once the child's condition is stabilized, nursing care shifts to preventative teaching. Partner with the child and parents to ensure their understanding of safety measures to prevent future injuries. Provide written materials, when available, to use as a reference when they return home.

Discuss the use of car safety restraint devices for riding in an automobile (see Chapters 11 through 15∞). If the child's injury was the result of a bicycle fall or crash, discuss the importance of the proper bicycle size and teach bike safety measures such as use of a helmet and knowledge and proper use of hand signals. Have the child practice safe biking habits at a bike rodeo sponsored by a local affiliate of the National SAFE KIDS Campaign.

■ Evaluation

Expected outcomes of nursing care of the child with abdominal trauma include:

- The child maintains fluid and hemodynamic stability.
- The child and family express their fears and concerns and acknowledge receiving adequate support.
- The child is free from infection.

INGESTION OF FOREIGN SUBSTANCES

Young children are at risk for ingestion of foreign substances because of their characteristic behaviors, which involve exploration of the environment. Ingestion of poisons (toxic substances) and ingestion of foreign objects are discussed in this section.

Ingestion of Poisons

Poisonings are the second leading cause of unintentional home-injury death and account for nearly one third of all unintentional home injuries (Home Safety Council, 2004a). Poisoning is a common cause of death and injury in children between 1 and 4 years of age. The American Association of Poison Control Centers reported approximately 1.2 million childhood poisonings in the United States in 2001.

Infants and toddlers commonly place objects in their mouths. Some household items are nontoxic and cause little harm, whereas other items contain caustic agents or toxic chemicals that can cause irreversible damage or death. Common causes of poisonings include medications, caustics and cleaning agents, cosmetics, plants, hydrocarbons, and insecticides and pesticides.

The Poison Prevention Packaging Act of 1970 mandates child protective devices for all potentially toxic substances, such as household cleansers and medications. However, many are still ingested by children; analgesics and hydrocarbons remain the two most common causes of poisoning deaths (Powers, 2000). Many other items commonly found in the home are less obvious sources of toxins. The leaves, stems, or flowers of many common household and garden plants are poisonous. Examples include Boston ivy, poinsettia, philodendron, lily-of-the-valley, daffodil (bulbs), azalea, and rhododendron. Nail care products, mothballs, weed and bug killers, and rodent killers are other potential hazards.

Most poisonings occur in the home (see Chapters 11 through 15∞ for more information about preventing hazardous conditions in the home). A child who has experienced a poisoning event is more likely to have another poisoning. Although 75% of poisons are ingested, other routes of contamination include dermal, inhalation, and ocular (Litovitz, Klein-Schwartz, White, et al., 2000).

Parents who suspect that their child has ingested a poison should immediately call the Poison Control Center (PCC). The PCC will advise parents about treatment to begin at home, and whether the child needs treatment in the emergency department. If the child has vomited, the vomitus should be brought to the emergency department. With older children, the possibility of intentional ingestion should be considered.

Clinical Manifestations

The manifestations of poisoning depend on the toxin. See page 1164 for clinical manifestations of commonly ingested toxic agents.

COLLABORATIVE CARE

Collaborative care focuses on identifying the source of poisoning, removing the offending agent, stabilizing the child's airway and blood pressure, and reducing the risk of recurrence.

Diagnostic Tests

Blood and urine toxicology screens, arterial blood gases, and electrolytes are performed. Testing of vomitus for presence of medication or other poisonings may be helpful in determining the amount ingested.

Clinical Therapy

In the emergency department the child's vital signs and level of consciousness are assessed and specific information about the poison is obtained from the parent. Box 30–8 summarizes emergency management for poisoning.

The goal of treatment is to prevent further absorption of the poison and to reverse or eliminate its effects. Potential complications of poisoning, depending on the type of poisoning, include respiratory and/or cardiac arrest, congestive heart failure, liver failure, renal failure, seizures, esophageal or tracheal corrosion with ingestion of caustic substances, and shock.

PRACTICE ALERT

After numerous years of syrup of ipecac serving as a mainstay in home treatment of poisonings, the American Academy of Pediatrics recommends that "syrup of ipecac should no longer be used routinely as a poison treatment intervention in the home" (AAP, 2003). The nurse informs families to avoid the use of ipecac and encourages disposal of ipecac kept in the home. Instruct the family to pour the ipecac down the drain or toilet and to discard the empty bottle.

NURSING MANAGEMENT

Nursing care focuses on initial emergent care and stabilization of the child with poisoning, followed by family education to reduce the risk of repeated poisoning.

MediaLink Poison Control Resources

Nursing Assessment and Diagnosis

Take a history from the family about the child's suspected ingestion substance, time, amount, and symptoms. Initial assessment focuses on airway, vital signs, and neurological status. Assess drooling, diaphoresis, and increased or depressed respirations. Assess for wheezing, respiratory distress, or stridor. Assess for decreased responsiveness and seizure activity. Assess heart rate, skin color, capillary refill, peripheral and central pulses, and blood pressure. Assess pupils (abnormally large or pinpoint pupils may be observed). Assess mouth, lips, and tongue for corrosive burns or edema. Assess breath for unusual odor. Assess the child for vomiting and diarrhea. Assess vomitus for presence of medication or other ingested substances. Determine the child's height and weight.

Nursing diagnoses for the child with ingestion of a toxic substance may include:

- Risk for Ineffective Airway Clearance related to effects of toxic substance
- Risk for Impaired Gas Exchange related to effects of toxic substance
- Risk for Aspiration related to depressed neurological status and vomiting
- Risk for Decreased Cardiac Output related to effects of toxic substance
- Risk for Injury related to repeated occurrence of poisoning
- Interrupted Family Processes related to poisoning of a family member

Planning and Implementation

Emergency care focuses on airway and hemodynamic stability, removal of toxic agent, and supporting the family. See

MediaLink Activated Charcoal Animation

CLINICAL MANIFESTATIONS of Commonly Ingested Toxic Agents

TYPE	SOURCES	CLINICAL MANIFESTATIONS	CLINICAL THERAPY
Corrosives (strong acids and alkaline products that cause chemical burns of mucosal surfaces)	Batteries Household cleaners Clinitest tablets Denture cleaners Bleach Toiletbowl cleaners	Severe burning pain in mouth, throat, or stomach; swelling of mucous membranes; edema of lips, tongue, and pharynx (respiratory obstruction); violent vomiting; hemoptysis; drooling; inability to clear secretions; signs of shock, anxiety, and agitation	Do not induce vomiting! Dilute toxin with water to prevent further damage Give activated charcoal
Hydrocarbons (organic compounds that contain carbon and hydrogen; most are distillates of petroleum)	Gasoline Kerosene Furniture polish Lighter fluid Paint thinners	Gagging Choking Coughing Nausea Vomiting Alteration in sensorium (lethargy) Weakness Respiratory symptoms of pulmonary involvement, tachypnea, cyanosis, retractions, grunting	Do not induce vomiting! (Aspiration of hydrocarbons places child at high risk for pneumonia.) Use gastric lavage if severe central nervous system and respiratory impairment are present Use of activated charcoal is controversial Provide supportive care Decontaminate skin by removing clothing and cleansing skin
Acetaminophen	Many over-the-counter products	Nausea Vomiting Sweating Pallor Hepatic involvement (pain in upper right quadrant, jaundice, confusion, stupor, coagulation abnormalities)	Induce vomiting or perform gastric lavage, depending on amount ingested Administer charcoal or NAC (concentrated form of Mucomyst), which binds with the metabolite, preventing absorption and protecting the liver
Salicylate	Products containing aspirin	Nausea Disorientation Vomiting Dehydration Diaphoresis Hyperpnea Hyperpyrexia Bleeding tendencies Oliguria Tinnitus Convulsions Coma	Depends on amount ingested Induce vomiting Administer intravenous sodium bicarbonate, fluids, and vitamin K
Mercury	Broken thermometers Chemicals Paints Pesticides Fungicides	Tremors Memory loss Insomnia Weight loss Diarrhea Anorexia Gingivitis	Similar to that for lead poisoning (see text discussion)
Iron	Multiple vitamin supplements	Vomiting Hematemesis Diarrhea Bloody stools Abdominal pain Metabolic acidosis Shock Seizures Coma	Induce vomiting Administer intravenous fluids and sodium bicarbonate Deferoxamine chelation therapy

Box 30–8 for a summary of emergency management for poisoning.

Once immediate care has been provided, nursing care shifts to providing emotional support and preventing recurrence.

Provide Emotional Support

Wait until the child is out of immediate danger before questioning parents in detail about the incident. Encourage parents to express feelings of anger, guilt, or fear about the incident.

Prevent Recurrence

Discuss with parents the need to supervise infants and young children at all times. Ask parents how medicines and cleaning agents are stored and whether the house contains any plants. Teach parents proper methods of childproofing the home. Have the PCC number readily available. Suggest measures for preventing recurrence of poisoning. (See Partnering with Families: Avoiding Childhood Poisoning.)

The toll-free number for the American Association of Poison Control Centers (AAPCC) is 1–800–222–1222. The num-

BOX 30–8 Emergency Management for Poisoning

1. Stabilize the child. Assess ABCs (airway, breathing, and circulation). Provide ventilatory and oxygen support.
2. Perform a rapid physical examination, start an IV infusion, draw blood for toxicology screen, and apply a cardiac monitor.
3. Obtain a history of the ingestion, including substance ingested, where child was found, by whom, position, when, how long unsupervised, history of depression or suicide, allergies, and any other medical problems.
4. Reverse or eliminate the toxic substance using the appropriate method:
   - **a.** *Antidotes and agonists*
     Mucomyst (for acetaminophen poisoning)
     Narcan (for opioid overdose)
     Romaxicon (for benzodiazepine overdose)
   - **b.** *Gastric lavage*
     - A gastric tube is inserted through the mouth.
     - Normal saline solution is instilled and aspirated until the return is clear. Reserved for children with central nervous system depression, diminished or absent gag reflex, or unwillingness to cooperate with other measures.
     - Contraindicated in children who have ingested alkaline corrosive substances, as insertion of the tube may cause esophageal perforation.
   - **c.** *Activated charcoal*
     Used in children who have ingested acids to decrease continued damage and potential perforation of stomach and intestines.
     - Given to absorb and remove any remaining particles of toxic substances.
     - Usual dosage administration is 1 g/kg of body weight.
     - A commercial preparation of activated charcoal is administered orally or through a gastric tube.
     - Available as a ready-to-drink solution in an opaque container.
     - May be mixed with apple juice or soda if protocol allows to encourage consumption.
     - A covered cup and straw is used for oral ingestion to prevent the child from seeing the black liquid and to minimize spillage.
     - Activated charcoal is administered only after the child has stopped vomiting, because aspiration of charcoal is damaging to lung tissue.
     - Should not be administered for ingestion of caustic substances or hydrocarbons.
   - **d.** *Cathartics*
     - Hasten excretion of a toxic substance and minimize absorption. The most commonly used cathartic is magnesium sulfate.

   Note: Syrup of ipecac. The use of ipecac is no longer recommended because it may not remove all poison and can be harmful in some situations. Encourage parents to remove it from their homes.
5. Other measures will depend on the child's condition, the nature of the ingested substance, and the time since ingestion. May include diuresis, fluid loading, cooling or warming measures, anticonvulsive measures, antiarrhythmic therapy, hemodialysis, or exchange transfusions.
6. The child's total condition is constantly evaluated to maintain airway, breathing, and circulation. Therapeutic management is adjusted as needed to treat evolving condition.
7. Consider the emotional status of the family. Provide information about the child, involve the child in care when possible, and arrange for support persons and services to be available to the child.

PARTNERING WITH FAMILIES

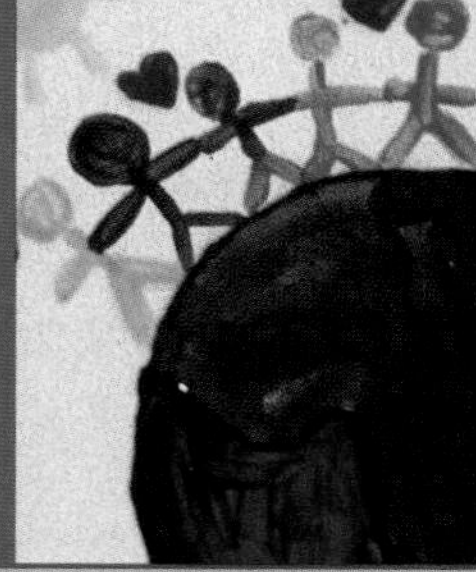

Avoiding Childhood Poisoning

Families with children require instructions for avoiding childhood poisoning. Teach family members the following interventions to help avoid childhood poisonings.

- Place household cleaners, medications, vitamins, and other potentially poisonous substances out of the reach of children or in locked cabinets.
- Use warning stickers such as Mr. Yuk on all containers.
- Buy products with childproof caps.
- Store products in their original containers.
- Never place household cleansers or other products in food or beverage containers.
- Remove all house plants from the child's play areas.
- Put poison control center phone number by every phone in the house.
- Use caution when visiting other settings that are not childproofed (e.g., grandparents' homes). Remember that visitors may have pills in their purses or pockets that are easily accessible.

ber can be accessed from anywhere in the United States and Puerto Rico, and the caller will be connected to the nearest poison control center.

Evaluation

Expected outcomes for nursing care of the child with poisoning include:

- The child maintains ventilatory function.
- The child maintains effective gas exchange and respiratory pattern.
- The child is free from wheezing, coughing, pneumonia, or other signs indicating aspiration.
- The child's heart rate and blood pressure remain stable and appropriate for age.
- The family and child (if older) verbalize understanding of preventive measures and demonstrate measures to improve home environment safety.

Ingestion of Foreign Objects

Approximately 80% of cases of ingestion of foreign objects occur in childhood. The majority of cases present in children between 6 and 36 months of age (Wahbeh, Wyllie, & Kay, 2002). The most common object ingested is coins, accounting for 27% to 70% of cases. Pins, parts of toys, batteries, and bones from foods are some other commonly ingested objects.

Clinical Manifestations

Adults often witness infants and young children ingesting foreign bodies, and older children will usually report swallowing a foreign object (Chen & Beierle, 2001). Most small, round, smooth objects may not cause clinical distress; however, if the foreign body is lodged in the esophagus, children may present with substernal pain, drooling, and dysphagia. Some children may exhibit respiratory symptoms including wheezing or coughing.

Serious complications can occur following foreign-body ingestion. These complications include perforation of the intestinal tract, the most serious sequelae of foreign-body ingestion. Sharp objects are associated with a higher perforation rate than dull objects. Approximately 75% of perforations occur in the region of the ileocecal valve. Development of strictures at the site of a retained foreign body may also occur (Wahbeh et al., 2002). Ingestion of a foreign body accounts for approximately 1,500 deaths in the United States annually (Chen & Beierle, 2001).

COLLABORATIVE CARE

Collaborative care centers on identifying the location of the ingested foreign body, supporting airway, removing foreign body, and educating child/family to reduce incidence of reoccurrence.

Diagnostic Tests

Since approximately 60% to 90% of foreign bodies ingested in children are radiopaque (Wahbeh et al., 2002), radiographs of the neck, chest, esophagus, and abdomen are useful tools in verifying ingestion and identifying the location of the object. Endoscopic examination and retrieval of the ingested foreign body may be necessary.

Approximately 5% to 10% of children will have the foreign body lodged in the oropharynx, 20% of foreign bodies will be located in the esophagus, 60% will be located in the stomach, and 10% will be located distal to the stomach, usually in the small intestine (Wahbeh et al., 2002).

Clinical Therapy

Most (80% to 90%) foreign bodies pass spontaneously through the gastrointestinal system and are eliminated through stool. However, foreign bodies may become lodged in the esophagus and pose a significant risk to the child.

Smooth, small, round objects that have passed into the stomach are generally allowed to pass through the bowel without intervention. Esophageal foreign bodies are removed or advanced into the stomach due to the risk for mucosal erosion and catastrophic perforation (Chen & Beierle, 2001).

Of children with foreign-body ingestion, 10% to 20% require endoscopic removal under general anesthesia and 1% or less ultimately require surgery for removal (Wahbeh et al., 2002).

NURSING MANAGEMENT

Nursing care centers on supporting the child, collaborative assistance in the identification and removal of the foreign body, and teaching the child and family measures to reduce reoccurrence.

■ Nursing Assessment and Diagnosis

Assess the child for drooling, wheezing, substernal pain, dysphagia, and coughing. Obtain a thorough history from family. Determine, if possible, what was ingested, when the ingestion occurred, and any symptoms that the child experienced. Assess breath sounds.

Nursing diagnoses that may apply to the child with ingested foreign body include:

- Risk for Ineffective Tissue Perfusion (gastrointestinal) related to pressure of foreign body on tissues
- Risk for Injury related to repeat occurrence of ingestion of foreign body
- Deficient Knowledge (family) related to home safety measures

■ Planning and Implementation

Prepare the child for radiologic studies. Explain the procedures and reassure the child and family during the studies. Prepare for endoscopic examination and/or retrieval if necessary.

If the foreign object is in the stomach and the child is to be observed for natural excretion of the object, explain monitoring of stools to parents. Suggest the use of tongue blades to examine stools for presence of the foreign body and to report if the object has not been passed within the expected time frame (generally 48 hours). Encourage the family to return for further radiologic examinations to determine progress of passage of foreign object.

Partner with the family and assist in establishing a safe home environment for the child. Encourage the family to keep all small items out of the child's reach and to ensure the child is monitored at all times.

■ Evaluation

Expected outcomes for nursing care of the child with ingested foreign body include:

- The foreign body is removed or excreted without evidence of compromised tissue perfusion.
- The child has a reduced incidence of ingestion of foreign bodies.
- The family and child (if older) verbalize understanding of preventative measures to reduce risk of ingestion of foreign bodies.

Lead Poisoning

Lead poisoning, an excessive accumulation of lead in the blood, has been successfully prevented in many areas of the United States, with a substantial decline in lead levels from the mid-1970s. The average serum lead level for children is now 0.6 mg/dL, down from 15 mg/dL in 1976. Approximately 434,000 children in the United States are above the recommended level of 10 mg/dL. Many of these children are poor and live in older houses in inner cities (CDC, 2003). Even children with levels below 10 mg/dL may experience cognitive defects due to lead exposure. Lead in paint is

BOX 30–9 Sources of Lead Exposure

Sources of lead exposure include the following:

- Lead-based paint
- Soil and dust
- Drinking water from coolers with lead-soldered or lead-lined tanks, from lead-soldered teapots, or from lead pipes or lead-soldered pipes
- Food grown in contaminated soil, stored in lead-soldered cans or leaded crystal, or prepared in improperly fired pottery
- Parental occupations and hobbies that involve exposure to lead (e.g., plumbing, battery manufacturing, highway construction, furniture refinishing, stained glass work, pottery making)
- Airborne lead in areas surrounding smelters and battery manufacturing plants

the most common source of lead exposure for preschool children. Children are also exposed to lead when they ingest contaminated food, water, and soil or when they inhale dust contaminated with lead. Box 30–9 summarizes several sources of lead exposure.

Children are at greater risk for lead poisoning because they absorb and retain more lead in proportion to their weight than adults do. Lead is particularly harmful to children under the age of 7 years.

Clinical Manifestations

Lead interferes with normal cell function, primarily of the nervous system, blood cells, and kidneys, and adversely affects the metabolism of vitamin D and calcium. Clinical manifestations depend on the degree of toxicity; see the table below.

CLINICAL MANIFESTATIONS of Lead Poisoning

MILD TOXICITY (10–15 μg/DL)	MODERATE TOXICITY (25–69 μg/DL)	SEVERE TOXICITY (>70 μg/DL)
Myalgia or paresthesia	Arthralgia	Paresis or paralysis
Mild fatigue	General fatigue	Encephalopathy may lead abruptly to seizures, changes in consciousness, coma, and death
Irritability, lethargy	Difficulty concentrating	Lead line (blue–black) on gingival tissue
Occasional abdominal discomfort	Muscular exhaustibility Tremor Headache Diffuse abdominal pain Vomiting Weight loss Constipation Anemia	Colic (intermittent, severe abdominal cramps)

Adapted from Agency for Toxic Substances and Disease Registry. (1990). Lead toxicity. Case studies in environmental medicine *(p. 11). Atlanta: Author.*

Neurologic effects include decreased IQ scores, cognitive deficits, impaired hearing, and growth delays. Impaired mental function can occur with blood levels even lower than 10 mg/dL. Lead ingestion by a woman during pregnancy can result in fetal malformations, reduced birth weight, and premature birth. Severe lead poisoning, which can result in encephalopathy, coma, and death, is now rare.

Once in the body, lead accumulates in the blood, soft tissues (kidney, bone marrow, liver, and brain), bones, and teeth. Lead that is absorbed by the bones and teeth is released slowly; thus, exposure to even small doses, over time, can result in dangerously high levels of lead in the body.

MediaLink Lead Poisoning

COLLABORATIVE CARE

The goals of collaborative care include reducing the risk of lead exposure in children, identifying lead toxicity, and implementing measures to remove lead.

Diagnostic Tests

The Centers for Disease Control and Prevention now recommends screening children at high risk, with reduced screening for those at low risk. In addition, all children enrolled in Medicaid should be tested, with follow-up management and care (Advisory Committee on Childhood Lead Poisoning Prevention, 2000).

A complete blood count reveals anemia. Iron deficiency is assessed by serum iron, total nonbinding capacity, and serum ferritin levels. Urinalysis, blood urea nitrogen (BUN), and creatine are performed to assess for renal damage. Abdominal radiograph reveals lead if present. A blood lead (Pb-B) level is the most useful screening and diagnostic test for lead exposure.

A Pb-B below 10 mg/dL is considered acceptable, although may still not screen out all children with impaired development due to lead. An environmental history should be obtained for children with Pb-B levels between 10 and 19 mg/dL to identify removable sources of lead. Follow-up testing is required. Children with Pb-B levels between 20 and 69 mg/dL require a full medical evaluation, including a detailed environmental and behavioral history, physical examination, and tests for iron deficiency. Interventions to remove sources of lead from the child's environment are necessary. For levels above 25 mg/dL, chelation therapy is also administered. Children with Pb-B levels greater than 70 mg/dL are critically ill from lead poisoning and require immediate chelation therapy and interventions to provide a lead-free environment.

Clinical Therapy

Chelation therapy involves the administration of an agent that binds with lead, increasing its rate of excretion from the body. Calcium disodium ethylenediamine tetraacetate ($CaNa_2$ EDTA), dimercaprol (BAL), d-penicillamine, or succimer (DMSA) may be used. Children with Pb-B levels between 25 and 69 mg/dL receive $CaNa_2$ EDTA for 5 to 7 days, followed by a rest period and then a second chelation treatment. Children with Pb-B levels greater than 70 mg/dL are given both BAL and

MediaLink Lead and Mercury Poisoning Prevention Resources

$CaNa_2$ EDTA, followed by a rest period and a second chelation treatment using $CaNa_2$ EDTA alone. Long-term follow-up of children receiving chelation therapy is essential. The child should never be discharged unless a lead-free home environment has been ensured.

NURSING MANAGEMENT

Nursing care centers on screening, education, and follow-up. Nurses often work with state and local health officials to plan screening for children at high risk of lead exposure. Ask parents about the child's development and eating habits and be alert for risk of lead exposure. Educate parents about sources of lead in the environment and techniques to reduce exposure. Emphasize the importance of housekeeping interventions to reduce exposure to lead dust. These interventions include damp mopping of hard surfaces, floors, window sills, and baseboards; washing the child's hands and face before meals; and frequent washing of toys and pacifiers.

Teach parents the importance of including foods high in iron and calcium in the child's diet to counteract losses of these minerals associated with lead exposure. The child should eat meals at regular intervals, as lead is absorbed more readily on an empty stomach.

Be sure that parents understand the importance of follow-up testing of lead levels. If the child is developmentally delayed, refer the family to an infant stimulation or child development program. Referral to social services and either a visiting nurse or home healthcare nurse may also be appropriate. See Developing Cultural Competence: Lead Sources.

DEVELOPING CULTURAL COMPETENCE
Lead Sources

Traditional medicines and cosmetics may contain large amounts of lead. Examples include azarcon and greta, preparations that are used by Mexican Americans to treat *empacho,* a coliclike illness; litargirio, used as a deodorant and for treatment of skin problems by some Hispanics; chifong tokuwan, pay-loo-ah, ghasard, bali goli, and kandu, used in some Asian communities; and alkohl, kohl, surma, saoott, and cebagin, used in some Middle Eastern communities.

Expected outcomes of nursing care for the child with lead or other poisoning include the following:

- The child displays normal growth and development, including cognition.
- The child's nutritional intake is adequate.
- The child's environment is free of lead or other poisons.
- Family expresses understanding of measures to establish a safe environment for the child.

Mercury Poisoning

Mercury poses another potential environmental health hazard to children. This metal is present in three forms: elemental mercury which is silver and liquid and was formerly used in thermometers and other medical and scientific equipment; inorganic salts that were formerly used in paints and a variety of other products; and organic mercury that is present in fish, breast milk in mothers who have consumed mercury in any form, and a variety of industrial wastes. The pathophysiology of disease depends on the type of mercury and its form of ingestion. Bronchitis and pneumonia may occur with respiratory ingestion; ulceration and hemorrhage of the gastrointestinal tract occur with oral ingestion; and cardiovascular collapse and mild to severe neurologic symptoms may occur with any form of ingestion. Intake by pregnant women can lead to cerebral palsy, seizures, and delayed development (Goldman & Shannon, 2001; Pike-Paris, 2004).

The major method for eliminating mercury poisoning is prevention. Medical equipment with mercury should be replaced by nonmercury alternatives. Encourage families to bring mercury thermometers to a safe site and replace them with alternative types of thermometers. Schools should not maintain mercury in science laboratories because of the risk of spillage and theft. Clean up mercury with care if spilled, such as when a thermometer breaks. Vacuums should never be used since mercury could then vaporize. Instead, use paper to move the mercury into a jar that can be securely covered and taken to a safe site for disposal. Contact local public health departments for further directions.

Another method of prevention is to lower levels of mercury ingestion from fish. See Chapter 9∞ for recommended maximum servings of fish for pregnant women and young children. Inform families about resources that can provide further information about mercury, in households, school, and medical facilities, as well as in local water supplies and fish.

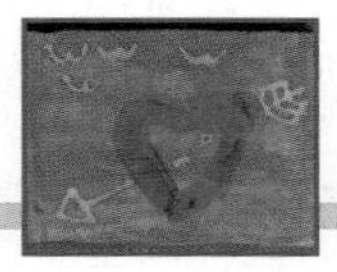

CHAPTER HIGHLIGHTS

- A variety of structural defects caused by fetal development alterations can affect the gastrointestinal system of infants.
- Cleft lip and palate are structural defects that often involve care by a team of providers such as plastic surgeon, pediatrician, nurse, audiologist, speech therapist, and orthodontist.
- A variety of defects of the esophagus and trachea can manifest as mild to life-threatening problems in the newborn period.
- Pyloric stenosis is a common cause of projectile vomiting in the newborn period.

- Intussusception, abdominal wall defects, and anorectal malformations are serious structural defects of infancy.
- Several of the intestinal problems of childhood necessitate temporary or permanent ostomy placement.
- Hernias can be present in the diaphragmatic area, umbilicus, or inguinal canal.
- Children with gastroesophageal reflux are irritable due to lack of food and discomfort when feeding.
- Common disorders of motility include vomiting, constipation, and encopresis.
- Hirschsprung disease, or aganglionic megacolon, leads to failure to pass normal stools and bloating of the abdomen.
- Gastroenteritis and parasitic disorders are common causes of gastrointestinal disturbance and distress in children, and may lead to fluid and electrolyte imbalance.
- The most common inflammatory disorder of the gastrointestinal tract is appendicitis.
- Necrotizing enterocolitis is a potentially life-threatening inflammatory disease of the intestines seen primarily in premature infants after enteral feedings are begun.
- Common inflammatory bowel diseases affecting primarily adolescent and young adult age groups are Crohn's disease and ulcerative colitis.
- Peptic ulcer may be primary (often caused by *H. pylori*) or secondary, in situations of stress, trauma, or other disease.
- Celiac disease is a malabsorption disorder caused by gluten sensitivity.
- Short bowel syndrome occurs when surgery is used to treat an intestinal disease and significant sections of the bowel are removed.
- Feeding disorders such as colic and rumination may require teaching and other nursing interventions.
- Biliary atresia and hepatitis are the most common liver diseases in young children. Hyperbilirubinemia can occur in newborns.
- Abdominal trauma most often occurs to children during motor vehicle crashes.
- Numerous medicines, plants, pesticides, and other household products are accidentally ingested by children each year. Parents must learn how to avoid these poisonings and how to contact the AAPCC in case of accidental exposure.

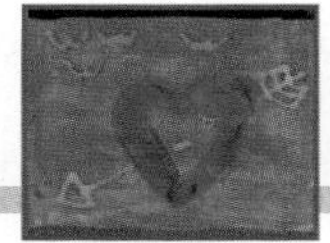

CRITICAL THINKING IN ACTION

INTRODUCTION

Recall 8-month-old Jerome from the chapter opening scenario. He was born with multiple gastrointestinal anomalies, including an imperforate anus and esophageal atresia. He has had two major surgeries, and currently has a colostomy and a gastrostomy feeding tube.

DESCRIPTION

Most of Jerome's care takes place within the home environment, where he lives with his mother and 6-year-old sister, Amanda. He is visited frequently by a home health nurse and an ostomy nurse. Jerome's mother is attentive to his needs and monitors his intake and output closely. Jerome is alert and smiles when elicited. His gastrostomy tube functions well and he is beginning to take oral fluids in increasing amounts. His colostomy is intact and functioning.

DISCUSSION

1. What growth and developmental tasks should Jerome exhibit at 8 months of age and how would you assess for achievement of those tasks? Why is Jerome at risk for delayed growth and development? Identify collaborative measures that would promote Jerome's achievement of developmental tasks and growth.
2. Consider Jerome's sister, Amanda. Based on her age, what thoughts might she be experiencing regarding her brother's condition? What suggestions can you make to the mother to include Amanda in Jerome's care and to promote Amanda's understanding of her brother's condition? How would you evaluate Amanda's response and understanding?
3. Jerome's mother has seemingly adapted well to his condition and provides attentive care to the child. Consider a discussion you might have with the mother regarding her feelings, stressors, and coping mechanisms. What advice would you provide to his mother in the event that she feels she is not coping well or is experiencing anxiety related to the task of caring for Jerome?
4. Consider Jerome's colostomy and tube feedings. Identify three risks to Jerome's safety associated with colostomy and tube feedings. What interventions can be taken to reduce those risks? How would you evaluate the effectiveness of the interventions?

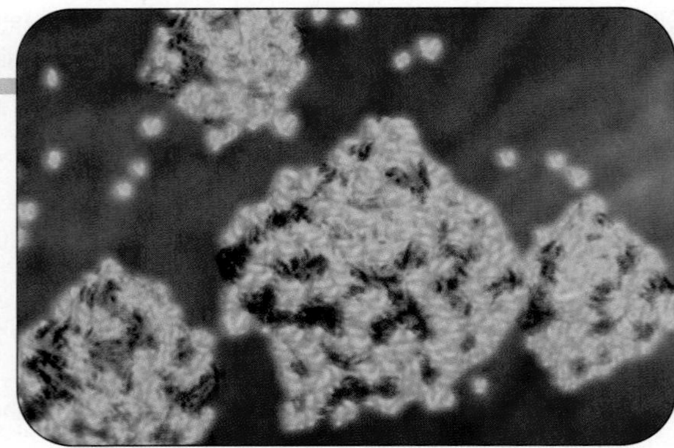

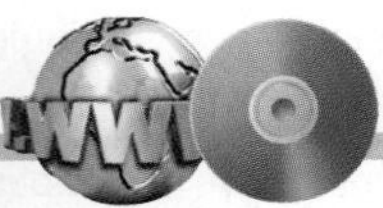

EXPLORE MediaLink

- NCLEX review, case studies, and other interactive resources for this chapter can be found on the Companion Website at **http://www.prenhall.com/ball.** Click on Chapter 30 to select the activities for this chapter.
- For animations, more NCLEX review questions, and an audio glossary, access the accompanying CD-ROM in this textbook.

http://www.prenhall.com/ball

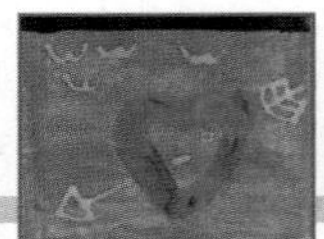

REFERENCES

Advisory Committee on Childhood Lead Poisoning Prevention. (2000). Recommendations for blood lead screening of young children enrolled in Medicaid: Targeting a group at high risk. *Morbidity and Mortality Weekly Report, 49*(RR14), 1–13.

Adzik, N. S., & Nance, M. L. (2000). Pediatric surgery: First of two parts. *The New England Journal of Medicine, 342,* 1651–1657.

American Academy of Pediatrics. (2004). Management of hyperbilirubinemia in the newborn infant 35 or more weeks of gestation. *Pediatrics, 114,* 297–316. http://aappolicy.aappublications.org/cgi/content/full/pediatrics;114/1/297.pdf, accessed 1/20/2005.

American Academy of Pediatrics and American College of Obstetricians and Gynecologists (ACOG) (2002). In L. C. Gilstrap & W. Oh (Eds.), *Guidelines for perinatal care* (5th ed., p. 221). Elk Grove Village, IL: Author.

Amiel, J., & Lyonnet, X. (2001). Hirschsprung disease, associated syndromes and genetics: A review. *Journal of Medical Genetics, 38,* 729–739.

Arce, D. A., Ermocilla, C. A., & Costa, H. (2002). Evaluation of constipation. *American Family Physician, 65,* 2283–2290.

Arguin, A. L., & Swartz, M. K. (2004). Gastroesophageal reflux in infants: A primary care perspective. *Pediatric Nursing, 30,* 45–52.

Ashburn, D. A., Pranikoff, T., & Turner, C. S. (2002). Unusual presentations of gastroschisis. *The American Surgeon, 68,* 724–727.

Bagolan, P., Casaccia, G., Crescenzi, F., Nahom, A., Trucchi, A., & Giorlandino, C. (2004). Impact of a current treatment protocol on outcome of high-risk congenital diaphragmatic hernia. *Journal of Pediatric Surgery, 39,* 313–318.

Barnard, N. D. (2003). The milk debate goes on and on and on! *Pediatrics, 112,* 448.

Baron, M. L. (2002). Crohn disease in children. *American Journal of Nursing, 102,* 26–34.

Barr, J. M. B. (2000). Chronic intestinal pseudo-obstruction: Pediatric case presentations and review of the literature. *Journal of the Society of Pediatric Nurses, 5,* 175–182.

Belkengren, R., & Sapala, S. (2002). Pediatric management problems. *Pediatric Nursing, 28,* 506–508.

Bell, E. F. (2005). Preventing necrotizing enterocolitis: What works and how safe? *Pediatrics, 115,* 173–175.

Blackburn, S. T. (2003). *Maternal, fetal, and neonatal physiology: A clinical perspective.* (pp. 656–669). St. Louis: Saunders.

Blum, J., Taubman, B., & Nemeth, N. (2004). During toilet training, constipation occurs before stool toileting refusal. *Pediatrics, 113,* 1791–1792.

Blumer, S. L., Zucconi, W. B., Cohen, H. L., Scriven, R. J., & Lee, T. K. (2004). The vomiting neonate: A review of the ACR appropriateness criteria and ultrasound's role in the workup of such patients. *Ultrasound Quarterly, 20*(3), 79–89.

Borkowski, S. (1998). Pediatric stomas, tubes, and appliances. *Pediatric Clinics of North America, 45,* 1419–1436.

Cash S. (2004, July). Guideline offers direction for prompt diagnosis, treatment of hyperbilirubinemia. *AAP News.* Elk Grove Village, IL: American Academy of Pediatrics.

Castiglia, P. T. (2001). Constipation in children. *Journal of Pediatric Health Care, 15,* 200–202.

Centers for Disease Control and Prevention. (2001). Blood and hair mercury levels in young children and women of childbearing age—United States, 1999. *MMWR, 50,* 140–143.

Centers for Disease Control and Prevention. (2001). Kernicterus in full-term infants—United States, 1994–1998. *Morbidity and Mortality Weekly Review, 50*(23), 491–494. www.cdc.gov/mmwr/preview/ mmwrhtml/mm5023a4.htm, accessed 1/22/2005.

Centers for Disease Control and Prevention. (2003). Childhood lead poisoning. www.cdc.gov/health/lead.htm

Centers for Disease Control and Prevention. (2004). Summary of notifiable diseases, 2002. *MMWR, 51,* 1–84. www.cdc.gov.mmwr/preview/mmwrhtml/mm5153a1.htm

Chen, M. K., & Beierle, E. A. (2001). Gastrointestinal foreign bodies. *Pediatric Annals, 30,* 736–742.

Chial, H. J., Camilleri, M., Williams, D. E., Litzinger, K., & Perrault, J. (2003). Rumination syndrome in children and adolescents: Diagnosis, treatment, and prognosis. *Pediatrics, 111,* 158–562.

Cho, S., Moore, S. P., & Fangman, T. (2001). One hundred three consecutive patients with anorectal malformations and their associated anomalies. *Archives of Pediatrics & Adolescent Medicine, 155,* 587–591.

Clayden, G., & Keshtgar, A. S. (2003). Management of childhood constipation. *Postgraduate Medical Journal, 79,* 616–621.

Cleft Palate Foundation. (2004). www.cleftline.org/aboutclp/, accessed 6/26/2004.

Committee on Nutrition, American Academy of Pediatrics. (2004). *Pediatric nutrition handbook* (5th ed.). Elk Grove Village, IL: AAP.

Corner, B. (2003). Intravenous atropine treatment in infantile hypertrophic pyloric stenosis. *Archives of Disease in Childhood, 88,* 87.

Coughlin, E. C. (2003). Assessment and management of pediatric constipation in primary care. *Pediatric Nursing, 29,* 296–302.

Cowden, J. D., & Hotez, P. J. (2001). A field guide to emerging enteric protozoa. *Contemporary Pediatrics, 18,* 440–447.

Daview, M. C., Creighton, S. M., & Wilcox, D. T. (2004). Long-term outcomes of anorectal malformations. *Pediatric Surgery Int, 20,* 567–572.

Estrada, B. (2000). Breast-feeding and vertical transmission of hepatitis C. *Infectious Medicine, 17,* 526–528.

Garrison, M. M., & Christakis, D. A. (2000). A systematic review of treatments for infant colic. *Pediatrics, 106,* 184–190.

Gereige, R. S., & Frias, J. L. (2002). Is it more than just constipation? *Pediatrics, 109,* 961–965.

Gokhale, R. (2001). Chronic abdominal pain: Inflammatory bowel disease and eosinophilic gastroenteropathy. *Pediatric Annals, 30,* 49–55.

Goldman, L. R., & Shannon, M. W. (2001). Technical report: Mercury in the environment: Implications for pediatricians. *Pediatrics, 108,* 197–205.

Hedrick, H. L., Crombleholme, T. M., Flake, A. W., Nance, M. L., von Allmen, D., Howell, L. J., Johnson, M. P., Wilson, R. D., & Adzick, N. S. (2004). Right congenital diaphragmatic hernia: Prenatal assessment and outcome. *Journal of Pediatric Surgery, 39,* 319–323.

Holst, B., & Ritter, D. (2001). Managing viral hepatitis. *Clinician Reviews, 11,* 51–62.

Home Safety Council. (2004a). www.homesafetycouncil.org/resource_center/resourcecenter.aspx, accessed 7/4/2004.

Home Safety Council. (2004b). Poisonings second leading cause of unintentional injury deaths in American homes (news release). www.prnewswire.com, accessed 7/4/2004.

Howard, E. R. (2001). Hirschsprung's disease and allied disorders. *Gut, 49*(5), 741–742.

Hyman, P. E., & Danda, C. E. (2004). Understanding and treating childhood bellyaches. *Pediatric Annals, 33,* 97–104.

Jadcherla, S., & Shaker, R. (2001). Esophageal and upper esophageal sphincter motor function in babies. *American Journal of Medicine, 111,* 64–68.

Jakubik, L. D., Colfer, A., & Grossman, M. B. (2000). Pediatric short bowel syndrome: Pathophysiology, nursing care, and management issues. *Journal of the Society of Pediatric Nurses, 5,* 111–121.

Joint Commission on Accreditation of Healthcare Organizations (JCAHO). (2001, April). Kernicterus threatens healthy newborns. *Sentinel Event Alert, 18.* www.jcaho.org/about+us/news+letters/sentinel+event+alert/sea_18.htm, accessed 1/23/2005.

Jung, A. D. (2001). Gastroesophageal reflux in infants and children. *American Family Physician, 64,* 1853–1850.

Katz, D. A. (2001). Evaluation and management of inguinal and umbilical hernias. *Pediatric Annals, 30,* 729–735.

Kazacos, K. R. (2000). Protecting children from helminthic zoonoses. *Contemporary Pediatrics* (Suppl.), 1–24.

Kelly, D. A. (2002). Managing liver failure. *Postgraduate Medical Journal, 78,* 660–667.

Kirschner, B. S. (2001). Management of abdominal pain. *Pediatric Annals, 30,* 12–14.

Klein, E. J., Kapoor, D., & Shugerman, R. P. (2004). The diagnosis of intussusception. *Clinical Pediatrics, 43,* 343–347.

Kliegman, R. M., & Willoughby, R. E. (2005). Prevention of necrotizing enterocolitis with probiotics. *Pediatrics, 115,* 171–172.

Kohli, R., & Li, B. U. K. (2004). Differential diagnosis of recurrent abdominal pain: New considerations. *Pediatric Annals, 33,* 113–122.

Kosloske, A. M., Love, C. L., Rohrer, J. E., Goldthorn, J. F., & Lacey, S. R. (2004). The diagnosis of appendicitis in children: Outcomes of a strategy based on pediatric surgical evaluation. *Pediatrics, 113,* 29–34.

Kotb, M. A., Kotb, A., Sheba, M. F., & El Koofy, N. M. (2001). Evaluation of the triangular cord sign in the diagnosis of biliary atresia. *Pediatrics, 108,* 416–420.

Lam, J. P. H., Eunson, G. J., Munro, F. D., & Orr, J. D. (2001). Delayed presentation of handlebar injuries in children. *British Medical Journal, 322,* 1288–1289.

Lembo, A., & Camilleri, M. (2003). Chronic constipation. *The New England Journal of Medicine, 349,* 1360–1368.

Letton, R. W. (2001). Pyloric stenosis. *Pediatric Annals, 30,* 745–750.

Levitzky, S., & Cooper, R. (2000). Infant colic syndrome—Maternal fantasies of aggression and infanticide. *Clinical Pediatrics, 39,* 395–400.

Levy, J. (2001). Gastroesophageal reflux and other causes of abdominal pain. *Pediatric Annals, 30,* 42–47.

Litovitz, T. L., Klein-Schwartz, W., White, S., Cobaugh, D. J., Youniss, J., Drab, A., & Benson, B. E. (2000). 1999 annual report of the American Association of Poison Control Centers Toxic Exposure Surveillance System. *American Journal of Emergency Medicine, 18,* 517–574.

Miller, K. E. (2003). Colic: Prevalence, risk factors, and potential sequelae. *American Family Physician, 67,* 2005–2006.

Mitchell, J. C., & Wood, R. J. (2000). Management of cleft lip and palate in primary care. *Journal of Pediatric Health Care, 14,* 13–19.

Morash, D. (2002). An interdisciplinary project that changed practice in feeding methods after pyloromyotomy. *Pediatric Nursing, 28,* 113–117.

Murdock, A. M., & Johnston, S. D. (2005). Diagnostic criteria for coelic disease: Time for change? *European Journal of Gastroenterology and Hepatology, 17,* 41–43.

Murray, K. F., & Christie, D. L. (2000). Vomiting in infancy: When should you worry? *Contemporary Pediatrics, 17,* 81–115.

National Institutes of Health. (2000). Hepatitis C. Community drug alert bulletin (NIH Publication No. 00–4663). Bethesda MD: Author.

National Safety Council. (2003). *Injury facts.* Itasca, IL: Author.

Nehring, W. M. (2004). Down syndrome. In P. L. Allen & J. A. Vessey, *Primary care of the child with a chronic condition* (pp. 445–468). St. Louis: Mosby.

Neidlinger, N. A., Madan, A. K., & Wright, M. J. (2001). Meckel's diverticulum causing cecal volvulus. *The American Surgeon, 67,* 41–43.

Orenstein, J. (2000). Update on intussusception. *Contemporary Pediatrics, 17,* 180–191.

Orlando, R. (2001). Overview of the mechanisms of gastroesophageal reflux. *American Journal of Medicine, 111,* 174–177.

Paulson, E. K., Kalady, M. F., & Pappas, T. N. (2003). Suspected appendicitis. *The New England Journal of Medicine, 348,* 236–242.

Pike-Paris, A. (2004). Mercury, 101. *Pediatric Nursing, 30,* 150–153.

Powers, K. S. (2000). Diagnosis and management of common toxic ingestions and inhalations. *Pediatric Annals, 29,* 330–343.

Ratan, S. K., Ratan, K. N., Pandey, R. M., Mittal, A., Magu, S., & Sodhi, P. K. (2004). Associated congenital anomalies in patients with anorectal malformations—a need for developing a uniform practical approach. *Journal of Pediatric Surgery, 39,* 1706–1711.

Reeves, J. J., Shannon, M. W., & Fleisher, G. R. (2002). Ondansetron decreases vomiting associated with acute gastroenteritis. *Pediatrics, 109*(4), e62.

Rogers, J. (2001). Hirschsprung's disease: Diagnosis and management in children. *British Journal of Nursing, 10,* 640–645.

Sadovsky, R. (2001). Meckel's diverticulum: Review and management. *American Family Physician, 64,* 2000–2001.

Salihu, H. M., Boos, R., & Schmidt, W. (2002). Omphalocele and gastrochisis. *Journal of Obstetrics and Gynecology, 22,* 489–492.

Sandberg, D. J., Magee, W. P., & Denk, M. J. (2002). Neonatal cleft lip and cleft palate repair. *Association of Operating Room Nurses (AORN) Journal, 75,* 490–506.

Sanders, H., Davis, M. F., Duncan, B., Meaney, F. J., et al. (2003). Use of complementary and alternative medical therapies among children with special health care needs in southern Arizona. *Pediatrics, 111,* 584–587.

Schulman, C. S. (2003). Emergency care focus: A FASTer method of deteching abdominal trauma. *Nursing Management, 34*(9), 47–49.

Scolapio, J. S. (2002). Short bowel syndrome. *Journal of Parenteral and Enteral Nutrition, 26,* S11–S16.

Shaw N. M. (2003). Assessment and management of the hematologic system. In C. Kenner & J. W. Lott (Eds.), *Comprehensive neonatal nursing: A physiologic perspective* (3rd ed., pp. 586–602). St. Louis: Saunders.

Shovein, J. T., Damazo, R. J., & Hyams, I. (2000). Hepatitis A: How benign is it? *American Journal of Nursing, 100,* 43–48.

Simpson, T., & Ivey, J. (2003). Pediatric management problems. *Pediatric Nursing, 29,* 310–311.

Singh, S., Behnde, M., & Kinnane, J. M. (2001). Delayed presentations of congenital diaphragmatic hernia. *Pediatric Emergency Care, 17,* 269–271.

Sondheimer, J. (2003). Gastroesophageal reflux. In W. Hay, A. Hayward, M. Levin, & J. Sondheimer (Eds.), *Current pediatric diagnosis St treatment* (16th ed., pp. 614–615). New York: Lange Medical Books/McGraw-Hill.

SPLIT Research Group. (2001). Studies of pediatric liver transplantation (SPLIT): Year 2000 outcomes. *Transplantation, 72,* 463–476.

Swenson, O. (2002). Hirschsprung's disease. *Pediatrics, 109,* 914—918.

Thielman, N. M., & Guerrant, R. L. (2004). Acute infectious diarrhea. *The New England Journal of Medicine, 350,* 38–47.

Thompson, J. (2001). Intussusception, pyloric stenosis and Hirschsprung's disease. *Community Practitioner, 74,* 312–313.

Tran, T. T., Nissen, N., Poordad, F. F., & Martin, P. (2004). Advances in liver transplantation: New strategies and current care expand access, enhance survival. *Postgraduate Medicine, 115*(5), 73–85.

Uhrich, K. S., & Mackin, A. L. (2001). Cleft lip and palate. *AJN, 101,* 24AA–24FF.

Van Rooij, I. A., Vermeij-Keers, C., Kluijtmans, J., Ocke, M. C., et al. (2003). Does the interaction between maternal folate intake and the methylenetetrahydrofolate reductase polymorphisms affect the risk of cleft lip with or without cleft palate? *Journal of Epidemiology, 157,* 583–591.

Vegunta, R. K., Ali, A., Wallace, L. J., Switzer, D. M., & Pearl, X. X. (2004). Laparoscopic appendectomy in children: Technically feasible and safe in all stages of acute appendicitis. *The American Surgeon, 70,* 198–202.

Wahbeh, G., Wylie, R., & Kay, M. (2002). Foreign body ingestion in infants and children: Location, location, location. *Clinical Pediatrics, 41,* 633–640.

Weir, E. (2003). Congenital abdominal wall defects. *Canadian Medical Association Journal, 169,* 809–810.

Wyllie, R. (2004). Stomach and intestines; Ileus, adhesions, intussusception, and closed loop obstructions. In R. E. Behrman, R. M. Kliegman, & H. B. Jenson, *Nelson textbook of pediatrics* (17th ed., pp. 1228–1232, 1241–1243). Philadelphia: Saunders.

Zelnik, N., Pacht, A., Obeid, R., & Lerner, A. (2004). Range of neurological disorders in patients with celiac disease. *Pediatrics, 113,* 1672–1677.

Ziegler, M. M. (2004). The diagnosis of appendicitis: An evolving paradigm. *Pediatrics, 113,* 130–132.

Zitsman. J. L. (2003). Current concepts in minimal access surgery for children. *Pediatrics, 111,* 1239–1245.

Chapter 31

Alterations in Genitourinary Function

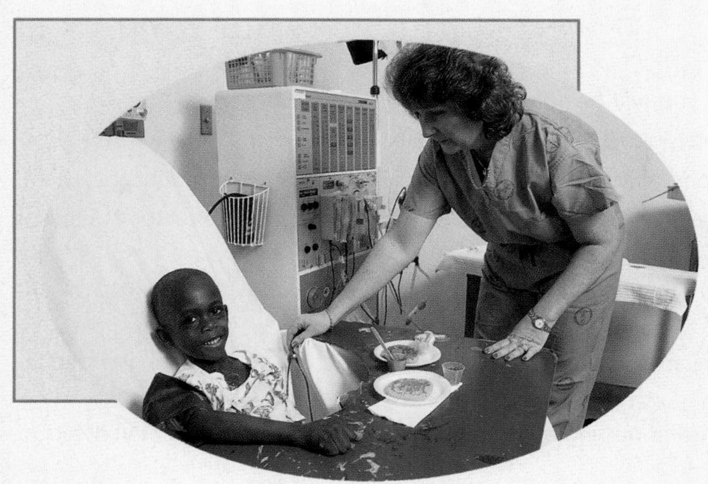

Terrell Thompson, who is now 5 years old, was born with posterior urethral valves, which caused damage to his kidneys. Despite undergoing surgery to correct the defect at 2 years of age, his kidney function continued to deteriorate. End-stage renal disease was diagnosed 2 years ago, and dialysis treatment was initiated. Terrell requires a kidney transplant; however, no family member is able or willing to donate a kidney. As a result, Terrell has been placed on the transplant list for a cadaver kidney.

Terrell was initially treated with peritoneal dialysis, but after experiencing several peritoneal infections in the first year, his healthcare team and family determined that hemodialysis would be the most beneficial method of treatment. Terrell visits the dialysis center three afternoons a week for treatments lasting approximately 3 to 4 hours. This schedule permits him to attend kindergarten classes in the morning.

What are the special concerns of the nurse in monitoring a child who is receiving hemodialysis treatment? Is Terrell at any higher risk for infection than other children? Does he require a special diet? What are the implications associated with schooling? What are the potential complications of this disease and of the hemodialysis treatments for Terrell's growth and development? If a donor kidney becomes available for transplant, what special teaching will Terrell and his family require to ensure the best survival of the kidney graft? What are the psychological effects of renal disease on the child and family? What role does the nurse have in the collaborative multidisciplinary approach to caring for Terrell? The answers to these questions and information about numerous other genitourinary conditions are presented in this chapter.

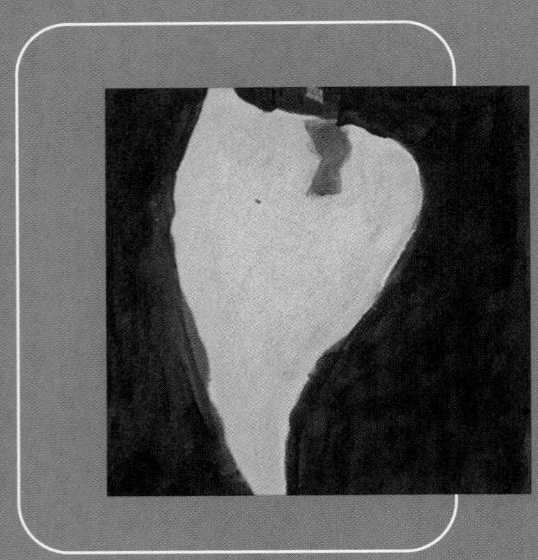

"I hope that I get a kidney soon. I'm tired of machines and needles and I want to be like other kids."

—Terrell, age 5

Key Terms

anuria/1198
azotemia/1198
balanitis/1222
bladder exstrophy/1177
chordee/1180
circumcision/1222
cryptorchidism/1223
cystitis/1186
dialysate/1210
disequilibrium syndrome/1213
diurnal enuresis/1189
end-stage renal disease (ESRD)/1203
enuresis/1189
epispadias/1180
glomerular filtration rate/1176
glomerulonephritis/1215
hydronephrosis/1182
hypospadias/1180
incarceration/1225
inguinal hernia/1224
kidney failure (renal failure)/1198
nephrotic syndrome/1192
neurogenic bladder/1188
nocturnal enuresis/1189
obstructive nephropathy/1182
obstructive uropathy/1182

Learning Outcomes

After completing this chapter, you will be able to:

- Describe the anatomy and physiology of the genitourinary system.
- Discuss the pathophysiology and clinical manifestations of alterations in the genitourinary system.
- Discuss the collaborative care and nursing management of the child with a structural defect of the genitourinary system.
- Discuss the collaborative care and nursing management of the child with a disorder of urinary elimination.
- Discuss the collaborative care and nursing management of the child with a renal disorder, including renal failure.
- Discuss the collaborative care and nursing management of the child with a structural defect of the reproductive system.
- Discuss the collaborative care and nursing management of the child with a sexually transmitted infection.

MediaLink  **http://www.prenhall.com/ball**

Resources for this chapter can be found on the CD-ROM accompanying this textbook and on the Companion Website at www.prenhall.com/ball. Click on Chapter 31 to select the activities for this chapter.

CD-ROM

Animations/Videos

- *Circumcision*
- *Furosemide*
- *Renal Function*
- *Sexually Transmitted Infections*

NCLEX Review

Audio Glossary

COMPANION WEBSITE

A & P Review

Clinical Manifestations Review

NCLEX Review

Case Study: A Child with Chronic Kidney Failure

Care Plan

- *A Child with Kidney Failure*
- *A Child with Nephrotic Syndrome*
- *A School-Age Child with Enuresis*

MediaLink Applications

- *Communication Strategy: Adolescents and Sexual Activity*

Key Terms *(continued)*

oliguria/1198
osteodystrophy/1204
paraphimosis/1222
phimosis/1222
pyelonephritis/1186
renal failure/1198
renal insufficiency/1184
renal replacement therapy/1210
testicular torsion/1226
uremia/1200
ureteral stent/1178
urethral stent/1178
urethritis/1186
vesicoureteral reflux (VUR)/1185

What are the consequences of urinary and renal disorders, such as end-stage renal disease or irreversible renal failure, in children? What specific and nonspecific signs alert parents and healthcare professionals to suspect these disorders?

Many infections, structural disorders, and disease processes can alter genitourinary function. Given that the kidneys and other urinary system organs perform numerous essential body functions, including removal of waste products and maintenance of fluid and electrolyte balance, disorders that affect these organs pose a significant threat to the health of children.

Although the reproductive system is functionally immature until puberty, disorders involving these organs may also have a significant impact on the health of children. Uncorrected structural defects and sexually transmitted infections can have both psychologic and physiologic implications on the developing child.

ANATOMY AND PHYSIOLOGY OF THE URINARY SYSTEM

The urinary system is comprised of the kidneys, ureters, bladder, and urethra (Figure 31–1 ■). Both kidneys are located in the intraperitoneal cavity and are on either side of the vertebral column. In children, the proportion of space occupied by the kidneys in the abdominal cavity is larger than the amount of space occupied in the adult. Within the *kidneys,* the glomeruli and tubules form urine through the processes of filtration, reabsorption, and secretion. The *ureters* carry the waste fluid from the kidneys to the bladder. The *bladder* is the muscular organ that stores urine until it is excreted through the *urethra.* The fetus begins to excrete urine at approximately the twelfth week of development.

The urinary system functions to excrete wastes and maintain acid–base and fluid and electrolyte balance. Other functions of the renal system include regulation of blood pressure, stimulation of production erythropoietin (for stimulation of erythrocyte development), and regulation of calcium metabolism in the body by activation of vitamin D.

The *nephrons* (Figure 31–2 ■), the structural and functional unit of the kidneys, perform filtration, reabsorption, and secretion functions. All of the nephrons which will comprise the mature

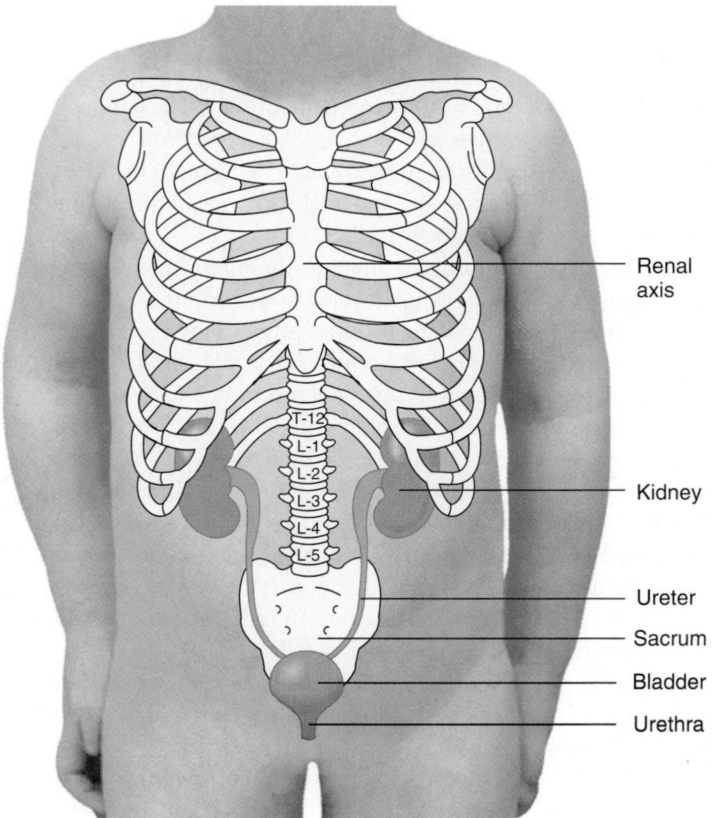

FIGURE 31–1 ■ The urinary system is comprised of the kidneys, ureters, bladder, and urethra. The kidneys are located between the twelfth thoracic (T12) and third lumbar (L3) vertebrae.

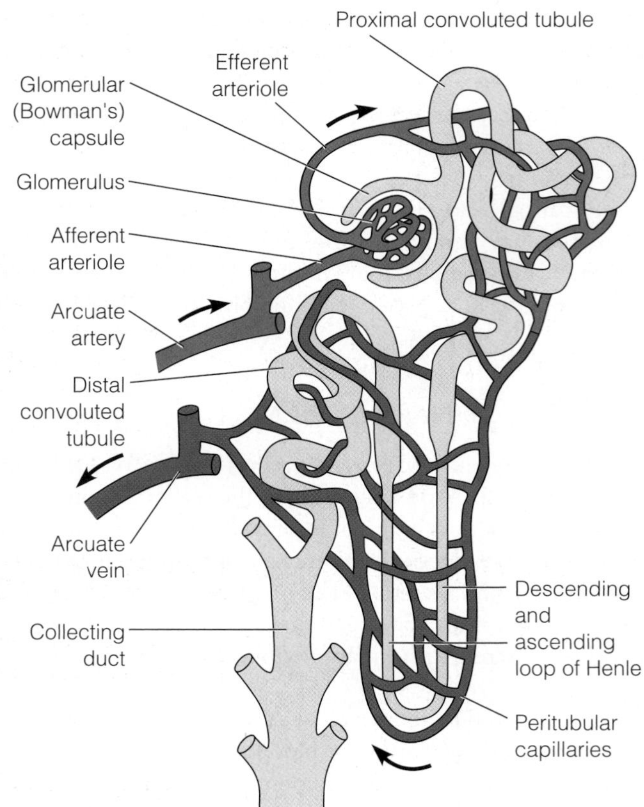

FIGURE 31–2 ■ The nephrons are the structural and functional unit of the kidneys. They filter water and wastes across the glomerular capillaries to maintain the body fluid level, electrolyte composition, and pH. A nephron holds six glomeruli, Bowman's capsule, proximal tubule, loop of Henle, distal tubule, and the collecting duct.

TABLE 31–1 Normal Glomerular Filtration Rates in Children and Adolescents

AGE AND GENDER	MEAN GFR ± SD (mL/min/1.73 m²)
1 week (males and females)	41 ± 15
2 to 8 weeks (males and females)	66 ± 25
> 8 weeks (males and females)	96 ± 22
2 to 12 years (males and females)	133 ± 27
13 to 21 years (males)	140 ± 30
13 to 21 years (females)	126 ± 22

**sd denotes standard deviation*

Data from National Kidney Foundation: The Kidney Disease Outcomes Quality Initiative. (2002). Clinical practice guidelines for chronic kidney disease: Evaluation, classification, and stratification. American Journal of Kidney Disease, *39(1), S1–S266.*

kidneys are present at birth. Filtration occurs at the glomerulus, Bowman's capsule, and the basement membrane. The basement membrane prevents passage of cells and large proteins. The proximal tubule reabsorbs approximately two-thirds of the filtered water and electrolytes, and reabsorbs all of the amino acids, glucose, proteins, and vitamins.

Glomerular filtration rate refers to the filtration of plasma and is mainly influenced by hydrostatic pressure in the glomerular capillaries. The hydrostatic pressure pushes blood against the walls as it circulates through the capillaries, forcing fluid to be filtered out. Proteins present in the blood promote the glomerular capillary osmotic pressure. The glomerular filtration rate is at approximately 30% to 50% of adult levels by age 1 year due to higher vascular resistance in infants (Huether, 2002a). See Table 31–1.

The loop of Henle contains sodium, potassium, and chloride co-transporters, which pump ions into the interstitium creating a high interstitial osmolarity in the renal medulla. Approximately 20% to 25% of the cardiac output is delivered to the kidneys by the renal arteries (Huether, 2002b).

Acid–base regulation is maintained through the kidneys by secretion of excess hydrogen (H^+) and by reabsorption and production of bicarbonate HCO_3^- See Chapter 23.

MediaLink Genitourinary A & P Review

Each kidney holds approximately 1 million nephrons. The kidneys grow and the tubular system matures gradually during childhood, reaching full size by adolescence. Most renal growth occurs during the first 5 years of life. This increase in size is due primarily to enlargement of the nephrons. The efficiency of the kidney also increases with age. During the first 2 years of life, the kidneys are less efficient at regulating electrolyte and acid–base balance (refer to Chapter 23) and eliminating some drugs from the body. After the age of 2 years, the kidneys' efficiency increases markedly. Because the kidney is less able to concentrate urine in infancy, urine output per kilogram of body weight is higher in infancy than in later childhood or adolescence (Box 31–1).

For the kidneys to function effectively, the following conditions need to be present.

- Unimpaired renal blood flow
- Adequate glomerular ultrafiltration
- Normal tubular function
- Unobstructed urine flow

Bladder capacity increases with age from 20 to 50 mL at birth to 700 mL in adulthood. Stimulation of "stretch receptors" within the bladder wall initiates urination. Simultaneous contraction of the detrusor muscle of the bladder and relaxation of the internal and external sphincters result in emptying of the bladder. Children less than 2 years of age cannot maintain bladder control due to insufficient nerve development. An important developmental consideration is that the child's kidneys are more susceptible to trauma due to the decreased amount of fat padding that offers protection in the adult.

BOX 31–1 Expected Urine Output According to Age

Urinary output per kilogram of body weight decreases as the child ages because the kidney becomes more efficient at concentrating urine. Expected output is:

- Infants 2 mL/kg/hr
- Children 0.5–1 mL/kg/hr
- Adolescents 40–80 mL/hr

CLINICAL TIP

A child's bladder capacity (in ounces) can be estimated by adding 2 to the child's age. For example, the normal bladder capacity of a 4-year-old child is 6 ounces.

See page 1222 for anatomic and physiologic differences of the reproductive system.

STRUCTURAL DEFECTS OF THE URINARY SYSTEM

Structural defects of the urinary system can result in obstructed or reduced urine flow, and may possibly affect reproductive function. Structural defects discussed in this section include bladder exstrophy, hypospadias, epispadias, obstructive uropathy, vesicoureteral reflux, and prune-belly syndrome. (See Chapter 29∞ for a discussion of Wilms' tumor.)

Bladder Exstrophy

Bladder exstrophy is a rare congenital defect in which the bladder wall extrudes through the lower abdominal wall (Figure 31–3 ■). The defect occurs in approximately 1 in 40,000 newborns and affects males more often than females (Sponseller, Jani, Jeffs, et al., 2001). In more extensive cases, epispadias is also present.

Etiology and Pathophysiology

Failure of the abdominal wall to close (fuse) during fetal development results in eversion and protuberance of the bladder wall, along with a wide separation of the rectus muscles and the symphysis pubis. The symphysis pubis is widened resulting in an external rotation of the pelvic bones. The upper urinary tract as well as the testes and ovaries are usually not involved in the disorder. Exposure of the bladder to air and trauma during delivery lead to inflammation, and renal damage can occur secondary to infection or obstruction.

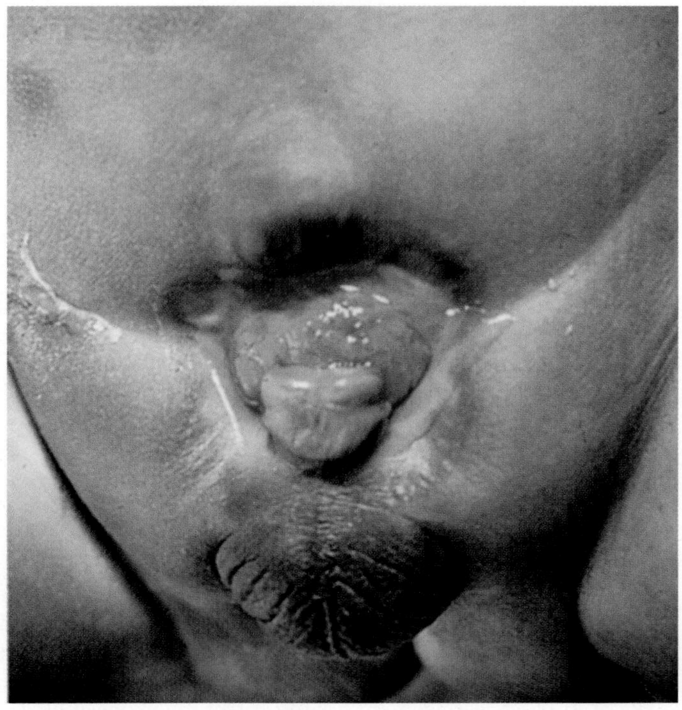

FIGURE 31–3 ■ This child has exstrophy of the bladder. Note the extrusion of the posterior bladder wall through the lower abdominal wall and deformity of the penis.

Clinical Manifestations

At the time of birth, the bladder mucosa appears as a mass of bright red tissue exposed through an abdominal opening, and urine continually leaks from an open urethra. The defect occurs in varying degrees of severity. Females may present with a bifid clitoris (divided into two parts), separated labia, or absent vagina. Males may demonstrate a short, stubby penis; and the glans may be flattened with dorsal chordee and a ventral prepuce. Epispadias and bilateral inguinal hernias (both defects are discussed later in the chapter) are also commonly associated with bladder exstrophy.

COLLABORATIVE CARE

The goal of collaborative care is to protect the exposed bladder from injury and prevent infection, as well as preserve renal and reproductive function.

Diagnostic Tests

Bladder exstrophy can be diagnosed by prenatal ultrasonography, and it is apparent at birth upon visual examination. Diagnostic studies that may be performed include urinalysis, urine culture, and radiological examinations, such as renal ultrasound, of the genitourinary tract. As the condition is treated, other diagnostic procedures will be used to evaluate the urinary system function. See Tables 31–2 and 31–3.

Clinical Therapy

Treatment is surgical reconstruction which has the following goals: (1) bladder and abdominal wall closure; (2) urinary continence, with preservation of renal function; (3) creation of functional and normal-appearing genitalia; and (4) improvement of sexual functioning. Surgical reconstruction is performed in several stages. Primary closure of the bladder and abdominal wall, the first stage, is usually completed within 24 to 48 hours after birth. Epispadias repair is often performed at the age of 1 or 2 years, before or at the same time as a continence surgical procedure. Surgery to reconstruct the bladder neck and reimplant the ureters is performed after the bladder has achieved adequate capacity. An osteotomy that rotates the innominate bones of the pelvis to approximate the symphysis pubis is usually performed to reduce tension on the closed bladder and lower abdominal wall, and to promote continence by restoring the sling of the pelvic floor muscles (Sponseller et al., 2001). Some children need urinary diversion to gain continence because a functional bladder cannot be reconstructed (Surer, Ferrer, Baker, et al., 2003). Cosmetic reconstruction may be required in later childhood.

Postoperatively (primary closure) the wound and pelvis are immobilized to facilitate healing. Internal (with sutures) and external immobilization techniques, such as Bryant's traction or

TABLE 31–2 Diagnostic Tests for Urinary System Conditions

DIAGNOSTIC TEST	INDICATION	NURSING INTERVENTIONS
Urinalysis	Detects the specific gravity and presence of glucose, ketones, protein, blood cells, casts, crystals, and microorganisms	Use a urine collection bag for infants and children who are not toilet trained. Give older children fluids if unable to void.
Urine culture	Indicates the presence of an infection in the urinary system	Explain the process for cleaning the peritoneum and collecting the urine in a sterile cup midstream. Clean the peritoneum and collect a catheter specimen midstream in a sterile container. Suprapubic tap may be performed in infants.
Voiding cystourethrogram or radionuclide cystography	Shows bladder structure and function, urethral anatomy, bladder masses; detects vesicoureteral reflux	Explain catheterization to child and that the bladder will be filled. Provide coaching strategies for parents accompanying the child to help the child cope. Assess for allergies as contrast media is used.
Renal and/or bladder ultrasound	Identifies large renal scars, renal anomalies, obstruction, abscesses, masses, and hydronephrosis	Noninvasive procedure. Fluids are administered as prescribed.
Intravenous pyelogram (intravenous urography)	Visualize kidney's collecting system, distal ureters, and bladder	Assess for allergies as contrast medium is used. Infants and children are NPO prior to the study. An IV is started for injection of contrast.
Diuretic renography	Helps distinguish between obstructive and nonobstructive hydronephrosis	Hydrate the child before the exam. An IV is started and diuretic is infused. The child is catheterized to drain urine during the procedure.
Radionuclide renal scan with DMSA	Detects renal parenchymal lesions, renal atrophy, scars, or pyelonephritis. Differentiates between hydronephrosis caused by obstructive lesions, reflux, or a cyst	Explain catheterization to child.
Renal biopsy	To determine presence and/or extent of renal involvement in specific disorders	NPO 6 hours (or as prescribed) before biopsy. Prep site and administer preprocedural sedation as prescribed. May require bowel evacuation before test.
Cystoscopy	To visualize interior urethra and bladder	Infants and children are NPO prior to the study. Sedation is administered. Children with cardiac anomalies need antibiotic prophylaxis. Fluids are forced after the procedure to detect problems with voiding.
CT (computed tomography)	Provides detailed visualization of structures of the urinary tract and major renal blood vessels	Infant or child may be NPO and require bowel evacuation prior to study. Prepare child for size of equipment. Assess for allergies if contrast medium is used. Sedation may be needed.
MRI (magnetic resonance imaging)	Provides detailed visualization of urinary structures	Prepare child for sounds, size of equipment, and tunnel. Ensure that the child has no metallic implants. Sedation may be neded.

Data from Kraus, S. J. (2001). Genitourinary imaging in children. Pediatric Clinics of North America, *48(6), 1381–1423; Hanson, K. A. (2003). Diagnostic tests and tools in the evaluation of urologic disease: Part II.* Urologic Nursing, *23(6), 405–415.*

spica cast (refer to Chapter 35∞), are used to promote pelvic closure. A suprapubic catheter is inserted during the surgical procedure, creating a urinary diversion to promote healing. Bilateral ureteral stents are utilized to promote effective drainage for approximately 1 week following the surgery, though they may be left in place for longer periods. Medication is provided to reduce urinary spasms that may stress the suture line.

CLINICAL TIP

A **ureteral stent** is a device used to maintain patency of the ureter allowing urine flow from the kidney to bladder. A **urethral stent** is a device used to maintain patency of the urethral canal and allow urine flow from the bladder through the urethra.

Postoperative complications include wound dehiscence and bladder prolapse (Sponseller, et. al., 2001) and bladder stone formation (Surer et al., 2003). Even with an anterior osteotomy and bladder neck reconstruction, not all children are able to achieve continence. However, creation of a urinary reservoir with a stoma that can be catheterized does result in a high rate of continence for children whose bladder has not grown sufficiently or when bladder neck repair failed (Surer et al., 2003).

Since the bladder epithelium is abnormal, it is prone to neoplasms. Periodic examination and cystoscopy after the age of 20 years are recommended to evaluate for possible malignancies.

NURSING MANAGEMENT

Goals of nursing management are to protect the exposed bladder until surgery is performed, prevent complications such as infection, and to provide the family with support.

TABLE 31–3 Normal Freshly Voided Urinalysis Results

MACROSCOPIC EXAMINATION	NORMAL RESULTS
Color	Pale yellow, clear
Odor	Ammonia-like smell
Specific gravity	≤1.010 in well hydrated child
pH	4.5–8
Protein	Negative; <150 mg/24 hr
Glucose	<130 mg/24 hr
Ketones	Negative
Bilirubin	Negative
MICROSCOPIC EXAMINATION	
Red blood cells	0–5 per high-powered field (HPF)
White blood cells	<2 per HPF
Casts (hyaline)	1 per every 10–20 low-powered fields (LPF)
Crystals	None

Data from Liao, J. C., & Churchill, B. M. (2001). Pediatric urine testing. Pediatric Clinics of North America, *48(6), 1425–1440.*

Nursing Assessment and Diagnosis

Nursing assessment includes immediate newborn assessment (see Chapter 8∞) and preoperative and postoperative assessments.

Newborn/Preoperative Assessment

Assess the newborn's renal function and hydration status by monitoring the adequacy of urine output and serum and urine chemistries. Measure the newborn's weight daily. Assess family support systems and coping mechanisms when the newborn is diagnosed with the defect.

Postoperative Assessment

Routinely empty and record urine output from each tube every 2 to 4 hours and note any change in urine output that could indicate an obstruction of the tube. Other signs of obstruction may include urine or blood draining from the urethral meatus or increased intensity of bladder spasms. Monitor for signs of pain (see Chapter 18∞). Monitor urine for blood or clots which are common in the first few days following surgery. Assess for wound dehiscence and bladder prolapse. Assess peripheral circulation of the lower limbs if a spica cast has been applied.

Family Assessment

Assess the parents for their response to the newborn's defect and the need for immediate surgery. Begin to identify family resources for support and care of an infant requiring long-term care and multiple surgeries.

Nursing diagnoses for the newborn with bladder exstrophy may include:

- Risk for Infection related to exposed bladder and surgical incision
- Impaired Skin Integrity related to exposed bladder and surgical incision
- Acute Pain related to surgical incision
- Risk for Impaired Parent/Infant Attachment related to newborn with genitourinary structural defect and immediacy of surgery

Planning and Implementation

Preoperative Care

Protect the bladder mucosa with a sterile saline-soaked dressing covered in sterile plastic wrap to prevent trauma and irritation. Do not allow the sterile dressing to become dry. The dry dressing will adhere to the exposed bladder, potentially causing damage to the tissue when removed. Clean the surrounding area according to guidelines and protect the skin from leaking urine with a skin sealant.

CLINICAL TIP

At the time of the newborn's delivery, the umbilical cord should be tied, rather than clamped, since a clamp could cause trauma to the bladder mucosa (Mollohan, 1999).

Postoperative Care

Maintain aseptic technique for wound care and monitor for signs of infection including redness, drainage, and edema. Additional nursing care includes maintaining proper body alignment. If the infant is not in a spica cast, avoid abduction of the infant's legs since this causes stress on the surgical area. Monitor for pain and promote comfort by administering pain medications and antispasmodic agents as needed. Administer antibiotics as prescribed.

Offer parents emotional support to assist them in coping with the infant's defect and the uncertainty of complete repair and achievement of urinary continence. To promote parent–infant bonding, encourage parents to partner with healthcare professionals in all aspects of the infant's care, including bathing, feeding, and wound care. Discharge teaching includes instructions regarding dressing changes and diapering and the need to immediately report any signs of infection or change in renal function. Help parents recognize complications and the need to seek immediate attention for the newborn. (See Partnering with Families: Recognizing Signs of Infection Following Repair.) Emphasize the importance of routine follow-up visits after surgery to assess urinary function and to ensure that the next stages of surgery for continence control are performed at the appropriate time and age in the child's development.

Care in the Community

Long-term care of the child with bladder exstrophy focuses on establishing continence and addressing social and sexual issues. The family should be aware that achievement of continence is more difficult in children with bladder exstrophy, and urinary diversion to achieve continence may be necessary if surgical procedures are not successful. However, parents should be encouraged to initiate

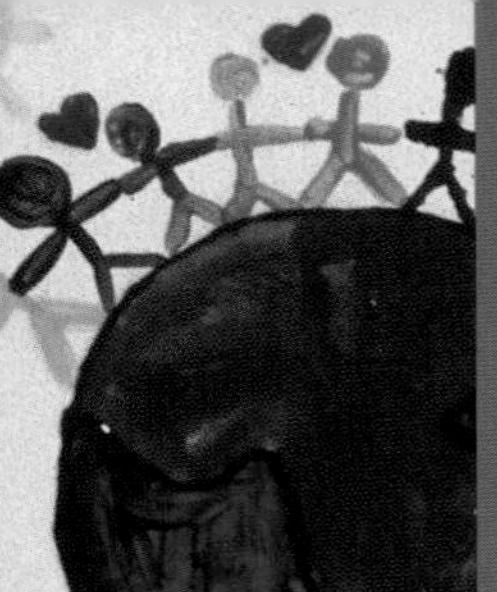

PARTNERING WITH FAMILIES

Recognizing Signs of Infection Following Surgery

Infants and children are often discharged the day of or the day following repair of genitourinary structural defects. Partner with parents to ensure they understand signs and symptoms of infection and to report any complications to the primary healthcare provider. Signs and symptoms of infection include:

- Cloudy urine
- Increased temperature
- Purulent drainage
- Foul odor from the incision
- Increased fussiness
- Decreased feeding

toilet training at the appropriate age for bowel movements. Until urinary continence is achieved, the nurse partners with the family to assist them in coping with the child's incontinence and identifying strategies to maintain skin integrity and promote the child's growth and development. Parents may require guidance to promote the child's self-esteem and self-confidence with sexual identity and function. Psychological counseling may be beneficial to the child during adolescence.

■ Evaluation

Expected outcomes of nursing care in the immediate postoperative period include the following:

- The child is free from infection.
- Skin integrity remains intact.
- The child's pain is effectively managed.
- Parent–newborn attachment occurs.

Hypospadias and Epispadias

Hypospadias and **epispadias** are congenital anomalies involving an abnormal location of the urethral meatus in males (Figure 31–4 ■). The reported incidence of hypospadias is 1 in 125 male births (Paulozzi, Erickson, & Jackson, 1997). Female epispadias occurs rarely, in approximately 1 in 150,000 to 300,000 live female births (Grady & Mitchell, 2002).

Etiology and Pathophysiology

Both defects result from failure of the urethral folds to fuse completely over the urethral groove. A familial tendency is recognized, in that about 9% of fathers and 14% of brothers of a boy with hypospadias also have the condition, but the specific genetic aspect to transmission is unknown (Stokowski, 2004). Hypospadias often occurs in conjunction with congenital inguinal hernias, undescended testes, and **chordee**—a fibrous line of tissue that results in ventral curvature of the penile shaft and can interfere with sexual function. Epispadias is most often seen with bladder exstrophy, but it may be an isolated defect in about 10% of cases (Caione & Capozza, 2001). Hypospadias and epispadias are classified according to the meatal location.

Clinical Manifestations

In hypospadias, the urethral meatus may be located anywhere along the course of the ventral surface of the penile shaft, from the perineum to the tip of the glans. A dimple or pit may be seen on the glans at the expected location of the meatus. Most cases of hypospadius are mild, with the meatus slightly off center from the tip of the penis; however, in severe cases, the meatus is located on the scrotum. Mild cases do not interfere with urinary function and they require no intervention. Severe cases, such as those located on the scrotum, require surgical correction. Chordee or curvature of the penis and an incomplete or hooded foreskin may also be present.

In epispadias, the meatal opening is located on the dorsal surface of the penile shaft, and may be at the level of the bladder neck. In severe cases there may be an absence of the dorsal aspect of the urethra and overlying skin.

COLLABORATIVE CARE

Collaborative care focuses on identification and correction of the defect, prevention of infection, and promotion of urinary elimination and sexual function.

Diagnostic Tests

Diagnosis is made prenatally by ultrasound or by physical examination at birth. Other diagnostic studies may include urinalysis and urine culture. Refer to the Skills Manual for guidelines related to collection of urine specimens. When the meatus is located on the perineum or scrotum, testing to rule out a chromosomal abnormality or problem in androgen metabolism will be conducted.

Clinical Therapy

Surgical correction of the structural defect is the treatment for hypospadias and epispadias. The defects are corrected, usually during the first year of life, to minimize psychologic effects when the child is older. The infant *should not be circumcised* because the foreskin tissue may be used for surgical repair. Surgery is generally performed in a single operation and often as an outpatient procedure. For more severe cases, however, surgical repair may require two stages. Goals of surgical repair are (1) placement of the urethral meatus at the end of the glans penis with satisfactory caliber and configuration for a urinary stream (enabling the child to void in a standing position); (2) release of chordee to straighten the penis (enabling future sexual function); and (3) satisfactory cosmetic appearance of the penis.

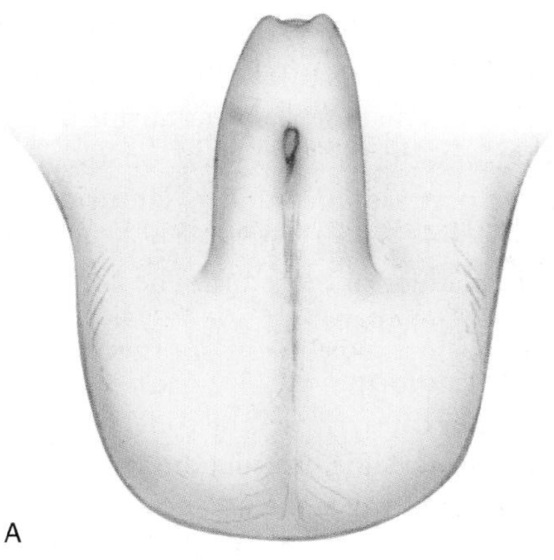

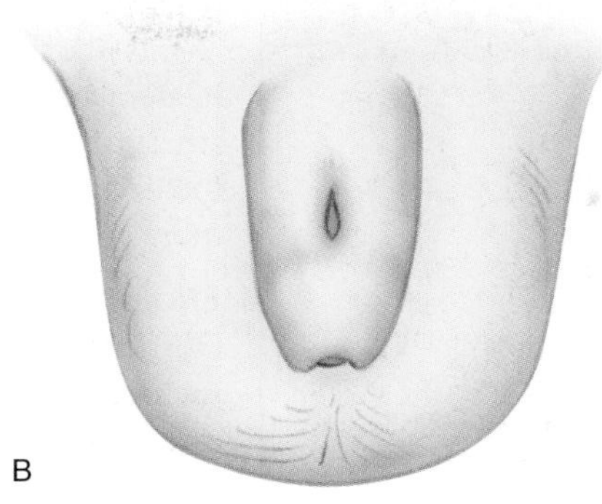

FIGURE 31–4 ■ Hypospadias and epispadias. *A,* In hypospadias, the urethral canal is open on the ventral surface of the penis. *B,* In epispadias the urethral canal is open on the dorsal surface.

A caudal nerve block is often used for initial postoperative pain relief. Anticholinergic medications such as oxybutynin or hyoscyamine may be prescribed to relieve bladder spasms. A urethral stent is placed to maintain patency of the new urethral canal opening.

A suprapubic or urethral urinary drainage catheter may be inserted to allow for urine flow without applying tension to the urethral sutures. The stent or catheter may either drain directly into the diaper or into a closed drainage collection bag.

NURSING MANAGEMENT

Goals of nursing management are to assist in collaborative identification of the defect, prevent potential complications such as infection and urethral obstruction, promote parental understanding and attachment to newborn, and promote normal voiding pattern.

■ Nursing Assessment and Diagnosis

Perform a thorough newborn assessment to detect the presence of genitourinary defects (see Chapter 8∞). Assess the newborn's flow of urine, exit site, and angle of urination. Assess family support systems and coping mechanisms when the newborn is diagnosed with this defect.

Assess the older child's level of understanding of the procedures and need for surgery. Postoperative assessment includes monitoring for penile swelling, dysuria, bleeding at the surgical site, infection, and evidence of pain.

Nursing diagnoses for the child with hypospadias and epispadias may include:

- Risk for Infection related to altered urinary elimination
- Risk for Injury related to dislodged stent or catheter
- Acute Pain related to surgical procedure
- Anxiety (parents) related to genitourinary defect in newborn infant and surgical procedures

■ Planning and Implementation

The nurse partners with the parents to address their concerns at the time of birth. Preoperative teaching may relieve some parental anxiety concerning the future appearance and functioning of the penis. For the older child undergoing surgical correction, the use of dolls and pictures to explain the procedure may help the child develop a better understanding. Address fear of mutilation in a manner appropriate to the developmental level of the child.

Postoperative care focuses on protecting the surgical site from injury. The infant or child returns from surgery with the penis wrapped in a simple dressing and a stent or catheter for urinary drainage. Partner with the family and plan care to ensure that the stent or catheter is not removed (Figure 31–5 ■).

Encourage fluid intake to maintain adequate urinary output appropriate for age and to maintain patency of the stent. Accurate and hourly documentation of intake and output is essential to detect postoperative urinary complications. Notify the primary healthcare provider if there is no urine drainage for 1 hour, as this may indicate kinks in the system or obstruction by sediment.

Pain may be associated with bladder spasms. Administer anticholinergic medications as prescribed. Once the caudal block wears off, administer acetaminophen or other mild analgesics for pain as ordered. Antibiotics are usually prescribed until the urinary stent falls out or is removed.

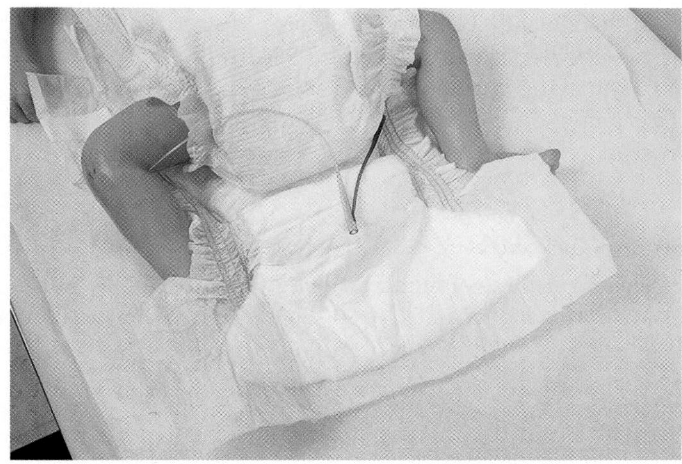

FIGURE 31–5 ■ A double diapering technique protects the urinary stent after surgery for hypospadias or epispadias repair. The inner diaper collects stool and the outer diaper collects urine.

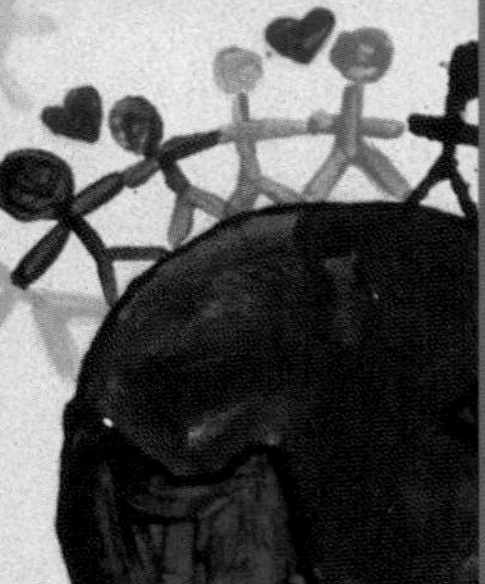

PARTNERING WITH FAMILIES

Care for the Child After Hypospadias and Epispadias Repair

Guidelines for the care of children at home following hypospadias or epispadias repair include the following:

- Use the double-diapering technique shown in Figure 31–5 to protect the stent (the small tube that drains the urine).
- Do not bathe the child in the tub until the stent or catheter is removed.
- Restrict the infant or toddler from activities (e.g., playing on riding toys) that put pressure on the surgical site. Avoid holding the infant or child straddled on the hip. Limit the child's activity for 2 weeks.
- Encourage the infant or toddler to drink fluids to ensure adequate hydration. Provide fluids in a pleasant environment or use a special cup. Offer fruit juice, fruit-flavored ice pops, fruit-flavored juices, flavored ice cubes, and gelatin.
- Administer the *complete course* of prescribed antibiotics to avoid infection.
- Observe for signs of infection: fever, swelling, redness, pain, strong-smelling urine, or change in flow of the urinary stream.
- The urine will be blood tinged for several days. Call the physician if urine is seen leaking from any area other than the penis.

The child is often discharged the day of surgery. Partner with the family to provide instructions regarding care of the reconstructed area, including catheter or stent care, incision care, penis care, emptying of the drainage bag, and securing the catheter. (See Partnering with Families: Care for the Child after Hypospadias or Epispadias Repair.) Inform parents that the urine will normally be blood tinged for several days following the surgery. Promote adequate fluid intake according to the child's age, and teach the family about medication administration—which may include antibiotics, pain medications, and antispasmodics. Emphasize to the parents the importance of follow-up visits as instructed by the surgeon for dressing and catheter or stent removal.

■ Evaluation

Expected outcomes of nursing care for the child with hypospadias or epispadias include:

- Postoperative infection does not occur.
- The catheter or stent remains intact until healing occurs.
- The child's pain is effectively managed.
- Parents manage their anxiety and support the infant or child having surgery.

Obstructive Uropathy

Obstructive uropathy refers to structural or functional abnormalities of the urinary system that interfere with urine flow and results in urine backflow into the kidneys. The uropathy may be bilateral or unilateral and partial or incomplete. The urinary obstruction may occur anywhere along the urinary tract, including the ureters, renal pelvis, bladder, and urethra. The condition is more common in males than females.

Etiology and Pathophysiology

Obstructive uropathy may be caused by several congenital lesions such as ureteropelvic junction (UPJ) obstruction, posterior urethral valves (PUVs), and narrowing at the ureterovesicular junction or ureteral hypoplasia (Figure 31–6 ■). Obstruction in the ureteropelvic junction may be caused by folds in the upper ureter or fibrotic stenosis. Posterior urethral valve, in which a congenital membrane completely or partially obstructs the posterior urethra, is the most common cause of bladder outlet obstruction and severe obstructive uropathy (Cooper, Andrews, Hansen et al., 2002). The incidence is 1 in 5,000 to 8,000 male births (Vogt, 2002). Obstruction at the ureterovesicular junction may be related to a ureterocele (cystic dilation at the distal end of the ureter), a ureter that inserts into an abnormal location within the urinary tract, or poor development of the distal ureteral muscle (Vogt, 2002).

Other congenital causes of obstructive uropathy include anterior urethral valves, urethral atresia, severe meatal stenosis, hypoplasia, agenesis, ectopic ureter, and ectopic ureterocele. Acquired causes of obstructive uropathy in children include crystal formation caused by certain drugs such as acyclovir, sulfa, anticholinergics, and methotrexate. Compression on the urinary tract at any point may also cause obstructive neuropathy such as nephrolithiasis (kidney stones), neuroblastoma, reproductive tract abnormalities, and gastrointestinal abnormalities (Roth, Koo, Spottswood, et al., 2002).

The pressure caused by urine backup often causes **hydronephrosis,** an accumulation of urine in the renal pelvis as a result of obstructed outflow, and compromises kidney function. Pathophysiologic changes that may occur as a result of hydronephrosis include the following:

- When pressure in the kidney pelvis equals the filtration pressure in the glomerular capillaries, glomerular filtration stops. In response, blood pressure increases as the body attempts to increase the glomerular filtration pressure. However, the increasing pressure on the glomeruli leads to cell death.
- Metabolic acidosis results when the distal nephrons are impaired in their ability to secrete hydrogen ions.
- Impairment of the kidney's ability to concentrate urine results in polydypsia and polyuria.
- Obstruction results in urinary stasis, promoting the growth of bacteria.
- Chronic renal failure results when the hydronephrosis damages the renal parenchyma causing **obstructive nephropathy** (Palmieri, 2002).

PATHOPHYSIOLOGY ILLUSTRATED

Obstruction Sites in the Urinary System

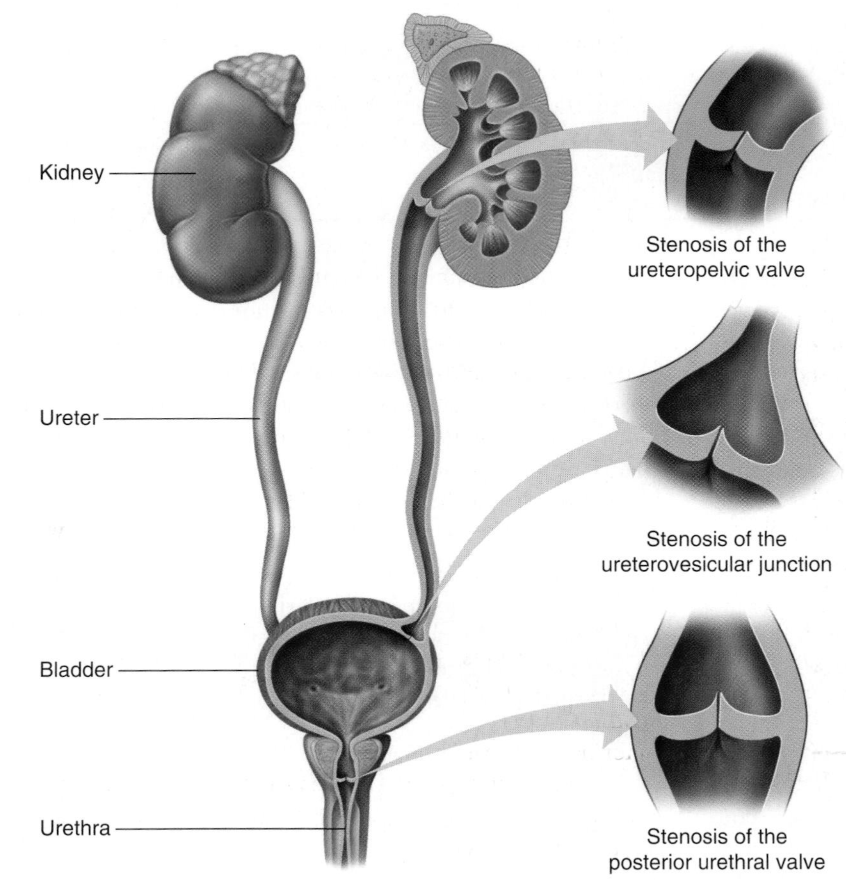

FIGURE 31–6 ■ Obstruction may occur in either the upper or lower urinary tract. Common sites of obstruction occur at the ureteropelvic valve, the ureterovesicular junction, or the posterior urethral valve. Why would damage from posterior urethral valves potentially be worse than other obstructions? Renal failure is most likely to occur when both kidneys are affected by hydronephrosis.

Approximately 30% of males with PUV diagnosed in infancy develop end-stage renal disease in childhood or adolescence (Vogt, 2002).

Clinical Manifestations

Clinical manifestations of obstructive uropathy may include an abdominal mass, palpable bladder, and alternating episodes of increased and decreased urinary output. Some clinical manifestations in infants and children are dependent on the location and severity of the obstructive lesion. See the clinical manifestations table on page 1184.

COLLABORATIVE CARE

Management of obstructive uropathy focuses on relieving the cause of obstruction to prevent or delay the development of renal failure.

Diagnostic Tests

Hydronephrosis may be detected by prenatal ultrasound; however, milder obstructions may not become apparent until later in infancy or childhood. An abnormal urinalysis may be present. A diuretic-enhanced radionuclide scan and a voiding cystourethrogram (VCUG) is performed when a ureteropelvic or ureterovesicular obstruction is suspected. Diagnosis of PUV is made on prenatal ultrasound or postnatal assessment, including distended bladder and signs and symptoms of renal insufficiency. A VCUG reveals a dilated posterior urethra, which is diagnostic for PUV. Serial serum creatinine and electrolyte levels are obtained to monitor renal function. Arterial blood gases may reveal metabolic acidosis due to improper renal function. See Table 31–2 on page 1178 for other diagnostic tests that may be performed.

Clinical Therapy

For acute obstructions, immediate intervention is required. Short-term management may include urethral or suprapubic

CLINICAL MANIFESTATIONS of Obstructive Lesions of the Urinary System

OBSTRUCTIVE LESION	ETIOLOGY	CLINICAL MANIFESTATIONS
Ureteropelvic junction obstruction	Folds of the upper ureter causing urinary stasis Fibrotic stenosis of the ureteropelvic junction	Infants: Abdominal mass (enlarged kidney), hypertension, urinary tract infection Children: Hematuria, pain, intermittent nausea and vomiting
Posterior urethral valves	Congenital membrane that partially or completely obstructs the posterior urethra	Infants: Abdominal mass (enlarged kidney), distended bladder, poor urinary stream, urinary tract infection, sepsis, low specific gravity, polyuria, increased creatinine level, failure to thrive Children: Urinary frequency and incontinence
Ureterovesicular junction obstruction	Maldevelopment of the distal ureteral muscle Ureterocele Ectopic ureter	Urinary tract infection (recurrent or chronic), hematuria, pain, abdominal mass (enlarged kidney), enuresis

catheterization for an obstructed PUV until surgical intervention is achieved (Woolf & Thiruchelvam, 2001). However, even with rapid intervention, as in the case of a newborn with hydronephrosis identified by prenatal ultrasound, damage to the kidneys is usually irreversible (Roth et al., 2002).

Goals of surgical correction or diversion are to lower the pressure within the collecting system, which prevents further renal parenchymal damage, and to prevent stasis, which decreases the risk of infection. Depending on the cause of the obstruction, surgical correction may necessitate pyeloplasty (removal of an obstructed segment of the ureter and reimplantation into the renal pelvis), valve repair, or reconstruction. Surgical interventions for PUVs include cutaneous vesicostomy, or valve ablation. Urinary incontinence resulting from sphincter incompetence, bladder dysfunction, and polyuria related to **renal insufficiency** (a decline in renal function that is about 25% of normal) is a common problem after surgery, and it can cause hydronephrosis due to urinary retention (Gatti & Kirsch, 2001; Yohannes & Hanna, 2002). Strategies to manage urinary incontinence in some cases include clean intermittent catheterization. In rare cases a urinary diversion with an ostomy may be necessary. This diversion may be either temporary or permanent. Antibiotic prophylaxis may be prescribed to reduce the risk for urinary tract infection.

For mild obstructions in the absence of significant complications such as urinary retention or urinary tract infections, correction is not emergent. Antibiotic prophylaxis to prevent urinary tract infections may be prescribed until vesicoureteral reflux is ruled out (see page 1185).

NURSING MANAGEMENT

The goal of nursing care is to collaborate in the identification of children with obstructive uropathy as well as in the prevention of further renal complications.

■ Nursing Assessment and Diagnosis

A thorough history and physical examination is performed on the child exhibiting any of the symptoms that are suggestive of this disorder. Palpate the abdomen for a mass or distended bladder. Monitor the urine output and observe the force of the urine stream. If hydronephrosis progresses and urine output diminishes, further manifestations may include peripheral edema and costovertebral angle tenderness.

Parents may be distressed, especially if hydronephrosis was detected on prenatal ultrasound. Assess the parents' coping and ability to hear and understand information presented about the infant's condition.

Nursing diagnoses for the child with obstructive uropathy may include:

- Impaired Urinary Elimination related to obstructed outflow
- Risk for Infection related to urinary retention
- Parental Anxiety related to infant's potential for progressive renal failure
- Acute Pain related to surgical procedure

■ Planning and Implementation

Preoperative nursing care focuses on preparing the parents and child for the procedure and addressing parental concerns about the postsurgical outcome. Provide parents with an opportunity to discuss concerns about the effect of the disorder on the child's long-term renal functioning.

Postoperative care involves monitoring vital signs, as well as intake and output and observing for signs of urine retention, such as decreased output and bladder distention. Administer medications as prescribed, including antibiotics and antispasmodics such as oxybutynin. An epidural catheter may have been placed for pain management. Once this is removed, provide prescribed pain medication.

Many children are discharged with stents or catheters (refer to previous section for discussion of care of the child with a stent or catheter). If a urinary diversion with an ostomy is present, ensure that the parents understand care of the stoma and proper diaper placement to collect the urine outflow. Partner with parents and provide instructions on dressing changes, care for catheters, assessing pain and administering analgesics, and recognizing signs of possible obstruction or infection.

Emphasize the importance of long-term monitoring of the child's renal function. Educate parents about the signs of urinary tract infection and impaired renal functioning. Provide guidelines for seeking healthcare promptly if signs are noted.

Encourage parents to promote growth and development with age-appropriate activities.

■ Evaluation

Expected outcomes for the child with obstructive uropathy include:

- The child remains free from infection.
- The child's postsurgical pain is effectively managed.
- Parents demonstrate understanding of home care instructions.

Congenital Hydronephrosis

Antenatal hydronephrosis is detected by prenatal ultrasound, demonstrating a dilated renal pelvis and calyces, in up to 1% of pregnancies. Up to 50% of newborns have persistence of hydronephrosis (Cooper et al., 2002). Anomalous ureteropelvic junction obstruction is the most common cause of significant congenital hydronephrosis (Vogt, 2002). Nonobstructive causes of hydronephrosis include vesicoureteral reflux, prune-belly syndrome, or physiologic dilation in the upper urinary system (Cooper et al., 2002).

Nursing care is the same as described for obstructive uropathy.

Vesicoureteral Reflux

Vesicoureteral reflux (VUR) results in backflow of urine from the bladder into the kidneys. This defect prevents complete emptying of the bladder and creates a reservoir for bacterial growth. The defect results from incomplete development of the ureterovesical junction (Vogt, 2002). Vesicoureteral reflux can also result from a structural anomaly in which the ureters insert in an abnormal position into the bladder. Vesicoureteral reflux is observed in 1% of all children, but in 50% of those affected with posterior urethral valves (Vogt, 2002). The disorder is also found in approximately 70% of infants treated for symptomatic urinary tract infections (Ellsworth, Cendron, & McCullough, 2000).

VUR has a genetic component, with increased incidence at 35% among siblings and other first degree relatives. A renal ultrasound and voiding cystourethrogram reveal the defect and permit grading the severity of reflux (to the ureter, renal pelvis, or causing some dilation of the ureter and renal pelvis). Sterile reflux does not seem to cause significant renal damage; however, reflux of infected urine may cause pyelonephritis and renal scarring (Ellsworth et al., 2000). Long-term complications include renal scarring, hypertension, and chronic renal failure (Vogt, 2002). The goal of treatment is to prevent pyelonephritis and renal scarring. Prophylactic antibiotics may be prescribed to prevent urinary tract infection. Surgical intervention, ureteral reimplantation, may be required depending on the grade of reflux. If a urinary tract infection is present 1 week before surgery, it must be treated to reduce the risk for postoperative complications.

Nursing Management

Following surgery to reimplant the ureters, a Foley catheter will be in place, and the urine will be bloody initially and clear within 2 to 3 days. Intravenous fluids will be administered at a higher rate than usual (1.5 times maintenance) to maintain a high urinary output to minimize clot formation and overcome the obstruction potentially caused by bladder swelling (Ellsworth et al., 2000). Monitoring urine output is important as clots may cause an obstruction. When urine output is diminished, notify the physician and follow orders for irrigating the Foley catheter.

Administer medications as prescribed, including antibiotics and antispasmodics such as oxybutynin. An epidural catheter may have been placed for pain management. Once this is removed, provide prescribed pain medication.

When the child has the Foley catheter removed and can void spontaneously, the child can be discharged. Educate the family about the administration of medications to include prophylactic antibiotics and antispasmodics if needed. Inform parents of the need for increased fiber in the diet to address the constipating effects of the antispasmodic medication. Guidelines for calling the physician include fever over 38.5°C (101.5°F), abdominal or back pain, or swelling and redness of the incision. The child may take a short shower or tub bath after discharge. The child should avoid active play for 3 weeks following surgery. Provide guidelines for annual follow-up and the potential need to resume prophylactic antibiotics if the child develops recurrent urinary tract infections.

Prune-Belly Syndrome

Prune-belly syndrome, also known as Eagle-Barrett syndrome, is a congenital defect characterized by failure of the abdominal musculature to develop. The skin covering the abdominal wall is thin and resembles a wrinkled prune. Other characteristics include urinary tract anomalies, poor ureteral peristalsis, enlarged bladder, high risk for recurrent urinary tract infection, vesicoureteral reflux, and bilateral cryptorchidism. Prune-belly syndrome occurs predominantly in males (95%), with an incidence of 1 in 35,000 to 50,000 live births (Vogt, 2002).

The etiology of prune-belly syndrome is unknown. However, it is thought to be related to a fetal urinary tract obstruction or a specific injury to the mesoderm before 10 weeks' gestation (Vogt, 2002). Common urinary tract abnormalities in these infants include renal dysplasia, vesicoureteral reflux, and a large capacity, poorly contractile bladder. The abdominal appearance is initially wrinkled, and later protruding. Cardiac, pulmonary, gastrointestinal, and orthopedic anomalies also occur. See Box 31–2.

Diagnosis is confirmed with abdominal ultrasound. An intravenous pyelogram is useful in assessing structural defects. Abdominal wall reconstruction and correction of genitourinary defects, including orchiopexy, are performed to repair defects. The mortality rate in infants has improved significantly in the past three decades with advances in surgical techniques. Mortality in the neonatal period is related to severe pulmonary hypoplasia. Approximately 30% of children with prune-belly syndrome will develop end-stage renal disease in childhood or adolescence because of inadequate renal function (Vogt, 2002).

BOX 31–2 Associated Anomalies of Prune-Belly Syndrome

- Genitourinary—cryptorchidism, renal dysplasia, vesicoureteral reflux
- Respiratory—pulmonary hypoplasia
- Cardiovascular—atrial septal defect, patent ductus arteriosus, tetralogy of Fallot, and ventricular septal defect
- Gastrointestinal—gastroschisis, imperforate anus, and malrotation with volvulus
- Musculoskeletal—club foot, congenital hip dysplasia, pectus excavatum or carinatum

Adapted from Prune Belly Syndrome Network, www.prunebelly.org., accessed 6/3/2004.

Nursing Management

Nursing management for the infant with prune-belly syndrome is the same as for other defects of the genitourinary system, including preoperative and postoperative management. Additional management includes psychosocial support for the child and family related to the numerous congenital anomalies, body image concerns, and long-term consequences of the defect.

DISORDERS AFFECTING URINARY ELIMINATION

Disorders affecting urinary elimination can range from basic complications of urinary tract infection and enuresis to renal disorders such as nephrotic syndrome or kidney failure. Disorders affecting urinary elimination discussed in this section include urinary tract infection and enuresis. The two major endocrine disorders affecting urinary elimination, diabetes insipidus (DI) and syndrome of inappropriate antidiuretic hormone (SIADH), are discussed in detail in Chapter 32∞. Renal disorders are discussed starting on page 1192.

Urinary Tract Infection

An infection of the urinary tract may be of bacterial, viral, or fungal origin, and can occur in the lower or upper urinary tract. Lower urinary tract infections (UTIs) may involve **cystitis,** an infection of the bladder, and **urethritis,** an infection of the urethra. **Pyelonephritis** is an upper UTI which involves the ureters, renal pelvis, and renal parenchyma. UTIs can be acute or chronic, and chronic UTIs can be either recurrent or persistent.

UTIs are one of the most common disorders of the genitourinary tract and a common infection in children. An estimated 3% of females and 1% of males will have a urinary tract infection (UTI) by the age of 11 (National Kidney and Urologic Diseases Information Clearninghouse, 2003). The higher percentage in females is attributed to the shorter female urethra (2 cm [1 in.] in young girls) and its proximity to the anus and vagina, which increases the risk of contamination by fecal bacteria. Urinary tract infections in newborns and infants may indicate an anatomic abnormality of the genitourinary tract.

Etiology and Pathophysiology

The urinary tract is normally sterile. The most common mechanism of infection is an organism entering the genitourinary tract and ascending from the urethra to the bladder and up toward the kidney. Three other mechanisms of infection include hematogenous (through the bloodstream of an infant or child with an immature or compromised immune system), direct extension through a fistula from the intestines or vagina to any location in the urinary tract, or through the lymphatic system (Chon, Lai, & Shortliffe, 2001). Many first UTIs are caused by *Escherichia coli,* a common gram-negative enteric bacterium. Other causative organisms include *Staphylococcus, Klebsiella, Proteus, Pseudomonas aeruginosa, Enterobacter,* and *Enterococcus* (Santen & Altieri, 2001).

Urinary stasis enhances the risk of UTI. Stasis may be caused by abnormal anatomic structures or functional abnormalities (e.g., a neurogenic bladder, which is common in children with myelomeningocele). Children normally void five to six times a day. Some children, however, develop the habit of urinating only once or twice a day, usually because they become preoccupied with play activities. This infrequent voiding results in incomplete emptying of the bladder, urinary stasis, and high urinary tract pressures. Other factors associated with increased risk of UTI include an irritated perineum, constipation, masturbation, sexual abuse, and sexual activity in adolescent females.

Renal scarring can result from hydronephrosis or pyelonephritis due to the inflammatory and ischemic effects of the infection. Renal scars have been associated with hypertension, proteinuria, and renal failure. The risk of renal damage increases in the following instances.

- UTI in infants under 1 year of age
- Delay in diagnosis and effective antibacterial treatment for an upper urinary tract infection
- Anatomic or neurologic obstruction
- Recurrent episodes of upper urinary tract infections

Clinical Manifestations

Symptoms depend not only on the location of the infection, but also on the age of the child. Symptoms in the newborn period tend to be nonspecific—unexplained fever, failure to thrive, poor feeding, vomiting and diarrhea, strong-smelling urine, change in voiding habit, and irritability. Since the thermoregulatory mechanism is unstable at birth, the neonate may not always present with fever (Santen & Altieri, 2001). Not until the toddler years with toilet training do the more "classic" symptoms of lower urinary tract infection appear. Many UTIs are asymptomatic and are discovered incidentally on routine examination. See the table on page 1187 for clinical manifestations of urinary tract infections.

COLLABORATIVE CARE

Collaborative care focuses on identifying the presence of a urinary tract infection, preventing associated complications, and preventing reinfection.

Diagnostic Tests

A urine specimen is collected by midstream clean-catch void, sterile catheterization, or suprapubic aspiration in a sterile con-

CLINICAL MANIFESTATIONS of Urinary Tract Infection

TYPE OF UTI	CLINICAL MANIFESTATIONS	CLINICAL THERAPY
Lower UTI—Cystitis		
Neonates	Poor feeding, vomiting, failure to gain weight, jaundice, abdominal distention, lethargy, fever may be present	Five- to 7-day course of trimethoprim or sulfamethoxazole or antibiotic matching organism sensitivity Encourage fluids
Infants	Fever, diarrhea, vomiting, irritability, lethargy, foul-smelling diapers, poor feeding, failure to gain weight	Analgesic such as acetominophen or pyridium
Preschooler	Fever, hematuria, urgency, dysuria, frequency, cloudy urine, foul-smelling urine, dehydration, abdominal pain, enuresis	Review voiding habits and establish a schedule for voiding if needed to increase voiding frequency
School-age	Dysuria, enuresis, hematuria, strong smelling urine, diarrhea, frequency or hesitancy, mood changes, abdominal pain, suprapubic or flank pain, dehydration	
Upper UTI—Pyelonephritis	High fever, chills, abdominal pain, nausea, vomiting, flank pain, costovertebral angle tenderness, moderate to severe dehydration	IV antibiotics initially then transitioned to oral antibiotics matching organism sensitivity for a total of 7–10 days Rehydration Antipyretics

tainer and tested for the presence of bacteria. Urine collection bags used on infants are unreliable because it is impossible to collect an uncontaminated specimen. Suprapubic and sterile catheterization collections are the most accurate methods to obtain a urine specimen for culture. See the Skills Manual for urine specimen collection methods. Diagnosis is confirmed with a urine culture. The criteria for infection, based on number of colony-forming units per milliliter, is dependent upon the method of specimen collection. Once the presence of bacteria is confirmed, antibiotic sensitivity for the specific organisms cultured is then determined. Urinalysis reveals white blood cells (WBCs) in the urine. A complete blood count reveals an elevated WBC count.

Radiologic studies are often performed to detect structural abnormalities and renal scarring in infants and children up to age 2 years. The most commonly performed tests are renal ultrasound and a voiding cystourethrogram (VCUG). A renal and bladder ultrasound is often obtained soon after diagnosis, and a voiding cystourethrogram is obtained to detect the presence of vesicoureteral reflux (VUR) (Mahant, To, & Friedman, 2001). Renal and bladder sonography and a cystogram (either VCUG or radionuclide) are the recommended imaging studies used to detect pyelonephritis and renal scarring (Kraus, 2001). See Table 31–2 on page 1178.

Clinical Therapy

Antibiotic therapy is initiated as soon as urine samples have been collected. Once the culture sensitivity information is obtained, the antibiotic is changed if necessary. Follow-up cultures are obtained 48 to 72 hours after drug therapy initiation, at which time the urine should be sterile. Children who appear ill and cannot tolerate oral antibiotics are often hospitalized because of the need for rehydration and initiation of parenteral antibiotic treatment. Fluid intake is provided according to recommended fluid intake for age. Intake and output is monitored.

Follow-up urine cultures may be obtained monthly for 3 months, every 3 months for 6 months, and then annually since subsequent infections may be asymptomatic. For children with vesicoureteral reflux or recurrent infections, a long-term suppressive dose of an antibiotic may be ordered for prophylaxis; however, there is limited evidence about the effectiveness of this therapy (Williams, Lee, & Craig, 2001). Children with renal scarring should have their blood pressure monitored periodically.

The immediate complications of urinary tract infections are sepsis, abscess formation, and death. A long-term complication of urinary tract infections is renal scar formation (Santen & Altieri, 2001). If a structural defect is identified, surgical correction may be necessary to prevent recurrent infections that could lead to renal damage.

NURSING MANAGEMENT

Goals of nursing care are to collaborate in the identification of the child with a urinary tract infection, to promote adherence to prescribed therapy, and to prevent reinfection.

■ Nursing Assessment and Diagnosis

Nursing assessment focuses on identifying signs and symptoms of urinary tract infections and related complications.

Physiologic Assessment

Obtain a history of urinary symptoms. Determine if there is a history of recurrent urinary tract infections. Assess the infant for toxic (very ill) appearance, fever, and poor feeding. Evaluate the child's oral fluid intake. Assess for quality, quantity, and frequency of voiding. This is an especially important assessment in infants and toddlers who cannot communicate. Observe the urinary stream if possible and perform a urinalysis, including specific gravity. Measure the child's height and weight and plot on a growth curve to identify any change in growth pattern. Assess the infant's or child's vital signs including blood pressure. Assess for behavioral changes such as bedwetting and loss of bladder control.

Palpate the abdomen and suprapubic and costovertebral areas for masses, tenderness, and distention. Assess for abdominal or flank pain, frequency, urgency, and dysuria. Palpate or percuss the bladder after voiding to evaluate bladder emptying. Assess bathing and toileting habits (e.g., determine whether the child takes bubble baths, wipes from front to back, and engages in adequate perineal hygiene). Also be alert for signs of sexual abuse such as bruising or scarring of the perineal region.

Psychosocial Assessment

Adolescents who are sexually active may deny experiencing symptoms because they fear disclosure of their sexual activity to their parents. Careful questioning and assurance of confidentiality may be necessary to elicit these concerns. The child and family are provided an opportunity to address their concerns during the psychosocial assessment. Refer to the section on sexually transmitted infections later in the chapter for a further discussion of assessment of the sexually active adolescent.

Following are common nursing diagnoses for the child with a UTI.

- Impaired Urinary Elimination related to urinary tract infection and altered voiding pattern
- Delayed Growth and Development related to effects of chronic infection
- Ineffective Health Maintenance related to lack of knowledge of preventive UTI measures (adequate fluid intake, proper hygiene, frequent voiding)
- Risk for Imbalanced Fluid Volume related to fever and inadequate fluid intake
- Acute Pain related to irritated urethra

Planning and Implementation

A clean-catch urine specimen may be obtained if the child is able to cooperate. If unable to obtain a clean-catch specimen, then obtain a catheterized sample. An early-morning urine specimen is preferred due to its higher concentration at this time. A blood culture may be obtained to assess for sepsis.

The child with an uncomplicated urinary tract infection is cared for in the home with antibiotics and oral fluids to treat dehydration. Nursing care for the hospitalized child with a complicated UTI centers on administering prescribed medications, promoting rehydration, assessing renal function, and partnering with parents and older children to establish methods to minimize the risk of future infection.

Administer antibiotics and antipyretics as prescribed to maintain therapeutic drug levels and reduce fever. Encourage fluid intake according to normal requirements for age to dilute the urine and flush the bladder. Frequent voiding minimizes urinary stasis.

Because bladder training is such an important milestone for young children, any disorder that affects voiding may have developmental implications. A toddler who has been toilet trained may regress and require diapers temporarily due to incontinence related to the pain and frequency associated with the UTI. Similarly, an older child might develop enuresis after a prolonged period of being dry at night. Partner with the family and offer reassurance that regression is normal and emphasize that the child requires support rather than disapproval. A preschooler may perceive the infection and any parental disapproval as punishment for an imagined wrong. Provide support and reassurance that the child is not being punished for any actions.

Care in the Community

The primary goal is to prevent reinfection. The child who has had one urinary tract infection is at increased risk for recurrent infections (Williams et al., 2001). Partner with the child and family and provide information on prevention through proper hygiene, especially for girls. See Partnering with Families: Preventive Strategies for Urinary Tract Infections.

Children with UTIs are usually cared for at home. Partner with parents and instruct them on the importance of administering antibiotics as prescribed and assist them to establish an effective administration schedule. Emphasize that antibiotics must be taken for the full course and that they may be continued even after the infection has cleared to prevent a recurrence. Provide parents specific guidelines for oral fluid intake. Ensure that the amount of fluids recommended for a 24-hour period equals the maintenance fluids for age plus any additional fluids required due to fever and diuresis (refer to Chapter 23∞) or as prescribed by primary healthcare provider. Recommend that the parents avoid giving the child caffeinated and carbonated beverages as these may potentially irritate the bladder mucosa.

Encourage the child to void more frequently even after the infection has cleared. A wristwatch with an alarm may be a helpful reminder. Partner with the family to ensure they recognize the signs and symptoms of recurrent infection and to seek care promptly. Instruct the sexually active female to void before and after intercourse and to engage in appropriate hygiene measures as previously described.

A **neurogenic bladder** occurs as a result of urinary tract obstruction related to an interrupted nerve supply to the bladder. Causes include myelomeningocele (refer to Chapter 33∞) and trauma to the spinal cord. The child with a neurogenic bladder requires a clean intermittent catheterization to be performed several times a day to reduce urinary stasis and the potential for UTI. See Partnering with Families: Clean Intermittent Catheterization on page 1190 for teaching guidelines.

Evaluation

Expected outcomes of nursing care may include the following:

- The child's urine is sterile after treatment.
- The child has catch-up growth once the infection is resolved.
- The child does not have a recurrent UTI.

Enuresis

Enuresis is repeated involuntary voiding by a child who has reached an age at which bladder control is expected, usually about 5 to 6 years of age. See Table 31–4 for bladder control milestones. Enuresis that occurs at night is called **nocturnal enuresis,** and accounts for approximately 50% of enuresis cases. Enuresis during the day is called **diurnal enuresis.** Both disorders can occur simultaneously. Nocturnal enuresis occurs more often in boys than in girls, with a 3.5:1 ratio, whereas diurnal enuresis is more common in girls. Approximately 5 to 7 million children older than 5 years are affected with primary nocturnal enuresis (Mercer, 2003).

Enuresis is further categorized as primary, intermittent, and secondary.

- *Primary enuresis*—child has never had a dry night; attributed to maturational delay and small functional bladder; not associated with stress or psychiatric cause.
- *Intermittent enuresis*—child has occasional nights or periods of dryness.
- *Secondary enuresis*—child begins bedwetting who has been reliably dry for 6 to 12 months; associated with stress, infections, and sleep disorders.

Etiology and Pathophysiology

Enuresis may result from neurologic or congenital structural disorders, illness, preoccupation with concerns, or stress. Nocturnal enuresis occurs with high frequency in children whose parents have a history of bedwetting. There is a 77% risk if both parents had enuresis, a 44% risk if one parent had enuresis, and a 15% risk if neither parent had enuresis (Tobias, 2000). Often children with nocturnal enuresis are harder to arouse and may fail to respond to full bladder signals.

In most children with primary enuresis, the bladder has a smaller functional capacity and neuromuscular maturation of the inhibitory fibers is delayed. Some children have been found to lack a normal circadian rhythm of vasopressin which helps concentrate the urine and reduce the urine volume produced during sleep. These children may produce more urine and exceed the functional bladder capacity (Jalkut, Lerman, & Churchill, 2001). Minor abnormalities of the bladder neck and urethra and unstable bladder contractions are also associated with enuresis. Some children affected with enuresis may have mild developmental delays. The majority of enuresis cases are not associated with structural or neurologic pathology. A recent study of 160 children undergoing a sleep study (polysomnography) for obstructive sleep apnea (OSA) revealed higher rates of enuresis in children with more severe respiratory distress during sleep (Brooks & Topol, 2003).

TABLE 31–4 Milestones in the Development of Bladder Control

AGE	DEVELOPMENTAL MILESTONE
1 1/2 years	Child passes urine at regular intervals.
2 years	Child announces when he or she is voiding.
2 1/2 years	Child makes known need to void; can hold urine.
3 years	Child goes to the bathroom by himself or herself; holds urge if preoccupied with play.
2 1/2–3 1/2 years	Child achieves nighttime control.
4 years	Child shows great interest in going to bathrooms when away from home (shopping centers, movies).
5 years	Child voids approximately seven times a day; prefers privacy; is able to initiate emptying of bladder at any degree of fullness.

PARTNERING WITH FAMILIES

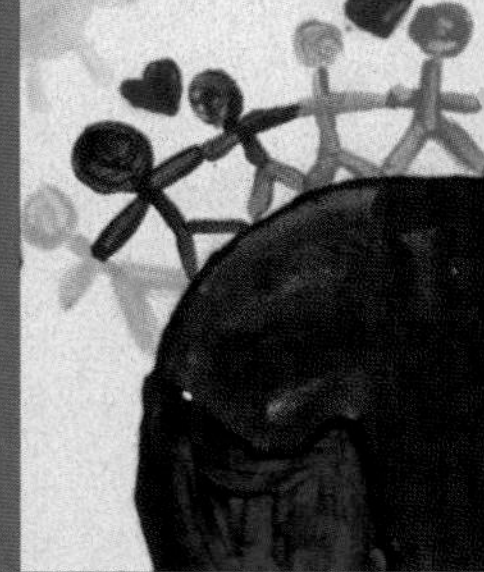

Preventive Strategies for Urinary Tract Infections

Provide education to parents about strategies to reduce the risk for future urinary tract infections, including the following:

- Teach proper perineal hygiene. Girls should always wipe the perineum from front to back after voiding.
- Encourage the child to drink plenty of fluids and avoid long periods of "holding urine."
- Caution against tight underwear; children should wear cotton rather than nylon underwear.
- Encourage the child to void more frequently and to fully empty the bladder.
- Discourage bubble baths and hot tubs, which can irritate the urethra.
- Encourage abstinence of sexual activity. However, if girls are sexually active, instruct them to void before and after sexual intercourse to prevent urinary stasis and flush out bacteria introduced during intercourse.

Clinical Manifestations

Children with diurnal enuresis may exhibit clinical manifestations of frequency, urgency, constant dribbling, and involuntary loss of control after voiding. Nocturnal enuresis is manifested by bedwetting.

COLLABORATIVE CARE

The goal of collaborative care is to identify and treat the cause of enuresis and to establish urinary control. Neurologic defects, structural defects, renal insufficiency, and disorders such as diabetes are ruled out.

Diagnostic Tests

A thorough history is taken to identify potential contributors to enuresis. See Box 31–3. Diagnostic laboratory tests include a urinalysis and urine culture. Further evaluation is needed when the child cannot concentrate the urine or achieve a specific

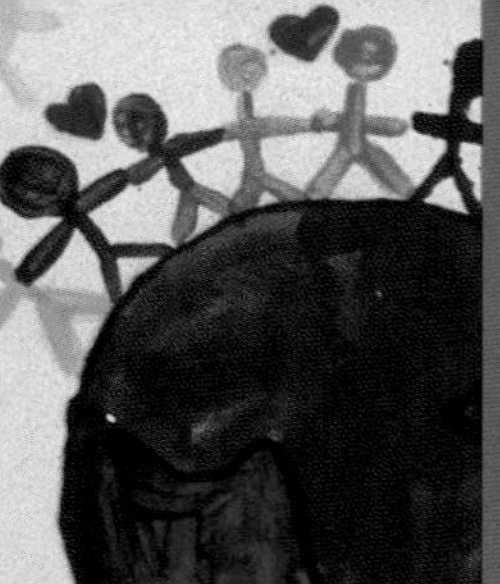

PARTNERING WITH FAMILIES

Clean Intermittent Catheterization

Clean intermittent catheterization (CIC) is performed to empty the bladder when nerves for bladder control are missing or damaged. Parents must learn to perform this procedure at home since it must be performed every 3 to 4 hours during the day, but is usually not done when the child sleeps at night. The child is ready to learn self-catheterization when he or she really wants to be dry and is learning independence. Until that time, parents usually perform CIC.

Equipment needed

- Four or five catheters of the size and type recommended—each catheter is used until it becomes hard and brittle (about 1 month)
- Water-soluble lubricant (not Vaseline)

How performed

- Usually clean technique is used. Wash hands with soap and water, then spread lubricant on the tip of the catheter. Hold the catheter like a pencil in one hand, about 8 cm (3 in.) from the tip. Position the other end of the catheter over the toilet or a container.

Females

- Spread the labia with the other hand and slide the catheter 5 to 8 cm (2 to 3 in.) into the urethra until urine begins to flow, then 2.5 cm (1 in.) further, up to 8 cm (3 in.) maximum.
- Hold the catheter in place until all urine flows out, then slowly remove it. If more urine begins to flow, let it drain before removal.

Males

- Hold the penis outward with the other hand and slide the catheter into the penis until urine begins to flow, then 2.5 cm (1 in.) further, up to 12 to 15 cm (5 to 6 in.) maximum. A sphincter muscle is located at the opening to the bladder, and it sometimes feels very tight. If the catheter will not slide into the bladder easily, use constant but gentle pressure on the sphincter muscle with the tip of the catheter. It will soon feel the pressure and gradually open up, allowing the catheter to slip in.
- Hold the catheter in place until all urine flows out, then slowly remove it. If more urine begins to flow, let it drain before removal.

Storage

- Wash the catheter with soap and water and shake out excess water. Store the catheter in a plastic bag after use.
- Keep a catheter in the car, bookbag, fanny pack, or at school. (The catheter can be carried to school in a toothbrush holder to avoid embarrassment.)

Adapted from Ball, J. W. (1998). Mosby's pediatric patient teaching guides. *St. Louis: Mosby.*

BOX 31–3 Questions to Ask When Taking an Enuresis History

FAMILY HISTORY

Is there a family history of renal or urinary structural abnormalities?
Is there a family history of bedwetting? At what age did bedwetting stop?

FAMILY MANAGEMENT OF ENURESIS

How serious is the problem for the family?
What happens when the child wets? (Who gets up and changes sheets?)
How is the child treated? Is the child punished or blamed for wetting?
What remedies have been tried?

TOILET TRAINING

When was it initiated and what method was used?
Has the child ever been dry during the day or night for an extended period?
How long was the child's longest dry period?
How often does the child void? Have a bowel movement?
Does the child have a history of constipation or encopresis?

STRESSORS

How is the child doing in school?
Are there any new or chronic stressors present in the child's life?
How does the problem interfere with play and social activities?

RISK FACTORS

Diabetes—Are there any signs of polyuria or polydypsia?
Urinary tract infection—Does the child have frequency, urgency, burning on urination?

gravity of 1.022 or greater, or if glucosuria is present. A urine culture may reveal that an asymptomatic urinary tract infection is present. Diagnostic studies include measurement of the child's functional bladder capacity. Other studies may include uroflow measurement, which identifies a slow urine stream, and bladder sonography, which measures postvoid residual (Jalkut et al., 2001).

Clinical Therapy

A spontaneous cure rate occurs in approximately 15% of children each year, regardless of intervention used or lack of intervention. When the child reaches age 6 to 7 years, intervention should be initiated when both the child and parents are motivated. A multitreatment approach is usually most effective. Approximately one third of children with nocturnal enuresis are treated with medications. See page 1191 for medications used to treat enuresis.

Common behavioral approaches such as fluid-intake programs, bladder training, and enuresis alarms are described in Table 31–5. Avoidance of foods believed to contribute to enuresis, such as those containing caffeine, milk, chocolate, and citrus, may be recommended (Tobias, 2000). Relapse often occurs when medications are stopped. Research suggests improved results when the enuresis alarm is used in conjunction with pharmacologic therapy (Jalkut et al., 2001).

MEDICATIONS Used in the Treatment of Enuresis

MEDICATION	ACTION/INDICATION	NURSING IMPLICATION
Desmopressin acetate (DDAVP) Oral or nasal administration	A vasopressin with an antidiuretic effect. It reduces urine production for 8–12 hours after dosing.	The use of DDAVP is primarily reserved for times when the child is away from home for a short period (e.g., sleep-over or camp). DDAVP may be administered as a nasal spray or in tablet form which has a more consistent dose. For nasal spray, sit the child upright so medication stays on nasal mucosa and not down the throat. Half of dose is administered to each nostril. Monitor blood pressure during initial dose-regulating period. Teach family to weigh child daily and report weight gain.
Oxybutynin (Ditropan) Oral administration, extended-release tablet available	An anticholinergic, relaxes smooth muscle of the bladder, allowing an increase in bladder capacity and a delay in the initial desire to void.	Educate family to monitor for responses to therapy, including effects on nocturia, urinary frequency, urge incontinence, and completeness of bladder emptying. May cause dry mouth. May be taken with food
Imipramine (Tofranil) Oral administration	Tricyclic antidepressant. Useful in nocturnal enuresis due to anticholinergic activity and nervous system stimulation, which result in earlier arousal to full bladder sensation.	Often used but requires close monitoring because of its effects on mood and sleep-arousal patterns and the associated dangers of overdoses. Monitor for mood changes, excess fatigue. Administer dose 1 hour before bedtime, or half dose is given in afternoon and half at bedtime. Give with food to lessen GI irritation. Educate parents to weigh child twice a week and monitor for edema. Over-the-counter medications are avoided while the child is on imipramine. Photosensitivity is a potential side effect; exposure to strong sunlight should be avoided. Effectiveness of drug may decrease with continued use.

Data from Mercer, R. (2003, February). Dry at night: Treating nocturnal enuresis. Advance for Nurse Practitioners, *26–32; Wilson, B. A., Shannon, M. T., & Stang, C. L. (2004).* Nurse's drug guide. *Upper Saddle River, NJ: Prentice Hall.*

NURSING MANAGEMENT

Goals of nursing include assisting the child and family in achieving the child's urinary control and promoting the child's self-esteem.

Nursing Assessment and Diagnosis

A thorough history can assist in identifying potential causes of enuresis. Review the child's elimination patterns, developmental milestones, toilet training history, and urinary symptoms. Assess for associated conditions by examining the child's lower spine for fistulas, sacral dimples, or tufts of hair that could be signs of occult spina bifida. Identify any potential stressors that may contribute to enuresis.

CLINICAL TIP

Enuretic children often have a history of constipation. Rectal pressure on the posterior bladder wall stimulates the bladder to empty.

Identify the perceived extent of the problem to the child and family. Determine if the parents and child are equally motivated to resolve the problem.

Nursing diagnoses that apply to the child with enuresis may include:

- Impaired Urinary Elimination related to dysfunctional voiding
- Readiness for Enhanced Therapeutic Regimen Management related to medication and behavioral interventions for enuresis

MediaLink Care Plan: A School-Age Child with Enuresis

TABLE 31–5 Nonpharmacologic Treatment Approaches for Enuresis

APPROACH	DESCRIPTION
Fluid intake program	The child's daily fluid requirements are calculated, then the fluid requirements are met by providing 40% of the fluid requirements in the morning (7 A.M. to 12 P.M.), 40% in the afternoon (12 P.M. to 5 P.M.), and 20% in the evening (after 5 P.M.). The benefits of this program include the promotion of adequate fluid intake and the decrease in urine production at nighttime.
Timed voiding	The child with diurnal enuresis is instructed to void every 2 hours and to use a double voiding pattern; this trains the bladder to empty completely and avoid overdistention.
Enuresis alarms	A detector strip is attached to the child's pants. The alarm sounds a buzzer that alerts the child when wetting occurs, so the child can get up and finish voiding in the bathroom. This works best for children over 7 years old.
Reward system/positive reinforcement	Set realistic goals for the child, offer praise, and reward the dry days or nights with stars and stickers on a calendar.

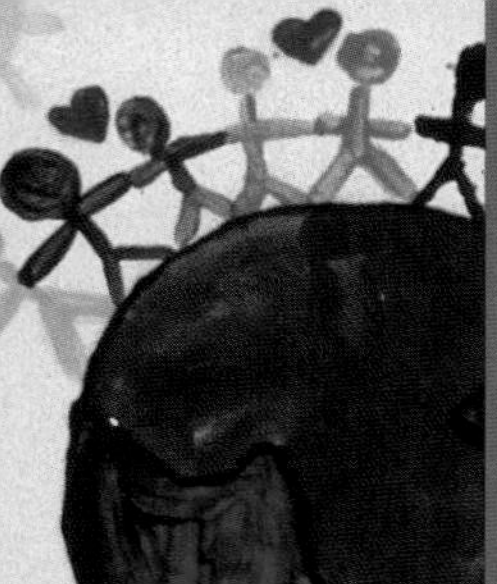

PARTNERING WITH FAMILIES

Guidelines for Using an Enuresis Alarm

The success of achieving urinary control at night by using an alarm is dependent on the family and child's understanding of the appropriate use of the alarm. Partner with parents to provide the following tips to help ensure their understanding.

- It takes 10 to 12 weeks for the average child to be consistently dry.
- Attach the alarm to close-fitting cloth underwear (not boxers or pajama bottoms) instead of disposable pants.
- Parents should respond to the alarm by going to the child's room and noting the child's response. Tell the child to put the feet on the floor and walk to the bathroom. Help the child if necessary. Turn the alarm off only after the child's feet are on the floor.
- Initially, the child will have emptied his or her bladder by the time he or she hears the alarm (or parent responds). Progress can be measured by recording the frequency of wetting episodes per night, the time of the wetting, and the size of the wet spot before the child responds.
- Many children wet more than one time per night initially. Reattach the alarm to clean underwear after each wetting episode. As they make progress, the nightly wetting episodes decrease.
- Use positive reinforcement by keeping charts to allow the child to track progress. Consider giving rewards (stickers, time for favorite activities, etc.) in recognition of cooperation, wearing the alarm and walking to the bathroom when parents arrive, as well as dry nights.
- Use the alarm until the child has had 2 weeks of consecutive dry nights, and then use the alarm every other night for 2 or more consecutive weeks of dryness. If wetting occurs during this process, start the 2-week weaning over again.
- Discontinuing the alarm prematurely can lead to a relapse of the wetting.

Adapted from Mercer, R. (2003, February). Dry at night: Treating nocturnal enuresis. Advance for Nurse Practitioners, *26–32.*

- Risk for Situational Low Self-Esteem related to embarrassment of lack of bladder control

Planning and Implementation

Partner with the child and parents and explain the physiologic development of bladder control and causes and treatment of enuresis. Explore parental and child feelings of guilt or blame. Ensure that the parents and child understand that the wetting cannot be controlled. Identify and discuss unsupportive strategies such as scolding or belittling the child and limiting daytime fluids.

Assess the parents' and child's motivation and readiness for interventions. Strategies for parents to implement include promoting regular stools, promoting most of fluid intake during the morning and afternoon, having the child double void before bed, offering praise and encouragement to the child, and maintaining a calendar to document progress. Discuss the use of an enuresis alarm to determine if the child and parents are willing to use it consistently long term, as many as 10 to 12 weeks before the child becomes consistently dry. Before parents purchase an enuresis alarm, suggest they use an alarm clock in the child's room for several nights to determine if the child will arouse. Establish whether the child shares a room with others who will be disturbed by the alarm. See Partnering with Families: Guidelines for Using an Enuresis Alarm.

Psychosocial support is an essential part of care since stress is a significant cause of secondary enuresis. Discuss potential strategies with the family to reduce stressors on the child or to help the child cope with the stressors.

Evaluation

Expected outcomes of nursing care may include the following:

- The family selects an intervention that is best suited for their lifestyle.
- The child has an increased number of dry nights.
- The child demonstrates satisfaction with progress and positive self-esteem.

RENAL DISORDERS

The following renal disorders are complex in nature, causing multisystem effects and potentially resulting in loss of kidney function. Renal disorders and therapies discussed in this section include nephrotic syndrome, renal failure, renal replacement therapy, hemodialysis, continuous renal replacement therapy, kidney transplantation, acute postinfectious glomerulonephritis, hemolytic uremic syndrome, and polycystic kidney disease.

Nephrotic Syndrome

Nephrotic syndrome (NS) is an alteration in kidney function secondary to increased glomerular basement membrane permeability to plasma protein (Figure 31–7 ■). Nephrotic syndrome refers not to a specific disease, but to a clinical state characterized by edema, massive proteinuria, hypoalbuminemia, hypoproteinemia, hyperlipidemia, and altered immunity. Primary nephrotic syndrome is present when only the kidney is involved. Secondary nephrotic syndrome results from a systemic disease, drugs, or toxins.

Approximately 85% of children with nephrotic syndrome have a type of primary disease called minimal change nephrotic syndrome (MCNS) (Huether, 2002a). MCNS usually occurs in children between the ages of 2 and 7 years, with an incidence of 2 per 100,000 children. African American and Hispanic children experience a greater incidence of nephrotic syndrome, and the disorder in these children is more virulent, progresses more rapidly to renal failure, and has a poorer prognosis (Robinson,

PATHOPHYSIOLOGY ILLUSTRATED

Nephrotic Syndrome

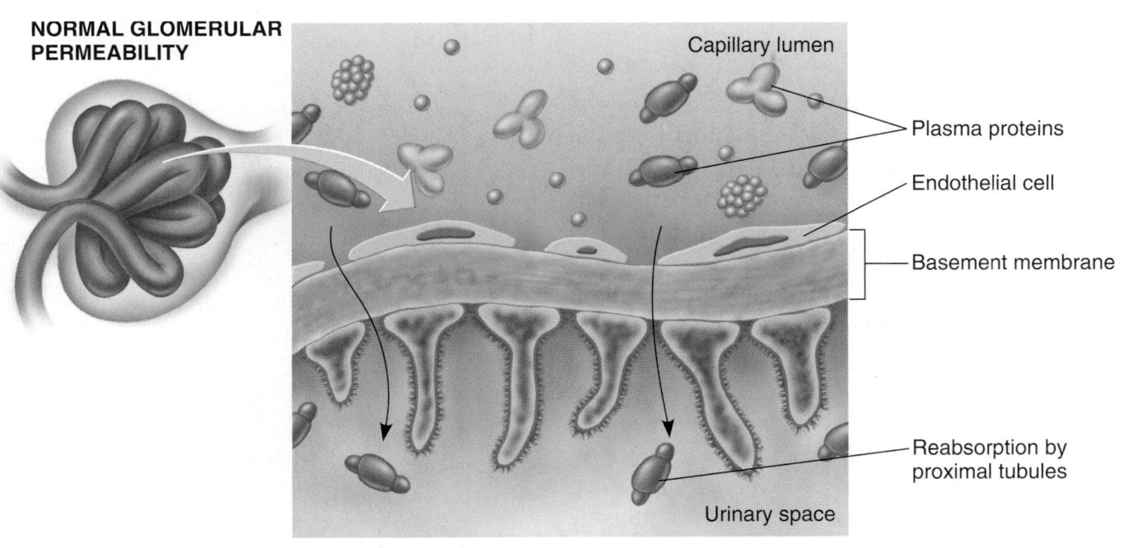

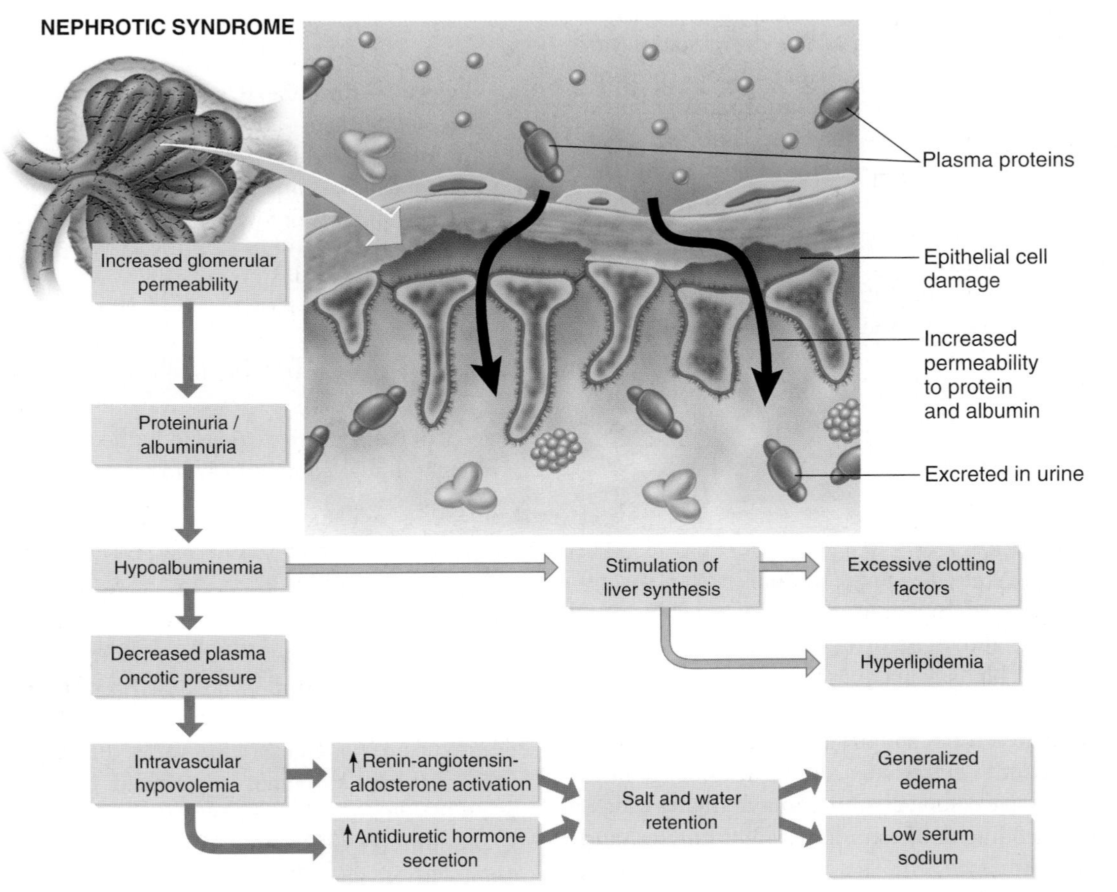

FIGURE 31–7 ■ Note the contrast between the normal glomerular anatomy and the changes that exist in nephrotic syndrome permitting protein to be excreted in the urine. The lower albumin blood level stimulates the liver to generate lipids and excessive clotting factors. Edema results from decreased oncotic plasma pressure, renin-angiotensin-aldosterone activation, and antidiuretic hormone secretion.

MediaLink Renal Function Animation

Nahata, Mahan, et al., 2003). The disorder is also more common in males than females.

MCNS derives its name from the fact that the glomeruli appear normal or show only minimal changes on light microscopic evaluation. Because MCNS is the most common form of nephrotic syndrome, it is the focus of the following discussion.

Etiology and Pathophysiology

The cause of primary MCNS is unknown, but an immune system role is strongly suspected as an upper respiratory infection often precedes the onset of edema by 2 to 3 days (Robinson et al., 2003). The mechanism of increased glomerular permeability is unknown as the glomeruli appear normal, although it may be related to the loss of a negative charge in the glomerular capillary wall (Huether, 2002a). Usually, a minute amount of protein is present in the urine. In MCNS, however, increased permeability of the glomerular membrane permits large negatively charged molecules such as albumin to pass through the membrane and be excreted in the urine. The proximal tubules are unable to reabsorb all the filtered proteins. Immunoglobulins are lost, resulting in altered immunity. Edema occurs as a result of decreased intravascular oncotic pressure secondary to urinary protein losses. Decreased plasma albumin levels result when the child cannot increase synthesis to compensate for the losses. The decreased plasma albumin results in decreased intravascular oncotic pressure and the development of edema, because fluid remains in the interstitial spaces instead of being pulled back into the vascular compartment (Robinson et al., 2003). The liver, stimulated perhaps by hypoalbuminemia or decreased osmotic pressure, responds by increasing synthesis of lipoprotein (cholesterol), resulting in hyperlipidemia.

Loss of antithrombin III and reduced levels of factors IX, XI, and XII due to urinary loss may lead to hypercoagulability, and hyperlipidemia may cause an increase in platelet count (Robinson et al., 2003). These conditions place the child at increased risk for thrombosis. Hypertension and renal failure may occur in children with progressive and virulent types of nephrotic syndrome.

Clinical Manifestations

In most children, edema develops gradually over several weeks. The child experiences a gradual or rapid weight gain, snug-fitting clothing, and tight-fitting shoes. Children may have a history of periorbital edema on waking that resolves during the day as fluid shifts to the abdomen and lower extremities. Medical treatment often is not sought until generalized edema develops on the child's extremities, abdomen, or genitals (Figure 31–8 ■). Massive edema resulting in a dramatic weight gain may occur, depending on the amount of albumin lost and the amount of sodium ingested. The child will generally feel malaise, irritable, fatigued, and weak.

Signs by body system are as follows:

- *Renal*—decreased urine output and dark, frothy urine
- *Cardiovascular*—hypertension, tachycardia

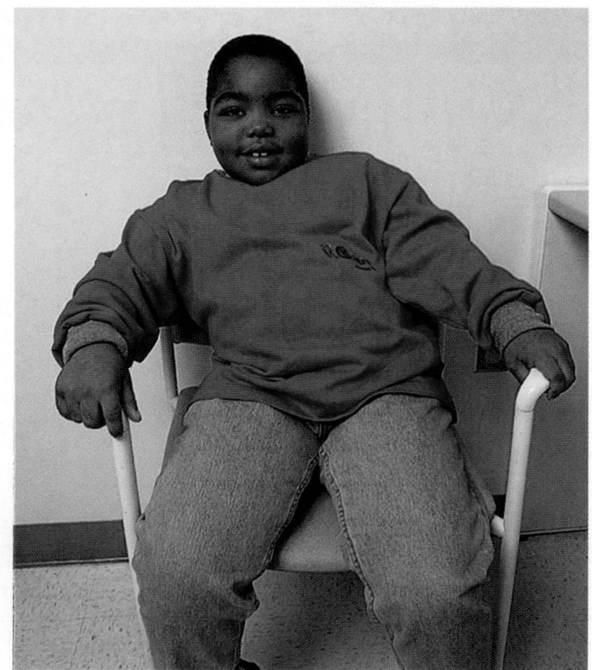

FIGURE 31–8 ■ This boy has generalized edema, a characteristic finding in nephrotic syndrome.

- *Vascular*—thrombosis
- *Gastrointestinal*—anorexia, abdominal pain, nausea and vomiting, diarrhea
- *Skin*—pallor, shiny with prominent veins, brittle hair, edema, skin breakdown
- *Pulmonary*—respiratory distress and pulmonary congestion in severe edema

COLLABORATIVE CARE

The goal of collaborative care is to induce remission, restore intravascular fluid volume, and avoid complications that may lead to progressive kidney dysfunction.

Diagnostic Tests

Diagnosis is based on the history, physical examination, presence of characteristic symptoms, and laboratory findings. Urinalysis reveals massive proteinuria (50 mg/kg/day), the primary indicator of nephrotic syndrome. A protein-to-creatinine (PR/CR) ratio is used to estimate protein excretion in children. Because urine protein excretion varies during the day, the first-morning voided specimen is preferred. Normal PR/CR ratios are <0.2 in children over 2 years and <0.5 in children 6 months to 24 months (Hogg, Furth, Lemley, et al., 2003). The serum creatinine, BUN, cholesterol, and albumin are also evaluated. Serum sodium levels are decreased and serum electrolytes will be altered and vary individually according to disease process. Renal ultrasonography may be performed in some cases. Though not routinely performed, a single-needle kidney biopsy for examination of glomeruli may be performed to assess for renal failure or other disorders.

Clinical Therapy

The child with nephrotic syndrome should be referred to a pediatric nephrologist for collaborative care along with the primary care provider. Clinical therapy focuses on decreasing proteinuria, relieving edema, managing associated symptoms, improving nutrition, and preventing infection. Children may be hospitalized when severe edema or a major infection is present. Treatment generally occurs on an outpatient basis. The child becomes malnourished as a result of protein loss in the urine. A diet that is normal for the child's age is recommended. No attempt should be made either to restrict or to increase protein intake. A "no added salt" diet is recommended during corticosteroid treatment.

In children with nephrotic syndrome, corticosteroids are the mainstay of treatment. See the medication table on page 1196. In most children, urine protein levels fall to trace or negative values within 2 to 3 weeks of the start of therapy. Approximately 90% of children experience complete remission with corticosteroid therapy. In addition to corticosteroids, pharmacologic agents prescribed in the treatment and management of nephrotic syndrome include diuretics, alkylating agents, cyclosporine, antihypertensive agents, and antibiotics. Pain medications may also be prescribed for the management of pain related to edema and flank pain associated with kidney infection. Albumin may occasionally be administered; however, because of the increased risks and short-term effects, it is reserved for use only in the child with severe edema who is resistant to diuretics (Robinson et al., 2003).

A relapse is commonly associated with a respiratory infection or live virus immunizations; however, relapses become less frequent or stop during puberty. Parents are encouraged to monitor body weight and use a urine dipstick to check for protein on a regular basis as this provides an indication of a relapse. Repeat therapy is administered to children who have a relapse after drug therapy is discontinued.

PRACTICE ALERT

Children with nephrotic syndrome who have not been immunized with varivax or who have not previously had chickenpox should have a varicella zoster titer drawn. If the child is exposed to chickenpox, varicella-zoster immune globulin should be administered within 72 hours of exposure to prevent or lessen the severity of the illness. These children should not receive vaccines containing live viruses because of the risk of disease from the vaccine. Live viruses are contained in the measles, mumps, and rubella (MMR) vaccine, and the varicella vaccine.

NURSING MANAGEMENT

Goals of nursing focus on managing the child's symptoms, including edema, preventing complications such as infection and impaired skin integrity, meeting nutritional needs, and addressing the emotional needs of the child and family.

Nursing Assessment and Diagnosis

Nursing assessment focuses on signs of fluid volume excess, complications related to the disorder, and the psychosocial impact of the condition on the child and family.

Physiologic Assessment

Carefully assess the child's hydration status. Monitor intake and output and vital signs at least every 4 hours and record these findings accurately. Signs of fluid volume excess include weight gain, local edema (facial, periorbital, and external genitalia), and ascites with taut shiny skin over the abdomen. Weigh the child daily using the same scale and measure abdominal girth to monitor changes in edema and ascites. Assess for respiratory distress associated with pulmonary congestion, pulmonary edema, and pleural effusion (refer to Chapter 25∞). Monitor for hypertension and signs of circulatory overload.

Test urine for proteinuria and specific gravity at least once each shift. Assess for skin breakdown resulting from edema. Assess the child for signs of hypovolemia during periods of diuresis. Monitor for signs of electrolyte imbalance such as arrhythmias, EKG changes, decreased or increased heart rate, hypotension, muscle weakness, and hyporeflexia.

Assess for indications of infection including fever and elevated white blood cell count as altered immunity is an adverse effect associated with corticosteroid therapy. Assess the child's comfort level and activity tolerance.

Psychosocial Assessment

Children and parents are often fearful or anxious on admission. Because edema often develops gradually, parents may feel guilty if they did not seek medical attention immediately. School-age children with generalized edema are often concerned about their appearance. Allow the child an opportunity to express feelings and concerns. The child who is hospitalized for a recurrence of nephrotic syndrome may be frustrated or depressed and may experience irritability or other changes in mood. Assess the child and family's coping mechanisms, support systems, and level of stress.

Following are examples of nursing diagnoses appropriate for the child with MCNS.

- Risk for Infection related to immunosuppressive therapy and loss of immunoglobulins in urine
- Excess Fluid Volume (extravascular) related to fluid and sodium retention
- Risk for Impaired Skin Integrity related to edema, lowered resistance to infection, injury, immobility, and malnutrition
- Imbalanced Nutrition: Less than Body Requirements related to loss of appetite and protein loss in urine

Planning and Implementation

Nursing care is mainly supportive and focuses on administering medications, preventing infection, preventing skin breakdown, meeting nutritional and fluid needs, promoting rest, and providing emotional support to the parents and child.

MediaLink Care Plan: A Child with Nephrotic Syndrome

MEDICATIONS Used to Treat Nephrotic Syndrome

MEDICATION	ACTION/IMPLICATION	NURSING CONSIDERATIONS
Corticosteroid Therapy		
Prednisone or prednisolone	Stimulates remission Prednisone reduces the excretion of protein in the urine	Children who respond successfully to therapy continue to take corticosteroids daily for 6 weeks and 6 weeks of alternate-day treatment. Monitor for infection, changes in blood pressure, and changes in growth and behavior. If long-term courses of corticosteroids are administered, observe for major side effects such as weight gain and moon face, obesity, gastrointestinal bleeding, growth retardation, hyperglycemia, hypertension, adrenal suppression, and bone demineralization. Educate parents about appetite-stimulating effect of corticosteroids and to limit calorie intake to prevent excessive weight gain. Administration of live vaccines should be delayed until child is no longer immunosuppressed.
Alkylating/Cytotoxic Agents		
Chlorambucil Cyclophosphamide	Stimulates remission and helps extend the interval between relapses Used when no response to corticosteroids or side effects are a problem	Monitor WBC count. Assess for gastrointestinal bleeding, alopecia, and impaired growth. Serious long-term side effects, include carcinogenesis and risk of sterility in males. Administer medications 1 hour before breakfast or 2 hours after evening meal. An antiemetic may be prescribed for nausea while taking medication. Encourage adequate hydration to reduce cystitis. Educate family to report unusual bleeding, bruising, chills, fever, or other signs of infection.
Cyclosporine Therapy (Immunosuppressant)		
	Used in children with corticosteroid refractory nephrotic syndrome by decreasing immunologic responses, decreasing the glomerular filtration rate, and affecting the glomerular basement membrane permeability to albumin	Monitor blood pressure for hypertension, and other side effects such as nausea, vomiting, anemia, and abdominal discomfort. Monitor electrolytes, cyclosporine serum concentrations, creatinine clearance, and serum creatinine levels to assess renal status. Educate family to administer medication with meals to reduce nausea, administer the medication at the same time each day, and use a glass rather than plastic container for mixing. May dilute with orange or apple juice. Do not use grapefruit juice.

Administer Medications

Administer the prescribed medications according to the scheduled time. Monitor closely for side effects of corticosteroids such as moon face, increased appetite, increased hair growth, abdominal distention, and mood swings. Monitor for adverse effects of corticosteroids such as hypertension, nausea, and hyperglycemia. Corticosteroids should be tapered rather than abruptly discontinued.

If the child is receiving albumin intravenously, monitor closely for hypertension or signs of volume overload caused by fluid shifts. Severe edema is treated with a loop, thiazide, or potassium-sparing diuretic. Hypovolemia may occur with diuretic administration. Though rarely done because of the associated risk factors, albumin infused simultaneously with diuretics may be required in order to reduce the risk of hypovolemic shock. Observe for signs of impending shock (refer to Chapter 26∞ for discussion of shock).

Prevent Infection

Children with MCNS are at risk for infection secondary to the loss of immunoglobulins in the urine and corticosteroid therapy. Implement careful handwashing and standard precautions. Strict aseptic technique is essential during invasive procedures. Monitor the child's white blood cell count when cytotoxic drugs are given since bone marrow suppression is a side effect. Monitor vital signs carefully to detect early signs of infection that may be masked by corticosteroid therapy. Decrease the child's social contacts during immunosuppressive treatment, and caution parents and children to avoid exposure to individuals with respiratory infections and communicable diseases. Partner with the family and educate them on the importance of avoiding shopping malls, sporting arenas, grocery stores, game stores, and other public areas where the risk of exposure to such infections is increased. Provide instructions to the parents on signs of infection, including fever and changes in behavior.

Prevent Skin Breakdown

Meticulous skin care is implemented to prevent skin breakdown and potential infection. Perform repeated skin assessments, turn the child frequently, and use therapeutic mattresses (e.g., egg crate, airflow mattress) to help prevent skin breakdown. Provide daily hygiene and maintain dry skin. Restrictive clothing or other items such as armbands and tape are avoided.

MediaLink Furosemide Animation

MEDICATIONS Used to Treat Nephrotic Syndrome (continued)

MEDICATION	ACTION/IMPLICATION	NURSING CONSIDERATIONS
Diuretics		
Loop diuretics Furosemide, bumetanide, torsemide *Thiazide diuretics*	Used for severe edema. Prevents reabsorption of water, sodium, and potassium by the renal tubules, thereby reducing massive edema Blocks the sodium-chloride transporter in the distal tubule, thereby reducing massive edema	May be administered orally or intravenously. Monitor for intravascular volume depletion (hypovolemia). Assess vital signs for tachycardia and hypotension. Monitor plasma concentration to identify child at risk for hearing loss. Monitor for other potential side effects including hyponatremia, hypokalemia, and other electrolyte imbalances.
Angiotensin-converting enzyme (ACE) inhibitor		
Vasotec (enalapril maleate)	Antihypertensive agent Some renal protective effects	Monitor blood pressure. Assess for transient hypotension, lightheadedness. Monitor serum potassium for side effect of hyperkalemia. If given in combination with NSAIDs, educate the family to avoid salt substitutes since they are high in potassium.
Antibiotics		
	Administered to children with *signs and symptoms* of infection Routine prophylaxis is not effective	Administer according to prescribed schedule. Monitor WBC count and assess for signs and symptoms of infection.
Antithrombotic Therapy		
Heparin, followed by oral anticoagulant therapy	Activates angiotensin III to reduce coagulation	Monitor clotting factors and platelet count. Assess for evidence of thrombosis. Assess for abnormal bleeding (oozing intravenous sites, nosebleeds).
NSAIDs		
	Promotes some decrease in protein excretion Analgesia	Establish a routine pain assessment schedule using a pain scale. Administer pain medications around the clock rather than prn.

Data from Robinson, R. F., Nahata, M. C., Mahan, J. D., & Batisky, D. L. (2003). Management of nephrotic syndrome in children. Pharmacotherapy, *22(8), 1021–1036; Hogg, R. J., Portman, R. J., Milliner, D., Lemley, K. V., Eddy, A., & Inglefinger, J. (2000). Evaluation and management of proteinuria and nephritic syndrome in children: Recommendations from a pediatric nephrology panel established at the National Kidney Foundation conference on proteinuria, albuminuria, risk, assessment, detection, and elimination (PARADE).* Pediatrics, *105(6), 1242–1249.*

Meet Nutritional and Fluid Needs

Keep the child's food preferences in mind when planning menus and allow the child to make dietary choices within the prescribed diet. The diet should be high in calories and low in sodium. Calcium supplementation may be given when the child is receiving corticosteroids. Encourage the child to eat by presenting attractive meals with small portions. Mealtimes should center on pleasurable socialization and be provided in a relaxed atmosphere. Encourage the child to eat meals with other children on the unit. Fluids are generally not restricted except during severe edema.

PRACTICE ALERT

Traditionally, a high-protein, low-salt diet was recommended for children with MCNS. Current data, however, suggest that the high-protein diet increases urinary protein loss and may accelerate the development of renal failure. On the other hand, low-protein diets may lead to protein deficiency. For these reasons, a regular-protein, low-salt diet is recommended.

Promote Rest

Provide opportunities for quiet play as tolerated, such as drawing, playing board games, listening to tapes, and watching videos. Adjust the child's daily schedule to allow rest periods after activities. Signs of fatigue may include irritability, mood swings, or withdrawal. Partner with the family and educate the parents and child about the importance of rest. Limiting visitors during the acute phase of the illness may be necessary. Telephone and e-mail contacts may be encouraged as an alternative to visitors. Encourage the child's peers to communicate by telephone calls, cards, computers, and letters. To provide a sense of control, encourage the child to set his or her own limits on activity.

Provide Emotional Support

Parents and children often require support to cope with this chronic disease. Provide parents with thorough explanations about the child's disease and treatment regimen. Parental anxiety in combination with the hospitalization may interfere with the child's independence. Partner with the parents and assist them in promoting the child's independence by allowing the child to select food from the menu or to select the daily activity schedule. Allowing choices when possible provides the child with some sense of control.

Children with MCNS may experience a distorted body image related to sudden weight gain and edema. Behavioral manifestations may include refusal to look in the mirror, refusal to participate in care, and decreased interest in appearance. Encourage children to express their feelings. Assist the child to maintain a normal appearance by promoting normal grooming routine and encouraging them to wear their own pajamas rather than hospital gowns. Scarves or hats may be used to lessen the child's edematous appearance.

Discharge Planning and Home Care Teaching

Provide parents and school-age children with explanations of the disease process, prognosis, and treatment plan. Partner with the family and ensure their understanding of medication administration and their ability to identify potential side effects. Educate parents about the need to monitor urine daily for protein, and instruct them to maintain a diary to record results. Monitoring the child's weight each week may help parents identify early stages of fluid retention and signs of relapse before edema occurs.

Care in the Community

Tutoring may be required for a short period after hospital discharge. Partner with the family in establishing a plan for the child to return to school and other normal activities once the acute episode has resolved. In consideration of the child's reduced immunity, emphasize the importance of avoiding contact with individuals who have infectious diseases. Reinforce to parents that as long as the child is receiving corticosteroid therapy or shows signs of MCNS, the no-added-salt diet should be followed. Caution the child and family about the appetite stimulant effects of steroids and to control food intake and weight gain. The schedule for immunizations for the child on immunosuppressive therapy is altered. Refer to Chapter 19∞ for further discussion of immunizations.

Most children do well with corticosteroid therapy; however, relapses commonly occur. Even those children with frequent relapses usually have a spontaneous resolution of MCNS before 30 years of age.

■ Evaluation

Expected outcomes of nursing care include the following:

- The child remains free from infection.
- The child's fluid, electrolyte, and acid–base balance is restored.
- The child's skin integrity remains intact.
- The child's nutritional requirements are met.

Renal Failure

Renal failure (also known as **kidney failure**) occurs when the kidney is unable to excrete wastes and concentrate urine. The two types of renal failure are acute and chronic. Acute renal failure occurs suddenly (over days or weeks) and may be reversible, whereas in chronic renal failure, kidney function diminishes gradually and permanently over months or years.

Both types of renal failure are characterized by **azotemia** (accumulation of nitrogenous wastes in the blood) and sometimes **oliguria** (urine output 0.5 to 1 mL/kg/hr), indicating the kidney's inability to excrete metabolic waste products. Chronic renal failure eventually results in **anuria** (absence of urine ouput). The degree of renal impairment is estimated by the glomerular filtration rate (Hogg et al., 2003).

Acute Renal Failure

Acute renal failure (ARF) occurs when kidney function abruptly diminishes and the kidneys are unable to maintain electrolyte and fluid balances. It may occur because of another serious systemic condition or obstructive disorder. ARF is seen in 2% to 3% of children cared for in pediatric intensive care units and up to 8% of infants cared for in neonatal intensive care units (Vogt & Avner, 2004).

Etiology and Pathophysiology. ARF occurs most frequently in neonates and children who are critically ill with asphyxia, shock, heart failure, and sepsis. It occurs in association with conditions that fall into one of three categories:

- *Prerenal acute renal failure* is a result of decreased blood flow and perfusion to an otherwise normal kidney in association with a systemic condition. Kidney damage is initially absent. Hypovolemia (hemorrhage or dehydration), septic shock, or cardiac failure may precipitate prerenal ARF. This is the most common type of ARF in infants and young children.
- *Intrarenal (intrinsic) acute renal failure* results from primary damage to the parenchymal cells of the kidneys. Damage can be caused by sustained hypoperfusion, infection, diseases such as hemolytic uremic syndrome or acute glomerulonephritis (Prakash, Sen, Kumar, et al., 2003), cortical necrosis, tumor lysis syndrome, prescribed drugs toxic to the kidneys such as aminoglycosides, or unintentional ingestion of drugs or poisons. The structure most susceptible to damage is the kidney tubule. Injury to the tubule resulting in acute tubular necrosis is the most frequent cause of intrinsic renal failure in children.
- *Postrenal acute renal failure* is caused by obstruction of the urinary flow from both kidneys, such as occurs in posterior urethral valves or a neurogenic bladder. Children may have oliguria, or normal or increased urine output. Renal failure without oliguria usually indicates a less severe renal injury. Children who recover from ARF may have residual kidney damage and compromised renal function Figure 31–9 ■.

Clinical Manifestations. With prerenal ARF, a healthy child suddenly experiences nonspecific symptoms that indicate a

PATHOPHYSIOLOGY ILLUSTRATED

Acute Renal Failure

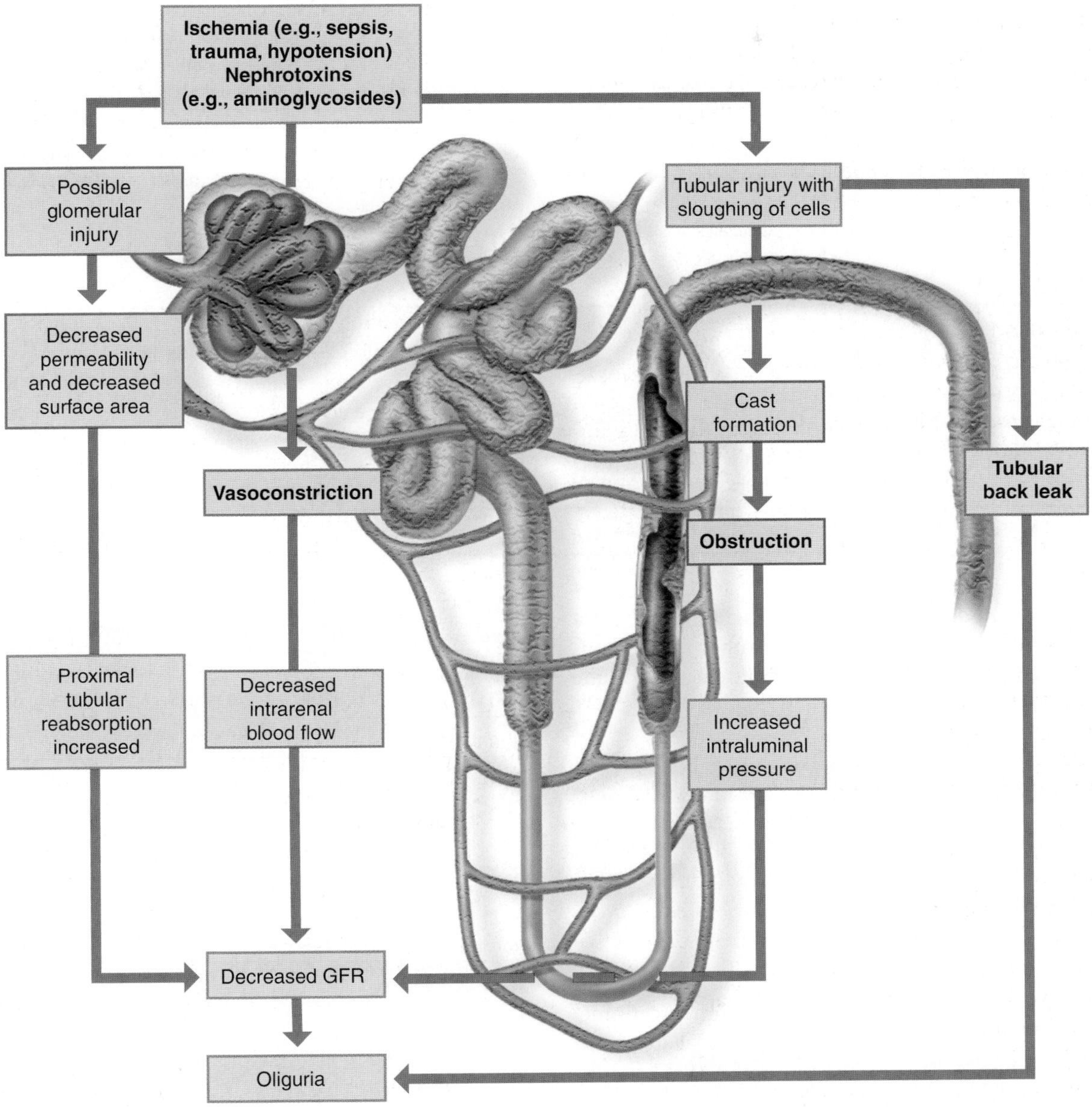

Ischemia (e.g., sepsis, trauma, hypotension) Nephrotoxins (e.g., aminoglycosides)
Possible glomerular injury
Decreased permeability and decreased surface area
Proximal tubular reabsorption increased
Vasoconstriction
Decreased intrarenal blood flow
Tubular injury with sloughing of cells
Cast formation
Obstruction
Increased intraluminal pressure
Tubular back leak
Decreased GFR
Oliguria

FIGURE 31–9 ■ The initial kidney injury is usually associated with an acute condition such as sepsis, trauma, and hypotension, or the result of treatment for an acute condition with a nephrotoxic medication. Injury to the kidney can occur because of glomerular injury, vasoconstriction of capillaries, or tubular injury. All consequences of injury lead to decreased glomerular filtration and oliguria.

significant illness or injury (fever, dehydration or hypovolemia, dry mucous membranes, tachycardia, and poor peripheral perfusion). With intrarenal and postrenal ARF, signs may include nausea, vomiting, lethargy, edema, crackles, gallop heart rhythm, gross hematuria, oliguria, and hypertension. These symptoms are a result of electrolyte imbalances, uremia, and fluid overload. The child appears pale and lethargic. A mass may be palpated in the flank area when cysts, tumors, or an obstructive disorder is present. See the clinical manifestations table on page 1200 for more information. Children with ARF are also more susceptible

CLINICAL MANIFESTATIONS of Electrolyte Imbalances in Acute Renal Failure

ELECTROLYTE IMBALANCE	CLINICAL MANIFESTATIONS	CLINICAL THERAPY
Hyperkalemia Results from inability to inadequately excrete potassium derived from diet and catabolized cells. In metabolic acidosis, there is also movement of potassium from intracellular fluid to extracellular fluid.	• Peaked T waves, widening of QRS on ECG. • Dysrhythmias: ventricular dysrhythmias, heart block, ventricular fibrillation, cardiac arrest • Diarrhea • Muscle weakness	• Eliminate all intake of potassium • Administration of alkalinizing agents • Kayexalate orally or in retention enema • Dialysis if other methods to reduce the potassium level are ineffective
Hyponatremia In the acute oliguric phase, hyponatremia is related to the accumulation of fluid in excess of solute.	• Change in level of consciousness • Muscle cramps • Anorexia • Abdominal reflexes, depressed deep tendon reflexes • Cheyne-Stokes respirations • Seizures	• Electrolyte replacement, sodium bicarbonate • Dialysis to correct severe electrolyte disturbance
Hypocalcemia Phosphate retention (hyperphosphatemia) depresses the serum calcium concentration. Calcium is deposited in injured cells. Hyperkalemia and metabolic acidosis may mask the common clinical manifestations of severe hypocalcemia.	• Muscle tingling • Changes in muscle tone • Seizures • Muscle cramps and twitching • Positive Chvostek sign (contraction of facial muscles after tapping facial nerve just anterior to parotid gland)	• Calcium gluconate • Dialysis to correct severe electrolyte disturbance

Data from Chan, J. C. M., Alon, U., & Oken, D. E. (1992). Acute renal failure. In C. M. Edelman, Jr. (Ed.), Pediatric kidney disease *(2nd ed., pp. 1923–1940). Boston: Little, Brown.*

to infection because of depressed immune functioning. **Uremia** occurs when there is an excess of urea and other nitrogenous waste products in the blood. Neurologic symptoms may include headache, seizures, lethargy, and confusion.

COLLABORATIVE CARE

The goal of collaborative care is to minimize or prevent permanent kidney damage while maintaining fluid and electrolyte balance and managing complications.

Diagnostic Tests

Diagnosis of renal failure is based primarily on urinalysis and blood chemistry results, including BUN, serum creatinine, sodium, potassium, and calcium levels (Table 31–6). Laboratory values vary depending initially on the cause of ARF. They may include anemia, leukopenia, thrombocytopenia, hyponatremia, hyperkalemia, elevated serum BUN and creatinine, and hypocalcemia. Urinalysis may reveal hematuria, proteinuria, and red blood cell or granular casts.

A chest radiograph may reveal pulmonary congestion. Renal ultrasound may reveal hydronephrosis or other structural defects such as cysts or a tumor. A renal biopsy may be required to diagnose ARF when the cause cannot be determined from other tests.

Clinical Therapy

A significant number of children with ARF are admitted to pediatric intensive care units because the disorder is often associated with multiple organ system failure (Williams, Sreedhar,

TABLE 31–6 Diagnostic Tests for Renal Failure

DIAGNOSTIC TESTS	NORMAL VALUES	FINDINGS IN RENAL FAILURE
Urinalysis		
pH	4.5–8	Lowered
Osmolarity	50–1,400 mOsm/L	>500 prerenal <350 intrinsic
Specific gravity	1.001–1.030	High: prerenal ARF Low: intrinsic ARF Normal: postrenal ARF
Protein	Negative	Positive
Serum Chemistry*		
Potassium	3.5–5.8 mmol/L	Elevated
Sodium	135–148 mmol/L	Normal, low, or high, depends solely on the amount of water in the body
Calcium	2.2–2.7 mmol/L	Low
Phosphorus	1.23–2 mmol/L	Increased
Urea nitrogen	3.5–7.1 mmol/L	Increased
Creatinine	0.2–0.9 mmol/L	Increased
pH	7.38–7.42	Low acidic
Hemoglobin	7.27–7.49	Decreased
Hematocrit	11–13.3 g/dL	Decreased
Platelet count	32.7%–39.3% 165–332 × 10^9/L	Decreased Decreased
Albumin	3.5–5.2	Decreased

Please refer to Appendix C ∞ for normal values for various ages

Mickell, et al., 2002). Treatment is dependent on the underlying cause of the renal failure. Initial emergency treatment of children with fluid depletion focuses on intravenous fluid replacement with boluses of normal saline or lactated Ringer's solution at 20 mL/kg given rapidly or over 5 to 10 minutes to ensure renal perfusion. In severe volume depletion, fluid boluses are repeated until circulation is stabilized. Albumin may also be administered when blood loss is the cause of circulatory depletion. If oliguria persists after restoration of adequate fluid volume, intrinsic renal damage is suspected.

Children with fluid overload, such as those with pulmonary edema, require diuretic therapy. If response to diuretics is poor, fluid restrictions are initiated. Fluid requirements are calculated to maintain zero water balance. Intake should equal output. All potential sources of potassium intake are eliminated until hyperkalemia is controlled. Kayexalate may be given orally or by enema to treat hyperkalemia. Other electrolyte imbalances may also need intervention, such as metabolic acidosis, hyponatremia, and hypocalcemia. Antibiotics are prescribed for infection. Nephrotoxic antibiotics such as aminoglycosides are avoided. Refer to the table below for medications used to treat complications of acute renal failure. Nutrition must be maintained with extra carbohydrate intake during the catabolic state.

Some children whose ARF is unresponsive to management require dialysis to correct severe electrolyte imbalances, manage fluid overload, and cleanse the blood of waste products. The clinical situation and age of the child will determine whether hemodialysis or peritoneal dialysis will be used. Refer to the section on renal replacement therapy later in this chapter.

Prognosis depends on the cause of ARF. When renal failure results from drug toxicity or dehydration that is rapidly treated, the prognosis is generally good. However, ARF that results from diseases such as hemolytic uremic syndrome or acute glomerulonephritis may be associated with residual kidney damage.

NURSING MANAGEMENT

Goals of nursing care for the child with acute renal failure are to promote fluid and electrolyte balance, prevent complications such as infection and injury, and support the child and family.

■ Nursing Assessment and Diagnosis

A complete history and physical examination are necessary to identify progression of symptoms and possible causes for renal failure.

Physiologic Assessment

Assess vital signs, level of consciousness, hydration status, peripheral perfusion, and signs of acute illness or injury. Assess for signs of electrolyte imbalance (see the clinical manifestations table on page 1200). Measurement of the child's weight on admission provides a baseline for evaluating changes in fluid status. Monitor urinalysis, urine culture, and blood chemistry studies. Inspect urine for color (Figure 31–10 ■). Cloudy urine may indicate infection; tea-colored urine suggests hematuria. Assess urine specific gravity and intake and output.

Psychosocial Assessment

The unexpected and acute nature of the child's hospitalization creates anxiety for parents and child. Assess for feelings of anger, guilt, or fear associated with the hospitalization. Assess the

MEDICATIONS Used to Treat Complications of Acute Renal Failure

COMPLICATION AND MEDICATION USED	ACTION OR INDICATION	NURSING CONSIDERATIONS
Hyperkalemia (> 5.8 mmol/L)		
Kayexalate	Exchanges sodium for potassium.	May require up to 4 hours to take effect.
Calcium gluconate 10%	Counteracts potassium-induced increased myocardial irritability.	Monitor for ECG changes. Intravenous infiltration may result in tissue necrosis.
Albuterol	Shifts potassium to the cells.	Give by inhalation.
Metabolic Acidosis		
Sodium bicarbonate or sodium citrate	Helps correct metabolic acidosis by exchanging hydrogen for potassium.	Do not mix with calcium. Complications include fluid overload, hypertension, and tetany.
Hypocalcemia (<2.2 mmol/L)		
Calcium gluconate 10%	Used in presence of tetany; provides ionized calcium to restore nervous tissue function to control serum phosphorus.	Administer slowly to prevent bradycardia. Monitor for ECG changes.
Malignant hypertension (blood pressure >95% for age)		
Sodium nitroprusside, nitroglycerin	Relaxes smooth muscle in peripheral arterioles.	Administer by continuous intravenous infusion; fall in blood pressure is seen within 10–20 minutes.

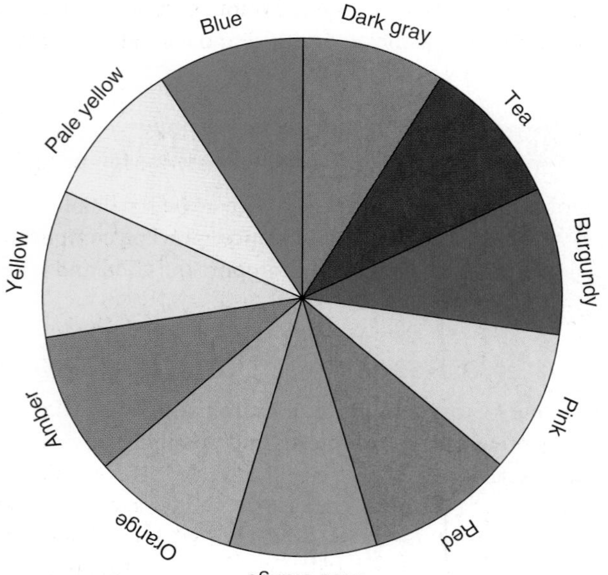

FIGURE 31–10 ■ A color wheel can be used as a guide to standardize descriptions of urine color. Normal urine is pale yellow. Changes in urine color can indicate the following alterations: *yellow*—concentrated urine, *amber*—bile in the urine, *orange*—alkaline or concentrated urine, *red orange*—acid pH, treatment with rifampin, *red*—blood, menses, *pink*—dilute blood, *burgundy*—laxatives, *tea*—melanin, hematuria, *dark gray*—medications, dyes, *blues*—dyes, medications.

From Cooper, C. (1993). What color is that urine specimen? American Journal of Nursing, *93, 97. Copyright © 1993 Connie Cooper, RN, MSN; graphics by Mike O'Grady, RN, MSN.*

child's and parents' coping abilities and the availability of support. Such feelings are likely if ARF developed as a result of dehydration, a preventable injury, or poisoning. Assess coping mechanisms, family support systems, and level of stress.

Examples of nursing diagnoses that may apply to the child with ARF include the following:

- Fluid Volume Excess related to renal dysfunction and sodium retention
- Imbalanced Nutrition: Less than Body Requirements related to anorexia, nausea, vomiting, and catabolic state
- Risk for Infection related to invasive procedures and monitoring equipment, and impaired immune functioning
- Compromised Family Coping related to sudden hospitalization and uncertain prognosis of child

MediaLink Care Plan: A Child with Acute Renal Failure

■ Planning and Implementation

Nursing care focuses on preventing complications, maintaining fluid balance, administering medications, meeting nutritional needs, preventing infection, and providing emotional support to the child and family.

Prevent Complications

Ensure adherence with the treatment plan to reduce potential for complications. Careful monitoring of vital signs, intake and output, serum electrolytes, and level of consciousness can alert the nurse to changes that indicate potential complications. Avoidance of nephrotoxic drugs such as aminoglycosides, aspirin, sulfonamides, tetracycline, and contrast dye with iodine is recommended.

PRACTICE ALERT

Nephrotoxic drugs include the following:

- Antimicrobials: aminoglycosides, cephalosporins, tetracycline, sulfonamides
- Radiographic contrast media with iodine
- Heavy metals: lead, barium, iron
- Nonsteroidal anti-inflammatory drugs (NSAIDs): indomethacin, aspirin

Maintain Fluid Balance

Estimate the child's fluid status by daily monitoring of weight on the same scale, intake and output, and blood pressure two or three times daily. Also monitor serum chemistry values, especially for sodium. The aim of maintaining fluid balance is to achieve a stable serum sodium concentration and a decrease in body weight by 0.5% to 1% a day. The child with renal insufficiency has a concentrating defect. In cases of acute gastrointestinal illness, children are at greater risk for dehydration.

If the child has oliguria, fluid intake—including parenteral nutrition—is limited to replacement of insensible fluid loss from the lungs, skin, and gastrointestinal tract (about one third the daily maintenance requirements in afebrile children). If the child is febrile, fluid administration is increased by 12% for each centigrade degree of temperature elevation.

CLINICAL TIP

If serum sodium concentration rises and weight falls, insufficient fluids are being administered. If the serum sodium level falls and the weight increases, excessive fluids are being administered.

Administer Medications

Antibiotics and antihypertensive agents may be prescribed. Because the kidney's ability to excrete drugs is impaired in ARF, review potential adverse effects of all medications and remain alert for signs of drug toxicity. Monitor drug levels to assess for drug toxicity. The actual dosage of the drug can be reduced or the time interval between doses can be increased to help adjust the dosage and to reduce adverse effects.

Meet Nutritional Needs

Children are at risk of malnutrition due to their high metabolic rate during acute renal failure. Parenteral or enteral feeding may be initially used to minimize protein catabolism. The diet is tailored to the individual child's need for calories, carbohydrates, fats, and amino acids or protein hydrolysates. Depending on the degree of renal failure, sodium, potassium, and phosphorus may be restricted. Oral feeding is initiated as soon as the child can tolerate consumption of foods.

Prevent Infection

The child with ARF is extremely susceptible to nosocomial infections as a result of altered nutritional status, compromised immunity, and numerous invasive procedures. Thorough handwashing and standard precautions are implemented to decrease the risk of infection. Sterile technique is utilized for all invasive procedures and when caring for central and other intravenous lines. Drainage from catheter sites is cultured to assess for the presence of infectious organisms.

Provide Emotional Support

The sudden onset of ARF presents parents with an unexpected threat to their child's life. Both the child and the parents experience anxiety related to the unexpected hospitalization and the uncertainty of the prognosis. Parents often feel guilty, regardless of the cause of renal failure. This guilt is intensified when renal failure is a result of dehydration or poisoning. Partner with parents and encourage verbalization of fears and assist them in working through feelings of guilt. Explain procedures and treatment measures to decrease anxiety. Encouraging parents and older siblings to participate in the child's care can increase their sense of control. Instruct the family that the child may participate in activities as tolerated with periods of rest as needed.

Discharge Planning and Home Care Teaching

Partner with the family to encourage parental involvement early in the child's hospitalization. Ensure that parents understand the importance of administering medications correctly. Educate family members in the proper technique for measuring blood pressure so they can monitor the child's blood pressure when home, if ordered. Make certain that the family can identify symptoms of progressive failure (refer to chronic renal failure discussion).

Nutritional counseling is a key component of discharge planning and is usually performed in collaboration with a nutritionist. Depending on the degree of renal failure, the child's diet may include restrictions on protein, water, sodium, potassium, and phosphorus. Partner with the parents, older child, and dietician to provide written guidelines identifying appropriate food choices and assist the family in menu planning. Ethnic and cultural preferences, as well as the child's food preferences, are considered in listing menu options. See Developing Cultural Competence: Sodium Intake.

Continued monitoring of kidney function during follow-up examinations is critical as deterioration may occur over time. Referral to support groups can be helpful for parents and children alike. The National Kidney Foundation is a source of numerous publications that are helpful to the child and family.

Evaluation

Expected outcomes of nursing care include the following:

- The child remains free from infection.
- The child's fluid, electrolyte, and acid–base balance is restored.
- The child's nutritional requirements are met.
- The child and family demonstrate effective coping.

DEVELOPING CULTURAL COMPETENCE
Sodium Intake

Special effort is often needed to reduce the sodium in the diet of a child of Asian descent. Sauces and seasonings for foods (soy sauce, mustards, monosodium glutamate, and garlic salt) are sodium rich even though the foods seasoned (rice, vegetables, shrimp, and chicken) are low in sodium. The child may ingest up to 18 g of sodium a day with these added sauces and seasonings whereas 4 g per day is the goal. The typical Mexican diet, high in sodium and potassium (avocados, tomatoes, beans) may also require significant modification. Individualized counseling and motivation are needed to encourage families to reduce the child's sodium intake and to use spices low in sodium when preparing meals.

Chronic Renal Failure

Chronic renal failure (CRF) is a progressive, irreversible reduction in kidney function that leads to end-stage renal disease (ESRD), the most advanced form of CRF. In **end-stage renal disease (ESRD),** less than 10% of the kidney is functioning and chronic dialysis treatment or kidney transplantation is required for survival. The prevalence of chronic renal failure in children is approximately 18 per 1 million (Vogt & Avner, 2004). Long-term complications from CRF and ESRD include hypertension, anemia, and bone disease. Children have growth and social developmental issues related to chronic renal disease and the needed treatments.

Etiology and Pathophysiology. In children, the major causes of chronic renal failure are congenital defects, obstructed urine flow and reflux, hereditary diseases such as polycystic kidney disease, glomerular diseases, and systemic diseases such as diabetes and lupus. Congenital defects, cystic, and hereditary diseases are the leading causes of renal failure in young children. In older children, ESRD is more often caused by glomerulonephritis, hereditary disorders, and acquired disorders such as hemolytic uremic syndrome (United States Renal Data System, 2004). Terrell, the child described at the beginning of the chapter, has ESRD resulting from posterior urethral valves, an obstructive defect that caused bilateral kidney damage.

The gradual, progressive loss of functioning nephrons that ultimately results in ESRD is thought to be caused by hyperfiltration injury. As nephrons are destroyed, the remaining nephrons undergo hypertrophy due to an increase in the glomerular blood flow. The nephrons compensate by hyperfiltration for a period to preserve renal function. Progressive damage to the remaining nephrons occurs through the elevated hydrostatic pressure on the capillary walls of the nephrons and increased proteinuria (Vogt & Avner, 2004). In ESRD, the kidneys can no longer maintain homeostasis and the child requires dialysis.

The kidneys function to excrete excess acid in the body and to regulate the body's fluid and electrolyte balance. Renal failure disrupts this fluid and electrolyte balance. As renal failure progresses, the kidneys are unable to excrete the acids that build up in the body and metabolic acidosis occurs. Retention of excessive sodium and water is a common cause of the elevated blood pressure associated with CRF. Insufficient calcium intestinal absorption and hypocalcemia stimulate excessive parathyroid hormone secretion in an effort to correct the hypocalcemia. As CRF

MediaLink Acute and Chronic Renal Failure Resources and Support progresses, phosphorus levels rise and further increase hypocalcemia and parathyroid hormone secretion. Renal **osteodystrophy** (increased resorption of bone caused by chronic hyperparathyroidism) can occur. Since the kidneys are also the site of production of erythropoietin (the growth factor responsible for the production and maturation of red cells), lack of erythropoietin and progressive renal disease are the underlying causes of the anemia of CRF.

Clinical Manifestations. Children with early stages of CRF may be asymptomatic initially. Symptoms do not manifest until the child is in advanced renal failure (refer to the clinical manifestations table for acute renal failure on page 1200). In the early stages, the child may appear pale and complain of headache, nausea, and fatigue. Decreased mental alertness and ability to concentrate may be seen. Anemia leading to tachycardia, tachypnea, and dyspnea on exertion may occur. As the disease progresses, the child experiences a loss of appetite and complications of renal impairment, including hypertension, edema, failure to thrive or short stature, osteodystrophy, delayed fine and gross motor development, and delayed sexual maturation. Growth retardation is caused by disturbances in the metabolism of calcium, phosphorus, and vitamin D; decreased caloric intake; and metabolic acidosis. Osteodystrophy increases the child's risk for spontaneous fractures, rickets, and valgus deformity of the legs.

In end-stage renal disease, the most advanced form of CRF, all body systems are adversely affected by kidney failure. As the severity of the clinical and biochemical disturbances resulting from progressive renal deterioration increase, uremic symptoms develop (see the clinical manifestations table below).

COLLABORATIVE CARE

The management goals for the child with chronic renal failure are to preserve remaining kidney function, slow progression to ESRD, maintain fluid and electrolyte balance, prevent associated complications, and promote growth and development.

Diagnostic Tests

The definitive lab value for determining the degree of chronic renal disease is the glomerular filtration rate (GFR) because it provides the best measure of overall kidney function. To accurately evaluate the stage of chronic renal failure, compare the normal GFR in Table 31–1 with those for stages of CRF in Table 31–7. The patient's GFR is calculated from prediction equations using the serum creatinine level and the patient's height and gender.

TABLE 31–7 National Kidney Foundation Classifications of Stages of Chronic Renal Disease

STAGE	GLOMERULAR FILTRATION RATE (GFR)*	DESCRIPTION
Stage 1	≥90	Kidney damage in the presence of normal or increased GFR
Stage 2	60–89	Kidney damage in the presence of mild reduction of GFR
Stage 3	30–59	Moderate reduction of GFR
Stage 4	15–29	Severe reduction of GFR
Stage 5	<15 (or dialysis)	Kidney failure

**Applies to children 2 years of age and above.*

Data from National Kidney Foundation: The Kidney Disease Outcomes Quality Initiative. (2002). Clinical practice guidelines for chronic kidney disease: Evaluation, classification, and stratification. American Journal of Kidney Disease, 39*(1), S1–S266.*

Additional laboratory tests of the blood and urine, as well as imaging studies, are used to identify kidney damage rather than a kidney biopsy. Serum electrolyte and phosphate levels, BUN, creatinine levels, and pH are used to monitor fluid and electrolyte status. See Table 31–6 for diagnostic findings related to renal failure.

Early recognition of chronic kidney disease is important so interventions can be initiated to slow progression of the disorder. The American Academy of Pediatrics (AAP) recommends urine screening (protein-to-creatinine ratio) at least twice during childhood, once before beginning school and then again during adolescence (Hogg et al., 2003).

Clinical Therapy

Goals of treatment are to slow the progression of kidney disease, prevent complications, and promote growth and development. Conservative treatment includes a combination of dietary and fluid and electrolyte management, control of hypertension, and if that fails and the child progresses to ESRD, dialysis is initiated.

CRF is irreversible; however, the course of the disease is variable. Some children progress quickly to renal failure, necessitating dialysis. Other children are managed with a combination of medication and diet therapy for some time before significant re-

CLINICAL MANIFESTATIONS of Uremic Syndrome

SYSTEM AFFECTED	CLINICAL MANIFESTATIONS	CLINICAL THERAPY
Gastrointestinal	Nausea, vomiting, anorexia, unpleasant (uremic) breath odor	Renal replacement therapy
Hematologic	Progressive anemia	Dietary restrictions of phosphorus, potassium, sodium
Integumentary	Uremic frost (urea crystals deposited on the skin), pruritis	Epoitin alfa
Neurologic	Malaise, headache, progressive confusion, tremors	Antihypertensive agents
Cardiovascular and pulmonary	Pulmonary edema, dyspnea, congestive heart failure	

nal impairment occurs. Frequent modifications in the treatment plan are often necessary to address the child's changing status.

Dietary management focuses on maximizing caloric intake for growth while limiting demands on the kidneys and minimizing fluid and electrolyte disturbances. Calories appropriate for age are recommended; however, restriction of dietary phosphorus, potassium, and sodium are tied to the child's electrolyte levels and fluid balance (Vogt & Avner, 2004). For example, children with renal insufficiency often have hyponatremia while those with progressive renal failure need sodium restrictions to reduce edema. Infants are often given special formula with less potassium, such as Similac 60/40, and the formula may be supplemented with extra carbohydrates, fat, and protein when tolerated. Overnight enteral feedings may be required to achieve adequate caloric intake when growth is impaired. This permits the infant or child to eat foods orally during the day. Children on peritoneal dialysis may lose significant amounts of protein in the dialysate. The child and family should meet with a dietitian who can develop a meal plan specific to the child's growth needs, fluid restrictions, and laboratory values. Vegetable oils, hard candy, sugar, honey, and jelly may be recommended to add calories to the child's diet.

CLINICAL TIP

When CRF is present, extra-high-quality protein, such as meat, fish, poultry, and egg whites, is needed to support growth. Optimal protein intake for infants is 2–2.5 g/kg/day; and for older children, 1.5–2 g/kg/day.

Growth in height and weight are often affected by CRF because of poor appetite and a growth hormone–resistant state. When poor growth is found despite adequate caloric intake and effective treatment of complications of CRF (anemia, renal osteodystrophy, and metabolic acidosis), growth hormone is administered to some children to help them achieve their target height (Pool & Korus, 2002).

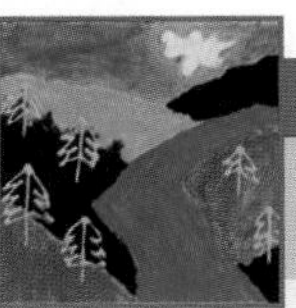

COMPLEMENTARY THERAPY

Avoiding Herbal Supplements in Children with Chronic Renal Failure

Herbal supplements should not be used in children with CRF as they may contain harmful minerals, such as potassium. The child's body is unable to clear waste products like healthy children. There is also the risk for interaction between the herbs and medications taken that could place the child at risk for rejection of a transplanted kidney (National Kidney Foundation, 2004).

Treatment for renal osteodystrophy is initiated early as it begins developing even before ESRD occurs. Phosphate binding agents, vitamin D, and calcium supplementation can help prevent some bone demineralization.

Medications used in the management of chronic renal failure are discussed in the medication table below. (See Complementary Therapy: Avoiding Herbal Supplements in Children with CRF.)

Children who progress to ESRD require renal replacement therapy (see page 1210). The timetable for dialysis or renal transplantation is different from that of adults; transplantation is the ultimate goal so that the child has an optimal chance for a more normal childhood. Earlier initiation of renal replacement therapy can prevent some complications of ESRD. Rather than use the absolute BUN or serum creatinine as the guide, in addition to GFR, nonspecific signs such as uremic syndrome, poorly controlled hypertension, renal osteodystrophy, failure of head circumference measurement to increase normally, developmental delay, and poor growth are used in determining when to initiate renal replacement therapy. Infection is the most common morbidity in children receiving renal replacement therapy, often requiring hospitalization

MEDICATIONS Commonly Used by Children with Chronic Renal Failure

MEDICATION	ACTION OR INDICATION	NURSING CONSIDERATIONS
Vitamin and mineral supplement (Nephrocaps)	Add vitamins and minerals missing from heavily restricted diet	Only prescribed vitamins should be used, over-the-counter brands may contain elements that are harmful.
Phosphate binding agents: Calcium carbonate (Tums), calcium acetate (PhosLo), or sevelamer hydrochloride (Renagel)	Reduce absorption of phosphorus from the intestines	Ensure that phosphate binding agent is aluminum free.
Calcitriol (Rocaltrol)	Replace the calcitriol that kidneys are no longer producing to keep calcium balance normal	Monitor serum calcium level. Ensure that calcium supplement is provided.
Epoetin alfa (Epogen, Procrit)	Stimulates bone marrow to produce red blood cells, treats anemia due to CRF	Given by IV or subcutaneous injection. Monitor blood pressure as hypertension is an adverse effect. Monitor hematocrit and serum ferritin level according to facility guidelines.
Iron supplementation	Treat iron deficiency when epoitin alfa is prescribed	May be administered orally or IV during hemodialysis.
Growth hormone (rhGH)	Used to stimulate growth in children with CRF	Record accurate height measurements at regular intervals.
Antihypertensive agents: Angiotensin-converting enzyme (ACE) inhibitor (enalapril, lisinopril) Loop diuretics	Used with proteinuric kidney disease as it slows the progression to ESRD Used when volume overload is present	Monitor renal function and electrolyte balance.

(United States Renal Data System, 2004). Long-term survival of children is often dependent on renal replacement therapy, with those having a kidney transplant (92%) having a better 5-year survival rate than children treated only with hemodialysis (81%) and peritoneal dialysis (83%) (United States Renal Data System, 2004).

NURSING MANAGEMENT

Goals of nursing care for the child with chronic renal failure are to promote fluid and electrolyte balance, prevent complications associated with renal dysfunction, and promote growth and development.

Nursing Assessment and Diagnosis

Nursing assessment focuses on identifying signs and symptoms of renal failure and associated complications, and assessing the psychosocial effects of renal failure on the child and family.

Physiologic Assessment

The initial and ongoing assessment of the child focuses on identifying complications of renal failure. Observe for signs of hypertension, edema, poor growth and development, and anemia. Assessment of vital signs helps to identify electrolyte alterations.

Psychosocial Assessment

As renal disease progresses, the number of stressors on the child and family increases. Denial and disbelief are common first reactions. A thorough family assessment can help to identify particular needs of the child and family. Preschoolers with progressive CRF are often hospitalized, which interferes with their normal socialization. The school-age child may experience peer prejudice (Pool & Korus, 2002) such as name calling related to appearance. The development of ESRD is particularly challenging during adolescence and the social, psychological, and physical issues related to this chronic illness should be addressed. Nonadherence with treatments can endanger the adolescent's life.

MediaLink Case Study: A Child with Chronic Renal Failure

Nursing diagnoses for the child with CRF are similar to those previously listed for ARF. Additional diagnoses may include the following:

- Delayed Growth and Development related to inadequate protein and caloric intake
- Excess Fluid Volume related to oral fluid intake that exceeds glomerular filtration rate
- Impaired Social Interaction related to hemodialysis schedule during school hours
- Activity Intolerance related to anemia and fatigue
- Disturbed Body Image related to short stature and visible external catheter for dialysis

Planning and Implementation

Children with CRF are frequently hospitalized for one of the following reasons: initial diagnostic evaluation, dialysis treatment initiation, infection, kidney transplant, or other problems. Nursing care for the hospitalized child with CRF focuses on monitoring for side effects of medications, preventing infection, meeting nutritional needs, and providing emotional support and anticipatory teaching.

Monitor for Side Effects of Medications

Assess for signs of electrolyte imbalance such as weakness, muscle cramps, dizziness, headache, and nausea and vomiting in children who are taking diuretics. Supervise the child's activities closely to prevent falls resulting from dizziness, especially at the beginning of diuretic therapy.

Prevent Infection

The child with CRF is extremely susceptible to infections. Use strict aseptic technique for all procedures. Be alert for signs of infection, such as elevated temperature; cloudy, strong-smelling urine; dysuria; cloudy dialysate; changes in respiratory pattern; or productive cough. Emphasize to the child and family the importance of good handwashing practices.

Meet Nutritional Needs

Maintaining adequate nutritional intake in a child with CRF who has dietary restrictions is challenging. See Table 31–8 for foods that children with CRF should avoid. Provide small, frequent feedings and present meals attractively to encourage the child to eat. Partner with the child and family to establish a meal plan with foods that meet the nutritional requirements and acknowledge the child's preferences.

Maintain Fluid Restrictions

Plan the child's oral intake through the entire 24 hours to ensure that the child has some fluids with meals, to take medications, and when thirsty. Keep in mind that many foods have a high fluid content (Jello, popsicles) and must be counted toward the daily fluid allowance. Use medicine cups or small cups for fluids given. Encourage parents and visitors to avoid drinking in the child's presence. Ensure that all visitors know and understand the importance of maintaining the child's fluid restriction.

Provide Emotional Support

Due to the nature of the disease and the complexity of the treatment regimen, the child is traumatized by frequent needle sticks, diagnostic procedures, and hospitalization that may involve periods of separation from the family. Keep the child with the parents as much as possible. Be prepared to offer immediate comfort following a procedure in the absence of the parents. Keep the child's security object close by or provide during comforting after a procedure.

The remainder of the child's family is also significantly affected. Development of progressive CRF requires a total lifestyle change for the child and family. Parents and child require opportunities to express and work through their feelings related to the disease, prognosis, and treatment restrictions. Children can be assisted to express their feelings through drawings or therapeutic play.

TABLE 31–8 Nutritional Information for the Child with Kidney Disease

Children with kidney disease have restricted diets, generally low in sodium, potassium, and phosphorus. A renal dietitian works with families of children with chronic renal failure to develop meal plans that fit a restricted diet. The nurse can help families remember that certain foods must be avoided or eaten in very small quantities by reviewing this table.

HIGH-SODIUM CONTENT FOODS	HIGH-POTASSIUM CONTENT FOODS	HIGH-PHOSPHORUS CONTENT FOODS
Soups and sauces: e.g., gravy, spaghetti and tomato sauce, barbeque sauce, steak sauce *Processed lunchmeats:* e.g., bologna, ham, salami, hot dogs *Smoked meat and fish:* bacon, chipped beef, corned beef, ham, lox Sauerkraut, pickles, and other pickled foods *Seasonings:* horseradish, soy sauce, Worchestershire sauce, meat tenderizer, and monosodium glutamate (MSG)	*Fruit:* apricots, avocados, bananas, citrus fruits, fresh pears, nectarines, dates, figs, canteloupe and other melons, prunes, and raisins *Vegetables:* celery, dried beans, lima beans, potatoes, leafy greens, spinach, tomatoes, winter squash *Whole grains:* especially those containing bran Sardines, clams Peanuts *Dairy products:* milk, ice cream, pudding, yogurt Potassium-containing salt substitutes	*Dairy products:* milk, cheese, yogurt, custard, pudding, ice cream Dried beans, peas Nuts, peanut butter Chocolate Dark cola Sausage, hot dogs

Discharge Planning and Home Care Teaching

Emphasize to the child and family the importance and necessity of long-term treatments and follow-up care. Partner with the family to develop a schedule for medication administration that fits with their routine. Give emphasis to the importance of consistency in administration times. Educate parents on how to recognize side effects of medications and complications associated with the disease.

Appropriate referrals are made to home care nursing agencies as indicated. Parents of children receiving peritoneal dialysis at home are taught how to perform the treatment and how to identify complications (see following section on page 1210). Strict aseptic technique is necessary to prevent infection at the catheter site.

Care in the Community

Children with CRF require frequent outpatient visits to monitor the progression of renal failure and complications, and to evaluate the effectiveness of current treatments. See Health Promotion and Maintenance Overview: The Child with Chronic Renal Failure on page 1208.

Anticipatory Teaching

Provide the child and family with timely information about the disease process, dialysis treatments, and issues related to kidney transplantation as the child's renal failure progresses. Make sure the child receives 23-valent pneumococcal and meningococcal vaccines in addition to usual childhood immunizations. The child should be immunized with live virus vaccines such as measles, mumps, and rubella prior to kidney transplantation.

Education and Socialization

Assist the family to register the child in an early education program to promote development and interaction with other children. Identify a schedule for dialysis that allows the child to participate in school. Encourage frequent handwashing for all children and adults in the classroom to reduce the spread of infection. Educate the school nurse and teachers about dialysis treatment and how to assist the child when a peritoneal dialysis exchange needs to occur during the day. When the child receives hemodialysis, inform the teacher that the child will become increasingly fatigued before the next hemodialysis treatment.

School-age children and adolescents are often embarrassed about being perceived as different from peers, which can occur due to any of the following:

- Short stature
- Dietary restrictions
- Baggy clothing to cover peritoneal dialysis bags
- Frequent absences due to treatments or infections
- Side effects of steroids and other medications to prevent rejection of the transplanted kidney

All children have a need for acceptance and self-esteem. The child with CRF or a kidney transplant may benefit from having a nurse visit the school to talk with the child's peers about the treatments the child requires. Partner with the child and family to assist the child in choosing clothing that can cover the dialysis shunt site and complement and enhance the child's physical appearance.

Psychosocial Support

The necessity for ongoing dialysis treatments and the wait for a suitable donor kidney are stressful for parents and child. Identification of effective coping methods and family support systems is necessary to promote treatment compliance. Partner with the child and family to determine stress factors and strategies for coping. Major stressors for the parents of the child treated with dialysis include appearance and limitations of the child, fluid and nutrition restrictions, education issues, care and emotional health of healthy children, and guilt about their child's illness (Cimete, 2002). The National Kidney Foundation and local support groups for kidney disease can provide the family with additional information and support. (See Evidence-Based Practice: Cultural Aspects of Living with End-Stage Renal Disease.)

Preparation for Kidney Transplant

Kidney transplantation is the optimal treatment for CRF. While the child is waiting for a transplant, remind the family to keep the transplant center informed of any changes in the child's

Health Promotion & Maintenance Overview

The Child with Chronic Renal Failure

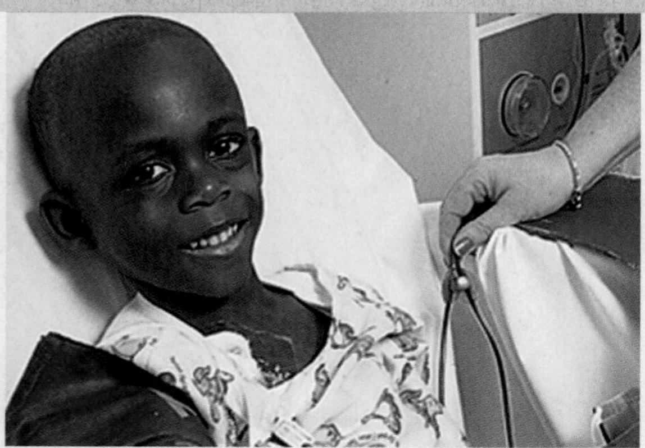

Growth and Development Surveillance

- Compare the child's height, weight, and head circumference to age-specific norms to identify growth retardation and to plot progress.
- Assess developmental progress using the Denver II or another screening tool (refer to Chapter 10∞).
- Educate parents on normal developmental milestones and measures to promote achieving those milestones.
- Assess the adolescent for signs of delayed sexual maturation and, in girls, amenorrhea.

Nutrition

- Review the dietary restrictions with the child and parents.
- Partner with the family to assist the child to make food selections and to restrict fluids and sodium as necessary, taking into account the child's likes and dislikes and cultural background. Encourage the child and family to take a list of a few favorite foods to the dietitian to see if they can be integrated into the child's meal plan.
- Make meal time pleasant and make foods taste more appealing with permitted spices.
- Discuss possible behavioral responses by older children and adolescents to dietary restrictions and limitations imposed by the treatment plan. Involve the child and adolescent in discussions about dietary restrictions and when possible integrate their recommendations for dietary restrictions and fluid management throughout the day.
- Emphasize to the school-age child that dietary and other restrictions are not punishment.
- Use enteral feeding at night to provide the needed calories for growth.
- Discuss a potential reward program that may be effective in motivating the child and adolescent to improve their nutritional habits and adherence to prescribed therapy (Ritz, 2002).

Physical Activity

- Encourage child to participate in developmentally appropriate activities as tolerated.
- Partner with the child to establish a routine plan for physical activity as tolerated that will help promote strong bones.

Oral Health

- Promote good dentition and oral hygiene.
- Schedule regular dental visits for examination and cleaning to reduce infections.
- Partner with the family to ensure they understand the need for antibiotic prophylaxis before certain invasive procedures, including dental care.

Mental and Spiritual Health

- Ask children how they feel about the need to follow a special diet, take medications, and undergo dialysis treatments. Ask what might make it easier for them to cope with the treatments and integrate at least one idea into the care plan.
- Encourage parents to promote their child's participation in age-appropriate activities to minimize the psychologic consequences of coping with a chronic disease.
- Adolescents often resent the dietary restrictions and ongoing dialysis treatments, which pose a threat to their independence, evolving sense of self, and their need for independence. Noncooperation, depression, and hostility are common responses.
- In preparation for transitioning to adult healthcare, encourage adolescents to participate in a program that assists them with transition to adult health services and job skill training (Myers, 2002).

Relationships

- Attendance at school and contacts with peers promotes normal growth and development.
- Work to promote the child's self-worth and a healthy self-esteem.
- Prepare the child for peer conflict.
- Ensure that parents understand the importance of encouraging normal socialization of their child.

Disease Prevention Strategies

- Partner with the child and family to establish plans to avoid large crowds, people with infections, crowds, or other risks that expose the child to infection.
- If possible, all immunizations should be provided before renal transplantation, as long-term immunosuppressive therapy will then be prescribed.
- Live vaccines should not be given to the child taking immunosuppressive agents.
- Encourage the family to maintain scheduled appointments for routine serum and urine diagnostic tests performed to monitor renal function.

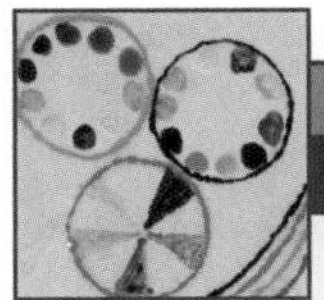

EVIDENCE-BASED PRACTICE

Cultural Aspects of Living with End-Stage Renal Disease

PROBLEM

End-stage renal disease is a serious chronic condition that requires significant adaptations in lifestyle and complex medical treatments that take a toll on the child and family. Children who develop end-stage renal disease are expected to develop adaptive functioning skills as well as cope with the consequences of the disease (physical trauma and operative scars, corticosteroid side effects, dietary restrictions, growth failure, and responses of peers). Parents must modify lifestyles and their hopes and dreams for their children's future. Strategies for managing the disease differ for every family.

EVIDENCE

A study of 35 adolescents, aged 13 to 18 years, was conducted to evaluate their perceptions of themselves and living with end-stage renal disease. Twenty-one of the adolescents provided responses that clustered into one of four groups:

- Normalization, n=8 (identified selves as independent and leading as normal a life as possible)
- Illness causes a barrier to normalcy, n=5 (the physical effects of the disease such as shortened stature affected how they looked and how they were treated by society), had psychological effects
- Illness management was parent focused, n=5 (adolescents wished to be independent but perceived that they were dependent upon parents to help care for them)
- Illness management was self-focused, n=3 (perceived that ongoing treatment for renal disease was very hard, and they perceived that they were different from their peers)

The study group of adolescents was 65.7% Caucasian and 28.6% African American. They were predominantly from intact families and 68.6% had positive treatment outcomes due to renal transplants (Snethen, Broome, Bartels, et al., 2001). Findings from this study vary significantly from others, perhaps due to the characteristics of the study population.

A study conducted in Turkey involving 31 parents of children aged 4.5 to 20 years who receive hemodialysis three times a week revealed stressors related to cultural issues as well as healthcare services available. Finances were a particular concern as the fathers often ended up in low-paying jobs because of the child's illness episodes. Excessively long hours were spent getting health treatments and authorized insurance coverage, and parents feared they would lose their children while waiting for initial dialysis treatment approvals. Other stressors were the concern over the growth and development of the ill children, fluid and dietary restrictions, jealousy of well siblings, and lack of social support. Mothers expressed a hopelessness that no change would occur because finding a kidney for transplant would only happen if they had money to pay for the kidney. Family members usually provided no support except to care for a younger child while the mother took the ill child for medical care. Coping strategies included crying, praying, sharing their feelings with the spouse or other parents, or looking at the positive side of matters (Cimete, 2002).

Another study compared the family resiliency of hemodialysis patients from three cultural groups—Anglo-Americans (n=35), Mexican Americans (n=20), and South Koreans (n=13). Differences in responses to dialysis care were noted by ethnic group. While this study population was adults, cultural values revealed are likely to be applicable to pediatric care. Anglo-Americans and Mexican Americans were similar in their family coping and family resiliency; however, resiliency scores were in the moderate range. South Koreans scored significantly lower in both categories. Anglo-Americans had significantly higher scores on social support, which indicated their greater integration in the community as a source of emotional and network support. Anglo-Americans often find ways to access care when they are chronically ill. The values and beliefs of Mexican Americans include family interdependence, being part of the family unit, and health is a matter of chance or God's will. South Koreans perceived the stressors imposed by their illness to be greater than patients in the other two ethnic groups. The Korean culture has a taboo against the expression of psychological symptoms, and the resulting hesitation to discuss the impact of the chronic illness may cause greater stress. These patients expect to turn to the family when an illness occurs; however, when the illness involves an internal organ and becomes chronic, the family may reject the patient (White, Richter, Koeckeritz, et al., 2002).

PRACTICE IMPLICATIONS

To provide effective nursing care, understanding the impact of culture on such family stress factors and coping strategies is important. End-stage renal disease often is a long-term condition that causes stress. Nurses need to talk with families to learn more about values and beliefs that need to be considered and integrated into care planning.

CRITICAL THINKING APPLICATION

Identify strategies to promote adolescent and family resiliency and coping in each of the ethnic groups described here.

health status, address, or phone number. This will enable the transplant center to notify the family immediately when a kidney is available for transplant.

Transition to Adult Services

As more children with CRF are surviving to adulthood, transition from pediatric to adult services needs to be carefully coordinated. Partner with the adolescent and family to establish a transition plan (refer to Chapter 20∞ for further discussion of the child with a chronic condition transitioning to adulthood). Begin educating the child during early adolescence about his or her health condition, including medications taken and their actions, how to access emergency help, and problems caused by not adhering to treatment. As the adolescent ages, have the family begin giving more responsibility for self-care, such as making appointments for medical care, taking responsibility for obtaining medication refills, and seeking out adult care professionals and dialysis programs. Assist the adolescent to apply for income assistance and Medicare.

■ Evaluation

Expected outcomes of nursing care include the following:

- The child achieves growth and developmental milestones.
- The child's social needs are met through social interaction.
- The child maintains a positive body image.
- The child completes self-care and other activities without fatigue.

Renal Replacement Therapy

Renal replacement therapy is the treatment for renal failure and includes both dialysis and kidney transplantation. In 2002, at least 6,982 children between birth and 19 years received some form of renal replacement therapy. Hemodialysis has emerged as the dominant form of dialysis therapy when treatment is initiated. By the eighteenth month of ESRD treatment, transplant is the dominant treatment method (United States Renal Data System, 2004).

Peritoneal Dialysis

In peritoneal dialysis, the peritoneum of the abdomen is the membrane through which the body's waste products pass from the blood to the abdominal cavity. A catheter is inserted through the abdominal wall into the peritoneal cavity. The dialysis solution that enters the abdomen contains dextrose and pulls body wastes and extra fluid into the abdominal cavity. These wastes and the extra fluid leave the body with the drained dialysate. This form of dialysis is beneficial for small children because it allows continuous removal of fluids and waste products. A continuous steady state of dialysis clearance occurs, decreasing the toxic effects of waste products on the child's developing body. The child can ambulate and interact with the environment. Dietary and fluid restrictions are less severe. The timing of the treatment can be set to minimize the interruption of school, play, or other social events. However, infection or peritonitis is a significant complication.

Two types of peritoneal dialysis are commonly used: continuous ambulatory peritoneal dialysis and automated peritoneal dialysis. Graduated cylinders are used to monitor the volume of fluid exchanged.

- Continuous ambulatory peritoneal dialysis (CAPD) uses gravity to instill prefilled bags of **dialysate** (dialysis solution) into the peritoneal cavity four or five times a day. The fluid remains in the cavity for 4 to 8 hours. The attached bag is folded under the child's clothes, permitting normal activity. After the allotted time, the dialysate is drained by hanging the bag lower than the pelvis. The repeated connections and disconnections with this method are time consuming for the child and family and increase the risk of infection.
- Automated peritoneal dialysis uses an automatic cycler to instill and drain the dialysate about five times over a 10-hour period, usually overnight. One additional exchange may be needed during the day. With this method, the number of connections and disconnections is minimized, which reduces demands on the family as well as the risk of infection. Of the peritoneal dialysis types, this method is preferred since a tailored schedule can be developed to meet the needs of the children to attend school (Verrina, Zacchello, Edefonti, et al., 2001).

The primary complications of peritoneal dialysis are peritonitis and abdominal hernia. See Table 31–9 for other complications. Chronic alterations in peritoneal membrane transport capacity may result from peritonitis, and may lead to peritoneal membrane failure (Warady, Schaefer, Holloway, et al., 2000). Peritonitis is treated with antibiotics infused in the dialysate.

PRACTICE ALERT

The predominant sign of peritonitis associated with peritoneal dialysis is cloudy dialysate. Other signs and symptoms may include fever, vomiting, diarrhea, abdominal pain, and tenderness. The nurse monitors for these symptoms and ensures that the child and family can recognize the symptoms and report immediately.

Nursing Management

Partner with the child and family to assist them in learning appropriate peritoneal dialysis methods and to use aseptic technique when performing dialysis and doing catheter care to reduce the risk for peritonitis. Wash the hands every time before and after touching the catheter. Clean the catheter exit site with antiseptic solution each day. Use sterile gloves to perform the exchanges.

Peritoneal dialysis is time consuming, and commitment by family members is required to manage this procedure daily. Assist the family to develop home routines that minimize disruptions to attending school and daily family life. Reinforce the importance of adhering to the prescribed exchanges every day to provide the child with the best clearance and general health status. For additional information, refer to the nursing care plan for the child receiving home peritoneal dialysis.

TABLE 31–9 Complications of Peritoneal Dialysis

COMPLICATION	MANIFESTATIONS	CAUSE
Peritonitis	Cloudy dialysate, abdominal pain, tenderness, leukocytosis, nausea or vomiting, fever (neonatal hypothermia), constipation	*Staphylococcus aureus, Staphylococcus epidermidis,* fungal infections, gram-negative rods (risk is proportional to duration of dialysis and inversely proportional to age)
Pain	During inflow	Too rapid a rate of infusion, too large a volume of dialysate, encasement of catheter in a false passage, extremes in temperature of dialysate
	During outflow at end of emptying	Omentum entering catheter at end of outflow
Leakage	Fluid around catheter, edema of penis or scrotum secondary to leakage into abdominal subcutaneous tissue, fluid leakage to pleural spaces through diaphragm	Overfilling of abdomen, catheter that has migrated from peritoneal cavity
Respiratory symptoms	Shortness of breath, decreased breath sounds in lower lobes, inadequate chest expansion	Abdominal fullness that compromises diaphragm movement, hole in diaphragm allowing dialysate into chest cavity

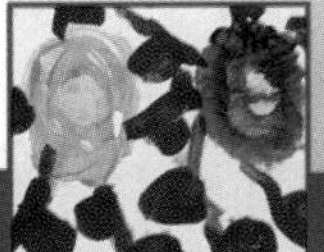

Nursing Care Plan

THE CHILD RECEIVING HOME PERITONEAL DIALYSIS

GOAL	INTERVENTION	RATIONALE	EXPECTED OUTCOME
1. Altered Nutrition: Less than Body Requirements related to poor appetite, feeling of fullness after a small amount, and loss of protein in dialysate			
	NIC Priority Intervention—*Nutrition Management:* Assistance with or provision of a balanced dietary intake of foods and fluids		**NOC Suggested Outcome—***Nutrition Status:* Food and fluid intake. Amount of food and fluid taken into the body over a 24-hour period.
The child will obtain adequate nutrients each day.	▪ With a dietitian, develop a meal plan to identify the amounts of essential nutrients needed. ▪ Provide small, frequent meals of needed nutrients. ▪ Make mealtimes pleasant and avoid battles over the child's intake. ▪ Provide supplements by tube feeding if oral intake is inadequate.	▪ Parents need concrete guidelines for food preparation. ▪ The child will feel full with smaller amounts of food because of the dialysate. ▪ The child will be more inclined to eat if there is less stress. ▪ Adequate nutrition is important for growth and development, and must be supported if oral intake is inadequate.	The child's intake is adequate for an expected growth pattern to be maintained.
2. Risk for Infection related to daily invasive procedure			
	NIC Priority Intervention—*Infection Control:* Minimizing the acquisition and transmission of infectious agents		**NOC Suggested Outcome—***Risk Control:* Actions to eliminate or reduce actual personal and modifiable health threats
The child will not develop peritonitis.	▪ Wash hands, use sterile gloves, and use aseptic technique for connection and disconnection of catheters. ▪ Perform daily catheter site care.	▪ Aseptic technique reduces chance of introducing bacteria into the abdomen. ▪ Skin around the catheter site will have fewer organisms that could potentially cause infection.	The child does not develop peritonitis.
If peritonitis occurs, it will be treated appropriately.	▪ Observe for signs of infection (fever, abdominal pain, cloudy dialysate). ▪ Report signs of infection to physician immediately.	▪ Early identification of infection will reduce complications. ▪ Rapid intervention may reduce need for hospitalization.	Hospitalization may not be needed for peritonitis due to early identification and prompt treatment.
3. Caregiver Role Strain related to daily dialysis treatments			
	NIC Priority Intervention—*Caregiver Support:* Provision of necessary information, advocacy, and support to facilitate primary patient care by someone other than a healthcare professional		**NOC Suggested Outcome—***Caregiver Performance:* Direct care: Provision by family care provider of appropriate personal and healthcare for a family member or significant other
The family copes with daily demands for the child's dialysis treatments.	▪ Discuss the importance of daily, consistent dialysis treatments for the child's overall health status. ▪ Collaborate with the family to identify strategies that could reduce the impact of dialysis on the family's life. ▪ Refer the family to local support groups for emotional support, treatment strategies, and respite care.	▪ If parents understand the need for consistent dialysis treatments, they are more likely to adhere to guidelines. ▪ When the family participates in planning care, compliance is more likely. ▪ Support groups may help the family develop effective coping strategies.	The family adheres with daily dialysis treatment guidelines.

(continued)

Nursing Care Plan THE CHILD RECEIVING HOME PERITONEAL DIALYSIS (continued)

GOAL	INTERVENTION	RATIONALE	EXPECTED OUTCOME
4. Body Image Disturbance related to small size and perception of being and looking different			
	NIC Priority Intervention—*Body Image Enhancement:* Improving a patient's conscious and unconscious perceptions and attitudes toward his/her body		**NOC Suggested Outcome—***Psychosocial Adjustment:* Life change: Psychosocial adaptation of an individual to a life change
The child will develop a sense of self-worth and self-esteem.	■ Identify and emphasize the child's strengths (e.g., interaction style, skills, or cognitive abilities) despite being smaller than peers.	■ Perception of personal strengths should increase self-esteem.	The child effectively interacts with peers and participates in age-appropriate activities.
	■ Assist the child and family to identify popular clothing styles that hide the protuberant abdomen, dialysate bag, and catheter.	■ Clothing that conforms to current styles will help the child feel less different from peers.	
	■ Increase the child's participation in self-care as appropriate for developmental age.	■ Ability to perform self-care increases the child's sense of control.	
	■ Promote participation in safe activities with peers.	■ Social interaction with peers helps reinforce similarities with others.	
	■ Encourage the child to participate in support groups with other children receiving dialysis when possible.	■ Interactions with other affected children provide a chance to express feelings and frustrations, and to develop successful coping strategies.	
5. Altered Health Maintenance related to chronic condition			
	NIC Priority Intervention—*Health System Guidance:* Facilitating a patient's location and use of appropriate health services		**NOC Suggested Outcome—***Health-seeking Behaviors:* Actions to promote optimal wellness, recovery, and rehabilitation
The child's routine health maintenance visits will be integrated with management of the chronic condition.	■ If a renal specialty team is not conveniently located and providing general healthcare, ensure the child has a primary care provider working in collaboration with the renal team.	■ A source of health maintenance and acute minor illness care is important, especially if the family lives a distance from the tertiary care center.	The child is fully immunized at appropriate intervals and the family has a source of regular care in the community.
	■ Assess the child regularly for height growth and developmental progress and signs that the chronic condition is being managed effectively.	■ Routine assessments will allow potential complications to be identified earlier.	
	■ Provide immunizations as recommended for the child with a chronic condition.	■ Immunizations may reduce the risk of potentially life-threatening infections in a child at high risk.	
	■ Provide anticipatory guidance related to safety, developmental progress, appropriate physical activities, and behavior management.	■ Information will help the family support the child's health status and promote development.	

Hemodialysis

In hemodialysis the blood flows through a machine with a special filter that removes body wastes and extra fluids. Blood is pumped out of the body and through a dialyzer, where waste products and extra fluids diffuse out across a semipermeable membrane. Dialysate is pumped in the direction opposite blood flow to promote waste extraction. Differences in osmolarity and concentration between the child's blood and the dialysate alter the intravascular electrolyte concentration and reduce the intravascular volume (Figure 31–11 ■).

Hemodialysis is once again emerging as the dominant initial dialysis therapy among children (United States Renal Data System, 2004). Hemodialysis is used in the critical care setting and for those children with CRF when peritoneal dialysis is not possible for technical reasons or when the family is unable to provide peritoneal dialysis safely. Hemodialysis for children is offered in a special dialysis center on an outpatient basis, or it can be performed at bedside during hospitalization. Treatment is usually performed three times a week, with each session lasting approximately 3 to 4 hours. In the opening scenario, Terrell's

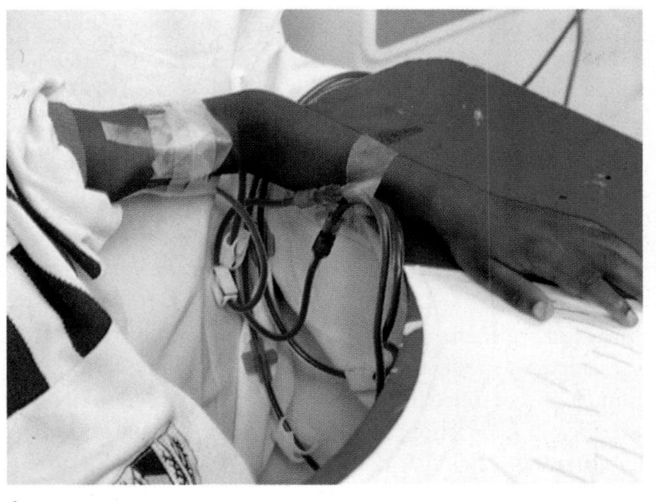

A

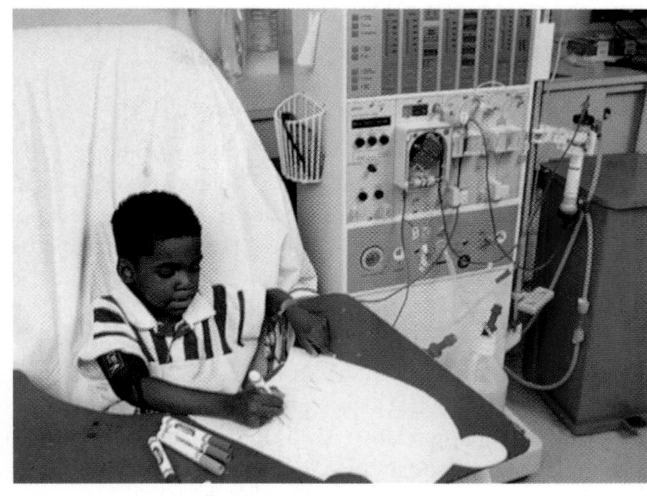

B

FIGURE 31–11 ■ This child is undergoing hemodialysis. *A,* Note the surgically implanted vascular graft. One needle is placed in the arterial end of the graft (red tubing), and one needle is placed in the venous end (blue tubing) for blood return. *B,* The child is able to draw or perform other quiet activities during dialysis treatment. Note that the child's blood pressure is carefully monitored throughout the treatment.

healthcare providers and his family made the decision to switch from peritoneal dialysis to hemodialysis after he developed several episodes of peritonitis in a single year.

Children over 20 kg (44 lb) often have an arteriovenous fistula (connection between an artery and a vein) created for long-term vascular access. Alternatively, a synthetic tube can be implanted under the skin creating a graft between the arterial and venous circulation to provide vascular access. Two needles are inserted into the arteriovenous fistula, one to carry blood to the dialyzer and one to return cleaned blood to the body. In emergency and for infants, a double-lumen cannula is inserted into a large vein (e.g., the femoral, jugular, or subclavian vein) for hemodialysis. With current technology, very-low-birth-weight infants can be safely hemodialyzed using a venous catheter for access.

Hemodialysis is more efficient than peritoneal dialysis but requires close monitoring for symptoms related to hypotension or rapid changes in fluid and electrolyte balance that may lead to shock. Uncommonly, a **disequilibrium syndrome** may occur during or soon after the dialysis procedure is first performed. Disequilibrium syndrome results from cerebral edema caused by a drop in plasma osmolality during dialysis. Symptoms of disequilibrium syndrome vary, but include nonspecific complaints of fatigue, nausea, vomiting, or tremors. More extreme cases may result in delirium, seizures, or coma. Symptoms begin during or shortly after dialysis and usually resolve within 24 hours (Hill, 2001). Other complications include access thrombosis and infection. Heparin is used to achieve an active clotting time of 150%, which reduces the risk of thrombosis.

Nursing Management

Monitor fluid balance in the child undergoing hemodialysis. Monitor vital signs and blood pressure every half hour. Monitor oral intake and urinary output every half hour while the child is on the dialysis equipment. Weigh the child before and after the dialysis to determine any fluid imbalances that require adjustment during the next hemodialysis session.

Nursing management also focuses on educating the child and family about the administration of heparin and the control of bleeding from minor trauma. Since dietary limitations are needed more often with hemodialysis than with peritoneal dialysis, partner with the family to ensure understanding of how to plan and provide for the child's daily nutritional needs. Methods to reduce the risk of infection are reviewed, including the provision of daily care to the catheter site. Encourage showering rather than tub baths. Activities such as swimming may be discouraged.

Continuous Renal Replacement Therapy

Continuous renal replacement therapy (CRRT) is a form of continuous hemodialysis treatment, used 24 hours per day when the child has acute renal failure, multiple organ failure, and hemodynamic instability. Advantages of CRRT include less risk of fluid overload, improved hemodynamic status, balanced lactic acid levels, decreased extravascular lung water, and lower rates of morbidity and mortality. Disadvantages of CRRT include the potential for filter clotting from hypoperfusion, risk of bleeding, possible air embolism, limited mobility related to catheter placement, and slower solute and fluid removal than hemodialysis (Kaplow & Barry, 2002). Contraindications for CRRT include coagulopathy, active bleeding, and liver disease.

Nursing Management

Nursing management focuses on monitoring the child's hemodynamic status, cardiac rhythm, mental status, breath sounds, and skin turgor. Admittance to the intensive care unit is required for constant observation, which may include central venous pressure and pulmonary artery pressure. Intake and output should be monitored hourly. Pharmacologic interventions may include sodium bicarbonate or other electrolytes and vasoactive agents. The nurse should constantly monitor for signs of hemorrhage.

Monitor for heat loss which occurs during filtration of the blood (Kaplow & Barry, 2002).

Kidney Transplantation

Kidney transplantation provides the only alternative to long-term dialysis for children with ESRD (Figure 31–12 ■). Kidney transplantation can normalize physiology and provide a potential for normal growth. Because of the adverse effects on growth and development resulting from delaying transplantation, children are often given priority over adults awaiting transplantation.

Blood type compatibility between the kidney donor and the recipient is necessary for a successful transplantation. A human leukocyte antigen (HLA) system match also improves survival of the graft. A living relative donor kidney has a higher survival rate than a cadaver (postmortem donation) kidney. Survival rate for living donor transplantation in children younger than 2 years is 85%, and for older children, the survival rate is 95%. Cadaveric kidney transplantation survival rates in children younger than 2 years are lower due to an increased risk of graft loss (Pool & Korus, 2002). See Developing Cultural Competence: Race and the Waiting List.

Children and their families are screened carefully prior to transplant in an effort to identify problems that could lead to rejection of the kidney or infection. For example, the child is screened for hepatitis, cytomegalovirus, varicella-zoster, Epstein-Barr virus, and HIV as these could be devastating infections once the immune system is suppressed. The child should be fully immunized prior to transplant. The child and family may be fully evaluated by a psychologist to identify strengths, weaknesses, and coping skills that would be important in adherence to the immune suppression treatment following transplant (Hillerman, Russell, Barry, et al., 2002).

After transplantation, the child receives immunosuppressive medications such as corticosteroids, azathioprine, cyclosporine, and antilymphocyte antibodies to suppress rejection. Immunosuppression regimens use various combinations and sequences of these drugs to reduce the incidence of acute and chronic rejection. Signs of rejection include fever, increased BUN and serum creatinine levels, pain and tenderness over the abdomen, irritability, and weight gain.

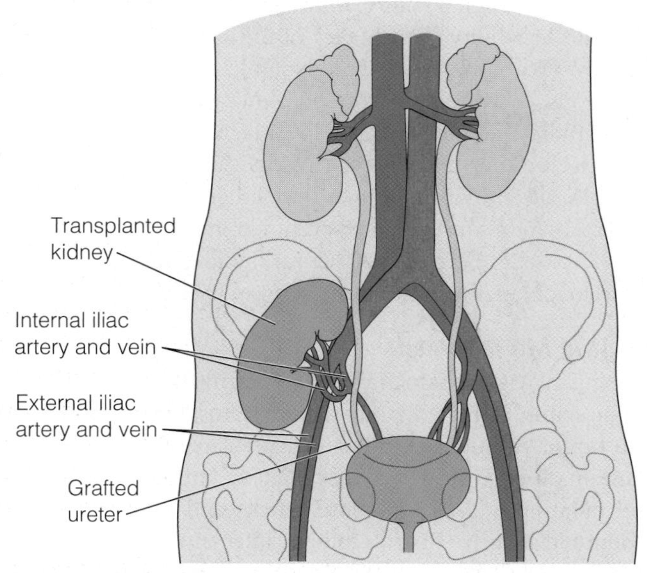

FIGURE 31–12 ■ The transplanted kidney is placed in the iliac fossa with anastomosis to the hypogastric artery, iliac vein, and bladder.

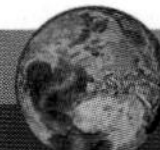

DEVELOPING CULTURAL COMPETENCE
Race and the Waiting List

Racial differences exist with regard to access to the renal transplant waiting list. Black children are 12% less likely to be placed on the waiting list than Whites at any point in time. It is unknown if these differences are due to physician bias in identifying transplant candidates, patient or family preference, or differences in the time before seeing a nephrologist (Furth, Garg, Neu, et al., 2000).

Complications of immunosuppression therapy include opportunistic infection, lymphomas and skin cancer, and hypertension. Nonadherence with therapy is the primary cause of transplanted kidney loss in 10% to 15% of all pediatric kidney transplant recipients. Nonadherence with immunosuppression management is highest among families with instability, adolescents, females, and in children with a previous kidney loss due to nonadherence (Griffin & Elkin, 2001). Adherence is higher in adolescents when their parents are knowledgeable and supportive, and when they promote the adolescent to become competent in self-care (Pool & Korus, 2002). Some primary kidney diseases, such as glomerulonephritis and hemolytic uremic syndrome, can also recur in the transplanted kidney.

In addition to the immunosuppression therapy, the child will need ongoing monitoring and management of anemia, renal osteodystrophy, and short stature. The steroids used for immunosuppression may have a similar impact on bone resorption and growth hormone suppression as renal osteodystrophy. Growth hormone therapy is often prescribed following kidney transplant in young children to promote height growth and new bone formation (Alon, 2001).

Nursing Management

Nursing management includes partnering with child and family to ensure understanding of the transplantation process before it occurs to help prepare them for the experience. The child and family experience rigorous protocols related to the complex medical history and the treatments related to the transplant. Discuss all aspects of the child's care that will have an impact on the family's life, including follow-up appointments, medications, and general health promotion. Emphasize that adherence with treatments is essential for the success of the transplant. Evaluate the child and parents' understanding of and adherence to the prescribed regimen. Education is ongoing, and requires frequent evaluation of child and parental understanding. Monitor adherence to immunosuppression treatment at each visit in an effort to identify any issues early. Families and children need to understand that nonadherence places them at risk for rejection of the kidney and return to dialysis. Special supports to the family and child, especially during periods of extra stress or family disruption, may be necessary to enable them to maintain the daily immunosuppression regimen (Bell, 2000). Ensure that the parents, and child if older, have the ability to recognize the signs of acute rejection and infection, and understand when and how to notify the child's physician if immediate care is required.

The burden of life-long treatment which includes changes in family lifestyle, financial obligations, frequent hospitalizations, and dependency on technology can lead to stress for the child and family (Cimete, 2002). The repeated hospitalizations, surgery, and medical procedures are stressful to children of all ages (Aley, 2002). Partner with the child and family in identifying stressors. Determine the child and family's coping mechanisms and availability of support. Promote the child's healthy responses to stress and their psychosocial well-being by encouraging therapeutic play during hospitalizations that is structured to the developmental age of the child.

Acute Postinfectious Glomerulonephritis

Glomerulonephritis is the most common inflammation of the glomeruli of the kidneys. In children, it is most often a response to a *group A beta-hemolytic streptococcal* infection of the skin or pharynx. Glomerulonephritis is also caused by other organisms including *Staphylococcus, Pneumococcus,* and coxsackievirus. The incidence of acute postinfectious glomerulonephritis (APIGN), also known as acute poststreptococcal glomerulonephritis (APG), is highest in children who are 2 to 12 years of age, and the disorder is more common in boys than in girls by a ratio of 2 to 1 (Lang & Towers, 2001). Early antibiotic therapy for streptococcal infection does not seem to prevent the development of APIGN. This disease is a significant cause of acute and chronic renal failure in children.

Etiology and Pathophysiology

The child with APIGN usually becomes ill after contracting a nephritogenic strain of group A beta-hemolytic streptococcal infection of the upper respiratory tract or the skin. Often the child contracts a streptococcal infection (e.g., strep throat), recovers, and then develops signs of APIGN after an interval of 8 to 14 days.

Glomerular damage occurs as a result of an immune complex reaction that localizes on the glomerular capillary wall (Figure 31–13 ■). Antibody–antigen complexes are deposited in the glomeruli, leading to inflammation and glomerular injury. Capillaries in the glomeruli are obstructed by damaged tissue cells and the glomerular filtration rate is reduced. Vascular permeability increases allowing red blood cells and red cell casts to be excreted. Sodium and water are retained, expanding the intravascular and interstitial compartments. As permeability increases, protein molecules escape into the filtrate. This process results in the characteristic finding of edema (Lang & Towers, 2001).

Clinical Manifestations

Half of all children affected are asymptomatic. In the remainder the onset is usually abrupt with flank or midabdominal pain, irritability, malaise, and fever. Microscopic hematuria is present in nearly all cases, while gross hematuria, resulting in smoky or tea-colored urine, is found in up to 50% of cases. Dysuria accompanies gross hematuria. Mild periorbital and dependent edema occurs as a result of glomerular inflammation and decreased filtration. Edema may progress in severity to cause dypsnea, cough, ascites, crackles, and a gallup rhythm (Lang & Towers, 2001). Acute hypertension may cause an encephalopathy that includes headache, nausea, vomiting, irritability, lethargy, and seizures. Oliguria may or may not be present. Costovertebral tenderness may occur and is related to stretching of the renal capsule from edema.

COLLABORATIVE CARE

The goal of collaborative care for the child with APIGN is to preserve renal function and prevent complications associated with the disorder.

Diagnostic Tests

A urinalysis reveals hematuria, proteinuria, leukocytes, and red and white cell casts. Serum studies may reveal elevated BUN and creatinine concentrations. Serum protein is decreased (hypoalbuminemia) due to mild to moderate proteinuria. The white blood cell count may be normal or slightly elevated. Hemoglobin and hematocrit reveals anemia, which is common in the acute phase and is generally caused by dilution of the serum by the extracellular fluid. Anemia during the late phase is a result of hematuria. The erythrocyte sedimentation rate is increased in the acute phase, and serum lipid levels are increased in approximately 40% of cases.

Serum IgG antibodies against Streptococcus may be noted if the illness was precipitated by a streptococcal infection. An elevated antistreptolysin O (ASO) titer reflects the presence of antibodies from a recent streptococcal respiratory infection, but the ASO level associated with a recent skin infection is low. The anti-DNAse B titer is helpful for detecting antibodies associated with recent skin infections. Serial tests may be performed to detect a rising titer. Up to 90% of children have reduced serum C3.

An electrocardiogram may reveal changes as a result of circulatory overload. A renal biopsy is not required for a diagnosis of APIGN but may be considered if clinical features are inconclusive (Lang & Towers, 2001).

Clinical Therapy

Treatment focuses on relief of symptoms and supportive therapy. Bed rest is a key component of the treatment plan during the acute phase.

Volume overload and mild to moderate hypertension are treated with medications and restriction of fluids as well as potassium and sodium intake. Initially, only insensible losses are replaced until the status of renal function is known. With severe azotemia, protein intake may have to be limited. Hypertension is generally managed with a combination of an antihypertensive medication such as hydralazine (Apresoline) and a diuretic such as furosemide (Lasix). For more severe hypertension, the child may be treated with intravenous diazoxide, nitroprusside, or hydralazine (Lang & Towers, 2001).

If laboratory results are positive for serologic evidence of streptococcal infection, a course of antibiotics is administered to treat the infection. Throat or skin cultures of close family contacts

PATHOPHYSIOLOGY ILLUSTRATED

Acute Postinfectious Glomerulonephritis

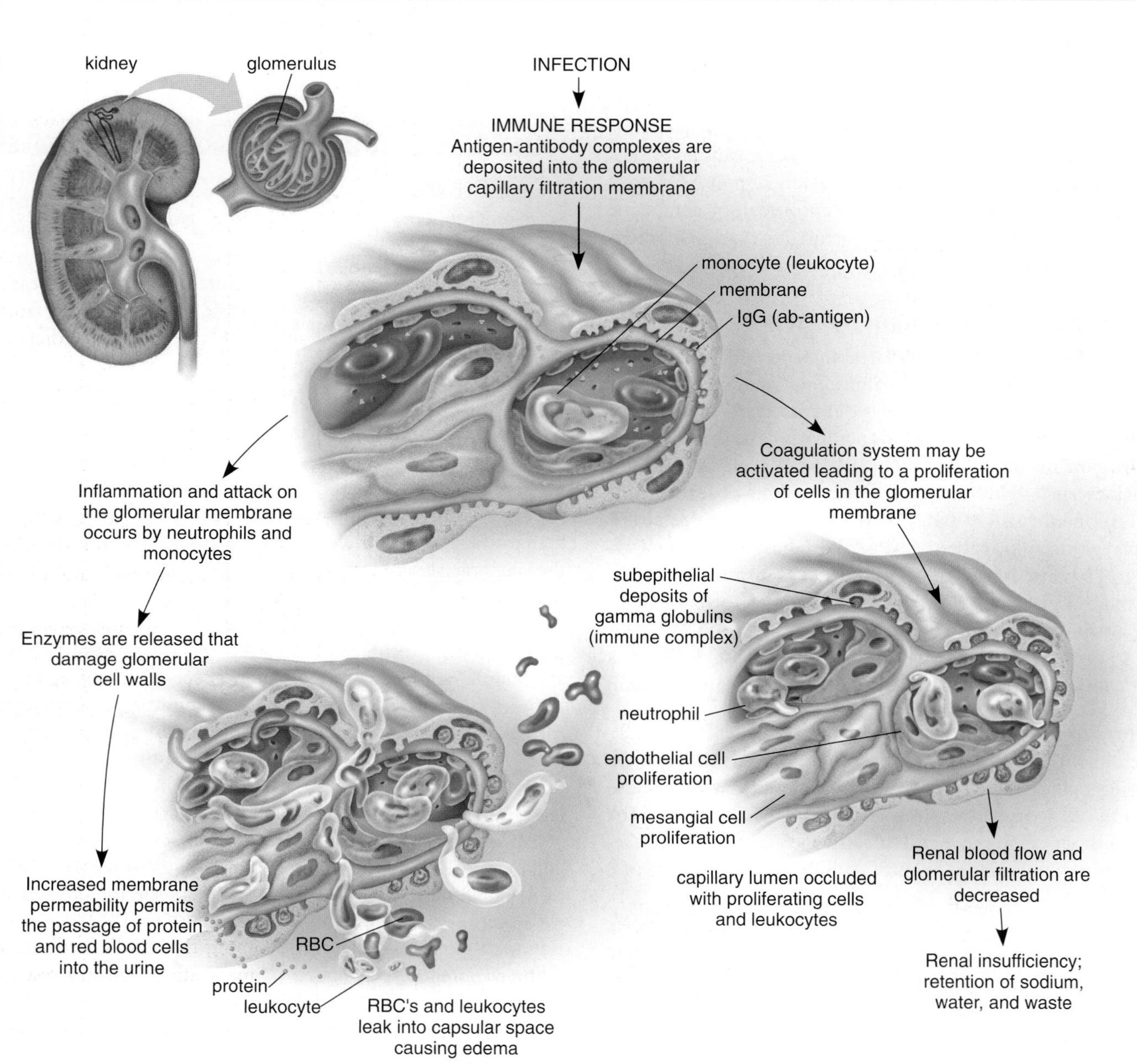
kidney
glomerulus
INFECTION
IMMUNE RESPONSE
Antigen-antibody complexes are deposited into the glomerular capillary filtration membrane
monocyte (leukocyte)
membrane
IgG (ab-antigen)
Coagulation system may be activated leading to a proliferation of cells in the glomerular membrane
Inflammation and attack on the glomerular membrane occurs by neutrophils and monocytes
subepithelial deposits of gamma globulins (immune complex)
Enzymes are released that damage glomerular cell walls
neutrophil
endothelial cell proliferation
mesangial cell proliferation
Renal blood flow and glomerular filtration are decreased
capillary lumen occluded with proliferating cells and leukocytes
Increased membrane permeability permits the passage of protein and red blood cells into the urine
RBC
protein
leukocyte
RBC's and leukocytes leak into capsular space causing edema
Renal insufficiency; retention of sodium, water, and waste

FIGURE 31–13 ■ Infection from group A beta-hemolytic Streptococcus causes an immune response that causes inflammation and damage to the glomeruli. Protein and red blood cells are allowed to pass through the glomeruli. Blood flow to the glomeruli is reduced due to obstruction with damaged cells and renal insufficiency results, leading to the retention of sodium, water, and waste.

should be performed and treatment with penicillin should occur when the culture is positive (Huether, 2002a).

CLINICAL TIP

Antibiotics are *not* a treatment for acute postinfectious glomerulonephritis (APIGN). Instead, antibiotics are prescribed to treat the original infection (such as strep throat or pyoderma).

The prognosis is good for >95% of children with APIGN. Gross hematuria and hypertension generally resolve in a few weeks, and proteinuria resolves over several months. Microscopic hematuria may persist for 1 to 2 years (Patel & Bissler, 2001). Recurrences are unusual. Approximately 2% of children progress to end-stage renal disease (Lang & Tower, 2001).

NURSING MANAGEMENT

Nursing care for the child with APIGN focuses on monitoring fluid status, preventing infection, preventing skin breakdown, meeting nutritional needs, and providing emotional support to the child and family.

Nursing Assessment and Diagnosis

Carefully monitor vital signs, fluid and electrolyte status, daily weight, and intake and output. Document urine specific gravity. Assess the urine color to detect hematuria. (See Figure 31–10.) Hypovolemia can occur as a result of fluid shifting from vascular to interstitial spaces despite the outward clinical signs of excess fluid retention. Assess edema, which may be periorbital or dependent and shifts as the child's position is changed. Monitor the degree of ascites by measuring abdominal girth. Auscultate heart and lung sounds every shift and note respiratory effort to detect signs of fluid overload. Assess for circulatory congestion (crackles, dyspnea, and cough).

Monitor blood pressure, which can rise as high as 200/120 mm Hg. When severe hypertension is present, assess for signs of central nervous system problems (headache, blurred vision, vomiting, decreased level of consciousness, confusion, and convulsions). Assess the child's and parents' level of understanding and the availability of support.

The accompanying nursing care plan lists several nursing diagnoses that may apply to the child with APIGN.

Planning and Implementation

Bed rest is generally required during the acute phase. Immediate emergency care is needed for severe hypertension with cerebral dysfunction; in these cases, antihypertensives are generally administered intravenously.

Maintain Fluid Status

Carefully plan the child's fluid intake over the entire day, including meals, so that some fluids are still available at the end of the day. Make sure parents and visitors understand the need to limit fluids to prevent inadvertent excessive intake. Make sure parents understand that Jello and popsicles are also fluid sources.

Prevent Infection

Impaired kidney function places the child at risk for infection. Monitor for signs of infection including fever, increased malaise, and an elevated white blood cell count. Screen family members for the presence of streptococcal infection and refer for treatment. Partner with the family to reduce exposure of child to infection. Instruct the family in good handwashing technique. Limit visitors, and screen for upper respiratory infections.

Prevent Skin Breakdown

Dependent areas or areas prone to pressure are vulnerable to skin breakdown. Reposition the child frequently. Pad bony prominences or susceptible areas with sheepskin, or protect skin with a transparent dressing. Elevate lower extremities on pillows when in the dependent position or when the child is lying in bed. Ensure the child's bed is free of crumbs or sharp toys. Maintain sheets tight and free of wrinkles. Maintain proper hygiene and dry skin. Diapers are changed frequently.

Meet Nutritional Needs

Partner with the family and multidisciplinary team, including the renal dietitian to establish a dietary plan to meet the child's nutritional needs. In most cases a no-added-salt and low-protein diet is implemented. This diet may be challenging since the child may refuse to eat foods that taste different. Anorexia presents the greatest challenge to meeting daily nutritional requirements during the acute phase of the disease. Encouraging parents to bring the child's favorite foods from home if they are in compliance with the prescribed diet, to serve foods in age-appropriate quantities, and to allow the child to eat with other children or with family members may increase the child's appetite.

Provide Emotional Support

Guilt is a common reaction for parents of a child with APIGN. Parents may blame themselves for not responding more quickly to the child's initial symptoms or may believe they could have prevented the development of glomerular damage. Discuss the etiology of the disease and the child's treatment, and correct any misconceptions. Emphasize that APIGN develops in only a few children with streptococcal or other infections. Provide the child and parents the opportunity to express their concerns. Explain the disease, treatment, and outcome, and allow for questions and further clarification.

Discharge Planning and Home Care Teaching

Children are hospitalized for a few days, although it may require 3 weeks for hypertension and gross hematuria to resolve and longer for complete resolution of the disorder. Discharge planning focuses on teaching parents about the child's medication regimen, potential side effects of medications, dietary restrictions, and signs and symptoms of complications.

Partner with parents and educate them in assessing the child's blood pressure and testing urine for albumin, if ordered. Evaluate the parent's ability by return demonstration of these procedures. Emphasize the importance of avoiding exposure of the child to individuals with upper respiratory tract infections. After discharge, partner with parents to plan for how to allow the child to return to normal routine and activities, with periods allowed for rest.

Evaluation

Expected outcomes of nursing care for the child with APIGN are listed on the nursing care plan.

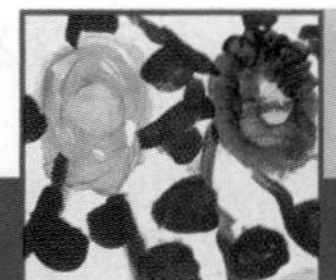

Nursing Care Plan

THE CHILD WITH ACUTE POSTINFECTIOUS GLOMERULONEPHRITIS

GOAL	INTERVENTION	RATIONALE	EXPECTED OUTCOME
1. Excess Fluid Volume related to decreased glomerular filtration and increased sodium retention			
	NIC Priority Intervention—*Fluid Management:* Promotion of fluid balance and prevention of complications resulting from abnormal and undesired fluid levels		**NOC Suggested Outcome—***Fluid Balance:* Balance of water in the intracellular and extracellular compartments of the body
The child will regain normal fluid balance.	■ Assess for edema (periorbital or dependent areas). ■ Calculate fluid intake and plan amounts to offer throughout the day. ■ Limit foods with moderate to high sodium content. ■ Document intake and output. ■ Perform daily weight measurement on same scale at the same time of day. ■ Administer prescribed medications (diuretics and antihypertensives).	■ Sodium and water retention leads to edema. ■ An intake/output ratio of 1:1 reflects normal hydration and kidney function. ■ Further reduction in sodium intake will help balance fluid and sodium retention. ■ Prevents excessive fluid intake. ■ Changes in weight can indicate fluid retention or improvement in condition. ■ Diuretics cause excretion of excess fluid by preventing reabsorption of water and sodium. Antihypertensives increase excretion of water and sodium and cause vasodilation.	The child maintains urine output that is balanced to urine intake. The child receives the appropriate amount of fluid each day.
2. Risk for Infection related to renal impairment and corticosteroid therapy			
	NIC Priority Intervention—*Infection Protection:* Prevention and early detection of infection in a patient at risk		**NOC Suggested Outcome—***Risk Control:* Actions to eliminate or reduce actual, personal, and modifiable health threats
The child will develop no secondary infection.	■ Assess temperature every 4 hours. Observe for signs of infection. ■ Obtain throat culture and other cultures as ordered.	■ The child is at risk for secondary infection. ■ Cultures can identify causative microorganisms in secondary infections or presence of residual streptococcal infection.	The child's temperature remains within normal limits and the child is free of secondary infection.
3. Risk for Impaired Skin Integrity related to tissue edema			
	NIC Priority Intervention—*Pressure Management:* Minimizing pressure to body parts		**NOC Suggested Outcome—***Risk Control:* Actions to eliminate or reduce actual, personal, and modifiable health threats.
The child's skin integrity will remain intact.	■ Assess skin for redness, abrasions, and breakdown secondary to edema, bed rest, and skin rubbing against sheets. ■ Encourage position changes every 1–2 hours. Provide skin care. Use a therapeutic mattress.	■ Ensures early identification and implementation of preventive measures. ■ Prolonged pressure leads to decreased circulation and skin breakdown.	The child develops no areas of redness, abrasions, or skin breakdown over pressure points.
4. Imbalance Nutrition: Less than Body Requirements related to loss of appetite			
	NIC Priority Intervention—*Nutrition Management:* Assistance with or provision of balanced dietary intake of foods and fluids		**NOC Suggested Outcome—***Food and Fluid Intake:* Amount of food and fluid taken into the body over a 24-hour period
The child will maintain adequate caloric intake.	■ Maintain meal schedule similar to that at home. Serve food in age-appropriate serving sizes. ■ Assess for food likes and dislikes. Provide favorite foods if allowed.	■ Normal routines and small frequent serving sizes help child feel less overwhelmed by calories needed. ■ Favorite foods may encourage child to eat.	The child maintains pre-illness body weight and tolerates the daily food intake that meets nutritional requirements.

Nursing Care Plan THE CHILD WITH ACUTE POSTINFECTIOUS GLOMERULONEPHRITIS (continued)

GOAL	INTERVENTION	RATIONALE	EXPECTED OUTCOME
5. Activity Intolerance related to fluid and electrolyte imbalance, infectious process, and altered nutrition			
	NIC Priority Intervention—*Energy Management:* Regulating energy use to treat and prevent fatigue and optimize function		**NOC Suggested Outcome—***Energy Conservation:* Extent of active management of energy to initiate and sustain activity
The child will progress in activity tolerance without excessive fatigue as the disease process improves.	■ Maintain bed rest during acute stage. Encourage gradual activity increase as the condition improves. ■ Provide quiet play for developmental stage of child (e.g., coloring books, music, videos, television).	■ Rest decreases the production of waste materials, which place increased stress on the kidneys. ■ Quiet activities minimize energy expenditure and stress on the kidneys.	The child avoids fatigue and exhibits the ability to tolerate activity for a longer period each day.
6. Effective Therapeutic Regimen Management related to parent's ability to manage child's medication schedule and treatment regimen at home			
	NIC Priority Intervention— *Anticipatory Guidance:* Preparation of patient for an anticipated developmental and/or situational crisis		**NOC Suggested Outcome—** *Compliance Behavior:* Actions taken on the basis of professional advice to promote wellness, recovery, and rehabilitation
The parents will state knowledge of the child's treatment regimen after discharge.	■ Assess parents' understanding of need for adherence to medication schedule, fluid limits, and dietary restrictions. ■ Collaborate on development of best schedule for giving medications to match child's and family's routines. ■ Inform parents about potential side effects of prescribed medication and signs of complications.	■ Diuretics, antihypertensives, fluid limits, and dietary restrictions in sodium and potassium are central to the treatment plan. ■ Partnering with the family improves adherence. ■ Allows for early intervention in case of problems to prevent complications.	The parents administer medications as prescribed. The child's sodium and potassium levels reflect adherence to dietary restrictions.

Hemolytic Uremic Syndrome

Hemolytic uremic syndrome (HUS) is an acute renal disease that is the most common cause of acute renal failure. HUS is also an important cause of chronic renal failure. It occurs most often in children under 4 years with a peak age between 1 and 2 years. The syndrome is characterized by a classic triad of signs: (1) hemolytic anemia, (2) thrombocytopenia, and (3) acute renal failure.

Etiology and Pathophysiology

The development of HUS is often linked to enterohemorrhagic *Escherichia coli* strain 0157:H7, which produces a verotoxin that binds to the glomeruli, collecting ducts, and distal tubules in young children. Contaminated beef is the vector in more than half of the epidemics. Other organisms responsible for the development of HUS include *Shigella dysenteriae, Salmonella, Yersinia,* and *Campylobacter.*

The verotoxin causes damage to the lining of the glomerular arterioles resulting in swelling of the endothelial cells. In response, clotting mechanisms deposit fibrin in the renal arterioles and capillaries. This partial occlusion damages the red blood cells passing through, resulting in hemolysis and subsequent hemolytic anemia when removed from circulation by the spleen. Platelets cluster in areas of vascular endothelial damage, causing thrombocytopenia. Acute renal failure develops as a consequence of blood clotting in the arterioles as well as the toxic effect of hemolyzed red blood cells on renal tubular cells leading to acute tubular necrosis. Autosomal recessive and dominant forms of HUS also exist and account for less than 5% of cases (Varade, 2000).

Clinical Manifestations

An episode of gastroenteritis with diarrhea, upper respiratory infection, or urinary tract infection precedes the development of HUS by 1 to 2 weeks. Signs and symptoms of HUS are described in the clinical manifestations table on page 1220.

COLLABORATIVE CARE

Care for the child with hemolytic uremic syndrome focuses on preservation of kidney function and prevention of complications associated with edema, thrombocytopenia, and gastrointestinal disturbances.

Diagnostic Tests

Diagnostic findings vary according to degree of kidney damage. Urinalysis reveals hematuria, casts, and proteinuria. BUN and creatinine are elevated. Hemoglobin, hematocrit, and platelet counts are decreased. White blood cells are increased due to infection. Serum electrolytes reveal hyponatremia and hyperkalemia. Calcium levels are decreased and phosphorus levels are increased. Serum albumin is decreased.

CLINICAL MANIFESTATIONS of Hemolytic Uremic Syndrome

STAGE	CLINICAL MANIFESTATIONS
Prodromal stage (1–7 days)	Upper respiratory illness Fever and irritability Lymphadenopathy Skin rash Edema Abdominal pain with nausea, vomiting, and bloody diarrhea
Acute stage	Hemolytic anemia Hypertension Pallor and purpura Neurologic involvement (irritability, seizures, altered level of consciouosness, hallucinations, cerebral edema, posturing, or blindness) Renal failure (hematuria and proteinuria, oliguria or anuria, edema and ascites)

Arterial blood gases reveal metabolic acidosis. Serum glucose levels may be elevated if the pancreas is affected by clot formation. A peripheral blood smear with fragments of red blood cells, fibrin split products, and a decreased platelet count (<140,000/mL[mm^3]) confirms the diagnosis. Chest radiographs may be performed to determine presence of pulmonary edema.

Clinical Therapy

Treatment is supportive and focuses on the complication of acute renal failure (see page 1198). Included are fluid restrictions and a high-calorie, high-carbohydrate diet that is low in protein, sodium, potassium, and phosphorus. Pharmacologic therapy may include calcium gluconate or calcium chloride to replace calcium levels, aluminum hydroxide gel to bind to phosphorus, kayexalate to remove excess potassium, and antihypertensive agents. Enteral nutritional support is sometimes needed. Insulin may be required to control hyperglycemia. The use of antibiotics is controversial. Use of an oral Shiga toxin-binding agent was recently evaluated and found to have no benefit in children with diarrhea-associated hemolytic uremic syndrome (Trachtman, Cnaan, Christen, et al., 2003).

CLINICAL TIP

Treatment of diarrhea with antimotility medications is contraindicated because they increase the risk of toxic megacolon or progression from hemorrhagic colitis to hemolytic uremic syndrome (Varade, 2000).

Dialysis is necessary for approximately 40% of children, and approximately 3% to 5% of those affected will die (Trachtman et al., 2003). Peritoneal dialysis is preferred unless the child has severe colitis and abdominal tenderness. Although most children with HUS recover with normal kidney function, chronic renal failure may develop in some children.

Transfusions of fresh-packed red blood cells may be ordered to treat severe anemia. Platelets are given if the child is bleeding or if surgery is needed. Transfusions are carefully administered to prevent hypertension caused by hypervolemia.

NURSING MANAGEMENT

The focus of nursing for the child with hemolytic uremic syndrome is to promote renal function, maintain fluid and electrolyte balance, promote adequate nutrition, prevent complications such as bleeding, and provide support to the child and family.

■ Nursing Assessment and Diagnosis

Monitor vital signs, neurologic signs, and laboratory values including electrolytes and blood counts. Monitor daily weights and calculate intake and output to assess fluid status. Observe the child carefully for evidence of progressive kidney impairment such as oliguria, elevated serum potassium, and creatinine. Monitor for signs of bleeding related to thrombocytopenia, including petechia and ecchymosis. Assess the coping strategies of the child and family and their availability of support. Monitor the child for abdominal discomfort from diarrhea or other gastrointestinal disturbances.

Nursing diagnoses for the child with hemolytic uremic syndrome may include:

- Fluid Volume Excess related to impaired kidney perfusion and function
- Risk for Impaired Skin Integrity related to edema
- Compromised Family Coping related to child's sudden severe illness

■ Planning and Implementation

Care for the child with hemolytic uremic syndrome is the same for care of the child with acute kidney failure (see page 1198). The child may be cared for in an intensive care unit while on dialysis. Carefully monitor neurologic signs, laboratory values, and fluid and electrolyte balance during treatment. Avoid invasive procedures when possible to prevent unnecessary bleeding.

Enteral nutrition may be necessary during the acute illness phase. When able to tolerate oral feeding, promote adequate nutritional intake by offering small, high-calorie, high-carbohydrate diet that is low in sodium, potassium, and phosphorus. Monitor bowel sounds and for vomiting and diarrhea.

Partner with the family and encourage parents to participate in the child's care. Explain the disease process and point out that 95% of children with the condition survive, but some children develop chronic renal failure. Encourage parents to monitor siblings for signs of diarrhea or hemolytic uremic syndrome.

Discharge planning focuses on teaching parents about medications and dietary and fluid restrictions and reducing risk of consumption of contaminated beef. (See Partnering with Families: Food Preparation.) Follow-up visits are necessary to evaluate the effectiveness of the treatment plan.

■ Evaluation

Expected outcomes for the care of the child with hemolytic uremic syndrome may include the following:

- The child maintains fluid and electrolyte balance.
- Skin integrity remains intact.
- Parents demonstrate coping and involvement in the child's care.

Polycystic Kidney Disease

Polycystic kidney disease (PKD) is a genetic disorder that has autosomal recessive and dominant forms. Liver abnormalities are associated with both forms of the disease. The incidence of the autosomal recessive form is 1 per 20,000 live births, and is most often detected in fetuses and at the time of birth (Guay-Woodford & Desmond, 2003). The autosomal dominant form is the most common inherited kidney disease, with a prevalence of 1 per 400 to 500 individuals. PKD affects both male and female equally.

Etiology and Pathophysiology

The autosomal dominant PKD results from mutations on the PKD1 locus on chromosome 16 and PKD2 on chromosome 4. The autosomal recessive gene (PKHD1) is located on chromosome 6 (National Kidney and Urologic Diseases Information Clearinghouse, 2004). Cellular hyperplasia of the collecting ducts causes dilation of the ducts. Fluid secreted into these ducts enables cyst sacs to form. Initially, cysts are usually less than 2 mm in size and do not obstruct urinary flow. As the child grows, however, the cysts become larger and fibrosis occurs. The cysts slowly replace much of the kidney's mass and reduce kidney function. Tubular atrophy may occur in some children, whereas others have minimal changes in renal function. Polycystic kidney disease can also cause cysts in the liver leading to bile duct proliferation and hepatic fibrosis, portal hypertension, and biliary infection, which progress in severity with age.

Newborns with polycystic kidney disease may have enlarged kidneys, detected at birth. Those with the most severe form of the disease die shortly after birth as a result of pulmonary hypoplasia.

Clinical Manifestations

Clinical manifestations in infants with autosomal recessive PKD include Potter facies (low-set ears, small jaw, and a flattened nose). Hypertension develops in early infancy and is often severe. The infant may have expected volume of urine output or oliguria. Polyuria and polydypsia develop with progressive renal insufficiency in which the kidneys' ability to conserve sodium and concentrate the urine decreases. As kidney function decreases, the child may have poor growth. Respiratory distress and feeding intolerance may develop from the enlarged kidneys. As uremia develops, infants and children experience progressive developmental delay and growth failure, as well as renal osteodystrophy. With this disorder, calcium levels are low, phosphorus levels are elevated, and there is an increase in parathyroid gland activity, all leading to disorders that resemble osteomalacia or osteoporosis.

PARTNERING WITH FAMILIES

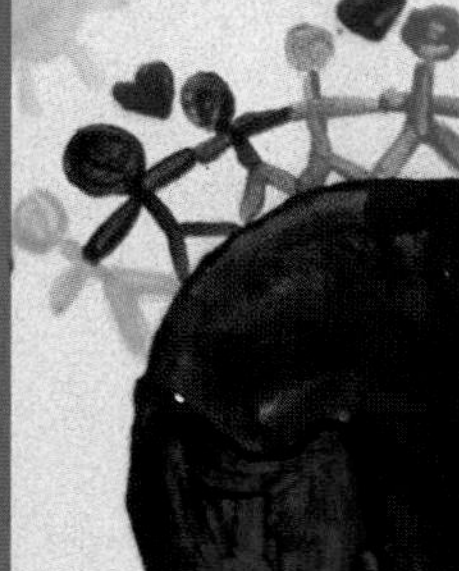

Food Preparation

Hemolytic uremic syndrome can be largely prevented by cooking of ground beef to 155°F throughout, meaning no more rare hamburgers. Teach the family to wash hands carefully when handling raw ground meats, and make sure utensils touching raw meat do not come into contact with cooked meats. Encourage the use of a meat thermometer since the absence of pink in the center of the meat does not ensure that the appropriate temperature has been achieved.

COLLABORATIVE CARE

The goal of management for the child with polycystic kidney disease is to detect the presence of the disorder, maintain fluid and electrolyte balance, prevent associated complications such as hypertension and anemia, and promote growth and development.

Diagnostic Tests

The disease is often diagnosed on prenatal ultrasound in which the fluid-filled cysts can be observed. At the time of birth enlarged kidneys may be palpated. Renal ultrasound detects enlarged kidneys with cysts. A liver biopsy may be performed and may reveal hepatic fibrosis. If identified, other family members should be screened for subclinical cases of the disease.

Clinical Therapy

Treatment is supportive. Ventilatory support is provided to newborns with pulmonary hypoplasia; however, many of these infants do not survive. Medications such as diuretics are prescribed for hypertension. Fluid and electrolyte abnormalities are managed. Antibiotics are utilized to treat urinary tract infection. Growth hormones may be administered to some children to promote growth. Approximately 50% of children develop end-stage renal failure by 10 years of age. Dialysis or a kidney transplant will prolong survival; however, liver problems may continue to complicate the child's health, even when the kidney condition is well controlled. As many as 20% to 30% of these children die by 15 years of age (Davis & Avner, 2004).

NURSING MANAGEMENT

Nursing care is the same as that for the child with renal insufficiency and chronic renal failure. Observe the child for signs of progressive renal impairment. Ensure that follow-up appointments are scheduled to assess growth, developmental progress, and the effectiveness of the treatment plan. Partner with the family to establish a home care management plan focusing on medications, diet adequate in protein and calories to support growth, management of acute gastrointestinal illnesses, and care for the child with progressive renal insufficiency and a liver disorder. Since the disease is inherited, the family should be referred for genetic counseling. See Chapter 4∞.

REPRODUCTIVE SYSTEM ANATOMIC AND PHYSIOLOGIC DIFFERENCES

The reproductive system consists of internal and external organs that at maturity function to promote the conception and healthy development of a fetus. The male reproductive system consists of the scrotum, testes, penis, prostate, and epididymis. The female reproductive system consists of the ovaries, fallopian tubes, uterus, vagina, and external genitalia.

The reproductive system in children is functionally immature until puberty. Throughout childhood the genitalia (with the exception of the clitoris in females) enlarge gradually. Anatomic and functional development accelerates with the hormonal changes of puberty (refer to Chapter 8∞ for an assessment of pubertal changes). In females, the mons pubis becomes more prominent and hair begins to grow. The vagina lengthens and the epithelial layers thicken. The uterus and ovaries enlarge, and the musculature and vascularization of the uterus also increase. In boys, hair begins to appear at the base of the penis, and the scrotum becomes increasingly pendulous. The penis increases in length and width. Discussion of the reproductive system in this chapter is specific to structural defects and sexually transmitted infections.

STRUCTURAL DEFECTS OF THE REPRODUCTIVE SYSTEM

Structural defects of the reproductive system may interfere with urinary flow or reproductive function. Defects discussed in this section are phimosis, cryptorchidism, inguinal hernia, hydrocele, and testicular torsion.

Phimosis

MediaLink Circumcision Video

In **phimosis,** the foreskin over the glans penis cannot be retracted. As a result of natural adhesion, phimosis is a normal finding in uncircumcised infants and young males. Generally the foreskin separates from the glans during childhood, and intermittent erections lead to physiologic foreskin retraction. Complications that arise from the narrowing of the preputial opening are related to the obstruction of urine flow. A dribbling stream may be noted. **Balanitis** (inflammation or infection of the glans penis) may occur as a result of the obstruction of urine flow.

The most serious complication of phimosis is **paraphimosis,** which occurs when the foreskin cannot be returned to its normal position over the glans, causing constriction of the penis. Paraphimosis results in swelling of the glans and obstructs penile blood flow. Ischemic injury to the glans penis occurs if the constriction is not relieved. Paraphimosis is a medical emergency and requires immediate intervention to preserve the glans penis.

COLLABORATIVE CARE

Circumcision, surgical removal of the foreskin, has long been a common practice performed in some countries and cultures during the newborn period to prevent phimosis, for ease of male hygiene, and to prevent urinary tract infections and penile cancer. See Developing Cultural Competence: Circumcision.

The procedure removes the skin covering the end of the penis. Circumcision is considered comparatively safe, although serious complications can result. Damage to the urethra and disfigurement to the penis, including amputation, hemorrhage, infection, meatal stenosis, and infection are potential complications (Kaufman, Clark, & Castro, 2001).

Analgesia for neonatal circumcision is necessary to prevent pain and physiologic stress on the neonate. Methods of analgesia for circumcision include sucrose pacifiers, EMLA cream, dorsal penile nerve block, and subcutaneous ring block (Lerman & Liao, 2001). Refer to Chapter 18∞ for further discussion on pain management.

Circumcision is contraindicated in newborns with blood dyscrasias, family history of bleeding disorder, and those who are premature. Anomalies such as hypospadias, epispadias, and chordee are other contraindications since the foreskin may be needed for later reconstruction (Lerman & Liao, 2001).

Recent studies indicate a decrease in the rate of neonatal circumcisions due to associations with infection, pain, and the potential for urethral injury, and the additional risk of anesthesia if utilized. The application of topical steroids, rather than circumcision, as the primary treatment of phimosis has been proven an effective, safe, and economical alternative measure (Ashfield, Nickel, Siemens, et al., 2003; Elmore, Baker, & Snodgrass, 2002). Therapy usually involves the application of betamethosone cream or another topical steroid to the outer prepuce twice daily for 4 to 8 weeks. Side effects from the use of betamethosone are not frequently observed (Elmore et al., 2002).

NURSING MANAGEMENT

Nursing initially focuses on partnering with parents on establishing proper hygiene care of the uncircumcised newborn male. This includes techniques in cleansing the foreskin and penis. Educate the parents to avoid forcibly retracting the foreskin to prevent complications such as scarring or paraphimosis. Avoid harsh

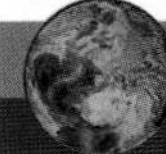

DEVELOPING CULTURAL COMPETENCE
Circumcision

The Jewish and Islamic faiths practice circumcision for religious and cultural reasons. Circumcision is an uncommon practice in Asia, Central America, South America, and most of Europe. There are few data to accurately estimate the rate of newborn circumcision in the United States; however, it is believed that the majority of newborn males are circumcised. The rate of circumcision varies by region, religion, and socioeconomic status. In the United States, Whites are more likely to be circumcised (81%) than Blacks (65%) or Hispanics (54%) (American Academy of Pediatrics, 1999).

soaps because they can irritate the penis. Frequent diaper changes help to prevent diaper rash and irritation. When the child is older, the foreskin separates from the penis and easily retracts. Once this occurs, the foreskin can be pulled back to allow for cleaning. Educate the child and family to always return the foreskin to its normal position to avoid constricting blood flow.

In the absence of medical necessity, the family requires adequate information when making an informed decision for routine circumcision of their newborn. Partner with the family and encourage them to discuss with their pediatrician the risks and benefits of circumcision, potential complications associated with circumcision, and pain relief for the infant during and following circumcision (Box 31–4). See Chapter 11∞.

If circumcision is requested by parents of the newborn or it is the method of treatment for phimosis, nursing care focuses on preoperative preparation of the infant, including the advocacy for and assistance in giving the newborn local anesthesia.

Postoperatively the nurse assesses the infant's vital signs and the operative site. Partner with the parents to ensure they understand proper care for the surgical site, as newborns are discharged within 24 hours of surgery. Inform parents that a yellow discharge on the glans is normal for several days following the circumcision. See Partnering with Families: Care Following Circumcision.

If topical steroids are prescribed as treatment, the nurse partners with the family to ensure the proper application of the medication, including the importance of adherence to the prescribed therapy. Additional instructions include methods of proper hygiene and the signs and symptoms of constriction and infection.

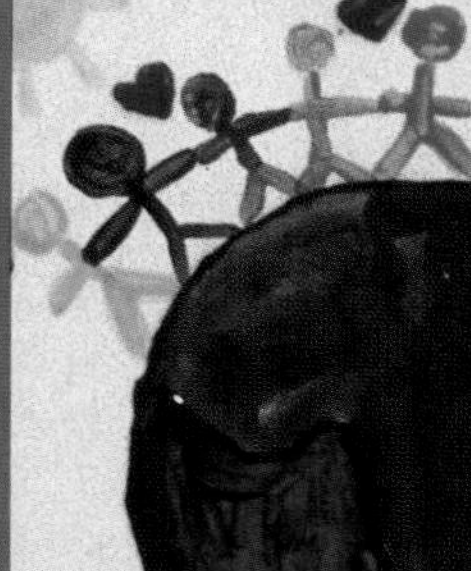

PARTNERING WITH FAMILIES

Care Following Circumcision

Instruct the family to wash hands well before and after each diaper change and to follow these instructions for care following circumcision:

- Cover the head of the penis with a generous amount of petroleum jelly with each diaper change until the redness goes away.
- A pale yellow crust around the incision site and on the glans is normal for several days after surgery.
- Use cotton balls moistened with tap water to gently clean the head of the penis.
- Contact the healthcare provider if there is increased redness, bleeding, or swelling of the head of the penis.

Adapted from Kaufman, M. W., Clark, J. Y., & Castro, C. L. (2001). Neonatal circumcision: Benefits, risks, and family teaching. Maternal Child Nursing, *26(1), 200.*

Cryptorchidism

Cryptorchidism, also called undescended testes, is a common disorder and occurs when one or both testes fail to descend through the inguinal canal into the scrotum. Normally, the testes descend during the seventh to ninth month of gestation. Approximately 3% of newborns are affected with the number significantly higher among preterm newborns. Testes spontaneously descend in a large number of these infants by 3 months of age (Koo, 2001a).

Etiology and Pathophysiology

Cryptorchidism may be the result of a testosterone deficiency, an absent or defective testis, or a structural problem such as a narrow inguinal canal, short spermatic cord, or adhesions, and is frequently associated with an inguinal hernia. It is thought that some spontaneous descent of the testes occurs due to the rise in plasma testosterone in the first 3 months of life (Koo, 2001a). The testes may be located in the inguinal canal, the abdomen, the perineum, or even the thigh. In some cases the testis is absent.

Exposure of the testis to a higher temperature in the abdomen compared to the scrotum results in morphologic changes to the testis that are apparent by 18 months of age and can lead to reduced sperm counts at sexual maturity (Koo, 2001b). Complications of uncorrected cryptorchidism include infertility, malignancy in undescended testis, torsion of the undescended testis, atrophy, and psychologic effects of "empty" scrotum.

BOX 31–4 Circumcision Decision Making

The American Academy of Pediatrics does not recommend circumcision as a routine procedure, as the benefits do not significantly outweigh the risks (American Academy of Pediatrics, 1999). Other studies have reported a lower incidence of urinary tract infections among circumcised male infants and make statements about circumcision having a preventive health benefit (Schoen, Colby, & Ray, 2000). Parents should discuss the risks and benefits of newborn circumcision with their pediatrician. Legitimate reasons for circumcision take into consideration cultural, religious, and ethnic traditions, as well as medical factors (such as phimosis and urinary tract infections).

Clinical Manifestations

Cryptorchidism is usually detected during the newborn examination when palpation of the scrotum fails to reveal one or both testes. It is not unusual for boys with cryptorchidism to have an inguinal hernia as well. In some cases the testes may retract into the inguinal canal but can be manipulated into the scrotum. After 1 year of age, the testes do not descend spontaneously.

COLLABORATIVE CARE

Care for the child with cryptorchidism focuses on identifying the defect, preserving testicular function, maintaining fertility, and maintaining a normal appearance of the scrotum.

Diagnostic Tests

Although diagnosis is made on physical examination, diagnostic studies including ultrasound, CT scan, and MRI are utilized to determine the location of the testes. When neither testis can be palpated, hormonal and chromosomal evaluation may be performed to detect an intersex disorder. A diagnostic laparoscopy may also be required to locate the testis.

Clinical Therapy

Management may include surgical or medical interventions. If spontaneous descent does not occur within the first year, some practitioners may consider prescribing human chorionic gonadotropin; however, this therapy is better accepted in Europe than in the United States (Koo, 2001b).

Surgical intervention, known as an orchiopexy, is performed prior to 2 years of age. The timing for surgery is crucial to preserve fertility and to avoid psychologic effects related to fear of castration and body-image issues in older children. With an orchiopexy, an incision is made at the location of the testis, either in the abdomen or in the inguinal area. Blood vessels are disentangled to allow the testis to reach into the lower scrotum. A second incision is made in the scrotum at the point where the testis is stitched to the inside wall to keep it in place. Goals of surgery are to position the testis for future accessibility to palpation, repair of any hernia, enhance the possibility of fertility, decrease the potential susceptibility for malignancy, and provide psychologic benefit of a normal-appearing scrotum. The orchiopexy also provides the opportunity to examine the testis for the presence of a tumor. The risk of testicular cancer is 35 to 50 times greater in men with a history of cryptorchidism (Ferrer & McKenna, 2000).

NURSING MANAGEMENT

Nursing care includes assessing the infant for undescended testes; implementing measures to reduce postoperative complications; educating parents on treatment, outcomes, and home care needs; promoting a positive body image in the older child; and teaching testicular self-examination to the adolescent.

■ Nursing Assessment and Diagnosis

Assess newborns and infants for undescended testes as described in Chapter 8∞. Inspect and then palpate the scrotum. One side or both sides of the scrotum may appear underdeveloped and may feel empty upon palpation. Inspect and palpate the area over the inguinal canal to determine if the testis is in the canal.

Nursing diagnoses that may be appropriate for the child with cryptorchidism include the following:

- Risk for Injury (reproductive function) related to undescended testes
- Risk for Infection related to surgical procedure
- Deficient Knowledge (child) related to understanding of testicular examinations
- Risk for Body Image Disturbance (older child) related to appearance of scrotum

■ Planning and Implementation

Preoperative nursing care includes preparing the parents and infant for the surgical procedure and addressing parents' concerns about the postsurgical outcome. Orchiopexy is often performed as an outpatient procedure. Postoperative nursing care focuses on maintaining comfort and preventing infection. Encourage bed rest and monitor voiding. Administer prescribed analgesics to relieve pain.

Parents will be anxious about the surgical correction and about future fertility. Assess parental level of coping and availability of support. Provide them with the opportunity to express concerns and offer thorough explanations regarding care and outcomes.

In preparation for discharge, educate parents on care of the incision. The incision should be cleaned gently with each diaper change to decrease chances of infection. Clothing should be loose to avoid pressure to the postoperative site. Provide parents with guidelines for recognition of pain and administration of pain medication. Instruct parents to identify signs of infection such as redness and swelling at the incision sites. Inform parents to avoid straddling the infant across the hip or placing on a riding toy for up to 2 weeks following surgery to promote healing and to prevent injury. Vigorous activity and rough play should also be avoided.

Care in the Community

Because the risk of testicular malignancy is greatly increased with cryptorchidism, long-term planning includes teaching the child to perform monthly testicular examinations after puberty to assist in the early detection of tumors. See Partnering with Families: Testicular Self-Examination. A discussion of fertility and the possible need for fertility testing is important since cryptorchidism increases the risk of infertility.

■ Evaluation

Expected outcomes of nursing care include the following:

- Postoperative infection does not occur.
- The child's pain is effectively managed.
- Parents demonstrate an understanding of postoperative care.
- Regular testicular self-examinations are performed upon the onset of puberty.

Inguinal Hernia and Hydrocele

An **inguinal hernia** is a painless inguinal or scrotal swelling of variable size that occurs when abdominal tissue, such as bowel, protrudes into the groin. Approximately 1% to 5% of full-term infants and up to 11% of preterm infants have an inguinal hernia, and inguinal hernias are up to 9 times more common in males than females (Burd & Burd, 2002).

A hydrocele is a fluid-filled mass in the scrotum. The condition is found in 1% to 5% of infants, more commonly in boys than girls by a 4:1 ratio and they are more often bilateral. Most hydroceles resolve spontaneously by reabsorption by the second year of life.

Etiology and Pathophysiology

During fetal development, a peritoneal sac precedes the testicle's descent to the scrotum. The lower sac enfolds the testis to become the tunica vaginalis, and the upper sac atrophies before birth. Fluid may become trapped in the tunica vaginalis and cause the hydrocele. When the tunica vaginalis does not atrophy, an abdominal structure may move into it. In males, the bowel is the most frequent organ protruding into the groin, and in females the ovaries or fallopian tubes are a common finding (Katz, 2001). Inguinal hernias are often associated with abdominal wall defects such as exstrophy of the bladder and prune-belly syndrome, and are a common occurrence with undescended testes.

Clinical Manifestations

On palpation of the scrotum, a round, smooth, nontender mass is noted with either a hernia or hydrocele. Parents may report noting an intermittent bulge in the groin or swelling in the scrotum that appears when the child is straining or crying. Some hernias spontaneously reduce in size during sleep or may be manually reduced by manipulation. Infants or children may have a painless enlargement of the scrotum that does not decrease in size.

The major complication of an inguinal hernia is **incarceration,** which occurs when the presence of intestine in the groin causes constriction of the blood supply to the scrotal sac. Incarceration can lead to intestinal strangulation and testicular ischemia. Manifestations of incarceration include acute onset of pain, abdominal distention, vomiting, and an irreducible mass. Other findings may include an edematous, erythematosus scrotum accompanied by abdominal distension, poor feeding, and bloody stools (Burd & Burd, 2002).

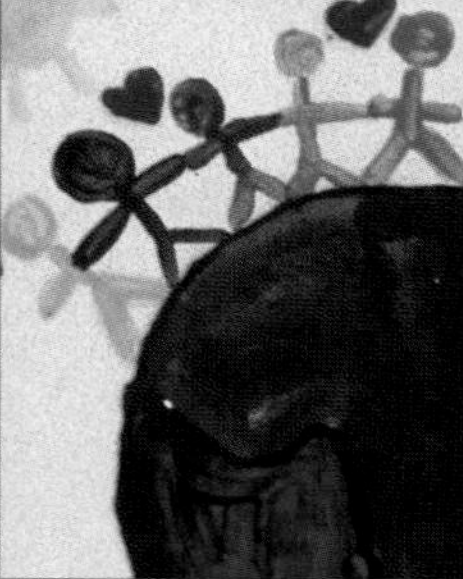

PARTNERING WITH FAMILIES

Testicular Self Examination

- Examine your testicles when you are taking a warm shower or bath, or just after if you prefer to use a mirror to compare size.
- The scrotum, testicles, and hands should be soapy to allow easy manipulation of the tissue.
- Gently roll each testicle between the thumb and fingers of each hand. If one testicle is substantially larger than the other, or if you feel any hard lumps, consult your physician immediately.
- Normal scrotal contents may be confusing. Just above and behind the testicle is the epididymis. It feels soft and tender overall, although parts of it may be rather firm. This is normal. The spermatic cord, a small, round, movable tube, extends up from the epididymis. It feels firm and smooth. Of greatest concern is any hard lump felt directly on the testicle, even if it is painless.
- Choose a day out of each month on which to examine yourself. Most men choose an easy day to remember, such as the first or last day of the month. Star this day on your calendar to help you remember.

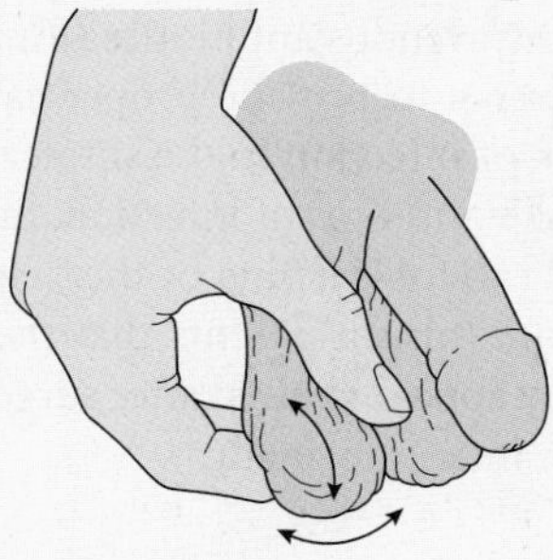

From LeMone, P. & Burke, K. (2004) Medical-Surgical Nursing: Critical Thinking in Client Care. *(3rd ed.) Upper Saddle River, NJ: Prentice Hall Health.*

COLLABORATIVE CARE

Care for the child with inguinal hernia and hydrocele focuses on identifying and correcting the defect, preventing complications, and promoting growth and development.

Diagnostic Tests

When the hernia appears intermittently, having the older child cough, cry, strain, or engage in vigorous movement increases the intraabdominal pressure and potentially enhances the ability to palpate a hernia. Transillumination may help determine whether the mass is a hernia or hydrocele. See Chapter 8∞.

Clinical Therapy

Outpatient surgery for repair of inguinal hernia is performed as an elective procedure at an early age (usually after 3 months of age to reduce anesthesia risks). A regional nerve block may be used to reduce postoperative pain. Surgical exploration of the contralateral side is controversial since bilateral involvement accounts for only about 10% of the cases. Major complications following routine inguinal hernia repair are uncommon; however, apnea and bradycardia secondary to the effects of anesthesia may be experienced in the premature infant. Most hydroceles without inguinal hernia resolve spontaneously as the fluid reabsorbs by the time an infant is 1 to 2 years of age, so surgical intervention is rarely required.

In the event of incarceration, attempts are made to reduce the hernia immediately to prevent strangulation, necrosis, and perforation of the intestine. Manual reduction involves positioning the child in a Trendelenburg position and applying gentle pressure to the mass. If attempts to reduce the hernia manually are unsuccessful, then immediate surgical intervention is required.

NURSING MANAGEMENT

Nursing care for hydrocele and inguinal hernia includes assessment, explaining the disorder and its treatment, and providing preoperative and postoperative teaching, care, and support.

Nursing Assessment and Diagnosis

Preoperative nursing assessment for the child with an inguinal hernia or hydrocele includes routine newborn assessment and monitoring for signs and symptoms of incarceration.

Postoperative care includes monitoring of vital signs and inspection of the incision for swelling, bleeding, or drainage. Assess the circulation in the leg on the side of the surgical repair to detect any potential blood flow obstruction resulting from edema of the groin. Assess for pain.

Nursing diagnoses for the child with an inguinal hernia or hydrocele may include the following:

- Acute Pain related to surgical incision (and possibly incarceration)
- Risk for Infection related to surgical incision in inguinal area

Planning and Implementation

The incision is covered with a protective sealant rather than a dressing and routine wound care is provided. Depending on the type of anesthesia utilized, pain medication requirements may be minimal, especially if spinal or regional block was used; however, provide pain medication as prescribed. For incarcerated hernias, postoperative care may include management of nasogastric tubes and intravenous antibiotics (Katz, 2001).

Educate the parents to provide proper care of the incision and reduce the risk of infection to the surgical site, as well as to recognize signs and symptoms of infection. Encourage frequent diaper change and careful cleaning of the diaper area to reduce the risk of infection. Inform parents that the scrotum may be edematous and may appear bruised after surgery. Encourage the parents to hold the infant normally.

Evaluation

Expected outcomes for nursing care of the child following surgery for an inguinal hernia may include the following:

- The skin remains intact and wound healing occurs.
- Postoperative infection does not occur.
- The child's pain is effectively managed.

Testicular Torsion

Testicular torsion is an emergency condition in which the testis suddenly rotates on its spermatic cord, obstructing its blood supply. The arteries and veins in the spermatic cord become twisted and interrupt the blood supply, leading to vascular engorgement and ischemia. Testicular torsion occurs in approximately 1 in 4,000 males before the age of 25 years, with the greatest incidence around puberty (Sessions, Rabinowitz, Hulbert, et al., 2003; McAndrew, Pemberton, Kikiros, et al., 2002).

Etiology and Pathophysiology

Often the testicles are positioned horizontally in the scrotum, a congenital anomaly known as a bell clapper deformity, which predisposes the male to this condition. Testicular torsion most often occurs as a result from trauma to the scrotum, but can occur during sporting activities, exercise, and sexual activity. The affected testis is positioned higher in the scrotum than the unaffected testis because of the shortened vascular pedicle.

Clinical Manifestations

Manifestations include severe pain and erythema in the scrotum, nausea and vomiting, abdominal pain, and scrotal swelling that is not relieved by rest or scrotal support. The testes are tender to palpation and become edematous. The cremasteric reflex is absent. There is a slight increase in incidence on the left side as compared to the right side (Sessions et al., 2003).

COLLABORATIVE CARE

Care for the child focuses on rapid diagnosis so that immediate interventions can be initiated to restore circulation to the testis and save the testicular function.

Diagnostic Tests

A testicular scan or Doppler flow sonogram may be performed to confirm the diagnosis; however, risk of inherent delay and misdiagnosis when using these studies should be considered (McAndrew et al., 2002).

Clinical Therapy

Torsion must be reduced within 4 to 6 hours to save the testis from damage as a consequence of lack of circulation to the organ. Manual reduction with an analgesic is sometimes attempted. More often, emergency surgery is performed. During surgery (orchiopexy), the testis is untwisted and stitched to the side of the scrotum in the correct position. The procedure is usually performed bilaterally to prevent future torsion in the other testis.

NURSING MANAGEMENT

The goal of nursing management is to recognize the urgency of the child's condition and to provide the necessary care and advocacy to obtain the emergency intervention.

Nursing Assessment and Diagnosis

Assess the child's symptoms and recognize that pain and swelling in the scrotum is a true emergency. Because the highest incidence of testicular torsion occurs in the adolescent and during sporting activities and trauma, the school nurse should be alert to the possibility of testicular torsion.

Nursing diagnoses that may be appropriate for the child with this condition include:

- Acute Pain related to swelling and constricted blood flow to the testis
- Anxiety related to urgent onset and fear of mutilation
- Ineffective Tissue Perfusion (testis) related to testicular rotation and twisting of blood vessels

■ Planning and Implementation

Provide analgesics as ordered and prepare the child for surgery. The adolescent may be especially anxious about the location of surgery and potential for mutilation. Answer questions the child and family have regarding the surgical procedure and need for rapid intervention.

Nursing management involves psychologic support for the child and family related to concern about the child's future fertility. Reassure parents that as only one testis is usually affected, fertility should not be affected. Explain that surgery is usually performed on the other testis to prevent a similar event from occurring.

The child often is discharged within a few hours following surgery; thus, the child and family require instructions regarding proper care of the incision and pain management. Partner with the family to ensure that the child does not lift heavy objects for 4 weeks or participate in strenuous activity for 2 weeks after surgery to promote healing. Educate the adolescent about the importance of testicular self-examination.

■ Evaluation

Expected outcomes for nursing care of the child following surgery for testicular torsion may include the following:

- The child's pain is effectively managed.
- The child's anxiety is reduced with information and answers to questions.

SEXUALLY TRANSMITTED INFECTIONS

Sexually transmitted infections (STIs) are a major national public health concern. Numerous organisms of bacterial, parasitic, and viral origin, including the human immunodeficiency virus (HIV), have been identified as causative agents of sexually transmitted infections. Human immunodeficiency virus is discussed in Chapter 27∞, and hepatitis B, another infection that can be transmitted sexually, is discussed in Chapter 30∞.

Federal, state, and local health departments have the combined responsibility to control and prevent STIs. On a national level, the Centers for Disease Control and Prevention (CDC) and the National Institutes of Health (NIH) coordinate control plans, provide surveillance, and fund basic science and clinical research. State and local health departments are responsible for controlling the spread of STIs through health promotion programs, staff training, reporting systems, diagnosis, treatment, patient counseling, and the notification of sex partners.

Sexually transmitted infections pose a significant health risk to the pediatric population. Children and adolescents can become infected with sexually transmitted organisms through sexual experimentation, sexual play, molestation, and sexual abuse. Some diseases, such as chlamydia, syphilis, and gonorrhea, acquired after the neonatal period are almost always indicative of sexual contact (CDC, 2002).

PRACTICE ALERT

When a child younger than 10 years is found to have gonorrhea or other sexually transmitted infection, consider the possibility of sexual abuse. When anorectal symptoms are found, suspect molestation (see Chapter 7∞).

Results from the Centers for Disease Control National 2003 Youth Risk Behavior Survey revealed that 46.7% of high school students had engaged in sexual intercourse and 37% of sexually active adolescents had not used a condom at last sexual intercourse (CDC, 2004a). Adolescents are considered an at-risk population related to their inexperience and lack of knowledge about STIs. Recent studies have determined that adolescents possess minimal knowledge about non-HIV sexually transmitted diseases, their treatments, and curability (Clark, Jackson, & Allen-Taylor, 2002). Many factors contribute to the adolescent's risk for an STI, including the following (American Academy of Pediatrics, 2003):

- Sexual contact with a person with known STI or history of STI
- Sexual intercourse with new partner during last 2 months
- Multiple sexual partners or more than two sexual partners in the last 12 months
- Homeless, has sex for survival
- Failure to use a contraceptive barrier

The adolescent who acquires an STI has a 40% chance of acquiring another STI within a year, especially if gonorrhea is the first infection (Stamm & McGregor, 2001).

Of the 15 million new STI cases each year, approximately 25% occur in adolescents (CDC, 2000a). The most frequently diagnosed STIs are chlamydia, genital herpes (herpes simplex type 2), gonorrhea, genital warts (human papillomavirus), trichomoniasis, and syphilis. Adolescents represent 0.5% of the population infected with HIV (CDC, 2000b). Refer to the table on page 1228 for clinical manifestations, clinical therapy, and nursing management of STIs.

Chlamydia

MediaLink ● Sexually Transmitted Infections Video

The causative organism of chlamydia is *Chlamydia trachomatis*. An estimated 3 million new chlamydia infections occur each year (U.S. Preventive Services Task Force, 2002). Chlamydia is the most frequently reported bacterial STI in the United States (CDC, 2004b). The risk for chlamydia is highest in young females under age 20 years (U.S. Preventive Services Task Force, 2002). *C. trachomatis* is the most frequent cause of nongonococcal urethritis with a prevalence of 6% to 12% in adolescents.

Chlamydia is transmitted during vaginal, anal, or oral sex. The infection may also be transmitted from an infected mother to the neonate during vaginal childbirth. Complications associated with chlamydia in females include pelvic inflammatory disease (PID), ectopic pregnancy, and infertility. Females are often reinfected if their sex partners are not treated or if they change sexual partners. Additionally, females infected with chlamydia are up to 5 times more likely to become infected with HIV, if exposed.

CLINICAL MANIFESTATIONS of Common Sexually Transmitted Infections

SEXUALLY TRANSMITTED INFECTION	CLINICAL MANIFESTATIONS AND COMPLICATIONS	CLINICAL THERAPY
Chlamydia	Adolescent female: asymptomatic, or yellow mucopurulent endocervical discharge, dysuria, pelvic pain, mild abdominal pain, vaginal spotting, cervicitis, salpingitis, pelvic inflammatory disease (PID). Adolescent male: asymptomatic, or urethritis, mucoid gray or clear discharge, dysuria, proctitis, epididymitis; 10% are asymptomatic.	Recommended medication therapy includes doxycyline, or erythromycin for 7 days, or single-dose azithromycin. HIV-positive persons with chlamydia receive the same treatment as those who are HIV negative. All sexual partners should be evaluated, tested, and treated. Abstain from sexual intercourse until they and their sex partners have completed treatment (approximately 7 days), otherwise reinfection is possible. Encourage use of condoms.
Genital herpes	Many persons infected with HSV-2 are not aware of their infection when no symptoms are present. Dull pain, itching, and small lesions or pimples on genitalia, buttocks, or thighs. Lesions may be fluid-filled blisters on an erythematous base or more commonly, painful papules and ulcers. Ulcers can appear between vaginal folds, in posterior cervix, on glans penis, or shaft of penis, in rectum, or in anus. Ulcers heal within 2–4 weeks. Lymph nodes closest to lesions are frequently enlarged. Disease frequently recurs four to five times a year with episodes lasting 5–10 days. Triggers include stress, menses, or trauma. Infection is lifelong. Individuals with immunosuppression may have systemic involvement.	There is no permanent cure. Recommended drug therapy to suppress the virus is an antiviral medication (acyclovir, valacyclovir, and famciclovir) given for 7–10 days. Treatment may also be used for recurrent episodes. Daily suppressive therapy for herpes can reduce or eliminate recurrences for the period of time taken. A cesarean delivery is usually performed for infected pregnant women with active lesions. Abstain from sexual activity of all types while lesions are present. Consistent and correct use of condoms may reduce the risk for transmission of genital herpes if the condom covers all lesions. Emphasize that the viral infection is lifelong and transmission can occur when lesions are present and during asymptomatic periods. Sexual partners of infected persons should be advised about the potential of becoming infected.
Gonorrhea	Symptoms and severity vary from mild to severe and are different for males and females. Signs or symptoms often appear 2–5 days after infection; symptoms can take as long as 30 days to appear. Females: 80% are asymptomatic. The classic sign is discharge from purulent vaginal discharge, dysuria, and vulvovaginitis. Males: may be asymptomatic, yellow purulent urethral discharge, erythematous meatus, frequency, dysuria, and painful or swollen testicles. Symptoms of rectal infection in both genders include discharge, anal itching, soreness, bleeding, or painful bowel movements. Infections in the pharynx may cause a sore throat but are usually asymptomatic.	For uncomplicated gonorrhea recommended drug therapy includes a single dose of cefixime, ciprofloxacin, ofloxacin, or levofloxacin PO, or a single dose of ceftriaxone IM. No follow-up is needed if symptoms resolve after treatment (CDC, 2002). All sexual partners within the past 60 days should be notified and treated. Sexual activity should be avoided until therapy has had time to resolve all symptoms. Encourage proper and consistent use of condoms or abstinence. If any genital symptoms such as discharge or burning during urination or unusual sore or rash are experienced, discontinue having sex and seek medical attention immediately.

Complications are rare in males, though infection sometimes spreads to the epididymis, causing pain, fever, and, rarely, sterility. Genital chlamydial infection can cause arthritis, though rarely, and is accompanied by skin lesions and inflammation of the eye and urethra.

Neonates born to infected mothers can contract chlamydial infections to their eyes and respiratory tracts. Chlamydia is a leading cause of early infant pneumonia and conjunctivitis (pink eye) in newborns.

Chlamydia may be cultured from endocervical, urethral, and urine specimens. When a urine specimen is used, the perineum or urethra is *not* cleaned first and the first part of the urine stream is collected (Blake & Woods, 2001). Annual screening for chlamydia is recommended for all sexually active females age 25 years and younger. Screening should potentially be performed at 6 to 12 months in previously infected women to determine if reinfection has occurred. All pregnant women should be screened for chlamydia.

Genital Herpes

Genital herpes is caused by the *herpes simplex virus* 1 (HSV-1) or 2 (HSV-2). HSV-2 is the most common cause of genital herpes. One of five adolescents have had a genital HSV infection, and the rate has increased significantly over the past 30 years. Genital HSV-2 infection is approximately 4 times more common in females than in males (CDC, 2004c). Because of the recurrent nature of the infection, it causes psychological distress.

HSV-1 and HSV-2 viruses are shed from open lesions as well as when the individual is asymptomatic. HSV-1 can cause genital herpes, though it more commonly causes infections of the mouth and lips. HSV-1 infection of the genitals may initially be caused by oral–genital sexual activity or by genital–genital contact with a person who has HSV-1 infection. HSV-2 infection generally occurs by genital–genital contact.

Diagnosis of genital herpes can be done by visual inspection if the outbreak is typical and by culture sample from the

CLINICAL MANIFESTATIONS of Common Sexually Transmitted Infections (continued)

SEXUALLY TRANSMITTED INFECTION	CLINICAL MANIFESTATIONS AND COMPLICATIONS	CLINICAL THERAPY
Human papillomavirus (HPV)	Females: small, flat, flesh-colored warts clustered or alone on the vulva, perineal area, vagina, or cervix; itching, bleeding, burning, irritation. A subclinical infection may be detected through a Pap smear. Males: small, flat, flesh-colored warts on the penis, near base of penis on scrotal skin, or near anus.	No cure exists. If left alone warts may resolve on their own, remain unchanged, or increase in size and number. Treatment includes cryotherapy, topical podophyllin or imiquimod cream, laser ablation, intralesional interferon, or chemical cautery with trichloroacetic acid. Encourage abstinence or condom use. The disorder is transmissible even after treatment.
Trichomoniasis	Females: pale yellow to gray-green discharge that may be frothy or have a fishy odor, dysuria, vulvar pruritis, occasional abdominal pain; symptoms worsen during menses, more commonly have symptoms than males. Males: mucoid or purulent urethral discharge, pruritis, dysuria; usually asymptomatic.	A single dose of metronidazole PO or alternatively metronidazole PO for 7 days. No follow-up test is needed if symptoms resolve after treatment. Treat both partners at the same time to eliminate the parasite. Sexual contact should be avoided until both partners are cured. Do not drink alcoholic beverages during treatment and until symptoms resolve.
Syphilis	Appearance of classic signs and symptoms of syphilis depends on stage of disease. *Primary stage:* ulcer on labia, within vagina, on penis, in anus, or on lips or tongue that appears at invasion site approximately 2 weeks to 3 months after infection. Ulcer has an indurated border and smooth base (chancre), and it is painless. Lymphadenopathy is usually present. Ulcer spontaneously heals within 5 weeks. *Second stage:* appears up to 10 weeks after initial infection with fever, malaise, lymphadenopathy, patchy alopecia, and diffuse rash. Rash can be macular, papular, papulosquamous, or bullous, and appearance on the palms and soles is classic. Flat mucous patches called condylomata latum appear on genitals. *Latent stage:* asymptomatic, follows the second stage by about 6 weeks. It can last for several years or be lifelong. *Tertiary stage:* occurs more than 2 years after onset and manifests as neurosyphillis, cardiovascular disease, ophthalmic, or congenital syphilis.	Recommended drug therapy includes single dose of benzathine penicillin G IM. Alternative treatment for those with penicillin allergy is doxycycline or tetracycline PO for 14 days (CDC, 2002). For children allergic to penicillin use erythromycin PO for 15 days. Follow-up with clinical examination and serology tests should be performed at 6 and 12 months following treatment to detect treatment failure or reinfection. Notify and treat all sexual contacts within the past 90 days to 1 year of diagnosis, depending on stage when diagnosed. During syphilis treatment, abstain from sexual contact with new partners until the syphilis sores are completely healed. Encourage abstinence or the correct and consistent use of condoms to prevent reinfection.

sore(s). A positive HSV-2 blood test is indicative of genital herpes infection.

Gonorrhea

Gonorrhea is caused by the organism *Neisseria gonorrhoeae.* The bacterium grows in warm, moist areas, including the cervix, uterus, and fallopian tubes in females and in the urethra in women and men. The bacterium can also grow in the eyes, mouth, throat, and anus.

In 2002, the rate of reported gonorrheal infections was 125 per 100,000 persons, or about 700,000 infected persons, making this a very common infection. The highest reported rates of infection in the United States are among sexually active teenagers, young adults, and African Americans (CDC, 2004d).

Gonorrhea is transmitted through contact with the penis, vagina, anus, or mouth. Ejaculation does not have to occur for gonorrhea to be transmitted or acquired. Gonorrhea can also be spread from mother to neonate during delivery. It is a common cause of pelvic inflammatory disease (PID). Individuals are often co-infected with Chlamydia.

Diagnosis is confirmed with a smear from cervix, urethra, rectum, or throat. Gonorrhea can also be diagnosed from urine sample.

Human Papillomavirus

Genital warts or genital human papillomavirus (HPV) infection is caused by one of more than 100 different strains of the *Human papillomavirus* organism (30 of which are sexually transmitted). This organism can infect the genitals of males and females, including the skin of the penis, vulva, or anus and the linings of the vagina, cervix, or rectum. Approximately 20 million people are currently infected with HPV, and about 6.2 million Americans contract the infection each year (CDC, 2004e).

Most individuals who become infected with HPV will be asymptomatic and the infection will clear spontaneously. Some

HPV viruses are high risk, leading to cancer of the cervix, vulva, vagina, anus, or penis. Others are low risk, causing genital warts, which are single or multiple growths appearing in the genital area that are sometimes cauliflower shaped.

HPV is spread primarily through genital contact. Most HPV are asymptomatic; therefore, most infected persons are unaware they are infected, and they can transmit the virus to a sexual partner. Rarely, a neonate can contract the HPV during vaginal delivery. The neonate that is exposed to HPV very rarely develops warts in the throat or voice box.

Most females are diagnosed with HPV on the basis of abnormal Pap tests. Also, a specific test is available to detect HPV DNA in females. No HPV tests are available for males (CDC, 2004e).

Trichomoniasis

Trichomoniasis is a common STI affecting both males and females, caused by the *Trichomonas vaginalis* organism. In young, sexually active females, trichomoniasis is the most common curable STI. It is estimated that 7.4 million new cases occur each year in both genders (CDC, 2004f).

The urethra is the most common site of infection in males and the vagina is the most common site of infection in females, although symptoms are more common in females. The organism is sexually transmitted through penis–vagina intercourse or vulva–vulva contact with an infected partner.

Syphilis

Syphilis is caused by the bacterium *Treponema pallidum.* In the United States, over 32,000 cases of syphilis were reported in 2002 with most cases involving adults over 20 years of age. A total of 412 cases of congenital syphilis in newborns were reported in 2002 (CDC, 2004g).

Transmission of the syphilis occurs during anal, oral, or vaginal sex through direct contact with a syphilitic sore or chancre that is found primarily on the external genitals, vagina, anus, or in the rectum. Sores may also be found on the lips and in the mouth. Sores may not be recognized as syphilis contributing to the transmission between unsuspecting individuals. The disease is transmissible to the fetus in utero.

Diagnosis may be confirmed through microscopic examination of chancre scrapings or through a blood test for serum antibodies for syphilis. Due to the risk of fetal disease and death, all pregnant women should be tested for syphilis. Those whose sexual behaviors put them at risk for syphilis and other STIs should be routinely screened.

NURSING MANAGEMENT

The goal of nursing is to reduce the transmission of STIs to the child and adolescent. Nursing care focuses on education, prevention, and collaborative treatment of sexually transmitted infections through partnership with the child or adolescent and family.

Nursing Assessment and Diagnosis

The nurse usually encounters the child or adolescent and family in the emergency department, outpatient clinic, or nursing unit. Nursing assessment focuses on identifying signs and symptoms indicative of STIs, assessing for the potential of an asymptomatic STI, and assessing the psychosocial impact on the child or adolescent with an STI.

Obtain a sexual history from the adolescent, specifically inquiring about the number and gender of sexual partners as well as any protection used during sexual activity. Maintain a nonjudgmental approach and conveying acceptance when discussing sexual health issues with the child or adolescent. To achieve the adolescent's cooperation, confidentiality must be assured.

During the physical examination, assess the child or adolescent for manifestations as described in the table on pages 1228–1229. Since many cases are subclinical or asymptomatic, routine screening of sexually active adolescents is recommended. When a child or adolescent is diagnosed with one STI, it is essential to screen for the presence of others as multiple infections may be present.

Assess the amount of anxiety or concern the adolescent expresses about a potential infection or fear that parents will be notified. Adolescents may postpone care due to feeling uncomfortable about genital examinations.

Nursing diagnoses that may apply to the child or adolescent with an STI include:

- Anxiety related to presence of sexually transmitted infection
- Acute Pain related to genital inflammation and discharge
- Deficient Knowledge related to cause, transmission, and treatments of sexually transmitted infection
- Potential for Disturbed Body Image related to genital lesions, presence of genital infection

Planning and Implementation

The nurse focuses on identifying adolescents at risk for STIs, providing appropriate education, and preventing transmission and complications. Partner with adolescents and encourage them to seek parental guidance and involvement. Abstinence from sexual contact is the best method to prevent an STI. However, methods to reduce the risk for STIs also include a long-term mutually monogamous relationship with a partner who has been tested for STIs and is known to be uninfected, and the proper use of condoms.

When the adolescent has a confirmed STI, provide information about the specific infection diagnosed, its treatment, potential adverse effects, and recommended follow-up. Encourage the adolescent to complete all prescribed medications if more than a single dose treatment is used. Provide psychological support as the adolescent may be upset, ashamed, embarrassed, or angry about having the infection.

When counseling the adolescent, reinforce the importance of treating all sexual partners involved. Partner notification is essential in order to provide treatment if the partner is infected, and to reduce the risk of reinfection. Adolescents with a better partner relationship are more likely to notify the partner (Fortenberry, Brizendine, Katz, et al., 2002). Encourage sexually active adolescents to receive hepatitis B immunization. Counsel the adolescent on ways to modify high-risk sexual behaviors.

Refer the child with signs of an STI for evaluation of sexual assault by a facility or healthcare provider specializing in collecting evidence and providing specialized care. Similarly refer any adolescent who has been sexually assaulted to a sexual assault nurse examiner or other healthcare provider who can collect evidence and coordinate mental health support.

Care in the Community

Education includes promoting abstinence, which means avoiding *any* type of sexual contact with a partner. (See Partnering with Families: Preventing STIs and Their Consequences.) The nurse, in partnership with schools and community organizations, should be active in promoting sexual health through schools, health clinics, community services, and groups or organizations.

Partner with the sexually active adolescent to identify methods of reducing the risk of contracting STIs. Suggestions include the use of latex condoms (though the possibility of STI transmission still exists even with the use of latex condoms), voiding immediately after sexual intercourse, and appropriate genital hygiene with soap and water. Encourage adolescents to discuss the choice of sexual partners and assist them to avoid those partners who are at higher risk for STIs, such as intravenous drug users and those who have multiple sexual partners. Emphasize to the adolescent that even with applying these measures, there is no guaranteed protection with the exception of abstinence. Explain to the adolescent that some STIs, such as chlamydia, are asymptomatic, and it is not possible to tell if a partner is "clean."

Take advantage of additional teaching opportunities to dispell myths of how STIs are spread. STIs are not contracted from sharing bath towels, clothing, and drinking glasses, or from sitting on toilet seats. Inform the adolescent female taking contraceptives that birth control offers no protection against STIs.

■ Evaluation

Expected outcomes for the child or adolescent with a sexually transmitted infection are as follows:

- The child remains free from pain.
- The child demonstrates an understanding of the transmission, prevention, and treatment of sexually transmitted infections.
- The child demonstrates a positive body image.
- The child displays reduced anxiety.

Pelvic Inflammatory Disease

Pelvic inflammatory disease (PID) is an infection of the upper genital tract caused by the ascending spread of organisms in the cervix and vagina. It is estimated that between 10% and 40% of untreated gonorrhea and Chlamydia infections result in PID (Bortot, Risser, & Cromwell, 2004).

Etiology and Pathophysiology

The majority of cases of PID are caused by *Chlamydia trachomatis* or *Neisseria gonorrhoeae,* although other organisms associated with the infection include *Gardnerella vaginalis, Hemophilus influenza, Mycoplasma hominis, Ureaplasma urealyticum,* and *Streptococcus agalactiae.* The infection ascends into the uterus and fallopian tubes during the menses when the cervix mucosal plug is open and retrograde menstrual blood can flow into the fallopian tubes. A significant complication is Fitz-Hugh-Curtis syndrome in which the anterior surface of the liver and adjacent parietal peritoneum become infected. The mechanism for spread of infection to these surfaces is unknown (Bortot et al., 2004).

Clinical Manifestations

Signs and symptoms of PID may include mild or dull bilateral lower abdominal pain, dysmenorrhea that is worse or longer lasting than usual, dysuria, vaginal discharge, pain with sexual activity, prolonged or increased menstrual bleeding, nausea and vomiting. Most cases are mild. Some females complain of right upper quadrant pain when Fitz-Hugh-Curtis syndrome is present.

PARTNERING WITH FAMILIES

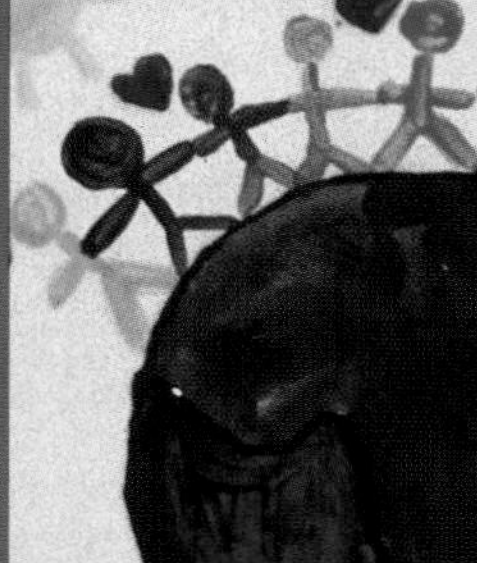

Preventing STIs and Their Consequences

It is important when talking with adolescents to give them information about the risks of STIs and strategies to protect themselves. One important strategy is to encourage the adolescent to talk with his/her partner about STI protection, even when the partner is perceived to be at no or little risk of having an STI. Important information to share includes the following:

- Abstinence is the best method to prevent STIs.
- Limit the number of sexual contacts; practice mutual monogamy.
- Always use condoms and spermicidal gels or foams for vaginal and anal intercourse.
- Refrain from oral sex if the partner has active sores in mouth, vagina, or anus or on the penis.
- Reduce high-risk sexual behaviors. Use of recreational drugs and alcohol can increase sexual risk taking.
- Seek care as soon as symptoms are noticed; make sure the partner gets treatment; and avoid sexual intercourse until the STI is cured.
- Seek annual screening for STIs as some can be present without symptoms.

COLLABORATIVE CARE

The goal of collaborative care is to diagnose and provide treatment for PID in an effort to reduce the potential consequences of infertility, ectopic pregnancy, and chronic pelvic pain.

Diagnostic Tests

PID is based on clinical findings as no specific laboratory test is specific for the disorder. A laparoscopy or endometrial biopsy can provide a definitive diagnosis, but they are rarely performed. During a pelvic examination, uterine or adnexal tenderness or tenderness with cervical motion is the minimal criterion for diagnosis when other potential causes of lower abdominal pain (ectopic pregnancy or appendicitis) are unlikely. Other criteria that help support the diagnosis of PID include a fever >38.3°C (101°F), mucopurulent discharge from the cervix or vagina, elevated erythrocyte sedimentation rate, elevated C-reactive protein level, white blood cells seen on microscopic examination of vaginal secretions, and documented cervical infection with gonorrhea or Chlamydia (CDC, 2002). A transvaginal sonogram may reveal thickened and fluid-filled fallopian tubes with or without free pelvic fluid. A pregnancy test, HIV test, and cultures for STIs should be performed.

Clinical Therapy

Parenteral antibiotic therapy is often used for the first 24 hours before converting to oral antibiotics for the remaining 14 days of treatment. Common intravenous antibiotics used include cefotetan or cefoxitin plus doxycycline or clindamycin plus gentamycin. Oral antibiotics may include ofloxacin, levofloxacin, and ceftriaxone or cefoxitin plus doxycycline. Follow-up physical examination is performed in 72 hours to ensure treatment adherence and to detect improvement in symptoms and reduced tenderness of the uterus, adnexae, and cervix. If improvement is not noted, IV antibiotics are initiated and hospitalization may be required. Male sexual partners should be examined and treated.

NURSING MANAGEMENT

Goals of nursing management are to identify the adolescent at risk for PID, provide medications for treatment, and provide education to reduce the risk for reinfection.

■ Nursing Assessment and Diagnosis

A sexual history should be obtained from all adolescent females to identify the risk for sexually transmitted infection and PID. Adolescents at greater risk for PID include those who have multiple sexual partners, have a history of a previous sexually transmitted infection, use sex for survival, lack consistent condom use, and use douching (Eissa & Cromwell, 2003). Less than 10% of adolescents with PID show signs of a severe infection. Encourage adolescents who are sexually active to have a pelvic examination to detect signs of a sexually transmitted infection and PID.

Nursing diagnoses that may be applicable for the adolescent with PID include the following:

- Acute Pain related to inflammation and swelling of uterus and fallopian tubes
- Health-seeking Behaviors (safe sexual practices) related to requested information on methods to reduce risk for sexually transmitted infections
- Effective Therapeutic Regimen Management related to adherence in completing all antibiotic doses and resolution of symptoms

■ Planning and Implementation

Administer medications intravenously for the first 24 hours, making arrangements for the adolescent to return for a second dose 12 hours after the first. Provide education for the ongoing treatment with oral antibiotics, ensuring that the adolescent understands the importance of taking all medications on schedule for the full 14 days. Provide signs of adverse effects and actions to take if they occur.

Determine if the adolescent's parents have been informed about the illness, and assist the adolescent to discuss the health problem with them. If parents are unaware of the health problem, discuss the importance of telling the parents so that they can help identify any problems that develop during treatment.

Provide counseling about methods to reduce the risk for reinfection with a sexually transmitted infection. Provide information about the potential consequences of infertility, ectopic pregnancy, and chronic abdominal pain for this infection and the increased risk for these consequences with subsequent infections. Encourage regular health visits with screening for sexually transmitted infections in the future. Chlamydia and gonorrhea infections may be asymptomatic.

■ Evaluation

Expected outcomes for the child or adolescent with PID are as follows:

- The child displays complete resolution of infection and pain through adherence to the treatment plan.
- The child conveys an understanding of methods to reduce the risk for future episodes of sexually transmitted infections and PID.

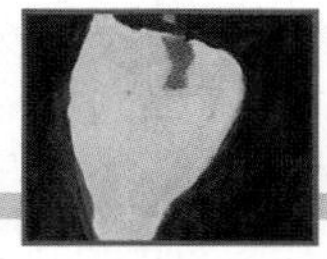

CHAPTER HIGHLIGHTS

- Functions of the urinary system include excretion of wastes, maintenance of acid–base and fluid and electrolyte balance, regulation of blood pressure, production of erythropoietin, and regulation of calcium metabolism.
- Bladder capacity increases with growth, from 20 to 50 mL in newborns to 700 mL in adults.
- Structural defects of the urinary system—including bladder exstrophy, hypospadias and epispadias, obstructive uropathy, vesicoureteral reflux, and posterior ureteral valves—generally require surgical treatment.
- Bladder exstrophy is a congenital defect in which the abdominal wall does not fuse during fetal development, leading to exposure of the bladder wall, a separation of the rectus muscles, and widening of the symphysis pubis.
- Surgical correction of hypospadias and epispadias generally occurs during the first year of life to minimize psychologic effects on the child.
- Obstruction of the urinary tract interferes with urine flow and results in hydronephrosis or urine backflow into the kidneys. This results in significant damage to the kidney and is a common cause of renal failure in children.
- Vesicoureteral reflux may result from a structural anomaly in which the ureters insert in an abnormal position into the bladder. Urinary tract infections are often a complication of this disorder.
- Eagle-Barrett (prune-belly) syndrome is a rare congenital disorder in which the skin covering the abdominal wall is thin and resembles a wrinkled prune. Anomalies associated with this syndrome include urinary tract anomalies, enlarged bladder, vesicoureteral reflux, and bilateral cryptorchidism.
- Urinary tract infections are common infections in children. Factors placing the child at risk for a UTI include urinary stasis, infrequent voiding, irritated perineum, constipation, masturbation, sexual abuse, and sexual activity in adolescent females.
- Nocturnal enuresis often occurs in children whose parents have a history of enuresis. Very few children have a structural or neurologic cause. Higher rates of enuresis have been noted in children with obstructive sleep apnea.
- Minimal change nephrotic syndrome is characterized by edema that develops over several weeks, weight gain, hypertension, irritability, hematuria, malaise, anorexia, and foamy or frothy urine.
- Acute renal failure occurs when kidney function diminishes abruptly and is often reversible. It may occur as a complication of trauma, sepsis, cardiac surgery, or drug toxicity. It is also seen in critically ill neonates with asphyxia, sepsis, or shock.
- Chronic renal failure is progressive and irreversible reduced function of the kidneys, eventually resulting in end-stage renal disease. It often results from developmental abnormalities of the kidneys or urinary tract.
- Children with end-stage renal disease are treated with renal replacement therapy, including hemodialysis, peritoneal dialysis, or kidney transplant.
- Acute postinfectious glomerulonephritis results from a beta-hemolytic group A streptococcal infection of the respiratory tract or skin. Most children have a complete recovery of kidney function.
- Hemolytic uremic syndrome is often associated with ingestion of *E. coli* strain 0157:H7 which produces a toxin that attacks the kidneys. The child develops hemolytic anemia, thrombocytopenia, and acute renal failure that can progress to chronic renal failure.
- Polycystic kidney disease is a genetic disorder with both autosomal recessive and autosomal dominant forms that lead to chronic renal failure. It may be detected prenatally or in young children by ultrasound.
- Structural defects of the male reproductive system include phimosis, cryptorchidism, inguinal hernia and hydrocele, and testicular torsion.
- Nursing care of sexually transmitted infections includes identifying the cause and organism, providing appropriate treatment, preventing transmission and complications, and educating the child, adolescent, and family.
- Pelvic inflammatory disease (PID) is an infection of the upper genital tract (uterus and fallopian tubes) caused by the ascending spread of organisms (usually Chlamydia or gonorrhea) in the cervix and vagina.

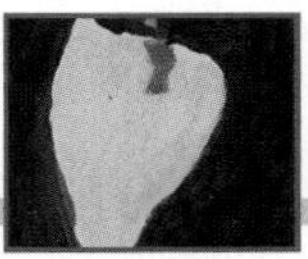

CRITICAL THINKING IN ACTION

INTRODUCTION

Recall Terrell, the child in the opening scenario with ESRD secondary to posterior ureteral valves. Terrell receives hemodialysis three times a week since peritonitis resulted after peritoneal dialysis. Terrell is on the transplant list for a cadaver kidney as no one in the family is able to donate a kidney.

DESCRIPTION

Terrell has been gaining weight and is edematous. Upon evaluation, his primary nurse at the dialysis center discovers that Terrell has been drinking juice and eating food the other children give him in kindergarten. Terrell asks the nurse not to tell his mother because she will be mad, but he just can't help eating and drinking what he isn't supposed to.

DISCUSSION

1. What is the immediate intervention for the nurse to take with Terrell?
2. What approach does the nurse take with discussing this nutritional issue with the family?
3. How does Terrell's growth and development level affect his adherence to the treatment regimen?
4. Terrell's family receives a call that a donor kidney is available and they immediately take Terrell to the medical center for a transplant. Following the transplant, what are the most important elements of teaching for Terrell and the family?
5. Establish three priority nursing diagnoses for Terrell's long-term post-transplant care. What interventions will be implemented? How will they be evaluated?

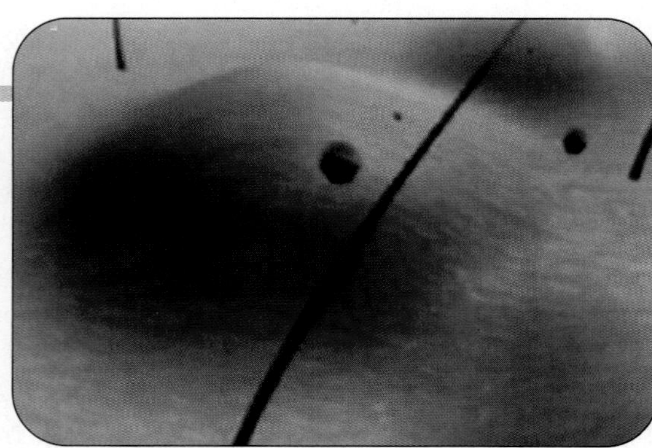

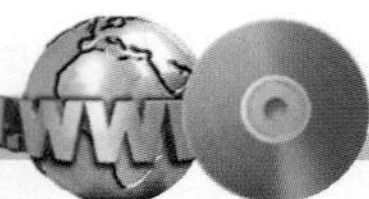

EXPLORE MediaLink

- NCLEX review, case studies, and other interactive resources for this chapter can be found on the Companion Website at **www.prenhall.com/ball**. Click on Chapter 31 to select the activities for this chapter.
- For animations, more NCLEX review questions, and an audio glossary, access the accompanying CD-ROM in this book.

http://www.prenhall.com/ball

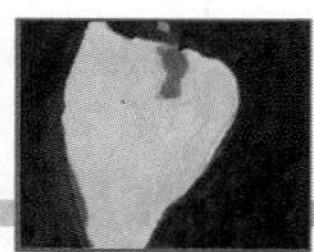

REFERENCES

Aley, K. E. (2002). Developmental approach to pediatric transplantation. *Progress in Transplantation, 12*(2), 86–91.

Alon, U.S. (2001). Preservation of bone mass in pediatric dialysis and transplant patients. *Advances in Renal Replacement Therapy, 8*(3), 191–205.

American Academy of Pediatrics. (2003). *Red book: Report of the committee on infectious diseases* (26th ed.). Elk Grove Village, IL: Author.

American Academy of Pediatrics, Task Force on Circumcision. (1999). Circumcision policy statement. *Pediatrics, 103*(3), 686–693.

Ashfield, J. E., Nickel, K. R., Siemens, D. R., MacNeily, A. E., & Nickel, J. C. (2003). Treatment of phimosis with topical steroids in 194 children. *The Journal of Urology, 169*(3), 1106–1108.

Ball, J. W. (1998). *Mosby's pediatric patient teaching guides.* St. Louis: Mosby.

Bell, F. (2000). Post-renal transplant compliance. *Journal of Child Health Care, 4*(1), 5–9.

Blake, D. R., & Woods, E. R. (2001). The future is here: Noninvasive diagnosis of STDs. *Contemporary Pediatrics, 18*(2), 71–87.

Bortot, A. T., Risser, W. L., & Cromwell, P. F. (2004). Coping with pelvic inflammatory disease in the adolescent. *Contemporary Pediatrics, 21*(4), 33–48.

Brooks. L. J., & Topol, H. I. (2003). Enuresis in children with sleep apnea. *The Journal of Pediatrics, 142*(5), 515–518.

Burd, A. J., & Burd, R. S. (2002). Inguinal hernia in the premature infant: Management of a common problem. *Neonatal Network, 21*(7), 39–47.

Caione, P., & Capozza, N. (2001). Evolution of male epispadias repair: 16-year experience. *The Journal of Urology, 165*(6, Part 2 of 2), 2410–2413.

Centers for Disease Control and Prevention. (2000a). Tracking the hidden epidemic: Trends in STDs in the United States 2000. Atlanta: Author.

Centers for Disease Control and Prevention. (2000b). *HIV/AIDS Surveillance Report, 12*(1). www.cdc.gov/hiv/stats

Centers for Disease Control and Prevention. (2002). Sexually transmitted diseases treatment guidelines 2002. *Morbidity and Mortality Weekly Report, 51*(RR-6), 1–82.

Centers for Disease Control and Prevention. (2004a). Youth risk behavioral surveillance—United States 2003. *Morbidity and Mortality Weekly Report, 53*(SS-2).

Centers for Disease Control and Prevention, National Center for HIV, STD and TB Prevention. (2004b). Chlamydia fact sheet. www.cdc.gov/std/Chlamydia/STDFact-Chlamydia.htm, accessed 12/28/2004.

Centers for Disease Control and Prevention, National Center for HIV, STD and TB Prevention. (2004c). Genital herpes fact sheet. www.cdc.gov/std/Herpes/STDFact-Herpes.htm, accessed 12/28/2004.

Centers for Disease Control and Prevention, National Center for HIV, STD and TB Prevention. (2004d). Gonorrhea fact sheet. www.cdc.gov/std/Gonorrhea/STDFact-gonorrhea.htm, accessed 12/28/2004.

Centers for Disease Control and Prevention, National Center for HIV, STD and TB Prevention. (2004e). Genital HPV infection fact sheet. www.cdc.gov/std/HPV/STDFact-HPV.htm, accessed 12/28/2004.

Centers for Disease Control and Prevention, National Center for HIV, STD and TB Prevention. (2004f). Trichomonas fact sheet. www.cdc.gov/std/Trichomonas/STDFact-Trichomoniasis.htm, accessed 12/28/2004.

Centers for Disease Control and Prevention, National Center for HIV, STD and TB Prevention. (2004g). Syphilis fact sheet. www.cdc.gov/std/Syphilis/STDFact-Syphilis.htm, accessed 12/28/2004.

Chon, C. H., Lai, F. C., & Shortliffe, L. M. D. (2001). Pediatric urinary tract infections. *Pediatric Clinics of North America, 48*(6), 1441–1459.

Cimete, G. (2002). Stress factors and coping strategies of parents with children treated by hemodialysis:

A qualitative study. *Journal of Pediatric Nursing, 17*(4), 297–306.

Clark, L. R., Jackson, M., & Allen-Taylor, L. (2002). Adolescent knowledge about sexually transmitted diseases. *Sexually Transmitted Diseases, 29*(8), 436–443.

Cooper, C. S., Andrews, J. I., Hansen, W. F., & Yankowitz, J. (2002). Antenatal hydronephrosis: Evaluation and outcome. *Current Urology Reports, 3,* 131–138.

Davis, I. D., & Avner, E. D. (2004). Anatomic abnormalities associated with hematuria. In R. E. Behrman, R. M. Kliegman, & H. B. Jenson, *Nelson textbook of pediatrics* (17th ed., pp. 1749–1750). Philadelphia: Saunders.

Eissa, M. A. H., & Cromwell, P. F. (2003). Diagnosis and management of pelvic inflammatory disease in adolescents. *Journal of Pediatric Health Care, 17*(3), 145–147.

Ellsworth, P. I., Cendron, M., & McCullough, M. F. (2000). Surgical management of vesicoureteral reflux. *AORN Journal, 71*(3), 498–513.

Elmore, J. M., Baker, L. A., & Snodgrass, W. T. (2002). Topical steroid therapy as an alternative to circumcision for phimosis in boys younger than 3 years. *The Journal of Urology, 168*(4, Part 2 of 2), 1746–1747.

Ferrer, F. A., & McKenna, P. H. (2000). Current approaches to the undescended testicle. *Contemporary Pediatrics, 17*(1), 106–111.

Fortenberry, J. D., Brizendine, E. J., Katz, B. P., & Orr, D. P. (2002). The role of self-efficacy and relationship quality in partner notification by adolescents with sexually transmitted infections. *Archives of Pediatric and Adolescent Medicine, 156*(11), 1133–1137.

Furth, S. L., Garg, P. P., Neu, A. M., Hwang, W., Fivush, B. A., & Powe, N. R. (2000). Racial differences in access to the kidney transplant waiting list for children and adolescents with end-stage renal disease. *Pediatrics, 106*(4), 756–761.

Gatti, J. M., & Kirsch, A. J. (2001). Posterior urethral valves: Pre- and postnatal management. *Current Urology Reports, 2,* 138–145.

Grady, R. W., & Mitchell, M. E. (2002). Management of epispadias. *Urologic Clinics of North America, 29,* 349–360.

Griffin, K. J., & Elkin, T. D. (2001). Non-adherence in pediatric transplantation: A review of the existing literature. *Pediatric Transplantation, 5,* 246–249.

Guay-Woodford, L. M., & Desmond, R. A. (2003). Autosomal recessive polycystic kidney disease: The clinical experience in North America. *Pediatrics, 111*(5), 1072–1080.

Hanson, K. A. (2003). Diagnostic tests and tools in the evaluation of urologic disease: Part II. *Urologic Nursing, 23*(6), 405–415.

Hill, M. B. C. (2001). Dialysis disequilibrium syndrome. *Nephrology Nursing Journal, 28*(3), 348–349.

Hillerman, W. L., Russell, C. L., Barry, D., Brewer, B., Bianchi. L., Cundiff, W., et al. (2002). Evaluation guidelines for adult and pediatric kidney transplant programs: The Missouri experience. *Progress in Transplantation, 12*(1), 30–35.

Hogg, R. J., Furth, S., Lemley, K. V., Portman, R., Schwartz, G. J., Coresh, J., Balk, E., Lau, J., Levin, A., Kausz, A. T., Eknoyan, G., & Levey, A. S. (2003). National Kidney Foundation's kidney disease outcomes quality initiative clinical practice guidelines for chronic kidney disease in children and adolescents: Evaluation, classification, and stratification. *Pediatrics, 111*(6), 1416–1421.

Hogg, R. J., Portman, R. J., Milliner, D., Lemley, K. V., Eddy, A., & Inglefinger, J. (2000). Evaluation and management of proteinuria and nephritic syndrome in children: Recommendations from a pediatric nephrology panel established at the National Kidney Foundation conference on proteinuria, albuminuria, risk, assessment, detection, and elimination (PARADE). *Pediatrics, 105*(6), 1242–1249.

Huether, S. E. (2002a). Alterations of renal and urinary tract function in children. In K. L. McCance & S. E. Huether, *Pathophysiology: The biologic basis for disease in adults and children* (4th ed., pp. 1217–1230). St. Louis: Mosby.

Huether, S. E. (2002b). Structure and function of the renal and urologic systems. In K. L. McCance & S. E. Huether, *Pathophysiology: The biologic basis for disease in adults and children* (4th ed., pp. 1170–1190). St. Louis: Mosby.

Jalkut, M. W., Lerman, S. E., & Churchill, B. M. (2001). Enuresis. *Pediatric Clinics of North America, 48*(6), 1461–1488.

Kaplow, R., & Barry, R. (2002). Continuous renal replacement therapies. *AJN, 102*(11), 26–34.

Katz, D. A. (2001). Evaluation and management of inguinal and umbilical hernias. *Pediatric Annals, 30*(12), 729–735.

Kaufman, M. W., Clark, J. Y., & Castro, C. L. (2001). Neonatal circumcision. *Maternal Child Nursing, 26*(4), 197–201.

The Kidney Disease Outcomes Quality Initiative. (2002). Clinical practice guidelines for chronic kidney disease: Evaluation, classification, and stratification. *American Journal of Kidney Disease, 39*(1), S1–S266.

Koo, H. P. (2001a). Is it really cryptorchidism? *Contemporary Urology, 13*(1), 12–16, 31.

Koo, H. P. (2001b). Management of the undescended testis. *Contemporary Urology, 13*(3), 20–26.

Kraus, S. J. (2001). Genitourinary imaging in children. *Pediatric Clinics of North America, 48*(6), 1381–1423.

Lang, M. M., & Towers, C. (2001). Identifying post-streptococcal glomerulonephritis. *The Nurse Practitioner, 26*(8), 34–49.

Lerman, S. E., & Liao, J. C. (2001). Neonatal circumcision. *Pediatric Clinics of North America, 48*(6), 1539–1557.

Liao, J. C., & Churchill, B. M. (2001). Pediatric urine testing. *Pediatric Clinics of North America, 48*(6), 1425–1440.

Mahant, S., To, T., & Friedman, J. (2001). Timing of voiding cystourethrogram in the investigation of urinary tract infections in children. *The Journal of Pediatrics, 139*(4), 568–571.

McAndrew, H. F., Pemberton, R., Kikiros, C. S., & Gollow, I. (2002). The incidence and investigation of acute scrotal problems in children. *Pediatric Surgery International, 18,* 435–437.

Mercer, R. (2003, February). Dry at night: Treating nocturnal enuresis. *Advance for Nurse Practitioners,* 26–32.

Mollohan, J. (1999). Exstrophy of the bladder. *Neonatal Network, 18*(2), 17–26.

Myers, P. S. (2002). Transitioning an adolescent dialysis patient to adult health care. *Nephrology Nursing Journal, 29*(4), 375–376.

National Kidney and Urologic Diseases Information Clearninghouse. (2003). *Urinary tract infections in children* (NIH Publication No. 04-4246). www.kidney.niddk.nih.gov/kudiseases/pubs/utichildren/index.htm, accessed 12/13/2004.

National Kidney and Urologic Diseases Information Clearinghouse. (2004). *Polycystic kidney disease* (NIH Publication No. 05-4008). www.kidney.niddk.nih.gov/kudiseases/pubs/polycystic/index.htm, accessed 12/19/2004.

National Kidney Foundation. (2004). Use of herbal supplements in chronic kidney disease. www.kidney.org/atoz/atozPrint.cfm?id=123, accessed 12/23/2004.

Palmieri, P. (2002). Obstructive nephropathy: Pathophysiology, diagnosis, and collaborative management. *Nephrology Nursing Journal, 29*(1), 15–23.

Patel, H. P., & Bissler, J. J. (2001). Hematuria in children. *Pediatric Clinics of North America, 48*(6), 1519–1537.

Paulozzi, L. J., Erickson, J. D., & Jackson, R. J. (1997). Hypospadias trends in two U.S. surveillance systems. *Pediatrics, 100*(5), 831–834.

Pool, R., & Korus, M. (2002). Pediatric kidney transplantation: Growth, development, and nursing implications. *Progress in Transplantation, 12*(2), 129–135.

Prakash, J., Sen, D., Kumar, N. S., Kumar, H., Tripathi, L. K., & Saxena R. K. (2003). Acute renal failure due to intrinsic renal diseases: Review of 1122 cases. *Renal Failure, 25*(2), 225–233.

Prune Belly Syndrome Network, Inc. www.prunebelly.org, accessed 6/3/2004.

Ritz, S. (2002). Pediatric hemodialysis and peritoneal dialysis: Report rewards program. *Journal of Renal Nutrition, 12*(3), 199–204.

Robinson, R. F., Nahata, M. C., Mahan, J. D., & Batisky, D. L. (2003). Management of nephrotic syndrome in children. *Pharmacotherapy, 23*(8), 1021–1036.

Roth, K. S., Koo, H. P., Spottswood, S. E., & Chan, J. C. M. (2002). Obstructive uropathy: An important cause of chronic renal failure in children. *Clinical Pediatrics, 41,* 309–314.

Santen, S. A., & Altieri, M. F. (2001). Pediatric urinary tract infection. *Emergency Medicine Clinics of North America, 19*(3), 675–690.

Schoen, E. J., Colby, C. J., & Ray, G. T. (2000). Newborn circumcision decreases incidence and costs of urinary tract infections during the first year of life. *Pediatrics, 105*(4), 789–793.

Sessions, A. E., Rabinowitz, R., Hulbert, W. C., Goldstein, M. M., & Mevorach, R. A. (2003). Testicular torsion: Direction, degree, duration, and disinformation. *The Journal of Urology, 169*(2), 663–665.

Snethen, J. A., Broome, M. E., Bartels, J., & Warady, B. A. (2001). Adolescent's perception of living with end-stage renal disease. *Pediatric Nursing, 27*(2), 159–167.

Sponseller, P. D., Jani, M. M., Jeffs, R. D., & Gearhart, J. P. (2001). Anterior innominate osteotomy in repair of bladder exstrophy. *Journal of Bone and Joint Surgery, 83*(A-2), 184–193.

Stamm, C. A., & McGregor, J. A. (2001). Diagnosing and treating STDs in young women. *Contemporary Pediatrics, 18*(2), 53–67.

Stokowski, L. A. (2004). Hypospadius in the neonate. *Advances in Neonatal Care, 4*(4), 206–215.

Surer, I., Ferrer, F. A., Baker, L. A., & Gearhart, J. P. (2003). Continent urinary diversion and the exstrophy-epispadias complex. *The Journal of Urology, 169*(3), 1102–1105.

Tobias, N. E. (2000). Management of nocturnal enuresis. *Nursing Clinics of North America, 35*(1), 37–60.

Trachtman, H., Cnaan, A., Christen, E., et al. (2003). Effect of an oral Shiga toxin-binding agent on diarrhea-associated hemolytic uremic syndrome in children. *Journal of American Medical Association, 290*(10), 1337–1344.

United States Renal Data System. (2004). 2004 annual data report. www.usrds.org/atlas.htm, accessed 12/13/2004.

U.S. Preventive Services Task Force. (2002). Screening for Chlamydial infection: Recommendations and rationale. *American Journal of Nursing, 102*(10), 87–92.

Varade, W. S. (2000). Hemolytic uremic syndrome: Reducing the risks. *Contemporary Pediatrics, 17*(9), 54–64.

Verrina, E., Zacchello, G., Edefonti, A., Sorino, P., Rinaldi, S., Gianoglio, B., Lavoratti, G., Maringhini, S., & Perfumo, F. (2001). A multicenter survey on automated peritoneal dialysis prescription in children. *Advances in Peritoneal Dialysis, 17,* 264–268.

Vogt, B. A. (2002). A newborn with a urinary tract anomaly: What role for the general pediatrician? *Contemporary Pediatrics, 19*(10), 131–153.

Vogt, B. A., & Avner, E. D. (2004). Renal failure. In R. E. Behrman, R. M. Kliegman, & H. B. Jenson, *Nelson textbook of pediatrics* (17th ed., pp. 1767–1775). Philadelphia: Saunders.

Warady, B. A., Schaefer, F., Holloway, M., Alexander, S., Kandert, M., Piraino, B., et al. (2000). Consensus guidelines for the treatment of peritonitis in pediatric patients receiving peritoneal dialysis. *Peritoneal Dialysis International, 20*(6), 610–624.

White, N., Richter, J., Koeckeritz, J., Lee, Y. A., & Munch, K. L. (2002). A cross-cultural comparison of family resiliency in hemodialysis patients. *Journal of Transcultural Nursing, 13*(3), 218–227.

Williams, D. M., Sreedhar, S. S., Mickell, J. J., & Chan, J. C. (2002). Acute kidney failure. *Archives of Pediatric and Adolescent Medicine, 156*(9), 893–900.

Williams, G., Lee, A., & Craig, J. (2001). Antibiotics for the prevention of urinary tract infection in children: A systematic review of randomized controlled trials. *The Journal of Pediatrics, 138*(6), 868–874.

Wilson, B. A., Shannon, M. T., & Stang, C. L. (2005). *Nurse's drug guide 2005.* Upper Saddle River, NJ: Prentice Hall.

Woolf, A. S. & Thiruchelvam, N. (2001). Congenital obstructive uropathy: Its origin and contribution to end-stage renal disease in children. *Advances in Renal Replacement Therapy, 8*(3), 157–163.

Yohannes, P., & Hanna, M. (2002). Current trends in the management of posterior urethral valves in the pediatric population. *Urology, 60*(6), 947–953.

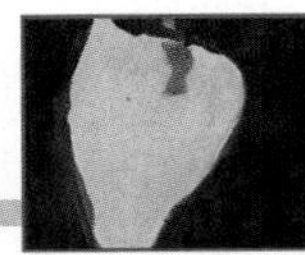

ADDITIONAL REFERENCES

Anderson, B., & Mitchell, M. (2001). Recent advances in hypospadias: Current surgical technique and research in incidence and etiology. *Current Urology Reports, 2,* 122–126.

Gonzalez, R., & Schimke, C. M. (2001). Ureteropelvic junction obstruction in infants and children. *Pediatric Clinics of North America, 48*(6), 1505–1517.

McEvoy, M., & Coupy, S. M. (2002). Sexually transmitted infection: A challenge for nurses working with adolescents. *Nursing Clinics of North America, 37*(3), 461–474.

Chapter 32

Alterations in Endocrine and Metabolic Function

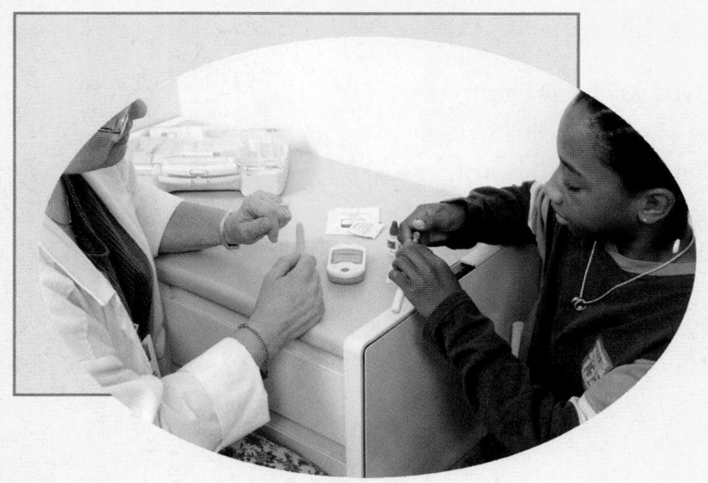

Anthony Maxwell, 12 years old, has just been diagnosed with diabetes mellitus. His parents sought medical attention from their family physician after Anthony complained of being constantly thirsty and hungry for over a week. Despite his vigorous appetite, he has lost 5 pounds since his last recorded weight. The family recalls that Anthony had a viral illness about 1 month ago but seemed to recover from the illness without difficulty. His mother says that Anthony has seemed lethargic for the last several days.

Anthony and his family must now learn to manage his diabetes using a combination of diet, exercise, and insulin therapy. Monitoring his serum glucose level is important in determining how much insulin he will require every day. Anthony and his mother will need to learn to schedule his meals and snacks, to have appropriate amounts of protein, fat, and carbohydrates at each meal. Anthony's meals and activities will be coordinated with his insulin doses. Anthony and his parents will need to monitor closely for signs of hypoglycemia. During his short hospitalization and follow-up sessions, the nurse partners with Anthony and his family in educating them regarding the cause, long-term implications, and management of diabetes.

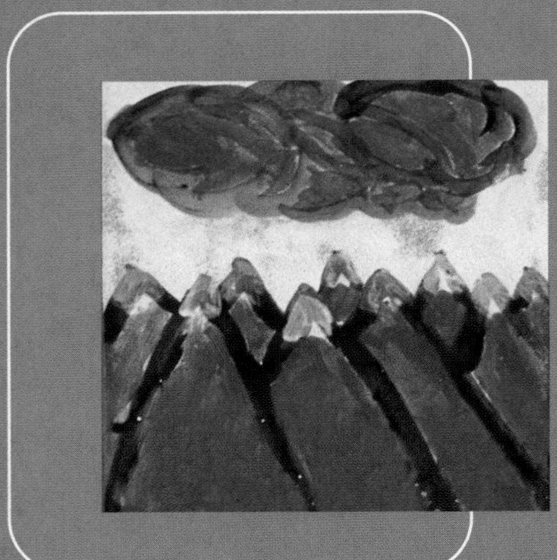

"I don't like this at all—I know I have to check my glucose levels and eat the right foods—but I still don't like it. Why doesn't my body make insulin like it's supposed to?"

—Anthony, 12 years old

Key Terms

acanthosis nigricans/1284
acromegaly/1244
bone age/1242
catecholamines/1257
euthyroid/1252
exophthalmos/1253
glucagon/1263
glucocorticoids/1257
glycogenolysis/1263
glycosuria/1265
goiter/1251
gynecomastia/1286
hormones/1239
hyperinsulinemia/1284
insulin/1263
insulin resistance/1283
karyotype/1260
Kussmaul respirations/1278
lipoatrophy/1273
mineralocorticoids/1257
myxedema/1251
negative feedback/1239
polydipsia/1245
polyphagia/1265
polyuria/1245
precursor/1250
pseudohermaphroditism/1259
puberty/1240
thyrotoxicosis/1253
virilization/1259
water intoxication/1247

Learning Outcomes

After completing this chapter, you will be able to:

- Describe the general function of the endocrine system.
- Identify signs and symptoms that may indicate a disorder of the endocrine system.
- Describe nursing management for general disorders of the endocrine system.
- Relate the pathophysiologic processes of diabetes to care of the child with type 1 and type 2 diabetes.
- Describe collaborative management for the child with diabetes.
- Describe nursing management of the child with inherited metabolic diseases.

MediaLink http://www.prenhall.com/ball

Resources for this chapter can be found on the CD-ROM accompanying this textbook and on the Companion Website at www.prenhall.com/ball. Click on Chapter 32 to select the activities for this chapter.

CD-ROM

Animations/Videos

Adolescent Diabetes and Quality of Life
Hormone Regulation and Secretion
Physiology of Diabetes
Responding to Hypoglycemia

NCLEX Review

Audio Glossary

COMPANION WEBSITE

A & P Review

NCLEX Review

Case Study: Child with Type 1 Diabetes Returning to Elementary School

MediaLink Applications

Develop a Peer Strategy: Child with Inborn Errors of Metabolism and Diet Management
Identify Strategies to Help Girls Understand Early Pubertal Development

The endocrine system controls the cellular activity that regulates growth and body metabolism through the release of hormones. **Hormones** are chemical messengers secreted by various glands that exert controlling effects on the cells of the body. Overlapping with all body systems, the general functions of the endocrine system include the following:

- Differentiation of the reproductive and central nervous systems in the fetus
- Regulation of the pace of growth and development in concert with the central nervous system throughout childhood and adolescence
- Coordination of the male and female reproductive systems, enabling sexual reproduction
- Maintenance of an optimal level of hormones for body functioning
- Maintenance of homeostasis, a healthy internal environment, in the presence of a constantly changing external environment

Inherited metabolic diseases—inherited biochemical abnormalities of the urea cycle and amino acid and organic acid metabolism—often have a significant impact on the endocrine system's ability to support growth and development. Some chromosomal abnormalities also result in disturbances in growth and sexual development. Endocrine disturbances result in alterations in metabolism, growth and development, and behavior that may have significant implications for children. If not diagnosed and treated early, these conditions can result in delays in growth and development, mental retardation, and, occasionally, death. However, treatment, which usually consists of supplementation of missing hormones, adjustment of hormone levels, or dietary measures, allows most children to live a normal life.

ANATOMY AND PHYSIOLOGY OF PEDIATRIC DIFFERENCES

The major organs of the endocrine system are the thyroid gland, pituitary gland, parathyroid glands, adrenal glands, pancreas, and the gonads (male and female reproductive glands). Figure 32–1 ■ illustrates the location of these glands.

The hypothalamic-pituitary axis produces several releasing and inhibiting hormones that regulate the function of many endocrine glands including the thyroid, adrenal, and the male and female reproductive glands. In addition, growth is regulated by hormones originating from this axis. Other endocrine glands include the parathyroid glands and islets of Langerhans in the pancreas. These glands secrete hormones into the bloodstream that are carried to target organs or tissues. Most hormones exert their influence through interaction with receptors in the target cells of specific tissues (Table 32–1).

The regulation of hormone secretion occurs through a **negative feedback** mechanism that functions to maintain an optimal internal environment in the body. Negative feedback occurs when an endocrine gland or secretory tissue receives a message that an adequate amount of hormone has been received by the target cells. In response, further secretion is inhibited. Secretion is resumed only when the secretory tissue receives another message indicating that levels of the hormone are low.

The endocrine system is responsible for sexual differentiation during fetal development and for stimulating growth and development during childhood and adolescence. This includes stimulating development of the reproductive system in both sexes.

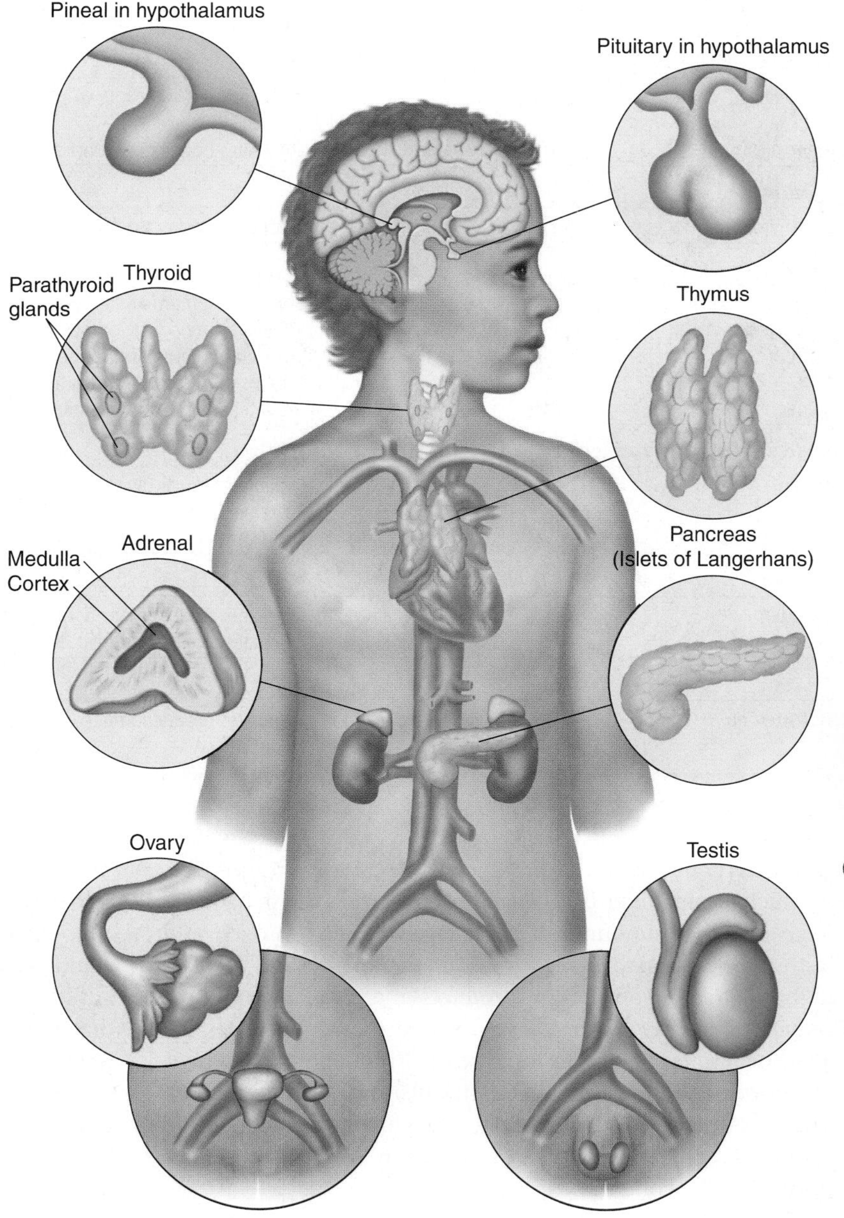

FIGURE 32–1 ■ Major organs and glands of the endocrine system.

MediaLink Endocrine System A & P Review

TABLE 32–1 Endocrine Glands and Their Functions

GLAND/HORMONE	FUNCTION
Anterior Pituitary	
Growth hormone (somadotropin)	Stimulates growth and metabolism of all body tissues
Thyroid-stimulating hormone (TSH)	Stimulates thyroid hormone secretion
Adrenocorticotropic hormone (ACTH) (corticotrophin)	Stimulates secretion of glucocorticoids and androgens
Follicle-stimulating hormone (FSH) (a gonadotropin)	Stimulates secretion of estrogen; stimulates follicle maturation in ovaries. Also critical for sperm production in males.
Luteinizing hormone (LH) and interstitial cell-stimulating hormone (ICSH) (male analog) (a gonadotropin)	Stimulates secretion of androgens in males and progesterone in females
Prolactin-releasing hormone	Stimulates secretion of prolactin which stimulates the secretion of milk during lactation
Melanocyte-stimulating hormone (MSH)	Stimulates skin pigmentation
Beta endorphins	Endogenous opioid involved in pain sensation
Posterior Pituitary	
Antidiuretic hormone (ADH)	Promotes water reabsorption back into blood, decreasing urine output
Oxytocin	Stimulates uterine contractions and breast milk letdown reflex
Thyroid	
Thyroxine (T_4) and triiodothyronine (T_3)	Regulates metabolic rate of all cells, body heat production; protein, fat, and carbohydrate catabolism in all cells
Thyrocalcitonin	Stimulates bone ossification and development
Parathyroid	
Parathyroid hormone	Regulates serum calcium levels and excretion of phosphorus
Adrenal	
Aldosterone	Conserves sodium and excretion of potassium
Androgens	Stimulates bone development and secondary sexual characteristics
Cortisol	Involved in maturation of the central nervous system, respiratory, gastrointestinal, and hepatic systems in the fetus. Stimulates anti-inflammatory reactions, maintains homeostasis
Epinephrine	Activates sympathetic nervous system; stimulates increase in blood pressure and blood glucose levels
Pancreas (islets of Langerhans)	
Insulin	Facilitates cellular glucose utilization
Glucagon	Increases blood glucose
Somatostatin	Stimulates inhibition of insulin and glucagon secretion; may prevent excess insulin secretion
Ovaries	
Estrogen	Stimulates development of breasts and ova
Progesterone	Stimulates breast glandular development; acts to maintain pregnancy
Testes	
Testosterone	Stimulates production of sperm, development of secondary sexual characteristics, and closure of epiphysis

Puberty, the period of life during which acquisition of reproductive capability is acheived, occurs when the gonads secrete increased amounts of the sex hormones estrogen and testosterone. At the average age of 10 years in girls and 11 years in boys, the hypothalamus produces increased amounts of *gonadotropin-releasing hormone.* This hormone stimulates the anterior pituitary gland to increase the production of luteinizing hormone (LH) and follicle-stimulating hormone (FSH). These hormones in turn stimulate the gonads to secrete more sex hormones (Figure 32–2 ■), resulting in the development of primary and secondary sex characteristics.

Disorders of pituitary, thyroid, adrenal, pancreatic, and gonadal function, as well as inherited metabolic diseases, are discussed in this chapter.

DISORDERS OF PITUITARY FUNCTION

The pituitary gland consists of two lobes, an anterior lobe and a posterior lobe. The functions of the posterior pituitary gland include regulation of fluid balance through release of antidiuretic hormone (ADH), which is stored in the hypothalamus; and production of oxytocin, which is also stored in the hypothalamus.

The anterior pituitary gland is considered to be the "master gland" of the body (Figure 32–3 ■). The major function of the anterior pituitary gland is the production and release of thyroid-stimulating hormone (TSH), adrenocorticotropic hormone (ACTH), luteinizing hormone (LH), follicle-stimulating hormone (FSH), growth hormone (GH), and prolactin (PRL). Most of these hormones regulate the secretion of other hormones.

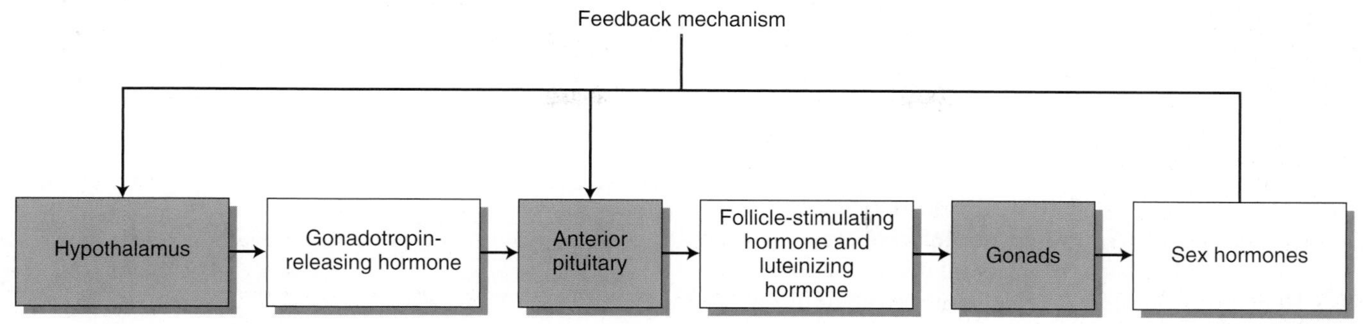

FIGURE 32–2 ■ Feedback mechanism in hormonal stimulation of the gonads during puberty.

- Growth hormone (GH) stimulates growth of all body tissues.
- Thyroid-stimulating hormone (TSH) stimulates the thyroid gland to produce thyroid hormone, which regulates body metabolism and is essential for normal growth.
- Adrenocorticotropic hormone (ACTH) stimulates the adrenal glands to produce cortisol (stress hormone) and other hormones that enable the body to respond to stress. Excess cortisol leads to growth failure in children.
- Luteinizing hormone (LH) stimulates secretion of androgens in males and progesterone in females.
- Follicle-stimulating hormone (FSH) stimulates secretion of estrogens; supports follicle development in ovaries.

Pituitary disorders such as growth hormone deficiency (hypopituitarism), hyperpituitarism, and precocious puberty directly affect the child's growth, while diabetes insipidus is a disorder affecting fluid balance. These disorders are discussed in the following section.

Growth Hormone Deficiency (Hypopituitarism)

Growth hormone deficiency (GHD) is a disorder caused by decreased activity of the pituitary gland. The primary characteristics of the disorder are growth retardation, short stature, and delayed bone maturation during infancy and childhood. The defect may occur in combination with a deficiency of other anterior pituitary hormones—thyroid-stimulating hormone, adrenocorticotropic hormone, luteinizing hormone, follicle-stimulating hormone, and prolactin. The disorder is diagnosed more often in males than in females because males are referred more often for evaluation of short stature than females.

Etiology and Pathophysiology

The release of growth hormone from the anterior pituitary gland is controlled by the hypothalamus, which secretes growth hormone-releasing (GRH) and inhibitory factors (somatostatin). Growth hormone (GH) stimulates linear growth and

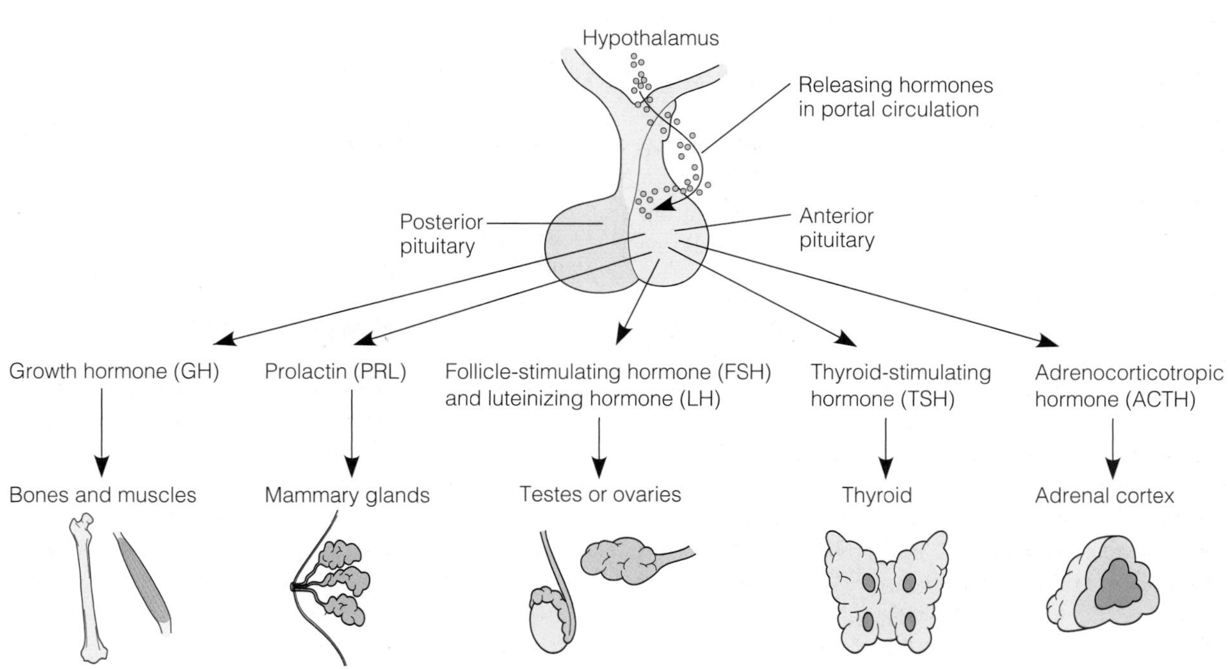

FIGURE 32–3 ■ Actions of the major hormones of the anterior pituitary.

MediaLink Hormone Regulation and Secretion Animation

bone mineral density, as well as the growth of all body tissues. Growth hormone also stimulates the synthesis of proteins in the liver, among them the somatomedins or insulinlike growth factors (IGFs), which promote glucose utilization by the cells and cell proliferation. In growth hormone deficiency, the pituitary fails to produce sufficient growth hormone.

Most often, the cause for the dysfunction is idiopathic. Known causes include central nervous infection, infarction of the pituitary gland (related to sickle-cell disease), central nervous system disease, tumors of the pituitary gland or hypothalamus (primarily craniopharyngiomas and gliomas), other brain tumors, cranial irradiation, brain trauma, and chemotherapy (Box 32–1). Additionally, psychosocial deprivation may cause growth hormone deficiency by interfering with the production or release of growth hormone. Deficiency of growth hormone or abnormalities of hormone receptors may be caused by dominant or recessive inheritance or by a genetic mutation (Witchel & Finegold, 2002).

Clinical Manifestations

Children with growth hormone deficiency have normal birth weights and lengths. By the age of 1 year, however, they are below the 3rd percentile on the growth chart. The child characteristically grows at a rate of less than 5 cm (2 in.) per year. Other characteristic findings in infants include hypoglycemic seizures, hyponatremia, neonatal jaundice, pale optic discs, micropenis, and undescended testes. Children with growth hormone deficiency tend to appear "cherubic" and exhibit youthful facial features, higher pitched voices, delayed dentition, "ripply" abdominal fat, decreased muscle mass, delayed skeletal maturation, and delayed sexual maturation. Slipped capital femoral epiphysis has been associated with growth hormone deficiency.

COLLABORATIVE CARE

Any child whose height is 2 to 3 standard deviations below the mean height for age or whose measurement is falling off the normal growth chart should be evaluated for short stature (Table 32–2). A child whose screening tests reveal low levels of insulinlike growth factors (IGF-1) requires further evaluation by a pediatric endocrinologist. A careful history, physical examination, assessment of pubertal development and unusual facies, and radiologic studies are necessary to rule out familial short stature and constitutional growth delay, which are normal variants, and skeletal dysplasias or psychosocial short stature, which requires further evaluation.

BOX 32–1 Major Causes of Short Stature

- Growth hormone deficiency
- Familial short stature
- Hypothyroidism
- Turner syndrome
- Constitutional growth delay
- Chronic renal failure
- Cushing syndrome
- Inborn error of metabolism
- Severe cardiac disease
- Pulmonary disease
- Gastrointestinal disease
- Failure to thrive

TABLE 32–2 Diagnostic Tests for Short Stature

TEST	PURPOSE RELATED TO SHORT STATURE
IGF-1 and IGFBP-3	Excludes growth hormone deficiency if normal
Radiographic views of the sella turcica (site of the pituitary gland)	Demonstrates size of the sella turcica or a tumor
Karotype (girls)	Detects Turner syndrome (see page 1287)
Thyroid function studies	Detects hypothyroidism (see page 1250)
Urine creatinine, pH, specific gravity, urea nitrogen, electrolytes	Detects chronic renal failure (see Chapter 31 ∞)
Bone age	Identifies other potential causes of delayed growth
Complete blood count and erythrocyte sedimentation rate	Screens for inflammatory bowel disease with anemia
Antigliadin antibodies	Screens for celiac disease

Data from D'Ercole, A. J., & Underwood, L. (1996). Anterior pituitary gland and hypothalamus. In A. M. Rudolph, J. I. E. Hoffman, & C. D. Rudolph (Eds.), Rudolph's pediatrics *(20th ed., p. 1692). Stamford, CT: Appleton & Lange. Modified.*

Diagnostic Tests

Early diagnosis and treatment are important to ensure attainment of maximum adult height potential. In some cases, the onset of puberty is delayed with gonadotropin-releasing hormone analogs to provide more time for growth hormone therapy to stimulate growth. Provocative growth hormone testing, in which various medications (arginine, clonidine, glucagon, insulin, L-dopa) are administered to stimulate release of growth hormone, is a diagnostic test that may be used to confirm growth hormone deficiency. Confirmation of the disorder is based on failure to demonstrate a growth hormone response (with a GH level > 10 ng/mL) after presentation of two provocative stimuli as previously mentioned. However, some endocrinologists believe this test is less reliable than other tests, such as low IGF-1 levels. Growth hormone defiency may occur alone or with one or more other pituitary hormone deficiencies. It may be total defiency (no growth hormone produced) or partial defiency (some growth hormone produced, but not enough to support normal growth).

Radiographic imaging of the hand or wrist bone is used to evaluate the stage of bone ossification, and thus the bone age of the child. Using standardized norms for bone ossification, radiologists can determine if the child's chronologic and bone ages match. **Bone age** (skeletal maturation) is used to evaluate the child with a growth problem. Significantly delayed (less than the child's age) or advanced (greater than the child's age) bone age may be indicative of a systemic chronic disease or hormone abnormality requiring investigation.

Clinical Therapy

For growth hormone deficiency, replacement therapy with growth hormone (GH) is administered to promote growth and development. Approved indications for growth hormone therapy are listed in Box 32–2. There has been concern that children without true growth hormone deficiency may be treated in order to achieve increased linear growth; however, the long-term consequences of this are unknown.

Multiple preparations of GH are available. There are no observable differences in the results obtained when using different preparations as long as the recommended injection regimen is followed. Most indications for growth hormone replacement require daily GH injections. The use of GH is being investigated for children with cystic fibrosis and other disorders (Wilson, et al., 2003).

The child receiving growth hormone experiences increased growth velocity for the first year of treatment, followed by a gradual decrease in growth for subsequent months or years. However, growth should progress at least at the normal growth rate for age while continued on growth hormone treatment. If growth is slower than anticipated, improper preparation and administration of growth hormone and poor adherence to therapy must be considered (Halec & Zimmerman, 2004b). Replacement therapy is continued until either the child achieves an acceptable height or growth velocity drops to less than 2 cm (1 in.) per year. Close monitoring of growth and endocrinology visits every 3 to 4 months is required.

PRACTICE ALERT

Slipped capital femoral epiphysis has been associated with hypothyroidism and growth hormone deficiency. Any child receiving growth hormone treatment who complains of hip pain, knee pain, or manifesting a limp must be evaluated for this disorder (Halec & Zimmerman, 2004b).

Side effects of growth hormone therapy include arthralgia, carpal tunnel syndrome, myalgia, reduced insulin sensitivity, slipped capital femoral epiphysis, gynecomastia, progression of scoliosis and hypothyroidism, and "benign" increased intracranial pressure (pseudotomor cerebri) (Miller & Zimmerman, 2004; Wilson et. al., 2003). Additional side effects include mild swelling and headaches. Peripheral edema is common in children with Turner syndrome treated with growth hormone. Though rare, lipoatrophy may occur at growth hormone injection sites if sites are not rotated. Growth hormone deficiency caused by psychosocial deprivation is reversible if the child is removed from the adverse environment.

BOX 32–2 FDA Approved Uses of Growth Hormone

- Growth Hormone deficiency/insufficiency
- Chronic renal insufficiency/pretransplanation
- Turner Syndrone
- Short stature from Prader-Willi Syndrome (PWS)
- Children with a history of intrauterine growth restriction (small for gestational age [SGA] who have not achieved normal height by two years of age
- Children with idiopathic short stature who are >2.25 SD below the mean in height and who are unlikely to catch up in height.
- Adults with growth hormone deficiency
- Adults with AIDS wasting

Data from Wilson, T. A., Rose, S. R., Cohen, P., et al. (2003). Update of guidelines for the use of growth hormone in children: the Lawson Wilkins pediatric endocrinology society drug and therapeutics committee. Journal of Pediatrics. 143*(4), 415–421.*

NURSING MANAGEMENT

Nursing care consists of monitoring and plotting growth, educating the child and family about the disorder and its treatment, and providing emotional support.

Nursing Assessment and Diagnosis

The child's height and weight are carefully measured and plotted on a growth chart (refer to Appendix A∞) to monitor growth changes over time. Assess the child's psychosocial adaptation to short stature. Assess parents for coping with child's short stature and treatment regimen.

Nursing diagnoses that apply to the child with growth hormone deficiency may include the following:

- Risk for Disproportionate Growth related to poor adherence to daily injection regimen.
- Disturbed Body Image related to short stature
- Risk for Chronic Low Self-esteem related to physical appearance

Planning and Implementation

Partner with the child and family in providing instructions regarding growth hormone replacement therapy and injection. Injections are given subcutaneously and parents must understand site selection and importance of site rotation. Some growth hormone preparations are available in pen form, which improves ease of preparation and delivery. Daily injections of growth hormone may be a source of major stress to the child. Assist the family in establishing techniques to minimize the trauma to the child who is receiving regular injections. Some growth hormone may require dilution before administration. Ensure parents utilize proper diluent techniques. Educate family about potential side effects and actions to take if noticed.

Partner with family members and direct them to educational resources such as the Magic Foundation or Human Growth Foundation. Replacement therapy is expensive (starting at approximately $35,000 per year) and may not be covered by insurance; therefore, parents may require financial assistance that is sometimes available from the growth hormone manufacturers and third-party payers.

Children with growth hormone deficiency, especially those due to tumors and trauma from radiation or surgery, may experience academic problems resulting from acquired learning disabilities. Before the child enters or returns to school, a comprehensive evaluation is performed to identify potential

MediaLink Growth Hormone Deficiency Resources and Support

problems. Partner with the family and school officials to ensure that the child is appropriately screened.

The best results occur when treatment is initiated at an early age, before psychologic effects of short stature become apparent. If growth hormone therapy is not initiated early enough, attainment of near normal height may not be reached. Often children are treated on the basis of their size rather than their age, and these children experience social prejudice related to height. Teasing is a common problem experienced by children with short stature. The teenage years may be particularly stressful due to the preoccupation with body image which is characteristic of adolescence. Partner with the adolescent and family to promote positive coping mechanisms.

Provide the child and family with information regarding normal growth and development patterns. Explain that developmental expectations are the same for a child with growth hormone deficiency as for children unaffected with the disorder. Encourage parents and teachers to treat the child in an age-appropriate manner. The child should dress in clothing that reflects his or her chronologic age. Encourage parents to emphasize the child's strengths, support independence, and promote participation in age-appropriate activities to assist in the development of a positive self-image. The child can participate in sports in which ability does not depend on size (e.g., swimming, gymnastics, wrestling, ice skating, and martial arts). The identification of positive role models, short-statured individuals who are successful in accomplishing their goals, is another approach that promotes a positive image. Refer the child and family for counseling if appropriate.

Evaluation

Outcomes of nursing care for the child with growth hormone deficiency may include the following:

- The child achieves linear growth that is near normal for adult height.
- The parents and child adhere to treatment regimen, can identify side effects, and can appropriately administer growth hormone.
- The child demonstrates a positive body image.
- The child demonstrates positive self-esteem.

Hyperpituitarism

Hyperpituitarism, a disorder in which excessive secretion of growth hormone increases the growth rate, is rare in children. Oversecretion of growth hormone is usually caused by a pituitary adenoma. If combined with precocious puberty, a tumor of the hypothalamus may be present. Affected children can grow to 7 or 8 feet in height when oversecretion occurs before closure of the epiphyseal plates. If the disorder occurs after closure of the epiphyseal plates, **acromegaly** occurs. In acromegaly, abnormal growth of the hands and feet occur as well as a protruding brow and lower jaw; the nasal bone enlarges, and spacing of the teeth increases.

Since tall stature is valued in our society, assessment of children, particularly males, with accelerated growth is often delayed. Any child with rapid linear growth whose predicted height exceeds that consistent with parental height should be evaluated for possible growth problems and underlying pathologic conditions.

A complete history is obtained, and physical examination and laboratory testing are performed. Increased levels of insulinlike growth factors (IGF-1) establish the diagnosis of hyperpituitarism. Radiologic examination for bone age is obtained to determine if the epiphyseal plates have begun to fuse. Radiological studies are conducted to detect the presence of a brain tumor. Thorough evaluation is required to differentiate hyperpituitarism from familial tall stature.

Treatment depends on the cause of the excessive growth and may involve surgical removal of a tumor or pituitary gland (hypophysectomy), radiation therapy, radioactive implants, or high doses of sex steroids given to close the epiphyseal plates. If the pituitary gland is removed, the child requires lifelong pituitary hormone replacement following surgery.

Nursing Management

Early identification of the child with excessive growth rate is essential. Monitor growth trends and refer children whose height growth rate exceeds expected development for further evaluation and treatment to retard the accelerated growth rate. Nursing care focuses on educating the parents and child about the disorder and its treatment, providing emotional support, and, if surgery is required, providing preoperative and postoperative teaching and care (refer to Chapter 17∞).

Tall stature, like short stature, can be stressful for children. Tall children are often treated as if they are older than their chronologic age. Tall adolescents may experience problems with self-image, and girls in particular may worry about their appearance. Partner with the child and family to promote a positive body image and self-esteem. Provide the child opportunities to express concerns regarding body image.

Diabetes Insipidus

Two forms of diabetes insipidus (DI), central DI and nephrogenic DI, exist. Diabetes insipidus is a disorder of the posterior pituitary gland, and can occur at any age. Both forms of the disorder involve antidiuretic hormone (ADH), a hormone secreted from the posterior pituitary gland. The most important function of ADH is to bind to the collecting ducts of the kidney and promote reabsorption of water back into the circulation. Diabetes insipidus can occur at any age and results from ADH or vasopressin deficiency (central diabetes insipidus) or inability of the collecting ducts to respond to ADH (neprogenic diabetes insipidus).

Etiology and Pathophysiology

Normally, fluid balance is maintained by actions of the hypothalamus, kidney, and pituitary gland by the following mechanisms.

- The antidiuretic hormone (ADH) is produced by the hypothalamus and is stored in the posterior pituitary gland.
- The hypothalamus detects dehydration, sends a message to the pituitary, which in turn releases antidiuretic hormone into the blood and it is carried to the kidney.
- In the kidney, antidiuretic hormone acts on the collecting and distal tubules to reabsorb water—promoting concentration of urine, and *retention* of fluids (decreased urine output) to restore fluid balance.

- When excess fluid volume occurs, the hypothalamus sends a message to the pituitary to inhibit secretion of antidiuretic hormone, promoting *excretion* of fluids to restore fluid balance.

Plasma osmolarity, or the concentration of solutes in the blood, is an important factor in ADH secretion. Osmolarity is sensed in the hypothalamus by osmoreceptor neurons, and those neurons provide feedback to the posterior pituitary gland to produce appropriate antidiuretic hormone.

- A low serum osmolality causes a reduction in antidiuretic hormone production, which leads to increased urine output and increased serum sodium (from hemoconcentration).
- An elevated serum osmolality causes an increase in antidiuretic hormone production, which leads to water retention and decreased urine output.

Antidiuretic hormone facilitates concentration of the urine by stimulating reabsorption of water from the distal tubule of the kidney. When antidiuretic hormone is inadequate or insufficient, as in diabetes insipidus, the tubules do not resorb water, leading to **polyuria** (passage of a large volume of urine in a given period). Therefore, the body is unable to conserve water, resulting in severe dehydration.

Central (or primary) diabetes insipidus is caused by a deficiency in production or release of antidiuretic hormone. This antidiuretic hormone deficiency in children is idiopathic or neurogenic.

Neurogenic causes that reduce the production of antidiuretic hormone include primary brain tumors, which account for 50% of central diabetes insipidus (Saborio, Tipton, & Chan, 2000). Other causes include central nervous system (CNS) trauma, infection, electrolyte imbalances, surgical procedures (such as hypophysectomy), hypoxic brain damage, neoplasm, vascular anomalies, or infiltrative diseases such as leukemia. Idiopathic etiology accounts for approximately 10% of children with central diabetes insipidus (Parks, 2004).

Nephrogenic diabetes insipidus, the less common form of diabetes insipidus, can be inherited or acquired. Inherited disorder occurs with either an X-linked, autosomal dominant, or autosomal recessive form. Acquired nephrogenic diabetes insipidus may also result from drug toxicity or adverse drug reactions. Drugs known to cause diabetes insipidus include lithium carbonate (Carbolith), demeclocycline (Declomycin), amphotericin, cisplatin, foscarnet, methicillin, and rifampin (Parks, 2004). In both inherited and acquired forms, the kidney is unable to respond to antidiuretic hormone. The actual amount of antidiuretic hormone produced is not deficient.

Clinical Manifestations

Polyuria (excess urine output) and **polydipsia** (excessive thirst) are the cardinal signs of diabetes insipidus. Polyuria in children is defined as urine volume excreted in excess of 150 mL/kg at birth, 110 mL/kg at 2 years, and 40 mL/kg/24h in the older child (Cheetham & Baylis, 2002). Polydipsia is the body's attempt to preserve fluid balance. Additional manifestations observed in children with diabetes insipidus include hypernatremia, dilute urine, and dehydration. See the table below for the clinical manifestations of diabetes insipidus associated with cause.

Although the onset of symptoms is usually sudden, diagnosis is often delayed if the child is outside of an intensive care unit where intake and output is monitored hourly. Children who are able to quench their thirst may not complain to parents about symptoms. In infants, symptoms may include failure to thrive, poor feeding, and irritability. Infants will suck vigorously during feeding; however, they vomit immediately afterwards (Saborio et al., 2000). Diapers are usually extremely saturated. Dehydration in the infant is manifested by sunken fontanels, sunken eyes, and mottled skin. Older children exhibit excessive fluid intake, nocturia, poor appetite, and delayed growth. Seizures may occur in response to extreme electrolyte imbalances. Hypotension, tachycardia, and poor perfusion due to dehydration may also occur.

In all forms of diabetes insipidus, the urine cannot be concentrated, regardless of the extent of dehydration experienced. Dehydration usually precipitates diagnosis. Serum sodium concentration and osmolality increase rapidly to pathologic levels. Often an unconscious child is admitted to the emergency department with dehydration accompanied by hypernatremia.

CLINICAL TIP

As dehydration occurs, serum sodium concentrations rise (hypernatremia). As fluid retention occurs, serum sodium concentrations decrease (hyponatremia).

COLLABORATIVE CARE

The goals of collaborative care include restoration and maintenance of fluid and electrolyte balance using fluid and pharmacologic management, identifying and correcting the underlying pathology, and preventing complications associated with the

Clinical Manifestations of Diabetes Insipidus

ETIOLOGY	CLINICAL MANIFESTATIONS	CLINICAL THERAPY
Central diabetes insipidus ADH deficiency Familial or idiopathic	Polyuria, polydipsia Nocturia, enuresis Irritable if fluids withheld Constipation, fever, dehydration	Desmopressin acetate
Nephrogenic diabetes insipidus Inherited or acquired Decreased responsiveness of kidneys to ADH	Polyuria, polydipsia Hypernatremia in neonatal period Dehydration, vomiting Mental status changes	Diuretics High fluid intake Salt and protein restricted diet

disorder. Early recognition and treatment is essential to prevent complications, such as secondary neurologic impairment associated with hypernatremic dehydration (see Chapter 23∞).

Diagnostic Tests

Serum electrolytes and both serum and urine osmolalities are tested. Urine osmolality is decreased (<200 mOsm/kg), urine specific gravity is decreased (< 1.005), serum sodium is elevated (> 145 mEq/L), and serum osmolality is elevated (> 285 mOsm/L) (Trimarchi, 2001). These values reflect that excessive urine has been inappropriately lost with resultant dehydration. Diagnosis in the acute care setting is often made based on these findings. Investigation of underlying causes of diabetes insipidus, such as brain surgery, brain trauma, tumor, infection, and a review of medications, is ongoing.

In the non-acute setting, diagnosis can be confirmed by measuring the plasma arginine vasopressin (AVP) level before and during a fluid deprivation test, which is usually conducted in the hospital or in a carefully controlled outpatient setting for up to 8 hours. During this procedure, fluid intake is prohibited. Weight, urine output, specific gravity, and osmolality are measured every 2 hours or per protocol. The child is monitored closely for surreptitious consumption of fluids.

Normally, the response to fluid deprivation is a decreased urine output with a high urine specific gravity. However, in diabetes insipidus, the child continues to excrete large amounts of dilute urine, and a low urine specific gravity which will remain less than 1.005 even after dehydration. After several hours of fluid deprivation, a dose of aqueous vasopressin is administered. A decreased urine output and increased urine concentration confirms the diagnosis of central or neurogenic diabetes insipidus. With nephrogenic diabetes insipidus, the kidney does not respond to the antidiuretic hormone (vasopressin); therefore, no response will be observed with the administration of vasopressin. Additional studies may include MRI to visualize the anterior and posterior pituitary glands.

Clinical Therapy

Water replacement therapy is essential to prevent severe hypotension and cardiovascular collapse. Rehydration with water is necessary, and if the child is unable to consume appropriate amounts orally, rehydration with intravenous fluids is implemented. In severely ill children, fluid boluses to overcome hypotension followed by fluid management of calculated insensible losses (400 ml/m2/day), plus hourly urine output replacement may be instituted.

Pharmacologic Treatment for Neurogenic Diabetes Insipidus. Pharmacologic treatment of neurogenic diabetes insipidus may require lifelong therapy and consists of the subcutaneous, intranasal, or oral desmopressin acetate (DDAVP) with an effect lasting 8 to 12 hours. Some cases of neurogenic diabetes insipidus, particularly post-operative, may be reversible. DDAVP reduces urinary output, enabling the child to live a more normal life with a decrease in thirst, urinary output, and nocturia. The dose of DDAVP must be titered for sufficient coverage of metabolic needs.

Administration of synthetic vasopressin (DDAVP) in small doses by intranasal insufflation (blowing the medication into the nasal cavity) in infants and young children often results in inconsistent absorption. If too large a dose is given, the child may swallow the medication, resulting in lack of absorption. Intravenous DDAVP is often administered to the hospitalized child with DI due to more predictable dose delivery. Side effects of DDAVP include hypertension and headaches due to water retention. Effects of DDAVP should be noted within the hour after administration of the medication; specifically, a rise in urine specific gravity and decrease in urine output (Trimarchi, 2001).

Intravenous fluids are adjusted after DDAVP has taken effect to prevent fluid overload and water intoxication. Serum sodium and serum osmolality are often measured frequently until the appropriate dose of DDAVP has been established. Therapeutic goals include urine output of 2-3ml/kg/hour, urine specific gravity of 1.010 to 1.020, and serum sodium of 140–145 mEq/L.

Other medications used to treat DI include clofibrate, which has an antidiuretic effect, chlorpropamide (Diabinese), and thiazide diuretics, which potentiate the action of vasopressin.

Pharmacologic Treatment for Nephrogenic Diabetes Insipidus. Since the actual amount of antidiuretic hormone produced is not deficient, DDAVP is not effective in controlling nephrogenic diabetes insipidus. Instead, children with nephrogenic diabetes insipidus are treated with thiazide diuretics, which act by enhancing sodium excretion and reducing the glomerular filtration rate, and prostaglandin inhibitors such as ibuprofen or indomethacin which have a similar effect. Additionally, a high fluid intake and a low sodium diet are essential (Cheetham & Baylis, 2002). The child's sodium and potassium levels are carefully monitored to prevent hypernatremia and hypokalemia (refer to Chapter 23∞).

NURSING MANAGEMENT

Nursing care centers on early detection of dehydration, promoting adequate hydration, administering medications, monitoring specific gravity, obtaining laboratory specimens, and providing parental education and support.

■ Nursing Assessment and Diagnosis

Assess for signs of fluid volume deficit. Weigh the child and compare to previous weight when healthy to detect fluid volume loss. Assess skin integrity and mucous membranes. Assess fontanels in infants. Monitor intake and output and assess thirst or water craving. Monitor vital signs to detect changes in blood pressure and heart rate. Assess level of consciousness or responsiveness as the child is usually irritable or lethargic as a result of hypernatremia and dehydration. Observe cardiac monitor for rhythm disturbances associated with electrolyte imbalances. Assess the child's sleeping pattern.

CLINICAL TIP

A weight loss of 2 pounds indicates a loss of 1 liter of fluid.

Nursing diagnoses that apply to the child with diabetes insipidus may include the following:

- Impaired Urinary Elimination related to polyuria
- Deficient Fluid Volume related to polyuria
- Sleep Pattern Disturbance related to nocturia and enuresis
- Risk for Impaired Skin Integrity related to incontinence
- Effective Therapeutic Regimen Management related to dietary and medication plan adherence

Planning and Implementation

Care in the hospital includes fluid replacement either orally or intravenously. Monitor urine specific gravity as indicated and report decreasing values. Monitor serum osmolality and sodium for increasing values. Keep fluids within child's reach at all times, with the exception of testing restrictions. Implement preventive measures for skin integrity if the child is incontinent.

Care in the Community

Parent education is of primary importance for the child with diabetes insipidus. For home care management, partner with the family in the management of the condition and how to recognize the signs of altered fluid status. Infants usually require fluid intake even during the night. Many infants have coexisting brain damage, requiring nasogastric or gastrostomy feeding to maintain adequate hydration and nutrition. Partner with the family to ensure proper feeding and safety precautions with nasogastric or gastrostomy feedings (refer to Chapter 9∞). Inform the family that treatment for diabetes insipidus may require lifelong medication therapy.

Instruct families about DDAVP administration, obtaining and recording daily weights, and measuring intake and output. The child should consume fluids equal to the amount of output unless otherwise instructed. Ensure that parents understand and can recognize signs of inadequate fluid intake (see Chapter 23∞) and are able to adequately adjust the child's fluid intake to prevent dehydration. Teach the parents that monitoring for excess fluid intake is also essential. When excessive fluid is consumed, the child will not have the ability to excrete the excess water load with DDAVP treatment.

When the child with nephrogenic diabetes insipidus has an acute illness, the child's physician should be notified immediately. An acute illness increases the child's metabolic activity and may cause dehydration and hypernatremia, resulting in seizures. Additional fluids during illness are required to prevent dehydration.

The child with chronic diabetes insipidus should always wear a medical alert identification (tag, bracelet, or necklace) to indicate the presence of the disorder. Partner with the parents and school officials to make arrangements to provide the child unrestricted access to toilet facilities and water.

Parents may require assistance to manage the child's care. Arrangements for a visiting nurse, a home health nurse, or respite care may be required. Assist the family in obtaining the appropriate support needed.

Evaluation

Outcomes of nursing care for the child with diabetes insipidus may include the following:

- The child's frequency of urination is decreased and fluid balance is restored.
- The child obtains adequate rest and sleep for optimal growth and development.
- The parents (and child if older) demonstrate an understanding of disease management, administer medication correctly, and monitor and record intake, output, and weight.
- The child's skin integrity remains intact.

Syndrome of Inappropriate Antidiuretic Hormone

Syndrome of inappropriate antidiuretic hormone (SIADH) results from an excessive amount of serum antidiuretic hormone (ADH). Syndrome of inappropriate antidiuretic hormone is caused by hypoxic or traumatic ischemic brain injury, and diseases of the hypothalamus, pituitary stalk, or posterior pituitary. It may also be noted in children with central nervous system (CNS) infections such as meningitis, pneumonia, or in those receiving positive pressure ventilation. In addition, some medications including diuretics and chemotherapy have been associated with SIADH. This disorder may be observed in critically ill infants and children.

Etiology and Pathophysiology

Failure of the normal mechanisms of feedback from the hypothalamus, pituitary gland, and kidney results in excessive secretion of antidiuretic hormone (ADH) resulting in water reabsorption despite the presence of low serum osmolality (refer to fluid balance regulation discussed in the diabetes insipidus section). ADH secretion causes increased permeability of the distal renal tubules and collecting ducts, resulting in water reabsorption, increased intravascular volume and decreased urine output (Trimarchi 2001). Elevated levels of antidiuretic hormone also cause suppression of the renin-angiotensin mechanism, resulting in renal excretion of sodium. The outcome is **water intoxication** (an abnormal proportion of water to sodium in the extracellular fluid), dilutional hyponatremia, and cellular edema. Dilutional hyponatremia results when more water is in the body and serum sodium levels drop. Cellular edema results as water shifts from the extracellular fluid compartment (see Chapter 23∞).

Clinical Manifestations

Manifestations of syndrome of inappropriate antidiuretic hormone are related to water intoxication and hyponatremia, and include elevated blood pressure, distended jugular veins, crackles auscultated in lung fields, and intake exceeding output. Other manifestations related to fluid and electrolyte imbalance include weight gain without edema, nausea, anorexia, abdominal cramps, weakness, fatigue, difficulty breathing, and concentrated amber urine with decreased urine output. As serum sodium levels continue to decline, symptoms including lethargy, confusion, headache, and progressive alteration in level of consciousness, seizures, and coma occur due to evolving cerebral edema.

COLLABORATIVE CARE

The goal of collaborative care is to restore fluid volume and electrolyte balance, and identify and correct the underlying cause of the disorder.

Diagnostic Tests

Urinalysis reveals a high urine osmolality (> 1200 mOsm/kg H_2O) secondary to increased water reabsorption and elevated specific gravity > 1.032. Serum osmolality is low (< 275 mOsm/kg) secondary to dilution, and hematocrit, BUN, and serum sodium (< 135 mEq/L) are also decreased as a result of expanding extracellular fluid volume.

Clinical Therapy

All fluids are restricted to prevent further hemodilution. The degree of restriction is dependent on the laboratory values. Urine osmolality, serum electrolytes, BUN, sodium, hematocrit, and serum osmolality are monitored. Serum sodium and osmolality levels should rise with fluid restriction. Diuretics such as furosemide (Lasix) are administered to eliminate excess body fluid. Demeclocycline (Declomycin) is administered to block the action of antidiuretic hormone (ADH) at the renal collecting tubules. Sodium supplementation may be required in severe cases and is achieved by intravenous infusion of hypertonic saline fluids administered at a slow rate.

NURSING MANAGEMENT

The goal of nursing care is to promote maintenance of fluid and electrolyte balance and prevent complications associated with the disorder.

Nursing Assessment and Diagnosis

Assess for changes in level of consciousness, mentation, and cognition, including headache and seizure activity. Monitor vital signs, and intake and output. Weigh the child daily to assess for weight gain, which may indicate a sign of water intoxication. Assess nutritional intake status and appetite.

Nursing diagnoses that apply to the child with SIADH may include the following:

- Fluid Volume Excess related to water retention
- Imbalanced Nutrition: Less than Body Requirements related to gastrointestinal symptoms
- Deficient Knowledge related to disease process and treatment regimen
- Risk for Injury related to the potential for seizures

Planning and Implementation

Nursing care focuses on preventing injury and monitoring fluid balance and nutritional intake. Implement seizure precautions. Weigh the child daily. Monitor intake and output, serum sodium, urine osmolality, and specific gravity. Monitor nutritional intake. Determine the child's food preferences and provide small, frequent meals to encourage intake.

Care in the Community

Partner with the family to ensure understanding of home care instructions. Include teaching the importance of daily weight and to report weight gain, which may indicate fluid retention. Refer the family to a nutritionist to assist in identifying hidden sources of water and fluids, such as popsicles, to prevent excessive fluid intake. See Partnering with Families: Food Sources of Fluids.

Depending on the cause of the disorder, lifelong medication may be required. If the child is prescribed demeclocycline, emphasize to the family the importance of follow-up care since the drug has nephrotoxic side effects. The child should wear a medical alert identification (tag, bracelet, or necklace) identifying the disorder and treatment.

Evaluation

Outcomes of nursing care for the child with syndrome of inappropriate antidiuretic hormone may include the following:

- The child's fluid balance is restored.
- The child has adequate nutritional intake to promote growth and development.
- The child and family demonstrate understanding of disorder, treatment regimen including fluid restriction and sources of sodium and water, and medication administration.
- The child is free from injury.

Precocious Puberty

Puberty normally occurs between 8 and 13 years in girls and between 9.5 and 14 years in boys. This change marks the development of reproductive capability and is characterized by the acquisition of secondary sexual characteristics. Pubertal development has started occurring earlier partly in response to better socioeconomic conditions, particularly improved nutrition. Racial differences also exist in the onset and progression of puberty, with secondary sexual characteristics occurring earlier in African American females than white females (Lalwani, Reindollar, Davis, 2003). Precocious puberty is defined as the appearance of any secondary sexual characteristics before 8 years in girls and 9 years in boys (Traggiai & Stanhope, 2003). The incidence of precocious puberty is approximately 1 in 5,000 to 10,000 children and is four to eight times more common in girls.

Etiology and Pathophysiology

Normally, puberty is initiated by an increase in nocturnal pulsatile gonadotrophin secretion of luteinizing hormone (LH) and follicle-stimulating hormone (FSH) from the pituitary gland. The secretion of LH and FSH is in response to pulsatile secretion of gonadotrophin-releasing hormone (GnRh) from the hypothalamus (Traggiai & Stanhope, 2003).

Early secretion of the normal hormones responsible for pubertal changes is not usually associated with abnormalities; however, a benign hypothalamic tumor may be present. Other causes include brain injury, brain tumor, postinfectious encephalitis or meningitis, congenital adrenal hyperplasia, tumors of the ovary, adrenal gland, or testicle, and exogenous hormone sources or androgens (i.e., anabolic steroids). Children with precocious puberty have an advanced bone age (premature skeletal maturation) and may appear unusually tall for their age. Their growth ceases prematurely, however, as the hormones stimulate closure of the epiphyseal plates, resulting in short stature.

Central precocious puberty (CPP) or gonadotropin-dependent precocious puberty occurs in premature activation of the hypothalamo-pituitary-gonadal axis, resulting in increased pulsatile release of luteinizing hormone (LH) and elevation of gonadal sex steroid concentration. In males, central precocious puberty is more likely the result of central nervous system disorders such as an intracranial tumor, while in females the cause is usually idiopathic (Traggiai & Stanhope, 2003).

Clinical Manifestations

Precocious puberty results in an accelerated growth rate, secondary sexual characteristics, advanced bone age, and behavioral changes such as mood swings and emotional lability. Typically, the child's psychosocial development is age appropriate.

Several other disorders are associated with premature pubertal development; however, these disorders require no treatment.

- Premature thelarche is characterized by breast development but no other signs of puberty. It is usually observed under the age of 2 years. The disorder is self-limiting over a few years.
- Isolated premature menarche is characterized by vaginal bleeding without other signs of sexual development. It is usually benign and self-limiting.
- Premature adrenarche (or pubarche) is characterized by the development of sexual hair (pubic, axillary) before 8 years of age in girls or 9 years of age in boys, without other signs of sexual maturation. Girls are usually taller than others their age, and an advanced bone age may be present. Early puberty may be an associated complication of this disorder.

COLLABORATIVE CARE

The goal of collaborative care is to determine the cause of precocious puberty, decrease the growth rate, stabilize development of secondary sexual characteristics, and promote optimal growth and development.

PARTNERING WITH FAMILIES

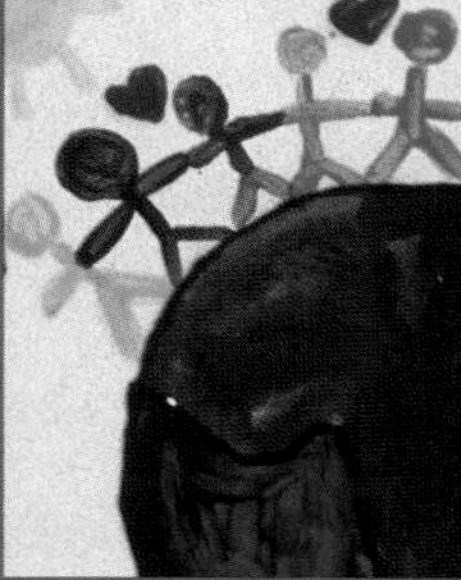

Food Sources of Fluids

Children with disorders such as syndrome of inappropriate antidiuretic hormone are placed on fluid restrictions. When parents are instructed to monitor and/or limit their child's fluid intake, they may not be aware of "hidden" sources of fluids. Partner with the family to ensure they can identify food sources containing significant fluid volume, such as the following:

- Ice cream
- Gelatin
- Popsicles
- Sherbet
- Watermelon

Diagnostic Tests

Radiologic imaging is performed to assess bone age. Serum diagnostic studies include luteinizing hormone, follicle-stimulating hormone, testosterone, or estradiol. Provocative testing includes gonadotropin-releasing hormone (GnRH) stimulation to confirm the diagnosis. Pelvic ultrasounds are performed on females to assess the uterus and ovaries. Computed tomography scans, MRI, or other radiologic studies are performed on males to assess for central nervous system abnormalities.

For isolated premature menarche, trauma, vaginal infections, unintentional estrogen ingestion, foreign bodies, and anal lesions should be ruled out.

Clinical Therapy

Therapy is focused on arresting the clinical signs of puberty, slowing the growth velocity, retarding skeletal maturation, and returning ovarian morphology and function to the prepubertal condition (Traggiai & Stanhope, 2003).

Central nervous system tumors require surgery, radiation, and/or chemotherapy. If precocious puberty begins before 6 years of age in girls, treatment is initiated immediately. For older girls, careful monitoring of growth patterns may be the initial step rather than beginning treatment. Currently, there are no definitive criteria for beginning treatment for children over the age of 6 years (Tato, Savage, Antoniazzi, et al., 2001).

Precocious puberty is treated with the administration of gonadotropin-releasing hormone analog (GnRHa) via subcutaneous, intramuscular, or intranasal route. Most commonly used are leuprolide acetate (Lupron) injections once a month or nafarelin acetate (Synarel) intranasally twice a day. The analog initially produces an increase followed by suppression of pituitary gonadotropin secretion. GnRHa results in decreased growth rate to age appropriate level and stabilization of secondary sexual development. Side effects of GnRHa include headache, local reactions, and photophobia.

NURSING MANAGEMENT

Nursing care focuses on educating the child and parents about the condition and its treatment, promoting growth and development, and providing emotional support.

Nursing Assessment and Diagnosis

A thorough history and physical examination are performed, including assessment of the child's secondary sexual characteristic development and sexual maturity rating using Tanner staging (see Chapter 8∞). Measure the child's height and weight and plot on a growth curve to detect changes in the growth rate from prior measurements. Assess the child's psychosocial adaptation to changes in body image. Assess for parental anxiety related to child's physical changes.

Nursing diagnoses that apply to the child with precocious puberty may include the following:

- Disturbed Body Image related to premature development of secondary sexual characteristics and rapid growth in height
- Risk for Disproportionate Growth related to accelerated growth and advanced bone age at an inappropriately early age
- Compromised Family Coping related to inappropriately early sexual maturation changes

Planning and Implementation

Promoting Positive Body Image

The goal of nursing care is to promote a positive body image in the child and to ensure proper medication administration. Partner with the child and family to explain to the child in age-appropriate terms that physiologic changes are normal but occurring at an earlier than usual age. Reassure the child that friends will experience the same stages of development eventually. Emphasize to the family that the child's social, cognitive, and emotional development corresponds with his or her age, even though the physical development is advanced.

Children with precocious puberty become self-conscious as body changes occur. Provide the child opportunities to express concerns and discuss issues related to body changes. The child may need to practice role playing as a coping mechanism to manage teasing by other children. Partner with family to encourage dressing the child in a manner appropriate to his or her chronologic age, even though the child may look older. Provide privacy during physical examinations. Advise parents that they may need to discuss issues of sexuality with the child at an earlier age than normal. Refer the child and family for counseling if appropriate.

Medication Administration

Teach the family proper medication administration and adherence to treatment regimen. Determine the family's ability to financially manage the cost of treatment. Assistance in covering the cost of therapy may be available through pharmaceutical companies and third-party payers. Refer the family to organizations that can assist them in obtaining support.

Evaluation

Expected outcomes of care for the child with precocious puberty include the following:

- The child demonstrates a positive body image.
- The child achieves growth stabilization and cessation of developing secondary sexual characteristics.
- The family and child demonstrate an understanding of the disorder and the treatment regimen.

DISORDERS OF THYROID FUNCTION

The function of the thyroid gland is to regulate the rate of cellular metabolism. In children, the hormones are responsible for normal development of the muscular, skeletal, and nervous systems.

Thyroxine, triiodothyronine, and calcitonin are hormones secreted by the thyroid. Thyroxine (tetraiodothyronine or T_4) and triiodothyronine (T_3) maintain metabolism and regulate growth and development. Their primary function is to control the cellular metabolic activity. T_4 is a **precursor**—a substance that precedes another substance or from which another substance is synthesized—to T_3. Calcitonin targets kidney and bone cells to regulate serum calcium ion concentrations. Thyroid-stimulating hormone (TSH), a hormone secreted by the pituitary gland, controls T_3 and T_4 production; therefore, thyroid-stimulating hormone function is evaluated in all thyroid disorders.

Some of the most common endocrine abnormalities are disorders of the thyroid gland. The two major disorders of the thyroid gland—hypothyroidism and hyperthyroidism—are discussed in this section.

Hypothyroidism

Hypothyroidism is a disorder in which levels of active thyroid hormones (TH) are decreased, leading to decreased metabolic rate, decreased heat production, and other effects on body systems. The disorder may be congenital or acquired. Hypothyroidism is the most common congenital endocrine disorder (Moreno, de Vijlder, Vulsma, et al., 2003). Premature infants often have transient alterations in thyroid function, with low T_4 and T_3 levels, along with low thyroxin-binding globulin (TBG) concentrations.

Congenital hypothyroidism occurs in approximately 1 in 4,000 live births and is twice as common in females as in males (Palma Sisto, 2004). Congenital hypothyroidism is less prevalent in African American infants more frequent in infants of Asian and Hispanic origin (1 in 2,000 births). The disorder also occurs more commonly in children with Down syndrome. It is also the leading cause of mental impairment in the world today (Palma Sisto, 2004).

Acquired hypothyroidism is more common in females than in males. A genetic predisposition to autoimmune thyroiditis exists and an autosomal dominant inheritance of thyroid autoantibodies has been found in the relatives of affected patients (Roberts & Ladenson, 2004).

Etiology and Pathophysiology

Thyroid hormones are important for growth and development and for the metabolism of nutrients and energy. When these hormones are not available for stimulation of other hormones or specific target cells, growth is delayed and mental retardation develops.

Congenital Hypothyroidism. Congenital hypothyroidism is usually caused by a spontaneous gene mutation, an autosomal recessive genetic transmission of an enzyme deficiency, hypoplasia or aplasia of the thyroid gland, failure of the central nervous system–thyroid feedback mechanism to develop, or iodine deficiency. The thyroid gland fails to produce T_3 and T_4 in response to elevated levels of thyroid-stimulating hormone (TSH). Mental retardation is irreversible if the disorder is not treated.

Acquired Hypothyroidism. Acquired hypothyroidism can be idiopathic or result from autoimmune thyroiditis (Hashimoto's thyroiditis), late-onset thyroid dysfunction, isolated thyroid-stimulating hormone (TSH) deficiency due to pituitary or hypothalamic dysfunction, or exposure to drugs or substances such as lithium that interfere with thyroid hormone synthesis.

Clinical Manifestations

Congenital Hypothyroidism. Infants with congenital hypothyroidism have few clinical signs of the disorder in the first weeks of life. In untreated infants, the characteristic cretinoid features (thickened protuberant tongue, thick lips, and dull appearance) appear during the first few months of life. Other signs include prolonged neonatal jaundice, hypotonia, respiratory distress, bradycardia, decreased pulse pressure, hypothermia, cool extremities, mottling, pallor, umbilical hernia, a posterior fontanel larger than 1 cm in diameter, difficulty feeding, lethargy, swollen eyelids, constipation, and a hoarse cry (Palma Sisto, 2004).

Acquired Hypothyroidism. Children with acquired hypothyroidism may demonstrate many of the same signs as adults with acquired hypothyroidism: decreased appetite, dry cool skin, thinning hair or hair loss, depressed deep tendon reflexes, bradycardia, constipation, sensitivity to cold temperatures, abnormal menses, and a **goiter** (a nontender enlarged thyroid gland). Manifestations unique to children include changes in past normal growth patterns with a weight increase, decreased height velocity, delayed bone and dental age, muscle hypertrophy with muscle weakness, and delayed or precocious puberty. However, children with acquired hypothyroidism may not exhibit the typical symptoms. The disorder should be suspected in the presence of a family history or other conditions, for example, another autoimmune disease such as diabetes, that predispose the child to acquired hypothyroidism.

A major complication associated with hypothyroidism is **myxedema,** a life-threatening crisis of hypothyroidism. Myxedema occurs when levels of thyroid hormone are extremely low. The disorder is characterized by nonpitting edema, puffy face and tongue, severe metabolic disorders, and hypothermia; with progression to hypoglycemia, hypotension, cardiovascular collapse, and coma (called myxedema coma). This complication is extremely rare in children.

COLLABORATIVE CARE

Goals of collaborative care include the early identification of the disorder, treatment with thyroid hormone for restoration of normalized thyroid function, and promotion of optimal growth and development.

Diagnostic Tests

Congenital hypothyroidism is usually detected during newborn screening of thyroxine (T_4) and thyroid-stimulating hormone (TSH) levels, which is mandatory in every state. Newborn screening has greatly reduced the morbidity of the disorder (Palma Sisto, 2004). A decreased T_4, normal T_3, and elevated thyroid-stimulating hormone level indicate hypothyroidism (Table 32–3). An elevated thyroid-stimulating hormone level indicates that the disease originated in the thyroid, not the pituitary. Ideally, the screening is performed at 3–5 days of life, as the TSH surge normally seen after birth has subsided to normal levels by that time. With earlier discharges from the hospitals, these samples are now often collected at 24 to 48 hours of life which can lead to false positive tests. Frequently, two separate evaluations are performed in order to identify the disorder early (Palma Sisto, 2004). The tests are conducted once before the newborn leaves the hospital and the second time at the first healthcare visit at 1 to 2 weeks of age. Rapid response from the laboratory that is testing the samples is important to reduce the time to diagnosis and the effects of hypothyroidism on the infant's development. Once there is notification of an abnormal screen the infant should be evaluated for symptoms. The infant should be retested with TSH, and free T_4 levels. Generally, the TSH will be above 50μU/L in congenital hypothyroidism (Palma Sisto, 2004). A thyroid scan or ultrasound of thyroid to confirm presence and position of the thyroid gland and radiologic examinations of bone growth may also be performed.

Antithyroid antibodies are measured in children with a goiter and suspected Hashimoto's thyroiditis, as increased titers of antithyroglobin and antimicrosomal antibodies are often found.

TABLE 32–3 Diagnostic Laboratory Values for Testing Thyroid Function

DIAGNOSTIC STUDY	HYPOTHYROIDISM	HYPERTHYROIDISM
Serum T_4 (tests level of thyroxine)	Decreased	Markedly elevated
Serum T_3 (tests level of triiodothyronine)	Normal	Markedly elevated
Serum TSH (tests level of thyroid-stimulating hormone)	Elevated	Decreased

*** Of note, normal values vary based on infant/child age.*

Clinical Therapy

If the T_4 level is below normal and the thyroid-stimulating hormone level is increased, the synthetic thyroid hormone levothyroxine (Synthroid) is prescribed. If imaging studies cannot be performed in a timely manner, the treatment should be initiated to avoid sequelae of hypothyroidism. The dose is increased gradually as the child grows to ensure a **euthyroid** (normal thyroid) state. Treatment is monitored by a pediatric endocrinologist. Periodic evaluation of T_4 and thyroid-stimulating hormone serum levels, bone age, and growth parameters is necessary to assess for signs of excess or inadequate thyroid hormone.

To ensure an adequate growth rate and prevent mental retardation, the hormone must be taken throughout life. Studies have shown that treated children with the most severe form of congenital hypothyroidism lose 6 to 15 IQ points, whereas less severely affected children have an IQ similar to their siblings (Van Vliet, 2001). Children with congenital hypothyroidism diagnosed before 3 months of age have the best prognosis for optimal mental development. Children with acquired hypothyroidism usually have normal growth following a period of catch-up growth. Many adolescents with Hashimoto's thyroiditis have a spontaneous remission.

Treatment of myxedema generally requires admission to an intensive care unit, and includes intravenous thyroid replacement and steroid therapy. Supportive therapy includes oxygen, assisted ventilation, fluid replacement, restoration of normothermia, and blood glucose monitoring.

NURSING MANAGEMENT

Nursing care focuses on educating the parents and child about the disorder and its treatment, monitoring the child's growth rate, and promoting optimal growth and development.

Nursing Assessment and Diagnosis

Routine neonatal screening is performed before discharge from the hospital and is often repeated at the infant's first health visit to evaluate levels of circulating thyroid hormones. If the nurse is making a home visit several days after discharge to assess the health of the mother and infant, the neonatal screening may be performed at that visit.

Serial measurements and recording of height and weight are performed at each follow-up visit with growth parameters plotted on a growth curve. Assess the child for signs of inadequate growth to determine if the dose of thyroid hormone requires adjustment and to monitor adherence with medication. Conduct developmental screenings to detect delays in achievement of developmental milestones.

Nursing diagnoses appropriate for the child with hypothyroidism may include the following:

- Risk for Delayed Development related to late initiation of thyroid replacement therapy
- Risk for Disproportionate Growth related to poor adherence to thyroid hormone therapy
- Disturbed Body Image related to physical changes associated with condition
- Fatigue related to inadequate dose of thyroid medication

Planning and Implementation

Lifelong medication therapy is required to promote the child's mental development. Partner with the family to ensure understanding of medication administration, including administering the dose consistently at the same time each morning, 1 hour before meals or 2 hours after a meal. Emphasize that doses should not be skipped.

Partner with the family to ensure proper assessment for an increased pulse rate, which could indicate the presence of too much thyroid hormone. Advise parents that the child may experience temporary sleep disturbances or behavioral changes in response to therapy. Ensure parental understanding to report problems such as fatigue, which could indicate an improper drug dose requiring readjustment. Additionally, parents are encouraged to monitor weight periodically to assess for weight gain, which could indicate the need for increased thyroid hormone dosage.

Since chilling increases metabolic rate, cardiac workload, and oxygen demand, caution parents to dress the child appropriately for the season to prevent hypothermia. Encourage modification of the child's diet by increasing the amount of fluids, fruits, and bulk if constipation is a problem.

Collaborate with the parents to plan activities for the child. The child is assessed for shortness of breath, dizziness, and fatigue during activities. Reassure the family that the child will develop normally with hormone replacement therapy. Reinforce the importance of follow-up visits to assess growth rate and response to therapy and to regulate medication dosages as the child grows.

Partner with the family and school officials to ensure periodic assessment of educational achievement. Even with good control, adolescents may have persistent visual-spatial deficits and memory and attention problems. Those with severe disease or who take longer to achieve a euthyroid status have the poorest academic achievement and more behavior problems. Close monitoring and regular follow-up is important to promote learning (Rovet & Ehrlich, 2000). When the cause is genetic, refer the family for genetic counseling (see Chapter 4∞).

Evaluation

Expected outcomes of nursing care of the child with hypothyroidism include the following:

- The child maintains adequate growth of height and weight, following a percentile curve throughout childhood.
- The child's cognitive development is appropriate for age.
- The child demonstrates a positive body image.
- The child participates in activities of daily living and other activities appropriate for age without experiencing fatigue.

- The parents (and child if older) demonstrate an understanding of the disorder and treatment regimen. Medications are administered properly and assessment for complications is ongoing.

Hyperthyroidism

Hyperthyroidism occurs when thyroid hormone levels are increased, resulting in excessive levels of circulating thyroid hormones. This leads to increased basal metabolic rate, cardiovascular function, gastrointestinal function, neuromuscular function, weight loss, heat intolerance, and metabolism of fats, proteins, and carbohydrates. Hyperthyroidism is rare in children and adolescents. The disorder is most common in adolescent girls and is almost always due to Graves' disease.

Etiology and Pathophysiology

Graves' disease, the most common cause of hyperthyroidism in children and adolescents (Nebesio, Siddiqui, Pescovitz, et al., 2002), is an autoimmune disorder in which the body produces antibodies that attack the cells of the thyroid gland. This disorder has a high familial incidence. Immunoglobulins produced by the B lymphocytes stimulate oversecretion of thyroid hormones, resulting in the clinical symptoms. Signs and symptoms are caused by hyperactivity of the sympathetic nervous system.

Other, more unusual forms of hyperthyroidism result from thyroiditis and thyroid hormone-producing tumors, including thyroid adenomas and carcinomas, and pituitary adenomas. Congenital hyperthyroidism can occur in infants of mothers with Graves' disease as a result of transplacental transfer of immunoglobulins.

Clinical Manifestations

Clinical manifestations vary according to the amount and time of hypersecretion. Characteristic findings include an enlarged, nontender thyroid gland (goiter), and prominent or bulging eyes (**exophthalmos**) (Figure 32–4 ■). The thyroid gland may be slightly enlarged or grow to 3 to 4 times its normal size; feel warm, soft, and fleshy; and have an auditory bruit on auscultation. See the table on page 1254 for clinical manifestations of hyperthyroidism.

Onset is subtle, and the condition often remains unrecognized for 1 to 2 years. The disorder can present in the preschool years, but occurs with an increased incidence during adolescence. The behavioral problems and declining performance manifested in children with Graves' disease result as they become easily frustrated in the classroom and overheated and fatigued during physical education class. Children with this disorder find it difficult to relax or sleep. These symptoms usually prompt parents to seek medical treatment for the child. Exophthalmos is less pronounced in children than in adults.

The most serious complication of hyperthyroidism is severe **thyrotoxicosis,** also called thyroid crisis or thyroid storm. It is a life-threatening emergency resulting from extreme hyperthyroidism, in which elevated circulating levels of TH result in a hypermetabolic state. The progression for thryotoxicosis to life-threatening thyroid storm can occur. This manifests as hyperpyrexia, mental status changes, tachycardia, hypertension, and multisystem organ failure (Goldberg & Inzucchi, 2003).

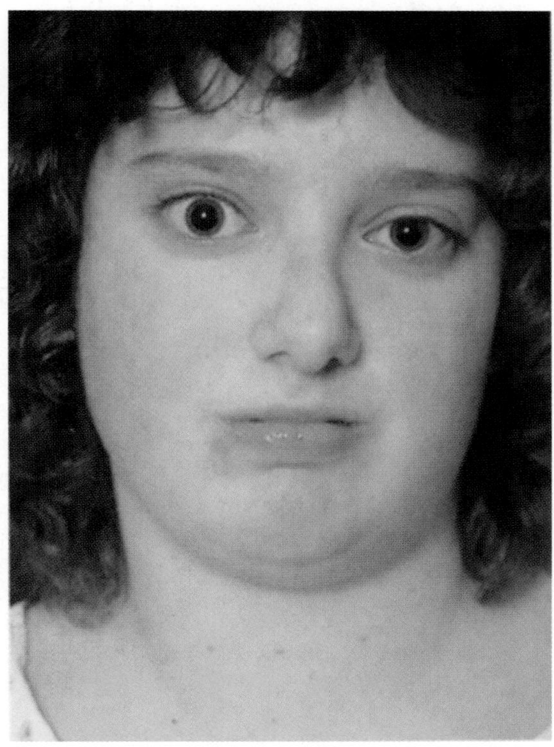

FIGURE 32–4 ■ Exophthalmos and an enlarged thyroid in an adolescent with Graves' disease.

From Zitelli, B. J., & Davis, H. W., (Eds.). (1997). Atlas of pediatric physical diagnosis *(3rd ed., p. 271). St. Louis: Mosby-White.*

PRACTICE ALERT

Clinical manifestations of thyroid storm include elevated temperature, tachycardia, hypertension, diaphoresis, tremors, confusion, seizures, agitation, abdominal pain, nausea, vomiting, and diarrhea. If untreated, shock progresses to death. Any child exhibiting these manifestations should be immediately evaluated to preserve life.

COLLABORATIVE CARE

Management includes identification of hyperthyroidism, inhibiting excessive secretion of thyroid hormones, and promotion of normal growth and development.

Diagnostic Tests

Diagnostic studies include laboratory evaluation of serum thyroid-stimulating hormone, T_3 (triiodothyronine) and T_4 levels, and a thyroid scan. T_3 and T_4 levels are markedly elevated. Thyroid-stimulating hormone levels are decreased since the increased levels of thyroid hormones inhibit production of thyroid-stimulating hormone from the anterior pituitary. Serum studies are also performed to detect autoantibodies specific for the various thyroid disorders. A radioactive iodine uptake scan and thyroid scan may be performed to determine the cause of hyperthyroidism.

CLINICAL MANIFESTATIONS of Hyperthyroidism (Graves' Disease)

SYSTEM	CLINICAL MANIFESTATIONS
Cardiovascular	Palpitations Tachycardia
Neuromuscular	Eyelid lag Fatigue Irritability Muscle weakness Nervousness, restlessness Pruritis Tremors
Endocrine	Diaphoresis Heat intolerance Increased growth rate Goiter Exophthalmos
Gastrointestinal	Frequent bowel movements Increased appetite Nausea Thirst Weight loss
Genitourinary	Urinary frequency, nocturia
Psychosocial	Anxiety Behavioral problems Declining school performance Emotional lability Inability to concentrate Insomnia

Clinical Therapy

The goal of clinical therapy is to inhibit excessive secretion of thyroid hormones. Treatment may include antithyroid medication therapy, radiation therapy, or surgery.

Medication Therapy. Medication therapy is most often used as the initial treatment modality, but adherence is often a problem due to medication side effects. Methimazole (Tapazole) or propylthiouracil (PTU) are administered to inhibit thyroid hormone secretion (Nebesio et al., 2002). See the medications table on page 1255.

PRACTICE ALERT

Propylthiouracil therapy can cause temporary side effects including skin rashes, urticaria, and lymphadenopathy. If fever or sore throat develops, the child should be evaluated by a healthcare professional to rule out granulocytopenia.

Treatment continues for 18 months to 2 years or longer until the thyroid decreases in size and immunologic remission has occurred (Ginsberg, 2003). Symptoms usually improve within weeks of starting treatment. Adjunct therapy with beta-adrenergic blocking agents such as propanolol (Inderal) may be administered to relieve symptoms, including tremors, tachycardia, and restlessness, associated with increased beta-adrenergic activity.

Radioactive Ablative Therapy. If medication therapy is ineffective, radiation therapy (radioactive ablative treatment) using oral radioactive iodine 1 is the next treatment choice. Historically, there has been reluctance to use radioactive ablative treatment in children. This reluctance was generated by the increased prevalence of posttreatment hypothyroidism requiring lifelong hormone replacement. Another concern has been the risk of causing leukemia or cancer. However, current data do not indicate a relationship between radioactive iodine and cancer or leukemia. Radioactive therapy also does not appear to increase the risk of birth defects in future offspring in those treated (Ginsberg, 2003).

Surgical Removal of Thyroid. Thyroidectomy, or subtotal thyroidectomy, is alternate treatment for hyperthyroidism. However, destruction or removal of the thyroid gland often results in permanent hypothyroidism, necessitating lifelong hormone replacement therapy (Boger & Perrier, 2004). Additionally, excess release of thyroid hormone during surgery may lead to thyrotoxicosis (thyroid storm). Treatment of thyrotoxicosis includes administration of antithyroid medications and propranolol.

Thyroidectomy provides immediate cure, avoids radiation and the possible long-term complications of radioactive iodine (Boger & Perrier, 2004). Inadvertent removal of the parathyroid gland may occur during surgical removal of the thyroid, resulting in the complication of hypocalcemia from lack of parathyroid hormone secretion. This hypoparathyroidism may be temporary or permanent (Boger & Perrier, 2004). Manipulation of the parathyroid gland during surgery can result in excess release of parathyroid hormone, leading to hypercalcemia. Monitoring of serum calcium levels following a thyroidectomy is essential.

NURSING MANAGEMENT

Nursing care focuses on educating the child and parents about the disorder and its treatment, promoting rest, providing emotional support, and, if the child requires surgery, providing preoperative and postoperative teaching and care.

■ Nursing Assessment and Diagnosis

Assess the child's vital signs, as blood pressure and pulse may be elevated, and respiratory effort may be increased. Measure and record the child's height and weight to establish a baseline allowing for identification of growth patterns. Assess for goiter and exophthalamos. Assess elimination pattern, nutritional status, fluid balance, and sleep pattern. Observe the child's behavior, activity, and level of fatigue.

If surgery is performed, assess the vital signs and monitor the child's surgical site. Assess the site postoperatively for bleeding, hoarseness, swelling, and difficulty breathing. Assess serum calcium levels. Monitor for signs of hypocalcemia by assessing Chvostek's and Trousseau signs (see Chapter 23∞) for numbness and tingling of extremities or lips, and assessing for muscle twitching. Assess for thyrotoxicosis, as it can be life-threatening.

MEDICATIONS Used in Management of Hyperthyroidism

MEDICATION	ACTION OR INDICATION	NURSING CONSIDERATIONS
Antithyroid medications methimazole (Tapazole) propylthiouracil (PTU)	Inhibits thyroid hormone secretion	Monitor for side effects including rash, mild leukopenia, arthralgia, and the more serious side effects including lupus-like syndrome, hepatitis, and glomerulonephritis Emphasize the importance of taking medication as prescribed and to take them at the same time each day Monitor for symptoms of hypothyroidism
Propanolol (Inderal)	Beta-blocking agent Decreases beta-adrenergic activity to relieve tremors, tachycardia, anxiety, heat intolerance, and restlessness	Monitor for side effects including hypotension Emphasize the importance of taking the medication as prescribed
Radioiodine Oral, in solution or capsule	Produces radiation thyroiditis and fibrosis, resulting in euthyroid state	Assess for allergy to iodine Antithyroid medications should be discontinued one week prior to treatment Liquid may be diluted in orange juice or other fluids to disguise taste Ensure adolescent is not pregnant before beginning treatment Partner with family to ensure avoidance of physical contact with secretions (urine, stool, saliva, sweat) for several days following the treatment Emphasize the importance of keeping follow-up appointments to monitor thyroid function Hypothyroidism is a potential complication

Common nursing diagnoses for the child with hyperthyroidism may include the following:

- Ineffective Thermoregulation (elevated) related to illness and excessive activity of the sympathetic nervous system
- Imbalanced Nutrition: Less than Body Requirements related to high metabolic needs
- Disturbed Body Image related to physical changes caused by illness (prominent eyes, excessive perspiration, and tremors)
- Fatigue related to hypermetabolic state and sleep deprivation

■ Planning and Implementation

Promote increased caloric intake by providing five or six moderate meals per day, considering the child's nutritional preferences. Encourage the child and family to express feelings and concerns about the disorder. Complimenting even slight improvement in the child's condition can increase adherence with therapy.

Promote Symptom Management

Children with hyperthyroidism are easily fatigued. Partner with the family and school officials to plan scheduled rest periods at school and to develop an education plan tailored to the child's needs during the state of hyperthyroidism. Emphasize to family and teachers that home and physical activities should be kept to a minimum until symptoms resolve. Encourage parents to provide a cool environment and allow the child to wear fewer clothes until symptoms subside.

If exophthalmos is present, teach the family about measures to protect the eye. Encourage regular eye examinations and eye protection measures such as safety tinted glasses, artificial tears as necessary, sleeping with head of bed elevated to minimize pressure on the optic nerve, and patching eyes at bedtime if eyelid does not completely cover eye. Report changes in vision or appearance of eye.

Preoperative and Postoperative Care

Children who have partial or total removal of the thyroid gland receive antithyroid medications, such as iodine, for approximately 2 weeks before surgery to reduce the vascularity and size of the thyroid gland and to decrease the risk of thyroid storm.

Instruct parents to observe for side effects of antithyroid medications, including fever, urticaria, and lymphadenopathy. Ensure the child and family understands the medication therapy. Provide routine preoperative teaching (refer to Chapter 17∞). Explain the procedure to the child using developmentally appropriate terms. Young children in particular may be fearful about having their throat "cut."

Postoperatively, elevate the head of bed to 30 degrees to promote patent airway. A tracheostomy kit, suction supplies, and IV calcium gluconate should be within immediate access for emergency treatment of tetany and respiratory complications. If thyroidectomy is performed, thyrotoxicosis does not immediately resolve because the half-life is 7 to 8 days. Antithyroid medications should be slowly tapered (Boger & Perrier, 2004).

Partner with the family to ensure their understanding of reportable symptoms including signs of hemorrhage, infection, respiratory difficulty, and discomfort. Promote pain relief by frequent assessment and regular administration of pain medications.

Discharge Planning and Home Care Teaching

Emphasize to the child and family the need for lifelong thyroid hormone replacement if radiation or surgery is performed. A medical alert identification (tag, bracelet, or necklace) should be worn at all times. Explain to the parents the importance of the child's scheduled follow-up visits for evaluation to ensure that the T_4 level is adequate to sustain growth and development.

Evaluation

Expected outcomes of nursing care for the child with hyperthyroidism may include the following:

- The child achieves balanced thermoregulation.
- The child maintains adequate nutritional intake to meet growth and development needs.
- The child participates in activities of daily living without experiencing fatigue.
- The child demonstrates a positive body image.

DISORDERS OF THE PARATHYROID

Children usually have four parathyroid glands located posterior to the thyroid gland. The primary function of the parathyroid hormone is to work in conjunction with vitamin D to regulate total body calcium. The parathyroid hormone (PTH) is the most important endocrine regulator of calcium and phosphorus concentration in the extracellular fluid. It is secreted from cells in the parathyroid glands and its major target organs are the bone and kidney. In response to hypocalcemia or hypomagnesemia PTH mobilizes calcium from bone (stimulating osteoclasts to reabsorb bone mineral and liberating calcium into blood). PTH also indirectly enhances absorption of calcium from the small intestine, and suppresses calcium loss in the urine. As the level of calcium increases in the extracellular fluid, the concentration of phosphorus is decreased by stimulating loss of phosphate ions in urine.

Hyperparathyroidism

Childhood hyperparathyroidism is rare (Doyle & DiGeorge, 2004). Primary hyperparathyroidism is most often the result of a tumor (adenoma) which secretes the hormone without proper regulation. It usually manifests after 10 years of age. Secondary hyperparathyroidism is due to disease outside of the parathyroid gland, leading to excessive secretion of parathyroid hormone (Rudock, 2002). This is commonly seen in chronic renal failure when the kidneys are unable to reabsorb calcium, causing low serum calcium levels and stimulating continual secretion of parathyroid hormone to maintain normal serum calcium levels. Secondary hyperparathyroidism can also result from malabsorption syndromes or diets deficient in calcium or Vitamin D, or which contain excessive phosphorus. Transient neonatal hyperparathyroidism has been reported in approximately 50 infants with a spectrum of symptoms from mild, resolving without treatment, to severe that may have a rapidly fatal course if not treated (Doyle & DiGeorge, 2004).

At any age, symptoms of primary hyperparathyroidism may include bone pain, nephrolithiasis (kidney stones), and pathologic bone fractures. Hypercalcemia may cause symptoms of muscle weakness, peptic ulcer disease, fatigue, volume depletion and subtle mental disturbance (Viera, 2002). Abdominal pain may be present and may indicate pancreatitis. In transient severe neonatal hyperparathyroidism, symptoms develop shortly after birth and consist of anorexia, lethargy, irritability, constipation and failure to thrive (Doyle & DiGeorge, 2004).

Collaborative Care

Serum calcium, ionized calcium, and serum levels of PTH are usually elevated. Radiographic images may reveal signs of rickets.

For patients with primary hyperparathyroidism, the recommendation is for surgical parathyroid exploration and removal of the adenoma. Surgical cure rate is estimated to be 90% (Viera, 2002). Management of secondary hyperparathyroidism focuses on prevention of hypercalcemia utilizing vitamin D replacement and phosphorus binders. Surgery is generally not required for these categories (Ahmad, & Hammond 2004).

Nursing Management

Nursing care centers on fluid management and electrolyte monitoring. Calcium supplementation may be required. In patients who require surgical intervention, post-operative monitoring includes assessment for expanding hematoma in the pretracheal space. If this situation occurs, it must be treated promptly with opening for the wound and evacuation of the hematoma. If left untreated, laryngeal edema may progress rapidly, causing airway obstruction.

Parent and child education is of primary importance to ensure their understanding of signs and symptoms of hypocalcemia and appropriate calcium supplementation. Families should be taught to avoid dehydration as well as inadequate or excessive calcium intake. If child has undergone surgical intervention, teach signs and symptoms of infection.

After diagnosis or after surgical intervention, follow-up is important to monitor serum calcium and phosphorus levels to detect persistence of hyperparathyroidism.

Hypoparathyoidism

Primary hypoparathyroidism is rare. It can result from congenital disorders (e.g., parathyroid aplasia, DiGeorge Syndrome), surgical removal of the parathyroid glands (e.g., parathyroid adenoma, thyroidectomy) or by disease processes that lead to destruction of the parathyroid glands (e.g., sarcoidosis, Wilson disease, hemochromatosis), medications (e.g., aluminum, asparagine, doxorubicin, cytosine, arabinoside), or can be idiopathic. The primary result is hypocalcemia and hyperphosphatemia in the blood.

Infants may display hyperirritability, muscle rigidity with normal mental status, seizures, vomiting, abdominal distention, apneic episodes, intermittent cyanosis or twitching. Muscle pain and cramps may be noted in children with progression to numbness, stiffness, and tingling of the hands and feet. Hyperreflexia may be noted in any age child. A positive Chvostek or Trousseau sign is classic. If hypocalcemia is severe, life threatening tetany and convulsions may occur (Doyle & DiGeorge, 2004).

Collaborative Care

Serum calcium and PTH levels are low and serum phosphorus is elevated. Radiographs often demonstrate increased bone density. A 12-lead ECG may demonstrate a prolonged QT interval.

In emergent situations, intravenous calcium and calcitriol must be administered to treat seizures, tetany, life threatening hypotension and cardiac arrhythmis. Both vitamin D in the form of calcitriol and calcium replacement may be necessary for an indefinite period time. (Palma Sisto, 2004). Foods with high phosphorus content (dairy products and eggs) are limited. Currently, studies to evaluate administration of injectable parathyroid hormone versus the use of calcitriol and calcium are being conducted (Winer, Ko, & Reynolds, et al., 2004).

PRACTICE ALERT

Dilute intravenous calcium per hospital protocol. Infiltration of IV calcium can cause extravasation and tissue sloughing. Always check patency of IV prior to administration.

Nursing Management

Assess and stabilize the airway, breathing, and circulation. In the acute care setting, children should be placed on a cardiorespiratory monitoring. Maintain seizure precautions until normal serum calcium levels are attained. Obtain intravenous access and administer calcium supplementation as ordered.

Partner with the family to ensure their understanding of the need for calcium supplementation and reduced intake of phosphorus. Teach the family that periodic monitoring of calcium levels is important. Inform the family that hypoparathyroidism may require lifelong therapy.

DISORDERS OF ADRENAL FUNCTION

The adrenal glands are composed of the inner cortex and the outer medulla. The adrenal medulla secretes the **catecholamines** epinephrine and norepinephrine which affect the nervous system, cardiovascular system, metabolic rate, temperature, and smooth muscles. The adrenal cortex produces the steroid hormones **glucocorticoids** (affects protein and carbohydrate metabolism and protects against stress) and **mineralocorticoids** (involved in regulation of fluid and electrolytes). Cortisol, the main glucocorticoid, affects the metabolism of proteins, glucose, and fats, stress responses, and inhibition of inflammation. The most important mineralocorticoid, aldosterone, maintains extracellular fluid volume and blood pressure by conserving sodium, chloride, water, and excretion of potassium by the kidneys.

Disorders of adrenal function discussed in this section are Cushing syndrome, congenital adrenal hyperplasia, adrenal insufficiency (Addison's disease), and pheochromocytoma.

Cushing Syndrome

Cushing syndrome, also called adrenocortical hyperfunction, is characterized by a group of symptoms resulting from excess levels of glucocorticoids (especially cortisol) in the bloodstream as a result of adrenal cortex hyperfunction. The disorder is uncommon in children and the true incidence is unknown.

Etiology and Pathophysiology

During infancy and childhood, most cases of endogenous Cushing syndrome are due to malignant adrenal or pituitary adenoma that causes adrenal cortex hyperfunction (Levine & White, 2004). The increased secretion of cortisol alters metabolism. Another cause is hyperplasia of one or both adrenal glands (adrenal hyperplasia is discussed later in the chapter).

Clinical Manifestations

The initial sign of Cushing syndrome in most children is gradual excessive weight gain and growth retardation. It generally takes up to 5 years for the child to develop the characteristic "cushingoid" appearance, which includes a moon face (chubby cheeks and a double chin) and fat pads over the shoulders and back (buffalo hump). See Box 32–3. Additional manifestations include obesity, hirsutism, muscle weakness, and growth retardation. See the table below for clinical manifestations caused by altered cortisol metabolism. Other signs include mental changes and delayed puberty.

COLLABORATIVE CARE

The goal of collaborative care is the surgical removal of any tumors, replacement of cortisol, restoration of normal physical appearance, and promotion of growth and development.

CLINICAL MANIFESTATIONS of Cushing Syndrome

ETIOLOGY	CLINICAL MANIFESTATIONS	NURSING CONSIDERATIONS
Catabolism of protein	Muscle weakness and wasting, capillary weakness and bruising, growth failure with delayed bone age, fatigue	Plan periods of rest for child Cluster nursing care Assess skin for bruising Assess and plot growth and development
Decreased absorption of calcium from the intestines	Demineralization of bones, osteoporosis	Monitor serum calcium levels
Increased appetite	Weight gain primarily on the trunk, striae on the abdomen, buttocks, thighs	Assist in meal planning Refer to nutritionist
Salt retention	Increased blood volume and hypertension	Teach family to monitor and record child's blood pressure

BOX 32–3 Causes of Cushingoid Features

The most common reasons for cushingoid features in children are (1) *excessive doses* of corticosteroids as treatment for other diseases, or (2) *prolonged use* of corticosteroids as treatment for a health condition, such as an organ transplant recipient. Corticosteroids suppress adrenal function when administered long term.

Diagnostic Tests

Diagnosis is based on characteristic physical findings and laboratory values, including elevated serum calcium, sodium, calcium, and potassium concentrations; increased 24-hour urinary levels of free cortisol and 17-hydroxycorticosteroid (17-OHC); and loss of diurnal rhythm in serum cortisol (usually elevated at night), and a positive ACTH suppression test. Additionally, the child has chronic hyperglycemia and an elevated glycosylated hemoglobin concentration. (Refer to Appendix C∞ for lab values).

The adrenal suppression test is used for the initial screening of children with suspected adrenocortical hyperfunction. If this test reveals that adrenal cortisol output is not suppressed overnight after a dose of dexamethasone, further diagnostic testing is necessary to determine the cause of hypercortisolism. CT and MRI are used to detect tumors in the adrenal and pituitary glands.

Clinical Therapy

Surgical removal is the current treatment of choice for adrenal tumors (adrenalectomy) or pituitary adenomas (transsphenoidal hypophysectomy). Lifelong cortisol replacement is required when both adrenal glands are removed. The prognosis for children with malignant adrenal tumors is poor because of frequent metastases to the liver and lungs.

NURSING MANAGEMENT

The nurse usually encounters a child with Cushing syndrome when the child is hospitalized for diagnostic evaluation or surgery. Nursing care focuses on assessment, management of symptoms, educating family, and providing support.

Nursing Assessment and Diagnosis

Nursing assessment includes monitoring the child's vital signs, fluid status, nutritional status, and weight. Additional assessment includes monitoring muscle strength and endurance during hospital play activities.

Perform postoperative assessments including vital signs, responsiveness, intake and output, level of pain, and signs of infection. Monitor electrolytes. Observe the incision site for signs of poor healing.

Nursing diagnoses that apply to the child with Cushing syndrome may include the following:

- Excess Fluid Volume related to elevated serum sodium and fluid retention
- Risk for Infection related to surgical incision
- Disturbed Body Image related to body changes
- Anxiety (child and parental) related to surgical procedure and serious disorder

Planning and Implementation

Partner with the child and family to ensure understanding of the disorder and its treatment, and, for children undergoing surgery, provide preoperative and postoperative teaching and care. Answer any questions the child and family may have and explain all laboratory and diagnostic tests. Explain to parents and child that the cushingoid appearance is reversible with treatment. Provide nutritional guidance or refer the child and parents to a nutritionist to promote maintenance of an appropriate weight. Encourage the child to discuss feelings regarding changes in physical appearance. Assist the child and family to identify effective coping strategies.

Preoperative and postoperative teaching and care are similar to those for the child undergoing surgery (see Chapter 17∞). Refer to Chapter 29∞ for general nursing care of the child with cancer. Postoperatively, elevate the head of the bed 30 degrees to promote effective breathing. Care is taken to prevent tension on the incision line during repositioning.

For children who require lifelong cortisol replacement therapy following the surgical removal of both adrenal glands, administering the medication early in the morning or every other day causes fewer symptoms and mimics the normal diurnal pattern of cortisol secretion. Carefully explain cortisol replacement in the postoperative period to the parents. Hydrocortisone (Cortef, Solu-Cortef, cortisone acetate) is available in liquid, tablet, or injectable form. Ensure the parents understand how and when to administer the injectable form, which is usually when the child is vomiting, has diarrhea, or cannot take the oral medication. It is imperative that children receive their medication when they are ill or it may lead to severe illness and cardiovascular collapse. See Partnering with Families: Hydrocortisone Instructions.

Oral cortisone preparations have a bitter taste and can cause gastric irritation. Administering the dose at mealtime helps reduce these side effects. Educate family to avoid over-the-counter medications including aspirin. These children may require chronic H2 blockers for gastric protection.

Teach the family to be alert to signs of acute adrenal insufficiency during the withdrawal of corticosteroid therapy, and to inform all healthcare providers of the child's condition and potential emergency medication needs (Box 32–4). A medical alert identification should be worn at all times.

Evaluation

Examples of outcomes of care for the child with Cushing syndrome include the following:

- The child achieves fluid volume balance.
- The child is free from infection.
- The child's appearance returns to normalized state and the child exhibits positive body image.

BOX 32–4 Signs of Acute Adrenal Insufficiency

Signs of acute adrenal insufficiency may include:

- Increased irritability, restlessness
- Headache, confusion
- Loss of appetite
- Lethargy
- Nausea and vomiting, diarrhea, dehydration
- Abdominal pain
- Fever

If untreated, the child will go into shock. In newborns, the symptoms include failure to thrive, weakness, vomiting, and dehydration. Hyponatremia and hyperkalemia are key signs.

- The family and child demonstrate understanding of the disease and treatment.
- The child and family are free from anxiety.

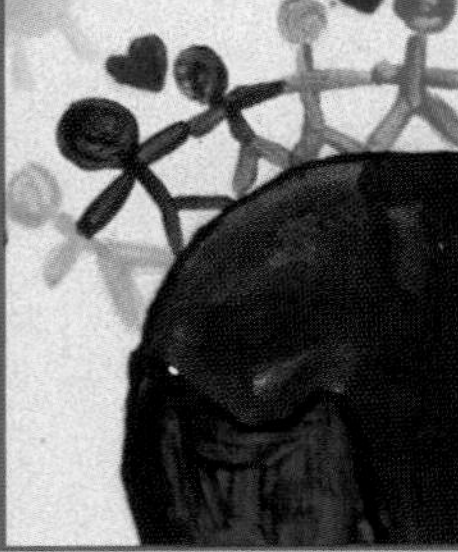

PARTNERING WITH FAMILIES

Hydrocortisone Instructions

Teach the family the following tips regarding hydrocortisone administration.

- Always have injectable hydrocortisone available at home and school and everywhere the child travels. An emergency kit should be available at all times to supply cortisol to the child during stressful situations.
- Always give the medication on time as scheduled since the schedule follows the body's normal cortisol release pattern.
- Never abruptly discontinue the medication.
- If the child has vomiting or diarrhea and is unable to take the medication by mouth, administer the injections as instructed.

Congenital Adrenal Hyperplasia

Congenital adrenal hyperplasia (CAH), sometimes called adrenogenital syndrome, adrenocortical hyperplasia, or congenital adrenogenital hyperplasia, results from a deficiency of one of the enzymes necessary for the synthesis of cortisol and aldosterone. The disorder occurs in 1 in 14,000 live births, and males and females are affected equally (Pang, 2003). The incidence is highest in Native Alaskans (American Academy of Pediatrics, 2000).

Etiology and Pathophysiology

The defective gene CYP21 is located on the short arm of chromosome 6. The most common defect is 21-hydroxylase (21-OH) deficiency, which accounts for more than 90% of all cases of CAH (Levine & White, 2004). This form has an autosomal recessive inheritance pattern. Approximately 10% of children have 11-hydroxylase deficiency. The remainder of cases involve deficiencies of five other enzymes. There are two classic forms of the disorder (Levine & White, 2004):

- 75% are salt losing, caused by the aldosterone deficiency, and
- 25% are non-salt losing, or simple **virilization**, the production of masculine secondary sex characteristics in females.

During fetal development, the lack of cortisol triggers the pituitary to continue secretion of adrenocorticotropic hormone. This in turn stimulates overproduction of the adrenal androgens. Virilization of the female external genitalia begins in week 10 of gestation. If untreated, the overproduction of androgens results in accelerated height, early closure of the epiphyseal plates, and premature sexual development with both pubic and axillary hair.

Clinical Manifestations

Congenital adrenal hyperplasia is the most common cause of **pseudohermaphroditism** (ambiguous genitalia) in newborn girls. The female infant is born with masculinized genitalia with an enlarged clitoris and partial or complete labial fusion; however, the uterus, ovaries, and fallopian tubes are normal (Figure 32–5 ■). The vagina usually has a common opening with the urethra (urogenital sinus). The enlarged clitoris may resemble a penis, and with the opening to the urethra below the clitoris, some females may be mistaken for males with hypospadias (Levine & White, 2004). Prenatal exposure of the brain to high levels of androgens may influence postnatal behavior with females more interested in masculine toys (Levine & White, 2004).

The male infant may appear normal at birth or may have a slightly enlarged penis and hyperpigmented scrotum. Signs of adrenal insufficiency may be the first indication of the disorder. The male may have tall stature and an adult-size penis by school age, but the testes are appropriately sized for age.

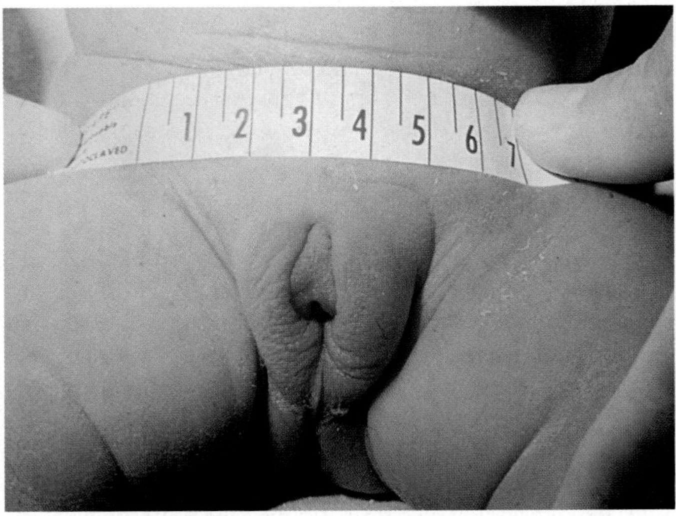

FIGURE 32–5 ■ Newborn girl with ambiguous genitalia. *Courtesy of Patrick C. Walsh, M. D.*

Partial enzyme deficiency produces less obvious symptoms. Precocious puberty, tall stature for age, acne, and excessive muscular development may be noted in both males and females as the child grows. Due to early epiphyseal fusion, adult stature is shorter than normal.

Recurrent vomiting, dehydration, metabolic acidosis, hypotension, and hypoglycemia are characteristic signs of the salt-wasting form of the disorder. These symptoms often develop rapidly and can lead to death if intervention is delayed. Hypertension with hypokalemic alkalosis is alternately found in children with 11-hydroxylase deficiency.

COLLABORATIVE CARE

The goal of collaborative care is to identify the newborn with congenital adrenal hyperplasia, suppress adrenal secretion of androgens, maintain homeostasis, and correct ambiguous genitalia.

Diagnostic Tests

Diagnosis in infants and children is usually confirmed by laboratory evaluation of serum 17-alpha-hydroxyl progesterone (17-OHP) level. Routine newborn screening for congenital adrenal hyperplasia is performed in 20 states (Lashley, 2002). Prenatal screening is available. In instances of ambiguous genitalia, a **karyotype** (a microscopic chromosome study in which the 46 chromosomes of the child are lined up in pairs from largest to smallest to detect errors in chromosome number, shape, and size) is obtained to determine the gender of the infant. (See Chapter 4∞.) Ultrasonography may be used to visualize pelvic structures.

In the salt-wasting form of the disorder, the child may have hyponatremia, hyperkalemia, a high urine sodium level, and low serum and urinary aldosterone levels. Serum concentrations of testosterone in girls and androstenedione in boys and girls are elevated in affected infants. Elevated adrenocorticotropic hormone (ACTH), with measurement of serum cortisol and 17-OHP levels, is necessary to confirm the diagnosis (American Academy of Pediatrics, 2000). Diagnosis may be delayed in the nonsalt-losing form until 3 to 7 years.

Clinical Therapy

The goal of treatment is to suppress adrenal secretion of androgens by replacing deficient hormones, which is accomplished by lifelong oral administration of glucocorticoids (dexamethasone, prednisone, or hydrocortisone). The glucocorticoid replacement leads to a reduction in secretion of adrenocorticotropic hormone which had overstimulated the adrenal cortex. As a result, excessive adrenal androgen production is suppressed. The dose is individualized by monitoring growth parameters, bone age, and hormone levels. In males with precocious puberty who are diagnosed in early childhood, treatment with gonadotropin-releasing hormone analogue may be prescribed (Levine & White, 2004).

If the infant has the salt-wasting form of the disorder, salt is added to the infant's formula and a mineralcorticoid (Florinef) is given to replace the missing hormone. Hormone dosage must be doubled or tripled during acute illnesses or injury and for surgery. Injectable hydrocortisone is administered for severe stress. Generally there are no side effects to the hormone; however, elevated doses can result in hypertension and growth impairment. Adrenalectomy is recommended only in cases in which medical therapy is ineffective (Pang, 2003).

Reconstructive surgery of the enlarged clitoris is often performed on girls during the first year of life. Vaginal reconstruction is performed in a later procedure.

NURSING MANAGEMENT

Nursing care of the newborn with congenital adrenal hyperplasia focuses on teaching parents about the disorder and its treatment, providing emotional support, and preoperative and postoperative teaching for parents of infants undergoing reconstructive surgery.

Nursing Assessment and Diagnosis

Assess the infant and child for signs of dehydration, electrolyte imbalance, and hypovolemic shock in the salt-wasting form of the disease. Monitor airway, breathing, circulation, and responsiveness. Assess vital signs and assess peripheral perfusion (capillary refill, distal pulses, color and temperature of the extremities) frequently to detect early changes in condition.

Assess the parents' emotional response to a newborn with ambiguous genitalia and a chronic condition. Explore their values and beliefs regarding gender roles and sexuality while awaiting results of the karyotype.

Nursing diagnoses for the child with congenital adrenal hyperplasia may include the following:

- Risk for Impaired Parenting related to a child with undetermined gender identity
- Risk for Deficient Fluid Volume related to failure of regulatory mechanisms and excess excretion of salt by the kidneys
- Risk for Disproportionate Growth related to accelerated growth and premature closure of epiphyseal plates
- Readiness for Enhanced Knowledge related to home care of an infant with lifelong medication requirements

Planning and Implementation

Parents are often concerned about the newborn's condition and appearance of the female's genitals. Provide information and respond to questions. In the newborn nursery, the infant should be referred to as "your infant" or "your baby," not "your son" or "your daughter," until gender identity is confirmed.

It is often difficult for parents to accept that their infant, whose genitalia look male, is really female. With medication and surgery, the genitalia can assume a female appearance and all organs necessary for future childbearing are usually functional. Several surgeries may be performed before 2 years of age and then during adolescence to dilate the vagina. Due to the risk for adrenal insufficiency, the child will most likely be hospitalized for surgery.

The administration of glucocorticoids and mineralcorticoids must be carefully controlled. Educate the family about the special problems that develop in the salt-wasting form of the disease during acute illness. Explain the medication regimen and help the family develop an emergency care plan. Emphasize the importance of the necessity for the child to wear a medical alert tag to identify the disorder and treatment. Ensure parents can properly administer intramuscular injections of hydrocortisone for emergencies. (See Partnering with Families: Hydrocortisone Instructions on page 1259.)

Inform parents that genetic counseling should be provided for the child during adolescence. Inform parents considering a future pregnancy that prenatal testing may detect congenital adrenal hyperplasia in the fetus. Refer the family for supportive counseling if indicated.

Care in the Community

Collaborate with parents to assist in educating the child's siblings, grandparents, other family members, and childcare providers about the condition. Ensure that parents have an emergency kit of injectable hydrocortisone at home and at school to be used when the child is vomiting or has diarrhea. Emphasize that the emergency kit should be carried wherever the child goes. If injectable hydrocortisone is not available, the child requires treatment in an emergency department. The child may become dehydrated quickly and require intravenous fluid and electrolyte replacement in addition to higher doses of hydrocortisone.

■ Evaluation

Expected outcomes of nursing care for the child with congenital adrenal hyperplasia may include:

- Parent/newborn attachment is achieved.
- The child maintains fluid volume balance.
- The child achieves age-appropriate growth and developmental milestones.
- The parents demonstrate understanding of treatment and respond appropriately when injectable medication is needed.

Adrenal Insufficiency (Addison Disease)

Adrenal insufficiency, also known as Addison disease, is a rare disorder in childhood characterized by a deficiency of glucocorticoids (cortisone) and mineralcorticoids (aldosterone). The result of this deficiency leads to a lack of glucocorticoids which aid the body's ability to handle stress (Gance-Cleveland, 2003).

Etiology and Pathophysiology

Adrenal insufficiency may be acquired after trauma; with tuberculosis, acquired immunodeficiency syndrome (AIDS), meningococcemia, or fungal infections that cause destruction of the adrenal glands. Autoimmune destruction of the adrenal gland is the main cause of Addison disease. Premature infants, especially those with chronic lung disease, may have associated adrenal insufficiency. Addison disease affects females two to three times more often than males (Gance-Cleveland, 2003). Since Addison disease can result from autoimmune destruction, the disorder should be considered in children with another autoimmune disease.

The adrenal glands are controlled by the pituitary gland, which stimulates the pituitary gland by increasing the production of adrenocorticotropic hormone (ACTH). Therefore, high serum levels of ACTH are detected in Addison disease (Gance-Cleveland, 2003).

Clinical Manifestations

Adrenal insufficiency usually develops slowly as the adrenal glands deteriorate. The early signs may not be noticed initially but include weakness with fatigue; lethargy and emotional lability; anorexia and salt craving; and poor weight gain or weight loss. Skin pigmentation changes as a result of increased ACTH include hyperpigmentation at pressure points, lip borders and gingival margins, nipples, palms and soles, body creases, and scarred areas of the body; and generalized bronzing of the skin or freckling without tan lines even in winter months. Additional manifestations include abdominal pain, nausea, vomiting and diarrhea, dehydration, and hypovolemia. Cardiovascular changes include tachycardia, dysrhythmias, and postural hypotension. Symptomatic hypoglycemia may also be present. Developmental delay and altered school performance may occur if diagnosis is delayed.

If the child experiences a stressful period (illness, injury, cold, stress, burns, or surgery), acute adrenal insufficiency may occur, leading to Addisonian crisis.

PRACTICE ALERT

Signs of Addisonian crisis include severe hypotension, weakness, fever, abdominal pain, hypoglycemia, seizures, dehydration, circulatory collapse, shock, and coma. Monitor the child for these symptoms as immediate interventions are required.

COLLABORATIVE CARE

The goal of collaborative care is to maintain fluid and electrolyte balance and establish normal levels of corticosteroids and mineralcorticoids.

Diagnostic Tests

Serum cortisol and urinary 17-hydroxycorticoid levels are measured in the early morning. Low levels of serum cortisol are associated with adrenal insufficiency. The adrenocorticotropic hormone (ACTH) stimulation test is used to detect adrenal gland reserve. Electrolyte values generally reveal low serum sodium, elevated serum potassium, and low fasting blood glucose levels. Computed tomography may be used to visualize the adrenal glands.

Clinical Therapy

Treatment involves replacement of the deficient corticosteroids and mineralcorticoids. Hydrocortisone is given in the lowest therapeutic dose to control symptoms and promote normal growth. Fludrocortisone acetate (Florinef) is administered to replace the missing mineralcorticoid in children with aldosterone deficiency.

Since Addisonian crisis can occur with stress, the dose of hydrocortisone is increased in the presence of any illness, trauma, surgery, or other stressor. Addisonian crisis is treated by fluid and electrolyte resuscitation, treatment of the precipitating illness or injury, adequate doses of glucocorticoid, and maintenance doses of mineralcorticoid.

NURSING MANAGEMENT

Nursing management focuses on restoring hemodynamic homeostasis in the acutely ill child. Educating the child and parents about the disorder, providing emotional support, and caring for the child during acute episodes are other aspects of nursing management.

Nursing Assessment and Diagnosis

Assess vital signs for changes in heart rate and blood pressure. Assess weight, skin turgor, and mucous membranes to determine the presence of dehydration. Monitor nutritional intake, elimination patterns, muscle strength, and level of consciousness. Monitor laboratory values, intake and output, and daily weight.

Nursing diagnoses that apply to the child with adrenal insufficiency may include the following:

- Deficient Fluid Volume related to dehydration
- Deficient Knowledge related to disease process and treatment regimen
- Disturbed Body Image related to changes in skin pigmentation

Planning and Implementation

Encourage fluid intake as prescribed. Administer intravenous fluids as indicated. Monitor serum electrolytes as ordered. Partner with the family to ensure proper medication and fluid administration is added to family routines. Educate the family and child to promote an understanding that the treatment for this disorder is lifelong replacement therapy.

If the child vomits within 1 hour of taking the medication, the dose is repeated. Parents may be instructed to double or triple medication in anticipation of stressful events, and to increase the medication in the event of illness. Since stress increases the body's need for cortisol, Solu-Cortef injections should be available on hand at home and in the school setting for emergencies. If the child is unable to take the medications orally or is unconscious, Solu-Cortef injections are indicated (Gance-Cleveland, 2003).

Discuss skin pigment changes with older children and adolescents. Encourage the child to identify clothing colors that are complimentary despite skin color changes. Help the child identify personal strengths and abilities to promote self-esteem.

Ensure the family recognizes symptoms that require reporting, including bleeding, dizziness, lethargy, weakness, changes in blood pressure or pulse, and weight gain. The child should wear a medical alert tag identifying the disorder and medications for treatment. As the child assumes independence, encourage the adolescent to share information about the disorder with at least one close friend who can provide assistance in an emergency. See Chapter 20∞.

Refer to the earlier discussion of congenital adrenal hyperplasia for further information on nursing care.

Evaluation

Expected outcomes for care of the child with adrenal insufficiency include the following:

- The child maintains hemodynamic stability.
- The child achieves fluid balance.
- The child and family demonstrate understanding of disease and treatment regimen.
- The child demonstrates a positive body image.

Pheochromocytoma

Pheochromocytoma is a tumor of the adrenal gland, but it may be extraadrenal with no anatomic connection. In most cases, these tumors are benign and curable, but approximately 10% are malignant (Failor, 2003). The tumor can occur in a familial pattern (autosomal dominant trait) with a 3:2 male to female ratio. The incidence is 1 to 500,000 children, and most tumors are diagnosed in children between the ages of 6 and 14 years (Reddy, O'Neill, Holcomb, et al., 2000). Pheochromocytomas occur in 1% to 2% of patients with neurofibromatosis (Von Recklinghausen disease).

The tumor results in excessive release of the catecholamines epinephrine and norepinephrine, leading to hypertension. The degree of hypertension is influenced by the level of circulating catecholamines, the level of sympathetic nervous system stimulation, and the cardiovascular response to those changes (Copstead & Banasik, 2000).

Clinical manifestations can be dramatic and labile. The degree of symptoms will depend on the amount of catecholamines being released from the tumor. Symptoms include labile hypertension with a systolic reading that may reach 250 mm Hg, tachycardia, arrhythmias, palpitations, profuse sweating with cool extremities, flushing, headache, abdominal pain, nausea and vomiting, weight loss, visual disturbances, tinnitus, weakness, and tremor. Additional symptoms include nervousness, fatigue, and fever as a result of the hypermetabolic state (Failor, 2003). Because release of catecholamines (norepinephrine and epinephrine) from the tumor is not continuous, these symptoms occur intermittently. Attacks may occur daily or monthly and generally last minutes to an hour (Failor, 2003). In some cases the condition may be silent until a stressor such as surgery causes a hypertensive crisis.

Collaborative Care

Diagnosis can be difficult to make since it is an uncommon tumor and symptoms may be episodic. Positive biochemical tests may have a high false-positive rate and localization procedures are sometimes unrevealing (Failor, 2003). Diagnosis is based on 24-hour urine studies to detect the presence of increased urinary catecholamines and VMA levels and serum catecholamines, metanephrine and normetanepheine levels (Failor, 2003). Ideally, serum levels are drawn in a fasting state without recent ingestion of caffeine. Imaging studies, including CT, PET scan, MRI, or ultrasound are required to localize the tumor in preparation for surgical removal. In 90% of cases, they are located in the adrenal glands, but they can also be located in the chest, bladder, head, and neck (Failor, 2003).

Initially, bed rest is prescribed and the head of the bed is elevated to promote an orthostatic decrease in blood pressure. The treatment of choice is surgical removal of the tumor and most likely an adrenalectomy; however, the procedure is dangerous and may result in pheochromocytoma crisis. Removal of the tumor during surgery may cause a release of stored epinephrine and norepinephrine, leading to elevated blood pressure and changes in heart rate (pheochromocytoma crisis). If this occurs, alpha-adrenergic blocking agents are administered.

PRACTICE ALERT

Pheochromocytoma crisis manifests with profound hypertension, seizures, shock, altered level of consciousness, disseminated intravascular coagulation, rhabdomyolysis (skeletal muscle destruction), and acute renal failure. This crisis can result in death. Monitor blood pressure frequently to detect changes.

Alpha- and beta-adrenergic blocking agents to control hypertension, tachycardia, and catecholamine release are administered for 10 to 14 days before surgery (Harris & Fawcett, 2002). Plasma catecholamines are used to measure the effectiveness of the preoperative adrenergic blockade. Postoperatively, for several days, a 24-hour urine collection is measured for catecholamines to determine if all tumor sites were removed. If a bilateral adrenalectomy was performed, lifelong corticosteroid replacement is required. With successful removal of all tumor sites, the prognosis is generally good, and catecholamine secretion should return to normal within one week. Follow-up is important to assess for recurrence of tumor.

Nursing Management

Nursing care is mainly supportive. Provide preoperative and postoperative teaching and care (refer to Chapter 17∞). Preoperatively, monitor vital signs and observe for signs of complications associated with pheochromocytoma crisis. Administer antihypertensives and observe for any signs of hyperglycemia (refer to page 1281). Provide emotional support to the child and family.

Postoperatively, the child may be managed initially in an intensive care unit. Monitor blood pressure and glucose levels. Hypoglycemia and hypotension may occur following the withdrawal of excessive amounts of catecholamines. Observe for changes in neurologic status, respiratory distress, and signs of shock.

Partner with the family to ensure understanding of lifelong follow-up care. Screening for hypertension and increased urinary catecholamine levels is required as symptoms have recurred in up to 20% of patients 2 to 7 years after surgery (Reddy et al., 2000).

DISORDERS OF PANCREATIC FUNCTION

The primary function of the pancreas is to regulate blood glucose metabolism. The islets of Langerhans of the pancreas consist of alpha, beta, and delta cells.

- Alpha cells secrete the hormone **glucagon,** which accelerates liver **glycogenolysis** (conversion of glycogen to glucose) to increase blood glucose. Glucagon acts as an antagonist to the hormone **insulin,** the hormone responsible for glucose metabolism.
- Beta cells produce insulin, which promotes glucose, protein, and fatty acid transport into the cells. Insulin also accelerates the movement of potassium and phosphate ions through the cell membranes with glucose, which reduces blood glucose levels and increases glucose metabolism.
- Delta cells produce somatostatin, the hormone that inhibits secretion of insulin and glucagons.

The pancreas normally secretes approximately 40 to 50 units of insulin per day. Normal blood glucose range in children is 60–105 mg/dL. Normally, after consumption of food, insulin secretion increases to move glucose from the blood into the liver, muscle, and fat cells for energy. When glucose is unavailable, as in lack of insulin, lipolysis (breakdown of fat), which results in the production of ketones, and proteolysis (breakdown of protein) occurs in order to meet the body's fuel demands for energy.

Other hormones that increase blood glucose levels are epinephrine, norepinephrine, cortisol, and growth hormone.

The major disorder of pancreatic function is diabetes mellitus types 1 and 2, which are discussed in the following section. Associated complications of diabetes, such as hypoglycemia and diabetic ketoacidosis, are also discussed.

Diabetes Mellitus

Diabetes mellitus, the most common metabolic disease in children and one of the most common chronic diseases in school-age children, is a disorder of carbohydrate, protein, and fat metabolism (Figure 32–6 ■). There are two main types of diabetes mellitus. The majority of children have immune-mediated type 1 diabetes, formerly called insulin dependent diabetes mellitus or juvenile diabetes. However, a disturbingly large number of children are being diagnosed with type 2 diabetes, formerly called noninsulin dependent diabetes (Alemzadeh, 2004).

In the United States, the prevalence of type I diabetes among all children 19 years and younger is 1.7 per 1,000 (CDC, 2004). Peak incidence of type 1 occurs in childhood, with a median age of 7 to 15 years, but it may be present at any age (Alemzadeh, 2004). Caucasians experience a higher incidence of type 1 diabetes than other racial groups. Approximately 75% of all newly diagnosed cases of type 1 diabetes occur in children younger than 18 years of age, and every year more than 13,000 children

PATHOPHYSIOLOGY ILLUSTRATED

Mechanism of Diabetes Mellitus

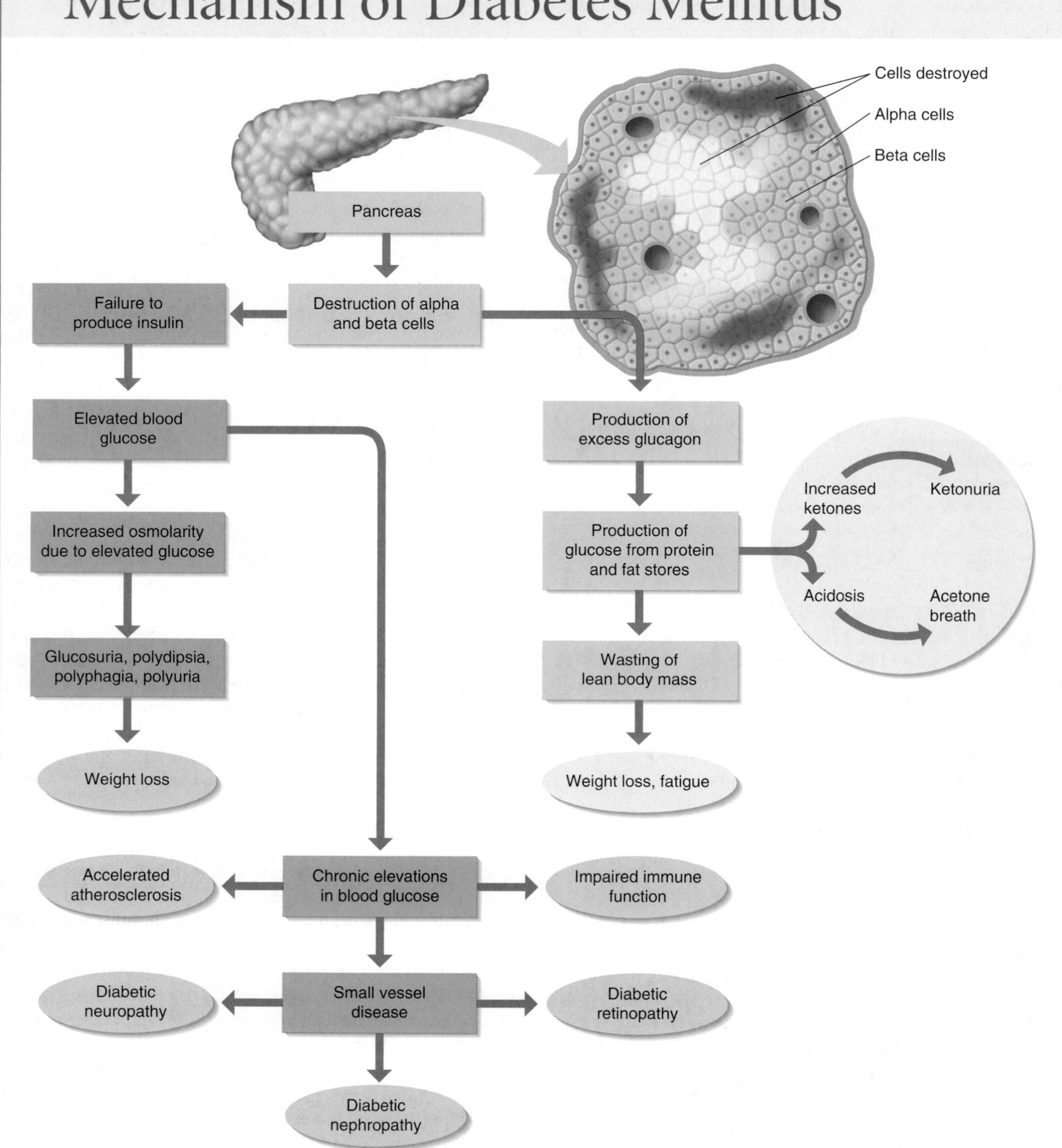

FIGURE 32–6 ■ Destruction of the alpha and beta cells in the islets of Langerhans produces multiple metabolic changes. Acute signs and symptoms are followed by short-term and long-term complications if the disease is not well managed. See Figure 32–7.

are diagnosed with type 1 diabetes (American Diabetes Association [ADA], 2004a). (See Box 32–5 for information on cystic fibrosis-related diabetes.)

Type 1 Diabetes

The majority of children with diabetes have immune-mediated type 1. This disorder results from destruction of pancreatic islet beta cells, which fail to secrete insulin. The body becomes dependent on exogenous sources of insulin.

Etiology and Pathophysiology. Insulin helps transport glucose into the cells so that this carbohydrate can be used as an energy source. It also prevents the outflow of glucose from the liver to the general circulation. It is hypothesized that type 1 diabetes may be caused by a genetic component, environmental influences, or an autoimmune response which damages the pancreatic beta cells (Alemzadeh, 2004). Type 1 diabetes has familial tendencies but does not show any specific pattern of inheritance. Approximately 5% of children with type 1 diabetes have a first- or second-degree relative with the type 1 diabetes (ADA, 2000). The child inherits a susceptibility to the disease rather than the disease itself. Females and males are equally affected (Alemzadeh, 2004).

Recent research reveals that children exposed to infections such as congenital Rubella and enterovirus may have a higher propensity towards developing Type 1 diabetes.

Environmental factors such as enteroviruses or toxins are believed to lead to an autoimmune destruction of the beta cells in the Islets of Langerhans. Antigens are generated which lead to production of antibodies that indicate ongoing destruction of the islet cells. As the destruction continues, the child develops glucose intolerance.

The preclinical stage may last up to 13 years as the autoimmune process begins early in life (Silverstein & Rosenbloom, 2000). Lack of insulin results in a rise in the serum glucose level and a decrease in the glucose level inside the cells. When the renal threshold for glucose (180 mg/dL) is exceeded, **glycosuria** (abnormal amount of glucose in the urine) occurs as a result of osmotic diuresis (Alemzadeh, 2004). Glucose is highly osmotic; therefore, fluids follow glucose and are excreted out of the body in large volumes of urine (polyuria).

When glucose is unavailable to the cells for metabolism, an alternate source of energy is provided by free fatty acids. The combination of insulin deficiency and elevated plasma levels of counter-regulatory hormones is also responsible for accelerated lipolysis and impaired lipid synthesis, resulting in increased total plasma lipids, cholesterol, triglycerides and free fatty acids. The hormonal interplay of insulin deficiency and glucagon excess shunts the free fatty acids into ketone body formation. Free fatty acids are metabolized at an increased rate by the liver, producing acetyl coenzyme A (CoA). The byproducts of acetyl CoA metabolism (ketone bodies) accumulate in the body at a higher rate than the body is capable of excreting, resulting in a state of metabolic acidosis, or ketoacidosis. (See Chapter 23∞ for discussion of metabolic acidosis; see page 1278 for ketoacidosis).

BOX 32–5 Cystic Fibrosis-Related Diabetes (CFRD)

Cystic fibrosis–related diabetes (CFRD) has similar features of types 1 and 2 diabetes; however, it is considered a separate condition. In cystic fibrosis, the pancreas does not produce sufficient insulin (as in type 1 diabetes), which is referred to as *insulin deficiency.* Another mechanism of CFRD is *insulin resistance,* in which the body fails to utilize insulin normally, requiring more insulin for metabolism. Insulin deficiency and insulin resistance combined in the patient with cystic fibrosis can lead to the development of diabetes more frequently than occurs in the general population (Cystic Fibrosis Foundation, 2004).

Clinical Manifestations. The classic signs of type 1 diabetes are polyuria, polydipsia, and **polyphagia** (excessive appetite) with significant weight loss (Figure 32–7 ■). Recall that Anthony, the child in the opening scenario, demonstrated these symptoms. See the table on page 1267 for clinical manifestations of type 1 and type 2 diabetes. Unexplained fatigue or lethargy, headaches, stomach aches, and occasional enuresis may also occur in a previously toilet-trained child. Adolescent girls may experience vaginitis caused by candida, which thrives in the hyperglycemic tissues. Symptoms develop gradually and insidiously but have usually been present less than a month when diagnosed. In severe cases, diabetic ketoacidosis (DKA), a type of metabolic acidosis, may develop rapidly.

Complications of type 1 diabetes, including retinopathy, atherosclerotic heart disease, renal failure, and peripheral vascular disease, result from long-term hyperglycemic effects on the blood vessels (Alemzadeh & Wyatt, 2004; Krantz, 2004). Without careful management, diabetic children may develop complications related to poor glucose control, including renal failure and loss of vision in adulthood. Intensive therapy is expected to reduce the risk for or delay the development of these complications. Risk may be further reduced if the adolescent does not begin smoking and if the blood pressure is controlled. See Table 32–4.

MediaLink Physiology of Diabetes Animation

COLLABORATIVE CARE

Care of the child with diabetes requires a multidisciplinary approach through collaboration with primary healthcare providers, an endocrinologist, nurse diabetic educator, nutritionist, behaviorist, school personnel, and counselors.

The management of diabetes, especially in children, is a complex process. The goal is to achieve optimal blood glucose control through medications and monitoring of glucose levels, adequate nutrition, and exercise; promotion of optimal growth and development; and prevention of long-term complications.

Diagnostic Tests

Fasting (no caloric intake for at least 8 hours) serum glucose levels at or above 126 mg/dL or a random (casual) serum glucose level of 200 mg/dL or greater, or an oral glucose tolerance test (OGTT) with the 2-hour plasma glucose > 200

PATHOPHYSIOLOGY ILLUSTRATED

Multisystem Effects of Diabetes

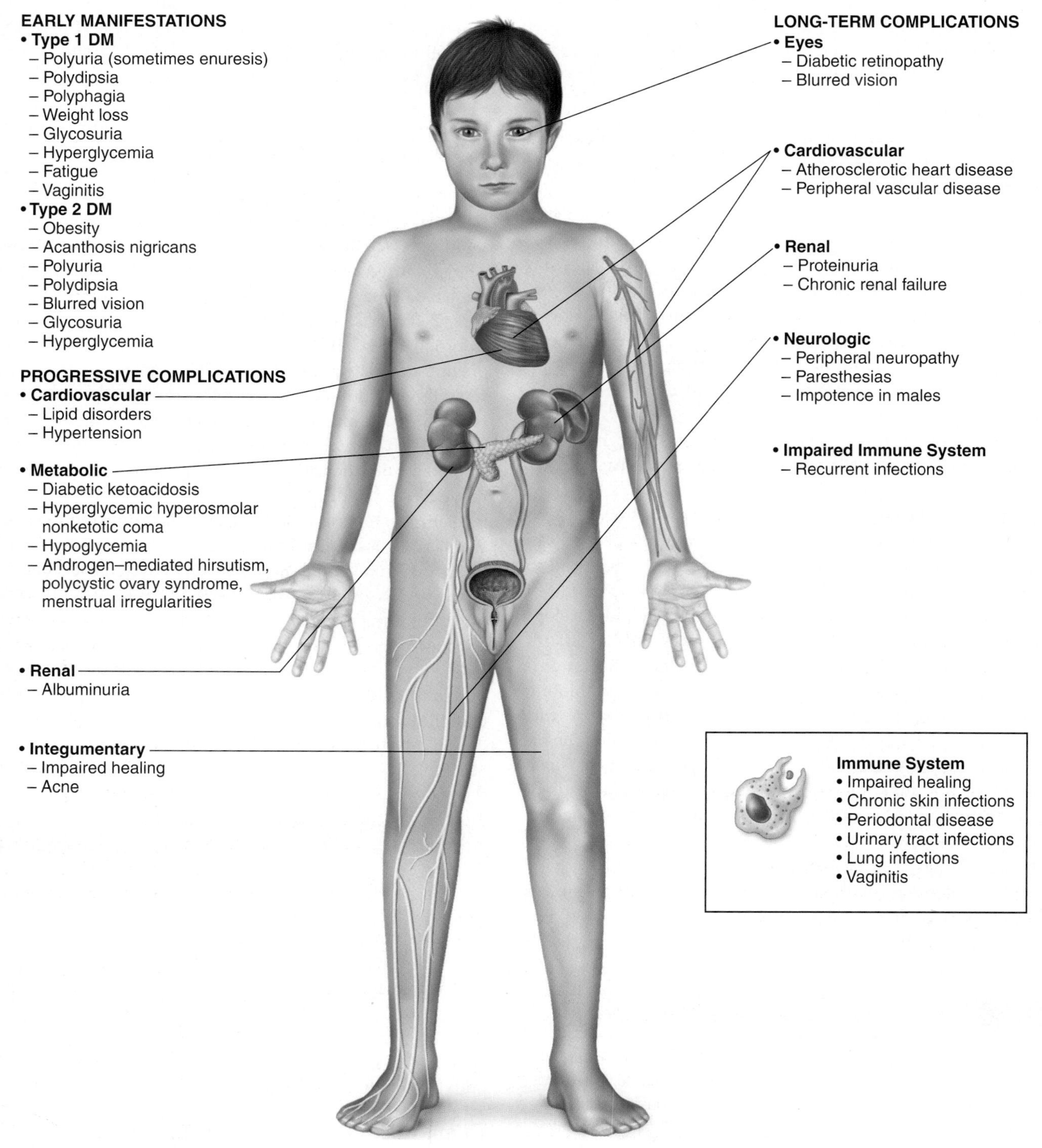
EARLY MANIFESTATIONS
• Type 1 DM
– Polyuria (sometimes enuresis)
– Polydipsia
– Polyphagia
– Weight loss
– Glycosuria
– Hyperglycemia
– Fatigue
– Vaginitis
• Type 2 DM
– Obesity
– Acanthosis nigricans
– Polyuria
– Polydipsia
– Blurred vision
– Glycosuria
– Hyperglycemia
PROGRESSIVE COMPLICATIONS
• Cardiovascular
– Lipid disorders
– Hypertension
• Metabolic
– Diabetic ketoacidosis
– Hyperglycemic hyperosmolar nonketotic coma
– Hypoglycemia
– Androgen–mediated hirsutism, polycystic ovary syndrome, menstrual irregularities
• Renal
– Albuminuria
• Integumentary
– Impaired healing
– Acne
LONG-TERM COMPLICATIONS
• Eyes
– Diabetic retinopathy
– Blurred vision
• Cardiovascular
– Atherosclerotic heart disease
– Peripheral vascular disease
• Renal
– Proteinuria
– Chronic renal failure
• Neurologic
– Peripheral neuropathy
– Paresthesias
– Impotence in males
• Impaired Immune System
– Recurrent infections
Immune System
• Impaired healing
• Chronic skin infections
• Periodontal disease
• Urinary tract infections
• Lung infections
• Vaginitis

FIGURE 32–7 ■ Multiple body systems are affected by metabolic changes reulting from diabetes.

CLINICAL MANIFESTATIONS of Diabetes by Type

ETIOLOGY	CLINICAL MANIFESTATIONS	CLINICAL THERAPY
Type 1—immune mediated, insulin deficiency due to pancreatic beta cell destruction	Polyuria, polydipsia Recent weight loss, but may be overweight Ketoacidosis on initial presentation in 30%–40% of cases, at continued risk for ketoacidosis Short duration of symptoms Ketosis Initial period of decreased insulin requirement, then need insulin for survival	Blood glucose monitoring Insulin Exercise Dietary management, balancing carbohydrate intake to insulin and exercise
Type 2—insulin resistance with relative insulin secretory defect	Obese, little or no weight loss, or may have significant weight loss Acanthosis nigricans Long duration of symptoms Polyuria, polydipsia may be mild or absent Glycosuria without ketonuria in 33% of cases on initial presentation Ketoacidosis on initial presentation in 5%–25% of cases Lipid disorders Hypertension Androgen-mediated problems such as acne, hirsutism, menstrual disturbances, polycystic ovary disease Excessive weight gain and fatigue due to insulin resistance	Diet with decreased calories and low-fat foods Decrease sedentary activity time or increase routine physical activity Blood glucose monitoring Oral medication (metoformin) to improve insulin sensitivity

mg/dL, are indicative of diabetes (ADA, 2004b). (See Box 32–6) Ketones, the waste product of fat metabolism, may be noted in the blood or urine.

Diagnosis is based on the presence of classic symptoms and serum glucose level as described previously. Additional laboratory tests for known autoantibodies that can indicate an autoimmune attack against the insulin-producing beta cells of the pancreas may be ordered such as glutamic acid decarboxylase (GAD-65), insulin autoantibodies, and islet cell cytoplasmic autoantibodies. A careful history is necessary to rule out the presence of a stress-related illness, corticosteroid usage, fracture, acute infection, cystic fibrosis, pancreatitis, or liver disease.

Clinical Therapy

Clinical therapy for type 1 diabetes combines insulin, medical nutrition therapy to support growth and to maintain blood glucose at near normal levels, an exercise regimen, and psychosocial support.

TABLE 32–4 Complications Associated with Diabetes Mellitus

ACUTE COMPLICATIONS	CHRONIC COMPLICATIONS	COMPLICATIONS RELATED TO GROWTH AND DEVELOPMENT
Diabetic ketoacidosis	Retinopathy	Delay in growth
Hypoglycemia	Nephropathy Neuropathy Peripheral vascular disease	Delay in puberty Emotional disturbances Menstrual disturbances

Insulin Therapy. Multiple approaches to insulin therapy for children and adolescents are available, and should be individualized according to the needs of the child and family. The American Diabetic Association (2004b) recommends that blood glucose levels be normalized using basal-bolus therapy for children and adolescents. The goal of initial basal-bolus therapy is to lower blood glucose levels, stabilize glucose levels, and to eliminate ketones. Insulin doses are adjusted according to frequent serum glucose monitoring, at least four times a day. Insulin can be administered by an insulin pump (subcutaneous insulin infusion, SCII) or by multiple daily injections (MDIs). The goal of insulin therapy is to maintain serum glucose levels from 80 to 120 mg/dL before meals and 100 to 140 mg/dL at bedtime (ADA, 2002). Glycemic goals for children younger than 6 years are generally less tight since they lack the cognitive capacity to recognize and respond to hypoglycemic symptoms (ADA, 2004b).

With basal-bolus therapy, basal insulin is administered once a day (Lantos or glargine), or twice daily (Humulin or Ultralente). Then a bolus of rapid-acting insulin is administered with each

BOX 32–6 Pre-Diabetes

The American Diabetic Association considers a fasting glucose of 100–125 mg/dL (5.6–6.9 mmol/L) to be an *impaired fasting glucose,* and a 2-hour postload glucose of 140–199 mg/dL to be an *impaired glucose tolerance.* Individuals with impaired fasting glucose and/or impaired glucose tolerance are now referred to as having "pre-diabetes," indicating that they have a relatively high risk for development of diabetes (ADA, 2004b).

meal and snack based on the carbohydrate grams consumed. The goal of basal-bolus insulin therapy is to maintain a blood glucose level as close to the target range as possible and to minimize episodes of hyperglycemia and hypoglycemia (see page 1281). Several forms of insulin are available, as identified in Table 32–5.

Studies of the effectiveness of inhaled insulin for administration before meals also are being conducted in adults with type 1 and 2 diabetes, with promising results (Alemzadeh, 2004). The goal is to find alternate methods of intensive insulin control without increasing injections (Silverstein & Rosenbloom, 2000).

CLINICAL TIP

Insulin is usually provided in prepackaged doses of 100 units/mL. Diluted insulin prepared by a pharmacist may be used for infants and toddlers who require a small insulin dosage. Insulin cartridges, disposable pens, and other devices, such as Innolet, are also available to make injections easier for active children and adolescents.

TABLE 32–5 Insulin Action, Subcutaneous Injection

TYPE	ONSET	PEAK	DURATION
Rapid acting			
Insulin Lispro/Humalog	5–15 minutes	1 hour	2–4 hours
Insulin aspart	10–20 minutes	1–3 hours	3–5 hours
Short acting			
Regular	½–1 hour	2–4 hours	4–6 hours
Intermediate acting			
NPH	1–2 hours	6–12 hours	18–26 hours
Lente	1–2 hours	6–12 hours	24–26 hours
Long acting			
Ultralente	4–8 hours	10–20 hours	16–24 hours
Lantos/insulin glargine	1–2 hours	None/slight	24 hours

Note: Intermediate-acting insulin mixed with short- or rapid-acting insulin (e.g., 70% NPH/30% regular, 50% NPH/50% regular, and 75% NPL/25% insulin lispro) are also available.

Basal-bolus therapy can be achieved with three or more insulin injections a day or a continuous subcutaneous insulin infusion (CSII) by an insulin pump. See Table 32–6 for criteria for selecting insulin pump therapy. Research reveals that the risk for developing retinopathy, microalbuminuria, and peripheral neuropathy is significantly lower with basal-bolus therapy over more conventional regimens. Advantages and disadvantages of an insulin pump are outlined in Table 32–7.

Basal-bolus therapy for type 1 diabetes includes:

- Monitoring blood glucose four to eight times a day and once a week at midnight and 3 A.M.
- Consistent carbohydrate counting
- Anticipating exercise in the routine

Stress, infection, and illness may either increase or decrease insulin needs. In addition, increased insulin doses are often required during growth and at puberty.

For some children, conventional insulin therapy may be used, requiring two or three insulin injections a day. One example of conventional insulin therapy consists of daily administration of a combination of a short-acting (regular) insulin and an intermediate-acting (NPH or Lente) or long-acting (Ultralente) insulin before breakfast and before the evening meal (Figure 32–8 ■). Older children may use a regimen of tighter control that includes two injections a day of intermediate or long-acting insulin and an injection of rapid-acting insulin with each meal to match carbohydrate intake. Advantages of rapid-acting insulin (Lispro) in therapy to achieve tight glucose control include:

- Decreased number of nocturnal hypoglycemic episodes
- Meal coverage for toddlers who have unpredictable food consumption
- Flexibility for adolescents concerned about weight gain who do not want to eat a mid-morning snack

TABLE 32–6 Age-Based Criteria for Selecting Insulin Pump Therapy

TODDLERS AND YOUNG CHILDREN	CHILDREN OVER 10 YEARS
Problems during therapy	Disease management readiness
➤ Recurrent episodes of moderate and severe hypoglycemia	➤ 3–6 months of intensive insulin therapy, including three or more injections per day.
➤ Persistent $HbA_{1c} \geq 9\%$ even with changes in insulin dosing	➤ 3–6 months of monitoring and recording blood glucose levels at least four times per day
➤ Unexplained erratic changes in blood glucose levels not resolved with insulin dosing changes	➤ 3–6 months of carbohydrate counting
➤ Recurrent diabetic ketoacidosis or severe hyperglycemia	➤ Ability to give abdominal injections and no fear of needles
Parents or caregivers available to provide constant supervision	➤ Diabetes identification medallion
➤ Understand pump functioning	➤ Ability to make small adjustments in treatment regimen appropriately between visits
➤ Able to adjust basal and bolus doses	➤ Evidence of diabetes team contact in emergency situations
➤ Monitor blood glucose levels four times daily	Psychosocial readiness
➤ Have collaborative working relationship with healthcare providers	➤ Child/adolescent responsibile for majority of diabetes self-care
Child can tolerate catheter and infusion set and refrain from touching the catheter and pump	

Adapted from Litton, J., Rice, A., Friedman, N., Oden, J., Lee, M. M., & Freemark, M. (2002). Insulin pump therapy in toddlers and preschool children with type 1 diabetes mellitus. Journal of Pediatrics, 141, *490–495; Cogen, F. R., Streisand, R., & Sarin, S. (2002). Selecting children and adolescents for insulin pump therapy: Medical and behavioral considerations.* Diabetes Spectrum, 15*(2), 72–75.*

TABLE 32–7 Advantages and Disadvantages of an External Insulin Infusion Pump

ADVANTAGES	DISADVANTAGES
➤ Delivers a continuous infusion of insulin to match the basal rate needed plus an insulin bolus at mealtime	➤ Requires highly motivated child and supportive parents and healthcare professionals
➤ Helps maintain blood glucose control between meals	➤ Requires willingness to live connected to a device (can be disconnected for short periods by removing or clamping the catheter; however, DKA can occur within hours of interruption of insulin flow)
➤ Decreased HbA_{1c}	➤ Hyperglycemia leading to ketoacidosis (which is the greatest risk associated with this therapy)
➤ Improves growth in children	➤ Site must be changed every 2–4 days, at least 1 inch from the last site
➤ Reduces number of injections	➤ Necessitates more time and energy to monitor blood glucose levels, dietary intake, and insulin bolus calculation
➤ Allows child to eat with less adherence to a schedule	➤ Involves changing syringe, catheter, and skin setup every 2–3 days
➤ Reduces number of injection sites, so variation in absorption decreases	➤ Infections can occur at the injection site
➤ More closely simulates normal pancreatic function	➤ Weight gain is common when blood sugar control improves
➤ Exact dosing of insulin since basal rates can be changed every 1/2 hour	
➤ Frequency of severe hypoglycemia has been decreased	
➤ Fewer incidences of diabetic ketoacidosis	
➤ More flexible lifestyle and meal timing is permitted	

Data from Saudek, C. D. (1997). Novel forms of insulin delivery. Endocrinology and Metabolism Clinics of North America, *26(3), 599–610; Maniatis, A. K., Klingensmith, G. J., Slover, R. H., Mowry, C. J., & Chase, H. P. (2001). Continuous subcutaneous insulin infusion therapy for children and adolescents: An option for routine diabetes care.* Pediatrics, *107(2), 351–356; Miller, M. M. (2003, November). Insulin pump therapy.* Advance for Nurse Practitioners, *61–66.*

Evaluation of Insulin Therapy. Laboratory evaluation of hemoglobin A_{1c} (HbA_{1c}) to measure glycosylated hemoglobin should be performed every 3 months. HbA_{1c} provides an objective measurement of glycemic control since it represents the amount of glucose irreversibly attached to the hemoglobin molecule over an extended period (the life span of the red blood cell, approximately 120 days), therefore predicting an index of glucose control over the prior 6 to 8 weeks (Haller, 2004). The HbA_{1c} is below 6.2% for individuals without diabetes, and the goal for children with diabetes is 7.5% to 8% depending on age and healthcare provider preferences. It is also important to determine if the HbA_{1c} matches recorded blood sugars.

Nutrition Therapy. The goal of nutrition therapy is to provide adequate calories for the child's normal growth and development. An evaluation of the child's food intake, metabolic status, and lifestyle are necessary before establishing a nutrition plan. Daily caloric requirements are individualized for each child according to need. To facilitate adherence to the nutritional plan, an individualized approach with considerations of the child and family's culture, lifestyle, and financial means should be incorporated. Careful instruction by a nutritionist is essential in the management of diabetes.

Carbohydrate counting provides flexibility in meal planning and is simple for children and adolescents to use. The carbohydrate requirements vary based on the needs of the child. Younger school-age children can consume two to four carbohydrate choices (one carbohydrate choice equals 15 g of carbohydrates) per meal and older children and adolescents can consume four to six carbohydrate choices per meal. Additional carbohydrate choices are necessary for older children who are more physically active. Between-meal snacks generally consist of one to two carbohydrate choices, depending on the type of insulin used (Evert, 2004). The number of units of insulin needed to cover the grams of carbohydrates eaten is determined based on the scale of 1 unit of insulin covering 8 g of carbohydrates. If additional carbohydrates are eaten at a meal or snack, the number of insulin units can also be adjusted, providing further flexibility.

The Food Guide Pyramid (see Chapter 9∞) is utilized to teach the child and family the correct portions and which foods are considered carbohydrates, fats, and proteins. A high fiber diet is recommended for improved control of blood glucose. Non-nutritive sweeteners such as aspartame and saccharin may be used in moderation. The child and family should understand how to read food labels. Daily caloric requirements are individualized for each child according to need.

CLINICAL TIP

Avoid use of sorbitol and zylitol as artificial sweeteners as they have been implicated in some diabetes complications (Alemzadeh & Wyatt, 2004).

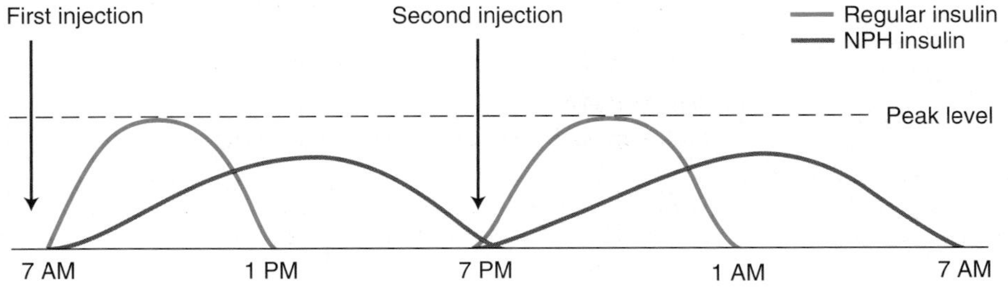

FIGURE 32–8 ■ Conventional therapy. Insulin levels vary over a 24-hour period in relation to injections and mealtimes.

Exercise Program. Physical activity is associated with increased insulin sensitivity. Regular exercise improves blood glucose control, reduces cardiovascular risk factors, contributes to weight loss, and improves overall well-being. Blood lipid levels are also positively affected. However, the child must have an adequate caloric intake to prevent hypoglycemia. An extra snack may help to prevent hypoglycemia. Excessive exercise associated with sports requires careful planning and management.

Islet-Pancreatic Transplantation. Pancreatic transplantation for patients requiring kidney transplant is an accepted procedure. With successful pancreatic transplantation, hyperglycemia is immediately reversed and there is some evidence of improved short-term outcomes (Eisenbrath, 2003). The surgery is extensive and there are multiple potential complications including chronic immunosuppression. Diabetes can recur because of recurrent autoimmune islet cell destruction due to rejection (Eisenbrath, 2003). Isolated pancreatic transplantation is not performed because immunosuppressive therapy is destructive to islet cells.

NURSING MANAGEMENT

Nursing care focuses on teaching the child and parents about the disease and its management—managing dietary intake, promoting growth and developmental milestones, providing emotional support, and planning strategies for daily management in the community.

Nursing Assessment and Diagnosis

Nursing assessment focuses on the child's physiologic status; child and parental psychosocial responses to the disease; and the child's developmental status.

Physiologic Assessment

Children are generally admitted to the hospital at the time of diagnosis. Assess the child's physiologic status, focusing on vital signs, fluid balance, and level of consciousness. Assess hydration by checking mucous membranes, skin turgor, and urine output. Blood initially is collected hourly to monitor blood gases, glucose, and electrolytes. Once the child is stable, assess dietary and caloric intake and the ability of the child or family to manage care.

Psychosocial Assessment

Parents may feel guilty at the time of diagnosis if they waited to seek care until the child began to experience symptoms of diabetic ketoacidosis. Assess coping mechanisms, ability to manage the disease, and educational needs of both the child and parents. Assess the child's understanding and ability to cope with the diagnosis of diabetes. Assess the child's previous experience with diabetes, for example, a relative with diabetes who experienced complications such as amputation or blindness. Examples of questions to use in assessing the family's strengths and limitations in the child's disease management are provided in Box 32–7. Assess the child's or adolescent's willingness and motivation to adhere to treatment regimen. See Evidence-Based Practice: Adolescent Diabetes and Quality of Life.

Developmental Assessment

Assess the child's developmental level, particularly fine motor skills, and cognitive level to determine delays in growth and development. Assess the child's height and weight and plot on growth chart to evaluate growth. Assess the child's cognitive development and fine motor skills to begin performing some aspects of self-care, such as obtaining and reading a blood glucose sample or injecting insulin. Children are usually able to perform some of these tasks with supervision by 6 to 8 years of age. Self-management is the

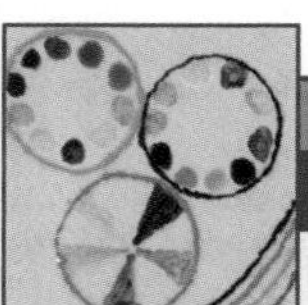

EVIDENCE-BASED PRACTICE

Adolescent Diabetes and Quality of Life

PROBLEM

Adolescents with type 1 diabetes not only experience the normal psychologic and physiologic changes that occur during the adolescent growth period, but they must also cope with the responsibility of increasing self-management of their disease, including insulin administration, exercise, nutrition, and self-esteem issues associated with a chronic illness.

EVIDENCE

A descriptive correlational study exploring the quality of life for 69 adolescents with type 1 diabetes versus 75 healthy adolescents revealed that adolescents with diabetes expressed lower life satisfaction and health perception controls. The mean age for both groups was 15 years. The adolescents with diabetes experienced psychologic and physiologic turmoil while attempting to balance their treatment regimen. Additionally, Caucasian middle adolescents (aged >15 years and <17 years) had lower life satisfaction than the younger (>13 years and <15 years) and older adolescents (>17 years and <19 years). Differences in level of metabolic control was not associated with worries of life satisfaction among youth with diabetes (Faulkner, 2003).

Another study explored the relationship between illness uncertainty, perceived control, and psychologic distress among 68 adolescents with type 1 diabetes aged 13 to 18 years. Adolescents completed three self-report measures that addressed each of the factors (Children's Uncertainty in Illness Scale, Perceived Control Scale, and Brief Symptom Inventory). Findings revealed that illness uncertainty was significantly associated with psychologic distress as well as perceived control. Thus, the extent to which adolescents view the treatment and prognosis of their disease as confusing and unpredictable likely increases their risk for negative emotional states or psychologic distress (Hoff, Mullins, Chaney, et al., 2002).

IMPLICATIONS

For the nurse, life satisfaction, illness uncertainty, perceived control, and worries associated with having diabetes are important considerations when counseling the adolescent and family about the therapeutic management of the disease.

CRITICAL THINKING APPLICATIONS

What are some possible reasons for adolescents in the middle-age range to perceive lower life satisfaction than younger and older teens? How will you address quality of life issues with adolescents in different age groups? With the family? What options can you explore with the adolescent and family that may improve the adolescent's view of quality of life?

BOX 32–7 Questions to Ask When Planning Diabetic Education

1. Do both parents work or does the single parent work? What hours?
2. Who else is involved in the child's care?
3. What is the child's usual daily schedule? Does the schedule vary on the weekend or any other days of the week?
4. Does the child have health insurance? What coverage exists for diabetes education, treatment, and home management?
5. Does the child have any cognitive, behavioral, motor, or visual problems coexisting with this condition?
6. What other family stressors coexist with the diagnosis?

eventual goal, and the child's responsibilities are gradually increased. Talk with adolescents and assess problem solving skills associated with daily condition management and ability to manage special circumstances such as illness or change in exercise routine.

Several nursing diagnoses that may apply to the child newly diagnosed with type 1 diabetes are provided in the accompanying nursing care plans. Additional diagnoses that may be appropriate are as follows:

- Risk for Deficient Fluid Volume related to active fluid loss associated with hyperglycemia
- Ineffective Breathing Pattern related to neuromuscular dysfunction associated with metabolic acidosis
- Ineffective Coping related to inability to admit impact of disease on lifestyle

Planning and Implementation

Refer to the accompanying nursing care plans, which summarize nursing care for the child who is hospitalized with newly diagnosed type 1 diabetes, and the child who is receiving care in the community. Many hospitals have developed clinical pathways to streamline and standardize diabetes care.

Provide Education

The nurse is an important member of the management team (physician, nurse, nutritionist, and social worker) and is usually responsible for educating the child and family. The majority of teaching often is performed by an advanced practice nurse or a certified diabetic nurse educator in the clinic setting, since children may be hospitalized only briefly following diagnosis.

The timing and amount of information provided are especially important in the first days following diagnosis. Both the child and parents are very tired, and they are often in a state of shock and disbelief. Information presented during this period requires repeated discussion. This time should be used to assess learning needs and to answer the family's questions. Initial teaching focuses on the survival skills necessary for home management (insulin administration, blood glucose testing, record keeping, dietary management, and the recognition and treatment of both hypoglycemia and hyperglycemia). Partner with the child and family to identify psychosocial barriers to management.

MediaLink: Adolescent Diabetes and Quality of Life Video

CLINICAL TIP

Ensure that children know to wash their hands before pricking fingers for blood glucose monitoring. Food contamination may lead to false test results.

Partner with the child and family to explain the goals of insulin therapy. Educate the child and parents on proper administration of insulin and to perform blood glucose tests (Figure 32–9 ■). Rotating the injection sites is important to decrease the chances of

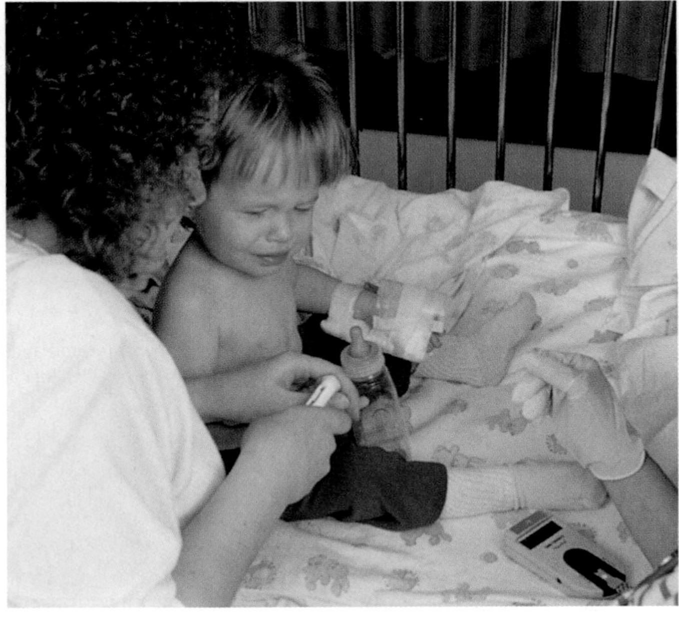
A

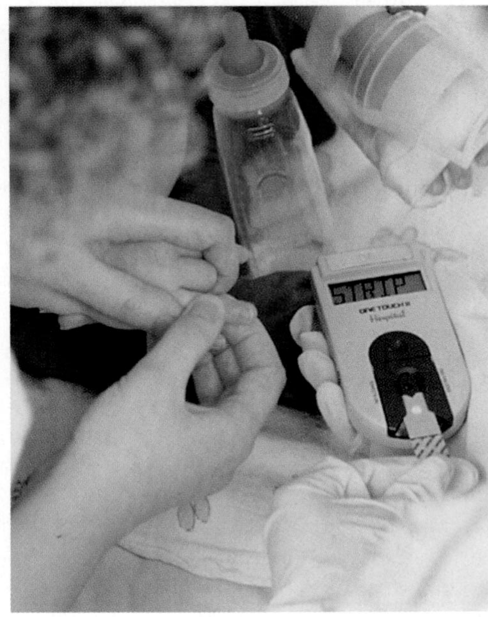

B

FIGURE 32–9 ■ This mother is being taught how to test her child's serum glucose level.

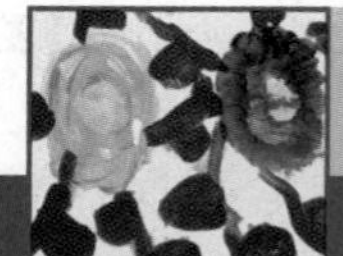

Nursing Care Plan

THE CHILD HOSPITALIZED WITH NEWLY DIAGNOSED TYPE 1 DIABETES MELLITUS

GOAL	INTERVENTION	RATIONALE	EXPECTED OUTCOME
1. Deficient Knowledge (child and parents) related to lack of exposure to diabetic management in the newly diagnosed child			
	NIC Priority Intervention— *Individual Teaching:* Planning, implementation, and evaluating a teaching program designed to address a patient's particular need.		**NOC Suggested Outcomes—** *Knowledge:* Extent of understanding conveyed about treatment regimen.
The child and parents will acquire survival skills for home management.	▪ Assess the child's developmental level and select an educational approach and self-care activities to match. ▪ Teach blood glucose monitoring, drawing up and injecting insulin, urine testing for ketones, record keeping, survival food guidelines, and when to call the physician. ▪ Use demonstration/return demonstration until the child and family are comfortable with procedures.	▪ Learning goals for the child must match knowledge and skill expectations appropriate for developmental stage. ▪ Diabetic management survival skills are needed for initial home management until more extensive education can be completed that permits more independent management. ▪ Evaluation permits positive reinforcement and guidance for modification of techniques.	The child and parents demonstrate proper technique for blood glucose monitoring, urine testing for ketones, drawing up insulin doses and injection and record keeping.
The child and parents will recognize signs and symptoms of hypoglycemia and hyperglycemia.	▪ Teach signs and symptoms of hypoglycemic and hyperglycemic reactions. ▪ Teach child to test blood glucose when feeling different than usual, and record the reading and symptoms felt.	▪ Recognition and treatment of poor glucose control will prevent progression of symptoms. ▪ Permits child to learn his/her specific symptoms of hyperglycemia and hypoglycemia.	The child and family can describe symptoms of hypoglycemia and hyperglycemia.
2. Risk for Injury related to periods of hypoglycemia and diabetic ketoacidosis			
	NIC Priority Intervention— *Hypoglycemia Monitoring:* Instituting special precautions with patient at risk for injury.		**NOC Suggested Outcomes—***Risk Control:* Actions to eliminate or reduce actual, personal, and modifiable health threats.
The child will experience few episodes of hypoglycemia during hospitalization.	▪ Assess the child at least every 2 hours for signs of hypoglycemia. If signs are present, check blood glucose to verify and administer source of quick sugar. ▪ When the child is NPO for a special procedure, verify with physician when food, fluids, and insulin are to be given, or if an intravenous infusion with dextrose is to be given. ▪ Have glucose paste or 50% dextrose solution readily available.	▪ Hypoglycemia commonly occurs during hospitalization because of change in diet, lack of food intake, or illness. ▪ Giving insulin without food intake can lead to hypoglycemia. Intravenous dextrose and insulin can be used when the child must be NPO. ▪ Dextrose is used for emergency intravenous treatment of severe hypoglycemia. Glucose paste is used for oral treatment.	The child and staff manage episodes of hypoglycemia without a crisis developing.
The child's condition is treated slowly but gradually to reverse hyperglycemia and ketoacidosis and to prevent cerebral edema.	▪ Assess the child's mental status for improvement or deterioration. ▪ Check blood glucose and urine ketones frequently to confirm reduction in blood glucose level and ketosis, to identify the insulin dose for administration.	▪ Improvement in mental status may indicate successful treatment. Deterioration may indicate onset of cerebral edema. ▪ Frequent blood glucose and ketone level determination helps assess progress in treating ketoacidosis.	The child's hyperglycemia and ketoacidosis resolves without additional complications.

Nursing Care Plan THE CHILD HOSPITALIZED WITH NEWLY DIAGNOSED TYPE 1 DIABETES MELLITUS (continued)

GOAL	INTERVENTION	RATIONALE	EXPECTED OUTCOME
2. Risk for Injury related to periods of hypoglycemia and diabetic ketoacidosis (continued)			
	■ Monitor and control IV fluid intake. Measure output.	■ The child with ketoacidosis will be dehydrated. IV fluid intake needs to be carefully controlled to prevent cerebral edema.	
	■ Have insulin doses checked by a second nurse.	■ Doses are frequently small, and the possibility of error is great.	
The child and parents will demonstrate emergency management of hypoglycemia.	■ Identify sources of glucose to give in case of hypoglycemic reaction. Tell the child and parent to carry glucose tablets or paste with them at all times.	■ Access to sources of glucose and its rapid administration are important for emergency care.	The child and family can identify several glucose sources for emergencies. The child and family have a source of glucose with them at each visit.
The child and parents will demonstrate management of sick days.	■ Teach the child and family to test blood glucose and urine for ketones with acute symptoms and notify the physician.	■ When the child is ill, hyperglycemia needs special management to prevent progression to ketoacidosis.	The child's hyperglycemic episodes do not progress to ketoacidosis.
3. Risk for Altered Nutrition: Less than Body Requirements related to glycosuria			
	NIC Priority Intervention—*Nutrition Management:* Assistance with or provision of a balanced dietary intake of foods and fluids		**NOC Suggested Outcomes—** *Nutritional Status:* Extent to which nutrients are available to meet metabolic needs.
The child will eat a well-balanced diet and maintain normal height and weight proportions.	■ Encourage and serve meals and snacks with consistent carbohydrates at the same time each day.	■ Keeps blood glucose levels stable during initial disease management stages.	The child regains weight lost and demonstrates normal growth and stable blood glucose levels.
	■ Initially provide a calorie nonrestricted diet.	■ Enables weight lost during onset of diabetes to be regained.	
The child and parents will state understanding of dietary management of diabetes mellitus.	■ Make an appointment with a nutritionist who can assess the child's favorite foods and promote their integration into the child's diet. Reinforce the dietary information taught.	■ The nutritionist can develop dietary recommendations that fit the specific needs of the child and include favorite foods, thereby increasing adherence with the food plan.	The child and parents describe nutritional needs of the child and select the dietary management best suited to the family's and child's eating habits.
	■ Provide sample menus and food exchanges, or teach the use of carbohydrate counting.	■ Assists the family and adolescent with meal planning.	

lipoatrophy, loss of subcutaneous tissue, or hypertrophy, in which collagen is replaced by fat cells (Figure 32–10 ■). The absorption rate of insulin varies by the site used. For example, normally insulin is absorbed most rapidly from the abdomen; however, insulin absorption is increased in extremities with exercise. An understanding of the different types of insulin and their actions is essential. Explain the "honeymoon phase" of insulin administration (Box 32–8). Discuss with patient and family other potential long-term consequences of type 1 diabetes, particularly if diabetes is poorly controlled (i.e., diabetic neuropathy, retinopathy, kidney disease).

Once the child and parents demonstrate understanding of this information, ensure they understand the guidelines for managing episodes of hyperglycemia during acute illness. The family also should learn "sick day" care guidelines to prevent diabetic ketoacidosis (Box 32–9). Caution parents to check the blood glucose level

BOX 32–8 The Honeymoon Phase

The family and child newly diagnosed with diabetes should be made aware of the "honeymoon phase." This is a period during "new onset" diabetes when the child has some residual β-cell function, which reduces exogenous insulin requirements. The child and family may assume this is an indication that the diabetes "is better." However, the insulin requirement does eventually return. The duration of the "honeymoon phase" varies among individuals.

BOX 32–9 Sick Day Guidelines

When the child with diabetes is sick, the following rules apply.

- Seek medical attention for fever or other signs of infection.
- Monitor the serum glucose levels more often than routine.
- The required dose of insulin may be increased.
- Do not skip doses of insulin.
- Continue to maintain food and fluid intake.
- Monitor urine for ketones.

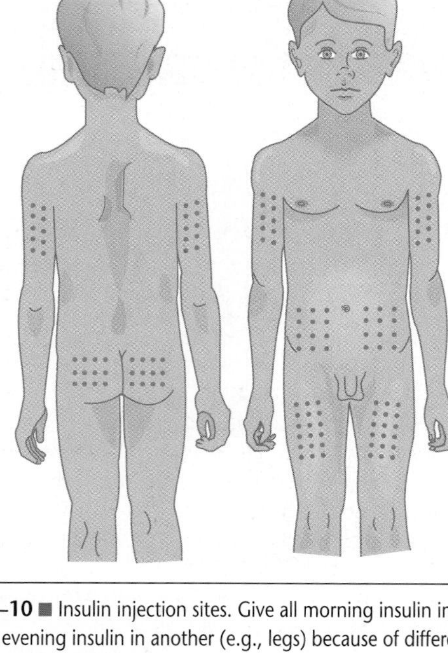

FIGURE 32–10 ■ Insulin injection sites. Give all morning insulin in one site (e.g., arms) and all evening insulin in another (e.g., legs) because of different rates of absorption from these sites. Space injections about 1.25 cm (0.5 in.) apart.

of the child who is extremely sleepy or irritable, as these can be signs of either hypoglycemia or hyperglycemia.

Inform the child that self-monitoring blood glucose, depending on the meter used, can now be assessed at sites other than fingertips, such as the upper arm, forearm, and thigh. Continuous glucose monitoring with a Gluco Watch can be used to track glucose levels over a 12-hour period, and it is especially helpful at night as the child sleeps (Cox, 2002). Partner with the child and family to determine the blood glucose monitoring system that best meets the child's ability and the needs of family. (See Partnering with Families: Minimizing Injection Pain.)

CLINICAL TIP

Children with type 1 diabetes must always have a rapid acting glucose source such as juice or glucose paste easily accessible in the event of hypoglycemia.

MediaLink Diabetes Resources and Support

Support Nutrition Adherence

Children with diabetes are ideally educated by a nutritional specialist or diabetes educator who is experienced in working with the pediatric population. Children with diabetes should consume a well-balanced diet, consisting of 55% carbohydrates, 30% fat, and 15% protein. The total amount of carbohydrates consumed is more important than whether it is a simple or complex carbohydrate. An increased ratio of polyunsaturated fats should be eaten to reduce the serum lipid levels. The child requires adequate calories to reach or maintain a desirable body weight. Usually at the time of diagnosis the child needs to regain lost weight, so calorie limitation is not recommended.

For conventional treatment, dietary intake should include three meals per day, eaten at consistent intervals, plus a mid-morning carbohydrate snack, a mid-afternoon carbohydrate snack, and a bedtime snack high in protein. A consistent intake of carbohydrates at each meal and snack is recommended.

CLINICAL TIP

Avoid the use of the term *diet* when discussing changes in food choices with the child or adolescent. *Diet* implies a temporary solution and not a lifelong change. Refer to the nutritional recommendations as a *food plan* (Evert, 2004).

Provide Emotional Support

The diagnosis of type 1 diabetes often comes as a shock to the family. If there is a familial history, parents may feel guilty about having caused the disease. Reassure parents that they did not cause their child's disease. The diagnosis of a chronic disease that requires daily management can be difficult to accept. Partner with the family and provide them with information about diabetes education programs, refer them to support groups with other parents of children with diabetes, and assist them in learning the role they can play in managing the disease.

Support for the child depends on age and developmental stage. Encourage the child to express feelings about the disease and its management. The adolescent may benefit from contact with other adolescents who have diabetes. Refer the family to organizations that focus on support for children with diabetes and their families.

Discharge Planning and Home Care Teaching

Partner with the family to identify and address home care needs before discharge. Initial survival skills as described are taught with the plans for ongoing outpatient education, often beginning the day after discharge.

Partner with the family to incorporate the diabetic regimen (insulin administration, food plan, blood glucose monitoring, and exercise) into the present lifestyle. Demonstrate and ensure return demonstration of injection administration. The fewer changes the family has to make, the greater the chance of adherence. Assist the family with the transition of the diabetic child going to school. Attending school can be a source of fear and concern for parents of young diabetic children as they experience concerns regarding insulin injections, glucose monitoring, nutrition, safety, and other associated issues. For adolescents, common fears include being perceived as different, the inconvenience of injections, self-monitoring of glucose, and dietary issues. The nurse can assist the family in collaboration with school personnel to establish a routine and plan.

Provide written materials and refer parents to books and other materials they can use in teaching the child about diabetes. The Juvenile Diabetic Research Foundation and the American Diabetes Association are excellent sources of information.

Care in the Community

During follow-up visits, ask the child or parents about signs indicating problems with diabetic control (Box 32–10). Maintain

BOX 32–10 Questions to Ask to Identify Problems in Diabetic Control

- Is the child hungry at meals? Between meals?
- How much fluid is the child drinking?
- Has the child been going to the bathroom frequently or had episodes of bedwetting?
- Does the child have dry skin?
- Are there sores on the feet? Do scratches or scrapes take a long time to heal?
- Has the child had any skin infections?
- Does the child have changes in mood (depression, unexplained sadness, irritability) or energy level from day to day or throughout the day?
- Have there been any changes in vision?

a record of the child's growth measurements and vital signs. Assess the child's secondary sexual characteristic development using Tanner staging guidelines (refer to Chapter 8∞). Puberty may be delayed if diabetic control is inadequate. Review the child's typical food intake and exercise regimens.

Partner with the child and family to ensure an ongoing shared responsibility of the child's care (see the Photo Story on pages 1276–1277). The child's developmental stage and cognitive level influence his or her readiness to assume responsibility for some aspects of self-care (Figure 32–11 ■). Ensure that parents and the adolescent understand the need for continued parental involvement in management of the diabetes. Assist the family in determining the responsibilities the adolescent will assume, and those that the parents will continue to take part in, such as supervising sick care problem solving. It is important for the adolescent's well-being that parents continue to be actively involved in the child's care. Summer camps and other programs for diabetic children are often helpful in providing education and support. Assist the family in identifying these programs.

The preschool child's need for autonomy and control can be met by allowing the child to choose snacks or to pick which finger to stick for glucose testing and by helping parents to gather necessary supplies. School-age children can learn to test blood glucose, administer insulin, and maintain records. Partner with school-age children and dieticians to assist the child in learning how to select foods and portion sizes appropriate for dietary management and how to plan an exercise program. Allowing the child to select the lunch menu increases the chance that the child will eat the meal served. Ensure that the school-age child can recognize the signs of hypoglycemia and hyperglycemia, and understand the importance of carrying a rapidly absorbed sugar product (refer to page 1284).

Although adolescents understand explanations about the potential complications of diabetes, they are present-time oriented and may rebel against the daily regimentation of insulin injections and medical nutrition therapy. Successful self-care depends in part on the adolescent's adjustment to the chronic nature of the disease and feelings of being different from peers.

PARTNERING WITH FAMILIES

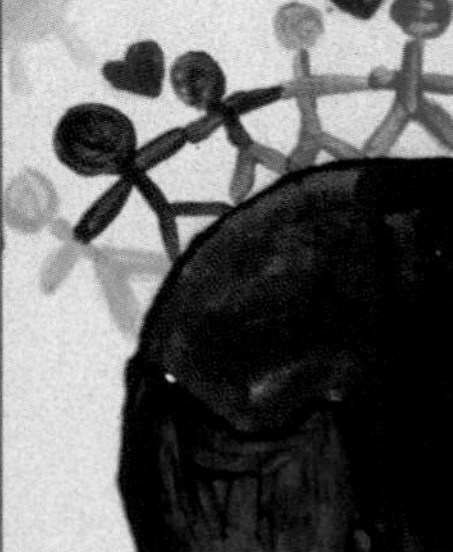

Minimizing Injection Pain

Children often fear pain associated with injections. For the child with type I diabetes, insulin injections may be a daily requirement. Partner with the family to establish techniques to minimize pain with injections. Recommend the following techniques (ADA, 2004).

- Inject the insulin at room temperature.
- Remove all bubbles from the syringe before injection.
- Let the alcohol (if used) evaporate before administering the injection.
- Tell the child to relax the muscles, not tense them, when injecting.
- When inserting the needle, penetrate the skin quickly.
- Do not change the direction of the needle during insertion or withdrawal.
- Do not reuse needles.

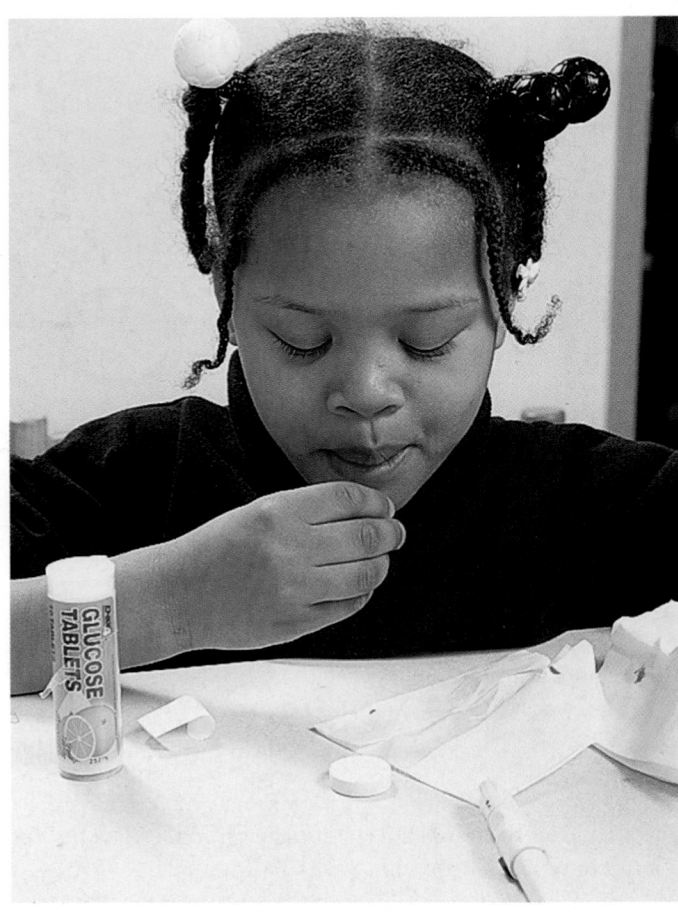

FIGURE 32–11 ■ This girl is old enough to understand the need to take glucose tablets or another form of a rapidly absorbed sugar when her serum glucose level is low.

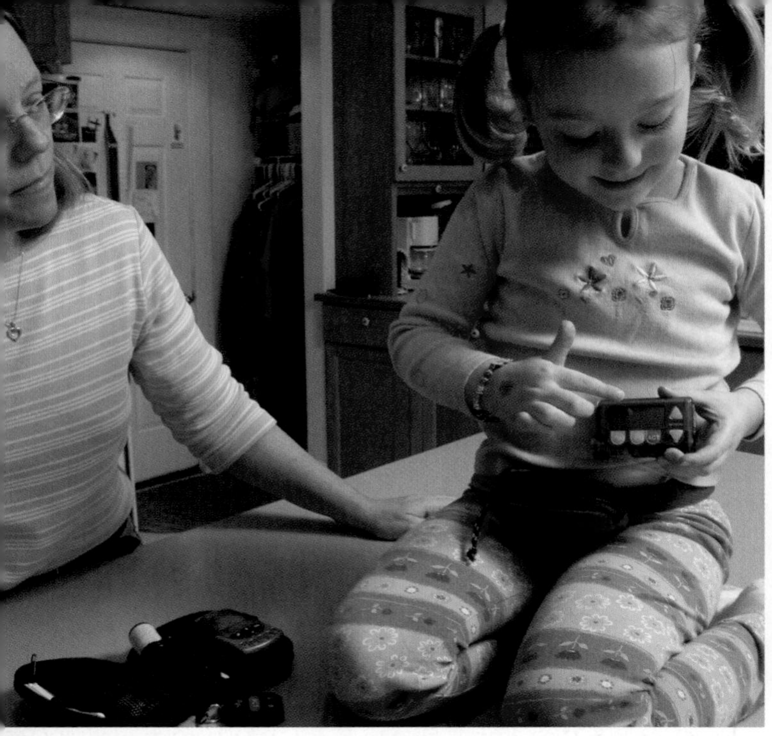

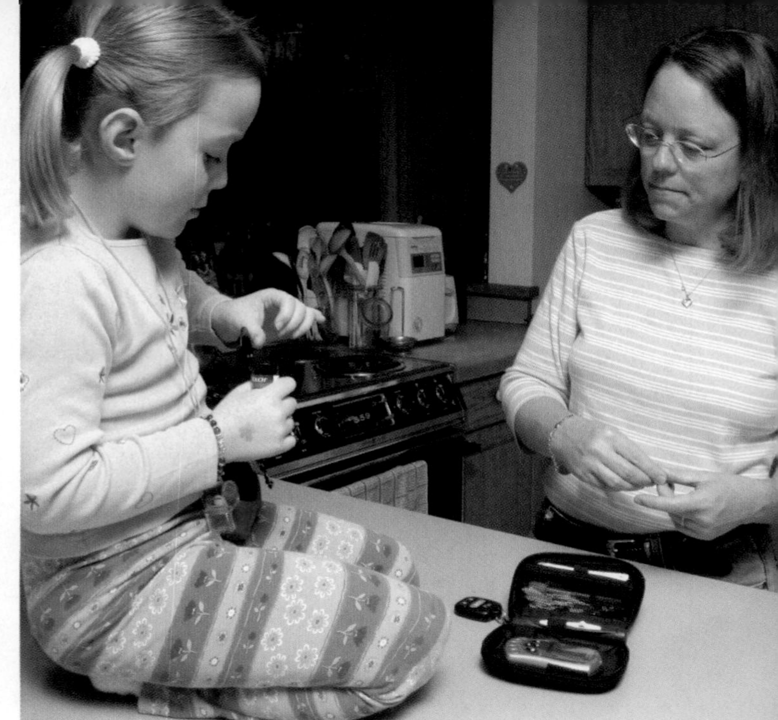

Anna is preparing to check her serum glucose level and insulin pump. ***(left)***

Anna prepares her equipment to perform self-glucose monitoring as her mother observes. ***(right)***

PHOTO Story...

Managing type 1 diabetes

Anna is a 5-year-old girl with type 1 diabetes. Following Anna's diagnosis of diabetes at age 2, her parents Cathy and Tom Deaver have been able to successfully manage her diabetes with an insulin pump and frequent glucose monitoring. Her mother also has type 1 diabetes, and uses an insulin pump. Anna is now able to participate in her disease management, learning about monitoring serum glucose levels and eating well-balanced meals.

Cathy started working with the diabetic nurse educator a few months ago to identify developmentally appropriate skills for Anna to learn. Cathy began by talking to Anna about each step while performing a serum glucose test on herself. Then she had Anna gather all the needed supplies. Now Anna is able to perform the finger stick and put the drop of blood on the test strip. As Anna grows older, she will learn to interpret the serum glucose reading. Anna is also learning about foods that are good for her to eat and foods she should ask about first.

Management of Anna's diabetes takes a considerable amount of time and supervision. However, Cathy and Tom ensure that Anna participates in activities typical for a 5-year-old to promote her growth and development. In addition to ballet and gymnastics, Anna attends a childcare center. Transitioning Anna into daycare required adaptations by both the family and the childcare center, but her parents emphasize that Anna's condition is manageable and should not interfere with her ability to engage in developmentally appropriate activities.

To ensure Anna's diabetes is managed at the childcare center, Anna, her parents, a community health nurse, and nutritionist met with the staff to discuss Anna's goals and needs. Although Anna is learning how to monitor her serum glucose levels, staff members are also trained, and Cathy and Tom provide the childcare center with phone numbers so that they can be reached anytime that the serum glucose level indicates additional treatment is needed.

Foods Anna can eat are sent with her each day to help keep her diabetes controlled. The child care center staff have also been told to contact her parents if there is a planned party so that Anna's meal plan is modified for the day and she can eat some party foods. ■

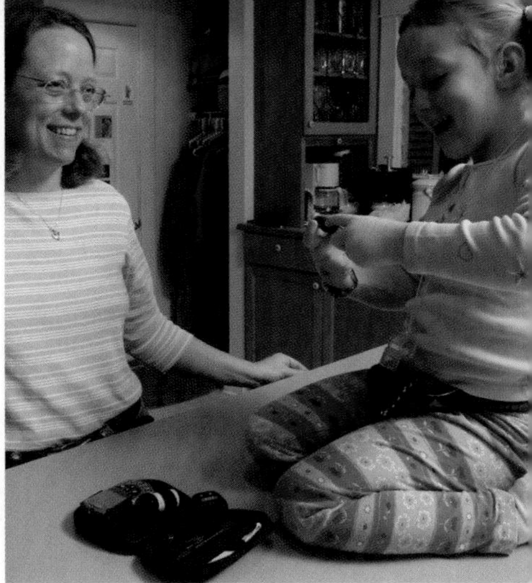

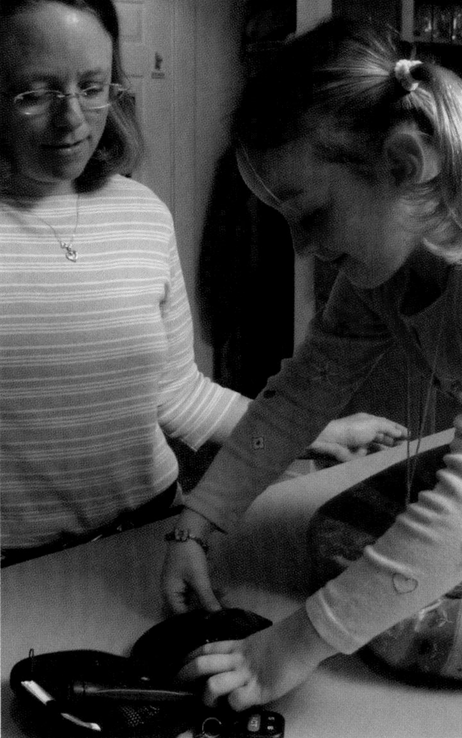

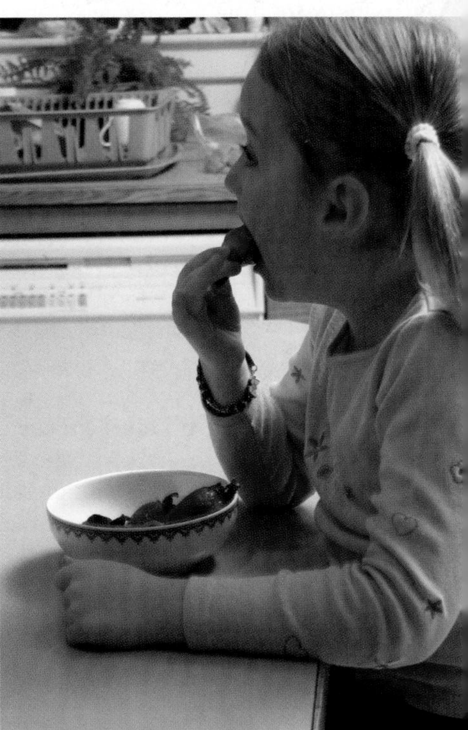

Anna performs her own glucose monitoring. She says, "It doesn't hurt a bit!" Note the waist pack on Anna, containing her insulin pump. ***(top)***

Anna and Cathy check the test results. ***(middle)***

Cathy ensures nutritious snacks are always available. ***(bottom)***

MediaLink Case Study: Child with Type 1 Diabetes

Although the adolescent is cognitively able to manage self-care, the desire to be like peers often interferes with treatment adherence. Adolescents perceive type 1 diabetes as a disability and often deny having the disease so they can be like their peers when eating and exercising. Talk with the adolescent to evaluate motivation to manage the food plan, exercise regimen, blood glucose testing, and insulin therapy. Identify and discuss how carbohydrate counting and insulin dose adjustment may provide the flexibility to participate in activities with peers. Collaborate with the adolescent in preparation to assume care, and assist parents in accepting the growing independence from adult supervision. The nurse partners with the family to discuss the hazards associated with being diabetic and the use of alcohol, drugs, and tobacco.

Observe the female adolescent's weight and eating behaviors for evidence of eating disorders as there is an increased frequency of eating disorders in this group (Alemzadeh & Wyatt, 2004). (Refer to Chapter 9∞ for further discussion of eating disorders).

Partner with families and emphasize that the child with diabetes should be treated as any other child without a chronic condition. Parents may find it difficult to discipline their child since they have a chronic condition; however, the parents should understand that all children require limit setting and consequences for unacceptable behavior. Children with type 1 diabetes may learn maladaptive behaviors. Teach parents to be alert to signs of maladaptation, such as helpless, demanding, or whining behaviors, and any evidence of poor coping. Additional behaviors may include skipping blood glucose testing and losing or damaging equipment. Food may become a battleground for toddlers who are picky eaters, but must have adequate intake for the insulin dose. Referral for counseling may be appropriate for some families.

The child with type 1 diabetes may develop complications associated with circulatory and neurologic changes over time (see Table 32–4 on page 1267). Emphasize the importance of good foot care from an early age, for example, wearing clean white cotton socks; changing socks and shoes when they are damp; washing, drying, and powdering feet; and keeping toenails short. Ensure the child and family understand the importance of inspecting feet daily for injuries. Emphasize the importance of wearing closed-toe shoes and to avoid walking barefoot.

Explain to parents that the child should wear some type of medical alert identification. Assist them in having an individualized health plan (IHP) developed (see Chapter 20∞) to ensure that the child can perform self-care and that school administrators and teachers can identify the signs of hypoglycemia or hyperglycemia and provide emergency management.

Emphasize to the parents the importance of the child receiving annual or more frequent evaluations for potential complications of diabetes. The tests to be performed include blood for lipid levels, blood pressure, liver and renal function, urine for albumin, an ophthalmologic examination for retinopathy, and a neurologic exam of the extremities for neuropathies. See the Health Promotion and Maintenance Overview on page 1279.

■ Evaluation

Expected outcomes of nursing care for children with type 1 diabetes can be found on the nursing care plans.

Diabetic Ketoacidosis

Diabetic ketoacidosis (DKA) is associated with severe metabolic, electrolyte, and fluid imbalances, manifested by hyperglycemia, dehydration, and metabolic acidosis. Diabetic ketoacidosis is a common and potentially life-threatening condition that occurs in children with type 1 diabetes when the body must burn fat and protein stores for energy because no insulin is available to metabolize glucose.

Etiology and Pathophysiology. Potential causes of DKA include the following:

- incorrect or missed insulin doses;
- incorrect insulin administration just under the skin; or
- illness, trauma, or surgery.

Insulin deficiency is accompanied by a compensatory increase in hormones (epinephrine, norepinephrine, cortisol, growth hormone, and glucagon—the counterregulatory hormones of insulin) which results from failure to deliver enough glucose to the cells. The muscle cells break down protein into amino acids that are then converted to glucose by the liver, leading to hyperglycemia. The adipose tissue releases fatty acids that are transformed by the liver into ketone bodies. Their accumulation leads to ketoacidosis. The hyperglycemia causes an osmotic diuresis resulting in dehydration, acidosis, and hyperosmolality. Altered consciousness occurs as symptoms progress (Hafeez & Vuguin, 2000).

Clinical Manifestations. Characteristic signs of diabetic ketoacidosis include dehydration, weight loss, tachycardia, flushed ears and cheeks, **Kussmaul respirations** (deep, rapid respirations in an attempt to rid the body of excess carbon dioxide and reduce the state of acidosis), acetone breath (fruity smell), altered level of consciousness varying from lethargy to coma, hypotension, and tachycardia. Hyperglycemia, glycosuria, acidosis, and ketonuria are also present. Polyuria, polydipsia, and polyphagia are premonitory signs of impending diabetic ketoacidosis. The child's response to metabolic acidosis includes complaints of abdominal or chest pain, nausea, and vomiting. The disorder may progress to electrolyte disturbances, arrhythmias, central nervous system depression, shock, and death if untreated. See the table on page 1281 for clinical manifestations of hypoglycemia and hyperglycemia.

Cerebral edema, which may result in increased intracranial pressure and decreased cerebral perfusion, is a life-threatening complication thought to be related to hyperosmolality. Signs and symptoms of cerebral edema include headache, lethargy, tachycardia or bradycardia, and widening pulse pressure. The healthcare provider must be notified immediately if any of these symptoms are noted, to prevent cerebral herniation and possible brain death.

COLLABORATIVE CARE

The immediate goal of collaborative care of management is to normalize the pH level, restore blood glucose to target level, and correct fluid and electrolyte imbalance. The long-term goal of management includes preventive education to reduce the risk of further diabetic ketoacidosis episodes.

Diagnostic Tests

See Table 32–8 for laboratory findings in diabetic ketoacidosis. CT scan of the brain, and possible intubation and implementation of ICP lowering strategies will be required. Diabetic coma occurs when the serum osmolality exceeds 350 mOsm/kg (normal serum osmolality is 275 to 295 mOsm/kg).

Clinical Therapy

The child with ketoacidosis is usually hospitalized. Medical management includes intravenous fluids and electrolytes for dehydration and acidosis. Regular insulin is administered by continuous intravenous infusion pump to decrease the serum glucose level at a rate not to exceed 100 mg/dL/hr. Glucose levels should not be lowered rapidly as rapid reduction of glucose increases the risk of cerebral edema and circulatory collapse. When glucose is lowered too rapidly, water is freed and attracted to the glucose, which has accumulated in large quantities in the brain. Mannitol is kept on standby for treatment of neurologic deterioration. Bicarbonate is no longer used for treatment of diabetic ketoacidosis as it places the child at risk for increased acidosis and hyperosmolality. Cerebral edema occurs in about 3% of children with DKA, but it accounts for 30% of DKA deaths and 20% of the overall childhood diabetes mortality (Felner & White, 2001).

As insulin is administered, potassium shifts into the cells, resulting in hypokalemia. Potassium supplement is indicated, but it is not administered until confirmation of renal function is established.

NURSING MANAGEMENT

Nursing care focuses on administering insulin, fluids, and electrolytes, and monitoring the child for signs and symptoms of associated complications. Once the child is stabilized, the shift of care focuses on educating the child and family on methods to prevent further diabetic ketoacidotic episodes.

Health Promotion & Maintenance Overview

The Child with Diabetes Mellitus

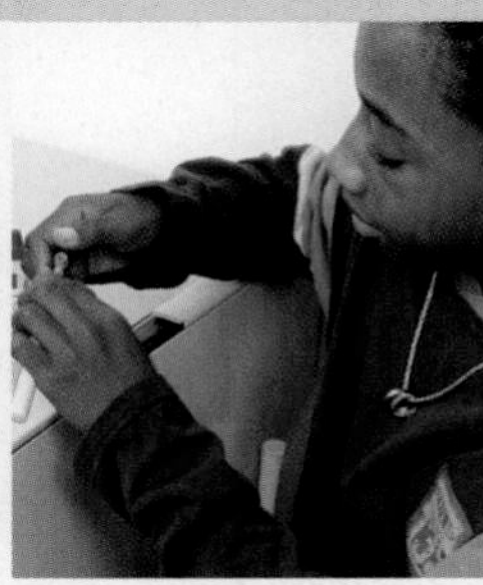

Growth and Development Surveillance

- Compare the child's height, weight, and head circumference to age-specific norms to determine if growth is meeting expectations for age.
- Assess developmental progress using the Denver II or another screening tool (refer to Chapter 10∞). Assess school performance.
- Assess for delays in development of sexual secondary characteristics and pubertal changes.

Nutrition

- Promote adherence to nutrition guidelines by including the child's personal preferences in the food plan.

Physical Activity

- Encourage regular physical activity and educate the child to modify insulin dosage or food intake for extra physical activity periods.
- Encourage the child to participate in sports when interested and work to balance exercise, food intake, and insulin dosage.

Oral Health

- Promote good dentition and oral hygiene.
- Regular dental visits are important to reduce risk of infections.
- The child with poorly controlled diabetes is at risk of gingivitis and cavities.

Mental and Spiritual Health

- Provide the child and adolescent an opportunity to discuss feelings regarding diabetes.
- Assess the adolescent for evidence of depression.

Relationships

- The child should attend school or childcare as any other child.
- Encourage the development of special friends who can be informed about the child's disorder and seek help when needed.

Disease Prevention Strategies

- Encourage family to maintain the child's active immunization status.
- Children with diabetes should receive an annual influenzae vaccine.
- Refer the child for an annual ophthalmologic examination.
- Maintain appointments for regular evaluation of $HgbA_{1c}$ to monitor glycemic control.

Injury Prevention Strategies

- Encourage the child to wear a medical identification tag.
- Encourage daily inspection of feet and footcare.
- Provide the family with strategies for safe disposal of needles and syringes.

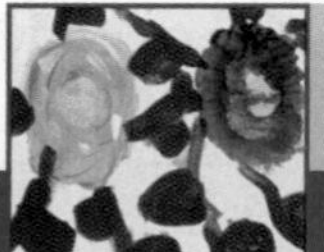

Nursing Care Plan

THE CHILD WITH PREVIOUSLY DIAGNOSED TYPE 1 DIABETES BEING CARED FOR AT HOME

GOAL	INTERVENTION	RATIONALE	EXPECTED OUTCOME
1. Risk for Altered Nutrition: Less Than Body Requirements related to chronic illness (diabetes mellitus)			
	NIC Priority Intervention—*Weight Management:* Assistance with or provision of a balanced dietary intake of foods and fluids		**NOC Suggested Outcomes—***Nutritional Status:* Nutrient Value: Adequacy of nutrients taken into body.
The child will eat a well-balanced diet that maintains weight proportional to height.	■ Assess height and weight regularly and plot on growth chart. ■ Make an appointment with a nutritionist who can assess the child's favorite foods and integrate them into a food plan that controls caloric intake. Encourage the child to keep a food diary.	■ Assesses change in body mass index to identify potential weight problem early. ■ Inclusion of child's favorite foods helps child adapt to changes in diet.	Diet records indicate meals and snacks have the appropriate distribution of carbohydrates, protein, and fats, and daily caloric intake goals are met.
2. Readiness for Enhanced Family Processes related to management of a chronic disease			
	NIC Priority Intervention—*Family Process Maintenance:* Minimization of family process disruption effects		**NOC Suggested Outcomes—**Not yet developed.
The child and family will manage the dietary modifications, exercise, blood glucose monitoring, and medications regimen.	■ Assess the family's lifestyle and attempt to fit the child's care needs into the family's schedule. ■ Discuss the family's routines for special occasions and vacations. Identify ways to modify the child's management for these occasions.	■ Fitting the care to the family's lifestyle promotes adherence with regimen. ■ It is important for the child to participate in special events with the family and peers as a normal child to promote psychologic development.	The child and family make minimal changes in usual lifestyle while managing the type 1 diabetes.
3. Ineffective Coping (individual) related to inadequate level of confidence in ability to cope			
	NIC Priority Intervention—*Coping Enhancement:* Assisting a patient to adapt to perceived stressors, changes, or threats which interfere with meeting life demands and roles.		**NOC Suggested Outcomes—***Coping:* Actions to manage stressors that tax an individual's resources.
The child will demonstrate enhanced coping skills.	■ Ask how the child has solved problems in the past. Review possible problems the child may encounter. Together evaluate the effectiveness of solutions. Suggest other solutions to consider.	■ Children's success in mastering maturational conflicts and daily psychosocial problems will influence their pattern of coping.	The child demonstrates enhanced coping skills and expresses positive attitude toward self. The child displays warmth and affection toward family.
The child will develop positive self-esteem.	■ Role-play ways to talk about diabetes with friends and teachers. Encourage the child to express feelings about diabetes to those he or she trusts. ■ Encourage the child to attend diabetes camp. ■ Encourage the child to continue previous social activities and hobbies.	■ Sharing information about the condition helps others understand changes in lifestyle needed by the child. Expressing feelings decreases anxiety. ■ Learning and support networks developed at camp can promote self-esteem. ■ Increased social interaction, especially in group sessions, improves self-esteem.	

Nursing Care Plan THE CHILD WITH PREVIOUSLY DIAGNOSED TYPE 1 DIABETES BEING CARED FOR AT HOME (continued)

GOAL	INTERVENTION	RATIONALE	EXPECTED OUTCOME
4. Health-Seeking Behaviors (child) related to learning self-management of chronic disorder			
	NIC Priority Intervention—*Self-Modification Assistance:* Reinforcement of self-directed change initiated by the patient to achieve personally important goals.		**NOC Suggested Outcomes—***Health Promotion:* Actions to sustain or increase wellness.
The child will develop independent ability to manage diabetes care.	■ Allow the child to perform as many self-care procedures as possible at each developmental stage.	■ Normal growth and development are ensured if the child is encouraged to participate in care from the beginning.	The child is able to perform as many diabetic care techniques as possible for age.
	■ Encourage the child to make decisions regarding care. Review decisions and discuss possible alternative solutions. Role-play possible scenarios.	■ Feelings of trust are developed when children sense that their decisions are respected or at least considered by others.	
	■ Encourage parents to stay involved even when the adolescent takes primary responsibility for care.	■ The adolescent's diabetic control is likely to be better when the parents continue to show interest and supervise care.	
	■ Provide 24-hour access to physician or diabetes nurse educator. Encourage the child to seek help early.	■ The child needs to overcome concerns about calling for guidance, and thus maintain better control.	

Nursing Assessment and Diagnosis

Continuously monitor the child's vital signs, respiratory status, perfusion, and mental status. Assess for changes in neurologic status, respiratory pattern, blood pressure, and heart rate. Monitor for cardiac arrhythmias associated with hypokalemia. Assess for signs of dehydration, including dry skin and mucous membranes, and depressed fontanels in infants.

Nursing diagnoses that apply to the child with diabetic ketoacidosis may include:

- Risk for Injury related to altered cerebral function
- Deficient Fluid Volume related to osmotic diuresis

CLINICAL MANIFESTATIONS of Hypoglycemia and Hyperglycemia

ETIOLOGY	CLINICAL MANIFESTATIONS	CLINICAL THERAPY
Hypoglycemia • Insulin dose too high for food eaten • Insulin injection into muscle • Too much exercise for insulin dose • Too long between meals/snacks • Too few carbohydrates eaten • Illness, stress	*Rapid onset* Irritability, nervousness, tremors, shaky feeling, difficulty concentrating or speaking, behavior change, confusion, repeating something over and over Unconsciousness, seizure, shallow breathing, tachycardia Pallor, sweating Moist mucous membranes, hunger Headache, dizziness, blurred vision, double vision, photophobia Numb lips or mouth	If conscious, give 15 g of carbohydrate. Wait 15 minutes and recheck blood glucose level. Give another 15 g of carbohydrate if ≤ 70 mg/dL. Recheck the blood glucose level in 15 minutes. If unconscious, give glucagon by injection.
Hyperglycemia • Insulin dose too low for food eaten • Illness or injury, stress • Too many carbohydrates eaten • Meals/snacks too close together • Insulin injected just under skin or into hypertrophied areas • Decreased activity	*Gradual onset* Lethargy, sleepiness, slowed responses, or confusion Deep, rapid breathing Flushed skin, dry skin Dry mucous membrances, thirst, hunger, dehydration Weakness, fatigue Headache, abdominal pain, nausea, vomiting Blurred vision Shock	Additional insulin given at usual injection time Sliding scale insulin doses for specific blood glucose levels when ill or injured. Extra injections if hyperglycemia and moderate to large ketones Increased fluids

MediaLink Responding to Hypoglycemia Animation

TABLE 32–8 Laboratory Findings in the Child with Diabetic Ketoacidosis

LABORATORY STUDY	RESULTS
Serum glucose	Greater than 300 mg/dL
Serum ketones	Positive
Arterial blood gas pH	Acidotic – pH ≤ to 7.3 and bicarbonate < 15 mEq/L
Urine	Positive for glucose (glycosuria), positive for ketones (ketonuria)
Potassium	Elevated
Chloride	Elevated
Sodium	Decreased
Phosphate	Decreased
Calcium	Decreased
Magnesium	Decreased
BUN and creatinine	Elevated due to dehydration
White blood cell count	Generally elevated due to presence of infection or dehydration
Serum osmolality	> 350 mOsm/kg (normal serum osmolality is 275 to 295 mOsm/kg)

- Imbalanced Nutrition: Less than Body Requirements related to catabolism of protein and fat for fuel
- Risk for Infection related to hyperglycemia and suppressed inflammatory response
- Deficient Knowledge related to recognition, treatment, and prevention of diabetic ketoacidosis

Planning and Implementation

Monitor blood glucose levels hourly or as indicated. Frequently monitor the electrolytes and acid–base status, as well as urine glucose and ketone levels as indicated. Intake and output are monitored hourly. Assess for signs of hypoglycemia which may occur during insulin infusion. Intravenous fluids are given in boluses of 10 to 20 mL/kg rapidly over 5 minutes if the child is in hypovolemic shock. Adequate fluids are given to reverse the fluid deficit. The insulin infusion must be carefully titrated to control the gradual reduction in hyperglycemia.

PRACTICE ALERT

Only regular insulin is administered intravenously for treatment of hyperglycemia or diabetic ketoacidosis. Do not use other insulin types.

The child is tapered off of intravenous insulin and transitioned to subcutaneous insulin when clinically stable. Oral feedings are reintroduced when the child is alert enough and the glucose level is stabilized. This plan varies according to the primary healthcare provider or endocrinologist.

CLINICAL TIP

Insulin binds to IV tubing. Run 50 to 100 mL of insulin through the new IV tubing to saturate all the binding sites. This ensures that the full dose of insulin reaches the child from the outset.

Electrolytes are replaced as needed. Potassium is not administered until the child has voided to confirm renal function. Monitor for signs and symptoms of hypokalemia, including hypotension and weak pulse, shallow respirations, and muscle weakness. Continuous cardiac monitoring is performed to detect cardiac conduction changes related to hypokalemia. Weigh the child daily. Provide emotional care and support to the child and family.

Care in the Community

The prevention of future episodes of diabetic ketoacidosis is important. Partner with the child and family to ensure they learn strategies to keep hyperglycemic episodes from progressing to diabetic ketoacidosis. (See Partnering with Families: Recognizing Signs of DKA.) For example, the child's urine should be tested for ketones if three or four consecutive blood glucose readings are higher than 200 mg/dL, or if the child is sick. If the child has an elevated blood glucose and moderate or large amounts of ketones, treatment with extra insulin and fluids can be initiated. Increased attention to blood glucose and urine ketone monitoring is especially important when the child has significant stressors such as an illness. It is important for the child and family to understand that insulin is required even when the child is not eating to counter the hormones secreted in response to the stressor.

Evaluation

Expected outcomes of care for the child with diabetic ketoacidosis include:

- The child is free from neurologic impairment.
- The child achieves fluid volume balance.
- The child's nutritional intake is adequate to support growth and development balanced to insulin administration.
- The child is free from infection.
- The child and family identify measures to reduce the risk or prevent DKA, the child and family recognize symptoms which require notification of healthcare provider, and the child experiences a reduced number of DKA episodes.

Hypoglycemia in the Child with Diabetes

Children receiving insulin for diabetes are at risk for hypoglycemia, which can develop within minutes. The symptoms outlined in the table on page 1281 may occur when there is a sudden drop in blood glucose levels or the serum glucose level is < 70 mg/dL. Children are at risk of hypoglycemia due to their rapid growth rates, unpredictable eating habits, and physical activity. Common causes of hypoglycemia include an error in insulin dosage, errors in injection technique, inadequate calories due to missed meals, or exercise without a corresponding increase in caloric intake.

Hypoglycemia is suspected on the basis of sudden onset of signs and symptoms. A serum glucose reading should be taken to confirm the diagnosis, because signs of hyperglycemia and hypoglycemia may be difficult to distinguish. Administer glucose immediately in the form of a low-fat carbohydrate-containing snack or drink, sugar gel, glucose tablets, or glucose paste.

If the child becomes unconscious, administer glucagon or if unavailable, administer sugar gel or glucose paste squeezed onto the gums. In the hospital setting, administer an intravenous infusion of dextrose to prevent progression of symptoms. Since the effects of dextrose and glucagon are temporary, additional snacks or a meal is provided. The child should be continually observed for several hours after treatment.

CLINICAL TIP

Do not use cake frosting or candy bars for treatment of hypoglycemia. The fat in the frosting and candy prevents the sugar from working quickly. Hard candy takes too long to dissolve to provide rapid treatment for hypoglycemia.

Nursing Management

Recognition of hypoglycemia is essential to quickly manage symptoms and prevent further reduction of glucose. Partner with the child and family to ensure they are able to recognize the signs of hypoglycemia and take appropriate action. (See Partnering with Families: Treating Hypoglycemic Episodes.) Parents are taught to give an intramuscular or subcutaneous dose of glucagon (a hormone produced by the pancreas that helps release stored glucose from the liver) for cases of severe hypoglycemia and to activate the emergency medical system (9-1-1).

Reinforce the importance of achieving a daily balance between food intake, insulin administration, and exercise. Partner with the family to educate school personnel about the signs and symptoms of hypoglycemia and appropriate interventions. The child should wear a medical alert identification indicating the disease and treatment. Expected outcomes include maintenance of optimal blood glucose level and a reduced number of episodes of hypoglycemia.

Neonatal Hypoglycemia. The neonate's serum glucose declines after a normal delivery (without complications) to a serum glucose concentration of 50 mg/dL by 2 hours of age, and then stabilizes at approximately 70 mg/dL at approximately 72 hours after birth.

Neonatal hypoglycemia occurs as a result of increased metabolic requirements during the initial newborn period. Causes of neonatal hypoglycemia are identified in Box 32–11. Signs and symptoms of neonatal hypoglycemia include apnea, cyanosis, hypotonia, tremors, abnormal cry, and cardiac arrest. Serum glucose < 45 mg/dL should be evaluated and treated to avoid permanent brain damage (Cowett & Loughead, 2002). Treatment includes administration of breastmilk or formula, or parenteral glucose if the neonate refuses oral fluids.

Type 2 Diabetes

Type 2 diabetes, formerly called noninsulin dependent diabetes, is a disease associated with **insulin resistance** (an alteration of the insulin receptor that signals the presence of insulin in the interior of cells). It may be connected with an insulin secretory defect in the pancreas (caused by a decrease in the beta cell weight and number) and insulin deficiency (Gungor, 2004). The single most important risk factor for type 2 diabetes is obesity, as approximately 80% of children diagnosed with type 2 diabetes are overweight (ADA, 2004a). Other significant risk factors include low physical exercise, a diet high in fat, minority race, polycystic ovary syndrome, and type 2 diabetes in a first-degree relative (Alemzadeh & Wyatt, 2004). Between 74% and 100% of children

PARTNERING WITH FAMILIES

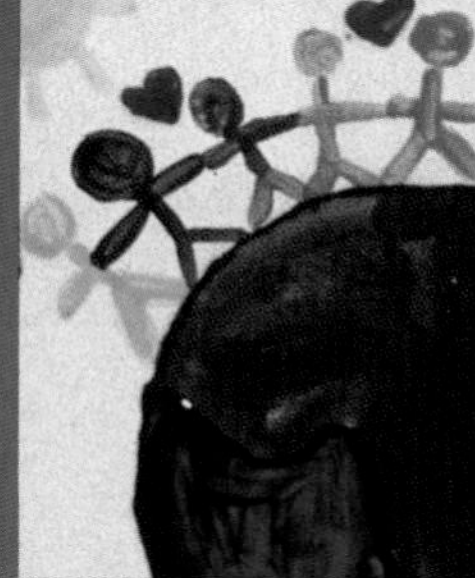

Recognizing Signs of DKA

The nurse should collaborate with the family and ensure that they can recognize symptoms that may indicate progressive development of diabetic ketoacidosis. The family should know to call the child's healthcare provider if the child has the following signs.

- Vomiting more than twice in a 6 hour period
- More than five diarrheal stools in 1 day
- Has illness (e.g., viral or other) and is unable to eat
- Change in mental status
- Temperature over 102°F (38.9°C) for 12 hours
- Blood glucose > 400 mg/dL on two separate readings, or > 200 mg/dL and moderate to large ketones
- Large ketones are present, acetone breath
- Evidence of a bacterial infection (e.g., fever, drainage)
- Difficulty breathing
- Decreased urine output
- Dysuria or other evidence of urinary tract infection

Data from Kaufman, F. R. & Halvorson, M. (1999). The treatment and prevention of diabetic ketoacidosis in children and adolescents with type 1 diabetes. Pediatric Annals, *28(9), 576–582; Boland, E. A., & Grey, M. (2000). Diabetes Mellitus (type 1). In P. L. Jackson & J. A. Vessey (Eds.),* Primary care of the child with a chronic condition *(3rd ed., pp. 426–444). St Louis: Mosby.*

BOX 32–11 Causes of Neonatal Hypoglycemia

- Intrauterine growth retardation
- Prematurity
- Cold stress
- Sepsis
- Hypoxia
- Congestive heart failure
- Inborn errors of metabolism
- Infant of diabetic mother
- RH incompatibility and subsequent exchange transfusion
- Adrenal insufficiency

Data From Cowett, R. M., & Loughead, J. L. (2002). Neonatal glucose metabolism: Differential diagnoses, evaluation, and treatment of hypoglycemia. Neonatal Network, *21(4), 9–19.*

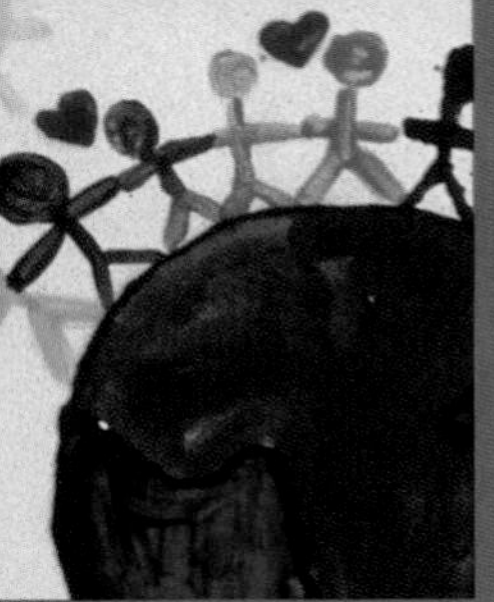

PARTNERING WITH FAMILIES

Treating Hypoglycemic Episodes

The nurse collaborates with the family to ensure that they can recognize symptoms indicating hypoglycemic episodes and the appropriate interventions.

- If the child shows signs of hypoglycemia (pallor, sweating, tremors, dizziness, numb lips or mouth, confusion, irritability, altered mental status), test the blood glucose level.
- Assist the child to perform the test, as skills needed to get an accurate reading deteriorate with the child's altered mental status.
- If the blood glucose reading is ≤ 70 mg/dL, give glucose rapidly. Use one of the following:
  - 1/2 cup orange juice
  - 3/4 cup of sugar-sweetened beverage
  - 1 small box raisins
  - 3–4 glucose tablets
- Wait 15 minutes and recheck the blood glucose level. Repeat the glucose if it is still ≤ 70 mg/dL. Recheck the blood glucose level in another 15 minutes.
- Once blood sugar has returned to at least 80 mg/dL, give a more substantial snack such as cheese and crackers if the next meal will be more than 30 minutes later or an activity or exercise is planned.
- If the child is unconscious, administer IM or SQ glucagon or spread glucose paste on the gums.

with type 2 diabetes have a first- or second-degree relative with the same type of diabetes (ADA, 2000). The peak age of onset in children is at the time of puberty, and females are affected more than males with a 1.7:1 ratio (Pinhas-Hamiel & Zeitler, 2001). The increasing number of children being diagnosed with type 2 diabetes has caused significant concern in the healthcare community. Up to 45% of children with a new diagnosis of diabetes have type 2. The true incidence in children is unknown as many children are undiagnosed. (See Developing Cultural Competence: Type 2 Diabetes Risk.)

Etiology and Pathophysiology. Type 2 diabetes is a complex metabolic disorder in which the child has insulin resistance, and therefore, insulin fails to transfer glucose into the cells and there is often a progressive defect in insulin secretion (Alemzadeh & Wyatt, 2004). With the increased weight, the visceral fat produces a cytokine hormone (tumor necrosis factor) that desensitizes the insulin receptor to insulin. The pancreatic cells produce more insulin in an attempt to facilitate glucose transfer and overcome the insulin resistance. This results in **hyperinsulinemia** (elevated insulin levels in the blood). The child maintains a balance between hyperinsulinemia and insulin resistance and a normal glycemic state. As insulin resistance worsens, the islet of Langerhans beta cells fail in their ability to hypersecrete insulin, thus leading to impaired glucose tolerance and overt diabetes. The growth hormone secretion may have a role during puberty in promoting insulin resistance.

DEVELOPING CULTURAL COMPETENCE
Type 2 Diabetes Risk

Children of African American, Native American, Hispanic, and Asian origins are at greater risk for developing type 2 diabetes (ADA, 2004a). The disease in children appears to follow the same racial and ethnic distribution as found in adults (Brosnan, Upchurch, & Schreiner, 2001). Particularly affected are members of some Native American tribes that historically have had a high level of exercise and hunter-gatherer types of diets. In some groups, such as the Pima Indians of the Southwest, the majority has diabetes and face complications from the disease.

Clinical Manifestations. Signs and symptoms of type 2 diabetes on initial presentation are very different from type 1. Presentation of type 2 DM is more insidious than type 1. A history of polyuria and polydipsia is rare in these patients (Alemzadeh & Wyatt, 2004). **Acanthosis nigricans** (Figure 32–12 ■), hyperpigmentation and thickening of the skin with velvety irregularities in the skin folds of the neck, axillae, elbows, knees, groin, and abdomen, is a common finding associated with chronic hyperinsulinemia. The child is usually obese, with truncal (or central) adiposity. Though rare in type 2

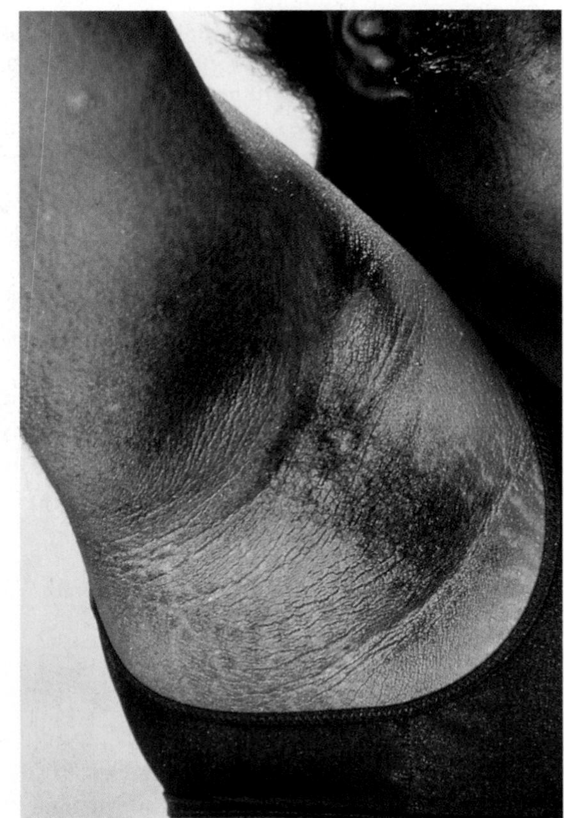

FIGURE 32–12 ■ Acanthosis nigricans.

Courtesy of Audrey Austin, M. D., Children's National Medical Center, Washington, D.C.

diabetes, the child may present in diabetic ketoacidosis. Other clinical manifestations can be found in the table on page 1267. Children with type 2 diabetes often come from home environments with a poor understanding of healthy eating habits. Common behaviors include skipping meals, heavy snacking, excessive television viewing, video game playing, and computer usage (Alemzadeh & Wyatt, 2004).

COLLABORATIVE CARE

The goal of management is to reduce risk factors associated with type 2 diabetes, promote normal physical and emotional development, maintain target glucose, reduce hypoglycemic and hyperglycemic episodes, and thus minimize long-term complications.

Diagnostic Tests

Obesity and the presence of acanthosis nigricans on physical exam are clues to the diagnosis. In some cases, a finding of glycosuria is discovered during routine physical examination. Blood glucose levels at or above 200 mg/dL without fasting or a fasting glucose at or above 126 mg/dL on two separate occasions is diagnostic of diabetes. Glycosylated hemoglobin (HbA_{1c}) provides an accurate indicator of the average serum glucose level for the previous 120 days (the life span of a red blood cell). Urine is tested and ketones are found in about 50% of children. Islet cell autoantibodies, insulin levels, glutamic acid decarboxylase autoantibody test (GAD-65), and fasting C-peptid level are used to differentiate between type 1 and type 2 diabetes. The child with type 2 diabetes has higher insulin and fasting C-peptid levels than the child with type 1 diabetes. Islet cell and GAD-65 autoantibodies will not be present. A fasting lipid profile is obtained since dyslipidemia (primarily elevated LDL-C and triglycerides) is usually present. Elevated fasting insulin levels are present (refer to Appendix C∞).

Clinical Therapy

Insulin therapy is occasionally required at the time of presentation in order to obtain glycemic control or when the child presents in ketoacidosis to reverse the metabolic decompensation. Insulin may not be required after the metabolic deterioration is resolved. Conditions such as illness, stress, surgery, and trauma may necessitate temporary insulin injections. The child and family may view this as a sign of worsening in condition and progression to type 1 diabetes. Assure the child and family that the use of insulin is temporary and is required during periods of increased stress (which increases glucose production).

Nutritional education is a cornerstone of therapy for children with type 2 diabetes. Management includes gradual sustained weight loss, medical nutrition therapy, metabolic control of blood glucose levels, exercise, and emotional support. Oral medication is used when the food plan and exercise efforts are inadequate to control hyperglycemia. Metformin enhances insulin sensitivity, slows the gastrointestinal absorption of glucose, and reduces the hepatic and renal glucose production. It can be used when there is normal liver and kidney function and no ketosis. If additional medication is needed, sulfonylurea or meglitinides may be used; however, they are not approved for use in children in the United States due to undue liver toxicity (Alemzadeh & Wyatt, 2004). The adolescent may ultimately require insulin for glycemic control.

NURSING MANAGEMENT

Nursing care focuses on promoting the child's blood glucose levels within target range if hospitalization is required and providing emotional support to the child and family. Assess growth and dietary intake, evaluate goals for weight loss and exercise programs, and review the child's knowledge about diabetes and strategies for management at home.

■ Nursing Assessment and Diagnosis

Because the child does not often present with an acute onset, assess any child with a BMI above the 85th percentile for age and gender for signs of insulin resistance (acanthosis nigricans, hypertension, and dyslipidemia). Family history of diabetes in an overweight child indicates a need to begin screening for the condition. Once the child has been diagnosed, monitor serum glucose levels, serum lipid levels, and blood pressure. Assess the child's diet and activity patterns to determine appropriate changes for disease management. Consider evaluating the siblings for diabetes.

Nursing diagnoses that may apply to the child with type 2 diabetes include the following:

- Imbalanced Nutrition: More than Body Requirements related to obesity and ethnic or cultural norms
- Activity Intolerance related to sedentary lifestyle and disease state (insulin resistance)
- Ineffective Therapeutic Regimen Management (family and individual) related to family conflict over changing eating patterns
- Situational Low Self-esteem related to situational crisis associated with diagnosis of new onset chronic illness

■ Planning and Implementation

The child with type 2 diabetes may be hospitalized at the time of diagnosis secondary to ketoacidosis. However, the nurse in an inpatient setting is more likely to encounter this child when hospitalized for another condition or during visits for healthcare in clinics or schools.

Care in the Community

Since the child is usually diagnosed with type 2 diabetes and managed on an outpatient basis, nursing care focuses on teaching the child and parents about the disease and its management, meal planning, providing emotional support, and planning strategies for daily management in the community.

Partner with the child and family to provide education about the disease and its management. Assist the child and family to establish lifestyle changes required for effective management of the condition. Focus on the need to increase activity with routine exercise of at least 30 to 60 minutes daily and decrease sedentary activity time, such as computer and television viewing, to no more than 2 hours daily. Customize the activity strategy for each child with motivation to develop a regular routine.

Collaborate with the family to substitute high-calorie and high-fat foods with a food plan that is sensitive to the family's resources and ethnic preferences. Suggestions include limiting fast foods and snacking on fruits and vegetables rather than foods high in fat and sugar.

Assess the child's height, weight, and body mass index (BMI) on each visit, and plot them on the appropriate growth curve for age and gender. A gradual sustained weight loss or decrease in BMI is the goal. If the child is experiencing a height growth spurt, maintenance of weight rather than weight loss is the goal. The child should receive a multivitamin daily. Since other family members are also at risk for developing type 2 diabetes, encourage the entire family to make dietary changes.

Partner with the child and family to ensure their ability to perform home serum glucose testing to monitor glycemic control. Documenting serum glucose levels will provide feedback to the child and family that efforts to manage the disease are successful. HbA_{1c} levels should be taken at each visit to determine the average blood glucose level for the past 3 months. An HbA_{1c} level of 7% or less is the goal. When the food plan and exercise are not successful in reducing blood glucose levels, teach the child and family about the prescribed oral medication.

Provide the child and family with opportunities to talk about the impact of the disease on their lives. Identify resources for information about strategies that have worked for other families. Identify local support groups and peer groups for the family and child.

Emphasize to the parents the importance of the child receiving annual or more frequent evaluations for potential complications of diabetes. The tests to be performed include blood for lipid levels, blood pressure, liver and renal function, urine for albumin, an ophthalmologic examination for retinopathy, and a neurologic exam of the extremities for neuropathies.

■ Evaluation

Examples of expected outcomes of nursing care for the child with type 2 diabetes include the following:

- The child achieves a balanced nutritional intake, resulting in body mass index reduction and a stable glucose level within target range.
- The child decreases sedentary activity time to under 2 hours a day and participates in exercise regimen and tolerates activity.
- The child and family demonstrate positive changes related to food plan management, incorporating the child's food preferences.
- The child demonstrates positive self-esteem.

DISORDERS OF GONADAL FUNCTION

The female gonads, or ovaries, regulate secondary sexual characteristics and reproduction in females. Estrogens are responsible for stimulating cells to develop secondary sexual characteristics, follicle maturation, and growth of uterine lining. The male gonads, or testes, regulate secondary sexual characteristics and reproduction in males. Androgens, primarily testosterone, are responsible for maturation of sperm, secondary sexual characteristics, and stimulation of cells for protein synthesis.

Gynecomastia, amenorrhea, and dysmenorrhea are the disorders of gonadal function presented in this section.

Gynecomastia

Gynecomastia is the presence of unilateral or bilateral enlarged breast tissue in males. This disorder is a common finding during adolescence and is sometimes confused with subcutaneous fat pads in obese males. Gynecomastia occurs when the ratio of estrogen to testosterone is greater than the usual male ratio. The amount of breast tissue varies among males. The condition usually resolves in 1 to 2 years as a result of growth and increasing testosterone levels.

Nursing Management

Nursing care focuses on reassuring the child and his parents that gynecomastia is a common and transient condition. Concerns about body image are common during adolescence and enlarged breast tissue can be a major source of embarrassment and anxiety in the male. Assure the child that the enlarged breasts are a temporary situation and the problem will resolve once the male hormones become active. Partner with the child and family to determine clothing styles and other methods to camouflage the enlarged breasts. Alerting the adolescent's teachers may be necessary if teasing becomes a problem.

Amenorrhea

Amenorrhea, or lack of menstruation, may be primary or secondary. Primary amenorrhea is defined as an absence of menarche by age 14.5 years in association with no growth or development of secondary sexual characteristics. Secondary amenorrhea is the absence of three or more consecutive menstrual cycles after menstruation has begun (Slap, 2003). Pregnancy is the most common cause of secondary amenorrhea in adolescents.

Primary amenorrhea is most often caused by structural defects of the reproductive system; chromosomal abnormalities (such as Turner syndrome); or hypothalamic or pituitary tumors, thyroid dysfunction, or polycystic ovary disease. No underlying pathologic condition is identified in some adolescents.

Primary or secondary amenorrhea may be identified in competitive athletes, particularly those who are pressured to be strong competitors. Girls competing in sports such as gymnastics, ballet, and long-distance running feel the need to maintain a low weight and specific body type. The inadequate nutrition and strenuous activity may cause hypothalamic dysfunction and a low estrogen level, resulting in amenorrhea. This, in turn, may increase the girl's risk of fractures and osteoporosis in young adulthood (see Chapters 9 and 35∞).

Collaborative Care

A thorough history (including sexual activity), physical examination, and laboratory evaluation are required to determine the cause of amenorrhea. The history focuses on asking questions about recent excessive weight loss or gain; excessive physical activity or sports training; chronic illness; use of illegal drugs, birth control pills, or phenothiazines; emotional problems; and age of the mother at menarche.

The physical examination focuses on evaluating the adolescent's stage of sexual development and assessing for hirsutism (refer to Chapter 8∞). A vaginal exam is performed to determine vaginal patency and if the vaginal mucosa is estrogenized. A pregnancy test is performed to rule out pregnancy. Bone age and hormone levels are evaluated (estrogen, LH, FSH, and prolactin).

Treatment of amenorrhea depends on the specific cause. The most common approach is to administer birth control pills containing both estrogen and progesterone.

Nursing Management

Nursing management for the adolescent with amenorrhea centers on education and providing emotional support. The goal is to promote normal growth and development.

The nurse partners with the adolescent to teach her that it is common to have irregular menstrual cycles and variable duration in menstrual periods for 1 to 2 years after menarche. A large number of cycles are anovulatory for the first 2 years after menarche. Athletic teenagers are encouraged to eat a well-balanced, high-calorie diet. Calcium supplements may be prescribed. Estrogen with progesterone in low doses may be prescribed for athletes to reduce the risk for osteoporosis.

If the adolescent female is or is considering becoming sexually active, the nurse should provide education about safe sex practices and birth control. Refer to obstetric or women's health textbooks for more information about birth control.

Dysmenorrhea

Dysmenorrhea (menstrual pain or cramping) is a common complaint of adolescent girls. Primary dysmenorrhea occurs in the absence of pathologic disorders. Dysmenorrhea accounts for more hours of missed school by females than any other cause. The prevalence increases from 38% to 39% at age 12 years or Tanner stage III, to 66% to 72% at age 17 years or Tanner stage V. Approximately 15% of adolescent females are incapacitated by dysmenorrhea for 1 to 3 days a month (Slap, 2003).

Primary dysmenorrhea is usually caused by an increased secretion of prostaglandins that are produced during the ovulatory cycle. Prostaglandin causes smooth muscle contraction in the uterus, leading to ischemia and pain. In secondary dysmenorrhea, a pathologic condition, such as endometriosis or pelvic inflammatory disease, has been identified.

Dysmenorrhea usually occurs prior to the beginning of the menstrual period and ends on the second day of the period. The cramping pain in the lower abdomen and pelvic region ranges from mild to severe and varies with the individual. Pain may also radiate to the back or thighs. Other symptoms may include nausea, headache, backache, vomiting, diarrhea, fatigue, and urinary frequency.

A gynecological examination may be conducted to rule out any structural abnormalities for primary and secondary dysmenorrhea. Uterine, rectovaginal, and adnexal tenderness is found in 76% of adolescents with endometriosis (Slap, 2003). Vaginal and cervical cultures are taken when a sexually transmitted infection is possible. See Chapter 31∞.

The treatment of choice is nonsteroidal anti-inflammatory drugs (NSAIDs) such as ibuprofen and naproxen sodium. These drugs inhibit prostaglandin synthesis, which leads to a reduction in uterine activity and pain. Oral contraceptives may be prescribed to prevent ovulation and to decrease prostaglandin production. An increase in protein, magnesium, calcium, and vitamin B_6 may help relieve symptoms.

Nursing Management

Nursing care centers on providing patient education and emotional support. For females with chronic dysmenorrhea, instruct the adolescent to keep a calendar and begin taking NSAIDs 1 day before the onset of the menstrual period, and that the medications should be taken with food to minimize side effects. See Complementary Therapy: Dysmenorrhea for non-pharmacologic interventions.

DISORDERS RELATED TO SEX CHROMOSOME ABNORMALITIES

Sex chromosome abnormalities are gender specific. Males inherit an X and a Y chromosome while females inherit two X chromosomes. Male abnormalities are the result of irregular numbers of either the X or the Y chromosome or both. Female abnormalities are the result of variations in the number of X chromosomes.

The two most common sex chromosome abnormalities, Turner syndrome in females and Klinefelter syndrome in males, are discussed in this section.

Turner Syndrome

Turner syndrome is a disorder caused by a complete loss, partial absence, or other abnormality of one X chromosome. The

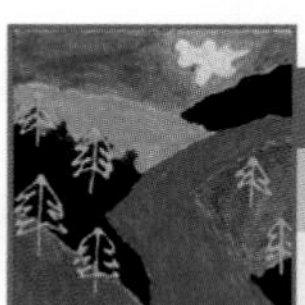

COMPLEMENTARY THERAPY

Dysmenorrhea

Guided imagery, hypnosis, meditation, chiropractic massage, and reflexology are non-pharmacologic methods that may be useful in the relief of dysmenorrhea. Application of a heating pad may also be helpful. Intake of vitamin B6 with B complex vitamins, vitamin E, calcium, and magnesium may help relieve symptoms of dysmenorrhea (Shuler, Huebscher, Miller, et al., 2004).

MediaLink Turner Syndrome Resources and Support

disorder occurs in approximately 1 in 2,000 to 5,000 live female births (Halec & Zimmerman, 2004c). The cause of the chromosomal error is unknown; the risk for this syndrome does not increase with maternal age. Approximately 99% of fetuses with the disorder are spontaneously aborted. Nearly half of females with Turner syndrome have 45 X chromosome complement (Rapaport, 2004). In the absence of one X chromosome, ovarian dysgenesis occurs in which the number of oocytes in the ovaries disappear rapidly and are nearly all gone by 2 years of age. Other specific clinical manifestations are related to specific genes missing.

Clinical Manifestations

Short stature is a significant finding. Growth usually proceeds at a normal rate for the first 2 to 3 years of life and then slows. Without treatment, final height is approximately 56 inches. Other characteristic findings include a short, webbed neck with a low posterior hairline; cubitus valgus (increased angle at the elbow); scoliosis, broad chest with widely spaced nipples; lymphedema; hyperconvex fingernails; dark, pigmented nevi; delayed or absent sexual development; amenorrhea; and infertility (Figure 32–13 ■). Few females present all of these features.

Many conditions may be associated with Turner syndrome, including the following: congenital heart disease; coarctation of aorta; hypertension, structural abnormalities of the kidney; congenital lymphedema; hypothyroidism or Hashimoto's thyroiditis; chronic or recurrent otitis media; strabismus, ptosis, myopia, or amblyopia (lazy eye); inflammatory bowel disease; idiopathic hypertension; and scoliosis.

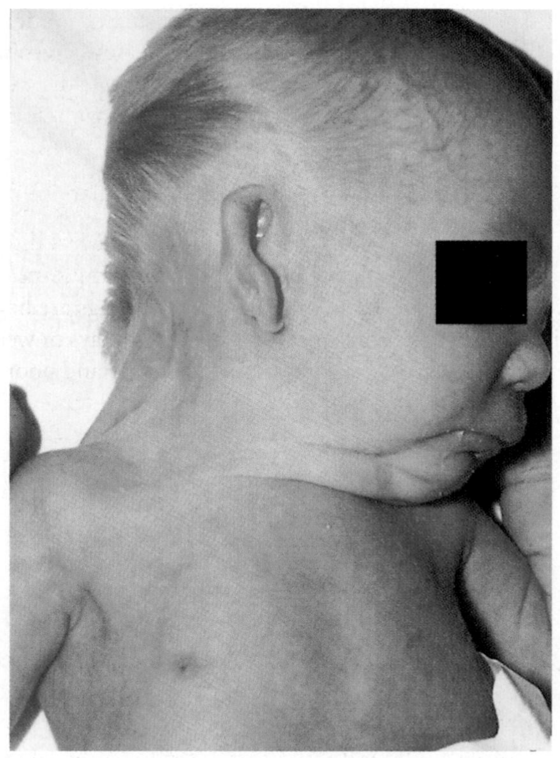

FIGURE 32–13 ■ What characteristic physical manifestation of Turner syndrome can you identify in this girl? *From Zittelli, B. J., & Davis, H. W. (Eds.) (1997). Atlas of pediatric physical diagnosis (3rd ed., p. 14). St. Louis: Mosby.*

Collaborative Care

The presence of characteristic physical findings may alert healthcare providers to suspect Turner syndrome. Some infants, however, have few of these characteristics and diagnosis is made only when short stature and delayed puberty become apparent during adolescence. The condition is diagnosed definitively by a karyotype, which reveals the classic 45,XO chromosome pattern or 46,XX pattern with one misshapen X chromosome.

Prenatal diagnosis includes the triple maternal marker screening of alpha-fetoprotein, estradiol, and HCG, maternal progesterone, and inhibin A levels. Fetal ultrasound may reveal nuchal thickening, aortic coarctation, renal abnormalities, short limbs, and growth retardation. However, definitive diagnosis for Turner syndrome is postnatal karyotyping (Halec & Zimmerman, 2004c)

The goal of collaborative care is to promote growth and development of the child. Treatment involves careful monitoring of the child's growth. A growth chart specifically for assessing the child with Turner syndrome is available from the Turner Syndrome Society of the United States. Growth hormone (GH) therapy may be prescribed to promote growth during childhood, and the therapy can begin at age 2 (Halec & Zimmerman, 2004c). Low-dose estrogen therapy is usually begun at around 15 years of age, with dosage increases over the next 2 to 3 years. Delaying treatment until the age of 15 years provides the child the opportunity to achieve maximum height before hormones cause the epiphyseal growth plates to close. This treatment produces pubertal changes such as breast development and pubic hair. Progesterone is added to the estrogen therapy to initiate menstrual periods.

Nursing Management

The goal of nursing care is to promote growth and development and positive body image. Assess for signs and symptoms of cardiac, renal, gastrointestinal, vision, hearing, musculoskeletal, or thyroid dysfunction associated with the disorder. Monitor growth rates using the Turner syndrome growth chart. Partner with the child and family to ensure proper administration of growth hormone and the monitoring of side effects. See page 1243.

The lack of growth and sexual development associated with Turner syndrome presents problems not only for physical growth but also for psychosocial development. Self-image, self-consciousness, and self-esteem are affected by the girl's perception of her body and how she differs from peers. Additionally, sexual inhibition or feelings of sexual inadequacy may also be experienced (Kagan-Krieger, 2001).

In the United States, cultural values place importance on attaining normal to tall stature. Short children tend to be treated according to their size rather than their age. Emphasis is also placed on sexual maturity. Television, advertisements, and movies encourage adolescents to dress and behave in a sexually mature manner. Females with Turner syndrome are often self-conscious, easily embarrassed, and suffer from low self-esteem. Even though their intelligence is generally normal, they have a higher incidence of learning problems related to visual-spatial deficits that affect performance on mathematical and manual dexterity tasks (Ranke & Saenger, 2001).

Partner with the child and family to promote adaptive skills and positive self-esteem. Active listening and reinforcement of abilities and skills that the child exhibits promotes self-esteem. Encourage parents to partner with the healthcare team to provide the child or adolescent with ongoing support. The Turner Syndrome Society can provide additional information about the disorder for parents and adolescents.

Klinefelter Syndrome

Klinefelter syndrome is a chromosomal disorder that occurs in males who have an extra X chromosome (usually 47, XXY). The disorder occurs in approximately 1 in 600 to 800 male births and is associated with increased maternal and paternal age. Klinefelter syndrome is the most common chromosomal abnormality in humans (Visootsak, Aylstock, & Graham, 2001) and is the single most common cause of hypogonadism (decreased secretory activity of the gonad) and infertility in males.

Clinical Manifestations

Most infants appear normal at birth. The condition is usually diagnosed during the school-age years when the child's behavior becomes disruptive in the classroom. Males with Klinefelter syndrome may experience emotional problems secondary to delayed language development and auditory processing problems causing frustration for the child. Intelligence quotient (IQ) scores are often 10 to 15 points below those of unaffected siblings, and IQs below 80 are not uncommon. The child with Klinefelter syndrome is tall and thin, with disproportionately long legs. The arm span to height ratio is normal. The onset of puberty may be delayed with an abnormal progression. Testicular size is decreased at all ages. Less facial and body hair may develop. Gynecomastia is a characteristic finding. Associated complications of Klinefelter syndrome may include cardiac abnormalities, pulmonary disease, dental abnormalities, and scoliosis.

Collaborative Care

Diagnosis is confirmed by chromosomal analysis revealing one or more extra X chromosomes. Often the diagnosis is not discovered until chromosomal evaluations are conducted during screenings for the school-age child with learning disabilities, behavioral problems, or language delay; and for the older child or adolescent for evaluation of delayed pubertal development (Visootsak et al., 2001).

The goal of treatment is to stimulate masculinization and the development of secondary sex characteristics when adolescence is delayed. Testosterone replacement is begun at puberty, when the male is 11 or 12 years of age. Depo-Testosterone is given by intramuscular injection every 3 to 4 weeks to maintain serum testosterone levels within the normal range. The dose is increased gradually until an adult dose is reached between 15 and 17 years of age.

The goal of replacement therapy is to maintain appropriate serum concentrations of testosterone, estradiol, follicle-stimulating hormone, and luteinizing hormone. Replacement therapy promotes normalization of body proportions, helps to prevent the development of gynecomastia, and promotes the development of normal secondary sex characteristics. Additionally, replacement therapy promotes general improvement in behavior, concentration, and learning ability (Visootsak et al., 2001).

Nursing Management

Assess secondary sexual characteristics, history, and height and weight. Nursing care consists of educating the parents and child about the syndrome, evaluating the child and family's coping mechanisms, assisting with school problems, and reinforcing the child's strengths.

Partner with the family and school officials to encourage an education environment tailored to the child's needs. The family may require assistance in coordinating an individualized developmental and educational program for their son. Language therapy to promote communication skills may be required. Refer the family to speech and communication specialists as indicated.

Encourage parents to channel their son's energy into areas that will provide opportunities for success and productive experiences. Emphasize the importance of rewarding the child's successes in school, sports, or hobbies. Encourage the child to express concerns related to body image. Genetic counseling should be made available to adolescents, if indicated, given that sexual functioning and fertility may be impaired.

Inherited Metabolic Diseases

Inherited metabolic diseases (also known as inborn errors of metabolism) include biochemical abnormalities of the urea cycle, amino acid, and organic acid metabolism. Therefore, protein, carbohydrate, fat, electrolyte, blood, and respiratory metabolism can be affected by inherited metabolic diseases. Individually they are rare disorders; however, as a group they are a significant health problem in infancy.

The biochemical defect usually causes an abnormal chemical by-product to accumulate in the blood, urine, or tissues or results in a decreased amount of normal enzymes. Most disorders are associated with protein intolerance, with symptoms developing shortly after formula or breast milk feedings are begun.

Clinical manifestations usually occur within days or weeks of birth. Signs and symptoms may include lethargy and poor feeding, persistent vomiting, abnormal muscle tone and seizures, apnea and tachycardia, and an unusual urine or body odor (musty, sweet odor of maple syrup or burnt sugar, or cheesy or sweaty feet).

In many states, neonatal screening is used to detect several of these conditions before symptoms develop. Four million newborns are screened each year for metabolic disorders (e.g., phenylketonuria), hematologic disorders (e.g., sickle-cell anemia), and endocrinopathies (e.g., hypothyroidism) (Centers for Disease Control and Prevention, 2001). See Chapters 4 and 11∞. However, most inherited metabolic diseases are not detected until signs and symptoms are present. Initial laboratory tests include measurement of serum glucose, electrolytes, blood gases, and serum ammonia. Results of these tests make it possible to classify the disorder by the presence of hypoglycemia, metabolic acidosis, hyperammonemia, or liver dysfunction. Further diagnostic laboratory tests are then performed.

Treatment, when available, focuses on replacing or reducing the amount of the substance causing the biochemical abnormality.

Four of the more common inherited metabolic diseases, phenylketonuria, galactosemia, fatty acid oxidation defects, and maple syrup urine disease, are presented in this section. Congenital hypothyroidism and congenital adrenal hyperplasia, also considered inherited metabolic diseases, were discussed earlier in this chapter.

Phenylketonuria

Phenylketonuria (PKU) is an autosomal recessive inherited disorder of amino acid metabolism that affects the body's utilization of protein. The disorder is caused by a mutation of the phenylalanine hydroxylase gene. The defect results in an accumulation of phenylalanine in the blood or phenylalanine metabolites in the urine. Phenylketonuria is rare, with an incidence of approximately 1:17,000 in the United States. Phenylketonuria is rare in Latin American, African American, Ashkenazi Jewish, and Japanese populations (Read & Charbonneau, 2004). If untreated, this disease leads to severe mental retardation, seizures, and death.

Etiology and Pathophysiology

Children with phenylketonuria have a deficiency of the liver enzyme phenylalanine hydroxylase that normally breaks down the essential amino acid phenylalanine into tyrosine. As a result, phenylalanine accumulates in the blood, causing a musty or mousey body and urine odor, irritability, vomiting, hyperactivity, hypertonic, hyperreflexive deep tendon reflexes, seizures, and an eczema-like rash (Revani, 2004). Persistence of elevated phenylalanine leads to disruption of cellular processes of myelination and protein synthesis and results in a seizure disorder and mental retardation without treatment.

Clinical Manifestations

Infants appear normal at birth except for a lighter skin complexion than their non-affected siblings (Revani, 2004). If diagnosis is delayed, a mousy or musty body odor is noticed and mental retardation may be severe. Microcephaly, prominent maxilla, and widely spaced teeth, enamel hypoplasia, and growth retardation are other common findings in untreated children (Revani, 2004).

COLLABORATIVE CARE

The goal of collaborative care is to diagnose the condition as soon as possible, before the toxic effect of phenylalanine has a chance to cause extensive harm to the body, and to begin treatment with medical formula and foods as soon as the diagnosis is made.

Screening for phenylketonuria is required by law in every state (Box 32–12). For best results, the newborn should have begun formula or breast milk feeding before specimen collection. Early hospital discharge places newborns at risk for false negative screening tests if screened within 24 hours of birth. Screening must occur no sooner than 48 hours after birth, or the test should be repeated at 1 to 2 weeks of age. If the test shows elevated levels of plasma phenylalanine, a repeat quantitative test is performed. If the second test is positive, the family is referred to an outpatient treatment center. Serum levels of phenylalanine should be measured periodically throughout life. Phenylalanine levels greater than 15 mg/dL are considered dangerous.

BOX 32–12 Neonatal Screening

Neonatal screening for hypothyroidism and phenylketonuria is mandated by state law in every state. When a state law exists, signed informed consent of the parents is not required. All states but South Dakota permit parents to refuse screening for religious or personal reasons. If parents refuse the test, obtain a signature of "informed dissent" to include in the child's medical record (American Academy of Pediatrics, 2001).

Clinical Therapy

Phenylketonuria is treated using special formulas (e.g., lofenalac, minafen, and albumaid XP) and a diet low in phenylalanine to maintain plasma phenylalanine levels between 2 and 6 mg/dL. The diet must also meet the child's needs for optimal growth. Breastfeeding is possible if phenylalanine levels are monitored. High-protein foods (meats and dairy products) and aspartame are avoided since they contain large amounts of phenylalanine. Elemental medical foods (modified protein hydrosylates in which the phenylalanine has been removed) are used instead.

The low-phenylalanine diet should be maintained for life. If dietary control is lost before 8 years of age, there is a significant impact on IQ. If adults go off the diet, there is no change in their IQ, but they may perform less well on tasks requiring attention and processing speed (National Institutes of Health, Consensus Statement, 2000). The low phenylalanine diet is especially important for adolescent females and women prior to conception and during pregnancy to prevent congenital anomalies (low birth weight, mental retardation, and microcephaly) in the fetus.

NURSING MANAGEMENT

Nursing care is mainly supportive and focuses on teaching parents about the disorder and its management.

■ Nursing Assessment and Diagnosis

Assess the infant and child for consequences of PKU, including neurologic findings such as tremor and hyperactive deep tendon reflexes, cognitive and behavioral problems, and atopic dermatitis (related to toxic effects of phenylalanine and its metabolites) (Read & Charbonneau, 2004). The severity of findings may provide a clue as to the dietary control maintained.

Nursing diagnoses that may be applicable to a child with PKU include the following:

- Risk for Delayed Development related to effects of disorder and less than optimal dietary control
- Noncompliance (PKU diet) related to desire to eat same foods as peers

- Risk for Impaired Parenting related to child with inherited disorder and need for lifelong special formula and foods.

Planning and Implementation

The low-phenylalanine diet is a rigid, strict diet that excludes many foods. Educate the family on sources of phenylalanine and refer the family to a nutritionist to establish a proper dietary plan. Parents and children require a great deal of support to promote adherence. The formula and elemental medical food costs are relatively expensive. The formula is usually reimbursed by insurance, but negotiations with health plans may help parents to obtain support for medical foods. Refer the family to services which may be able to provide financial assistance for responsibilities of treatment.

Like children with diabetes mellitus, children with phenylketonuria may rebel against the dietary limitations in an effort to be like their peers. Reinforcement of education is imperative during this time. The current recommendation is that all patients remain on a phenylalanine-restricted diet for life (Revani, 2004).

During health promotion visits, encourage parents to promote the child's development and gain new skills.

Parents of an affected child who are considering a future pregnancy and adolescents with the disorder should be referred for genetic counseling. See Chapter 4∞.

Evaluation

Examples of expected outcomes of nursing care for the child with PKU include the following:

- The child demonstrates age-appropriate development.
- The child adheres to special dietary requirements at school.
- The parents adapt by integrating the child's special care needs into the family's routines.

Galactosemia

Galactosemia is a disorder of carbohydrate metabolism that has an autosomal recessive inheritance pattern. The disorder occurs in 1 in 50,000 live births (Larsson & Therrell, 2002).

Galactosemia results from a deficiency of the liver enzyme galactose-1–phosphate uridyltransferase (GALT), one of three enzymes needed to convert galactose to glucose. Galactosemia is the most severe of the disorders of galactose metabolism (Larsson & Therrell, 2002). The lack of enzyme leads to an accumulation of galactose metabolites in the eyes, liver, kidney, and brain, rapidly damaging the organs and causing life-threatening problems. Children become susceptible to gram-negative sepsis.

Early signs include poor sucking and nutritional intake, failure to gain weight due to vomiting followed by diarrhea, hypoglycemia, and an enlarged liver. Later signs include mental retardation, jaundice, ascites, sepsis, lethargy, seizures, hypotonia, cataracts, and coma. Death, usually due to sepsis, may occur within 1 month of birth without treatment. When the diagnosis is not made at birth, damage to the liver (cirrhosis) and brain (mental retardation) become progressively more severe and irreversible.

Collaborative Care

Routine newborn screening for galactosemia is performed in almost all U.S. newborn screening programs (Larsson & Therrell, 2002). Infants not initially screened are identified once they become symptomatic. The diagnosis is based on history, physical examination, and laboratory tests (galactose, SGOT, and SGPT are abnormally high). Urine specimens are checked for reducing substances (the clinitest is positive and the clinistix is negative) in several specimens while the patient is receiving human milk, cow's milk, or another lactose containing formula.

Treatment requires the elimination of galactose from the diet. Infants with galactosemia are placed on a lactose- or galactose-free formula (e.g., nutramigen, a meat-based or soybean formula), which remains the child's milk substitute for life. Improvement in the infant's condition is generally observed within 24 hours. A galactose-free diet (no milk or cheese products, including foods with dry milk products) is prescribed when the infant is ready for consumption of solid foods. Despite adherence to the diet, complications, such as learning disabilities, speech defects, ovarian failure, and neurologic syndromes, develop in many children.

Nursing Management

Nursing care focuses on educating the parents and child about the disorder and required diet, assessing coping abilities, and providing emotional support. Partner with the family and nutritionist for diet counseling. Families must learn to screen foods for added milk solids and to avoid medications, such as antibiotics, that have lactose fillers. Calcium supplementation may be required. Advise parents that several galactose-free cheeses are sold commercially. Because the disorder is inherited, the family should be referred for genetic counseling.

Fatty Acid Oxidation Disorders

Mitochondrial oxidation of fatty acids is an imperative energy producing pathway. This pathway becomes essential during periods of starvation when the body changes its fuel from primarily carbohydrate to fat utilization. Gene defects can occur in nearly every stage in the fatty acid oxidation pathway. Therefore, there are many subclasses of fatty acid oxidation defects. All of these defects are autosomal recessive traits that occur in both males and females. Most patients have a northwestern European ancestry (Venditti & Stanley, 2004).

There is a wide variation in presentations of fatty acid oxidations disorders, even within the same family. Screening has revealed that fatty acid oxidation disorders are among the most common inborn errors of metabolism. Some of these defects include medium-chain acyl-CoA dehydrogenase (MCAD) deficiency (most common), long-chain acyl-CoA dehydrogenase (LCHAD) deficiency, and plasma carnitine deficiency. If undiagnosed, these disorders can lead to serious complications affecting the heart, liver, eyes, muscular system, and even death.

The most common presentation is an acute onset life threatening coma and hypoglycemia induced by a period of fasting. Other manifestations often include cardiomyopathy, hepatomegaly, and muscle weakness. Infants and children can by asymptomatic except for times during fasting or stress.

Collaborative Care

Diagnosis can occur during routine newborn screening when laboratories use mass spectrometry. Most cases are identified during an acute presentation of symptoms when laboratory evaluation may include blood gases, electrolytes, hepatic profile, plasma lactate, plasma amino acids, urine organic acids, acylcamitine profile, quantitative carnitine levels and urine for ketones. Hypoglycemia is usually present and ketone levels are unusually low. Liver function tests demonstrate elevated transaminases, urea, and ammonia. Plasma and tissue concentrations of total carnitine are reduced. Skin biopsies are often obtained for fibroblast analysis. Physical examination may reveal hepatomegaly due to fatty infiltration.

Treatment of acute illnesses with 10% dextrose is needed to suppress lipolysis. Chronic therapy is to avoid fasting, ensuring that no more than 10 hours passes before food is eaten. Carnitine supplementation may be required in some disorders as it is useful in preventing low blood sugar and assists in removing metabolic waste from cells.

Nursing Management

Nurses can partner with parents to educate about the importance of frequent feedings and avoidance of fasting. Teach parents that these children should go no longer than 8 to 12 hours without food. Infants should be fed around the clock every 2 to 4 hours. If the infant or child is unable to sustain oral intake during an acute illness, they must be referred to the hospital for intravenous dextrose supplementation. Even simple infections such as an ear infection or influenza can become life-threatening for these children. Several snack foods and meals of low fat and high carbohydrate foods (i.e. cereal, pasta) are recommended throughout the day. Genetic counseling should be offered to the family. If one child in the family is diagnosed with the disorder, their siblings should also be tested, even if they are asymptomatic.

Maple Syrup Urine Disease

Maple syrup urine disease (MSUD) is a disorder of amino acid metabolism that has an autosomal recessive inheritance pattern. Maple syrup urine disease is a rare disorder found in 1 in 225,000 live births, but has a high incidence in some Pennsylvania Mennonites at 1 in 380 live births (Robinson & Drumm, 2001).

In maple syrup urine disease, three essential amino acids (leucine, isoleucine, and valine) cannot be broken down because of absent or defective enzyme branched chain alpha-ketoacid dehydrogenase. This results in alpha ketoacidosis. All three amino acids are essential to form normal structures such as the hair, skin, and muscle. Leucine has the potential to accumulate in the brain and cause cerebral edema, progressive neurologic impairment, and death.

Within 3 to 7 days of life, the newborn develops symptoms of poor appetite, lethargy, vomiting, variable muscle tone, irritability, seizures, high-pitched cry, severe ketoacidosis, and a sweet odor of maple syrup in bodily fluids. The symptoms may quickly progress to coma and death if not treated (Larsson & Therrell, 2002).

Collaborative Care

Not all states require newborn screening for this condition. Diagnosis is made with laboratory tests of the urine for positive ketones and blood tests for elevated leucine, isoleucine, alloisoleucine, (a stereoisomer of isoleucine not normally found in blood) and valine.

Early treatment is required to prevent neurological impairment or death (Larsson & Therrell, 2002). In the acute state, treatment is to remove the branch-chained amino acids and their metabolites from the tissues and body fluids. Renal clearance of these compounds is poor and some critically ill infants may require peritoneal or hemodialysis to remove these compounds. The infant's catabolic state can then be reversed by providing sufficient calories intravenously and orally.

Life long treatment involves specially designed medical formulas and foods rich in amino acids, calories, vitamins, minerals, and other nutrients as prescribed. These special medical foods have the three amino acids removed. Small amounts of these amino acids are added to the diet as the body cannot generate them. The child requires special low-protein foods that are adequate for growth with enough calories to support twice the child's basal metabolic rate. Daily urine testing is required to determine if ketones are being excreted, an indication that the body is in a catabolic state. A liver transplant has been performed in a few affected children who were subsequently able to tolerate a normal diet (Rezvani & Rosenblatt, 2004).

Long-term prognosis of affected children remains guarded. Severe ketoacidosis, cerebral edema, or death may occur during any stressful situation, including infection or surgery. Affected children commonly have neurologic and mental sequalae.

Nursing Management

Nursing care includes educating the families about the disorder and special dietary requirements. Partner with the family to ensure their understanding of how to mix the child's special formula with natural protein source, amino acid supplements, and water. The child requires formula even when ill, and a sick day plan should be provided to prevent ketoacidosis. Refer the family to a nutritionist for diet counseling. The child should be permitted moderate exercise only to prevent increases in leucine levels. Help families identify sources of information or support groups who can share recipes and tips for managing the child's condition.

Partner with the family, nutritionist, and school or childcare officials to ensure their understanding of foods the child should avoid. Assist in the establishment of a list of snacks for special occasions. The child should have formula and other supplements available to ensure a steady intake of calories during the day. An individual school health plan should be developed with the school nurse so that teachers and other school personnel are informed.

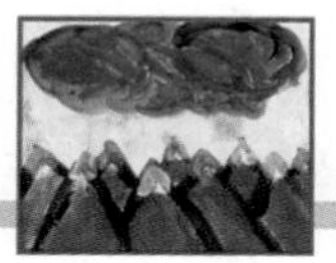

CHAPTER HIGHLIGHTS

- Puberty is the process of sexual maturation that occurs when the gonads secrete increased amounts of the sex hormones estrogen and testosterone, resulting in the development of primary and secondary sexual characteristics.
- The anterior pituitary gland is considered to be the "master gland" of the body because of its role in the production of hormones that regulate the secretion of other hormones.
- Children with hypopituitarism have short stature as a result of growth hormone deficiency. Treatment with growth hormone early in life enables these children to have near normal heights.
- An excessive secretion of growth hormone or hyperpituitarism may cause children to have tall stature, growing up to 7 or 8 feet in height if no intervention is provided before the epiphyseal plates close.
- In diabetes insipidus, the urine cannot be concentrated, no matter how dehydrated the child becomes. Diagnosis rarely occurs until the child experiences hypernatremic dehydration.
- Syndrome of inappropriate antidiuretic hormone (SIADH) results from an excessive amount of serum antidiuretic hormone (ADH) leading to water intoxication and hyponatremia.
- Precocious puberty is defined as the appearance of any secondary sexual characteristics before 8 years in girls and 9 years in boys. If no treatment is provided, the hormones will stimulate closure of the epiphyseal plates and the child will have short stature as an adult.
- Untreated or ineffectively treated congenital hypothyroidism results in impaired growth and mental retardation.
- Signs of hyperthyroidism include an enlarged, nontender thyroid gland (goiter), prominent eyes, eyelid lag, tachycardia, nervousness, restlessness or irritability, increased appetite with weight loss, emotional lability, heat intolerance, increased sweating, insomnia, tremor, and muscle weakness.
- During infancy and childhood, most cases of Cushing syndrome are due to a malignant adrenal tumor. It generally takes up to 5 years for the child to develop the characteristic cushingoid appearance.
- Congenital adrenal hyperplasia has two forms, salt losing or simple virilization. Approximately 65% to 75% of children have a disturbance in mineralcorticoid regulation that can lead to acute adrenal insufficiency with any serious illness or injury.
- Adrenal insufficiency, though rare in children, is characterized by weakness with fatigue, anorexia and salt craving, poor weight gain or weight loss, hyperpigmentation at pressure points, generalized bronzing of the skin, abdominal pain, nausea and vomiting, and diarrhea.
- Congenital adrenal hyperplasia is the most common cause of pseudohermaphroditism (ambiguous genitalia) in newborn girls.
- Pheochromocytoma is a rare benign tumor of the adrenal gland which causes labile hypertension and intermittent signs associated with epinephrine and norepinephrine secretion.
- Diabetes mellitus type 1 is the most common metabolic disease in children and one of the most common chronic diseases in school-age children. It is a disorder of carbohydrate, protein, and fat metabolism.
- Treatment of the child with diabetic ketoacidosis includes intravenous fluids and electrolytes for dehydration and acidosis. Insulin is given by continuous infusion pump to decrease the serum glucose level at a slow but steady rate to prevent the development of cerebral edema.
- Common causes of hypoglycemia in children with type 1 diabetes include an error in insulin dosage, errors in injection technique, inadequate calories because of missed meals, or exercise without a corresponding increase in caloric intake.
- Type 2 diabetes mellitus is an emerging condition among children and adolescents that results from insulin resistance. Children most commonly affected are obese and many have family members with the same type of diabetes.
- Secondary amenorrhea is the cessation of spontaneous menstrual periods for at least 120 days and occurs 6 months or three cycles after menarche.
- Turner syndrome is diagnosed definitively by a karyotype, which reveals the classic 45,XO chromosome pattern or 46,XX pattern with one misshapen X chromosome.
- Signs of Klinefelter syndrome include a gynecomastia, delayed onset of puberty with an abnormal progression, decreased testicular size, and less facial and body hair than normal.
- Inherited metabolic diseases—inherited biochemical abnormalities of the urea cycle and amino acid and organic acid metabolism—often have a significant impact on the endocrine system's ability to support growth and development. These disorders include phenylketonuria, galactosemia, defects in fatty acid oxygenation, and maple syrup urine disease.
- Children with phenylketonuria (PKU) have a deficiency of the liver enzyme phenylalanine hydroxylase that normally breaks down the essential amino acid phenylalanine into tyrosine. It is treated with special formula and engineered foods.
- Galactosemia results from a deficiency of a liver enzyme needed to convert galactose to glucose. This leads to an accumulation of galactose metabolites in the eyes, liver, kidney, and brain, rapidly damaging the organs and causing life-threatening problems.
- In the inborn error of metabolism involving a defect in fatty acid oxygenation, the most common presentation is an acute onset life-threatening coma and hypoglycemia induced by a period of fasting.
- Maple syrup urine disease is a rare inherited enzyme deficiency that results in ketoacidosis unless special formula, engineered foods, and extra calories are eaten.

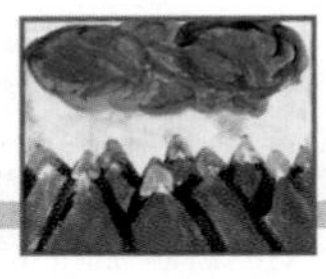

CRITICAL THINKING IN ACTION

INTRODUCTION

Recall Anthony, the 12-year-old in the opening scenario, who is newly diagnosed with type 1 diabetes. His glucose is now stabilized and he is receiving basal-bolus insulin therapy.

DESCRIPTION

Anthony is learning to check his own serum glucose and demonstrates the correct technique. He states that he is afraid of giving himself a "shot" and becomes anxious when he receives injections. Anthony will soon be discharged from the hospital and will receive further diabetes education on an outpatient basis. Anthony's parents are eager to learn about caring for him, but express concerns now that he will not be able to participate in sports activities as he has in the past.

DISCUSSION

1. Considering Anthony's age and developmental level, how will the nurse explain type 1 diabetes to Anthony?
2. How will the nurse address Anthony's reluctance to self-administer his insulin? What are some potential causes of Anthony's reluctance?
3. What are the most important instructions to ensure that Anthony and his parents understand before he is discharged and receives further education on an outpatient basis?
4. What will the nurse explain to Anthony and his parents regarding activity, exercise, and participation in sports?

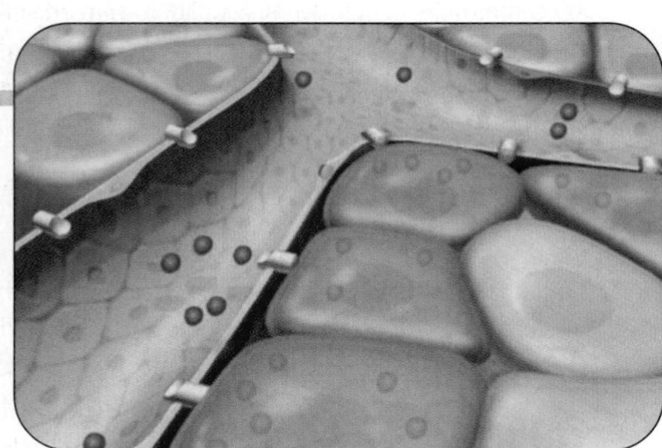

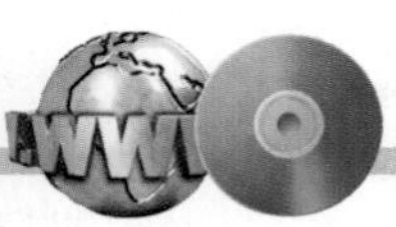

EXPLORE MediaLink

- NCLEX review, case studies, and other interactive resources for this chapter can be found on the Companion Website at **www.prenhall.com/ball**. Click on Chapter 32 to select the activities for this chapter.
- For animations, more NCLEX review questions, and an audio glossary, access the accompanying CD-ROM in this book.

http://www.prenhall.com/ball

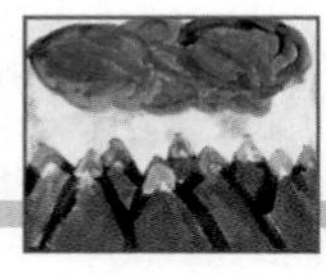

REFERENCES

Ahmad, R., Hammond, J. M. (2004). Primary, secondary, and tertiary hyperparathyroidism. *Otolaryngologic Clinics of North America, 37*(4), 701–713, vii–viii.

Alemzadeh, R., & Wyatt, D. T. (2004). Diabetes mellitus in children. In R. E. Berhman, R. M. Kliegman, & H. B. Jenson (Eds.), *Nelson textbook of pediatrics* (17th ed., pp. 1947–1972). Philadelphia: Saunders.

American Academy of Pediatrics Committee on Bioethics. (2001). Ethical issues with genetic testing in pediatrics. *Pediatrics, 107*(6), 1451–1455.

American Academy of Pediatrics Section on Endocrinology and Committee on Genetics. (2000). Technical report: Congenital adrenal hyperplasia. *Pediatrics, 106*(6), 1511–1518.

American Diabetes Association. (2000). Type 2 diabetes in children and adolescents. *Diabetes Care, 23*(3), 381–389.

American Diabetes Association. (2002). Clinical practice recommendations. *Diabetes Care, 25*(1).

American Diabetes Association. (2004a). Statistics. www.diabetes.org/diabetes-statistics.jsp

American Diabetes Association. (2004b). Clinical practice recommendations. www.diabetes.org/for-health-professionals-and-scientists/cpr/jsp

Boger, M. S. & Perrier, N. D. (2004). Advantages and disadvantages of surgical therapy and optimal extent of thyroidectomy for the treatment of hyperthyroidism. *Surgical Clinics of North America, 84,* 849–874.

Boland, E. A., & Grey, M. (2000). Diabetes mellitus (type 1). In P. J. Allen & J. A. Vessey (Eds.), *Primary care of the child with a chronic condition* (4th ed., pp. 426–444). St. Louis: Mosby.

Brosnan, C. A., Upchurch, S., & Schreiner, B. (2001). Type 2 diabetes in children and adolescents: An emerging disease. *Journal of Pediatric Health Care, 15*(4), 187–193.

Carel, J. C., Chatelain, P., Rochiccioli, P., & Chaussain, J. L. (2003). Improvement in adult height after growth hormone treatment in adolescents with short stature born small for gestational age: Results of a randomized controlled study. *Journal of Clinical Endocrinology and Metabolism, 88*(4), 1587–1593.

Centers for Disease Control and Prevention. (2001). Using tandem mass spectrometry for metabolic disease screening among newborns: A report of a work group. *Morbidity and Mortality Weekly Report, 50*(RR-31), 1–34.

Centers for Disease Control and Prevention. (2004). Diabetes projects. www.cdc.gov/diabetes/projects/cda2.htm

Cheetham, T., & Baylis, P. H. (2002). Diabetes insipidus in children. *Pediatric Drugs, 4*(12), 785–796.

Cogen, F. R., Streisand, R., & Sarin, S. (2002). Selecting children and adolescents for insulin pump therapy: Medical and behavioral considerations. *Diabetes Spectrum, 15*(2), 72–75.

Copstead, L. C., & Banasik, J. L. (2000). *Pathophysiology: Biological and behavioral perspectives* (2nd ed.) Philadelphia: Saunders.

Cowett, R. M., & Loughead, J. L. (2002). Neonatal glucose metabolism: Differential diagnoses, evaluation, and treatment of hypoglycemia. *Neonatal Network, 21*(4), 9–19.

Cox, M. (2002). A better mousetrap: What's new in blood glucose monitoring? *Journal of Pediatric Health Care, 16*(6), 314–316.

Cystic Fibrosis Foundation. (2004). www.cff.org

Doyle, D. A., & DiGeorge, A. M. (2004). Disorders of the parathyroid. In R. E. Berhman, R. M. Kliegman, & H. B. Jenson (Eds.), *Nelson textbook of pediatrics* (17th ed., pp. 1890–1898). Philadelphia: Saunders.

Dveirin, K., & Tunnessen, W. W. (2000). A 14-month-old with polyuria and polydipsia: Searching for buried treasure. *Contemporary Pediatrics, 17*(10), 23–30.

Eisenbrath, G. S., Polonsky, K. S., & Buse, J. B. (2003). In P. R. Larsen, H. Kronenberg, S. Melmed, & K. Polonsky (Ed.), *Williams textbook of endocrinology* (10th ed., pp. 1485–1504). Philadelphia: Saunders.

Evert, A. B. (2004). Tools and techniques for working with young people with diabetes. *Diabetes Spectrum, 17*(1), 8–13.

Failor, R. A., Capell, P. T. (2003). Hyperaldosteronism and pheochromocytoma: New tricks and tests. *Primary Care: Clinics in Office Practice, 30*(4), 801–820, viii.

Faulkner, M. S. (2003). Quality of life for adolescents with type 1 diabetes: Parental and youth perspectives. *Pediatric Nursing, 29*(5), 362–368.

Felner, E. I., & White, P. C. (2001). Improving management of diabetic ketoacidosis in children. *Pediatrics, 108*(3), 735–740.

Gance-Cleveland, B. (2003). Adaptation to Addison's disease in a child: A case study. *Journal of Pediatric Health Care, 17*(6), 301–310.

Goldberg, P. A., & Inzucchi, S. E. (2003). Critical issues in endocrinology. *Clinics in Chest Medicine, 24*(4), 583–606, vi.

Gruters, A., Biebermann, H., & Krude, H. (2003). Neonatal thyroid disorders. *The Neonate and Endocrine Disease, 59*(1), 24–29.

Gungor, N., & Arslanian, S. (2004). Progressive beta cell failure in type 2 diabetes mellitus of youth. *Journal of Pediatrics, 144*(5), 656–659.

Hafeez, W., & Vuguin, P. (2000). Managing diabetic ketoacidosis: A delicate balance. *Contemporary Pediatrics, 17*(6), 72–83.

Halec, I., & Zimmerman, D. (2004a). Evaluating short stature in children. *Pediatric Annals, 33*(3), 170–176.

Halec, I., & Zimmerman, D. (2004b). Managing growth hormone treatment in pediatric patients. *Pediatric Annals, 33*(3), 183–190.

Halec, I., & Zimmerman, D. (2004c). Coordinating care for children with Turner syndrome. *Pediatric Annals, 33*(3), 189–196.

Haller, M. J., Stalvey, M. S., & Silverstein, J. H. (2004). Predictors of control of diabetes: Monitoring may be the key. *Journal of Pediatrics, 144*(5), 660–661.

Harris, G. D., & Fawcett, G. F. (2002). Hypertensive endocrine disorders. *Clinics in Family Practice, 4*(3), 585–600.

Hoff, A. L., Mullins, L. L., Chaney, J. M., Hartman, V. L., & Domek, D. (2002). Illness uncertainty, perceived control and psychological distress among adolescents with type 1 diabetes. *Research and Theory for Nursing Practice: An International Journal, 16*(4), 223–236.

Ismail, A. A. A., & Barth, J. H. (2001). Endocrinology of gynaecomastia. *Annals of Clinical Biochemistry, 38*(6), 596–607.

Kagan-Krieger, S. (2001). Factors that affect coping with Turner syndrome. *Journal of Nursing Scholarship, 33*(1), 43–45.

Kaplowitz, P. A., Slora, E. J., Wasseman, R. C., Pedlow, S. E., & Herman-Giddens, M. (2001). Earlier onset of puberty in girls: Relation to increased body mass index and race. *Pediatrics, 108*(2; Part 1), 347–353.

Kaufman, F. R., & Halvorson, M. (1999). The treatment and prevention of diabetic ketoacidosis in children and adolescents with type 1 diabetes. *Pediatric Annals, 28*(9), 576–582.

Kim, L., & Nwariaku, F. (2004). Hyperparathyroidism. www.emedicine.com, accessed 12/3/2004.

Krantz, J. S., Mack, W. J., Hodis, H. N., Liu, C. R., & Kaufman, F. R. (2004). Early onset of subclinical atherosclerosis in young persons with type 1 diabetes. *Journal of Pediatrics, 145*(4), 452–457.

Lalwani, S., Reindollar, R. H., & Davis, A. J. (2003). Normal onset of puberty. Have the definitions changed? *Obstetrics and Gynecology Clinics, 30*(2), 279–286.

Larsson, A., & Therrell, B. L. (2002). Newborn screening: The role of the obstetrician. *Clinical Obstetrics and Gynecology, 45*(3), 697–732.

Lashley, F. R. (2002). Newborn screening: New opportunities and new challenges. *Newborn and Infant Nursing Reviews, 2*(4), 228–242.

Levine, L. S., & White, P. C. (2004). Disorders of the adrenal glands. In R. E. Berhman, R. M. Kliegman, & H. B. Jenson (Eds.), *Nelson textbook of pediatrics* (17th ed., pp. 1898–1921). Philadelphia: Saunders.

Litton, J., Rice, A., Friedman, N., Oden, J., Lee, M., & Freemark, M. (2002). Insulin pump therapy in toddlers and preschool children with type 1 diabetes mellitus. *The Journal of Pediatrics, 141*(4), 490–495.

Maniatis, A. K., Klingensmith, G. J., Slover, R. H., Mowry, C. J., & Chase, H. P. (2001). Continuous subcutaneous insulin infusion therapy for children and adolescents: An option for routine diabetes care. *Pediatrics, 107*(2), 351–356.

Merke, D. P., & Cutler, G. B. (1997). New approaches to the treatment of congenital adrenal hyperplasia. *Journal of the American Medical Association, 277*(13), 1073–1076.

Miller, B. S., & Zimmerman, D. (2004). Idiopathic short stature in children. *Pediatric Annals, 33*(3), 177–181.

Miller, M. M. (2003, November). Insulin pump therapy. *Advance for Nurse Practitioners,* 61–66.

Moreno, J. C., de Vijlder, J. M., Vulsma, T., & Ris-Stalpers, C. (2003). Genetic basis of hypothyroidism: Recent advances, gaps and strategies for future research. *Trends in Endocrinology and Metabolism, 14*(7), 318–326.

Nebesio, T. D., Siddiqui, A. R., Pescovitz, O. H., & Eugster, E. A. (2002). Time course to hypothyroidism after fixed-dose radioablation therapy of Graves' disease in children. *The Journal of Pediatrics, 141*(1), 99–103.

NIH Consensus Statement. (2000, October 16–18). *Phenylketonuria: Screening and management, 17*(3), 1–33.

Palma Sisto, P. A. (2004). Endocrine disorders in the neonate. *Pediatric Clinics of North America, 51*(4), 1141–1168.

Pang, S. (2003). Newborn screening for congenital adrenal hyperplasia. *Pediatric Annals, 32*(8), 516–523.

Parks, J. S. (2004). Disorders of the hypothalamus and pituitary gland. In R. E. Berhman, R. M. Kliegman, & H. B. Jenson (Eds.), *Nelson textbook of pediatrics* (17th ed., pp. 1845–1853). Philadelphia: Saunders.

Pinhas-Hamiel, O., & Zeitler, P. (2001). Type 2 diabetes: Not just for grownups anymore. *Contemporary Pediatrics, 18*(1), 102–125.

Ranke, W. B., & Saenger, P. (2001, July 28). Turner's syndrome. *The Lancet, 358,* 309–314.

Rapaport, R. (2004). Disorders of the gonads. In R. E. Berhman, R. M. Kliegman, & H. B. Jenson (Eds.), *Nelson textbook of pediatrics* (17th ed., pp. 1921–1946). Philadelphia: Saunders.

Read, C. Y., & Charbonneau, R. M. (2004). Phenylketonuria. In P. J. Allen & J. A. Vessey (Eds.), *Primary care of the child with a chronic condition* (4th ed., pp. 667–681). St. Louis: Mosby.

Reddy, V. S., O'Neill, J. A., Holcomb, G. W., Neblett, W. W., Pietsch, J. B., & Morgan, W. M. (2000). Twenty-five year surgical experience with pheochromocytoma in children. *American Surgeon, 66*(12), 1085–1091.

Rezvani, I. (2004). Defects in metabolisim of amino acids. In R. E. Berhman, R. M. Kliegman, & H. B. Jenson (Eds.), *Nelson textbook of pediatrics* (17th ed., pp. 398–402). Philadelphia: Saunders.

Rezvani, I., & Rosenblatt, D. S. (2004). Valine, leucine, isoleucine and related organic acidemias. In R. E. Berhman, R. M. Kliegman, & H. B. Jenson (Eds.), *Nelson textbook of pediatrics* (17th ed., pp. 409–421). Philadelphia: Saunders.

Roberts, C. G. P., & Ladenson, P. W. (2004). Hypothyroidism. *The Lancet, 363*(9411), 793–803.

Robinson, D., & Drumm, L. (2001). Maple syrup urine disease: A standard of nursing care. *Pediatric Nursing, 27*(3), 255–264, 270.

Rovet, J. F., & Ehrlich, R. (2000). Psychoeducational outcome in children with early-treated congenital hypothyroidism. *Pediatrics, 105*(3), 515–522.

Rudock, A. S. (2002). Secondary hyperparathyroidism—current concepts and controversies. *Clinics in Family Practice, 4*(3), 639–642.

Saborio, P., Tipton, G. A., & Chan, J. C. M. (2000.) Diabetes insipidus. *Pediatrics in Review, 21*(4), 122-129.

Saudek, C. D. (1997). Novel forms of insulin delivery. *Endocrinology and Metabolism Clinics of North America, 26*(3), 599–610.

Shuler, P., Huebscher, R., Miller, H., & Rauckhorst, L. (2004). Genitourinary concerns. In R. Huebscher & P. A. Shuler (Eds.), *Natural, alternative and complementary health care practices* (pp. 567–658). St. Louis: Mosby.

Shulman, D. I., & Bercu, B. B. (1998). Growth hormone therapy: An update. *Contemporary Pediatrics, 15*(8), 95–110.

Silverstein, J. H., & Rosenbloom, A. L. (2000). New developments in type 1 (insulin dependent) diabetes. *Clinical Pediatrics, 39*(5), 257–266.

Slap, G. B. (2003). Menstrual disorders in adolescence. *Best Practice and Research Clinical Obstetrics & Gynecology, 17*(1), 75–92.

Tato, L., Savage, M. O., Antoniazzi, F., Buzi, F., Di Maio, S., Oostdijk, W., Pasquino, A. M., Raiola, G., Saenger, P., Gonini, G., & Voorhoeve, P. G. (2001). Optimal therapy of pubertal disorders in precocious/early puberty. *Journal of Pediatric Endocrinology & Metabolism, 14,* 985–995.

Traggiai, C., & Stanhope, R. (2003). Disorders of pubertal development. *Best Practice & Research Clinical Obstetrics & Gynecology, 17*(1), 41–56.

Trimarchi, T. (2001). Endocrine critical care problems. In M. A. Q. Curley & P. A. Moloney-Harmon (Eds.), *Critical care nursing of infants and children* (2nd ed., pp. 805–819). Philadelphia: Saunders.

Van Vliet, G. (2001, July 14). Treatment of congenital hypothyroidism. *The Lancet, 358,* 86–87.

Venditti, C. P., & Stanley, C. A. (2004). Defects in metabolism of lipids. In R. E. Berhman, R. M. Kliegman, & H. B. Jenson (Eds.), *Nelson textbook of pediatrics* (17th ed., pp. 433–438. Philadelphia: Saunders.

Viera, A. J. (2002). Hyperparathyroidism. *Clinics in Family Practice, 4*(3), 627–638.

Visootsak, J., Aylstock, M., & Graham, J. M. (2001, December). Klinefelter syndrome and its variants: An update and review for the primary pediatrician. *Clinical Pediatrics,* 639–651.

Wilson, T. A., Rose, S. R., Cohen, P., Rogol, A. D., Backeljauw, P., Brown, R., et al. (2003). Update of guidelines for the use of growth hormone in children: the Lawson Wilkins pediatric endocrinology society drug and therapeutics committee. *Journal of Pediatrics, 143*(4), 415–421.

Winer, K. K., Ko, C. W., Reynolds, J. C., Dowdy, K., Keil, M., Peterson, D., Gerber, L. H., et al. (2004). Long-term treatment of hypoparathyroidism : A randomized controlled study comparing parathyroid hormone (1–34) versus calcitriol and calcium. *The Journal of Clinical Endocrinology & Metabolism, 88*(9), 4214–4220.

Wisniewski, A. B., & Migeon, C. J. (2002). Gender identity/role differentiation in adolescents affected by syndromes of abnormal sex differentiation. *Adolescent Medicine, 13*(1), 119–128.

Witchel, S. F., & Finegold, D. N. (2002). Endocrinology. In B. J. Zitelli & H. W. Davis, *Atlas of pediatric physical diagnosis* (4th ed., pp. 315–336). St. Louis: Mosby.

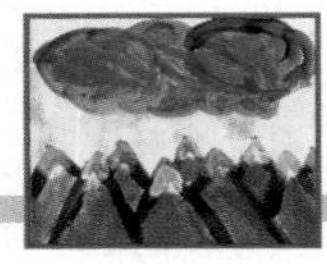

ADDITIONAL REFERENCES

Felner, E. I. (2003). Human insulin-induced lipoatrophy. *Journal of Pediatrics, 142,* 448.

Ginsberg, J. (2003). Diagnosis and management of Graves' disease. *Canadian Medical Association Journal, 168*(5), 575–579.

Lazar, L., Dan, S., & Phillip, M. (2003). Growth without growth hormone: Growth pattern and final height of five patients with idiopathic combined pituitary hormone deficiency. *Clinical Endocrinology, 59,* 82–88.

Moshang, T. (2003). Cushing's disease, 70 years later . . . and the beat goes on. *The Journal of Clinical Endocrinology & Metabolism, 88*(1), 31–33.

Peregrin, T. (2002). P. E. D. S.: A curriculum for diabetes care in the schools. *Journal of the American Dietetic Association, 102*(8), 1502–1053.

Chapter 33

Alterations in Neurologic Function

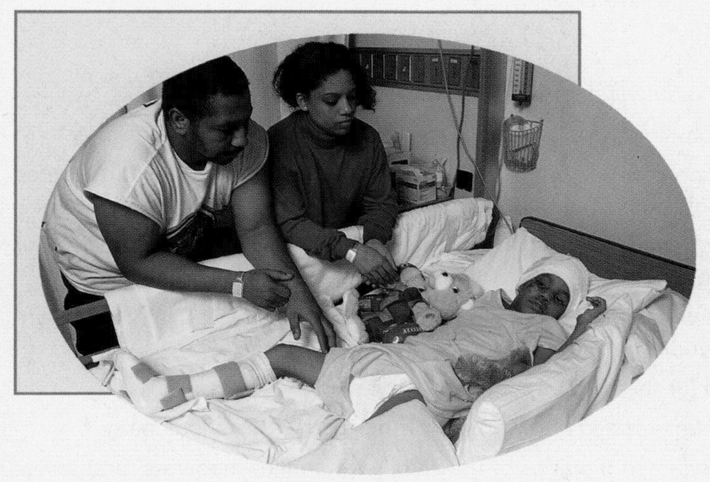

Antwan Baxter, 7 years old, was injured when struck by a car and thrown several feet into the air. He was unconscious upon admission to the emergency department and showed some signs of increased intracranial pressure (dilated and fixed pupils). He was treated for shock, and his neurologic status and vital signs were frequently assessed. The initial evaluation revealed that Antwan had sustained several contusions of the brain, but no skull fracture. He was intubated and medicated to manage the increased intracranial pressure.

Antwan's intracranial pressure has now stabilized, but he still has not totally regained consciousness. He is restless and agitated, and unable to follow directions. His parents stay at his bedside and provide auditory and tactile stimulation, hoping he will eventually respond. Physical therapy has been initiated to prevent contractures and to maintain function. Long-term rehabilitation will be needed to help Antwan and his family achieve the best outcome possible after this injury.

What is the role of the nurse in acute care of the child who has a brain injury? What support does the family need to contribute to the child's care? How does the nurse work with other healthcare professionals to plan the long-term care of a child such as Antwan?

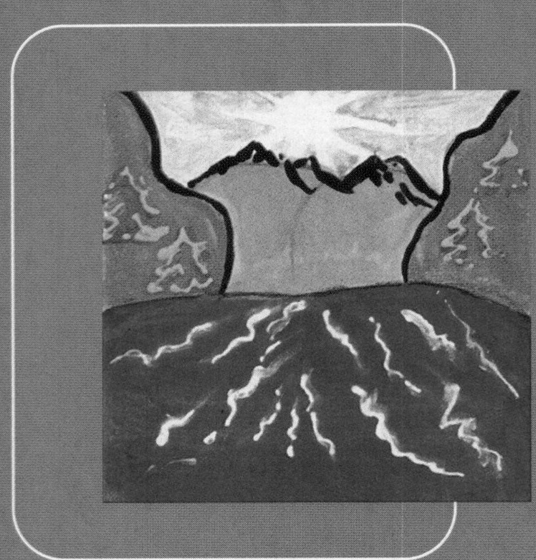

"I wish Antwan would wake up and talk to me. I want to tell him how sorry I am that he got hurt. I didn't mean the things I said would happen to him. I just got mad at him because he was messing with my stuff."

—Janet, age 10

Key Terms

alertness/1300
anencephaly/1328
areflexia/1348
assistive technology/1343
aura/1308
autonomic dysreflexia/1358
Brudzinski sign/1315
cerebral edema/1350
cerebral perfusion pressure/1300
clonic/1307
cognitive power/1300
coma/1300
consciousness/1300
contrecoup injury/1347
coup injury/1347
Cushing's triad/1302
drowning/1360
encephalocele/1328
encephalopathy/1320
fontanels/1300
herniation/1350
intracranial pressure/1300
intractable seizure/1309
Kernig sign/1315
level of consciousness (LOC)/1300
meningocele/1328
meningomyelocele/1328

Learning Outcomes

After completing this chapter, you will be able to:

- Describe the anatomy and physiology of the neurologic system.
- Describe the nursing assessment process and tools used for infants and children with altered levels of consciousness and other neurologic conditions.
- Differentiate between the signs of infants and children with epilepsy and status epilepticus, and describe appropriate nursing management for each condition.
- Differentiate between signs of bacterial meningitis, viral meningitis, encephalitis, Reye syndrome, and Guillain-Barré syndrome in infants and children.
- Develop a nursing care plan for the child with myelodysplasia and hydrocephalus.
- Describe the focus of community-based nursing care for the child with cerebral palsy.
- Distinguish between the assessment findings of the child with a mild, moderate, and severe traumatic brain injury and plan the appropriate initial nursing management for the child with mild and severe traumatic brain injury.

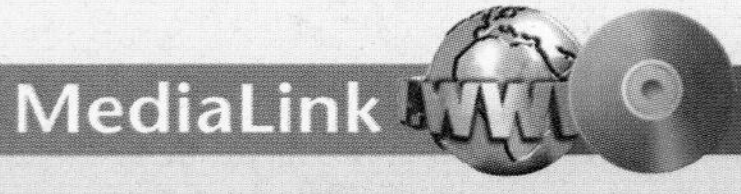

MediaLink http://www.prenhall.com/ball

Resources for this chapter can be found on the CD-ROM accompanying this textbook and on the Companion Website at www.prenhall.com/ball. Click on Chapter 33 to select the activities for this chapter.

CD-ROM

Animations/Videos

3D Brain and Brainstem
Components of a Reflex Arc
Coup-Contracoup Injury
Diazepam
Living with Spina Bifida
Seizures
Synaptic Transmission

NCLEX Review

Audio Glossary

COMPANION WEBSITE

A & P Review

Clinical Manifestations Review

Medication Match-Up

NCLEX Review

Case Study: Assessing a Child with a Concussion for Return to Competitive Play

Care Plan: Newborn with Neonatal Abstinence Syndrome

MediaLink Applications

Critical Thinking: Traumatic Brain Injury Death Prevention

Key Terms *(continued)*

Why do certain neurologic disorders occur more often in children than in adults? What effect do these disorders have on a child's growth and development? Why are some neurologic injuries more likely to be seen in children? What role do nurses play in ensuring early diagnosis and treatment of neurologic disorders? This chapter will answer these questions by examining some of the more common disorders of neurologic function in children.

ANATOMY AND PHYSIOLOGY OF PEDIATRIC DIFFERENCES

Knowledge of the anatomy of the nervous system makes neurologic symptoms easier to understand. The brain, spinal cord, and nerves are the major structures of the nervous system (Figure 33–1 ■). The spinal cord transmits impulses to and from the brain, conveying sensory information and relaying impulses that stimulate motor responses. Because the nervous system helps to control and coordinate many body functions, alterations in neurologic function can have widespread effects on the body's metabolism.

The brain and spinal cord are formed early in gestation from the neural plate which evolves into the neural groove and neural folds by the third week of gestation. The neural groove deepens and the neural folds develop laterally and close to form the neural tube which becomes the central nervous system. The neural folds close first in the cervical region. Closure then progresses in both the cranial and caudal directions. The brain develops from the cranial end of the neural tube, and the spinal cord develops from the other end (Padgett, 2002). Any insult (such as inadequate folic acid) or critical event (teratogen, infection, substance abuse, or trauma) during this early period of gestation can result in a central nervous system (CNS) malformation. Such defects account for approximately one third of all apparent congenital malformations in live infants, and 90% of these are neural tube defects. CNS defects are responsible for 40% of infant deaths in the first year of life (Padgett, 2002).

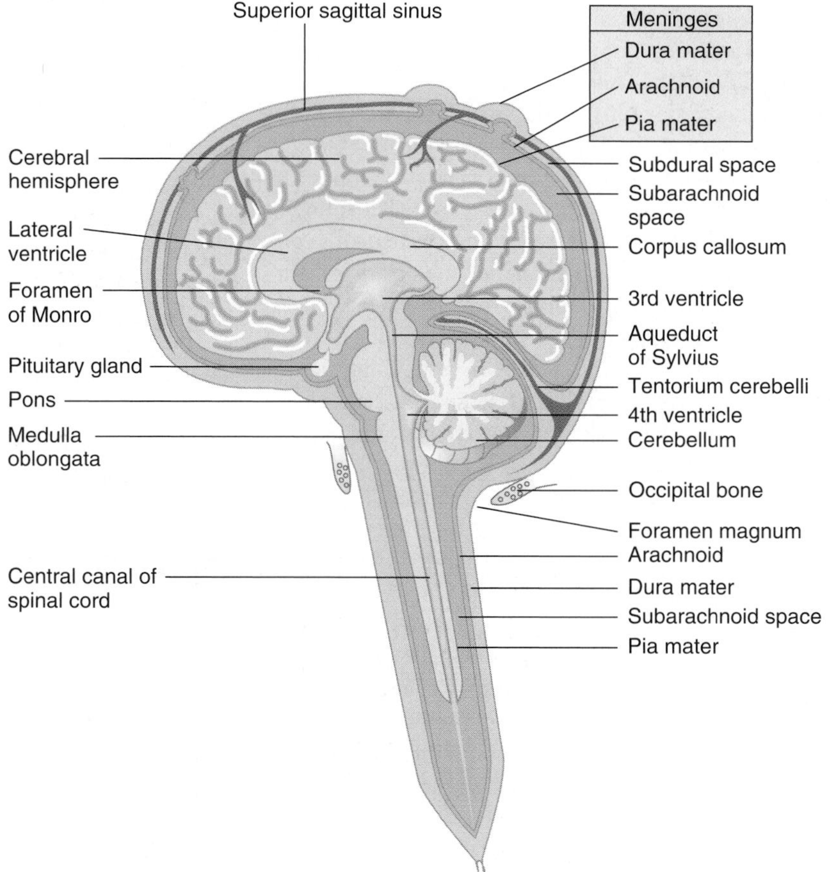

FIGURE 33–1 ■ Transverse section of the brain and spinal cord. Knowledge of brain anatomy is helpful in understanding the symptoms of neurologic dysfunction.

MediaLink Neurology A & P Review

At birth, the nervous system is complete but immature. The infant is born with all of the nerve cells that will exist throughout life, but maturation of these nerve cells continues after birth. The number of glial cells and dendrites, which enable receipt of nerve impulses, continues to increase until approximately 4 years of age. This brain growth results in the increasing head circumference in infants and toddlers. Brain growth continues until the child is 12 to 15 years of age.

Myelination, the progressive covering of axons with layers of myelin or a lipid protein sheath, is also incomplete at birth. Lack of myelination is associated with the presence of primitive reflexes. As the myelination progresses the primitive reflexes disappear. See Table 8–23∞ for the expected appearance and disappearance of primitive reflexes during early infancy. This process continues throughout childhood, proceeding in a cephalocaudal direction, permitting voluntary movement. The myelination process accounts for the progressive acquisition of fine and gross motor skills and coordination during early childhood, and it is ultimately responsible for the speed and accuracy of nerve impulses.

The brain depends on a continuous blood flow to meet its high demands for oxygen. Through an autoregulatory process, the cerebral blood vessels dilate to maintain the cerebral blood flow in response to physiologic changes such as fluctuating cerebral perfusion pressure from decreased cardiac output, increased intracranial pressure, or constriction of the neck's blood vessels due to positioning. When blood flow and oxygenation is not maintained, the brain cells become damaged in a very short time.

The peripheral nervous system arises from the neural crest which evolves into the cranial and spinal ganglia. The peripheral nerves permit transmission of impulses from the nerve pathways to the cerebral cortex through simple spinal reflex arcs. The upper motor neurons consist of the fibers originating in the anterior horn of the spinal cord that travel to the brainstem and the nerve cells in the cerebral cortex. The lower motor neurons consist of the peripheral nerves and branches that transmit impulses to the anterior horn of the spinal cord.

The anatomic and physiologic differences between the nervous systems of children and adults help explain why children and adults have different neurologic problems (Figure 33–2 ■). For example, the brain and spinal cord are protected by the skeletal structures of the skull and vertebrae. In infants, however, the cranial bones and vertebrae are not completely ossified. The infant's brain and spinal cord are thus at greater risk for injury resulting from trauma. The bones of the skull are separated but held together with bands of connective tissue to allow for normal brain growth. **Fontanels** are spaces of connective tissue covering the brain at the junction of skull bones, which gradually close and ossify. The posterior fontanel closes at 3 months of age and the anterior fontanel closes at about 18 to 24 months of age. See Figure 8–16∞. The suture lines between skull bones interlock as early as 6 months of age, and by 12 years of age the sutures are completely ossified and cannot be separated (Padgett, 2002).

MediaLink 3-D Brain Animation

ALTERED STATES OF CONSCIOUSNESS

Level of consciousness (LOC) is perhaps the most important indicator of neurologic dysfunction. Altered levels of consciousness range from consciousness to coma. **Consciousness,** the responsiveness of the mind to sensory stimuli, has two components: **alertness,** or arousal, the ability to react to stimuli, is controlled by the reticular activating system; and **cognitive power,** the ability to process the data and respond either verbally or physically, is controlled by cerebral function. **Unconsciousness,** on the other hand, is depressed cerebral function, or the inability of the brain to respond to stimuli. Altered levels of consciousness can be further categorized as follows:

- *Confusion:* disorientation to time, place, or person. The child may seem alert. Answers to simple questions may be correct, but responses to complex ones may be inaccurate.
- *Delirium:* a state characterized by confusion, fear, agitation, hyperactivity, or anxiety.
- *Obtunded:* limited response to the environment. The child falls asleep unless given verbal or tactile stimulation.
- *Stupor:* response to vigorous stimulation only. The child returns to the unresponsive state when the stimulus is removed. For example, the child may react to a needle stick but not respond to a milder stimulus such as touching the skin.
- ***Coma:*** a state characterized by severely diminished response. The child is unresponsive and cannot be aroused, even by painful stimuli.

Etiology and Pathophysiology

Trauma, infection, poisoning, seizures, or any other process that affects the CNS may alter the level of consciousness (Box 33–1). Any of these pathologic processes can also cause increased **intracranial pressure** (force exerted by brain tissue, cerebrospinal fluid, and blood within the cranial vault). Decreased **cerebral perfusion pressure,** the amount of pressure needed to ensure that adequate oxygen and nutrients will be delivered to the brain, often results when the arterial blood flow to the brain is reduced due to the increase in intracranial pressure. Discovering the cause of an altered level of consciousness is essential so that immediate treatment can begin, to prevent possible secondary effects of the illness or injury.

Clinical Manifestations

Decline in a child's level of consciousness often follows a sequential pattern of deterioration. A child may first appear awake and alert, and may respond appropriately. Initial changes may be sub-

BOX 33–1 Causes of Altered Consciousness

- Hypoxia
- Trauma
- Infection
- Poisoning
- Ventriculoperitoneal shunt malfunction or infection
- Seizures
- Endocrine or metabolic disturbances (e.g., hypoglycemia)
- Electrolyte, acid–base, or biochemical imbalance
- Central nervous system pathology (e.g., neoplasms or degenerative disorders)
- Congenital structural defect

AS THEY GROW

Anatomic Differences in the Structures of the Nervous System Between Children and Adults

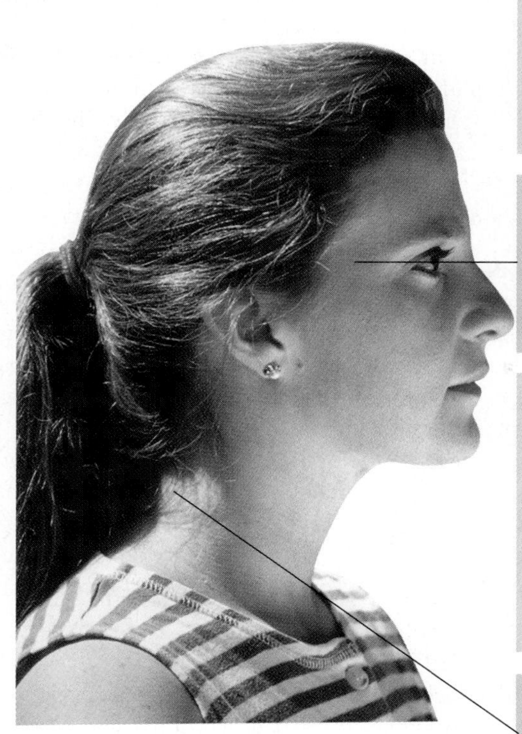

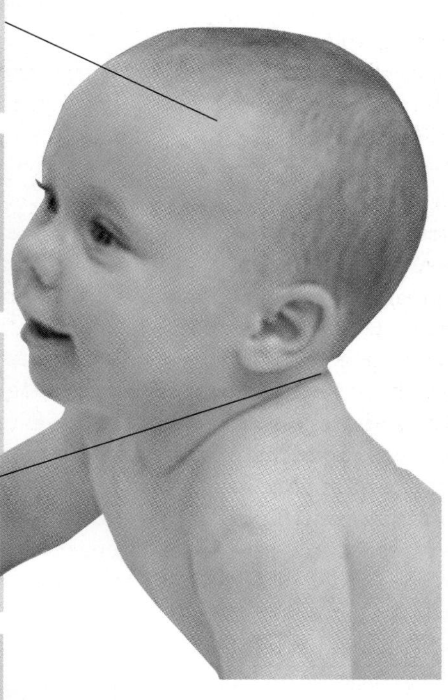

Top heavy, head is large in proportion to body; neck muscles poorly developed; thin cranial bones not well developed; unfused sutures; skull expands until age 2 years. *Prone to brain injury and skull fracture with falls.*
Head size proportional to body; neck muscles well developed, can reduce risk for brain injuries; sutures are ossified by age 12 years; no expansion of skull after 5 years.
Excessive spinal mobility; immature muscles, joint capsule, and ligaments of cervical spine; wedge-shaped, cartilaginous vertebral bodies; incomplete ossification of vertebral bodies. *Greater risk for high cervical spine injury at C1-C2 level or vertebral compression fractures with falls.*
Well developed muscles and ligaments reduce spinal mobility; vertebral bodies completely formed and ossified.

FIGURE 33–2 ■ Infants and young children are at higher risk for injury to the brain and spinal cord because of developing bones and muscles.

tle: a slight disorientation to time, place, and person. The child may become restless or fussy, and actions that normally calm or soothe the child only increase irritability. As responsiveness decreases, the child may become drowsy but still respond to loud verbal commands and withdraw from painful stimuli. Keeping the child awake is sometimes difficult. The response to pain progresses from purposeful to nonpurposeful. Decorticate or decerebrate **posturing,** the abnormal positions assumed after injury or damage to the brain, may occur (Figure 33–3 ■).

Detection of an altered level of consciousness in newborns is more difficult due to the time they spend sleeping. Newborns may have lethargy, irritability, or hyperalertness as key findings of altered consciousness.

Clinical manifestations of increased intracranial pressure are provided in Table 33–1.

COLLABORATIVE CARE

The goal of collaborative care is to rapidly identify the cause for an altered level of consciousness and to provide therapy to prevent further insult to the central nervous system.

Diagnostic Tests

The Glasgow Coma Scale is used to quantify the level of consciousness, thus enabling future comparison of improvement or deterioration in the child's condition (see Skills Manual). Pediatric criteria, which take into account the child's developmental age for each category of the test, have been established to assess responses (Table 33–2).

Laboratory tests include a complete blood cell count, blood chemistry, clotting factors, and blood culture; toxicology

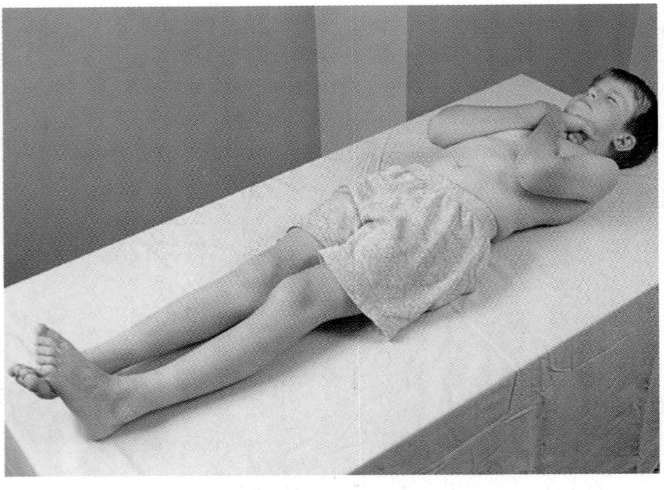

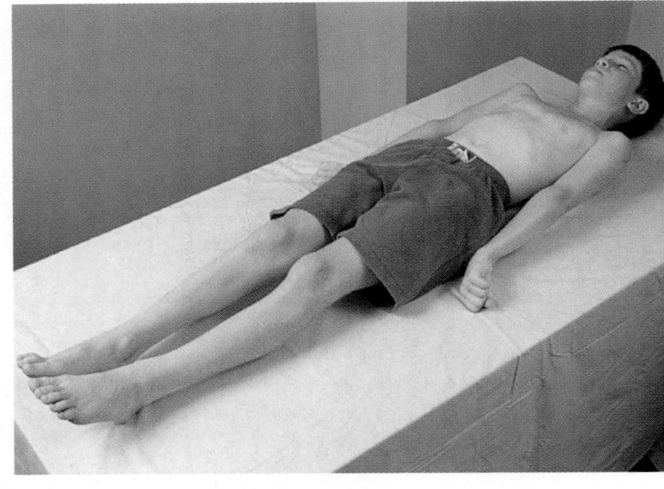

A B

FIGURE 33–3A ■ *A,* Decorticate posturing, characterized by rigid flexion, is associated with lesions above the brainstem in the corticospinal tracts. *B,* Decerebrate posturing, distinguished by rigid extension, is associated with lesions of the brainstem.

assessments of both blood and urine; and urinalysis with culture. A lumbar puncture may be performed to assess the cerebrospinal fluid for protein, glucose, or blood cells as well as pressure level. An electroencephalogram (EEG) identifies damaged or nonfunctioning areas of the brain. Computed tomography (CT) or magnetic resonance imaging (MRI) is used to detect any lesions, structural abnormalities, vascular malformations, or edema. Skull radiograph studies are used to detect fractures or bony malformations. Intracranial pressure monitoring is discussed on page 1350. A summary of diagnostic procedures used in children with neurologic conditions is provided in Table 33–3.

TABLE 33–1 Signs of Increased Intracranial Pressure

TIMING OF SIGNS	SIGNS
Early signs	Headache Visual disturbances, diplopia Nausea and vomiting Dizziness or vertigo Slight change in vital signs Pupils not as reactive or equal Sunsetting eyes Seizures Slight change in level of consciousness
Additional signs in infants	Bulging fontanel Wide sutures, increased head circumference Dilated scalp veins High-pitched, catlike cry
Late signs	Significant decrease in level of consciousness **Cushing's triad** ➤ Increased systolic blood pressure and widened pulse pressure ➤ Bradycardia ➤ Irregular respirations Fixed and dilated pupils

Clinical Therapy

Clinical therapy focuses on early diagnosis, intervention, and prevention of complications. The child is treated with oxygen, and assisted ventilation is provided when gas exchange is inadequate. Any metabolic, acid–base, or electrolyte imbalances are corrected. Antibiotics are initiated for suspected infection.

Efforts are made to maintain the cerebral perfusion pressure. In cases of hypovolemia, intravenous fluids are given. In cases of poor perfusion and fluid overload, dopamine or dobutamine is administered. If the intracranial pressure is markedly increased and results from the accumulation of cerebrospinal fluid because of obstruction, a ventricular catheter can be inserted to drain cerebrospinal fluid and to decrease the intracranial pressure.

NURSING MANAGEMENT

Nursing care is focused on assessing potential causes of altered consciousness, monitoring the child's condition, and providing support to the child and family with altered level of consciousness.

■ Nursing Assessment and Diagnosis

Take a thorough history to identify a potential cause of altered consciousness. Assess whether the child had a recent head trauma, has an infection, has ingested toxins, or has a shunt, tumor, or other condition that could affect the level of consciousness.

Initially assess the child's physiologic status, focusing on the child's responsiveness to the environment or stimuli, ability to maintain the airway, vital signs, head circumference, and breathing patterns. See Box 33–2 and Chapter 8∞ for additional tips in assessing the responsiveness of an infant. Use the Glasgow Coma Scale to assess the child at specified intervals.

TABLE 33–2 Glasgow Coma Scale for Assessment of Coma in Infants and Children

CATEGORY	SCORE*	INFANT AND YOUNG CHILD CRITERIA	OLDER CHILD AND ADULT CRITERIA
Eye opening	4	Spontaneous opening	Spontaneous
	3	To loud noise	To verbal stimuli
	2	To pain	To pain
	1	No response	No response
Verbal response	5	Smiles, coos, cries to appropriate stimuli	Oriented to time, place, and person; uses appropriate words and phrases
	4	Irritable; cries	Confused
	3	Inappropriate crying	Inappropriate words or verbal response
	2	Grunts, moans	Incomprehensible words
	1	No response	No response
Motor response	6	Spontaneous movement	Obeys commands
	5	Withdraws to touch	Localizes pain
	4	Withdraws to pain	Withdraws to pain
	3	Abnormal flexion (decorticate)	Flexion to pain (decorticate)
	2	Abnormal extension (decerebrate)	Extention to pain (decerebrate)
	1	No response	No response

**Add the score from each category to get the total. The maximum score is 15, indicating the best level of neurologic functioning. The minimum is 3, indicating total neurologic unresponsiveness.*

From Teasdale, G., & Jennett, B. (1974). Assessment of coma and impaired consciousness. Lancet, 2, *81–84; James, H. E. (1986). Neurologic evaluation and support in the child with acute brain insult.* Pediatric Annals, *15(1), 17.*

CLINICAL TIP

Performing the Glasgow Coma Scale Assessment in Infants and Young Children

- *Eye opening.* Note if eye opening is spontaneous or occurs in response to stimuli.
- *Verbal response.* Crying in an infant is a positive response. The 2-year-old who says *no* to each command is also responding in an age-appropriate way.
- *Motor response.* Motor score is probably the most critical aspect of this test, since the child cannot control reflexes. A fearful toddler may refuse to open the eyes or talk to strangers, but the child's reflexes should automatically respond to appropriate stimuli. To help the toddler feel less threatened when assessing motor skills, ask the child to reach for a finger puppet or doll rather than your hand. The toy can serve as a reward.

Assess the child's cranial nerves (see Table 8–22∞). The child's responses may differ significantly when stress and anxiety are reduced. Encourage the parents to take part in the examination to reduce the child's anxiety. In the unconscious child, cranial nerve assessment and interpretation are more challenging. See Table 33–4 for cranial nerve assessment guidelines in the unconscious child.

Assess the child's respiratory effort and color. Monitor pulse oximetry or arterial blood gas measurements. Adequate air exchange to keep oxygen and carbon dioxide levels within normal ranges is critical to reduce the risk of increased intracranial pressure. If the child cannot maintain an adequate respiratory effort, mechanical ventilation will be necessary.

Perform routine neurologic checks to monitor neurologic status, including assessment of pupil size and reactivity, eye movements, and motor function (Figure 33–4 ■). Monitor vital signs: Increased systolic blood pressure, a wide pulse pressure, and bradycardia indicate increased intracranial pressure. Observe for other physiologic signs of increased intracranial pressure listed in Table 33–1.

TABLE 33–3 Diagnostic Tests Used for the Neurologic System

DIAGNOSTIC PROCEDURE	PURPOSE
Lumbar puncture	Collects cerebrospinal fluid for culture and lab analysis, measures pressure of cerebrospinal fluid in spinal column
Electroencephalogram	Measures electrical activity in various lobes of the brain to identify the potential for seizures, and to determine brain death
Radiograph	Evaluates the bones of the skull for fractures, spreading suture lines, unexpected characteristics such as bone erosion or degeneration Evaluates the bones of the vertebrae for alignment, fractures, unusual separation, or bony defects
Computed tomography	Evaluates the density of intracranial tissues and structures to identify congenital anomalies, hemorrhage, tumors, and infection
Magnetic resonance imaging	Examines specific characteristics of brain tissue on multiple planes for detailed imaging and to identify anatomic cause of disorders, may also permit study of cerebrospinal fluid flow dynamics
Positron emission tomography (PET)	Evaluates blood flow, metabolic activity, and biochemical changes within the brain
Ventricular catheter insertion	Measures intracranial pressure
Ultrasonography	Visualizes anatomic structure of brain, primarily used in newborns and infants when the anterior fontanel is open

BOX 33–2 Assessment of Responsiveness

When initially checking the responsiveness of infants, the acronym AVPU provides a method for rapid assessment.

Alert, responsive to parents, cuddles, coos or babbles, smiles

Verbal, responsive to verbal stimulation

Pain, responsive to painful stimulation only

Unresponsive to painful stimulation

Additionally assess the infant for a loud energetic quality to the cry, feeding for a strong suck and suck-swallowing coordination, and the presence of appropriate primitive reflexes for age. These signs all indicate intact mental status.

Following are nursing diagnoses that may be appropriate for the child with an altered level of consciousness.

- Ineffective Breathing Pattern related to neuromuscular dysfunction associated with increased intracranial pressure
- Risk for Aspiration related to decreased level of consciousness
- Risk for Impaired Skin Integrity related to decreased level of consciousness and impaired mobility
- Impaired Verbal Communication related to physiologic condition of decreased level of consciousness
- Interrupted Family Processes related to care of a child with an acquired disability

Planning and Implementation

Nursing care of the child with altered consciousness or increased intracranial pressure focuses on maintaining airway patency, monitoring neurologic status, performing routine care, providing sensory stimulation, and providing emotional support to parents. Nursing care for the child with increased intracranial pressure is described beginning on page 1352.

Maintain Airway Patency

Make sure the airway of the infant or child is clear at all times. If the child does not have a gag reflex or has difficulty swallowing secretions, intubation or a tracheostomy is performed. Frequent suctioning may be required. Keep suction apparatus with catheters at the bedside along with oxygen, resuscitation bag and mask, and extra tracheostomy tubes (if applicable). (See Skills Manual.)

Pulse oximetry or arterial blood gas analysis is performed at regular intervals to ensure that gas exchange is adequate. Mechanical ventilation may be required.

Anticipate that seizures may occur. Pad the side rails to protect the child from injury.

Perform Routine Care

If the corneal reflex is absent, place an approved ophthalmologic ointment or artificial tears in the eyes and cover with gauze, taping over so they remain closed. Perform routine mouth care by brushing the teeth and using glycerine swabs. Gently clean the oral mucosa in newborns and keep secretions from accumulating.

Provide adequate nutrition. Initially, nutrients may be supplied intravenously. A nasogastric or gastrostomy tube may be inserted if the infant or child remains unconscious or is not alert enough to take food by mouth.

Prevent complications associated with immobility (muscle atrophy, contractures, and skin breakdown) as described in

TABLE 33–4 Assessment of Cranial Nerves in the Unconscious Child

CRANIAL NERVES	REFLEX ASSESSMENT PROCEDURE AND *NORMAL FINDINGS*
II, III Pupillary	Shine a light source in eye. *Rapid, concentrically constricting pupils indicate intact cranial nerves II, III.*
II, IV, VI Oculocephalic	Should be performed with eyes held open (doll's eyes) and head turned from side to side. *Eyes gazing straight up or lagging slightly behind head motion indicates intact cranial nerves.* Precaution: Cervical spine injury must be ruled out before this assessment is performed.
III, VIII Oculovestibular	Place the head in a midline and slightly elevated position. Inject ice water into ear canal. *Eyes deviating toward the irrigated ear indicate intact cranial nerves III, VIII.* Precautions: Cervical spine injury must be ruled out before this assessment is performed. Tympanic membrane must be intact; otherwise brain may be filled with bacteria-laden fluid. Note: This assessment is usually performed by a physician.
V, VII Corneal	Cornea is gently swabbed with sterile cotton swab. *A blink indicates intact cranial nerves V, VII.*
IX, X Gag	Pharynx is irritated with tongue depressor or cotton swab. *Gagging response indicates intact cranial nerves IX, X.*

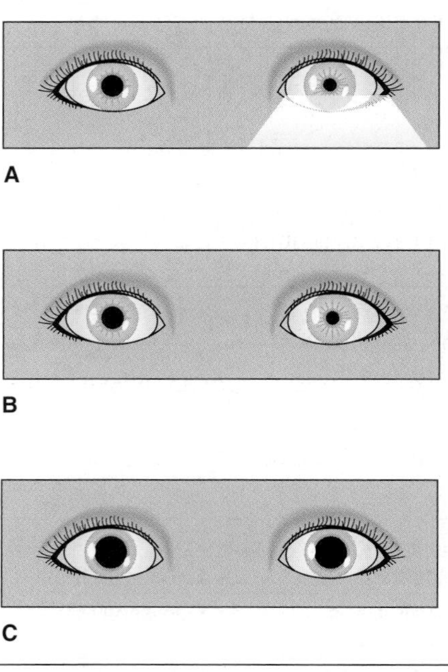

FIGURE 33–4 ■ Pupil findings in various neurologic conditions with altered consciousness. *A,* A unilateral dilated and reactive pupil is associated with an intracranial mass. *B,* A fixed and dilated pupil may be a sign of impending brainstem herniation. *C,* Bilateral fixed and dilated pupils are associated with brainstem herniation from increased intracranial pressure.

Box 33–3. With Antwan, as discussed in the chapter opener, nurses support physical therapy efforts with extra passive range of motion exercises.

Provide Sensory Stimulation

Explain all procedures and actions. Because the child with a severely altered level of consciousness may still be able to hear, it may be beneficial to talk, play music, or play tapes of stories. Encourage the parents to stroke and touch the child in a soothing manner.

When the child becomes more alert, orient the child to time, place, and person. Use information that corresponds to the child's age and level of understanding. Encourage parents to bring objects or toys from home to make the environment more familiar and promote a feeling of security. Listening to music or tapes of family members talking or reading can soothe a child who has an altered level of consciousness.

Provide Emotional Support

Explain the child's condition to the family in simple terms. Encourage parents to take part in the child's care and therapy as much as possible. If the child's normal functioning has been permanently impaired, refer the family to the appropriate psychologic and social services for emotional support. (See Chapter 21∞ for more information about helping families cope with a child's life-threatening illness.) Provide family members with opportunities to express their feelings.

Discharge Planning and Home Care Teaching

The child's transition from the hospital to home, a long-term care facility, or inpatient rehabilitation center must be planned well in advance of discharge. A case manager or social worker who can help plan the child's long-term care needs, including home health nursing, adaptation of the home, and the purchase of special equipment, should be identified.

Care in the Community

Home care nurses play a vital role in the care of such children as Antwan who have an acquired neurologic dysfunction and prolonged altered consciousness. Teach the family how to care for the child with severe neurologic dysfunction and to perform routine procedures such as suctioning and maintaining the airway, skin care, feeding, positioning, range of motion exercises, and stimulation. See Chapter 36∞ for recognition of pressure areas needing intervention. Regular follow-up visits are needed to assess the child's progress and to modify the treatment plan.

The child also needs to be linked with community rehabilitation services through an early intervention program or school-based program. The home health nurse or case manager should assist the family to have an individualized education plan developed for the child (see Chapter 20∞).

BOX 33–3 Care of the Immobile Child

- Help keep body in proper alignment with splints or rolls made of towels or blankets.
- Perform passive or gentle range of motion exercises 3–4 times per day according to physician's orders.
- Maintain skin integrity:
  - Change position every 2 hours.
  - Place child on foam or egg-crate mattress or sheepskin covering.
  - Massage child gently using lotion.
  - Place transparent dressing over surfaces exposed to frequent friction.

■ Evaluation

Expected outcomes of nursing care include the following:

- The child's airway is maintained and the cerebral perfusion pressure is maintained to oxygenate the brain.
- The child develops no complications related to immobility.
- The family is supported to provide care and stimulation to the nonresponsive child.
- The child with prolonged altered consciousness receives care from a multidisciplinary team to minimize long-term disabilities..

SEIZURE DISORDERS

Seizures are periods of abnormal electrical discharges (excessive concurrent firing) of the cortical neuronal network of cells on the surface of the brain that cause involuntary movement, and behavior and sensory alterations. They are a common neurologic disorder in children. Epilepsy is a chronic disorder characterized by recurrent, unprovoked seizures secondary to an underlying brain abnormality. One in 100 people have epilepsy (Valente, 2000). Infants are susceptible to developing seizures in the first year of life with an incidence of 1 per 1,000. The incidence decreases with age. The median age for development of epilepsy is 5 to 6 years of age. In the United States, approximately 150,000 to 325,000 children between 5 and 14 year of age have epilepsy (Blair & Selekman, 2004). See Developing Cultural Competence: Seizures.

Etiology and Pathophysiology

Seizures are believed to be the result of abnormal excessive concurrent electrical discharges of the cortical neuronal network of cells on the surface of the brain. Chemical changes (potassium, sodium, chloride) within the neurons create an electrical negativity that enables the transfer of information between neurons. When an excessive number of the cells become excited, they discharge abnormally. These cells can be triggered by either environmental or physiologic stimuli such as emotional stress, anxiety, fatigue, infection, or electrolyte or metabolic disturbances. The most common cause in children is an acute brain insult such as a central nervous system infection, hypoxia, or brain injury.

Some seizures are idiopathic, or not provoked by known stimuli. Genetic factors may lower the seizure threshold by making brain cells more vulnerable to abnormal electrical discharges. Acquired seizures may be caused by underlying pathologic conditions such as trauma, infection, hypoglycemia, endocrine dysfunction, toxins, tumors, or lesions that may be manifested at

MediaLink Seizure Disorders Video

CLINICAL MANIFESTATIONS of Seizures

TYPE OF SEIZURE AND ETIOLOGY	CLINICAL MANIFESTATIONS
Partial Seizures ***Complex Partial Seizures*** (psychomotor seizures) Lesions, cysts, or tumors Perinatal trauma Focal sclerosis, i.e. scarring of the mediotemporal lobe from prolonged febrile seizures Vascular anomalies, i.e. arteriovenous malformations Brain trauma	*Onset:* 3 years of age to adolescence Consciousness is impaired immediately or gradually after a simple partial onset, lasts 30 seconds up to 5 minutes, post-seizure amnesia or confusion May have abnormal motor activity, twitching, loss of tone, sensory changes such as tingling or numbness, may progress to a generalized seizure Aura frequently present, unusual taste or odor (may actually be a simple partial seizure) Feelings of anxiety, fear or déjà vu (sensation that event occurred before) Abdominal pain Staring into space, mental confusion Posturing Automatisms— lip smacking, lip chewing, sucking
Simple Partial Seizures (focal seizures) Focal damage (e.g., with cerebral palsy) Tumors or lesions Arteriovenous malformation Brain abscesses	*Onset:* any age No loss of consciousness. Lasts less than 30 seconds. No postseizure confusion No aura Occurs many times a day Motor responses may involve one extremity, part of extremity, or ipsilateral extremities with eyes and head turning in opposite direction Sensory responses involve paresthesias (decreased sensation or tingling); auditory, olfactory, or visual sensations; autonomic (sweating, papillary dilation) or psychic symptoms Motor and sensory involvement may be combined and progress to a generalized seizure Jacksonian march (rare in children): tonic contractions of either fingers of one hand, toes of one foot, or one side of face become clonic or tonic-clonic movements; activity then "marches" up to adjacent muscles of either affected extremity or same side of body (such as face)
Generalized Seizures ***Tonic-clonic Seizures*** (grand mal seizures) Cerebral damage from perinatal trauma, brain trauma, tumors, structural lesions Metabolic and neuromuscular degenerative disorders Genetic link Many are idiopathic	*Onset:* any age, rare before 6 months of age, strong familial incidence Abrupt onset seizure, 1–2 minute loss of consciousness, postseizure confusion (few minutes to hours) May or may not have aura Body becomes stiff and rigid when all muscles contract (tonic phase), followed by rhythmic jerking motions (clonic phase) Eyes roll upward or deviate to one side with pupils dilated Drooling or foaming at mouth as secretions are not swallowed Abdominal or chest wall rigidity with leg, head, and neck extended, and arms flexed or contracted Cry or grunt as air is forced out when diaphragm and chest muscles contract Urinary or bowel incontinence as muscles become flaccid during clonic phase Characterized by sleepiness, difficulty in arousal; hypertension; diaphoresis; headache, nausea, vomiting; poor coordination, decreased muscle tone; confusion, amnesia; slurred speech; visual disturbances; combativeness

any time. See the clinical manifestations table above and on the following page for the etiology of various types of seizures.

Partial or focal seizures are caused by abnormal electrical activity in one hemisphere or a specific area of the cerebral cortex, most often the temporal, frontal, or parietal lobes. The symptoms that are displayed depend on the region of the cerebral cortex affected.

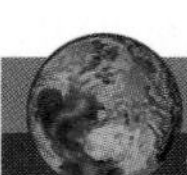

DEVELOPING CULTURAL COMPETENCE Seizures

Seizures may have a special meaning to different cultural groups. For example, the Hmong believe the child is experiencing quag dab peg, or "the spirit catches you and you fall down." Traditional Hmong view the condition as serious, but take pride in the child who has the condition, as they have a link to the spirit world. In 1997, Anne Fadiman wrote a compelling story about the cultural conflict between a Hmong family and healthcare providers over the treatment of their daughter's seizures, *The Spirit Catches You and You Fall Down* (Fadiman; 1997, Spector, 2000).

In contrast, generalized seizures are the result of diffuse electrical activity that begins in both hemispheres of the brain simultaneously and spreads throughout the cortex into the brainstem. As a result, movements and spasms displayed by the child are bilateral and symmetric.

The length of a seizure, especially a generalized seizure, is important because the airway may be compromised during the tonic phase. The basal metabolic rate rises during the peak of seizure activity. This change, in turn, increases the demand for oxygen and glucose. During a seizure the child may become pale or cyanotic as a result of hypoxia or hypoglycemia.

Febrile seizures occur in connection with a sudden rise in temperature in association with an acute illness. No evidence of intracranial infection or other defined cause is found. They are usually seen between 3 months and 5 years with a peak incidence between 17 to 24 months of age. There is often a family history

CLINICAL MANIFESTATIONS of Seizures (continued)

TYPE OF SEIZURE AND ETIOLOGY	CLINICAL MANIFESTATIONS
Absence Seizures (petit mal, or lapse seizures) Hyperventilation Genetic predisposition	*Onset:* age 3–12 years with remission in adolescence More prevalent in females Hyperventilation or flashing lights may trigger a seizure May go on to develop other generalized seizures Brief loss of consciousness, usually lasts 5–10 seconds, rarely exceeds 30 seconds, no postseizure confusion, lethargy, or sleepiness Frequent attacks (50–100 or more per day), may cluster, interfere with learning No aura Child may continue simple movements such as walking or looking, but ceases activities such as reading Staring, usually a glazed eye appearance, episodes may be confused with daydreaming or inattentiveness Cannot be interrupted by verbal or touch stimulation Rolling of eyes, eye blinking, ptosis or fluttering of eyelids Slight increase or loss of muscle tone (head may droop, handheld objects may be dropped) Amnesia
Myoclonic Seizures Progressive or degenerative encephalopathy like Tay-Sachs disease	*Onset:* as early as 2 years, but more prevalent in school-age child or adolescent No loss of consciousness, child recovers in seconds, no postictal period Attacks occur most often upon falling asleep or awakening Quick involuntary muscle jerks, may appear to drop or throw object; sudden flexion and bending of upper torso and head, extremity, or body contractions, may be limited to one body part or whole body
Infantile Spasms (myoclonic epilepsy of infancy, salaam seizures) Prenatal and perinatal encephalopathy Brain malformation Metabolic disorder Tuberous sclerosis Microcephaly Evolve into Lennox-Gaustaut syndrome	*Onset:* begin at age 3 months and resolve by 2 years Positive history of gestational difficulties, developmental delays or other neurologic abnormalities May occur with altered consciousness as part of a complex partial seizure Occur in clusters, 5 to 150 per day Episodes of abrupt flexor (jackknife seizures), extensor or mixed jerks occurring in flurries when infant is awakening or throughout wakefulness Eye rolling, either upward or downward Crying, pallor, or cyanosis Seizure activity increases in intensity and severity over time Regression in development milestones and irritability
Akinetic or Atonic Seizures (drop attacks) Gray matter degenerative diseases and subacute seizures Sclerosing panencephalitis Many are idiopathic	*Onset:* first seen at 2 years, disappear by 6 years Momentary loss of consciousness Falls to ground with sudden loss of postural tone, inability to break fall, is limp for period of time Quickly regains consciousness

of febrile seizures. In addition, children who have one febrile seizure have a 30% to 40% greater chance of having future seizures (Gill & Gieron-Korthals, 2002). The lower convulsive threshold of infants may explain this type of seizure.

Newborn seizures usually occur because of primary central nervous system disease (intraventricular or other hemorrhage), infection, inborn error of metabolism, asphyxia, metabolic insult, electrolyte disorder, or other underlying disease. Cortical seizures (like a myoclonic seizure) are rare in newborns because they have more inhibitory rather than excitatory synapses.

Children with seizure disorders have been found to have more behavior problems than their siblings and children with other chronic conditions, particularly attention deficit problems. There is some speculation that the association of behavioral disturbances and epilepsy may be a transient cognitive impairment caused by subclinical epileptiform discharges that interfere with normal brain functioning (Austin, Harezlak, Dunn, et al., 2001).

Clinical Manifestations

The symptoms of a seizure depend on its type and duration. Seizures are classified into two types: partial (focal) seizures and generalized seizures of nonfocal origin. The specific characteristics of the various types of partial and generalized seizures are presented in the clinical manifestations table above and on the previous page.

Partial seizures are the most common type and often start with an aura or abrupt unprovoked alteration in behavior. Generalized seizures often begin with a **tonic** phase characterized by unconsciousness, continuous muscular contraction, and sustained stiffness. The tonic phase is followed by the **clonic** phase, characterized by alternating muscular contraction and relaxation as a rhythmic repetitive jerking. Tonic-clonic seizures are the most common seizure type in children, accounting for about 25% of seizures in individuals of all ages (Weinstein, 2002). The **postictal period** following seizure activity is a phase during which the level of consciousness is decreased. The length of the postictal period varies among children. Children may have a partial seizure and progress to a generalized seizure.

An **aura** is a sensation (visual, auditory, taste, or motor) that gives warning of an impending seizure. Some practitioners consider an aura associated with epilepsy to be a simple partial seizure (Blair, & Selekman, 2004). When the child recognizes the pattern of an aura, he or she may have time to avoid injury by getting to the floor.

Febrile seizures—generalized seizures that usually occur in children as the result of rapid temperature rise above 39°C (102°F)—involve generalized tonic-clonic movements that last less than 15 minutes. Most often the seizure lasts 1 to 2 minutes. A complex form of febrile seizures may be partial (focal) or generalized. It may last longer than 15 minutes (see status epilepticus below) and recur within 24 hours.

Newborn seizures are more subtle (horizontal deviation of eye, repetitive blinking, sucking or lip smacking/tongue thrusting, rhythmic repetitive movement of an extremity [like bicycling of the legs]).

COLLABORATIVE CARE

The goal of collaborative care is to identify the underlying cause of the seizure and identify the appropriate clinical therapy to interrupt a prolonged seizure and to prevent future seizures.

Diagnostic Testing

After the child's first seizure, it is essential that a thorough history be taken from the parent, primary caretaker, or witnesses to the event. Box 33–4 lists appropriate questions to ask. Details such as the description and length of the seizure, presence or absence of an aura, and if the child lost consciousness should be noted. This information is used to identify the type of seizure according to the International Classification of Epileptic Seizures described in the previous clinical manifestations table.

Based on the physical findings and history, diagnostic tests ordered may include a complete blood cell count, blood chemistry, urine culture, and lumbar puncture (if the child is febrile). If the child is taking any anticonvulsants, a medication blood level is checked. An electroencephalogram (EEG) is often performed at a follow-up visit between seizures. Other potential screening tests that may be considered include a lead level, toxicology screening, and tests for inborn errors of metabolism. Radiologic tests such as a CT scan or an MRI may be performed to identify a cerebral lesion or to identify metabolic derangements of the brain.

BOX 33–4 Questions to Ask about Seizures

- Did the child complain of not feeling well or feeling "funny" just before the seizure?
- Did the child complain of headache, nausea, muscle pain? Did the child vomit?
- Did the child suffer any trauma before the seizure?
- Did the child get into any medications or poisons before the seizure?
- Was the child sick or feverish before the seizure?
- What movements of the arms and legs were seen? Were the movements on one side of the body or in one extremity only?
- Was the child's vision normal?
- Were the pupils dilated or the eyes deviated to one side?
- Was the child aware of surroundings? Could the child respond to questions?
- Was the child incontinent of urine or stool?
- How long did the episode last? When did the child begin to wake up?
- Was the child lethargic, weak, or uncoordinated upon arousal?
- Was the child injured during the convulsion?
- Did the child's color change (pale, red, blue)?

Clinical Therapy

Many convulsions are self-limiting and require no emergency intervention.

Febrile Seizures. Children with febrile seizures may be treated with an anticonvulsant for the remainder of the presenting febrile illness. Some practitioners offer intermittent anticonvulsants to be given at the time of a fever or continuous anticonvulsant therapy if the child has had more than one febrile seizure and if parents are especially anxious (Gill & Gieron-Korthals, 2002). However, the American Academy of Pediatrics (1999) recommends that no long-term anticonvulsant therapy be given for febrile seizures. Instead, parents are taught to lower fevers by using nonaspirin antipyretics and keep the child cool with light clothing. Parents are also taught to protect the child from injury in the event of a subsequent seizure.

Status Epilepticus. The child with a generalized seizure lasting longer than 10 minutes needs to have electrolytes, glucose, blood gases, increasing fever, and abnormal blood pressure monitored. Anticonvulsants such as diazepam are given intravenously or rectally in an effort to end the seizure. Monitor for continued motor activity and the potential for **status epilepticus** (a continuous seizure that lasts for more than 30 minutes or a series of seizures during which consciousness is not regained). Motor activity may become less apparent after anticonvulsants are given, even though the child is still unconscious (Altmeier, 1999). The postictal period ranges from 30 minutes to 2 hours. Management of the child in status epilepticus is described in Table 33–5.

Medications. Most seizure disorders are treated with anticonvulsants. A single medication (monotherapy) is preferred for seizure control to minimize side effects that can be significant (sleepiness, decreased attention and memory, difficulty with speech, ataxia, and diplopia). Monotherapy works for 60% to 70% of children with new onset epilepsy (Blair & Selekman, 2004). If seizure control is not accomplished with the first antiepileptic medication, another medication is used to see if the response is better. Medications may also be changed if unacceptable side effects occur. See the medication table on page 1310 for a listing of antiepileptic medications. Serum drug levels are monitored to achieve therapeutic levels or when toxicity is possible. Therapeutic ranges of medications may be exceeded when tolerated by the child to achieve seizure control. Medication dosage adjustments are often needed as the child grows.

TABLE 33–5 Collaborative Care for Status Epilepticus

TYPE OF CARE	COLLABORATIVE CARE
Emergency assessment and interventions	➤ Maintain a patent airway. Muscle rigidity may compromise the airway. ➤ Perform a jaw thrust maneuver if the airway is obstructed. ➤ Keep suction equipment at bedside to clear secretions. ➤ Give oxygen by mask, as increased metabolic demands deplete oxygen stores. ➤ Monitor vital signs and circulation with pulse oximeter and cardiorespiratory monitor. ➤ Assess neurologic level.
Ongoing urgent management	➤ Establish an intravenous line to administer any necessary fluids or medications. ➤ Assess blood glucose level and administer glucose if the child is hypoglycemic; the physical stress of the seizure may result in declining glucose levels. ➤ Insert a nasogastric tube to reduce risk of aspiration due to vomiting. ➤ Protect the child from injury. ➤ Manage thermoregulation.
Medications	➤ Administer benzodiazepines such as diazepam, lorazepam, or midazolam. If there is no response, the dose may be repeated. Phenytoin or phenobarbital may be necessary if seizure activity continues. ➤ Cumulative doses of drugs may produce apnea, so be prepared to assist with intubation and ventilations.

Approximately 25% to 30% of children have refractory or **intractable seizures,** which continue to occur even with optimal medical management (Danielpour & Peacock, 2000). These children are often treated with multiple anticonvulsants. Some children have multiple seizure types and are also treated with multiple anticonvulsants. Regular blood testing is performed to identify any developing hematologic or liver problems, as well as to determine if therapeutic ranges of medications are maintained.

CLINICAL TIP

Herbal preparations with ginkgo may decrease the effectiveness of anticonvulsants.

A trial of medication withdrawal is often attempted for children who have been seizure free for at least 2 years. Approximately 60% to 75% of children are successfully weaned from antiepileptic medications and have no seizures (Blair & Selekman, 2004).

Invasive Procedures. Surgery may occasionally be performed to remove a tumor, lesion, or portion of the brain that has been identified as causing the seizures, particularly when the seizures are not responsive to medication. When the precise seizure focus can be determined, surgical resection of that area can be performed. A temporal lobectomy (removal of the temporal lobe) or hemispherectomy (complete or partial removal of most of one side of the brain) may be used for certain seizure disorders. Another option is a corpus callosotomy in which the corpus callosum is divided to stop the spread of seizures from one side of the brain to the other.

A vagal nerve stimulator is another option for children who are unable to tolerate several antiepileptic medications and are not candidates for surgery. A pulse generator is implanted in the chest and leads are threaded under the skin and wrapped around the left vagus nerve. The pulse generator is programmed to stimulate the vagus nerve. A strong magnet can be passed across the skin over the pulse generator to prevent or stop a seizure (Blair & Selekman, 2004).

Ketogenic Diet. A ketogenic diet is occasionally used for children with myoclonic and absence seizures. This diet involves a high intake of fat (90%), an adequate intake of protein (1 gm/kg), and very low intake of carbohydrates (Figure 33–5 ■). Caloric intake is calculated at 75% and fluids are restricted to 80% of usual (Freeman, 2003). The ketosis caused by the diet is believed to produce the anticonvulsant effects. The diet is adjusted and customized to the child to maintain the ideal body weight, maximize ketosis, and achieve optimal seizure control. Family motivation must be high to maintain the diet for 2 to 3 years and to frequently monitor the child's urine ketone values (Katyal, Koehler, & McGhee, et al., 2000). The most common complications are constipation and kidney stones. Constipation can be treated with medium-chain triglycerides (MCT oil) and increasing fluids. Kidney stones occur in 6% to 7% of children on the ketogenic diet and they are treated with increased fluid

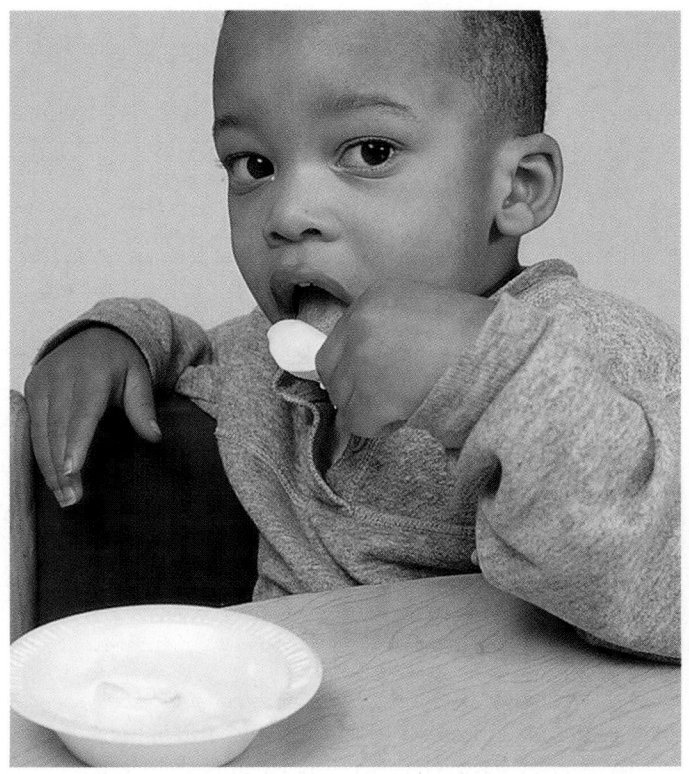

FIGURE 33–5 ■ The family must make an effort to make the high-fat diet appealing to the child on a ketogenic diet, despite their personal feelings about eating large amounts of food such as mayonnaise, as this child is doing.

MEDICATIONS Used to Treat Seizures

MEDICATION	ACTION	NURSING CONSIDERATIONS
Diazepam IV	Anticonvulsant agent used for status epilepticus.	➤ IV push medication is administered very slowly as close to vein as possible. ➤ Monitor vital signs for hypotension, tachycardia, and respiratory depression.
Phenobarbital PO, IV, IM	Limits spread of seizure activity by increasing threshold for motor cortex stimuli; used for generalized and partial seizures, and status epilepticus.	➤ IV medication must be administered slowly. ➤ Monitor child's vital signs frequently when given IV. ➤ May crush tablets and mix with food or fluid.
Phenytoin PO, IV	Inhibits seizure activity, reduces voltage, frequency, and spread of electrical discharges within motor cortex; used for generalized, psychomotor, and nonepileptic seizures.	➤ Educate family to ensure adequate intake of vitamin D, folic acid, and calcium. ➤ Promote frequent dental care for gingival hyperplasia. ➤ Ginkgo may decrease anticonvulsant effectiveness.
Carbamazepine PO	Action similar to phenytoin; used for generalized, psychomotor, and mixed seizures.	➤ Give with food to enhance absorption. ➤ Do not administer suspension simultaneously with another liquid medication to prevent formation of a precipitate. ➤ Causes photosensitivity reactions.
Valproic acid PO	Anticonvulsant, mechanism of action unknown; used for absence and mixed seizures.	➤ Do not use carbonated beverage to dilute syrup. ➤ Tablets and capsules should not be chewed. ➤ Give with food to decrease GI irritation. ➤ Monitor platelet count and bleeding times. ➤ Drug should not be used in combination with aspirin, sedatives, and allergy medications.
Ethosuximide PO	Depresses motor cortex and increases CNS threshold to stimuli; used for absence, myoclonic, and akinetic seizures.	➤ Monitor for weight loss or anorexia. ➤ Give with food if GI upset occurs.
Primidone PO	Raises seizure threshold and changes seizure patterns, similar to barbiturate action; used for complex partial and generalized seizures.	➤ Tablet may be crushed and given with fluid; may be given with food. ➤ Do not combine with OTC medications unless approved by healthcare provider. ➤ Educate family to ensure adequate intake of vitamin D, folic acid, calcium, and vitamin B_{12}.
Clonazepam PO	Suppresses spike and wave pattern in absence seizures, decreases spread of discharge in minor motor seizures; used for absence, myoclonic, and akinetic seizures.	➤ Monitor for signs of overdose (confusion, irritability, sleepiness, sweating, muscle cramps, diminished reflexes). ➤ Do not combine with OTC medications unless approved by healthcare provider.
Felbamate PO	Blocks repetitive firing of neurons and increases seizure threshold; used for partial seizures and Lennox-Gastaut syndrome.	➤ Monitor weight for gain or loss. ➤ Child needs regular monitoring for hematologic and liver problems. ➤ Careful dosing is needed when combined with other anticonvulsants.
Gabapentin PO	GABA neurotransmitter analog; used with other anticonvulsants for control of partial seizures.	➤ Vision, concentration, and coordination may be impaired by the medication. ➤ Do not take medication within 2 hours of an antacid.
Lamotrigine PO	Inhibits release of glutamate (neurotransmitter) in brain tissue; used for partial, generalized, and absence seizures.	➤ Drug increases photosensitivity. ➤ Monitor for adverse effects if used with valproic acid.
Tiagabine PO	GABA inhibitor; used for partial seizures.	➤ Give with food. ➤ Monitor for signs of central nervous system depression. ➤ Avoid using with OTC medications that cause drowsiness.
Topiramate PO	GABA inhibitor; used for partial seizures.	➤ Increase fluid intake to reduce risk of kidney stones. ➤ Psychomotor slowing as well as speech and language problems may develop with use of medication.

Data from Wilson, B. A., Shannon, M. T., & Stang, C. L. (2005). Nurse's drug guide 2005. *Upper Saddle River, NJ: Prentice Hall Health.*

intake and alkalinization of the urine. Evaluation of the effectiveness of the diet is determined by lack of seizures or significant reduction in frequency. Sometimes the medications can be reduced so that side effects are minimized. Some children have discontinued the diet after 2 years with no seizures and no antiepileptic medications needed.

NURSING MANAGEMENT

Nursing care at the time of a seizure focuses on maintaining airway patency, ensuring safety, administering medications, and providing emotional support. The nurse also assists the family to manage the condition long term.

■ Nursing Assessment and Diagnosis

Nursing assessment first focuses on assessing the child with a seizure to identify immediate care needed. For the child with known seizures, assessment focuses on adaptation of the child and family to the seizure disorder.

Assess and monitor the child's physiologic status. Observe the specific seizure activity, level of consciousness, vital signs, and signs of hypoxia. Once the child is stable, a more definitive assessment can be made. Level of consciousness is a vital indicator of neurologic function. Remember that the child's lack of response may be the result of the postictal state.

Collect and analyze historical information about the seizure activity, clustering, aura, description of motor activity or changes in muscle tone, automatisms, and any changes in development or school performance to help determine the type of seizures the child experiences.

Assess the family's adaptation to the seizure disorder as epilepsy is a disorder with a stigma associated with it. Identify how well the family is coping with the uncertainty of when the next seizure will occur. Identify how well the child is coping with a visible condition when a seizure happens at school. See Evidence-Based Practice: Supporting Children with Epilepsy.

Common nursing diagnoses for the child with a seizure disorder include the following:

- Ineffective Breathing Pattern related to neuromuscular dysfunction during the tonic phase of a seizure
- Ineffective Airway Clearance related to inability to control secretions during seizure
- Risk for Trauma related to seizure activity
- Chronic Low Self-esteem related to refractory seizures and loss of bowel and bladder control during seizure activity
- Anxiety related to unpredictable nature of seizure disorder
- Ineffective Therapeutic Regimen Management related to poor adherence with pharmacologic management of seizures
- Readiness for Enhanced Family Processes related to care of a child with a chronic disorder

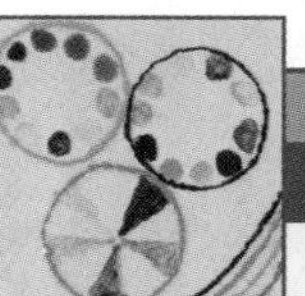

EVIDENCE-BASED PRACTICE
Supporting Children with Epilepsy

PROBLEM

Children who develop epilepsy during childhood are faced with many issues, such as making an adjustment to living with a chronic condition, managing their condition, and telling friends about the seizures. What information and support do school-age children need to live with epilepsy and to manage their lives?

EVIDENCE

A scale developed to measure the psychosocial care needs of children with seizures has three sections; feelings about information received, need for information or support, and concerns and fears (Austin, Dunn, Huster, et al., 1998). The scale was tested with a total of 63 children with an average age of 10.5 years at both 3 months and 6 months after the first seizure. Children were most satisfied with explanations they received from healthcare providers about their condition, but they had the least satisfaction with an opportunity to ask questions 3 months after the first seizure. Children reported that they needed more information about activity restrictions, protection from injury, and handling future seizures. They also indicated a great need to talk with other children their age with seizures and how to handle seizures at school (McNelis, Musick, Austin, et al., 1998). When interviewing eight school-age children who had lived with epilepsy for at least a year, various themes emerged. Children understood the need for medications, knew the medication name and dosage schedule, but six of the children did not like taking the medication or its side effects. They did not like having seizures. Most of the children had found a way to educate their peers and to fit in with their peer group. Some of these children had identified patterns that were warning signs of an impending seizure, and they also took preventive measures to avoid future seizures such as getting plenty of sleep, drinking adequate fluids, exercising appropriately, staying out of the sun, and avoiding getting angry (Hightower, Carmon, & Minick, 2002). While the sample sizes for these studies are not large, important information about living with a chronic disease such as epilepsy from the child's perspective is important. Information gained supports the importance of regular assessment of the child's understanding about epilepsy and providing education to address their questions.

IMPLICATIONS

Learning how a child understands and copes with a chronic condition helps the nurse to determine strategies that may help the child cope more effectively and to enhance development of self-esteem. As the child grows, self-management of the condition is important, including preventive measures that can become part of the child's daily routine, such as sleep, hydration, nutrition, and avoiding certain types of stimulation. Finding ways to support the child, such as identifying other children with seizures with whom the child can talk, may help these children recognize that they are not so different than their peers.

CRITICAL THINKING APPLICATION

Develop a teaching plan for an adolescent with generalized seizures who is beginning to assume more responsibility for daily care. After reviewing the information about type of seizure and clinical therapy, identify the key points in the teaching plan addressing nutrition, hydration, medication administration, and safe activities that will enhance the adolescent's self-esteem.

■ Planning and Implementation

Maintain Airway Patency

Be sure that nothing is placed in the child's mouth during a seizure. Monitor the child to ensure adequate oxygenation: The child's color should be pink, the heart rate at a normal or slightly elevated rate for age, and the pulse oximetry reading greater than 95%. Oxygen is usually given at SpO_2 levels below 95%.

Ensure Safety

Protect the child from self-harm during violent seizures (Figure 33–6 ■). Any child with a seizure history should have the bedside rails padded to prevent injury. During the postictal period, monitor the child's vital signs, perform neurologic checks, and keep the environment safe.

Administer Medications

Take special precautions when administering intravenous medications for the acute management of seizures. These medications should be given very slowly to minimize the risk of respiratory or circulatory collapse.

Medications for the management of chronic seizures are given orally. Crushing pills and mixing them in a teaspoonful of applesauce, pudding, or other soft food make them more palatable and easier for the child to swallow. For some medications elixirs and flavored chewables are available.

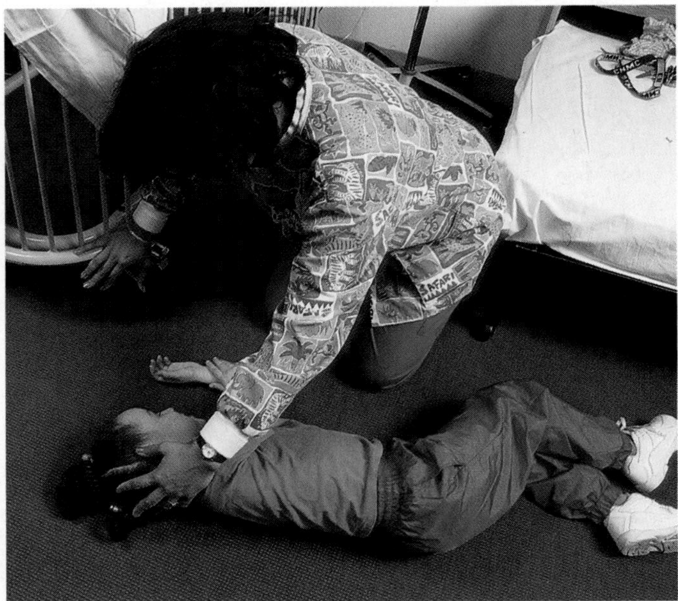

FIGURE 33–6 ■ A child who has a seizure when standing should be gently assisted to the floor and placed in a side-lying position. Clear the area of any objects that might cause harm to the child.

When a child is NPO due to illness or on the day of surgery, seizure medications are usually given with a swallow of water. Obtain medication orders for these cases.

Provide Emotional Support

The loss of control of body movements and possible loss of consciousness make seizures frightening and difficult to accept for the child, parents, and other family members. Make sure that parents are informed about the cause of the seizures when possible to allay concerns about a potential brain tumor and prognosis. Parents may also be concerned about the effect of epilepsy on the child's intelligence.

Parents often feel guilty about the child's seizure disorder and compensate by not disciplining or restricting the child appropriately. Stress the need to treat the child as normally as possible. Refer the child and family to support groups and counseling services if indicated. See Box 33–5.

MediaLink Epilepsy and Seizure Resources and Support

BOX 33–5 Research: Depression in Mothers of Children with Epilepsy

A study of 115 mothers of children with epilepsy with a mean age of 14.4 years was conducted to identify factors associated with maternal depression. A variety of tools were used to assess the severity of the child's seizure condition, child behavior problems, the mother's satisfaction with family relationships, perception of stigma, and maternal depression. Maternal depression was found to be significantly associated with the severity of the child's seizure condition, mother's perception of stigma, and greater number of child behavior problems. However, satisfaction with family relationships, greater family income, and social support were negatively associated with maternal depression (Shore, Austin, Huster, et al., 2002). Identifying problems with maternal depression or concerns may help identify those families that are in need of further nursing interventions.

Discharge Planning and Home Care Teaching

Encourage parents to express their fears and anxieties. Answer their questions honestly, and refer them to organizations, such as the Epilepsy Foundation of America, where they can obtain more information about the child's disorder. Be sure parents know how to administer medications and provide for the child's safety. Discuss with them whom to call with questions and when to return for follow-up. See Box 33–6 for resources that may be used for family and child education.

Care in the Community

Ensure that parents and children have an opportunity to receive current information about the conditions and to ask questions about their concerns and fears.

MEDICATION EDUCATION

Educate the child and parents about medication regimens. Explain the purpose of each drug, its schedule for administration, and the importance of giving all doses. As the child grows older, ensure that information is shared directly with the child so that the child can begin to take more responsibility for condition management. Teaching the older child to take medications without parental intervention provides a sense of self-control.

Provide information about the side effects of medications ordered, and alert parents to the signs of toxic reactions or undermedication. Regular dental care is important because some anticonvulsants cause gingival hyperplasia. Explain the importance of follow-up visits to healthcare providers so the effectiveness of the child's medications can be monitored. Ensure that the family knows that dosage adjustments will be needed as the child grows, particularly during time of growth spurts.

Parents of children with recurrent febrile seizures should be taught how to give antipyretics in the proper dose. Antipyretic doses will need to be updated as the child grows. Parents must know that antipyretics and anticonvulsants may not prevent a future febrile seizure associated with an acute illness. The potential toxicity and side effects of an anticonvulsant in a child with febrile seizures often outweigh the risk of the seizures, and parents can be reassured that complications from febrile seizures are rare.

Adolescent females need to be educated about the potential teratogenicity of some antiepileptic medications. Valproic acid and carbamazepine are associated with neural tube defects. If sexually active, contraception should be used until such time as a planned pregnancy is desired; however, because some anticonvulsants interfere with the effectiveness of certain contraceptive choices, refer the adolescent to a healthcare provider who can help select an effective contraceptive. When pregnancy is desired, the female

BOX 33–6 Epilepsy Resources for Families

- *Seizures and Epilepsy in Childhood: A Guide for Parents,* by John M. Freeman, E. P. Vining, and D. Pillas, Johns Hopkins University Press, 1997.
- *Epilepsy: Patient and Family Guide,* by O. Devinsky, F. A. Davis Co., 2001.
- The Brainstorms series, edited by S. C. Schachter, Lippincott-Raven.

should work closely with her primary care provider to select the appropriate medication and dosage to reduce the risk of birth defects.

KETOGENIC DIET

When families choose to follow the ketogenic diet, help coordinate their care with a dietician who can customize the diet to the child's growth and activity needs. Ensure that vitamins and other medications used are carbohydrate-free so ketosis is maintained. Alert parents that sunscreen lotions and shampoos with sorbitol should not be used; sorbitol is a carbohydrate that can be absorbed through the skin. When it is time to discontinue the ketogenic diet, it should be tapered by slowly decreasing the ratio of fats to protein and carbohydrates.

FAMILY AND CHILD SUPPORT

Families of children with severe seizure disorders need to develop an emergency care plan so that emergency personnel are informed about their needs for care in advance (see Chapter 16∞). See Partnering with Families: Safety for the Child with a Seizure Disorder.

Assist the family to develop an individual school health plan so the child can receive medications during school hours, if necessary. If it is likely that the child could have a seizure while at school, it may be desirable to provide students with information about seizures, what happens, and how they can help the child. Parents may also want to provide a towel and change of clothing for the child to use if incontinence occurs with the seizures. Teachers and school administrators should know what actions to take if the child has a seizure and what information to report about the seizure.

Physical activity and exercise are important for all children. Encourage participation in sports when supervision is provided. Some activities are potentially more dangerous for children, especially when seizures are not completely controlled, such as rope climbing, rock or mountain climbing, tree climbing, snow skiing, scuba diving, and sky diving. Swimming and water sports should only be allowed when there is an adult who can provide one-to-one supervision.

The child may be afraid of having a seizure in front of friends. Reassure the child and family that taking medications regularly should control seizures. Children should explain to peers what a seizure is and what to do if they are present when one occurs. Summer camps for children with seizures can be a safe and comfortable place for the child to enjoy outdoor activities. Tell parents to boost the child's self-image by emphasizing what the child can do, rather than focusing on contraindicated activities. Depending on state laws, most adolescents can drive after they have been seizure free for at least 2 years.

Evaluation

Expected outcomes of nursing management include the following:

- The child achieves good seizure control with medication, ketogenic diet, or surgical intervention.
- The child experiences no injuries when seizures occur because of effective safety measures used by the child and family.
- The family learns to manage seizures and maintain a healthy life.
- The child's self-esteem is enhanced through participation in well-supervised sports and activities.

PARTNERING WITH FAMILIES

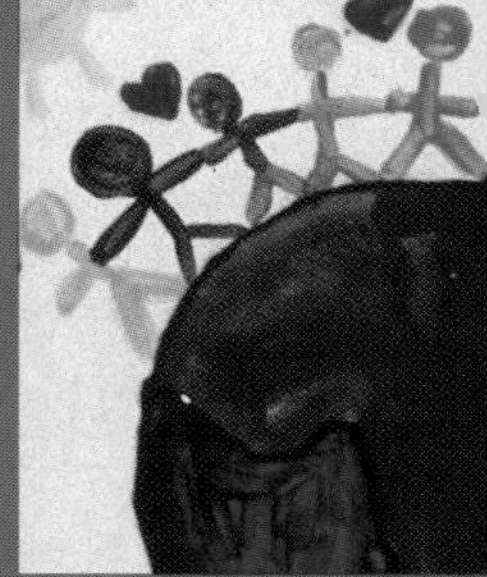

Safety for the Child with a Seizure Disorder

First-aid techniques to care for the child who has a seizure include the following:

- Place the child on the floor or bed, lying on one side so that saliva or vomit can drain out of the mouth.
- Loosen the clothing around the neck.
- Move objects away from the child so that they are not close enough to cause injury.
- Put no objects into the child's mouth or between the teeth. Loose teeth may be knocked out and aspirated.
- Stay with the child until he or she is fully awake.
- Call 9-1-1 or your emergency number if the child's seizure lasts longer than 5–10 minutes, if a second seizure occurs, or if the child does not become conscious immediately after the seizure. Have a completed and current emergency medical information form available for the emergency care personnel.

Children with epilepsy have more injuries of all sorts, including burns, falls, and drowning. Children are at increased risk for death due to drowning. Planning for safety includes the following:

- Do not leave the child alone in the bathtub.
- Children who bathe alone should use the shower.
- A buddy and lifeguard should always be present when the child swims.
- A life vest should always be worn when boating.
- The child with frequent seizures should wear a helmet to protect the head in case of a fall.
- The child should not play or stand around open flames or outdoor grills.
- The child should avoid areas where fall risks are increased.
- A form of medical identification should be worn (e.g., medic alert bracelet).

INFECTIOUS DISEASES

Bacterial Meningitis

Meningitis, an inflammation of the meninges, can be caused by either bacterial or viral agents. Bacterial meningitis is more virulent than viral meningitis and is sometimes fatal. Newborns and infants are at greatest risk for acquiring bacterial meningitis. Infants and children who develop meningitis have the potential for acute complications and long-term morbidity.

PATHOPHYSIOLOGY ILLUSTRATED

Central Nervous System Infection

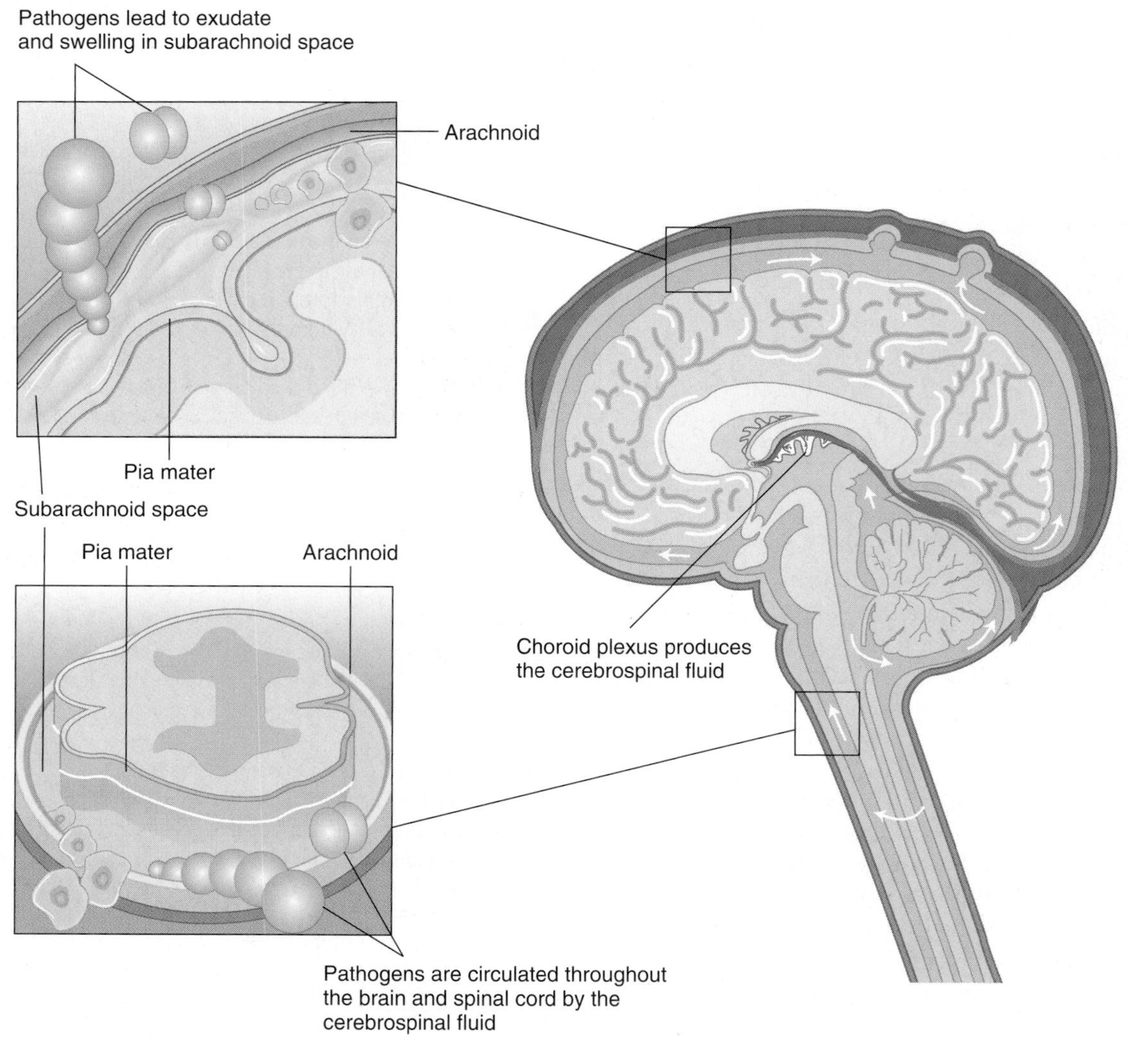
Pathogens lead to exudate and swelling in subarachnoid space
Arachnoid
Pia mater
Subarachnoid space
Pia mater
Arachnoid
Choroid plexus produces the cerebrospinal fluid
Pathogens are circulated throughout the brain and spinal cord by the cerebrospinal fluid

FIGURE 33–7 ■ After bacteria reach the central nervous system, the pia mater, the arachnoid, and the cerebrospinal fluid–filled subarachnoid space become infected. The cerebrospinal fluid then circulates the pathogens throughout the brain and spinal cord.

Etiology and Pathophysiology

Meningitis may occur secondary to other infections such as otitis media, sinusitis, pharyngitis, cellulitis, pneumonia, or septic arthritis; head trauma; or a neurosurgical procedure. Three organisms cause the majority of cases in children between 2 months and 12 years of age: *Haemophilus influenzae* type b, *Neisseria meningitidis,* and *Streptococcus pneumoniae.* The organisms responsible for meningitis in newborns include these and group B streptococcus (Prober, 2004). Fortunately, immunization of infants with the pnemococcal vaccine is reducing the incidence of invasive disease such as meningitis caused by S. *pneumoniae* (Black, Shinefield, Baxter, et al., 2004).

In many cases, bacteremia spreads the infectious agent to the CNS (Figure 33–7 ■). An inflammatory response follows. White blood cells accumulate, covering the surface of the brain with a thick, white, purulent exudate. The brain then becomes hyperemic and edematous. If the infection spreads to the ventricles, they can become obstructed and impede the flow of cerebrospinal fluid, causing increased intracranial pressure and hydrocephalus as an acute complication. Inflammation of the spinal nerves and roots causes the classic meningeal signs of a headache and stiff neck.

Clinical Manifestations

Symptoms are variable and depend on the child's age, the pathogen, and the length of the illness before diagnosis. Onset may be sudden or may develop over approximately a 1-week period.

Symptoms in the young infant may include fever, change in feeding pattern, vomiting, or diarrhea. The anterior fontanel may be bulging or flat. The infant may be alert, restless, lethargic, or irritable. Rocking or cuddling, which normally calms a fussy infant, only irritates the infant with meningitis.

Older children are usually febrile for several days with an upper respiratory tract or gastrointestinal tract illness. This is followed by increasing irritability and lethargy. The child may be confused, have vomiting, and complain of muscle or joint pain. A hemorrhagic rash, first appearing as petechiae and changing to purpura or large necrotic patches, may be seen in meningococcal meningitis. The child displays other symptoms consistent with meningeal irritation: headache (most often frontal), photophobia, esotropia, and **nuchal rigidity** (resistance to neck flexion). The child is comfortable only in an **opisthotonic position** (hyperextension of the head and neck to relieve discomfort; see Figure 33–8 ■). The child may have a positive Kernig or Brudzinski sign, or both, on examination (Figure 33–9 ■).

Symptoms can progress to include seizures, apnea, cerebral edema, photophobia, altered mental status, subdural effusion, hydrocephalus, disseminated intravascular coagulation (DIC), and shock. The bacteria may also colonize within a joint, causing septic arthritis.

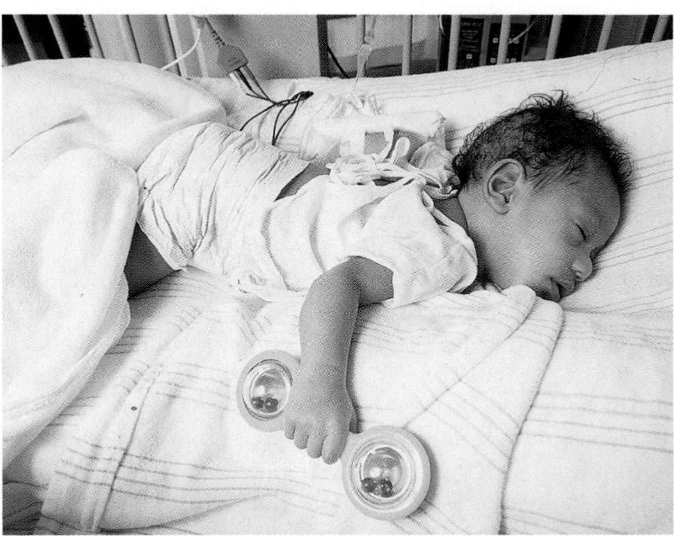

FIGURE 33–8 ■ The child with bacterial meningitis assumes an opisthotonic position, with the neck and head hyperextended, to relieve discomfort.

COLLABORATIVE CARE

The goal of collaborative care is to identify the causative organism and rapidly begin clinical therapy in an effort to reduce the risk for complications.

Diagnostic Testing

Diagnosis is based on the history, clinical presentation, and laboratory findings. Laboratory tests include a complete blood count, blood cultures, serum electrolytes and osmolality, and clotting factors. Blood cultures usually identify the responsible bacteria causing meningitis. A lumbar puncture is performed to evaluate the cerebrospinal fluid for number of white blood cells and protein and glucose levels. A Gram stain and culture are done on the cerebrospinal fluid. CT scanning may be performed when increased intracranial pressure or a brain abscess is suspected. Repeat assessment of cerebrospinal fluid analysis may be performed to evaluate response to treatment.

Clinical Therapy

Antibiotics are administered as soon as diagnostic tests are obtained. Those commonly used to treat bacterial meningitis include ampicillin, aminoglycosides, cefotaxime, ceftriaxone, and penicillin G. Antibiotics are often changed once culture and sensitivity results are known, especially as many organisms have resistance to certain antibiotics. These medications

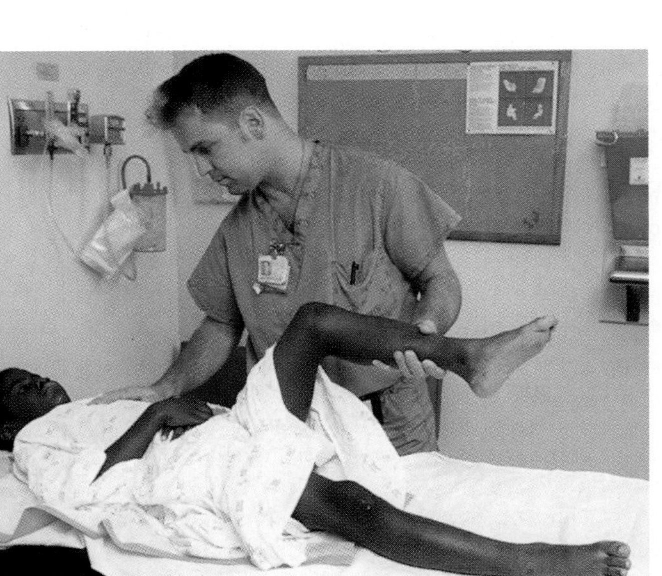

A

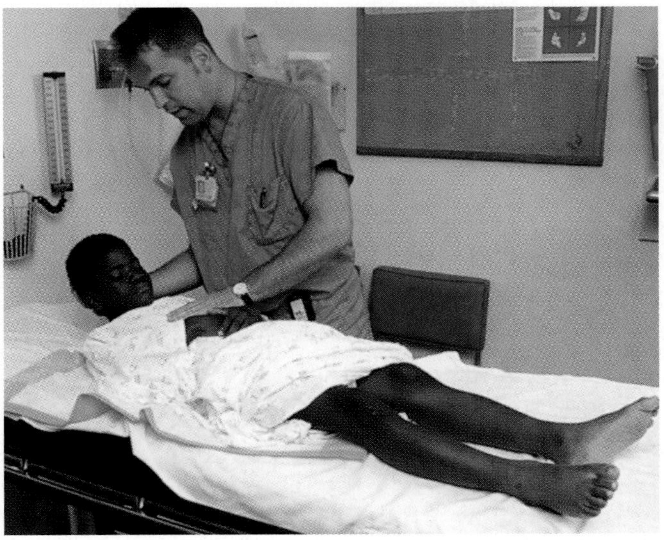

B

FIGURE 33–9 ■ *A,* To test for **Kernig sign,** raise the child's leg with the knee flexed. Then extend the child's leg at the knee. If any resistance is noted or pain is felt, the result is a positive Kernig sign. This is a common finding in meningitis. *B,* To test **Brudzinski sign,** flex the child's head while in a supine position. If this action makes the knees or hips flex involuntarily, a positive Brudzinski sign is present. This is a common sign in meningitis.

are administered intravenously for 7 to 21 days, depending on the organism and the child's clinical response. Depending on the causative organism, the disease may need to be reported to the local health department, and contacts may need to take prophylactic antibiotics, such as rifampin or ciprofloxacin. Corticosteroids (dexamethasone) are given as an adjunct to children over 6 weeks of age to reduce the risk of severe neurologic sequelae such as sensorineural hearing loss. In some cases, anticonvulsants and antipyretics are given (American Academy of Pediatrics, 2003a).

Infants and children receive nothing by mouth and are started on IV fluids. The IV fluids may be initially restricted to two-thirds maintenance as careful monitoring for increased intracranial pressure and syndrome of inappropriate antidiuretic hormone (SIADH) is initiated. See Chapter 32∞. If the child is in shock, aggressive fluid resuscitation occurs to maintain the cerebral perfusion pressure. Intensive care monitoring will be required in children with shock, increased intracranial pressure, coma, and seizures unresponsive to therapy. Care of the child in septic shock is described in Chapter 26∞.

Some infants and children who have had bacterial meningitis suffer neurologic damage despite early, aggressive management. The most common sequelae involve cranial nerves, especially the eighth, resulting in hearing loss. In addition, seizures, developmental delay, and other complications may occur, as described in Box 33–7. Another potential complication is meningococcal septicemia, which is characterized by high fever, hypotension, disseminated intravascular coagulation, and multisystem organ failure (Harrison, 2001). See the discussion about meningococcus in Chapter 19∞.

NURSING MANAGEMENT

The goal of nursing care is to carefully monitor the child for signs of illness progression or development of complications, support the family, administer medications, and manage pain.

Nursing Assessment and Diagnosis

Assess the child's physiologic status, including vital signs and level of consciousness. Measure head circumference frequently in infants during hospitalization and compare to previous measurements because of the potential for hydrocephalus to develop. Be alert for signs of a change in the child's condition and response to treatment. Monitor the child's ability to control secretions and to drink sufficient fluids. Monitor intake and output. Assess for any sensory deficits. Identify parents' concerns related to this potentially life-threatening condition.

Several nursing diagnoses that may apply to the child with bacterial meningitis are given in the accompanying nursing care plan. Additional nursing diagnoses may include the following:

- Risk for Aspiration related to altered level of consciousness and poor secretion control
- Risk for Deficient Fluid Volume related to poor oral fluid intake
- Anticipatory Grieving (parent) related to the child's potentially life-threatening condition
- Caregiver Role Strain related to a hospitalized child and other family responsibilities

BOX 33–7 Complications of Bacterial Meningitis

- Syndrome of inappropriate antidiuretic hormone (SIADH) secretion
- Disseminated intravascular coagulation (DIC)
- Subdural effusion
- Septicemia
- Septic arthritis
- Seizures
- Sensorineural hearing loss
- Hydrocephalus
- Behavior problems
- Learning problems

Planning and Implementation

The nursing care plan on pages 1317–1319 summarizes care for the child with bacterial meningitis. Nursing care begins with emergency treatment and continues as the child's condition stabilizes. Monitor respiratory and neurologic status, maintain hydration, administer medications, and prevent complications. Promote the child's comfort with reduced stimulation (dim lights, quiet room) and by placing the child in a side-lying position. Isolate the child and use standard and droplet precautions until the causative organism is identified and effective treatment is underway.

PRACTICE ALERT

Maintenance and replacement fluids are usually given to children with bacterial meningitis. However, it is important to monitor the serum sodium concentration and urine specific gravity, because these children are at risk for developing the syndrome of inappropriate antidiuretic hormone (SIADH; see Chapter 32∞). Fluids are restricted. Sodium chloride, potassium, and acetate or lactate are administered intravenously to balance sodium excretion.

Monitor the child's response to antibiotic therapy. Remember that gastrointestinal bleeding is a potential complication of corticosteroid use. Monitor the child receiving these drugs for signs of intestinal discomfort and for blood in the stools.

Respond to parents' concerns about their child's condition, explaining all measures to reduce the child's discomfort and provide adequate treatment. Identify ways parents can participate in meeting the child's comfort needs. Parents may also need assistance in identifying the best strategies for meeting the needs of other children at home while spending time with the hospitalized child.

A major role of nurses is prevention. Parents should be encouraged to get their infants and children fully immunized, especially the HIB and pneumococcal vaccines. Adolescents entering college who will live in dormitories should be encouraged to get the meningococcal vaccine to prevent meningococcal meningitis (see Chapter 19∞).

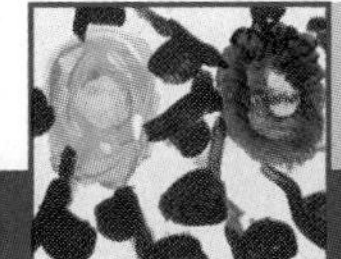

Nursing Care Plan

THE CHILD WITH BACTERIAL MENINGITIS

GOAL	INTERVENTION	RATIONALE	EXPECTED OUTCOME
1. Impaired Spontaneous Ventilation related to decreased level of consciousness.			
	NIC Priority Intervention— *Respiratory Monitoring:* Collection and analysis of patient data to ensure airway patency and adequate gas exchange.		**NOC Suggested Outcome—***Vital Sign Status:* Pulse, respiration, and blood pressure are within expected range for age.
The child's respiratory failure does not progress to respiratory arrest.	▪ Place the child on a cardiorespiratory monitor with a 20-second alarm.	▪ The alarm on the monitor alerts staff that the child is having bradycardia or an apneic spell.	The child's respiratory failure is managed with prompt assessment and treatment.
	▪ Have resuscitation equipment, including oxygen, resuscitation bag with mask, and suction apparatus at the bedside.	▪ Equipment should be at the bedside in case of respiratory arrest. Bag-valve-mask ventilation is recommended as the child's respiratory secretions contain bacteria.	
	▪ Stimulate the child if apneic. If no response, begin assisted ventilations and call for the resuscitation team.	▪ Stimulation may encourage spontaneous respirations; if not, ventilation is necessary. Calling for the emergency resuscitation team ensures help in managing the child in a timely manner.	
	▪ Monitor heart rate and perform compressions if necessary.	▪ The apneic child may have bradycardia resulting from cardiac hypoxia.	
2. Ineffective Protection related to infection of cerebrospinal fluid and potential sequelae			
	NIC Priority Intervention—*Safety Surveillance:* Purposeful and ongoing collection and analysis of information about the patient and the environment for use in promoting and maintaining patient safety.		**NOC Suggested Outcome—***Immune Status:* Adequacy of natural and acquired appropriately targeted resistance to internal and external antigens.
The child will suffer minimal central nervous system injury secondary to infection.	▪ Administer prescribed antibiotics and corticosteroids as scheduled.	▪ Administration of antibiotics helps eradicate the pathogen and prevents cerebral edema. Administration of corticosteroids diminishes inflammatory response and reduces the chance of neurologic sequelae.	The child's condition improves significantly within 48–72 hours (fever decreases and no signs of neurologic sequelae are detected).
	▪ Note return of fever, nuchal rigidity, or irritability. Monitor vital signs, assess for signs of increased intracranial pressure, measure head circumference once or twice daily, note changes in responsiveness. Notify the physician immediately if any signs are detected.	▪ Watching for common sequelae such as subdural effusions, hydrocephalus, or septic arthritis ensures prompt treatment.	
The child will not develop cerebral edema as a result of water retention.	▪ Monitor for syndrome of inappropriate antidiuretic hormone (SIADH) secretion and watch for signs of increased intracranial pressure (ICP).	▪ SIADH can be either avoided or quickly managed if early recognition is achieved.	Cerebral edema does not develop. If SIADH or increased ICP occurs, the condition is treated promptly so effects on the child are minimal.
	▪ Perform strict intake and output measurements. Determine urine specific gravity. Check electrolytes and osmolality of both serum and urine. Weigh the child daily. Restrict fluids and give sodium chloride as ordered.	▪ Low urine output with a high specific gravity is a sign of fluid retention and SIADH. The child is maintained with lower fluids and provided sodium supplements to reduce the possibility for cerebral edema.	

(continued)

Nursing Care Plan THE CHILD WITH BACTERIAL MENINGITIS (continued)

GOAL	INTERVENTION	RATIONALE	EXPECTED OUTCOME
2. Ineffective Protection related to infection of cerebrospinal fluid and potential sequelae (continued)			
The child will be free of injury resulting from disseminated intravascular coagulation (DIC).	■ Be aware of needle sticks that continue to bleed and lesions that continue to ooze. Monitor clotting times. ■ Administer blood products, vitamin K, or heparin as ordered.	■ Prompt recognition leads to management of the coagulopathy. ■ Prompt recognition allows for early initial treatment of DIC. The child may bleed to death if treatment is delayed.	The child does not sustain injury from DIC.
The child will be free of injury secondary to shock.	■ Monitor vital signs including pulse, respirations, and blood pressure. Note perfusion (capillary refill, central versus proximal pulses). Check level of consciousness. Note urine output. ■ Begin fluid resuscitation as ordered. ■ Administer inotropes if ordered.	■ Monitoring allows for prompt diagnosis of shock based on clinical signs. ■ Intravenous fluid bolus may improve perfusion. ■ Inotropes enhance perfusion when response to fluid challenge is minimal.	The child recovers from shock quickly with no complications. Prompt management of shock can enhance the child's recovery, since it prevents complications associated with poor perfusion (tissue acidosis and ischemia).
3. Impaired Social Interaction related to decreased level of consciousness, hospitalization, and isolation			
	NIC Priority Intervention— *Socialization Enhancement:* Facilitation of the child's ability to interact with others.		**NOC Suggested Outcome—***Role Performance:* Congruence of the child's role behavior with role expectations.
The child's social interaction will be near normal despite isolation.	■ Educate parents and other visitors to use proper infection control techniques. ■ Encourage parents to help with daily activities such as feeding and bathing. ■ Have age-appropriate games and toys in the room. Play with the child. When the child is feeling better, encourage watching television/videotape or listening to the radio/audiotape.	■ Family members help fulfill the emotional and social needs of the ill and contagious child. ■ Parental involvement in the child's care provides the child with a sense of security and emotional well-being. Parents have a sense of control and a feeling that they are doing something to enhance the child's recovery. ■ Providing the child with toys and games as well as sensory stimulation helps the child achieve a sense of well-being.	The child's social and developmental needs are met by family members despite the child's illness and hospitalization.
The child with any degree of hearing loss will be identified.	■ Arrange for hearing assessment prior to discharge.	■ Hearing loss is a common complication. Early intervention is needed to promote growth and development.	The child with identified hearing loss is referred to appropriate specialist or program for intervention.
4. Acute Pain related to meningeal irritation			
	NIC Priority Intervention—*Pain Management:* Alleviation of pain or reduction in pain to a level of comfort that is acceptable to patient.		**NOC Suggested Outcome—***Comfort Level:* Feelings of physical and psychologic ease.
The child will be as comfortable as possible.	■ Provide pain medication ordered for the child. ■ Minimize tactile stimulation.	■ Pain medication is appropriate for acute discomfort associated with illness. ■ Sensory stimulation during acute illness increases discomfort.	The child is calm and expresses increased comfort.

Nursing Care Plan THE CHILD WITH BACTERIAL MENINGITIS (continued)

GOAL	INTERVENTION	RATIONALE	EXPECTED OUTCOME
4. Acute Pain related to meningeal irritation (continued)			
	■ Allow the child to assume a position of comfort.	■ The child determines the most comfortable position. Opisthotonic position, with the head and neck hyperextended, may be the most comfortable.	
	■ Keep the lights dim.	■ Dim lights reduce the discomfort from photophobia.	
	■ Maintain a quiet environment. Keep doors closed.	■ Noise can disturb the child.	
5. Risk for Infection (family and close contacts) related to pathogens in the cerebrospinal fluid			
	NIC Priority Intervention—*Infection Control:* Minimizing the acquisition and transmission of infectious agents.		**NOC Suggested Outcome—***Risk Control:* Actions to eliminate an actual health threat.
Caretakers or family members will have no apparent evidence of infection.	■ Explain rationale and dose schedule for taking rifampin or ciprofloxacin.	■ Rifampin and ciprofloxacin provide prophlylaxis for many bacterial pathogens responsible for meningitis.	Family members and other close contacts verbalize schedule for rifampin or ciprofloxacin therapy.
	■ Instruct family members about signs and symptoms associated with acute infection.	■ Family members may need a review of important signs of infection in older children and adults.	

Discharge Planning and Home Care Teaching

Home care needs should be identified and addressed well in advance of discharge. Follow-up visits are important to monitor for complications and sequelae. Help parents deal with any physical requirements resulting from the child's illness and any emotional, social, and financial repercussions of the child's condition. Teach parents what to do if the child has a seizure.

Infants and toddlers with neurologic sequelae should be referred to an early intervention program. If the child has had a hearing loss, referral to an otolaryngologist and speech and language specialist should be made. Early identification of other neurologic sequelae, such as learning problems, should be encouraged.

■ Evaluation

Expected outcomes of nursing care are provided on the nursing care plan.

Viral (Aseptic) Meningitis

Viral meningitis is an inflammatory response of the meninges characterized by an increased number of blood cells and protein in the cerebrospinal fluid. In the United States, an enterovirus is the cause of more than 80% of viral meningitis cases (Prober, 2004). Other organisms that may cause viral meningitis include arboviruses, herpes simplex, and varicella zoster. Viral meningitis due to enteroviruses occurs more frequently in the summer and fall.

Generally, the child with aseptic meningitis does not appear to be as ill as the child with bacterial meningitis. The child may be irritable or lethargic and usually has a fever. Other symptoms include general malaise, headache, photophobia, gastrointestinal distress, upper respiratory symptoms, and a maculopapular rash. The child may also show signs of meningeal irritation such as stiff neck, back pain, and positive Kernig and Brudzinski signs (see Figure 33–9 ■). The infant may have a tense anterior fontanel. Seizures are rare. Symptoms usually resolve spontaneously within 3 to 10 days.

The child with fever and meningeal signs is hospitalized. Blood, urine, and cerebrospinal fluid analyses are performed. A polymerase chain reaction test of the cerebrospinal fluid is performed for diagnosis of viral meningitis, and is often available within 24 hours. Until the diagnosis of aseptic meningitis is confirmed, the child is treated aggressively, as if he or she has bacterial meningitis. Acyclovir is used to treat meningitis caused by a herpes simplex virus. Other treatment is supportive of symptoms.

Nursing Management

Initial nursing care focuses on providing supportive care as described for the child with bacterial meningitis. Give acetaminophen as ordered to reduce fever, headache, and muscle or joint pain. Keep the room dark and quiet (to decrease stimuli and meningeal irritation), give fluids either intravenously or orally, and promote comfort with proper positioning. Prepare to manage seizures that can occur with the disorder.

The child and family need information about the disease. Explain medical and nursing procedures in terms that the child and family can understand. Keep parents informed about the child's progress. Once the diagnosis of viral meningitis is made, discharge planning and teaching for home care must begin immediately. Explain that recovery may take several weeks but that complete recovery is expected.

Encephalitis

Encephalitis is an inflammation of the brain usually caused by a viral infection. Inflammation of the meninges is also common.

Viruses are believed to cause most cases of encephalitis (Box 33–8). Herpes simplex type I is the most common cause after the newborn period, and it is associated with a high mortality rate. Those who survive often have significant neurologic sequelae (American Academy of Pediatrics, 2003a).

Signs and symptoms depend on the causative organism and the location of the infection within the brain. An acute onset of a febrile illness with neurologic signs is the classic manifestation of encephalitis. Initially the child may have a severe headache, fever, signs of an upper respiratory infection, malaise, and nausea or vomiting. Meningeal irritation signs such as nuchal rigidity, photophobia, and positive Kernig and Brudzinski signs are uncommon. Other neurologic signs vary. The child may be disoriented or confused, with behavioral or personality changes. Speech disturbances; motor dysfunction such as hemiparesis, ataxia, or weakness; cranial nerve deficits; or alterations in reflex response may be present. Focal or generalized seizures may occur, alternating with periods of screaming, hallucinating, and moving in a bizarre fashion. The child's level of consciousness may deteriorate from stupor to coma.

Diagnosis is based on history and laboratory findings. Information about recent immunizations, insect bites, and residing in or travel to areas where vectors are present should be obtained (e. g., cases of West Nile virus or eastern equine encephalitis). Cerebrospinal fluid analysis, blood serologic tests, and nasopharyngeal and stool specimens are evaluated to identify viral pathogens. Testing for virus specific immunoglobulin M antibodies with an enzyme-linked immunosorbent assay (ELISA) is performed after 5 days of the acute illness. A CT scan, MRI, and EEG may also be performed. The nucleic acid detection test is used to assay for herpes DNA in the spinal fluid. Brain biopsy may be performed to diagnose herpes simplex and parasitic infections.

BOX 33–8 Causative Viruses of Encephalitis

- Enteroviruses
  - Poliovirus
  - Echovirus
  - Coxsackievirus
- Adenoviruses and herpes viruses
- Arboviruses
- Measles
- Mumps
- Rubella
- Rabies
- Hepatitis B

The child with encephalitis is at risk for seizures, respiratory failure, and increased intracranial pressure and should be cared for in an intensive care unit. Treatment is both pharmacologic and supportive. The child with a suspected bacterial infection should be treated with antibiotics until bacterial pathogens have been ruled out. Acyclovir may be used for herpes viral infections.

Children with encephalitis have many permanent neurologic sequelae. Although some children recover completely, many more are left with cognitive, motor, visual, or auditory deficits. The cardiovascular system, lungs, or liver may also be affected. The younger child generally has a more serious illness and more severe residual effects.

Nursing Management

Nursing care focuses on monitoring cardiorespiratory function, preventing complications resulting from immobility, reorienting the child, and teaching the parents about the child's condition.

Monitor the child's cardiorespiratory function. Check the child's airway and ability to handle secretions. Monitor respiratory status by observing color, pulse oximetry readings, and arterial blood gas values. Observe cardiopulmonary status by monitoring heart rate, blood pressure, capillary refill time, and urine output. Provide seizure precautions, and have appropriate equipment for managing seizures at bedside.

Prevent complications resulting from immobility as described in Box 33–3 on page 1305. Maintain skin integrity. Proper positioning with frequent turning is important. When indicated by the physician, perform chest physiotherapy to prevent pneumonia. (See Skills Manual.)

As the level of consciousness begins to improve, the child may at first be confused and disoriented and have residual effects of the disease. Orient the child to the hospital environment. Have the family help to reorient the child by bringing favorite stuffed animals or music from home. Engage in therapeutic play (refer to Chapter 17 for techniques). Give the child age-appropriate toys to encourage a return to normal behavior.

Provide the parents with information about their child's condition and prognosis. If the child receives physical, occupational, or speech therapy, explain the treatment regimen to the parents.

Discharge Planning and Home Care Teaching. Encourage parents to take an active role in the child's physical and emotional care in the hospital, and give them written instructions concerning care for their child at home. Encourage the parents to learn specific physical, occupational, and speech therapies so they can work with their child at home between home care visits. Refer parents to home care, social services, family counseling, and support groups. Plan follow-up visits so the child can be evaluated for neurologic sequelae.

Reye Syndrome

Reye syndrome is an acute **encephalopathy,** a cerebral dysfunction caused by a toxic, injury, inflammatory, or anoxic insult that may result in permanent tissue damage, although the dysfunction may improve over time. In 1980, researchers reported an association between the use of aspirin for a mild viral illness and the subsequent development of Reye syndrome. Because most parents now give children acetaminophen rather than aspirin for flulike symptoms and varicella, Reye syndrome has become rare. Between 1994 and 1997, only two cases were reported each year (Belay et al., 1999). The mortality and neurologic morbidity rates for children who develop the condition are high.

The etiology of Reye syndrome is unclear. The encephalopathy usually develops after a mild viral illness, such as varicella, influenza, echovirus 2, coxsackievirus A, or Epstein-Barr virus. The disorder also affects the liver with an elevation of the short-chain fatty acid levels and hyperammonemia. The disorder is characterized by cerebral edema and an enlarged, fatty, poorly functioning liver.

Reye syndrome begins with nausea and vomiting, mental status changes, seizures, and progressive unresponsiveness (Ressler & Nelson, 2000). The condition has five stages that demonstrate increasing signs of cerebral edema and neurologic dysfunction. See the clinical manifestation table below for the signs associated with each stage.

The diagnosis of Reye syndrome is based on an abrupt change in the child's level of consciousness and diagnostic laboratory tests. The child has often progressed to coma or stage III by the time of diagnosis. Liver enzyme and ammonia levels are elevated, blood glucose levels are below normal, and prothrombin time is prolonged. A liver biopsy is sometimes performed to confirm the diagnosis.

The child with Reye syndrome should be placed in a pediatric intensive care unit due to the potential for rapid deterioration in his or her condition. The goal of medical management is to provide supportive treatment and to prevent the secondary effects of cerebral edema and metabolic injury. Mechanical ventilation is often needed once the child is comatose. Arterial and venous pressure monitoring are performed. The child is carefully monitored for signs of increased intracranial pressure, which can be secondary to cerebral edema. Hypoglycemia is treated with intravenous glucose; and electrolytes, blood chemistry, and blood pH are monitored.

CLINICAL MANIFESTATIONS of Reye Syndrome by Stages

STAGE	CLINICAL MANIFESTATIONS
I	Vomiting; lethargy; appropriate responses to verbal commands; purposeful responses to pain; brisk pupillary reaction
II	Combativeness; stupor; inappropriate language; confusion; anxiety, fear; purposeful and nonpurposeful responses to pain; sluggish pupillary reaction; conjugate deviation with oculocephalic reflex; hyperactive reflexes; progresses to coma but interrupted by periods of screaming and ranting
III	Coma; decorticate rigidity; conjugate deviation with diminished oculocephalic reflex; sluggish pupillary reaction; decorticate posturing
IV	Coma with brainstem dysfunction; decerebrate rigidity; inconsistent or absent oculocephalic reflex; loss of corneal reflex; sluggish pupillary reaction; decerebrate posturing
V	Coma with seizures; flaccidity; loss of deep tendon reflexes; respiratory arrest

MediaLink National Reye Syndrome Foundation

Nursing Management

Nursing care focuses on monitoring the child's physical status, providing emotional support, and teaching parents about disease prevention.

PRACTICE ALERT

Ensure all parents know that aspirin must not be given when the child has a viral illness such as chickenpox or influenza, because aspirin is associated with the development of Reye syndrome. Instruct parents to check all over-the-counter medicines for the presence of aspirin compounds. Examples of nonprescription medications that contain aspirin are Alka Seltzer, Anacin, Ascriptin, Bufferin, Pamprin, Pepto-Bismol, Sine-Off, and Vanquish. Many prescription medications also contain aspirin. See the National Reye Syndrome Foundation website for updated information about aspirin or salicylate-containing medications. Emphasize the importance of obtaining healthcare when a child's condition worsens at the end of a viral illness

Check the child's respiratory and neurologic status frequently, and note any signs of improvement or deterioration. Orient the child who awakens from coma. Refer to the discussion of nursing management of altered states of consciousness at the beginning of this chapter for specific nursing interventions. Look for changes in laboratory values that indicate acidosis, an elevation of ammonia levels, or hypoglycemia. Carefully monitor the child's intake and output. Correct imbalances by administering fluids, electrolytes, or medications as ordered. Prevent complications associated with immobility.

Provide emotional support to the parents, who may feel guilty because they did not seek medical attention sooner. Keep them informed about the child's condition, and prepare them for potential deterioration in the course of the disease. Explanations of treatments can help reduce anxiety. Encourage the parents to participate in the child's care when possible.

If the child recovers and is discharged, monitoring is needed to observe for sequelae of the illness. Developmental and neurologic deficits may occur and are more severe in children under 2 years of age. Arrange for home nursing visits during the recovery period so that developmental and neurological status monitoring can be assessed. Be sure the parents are informed about resources in the community that can assist them in dealing with the child's recovery.

Guillain-Barré Syndrome (Postinfectious Polyneuritis)

Guillain-Barré syndrome is an acute inflammatory demyelinating polyradiculoneuropathy. This condition may lead to deteriorating motor function, weakness, and paralysis that progresses in an ascending pattern, as well as paresthesia and areflexia. It is the most common cause of acute flaccid paralysis in infants and children (Jones, 2000).Guillain-Barré syndrome is caused by an autoimmune response to an infectious organism, usually from a gastrointestinal or respiratory illness about 10 days prior to onset. It has also been associated with immunizations and cytomegalovirus (Jones, 2000).

Infants have an onset of rapidly progressive severe hypotonia, possible respiratory distress, and feeding difficulties. Older children have rapidly progressive symmetric weakness and muscle pain with varying degrees of distal paresthesia and numbness that begins in the legs. This weakness spreads to the upper extremities, trunk, chest, neck, face, and head. Deep tendon reflexes may be diminished or absent. The child may develop acute ataxia. Difficulty swallowing and facial weakness are signs of impending respiratory failure. Respiratory effort may be inadequate to ensure proper ventilation. Cranial nerves may be affected, thus causing, for example, Bell's palsy. A dysfunctional autonomic nervous system may cause such symptoms as hypertension, postural hypotension, sinus tachycardia or bradycardia, excessive diaphoresis, urinary and bowel incontinence, and facial flushing.

COLLABORATIVE CARE

Diagnostic criteria of Guillain-Barré syndrome include progressive motor weakness (minimal weakness of the legs to total paralysis of all extremities), and areflexia of varying degrees. Two tests are used to diagnose. Lumbar puncture is performed to obtain cerebrospinal fluid; twice the upper limit of normal protein levels, normal glucose level, and fewer than 10 white blood cells per cubic millimeter are a positive indicator of the condition (Sarnat, 2004). Electroconduction tests such as electromyography show acute muscle denervation. Muscle biopsy is not required.

Clinical therapy for rapidly progressive ascending paralysis of Guillain-Barré syndrome is plasmapheresis or intravenous immune globulin if the child is unable to ambulate. Guidelines for administration of intravenous immune globulin can be found in Chapter 27∞. Responses to intravenous immune globulin are dramatic, often within days. If the child is able to ambulate, physical therapy and supportive care are provided. The condition is rarely fatal. Supportive care is also provided.

NURSING MANAGEMENT

Nursing care focuses on monitoring respiratory status, meeting nutritional needs, managing autonomic nervous system dysfunction, preventing complications associated with immobility, providing emotional support, and teaching the parents how to care for the child after discharge.

Monitor Respiratory Status

Monitor the child's respiratory status closely, especially in the early phase of illness. Look for such signs as dyspnea, inability to handle secretions, inadequate respiratory effort, and color changes that may indicate the need for endotracheal intubation and mechanical ventilation.

Manage Autonomic Nervous System Dysfunction

Monitor the child's vital signs closely for episodes of tachycardia, bradycardia, and hypotension. Blood pressure fluctuations and autonomic instability are linked to fatal cardiac arrhythmias (Jones, 2000). Observe frequently for decreased responsiveness. Intervene promptly if these or other signs of autonomic nervous system dysfunction are noted.

Meet Nutritional Needs

Assess whether the child is having difficulty swallowing. If the child has no gag reflex, nutritional needs are maintained with intravenous supplements or nasogastric tube feedings.

Prevent Complications

Prevent complications associated with immobility (see Box 33–3 on page 1305). Ensure good postural alignment, and turn the child every 2 hours. Maintaining skin integrity is also important.

Evaluate the child's muscle tone, strength, and symmetry. When the child's condition begins to improve, recovery of lost strength is the priority. Active exercise is emphasized in physical therapy. Encourage family members to participate in the child's care, especially during the recovery phase. They can help with the activities of daily living and reinforce what the child has learned in physical therapy.

Provide Emotional Support

Explain the progression of Guillain-Barré syndrome to the parents during the initial stages. Witnessing a rapid deterioration in their child's physical status can be frightening; therefore, preparation is essential to reduce their anxieties. Be honest when discussing recovery and prognosis for the child.

Have parents bring in favorite toys, dolls, or books to make the child feel more secure. Playing with or reading to the child can be comforting.

Discharge Planning and Home Care Teaching

Home care needs should be identified and addressed well in advance of discharge. Support the parents as they prepare for the child's return home. Provide referral to home care nurses who can manage all aspects of treatment, rehabilitation, and follow-up. Refer the parents to social workers who can help with financial arrangements and school considerations.

Care in the Community

Help the child to adjust to any residual effects of Guillain-Barré syndrome. Help the child practice exercises learned in physical therapy sessions, and encourage the child to perform activities of daily living, such as brushing the teeth or combing the hair. Refer the child to outpatient rehabilitation programs to promote recovery.

To promote a positive self-image, praise any effort the child makes to be self-sufficient. The child may have feelings of frustration and anger. Allow the child to express these feelings in an appropriate way, either during play or in conversation.

HEADACHES

Children commonly experience headaches. They may be the cause of school absence, decreased extracurricular activity, and poor academic achievement. Up to 82% of children experience a headache by late adolescence (O'Hara & Koch, 1998). Migraine headaches occur in 1% to 3% of children under 5 years of age, and 5% to 10% of children under 15 years (Rosenblum & Fisher, 2001).

Headaches have both benign (migraine, inflammatory, and tension) and structural causes (tumors and increased intracranial pressure). Causes and clinical manifestations for various headaches can be found in the table below.

- Migraines may be triggered by stress; foods containing nitrates, glutamate, caffeine, tyramine, and salt; menses; oral contraceptives; stress; fatigue; and hunger. Another family member often has similar headaches, so genetic predisposition may also be a factor. Children with classic migraines have an aura (auditory, visual, or taste sensation) that provides a warning of an impending headache. When the aura occurs, taking abortive medication may abort or diminish the severity of the headache.
- Tension headaches may be associated with stresses associated with school, insecurity, or conflict in the family.
- Medication overuse headaches are associated with the frequent use of medications for headaches, more than two to three times a week. Medications associated with this disorder include acetaminophen, nonsteroidal anti-inflammatory drugs (NSAIDs), triptans, caffeine, opiates, benzodiazepines, barbiturates, and ergotamines (Reimschisel, 2003).

CLINICAL MANIFESTATIONS and Management of Headaches

TYPE OF HEADACHE AND ETIOLOGY	CLINICAL MANIFESTATIONS	CLINICAL THERAPY
Migraine—vascular Acute recurrent	• Unilateral or bilateral pulsatile throbbing pain lasting for hours or days • Pain often in retro-orbital frontal and temporal region • Preschool-age children may have irritability, malaise, head banging, head holding, and sensitivity to light and sound • Nausea and vomiting • Photophobia and phonophobia • Visual or motor aura several minutes before headache starts • Recurrent abdominal pain • Increased pain with activity • Relief with sleep	• Food elimination trial to identify food triggers • Caffeine avoidance • Noise and light avoidance • Medications to abort migraine (e.g., ergot, esometheptene, supatriptan) • Analgesic medication (e.g., ibuprofen, acetaminophen) • Relaxation techniques and biofeedback
Tension—muscular contraction Acute recurrent or chronic nonprogressive	• Dull, achy pain in band around head, in temporal or occipital areas, in neck and shoulders that may last for days • Intermittent or constant pain with fluctuations in degree of pain • Nausea and vomiting are rare • Dizziness and fatigue may be present • Sensitive to light or sound • Pain may be aggravated with increased physical activity	• Relaxation techniques • Analgesic and anti-inflammatory medications • Ice pack • Rest
Medication overuse	• Dull, bilateral or unilateral pain in frontal area • Occur at least 2–4 times a week or almost daily • Can vary in character, location, and severity from time to time • Usually increases in frequency and severity over time, paralleling the increase in medication use • Recur with the abortive therapy or medication wears off	• Discontinuation of all medications for headaches (e.g., caffeine, acetaminophen, NSAIDs, and triptans) • Clonidine may be used to treat withdrawal symptoms
Inflammatory—sinusitis or dental abscess Acute localized	• Facial pain or tenderness over affected sinus • Dull, constant pressure • Severity of pain varies with position of head • Fever	• Analgesic, antipyretic, and anti-inflammatory medications • Antibiotic medications • Cold or heat application
Structural—space-occupying lesion, hemorrhage, increased intracranial pressure Chronic progressive	• Pain that awakens child in morning • Pain worse in morning, with coughing, sneezing, or straining • Morning vomiting, no nausea • Worsening pain with exertion or position changes, increasing frequency • Abnormal neurologic signs within 2–6 months of headache onset (i.e., double vision, papilledema)	• Surgery • Analgesic medications

MediaLink Headache Resources and Support

Collaborative Care

Diagnosis is usually made by obtaining a detailed history of the following headache characteristics: onset, warning signs, duration, time of day, severity and location of pain, and associated symptoms such as blurred vision, and photophobia. Laboratory tests are not useful for diagnosing the most common headaches. The child is assessed for neurologic signs such as altered consciousness, abnormal cranial nerves, papilledema, and motor or sensory deficits. Radiological studies (CT scan or MRI) are used only if a structural problem is suspected. A lumbar puncture is performed if an infection or inflammatory process is suspected.

Treatment includes relaxation techniques, acetaminophen, and anti-inflammatory medications. Food elimination diet trials may be initiated in an effort to identify foods that trigger headaches; however, they are often unsuccessful. Medications to abort migraines (ergot or isometheptene) are used in children old enough to identify an aura, or warning. Sumatriptan in oral, nasal spray, or subcutaneous injectable form may be used to abort migraines in adolescents. Cyproheptadine, beta-blockers, tricyclic antidepressants, and anticonvulsants (valproic acid, topiramate, and gabapentin) may be used prophylactically if headaches significantly interfere with usual activities (Lewis, Scott, & Rendin, 2002).

Nursing Management

Nursing management involves assessing the child for potential neurologic signs associated with headaches. Encourage the child to keep a calendar or diary of headaches, including the events and stresses occurring at the time. This will help to identify the recurrence pattern of headaches and potential triggers. When a food elimination trial is implemented, educate the child and family about foods to eat and not eat, and how to gradually add foods to identify offending chemical triggers. Assist the child and family to identify strategies for relieving the headaches. Make sure the child learns to take analgesics early and other prescribed medications appropriately. Teach children and parents that medications should not be taken in any combination for more than 2 to 3 days a week. Using them more frequently can result in medication overuse headaches. Assist the child to see patterns of stress that appear in the headache diary and discuss strategies that may help reduce that stress. See Complementary Therapy: Treating Headaches.

See Chapter 29∞ for care of the child with a brain tumor.

STRUCTURAL DEFECTS

Microcephaly

Microcephaly is a small brain with a head circumference greater than 3 standard deviations below the mean for age and sex, or below the 3rd percentile on growth curves (Vannucci, 2002). It may be caused by chromosomal abnormalities, fetal insult, maternal infection, or destructive insult during the infancy, such as infection, metabolic disorder, or anoxia. There is a relationship between microcephaly and cognitive impairments. See Chapter 34∞ for care of the child with mental retardation.

> **COMPLEMENTARY THERAPY**
> **Treating Headaches**
>
> Mind-body therapies that include biofeedback, self-hypnosis, progressive relaxation, meditation, and cognitive-behavioral therapy have been studied in children and found to be effective in treating the pain associated with headaches. In biofeedback, instruments (α-electroencephalography, muscle electromyography, skin temperature, and temporal pulse feedback) can be used to raise the awareness of physical states in the body and to make changes in cranial blood flow, thus helping to control pain. Most children reported a 50% reduction in headache pain with the use of biofeedback. Other therapies are often used with biofeedback to enhance the effect (Scharff & Kemper, 2003).

Hydrocephalus

Hydrocephalus is the body's response to an imbalance between the production and absorption of cerebrospinal fluid, leading to an increase in the volume of cerebrospinal fluid. The condition is often congenital and associated with other central nervous system malformations. The overall incidence is estimated to be 1 per 2,000 births (Ditmyer, 2004). It is commonly associated with **myelomeningocele**, a spinal fluid–filled meningeal sac that contains a portion of the spinal cord and nerves protruding through a vertebral defect. Hydrocephalus can develop as a complication of illness (e.g., meningitis or brain tumor) or injury (intraventricular hemorrhage and brain injury).

Etiology and Pathophysiology

Cerebrospinal fluid is produced by the choroid plexus within the lateral, third, and fourth ventricles at a rate of about 500 mL per day after 1 year of age (Ditmyer, 2004). In usual circumstances, the same amount of cerebrospinal fluid is absorbed by the subarachnoid space into the venous circulation. Cerebrospinal fluid must pass through a number of channels and pathways between the ventricles, around the brainstem and spinal cord, and to the surface of the brain until it reaches the subarachnoid space. Hydrocephalus may be either communicating or noncommunicating, and congenital or acquired.

In communicating hydrocephalus the cerebrospinal fluid flows freely between normal channels and pathways, but absorption of cerebrospinal fluid in the subarachnoid space and the arachnoid villi is impaired. This form of hydrocephalus is often acquired from postinfectious meningitis, trauma, or intraventricular hemorrhage, or it may be a congenital malformation of the subarachnoid spaces.

Noncommunicating hydrocephalus is responsible for the majority of cases in children. It results from an obstruction in the channels or pathways that impede the flow of cerebrospinal fluid and prevent it from entering the subarachnoid space (Figure 33–10 ■). Enlargement of one or more of the ventricles occurs. This obstruction can be caused by infection, ventricular hemorrhage, tumor, or structural deformity. Congenital structural defects include the Chiari II malformation (found in most children with myelomeningocele), aqueduct of Sylvius stenosis, and the Dandy-Walker syndrome.

PATHOPHYSIOLOGY ILLUSTRATED

Hydrocephalus

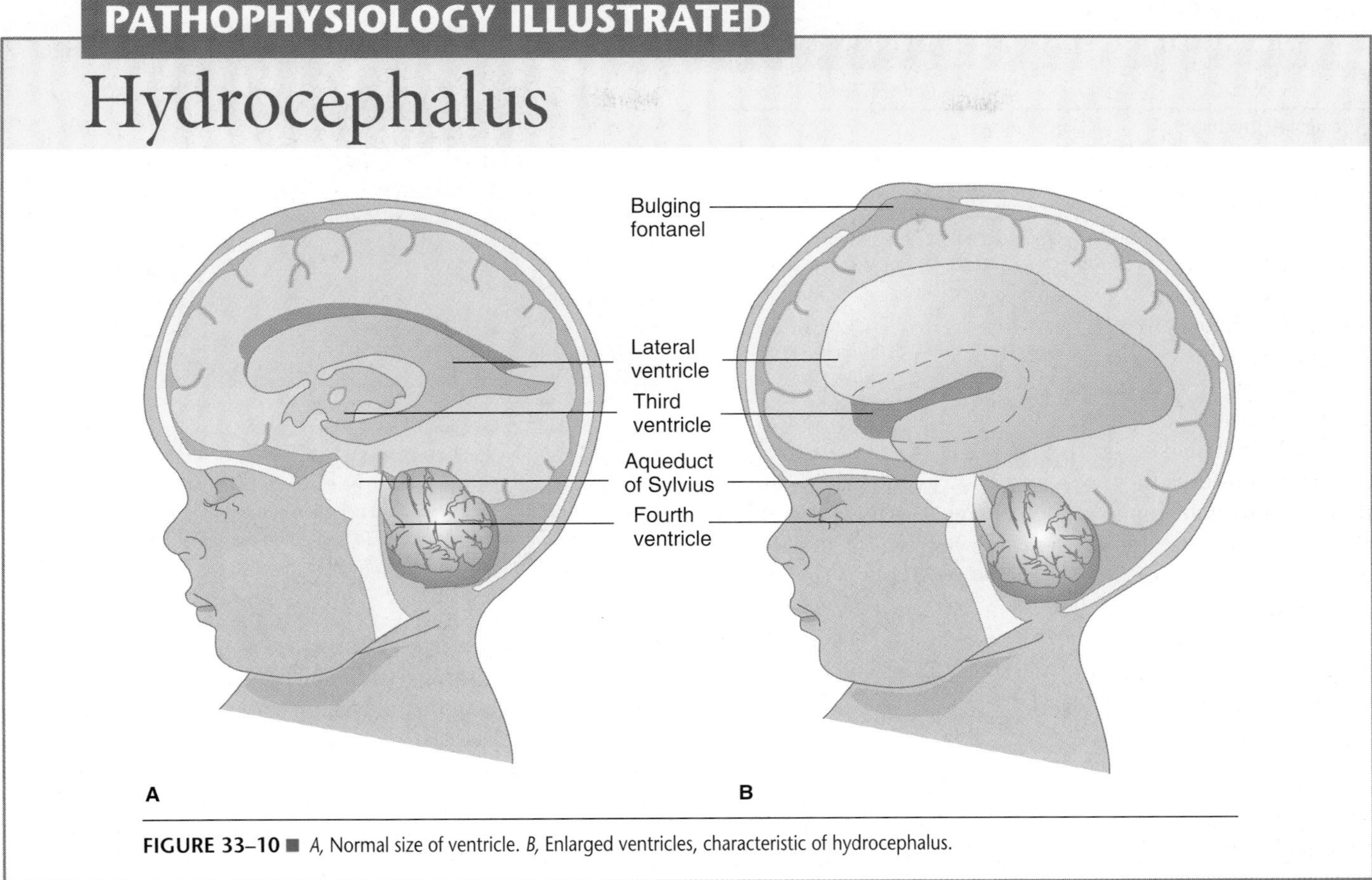

FIGURE 33–10 ■ *A,* Normal size of ventricle. *B,* Enlarged ventricles, characteristic of hydrocephalus.

The development of Chiari II malformation may be associated with the low pressure in the hindbrain that occurs with leakage of cerebrospinal fluid from the back during fetal development (Liptak, 2002). See Box 33–9. Stenosis of the aqueduct of Sylvius is usually a recessive X-linked cause of hydrocephalus. In Dandy-Walker syndrome, the fetal brain does not develop as expected and the fourth ventricle enlarges into an ependymal cyst.

Very premature infants are at great risk for an intraventricular hemorrhage within a week after birth. Hydrocephalus is a major complication of intraventricular hemorrhage.

BOX 33–9 Chiari II Malformation

The Chiari II malformation involves a downward displacement of the cerebellum, brainstem, and fourth ventricle and herniation through the foramen magnum into the cervical spaces. Because these structures control respiration and the protective reflexes, as well as house the cranial nerves, the displacement can have varying effects such as sudden death, respiratory difficulty, swallowing difficulties, and the need for assisted ventilation. Signs and symptoms may occur at any time. Rapid surgical decompression is needed to reduce brainstem compression and to prevent death. Approximately 15% of children with this malformation die by the age of 3 years, and another third have permanent neurologic disability (Stevenson, 2004). Another period when there is progression of clinical signs occurs in adolescents and young adults (Lazzaretti & Pearson, 2004).

Clinical Manifestations

The signs and symptoms of hydrocephalus, which vary depending on the age of the child, are listed in the clinical manifestations table on page 1326. The predominant manifestation of the condition in infants is a rapidly increasing head circumference (Figure 33–11 ■). Once the skull sutures have closed, children develop signs of increased intracranial pressure (see Table 33–1).

COLLABORATIVE CARE

The goal of collaborative care is to rapidly diagnose the hydrocephalus and perform surgery to reduce the consequences of excessive cerebrospinal fluid on the child's developing cognitive and motor function.

Diagnostic Testing

Diagnosis is based on physical examination and neuroimaging studies. A rapidly increasing head circumference that crosses percentile lines on a growth curve raises early suspicions. In the hospital setting, daily measurements of the infant's head circumference are critical in any infant at risk of developing hydrocephalus. In older children, signs of increased intracranial pressure are noted. CT scanning and MRI are used to diagnose hydrocephalus, and in some cases the anatomic cause is revealed. In the infant whose fontanel is still open, ultrasonography or echoencephalography may be used to confirm the diagnosis.

CLINICAL MANIFESTATIONS of Hydrocephalus

ETIOLOGY	CLINICAL MANIFESTATIONS
Congenital structural defect in infancy Dandy-Walker syndrome Arnold-Chiari II malformation Aqueductal stenosis Acquired injury in infancy Intraventricular hemorrhage	Early signs Rapidly increasing head circumference Tense, full, or bulging fontanel; split sutures Bossing (protrusion) of frontal area, face is disproportionate to the skull size Macewen's or "cracked-pot" sign with percussion of the skull indicates split sutures **Sunsetting eyes** (sclera visible above iris), sixth cranial nerve palsy Prominent, distended scalp veins Translucent scalp skin Increased tone or hyperreflexia, brisk deep tendon reflexes, Babinski sign Irritability or lethargy, poor feeding Decline in level of consciousness Difficulty holding the head up Late signs Apnea Shrill, high-pitched cry Difficulty swallowing or feeding Vomiting Cardiopulmonary depression (severe cases)
Acquired hydrocephalus in older child after closure of sutures Postinfectious Tumor Hemorrhage	No head enlargement Irritability, lethargy, poor appetite Headache upon arising with vomiting Fussiness, sleepiness, confusion, or apathy Altered level of consciousness Personality change, loss of interest in daily activities Poor judgment or verbal incoherence, worsening school performance, memory loss Ataxia, spasticity, or other alterations in motor development Visual defects secondary to pressure on second, third, and sixth cranial nerves; papilledema Signs of increased intracranial pressure

CT scanning and MRI are also used to evaluate shunt failure. Other studies used to evaluate shunt function include lateral radiographs of the skull, neck, chest, and abdomen to view all the apparatus components, a radionucleotide cerebrospinal fluid study, and a culture of the cerebrospinal fluid obtained by tapping the shunt.

Clinical Therapy

For some children, treatment with medications (furosemide and acetazolamide) helps reduce the rate of cerebrospinal fluid production by about 50% to 75% on a temporary basis until surgery is performed. A ventricular access device may alternately be inserted prior to shunt placement, enabling withdrawal of cerebrospinal fluid. Surgery is performed to remove the obstruction (e.g., surgical removal of a tumor) or to create a new cerebrospinal fluid pathway. When the obstruction to cerebrospinal

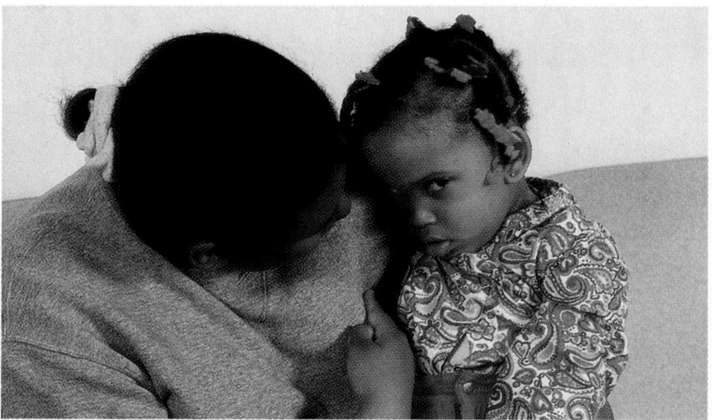

FIGURE 33–11 ■ In communicating hydrocephalus, an excessive amount of cerebrospinal fluid accumulates in the subarachnoid space, producing the characteristic head enlargement seen here. When observing the child with hydrocephalus, look for a downward deviation of the eyes in which the lower half of the iris is hidden by the lower eyelid (sunsetting eyes). This finding occurs in severe hydrocephalus, but it is not present in this child.

fluid flow cannot be removed, a catheter or shunt is placed in the ventricle to divert the cerebrospinal fluid to the peritoneal cavity, atrium of the heart, or the pleural spaces. Ventriculoperitoneal shunts (Figure 33–12 ■) are commonly used. In some older children a ventriculoatrial shunt is used, draining the cerebrospinal fluid into the right atrium of the heart. The reservoir is palpable at the burr hole placed into the skull, providing access for evaluation of function. The tubing may be palpated from the burr hole to the insertion point into the chest or abdomen. Adequate distal tubing is now inserted to accommodate the child's growth and reduce the need for future surgery. See Box 33–10.

Mechanical complications may include blockage at either the proximal or the distal end of the catheter, kinking of the tubing, or valve breakdown. Infants or children with shunt failure show signs and symptoms of recurrent hydrocephalus and increased intracranial pressure. Shunt failure and ventricular size are confirmed by CT scanning or MRI. Shunt materials and systems continue to be refined in an attempt to reduce mechanical problems.

The most serious complication is shunt infection, which may occur at any time but is most prevalent in the first few

BOX 33–10 Research: New Techniques for Hydrocephalus Management

Researchers in neuroendoscopy are developing techniques to create a new pathway for cerebrospinal fluid to flow between the ventricles and spinal cord in individuals with obstructive hydrocephalus. The new endoscopy procedure in which a hole is placed in the floor of one of the ventricles to drain cerebrospinal fluid from the brain seems to have a higher success rate over 18 months in infants newly diagnosed with hydrocephalus and in children diagnosed with aqueductal stenosis. It is unknown if a shunt will ultimately need to be placed in these children due to long-term treatment failure. Continuing research is needed to identify the types of hydrocephalus in which the procedure may be most successful (Ditmyer, 2004).

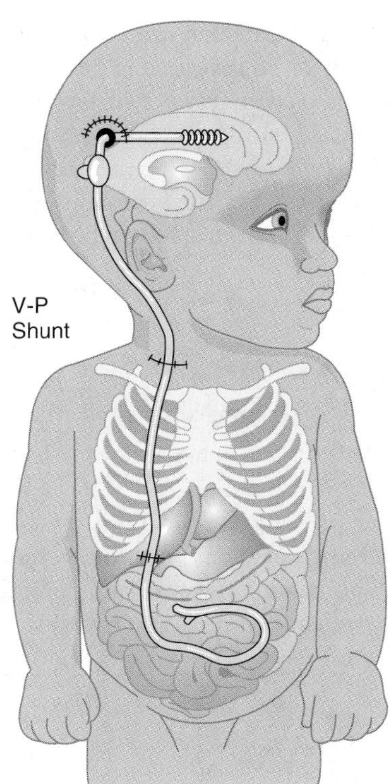

FIGURE 33–12 ■ A ventriculoperitoneal shunt, commonly used to treat children with hydrocephalus, is often placed at about 3–4 months of age; however, it may be placed at any age as needed to treat secondary hydrocephalus from conditions such as meningitis or tumors. The shunt systems consist of four parts: a ventricular catheter, a pumping chamber or reservoir, a one-way pressure valve, and a distal catheter. The tubing drains the excess cerebrospinal fluid from the ventricles to the abdomen. The main goal of treatment is to reduce the intracranial pressure and to preserve central nervous system function.

months after placement. The infection rate is 4% per year, with infants under 6 months having the highest rates (Ditmyer, 2004). The infection may be confirmed by culture of the cerebrospinal fluid obtained from the reservoir located in the burr hole. Antibiotics are usually prescribed. The shunt is surgically removed and an external ventricular drainage device is placed. The positioning of the external collection device, usually at the level of the external auditory meatus, is important to allow the appropriate amount of cerebrospinal fluid to flow by gravity. A new shunt is inserted when the cerebrospinal fluid cultures are sterile.

Some children, especially those with ventriculoatrial shunts, are placed on the same prophylactic antibiotic treatment regimen used for children with cardiac anomalies to reduce the risk of shunt infections (refer to Chapter 26∞).

NURSING MANAGEMENT

The goals of nursing management are to monitor infants for signs of unexpected increases in head circumference and increased intracranial pressure, and to provide nursing care during the recuperation from surgery and community follow-up.

Nursing Assessment and Diagnosis

It is important for nurses to become familiar with the clinical manifestations of hydrocephalus to ensure prompt identification and treatment of children with this condition. Head circumference of all infants is measured at each well-child visit and plotted on a growth curve to detect the condition at an early stage. (See Skills Manual.)

Following surgery to place a shunt, the child's vital signs and levels of responsiveness and irritability are assessed frequently to monitor the functioning of the shunt and for signs of increased intracranial pressure. Surgical sites are evaluated for signs of drainage and infection; redness and swelling of the shunt tract; leakage of cerebrospinal fluid from a surgical site; nuchal rigidity; neck or back pain; headache; and photophobia (Ditmyer, 2004). Carefully assess respiratory status. Assess intake and output in the immediate postoperative period. Assess pain in the postoperative period.

Following surgery and at each healthcare visit, assess the child with a ventriculoperitoneal shunt for shunt failure and infection. Signs and symptoms include changes in responsiveness, irritability after fever is controlled, low-grade fever, malaise, headache, and nausea.

Daily measurement of the infant's head circumference and comparison with the previous day's measurement is performed when shunt failure is suspected. Report any abnormalities to the physician immediately.

Nursing diagnoses that may be appropriate for the child with hydrocephalus include the following:

- Risk for Infection related to presence of shunt
- Impaired Physical Mobility related to decreased muscle mass to lift the increased weight of head
- Risk for Caregiver Role Strain related to care of a child with a chronic condition or life-threatening illness
- Anxiety (parent) related to repeated surgeries and life-threatening illness
- Risk for Delayed Development related to compression of brain tissue with excess cerebrospinal fluid

Planning and Implementation

Nursing care in the hospital setting focuses on providing postoperative care and providing emotional support.

The child is usually placed in a flat position to prevent rapid cerebrospinal fluid drainage. The head of the bed is elevated gradually. Position the child carefully; do not stretch or strain the neck muscles, as they must support the large head. Holding the child may be awkward because of the additional weight of the head.

Provide good skin care. Reduce the chances for skin breakdown by the use of an air mattress or by placing sheepskin or a lamb's wool blanket under the head. Prevent any other complications associated with immobility (see Box 33–3 on page 1305).

Attend to the child's special nutritional needs. Because the infant is prone to vomiting, frequent small feedings with frequent burping are beneficial.

Provide Emotional Support

Provide parents with explanations about the child's condition and all procedures to be performed. Encourage parents and family to help with the child's care in the hospital when appropriate. Be sympathetic and understanding, and allow parents to express their concerns. If hydrocephalus occurs during early infancy, the parents will be anxious about the impact of the chronic condition and subsequent surgical procedures. If hydrocephalus is secondary to neoplasm, however, the parents' anxieties are compounded by their child's life-threatening illness.

Assure parents that most children with shunts lead normal lives, attending school and interacting with others no differently than their peers.

Discharge Planning and Home Care Teaching

MediaLink Hydrocephalus Resources and Support

Address home care needs well in advance of discharge. Parents must know how to care for a child with a shunt. Educate parents and other family members about important signs and symptoms of both shunt failure (signs of increased intracranial pressure) and infection (changes in responsiveness, irritability, personality change, malaise, headache, diplopia, nausea, loss of developmental milestones or loss of coordination and balance, and low-grade fever) and the need to inform the healthcare provider immediately. Alert parents that the child may also develop a seizure disorder, and how to care for the child if a seizure occurs. Provide telephone numbers of the pediatrician and the neurosurgeon, and instruct parents to contact a physician immediately if the child develops seizures or if a problem is suspected with the shunt. Inform them that the shunt may need to be replaced if an infection occurs.

Infants with poor head control due to an enlarged head should not be placed in forward-facing car safety seats, regardless of their age. This position increases the risk of cervical spine injury and death to these children in the event of a car crash.

Appropriate home care referrals should be arranged. Refer families to the support groups and appropriate social services, including the Hydrocephalus Association.

Care in the Community

Infants and children need frequent monitoring to ensure proper functioning of the shunt. Head circumference is measured at each visit and compared to expected growth curves to monitor growth. Assess the child for visual problems and cognitive, speech, and motor developmental delays that are often associated problems. The child and family should be referred to an early intervention program to promote developmental progress. School-age children may need to have an individualized education plan developed (see Chapter 20∞). Intellectual functioning outcomes may be associated with the cause of the hydrocephalus and age at diagnosis. For example, children with uncomplicated congenital causes do better than those who have brain injury, infection, or intraventricular hemorrhage.

Parents seeking childcare for their infant should be encouraged to use a setting with fewer children to decrease exposure to infection. Review the signs of shunt failure and infection with parents at each visit and make sure they have a plan to manage the emergency of a shunt failure. An emergency information form should be completed and up to date that can be provided to emergency department personnel who may need to care for the child.

Continue to support parents who will have ongoing concerns about shunt failure. Encourage parents not to be overprotective and to allow the child to develop normally. Participation in sports with a high potential for head and abdominal impact should be discouraged. A helmet should be used for bicycle riding and skateboarding.

Evaluation

Expected outcomes of nursing care include the following:

- The child develops adequate neck muscle control to interact with the environment.
- Shunt infections and malfunctions are identified by the parents and medical attention is sought quickly.
- The child's potential for growth and development is maximized by care and a stimulating environment.

Neural Tube Defects

The neural tube is the tissue that ultimately develops the central nervous system, including the brain and spinal cord. The incidence of neural tube defects is 0.7 to 1 per 1,000 live births in the United States (Padgett, 2002). See Box 33–11 for types of neural tube defects.

Myelodysplasia or Spina Bifida

Myelodysplasia refers to a malformation of the spinal cord and spinal canal while **spina bifida** refers to a defect in one or more vertebrae through which spinal cord contents can protrude. It is often associated with a protrusion of meningeal sac filled with a portion of the spinal cord. The malformation can occur anywhere along the vertebral column, but is most common at the lumbar or sacral portion of the spine. This is the most common developmental disorder of the central nervous system. The condition occurs in about 1 per 2,000 births in the United States each year, but varies by region of the country (Northrup & Volcik, 2000). See Developing Cultural Competence: Spina Bifida Occurrence.

Etiology and Pathophysiology. Neural tube defects occur within 1 month of conception during the initial formation of

BOX 33–11 Types of Neural Tube Defects

Anencephaly—no development of the brain above the brainstem

Encephalocele—protrusion of meningeal tissue or meningeal-covered brain through a defect in the skull

Spina bifida occulta—a vertebral defect without visible protrusion of the meninges or spinal cord tissue; the area lying over the defect may have an abnormal growth of hair, a dimple or sinus tract, a subcutaneous mass such as a lipoma, or a vascular skin lesion

Meningocele—a spinal fluid–filled meningeal sac protruding through a vertebral defect, associated with no abnormalities of the spinal cord

Meningomyelocele—a spinal fluid–filled meningeal sac that contains a portion of the spinal cord and nerves protruding through a vertebral defect

DEVELOPING CULTURAL COMPETENCE
Spina Bifida Occurrence

The rate of spina bifida varies with ethnicity and geographic location in the United States. Hispanic persons, especially those in Texas, have the highest rate. The rates of other ethnic groups in descending order are Caucasians, African Americans, and Asian Americans. This may be due to parental environmental exposures and genetic factors as neural tube defects are known to cluster in families (Northrup & Volcik, 2000).

the central nervous system. During this period, the neural groove folds over to become the neural tube, from which the spinal cord and vertebral arches develop. If the neural groove does not close completely, a neural tube defect develops.

The cause of myelodysplasia is unknown, although environmental factors such as chemicals (excessive use of alcohol), medications (e.g., valproic acid and carbamazepine used for seizures, isotretinoin for acne), genetic factors, and maternal health conditions (insulin-dependent diabetes mellitus, gestational diabetes, folic acid deficiency, and maternal obesity) have been implicated. The increased incidence of the condition in families indicates a possible genetic influence. The U.S. Food and Drug Administration mandated fortification of all enriched grain products with folate by January 1998, which has resulted in significant reduction in both spina bifida and anencephaly. See Table 33–6.

Clinical Manifestations. There are several different types of spina bifida (Figure 33–13 ■). A saclike protrusion on the infant's back indicates meningocele or myelomeningocele. The clinical manifestations seen depend on the location of the defect: The higher the defect, the greater the neurologic dysfunction.

- *Thoracic or lumbar 1–2 level:* paralysis of the legs, weakness and sensory loss in the trunk and lower body region
- *Lumbar 3:* can flex hips, extend the knees, ankle and toe paralysis
- *Lumber 4–5 level:* can flex hips, extend knees, weak or absent ankle extension, toe flexion, and hip extension

TABLE 33–6 The Declining Incidence of Neural Tube Defects Since Fortification of Enriched Grain Products with Folate Beginning in 1996

YEAR	MYELODYSPLASIA RATE (PER 100,000 LIVE BIRTHS)	ANENCEPHALY RATE (PER 100,000 LIVE BIRTHS)
2001	20.05	9.42
2000	20.85	10.33
1999	20.72	10.81
1998	22.45	9.92
1997	24.70	12.51
1996	26.36	11.96
1995	27.98	11.71

From Mathews, T. J. (2003). Trends in spina bifida and anencephalus in the United States, 1991–2001. *National Center for Health Statistics Health and Stats.* www.cdc.gov/nchs/products/pubs/pubd/hestats/spine_anen.htm, *accessed 7/17/2003.*

- *Sacral level:* mild weakness in ankles and toes, bladder and bowel function may be affected

Sensory loss is often more pronounced on the back of the legs, and the loss of motor and sensory function may not be symmetric between the lower extremities. Sensory loss around the anus, genitalia, and feet is common. Bowel and bladder sphincters may be affected. Renal involvement may result from neurologic impairment and urinary retention. Hydrocephalus is usually present in children with myelomeningocele due to the Chiari II malformation that is found in nearly all children with the defect above the sacral level. See the clinical manifestations table below for the range of potential problems in the child with myelodysplasia.

Children have many associated disabilities as a result of myelodysplasia, including mobility problems, cognitive impairment, seizure disorders, and visual impairment such as strabismus. Complications can develop such as spinal curvatures, musculoskeletal and joint abnormalities, skin sores, urinary dysfunction, and sexual dysfunction.

PRACTICE ALERT

Between 18% and 40% of children with myelodysplasia have a latex allergy. Cases in which latex exposure has caused anaphylaxis in a child have been reported. All children with latex allergy need to carry a kit with premeasured adrenaline for emergency treatment of anaphylaxis. Use nonlatex materials when providing care to the child in the hospital, in the outpatient setting, or at home. The Spina Bifida Association maintains an updated list of products containing latex and potential substitutes (Table 27–10∞).

CLINICAL MANIFESTATIONS of Myelodysplasia

CAUSE	CLINICAL MANIFESTATIONS
Interruption of the spinal cord at site of the spinal defect	Loss of motor and sensory function of the abdomen and lower extremities, dependent on defect level Scoliosis or kyphosis Incontinence of urine or urinary retention Incontinence of feces or constipation Sensory loss around genitalia
Muscle imbalance	Hip abnormalities, hip dysplasia Foot deformities, e.g., clubfoot
Chiari II malformation	Hydrocephalus *Infants:* Difficulty swallowing Apnea, respiratory difficulty, inspiratory stridor Weak or poor cry Sustained backward arching of the head (opisthotonos) *Older children:* Choking, hoarseness, vocal cord paralysis Disordered breathing during sleep Stiffness or spasticity of arms and hands Loss of feeling or sensation
Brain and spinal cord abnormalities	Learning problems, attention deficit disorder Problems with perceptual motor skills Memory and organization problems Problems with numerical reasoning

MediaLink Living with Spina Bifida Video

PATHOPHYSIOLOGY ILLUSTRATED

Types of Spina Bifida

Spina bifida occulta Failure of posterior vertebral arches to fuse, most commonly at fifth lumbar or first sacral vertebrae; spinal cord and meninges entirely within vertebral canal; condition usually not visible externally; tuft of hair, a dermoid cyst, or hemangioma may be found over the site; mildest form

Spina bifida cystica Defect in closure of posterior vertebral arch with protrusion through bony spine

Meningocele Saclike protrusion through bony defect containing meninges and cerebrospinal fluid; sac covering defect may be translucent or membranous; spinal cord and spinal root in normal position

Myelomeningocele Saclike herniation through bony defect holding meninges, cerebrospinal fluid, and a portion of spinal cord or nerve roots; fluid leakage may also occur; lesion poorly covered with imperfect tissue; handicap 99% of time; more common than meningocele

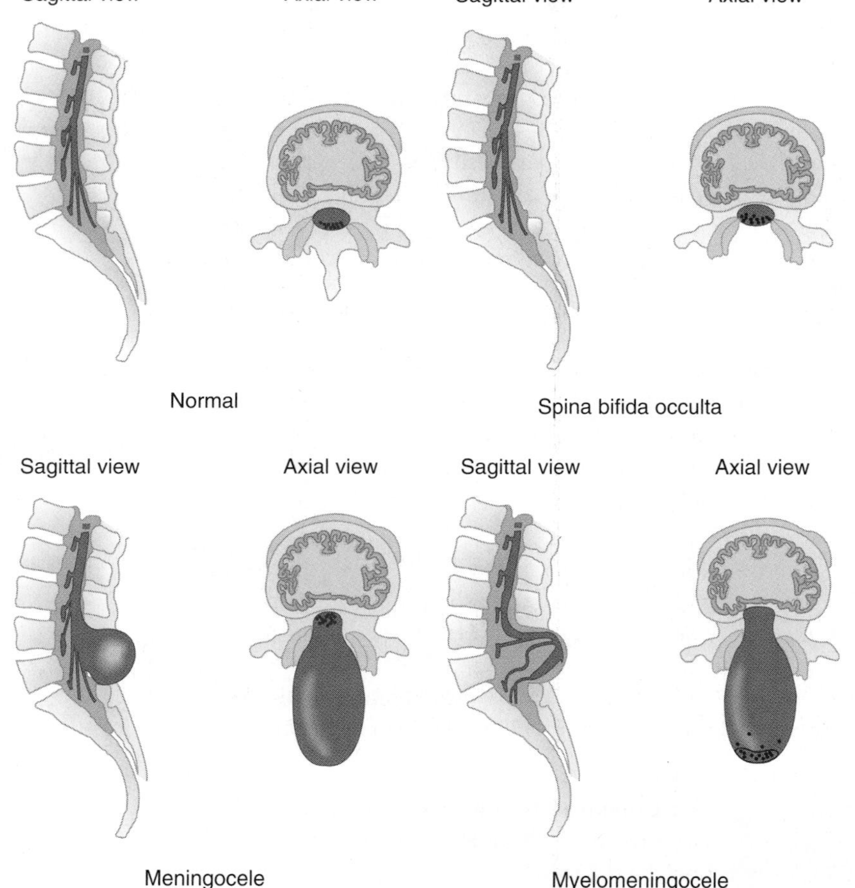

FIGURE 33–13 ■ Note the different conditions that result from a vertebral bony defect.

COLLABORATIVE CARE

The goal of collaborative care is to close the defect to reduce infection and evaluate the neurologic complications resulting from the defect. Clinical therapy is then focused on managing the complications of the disorder while promoting the child's growth and development.

Diagnostic Testing

Prenatal maternal serum tests for alpha-fetoprotein that are elevated raise suspicion that the newborn will have a neural tube defect and a high resolution fetal ultrasound may aid diagnosis. After birth a multidisciplinary team examines the lesion and evaluates neurologic status. Ultrasonography, radiologic imaging by CT scan, MRI, and flat films of the spinal column can pinpoint the bony defect. Subsequent testing is performed to evaluate bladder and bowel function, neurologic and motor function, and cognitive function.

Clinical Therapy

Surgery to close and repair the meningocele or myelomeningocele lesion usually occurs within 24 to 48 hours of the infant's birth to reduce infection. Depending on the size of the defect, the excision area may be extensive. In some cases, uteromyelomeningocele repairs are performed. In cases of spina bifida occulta, surgical intervention is rarely needed.

Braces are used to support joint position and mobility. Assistive devices such as walkers, crutches, and wheelchairs are used to enhance mobility. To minimize the risk for osteoporosis, the diet should ensure adequate calcium and vitamin D and weight-bearing activities should be encouraged. Surgery or an orthotic jacket may correct spinal deformities that affect lung capacity and interfere with mobility and sitting.

Bladder interventions are initiated early to prevent kidney damage and to maintain bladder function and urinary continence. When clean intermittent catheterization is not totally effective in promoting continence, surgical interventions may be performed. Stools softeners and glycerin or bisacodyl suppositories are prescribed for bowel evacuation.

Prognosis depends on the type of defect, the level of the lesion, and the presence of other complicating factors. Children need multiple surgeries and invasive procedures. A team of physicians, nurses, and therapists from the neurosurgery, orthopedic, urology, and physical therapy departments will work with the child and family to form a comprehensive care plan. Pediatric referral centers often establish a clinic for children with myelodysplasia in which services by all disciplines are coordinated in a single visit. Parents and their children often need to travel to these centers to obtain needed care. With the improved care and survival of these children, the majority survive into adulthood.

NURSING MANAGEMENT

Nursing care of the infant or child in the hospital focuses on providing preoperative and postoperative care, promoting mobility, and providing emotional support.

■ Nursing Assessment and Diagnosis

Newborn

Monitor the newborn for integrity of the sac and leakage of cerebrospinal fluid. (Figure 33–14 ■). Assess the extremities for deformities. Frequently assess the vital signs and stay alert for signs of infection. Following surgery, observe the wound healing. Note any signs of infection and cerebrospinal fluid leakage. Measure the head circumference daily after surgery to assess for potential hydrocephalus. Assess intake and output.

Child

Assess the child's vital signs, growth, and head circumference. Assess neurologic status for any deterioration in function that could be associated with shunt failure or problem with the spinal cord. Assess the range of motion of joints and mobility status.

The child with myelodysplasia may be hospitalized for surgery to correct deformities. Assess the child's vital signs, responsiveness, and level of pain. Assess dressing sites for bleeding and draining. Monitor the distal extremities for swelling and circulation. Assess intake and output.

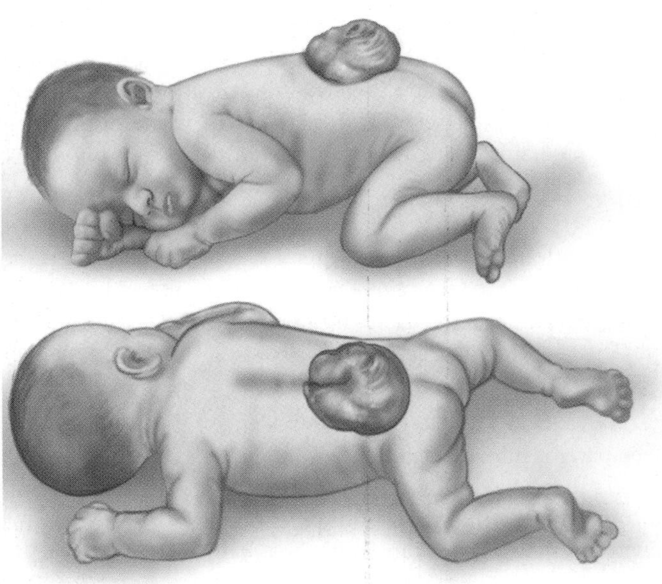

FIGURE 33–14 ■ Lumbrosacral myelomeningocele is caused by a neural tube defect that results in incomplete closure of the vertebral column. As shown here, the meninges (and sometimes the spinal cord) protrude as a saclike structure. Observe for leakage of cerebrospinal fluid.

Examples of nursing diagnoses for the child with myelodysplasia include:

- Impaired Physical Mobility related to neuromuscular impairment
- Impaired Urinary Elimination related to sensory impairment
- Risk for Latex Allergy Response related to multiple surgical procedures
- Risk for Disproportionate Growth related to caloric intake in excess of needs due to limited mobility
- Risk for Impaired Skin Integrity associated with use of braces and wheelchair
- Risk for Infection related to urinary retention

■ Planning and Implementation

Newborn

Cover the sac with a sterile saline dressing to protect its integrity. Protect the defect from pressure, infection, and trauma until surgery can be performed. Place the newborn in a prone position with hips slightly flexed and legs abducted to minimize tension on the sac. Maintain this position using towel rolls placed between the knees. Assess the neonate regularly for motor deficits as well as bladder and bowel involvement.

The newborn is difficult to handle before surgery. Feed the newborn with the head turned to one side until surgery has been performed. Comfort the neonate before surgery with tactile stimulation such as touching, patting, and cuddling.

Monitor the infant's vital signs carefully during the postoperative period. Watch closely for symptoms of infection, especially meningitis. If a ventriculoperitoneal shunt is placed, watch for hydrocephalus, increased intracranial pressure, or infection. Inspect the surgical site for cerebrospinal fluid leakage.

MediaLink Spina Bifida Resources and Support

The infant should be placed in the prone position for sleep until healing has occurred (despite guidelines to put infants to sleep on their backs), and then a supine position for sleep may be used. Keep the diaper away from the incision site. Splints may be used to maintain extremity alignment.

Promote Mobility

Begin gentle range of motion exercises as soon as possible to prevent muscle contractures and atrophy. Extreme caution should be used because these children have brittle bones and are subject to idiopathic fractures.

Provide Emotional Support

Keep parents informed about their infant's status. Allow them to express their frustrations and anger. As soon as parents are able to cope with the infant's condition, encourage them to become involved in the infant's care in the hospital.

Discharge Planning and Home Care Teaching

Home care needs should be identified and addressed well in advance of discharge. Make sure family members understand how to care for the infant or child at home. Help them obtain special devices such as splints, wedges, and rolls, if indicated, to prevent complications. Instruct parents how to position, handle, feed, and perform range of motion exercises. Teach parents the signs and symptoms of increased intracranial pressure, hydrocephalus, shunt infection or malfunction, and urinary tract infection. Home care nursing should be arranged, if necessary. The home care nurse will reinforce the skills learned in the hospital setting and coordinate the numerous healthcare professionals who will be working with the child and family. Refer parents to resource groups such as the Spina Bifida Association of America.

Care in the Community

To reduce complications and promote optimal development, children with myelodysplasia require comprehensive care that is planned and coordinated by a knowledgeable team of healthcare professionals at a pediatric referral center. This care may be provided in partnership with the primary care physician. The nurse has an important role in ensuring that the families with limited financial resources are linked with social services for assistance with transportation, housing, and other care needs. See the Photo Story on pages 1334–1335.

Promote safety and independent mobility with proper use of braces, walkers, crutches, canes, and in some cases custom-designed wheelchairs and car safety seats (Figure 33–15 ■). Encourage the use of latex-free products as the child is at risk for latex allergy (see Chapter 27 ∞). Other safety guidelines are provided later in the chapter.

Parents need to learn how to catheterize the child and then at an appropriate age teach the child intermittent self-catheterization to prevent urinary tract infections and other renal complications (see Chapter 31 ∞). Good nutrition planning is important to prevent obesity and to reduce constipation and complications such as fecal impaction. Bowel training is initiated to control bowel evacuation at appropriate times and places. A diet high in

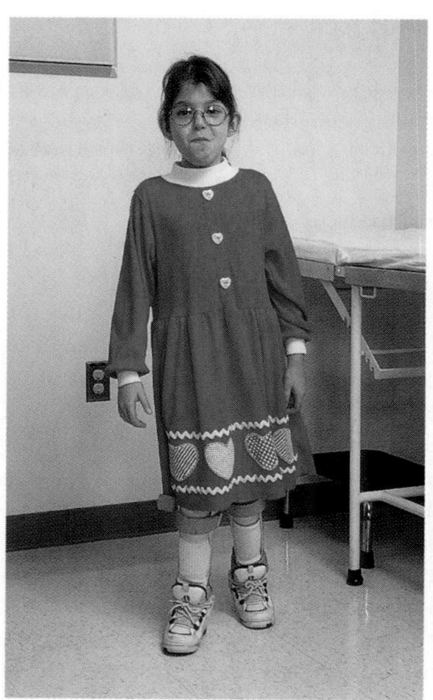

A

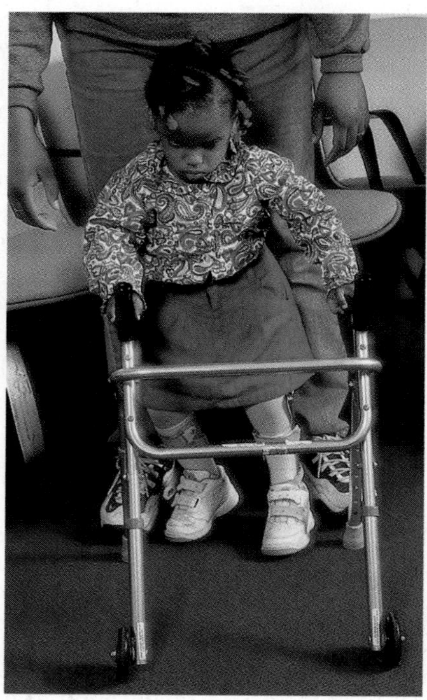

B

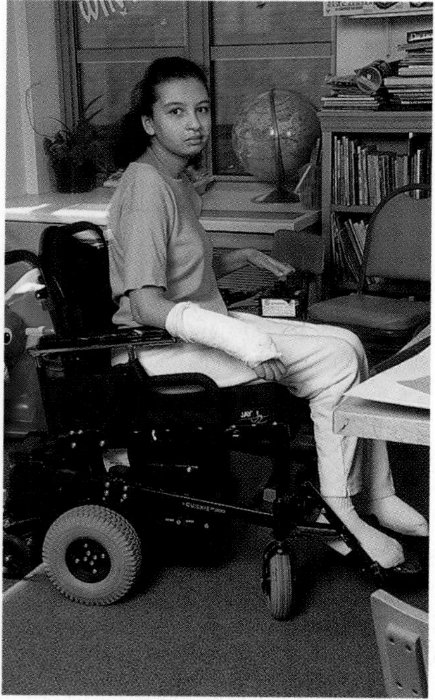

C

FIGURE 33–15 ■ Help determine the best assistive device for the child to gain the most independence for mobilizing and to promote development. The child may change devices in different settings to promote optimal independence. *A* and *B*, Braces and walkers may be best for young children to promote an upright posture that encourages a normal interaction with the environment. *C*, A motorized wheelchair can assist the child with a significant neurologic impairment to achieve independence and mobility.

fiber helps ensure adequate stool. At a convenient time, either morning or night, a glycerin or bisacodyl suppository can be given. Consistency in time of day for bowel evacuation is important. Surgery to create a channel between the skin and bowel (Malone antegrade continence enema) is sometimes performed. Children must learn to assume greater responsibility for self-care as they get older.

Promote good skin care to reduce the risk for skin injury. Encourage daily inspection of all skin areas under braces and splints (see Partnering with Families: Safety for the Child with Myelodysplasia, and Chapter 36∞).

Treat older children according to their intellectual level, not their motor development. Encourage them to take responsibility for self-care, and recognize their need to control their bodily functions. Educational services must be coordinated. An individualized education plan needs to be developed for the child that addresses learning needs and mobility. Adaptive equipment may be needed. Monitor the adolescent for depression and need for counseling services, particularly at this time when differences and challenges in lifestyle become more of concern. Planning for vocational and transition services are important for the adolescent.

Parents are faced with the long-term financial issues of caring for the child who needs regular new adaptive equipment to match growth, as well as other medical supplies. At least 75% of children born with myelodysplasia generally survive to at least the early adult years (Bowman, McLone, Grant, et al., 2001). Parents thus need to learn how to act as the child's case manager, or to work effectively with another individual in this role.

Evaluation

Expected outcomes of nursing interventions include:

- The child maintains weight bearing and mobility with a walker and crutches as much as possible.
- The parents identify signs of neurologic impairment quickly and seek care immediately.
- Daily skin inspection and care prevents pressure ulcers.
- Urinary elimination is managed appropriately, minimizing the risk for kidney damage.
- The child develops self-esteem and is integrated into peer groups and social activities.

PARTNERING WITH FAMILIES

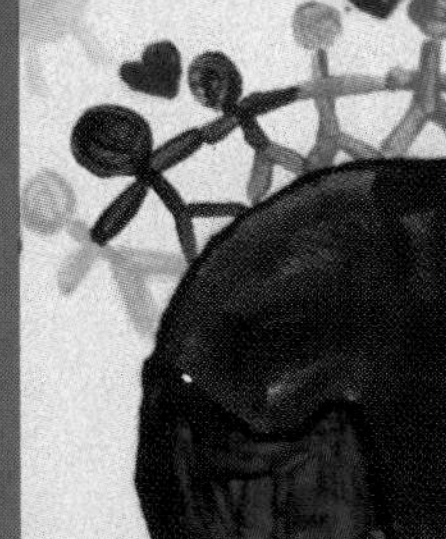

Safety for the Child with Myelodysplasia

Due to the loss of sensation in the lower extremities, the child may not notice injuries to the skin.

- Perform a daily check of all skin surfaces and pressure points associated with sitting, braces, and shoes for abrasions, scrapes, reddened areas, and other lesions.
- Keep all skin surfaces clean and dry.
- Use a gel-filled cushion and teach the child to perform position shifts when in the wheelchair to avoid pressures sores.
- Avoid burns to the lower extremities by checking the temperature of bath water and car safety seats during hot weather.
- Take latex precautions as the child is at high risk for latex allergy. Inform all healthcare providers about the child's latex allergy.
- Use safe ambulation techniques with walkers, canes, and crutches.

Craniosynostosis

Craniosynostosis is the premature closing of the cranial sutures during the first 18 months of life. This condition occurs in up to 1 in 2,000 births (Renier, Lajeunie, Arnaud, et al., 2000). Boys make up two thirds of all cases (McGee & Burkett, 2000). Most children have no family history of the condition, although 15% have autosomal dominant inherited syndromes such as Alpert syndrome and Crouzon syndrome (McGee & Burkett, 2000).

The cause of craniosynostosis is unknown. Closure of the sutures usually takes place at predetermined times during the child's development. Problems arise if one or more sutures close early. Bone growth continues in a direction parallel to the suture line, which leads to compensatory overgrowth at normal suture lines and the classic skull deformities associated with craniosynostosis (Figure 33–16 ■). Sagittal synostosis accounts for 50% of all cases. The infant typically has an elongated head and bilateral bossing on the frontal and occipital areas. The parietal bones appear flattened. A ridge over the sagittal suture is palpable. Facial symmetry is apparent. The head circumference is often greater than 98th percentile. When one coronal suture is involved, facial and skull asymmetry is apparent with eyes and ears out of alignment. Bicoronal synostosis is associated with Alpert or Crouzon syndrome.

Positional plagiocephaly, a totally flat occiput, is seen increasingly in healthy infants because they are put to sleep on their backs to prevent sudden infant death syndrome. Since the infant's sleep position does not change, the weight of the head sometimes flattens the skull. Positional plagiocephaly may also be seen as a result of intrauterine positioning or in premature infants due to side-to-side positioning in the neonatal intensive care unit.

Diagnosis is made by clinical appearance. Palpation of the skull reveals a bony ridge along a suture. A skull radiograph, CT scan, and MRI confirm the diagnosis. The hands and feet should be carefully examined to detect any skeletal defect that could be associated with a syndrome (Renier et al., 2000).

Reconstructive surgery, the most common form of treatment, is performed to protect mental development and vision. Some children need multiple procedures. Children having surgery before 1 year of age have a better outcome. After surgery, it is important for the incision to remain dry and intact. The nurse should also observe the child for symptoms of

PHOTOStory...

Managing myelodysplasia

Sam is a 7-year-old child with myelodysplasia. Sam and his parents are seen every few months in the multidisciplinary spina bifida clinic located in the university medical center about 100 miles from his home. The health professionals in this clinic help the family coordinate care for Sam with his local pediatrician and physical therapy center. An important part of the health visit is to measure his height and weight and to determine that growth is occurring as expected. In particular, it is important to monitor for signs of excessive weight gain as this would potentially reduce his mobility.

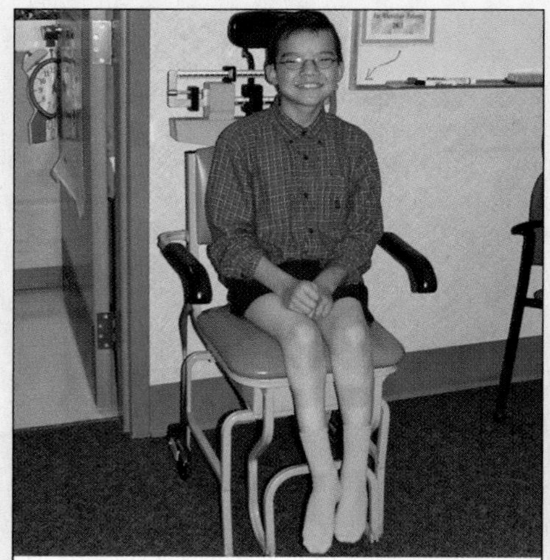

A scale with a chair attached is often used to measure the weight of children with an inability to stand without support.

Sam's lesion is at the L4 to L5 level, so he can flex his hips and extend his knees, but he has weak ankle extension, toe flexion, and hip extension. He has minimal sensation in his lower legs and feet. His bladder and bowel sphincters are also affected. Sam and his parents have worked hard to establish bowel control with a high fiber diet and to establish a specific

increased intracranial pressure (see Table 33–1). A special molding helmet may be used after surgery to promote proper cranial growth. Explain to parents that surgery will improve the child's appearance. Assure them that most children with craniosynostosis are healthy, and that their brains develop normally.

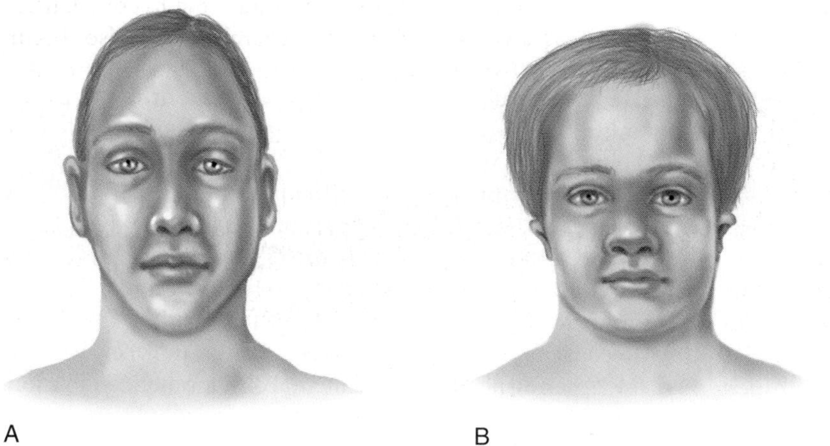

FIGURE 33–16 ■ In craniosynostosis, the head shape is dependent on which sutures are involved. Examples of different head shapes include those shown in *A* and *B*.

A helmet device may also be used to correct severe cases of positional plagiocephaly. It is most effective when used in infants under 9 months of age and when treatment is initiated at 3 months of age. The helmet is worn 23 hours a day for 3 months. Remolding of the head shape continues after that treatment period because the infant spends more hours awake and upright.

Neurofibromatosis

Neurofibromatosis 1, or von Recklinghausen disease, is an autosomal dominant genetic disorder in which tumors grow along nerves. Skin changes and bone deformities also occur. The incidence of the disorder is 1 per 3,000 live births. Between 30% and 50% of new cases result from a mutation (National Institute of Neurologic Disorders and Stroke, 2000). The condition varies in severity with most individuals having the milder form of the disease, but it can be debilitating when the severe form of the disease is present.

time of day for bowel evacuation. Sam has learned to perform intermittent self-catheterization for bladder control to reduce the risk for kidney damage.

During the health visit, Sam's general health is reviewed, along with changes in muscle tone, joint range of motion, and any signs of damage to his skin. As this visit is completed, his socks will be removed to check for signs of redness or breaks on his feet and lower extremities, especially where braces may rub.

The health professionals at the spina bifida clinic are encouraging Sam to be as mobile as possible. Daily exercise using crutches is important for him to maintain the strength to continue bearing weight and walking independently. This enables Sam to interact with his environment and other children in school. As the visit is finishing, Sam's mobility is evaluated by watching him walk down the hall with his crutches. ■

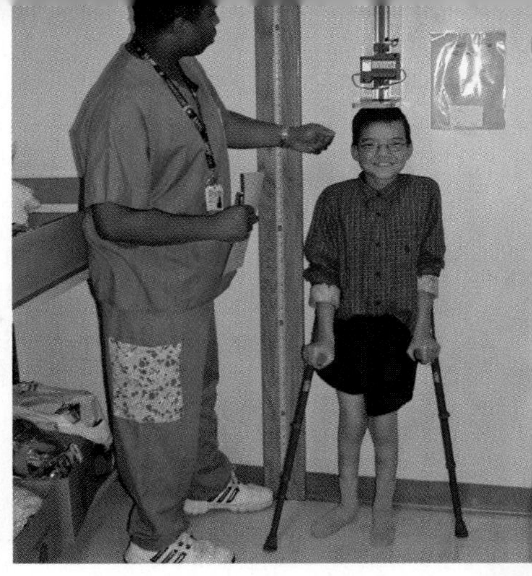

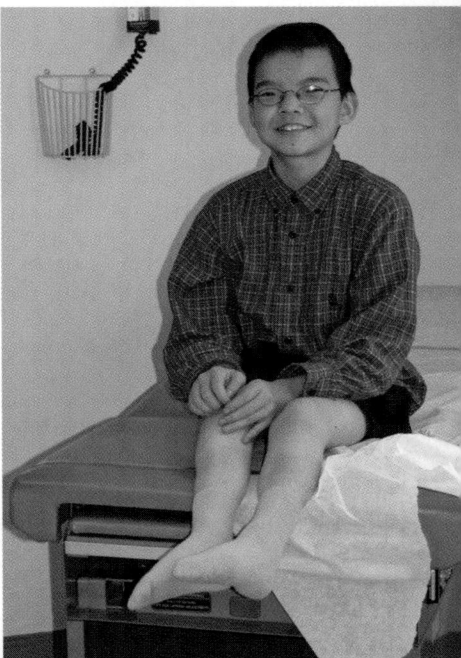

Assessing height is also important to contrast with weight and to calculate a body mass index. In this case Sam is using crutches to stand erect. ***(top)***

Sam has been placed on the examining table so that his lower extremities can be evaluated. Next his socks will be removed so his feet can be inspected. ***(bottom)***

Etiology and Pathophysiology

The NF1 gene responsible for neurofibromatosis 1 is located on chromosome 17. This gene encodes a large protein called neurofibromin. This protein and another family of proteins called Ras-GAP suppress the action of a tumor growth-promoting protein. It is thought that defects in the gene may interfere with the normal output of neurofibromin, allowing abnormal cell growth and tumor development to occur (National Institute of Neurologic Disorders and Stroke, 2001).

Clinical Manifestations

The disorder is characterized by multiple, light tan–colored café-au-lait spots 5 mm or larger seen at birth or by 2 years of age. In darker skinned children, the spots are darker than surrounding skin. The spots grow to 15 mm or larger in diameter by adulthood. Multiple neurofibromas or benign tumors, composed of nervous system tissue and fibrous tissue, grow on or under the skin beginning during puberty. Other findings include plexiform neurofibromas, freckling in the axillary or inguinal areas (Figure 33–17 ■). See the clinical manifestations table on page 1337. Pain may occur when tumors grow around and compress a nerve or when a tumor grows in the spinal cord. Tumors may develop in the optic nerve (optic glioma) and cause various vision deficits or blindness. Children may grow normally until puberty, but at puberty the height velocity decreases and the ultimate final height is often lower than expected. Precocious puberty may occur with neurofibromatosis 1 when an optic glioma exists and invades the hypothalamus. Delayed puberty with delayed menarche may also occur (Virdis, Street, Bandello, et al., 2003). Hypertension may develop in association with renal vascular stenosis or a pheochromocytoma. There is a rare chance that tumors will become malignant.

COLLABORATIVE CARE

The goal of collaborative care is to accurately diagnose the condition and monitor for complications that arise from the development of neurofibromas in different body sites.

Diagnostic Testing

Diagnosis is made in infancy or early childhood by the presence of six or more café-au-lait spots, Lisch nodules, small

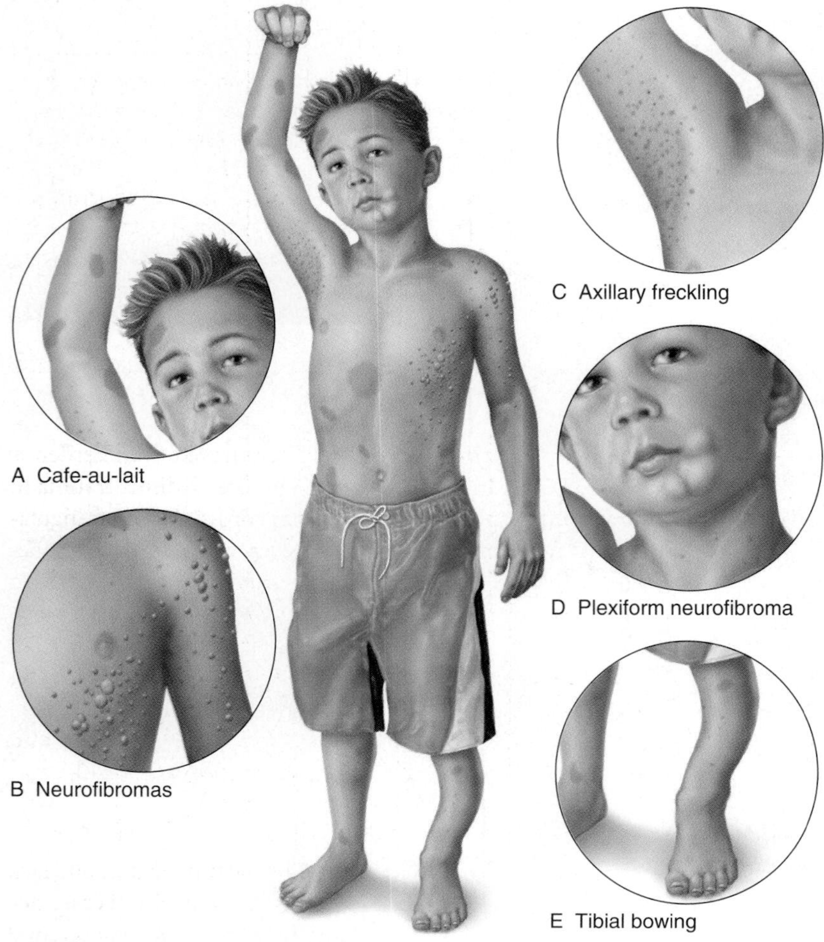

FIGURE 33–17 ■ Physical signs of neurofibromatosis 1 become more apparent during adolescence. Café-au-lait spots enlarge, axillary freckling appears, and multiple neurofibromas develop. Some children develop plexiform neurofibromas.

skin tumors, and a positive family history of neurofibromatosis. See Box 33–12 for diagnostic criteria. Prenatal diagnosis using amniocentesis or chorionic villus sampling procedures is possible. Genetic testing is available in families with documented cases; however, genetic testing is not helpful when the disorder is caused by a mutation.

BOX 33–12 Diagnostic Criteria for Neurofibromatosis 1

Diagnostic criteria for neurofibromatosis 1 include the presence of two or more of the following characteristics (Haslam, 2004):

- Six or more café-au-lait spots over 5 mm in diameter in prepubetal children and over 15 mm in diameter in postpubertal individuals
- Two or more neurofibromas of any type or one plexiform neurofibroma (grow diffusely under the skin or in deeper areas of the body)
- Freckling in the axillary or inguinal regions
- Optic glioma (a tumor of the optic nerve)
- Two or more Lisch nodules
- A distinctive osseous lesion such as sphenoid dysplasia or thinning of the long bone cortex with or without incomplete healing associated with fractures
- A first degree relative (parent, sibling, offspring) with neurofibromatosis 1 by the above criteria

Clinical Therapy

Clinical therapy focuses on monitoring the child for signs of developing problems associated with the condition. Regular health visits focusing on growth, developmental screening, blood pressure monitoring, scoliosis screening, timing of sexual development, and development of neurofibromas are encouraged. Radiologic imaging (MRI of the brain and radiographs of the spine and other bones) is performed when problems are detected. Ophthalmic examinations should be performed at least annually during childhood to detect optic gliomas, to monitor Lisch nodules, and to detect vision deficits. Genetic counseling is offered. Most children and adults with mild symptoms can live a normal, productive life.

When neurofibromas are disfiguring or cause problems because of their location, surgery may be performed to remove the tumor. The plexiform neurofibromas are challenging to remove surgically, and they may grow back. Surgical removal is more often attempted when tumors are painful, disfiguring, cause paralysis, or life-threatening problems develop.

NURSING MANAGEMENT

The goal of nursing management is to assess the child and identify emerging problems with the disorder and to provide support to the child and family living with the condition.

Nurses assess the child to identify signs of neurofibromatosis, including café-au-lait spots, axillary and inguinal freckling, and small tumors on the body. Vital signs with blood pressure are monitored for hypertension. Vision screening to detect any vision impairment is performed. Monitor growth and development to detect any unusual patterns, identifying signs of early or late pubertal development. Perform scoliosis screening on a frequent basis. Note any evidence of tibial bowing or thinning. School performance should be monitored as learning disabilities and hyperactivity may occur. Pay attention to any mass that is rapidly enlarging or causing new pain.

Provide psychological support to the child and family. In children with moderate to severe conditions, the tumors will cause cosmetic problems. As tumor development increases during adolescence, problems with self-image and self-esteem are common. The adolescent may have a difficult adjustment to the disorder. Adolescents may fear the response of peers to the tumors and

CLINICAL MANIFESTATIONS of Neurofibromatosis Type 1

SYSTEM INVOLVED	CLINICAL MANIFESTATIONS
Skin	Six or more café-au-lait spots, dark macules that range in size from 5 mm to several centimeters. Café-au-lait spots grow to 15 mm in diameter by adulthood Dermal neurofibromas, benign tumors that grow around nerves under the skin Plexiform neurofibromas, tumors involving multiple nerves that can be disfiguring Freckling in the axillary and inguinal areas is common
Eye	Lisch nodules, tan or brown benign tumors on the iris of the eye Vision deficits in one eye or blindness
Bones	Thinning or bowing of the tibia resulting in fractures that fail to heal properly Scoliosis
Cardiovascular	Hypertension
Central nervous system	Optic glioma, tumor along the optic pathway, found in 20% of children Learning disability, hyperactivity, and speech abnormalities Seizures Pain
Endocrine	Precocious puberty, associated with the tumor along the optic pathway Delayed puberty with delayed menarche

isolate themselves. Identify peers or refer the adolescent to a support group. Assist children and adolescents to learn to live with the disorder. Focus on the child's strengths and encourage continuing development of those strengths.

CEREBRAL PALSY

Cerebral palsy is a disorder of movement and posture that results from a nonprogressive abnormality of the immature brain occurring in the prenatal, perinatal, or postnatal (up to 2 years) periods. Cerebral palsy is the most common chronic disorder of childhood, occurring in an estimated 2 to 3 per 1,000 births (Nehring, 2004). The four types of motor dysfunction seen with cerebral palsy—spastic, dyskinetic, ataxic, and mixed—are related to the location of brain insult.

Etiology and Pathophysiology

Most cases of cerebral palsy are caused by intrauterine insults or structural abnormalities of the CNS (Nelson & Grether, 1999). During gestation, insufficient nutrients and oxygen can cause damage to the developing brain of the fetus. Very premature infants are at high risk because of their immature CNS and the measures taken at birth to promote their survival. Cerebral palsy related to prematurity is most often caused by injury to the white matter of the brain by conditions such as intraventricular hemorrhage. The risk for cerebral palsy is increased when intrauterine infection (chorioamnionitis) is documented (Van Eerden & Bernstein, 2003). Injury at birth may be due to direct trauma to the brain or to asphyxia resulting from cord collapse, strangulation, or meconium aspiration; however, birth asphyxia is believed to account for only 9% of the cerebral palsy cases. No reduction of incidence of cerebral palsy was noted since the implementation of electronic fetal heart rate monitoring (Van Eerden & Bernstein, 2003). Neonatal sepsis and hyperbilirubinemia place the child at higher risk. In young children, CNS infection and head trauma are the major sources of acquired brain injury and subsequent motor dysfunction. See Box 33–13.

BOX 33–13 Ethical Considerations

As the healthcare of women in labor and newborns has improved, new health issues have emerged. Fetal monitoring has led to the early diagnosis of fetal distress and improved the mortality rate of newborns. However, as more premature infants survive, more anoxic episodes also occur. Thus, the incidence of cerebral palsy has not decreased, and indeed the incidence of spastic diplegia has increased with technology improvements (Nelson & Grether, 1999). How should healthcare practitioners weigh the benefits and risks of certain procedures or interventions? Are parents always well informed about the benefits and risks of procedures involving their newborns? How can nurses deal with their feelings about these issues?

Clinical Manifestations

Cerebral palsy is characterized by abnormal muscle tone and lack of coordination with spasticity found in the majority of cases. See Table 33–7 for descriptions of different characteristics of cerebral palsy. Children have a variety of symptoms depending on their ages. See the table on page 1338 for clinical manifestations by type of CNS injury. There is wide variability in symptoms depending on the area of the brain involved and the degree of anoxia.

TABLE 33–7 Clinical Characteristics of Cerebral Palsy

CLINICAL CHARACTERISTICS	DEFINITIONS
Hypotonia	Floppiness, increased range of motion of joints, diminished reflex response
Hypertonia	
Rigidity	Tense, tight muscles
Spasticity	Uncoordinated, awkward, stiff movements; scissoring or crossing of the legs; exaggerated reflex reactions
Ataxia	Irregularity in muscle coordination or action
Athetosis	Constant involuntary writhing motions that are more severe distally
Hemiplegia	Involvement of one side of the body with the upper extremities being more dysfunctional than the lower extremities
Diplegia	Involvement of all extremities, but the lower extremities are more affected than the upper, usually spastic
Quadriplegia	Involvement of all extremities with the arms in flexion and legs in extension

CLINICAL MANIFESTATIONS of Cerebral Palsy by Type of Insult

CLASSIFICATION AND TYPE OF INSULT	CLINICAL MANIFESTATIONS	CLINICAL THERAPY
Spastic Cerebral cortex or pyramidal tract injury 75% of cases	Persistent hypertonia, rigidity Exaggerated deep tendon reflexes Persistent primitive reflexes Leads to contractures and abnormal curvature of the spine	Braces and splints to prevent contractures Tone-reducing casts to keep spastic muscles in stretched position Nerve blocks Static positioning devices Surgery to lengthen tendons, reduce spasticity Braces to manage scoliosis Diazepam, baclofen, dantrolene to control spasticity Physical and occupational therapy to promote improved muscle tone and better motor control for function Mobility options – tricycle, walker, wheelchair Early intervention program Individualized education plan Assistive technology such as a computer
Dyskinetic Extrapyramidal, basal ganglia injury 10%–15% of cases	Impairment of voluntary muscle control Bizarre twisting movements Tremors, difficulty with fine and purposeful motor movements Exaggerated posturing Rigid muscle tone when awake and normal or decreased muscle tone when asleep Inconsistent muscle tone that may change hour to hour or day to day	
Ataxic Cerebellar (extrapyramidal) injury 5%–10% of cases	Abnormalities of voluntary movement involving balance and position of the trunk and limbs Difficulty controlling hand and arm movements during reaching Increased or decreased muscle tone Hypotonia in infancy Muscle instability and wide-based unsteady gait	
Mixed Injuries to multiple areas	No dominant motor pattern Unique compensatory movements and posture to maintain control over specific neuromotor deficits Combination of characteristics from other types	

Children with cerebral palsy usually are delayed in meeting developmental milestones (Figure 33–18 ■). For example, after 6 months of age, they may be unable to sit up, have persistent back arching, and little spontaneous movement. They frequently have other problems, including visual defects such as strabismus, nystagmus, or refractory errors; hearing loss; language delay; speech impediment; seizures; or mental retardation. They have difficulty feeding because of oral motor involvement. Behavior problems such as attention deficit hyperactivity disorder and self-injurious behavior may be seen in some children.

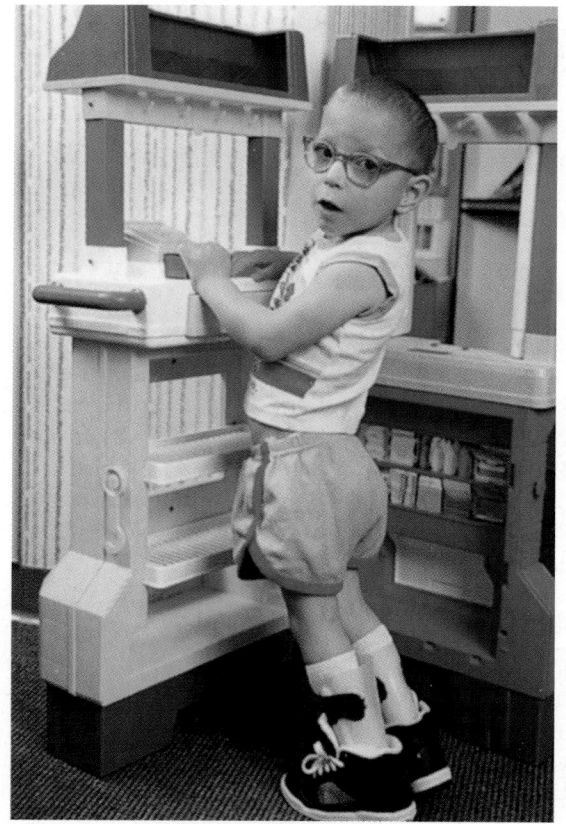

FIGURE 33–18 ■ A child with cerebral palsy has abnormal muscle tone and lack of physical coordination.

COLLABORATIVE CARE

The goal of collaborative care is to cautiously diagnose cerebral palsy and to promote motor function and provide specific therapies that enable the child to develop the greatest amount of independence possible.

Diagnostic Testing

Diagnosis is usually based on clinical findings. Generally cerebral palsy is difficult to diagnose in the early months of life as it must be distinguished from other neurologic conditions and signs may be subtle. Suspicious historical findings include an infant who is from a multiple gestation; has a history of prematurity; a low Apgar score (0–3 at 5 minutes); and an inflammatory, traumatic, or anoxic event (Van Eerden & Bernstein, 2003). However, 75% of children who develop cerebral palsy have normal Apgar scores at birth. Ultrasonography can be used to detect fetal and neonatal abnormalities of the brain, such as intraventricular hemorrhage. Neuromotor tests that evaluate the presence of normal movement patterns and the absence of primitive reflexes and abnormal tone in young infants have been developed. Infants at high risk for cerebral palsy should be referred to specialists who can conduct assessments with these tests. Once cerebral palsy is suspected, CT scans and MRI provide information about anatomical structures, and positron emission tomography (PET) provides information about brain metabolic functioning.

Clinical Therapy

It is not uncommon for children who are delayed in meeting developmental milestones or have neuromuscular abnormalities at 1 year of age to show gradual improvement in function. Half of the infants suspected to be at risk for cerebral palsy at 1 year of age are unimpaired neurologically by 2 years of age due to physical maturation (Pelligrino, 2002). Therefore, careful monitoring and early referral for evaluation is important.

Clinical therapy focuses on helping the child develop to his or her maximum level of independence. Referrals are made for physical, occupational, and speech therapy, as well as special education to improve motor function and ability. Braces and splints are used to maintain an adequate range of motion, stability, control of involuntary movements, and to prevent contractures. Serial casting may be performed to increase the range of motion gradually when joint contractures have occurred, and then casting is used intermittently to maintain the range of motion. Positioning devices (prone wedges, standers, and sidelyers) are used to promote skeletal alignment and to compensate for abnormal postures. Mobility devices such as scooters, tricycles, and wheelchairs help the child to move independently and explore the environment.

Surgical interventions may be required to improve function by balancing muscle power and stabilizing uncontrollable joints. The Achilles tendon may be lengthened to increase range of motion in the ankle, which allows the heel to touch the floor and thus improves ambulation. The hamstrings may be released to correct knee flexion contractures. Other procedures may be performed to improve hip adduction or correct the natural position of the foot. A dorsal rhizotomy may be performed for spastic diplegia to cut the afferent fibers that contribute to spasticity; however, some muscle weakness may result from the procedure (Pelligrino, 2002). Physical and occupational therapy are provided to promote optimal independent functioning.

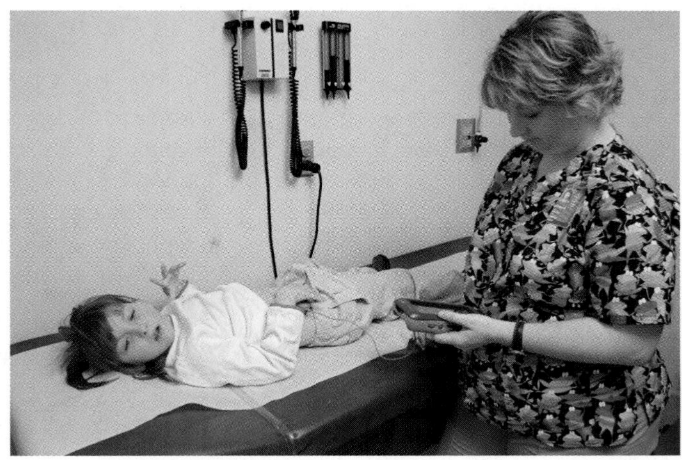

FIGURE 33–19 ■ Child having baclofen pump filled.

Medications are given to control seizures, to control spasms (skeletal muscle relaxants, baclofen, and benzodiazepines), and to minimize gastrointestinal side effects (cimetidine or ranitidine). See the medication table below. Baclofen is administered by intrathecal pump to decrease muscle tone and vasospasms when oral administration is ineffective or causes side effects (Pellegrino, 2002). See Figure 33–19 ■. Botulinum

MEDICATIONS Used to Treat Cerebral Palsy

MEDICATION	ACTION	NURSING CONSIDERATIONS
Diazepam, lorazepam, clonazepam *Oral*	Control spasticity and rigidity	Can cause drowsiness and excessive drooling May interfere with feeding and speech Physiologic dependence can develop, so taper drug when discontinued
Dantrolene *Oral*	Calcium channel blocker that inhibits muscle contraction	Can cause drowsiness, muscle weakness, and increased drooling May cause liver damage, so liver function testing should be performed periodically
Baclofen *Intrathecal* *Oral*	Inhibits motor nerve conduction at the level of the spinal cord Delivered intrathecally to the cerebrospinal fluid by a pump placed in the abdomen	Adjustable dosing is possible May cause hypotonia, increased seizures in children with known epilepsy, sleepiness, and nausea and vomiting Monitor for pump failure and signs of infection
Botulinum toxin type A *Injection*	Used to treat spasticity in lower extremities When injected into the muscle it blocks neuromuscular conduction, inhibits acetylcholine release. Leads to partial chemical denervation and localized paralysis lasting 3–6 months	Used to improve walking in children with equinus gait, may be used in hip adductors and hamstrings to improve positioning May have stumbling, leg cramps, leg weakness, and calf atrophy Repeated injections needed to continue effect

toxin injections into specific muscles is a new therapy used to help control spasticity (Buck, 2003).

The prognosis for infants and children with cerebral palsy depends on the level of physical involvement and on the presence of intellectual, visual, or hearing deficits. Intelligence may be intact but difficult to assess due to communication difficulties. Many children with hemiplegia or ataxia show some improvement with maturation and are able to ambulate. Others will need assistance with mobility and activities of daily living. They are usually cared for in their homes, but in some cases receive care in long-term care facilities.

NURSING MANAGEMENT

The goal of nursing care is to support the early identification of children with cerebral palsy and then to provide supportive care to promote cognitive, motor, and social functioning.

Nursing Assessment and Diagnosis

Be alert for children whose histories indicate an increased risk for cerebral palsy. Assess all children at each healthcare visit for developmental delays (see Chapters 12 and 13∞). Any orthopedic, visual, auditory, or intellectual deficits should be noted. Assess for the presence of newborn reflexes, which may persist beyond the normal age in a child with cerebral palsy (see Chapter 8∞). Identify infants that appear to have an abnormal muscle tone or abnormal posture (arched back, becomes stiff when moving against gravity, neck or extremities have increased or decreased resistance to passive movement). See Box 33–14. Asymmetric or abnormal crawling by using two or three extremities indicates a motor problem. Hand dominance before the preschool years is another sign of a motor problem. Record dietary intake and height and weight percentiles for children suspected to have or diagnosed with the condition.

Nursing diagnoses for the child with cerebral palsy vary, depending on the type, the particular child's symptoms and age, and the family situation. The accompanying nursing care plan includes several diagnoses that may be appropriate for the child with cerebral palsy. Additional nursing diagnoses may include the following:

- Constipation related to low intake of fiber and fluids and insufficient physical activity
- Impaired Tissue Integrity related to decreased physical mobility and limited self-care ability
- Impaired Verbal Communication related to hearing and/or speech impairment
- Impaired Home Maintenance related to child's developmental disability and inadequate support system
- Delayed Growth and Development related to lack of muscle strength or limited social interaction

BOX 33–14 Assessment of High-Risk Infants

All infants who show symptoms of developmental delays, feeding difficulties caused by poor sucking, or abnormalities of muscle tone should be evaluated. Two simple screening assessments are as follows:

- Place a clean diaper on the infant's face. The normal infant will use two hands to remove it, but the infant with cerebral palsy will either use one hand or not remove the cloth at all.
- Turn the infant's head to one side. A persistent asymmetric tonic neck reflex (beyond 6 months of age) is an indicator of a pathologic condition. Cerebral palsy should be suspected in any infant who has persistent primitive reflexes.

Planning and Implementation

The accompanying nursing care plan summarizes care for the child with cerebral palsy. Because the condition can range from mild to severe and involve numerous manifestations, interventions need to be adapted to the particular child and family. Nursing care focuses on providing adequate nutrition, maintaining skin integrity, promoting physical mobility, promoting safety, promoting growth and development, teaching parents how to care for the child, and providing emotional support.

Provide Adequate Nutrition

Children with cerebral palsy require high-calorie diets or supplements to the diet because of feeding difficulties associated with spasticity. Many children have difficulty chewing and swallowing. Give the child small amounts of soft foods at a time. Feeding utensils with large, padded handles may be easier for the child to use.

Maintain Skin Integrity

Take special care to protect the bony prominences from skin breakdown. Monitor the skin under splints and braces for redness.

Proper body alignment should be maintained at all times. Support the child with pillows, towels, and bolsters whether the child is in bed or in a chair. Use splints and braces to help support the child and reduce the risk for contractures. Support the head and body of a floppy infant. A spastic child with scissored, extended legs or an athetoid child who writhes constantly is difficult to carry and transport.

Promote Physical Mobility

Range of motion exercises are essential to maintain joint flexibility and to prevent contractures. Consult with the physical therapists that work with the child and assist with recommended exercises. Teach parents to position the child to foster flexion rather than extension so that interaction with the environment can be enhanced (e.g., the child can bring objects closer to the face). Encourage parents to bring the child's adaptive appliances (e.g., customized wheelchairs, braces, positioning devices) to the hospital to prevent deterioration during hospitalizations. Refer parents to the appropriate resources for help with the acquisition of adaptive devices.

Promote Safety

Teach parents the importance of using safety belts with children in strollers and wheelchairs. Determine if an adaptive car safety seat is needed so the child can be safely transported. A helmet

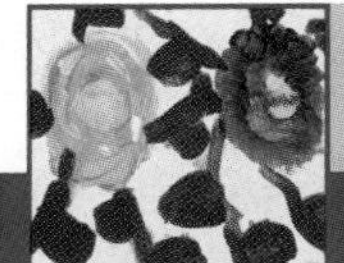

Nursing Care Plan

THE CHILD WITH CEREBRAL PALSY

GOAL	INTERVENTION	RATIONALE	EXPECTED OUTCOME
1. Impaired Physical Mobility related to decreased muscle strength and control			
	NIC Priority Intervention—*Exercise Therapy, Joint Mobility:* Use of active and passive body movement to maintain joint flexibility.		**NOC Suggested Outcome—***Joint Movement–Active:* Range of motion of joints with self-limited movement.
The child will attain maximum physical abilities possible.	■ Perform developmental assessment and record age that milestones were achieved (e.g., reaching for objects, sitting).	■ Delayed developmental milestones are common with cerebral palsy. Once one milestone is achieved, interventions can be planned to assist in the next skill acquisition.	The child reaches maximum physical mobility and all developmental milestones.
	■ Plan activities to use gross and fine motor skills (e.g.,holding pen or eating utensils, toys positioned to encourage reaching and rolling over).	■ Many activities of daily living and play activities promote physical development.	
	■ Allow time for the child to complete activities.	■ The child may perform tasks more slowly than most children.	
	■ Perform range of motion exercises every 4 hours for the child unable to move body parts. Position the child to promote tendon stretching (e.g., foot plantar flexion instead of dorsiflexion, legs extended instead of flexed at knees and hips).	■ Promotes mobility and increased circulation, and decreases the risk of contractures.	
	■ Arrange for and encourage parents to keep appointments with a rehabilitation therapist.	■ A regular and frequently reevaluated rehabilitation program assists in promoting development.	
	■ Teach the family to maintain appropriate brace wear.	■ Adaptive devices are often necessary to maximize physical mobility.	
2. Disturbed Sensory Perception: Visual or Auditory related to cerebral damage			
	NIC Priority Intervention—*Communication Enhancement:* Visual deficit or auditory deficit: Assistance with accepting or learning alternative methods for living with diminished vision or hearing.		**NOC Suggested Outcome—***Body Image:* Positive perception of own appearance and body functioning.
The child will receive and benefit from varied forms of sensory and perceptual input.	■ Facilitate eye and auditory examinations by specialist. Promote the use of adaptive devices (glasses, contact lenses, hearing aids), and encourage recommended return visits to specialists.	■ Adaptive devices often enhance sensory input. These devices need frequent changes as the child grows.	The child receives adequate sensory/perceptual input to maximize developmental outcome.
	■ Maximize the use of intact senses (e.g., describe verbally the surroundings to a child with poor vision, allow touching of objects, provide visual materials to enhance learning in the child with impaired hearing, use computers to promote communication).	■ Other senses can help compensate for those that are impaired.	
3. Imbalanced Nutrition: Less than Body Requirements related to difficulty in chewing and swallowing and high metabolic needs			
	NIC Priority Intervention—*Weight Gain Assistance:* Facilitation of body weight gain.		**NOC Suggested Outcome—***Nutritional Status:* Extent to which nutrients are available to meet metabolic needs.
The child will receive nutrients needed for normal growth.	■ Monitor height and weight and plot on a growth grid. Perform hydration status assessment.	■ Insufficient intake can lead to impaired growth and dehydration.	The child shows normal growth patterns for height, weight, and other physical parameters.

(continued)

Nursing Care Plan THE CHILD WITH CEREBRAL PALSY (continued)

GOAL	INTERVENTION	RATIONALE	EXPECTED OUTCOME
3. Imbalanced Nutrition: Less than Body Requirements related to difficulty in chewing and swallowing and high metabolic needs (continued)			
	▪ Teach the family techniques to promote swallowing and caloric and nutrient intake. ▪ Position the child upright for feedings. ▪ Place foods far back in the mouth to overcome tongue thrust. ▪ Use soft and blended foods. ▪ Allow extra time and quiet environment for meals.	▪ Special feeding techniques to promote swallowing and soft foods can facilitate food intake.	
	▪ Perform frequent respiratory assessment. Teach the family to avoid aspiration pneumonia. Teach care of gastrostomy and tube feeding technique as appropriate.	▪ Aspiration pneumonia is a risk for the child with poor swallowing. Special feeding techniques may be needed.	
4. Ineffective Therapeutic Regimen Management: Family related to excessive demands made on family with child's complex care needs			
	NIC Priority Intervention—*Family Process Maintenance:* Minimization of family process disruption effects.		**NOC Suggested Outcome**—Not yet developed.
The family will adapt to growth and development needs of the child with cerebral palsy.	▪ Allow opportunities for parents to verbalize the impact of cerebral palsy on the family. Provide referral to other parents and support groups.	▪ The family needs an opportunity to explore the emotional and social impact of the child's care in order to integrate and grow from the experience.	The family continues its development and provides support for all of its members.
	▪ Explore community services for rehabilitation, respite care, childcare, early intervention program, and other needs and refer family as appropriate.	▪ Diverse services are available and will be needed due to the multiple impacts of cerebral palsy on the child.	
	▪ During home and office visits review the child's achievements and praise the family for care provided.	▪ The child's achievements are positive reinforcement of the family's efforts.	
	▪ Teach the family skills needed to manage the child's care (e.g., medication administration, physical rehabilitation, seizure management).	▪ Complex skills must be learned before they can be performed with efficiency.	
	▪ Teach case management techniques.	▪ The child requires care by many specialists. Many parents become case managers to coordinate care.	
	▪ Involve siblings in the care for the child with cerebral palsy. Review for parents the needs of all children in the family.	▪ Siblings of the child with cerebral palsy may feel left out because of the care provided. Special efforts contribute to meeting the developmental needs of all family members.	
5. Deficient Diversional Activity (child) related to poor social skills			
	NIC Priority Intervention—*Recreation Therapy:* Purposeful use of recreation to promote relaxation and enhancement of social skills.		**NOC Suggested Outcome**—*Play Participation:* Use of activities as needed for enjoyment, entertainment, and development by children.
The child will engage in adequate diversional activity to maximize growth and development.	▪ Refer the family to early childhood intervention programs. Encourage contact with other children. When hospitalized, place the child in a room with other children when possible.	▪ The child needs a variety of activities and contact with other children and adults to maximize development.	The child engages in activities that maximize development.
	▪ Work with the local school to develop an individualized education plan that allows the child contact with other children and a variety of activities.	▪ Public schools must provide an individualized education plan. Parents may need assistance to interact effectively with the school system.	
	▪ Investigate recreational programs for children with disabilities and share information with the parents.	▪ Recreational programs for children with disabilities may promote social experiences and physical activity.	

should be worn by the child with chronic seizures to protect from further injury during seizures.

Promote Growth and Development

Remember that many children with cerebral palsy are physically but not intellectually disabled. Use terminology appropriate for the child's developmental level. Help the child develop a positive self-image to ensure emotional health and social growth. Children with a hearing impairment may need referral to learn American Sign Language or other communication methods. Adaptive and assistive technology may be needed to promote mobility and communication. **Assistive technology** is any item, piece of equipment, or product system modified or customized for use to improve or maintain functional capabilities of individuals with disabilities so that they are as independent as possible. Items such as customized wheelchairs and computers help to promote contact with the world when speech is a problem.

Foster Parental Knowledge

Teach parents about the disorder and arrange sessions to teach them about all of the child's special needs. Teach administration, desired effects, and side effects of medications prescribed for seizures. Make sure parents are aware of the need for dental care because enamel defects and malocclusion commonly occurs in children with cerebral palsy and for hyperplasia when anticonvulsants are prescribed.

Provide Emotional Support

Refer parents to individual and family counseling if appropriate. Listen to the parents' concerns and encourage them to express their feelings and ask questions. Explain what they can expect regarding future treatment. Work with other healthcare professionals to help families adjust to this chronic disease.

Care in the Community

Children with cerebral palsy need continuous support in the community. A case manager such as the parent or nurse will likely be needed to coordinate care. As they grow, these children will need new adaptive devices, ongoing developmental assessment and care planning, and possibly surgery. Although the brain lesion does not change, it manifests itself in different ways as the child grows. For example, once the child begins to walk, the extensor tone may cause Achilles cord tightening. Braces may be used to decrease deformities, but surgery may eventually be needed. Later, surgery may be needed to loosen tight tendons in the knees or hips. Speech therapy may be needed, as well as new glasses and eye examinations as the child grows. Other parents of children with cerebral palsy can provide needed support.

Schedule regular appointments for vision and hearing screening. Give immunizations according to the recommended schedule, even though children who already have a seizure disorder are at higher risk of seizures in association with the pertussis vaccine and the measles-mumps-rubella vaccine. Educate parents about the possible risk for a seizure associated with the vaccines.

Early intervention programs can help parents learn how to meet their child's special needs, including physical, occupational, and speech therapy, as well as educational needs. Parents may need financial assistance to provide the care that the child needs and to obtain appliances such as braces, wheelchairs, or adaptive utensils. Technology offers many new strategies to promote communication and self-care by these children. The nurse can be instrumental in helping parents meet the needs of the child with cerebral palsy in preschools, schools, offices, clinics, and other settings. In addition, the nurse makes referrals as appropriate to early intervention programs, support groups, and organizations such as the United Cerebral Palsy Association and Shriners Hospitals. Recreational activities may be identified through the National Association of Sports for Cerebral Palsy.

MediaLink Cerebral Palsy Resources and Support

Individualized education plans are needed for the child entering school. Both the special mobility needs and educational support needed by the child must be addressed. The majority of children with cerebral palsy have a normal intelligence quotient (IQ), but behavior problems, perceptual problems, and speech difficulties create challenges for learning. (See Chapter 20∞).

Transition programs assist the family and adolescent with cerebral palsy to develop plans for adult living. The young adult (18 to 21 years) may be able to move into a group home or live independently if desired. Vocational training options can be explored. Nurses in hospital programs may coordinate transition into smaller communities and settings and to assist the family in gaining access to available resources.

■ Evaluation

Expected outcomes of nursing care for the child with cerebral palsy are provided on the nursing care plan.

NEONATAL ABSTINENCE SYNDROME

While the exact number of newborns exposed to illicit substances in utero is unknown, it is estimated that 3.7% of women used illicit drugs during pregnancy; and rates of drug use were similar for White, Black, and Hispanic pregnant women (Substance Abuse and Mental Health Services Administration, 2002). Other reports have identified an even higher number of women (10.7%) who used illicit substances during pregnancy (Lester et al., 2001). Illicit substances that may cause neonatal abstinence syndrome when used by the mother during pregnancy include opiates (heroine, meperidine, methadone), CNS stimulants (cocaine, propoxyphene, amphetamines), and CNS depressants (barbiturates, alcohol, and marijuana). Cocaine and marijuana are the most common illicit substances used by expectant mothers (Robinson, 1999). See Chapter 34∞ for information about fetal alcohol syndrome.

Etiology and Pathophysiology

Cocaine is a central nervous system stimulant that causes feelings of well-being, euphoria, and excitement in the mother. It comes in many forms, and crack cocaine is often preferred because it is affordable and quick acting. Cocaine acts on the developing fetus by decreasing placental blood flow that deprives the fetus of essential oxygen and nutrients while elevating the fetal blood pressure and heart rate. Repeated use of narcotics and other substances leads to tolerance and physical dependence. All narcotics, regardless of their mode of administration, readily cross the placenta, enter the fetal circulation, and have the same effects on the fetus that they do in the mother. When the mother stops taking drugs during pregnancy, both she and the fetus have withdrawal symptoms. If the infant is born to a mother who is still actively using drugs, then the neonate has signs of abrupt withdrawal from the illicit substance shortly after birth. Between 50% and 90% of infants born to drug-addicted mothers suffer withdrawal. See Chapter 18∞ for information about opioid withdrawal.

Clinical Manifestations

Prematurity, intrauterine growth retardation, microcephaly, and low birth weight are common results of prenatal cocaine exposure. In the newborn, jitteriness, seizures, hyperexcitability, and poor feeding are often seen and may be related to the direct effects of cocaine on the developing central nervous system rather than signs of drug withdrawal (Kuehne & Reilly, 2004). These infants may also exhibit the following signs: hypertonia, tremors, extensor leg posture, poor sucking and feeding difficulties, less time in quiet sleep, more stressed behaviors such as mouthing and clenched fists, and difficulty regulating their behaviors. Long-term issues for children with cocaine exposure in utero include potential difficulties with language development, attention span, memory, and motor skills (Campbell, 2003). See Box 33–15.

BOX 33–15 Research: Cocaine Exposure

A metaanalysis of 36 studies was performed to identify specific effects of uterine cocaine exposure. Less than optimal motor scores were found up to 7 months of age. No consistent negative associations were found between prenatal cocaine exposure and physical growth, developmental test scores, and receptive or expressive language. An association between cocaine exposure and decreased attentiveness and emotional expressivity was found possible. Actual long-term outcomes may be associated with the exposure dose (Frank, Augustyn, Knight, et al., 2001).

A longitudinal prospective study of infants confirmed to have prenatal cocaine exposure compared with infants without exposure was conducted to identify differences in cognitive and motor outcomes between the two groups. A total of 218 cocaine-exposed infants and 197 unexposed infants were followed and evaluated at 6 months, 12 months, and 24 months of age with the Bayley Mental and Motor Scales of Infant Development. The Bayley is a standardized test for assessment of infant development that is predictive of future cognitive development. No significant differences in the Bayley Motor Scales were noted between the two groups at 24 months of age. Significant cognitive deficits were found using the Bayley Mental Scales in the cocaine-exposed group of infants at 24 months of age even after other confounding variables were controlled. The infants with higher amounts of cocaine were found to have poorer cognitive performance. However, it is not known if the compounded exposure to alcohol, marijuana, and tobacco could have impacted the negative outcome of higher cocaine exposure (Singer, Arendt, Minnes, et al., 2002).

The newborn with drug withdrawal from other illicit substances may have irritability and jitteriness. These infants may have excoriated skin, especially on the heels, toes, hands, elbows, nose, or chin, as a result of their continuous movements on the crib sheets. See the clinical manifestations table on page 1345.

The onset of symptoms may be attributed to the type and amount of drug taken by the mother and how soon before birth it was taken. Withdrawal symptoms for opiates usually appear 24 to 48 hours after birth; however, it is not uncommon for barbiturate withdrawal symptoms to appear between 4 and 14 days after birth, or up to 7 days after birth if the mother was using cocaine or amphetamines. Opiates cause the most withdrawal symptoms, but consider the possibility of multiple drug use by the mother. Long-term exposure to these substances can result in intrauterine growth retardation, prematurity, small head circumference, shorter length, and low Apgar scores.

COLLABORATIVE CARE

The goal of collaborative care is to identify the newborn with neonatal abstinence syndrome and to initiate supportive care during the withdrawal process.

Diagnostic Testing

Diagnosis is based on the history of maternal substance abuse and physical signs in the infant. EEG abnormalities may be noted. Identification of the drug may be determined in some cases from maternal and infant urine. Because only recent use of cocaine can be detected in urine samples, meconium toxocologic screening may be performed. The hair of the infant may also be tested. Urine testing provides information on drug use immediately prior to labor, and meconium screening provides information of drug use by the mother for the last half of the pregnancy. If urine is positive, compare results with medications used during labor and delivery. Chain of custody for specimens may be needed.

Behavioral and neurologic functioning may also be assessed with diagnostic tools such as the Brazelton Neonatal Behavioral Assessment Scale that evaluates infants on habituation (ability to respond to and then inhibit response to discrete stimuli when asleep), general arousal level, orientation, quality of movement and tone, autonomic stability, reflexes, and responsiveness when aroused (Campbell, 2003).

Clinical Therapy

Treatment is generally supportive. Infants with cocaine exposure need to have reduced environmental stimuli and swaddling. Medications such as phenobarbitol, diazepam, methadone, clonidine, and paregoric may be prescribed to alleviate symptoms of drug withdrawal. If the mother is still using illicit drugs, breastfeeding is discouraged as the drugs cross over into milk.

The most serious and prevalent complication for the neonate whose mother used illicit drugs is congenital infection, such as

CLINICAL MANIFESTATIONS of Neonatal Abstinence Syndrome

SYSTEM INVOLVED	CLINICAL MANIFESTATIONS	CLINICAL THERAPY
Central nervous system	Irritability, restlessness, tremors, seizures, high-pitched cry, abnormal sleep patterns, drowsiness, yawning, and hypertonicity	Phenobarbitol, diazepam, methadone, clonidine, or paregoric are prescribed to relieve symptoms of drug withdrawal Skin care to protect skin surfaces that rub against sheets
Autonomic nervous system	Sneezing, stuffy nose, sweating, tachycardia, and tachypnea	Keep the newborn's nasal passages clear Bathe skin with warm water Swaddle the newborn to reduce stimuli
Gastrointestinal system	Diarrhea, vomiting, and poor feeding	Small frequent feedings Monitor weight gain

with human immunodeficiency virus (HIV), hepatitis B, hepatitis C, and syphilis. Assessment and treatment for these conditions is implemented. See Chapters 27, 30, and 31∞ for treatment of these infections.

NURSING MANAGEMENT

Nursing care focuses on monitoring withdrawal symptoms, administering prescribed medications, and meeting the infant's emotional needs.

■ Nursing Assessment and Diagnosis

Crying accompanied by poor feeding constitutes clinical signs that should increase the nurse's suspicion of neonatal abstinence syndrome. The drug-addicted infant should be observed closely for poor sucking, seizures, vomiting and diarrhea, dehydration, and an increased metabolic rate. Many withdrawal symptoms are identical to those seen in other conditions such as infection, bowel obstruction, electrolyte disorder, hydrocephalus, and intracranial anomaly. The infant could potentially have both neonatal abstinence syndrome and another condition. Monitor the condition of the skin to identify abrasions associated with rubbing against sheets.

Assess the strengths, safety, and competence of the mother and other potential caregivers. Determine if the mother is still using illicit drugs and identify other family supports that may help provide the care and safety needed by the newborn.

Examples of nursing diagnoses may include:

- Ineffective Infant Feeding Pattern related to prematurity and oral hypersensitivity
- Disorganized Infant Behavior related to prenatal cocaine exposure
- Delayed Growth and Development related to intrauterine exposure to illicit substances
- Risk for Impaired Parenting related to infant with altered behavior organization and mother who uses illicit substances

■ Planning and Implementation

Provide Supportive Care

Provide frequent, small, high-calorie feedings, which are more readily tolerated by these infants. Special attention is given to dietary intake during hospitalization and at home for several months, as the infant may not eat well. Breastfeeding is not recommended for mothers continuing to use cocaine and other illicit drugs, as the substance is excreted in the breast milk. Infants suffering from withdrawal need increased calories; a formula with 24 calories per ounce may be recommended. Be patient with feeding as these infants often have poor coordination of sucking and swallowing. Teach parents to use a calm approach and soothing voice when feeding. Newborns may initially feed better in side-lying position while swaddled.

Administer prescribed medications, if ordered, for drug withdrawal and monitor the infant's response. However, many infants are managed without drugs, using the following techniques to calm and soothe the newborn.

- Keep the infant in a quiet environment, away from monitors that beep and paging speakers. Keep the lighting subdued and minimize stimulation to promote rest and sleep.
- Provide comfort and pacify the infant with swaddling and a pacifier for sucking needs. Rocking and soothing music may also be calming.
- Infant massage may also be beneficial in some infants.

Satisfy the emotional needs of the neonate by rocking, holding, and cuddling along with decreased light and noise. Hold the infant with the spine flexed to decrease extensor tone. Volunteers or hospital-based foster grandparents, if available, may help fulfill these needs. Such positive interaction with adults promotes comfort and supplies necessary emotional support for the infant. Protect the newborn's skin.

Begin working with the mother and other family members to demonstrate strategies for promoting parent–infant interaction, minimizing stimulation, and promoting feeding. Make plans for careful follow-up by health professionals (social services, physicians, and nurses) so that the infant's safety is assured and the growth and development are monitored and promoted.

Care in the Community

Long-term follow-up care of the child should be planned to ensure regular developmental testing and assessment for catch-up growth, neurobehavioral problems, and fetal alcohol syndrome (as multiple substances could have been used by the mother). Interventions for any identified problem will need to be initiated. In

MediaLink Case Study: Newborn with Neonatal Abstinence Syndrome

Health Promotion & Maintenance Overview

The Infant with Prenatal Exposure to Cocaine

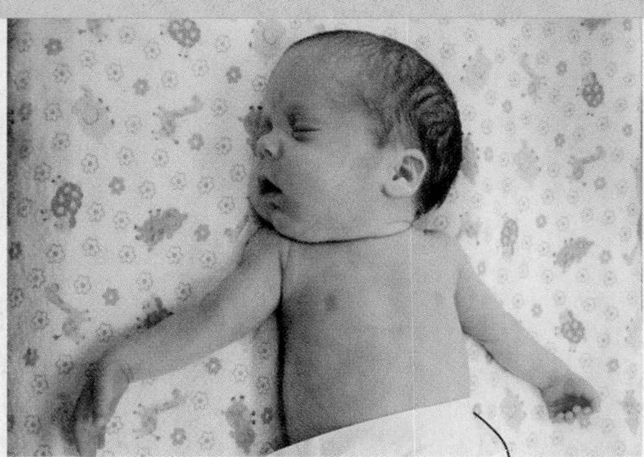

Growth and Development Surveillance

- Monitor the child's motor, psychosocial, and language development and refer the infant for a complete assessment if a developmental delay or other problem is suspected.
- Enroll the infant in an early intervention program to assist the parents or caregivers to promote the infant's development.
- Encourage enrollment in Head Start programs when the child is old enough as this may help later school performance.

Nutrition

- Monitor the infant's dietary intake. Assess the number of calories ingested and determine if calories are adequate for growth.
- Provide guidance about introduction of solid foods as the infant may have a strong tongue thrust and oral hypersensitivity. An occupational therapy feeding specialist referral may be helpful if the parent is having difficulty successfully feeding the infant.

Sleep and Rest

- Encourage parents or caregivers to establish a regular sleeping pattern. Use swaddling, low lighting, low noise, infant massage, rocking the infant in a flexed position, and a pacifier to relax the infant and promote sleep.
- Make sure the infant is placed to sleep on the back to reduce the risk for sudden infant death syndrome, as these infants may be at increased risk.

Relationships

- Monitor the parent for continued use of drugs to determine the safety of the infant and the ongoing ability of the parents to provide care. Monitor for potential signs of child abuse or neglect.
- Conduct home visits if ongoing use of drugs is suspected. Coordinate care with social services as necessary to determine if the infant needs foster care placement.
- Assess the patience and ability of the parents or caregivers to care for and have patience with an infant having behaviors such as irritability, excessive crying, and hyperactivity. Provide support to the parents or caregivers with education, support groups, or respite care to enable them to continue effective parenting of the infant.

Disease Prevention Strategies

- Work with the parents to ensure that the infant receives all immunizations according to the recommended schedule. Hepatitis B vaccine is especially important to administer as recommended because many mothers using illicit drugs acquire the infection through needle sharing or as a sexually transmitted disease.
- Perform all recommended screening tests to identify health problems.
- Weigh and measure the infant regularly to monitor catch-up growth. Monitor head circumference, as microcephaly is a potential complication of cocaine exposure.

some cases referral to child protective services may be made. The mother will also need follow-up to determine if her drug use continues and if the infant is safe from neglect or other harmful situations. See the Health Promotion and Maintenance Overview above to identify key areas for attention during follow-up visits.

Infants with neonatal abstinence syndrome are at a significantly higher risk (5–10:1) for sudden infant death syndrome when their mother used heroin or cocaine. Be sure to teach the caregiver to place the infant to sleep on the back. Home apnea monitoring may be used in some high-risk situations (Blatt, Meguid, & Church, 2000).

Care of the infant with neonatal abstinence syndrome and the substance-abusing mother often present complex family situations, and support from social services is often needed. The infant is at risk for neurobehavioral problems that a substance-abusing parent has difficulty meeting. Family resources and foster care may need to be considered if the infant does not have adequate growth. The long-term effects of this condition on cognitive function are not known at this time.

Evaluation

Expected outcomes of nursing intervention include:

- The parent establishes a routine so the infant has times during the day when receptive to interaction.
- The parent bonds and nurtures the infant.
- The infant receives regular healthcare in which growth and development is monitored.

INJURIES OF THE NEUROLOGIC SYSTEM

Traumatic Brain Injury

Traumatic brain injury is defined as trauma sufficient to cause a change in level of consciousness and/or an anatomical abnormality of the brain. The injury may be caused by blunt force or penetration. Traumatic brain injuries are the most common injuries in childhood. Among children 0 to 14 years, approximately 400,000 require emergency department visits, 29,000 require hospitalization, and 3,000 die (Centers for Disease Control, 2003). Children are at greater risk when under 5 years or during adolescence. Children and adolescents with a moderate or severe injury may develop a permanent disability such as epilepsy, cognitive impairment, learning problems, and behavioral or emotional problems. Traumatic brain injuries are responsible for nearly a third of all injury-related deaths (Adekoya, Thurman, White, et al., 2002).

Children are prone to skull fractures, often resulting in hematomas and brain injury. They may suffer from the secondary effects of trauma, such as diffuse cerebral edema, malignant brain edema, and increased intracranial pressure.

Young children with moderate and severe traumatic brain injury are at risk for long-term cognitive deficits. Most recovery occurs in the first 12 months following injury. With fewer well-established skills and knowledge and the slowed processing of information and attention impairment following the brain injury, the child has more challenges to develop cognitive and social competence (Anderson, Catroppa, Morse, et al., 2000).

Etiology and Pathophysiology

Falls are a major cause of unintentional brain injuries in young children.

- Infants fall from dressing tables, beds, and sofas and also tumble down stairs, especially in walkers (American Academy of Pediatrics Committee on Injury and Poison Prevention, 2001). Child abuse and shaken baby syndrome account for a large number of traumatic brain injuries in children under 1 year of age.
- Toddlers and preschoolers lack good judgment, and so may run haphazardly into the street or lean out of windows and fall.
- School-age children may be injured in motor vehicle crashes, either as passengers or pedestrians, and they may also be injured in bicycle, roller-blading, scooter, or skateboard mishaps.
- Adolescents are frequently the drivers in motor vehicle crashes; often alcohol or drugs are involved. Adolescents are also injured in sports-related accidents (see Chapter 15∞). An increasing number of traumatic brain injuries in adolescents are the result of firearm injuries.

Brain injuries can be categorized as either primary or secondary. Primary injuries occur at the time of the insult when the initial cellular damage occurs. These injuries result from either a direct blow to the head (**coup injury**) or inertial forces, the acceleration-deceleration movement of the brain within the skull (**contrecoup injury**; Figure 33–20 ■). At the time of impact, scalp injuries, skull fractures, contusions, and hematomas of brain tissue may occur. The inertial forces resulting when the head and skull stop moving, but the brain tissues within the skull continue moving, cause tearing of nerves, fibers, and blood vessels. Altered level of consciousness results due to concussions, diffuse axonal injuries, and subdural hematomas. These injuries usually occur simultaneously.

The secondary phase of brain trauma is a biochemical and cellular response to the initial insult, and can be manifested immediately or over hours, days, or weeks. Excitatory neurotransmitters are released in toxic amounts and may intensify the brain damage following traumatic brain injury. Damage usually results from destruction of brain tissue secondary to hypoxia, hypotension, edema, change in the blood-brain barrier, or hemorrhage. The result is increased arterial and intracranial pressure.

See the clinical manifestations table below for information about specific types of injury associated with traumatic brain injury.

Clinical Manifestations

The signs and symptoms of brain injuries in children depend on the pathologic features and severity of the injury. The child with a mild brain injury may remain conscious or have a brief loss of consciousness (seconds to a few minutes) or amnesia. The child with a moderate brain injury loses consciousness for 5 to 10 minutes. Following mild and moderate brain injuries, children may have amnesia about the event, headache, nausea, and vomiting. A child with a severe brain injury, such as Antwan in the opening

CLINICAL MANIFESTATIONS of Traumatic Brain Injury by Severity

TYPE OF BRAIN INJURY	CLINICAL MANIFESTATIONS
Concussion or mild brain injury	Low-grade headache that will not go away Slowness in thinking, acting, speaking, reading Memory problems Loss of balance, unsteady walking Difficulty paying attention or concentrating, change in performance at school Feeling tired all the time, change in sleeping pattern Change in eating patterns Increased sensitivity to lights, sounds, distractions Easily irritated Lack of motivation or interest in favorite toys
Moderate brain injury	Glasgow Coma Scale score of 9–12 Posttraumatic amnesia for 1–24 hours Loss of consciousness
Severe brain injury	Glasgow Coma Scale score of 8 or less Posttraumatic amnesia greater than 24 hours Coma Increased intracranial pressure

PATHOPHYSIOLOGY ILLUSTRATED

Brain Injury

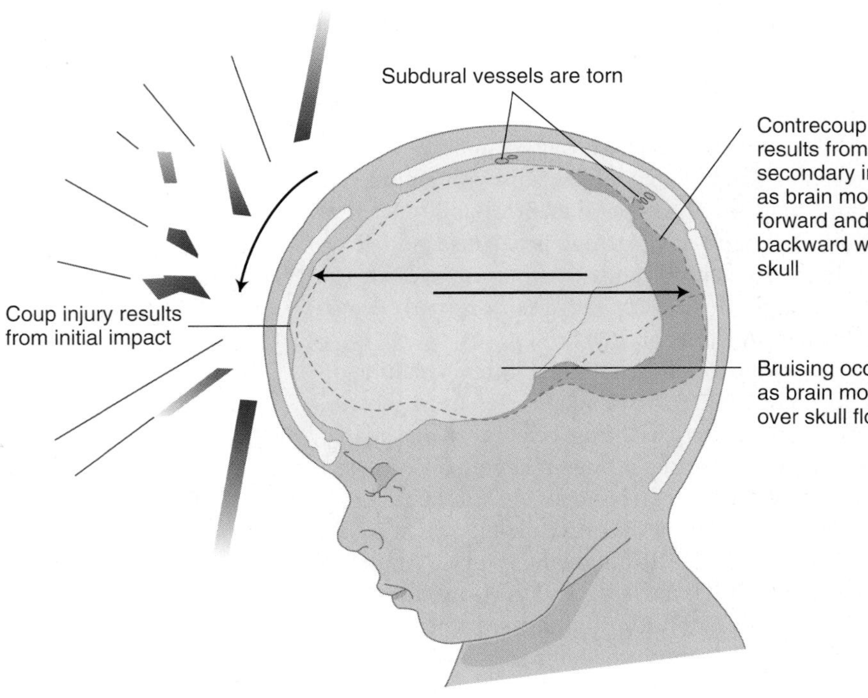
Subdural vessels are torn
Contrecoup injury results from secondary impact as brain moves forward and then backward within skull
Coup injury results from initial impact
Bruising occurs as brain moves over skull floor

FIGURE 33–20 ■ Brain injury can result from a direct blow to the head just under the skull where the initial impact occurs (coup injury). The acceleration-deceleration movement of the brain within the skull also results in an injury where the brain strikes the skull (contrecoup injury).

scenario, is usually unconscious for more than 10 minutes and may rapidly show signs of increased intracranial pressure.

Unconsciousness may result from increased intracranial pressure, edema, hemorrhage, or parenchymal damage to the cortex in both cerebral hemispheres or the brainstem. Posttraumatic seizures are common. Retinal hemorrhages are seen in 65% to 90% of children with inflicted traumatic brain injury (Schutzman & Greenes, 2001).

Vital signs are important indicators of brain injury. Changes in respiratory effort or periods of apnea may result from shock, injury to the spinal cord above C4, or damage to or pressure on the medulla. Heart rate and blood pressure are indices of brainstem function. Tachycardia can be a sign of blood loss, shock, hypoxia, anxiety, or pain. Cushing's triad, associated with increased intracranial pressure or compromised blood flow to the brainstem, is characterized by hypertension, increased systolic pressure with wide pulse pressure, bradycardia, and irregular respirations. Refer to the earlier discussion of altered states of consciousness for more information about increased intracranial pressure.

Reflexes may be hyporesponsive, hyperresponsive, or nonexistent. The child may be **areflexic** (no response to verbal, sensory, or pain stimulation) and assume a decorticate, decerebrate, or flaccid posture (see Figure 33–3).

See the clinical manifestations table on pages 1349–1350 for specific types of complications of traumatic brain injury.

MediaLink Coup-Contrecoup Injury Animation

COLLABORATIVE CARE

The goal of collaborative care is to rapidly identify the brain injuries that may lead to serious morbidity or mortality if untreated, and to initiate aggressive interventions to reduce increased intracranial pressure and minimize complications in those with potential for greater injury severity.

Diagnostic Testing

Identifying the severity of a brain injury involves history, observation, examination, and diagnostic testing. Ask questions about how the injury occurred, the child's initial responses and current responses, any loss of consciousness, and the child's memory of the event.

PRACTICE ALERT

Any infant who arrives in the emergency department with seizures, failure to thrive, vomiting, lethargy, respiratory irregularities, or coma should be evaluated for child abuse, particularly shaken child syndrome. The infant has a relatively large head with relatively weak neck muscles. An extremely frustrated adult can shake an infant and cause inertial injuries (acceleration and deceleration) to the head that cause diffuse tearing of the nerve fibers in the brain.

Neurologic evaluation with the pediatric Glasgow Coma Scale is performed frequently to describe the severity of the

CLINICAL MANIFESTATIONS of Specific Brain Injuries

BRAIN INJURY AND ETIOLOGY	CLINICAL MANIFESTATIONS	CLINICAL THERAPY
Subdural Hematoma Result of severe head trauma such as falls, assaults, motor vehicle crashes, or shaken child syndrome Occurs most frequently in children less than 1 year of age Inertial forces cause laceration of the bridging veins; venous hematoma forms beneath the dura and presses directly on brain Subdural hematoma Dura Bleeding occurs between dura and brain	Symptoms (may not appear until 48–72 hours after the injury) include: • Change in level of consciousness (confusion, agitation, or lethargy) • Nausea or vomiting • Headache • Retinal hemorrhages in both eyes • Pupil on side of injury may be fixed and dilated • Seizures • Fever	Diagnosis confirmed by CT scan Hematoma is evacuated surgically Management of increased intracranial pressure; subdural taps may be needed Morbidity and mortality rates are high Damage from the initial inertial injury is compounded by the hematoma Surviving children have a 75% chance of developing seizures
Epidural Hematoma Rare in children and almost never occurs in children less than 4 years of age Results from blunt trauma (most often falls), motor vehicle crashes, assaults, or baseball to temporal area Temporal and parietal areas are most common sites May be associated with linear skull fracture Arterial or venous bleeding occurs between the skull and the dura Epidural hematoma Dura Bleeding occurs between dura and skull	• Delayed onset, minimal or absent symptoms from initial impact • Rapid deterioration • Sleepiness or lethargy • Headache • Full fontanel • Paresis of cranial nerves III and VI • Papilledema • Fixed and dilated pupil • Signs of increased intracranial pressure	Diagnosis confirmed by CT scan Treatment involves immediate surgical intervention; craniotomy is performed followed by evacuation of the hematoma Prognosis is good, although 25% of children have seizures May be fatal if bleeding is arterial
Cerebral Contusion Bruising of brain tissue secondary to blunt trauma that can occur with either coup or contrecoup injuries The temporal or frontal sections of the skull are the most common sites of this injury May involve damage to the parenchyma with tears in vessels or tissue, pulping, and subsequent areas of necrosis or infarction	• Altered levels of consciousness range from confusion and disorientation to being obtunded • Focal symptoms depending on the area of injury	Diagnosis is confirmed by CT scan The child is observed in the hospital to rule out other injuries. Surgical treatment is rarely necessary Sequelae are focal and specific to the area of the brain that is injured, i.e., injury to the left temporal area may affect speech
Diffuse Axonal Injury Results from tearing of nerve fibers throughout the brain through violent inertional forces Accompanying trauma to other organ systems or to the spine is frequent	• Immediate loss of consciousness • Unconsciousness lasting longer than 6 hours • Abnormal movements or posturing • Seizures • Increased intracranial pressure • Difficulty regulating blood pressure and breathing	Diagnosis is confirmed by CT and MRI scans that show brain tissue tears and hemorrhages Long-lasting impairments may include motor, cognitive, communication, and behavior problems A small number remain in a chronic unresponsive state (continued)

CLINICAL MANIFESTATIONS of Specific Brain Injuries (continued)

BRAIN INJURY AND ETIOLOGY	CLINICAL MANIFESTATIONS	CLINICAL THERAPY
Subarachnoid Hemorrhage Associated with severe head injuries such as intracranial hematomas or contusions, result from laceration of arteries or veins in the subarachnoid space	• Decreased level of consciousness • Ipsilateral pupil dilation • Diplopia • Hemiparesis • Nausea and vomiting • Nuchal rigidity • Headache	Diagnosis is confirmed by CT scan General supportive treatment for brain injuries Clinical course depends on associated injuries
Intracerebral Hematoma Result of deep contusion or intracerebral laceration (secondary to foreign body or bony penetration or impalement) Causes diffuse bleeding in parenchyma; there may be a hematoma with associated small areas of bleeding Intracerebral hematoma Bleeding occurs within cerebrum	• Symptoms depend on size and location of hematoma as well as if size is increasing due to uncontrolled bleeding • Altered consciousness	Diagnosis confirmed by CT scan Surgical treatment not indicated Neurologic effects depend on size and location of lesion and whether bleeding can be controlled Hemiplegia or visual loss may result

brain injury and to detect changes in the child's condition (see Table 33–2). Cranial nerves are assessed (see Table 8–22∞ and Table 33–4).

Laboratory tests include a complete blood cell count, blood chemistry, toxicology screening, and urinalysis. Radiologic examination is performed to identify the specific injury (Box 33–16). Most children with head injuries are the victims of multiple trauma, and even though cervical spine injuries are rare, all children should be suspected of having a cervical spine injury until this possibility has been ruled out by radiologic examination. Intracranial pressure monitoring can be performed after insertion of a catheter into the ventricle or a bolt into the subarachnoid space.

Clinical Therapy

The initial management of a child with a brain injury is based on the child's physiologic status. When the child has altered consciousness, ensure that the airway is clear and stable. Administer oxygen to prevent hypoxemia. If indicated, the child is intubated to protect the airway and prevent aspiration. Assisted ventilation may be used to prevent hypoxemia and hypercarbia. Perfusion of the brain must be maintained to ensure that it gets adequate oxygen and nutrients, and so the accumulation of neurotoxins is removed.

BOX 33–16 Radiographic Diagnostic Procedures for Brain Injury

- Skull radiograph—detect skull fracture
- Cervical spine radiograph—detect fracture of the cervical vertebrae
- CT scan—diagnose intracranial hemorrhage, swelling, diffuse axonal injury, skull fractures
- MRI scans—used during recovery to identify extent of residual brain damage
- PET scans—measure blood flow in the brain

PRACTICE ALERT

In the child with moderate head injury, the oxygen saturation should remain over 95%. For the severely injured child who is intubated, monitor arterial blood gas results. The PaO_2 should be 70–100 mm Hg

Hypovolemic Shock Therapy. Shock is treated aggressively with fluid boluses. Keep the head of the bed flat until adequate cerebral perfusion pressure is ensured. Inotropic medications may be used to maintain the blood pressure and ensure perfusion if **cerebral edema** (the increase in intracellular and extracellular fluid in the brain that results from anoxia, vasodilation, or vascular stasis) is present. A continuous infusion of hypertonic saline (3%) is sometimes used for control of increased intracranial pressure (Chestnut et al., 2003). Fluid administration is focused on maintaining the blood pressure level.

Increased Intracranial Pressure Management. Increased intracranial pressure must be controlled. Brain swelling can lead to worsening cerebral ischemia and more brain swelling. If this is unrelieved, brain shifting in the cranium begins, which may be a precursor of **herniation** (protrusion of brain contents into the brainstem area). Hypoxia and hypercapnia have disastrous effects on cerebral function, as they can cause vasodilation and increased intracranial pressure. Mechanical ventilation with 100% oxygen at the child's normal respiratory rate is used in the first 24 hours after injury to maintain oxygenation levels. Hyperventilation may be used for a short period in cases of severe increased intracranial pressure, but prolonged use may cause cerebral ischemia (Chestnut et al., 2003).

In children with severe brain injury, invasive intracranial pressure monitoring may be initiated, particularly if the child is sedated and cannot be evaluated by physical signs. Treatment for increased intracranial pressure is started when the intracranial pressure is ≥ 20 mm Hg. Cerebral perfusion pressure should be maintained at ≥ 40 mm Hg (Chestnut et al., 2003). Mannitol may be administered to decrease the intracranial pressure. Pain and sedation medications are used to facilitate mechanical ventilation support, promote intracranial pressure management, and promote comfort. The child may be placed in a chemically induced coma to reduce brain activity during this acute care phase. Corticosteroids are not recommended for reducing intracranial pressure. See the medication table below.

Invasive procedures may be necessary to reduce increased intracranial pressure. Burr holes may be made or more extensive surgery performed as a method of evacuating a lesion or hematoma. A ventriculostomy catheter may be placed to drain cerebrospinal fluid and to monitor pressure when brain swelling reaches dangerous heights. Decompressive craniectomy may be considered as a last resort when intracranial pressure cannot be otherwise controlled. Therapeutic hypothermia is being investigated as a treatment to protect the brain.

If there is no cervical spine injury, the head of the bed is elevated up to 30 degrees. The child's head is kept in the midline to promote venous (jugular) drainage. Hip flexion is avoided. The child's body temperature is kept within normal limits. The environment is kept as quiet as possible. Fluids may be restricted only after the child is hemodynamically stable. Diuretics such as mannitol or furosemide may be given to shrink brain volume. A urinary catheter is inserted to monitor output, and electrolytes should be checked frequently. Nutritional support should be started within 72 hours with total parenteral nutrition or enteral nutrition.

Rehabilitation Care. Aggressive support continues until the child regains consciousness and rehabilitation can be initiated. Initial stages of rehabilitation are made during the acute phase of management to prevent complications from immobilization, disuse, and neurologic dysfunction. When long-term rehabilitation is needed, the primary goal is to improve basic self-care skills of bathing, grooming, dressing, and feeding. Disabilities that often result from a severe brain injury include motor impairments, feeding disorders, hearing and vision impairments, communication problems, and cognitive impairments. Physical therapy, occupational therapy, speech-language specialists, and social workers all play vital roles in the rehabilitation process.

NURSING MANAGEMENT

The child with a moderate or severe traumatic brain injury is hospitalized. A severe traumatic brain injury can be life threatening, so care is provided in a critical care unit. Nursing management of

MEDICATIONS Used for Increased Intracranial Pressure (ICP)

MEDICATION	ACTION	NURSING ACTION
Analgesics and sedatives	Neuromuscular blockade causes muscular paralysis that helps with ventilatory control, prevents increases in arterial blood pressure associated with isometric muscle contractions due to decerebrate or decorticate posturing, and minimizes anxiety and pain.	Mechanical ventilation is needed, monitor airway for secretions that need suctioning Monitor respiratory status with pulse oximetry and blood gases Monitor physiologic responses (heart rate, blood pressure, and ICP) to assess adequacy of pain management
Mannitol	Osmotic agent that reduces blood viscosity and lowers ICP as fluid is moved out of brain tissue into the circulation. Cerebral blood volume is maintained as less viscous blood reduces resistance to blood flow.	Carefully monitor ICP as well as intake and output Monitor serum osmolality to ensure that the value stays at the target value, just above high normal range (300–310 mOsm/L) Monitor serum and urine electrolytes to detect syndrome of inappropriate antidiuretic hormone secretion
Furosemide	A diuretic that works to reduce cerebrospinal fluid production and reduction of sodium transport to the brain. It also causes a reduction in total body fluids.	Monitor intake and output to prevent hypovolemia that could compromise cerebral blood flow Same as with mannitol
Hypertonic saline (3%) infusion	Osmotic agent that moves fluid out of the brain tissue into the circulation to lower ICP.	Same as with mannitol
Barbiturates Pentobarbitol	In high doses, barbiturate coma is induced to lower the resting cerebral metabolic rate for oxygen. Used when other therapies have not been successful.	Use a cardiorespiratory monitor to detect dysrhythmias Monitor mean arterial blood pressure as the medication can cause decreased cardiac output and hypotension
Anticonvulsants	Used to treat status epilepticus or prevent breakthrough seizures that can cause spikes in ICP.	Monitor the child for seizures. Immediate medications are needed to stop seizure activity

the child with a severe traumatic brain injury focuses on assessment of changes in neurologic status and vital signs, management of clinical therapies, prevention of complications, and support for the family.

Nursing Assessment and Diagnosis

Assess the child's ability to maintain an open airway, regulate breathing, and circulation. As level of consciousness drops, protective gag and cough reflexes are lost, and the tongue obstructs the airway. If the child is intubated, assess the CO_2 monitor on the endotracheal tube to confirm tube placement in the trachea.

Neurologic Assessment

Assess the child's neurologic status frequently. Quantify the child's level of consciousness using the pediatric Glasgow Coma Scale for future comparison (see Table 33–2). Assess the pupils for size and reactivity. Check the cranial nerves for impaired functioning. Note decerebrate or decorticate posturing. The child's neurologic status is compared with his or her previous state, with improvement, stability, or deterioration documented. The cause of any deterioration must be quickly identified and appropriate interventions taken.

CLINICAL TIP

A child who has a decreased level of consciousness shortly after a brain injury may have had a posttraumatic seizure and may still be in the postictal state.

Monitor vital signs closely. Stay alert for changes in vital signs and behavior that indicate increased intracranial pressure (see Table 33–1) and potential progression to Cushing's triad (bradycardia, irregular respirations, and increased systolic blood pressure with a widening pulse pressure). Changes in vital signs may indicate hypoxia, decreased perfusion, shock, or increased intracranial pressure. If a ventricular catheter or bolt is inserted, monitor the actual intracranial pressure readings.

Suspect that the child with increased intracranial pressure is in pain, even when unresponsive. Observe for physiologic and behavioral signs of pain. See Chapter 18∞.

Psychological Assessment

Assess the family's coping with the uncertainty of the child's severe injury and the support systems available to them. Assess their ability to understand the information about the child's status. They may feel guilty if the child was in their care when the life-threatening injury occurred. Refer to Chapter 21∞.

The following nursing diagnoses may be appropriate for the child with a serious traumatic brain injury.

- Ineffective Cerebral Tissue Perfusion related to hypoventilation, hypovolemia, and/or reduction of arterial blood flow to the brain due to increased intracranial pressure
- Ineffective Breathing Pattern related to decreased level of consciousness and brain trauma
- Risk for Aspiration related to decreased level of consciousness and loss of protective reflexes
- Risk for Impaired Skin Integrity related to bed rest and immobility
- Risk for Imbalanced Fluid Volume related to therapies for reducing intracranial pressure
- Compromised Family Coping related to life-threatening injury to child
- Interrupted Family Processes related to shift in health status of child

Planning and Implementation

Critical Care

Nursing care focuses on maintaining cardiopulmonary function and cerebral perfusion, preventing complications, promoting recovery, and providing emotional support. The goal of nursing management is to prevent secondary injury and to promote return to an optimal level of function.

MAINTAIN CEREBRAL PERFUSION

In the severely injured child, measures are taken to reduce or minimize increases in the intracranial pressure. Maintain oxygenation and ventilation to prevent hypoxemia. Keep the airway clear and cautiously suction the airway only when excessive secretions are present, as suctioning can increase the ICP. Administer intravenous fluids at the rate that maintains hydration and blood pressure thus ensuring an adequate cerebral perfusion pressure. Monitor the effects of medications on hydration status. Report any sign of decreased oxygenation, bradycardia, and lowered blood pressure to the physician immediately.

When an intraventricular catheter or bolt is inserted, stabilize and protect the catheter or bolt to keep it from becoming displaced. Position the child with head at midline position either on a flat surface or with bed elevated 15 to 30 degrees to prevent compression of the neck blood vessels. Elevating the head may help promote venous drainage from the cerebral circulation; however, elevation should only be used if the cerebral perfusion pressure is maintained. Avoid excessive flexion of the hips and neck that could slow venous circulation. The child may also be placed in a side-lying position with the head in neutral position (not flexed or extended). Logroll the child for turning to prevent intraabdominal and intrathoracic pressure that could cause an increase in ICP.

REDUCE INTRACRANIAL PRESSURE

Provide careful thermoregulation to reduce the physiologic stress on the body that could further increase the intracranial pressure. Minimize unpleasant stimuli when possible. Keep the environment quiet and avoid jarring the bed. Minimize pain associated with painful procedures and control pain associated with increased intracranial pressure. Monitor the effect of nursing procedures on the level of ICP and determine if clustering procedures is better than spreading procedures over time.

Promote Nutrition

Nutrition is implemented as soon as possible to promote wound healing. Initial feeding may be by total parenteral nutrition or enteral feeding, slowly progressing to oral foods as tolerated.

Provide Routine Care

Provide oral care to keep mucous membranes moist and intact. Provide skin care. Pad and cushion bony prominences and change the child's position frequently. Protect the eyes from corneal irritation with ophthalmic ointment and patching. Prevent constipation with stool softeners and suppositories as needed.

Perform passive range of motion exercises to prevent contractures. Splints may be used to position extremities in functional positions (Figure 33–21 ■). Ensure that the side rails of the bed are padded to protect the child if a seizure occurs.

Promote Recovery

Physical, occupational, and speech therapy should begin in the hospital. Work with therapists to reinforce exercises and help teach parents the techniques so they can work with the child in the hospital and at home. The nurse can reinforce what has been done during these sessions, noting positive changes. Provide stimulation based on the child's age and ability using toys, books, music, or games.

Provide Emotional Support

Nurses, social workers, physicians, psychologists, rehabilitation therapists, and members of the clergy can support and help parents adjust to having a child with a new disability. Encourage parents to participate in the child's care. Encourage parents to bring in favorite toys, stuffed animals, and tape recordings of the child's favorite music or of family members talking.

Despite all care, the child with a serious brain injury may die due to herniation and brain death. See Table 22–2∞ for brain death criteria. Provide support to the family while testing for brain death criteria is performed. Allow the family to have time with the child to make important decisions regarding termination of life support and potential organ donation. See Chapter 22∞.

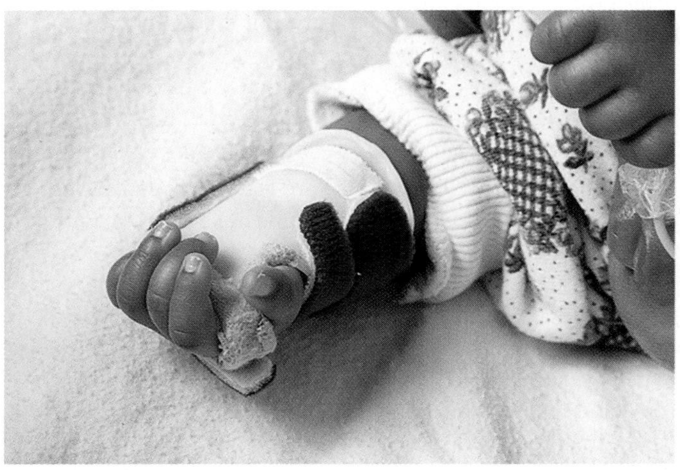

FIGURE 33–21 ■ Splints are often used to prevent contractures, thus maintaining optimal functioning of the child's hands or feet.

Discharge Planning and Home Care Teaching

Home care needs should be identified and addressed well in advance of discharge. Children with serious traumatic brain injuries will benefit from inpatient or outpatient rehabilitation to promote optimal achievement of function. If the child's condition qualifies for inpatient rehabilitation, encourage the family to visit the rehabilitation center to learn more about the care that will be provided, and the family's role in the child's care. Rehabilitation focuses on augmenting abilities regained during recovery and teaches adaptive compensation for lost function. An initial focus will be on self-care skills such as toileting, bathing, dressing, grooming, and feeding. A case manager may be needed to coordinate services and resources during rehabilitation.

Give parents information about caring for children with mild and moderate brain injuries at home and possible behaviors to expect from the child. For children with disabilities, determine what adaptations and assistive technology are needed in the home to care for the child, such as a wheelchair, walker, braces, or special bed. Social work and home health agencies can often help the parents make special arrangements for needed resources. Many children with severe brain injuries are disabled enough to qualify for Social Security's Supplemental Security Income (SSI) benefits or the state program for children with special healthcare needs.

MediaLink Traumatic Brain Injury Resources and Support

Care in the Community

Home care nurses play a vital role in the care of such children as Antwan who have an acquired neurologic dysfunction and prolonged altered consciousness. The home care nurse can assume the role of case manager for the disabled child and make sure the environment is safe. Nurses can also teach the family how to care for the child with severe neurologic dysfunction and to perform routine procedures such as suctioning and maintaining the airway, skin care, feeding, positioning, range of motion exercises, and stimulation. The skin over pressure areas must be protected and observed carefully for redness or other signs of damage. See Chapter 36∞ for recognition of pressure areas needing intervention. The home health nurse can assist the parents to monitor the child's intake of food and fluids to ensure that adequate nutrition and fluids are received. During the acute rehabilitation phase, physical therapy may be provided in the home to help educate the parents to appropriately position the child and exercise the muscles to reduce contractures and to promote improved functioning. Regular follow-up visits are needed to assess the child's progress and to modify the treatment plan.

Mild Brain Injury

Parents of children with mild or moderate traumatic brain injuries need to be prepared for altered behavior until full recovery has occurred. Even though the child looks normal within days of a mild or moderate injury, brain healing takes up to 6 weeks. Parents and teachers should be made aware that typical behavior during this period may include any of the following: tiring easily, memory loss or forgetfulness, easy distractibility, difficulty concentrating, difficulty following directions, irritability or short temper, and needing help starting and finishing tasks. Educational assessment should be initiated if recovery takes longer than 6 weeks.

Moderate and Severe Brain Injury

Children with moderate or severe traumatic brain injuries may require academic accommodations. Children with moderate injuries commonly have problems with attention, problem solving, and speed of information processing that compromise their school performance, as well as behavior problems. Neuropsychological testing is needed to identify the subtle learning disabilities that are not usually revealed on standardized school achievement tests. Educational accommodations needed are usually different from those made for children with other learning disabilities. Future neuropsychological testing is often needed as the child progresses to different developmental stages or when educational demands increase, such as deductive reasoning and organizational abilities needed in middle school and high school. The brain injury impairs new learning more than the retention of prior learning. Children who experience a brain injury at a young age may be at a special disadvantage because they have not had the time to store knowledge and develop learning strategies.

Children with moderate to severe brain injuries may experience behavioral problems that include inattention, increased or decreased activity, impulsivity, irritability, lowered frustration tolerance, emotional lability, apathy, aggression, and social withdrawal (Michaud, Semes-Concepcion, Duhaime, et al., 2002).

Arrangements to return the child with a severe brain injury to the school setting should include evaluation for special needs and development of an IEP to address those needs. The severity of deficits and functional capabilities may influence whether the best resources for the child are in a mainstreamed or separate classroom. Examples of behavior challenges in children with some severe brain injuries include social inappropriateness, lack of awareness, and decreased control of attention, memory, or strategic thinking. Other long-term functional deficits may include limitations in self-care skills such as walking, dressing, and self-feeding (Agency for Healthcare Research and Quality, 1999).

The family of a child with a significant brain injury will need continuing psychological support, case management, and linkage to rehabilitation services that may help promote improvements in the child's functioning. Public Law 104-166, the Traumatic Brain Injury Act, was enacted by Congress in 1996 to prevent brain injuries and to minimize the severity of dysfunction as a result of brain injury by providing funding to states to identify mechanisms to improve access to services (U.S. Congress, 1996).

The child or adolescent who is facing long-term rehabilitation requires support to adjust to the disability and to find the strength to maximize his or her abilities. Identify recreational opportunities for the child with disabilities to promote exercise and self-esteem. The adolescent may need to gain vocational skills and learn to live independently. Refer parents to the Brain Injury Association for further information.

Evaluation

Examples of expected outcomes of nursing care for the child with traumatic brain injury include the following:

- Cerebral perfusion pressure is maintained at an adequate rate to sustain oxygenation of the brain.
- The child regains consciousness and begins the process of regaining function.
- Muscle function is maintained and physical deformities are prevented with range of motion exercises and splinting during the recovery stages of the brain injury.
- Parents are supported through the child's acute recovery phase and learn to provide appropriate care at home.
- The child's school performance is monitored and appropriate educational resources are provided to support the child's learning.

Specific Head Injuries

Intraventricular Hemorrhage

Low-birth-weight and premature infants are at increased risk for brain injury from birth trauma and conditions such as respiratory distress syndrome, hypoxic-ischemic injury, and infection. Such stressors lead to rupture of blood vessels in the developing brain. Bleeding often involves the ventricles.

Common signs and symptoms include diminished or absent Moro reflex, poor muscle tone, lethargy, and apnea. The newborn may deteriorate in the early days of life with apnea, poor sucking, high-pitched cry, muscular twitching and seizures, decreased muscle tone, shock, and coma.

Diagnosis is based on history, physical findings, and a cranial ultrasound or CT scan. Evaluation of the hematocrit may reveal anemia. Newborns with massive hemorrhage often die after rapid deterioration. Seizures are treated with anticonvulsant drugs. Hydrocephalus may develop in some newborns and require placement of a ventriculoperitoneal shunt. Motor and neurologic deficits often result and require long-term care.

Scalp Injuries

Injuries to the scalp, which can be caused by falls, blunt trauma, or penetration of a foreign body, are usually benign. Although bleeding may be extensive, hypovolemia or shock is uncommon unless the patient is an infant.

Lacerations should be irrigated with copious amounts of sterile normal saline solution and inspected for bony fragments or depressions, cerebrospinal fluid leakage with a tear of the dura mater, or debris. If the injury is simple, the laceration can be sutured and the child discharged from the emergency department. If not, a neurosurgeon should be consulted.

Concussion

A concussion can involve transient impairment of consciousness that usually results from blunt trauma to the head. Sports with a high risk for concussion include boxing, field hockey, football, ice hockey, lacrosse, martial arts, soccer, rodeo, wrestling, rugby, baseball, rollerblading, trampolining, and basketball. An estimated 62,800 high school athletes experience a concussion each year, and the concussion is related to football in approximately 63% of cases (Lovell, Collins, Iverson, et al., 2003).

Concussions are secondary to stretching, compression, or shearing of nerve fibers from an impact injury to the head. There is usually no gross structural damage or focal injury. The child will have an alteration in mental status (e.g., amnesia, dizziness, memory or orientation impairment, unsteady gait), but not necessarily loss of consciousness. Athletes who sustain a concussion are nearly three times as likely to have a second concussion in the same season (Guskiewicz, Weaver, Padua, et al., 2000).

Clinical manifestations of concussions, categorized by three levels of severity, are listed in the table below.

Treatment is supportive. Children are observed in the emergency department for several hours before being sent home with instructions to the parents to watch the child closely for decreased responsiveness. Any child who is unconscious for more than 5 minutes or has amnesia of the event may be admitted to the hospital or observed in a short-stay unit to rule out other injury.

Pediatric concussive syndrome, believed to be caused by an injury to the brainstem, is seen in children who are under 3 years of age. Toddlers seem stunned at the time of injury, but do not lose consciousness. Later, however, these children become pale, clammy, and lethargic, and they may vomit. They are usually brought to the hospital for treatment when such symptoms appear. These children may be placed in a short-stay unit for observation and usually recover within 24 hours.

Postconcussive syndrome, common in both children and adults, may occur anytime after the initial brain injury. Signs and symptoms can include headache, dizziness or vertigo, fatigue, irritability, photophobia, subtle changes in personality, poor concentration, poor memory, and ataxia. Treatment is supportive. Symptoms usually disappear within several weeks but may last up to 6 months. Parents and teachers should be informed to expect altered behavior in the child. They should be encouraged to help the child maintain self-esteem.

CLINICAL MANIFESTATIONS by Concussion Severity Level

SEVERITY GRADE	CLINICAL MANIFESTATIONS
Grade 1	Transient confusion, no loss of consciousness, and a duration of mental status abnormalities of less than 15 minutes
Grade 2	Transient confusion, no loss of consciousness, and a duration of mental status abnormalities of 15 minutes or longer
Grade 3	Loss of consciousness, either brief (seconds) or prolonged (minutes or longer)

Adapted from Quality Standards Subcommittee, American Academy of Neurology. (1997). Practice parameters: The management of concussion in sports. Neurology, 48, *581–585.*

Young athletes suffering a second concussion before complete recovery from the first may develop second impact syndrome. This injury results in acute brain swelling, neurologic or cognitive deficits, and sometimes death from the cumulative effect of these concussions. Recommendations should be followed for the management of sports-related concussions to reduce the risk of disability and death. Removal from sports participation ranges between 7 days to the entire season, depending on the severity of concussion and neurologic symptoms (Guskiewicz et al., 2000). A postconcussion symptom scale is now commonly used for amateur and professional sports to provide uniform information about the actual recovery time from the concussion. It also reduces the risk of athletes who try to minimize symptoms to get back in the game of being returned to play too soon. Those with a history of multiple concussions have a significantly longer recovery time (Guskiewicz & McCrea, 2003)

MediaLink Case Study: Post-Concussion Return to Competitive Play

Skull Fractures

A fracture to any of the eight cranial bones is caused by a considerable force to the head. Any area of the skull with swelling or a hematoma should be evaluated for possible fracture. The skull fracture of a newborn in association with a traumatic birth is often a linear fracture or a depressed "ping-pong" fracture (McGee & Burkett, 2000). Diagnosis is made by visual inspection, palpation, radiologic study, or CT scan. Treatment should always include neurosurgical consultation.

Management of skull fractures depends on the type and extent of injury (Figure 33–22 ■). See Table 33–8.

Penetrating Injuries

Gunshot wounds to the head can damage tissue, bone, and vessels. Low-velocity bullets enter but do not exit the skull; instead

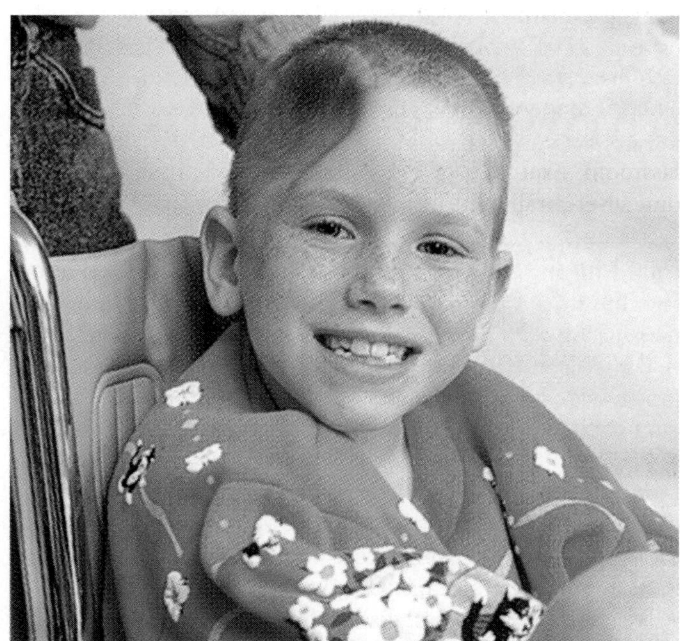

FIGURE 33–22 ■ This child has had a significant depressed skull fracture that required removal of bony fragments over a section of the skull.

TABLE 33–8 Skull Fractures

INJURY	DIAGNOSIS AND CLINICAL THERAPY
Linear Fracture Results from impact to large area of the skull. Usually no symptoms. May have overlying hematoma or soft tissue swelling. Such fractures in newborns may result from pressure from forceps or from maternal pelvic bones.	If fracture is on temporal bone or crosses sagittal suture line a CT scan is performed to detect potential epidural hematoma. Consider the possibility of an inflicted injury. No treatment is commonly needed.
Depressed Fracture Break in skull itself or an area shattered into many fragments. Pieces of bone may be depressed into brain tissue with hematoma forming on top. This type of fracture in a newborn may be the result of a forceps injury.	Plain radiographic film or CT scan. Surgery to elevate bone fragments when depression is greater than 5 mm. Tetanus prophylaxis is given as needed. Many are associated with intracranial injury and posttraumatic epilepsy.
Compound Fracture Combination of a full thickness scalp laceration and depressed skull fracture with the bone exposed, considered penetrating fractures if the dura is torn.	Visual diagnosis along with radiographic studies. Surgical debridement, a search for foreign bodies, and copious irrigation is performed. Parenteral antibiotics and tetanus prophylaxis are provided as needed.
Basilar Fracture Fracture at the base of the skull that may involve the frontal, ethmoid, sphenoid, temporal, or occipital bones. A dural tear may be present.	Diagnosis is confirmed by signs of blood behind the tympanic membranes, cerebrospinal fluid leakage from the nose or ears, periorbital ecchymosis (raccoon eyes) or bruising of the mastoid (Battle sign). Radiographic imaging locates the fracture site. Antibiotics may be prescribed. Surgical repair of the site of the cerebrospinal fluid lead is performed if the leak persists after 7–10 days. Transient or permanent cranial nerve injuries occur (e.g., hearing loss).

Data from Rosman, N. P. (1999). Acute head trauma. In J. A. McMillan, C. D. DeAngelis, R. D. Feigin, & J. B. Warshaw, Oski's pediatrics: Principles and practice, *(3rd ed., pp. 603–617). Philadelphia: Lippincott, Williams & Willkins.*

they ricochet within the cranial vault, destroying brain tissue and vessels. Although the child may be conscious just after the injury, the level of consciousness quickly deteriorates due to the edema surrounding the penetration tract. High-velocity bullets, on the other hand, cause immediate, severe damage on impact. (See Chapter 7∞ for a discussion of violence in childhood.) CT is used to evaluate gunshot trauma and to pinpoint the location of bullet and bone fragments as well as parenchymal damage. Treatment involves surgical debridement of the tract, evacuation of any hematomas, and removal of accessible bone or bullet particles. Approximately 50% of children with gunshot wounds to the head die. Those who survive may suffer multiple focal deficits and seizures.

Impalement injuries frequently occur in children in association with lawn darts or dog bites. All objects must be left in place and removed in the operating room by a neurosurgeon. The child with an impalement injury is at high risk for focal injury and infection. After surgery, children with this type of injury are managed as with other postoperative head injuries, with attention focused on level of consciousness, increased intracranial pressure, and infection control.

Spinal Cord Injury

Less than 5% of all spinal cord injuries occur annually in children under 16 years of age (Massagli, 2000). Many children with these injuries die within the first hour of trauma or during the first 3 months after trauma. A high proportion of children under 15 years of age with a spinal cord injury die immediately or within the first hour of injury. Even when the child survives the first hours, mortality rates are high (Moloney-Harmon & Adams, 2001).

Etiology and Pathophysiology

Motor vehicle crashes are the leading cause of spinal cord injuries, either pedestrian–vehicular, bicycle–vehicular, passenger, or driver related. Other causes of spinal injuries, especially in toddlers and young children, are falls and child abuse. Recreation or sports-related trauma accounts for more spinal cord injury in older children and adolescents. Penetrating injuries such as stabbings and gunshot wounds are becoming more prevalent.

The mechanism of injury and the direction of forces determine the type of lesion that occurs (Figure 33–23 ■). Hyperflexion injuries produce tears or avulsions and fractures of vertebral bodies, as well as subluxation and dislocation. Lateral flexion (rotation) may cause joint dislocations or unstable spinal fractures. Extension may result in the so-called hangman's fracture, ligament tears, avulsion fractures of vertebral bodies, and central or posterior spinal cord syndrome. Compression injuries cause anterior cord syndrome.

Children are prone to specific kinds of spinal cord injuries due to the extreme mobility and flexibility of their spinal column. The upper cervical region (C1 to C4) is the most mobile section of the spine. The vertebrae are incompletely ossified in children under 9 years. The facet joints are more shallow and horizontal. The young child's head is relatively large compared with the strength of the neck muscles. The fulcrum is at the C2–C3 level so injuries are more likely to occur at the C1–C3 level under 9 years and at the C4–C6 level for children 9 to 15

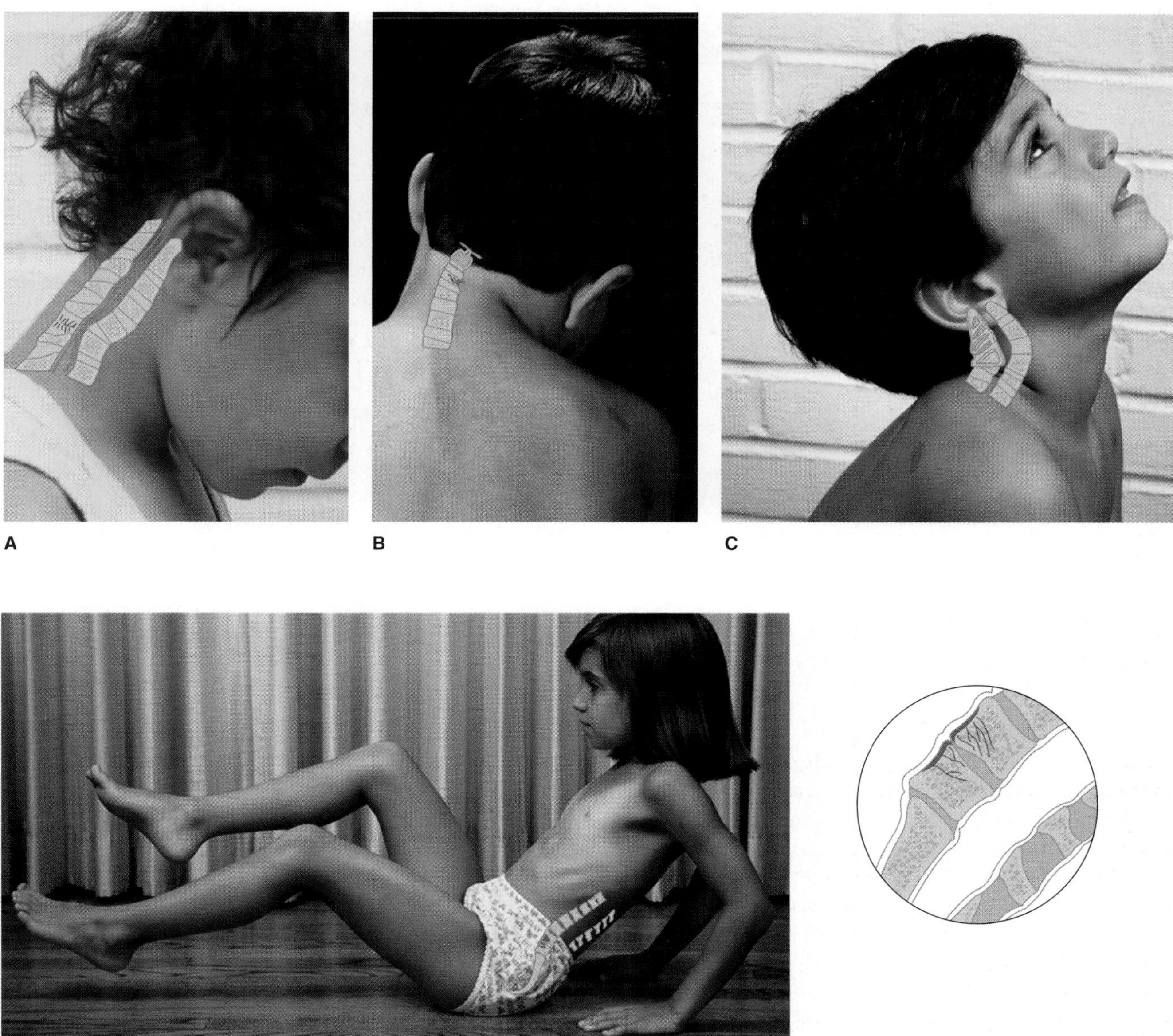

FIGURE 33–23 ■ Mechanics of injury to the spinal cord: *A*, hyperflexion; *B*, lateral flexion; *C*, hyperextension; *D*, compression.

years (Massagli, 2000). Atlanto-occipital dislocation occurs more frequently in infants and young children because of the flat articulation between the occiput and the atlas, and the ligaments supporting the junction between the occiput and cervical vertebrae are underdeveloped and have more laxity. A combination of forces (hyperextension, lateral flexion, and/or hyperflexion) is believed to be responsible for this dislocation (Steinmetz, Lechner, & Anderson, 2003). Table 33–9 describes the spinal cord injuries most common in children.

Spinal shock may occur as there is loss of sympathetic nervous system innervation below the level of the injury that maintains muscle tone. A temporary loss of segmental reflex activity may occur. Edema of the cord and resulting ischemia may cause physiologic transection even when no actual severance of the cord has occurred.

Clinical Manifestations

Spinal cord injuries are classified as complete or incomplete. Complete lesions are irreversible and involve a loss of sensory, motor, and autonomic function below the level of the injury. Incomplete lesions involve varying degrees of sensory, motor, and autonomic function below the level of injury.

At the time of injury, the child is flaccid and areflexic below the lesion and has loss of sensation because of spinal shock (hypotension, bradycardia, and hypothermia). Hypotension, loss of bladder and bowel control, and loss of environmental

TABLE 33–9 Spinal Cord Injuries in Children

SPINE REGION	INJURY CHARACTERISTICS
Cervical	➤ Site of 60% of spinal injuries in children under 10 years ➤ Injury above C3 segment causes respiratory arrest and death without ventilatory support; many of these injuries are fatal ➤ Diaphragm function is present when injury is at C5 level ➤ Quadreplegia, some function of upper extremities when injury is at C6–C7 level ➤ Loss of sphincter function ➤ Sensory level lost below the sternum
Thoracic	➤ Site of 20% of spinal injuries usually between 8 and 14 years ➤ Full control of upper extremities including hands ➤ Poor trunk balance
Thoracolumbar	➤ Full control of muscles in abdomen and upper back ➤ Good trunk balance
Lumbar	➤ Most injuries occur at the L2–L4 level; second most common area of injury, probably a result of improperly placed lap belts ➤ Below L3 may have functioning of muscles in upper leg ➤ Loss of ankle and foot control

thermoregulatory function are associated with autonomic dysfunction. Priapism may be seen. Respiratory compromise may be present due to paralysis of the diaphragm. The higher the level of spinal cord injury, the more severe the neurologic damage.

As neurologic recovery begins, spinal reflex activity returns and increasing spasticity below the level of the lesion is seen. **Autonomic dysreflexia** is a condition in which hypertension, bradycardia, severe headaches, pallor below and flushing above the level of the spinal cord lesion, and seizures occur due to an impaired autonomic nervous system. A full bladder can trigger this response.

The child with a spinal cord injury is often a victim of multiple trauma and may display signs of hypovolemic shock resulting from other injuries, increased intracranial pressure, or respiratory depression. Children can also experience neurogenic or spinal shock (see Chapter 26∞).

COLLABORATIVE CARE

The goal of collaborative care is to determine the extent of spinal cord injury and to aggressively treat the injury to reduce the potential for permanent disability.

Diagnostic Testing

Diagnosis is made by observation, neurologic examination, and radiographic studies. Radiographic studies include lateral cervical spine and anteroposterior and lateral views of the thoracic and lumbosacral spine to determine if a vertebral fracture or compression on the spinal cord is present. The child's immobilized position is unchanged until radiographs read by a radiologist have cleared the spine for any injury. In addition, CT scanning, MRI, fluoroscopy, or myelography may be performed. See Box 33–17.

Clinical Therapy

Spinal injuries are managed aggressively. Immediate stabilization and immobilization of the child with a suspected spinal injury is essential. Immobilization of infants and young children is more difficult due to the large occiput and short neck. Immobilizing the child with head in midline with cervical spine straight is the goal. Once the child arrives at the hospital, the child with a spinal cord injury may be placed in skeletal traction or a halo device. Surgery to reduce and internally fixate the fracture is performed for unstable fractures and dislocations. Decompression of the spinal cord and nerve roots may also be performed if transection is not complete.

Methylprednisolone is administered in high doses to children with motor deficits to decrease neurologic sequelae. Administration must be started within 8 hours of the injury. Other medications such as atropine and norepinephrine may be given to manage spinal shock. Intravenous fluid resuscitation is also performed if the child could have hypovolemic shock from other injuries. Complications of spinal cord injury include the following:

- Scoliosis if injury occurs before the skeleton is immature
- Impaired respiratory function due to a paralyzed diaphragm or diminished vital capacity
- Hip instability due to poor acetabular development
- Pathologic fractures of the long bones due to immobilization hypercalcemia
- Pressure ulcers
- Deep-vein thrombosis
- Autonomic dysreflexia

An interdisciplinary approach is required to manage the rehabilitation and long-term care needs of the child and family. Physical therapy and occupational therapy assessments and interventions begin during the acute phase of care so that planning for long-term rehabilitation can begin.

BOX 33–17 SCIWORA

Up to 15%–25% of children have spinal cord injury without radiographic abnormality (SCIWORA), because the initial radiographic films and CT scan show no bony deformity. The child is believed to be free of injury; however, profound or progressive paralysis occurs either immediately or within 48 hours. This diagnostic challenge occurs because the spine and ligaments are continuously developing throughout childhood. The vertebral facets are more horizontal and become more vertical as ossification occurs. The horizontal nature of the vertebrae provides less stability to the spine. Paravertebral muscles are less developed, and the ligaments and soft tissues are more elastic. All of these features contribute to the lack of radiographic abnormalities (Moloney-Harmon & Adams, 2001). An MRI can detect the injury.

NURSING MANAGEMENT

Nursing care focuses on monitoring vital signs, meeting nutritional needs, maintaining skin integrity, promoting independent functioning, encouraging therapeutic play, providing emotional support, and promoting rehabilitation.

■ Nursing Assessment and Diagnosis

Monitor Physiologic Status

Be alert for any changes in vital signs, especially those that may signify spinal shock (hypotension, bradycardia, and hypothermia), increased intracranial pressure (see Table 33–1), or autonomic dysreflexia. Monitor the child's respiratory status and vital capacity to determine the functioning of the diaphragm. Notify the physician immediately if autonomic dysreflexia occurs. Monitor intake and output. Monitor for bladder function and constipation. Assess the skin for integrity.

Monitor Neurologic Functioning

With higher cervical injuries, assess cranial nerves as they may be affected by swelling around the cord. Assess for the return of segmental reflex function and change from flaccid tone to spasticity. Note any changes in level of sensation and motor function. Carefully check the immobilizing devices to ensure that the spine remains stable.

Family Coping

Assess the family's understanding of the child's injury and coping. Begin identifying family resources and needs for future home management of the child.

Examples of nursing diagnoses for the child with a spinal cord injury include:

- Ineffective Breathing Pattern related to lack of spinal innervation of diaphragm
- Risk for Constipation related to immobility and loss of sphincter innervation
- Risk for Autonomic Dysreflexia related to spinal cord injury
- Ineffective Thermoregulation related to spinal shock
- Risk for Impaired Skin Integrity related to immobility
- Impaired Urinary Elimination related to loss of sphincter innervation

■ Planning and Implementation

Some children with cervical lesions have tracheostomies performed to help maintain airway patency; others with very high lesions are dependent on ventilators. Keep suctioning equipment and other emergency equipment at bedside at all times.

Meet Nutritional Needs

Ensure adequate nutrition. A child with complete paralysis may require a gastrostomy tube. When the child is able to begin eating, feed soft foods slowly as the child may have some swallowing problems. Work with occupational therapists when the child is able to begin some self-feeding.

Maintain Skin Integrity

Provide skin care to prevent skin breakdown and pressure sores. See Chapter 36∞. Observe surgical sites and traction pin sites for signs of infection or inflammation. Perform regular traction pin site skin care according to institutional guidelines.

Promote Independent Functioning

Reinforce the exercises and skills learned in physical and occupational therapy. Use supports, boots, footboards, splints, and braces as recommended by therapists to prevent contractures. If hand mobility is limited, explore options for independence. Encourage the child to be as independent as possible in a wheelchair. An important mobility goal is to achieve wheelchair transfer and to perform self-care. Identify adaptive equipment that makes it possible to achieve those goals.

When bladder and bowel sphincter control is impaired, bowel and bladder control may be hard to achieve. When urinary retention occurs, perform intermittent catheterizations on a regular schedule to prevent hydronephrosis, urinary tract infection, and kidney damage (see Chapter 31∞). Anticipate that constipation will occur and initiate bowel training with a diet high in fiber and the use of stool softeners.

Encourage Therapeutic Play

Therapeutic play appropriate for the child's developmental level is an important part of the healing process. Provide as many normal activities for the child as possible, but do not assign tasks that the child will have difficulty completing. Child life teachers or tutors can help the child keep up with schoolwork.

Television, videotapes, and music can offer diversion for prolonged hospitalization. Paraplegic children can learn to use their arms and hands to play interactive games. Devices can also be adapted so that the child can play video games or manipulate the television or radio. Assistive devices to provide recreation for the child with quadraplegia should also be identified.

Provide Emotional Support

Support the child emotionally. Encourage the child to meet small, short-term goals, including those that involve self-care. Encourage the child to express fears and frustrations.

Be compassionate and understanding. Encourage siblings to visit, answer their questions honestly, and help them to discuss their feelings. Involve the parents and siblings in the care of the child as much as possible. When appropriate, encourage them to help with activities of daily living.

Discharge Planning and Home Care Teaching

Many children are discharged to inpatient rehabilitation facilities. Assist with arrangements for the child's transfer from the hospital to the rehabilitation facility. Work closely with the child,

MediaLink Spinal Cord Injury Support

parents, and other members of the healthcare team concerning placement. Home care needs, reintegration into educational programs, and safety issues should be identified and addressed well in advance of discharge from the rehabilitation facility. Refer families to social services, family counseling, and support groups if indicated.

The young child's ultimate functioning will be related to cognitive development, the amount of upper body strength, and the family's expectations (Massagli, 2000).

Evaluation

Expected outcomes of nursing care include the following:

- Complications such as pressure ulcers and contractures are prevented.
- The child's nutritional needs are met.
- Bowel and bladder control is established.
- The child and family are supported in adaptation to the disability.

Hypoxic-Ischemic Brain Injury (Drowning and Near Drowning)

Drowning is defined as death within 24 hours of a submersion incident. **Near drowning** is survival for at least 24 hours after submersion. Between 40% and 50% of children who are injured in drowning incidents are less than 4 years of age, with peak incidence between 1 and 2 years. The majority of infant drowning deaths (55%) occur in bathtubs. The most common drowning locations for children 1 to 4 years are artificial pools (56%) and other bodies of fresh water (26%). Among older children, 63% of drownings occur in natural bodies of fresh water (Brenner, Trumble, Smith, et al., 2001). Boys are five times more likely than girls to die from drowning. Groups at high risk include toddlers due to their inability to escape from the water and adolescent boys because of risk-taking behavior. Children with seizure disorders are also at high risk because they may experience a sudden and uncontrollable loss of body position that places them at a significantly higher risk for drowning. Over 90% of drowning incidents occur in fresh water such as ponds and residential swimming pools (Zuckerman & Conway, 2000).

Most drownings occur in the child's home pool or at the residence of a neighbor, friend, or relative. Usually the child is playing, is not wearing a swimsuit, and is briefly unsupervised before the immersion. Other common drowning sites for young children include bathtubs, hot tubs, toilets, and even large water-filled buckets.

Etiology and Pathophysiology

A child can drown in as little water as it takes to cover the nose and mouth. The events preceding drowning follow a sequential pattern. The child trapped in water panics, struggles, attempts to move using swimming motions, and holds his or her breath. Then the child swallows a small amount of fluid, vomits, and then aspirates the vomitus. This leads to a brief period of laryngospasm, which lasts no more than 2 minutes. Because of the increasing panic and hypoxia, the child swallows more liquid. Then either the child goes into profound laryngospasm, becomes severely hypoxic, has a seizure, and dies (dry drowning), or the child becomes unconscious, the laryngospasm relaxes as reflexes are lost, and the child passively aspirates even greater amounts of water into the airway and stomach (wet drowning). Hypothermia may result because the child's body cools more quickly in water than in air. See Chapter 36 for more information on hypothermia. As the child becomes hypoxic, the cardiac muscle becomes impaired and ultimately the heart stops.

Hypoxemia begins within seconds and irreversible central nervous system damage begins within 4 to 6 minutes. If resuscitation is successful, restoring the circulation leads to cerebral edema and increasing intracranial pressure, secondary damage from the submersion incident. Little can be done to resuscitate the brain, but with aggressive cardiopulmonary resuscitation, more severely brain-injured children are surviving in a permanent vegetative state.

When the child is resuscitated, water in the airway inactivates the surfactant and damages the alveolar basement membrane. Pulmonary edema and acute respiratory distress syndrome (ARDS) develop. Pneumonia may develop. (See Chapter 25 for care of the child with ARDS and pneumonia.) Hypovolemia develops because of damage to the alveoli that causes excessive capillary permeability.

Clinical Manifestations

The child who has been immersed exhibits a wide variety of signs and symptoms depending on the length of time underwater, the temperature of the water, the response to the episode, and the initial treatment performed at the scene. The child may be pulseless and apneic. Children who are submerged for short periods are resuscitated and have few symptoms and recover without complication. The child with a longer submersion can experience the following symptoms after resuscitation: decreased level of consciousness ranging from stupor to total unresponsiveness, cerebral edema, increased intracranial pressure, seizures, respiratory acidosis, irregular respirations, apnea, and gastric distention.

COLLABORATIVE CARE

The goal of collaborative care is to begin resuscitation and provide supportive diagnostic and clinical care to promote the child's recovery.

Diagnostic Testing

Initial diagnosis is made from physical assessment signs of spontaneous breathing and a heart rate. Once the child arrives in the emergency department, monitoring equipment is applied to assess for arrhythmias and oxygen saturation. Pupils are assessed for reactivity. The Glasgow Coma Scale is used to quantify and monitor the level of consciousness. Arterial blood gases are obtained to detect changes in gas exchange and pH. A chest radiograph may be ordered to establish baseline information about lung expansion and pulmonary integrity.

Clinical Therapy

Initial care of the child at the scene involves clearing the mouth of foreign matter and initiating cardiopulmonary resuscitation (CPR) as soon as the child is removed from the water. The sooner CPR is initiated, the better the child's chance for a favorable outcome. It is hoped that spontaneous respiratory effort by the child will begin within 5 minutes after removal from the water. Emergency transport to a hospital should occur as soon as possible, even if spontaneous breathing is initiated. Children still requiring CPR upon arrival at the emergency department are most likely to die or have significant neurologic impairment (American Academy of Pediatrics Committee on Injury, Violence, and Poison Prevention, 2003).

Initial treatment is 100% oxygen given by nonrebreather face mask and rewarming. Intravenous fluids are administered to address hypovolemia. If the child is unconscious, an airway is secured with an endotracheal tube. Positive end-expiratory pressure (PEEP) may be used to keep the alveoli open. Once hypovolemia is corrected, fluids may be restricted and diuretics may be used to help reduce the risk of cerebral edema. Vasopressor medications may be used to maintain a normal blood pressure. Antibiotics may be used if signs of pneumonia develop.

PRACTICE ALERT

All near drowning victims should be admitted to the hospital for at least 24 hours or observed in a short-stay observation unit for several hours, even when asymptomatic. Many life-threatening complications, including respiratory distress and cerebral edema, may not become evident for at least 12 hours after the incident.

Near drowning may result in complete recovery, severe brain injury, or variable neurologic deficits. Prognosis and outcome are highly individual. Anoxic brain injury is the leading cause of mortality. Predictors of good outcome are submersion less than 5 minutes and cardiopulmonary resuscitation for less than 10 minutes (Zuckerman & Conway, 2000).

NURSING MANAGEMENT

Nursing care of the child who survives a submersion incident focuses on monitoring the child's neurologic and cardiopulmonary status, providing emotional support to the family, and implementing needed therapies.

Nursing Assessment and Diagnosis

Assess the child's responsiveness, spontaneous respiratory efforts, and pulse. As resuscitation proceeds, monitor the child's respiratory status, oxygenation, cardiopulmonary function, and neurologic status. Frequent neurologic monitoring with the Glasgow Coma Scale, pupil checks for reactivity, and assessment of vital signs are performed.

Attach a cardiorespiratory monitor and pulse oximetry to provide continuous assessment information about the child's oxygenation status. Once the child has been resuscitated, the child is monitored frequently for signs of potential complications of the near drowning such as respiratory distress and worsening mental status indicating potential cerebral edema. Assess intake and output.

Parents and family members are assessed for their response and need for support associated with the child's life-threatening injury.

Examples of nursing diagnoses that may be appropriate for the child with near drowning include:

- Ineffective Cerebral Tissue Perfusion related to interruption of arterial blood flow
- Risk for Infection related to aspiration and trauma to the respiratory system
- Impaired Gas Exchange related to damage to the alveolar-capillary membranes of the lungs
- Decisional Conflict (parents) related to continuing life support for a dying child
- Interrupted Family Processes related to situational crisis of child with life-threatening injury

Planning and Implementation

Nursing management focuses on observation and support of cardiopulmonary and central nervous system function. The child with seriously compromised respiratory and neurologic status will be cared for in the intensive care unit. Oxygen and positive end-expiratory pressure or mechanical ventilation will be needed if acute respiratory distress develops. Position the child properly to promote respiratory function. Note any change in respiratory status and blood gases, and notify the physician promptly.

Implement other nursing interventions for the child with altered states of consciousness as described on page 1302. If cerebral edema develops, implement nursing interventions as described on page 1352.

Family Support

Provide emotional support to the family. Be nonjudgmental and provide a forum for parents to express their feelings. Reassure parents who exhibit guilt reactions that their child is receiving all possible medical treatment. Parents may be faced with an unknown prognosis. Encourage parents to seek assistance from social workers, clergy, close friends, and relatives. Arrange for appropriate referrals. The child and family need support to work through the feelings surrounding the near drowning incident, the unexpected hospitalization, and an uncertain prognosis that may mean the child will not return to normal functioning. If the child's prognosis is poor, an ethical consult may be offered to educate the family about options for decision making regarding sustaining or terminating life support.

Prevention

Another significant nursing role is prevention. Drowning can be prevented through education, legislation, and changes in the environment. Provide education to the family about strategies to protect the child from other drowning episodes. Become involved in community efforts to reduce the incidence of drowning and near drowning through education, enforcement of regulations for fencing around all four sides of swimming pools, and organizations such as a local Safe Kids chapter. Encourage parents with private pools to become trained in cardiopulmonary resuscitation and to keep a phone at poolside so that emergency care providers can be called immediately. Educate adolescents about the dangers of mixing alcohol and swimming. Inform families to keep 5- and 10-gallon buckets empty when not in use. The nurse should emphasize the importance of closely supervising children when near or in the water, whether at pools, at the beach, or in the bathtub.

Discharge Planning

Home care needs should be identified and addressed well in advance of discharge. Assist with arrangements for the child with minor deficits. Assign a case manager to the child with significant neurologic impairments so that long-term care options can be explored. Inpatient or outpatient rehabilitation services should be matched to the child's needs and family resources.

Evaluation

Expected outcomes of nursing care for the child with a near drowning episode include the following:

- The child responds to cardiopulmonary resuscitation and regains consciousness rapidly.
- Any change in mental status or respiratory distress are detected and immediately managed.
- Parents take preventive steps to reduce the risk of drowning for all children in the family.

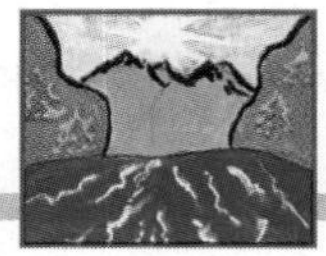

CHAPTER HIGHLIGHTS

- The nervous system is complete with all nerve cells at birth, but the number of glial cells and dendrites continues to increase until 4 years of age. Myelination continues throughout childhood.
- Altered level of consciousness is caused by trauma, infection, poisoning, seizures, or any other process that affects the CNS. Cerebral perfusion pressure (the amount of pressure needed to ensure that adequate oxygen and nutrients will be delivered to the brain) is decreased with hypovolemia and increased intracranial pressure.
- The most common type of seizure in children are tonic-clonic generalized seizures. Most seizures last 1 to 2 minutes.
- Monitor any child with a generalized seizure lasting longer than 10 minutes for electrolytes, glucose, blood gases, increasing fever, and abnormal blood pressure to identify any conditions that can be treated and reduce the risk of significant CNS injury. Carefully document the duration of the seizure or series of seizures to detect status epilepticus.
- Neurologic damage from bacterial meningitis often occurs in infants and young children despite early, aggressive management. The most common sequelae involve cranial nerves, especially the eighth, resulting in hearing loss, seizures, and developmental delay.
- Viral (aseptic) meningitis in most cases is not as virulent as bacterial meningitis; and the child with aseptic meningitis appears less ill than the child with bacterial meningitis.
- Encephalitis is usually caused by a virus, often herpes simplex I, and has a high mortality rate. Presenting signs include a severe headache, fever, signs of an upper respiratory infection, malaise, nausea, and vomiting.
- Reye syndrome is an encephalopathy with a high mortality rate that is associated with aspirin use for a mild viral illness. Because most parents give children acetaminophen or ibuprofen rather than aspirin for flulike symptoms and varicella, Reye syndrome has become rare.
- Guillain-Barré syndrome is the most common cause of flaccid paralysis in infants and children. It is caused by an immune response to an infectious organism, usually from a gastrointestinal or respiratory illness 2 to 3 weeks prior to onset.
- More than 80% of children experience a headache by late adolescence, and migraine is the most common type of benign headache in children. Other benign headache types are inflammatory (sinusitis) and tension.
- Microcephaly is a small brain that may be caused by chromosomal abnormalities, fetal insult, maternal infection, or destructive insult during the infancy, such as infection, metabolic disorder, or anoxia.
- Hydrocephalus is caused by the blocked cerebrospinal fluid flow through normal channels and pathways or the impaired absorption of cerebrospinal fluid in the subarachnoid space and the arachnoid villi. It can be associated with a congenital condition or acquired from meningitis or intraventricular hemorrhage, tumor, or structural deformity.
- The more common types of neural tube defects include anencephaly (no development of the brain above the brainstem), encephalocele (protrusion of meningeal or skin-covered brain through the skull), and myelodysplasia or spina bifida.
- Myelodysplasia or spina bifida is a malformation of the spinal cord and spinal canal that may be associated with a protrusion of a meningeal sac filled with a portion of the spinal cord, and is the most common devel-

opmental disorder of the CNS. Its prevalence is decreasing due to the fortification of all enriched grain products with folate.

- Neurofibromatosis 1 is characterized by multiple café-au-lait spots, darker than the surrounding skin, that are 5 mm or larger in infants but grow to 15 mm in diameter during adolescence. Multiple benign tumors grow on or under the skin beginning during puberty.
- Positional plagiocephaly, a totally flat occiput, is seen increasingly when infants who are placed on their backs to prevent sudden infant death syndrome do not change the position of the head. The weight of the infant head sometimes flattens the skull. It may be treated with a helmet device to help remold the skull.
- Most cases of cerebral palsy are characterized by spasticity and a lack of coordination. The risk for cerebral palsy is increased when an intrauterine infection is documented. Neonatal sepsis and hyperbilirubin increase the child's risk of developing cerebral palsy.
- Jitteriness, seizures, hyperexcitability, and poor feeding in the newborn may be related to the direct effect of cocaine on the developing central nervous system. Irritability and jitteriness may also be seen with withdrawal from other illicit substances. The infant may also have excoriated skin, especially on the heels, toes, hands, elbows, nose, or chin, because of continuous rubbing against the crib sheets.
- Traumatic brain injuries are the most common injuries during childhood. They result from falls, motor vehicle crashes, sports injuries, and child abuse. Traumatic brain injuries are responsible for nearly a third of all injury-related deaths in children.
- Concussions are associated with a transient impairment of consciousness resulting from the stretching, compression, and shearing of nerve fibers after an impact injury to the head. Impairment in consciousness may include amnesia, dizziness, memory or orientation impairment, and unsteady gait.
- Spinal cord injuries, although relatively rare in children, often result from significant forces such as from motor vehicle crashes. Because of the child's larger and heavier head and weaker neck muscles, cervical spine injuries are more common.
- Children who have the best outcomes following a near drowning include those submerged less than 5 minutes and those who need cardiopulmonary resuscitation for less than 10 minutes.

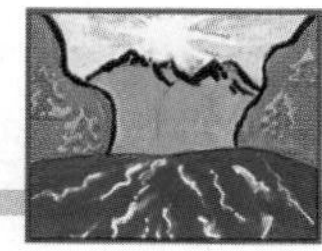

CRITICAL THINKING IN ACTION

INTRODUCTION

Return to 7-year-old Antwan at the beginning of the chapter. He experienced a serious brain injury after being struck by a car. He is about 2 weeks postinjury and planning for his rehabilitation has begun.

DESCRIPTION

One of Antwan's parents has been at his side since he was transferred from the intensive care unit 4 days ago. They were very much afraid that he would die as a result of his injuries; now they are looking at a long recuperation. They want the best care for Antwan, but are somewhat limited in their choices because of their health insurance and limited pediatric rehabilitation beds in their state. A case manager has been assigned by the health plan to identify the health services that Antwan will need. A short stay in an inpatient rehabilitation hospital will be possible, and then Antwan will return home and have outpatient rehabilitation services. Both of Antwan's parents have jobs, and the difficult decision needs to be made about how Antwan will be cared for at home. In addition, Antwan has a 10-year-old sister, Janet, and a 14-year-old brother, Manny, who have been supervised over the past couple of weeks by a family friend. Members of their church have been very helpful in providing meals and transportation for the older children. Janet has asthma, but fortunately has not been ill over the past 2 weeks. She is very upset because the last time she spoke to Antwan, she yelled at him for getting into her things.

DISCUSSION

Antwan's family has been totally disrupted by the life-threatening nature of his injury. Antwan is not expected to make a full recovery from his injuries, but the level of impairment cannot yet be predicted.

1. Using the tools described in Chapter 2∞, identify the strengths and coping strategies in this family. Identify those factors that will be most helpful as the nursing care plan is developed.
2. Describe the pathophysiology that could account for Antwan's prolonged diminished responsiveness.
3. Develop a nursing care plan for Antwan taking into account his diminished responsiveness. Be sure to address nutrition and hydration, care needs associated with immobility, and sensory stimulation.
4. Develop an education program for the parents to begin practicing now that will introduce them to the types of care they will become responsible for when Antwan goes home.
5. Assist the parents to begin thinking about how they will tell Janet and Manny about the challenges and potential disabilities Antwan will have as a result of his injuries, and how this will lead to changes in family routines and lifestyle over the next several months.

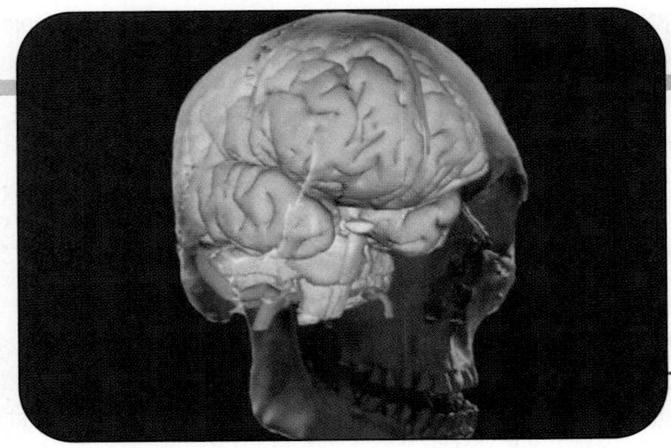

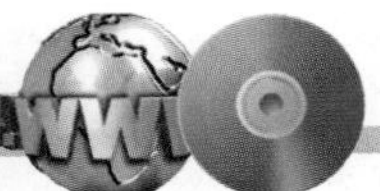

EXPLORE MediaLink

- NCLEX review, case studies, and other interactive resources for this chapter can be found on the Companion Website at **www.prenhall.com/ball**. Click on Chapter 33 to select the activities for this chapter.
- For animations, more NCLEX review questions, and an audio glossary, access the accompanying CD-ROM in this book.

http://www.prenhall.com/ball

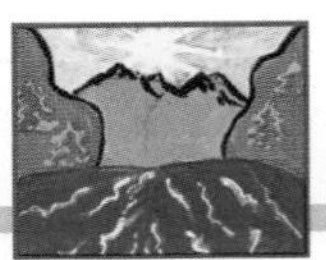

REFERENCES

Adekoya, N., Thurman, D. J., White, D. D., & Webb, K. W (2002). Surveillance for traumatic brain injury deaths—United States, 1989–1998. *Morbidity and Mortality Weekly Report, 51*(SS-10), 1–14.

Agency for Healthcare Research and Quality. (1999). Rehabilitation for traumatic brain injury in children and adolescents. *Summary, Evidence Report/Technology Assessment, 2* (Suppl). www.ahrq.gov/clinic/epcsums/tbisum2.htm, accessed 6/10/2004.

Altmeier, W. A. (1999). Status epilepticus. *Pediatric Annals, 28*(4), 206–208.

American Academy of Pediatrics Committee on Infectious Disease. (2003a). *Red book: Report of the committee on infectious disease* (26th ed.). Elk Grove Village, IL: Author.

American Academy of Pediatrics Committee on Injury and Poison Prevention. (2001). Injuries associated with infant walkers. *Pediatrics, 108*(3), 790–792.

American Academy of Pediatrics Committee on Injury, Violence, and Poison Prevention. (2003). Prevention of drowning in infants, children, and adolescents. *Pediatrics, 112*(2), 440–445.

American Academy of Pediatrics Committee on Quality Improvement, Subcommittee on Febrile Seizures. (1999). Practice parameter: Long-term treatment of the child with simple febrile seizures. *Pediatrics, 103*(6, Pt 1), 1307–1309.

Anderson, V., Catroppa, C., Morse, S., Haritou, F., & Rosenfeld, J. (2000). Recovery of intellectual ability following traumatic brain injury in childhood: Impact of injury severity and age at injury. *Pediatric Neurosurgery, 32*(6), 282–290.

Austin, J., Dunn, D., Huster, G., & Rose, D. (1998). Development of scales to measure psychosocial care needs of children with seizures and their parents. *Journal of Neuroscience Nursing, 30*(3), 155–160.

Austin, J. K., Harezlak, J., Dunn, D. W., Huster, G. A., Rose, D. F., & Ambrosius, W. T. (2001). Behavior problems in children before first recognized seizure. *Pediatrics, 107*(1), 115–122.

Belay, E. D., et al. (1999). Reye's syndrome in the United States from 1981 through 1997. *New England Journal of Medicine, 340*(18), 1377–1382.

Black, S., Shinefield, H., Baxter, R., Austrian, R., Bracken, L. et al. (2004). Postlicensure surveillance for pneumococcal invasive disease after use of pneumococcal conjugate vaccine in Northern California Kaiser Permanente. *Pediatric Infectious Disease Journal, 23*(6), 485–489.

Blair, J., & Selekman, J. (2004). Epilepsy. In P. J. Allen & J. A. Vessey (Eds.), *Primary care of the child with a chronic condition* (4th ed., pp. 469–497). St. Louis: Mosby.

Blatt, S. D., Meguid, V., & Church, C. C. (2000). Prenatal cocaine: What's known about outcomes? *Contemporary Pediatrics, 17*(5), 43–57.

Bowman, R. M., McLone, D. G., Grant, J. A., Tomita, T., & Ito, J. A. (2001). Spina bifida outcome: A 25-year perspective. *Pediatric Neurosurgery, 34*(3), 114–120.

Brenner, R. A., Trumble, A. C., Smith, G. S., Kessler, E. P., & Overpeck, M. D. (2001). Where children drown, United States, 1995. *Pediatrics, 108*(1), 85–89.

Buck, M. L. (2003). Clinical applications for botulinum toxin type A in pediatric patients. *Pediatric Pharmacology, 9*(3). www.medscape.com/viewarticle/451626, accessed 4/18/2003.

Campbell, S. (2003). Prenatal cocaine exposure and neonatal/infant outcomes. *Neonatal Network, 22*(1), 19–21.

Centers for Disease Control. (2003). Traumatic brain injury incidence and distribution. www.cdc.gov/node/do?id=0900f3ec8000dbdc&aspectId=A0400020&print=on, accessed 2/25/2004.

Chestnut, R. A, et al. (2003). Threshold for treatment of intracranial hypotension: Guidelines for management of severe traumatic brain injury. *Pediatric Clinical Care Medicine, 4*(3), S25–S27.

Danielpour, M., & Peacock, W. J. (2000). Epilepsy surgery in children. *Clinical Neurosurgery, 47*, 400–421.

Ditmyer, S. (2004). Hydrocephalus. In P. J. Allen & J. A. Vessey (Eds.), *Primary care of the child with a chronic condition* (4th ed., pp. 543–560). St. Louis: Mosby.

Fadiman, A. (1997). *The spirit catches you and you fall down.* New York: Farrar, Strauss, Giroux.

Frank, D. A., Augustyn, M., Knight, W. G., Pell, T., & Zuckerman, B. (2001). Growth, development, and behavior in early childhood following prenatal cocaine exposure: A systematic review. *JAMA, 285*(12), 1613–1627.

Freeman, J. M. (2003). What every pediatrician should know about the ketogenic diet. *Contemporary Pediatrics, 20*(5), 113–127.

Gill, J. K., & Gieron-Korthals, M. (2002). What pediatricians—and parents—need to know about febrile convulsions. *Contemporary Pediatrics, 19*(5), 139–144.

Guskiewicz, K. M., & McCrea, M. (2003). Increased recovery time with multiple sports-related traumatic brain injuries. *Journal of American Medical Association, 290*, 2549–2563.

Guskiewicz, K. M., Weaver, N. L., Padua, D. A., & Garrett, W. E. (2000). Epidemiology of concussion in collegiate and high school football players. *American Journal of Sports Medicine, 28*(5), 643–650.

Harrison, L. H. (2001, Spring). Meningococcal infection in adolescents and young adults. *Contemporary Pediatrics*, 4–15.

Haslam, R. H. A. (2004). Neurocutaneous syndromes. In R. E Behrman, R. M. Kliegman, & H. B. Jenson, *Nelson textbook of pediatrics* (17th ed., pp. 2015-2017), Philadelphia: Saunders.

Hightower, S., Carmon, M., & Minick, P. (2002). A qualitative descriptive study of the lived experiences of school-aged children with epilepsy. *Journal of Pediatric Health Care, 16*(3), 131–137.

Honein, M. A., Paulozzi, L. J., Matthews, T. J., Erickson, J. D., & Wong, L. Y. (2001). Impact of folic acid fortification of the U.S. food supply on the occurrence of neural tube defects. *Journal of the American Medical Association, 285*(23), 2981–2986.

Jones, H. R. (2000). Guillain-Barre syndrome: Perspectives with infants and children. *Seminars in Pediatric Neurology, 7*(2), 91–102.

Katyal, N. G., Koehler, A. N., McGhee, B., Foley, C. M., & Crumrine, P. K. (2000). The ketogenic diet in refractory epilepsy: The experience of Children's Hospital of Pittsburgh. *Clinical Pediatrics, 39*(3), 153–159.

Kuehne, E. A., & Reilly, M. W. (2004). Prenatal cocaine exposure. In P. J. Allen & J. A. Vessey (Eds.), *Primary care of the child with a chronic condition* (4th ed., pp. 708–721 St. Louis: Mosby.

Lazzaretti, C. C., & Pearson, C. (2004). Myelodysplasia. In P. J. Allen & J. A. Vessey (Eds.), *Primary care of the child with a chronic condition* (4th ed., pp. 630–643). St. Louis: Mosby.

Lester, B. M., et al. (2001). The maternal lifestyle study: Drug use by meconium toxicology and maternal self-report. *Pediatrics, 107,* 309–317.

Lewis, D. W., Scott, D., & Rendin, V. (2002). Treatment of pediatric headache. *Expert Opinion in Pharmacotherapeutics, 3*(10), 1433–1441.

Liptak, G. S. (2002). Neural tube defects. In M. L. Batshaw (Ed.), *Children with disabilities* (5th ed., pp. 467–492). Baltimore: Paul H. Brooks Publishing Co.

Lovell, M. R., Collins, M. W., Iverson, G. L., Field, M., & Maroon, J. C., et al. (2003). Recovery from mild concussion in high school athletes. *Journal of Neurosurgery, 98*(2), 296–301.

Massagli, T. L. (2000). Medical and rehabilitation issues in the care of children with spinal cord injury. *Physical Medicine and Rehabilitation Clinics of North America, 11*(1), 169–182.

Mathews, T. J. (2003). Trends in spina bifida and anencephalus in the United States, 1991–2001. National Center for Health Statistics Health and Stats. www.cdc.gov/nchs/products/pubs/pubd/hestats/spine_anen.htm, accessed 7/17/2003.

McGee, S., & Burkett, K. W. (2000). Identifying common pediatric neurosurgical conditions in the primary care setting. *Nursing Clinics of North America, 35*(1), 61–85.

McNelis, A., Musick, B., Austin, J., Dunn, D., & Creasy, K. (1998). Psychosocial care needs of children with new-onset seizures. *Journal of Neuroscience Nursing, 30*(3), 161–165.

Michaud, L. J., Semes-Concepcion, J., Duhaime, A. C., & Lazar, M. F. (2002). Traumatic brain injury. In M. L. Batshaw (Ed.), *Children with disabilities* (5th ed., pp. 525–545). Baltimore: Paul H. Brooks Publishing Co.

Moloney-Harmon, P. A., & Adams, P. (2001). Trauma. In M. A. Q. Curley & P. A. Moloney-Harmon, *Critical care nursing of infants and children* (2nd ed. pp. 947–979). Philadelphia: W. B. Saunders.

National Institute of Neurologic Disorders and Stroke. (2000). NINDS Workshop: Defining the future of neurofibromatosis research. www.ninds.nih.gov/news_and*events/neurofibromatosis*workshop.htm, accessed 1/26/2004.

National Institute of Neurologic Disorders and Stroke. (2001). NINDS Neurofibromatosis information page. http://ninds.nih.gov/health_and_medical/disorders/neurofibro.htm, accessed 1/26/2004.

Nehring, W. M. (2004). Cerebral palsy. In P. J. Allen & J. A. Vessey (Eds.), *Primary care of the child with a chronic condition* (4th ed., pp. 327–346). St. Louis: Mosby.

Nelson, K. B., & Grether, J. K. (1999). Causes of cerebral palsy. *Current Opinion in Pediatrics, 11*(6), 487–491.

Northrup, H., & Volcik, K. A. (2000). Spina bifida and other neural tube defects. *Current Problems in Pediatrics, 30*(10), 317–331.

O'Hara, J., & Koch, T. K. (1998). Heading off headaches. *Contemporary Pediatrics, 15*(3), 97–116.

Padgett, K. (2002). Alterations in neurologic function in children. In K. L., McCance & S. E. Huether, *Pathophysiology: The biologic basis for disease in adults and children* (4th ed., pp. 566–596). St. Louis: Mosby.

Papile, L. A. (2002). Intracranial hemorrhage. In A. A. Fanaroff & R. J. Martin, *Neonatal-perinatal medicine: Diseases of the fetus and infant* (7th ed., pp. 879–887). St. Louis: Mosby.

Pellegrino, L. (2002). Cerebral palsy. In M. L. Batshaw (Ed.), *Children with disabilities* (5th ed., pp. 443–466). Baltimore: Paul H. Brooks Publishing Co.

Prober, C. G. (2004). Central nervous system infections. In R. E. Behrman, R. M. Kliegman, & H. B. Jenson, *Nelson textbook of pediatrics* (17th ed., pp. 2038–2047). Philadelphia: Saunders.

Reimschisel, T. (2003). Breaking the cycle of medication overuse headache. *Contemporary Pediatrics, 20*(10), 101–114.

Renier, D., Lajeunie, E., Arnaud, E., & Marchac, D. (2000). Management of craniosynostosis. *Children's Nervous System, 16,* 645–658.

Ressler, J. A., & Nelson, M. (2000). Central nervous system infections in the pediatric population. *Neuroimaging Clinics of North America, 10*(2), 427–443.

Robinson, T. M. S. (1999). Perinatal substance abuse: Working with neonates and families. *Neonatal Network, 18*(2), 68–70.

Rosenblum, R. K., & Fisher, P. G. (2001). A guide to children with acute and chronic headaches. *Journal of Pediatric Health Care, 15*(5), 229–235.

Rosman, N. P. (1999). Acute head trauma. In J. A. McMillan, C. D. DeAngelis, R. D. Feigin, & J. B. Warshaw, *Oski's pediatrics: Principles and practice* (3rd ed., pp. 603–617). Philadelphia: Lippincott, Williams, & Wilkins.

Sarnat, H. B. (2004). Guillain-Barre syndrome. In R. E. Behrman, R. M. Kliegman, & H. B. Jenson, *Nelson textbook of pediatrics* (17th ed., pp. 2080–2081). Philadelphia: Saunders.

Scharff, L., & Kemper, K. J (2003). For chronic pain, complementary and alternative medical approaches. *Contemporary Pediatrics, 20*(10), 117–141.

Schutzman, S. A., & Greenes, D. S. (2001). Pediatric minor head trauma. *Annals of Emergency Medicine, 27*(1), 65–74.

Selekman, J. (2003). Preventing meningitis. *Pediatric Nursing, 29*(6), 467–469.

Shore, C., Austin, J., Musick, B., Dunn, D., McBride, A., & Creasy, K. (1998). Psychosocial care needs of parents of children with new-onset seizures. *Journal of Neuroscience Nursing, 30*(3), 169–174.

Shore, C. P., Austin, J. K., Huster, G. A., & Dunn, D. W. (2002). Identifying risk factors for maternal depression in families of adolescents with epilepsy. *Journal of the Society of Pediatric Nurses, 7*(2), 71–80.

Singer, L. T., Arendt, R., Minnes, S., Farkas, K., Salvator, A., Kirchner, H. L., & Kliegman, R. (2002). Cognitive and motor outcomes of cocaine-exposed infants. *Journal of the American Medical Association, 287*(15), 1952–1960.

Spector, R. E. (2000). *Cultural diversity in health and illness* (5th ed., p. 71). Upper Saddle River, NJ: Prentice Hall Health.

Steinmetz, M. P., Lechner, R. M., & Anderson, J. S. (2003). Atlantooccipital dislocation in children: Presentation, diagnosis, and management. *Neurosurgery Focus, 14*(2). www.medscape.com/viewarticle/449884_print, accessed 3/11/2003.

Stevenson, K. L. (2004). Chiari type II malformation: Past, present, future. *Neurosurgical Focus, 16*(2). www.medscape.com/viewarticle/470602_print, accessed 3/25/2004.

Substance Abuse and Mental Health Services Administration, Office of Applied Statistics. (2002). *Preliminary results from the 2001 National Household Survey on Drug Abuse.* Washington, DC: U.S. Department of Health and Human Services. www.samhsa.gov/oas/nhsda/2k1nhsda/vol1/highlights.htm.

Sutton, L., Adzick, N. S., Belaniuk, L. T., Johnson, M. P., Crombleholme, T. M., & Flake, A. W. (1999). Improvement of hindbrain herniation demonstrated by serial fetal magnetic resonance imaging following fetal surgery for myelomeningocele. *JAMA, 282*(19), 1826–1831.

Task Force for the Determination of Brain Death in Children. (1987). Guidelines for the determination of brain death in children. *Neurology, 37,* 1077–1078.

United States Congress. (1996, July 29). Traumatic brain injury act of 1996. *Congressional Record, 142,* 110 STAT, 1445–1449.

Valente, L. R. (2000). Seizures and epilepsy: Optimizing patient management. *Clinician Reviews, 10*(3), 79–104.

Van Eerden, P., & Bernstein, P. S. (2003). Neonatal encephalopathy and cerebral palsy: Defining the pathogenesis and pathophysiology. ACOG Task Force on Neonatal Encephalopathy and Cerebral Palsy. *Medscape OB/GYN & Women's Health, 8*(2). www.medscape.com/viewarticle/457882_, accessed 7/10/2003.

Vannucci, R. C. (2002). Disorders in the head size and shape. In A. A. Fanaroff & R. J. Martin, *Neonatal-perinatal medicine: Diseases of the fetus and infant* (7th ed., pp. 911–917). St. Louis: Mosby.

Virdis, R., Street, M. E., Bandello, M. A., Tripodi, C., Donadio, A., Villani, A. R., Cagozzi, L., Garavelli, L., & Bernasconi, S. (2003). Growth and pubertal disorders in neurofibromatosis type 1. *Journal of Pediatric Endocrinology Metabolism, 16*(Supp 2), 289–292.

Weinstein, S. (2002). Epilepsy. In M. L. Barshaw (Ed.), *Children with disabilities* (5th ed., pp. 493–523). Baltimore: Paul H. Brooks Publishing Co.

Wilson, B. A., Shannon, M. T., & Stang, C. L. (2005). *Nurse's drug guide 2005.* Upper Saddle River, NJ: Prentice Hall Health.

Zuckerman, G. B., & Conway, E. E. (2000). Drowning and near-drowning: A pediatric epidemic. *Pediatric Annals, 29*(6), 360–366.

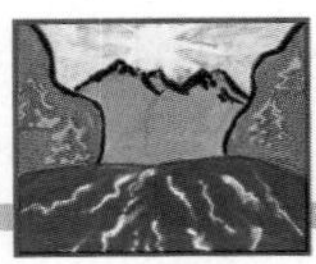

ADDITIONAL REFERENCES

Arbuckle, H. A., & Morelli, J. G. (2000). Pigmentary disorders: Update on neurofibromatosis 1 and tuberous sclerosis. *Current Opinion in Pediatrics, 12,* 354–358.

Forti, R., & Delgado, A. (2000). Short course: Near drowning. *Office and Emergency Pediatrics, 13*(3), 81–85.

Gonzalez, R. & Schimke, C. M. (2002). Strategies in urological reconstruction in myelomeningocele. *Current Opinion in Urology, 12*(6), 485–490.

Hymel, K. P. (2002). Inflicted traumatic brain injury in infants and young children. *Infants and Young Children, 15*(2), 57–65.

Keenan, H. T., Runyan, D. K., Marshall, S. W., Nocera, M. A., Merten, D. F., & Sinal, S. H. (2003). A population-based study of inflicted traumatic brain injury in young children. *Journal of the American Medical Association, 290*(5), 621–626.

Chapter 34

Alterations in Mental Health and Cognition

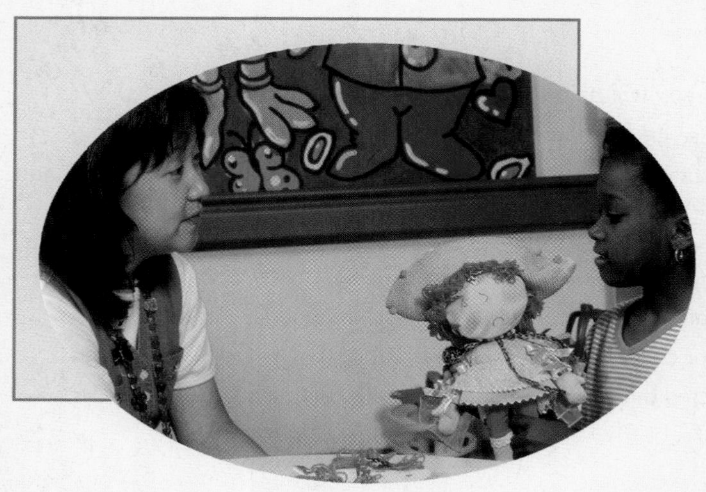

Cassandra Nielsen is a 9-year-old girl who has recently become fearful about attending school and awakens crying each night. She is in the third grade at a school she has attended for 2 years. A few weeks ago she was in a car crash as her mother drove her to school. She received only minor injuries and returned to school the next day. Her mother believes that Cassandra's behavior has been worsening since the car crash. She spoke with the school nurse, who is aware of no trauma at school, but did learn from the teacher that Cassandra has not been paying attention in class. Cassandra cannot explain why she does not want to go to school, only that her stomach aches or some other part of her body hurts each morning.

Cassandra visited her pediatrician who ruled out any physical cause for her complaints, and referred her to a child psychologist. The psychologist has scheduled several sessions with Cassandra to help her learn to verbalize her fears and learn strategies to deal with them. She uses dolls in an attempt to help Cassandra act out her fears and gain some understanding. The psychologist communicates Cassandra's progress to the school nurse, who verifies her attendance and helps to support her throughout each day.

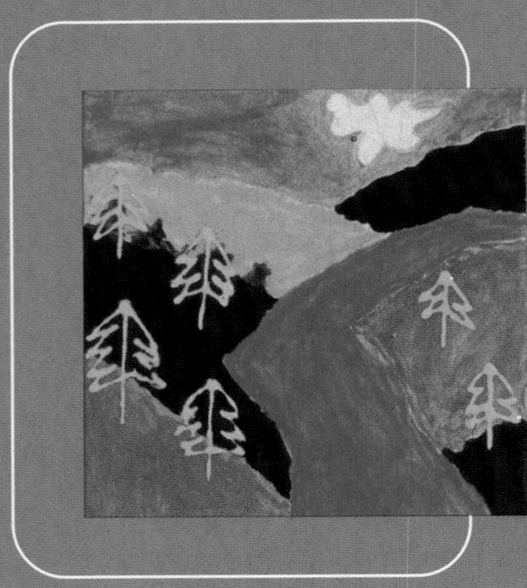

"It was so scary when our car was hit. I didn't know what was happening and can't stop thinking about it."

—Cassandra, age 9

Key Terms

adaptive functioning/1397
affect/1396
agoraphobia/1390
anhedonia/1384
behavior modification/1372
cognitive therapy/1370
coprolalia/1395
copropraxia/1395
developmental disability/1397
echolalia/1375
learning disabilities/1396
mental health/1369
mental retardation/1397
pervasive developmental disorder (PDD)/1374
play therapy/1371
stereotypy/1374

Learning Outcomes

After completing this chapter, you will be able to:

- Define mental health and describe major mental health disruptions in childhood.
- Discuss the clinical manifestations of the major mental health disorders of childhood and adolescence.
- Plan for the nursing management of children and adolescents with mental health disruptions in the hospital and community settings.
- Describe characteristics of common cognitive disorders of childhood.
- Plan nursing management for children with cognitive disorders.
- Establish and evaluate expected outcomes of care for the child with a cognitive disorder.

MediaLink 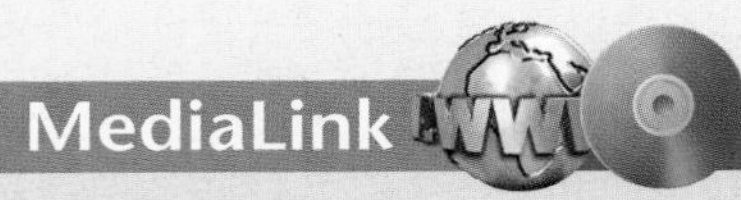 **http://www.prenhall.com/ball**

Resources for this chapter can be found on the CD-ROM accompanying this textbook, and on the Companion Website at www.prenhall.com/ball. Click on Chapter 34 to select the activities for this chapter.

CD-ROM

Animations
- *ADD/ADHD*
- *Down Syndrome*

NCLEX Review

Audio Glossary

COMPANION WEBSITE

A & P Review

Clinical Manifestations Review

Medication Match-Up

NCLEX Review

Case Study: Calculate SSRI Dosage

Critical Thinking: Females and Posttraumatic Stress Disorder

MediaLink Applications
- *Help Families Evaluate Mental Health Information on the Internet*
- *Nursing Practice: Put National Goals into Community Practice*

How can the school nurse partner with the psychologist and family to provide care for Cassandra? What support does she need to deal with the stress of the car crash? This chapter provides the knowledge and tools that can help you to plan and implement care for children with alterations in mental health or cognition. Much of the care for mental health disruptions is provided by psychiatric–mental health specialists such as Cassandra's psychologist, so the nurse partners with these specialists to identify problems, support and carry out the therapy, provide education to the family, and refer the family to appropriate resources.

Cognitive conditions are commonly managed by the family and the school personnel. The nurse forms partnerships with families and school personnel to plan and evaluate care for the child with cognitive conditions such as mental retardation. A thorough knowledge of development is a prerequisite to understanding mental health disruptions and cognitive conditions since developmental status is often altered in both.

Some mental health and cognitive conditions in children originate from genetic or physiologic causes. Examples include mental retardation and childhood schizophrenia. The environments in which children live also influence their characteristics and can contribute to mental dysfunctions such as anxiety, depression, and posttraumatic stress disorder.

Most mental health and cognitive conditions are treated in community settings, and nurses in these settings play an active role in the treatment and support of the child and family. Nurses may function as case managers, assisting a family to deal with all areas of the child's care. Occasionally a child is hospitalized for treatment of a significant mental health disruption, or is hospitalized for treatment of another health problem and requires continued mental health services. Cognitive and developmental characteristics must be considered and integrated into care for all children. In this chapter mental health disruptions will be discussed first, with cognitive conditions following. Children can manifest both mental health and cognitive alterations, necessitating integration of concepts from both areas to plan care.

ALTERATIONS IN MENTAL HEALTH

Mental health is foundational to a sense of personal well-being. It involves successful engagement in activities and relationships and the ability to adapt to and cope with change. However, 25% of children in the United States suffer from mental illness that is severe enough to impair functioning at home or school, and only 30% of those children receive any mental health services (Melnyk, Brown, Jones, et al., 2003; Melnyk, Feinstein, Tuttle, et al., 2002). Further, some of the services received are not comprehensive or multidisciplinary, leading to unmet mental health needs (Navon, Nelson, Pagano, et al., 2001). In other cases, the interventions used are not established on evidence-based practice (Hoaglund, Burns, Kiser, et al., 2001).

The surgeon general is leading an initiative to examine mental health in the United States and has identified a series of goals and steps toward improving mental healthcare for children (Department of Health and Human Services, 2000). From the ages of 10 to 21 years, mental health issues are among the top two leading causes of hospitalization in all age groups (see Chapter 1∞). This high rate of hospitalization infers that children are not receiving mental health services early, when outpatient care is appropriate and prognosis is best. To confront this childhood mental health crisis, the surgeon general's agenda has established a commitment to promote mental health as an essential part of child health, to integrate mental health services into all health services provided to children, to engage families and youth in planning for mental healthcare, and to develop and enhance the infrastructure to support child and youth mental health services (Department of Health and Human Services, 2000). See Box 34–1 for a list of the goals established in the surgeon general's report.

Nurses have been leaders in the field of pediatric mental healthcare. An initiative known as KySS (Keep your children/yourself Safe and Secure) was launched by nurses in 2001 and was the subject of a summit for health professional collaboration in 2003. The goals of the summit included identification of assessment, implementation, and dissemination strategies for promoting the mental health of children and teens in primary care and alternative care settings, and review of evidence-based practice to make recommendations for interventions and needed research areas (Melnyk, Moldenhauer, Tuttle, et al., 2003). Recommendations regarding screening for certain mental health conditions will be found throughout this chapter.

MediaLink National Mental Health Goals and Resources

NURSING MANAGEMENT

Nursing Assessment and Diagnosis

Mental health conditions often escalate to a level of crisis for families because they are not identified early. To avoid serious mental health problems, ongoing assessment of all children for risks is imperative. During all health visits, mental health screening

BOX 34–1 Goals of the Surgeon General's National Action Agenda for Children's Mental Health

1. Promote public awareness of children's mental health issues and reduce stigma associated with mental illness.
2. Continue to develop, disseminate, and implement scientifically proven prevention and treatment services in the field of children's mental health.
3. Improve the assessment and recognition of mental health needs in children.
4. Eliminate racial/ethnic and socioeconomic disparities in access to mental healthcare services.
5. Improve the infrastructure for children's mental health services, including support for scientifically proven interventions across professions.
6. Increase access to and coordination of quality mental healthcare services.
7. Train frontline providers to recognize and manage mental health issues and educate mental healthcare providers in scientifically proven prevention and treatment services.
8. Monitor the access to and coordination of quality mental healthcare services.

Note: From Department of Health and Human Services. (2000). Report on the surgeon general's conference on children's mental health: A national action agenda. *Washington, DC: U.S. Department of Health and Human Services.*

should be integrated into care so that disruptions can be identified. See Chapters 10 to 15 for specific questions to ask during health promotion and health maintenance visits. When a potential mental health condition exists, the child receives further assessment from a mental health specialist. A resource commonly used is the *Diagnostic and Statistical Manual of Mental Disorders,* which lists diagnostic criteria for known mental health conditions. The current edition is the *DSM IV-TR* (American Psychiatric Association, 2000) and its criteria for several conditions are listed throughout this chapter and other chapters in this book.

Once a mental health problem is identified, the nurse assesses the child for related issues and conditions. Mental health is linked to development, so developmental screening tests are administered. Mental health status can influence activity level, physiological parameters, and risk for certain conditions. Therefore, height and weight, review of systems, vital signs, and medication/substance use history are important to perform. Family interactions, stressors, and methods of coping are assessed (see Chapter 2 for further detail on family assessment). See Table 34–1.

Many nursing diagnoses can be formulated based on particular mental health conditions and child situations. Examples include:

- Impaired Adjustment related to multiple stressors
- Anxiety related to situational or maturational crises
- Ineffective Coping related to inadequate social support
- Dysfunctional Grieving related to difficulty expressing loss of significant other
- Ineffective Role Performance related to inadequate support system and inadequate linkage with healthcare system

Planning and Implementation

The primary treatment goal in the management of children and adolescents with mental health disruptions is to assist the child and family to achieve and maintain an optimal level of functioning through interventions designed to reduce the impact of risk factors and to enhance protective factors such as coping ability. Therapeutic interventions and communication are tailored with the recognition that feelings motivate behaviors. Parents and others who are close to the child may react to the child's behaviors rather than trying to find out what feelings may be precipitating the undesirable actions. Although behaviors may be considered in treatment, feelings and life experiences are often explored to provide insight and to maximize potential for behavior change. Medication may be used to enhance and support other therapy, or may be a major therapeutic measure.

Three basic treatment modes are used: individual, family, and group therapy. These treatments are often performed collaboratively by mental health specialists. For example, a psychologist or advanced practice nurse may prescribe the treatment modes, while a nurse trained in mental health is the therapist. The choice of treatment mode takes into account the child's age and developmental stage as well as the family situation and access to care. Most therapists incorporate several intervention strategies simultaneously within these modes. Different strategies are more or less effective and appropriate for children and adolescents in various stages of development. A thorough understanding of developmental needs, expectations, and abilities is therefore essential for mental health professionals. Treatment modes and therapeutic strategies commonly used with children and adolescents are described below.

Individual Therapy

Individual therapy involves only the child and the therapist. Treatment of specific emotional problems or disorders may involve various techniques such as play therapy, psychodrama, art therapy, and **cognitive therapy** (a technique used to help a person recognize automatic negative thinking). Individual therapy may be short term (four to six sessions) or long term (lasting for several years).

Family Therapy

Family therapy involves the exploration of a particular emotional problem and its manifestations among the family members. Family therapy is based on the idea that the emotional symptoms or problems of an individual are an expression of emotional symptoms or problems in the family. The focus is on

TABLE 34–1 Mental Health Assessment

The nurse gathers information about the child's mental health by asking questions and making observations. The following components may be helpful.

APPEARANCE	BEHAVIOR	DEVELOPMENT	LIFE EVENTS	HISTORY
➤ Clothing appropriate for age, setting, and developmental level ➤ Facial expression and response to nurse ➤ Body size and posture ➤ Interactions with parents or others ➤ Interest in surroundings	➤ Level of consciousness and interaction with surroundings ➤ Recent reported changes in behavior (e.g., sleep, eating patterns, communication with others, school performance, friendships, risky activities) ➤ Problem behaviors identified by child or parent ➤ Events associated with problem behaviors	➤ Results of developmental testing ➤ Progression of skills reported by family ➤ Unusual capabilities or deficits ➤ Progression in school and extracurricular activities	➤ Recent stress or trauma ➤ Changes in family structure ➤ Chronic health conditions in family members	➤ Prenatal events or birth trauma ➤ Diagnosed mental health disorder in child or other family members ➤ Neurological injuries or diseases ➤ Alterations in mental health function

the relationships among the family members, not the psychologic conflict within each individual member.

Group Therapy

Group therapy involves an ongoing or limited number of sessions in which several individuals participate. The emphasis is on the interpersonal styles of relating to one another in the group. Group therapy is particularly effective with adolescents because of the importance of the peer group at this age. An advantage of group therapy is that stimuli and feedback come from multiple sources (the group members) instead of just one person (the therapist).

In addition to treatment modes, the following therapeutic strategies can be integrated into therapy.

Play Therapy

Play is often called the language or work of the child. From a developmental perspective, children progressively learn to express feelings and needs through action, fantasy, and, finally, language. The special quality of play buffers children against the pressures and demands of daily life. Play facilitates mastery of developmental stages by strengthening physical and neurologic processes. Play also assists in cognitive learning, setting the stage for problem solving and creativity.

Play therapy is a technique that reveals problems on a fantasy level through the use of toys, dolls, clay, art, and other creative objects. It is often used with preschool and school-age children who are experiencing anxiety, stress, and other specific nonpsychotic mental disorders. Play therapy encourages the child to act out feelings such as anger, hostility, sadness, and fear. It also provides the opportunity for the therapist to help the child understand, on a conscious or unconscious level, personal responses and behavior in a safe, supportive environment. This type of therapy was helpful for Cassandra, in the opening scenario, who was able to gain some control over a frightening environment by acting out fears and trying solutions during play with a therapist.

CLINICAL TIP

Play therapy, a technique used with children who have psychosocial disorders, is different from therapeutic play, which may be used with many hospitalized children (see Chapter 17∞). Although some techniques overlap, only a specialist is qualified to provide play therapy as a treatment for mental health disruption, while anyone with a basic knowledge of development can plan therapeutic play approaches.

Art Therapy

Children who may be apprehensive about playing can sometimes be encouraged to participate in art therapy, using brief drawing exercises. This technique is appropriate for children of all ages, including adolescents. The drawings can help the therapist gain information about the child, the family, and the interactions between the child and family. However, children's drawings should never be used solely to form a definitive diagnosis.

When used in conjunction with a thorough history and appropriate psychologic testing information, art therapy can guide the child's treatment. These drawing exercises provide an opportunity to help in the healing process. The therapist can assist the child to release feelings of anger, pain, or fear onto paper, where they can be examined objectively. Figures 34–1 ■ to 34–4 ■ present examples of this technique.

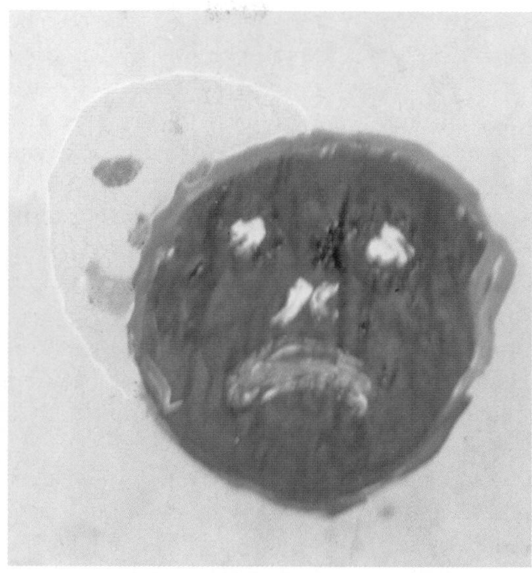

FIGURE 34–1 ■ "Me." Drawn by a 14-year-old girl with major depression, anxiety, and school phobia who had experienced multiple losses over several years. Her mother had severe chronic lung problems and diabetes, and the girl had stopped attending school for fear that something would happen to her mother. This drawing represents the girl's obvious feelings of sadness and depression, but also indicates a glimmer of hope (represented by the yellow mask coming from behind the dark mask of depression).

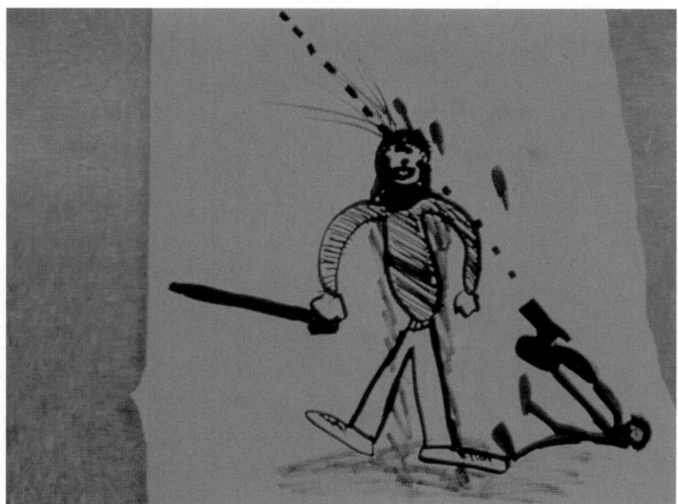

FIGURE 34–2 ■ "Self-Portrait." Drawn by a 15-year-old boy who was admitted through the emergency department after a failed suicide attempt by hanging. He had a psychiatric diagnosis of depression and polysubstance abuse (including inhalants and alcohol) and insisted that he was a member of a satanic cult in his hometown. Most of his drawings depicted a preoccupation with violence and suicide. The boy said he always felt a "darkness" like a shadow that followed him around and wanted him dead. His family history was significant for depression and suicide on both his mother's and his father's side. His father also had a lengthy history of polysubstance abuse and alcoholism. The boy was discharged to a long-term residential treatment facility for adolescents.

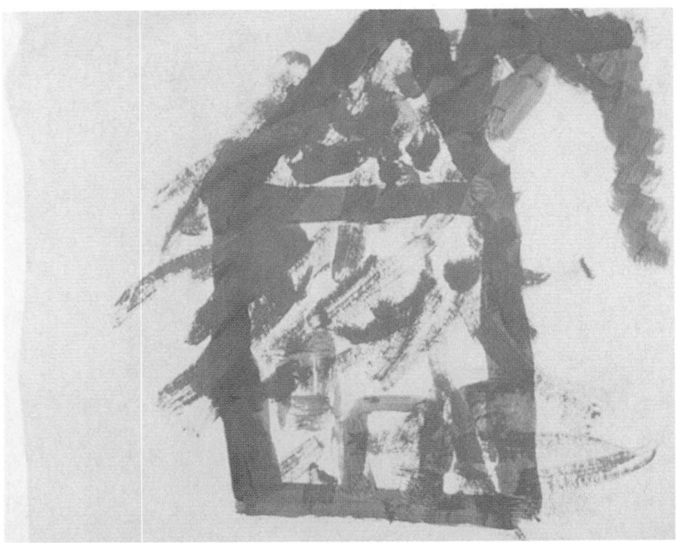

FIGURE 34–3 ■ "An Activity." Drawn by an 8-year-old boy who was initially admitted to the medical-surgical floor of a pediatric hospital for dehydration resulting from vomiting and diarrhea. Psychiatric evaluation was ordered for extreme anxiety. These drawings, completed during the initial interview, led to further investigation, which revealed that the child had started a house fire in which his grandmother was killed. The family's home and all their belongings were lost. No one knew that the child had set the fire. Further sessions indicated that he had been setting neighborhood garage fires and watching them burn from a distance.

Behavior and Cognitive Therapy

Behavior modification is a therapeutic technique that uses stimulus and response conditioning to alter inappropriate behaviors. It is used to reinforce desirable behaviors, helping the child to replace maladaptive behaviors with more appropriate ones. This technique is based on the assumption that any learned behavior can be unlearned. Thus, if parents, nurses, teachers, and other adults consistently reinforce desirable behaviors, the child will eventually alter or discontinue undesirable behaviors.

Behavior modification may include (1) removing the child from the home to a more structured environment, such as a hospital, for a brief time, and (2) instructing the parents, teachers, and other appropriate adults to be agents of behavioral change. Several ongoing sessions may be required with the adults involved, using role play and other techniques. Consistency is the most important principle in the successful use of behavior modification.

Cognitive therapy teaches thinking patterns to change reactions to situations that cause anxiety or undesirable behaviors. Children are taught how their brain and body are working; this understanding assists them in having control over the experience. Often a combination of cognitive and behavioral approaches is useful in treating children.

Visualization and Guided Imagery

The techniques of visualization and guided imagery begin with specific directions for progressive relaxation according to the child's ability. This form of therapy uses the child's own imagination and positive thinking to reduce stress and anxiety, decrease the experience of pain or discomfort, and promote healing. The techniques are especially useful in the management of anxiety disorders and chronic pain. It is not easy for every child to use his or her imagination in this way, so the technique may not work or be appropriate for every child.

Hypnosis

Hypnosis involves varying degrees of suggestibility and deep relaxation effects. This technique is useful for children and adolescents because they can usually be hypnotized more easily than adults. Hypnosis is especially helpful in treating physical symptoms with a psychologic component, anxiety, and phobias and in managing severe physical symptoms or discomfort (pain or nausea) associated with a physiologic disorder or its treatment (e.g., cancer or juvenile rheumatoid arthritis).

Care in the Hospital

Although most mental health disorders are managed effectively with therapy and/or medication on an outpatient basis, some necessitate admission to an inpatient psychiatric setting. In addition, you may encounter the child with a mental health disorder during hospitalization for a concurrent physiologic problem requiring hospitalization. If hospitalized for a concurrent problem, the child's current level of mental health functioning needs to be assessed in addition to the admitting diagnosis in order to plan appropriate interventions.

Nursing care includes carrying out the prescribed treatment plan and administering psychotropic medications. The child's medication regimen should be evaluated for administration schedule, dosage, side effects, and effectiveness. Inform the therapist of the child's hospitalization if the child has been hospital-

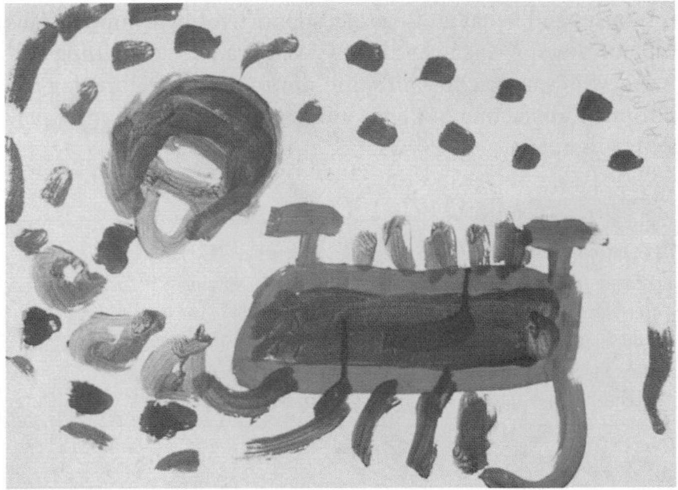

FIGURE 34–4 ■ "A Family Activity." By the same boy who drew Figure 34–3. This drawing depicts a recurring incident of physical and emotional abuse by his mother's live-in boyfriend. It shows the family bathtub with feces and blood smeared on the floor and walls. The boy reported that when either he or his 3-year-old brother had a toileting accident the boyfriend would make them go into the bathroom and stand in the bathtub while he smeared the feces on the walls. He would then hit the children and make them clean up the mess. The boy had previously been removed from the mother's custody for neglect. He was transferred from the medical-surgical area to the inpatient children's psychiatric unit, where he received a diagnosis of depression, anxiety disorder, and child abuse (physical and emotional). Charges were filed against the mother's boyfriend and custody of both children was temporarily revoked.

ized for a concurrent condition, and consult with the therapist regarding appropriate approaches for the child.

An important nursing intervention is to ensure safety of the child. Actions begin in the emergency department if a child is admitted for a mental health crisis. Remove or lock potentially dangerous material in the room such as medications, tubing, and sharps container. Parent, guardian, or health professional should remain with the child at all times. Inform the family member of the need to stay with the child and how to immediately notify the nurse if the adult needs to leave or if the child's condition changes. Part of the initial care is to evaluate risk by asking if the child has tried or has been thinking about self-harm. Ask about recent stresses, thoughts of hurting others, and why the child thinks he or she has been brought to the emergency room (Meunier-Sham, 2003). If the child is admitted to the psychiatric unit, follow unit policies for ensuring safety for children who are at risk of hurting themselves or others.

Psychiatric hospitalization is a stressful event for all families and both the family and child need supportive care. Continuation of family involvement is critical. See Evidence-Based Practice: Family Needs During Hospitalization for Mental Healthcare.The nurse frequently is the liaison between the family and the therapist in making follow-up arrangements at the time of discharge. The nurse must be aware of the meaning of mental illness in various cultural groups and the treatments that may be commonly used. These complementary therapies should be integrated within the care plan when considered safe and families must feel that their responses and approaches to the child with a mental disorder are not judged by health professionals. See Developing Cultural Competence: Mental Health Definition and Treatments.

Care in the Community

The nurse in the community conducts therapy sessions and performs ongoing evaluation and updates of the child's level of functioning. Changes in the child and family stressors and coping mechanisms are identified. Since many children do not receive adequate mental health services, nurses need to be knowledgeable about resources for mental health care and facilitate their use by child and family. The nurse in the community often acts as a partner to inform other health professionals such as psychiatrists, psychologists, psychiatric nurse practitioners, school counselors, teachers, and hospital nurses about the child's mental health status.

■ Evaluation

Desired outcomes for mental healthcare depend on the particular condition and the child's situation. Examples are:

- Ability to self-restrain compulsive or impulsive behaviors
- Psychosocial adaptation to change in family structure
- Verbalization regarding feelings of productivity and self-worth
- Identification and use of available social support
- Ability to draw on spiritual beliefs for comfort

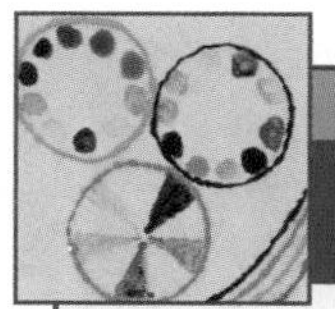

EVIDENCE-BASED PRACTICE

Family Needs During Hospitalization for Mental Health Care

PROBLEM

Hospitalization for mental health care is always a stressful event. Families frequently do not understand treatment procedures or the child's condition and diagnosis. Treatment may last for several days to months, causing disruption in family roles and routines. Family stresses must be understood so that the nurse can adequately support both the child and the family.

EVIDENCE

A nursing study involved interviews with 38 parents of 29 children who had recently been hospitalized for psychiatric illness. In this qualitative study, themes that emerged during the interviews were analyzed and categorized into categories. Three major categories were identified (Scharer, 2002).

The first was a need for *information.* Parents often did not receive information about admission and unit procedures. Many felt that the physicians and other therapists were hard to reach and did not provide adequate information about the child's condition and treatment. Parents identified a need to have access to hospital records and the child's diagnosis. Such information was viewed as important to link to outpatient facilities where the child was also treated.

The second set of needs was for *instrumental support.* These items included reasonably priced lodging near the hospital, ready access to the hospitalized child, assistance with providing physical care for the hospitalized child, and improved physical environment of the hospital unit and rooms. Some parents voiced a lack of mental health services in their own communities, resulting in lack of care both before and after hospitalization.

The third need was for *emotional support.* Parents often felt isolated and did not know where to turn. They suggested that staff could provide additional emotional support, and that having a parent to call who had similar experiences would have been helpful.

IMPLICATIONS

The nurse in a psychiatric facility is in a unique position to offer support to the family of the child or adolescent. Information about the unit can be provided by videotape, tour, and written materials. Daily updates on the child's condition and treatment plan are needed. Families must be viewed as partners in the treatment, along with the child and health professionals. Provide an opportunity for parents to ask questions and be sure they understand the diagnosis and treatment.

Consider visiting hours and access to children. If they are limited to certain times, explain the reason to parents. Provide access to Ronald McDonald House or other low-cost facilities if the parent is from out of town. Provide assistance and instruction with any physical care the child needs. Consider changes that can be made to make the unit more welcoming and pleasant, such as color of walls, presence of posters and brochures, and general cleanliness.

Facilitate parent-to-parent communication. Ask parents each day about how they feel and what can be done for them. Use empathy and interest to convey support.

CRITICAL THINKING APPLICATION

Why do you think that families find psychiatric facilities frightening or strange? How can you explain the need to remove items with which children could injure themselves or others? What questions will you ask early in the hospitalization to learn about facilities that are present in the home community that can be used for referral upon discharge? How could you locate available treatment options for a family from a community several miles from the hospital? How could support by the family members influence the care and condition of their child or adolescent?

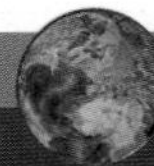

DEVELOPING CULTURAL COMPETENCE
Mental Health Definition and Treatments

Mental health is defined in different ways by various cultural groups. For most it is a sense of well-being, peace, and productive use of the mind. In many cultures care of the "spirit" is believed necessary to promote mental health. An array of therapies is used to support and restore mental health. They may include healers, family and community support, relaxation or meditation, storytelling, singing, rites of passage, teas and other herbal products, and exorcism. Find out how individuals and groups define mental health and how they believe health is maintained. Be alert to learn if mental disorders are viewed as a negative stigma or are openly accepted and discussed within the culture.

DEVELOPMENTAL AND BEHAVIORAL DISORDERS

Pervasive Developmental Disorders

It is estimated that 12% to 16% of children have a developmental or behavioral disorder. One of the most common types of disorders is pervasive developmental disorders. **Pervasive developmental disorders (PDDs)** begin in early childhood and are characterized by impaired social interactions and communication, with restricted interests, activities, and behaviors (Baird, Charman, Cox, et al., 2001). The disorders are called "autistic spectrum disorders" and are classified into five types:

- Autistic disorder
- Asperger's syndrome
- Rett's disorder
- Childhood disintegrative disorder
- Pervasive developmental disorder not otherwise specified

About two or more children in 1,000 have autistic spectrum disorder, with about half of the cases comprised of autistic disorder (commonly called autism) (Committee on Children with Disabilities, 2001). This incidence represents an increase from formerly described levels. Before 1985, about 0.4 to 0.5 children in 1,000 were diagnosed with autistic disorder (Hudson & Dixon, 2003). It is unclear whether there is a true increase in cases or simply improved techniques in making the diagnosis (Jick & Kaye, 2003). The disorder is about four times more common in males than females. Males frequently have mild forms of the disorder and females commonly have associated mental retardation.

Etiology and Pathophysiology

The etiology of autistic spectrum disorders in unclear but several theories have been proposed. Genetic transmission, immune responses, and neuroanatomy are being investigated as causes (Williams, Dalrymple, & Neal, 2000). Occurrence in siblings is 3% to 7%, supporting theories of genetic links (Committee on Children with Disabilities, 2001). Neurotransmitters such as dopamine, serotonin, and opioids are abnormal in some children and are a focus of present research (Cade & Tidwell, 2001). Congenital rubella syndrome, fragile X syndrome, phenylketonuria, Down syndrome, and tuberous sclerosis are all associated with a higher than normal incidence (American Academy of Pediatrics, 2001; Hudson & Dixon, 2003). Some earlier research studies suggested a relationship with measles-mumps-rubella vaccine (Kaye, Melero-Montes, & Jick, 2001), but more recent research has indicated that there is no connection between the vaccine and reported cases of the disorder (Dales, Hammer, & Smith, 2001; Bechtel, 2003).

Clinical Manifestations

The essential features typically become apparent by the time a child is 3 years of age. They involve three areas, including impairments in:

- Social reciprocity
- Communication
- Behavior

(Towbin, Mauk, & Batshaw, 2002)

Social interactions are always complex and involve perceptions of the other person as well as social behaviors. The autistic child does not learn the common characteristics of these social interchanges. The child may be unable to converse normally, fail to initiate conversations, and have impaired observations of nonverbal behavior. Autistic children are often unable to relate to people or to respond to social and emotional cues. In addition, they engage in **stereotypy,** or rigid and obsessive behavior. Characteristically these repetitive behaviors in affected children include head banging, twirling in circles, biting themselves, and flapping their hands or arms. Frequently a child's behavior is self-stimulating or self-destructive. Responses to sensory stimuli are frequently abnormal and include an extreme aversion to touch, loud noises, and bright lights. Emotional lability is common (Figure 34–5 ■).

Communication difficulties or delays in speech and language are common and are often the first symptoms that lead to diagnosis. Absence of babbling and other communication by 1 year,

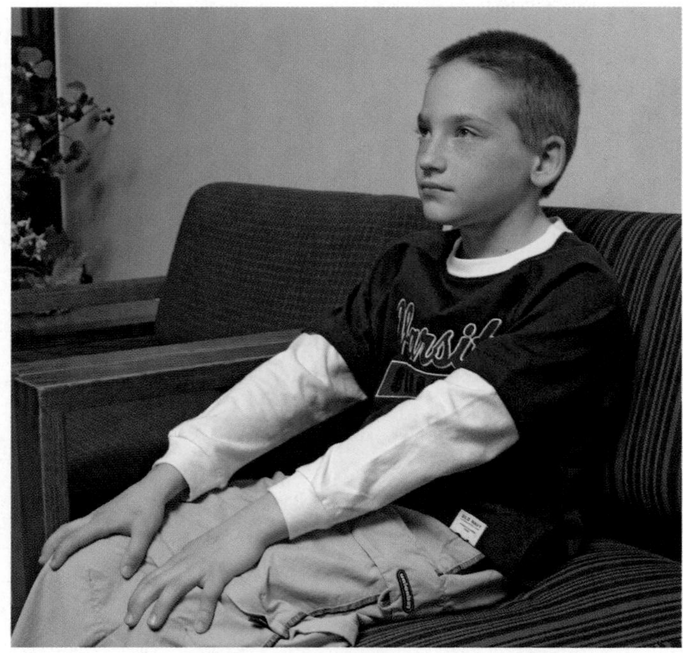

FIGURE 34–5 ■ This child with autism sits stiffly in the chair and engages in rhythmic rocking behavior. He has a disengaged look and does not readily interact with other children or adults who are in his environment.

absence of two-word phrases by 2 years, and deterioration of previous language skills are characteristic. Abnormal communication patterns include both verbal and nonverbal communication. Autistic children may eventually learn to talk, in some cases well, but their speech is likely to show certain abnormalities: use of "you" in place of "I"; **echolalia** (a compulsive parroting of what is heard); repeating questions rather than answering them; and fascination with rhythmic, repetitive songs and verses.

Behaviors of affected children show several differences from others. They do not commonly explore objects but have stereoptyped behaviors. They may line up objects, play with the same objects over and over, and have certain rituals that must be performed. They often become upset if these normal routines are disrupted. Rituals may involve eating only certain types or colors of foods or eating in specific patterns. Autistic children may manifest disturbances in the rate or sequence of development. They are frequently cognitively impaired but can demonstrate a wide range of intellectual ability and functioning. Cognitive impairment may become manifested early in life by slow developmental progression, particularly in social skills. Some children are impaired in particular areas of development while others are above normal. While 25% have microcephaly, most children have normal appearance.

The specific differences in clinical manifestations of the types of autistic spectrum disorder are listed in the clinical manifestations table below.

No specific physical examination parameter is clearly diagnostic of autistic spectrum disorders, but growth measurements may provide clues (Box 34–2).

BOX 34–2 Research: Brain Growth and Autism

In an effort to obtain clearly measurable signs of developing autism, researchers have examined many criteria. It is known that increased brain volume is seen in the disorder. In a study of 48 children with autism spectrum disorder, it was noted that the infants had low occipital frontal circumference at birth but had a significant increase in head size at 1–2 months and again at 6–14 months (Courchesne, Carper, & Akshoomoff, 2003). Since head circumference is easily and routinely measured by nurses in health promotion visits, attention to patterns of accelerated growth during infancy may help to identify some cases of the disorder. Measure head circumference at every visit, place results on a growth chart, and evaluate for babies who have changing percentile channels. See Chapter 9∞ for more information about interpretation of channels on growth grids.

COLLABORATIVE CARE

Nurses partner with families and other health professionals to identify children with autistic spectrum disorders. Care involves collaborative efforts of many resources, including speech therapy, psychologists, teachers, and mental health therapists.

Diagnostic Tests

Diagnosis is based on the presence of specific criteria, as described in the American Psychiatric Association's *Diagnostic and Statistical Manual of Mental Disorders,* 4th edition (*DSM-IV-TR*). See the specific criteria for autistic disorder (autism) in Box 34–3; consult *DSM-IV,* which lists similar criteria for other autistic syndrome disorders. Symptoms may emerge as early as

CLINICAL MANIFESTATIONS of Autistic Spectrum Disorders (Pervasive Developmental Disorders)

DISORDER	CLINICAL MANIFESTATIONS	CLINICAL THERAPY
Autistic disorder	Impaired social, communicative, and behavioral development, usually noted in first year of life.	Early intervention is key to maximal performance. Interventions focus on improving behaviors and communication skills, providing physical and occupational therapy, structuring play interactions with other children, and educating parents about the child's needs.
Asperger syndrome	Impaired social interactions with normal language development for age; pitch, tone, and other speech characteristics may be abnormal. Verbal skills involving spelling and vocabulary are high with concept formation, language flexibility, and comprehension low.	Social interactions are focus of therapy.
Rett's disorder	Early development appears normal and symptoms emerge at 6–18 months. Ataxia, handwringing, intermittent hyperventilation, dementia, and growth retardation show progressive increase. Appears only in females as an X-linked dominant disorder; mutations occur in the gene MeCP2, affecting methyl-CpG-binding protein 2 which is important in brain development.	Early intervention in areas of abnormal behaviors.
Childhood disintegrative disorder	First 2–5 years of development appear normal followed by deterioration in many areas of functioning. Behaviors finally stabilize at some point without further deterioration.	Focus on areas of developmental function that show abnormality. Individualized education plans are needed in school to deal with communication, play, physical therapy, and teaching management skills to parents. Regression in toileting and other skills may occur.
Pervasive developmental disorder not otherwise specified	Severe social impairment without meeting DSM criteria for other types of autistic spectrum disorder.	Behavioral therapy focuses on building social skills.

BOX 34–3 ***DSM-IV-TR* Diagnostic Criteria for Autistic Disorder**

A. A total of six or more items from 1, 2, and 3, with at least two from 1, and one each from 2 and 3:
   1. Qualitative impairment in social interaction, as manifested by at least two of the following:
      a. Marked impairment in the use of multiple nonverbal behaviors such as eye-to-eye gaze, facial expression, body posture and gestures to regulate social interaction
      b. Failure to develop peer relationships appropriate to developmental level
      c. A lack of spontaneous seeking to share enjoyment, interests, or achievements with other people
      d. Lack of social or emotional reciprocity
   2. Qualitative impairments in communication as manifested by at least one of the following:
      a. Delay in, or total lack of, the development of spoken language (not accompanied by an attempt to compensate through alternative modes of communication such as gesture or mime)
      b. In individuals with adequate speech, marked impairment in the ability to initiate or sustain a conversation with others
      c. Stereotyped and repetitive use of language or idiosyncratic language
      d. Lack of varied, spontaneous make-believe play or social imitative play appropriate to developmental level
   3. Restricted repetitive and stereotyped patterns of behavior, interests, and activities, as manifested by at least one of the following:
      a. Encompassing preoccupation with one or more stereotyped and restricted patterns of interest that is abnormal either in intensity or in focus
      b. Apparently inflexible adherence to specific, nonfunctional routines or rituals
      c. Stereotyped and repetitive motor mannerisms (e.g., hand or finger flapping or twisting, or complex whole-body movements)
      d. Persistent preoccupation with parts of objects

B. Delays or abnormal functioning in at least one of the following areas, with onset prior to age 3 years: (1) social interaction, (2) language as used in social communication, or (3) symbolic or imaginative play.

C. The disturbance is not better accounted for by Rett's Disorder or Childhood Disintegrative Disorder.

6 months for some disorders, or later for others. However, diagnosis is often delayed and parents may later state that they knew something was abnormal in the child's responses to interactions even during infancy. Several screening tests are available for use in health maintenance visits if autistic disorder is suspected (Table 34–2). It is important to note that screening tests may be helpful in diagnosis but none have reliability and validity strong enough to rule out over- or underdiagnosis. Additional testing is done to rule out other causes of the child's behavior. Tests may include neuroimaging (CT scan or MRI), lead screening, metabolic studies, DNA analysis, and electroencephalogram. See Chapters 8 and 33∞ for further descriptions related to the neurological system.

Clinical Therapy

Early intervention assists in maximizing the child's potential and establishing helpful support for parents. Treatment focuses on behavior management to reward appropriate behaviors, foster positive or adaptive coping skills, and facilitate effective communication. The goals of treatment are to reduce rigidity or stereotypy (repetitive, obsessive, machinelike movements) and other maladaptive behaviors. Often the child must be physically restrained from aggressive or self-destructive behaviors. Some parents choose to use complementary therapies such as vitamin supplements and dimethylglycine. Foods such as sugar, aspartame, milk products, and wheat are sometimes eliminated from the diet (Hyman & Levy, 2000). See Complementary Therapy: Autism.

Medications are used with some children to treat associated disorders but are not effective in treatment of these disorders. They may include stimulants, selective serotonin reuptake inhibitors (SSRIs), and mood stabilizers.

The overall prognosis for autistic children to become functioning members of society is guarded. The extent to which adequate adjustment is achieved varies greatly. Successful adjustment is more likely for children with higher IQs, adequate speech, and access to specialized programs.

NURSING MANAGEMENT

Nursing Assessment and Diagnosis

The nurse may encounter the autistic child when parents seek care for a suspected hearing impairment, speech difficulty, or developmental delay. Early and frequent developmental screening of all children can help in referral for thorough assessment and identification of cases. Parents may report abnormal interaction such as lack of eye contact, disinterest in cuddling, minimal facial responsiveness, and failure to talk. Be alert to parental observations that the baby or young child does not look at them or provides other developmental or behavioral cues of aversion to contact (Beauchesne & Kelley, 2004). Initial assessment focuses on language development, response to others, and hearing acuity (see Chapters 8 and 24∞). Carefully evaluate the child for history of developmental milestones and refer for abnormalities. Perform developmental screening that considers several areas of development including motor activity, social skills, and language. Recall that the child may have normal performance in one area such as motor skills and delayed development in another area such as language skills. Likewise, language may be normal for age but social interactions may be delayed. Include questioning about adaptive skills such as toilet training and feeding patterns. Inquire about school performance since some areas may be normal while others are delayed. Observe the child in play situations and evaluate the use of creative and exploratory play versus more repetitive patterns. Perform hearing and vision screening to rule out sensory problems. When a child with a diagnosis of autistic disorder is hospitalized for a concurrent problem, obtain a history from the parents regarding the child's routines, rituals, and likes and dislikes, as well as ways to promote interaction and co-

TABLE 34–2 Screening Tests for Autism

TEST	SOURCE
Clinical Practice Guidelines—Early Intervention Program of the New York State Department of Health	www.health.state.ny.us
Checklist for Autism in Toddlers (CHAT) or Modified Checklist for Autism in Toddlers (MCHAT)	Scambler, D., Rogers, S. J., & Wehner, E. A. (2001). Can the checklist for autism in toddlers differentiate young children with autism from those with developmental delays? *Journal of the American Academy of Child and Adolescent Psychiatry, 40,* 1457–1463.
Autism Diagnostic Interview—Revised	Lord, C., Rutter, M., & LeConteur, A. (1994). Autism Diagnostic Interview—Revised: A revised version of a diagnostic interview for caregivers of individuals with possible pervasive developmental disorder. *Journal of Autism and Developmental Disorders, 24,* 659–685.
Detection of Autism by Infant Sociability Interview (DAISI)	Hopson, R. P. (1993). *Autism and the development of mind.* Hillsdale, NJ: Erlbaum.
Screening Tool for Autism in Two-Year-Olds	Stone, W. L., Coonrod, E., & Osley, O. (2000). Brief report: Screening Tool for Autism in Two-Year-Olds (STAT): Development and preliminary data. *Journal of Autistic and Developmental Disorders, 30,* 607–612.
Autism Behavior Checklist	Gillberg, C., Nordin, V., & Ehlers, S. (1996). Early detection of autism: Diagnostic instruments for clinicians. *European Child and Adolescent Psychiatry, 5*(2), 67–74.
Autism Diagnostic Observation Schedule—Generic (ADOS-G)	Lord, C., Risi, S., Lambrecht, L., et al. (2000). The Autism Diagnostic Observation Schedule—generic: A standard measure of social and communication deficits associated with the spectrum of autism. *Journal of Autism and Developmental Disorders, 30,* 205–233.
Childhood Autism Rating Scale (CARS)	Schopler, E., Reichler, R. J., & Renner, B. R. (1988). *The Childhood Autism Rating Scale (CARS).* Los Angeles: Western Psychological Services.

operation. Autistic children may carry a special toy or object that they play with during times of stress. Ask parents about these objects and their use.

Ask about the child's behaviors as well as observing them on admission. Obtain a history of acute and chronic illnesses and injuries. Ask about eating patterns and food restrictions. Inquire about complementary therapies used in a nonjudgmental and supportive manner.

Nursing diagnoses must be tailored to fit the individual needs of the child. Examples of diagnoses that may be appropriate for autistic children or those with other pervasive developmental disorders include the following:

- Impaired Verbal Communication related to psychological condition
- Impaired Social Interaction related to developmental disability
- Disturbed Thought Processes related to mental disorder
- Risk for Injury related to cognitive impairment
- Risk for Caregiver Role Strain related to chronicity and demands of child's condition
- Disabled Family Coping: Compromised related to having a child with prolonged disability

COMPLEMENTARY THERAPY

Autism

Some parents who have a child with autism will choose to use CAM in an attempt to help the child. Some CAM approaches include vitamin therapy with vitamin A, C, or B; elimination of some additives from the diet; or providing medicines such as secretin (a pancreatic hormone), Pepcid, or other antacids. Nurses can help parents to evaluate studies on CAM and encourage them to initiate only one treatment at a time to measure effectiveness (Hyman & Levy, 2000).

Planning and Implementation

Nursing care focuses on stabilizing environmental stimuli, providing supportive care, enhancing communication, maintaining a safe environment, and offering the parents anticipatory guidance.

Stabilize Environmental Stimuli

Autistic children interpret and respond to the environment differently from other individuals. Sounds that are not distressing to the average person may be interpreted by autistic children as louder, more frightening, and overwhelming. The child needs to be oriented to new settings such as a classroom or the hospital room and may adjust best to a small classroom or a hospital room with only one other child. Encourage parents to bring the child's favorite objects from home, and try to keep these objects in the same places, because the child often does not cope well with changes in the environment.

Provide Supportive Care

Developing a trusting relationship with the autistic child is often difficult. Adjust communication techniques and teaching to the child's developmental level. Ask parents about the child's usual home routines, and maintain these routines as much as possible if the child is not in the home setting. Because self-care abilities are often limited, the child may need assistance to meet basic needs. When possible, schedule daily care and routine procedures at consistent times to maintain predictability. Encourage parents to remain with the hospitalized child and to participate in daily care planning. Parents are integral parts of the treatment team when

MediaLink Autism Resources and Support

the child's learning goals are established in early intervention or school programs. Identify rituals for naptime and bedtime, and maintain them to promote rest and sleep. Integrate patterns that facilitate intake of nutritious foods at mealtimes.

School programs, behavioral therapy, and individualized education plans (see Chapter 20∞) can help the child to learn self-care skills within community settings. See additional suggestions for family support in the community care section.

Enhance Communication

Because children with autism have impaired communication, nursing care focuses on utilizing and improving communication with the child (Cade & Tidwell, 2001). Speech is used when possible. If the child responds well to visual cues, then pictures, computers, and other visual aids may form an important part of interaction. Sign language is used with some children.

Maintain a Safe Environment

Monitor autistic children at all times, including bathtime and bedtime. Close supervision is needed to ensure that the child does not obtain any harmful objects or engage in dangerous behaviors. For the child who engages in head banging or other abusive behaviors, bicycle helmets and hand mitts can be the least restrictive method to provide safety. They enable the child to participate in activities and engage in a social environment to the degree possible.

Provide Anticipatory Guidance

Approximately half of all children with autistic disorder require lifelong supervision and support, especially if the disorder is accompanied by mental retardation. Some children may grow up to lead independent lives, although they will have social limitations with impaired interpersonal relationships. Encourage parents to promote the child's development through behavior modification and specialized educational programs. The overall goal is to provide the child with the guidance, education, and support necessary for optimal functioning. Parents need support over a long period of time and may benefit from contact with other families in similar situations. They may be vulnerable to "quick cures" offered on the Internet and other sources, and need reliable materials and opportunities to discuss what they have read or heard.

Care in the Community

Families of autistic children need a great deal of support to cope with the challenges of caring for the autistic child. Help them to identify resources for childcare, such as special toddler programs and preschools. The child will need an individualized education plan. The parent or primary caretaker often has difficulty obtaining respite care and may need assistance to find suitable resources. Siblings of the autistic child may need help to explain the disorder to their friends or teachers. Family support programs are available in some states to provide assistance to parents. School nurses partner with health professionals in other settings to implement communication plans and other strategies for the autistic child.

Genetic counseling should be offered to the family. Information on immunizations is necessary, because parents may have heard about a potential connection between immunization and the disorder. They should be encouraged to have the child immunized on the recommended schedule. Parents may have questions about where to find information on complementary and alternative therapies.

Local support groups for parents of autistic children are available in most areas. Parents can also be referred to the Autism Society of America for information.

■ Evaluation

Expected outcomes of nursing care for the child with autism are as follows:

- Management of behavioral symptoms
- Maximization of self-care
- Maintenance of safe environment
- Consistent developmental progression
- Successful communication strategies

Attention Deficit Disorder and Attention Deficit Hyperactivity Disorder

Attention deficit disorder (ADD) is a variation in central nervous system processing characterized by developmentally inappropriate behaviors involving inattention. When hyperactivity and impulsivity accompany inattention, the disorder is called attention deficit hyperactivity disorder (ADHD). The latter is the more common condition and affects from 4% to 12% of all school-age children, boys almost four times more commonly than girls (National Initiative for Children's Healthcare Quality, 2003). It is now known to affect adolescents and adults; those with the disorder often continue to manifest at least some of the symptoms as they grow into adulthood. Hyperactivity and impulsivity may improve as the child nears adulthood, with inattentiveness the most persistent characteristic (McDonnell, Doyle, & Surman, 2003).

Etiology and Pathophysiology

Although a variety of physical and neurologic disorders are associated with ADHD, children with identifiable causes represent a small proportion of this population. Examples of known associations include exposure to high levels of lead or mercury in childhood and prenatal exposure to alcohol or tobacco smoke. Other prenatal factors associated with a higher incidence of ADHD include preterm labor, impaired placenta functioning, and impaired oxygenation. Seizures and serious head injury are other potential associations. Genetic factors may be important, as well as family dynamics and environmental characteristics. Although ADHD occurs more commonly within families (25% have a first-degree relative with the disorder), a single gene has not been located and a specific mechanism of genetic transmission is not known. It is believed that a genetic predisposition interacts with the child's environment, so that both factors contribute to the appearance of the condition. Family stress, poverty, and poor nutrition may also be contributing factors. Daily television exposure at ages 1 to 3 years is associated with attentional symptoms of the condition at 7 years (Christakis, Zimmerman, DiGiuseppe, et al., 2004). It is likely that there are many types of attention deficit, resulting from several different mechanisms that involve interaction of genetic, biological, and environmental risk factors (Gottesman, 2003).

The pathophysiology of ADD/ADHD is unclear, but certain brain characteristics provide clues. Some children may exhibit a deficit in the catecholamines dopamine and norepinephrine, lowering the threshold for stimuli input. The disorder is marked by brain maturation delay in the area of self-regulation. Increased input from stimuli and decreased self-regulation cause the hallmark inability to inhibit stimuli and motor activity. Some children exhibit additional problems such as aggressive behaviors, learning disabilities, and motor disorders.

Clinical Manifestations

Children with ADD and ADHD have problems related to decreased attention span, impulsiveness, and/or increased motor activity (Figure 34–6 ■). Symptoms can range from mild to severe. The disorders often coexist with various developmental learning disabilities. The child has difficulty completing tasks, fidgets constantly, is frequently loud, and interrupts others. Sleep disturbances are common. Because of these behaviors, the child often has difficulty developing and maintaining social relationships and may be shunned or teased by other children. This only increases the anxiety of the already compromised child, whose behavior is set on a downward spiraling course (American Academy of Pediatrics, 2000).

Typically, girls with ADHD show less aggression and impulsiveness than boys, but far more anxiety, mood swings, social withdrawal, rejection, and cognitive and language problems. Girls tend to be older at the time of diagnosis. Children are frequently diagnosed with the disorder soon after beginning school, when demands increase for attentive behavior. See Box 34–4 for the *DSM-IV-TR* diagnostic criteria for attention deficit hyperactivity disorder.

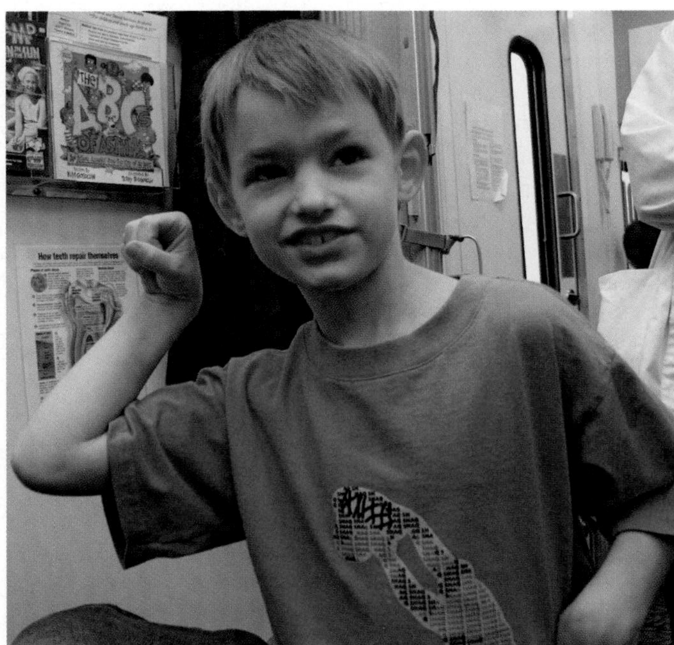

FIGURE 34–6 ■ This child with ADHD is challenged by a visit to a healthcare facility for dental care. He found it difficult to remain in the chair for the examination, and once it was over, he rapidly ran from one piece of equipment to another in the facility. He asked what things were for, but did not wait for answers. His engaging personality can be seen as he poses briefly for a picture. Such behaviors can be exhausting for parents to manage, and may create safety hazards in the healthcare setting.

BOX 34–4 *DSM-IV-TR* Diagnostic Criteria for Attention Deficit Hyperactivity Disorder

A. Either 1 or 2:

1. Inattention: Six (or more) of the following symptoms of inattention have persisted for at least 6 months to a degree that is maladaptive and inconsistent with developmental level:
   - **a.** Often fails to give close attention to details or makes careless mistakes in schoolwork, work, and other activities
   - **b.** Often has difficulty sustaining attention in tasks or play activities
   - **c.** Often does not seem to listen when spoken to directly
   - **d.** Often does not follow through on instructions and fails to finish schoolwork, chores, or duties in the workplace (not due to oppositional behavior or failure to understand instructions)
   - **e.** Often has difficulty organizing tasks and activities
   - **f.** Often avoids, dislikes, or is reluctant to engage in tasks that require sustained mental effort (such as schoolwork or homework)
   - **g.** Often loses things necessary for tasks or activities (e.g., toys, school assignments, pencils, books, or tools)
   - **h.** Is often easily distracted by extraneous stimuli
   - **i.** Is often forgetful in daily activities
2. Hyperactivity-impulsivity: Six (or more) of the following symptoms of hyperactivity-impulsivity have persisted for at least 6 months to a degree that is maladaptive and inconsistent with developmental level:

Hyperactivity
   - **a.** Often fidgets with hands or feet or squirms in seat
   - **b.** Often leaves seat in classroom or in other situations in which remaining seated is expected
   - **c.** Often runs about or climbs excessively in situations in which it is inappropriate (in adolescents or adults, may be limited to subjective feelings of restlessness)
   - **d.** Often has difficulty playing or engaging in leisure activities quietly
   - **e.** Is often "on the go" or often acts as if "driven by a motor"
   - **f.** Often talks excessively

Impulsivity
   - **a.** Often blurts out answers before questions have been completed
   - **b.** Often has difficulty awaiting turn
   - **c.** Often interrupts or intrudes on others (e.g., butts into conversations or games)

B. Some hyperactive-impulsive or inattentive symptoms that caused impairment were present before age 7 years.

C. Some impairment from the symptoms is present in two or more settings (e.g., at school [or work] and at home).

D. There must be clear evidence of clinically significant impairment in social, academic, or occupational functioning.

E. The symptoms do not occur exclusively during the course of a Pervasive Developmental Disorder, Schizophrenia, or other Psychotic Disorder and are not better accounted for by another mental disorder (e.g., Mood Disorder, Anxiety Disorder, Dissociative Disorder, or a Personality Disorder).

MediaLink ADD/ADHD Video

COLLABORATIVE CARE

Families and professionals collaborate to make the diagnosis and ensure adequate treatment for the child with ADHD. Parents often refer the child to a pediatrician or other primary care provider. A specialist in the disorder should then be consulted for the diagnosis. School personnel will be asked for their observations in order to meet diagnostic criteria. Parents and professionals in healthcare and school partner to plan and provide care for the child.

Diagnostic Tests

Children are usually brought for evaluation when behaviors escalate to the point of interfering with the daily functioning of teachers or parents. When children have learning disabilities or anxiety disorders, the problem is commonly misdiagnosed as ADHD if full and accurate evaluation of the child's symptoms is not performed. Obtaining an accurate diagnosis by a pediatric mental health specialist is vital (American Academy of Pediatrics, 2000). Specific diagnostic criteria must be applied to all children with the potential diagnosis (see DSM criteria in Box 34–4). The diagnosis of ADD is often difficult due to the absence of hyperactivity behaviors. Behaviors both at home and school or childcare must be evaluated, because abnormal patterns in two settings are needed for diagnosis. A variety of tests are available for use by the trained professional in establishing the diagnosis.

Diagnosis begins with a careful history of the child, including family history, birth history, growth and developmental milestones, behaviors such as sleep and eating patterns, progression and patterns in school, social and environmental conditions, and reports from parents and teachers. A physical examination should be performed to rule out neurological diseases and other health problems. The mental health specialist then performs testing of the child and administers questionnaires to the parent and teacher. See Table 34–3 for examples of comprehensive testing resources. It is important to identify other conditions that may either mimic as ADD/ADHD or exist in conjunction with the disorders. These might include depression, anxiety, learning disorder, conduct disorder, or oppositional defiant disorder (Adesman, 2003).

Clinical Therapy

Treatment is established to meet the desired behavioral outcomes, and includes a combination of approaches, such as environmental changes, behavior therapy, and pharmacotherapy (American Academy of Pediatrics Committee on Quality Improvement, 2001). It is expected that treatment will be long term.

Children often benefit from environmental changes. Decreasing stimulation, for example, by turning off television, keeping the environment quiet, and maintaining an orderly and clutter-free desk or study area without distractions, may help the child to stay focused on the task at hand. Another relatively simple change is appropriate classroom placement, preferably in a small class with a teacher who can provide close supervision and a structured daily routine. Consistent limits and expectations should be set for the child. Children living in chaotic homes and communities may function better if the environment can be simplified. When aggressive behaviors occur, therapeutic approaches such as play and group therapy may be useful.

Behavior therapy involves rewarding the child for desired behaviors and applying consequences for undesirable behaviors. Children may be rewarded by praise or earn points toward a movie or other desired outing for staying seated during meals or quietly listening in a classroom. Cues are established so that a child can subtly be reminded when impulsive or hyperactive behaviors are escalating. All adults who are in close contact with the child, such as parents and teachers, must be informed and involved in the established behavioral program.

Children with moderate to severe ADD/ADHD are treated with pharmacotherapy. Methylphenidate (Ritalin, Concerta) is most often prescribed. Usually a favorable response (a decrease in impulsive behaviors and an increase in the ability to sit still and attend to an activity for at least 15 minutes) is seen in the first 10 days of treatment and frequently with the first few doses (Box 34–5). Other medications that may be used include dextroamphetamine (Dexedrine or Adderall) and the nonstimulant medication Atomoxetine. Occasionally the tricyclic antidepressants desipramine and imipramine, and the antidepressant bupropion (Wellbutrin) are helpful, particularly with presence of comorbitities (other mental health disorders) (American Academy of Pediatrics Committee on Quality Improvement, 2001).

See the medication table on page 1382 for a listing of common pharmacologic treatments.

A variety of other treatments have been attempted for ADHD, and are used by families. Chiropractic manipulation, biofeedback, and dietary interventions (both elimination diets

TABLE 34–3 Screening Tests for ADD/ADHD

TEST	SOURCE
Vanderbilt Parent and Teacher Scales	Wolraich, M. L. (1998). *Journal of Abnormal Child Psychology, 26,* 141; Wolraich, M. L. (2003). *Journal of Pediatric Psychology, 28,* 559.
Connors' Parent and Teacher Rating Scales—Revised—Long Form	Connors, C. K. (1998). Journal of Abnormal Child Psychology, 26, 257, 279.
Swanson, Nolan and Pelham Questionnaire II Teacher and Parent Rating Scale (SNAP-IV)	Swanson, J. M. (1992). *School-based assessments and interventions for ADD students.* Irvine, CA: KC Publications.
Disruptive Behavior Disorder Scale	Pelham, W. E. (1992). *Journal of the American Academy of Child and Adolescent Psychiatry, 31,* 210.
ADHD Rating Scale	DuPaul, G. J. (1991). *American Academy of Child and Adolescent Psychiatry, 20,* 245.

Data from Liu, Y. H., & Leslie, L. K. (2003). Diagnosing ADHD: Putting AAP guidelines to the test—and into practice. Contemporary Pediatrics, 20*(12), 51–73.*

BOX 34–5 Research: Stimulant Treatment of ADHD and Future Risk of Substance Abuse

Data from six studies of people with ADHD were combined and analyzed. A total of 647 children with ADHD treated with stimulants during childhood and 360 who were not treated with these medications were evaluated in adulthood. Those treated with stimulants in childhood had significantly less substance abuse as adults than did those children not treated. This should be reassuring for parents who are concerned about the possible harmful effects of stimulant use for children with ADHD (Wilens, 2003). In addition, the recent introduction of the first nonstimulant medication for ADHD treatment, Atomoxetine, introduces a new and novel way to treat the disorder and may be more acceptable to some parents.

and supplement use) are examples of common complementary or alternative therapies.

Although ADHD was once thought to be a disorder of childhood that gradually improved with age, it is now believed that symptoms continue into adulthood and that careful management in childhood assists in lessening problems of social functioning later in life.

NURSING MANAGEMENT

Nursing management consists of referring children with possible ADHD for appropriate screening, monitoring the child's growth and development, following progress in behavioral manifestations, and partnering with parents and other professionals in the treatment of the disorder.

Nursing Assessment and Diagnosis

The nurse often encounters the family who is concerned about the child's behavior before a diagnosis has been made. Ask about family and birth history and have the parents describe the child's behaviors. Perform developmental testing and look specifically for attention span and physical activity. Refer the family to their pediatric healthcare home for further assessment, and then to a mental healthcare specialist who is experienced in diagnosing ADHD.

The nurse may encounter the child with known ADHD in the hospital when parents bring the child for treatment of an injury (e.g., fracture) or other problem. Explore the parents' report of the child's attention span in detail. Usually within a few minutes in an unstructured setting or waiting area, the child with ADHD becomes restless and searches for distraction. Gather information about the child's activity level and impulsiveness. Be alert for information that reveals a serious problem, such as hurting animals or other children. Obtain information about distractibility, attention deficit in activities of daily living, characteristic ways of reacting, and the extent of impulsiveness when the child is receiving medication. Find out how the family manages at home and what treatment is being used.

Examples of nursing diagnoses that may be appropriate for a child with ADD/ADHD include the following:

- Impaired Verbal Communication related to altered perceptions
- Impaired Social Interaction related to chronic episodes of impulsive behavior
- Chronic Low Self-Esteem related to behaviors associated with ADD/ADHD
- Risk for Injury related to high level of impulsiveness and excitability
- Risk for Caregiver Role Strain related to management of child with unpredictable moods and high energy

Planning and Implementation

Nursing care of the hospitalized child with ADD/ADHD focuses on administering medications, managing the child's environment, implementing behavioral management plans, providing emotional support to the child and family, promoting self-esteem, and ensuring ongoing care. Care in the community includes the same components along with guiding parents to appropriate resources when needed. Prevention can focus on discouraging regular television exposure for young children from 1 to 3 years and encouraging daily vigorous physical activity for all children.

Administer Medications

Stimulant and nonstimulant medications increase the child's attention span and decrease distractibility. Be alert for the common side effects of these medications, including anorexia, insomnia, and tachycardia. Administering medication early in the day helps to alleviate insomnia. Anorexia can be managed by giving medication at mealtimes. Careful periodic monitoring of weight, height, and blood pressure is necessary. Instruct families about the abuse potential of stimulant drugs; they should be kept locked and administered only as directed.

Minimize Environmental Distractions

The child may need to be placed in an environment with minimal distractions. When hospitalized, this may mean a room with only one other child. Potentially harmful equipment should be kept out of reach. Television and video game time needs to be monitored and limited. Use shades to darken the room during naps or at bedtime and minimize noise. Integrate plans for physical activity into the day and limit television and video games.

Implement Behavioral Management Plans

Behavior modification programs can help to reduce specific impulsive behaviors. An example is setting up a reward program for the child who has taken medication as ordered or completed a homework assignment. The rewards may be daily as well as weekly or monthly, depending on the child's age. For example, one completed homework assignment might be rewarded with 30 minutes of basketball or a bike ride; assignments completed

MEDICATIONS Used to Treat ADHD

MEDICATION	ACTION AND INDICATION	NURSING IMPLICATIONS
Methylphenidate	A derivative of piperidine that acts like amphetamine. May work in ADHD treatment by enhancing catecholamine effects in the NS, improving attention span and task performance. Schedule II drug in Schedule of Controlled Substances.	Available in short-acting forms of 5, 10, and 20 mg as Ritalin and Methylin, and in 2.5, 5, and 10 mg forms as Focalin. Also in intermediate-acting forms of 20 mg (Ritalin SR), 10 and 20 mg (Metadate ER and Methylin ER). Available in long-acting forms of 18, 27, 36, and 54 mg (Concerta), 20 mg (Metadate CD), and 20, 30, and 40 mg (Ritalin LA). The variety of available forms makes it important to read labels carefully and inform families about proper administration of the child's specific type of drug. Periodic growth measurements are needed. Behavior and school performance are monitored.
Amphetamine preparations	Synthetic sympathomimetic amine with stimulant effect on CNS. Increases release of norepinephrine and dopamine by blocking their reuptake. Schedule II drug in Schedule of Controlled Substances.	Available in short-acting forms of 5 mg (Dexedrine), 5 and 10 mg (CextroStat) and 5 and 7.5 mg (Adderall). Intermediate-acting forms include 10, 12.5, 15, 20 and 30 mg Adderall, and 5, 10 and 15 mg Dexedrine Spansules. A long-acting form is 5, 10, 15, 20, 25, or 30 mg Adderall-XR. Read labels and instruct in proper administration. Monitor vital signs and growth measurements periodically.
Atomoxetine	This is the first nonstimulant drug for treatment of ADHD. It inhibits norepinephrine reuptake. Decreases hyperactivity and impulsivity of ADHD and may assist with improving mood and decreasing anxiety.	Available in 10, 18, 25, 40, and 60 mg capsules. Recommended starting dose for children is 0.5 mg/kg/day. Has been shown to have long-lasting effect of 1 day or longer. Side effects are uncommon and transient, with dyspepsia or vomiting, fatigue, decreased appetite, and dizziness most common. Have the child change position slowly if dizziness occurs; caution teen not to drive until effects of drug are clear. Perform periodic growth measurements.

Data from Buck, M. L. (2003). Atomoxetine: A new alternative for the treatment of attention-deficit/hyperactivity disorder. Pediatric Pharmcology, *9(2). www.medscape.com/viewarticle/452714, accessed 5/7/2003; Stein, J. A., & Baren, M. (2003). Welcome progress in the diagnosis and treatment of ADHD in adolescence.* Contemporary Pediatrics, *20(8), 83–107.*

for a week might be rewarded with participation in an activity of the child's choice on the weekend. Find out what behavioral rewards are being used at school and home and integrate them as much as possible into hospital routines.

If punishment is necessary, the behavior should be corrected while simultaneously supporting the child as a person. Punishment is generally withdrawal of a privilege, and should follow the offense quickly as the child may not otherwise connect the punishment with the behavior.

Provide Emotional Support

Children with ADD or ADHD offer a special challenge to parents, teachers, and healthcare providers. Parents must cope simultaneously with managing the difficult needs and demands of a hard-to-handle child, obtaining appropriate evaluation and treatment, and understanding and accepting the diagnosis, even when the child exhibits different behaviors with different people. Family support is essential. Educate both the parents and the child about the importance of appropriate expectations and consequences of behaviors. Teach skills that will help as the child grows older: making lists of tasks to accomplish; implementing routines for eating, sleeping, recreation, and schoolwork; minimizing stimuli in the environment when completing work; and asking teachers and friends to identify when behavior is inappropriate. When the child is hospitalized for another condition, the time may provide a brief respite from constant care by the parent. The activity, impulsivity, and general high energy of children with ADHD can fatigue parents. They may wish to spend a few hours each day at home or a nearby residence for families when the child is hospitalized. Ask them how they manage at home and offer ideas for respite care.

Promote Self-Esteem

Help the child to understand the disorder at an appropriate developmental level, and facilitate a trusting relationship with healthcare providers. Assist the child with social skills through the use of role play, small-group play, and modeling. Promote the child's self-esteem by emphasizing the positive aspects of behavior and treating instances of negative behavior as learning opportunities. Help the child to develop ego strengths (the conscious ability to screen outside stimuli and to control internal demands), which will result in better impulse control and thus increase self-esteem over time. Praise the child for lying still for a procedure, taking a medication on time, or helping a staff member to carry toys around to other children.

Care in the Community

Most children with ADD or ADHD are only hospitalized when needing care for another condition. Parents need support to understand the diagnosis and to learn how to manage the child so this will usually be accomplished in the pediatric healthcare home or in the office of a mental health specialist. Explain the diagnosis and what is known about attention deficit disorders. Provide written materials and Internet sites, and an opportunity to ask questions. See Developing Cultural Competence: ADHD and Sensitivity.

Emphasize the importance of a stable environment, at home as well as at school. At home, the child may have difficulty staying on task. Teach parents to minimize distractions at home during periods when the child needs to concentrate, for example, when doing schoolwork. Visits to areas such as shopping malls and playgrounds may need to be limited, especially on school days. Ensure daily physical activity and frequent activity breaks during school and homework sessions. Limit television, video, and com-

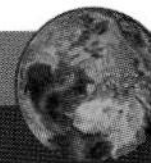

DEVELOPING CULTURAL COMPETENCE
ADHD and Sensitivity

Many families who have a child with ADHD or another mental health disorder are embarrassed and feel shame because of the diagnosis, especially in certain cultures such as some Asian groups, and in very structured and highly achieving families. When taking histories from family members, it is best to be sensitive to the stigma they may feel. Ask questions in a private setting and ask about the family's feelings regarding a mental health disorder. Is there someone in their family who they can talk to about the diagnosis? Provide information in a nonjudgmental manner and offer support if appropriate from other families with similar experiences.

puter use to less than the usual recommended daily maximum of 2 hours. Parents need to consider age and developmental appropriateness of tasks, give clear and simple instructions, and provide frequent reminders to ensure completion. Routines in the evening can promote good sleep patterns (Figure 34–7 ■).

The nurse can serve as a liaison to teachers and school personnel, or as the case manager for the child. An individualized education plan may be needed (see Chapter 20∞), with clear expected outcomes stated for the child's behaviors. Special classrooms or periods of instruction free from the distractions of the entire class may enable the child to improve school performance. Parents may have difficulty understanding the need for these approaches because the child often tests with above-average intelligence. Reinforce the importance of providing a structured environment free from unnecessary external stimuli. Be sure that parents understand behavioral approaches that will help the child, how to administer prescribed medications, and the importance of returning for healthcare visits to monitor for side effects. (See Partnering with Families: School Suggestions for Children with ADD/ADHD.) Ensure that medication is locked safely away at home and school to

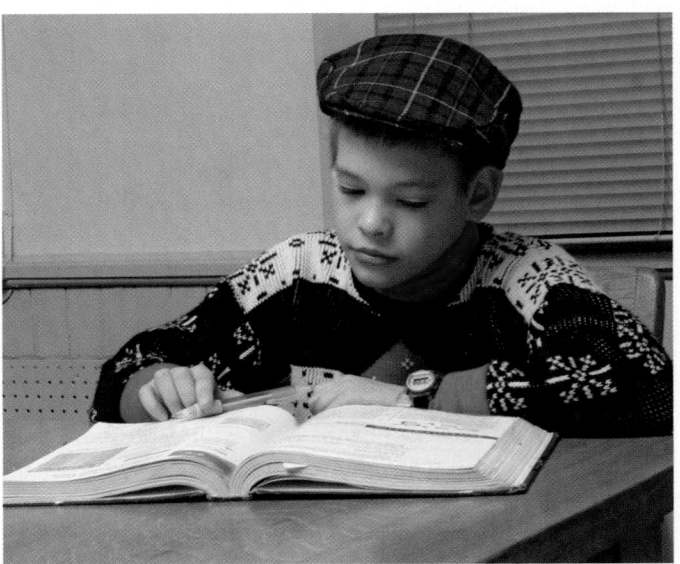

FIGURE 34–7 ■ Managing the environment to provide quiet places with minimal distractions is often necessary for the child with ADHD. This boy reads and does homework in a room with few pictures, no music, and has only the book with homework on the table. He is also assisted by structure such as a scheduled time for homework, with short breaks to walk around every 10–15 minutes.

PARTNERING WITH FAMILIES

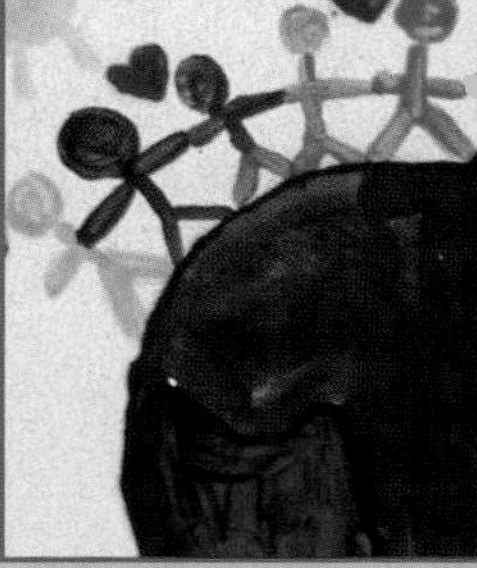

School Suggestions for Children with ADD/ADHD

Parents can work with teachers to provide for a school environment that fosters attention and learning. Ideas that may be helpful include:

- Having the child sit near the front of the class.
- Plan a reminder that is apparent to teacher and student but not to other children when the child needs to concentrate on attention. This might be an object placed on the student's desk or hand placed gently on the shoulder or arm.
- Give instructions verbally and in written form and repeat them more than once.
- Provide opportunities to take notes and make lists of assignments and mark them off when accomplished.
- Computers may be useful for making lists and taking notes. The child may need to listen in class, record the teacher, and take notes later from the recording.
- If the child has well-developed fine or gross motor skills, integrate motor movement into learning situations when possible.
- Provide quiet places with minimal distraction for examinations. Offer additional time.
- Go over assignments and tests with the child in person to explain areas that are understood and those that need attention.
- Find the child's areas of excellence and allow for performance in these ways. Some children are talented in dance, others in art or extemporaneous speech.
- Never call the child names, make fun of behavior or performance, or call them "hyperactive" in front of other children, teachers, or parents.

Adapted from Stein, J. A., & Baren, M. (2003) Welcome progress in the diagnosis and treatment of ADHD on adolescence. Contemporary Pediatrics, 20, *83–107.*

keep it away from other children and prevent illegal use of this controlled substance. An individualized school health plan may be needed for medication management.

Children with ADD or ADHD may have few friends due to their impulsivity, lack of connectedness with other children, and other behaviors. Ask about social interactions and recommend participation in school and community sports and clubs where the rules of working with others can be learned.

Parents may have heard about attention deficit disorders in the media and can have many questions about its cause and management. Providing information about complementary and alternative treatments is a nursing role (see Complementary Therapy: ADD/ADHD).

As the child grows older, provide explanations about the disorder and information about techniques that will assist in dealing with problems. Emphasize the importance of doing homework or other tasks requiring concentration in a quiet environment without

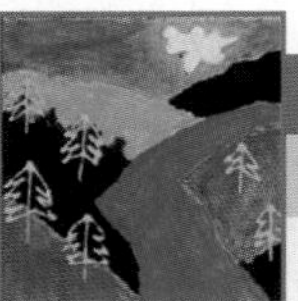

COMPLEMENTARY THERAPY

ADD/ADHD

ADD and ADHD are common diagnoses and there are many claims in the media about what causes these conditions. Parents may wish to try a variety of approaches in addition to or instead of traditional behavioral therapy and medication. Some common alternative therapies include elimination of dietary components such as highly processed foods, sugar, aspartame, or yeast. Other therapies include use of supplements such as iron, magnesium zinc, and vitamin B_6. Herbs such as pycnogenol, melatonin, Echinacea, St. John's wort, and gingko biloba are sometimes used, as are visual and auditory training. Parents do not typically tell healthcare providers about use of herbs; 70%–75% have not discussed their use during healthcare visits. Ask parents about alternative therapies used and investigate what is known about them in order to share this information with parents (Cala, Crismon, & Baumgartner, 2003).

background noise from a television or radio. Encourage children with ADD/ADHD to keep assignment notebooks and use checklists to help them accomplish specific tasks. Such interventions lead to establishment of a positive self image and confidence in the ability to manage the condition successfully.

Evaluation

Expected outcomes of nursing care for the child with ADD or ADHD include the following:

- Understanding of disorder by parents and child
- Management of medication administration
- Increase in attentiveness and decrease in hyperactivity, impulsivity, and sleep disturbance
- Formation of positive self-image in the child
- Formation of healthy social interactions with peers and family
- Educational performance to maximum potential

MOOD DISORDERS

The major mood disorders in children are depression and bipolar disease, both of which are discussed in this chapter. A third disorder, dysthmic disease, is less common in children but represents an additional mood disorder. It has similar but milder symptoms than depression; however, it lasts longer with a mean duration of 3 years.

Depression

Depression is psychological distress that can range from mild to severe. Only in recent years has depression in children been recognized as a clinical condition. Many children referred to child guidance centers and mental health professionals due to behavioral difficulties or poor achievement actually suffer from depression. The incidence of major depression is estimated to be about 2% in prepubertal children and about 4% to 8% in adolescents. Males and females are equally affected until adolescence when the incidence in girls rapidly increases until they are twice as commonly afflicted (Shugart & Lopez, 2002; Castiglia, 2000a and 2000b).

Etiology and Pathophysiology

Many theories have been proposed to explain the cause of depression in children and adolescents. Depression may be biologic in origin or a result of learned helplessness, cognitive distortion, social skills deficit, or family dysfunction. The physiological theory focuses on monoamine neurotransmission. These amines include indolamine, serotonin, norepinephrine, and dopamine, and decreases are sometimes found in depression. Childhood depression sometimes occurs secondary to parental depression, because the parent with depression is unable to provide the child with effective parenting. Abuse and neglect predispose children to depression, especially very young children. In about half of all children with depression, at least one other psychiatric diagnosis is made; these include conditions such as ADHD, anxiety disorder, or another personality disorder. Depressive disorders may contribute to other mental illness such as disturbed relationships, substance abuse, and suicide (Lyon & Morgan-Judge, 2000). Obesity is more common in depressed adolescents.

Clinical Manifestations

Characteristic findings of major depression in children and adolescents include declining school performance; withdrawal from social activities; sleep disturbance (either too much or too little); appetite disturbance (too much or too little); multiple somatic complaints, especially headaches and stomachaches; decreased energy; difficulty concentrating and making decisions; low self-esteem; and feelings of hopelessness. There is much variation among children in the symptoms displayed, and they often have some but not all of the major criteria (Williamson, Birmaher, Brent, et al., 2000).

Symptoms of depression in children vary according to their developmental levels. Infants may fail to eat and grow, toddlers can show regressive behaviors in toileting and other activities, and school children may show a decrease in academic performance, increased or decreased activity, somatic complaints, and loss of friends. Children may be irritable and manifest frequent death themes in their play. The adolescent can have a wide array of symptoms such as anxiety, decreased social contact, poor school performance, lack of prior involvement in activities, poor self-care, difficulty with parents and teachers, or focus on violence. Sadness and **anhedonia** (inability to experience pleasure) are common at all ages.

COLLABORATIVE CARE

Nurses partner with families and other health professionals to ensure adequate treatment of the child with depression. They may include parents, school nurses and teachers, pediatricians, and mental health specialists.

Diagnostic Tests

Initial assessment is performed by a child psychologist or child psychiatrist. A variety of scales and techniques are used; however, very little guidance is available relating to evaluation of children under 6 years of age. Examples of useful tools are:

- Children's Depression Inventory (CDI)
- Revised Children's Manifest Anxiety Scale

- Beck Depressive Inventory
- Reynolds Child Depression Scale
- Reynolds Adolescent Depression Scale
- Center of Epidemiologic Studies Depression Scale of Children (CES-DC)

The child is tested for various mental health problems since comorbidities or combination with other disorders is common. (Jellinek, Patel, & Froehle, 2002).

Clinical Therapy

Treatment may include psychotherapy in combination with psychotropic medication. Often a combination of individual, family, and group therapy provides the greatest benefit for young children and adolescents. Involving parents and other family members in the treatment plan is essential. Group therapy is an effective treatment measure for adolescents because of the importance of peer group relationships during the teenage years. Cognitive therapy may be used with adolescents, and play therapy with younger children, as demonstrated in the case of Cassandra in the opening scenario (see discussion of play therapy earlier in this chapter).

Antidepressant medications, most commonly the selective serotonin reuptake inhibitors (SSRIs); tricyclic antidepressants (TCAs) such as imipramine (Tofranil) and desipramine (Norpramin); and amitriptyline (Elavil), may be prescribed. Analysis of TCA studies have demonstrated their usefulness in adolescents but not in children (Hazell, O'Connell, Heathcote, et al., 2002).

PRACTICE ALERT

Sudden cardiac death has occurred in several children on tricyclic antidepressants (TCAs). Due to this risk, serum levels should be monitored and electrocardiograms (ECGs) performed. Specific ECG changes along with a resting heart rate above 100, systolic blood pressure above 130 mm Hg, and diastolic blood pressure above 85 mm Hg necessitate immediate report to the prescriber.

The SSRIs act to block reuptake of serotonin in the synapse, so that serotonin levels (which influence mood) increase. Although the SSRIs are generally considered safer than some other types of antidepressants, their use in children has been limited; there have been reports of increased suicidal ideation, and cautions must be taken. Fluoxetine is the only SSRI approved for use in children and adolescents for treatment of depression by the U.S. Food and Drug Administration; the other SSRIs have been used clinically but adequate research has not demonstrated their safety or efficacy in children. A major serious side effect is serotonin syndrome, and potential increase in suicidality and agitation are of great concern.

PRACTICE ALERT

Serotonin syndrome, the serious and life-threatening side effect of SSRIs, is caused by overstimulation of serotonin receptors. It is more likely to develop when the child or adolescent is also taking St. John's wort, other antidepressants, alcohol, diet pills, or abuse drugs such as ecstasy and LSD (Lyon & Morgan-Judge, 2000). Be certain to ask questions in a nonjudgmental way about intake of any alternative therapies, other medications, or substance use to identify those most at risk.

Serotonin syndrome is characterized by agitation, muscle twitching, gastric upset, chills, fever, confusion, and dizziness. Generally the child is started with a low dose and it is increased slowly to minimize chance of side effects. There have been recent reports of children who developed suicidal thoughts and committed suicide while taking SSRIs. Because of these reports and the lack of efficacy evidence, the FDA has cautioned against use of paroxetine in children under 18 years and boxed warnings are provided on antidepressants as described below (National Institute of Mental Health, 2004).

PRACTICE ALERT

There have been reports of increased suicidal ideation and other behavioral changes in children and adolescents taking antidepressant medications. In both the United States and Canada, the medications are now accompanied by clear warnings for use in these age groups. Agencies in both countries have alerted healthcare providers and families of the risks, but leave decisions about medications to the prescribers and families, since the risk of depressive illness in itself carries a risk of harm to the individual.

In the U.S., the Food and Drug Administration recommends that a Patient Medication Guide (MedGuide) be provided to each patient explaining the risks of the drug and precautions to take. In addition, the following information should be in a boxed warning on the drug labels:

- Antidepressants increase the risk of suicidal thinking and behavior in children and adolescents with major depressive disorder and other psychiatric disorders.
- Anyone considering the use of an antidepressant in a child or adolescent for any clinical use must balance the risk of increased suicidality with the clinical need.
- Patients who begin medication therapy should be observed closely for clinical worsening, suicidality, or unusual changes in behavior.
- Families and caregivers should be advised to closely observe the patient and to communicate with the prescriber.
- A statement regarding whether the particular drug is approved for any pediatric indication and if so, which one(s).

Note: The only antidepressant approved to treat major depressive disorder in pediatric patients is fluoxetine HCL (Prozac). Drugs approved for obsessive-compulsive disorder (see discussion later in this chapter) in pediatrics include Fluoxetine HCL (Prozac), sertraline HCL (Zoloft), fluvoxamine maleate (Luvox), and clomipramine HCL (Anafranil).

In Canada, a Therapeutic Products Directorate has been issued by Health Canada. It notes that SSRIs and other new antidepressants in patients under 18 years may be associated with behavioral and emotional changes, including severe agitation-type adverse events coupled with self-harm or harm to others. The agitation-type events include akathisia, agitation, disinhibition, emotional lability, hostility, aggression, depersonalization, often within several weeks of starting treatment.

Nurses must reinforce this important teaching for all families when the child or adolescent receives medication, and emphasize the importance of follow-up visits and prompt reporting of any changes in the child/adolescent behavior.

Data from U.S. Food and Drug Administration (2004). FDA Public Health Advisory, October 15, 2004. Accessed on March 25, 2005 from http://www.fda.gov.cder/drug/antidepressants/SSRIPHA200410.htm and Health Canada (2004). Therapeutic Products Directorate: TPD-Web, June 2, 2004. Accessed on March 25, 2005 from http://www.hc-sc.gc.ca/hpfb-dgpsa/tpd-dpt/paxil_hpc_e.html

NURSING MANAGEMENT

Nursing management focuses on encouraging the child and family to participate in therapy and to report side effects to drugs and any changes in condition.

Nursing Assessment and Diagnosis

A thorough history and physical examination, including observation of behavior, are obtained at the time of admission. Assess the child for common risk factors for depression (Table 34–4).

Several nursing diagnoses that may be appropriate for the child or adolescent hospitalized with depression are included in the accompanying nursing care plan. Other diagnoses may include the following:

- Imbalanced Nutrition: More than Body Requirements related to eating in response to internal cues other than hunger
- Powerlessness related to sense of helplessness
- Chronic Low Self-Esteem related to negative self-evaluation

Planning and Implementation

Nursing care of the child or adolescent hospitalized for depression includes administering medications and other therapy, and providing supportive care. Monitor vital signs of youth receiving antidepressant medications. Watch for common side effects of the agent(s) used. Carefully monitor for serious side effects of TCAs or SSRIs and be aware that lower doses are used at initiation with doses increasing slowly to desired level. All behavior and ideation changes are noted with alterations in dosages. Monitor cardiovascular status, including hypertension and tachycardia, observe motor movement, and record dietary intake. Help parents to evaluate inpatient settings to be certain the care provided will best meet the needs of the child or adolescent. See Partnering with Families: Selecting Residential and Inpatient Care for the Child with Mental Illness. Refer to the nursing care plan for specific nursing interventions for the child or adolescent hospitalized with depression.

Discharge Planning and Home Care Teaching

When the child has been hospitalized and is returning home, teach parents to recognize signs and symptoms of worsening depression. Parents should also be taught dosages and side effects of any prescribed medications. Review data in the MedGuide for any medications with the family. Caution not to alter dose or discontinue drug without guidance and monitoring of prescriber. Refer the family to appropriate healthcare professionals and to support groups for family members dealing with depression. Instruct to remove guns and other potentially harmful items from the home.

Care in the Community

Most children with depression are cared for in the community. Maintain regular contact with family members through their healthcare visits to outpatient agencies and by making home visits. Monitor the child's affect, activity, and food intake. School teachers and counselors often are aware of the child's ability to perform in the school setting. Have the family schedule afterschool care so young children with depression are not left at home alone for extended periods. Assist the family in finding support for financial and emotional needs related to managing the child's depression.

Evaluation

Expected outcomes for nursing care of the child with depression are found in the accompanying nursing care plan.

Bipolar Disorder (Manic Depression)

Bipolar disorder is a mental illness in which extreme changes in affect and energy are manifested. Moods most often alter between mania and depression. Children often present with irritability or hyperactivity. About 1.5% of the total population and 1% of children suffer from bipolar illness, although diagnosis and accurate numbers are difficult to obtain due to the frequency of accompanying additional mental illness and the lack of clear diagnostic criteria in childhood. Twenty percent of patients with bipolar disorder have the first manic episode in adolescence (Jellinek et al., 2002). About 10% to 20% of individuals with bipolar illness commit suicide. The average age for children to demonstrate bipolar disorder is 11 years, but an initial manic episode at 5 years is not uncommon. Children may show mainly depressive symptoms, and then develop mania in adolescence, or may have episodes of both mania and depression in the same day.

Little is known about the etiology and pathophysiology of bipolar disease. The manic phase of bipolar illness is characterized by hyperactivity and high energy, irritability, aggression, and sometimes hallucinations. In the depressive phase, the child is sad, has alterations in sleep and eating patterns, and is socially withdrawn, similar to any depressive illness. The presence of comorbidities makes diagnosis difficult. Disorders that often present in the same children include conduct disorder, attention deficit hyperactivity disorder, depression, anxiety, autistic disorder, mental retardation, and Tourette's syndrome (Mohr, 2001).

TABLE 34–4 Risk Factors for Child and Adolescent Depression

CHILD	FAMILY	SCHOOL AND SOCIAL SITUATIONS
➤ Frequent feelings of sadness, sleep problems, loss of interest in activities ➤ Increase in risk taking and impulsivity ➤ Previous suicide attempt ➤ Alcohol or substance abuse ➤ Diagnosed psychotic disorder ➤ Chronic illness and frequent hospitalization	➤ Parental neglect, abuse, or loss ➤ Dysfunctional family relationships ➤ Family history of depression, suicide, substance abuse, alcoholism, other psychopathology	➤ Academic pressures and underachievement ➤ Stressful social relationships ➤ Declining participation in social events

COLLABORATIVE CARE

Collaborative care focuses on early identification of bipolar illness so that treatment can begin when it is most effective.

Diagnostic Tests

Diagnosis and treatment of bipolar disorder should be performed by mental health specialists. Use of alcohol or illegal drugs should be ruled out as a cause of symptoms, even in children. Since the manic phase is often manifested by hyperactivity, the child may incorrectly be treated with stimulants (see discussion of ADHD earlier in this chapter), and the disease can be worsened. There are not specific criteria for diagnosis of bipolar disease in children, and yet they are unique in presentation. More often the determining characteristic is severe irritability rather than euphoria.

Clinical Therapy

The treatment of bipolar disease involves a variety of drugs used to stabilize mood. Lithium, valproate (Depakote), and carbamazepine (Tegretol) are most frequently used (Weller, Calvert, & Weller, 2003). Individual and family education and therapy can be helpful. The most important measure in preventing serious further illness is early recognition and treatment so referral to mental health specialists is essential.

NURSING MANAGEMENT

Nurses are instrumental in identifying children with the disorder, providing information to families, and monitoring the drugs and psychotherapy for the child.

Nursing Assessment and Diagnosis

The nurse is aware of children with symptoms of bipolar disorder when they appear in any setting. Be alert for the child described as having wide mood swings and irritability. A low tolerance for frustration and overactive stress and startle response may occur. Ask about response to stressful situations and change in behavior over time. Be alert for substance abuse and other mental health disorders. Based on the assessment, several diagnoses may be established, including:

- Risk for Injury related to behaviors in manic phase and potential suicide in depressive phase
- Impaired Social Interaction related to irritability and frustration
- Powerlessness related to mood instability

Planning and Implementation

The child with bipolar disorder needs ongoing care to ensure implementation of therapy and return to function. The nurse administers medications in some settings and instructs parents, the child, and other family members in other settings. Observe for side effects specific to the drug regimen used. Assist parents to find resources for healthcare since medications and other treatments may be costly. Parents and children need information about the disorder as it may recur several times throughout the child's life. Assist the child to find social events and groups that build a sense of self-esteem.

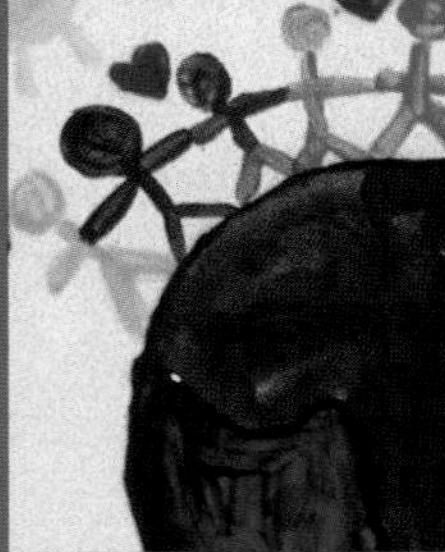

PARTNERING WITH FAMILIES

Selecting Residential and Inpatient Care for the Child with Mental Illness

Families need guidelines to assist them in evaluating inpatient facilities when a child with a mental disorder must be placed in an institution. They can be referred to the National Alliance for the Mentally Ill website. Nurses can provide questions for the families to ask:

- What is the staff-to-youth ratio?
- What are the guidelines for chemical and physical restraint?
- Are children isolated when behaviors are inappropriate?
- Are children constantly monitored visually when in restraint or when potentially dangerous to self or others?
- Does the child have a full physical and psychological evaluation by a specialist within 24 hours of entry to the facility?
- What professionals review the plan of care and how often?
- To whom can the family speak for regular updates on the child?
- How often can the family visit?
- What services will be covered by insurance?
- What subjective feelings does the family member have when visiting the unit and facility?
- What services will be offered on an ongoing basis upon discharge?

Evaluation

The desired outcomes for a child with bipolar disorder include:

- Interest in school, family, and other life events
- Successful family management of stressors that challenge resources
- Personal conviction of child related to managing life and its stresses
- Congruence with expected role behaviors for developmental age

ANXIETY AND RELATED DISORDERS

A large group of anxiety disorders can affect youth as well as adults. Some of the more common types seen in children and adolescents are described in this section, with detailed nursing management described after the last condition, posttraumatic stress disorder.

Generalized Anxiety Disorder

Anxiety is a subjective feeling of uncertainty, worry, and helplessness, usually accompanied by CNS signs, including restlessness,

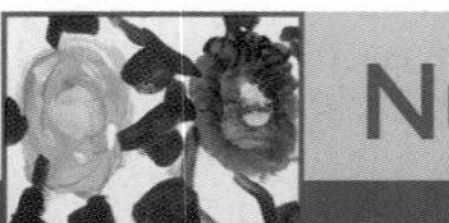

Nursing Care Plan

THE CHILD OR ADOLESCENT HOSPITALIZED WITH DEPRESSION

GOAL	INTERVENTION	RATIONALE	EXPECTED OUTCOME
1. Hopelessness related to long-term stress			
	NIC Priority Intervention—*Hope Instillation:* Facilitation of the development of a positive outlook		**NOC Suggested Outcome**— *Hope:* Presence of internal state of optimism that is personally satisfying and life supporting.
The child or adolescent will discuss feelings of hopelessness.	■ Encourage open expression of feelings. Explore hopeless, sad, or lonely feelings. Point out the connection between feelings and behavior. Assess the child or adolescent to identify the precipitating event when feelings of sadness arose. ■ Encourage the child or adolescent to take part in self-care and unit activities. Use routines to establish feelings of control. ■ Medicate as ordered and document results.	■ Expressing feelings may help to relieve sadness, loneliness, despair, and hopelessness. An accepting and nonjudgmental attitude must be maintained regarding any feelings expressed by the child. ■ An active role in self-care and treatment helps the child or adolescent to feel more in control. ■ Antidepressants modify mood to a more hopeful outlook.	By discharge, the child or adolescent expresses an interest in the future.
2. Ineffective Individual Coping related to inadequate social support or disturbance in pattern of appraisal of threat			
	NIC Priority Intervention—*Coping Enhancement:* Assisting a patient to adapt to perceived stressors, changes, or threats which interfere with meeting life demands and roles.		**NOC Suggested Outcome**—*Coping:* Actions to manage stressors that tax an individual's resources.
The child or adolescent will use effective coping skills.	■ Teach positive, effective coping strategies such as guided imagery and relaxation. Assist the child or adolescent to focus on strengths rather than weaknesses. ■ Assist the child or adolescent to identify friends, family members, and others who are positive and supportive.	■ Therapeutic techniques can help the child or adolescent to replace negative thoughts and images with more positive and effective beliefs and Images. These interventions foster resilience. ■ Helps the child or adolescent to become aware that people can be caring and supportive (thus validating self-esteem).	The child or adolescent verbalizes and demonstrates ability to cope appropriately for his or her age.

trembling, perspiration, and rapid pulse. The disorder is often manifested in children with restlessness, excessive fatigue, poor concentration, irritability, muscle tension, and sleep disturbance (American Psychiatric Association, 2000). Anxiety disorder affects about 4% of high school students and is second to only substance abuse (see Chapter 7∞) in incidence for mental disorders (Smoller, Finn, & White, 2000). While all children experience anxiety at certain times, those with anxiety disorder are excessively worried about many things and are difficult to reassure. They are not able to distract themselves from the worry. Many youth have accompanying physical complaints, such as headache or stomachache.

Anxiety disorders are strongly linked to familial and genetic factors. They may coexist with other mental health disorders, or children sometimes have more than one type of anxiety (Walsh, 2002). Diagnosis is performed by a mental health specialist and treatment is usually medication and individual therapy. While a variety of medications have been used to treat adults, studies are lacking in children. One medication that has been reported as safe and effective in children in at least one study is sertraline 50 mg/day (Rynn, Siqueland, & Rickels, 2001).

Separation Anxiety Disorder

Separation anxiety disorder is characterized by an extreme state of uneasiness when in unfamiliar surroundings and often by refusal to visit friends' homes or attend school for at least 2 weeks. Approximately 75% of children with separation anxiety disorder refuse to attend school (see "School Phobia" later in the chapter). Many children worry about losing a parent or significant other. They may have physical complaints, nightmares, and other sleep disturbance. This disorder occurs in approximately 4% to 5% of children and in twice as many girls as boys (Masi, Mucci, & Millepiedi, 2001). The peak age for occurrence is 7 to 9 years (Walsh, 2002). It may be recurrent and become worse at certain times.

Children with separation anxiety disorder tend to be perfectionistic, overly compliant, and eager to please. They appear to

Nursing Care Plan THE CHILD OR ADOLESCENT HOSPITALIZED WITH DEPRESSION (continued)

GOAL	INTERVENTION	RATIONALE	EXPECTED OUTCOME
3. Impaired Social Interaction related to self concept disturbance			
	NIC Intervention—*Socialization Enhancement:* Facilitation of ability to interact with others.		**NOC Outcome**—*Social Interaction Skills:* An individual's use of effective interaction behaviors.
The child or adolescent will participate in and initiate activities and conversation.	■ Assist the child or adolescent to identify topics and activities of interest. ■ Encourage interaction with peers and staff. ■ Facilitate visits from family and friends. ■ Provide guidance to family regarding interaction that promotes self-esteem.	■ The more the child or adolescent focuses on areas of interest, the less he or she will focus on internal anxiety and depression. ■ Each positive interaction reinforces feelings of success. Each success reinforces the desire for future social interaction. ■ Reinforces positive and rewarding relationships. ■ The family's existing interaction style is often negative.	By discharge, the child or adolescent initiates conversation and activities with staff and peers.
4. Imbalanced Nutrition: Less than Body Requirements related to loss of appetite secondary to depression			
	NIC Intervention—*Nutrition Management:* Assistance with or provision of a balanced dietary intake of foods and fluids.		**NOC Outcome**—*Nutritional Status:* Amount of food and fluid taken into the body over a 24-hour period.
The child or adolescent's daily intake will be adequate to maintain optimal nutritional status.	■ Offer nutritious finger foods, sandwiches, and high-calorie liquid supplements frequently throughout the day. ■ Offer easy-to-carry drinks that are high in vitamins, minerals, and calories. ■ Encourage daily vigorous physical activity of at least 30 minutes.	■ Convenient easy-to-eat foods encourage the child or adolescent to eat and maintain nutritional status. ■ These are a convenient method for meeting hydration and electrolyte needs. ■ Physical activity stimulates appetite.	The child or adolescent's daily intake will be adequate to maintain optimal nutritional status by discharge.

cling to the parent or caretaker. They may use physical complaints such as headaches, abdominal pain, nausea, and vomiting in an attempt to avoid being away from the parent. Depression frequently accompanies separation anxiety disorder. The resulting avoidant behaviors can interfere with personal growth and development, academic achievement, and social functioning.

CLINICAL TIP

The separation anxiety experienced by a toddler differs from the psychiatric disorder in age appropriateness, duration, and severity. Separation anxiety disorder affects children of preschool age or older, lasts for at least 2 weeks, and is characterized by excessive anxiety. In contrast, the separation anxiety experienced by the toddler directly follows a separation from a familiar caretaker, lasts only for a short time after the separation, and is a normal developmental response in toddlers.

Diagnosis is made by a mental health specialist. Treatment includes both child and parents. Parents learn about the disorder and how to structure the setting so that the child is expected to attend school. Consistency in expectations is necessary; if the child is permitted to stay home some days or has missed school and other activities for longer periods, treatment is more difficult. Both parents and child work out the expectations for behavior for the child with the mental health therapist. Medication has occasionally been used if other therapy is not helpful. The SSRI fluoxetine has been used with a dose of 24 mg/day for children and 40 mg/day for adolescents (Walsh, 2002). See the medication table on page 1390.

Panic Disorder

Panic disorder is the presence of recurrent, unexpected panic attacks. These attacks are periods of intense fear and discomfort in the absence of real danger. The risk of panic disorder ranges from 1.5% to 3.5% of the population (Smoller et al., 2000), with adolescence a common age for the onset of symptoms. The risk of panic disorder is 20 times more likely when there is a family history of the disorder (American Psychiatric Association, 2000).

MediaLink Case Study: Calculate SSRI Dosage

MEDICATIONS Used to Treat Depression

Selective Serotonin Reuptake Inhibitor (SSRI) Drugs Used to Treat Depression

MEDICATION	PEDIATRIC DOSE	ADOLESCENT DOSE	SELECTED SIDE EFFECTS
Fluoxetine (Prozac)	2.5-40 mg qd or 0.5-1 mg/kg/day	10–60 mg qd	Restlessness, headaches, akathesia
Sertraline (Zoloft)	25–125 mg qd or 1.5-3 mg/kg/day	50–200 mg qd	Dry mouth, gastric upset
Paroxetine (Paxil)	5–40 mg qd or 0.25-0.7 mg/kg/day	20–40 mg qd	Dry mouth, weight gain
Fluvoxamine (Luvox)	50–100 mg bid or 1.5-4.5 mg/kg/day	50-300 mg qd	Dry mouth, gastric upset
Citalopram (Celexa)	Little data available	10–40 mg qd	Dry mouth, nausea, sleep disturbance

Note: Data from Shugart, M. A., & Lopez, E. M. (2002). Depression in children and adults. Postgraduate Medicine, 112*, 53–61; Walsh, K. H. (2002). Welcome advances in treating youth anxiety disorders, 19(9), 66–82.*

Note: Although a variety of SSRIs are used in treatment of children and adolescents, the only approved U.S. FDA medication for major depressive disorder in this age group is Prozac, and the only approved FDA medications for OCD in pediatric age group are Prozac, Zoloft, Luvox, and Anafranil.

Examples of the physical symptoms experienced are palpitations, sweating, chills, hot flashes, shaking, shortness of breath, choking, chest pain, nausea, and dizziness. The person describes feelings of danger or doom. There may be accompanying agoraphobia in some people. **Agoraphobia** is an anxiety of being in places or situations from which escape may be difficult or embarrassing, or in which help may not be available. The attacks may be continuous or episodic, but generally are chronic in nature.

Diagnosis is made by a mental health specialist. Similar to anxiety, treatment may involve individual and family therapy, with use of medication (SSRIs) in some cases (Carson, 2000).

Obsessive-Compulsive Disorder

Individuals with obsessive-compulsive disorder (OCD) may be mildly or severely affected. One in about 200 children is affected, and there may be associated conditions such as tic disorders or attention deficit hyperactivity (Leonard, Freeman, Barcia, et al., 2001). Affected children have recurrent ritualistic thoughts or actions; these obsessions or compulsions interfere with daily life. Examples of behaviors and concerns are obsessions about dirt or germs, worries about harm, and sexual thoughts. Common behaviors are excessive handwashing, counting objects, and hoarding substances. These practices may take 1 or more hours each day. Children with OCD differ from adults in several ways. They have more aggressive obsessions, such as fears of catastrophe, more commonly hoard objects, and are more likely to have religious obsessions. The presence of additional mental health disorders is common (Geller, Biederman, Farone, et al., 2001).

Causes of OCD are not clear. The basal ganglia of the brain are affected and a genetic link is observed. Poststreptococcal autoimmune disorder may be a cause in some cases (Box 34–6).

Diagnosis is made by a mental health specialist. The disorder may have been present for some time before diagnosis since parents tend to overlook or deny the symptoms, and children may hide the behaviors. Treatment may involve cognitive-behavioral therapy, where the feared occurrence is presented and the person learns that no harm will occur. Medications, such as clomipramine and the SSRIs, are effective in most children and adolescents. Nurses can identify cases and refer for psychiatric evaluation. Families need detailed instruction about medications and potential side effects (see Practice Alert on page 1385).

School Phobia

School phobia (also called school avoidance or school refusal) is a persistent, irrational, or excessive fear of attending school. The child may fear being harmed or losing control. School phobia is common in children between 5 and 12 years of age, but can occur in children up to 16 years. The child's avoidance of school is often a manifestation of fear of leaving the parent or primary caretaker. Children commonly report that teachers and peers "pick on" them. Somatic complaints are similar to those in children with separation anxiety disorder. Characteristically, symptoms are present only on school days and not on weekends or holidays.

Treatment includes the family and child, and establishes firm limits for behavioral expectations and consequences, similar to treatment for separation anxiety disorder. Antidepressant medications may sometimes be needed to promote the child's feelings of comfort. The longer a child is out of school, the greater the likelihood that a chronic, treatment-resistant condition will result. Referral for psychiatric evaluation is indicated for persistent symptoms.

Conversion Reaction

Conversion reaction is a disorder in which a disturbance or loss of sensory, motor, or other physical functions suggests neurologic or other somatic disease. The disturbance or loss cannot be explained by any known pathophysiologic mechanism. Instead, psychologic factors are involved. About 3% of the population

BOX 34–6 Research: PANDAS

Pediatric autoimmune neuropsychiatric disorders (PANDAS) are characterized by obsessive-compulsive and/or tic disorder, childhood onset, association with Group A beta hemolytic streptococcal infection, and neurological abnormalities. It is believed that in certain children, the strep infection leads to a neural autoimmune response, resulting in the psychiatric disorder. Research continues to identify possible mechanisms, results, and treatments for this cause of OCD (March, 2004).

experiences conversion reactions at some time (American Psychiatric Association, 2000). Adolescence and early adulthood are common times for the onset to occur.

Conversion reactions develop in response to a catastrophic event such as threat, loss, or harm. Clinical manifestations include altered sensations such as blindness or deafness; paralysis or ataxia, including inability to stand or walk and loss of ability to speak (aphonia); involuntary movements, such as pseudoepileptic convulsions; and constant complaints of pain with no physical basis (psychogenic pain). Children under 10 years usually present with gait abnormalities or seizures. The onset of conversion symptoms is usually dramatic and sudden. Symptoms often appear to be neurologic, but on careful examination obvious discrepancies are found. The person is usually calm about the symptoms even though they are serious. Often the child or family members appear indifferent or unconcerned over what healthcare providers consider an overwhelming physical disability.

Children suspected of having a conversion reaction require a complete physical and neurologic evaluation to rule out any possible physiologic basis for the symptoms. Individual and family therapy is usually necessary to identify the source of the psychologic conflict, pain, or need resulting in the conversion symptoms.

Posttraumatic Stress Disorder

Etiology and Pathophysiology

Posttraumatic stress disorder (PTSD) patients have experienced or witnessed a life-threatening event that could potentially result in death or severe injury (Meltzer-Brody, Hidalgo, Connor, et al., 2000). The event is persistently reexperienced through thoughts, dreams, or memories. Although accurate statistics are not available on children, about 1% to 2% of children are probably affected, with increasing numbers as more children are exposed to war and other violence (Kessler, 2000). The child or adolescent with the disorder has feelings of fear, terror, and helplessness, and may relive the event frequently in thought and nightmares. The child may become emotionally numb in a subconscious attempt to protect the self, but may have a persistently increased state of arousal (Kent, Sullivan, & Rauch, 2000). Examples of events that are associated with posttraumatic stress include sexual or other child abuse, rape, car crash, fire, witnessing violence, and having experience in war. The events which occurred in the United States on September 11, 2001, are potential causes of posttraumatic stress in children who either had a family member involved, lived near the events, or in some other way were profoundly affected.

Cassandra, described in the opening scenario, was experiencing PTSD due to a car crash as she was driven to school. She was too young to describe her feelings verbally to her mother or school personnel; however, she manifested sleep abnormalities and other complaints common in the disorder (Figure 34–8 ■). Even children of Holocaust victims experience PTSD, leading mental health professionals to believe that the condition can be transmitted from parent to child (Yehud, Hallig, & Grossman, 2001). There is a relatively high incidence of PTSD among incarcerated youth (Lamberg, 2001). (See Chapter 7∞.)

The disorder involves both a traumatic event and the child's reaction to this event. It is believed that brain changes occur in trauma, leading to neurobiological alterations that cause dysfunction of memory. Females, those with other psychiatric disorders, a family history of psychiatric illness, and severe or lengthy trauma are all risk factors. The incidence ranges from 1% to 9% (Meltzer-Brody et al., 2000).

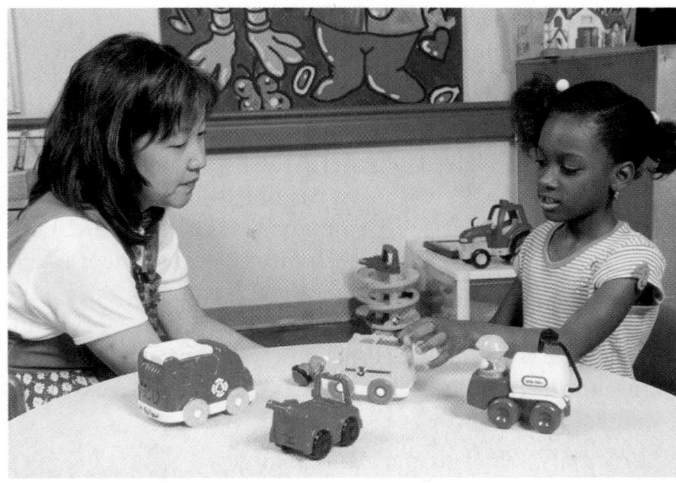

FIGURE 34–8 ■ The psychologist uses play therapy to help Cassandra reenact her car crash. This helps her gain control over the event so that it is not so frightening.

Clinical Manifestations

The child with PTSD is often irritable, and has sleep problems and inattentiveness. There is a state of hypervigilance and exaggerated startle response, such as to touch or loud noises. The person feels detached from others and alone. Immediately after the event the child may appear to have adapted and functions normally. However, after several weeks or even months, the symptoms of the disorder begin to appear.

COLLABORATIVE CARE

Collaborative care for children with PTSD involves identification of the condition and treatment so that long-term consequences can be avoided.

Diagnostic Tests

The diagnosis is made by a mental health specialist. A history of traumatic event with normal childhood developmental behaviors before the event is characteristic.

Clinical Therapy

Counseling by a mental health specialist is the main therapy for PTSD. A variety of antidepressants and SSRIs can be used for pharmacologic treatment. Cassandra's clinical psychologist used play therapy to help her to communicate her fears related to the car crash. Once the fears are clearly communicated, they often lose their power over the person, so that normal behaviors can resume.

NURSING MANAGEMENT

Nursing management for PTSD patients and other anxiety disorders focuses on partnering with other health professionals

MediaLink Critical Thinking: Females and PTSD

and families to relieve the child's anxiety and return the child to a normal, developmentally appropriate level of functioning.

Nursing Assessment and Diagnosis

Nurses often help to identify PTSD patients and others with anxiety disorders so that care can be obtained. Ask about traumatic events in the past and how the child reacted. Inquire about recent changes in the child's behavior. Include school attendance, complaints of physical illness, sleep patterns, and rituals in behavior. A family history of mental disorders may be useful. Based on the data gathered, the child's symptoms, and the mental health diagnosis, the nurse determines nursing diagnoses. Examples include:

- Anxiety related to unconscious conflict
- Ineffective Coping related to perceived high degree of threat
- Powerlessness related to chronic mental illness
- Disturbed Sleep Pattern related to anxiety
- Posttrauma Syndrome related to motor vehicle or other accidents

Planning and Implementation

Nursing care for anxiety disorders focuses on behavioral and cognitive therapies to enhance coping skills. Mental health nurses may conduct group therapy sessions both in inpatient and community settings (Figure 34–9 ■). Group sessions for children often provide a forum for discussion of fears, an opportunity to enhance skills of working together, and an opportunity to learn coping skills. Being a member of a group with other children experiencing anxiety or trauma can remove the stigma and allow the child the freedom to explore feelings, behaviors, and their causes. Several of the techniques described earlier in the chapter, such as drawing pictures and discussing them or telling stories, are techniques used by mental health nurses in child therapy groups.

Children need to learn relaxation techniques and nurses may teach such techniques or recommend that the child consider participation in yoga or guided imagery classes. Inquire about alternative therapies that the child and family are using or have an interest in beginning, and refer as needed. See Complementary Therapy: Selected Methods for Anxiety Disorders.

> **COMPLEMENTARY THERAPY**
> **Selected Methods for Anxiety Disorders**
>
> - Herbal therapy—e.g., St John's wort
> - Self-hypnotic relaxation—to reduce pain and anxiety
> - Acupuncture—for anxiety, depression
> - Massage therapy—for anxiety, anger, grief
> - Reflexology (manual stimulation of specific points on the foot)—for anxiety
> - Guided imagery—to relieve anxiety
> - Biofeedback (use of machines to watch muscle or skin responses)—for anxiety

Parents or other significant people should be included in the treatment program. Nurses often teach them basic information about the child's diagnosis and therapy. They should be in at least some therapy sessions with the child. Provide resources that they need for relief from worry about the child, guilt about causing an accident that triggered the child's symptoms, or other feelings related to the diagnosis. See Partnering with Families: Talking with Children about Traumatic Events.

Insurance companies may provide limited payment for mental health services. Help the family to see the importance of recommended therapy and assist them to find resources for care if needed.

School personnel may need to know about the child's treatment. Partner with the families to provide needed information. Some schools have counselors that can be instrumental in carrying out treatment plans at school and acting as a resource in that setting. School personnel may be asked to provide feedback about the child's attendance, performance, and social skills as a measure of the success of therapy and the community or school nurse can relay this information.

Nurses often administer medications to children being treated for anxiety. Be alert for side effects and ensure the fam-

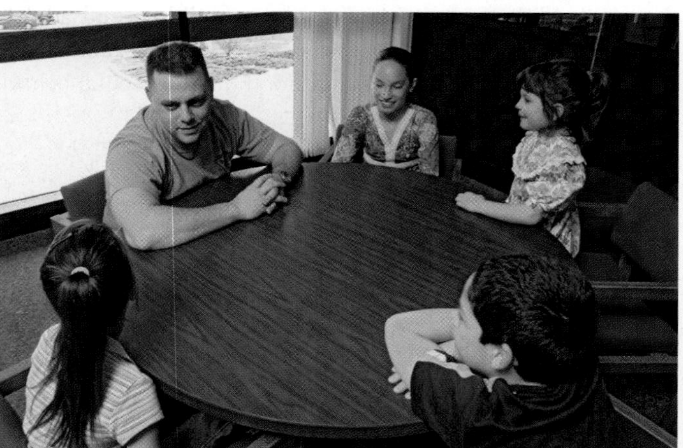

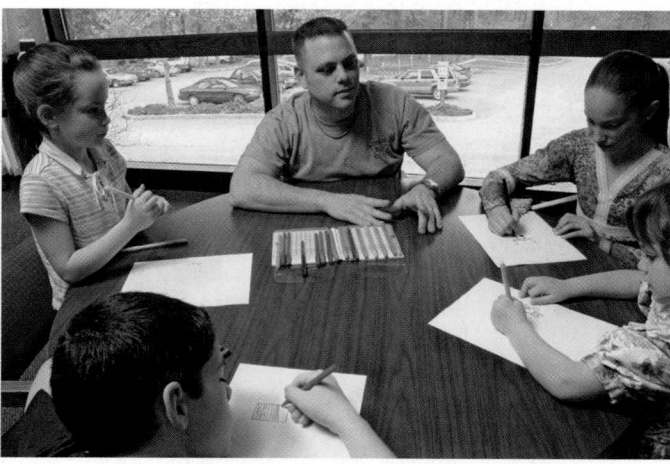

FIGURE 34–9 ■ This nurse conducts a group therapy session for children who have experienced traumatic events and have resulting anxiety disorders. He is clearly engaged, has a positive rapport, and fosters exchanges among the children. Games and drawing are frequent techniques used in the group.

ily knows how to safely administer the drugs. They should be kept locked securely. Have the child return for follow-up as needed since some medications may take several weeks to achieve effects, and close monitoring is essential. The child should have a medication alert tag for drugs being taken.

Evaluation

The outcomes of nursing care for the child with anxiety disorder center on return to normal developmental activities, engagement in social relationships, learned coping skills for dealing with stress, and maintenance of safety.

SUICIDE

Suicide is the third leading cause of death in adolescents between 15 and 19 years of age. Over the past 40 years, teenage suicide has nearly tripled (Fish, 2000; National Strategy for Suicide Prevention, 2001). Suicide accounts for about 14% of deaths in teens. About 9% of teens and 1% of prepubertal children have attempted suicide. Many more children have suicidal thoughts; 12% of 6- to 12-year-olds and 53% of adolescents have had suicidal thoughts (Horowitz, Wang, Koocher, et al., 2001). See Developing Cultural Competence: Suicide and Ethnicity.

Males die as a result of suicide four times more often than females. This statistic is reversed for suicide attempts, perhaps because boys use lethal methods such as guns, hanging, and jumping more often than girls, who more commonly use drug overdose and wrist cutting. There may be different triggers for suicide in female and male adolescents. Female adolescents consider suicide more frequently when their situations are unstable, and it is often an impulsive act. Male adolescents think of suicide when they are depressed and when their social environment is unsatisfactory.

It is not unusual for healthcare professionals and parents to label suicide attempts by children and adolescents as accidents. Up to half of childhood suicides may be recorded as accidents; suicide data for children under age 10 years are not maintained.

DEVELOPING CULTURAL COMPETENCE
Suicide and Ethnicity

Some ethnic groups have a high rate of suicide. For example, Native Americans and Alaskan Natives have a rate of suicide at 1.5 times the national average. Many youth in this group are suicide victims; it is the third major cause of death in Native American youth. The historic pain experienced by this ethnic group and lack of opportunities for many youth may be some of the reasons for a high suicide rate. Hispanic females have a higher rate of suicide than other gender and ethnic groups. White males have traditionally had highest rates of suicide, but recently Blacks have had greatly increasing numbers of suicides (Rew, Thomas, Horner, et al., 2001; Centers for Disease Control and Prevention, 2004a). *Healthy People 2010* goals focus on eliminating such health disparities by finding the causes, setting up prevention programs, and providing more support and opportunities for native populations.

PARTNERING WITH FAMILIES

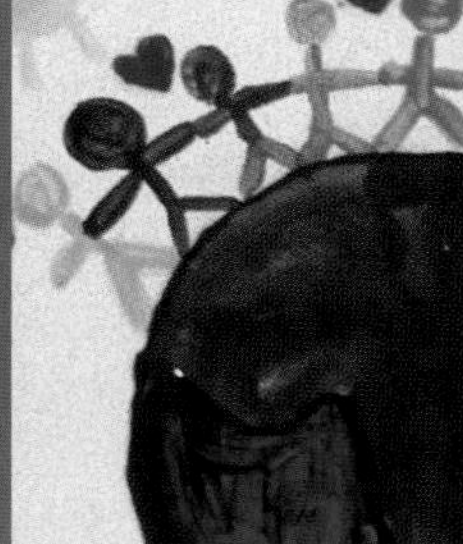

Talking with Children about Traumatic Events

Whether a child or adolescent experiences trauma from a car crash, abuse, or environmental event, parents can help to decrease the effects of the stress and prevent the appearance of posttraumatic stress disorder by doing the following:

- Be sure children feel comfortable asking parents, teachers, or others about the events and their feelings.
- Assure children that their feelings are normal and may return over time.
- Be honest and open in responses, without overloading the child with more details than they need.
- Be prepared to repeat answers and discuss the same topics many times.
- Get help from counselors who can suggest how to talk with the child.
- Use communication methods appropriate at various ages, such as reading books, doing art projects, or drawing.
- Show children that they are loved by spending time and planning activities with them.
- Limit the television and other media time where the child is exposed to violence and traumatic events. Do not have television on so often that children repeatedly view a traumatic event.
- Restore a sense of normal routines into the child's life.
- Be alert for increasing signs of distress and seek care from a professional if they occur.

Adults may have difficulty believing that young children, in particular, would have any reason to want to end their lives. For this reason, many children who are brought to the emergency department with indications of a suicide attempt are often classified as unintentional injury victims and released without arrangements for appropriate follow-up care.

Many risk factors for suicide exist in children and adolescents, and there are also known protective factors (Table 34–5). The most common precursor to adolescent suicide is depression (see previous discussion). Common signs or symptoms of an underlying depression that could lead to suicide include boredom, restlessness, problems with concentration, irritability, lethargy, intentional misbehavior, preoccupation with one's own body or health, and excessive dependence on or isolation from others (especially adults or caregivers). The depression may be exacerbated by a recent psychosocial stress such as loss or perceived rejection or ridicule. Youth who are gay or lesbian may feel stigmatized, and have a higher risk of suicide (Russell & Joyner, 2001). A previous attempt is also a common risk factor (Zametkin, Alter, & Yemini, 2001).

The child or adolescent found to be at high risk for suicide may be admitted to a psychiatric unit for care or cared for in a community mental health facility. When a suicide attempt is

TABLE 34–5 Risk and Protective Factors for Suicide in Children and Adolescents

RISK FACTORS	PROTECTIVE FACTORS
History of previous attempted suicide	Emotional well-being
Friend committed or attempted suicide	Satisfactory school performance
School problems or changes in grades	Participation in sports or other group events
Pregnancy	Weight satisfaction
Drug use or abuse	Parent/family connectedness
Problems with a romantic relationship	Frequent discussions of important issues with family
Minority sexual practice	School connectedness
Loneliness, withdrawal	Safe school
Feelings of anxiety	Safe neighborhood
History of chronic family problems	Caring adult presence at school or elsewhere
Chronic illness	Availability of school counseling
Physical, emotional, or sexual abuse	School policies to limit and cope with fighting, bullying
History of suicide in a family member	
History of depression	
Chronic low self-esteem	
Change in behavior	
Change in weight	
Giving away special possessions	
Access to firearms and ammunition	

made, the child or adolescent may be hospitalized for 24 hours, kept in a short-term monitoring unit, or sent home under close observation to ensure adequate assessment and monitoring. It is important to provide crisis intervention at the time of the suicide attempt to minimize the opportunity for repeat attempts and to begin a therapeutic treatment plan.

Treatment may include individual, group, or family therapy. Negotiating a no-suicide contract is an important first step in therapy. In the contract, the child agrees not to attempt suicide during a specified time period. The presence of a contract is not a guarantee of child safety so vigilant monitoring of the youth's condition continues. Comorbidities such as depression or substance abuse must also be addressed for treatment to be successful.

MediaLink Suicide Prevention Resources and Support

NURSING MANAGEMENT

Nursing Assessment and Diagnosis

The major nursing role is in prevention of suicide. All children and adolescents in health promotion visits and emergency rooms should be evaluated for risk. Health promotion visits are an opportunity to be alert for children with depression (see previous discussion), substance abuse, recent stresses, and changes in behavior. Gather a family history of mental health disorders, suicide attempts, and stresses. Ask about how often the youth talks with or has meals with the family. Most suicides are committed with firearms present in the home. At each healthcare visit determine if the family has firearms. Encourage them to keep the guns unloaded, with ammunition and firearms locked in separate locations. Be sure that children and adolescents do not have access to the keys for the locked firearms.

The most important questions to ask of a youth admitted to the emergency room for a suicide attempt are as follows:

- Are you here because you tried to hurt yourself?
- In the past week, have you been having thoughts about hurting yourself?
- Have you ever tried to hurt yourself in the past other than this time?
- Has something very stressful happened to you in the past few weeks?

(Horowitz et al., 2001)

Possible nursing diagnoses for the child at risk of suicide are:

- Risk for Suicide related to hopelessness and substance abuse
- Risk for Self-directed Violence related to history of suicide attempts, present suicidal ideation, and recent failure in school
- Readiness for Enhanced Family Coping related to recent teen attempted suicide

Planning and Implementation

Care in the Hospital

Many children at risk for suicide or who have just attempted to commit suicide will be admitted to the hospital for a period of monitoring. Therapy is initiated and medications can be given under close supervision.

Nursing care centers on taking appropriate precautions to ensure the safety of a child or adolescent at risk of suicide. The child and the environment of the hospital or other setting are monitored for any object that could be used for self-harm. All potentially harmful objects, such as shoestrings, belts, pantyhose, and hair ribbons, are removed. All personal care items (including toothbrush and shampoo) are kept locked at the nursing station and monitored constantly when used by the child.

Children or adolescents who are considered at high risk for suicidal behaviors are attended by a nursing staff member at all times, including while using the bathroom and sleeping. It may be necessary for the child to dress in a plain hospital gown, be kept in a visually monitored seclusion room, or (if seriously impaired and self-abusive) be medicated for restraint for a period of time. Restraints are used only when ordered by the physician and interdisciplinary team caring for the youth. Physical restraint is only a short-term approach to provide immediate safety if necessary. Chemical restraint (medication) may need to be used to prevent self-injury by the suicidal person. See page 1387 for information to help families consider when choosing care for their suicidal child.

Hospitalization continues as long as the child's behavior is self-destructive. Children are referred for intensive individual and family therapy to begin in the hospital and continue after discharge.

Care in the Community

Encourage parents to keep follow-up clinic appointments, to watch for self-destructive behaviors, and to administer any prescribed medications according to the treatment schedule. Arrange home visits and other community resources for families.

Education in all school settings is appropriate to assist children in awareness of resources for help when needed and in identifying peers at risk. Be alert for children and adolescents at risk for suicide in any setting. Assess children and adolescents in schools, outpatient settings, and emergency rooms for the possibility of suicidal behavior. Report threats of suicide and depressive behavior. Recognize that when one suicide has occurred, there may be an increased risk for friends of the victim. Teach students to report to teachers, nurses, or counselors about friends who have threatened suicide or seem depressed or display behaviors different than usual. Nurses often plan with mental health specialists to implement suicide prevention programs in schools and communities (King, 2001). Provide supportive services to family and friends when suicide occurs. Consult websites and refer parents as appropriate. The Suicide Prevention Resource Center has helpful regional offices to facilitate networks at national, state, territorial, community, and tribal levels.

Evaluation

Desired outcomes related to suicide risk include:

- Family develops coping strategies to support suicidal member.
- Child or adolescent takes actions to decrease sadness and increase interest in life events.
- Child or adolescent remains safe with no further suicide attempts or ideation.

TIC DISORDERS AND TOURETTE'S SYNDROME

Tics are sudden, rapid, recurrent, nonrhythmic, and brief motor movements or vocalizations. They may involve movement of the head or upper body, blinking of eyes, or a variety of verbal noises. They may be worse during periods of stress or tiredness. Many children have mild motor tics at some time which gradually disappear with no intervention. Midadolescence is the most common age for tics to appear. When the tics are severe or last over 1 year, they are considered chronic and may require attention from a mental health provider (Snider, Seligman, Ketchen, et al., 2002).

Severe motor tics accompanied by verbal utterances are known as Tourette's syndrome. The syndrome is often accompanied by other diagnoses such as attention deficit and learning disabilities (Kurlan, McDermott, & Deeley, et al., 2001). Children with Tourette's syndrome may exhibit **coprolalia,** the involuntary utterance of obscenities, profanities, and racial slurs, or **copropraxia,** the involuntary use of obscene gestures.

There is an underlying genetic cause for tic disorders since about 75% have a family history. Boys are more affected than girls suggesting an autosomal dominant transfer. The direct pathophysiology of the disorder is unknown but dopamine, serotonin, and other neurotransmitter and neuropeptide levels are disrupted. Comorbidity commonly involves obsessive compulsive disorder. The disorders have been treated with haloperidol in adults; pimozide (Orap), a dopamine receptor antagonist, is approved for treatment of childhood tics. Other treatments involve self-monitoring and progressive relaxation (Kuperman, 2002).

CLINICAL TIP

Children with Tourette's syndrome may initially be diagnosed with ADHD due to their increased activity. If they are medicated with a drug such as methylphenidate (Ritalin, Concerta), their activity will worsen. Monitor symptoms carefully after the child begins taking medication and be sure the child is seen regularly for ongoing care.

Nursing care involves supporting parents and encouraging normal developmental progression for the child. Stress should be minimized and relaxation techniques taught. Administer medications and teach families about desired and side effects. If the child's verbal utterances are disruptive in the classroom, partner with families and school to arrange for home tutors for a while if needed. The nurse can be instrumental in teaching school personnel and other children about the disorder so that they understand the child's behaviors.

Trichotillomania

Trichotillomania, or chronic hair pulling, can affect children and adolescents. Head hair is most commonly pulled, leaving patches of baldness, but eyebrows, eyelashes, pubic and other body hair may be involved. Incidence is greatest in middle childhood but it can occur earlier or later. Hair pulling may occur in brief periods of stress or over longer periods during sedentary activities.

Trichotillomania is classified as an impulse control disorder. It has similarities to both obsessive-compulsive disorder and Tourette's syndrome, described earlier in the chapter (Whitaker, Wolf, & Keuthen, 2003). Behavioral therapy, hypnosis, and SSRI medication therapy are generally used in treatment. Group therapy may be an effective support mechanism that helps to decrease guilt and feelings of isolation.

People affected by the disorder usually feel shame and guilt. They try to hide the disorder and may not seek help for an extended period. The nurse should be alert for the disorder when head or body hair is missing, someone is wearing a wig, or eyebrows are heavily penciled. An appropriate way to question is to say, "Some people pull out their hair. I notice that you have no eyebrows or eyelashes. Is pulling them out something you do?"

Refer the child or adolescent to a healthcare professional. Try to establish a trusting atmosphere that fosters communication about the disorder. Encourage participation in the treatment plan. Ensure follow-up for care so effectiveness of treatment can be measured.

SCHIZOPHRENIA

Schizophrenia is a psychotic disorder that is relatively rare in young children and adolescents, although it can occur in children as young as 5 years of age. The prevalence of schizophrenia increases after puberty and reaches adult levels by late adolescence. About 1 in 10,000 children develop schizophrenia (Lambert, 2001).

The cause of schizophrenia is unknown, but genetic predisposition or a neurovirus during the mother's pregnancy may play a role in its occurrence (Lambert, 2001). The brain is altered in the disease, with progressively enlarged ventricles and nervous system arousal. Impaired glucose metabolism is often present. The disorder most often manifests between 15 and 20 years of age. Onset is usually slow with increasing intensity over time. Most often the child demonstrates restlessness, poor appetite, and social withdrawal over a period of several weeks to months. Behavioral problems, slowed development, and minor neurologic symptoms may occur.

The clinical manifestations of schizophrenia are the same in children as in adults. Characteristic behaviors of the schizophrenic individual include social withdrawal, impaired social relationships, flat **affect** (outward appearance of feeling or emotion), regression, loose associations (thought characterized by speech in which ideas shift from one subject to another that is unrelated), poor judgment and problem solving, anxiety, delusions, and hallucinations. Motor abnormalities may include rocking and arm flapping.

During adolescence, acute schizophrenia can occur suddenly while the teenager is making plans to leave home to attend college, marry, or work in another area. Onset of symptoms may be triggered by an important loss (death of a significant other, parent, child, or friend).

Prompt diagnosis can lead to early treatment and more positive outcomes. Clinical therapy for childhood schizophrenia is multifaceted, including individual psychotherapy, family therapy, and various psychotropic medications (antipsychotics such as haloperidol [Haldol], antianxiety agents such as lorazepam [Ativan], antidepressants such as imipramine [Tofranil], and newer antipsychotics such as dozapine, olanzapine, and risperidone). Drugs are only moderately effective at controlling hallucinations and delusions, responses vary considerably among individuals, and children may have different responses than adults. Side effects will determine what drugs are used and their duration. Antipsychotic medication is continued for at least 4 to 6 weeks before effectiveness can be determined. Medications often must be continued for several months or years after recovery from an acute schizophrenic episode, although medication-free trials may be attempted in children who have shown an absence of symptoms for 6 to 12 months (American Academy of Child and Adolescent Psychiatry, 2001; Bryden, Carrey, & Kutcher, 2001).

Episodes of acute schizophrenia often require inpatient hospitalization on a psychiatric unit for thorough diagnosis and beginning management. Treatment may include an intensive school-based program in a structured, supervised setting with specially trained professionals. The goal of initial treatment is to reduce or control psychotic episodes and provide a safe, structured environment for the child or adolescent, enabling the child to live each day at an optimal level of functioning. Outpatient care is provided following initial diagnosis and establishment of treatment regimen.

Most children require long-term treatment, including intermittent periods of hospitalization. Children or adolescents whose symptoms are difficult to control and who present a safety risk to themselves or others may require long-term residential treatment. Earlier age at diagnosis and delay in treatment lead to poorer prognosis.

NURSING MANAGEMENT

The nurse may encounter the child or adolescent with schizophrenia during hospitalization for an acute episode, for treatment of another problem, or while working with the individual in the community. Nursing care centers on providing for physical safety and psychologic care, and normal growth and development for the child.

Family education and involvement in the treatment plan are essential. The family is taught to monitor the child's symptoms and progression. Educating the child and parents about the risk of recurrence and methods to alleviate side effects of prescribed medications may increase compliance with the treatment plan. The nurse performs assessments of the child for common medication side effects. For example, when excess weight is a potential side effect, frequent growth measurements are made. Neurological assessment and laboratory studies may be needed with some medications.

The family is assisted in establishing educational plans for the child and for integration within the school system. The nurse communicates with school personnel to ensure understanding of the child's condition and ongoing management of the individualized education plan.

Desired outcomes for nursing care of the child with schizophrenia include physical and psychological security, normal growth and development, and decrease in psychotic symptoms (Lambert, 2001).

COGNITIVE DISORDERS

A wide array of cognitive conditions occur in childhood. Some are mild and not diagnosed until a child has difficulty in school, while others may be associated with physical signs which are visible at birth.

Learning Disabilities

Learning disabilities are a common problem of young children, affecting about 5% of school children. They involve neurological conditions in which the brain cannot receive or process information in the normal manner. Often the impairment is only in one or

CLINICAL MANIFESTATIONS of Various Learning Disabilities

DISORDER	CLINICAL MANIFESTATIONS
Dyslexia	Difficulty with writing, reading, spelling
Dyscalculia	Mathematics and computation problems
Dysgraphia	Difficulty with writing, spelling, and composition
Dyspraxia	Problems with manual dexterity and coordination

two types of learning, making diagnosis difficult. Common types of learning disorders are listed in the clinical manifestations table below. Children may have difficulty in processing visual information, which may be manifested in reading, writing, and mathematics performance. Others may have more difficulty with oral information, leading to problems in language development and reading (National Center for Learning Disabilities, 2004).

The causes of learning disorders are complex. Sometimes they are related to low birth weight or problems during the perinatal period. There may be a genetic component since their occurrence is more common when other family members are affected. The disabilities should be diagnosed by a learning specialist such as a psychologist with specialty training. A series of cognitive and developmental tests are most commonly used. Brain scanning with magnetic resonance imaging (MRI) is showing promise for diagnostic clues in the future. Treatments involve learning how to compensate for the difficulties by using capabilities that are intact. Some children need to have all material written for them, and others need verbal presentations. Specific learning goals are established with the assistance of learning specialists. Children with learning disabilities should have individualized education plans (IEPs) established with realistic goals for school performance (see Chapter 20∞ for further information about IEPs).

Nurses play a major role in identification of children with learning disabilities. You may be in contact with families during health promotion visits or other settings when parents relay concern about the child's performance or difficulty in some aspect of school. Assess the child for the following developmental milestones, which can indicate learning disability:

- Inability to phrase sentences together by 2 1/2 years
- Inability to use speech that is understandable at least 50% of the time by 3 years
- Unable to ties shoes, button, hop, or cut by kindergarten
- Inability to sit for a short story by 3 to 5 years

(American Academy of Pediatrics, 2000)

When a child may have a learning disability, refer the family to the school or other testing resource. Partner with the family to plan for the child's learning needs. Help the family to work closely with the child, provide a setting at home to maximize potential for learning, and build healthy self-esteem in the child. Assist the family to work with the school to establish annual goals for the child. Most children with learning disabilities can learn to perform well in their areas of strength and compensate for areas of difficulty. Early intervention is key to success and building positive self-image regarding abilities.

Mental Retardation

Mental retardation is defined as significant limitation in intellectual functioning and adaptive behavior. It is manifested in differences in conceptual, social, and practical life skills, and begins before the age of 18 years (American Association of Mental Retardation, 2004). Events after that age that lead to limitations in function are generally referred to as brain injury. Intellectual functioning is generally characterized by an IQ below 70 to 75, with significant impairments in **adaptive functioning** (the ability of an individual to meet the standards expected for his or her cultural group). The child with mental retardation has adaptive deficits in at least two areas such as communication, self-care, home living, social/interpersonal skills, use of community resources, self-direction, functional academic skills, work, leisure, health, or safety. A low IQ score by itself does not necessarily correlate with impairment in the ability to carry out adaptive skills. The child should be evaluated within the contexts of the individual cultural and community environment. The IQ score and the level of adaptive skills together determine the degree of severity of mental retardation.

Mental retardation is one type of **developmental disability,** any of a variety of chronic conditions that are characterized by mental and/or physical impairments. Other examples include pervasive developmental disorder, cerebral palsy, and sensory loss. A developmental disability can manifest up to the age of 21 years, and lasts throughout the lifetime (Centers for Disease Control and Prevention, 2004b).

Etiology and Pathophysiology

Mild retardation occurs in 3 to 6 per 1,000 people, and mental retardation affects about 3% of the population (Baralle, 2001). The causes of mental retardation can be grouped into three general categories: prenatal errors in the development of the CNS, prenatal or postnatal changes in the biologic environment of the person, and external forces leading to CNS damage. In each instance, the precipitating factor causes a change in the form, function, and adaptation of the CNS. Table 34–6 provides examples of common causes of mental retardation for each category.

Three conditions associated with mental retardation from prenatal conditions are Down syndrome, fragile X syndrome, and fetal alcohol syndrome. They will be discussed in greater detail in this section. See Table 34–7 for physical characteristics of children with each of these conditions.

TABLE 34–6 Common Conditions Associated with Mental Retardation

PRENATAL CONDITIONS	BIOLOGIC ENVIRONMENT	EXTERNAL FORCES
Down syndrome Fragile X syndrome Fetal alcohol syndrome Maternal infection (e.g., rubella, cytomegalovirus)	Inborn errors of metabolism (e.g., phenylketonuria, hypothyroidism)	Traumatic brain injury (e.g., accident) Poison ingestion (acute or chronic) Hypoxia/anoxic insult Infection (e.g., meningitis) Environmental deprivation

MediaLink Down Syndrome Video

TABLE 34–7 Characteristics of Three Common Conditions Associated with Mental Retardation

DOWN SYNDROME	FRAGILE X SYNDROME	FETAL ALCOHOL SYNDROME
(see Figure 39–10) Small head (microcephaly) Flattened forehead Wide, short neck Epicanthal eye folds White spots on eye iris (Brushfield spots) Congenital cataracts Flat nose Small, low-set ears Protruding tongue Short broad hands Simian line on palm Wide space between first and second toes Hearing loss Increased incidence of diabetes, congenital heart defect, and leukemia Hypotonia	Long face Prominent jaw Large ears Frequent otitis media Large testicles Epicanthal eye folds Strabismus High-arched palate Scoliosis Pliable joints	(see Figure 39–11) Flat midface Low nasal bridge Long philtrum with narrow upper lip Short upturned nose Poor coordination Failure to thrive Skeletal and joint abnormalities Hearing loss

In the United States, about 1 in 1,000 infants, or 4,000 infants each year, are born with Down syndrome (Roizen, 2002). The condition is caused by an extra chromosome; the child has 47 rather than 46 chromosomes (see discussion of genetic transmission in Chapter 4∞). The most common chromosome affected is 21, so that the child often has trisomy 21, or three instead of two copies of chromosome 21. In addition to mental retardation and physical signs, the child with Down syndrome is at higher risk of developing other conditions such as cardiac defects, hearing loss, thyroid disease, and leukemia (van Riper & Cohen, 2001). See Figure 34–10 ■.

Fragile X syndrome is caused by a single recessive gene abnormality on the X chromosome. A permutation to the X chromosome may occur in males or females. When a father or mother passes the faulty X chromosome to a daughter, it may remain as a permutation or may change into a true mutation. The daughter has two X chromosomes and therefore does not manifest this recessive disorder; however, she can give the mutated X chromosome to her son who becomes affected with fragile X. The mutation of fragile X is on gene FMRP-1, which instructs cells to make a protein necessary for normal brain development (Bailey, Roberts, & Mirrett, et al., 2001).

Fetal alcohol syndrome (FAS) is caused by the effect of ethyl alcohol on the developing fetus. Alcohol ingestion by the pregnant woman can influence development of many body organs and effects can range from mild to severe.

Chapter 32∞ discusses phenylketonuria and hypothyroidism, two common biochemical causes of mental retardation. Other causes involve traumatic brain injury and infections of the CNS (see Chapter 33∞).

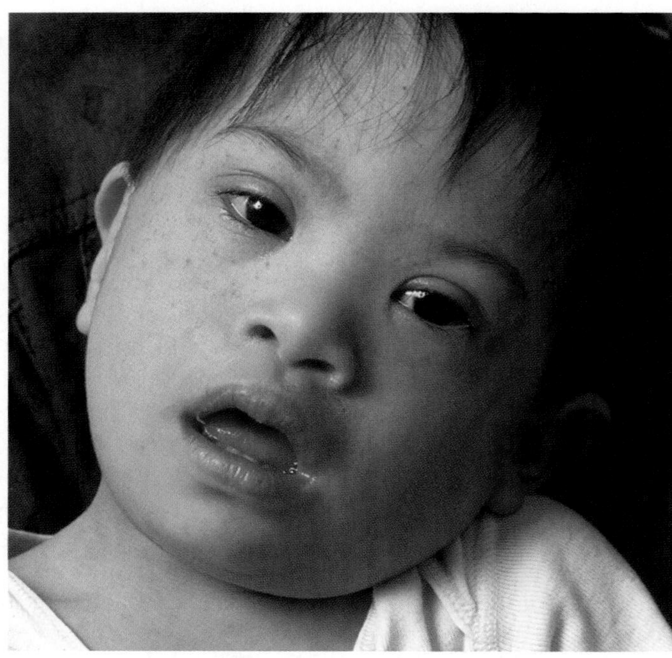

FIGURE 34–10 ■ A child with Down syndrome.

Clinical Manifestations

Mild mental retardation was originally described as an intelligence quotient (IQ) between 50 and 70, moderate retardation with IQ of 35 to 50, severe retardation with IQ of 20 to 35, and profound retardation with IQ below 20. Although an IQ below 70 is generally considered indicative of retardation, the functional assessment of the child is now considered to be a more accurate identification of children's performance and needs. Children who are mentally retarded manifest delays in several areas of development, including motor movement, language, and adaptive behavior. They usually achieve developmental milestones more slowly than the average child. These developmental delays may be the first indication to parents and care providers of the child's condition.

Mental retardation is sometimes accompanied by sensory impairment, speech problems, motor and orthopedic disabilities, and seizure disorders. Of children with mental retardation, 10% to 30% manifest one such disorder. See Table 34–7 for several physical characteristics associated with Down syndrome, fragile X syndrome, and fetal alcohol syndrome (Figure 34–11 ■).

COLLABORATIVE CARE

Many professionals, family members, and community partners work together to provide a nurturing environment for children with mental retardation. See Developing Cultural Competence: Culture and Alcohol Use.

Diagnostic Tests

Mental retardation is diagnosed and initial treatment is planned in a multistep process involving a multidisciplinary

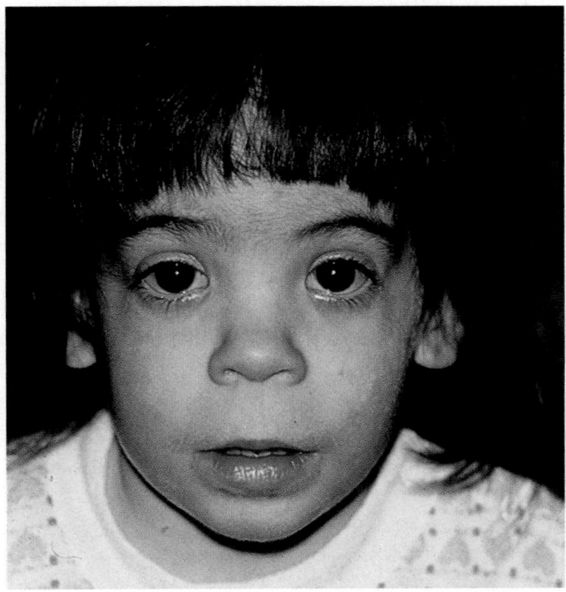

FIGURE 34–11 ■ A child with fetal alcohol syndrome.

Courtesy of Dr. Sterling Clarren, Seattle, WA. From Clarren, S. K. & Smith, D. W. (1978). The fetal alcohol syndrome. New England Journal of Medicine 298, *1063–1067.*

team. Members of the team are commonly a developmental specialist, physician, geneticist, nurse, teacher, language therapist, occupational therapist, and physical rehabilitation specialist. See Box 34–7 for a description of the *DSM-IV-TR* for mental retardation.

First, a comprehensive history and evaluation of the child's physical characteristics, developmental level, and intellectual and adaptive functioning is carried out. Laboratory tests such as chromosome analysis, blood enzyme levels, lead levels, or cranial imaging provide valuable information in some circumstances.

Developmental screening using a test such as the Denver II (see Chapter 10∞) can help to identify children who may be at risk. Tests of intellectual and adaptive functioning are performed when mental retardation is suspected. A neurologic examination may indicate asymmetry of movement or strength, irritability or lethargy, or abnormal pitch to an infant's cry. Because mental retardation may be accompanied by physical abnormalities, it is important to observe the child for facial symmetry, distance between the eyes, level of the ears, hair growth, and palmar creases. These abnormalities may be cues to other health problems.

DEVELOPING CULTURAL COMPETENCE
Culture and Alcohol Use

Fetal alcohol syndrome is more common in groups with higher intake of alcohol. Because some Native American tribes have a high rate of alcoholism, the federal government and some tribes have joined to lower that risk among this ethnic group. On reservations such as the Yakama Nation in Washington state, alcoholic beverages are not sold and educational programs are in place.

BOX 34–7 *DSM-IV-TR* Diagnostic Criteria for Mental Retardation

A. Significantly subaverage intellectual functioning: an IQ of approximately 70 or below on an individually administered IQ test (for infants, a clinical judgment of significantly subaverage intellectual functioning)
B. Concurrent deficits or impairments in present adaptive functioning (i.e., the person's effectiveness in meeting the standards expected for his or her age by his or her cultural group) in at least two of the following areas: communication, self-care, home living, social/interpersonal skills, use of community resources, self-direction, functional academic skills, work, leisure, health, and safety
C. The onset is before age 18 years

Clinical Therapy

Based on results of the evaluation, the multidisciplinary team plans the support needed to maximize the child's potential for development. Management focuses on early intervention to improve the degree of adaptive functioning. Simultaneous treatment of associated physical, emotional, and behavioral problems is provided. Depending on the child's condition, special education programs and physical or occupational therapy may be necessary (Figure 34–12 ■). The Education for All Handicapped Children Act, PL. 94-142, provides free appropriate education to all handicapped children between 2 and 21 years of age. Amendments to this act in 1986 (PL. 99-457) encouraged states to provide early intervention services for infants and toddlers with developmental delay conditions through federal funding.

The child may require supportive care and assistance with ADLs. The plans for intervention change as the child grows and family situations evolve. Some classes and community agencies offer transitional classes when children who are mentally retarded reach adolescence and young adulthood. These services help to teach self-care skills that may enable some youth to live in group homes or other community settings. Families receive help in planning for the child's future as parents look toward retirement. Information is provided on living options, health insurance, work opportunities, and other needs. This can also provide respite services for parents and other family members who have spent much time with the child for many years.

NURSING MANAGEMENT

Nursing management of the child with mental retardation focuses on prevention when possible, and support of the child and family to enhance development throughout the life span.

■ Nursing Assessment and Diagnosis

Nurses can help to identify children with mental retardation through history taking, observation, and developmental screening during early childhood. The history should provide information about the mental and adaptive functioning of birth

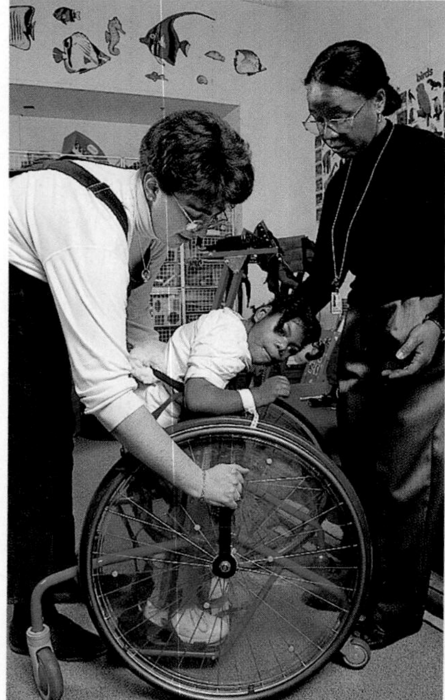

A

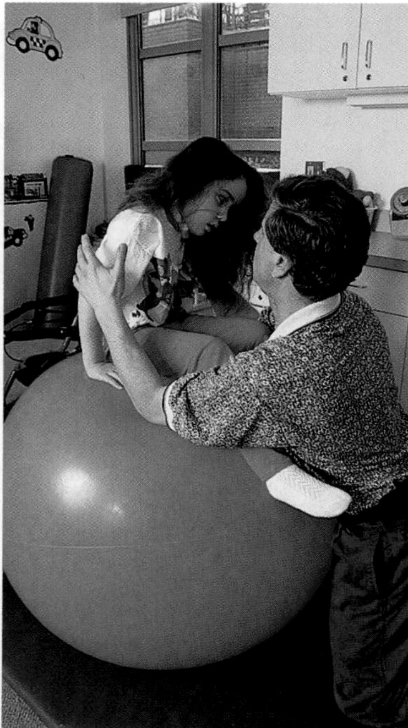

B

FIGURE 34–12 ■ Physical therapy is an important component of medical management for many children who are mentally retarded. *A,* This girl with severe retardation who uses a wheelchair is being positioned in a mobile prone stander, which enables her to interact in a different manner with her therapists and the environment. *B,* Physical therapists also provide outpatient care in the community to children with varying degrees of disability.

parents and other family members, as mental retardation may cluster in some families and conditions such as fragile X syndrome are genetic in origin. The pregnancy and birth history can provide important information relating to alcohol and drug use by the mother during pregnancy. Be alert for a history of difficult pregnancy and problems during delivery.

> **CLINICAL TIP**
>
> Prematurity places the child at risk of displaying below normal cognitive development. The premature infant needs frequent, thorough neurologic and developmental examinations, particularly in the first 2 years of life. Premature infants are expected to reach developmental milestones at approximately the same age they would reach them if they were born at normal gestational age. For example, an infant born two months prematurely should be evaluated on milestones of an infant two months younger than the infant's current age.

When genetic conditions in the family predispose family members to mental retardation, careful assessment of the child is needed. Children from deprived environments or those at risk because of environmental factors such as lead poisoning (see Chapter 30∞) are more likely to manifest mental retardation.

Many children with mental retardation are not diagnosed with the condition until they reach school age, particularly if the condition is mild or moderate. Early intervention, however, can help to enhance the child's functioning later. During home visits, clinic appointments, in childcare centers, and during hospitalization, be alert for signs of developmental delays, multiple (more than three) physical anomalies associated with a specific condition, or neurologic alterations. Developmental assessment should be part of each health promotion/health maintenance visit to aid in early identification.

MediaLink Mental Retardation Resources and Support

Once the diagnosis of mental retardation has been made, assess the adaptive functioning of the child and family. A functional assessment of the child should be performed, including toileting, dressing, and feeding skills. Assess the child's language, sensory, and psychomotor functioning. Assess the home and community for safety hazards. Observe how the family is managing with the child. To determine the impact of the child with mental retardation on the family, ask parents to describe (1) family activities that include the child, (2) strategies that parents and siblings use to deal with community attitudes about the child, and (3) in the case of a child with other disabilities, methods of managing the child's care and planning for future care needs.

Assess the availability of services such as support groups for parents and special education opportunities for children. Evaluate the coping skills of family members.

Several nursing diagnoses may be appropriate for the child with mental retardation, depending on the degree, cause, and outcome of the condition. Diagnoses that relate to impairments in adaptive functioning and family impact include the following:

- Delayed Growth and Development related to neonatal disease or condition
- Imbalanced Nutrition: Less than Body Requirements related to inability to ingest sufficient food
- Self-Care Deficit: Dressing, Toileting, Bathing related to developmental disability
- Impaired Verbal Communication related to developmental disability
- Risk for Injury related to lack of understanding of environmental hazards
- Compromised Family Coping related to the child's developmental variations

Planning and Implementation

Prevention is important for some types of mental retardation. All pregnant women or those who may become pregnant should stop ingestion of alcohol and nonprescription drugs. Encourage regular prenatal visits; this helps to prevent premature births, which have a higher association with mental retardation than birth at term.

Nearly all children who are mentally retarded are cared for in the community; however, they may have conditions that require periodic hospitalization or frequent healthcare visits. When needed, nursing care focuses on providing emotional support and information to family members, assisting the child with adaptive functioning, and fostering parental management of the child's activities.

Provide Emotional Support and Information

Family members need empathy and support both at the time of diagnosis and in the ensuing years. Parents may be in an acute or chronic state of grief over the loss of the perfect child. Encourage them to verbalize their feelings. Introducing them to parents of other mentally retarded children may provide assistance and support as they learn how to manage the child's needs. Discuss the availability of respite care to provide parents with a break from caretaking. Other family members such as grandparents and siblings may also be experiencing grief or guilt and should be given an opportunity to talk about their feelings.

Parents need honest information and answers to their questions about the child's condition. Reinforce information provided by genetic counselors and other healthcare professionals. Parents need to be informed about community resources designed to assist children with mental retardation. Such resources include the Zero to Three Project, special education preschools and schools, county health services, and respite care. Ask parents if they have questions about individualized education plans (IEPs). Refer parents to Internet sources, and help them to interpret information received and analyze its strengths and limitations. Review federal and state laws and services that might be helpful to the family. Examples are as follows:

- Public Law (PL) 94-142 of 1975 mandated that all children be provided with public education and related services.
- Public Law (PL) 99-457 of 1986 expanded the services of PL 94-142 to include children from birth to 5 years who need special education. It focused on the importance of fostering development and enhancing the capacity of families to meet the needs of children.
- Public Law (PL) 101-336 of 1990 is known as the American Disabilities Act (ADA). It prohibits discrimination and ensures equal opportunity for persons with disabilities in employment, state and local government services, public accommodations, commercial facilities, and transportation.
- Individuals with Disabilities Education Act Amendments (IDEA) of 1997 strengthened the academic expectations and accountability for children with disabilities.
- Administration on Developmental Disabilities (ADD) is the U.S. organization that ensures that the Developmental Disabilities (DD) Act goals are met. The DD Act implemented the Developmental Disabilities and Bill of Rights Act of 2000 and seeks to enhance life through training activities, community education, eliminating barriers, and influencing policy (Administration for Children & Families, 2004).
- State Councils on Developmental Disabilities (SCDD) are present in each state to increase integration of children with developmental disabilities into their communities.

Maintain a Safe Environment

Children with mental retardation require close supervision because they may lack an understanding of common hazards. Ensure safety in the hospital environment. Assist parents to provide safety at home and school and to teach their child necessary skills such as pedestrian safety. Consider both physical and emotional safety. The child with mental retardation may be trusting of others and sometimes is at risk for physical or sexual abuse.

Provide Assistance with Adaptive Functioning

Encourage parents' efforts to maximize the child's areas of strength and identify needs related to adaptive behaviors. Refer them to resources to assist in the areas of adaptive functioning in which the child has impairment, such as communication, self-care activities, or social skills. During hospitalization, support parents' efforts to maintain the child's skills in toileting, dressing, and self-care by planning interventions to use the skills being taught at home.

Care in the Community

The child with mental retardation needs ongoing care throughout childhood, and adaptation of interventions as development occurs and the family's needs evolve. Parents often act as case managers for the child's care. Partner with parents as necessary to acquire the skills required to coordinate the child's plan of care. Evaluate the child's needs regularly and assist parents with the treatment plan as necessary. Collaborate with the family and other health care professionals to provide for education and for services such as physical or speech therapy. Most children with mental retardation have an individualized education plan (IEP) designed to meet their specific learning needs. Parents, nurses, and others such as teachers and language therapists are part of the team that establishes this plan. Promote optimal development and socialization. As the child reaches adolescence, education is directed toward a vocation, issues of sexuality, and the goal of independent living, when appropriate.

Specific guidelines for care are available for the child with Down syndrome. These guidelines suggest specific times for evaluation of hearing, growth, cardiac function, and other areas designed for early identification and treatment of associated disorders (van Riper & Cohen, 2001). There are specific growth grids for children with Down syndrome, and specific topics to suggest for anticipatory guidance during healthcare visits (American Academy of Pediatrics Committee on Genetics, 2001).

Evaluation

The expected outcomes of nursing care depend on the child's needs and developmental level. Early in the diagnostic phase, desired outcomes may involve the family's understanding of the diagnosis and the child's special needs. Later outcomes may focus on the child's communication or self-help skills. Outcomes related to cognitive performance and adaptive skills may be developed during childhood.

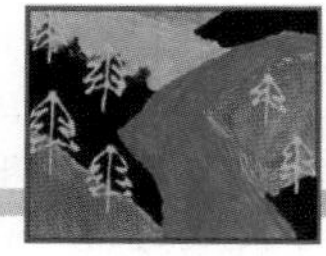

CHAPTER HIGHLIGHTS

- Major treatment modes for children with mental health disorders include individual therapy, family therapy, and group therapy.
- Therapeutic strategies for treatment of children and adolescents with mental health disorders include play therapy, art therapy, behavior therapy, visualization, and hypnosis.
- Families often attempt to treat mental health conditions with use of alternative and complementary therapy; nurses can provide information to assist families in evaluating the results of these therapies.
- Nurses are involved in conducting mental health assessments, preventing disorders when possible, participating in intervention to treat disorders, and evaluating success of treatments.
- Autistic spectrum disorder is the major type of pervasive developmental disorder, and is manifested by abnormal behavior, social interaction, and communication.
- Attention deficit disorder (ADD) and attention deficit hyperactivity disorder (ADHD) are characterized by developmentally inappropriate behaviors involving inattention, and sometimes hyperactivity.
- ADD and ADHD must be diagnosed using recommended criteria and are commonly treated with a combination of behavioral, environmental, and medication therapies.
- Schizophrenia is a psychotic disorder manifested by social withdrawal, delusions, and hallucinations.
- Mood disorders in childhood and adolescents are commonly manifested as depression or manic depression (bipolar disorder).
- Several anxiety disorders occur in children and adolescents, most notably generalized anxiety, separation anxiety, panic, obsessive-compulsive disorder, school phobia, conversion reaction, and posttraumatic stress disorder.
- Behavioral therapy and selective serotonin reuptake inhibitors (SSRIs) are used in treatment of anxiety disorders; their use in children must be closely monitored.
- Posttraumatic stress disorder may occur as victims relive the terror of traumatic events.
- Suicide is a frequent cause of death among youth.
- Nurses are key health professionals in identifying youth at risk of suicide, instituting suicide prevention programs, and counseling family and friends of suicide victims.
- Children may experience tic disorders that impair development and social interactions; medications are helpful in treatment of these disorders.
- Childhood schizophrenia presents a crisis for families and may require inpatient hospitalization for youth affected.
- Nurses play a role in identifying children with potential learning disabilities, referring for diagnosis, and partnering with the family to provide a positive learning environment for the child.
- Mental retardation is defined as subaverage intellectual and adaptive functioning, and is caused by chromosomal, genetic, or environmental factors.
- Nurses identify children with possible mental retardation by careful evaluation of development.
- A multidisciplinary team plans the care for children with mental retardation and periodically evaluates the child's progress and the family's needs.
- Nurses play a vital role in maintaining the mental health of children, preventing mental health problems, identifying children at risk of mental health disorders, and providing care or referring families for mental health services.

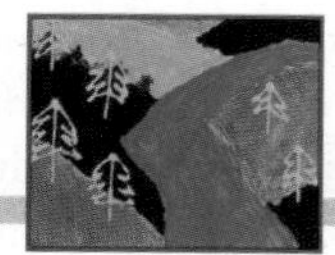

CRITICAL THINKING IN ACTION

INTRODUCTION

Recall 9-year-old Cassandra Nielsen who was in a car accident and subsequently manifested posttraumatic stress disorder. She managed well after the crash, but began developing somatic complaints, school phobia, and sleep disturbance. Cassandra is being seen by a psychologist to assist her in dealing with her fears.

DESCRIPTION

It appears that Cassandra is receiving the assistance she needs. However, a schoolmate, 11-year-old Daniel Barrington, had a sibling who died from an accidental gunshot wound in the previous year. Daniel has regularly attended school but has become more aggressive with friends and is now known as a bully. He has been referred to the office and the school nurse several times due to fighting or complaints of "feeling sick." Daniel appears very bright and almost carefree. He rarely talks of his sibling who died at age 13 years. When he does, it is in a joking manner.

DISCUSSION

1. Is Daniel manifesting signs of PTSD? If so, what are they?
2. What symptoms are the same and which are different from those of Cassandra?
3. What assessments can the school nurse complete on children such as Cassandra and Daniel?
4. What types of specialists can help children deal with challenges of PTSD?
5. How could you explain to the parents the effect on a child of an accident such as Cassandra's or a family death such as that experienced by Daniel? List several nursing diagnoses for Cassandra and establish desired outcomes for each.
6. How will you integrate knowledge of Cassandra's developmental stage into possible nursing interventions? List the stages of developmental theorists such as Piaget and Erikson which should be considered (see Chapter 5∞).

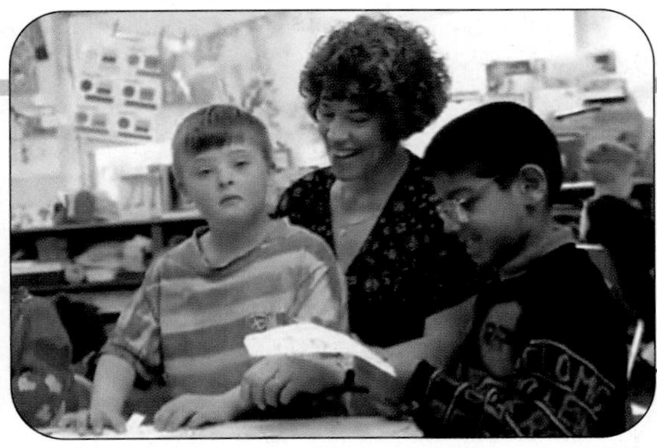

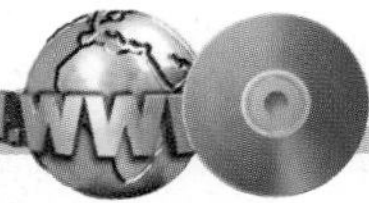

EXPLORE MediaLink

- NCLEX review, case studies, and other interactive resources for this chapter can be found on the Companion Website at **www.prenhall.com/ball**. Click on Chapter 34 to select the activities for this chapter.
- For animations, more NCLEX review questions, and an audio glossary, access the accompanying CD-ROM in this book.

http://www.prenhall.com/ball

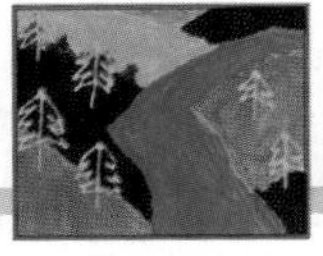

REFERENCES

Adesman, A. (2003). A diagnosis of ADHD? Don't overlook the probability of comorbidity! *Contemporary Pediatrics, 20*(12), 91–106.

Administration for Children & Familie. (2004). About ADD. www.acf.dhhs.gov/programs/add/about/htm, accessed 7/15/2004.

American Academy of Child and Adolescent Psychiatry. (2001). The practice parameter for the assessment and treatment of children and adolescents with schizophrenia. *Journal of the American Academy of Child & Adolescent Psychiatry, 40*(7), 4S–23S.

American Academy of Pediatrics. (2000). Types of learning disabilities. www.medem.com/melb/article_detaillb_for_printer.cfm?article_ID=ZZZ0QSFNQ, accessed 5/25/2004.

American Academy of Pediatrics. (2001). Diagnosis and management of autistic spectrum disorder. *Pediatrics, 107,* 1221–1226.

American Academy of Pediatrics, Committee on Genetics. (2001). Health supervision for children with down syndrome. *Pediatrics, 107,* 442–449.

American Academy of Pediatrics, Committee on Quality Improvement, Subcommittee on Attention-Deficit/Hyperactivity Disorder. (2000). Diagnosis and evaluation of the child with attention-deficit/hyperactivity disorder. *Pediatrics, 105,* 1158–1170.

American Academy of Pediatrics, Committee on Quality Improvement, Subcommittee on Attention-Deficit/Hyperactivity Disorder. (2001). Clinical practice guideline: Treatment of the school-aged child with attention-deficit/hyperactivity disorder. *Pediatrics, 108,* 1033–1044.

American Association of Mental Retardation. (2004). Definition of mental retardation. www.aamr.org/Policies/faq_mental_retardation.shtml, accessed 7/15/2004.

American Psychiatric Association. (2000). *Diagnostic and statistical manual of mental disorders* (4th ed., revised). Washington, DC: American Psychiatric Association.

Bailey, D. B., Roberts, J. E., Mirrett, P., & Hatton, D. D. (2001). Identifying infants and toddlers with fragile X syndrome: Issues and recommendations. *Infants and Young Children, 14,* 24–33.

Baird, G., Charman, T., Cox, A., Baron-Cohen, S., Swettenham, J., Wheelwright, S., & Drew, A. (2001). Screening and surveillance for autism and pervasive developmental disorders. *Archives of Disease in Childhood, 84,* 468–475.

Baralle, D. (2001). Chromosomal aberrations, subtelomeric defects, and mental retardation. *Lancet, 358,* 7–8.

Beauchesne, M. A., & Kelley, B. R. (2004). Evidence to support parental concerns as an early indicator of autism in children. *Pediatric Nursing, 30,* 57–67.

Bechtel, B. (2003, September). New research offers inroads to better understanding of autism. *Infectious Diseases in Children,* 14–16.

Bryden, K. E., Carrey, N. J., & Kutcher, S. P. (2001). Update and recommendations for the use of antipsychotics in early-onset psychosis. *Journal of Child and Adolescent Psycho-Pharmacology, 11,* 113–130.

Buck, M. L. (2003). Atomoxetine: A new alternative for the treatment of attention-deficit/hyperactivity disorder. *Pediatric Pharmcology, 9*(2). www.medscape.com/viewarticle/452714, accessed 5/7/2003.

Cade, M., & Tidwell, S. (2001). Autism and the school nurse. *Journal of School Health, 71,* 96–100.

Cala, S., Crismon, M. L., & Baumgartner, J. (2003). A survey of herbal use in children with attention-deficit-hyperactivity disorder or depression. *Pharmacotherapy, 23,* 222–230.

Carson, V. B. (2000). *Mental health nursing* (2nd ed.). Philadelphia: WB Saunders.

Castiglia, P. T. (2000a). Depression in adolescents. *Journal of Pediatric Health Care, 14,* 180–182. www.cdc.gov.ncipc.factsheets.suifacts.htm, accessed 7/15/2004.

Castiglia, P. T. (2000b). Depression in children. *Journal of Pediatric Health Care, 14,* 73–75.

Centers for Disease Control and Prevention. (2004a). Suicide: Fact Sheet. http://www.cdc.gov/ncipc/factsheets/suifacts.htm

Centers for Disease Control and Prevention. (2004b). Developmental disabilities. www.cdc.gov.ncbddd.dd.default.htm, accessed 7/15/2004.

Christakis, D. A., Zimmerman, F. J., DiGiuseppe, D. L., & McCarty, C. A. (2004). Early television exposure and subsequent attentional problems in children. *Pediatrics, 113,* 708–713.

Committee of Children with Disabilities, American Academy of Pediatrics. (2001). The pediatrician's role in the diagnosis and management of autistic spectrum disorder in children. *Pediatrics, 107,* 1221–1226.

Courchesne, E., Carper, R., & Akshoomoff, N. (2003). Evidence of brain overgrowth in the first year of life in autism. *Journal of the America Medical Association, 290,* 337–344.

Dales, L., Hammer, S. J., & Smith, N. J. (2001). Time trends in autism and in MMR immunization coverage in California. *Journal of the American Medical Association, 285,* 1183.

Department of Health and Human Services. (2000). *Report of the surgeon general's conference on children's mental health: A national action agenda.* Washington, DC: U.S. Department of Health and Human Services.

Fish, K. B. (2000). Suicide awareness at the elementary school level. *Journal of Psychosocial Nursing, 38,* 20–23.

Geller, D. A., Biederman, J., Farone, S., Agranat, A., Cradock, K., Hagermoser, L., Kim, G., Frazier, J., & Coffey, B. (2001). Developmental aspects of obsessive compulsive disorder: Findings in children, adolescents and adults. *Journal of Nervous and Mental Disease, 189,* 471–477.

Gottesman, M. M. (2003). Helping parents make sense of ADHD diagnosis and treatment. *Journal of Pediatric Health Care, 17,* 149–154.

Hazell, P., O'Connell, D., Heathcote, D., & Henry, D. (2002). Tricyclic drugs for depression in children and adolescents (Cochrane Review). In *The Cochrane Library,* Issue 2. Oxford: Update Software.

Hoagland, K., Burns, B. J., Kiser, L., Rindeisen, H., & Schoenwald, S. K. (2001). Evidence-based practice in child and adolescent mental health services. *Psychiatric Services, 52,* 1179–1189.

Horowitz, L. M., Wang, P. S., Koocher, G. P., Burr, B. H., Smith, M. F., Klavon, S., & Cleary, P. D. (2001). Detecting suicide risk in a pediatric emergency department: Development of a brief screening tool. *Pediatrics, 107,* 1133–1137.

Hudson, G. T., & Dixon, D. (2003). Autism: Challenges in diagnosis and treatment. *Clinician Reviews, 13,* 45–52.

Hyman, S. L., & Levy, S. E. (2000). Autistic spectrum disorders: When traditional medicine is not enough. *Contemporary Pediatrics, 17,* 101–116.

Jellinek, M., Patel, B. P., & Froehle, M. C. (2002). *Bright futures in Practice: Mental health* (Vol. II). Arlington, VA: National Center for Education in Maternal and Child Health.

Jick, H., & Kaye, J. A. (2003). Epidemiology and possible causes of autism. *Pharmacotherapy, 23,* 1524–1530.

Kaye, J. A., Melero-Montes, M. M., & Jick, H. (2001). Mumps, measles, and rubella vaccine and the incidence of autism recorded by general practitioners: A time-trend analysis. *British Medical Journal, 322,* 460–463.

Kent, J. M., Sullivan, G. M., & Rauch, S. L. (2000). The neurobiology of fear: Relevance to panic disorder and posttraumatic stress disorder. *Psychiatric Annals, 30,* 733–742.

Kessler, R. C. (2000). Posttraumatic stress disorder. *Journal of Clinical Psychiatry, 61* (Suppl. 15), 4–12.

King, K. A. (2001). Developing a comprehensive school suicide prevention program. *Journal of School Health, 71,* 132–137.

Kuperman, S. (2002). Tic disorders in the adolescent. *Adolescent Medicine, 13,* 537–551.

Kurlan, R., McDermott, M. P., Deeley, C., Como, P. G., Brower, C., Eapen, S., Adresen, E. M., & Miller, E. M. (2001). Prevalence of tics in school children and adolescents associated with placement in special education. *Neurology, 57,* 1383–1388.

Lamberg, L. (2001). Psychiatrists explore the legacy of traumatic stress in early life. *Journal of the American Medical Association, 286,* 523–526.

Lambert, L. T. (2001). Identification and management of schizophrenia in childhood. *Journal of Child and Adolescent Psychiatric Nursing, 14,* 73–80.

Leonard, H. L., Freeman, J., Barcia, A., Garvey, M., Snider, L., & Swedo, S. E. (2001). Obsessive-compulsive disorder and related conditions. *Pediatric Annals, 30,* 154–160.

Liu, Y. H., & Leslie, L. K. (2003). Diagnosing ADHD: Putting AAP guidelines to the test—and into practice. *Contemporary Pediatrics, 20*(12), 51–73.

Lyon, D. E., & Morgan-Judge, T. (2000). Childhood depressive disorders. *Journal of School Nursing, 16*(3), 29–31.

March, J. S. (2004). Pediatric Autoimmune neuropsychiatric disorders associated with streptococcal infection (PANDAS): Implications for clinical practice. *Archives of Pediatric and Adolescent Medicine 158,* 927–929.

Masi, G., Mucci, M., & Millepiedi, S. (2001). Separation anxiety disorder in children and adolescents: Epidemiology, diagnosis and management. *CNS Drugs, 15,* 93–104.

McDonnell, J. A., Doyle, R., & Surman, C. (2003). *Clinician Reviews, 13,* 110–117.

Melnyk, B. M., Brown, H. E., Jones, D. C., Kreipe, R., & Novak, J. (Eds.). (2003). Improving the mental/psychosocial health of US children and adolescents: Outcomes and implementation strategies from the National KySS Summit. *Journal of Pediatric Health Care, 17,* S1-S245.

Melnyk, B. M., Feinstein, N. F., Tuttle, J., Moldenhauer, Z., Herendeen, P., Veenema, T. G., et al. (2002). Mental health worries, communications, and needs of children, teens, and parents during the year of the nation's terrorist attack: Findings from the national KySS survery. *Journal of Pediatric Health Care, 16,* 222–234.

Melnyk, B. M., Moldenhauer, Z., Tuttle, J., Veenema, T. G., Jones, D., & Novak, J. (2003, February). Improving child and adolescent mental health: An evidence-based approach. *Advance for Nurse Practitioners,* 47–52.

Meltzer-Brody, S., Hidalgo, R., Connor, K. M., & Davidson, J. R. T. (2000). Posttraumatic stress disorder: Prevalence, health care use and costs, and pharmacologic considerations. *Psychiatric Annals, 30,* 722–730.

Meunier-Sham, J. (2003). Increased volume/length of stay for pediatric mental health patients: One ED's response. *Journal of Emergency Nursing, 29,* 229–239.

Mohr, W. K. (2001). Bipolar disorder in children. *Journal of Psychosocial Nursing & Mental Health Services, 39*(3), 12–23.

Moldenhauer, Z., & Melnyk, B. M. (1999). Use of antidepressants in the treatment of child and adolescent depression: Are they effective? *Pediatric Nursing, 25,* 643–645.

National Center for Learning Disabilities. (2004). Learning disability. www.ldanatl.org/, accessed 5/25/2004.

National Initiative for Children's Healthcare Quality. (2003). *Improving care for children with ADHD.* Boston: Author.

National Institute of Mental Health. (2004). Antidepressant medications for children: Information for parents and caregivers. www.nimh.nih.gov/press/StmntAntidepmeds.cfm?Output=Print, accessed 5/25/2004.

National Strategy for Suicide Prevention. (2001). www.mentalhealth.org/suicideprevention, accessed 11/5/2001.

Navon, M., Nelson, D., Pagano, M., & Murphy, M. (2001). Use of the pediatric symptom checklist in strategies to improve preventive behavioral health care. *Psychiatric Services, 52,* 800–804.

Rew, L., Thomas, N., Horner, S. D., Resnick, J. D., & Beuhring, T. (2001). Correlates of recent suicide attempts in a triethnic group of adolescents. *Journal of Nursing Scholarship, 33,* 361–367.

Rohde, P., Seeley, J. R., & Mace, D. E. (1997). Correlates of suicidal behavior in a juvenile detention center. *Suicide and Life-Threatening Behavior, 27,* 164–175.

Roizen, N. J. (2002). Down syndrome. In M. L. Batshaw (Ed.), *Children with disabilities* (5th ed.). Baltimore: Paul H. Brookes Publishing Co.

Russell, S. T., & Joyner, K. (2001). Adolescent sexual orientation and suicide risk: Evidence from a national study. *American Journal of Public Health, 91,* 1276–1281.

Rynn, M. A., Siqueland, L. & Rickels, K. (2001). Placebo-controlled trial of sertraline in the treatment of children with generalized anxiety disorder. *American Journal of Psychiatry 158,* 2008–2014.

Scharer, K. (2002). What parents of mentally ill children need and want from mental health professionals. *Issues in Mental Health Nursing, 23,* 617–640.

Shugart, M. A., & Lopez, E. M. (2002). Depression in children and adolescents. *Postgraduate Medicine, 112*(3), 53–61.

Smoller, J. W., Finn, C., & White, C. (2000). The genetics of anxiety disorders: An overview. *Psychiatry Annals, 30,* 745–753.

Snider, L. A., Seligman, L. D., Ketchen, B. R., Levitt, S. J., Bates, L. R., Garvey, M. A., & Swedo, S. E. (2002). Tics and problem behaviors in schoolchildren: Prevalence, characterization, and associations. *Pediatrics, 110,* 331–336.

Stein, J. A., & Baren, M. (2003). Welcome progress in the diagnosis and treatment of ADHD in adolescence. *Contemporary Pediatrics, 20*(8), 83–107.

Towbin, K. E., Mauk, J. E., & Batshaw, M. L. (2002). Pervasive developmental disorders. In M. L. Batshaw (Ed.), *Children with disabilities* (5th ed.). Baltimore: Paul H. Brookes Publishing Co.

Van Riper, M., & Cohen, W. I. (2001). Caring for children with Down syndrome and their families. *Journal of Pediatric Health Care, 15,* 123–131.

Walsh, K. H. (2002). Welcome advances in treating youth anxiety disorders. *Contemporary Pediatrics, 19*(9), 66–82.

Weller, E. B., Calvert, S. M., & Weller, R. A. (2003). Bipolar disorder in children and adolescents: Diagnosis and treatment. *Current Opinions in Psychiatry, 16,* 383–388.

Whitaker, H., Wolf, K. A., & Keuthen, N. (2003). Chronic hair pulling: Recognizing trichotillmania. *Clinician Reviews, 13*(3), 37–44.

Wilens, T. E., et al. (2003). Does stimulant therapy of attention-deficit/hyperactivity disorder beget later substance abuse? A meta-analytic review of the literature. *Pediatrics, 111,* 179–185.

Williams, P. G., Dalrymple, N., & Neal, J. (2000). Eating habits of children with autism. *Pediatric Nursing, 26,* 259–264.

Williamson, D. E., Birmaher, B., Brent, D. A., Bolach, L., Dahl, R. E., & Ryan, N. D. (2000). Atypical symptoms of depression in a sample of depressed child and adolescent outpatients. *Journal of the American Academy of Child and Adolescent Psychiatry, 39,* 1253–1259.

Yehud, R., Hallig, S. L., & Grossman, R. (2001). Childhood trauma and risk for PTSD: Relationship to intergenerational effects of trauma, parental PTSD, and cortisol excretion. *Developmental Psychopathology, 13,* 733–753.

Zametkin, A. J., Alter, M. R., & Yemini, T. (2001). Suicide in teenagers. *Journal of the American Medical Association, 286,* 3120–3125.

Zickler, C. F., Morrow, J. D., & Bull, M. J. (1998). Infants with down syndrome: A look at temperament. *Journal of Pediatric Health Care, 12,* 111–117.

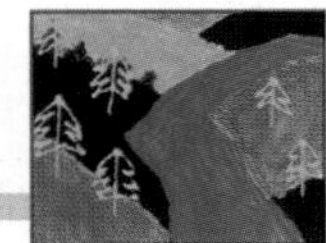

ADDITIONAL REFERENCES

Blondis, T. A. (1999). Motor disorders and attention-deficit/hyperactivity disorder. *Pediatric Clinics of North America, 46,* 899–914.

Brent, D. A., & Birmaher, B. (2002). Adolescent depression. *New England Journal of Medicine, 347,* 667–671.

Butter, E. M., Wynn, J., & Mulick, J. A. (2003). Early intervention critical to autism treatment. *Pediatric Annals, 32,* 677–684.

Elder, J. H. (2002). Current treatments in autism: Examining scientific evidence and clinical implications. *Journal of Neuroscience Nursing, 34*(2), 67–73.

Fletcher, J. M., Shaywitz, S. E., & Shaywitz, B. A. (1999). Comorbidity of learning and attention disorders: Separate but equal. *Pediatric Clinics of North America, 46,* 885–898.

Frederic, D. W., & Williams, S. L. (1998). New definition of mental retardation for the American Association of Mental Retardation. *Image, 30,* 53–56.

Freeman, B. J., & Cronin, P. (2002). Diagnosing autism spectrum disorder in young children: An update. *Infants and Young Children, 14*(3), 1–10.

Hunt, R. D., Paguin, A., & Payton, K. (2001). An update on assessment and treatment of complex attention-deficit hyperactivity disorder. *Pediatric Annals, 30,* 162–172.

Kaplan, E. L. (2000). PANDAS? Or PAND? Or both? Or neither? *Contemporary Pediatrics, 17,* 81–96.

Koenig, K. (1998). Pervasive developmental disorders: Diagnosis, intervention and education. *American Journal for Nurse Practitioners, 2*(8), 15–28.

Koenig, K., & Scahill, L. (2001). Assessment of children with pervasive developmental disorders. *Journal of Child and Adolescent Psychiatric Nursing, 14,* 159–166.

Sivberg, B. (2003). Parents' detection of early signs in their children having an autistic spectrum disorder. *Journal of Pediatric Nursing, 18,* 433–439.

Chapter

35

Alterations in Musculoskeletal Function

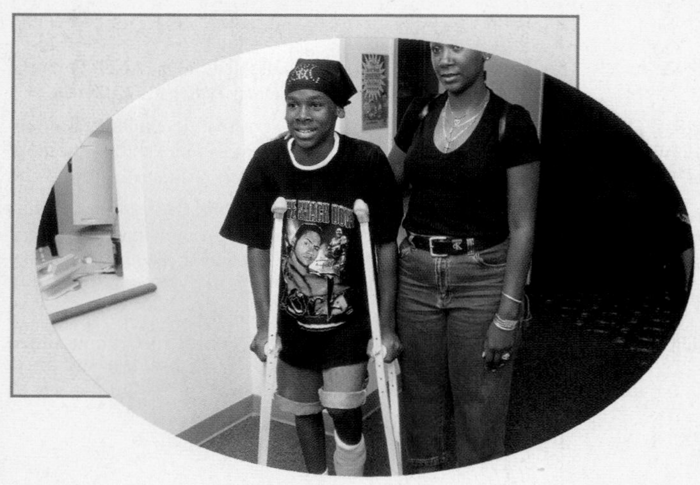

Douglass Langlois was admitted to the clinic today for application of a short leg cast. He broke his left lower fibula nearly a week ago when he was on a trampoline with three friends, trying to see who could jump the highest. Douglass slipped and his lateral leg hit the frame on the side. His friends helped him off the trampoline and called his mother, who transported Douglass to the emergency room.

His mother states that he is now 12 years old and in middle school. He has been going to a friend's house nearly every day after school and spending time on activities such as the trampoline and roller blading, as well as watching television and playing video games. She felt this was safer than him being at home alone during her work hours, but is now starting to wonder about whether to allow Douglass to engage in activities with his friend. In the emergency room after the accident, a splint was used to provide support for a few days and allow the swelling to decrease before today's cast application. Douglass has been non-weight bearing on his leg and has been using crutches.

"How am I going to go back to school? There are stairs and you wouldn't believe all the kids in the hallways between classes."

—Douglass, age 12

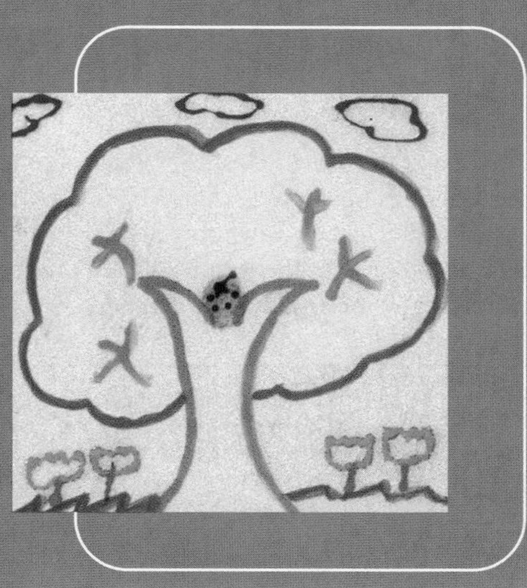

Learning Outcomes

After completing this chapter, you will be able to:

- Describe pediatric variations in the musculoskeletal system.
- Plan nursing care for children with structural deformities of foot, hip, and spine.
- Recognize signs and symptoms of infectious musculoskeletal disorders and refer for appropriate care.
- Partner with families to plan care for children with musculoskeletal conditions that are chronic or require long-term care.
- Plan nursing interventions to promote safety and developmental progression in children who require braces, casts, traction, and surgery.
- Provide nursing care for fractures, including teaching for injury prevention and nursing implementations for the child who has sustained a fracture.

Key Terms

Blount's disease/1415
chondrolysis/1422
compartment syndrome/1444
dislocation/1416
dwarfism/1433
dysplasia/1416
equinus/1412
ossification/1409
osteopenia/1409
osteoporosis/1409
osteotomy/1415
pseudohypertrophy/1437
rickets/1415
sprain/1410
subluxation/1416
valgus/1415
varus/1412

MediaLink http://www.prenhall.com/ball

Resources for this chapter can be found on the CD-ROM accompanying this textbook, and on the Companion Website at www.prenhall.com/ball. Click on Chapter 35 to select the activities for this chapter.

CD-ROM

Animations

Muscle Physiology

NCLEX Review

Audio Glossary

COMPANION WEBSITE

A & P Review

Clinical Manifestations Review

NCLEX Review

Case Study: Fracture Assessment

Care Plan: Home Care of an Infant in a Spica Cast

MediaLink Applications

Critical Thinking: Autosomal Dominant Disorders

What teaching does Douglass need to keep the cast intact and to ensure his safety? What special adaptations will be needed in his home and school? How can the clinic nurse partner with the school nurse to provide for Douglass's transition back to school? Is there any way his injury could have been avoided? The information in this chapter will discuss issues such as these and help you to provide effective care for children like Douglass who have musculoskeletal disorders.

The musculoskeletal system helps the body to protect its vital organs, support weight, control motion, store minerals, and supply red blood cells. *Bones* provide a rigid framework for the body, and *joints* are the articulations or places where adjoining bones

TABLE 35–1 Components of the Musculoskeletal System

BONES	JOINTS	MUSCLES	LIGAMENTS	TENDONS
Dense connective osseous tissue giving support to the body. ➤ Long bones—major parts are diaphysis and epiphysis. Examples include femur, fibula, tibia, humerus, radius, ulna ➤ Short or cuboid bones—a combination of spongy (cancellous) and compact bone. Examples include wrist and some foot bones ➤ Flat bones—combination of spongy (cancellous) and a thin layer of compact bone, usually curved in shape. Examples include skull, sternum, and ribs ➤ Irregular bones—variable thicknesses and shapes of spongy (cancellous) and compact bone. Examples include vertebrae, scapula, and pelvis	Articulation or point of juncture between two bones. The joint capsule is covered with articular cartilage, and free spaces are filled with synovial fluid. Classifications are: ➤ Synarthrosis—immovable joints such as cranial sutures ➤ Amphiarthrosis—slightly movable joints such as vertebrae and symphysis pubis ➤ Diarthrosis—freely movable joints such as knee, hip, elbow, shoulder (the joint with the most movements possible) Joint types are classified as: ➤ Hinge—allow movement in only one plane such as elbow, fingers, knee, ankle ➤ Pivot—one bone pivots in a ring allowing rotary movement such as between C1 and C2 ➤ Gliding—one bone glides against another such as many small bones of wrist and ankle ➤ Ball and socket—a rounded end of one bone moves within a concavity on the adjoining bone such as head of femur into hip ➤ Condyloid—an oval end of one bone moves within an elliptical concavity on the adjoining bone such as connection of radius to carpal bones ➤ Saddle—allows movement to switch in different directions such as thumb Joint motions are classified as: ➤ Gliding—bones are flat or slightly curved and glide over each other such as in wrist and ankle bones ➤ Angular—movements between long bones adjacent to each other such as radius and humerus ➤ Circumduction—motion of a long bone in a cavity such as hip joint ➤ Rotation—bone moves in a central axis such as the shoulder	Fibers or bundles of cells that contract, causing movement. Types are: ➤ Skeletal—striated, voluntary muscles grouped in bundles; examples are triceps, biceps, quadriceps ➤ Smooth—nonstriated, involuntary muscles with spindle-shaped cells; examples are those in digestive, respiratory, urinary and vascular systems ➤ Cardiac—striated, involuntary network of muscles in the heart	Fibrous tissue connecting bones or cartilage; support and strengthen synovial joints or those able to move.	Band of strong fibrous tissue connecting muscles to bone. As a muscle contracts, it pulls the tendon, thus moving the attached bone.

MediaLink Musculoskeletal A & P Review

meet. *Muscles* are fibrous tissue that provide for movement, while *ligaments* are bands of connective tissue holding bones together and *tendons* are connective tissue that connects bones and muscles. Bones, muscles, and supporting structures are needed for gross and fine motor development, and therefore alterations in musculoskeletal functioning can have a significant impact on a child's growth and development (Table 35–1).

Musculoskeletal disorders may be congenital, such as clubfoot, or acquired, such as osteomyelitis. They may require short- or long-term management, and may be treated on an outpatient basis or require hospitalization. Many musculoskeletal disorders require surgical correction, casting, or braces.

Figure 35–1 ■ reviews several terms used throughout this chapter in describing the positioning of a child's limbs and possible joint motions.

ANATOMY AND PHYSIOLOGY OF PEDIATRIC DIFFERENCES

Bones

Several differences exist between the bones of children and those of adults. Although primary centers of **ossification** (bone formation) are nearly complete at birth, a fibrous membrane still exists between the cranial bones (fontanels) (see Figure 8–16∞). The posterior fontanel closes between 2 and 3 months of age. The anterior fontanel does not close until approximately 12 to 18 months of age, allowing for growth of the brain and skull. In addition, the ends of the long bones (epiphyses) remain cartilaginous (Figure 35–2 ■). Long bone growth continues until approximately age 20 years, when skeletal maturation is complete.

Secondary ossification occurs as the long bones grow. Cartilage cells at the epiphyses are replaced by osteoblasts (immature bone cells), resulting in the deposition of calcium. Premature infants are at risk of decreased bone mineralization due to a shortened gestation and nutritional intake challenges in the newborn period (Abad-Sinden, Verbrugge, & Buck, 2001). Calcium intake during childhood and adolescence is essential to provide adequate bone density that will prevent osteoporosis and fractures in adulthood. Inadequate bone mineralization can cause **osteopenia** (decreased mineralization and bone mass) or **osteoporosis** (softening of bone due to marked decrease in mineralization and bone mass). See Chapter 9∞ for a discussion of inadequate calcium intake during school age and adolescence and its contribution to osteoporosis.

Varus
An abnormal position of limb that involves bending inward toward the mindline of the body

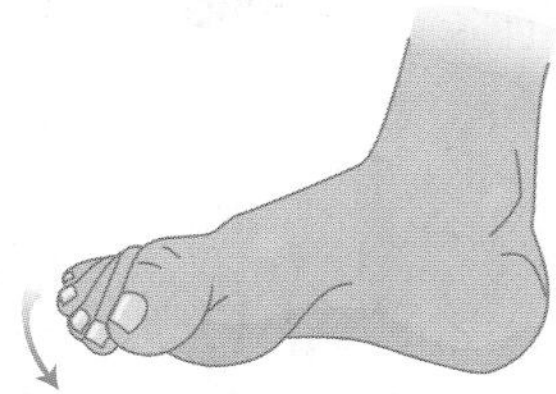

Valgus
An abnormal position of a limb that involves bending outward away from the midline of the body

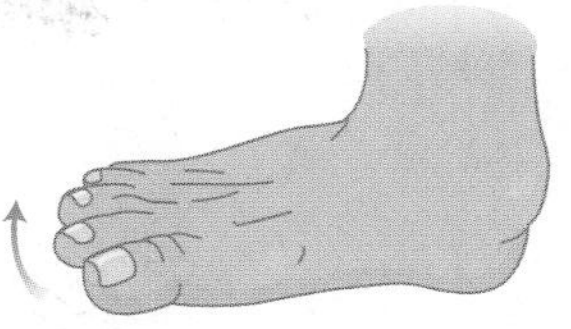

Adduction
Lateral movement of limbs toward the midline of the body

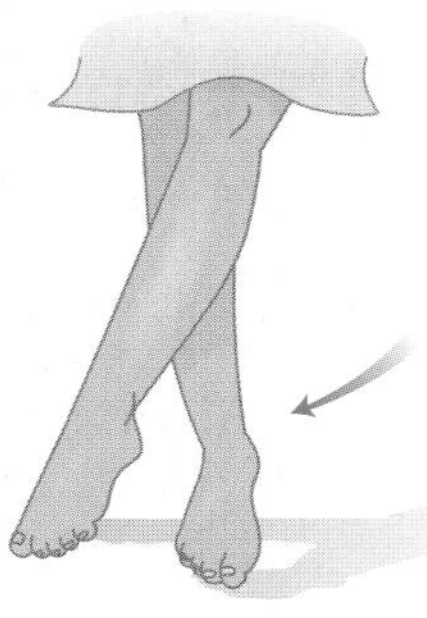

Abduction
Lateral movement of limbs away from the midline of the body

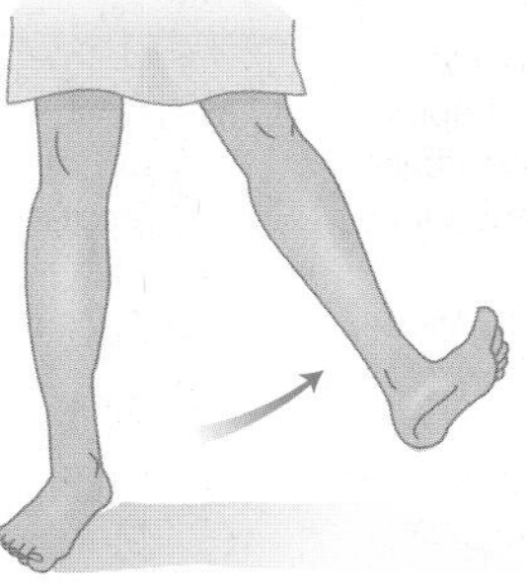

Inversion
Turning inward, usually more than normal

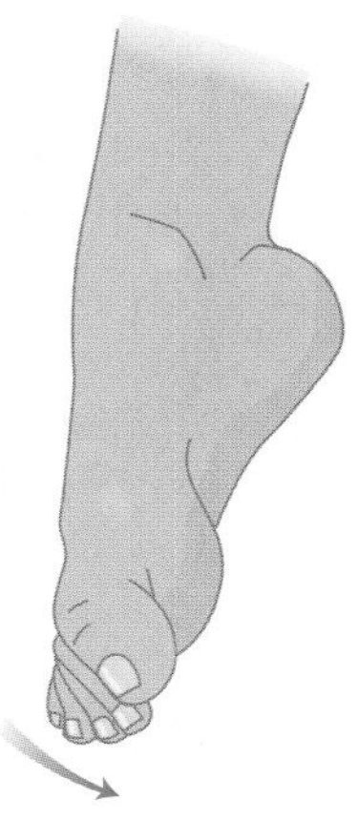

Eversion
Turning outward

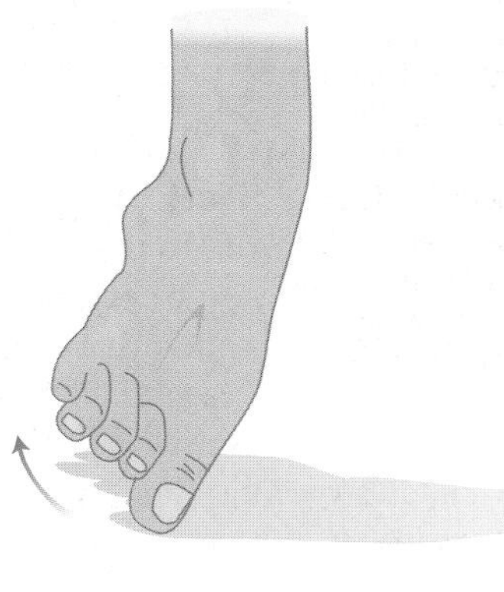

Supination
Lying on the back or placing the hand so that palm faces upward

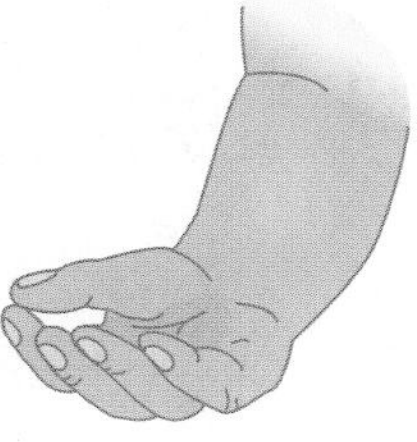

Pronation
Lying on the stomach or placing the hand so the palm faces downward

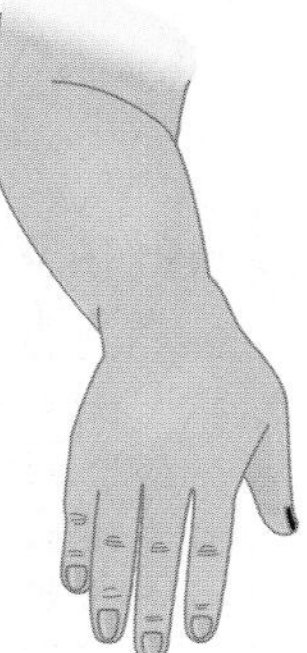

FIGURE 35–1 ■ Musculoskeletal positions and joint motions.

MediaLink Muscle Physiology Animation

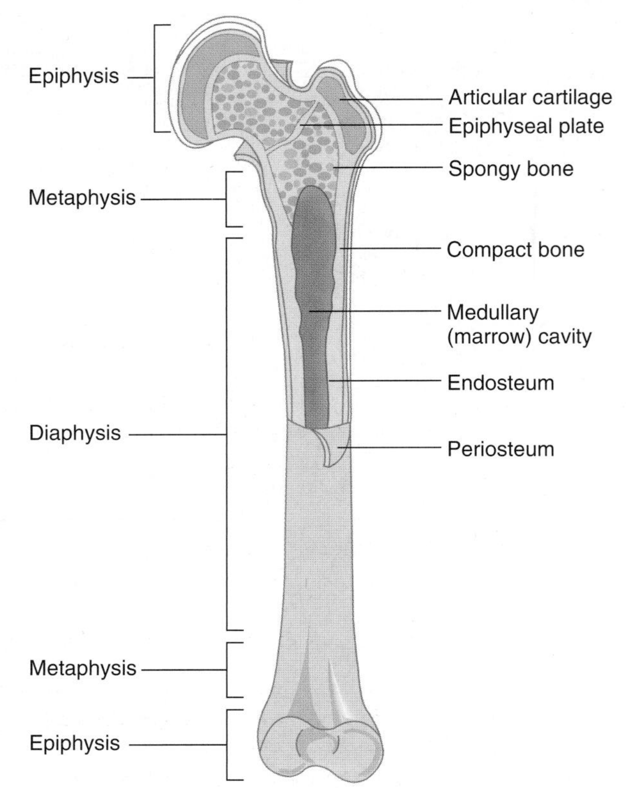

FIGURE 35–2 ■ The parts of long bones.

Children and adolescents may suffer injuries to the musculoskeletal system from falls, car crashes, and sports. Fractures are one type of common injury. Because growth takes place at the epiphyseal plates, injuries to this portion of a long bone are of particular concern in young children.

The long bones of children are porous and less dense than those of adults. For this reason, children's bones can bend, buckle, or break as a result of a simple fall. Children's bones are growing which facilitates healing after fractures, but may also lead to "growing pains" as muscles are pulled when bones grow quickly.

In addition to the structural differences between the bones of children and adults, there are functional differences in the skeletal system of children (see Figure 8–2∞). Before birth, the thoracic and sacral regions of the spine are convex curves. As the infant learns to hold up the head, the cervical region becomes concave. When the child learns to stand, the lumbar region also becomes concave. Failure of the spine to assume these final curves results in an abnormal curvature of the spine (kyphosis or lordosis).

Muscles, Tendons, and Ligaments

The muscular system, unlike the skeletal system, is almost completely formed at birth. As a child grows, muscles do not increase in number, but rather in length and circumference. Until puberty, both ligaments and tendons are stronger than bone. When these structural differences are not recognized, a childhood fracture is sometimes mistaken for a sprain. A **sprain** is a tearing of ligaments, the structural support connecting bones, usually caused when a joint is twisted or otherwise traumatized. Tendons, which connect bones to muscles, grow in length and fibrous tissue as mechanical pressure is placed on them.

DISORDERS OF THE FEET AND LEGS

Metatarsus Adductus

Metatarsus adductus, the most common congenital foot deformity, is characterized by an inward turning of the forefoot at the tarsometatarsal joints (Figure 35–3 ■). Often referred to as "intoeing," metatarsus adductus affects male and female infants equally and occurs in approximately 1 in 1,000 births, with more common incidence among siblings. This condition is most likely caused by both intrauterine positioning and genetic factors (Ryan, 2001). See Box 35–1.

Foot radiographs may be taken and physical assessment of the foot is performed. Treatment depends on the degree of foot flexibility. If the foot can be readily maneuvered past the neutral position, simple exercises may correct the problem. (See Partnering with Families: Stretching Exercises for Metatarsus Adductus.) Most cases will resolve spontaneously by the time the infant is about 3 months of age. Serial casting is the treatment of choice for curvature angles greater than 15 degrees, or in cases that do not improve. The infant's feet are placed in a position as close to neutral as possible and are held secure with casts. Casts are changed weekly until the desired correction is achieved. Braces and orthopedic shoes may also be used to maintain correction after casting.

NURSING MANAGEMENT

Reassure parents that the child's condition can be corrected. If the deformity is mild, teach parents simple stretching exercises that can be performed at each diaper change. If casting is necessary, provide cast care and teach parents how to care for the child in a cast at home (Box 35–2). See Partnering with Families: Care of the Child with a Cast. If metatarsus adductus persists into

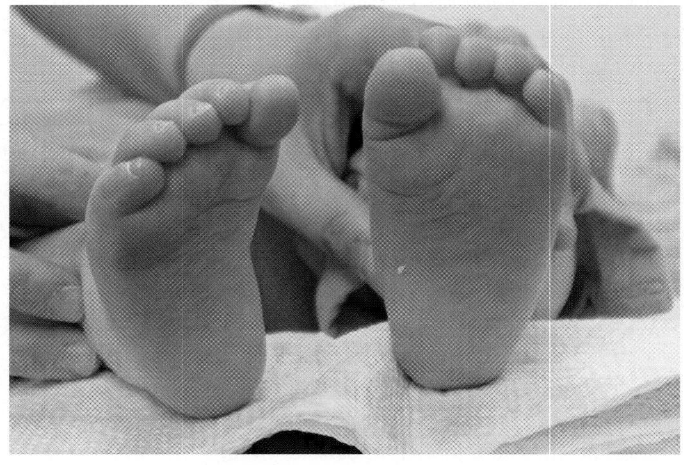

FIGURE 35–3 ■ Metatarsus adductus is characterized by convexity (curvature) of the lateral border of the foot. The child's right foot demonstrates the disorder. Note that the forefoot turns inward and appears out of alignment with the remainder of the foot.

BOX 35–1 Intoeing

Metatarsus adductus is one cause of intoeing. There are other potential causes that should be considered; some are more likely at certain ages in development. If intoeing is first observed when the child walks (12–18 months), internal tibial torsion may be the cause. This generally improves with walking. Intoeing that persists until 2–4 years may be related to femoral anteversion. Stretching exercises, ballet, and ice skating may help to decrease intoeing (Ryan, 2001).

childhood without correction, the challenge is to find shoes that accommodate the unusual shape of the foot.

Clubfoot

Clubfoot is a congenital abnormality in which the foot is twisted out of its normal position. It occurs in approximately 1 in 1,000 births, affects boys nearly twice as often as girls, and is bilateral in about half of affected infants (Gilmore & Thompson, 2003).

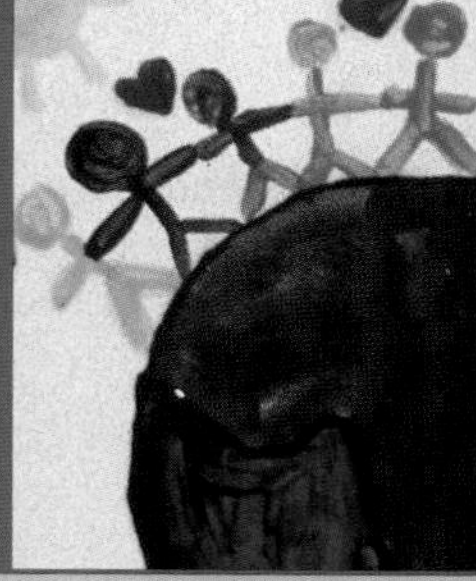

PARTNERING WITH FAMILIES

Stretching Exercises for Metatarsus Adductus

- Hold the infant's foot securely by the heel. Maintain the heel in this position.
- Move the forefoot outward away from the body with the other hand.
- Hold the foot in this position for 5 seconds.
- Repeat five times during each diaper change.

BOX 35–2 Nursing Care of the Child in a Cast

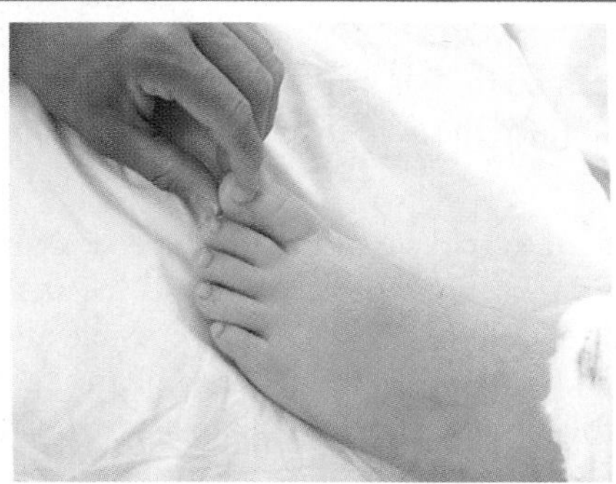

A

- A plaster cast takes anywhere from 24–48 hours to dry. When handling the cast, be gentle and use the palms of your hands, as fingertips can indent plaster and create pressure areas.
- After the cast is applied, elevate the extremity on a pillow above the level of the heart. Elevation helps to reduce swelling and increases venous return.
- If the cast is applied after surgery, there may be drainage or bleeding through the cast material. Circle the stain and note the date and time on the cast to provide a means of assessing the amount of fluid lost. Once a cast is dry a "window" or opening is sometimes cut so that a wound can be viewed or in order to allow the stomach to expand more comfortably.
- Assess the distal pulses, and check the fingers and toes for color, warmth, capillary refill, and edema. Assess sensation as well as movement. Any deviation from normal may indicate nerve damage or decreased blood supply.
- During the first 24 hours, the casted extremity should be checked every 15–30 minutes for 2 hours, then every 1–2 hours thereafter. The skin should be warm. It should blanch when slight pressure is applied and then return to its normal color within 3 seconds (**A**). For the next 2 days, the casted extremity should be assessed at least every 4 hours.
- Check the edges of the cast for roughness or crumbling. If necessary, pull the inner stockinette over the edge of the cast and tape.
- The rough edges of the cast may also be alleviated by "petaling." This is done by securing adhesive tape to the inside of the cast and pulling it over the edge, covering the jagged or broken pieces of plaster, and securing it to the outer surface of the cast (**B, C, D**). Moleskin may be used on the cast as well. Petal the opening around a window in the cast if one is present.

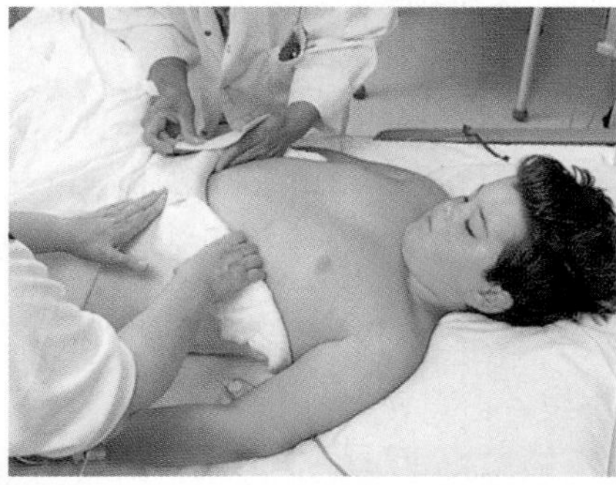

B

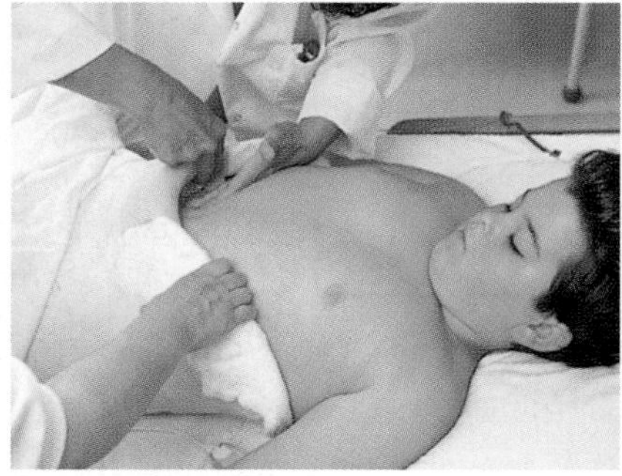

C

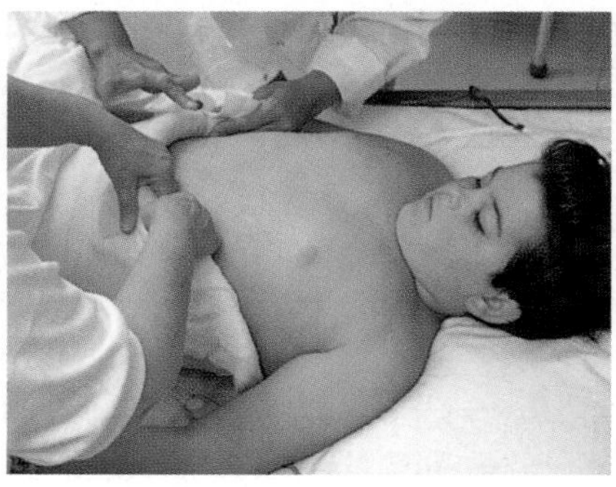

D

- Keep the cast as clean and dry as possible. Cover the cast with a plastic bag or plastic wrap when the child bathes or showers.
- The skin under the cast may itch; however, do not use powders or lotions near the edges or under the cast as they can cause skin irritation.
- Be sure that children do not put small objects between the casts and their extremities; these actions can cause skin irritation as well as neurovascular compromise.

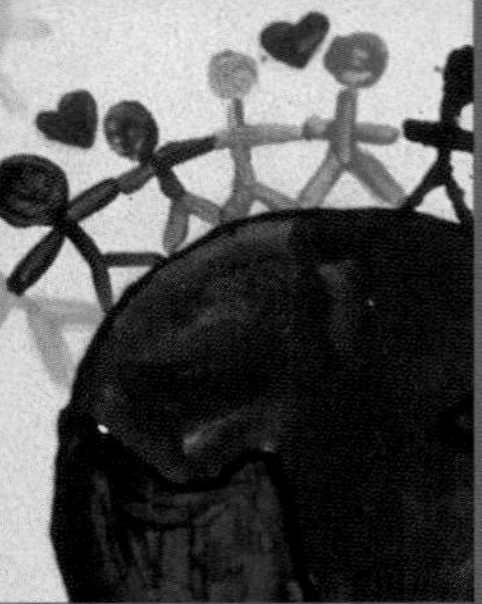

PARTNERING WITH FAMILIES

Care of the Child with a Cast

Skin care

- Check the skin around the cast edges for irritation, rubbing, or blistering. The skin should be clean and dry.
- Cleanse the skin just under the cast edges and between the toes or fingers with a cotton-tipped applicator and rubbing alcohol. Avoid using lotions, oils, and powders near the cast as they may collect on and irritate the skin.
- Avoid poking sharp objects down inside the cast as this may result in sores.

Cast care

- Keep the cast dry. Protect plaster with a cast shoe, thick sock, or sling.
- Allow a new, wet cast to air dry for 24 hours.
- Begin walking on a leg cast only when the physician gives permission.

Be alert for possible complications

- Toes or fingers should be pink, not blue or white.
- Skin should be warm and the tips of the toes should blanch when pinched.
- Raise the casted arm or leg above heart level and rest it on pillows to prevent or reduce any swelling.

Notify the healthcare provider if any of the following occur

- Unusual odor beneath the cast
- Tingling
- Burning or numbness in the casted arm or leg
- Drainage through the cast
- Swelling or inability to move the fingers or toes
- Slippage of the cast
- Cast cracked, soft, or loose
- Sudden, unexplained fever
- Unusual fussiness or irritability in an infant or child
- Fingers or toes that are blue or white
- Pain that is not relieved by any comfort measures (e.g., repositioning or pain medication)

Note: Courtesy of Shriners Hospital for Children, Spokane, WA.

Etiology and Pathophysiology

The exact cause of clubfoot is unknown; however, several possible etiologies have been proposed. Some authorities believe abnormal intrauterine positioning causes the deformity, others suspect neuromuscular or vascular problems. Yet other experts believe there is a genetic component, either at the chromosomal level or by the arrest of normal fetal development. A positive family history increases the chance of the deformity. See Developing Cultural Competence: Ethnic Influence on Clubfoot Incidence.

Clinical Manifestations

A true clubfoot (talipes equinovarus) involves three areas of deformity: the midfoot is directed downward (**equinus**), the hindfoot turns inward (**varus**), and the forefoot curls toward the heel (adduction) and turns upward in partial supination. Muscles, tendons, and bones are involved in the abnormality and it cannot be corrected by exercise. Most children have this combination of findings. The foot is small with a shortened Achilles tendon. Muscles in the lower leg are atrophied, but leg lengths are generally normal. Clubfoot is bilateral in 50% of cases (Figure 35–4 ■). Clubhand is a rare occurrence that has similar characteristics to the foot deformity (Figure 35–5 ■).

COLLABORATIVE CARE

The goal of collaborative care for the child with clubfoot is successful treatment to facilitate normal ambulation.

Diagnostic Tests

Diagnosis is made at birth on the basis of visual inspection. Radiographs are used to confirm the severity of the condition.

Clinical Therapy

Early treatment is essential to achieve successful correction and reduce the chance of complications. Serial casting is the treatment of choice. Casting should begin as soon as possible after birth. Timing is critical, because the short bones of the foot, which are primarily cartilaginous at birth, begin to ossify shortly thereafter. The foot is manipulated to achieve maximum correction first of the varus deformity and then of the equinus deformity. A long leg cast is applied to hold the foot in the desired position. The cast is changed every 1 to 2 weeks. This regimen of manipulation and casting continues for approximately 8 to 12 weeks until maximum correction is achieved. If the deformity has been corrected, the child may begin wearing a splint with a crossbar between shoes (most commonly called a Denis Browne splint) or reverse last corrective shoes (shoes with the toes pointing outward rather than inward) to maintain the correction (Gilmore & Thompson, 2003; Morcuende, Dolan, Dietz, et al., 2004). If the deformity has not been corrected, surgical intervention is required. Casting is maintained to hold the foot in position until surgery is performed (Figure 35–6 ■).

The age at which a child undergoes clubfoot surgery varies among surgeons. However, most children have surgery between

DEVELOPING CULTURAL COMPETENCE
Ethnic Influence on Clubfoot Incidence

The incidence of talipes equinovarus (clubfoot) varies among ethnic groups. The condition is least common in Asian groups and Whites, with a higher incidence in groups from the Middle East, South Africa, and Mexico. It is most common in Polynesian groups (Blakeslee, 1997).

3 and 12 months of age. The one-stage posteromedial release procedure, which involves realignment of the bones of the foot and release of the constricting soft tissue, is most commonly performed. The foot is held in the proper position by one or more stainless steel pins. A cast is then applied with the knee flexed to prevent damage to the pin and to discourage weight bearing. Casting continues for 6 to 12 weeks. The child may then need to wear a brace or corrective shoes, depending on the severity of the deformity and the surgeon's preference.

More severe cases or those not corrected in infancy may require more than one surgery to correct the foot.

PATHOPHYSIOLOGY ILLUSTRATED

Bilateral Clubfoot Deformity

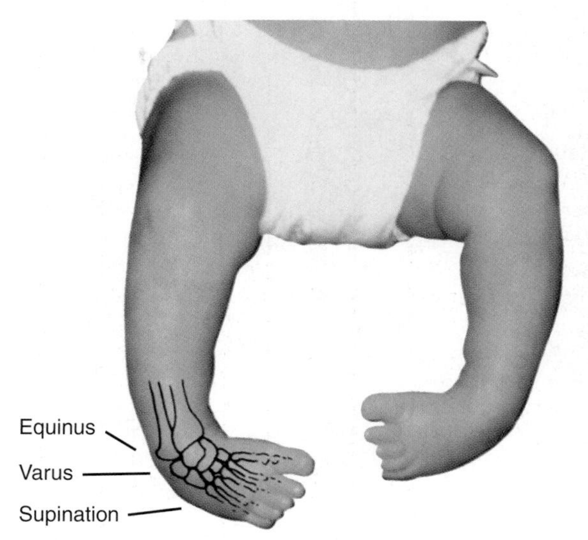

FIGURE 35–4 ■ Parents of a child with clubfoot will have many questions. Can the condition be treated? Will the child be able to walk normally after surgery? Will they need help caring for the infant? How much will surgery and other care cost? Will any subsequent children have a clubfoot?

Modified from Staheli, L. T. (1992). Fundamentals of pediatric orthopedics *(p. 5.10). New York: Raven Press.*

NURSING MANAGEMENT

The goals of nursing care for the child with a clubfoot are to provide necessary information to parents and ensure adequate healing during the treatment process.

■ Nursing Assessment and Diagnosis

Nursing assessment, which begins at birth and continues throughout the child's subsequent outpatient casting visits and hospitalization for surgery, includes taking a genetic and birth history, performing a physical examination (including position and appearance of the foot), and assessing the child's motor development and family's coping mechanisms. Because parents will need to bring the child for frequent cast changes, assess the family's access to transportation and other arrangements that are necessary to facilitate these visits.

Nursing diagnoses that may apply to the child with a clubfoot deformity are as follows:

- Impaired Physical Mobility related to restricted movement due to cast
- Risk for Impaired Skin Integrity related to pressure from cast
- Risk for Impaired Parenting related to birth of a child with a physical defect
- Health-Seeking Behaviors related to lack of information about deformity, treatment, and home care

■ Planning and Implementation

Nursing management involves providing emotional support, educating the family about home care of the child in a cast and the importance of keeping appointments at the outpatient facility for cast changes, preparation of the family for the child's hospitalization if surgery is to occur, and providing postsurgical care.

Provide Emotional Support

Clubfoot is a condition that affects both the child and the family. The child's foot deformity may be upsetting to parents, and they need emotional support to allay their fears. Helping parents understand the condition and its treatment is essential.

Encourage parents to hold and cuddle the child and to take an active role in the child's care to help promote bonding. Explain that, with treatment, the child will grow and develop normally.

Provide Cast and Brace Care

Routine cast care is important to ensure skin and neurovascular integrity. (See Box 35–2.)

CLINICAL TIP

When an infant is receiving serial casting for clubfoot, the physician often recommends that the parent soak the cast off the night before a scheduled cast change. Teach the parents how to remove the plaster cast. The infant can be placed in a warm bath, and the cast will start to disintegrate and can be unrolled. This avoids exposure of the infant to the loud sound of the cast cutter, and allows for the infant's leg to be washed and out of the cast overnight. Parents can also be encouraged to bring a bottle to the clinic. If the infant is hungry and feeding, the foot is more easily kept still for the cast application.

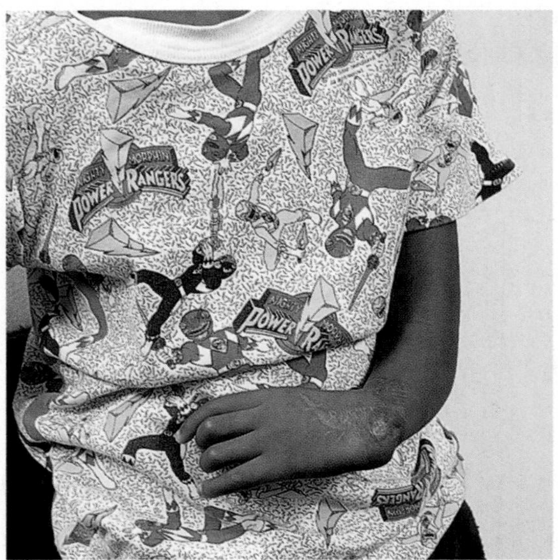

FIGURE 35–5 ■ A clubhand deformity is a less common condition than clubfoot.

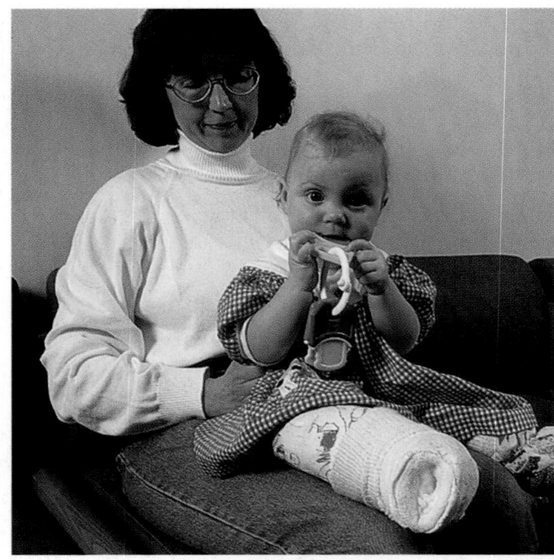

FIGURE 35–6 ■ This girl has a long leg cast, which was applied after surgery to correct her clubfoot.

After serial casting is complete, or following surgery, the child may progress to wearing a brace or special shoe for 6 to 12 months. Braces should fit snugly but should not interfere with neurovascular function. Before the child begins to wear a brace, check the skin for any areas of redness or breakdown. Provide parents with guidelines for brace wear as outlined later in the chapter. (See Partnering with Families: Guidelines for Brace Wear.) Emphasize that proper skin care is essential. If skin redness develops, arrange to have the fit of the brace evaluated and modified if necessary.

Provide Postsurgical Care

Routine postoperative care after surgical correction includes neurovascular status checks every 2 hours for the first 24 hours and observing for any swelling around the cast edges (see Box 35–2). Apply ice bags to the foot, and keep the ankle and foot elevated on a pillow for 24 hours to promote healing and help with venous return. Keep the cast open to air to facilitate drying. Check for drainage or bleeding. Administer pain medication routinely for 24 to 48 hours. Popliteal or epidural blocks may be placed during surgery and used in the immediate postsurgical period for pain control (Figure 35–7 ■). The nurse monitors these blocks for effectiveness and any undesired effects (see Chapter 18∞ for detailed instructions on pain management). See the Skills Manual for detail on monitoring nerve blocks.

Discharge Planning and Home Care Teaching

Parents should be given written instructions for care of the child with a cast (see page 1412). In addition, assist them in the following ways.

- Demonstrate the use of a sponge bath to protect the cast from water breakdown.
- Discuss several options for clothing that accommodate a cast, for example, one-piece snap suits or sweatpants.
- Discuss potential safety hazards that may result from awkward positioning. Be sure the child is properly situated in a car safety seat for the trip home.
- Suggest that parents make an effort to place toys within the child's reach, because movements of a child in a cast may be slowed.
- Have parents avoid use of "umbrella" strollers and infant swings since they do not provide adequate support for the casted leg.

■ Evaluation

Expected outcomes of nursing care include maintenance of skin integrity, recovery without complications after surgery, normal

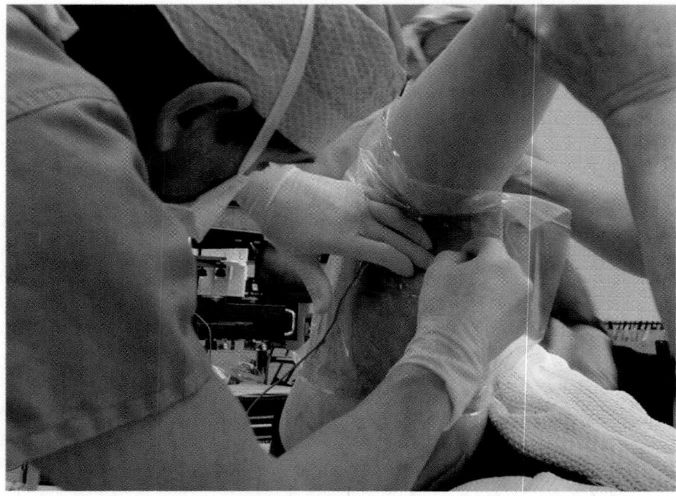

FIGURE 35–7 ■ The insertion of a popliteal block during surgery. The site will be wrapped and the tubing connected to an infusion pump. The nurse will monitor the infusion and pain control after surgery.

Courtesy of Shriners Hospital, Spokane, WA.

developmental progression of the child, and demonstrated knowledge by parents for care of braces or casts, as needed.

Genu Varum and Genu Valgum

Genu varum (bowlegs) is a deformity in which the knees are widely separated while the ankles are close together and the lower legs are turned inward (varus). In genu valgum (knock-knees), the knees are close together while the ankles are widely spaced so that the lower legs are directed outward (**valgus**) (Figure 35–8 ■).

At certain stages of a child's development, the appearance of bowlegs or knock-knees is normal. Until 2 to 3 years, the knees are normally bowed, showing varus alignment, and by 4 to 5 years, some knock-knee or valgus alignment commonly emerges (see Figure 8–61∞). Chapter 8∞ discusses the assessment of bowlegs and knock-knees in children.

If bowlegs are pronounced or have not improved by 2 years of age, the child should be evaluated by an orthopedist. Blount's disease and rickets are two pathological causes of bowlegs and should be ruled out. **Blount's disease** is characterized by abnormal growth on the medial side of the proximal tibia which causes an increasing varus deformity. It is believed to be due to increasing compression forces across the medial knee and is more common in overweight, Black, and female children (Thompson, 2004c). **Rickets** is a result of inadequate bone mineralization, usually caused by a deficiency of calcium and/or vitamin D. (See Chapter 9∞ for a description of the association between rickets and diet.) Since the bones are decalcified or softened, long bones such as those in the legs may bend into a bowed position. Occasionally rickets is congenital and is caused by an X-linked autosomal dominant or recessive gene with the chromosomal location Xp22.31-p21.3. It results in an enzyme deficiency of alkaline phosphatase which in turn leads to excessive inhibitors of bone mineralization. This type of rickets is rare and is called familial hypophosphatemic rickets (FHR).

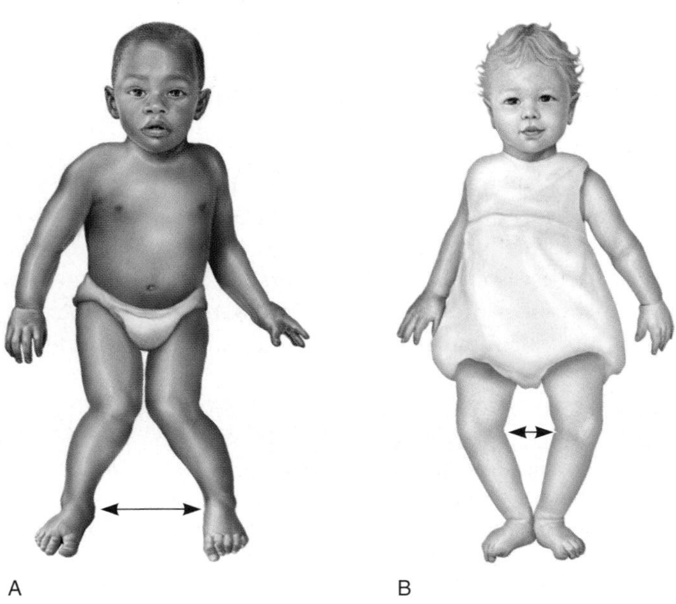

FIGURE 35–8 ■ *A,* Genu valgum, or knock-knees. Note that the ankles are far apart when the knees are together. *B,* Genu varum, or bowlegs. The legs are bowed so that the knees are far apart as the child stands.

PARTNERING WITH FAMILIES

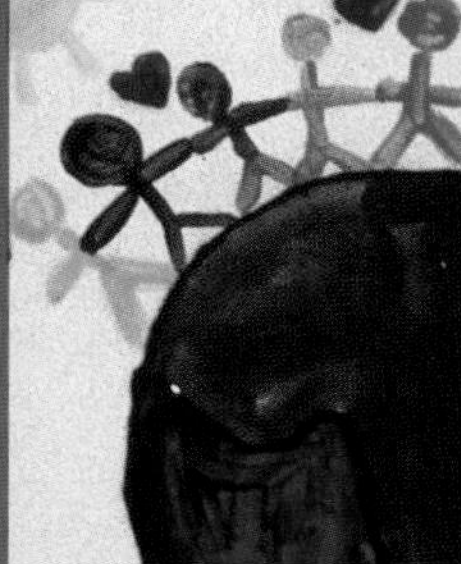

Guidelines for Brace Wear

- Braces should be as comfortable as possible and the child should have adequate mobility while wearing the brace.
- Begin wearing the brace for periods of 1–2 hours and then progress to 2–4 hours.
- Check the skin at 1–2-hour intervals initially, then lengthening to every 4 hours once skin has been clear for several days. If redness is apparent, leave the brace off and allow the skin to clear. If breakdown has occurred, the brace cannot be replaced until healing is complete. (See Chapter 36∞ for a discussion of pressure ulcers.)
- Always have the child wear a clean white sock, T-shirt, or other thin white liner beneath the brace. Be sure the liner is wrinkle free under the brace. Avoid using powders or lotions that can cause skin to break down. Toughen any sensitive areas using alcohol wipes 3–4 times daily.
- Reapply the brace when the skin returns to its normal color.
- Return to the physician or orthotic specialist if discomfort or red areas persist or if the brace needs adjustment or repair or is outgrown.
- Check the brace daily for rough edges

Excessive or continued knock-knees should also be evaluated by an orthopedist although, unlike genu varum, the condition has no pathologic causes.

Careful measurements and radiographic studies are used for accurate diagnosis of varus and valgus conditions. Arthrography (joint radiograph), MRI, and CT imaging may be added as needed for accurate diagnosis.

Braces are often used to correct mild varus and valgus deformities that could worsen as the child grows. Braces for varus deformities (bowlegs) are worn at night; those for valgus deformities (knock-knees) are worn both day and night. Duration of brace wear is determined by the severity of the deformity. If the deformity continues to worsen, surgical intervention is necessary.

When dietary rickets is the cause of varus deformity, supplementation with calcium and vitamin D are needed. FHR is treated with calcium and phosphorus in five to six daily doses. Surgery may be needed, particularly in treatment of Blount's disease. An **osteotomy** (cutting of the bone) is performed and the tibiofemoral angle surgically corrected. The child is then placed in a cast for approximately 6 to 10 weeks, or until full healing has occurred.

Nursing Management

Reassure parents that bowlegs and knock-knees are usually a normal part of a child's growth and development. These conditions often resolve on their own and require no treatment other than monitoring. Encourage them to ask for evaluation at each health promotion visit to be sure the condition is not worsening. Ask about familial bone diseases.

Nursing care focuses on educating the parents and child about the conditions and their treatment. Provide the child and family with guidelines for brace wear and maintenance (see page 1415). Instruct about intake of calcium and vitamin D when there is a deficiency and partner with parents to plan for dietary supplements in children with dietary rickets or FHR. Provide postoperative care and cast care as needed for the child who undergoes surgery.

Desired outcomes for nursing care include establishment of normal gait patterns and activities for the child, maintenance of intact skin and neurovascular status during treatment, and understanding by the parent of assessment and intervention when needed.

DISORDERS OF THE HIP

Developmental Dysplasia of the Hip

Developmental dysplasia of the hip (DDH) refers to a variety of conditions in which the femoral head and the acetabulum are improperly aligned. These conditions include hip instability, **dislocation** (displacement of the bone from its normal articulation with the joint), **subluxation** (in this instance, a partial dislocation), and acetabular **dysplasia** (abnormal cellular or structural development) (American Academy of Pediatrics, 2000). In the past, DDH was referred to as congenital dislocated hip (CDH). The revised name of the disorder emphasizes that many cases of dislocation, subluxation, and dysplasia occur well after the neonatal period and involve more than a simple dislocation.

Hip instability is present in 1 in 100 newborns, while dislocation occurs in 1 to 2 in 1,000 births, and the condition affects girls four times as often as boys. It is unilateral in 80% of affected children, and the left hip is affected three times as often as the right (American Academy of Pediatrics, 2000).

Etiology and Pathophysiology

Some types of DDH are linked to early gestational events at 12 and 18 weeks' gestation, as the lower limbs rotate and surrounding muscles develop. On the other hand, milder cases may be influenced by mechanical forces in the last month of pregnancy such as breech position or fetal size, and some cases develop after birth as the hip assumes an extended rather than flexed posture (Witt, 2003).

Although the exact cause of DDH is unknown, genetic factors appear to play a role. DDH is 20 to 50 times more common in first-degree relatives of an infant with the condition than in the general population. If one child of a set of identical twins has DDH, the other twin is affected 30% to 40% of the time.

The left hip is involved more often than the right hip as a result of intrauterine positioning of the left side of the fetus against the mother's sacrum. Maternal estrogen may cause laxity of the hip joint and capsule, leading to joint instability, especially in females who respond more than males to these estrogen levels. DDH is more common in infants born in the breech position, when oligohydramnios occurs, and in babies that are large for gestational age (Witt, 2003). Cultural factors may also be associated with DDH. (See Developing Cultural Competence: Developmental Dysplasia of the Hip.)

Clinical Manifestations

Common signs and symptoms of DDH include limited abduction of the affected hip, asymmetry of the gluteal and thigh fat folds, and telescoping or pistoning of the thigh (Figure 35–9 ■). The older child with untreated DDH walks with a significant limp, which results from telescoping of the femoral head into the pelvis. The longer the disorder goes untreated, the more pronounced the clinical manifestations become, and the worse the prognosis.

COLLABORATIVE CARE

The purpose of care is to identify all children with DDH early in infancy, when treatment is most successful. Partnership between many health professionals is needed to provide care and ensure normal mobility.

Diagnostic Tests

Physical examination of all newborns and infants is important to identify DDH. Both the United States and Canada recommend such screening for all newborns and infants/young children until walking is well established (American Academy of Pediatrics, 2000; Patel, 2001). Specific tests include Allis' sign (one knee lower than the other when the knees are flexed) and positive Ortolani-Barlow maneuver. Refer to Chapter 8∞ for a discussion and photographs of the assessment for hip dysplasia in newborns and infants. Radiographs are generally not reliable until approximately 4 months of age, because the pelvis in a newborn is still primarily cartilaginous. Before 4 months, ultrasonography may be useful for diagnosis. After that age, radiographs are used for diagnosis.

Clinical Therapy

Treatment plans vary according to the child's age. For infants younger than 3 months, the Pavlik harness is the most commonly used method for hip reduction (Figure 35–10 ■). The Pavlik harness is a dynamic splint, that is, a splint that allows movement. It ensures hip flexion and abduction but does not allow hip extension or adduction. For infants older than

> **DEVELOPING CULTURAL COMPETENCE**
> **Developmental Dysplasia of the Hip**
>
> Infants who are positioned on cradleboards or traditionally swaddled, as in some Native American cultures, have a high incidence of developmental dysplasia of the hip (DDH). Canadian Indian babies have an incidence of 188 per 1,000 births and Navaho Indians in the southwest United States have an incidence of 20 per 1,000. On the other hand, among cultures in which mothers carry infants on their hips or backs with the infants' legs abducted—as in Korean, Chinese, and some African groups—the incidence of DDH is rare (Witt, 2003).

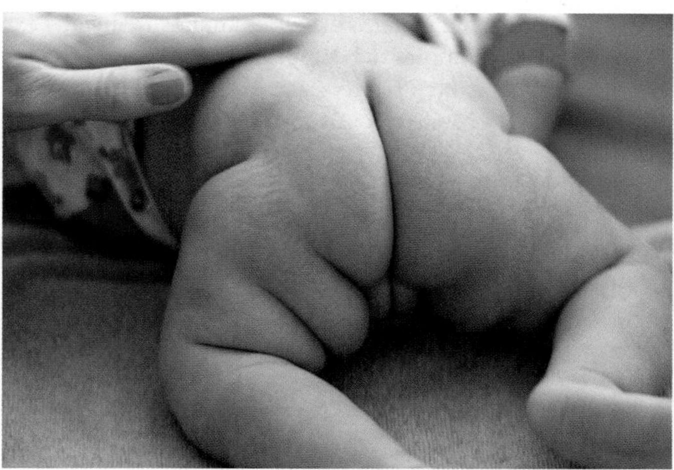

FIGURE 35–9 ■ The asymmetry of the gluteal and thigh fat folds is easy to see in this child with developmental dysplasia of the hip.

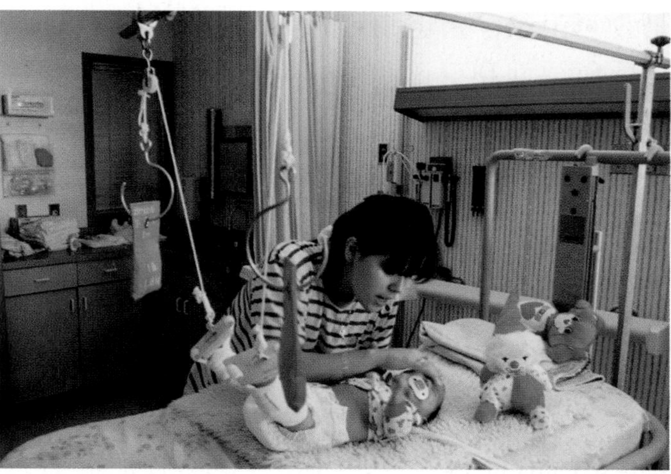

FIGURE 35–11 ■ For infants older than 3 months of age, skin traction is commonly used for treatment of DDH.

3 months, skin traction is used (Figure 35–11 ■). Correct positioning, which involves relocating the femoral head into the acetabulum while gently stretching the restrictive soft tissue, is essential. Surgery and the application of a hip spica cast may be necessary. In children over 18 months of age, surgery and casting are usually necessary and bracing may also be required.

Early screening, detection, and treatment enable the majority of affected children to attain normal hip function.

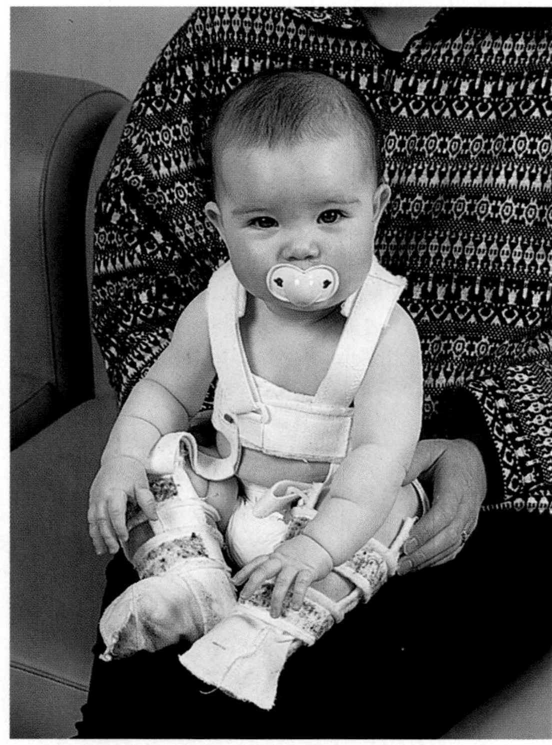

FIGURE 35–10 ■ The most common treatment for DDH in a child under 3 months of age is a Pavlik harness. A shirt should be worn under the harness to prevent skin irritation (it was omitted for clarity in this photograph).

NURSING MANAGEMENT

The goal of nursing management is to promote early identification of DDH and to provide safe care for the child using a brace or traction, requiring surgery, or wearing corrective shoes.

■ Nursing Assessment and Diagnosis

Assessment for DDH begins at delivery and continues through all health promotion visits. The specific family history or birth data may indicate a high-risk infant, as does oligohydramnios, large-for-gestational-age infant, or breech birth. Instructions for performing the physical examination to assess the infant for DDH are given in Chapter 8∞. Further assessments are determined by the treatment provided. Skin assessments are performed on the child in traction or a cast, every few minutes in the immediate postoperative period and progressing to once or twice daily at home. Respiratory and circulatory assessments are included when the child is immobilized. Ongoing assessments of the child's growth and development are needed when mobility is impaired. Weigh the casted child once the cast is dry so a baseline casted weight can be used for comparison during the weeks and months while the cast remains in place.

The following nursing diagnoses may apply to the child with DDH.

- Impaired Physical Mobility related to prescribed movement restriction (Pavlik harness, traction, spica cast, brace)
- Risk for Impaired Skin Integrity related to irritation from harness straps or skin traction
- Risk for Altered Urinary Elimination or Constipation related to immobility caused by treatment
- Risk for Imbalanced Nutrition related to decreased appetite
- Risk for Delayed Growth and Development related to limited mobility and potential decreased exposure to stimulation
- Health-Seeking Behavior (parental) related to lack of information about disease process and treatment

Planning and Implementation

The infant with DDH is often cared for at home and in outpatient facilities. If surgery is performed, the child is hospitalized for surgery and the immediate postoperative period. Nursing care varies according to the medical treatment and the child's age. Management includes maintaining traction, if ordered; providing cast care; preventing complications resulting from immobility; promoting normal growth and development; and teaching parents how to care for a child in a cast, traction, or a Pavlik harness at home. Because treatment may interfere with the child's normal movement, the treatment plan should take into consideration the age and developmental stage of the child.

Maintain Traction

Bryant skin traction is the most common form of traction used in the treatment of DDH. (Types of traction are discussed later in the chapter and presented in Table 35–4.) Check the traction apparatus frequently to ensure that proper alignment and healing occur. Traction may also be used as a treatment in the home. The family needs to be given careful instruction in how to care for the child in traction. In addition, arrangements should be made for a nurse to make several home visits to set up the traction apparatus and monitor the child's progress after discharge.

Provide Cast Care

The principles of routine cast care presented in Box 35–2 apply to the care of hip spica casts. Special techniques should be used to help keep the cast clean and dry in children who are not toilet trained. Female and male urinals can be used for older children. Use a plastic lining to protect the cast edges during elimination for older children and use a small disposable diaper to cover the perineum in babies, tucking edges beneath the cast. Be sure to change the diaper frequently to prevent soiling of the cast.

Control Pain

If the child has surgery to correct DDH, pain control in the immediate postoperative period is needed. Assess the child's pain frequently in a method appropriate for age (see Chapter 18∞). Administer intravenous and then oral pain medications as ordered. Use methods such as holding, rocking, and gentle music to calm the child. An ice bag placed on top of the cast at the operative site may be helpful. Encourage parents to be present and provide care when possible.

> **CLINICAL TIP**
>
> If pain is not controlled or if it increases over time, compression at the surgical site may be occurring; promptly report this to the physician. Pain in the infant may be manifested by a combination of physiological and behavioral changes.

Prevent Complications Resulting from Immobility

Immobilization from traction or a cast can cause alterations in physiologic functioning. Take the following actions to prevent complications.

- Assess breathing patterns and lung sounds frequently for congestion or respiratory compromise.
- Perform skin and neurovascular assessments approximately every 2 hours.

> **CLINICAL TIP**
>
> Neurovascular assessment involves evaluation of temperature, movement, color, capillary refill, and sensation. Even if the child is not old enough to respond to questions about feeling, usually brushing the hands or sheets along the toes elicits a movement from the child indicating sensation. Report any abnormalities immediately. Keep limbs aligned as ordered during traction. For the child in a hip spica, immediately after surgery elevate the lower body on pillows to decrease edema under the cast at the operative site.

- Use adequate padding and skin wrapping to avoid placing pressure on the popliteal space. Such pressure could lead to nerve damage.
- For the child in a cast, change the child's position every 2 to 3 hours while awake to help avoid areas of pressure and promote increased circulation. The child can be placed either prone or supine or positioned on the floor and supported with pillows.
- Help prevent skin irritation and breakdown in the child with a cast. Use moleskin to provide protection from rough edges. Place tape around the perineal opening of the cast to prevent soiling.
- Increase fluids and fiber in the child's diet, as a change in bowel or bladder status is commonly associated with immobility.
- If permitted by physician's orders, release the child from traction for meals and daily care. The time out of traction should not exceed 1 hour per day. Encourage parents to hold and cuddle the child at this time to promote comfort and bonding.

Promote Normal Growth and Development

Engage the child in activities that stimulate the upper extremities and all five senses. Provide stimulating toys such as stacking blocks, brightly colored mobiles, Koosh balls, or musical toys. Position toys within the child's reach and interact with the child as much as possible.

> **PRACTICE ALERT**
>
> Use caution in selecting toys appropriate for the child's developmental age. If the child is in a cast, be sure that toys or parts cannot be swallowed or inserted under the edges of the cast. Place a T-shirt over the cast so that the edges are securely covered and it is difficult for the child to place something under them.

Discharge Planning and Home Care Teaching

Parents must learn how to care for a child in a hip spica cast at home. The active participation of family members in the daily care of the child while hospitalized gradually increases confidence in their ability to provide care at home. Home care needs should be identified and addressed early in hospitalization. Before discharge, be sure the parents have the following information.

- Instructions about general cast care (see page 1412), positioning, bathing, toileting, and age-appropriate diversional activities (Emphasize the importance of performing neurovascular checks and reporting any abnormalities immediately. Be sure that parents understand that the bar between the legs on the cast is not to be used for holding or turning the child. The bar is used to position the legs at the proper distance; using it to lift can cause the cast to fracture, weaken, or disintegrate.)
- Appropriate referrals for periodic assessment by a visiting nurse or home health nurse
- Family resources to care for the child

Before discharge, have parents demonstrate how to dress and feed a child in a hip spica cast. Ensure that safe travel arrangements have been made for the day of discharge (see Partnering with Families: Transporting the Child with an Orthopedic Device). Help parents to obtain an appropriate car safety seat in advance of discharge. Some agencies have loaner programs for families. Encourage parents to let the child interact with other children at home, and to provide the child in a cast opportunities for play and social activities.

Care in the Community

Have parents of an infant in a Pavlik harness demonstrate proper application of the harness and care of the infant while in the harness (see Partnering with Families: Guidelines for Pavlik Harness Application). Teach family members about daily care (bathing, dressing, and feeding) of the infant. Ideally, the harness is worn 23 hours per day and is removed only for skin checks and bathing. The hips and buttocks should be supported carefully when the infant is out of the harness. Demonstrate how to feed the infant in an upright position to maintain abduction and how to change a diaper without removing the harness.

Instruct the parents of an infant with a harness to look for any reddened or irritated areas near the harness or cast edges and to check toes frequently for proper circulation. Frequent repositioning reduces the risk of pressure sores or circulatory compromise. The infant should wear an undershirt and socks under the harness to prevent rubbing of the skin.

Safety precautions are important as the child will not have normal mobility. Parents will need to use a specially designed car seat that accommodates the child with abducted hips (see guidelines on this page). Strollers and cribs should provide sufficient room to protect the legs from injury and to prevent hip adduction.

Evaluation

Expected outcomes for nursing care of the child with developmental dysplasia of the hip include the following:

- Maintenance of skin integrity
- Absence of complications related to immobility
- Knowledge of parents regarding the condition, treatment, and necessary home care
- Maintenance of a safe environment for the child
- Eventual attainment of normal mobility

PARTNERING WITH FAMILIES

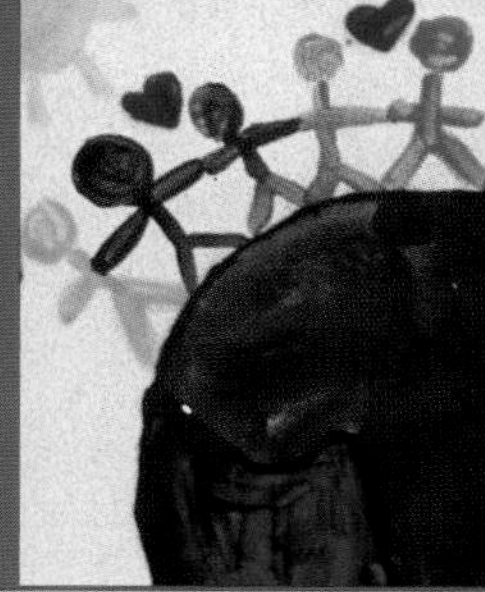

Transporting the Child with an Orthopedic Device

The American Academy of Pediatrics has established guidelines for transporting children with special healthcare needs.

- Placement in the rear seat is preferable.
- If the front seat must be used, the front passenger airbag should be disconnected.
- Use only approved car seat transport systems approved for use with children with special needs.
- Install and use seats as instructed.
- A child should be moved from a wheelchair or other special device to be placed in the vehicle safety seat when reasonable.
- Pieces of medical equipment required during transportation (such as monitors or oxygen) or that are being transported with the child (such as wheelchair or walker) should be secured to the floor of the vehicle.
- If the child is transported by school bus, state and federal recommendations for school bus transportation of children with special needs should be followed.

Data from American Academy of Pediatrics, Committee on Injury and Poison Prevention. (1999). Transporting children with special healthcare needs. Pediatrics, 104, *988–992.*

Legg-Calvé-Perthes Disease

Legg-Calvé-Perthes disease (often called Perthes disease) is a self-limiting condition in which there is avascular necrosis of the femoral head. The disease occurs in approximately 1 in 12,000 children and affects boys four to five times more often than girls. It usually occurs between the ages of 2 and 12 years, with an average age of 7 years at onset. The disease is bilateral in 20% of cases (Thompson, 2004b).

Etiology and Pathophysiology

The necrosis associated with Legg-Calvé-Perthes disease results from an interruption of the blood supply to the femoral epiphysis. How and why this occurs is not completely understood, but several predisposing factors have been identified. One theory is that a coagulation system disorder causes repeated vascular interruptions to the proximal femur (Eldridge, Dilley, Austin, et al., 2001). The incidence of this disease is up to 20% higher in families with

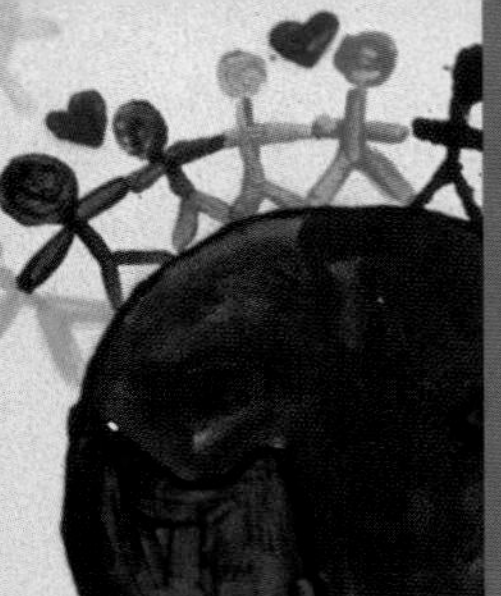

PARTNERING WITH FAMILIES

Guidelines for Pavlik Harness Application

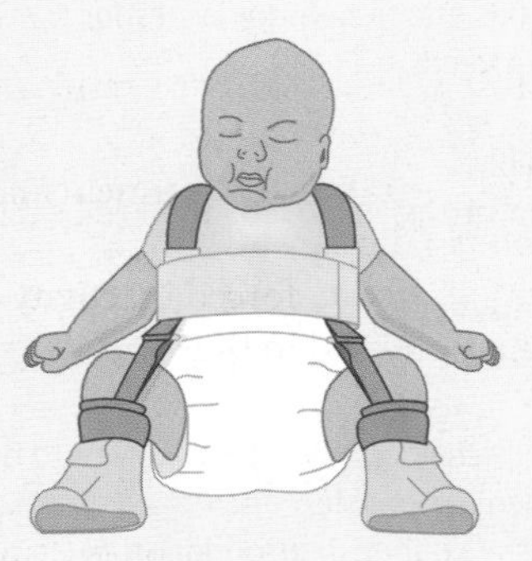

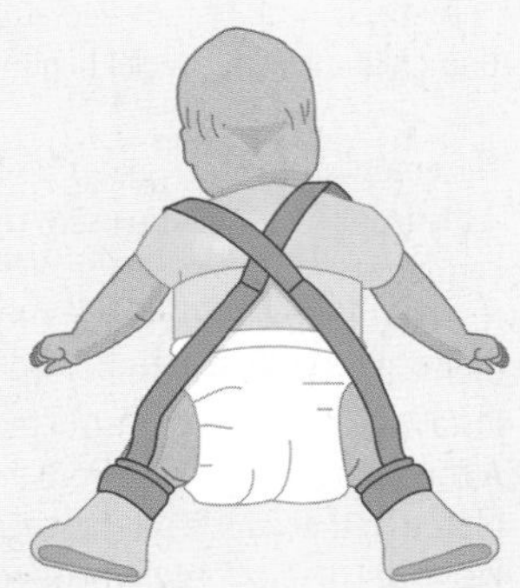

1. Position the chest halter at nipple line and fasten with Velcro.
2. Position the legs and feet in the stirrups, being sure the hips are flexed and abducted. Fasten with Velcro.
3. Connect the chest halter and leg straps in front.
4. Connect the chest halter and leg straps in back.

All the straps are marked at the first fitting with indelible ink so they can be reattached easily after the harness is rinsed and dried.

a history of the disease than in the general population, which suggests that genetic factors may play a role. In 25% of the cases, onset of the disease is preceded by a mild traumatic injury. Trauma may cause a subchondral fracture and resultant synovitis, which in turn causes pressure that occludes the blood supply. Children with Legg-Calvé-Perthes disease often have delayed skeletal maturation, increased thyroid levels, and low somatomedin C (insulin-like growth factor). It is more common in those with low birth weight, increased parental age, and exposure to environmental tobacco smoke (Roy, 1999). (See Developing Cultural Competence: Legg-Calvé-Perthes Disease.)

DEVELOPING CULTURAL COMPETENCE
Legg-Calvé-Perthes Disease

Legg-Calvé-Perthes disease is most common among White, Chinese, and Japanese children. It is less common among Blacks and Native Americans. This suggests a genetic link to the disease, as does the more frequent occurrence in certain families. However, the cause of the disease is not known so the reason for ethnic variation in incidence is not certain (Thompson, 2004b).

Clinical Manifestations

Legg-Calvé-Perthes disease progresses through four distinct stages after the original insult (usually unidentified) occurs, over a period of 1 to 4 years. Early symptoms of the disease include a mild pain in the hip or anterior thigh and a limp, which are aggravated by increased activity and relieved by rest. The child favors the affected hip and limits hip movement to avoid discomfort (Davids, 1998). See the clinical manifestations table below.

As the disease progresses, range of motion becomes limited and weakness and muscle wasting develop. The affected thigh is 2 to 3 cm smaller than the unaffected thigh. Prolonged hip irritability may produce muscle spasms and pain increases. This period of the disease varies from 1 to 4 years. Gradually, revascularization begins and pain decreases.

COLLABORATIVE CARE

Medical management and prognosis depend on the degree of femoral involvement. Early detection is important. The desired outcome is a pain-free hip that functions properly.

Diagnostic Tests

Because the child's initial symptoms are so mild, parents often do not seek medical attention until symptoms have been present for several months. Diagnosis is made using standard anteroposterior and frog-leg radiographs. As noted, radiographs taken early in the course of the disease may be normal or show vague widening of the cartilage space. Bone scans and MRI may show the disease process earlier than radiographs. Laboratory studies of the blood, such as white blood cell count, help to rule out inflammatory synovitis of the hip. Protein C, protein S, and APC-R (resistance to activated protein C) may sometimes be performed to evaluate if a coagulation abnormality is present (Eldridge et al., 2001).

CLINICAL MANIFESTATIONS of Legg-Calvé-Perthes Disease

STAGE	CLINICAL MANIFESTATIONS
Prenecrosis	An insult or coagulation disorder causes loss of blood supply to the femoral head.
I—Necrosis	Avascular stage (3–6 months); the child is asymptomatic, bone radiographs are normal, and the head of the femur is structurally intact but avascular.
II—Revascularization	Period of 1–4 years characterized by pain and limitation of movement. Bone radiographs show new bone deposition and dead bone resorption. Fracture and deformity of the head of the femur can occur.
III—Bone healing	Reossification takes place; pain decreases.
IV—Remodeling	The disease process is over, pain is absent, and improvement in joint function occurs.

Clinical Therapy

The femoral head must be contained within the hip socket until ossification is complete to promote healing and prevent deformity. Adequate containment will be best achieved if the hips remain in an abducted position. At the beginning of treatment, traction can be used to maintain the hips in an abducted and internally rotated position. Once abduction is accomplished, treatment consists of Petrie (leg abduction) casting, or surgical soft tissue releases such as adductor tenotomy, followed by bracing. Toronto (Figure 35–12 ■) and Scottish-Rite braces are most commonly used. Prognosis is good if the femoral head can be contained long enough for proper healing to occur. Severe disease may be treated by surgery to release adductor muscles, treat the acetabulum or femur, and restore range of motion. Children with untreated disease or those diagnosed late in the disease process occasionally develop osteoarthritis and hip dysfunction later in life (Roy, 1999).

NURSING MANAGEMENT

Goals of nursing management include early identification of Perthes disease and ensuring maintenance of the treatment regimen in active children.

■ Nursing Assessment and Diagnosis

Legg-Calvé-Perthes disease should be suspected in any child, especially a boy age 2 to 12 years, who complains of hip discomfort accompanied by a limp. The school nurse may be the first health professional to observe the child with symptoms of the disease. The child may complain of pain and have to rest during physical education classes. Immediate referral should be made to the healthcare provider. Question the child who has an apparent limp about pain, and assess the child's range of motion. Ask if the child previously injured the hip. Nursing diagnoses for the child with diagnosed Legg-Calvé-Perthes Disease center on altered activities and compliance, and may include the following:

- Impaired Physical Mobility related to restriction of brace or cast
- Risk for Injury related to potential complications resulting from noncompliance with the treatment regimen
- Impaired Adjustment related to duration of treatment and non-adherence to recommended therapy
- Deficient Diversional Activity related to forced inactivity
- Potential Disturbed Body Image related to brace

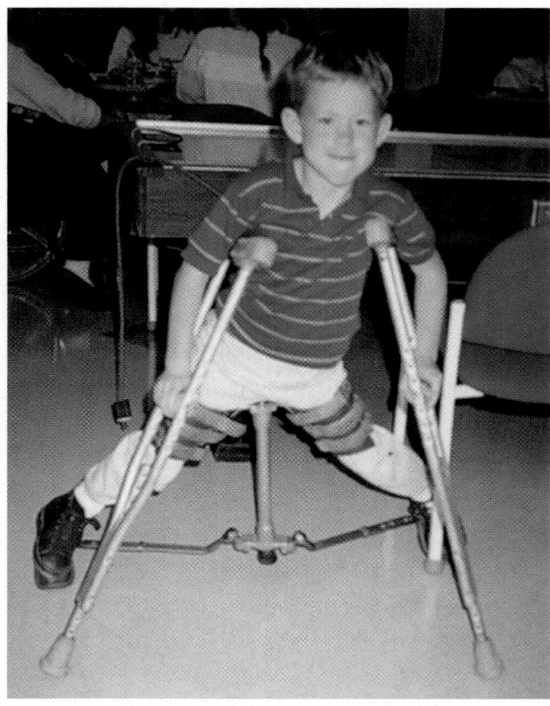

FIGURE 35–12 ■ Although the Toronto brace may seem formidable for a child to wear, you can see by this photograph that, as usual, children adapt quite well to it.

■ Planning and Implementation

Children with Legg-Calvé-Perthes disease often receive all of their treatment at home. Helping the child and family adhere to the prescribed treatment plan may be challenging, because children develop the disease at an age when they are usually very active. The child, who may have little pain, often finds immobilization difficult.

Promote Normal Growth and Development

Parents should be given suggestions to help redirect the child's energy within the limitations in mobility imposed by treatment. A return to school promotes a feeling of normalcy. Coordinate the return to school by facilitating the child's use of elevator or ramp as needed in that setting. Partner with the family to provide instruction for school personnel and other children to foster understanding of the child's condition and treatment. Activities that involve peers also help the child achieve developmental milestones. Help the child adjust to wearing a brace. Legg-Calvé-Perthes disease primarily affects boys with an average age of 7 years. These school-age children are industrious and independent. Offer suggestions for activities that redirect energy and promote normal development. These may include horseback riding, which promotes hip abduction; swimming to increase mobility; handcrafts to promote fine motor skills; and computer activities to stimulate cognitive development.

Care in the Community

Both the child and the family should be aware that treatment generally takes approximately 2 years. Emphasize the importance of following the treatment plan to ensure adequate hip containment and proper healing. Teach the family how to care for a child in traction and how to check the child's skin for breakdown. Follow-up visits should be arranged at regular intervals, in addition to home care visits during the period of traction.

Evaluation

Expected outcomes of nursing care are elimination of hip pain and discomfort, normal development during the period of immobilization, parent and child knowledge of treatment regimen, and eventual normal proximal femur without joint deformity.

Slipped Capital Femoral Epiphysis

Slipped capital femoral epiphysis (SCFE) occurs when the femoral head is displaced from the femoral neck. This condition is commonly seen during the adolescent growth spurt, between the ages of 12 and 15 years in boys and 10 and 13 years in girls. Boys are more often affected than girls. Blacks are affected more often than other ethnic groups, as are children who are overweight, those with sports injuries or other trauma, a history of radiation therapy, or endocrine disease (Acosta, Vade, Lomasney, et al., 2001).

Etiology and Pathophysiology

The cause of SCFE is unknown. Predisposing factors include obesity, malnutrition, a recent growth spurt, sports injuries or other trauma, history of radiation therapy, and endocrine disorders such as hypothyroidism, hypopituitarism, and hypogonadism. There may be a genetic predisposition to the development of the disorder (Acosta et al., 2001).

Slippage of the femoral head occurs at the proximal epiphyseal plate, and the femur displaces from the epiphysis (Figure 35–13 ■). Slippage is usually gradual (chronic), but may also result from acute trauma. The synovial membrane becomes inflamed, edematous, and painful. If untreated, callous formation occurs, resulting in a deformed hip with limited range of motion.

PATHOPHYSIOLOGY ILLUSTRATED

Slipped Epiphysis

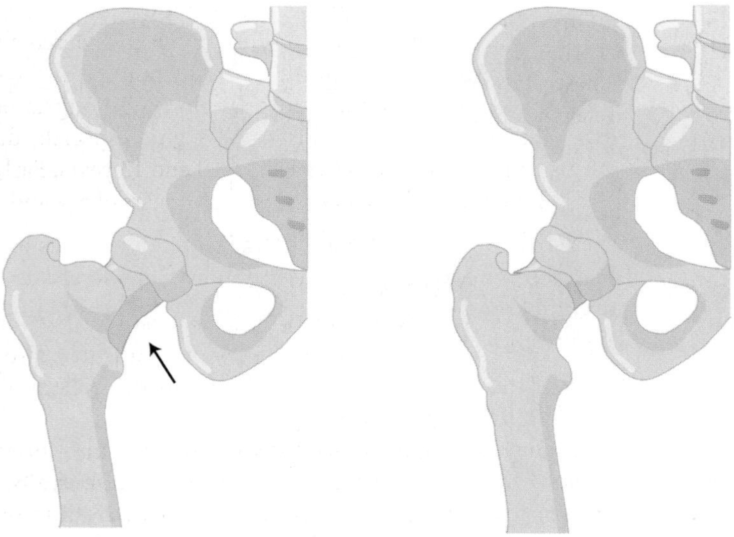

Slipped epiphysis

Normal hip

FIGURE 35–13 ■ In slipped capital femoral epiphysis, the femoral head is displaced from the femoral neck at the proximal epiphyseal plate.

Clinical Manifestations

Symptoms include limp, pain, and loss of hip motion. The condition is categorized as acute, chronic, or acute-on-chronic. *Acute* SCFE has a sudden onset of less than 3 weeks' duration. The child with an acute slip has sudden, severe pain and cannot bear weight. This may be associated with traumatic injury.

Chronic SCFE has a duration of longer than 3 weeks. It involves persistent hip pain, which is generally aching or mild and can be referred to the thigh, knee, or both. A limp and decreased range of motion may also occur.

Acute-on-chronic SCFE is an additional slippage in a child with a chronic condition. The child with a chronic slip sustains a traumatic incident that causes further slippage of the femoral head, causing sudden, severe pain.

COLLABORATIVE CARE

The goal of medical management is to stabilize the femoral head while keeping displacement to a minimum and retaining as much hip function as possible.

Diagnostic Tests

A complete history provides information about risk factors and the development of the condition. Radiographs are used to confirm the diagnosis. A bone scan, ultrasound, CT, and MRI are sometimes performed to verify the extent of injury.

Clinical Therapy

Surgical treatment is usually necessary; this involves fixation of the epiphysis with screws or pins. If treated early, a single screw into the hip in an outpatient procedure may be sufficient for stabilization. More commonly, surgery involves placement of two or three pins placed through the physis into the epiphysis to stabilize the femoral head (Acosta et al., 2001). Medical treatment, which is occasionally used, includes a regimen of no weight bearing, bed rest, a spica cast, and Buck or Russell traction (see Table 35–4 later in the chapter).

Prognosis is related to the severity of the deformity and the occurrence of complications, such as avascular necrosis of the femoral head or **chondrolysis** (the breaking down and absorption of cartilage).

NURSING MANAGEMENT

The goals of nursing management are early detection and referral of potential slipped epiphysis and providing care for the surgically treated adolescent.

Nursing Assessment and Diagnosis

The child usually presents with hip pain or referred pain to the groin, thigh, or knee, and limited mobility. If pain of any joint or part of the leg is present, examine the entire leg carefully from hip to foot. Assess the child's range of motion, pain, and limp, if apparent. Take a thorough history to assess for injury, radiation therapy, or underlying endocrine disorder as a cause. Refer the child for treatment immediately if SCFE is suspected. This condition is considered to be an emergency, and it is essential that the child be treated immediately to keep weight off the affected joint.

Nursing diagnoses that may apply to the child with SCFE are as follows:

- Impaired Physical Mobility related to treatment
- Pain related to hip injury
- Risk for Disturbed Body Image related to treatment
- Risk for Delayed Growth and Development related to mobility restrictions
- Risk for Imbalanced Nutrition: More than Body Requirements related to immobility
- Ineffective Tissue Perfusion: Peripheral related to traction, casting, and other treatments
- Health-Seeking Behaviors (child and parent) related to disease process and treatment

Planning and Implementation

Nursing management involves caring for the child in traction or after surgery, administering medications and other pain control interventions, maintaining mobility within the limits imposed by treatment, providing adequate nutrition, educating the child and family about the disorder, providing emotional support, and promoting compliance with the treatment plan.

Encourage Appropriate Nutritional Intake and Physical Activity

A growing adolescent needs increased amounts of proteins, carbohydrates, and calcium to promote skeletal healing. Provide written instructions about nutritional requirements necessary to promote bone healing and maintain an ideal body weight. If a child is overweight, encourage weight loss by decreasing percent of fat and carbohydrate in the diet and by increasing physical activity as appropriate. This decreases pressure on the femoral epiphysis and can also lead to a more positive self-image. Incorporate upper body exercises into treatment, both to assist in weight control and to build muscle. A few visits to physical therapy may facilitate a program of upper body exercise and teach safe ways of increasing total amount of physical activity.

Provide Emotional Support

Because the onset of SCFE is usually unexpected, the child and family may find themselves facing surgery with little warning. Explain the treatment plan simply and thoroughly. Reassure the child and family that with proper compliance, treatment should be successful.

Discharge Planning and Home Care Teaching

Partner with the family to help them plan for the child's return to school. If attendance is not possible for a period of time due to traction or surgery, suggest tutors and computer communication with the school as needed. Follow-up visits are necessary until the child's epiphyseal plates close. It is not uncommon for SCFE to occur in the other hip. Make sure the child and family are aware of symptoms such as decreased range of motion or pain that could indicate onset of the disorder in the other hip. Tell parents to contact their healthcare provider immediately if these symptoms occur.

Evaluation

Expected outcomes of nursing care for the child with SCFE include maintenance of normal weight and recommended nutritional intake, absence of complications of immobility, successful adaptation to school following treatment, and family recognition of need for ongoing monitoring for complications.

DISORDERS OF THE SPINE

Scoliosis

Scoliosis is a lateral S- or C-shaped curvature of the spine that is often associated with a rotational deformity of the spine and ribs. Many individuals exhibit some degree of spinal curvature, but curvatures of more than 10 degrees are considered abnormal. Curves are either structural or compensatory, as the spine curves to compensate for a structural deformity along its length. Idiopathic scoliosis occurs most often in girls, especially during the growth spurt between the ages of 10 and 13 years. Early onset of idiopathic scoliosis occurs before 10 years of age and comprises 15% of cases (Thompson, 2004b).

Etiology and Pathophysiology

The cause of scoliosis is complex. Structural scoliosis may be congenital, idiopathic, or acquired (associated with neuromuscular disorders such as muscular dystrophy or myelodysplasia, or secondary to spinal cord injuries).

In idiopathic structural scoliosis (the most common type), the spine for unknown reasons begins to curve laterally, with vertebral rotation. The most common curve is a right thoracic and left lumbar deformity. As the curve progresses, structural changes occur. The ribs on the concave side (inside of the curve) are forced closer together, while the ribs on the convex side separate widely, causing narrowing of the thoracic cage and formation of the rib hump. The lateral curvature affects the vertebral structure. Disk spaces are narrowed on the concave side and spread wider on the convex side, resulting in an asymmetric vertebral canal (Figure 35–14 ■).

Scoliosis can also occur in congenital diseases involving the spinal structure and in the musculoskeletal changes seen in conditions such as myelomeningocele, cerebral palsy (see Chapter 33∞), or muscular dystrophy. It can also be acquired after injury to the spinal cord. The child in Figure 35–15 ■ acquired scoliosis after chemotherapy and radiation to the chest during treatment for cancer.

Clinical Manifestations

The classic signs of scoliosis include truncal asymmetry, uneven shoulders and hips, a one-sided rib hump, and a prominent scapula. The child does not complain of pain or discomfort. If diagnosis does not occur before the curvature reaches about 40 degrees, some compensatory problems may develop. Hip and back pain can result, and lung compromise can lead to fatigue or dyspnea with exertion.

COLLABORATIVE CARE

The goal of medical management is to limit or stop progression of the curvature. School and office nurses often screen children for scoliosis and refer abnormalities for further evaluation. Many professionals such as physical therapists, physicians, and nurses partner with families to treat the adolescent with scoliosis.

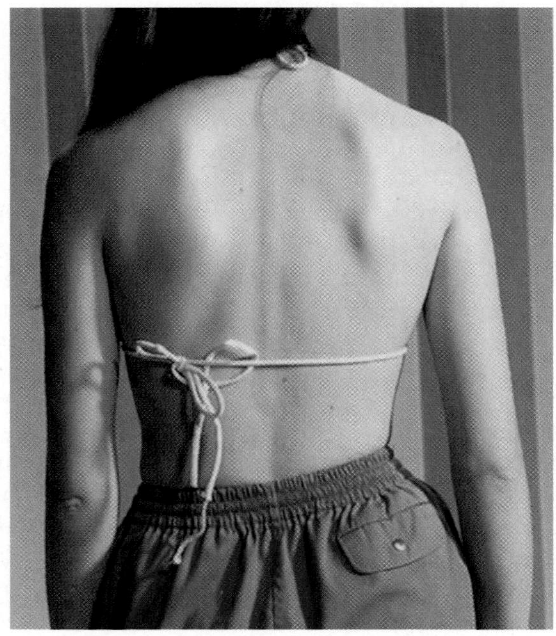

FIGURE 35–14 ■ A child may have varying degrees of scoliosis. For mild forms, treatment will focus on strengthening and stretching. Moderate forms will require bracing. Severe forms may necessitate surgery and fusion. Clothes that fit at an angle, such as this teenage girl's shorts, and anatomic asymmetry of the back provide clues for early detection.

Diagnostic Tests

Generally, observation and radiographic examination are used to diagnose scoliosis. Additional diagnostic studies include MRI, CT scan, and bone scan, which are used occasionally to assess the degree of curvature.

Clinical Therapy

Early detection is essential to successful treatment. Adequate treatment and follow-up maximize the child's chances for proper spinal alignment. The treatment regimen chosen depends on the degree and progression of the curvature and the response of the child and family to medical management.

Treatment of children with mild scoliosis (curvatures of 10 to 20 degrees) consists of exercises to improve posture and muscle tone and to maintain, or possibly increase, flexibility of the spine. Emphasis is placed on building strength toward the outside of the curve while stretching the inside of the curve. These exercises are not a cure, however, and the child should be evaluated by a physician at 3-month intervals, with radiographic evaluation every 6 months.

Medical management of moderate scoliosis (curvatures of 20 to 40 degrees) includes bracing with either a Boston or Milwaukee brace. The goal of wearing a brace is to maintain the existing spinal curvature with no increase. Brace wear begins immediately after diagnosis. To achieve maximum effectiveness, the brace should be worn 23 hours per day. Brace treatment is lengthy and requires a high degree of compliance, which can be difficult for adolescents who view body image or sports involvement as important (Box 35–3).

Electrical stimulation is used occasionally as an alternative treatment. An electric current stimulates the back muscles to contract, thus helping to correct the spinal curvature. This

BOX 35–3 Research: Adolescent Self-Image and Braces

A comparison of 150 adolescents wearing a brace for scoliosis with 150 adolescents without scoliosis revealed that those wearing the brace had poorer perception of self-image when completing the Piers-Harris scale, "How I feel about myself." In addition, only 5% of youth with scoliosis had opportunities to discuss their feelings with health professionals and 90% stated that they wanted more opportunities to do so (Sapountzi-Krepia, Valavanis, Panteleakis, et al., 2001). The findings that adolescents are concerned with body image is not surprising, considering a developmental stage that focuses on appearance and fitting in with others. It is surprising that this is not acknowledged and discussed during healthcare. Health professionals should realize that wearing a brace can be difficult for adolescents and provide a chance for youth to discuss how they feel about the diagnosis and treatment. Consider interventions that aid in improving body image. For example, some department stores sponsor fashion shows for adolescents with scoliosis who must wear braces. Children with braces in place model and demonstrate how popular clothing can be worn to disguise the wearing of the brace. These events can have a positive impact on the self-esteem of adolescents who participate in and view the shows.

treatment, which is performed at night, eliminates the need for bracing.

Children with severe scoliosis (curvatures of 40 degrees or more) require surgery, which involves spinal fusion. The majority of spinal fusions are performed using instrumentation with Luque wires, Coutrel-Dubosset (CD) instrumentation, Texas Scottish Rite Hospital system, and Moss-Miami system (Slote, 2002). These treatments stabilize the spine well during surgery, may be accompanied by bone grafting to the spine, and require no long-term therapy or postoperative casting. Following surgery with wires or instrumentation, the child is on bed rest during a recovery period and then is generally fitted with anteroposterior plastic shells (also called thoracolumbar sacral orthotics) that are worn for several months to provide stability for the spine. The wires will remain in the back forever. Occasionally in severe cases, halo traction is used postoperatively to provide support for the unstable spine (see Figure 35–15 ■).

NURSING MANAGEMENT

Nursing management focuses on screening and early detection, teaching about brace wear, caring for the adolescent having surgery for scoliosis, and partnering with the adolescent and family to provide support during all treatments.

■ Nursing Assessment and Diagnosis

School nurses often screen children for scoliosis, generally in the fifth and seventh grades. This screening is mandated by law in several states. When abnormalities are noted, the child is referred to an orthopedic center for further evaluation. Children should be examined every 6 to 9 months thereafter. If scoliosis is detected, the child's brothers and sisters should be examined and observed closely. Scoliosis screening involves the following:

From the Front

- Is the head midline?
- Are the shoulders at the same height?

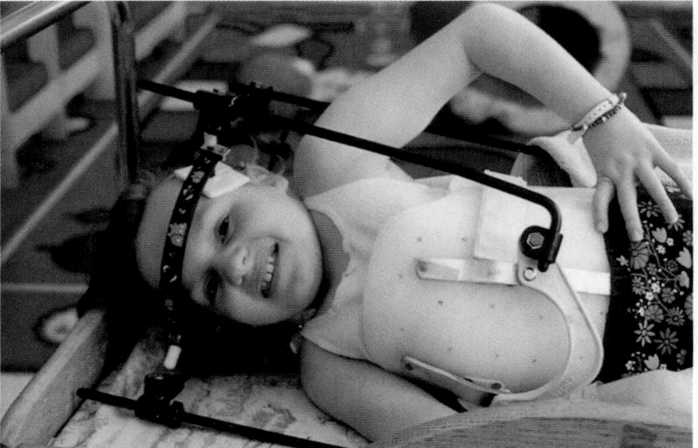

FIGURE 35–15 ■ In severe scoliosis, the child may wear a halo brace, shown here, to hold the body in position after surgery.

- Is there the same amount of space between arms and body on each side?

From the Back

- Is the head midline?
- Are the shoulders at the same height?
- Are the scapula equally prominent and at the same height?
- Is the spine straight?
- Is there the same amount of space between arms and body on each side?
- Are the hips at the same height?

With the Adolescent Holding Hands Together and Bent Over Slightly

- Are the scapular humps even?

With the Adolescent Holding Hands Together and Bent Over Toward Floor

- Are the flank humps even?
- Is the spine straight?
- Is there a marked roundness when viewed from the side (evidence of kyphosis)?

Once scoliosis has been identified, the nurse's focus becomes education and follow-up. Any child with scoliosis should have a comprehensive neurologic, cardiac, and respiratory examination, since the rib cage deformity can influence the functioning of these systems.

The following nursing diagnoses may apply to the child with scoliosis who is not undergoing surgery.

- Risk for Impaired Adjustment to the Exercise Program related to duration and intensity of exercise
- Impaired Physical Mobility related to brace
- Risk for Impaired Skin Integrity related to brace
- Ineffective Breathing Pattern related to rib cage deformity
- Health-Seeking Behaviors (child and parent) related to unfamiliarity with disease process
- Disturbed Body Image related to deformity and brace wear

Common nursing diagnoses for the child who is having surgery can be found in the accompanying nursing care plan.

■ Planning and Implementation

An important aspect of nursing care is patient education. Patient compliance is critical to the success of treatment. Children and their families need to understand the condition and the stages of treatment, particularly adolescents who are undergoing treatment for scoliosis. Children or adolescents facing surgery require education, reassurance, and support. Teach about pain control and the PCA (patient-controlled analgesia) pump. Often the child donates some of his or her own blood prior to surgery and the family may also donate so blood transfused in surgery is the child's or a family member's. Explain to the child the safety that this ensures. The adolescent will benefit from learning about deep breathing, positioning, surgical incision, and all other aspects of postoperative care. The accompanying nursing care plan summarizes nursing care for the child undergoing surgery for scoliosis.

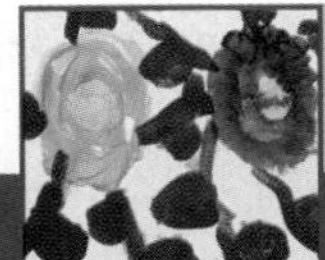

Nursing Care Plan

THE CHILD UNDERGOING SURGERY FOR SCOLIOSIS

GOAL	INTERVENTION	RATIONALE	EXPECTED OUTCOME
1. Deficient Knowledge (child and parents) related to lack of information about surgery			
	NIC Priority Intervention—*Teaching, Disease Process and Preoperative:* Assisting the patient to understand information and mentally prepare for surgery and postoperative recovery.		**NOC Suggested Outcome—***Knowledge:* Extent of understanding conveyed about scoliosis treatment.
The child and parents will verbalize understanding of the disease, its treatment, and the surgical procedure.	▪ Teach the child and family about the course of the disease, its signs and symptoms, and treatment. Provide appropriate handouts. Encourage the child and parents to ask questions. ▪ Begin preoperative teaching at the time of admission. Orient the child to hospital and postoperative procedures. Before surgery, have the child demonstrate log-rolling, range of motion exercises, and the use of an incentive spirometer. Discuss pain management.	▪ Understanding and involvement increase motivation and compliance while reducing fear. ▪ Preoperative teaching and familiarity with hospital procedures reduces the stress related to surgery and postoperative complications.	The child and family accurately verbalize knowledge about the disease and its treatment. The child and family ask appropriate questions about postoperative care.
2. Ineffective Breathing Pattern related to hypoventilation syndrome			
	NIC Priority Intervention—*Airway Management and Respiratory Monitoring:* Facilitation of patency of air passages and analysis of patient data.		**NOC Suggested Outcome—***Respiratory Status: Ventilation:* Movement of air in and out of the lungs.
The child will show no signs of respiratory compromise.	▪ Monitor respiratory status, especially after the administration of analgesics. Apply pulse oximeter. ▪ Administer oxygen if ordered. ▪ Have the child use an incentive spirometer. ▪ Monitor intake and output. ▪ Reposition the child at least every 2 hours.	▪ Evaluation of the child's respiratory condition anticipates and avoids complications. Analgesics such as morphine may increase or potentiate respiratory compromise. ▪ Oxygen increases peripheral oxygen saturation to 95%–100%. ▪ Spirometry increases lung expansion and aeration of the alveoli. ▪ Good hydration promotes loose secretions and helps prevent infection. ▪ Repositioning ensures inflation of the lung fields.	The child has no respiratory complications.
3. Risk for Injury related to neurovascular deficit secondary to instrumentation			
	NIC Priority Intervention—*Injury Prevention:* Instituting special precautions with patient at risk.		**NOC Suggested Outcome—***Risk Control:* Actions to eliminate or reduce modifiable health risks.
The child's neurovascular system will remain intact as evidenced by circulation, sensation, and motor checks. The child will feel no numbness or tingling.	▪ Monitor the child's color, circulation, capillary refill, warmth, sensation, and motion in all extremities, Perform neurovascular checks every 2 hours for the first 24 hours and then every 4 hours for the next 48 hours. Record presence of pedal and distal tibial pulses every hour for 48 hours. Report changes and abnormal findings immediately.	▪ When the spinal column is manipulated during surgery, altered neurovascular status, thrombus formation, and paralysis are possible complications. Postoperative risks include loss of bowel or bladder control, weakness or paralysis, and impaired vision or sensation.	The child exhibits only temporary alteration (pale skin, faint pulse, and edema occur, but then resolve within the initial postoperative phase). The child returns to the preoperative baseline state by discharge.

Nursing Care Plan THE CHILD UNDERGOING SURGERY FOR SCOLIOSIS (continued)

GOAL	INTERVENTION	RATIONALE	EXPECTED OUTCOME
3. Risk for Injury related to neurovascular deficit secondary to instrumentation (continued)			
	■ Have the child wear antiembolism stockings until ambulatory. The stockings may be removed for 1 hour 2–3 times daily. ■ Check for any pain, swelling, or a positive Homans' sign in the legs. Record any evidence of edema. ■ Monitor input and output. ■ Encourage and assist the child with range of motion exercises, both passive and active.	■ Antiembolism stockings prevent blood clots and promote venous return. Thrombus formation is a postoperative risk. ■ Swelling may indicate a tight dressing and tissue damage. A positive Homans' sign and pain may indicate thrombus formation. ■ Abnormalities may indicate a fluid shift problem. ■ Activity promotes mobility and reduces risk of thrombus formation.	
4. Pain related to spinal fusion with Instrumentation			
	NIC Priority Intervention—*Pain Management:* Alleviation of pain or a reduction of pain to a level of comfort acceptable to the patient.		**NOC Suggested Outcome—***Pain Level:* Amount of reported or demonstrated pain.
The child will verbalize an adequate level of comfort or show absence of pain behavior within 1 hour of a specific nursing intervention.	■ Assess the level of pain and initiate pain management strategies as soon as possible. Use patient-controlled analgesics if ordered. ■ Administer pain medication around the clock to help ensure pain relief, especially during the first 48 hours. Monitor epidural blocks and patient-controlled analgesia or other methods used for pain control. ■ Use nonpharmacologic pain management techniques, such as imagery, relaxation, touch, music, application of heat and cold, and reduced environmental stimulation to supplement medications (see Chapter 18∞). ■ Document pain assessment, interventions, and the child's reactions. ■ Reassure the child that some discomfort is expected and that a variety of measures can be tried to reduce discomfort.	■ Adequate pain management allows for faster healing and a more cooperative patient. Patient-controlled analgesics may be effective. ■ Medicating around the clock helps to maintain comfort. Monitoring ensures patient safety. ■ Alternative treatments also interrupt the pain stimulus and provide relief. Nonpharmacologic methods can be an effective adjunct to pain management. ■ Proper documentation guides the selection of the most effective means of pain control. ■ Realistic expectations decrease anxiety and give the child a sense of control.	The child experiences pain relief early in the postoperative period.
5. Impaired Physical Mobility related to movement restrictions and pain			
	NIC Priority intervention—*Positioning and Ambulation:* Moving the patient to provide comfort and promote healing, assist with walking.		**NOC Suggested Outcome—***Ambulation:* Ability to walk from place to place.
The child will maintain proper body alignment and progress with activity as ordered by the physician. If no anteroposterior shell bracing is required the child will have active mobility by the third to fifth postoperative day.	■ Resposition the child every 2 hours using the log-roll technique. Support the back, feet, and knees with pillows. ■ Have the child perform passive and active range of motion exercises every 2 hours for 48 hours and then every 4 hours while awake. Have the child (continued)	■ Proper positioning prevents twisting or turning the spine. ■ Exercises help maintain strength, circulation, and muscle tone. If the spine is stable and the physician has ordered no external support, the (continued)	The child is as mobile as appropriate for condition within 3–5 days after surgery.

(continued)

Nursing Care Plan THE CHILD UNDERGOING SURGERY FOR SCOLIOSIS (continued)

GOAL	INTERVENTION	RATIONALE	EXPECTED OUTCOME
5. Impaired Physical Mobility related to movement restrictions and pain (continued)			
	dangle his or her legs at beside by the second to fourth postoperative day or as ordered by surgeon. Begin ambulation generally by the third to fifth postoperative day. Note any complaints of dizziness, pallor. Proceed slowly.	child may progress to full ambulation as tolerated. If the spine is not stable, great care must be taken until external supportive devices are used.	
6. Risk for Disturbed Body Image related to treatment			
	NIC Priority Intervention—*Body Image Enhancement:* Improving conscious and unconscious perceptions toward the body.		**NOC Suggested Outcome—***Body Image:* Positive perception of own appearance and body.
The child will verbalize feelings about body image and self-esteem in relation to the disease and its treatment. The child will be informed about available support services and use them as needed.	■ Encourage independence in daily activities within allowable limits. Use positive reinforcements. Encourage the child to participate in community activities, if possible. Involve the child in scoliosis support groups. ■ Provide contact with a peer resource person who has undergone treatment for scoliosis.	■ Involvement in activities demonstrates that a "normal" life is realistic. ■ Peers are an effective means of support.	The child has a positive self-image and is involved in community activities or support groups.
7. Risk for Deficient Knowledge (child and parent) related to lack of information about home care			
	NIC Priority Intervention—*Teaching: Prescribed Treatment:* Preparing family to understand and perform prescribed treatment.		**NOC Suggested Outcome—***Knowledge:* Extent of understanding conveyed about postoperative treatment and follow-up care.
The child and family will verbalize reduced anxiety about home care. The child will demonstrate knowledge of self-care and permitted activities.	■ Teach cast or brace care as appropriate (see pp. 1412 and 1415). Provide oral and written instructions and a list of activity limitations. Have the child and family demonstrate adequate knowledge. ■ Arrange for follow-up appointments as ordered by the physician. Encourage the child and family to notify the nurse or physician if they have any questions or concerns.	■ Providing education decreases anxiety and increases compliance with treatment plan. Demonstration reinforces the learning process. ■ Follow-up visits help the nurse and physician evaluate the effectiveness of the treatment plan and patient adjustment to recommended therapy.	The child and family demonstrate home care and implementation of discharge teaching.

Promote Compliance with the Treatment Plan

Provide instructions about exercises that will help to decrease the severity of the spinal curvature. Demonstrate the exercises, and explain their purpose (e.g., to strengthen back muscles). Help the child adjust to wearing a brace. Adolescents, in particular, may be reluctant to wear an external device such as a brace. To promote a sense of control, allow the adolescent to choose when to exercise and when to be out of the brace, within the treatment guidelines. Provide reassurance and encouragement and promote interaction with peers. Consider suggesting that the adolescent work with a peer support person who is being treated for scoliosis or has had the condition in the past. Provide information about fashionable clothing that can be worn with the brace.

Discharge Planning and Home Care Teaching

Home care needs should be identified and addressed well in advance of discharge after spinal surgery. The child must learn to adapt to a new set of body mechanics. Show the child how to perform simple tasks without bending or twisting the torso. Have the child demonstrate the ability to perform activities of daily living before discharge from the hospital. Partner with physical therapy/rehabilitation to plan for the youth's needs related to safe and effective movement with the brace.

Activities for the child who has had spinal surgery are commonly limited for a period of time. Restrictions usually should be followed for 6 to 8 months, depending on the type of surgery and the surgeon's choice. Emphasize to both the child and the family the importance of adhering to therapy, and give them written discharge instructions. Follow-up visits are important. The child should be examined 4 to 6 weeks after discharge, then every 3 to 4 months for 1 year, and every 1 to 2 years thereafter (see Partnering with Families: Postoperative Activities after Spinal Surgery).

Several organizations provide information and assistance to families of children with scoliosis. Referrals can be made as appropriate.

Evaluation

Expected outcomes of nursing care for the child with scoliosis treated by brace are maintenance of intact skin and compliance with prescribed therapy. Expected outcomes after surgical correction are listed on the accompanying nursing care plan.

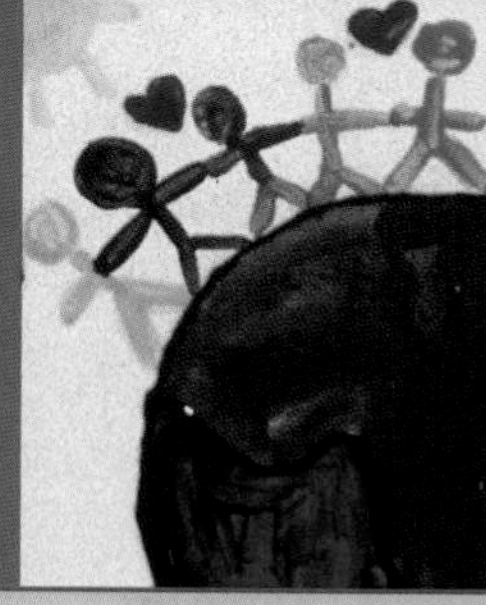

PARTNERING WITH FAMILIES

Postoperative Activities After Spinal Surgery

Recommended

- Lying
- Sitting
- Standing
- Walking (including normal stair climbing)
- Swimming, gentle (not with a cast); diving is not permitted

Note. People with metal hardware in their back after scoliosis surgery need to carry an explanation from the physician on airplane flights as they will set off metal detectors in airports. Have families call airlines before flights to be certain what documentation will be needed.

Not recommended

- Bending or twisting at the waist
- Lifting more than 10 pounds
- Household chores such as vacuuming, unloading groceries, mowing the lawn, taking out the garbage
- Sports such as bicycle riding, horseback riding, skiing, roller blading, skating
- Physical education classes

Torticollis, Kyphosis, and Lordosis

Torticollis is tilt of the head caused by rotation of the cervical spine. The cause is generally an injury sustained to the sternocleidomastoid muscle at the time of birth or to a cervical spine abnormality. Stretching exercises or surgical lengthening of the sternocleidomastoid muscle are usual treatments. Occasionally the cause of torticollis is visual impairment, leading to constant turning in one direction in order to see with the better eye.

Kyphosis (hunchback) and lordosis (swayback) are two other types of spinal curvature that may occur in children. The type of kyphosis in adolescence is most commonly Scheuermann kyphosis, an abnormality in ossification of anterior vertebral bodies; it differs from the degenerative kyphosis sometimes seen in the elderly. Postural lordosis is a characteristic finding in toddlers, but should disappear by the school-age years.

Nurses perform thorough musculoskeletal assessments of children (see Chapter 8∞) and refer any children with abnormalities for further evaluation. Clinical therapy depends on the cause and degree of the curvature, and the age of the child at onset. Refer to the table on page 1430 for clinical manifestations, treatment, and nursing management of kyphosis and lordosis.

ADDITIONAL DISORDERS OF THE BONES AND JOINTS

Osteoporosis and Osteopenia

Osteoporosis, a condition in which there is decreased density and mass of bone, promotes the risk of fractures and is commonly associated with aging. However, children can have osteoporosis (also known as metabolic bone disease or a bone mineral density more than 2.5 standard deviations below the norm) related to imbalanced nutrition or other pathological conditions. Osteoporosis is proceeded by osteopenia or low bone mass which is between 1 and 2.5 standard deviations below norm (Bowman & Russell, 2001; Chan & Bishop, 2002).

Etiology and Pathophysiology

Very-low-birth-weight infants who are premature often have osteopenia of prematurity because much of bone mass is usually acquired in the latter weeks of pregnancy. In addition, they may have other health problems after birth and be unable to ingest enough nutrients to meet metabolic needs for bone growth. Prematures are often less active than other infants which decreases the amount of mechanical loading on their bones, a factor known to increase bone resorption and decrease bone mass (Moyer-Mileur, Brunstetter, McNaught, et al., 2000; Abad-Sinden et al., 2001).

A group of children who may show signs of osteoporosis are those who have decreased mechanical loading. Children with spina bifida or cerebral palsy, conditions that interfere with ambulation, have limited pressure on bones and lowered bone mass in affected extremities and spine. Other conditions associated with lower bone mass include Turner syndrome, growth hormone deficiency, osteogenesis imperfecta, juvenile rheumatoid arthritis, and diabetes. Children who are treated for disorders or injuries with casting and bracing are also at high risk of osteoporosis due to immobilization.

Lastly, adolescence is a period when adequate intakes of calcium and vitamin D are needed to maximize bone formation and prevent osteoporosis later in life. Adolescents, particularly

MediaLink Scoliosis Resources and Support

CLINICAL MANIFESTATIONS of Kyphosis and Lordosis

CONDITION	CLINICAL MANIFESTATIONS	CLINICAL THERAPY
Kyphosis Excessive convex curvature of the cervical thoracic spine. (Scheuermann kyphosis is a common type)	*Clinical manifestations:* Visible hunchback or rounded shoulders; shortness of breath or fatigue; pain; abdominal creases and light hamstrings in severe cases. *Diagnostic tests:* Spinal curvature is assessed by having the child bend 90 degrees at the waist and noting roundness at the scapular area from side. Sharp angulation is visible. Diagnosis is confirmed by radiograph.	*Medical therapy:* Exercises are prescribed for mild condition; bracing is commonly used; spinal fusion surgery is performed in severe cases. *Nursing management:* Provide support. Encourage exercises and diligent brace wear. Help the child to deal with the psychologic stress of altered body image.
Lordosis Excessive concave curvature of the lumbar spine with an angle of more than 60 degrees; most common in prepubescent girls and Blacks.	*Clinical manifestations:* Presence of sway-back; prominent buttocks; hip flexion contractures; tight hamstrings. *Diagnostic tests:* Spinal curvature is assessed by looking at the standing child from the side. Lumbar lordosis is confirmed by visualizing the spine on standing, lateral radiograph.	*Medical therapy:* Treatment focuses on exercises and postural awareness. Bracing and surgery are rarely prescribed. *Nursing management:* Provide support. Reassure the child and family that the condition is often outgrown as the child matures. Encourage physical conditioning exercises and follow-up examinations on a yearly basis.

females, often do not meet the RDA for these nutrients and are at risk for osteoporosis even though it may not be manifested for years. Other lifestyle patterns of youth that decrease bone formation are smoking, alcohol use, and keeping weight at a very low level (Durst, 2000). Those with anorexia nervosa are clearly at risk for osteoporosis.

Clinical Manifestations

Osteoporosis is a silent disease, as is its precursor osteopenia; those who have the disorders are often without signs or symptoms for years. The problem may become apparent when a baby or child has a fracture and radiologic studies make the problem evident.

COLLABORATIVE CARE

All health professionals should partner with parents and children to increase awareness of the silent and insidious disease of osteoporosis. The goal of care is to prevent the disease in all youth, and to direct special attention to those conditions that may contribute to its occurrence.

Diagnostic Tests

Bone mineral content and density are measured by single photon absorptiometry (SPA), dual photon absorptiometry (DPA), or dual-energy X-ray absorptiometry (DEXA). Although uncommonly used, serum studies such as bone-specific alkaline phosphatase, phosphorus, and type I collagen can be used to measure osteoblastic and osteoclastic activity. Recall that over 90% of the body's calcium is stored in bone so serum calcium is not reflective of bone density.

Clinical Therapy

Premature newborns at risk of osteopenia of prematurity need collaborative management by neonatologists, neonatal nutritionists, and neonatal nurses. Breast milk is enhanced by adding special fortifiers; premature formula should be used rather than regular baby formula. When babies need enteral or parenteral feedings, calcium to phosphorus ratios are carefully balanced to enhance osteoblastic activity. Extremity range of motion for very-low-birth-weight newborns can decrease bone loss in the period after birth (Litmanovitz, Dolfin, Friedland, et al., 2003).

For older children at risk of developing osteoporosis, calcium and vitamin D intake is encouraged and oral supplements may be given. Standing therapy for those who are nonambulatory can provide mechanical weight and enhance bone density (Caulton, Ward, Alsop, et al., 2004). Biphosphanates, calcitonin, fluoride and parathyroid hormone have been use but there are no clear data to indicate their effectiveness in children (Chan & Bishop, 2002). When a cast or other immobilizing device is removed from a child, a gradually increasing program of exercise in collaboration with physical rehabilitation professionals promotes bone strengthening and lowered risk for fractures or related sequellae.

NURSING MANAGEMENT

The goal of nursing care is to prevent osteopenia, osteoporosis, and resultant fractures in all children, from newborns through adolescence and on into adulthood.

■ Nursing Assessment and Diagnosis

Nurses identify newborns, children, and adolescents at risk of developing low bone mass and density. This is accomplished by identifying diseases putting the child at risk. Ask about exercise and activity patterns, and physical therapy for children who are nonambulatory. Dietary intake is measured periodically for all youth at health promotion visits, and RDAs for calcium, phosphorus, and vitamin D are compared to intake.

Nursing diagnoses that may apply to the child with osteoporosis include the following:

- Imbalanced Nutrition related to inability to consume essential nutrients
- Risk for Injury to Bones related to decreased bone mass and density

- Ineffective Health Maintenance related to inadequate dietary intake

Planning and Implementation

Perform dietary analysis of children at risk (see Chapter 9∞ for detailed methods for diet assessment). Refer children at risk to nutritionists and physicians for further education and diagnosis. Suggest referrals to physical rehabilitation to recommend weight-bearing exercise. Administer nutritional supplements when prescribed and teach families how to give these medications. Partner with families to provide therapy for nonambulatory children that stimulates weight bearing. Teach parents how to recognize fractures in children who may not have normal sensation and are unable to report them. Swelling, unusual shape of a limb, fussiness of the child, and falls should be reported promptly.

Effects of Immobility

When osteoporosis is due to immobility, many other symptoms occur as well. Be alert for these problems and integrate physical activity in care as much as possible to minimize their effects.

Evaluation

Expected outcomes for the child with a potential for osteoporosis include adequate intake of recommended amounts of nutrients, absence of fractures, and normal findings on studies of bone mineral content and density.

Osteomyelitis

Osteomyelitis is an infection of the bone, most often one of the long bones of the lower extremity. It may be acute or chronic and may spread into surrounding tissues. Although osteomyelitis may occur at any age, it is most common in children between the ages of 1 and 12 years. Boys are affected two to three times as often as girls, primarily because they have a greater incidence of trauma (Carek, Dickerson, & Sack, 2001).

Etiology and Pathophysiology

Osteomyelitis is caused by a microorganism, which is usually bacterial but can be viral or fungal. *Staphylococcus aureus* is the most common causative pathogen, followed by *Escherichia coli*, group B streptococci, *Streptococcus aureus*, *Streptococcus pyogenes*, and *Haemophilus influenzae*. *S. aureus* is able to bind to bone proteins and injury or surgery of bone may expose those sites to the organism. Trauma to the bone or surgical interventions are thus other common causes of infection. Osteomyelitis may follow another infection in the body, such as upper respiratory infection.

The infecting organism spreads through the bloodstream or via a penetrating injury to the bone, where it becomes established. Most infections in children begin in the metaphysis of long bones (see Figure 35–2), which has a sluggish blood supply. Eventually the infection may penetrate the bone cortex and periosteum. Inflammation and abscess formation can lead to interruption of the blood supply to the underlying bone, involvement of the surrounding soft tissue, and, if the infection is left untreated, to necrosis. Other types of bone may be affected as well, such as vertebrae and scapulae.

PRACTICE ALERT

Osteomyelitis in a newborn is of great concern, as before 18 months of age the blood vessels cross the growth plates. This creates a higher risk of epiphyseal involvement with resultant limb length discrepancy and other problems. Be alert for the newborn who exhibits poor feeding, fussiness when moved, or refusal to move a limb. Fever and other signs of infection are less often seen in newborns.

Clinical Manifestations

Symptoms include constant bone pain, edema, decreased mobility of the infected joint, and fever. Redness over the area may occur. The child may refuse to walk or may limp (Fernandez, Carrol, & Baker, 2000). Because the onset of acute osteomyelitis is generally rapid, it is sometimes misdiagnosed as a sports injury.

COLLABORATIVE CARE

The goal of treatment is eradication of the causative organism and prevention of any complications or long-term sequelae from the infection.

Diagnostic Tests

A history suggestive of osteomyelitis includes an upper respiratory infection or blunt trauma followed by pain at the area of a growth plate. Laboratory evaluation shows leukocytosis and an elevated erythrocyte sedimentation rate (ESR) and C-reactive protein (Carek et al., 2001). The degree of ESR elevation is directly related to the severity of the infection. Radiographs and bone scans may identify the area of involvement. A needle aspiration of the site or a blood culture can confirm the diagnosis and provide a culture of the causative organism.

Clinical Therapy

In children with extensive orthopedic surgery, or in those with immunosuppression, a short course of prophylactic antibiotic may be administered after surgery to prevent infection.

Medical management of infection begins with the intravenous administration of a broad-spectrum antibiotic, even before culture results are available. Because *S. aureus* is a common cause of infection, the antibiotic should be effective against this organism. Treatment is influenced by the possibility of methicillin-resistant *S. aureus* (MRSA) so beginning antibiotics are usually vancomycin or clindamycin, drugs effective against MRSA. Once the culture results are obtained, the antibiotic may be altered. Intravenous antibiotics may be changed to oral forms once an adequate response has occurred. However, extended intravenous home therapy may be used. Antibiotic therapy continues for about 3 to 6 weeks. The cause of infection is not always identified from culture so ESR and

C-reactive protein are followed carefully in these cases to identify if treatment is successful. Some clinicans treat with antibiotics until the ESR is < 25 to 30 mm/hour (Givner & Kaplan, 2003). When an adequate response to antibiotic is not obtained within 2 to 3 days, the area may be aspirated again, or surgical drainage may be performed. Intravenous fluids may be administered to ensure adequate hydration. Prompt diagnosis and treatment usually result in complete resolution of the infection. The prognosis is related to the initiation of therapy—the earlier treatment begins, the better the outcome. Long-term unfavorable outcomes include disruption of the growth plate, which can interrupt growth, damage the joints from septic arthritis, and recurrent infection.

NURSING MANAGEMENT

The goals of nursing management include early identification of osteomyelitis and careful monitoring for outcomes of treatment.

Nursing Assessment and Diagnosis

A thorough history, including information about the onset of symptoms and a history of recent infections or trauma, is essential. Ask about immunization status, especially tetanus. Assess the affected area for signs of redness, swelling, pain, and decreased range of motion. Measure vital signs; increased temperature and pulse in particular may provide clues about worsening infection.

Nursing diagnoses that may apply to the child with osteomyelitis are as follows:

- Acute Pain related to biologic injury
- Impaired Physical Mobility related to discomfort
- Risk for Infection (sepsis) related to spread of infection
- Risk for Imbalanced Nutrition: Less than Body Requirements related to anorexia
- Health-Seeking Behaviors (child and parent) related to lack of information about disease process

Planning and Implementation

Nursing management focuses on performing cultures and obtaining blood samples, administering antibiotics, protecting the child from spread of the infection, and encouraging generous amounts of fluid and a well-balanced diet. Standard precautions should be used, with transmission-based precautions for any drainage from the site of infection.

Obtain Cultures and Blood Work

Blood cultures and cultures of any open wound must be performed before the first dose of antibiotic when osteomyelitis is suspected. Obtain continuing blood samples as needed to monitor ESR and C-reactive protein.

Administer Fluids and Medications

Administer intravenous fluids as ordered to maintain the hydration status of the child. Offer oral fluids that will encourage oral intake by affected young children. Antibiotics are administered intravenously at first, then orally. Monitor the intravenous site and provide care for the central line, if used (refer to the Skills Manual). In the early stages of the infection, analgesics are prescribed to relieve the associated pain and joint tenderness.

Protect from the Spread of Infection

Strict aseptic technique and transmission-based precautions should be used during all dressing changes. Children and family members should avoid direct contact with any dressings or drainage. Teach good hygiene practices, including handwashing, to maintain infection control. Take vital signs and evaluate the child frequently for symptoms indicating the spread of infection (e.g., increasing pain, difficulty breathing, increased pulse rate, fever).

Encourage a Well-Balanced Diet

Educate both the child and the parents about healthy dietary choices that promote the healing process. Providing a high-protein diet and extra vitamin C will contribute to this process. Encourage increased fluid intake to provide adequate hydration and circulation.

Discharge Planning and Home Care Teaching

Emphasize the importance of completing the full course of antibiotic therapy, especially for children who have undergone surgical drainage of an abscess or lesion. Some children may be discharged on intravenous antibiotics if the family is willing to learn the procedure for medication administration and care of the central line. Several sessions of demonstration and return demonstration are needed to ensure safe administration. If the family is unable to perform antibiotic therapy, a home infusion company may be available to come to the home and administer the medication. Explain that failure to follow the prescribed antibiotic therapy may result in chronic infection. Emphasize the importance of returning for blood analysis to monitor progression of healing.

Consider the child's age and developmental level and partner with the family to plan quiet activities and access to school work if the child will be immobilized at home. If the child is homebound for a period of time during treatment, assist the family in planning for completion of school tasks.

- Contact the school and ask that work be sent home.
- Arrange for a tutor if needed.
- Facilitate computer communication between child, teacher, and other students.
- Help family members to plan for help at home, to monitor the child when they are at work or performing other tasks.
- Refer to financial resources as appropriate for the services the child needs.
- Suggest activities that the child can do at home to foster developmental progression.

Evaluation

Expected outcomes of nursing care for the child with osteomyelitis include the following:

- Absence of signs of infection or sepsis
- Completion of prescribed course of antibiotics
- Prevention of infection in contacts
- Adequate intake of fluids and nutrients
- Absence of pain
- Return to normal activities of daily living

Skeletal Tuberculosis and Septic Arthritis

Skeletal tuberculosis (Figure 35–16 ■) and septic arthritis are two infections that, although infrequent, may affect children and adolescents. See page 1434 for clinical manifestations, diagnostic tests, and medical and nursing management for these infections.

Osgood-Schlatter Disease

Osgood-Schlatter disease is an inflammation of the proximal tibial physis as it inserts into the patellar tendon. The condition is painful and is associated with repeated stress on the site resulting from sports such as hockey, gymnastics, or basketball. The child presents with knee pain centered at the tibial tubercle, particularly during sporting activities. Swelling or prominence of the tubercle may be present. The condition is observed in preadolescents and adolescents. The condition is diagnosed by its history, localization of pain, and radiographs.

The condition is treated conservatively by resting the limb from vigorous activity for several weeks. Anti-inflammatory medications may provide comfort. Exercises to stretch and strengthen the quadriceps may be helpful. Wrapping the knee during activities and application of ice after can be recommended. If the condition does not improve, a brace to immobilize the knee is occasionally used. After several weeks the condition generally improves. It may recur while growth continues but disappears after full growth has occurred.

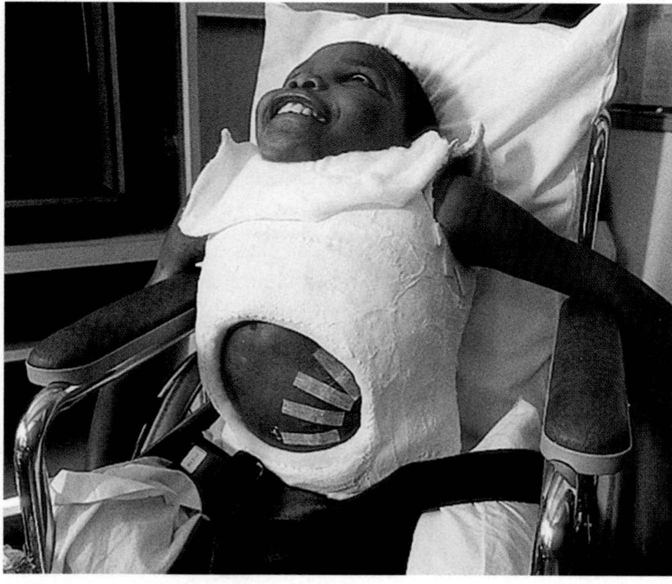

FIGURE 35–16 ■ This boy from Kenya had surgery to correct severe kyphosis and scoliosis, caused by tuberculosis of the spine. A Risser cast has been applied to maintain stability of the spine and thoracic cage during healing. Notice the area cut out of the cast to allow for auscultation of the abdomen, as well as to facilitate the child's comfort and adequate intake of food.

Nursing management consists of recognizing recurrent knee pain and referring for diagnosis so that Osgood-Schlatter can be differentiated from other abnormalities such as Legg-Calvé-Perthes disease, slipped capital femoral epiphysis, osteomyelitis, and arthritis. Explain to the family the chronic nature of Osgood-Schlatter during the growth period and the need to rest the limb for several weeks to decrease the inflammation. Teach the child to wrap the knee and apply ice after activities resume.

Achondroplasia

Dwarfism is a genetic condition usually resulting in an adult height of 58 inches or less. The most common cause of dwarfism is achondroplasia which causes short arms and legs. The torso and head are approximately normal size but decreased growth of long bones causes short stature. This is known as disproportionate short stature. Achondroplasia is caused by an abnormal gene of chromosome 4 and occurs in 1 in 26,000 births (March of Dimes, 2004). The gene is coded to produce proteins called fibroblast growth factor receptors. When less receptors are produced the cells cannot respond normally to signals from growth factors. Achondroplasia may occur as a new genetic mutation with no previous family history or can occur when one or both parents are also dwarfs. There are other less common forms of dwarfism with about 200 identified types.

Children with achondroplasia have short legs and arms; short fingers with a separation between middle and ring fingers, and a large, prominent forehead. Hydrocephalus sometimes occurs in children with achondroplasia (see Chapter 33∞ for a description of hydrocephalus). Most children with the disorder inherit the gene from one parent. Since only one faulty gene must be present for manifestation of the disorder, it is a dominant characteristic (review as needed the genetic transfer described in Chapter 4∞). When a child inherits two copies of the gene from two affected parents, a fatal form of achondroplasia occurs which is characterized by a small thorax, respiratory failure, and death in infancy.

Children with the disorder are diagnosed at birth or shortly after. When there is a family history, genetic testing before or after birth identifies the presence of the faulty gene. Characteristics common in the growth disorder during childhood include frequent otitis media, dental malocclusion, bowing of legs, sleep apnea, and marked lordosis. Low back and leg pain are common as the child grows into adulthood. Perhaps the greatest challenge for families is helping the child to establish a positive self-image in a society that values tall height.

There is no treatment for the disorder at this time. Gene therapy and human growth hormone therapy are being explored as possible treatments for the future. Some children and adults with dwarfism have undergone limb lengthening procedures, described later in this chapter. Other orthopedic interventions may be needed to treat back pain or bone problems. For those

CLINICAL MANIFESTATIONS and Treatment of Skeletal Tuberculosis and Septic Arthritis

CONDITION	CLINICAL MANIFESTATIONS	DIAGNOSTIC TESTS AND CLINICAL THERAPY	NURSING MANAGEMENT
Skeletal Tuberculosis Rare mycobacterial infection that can be destructive. The spine is the most frequent site of infection (Pott's disease), with joints and other sites sometimes affected.	Depending on the site, pain, limp, severe muscle spasms, kyphosis, muscle atrophy, "doughy" swelling of joints, decreased joint motion, changes in reflexes, low-grade fever.	*Diagnostic tests:* Diagnostic studies include tuberculosis skin test, complete blood count, synovial fluid analysis, and radiographs of affected limb or joint. *Clinical Therapy:* Antibiotic therapy (using a combination of drugs) for 6–9 months is the treatment of choice. The affected site is immobilized. Disease may become resistant to these drugs, and additional drug therapy may be necessary.	Educate the child and family about the disorder and stress the importance of complying with long-term antibiotic therapy. Test all members of the family for tuberculosis. Report the disease to the local health department. Facilitate the immobilization and physical therapy of the child at home.
Septic Arthritis Joint infection of the synovial space most often caused by *Haemophilus influenzae, Staphylococcus,* and *Steptococcus.* The most common site of infection is the knee, followed by the hip, ankle, and elbow. Most common in children < 3 years of age.	Fever, pain and local inflammation, joint tenderness, swelling, loss of spontaneous movement. Infant may be irritable, cries when handled, refuses food.	*Diagnostic tests:* CBC with differential ESR, blood cultures. Diagnosis is made based on joint aspiration findings. Results are commonly 100,000 WBCs and 75% neutrophils. Radiographic changes may not be evident until later in the disease process. *Clinical Therapy:* This is a medical emergency requiring prompt treatment to avoid permanent disability. Treatment involves joint aspiration, open drainage, and irrigation, followed by intravenous antibiotic therapy for 3–4 weeks and then oral antibiotics. If the full course of antibiotic treatment is not completed, the child risks recurrent infection and further degeneration of the infected joint.	Educate the child and family about the disorder and emphasize the importance of proper antibiotic therapy. Carefully position the painful joint. Administer antibiotics as ordered. Use transmission-based precautions.

MediaLink Achondroplasia Resources and Support

children who develop hydrocephalus, insertion of a shunt to divert excess fluid may be needed. Treatment of conditions such as otitis media and malocclusion of teeth is provided.

Nursing Management

Nurses play an important role in helping families when a child is diagnosed with achondroplasia. If a parent is a dwarf or a family has a positive history of dwarfism, genetic counseling should be offered prenatally. Explain findings of testing and provide assistance with decision making about pregnancy if needed. Nurses assist parents who have a child with achondroplasia to adjust to the diagnosis, particularly if the parents have had no previous experience with the condition. They may feel guilt and anxiety; contact with other families who have children with achondroplasia can be a supportive intervention.

Nurses help the child with achondroplasia to develop a positive self-concept during childhood. Many resources are available, such as the Little People of America, that provide suggestions about how to foster a positive self-concept, adjust the home to facilitate the dwarf, and assist the child with adjustments in school settings. Partner with school nurses to ensure the child's successful inclusion in all school facilities. An individualized education plan (IEP) will likely be needed. Frequent otitis media and related disorders may create a need for adaptation in communication methods (Haga, 2004). While some families decide to explore limb lengthening procedures, most organizations encourage a focus placed on development of a healthy self-image rather than limb lengthening.

Nurses provide careful assessments of children throughout childhood. Head circumference is especially important in early childhood to identify hydrocephalus if it should occur. Carefully evaluate growth with specialized growth grids for achondroplasia, evaluate dental health at each visit, and perform developmental assessment with special emphasis on gross motor skills. Suggest activities such as swimming and biking that provide activity with little stress on bones. Assist the family by providing resources to help with planning for car safety seats, methods of adjusting the home, and partnering with the school to provide a supportive atmosphere for the child. Helpful organizations include Little People of America, Dwarf Athletic Association of America, Human Growth Foundation, The Magic Foundation for Children's Growth and Related Adult Disorders, and March of Dimes. Refer for care for otitis media and provide postoperative care if ear tubes are inserted (see Chapter 24∞). Refer to dentists and orthodontists and encourage regular dental care.

Marfan Syndrome

Marfan syndrome is another example of a condition inherited in an autosomal dominant manner. About 1 in 5,000 children are affected with the syndrome which manifests with several conditions of connective tissue. The most common problems are cardiac (mitral valve prolapse, aortic regurgitation, abnormal aortic root dimensions), skeletal (pectus excavatum, long arms and digits, scoliosis, elongated head, high arched palate), ocular (lens subluxation), and respiratory (pneumothorax) (Yetman, Huang, Bornemeier, et al., 2003). The average age for diagnosis is 3 years, with a heart murmur the usual finding. Careful assessment identifies additional characteristics of the condition along with a positive family history.

There is no treatment for the syndrome which causes abnormal formation of fibrillin matrix in connective tissue. However, early diagnosis can be successful in treating the cardiac abnormalities with medication or surgery to prevent dissection of the aorta, the major cause of death (Holcomb, 2000). Surgery may be needed to correct scoliosis, pectus excavatum, or pneumothorax. Careful monitoring throughout life is needed to prevent and treat abnormalities associated with the disorder.

Nursing management of Marfan syndrome begins with identification of infants and children with symptoms of the disorder. Once diagnosed, collaboration with a cardiologist, ophthalmologist, and orthopedist are needed throughout life. The child may require surgery for one or more conditions, can require antibiotics during elective procedures or dental care if the mitral valve is affected, and needs echocardiogram and other cardiac studies regularly. The nurse may need to explain the disorder to the family and provide referrals for genetic counseling. The child needs support during childhood to learn about the disorder and to manage the medication and monitoring required.

Osteogenesis Imperfecta

Osteogenesis imperfecta, also known as brittle bone disease, is a connective tissue disorder that primarily affects the bones. Children with this condition have fragile bones that are more likely to fracture. The major type of osteogenesis imperfecta (OI) occurs in 1 in 30,000 live births and affects boys and girls equally. Prognosis depends on the type of disease, as described in this section.

Etiology and Pathophysiology

The underlying disorder is a biochemical defect in the production of collagen. The disease is genetically transmitted, generally in an autosomal dominant inheritance pattern, although some types are transmitted in a recessive pattern. The most common types are caused by mutations on the COLIA1 or COLIA 2 genes on chromosomes 17 and 7 (Astrom & Soderhall, 2002).

Clinical Manifestations

Clinical manifestations include multiple and frequent fractures; blue sclerae; thin, soft skin; increased joint flexibility; enlargement of the anterior fontanel; weak muscles; soft, pliable, brittle bones; and short stature. Conductive hearing loss can occur by adolescence or young adulthood (Paterson, Monk, & McAllion, 2001).

The disease is classified into four types. In type I disease, the most common form, children have fragile bones, blue sclerae, weakened tooth dentin, and hearing loss that manifests in adolescence. In type II disease, the ribs and skeleton are extensively involved; most children with this form of the disease die in utero or shortly after birth. Type III disease is identified in the newborn period or in infancy when the child sustains numerous fractures and manifests blue sclera. Severe bone fragility and kyphoscoliosis are observed. Most children with type III disease die in childhood as a result of cardiorespiratory failure. Type IV disease is characterized by fractures without other symptoms of the disease. Bowing of the legs and other structural deformities can occur; however, the incidence of fractures decreases beginning in puberty. Most children with OI are short in height and may have decreased range of motion in several joints.

COLLABORATIVE CARE

There are many goals for the child and family with osteogenesis imperfecta. Genetic counselors work with the family to explain the transmission. Physicians perform surgery and ongoing management. Nurses and physical rehabilitation unite to plan for health promotion, physical activity, developmental stimulation, and partner with the school for an individualized education plan.

Diagnostic Tests

Improved knowledge about the genetic transmission of this disease means that some cases of osteogenesis imperfecta can be identified before birth using ultrasound or collagen analysis of chorionic villus cells. In many cases, however, diagnosis of osteogenesis imperfecta is made only when the child has a delay in walking or sustains a fracture. Radiographic evaluation may detect both old and new fractures.

CLINICAL TIP

Multiple fractures in various stages of healing may be seen in infants or young children with both child abuse and osteogenesis imperfecta. Collect data to assist in determining the cause. Ask about family history of diseases, stress to the family, and other pertinent factors.

Tests such as dual energy X-ray absorptiometry (DEXA) can be used to measure bone density. Serum alkaline phosphatase may be elevated; other measures of bone metabolism such as serum osteocalcin, procollagen 1 C-terminal peptide, collagen 1 teleopeptide, and urine deoxypyridinoline may be performed occasionally to measure effects of experimental medication.

Clinical Therapy

There is no cure for osteogenesis imperfecta. Medical management consists primarily of fracture care and prevention of

MediaLink OI Resources and Support

deformities. The goal is to maximize the child's independence and mobility while minimizing the risk of fractures. Treatment includes physical therapy; casting, bracing, or splinting; surgical stabilization; nutritional management with high vitamin D and calcium; and biphosphanate medication such as pamidronate. Surgery to insert telescoping rods in long bones may be helpful to stabilize bones. Hematologic stem cell transplant has been used successfully in some children with severe osteogenesis imperfecta and is under further research (Horwitz, Prockop, Gordon, et al., 2001) (Box 35–4).

NURSING MANAGEMENT

Nursing care is primarily supportive and focuses on educating the parents and child about the disease and its treatment.

Nursing Assessment and Diagnosis

The child with OI is assessed carefully and frequently for signs of fractures. Ask about favorite activities of the child since these will need to be integrated into plans for physical activity and developmental progression. Perform careful growth measures and developmental screening.

Nursing diagnoses that may apply to the child with OI include the following:

- Risk for Falls related to learning to walk and other developmental tasks
- Imbalanced Nutrition: Less than Body Requirements related to frequent increased needs to heal fractures
- Impaired Walking related to frequent immobility and bone changes

Planning and Implementation

Nursing care focuses on fostering safety and minimizing chance of fractures, encouraging healing of fractures, reducing pain, supporting the family during the management of this chronic condition, providing care when surgery is required, along with rehabilitation after surgical interventions, and fostering normal growth and development (McLean, 2004).

Foster Safety

To prevent fractures, children with osteogenesis imperfecta must be handled gently. The trunk and extremities should be supported when the child is moved. Tasks such as bathing and diapering may cause fractures and should be performed carefully. Newborns and infants are at particular risk. Use a blanket or pillow under the child for additional support when lifting and moving the child. Do not pull the legs upward when changing a diaper as this can cause a fracture. Instead, slip a hand under the hips to raise the child, sliding the diaper carefully in, and then bringing it up as the legs are slightly abducted.

Partner with families to provide safe activities for the child. Discourage contact sports and other activities that are likely to lead to fractures.

Encourage Healing

Children usually have several or many fractures during childhood. The period of immobility and casting causes further bone breakdown due to decreased mechanical loading, further increasing chance of fracture. The child should eat a well-balanced diet with additional vitamin C, vitamin D, and calcium to encourage healing and bone growth. Calories should be limited to maintain weight at recommended levels since immobility can lead to overweight and the child is generally short for age. Partner with parents if the child is receiving experimental biphosphanate medication, so that doses are properly administered and serum/urine samples are obtained for monitoring.

Family Support

The family may have been suspected of child abuse before the disease was diagnosed, and they should be given an explanation about the similar presenting symptoms if this occurred. Parents should be offered access to genetic counseling.

Parents may initially feel guilt or anger about the diagnosis. As time progresses and they focus on care of the child, they must deal with the disappointment that occurs with each fracture, and a rehabilitation period after. The Osteogenesis Imperfecta Foundation provides information about the disease and can put families in touch with others who have the disease.

For parents who have a child with type II or III OI, the terminal nature of the condition necessitates psychological support, linkage to potential resources, and assistance with managing other tasks of family life (see Chapters 20 and 21∞ for management of chronic conditions and end-of-life care). The siblings and extended family will need support to understand the disease and deal with their feelings and the affected child.

Surgical Care and Rehabilitation

When the child needs a fracture stabilized in surgery, or is having rods inserted to strengthen bones, surgical care management is important. Assess the child's vital signs and growth measurements. Obtain accurate weight before surgery and again after with the cast in place. Administer fluids and use pain control techniques such as medication and other comfort measures. Be alert for signs of infection such as osteomyelitis, or respiratory or urinary tract infection. Begin fluids and perform dietary teaching before discharge to promote intake that fosters healing. Follow activity orders precisely to minimize safety hazards for the family. Partner with physical and occupational rehabilitation to

BOX 35–4 Research: Pamidronate

Pamidronate is a bone resorption inhibitor that absorbs calcium phosphate crystals in bone and is used in adults to treat hypercalcemia of cancer and Paget's disease. It is being used experimentally in children with osteogenesis imperfecta. Low-dose medication is given intravenously every 6 months, and appears to significantly reduce bone fractures and pain. Density of lumbar bones was improved in children receiving the medication (Gonzalez, Pavia, Ros, et al., 2001). The medication does not decrease children's linear growth, but shows signs of promoting bone growth similar to that seen in unaffected children (Zeitlin, Rauch, Plotkin, et al., 2003).

plan for the child's return home and to school and to ensure the family can perform range of motion exercises and other therapies. Ensure that the family has an approved car safety seat to transport the child.

Foster Normal Growth and Development

Emphasize the importance of maintaining normal patterns of growth and development. Toddlers should be helped to explore and interact safely in their environment. Socialization is essential during the school-age and adolescent years. Encourage exercise, such as swimming, to improve muscle tone and prevent obesity. Independent functioning is promoted by the use of adaptive equipment and motorized wheelchairs. Maintenance of function can depend on proper rehabilitation services. The nurse can arrange and manage such services for the family. If the child is hospitalized or must remain out of school for a period of time, partner with the family to provide for continuing learning at home and for safe transition back to the school setting.

■ Evaluation

Expected outcomes for the child with osteogenesis imperfecta include the following:

- Minimal fractures with optimal healing
- Normal range of motion
- Maintenance of normal weight with a diet rich in vitamins and calcium
- Meeting of expected developmental milestones
- Family support
- Adequate family resources to provide rehabilitation and other treatments for the child

---

MUSCULAR DYSTROPHIES

The muscular dystrophies are a group of inherited diseases characterized by muscle fiber degeneration and muscle wasting. These disorders can begin early or late in life, and onset can be at birth or gradual. They are all terminal disorders but the progression can vary from a few to many years.

Etiology and Pathophysiology

Many types of muscular dystrophies affect children and adults. The most common form of childhood muscular dystrophy is Duchenne muscular dystrophy (pseudohypertrophic), which occurs in 1 in 3,500 live male births (Metules, 2002). **Pseudohypertrophy** refers to enlargement of the muscles as a result of their infiltration with fatty tissue. The gene for Duchenne muscular dystrophy was identified in 1987; it is carried in the Xp21.2 region of the chromosome and is either absent or deleted in affected children. This area codes for a protein call dystrophin which is needed as a muscle membrane stabilizer. A cascade of cellular events occurs, leading to necrosis in the fibers and their replacement by connective tissue and fat (Papazian & Alfonso, 2002). Because this is an X-linked disorder it is seen only in males. There is similar incidence in various ethnic groups.

Becker muscular dystrophy is also X-linked and affects 1 in 20,000 males. Although the gene mutation is similar to Duchenne, it is milder in form. Other rare muscular dystrophies manifest in infancy, later childhood, or adolescence. There are a variety of genetic mutations ranging from X-linked to autosomal.

Clinical Manifestations

With Duchenne muscular dystrophy, muscle weakness begins in the lower extremities in early childhood. The parents may notice the child tripping, toe walking, and displaying enlargement of the calf muscles. In fact, the calf is not enlarged but muscle is replaced by fat. By the middle teen years, the child's condition has usually progressed so that walking is not possible. The disease continues to rise, potentially causing conditions such as scoliosis, other musculoskeletal conditions, cardiomyopathy, and respiratory difficulty. Fractures may occur when the child falls due to weakness. The child's life expectancy is the early 20s (Driscoll, 2001). Becker dystrophy is similar but emerges later and more slowly.

The dystrophies of infancy are manifested by generalized weakness and hypotonia. The baby may have difficulty with sucking and swallowing. Ocular problems may be present. Adolescent onset disease is generally milder and slower to progress. Some individuals may live into middle adulthood. See the table below for a summary of clinical manifestations and treatment for some of the more common muscular dystrophies.

COLLABORATIVE CARE

The goal of medical management is to provide support and prevent complications such as infection or spinal deformities.

Diagnostic Tests

Diagnosis and classification are most often based on clinical signs and the pattern of muscle involvement. Children with muscular dystrophy have generalized muscle weakness. They compensate for weak lower extremities by using the upper extremity muscles to raise themselves to a standing position (Gower's maneuver) (Figure 35–17 ■). Biochemical examinations such as serum enzyme assay, muscle biopsy, and electromyography confirm the diagnosis. Serum creatine kinase (CK) is elevated early in the disease. Dystrophin, the muscle protein that is deficient in muscular dystrophy, can be measured by muscle biopsy. Genetic testing establishes the specific abnormality and type of disease present. Testing of newborns may be offered to families who have one child with the disease since this helps some families to adapt and prepare to the care the child will need (Parsons, Clarke, Hood, Lycett & Bradley, 2002). Respiratory function is measured periodically with pulmonary function tests and overnight pulse oximetry (Sobus, Horan & Warren, 2000).

Clinical Therapy

There is no effective treatment for childhood muscular dystrophy. At the present time, research is being directed at several techniques to repair mutations by gene therapy and stem cell therapy (Takeda & Miyagoe-Suzuki, 2001; Papazian & Alfonso, 2002). The steroids prednisone and deflazacort may preserve

CLINICAL MANIFESTATIONS of Muscular Dystrophies of Childhood

TYPE OF DYSTROPHY	CLINICAL MANIFESTATIONS	CLINICAL THERAPY
Duchenne's Muscular Dystrophy X-linked recessive disorder seen in boys (on Xp21 gene); however, 30%–50% of affected children have no family history. Onset: within the first 3–4 years of life.	Delayed walking; frequent falls; easily tired when walking, running, or climbing stairs; toe walking, hypertrophied calves; waddling gait; lordosis; positive Gower's maneuver; mental retardation frequently seen.	Supportive care; physical therapy and braces to help maintain mobility and prevent contractures. Most children are wheelchair bound by 12 years of age; death usually occurs during adolescence from respiratory or cardiac failure.
Becker's Muscular Dystrophy X-linked recessive disorder. Onset: usually after 5 years.	Symptoms are similar to those of Duchenne's muscular dystrophy, but milder and delayed; child is mobile until late teens; normal intelligence; congestive heart failure; contractures.	Supportive care, same as for Duchenne's muscular dystrophy. Slow progression (same as for Duchenne's muscular dystrophy); death usually occurs by 30–50 years of age.
Fascioscapulohumeral Muscular Dystrophy Autosomal dominant disorder (on 4q35 chromosome). Onset: later childhood and adolescence.	Face, shoulder girdle, lower limbs affected; unable to raise arms over head; lordosis; cannot close eyes, whistle, smile, or drink from a straw because of inability to move face; characteristic appearance includes facial weakness, winging of the scapula, thin arms, well-developed forearms.	Physical therapy Slow progression; confined to wheelchair as older adult, but usually attains normal life span.
Emery-Dreifuss Muscular Dystrophy X-linked recessive disorder (on Xq28 gene). Onset: childhood.	Early onset of contractures followed by weakness; Achilles tendon, elbow, and spine affected; muscle weakness in upper body follows, with lower body weakness occurring later; cardiac conduction defect may occur.	Physical therapy Surgery Pacemaker insertion
Congenital Muscular Dystrophies Autosomal recessive group of disorders. Onset: present at birth.	Muscle weaknesses present at birth; motor development delay; contractures and joint deformities; hypotonia.	Correction of skeletal deformity (orthosis or surgery). Usually nonprogressive.

muscle function, preserving walking for a longer period (Biggar, Gingras, Feblings, et al., 2001).

Progressive weakness and muscle deformity result in chronic disability (Figure 35–18 ■). Foot deformity, scoliosis, and respiratory problems are common. Surgery may be used to correct scoliosis to facilitate lung expansion. Respiratory infections are vigorously treated with deep breathing, coughing, nebulizer treatments, and antibiotics when indicated.

Children and families can benefit from mental health support due to the progressive and terminal nature of the disease. The team approach to managing the child with muscular dystrophy ensures collaborative partnering of parents with all health professionals and a comprehensive management plan. Team members should include parents, child when able, physicians (pediatrician, orthopedic surgeon, neurologist), nurses, physical and occupational therapists, a nutritionist, psychologist or mental health therapist, and a social worker.

NURSING MANAGEMENT

Nursing care focuses on promoting independence and mobility and providing psychosocial support that helps the child and family deal with this progressive, incapacitating disease.

■ Nursing Assessment and Diagnosis

Monitor all vital signs as well as cardiac and respiratory functioning. Assess urinary function and frequency of bowel movements. Periodically measure strength and range of motion. Assess mobility via ambulation or assisted device. Perform periodic developmental assessments. Evaluate the family's risk and protective factors for dealing with this chronic and fatal disorder.

Nursing diagnoses that may apply to the child and family with muscular dystrophy include the following:

- Caregiver Role Strain due to increasing dependence of child on care
- Activity Intolerance related to weakness
- Anxiety, Hopelessness, and Powerlessness (child and family) related to diagnosis of terminal disease
- Compromised Family Coping related to a family member with chronic disease and worsening condition
- Risk for Infection related to impaired respiratory system and stasis in urinary system
- Risk of Constipation related to immobility
- Imbalanced Nutrition: Less than Body Requirements related to inability to ingest adequate nutrients
- Anticipatory Grieving (child and family) related to terminal illness

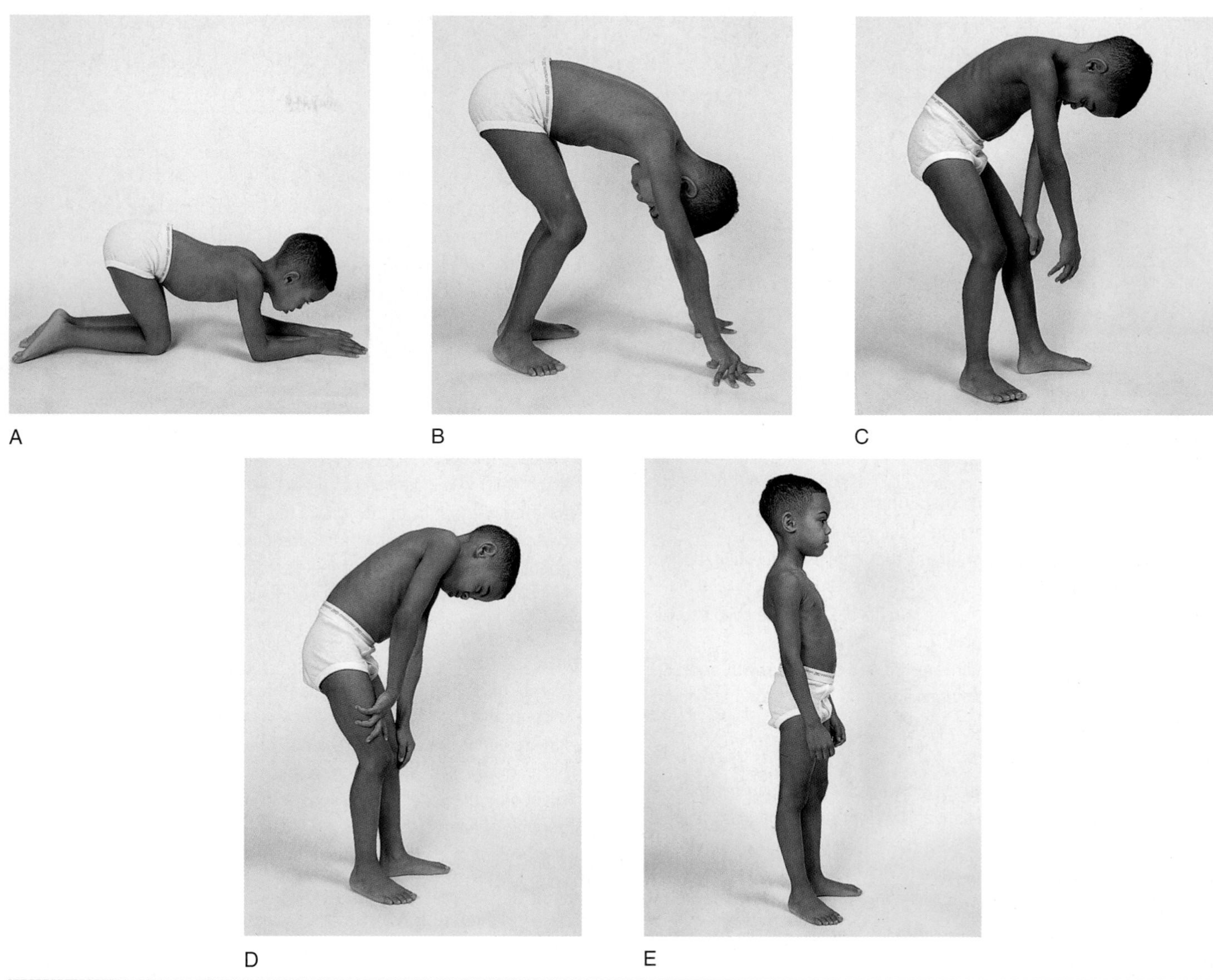

FIGURE 35–17 ■ Because the leg muscles of children with muscular dystrophy are weak, they must perform the Gower's maneuver to raise to a standing position. *A* and *B*, The child first maneuvers to a position supported by arms and legs. *C*, The child next pushes off the floor and rests one hand on the knee. *D* and *E*, The child then pushes himself upright.

■ Planning and Implementation

Care for the child with muscular dystrophy is usually long term and offers challenges to maintain both physical and emotional health of the entire family. Periods of crisis occur when the child is diagnosed and at any time the condition worsens. Nurses often provide home healthcare services to such children, work with them in school nursing positions, and partner with parents in clinics and other facilities to provide health promotion and maintenance as the child grows; this is often a close and meaningful relationship for child, family, and nurse. See the Health Promotion and Maintenance Overview on page 1440 for detailed nursing activities. Provide other therapies to maintain function of body systems and support the family as needed.

Maintenance of Body Systems

Administer oxygen or respiratory therapy as ordered. Soft foods or enteral tube feedings may be needed to promote nutrition. The infant with a rare dystrophy in infancy may need gavage feedings. Maintain bowel function with fluids, high-fiber foods, and medications as needed. Monitor and ensure adequate fluid output. Watch for signs of infection. Perform range of motion and provide for physical activity to level of ability. Physical therapy helps the child ambulate and prevents joint contractures. It is important to provide good back support and posture by keeping the child's body in alignment when confined to a wheelchair. Splints may be needed to maintain extremities in proper position.

Health Promotion & Maintenance Overview

The Child with Muscular Dystrophy

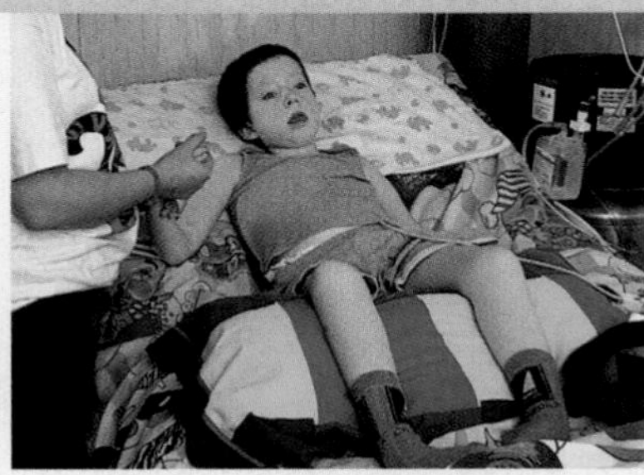

The child with muscular dystrophy needs close monitoring and intervention to foster growth and development in spite of a chronic and terminal disease. The nurse in health promotion can assist the child and family in many ways.

Growth and Development Surveillance

- Perform developmental screening of the young child.
- Refer to early intervention programs that establish educational plans to foster development.
- Provide resources and ideas for the parents based on the child's status rather than expected age norms.
- Measure growth at each healthcare visit and plot on growth grids. Be alert for the child who is gaining weight due to decreased activity in order to avoid overweight.

Nutrition

- Perform 24-hour analysis and evaluate for all essential nutrients. Base the analysis on the child's height and weight rather than chronological age.
- Ask about appetite and food likes and dislikes.
- Encourage adequate fluid, whole grains, fruits, and vegetables to maintain bowel function.
- For the infant with muscular dystrophy, evaluate intake carefully; gavage feeding or nutritional supplementation such as with high-calorie formula may be needed.

Physical Activity

- Carefully monitor physical ability at each visit. Observe for decreases in movement, difficulty ambulating, or a history of falls.
- Partner with physical therapists to ensure range of motion and proper positioning of extremities.
- Explore activities that the child can do as mobility decreases. Swimming and upper body exercise may be good options.
- If the child is using a wheelchair, evaluate fit, safety, and ability to move the chair by arm controls.
- Physical activity should be regular and daily. Ensure that the family has resources to accomplish this need.

Activities of Daily Living

- Partner with occupational therapy to evaluate the child's ability to feed, bathe, dress, and provide own oral care. Provide adaptive devices as needed.
- Encourage the family to provide time for the child to perform own self-care as much as possible.
- Make a home visit or discuss with the family adaptations that could make it easier for the child to be independent in activities of daily living. Low drawers for clothing, or open shelves that do not require pulling out to get items are examples of important adaptations.

Mental and Spiritual Health

- Inquire about the child's general mood.
- Ask the parents what is best and worst about their lives at this time. Use the information to establish a list of their meaningful activities and to identify the areas most in need of support.
- Ask about sources of support such as a group for parents of a child with muscular dystrophy, family participation in faith-based activity, and extended family or neighbors.
- Be alert for signs of depression in child or family (see Chapter 34∞).
- Assist the family to establish activities to increase self-esteem in the youth. The youth should be able to make choices appropriate for developmental age.
- If the child was diagnosed at a younger age, ask what the parents have now told him or her about the disease. Provide support and role-playing opportunities for parents who wish to tell the child about the terminal nature of the disorder.
- Refer for services such as genetic counseling, grief counseling, or other supportive interventions.

Relationships

- Ask about siblings and their relationship with the child with muscular dystrophy.
- Inquire about the child's participation in early intervention or school programs, and community groups. Refer the family to resources that encourage the child's interactions with peers. This is particularly important for teens.
- Ask the parents if and how often they are able to spend time with other adults.

Disease Prevention Strategies

- Immunize the child at recommended times. If the child is ill and immunization is delayed, be sure to call the family back promptly so that infectious diseases can be avoided. Annual influenza vaccine is needed. If the child is treated with steroids for the disease, follow recommendations for immunization of children on steroids.
- Teach the family to avoid crowds and known infectious persons. The child may need to be out of school for a few days or weeks if there is influenza or other diseases in the school population.
- Teach the family signs of infection, especially of the respiratory tract. Have them report these symptoms promptly.
- Monitor effects of antibiotics when administered for infection.
- Encourage daily activities that encourage deep breathing. Swimming, blowing into an incentive spirometer, or playing with a pinwheel are examples.

Injury Prevention Strategies

- Inquire about whether the family has an emergency evacuation plan for the child in case of house fire or other emergency. Assist them to develop a plan.
- If the child is using oxygen, teach about fire safety.
- When mechanical ventilation is used at home, help the family establish emergency backup systems for power outage, such as portable generators.
- Assist the family to learn proper body mechanics to safely transfer and provide care for the child.

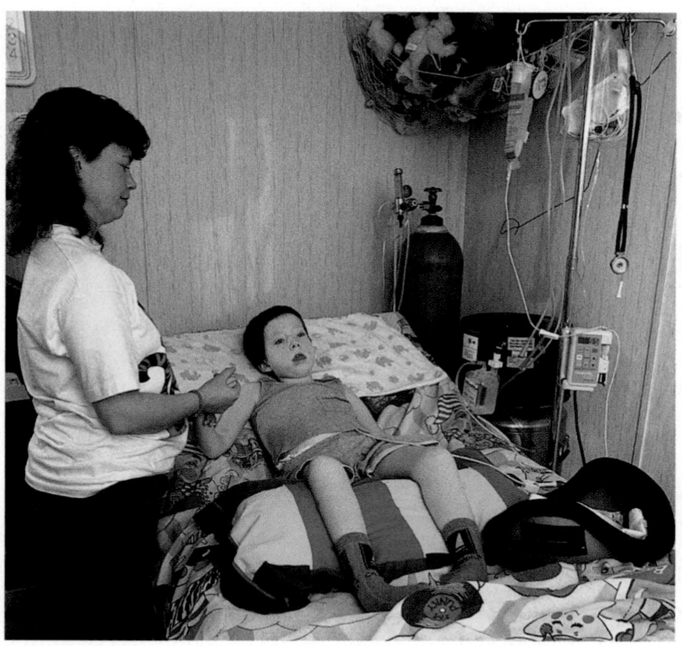

FIGURE 35–18 ■ This young boy with muscular dystrophy needs to receive tube feedings and home nursing care. He attends school when possible and is able to use an adapted computer.

Child and Family Support

Perform periodic developmental assessments and provide parents with suggestions for encouraging the child's development. Meet with teachers to evaluate the child's learning needs and functioning in the classroom. An individualized education plan should be established. Partner with the school to provide tutors or home computers if needed. Young children should be enrolled in early intervention programs before they are old enough for school.

Encourage the child to be independent for as long as possible. Concentrate on what the child can accomplish and do not ask the child to complete tasks that may prove frustrating. Reading books to the child, listening to tapes, and watching television offer the child stimulation during hospitalization. Exercise as tolerated contributes to muscle strength and a general sense of well-being.

Families may be challenged by the care the child needs. Surgery, hospitalization for respiratory infection, visits to physical therapy, and constant daily care are examples of the challenges faced. Managing this care, providing a nurturing environment for other children and family members, and obtaining necessary financial resources over many years creates a need for assistance from various resources. Refer the family to respite care, assist them in finding resources, and be certain that either a family member or health professional acts as case manager to coordinate various services needed. Refer family members to resource and support groups such as the Muscular Dystrophy Association.

Parents may exhibit feelings of guilt and hopelessness. The mother who learns she has carried the gene that affects her son can be devastated. Encourage parents to express their feelings. Genetic counseling is recommended for the entire family, and it is especially important to identify women who are carriers of one of the X-linked disorders. Siblings may feel neglected because their brother or sister is receiving so much attention. They may be concerned that they will develop the disease. Sometimes multiple children in a family are affected with the condition and as one child worsens, the effect on siblings is profound. On the other hand, siblings without the disease may feel guilty for their good health. Encourage the parents to involve siblings in the affected child's care to reassure them of their importance.

As the child's condition weakens, the family again needs additional support. They experience grieving, each person in their own way. They have lived with chronic sorrow and now need to prepare for the child's death. The child is usually old enough to recognize the deteriorating condition. See Chapter 22∞ for further discussion of bereavement and end-of-life care.

■ Evaluation

Expected outcomes for nursing care of the child with muscular dystrophy include maintenance of optimal mobility and development, positive self-image for the affected child, and positive management of the emotional challenges by all family members.

INJURIES TO THE MUSCULOSKELETAL SYSTEM

Musculoskeletal injuries are classified according to the mechanism, the location, and the force of the injury. Strains, sprains, dislocations, and fractures are the most common musculoskeletal injuries in children. Distinguishing among these injuries is often difficult. Athletic participation and injuries in car crashes are frequent causes of strains, sprains, dislocations, and fractures. (See Evidence-Based Practice: Backpacks and Pain.) Serious injuries affecting the brain and spinal cord are discussed in Chapter 33∞. See page 1443 for clinical manifestations and management of strains, sprains, and dislocations. A detailed discussion of fractures follows.

Fractures

A fracture is a break in a bone that occurs when more stress is placed on the bone than the bone can withstand. Fractures, which may occur at any age, occur frequently in children because their bones are less dense and more porous than those of adults.

Etiology and Pathophysiology

Fractures in children may result from direct trauma to a bone (falls, sports injuries, abuse, motor vehicle crashes) or bone diseases (osteogenesis imperfecta) that result in weakening of the bone. Due to their porous nature, the bones of children may bow leading to more common greenstick or spiral fractures in children (Eiff & Hatch, 2003) (Table 35–2). Trauma may be caused by an acute injury, direct and forceful impact, or overuse such as in chronic and repetitive activities. In the opening scenario of this chapter, Douglass experienced an acute injury when his leg forcefully hit the trampoline frame, suffering a closed fracture of the fibula.

MediaLink Muscular Dystrophy Resources and Support

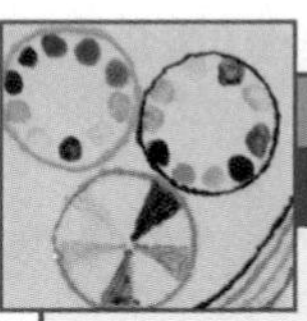

EVIDENCE-BASED PRACTICE
Backpacks and Pain

PROBLEM

Many children wear backpacks that are heavy and carry them for large parts of the day. Low back, neck, and shoulder pain seem to be increasing in children and a possible connection with backpacks has been suggested.

EVIDENCE

Several studies have now investigated the relationships between backpack use and complaints of pain. In one study 1,126 youth from 12 to 18 years completed a questionnaire about backpack use, their health, and had physical measurements completed. Almost 75% of the youth had back pain, and the pain was associated with poorer general health, being overweight, being female, and carrying heavy backpacks (Sheir-Neiss, Kruse, Rahman, et al., 2003). In another study of 745 adolescents, 45% had back pain and severe neck discomfort, while shoulder pain was suffered by 6%. The weight of backpacks was not associated with incidence of pain reports in this study (van Gent, Dols, de Rover, et al., 2003).

IMPLICATIONS

A clear association between backpack use and weight and complaints of pain is not evident. Therefore, nurses should ask about backpack use at health promotion visits and advise on how to wear them. The American Academy of Pediatrics lists recommendations for backpack use:

- Have wide, padded shoulder straps and wear the pack on both shoulders, close to the body.
- Use a padded back and waist strap.
- Be sure the backpack is lightweight (no more than 10%–20% of the youth's weight) or consider a rolling pack if it is heavy.
- Practice back strengthening exercises and learn to bend at the knees.

CRITICAL THINKING APPLICATION

How will you partner with youth who are in sports after school to plan how to carry school items and sports gear safely? What exercises can you plan to help strengthen the back and thighs for carrying a pack?

Clinical Manifestations

Signs and symptoms of fractures vary depending on the location, type, and nature of the causative injury. Fractures are generally characterized by pain, abnormal positioning, edema, immobility or decreased range of motion, ecchymosis, guarding, and crepitus. Childhood fractures most often involve the clavicle, tibia, ulna, and femur, with distal forearm fractures the most common type. Fractures to the pelvis are often associated with motor vehicle crashes. Epiphyseal (growth plate) injuries are dangerous in children as they can interfere with future growth at the site. These constitute about 30% of childhood fractures (Eiff & Hatch, 2003). Types of fractures are described using the Salter-Harris classification system (Figure 35–19 ■).

COLLABORATIVE CARE

Medical management consists of two basic steps: reduction to realign displaced or fragmented bones, and immobilization so that healing can take place. Some fractures have sides that are properly aligned and no reduction is needed.

Diagnostic Tests

Radiographs are useful for determining the exact location and type of fracture.

Clinical Therapy. Immobilization is essential for the bone healing process to take place. A closed reduction aligns the bone by manual manipulation or traction. Sedation or other pain management techniques are used during closed reduction. An open reduction requires surgical alignment of the bone, often using pins, plates, wires, or screws. For open fractures, surgery must also be performed for debridement, to remove dead tissue and clean the wound. Casting is the most common external method of immobilization. Casts may be placed on extremities (short or long leg or arm cast) or the upper body to immobilize the spine, or may be applied from chest to legs to stabilize pelvis or hips (hip spica cast). Leg casts may be walking or nonwalking casts. Cast material is either plaster or a synthetic fabric. Other external methods of stabilization include traction and splinting (see Table 35–4 later in the chapter for types of traction). Pins may be inserted to stabilize the fracture, and can be used with or without casts or traction. A combination of treatments may be needed in the child with multiple fractures following a car crash or other trauma.

Healing of fractures is influenced by factors including age, size of the involved bone, and fracture site. The healing process progresses from cartilaginous callous formation to bone remodeling and bony callous formation (Figure 35–20 ■). Fractures heal in less time in children than in adults, because the periosteum or vascular outer layer of bone is thicker and remains intact even during a fracture (Scudder, 2004). This blood supply enhances the healing process. Immobilization is essential for the bone healing process to take place. If a fracture is properly reduced, complications should be minimal (Table 35–3).

Fractures involving the epiphyseal plate disrupt the growth process in children. These injuries require ongoing care to evaluate for outcomes such as limb length discrepancy, joint incongruity, and angular deformities. Further surgery or treatment may be needed in such cases.

NURSING MANAGEMENT

The goals of nursing management are early identification and immobilization of fractures, and providing care to promote safety during the healing process.

■ Nursing Assessment and Diagnosis

Assess the diets of all youth who might be at risk for fractures and insert dietary teaching in health promotion visits (Box 35–5).

When dealing with an injured child, be alert to the signs and symptoms of fractures before moving the child. Try to identify

CLINICAL MANIFESTATIONS of Strains, Sprains, and Dislocations

CONDITION	CLINICAL MANIFESTATIONS	CLINICAL THERAPY
Strain • Stretching or tearing of either a muscle or a tendon, usually from overuse (e.g., back strain resulting from improper or overly heavy lifting, shoulder and elbow tears from baseball).	• Vary according to the type and severity of the strain. Pain can be acute or chronic.	• Rest and support of the injured part until the muscle or tendon heals and normal activity can occur.
Sprain • Stretching or tearing of a ligament, usually caused by a fall, sports injury, or motor vehicle crash (e.g., anterior cruciate ligament [ACL] tear requiring reconstruction).	• Edema, joint immobility, and pain.	• For the first 24–36 hours: **R**est **I**ce **C**ompression **E**levation • After the first 24–36 hours, mobility is gradually increased.
Dislocation • Complete displacement of an articular joint surface, usually associated with a fall, sports injury, or motor vehicle crash. Although almost any joint may be dislocated, most dislocations occur in the shoulder, knee, and hip.	• Pain and tenderness, swelling and obvious deformity, and instability of the joint.	• Varies according to the site and severity of the injury, and consists of: Shoulder: Open or closed reduction followed by the application of a sling. Knee: Closed reduction with gentle traction, then immobilization with a splint. Hip (posterior): Immediate closed reduction or possibly open reduction, traction, or hip spica cast. Hip (anterior): Immediate closed reduction, extension traction, and hip spica cast.

the cause of the injury by asking the child, parents, or other family members what happened.

CLINICAL TIP

When in doubt about the nature of an injury, apply a splint. Splinting immobilizes the site, prevents further damage, and decreases pain. Be sure to immobilize both the joints above and below the injury.

Evaluate pain, swelling, and any abnormal positioning of the injured area. When a child is admitted to the emergency department or hospital, nursing assessment includes the extent of the injury, the degree of pain, and the child's vital signs (respiratory status, pulse, blood pressure).

The following nursing diagnoses may apply to the child with a fracture:

- Pain related to injury
- Risk for Impaired Skin Integrity related to treatment
- Risk for Infection related to open fracture or trauma
- Impaired Physical Mobility related to treatment
- Health-Seeking Behaviors related to lack of information about treatment and expected outcome

Planning and Implementation

Nurses may be in community settings when children experience a fracture, and need to provide emergency care and arrange for transport. Emergency personnel are informed of the assessment data to provide for safe care. In addition, nurses are aware that repeated fractures in the same child can be a sign of other healthcare conditions.

PRACTICE ALERT

It is uncommon for children to have repeated fractures. If they occur, make further assessments for their cause. The child may suffer from osteogenesis imperfecta. If attention deficit hyperactivity disorder (ADHD) is present or if the child has a mental health problem, excessive risky behavior may be the cause of fractures. When children are found on radiograph to have several old and healing fractures, or multiple fractures of the same or different bones, they may be victims of physical abuse, particularly if the caretaker explanation of fracture does not match the clinical picture. An example could be the parent who claims the child fell from a chair, but there is a severe arm fracture and skull fracture. See Chapter 7 ∞ for a description of child abuse and Chapter 34 ∞ for a discussion of ADHD.

TABLE 35–2 Common Fractures

FRACTURE TYPE	DESCRIPTION	COMMENTS
Closed	Bone breaks cleanly but does not penetrate skin.	Also called a simple fracture.
Open	Broken ends of bone protrude through soft tissues and skin.	Serious; may result in osteomyelitis. Also called a compound fracture.
Comminuted	Bone fragments into many pieces.	Common in those with conditions causing brittle bones, such as osteogenesis imperfecta
Compression	Bone is crushed.	Common in clients with osteoporosis.
Impacted	Broken ends of bone are forced into each other.	Commonly results from falls; also common in hip fracture.
Depressed	Broken bone is pressed inward.	Common in skull fractures.
Spiral	Jagged break due to twisting force applied to bone.	Common fracture due to sports injuries.
Greenstick	Bone breaks incompletely, much in the way a green twig breaks.	Common in children, whose bones have proportionally more organic matrix and are more flexible than those of adults.

Adapted from Marieb, E. N. (1998). Human anatomy and physiology *(4th ed., (p. 180). Menlo Park, CA: Benjamin Cummings.*

Nursing care focuses on care of the child before and after fracture reduction, encouraging mobility as ordered, maintaining skin integrity, preventing infection, and teaching the parents and child how to care for the fracture. If conscious sedation or pain blocks are used, nursing care for these procedures is needed. When caring for a child who has undergone fracture reduction, it is important to be aware of the signs of complications (Table 35–3). Notify the physician immediately if these signs occur. The major serious complication is **compartment syndrome,** or a condition of increased pressure in a limited space such as the soft tissue of an extremity, which compromises circulation and nervous innervation (Harvey, 2001). See the clinical manifestations table on page 1445.

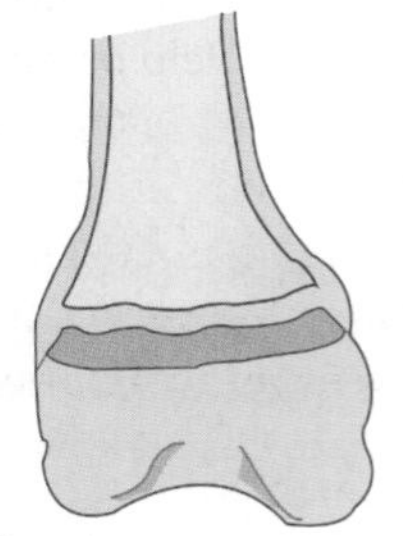

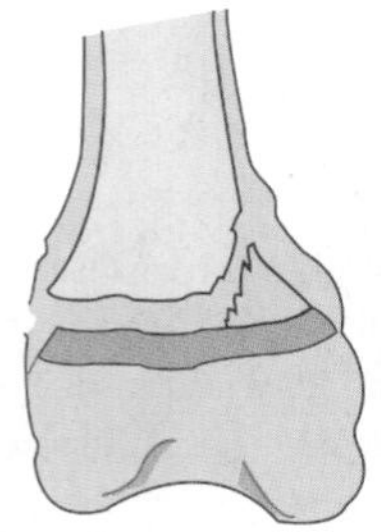

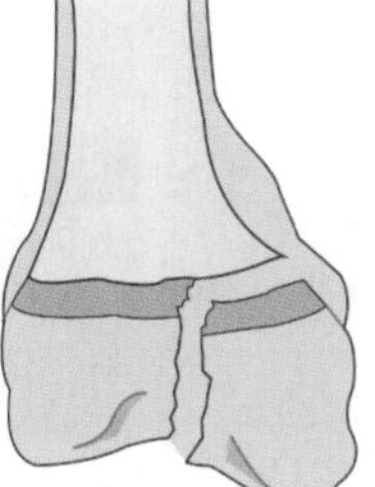

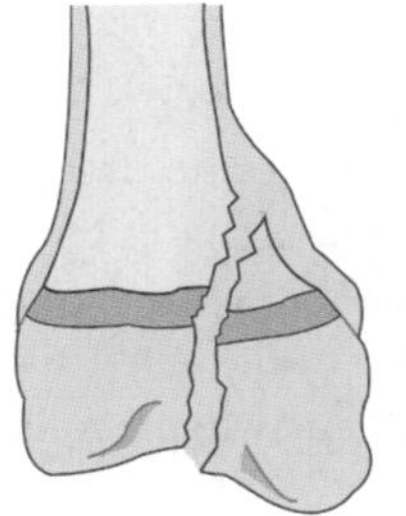

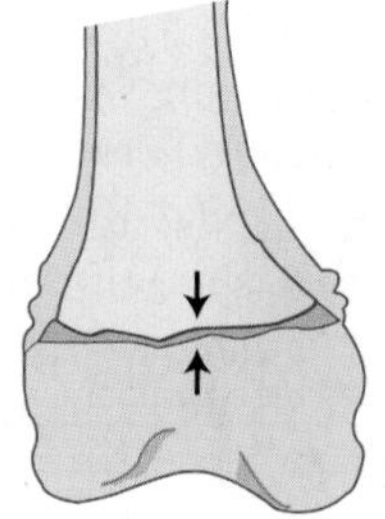

Type V
Rare
Crush injury causes cell death in growth plate, resulting in arrested growth and limited bone length
If growth plate is partially destroyed, angular deformities may result

FIGURE 35–19 ■ The Salter-Harris classification system is based on the angle of the fracture in relation to the epiphysis.

BOX 35–5 Stress Fractures

Stress fractures are becoming more common in adolescents who limit their intake of calories and calcium in an attempt to remain lean for sports such as distance running or gymnastics. These fractures may present with chronic pain that changes in intensity. Be alert to this possibility when teenagers' diets and athletic activities place them at risk. In addition, the risk of bone fractures in adolescent females who consume carbonated beverages is three times higher than in those who do not consume such drinks. It is thought that the high phosphorus content of carbonated beverages fosters bone loss and that these beverages displace milk, a major calcium source, in the diet (Wyshak, 2000).

Maintain Proper Alignment

Immobilization is used to maintain proper alignment of the fracture. Casts and traction are methods used for immobilizing an injured child. Cast care guidelines are included on page 1411.

Different types of traction are used, depending on the location and type of fracture (Table 35–4). Nursing care for the child in traction is described in Box 35–6 on page 1449.

Monitor Neurovascular Status

Neurovascular assessment is used for early detection of compartment syndrome, which may occur with a crush injury or when a fracture is reduced. Swelling associated with inflammation reduces blood flow to the affected area, and casting causes further constriction of blood flow. Douglass, in the opening scenario, had a splint applied for several days, with casting later, to allow swelling to decrease and to minimize risk for compartment syndrome. Monitor the child's sensation to touch, temperature, movement, strength of the pulse, and capillary refill time in the extremity distal to the injury. Monitor every 15 minutes after the cast is applied for at least 2 hours and then every 1 to 2 hours, depending on the care facility's policy and the child's condition. Keep the cast elevated above heart level to minimize edema.

TABLE 35–3 Complications of Fracture Reduction

COMPLICATION	CLINICAL THERAPY
Infection Acute (may occur with open fractures) Chronic (osteomyelitis)	Debridement, drainage, culture, and treatment with antibiotics
Neurovascular injury resulting from physical nerve damage	Nerve repair
Vascular injury	Vascular repair, amputation, tendon lengthening
Malunion (undesired healed alignment of bone) or delayed union	Corrective osteotomy; prolonged immobilization
Nonunion	Surgical intervention; internal fixation
Leg length discrepancy	Shoe lift

CLINICAL MANIFESTATIONS of Compartment Syndrome

CLINICAL MANIFESTATIONS	ASSESSMENT
Clinical manifestations begin about 30 minutes after tissue ischemia starts. Major manifestations are: • Paresthesia (tingling, burning, loss of two-point discrimination) • Pain (unrelieved by medication, characterized by crying in the young child) • Pressure (skin is tense, cast appears tight) • Pallor* (pale, gray, or white skin tone) • Paralysis* (weakness or inability to move extremity) • Pulselessness* (weak or absent pulse)	Check extremities for: • Color • Temperature • Capillary refill • Peripheral pulses • Edema • Sensation • Motor ability • Pain

Document results and report changes or abnormal results immediately.

** = late sign*

Adapted from Kunkler, C. E. (1999). Neurovascular assessment. Orthopaedic Nursing, *18(3), 63–71; Harvey, C. (2001). Compartment syndrome: When it is least expected.* Orthopaedic Nursing, *20(3), 15–26.*

MediaLink Case Study: Fracture Assessment

Promote Mobility

The amount of mobility the child is allowed is ordered by the physician and restrictions depend on the extent and site of the fracture. Fractures of the hip or pelvis may involve body casts, and providing wheeled carts makes mobility possible. Children with leg fractures can sometimes bear weight on the cast; but if they cannot bear weight, they move around with crutches, walkers, or wheelchairs. See the Skills Manual for information on crutch walking.

Discharge Planning and Home Care Teaching

Most fractures can be easily managed at home. Activities are generally limited for approximately 8 weeks. Teach the parents and child cast care, activity restrictions, and how to identify problems that should be reported (see page 1412). Help parents to identify any modifications that may be needed at home and school. The child who has to manage steps at home or school may need special training with crutches or a temporary ramp. Refer parents to home health nurses or home teaching services if indicated. Provide pertinent teaching to prevent future injuries.

PRACTICE ALERT

When a child has a fracture from sports or other activities, ask details about how the injury occurred. If protective gear is recommended and was not worn, reinforce the need for protection. Suggest financial resources as necessary.

Sports Injuries

Sports injuries are the most common type of injury in youth from 13 to 19 years. Football, wrestling, soccer, and gymnastics

PATHOPHYSIOLOGY ILLUSTRATED

Process of Bone Healing

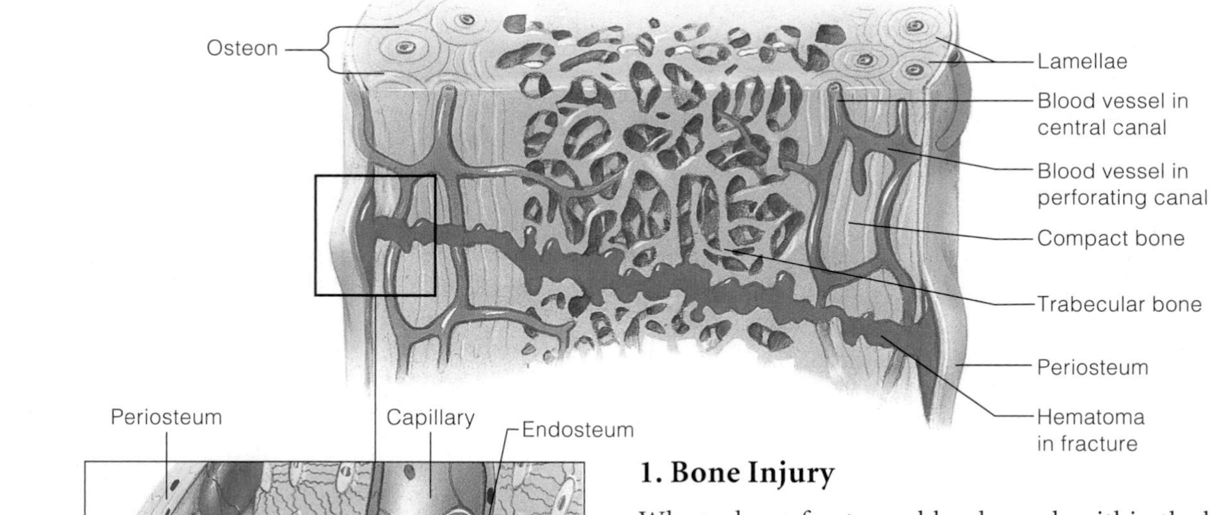

1. Bone Injury

When a bone fractures, blood vessels within the bone and surrounding soft tissues tear and begin to bleed, forming a hematoma. Necrotic bone tissue adjacent to the fracture causes an intense inflammatory response characterized by vasodilation, exudate formation, and white cell migration to the fracture site.

2. Fibrocartilaginous Callus Formation

Clotting factors within the hematoma form a fibrin meshwork. Within 48 hours, fibroblasts and new capillaries growing into the fracture form granulation tissue that gradually replaces the hematoma. Phagocytes begin to remove cell debris.

Osteoblasts, bone-forming cells, proliferate and migrate into the fracture site, forming a fibrocartilaginous callus. The osteoblasts build a web of collagen fibers from both sides of the fracture site that eventually unites to connect bone fragments, thus splinting the bone. Chondroblasts lay down patches of cartilage that provide a base for bone growth.

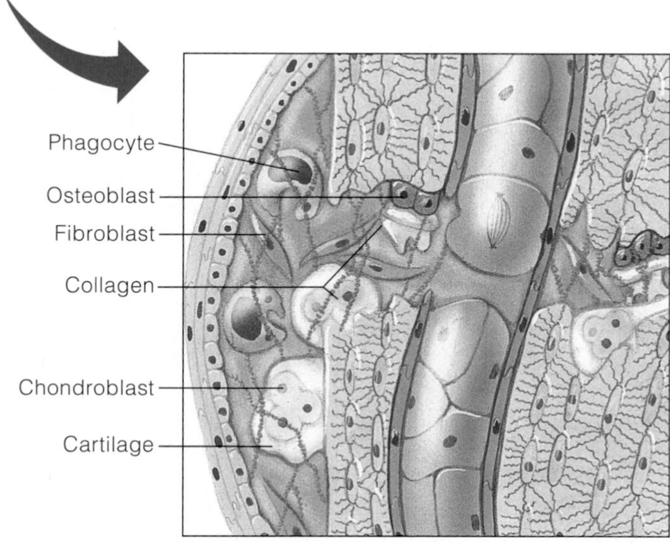

FIGURE 35–20 ■ Metatarsus adductus is characterized by convexity (curvature) of the lateral border of the foot, as shown by the red line.

PATHOPHYSIOLOGY ILLUSTRATED

Process of Bone Healing (continued)

4. Bone Remodeling

Osteoblasts continue to form new woven bone, which is in turn organized into the lamellar structures of compact bone. Osteoclasts resorb excess callus as it is replaced by mature bone.

As the bone heals and is subjected to the mechanical stress of everyday use, osteoblasts and osteoclasts respond by remodeling the repair site along the lines of force. This ensures that the repaired section of bone eventually resembles the structure of the uninjured part.

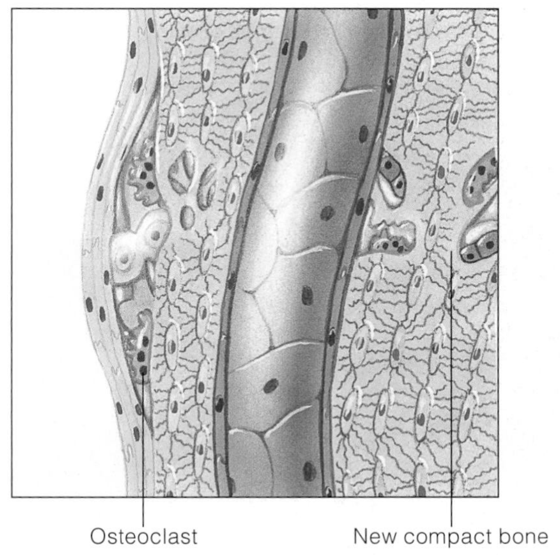

3. Bony Callus Formation

Osteoblasts continue to proliferate and synthesize collagen fibers and bone matrix, which are gradually mineralized with calcium and mineral salts to form a spongey mass of woven bone. The trabeculae of woven bone bridge the fracture. Osteoclasts migrate to the repair site and begin removing excess bone in the callus. Bony callus formation usually continues for 2 to 3 months.

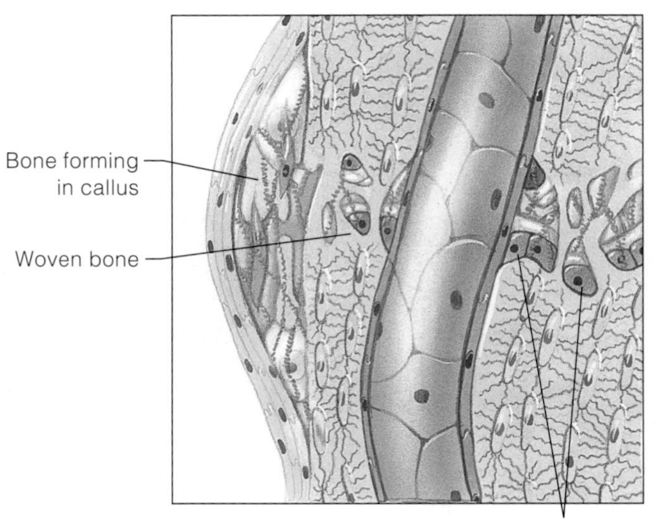

FIGURE 35–20 ■ (continued)

TABLE 35–4 Types of Traction

TYPE

Skin Traction

Pull is applied to the skin surface, which puts traction directly on the bones and muscles. Traction is attached to the skin with adhesive materials or straps, or foam boots, belts, or halters.

Dunlop Traction (can be either skeletal or skin)

Used for fracture of the humerus. The arm, which is flexed, is suspended horizontally with straps placed on both the upper and lower portions for pull from both sides.

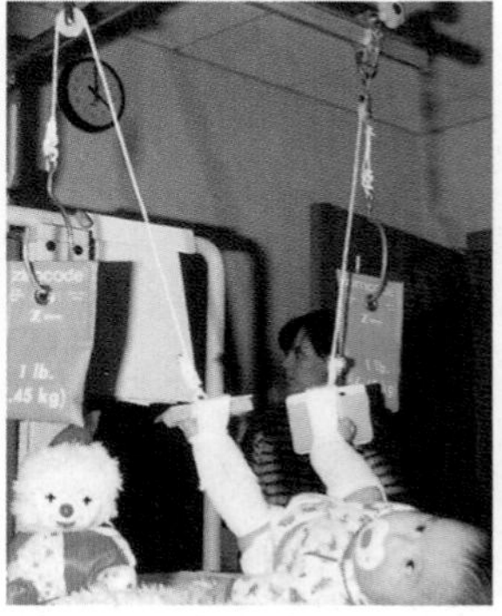

(1)

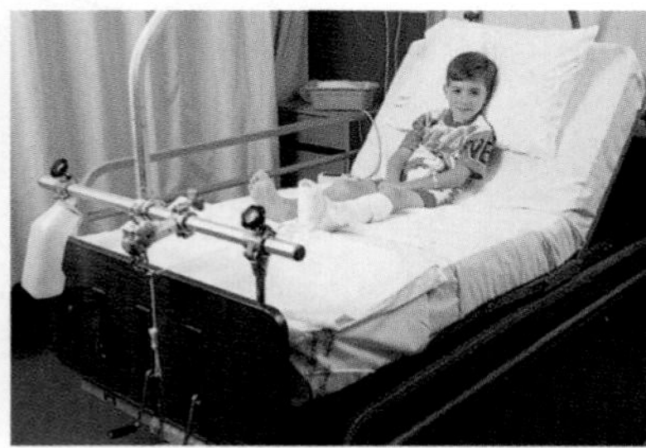

(2)

Bryant Traction (1)

Used specifically for the child under 3 years of age and weighing less than 17.5 kg (35 lb), who has developmental dysplasia of the hip or a fractured femur. This bilateral traction is applied to the child's legs and kept in place by wrapping the legs from foot to thigh with elastic bandages. The hips are flexed at a 90-degree angle, with knees extended. This position is maintained by attaching the traction appliance to weights and pulleys, which are suspended above the crib. The buttocks do not rest on the mattress, but are slightly elevated off the bed.

Buck Traction (2)

Used for knee immobilizattion; to correct contractures or deformities; or for short-term immobilization of a fracture. It keeps the leg in an extended position, without hip flexion. Traction is applied to the extremity in one direction (straight line) with a single pulley system.

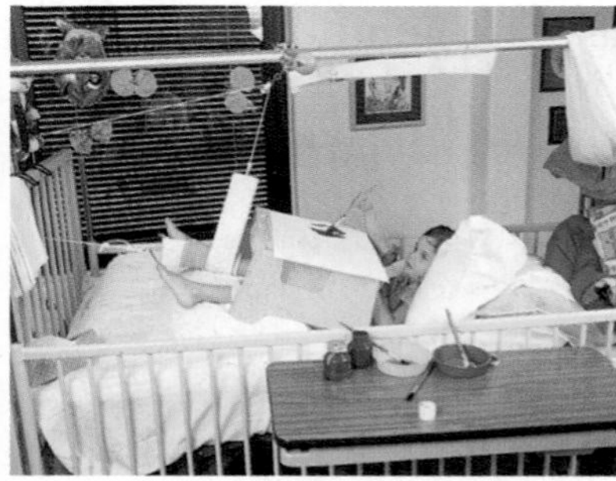

(3)

Russell Traction (3)

Used for fractures of the femur and lower leg. Traction is placed on the lower leg while the knee is suspended in a padded sling. The hips and knees, which are slightly flexed, are immobilized. One force is applied by a double pulley to the foot and another force is applied upward using a sling under the knee and an overhead pulley.

Skeletal Traction

Pull is directly applied to the bone by pins, wires, tongs, or other apparatus that have been surgically placed through the distal end of the bone.

Skeletal Cervical Traction

Used for cervical spine injuries to reduce fractures and dislocations, Crutchfield Gardner-Wells, or Vinke tongs are placed in the skull with burr holes. Weights are attached to the apparatus with a rope and pulley system to the hyperextended head.

Halo Traction

Used to immobilize the head and neck after cervical injury or dislocation. Also used for positioning and immobilization after cervical injury.

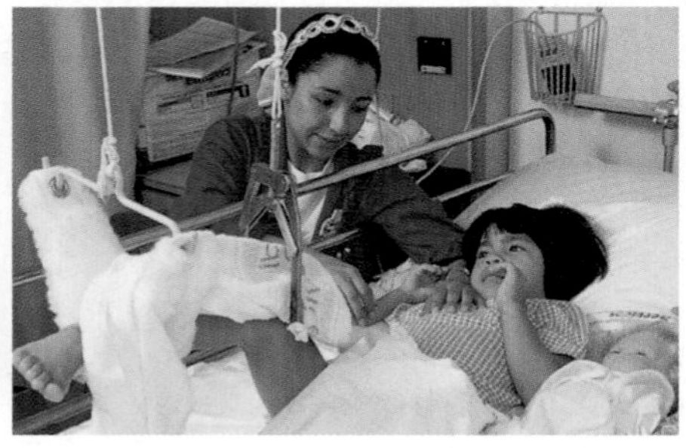

(4)

90-90 Traction (4)

Used for fractures of the femur or tibia. A skeletal pin or wire is surgically placed through the distal part of the femur, while the lower part of the extremity is in a boot cast. Traction ropes and pulleys are applied at the pin site and on the boot cast to maintain the flexion of both the hip and knee at 90 degrees. This traction can also be used for treatment of an upper extremity fracture.

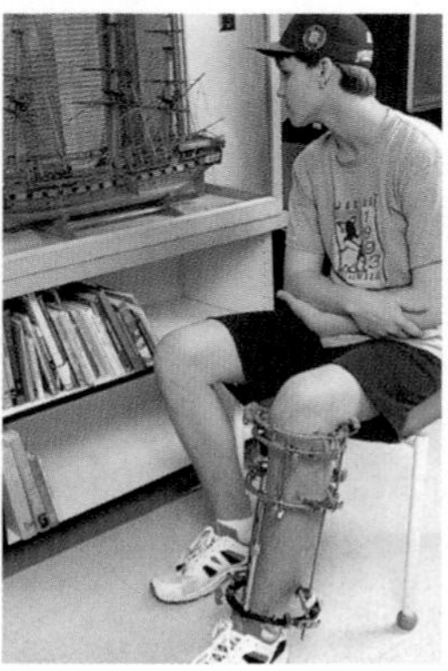

(5)

External Fixators (5)

These devices can be used in the treatment of simple fractures, both open and closed; complex fractures with extensive soft tissue involvement; correction of bony or soft tissue deformities; pseudoarthroses; and limb length discrepancy. They are attached to the extremity by percutaneous transfixing of pins or wires to the bone.

BOX 35–6 Nursing Care of the Child with Traction or External Fixator

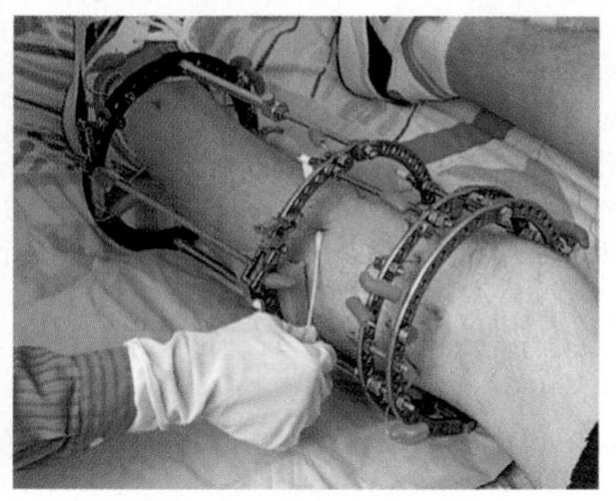
Providing pin care for external fixator

1. Assess the child in traction by first checking the equipment. Make sure that the equipment is in the proper position. Observe both the body appliance and the attached weights and pulleys. Make certain that the child's body is in proper alignment.
2. Assess the skin under the straps and pin insertion sites for any signs of redness, edema, or skin breakdown.
3. Assess the extremity by checking neurovascular status frequently (check warmth, color, distal pulses, capillary refill time, movement, sensation).
4. Provide pin care when ordered using sterile technique. Clean the area surrounding the pin with cotton-tipped applicators saturated with normal saline or half-strength hydrogen peroxide. Clean the area again with sterile water or more saline. Apply an antibacterial ointment, if ordered, using another cotton-tipped applicator.
5. When the traction equipment can be removed, skin care should be performed every 4 hours.
6. Place a sheepskin pad under the child's extremity if orders permit.

are the sports most frequently associated with injury (Stracciolini & Metzel, 2000). Fractures, as described, are common sports injuries of young athletes. Douglass, in the opening scenario, is an example of a child with this type of injury. However, a variety of other injuries that affect the musculoskeletal system are common in sports. Children and adolescents have characteristics that put them at risk for injury. These include:

- Vulnerability of growth plates to injury, especially distal tibia and fibula
- Increased joint mobility from lax tendons and ligaments, leading to injury of knee, ankle, and hip
- More porous bones that lead to fractures and more common injury to underlying organs
- Lack of experience in the sport and inadequate training
- Lack of acceptance of protective gear
- Impatience with taking the time to heal after injury

Common sports injuries are listed in Table 35–5. Treatments for sprains, strains, dislocations, and fractures are described in the previous sections. Head and neck injuries are discussed in Chapter 33∞ and dental emergencies in Chapter 24∞. General approaches to minimize and treat injuries for youth athletes follow.

Athletes can benefit from teaching that enhances performance of their sports and also minimizes chance of injury. They should receive instruction in correct techniques from a person qualified to coach and supervise children. Encourage youth to gradually increase time and intensity at a sport, rather than immediately playing a new sport for long periods of time. Have parents inquire about the coach's experience and also verify that the coaching staff is prepared in emergency care.

The nurse should be alert for sports injuries during contacts with children and adolescents in health promotion visits. Ask about sports participation for all youth, but especially when there are complaints of sore muscles, edema of body parts, and bruises. Perform neurovascular assessment of extremities, including color, temperature, capillary refill time, edema, pulses, sensation, and pain. Phrase questions so that you identify sports such as skate boarding or snow boarding which may not be performed under supervision or in organized sports programs. Youth may not consider these "sports."

Teach the importance of warming up for 10 to 15 minutes before participation, and to cool down for a corresponding period at the end of activity. Encourage wearing recommended safety gear for the sport including equipment such as well-fitted protective helmet, face masks, eye protection, mouth guards, elbow and wrist guards, gloves, knee pads, and shin pads. Parents may need assistance to learn recommended equipment and resources for purchase. Frequent updates are needed as the child grows. Teach the child not to ignore pain.

Injuries such as muscle strains should be treated promptly. They involve several steps.

- Resting the injury for 24 to 48 hours; applying ice for 20 minutes four times daily; compression with an elastic wrap

TABLE 35–5 Common Sports Injuries

SPORT	TYPE OF INJURIES
Baseball	➤ Hand and finger fractures and sprains ➤ Contusions and sprains of upper or lower extremities; wrists, elbows, knees, and ankles are common sites ➤ Injury to body parts when hit by a ball, e.g., broken teeth, face, head, eye, and chest injuries
Football	➤ Head and neck injury such as skull or cervical vertebrae fracture ➤ Pulled muscles or dislocations in shoulders and legs
Gymnastics	➤ Wrist and elbow fractures and strains ➤ Tendonitis in elbows and ankles/legs
Hockey (ice and inline)	➤ Dental injury ➤ Leg fractures ➤ Head and neck injuries
Soccer	➤ Head and neck injury ➤ Strains and fractures of legs
Wrestling	➤ Fractures and dislocations of upper and lower extremities

to provide comfort and decrease edema; elevating the part affected above heart level
- Gradually increasing motion to the part
- Adding flexibility and resistance or strengthening exercises
- Returning gradually to the sport, usually in 2 to 3 weeks after injury

(Harper, 2002)

Partner with the child, family, and other health professionals to plan for activity when an injury has occurred. Praise the family and youth for physical activity, an important part of a healthy lifestyle. Provide community resources to foster sports participation.

Amputations

Amputation—the complete absence of a body extremity—can be either congenital or acquired. Approximately two thirds of amputations in children are congenital and one third are acquired. Congenital amputations can be caused by constrictive amniotic bands, drugs, or irradiation. Acquired amputations are generally associated with trauma or the result of a disease or disorder.

The child with an absent limb should be fitted with a prosthesis as soon as feasible, to foster a positive body image, independence, and self-confidence and to ensure that the child's motor skills develop as normally as possible. The prosthetic device should be reevaluated as the child progresses physically and developmentally. Periodic stump reconstructions may be necessary in children with traumatic amputations, because as children grow, so do their bones, and the skin tends to adhere to the bone. Bone may need to be cut and soft tissue added to keep the stump rounded. Joint fusions or stump lengthenings may also be needed to allow for the effective use of a prosthesis.

NURSING MANAGEMENT

Nursing care focuses on providing emotional support regarding altered body image, managing pain, maintaining skin integrity, and encouraging maximal independent functioning.

Recovering from the loss of a limb is one of the most difficult challenges facing a child. Emphasize what the child can do rather than what he or she cannot do. Good listening skills are important.

The child who has had surgery or a traumatic injury experiences pain. Many of the techniques discussed in Chapter 18∞ are useful interventions. After surgery, an epidural may be the treatment of choice. Oral analgesics are used during the period of adaptation to a prosthesis if tenderness is present. Children can experience "phantom" limb pain in the lost extremity, although this phenomenon is less common in children than adults (Ray, 2000).

The child usually begins wearing the prosthetic device for 1 to 2 hours at a time. Check the skin for any redness or breakdown. If such conditions develop, leave the prosthesis off and allow the skin to clear before reapplying. Have the prosthesis adjusted if necessary, and increase wearing time as tolerated by the child.

Children with amputated limbs quickly learn how to accommodate to the prosthetic device. Make use of physical therapy programs that are specifically designed to help the child perform activities of daily living.

Answer any questions the family has about how to care for the prosthetic device and how to perform skin checks. Encourage parents to allow the child to participate in peer activities that are physically and emotionally challenging. Sporting activities that enable the child to participate using modified equipment are a good way to build self-confidence and motivation. For example, ski centers may offer programs that teach children with physical disabilities how to ski, and Special Olympics is a motivating option for some children. Assess the need for counseling and offer referrals as appropriate.

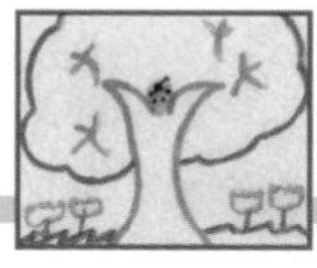

CHAPTER HIGHLIGHTS

- Children may develop musculoskeletal conditions as a result of congenital conditions, developmental variations, or trauma.
- Talipes equinovarus (clubfoot) is a common unilateral or bilateral variation in newborns that is treated by casting, traction, and/or surgery.
- Genu varum and genu valgum are normal variations at certain times in development that may need treatment if they persist.
- The nurse may identify developmental dysplasia of the hip (DDH) during newborn assessments and must refer the child for care to a specialist.
- Mild DDH may be treated by a harness, but more severe cases may require surgery for the child to walk normally.
- Legg-Calvé-Perthes is a reversible disease most commonly seen in school-age boys, and causes necrosis of the femoral head.
- Slipped capital femoral epiphysis is treated by casting, traction, or more commonly surgery with pinning, to stabilize the epiphysis.
- Scoliosis is a lateral curvature of the spine, and nurses commonly screen adolescents to identify the disorder.
- Scoliosis may require exercises, bracing, or surgery with instrumentation and spinal fusion.

- Osteoporosis can occur in premature infants, children with conditions that lead to immobility and decreased weight bearing, and in youth with inadequate calcium or vitamin D intake.
- Osteomyelitis most commonly follows another infection and requires prompt treatment to prevent sepsis and serious injury to the bone.
- The child with osteogenesis imperfecta (brittle bone disease) requires careful handling by the nurse and parents to prevent fractures while fostering developmental progression.
- Muscular dystrophies are inherited diseases characterized by muscle wasting and degeneration.
- Children can experience a variety of fractures due to sports, car crashes, and other injuries.
- Many sports injuries experienced by youth can be avoided by proper equipment and training.
- Casts, braces, and traction are common interventions for musculoskeletal disorders; nursing interventions minimize development of problems related to these treatments.

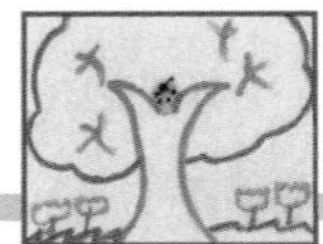

CRITICAL THINKING IN ACTION

INTRODUCTION

Recall the opening scenario. Douglass, 12 years old, has a fractured fibula from a fall while jumping on a trampoline. He talks openly in the office about how much fun he has at his friend's house after school and shares that he hopes his mother will still let him go there. He is also nervous about returning to his busy school with a cast and crutches.

DESCRIPTION

Douglass has normal vital signs and neurovascular checks of the lower extremities. He ambulates well with crutches but appears slow and careful. Douglass admits that he has been pretty "crazy" at his friend's house and takes chances on the trampoline that he should not take. He is worried that his friends at school will make fun of him now that he has a cast and crutches.

DISCUSSION

1. Douglass's fracture did not disrupt the growth plate. What is the type of his fracture according to the Salter-Harris classification? If his growth plate had been disturbed what are some possible long-term outcomes?
2. What is Douglass's developmental stage according to Erikson? Can that explain his risk-taking behaviors at his friend's house?
3. Douglass's mother is worried about whether she should allow her son to continue going to his friend's house. What questions can you help her to ask the friend's parents about supervision, activities allowed, and plans for emergencies?
4. What are some of the microsystems you can identify in Douglass's life? How are these supportive or offering challenges to him?
5. List two nursing diagnoses dealing with the physical systems and two focusing on psychosocial systems for Douglass.
6. What nursing interventions can you establish for each nursing diagnosis?

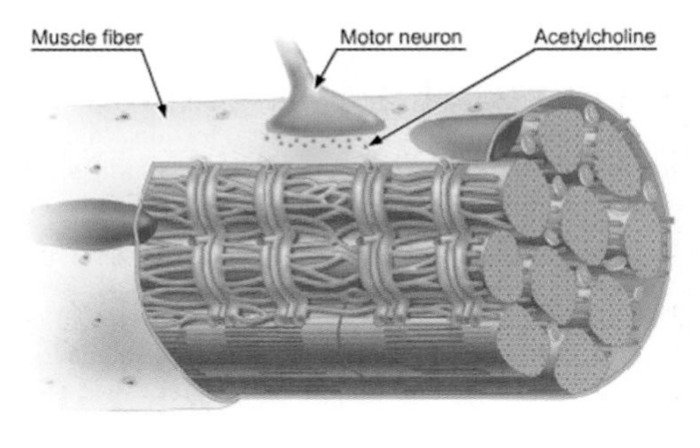

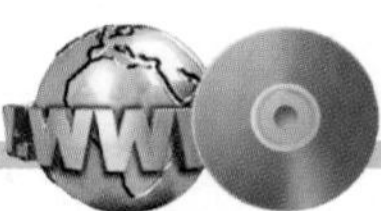

EXPLORE MediaLink

- NCLEX review, case studies, and other interactive resources for this chapter can be found on the Companion Website at **www.prenhall.com/ball**. Click on Chapter 35 to select the activities for this chapter.
- For animations, more NCLEX review questions, and an audio glossary, access the accompanying CD-ROM in this book.

http://www.prenhall.com/ball

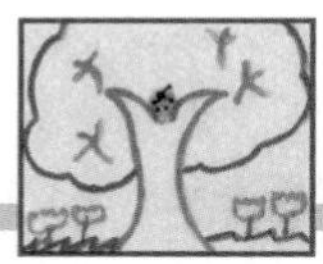

REFERENCES

Abad-Sinden, A., Verbrugge, K. C., & Buck, M. L. (2001). Assessment, prevention and management of metabolic bone disease in very low birthweight infants: The role of the neonatal nutritionist. *Nutrition in Clinical Practice, 16*, 13–19.

Acosta, K., Vade, A., Lomasney, L. M., Demos, T. C., & Bielski, R. (2001). Radiologic case study. *Orthopedics, 24*, 737–745.

American Academy of Pediatrics, Committee on Quality Improvement and Subcommittee on Developmental Dysplasia of the Hip. (2000). *Pediatrics, 105*, 896–905.

Astrom, E., & Soderhall, S. (2002). Beneficial effect of long term intravenous bisphosphonage treatment of osteogenesis imperfecta. *Archives of Disease in Childhood, 86*, 356–361.

Biggar, W. D., Gingras, M., Feblings, D. L., Harris, V. A., & Steele, C. A. (2001). Deflazacort treatment of Duchenne muscular dystrophy. *Journal of Pediatrics, 138*, 45–50.

Blakeslee, T. J. (1997). Congenital talipes equinovarus (clubfoot). *Clinics in Pediatric Medicine and Surgery 14*, 9–55.

Bowman, B. A., & Russell, R. M. (2001). *Present knowledge of nutrition* (8th ed.). Washington, DC: International Life Sciences Institute.

Carek, P. J., Dickerson, L. M., & Sack, J. L. (2001). Diagnosis and management of osteomyelitis. *American Family Physician, 63*, 2413–2420.

Caulton, J. M., Ward, K. A., Alsop, C. W., Dunn, G., Adams, J. E., & Mughal, M. Z. (2004). A randomized controlled trial of standing programme on bone mineral density in non-ambulant children with cerebral palsy. *Archives of Disease in Childhood, 89*, 131–135.

Chan, Y. Y., & Bishop, N. J. (2002). Clinical management of childhood osteoporosis. *International Journal of Clinical Practice, 56*, 280–286.

Davids, J. R. (1998). Limping. In L. T. Staheli (Ed.), *Pediatric orthopedic secrets* (pp. 195–199). Philadelphia: Hanley & Belfus.

Driscoll, D. A. (2001, October). Duchenne and Becker muscular dystrophies. *Contemporary OB/GYN*, 97–102.

Durst, E. S. (2000). The A, B, C's of bone building in adolescence. *Journal of the American Academy of Nurse Practitioners, 12*, 135–140.

Eiff, M. P., & Hatch, R.L. (2003). Boning up on common pediatric fractures. *Pediatrics, 20*(11), 30–59.

Eldridge, J., Dilley, A., Austin, H., EL-Jamil, M., Wolstein, L., Doris, J., Hooper, C., Meehan, P. L., & Evatt, B. (2001). The role of protein C, protein S, and resistance to activated protein C in Legg-Perthes disease. *Pediatrics, 107*, 1329–1334.

Fernandez, J., Carrol, C. L., & Baker, C.J. (2000). Discitis and vertebral osteomyelitis in children: An 18-year review. *Pediatrics, 105*, 1299–1304.

Gilmore, A., & Thompson, G.H. (2003). Common childhood foot deformities. *Consultant for Pediatricians, 2*, 63–71.

Givner, L. B., & Kaplan, S. L. (2003). *Bone and joint infections: Pediatrics*. Presented at the 40th annual meeting of the Infectious Diseases Society of America in October 2002. As reported in *Infectious Diseases in Children* (2003, February), 82.

Gonzalez, E., Pavia, C., Ros, J., Villaronga, M., Valls, C., & Exxcola, J. (2001). Efficacy of low dose schedule pamidronate infusion in children with osteogenesis imperfecta. *Journal of Pediatric Endocrinology and Metabolism, 14*, 529–533.

Haga, N. (2004). Management of disabilities associated with achondroplasia. *Journal of Orthopaedic Science, 9*, 103–107.

Harper, R. S. (2002, December). Back in the game: Preventing and treating athletic injuries in adolescents. *Advance for Nurse Practitioners*, 55–66.

Harvey, C. (2001). Compartment syndrome: When it is least expected. *Orthopaedic Nursing, 20*(3), 15–26.

Holcomb, S. S. (2000). Marfan syndrome: A review. *Dimensions of Critical Care Nursing, 19*(4), 22–24.

Horwitz, E. M., Prockop, D. J., Gordon, P. L., Koo, W. W., Fitzpatrick, L. A., Neel, M. D., McCarville, M. E., Orchard, P. J., Pyeritz, R. E., & Brenner, M. K. (2001). Clinical responses to bone marrow transplantation in children with severe osteogenesis imperfecta. *Blood, 97*, 1227–1231.

Kunkler, C. E. (1999). Neurovascular assessment. *Orthopaedic Nursing, 18*(3), 63–71.

Litmanovitz, I., Dolfin, T., Friedland, O., Arnon, S., Regev, R., Shainkin-Kestenbaum, R., Lis, M., & Eliakim, A. (2003). Early physical activity intervention prevents decrease of bone strength in very low birth weight infants. *Pediatrics, 112*, 15–19.

March of Dimes. (2004). *Achondroplasia*. www.marchofdimes.com/professionals/681_1204.asp. 3, accessed 6/1/2004.

McLean, K. R. (2004). Osteogenesis imperfecta. *Neonatal Network, 23*(2), 7–14.

Metules, T. (2002). Duchenne muscular dystrophy. *RN, 65*(10), 39–48.

Morcuende, J. A., Dolan, L. A., Dietz, F. R., & Ponseti, I. V. (2004). Radical reduction in the rate of extensive corrective surgery for clubfoot using the Ponseti method. *Pediatrics, 113*, 376–380.

Moyer-Mileur, L. J., Brunstetter, V., McNaught, T. P., Gill, G., & Chan, G. M. (2000). Daily physical activity program increases bone mineralization and growth in preterm very low birth weight infants. *Pediatrics, 106*, 1088–1092.

Papazian, O., & Alfonso, I. (2002). Adolescents with muscular dystrophies. *Adolescent Medicine, 13*, 511–532.

Patel, H. (2001). Preventive health care, 2001 update: Screening and management of developmental dysplasia of the hip in newborns. *Canadian Medical Association Journal, 164*, 1669–1681.

Paterson, C. R., Monk, E. A., & McAllion, S. J. (2001). How common is hearing impairment in osteogenesis imperfecta? *Journal of Laryngology and Otolaryngology, 115*, 280–282.

Ray, R. L. (2000). Complications of lower extremity amputations. *Topics in Emergency Medicine, 22*(3), 35–43.

Roy, D. R. (1999). Current concept in Legg-Calvé-Perthes disease. *Pediatric Annals, 28*, 748–754.

Ryan, D. J. (2001). Intoeing: A developmental norm. *Orthpaedic Nursing, 20*(2), 13–18.

Sapountzi-Krepia, D. S., Valavanis, J., Panteleakis, G. P., Zangana, D. T., Vlachojiannis, P. C., & Sapkas, G.S. (2001). Perceptions of body image, happiness and satisfaction in adolescents wearing a Boston brace for scoliosis treatment. *Issues and Innovations in Nursing Practice, 35*, 683–690.

Scudder, L. (2004). How should I evaluate fractures in children? *Medscape Nurses*. www.medscape.com/viewarticle/465797_print, accessed 1/13/2004.

Sheir-Neiss, G. I., Kruse, R. W., Rahman, T., Jacobsen, L. P., & Pelli, J. A. (2003). Association of backpack use and back pain in adolescents. *Spine, 28*, 922–930.

Slote, R. J. (2002). Psychological aspects of caring for the adolescent undergoing spinal fusion for scoliosis. *Orthopedic Nursing, 21*, 19–32.

Sobus, K. M. L., Horan, S. M., & Warren, R. H. (2000). Respiratory management of neuromuscular diseases in children. *Physical Medicine and Rehabilitation, 14*, 285–299.

Stracciolini, A. & Metzl, J. D. (2000). Pediatric sports emergencies. Physical Medicine and Rehabilitation Clinics of North America 11, 961–979.

Takeda, S., & Miyagoe-Suzuki, Y. (2001). Gene therapy for muscular dystrophies: Current status and future prospects. *Biodrugs, 15*, 635–644.

Thompson, G. H. (2004a). The hip. In R. E. Behrman, R. M. Kliegman, & H. B. Jenson, *Nelson textbook of pediatrics* (17th ed., pp. 2273–2280). Saunders: Philadelphia.

Thompson, G. H. (2004b). The spine. In R. E. Behrman, R. M. Kliegman, & H. B. Jenson, *Nelson textbook of pediatrics* (17th ed., p. 2280–2287). Saunders: Philadelphia.

Thompson, G. H. (2004c). Torsional and angular deformities. In R. E. Behrman, R. M. Kliegman, & H. B. Jenson, *Nelson textbook of pediatrics* (17th ed., pp. 2261–2269). Saunders: Philadelphia.

Van Gent, C., Dols, J. J., de Rover, C. J., Hira Sing, R. A., & de Bet, H. C. (2003). The weight of schoolbags and the occurrence of neck, shoulder, and back pain in young adolescents. *Spine, 28*, 916–921.

Witt, C. (2003). Detecting developmental dysplasia of the hip. *Advances in Neonatal Care, 3*, 65–75.

Wyshak, G. (2000). Teenaged girls, carbonated beverage consumption, and bone fractures. *Archives of Pediatrics and Adolescent Medicine, 154*, 610–613.

Yetman, A. T., Huang, P., Bornemeier, R. A., & McCrindle, B. W. (2003). Comparison of outcome of the marfan syndrome in patients diagnosed at age ≤ 6 years versus those diagnosed at 6 years of age. *American Journal of Cardiology, 91*, 102–103.

Zeitlin, L., Rauch, F., Plotkin, H., & Glorieux, F. H. (2003). Height and weight development during four years of therapy with cyclical intravenous pamidronate in children and adolescents with osteogenesis imperfecta types I, III, and IV. *Pediatrics, 111*, 1030–1036.

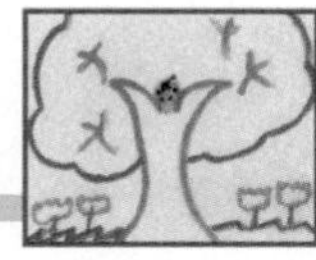

ADDITIONAL REFERENCES

Apkon, S. D. (2002). Osteoporosis in children who have disabilities. *Physical Medicine and Rehabilitation Clinics of North America, 13*, 839–855.

Chin, K. R., Price, J. S., & Zimbler, S. (2001). A guide to early detection of scoliosis. *Contemporary Pediatrics, 18*, 77–98.

Cushing, V., & Slocumb, E. (2004). Identification of Marfan syndrome in primary care. *Advance for Nurse Practitioners, 12*(3), 87–90.

DiFazio, R. (2003). Creating a halo traction wheelchair resource manual: Using the EBP approach. *Journal of Pediatric Nursing, 18*, 148–151.

Engelbert, R. H., Gulmans, V. A., Uiterwaal, C. S., & Helders. P. J. (2001). Osteogenesis imperfecta in childhood: Perceived competence in relation to impairment and disability. *Archives of Physical Medicine and Rehabilitation, 82*, 943–948.

Fernbach, S. A. (1998). Common orthopedic problems of the newborn. *Nursing Clinics of North America, 33*, 583–596.

Frye, K. E., & Luterman, A. (1999). Burns and fractures. *Orthopaedic Nursing, 18*(1), 30–35.

Harper, R. S. (2002, December). Back in the game: Preventing and treating athletic injuries in adolescents. *Advance for Nurse Practitioners*, 55–66.

Ilardi, D. (2001). Scoliosis. *School Nurse News, 18*(3), 2.

Iyer, S. R. (2002). Backpacks and musculoskeletal pain: Do children with idiopathic scoliosis face a greater risk? *Journal of School Health, 72*, 270–271.

Kautz, S. M., & Skaggs, D. L. (1998). Getting an angle on spinal deformities. *Contemporary Pediatrics, 15*, 111–128.

Killian, J. T., Mayberry, S., & Wilkinson, L. (1999). Current concepts in adolescent idiopathic scoliosis. *Pediatric Annals, 28*, 755–761.

LaMontagne, L. L., Hepworth, J. T., Cohen, F., & Salisbury, M. H. (2003). Cognitive-behavioral intervention effects on adolescents' anxiety and pain following spinal fusion surgery. *Nursing Research, 52*, 183–190.

Muscari, M. E. (1998). Preventing sports injuries. *American Journal of Nursing, 98*, 58–60.

O'Connor, D. L. (1998). Preventing sports injuries in kids. *Patient Care Nurse Practitioner, 1*(4), 24–36.

Parsons, E. P., Clarke, A. J., Hood, K., Lycett, E., & Bailey, D. M. (2002). Newborn screening for Duchenne muscular dystrophy: A psychosocial study. *Archives of Disease in Childhood, 86*, F91–F95.

Taft, E. (2003). Evaluation and management of scoliosis. *Journal of Pediatric Health Care, 17*, 42–44.

Van Karnebeek, C. D. M., Naeff, M. S. J., Mulder, B. J. M., Hennekam, R. C. M., & Offringa, M. (2001). Natural history of cardiovascular manifestations in Marfan syndrome. *Archives of Diseases in Children, 84*, 129–137.

Chapter

36

Alterations in Skin Integrity

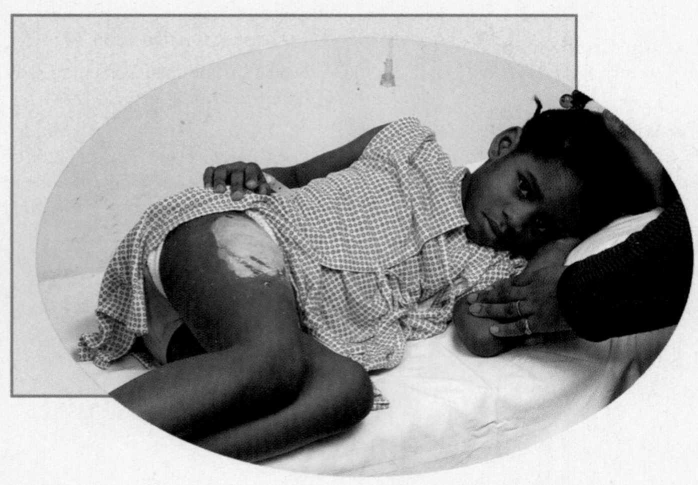

Sherray Davidson, 6 years old, was admitted to the hospital with a deep partial thickness burn after dropping a bowl of soup on her leg. By her second day of hospitalization, it is clear that Sherray's burn is not full thickness and that no skin grafting is needed. The amount of scarring she will have cannot be anticipated at this time.

Sherray's treatment includes a bath with wound debridement and dressing changes twice a day. Although pain medication is provided, the debridement and dressing changes cause her much anxiety and pain. Sherray needs a high-protein, high-calorie diet to promote wound healing. She has a hard time extending her leg and walking, because movement stretches the burned skin, so she needs assistance to get out of bed and participate in child life activities.

Sherray's mother is rooming in, and remains at her side during the dressing changes. Her greatest concern now is to help Sherray deal with the burn injury and to reduce the chance of infection. Over the next couple of days, Sherray's mother will take more responsibility for the dressing changes in anticipation of continuing her daughter's care at home.

"I want to stay in the playroom longer. Cleaning the cream off my leg really hurts. Why do you have to change it now? I'll eat all my dinner and work harder to straighten my leg and walk if you don't change the bandage."

—Sherray, 6 years old

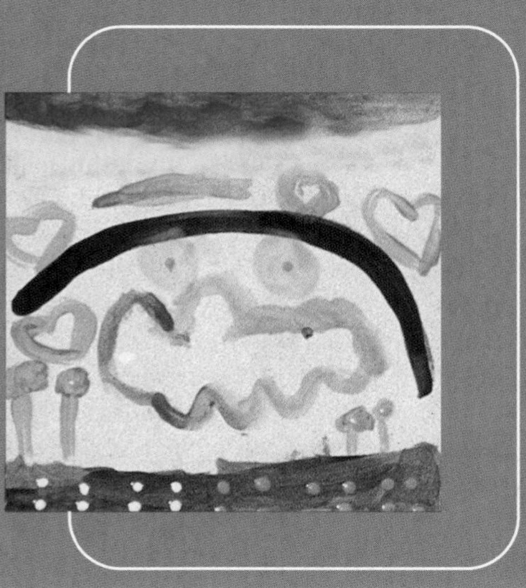

Learning Outcomes

After completing this chapter, you will be able to:

- Identify the characteristics of different skin lesions by their cause, including those caused by irritants, drug reactions, mites, infection, and injury.
- Identify the skin conditions that have a hereditary cause or hereditary predisposition.
- Describe nursing education for adolescents with acne to promote self-care.
- Describe the nursing care for the child with various alterations in skin integrity, including dermatitis, infectious disorders, infestations, and injuries to the skin.
- Identify important teaching points for families to help prevent and manage integumentary alterations.

Key Terms

allograft/1493
atopy/1460
autografting/1493
cellulitis/1475
circumferential/1490
collagen/1459
comedone/1470
debridement/1493
dermatophytoses/1478
epithelialization/1458
eschar/1490
escharotomy/1492
hemangioma/1484
intertriginous areas/1468
involution/1484
keloid/1460
kerion/1479
lichenification/1458
melanin/1501
paronychia/1477
phototoxic/1472
probiotic/1462
rebound effect/1462
stratum corneum/1456
telangiectasia/1458
xerosis/1460

MediaLink http://www.prenhall.com/ball

Resources for this chapter can be found on the CD-ROM accompanying this textbook and on the Companion Website at www.prenhall.com/ball. Click on Chapter 36 to select the activities for this chapter.

CD-ROM

Animations/Videos

- *Integumentary Repair*
- *Layers of the Skin*

Nursing in Action: Topical Medication: Burn Wound Care

NCLEX Review

Audio Glossary

COMPANION WEBSITE

A & P Review

Clinical Manifestations Review

Medication Match-Up

NCLEX Review

Care Plan: Atopic Dermatitis

MediaLink Applications

- *Adolescents and Acne Management*
- *Develop an Educational Program: Scald Burn Reduction in Children*
- *Develop a Community Education Program: Dog Bite Reduction*

What is the role of the nurse in providing care to the child with a burn injury? What nursing support may help the child deal with painful dressing changes and a disfiguring injury? What other healthcare team members are important in ensuring an optimal recovery for Sherray? What teaching must be provided to her mother to enable her to provide care at home? The information in this chapter will prepare you to answer these questions and to provide care to children such as Sherray with burn injuries or other alterations in skin integrity.

Skin disorders are seen frequently by nurses who work in outpatient clinics, schools, emergency departments, and pediatric units of hospitals. Many of these disorders are not unique to children, but children are at greater risk for some skin conditions for reasons that are discussed in this chapter.

ANATOMY AND PHYSIOLOGY OF PEDIATRIC DIFFERENCES

Function of the Skin

The skin is the largest organ in the body. It performs several essential functions.

- *Protection*—The outer layer of the skin when intact provides a barrier against microorganisms, ultraviolet radiation, and loss of body fluids. It also protects the underlying tissues from trauma.
- *Temperature regulation*—When the central nervous system detects that the body is too warm, blood vessels and sweat glands are dilated to release body heat. When the central nervous system detects that the body is too cool, blood vessels and sweat glands are constricted to conserve heat.

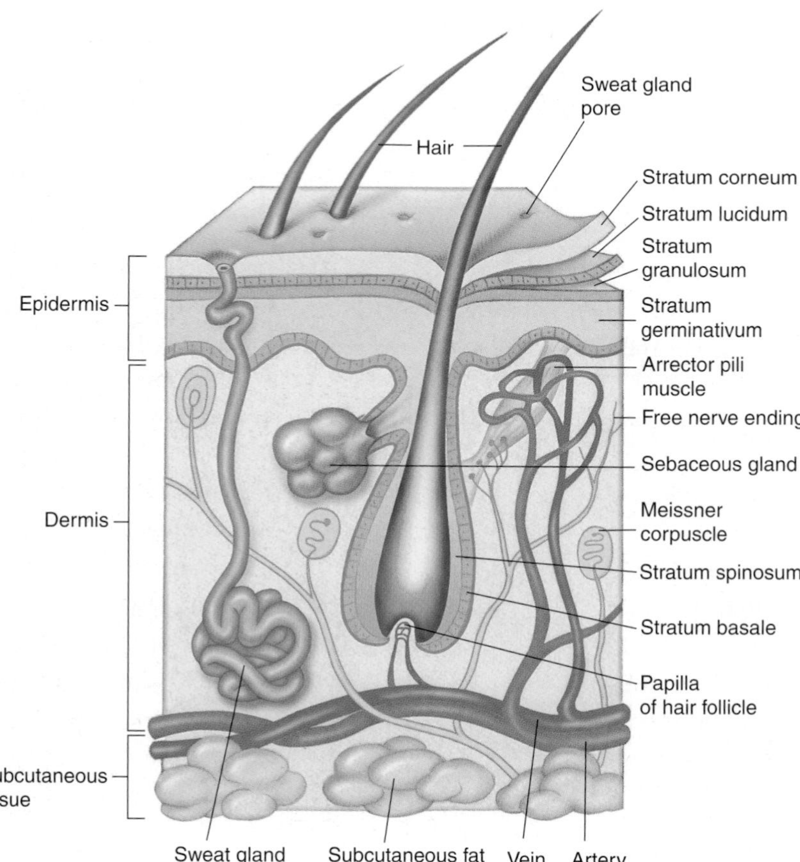

MediaLink Layers of the Skin

FIGURE 36–1 ■ Layers of the skin with accessory structures.

- *Vitamin D synthesis*—The skin supplements the body's intake of vitamin D by synthesizing this vitamin when exposed to small amounts of ultraviolet light.
- *Excretion*—Excretion is performed by the sweat glands, which secrete a solution of water, electrolytes, and urea, thus helping to rid the body of toxins.
- *Sensation*—The skin is a sensory organ with nerves that enable the person to perceive touch, pressure, pain, heat, and cold.

The skin consists of three distinct layers: the epidermis, dermis, and subcutaneous fatty layer that separates the skin from the underlying tissue (Figure 36–1 ■).

The epidermis is the superficial and most important layer of skin. It is typically very thin at 0.12 mm, but it can thicken with pressure or friction. The epidermis grows continuously by shedding the cells of the **stratum corneum,** the tough outer layer covering the body composed of flat keratinized, nonnucleated cells. Skin cells (keratinocytes) are produced by the deeper stratum germinativum and gradually move up through the other layers to replace the skin cells in the epidermis about every 30 days (Huether, 2002). Within the epidermis are melanocytes, Langerhans cells, and Merkel cells. Melanocytes synthesize and secrete melanin with exposure to sunlight that helps provide a shield again ultraviolet radiation. Langerhans cells help initiate the immune response to antigens. Merkel cells are mechanical receptors of touch stimulated by pressure on the epidermis.

The dermis is a connective tissue layer with nerves, muscles, connective tissue, hair follicles, sebaceous and sweat glands, lymph channels, and blood vessels. It is generally 1 to 4 mm in thickness. The fibrous connective tissues of the dermis provide the elasticity to the skin permitting it to stretch and contract with body movement. Cells in the dermis include fibroblasts, mast cells, and macrophages. The fibroblasts contribute to the development of the connective tissues. The mast cells release histamine and contribute to hypersensitivity reactions by the skin. The macrophages play a role in immune responses.

The subcutaneous layer of the skin contains the hair, sebaceous glands, as well as the eccrine and apocrine sweat glands. The blood supply and the nerves of the autonomic nervous system supporting the dermis also are found in the subcutaneous layer. A cushioning layer of fat is also present that helps insulate the body from cold temperatures.

Hair follicles arise from the bulb located deep in the dermis and extend from the dermis at an angle. Hair growth begins in the bulb and cells mature and differentiate as hair progresses toward the skin surface within the follicle.

Sebaceous glands form in connection with hair follicles, and they open on the skin surface through a canal. They vary in size and appear all over the body except on the hands and soles of the feet. Sebum, a lipid substance produced and secreted into the hair follicle or directly onto the skin, provides lubrication to the skin and hair. By helping to keep the skin supple, sebum has a role in reducing water loss. Sebaceous gland growth is stimulated by testosterone, and these glands become enlarged during puberty.

Eccrine sweat glands, located in the dermis, open onto the skin surface. The skin surfaces with the greatest number include the palms of the hands, soles of the feet, and forehead. They secrete an odorless, watery fluid, primarily in response to emotional stress. They also respond to changes in body temperature. As body temperature increases, the glands increase production of sweat. The result is decreased heat as the sweat evaporates. Because the eccrine sweat glands usually are not fully functional until middle childhood, infants and young children are unable to regulate temperature as effectively as older children and adults.

Apocrine sweat glands, located mainly in the axillary and genital areas, do not function until puberty. Decomposition of the fluid secreted by these glands leads to body odor. Their biologic function, however, is unknown.

Nails are protective keratinized plates that appear at the ends of fingers and toes. They grow at a rate of 1 mm or less a day.

Newborn Skin Characteristics

At birth the skin is thin, with little underlying subcutaneous fat. Because of this the newborn loses heat more rapidly, has greater difficulty regulating body temperature, and becomes more easily chilled than an older child or an adult. The thinner skin also leads to increased absorption of harmful chemical substances. The newborn's skin contains more water than an adult's skin and has loosely attached cells. As the infant grows, the skin toughens and becomes less hydrated, making it less susceptible to bacteria (Figure 36–2 ■).

AS THEY GROW

Integumentary System Changes

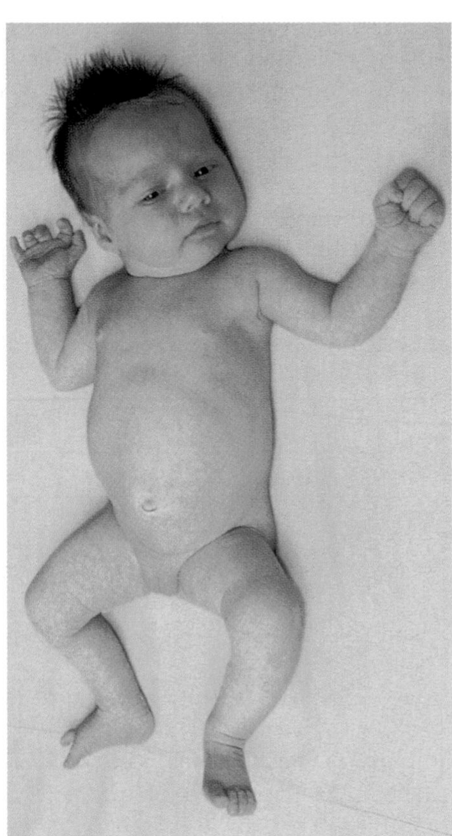

Newborns
Skin is very thin
Epidermis is loosely bound to the dermis, friction can cause separation of the layers with blistering
Eccrine sweat glands function, produce sweat in response to heat and emotional stimuli
Apocrine sweat glands are small and nonfunctional
Less melanin is present at birth so skin is lighter colored

Adolescents
Skin thickens
Epidermis and dermis are tightly bound, increasing resistance to infection and irritation
Eccrine sweat glands achieve full function, after puberty males sweat more than females
Apocrine sweat glands mature during puberty
Melanin is at adult levels, determining skin color and serving as a shield against ultraviolet radiation

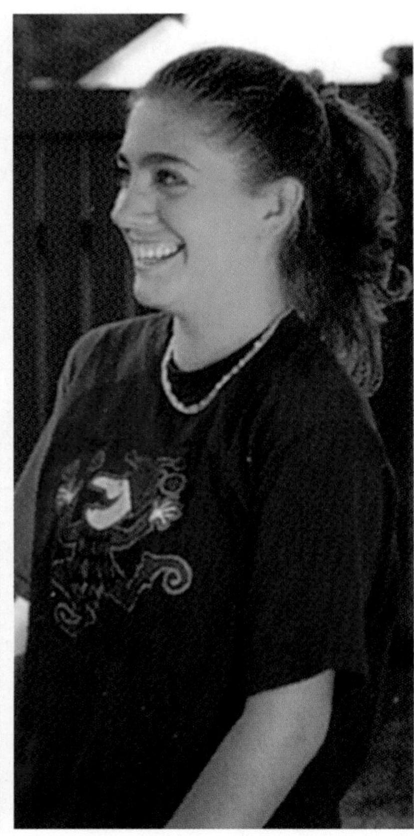

FIGURE 36–2 ■ The structures of the skin mature during childhood, reaching adult function at puberty.

PRACTICE ALERT

Newborn bathing should be performed with warm water and no soap during the first week of life to reduce dryness and irritation. When cleansing agents are needed, choose one with a neutral pH, but make sure the skin is well rinsed. Emollients help prevent desquamation of the skin.

Avoid or minimize the use of adhesive tape with newborns and preterm infants as tape removal causes injury to the skin. Solvents are toxic and are absorbed through the newborn's skin.

At birth, the newborn may have soft, downy hair, called lanugo, on the shoulders and back. Lanugo is usually shed by 2 to 3 weeks of age. The amount of hair on the head varies. Scalp hair usually is shed within a few months and replaced, sometimes with hair of a different color. The accessory structures of the skin (sebaceous glands, eccrine glands, and apocrine glands) are present at birth. Like other body structures, however, they are still immature.

SKIN LESIONS

Skin lesions vary in size, shape, color, and texture characteristics. The two major types of skin lesions are primary lesions and secondary lesions. Primary lesions arise from previously healthy skin and include macules, patches, papules, nodules, tumors, vesicles, pustules, bullae, and wheals (see Figure 8–12∞). Secondary lesions result from changes in primary lesions. They include crusts, scales, **lichenification** (thickening of the skin), scars, keloids, excoriation, fissures, erosion, and ulcers (Table 36–1). It is important for the nurse to be able to identify and describe the primary and secondary skin lesions and understand their underlying cause and treatment. Some families may use complementary therapies to treat skin lesions. See Complementary Therapy: Skin Lesions.

Wound Healing

Wound healing is a process that occurs in three overlapping phases: inflammation, reconstruction, and maturation (Figure 36–3 ■) (Rote, 2002; Valencia, Falabella, & Schachner, 2001).

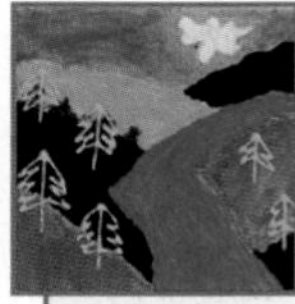

COMPLEMENTARY THERAPY

Skin Lesions

CONDITION	COMPLEMENTARY THERAPY	USE
Poison ivy	Aloe, calendula, oatmeal (topical)	Relief from itching
Atopic dermatitis	Evening primrose oil (oral)	Decreases excoriations and lichenification Decreases need for antihistamines for itching
Accelerated wound healing, burns, abrasions	Aloe vera gel (topical)	Antimicrobial effects, bacteriostatic, bacteriocidal
Skin inflammation	Chamomile (topical)	Wound drying, antimicrobial properties
Acne	5% tea tree oil (topical)	Antibiotic, decreases open and closed comedomes

Adapted from Gardner, P., Coles, D., & Kemper, K. J. (2001). The skinny on herbal remedies for dermatologic disorders. Contemporary Pediatrics, *18(7), 103–114.*

Inflammation, the initial response at the injury site, lasts approximately 3 to 5 days. This phase prepares the injury site for the repair process. Coagulation occurs as platelets, red blood cells, and fibrin gather to form a clot. This seals the wound, preventing bacterial invasion and joining the wound edges. Vasodilation, which occurs shortly after injury, allows leukocytes and neutrophils to travel to the injury site, where they ingest bacteria and debris.

Reconstruction or **epithelialization** (the process by which epithelial cells grow into the wound from surrounding healthy tissue), the second phase, may last from 4 days to 2 weeks, depending on the extent of the injury. Capillary budding to reestablish the blood flow and natural debridement (enzyme action to clean the

TABLE 36–1 Common Secondary Skin Lesions and Associated Conditions

LESION NAME	DESCRIPTION	EXAMPLE
Crust	Dried residue of serum, pus, or blood	Impetigo
Scale	Thin flake of exfoliated epidermis	Dandruff, psoriasis
Lichenification	Thickening of skin with increased visibility of normal skin furrows	Eczema (atopic dermatitis)
Scar	Replacement of destroyed tissue with fibrous tissue	Healed surgical incision
Keloid	Overdevelopment or hypertrophy of scar that extends beyond wound edges and above skin line due to excess collagen	Healed skin area following traumatic injury
Excoriation	Abrasion or scratch mark	Scratched insect bite
Fissure	Linear crack in skin	Tinea pedis (athlete's foot)
Erosion	Loss of superficial epidermis; moist but does not bleed	Ruptured chickenpox vesicle
Ulcer	Deeper loss of skin surface; bleeding or scarring may ensue	Chancre
Comedone	A plug of sebaceous and keratin material in a hair follicle opening	Acne
Burrow	A narrow, raised irregular channel caused by a parasite	Scabies
Telangiectasia	Dilated, superficial blood vessels	Birthmark

PATHOPHYSIOLOGY ILLUSTRATED

Phases of Wound Healing

Inflammation (3–5 days)

Clot formation that seals the wound with fibrin and trapped cells and platelets
Increased blood flow to area carrying exudate with phagocytes and lymphocytes to the site
Increased capillary permeability, causing swelling
Dilute toxic products released by dying cells
Phagocytosis

Inflammation

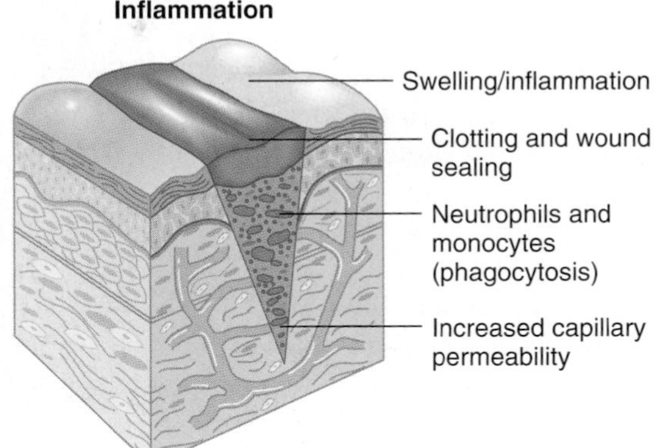

FIGURE 36–3 ■ Wound healing occurs in three overlapping phases.

Data from Rote, N. S. (2002). Inflammation. In K. L. McCance & S. E. Huether (Eds.), Pathophysiology: The basis for disease in adults and children *(4th ed., pp. 197–226). St. Louis: Mosby.*

Reconstruction (4 days to 2 weeks)

Debridement or cleanup of the site, fibrinolytic enzymes dissolve the fibrin clots
Regeneration of destroyed cells if injury is minor
Collagen production for scar formation occurs when tissue is too injured to regenerate
Epithelialization with granulation tissue that includes capillary budding and becomes scar tissue
Wound contraction, inward movement of the wound edge

Reconstruction

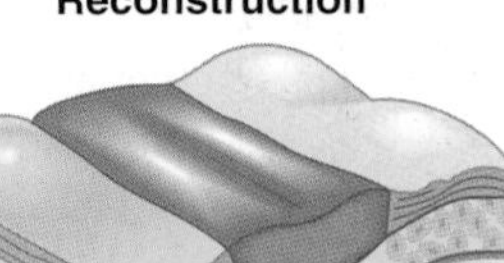

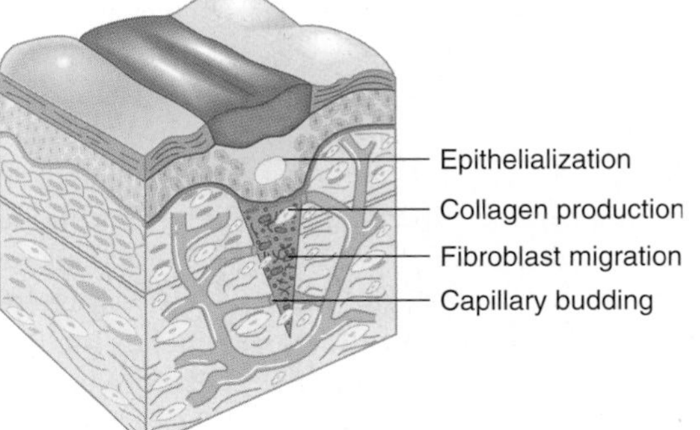

Maturation (Months to 2 Years)

Remodeling of the site as scar tissue forms
Scar formation and strengthening
Capillary disappearance from scar tissue

Maturation

Scar formation and strengthening
Granulation tissue
Capillary disappearance

MediaLink Integumentary Repair Animation

lesion and dissolve the clot or scab) occur. The wound contracts as the wound edges grow toward each other. Fibroblasts migrate to the site and multiply, producing **collagen** (a protein that is the material of tissue repair) and granulation tissue to fill the wound to skin level. The granulation tissue is red and shiny. Leukocytes gradually disappear from the site. A fine layer of epithelial cells forms over the site. The wound is fragile at this stage of healing.

Maturation or remodeling, the third phase, involves continued collagen production for scar production. Fibroblasts disappear and their movement further contracts the healing site, bringing the edges closer together. A mature scar forms and gradually strengthens and devascularizes, although it will never be as strong as normal skin. Maturation can take months to years, depending on the extent of the injury.

Wounds that heal well with minimal tissue loss are those that heal by *primary intention*. An example is the wound healing after an incision in which there is little tissue loss, wound edges are joined together, and little epithelialization and contraction are needed. Wounds that are open and require a lot of tissue regeneration heal by *secondary intention*. See Box 36–1.

Formation of a **keloid,** a scar that extends beyond the original boundaries of the wound, is caused by an imbalance between collagen synthesis and collagen lysis or breakdown. The cause is unknown, but a familial tendency for keloid scarring is reported. The incidence is greater in Blacks than in Whites (Rote, 2002).

DERMATITIS

Many skin inflammations occur in early childhood. Most are easily treated and have no long-term consequences. Dermatitis is a broad term describing changes that occur in the skin in response to various stimuli. The four most common types of dermatitis that occur in infants, children, and adolescents are contact dermatitis, diaper dermatitis, seborrheic dermatitis, and eczema (atopic dermatitis). It is important for the nurse to understand that these skin disorders bring with them emotional problems for the family and child. Be sympathetic; remember that the family and child can see the skin condition and need to be reassured that the child is not infectious.

Atopic Dermatitis (Eczema)

Atopic dermatitis, also called eczema, is a chronic, superficial inflammatory skin disorder characterized by intense pruritus (Figure 36–4 ■). The condition affects infants, children, and adolescents. It is a common skin condition, believed to affect 10% to 20% of children (Paller, 2001). Up to 75% of children who develop the condition do so during the first 6 months of life, and 80% to 90% develop it by 5 years of age (Nicol, 2000). An increasing prevalence has been noted in developed countries over the last 30 to 40 years that also exhibit an increased rate of asthma, demonstrating the allergic tendency for this condition (Raimer, 2000).

Etiology and Pathophysiology

The etiology of atopic dermatitis is unknown, but an immune dysfunction of the skin that is influenced by genetic predisposition and external triggers may be involved. Children have T-cell activation and excessive production of IgE (Paller, 2001). See Chapter 26∞ for a discussion of IgE. The epidermis has a genetic inability to bind water. The disorder tends to occur in children with hereditary allergic tendencies (**atopy**). When one parent has allergies (e.g., hay fever, asthma, or contact dermatitis), the child has a 60% greater chance of having allergies. This chance increases to 80% if both parents have allergies (Cheigh, 2003). Therefore, a family history of asthma or hay fever frequently predisposes a child to eczema. Infantile eczema is more likely to be food induced when the condition is severe (Hebert, Rakes, Loach, et al., 1997). Several factors exacerbate the condition: triggers (house mites, animal dander, pollens), food allergies, irritants (soaps, detergents, chemicals, solvents, abrasive clothing), hormonal changes, and emotional stress.

BOX 36–1 Causes of Dysfunctional Wound Repair and Healing

- Predisposing condition—e.g., diabetes
- Hypoxemia—insufficient oxygen in the tissues making them susceptible to infection
- Hypovolemia—inflammation is inhibited because of low circulating blood volume
- Steroids—macrophages are prevented from migrating to the site of injury and epithelialization is suppressed
- Poor nutrition—hypoproteinemia impairs fibroblast proliferation and collagen synthesis

Data from Rote, N. S. (2002). Inflammation. In K. L. McCance & S. E. Huether (Eds.), Pathophysiology: The basis for disease in adults and children *(4th ed., pp. 197–226). St. Louis: Mosby.*

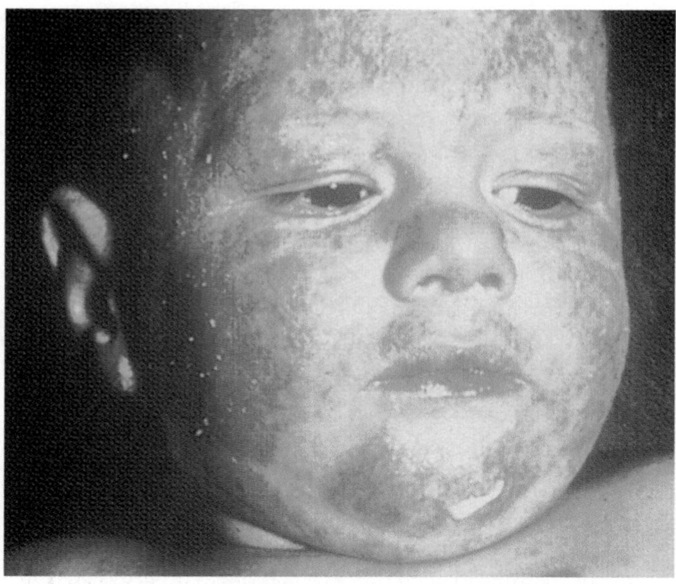

FIGURE 36–4 ■ Chronic atopic dermatitis.

Children with atopic dermatitis have **xerosis,** generally dry skin that is more likely to crack and fissure. The lipid barrier function of the skin is impaired, leading to increased water loss from the epidermis and decreased elasticity. When the skin is chronically dry, irritants have a greater chance to penetrate, and the child is more susceptible to infection.

Due to impaired skin barrier function and cutaneous immunity, children are also at greater risk for the development of skin infections by organisms such as staphylococcus, herpes simplex, and molluscum contagiosum.

Clinical Manifestations

Acute atopic dermatitis is characterized by pruritus and erythematous patches with vesicles, exudate, and crusts. Subacute cases are characterized by scaling with erythema and excoriation. There are often postinflammatory pigment changes. Symptoms of chronic atopic dermatitis are pruritus, dryness, scaling, and lichenification (thickening of the skin with increased visibility of normal skin furrows). Symptoms are often worse in dry and cold weather. Inflammation usually occurs on the face, upper arms, back, upper thighs, and back of the hands and feet. Skinfolds such as the antecubitus and popliteal areas are often affected. The itching interferes with sleep, causes irritability, and the perception of hyperactivity in affected children because the children move so much due to itching discomfort. Exacerbations of atopic dermatitis are related to factors such as allergies, dry skin, high and low ambient temperatures, perspiring, scratching, and skin irritants (detergents, wool, other rough fabrics, anxiety, and stress). Erythema and warmth may indicate a secondary bacterial skin infection. Children typically have numerous relapses.

Atopic dermatitis occurs in three forms: infantile (ages 2 months to 2 years), childhood (ages 2 years to puberty), and adolescent (puberty and onward). See the clinical manifestations table below.

COLLABORATIVE CARE

The goal of collaborative care is to identify potential triggers for atopic dermatitis, to keep the skin hydrated and lubricated, and to treat flare-ups aggressively and reduce the risk for infection.

Diagnostic Tests

Atopic dermatitis is distinguished from other forms of dermatitis by its history and clinical manifestations. See Box 36–2 for diagnostic criteria. No laboratory tests are diagnostic. Eczema is more likely to have a generalized distribution with no known exposure to an allergen. Cultures of the skin may be used when a secondary infection is suspected.

Infants under 2 years of age who have severe eczema and a poor response to therapy may have food allergies. A food elimination test may be suggested for these children to see if improvements in the skin condition occur. Cow milk, wheat, eggs, soy products, citrus, and peanuts are the foods most often withheld for 2 or more weeks to determine if any change in skin condition occurs. Foods withheld are then introduced one at a time to determine which ones are the allergens. A radioallergosorbent test (RAST) is sometimes used to exclude allergens (see Chapter 26∞). Allergens often change over time with one causing less significant reactions as new allergens begin to cause a reaction.

BOX 36–2 Diagnostic Criteria for Atopic Dermatitis (Eczema)

Itching skin condition with three additional factors from the following list:

- History of flexural dermatitis (knees, ankles, neck, or cheeks) if less than 4 years old
- History of asthma or hay fever in a child, or in a first-degree relative, if less than 4 years old
- History of dry skin in past year
- Skin rash occurring before 2 years of age
- Visible flexural dermatitis; dermatitis on cheeks, forehead, and outer limbs if less than 4 years old

Adapted from Raimer, S. S. (2000). Managing pediatric atopic dermatitis. Clinical Pediatrics, *39(1), 1–14.*

Clinical Therapy

As there is no cure, the goals of treatment are to hydrate and lubricate the skin, reduce pruritus, minimize inflammatory changes, and try to determine what triggers flare-ups. The cardinal principle of topical therapy for oozing or weeping is "wet on wet." If lesions are weeping, wet compresses (cotton cloths) soaked in aluminum acetate solution sometimes are used. Lubrication is achieved by applying occlusive topical ointment after bathing to trap moisture and prevent drying of the skin. Moisturizing ointments and creams should be applied three to four times a day or whenever the skin feels dry. Numerous types of medications are used to treat atopic dermatitis. See the medications table on page 1462.

CLINICAL MANIFESTATIONS of Atopic Dermatitis

TYPE	CLINICAL MANIFESTATIONS
Infantile (2 months to 2 years) 50% of cases resolve by age 2–3 years	Exudative, crusty, papulovesicular, and erythematous lesions on cheeks, scalp, forehead, neck, trunk, and extensor surfaces of extremities. Areas spared: diaper area because the area is damp, and the diaper protects the area from scratching; folds of neck and flexor surfaces of elbows and knees. Some patches may weep. Intensely pruritic, child wiggles to rub or scratch areas out of reach. Secondarily infected lesions. Lichenification after the child can scratch at about 2 months of age.
Childhood (2 years to puberty) Subacute and chronic 75% of cases have no recurrence after adolescence	Erythematous, dry scaly or weeping, well-circumscribed, papular. Flexor surfaces become more involved, including the wrists and ankles. Once toilet trained the buttocks become excoriated. More thickened and lichenified lesions on antecubital, popliteal, and extensor surfaces of extremities, neck, and retroauricular folds. Pruritis Dry skin Secondarily infected lesions
Adolescent (puberty and onward) May recur often as it is primarily a chronic inflammation	Much the same as childhood eczema, but the generalized form is less acute. Antecubital fossa, neck folds, upper posterior thighs, knee folds and ankles often involved. Localized areas affected may include the eyelids, where the earlobe touches the face, fingertips, toes, nipple, and the vulvar area.

MEDICATIONS Used to Treat Atopic Dermatitis

MEDICATIONS	ACTION	ADVERSE EFFECTS
Emollients Eucerin cream Aquaphor ointment Vanicream Cetaphil cream SBR-Lipocream White petrolatum	Helps lubricate the skin when applied immediately after bathing.	Fragrances and preservatives in products may cause irritation. Fragrance-free or bland emollients should be used.
Oral antihistamines	Control of itching and sedating effect when given at night.	Sleepiness and interference with learning if given during the day.
Antibiotics Topical Oral	Treat cutaneous skin superinfections.	Hypersensitivity reaction.
Corticosteroids Topical Oral	Anti-inflammatory	Skin atrophy, suppression of the hypothalamic-pituitary-adrenal axis (see Chapter 32∞). Can induce glaucoma or cataract formation if used around eyes.
Immunomodulators (second-line drug) Tacrolimus ointment Pimecrolimus (Elidel, SDZ ASM 981)	Inhibiting T lymphocyte activation. Inhibit release of cytokines and inflammatory mediators from anti-IgE-activated skin mast cells and basophils. Often used on face rather than topical corticosteroids.	Pruritis, burning or stinging sensation for up to 20 minutes in some children, but this response may be longer in the first week of therapy (Buck, 2002). Potential increased risk for lymphoma and skin cancer with respect to dose duration (FDA, 2005). Approved for children over 2 years of age.

Topical corticosteroids are used to reduce inflammation. Ointments are preferred over creams because of their occlusive effect, which ensures a stronger barrier and absorption into the skin, especially when lichenification is present. Hydrocortisone 1% to 2.5% or triamcinolone 0.1% is usually the drug of choice; however, many different preparations and seven categories of corticosteroid strength exist. See the medications table on page 1463 for topical corticosteroid preparation categories. Newer corticosteroid ointments such as fluticasone propionate bind better with the glucocorticoid receptor. This maximizes the penetration and its anti-inflammatory properties. They also have fewer adverse effects (Nicol, 2000). Corticosteroids are used twice daily for 2 weeks and must be applied before the skin moisturizer is used. Lower potency nonfluorinated ointments are used for infants and for thinner skin areas, such as the face, diaper area, and skinfolds. A higher potency ointment is used for flare-ups, with tapering to lower potency as the dermatitis improves. When the dermatitis resolves, the corticosteroids are discontinued and only moisturizers are used. Topical steroids are not used on healthy skin to reduce the risk of steroid side effects. Oral corticosteroids may be used for a severe acute exacerbation; however, there is often a **rebound effect** (i.e., after the medication is discontinued, the rash returns).

PRACTICE ALERT

The percentage following the topical corticosteroid preparation is not an indication of its strength. The strength is based on the type of preparation (ointment, lotion, or cream), and whether it is fluorinated. See the medication box on page 1463.

Avoid the use of fluorinated corticosteroids on the face, genitalia, and intertriginous (skinfold) areas where absorption of the medication may be increased because of the thinness of the stratum corneum. Occlusive dressings, such as may occur with a tight-fitting diaper, further increase the potential absorption. The lowest concentration of topical corticosteroids should also be used in these areas. Posterior cataracts and glaucoma are a potential adverse effect of topical corticosteroid exposure in the periorbital area. Other adverse effects may include skin atrophy due to decreased collagen synthesis and striae after 3–4 weeks of therapy.

Topical antibiotics are used to treat excoriated, open lesions and those that appear infected. Oral antibiotics are often given to reduce the *Staphylococcus aureus* population as these organisms can trigger an immune cascade that increases pruritis. Oral and topical antibiotics are often used in 7- to 10-day intervals rather than continuously to reduce the risk of drug-resistant organisms getting established (Shwayder, 2003). Superinfections with herpes simplex may be treated with acyclovir.

Immunomodulator ointments are increasingly used as a second-line treatment for some children; however, the expense of the medication may be prohibitive for some families. The medication has been approved by the FDA for children over 2 years of age. Using these therapies helps reduce the steroid side effects. Immunomodulators may also be used in children under age 2 years and older who are not responsive to or intolerant of conventional therapy. Recent warnings of the potential for increased risk of cancer may be of concern to parents (FDA, 2005). Complementary therapy may also be beneficial (see Complementary Therapy: Chinese Medical Herbs for Atopic Dermatitis). See Box 36–3.

BOX 36–3 Research: Probiotics and Atopic Dermatitis

Giving a **probiotic** (a product with a sufficient number of microorganisms to alter the infant's microflora to produce beneficial health effects), such as Lactobacillus GG, in the perinatal period may potentially help prevent the development of atopic dermatitis in many children. A recent case control study of 107 children who received the probiotic and the remainder who received a placebo, cut in half the development of atopic dermatitis during the first 2 years of life in children receiving the probiotic at high risk of atopy. Lactobacillis GG was considered safe to give during infancy. Reactivity to food and other allergens was similar in both groups at 4 years of age. The use of probiotics may be a significant treatment of the future preventive treatment for atopic dermatitis (Kalliomäki, Salminen, Poussa, et al., 2003)

MEDICATIONS Used for Topical Corticosteroid Potency

GROUPS (IN DECREASING ORDER OF POTENCY)	MEDICATION EXAMPLES
Group 1 (most potent)	Betamethasone dipropionate 0.05%, ointment and cream Clobetasol propionate 0.05% Halobetasol propionate 0.05%
Group 2	Fluocinonide 0.05% Mometasone furoate 0.1%, ointment Halcinonide 0.1%
Group 3	Betamethasone valerate 0.1%, ointment Triamcinolone acetonide 0.1%, ointment
Group 4	Hydrocortisone valerate 0.2% Mometasone furoate 0.1%, cream
Group 5	Betamethasone dipropionate 0.05%, lotion Fluticasone propionate 0.05%
Group 6	Triamcinolone acetonide 0.1%, cream Fluocinolone acetonide 0.01%, cream
Group 7 (least potent)	Hydrocortisone hydrochloride 2.5% or 1% Hydrocortisone acetate 1%

From Bell, E. A. (2004, March). Minimize the potential for side effects with topical corticosteroids. Infectious Diseases in Children, 12, *15.*

Antihistamine agents such as diphenhydramine (Benadryl) or hydroxyzine (Vistaril and Atarax) have a limited effect on itching, but the sedative effect is beneficial for promoting sleep. Topical antihistamines are not used because they may cause skin irritation. Methods to reduce pruritus include environmental controls, such as humidification in the winter and air conditioning in the summer. Use of a humidifier counteracts dryness of the surrounding air, minimizing loss of skin moisture. Air conditioning limits unnecessary sweating that can exacerbate inflamed areas.

Breast milk is hypoallergenic, and exclusive breastfeeding for the first 3 months of life may be associated with a lower incidence of atopic dermatitis in infants with a positive family history. Introduction of solid foods at a later age, after 4 months of age, can result in decreased atopic dermatitis during the first 4 years of life. In some children, avoidance of highly allergenic foods such as eggs, wheat, milk, and peanuts from the diets of infants and lactating mothers may improve the skin condition (Cheigh, 2003). When regular therapy does not result in improvements in the skin condition, collaboration with an allergy specialist may help identify food or other environmental allergens that trigger the eczema.

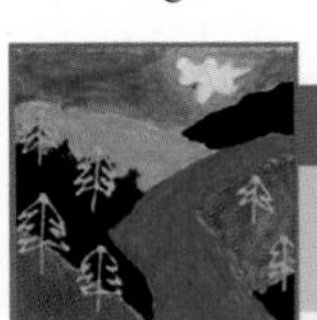

COMPLEMENTARY THERAPY
Chinese Medical Herbs for Atopic Dermatitis

One or more of the components of Zemaphyte, a mixture of plant extracts based on Chinese herbal therapy, has been found effective in treatment of children with atopic dermatitis (Latchman, Xu, Poulter, et al., 2002).

The mixture contains 10 primary herbs that are ground, placed in teabags, and boiled for 90 minutes. The herbs include the following: Ledebouriella seseloides, Potentilla chinensis, Clematis armandii, Rehmannia glutinosa, Paeonia lactoflora, Lophatherum gracile, Dictamnus dasycarpus, Tribulus terrestris, Glycyrrhiza uralensis, and Schizonepeta tenuifolia.

Children should not eat food 1 hour prior to drinking the warm mixture. If the liquid is too unpleasant tasting to drink, it can be freeze-dried into granules to put into a capsule. Significant improvements in skin lesion severity were noted in children who completed a year of treatment without significant adverse effects.

NURSING MANAGEMENT

The goal of nursing management is to provide support and education to the family to manage the child's skin condition and reduce the number of flare-ups requiring medical intervention.

Nursing Assessment and Diagnosis

A thorough history, including any family history of allergy, environmental or dietary factors, and past exacerbations, is necessary. Note the distribution and type of lesions. Note the presence of weeping lesions or signs of infection.

Identify the potential impact that the skin disorder is having on the child and family. Do the child, sibling, or other family members have disturbed sleep? Is the child's self-esteem disturbed? What stresses have the child's skin condition imposed on the family?

Common nursing diagnoses that may be appropriate for the child with eczema include the following:

- Impaired Tissue Integrity related to chemical irritants and mechanical factors (abrasive clothing)
- Disturbed Sleep Pattern related to prolonged physical discomfort (itching)
- Risk for Infection related to dry skin and breaks in skin barrier
- Chronic Low Self-Esteem related to chronic illness and peer reaction to visible skin lesions
- Ineffective Therapeutic Regimen Management (families) related to excessive demands made on the family to keep the condition under control

MediaLink Care Plan: Atopic Dermatitis

Planning and Implementation

Nursing management focuses on education and emotional support. Although no cure has been found for eczema, the condition can be controlled. Advise parents that the lesions are not contagious and will not usually result in scarring.

Help parents and children of all ages deal with the frustration of the acute flare-ups of the condition by reinforcing that remissions do occur with good home care. Parents may feel guilty or embarrassed because of their inability to clear the child's skin and to keep it clear. Make an effort to have the child return for follow-up visits about 2 weeks after a flare-up to monitor progress in controlling the skin inflammation. Provide encouragement and positive reinforcement for improvements in the child's skin.

The child, parents, and siblings may be tired because of lost sleep caused by the scratching child. This may affect school performance if the child has sleep deprivation or if the child has physical discomfort that interferes with learning. If an oral antihistamine has been ordered, make sure the parents understand when to give the medication to maximize the effectiveness of the medication to produce a full night of sleep.

Patient Education

Instruct parents or adolescents to avoid using harsh or perfumed soaps or bubble baths. Bathing with tepid water once or twice a day with a mild soap such as Dove or Tone is recommended. Washing clean skin with soap and hot water only dries it out and may increase itching. Use wet wraps for severely affected skin to replace moisture. Pat the skin dry or air-dry afterward. Moisturizers should be applied within 3 minutes of exiting the bath to help promote absorption and the retention of moisture. See recommended moisturizers in the medication table on page 1462. This should be performed once or twice daily. Wool clothing and clothing washed in harsh laundry detergents should be avoided because it can increase skin irritation and pruritus. Encourage the wearing of loose cotton clothing.

Teach parents and children appropriate application of topical ointments or creams. A thin layer over the entire area should be applied twice daily. The medication should be rubbed in gently and completely. Treatment should continue until the skin clears. Medications should be applied first, and then lubricants applied on top. Instruct parents to place clean cotton gloves or socks over the infant or young child's hands and to keep the child's fingernails cut short to decrease scratching and reduce the chance of secondary infection. See Partnering with Families: Skin Care for Atopic Dermatitis for additional tips for skin care.

MediaLink Eczema Resources and Support

Emotional Support

Allow parents to talk about their feelings about having a child with visible skin lesions, and the types of comments they hear from family, friends, and strangers. Reassure parents that the condition does improve with age in most cases, and generally does not leave scars.

Eczema produces visible changes that can affect a child's self-confidence and self-esteem. Identify activities that the child can participate in to improve self-esteem. See Complementary Therapy: Massage and Atopic Dermatitis. Even though humidity and sweating can make eczema worse, have the child shower after a sporting event or strenuous activity to clean the skin. Needed medications and lubricants can then be applied.

Atopic dermatitis that is difficult to manage is more stressful and has a profound effect on the child's and family's quality of life. The use of immunomodulators in children with moderate to severe atopic dermatitis significantly improve the quality of life in children and adults as measured by daily activities, feelings, relationships, and sleep (Drake & Prendergast, 2001; Whalley, Huels, McKenna, et al., 2002).

Food Allergy Management

Once the condition is under control, counsel the parents about the method for introducing a food that was previously eliminated when an allergen cause of atopic dermatitis was suspected (see Chapter 26∞). Emphasize that increased itching within hours of eating a food may be associated with the eczema flare-up. Teach parents how to control the skin inflammation that results, as described. Once a specific food allergy has been identified, refer the parents to a nutritionist for counseling related to alternative food options that will fulfill daily nutritional requirements. Caution parents that food allergies can change, so foods connected with atopic dermatitis can sometimes be safely eaten at a later age. Different food sensitivities may also develop. Refer the family to the Food Allergy Network.

Evaluation

Expected outcomes of nursing care include the following:

- Control of the child's eczema is maintained and no infection occurs.
- Parents identify triggers of the child's eczema and avoid or eliminate them.
- The child's sleep is minimally disturbed by itching.

Contact Dermatitis

Contact dermatitis is an inflammation of the skin that occurs in response to direct contact with an allergen or irritant. Up to 35% of

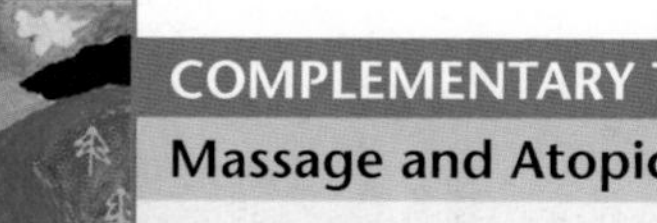

COMPLEMENTARY THERAPY

Massage and Atopic Dermatitis

A study of the effectiveness of massage in treating eczema showed positive benefit for the child and parent. Daily massage of the child for 20 minutes over 1 month resulted in improvements in redness, scaling, lichenification, excoriation, and pruritis. The child's activity level and disposition also improved. Parents performing the massage reported decreased anxiety (Schachner, Field, Hernandez-Ruif, et al., 1998).

the infant population is affected, most commonly between 9 and 12 months of age (Kazaks & Lane, 2000). At least 20% of children are at risk for allergic contact dermatitis (Weston & Bruckner, 2000).

Etiology and Pathophysiology

In the case of contact dermatitis caused by external irritants, an inflammatory reaction occurs, but no memory T-cell function or antigen-specific immunoglobulins are involved. Common irritants include soaps, detergents, fabric softeners, bleaches, lotions, urine, and stool. Sweating and friction enhance the absorption of the allergen or irritant. Photodermatitis can result when the child has contact with citrus rinds and juice or fig leaves followed by sun exposure. The child develops erythema and blistering at the site of the exposure that then becomes hyperpigmented. The hyperpigmentation fades over time (Friedlander, 1998).

In allergic contact dermatitis, an antigen is absorbed from the skin surface during the initial sensitization phase, and the Langerhans cells process the antigen and carry it to the T lymphocytes to create an immune memory. Generally, repeated or a long-term exposure is required to cause the immune response and the resulting dermatitis. However, when the antigen is strong, such as with poison ivy, only one to two exposures is needed to cause the immune response. See Chapter 27∞ for a complete explanation of the immune response to allergens. Common allergens include nickel, poison ivy, poison oak, lanolin, neomycin, rubber, potassium dichromate (leather tanning agent), thimersol, fragrances, and latex. Both irritant and allergic reactions to latex, which can be found in many types of hospital equipment and supplies, as well as in products in the home and community, have been reported (see Chapter 27∞).

Clinical Manifestations

Erythema, edema, pruritis, vesicles, or bullae that rupture, ooze, and crust characterize the rash of allergic contact dermatitis (Figure 36–5 ■). The rash is usually limited to the area of contact. Symptoms of allergic contact dermatitis can develop within 12 to 24 hours after exposure and peak in 3 to 5 days (Weston & Bruckner, 2000). No fever is present. A more generalized dermatitis may develop distal to the original site about 1 week after the initial localized dermatitis. Symptoms can last up to 3 to 4 weeks without treatment. Less potent allergens may cause a subacute nonvesicular rash that is erythematous with scaling and lichenification.

In contrast, irritant contact dermatitis is a discrete area of redness that corresponds to the exposure location. The rash usually develops within a few hours of contact, peaks within 24 hours, and quickly resolves with removal of the irritant. Reactions to irritants include painful erythema, edema, vesiculation, dryness of the skin, scaling, fissuring, and necrosis.

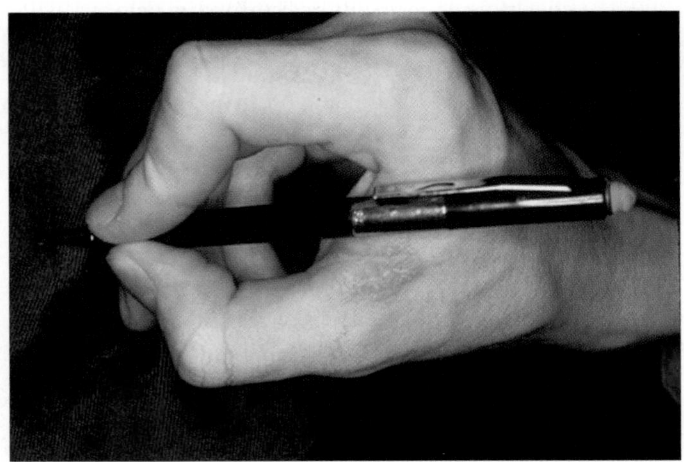

FIGURE 36–5 ■ Contact dermatitis.

PARTNERING WITH FAMILIES

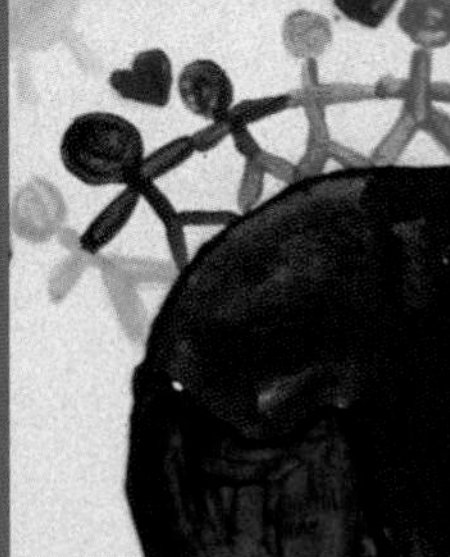

Skin Care for Atopic Dermatitis

- Help select an appropriate ointment or cream for the family to use. Because lotions contain less oil, they are less effective. Avoid ointments and creams with a fragrance as these may irritate the skin.
- Consider the cost of ointments and creams, as large quantities are needed to cover the body at least twice a day. Petrolatum or Vaseline is inexpensive, safe, and easily applied.
- Help ensure that parents receive adequate amounts of corticosteroids for effective treatment. It takes 5–8 g to cover the entire body of a child who weighs 10 kg, so a 15 g tube of corticosteroid ointment is enough for only 1 day. It takes 45 g to cover the entire body of an adolescent once (Hansen, 2003). Fortunately most children do not have atopic dermatitis over the entire body, and the steroid is only used where there is inflammation.
- For immunomodulators, a pea-size amount should cover a 2 in. circle.
- Bathe and let the child soak in tepid water for 5–15 min once or twice a day. Use mild soap only on areas that are dirty. Rinse well. Pat the child dry with a towel rather than rubbing the skin. Immediately apply the medication (corticosteroid, topical antibiotic, or immunomodulator) to the inflamed area and then the lubricant on top. Apply the lubricant to the entire body.
- In areas where the humidity is low, more frequent application of lubricants to the skin is needed. Corticosteroids should be applied no more than twice a day.
- With a skin flare-up, wet occlusive dressings increase penetration of corticosteroid ointments and help decrease itching. Apply the topical ointment and then wrap the child in a wet towel for 10 min, then reapply the topical ointment followed by an emollient (Raimer, 2000).
- Educate children about the disorder and skin care. Emphasize the importance of following the treatment plan to promote healing of existing lesions and to reduce the risk of secondary infections.

COLLABORATIVE CARE

The goal of collaborative care is to remove the irritant or allergen causing the skin reaction and to promote reduced itching and healing.

Diagnostic Tests

The distribution of the lesions provides clues about the source and identity of the allergen or irritant (Table 36–2). In some cases patch testing is needed to identify the antigen causing the allergic contact dermatitis. Patch testing monitors the T lymphocyte response to the placement of suspected allergens on the skin surface and development of contact dermatitis.

Clinical Therapy

Treatment involves removing the offending agent (e.g., clothes, plant, soap). Calamine lotion can be applied to the affected skin. Cool compresses with aluminum acetate (Burow's solution) promote drying. Wet dressings or colloidal oatmeal soaks relieve itching. Antihistamines may be given to reduce itching or for a sedative effect when the child is too irritable to sleep.

Acute allergic contact dermatitis is managed with medium potency topical corticosteroids when less than 10% of the body surface area is affected. The topical corticosteroids limit the production of cytokines, stop lymphocyte proliferation, and limit the inflammatory response to the allergens. The topical corticosteroid must be continued for 2 to 3 weeks as stopping it too quickly can cause rebound dermatitis. Reducing twice daily application to once daily application near the end of treatment may also be helpful in reducing rebound dermatitis. Reactions to poison ivy or other allergens covering more than 10% of the body surface area require treatment with oral corticosteroids. The oral corticosteroid is given for 7 to 10 days with subsequent tapering of the dose over another 7 to 10 days.

NURSING MANAGEMENT

Patient education for home care management focuses on care of the skin and on prevention of future exposures.

Topical corticosteroids are applied to the affected area twice a day for 2 to 3 weeks. Advise parents to continue use of the ointments even when the skin shows signs of healing to prevent rebound dermatitis. When oatmeal soaks are used, caution parents that the tub will be slippery. Inform them to pat the child dry to leave the oatmeal film in place. Wet dressings may be soothing and they help to loosen crusts. Burrows or Domeboro solution applied to blistered or oozing lesions for 20 minutes daily helps dry lesions (Allen, 2004). The child can wear these wet dressings to bed or for up to 8 hours during the day before changing them. Familiarize parents with the symptoms of infection in the affected area (e.g., increased redness, oozing, fever) and tell them when to return for follow-up care.

Teaching the child and family how to avoid exposure to the allergen or irritant is an important nursing role. See Partnering with Families: Exposure to Poison Ivy or Poison Oak.

- Advise parents to wash all clothes before the first wearing and to rinse clothes an extra time to remove all soap. Mild soap should be used to clean the skin.
- Place a barrier between the allergen and the skin. For example, cover all metal snaps on clothing with cloth, and wear socks to avoid exposure to tanning chemicals left on shoe leather. If barriers do not reduce the dermatitis, then efforts to find clothing without nickel or shoes with specific tanning chemicals may be necessary.
- Make sure nickel jewelry and belt buckles are not used if a nickel allergy exists.
- Children should remove clothing worn after outside activities and shower. Clean clothes should then be worn.

TABLE 36–2 Distribution of Lesions by Type of Allergen

DISTRIBUTION OF LESION	ALLERGEN
Linear	Plant exposure
Ear lobes, neck	Nickel
Dorsal aspects of toes and feet	Rubber or leather chemical in shoes
Face, eyelids	Cosmetic preservatives
Subumbilical	Snaps on pants
Axillary	Deodorants

Adapted from Weston, W. L., & Bruckner, A. (2000). Allergic contact dermatitis. Pediatric Clinics of North America, *47(4), 897–907.*

Diaper Dermatitis

Diaper dermatitis, one of the most common causes of irritant contact dermatitis, occurs in approximately one third of young children, usually in a mild form. It is most common in infants from 4 to 12 months of age.

Etiology and Pathophysiology

Diaper dermatitis is a primary reaction to urine, feces, moisture, or friction. Urine and feces interact with the skin to cause dermatitis. The urine increases the wetness and pH of the skin, increasing abrasion and its permeability to irritants and microbes. Fecal enzymes are activated by the alkalinity of the urine and cause the skin irritation. Breastfed babies have stools with a lower pH, which helps reduce the incidence of diaper rash (Kazaks & Lane, 2000). *Candida albicans,* a secondary infection, is a common complication of diaper dermatitis or antibiotic therapy for another condition. It is frequently the underlying cause of severe diaper rash. Diaper candidiasis often occurs simultaneously with oral candidiasis (see later discussion).

Clinical Manifestations

The primary irritant rash is characterized by glazed red plaques over the skin in direct contact with the diaper area. Usually the perineum, genitals, and buttocks are affected, and the skinfolds are spared. In severe cases, the infant develops a rash that is fiery red, raised, and confluent. Pustules with tenderness can also be present (Figure 36–6 ■).

When a primary or secondary infection with *Candida albicans* occurs, the rash has bright red scaly plaques with sharp margins. Small papules and pustules may be seen, along with satellite lesions. Skinfolds and the convex surfaces of the diaper area are involved.

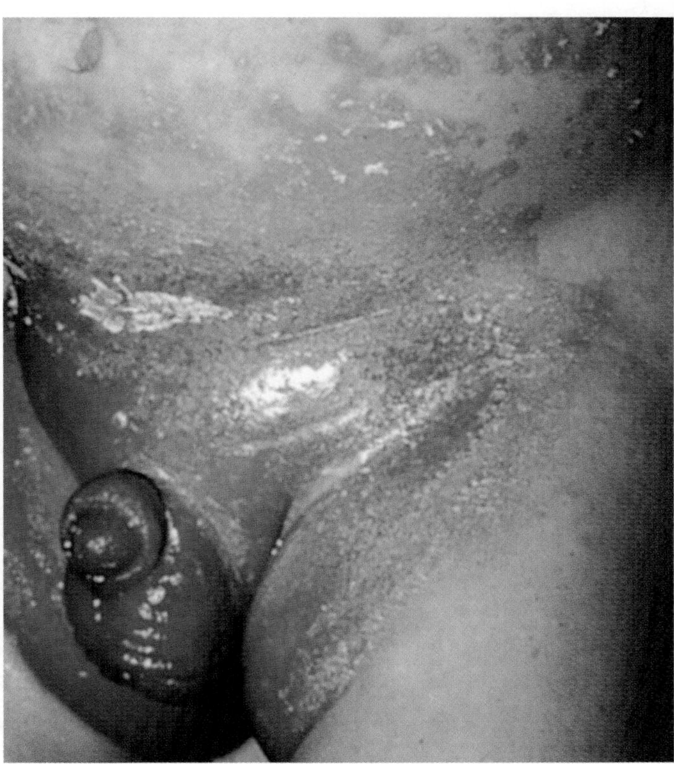

FIGURE 36–6 ■ Diaper dermatitis. *Note the skinfold that is free of inflammation.*
Courtesy of the Centers for Disease Control, Atlanta, GA.

COLLABORATIVE CARE

The goal of collaborative care is to correctly distinguish between types of diaper dermatitis, and provide appropriate ointments to promote healing and improve the infant's comfort.

Diagnostic Procedures

When *Candida albicans* is suspected as a cause of the diaper rash, a skin scraping is sometimes taken for microscopic examination with KOH (potassium hydroxide).

Clinical Therapy

Mild diaper dermatitis is treated with a barrier or protective sealant such as zinc oxide paste, Desitin, or Balmex. Treatment for moderate or severe diaper dermatitis involves application of low to moderate potency (0.25% to 1%) hydrocortisone cream with each diaper change for 5 to 7 days and good basic hygiene. The cream must be applied before any protective sealant is used.

Diaper candidiasis is treated with alternating applications of 1% hydrocortisone cream and antifungal creams (clotrimazole or nystatin) applied to the affected areas at each diaper change, so that each medication is applied several times a day. An oral antifungal agent may occasionally be given to clear the candidiasis from the intestines. Fluorinated topical corticosteroids should not be used because of the higher rate of absorption through damaged skin.

PARTNERING WITH FAMILIES

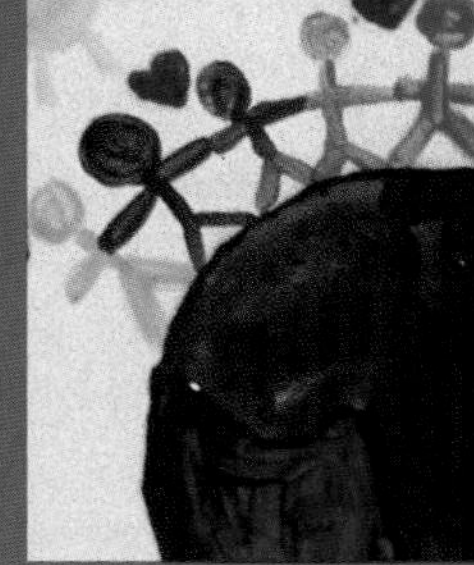

Exposure to Poison Ivy or Poison Oak

- The rash is caused by contact with the oils from the sap of the plants, either from the plants directly or indirectly, such as on animal fur or clothing.
- React quickly after contact. Wash the skin with cold water from a stream, lake, or garden hose as soon as possible.
  - Wash off sap with soap and water within 10 minutes if possible. Remember to scrub under the nails.
  - Do not rub fingers exposed to poison ivy or poison oak against broken skin or in eyes.
  - Avoid hugging a pet exposed to poison ivy until after it has been bathed.
  - Launder clothing worn during exposure, and wash hands after handling exposed clothing.
- Wear vinyl gloves to handle plants (cloth and rubber gloves allow sap to penetrate).
- Search the yard and remove all plants. Do not burn the plants. An individual with sensitivity may inhale the oil particles in the smoke and develop airway inflammation.
- For children with sensitivity to poison ivy or poison oak, some over-the-counter barrier creams such as IvyBlock can help prevent skin penetration by the plant oil.

NURSING MANAGEMENT

Severe diaper dermatitis can be a major source of stress for parents who must deal with a child in constant discomfort. Instruct parents to change the diaper as soon as the infant is wet, or at least every 2 hours during the day and once during the night.

Encourage parents to use superabsorbent disposable diapers, which tend to reduce the frequency and severity of diaper dermatitis. When wet, these diapers form a gel that keeps the skin drier than cloth diapers. However, this should not be an excuse for waiting until the diaper is saturated to change it. Tell parents to avoid using tight diapers and waterproof pants. A&D ointment, zinc oxide, Desitin, and Balmex can be used to protect the skin from urine and stool.

Advise parents to wash the perianal area with warm water and a mild soap (such as unscented Dove or Tone) or a cleanser not needing water (Acquanil HC lotion or Cetaphil) only after a bowel movement. Soft paper towels with warm tap water may substitute for baby wipes. If baby wipes are preferred, advise parents to use those without alcohol (Box 36–4). Mineral oil may be used to help remove the zinc oxide from the skin. Cornstarch or zeaSORB powder helps to decrease friction and moisture, but it is important to keep these powders away from the infant's face. Encourage parents to use powders only after the

BOX 36–4 Research: Use of Disposable Baby Wipes

Disposable baby wipes were compared with cotton washcloths and water for the routine daily use in cleaning the diaper area of 82 infants. Prior to the start of the study, use of any lotions, creams, and powders were discontinued and all infants used the same disposable diaper. Parents were given an adequate supply of either the baby wipes or cotton washcloths to use for an 8-day period. At the end of the study period, skin was evaluated for amount of erythema, transepidermal water loss (method to evaluate the skin barrier function), and skin surface roughness. Results indicated that baby wipes were comparable to cotton washcloths and water for maintenance of skin barrier and amount of erythema in the genital area. Baby wipes were associated with significantly less erythema severity in the perianal area and less skin roughness. Baby wipes were also found to be gentler than cotton washcloths and water on irritated skin, enabling normal healing process of the skin barrier to proceed more rapidly (Odio, Streicher-Scott, & Hansen, 2001).

skin has healed. Exposing the diaper area to air helps aid healing, for example, allowing the child to go without a diaper while lying on an absorbable pad or cloth. Observe for signs of infection since the skin is damaged and can allow infectious organisms to grow. If significant improvement in the infant's skin is not seen within a week, encourage the parents to return for further assessment and care.

Seborrheic Dermatitis

Seborrheic dermatitis is a recurrent inflammatory skin condition thought to be caused by an overgrowth of Pityrosporum yeast, commonly found in areas of sebaceous gland activity. The condition is also thought to be influenced by hormones and associated with an oily complexion. The rash is found over the areas of the body where the sebaceous glands are most plentiful: scalp (cradle cap), forehead, and postauricular and periorbital areas. It may also occur on the skin of the eyelids, inguinal area, or nasolabial folds. The condition is frequently seen in infants up to 3 months of age and in adolescents.

Common symptoms are a mildly erythematous, adherent waxy scaling of the scalp (or "dandruff"). Yellow-red patches with greasy scaling may be present, typically on the scalp and nasolabial folds on the face, behind the ears, on the upper chest, and sometimes the **intertriginous areas** (skinfolds of the neck, axillae, antecubital fossa) (Figure 36–7 ■). The rash itches less than in atopic dermatitis.

Treatment for seborrheic dermatitis consists of daily shampooing with baby shampoo in young infants and with a medicated shampoo in adolescents (e.g., Selsun or Head and Shoulders). An emollient is left on the scalp for about 20 minutes to soften the crusts. The scales are removed by brushing with the fingertips, a baby hairbrush, or a soft toothbrush. The hair is then rinsed thoroughly. Lesions on the body of adolescents can be treated with shampoos containing selenium sulfide or salicylic acid. Use baby shampoo to wash lesions on the eyelids and eyelashes. Treatments are continued for several days after the lesions disappear. Topical corticosteroids are often used to treat seborrhea that is not on the scalp.

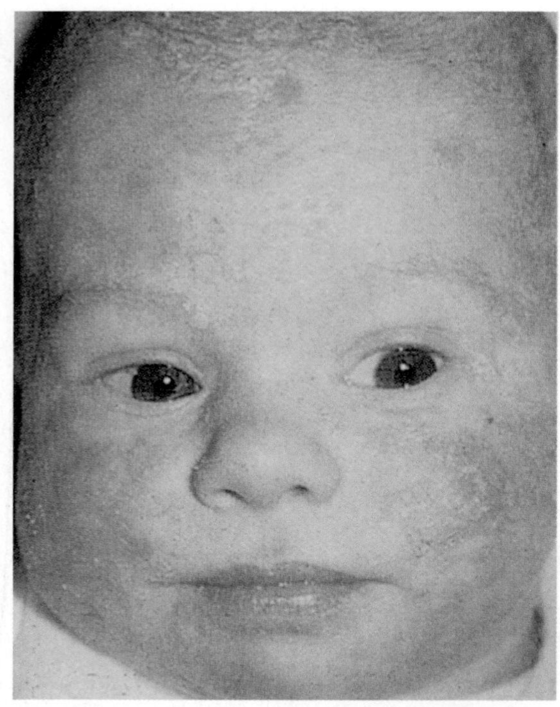

FIGURE 36–7 ■ Seborrheic dermatitis.

Nursing Management

Teach new parents that the infant's hair should be washed regularly with each bath to reduce the risk for seborrheic dermatitis. Reassure parents that gentle cleansing will not harm the infant's "soft spot." Provide a bath demonstration to show them the proper technique, if necessary. Follow-up is seldom necessary, as the condition resolves with treatment.

Educate adolescents about the daily use of shampoo and topical corticosteroid ointment or cream application. Advise adolescents that emotional distress may trigger future flare-ups and to initiate treatment promptly when symptoms begin.

Drug Reactions

Adverse reactions to over-the-counter or prescription medications are relatively common. Children with drug allergies usually have reactions after ingestion (e.g., aspirin, antibiotics, sedatives), injection (e.g., penicillin), or direct skin contact with medications. Drug sensitivities may result from variations in an individual's ability to tolerate a particular drug or concentration of a drug or from allergic responses. (See Chapter 27∞ for a description of allergic reactions.)

Sensitivity reactions to a drug not previously administered may take up to 7 days to develop. If the child has been sensitized to a drug, the reaction is almost immediate. The most common reactions in children are the development of erythematous macules and papules or urticaria, which may be pruritic. Drugs most likely to cause maculopapular eruptions, urticaria, and pruritis include the following: amoxicillin, ampicillin, cephalosporins, erythromycin, penicillin G, semisynthetic penicillins, sulfamethoxazole, and trimethoprim (Vanderhooft, 1998). Some drug reactions can be life threatening. Be alert to the possibility of serious drug reactions that may become a medical emergency. See the clinical manifestation table below for signs associated with drug reactions of varying severity.

The treatment of choice for most drug sensitivity reactions is discontinuation of the causative drug. In rare cases, a drug may be continued with careful monitoring when the child has a sensitivity reaction because it is the best treatment choice. Supportive measures should be taken to decrease the intensity of the

CLINICAL MANIFESTATIONS of Drug Reactions

TYPE OF REACTION	CLINICAL MANIFESTATIONS	CLINICAL THERAPY
Allergic drug reaction Most common offending drugs include sulfonamides, tetracyclines, NSAIDs, oral contraceptives, barbiturates, and phenolphthalein.	Erythematous macules and papules Pruritis Urticaria, moves from one part of body to another A fixed drug reaction may commonly involve the face, genitals, sacrum Recurrent localized target lesions may be seen with repeated exposure. Healing with hyperpigmentation of the center may be seen (Cohen, 2002).	Remove offending drug Topical antipruritics Oral antihistamines Lubricate skin when scaly Systemic corticosteroids if no response to other treatment
Stevens-Johnson syndrome (erythema multiforme major) Hypersensitivity reaction to the drug (sulfonamides, anticonvulsants, and NSAIDs) or reaction to an infectious agent. Cause has also been related to herpes simplex and mycoplasma pneumoniae (Forman, Koren, & Shear, 2002)	Prodrome of an upper respiratory infection for 1–7 days with cough, coryza, sore throat, fever, malaise, headache, muscle aches, joint pain. Vomiting and diarrhea may be seen. Skin lesions are then seen as blistering and crusting on the mucous membranes and redness in the eyes. Blisters spread in some cases to the entire skin surface. If this happens red macules progress to edematous papules and plaques, target lesions with vesicular dusty centers. Pruritis	Remove offending drug Balance intake and output Gentle debridement of crusts Provide topical anesthetics for oral lesions Oral antihistamines Topical antipruritics Nutritional support Ophthalmic consultation Corticosteroid use is controversial; no studies have demonstrated its effectiveness. Corticosteroids may delay wound healing and increase risk of secondary infection or sepsis IV immune globulin use is controversial, as no studies have demonstrated its effectiveness.
Toxic epidermal necrolysis Acute life-threatening hypersensitivity reaction to NSAIDs, sulfa, antibiotics, and anticonvulsants	Rash similar to Stevens-Johnson syndrome Appearance of tender skin, then bullae or erosions occur over more than 20% of body surface area Full thickness epidermis peels off in sheets easily with tangential pressure (Nikolski's sign). Respiratory tract may be involved with mucosal sloughing Causes hypopigmentation in children with dark skin, but hyperpigmentation in children with white skin. Hyperpigmentation fades over time. Signs of sepsis	May be cared for in a burn center Debridement of blisters and necrotic epidermis may be performed Gentle cleaning with saline or Burrows solution (aluminum acetate) compresses Topical antibiotic ointment, but no sulfa as this may be the original cause of toxicity Sterile nonadherent dressings Wounds may be covered with biosynthetic dressing, hydrogel, human allografts to reduce infection and pain IV immunomodulators have shown some success, but prospective studies are needed Intensive nutritional support Ophthalmic consultation and eye care No corticosteroids
Erythema multiforme minor Hypersensitivity reaction to anticonvulsants, penicillins, salicylates, sulfa antibiotics, barbiturates, and phenytoin; infectious agents	May have prodromal symptoms of a mild respiratory infections (malaise, fever, weakness, sore throat, cough) Target lesions with dusky centers (papules, vesicles, or bullae in a pale ring with an erythematous border) Lesions may or may not be present on the mucosa, common on palms and soles. Edema Burning, pruritis, or tenseness of the skin	Remove offending drug Oral antihistamines Topical antipruritics Analgesics Cool compresses or baths Topical corticosteroids are sometimes prescribed.

Data from Vanderhooft, S. L. (1998). Is the rash really an adverse drug reaction? Contemporary Pediatrics, *15(5), 118–137; Valencia, I. C., Falabela, A. F., & Schachner, L. A. (2001). New developments in wound care for infants and children.* Pediatric Annals, *30(4), 211–218; Schmidt, C. E. (2003). A 12-month-old girl with maculopapular lesions and lower extremity edema.* Journal of Emergency Nursing, *29(3), 204–207; Cohen, B. A. (2002). Plaques: Oval, itchy, and red: What's your diagnosis?* Contemporary Pediatrics, *19(4), 36, 41; Spies, M., Sanford, A. P., Low, J. F. A., Wolf, S. E., & Herndon, D. N. (2001). Treatment of extensive toxic epidermal necrolysis in children.* Pediatrics, *108(5), 1162–1168.*

reaction. An antihistamine may be used to block the release of histamine, which causes the rash. Topical corticosteroids, cool compresses, and baths may also be prescribed for pruritis. For some severe drug reactions the child must be hospitalized and treated on a burn unit.

CLINICAL TIP

Children with a true drug allergy (having a past serious systemic reaction) should not be treated with that drug again. The child should wear a medic alert tag.

Therapies for differing types of drug reactions are identified in the clinical manifestations table on page 1469.

Nursing Management

Nurses can play an important role by teaching parents to be alert for the signs of drug sensitivity reactions. Obtain a careful history of the child's past reactions to medications before starting new therapies. If a reaction occurs, discontinue the medication until the physician is notified. Prominently mark the child's records so that all allergies are easily identified. See nursing care for the burned child on page 1494 for additional nursing interventions for the care of damaged skin due to severe drug reactions.

ACNE

Acne is a chronic inflammatory disorder of the pilosebaceous hair follicles located on the face and trunk. It is the most common skin disorder in the pediatric population. It is believed to be triggered by the increased androgen production of puberty and the overproduction of sebum. The prevalence in adolescents aged 12 to 16 is estimated to approach 50% to 85% (Rudy, 2003). Acne is found in all ethnic groups and is present equally in males and females. Acne may also occur in 20% of neonates in response to maternal androgen hormones. This form of acne usually develops between 2 and 4 weeks of age and resolves by 4 to 6 months.

Etiology and Pathophysiology

Acne is caused by the interaction of several factors: an overgrowth of residential bacteria on the skin, increased sebum production, and abnormal follicular skin cell shedding that is more adherent than normal. The pilosebaceous unit consists of the sebaceous gland that produces an oily substance called sebum. The sebaceous gland has a duct to the keratinocyte-lined follicular canal that opens onto the skin surface. The keratin initially plugs the follicular canal. The extra sebum caused by androgen hormone secretion mixes with the shed skin cells and causes them to clump together. The keratin and sebum that usually flow to the skin surface are obstructed in the follicular canal, causing **comedones** (whiteheads and blackheads). The sebum behind the comedone is an ideal environment for the anerobic *Propionibacterium acnes,* and this bacterium metabolizes the sebum causing an inflammatory reaction. When the inflammatory reaction is close to the surface, a papule or pustule develops. If the inflammatory reaction is deeper, a larger papule or nodule develops. Although familial trends are recognized, hard data to define a pattern of inheritance are not conclusive.

Drugs such as androgens, glucocorticoids, phenytoin, lithium, and isoniazid are reported to cause acne (Rudy, 2003). Other factors that can help trigger acne include friction of the skin from hairbands, helmets, and hats, as well as oil-based cosmetics.

Clinical Manifestations

Noninflammatory acne involves a follicular plug that precedes inflammatory acne lesions. It has both closed and open comedones. Closed comedones are flesh-colored papules with tiny follicular openings called whiteheads. Open comedones are found when the follicular plug has enlarged and dilated the follicular opening, called blackheads. The three main types of acne are comedomal (characterized by open and closed comedones), papulopustular (characterized by red papules and pustules) (Figure 36–8 ■), and cystic (characterized by nodules and cysts). Noninflammatory lesions are commonly found with the moderate and severe forms of acne. Lesions occur most often on the face, upper chest, shoulders, and back. Scars form when the surrounding dermis is damaged. See Developing Cultural Competence: Acne Lesions in Individuals with Dark Skin. The types of scars that may be seen include (Woodard, 2002):

- Ice pick (small, deep, punched out pits)
- Atrophic macules
- Hypertrophic scars or keloids
- Broad sloping depressions

COLLABORATIVE CARE

The goal of collaborative care is to identify the therapy to match the severity of the adolescent's acne and to provide guidelines for safe and effective use of these treatments.

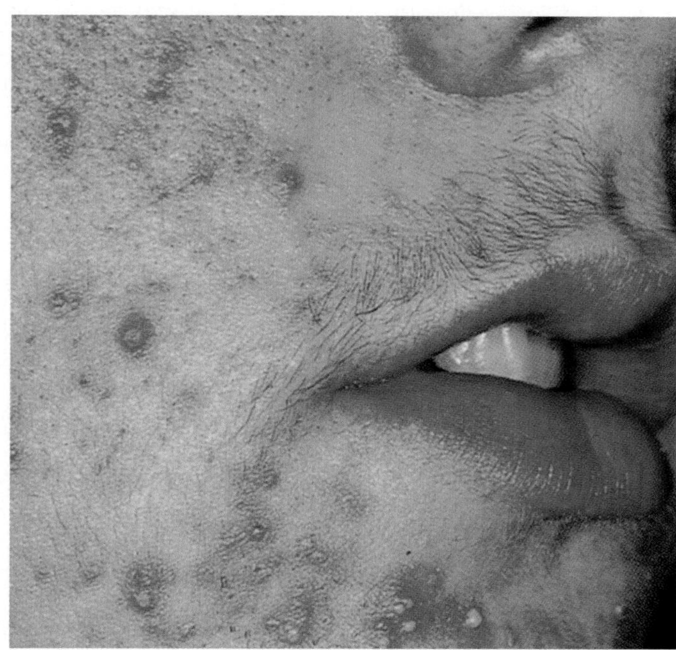

FIGURE 36–8 ■ Pustular acne can have a significant effect on an adolescent's self-esteem.

From Habif, T. P. (1990). Clinical dermatology: A color guide to diagnosis and therapy *(2nd ed., p. 113). St. Louis: Mosby-Year Book.*

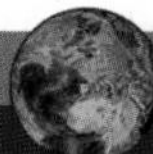

DEVELOPING CULTURAL COMPETENCE
Acne Lesions in Individuals with Dark Skin

Inflammatory acne in adolescents with darker skin color is associated with a hyperpigmented macule. Extra pigment gets deposited in the areas of inflammation and this color change can last for 4 months or longer. If inflammation is controlled with acne therapy, the hyperpigmented areas may fade over time; however, keloid scars that can develop will not recede (Rudy, 2003).

Diagnostic Tests

Diagnosis is based on examination of the skin. The most predominant type of lesion present is identified and the severity of skin lesions is graded.

Clinical Therapy

Treatment is customized to the predominant type of lesion present and general severity of lesions. See the medications table below. Therapeutic options include keratolytics, retinoids, and oral antibiotics. The goal of treatment is to suppress lesions until the condition is outgrown, thus preventing infection, scarring, and minimizing psychologic distress. Thus the treatment is long term. Acne will generally recur gradually if treatment is stopped, although adolescents treated with isotretinoin have fewer recurrences.

Topical keratolytics are used, such as benzoyl peroxide that has both a bacteriocidal action and an effect on follicular hyperkeratosis. When used in combination with topical antibiotics, bacterial resistance is reduced. Other topical keratolytics include azelaic acid 20%, salicylic acid, and sulfur. Topical antibiotics are used to reduce the colonization of bacteria and to reduce inflammation.

Topical retinoids slow the desquamation and decrease the adherence of shed cells within the follicles that reduces follicular plugging. Topical retinoids include tretinoin, adapalene, and tazarotene. Dryness and scaling of the skin are typical after several days of treatment. The initial response may look like the condition is worsening for the first 1 to 3 weeks of treatment, but with continued used, the skin adapts (Rudy, 2003). Thinning of the stratum corneum leads to the irritant reaction, but the skin thinning assists in the penetration of other topical acne medications.

Irritant contact dermatitis is a frequent problem experienced by adolescents with dry or sensitive skin, or by adolescents with darker colored skin. Increased sun sensitivity is noted. Creams are used for adolescents with more sensitive skin while adolescents with more oily skin or those who live in a hot and humid climate should use gels.

Oral antibiotics are used for moderate to severe acne. Generally 3 months are needed for the medication to be effective. After a good response to oral antibiotics and topical acne medications is achieved, the antibiotic dose is tapered to the lowest dose that maintains acne control when used in combination with topical acne medications. Increasing numbers of cases of bacterial resistance to antibiotics have been noted. A recurrence or flare-up of acne after control has been achieved may be an indication that the bacteria have developed resistance to the antibiotic. The antibiotic may need to be replaced to find one that is effective.

Isotretinoin (Accutane) is reserved for the most serious cases of acne that are not responsive to other therapies. A 5-month course of treatment is given. Because the medication causes sebaceous gland atrophy, the improvement in acne is permanent in 70% to 75% of those treated. Individuals taking isotretinoin often experience dry skin and mucous membranes.

PRACTICE ALERT

Isotretinoin Precautions

Because of its teratogenicity and potential adverse reactions, the Food and Drug Administration requires that individuals taking isotretinoin sign informed consent about teratogenicity, monthly blood testing, and the potential for depression or suicide ideation (Woodard, 2002). A recent study examining the association between isotretinoin (Accutane) and mental health problems found no increased risk for depression, suicide, or other psychologic problems (Jick, Kremers, & Vasilakis-Scaramozza, 2000). However, press reports have linked isotretinoin to depression and suicide.

Adolescent females need two negative pregnancy tests before starting on isotretinoin and a monthly pregnancy test during treatment. Two forms of contraception must be used when taking isotretinoin (Buck, 2001). Contraception must be used 1 month prior to treatment, during, and 1 month after therapy is completed. Because of potential adverse reactions of hepatotoxicity and increased levels of triglycerides, monthly laboratory monitoring of liver function, cholesterol, and triglycerides is also required. A 1-month supply of isotretinoin is provided to promote compliance.

MEDICATIONS Used to Treat Acne Based on Severity

MEDICATION	SEVERITY AND APPEARANCE
Tretinoin (Retin-A) 0.025% cream daily (to comedones only), in the evening Salicylic acid, adapalene, tazarotene	Grade I (mild) Comedonal acne
2.5% benzoyl peroxide gel Tretinoin (Retin-A) in evening Topical antibiotics (clindamycin, erythromycin, tetracycline) twice a day Azelaic acid cream twice a day	Grade II (moderate) Papulopustular acne (red papules, pustules)
Tretinoin (Retin-A) and benzoyl peroxide twice a day Oral antibiotics (tetracycline, minocycline, or doxycline)	Grade III (severe) Cystic acne (red papules, many pustules, cysts)
Isotretinoin (Accutane) given twice a day for 15–20 weeks. A second course of treatment for 8 weeks may be given to those who do not have a good response.	Grade IV Pustulocystic nodular (severe, resistant to other treatment)

Oral contraceptives with norgestimate and ethinyl estradiol are FDA approved for the treatment of acne (Sidbury & Paller, 2000). This therapy is beneficial to adolescent females who have acne flares with menstruation or elevated serum androgens. Improvement in skin appearance can take 3 to 6 months with oral contraceptives. Spiralatone is sometimes prescribed due to its action in decreasing sebum production, and when prescribed with oral contraceptives, the effectiveness of both medications is enhanced (Woodard, 2002).

NURSING MANAGEMENT

The goal of nursing management is to support the adolescent with the psychological impact of acne, and education about potential triggers, appropriate medication use, and skin care for optimal treatment outcomes.

Nursing Assessment and Diagnosis

Physical assessment should include documentation regarding distribution, predominant type, and severity of acne lesions. Assess the adolescent's and parents' knowledge about the cause and treatment of acne, and home therapies used. Adolescents with acne have reported social, psychological, and emotion problems such as those caused by other chronic disorders such as asthma, epilepsy, and diabetes, regardless of the level of acne severity (Woodard, 2002). Explore the amount of emotional distress the acne is causing the adolescent. Adolescents with acne have reported social, psychological, and emotional problems as great as those caused by other chronic disorders such as asthma, epilepsy, and diabetes, regardless of the level of acne severity (Woodard, 2002).

Common nursing diagnoses are presented in the accompanying nursing care plan.

Planning and Implementation

Nursing care for the adolescent with acne is summarized in the accompanying nursing care plan. Nursing management focuses on educating the child and parents about acne and its treatment. See Partnering with Adolescents: Caring for Acne. Advise adolescents to wash their hands before touching the affected areas and to avoid picking or squeezing the lesions. Remind them that the inflammation occurs with the rupture of lesions below the skin surface, which picking and squeezing may cause. In addition, advise them to avoid using any cleansing products that have a greasy base, to shampoo hair regularly (to treat seborrhea that can accompany acne), to expect flare-ups despite treatment, and to eat a well-balanced diet.

Correct any misconceptions adolescents and their family have about dietary causes of acne. Although no food has been found to cause acne or to increase the severity of lesions, good nutrition is important to help the skin heal. Teach parents and children that increased sweating, as well as heat and humidity, may exacerbate acne. Emotional stress may increase adrenal androgen production, resulting in increased sebum production and acne flare-ups.

Instruct adolescents to wash the face no more than two to three times a day with a mild soap, then wait about 20 to 30 minutes before applying tretinoin (Retin-A), if prescribed. Use a pea-sized dose of topical medications to spread in a thin film over the skin. Avoid getting the topical medications near the eyes, lips, and mucous membranes. Alert the adolescent that treatment may seem to worsen the acne as the comedones are being pushed out. This is a sign that the medication is working. Emphasize that treatment is often long term. Significant improvement may not be seen until at least 6 to 12 weeks after the start of treatment. Make sure the adolescent knows to take tetracycline on an empty stomach to promote absorption.

Caution patients who are using tretinoin that this medication is **phototoxic.** It causes a rapid nonimmunologic reaction of the skin when exposed to sunlight, resulting in sunburn with even minimal exposure. Teach correct procedures for taking other prescribed drugs, such as tetracycline and isotretinoin (Accutane), and discuss possible side effects. Emphasize the importance of return visits to the adolescent's healthcare provider to monitor side effects of medications.

Psychologic support is an important aspect of care. Because adolescents are preoccupied with their body image and peer relationships, they often find having acne embarrassing. Encourage them to express their feelings and refer for counseling, if necessary.

Evaluation

Expected outcomes of nursing care can be found in the accompanying nursing care plan.

INFECTIOUS DISORDERS

Bacterial Infections

Impetigo

Impetigo is a highly contagious, superficial (epidermal) infection caused by streptococci, staphylococci, or both. The most common sites are the face, around the mouth, the hands, the neck, and the extremities. It is an extremely common bacterial skin condition in children.

Etiology and Pathophysiology. Minor skin abrasions, lacerations, insect bites, burns, and dermatitis provide the portal for the infectious agent commonly present in the environment. For these reasons, impetigo is more common in the summer months. Because the bacteria that cause impetigo live in the nose, the nose is a common location for impetigo lesions. *Streptococcus pyogenes* and *Staphylococcus aureus* are usually responsible for the infection. Staphylococcus aureus colonizes on the skin and mucous membranes, particularly in the anterior nares and throat. Children commonly touch or pick their nose and can spread the organism to a break in the skin. This infection occurs more commonly in children who are in close physical contact with others, such as in childcare settings, or who have poor hygiene.

Bullous impetigo results from *Staphylococcus aureus* that produces a bacterial toxin.

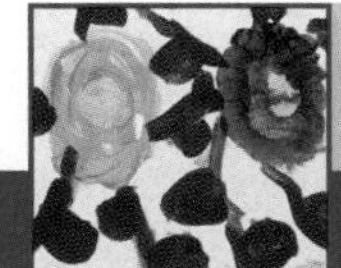

Nursing Care Plan

THE ADOLESCENT WITH ACNE

GOAL	INTERVENTION	RATIONALE	EXPECTED OUTCOME
1. Effective Individual Therapeutic Regimen Management related to daily skin care			
	NIC Priority Intervention— *Anticipatory Guidance:* Preparation of patient for an anticipated developmental and/or situational crisis.		**NOC Suggested Outcome—** *Symptom Control Behavior:* Personal actions to minimize perceived adverse changes in physical and emotional functioning.
The adolescent will verbalize proper hygiene, nutrition, and treatment of acne.	■ Teach good skin care: ■ Wash skin with mild soap and water twice a day. ■ Do not use astringents. ■ Avoid vigorous scrubbing.	■ Good hygiene and appropriate skin care reduce irritation, surface oils and bacteria, which intensify inflammatory reactions.	The adolescent exhibits habits of good hygiene.
	■ Praise good habits.	■ Positive reinforcement encourages continued effort.	
	■ Advise the adolescent to wash hair with antiseborrheic shampoo, avoid oil-based cosmetics or lotions; avoid hats and other items close to face.	■ Treats seborrhea, which frequently accompanies acne. Oil-based preparations can obstruct sebaceous glands, exacerbating acne.	
	■ Encourage a balanced diet, adequate fluids, exercise, and adequate rest.	■ Adequate nutrients, water, and exercise promote healthy skin.	
	■ Encourage the adolescent to keep a diary of health and diet habits.	■ A record may help identify associations with flare-ups that can be avoided in the future.	
The adolescent will verbalize understanding of treatment regimen.	■ Educate the adolescent about medications (action, side effects, dosage, and method of application).	■ Proper application of medication enhances healing of lesions.	The adolescent implements the treatment regimen as outlined, resulting in a noticeable reduction in lesions.
	■ Encourage application of tretinoin at night. Encourage use of non-comedonic sunscreens of at least SPF 15.	■ Helps reduce sensitivity to sun and avoid sunburn.	
	■ Educate the adolescent about time needed for response and importance of adherence to daily regimen.	■ May take up to 3 months for significant improvement to occur. The adolescent needs a reason to continue with the care plan.	
2. Disturbed Body Image related to biophysical factors (visible facial lesions)			
	NIC Priority Intervention—*Body Image Enhancement:* Improving a patient's conscious and unconscious perceptions and attitudes toward his/her body.		**NOC Suggested Outcome—***Self-esteem:* Personal judgment of self-worth.
The adolescent will demonstrate increased self-confidence and self-esteem.	■ Establish a rapport with the adolescent.	■ A trusting relationship promotes verbalization of concerns and fears.	The adolescent freely discusses concerns and fears.
	■ Provide education about the condition and therapy modalities.	■ Providing information better enables the adolescent to take control of the condition.	The adolescent demonstrates active involvement in own care.
	■ Encourage the adolescent to be responsible for treatment and follow-up, and give positive reinforcement.	■ Responsibility reinforces sense of self-esteem.	
	■ Encourage the adolescent to become involved with school activities and peers.	■ Involvement in activities helps enhance self-esteem and allows the adolescent to explore new experiences and friendships.	The adolescent shows increased confidence, as demonstrated by involvement in extracurricular activities.

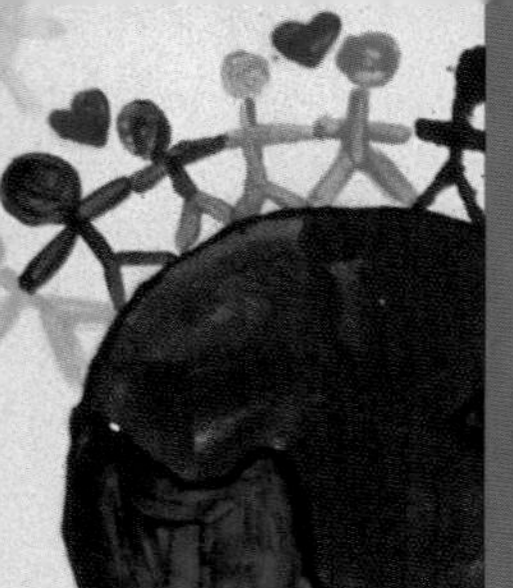

PARTNERING WITH FAMILIES

Caring for Acne

- ➤ Avoid picking and squeezing pimples. Wash your hands often and avoid touching your face to reduce the transfer of oils and bacteria to the face.
- ➤ Use gentle skin cleansers to wash the face twice a day. Do not use abrasive sponges or cloths. Wait 20 minutes until the skin is thoroughly dry before applying topical retinoid.
- ➤ Avoid the use of astringents and aftershaves that contain alcohol. They may further dry the skin and make it difficult to tolerate the prescribed treatments.
- ➤ Avoid hats or gear that can cause friction and occlusion of the skin.
- ➤ Greasy foods may leave a residual oil on the face and hands that can be occlusive. Wash your hands after handling greasy foods.
- ➤ Limit the use of pomades or petrolatum-based hair products. Keep hair spray and mousse away from the face.
- ➤ Use noncomedonic (for acne-prone skin) moisturizers to reduce irritation.
- ➤ Use oil-free or water-based makeup. Avoid waterproof makeup.
- ➤ Use noncomedonic sunscreen and protective clothing even on cloudy days as the medications used make the skin more sensitive to sun exposure.
- ➤ Protect the face from cold, windy weather.
- ➤ Do not get discouraged with daily treatments, as it will take 6–8 weeks before improvement is seen.
- ➤ Continue daily topical therapies, even when acne has improved significantly, so that acne does not return.

Staphylococcus scalded skin syndrome results from group II staphylococcus that produces a toxin that spreads systemically, causing the skin to separate below the granular layer of the epidermis. Newborns are at the highest risk as they have no immunity because of no prior exposure to the organism. Staphylococcus scalded skin syndrome in the newborn is known as Ritter syndrome, in which there is generalized exfoliation.

Clinical Manifestations. Impetigo lesions begin as a vesicle or pustule that is surrounded by edema and redness, usually at a site that has been injured. This progresses to an exudative and crusting stage. The initially serous vesicular fluid becomes cloudy, and the vesicle ruptures, leaving a honey-colored crust covering an ulcerated base (Figure 36–9a ■). Pruritus and regional lymphadenopathy may be present. Common sites include the intertriginous areas. The rash may spread to the face and extremities by self-innoculation.

In bullous impetigo, vesicles stimulated by the bacterial toxin enlarge and coalesce to form the bullae in a few lesions or scattered over the entire body (Figure 36–9b ■). A thin, honey-colored crust forms when the bullae rupture. When the crust is removed, a moist, erythematous lesion with a collar of skin around the shining, superficial erosion is seen. Lesions seem to occur more frequently in moist skinfold areas.

In staphylococcus scalded skin syndrome, the infant or child may have fever, malaise, runny nose, and irritability. This is followed by generalized erythema and skin tenderness. Within 48 hours, blisters and bullae (large blisters) form and the severe pain are present. In severe cases, the skin of the entire body may separate and slough. Bacteremia is rare, but dehydration and superinfections may occur with extensive exfoliation. Healing occurs over 10 to 14 days without scarring when there is no secondary infection.

COLLABORATIVE CARE

The goal of collaborative care is to diagnose the organism causing the infection and to implement effective antibiotic therapy.

Diagnostic Tests

Impetigo is diagnosed by a Gram stain and bacterial culture. For staphyolococcal scalded skin syndrome, bacterial culture, histol-

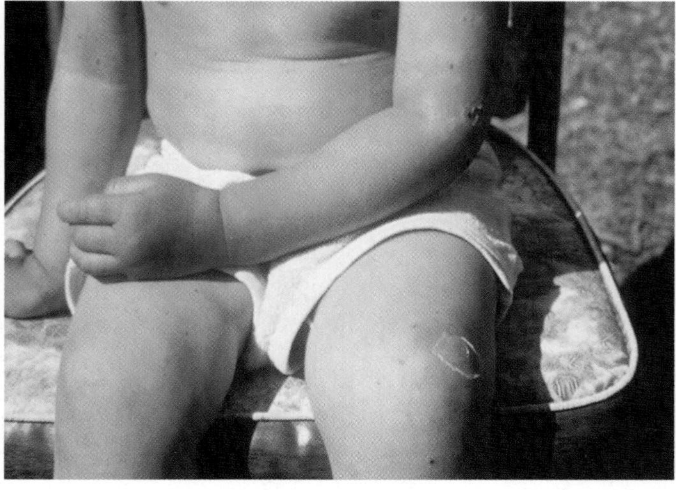

A

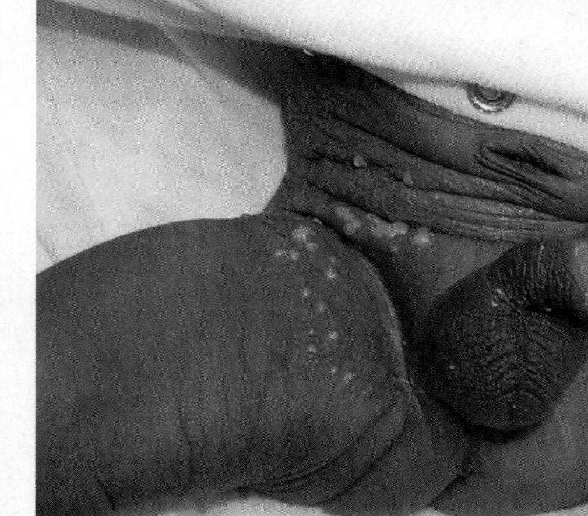

B

FIGURE 36–9 ■ Characteristic lesions of *A*, impetigo on elbow and knee, and *B*, bullous impetigo.

A, Courtesy of the Centers for Disease Control, Atlanta, GA. B, Courtesy of Dr. William H. Sorey, University of Mississippi Medical Center.

ogy, and exfoliated skin cytology testing are performed to distinguish the condition from toxic epidermal necrolysis (see the clinical manifestations table on page 1469). Methicillin-resistant *Staphylococcus aureus* is becoming more common and identifying the appropriate antibiotic to which the organism is sensitive is critical when there is poor response to initial topical or systemic antibiotics.

Clinical Therapy

Local treatment involves removal of the crusts and application of a topical antibiotic. Crusts are soaked in warm water and gently scrubbed off with an antiseptic soap. A topical bactericidal ointment (such as bacitracin or mupirocin) is applied for 5 to 7 days. If there is no response to topical antibiotics, a skin culture and a systemic antibiotic (e.g., dicloxacillin or erythromycin) may be needed. In children with bullous impetigo, an oral antibiotic may be used. The infection continues to be communicable for 48 hours after antibiotic ointment treatment is begun.

PRACTICE ALERT

If the child has a history of recurrent impetigo, determine if a caregiver or family member is a nasal carrier of *Staphylococcus aureus.* The carrier can be effectively treated with topical mupirocin ointment applied to the nares four times daily (Mancini, 2000).

Staphylococcal scalded skin syndrome in infants and children with extensive skin involvement is treated with IV antibiotics. The affected skin is treated like other burn injuries, as described later in the chapter.

NURSING MANAGEMENT

Advise parents that oral or topical medications must be continued for the full number of days prescribed. Tell the parents to observe all close contacts and family members for the development of lesions. Caution parents that an infected child should not share towels or toiletries with others and that all linens and clothing used by the child should be washed separately with detergent in hot water. Fingernails should be kept short and clean to prevent the spread of infection from scratching. Inform the childcare center about the child's infection, so toys and surfaces can be sanitized. Assist childcare centers in establishing guidelines for regular toy and surface sanitation, and for an exclusion policy for infected children.

Prevention of skin infections with methicillin-resistant *Staphylococcus aureus* is an important nursing role. An increased number of cases have been reported among athletes in high school, particularly when skin trauma occurs or when items are shared. Educate parents, adolescents, coaches, and teachers about the importance of a regular schedule for cleaning equipment, showers with soap and hot water after all practice sessions, discouraging sharing towels and clothing, covering wounds, and recognizing infections that need treatment (Centers for Disease Control, 2003a).

Folliculitis

Folliculitis is a superficial inflammation of the pilosebaceous follicle caused by infection, trauma, or irritation. The causative organism is usually *Staphylococcus aureus,* but *Pseudomonas aeruginosa* may also be a cause. The condition is common in children and teenagers because of increased sweat production. Folliculitis may be associated with Pseudomonas exposure in an inadequately chlorinated pool or hot tub. Lesions develop 8 to 48 hours after exposure.

Symptoms include tenderness, localized swelling, and the formation of tiny dome-shaped, yellowish pustules and red papules at follicular openings with surrounding erythema. Itching may be noted. Individual lesions may become deeper and form an abscess (furuncle). Lesions are usually seen in clusters on the face, scalp, trunk, and extremities. Ruptured lesions heal with hyperpigmentation and no scarring. Folliculitis caused by pseudomonas associated with hot tubs may develop on areas covered by bathing suits. Pustules may be isolated or separated from each other. While many children only have a rash, some children have fever, aching, and flulike symptoms.

Treatment of inflamed follicles consists of washing the affected area with a topical antibiotic cleanser and water, followed by application of hot compresses for 20 minutes, four times a day. In the case of Pseudomonas folliculitis, avoiding the contaminated water source will eliminate the folliculitis as pseudomonas needs a moist environment. A benzoyl peroxide gel or wash or another drying agent will also help clear the infection. Complications are rare. If lesions do not resolve within 1 week, the child may need systemic antibiotics (e.g., cephalexin or dicloxacillin) and, if the infection is deep, incision and drainage.

Nursing Management. Nursing management focuses on educating the parents and child about prevention. Advise children to shower daily and shortly after exercise, to cleanse with an antibacterial soap, and to wear loose cotton clothing. Talk with parents about the importance of maintaining the correct pH level and chlorine concentration in swimming pools, whirlpools, and hot tubs. Bathing suits of affected children should be laundered and well dried before the next use.

Cellulitis

Cellulitis is an acute inflammation of the dermis and underlying connective tissue characterized by red or lilac, tender, warm, edematous skin that may have an ill-defined, nonelevated border. The condition usually occurs on the face and extremities as a result of trauma or compromise of the skin barrier.

Etiology and Pathophysiology. Children with cellulitis often have a history of trauma, impetigo, folliculitis, or recent otitis media. Common causative organisms are *Staphylococcus aureus, Streptococcus pneumoniae, Hemophilus influenza,* and beta-hemolytic and group A streptococcus. The condition may also result from a nearby abscess or sinusitis. Onset is usually rapid.

Clinical Manifestations. Children with cellulitis have a rapid onset and they appear ill. Classic signs and symptoms include erythema, edema of the face or infected limb, warmth, and tenderness around the infected site (Figure 36–10 ■). Other symptoms include fever, chills, malaise, and enlargement and tenderness of regional lymph nodes. Lymphangitis may be present. In some cases, a rapidly progressive lesion may result in septicemia.

COLLABORATIVE CARE

The goal of collaborative care is to initiate rapid effective antibiotic treatment of the infection to prevent progression of the infection into deeper tissues.

Diagnostic Tests

A complete blood count with differential may show an increase in white blood cells. Cultures may be taken by needle aspiration to identify the causative organisms. Blood cultures are taken if the child has a toxic (very ill) appearance.

Clinical Therapy

If the face is involved, IV antibiotic therapy is administered to avoid serious complications. (Periorbital cellulitis is discussed in Chapter 32∞.) Children with severe cases or a large affected surface area are hospitalized to prevent sepsis. Systemic antibiotics and analgesics are administered.

Children with cellulitis on the trunk, limbs, or perianal area may be treated on an outpatient basis with oral antibiotics. Recovery begins within 48 hours, but therapy should continue for at least 10 days. Untreated cellulitis or cellulitis that does not respond to treatment can lead to osteomyelitis, arthritis, or serious systemic infection.

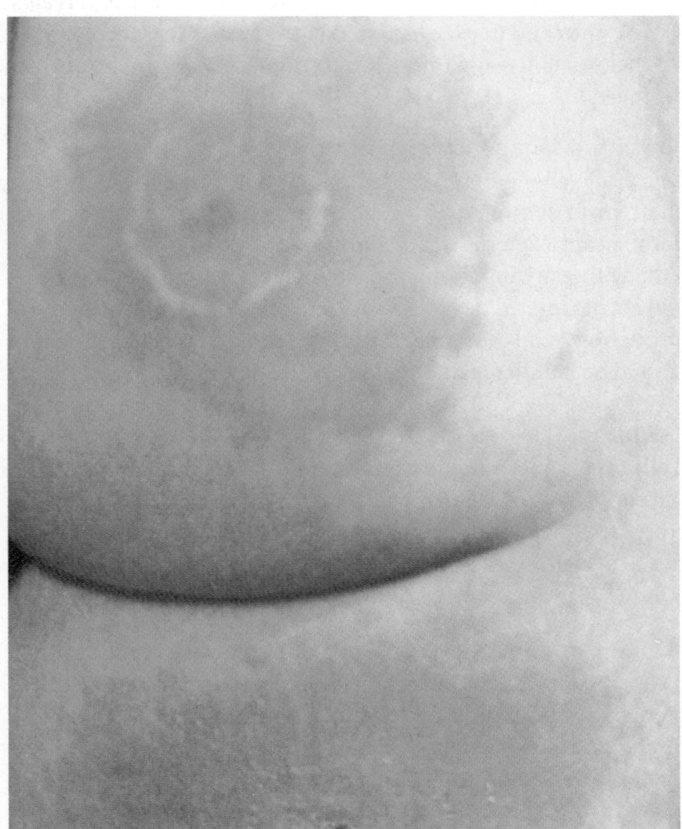

FIGURE 36–10 ■ Characteristic appearance of cellulitis.

From Ben-Amitai, D., & Ashkenazi, S. (1993). Common bacterial skin infections in children. Pediatric Annals, 22(4), 226. Photograph courtesy of Dr. Aryeh Metzker.

NURSING MANAGEMENT

The goal of nursing management is to recognize the seriousness of the infection and to provide support and education to the family for effective home care and recognition of complications.

■ Nursing Assessment and Diagnosis

Assessment centers on recognition of infection, documentation of location and related symptoms, and monitoring of vital signs and response to therapy.

Examples of nursing diagnoses that may be appropriate for the child with cellulitis are as follows:

- Impaired Skin Integrity related to mechanical factors (injury, the inflammatory process, and presence of infection)
- Acute Pain related to injury agents (swelling and inflammation of the skin)
- Readiness for Enhanced Knowledge related to home care needs of child with an infection

■ Planning and Implementation

While hospitalization is common, many children are treated on an outpatient basis. Because of the risk of sepsis, cellulitis should be managed carefully. Administer prescribed oral or IV antibiotics as scheduled. Supportive care includes warm compresses to the affected area four times daily, elevation of the affected limb, and bed rest. Outpatient follow-up is crucial to ensure appropriate response to therapy.

Advise parents about possible complications, such as abscess formation. Instruct parents of children who are treated at home to contact their healthcare provider if the child displays any of the following:

- Spread of the infected area in the 24- to 48-hour period after the start of treatment
- Temperature over 38.3°C (101°F)
- Increased lethargy

Reinforce to parents the importance of adherence to the treatment regimen and the seriousness of complications.

■ Evaluation

Expected outcomes of nursing care include pain control, adherence to administration of antibiotics, and resolution of the infection without progression to systemic infection.

Viral Infectious Disorders

Molluscum Contagiosum

Molluscum contagiosum is a viral infection of the skin caused by the pox virus transmitted by direct contact or by contact with the virus on surfaces. The individual lesions are pearl-like, skin-colored smooth papules about 1 to 5 mm in size. The lesion has a central depression and a plug of cheesy material that can be expressed when punctured. Lesions may appear anywhere on the body, but tend to be seen more commonly on the face, eyelids, axillae, cubital creases, thighs, and genitoanal region. The palms and soles are not involved. Children generally have 11 to 20 lesions that appear singly or in groups. Immunosuppressed and immunodeficient children often have larger and more numerous lesions. Children with atopic dermatitis treated with topical corticosteroids may have more numerous lesions. The lesions often disappear spontaneously in 6 to 9 months, but the condition can continue for several years.

Clinical therapy may involve the application of tretinoin to irritate the skin and stimulate the immune system to recognize that a viral condition is present and then respond. Curettage after topical anesthesia application may be performed by dermatologists. Cryotherapy, freezing each lesion with liquid nitrogen, is an alternate procedure. Care must be taken in reducing the pain and trauma associated with treating children. Scarring often results from any of the clinical therapies. Secondary infections are a potential complication. In mild cases, the lesions may be permitted to resolve without intervention.

Nursing Management. Nursing education focuses on reducing disease transmission. Public swimming pools, hot tubs, and other joint bathing should be avoided as children more easily transmit the virus when the skin is wet. Transmission of the virus among members of the household is high. Towels and sponges should not be shared.

The parents or child should wash the skin daily with gentle fragrance-free cleansers. A hypoallergenic moisturizer or emollient is then applied to the entire skin surface. If tretinoin is selected as a therapy, educate the parents to apply the lotion. Educate parents to recognize potential secondary infections.

When intervention such as curettage or cryotherapy is performed, provide information to help the child understand what will happen, and then provide distraction during the procedure to reduce anxiety. Ensure that the child has adequate topical anesthetic to minimize any pain from the intervention.

Warts (Papillomavirus)

Warts in children are a common cause of healthcare visits. Several types of human papillomavirus infect epithelial cells and causes benign epithelial tumors called warts. Various types of warts are found in children: common warts that appear on any skin surface and plantar warts found on the feet. The human papillomavirus is commonly transmitted by direct skin-to-skin contact or mucous membrane contact. The virus may well survive on various surfaces, and transmission can occur with contact, such as plantar warts from locker room floors. The incubation period may be 2 to 6 months; however, a latency period may exist in some cases. Children with immune compromise are more susceptible to the human papillomavirous and often have numerous warts.

Common warts appear as skin-colored, rough, scaly papules and nodules on exposed skin surfaces. Individual and multiple warts may be seen, but they may form large plaques if autoinoculation occurs. Warts usually cause no pain or itching unless in skin surface areas or creases that becomes irritated. Plantar warts appear as papules and plaques on the bottom of feet that grow inward and cause pain. Small black dots result from thrombosed vessels on the surface of the warts caused by weight bearing.

Clinical therapy for warts varies from no treatment to some form of destructive therapy which is individualized to the location, number, and type. Examples of treatments include cryotherapy, application of caustic substances or peeling agents, duct tape, electrocautery, and laser therapy. Treatment is not always successful and may result in scarring; however, warts tend to disappear spontaneously over a couple of years.

Nursing Management

Educate the parents and child about the application of peeling agents and caustic substances when prescribed for home use. If the reaction to the substance is painful, encourage the parents to reduce the frequency of the treatment until the pain subsides and then to resume the original treatment schedule. Successful treatment may take several months, and parents may need encouragement to continue the therapy and remain optimistic.

Other viral skin conditions are described in Chapter 19∞.

Fungal Infections

Oral Candidiasis (Thrush)

Oral candidiasis (moniliasis or thrush) is a fungal infection that occurs as an acute condition in newborns (usually acquired during birth from the vaginal canal of an infected mother). It is also a chronic condition in young children who have an immune disorder, regularly use a corticosteroid inhaler, or are receiving antibiotics, which have disturbed the normal flora, allowing the growth of the fungus.

Candida albicans causes 50% to 60% of the infections (American Academy of Pediatrics [AAP], 2003). Newborns may become infected in utero, during passage through the vagina, or postnatally. Transmission rarely occurs from person to person. Individuals at risk for invasive candida infection include those with impaired immune status, immunodeficiency, prolonged hyperalimentation, and receiving broad-spectrum antibiotics.

Oral thrush is characterized by white patches that resemble coagulated milk on the oral mucosa and may bleed when removed (Figure 36–11 ■). The white patches of candidiasis are easily differentiated from coagulated milk. Milk residue can be removed from the oral mucosa with gentle swabbing. With candidiasis, however, attempts at gentle removal are unsuccessful. (Avoid scraping the patches, as this will result in bleeding.) The infant may refuse to nurse or feed because of discomfort and pain. The infant may also have diaper dermatitis superinfection with candidiasis. Fever is usually not present.

Candida lesions may also be seen in the diaper area or various skinfolds of the neck, groin, axillae, and **paronychia** (infection in the tissue surrounding the nail). (See page 1466 for the discussion on candida diaper rash.)

Diagnosis is made by clinical appearance or by microscopic examination of a skin scraping suspended in potassium hydroxide. The appearance of yeast cells and threadlike structures of the fungus is diagnostic. A fungal culture may also be taken.

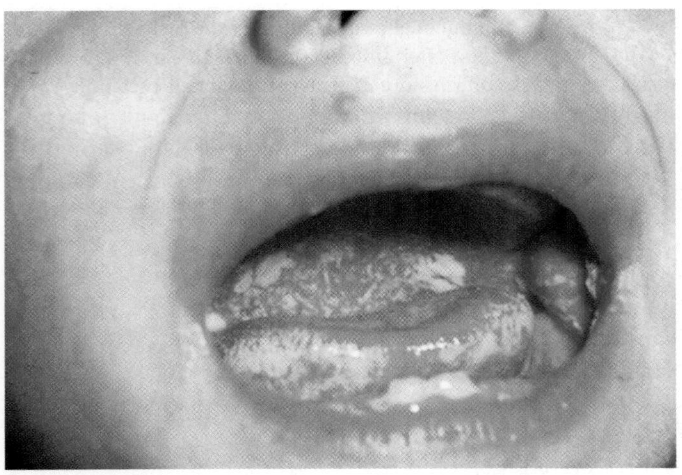

FIGURE 36–11 ■ Thrush, an acute pseudomembranous form of oral candidiasis, is a common fungal infection in infants and children.

From Zitelli, B. J., & Davis H. W. (Eds.). (1997). Atlas of pediatric physical diagnosis *(3rd ed., p. 104). St. Louis: Mosby.*

Treatment involves oral nystatin suspension or clotrimazole, which is applied to the mouth and tongue after feedings. Fluconazole or itraconazole may be beneficial for immunocompromised patients with oropharyngeal candidiasis.

Skin infections are treated with nystatin or one of many other antifungal topical agents such as clotimazole, miconazole nitrate, or ketoconazole.

If infection is severe, occurs in the esophagus, or invades other body systems, then oral fluconazole or itraconazole is required for a minimum of 21 days. Intravenous amphotericin B is used for invasive and systemic candida infections. Duration of treatment depends on severity of illness, the age of the child, and the extent of compromise to the immune status.

Nursing Management. Nurses educate the family to give oral nystatin to infants and children. For infants, instruct parents to use a swab to apply the suspension to the buccal mucosa and tongue surfaces, and then allow the infant to swallow the remaining suspension. Instruct older children to swish the solution around in the mouth before swallowing.

A significant nursing role is in prevention of candida infections, especially in infants and children at risk.

- Educate parents about the appropriate sterilization technique for bottle nipples and pacifiers the infant puts in the mouth.
- A commercial antiseptic spray may be used on toys that cannot be autoclaved, but follow directions carefully so the child does not ingest any harmful residue.
- Teach parents and older children with asthma to rinse the mouth well with water after using a corticosteroid inhaler to prevent candidiasis. If the child uses a spacer, that should also be rinsed with water after use.
- Meticulous nursing care for central or intravascular lines in children with impaired immune status or in those receiving prolonged hyperalimentation is critical in reducing the risk of invasive candida infections.

Dermatophytoses (Ringworm)

Dermatophytoses are fungal infections that affect the skin, hair, or nails. Children of all ages may be affected. The most common infections are as follows:

- Tinea capitis, involving the hair of the scalp, usually seen in prepubertal children between 1 and 10 years
- Tinea corporis, involving the skin of the body, except the scalp, beard, groin, hands, or feet; seen in children and adolescents
- Tinea cruris, jock itch or involving the inner thighs, inguinal creases, or perianal area; rare before adolescence
- Tinea pedis, athlete's foot or involving the webbed areas of the toes and feet

Etiology and Pathophysiology

Dermatophytoses may be spread from person to person or from animal to person, or by contact with an inanimate object such as the clothing, furniture, and bed linen of another infected individual. A carrier state for tinea capitis is suspected as some individuals are colonized but remain asymptomatic, particularly among family members of the affected child. These carriers may serve as reservoirs for infection and reinfection within families, schools, and communities. See Developing Cultural Competence: Tinea Capitis.

Clinical Manifestations

The clinical manifestations table on page 1479 compares and contrasts these infections. See Figure 36–12 ■ to contrast tinea capitis with tinea corporis.

COLLABORATIVE CARE

The goal of collaborative care is the accurate diagnosis of the lesions and effective therapy to treat the condition.

Diagnostic Tests

Diagnosis is confirmed through microscopic examination of the hair and scalp scrapings using a potassium hydroxide (KOH) wet mount to reveal rows and chains of spores within the hair shaft. A fungal culture can also be taken. To take a fungal culture from a scalp lesion, rub a cotton-tipped applicator across the scalp and place in a throat culture tube. A Wood's lamp, historically useful in identifying some forms of tinea that fluoresce under ultraviolet light, rarely is helpful as the more common cause

DEVELOPING CULTURAL COMPETENCE
Tinea Capitis

While tinea capitis can occur in any racial or ethnic group, it is most prevalent in African American children. This is believed due to immunological factors, genetic factors, or hair care practices. For this reason, any African American child with scaling in the scalp should be screened for tinea capitis (Elewski & Krowchuk, 2001).

CLINICAL MANIFESTATIONS of Tinea Infections

SITE AND COMMON DERMATOPHYTE	CLINICAL MANIFESTATIONS	CLINICAL THERAPY
Tinea capitis (scalp) *Trichophyton tonsurans*	*Noninflammatory lesions* • Circumscribed hair loss, erythema • Broken hairs; dotted stubbed appearance the color of the child's hair is seen where weakened hair has broken off • Diffuse fine scaling, may appear as seborrhea, with yellow, greasy scales • Mild itching • **Kerion**—large purulent tender boggy mass on scalp with drainage *Inflammatory lesions* • Papules, pustules, and crusting on scalp • Suboccipital or posterior cervical nodes	Griseofulvin orally for 6–8 weeks, or 2 weeks after symptoms disapper Selenium sulfide shampoo 2–3 times weekly, leave on for 10 minutes before rinsing to help eliminate scalp spores Alternate antifungal agents used when children do not tolerate or do not respond to griseofulvin include fluconazole, itraconazole, and terbinafine (not FDA approved in children < 12 years of age)
Tinea corporis *Trichophyton tonsurans* *Trichophyton rubrum* *Microsporum canis*	• Pink, scaly circular patch with an expanding border, may be scaly or erythematous throughout • Slightly raised borders with a clearing center • Multiple lesions on the face, neck, and arms may be associated with cuddling an infected kitten	Topical cream (e.g., clotrimazole, miconazole, ketoconazole, naftifine, terbinafine) twice a day for 4 weeks Wash body area with selenium sulfide shampoo An oral antifungal agent may be needed when lesions are extensive, involve hair follicles, or there is no response to topical therapy
Tinea cruris *Epidermophyton floccosum* *Trichophyton rubrum*	Annular lesions Scaly, erythematous eruption symmetric bilaterally, may spread to abdomen, buttocks, and upper thighs, usually spare the penis and scrotum Possible elevated lesions, possible papules or vesicles Can be associated with presence of tinea pedis, may have been spread by hand to groin area More common in summer months and in tropical areas	Topical antifungal agent such as imidazole for 2 weeks or butenafine, naftifine, or terbinafine for 1 week Wash body area with selenium sulfide shampoo Decrease moisture and occlusion in area
Tinea pedis *Trichophyton rubrum* *Trichophyton mentagrophytes* *Epidermophyton floccosum*	Itching Vesicles or erosions on instep or between toes (fissures, red scaly) Peeling maceration and fissures in lateral toe web spaces indicate a secondary bacterial involvement Dry scaly patches or plaques with mild erythema on plantar and lateral surfaces of foot	Broad-spectrum topical antifungal agent that has antibacterial properties, such as econazole or ciclopirox Keep feet dry with absorbent talc Allow feet to air dry Use 100% cotton socks, change twice daily

of tinea capitis and corporis (*Trichophyton tonsurans*) does not fluoresce with a Wood's lamp (Brodell & Vescera, 2002). Tinea caused by a microsporum infection fluoresces a brilliant green under the Wood's lamp (AAP, 2003).

Clinical Therapy

An oral antifungal agent (e.g., griseofulvin) is usually prescribed for tinea capitis, but resistance is developing. As the medication is still effective in higher doses, it remains the drug of choice. Medication must be taken for at least 6 weeks to be effective. Absorption of the medication is enhanced if given with a high-fat meal. Other drugs not yet approved for use in children include itraconazole, fluconazole, and terbinafine (AAP, 2003). Antifungal shampoo is often recommended. The child should be evaluated periodically during treatment to ensure that an appropriate response is noted. Kerions are initially treated with oral antifungal agents, but corticosteroid therapy may be needed if response is poor. Refer to the clinical manifestations table above for addition therapy guidelines.

PRACTICE ALERT

A large number of children treated for tinea capitis will develop an extensive, itchy rash on the trunk, extremities, and face similar to atopic dermatitis. This is called the "id" reaction, and it is a hypersensitivity reaction to the fungal antigen, not an allergic reaction to the oral medication. True allergic reactions to griseofulvin occur, but they are rare. Mild topical corticosteroids can be applied to the skin and a systemic antihistamine may be given for itching. Continuing therapy with the antifungal agent is critical to resolving the fungal infection (Williams, Godfrey, & Friedlander, 2003).

Topical antifungal agents are used for tinea corporis, tinea cruris, and tinea pedis. Oral therapy is required if tinea capitis is also present or if the response to topical agents is poor after

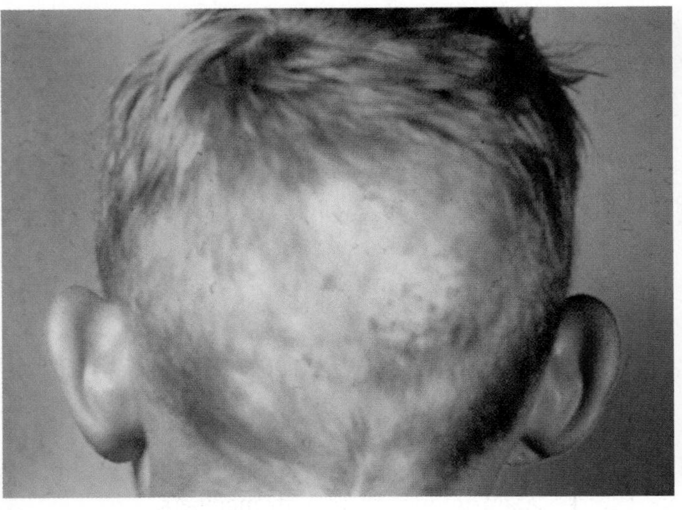

A

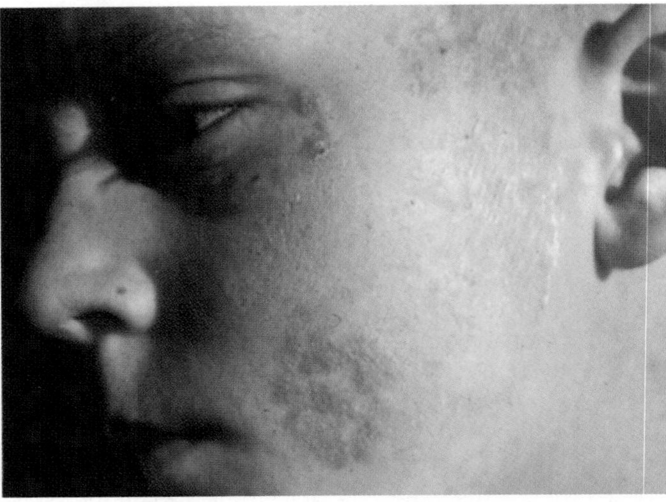

B

FIGURE 36–12 ■ *A,* Tinea capitis; *B,* tinea corporis.
Courtesy of the Centers for Disease Control and Prevention, Atlanta, GA.

the recommended length of treatment. Treatment should continue for 1 to 2 weeks after the skin lesions have cleared to ensure that the infection is fully treated. Topical medications with corticosteroids should not be used as first-line agents. The resolution of the inflammation may confuse families who think the infection is cleared earlier than expected. They may discontinue treatment too soon, resulting in a recurrence of the infection.

NURSING MANAGEMENT

All members of the family and household pets should be assessed for fungal lesions. Because person-to-person transmission is common, personal contact with hair and the sharing of hair accessories, brushes, and hats should be avoided. In some cases, there may be an asymptomatic carrier among the family, in which case all members of the family should be treated. Teach parents and children that fungi are found in soil and animals and are transmitted through direct contact.

Advise parents to give oral griseofulvin with fatty foods such as whole milk or peanut butter to enhance absorption. The medications must be used for the entire prescribed period, even if the lesions are gone, to prevent recurrence of the infection. Alert parents to the possibility of the "id" reaction rash so that they do not stop the medication.

For children with tinea cruris, encourage the use of cotton underwear and loose-fitting undergarments to promote dryness. An antifungal powder may help promote dryness and serve as a prophylaxis.

With tinea pedis, feet should be kept clean and dry and nails clipped short. Use of 100% cotton socks that wick moisture away from the skin is helpful in reducing the maceration and potential for secondary infection. Socks should be changed frequently. To help prevent tinea pedis, encourage children to wear shower shoes in public showers and the locker room.

Parents of children with tinea capitis should be told that hair regrowth is slow and may take 6 to 12 months. In rare cases hair loss is permanent, which can be particularly stressful for older children or adolescents. Provide emotional support and suggestions for hairstyles.

INFESTATIONS

Pediculosis Capitis (Lice)

Pediculosis capitis is an infestation of the hair and scalp with lice common in children between 3 and 12 years of age. Approximately 6 to 12 million infestations occur each year (Frankowski, Weiner, Committee on School Health, et al. 2002). Infestation occurs among children of all socioeconomic levels. The presence of lice may be noted by parents or teachers or by healthcare providers during routine examination of the child (see Chapter 8∞). Outbreaks occur periodically among preschool and school-age children, particularly those in childcare and elementary school.

Etiology and Pathophysiology

Head lice live and reproduce only on humans and are transmitted by direct hair-to-hair contact or indirect contact by sharing hair accessories, brushes, hats, towels, and bedding. Lice do not fly or jump, but they can crawl quickly. The female louse lays her eggs (nits) on the hair shaft, close to the scalp. The incubation period for eggs to hatch is 8 to 10 days. Children between 3 and 10 years are most often affected.

Clinical Manifestations

Classic signs include intense pruritus and complaints of "dandruff" that sticks to the hair (actually the nits) and "bugs" in the hair. Open sores from scratching may be noted. Nits look like silvery-white, yellow, or darker 1 mm teardrops adhering to one side of the hair shaft. See Figure 36–13 ■. Secondary effects of scratching include inflammation, pustules, and bacterial infec-

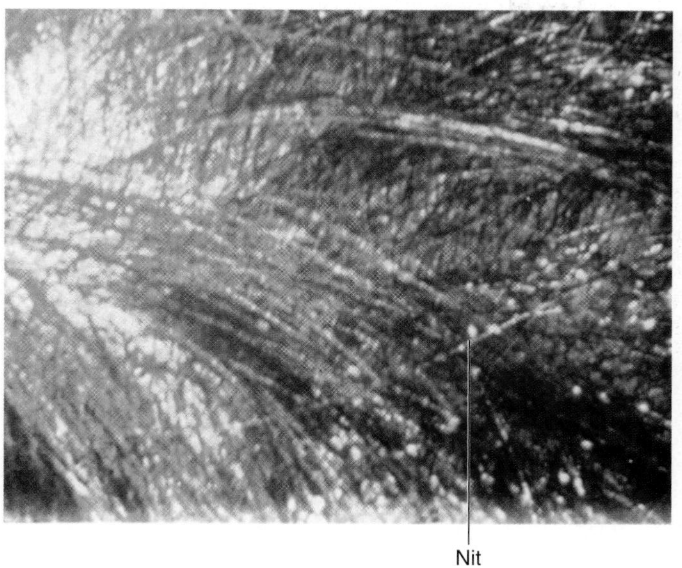

FIGURE 36–13 ■ Note the presence of nits adhereing to hair shafts.

tion. Nits are found most commonly behind the ears and at the base of the head. Lice are wingless insects about the size of sesame seeds. Lice move quickly away from light and are not commonly seen. Posterior cervical nodes are frequently palpable.

COLLABORATIVE CARE

Treatment involves the use of a pediculicide shampoo, such as pyrethrin with an enzymatic lice egg remover, or an ovicidal rinse, such as permethrin (Nix). See the medications table on page 1482. Pediculocides act on the nervous system of the lice, but are ineffective on the nits, as the eggs do not yet have a nervous system. Permethrin resistance has been reported at a 1% concentration, and evidence of the effectiveness of a 5% concentration in the case of resistance to 1% is unconfirmed. Permethrin products may cause an allergic reaction in children allergic to ragweed or chrysanthemums. A second line or alternate therapy is malathion (ovide); however, toxicity, flammability, odor, and higher cost are associated. Lindane shampoo is a last resort in the case of treatment failures. It is not recommended because of lice resistance and toxicity (Angel, Nigro, & Levy, 2000).

PRACTICE ALERT

Lindane is a second-line treatment for head lice, and it must be used with caution because of neurotoxicity. It should only be used when other treatments are not tolerated or other approved therapies have failed. It should not be used in infants and it is contraindicated in premature infants. Lindane is absorbed through the skin, and because infants and children have a larger skin surface area for weight, they may absorb more of the pesticide than adults. Most adverse effects have been associated with misuse or overuse of the product (FDA, 2003).

Permethrin cream rinse is applied to washed and towel-dried hair. The preparation is applied, left in place for 10 minutes, and then rinsed. The hair is towel dried, and the nits are removed with a fine-toothed comb. Distilled white vinegar or an over-the-counter formic acid solution helps loosen the nit's bond to the hair shaft. A second treatment is needed in 7 days, as the neurotoxin is ineffective on nits. If live lice still persist after two treatments, a prescription pediculocide such as malathion may be ordered,

NURSING MANAGEMENT

The goal of nursing management is to educate parents about the shampoo and combing of the hair to eradicate lice, and ways to prevent infestation among other family members.

Nursing Assessment and Diagnoses

Carefully assess children who have been exposed to head lice (see Chapter 8∞). Use a bright light and magnifying glass to see the lice and nits along the hair shaft close to the scalp. Make sure to distinguish lice and nits from dandruff flakes. To avoid potential reinfestation of other children, change gloves frequently when assessing several children in a classroom setting. If lice are hard to find, apply about 300 mL of isopropyl alcohol into the hair. Rub with a white towel for about 30 seconds. Check the towel for lice. The alcohol will intoxicate the lice forcing them to release from the hair.

Examples of nursing diagnoses that might apply with the child who has a lice infestation include:

- Risk for Impaired Skin Integrity related to scratching
- Effective Individual Therapeutic Regimen Management related to proper use of pediculocide and removal of nits
- Social Isolation related to exclusion from school until all nits associated with lice infestation are removed

Planning and Implementation

Infestation with lice can be upsetting for both the child and family. Emphasize to the family that anyone can get lice. Thorough interventions and education are essential for effective treatment. All family members and contacts of the child should be examined for infestation and should be treated as necessary. Teach the child not to share clothing, headwear, or combs.

Explain to parents that the shampoo and rinses prescribed are pesticides and must be used as directed. Keep these products out of the eyes, nose, and mouth of the child during their application as they will irritate the mucous membranes. Caution parents to use the pediculocide for the time specified on the directions. This ensures the product is used long enough for adequate treatment, but limits the child's exposure to the neurotoxin. If the child has extra long hair, a second bottle of pediculocide may be needed. No crème rinse or shampoo conditioner should be used before the pediculocide, but a crème rinse or oil after the treatment may make the combing easier.

MEDICATIONS and Preparations for Head Lice

NAME OF MEDICATION/PREPARATION	NURSING CONSIDERATIONS
Insecticide Free	
Lice B Gone Lice Away Enzyme Shampoo Hair Clean 1-2-3	Apply all products to *dry hair.*
Oil, petrolatum jelly, mayonnaise,	Cover with shower cap overnight.
Distilled white vinegar used as a rinse	Used as a rinse to loosen nits.
Formic acid used as a rinse	Used as a rinse to loosen nits.
First-line Pesticide Treatment	
Permethrin 1% Crème Rinse – Nix Pyrethrin shampoo (0.17% to 0.33%) or Piperonyl butoxide (2% to 4%)—Rid, A-200, R&C, Triple X, Pronto, Tegrin-LT, InnoGel Plus	Should be applied to *dry hair and scalp.* Massage into the hair one section at a time. Wet hair dilutes the product and may contribute to treatment failure.
Second-line Pesticide Treatment	
Malathion 0.5%—Ovide lotion Lindane 1% or "lindano"—Kwell, limited effectivnenss due to resistance	Apply to *dry scalp and hair* until soaked and allowed to dry naturally. Leave on for 8–12 hours. Do not expose the child to electric heat sources as the malathion treatment contains flammable alcohol.
Non-FDA Approved	
Trimethoprim/sulfamethoxazole Ivermectin—antiparasitic	Drug in bloodstream is ingested by louse, destroys bacterial flora in louse intestine. Does not treat the nits.

Because lice move so quickly, they should be killed before combing out the nits.

To remove the nits, use a small-toothed comb, tweezers, and a basin filled with water or isopropyl alcohol to dip and clean the comb and tweezers. Have blunt-nosed scissors available. Comb 1-inch sections from the scalp outward and pin these out of the way when done. All nits should be removed. Put the child under a bright light and use techniques such as a video to keep the child entertained during the procedure. Nits adhere to the hair shaft and must be manually pulled down the hair shaft with the comb, tweezers, or fingernails. If the nit cannot be removed, cut the hair shaft below the level of the nit. Make sure the parents know how long it may take for all the lice and nits to be removed from the hair shafts because they are firmly cemented to the hair shaft. The hair should be checked every 2 to 3 days and remove any lice or nits seen.

Some parents choose to use nonpesticide products to suffocate the lice, such as mayonnaise, petroleum jelly, margarine, olive oil, or baby oil. Flammable products such as kerosene, turpentine, and gasoline should not be used. Other products contain plant oils, isopropyl alcohol, and enzyme products to dissolve the outer shell of the lice and nits. No scientific evidence for the effectiveness of these alternative therapies has been reported. An alternate therapy for boys is to cut off all the hair, such as a close buzz cut. For girls, a shorter hair cut may help with nit removal.

Although lice can survive for only about 3 days away from a human host, nits that are shed are capable of hatching 8 to 10 days later. Even with appropriate pediculocide use, some of the nits will still hatch in 6 to 8 days. Repeat treatment is needed a week later. For this reason, bedding and clothing used by the child should be changed daily, laundered in hot water with detergent, and dried in a hot dryer for 20 minutes. Nonessential bedding and clothing can be stored in a tightly sealed bag for 2 to 3 weeks and then washed. Hair accessories, brushes, and combs should be discarded or soaked in hot soapy water (54.4°C [130°F]) for 10 minutes. Furniture and carpets should be vacuumed and treated with a hot iron when possible. Seal toys and other personal items that cannot be washed or dry-cleaned in a plastic bag for 2 weeks. Use of an insecticide in the home to kill the lice on carpets, furniture, and other items with which young children and pets come into contact is not recommended. Some families are challenged to adhere to these guidelines, such as those who are living in crowed conditions, having many stresses in their lives, and being homeless. Consider if a home visit would be helpful, and explore the complementary and alternative therapies the families use.

Instruct parents that children infested with lice should not return to childcare or school until after the first pediculicide treatment is completed. Despite recommendations to the contrary by the American Academy of Pediatrics, some schools and childcare centers have "no nits" policies, meaning the child cannot return until all nits have been removed (AAP, 2002). Parents of other children exposed to the infested child should be notified so they can watch for signs of lice.

If treatment failure is found, discuss the following issues with the parents to determine a strategy for improved outcomes.

- Review the application and use of selected products with the parents to ensure proper use.
- Review any potential sources for continued infestation.
- Make sure lice is the proper diagnosis.
- Actual resistance to pediculocides may be present and the next line of pediculocide may be needed.

■ Evaluation

Expected outcomes of nursing care include:

- Parents successfully remove nits after pediculocide treatment.
- Prevention measures used by the child and family are successful in keeping the child from becoming reinfested.

Scabies

Scabies is a highly contagious infestation caused by the mite *Sarcoptes scabei.* It is spread by skin-to-skin contact, and transmission within a household is very common. Adults often pass scabies on to their children. The highest prevalence is in children under 2 years of age (Angel et al., 2000).

The female mite burrows into the outer layer of the epidermis (stratum corneum) to lay her eggs, leaving a trail of debris and feces. The larvae hatch in approximately 2 to 4 days and proceed toward the surface of the skin. The cycle is repeated 14 to 17 days later. The irritation and intense pruritus is caused by hypersensitivity to the ova and mite feces, which occurs approximately 1 month after infestation. Nodules, which can persist for weeks after effective treatment, develop as a granulomatous response to the dead mite antigens and feces. Because the mite usually takes at least 45 minutes to burrow into the skin, transient contact is unlikely to cause infestation.

Symptoms include a rash with various types of lesions, severe pruritus that worsens at night, and restlessness. Papules on the hands may be seen in early stages. Lesions are usually located in the webs of the fingers, in the intergluteal folds, around the axillae, or on the palms, wrists, head, neck, legs, buttocks, chest, abdomen, and waist (Figure 36–14 ■). In infants pustules or water blisters on the palms and soles of the feet may be seen. The scalp and face can also be affected. Occasionally lesions appear as linear, threadlike, grayish burrows 1 to 10 cm in length, which may end in a pinpoint vesicle. The child's scratching and secondary infection may obliterate the lesions.

Diagnosis is confirmed by examination under the microscope of scrapings from a burrow, which reveals actively moving mites, fecal pellets, and eggs or nits.

Treatment involves application of a scabicide, such as 5% permethrin lotion, over the entire body from the chin down. Apply scabicide to the scalp and forehead of infants, avoiding the face. The lotion can be applied to the face of older children if lesions are present.

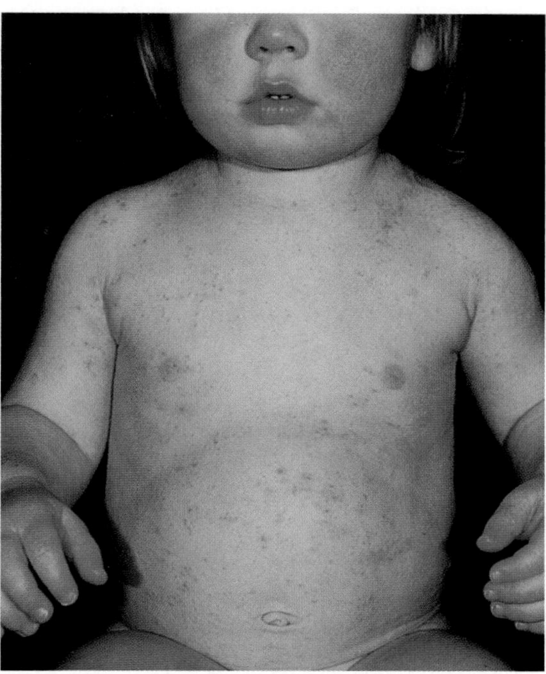

FIGURE 36–14 ■ Diffuse scabies in an infant. The lesions are most numerous around the axillae, chest, and abdomen.

From Habif, T. P. (1990). Clinical dermatology: A color guide to diagnosis and therapy *(2nd ed., p. 298). St. Louis: Mosby-Year Book.*

Application of 5% permethrin lotion or malathion (ovide) is preceded by a warm soap and water bath. Lindane is no longer recommended for full-body application in infants and young children because of toxicity (Angel et al., 2000). The skin must be cool and dry before the lotion is applied. The lotion is left in place for 8 to 12 hours (overnight) before washing it off. A second treatment is used 1 week later. Topical and oral invermectin is a new antiparasitic product with FDA approval for children over 5 years of age. All members of the household and all child caregivers should be treated at the same time, even if not symptomatic. Precipitated sulfur in petrolatum for 3 successive nights is used to treat scabies in infants less than 2 months of age who should not be exposed to the more toxic scabicide lotions (Metry & Hebert, 2000). It is malodorous, messy, and stains the bedding and clothing, so parents do not like using it.

Itching may persist for 1 to 2 weeks after treatment. An oral antihistamine (e.g., Benadryl, Atarax) may be prescribed to help relieve itching. Antibiotics may be needed when a secondary infection occurs. The treatment also dries the skin, further increasing itching. Encourage the use of emollients to moisturize the skin.

Nursing Management

Advise parents that scabies is transmitted by close contact and is highly contagious. All clothing, bedding, and pillowcases used by the child should be changed daily, washed with hot water, and ironed before reuse. Nonwashable toys and other items should be sealed in plastic bags for 5 to 7 days.

Family members who are not infected should avoid touching the affected child until after treatment is completed. If contact is made, hands should be washed well. Inform the parents about signs of secondary infections and that itching and nodules may persist for weeks after effective treatment.

Scabies, like pediculosis, can be embarrassing or upsetting for the child and family. Educate them about the condition, its spread, and treatment measures to prevent recurrence.

OTHER SKIN CONDITIONS

Birthmarks

Children are born with a variety of birthmarks or congenital problems that affect the integumentary system. Congenital nevi and vascular birthmarks are among the more common conditions. See the table below for clinical manifestations and clinical therapy.

Parents are very distressed by the presence of birthmarks on their newborn, especially when it is on the face and is viewed as disfiguring. Encourage parents to discuss their concerns and feelings. Provide education about the birthmark, expected changes, and when intervention might be appropriate. Since some birthmarks spontaneously improve, parents should be encouraged to be patient. Help them identify ways to discuss the birthmark with other family members and friends to gain support rather than pressure to treat the skin lesion.

Vascular Tumors (Hemangiomas)

A vascular tumor, or **hemangioma,** occurs in 1% to 3% of all neonates; however, by the age of 1 year, approximately 10% of infants are affected. An increased incidence has been noted in girls and preterm infants weighing less than 1,500 g. The risk for a hemangioma is greater in children of women who had chorionic villus sampling during pregnancy (Dinehart, Kincannon, & Geronemus, 2001).

Etiology and Pathophysiology

Vascular tumors are neoplasms of endothelial cells and increased numbers of small blood vessels that undergo rapid growth and proliferation during the first 6 to 10 months during infancy. This phase is followed by a slow **involution** (process of decreasing in size) phase that lasts years. It is estimated that 50% of vascular tumors have involuted by 5 years of age, 70% by 7 years of age, and the remainder have completed involution by 12 years of age (Dinehart et al., 2001). The tumor cellularity and vascular channels are replaced by increased fibrous and fatty deposits, tissue fibrosis, and fewer but larger vascular channels. Hemangiomas may be superficial (located in the epidermis), deep (located in the dermis or subcutaneous tissue), or mixed superficial and deep. Multiple hemangiomas or a large facial hemangioma are associated with hemangiomas in major organs such as the liver. Complications of hemangiomas are caused by their location as the rapid growth may press against or obstruct vital structures, such as the airway, eye, or ear canal. Ulceration of the vascular tumor may occur during the rapid growth phase.

Clinical Manifestations

Superficial hemangiomas are bright red vascular cutaneous plaques that resemble strawberries. Deep hemangiomas appear as bluish tumors covered with normal-appearing epidermis. Mixed hemangiomas have features of both superficial and deep tumors. The lesions, appearing any place on the body, are minimally compressible and have no bruit or thrill. Some chil-

CLINICAL MANIFESTATIONS of Common Birthmarks

CONDITION	CLINICAL MANIFESTATIONS	CLINICAL THERAPY
Salmon patch (stork bite)	Pink blanching patch on the forehead or neck; may also appear on nose, upper eyelids, or upper lip.	Usually disappears within 2 years without therapy, few if any cosmetic problems
Vascular formations (port-wine stain)	Purplish-red patches that progressively darken with age becoming deeper red or blue; usually on one side of the face. They stay flat and grow proportionately as the child grows. If patch is on face above the lateral canthus of the eye (in distribution of the ophthalmic branch of the fifth cranial nerve), the child may have Sturge-Weber syndrome with associated cerebral atrophy, seizures, mental retardation, hemiplegia, vision loss, or glaucoma.	Flashlamp-pulsed dye laser therapy on the small blood vessels of the patch to destroy the vasculature and lighten the discoloration. Early treatment is encouraged and may be more effective when young. In cases of Sturge-Weber syndrome, • regular ophthalmic assessments for glaucoma beginning at birth. • Magnetic resonance imaging is performed to detect vascular problems or atrophic changes of the central nervous system
Congenital nevus	Uniformly pigmented plaque that covers a large area of the skin. May have papillated surface and dense hair growth. Giant congenital nevi are rare and cover 20 cm or more skin surface area.	Full thickness excision and skin grafting is often performed due to high lifetime risk of melanoma. If surgical excision is not possible, perform regular examination (inspection and palpation) and comparison to photographs at 6-month intervals.
Café-au-lait spots	Tan macules that may have smooth or irregular borders. May vary from a few mm to 10 cm in size. May be an indication of neurofibromatosis (see Chapter 33∞) or Albright disease.	Monitor child for increase in size and number of café-au-lait spots and development of tumors indicative of neurofibromatosis.

dren have multiple lesions. As the vascular tumors involute, signs of tissue atrophy, wrinkles, telangiectasias, and hypopigmentation may be residual clinical manifestations. Ulceration of the vascular tumor may occur during the period of rapid growth.

COLLABORATIVE CARE

The goal of collaborative care is focused on evaluating the infant for potential complications and providing clinical therapy that will result in the best cosmetic appearance.

Diagnostic Tests

Initial diagnosis is by physical examination and monitoring the growth of the vascular tumor. In cases where the location of the vascular tumor suggests the potential for complications associated with pressure on vital organs or other abnormalities, additional diagnostic tests are performed, such as ultrasound, computed tomography scanning, or magnetic resonance imaging. If the airway is potentially compromised, a laryngoscopy may be performed. Complete blood count, platelets, and coagulation studies are obtained if the child is suspected of having the Kasabach-Merritt phenomenon, a condition associated with a rapidly enlarging vascular lesion characterized by hemolytic anemia, consumption of platelets, thrombocytopenia, and coagulopathy. Children suspected of having hemangiomas in the liver receive an abdominal ultrasound and Doppler studies.

Clinical Therapy

Various therapies are used for vascular lesions. Systemic corticosteroids are used during the proliferation phase for infants with extensive facial hemangiomas, including those in the periorbital area, as well as infants with Kasabach-Merritt phenomenon. One dose a day of oral prednisone is given for 7 to 10 days when a response is noted, and the dose is then tapered to the lowest effective dose for a 4- to 6-week course of treatment. Two- to 4-week rest periods between courses of corticosteroid treatment may be prescribed (Dinehart et al., 2001). Treatment often needs to continue throughout the proliferative phase so that rebound growth does not occur (Drolet, Esterly, & Frieden, 1999). Injections of corticosteroids into small localized hemangiomas are sometimes performed.

Pulsed dye laser treatment is beneficial for superficial hemangiomas during the proliferative phase. The proliferative phase is often minimized or halted with laser treatments at 2- to 3-week intervals. Laser treatment is also effective for treating hemangiomas that ulcerate, leading to decreased pain and faster healing.

Recombinant interferon alpha has been used in the treatment of life-threatening hemangiomas that failed to respond to corticosteroids. This medication works by inhibiting the rapid growth of blood vessels. Common side effects include irritability, neutropenia, and liver enzyme abnormalities. A significant adverse effect is neurotoxicity and potentially irreversible spastic diplegia that has been reported in 20% of children (Dinehart et al., 2001; Drolet et al., 1999).

NURSING MANAGEMENT

The goal of nursing care is to support families through the period of rapid hemangioma growth and treatment, helping them to deal with emotional responses to the infant's appearance.

■ Nursing Assessment and Diagnoses

Assess the distribution of the hemangioma and consider the potential for complications as it goes through a rapid growth stage. Monitor the child during regular visits for development of any complications, such ulceration or stridor that could be associated with compression on the airway. Monitor the infant's growth to identify periods of slowed growth associated with corticosteroid treatment.

Assess the parents' response to the infant's appearance and how they are managing interactions with friends and family about the infant's changing appearance. Take photos of the infant at each visit so that parents have a record of improvements once therapy is initiated.

Examples of nursing diagnoses that might apply with the infant who has a hemangioma include:

- Risk for Impaired Parent Attachment related to birth of an infant with an extensive vascular lesion on the face
- Impaired Skin Integrity related to presence of rapidly growing vascular lesion
- Risk for Infection related to potential ulceration of hemangioma

■ Planning and Implementation

Provide education to parents about the type of vascular lesion and potential treatment options. When corticosteroids are prescribed, teach the parents about administration and need to take full course as prescribed. Inform the parents about potential side effects, including gastrointestinal upset, sleep disturbance, temporary growth retardation, decreased appetite, and transient facial edema. Reassure parents that growth catch-up will occur once corticosteroid treatment ends.

Educate parents about the possibility of ulceration as the hemangioma grows rapidly and what signs to expect. Provide guidelines for covering and protecting the skin from infection until the infant can be seen in the outpatient setting. Provide education on appropriate care for the ulcerated area.

Listen to parents as they describe challenges with family and friends who comment about the infant's appearance. Role-play possible responses that parents can make to these individuals. Help the parents see positive characteristics in the infant, such as responsiveness to interaction and smiling, to promote attachment. Show parents photos of other children with similar lesions who have completed therapy. Demonstrating that improvements in appearance are gradual, but possible, is encouraging to parents overwhelmed with the infant's current appearance.

Prepare parents for changes to the child's appearance with pulsed dye laser therapy. Explain that the initial appearance will be darkening of the hemangioma for 1 to 2 weeks, and then the darkness will fade to red and eventual lightening of the treated skin surface. Following treatments protect the skin surface from trauma and keep the infant's nails short to prevent scratching. Cleanse the area treated with water and pat it dry. Inform parents to avoid sun exposure for several weeks following the treatments, and to use sunscreen on the area in the future to protect the skin from sunburn.

Evaluation

Expected outcomes of nursing care include:

- Parents form a close attachment with the infant.
- Parents are able to cope with comments about the infant's appearance.
- The hemangioma is effectively treated and additional injury to the treated skin is prevented.

Epidermolysis Bullosa

Epidermolysis bullosa is a rare and severe chronic blistering skin disorder of genetic origin. (See Chapter 4∞.) The most common form has blistering that is limited to the hands and feet, but blistering can occur on any skin surface area. In some cases the mucosal linings of the body may be affected.

Three general classifications are simplex, junctional, and dystrophic. The classifications for this disorder are distinguished by the inheritance pattern (autosomal dominant or recessive) and skin layer in which the split or blister occurs. Some forms of the disorder are life threatening and result in death at early ages. Within each classification of the disorder there are milder and more severe forms.

Children have extremely fragile skin and blisters form with minor trauma, friction, or heat applied to the skin. Blistering may occur in the mouth or throat, as well as the entire gastrointestinal tract. In severe forms, the blistering can be extensive and damage to the skin is apparent. Fingers and toes may fuse and contract leading to malformations. Children experience pain with blisters and may have difficulty walking when feet are affected.

The condition is managed by wound care, good nutrition, and minimizing the risk for infection. In the more common form of the disorder, blisters generally heal without scarring, and the condition may gradually improve with age. Open wounds increase the risk of infection so wound care is important. Blisters are lanced with a sterile blade or needle each day and drained so that they do not extend. The blister roof is not removed as it acts as a natural biological dressing. Antibiotic ointments are used when an infection is present.

These infants need two to four times as much protein and calories as healthy children because of the chronic wound healing. Additional vitamin A, C, zinc oxide, B_6, B_{12}, and iron are needed to sustain wound healing (Scober-Flores, 2003). Collaboration with a nutritionist and gastroenterologist may be essential to prevent malnutrition.

NURSING MANAGEMENT

Teach the family to provide wound care at home; it can be quite time consuming. In newborns, dressing changes need to be performed at a time that is good for the parents and the infant. The process needs to become a daily part of the care routine. Give new parents tips on aspects of dressing changes, such as gathering all supplies together first and then removing the dressings from one location at a time rather than removing all dressings at once as exposure of the wounds to the air is painful. The infant may be placed in a bath with dressings intact, and then when wet remove them one at a time. A second person is needed to assist the parent by carefully preventing the movement of an extremity while blisters are lanced and the dressing is reapplied. Holding or grabbing the extremity too tightly can cause further injury. Use soft music and distraction to help calm the infant.

Parents must learn to inspect the skin each day, to lance the blisters with a sterile needle, and to drain the fluid. A mild cleanser is used to wash and rinse the skin. Dressings that are stuck to the skin need to be soaked off. The skin is dried gently without rubbing. Nonadherent dressings that can absorb the fluid from blisters is helpful in preventing dressings from sticking to the skin. A bulky cover over the dressing (roller gauze or elastic tube dressings) is often used to protect the skin and promote healing. Fingers and toes must be wrapped separately so they do not fuse together with healing. Provide information about the signs of infection that the parents should monitor for on a daily basis. Determine if financial support is needed to ensure that parents have the dressing supplies needed to effectively manage the child's wounds.

Help the parents to identify ways to prevent or reduce the blistering of the skin but still permit the child to interact with other children and have opportunities for development. The child will learn to avoid situations that cause injury and blisters.

Promote good nutrition with adequate calories and nutrition to meet their growth needs. Protein is lost with blisters and chronic wound healing requires extra calories, so ensure that high-protein meals are provided. In infants, blistering in the mouth may interfere with feeding. A premie nipple is softer and may be easier for the infant to use. Vaseline on the lips may help reduce trauma to the mouth. If mucosal linings are affected in older children, provide liquid and soft foods. In some cases a gastrostomy tube is inserted for nutritional supplementation. Regularly measure height and weight and plot measurements on a growth curve to monitor growth and to identify growth deficiencies early.

Help parents and the child manage the psychological impact of this disfiguring disorder and the inability to fully participate in all activities. An individual education plan with an individual health plan will be necessary. Because the hands and feet are often involved, writing and test taking may be challenging. Mobility and walking throughout the school may also be challenging. Adaptations to achieve the most appropriate education are still possible in the school setting. Information needs to be provided to classroom teachers and classmates to help minimize injury.

INJURIES TO THE SKIN

Pressure Ulcers

An increasing number of children with disabilities are cared for in hospital, community, and home care settings. Many of these children are at risk for skin breakdown and pressure ulcer formation. Children at greatest risk are those with paralysis, limited mobility or high activity, sensory deficits, the inability to change positions, or chronic fecal or urinary soiling (Table 36–3). While the incidence of pressure ulcers in children is not fully known, 27% in a pediatric critical care setting and 14.6% in an outpatient setting have been reported (Curley, Razmus, Roberts, et al., 2003; Samaniego, 2003).

TABLE 36–3 Sites and Potential Causes of Pressure Ulcers

SITES	POTENTIAL CAUSES
Occipital region of scalp	Inability to lift head
Sacrum and buttocks	Confinement to bed or wheelchair
Legs and feet	Orthotics, leg braces, casts
Spine and neck	Scoliosis brace
Knees and elbows	Rubbing against bed sheet

Etiology and Pathophysiology

Soft tissues and capillary beds can be compressed for a prolonged period between a bony prominence and another surface. Tissue ischemia occurs when high pressure is maintained over a short period or low pressure is maintained over a prolonged time. The cells are deprived of oxygen and nutrients, and metabolic waste products accumulate, resulting in soft tissue injury. Without appropriate intervention, the injury becomes rapidly progressive and a pressure ulcer forms.

Clinical Manifestations

Pressure ulcer severity is defined in four stages (Figure 36–15 ■). Stage 1 is associated with the earliest sign of skin damage, an area of redness that does not dissipate within 30 minutes of removing

A

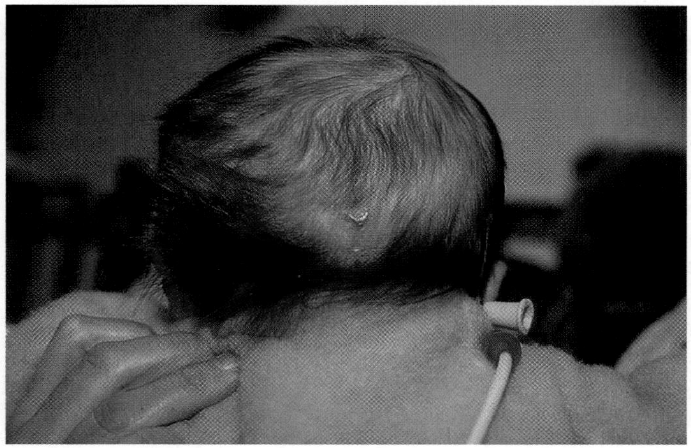
B

C

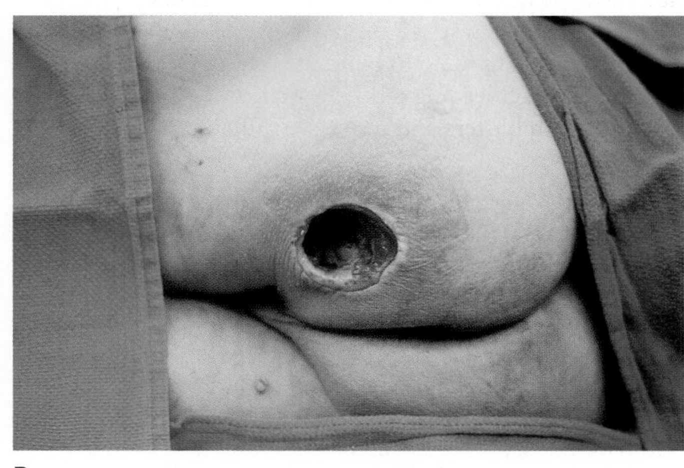
D

FIGURE 36–15 ■ The four stages of ulcer formation. *A,* Stage 1, nonblanchable erythema of intact skin that does not resolve within 30 minutes of pressure relief. *B,* Stage 2, a partial thickness injury, such as a blister involving the epidermis or partly into the dermis. *C,* Stage 3, full thickness injury through the dermis and into the subcutaneous tissue; deep crater with or without undermining of adjacent tissue. *D,* Stage 4, extensive tissue destruction through the subcutaneous tissue and fascia that may extend to the muscle, bone, or supporting tissues.

Courtesy of Sandra Quigley, Children's Hospital, Boston, MA.

the pressure or skin irritant. Children with dark skin may have persistent red, blue, or purple discoloration. In stage 2, the skin looks rubbed or raw (superficial or partial thickness injury), similar to an abrasion or blister. If intervention does not occur, the skin damage extends through the epidermis and dermis (full thickness injury) and an ulcer forms in stage 3. Injury deepens to underlying tissue (muscles, bone, or connective tissue) in stage 4 (Curley et al., 2003). The site of greatest pressure in infants and young children is the occiput. Older children have increased pressure on the sacral and occipital areas.

COLLABORATIVE CARE

No laboratory diagnostic tests are needed. Tools to assess the risk for development of pressure ulcers exist for adults and modification of the Braden Scale (which assesses risk associated with sensory perception, moisture, activity, mobility, nutrition, friction, and shear) has been proposed and is being validated for use in children (Curley et al., 2003).

Initial treatment for early stages of skin damage involves removing pressure from the affected site until the skin has healed. Children who use leg braces for alignment and mobility are often put in wheelchairs. Children who use wheelchairs are often put on bed rest on a pressure-reducing surface. Frequent repositioning is needed. A transparent film may be applied to affected red skin to minimize friction. Pressure ulcers are treated with various dressings, such as hydrocolloids, gels or hydrogels, and calcium alginates.

NURSING MANAGEMENT

The goal of nursing care is the prevention of pressure ulcers by regular assessment, skin care, and position change.

Nursing Assessment and Diagnosis

Carefully inspect the dependent skin surfaces of all infants and children confined to bed at least three times in each 24-hour period. Evaluate the risk for skin damage based on factors that can contribute to skin breakdown. See Box 36–5 for risk factors.

Identify the size (diameter and depth) and character of the skin lesion. Note any signs of infection, the appearance of wound edges, and the type of tissue at the wound base. Describe drainage amount, color, and type.

Examples of nursing diagnoses that may be appropriate for the child at risk for pressure sores are as follows:

- Risk for Impaired Skin Integrity related to infant's heavy head and inability to shift position
- Risk for Injury related to sensory/perceptual alterations
- Impaired Physical Mobility related to decreased muscle strength and control

Planning and Implementation

Develop protocols for pressure ulcer prevention so that children at high risk are identified and appropriate interventions are initiated.

BOX 36–5 Factors that Place the Child at Greater Risk for Skin Breakdown

- Prolonged pressure over a bony prominence
- Decreased mobility and activity
- Decreased sensory perception of pressure-related discomfort or injury
- Perspiring or exposure to moisture
- Incontinence of urine and feces
- Excessive movement that can lead to friction injury
- Edema
- Poor nutritional status
- Use of orthotics, braces, or prosthetics
- Extended pediatric intensive care stay
- Conditions causing vasoconstriction, such as low cardiac output, in which blood is shunted away from nonvital organs like the skin
- Impaired tissue perfusion and oxygenation requiring ventilator support

Such interventions may include increased ambulation, posting a turning schedule or encouraging frequent position changes, use of pressure-reducing surfaces such as sheepskin, and use of moisture barriers. If the child is incontinent, change the diaper frequently to keep the skin clean and dry. A nutrition consultation may be helpful to ensure adequate intake of fluids, proteins, and vitamins.

Provide wound care and dressing changes according to agency guidelines. These guidelines may include irrigating the site with saline, debridement, and the application of a dressing appropriate for the wound condition. Avoid the use of tape to hold dressings in place unless a protective skin barrier is used.

Care in the Community

Teach parents of children with impaired mobility and diminished pain sensation to inspect the braces and skin under the braces daily for signs of irritation (redness or blisters). Take the braces off and help the child to use a mirror with a long handle to inspect skin on the bottom and sides of the feet, behind the knees, and lower legs. Check all edges of the braces for roughness or breakage that can pinch or scrape the skin. If any sign of skin irritation is seen and redness does not diminish within 30 minutes, do not wear the brace until the skin heals. Inform the child's physician so that an appropriate treatment regimen can be started immediately. To prevent braces from rubbing on bare skin, have the child wear cotton socks under the braces. To avoid irritation of the foot, shoes should be purchased that are large enough to accommodate the brace and the foot in the shoe. Advise parents to return to a prosthetist regularly for refitting as the child grows. See Chapter 35∞ and the Skills Manual for further information on the care of the child with braces.

Children who are confined to a wheelchair are at risk for skin breakdown on the buttocks and lower back because of the pressure from sitting for hours. A wheelchair cushion can distribute and shift the child's weight when sitting in the chair. Frequent position changes are needed to relieve the pressure on the skin. Teach the child to do wheelchair push-ups or to shift the weight by leaning to the side or forward for several minutes every 10 to 15 minutes. Make sure the child wears a safety belt when sitting in the wheelchair. Teach school personnel about the child's recommended protocol so they can provide opportunities in school to change positions and reinforce the routine.

Burns

Burns are the third leading cause of injury deaths in children between 5 and 19 years of age (Murphy, 2000). See Figure 1–13∞. Boys between the ages of 1 and 4 years are twice as likely as girls to be burned; however, the national average age of pediatric burn patients is 32 months. In 1999, 99,500 children less than 15 years of age were treated in U.S. emergency departments for burns (Perry, 2003). In Canada, burns to children under 5 years of age accounted for 54.3% of cases reported to the Canadian Hospitals Injury Reporting and Prevention Program (Health Canada, 2002).

PRACTICE ALERT

A full thickness burn can occur in adults after only a 2-second immersion in water with a temperature of 65°C (149°F). The amount of time for a burn to occur increases to 10 minutes when water temperature is 50°C (122°F). Because infants and children have more sensitive skin, less time is needed for them to receive a serious burn (Stewart, 2000).

The four main types of burns are thermal, chemical, electrical, and radioactive. Thermal burns, the most common burns in children, may occur through exposure to flames or scalds (such as coffee or grease), or contact with a hot object (such as a wood stove or curling iron). Sherray, described in the opening vignette, sustained a scald burn when a bowl of hot soup fell onto her leg. Chemical burns occur when children touch or ingest caustic agents. Electrical burns occur from exposure to direct or alternating current in electrical wires, appliances, or high-voltage wires. Radiation burns result from exposure to radioactive substances or sunlight. About 10% of all burns in children are due to child abuse (Rodgers, 2000). See Chapter 7∞ for a description of child abuse.

Etiology and Pathophysiology

Children at different developmental stages are at risk for different types of burns.

- Infants are most often injured by thermal burns (scalding liquids, house fires) (Figure 36–16 ■).
- Toddlers are at risk for thermal burns (pulling hot liquids or grease onto themselves), electrical burns (biting electrical cords or chewing through insulation of electric cords) (Figure 36–17 ■), contact burns, and chemical burns (ingesting cleaning agents and other substances) associated with exploring the environment.
- Preschool-age children are most often injured by scalding or contact with hot appliances (curling irons, ovens).
- School-age children are at risk for thermal burns (playing with matches, fireworks), electrical burns (climbing high-voltage towers, climbing trees, and contact with electrical wires), and chemical burns (combustion experiments) associated with their curiosity and interest in experimentation (Figure 36–18 ■).
- Adolescents also experience thermal, chemical, and electrical burns.

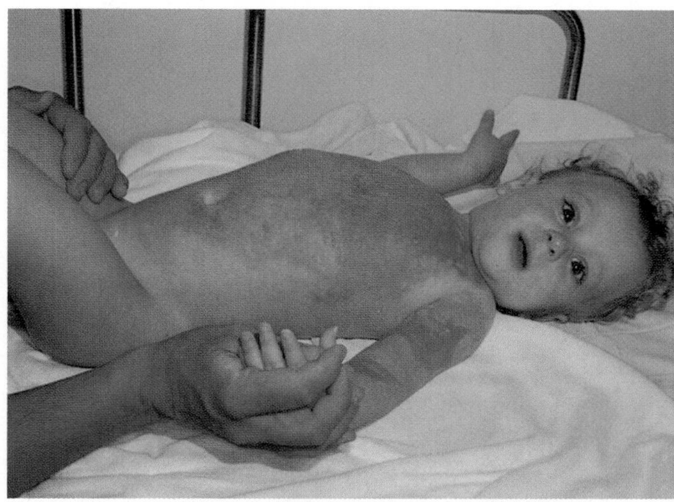

FIGURE 36–16 ■ Thermal (scald) burns are the most common burn injury in infancy.

Immediately after the burn, intense vasoconstriction occurs in response to substances released by the injured cells. Ischemia due to vasoconstriction may increase the depth of the burn injury. Vasoactive hormones are then released, which increases capillary permeability. This permits fluid and plasma to shift into the interstitial spaces causing edema and decreased volume circulating in the vascular beds. Water is also lost through the injured skin. Capillary integrity is not restored for 18 to 36 hours after the burn injury. If fluids are not replaced, hypovolemia,

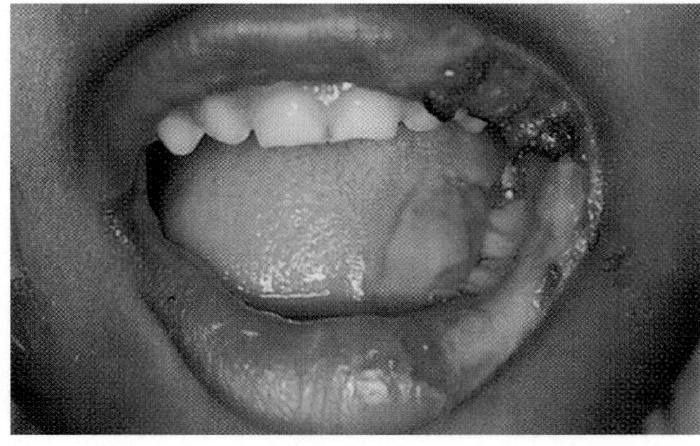

FIGURE 36–17 ■ Electrical burn caused by biting an electric cord. The burn is caused when the current arcs through the lips, often causing a full thickness injury through the mucosa, submucosa, muscle, nerves, and blood vessels. The labial artery may be injured and cause significant bleeding once the eschar falls off after 2 to 3 weeks.

Courtesy of Dr. Lezley McIlveen, Department of Dentistry, Children's National Medical Center, Washington, DC.

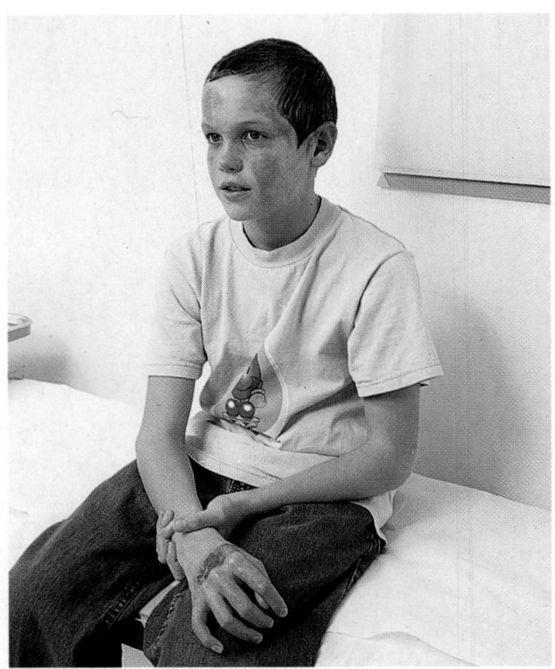

FIGURE 36–18 ■ The burns on the face and hands of this school-age boy were the result of a flash burn caused by igniting gasoline.

shock, and renal failure can occur (Milner, Mottar, & Smith, 2001). The child also experiences heat loss through the injured epidermis. The child's metabolic rate and need for calories increases as the child tries to maintain body temperature.

Clinical Manifestations

Burns are classified by depth. Burn depth may be defined as partial thickness or full thickness. Partial thickness burns, in which the injured tissue can regenerate and heal, encompass first and second degree burns. Full thickness burns, in which the injured tissue cannot regenerate, are known as third degree burns. The depth of the burn depends on the temperature and duration of the heat application, and on the ability of tissues to dissipate the transferred energy. See Figure 36–19 ■ for pathophysiology and clinical manifestations by burn depth. Severe pain is associated with partial thickness burns.

In burns from electric cords, the painless lesion appears as a white to yellow patch or depression surrounded by erythema. Edema develops in a few hours but subsides in 5 to 12 days. The necrotic **eschar** (the tough leathery scab that forms over severely burned areas) sloughs between 2 and 4 weeks after injury. Bleeding from the labial artery can occur when the eschar separates (Milano, 1999).

Signs of infection include purulent drainage, focal areas of necrosis, edema, erythema, discoloration of wound margins, and conversion from partial thickness to full thickness injury depth (Rodgers, 2000).

COLLABORATIVE CARE

The goal of therapy is to promote optimal functioning with minimal scarring, and minimal psychologic impact. Physical therapy and occupational therapy are important in promoting joint and muscle function with passive and active range of motion, as well as self-care skills. Splints may be needed to prevent contractures and to reduce scarring. Child life specialists can help the child cope with the stress and anxiety of the hospitalization through play activities.

Diagnostic Tests

Assessment of Burn Severity. Burn severity is determined by the depth of the burn injury, percentage of body surface area (BSA) affected, and involvement of specific body parts (Table 36–4). A Lund and Browder Chart with BSA distributions for various body parts at different ages is used to calculate the area affected by the burn injury (Figure 36–20 ■). Alternatively the palm of a child's hand can be used to assess the BSA to make a quick estimate of the burn size. The palmar surface (without fingers and thumb) is equal to 1% BSA.

Once the affected BSA is calculated, the burn can be classified as minor, moderate, or major. Reassessment of the extent of thermal injury is performed after 24 to 48 hours when the true extent of the injury can be identified. Children with moderate and major burns require hospitalization, and those with major burns should be transferred to a specialized burn center.

The involvement of specific body parts or specific burn distributions increases the burn severity, regardless of the percentage of BSA affected. Burns to the face, hands, feet, or perineal area are treated as major injuries because of the potential for functional and cosmetic impairment. **Circumferential** burns (injury completely surrounding the thorax or an extremity), anterior chest burns, and smoke inhalation are also classified as major burns.

Clinical Therapy

Initial Treatment. The first step is to ensure that the child has an airway, is breathing, and has a pulse. Then stop the burning

TABLE 36–4 Classification of Burn Severity in Children

Minor	
Can usually be treated as an outpatient	Partial thickness < 10% BSA Full thickness < 2% BSA
Moderate	
Can be treated in burn unit or general hospital	Partial thickness 10%–20% BSA Full thickness 3%–10% BSA
Major	
Should be treated in a specialized burn center	Partial thickness > 20% BSA Full thickness ≥10% BSA All burns involving face, eyes, ears, hands, feet, and perineum that may result in cosmetic or functional impairment All burns complicated by inhalation injury, major trauma, and preexisting chronic conditions

Adapted from Perry, C. M. (2003). Thermal injuries. In P. A. Moloney-Harmon, & S. J. Czerwinski (Eds.), Nursing care of the pediatric trauma patient *(p. 279). St. Louis: Saunders.*

PATHOPHYSIOLOGY ILLUSTRATED

Classification of Burns

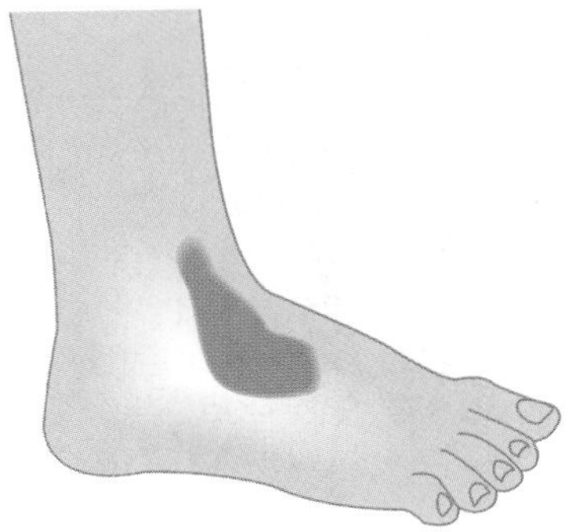

Superficial Partial Thickness (first degree)
Damages only outer layer of skin; burn is painful and red; heals in a few days (e.g., sunburn)

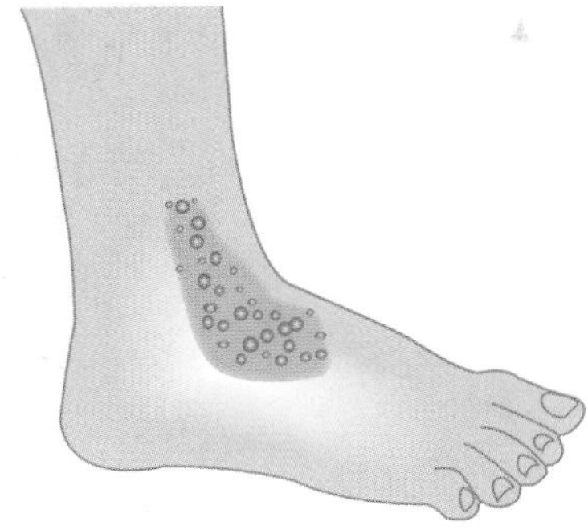

Partial Thickness (second degree)
Involves epidermis and upper layers of dermis; may have sparing of sweat gland and sebaceous glands; heals in 10–14 days

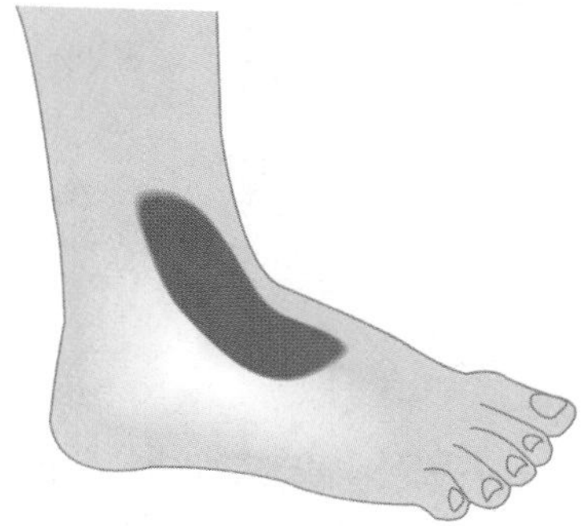

Full Thickness (third degree)
Involves all of epidermis and dermis; may also involve underlying tissue; nerve ending usually destroyed; requires skin grafting

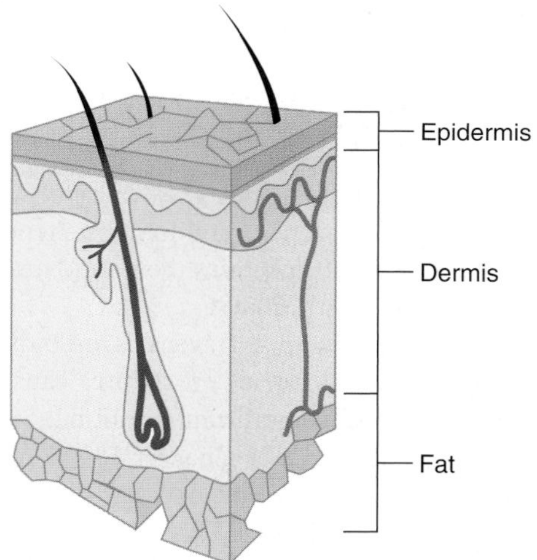

Erythema, blanches on pressure, no bullae, peeling after a few days due to premature cell death

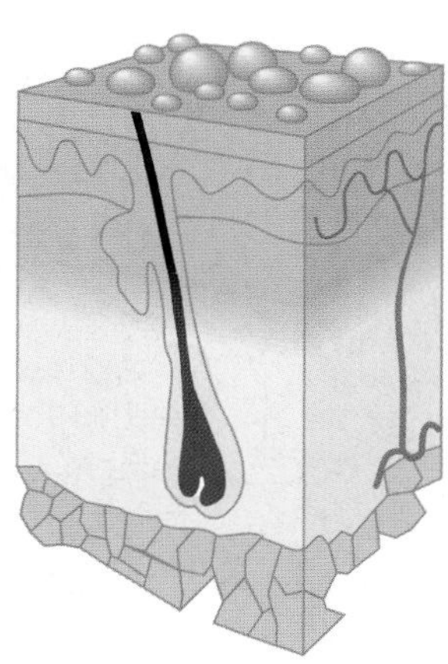

Blisters or bullae, erythema, blanches on pressure, pain and sensitivity to cold air, minimal scar formation

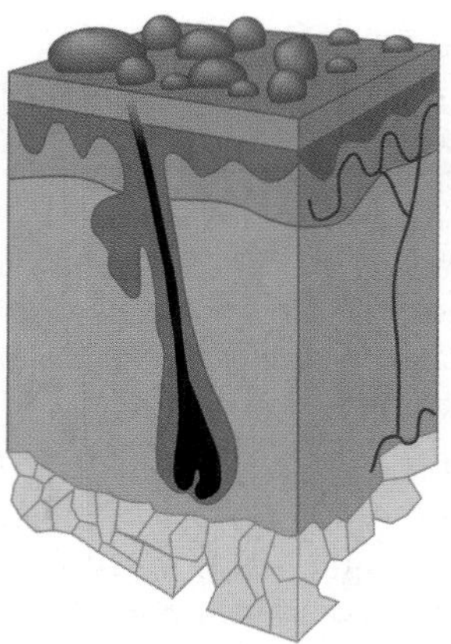

Skin may appear brown, black, deep cherry red, white to gray, waxy or translucent, usually no pain, injured area may appear sunken

FIGURE 36–19 ■ Characteristics of burns by depth of thermal injury.

process by removing any jewelry and all clothing. Moist soaks or ice (if small surface area is affected) are used to stop the burning process and to relieve pain. A tetanus vaccine booster is given if more than 5 years have passed since the last vaccine, or when the child has not completed the full vaccine series.

If the child has been struck by lightening, immediate resuscitation is initiated even if the child is not breathing and has no pulse. Begin cardiopulmonary resuscitation and give oxygen as soon as possible as the effect of the electric shock may be reversible. Once the child has been resuscitated, then entrance and exit injuries associated with the electrical burn can be identified and cared for.

Treatment of Major Burns. Treatment focuses on decreasing burn fluid losses, preventing infection, controlling pain, promoting nutrition, and salvaging all viable burned tissue.

Fluid replacement is necessary to maintain the cardiovascular and renal systems and to prevent hypovolemic shock in cases of major burn injury. Fluid shifts from the vasculature to the interstitial spaces (third spacing) occur soon after the burn. Fluid replacement for the first 24 hours after the injury is based on a fluid volume formula calculated from the child's body weight, affected BSA, and normal maintenance needs. The Parkland and Galveston formulas are two examples used to calculate the amount of fluid needed (Milner et al., 2001).

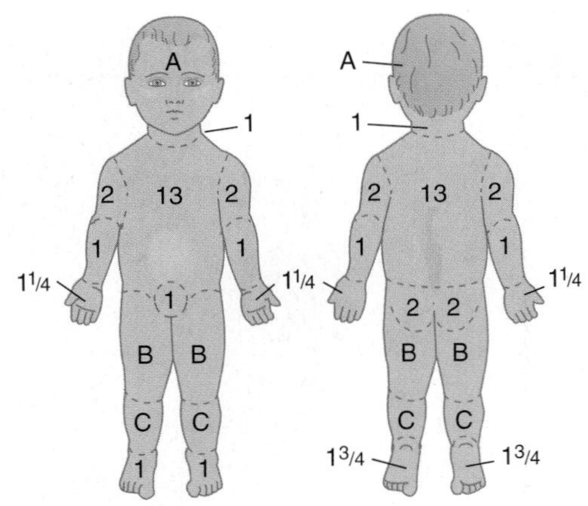

Relative Percentages of Areas Affected by Growth

Area	Age in years 0	1	5	10	11	Adult
A = 1/2 of head	9 1/2	8 1/2	6 1/2	5 1/2	4 1/2	3 1/2
B = 1/2 of one thigh	2 3/4	3 1/4	4	4 1/2	4 1/2	4 3/4
C = 1/2 of one lower leg	2 1/2	2 1/2	2 3/4	3	3 1/4	3 1/2

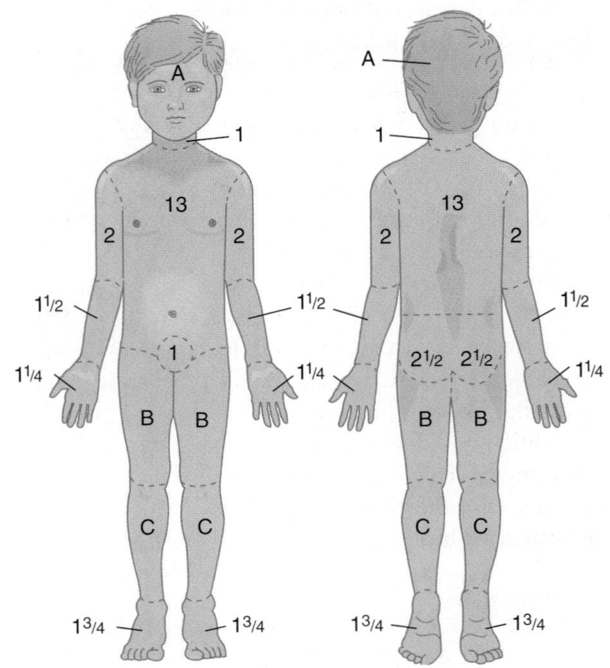

FIGURE 36–20 ■ Lund and Browder Chart for determining percentage of body surface areas in pediatric burn injuries.

Adapted from Artz, C. P., & Moncrief, J. A. (1969). The treatment of burns *(2nd ed.). Philadelphia: Saunders.*

CLINICAL TIP

- Parkland Formula: 4 mL × body weight (kg) × percentage of total body surface area = total 24 hour fluid requirement in mL. Maintenance fluids must be added to the amount of fluid calculated with this formula.
- Carvajal or Galveston Formula: 5,000 mL/m^2 burned area + 2,000 mL/m^2 of total body surface area = total 24 hour fluid requirement in mL.

Lactated Ringer's or normal saline solution is the preferred fluid. Hypotonic intravenous solutions such as D5W increase the risk of hyponatremia and subsequent cerebral edema and seizures (Stewart, 2000). Half of the total volume calculated for the 24-hour period is infused over the first 8 hours, starting at the time of the burn, not the time of arrival in the emergency department. The remainder is then distributed evenly over the next 16 hours. Fluid volume is reduced after 24 to 48 hours once the capillary integrity is restored.

Resuscitation efforts are also focused on maintaining the child's temperature, because heat is lost rapidly through burned skin. Vascular integrity is usually restored after the first 24 hours.

Fever is a normal, expected outcome of any significant thermal injury, but it is not always a sign of infection. Treatment may include analgesics, ice packs, cooling blankets, or cool hydrotherapy sessions. Infection of the burned area is, however, a frequent complication, and can cause a partial thickness burn to convert to full thickness (Rodgers, 2000).

Continuous enteral feedings are often initiated within 6 hours of the burn injury to support the child's increased nutritional requirements, which result from the increased metabolic rate needed to support healing and the body's stress response to injury (Herndon & Spies, 2001). These children often need nearly twice the basal metabolic caloric requirements and nearly 2 g/kg body weight of protein (Smith, 2000).

Aggressive pain management with intravenous opioids is needed for pain management and for all procedures causing pain. In addition, the burns cause a significant emotional overlay that increases the pain perceived. See Chapter 18 for a discussion of pain management. Cimetidine or other H_2 blockers may be ordered to prevent a burn stress ulcer.

Special consideration is needed when burns involve certain areas of the body:

- Deep partial thickness and full thickness burns develop eschar with no elasticity. When the burn is circumferential, blood flow can become restricted due to edema and result in tissue hypoxia. An **escharotomy** (incision into the constricting tissue) may be necessary to restore peripheral circulation.
- Facial burns usually cause significant edema. Care must be taken to ensure airway patency. For burns to the eye, an ophthalmologist should be consulted to assess damage and prescribe treatment. If the lips are burned, an infant may be unable to suck.
- Burns of the hands require careful management to maintain function. Special splinting and physical therapy are usually necessary.
- Perineal burns are at higher risk for infection because of frequent contamination with urine and stool. Frequent dressing changes are required. A urinary catheter is usually

inserted but is removed once hydration status is stable to minimize the risk of urinary tract infection.

Wound Management. Burn wound care has several goals: (1) to speed wound debridement, (2) maintain moist wound conditions and adequate circulation, (3) to conserve body heat and fluids, (4) to protect from infection, and (5) to control scarring and prevent scar contracture. Several treatment regimens are used to achieve these goals.

The entire body is bathed to initiate **debridement** (removal of dead tissue to speed the healing process). Conscious sedation and anesthesiology support are often ordered for pain management during debridement. Intact blisters provide a natural, pain-free, sterile dressing; however, some healthcare providers believe the fluid provides a medium for bacterial infection. Some burn centers keep blisters intact while others break blisters open. In either case the tissues should be carefully cut away when the blisters are broken.

CLINICAL TIP

Be sure to follow all agency guidelines for assessment and monitoring of child when conscious sedation is used during the debridement process (see Chapter 18∞).

Various options are used for wound management after debridement. Traditional burn care for a partial thickness injury involves the use of antibacterial agents, such as silver sulfadiazine, sulfamylon, or bacitracin after initial cleansing. The topical medication is applied to prevent bacterial infection and dressings are added to cover the burned area. Dressing changes are performed once or twice daily. These dressing changes are often very painful. When an old dressing is removed, a layer of eschar is also debrided.

Hydrotherapy (whirlpool) baths are given twice daily to help cleanse the wound before debridement, to increase vasodilation and circulation and to speed healing. The water loosens exudates, topical medications, and dead tissue (Figure 36–21 ■). As a rule, tap water is used for debridement. Gentle washing is necessary to protect new epithelial cells. Granulation tissue forms as a result of daily debridement. Superficial second degree burns reepithelialize within 3 weeks.

Skin grafting is necessary with any deep second or third degree burn. Often a temporary skin substitute or **allograft** (cadaver skin from a skin bank) is used to cover a second degree burn until healing occurs. See Table 36–5. The allograft closes the wound and allows healing or improves the condition of the underlying skin of a deep second and third degree burn until **autografting** (use of healthy skin taken from a nonburned area of the child's body) can be performed. The major concern over the use of cadaver skin allografts is the potential for disease transmission. The graft or skin replacement product is placed after the wound is debrided in the operating room to reveal healthy, bleeding tissue. This forms a protective barrier over the wound surface to decrease infection risk and to protect against fluid loss (Figure 36–22 ■). It is applied with a surgical adhesive or staples and covered with a bulky dressing or pressure dressing. See Box 36–6.

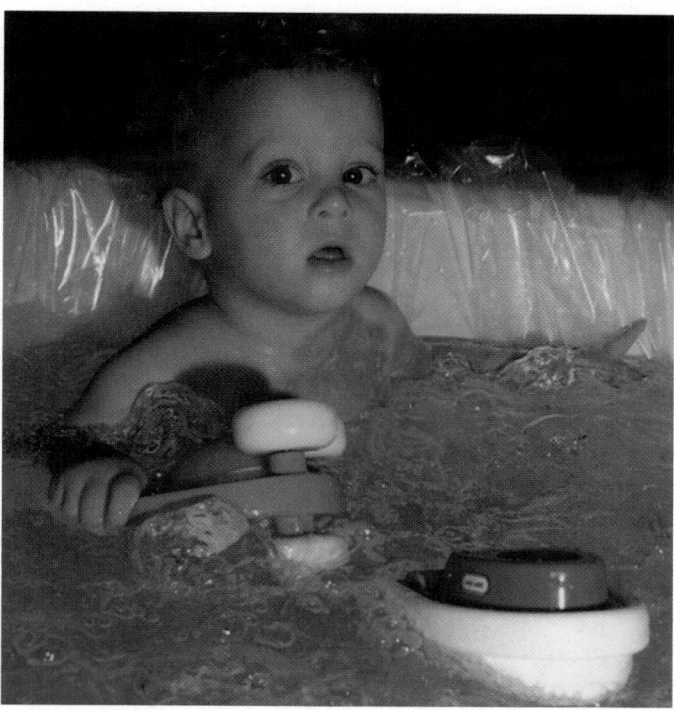

FIGURE 36–21 ■ A whirlpool bath is being used to increase this child's vasodilation and circulation, and to speed the healing of his burns.

An autograft is permanent. The donor site (where the autograft was harvested) is a new wound, causing pain and requiring close monitoring for signs of infection. A temporary skin substitute may be used to cover the donor site until healing occurs. Skin replacements may also be used to cover the burn and to promote healing (see Table 36–5).

The goal of therapy is to promote optimal functioning with minimal scarring and minimal psychologic impact. Physical therapy and occupational therapy are important in promoting joint and muscle function with passive and active range of motion, as well as self-care skills. Splints may be needed to prevent contractures and to reduce scarring. Child life specialists can help the child cope with stress and anxiety of the hospitalization through play activities.

During the rehabilitation stage, Jobst® or pressure garments are used to reduce development of hypertrophic scarring and contractures. Such garments are worn 24 hours a day for 6 to 8 months to shorten the time of scar maturation and to reduce the thickness of the scars (Perry, 2003). Cosmetic surgery may be needed to improve the child's appearance.

BOX 36–6 Research: Trans-Cyte

Trans-Cyte is a temporary skin substitute approved by the Food and Drug Administration that is bioengineered from newborn foreskin tissue. Research conducted in children indicates that it promotes healing more rapidly than silver sulfadiazine, decreases infection risk, avoids painful burn dressings, and reduces length of hospital stay (Wiebelhaus & Hansen, 2001; Lukish, Eichelberger, Newman, et al., 2001).

TABLE 36–5 Skin Replacement Products Used for Burn Injuries

TYPE OF DRESSING	CHARACTERISTICS	NURSING CONSIDERATIONS
Beta-glucagons collagen matrix Used for partial thickness injuries	Semiocclusive wound covering Decreases evaporative heat loss Nerve endings are covered so pain is reduced Effective barrier against bacteria	Is applied to wounds immediately after cleansing and debridement If it adheres well, it can serve as the protective dressing until the wound is healed
Biobrane Use for partial thickness injuries	Knitted nylon mesh bonded to a thin silicone membrane that provides a protective barrier against bacteria and water loss Placed over clean, debrided surfaces and donor sites May be used as a cover for autografts Provides a moist environment to allow for rapid healing	Minimizes dressing changes and associated pain May be left open to the air or covered with thick dressing Trimmed away as the wound heals Fluid accumulation under the membrane can occur Enables children to be treated as outpatients, reducing costs of care
TransCyte (see Figure 36–22) For partial thickness injuries	Human fibroblast-derived temporary skin substitute with polymer membrane and cultured human fibroblast cells Semipermeable temporary covering, allows for fluid and gas exchange Placed over clean, debrided surfaces May be used as a cover for full thickness burns prior to autografting	Minimizes dressing changes and associated pain Use adhesive strips and surgical adhesives to keep in place Cover with a bulky dressing for first 24 hours Fluid accumulation under membrane may occur Remains in place until the wound has healed, trim away as the wound heals Use is associated with less hypertrophic scarring Contraindicated in cases of known porcine dermal collagen or bovine serum albumin hypersensitivity

Data from Delatte, S. J., Evans, J., Hebra, A., Adamson, W., Othersen, H. B, & Tagge, E. P. (2001). Effectiveness of beta-glucagon collagen for treatment of partial thickness burns in children. Journal of Pediatric Surgery, *36(1), 113–118; Hansen, S. L., Voight, D. W., Wiebelhaus, P., & Paul, C. N. (2000). Using skin replacement products to treat burns and wounds.* Advances in Skin and Wound Care, *14(1), 37–44.*

NURSING MANAGEMENT

The goals of nursing care include prevention of burns, the careful assessment and monitoring of the child's condition and burn injury, pain management, psychosocial support of the child and family, treatment of the burn injury, and prevention of complications.

Nursing Assessment and Diagnosis

Emergency assessment is based on the ABCs of basic life support (airway, breathing, and circulation). Assessment of the airway patency is necessary, especially when signs of smoke inhalation or burns to the face and neck are present. The child is assessed for other potential injuries when the mechanism of injury also includes a fall or explosion. Additional injuries, such as from an ex-

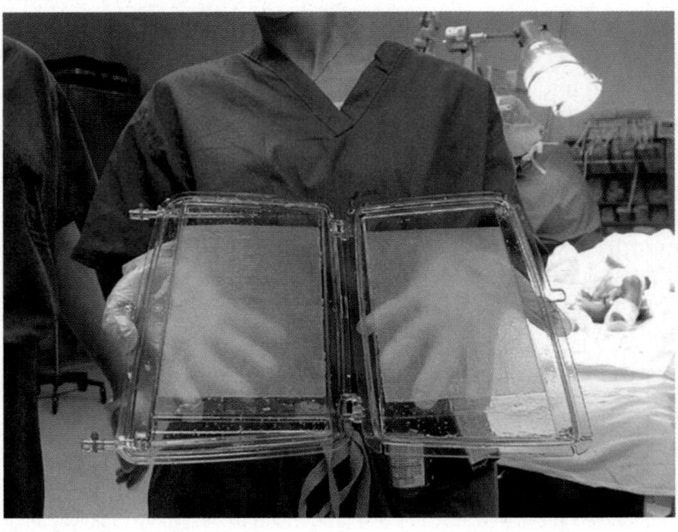
A

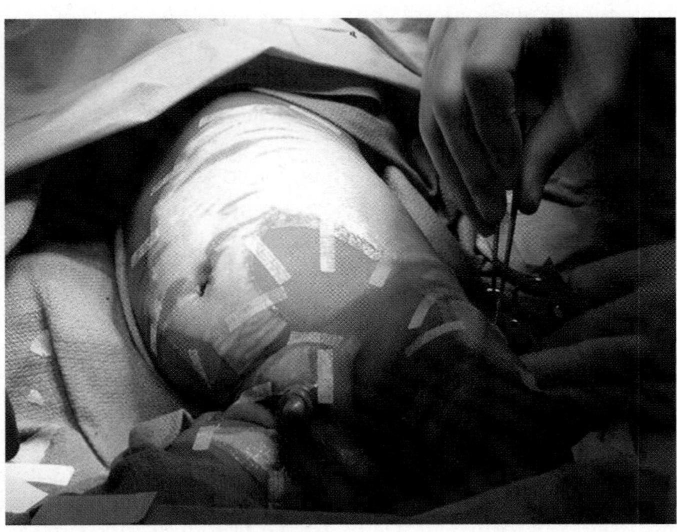
B

FIGURE 36–22 ■ *A*, Trans-Cyte, a temporary skin substitute, prior to application. *B*, Application of Trans-Cyte after debridement of a scald burn.

Courtesy Martin R. Eichelberger, M.D., Children's National Medical Center, Washington, DC.

plosion or fall, compound the severity of the burn injury. Identify signs of respiratory distress and any potential bleeding source. A weak, thready pulse, tachycardia, and pallor are important signs of early shock that may provide clues to an internal injury.

PRACTICE ALERT

Assess for increases in cyanosis, deep tissue pain, and capillary refill time, and a decreased pulse distal to a circumferential burn, signs of impaired circulation. Detection of these signs requires immediate notification of the physician.

Obtain information about the type of burn (e.g., thermal, electrical, chemical) and a complete history. If a burn injury was preventable, parents may be emotionally stressed by feelings of guilt. Caution is needed to avoid sounding accusatory when questioning parents about the injury. Be alert to signs of child abuse (e.g., glove and stocking burns, burns that spare flexor surfaces, contact burns from cigarettes or irons, zebra burn lines from contact with a hot grate) (Figure 36–23 ■). Child neglect can be a factor in the burn of a child who was not adequately supervised. When taking a burn history, carefully document the following:

- Type of injury
- Time of injury
- People present at the time of injury
- First aid administered
- History of other unusual injuries or emergency department visits

Physical assessment should be thorough, including frequent monitoring of vital signs, pain control, and daily weight measurement. Monitor the child's circulatory and respiratory status to identify signs of hypovolemia in the first 24 hours or fluid overload as capillary integrity is restored. A head-to-toe assessment is performed at the beginning of every shift followed by system-specific assessments, depending on clinical findings and changes in the child's status. Be alert to signs of infection such as purulent drainage and edematous, red, or discolored wound margins. Monitor the child for pain with an appropriate pain scale. Intake and output must be monitored closely. A urinary catheter may be inserted to enable close monitoring of urine output.

Assess the child's concerns over appearance and the stress of hospitalization. Determine if the child has memories or nightmares about the burn so psychologic support can be provided as needed. Identify how well the family is coping with the child's injury and other family stressors.

Common nursing diagnoses for the child with a major burn injury are included in the accompanying nursing care plan. Additional nursing diagnoses for the child with a major burn may include the following:

- Impaired Physical Mobility related to prescribed movement prescriptions (limb immobilization) and pain
- Disturbed Body Image related to burn injury
- Anxiety related to situational crisis and threat of death or disfigurement

■ Planning and Implementation

Care of the burned child involves various treatments designed to promote healing and prevent complications. These include

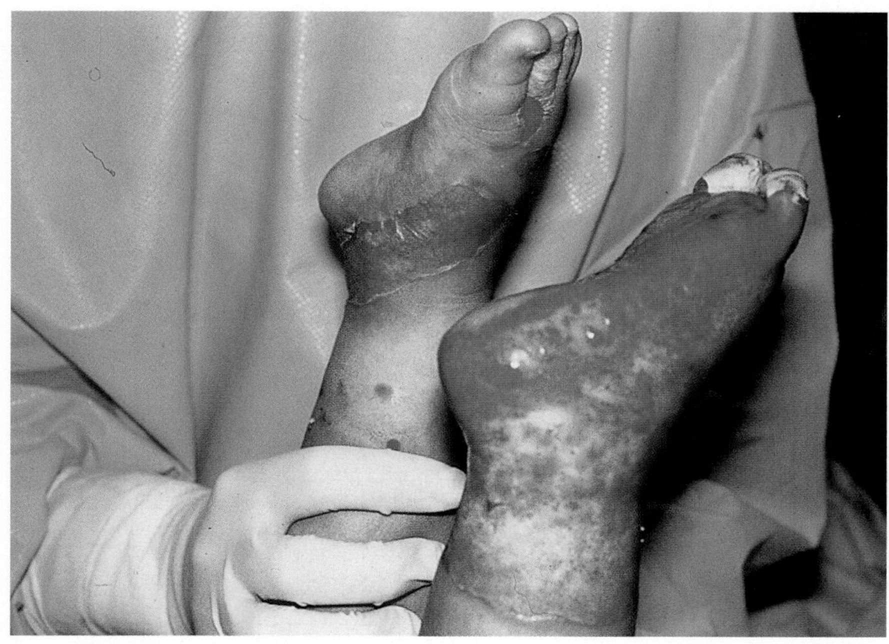

A

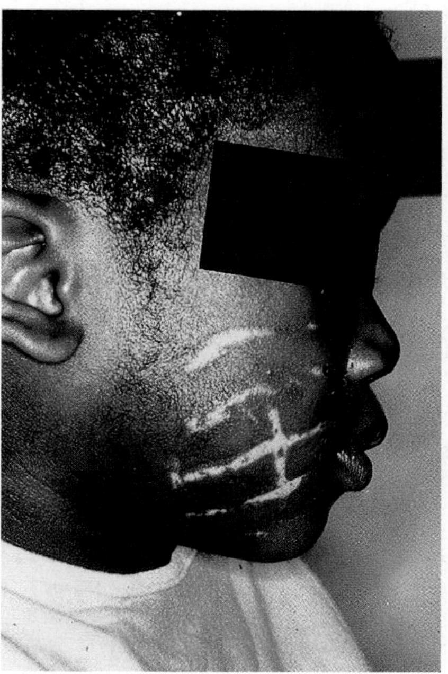

B

FIGURE 36–23 ■ Burn injuries associated with child abuse. *A,* Burns of the hands or feet that are distributed like gloves or stockings. *B,* Zebra burns from a grate.

Courtesy of the American Academy of Pediatrics, Elk Grove, IL; and the Kempe Children's Center.

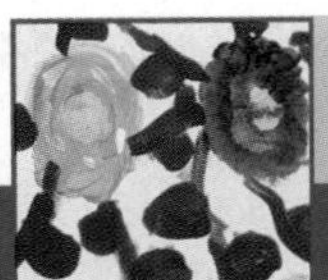

Nursing Care Plan

THE CHILD WITH A MAJOR BURN INJURY

GOAL	INTERVENTION	RATIONALE	EXPECTED OUTCOME
1. Acute Pain related to physical injury agents			
	NIC Priority Intervention—*Pain Management:* Alleviation of pain or a reduction in pain to a level of comfort that is acceptable to the patient.		**NOC Suggested Outcome—***Comfort Level:* Feelings of physical and psychological ease.
The child will verbalize adequate relief from pain and will be able to perform activities of daily living (ADLs).	■ Assess the level of pain frequently using pain scales (see Chapter 18).	■ Pain scale provides objective measurement. Pain is always present, but changes in location and intensity may indicate complications.	The child verbalizes adequate relief from pain and is able to perform ADLs.
	■ Cover burns as much as possible.	■ Temperature changes or movement of air causes pain.	
	■ Change the child's position frequently. Perform range of motion exercises.	■ Reduces joint stiffness and prevents contractures.	
	■ Encourage verbalization about pain.	■ Provides outlet for emotions and helps the child cope.	
	■ Provide diversional activities and complementary therapies such as imagery and music.	■ Helps lessen focus on pain.	
	■ Promote uninterrupted sleep with use of medications.	■ Sleep deprivation can increase pain perception.	
	■ Use analgesics before all dressing changes and burn care. Use sedation when appropriate for major debridement.	■ Helps to reduce pain and decreases anxiety for subsequent dressing changes.	
2. Risk for Infection related to trauma and destruction of skin barrier			
	NIC Priority Intervention—*Infection Protection:* Prevention and early detection of infection in a patient at risk.		**NOC Suggested Outcome—***Risk Control:* Actions to eliminate or reduce actual, personal, and modifiable health threats.
The child will be free of infection during healing process.	■ Take vital signs frequently.	■ Increased temperature is an early sign of infection.	The child either stays free of secondary infection, or has infection diagnosed and treated early.
	■ Use standard precautions (gown, gloves, mask) when wounds of a major burn are exposed. Limit visitors (no one with an upper respiratory infection or other contagious disease).	■ Reduces risk of wound contamination.	
	■ Clip hair around burns.	■ Hair harbors bacteria.	
	■ Keep biosynthetic burn dressing dry.	■ Helps reduce the number of bacteria introduced to the burned site.	
	■ Do not place the IV in any burned area.	■ Reduces risk of wound contamination	
	■ Administer oral or IV antibiotics for diagnosed infections as prescribed.	■ Antibiotics administered as prescribed help to clear the infection quickly.	
3. Risk for Imbalanced Fluid Volume related to loss of fluids through wounds and to subsequent excess fluid intake			
	NIC Priority Intervention—*Fluid Management:* Promotion of fluid balance and prevention of complications resulting from abnormal or undesired fluid levels.		**NOC Suggested Outcome—***Fluid Balance:* Balance of water in intracellular and extracellular compartments of the body.
The child will maintain adequate urine output.	■ Monitor vital signs, central venous pressure, capillary refill time, pulses. (continued)	■ The child is initially at risk for hypovolemic shock and needs fluid resuscitation (see Chapter 26). (continued)	The child maintains normal urine output and burn site edema is not excessive.

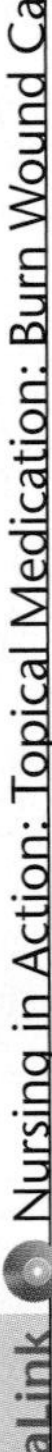

Nursing Care Plan THE CHILD WITH A MAJOR BURN INJURY (continued)

GOAL	INTERVENTION	RATIONALE	EXPECTED OUTCOME
3. Risk for Imbalanced Fluid Volume related to loss of fluids through wounds and to subsequent excess fluid intake (continued)			
	▪ Administer IV and oral fluids as ordered. ▪ Estimate insensible fluid losses. ▪ Monitor intake and output. ▪ Weigh child daily. ▪ Insert urinary catheter. ▪ Monitor for hyponatremia and hypercalcemia (see Chapter 23∞).	▪ Careful calculation of fluid needs and ensuring proper intake helps keep the child properly hydrated. ▪ Losses are increased during the first 72 hours after burn injury; may need replacement. Plasma is lost through burn site because of capillary damage. ▪ The child is at risk for fluid overload during hydration, and for edema in the tissues at the burn site. ▪ Significant weight loss or gain can help determine fluid imbalances. ▪ Helps maintain accurate output measurement during critical care stage. ▪ Sodium is lost with burn fluid and potassium is lost from damaged cells, causing electrolyte imbalances.	
4. Ineffective Peripheral Tissue Perfusion related to mechanical reduction of venous and/or arterial blood flow (edema) of circumferential burns			
	NIC Priority Intervention— *Circulatory Care:* Promotion of arterial and venous circulation.		**NOC Suggested Outcome—***Tissue Perfusion (Peripheral):* Extent to which blood flows through the small vessels of the extremities and maintains tissue function.
The child will maintain adequate perfusion in burned extremities.	▪ Elevate extremities. Perform hourly distal pulse checks. Notify the physician of decreased or absent pulses. ▪ Assess eschar.	▪ Elevation helps to reduce dependent edema by promoting venous return. Dependent edema can constrict peripheral circulation. ▪ Eschar can constrict peripheral circulation in edematous extremity.	The child has no episodes of poor perfusion in the burned extremity.
5. Ineffective Breathing Pattern related to respiratory muscle fatigue due to smoke inhalation and airway edema			
	NIC Priority Intervention— *Respiratory Monitoring:* Collection and analysis of patient data to ensure airway patency and adequate gas exchange.		**NOC Suggested Outcome—***Vital Signs Status:* Temperature, pulse, respiration, and blood pressure within expected range for the individual.
The child will maintain or demonstrate improvement in breathing pattern.	▪ Closely monitor quality of respirations, breath sounds, mucous secretions, pulse oximetry. ▪ Provide thorough pulmonary care. ▪ Elevate head of bed. Keep resuscitation equipment at bedside. ▪ Administer corticosteroids, as prescribed. ▪ Encourage use of activities that facilitate breathing, such as blowing bubbles.	▪ Excess fluid replacement can cause pulmonary edema; toxins from burning products can cause airway inflammation. ▪ Pulmonary care assists in removal of secretions to prevent infection. ▪ Dyspnea, nasal flaring, air hunger (respiratory distress) may develop. ▪ Reduces airway edema. ▪ Encourages child to expand the lungs and reduce risk for infection.	The child has regular and unlabored breathing pattern.
6. Impaired Physical Mobility related to joint stiffness due to burns			
	NIC Priority Intervention—*Exercise Therapy, Joint Mobility:* Use of active or passive body movement to maintain or restore joint flexibility.		**NOC Suggested Outcome—***Joint Movement (Active):* Range of motion of joints with self-initiated movement.
The child will maintain maximum range of motion.	▪ Arrange physical and occupational therapy twice daily for stretching and range of motion exercises. Splint as ordered. Encourage independent ADLs.	▪ Good positioning, range of motion exercises, and alignment prevent contractures.	(continued)

Nursing Care Plan THE CHILD WITH A MAJOR BURN INJURY (continued)

GOAL	INTERVENTION	RATIONALE	EXPECTED OUTCOME
6. Impaired Physical Mobility related to joint stiffness due to burns (continued)			
	■ Encourage activities to promote range of motion (toss a bean bag, mimic animal movements).	■ Fun activities help the child with diversion and promote movement.	The child maintains maximum range of motion without contactures.
7. Imbalanced Nutrition: Less than Body Requirements related to high metabolic needs			
	NIC Priority Intervention—*Nutrition Management:* Assistance with or provision of balanced dietary intake of foods and fluids.		**NOC Suggested Outcome—***Nutritional Status:* Extent to which nutrients are available to meet metabolic needs.
The child will maintain weight and demonstrate adequate serum albumin and hydration.	■ Provide an opportunity to choose meals. Offer a variety of foods. Provide snacks and finger foods. ■ Encourage the child to have meals with other children. ■ Substitute milk and juices for water. Provide a multivitamin supplement. ■ Provide nasogastric feedings as needed. ■ Weigh the child daily.	■ Encourages intake. General malaise and anorexia lead to poor healing. ■ Socialization improves intake. ■ Vitamin C aids zinc absorption; zinc aids in healing. ■ A child with a burn greater than 10% of BSA cannot usually meet nutrition requirements without assistance. ■ Provides objective evaluation.	The child maintains weight, adequate hydration, normal serum albumin.
8. Anxiety (child) related to threat to or change in health status			
	NIC Priority Intervention—*Anxiety Reduction:* Minimizing apprehension, dread, foreboding, or uneasiness related to an unidentified source of anticipated danger.		**NOC Suggested Outcome—***Coping:* Actions to manage stressors that tax an individual's resources.
The child will verbalize reduced anxiety.	■ Provide continuity of care providers. ■ Encourage parents to stay with the child; calls from home; pictures from classmates. ■ Group tasks and activities. ■ Use art, music, relaxation activities, touch, and massage to provide diversion.	■ Helps to build a trusting relationship. ■ Familiar surroundings, people, and items encourage relaxation. ■ Reduces overstimulation and encourages rest. ■ Complementary therapies help divert the child's attention away from treatments and pain.	The child expresses and shows signs of reduced anxiety.
9. Anxiety (parent) related to situational crisis			
	NIC Priority Intervention—*Anxiety Reduction:* Minimizing apprehension, dread, foreboding, or uneasiness related to an unidentified source of anticipated danger.		**NOC Suggested Outcome—***Anxiety Control:* Ability to eliminate or reduce feelings of apprehension and tension from an unidentified source.
Parents will verbalize decreased anxiety.	■ Provide educational materials about healing, grafting, dressing changes, and course of action. ■ Be flexible when teaching parents about wound care. ■ Allow parents to talk about their feelings, concerns, and frustrations. Provide referral to social services or parent support group. ■ Encourage parents to participate in the child's care and development of the care plan.	■ Knowledge reduces anxiety. ■ Adults learn in many different ways. ■ Allows for venting of fears and guilt feelings, and provides exchange of ideas on dealing with hospitalization and long-term care. ■ Actual role in planning the child's care helps them gain some control and comfort in setting.	Parents state decreased anxiety.

dressing changes, hydrotherapy, antibiotic therapy, fluid and nutrition management, analgesic support, physical therapy, play therapy, and possibly skin grafting.

Severe morbidity is likely with major burns. Significant scarring may occur regardless of autografting and the use of pressure garments. Contractures and loss of function are also possible. If fluid replacement is inadequate, irreversible renal damage or cardiac damage may ensue, necessitating close follow-up unrelated to the actual burn injury. Children with major burns require comprehensive follow-up, sometimes involving repeated hospitalizations for surgery to release burn contractures, perform new grafting, or cosmetic surgery for scar revision.

Prevent Complications

Severe complications of burns include infections, pneumonia, and renal failure, as well as possible irreversible loss of function of the burned area. The goal of the healthcare team is to prevent complications. Parents need to be involved in their child's care and to learn how to change dressings, assess for infection and dehydration (see Chapter 23), and perform range of motion exercises to aid in the child's recovery.

Wound Care

See Box 36–7 for the cleansing and dressing change procedure for the child with a burn.

When a synthetic skin cover such as Trans-Cyte is used, regular dressing changes are not needed. The area must be protected from moisture and ointments, as these interfere with adherence. Trans-Cyte is transparent, so the site can be monitored for signs of infection and wound healing. The skin covering is assessed for air bubbles or fluid, which are aspirated or drained as ordered. If the covering is used over a joint, a splint will prevent movement. When healing occurs, the skin covering loosens, permitting it to be trimmed.

Provide Emotional Support

Burned children have received a profound insult to their body and their self-image. Fear and anxiety related to disfigurement and scarring are common responses, especially among adolescents.

BOX 36–7 Burn Wound Care

PREPARATION

1. Check the physician's orders. Since burn care is often a painful procedure, check for pain medication orders and administer medication at least 30–60 minutes before starting burn care. Conscious sedation may be used for some debridement procedures.
2. Wash your hands. Gather supplies, including gloves (clean and sterile), a basin, sterile normal saline solution, a large supply of 4 × 4 gauze pads, forceps, scissors, a sterile tongue blade, the prescribed topical medication, tape, and an absorbent pad.
3. You may need an assistant to hold the child and the burned extremity during care.

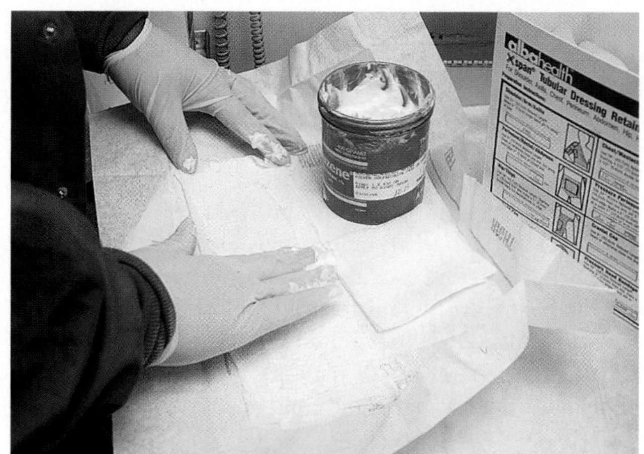

PROCEDURE

1. Place the absorbent pad under the area to be cleaned. Put on clean gloves. Soak the wound for about 10 minutes in normal saline solution, or apply a wet dressing to the area. Hydrotherapy may also be used for this stage. This will soften the wound. Remove the gloves.
2. After approximately 10 minutes, put on sterile gloves and wash the burn with the gauze pads using a firm, circular motion, moving from the inside to the outer edges. As you do this, be sure to remove any medication or crusting. Bleeding may occur, but this is a sign of healing, healthy tissue. Rinse with more normal saline solution. Pat dry with sterile gauze.
3. Remove (per physician's orders) any loose or dead skin around the edges of the burn by gently lifting it with the forceps and snipping it. This is not painful to the child. You may rinse and dry again.
4. Place a thin layer of prescribed medication (about 1/8 in. thick) on the burn or gauze with fingers or a tongue blade. Place the medicated gauze on the burn and cover with a dry, sterile dressing.

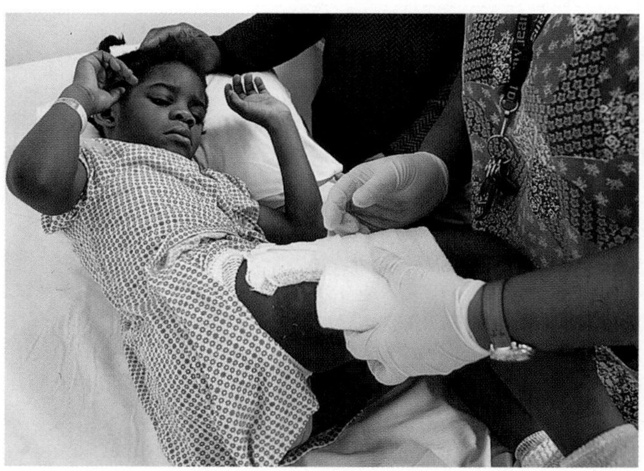

Burn wound care written by Marcia Wellington, R. N., M. S.

Increased stress occurs as a result of the shock and pain of the injury, as well as the unfamiliar surroundings and presence of healthcare providers.

An attitude of genuine interest and concern on the part of the nurse is essential. The child should be oriented to his or her surroundings frequently and given ample preparation for procedures, when possible. Continuity of care providers is important in developing a trusting relationship and partnership with the child and family. Encourage the child and parents to voice concerns, and show understanding and support. Play therapy is encouraged for children, even if they can only observe initially. Play therapy serves several purposes for the child with a major burn.

- Provides an outlet for frustration, independence, and creativity.
- Promotes activities that challenge range of motion.
- Normalizes the child's daily routine.
- Encourages the child, who sees the progress that other children make day by day.

Families are at risk for emotional stress. They should be forewarned about the expected edema and the resulting major changes in the child's body. Parents often feel guilty and responsible for the child's injury. It is important to help parents focus on recovery rather than on past actions. Fear usually results from lack of knowledge about the severity of the burn and the child's status, especially in the early stages of burn care and admission to the hospital ICU. Include the family in the child's care when possible. The family must be given information and frequent updates to promote the development of trust between the family and the healthcare team.

Autografting procedures enable the child to recover from major burns, but the operation leaves visible scarring. Psychologic support is therefore essential to the child's recovery. Social workers, chaplains, art therapists, child life specialists, and play therapists are trained to help the child and partner with the family to deal with the stressors of recovery. Appropriate referrals should be made to ensure that the child and family receive necessary services.

MediaLink Burn Resources and Support

Discharge Planning and Home Care Teaching

Home care needs should be identified and addressed well in advance of discharge. Thorough assessment is necessary to identify the family's needs related to the child's discharge home or to a rehabilitation facility. Discharge planning may include instructing parents in nutrition and diet needs, safety in the home, burn wound care, use of pressure garments, and range of motion exercises to prevent contractures.

Provide support and encouragement to parents when they are learning how to care for the burned child. Many parents find it difficult to perform dressing change procedures they know will inflict pain on their child. Provide pain medication for dressing changes, and give guidelines about how soon before the dressing change to give the medication. Outline specific guidelines for dressing changes so that parents and healthcare team members will have the same focus. Parents should first observe care being performed and then provide repeat demonstrations until competent.

Care in the Community

A major role of nurses in the community is prevention. Provide burn prevention information to parents at each health promotion visit. Examples of prevention messages include the following:

- Appropriate temperature settings for hot water heaters
- Keeping the handles of pots on the stove turned toward the wall and dishes with hot liquids out of the toddler's reach
- Keeping infants and toddlers off the lap when drinking hot beverages or eating soup
- Keeping matches, lighters, and flammable materials away from children
- Installing smoke detectors and replacing the batteries annually.

Become involved with a Safe Kids coalition and local firefighters to help educate families and caregivers about ways to prevent scald burns and house fires. Encourage families to develop and practice escape plans from the home in case of a house fire. Look for burn hazards when making home visits. Provide adolescents and parents with first-aid training so that they can provide appropriate care when a child or other family member becomes injured.

Care of the child with a serious burn requires long-term therapy and rehabilitation. Nurses in clinic and home care settings continue the care provided during hospitalization. Long-term care commonly occurs in the home, with frequent visits to healthcare professionals. In some cases, children return to the hospital clinic for dressing changes on a regular basis. Children with extensive burns or with burns in locations that have the potential to cause functional limitations related to scarring must often wear a pressure garment, and sometimes a facemask if the face was burned. The pressure garment may present a threat to the child's body image, but it is an important means of decreasing scarring. Scar management may also be handled through drug injections or surgery (e.g., revision, grafting, or Z-plasty). Help families understand the need for the special garments and masks and how to clean and care for them.

Continued physical therapy and occupational therapy are often needed to increase strength and dexterity in performing self-care skills and to prevent contractures. Emphasis is placed on returning to normal activities of daily living as soon as possible, such as returning to school as soon as health permits. Some children have home tutors and are provided with computer connections to school activities for a time to ensure learning while decreasing their exposure to infection.

School reentry is often a traumatic experience, especially for older children and adolescents, because of the fear of rejection, decreased self-esteem, and impaired body image. The child's primary nurse, social worker, and child life specialist may visit the school of a child with a burn injury before the child returns to school—bringing photographs of the child, pressure garments, or other items—to inform the classmates and allow them to explore their emotions relating to the child's burn injury. Several communities offer support groups for families and children with burn injuries. Referral to these groups may be beneficial.

Management of Minor Burns

Many children with minor burns are cared for at home after an initial visit to the emergency department or urgent care clinic. Discuss home remedies for minor burn care. See Developing Cultural Competence: Litargirio Use. Any open blisters are debrided, and a thin layer of silver sulfadiazine is applied over the burn. Do not place this medication close to the eyes or mouth. Bacitracin is often used for burns on the face. The burn is then covered with one or two layers of gauze. Burn dressings should be changed once or twice daily. This involves cleaning the burn and reapplying antibiotic cream. See Partnering with Families: Caring for Minor Burns.

CLINICAL TIP

For superficial burns covering a small area, use moist soaks or ice to stop the burning process and to relieve pain. Pain management is initiated as soon as possible. Soak charred clothing off with sterile saline and clip any hair within 2 in. of the burn to keep it out of the burn site. Cleanse the burn with mild soap and water and remove any foreign matter. If a chemical is the burning agent, remove the clothing and wash with lots of water. Elevate burned extremities.

Instruct parents to increase the child's fluid intake to compensate for loss of fluid through damaged skin. A high-calorie, high-protein diet is necessary to meet the increased nutritional requirements of healing. Acetaminophen (Tylenol) with codeine is often given, especially before dressing changes. Infection is a common complication. The child should be seen within 48 hours of treatment to monitor progress. Educate the parents to observe for the following signs of infection: inflammation extending under the dressing, bad odor, excessive exudates, and fever, and to notify the healthcare provider immediately. Reinforce to parents the importance of follow-up appointments.

Moisturizing creams can be used after healing to relieve residual drying. The healed skin is highly sensitive to sunburn, so cover the area or use a sunscreen. Use of a sunscreen will also help prevent hyperpigmentation after burn healing.

Evaluation

Examples of expected outcomes of nursing management are as follows:

- Pain is effectively managed from acute injury and for subsequent dressing changes.

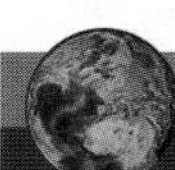

DEVELOPING CULTURAL COMPETENCE
Litargirio Use

When taking a history about methods used to treat minor burns in children, inquire about the use of "litargirio." This is a traditional remedy used for burn and wound healing and as a deodorant and foot fungicide in the Dominican Republic. The powder is sold in small packets at specialty stores that cater to Spanish-speaking populations. It contains up to 79% lead and can cause lead toxicity in children (FDA, 2003).

PARTNERING WITH FAMILIES

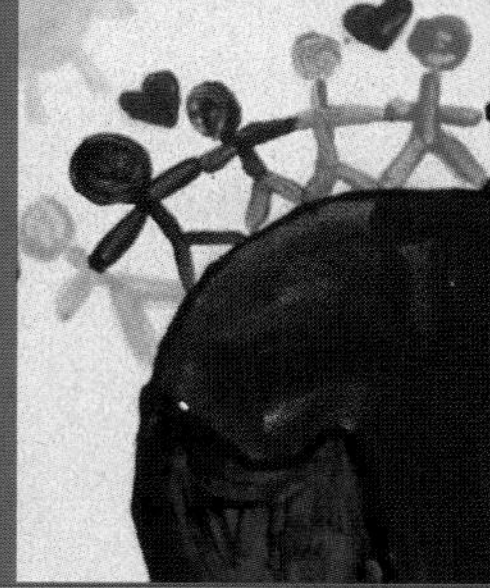

Caring for Minor Burns

- Place burn under cool, running water to stop the burning process and to help pain.
- Do not use ice as it can cause more damage to the injured skin.
- Remove all clothing and jewelry from the burned area.
- Apply a topical antibiotic such as Neosporin.

- Fluid management prevents shock and later fluid overload.
- Wound management is performed to reduce infection and pain.
- Other outcomes are listed in the nursing care plan.

Sunburn

Sunburn is a burn injury to the outer layer of skin caused by excess ultraviolet light exposure, or sun exposure after taking phototoxic drugs (acne medication, chlorpheniramine, diphenylhydramine, sulfonamides, tetracycline) (Laughlin-Richard, 2000). It is estimated that 80% of a person's lifetime exposure to sunburns occurs before 21 years of age because there is more time for sun exposure during childhood (Centers for Disease Control, 2002). This exposure occurs at a time when the epidermis is relatively thin. **Melanin** (skin pigment) is also present in low levels during infancy and childhood (Laughlin-Richard, 2000). For these reasons, it is recommended that children of all ages use a sunscreen with an SPF of 15 or higher during outdoor activities. However, use of sunscreen does not ensure that sunburn will be prevented, especially during lengthy sun exposure.

Sunburn occurs more often in children with red or blond hair and fair skin that freckles easily. These children have less melanin to protect their skin against these harmful ultraviolet (UV) rays. UV-B rays burn and tan the skin. UV-A rays deeply penetrate the skin to cause premature aging and potential suppression of the immune system. Repeated sunburns during childhood correlate strongly with the development of moles during childhood and adolescence, and with the development of skin cancer (basal cell carcinoma, squamous cell carcinoma, and melanoma) in adulthood. Melanoma is one of the most common cancers found in individuals less than 30 years of age (CDC, 2002). The risk for melanoma and basal cell carcinoma is strongly related to a history of one or more severe blistering sunburns during childhood or adolescence. The incidence of melanoma is significantly higher for Caucasians than for African Americans and Hispanics.

Erythema and skin tenderness usually develop between 30 minutes and 4 hours after exposure to sunlight. Increased

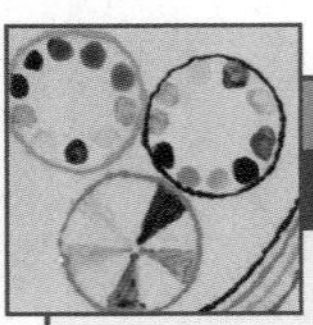

EVIDENCE-BASED PRACTICE
Sunburn Prevention Education

PROBLEM

Excessive exposure to ultraviolet (UV) radiation during childhood and adolescence is associated with the development of skin cancer during adulthood. Primary prevention strategies to reduce childhood exposure are needed to reverse the dramatic increase in skin cancer attributed to UV radiation exposure. What prevention strategies successfully promote reduced sun exposure in children and adolescents?

EVIDENCE

A survey of 10,000 adolescents 12 to 18 years of age in the United States revealed the following information: Girls used sunscreen more routinely than boys, but they were more likely to have received at least three sunburns the previous summer. Girls believed it was worth burning to get a good tan, and girls were more likely than boys to have used a tanning booth in the past year. Tanned skin was more strongly preferred by girls than boys. Only one third of survey respondents reported routine use of sunscreen. Responses did not vary by geographic location (Geller, Colditz, Oliveria, et al., 2002). The parents of 77 children seen in a medical clinic in Florida were surveyed about current methods of sun protection for their children and their attitudes and knowledge about sun protection. Fewer than half of the parents reported regular use of sun protection for their children despite some knowledge of sun protection measures and potential consequences of sun exposure. The majority of parents reported that their children were outside 1–4 hours a day. Sunscreen was the most common reported sun protection measure; however, half of the parents indicated it was okay to stay outside longer when sunscreen was used. This potentially increased the overall sun exposure for these children (Johnson, Davy, Boyett, et al., 2001). When this same population was asked about sun protection counseling received by the child's physician, those who received enthusiastic counseling perceived that sun protection was important for their children. Of the 21 parents who had received enthusiastic counseling, more than 40% of them stated that they had increased sun protection habits and were more likely to teach their child safe sun habits. More than half indicated a desire to have more information about sun protection (Davy, Boyett, Weathers, et al., 2002). A national telephone survey of 651 parents of children ages 5 to 12 years was conducted to assess the parent's skin cancer knowledge, sun protection behavior, and perceived risk of skin cancer, as well as the child's sun protection behavior, and the parent's and child's vigilance in sunscreen use. Results indicated that parents were more likely than their children to wear sunglasses and to adopt sun avoidance habits while children more often than parents used sunscreen. Children were more likely to sunburn when parents also got sunburned. When both parents and children were vigilant in using sunscreen, children were less likely to get sunburns. The importance of parents to be role models in sun protection behavior is essential (O'Riordan, Geller, Brooks, et al., 2003). The Task Force on Community Preventive Services on reducing exposure to UV light found sufficient evidence to recommend only two interventions for sun protection or covering up behavior: educational and policy approaches in primary schools and recreational or tourist sites (Centers for Disease Control, 2003b). A 1–2 hour education program developed by the Environmental Protection Agency was used and evaluated in 85 schools across the country. Children aged 5 to 15 years participated. When compared to children in schools who did not receive the education, study children were more likely to report a change in attitude about the healthier look with a suntan, and intentions to play in the shade more frequently; however, there was no change in plans to wear sunscreen, sunglasses, or protective clothing (Geller, Rutsch, Kenausis, et al., 2003).

IMPLICATIONS

Successful strategies to reduce UV exposure have not yet been identified. Policy changes may be a better strategy than education to reduce sun exposure in childcare and school settings. Information about sun protection behaviors indicates a need for education and behavior change by parents and children. Alternate behaviors such as regularly wearing a hat, sunglasses, covering skin, and staying in the shade should also be encouraged. Guidelines exist for skin cancer prevention efforts in the school setting that the nurse should help implement.

CRITICAL THINKING IN ACTION

Develop guidelines that a childcare center could use for the reduction of UV radiation exposure by enrolled infants and children.

vasodilation and vascular permeability result in the extravasation of fluid to the tissues and white blood cell migration to the damaged skin. The erythema peaks at 24 hours. Prolonged exposure can result in edema, vesiculation, bullae, or ulceration. Systemic complaints include malaise, insomnia (because of skin tenderness), fatigue, headaches, and chilling (because of rapid heat loss).

Treatment is generally supportive. Increased oral fluids are encouraged. Pain can be relieved by cool compresses followed by the application of a low-potency topical corticosteroid (on unblistered skin) to relieve discomfort. Children with severe sunburn may require nonsteroidal anti-inflammatory drugs for pain relief and to reduce inflammation (see Chapter 18∞).

NURSING MANAGEMENT

Educate parents and children about ways to prevent sunburn. See Box 36–8 for the *Healthy People 2010* objectives for the reduction of sun exposure and melanoma. Advise that repeated sunburns may lead to permanent skin damage, skin cancer, cataracts, premature aging of the skin, and possible suppression of the immune system. Recommend to parents that children use sunscreens with at least sun protection factor (SPF) ≥ 15, reapplied several times daily or use a sun block agent such as zinc oxide, wear protective clothing, and limit the amount of time in the sun. Children should also wear sunglasses with 99% ultraviolet blockage; see Evidence-Based Practice: Sunburn Prevention Education. Sunscreen should be applied 30 minutes prior to sun

BOX 36–8 *Healthy People 2010* Skin Cancer Prevention Objective

Increase the proportion of persons who use at least one of the following protective measures that might reduce the risk for skin cancer.

- Avoid the sun between 10 A.M and 4 P.M.
- Wear sun-protective clothing when exposed to the sun.
- Use sunscreen with sun protection factor (SPF) ≥ 15.
- Avoid artificial sources of UV light.
- Reduce deaths from melanoma to < 2.5 per 100,000 persons.

From U.S. Department of Health and Human Services. (2000). Healthy People 2010 *(2nd ed.). Washington, DC: U.S. Government Printing Office. www.healthypeople.gov*

exposure to permit the ingredients to activate with the skin, and it should be reapplied every 2 hours as sweating may diminish the protective effects of the sunscreen. Participate in policy changes for sun exposure in school settings (CDC, 2002). Teach adolescents how to monitor for changes in moles that could signal the development of skin cancer and to seek care immediately. Characteristics of moles that indicate a need for evaluation include those that are asymmetric and have an irregular border, color variations, and a diameter greater than 0.6 cm. See Partnering with Families: Preventing Sunburn.

Hypothermia

Hypothermia is a condition in which the core body temperature falls below 35°C (95°F). This occurs when the body heat production is less than the body heat lost. Hypothermia is a life-threatening emergency that can occur in any season and any geographic location. Infants and young children are at risk because of immature thermoregulatory mechanisms, thinner skin, limited subcutaneous fat, and higher surface area to body mass ratio. Adolescents are at risk due to risk-taking behaviors such as drug and alcohol use, and engaging in remote outdoor activities without proper equipment.

Etiology and Pathophysiology

Primary hypothermia results from environmental exposure. Heat is lost through four primary mechanisms (Deegan, 2000).

- *Radiation*—heat transfers from the body to cooler surfaces not in direct contact with the skin, accounting for about 60% of body heat loss. Most heat is lost from an uncovered head.
- *Convection*—loss of heat to cooler air currents, accounting for about 12% of body heat loss. The rate of heat loss can be increased dependent on wind speeds or the wind chill factor.
- *Conduction*—transfer of heat from the body to a cooler surface in direct contact with the skin, accounting for about 2% to 3% of body heat loss. This mechanism of heat loss is increased when clothing is wet or the child is submerged in water.
- *Evaporation*—loss of heat when water is converted to a vapor, accounting for about 15% of body heat loss.

Hypothermia is associated with near drowning episodes, because body heat is lost quickly in water, as compared with air. As the core temperature falls, the body tries to conserve this temperature at the expense of the extremities. Increased muscle tone and an increased metabolic rate occur. Shivering occurs to try to rewarm the blood before it returns to the core of the body. Other causes of hypothermia include ingestion of alcohol or barbiturates, trauma or a brain disorder that interferes with temperature regulation, and overwhelming sepsis.

Clinical Manifestations

Symptoms of hypothermia are associated with severity.

- Mild hypothermia (32°–35°C) signs include slurred speech, poor coordination, confusion, poor judgment and inappropriate behavior, and shivering. Tachycardia and peripheral vasoconstriction maintain the cardiac output and blood pressure. Tachypnea with increased secretions and bronchospasm are also present. The kidneys respond with increased urine production.
- Moderate hypothermia (29°–32°C) signs include depressed respirations, bradycardia, low blood pressure, pale or cyanotic color, shivering, and pupillary reflexes and dilation are decreased. Atrial and ventricular arrhythmias may occur. Lethargy, hallucinations, and coma develop as the central nervous system becomes depressed. As the child becomes colder, the gag and cough reflexes are lost, breathing is hard to detect, shivering stops, and muscle rigidity occurs.
- Profound hypothermia (body temperature below 28°C) is characterized by coma, dilated and unresponsive pupils, apnea, reduced cardiac output and blood pressure, ventricular fibrillation, and asystole. It may be impossible to distinguish between severe hypothermia and death.

PARTNERING WITH FAMILIES

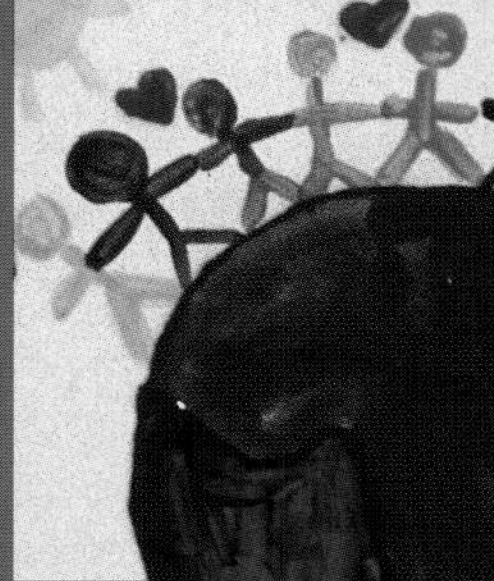

Preventing Sunburn

- Keep children out of direct sunlight as much as possible, especially the midday sun. Avoid scheduling outdoor activities during the hours of maximum exposure (10 A.M. to 2 P.M.).
- When outdoors, minimize exposed areas by wearing hats and long-sleeves, closely woven cotton clothing and pants; wear T-shirts while swimming. Special sun protection clothing is now available from some manufacturers.
- Be aware that water, concrete, and sand reflect sunlight and increase exposure up to 90% by reflecting up to 85% of the ultraviolet rays.
- Use sunscreen with at least 15 SPF. For optimal protection, apply as thickly as directed to all exposed areas 30–45 minutes before sun exposure. Reapply every 2 hours as needed, or sooner if swimming, toweling off, or perspiring heavily.
- Use a waterproof sunscreen when swimming; this provides protection in water for approximately 60–80 minutes. Then reapply. Avoid placing waterproof sunscreen in the eyes as it causes severe pain and a chemical burn. Call the poison control center immediately for guidance.
- Avoid using sunscreens in infants less than 6 months of age because of the possibility of absorption of the chemicals through their skin.
- Remember that a child can be burned even on a cloudy day. Up to 80% of ultraviolet rays can penetrate the cloud cover.
- If the child is taking any medications, check with the healthcare practitioner before exposure (some medications cause hypersensitivity to sunlight).

COLLABORATIVE CARE

Clinical therapy focuses on resuscitation, if necessary, and gradual core body rewarming. If the child was immersed or submerged in water, remove the wet clothing and wrap in a blanket. The child who has profound hypothermia should receive CPR until the body temperature returns to normal because the hypothermia may have preserved vital organs. Volume expanders are needed to promote cardiac output. Body temperature is monitored with a deep rectal probe inserted about 15 cm. Aggressive techniques for rewarming include the use of humidified, warm oxygen; warmed intravenous fluids; warm packs to the core circulation areas (axillae, groin, and posterior neck); and peritoneal lavage or hemodialysis. Hypoglycemia is a common complication and should be treated with IV glucose.

PRACTICE ALERT

The diving reflex occurs when the face and nose are immersed in cold water. The response is breath holding, intense peripheral vasoconstriction, bradycardia, decreased cardiac output, and increased mean arterial pressure. The bradycardia is inversely proportional to the water temperature, and drops to about 18 beats per minute when water is 10°C. The brain and heart are selectively oxygenated. The breath holding prevents or delays aspiration or ventilation of cold water until the body has cooled to the point that hypothermia protection has occurred. Rapid hypothermia cools the brain and provides an opportunity for resuscitation of children submerged in cold water for short periods of time (Giesbrecht, 2000).

For mild hypothermia (temperature above 35°C [95°F]), external heat lamps, immersion in warm water, and an electric blanket may be all that are necessary.

If a child becomes hypothermic during an outing such as a camping trip, a warm person should get into a sleeping bag (or under the blankets) next to the child. This action will warm the child and prevent further heat loss.

NURSING MANAGEMENT

Prevention of hypothermia is an important nursing education role. Educate parents to layer children's clothing in cold climates, recognize signs of hypothermia, decrease time of exposure to cold, and be aware of actions to take for mild hypothermia. Teach school-age children and adolescents who go on camping and hunting trips how to recognize and manage hypothermia in themselves and others. Teach preventive techniques such as not riding snowmobiles or walking on ice that may be thin.

The child with moderate or profound hypothermia will be treated in the emergency department and critical care unit as efforts are made to stabilize the child's temperature and manage potential complications. Monitor vital signs, including the core body temperature, and urine output during rewarming. Avoid excessive manipulation and stress on the child as arrhythmias can be triggered. Care must be taken in giving medications as they may not be metabolized during the rewarming period, leading to potential toxicity once the circulation is reestablished when extra doses were administered during resuscitation.

If mild hypothermia occurs at home, move the child to a dry area and remove any wet clothing. Replace with warm, dry clothing, and encourage the child to drink a warm, high-calorie liquid, if able.

Frostbite

Frostbite is a cold injury that results from the overexposure of skin cells to temperatures low enough to cause crystal formation. Skin cells have a high concentration of water.

Frostbite develops in tissues exposed to temperatures below freezing, such as −2°C, for more than 1 hour when environmental protection is inadequate. Wind velocity, altitude, wetness of tissue, the child's vascular status, and previous exposure to cold injury are factors in the severity of the cold injury. Areas of the body at high risk for frostbite include the hands, feet, cheeks, nose, and ears. Ice crystallizes in the tissues, resulting in cellular dehydration and ischemic damage.

Clinical manifestations depend on the severity and depth of the cellular damage (von Heimburg, Noah, Sieckmann, et al., 2001).

- Superficial skin affected—pallor and waxy skin with a spongy texture, decreased sensation; upon rewarming the skin is erythematous and edematous with hyperemia of affected tissues
- Full thickness skin affected—erythema, vesicle formation with clear or pink fluid, numbness
- Full thickness and subcutaneous skin affected—local edema, grayish-blue discoloration
- Deeper cold injury—deep cyanosis, no vesicles or local edema, necrosis of subcutaneous tissue or lower, possibly involving the muscles or tendons

Get the child to a warmer environment. If frostbite is suspected, loosen all constricting clothing and remove any wet clothes. Because the frostbitten area is numb, extreme caution is needed to protect it from any trauma. Obtain healthcare as soon as possible. Rewarming is done slowly to decrease the chance of cellular damage. Immerse the affected part for 10 to 15 minutes in water warmed to between 38° and 40°C (100.4° and 104°F). Analgesics are given as the rewarming process will cause severe pain. Gently clean the affected skin with saline. Cover the exposed skin with sterile dressings. The erythema and mild swelling develop into bullae. The extent of injury usually is not initially apparent. Elevate the affected part, if possible, to improve venous return. Encourage the child to drink warm fluids to aid in the warming process. As the extent of the cold injury is gradually revealed, the ruptured vesicles and eschar are debrided. Whirlpool and physical therapy treatment is important to improve circulation and maintain function. Amputation may be needed when circulation is not restored. Physical therapy will then be needed for rehabilitation.

Nursing Management

As with hypothermia, the goal of management is prevention. Teach parents to layer children's clothing for warmth and to pack extra blankets and clothing if cold temperatures are expected during outdoor activities. Teach adolescents how to avoid frostbite during hunting and other cold weather expeditions. Wet clothing should be changed quickly. Early care is instrumental in minimizing permanent injury.

The nurse plays an important role in rewarming the extremity with a cold injury and protecting the extremity from additional injury. Assess the need for and provide pain medication. Monitor the extremity for warmth, circulation, and sensation. Severe frostbite will require hospitalization, with fluid management, dressing changes, antibiotic therapy, and careful attention to diet. Provide emotional support to the child and family during the waiting time needed to learn the full extent of injury and disability.

BITES

Animal Bites

Each year, 5 million people are bitten by animals in the United States, of which 80% are dog bites. Other animals that may bite include cats, birds, turtles, and wild animals such as bats, squirrels, and raccoons. Children, especially less than 8 years old, are at higher risk for animal bites, and boys are bitten more than twice as often as girls (Bernardo, Gardner, O'Connor, et al., 2000). In the majority of cases the dog is known by the child.

Dog bites tend to be crushing, rather than clean, sharp lacerations. Cat bites tend to be puncture wounds. Dog bites are more commonly on the upper torso, face, and scalp in children, rather than on the arms and legs. Bites are commonly associated with inappropriate behavior by the child, such as teasing, playing, or interfering with feeding.

Collaborative Care

Immediate care includes noting location and number of puncture wounds, abrasions, lacerations, and crushing injuries, redness or swelling at entry sites, redness extending from site (possible cellulitis), and any drainage related to the bite. Cat bites tend to be puncture wounds and associated with a higher rate of infection, cellulitis, and abscesses. Damage to nerves, muscles, tendons, and vascular structures is identified. Head and neck bites require radiographic examination to rule out any associated injury, such as trauma to the airway or breathing structures or a depressed skull fracture.

Initial treatment includes irrigation of the wound, removal of devitalized tissue, and a clean dressing. Conscious sedation and pain management may be needed for some children. Small wounds may be closed with adhesive strips rather than suturing because of the potential for infection. Severe bites sometimes require surgical closure or reconstruction. Wounds over joints should be immobilized and elevated. Puncture wounds should not be irrigated or sutured. The major complication of bites is infection such as cellulitis. Cat bites can result in septic arthritis and osteomyelitis if a bone or joint is punctured. Antibiotics and early treatment of the wound can greatly decrease these sequelae.

Dog bites should be reported to the police, and the dog should be observed for 10 days for signs of rabies. Cat bites are also dangerous because fewer cats are immunized against rabies. Bites by wild animals in areas with endemic rabies will require rabies prophylaxis.

PRACTICE ALERT

Human rabies immune globulin (HRIG) or human diploid cell rabies (HDCV) vaccine should be given to all children bitten by wild animals in which rabies cannot be excluded, as well as to children bitten by domestic animals (cats and dogs) suspected or proven to be rabid. See Chapter 19∞ for a description of rabies treatment.

Nursing Management

If a child sustains an animal bite, a complete and accurate history is essential. The following items should be documented.

- Extent of injury
- Circumstances surrounding attack
- Present location of animal
- Attempts to assess animal's health

Wound care is an important nursing intervention. To decrease infection, high-pressure wound irrigation with large quantities of sterile saline or lactated Ringer's solution is performed rather than scrubbing. A 19-gauge needle on a 60 cc syringe may be used. A clean pressure dressing is applied, and the affected part is elevated to reduce bleeding. Instruct parents about how to care for the wound and signs of infection that indicate a need to return for care.

Review the child's immunization record to determine if a tetanus booster is necessary. Refer to Chapter 19∞ for immunization information.

Children who receive traumatic animal bites often experience significant psychologic trauma. They may develop a fear of strange animals and a decreased capacity to enjoy the presence of household pets. Counseling and follow-up may be necessary to evaluate such concerns.

Prevention of animal bites is another important nursing role. See education recommendations in Partnering with Families: Preventing Animal Bites.

Human Bites

Human bites are more common than most people realize. They usually occur in toddlers and young children. Because the mouth harbors many bacteria, infection is fairly common. Assess the risk for hepatitis B and HIV infection. Antibiotics may be prescribed to prevent systemic complications. Initial treatment includes irrigating with sterile saline and debridement. Instruct parents about how to care for the wound. Follow-up is important to watch for infection.

Nursing Management

Educate parents about ways to prevent human bites and the importance of teaching children appropriate behavior around other children. When these bites occur in a childcare or school setting, inform parents about the human bite so they can discuss potential risks and follow up with a healthcare provider.

As these children are often cared for at home, teach the parents about the normal healing process, proper wound care, and

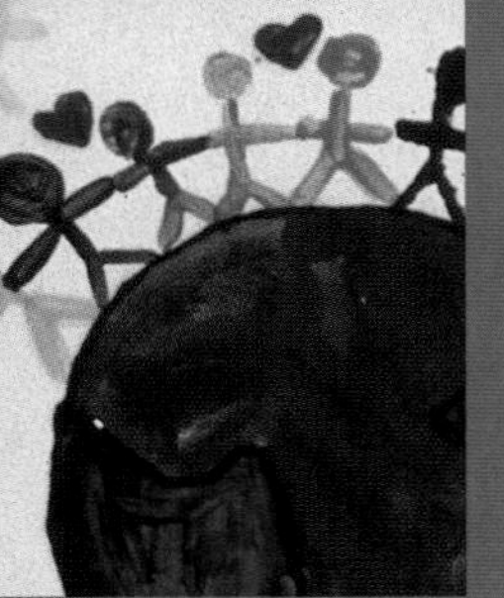

PARTNERING WITH FAMILIES

Preventing Animal Bites

General guidelines for pets in the home

- Never leave a young child alone with an animal.
- Do not buy or adopt a pet unless you are confident of your child's ability to respect it.
- Spay or neuter the pet to reduce aggression.

If an animal (wild or unknown) is sick or acting strangely, notify the health department.

Teach children the following rules

- Avoid all unfamiliar animals and report them to a parent.
- Avoid contact with all wild animals.
- Do not touch an animal when it is eating, sleeping, or nursing.
- Never overexcite an animal, even in play. Do not rough house or play games that stimulate aggressive behavior.
- Never tease or throw objects at an animal.
- Never put your face close to an animal. Seek permission before hugging or petting an animal.
- If approached by a dog, stay calm, stand still, talk softly, and back away slowly until the dog loses interest; do not run.
- If attacked, pretend to be a tree or a log and protect the face.

the signs and symptoms of infection. Assist childcare centers and schools to set up policies related to human bites. Parents should be informed when their child has been bitten by another child and recommendations for care should be provided.

Insect Bites and Stings

Insect bites and stings occur frequently in children and usually are not a cause for concern. Exceptions include bites or stings by insects that carry parasites or communicable diseases (ticks, mosquitoes), those of venomous nature (spiders), and those that produce an allergic reaction. About 4% of the population is sensitized to Hymenoptera (bees, wasps, fire ants) stings (White, Stewart, & Murdock, 2001). For a discussion of Lyme disease and Rocky Mountain spotted fever, see Chapter 19∞.

Clinical manifestations and clinical therapy for various insect and spider bites can be seen in the clinical manifestations table on page 1507.

- Reactions to bites of mosquitoes and fleas can be localized or systemic.
- Reactions to either bee stings or fire ant bites may be local inflammation or a systemic allergic response (wheezing, urticaria, diarrhea, vomiting, and dizziness). In some cases an anaphylactic response occurs. Desensitization for the Hymenoptera group may be considered when the child has a systemic reaction.
- Black widow spiders can be recognized by the red and orange hourglass-shape markings on its underside. It usually bites in self-defense and avoids light areas. If large doses of venom are absorbed, the bite may lead to paralysis and death. Antivenom (produced in horse serum) is used only in severe or high-risk cases because of the risk for anaphylaxis (Metry & Hebert, 2000).
- The brown recluse spider is recognized by the fiddle-shape marking on its head. It is usually unaggressive and bites only when provoked. Serious bites can cause necrosis that can extend into the muscle tissue. Hemolysis and systemic responses to the venom are sometimes seen.

Nursing Management

The goal of nursing care is prevention. Become familiar with the harmful insects in your geographic area so you can identify them and recognize their effects. Children should be taught to avoid spiders and other biting or stinging insects. Many commercial repellents (OFF, Cutter's, Deep Woods OFF) are available. Most products contain DEET (diethyltoluamide) and are effective against many insects including mosquitoes, fleas, ticks, and chiggers. The insect repellent produces a vapor layer that is malodorous and distasteful to insects. DEET does not repel stinging insects such as bees. Teach children to stay calm when a bee or wasp approaches and to slowly walk away without swatting.

PRACTICE ALERT

Insect repellent containing DEET (diethyltoluamide) should not be used in concentrations greater than 10% for children. Avoid application to the child's hands, near the eyes, lips, or broken skin. Wash DEET off of the skin with soap and water once the child is back indoors. Caution parents to avoid overuse of products containing DEET, especially with infants and small children. Cases of toxicity (behavioral changes, ataxia, encephalopathy, seizures, and coma) have been reported following repeated use on children's bedding and clothing (Metry & Hebert, 2000). It is believed that a combination of DEET with sunscreens may decrease the effectiveness of the sunscreen, so limit the sun exposure for these children.

Warn parents against using heavily perfumed shampoos, powders, soaps, or lotions, or dressing children in bright-colored or floral-print clothing when outdoors, as these may attract insects. Light-colored and smooth-textured clothing is less attractive to bees and wasps. Long sleeves and pants and loose-fitting clothing reduce the risk for stings and bites. Wear gloves for working in the garden and around shrubs.

Avoid eating sweet foods and beverages outdoors as these will attract bees and wasps. Bees and wasps may crawl into a canned beverage and not be seen. Pour beverages into a cup rather than drinking them from the can to prevent stings to the mouth and lips.

Household pets may be a source of fleas or ticks. Encourage frequent inspection of pets and preventive treatments against fleas and ticks before pets are allowed prolonged contact with children.

CLINICAL MANIFESTATIONS of Insect Bites and Stings

TYPE	CLINICAL MANIFESTATION	CLINICAL THERAPY
Mosquitoes and fleas Local inflammation results from injected foreign protein or chemicals.	Local reactions: • Discrete, red papules and edema at the bite site • Itching, burning, pain, and hives • Minimal discomfort • Pruritic wheals and bullae tend to develop with repeat exposure Systemic reactions: • Wheezing, urticaria • Laryngeal edema • Shock	Treatment is supportive for local reactions • Cold compresses or ice applied to the site • Antihistamine medication Systemic reactions need emergency medical treatment
Bee or wasp sting Venoms contain enzymes that affect vascular tone and permeability.	Local reaction: • Mild, local pain • Erythema and edema Systemic reaction: • Generalized urticaria, flushing, angioedema, pruritis • Wheezing • Anaphylaxis is rare	Local reactions: • Remove stinger if present as quickly as possible • Ice or cold compresses • A dash of meat tenderizer (papain powder) and a drop of water massaged into the skin for 5 minutes quickly relieves the pain of most insect bites and stings • Elevate extremity • Antihistamine medication Systemic reactions are treated with glucocorticoids and antihistamines or epinephrine Desensitization for severe reactions
Fire ants Venom is hemolytic and neurotoxic, causing a histamine-like response.	• A black center at the point of the bite, or trail of lesions across skin • Initial wheal turns into a vesicle within a few hours. In 24 hours the fluid is cloudy and the vesicle is surrounded by a red halo. • Pruritis • Erythema, edema, induration Systemic and anaphylactic reactions can occur	Local reactions: • Ice or cold compresses • Antihistamine medication • Elevate extremity Systemic reactions—same as bees and wasps
Black widow spider Venom is neurotoxic.	• Stinging sensation at time of bite • Localized edema and erythema • Two fang marks • Petechiae branching from site Systemic reaction in 1–3 hours • Muscle rigidity of torso and abdomen, priapism, muscle cramps near the bite • Malaise, sweating, nausea, vomiting, dizziness • Hypertension and arrhythmias • Oliguria • Restlessness and insomnia • Symptoms peak in 3–12 hours and diminish within 72 hours	Ice Diazepam and opioids Antivenom IV is used in severe reactions after negative skin test for hypersensitivity to horse serum Antihistamine medication Hydrocortisone may decrease the inflammatory response
Brown recluse spider Venom contains proteolytic enzymes and sphingomyelinase D, a cytotoxic factor.	• Erythema and edema evolving to purple bull's eye lesion with an outer white zone of induration • Progresses to severe necrosis that hardens and falls off in 7–14 days when ulcerated depression is seen that heals in 6–8 weeks with scarring • Necrosis is more extensive on adipose tissue • Severe progressive reactions may occur in 12–72 hours, including fever, chills, restlessness, malaise, joint pain, and nausea and vomiting • Intravascular hemolysis may also occur with a severe reaction that results in anemia	Ice Cleanse the wound and good wound care Analgesics Antibiotics for secondary infection Excision and skin grafting in cases of severe necrosis

When a severe allergic reaction to Hymenoptera has occurred, the child should wear a medical alert identification and carry an emergency kit with epinephrine. Teach parents how to monitor the expiration date of the epinephrine and to check the medication weekly for discoloration or a precipitate, indicating a need for replacement. Teach the child, parents, and school personnel how to administer epinephrine. Make sure the school nurse receives the written order for the epinephrine injector so that it can be administered if necessary. Desensitization injections may be given to children with an anaphylactic reaction or severe systemic reaction.

Snakebites

Venomous snakes are found in most areas of the country. During warm months of the year, snakes are active and likely to bite if disturbed. Fortunately many bites are dry, delivering no venom. Fatalities are rare. The United States has several types of venomous snakes that children may encounter. Rattlesnakes, copperheads, and cottonmouths are members of the Crotalidae family of snakes with similar venom characteristics, and they account for 95% of snakebites (Herman & Skokan, 1999). Coral snakes are members of the Elapidae family of snakes that also includes cobras and mambas.

Etiology and Pathophysiology

Rattlesnake, copperhead, and water moccasin venom is composed of proteolytic enzymes that break down proteins, fats, and connective tissue, as well as components that cause hemolysis and vacular permeability. Neurotoxin and cardiotoxin components are also present (Cordasco, Jones, & Lindell, 2001). Loss of vascular integrity permits blood cells, plasma, and albumin to move into surrounding soft tissues, depleting vascular volume. Cardiotoxins may depress cardiac contractility. The child may be at risk for shock. Coral snake venom is a neurotoxin that blocks nerve impulses to the muscle tissue. They deliver venom by biting, hanging on, and chewing repeatedly. If untreated, respiratory and cardiac failure are a common cause of death (Pitman, 2002). The amount and toxicity of the venom injected has an impact on the morbidity and mortality associated with the snakebite. Because children usually receive a higher concentration of venom relative to body mass, their response to snake bite may be greater than an adult's. Envenomation may be life threatening in small children who receive a full dose of venom.

Clinical Manifestations

Bites by the Crotalidae family snakes will result in puncture marks, a white wheal, and a burning sensation at the site. Erythema, ecchymosis, and edema rapidly develop and extend from the site, as the vascular integrity is lost. Edema and erythema may spread for up to 24 hours. Local areas become swollen and tense, but true compartment syndrome does not usually occur. Autonomic signs may include dizziness, tachycardia, sweating, nausea, vomiting, and diarrhea, and the severity is associated with amount of venom injected. With significant envenomation, systemic signs will potentially include hypotension, altered mental status, bleeding from multiple sites (if disseminated intravascular coagulation develops), dyspnea, cough and frothy pink secretions (pulmonary edema due to capillary leaks into the lungs), and renal failure.

Bites from the coral snake are accompanied by numbness and mild soft tissue swelling. Neurologic signs include diplopia and ptosis, difficulty speaking and swallowing, hypersalivation, and altered mental status (lethargy, drowsiness, or euphoria). If untreated, signs progress to pharyngeal spasm, cyanosis, hypotension, and tachycardia, heralding the onset of respiratory failure.

COLLABORATIVE CARE

The goal of collaborative care is to identify the snake, treat systemic signs of envenomation, and care for the resulting integumentary injury.

Diagnostic Tests

Laboratory studies include complete blood count, platelet count, coagulation studies, electrolytes, and renal function. Attempt to determine the identity of the snake causing the bite to determine if it was venomous. The poison control center can provide guidelines for treatment.

Clinical Therapy

Clinical therapy involves immediate immobilization of the extremity and a cold compress to slow the spread of the venom during transport to the emergency department. Remove rings or constricting items as soon as possible. A compression bandage at the bite site (ace wrap) and extended proximally may help slow the spread of the venom to the circulation. This bandage should not obstruct venous or arterial blood flow. Tourniquets and excision of the bite are no longer recommended.

The bite site should be cleaned with germicidal soap and water. Antibiotics are not indicated unless a secondary infection develops. Give a tetanus booster if the vaccination status is unknown or if the tetanus series is incomplete.

In severe envenomations, antivenom is the treatment of choice when there is rapid progression of swelling or the presence of systemic signs. Antivenom works best if administered within 4 to 6 hours of the bite. Because antivenom is a hyperimmune horse serum product, it can cause anaphylaxis or delayed serum sickness reaction. A skin test may be performed first to detect hypersensitivity, but false positives and false negatives are common. Antihistamines are given in preparation for a hypersensitivity reaction. Antiserum is diluted in saline and slowly infused intravenously while carefully monitoring for a hypersensitivity reaction. Response to antivenom (increased swelling of the extremity or coagulation defects) is monitored to determine when to continue or discontinue antivenom administration. Because of the amount of venom potentially injected into a child, a larger amount of antivenom may be needed. See Chapter 26∞ for information on anaphylaxis and serum sickness.

A fasciotomy for true compartment syndrome may be needed, and surgical debridement is performed to remove necrotic tissue once it is clearly demarcated.

NURSING MANAGEMENT

The goals of nursing management include reducing the consequences of the snakebite, carefully monitoring the child receiving antivenom treatment, and educating parents to care for the child at home following discharge.

Nursing Assessment and Diagnosis

Assess families for knowledge of poisonous snakes that are present in specific geographic areas during health promotion/health maintenance visits. When families are visiting other countries or different sections of their home country, ask if they know about snakes or other hazards, particularly if outdoor activities are planned.

Nursing care involves assessment of the child for initial and progressive signs of envenomation. Monitor vital signs according to hospital guidelines. Assess the need for emergency airway, breathing, and circulatory interventions. Assess pain and the child's response to pain medication. Measure the circumference of the extremity with the bite every 20 to 30 minutes to track progression in swelling and response to treatment.

Examples of nursing diagnoses that might be appropriate in the child with a snakebite include:

- Fear related to separation from support system in the stressful situation associated with emergency treatment of the snakebite
- Decreased Cardiac Output related to loss of vascular integrity associated with envenomation
- Ineffective Breathing Pattern related to neuromuscular dysfunction associated with envenomation
- Impaired Skin Integrity related to altered circulation associated with envenomation

Planning and Implementation

First aid involves immobilizing the extremity, keeping it in dependent position to slow the spread of venom, and applying cold compresses. Remove any jewelry or constricting items from the injured extremity. Keep the child quiet and calm to slow the circulation and spread of the venom. Help the child identify the snake from pictures of snakes common to the geographic area; however, keep in mind that other venomous snakes may be kept as exotic pets.

The child receiving antivenom treatment is usually cared for in a critical care unit. Administer the antihistamines and intravenous antivenom after tests for sensitivity to horse serum are completed. Have resuscitation equipment at hand in preparation for anaphylactic reaction. Monitor the child for progressive signs of envenomation and for hypersensitivity responses to antivenom. Assist in locating additional antivenom if the hospital does not have an adequate supply.

Provide emotional support to the child and family.

Provide skin care to the swollen and tense skin to prevent abrasions or skin breakdown. Monitor the bite area for necrosis and secondary infection. Protect the injured extremity from further injury once the child is well enough to mobilize.

Discharge Planning and Home Care Teaching

Provide information about the potential for development of delayed serum sickness up to 2 weeks after administration of antiserum, and signs to watch for (joint pain, skin rash, swollen lymph nodes, urinary symptoms, or mental status changes). Provide guidelines for seeking care if symptoms develop. Additionally provide information to care for the child's skin and bite injury.

Teach the child and family how to avoid future snakebites. Children venturing into areas where snakes inhabit should wear protective clothing, avoid reaching into areas where snakes may hide, and avoid threatening a snake. If a snake is seen, the child should slowly retreat and give the snake lots of room.

Evaluation

Expected outcomes of nursing care include the following:

- Hypersensitivity reactions to antivenom are quickly identified and treated effectively.
- The injured extremity heals without secondary infection.
- Signs of delayed serum sickness are quickly identified by the family and prompt care is obtained.

Scorpion Bites

Scorpions are an arthropod with a stinger on the tail. One species of scorpion, found in the Southwest, is potentially dangerous to humans. Scorpions are not aggressive and they sting in self-defense. Stings cause intense pain that worsens with light pressure on the sting site. Neurologic signs may include neuromuscular excitation, paresthesias, tachycardia, and hypertension. Pain usually resolves in 4 hours and symptoms resolve in 24 hours. Stings rarely result in death, except in small children who may experience respiratory failure.

No diagnostic procedures are performed. Efforts to capture the scorpion for identification should be attempted. Treatment involves supportive measures such as intravenous access, oxygen, pulse oximetry, and cardiac monitoring. Sedation may be required for neuromuscular symptoms. Narcotics are not used as they may worsen the neurotoxicity. Antivenom is available for some species and is sometimes used.

Nursing Management

Nursing care involves supportive care during the day after the bite. Carefully monitor vital signs, oxygen saturation, and cardiac rhythm. Clean the sting site with warm soap and water. Apply ice to the sting site and keep the extremity elevated. Monitor intake and output. If antivenom is used, provide care as described for snakebite antivenom. Provide reassurance to the child and family that the pain and reaction will be gone within 24 hours.

MINOR SKIN INJURIES

Contusions

Contusions are soft tissue injuries that result from a variety of causes. Often it is difficult to assess whether an injury has caused underlying tissue damage. An injury does not have to break the skin to result in internal damage. Radiographic examination may be necessary to rule out broken bones or further tissue damage. Signs and symptoms that indicate a need for treatment include swelling that does not subside within 72 hours, intense pain, inability to move the injured part, and infection. Elevate the injured extremity and apply ice as soon as possible after injury to reduce inflammation and swelling in the area.

Foreign Bodies

Many skin injuries result from penetration of foreign particles. Common substances include gravel from abrasions, bee stingers, and splinters. Treatment of superficial foreign bodies involves irrigating the wound to try to forcibly dislodge the debris. A deeply embedded foreign body is best removed under medical supervision to avoid permanent injury or scarring.

Lacerations

Lacerations are caused by cuts or tears to the skin. In many cases the cut is minor and can be managed at home with gentle cleansing, antibiotic ointment, and a bandage. More extensive lacerations, and those on the face or over joints, often need suturing to promote healing and reduce scarring. Laceration repair is performed after wound cleansing and appropriate local analgesia to control pain. Sutures are usually removed about 7 days later.

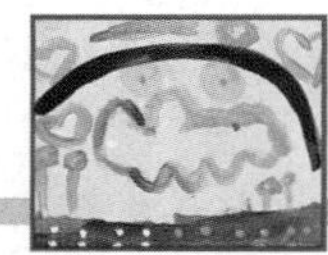

CHAPTER HIGHLIGHTS

- The skin has several essential functions: perception of pain, heat, and cold; protective barrier against microorganisms, ultraviolet radiation, and loss of body fluids; temperature regulation; vitamin D synthesis; and excretion.
- Wound healing has three overlapping phases: inflammation, reconstruction, and maturation.
- Treatment of atopic dermatitis involves hydration and lubrication of the skin with moisturizing ointments. Inflammation is treated with wet compresses, corticosteroid ointments, and emollients.
- Contact dermatitis is an inflammation of the skin that occurs in response to direct contact with either an allergen, causing an immune response, or with an irritant, resulting in no immune response.
- Superabsorbent disposable diapers reduce the frequency and severity of diaper dermatitis because, when wet, a gel forms and keeps the skin drier than cloth diapers.
- Seborrheic dermatitis is an inflammatory skin condition due to an overgrowth of *Pityrosporum* yeast in areas of sebaceous gland activity. It is commonly found on the scalp, forehead, and postauricular and periorbital areas.
- Drug reactions vary in severity from a simple allergic reaction and erythema multiforme minor to potentially life-threatening responses such as erythema multiforme major (Stevens-Johnson syndrome), and toxic epidermal necrolysis.
- Acne medications, tretinoin or isotretinoin, are phototoxic, resulting in sunburn with even minimal exposure. Avoidance of sun exposure or the use of sunscreen is important to prevent significant sunburn.
- The classic impetigo lesion begins as a vesicle surrounded by edema and redness. The vesicle fluid turns cloudy and ruptures, leaving a honey-colored crust on an ulcerated base.
- Folliculitis, a superficial inflammation of the pilosebaceous follicle, may be associated with *Pseudomonas* exposure in a poorly chlorinated pool or hot tub.
- Children with cellulitis appear ill with fever, chills, malaise, and enlarged lymph nodes. The infected site is red or lilac in color, warm, edematous, and tender.
- Viral skin infections include molluscum contagiosum and warts.
- Children regularly using oral inhalers with corticosteroids are at risk for thrush (oral candidiasis). Rinsing the mouth and spacer well with water after using the inhaler helps to prevent thrush.
- Treatment for tinea capitus involves 8 to 12 weeks of oral griseofulvin. Giving this medication with fatty foods such as whole milk or peanut butter enhances its absorption. Children being treated may develop an "id" hypersensitivity reaction rash to the fungal antigen, not an allergic reaction to the medication.
- Treatment for lice includes a pediculicide shampoo or an ovicidal rinse, distilled white vinegar to loosen the nits' bonds to the hair shafts, and combing the hair with a fine-toothed comb to remove all the nits. A second treatment is needed in 7 days.
- Scabies is an infestation caused by direct contact in which the female mite burrows under the skin to lay eggs. The eggs, feces, and debris left behind causes irritation and intense itching. Often the child's scratching and secondary infection result in lesions with no distinct appearance.
- Hemangiomas undergo a period of rapid growth during infancy before involuting. The rapid growth may cause complications, such as pressure on the airway, eye, or ear canal.
- Birthmarks or skin lesions that can indicate an underlying condition include a port-wine stain (Sturge-Weber syndrome) and café-au-lait spots (neurofibromatosis).
- Children at greatest risk for pressure ulcers are those with limited mobility, sensory deficits, or the inability to change positions. Tissue ischemia occurs when the soft tissues and capillary beds are compressed between a bony prominence and another surface.
- Of the four main types of burns (thermal, chemical, electrical, and radioactive), thermal burns are most common in children. Infants, toddlers,

and preschool-age children most commonly suffer scald burns. Other types of thermal burns include flames and contact with a hot object.

- Initial treatment for a child with a significant burn injury includes emergency assessment of the airway, breathing, and circulation; and stopping the burning process by removing jewelry, clothing, and applying moist soaks or ice.
- Up to 80% of a person's lifetime exposure to the sun occurs before 21 years of age. Repeated sunburns during childhood increase the risk for development of malignant melanoma in early adulthood.
- Children are at greater risk for hypothermia because of their thinner skin, limited subcutaneous fat, and high surface area to body mass ratio. Body heat is lost more quickly in water or when clothing is wet.
- Frostbite occurs when ice crystallizes in the tissues, causing cellular dehydration and ischemic damage.
- Dog bites account for 80% of animal bites treated in the United States. Children at greater risk for animal bites are boys less than 8 years old. Most children know the dog that bites them.
- Insects and spiders with venomous bites include bees, fire ants, black widow spiders, and brown recluse spiders.
- Venomous snakes living in the wild in the United States include rattlesnakes, copperheads, water moccasins, and coral snakes. Initial treatment includes immobilization of the extremity and cold compresses to slow the spread of the venom.
- Minor skin injuries that may need clinical therapy include contusions, foreign bodies, and lacerations.

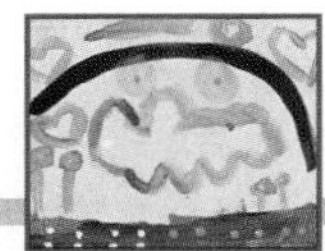

CRITICAL THINKING IN ACTION

INTRODUCTION

Return to the scenario at the beginning of the chapter. As mentioned, Sherray has a wound debridement and a dressing change twice a day that causes pain. Consider the physical and psychological issues in the nursing care of Sherray.

DESCRIPTION

Sherray will be discharged in the next day and continuing care of her wound will be performed at home by her mother with frequent visits to the burn clinic.

DISCUSSION

1. Sherray has no intravenous line, so what is the appropriate method to administer pain medication? How soon in advance of the wound debridement should the pain medication be administered?
2. Describe complementary interventions that could further reduce Sherray's pain and anxiety. Describe other interventions that could potentially reduce the psychological impact of the burn injury.
3. Develop a teaching plan to ensure that Sherray's mother is prepared to change Sherray's dressings.
4. Discuss food choices with Sherray's mother and help her plan a high-calorie diet, that includes foods Sherray enjoys, to promote healing.

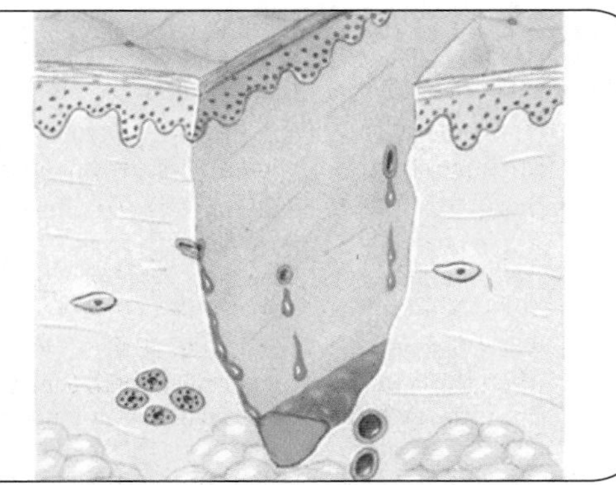

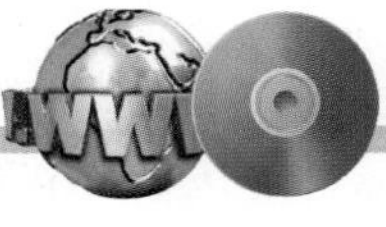

EXPLORE MediaLink

- NCLEX review, case studies, and other interactive resources for this chapter can be found on the Companion Website at **www.prenhall.com/ball**. Click on Chapter 36 to select the activities for this chapter.
- For animations, more NCLEX review questions, and an audio glossary, access the accompanying CD-ROM in this book.

http://www.prenhall.com/ball

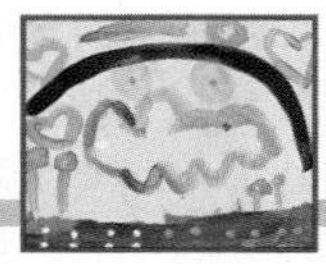

REFERENCES

Allen, P. L. J. (2004). Leaves of three, let them be: If it were only that easy! *Pediatric Nursing, 30*(2), 129–135.

American Academy of Pediatrics Committee on Infectious Disease. (2003). *Red book: Report of the committee on infectious disease* (26th ed). Elk Grove Village, IL: Author.

American Academy of Pediatrics Committee on School Health. (2002). Head lice. *Pediatrics, 110*(3), 638–643.

Angel, T. A., Nigro, J., & Levy, M. L. (2000). Infestations in the pediatric patient. *Pediatric Clinics of North America, 47*(4), 921–935.

Bell, E. A. (2004, March). Minimize the potential for side effects with topical corticosteroids. *Infectious Diseases in Children*, 12, 15.

Bernardo, L. M., Gardner, M. J., O'Connor, J., & Amon, N. (2000). Dog bites in children treated in a pediatric emergency department. *Journal of Society of Pediatric Nurses, 5*(2), 87–95.

Brodell, R. T., & Vescera, G. (2002). Black-dot tinea capitus. *Postgraduate Medicine, 111*(4), 123–126.

Buck, M. L. (2001). Isotretinoin: Improving patient education and reducing risk. *Pediatric Pharmacology, 7*(7), 1–6.

Buck, M. L. (2002). Topical macrolactam immunomodulators for atopic dermatitis in children. *Pediatric Pharmacology, 8*(5). www.medscape.com/viewarticle/441911_print, accessed 11/12/2002.

Centers for Disease Control and Prevention. (2002). Guidelines for school programs to prevent cancer. *Morbidity and Mortality Weekly Report, 51* (RR-4), 1–18.

Centers for Disease Control and Prevention. (2003a). Methicillin-resistant Staphylococcus aureus infections among competitive sports participants—Colorado, Indiana, Pennsylvania, and Los Angelos County, 2000–2003. *Morbidity and Mortality Weekly Report, 52*(33), 793–795.

Centers for Disease Control and Prevention. (2003b). Preventing skin cancer: Recommendations and reports. *Morbidity and Mortality Weekly Report, 52* (RR-15), 1–12.

Cheigh, N. H. (2003). Managing a common disorder in children: Atopic dermatitis. *Journal of Pediatric Health Care, 17*(2), 84–88.

Cohen, B. A. (2002). Plaques: Oval, itchy, and red: What's your diagnosis? *Contemporary Pediatrics, 19*(4), 36, 41.

Cordasco, R., Jones, W., & Lindell, W. (2001). Treatment of the pediatric snakebite victim. *Air Medical Journal, 20*(2), 32–34.

Curley, M. A. Q., Razmus, I. S., Roberts, K. E., & Wypij, D. (2003). Predicting pressure ulcer risk in pediatric patients. *Nursing Research, 52*(1), 22–31.

Davy, L., Boyett, T., Weathers, L., Campbell, R. J., & Roetzheim, R. B. (2002). Sun protection counseling by pediatricians. *Ambulatory Pediatrics, 2*(3), 207–211.

Deegan, T. (2000). Pediatric perspective: Accidental hypothermia. *AirMed, 6*(6), 6–9.

Delatte, S. J., Evans, J., Hebra, A., Adamson, W., Othersen, H. B., & Tagge, E. P. (2001). Effectiveness of beta-glucagon collagen for treatment of partial thickness burns in children. *Journal of Pediatric Surgery, 36*(1), 113–118.

Dinehart, S. M., Kincannon, J., & Geronemus, R. (2001). Hemangiomas: Evaluation and treatment. *Dermatologic Surgery, 27*(5), 475–485.

Drake, L., & Prendergast, M. (2001). The impact of tacrolimus ointment on health-related quality of life of adult and pediatric patients with atopic dermatitis. *Journal of American Academy of Dermatology, 44*, S65–S72.

Drolet, B. A., Esterly, N. B., & Frieden, I. J. (1999). Hemangiomas in children. *New England Journal of Medicine, 341*(3), 173–181.

Elewski, B. E., & Krowchuk, D. P. (2001). Update on tinea capitus: Reaching consensus. *Contemporary Pediatrics*, S11–S14.

Food and Drug Administration. (2005). FDA public health advisory: Elidel (pimecrolimus) cream and Protopic (tacrolimus) ointment. www.fda.gov/cder/drug/advisory/elidel_protopic.htm, accesed 4/3/2005.

Food and Drug Administration. (2003). FDA issues health advisory regarding labeling changes for lindane products. www.fda.gov/bbs/topics/ANSWERS/2003/ANS01205.html, accessed 3/31/2003.

Forman, R., Koren, G., & Shear, N. H. (2002). Erythema multiforme, Stevens-Johnson syndrome, and toxic epidermal necrolysis in children. *Drug Safety, 25*(13), 965–972.

Frankowski, B., Weiner, L., Committee on School Health, Committee on Infectious Diseases, & American Academy of Pediatrics. (2002). Head lice. *Pediatrics, 110*(3), 638–643.

Friedlander, S. F. (1998). Contact dermatitis. *Pediatrics in Review, 19*(5), 166–170.

Gardner, P., Coles, D., & Kemper, K. J. (2001). The skinny on herbal remedies for dermatologic disorders. *Contemporary Pediatrics, 18*(7), 103–114.

Geller, A., Rutsch, L., Kenausis, K., & Zhang, Z. (2003). Evaluation of the SunWise school program. *Journal of School Nursing, 19*(2), 93–99.

Geller, A. C., Colditz, G., Oliveria, S., Emmons, K., Jorgensen, C., Aweh, G. N., & Frazier, A. L. (2002). Use of sunscreen, sunburning rates, and tanning bed use among more than 10,000 children and adolescents. *Pediatrics, 109*(6), 1009–1014.

Giesbrecht, G. G. (2000). Cold stress, near drowning, and accidental hypothermia: A review. *Aviation, Space, and Environmental Medicine, 71*(7), 733–752.

Hansen, R. C. (2003). Atopic dermatitis: Taming the "itch that rashes." *Contemporary Pediatrics, 20*(7), 79–97.

Hansen, S. L., Voight, D. W., Wiebelhaus, P., & Paul, C. N. (2000). Using skin replacement products to treat burns and wounds. *Advances in Skin and Wound Care, 14*(1), 37–44.

Health Canada. (2002, September). Burns and scalds in the 1999 CHIRPP database. *CHIRPP News, 21.* www.hc-sc.gc.ca/pphb-dgspsp/publicat/chirpp-schirpt/21se02/index.html, accessed 7/2/2003.

Hebert, P. W., Rakes, G. P., Loach, T. C., & Murphy, D. D. (1997). Recognizing the young atopic child. *Contemporary Pediatrics, 14*(4), 131–139.

Herman, B. E., & Skokan, E. G. (1999). Bites that poison: A tale of spiders, snakes, and scorpions. *Contemporary Pediatrics, 16*(8), 41–65.

Herndon, D. N. & Spies, M. (2001). Modern burn care, *Seminars in Pediatric Surgery, 10*(1). 28–31.

Huether, S. E. (2002). Structure, function, and disorders of the integument. In K. L. McCance & S. E. Huether, *Pathophysiology: The biologic basis for disease in adults and children* (4th ed., pp. 1434–1468). St. Louis: Mosby.

Jick, S. S., Kremers, H. M., & Vasilakis-Scaramozza, C. (2000). Isotretinoin use and risk of depression, psychotic symptoms, suicide, and attempted suicide. *Archives of Dermatology, 136*(10), 1231–1236.

Johnson, K., Davy, L., Boyett, T., Weathers, L., & Roetzheim, R. G. (2001). Sun protection practices for children: Knowledge, attitudes, and parent behaviors. *Archives of Pediatric and Adolescent Medicine, 155*(8), 891–896.

Kalliomäki, M., Salminen, S., Poussa, T., Arvilommi, H., & Isolauri, E. (2003). Probiotics and prevention of atopic disease: 4 year follow-up of randomized placebo-controlled trial. *Lancet, 361*(9372), 1869–1871.

Kazaks, E. L., & Lane, A. T. (2000). Diaper dermatitis. *Pediatric Clinics of North America, 47*(4), 909–919.

Latchman, Y. E., Xu, X. J., Poulter, L. W., Ruston, M. H. A., & Brostoff, J. (2002). Chinese medical herbs in the treatment of atopic dermatitis. *ACI International, 14*(1), 4–9.

Laughlin-Richard, N. (2000). Sun exposure and skin cancer prevention in children and adolescents. *Journal of School Nursing, 16*(2), 20–26.

Lukish, J. R., Eichelberger, M. R., Newman, K. D., Pao, M., Nobuhara, K., Keating, M., et al. (2001). The use of a bioactive skin substitute decreases length of stay for pediatric burn patients. *Journal of Pediatric Surgery, 36*(8), 1118–1121.

Mancini, A. J. (2000). Acne vulgaris: A treatment update. *Contemporary Pediatrics, 17*(12), 122–133.

Metry, D. W., & Hebert, A. A. (2000). Insect and arachnid stings, bites, infestations, and repellents. *Pediatric Annals, 29*(1), 39–48.

Milano, M. (1999). Oral electrical and thermal burns in children: Review and report of case. *Journal of Dentistry for Children, 66*(2), 116–119.

Milner, S. M., Mottar, R., & Smith, C. E. (2001). The burn wheel: An innovative method for calculating the need for fluid resuscitation in burned patients. *American Journal of Nursing, 101*(11), 35–37.

Murphy, S. A. (2000). Deaths: Final data for 1998. *National Vital Statistics Reports, 48*(11). Hyattsville, MD: National Center for Health Statistics.

Nicol, N. H. (2000). Managing atopic dermatitis in children and adults. *The Nurse Practitioner, 25*(4), 54–76.

Odio, M., Streicher-Scott, J., & Hansen, R. C. (2001). Disposable baby wipes: Efficacy and skin mildness. *Dermatology Nursing, 13*(2), 107–121.

O'Riordan, D. L., Geller, A. C., Brooks, D. R., Zhang, Z., & Miller, D. R. (2003). Sunburn reduction through parental role modeling and sunscreen vigilance. *Journal of Pediatrics, 142,* 67–72.

Paller, A. S. (2001). Use of nonsteroidal topical immunomodulators for the treatment of atopic dermatitis in the pediatric population. *Journal of Pediatrics, 138*(2), 163–168.

Perry, C. M. (2003). Thermal injuries. In P. A. Moloney-Harmon, & S. J. Czerwinski, (Eds.), *Nursing care of the pediatric trauma patient* (pp. 277–294). St. Louis: Saunders.

Pitman, H. J. (2002). Once bitten: The keys to coral snakebite management. *American Journal of Nursing, 102*(4), 24DD-24GG.

Raimer, S. S. (2000). Managing pediatric atopic dermatitis. *Clinical Pediatrics, 39*(1), 1–14.

Rodgers, G. L. (2000). Reducing the toll of childhood burns. *Contemporary Pediatrics, 17*(4), 152–173.

Rote, N. S. (2002). Inflammation. In K. L. McCance & S. E. Huether (Eds.), *Pathophysiology: The basis for disease in adults and children* (4th ed., pp. 197–226). St. Louis: Mosby.

Rudy, S. J. (2003). Overview of the evaluation and management of acne vulgaris. *Pediatric Nursing, 29*(4), 287–293.

Samaniego, I. A. (2003). A sore spot in pediatrics: Risk factors for pressure ulcers. *Pediatric Nursing, 29*(4), 278–282.

Schachner, L., Field, T., Hernandez-Ruif, M., Duarte, A. M., & Krasnegor, J. (1998). Atopic dermatitis symptoms decreased in children following massage therapy. *Pediatric Dermatology, 15*(5), 390–395.

Schmidt, C. E. (2003). A 12-month-old girl with maculopapular lesions and lower extremity edema. *Journal of Emergency Nursing, 29*(3), 204–207.

Schober-Flores, C. (2003). Epidermolysis bullosa: The challenges of wound care. *Dermatologic Nursing, 15*(2), 135–138.

Shwayder, T. (2003). Five common skin problems—and a string of pearls for managing them. *Contemporary Pediatrics, 20*(7), 34–54.

Sidbury, R., & Paller, A. S. (2000). The diagnosis and management of acne. *Pediatric Annals, 29*(1), 17–24.

Smith, M. L. (2000). Pediatric burns: Management of thermal, electrical, and chemical burns and burnlike dermatologic conditions. *Pediatric Annals, 29*(6), 367–378.

Spies, M., Sanford, A. P., Low, J. F. A., Wolf, S. E., & Herndon, D. N. (2001). Treatment of extensive toxic epidermal necrolysis in children. *Pediatrics, 108*(5), 1162–1168.

Stewart, C. (2000). Emergency care of pediatric burns. *Pediatric Emergency Medicine Reports, 5*(10), 101–112.

U.S. Department of Health and Human Services. (2000). *Healthy People 2010* (2nd ed.). Washington, DC: U.S. Government Printing Office. www.healthypeople.gov

Valencia, I. C., Falabella, A. F., & Schachner, L. A. (2001). New developments in wound care for infants and children. *Pediatric Annals, 30*(4), 211–218.

Vanderhooft, S. L. (1998). Is the rash really a drug reaction? *Contemporary Pediatrics, 15*(5), 118–137.

von Heimburg, D., Noah, E. M., Sieckmann, U. P. F., & Pallua, N. (2001). Hyperbaric oxygen treatment in deep frostbite of both hands in a boy. *Burns, 27,* 404–408.

Weston, W. L., & Bruckner, A. (2000). Allergic contact dermatitis. *Pediatric Clinics of North America, 47*(4), 897–907.

Whalley, D., Huels, J., McKenna, S. P., & van Assche, D. (2002). The benefit of pimecrolimus on parents' quality of life in the treatment of pediatric atopic dermatitis. *Pediatrics, 110*(6), 1133–1136.

White, G. L., Stewart, J. S., & Murdock, R. T. (2001). Hymenoptera stings: Treatment and prevention. *Physician Assistant, 25*(2), 15–23.

Wiebelhaus, P., & Hansen, S. L. (2001). Another choice for burn victims. *RN, 64*(9), 34–37.

Williams, J. V., Godfrey, J. C., & Friedlander, S. F. (2003). Superficial fungal infections: Confronting the fungus among us. *Contemporary Pediatrics, 20*(1), 58–80.

Woodard, I. (2002). Adolescent acne: A stepwise approach to management. *Topics in Advanced Practice Nursing eJournal, 2*(2). www.medscape.com/viewarticle/430534, accessed 9/24/2003.

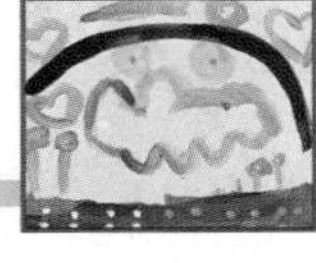

ADDITIONAL REFERENCES

Armsmeier, S. L., & Paller, A. S. (1997). Getting to the bottom of diaper dermatitis. *Contemporary Pediatrics, 14*(11), 115–129.

Ball, J. W. (1998). *Mosby's pediatric patient teaching guides.* St. Louis: Mosby.

Darmstadt, G. L. (1997). A guide to superficial strep and staph skin infections. *Contemporary Pediatrics, 14*(5), 95–116.

Dohil, M. A., Baugh, W. P., & Eichenfield, L. F. (2000). Vascular and pigmented birthmarks. *Pediatric Clinics of North America, 47*(4), 783–812.

Ebling, A. M. (2001). Effectiveness of oral antibiotics and topical retinoid therapy in the treatment of acne in adolescents. *Pediatric Nursing, 27*(4), 410–411, 421.

Hernandez-Reif, M., Field, T., Largie, S., Hart, S., Redezepi, M., Nierenberg, B., & Peck, M. (2001). Children's distress during burn treatment reduced by massage therapy. *Journal of Burn Care Rehabilitation, 22*(2), 191–195.

Martin-Herz, S. P., Patterson, D. R., Honari, S., Gibbons, J., Gibran, N., & Heimbach, D. M. (2003). Pediatric pain control practices of North American burn centers. *Journal of Burn Rehabilitation, 24*(1), 26–36.

Quigley, S. M., & Curley, M. A. Q. (1996). Skin integrity in the pediatric population: Preventing and managing pressure ulcers. *Journal of the Society of Pediatric Nurses, 1*(1), 7–18.

Schachner, L. A. (2000, May). Sun protection in three ways. *Contemporary Pediatrics,* S8–S11.

Silverberg, N. B. (2003). Pediatric molluscum contagiosum: Optimal treatment strategies. *Pediatric Drugs, 5*(8), 505–512.

Silverberg, N. B., Licht, J., Friedler, S., Sethi, S., & Laude, T. A. (2002). Nickel contact hypersensitivity in children. *Pediatric Dermatology, 19*(2), 110–113.

Su, J. C., Kemp, A. S., Varigos, G. A., & Nolan, T. M. (1997). Atopic eczema: Its impact on the family and financial cost. *Archives of Diseases in Children, 76*(2), 159–162.

Taylor, K. (2001). The management of minor burns and scalds in children. *Nursing Standard, 16*(11), 45–51.

Yetman, R. J., & Parks, D. (2002). Diagnosis and management of atopic dermatitis. *Journal of Pediatric Health Care, 16*(3), 143–145.

Young, R. J., & Huffman, S. (2003). Probiotic use in children. *Journal of Pediatric Health Care, 17*(6), 277–283.

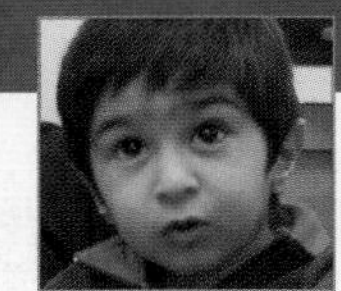
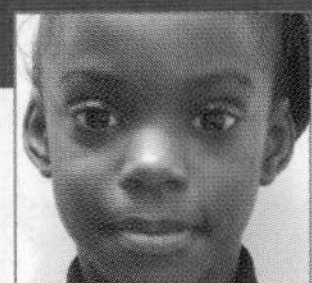
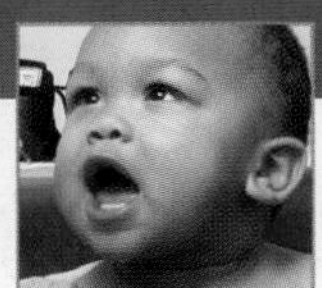
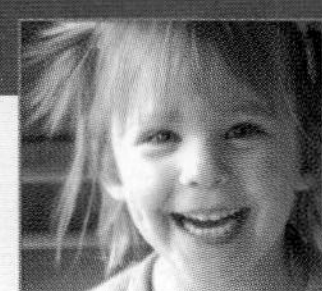

APPENDIX A
Physical Growth Charts

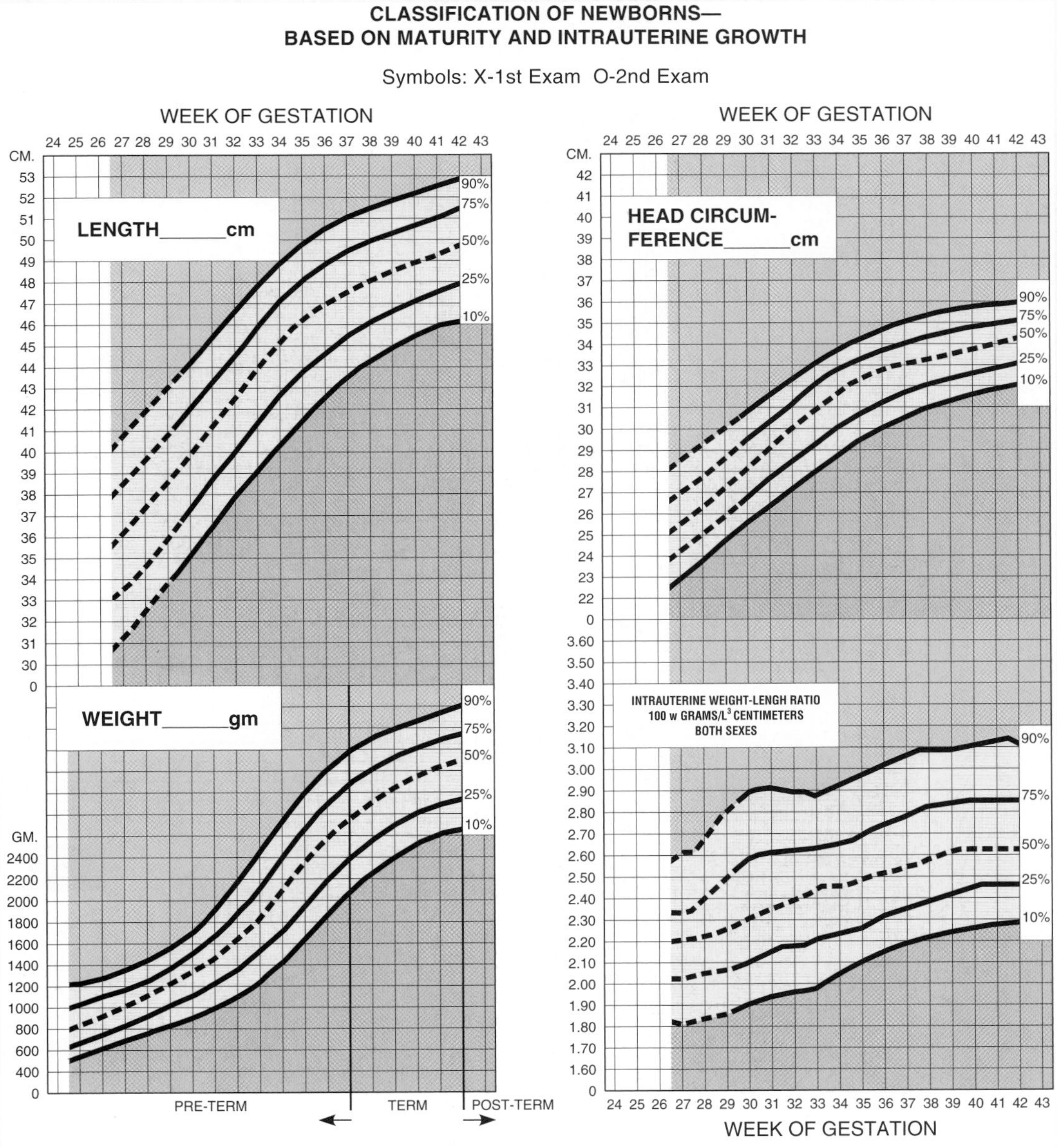

CLASSIFICATION OF NEWBORNS—
BASED ON MATURITY AND INTRAUTERINE GROWTH

Symbols: X-1st Exam O-2nd Exam

WEEK OF GESTATION

24 25 26 27 28 29 30 31 32 33 34 35 36 37 38 39 40 41 42 43

CM.

LENGTH______cm

90% 75% 50% 25% 10%

WEIGHT______gm

90% 75% 50% 25% 10%

GM.

PRE-TERM TERM POST-TERM

WEEK OF GESTATION

HEAD CIRCUM-
FERENCE______cm

90% 75% 50% 25% 10%

INTRAUTERINE WEIGHT-LENGH RATIO
100 w GRAMS/L^3 CENTIMETERS
BOTH SEXES

90% 75% 50% 25% 10%

24 25 26 27 28 29 30 31 32 33 34 35 36 37 38 39 40 41 42 43

WEEK OF GESTATION

	1st Exam (X)	2nd Exam (O)
LARGE FOR GESTATIONAL AGE **(LGA)**		
APPROPRIATE FOR GESTATIONAL AGE **(AGA)**		
SMALL FOR GESTATIONAL AGE **(SGA)**		
Age at Exam	hrs	hrs
Signature of Examiner	M.D.	M.D.

FIGURE A–1 ■ Classification of newborns based on maturity and intrauterine growth.

Sources: Adapted from Lubchenco, L. O., Hansman, C., & Boyd, E., (1966). Intrauterine growth in length and head circumference as estimated from live births at gestational ages from 26 to 42 weeks. Pediatrics, *37, 403–408; Battaglia, F. C., & Lubchenco, L. D. (1967). A practical classification of newborn infants by weight and gestational age.* Journal of Pediatrics, *71, 159.*

FIGURE A–2 ■ Physical growth percentiles for length and weight—boys: birth to 36 months.

From CDC, 2001. www.cdc.gov/growthcharts

Birth to 36 months: Boys
Length-for-age and Weight-for-age percentiles

NAME ______________________

RECORD # ____________

AGE (MONTHS): Birth 3 6 9 12 15 18 21 24 27 30 33 36

LENGTH (in / cm) — percentiles 97, 90, 75, 50, 25, 10, 3

WEIGHT (lb / kg) — percentiles 97, 90, 75, 50, 25, 10, 3

Mother's Stature ____________ Gestational

Father's Stature ____________ Age: ______ Weeks

Date	Age	Weight	Length	Head Circ.	Comment
	Birth				

Revised April 20, 2001.
SOURCE: Developed by the National Center for Health Statistics in collaboration with the National Center for Chronic Disease Prevention and Health Promotion (2000).
http://www.cdc.gov/growthcharts

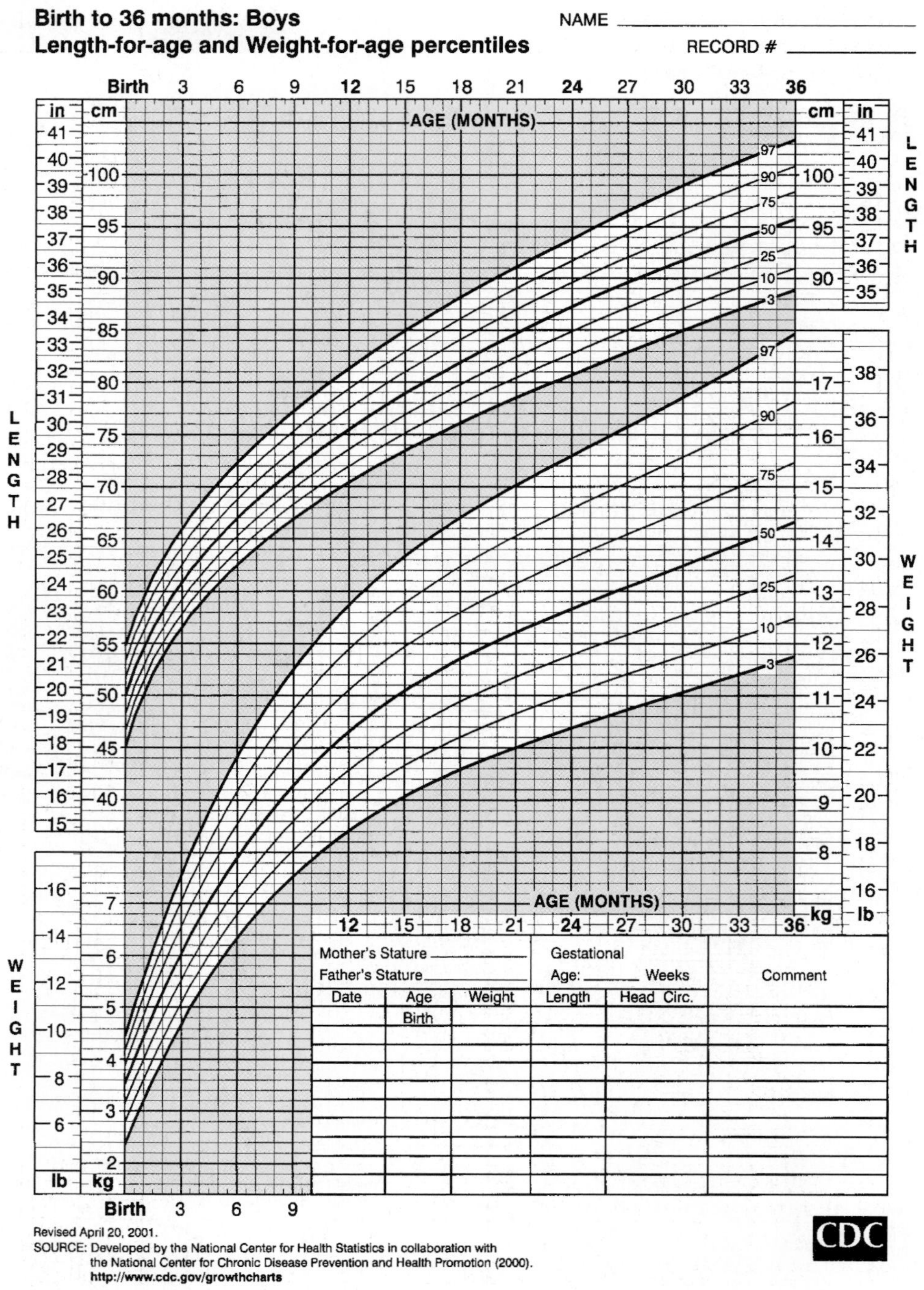

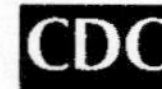

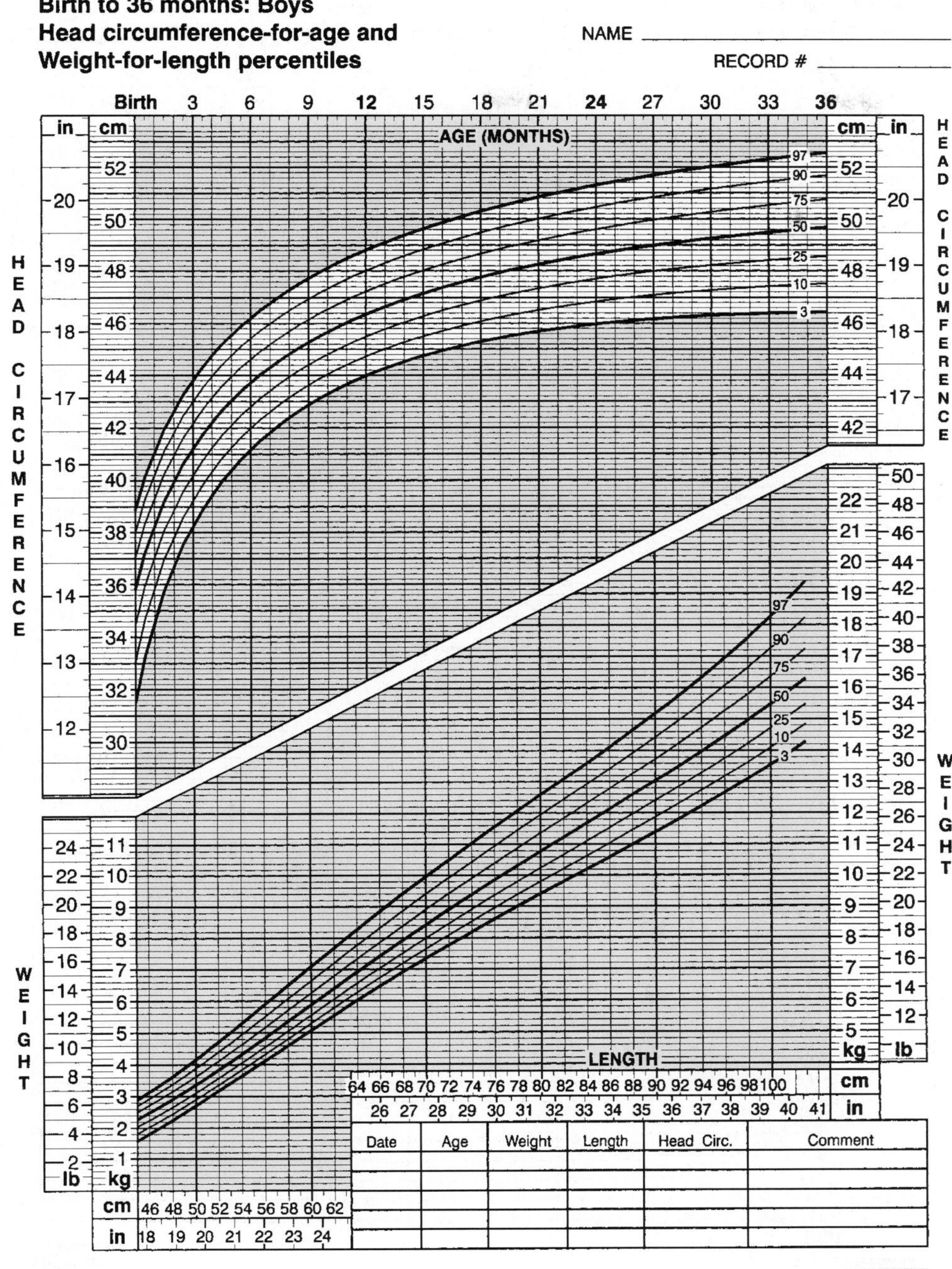

FIGURE A–3 ■ Physical growth percentiles for head circumference, weight for length—boys: birth to 36 months.

From CDC, 2001. www.cdc.gov/growthcharts

FIGURE A–4 ■ Physical growth percentiles for length and weight—girls: birth to 36 months.

From CDC, 2001. www.cdc.gov/growthcharts

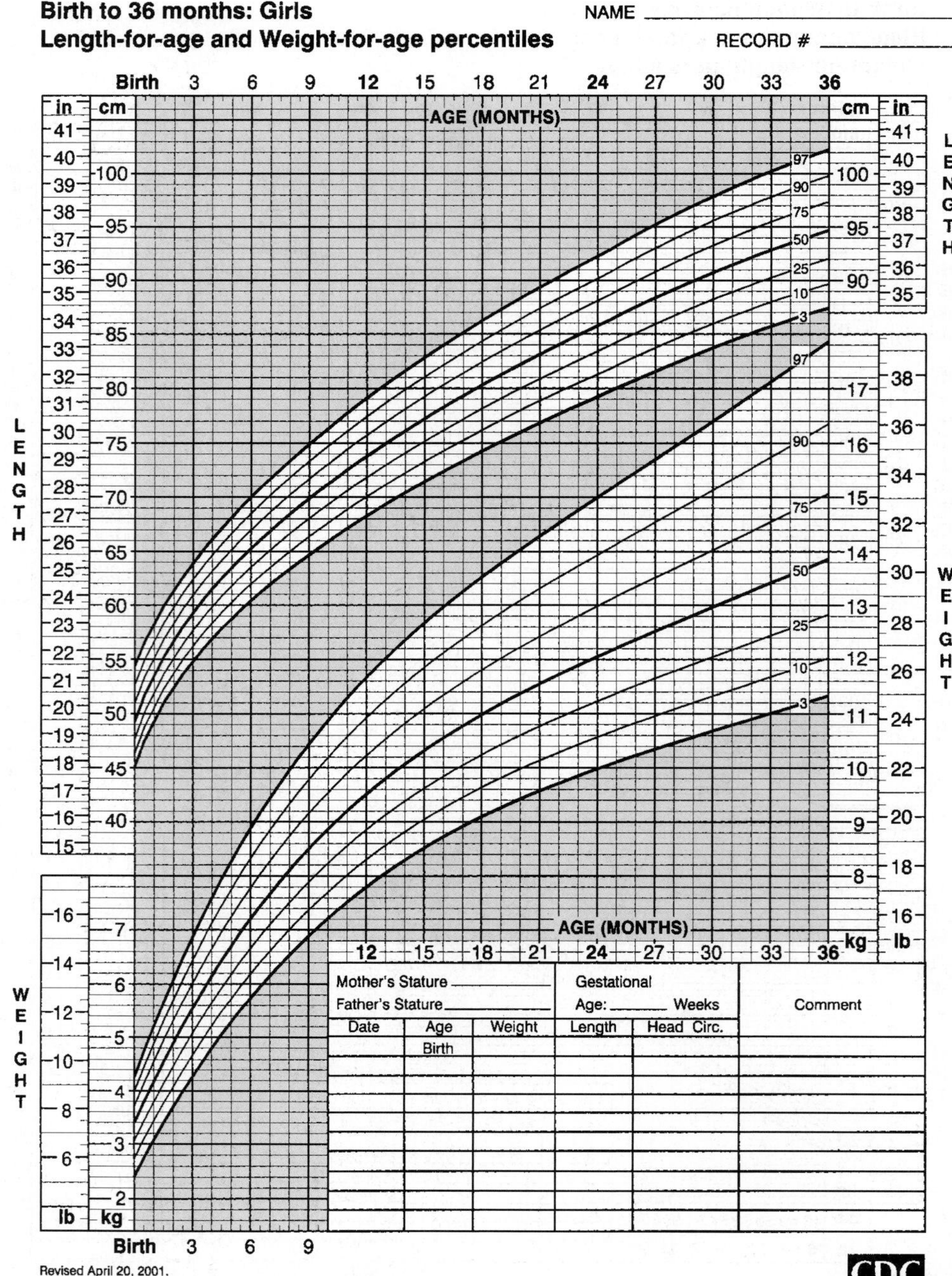

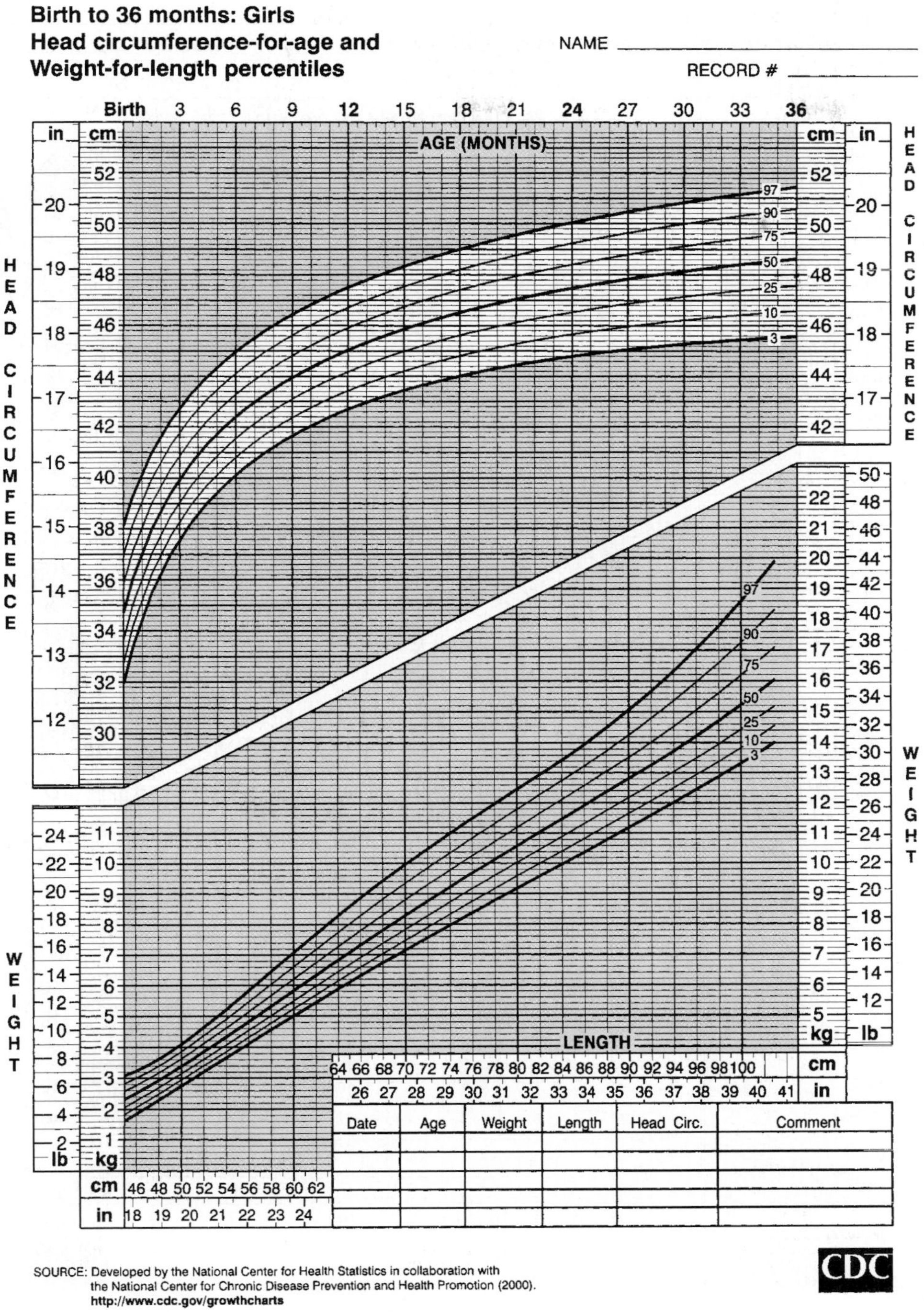

FIGURE A–5 ■ Physical growth percentiles for head circumference, weight for length—girls: birth to 36 months.

From CDC, 2001. www.cdc.gov/growthcharts

Birth to 36 months: Girls
Head circumference-for-age and
Weight-for-length percentiles

NAME ______________________

RECORD # ______________

Birth 3 6 9 12 15 18 21 24 27 30 33 36

AGE (MONTHS)

HEAD CIRCUMFERENCE

in: 12 13 14 15 16 17 18 19 20

cm: 30 32 34 36 38 40 42 44 46 48 50 52

Percentiles: 97 90 75 50 25 10 3

WEIGHT

kg: 1 2 3 4 5 6 7 8 9 10 11 12 13 14 15 16 17 18 19 20 21 22

lb: 2 4 6 8 10 12 14 16 18 20 22 24 26 28 30 32 34 36 38 40 42 44 46 48 50

LENGTH

cm: 46 48 50 52 54 56 58 60 62 64 66 68 70 72 74 76 78 80 82 84 86 88 90 92 94 96 98 100

in: 18 19 20 21 22 23 24 25 26 27 28 29 30 31 32 33 34 35 36 37 38 39 40 41

Date	Age	Weight	Length	Head Circ.	Comment

SOURCE: Developed by the National Center for Health Statistics in collaboration with the National Center for Chronic Disease Prevention and Health Promotion (2000). http://www.cdc.gov/growthcharts

FIGURE A–6 ■ Physical growth percentiles for stature and weight according to age—boys: 2 to 20 years.

From CDC, 2001. www.cdc.gov/growthcharts

2 to 20 years: Boys
Stature-for-age and Weight-for-age percentiles
NAME
RECORD #
Mother's Stature
Father's Stature
Date
Age
Weight
Stature
BMI*
*To Calculate BMI: Weight (kg) ÷ Stature (cm) ÷ Stature (cm) x 10,000
or Weight (lb) ÷ Stature (in) ÷ Stature (in) x 703
AGE (YEARS)
STATURE
WEIGHT
in
cm
lb
kg
97
90
75
50
25
10
3
Revised and corrected November 21, 2000.
SOURCE: Developed by the National Center for Health Statistics in collaboration with
the National Center for Chronic Disease Prevention and Health Promotion (2000).
http://www.cdc.gov/growthcharts
CDC

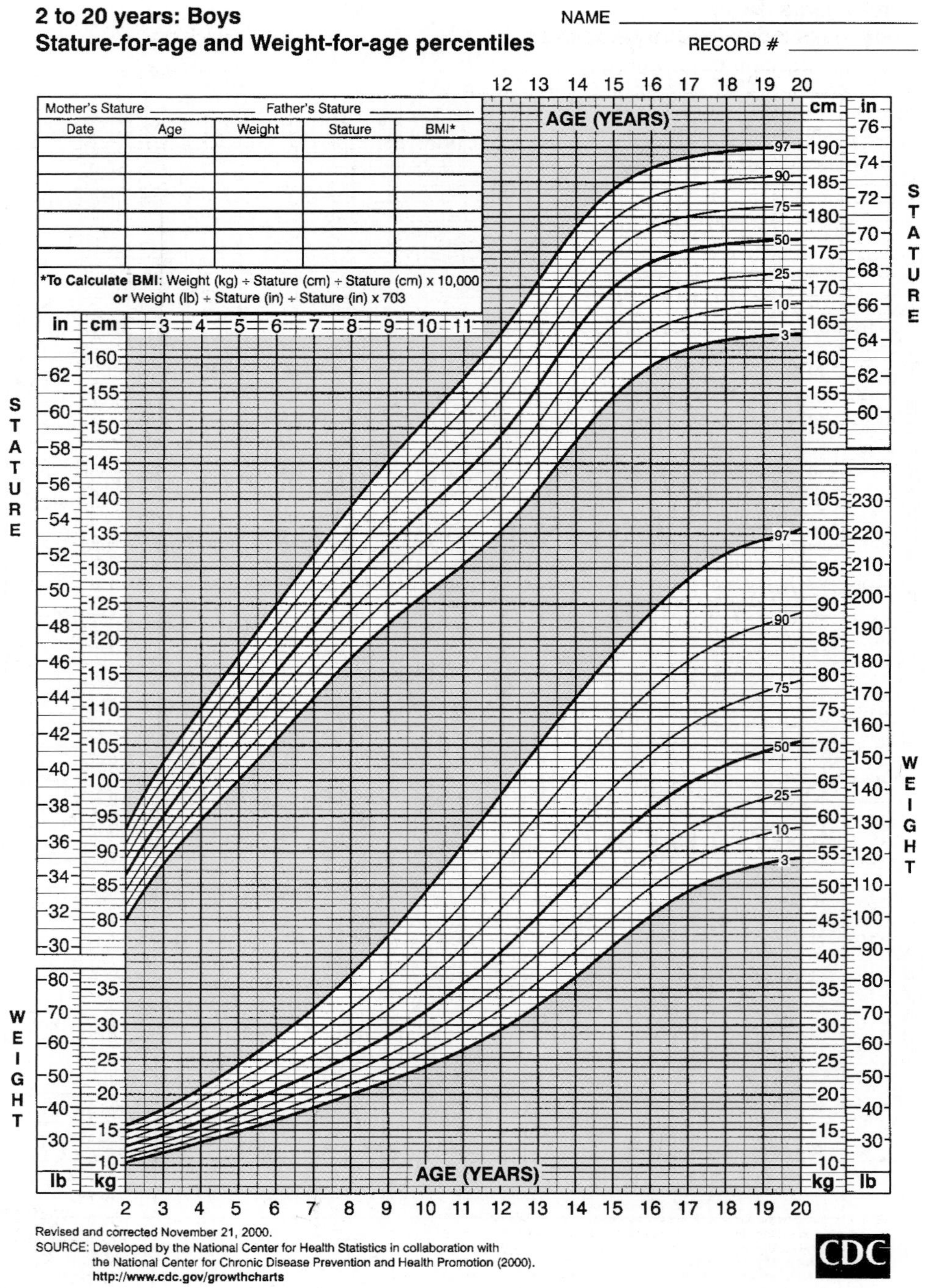

2 to 20 years: Boys
Body mass index-for-age percentiles

NAME ______________________

RECORD # ______________

Date	Age	Weight	Stature	BMI*	Comments

***To Calculate BMI:** Weight (kg) ÷ Stature (cm) ÷ Stature (cm) x 10,000
or Weight (lb) ÷ Stature (in) ÷ Stature (in) x 703

BMI

35 34 33 32 31 30 29 28 27 26 25 24 23 22 21 20 19 18 17 16 15 14 13 12

97 95 90 85 75 50 25 10 3

kg/m² AGE (YEARS) kg/m²

2 3 4 5 6 7 8 9 10 11 12 13 14 15 16 17 18 19 20

SOURCE: Developed by the National Center for Health Statistics in collaboration with the National Center for Chronic Disease Prevention and Health Promotion (2000).
http://www.cdc.gov/growthcharts

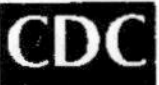

FIGURE A–7 ■ Physical growth percentiles for body mass index according to age—boys: 2 to 20 years.

From CDC, 2001. www.cdc.gov/growthcharts

FIGURE A–8 ■ Physical growth percentiles for weight for stature—boys: 2 to 20 years.

From CDC, 2001. www.cdc.gov/growthcharts

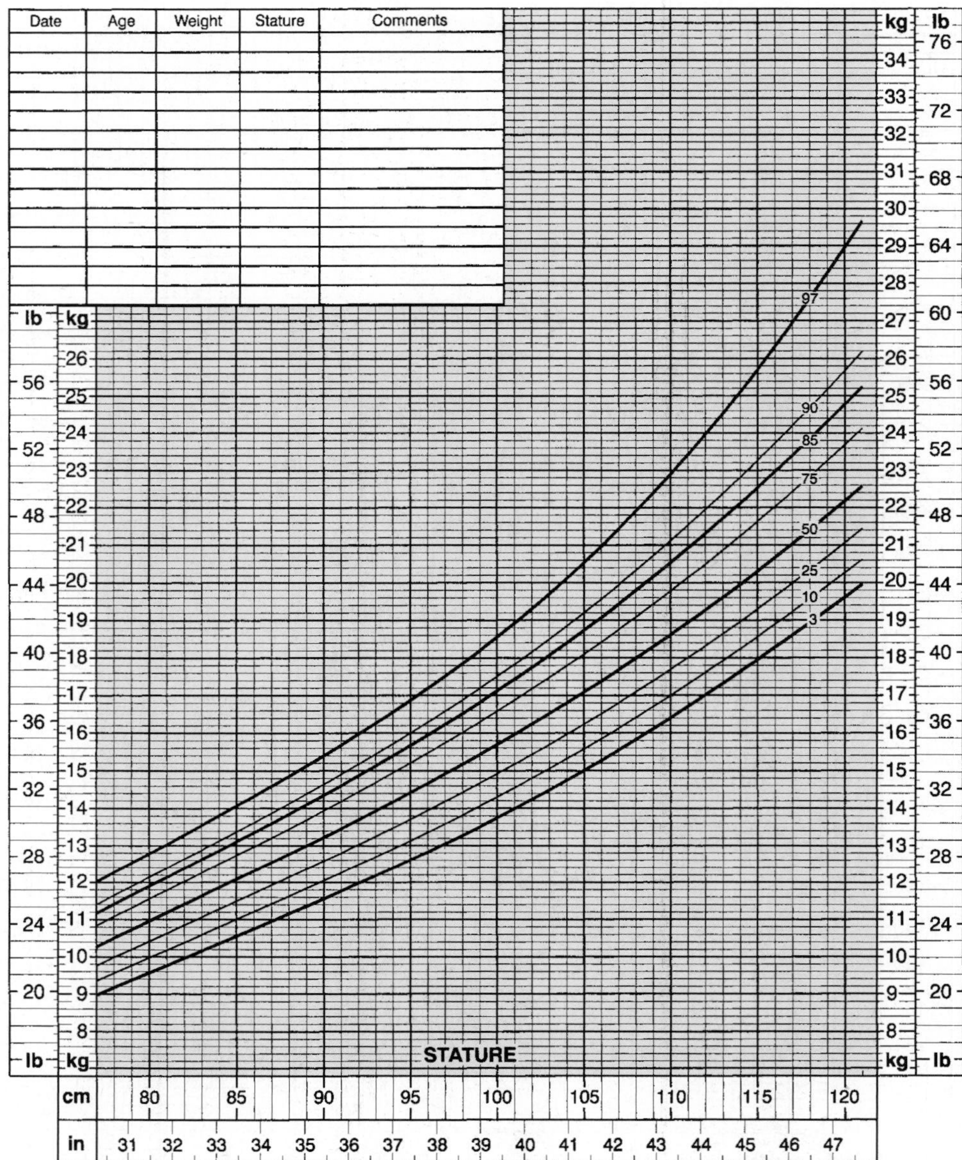

SOURCE: Developed by the National Center for Health Statistics in collaboration with the National Center for Chronic Disease Prevention and Health Promotion (2000). http://www.cdc.gov/growthcharts

CDC

FIGURE A–9 ■ Physical growth percentiles for stature and weight according to age—girls: 2 to 20 years.

From CDC, 2001. www.cdc.gov/growthcharts

2 to 20 years: Girls
Stature-for-age and Weight-for-age percentiles

NAME ____________

RECORD # ____________

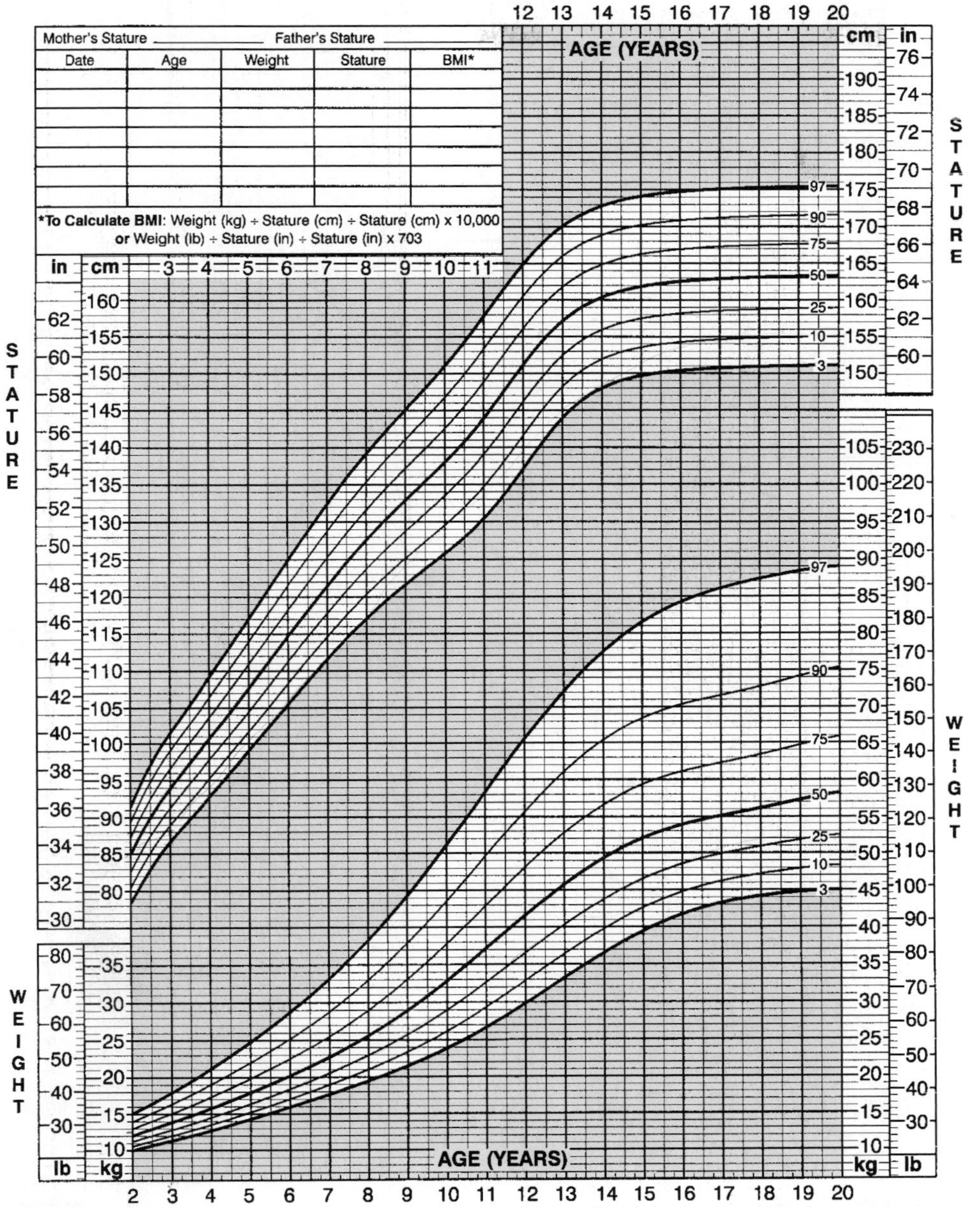

Mother's Stature ________ Father's Stature ________

Date	Age	Weight	Stature	BMI*

*To Calculate BMI: Weight (kg) ÷ Stature (cm) ÷ Stature (cm) x 10,000 or Weight (lb) ÷ Stature (in) ÷ Stature (in) x 703

AGE (YEARS)

STATURE

WEIGHT

Revised and corrected November 21, 2000.
SOURCE: Developed by the National Center for Health Statistics in collaboration with the National Center for Chronic Disease Prevention and Health Promotion (2000).
http://www.cdc.gov/growthcharts

CDC

FIGURE A–10 ■ Physical growth percentiles for body mass index according to age—girls: 2 to 20 years.

From CDC, 2001. www.cdc.gov/growthcharts

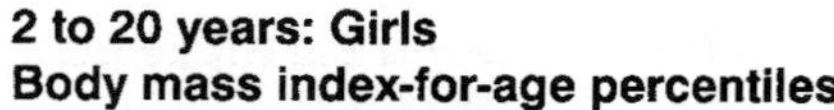

NAME ____________________

RECORD # ____________

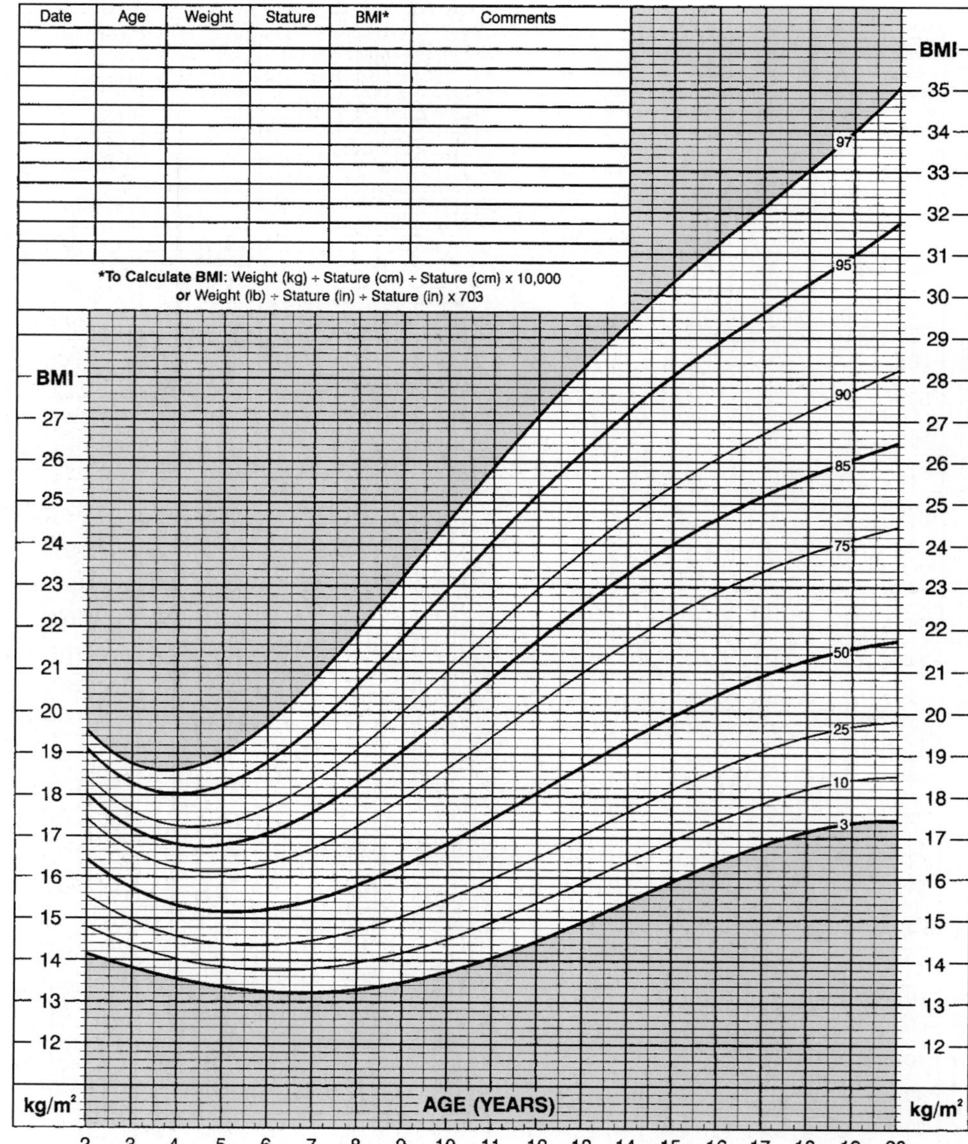

SOURCE: Developed by the National Center for Health Statistics in collaboration with the National Center for Chronic Disease Prevention and Health Promotion (2000). http://www.cdc.gov/growthcharts

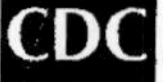

FIGURE A–11 ■ Physical growth percentiles for weight for stature—girls: 2 to 20 years.

From CDC, 2001. www.cdc.gov/growthcharts

NAME ______________

Weight-for-stature percentiles: Girls

RECORD # ______________

Date	Age	Weight	Stature	Comments

SOURCE: Developed by the National Center for Health Statistics in collaboration with the National Center for Chronic Disease Prevention and Health Promotion (2000). http://www.cdc.gov/growthcharts

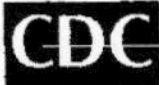

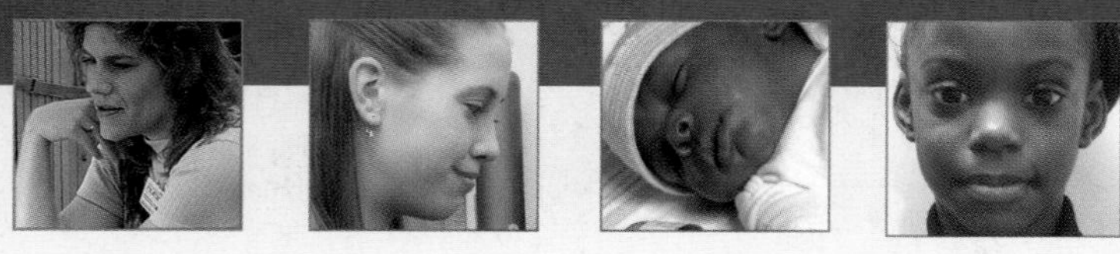

APPENDIX B

Dietary Reference Intakes

TABLE B–1 Dietary Reference Intakes

	AGE	VITAMIN A (mcg/d)	VITAMIN D (mcg/d)	VITAMIN E (mg/d α-tocopherol)	VITAMIN K (mcg/d)	VITAMIN C (mg/d)	THIAMIN (mg/d)	RIBOFLAVIN (mg/d)	NIACIN (mg/d)	VITAMIN B_6 (mg/d)
Infants	0–6 months	400*	5*	4*	2.0*	40*	0.2*	0.3*	~0.2*	0.1*
	7–12 months	500*	5*	5*	2.5*	50*	0.3*	0.4*	~0.4*	0.3*
Children	1–3 years	300	5*	6	30*	15	0.5	0.5	6	0.5
	4–8 years	400	5*	7	55*	25	0.6	0.6	8	0.6
Males	9–13 years	600	5*	11	60*	45	0.9	0.9	12	1.0
	14–18 years	900	5*	15	75*	75	1.2	1.3	16	1.3
Females	9–13 years	600	5*	11	60*	45	0.9	0.9	12	1.0
	14–18 years	700	5*	15	75*	65	1.0	1.0	14	1.2

Values are Adequate Intakes (AI) rather than Recommended Dietary Allowances (RDAs). All other values on chart are RDAs. See Chapter 9 for a discussion of nutrient requirements.

Note: All data from Institute of Medicine. (1997–2004). Dietary reference intakes. *Washington, DC: National Academy Press. Available also at http://www.nas.edu/lam*

TABLE B–2 Dietary Reference Intake for Water (L/d)

	AGE	FROM FOOD	FROM BEVERAGES	TOTAL
Infants	0–6 months	0	0.7	0.7*
	7–12 months	0.2	0.6	0.8*
Children	1–3 years	0.4	0.9	1.3*
	4–8 years	0.5	1.2	1.7*
Males	9–13 years	0.6	1.8	2.4*
	14–18 years	0.7	2.6	3.3*
Females	9–13 years	0.5	1.6	2.1*
	14–18 years	0.5	1.8	2.3*

Values are Adequate Intakes.

FOLATE (mcg/d)	VITAMIN B_{12} (mcg/d)	CALCIUM (mg/d)	PHOSPHORUS (mg/d)	MAGNESIUM (mg/d)	IRON (mg/d)	ZINC (mg/d)	IODINE (mcg/d)	SELENIUM (mcg/d)	POTASSIUM (g/d)	SODIUM (g/d)
65*	0.4*	210*	100*	30*	0.27*	2.0*	110*	15*	0.4*	0.12*
80*	0.5*	270*	275*	75*	11	3	130*	20*	0.7*	0.37*
150	0.9	500*	460	80	7	3	90	20	3*	1*
200	1.2	800*	500	130	10	5	90	30	3.8*	1.2*
300	1.8	1300*	1250	240	8	8	120	40	4.5*	1.5*
400	2.4	1300*	1250	240	11	11	150	55	4.5*	1.5*
300	1.8	1300*	1250	410	8	8	120	40	4*	1.5*
400	2.4	1300*	1250	360	15	9	150	55	4.7*	1.5*

TABLE B–3 Recommended Dietary Allowances

	AGE	PROTEIN	CARBOHYDRATE	POLYUNSATURATED FATTY ACIDS n-6	POLYUNSATURATED FATTY ACIDS n-3	TOTAL FAT	FIBER
Infants	0–6 months	9.1 g/d or 1.52 g/kg/d*	60 g/d*	4.4 g/d	0.5 g/d	31 g/d	NE
	7–12 months	1.5 g/kg/d	95 g/d*	4.6 g/d	0.5 g/d	30 g/d	NE
Children	1–3 years	1.1 g/kg/d or 13 g/d	130 g/d	7 g/d (linoleic)	0.7 g/d (α-linolenic)	NE	19 g/d
	4–8 years	0.95 g/kg/d or 19 g/d	130 g/d	10 g/d (linoleic)	0.9 g/d (α-linolenic)	NE	25 g/d
Males	9–13 years	0.95 g/kg/d or 34 g/d	130 g/d	12 g/d (linoleic)	1.2 g/d (α-linolenic)	NE	31 g/d
	14–18 years	0.85 g/kg/d or 52 g/d	130 g/d	16 g/d (linoleic)	1.6 g/d (α-linolenic)	NE	38 g/d
Females	9–13 years	0.95 g/kg/d or 34 g/d	130 g/d	10 g/d (linoleic)	1.0 g/d (α-linolenic)	NE	26 g/d
	14–18 years	0.85 g/kg/d or 46 g/d	130 g/d	11 g/d (linoleic)	1.1 g/d (α-linolenic)	NE	26 g/d

**Values are Adequate Intakes (AIs) rather than Recommended Dietary Allowances (RDAs). All other values on charts are RDAs.*

NE = not established

All data from Institute of Medicine. (2002). Dietary Reference Intakes. *Washington DC: National Academy Press.* www.nap.edu/iom

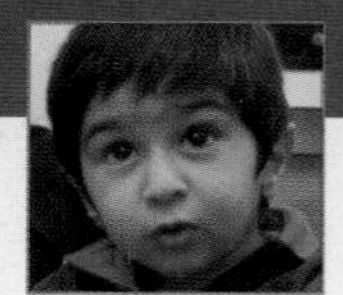 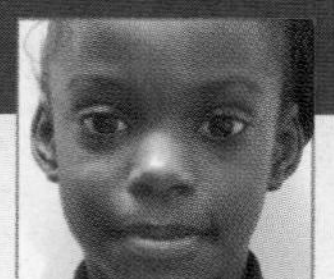 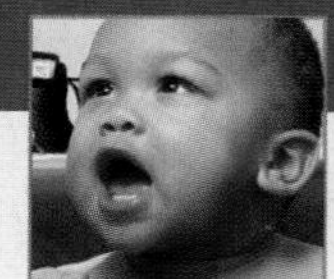 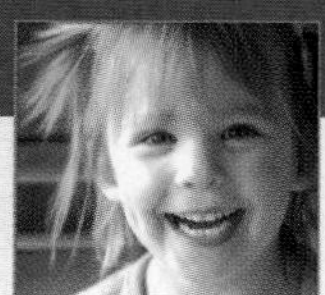

APPENDIX C

Normal Laboratory Values

All laboratory values listed are approximate. Consult your local laboratory for guidelines as to normal values for the specific testing procedures used.

NORMAL VALUES: BLOOD

Albumin (S)[1]

Newborn: 2.6–4.1 g/dL
1 mo–1 year: 2.8–4.8 g/dL
1–18 years: 3.2–4.7 g/dL

Aldolase (S)[1]

10–24 mo: 3.4–11.8 Units/L
2–16 years: 1.2–8.8 Units/L
Adult: 1.7–4.9 Units/L

Aldosterone (S)[1]

6–9 years: 28–666 pmol/L
10–11 years: 55–416 pmol/L
12–14 years: 28–610 pmol/L
15–17 years: 28–888 pmol/L

Alkaline Phosphatase (S)[1]

Age	Males Units/L	Females Units/L
Newborns (1–30 days)	75–316	48–406
1–3 years	104–345	108–317
4–6 years	93–309	96–297
7–9 years	86–315	69–325
10–12 years	42–362	51–332
13–15 years	74–390	50–162
16–18 years	52–171	47–119

α_1 Antitrypsin (S)[1]

Newborn:	79.4–222.7 mg/dL
1–6 mo:	71–190.1 mg/dL
6 mo–2 years:	60.1–160.6 mg/dL
2–19 years:	70.4–178.6 mg/dL

Alpha-fetoprotein (AFP) (S)[1]

Newborn:	50–100,000 ng/mL
1–3 mo:	40–1000 ng/mL
4 mo–18 years:	0–12 ng/mL

Ammonia (P)[3]

Newborn:	90–150 mcg/dL
Child:	45–80 mcg/dL

Amylase (S)[1]

1–19 years:	30–100 Units/L

Base Excess (B)[1]

Newborn:	−10 to −2 mmol/L
Infant:	−7 to −1 mmol/L
Child:	−4 to +2 mmol/L
Thereafter:	−3 to +3 mmol/L

Bicarbonate, Actual (P)[2]

Calculated from pH and Pa_{CO_2}

Newborn:	17.2–23.6 mmol/L
2 mo–2 years:	19–24 mmol/L
Child:	18–25 mmol/L
Adult male:	20.1–28.9 mmol/L
Adult female:	18.4–28.8 mmol/L

Bilirubin, Conjugated (S)[3]

Child (past newborn stage): 0–0.4 mg/dL

Bilirubin, Total (S)[3]

Neonate:	1–16 mg/dL
Child:	0.1–1 mg/dL

Bleeding Time (Simplate)[2]

2–9 min

Blood Volume[2]

Premature infant:	98 mL/kg
At 1 year:	86 mL/kg (range, 69–112 mL/kg)
Older child:	70 mL/kg (range, 51–86 mL/kg)

Calcium (P,S)[1]

Newborn:	8.5–10.6 mg/dL
Thereafter:	8.7–10.6 mg/dL

Carbon Dioxide, Partial Pressure (pco_2) (B)[1]

Newborn:	27–40 mm Hg (3.6–5.5 kPa)
Infant:	27–41 mm Hg (3.6–5.5 kPa)
Child:	32–48 mm Hg (4.3–6.4 kPa)

Carbon Dioxide, Total (P)[1]

Cord blood:	13–29 mmol/L
<1 year:	17–31 mmol/L
Adult:	24–30 mmol/L

Chloride (S, P)[1]

<1 year:	96–111 mmol/L
1–17 years:	102–112 mmol/L

Cholesterol, High-density Lipoprotein (S)[4]

<35 mg/dL

Cholesterol, Low-density Lipoprotein (S)[4]

Borderline:	>110 mg/dL
Elevated:	>130 mg/dL

Cholesterol, Total (S, P)[4]

Borderline:	>170 mg/dL
Elevated:	>200 mg/dL

Complement (S)[1]

	Newborn	1–18 years
C1r:	27–65 mg/L	25–140 mg/L
C2:	12–24 mg/L	18–40 mg/L
C3a:	4–255 mcg/L	0–161 mcg/L
C4:	5–33 mg/dL	7–40 mg/dL

C-Reactive Protein (CRP) (P, S)[1]

Newborn:	13–444 mcg/L
Adult:	86–10406 mcg/L

Creatine Kinase (S, P)[1]

Birth–90 days:	29–474 Units/L
1–2 years:	25–177 Units/L
3–14 years:	31–177 Units/L
15–18 years:	28–147 Units/L

Creatinine (S, P)[1]

Values in mg/dL (mmol/L)

1–7 days:	0.7–1.2 (0.06–0.11)
7–30 days:	0.3–0.8 (0.03–0.07)
1 mo-1 year:	0.2–0.5 (0.02–0.04)
1–9 years:	0.2–0.8 (0.02–0.07)
10–18 years:	0.5–1.1 (0.04–0.10)

Erythropoietin (P)[1]

Values in mIU/mL

	Males	Females
1–3 years:	1.7–17.9	2.1–15.9
4–6 years:	3.5–21.9	2.9–8.5
7–9 years:	1–13.5	2.1–8.2
10–12 years:	1–14	1.1–9.1
13–15 years:	2.2–14.4	3.8–20.5
16–18 years:	1.5–15.2	2–14.2

Ferritin (P, S)[1]

Newborn:	47–554 ng/mL
1–6 mo:	47–449 ng/mL
Thereafter:	47–110 ng/mL

Fibrinogen (P)[2]

200–500 mg/dL

Galactose (S, P)[2]

1.1–2.1 mg/dL (0.06–0.12 mmol/L)

Galactose-1-Phosphate (RBC)[2]

Normal: 1 mg/dL of packed erythrocyte lysate; slightly higher in cord blood

Infant with congenital galactosemia on a milk-free diet: <2 mg/dL

Infant with congenital galactosemia taking milk: 9–20 mg/dL

Galactose-1-Phosphate Uridyl Transferase (RBC)[2]

Normal: 308–475 mIU/g of hemoglobin

Heterozygous for Duarte variant: 225–308 mIU/g of hemoglobin

Homozygous for Duarte variant: 142–225 mIU/g of hemoglobin

Heterozygous for congenital galactosemia: 142–225 mIU/g of hemoglobin

Homozygous for congenital galactosemia: <8 mIU/g of hemoglobin

Glucose (S, P)[1]

0–7 days: 47–110 mg/dL (2.61–6.11 mmol/L)

Thereafter: 54–117 mg/dL (3–6.49 mmol/L)

Glucose 6–Phosphate Dehydrogenase (RBC)[2]

150–215 units/dL

Glucose Tolerance Test Results in Serum[a 2]

	Glucose		Insulin	
Time	**mg/dL**	**mmol/L**	**mU/mL**	**pmol/L**
Fasting	59–96	3.11–5.33	5–40	36–287
30 min	91–185	5.05–10.27	36–110	258–789
60 min	66–164	3.66–9.10	22–124	158–890
90 min	68–148	3.77–8.22	17–105	122–753
2 hr	66–122	3.66–6.77	6–84	43–603
3 hr	47–99	2.61–5.49	2–46	14–330
4 hr	61–93	3.39–5.16	3–32	21–230
5 hr	63–86	3.50–4.77	5–37	36–265

[a]Normal levels based on results in 13 normal children given glucose, 1.75 g/kg orally in one dose, after 2 weeks on a high-carbohydrate diet.

Growth Hormone (S)[1]

During the newborn period (fasting specimen): GH levels are high (6–56 ng/mL)

After newborn period: <6 ng/mL

In response to natural and artificial provocation (e.g., sleep, arginine, insulin, hypoglycemia): >6 ng/mL

Hematocrit (B)[1]

Values in %

Age	Males	Females
Newborns	43.4–56.1	37.4–55.9
6 mo–2 years	30.9–37	31.2–37.2
2–6 years	31.7–37.7	32–37.1
6–12 years	32.7–39.3	33–39.6
12–18 years	34.8–43.9	34–40.7
>18 years	33.4–46.2	33–41

Hemoglobin (B)[1]

Values in g/dL

Age	Males	Females
Newborns	14.7–18.6	12.7–18.3
6 mo–2 years	10.3–12.4	10.4–12.4
2–6 years	10.5–12.7	10.7–12.7
6–12 years	11–13.3	10.9–13.3
12–18 years	11.5–14.8	11.2–13.6
>18 years	10.9–15.7	10.7–13.5

Hemoglobin A1c (B)[1]

Normal: 4%–7%

Stable diabetic patient: 8%–10%

Young and unstable diabetic patient: 8%–18%

Pregnant woman: 5%–8%

Hemoglobin Electrophoresis (B)[2]

A_1 hemoglobin: 96%–98.5% of total hemoglobin

A_2 hemoglobin: 1.5%–4% of total hemoglobin

Hemoglobin, Fetal (B)[2]

At birth: 50%–85% of total hemoglobin

At 1 year: <15% of total hemoglobin

Up to 2 years: Up to 5% of total hemoglobin

Thereafter: <2% of total hemoglobin

Immunoglobulins (P, S)[1]

Values in mg/dL

Age	IgG	IgA	IgM
1–30 days	197–872	1–17	0–65
1–6 mo	140–664	1–49	9–127
7–12 mo	130–647	8–89	15–130
1–3 years	413–1202	15–142	30–184
4–6 years	468–1328	39–192	31–184
7–9 years	485–1473	34–209	21–165
10–12 years	586–1620	51–223	27–211
13–15 years	590–1640	35–252	26–225
16–18 years	522–1817	74–267	28–224

Immunoglobulin D (S)[1]

Newborn: 0

Thereafter: 0–8 mg/dL

Immunoglobulin E (S, P)[1]

	Male	Female
0–12 mo:	<20 KIU/L	<17 KIU/L
1–3 years:	<85 KIU/L	<33 KIU/L
4–10 years:	<146 KIU/L	<124 KIU/L
11–18 years:	<159 KIU/L	<177 KIU/L

Iron (S, P)[1]

All ages 5–11 AM: 20–105 mcg/dL (3.6–18.8 μmol/L)

All ages 5–11 PM: 20–145 mcg/dL (3.6–26 μmol/L)

Iron-binding Capacity (S, P)[1]

1–5 years: 268–441 mcg/dL (48–79 μmol/L)

6–9 years: 240–508 mcg/dL (43–91 μmol/L)

10–14 years: 302–575 mcg/dL (54–103 μmol/L)

14–19 years: 290–570 mcg/dL (52–101 μmol/L)

Lactate Dehydrogenase (LDH) (S, P)[1]

Values using lactate substrate (kinetic)

Newborn:	178–629 Units/L
1–12 mo:	158–373 Units/L
1–3 years:	164–286 Units/L
4–6 years:	155–280 Units/L
7–13 years:	141–237 Units/L
Thereafter:	117–217 Units/L

Lead (B)[1]

0–15 years: <5 mcg/dL

Magnesium (P, S)[1]

Values in mg/dL (mmol/L)

Newborn:	1.3–2.7 (0.5–1.1)
1 mo–2 years:	1.7–2.7 (0.7–1.1)
2–5 years:	1.6–2.5 (0.7–1)
6–14 years:	1.7–2.4 (0.7–1)
15–18 years:	1.6–2.4 (0.7–1)

Osmolality (S)[1]

Birth to 1 mo:	275–305 mOsm/kg
Thereafter:	280–300 mOsm/kg

Oxygen, Partial Pressure (po_2) (B)[1]

Birth:	8–24 mm Hg	1.1–3.2 kPa
>1 hour:	55–80 mm Hg	7.3–10.6 kPa
>1 day:	83–108 mm Hg	11–14.4 kPa

Oxygen Saturation (B)[1]

Newborn:	85%–90%
Thereafter:	95%–99%

Partial Thromboplastin Time (P)[2]

Child: 42–54 sec

pH (B)[1]

0–6 mo:	7.18–7.50
6–12 mo:	7.27–7.49

Phenylalanine (S, P)[2]

0.7–3.5 mg/dL (0.04–0.21 mmol/L)

Phosphorus, Inorganic (S, P)[1]

Newborn:	2.7–8 mg/dL (0.87–2.58 mmol/L)
1 year:	2.5–6.5 mg/dL (0.81–2.1 mmol/L)
2–12 years:	2.5–6 mg/dL (0.97–1.94 mmol/L)
13–18 years:	3–5.6 mg/dL (0.97–1.81 mmol/L)

Platelet Count (RBC)[1]

Value × 10^9/L

Age	Males	Females
Newborn	218–586	144–571
1–2 mo	229–562	331–597
2–6 mo	244–529	247–580
6 mo–2 years	206–445	214–459
2–12 years	202–403	189–394
12–18 years	175–332	194–345

Potassium (S, P)[1]

Full-term infant:	3.2–5.7 mmol/L
>1 year:	3.3–4.7 mmol/L

Protein, Total (P, S)[1]

Age	Male	Female
1–30 days	41–63 g/L	42–64 g/L
31–182 days	47–67 g/L	44–66 g/L
7–12 mo	55–70 g/L	56–79 g/L
1–18 year	57–80 g/L	57–80 g/L

Prothrombin Time (P)[2]

Child: 11–15 sec

Protoporphyrin, "Free" (FEP, ZPP)(B)[2]

Values for free erythrocyte protoporphyrin (FEP) and zinc protoporphyrin (ZPP) are 1.2–2.7 mcg/g of hemoglobin

Red Blood Cell Count (B)[1]

Values × 10^{12}/L

Age	Males	Females
Newborn	4.1–5.55	4.12–5.74
6 mo–2 years	4.03–5.07	3.97–5.01
2–12 years	3.96–5.03	3.90–4.96
12–18 years	4.03–5.29	3.93–4.9
>18 years	4.18–5.48	3.70–4.87

Sedimentation Rate (Micro) (B)[2]

<2 years: 1–5 mm/hr

>2 years: 1–8 mm/hr

Sodium (P, S)[1]

Newborn: 131–144 mmol/L

> 1 year: 132–141 mmol/L

Thrombin Time (P)[2]

Child: 12–16 sec

Thyroid-stimulating Hormone (TSH) (P,S)[1]

Values in mUnit/mL

Age	Males	Females
1–30 days	0.52–16	0.72–13.1
1 mo–5 years	0.55–7.1	0.46–8.1
6–18 years	0.37–6	0.36–5.8

Thyroxine (T4) (S, P)[1]

Values in mg/dL (nmol/L)

Age	Males	Females
1–30 days:	5.9–21.5 (76–276)	6.3–21.5 (81–276)
1–12 mo:	6.4–13.9 (82–179)	4.9–13.7 (63–176)
1–3 years:	7–13.1 (90–169)	7.1–14.1 (91–180)
4–6 years:	6.1–12.6 (79–162)	7.2–14 (93–180)
7–12 years:	6.7–13.4 (86–172)	6.1–12.1 (79–156)
13–15 years:	4.8–11.5 (62–148)	5.8–11.2 (75–144)
16–18 years:	5.9–11.5 (76–148)	5.2–13.2 (67–170)

Thyroxine, "Free" (Free T4) (S, P)[1]

Newborn: 0.8–2.78 ng/dL (10–36 pmol/L)
1–12 mo: 0.76–2 ng/dL (10–26 pmol/L)
1–5 years: 0.9–1.72 ng/dL (12–22 pmol/L)
6–10 years: 0.81–1.68 ng/dL (10–22 pmol/L)
11–15 years: 0.79–1.57 ng/dL (10–20 pmol/L)
16–18 years: 0.83–1.53 ng/dL (11–20 pmol/L)

Throxine-binding Globulin (TBG) (P)[1]

1–12 mo: 16.2–32.9 mg/L
1–3 years: 16.4–33.8 mg/L
4–6 years: 16.6–30.8 mg/L
7–12 years: 15–29.2 mg/L
13–18 years: 13.4–28.7 mg/L

Triglycerides (S)[4]

<150 mg/dL

Triiodothyronine (T3) (S)[1]

1–3 days: 60–300 ng/dL
3–365 days: 90–260 ng/dL
1–6 years 90–240 ng/dL
7–11 years 90–230 ng/dL
12–18 years 100–210 ng/dL

Urea Clearance[2]

Premature infant: 3.5–17.3 mL/min/1.73 m^2
Newborn: 8.7–33 mL/min/1.73 m^2
2–12 mo: 40–95 mL/min/1.73 m^2
≥2 years: >52 mL/min/1.73 m^2

Urea Nitrogen (S, P)[1]

< 1 year: 1–16 mg/dL (0.3–4.3 mmol/L)
1–3 years: 4–17 mg/dL (1.1–4.6 mmol/L)
4–13 years: 6–17 mg/dL (1.6–4.6 mmol/L)
14–19 years: 7–21 mg/dL (1.9–5.7 mmol/L)

Uric Acid (S, P)[1]

< 1 year: 1.4–6.7 mg/dL (71–399 mmol/L)
1–3 years: 1.7–5 mg/dL (101–297 mmol/L)
4–6 years: 2.2–4.7 mg/dL (131–280 mmol/L)
7–9 years: 1.9–5 mg/dL (113–297 mmol/L)
10–15 years: 2.3–7.9 mg/dL (137–470 mmol/L)
16–19 years: 3–8.7 mg/dL (178–518 mmol/L)

White Blood Cell Count (B)[1]

Values × 10^9/L

Age	Males	Females
Newborn	6.8–13.3	8–14.3
6 mo–2 years	6.2–14.5	6.4–15
2–12 years	5.3–11.5	5.3–11.5
12–18 years	4.5–10	4.8–10.1
>18 years	4.4–10.2	4.9–10

NORMAL VALUES: URINE

Addis Count[2]

Red cells (12-hr specimen): <1 million
White cells (12-hr specimen): <2 million
Casts (12-hr specimen): <10,000
Protein (12-hr specimen): <55 mg

Albumin[2]

First mo: 1–100 mg/L
Second mo: 0.2–34 mg/L
2–12 mo: 0.5–19 mg/L

Ammonia[2]

2–12 mo: 4–20 microEq/min/m^2
1–16 years: 6–16 microEq/min/m^2

Calcium[2]

4–12 years: 4–8 mEq/L (2–4 mmol/L)

Catecholamines (Norepinephrine, Epinephrine)[1]

Values in mmol/mol creatinine

Age	Norepinephrine	Epinephrine
<1 year	0.017–0.207	0–0.232
1–4 years	0.017–0.194	0–0.051
4–10 years	0.018–0.072	0.003–0.057
10–18 years	0.003–0.070	0.001–0.027

Chloride[2]

Infant:	1.7–8.5 mmol/24 hr
Child:	17–34 mmol/24 hr
Adult:	140–240 mmol/24 hr

Creatine[2]

18–58 mg/L (1.37–4.42 mmol/L)

Creatinine[1]

3–8 years:	0.11–0.68 g/24 hr
9–12 years:	0.17–1.41 g/24 hr
13–17 years:	0.29–1.87 g/24 hr
Adult:	0.63–2.50 g/24 hr

Growth Hormone[1]

2.2–13.3 years (Tanner 1):	0.4–6.3 ng/24 hr (0.9–12.3 ng/g creatinine)
10.3–14.6 years (Tanner 2):	0.8–12 ng/24 hr (1–14.1 ng/g creatinine)
11.5–15.3 years (Tanner 3):	1.7–20.4 ng/24 hr (1.9–17 ng/g creatinine)
12.7–17.1 years (Tanner 4):	1.5–18.2 ng/24 hr (1.3–14.4 ng/g creatinine)
13.5–19.9 years (Tanner 5):	1.2–14.5 ng/24 hr (0.8–11 ng/g creatinine)

Homovanillic Acid[1]

0–1 years:	<32.6 mg/g creatinine
2–4 years:	<22.0 mg/g creatinine
5–9 years:	<15.1 mg/g creatinine
10–19 years:	<12.8 mg/g creatinine

Osmolality[2]

Infant:	50–600 mOsm/L
Older child:	50–1400 mOsm/L

Phosphorus, Tubular Reabsorption[2]

78%–97%

Porphyrins[2]

δ-Aminolevulinic acid:	0–7 mg/24 hr (0–53.4 micromol/24 hr)
Porphobilinogen:	0–2 mg/24 hr (0–8.8 micromol/24 hr)
Coproporphyrin:	0–160 mcg/24 hr (0–244 nmol/24 hr)
Uroporphyrin:	0–26 mcg/24 hr (0–31 nmol/24 hr)

Potassium[2]

26–123 mmol/L

Sodium[2]

Infant:	0.3–3.5 mmol/24 hr (6–10 mmol/m^2)
Child and adult:	5.6–17 mmol/24 hr

Specific Gravity

1.010–1.030

Urobilinogen[2]

<3 mg/24 hr (<5.1 micromol/24 hr)

Vanillylmandelic Acid (VMA)[1]

1–3 mo:	5.9–37 mg/g creatinine
3–12 mo:	8.4–43.8 mg/g creatinine
1–2 years:	7.9–23 mg/g creatinine
2–5 years:	2.9–23 mg/g creatinine
5–10 years:	5.8–18.7 mg/g creatinine
10–15 years:	1.6–10.6 mg/g creatinine
>15 years:	2.8–8.3 mg/g creatinine

NORMAL VALUES: FECES

Fat, Total[2]

2–6 mo:	0.3–1.3 g/d
6 mo–1 year:	<4 g/d
Child:	<3 g/d
Adolescent:	<5 g/d
Adult:	<7 g/d

NORMAL VALUES: SWEAT

Electrolytes[1]

Normal: <40 mmol/L for both sodium and chloride

Patient with cystic fibrosis: >60 mmol/L for both sodium and chloride

NORMAL VALUES: CEREBROSPINAL FLUID

Protein[1]

< 1 mo: 15–153 mg/dL

< 3 mo: 15–93 mg/dL

>3 mo: 15–45 mg/dL

Glucose[1]

All ages: 60%–80% of blood glucose

***S**, serum; **B**, whole blood; **P**, plasma; **RBC**, red blood cells*

Modified from:

[1] *Soldin, S. J., Brugnara, C., & Wong, E. C. (2003).* Pediatric reference ranges *(4th ed.). Washington, DC: AACC Press.*

[2] *Hay, W. W., Hayward, A. R., Levin, M. J., & Sondheimer, J. M. (2003).* Current pediatric diagnosis and treatment *(16th ed.). New York: Lange Medical Books/McGraw Hill.*

[3] *Corbett, J. V. (2004).* Laboratory tests and diagnostic procedures with nursing diagnoses *(6th ed.). Upper Saddle River, N.J.: Prentice Hall Health.*

[4] *Kavey, R. W., Daniels, S. R., Lauer, R. M., Atkins, D. L., Hayman, L. L., & Taubert, K. (2003). American Heart Association guidelines for primary prevention of atherosclerotic cardiovascular disease beginning in childhood.* Journal of Pediatrics, 142, *368–372.*

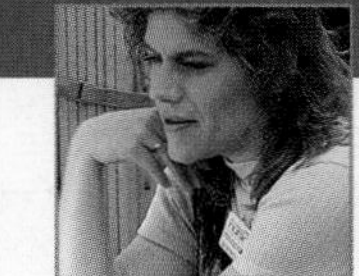 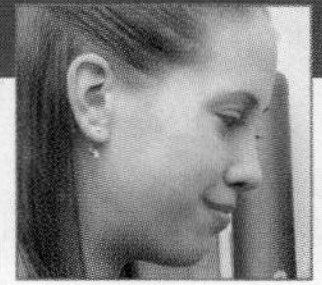 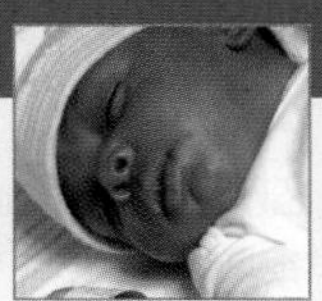 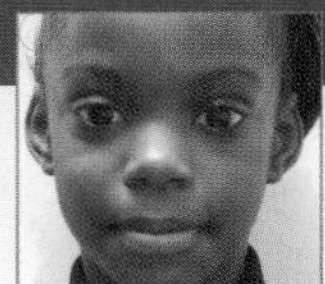

APPENDIX D

West Nomogram-Body Surface Area

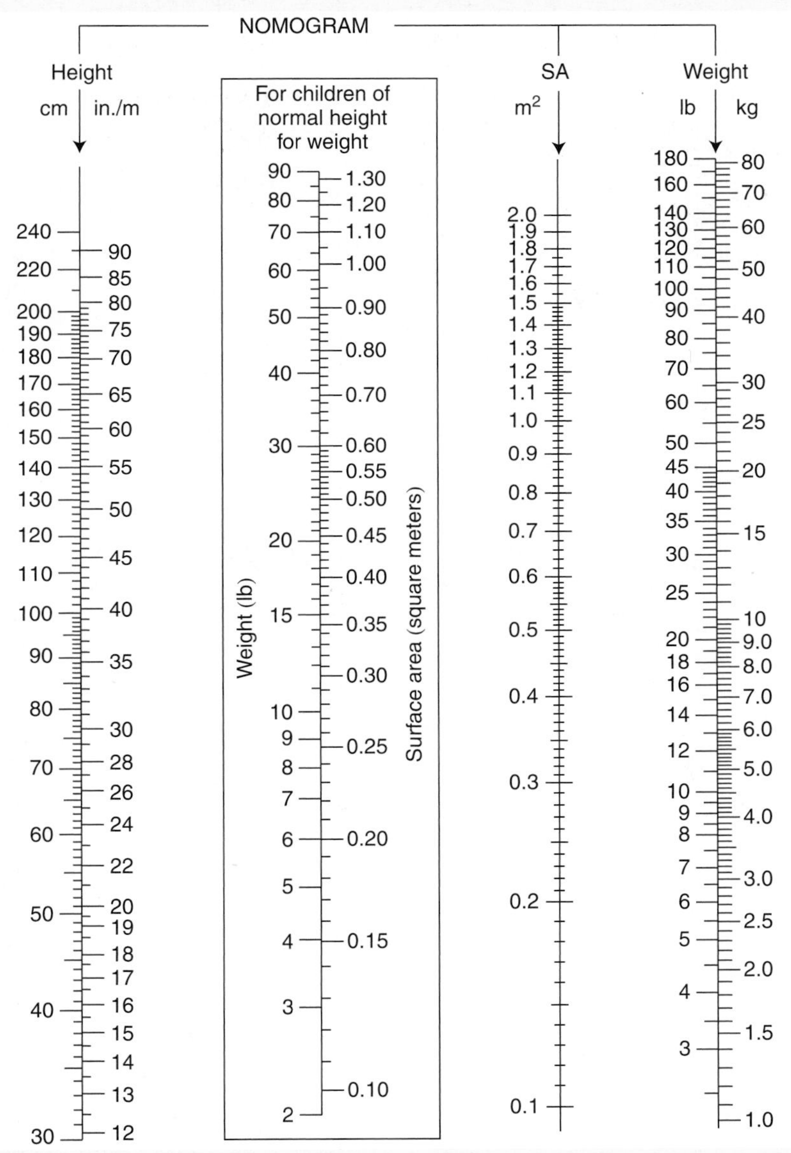

Note: Nomogram modified from data of E. Boyd by C. D. West; from Behrman, R. E., Kliegman, R. M., & Jenson, H. B. (Eds.). (2004). Nelson textbook of pediatrics *(17th ed.). Philadelphia: W. B. Sounders.*

Pediatric doses of medications are generally based on body surface area (BSA) or weight. To calculate a child's BSA, draw a straight line from the height (in the left-hand column) to the weight (in the right-hand column). The point at which the line intersects the surface area (SA) column is the BSA (measured in square meters [m^2]). If the child is of roughly normal proportion, BSA can be calculated from the weight alone (in the enclosed area).

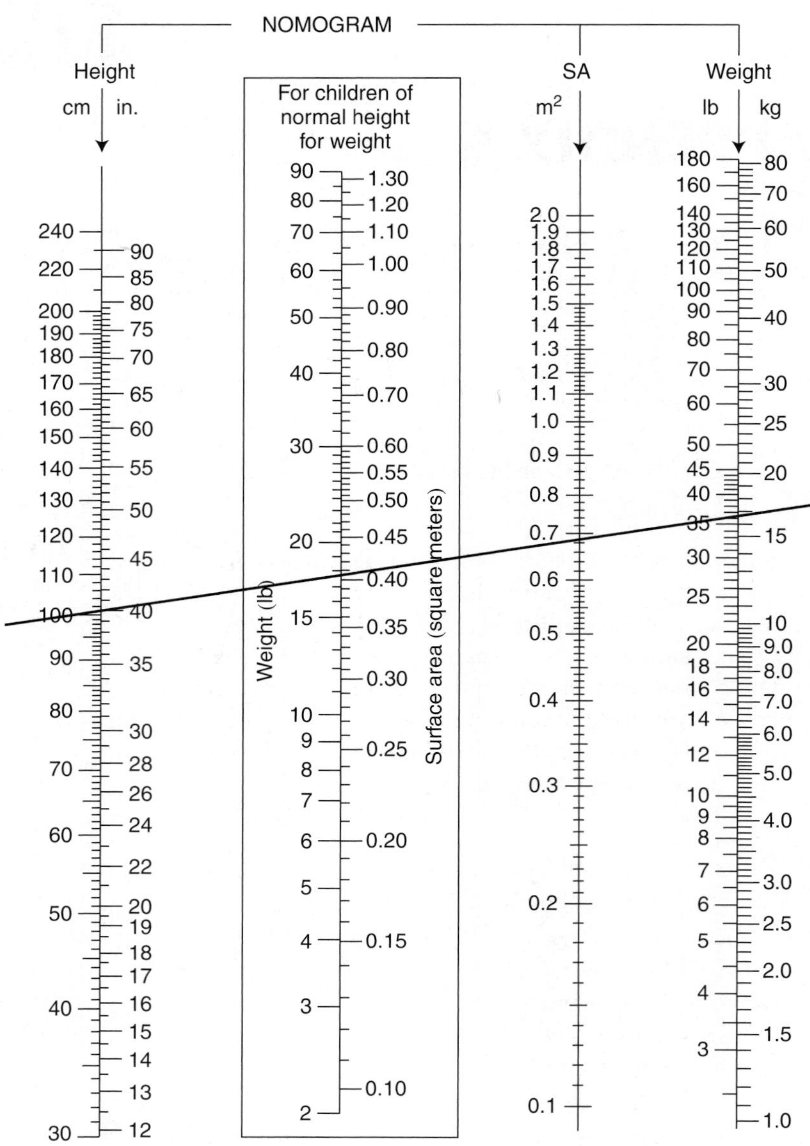

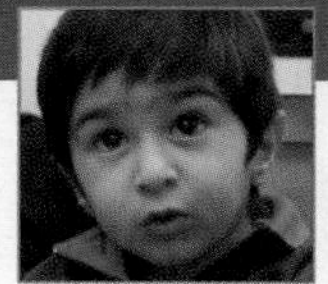 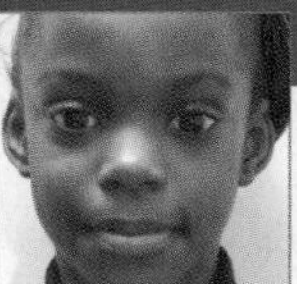 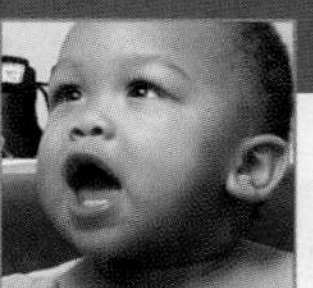 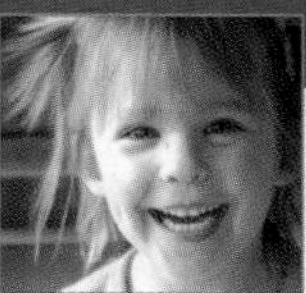

APPENDIX E

Emergency Assessment and Initial Management

EMERGENCY ASSESSMENT OF THE CHILD

Initial Assessment

An initial assessment begins as soon as the child comes in to view. It is important to gain an initial impression of the severity of the child's condition. Experienced healthcare providers use visual and auditory clues (based on appearance, breathing effort, and circulation of the skin) to make a rapid judgment about the urgency of the child's condition. This may take only 5 to 10 seconds to perform. It is not necessary to touch or disturb the child to make these assessments.

Appearance

Before touching the child, quickly look at the following characteristics and behavior of the infant or child.

- Observe for alertness, eye contact and interaction with parent or caregiver, and interest in toys or objects.
- Observe for spontaneous movement and good muscle tone.
- Observe consolability.
- Note quality of speech or cry.

Be concerned when the infant or child does not make eye contact with parent or caregiver, is uninterested in toys or objects, is limp or flaccid, is inconsolable, or has a weak, hoarse, or muffled cry.

Breathing Effort

Increased effort associated with breathing indicates an attempt by the child to overcome hypoxia, especially when some airway obstruction or problem with ventilation exists.

- Observe for nasal flaring, retractions, and head bobbing.
- Listen for abnormal airway sounds such as stridor, wheezing, grunting, snoring, or muffled or hoarse speech.
- Observe for tripod positioning, sitting with the head and neck extended, or refusal to lie down.

Presence of any of the signs may be associated with respiratory distress.

Circulation of the Skin

Constriction of the blood vessels occurs when the child has reduced circulating volume due to hemorrhage or dehydration. This action shifts blood flow to the vital organs to keep them oxygenated.

- Observe the color of the skin and mucous membranes.
- Inspecting the mucous membranes is especially important in children of darker skin because the mucous membranes are usually pink, regardless of skin color.

Pallor is an early sign of poor tissue perfusion. Mottling, caused by constriction of the blood vessels to the skin, indicates poor tissue perfusion (Figure E–1 ■). Cyanosis, a blue discoloration of the skin and mucous membranes, indicates severely impaired tissue perfusion.

To make a judgment about the child's physiologic stability, integrate the impressions from the appearance, breathing effort, and circulation of the skin. The greater the number of abnormal findings present, the more serious the child's condition. See Figure E–2 ■ for an example of an infant with poor physiologic stability that is characterized by an insecure airway, respiratory distress, impaired circulation, or unresponsiveness.

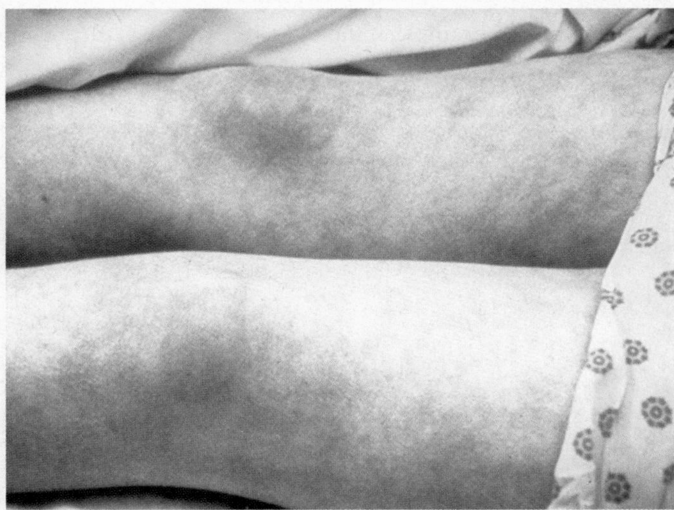

FIGURE E–1 ■ Mottling of the skin indicates vasoconstriction and poor tissue perfusion.

Courtesy of Health Resources and Services Administration, Maternal and Child Health Bureau, EMSC Program.

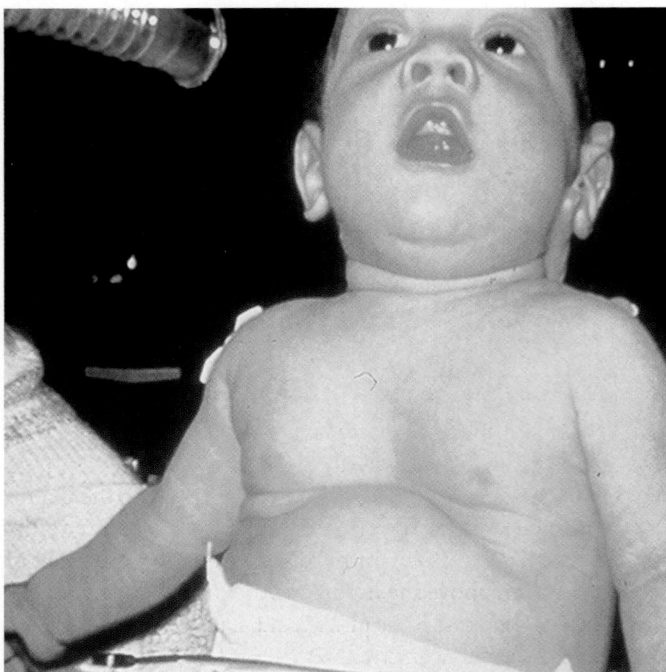

FIGURE E–2 ■ Using the initial assessment of appearance, breathing effort, and circulation of the skin, this infant is determined to have an emergency condition. *What are the visual clues that resulted in this assessment?*

Courtesy of Health Resources and Services Administration, Maternal and Child Health Bureau, EMSC Program.

Forming an Initial Impression

When the initial impression of a child's condition indicates an emergency due to an injury or acute medical condition, an altered sequence of assessment is implemented to quickly identify the presence of a life-threatening condition. This sequence is focused on recognizing physiologic changes that require immediate care to save the child's life. The physiologic changes that are most critical for survival are assessed first:

- *A*irway (for example, if the child's airway is obstructed, no oxygen can enter the child's system)
- *B*reathing (for example, if there is damage to the child's lungs or the bronchioles are constricted, the child may be unable to ventilate and support gas exchange)
- *C*irculation (for example, hemorrhage may reduce blood volume to the extent that it is inadequate to circulate oxygen to the brain and other vital organs)

As soon as a potential life-threatening physiologic condition is identified, the assessment is interrupted to provide the needed care. Only when the physiologic condition is stabilized does the assessment continue to the next physiologic assessment, or on to other body systems. When a child has an emergency condition, the physiologic status of the airway, breathing, and circulation are assessed frequently (every 5 minutes) because the child's condition can change and deteriorate rapidly.

ASSESSING THE ABCS

Airway Assessment

Is the infant or child crying or talking?	Crying or talking indicates an open airway at that point in time.
Are there any airway sounds?	Their presence may indicate an upper or lower airway obstruction due to a foreign body, inflammation, secretions, or blood.
Could the tongue be blocking the airway?	When a child is unresponsive and lying supine, the tongue can fall back into the pharynx and obstruct the airway.
Is there chest rise?	Chest rise indicates movement of air within the airway.

Airway Management

If there is an obstruction in the airway, then take immediate actions to open the airway.

- Perform a chin lift or a jaw thrust to lift the tongue out of the pharynx (see Figure E–3 ■ for guidance in performing these maneuvers).

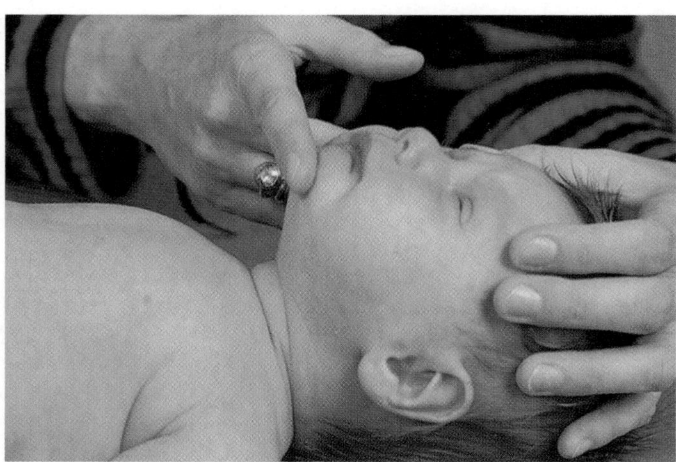

A

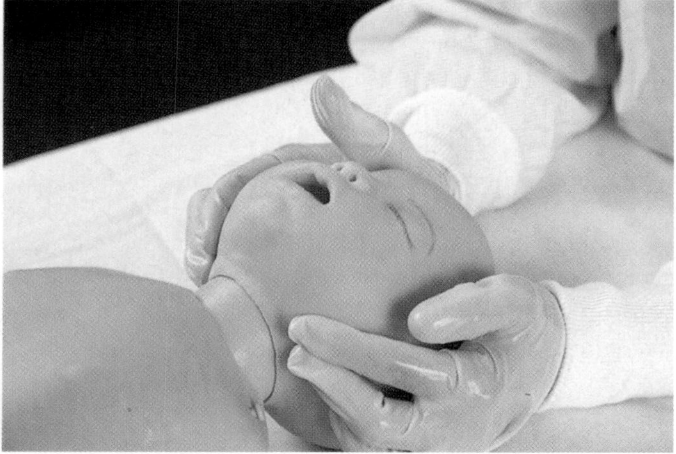

B

FIGURE E–3 ■ Opening the airway of an infant. For both techniques place the child's head in sniffing position (as if to move the head forward slightly to smell a flower). Avoid hyperextending the neck. Place a small towel under the shoulders of an infant and young child to maintain the head position. This helps offset the child's large occiput. *A,* Perform the chin lift by tilting the head back (as described) and lifting the chin up and out. *B,* Perform the jaw thrust by placing two fingers under each side of the jaw at its angle and lift the jaw upward and outward.

- An oropharyngeal airway may be inserted to maintain the airway in an unconscious child. Secretions and blood should be gently suctioned to clear the airway. An endotracheal tube may be inserted to maintain and secure the airway. The endotracheal tube placement needs to be monitored to make sure it does not become dislodged from the trachea. End-tidal CO_2 monitoring can be used to confirm endotracheal tube placement. Once placement is confirmed, the tube is secured and level of the tube at the teeth is recorded.
- If the chest does not rise and fall, use a bag-valve mask or perform rescue breathing with a pocket mask, and give two slow breaths.
- If the chest does not rise, check the child's head position with the chin lift or jaw thrust. Give two slow breaths again. If the chest does not rise, initiate procedures for removing a foreign-body obstruction.

Removing a Foreign-Body Obstruction

Follow the most current guidelines for foreign-body obstruction and cardiopulmonary resuscitation (CPR) from the American Heart Association.

Infant

- Position the infant face down on your arm supporting the head.
- Perform five back blows with the heel of the hand between the infant's shoulder blades. Then rotate the infant to be face up on your forearm.
- Place the fingers on the lower half of the sternum, avoiding the ziphoid process (the same position used for CPR). Give five chest thrusts near the center of the sternum (Figure E–4 ■).
- Place your index finger on the bony prominence of the infant's chin and your thumb in the mouth on the tongue. Pull up and out to open the mouth. Look in the infant's mouth for the foreign body and remove it if seen. *Do not perform a blind finger sweep.*
- If no object is found, try to ventilate the infant again. If the obstruction is still present, reposition the infant's head and attempt to ventilate again. If the obstruction remains, begin another series of back blows and chest thrusts. Look in the mouth, try to ventilate, reposition the head, and attempt to ventilate again. Continue repeating this sequence until the airway is clear. If the airway clears, give two slow breaths and continue the emergency assessment of the infant.
- If the infant becomes unconscious, begin CPR.

Child Between 1 and 8 Years

Conscious Child

- When the child is conscious, perform abdominal thrusts with the child in either a sitting or standing position.
- Stand behind the child, with your arms under the child's axilla and around the chest. Place the thumb of one fist against the abdomen in the midline, under the xiphoid process and above the umbilicus.
- Grasp your fist with the other hand. Deliver up to five quick upward thrusts against the abdomen (Figure E–5 ■). Each thrust should be a distinct effort to remove the obstruction.
- After the thrusts, assess the ability of the child to breathe. Repeat the series of five thrusts until the obstruction is cleared.
- If the child becomes unconscious, continue using the abdominal thrust procedure for the unconscious child.

Unconscious Child

- When the child is unconscious, place the child in supine position and kneel, straddling the child's body at the hips and facing the child's head.
- Place the heel of your hand on the child's abdomen at midline, between the xiphoid process and the umbilicus. Place your other hand over the wrist (Figure E–6 ■). Press into the abdomen, using both hands in quick upward strokes. Deliver up to five thrusts. Make each thrust distinct in an effort to remove the obstruction.

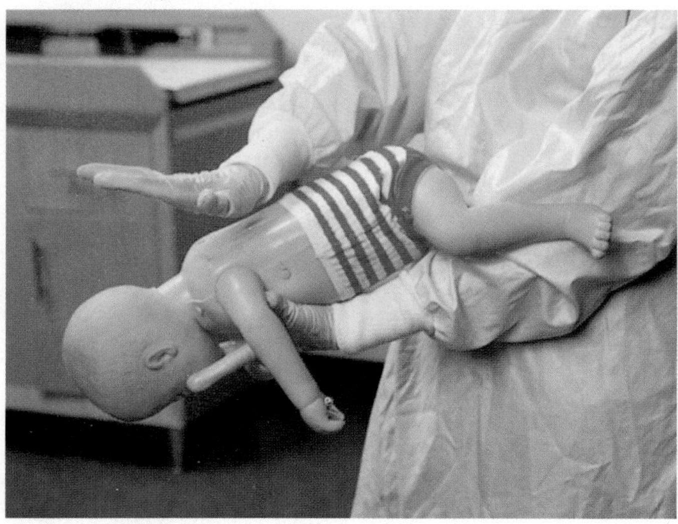

A

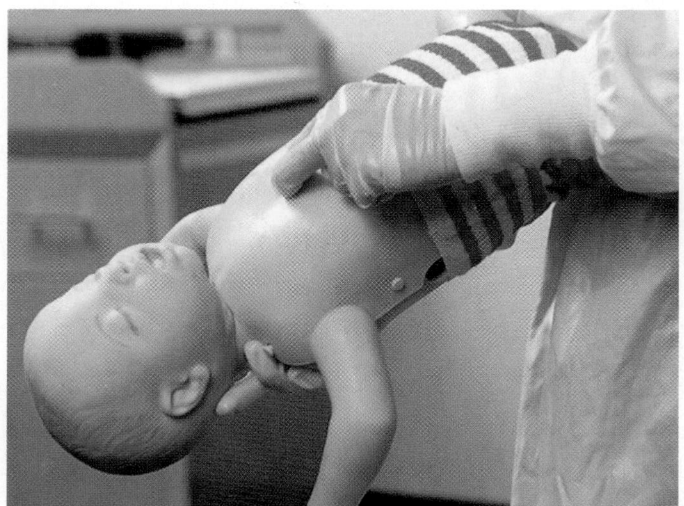

B

FIGURE E–4 ■ *A,* Performing back blows. *B,* Performing chest thrusts.

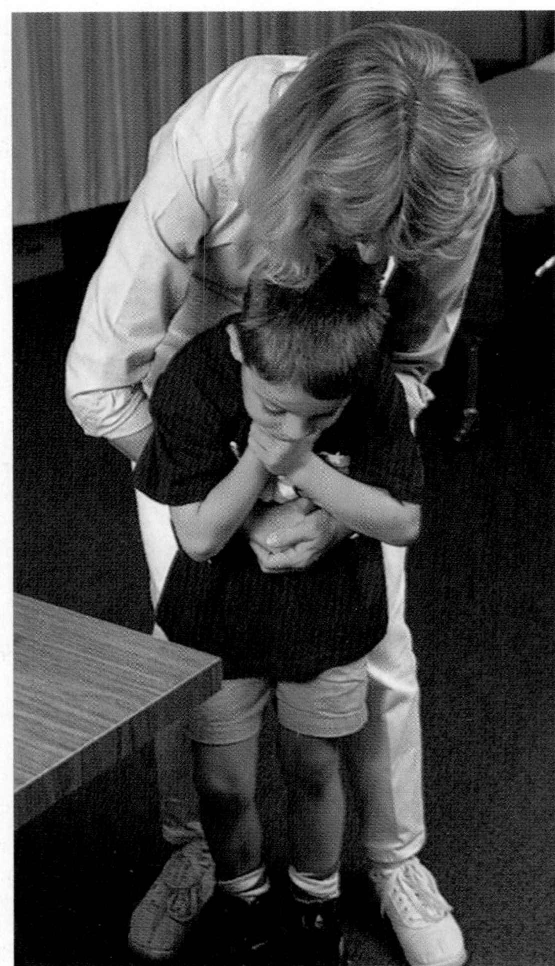

FIGURE E–5 ■ Hand positioning for abdominal thrusts when the child is standing.

- Use the tongue-jaw lift to open the mouth of the child to look for the foreign body. Remove it if seen, but *do not perform a blind finger sweep.* If the foreign body is not seen, open the airway and attempt to ventilate the child. If the airway is still obstructed, reposition the child's head and attempt to ventilate again. If the child's airway is still obstructed, begin another series of abdominal thrusts. Continue repeating this sequence until the airway is clear. If the airway clears, give two slow breaths and continue the emergency assessment of the child.

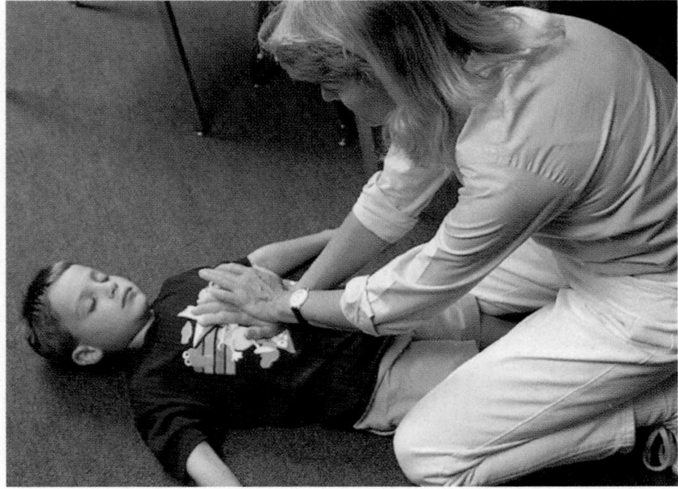

FIGURE E–6 ■ Hand positioning for abdominal thrusts when the child is supine.

Additional information about management of the child with a foreign-body airway obstruction, croup, or asthma can be found in Chapter 25∞.

Breathing Assessment

What is the effort associated with breathing?	The presence of retractions, nasal flaring, stridor, wheezing, or grunting are signs of respiratory distress.
What is the respiratory rate and how does it compare with the expected rate by age?	See Table E–1 for expected respiratory rates by age. A rate higher than expected may be a sign of respiratory distress, especially when accompanied by increased breathing effort. A rate lower than expected may indicate respiratory failure, an ominous sign that could mean the child may stop breathing.
What sounds are heard when auscultating the chest?	Absent or decreased breath sounds with respiratory effort are associated with an airway obstruction such as asthma or a foreign body. Identify any adventitious sounds such as wheezes, crackles, grunting, and rhonchi. Adventitious sounds may indicate an injury, aspiration, or inflammatory process.
Are there any penetrating chest injuries? Are there any rib fractures? Are there any marks on the chest indicating an injury?	Any obvious openings on the anterior and posterior chest wall, and sounds that could be air sucked into or escaping from the chest, are indications of a penetrating chest injury. An open chest wound can develop into a life-threatening tension pneumothorax. Rib fractures are uncommon in children, but if present interfere with the ability to adequately ventilate the child. Bruises on the chest wall may indicate a deeper injury to the lung tissue such as a pulmonary contusion or pneumothorax.

Breathing Management

High-concentration oxygen is provided to most infants and children with emergency conditions. A nonrebreather mask has a face mask and a reservoir bag that enables delivery of 60% to 90% oxygen at a flow rate of 12 to 15 L/min when the mask maintains a tight seal on the face. High-concentration oxygen can also be delivered through a bag-valve mask (used to assist ventilations). In some cases, low-concentration oxygen is provided to the infant or

TABLE E–1 Normal Respiratory Rate Ranges by Age

AGE	RESPIRATORY RATE PER MINUTE
Newborn	30–60
1 year	20–40
3 years	20–30
6 years	16–22
10 years	16–20
17 years	12–20

child using a simple face mask, nasal cannula, or blow-by tubing. See the Skills Manual for additional information.

Assisted Ventilation

When the child has minimal or no respiratory effort, assisted ventilation is initiated with a bag-valve mask.

Select the appropriate size mask for the child, one that extends from the bridge of the nose to the cleft of the chin.

- Select the appropriate size resuscitation bag to ensure that adequate tidal volume is delivered. A pediatric bag has a volume of 450 to 759 mL, while an adult bag has a volume of 1,200 mL.
- Connect the bag to the oxygen tubing and set the flow rate at 15 mL/min.
- Apply the mask to the face and get an airtight seal. Hold the mask securely to the face to maintain the seal. Form a C with the thumb and index finger to hold the mask securely over the face to cause an airtight seal. Place the remaining fingers of the hand against the mandible to secure the mask to the face (Figure E–7 ■).
- When assisting ventilation with the resuscitation bag, use reminder words like "squeeze, release, release" to provide an inspiratory phase to expiratory phase ratio of 1:2 (Dieckmann, Brownstein, & Gaushe-Hill, 2000). Make sure the chest rises with each ventilation, but use only enough pressure and air volume to make the chest rise.

Assisted ventilation often causes gastric distention because more air is forced into the airway than is needed to inflate the lungs. The extra air enters the stomach, and over a short period of time the stomach becomes distended and presses against the diaphragm. A nasogastric or orogastric tube may be inserted to keep the stomach deflated and improve ventilation. The nasogastric tube also reduces the risk for vomiting which can compromise the airway.

Managing a Chest Injury

An open chest wound is immediately covered with an occlusive dressing and taped on three sides. This prevents air from entering the chest while permitting an outlet for air escaping from the chest. A chest tube is inserted when a pneumothorax is present to reduce the elevated pressure in the chest and to help reexpand the lung.

Additional information for the management of respiratory conditions and injuries, such as croup, asthma, and pneumothorax, can be found in Chapter 25.

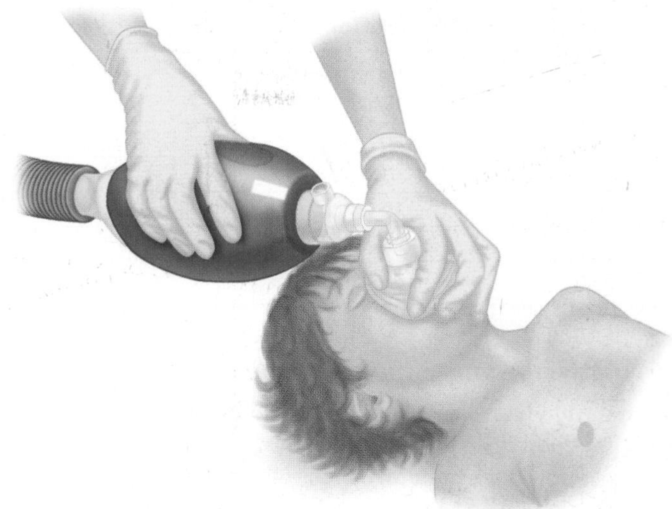

FIGURE E–7 ■ Proper placement of the hand to hold the mask of a resuscitation bag. Note the C formed by the thumb and index finger and the three fingers forming an E on the mandible to become the E-C clamp. This helps promote a tight seal with the face and prevents the remaining fingers from occluding the airway by pressing on the soft tissue of the neck.

Circulatory Assessment

What is the circulation to the skin?	When the skin is warm and the child's color is pink, tissue perfusion is good. Cool extremities accompanied by pallor, mottling, or cyanosis is associated with poor tissue perfusion.
What is the capillary refill time?	Delayed capillary refill > sec 2 is associated with poor tissue perfusion.
Is there any bleeding or potential internal bleeding? How much blood has been lost?	Estimation of blood loss from all sites is helpful in determining the potential for hypovolemic shock. Consider if there could be bleeding into the chest or abdomen from the type of injury sustained and presence of bruises or abrasions in those areas.
Is the child possibly dehydrated?	Dehydration also reduces the volume of circulating blood.
What is the heart rate?	Check the brachial pulse in infants and the carotid pulse in children and adolescents. Check the pulse for 10 sec before determining absence of a pulse. See Table E–2 for the expected heart rates by age. A sustained and increasing heart rate >130 beats/min is associated with continuing blood loss and hypovolemia.
What is the child's blood pressure?	The child's systolic blood pressure often does not reveal changes until uncompensated shock is present. See Table 8–16 for expected blood pressure by age, height, and sex. A drop in the systolic blood pressure is a serious sign that the circulatory volume is depleted by 20% to 25% (American Heart Association, 2002).

TABLE E–2 Normal Heart Rate Ranges by Age

AGE	HEART RATE RANGE (BEATS/MIN)
Newborn	120–160
Infant to 2 years	80–130
2–6 years	70–120
6–10 years	70–110
10–16 years	60–100

Circulation Management

When the bradycardia is present, provide oxygen and assist ventilations as described under the breathing management section. A cardiorespiratory monitor is attached to the child. Monitor the heart rate during interventions to see if the heart rate increases and stabilizes. An intravenous line is established to provide medications that stimulate and support myocardial function, as well as to treat arrhythmias and to correct metabolic acidosis. If an IV line cannot be started, but an endotracheal tube is in place, small amounts of medication can be administered down the endotracheal tube. See the commonly used resuscitation medications on page 1543–1544.

Pulselessness

If no pulse can be palpated or the pulse rate is less than 60 beats/min in an infant or child with poor tissue perfusion, cardiac compressions are initiated (American Heart Association, 2002).

Infants

- Find the finger position near the lower half of the sternum, making sure the fingers are not over the xiphoid process.
- Perform five compressions and one breath at a rate that provides 100 compressions and 20 breaths per minute. The depth of compressions is 0.5 to 1 inch. Perform 20 cycles of compressions and breaths and then reassess the infant.
- Palpate the brachial pulse for 5 seconds. If the pulse is absent, continue the cycle for another 3 to 5 minutes. Reassess the infant. Repeat the cycle of compressions and breaths until signs of circulation return or until help arrives. If the infant has return of a pulse and spontaneous respirations and is not a trauma victim, place the infant in a side-lying position to protect the airway.

Children Between 1 and 8 Years

- Place the heel of the hand on the lower half of the sternum, making sure the hand is not over the xiphoid process.
- Perform five compressions and one breath at a rate that provides 100 compressions and 20 breaths per minute. Compression depth is 1 to 1.5 inches. At the end of each compression allow the chest to return to the normal position before beginning the next compression. Maintain the head tilt position so the airway remains open. Reassess the child after 20 cycles of compressions and breathing.
- Palpate the carotid pulse for 5 seconds. If the pulse is still absent, continue the cycle of compressions and breaths for 3 to 5 minutes before reassessment. Repeat the cycle of compressions and breaths until circulation returns. If the child has return of pulse and spontaneous respirations and is not a trauma victim, place the child in a side-lying position.

Defibrillation

Defibrillation of the pulseless infant or child with ventricular fibrillation or pulseless ventricular fibrillation is performed within healthcare and community settings. The shock causes a sudden depolarization of the myocardial cells and terminates the ventricular fibrillation rhythm long enough for a more organized myocardial rhythm to start.

- Place the appropriate size pads or electrodes on the child's chest. Use small paddles or electrode pads (4.5 cm) for infants up to 1 year of age. Use adult paddles or electrode pads (8 to 13 cm) for all children over 1 year of age. Place the paddles or pads so that the heart is between them—one on the right upper sternal border and one on the left chest under the arm at the level of the left nipple. Alternatively, one paddle may be placed along the left sternal border and one on the back.
- A starting does of 2 joules/kg is recommended. The dose may be increased up to 4 joules/kg if ventricular fibrillation persists after the first shock (American Heart Association, 2002). Make sure no one is touching the child, bed, or attached equipment when the shock is delivered. The shocks are delivered in quick succession, with only enough time in between to check the rhythm. Up to three shocks may be provided. Automatic external defibrillators are also available in many public settings, and can be used on a child.

Hypovolemic Shock

Control bleeding with direct pressure using a gloved hand and elevate the body part if it is safe to do so. In the case of hemorrhage, apply pressure to an arterial pressure point proximal to the injury to slow the flow of bleeding.

Two intravenous lines are usually established when the child has signs of uncompensated shock, meaning there are signs of shock plus a drop in the systolic blood pressure. See the clinical manifestations table on page 945. A bolus (20 mL/kg) of crystalloid fluids (lactated Ringer's or normal saline) are administered quickly to increase the volume of circulating blood so that remaining blood can get to and oxygenate the vital organs. The heart rate, capillary refill, and responsiveness are reassessed frequently over the next 5 to 15 minutes to determine the child's response to the extra fluid volume and to determine the need for additional crystalloid IV fluid, albumin, or blood. Additional fluids or blood are given until the circulatory system is stabilized. See Chapter 28∞ for blood administration guidelines.

Additional information for the management of the child with dehydration and hypovolemic shock can be found in Chapters 23 and 26∞.

Pediatric Advanced Life Support Medications for Cardiac Arrest and Symptomatic Arrhythmias

DRUG	DOSAGE (PEDIATRIC)	REMARKS
Adenosine	0.1 mg/kg Repeat dose: 0.2 mg/kg Maximum single dose: 12 mg	Rapid IV/IO bolus Rapid flush to central circulation Monitor ECG during dose.
Amiodarone for pulseless VF/VT Amiodarone for perfusing tachycardias	5 mg/kg IV/IO Loading dose: 5 mg/kg IV/IO Maximum dose: 15 mg/kg per day	Rapid IV bolus IV over 20 to 60 minutes Routine use in combination with drugs prolonging QT Interval is *not* recommended. Hypotension is most frequent side effect.
Atropine sulfate*	0.02 mg/kg Minimum dose: 0.1 mg Maximum single dose: 0.5 mg in child, 1.0 mg in adolescent. May repeat once.	May give IV, IO or ET. Tachycardia and pupil dilation may occur but *not* fixed dilated pupils.
Calcium chloride 10% = 100 mg/mL (=27.2 mg/mL elemental Ca)	20 mg/kg (0.2 mL/kg) IV/IO	Give slow IV push for hypocalcemia, hypermagnesemla, calcium channel blocker toxicity, preferably via central vein. Monitor heart rate; bradycardia may occur.
Calcium gluconate 10% = 100 mg/mL (= 9 mg/mL elemental Ca)	60–100 mg/kg (0.6–1 mL/kg) IV/IO	Give slow IV push for hypocalcemia, hypermagnesemia, calcium channel blocker toxicity, preferably via central vein.
Epinephrine for symptomatic bradycardia* Epinephrine for pulseless arrest*	IV/IO: 0.01 mg/kg (1:10 000, 0.1 mL/kg) ET: 0.1 mg/kg (1: 1000, 0.1 mL/kg) First dose: IV/IO: 0.01 mg/kg (1:10 000, 0.1 mL/kg) ET: 0.1 mg/kg (1:1000, 0.1 mL/kg) Subsequent doses: Repeat initial dose or may increase up to 10 times (0.1 mg/kg, 1:1000, 0.1 mL/kg) Administer epinephrine every 3 to 5 minutes. IV/IO/ET doses as high as 0.2 mg/kg of 1:1000 may be effective.	Tachyarrhythmias, hypertension may occur.
Glucose (10% or 25% or 50%)	IV/IO 0.5–1 g/kg •1–2 mL/kg 50% •2–4 mL/kg 25% •5–10 mL/kg 10%	For suspected hypoglycemia; avoid hyperglycemia.
Lidocaine* Lidocaine Infusion (start after a bolus)	IV/IO/ET: 1 mg/kg IV/IO: 20–50 mcg/kg per minute	Rapid bolus 1 to 2.5 mL/kg per hour of 120 mg/100 mL solution
Magnesium sulfate (500 mg/mL)	IV/IO: 25–50 mg/kg, Maximum dose: 2 g per dose	Rapid IV Infusion for torsades or suspected hypomagnesemia; 10- to 20-minute infusion for asthma that responds poorly to β-adrenergic agonists.
Naloxone*	≤5 years or ≤20 kg: 0.1 mg/kg >5 years or >20 kg: 2 mg	For total reversal of narcotic effect. Use small repeated doses (0.01 to 0.03 mg/kg) titrated to desired effect.
Procainamide for perfusing tachycardias (100 mg/mL and 500 mg/mL)	Loading dose: 15 mg/kg IV/IO	Infusion over 30 to 60 minutes; routine use in combination with drugs prolonging QT interval is *not* recommended.
Sodium bicarbonate (1 mEq/mL and 0.5 mEq/mL)	IV/IO: 1 mEq/kg per dose	Infuse slowly and only if ventilation is adequate.

IV indicates intravenous; IO, intraosseous; and ET, endotracheal.

*For endotracheal administration use higher doses (2 to 10 times the IV dose); dilute medication with normal saline to a volume of 3 to 5 mL and follow with several positive-pressure ventilations.

Pediatric Advanced Life Support Medications to Maintain Cardiac Output and for Postresuscitation Stabilization

MEDICATION	DOSE RANGE	COMMENT
Amrinone	IV/IO loading dose: 0.75–1 mg/kg IV over 5 minutes; may repeat 2 times IV/IO infusion: 5–10 mcg/kg per minute	Inodilator
Dobutamine	IV/IO infusion: 2–20 mcg/kg per minute	Inotrope; vasodilator
Dopamine	IV/IO influsion: 2–20 mcg/kg per minute	Inotrope; chronotrope; renal and splanchnic vasodilator in lower doses; pressor in higher doses
Epinephrine	IV/IO influsion: 0.1–1 mcg/kg per minute	Inotrope; chronotrope; vasodilator in lower doses and pressor in higher doses
Lidocaine	IV/IO loading dose: 1 mg/kg IV/IO influsion: 20–50 mcg/kg per minute	Antiarrythmic, mild negative inotrope. Use lower infusion rate if poor cardiac output or poor hepatic function.
Milrinone	IV/IO loading dose: 50–75 mcg/kg IV/IO influsion: 0.5–0.75 mcg/kg per minute	Inodilator
Norepinephrine	IV/IO influsion: 0.1–2 mcg/kg per minute	Vasopressor
Prostaglandin E_1	IV/IO influsion: 0.05–0.1 mcg/kg per minute	Maintains patency of ductus arteriosus in cyanotic congenital heart disease. Monitor for apnea, hypotension, and hypoglycemia.
Sodium nitroprusside	IV/IO influsion: 1–8 mcg/kg per minute	Vasodilator Prepare only in dextrose in water

IV indicates intravenous,; IO, intraosseous.

* Most infusions may be calculated on the basis of the "Rule of 6" as illustrated in the table. Alternatively, a standard concentration may be used to provide more dilute or more concentrated drug solution, but then an individual dose must be calculated for each patient and each infusion rate as follows: Infusion rate (mL/h) = [weight (kg) × dose (µg/kg per minute) × 60 min/h]/concentration (µg/mL). Diluent may be 5% dextrose in water, 5% dextrose in half-normal saline, normal saline, or flinger's lactate unless noted otherwise.

Disability (Neurologic) Assessment

What is the infant's or child's level of responsiveness using AVPU? What is the Glasgow Coma Scale score?	See Box 33-2 and Table 33-2 for assessment guidelines. When the child is alert or responsive to verbal stimuli, a mild injury or condition may be present. When the child is responsive only to pain or unresponsive, a severe injury or condition is usually present.
Check the pupils for size, symmetry, and reactivity to light.	Dilated or asymmetric pupils that do not react to light may indicate the development of increased intracranial pressure. Pupillary response may also be abnormal in the presence of drugs, seizures, or hypoxia.
Has the child had a seizure?	Seizures may happen when the infant or child has had a brain injury or a hypoxic event. Seizures may also be due to hypoglycemia or a metabolic disorder.
Is the child moving spontaneously? Is the child flaccid? Is any abnormal posturing present?	Spontaneous movement of the extremities is a positive sign of neurologic integrity. Limpness accompanied by decreased responsiveness may indicate hypoxia or a brain injury. Total loss of flexor and extensor tone may indicate a spinal cord injury. Decerebrate or decorticate posturing indicates a significant brain injury.

Disability Management

Initial management of the child with a brain injury is to ensure oxygenation with assisted ventilation at the appropriate respiratory rate for the infant or child. Hyperventilation is not routinely recommended, but it may be used in cases of an acute elevation in intracranial pressure or signs of brainstem herniation (asymmetric or fixed dilated pupils, bradycardia, hypertension, and irregular respirations) (American Heart Association, 2002). See Chapter 33∞ for management of the child with a brain injury.

When a seizure occurs following a brain injury or other hypoxic event, a benzodiazepine medication is usually administered. See Chapter 33∞ for management of the child with a seizure.

If spinal cord injury is suspected, immobilize the head in neutral position and prevent movement of other parts of the body. This helps protect the child from additional injury. Radiographs and often CT scanning are required to determine if a spinal cord injury is present.

Exposure

Full Body Inspection

When the child's condition is stabilized, a rapid inspection of the entire body is conducted to identify any additional injuries such as fractures of the extremities or soft tissue injuries. Check for the presence of pulses in extremities distal to the injury. Any object impaling a part of the body is stabilized in place until it can be surgically removed. Assess the child's pain level.

Temperature Management

Temperature control is important in children who have experienced an emergency. Remember that the infant and child have a larger body surface area and lose body heat quickly. Often the clothes have been removed to assess and provide treatment. Keep the child warm with heat lamps and warmed IV fluids. Maintaining a neutral temperature is beneficial for management of the child's emergency condition.

HISTORY

An abbreviated history of the event leading to the emergency is collected from the parent, caregiver, or witness by another healthcare provider while the emergency assessment and resuscitation is occurring. The acronym for this history is SAMPLE.

- *Signs and symptoms*—onset and nature of the symptoms
- *Allergies*—any known allergies
- *Medications*—names and doses of prescribed and over-the-counter medications, including aerosol medications and complementary therapies
- *Past medical problems*—any significant health conditions, past hospitalizations, immunizations
- *Last food or liquid*—when the infant or child last ate or had liquids, including breast or bottle feeding
- *Events leading to the injury or illness*—progression of illness over time, activities contributing to injury

QUICK REVIEW

- Use the initial assessment guidelines to quickly identify the need for emergency intervention.
- Always start by ensuring that the child has a patent airway.
- Assess breathing and provide assisted ventilation as needed.
- Check the circulation and intervene as needed with chest compressions or IV fluids.
- Repeat the assessment of ABCs every 5 minutes and intervene immediately if any deterioration in status is noted.
- Continue with other parts of the physical examination only when the infant's or child's condition is stabilized.

REFERENCES

American Heart Association. (2002). *PALS provider manual.* Dallas, TX: Author.

Bindler, R. C., & Ball, J. W. (2003). *Clinical skills manual for pediatric nursing: Caring for children* (3rd ed.). Upper Saddle River, NJ: Prentice Hall.

Dieckmann, R., Brownstein, D., & Gaushe-Hill, M. (Eds.). (2000). *American Academy of Pediatrics' pediatric education for prehospital professionals.* Sudbury, MA: Jones & Barlett Publishers.

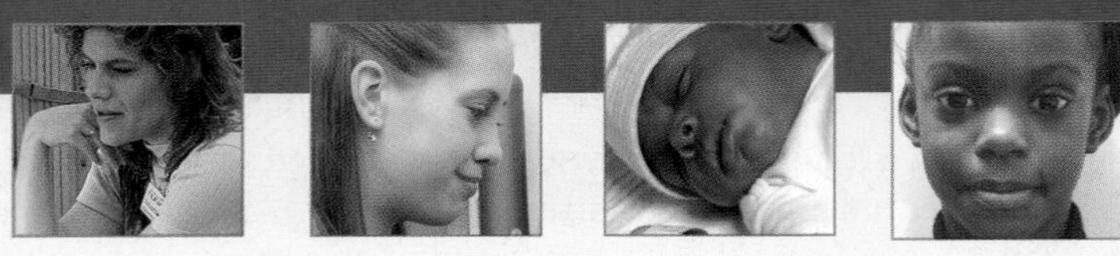

APPENDIX F

Diagnostic Tests and Procedures

As with all procedures in children, a discussion appropriate to the growth and developmental level of the child is optimal to meet the needs of both the child and the family. Parents need to complete a signed consent with an understanding of the procedure, results, and risk factors. Allow the child and family to express concerns. Support child and family before, during, and after the procedures.

Test/Procedure	Description/Purpose	Nursing Implications
Arteriography/angiogram	A contrast dye is injected to allow visualization of blood vessels. Useful in evaluating patency of blood vessels and identifying abnormal vasculature resulting from tumors.	• Obtain history of hypersensitivity to iodine, seafood, or contrast dye from other radiographic procedures. • Explain to child that there may be a warm, flushing feeling that could last a few minutes. It may feel uncomfortable, but there will be no pain. • Ensure child remains still during procedures so that pictures are clear. • During and after test, monitor vital signs; assess for vasovagal and allergic reactions.
Biopsy	Removal and examination of tissue from the body. Usually performed to detect malignancies or identify disease presence. Biopsies can be obtained in several ways: • Brush method, scraping cells and tissue with stiff bristles • Surgical excision at tissue site • Needle aspiration at tissue site, with or without ultrasound • Needle insertion into skin	• Prepare necessary instruments and specimen containers. • Label specimens accurately and arrange for transport as recommended for the particular specimen. • Monitor vital signs during and following the procedure. • Prepare surgical site. • Adhere to sedation and analgesia monitoring guidelines. • Ensure that child remains still during procedure. • Apply dressing if appropriate to the site after procedure. • Teach family to monitor site for infection and to care for wound.
Bone marrow aspiration	May be performed for diagnostic purposes (to diagnose anemias or cancers) or for harvesting for transplant. Common sites for bone marrow aspiration are the iliac crest and sternum.	• Bone marrow aspirations are painful and the child is generally sedated. • The site is prepped with a cleansing agent according to practitioner's protocol. • Positioning is determined according to the site used, side-lying for the ileac crest, and supine for the sternum. • The child should not move during this procedure since the needle may become dislodged. For this reason, infants and small children are given sedation and analgesia. Monitor the child during the procedure according to agency guidelines. • If the child is awake during the procedure, inform the child that pressure may be felt. • After the procedure is complete, maintain the child on bed rest for at least 1 hour. Assess vital signs following agency protocol. Monitor for signs of bleeding such as tachycardia and hypotension. Mild analgesics are provided for pain at the harvest site.

Test/Procedure	Description/Purpose	Nursing Implications
Cardiac catheterization Chapter 26∞	An invasive procedure that passes a radiopaque catheter through a large vein or artery in an arm or leg to the heart. The catheter is threaded to the heart chambers or coronary arteries, or both, guided by fluoroscopy, which enables precise measurement of oxygen saturation within the heart's chambers and great arteries and pressure gradients in the pulmonary vessels or heart chambers. This helps identify: • Congenital heart defects • Cardiac valvular disease • Coronary artery disease In some cases a biopsy of the heart muscle may also be obtained to evaluate muscle function problems, inflammation, or heart transplant rejection. Also, cardiac catheterization can aid in evaluation of artificial valves.	• No food or fluid 6–8 hours prior to test. • Take the child and parents on a tour of the catheterization lab and inform the child about the equipment that will be used and sensations that will be felt. • Obtain history of hypersensitivity to iodine, seafood, or contrast dye from other radiographic procedures. If allergic reaction is suspected, antihistamines and/or steroids may be ordered prior to procedure. Assess for allergic reaction during procedure. • Anticoagulant therapy is discontinued prior to the test. • Have the child void before the procedure. • An IV is started for administration of emergency drugs, as needed. • Position child on a padded table. Sedation is given to help the child remain still. • ECG leads are applied to the chest to monitor heart activity. Vital signs and heart rhythm are monitored. • Once the catheter and guidewires are removed, apply direct pressure on the catheterization site for 15 minutes and then apply a pressure dressing for 6 hours. • Monitor the site for bleeding and assess the distal extremity for pulse, capillary refill, and temperature according to agency guidelines. • After the procedure, maintain the child on bed rest for 6 hours and then limit acitivities for 24 hours. • Monitor intake and output as the contrast dye causes diuresis
Cerebral spinal fluid (CSF) analysis Chapter 33∞	CSF is obtained during a lumbar puncture performed at the L3–4 or L4–5 level. CSF pressure is measured, then fluid is collected and placed in sterile test tubes. Data obtained is used to diagnose spinal cord and brain disease processes.	• The infant or child is held in knee-chest position and kept still during this procedure. • Specimens must be collected in numerical order of tubes. • Assess vital signs before and after procedure at specified times. • Assess for changes in neurological function. • Administer analgesics as ordered for headache.
Computed tomography (CT)	The CT scan produces a narrow X-ray beam that examines body sections from different angles, producing a two-dimensional cross section of the structures. It can be performed with or without iodine contrast media; it is not invasive unless contrast dye is used. CT scanning usually takes 5–15 minutes. CT is used to screen for coronary artery disease; head, liver, and renal lesions; tumors; edema; abscess; bone destruction; and to locate foreign objects in soft tissue, such as the eye.	• Depending upon body system evaluated the infant or child may be NPO and require bowel evacuation prior to study. • If contrast medium is used, obtain history of hypersensitivity to iodine, seafood, or contrast dye from other radiographic procedures. If allergic reaction is suspected, antihistamines and/or steroids may be ordered prior to procedure. Assess for allergic reaction during procedure. • Prepare child for the procedure by describing size of equipment, noises, and other sensations that will be experienced, and how the child can help during the procedure. • Sedation may be required for infants and small children to keep them still. Monitor sedated children according to agency guidelines.

Test/Procedure	Description/Purpose	Nursing Implications
Cultures See Skills Manual	Cultures are taken to isolate microorganisms causing body tissue or body fluid infection, and often to isolate the specific antibiotics to which the organisms are sensitive. The culture specimen is taken to the laboratory immediately after collection, where it will take 24–36 hours to grow the organisms. Cultures commonly used with children include: • Blood • Sputum • Stool • Throat • Wound • Urine • Cerebrospinal fluid See the Skills Manual for details on performing each culture.	• Do not administer newly prescribed antibiotics until after specimen collection, as they may cause false results. If these drugs have been given, list on laboratory slip. • Deliver all specimens immediately to the laboratory, or refrigerate the specimen. • Handle the specimen using strict aseptic technique. • Keep lids on sterile specimen containers.
Dual energy X-ray absorptiometry (DEXA)	DEXA is a noninvasive procedure that measures bone mineral density. The child will lie on an imaging table with a radiation source below and a detector above, which measure the bone's radiation absorption.	• Obtain family history of osteoporosis and skeletal problems. • Remove metal objects from area to be scanned.
Echocardiography	Ultrasound (see below) of the heart. This noninvasive test is used to identify abnormal heart size, structure, and function, and valvular disease. There are several types of echocardiographic studies.	• Obtain baseline vital signs and an ECG recording as indicated. • Obtain history of physical complaints. • Explain procedure to parents and child. • Inform the child of the need to hold still for the procedure. • Inform the child that a gel will be applied to the skin and a transducer will move over the area, but that the test causes no pain.
Electrocardiography (ECG or EKG)	An electrocardiogram (ECG) records the electrical impulses of the heart via electrodes and a galvanometer (ECG machine). Purposes of this procedure include: • Detection of cardiac dysrhythmias • Identification of electrolyte imbalances • Monitoring ECG changes during the stress test and post MI Electrodes with electropaste or pads are strapped to the four extremities, and chest electrodes are applied. The lead selector is turned to read the 12 standard leads.	• Obtain list of current medications and the last time they were taken. • When applying the chest leads, explain to the child that the procedure is not painful and they will need to hold still for a very short time. • Teach methods to relieve anxiety and remain relaxed.
Electroencephalogram (EEG)	Measures electrical activity in various lobes of the brain to identify the potential for seizures, and to determine brain death. Electrodes are applied to the scalp to record brain-wave activity. EEGs are used to: • Detect seizure disorder • Identify a brain tumor, abscess, intracranial hemorrhage, or other abnormality • Determine brain death	• Obtain a list of current medications and when last taken to identify any that could alter the EEG result. • Hair must be clean and dry, and free from mousse or gel. • EEGs are usually performed with the child lying down or seated in a reclining chair. • When applying the electrodes, explain to the child that the procedure is not painful. • Observe for seizures and describe seizure activity. • Inform parents to wash the child's hair to remove electrode gel.

Test/Procedure	Description/Purpose	Nursing Implications
Electromyography (EMG)	Measures the electrical activity of skeletal muscles at rest and during voluntary muscle contraction. A needle is inserted to detect electrical activity. This test is used to diagnose neuromuscular disorders such as muscular dystrophy, and can also be used to differentiate between myopathy and neuropathy.	• Be alert to medications that could affect EMG results. • Draw blood for serum enzymes prior to test if ordered. • Inform child that there may be slight pain when the needle electrodes are inserted. Support the child with age-appropriate relaxation techniques or distraction techniques. If pain persists, inform technician. • Administer analgesic as need for pain.
Endoscopy	A flexible, fiber-optic endoscope is used to visualize the internal structures of the esophagus, stomach, and duodenum. This procedure is also used to collect cytologic specimens and to confirm GI pathology.	• Maintain NPO status preprocedure. • The child will be sedated for the procedure and monitor the child according to agency guidelines. • Inform child that some pressure will be felt upon endoscope insertion. • Postoperatively monitor vital signs per protocol. Resume oral feedings as prescribed.
Genetic testing	Testing for chromosomal abnormalities and genetically linked diseases with specimens from: • Fetal cells collected from amniotic fluid before birth to analyze DNA and metabolic substances • After birth scrapings from the child's buccal mucosa used for DNA analysis.	• Arrange for explanations and genetic counseling for the family as needed to explain results and the implications for them and the child.
GI series See Chapter 30∞	Upper GI and small bowel series are fluoroscopic and radiographic examinations of the esophagus, stomach, and small intestine. Oral barium meal or water-soluble contrast agent is swallowed. The barium is observed as it passes through the digestive tract and films are taken. This series identifies: • Esophageal, gastric, or dudodenal ulcers • Polyps, tumors, or hiatal hernias in the GI tract • Foreign bodies, varices, or strictures	• Maintain NPO status preprocedure. A low-residue diet may be ordered before the test. • Withhold medications as ordered. • Record vital signs; note epigastric pain or discomfort. • Inform child that all of the liquid must be swallowed, but that the test will not cause pain or discomfort.
Intraesophageal pH probe monitoring	Considered the gold standard test for diagnosing gastroesophageal reflux disease and for evaluating atypical symptoms such as apnea, stridor, or cough. Place probe in the distal esophagus to detect pH changes below 4. pH is measured and recorded every 4–8 seconds; acid reflux is defined by a pH of <4 for at least 15–30 seconds.	• Ensure pH probe is secured. • Prevent infant or child from inadvertent removal of probe. • Probe is left in place to measure pH for 24 hours. • Monitor and record pH measurements per protocol.
Intravenous pyelogram See Chapter 31∞	Visualizes kidney's collecting system, distal ureters, and bladder. A radiopaque substance is injected IV, and a series of radiographs is obtained. IVP is useful for locating stones and tumors, and for diagnosing kidney disorders.	• Explain procedure to parents and child. Inform them that a transient flushing or burning sensation may occur. • Assess for allergies as contrast medium is used. • If BUN levels are greater than 40 mg/dL prior to the test, notify primary care provider. • Infants and children are NPO prior to the study. An IV is started for injection of contrast.

Test/Procedure	Description/Purpose	Nursing Implications
Magnetic resonance imaging (MRI)	Produces results similar to those of CT; however, it does not use ionizing radiation. The MRI scanner is a large, doughnut-shaped cylinder. The child lies on a table and is guided into the cylinder until the body part to be imaged is within the magnetic field.	• Prepare child for sounds, size of equipment, and tunnel. • Ensure that the child has no metallic objects or implants, and is not connected to metal equipment (e.g., oxygen tank). • Sedation may be needed to keep the infant or child still. Monitor the child according to agency guidelines.
Polysomnography (sleep study)	To identify apnea during sleep and to determine the cause of sleep disorders. Sleep studies include, but all may not be indicated, ECG or EKG, pulse oximetry, EEG, EOG, EMG, airflow monitoring, and snoring sensor. Testing for sleep disorders is performed at a sleep laboratory over an 8-hour period.	• Instruct family to keep sleep log 1 to 2 weeks prior to sleep studies, including notes about snoring and sleepiness during the day. Review sleep log. • Instruct patient/family to avoid caffeine products, sedatives, and naps 1 to 2 days prior to testing. • Obtain a history related to medications, head injury, headache, and seizures. • Explain procedure to parents and child. • Check vital signs. Observe for respiratory distress.
Positron emission tomography (PET) scan	PET measures areas of positron-emitting isotope concentration. PET is most effective in determining blood flow and can detect: • Decreased oxygen and blood flow in the brain • Tumors, nodules, and colorectal metastasis • Decreased blood flow in coronary arteries • Transient ischemia	• Monitor vital signs. • Two IVs are started; one for contrast and the other to draw blood gases. • Assess for allergies as contrast medium is used.
Pulmonary function tests	Used to differentiate between mild and obstructive lung disease, and in quantifying the degree of a disorder such as asthma or cystic fibrosis. These tests are also used to establish baselines for comparison, to detect pulmonary dysfunction, to evaluate pulmonary status prior to surgery, and to assess response to therapy. Tests include: • Slow vital-capacity tests • Lung-volume measurements • Forced vital capacity • Flow-volume loop • Diffusion capacity test • Bronchial provocation studies • Exercise studies • Pulse oximetry • Nutritional studies	• Obtain a list of any bronchodilators and steroids the child is taking. • Record child's age, height, weight, and vital signs. • Assess for signs and symptoms of respiratory distress. • Explain the purpose of tests and procedures; provide teaching as needed to enable the child to have an optimal performance. • Child may need to practice breathing patterns required for test.
Radiograph (X-ray)	The most common form of imaging, radiographs use irradiation to obtain images and capture them on film for diagnostic and screening purposes. Radiographs are commonly used to: • Identify bone structure and tissue • Detect abnormalities in size, structure, and shape of bone and body structures	• Explain procedure to parents and child. Inform them that the radiographic test usually takes 10–15 minutes, and that there may be several taken from different angles. Explain that modern equipment decreases radiation exposure. • Tell child about the need to hold still for the procedure. Have the child practice holding still and holding a breath in preparation for the test. • Radiopaque materials for IVP and GI studies administered within 3 days of radiograph may distort pictures.

Test/Procedure	Description/Purpose	Nursing Implications
Radionucleotide testing (nuclear scans)	Nuclear medicine is the clinical field concerned with diagnostic and therapeutic uses of radioactive isotopes. A radioactive isotope is an unstable isotope that decays or disintegrates, emitting radiation. Radioisotopes, known as radionuclides, concentrate in certain parts of the body. Scintillation (gamma) camera detectors are used for imaging. Uniform gray distribution indicates normal function, but lighter areas known as hot spots indicate hyperfunction, and dark areas or cold spots indicate hypofunction. Planar and single photon emission computed tomography are both utilized. Children may require bone, brain, renal, and thyroid scans.	• Obtain brief history related to recent exposure to radioisotopes, and allergies that could cause a reaction. • List on the request slip restricted drugs containing iodine that the child is taking on the order form. • Explain procedure to parents and child. Inform them that the amount of radiation received from radionuclide imaging is usually less than that received from a radiograph, and that there will be no discomfort. • Inform child and family that radionuclide is excreted from the body in 6–24 hours. • Jewelry and clothing should be removed. • An IV is started for injection of contrast.
Ultrasound	Ultrasound is a noninvasive procedure used to detect tissue abnormalities by visualizing body tissue structure or wave-form analysis of Doppler studies. An ultrasound probe (transducer) is held over the skin or body cavity to produce an ultrasound beam to the tissues. The reflected sound waves or tissues are then transformed into scans graphs, or sounds (Doppler).	• Administer sedation as prescribed. • Maintain NPO status preprocedure for abdominal studies. • Explain procedure to parents and child. Inform them that the procedure is painless, and there is no exposure to radiation. • Confirm the child has not received any tests that will interfere with results, e.g., upper GI series. • Instruct child to remain still during the procedure.

Data from Corbett, J. V. (2004). Laboratory Tests and Diagnostic Procedures with Nursing Diagnosis *(6th ed.). Upper Saddle River, NJ: Prentice Hall Health; Kee, J. L. (2005).* Handbook of Laboratory & Diagnostic Tests with Nursing Implications (5th ed.). *Upper Saddle River, NJ: Prentice Hall Health.*

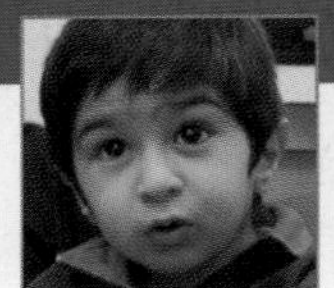 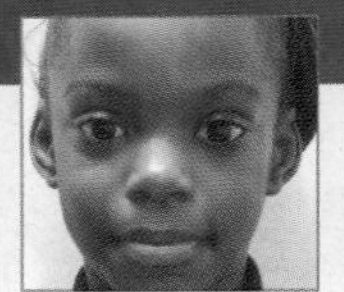 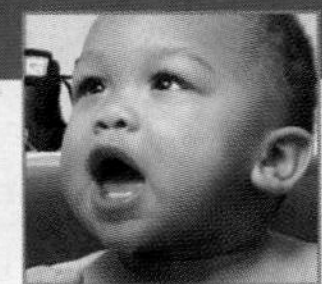 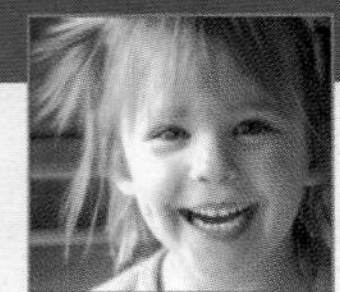

APPENDIX G

Temperature and Weight Conversion

°C	°F
35	95
35.2	95.4
35.3	95.7
35.6	96.1
35.8	96.4
36	96.8
36.2	97.2
36.4	97.5
36.6	97.9
36.8	98.2
37	98.6
37.2	99
37.4	99.3
37.6	99.7
37.8	100
38	100.4
38.2	100.8
38.4	101.1
38.6	101.5
38.8	101.8
39	102.2
39.2	102.6
39.4	102.9
39.6	103.3
39.8	103.6
40	104
40.2	104.4
40.4	104.7
40.6	105.1
40.8	105.4
41	105.8

Temperature Conversion Formula

°F = (°C × 9/5) − 32 or (°C × 1.8) + 32

°C = (°F − 32) × 5/9 or (°F − 32) × 0.55

Weight Conversion Formula

lb/2.2 = kilograms

kg × 2.2 = pounds

Example:

40 lb = 40/2.2 = 18.2 kg

20 kg = 20 × 2.2 = 44 lb

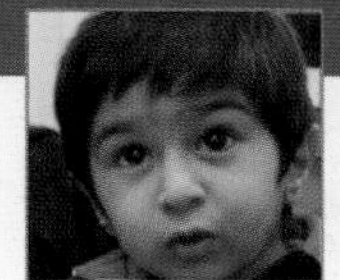
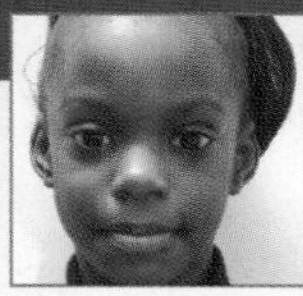
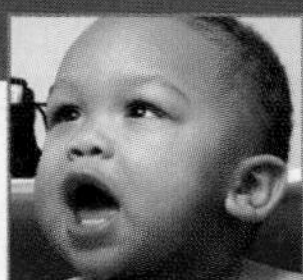
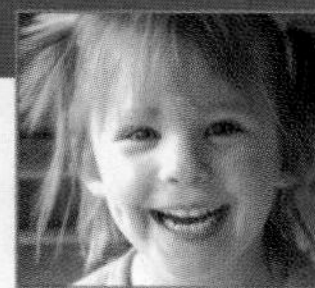

Index

Page numbers followed by italic *f* indicate figures and those followed by italic *t* indicate tables or boxes.

Pearson Education, Inc.

YOU SHOULD CAREFULLY READ THE TERMS AND CONDITIONS BEFORE USING THE CD-ROM PACKAGE. USING THIS CD-ROM PACKAGE INDICATES YOUR ACCEPTANCE OF THESE TERMS AND CONDITIONS.

Pearson Education, Inc. provides this program and licenses its use. You assume responsibility for the selection of the program to achieve your intended results, and for the installation, use, and results obtained from the program. This license extends only to use of the program in the United States or countries in which the program is marketed by authorized distributors.

LICENSE GRANT

You hereby accept a nonexclusive, nontransferable, permanent license to install and use the program ON A SINGLE COMPUTER at any given time. You may copy the program solely for backup or archival purposes in support of your use of the program on the single computer. You may not modify, translate, disassemble, decompile, or reverse engineer the program, in whole or in part.

TERM

The License is effective until terminated. Pearson Education, Inc. reserves the right to terminate this License automatically if any provision of the License is violated. You may terminate the License at any time. To terminate this License, you must return the program, including documentation, along with a written warranty stating that all copies in your possession have been returned or destroyed.

LIMITED WARRANTY

THE PROGRAM IS PROVIDED "AS IS" WITHOUT WARRANTY OF ANY KIND, EITHER EXPRESSED OR IMPLIED, INCLUDING, BUT NOT LIMITED TO, THE IMPLIED WARRANTIES OR MERCHANTABILITY AND FITNESS FOR A PARTICULAR PURPOSE. THE ENTIRE RISK AS TO THE QUALITY AND PERFORMANCE OF THE PROGRAM IS WITH YOU. SHOULD THE PROGRAM PROVE DEFECTIVE, YOU (AND NOT PRENTICE-HALL, INC. OR ANY AUTHORIZED DEALER) ASSUME THE ENTIRE COST OF ALL NECESSARY SERVICING, REPAIR, OR CORRECTION. NO ORAL OR WRITTEN INFORMATION OR ADVICE GIVEN BY PRENTICE-HALL, INC., ITS DEALERS, DISTRIBUTORS, OR AGENTS SHALL CREATE A WARRANTY OR INCREASE THE SCOPE OF THIS WARRANTY.

SOME STATES DO NOT ALLOW THE EXCLUSION OF IMPLIED WARRANTIES, SO THE ABOVE EXCLUSION MAY NOT APPLY TO YOU. THIS WARRANTY GIVES YOU SPECIFIC LEGAL RIGHTS AND YOU MAY ALSO HAVE OTHER LEGAL RIGHTS THAT VARY FROM STATE TO STATE.

Pearson Education, Inc. does not warrant that the functions contained in the program will meet your requirements or that the operation of the program will be uninterrupted or error-free.

However, Pearson Education, Inc. warrants the diskette(s) or CD-ROM(s) on which the program is furnished to be free from defects in material and workmanship under normal use for a period of ninety (90) days from the date of delivery to you as evidenced by a copy of your receipt.

The program should not be relied on as the sole basis to solve a problem whose incorrect solution could result in injury to person or property. If the program is employed in such a manner, it is at the user's own risk and Pearson Education, Inc. explicitly disclaims all liability for such misuse.

LIMITATION OF REMEDIES

Pearson Education, Inc.'s entire liability and your exclusive remedy shall be:

1. the replacement of any diskette(s) or CD-ROM(s) not meeting Pearson Education, Inc.'s "LIMITED WARRANTY" and that is returned to Pearson Education, or
2. if Pearson Education is unable to deliver a replacement diskette(s) or CD-ROM(s) that is free of defects in materials or workmanship, you may terminate this agreement by returning the program.

IN NO EVENT WILL PRENTICE-HALL, INC. BE LIABLE TO YOU FOR ANY DAMAGES, INCLUDING ANY LOST PROFITS, LOST SAVINGS, OR OTHER INCIDENTAL OR CONSEQUENTIAL DAMAGES ARISING OUT OF THE USE OR INABILITY TO USE SUCH PROGRAM EVEN IF PRENTICE-HALL, INC. OR AN AUTHORIZED DISTRIBUTOR HAS BEEN ADVISED OF THE POSSIBILITY OF SUCH DAMAGES, OR FOR ANY CLAIM BY ANY OTHER PARTY.

SOME STATES DO NOT ALLOW FOR THE LIMITATION OR EXCLUSION OF LIABILITY FOR INCIDENTAL OR CONSEQUENTIAL DAMAGES, SO THE ABOVE LIMITATION OR EXCLUSION MAY NOT APPLY TO YOU.

GENERAL

You may not sublicense, assign, or transfer the license of the program. Any attempt to sublicense, assign or transfer any of the rights, duties, or obligations hereunder is void.

This Agreement will be governed by the laws of the State of New York.

Should you have any questions concerning this Agreement, you may contact Pearson Education, Inc. by writing to:

Director of New Media
Higher Education Division
Pearson Education, Inc.
One Lake Street
Upper Saddle River, NJ 07458

Should you have any questions concerning technical support, you may contact:

Product Support Department: Monday–Friday 8:00 A.M. –8:00 P.M. and Sunday 5:00 P.M.-12:00 A.M. (All times listed are Eastern). 1-800-677-6337

You can also get support by filling out the web form located at http://247.prenhall.com

YOU ACKNOWLEDGE THAT YOU HAVE READ THIS AGREEMENT, UNDERSTAND IT, AND AGREE TO BE BOUND BY ITS TERMS AND CONDITIONS. YOU FURTHER AGREE THAT IT IS THE COMPLETE AND EXCLUSIVE STATEMENT OF THE AGREEMENT BETWEEN US THAT SUPERSEDES ANY PROPOSAL OR PRIOR AGREEMENT, ORAL OR WRITTEN, AND ANY OTHER COMMUNICATIONS BETWEEN US RELATING TO THE SUBJECT MATTER OF THIS AGREEMENT.

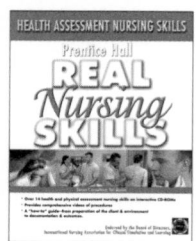

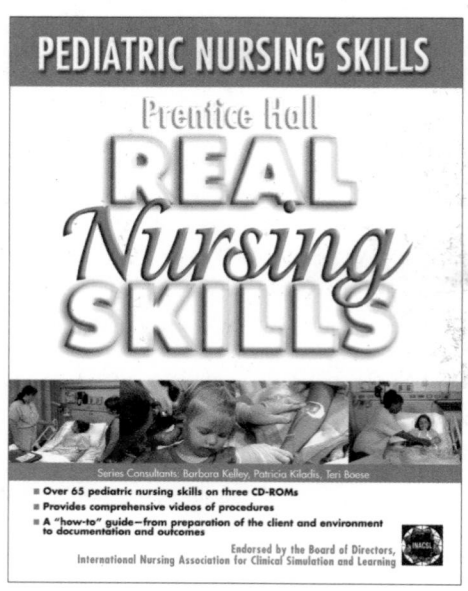

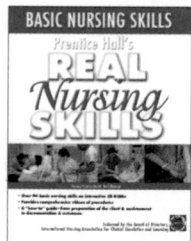

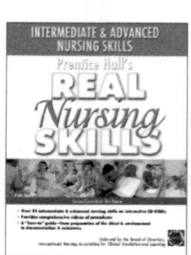

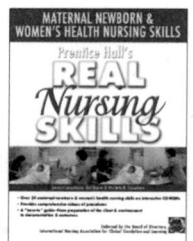

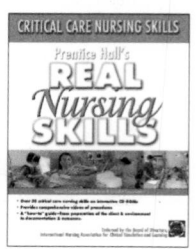